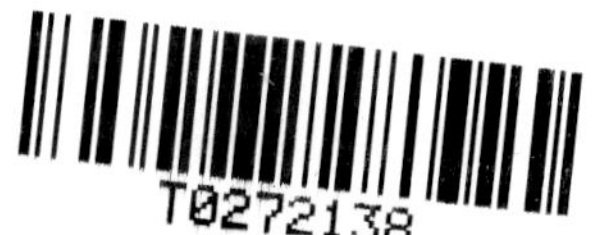

Herbs & Natural Supplements

An evidence-based guide

4TH EDITION

VOLUME 2

Herbs & Natural Supplements

An evidence-based guide

4TH EDITION

VOLUME 2

Lesley Braun

PhD, BPharm, DipAppSciNat

Associate Professor of Integrative Medicine (Hon) National Institute of Complementary Medicine, University of Western Sydney, NSW
Senior Research Fellow (Hon), Monash/Alfred Psychiatric Research Centre, Melbourne, VIC, Australia

Marc Cohen

MBBS(Hons), PhD, BMedSc(Hons), FAMAC, FICAE

Professor of Health Sciences, School of Health Sciences, RMIT University, Melbourne, VIC, Australia

ELSEVIER

indicates a herb or supplement action with particular significance for pregnant women.

indicates a warning or cautionary note regarding the action of a herb or supplement.

indicates FAQs about the herb or supplement.

ELSEVIER

Elsevier Australia. ACN 001 002 357
(a division of Reed International Books Australia Pty Ltd)
Tower 1, 475 Victoria Avenue, Chatswood, NSW 2067

National Library of Australia Cataloguing-in-Publication Data

---

Braun, Lesley, author, editor.

Herbs and natural supplements : an evidence-based guide.
Volume 2 / Lesley Braun (main editor);
Marc Cohen ; associate editors, Rachel
Arthur, Gina Fox, Brad McEwen, Liza
Oates, Evelin Tiralongo, Louise Zylan.

Fourth edition.

9780729541725 (paperback)

Herbs — Therapeutic use — Textbooks.
Dietary supplements — Textbooks.
Alternative medicine — Textbooks.

Cohen, Marc, author.
Arthur, Rachel, editor.
Fox, Gina, editor.
McEwen, Brad, editor.
Oates, Liza, editor.
Tiralongo, Evelin, editor.
Zylan, Louise, editor.

615.321

Content Strategist: Larissa Norrie
Senior Content Development Specialist: Neli Bryant
Project Managers: Devendran Kannan and ShriVidhya Shankar
Edited by Margaret Trudgeon & Liz Williams
Proofread by Tim Learner
Cover and internal design by Tania Gomes
Index by Robert Swanson
Typeset by Toppan Best-set Premedia Limited
Printed in Malaysia by Papercraft.

About the cover image (Gustoimages/Science Photo Library): Passion flower (Passiflora incarnata), Passion flower (*Passiflora incarnata*) flower head. As well as being cultivated for use as a decoration due to its impressive flowers, the passion flower is also used medicinally. It has a sedative effect and can be used as a hypnotic (sleep inducer) and an anti-spasmodic (relaxes involuntary muscles). When used as a compress, passion flower can ease minor skin irritations. It is usually used as an infusion or as a tincture (alcohol extract).

CONTENTS

Appendixes

ORGANISATION OF THIS BOOK

This fourth edition of *Herbs and Natural Supplements: an evidence-based guide* is organised into four sections. The first volume provides a basic introduction to complementary medicine in general and then, more specifically, to herbal medicine, clinical nutrition, aromatherapy and food as medicine. It is hoped that many of your general questions will be answered here. In this first volume, we have also included the chapters relating to clinical practice and explore the relatively new fields of integrative medicine and wellness as it relates to health. These areas are gaining popularity around the globe and complementary medicine philosophy and treatments are often an integral part of the approach. We have also included chapters with a focus on safety because the wise clinical use of all interventions must be based on a benefit versus risk assessment. There are general chapters discussing the safety of herbs and natural supplements and drug interactions, and then specific chapters focusing on safety in pregnancy, before surgery and for people undertaking treatment for cancer. These topics are discussed in both a theoretical and a practical way to clarify the key concerns and produce some general guidelines that can be used to inform practice.

The second part of this volume consists of ready-reference appendices, the largest of which is a table outlining the interactions possible between the complementary medicines reviewed and pharmaceutical drugs. Although investigation into this area is still in its infancy, we have provided a brief explanation for each possible interaction and a general recommendation based on what is currently known or suspected. It is intended as a guide only, to be used to inform practice when clinicians take a medical and medication history; obviously it should be interpreted within the individual patient's context. It is anticipated that this section will continue to change in future editions as more clinical studies are published and theoretical predictions are tested.

The second volume comprises of 132 evidence-based reviews of some of the most popular herbs and natural supplements available over the counter. Exhaustive reviews of the peer-reviewed literature have been undertaken by the author team to update, modify and expand information from the previous edition. Common names, chemical components, main actions, clinical uses, dosage range and safety issues are included for each herbal medicine. For nutritional supplements, background information and pharmacokinetics, food sources, deficiency signs and symptoms and the new Australian and New Zealand recommended daily intakes (RDIs) are also included where appropriate. Although technical language is frequently used, there is also a summary in non-technical language (Practice Points/Patient Counselling) and answers to key questions patients may have about the product (Patients' FAQs). A Historical note is included where appropriate and occasionally there are also Clinical note boxes that provide further information.

ACKNOWLEDGMENTS

Each edition of *Herbs and Natural Supplements* is bigger than the last and has required even more effort to produce. This is certainly true of this, our fourth edition, which has been expanded to two volumes and is now also available as an eBook.

The increase in size is chiefly due to the enormous amount of new material we have uncovered and felt important enough to include in this completely revised edition. Between Medline, Science Direct and the Cochrane database, there are tens of thousands of peer-reviewed articles that are now available to help us uncover the potential of herbs and natural supplements.

Identifying, interpreting, collating and synthesizing this information is an important and challenging task. For this edition, we significantly expanded our contributor team and searched for people with a range of backgrounds, training and skills. Some contributors are research academics with an expertise in complementary medicine; others are university lecturers working at the interface with students, whereas others are clinicians that bring a real-world perspective to the task. As always, I believe the author team to be among the brightest and most talented technical CM writers in the country. Their dedication, tenacity and enthusiasm have been integral to this project and I am privileged to have them on the team.

On a personal note, undertaking such a major project as this book means many hours dedicated to working in the home office, away from family and friends. It also means mentally retreating from everyday life as thoughts about the book and the issues raised, permeate nearly everything.

I'd like to thank my husband Gary, who is my biggest support, greatest teacher and best friend. His understanding and patience are always given without a second thought and forever appreciated. My three daughters Sarah, Lori and Jaimie are wonderful, warm and intelligent people who have found a genuine interest in health and helping others. I am so proud and thank you for your understanding and support during my busy and distracted writing periods.

I'd also like to thank all my parents Shana and Fred Green, Judy Braun for their emotional and hands-on support; my late grandfather Leon Kustin and father-in-law Emil Braun, who continue to serve as reminders to me to have courage and persevere; and the rest of my wonderful extended family and friends who accept that I'm off the radar every now and again, working on another book.

I'd like to make a special mention of my late father, Magenesta, who passed away between editions. Without him I would not have finished my pharmacy degree or started my life long journey into natural medicine — you have been my mentor and guide from the beginning.

I'd like to thank associate editors Liza Oates, Rachel Arthur, Gina Fox, Evelin Tiralongo, Louise Zylan and Brad McEwan for helping to guide the newer contributors with their patience, experience and wisdom. I'd like to thank returning contributors Ondine Spitzer, Leah Hechtman, Emily Bradley, Trisha Dunning and Surinder Baines for their continued commitment and professionalism and Marc Cohen for your unwavering vision. We also have a large number of new contributors who have been important additions to the author team; without you, this book simply would not have been possible — thank you.

I'd like to thank the team at Elsevier, especially Neli Bryant, for her energy and co-ordination, and my inspiring work colleagues at The Alfred Hospital (especially Prof Frank Rosenfeldt), Monash University (esp. Prof Paul Komesaroff), National Institute of Complementary Medicine (esp Prof Alan Bensoussan) and most recently, Blackmores (esp Christine Holgate and Marcus Blackmore) and the wonderful Blackmores Institute.

Finally, thank you to all the health care professionals that have told me they use this book every day to guide their clinical practice. Knowing this helps make the difficult journey easier and is an important reminder of why our work is important, because the information within helps improve people's lives through you.

ABOUT THE AUTHORS

EDITORS

Lesley Braun, PhD, BPharm, DipAppSciNat
Associate Professor of Integrative Medicine (Hon) National Institute of Complementary Medicine, University of Western Sydney, NSW, Senior Research Fellow (Hon), Monash/Alfred Psychiatric Research Centre, Melbourne, VIC, Australia

Senior Research Fellow (Hon), Monash/Alfred Psychiatric Research Centre, Vic, Australia

Dr Lesley Braun is a registered pharmacist and naturopath. She holds a PhD from RMIT University, Melbourne, in which she investigated the integration of complementary medicine into hospitals in Victoria. Dr Braun is an Adjunct Associate Professor of Integrative Medicine at the National Institute of Complementary Medicine (NICM) at the University of Western Sydney. NICM provides leadership and support for strategically directed research into complementary medicine and translation of evidence into clinical practice and relevant policy to benefit the health of all Australians.

Dr Braun serves on the Australian Therapeutic Goods Advisory Council, which oversees the implementation of TGA reforms and provides general strategic guidance to the TGA, advice on relationships and communication with stakeholders. She is also on the executive for the Complementary and Integrative Therapies interest group of the Clinical Oncology Society of Australia and is an advisory board member to the Australasian Integrative Medicine Association. As of 2014, she is also Director of Blackmore's Institute, the academic and professional arm of Blackmores, which entails engaging with a broad range of academics, government and industry bodies and overseeing a comprehensive academic and research program.

Since 1996 Lesley has authored numerous chapters for books and more than 100 articles, and since 2000 has written regular columns for the *Australian Journal of Pharmacy* and *Journal of Complementary Medicine*. She lectures to medical students at Monash University and to chiropractic students at RMIT University, and is regularly invited to present at national and international conferences about evidence-based complementary medicine, drug interactions, complementary medicine safety and her own clinical research.

Her role as the main author of *Herbs and Natural Supplements: an evidence-based guide* represents a continuation of a life-long goal to integrate evidence-based complementary medicine into standard practice and improve patient outcomes safely and effectively.

Marc Cohen, MBBS(Hons), PhD, BMedSc (Hons), FAMAC, FICAE
Professor of Health Sciences, School of Health Sciences, RMIT University, Melbourne, VIC, Australia

Professor Marc Cohen is one of Australia's pioneers of integrative and holistic medicine who has made significant impacts on education, research, clinical practice and policy. He is a medical doctor and Professor of Health Sciences at RMIT University, where he leads postgraduate wellness programs and supervises research into wellness and holistic health, including research on yoga, meditation, nutrition, herbal medicine, acupuncture, lifestyle and the health impact of pesticides, organic food and detoxification. Professor Cohen sits on the board of a number of national and international associations, including the Australasian Integrative Medicine Association, the Global Spa and Wellness Summit and the Australasian Spa and Wellness Association, as well as serving on the editorial boards of several international peer-reviewed journals. Professor Cohen has published more than 80 peer-reviewed journal articles and co-edited *Understanding the Global Spa Industry*, along with more than 10 other books on holistic approaches to health. He is a frequent speaker at many national and international conferences where he delivers inspiring, informative and uplifting presentations. His impact on the field has been recognised by four consecutive RMIT Media Star Awards, as well as the inaugural Award for Leadership and Collaboration from the National Institute of Complementary Medicine.

ASSOCIATE EDITORS

Rachel Arthur, BHSc BNat(Hons)
Rachel Arthur Nutrition

Rachel is a naturopath, lecturer, researcher and author. Graduating with a Bachelor of Health Science (Naturopathy) from the Southern School of Natural Therapies, Melbourne, she now lectures in clinical nutrition and naturopathic practice at a number of institutions, including Southern Cross University. In addition to this, Rachel is frequently asked to speak on nutrition by a variety of organisations, including professional medical organisations across Australia and overseas. A contributing author for the previous editions, Rachel is also a regular contributor to a range of complementary medicine publications. In this edition, Rachel was involved with updating the Zinc monograph and was also an associate editor.

Gina Fox, BHSc(Nat), GradCert (ReproMed)
Gina is a clinician, writer, lecturer and speaker. She qualified as a naturopath in 2001 and has been specialising in pre-conception health, infertility, fertility and pregnancy since starting practice at Fertile Ground Health Group in Melbourne in 2003. Gina is an educator and lecturer and enjoys supervising student naturopaths at Endeavour College of Natural Health. She is also a meditation teacher and has co-written a Be Fertile series of guided relaxation CDs for women around conception, IVF support and pregnancy. Gina is currently undertaking a master degree in Reproductive Medicine with UNSW. In this edition, Gina has been involved in updating a number of monographs and was an associate editor.

Bradley McEwen, PhD, MHSc(HumNutr), BHSc(ComplMed), GCertHSc (HumNutr), AdvDip (Natur), DipBotMed, DipHom, DipNutr, Dip-SpMed, DipRMed
PhD, MHlthSc (Hum. Nutr.), BHlthSc (ComplMed), Grad. Cert. HlthSc (Hum. Nutr.), N.D. (Adv.), D.B.M., D.Hom., D.Nutr., D.S.M., D.R.M
Lecturer, Clinic Supervisor, and Research and Curriculum Developer — Endeavour College of Natural Health

Dr Bradley McEwen is a naturopath, nutritionist, herbalist and educator. He has a PhD from the University of Sydney and a Master of Health Science (Human Nutrition) from Deakin University. His doctoral research investigated the effect of omega-3 on platelet function and coagulation in healthy subjects and cardiovascular patients.

Bradley has a passion for education and research. He has 15 years clinical experience and 10 years lecturing experience and currently lectures and supervises student clinic. In addition, he presents at seminars and conferences, both nationally and internationally. Bradley's research focus is on the effects of nutrition on chronic disease, particularly cardiovascular disease, omega-3 PUFA, and public health. He has a number of original research and review articles published in peer-reviewed international journals.

Liza Oates, PhD, GCertECompMed, BHSc (Natr)
Course co-ordinator Food as Medicine, and Wellness Practices & Perspectives, Postgraduate Wellness Program, RMIT University, Melbourne, Australia

Naturopathic Clinical Supervisor, Southern School of Natural Therapies and Endeavour College of Natural Health

Teaching Associate, Department of General Practice, Monash University

Dr Liza Oates is a naturopathic practitioner, educator and writer. Having initially graduated with a Bachelor of Health Science (Naturopathy) she later completed a Graduate Certificate in Evidence-based Complementary Medicine (University of Queensland and Southern Cross University), and a PhD (RMIT University). Her doctoral research investigated the health and wellness effects of organic diets and the findings have been presented at conferences in Australia, Poland, South Korea and the Czech Republic.

Liza is the course co-ordinator for Food as Medicine and Wellness Practices & Perspectives in the online Postgraduate Wellness program at RMIT University, and she supervises naturopathic student clinics. She has taught Nutrition, Complementary Medicine in Chronic Diseases and Health Enhancement to naturopathic and medical students.

Liza was a contributing author on the first three editions of *Herbs & Natural Supplements: an evidence-based guide*, and has published over 35 peer-reviewed journal articles in the complementary medicine field. Journal publications include *Australian Pharmacist, The Journal of Complementary Medicine, Journal of the Science of Food and Agriculture, Environmental Research, The International Journal of Environmental Research and Public Health* and *The Journal of Organic Systems*.

Evelin Tiralongo, PhD, BPharm, GradCert (HigherEd)
Associate Professor and Discipline Head in Complementary Medicine, School of Pharmacy, Griffith University, Gold Coast, QLD, Australia

Developer and Presenter, Short Course in Integrative Medicine, Griffith University School of Pharmacy

Associate Professor Evelin Tiralongo is a foundation member of Griffith University's Pharmacy School and is the discipline head for complementary medicine (CM) teaching and research at the School. She has an Honours degree in herbal medicine and a PhD in biochemistry. She gained extensive practical experience in integrative medicine as a registered pharmacist in German pharmacy practice, and has also completed her Australian registration as a pharmacist.

Her research focuses on CMs and natural products, and spans from laboratory to practice-based and clinical projects. As a chief investigator she has won over $1.3 million in research funding and has co-authored 38 peer-reviewed publications and one patent, and designed online CM resources for *Pharmacology for Health Professionals* by Bryant et al.

She is a member of the NHMRC Homeopathy Advisory Committee, acts as a reviewer and editor for several internationally recognised CAM journals (eCAM) and has served on the scientific board of international conferences and forums (ICMAN5).

Evelin conducts continuous professional development seminars on CMs to pharmacists and other healthcare professionals and is co-founder of the Short Course in Integrative Medicine. http://www.integramedshortcourses.com/

Louise Zylan, PhD (candidate), MNutrMed, BHScNat

Louise is the Head of Academic Studies for Natural and Nutritional Health and has over 25 years work experience in health and education. She ran a busy private practice for 10 years, specialising in reproductive health.

Louise holds a Master degree in Nutritional Medicine and is currently undertaking a PhD in Public Health at Torrens University, where she is exploring the nutritional status of intellectually disabled adults in residential accommodation within Australia.

CONTRIBUTORS

Ayesha Amos, GCertEvidCompMed, GCertHigherEd, AdvDipAppSci(Nat)
Program Manager Naturopathy, Southern School of Natural Therapies, Victoria, Australia
Monographs contributed: Black Cohosh; Gymnema; Hawthorn; Valerian

Rachel Arthur, BHSc BNat(Hons)
Rachel Arthur Nutrition
Monograph contributed: Zinc

Surinder K. Baines, APD, PhD, BSc(Hons), GDip(Diet), GDip(Nutr)
Associate Professor of Nutrition and Dietetics, Faculty of Health and Medicine, University of Newcastle, NSW, Australia
Monographs contributed: Arginine; Carnitine; L-Glutamine; L-Lysine, Taurine

Liesl Blott, BPharm, PGDip(MM), BHSc(WHerbalMed), AdvDip(Nat)
School of Pharmacy, Curtin University, Perth, Australia
Monographs contributed: Andrographis; Calcium; Honey; Iodine; Iron; Nigella; New Zealand green-lipped mussel; Tea tree

Emily Bradley, MNM, BHSc (Natr)
Southern School of Natural Therapies, Endeavour College of Natural Medicine, Victoria, Australia
Monographs contributed: CoQ10; Creatine

Lesley Braun, PhD, BPharm, DipAppSciNat
Associate Professor of Integrative Medicine (Hon), National Institute of Complementary Medicine, University of Western Sydney, NSW, Senior Research Fellow (Hon), Monash/Alfred Psychiatric Research Centre, Melbourne, VIC, Australia
Senior Research Fellow (Hon), Monash/Alfred Psychiatric Research Centre, VIC, Australia
Monographs contributed: Bergamot; Brahmi; Hops; Horseradish; Pelargonium; Policosanol; Rhodiola; Saffron; Shark Cartilage; Stinging Nettle

Marc Cohen, MBBS(Hons), PhD, BMedSc (Hons), FAMAC, FICAE
Professor of Health Sciences, School of Health Sciences, RMIT University, Melbourne, VIC, Australia
Monographs contributed: Beta carotene; Chondroitin; Dunaliella; Glucosamine; Rosehip; Tulsi

Stacey Curcio, BHSc(ND)
Practitioner, Gladstone Holistic Health, QLD
Monographs contributed: Elderflower; Noni; Quercetin; Thyme

Helene de la Follye de Jeux, BNatr
Monographs contributed: Alpha lipoic acid; Chromium; Cloves; Perilla

Trisha Dunning, AM, RN, CDE, MEd, PhD
Chair, Nursing; Director Centre for Nursing and Allied Health Research, Deakin University and Barwon Health, Vic, Australia
Monographs contributed: Citrus aurantium; Eucalyptus oil; Lavender

Gina Fox, BHSc(Nat), GradCert (ReproMed)
Monographs contributed: Cranberry; Ginkgo Biloba; Green tea

Elizabeth Hammer, BHSc(CompMed/Nurs), AdvDipWHM, CertIVWTA(TAE)
Western Herbalist/ RN, Vice President National Herbalists Association of Australia, Tasmania, Australia
Monographs contributed: Bilberry; Garlic; Pygeum; Saw Palmetto; Withania

Jason Hawrelak, PhD, BNat(Hons), DipN
Senior Lecturer, Course Coordinator, Graduate Certificate in Evidence-based Complementary Medicine, School of Medicine, University of Tasmania, Australia
Adjunct Lecturer, Master of Science in Human Nutrition and Functional Medicine program, University of Western States, Oregon, USA, Naturopathic practitioner, Goulds Naturopathica, Tasmania, Australia
Monographs contributed: Prebiotics; Probiotics; Psyllium

Leah Hechtman, PhD(candidate), MSciMed(RHHG), BHSc(Nat), DipN
Director and Clinician, The Natural Health and Fertility Centre
PhD candidate — University of Sydney, Department of Obstetrics, Gynaecology and Neonatology, Faculty of Medicine, President, National Herbalists Association of Australia, NSW, Australia
Monograph contributed: Vitamin C

Rebecca Hughes, BNatr
Naturopathic practitioner at ReMed and The Well Room, Victoria, Member of National Herbalists Association of Australia, Victoria, Australia
Monographs contributed: Astragalus; Baical skullcap; Coriolus versicolour; Siberian ginseng

Kate Levett, BEd(Hons), AdvDipAppSci(Acup), GradCertJapAcup, MPH(Merit), PhD
University of Notre Dame, School of Medicine, NSW, Australia
Monographs: Colostrum; Flaxseed oil; Korean ginseng; Vitamin D

Sally Mathrick, BNat, BArts, DipRemMass
Principal Naturopath Sound Medicine; author *Sparkle Wellness & Detox Guide*, Bendigo, Victoria, Australia
Monographs contributed: Cinnamon; Dandelion; Fenugreek; Maca; Myrrh

Bradley McEwen, PhD, MHSc(HumNutr), BHSc(ComplMed), GCertHSc (HumNutr), AdvDip (Natur), DipBotMed, DipHom, DipNutr, Dip-SpMed, DipRMed, PhD, MHlthSc (Hum. Nutr.), BHlthSc (ComplMed), Grad. Cert. HlthSc (Hum. Nutr.), N.D.(Adv.), D.B.M., D.Hom., D.Nutr., D.S.M., D.R.M
Lecturer, Clinic Supervisor, and Research and Curriculum Developer — Endeavour College of Natural Health
Monographs contributed: Turmeric; Feverfew; Horsechestnut; Willowbark; Meadowsweet; Rosemary; Goldenrod; Fish Oil; Appendix 2: Herb/Nutrient-Drug Interactions

Amelia June McFarland, MPharm(Hons), BPharmSci
Registered Pharmacist, Clinical Tutor, School of Pharmacy, Griffith University, Queensland, Australia
Monographs contributed: Aloe vera; Celery; Cocoa; Folate; Golden seal; Licorice; Lutein; Selenium; Vitamin A; Vitamin B_{12}

Teresa Mitchell-Paterson, AdvDipNatr, BHSc(CompMed), MHSc (HumNutr), DipCompMedSci
Senior Lecturer Bachelor of Health Science Naturopathy, Nutrition and Western Herbal Medicine Australasian College of Natural Therapies Sydney, NSW, Australia
Integrative Natural Therapies Practitioner, Sydney Integrative Medicine, Sydney, Australia
Health and Medical Panellist, The Memorial Winston Churchill Trust Fund, Nutritional Advisor Bowel Cancer Australia
Monographs contributed: Magnesium; Vitamin E

Kathleen Murphy, BA, BHSci
Clinical Naturopath, Sydney Integrative Medicine, Surry Hills, NSW, Australia
Sessional lecturer, Endeavour College of Natural Health, Sydney, NSW, Australia
Monographs contributed: Grapeseed; Guarana; Wild yam

Vijayendra Murthy, BNat, BAyu(MedSurg), MSci, MPH
Ayurvedic physician, Ayuwave Natural Health, London, UK
Research collaborator, Australian Research Centre in Complementary and Integrative Medicine (ARCCIM), Faculty of Health, University of Technology, Sydney, NSW, Australia
Monographs contributed: Adhatoda; Bitter melon; Oats; Shatavari

Miranda Myles, MAppSc(Acu), BHSc(Nat), BA(Psych), CertNatFert, CertClinIntern, CertEsotAcu, CertIVEdTrain
Educator and Contract Lecturer at Southern School Natural Therapies and Endeavour College of Natural Health
Guest Lecturer, RMIT, Bundoora and La Trobe University, Bendigo, Victoria, Australia
Monographs contributed: Soy; Vitamin B_1; Vitamin B_2; Vitamin B_5; Vitamin B_6

Ses Salmond, PhD, BA, DipN, DipBotMed, DipHom, DipNutr
Herbalist/Naturopath, Leichhardt Women's Community Health Centre, Sydney
Local Health District and Liverpool Women's Health Centre, South Western Local Health District, Private Practitioner, NSW, Australia
Monographs contributed: Gentian; Globe artichoke; Red rice yeast extract; St Mary's thistle

Kate Savage, BPharm, BNat
Analytical Chemist (Phytochem), Southern Cross Plant Science, Southern Cross University, Lismore, NSW, Australia
Monographs contributed: Calendula; Damiana; Mullein

Ondine Spitzer, MSocH, BHSci, BA, DipAppSciNat
Monographs contributed: Passionflower; Raspberry leaf; Red clover; Sage; Vitex

Kate Sullivan, BNat, MPharm(candidate)
Monographs: Chickweed; Chitosan; Peppermint; Tribulus

Evelin Tiralongo, PhD, BPharm, GradCert (HigherEd)
Associate Professor, School of Pharmacy, Griffith University
Monographs contributed: St John's Wort; Echinacea; Kava

Quilla Watt, BNat(Hons)
Monographs contributed: Albizzia; Goji; Lemon balm; Schisandra; Slippery elm

Tanya Wells, BSc(Hons), BHSci(Nat), GCertHealthProfEd
Integrative Medicine Naturopath, Lecturer Synergy Health — Consulting, Seminars and Training — Drug–Herb/Nutrient Interaction Seminars for Medical and Nursing Practitioners, Vic, Australia
Monographs contributed: Devil's claw; Ginger; SAMe; Tyrosine

REVIEWERS

Robyn Carruthers, PGDip(HSci), BEd, DipTeach, BHSci(CompMed), AdvDipNat, AdvDipHerbMed
Deputy Director, Clinical and Research South Pacific College of Natural Medicine

Sandy Davidson, MPH, DipNat, AdvDipNat, DipNutr
Associate Program Leader — Nutritional Medicine, Endeavour College of Natural Health

Lauren Frail, Critical Care RN
Nurse Educator, Melbourne IVF, East Melbourne, Vic, Australia

Chandrika Gibson, DipNat, MWell
Naturopathic practitioner, yoga therapist and project officer at Cancer Council WA, Australia
Former lecturer and clinical supervisor at Endeavour College of Natural Health and Paramount College of Natural Medicine, Perth, WA, Australia

Mara Goodridge, BHSc (Nat), ND, AdvDipAppSci(Nut), AdvDipHom, AdvDipWHM
Lecturer, Australasian College of Natural Therapies (ACNT), Think Education, NSW, Australia

Myfanwy Graham, MPharm
Associate Lecturer, School of Biomedical Sciences and Pharmacy, Faculty of Health and Medicine, University of Newcastle, NSW, Australia

Margot Jensen, AdvDipNat, BHSc(CompMed), BA/LLB
Population Health Coordinator, Canberra Institute of Technology, ACT, Australia

Elizabeth MacGregor, MEd(HighEd), BHSc(Nat)
Naturopathic Practitioner, Senior Lecturer of Naturopathic Medicine, Endeavour College, Perth, WA, Australia

Amanda Richardson, AdvDipNat, AdvDipWHM
Lecturer, Australasian College of Natural Therapies, Pyrmont, NSW, Australia

Kylie Seaton, BHSc(Nat), BA(Jour), PGDipComm, AdvDipNat, AdvDipHomeop, AdvDipWHM, DipNutr/Cert Iridology, Primary modules NutrEnvMed (ACNEM), IntegHeal(Kines), CertIV(TAE)
Owner, Kylie Seaton Naturopath Homeopath

Caroline van der Mey, BHSc(Comp Med), PGDip(Phyto), AdvDipNat, DipHomeop
Private practitioner Naturopathy, WA, Australia

Karen Wallace, BHSc(Nat), BBus(HAdm)
Naturopathic Practitioner, Lecturer, Endeavour College of Natural Health, Perth, WA, Australia

PREFACE

Welcome to the fourth edition of *Herbs and Natural Supplements: an evidence based guide*. Due to the exponential growth in the peer-reviewed literature, we have had to expand our team of contributors significantly since the last edition. We have contributions from experts with a range of backgrounds such as nutrition and naturopathy, herbal medicine, pharmacy, dietetics and medicine and also a number of research active academics and university lecturers.

I started writing the first edition, together with Prof Marc Cohen, nearly 10 years ago, and it is very heartening to see the enormous growth in the evidence base that has occurred since that time. We now have far more information available in the peer-reviewed literature about key active components in herbal medicines, pharmacological activity in vivo and clinical trials. In particular, the complexity of herbal medicines has become more evident as nearly all have multiple mechanisms of action and we have well and truly moved beyond using solely traditional evidence to guide their use. Unfortunately, some authors of meta-analyses still continue to pool information from studies that have tested different plant parts and even species. This is like lumping apples and oranges together, and thereby compromises the usefulness of these reviews. However, overall reporting in herbal medicine studies has improved and where possible, we state the extract used, dose and administration form to help guide you in your practice.

The area of drug-herb interactions was of particular concern in the early-mid 2000s and there is now far more information about interactions that are clinically relevant. You will notice that we place most importance on drug interactions that have been demonstrated in vivo because in vitro testing has led us all astray in the past with false positives.

Probably the biggest growth area has been in nutritional science and research. In this edition, the fish oil, vitamin D and probiotic monographs in particular have expanded significantly. They are among the most popular supplements being bought in retail stores today. Fish oils are being intensively investigated for health conditions beyond cardiovascular disease, and there is work being done in mental health, neurological diseases, neonates and children and even cancer. Unfortunately, some researchers still use olive oil as a placebo, which is unfortunate because this is not an inert substance and could be compromising results. Vitamin D is also being investigated for conditions unrelated to the musculoskeletal system, and population studies are indicating low vitamin D status is rife. Probiotics has been another area to explode with new information about potential effects beyond the gastrointestinal tract. The effect of the microbiome on multiple diseases is only starting to be understood and the role of pre- and probiotics in influencing it is slowly being uncovered. In contrast, there have been relatively fewer studies published on vitamins E and C than in the past.

Our team of contributors have systematically searched the main medical databases, using primary literature where possible, to capture, collate and synthesise the best and most relevant information for busy clinicians. We used Medline, Science Direct and the Cochrane database as a starting point to identify articles published since our last edition. This means having access to over 24 million peer-reviewed articles. Despite our best efforts, no doubt we will have missed something. This is due to the intense research activity underway and almost weekly publication of new information making it extremely difficult to keep up.

In this book, we report on positive, negative and inconclusive results and try to put forward theories as to why results are inconsistent. I think that in the future, we will better understand these differences. In particular, I wonder how much individual genetics is playing a role which we have not fully explored at this time.

Most adults in Western countries are using over-the-counter herbal and nutritional supplements, and informed advice from their healthcare practitioner is important and expected. I hope that this book will help expand your practice by unlocking the potential of natural medicines and safely guide your patients to use them appropriately.

Adhatoda

HISTORICAL NOTE An important herb in Ayurvedic medicine for over 2000 years (Singh et al 2011), adhatoda is used traditionally in productive cough, asthma, haemoptysis and tuberculosis (Caldecott 2006). Adhatoda is a popular plant for digestion due to its extreme bitter taste (Caldecott 2006). The Sanskrit language term for adhatoda is *vasaka*, meaning a plant with characteristic unpleasant odour (Caldecott 2006, Pa & Mathew 2012). Adhatoda is an evergreen perennial shrub that grows all over the plains of India and Sri Lanka (Pole 2006).

Clinical note

One of the alkaloids found in the herb (vasicine) has been chemically modified and is referred to as RLX (6,7,8,9,10,12-hexahydro-azepino-[2,1-b]-quinazoline-12-one) in the medical literature (Johri & Zutshi 2000). It has been shown in animal studies to inhibit antigen-induced mast cell degranulation and histamine release and to exert bronchodilator activity. It is the lead molecule for bromhexine and ambroxol (Gurib-Fakim 2006).

COMMON NAMES

Adhatoda, Malabar nut tree, vasa, vasaka

OTHER NAMES

Adhatoda zeylanica, *Justicia adhatoda*, arusha, bakash, *Justicia adhatoda-Folium*, vasaka, vasa, adusa, Bagabahouk

BOTANICAL NAME/FAMILY

Adhatoda vasica (family Acanthaceae)

PLANT PARTS USED

Leaves, root, bark, flower

CHEMICAL COMPONENTS

The leaves contain several different alkaloids, including vasicine, vasicinone, vasicinol, adhatodine, adhatonine, adhavasinone, anisotine, peganine, 7-methoxyvaicinone, desmethoxyaniflorine, 3-hydroxyanisotine, vasnetine, betaine, steroids and alkanes (Claeson et al 2000, Kamal et al 2006, Mhaske & Argade 2006). The root also contains alkaloids (vasicinol, vasicinolone, vasicinone, adhatonine), a steroid (daucosterol), carbohydrates and alkanes (Claeson et al 2000).

MAIN ACTIONS

Indigenous usage in India was as an antispasmodic, antiseptic and insecticide (Claeson et al 2000). Current application focuses on the herb's antispasmodic, oxytocic and cough-suppressant activities (Gurib-Fakim 2006). It is an ingredient in the Rasayana preparation called chyavanprash, which is used widely as a health-promotive and disease-preventive tonic and is believed to be hepatoprotective and immunomodulating (Govindarajan et al 2007).

As with many Ayurvedic herbs, most investigation has been undertaken in India and locating original research from these sources is difficult.

Antitussive effects

Results from animal studies show that *Adhatoda vasica* extract exerts considerable antitussive activity when administered orally and is comparable to codeine when cough is due to irritant stimuli (Dhuley 1999). The antitussive activity may be due to the action of vasicinone and vasicinol, which have activity in the cerebral medulla. In Ayurvedic medicine, adhatoda is prescribed in combination with *Curcuma longa*, *Zingiber officinale*, *Glycyrrhiza glabra*, *Terminalia chebula* and *Ocimum sanctum* to control cough and shortness of breath, especially for lung cancer patients (Balachandran & Govindarajan 2005).

Anti-inflammatory

Vasicine, vasicinone, vasicine acetate, 2-acetyl benzyl amine and vasicinolone, the most bioactive constituents in adhatoda, showed strong anti-inflammatory activity in carrageenan-induced oedema in rats (Singh & Sharma 2013). Potent anti-inflammatory activity has also been demonstrated for the alkaloid fraction deoxyvasicinone, the naturally occurring quinazolinone alkaloid (Mhaske & Argade 2006). This has been shown to be equivalent to the anti-inflammatory effect of hydrocortisone in one study (Chakraborty & Brantner 2001).

Bronchodilator and antiasthmatic activity

According to a 2002 review, both vasicine and vasicinone possess in vitro and in vivo bronchodilatory activity and inhibit allergen-induced bronchial obstruction in a manner comparable to that of sodium cromoglycate (Dorsch & Wagner 1991, Jindal et al 2002).

OTHER ACTIONS

Hepatoprotective and antioxidant activity

Traditionally adhatoda was used to treat liver disease: the juice of fresh leaves (5–10 g) was mixed with honey and orally ingested three times daily for 2–3 weeks (Kotoky & Das 2008). *A. vasica* leaf (50–100 mg/kg) was shown to protect against induced liver damage in rats (Bhattacharyya et al 2005);100 mg/kg of *A. vasica* was comparable to the hepatoprotective ability of silymarin at 25 mg/kg. An earlier study showed that *A. vasica* (100–200 mg/kg) protected against carbon tetrachloride-induced liver damage in rats (Pandit et al 2004). The leaf extract significantly enhanced the protective enzymes superoxide dismutase and catalase in the liver: 200 mg/kg of *A. vasica* was shown to be comparable to 25 mg/kg of silymarin. In rats pretreated with aqueous extract of *Adhatoda vasica* an antioxidant effect against D-galactosamine-induced hepatic damage was shown (Jayakumar et al 2009). In vivo tests on mice also showed the extract is effective in inducing glutathione-*S*-transferase and DT-diaphorase in lungs and forestomach, and superoxide dismutase and catalase in kidneys (Singh et al 2000).

Protection against radiation damage

Adhatoda vasica (800 mg/kg) protects haematopoietic stem cells against radiation damage by inhibiting glutathione deletion, reducing lipid peroxidation and increasing phosphatase activity in mice (Kumar et al 2005). Animals pretreated with oral doses of adhatoda showed an 81.25% survival rate at 30 days as compared to control animals, who could not survive past 25 days. In additional studies on mice, adhatoda exhibited highly significant increases in glutathione content and significant decrease in lipid peroxidation (Samarth et al 2008). A cyto-geno analysis of 50% methanolic extract of adhatoda leaves on human peripheral lymphocytes showed radioprotective activity against therapeutically induced mutations, therefore demonstrating a potential as an adjuvant to cancer treatment (Sharma et al 2011).

Enzyme induction

In vitro tests show that *A. vasica* acts as a bifunctional inducer, since it induces both phase I and phase II enzyme systems (Singh et al 2011). The clinical significance of this finding is unclear and remains to be tested.

Abortifacient

One of the traditional uses of the herb is as an abortifacient and anti-fertility; however, inconsistent results from in vivo studies have made it difficult to determine whether adhatoda has significant abortifacient activity. One animal study investigating oral administration of leaf extracts showed 100% abortive rates at doses equivalent to 175 mg/kg of starting dry material (Nath et al 1992). Another study found that an *A. vasica* extract had anti-implantation activity in 60–70% of test animals (Prakash et al 1985).

Antispasmodic

The essential oil from the leaves exerts antispasmodic action, as demonstrated in an animal model of guinea pig tracheal chain (Claeson et al 2000).

Nematocidal/anticestodal activity

Naga tribes in India have traditionally used adhatoda for curing intestinal worm infestations. In an experimental study *Adhatoda latibracteata* was shown to have high antiplasmodial activity (Lekana-Douki et al 2011). Animal studies indicate that crude aqueous root extracts of 3 g/kg body weight exhibit 37.4% reduction of mixed gastrointestinal nematode infestations in sheep, as a result of the alkaloid and glycoside content of adhatoda (Githiori et al 2006, Lateef et al 2003). In one animal study, adhatoda exhibited significant anticestodal efficacy, greater than that of praziquantel (Yadev & Tangpu 2008).

Antidiabetic activity

Ethanolic extract of *Justicia adhatoda* leaves and roots in doses of 50 and 100 mg/kg body weight, when administered to alloxan-induced diabetic rats showed reduction in blood glucose levels and at doses of 100 mg/kg body weight, hypoglycaemic activity was more pronounced than glibenclamide (Imran et al 2011).

Other

Deoxyvasicinone, the naturally occurring quinazolinone alkaloid, exhibits antimicrobial and antidepressant activities (Mhaske & Argade 2006). Antimicrobial activity was specific to certain strains of penicillin- and ciprofloxacin-resistant *Neisseria gonorrhoeae* (Shokeen et al 2009). Vasicinone isolated from adhatoda showed in an in vitro study antimycobacterial and anticancer activities (Balachandran et al 2012). In an in vitro study, aqueous extract of adhatoda leaves showed antituberculosis activity against two multidrug-resistant isolates of *Mycobacterium tuberculosis*, DKU-156 and JAL-1236 (Gupta et al 2010).

CLINICAL USE

Adhatoda has not been significantly investigated under clinical trial conditions, so evidence largely comes from traditional use; in vitro and in vivo studies providing preliminary support for its uses.

Cough

The antitussive activity of adhatoda extract has been compared to that of codeine in two different models of coughing and in two different animal species (Dhuley 1999). When administered orally, *A. vasica* extract produced antitussive effects comparable to those of codeine against coughing induced by peripheral irritant stimuli. When coughing was induced by electrical stimulation of the tracheal mucosa, adhatoda extract was only one-quarter as active as codeine. Intravenous administration was far less effective in both cough models.

IN COMBINATION

A double-blind, randomised, controlled trial of *Adhatoda vasica* in combination with *Echinacea purpurea* and *Eleutherococcus senticosus* was compared with an *Echinacea* and *Eleutherococcus* mixture and bromhexine (Narimanian et al 2005). Bromhexine is a semisynthetic derivative of the alkaloid vasicine found in *A. vasica* (Grange & Snell 1996) and is found in some pharmaceutical cough mixtures. Compared with the other two formulas, the *A. vasica* combination reduced the severity of cough, increased mucus discharge and reduced nasal congestion. Both herbal mixtures reduced the frequency of cough compared with bromhexine. Furthermore, Grange and Snell (1996) identified pH-dependent growth-inhibitory effects on *Mycobacterium tuberculosis*, which further supports its usage as a mucolytic.

Asthma

Although *A. vasica* is used for asthma in combination with other herbs, clinical evidence is limited. Evidence of bronchodilator activity from in vitro and animal studies provides a theoretical basis for use in treating asthma.

One 12-week randomised, double-blind, placebo-controlled clinical trial was undertaken to assess the efficacy of an Ayurvedic herbal formula in asthmatic patients. While the formula contained 15 different herbs, almost half the total weight consisted of adhatoda. Active herbal treatment increased the efficacy of medication (salbutamol and theophylline) in bronchodilation, thus increasing forced expiratory volume in the first second. In addition, the herbal combination significantly improved other clinical parameters, resulting in reductions in dyspnoea, wheezing, expectoration, disability and respiratory rate when compared to a placebo (Murali et al 2006). Although these results are promising, the role of adhatoda as a stand-alone treatment remains unclear.

OTHER USES

Adhatoda is traditionally used to treat cough, asthma, bronchitis and colds, but has also been used to treat fever, dysentery, diarrhoea, jaundice, tuberculosis and headache, to stimulate the birthing process and aid healing afterwards, and as an antispasmodic (Claeson et al 2000). It has also been used as an abortifacient in some Indian villages.

Leaves that have been warmed on the fire are applied topically in the treatment of joint pain, lumbar pain and sprains.

Use of the powder is reported as a poultice on rheumatic joints, a counterirritant for inflammatory swelling, a treatment for fresh wounds, and in urticaria and neuralgia (Dhuley 1999).

DOSAGE RANGE

As clinical research is lacking, the following dosages come from Australian manufacturers' recommendations.

- Liquid extract tincture (1:2): 1–3 mL/day (Pole 2006).
- Dried herb/powdered leaf: 2.0–5.0 g/day (Caldecott 2006).

ADVERSE REACTIONS

Insufficient reliable information is available.

SIGNIFICANT INTERACTIONS

Controlled studies are not available, so interactions are based on evidence of activity and are largely theoretical and speculative.

Codeine and other antitussive drugs

Theoretically, adhatoda may increase the antitussive effects of these drugs — beneficial interaction may be possible under professional supervision.

Practice points/Patient counselling

- Adhatoda is an important Ayurvedic medicine used in the treatment of cough, asthma, bronchitis and colds.
- Traditional use further includes fever, dysentery, diarrhoea, jaundice, skin disorders, tuberculosis and headache.
- Preliminary evidence suggests that adhatoda may have bronchodilator activity and inhibit allergen-induced bronchoconstriction; however, clinical studies are unavailable to determine clinical significance.
- Antitussive effects comparable to those of codeine have also been reported in animal studies in which cough has been peripherally induced.
- Adhatoda has been used to stimulate the birthing process and aid healing afterwards, and may have abortifacient activity.
- Overall, little clinical evidence is available. Much of the available information is therefore speculative and based on in vitro and animal research and traditional use.

CONTRAINDICATIONS AND PRECAUTIONS

Insufficient reliable information is available.

PREGNANCY USE

Adhatoda is contraindicated in pregnancy, as the herb may have abortifacient activity. In Ayurvedic medicine it is considered safe postpartum (Pole 2006), and is used in combination with *Bacopa monniera* and 12 other herbal medicines in the treatment of vaginal discharge, pregnancy pain and pregnancy fever (Jadhav & Bhutani 2005).

PATIENTS' FAQs

What will this herb do for me?

Because adhatoda has been investigated mainly in animal and test tube studies, its effects on humans are uncertain. Based on preliminary information and historical use, it may suppress cough and have some beneficial effects in asthma.

When will it start to work?

This is uncertain because insufficient research data are available.

Are there any safety issues?

Some research suggests that adhatoda may stimulate uterine contractions, so it is not recommended in pregnancy.

REFERENCES

Balachandran P, Govindarajan R. Cancer — an ayurvedic perspective. Pharmacological research. 2005;51(1):19–30.

Balachandran C, et al. Antimycobacterial and cytotoxic (A549) properties of Vasicinone isolated from *Adhatoda vasica* (L.) Nees. Asian Pacific Journal of Tropical Biomedicine. 2012;1:1–4.

Bhattacharyya D, et al. Hepatoprotective activity of *Adhatoda vasica* aqueous leaf extract on Dgalactosamine-induced liver damage in rats. Fitoterapia. 2005;76(2):223–5.

Caldecott T. Vāsaka. Ayurveda. Edinburgh: Mosby; 2006. p. 290–2.

Chakraborty A, Brantner A. Study of alkaloids from *Adhatoda vasica* Nees on their antiinflammatory activity. Phytotherapy research. 2001;15(6):532–4.

Claeson UP, et al. *Adhatoda vasica*: a critical review of ethnopharmacological and toxicological data. Journal of ethnopharmacology. 2000;72(1):1–20.

Dhuley JN. Antitussive effect of *Adhatoda vasica* extract on mechanical or chemical stimulation-induced coughing in animals. Journal of ethnopharmacology. 1999;67(3):361–5.

Dorsch W, Wagner H. New antiasthmatic drugs from traditional medicine? Int Arch Allergy Appl Immunol. 1991;94(1–4):262–5.

Githiori J, et al. Use of plants in novel approaches for control of gastrointestinal helminthes in livestock with emphasis on small ruminants. Vet Parasit 2006;139:308–20.

Govindarajan R, et al. High-performance liquid chromatographic method for the quantification of phenolics in 'Chyavanprash', a potent Ayurvedic drug. Journal of pharmaceutical and biomedical analysis. 2007;43(2):527–32.

Grange JM, Snell NJ. Activity of bromhexine and ambroxol, semi-synthetic derivatives of vasicine from the Indian shrub *Adhatoda vasica*, against *Mycobacterium tuberculosis* in vitro. Journal of ethnopharmacology. 1996;50(1):49–53.

Gupta R, et al. Anti-tuberculosis activity of selected medicinal plants against multi-drug resistant *Mycobacterium* tuberculosis isolates. Indian Journal of Medical Research. 2010;131:809–813.

Gurib-Fakim A. Medicinal plants: traditions of yesterday and drugs of tomorrow. Molecular aspects of Medicine. 2006;27(1):1–93.

Imran M, et al. Antidiabetic activities of leaves and root extracts of *Justicia adhatoda* Linn against alloxan induced diabetes in rats. African Journal of Biotechnology. 2011;10(32):6101–6.

Jadhav AN, Bhutani K. Ayurveda and gynecological disorders. Journal of ethnopharmacology. 2005;97(1):151–9.

Jayakumar T, et al. Protective effect of *Adhatoda vasica* on D-galactosamine induced liver damage in rats with reference to lipid peroxidation and antioxidant status. Journal of Natural Remedies. 2009;9(1):91–8.

Jindal DP, et al. Synthesis and bronchodilatory activity of some nitrogen bridgehead compounds. European journal of medicinal chemistry. 2002;37(5):419–25.

Johri R, Zutshi U. Mechanism of action of 6, 7, 8, 9, 10, 12-hexahydro-azepino-[2, 1-b] quinazolin-12-one-(RLX) — a novel bronchodilator. Indian journal of physiology and pharmacology. 2000;44(1):75.

Kamal A, et al. Solid-phase synthesis of fused [2,1- *b*] quinazolinone alkaloids. Tetrahedron letters. 2006;47(51):9025–8.

Kotoky J, Das P. Medicinal plants used for liver diseases in some parts of Kamrup district of Assam, a North Eastern State of India. Fitoterapia. 2008;79(5):384–7.

Kumar A, et al. Modulatory influence of *Adhatoda vasica* Nees leaf extract against gamma irradiation in Swiss albino mice. Phytomedicine. 2005;12(4):285–93.

Lateef M, et al. Anthelmintic activity of *Adhatoda vasica* roots. Int J Agric Biol 2003;5:86–90.

Lekana-Douki JB, et al. Invitro antiplasmodial activity and cytotoxicity of nine plants traditionally used in Gabon. Journal of Ethnopharmacology. 2011;133:1103–108.

Mhaske SB, Argade NP. The chemistry of recently isolated naturally occurring quinazolinone alkaloids. Tetrahedron. 2006;62(42): 9787–826.

Murali P, et al. Plant-based formulation for bronchial asthma: A controlled clinical trial to compare its efficacy with oral salbutamol and theophylline. Respiration. 2006;73(4):457–63.

Narimanian M, et al. Randomized trial of a fixed combination (Kan Jang) of herbal extracts containing *Adhatoda vasica*, *Echinacea purpurea* and *Eleutherococcus senticosus* in patients with upper respiratory tract infections. Phytomedicine. 2005;12.8:539–47.

Nath D, et al. Commonly used Indian abortifacient plants with special reference to their teratologic effects in rats. Journal of ethnopharmacology. 1992;36(2):147–54.

Pa R, Mathew L. Antimicrobial activity of leaf extracts of *Justicia adhatoda* L. in comparison with vasicine. Asian Pacific J Trop Biomed (2012):S1556–S1560.

Pandit S, et al. Prevention of carbon tetrachloride-induced hepatotoxicity in rats by *Adhatoda vasica* leaves. Indian journal of pharmacology. 2004;36(5):312.

Pole S. Ayurvedic medicine: the principles of traditional practice: Elsevier Health Sciences, Philadelphia, 2006.

Prakash AO, et al. Anti-implantation activity of some indigenous plants in rats. Acta europaea fertilitatis. 1985;16(6):441.

Samarth RM, et al. Evaluation of antioxidant and radical-scavenging activities of certain radioprotective plant extracts. Food chemistry. 2008;106(2):868–73.

Sharma P, et al. Radiation protective potentiality of *Adhatoda vasica*. International Journal of Phytomedicine. 2011;1(1).

Shokeen P, et al. Evaluation of the activity of 16 medicinal plants against *Neisseria gonorrhoea*. International Journal of Antimicrobial Agents. 2009;33(1):86–91.

Singh B, Sharma RA. Anti-inflammatory and antimicrobial properties of pyrroloquinazoline alkaloids from *Adhatoda vasica* Nees. Phytomedicine. 2013;20 (5): 441–5.

Singh RP, et al. Modulatory influence of *Adhatoda vesica* (*Justicia adhatoda*) leaf extract on the enzymes of xenobiotic metabolism, antioxidant status and lipid peroxidation in mice. Molecular and cellular biochemistry. 2000;213(1):99–109.

Singh TP et al. Adhatoda vasica Nees: Phytochemical and Pharmacological Profile. The Natural Products Journal. 2011;1: 29–39.

Yadav AK, Tangpu V. Anticestodal activity of *Adhatoda vasica* against *Hymenolepis diminuta* infections in rats. Journal of ethnopharmacology. 2008;119(2):322–4.

Albizia

HISTORICAL NOTE It is believed that albizia received its name because Filipo del Albizi, an 18th-century Florentine nobleman, introduced the species into cultivation (The Plants Database 2004). It has been used in Ayurvedic medicine for many years and is still a popular treatment for asthma, allergy and eczema.

COMMON NAME

Albizia

OTHER NAMES

Pit shirish shirisha

BOTANICAL NAME/FAMILY

Albizia lebbeck (family Fabaceae)

PLANT PARTS USED

Leaves and stem bark

CHEMICAL COMPONENTS

These are poorly understood, but albizia has been reported to contain alkaloids, steroids, terpenoids, coumarins, tannins, flavanoids, glycosides including anthraquinones, epicatechin, procyanidins, stigmastadienone, haemolytic proteins including lebbeckalysin and saponins including albiziasaponins A, B and C (Babu et al 2009, Bobby et al 2012a, Lam & Ng 2011).

MAIN ACTIONS

Albizia has not been significantly investigated in clinical studies; therefore, information is generally derived from in vitro and animal studies.

Anti-inflammatory, antiarthritic

Albizia has demonstrated anti-inflammatory, analgesic and antiarthritic activity in several animal models (Akilandeswari et al 2009, Babu et al 2009, Yadav et al 2010). Saha and Ahmed (2009) suggest that albizia's anti-inflammatory and analgesic activity may be due to inhibition of cyclooxygenase activity and prostaglandin synthesis. Pandey et al (2010) suggest that albizia's antiarthritic activity may also be due to its antioxidant capacity, as they observed an increase in superoxide dismutase and catalase, and a decrease in lipid peroxidation in arthritic rats treated with albizia.

Antibacterial

Albizia has demonstrated antibacterial activity against *Bacillus subtilis, Escherichia coli, Klebsiella pneumoniae, Proteus vulgaris, Pseudomonas aeruginosa, Salmonella typhi* and *Staphylococus aureus, Vibrio cholerae* and *Aeromonas hydrophila* in vitro (Acharyya et al 2009, Bobby et al 2012b, Mahmood et al 2012) in all but one study (Seyydnejad et al 2010).

Antiprotozoal

Methanolic extracts of albizia demonstrated antitrypanosomal activity against *Trypanosoma cruzi* (Al-Musayeib et al 2012).

Antiallergic

Both in vitro and in vivo tests have reported significant mast cell stabilisation effects similar to those of cromoglycate (Johri et al 1985, Tripathi et al 1979). One study found that degranulation was inhibited by 62% (Tripathi et al 1979). The saponin fraction is believed to be the key group responsible for activity. An in vitro study compared the effects of albizia leaf, albizia stem bark and disodium cromoglycate on mast cell stabilisation. All three extracts were found to be equally potent (Shashidhara et al 2008). A more recent study confirmed dose-dependent mast cell stabilisation activity and inhibition of histamine release in mice with induced systemic anaphylaxis for the bark extract of albizia stem (Venkatesh et al 2010). Another study noted that albizia bark extract acted by suppressing histamine H_1 receptor (H_1R), histidine decarboxylase (HDC), interleukin-4 (IL-4), IL-5 and IL-13 mRNA elevations in sensitised allergy model rats. It also decreased HDC activity and histamine content in the nasal mucosa, and significantly decreased the incidence of sneezing and nasal rubbing (Nurul et al 2011). In addition, albizia was found to prevent phorbol-12-myristate-13-acetate or histamine-induced increases in H_1R mRNA in HeLa cells (Nurul et al 2011).

Altering neurotransmitter activity

Albizia has an influence on γ-aminobutyric acid (GABA), serotonin and dopamine levels, according to in vivo studies (Chintawar et al 2002, Kasture et al 2000). It appears that different fractions within the herb exert slightly different effects on neurotransmitters. In one study, a saponin-containing fraction from the extract of dried leaves of albizia was shown to decrease brain concentrations of GABA and dopamine, whereas serotonin levels increased. Another study that tested the methanolic fraction of an ethanolic extract of albizia leaves found that it raised brain levels of GABA and serotonin (Kasture et al 2000). Additionally, anticonvulsant activity has been demonstrated in vivo for this fraction.

Memory enhancement

Saponins isolated from albizia have been shown to improve the memory retention ability of normal and amnesic mice significantly, compared with their respective controls (Une et al 2001).

Reduces male fertility

Three studies using animal models have demonstrated that albizia significantly reduces fertility in males (Gupta et al 2004, 2005, 2006).

Albizia saponins A, B and C (50 mg/kg) isolated from the stem bark have been shown to reduce the weight of the testis, epididymides, seminal vesicle and ventral prostate of male rats significantly (Gupta et al 2005). A significant reduction in sperm concentration was also noted and albizia reduced fertility by 100% after 60 days. A follow-up study administered oral doses of methanolic bark extract (100 mg/day) for 60 days (Gupta et al 2006). Testis, epididymides, seminal vesicle and ventral prostate weights along with sperm motility and density were all significantly decreased compared to controls, also resulting in a 100% drop in male fertility. The methanolic extract of albizia pods (50, 100 and 200 mg/kg) was also shown to decrease fertility significantly and arrest spermatogenesis in rats after 60 days (Gupta et al 2004).

OTHER ACTIONS

Other actions seen in vitro and in vivo include antioxidant and antifungal actions, antispasmodic effect on smooth muscle, positive inotropy and an immunostimulant effect (Barua et al 2000, Bone 2001, Kasture et al 2000, Resmi et al 2006, Yadav et al 2011). Cholesterol-lowering activity has been demonstrated in vivo (Tripathi et al 1979).

Lebbeckalysin, a haemolytic protein isolated from albizia seeds, inhibited proliferation of breast cancer cells and hepatic cancer cells, and inhibited the growth of *Escherichia coli* and the fungus *Rhizoctonia solani* in vitro. However, it was also found to reduce the viability of murine splenocytes (Lam & Ng 2011).

CLINICAL USE

Albizia has not been significantly investigated under clinical trial conditions, so evidence is mainly derived from traditional, in vitro and animal studies, providing preliminary support for its use.

Allergy and asthma

Albizia is mainly used to treat allergic rhinitis, urticaria and asthma in clinical practice. In vitro and in vivo evidence of mast cell stabilisation provides a theoretical basis for its use in allergic conditions; however few clinical studies exist to confirm its significance. In a single-blind study 81 participants with asthma were given 50 mL of albizia stem bark decoction three times daily for 6 weeks. At 6 weeks, there was a significant increase in lung function and a decrease in total leucocyte count, eosinophil count and erythrocyte sedimentation rate. Of the 50 participants who completed the trial, 56% reported symptom reduction of >75%, 38% reported symptom reduction of 50–75% and 6% reported symptom reduction of less than 50% (Kumar et al 2010).

OTHER USES

Traditionally, a juice made from the leaves has been used internally to treat night blindness. The bark and seeds have been used to relieve diarrhoea and dysentery and treat haemorrhoids, most likely because of their astringent activity. The flowers have been used as an emollient to soothe eruptions, swellings, boils and carbuncles. In Ayurvedic medicine, albizia is used to treat bronchitis, asthma, allergy and inflammation.

DOSAGE RANGE

Australian manufacturer recommendations

- Liquid extract (1 : 2): 3.5–8.5 mL/day or 25–60 mL/week.
- Dried herb: 3–6 g/day.
- Based on clinical trials:
  - Asthma: 50 mL of albizia stem bark decoction three times daily for 6 weeks (Kumar et al 2010).

TOXICITY

This is unknown; however, research with the methanolic fraction of albizia extract has identified a median lethal dose of 150 mg/kg (Kasture et al 2000).

ADVERSE REACTIONS

Insufficient reliable information available.

SIGNIFICANT INTERACTIONS

Controlled studies are not available; therefore, interactions are based on evidence of activity and are largely theoretical and speculative.

Barbiturates

Additive effects are theoretically possible, as potentiation of pentobarbitone-induced sleep has been observed in vivo — use with caution.

Antihistamines and mast cell-stabilising drugs

Additive effects are theoretically possible because both in vitro and in vivo tests have identified significant mast cell-stabilisation activity similar to that of cromoglycate — potentially beneficial interaction.

Tricyclic and selective serotonin reuptake inhibitor antidepressant drugs

Increased risk of serotonin syndrome is theoretically possible, as albizia increases serotonin levels, according to in vivo studies — observe patient.

CONTRAINDICATIONS AND PRECAUTIONS

Significant reductions in male fertility have been reported in tests using animal models; however, it is not known whether the effects also occur in humans. Until further research is conducted, caution is advised.

PREGNANCY USE

Insufficient reliable information available. Based on animal studies indicating a significant effect on male fertility, males with low sperm counts or poor sperm motility should avoid this herb if attempting to father a child.

Practice points/Patient counselling

- Albizia is a traditional Ayurvedic herb used to treat allergies, asthma, eczema and inflammation.
- Preliminary research has shown that it has significant mast cell-stabilisation activity comparable to cromoglycate, and has also identified memory enhancement activity and possible anticonvulsant effects.
- Preliminary human research suggests a possible role in asthma; however more research is required to clarify its role.
- Overall, little clinical evidence is available; therefore, much information is speculative and based on in vitro and animal research.

PATIENTS' FAQs

What will this herb do for me?

Albizia is a traditional Ayurvedic medicine used to reduce allergic conditions, such as allergic rhinitis and urticaria. It is also used for atopic conditions, such as eczema and asthma, when indicated. Controlled trials have not been conducted, so it is uncertain whether it is effective.

When will it start to work?

This is uncertain because insufficient research data are available.

Are there any safety issues?

This is uncertain because insufficient research data are available. It is advised that people with asthma be monitored by a healthcare professional. Males with low sperm counts or poor sperm motility should avoid this herb if attempting to father a child.

REFERENCES

Acharyya S, et al. Evaluation of the antimicrobial activity of some medicinal plants against enteric bacteria with particular reference to multi-drug resistant *Vibrio cholerae*. Tropical Journal of Pharmaceutical Research 8.3 (2009).

Akilandeswari S et al. Evaluation of anti-inflammatory and anti-arthritic activity of *Albizia lebbeck* and *Albizia amara* extracts. Biomed 4.3 (2009): 295–302.

Al-Musayeib NM et al. Study of the in vitro antiplasmodial, antileishmanial and antitrypanosomal activities of medicinal plants from Saudi Arabia. Molecules 17.10 (2012): 11379–90.

Babu NP, et al. Anti-inflammatory activity of *Albizia lebbeck* Benth., an ethnomedicinal plant, in acute and chronic animal models of inflammation. Journal of Ethnopharmacology 125.2 (2009): 356–60.

Barua CC et al. Immunomodulatory effects of *Albizia lebbeck*. Pharmaceut Biol 38.3 (2000): 161–166.

Bobby M, et al. High performance thin layer chromatography profile studies on the alkaloids of *Albizia lebbeck*. Asian Pacific Journal of Tropical Biomedicine 2.1 (2012a): S1–S6.

Bobby M, et al. In vitro anti-bacterial activity of leaves extracts of *Albizia lebbeck* Benth against some selected pathogens. Asian Pacific Journal of Tropical Biomedicine 2.2 (2012b): S859–S62.

Bone K. Clinical Applications of Ayurvedic and Chinese Herbs. Warwick, Qld: Phytotherapy Press, 2001.

Chintawar SD et al. Nootropic activity of *Albizia lebbeck* in mice. J Ethnopharmacol 81.3 (2002): 299–305.

Gupta RS, et al. Antifertility effects of methanolic pod extract of *Albizia lebbeck* (L.) Benth in male rats. Asian J Androl 6.2 (2004): 155–159.

Gupta RS et al. Effect of saponins of *Albizia lebbeck* (L.) Benth bark on the reproductive system of male albino rats. J Ethnopharmacol 96.1–2 (2005): 31–36.

Gupta RS, et al. Antispermatogenic, antiandrogenic activities of *Albizia lebbeck* (L.) Benth bark extract in male albino rats. Phytomedicine 13.4 (2006): 277–283.

Johri RK et al. Effect of quercetin and *Albizia* saponins on rat mast cell. Indian J Physiol Pharmacol 29.1 (1985): 43–46.

Kasture VS, et al. Anticonvulsive activity of *Albizia lebbeck*, *Hibiscus rosa sinensis* and *Butea monosperma* in experimental animals. J Ethnopharmacol 71.1–2 (2000): 65–75.

Kumar S et al. The Clinical Effect of *Albizia lebbeck* Stem Bark Decoction on Bronchial Asthma. International Journal of Pharmaceutical Sciences and Drug Research 2.1 (2010): 48–50.

Lam SK & Ng TB. First report of an anti-tumor, anti-fungal, anti-yeast and anti-bacterial hemolysin from *Albizia lebbeck* seeds. Phytomedicine 18.7 (2011): 601–8.

Mahmood A, et al. Antimicrobial activities of three species of family mimosaceae. Pakistan Journal Of Pharmaceutical Sciences 25.1 (2012): 203–6.

Nurul IM et al. *Albizia lebbeck* suppresses histamine signaling by the inhibition of histamine H1 receptor and histidine decarboxylase gene transcriptions. International Immunopharmacology 11.11 (2011): 1766–72.

Pandey S, et al. Biological evaluation of free radical scavenging activity of *Albizia lebbeck* methanolic extract in arthritic rats. Annals of Biological Research 1.1 (2010): 116–23.

Resmi CR, et al. Antioxidant activity of *Albizia lebbeck* (Linn.) Benth. in alloxan diabetic rats. Indian J Physiol Pharmacol 50.3 (2006): 297–302.

Saha A & Ahmed M. The analgesic and anti-inflammatory activities of the extract of *Albizia lebbeck* in animal model. Pak. J. Pharm. Sci 22.1 (2009): 74–7.

Seyydnejad SM et al. Antibacterial Activity of Hydroalcoholic Extract of *Callistemon citrinus* and *Albizia lebbeck*. American Journal of Applied Sciences 7.1 (2010): 13–6.

Shashidhara S, et al. Comparative evaluation of successive extracts of leaf and stem bark of *Albizia lebbeck* for mast cell stabilization activity. Fitoterapia 79.4 (2008): 301–302.

The Plants Database. Online. Available: www.plantsdatabase.com March 2004.

Tripathi RM, et al. Studies on the mechanism of action of *Albizia lebbeck*, an Indian indigenous drug used in the treatment of atopic allergy. J Ethnopharmacol 1.4 (1979): 385–396.

Une HD et al. Nootropic and anxiolytic activity of saponins of *Albizia lebbeck* leaves. Pharmacol Biochem Behav 69.3–4 (2001): 439–444.

Venkatesh P et al. Anti-allergic activity of standardized extract of *Albizia lebbeck* with reference to catechin as a phytomarker. Immunopharmacology and immunotoxicology 32.2 (2010): 272–6.

Yadav SS et al. Anti-inflammatory activity of Shirishavaleha: An Ayurvedic compound formulation. International Journal Of Ayurveda Research 1.4 (2010): 205–7.

Yadav SS et al. Evaluation of immunomodulatory activity of "Shirishavaleha" — An Ayurvedic compound formulation in albino rats. Journal Of Ayurveda And Integrative Medicine 2.4 (2011): 192–6.

Aloe vera

HISTORICAL NOTE *Aloe vera* has been used since ancient times as a medicinal plant. In fact, evidence of use has been found on a Mesopotamian clay tablet dating back to 2100 BC (Atherton 1998). It has been used as a topical treatment for wounds, burns and other skin conditions and internally as a general tonic, anti-inflammatory agent, carminative, laxative, aphrodisiac and anthelminthic by the ancient Romans, Greeks, Arabs, Indians and Spaniards. According to legend, Alexander the Great captured an island in the Indian Ocean in order to access the *Aloe vera* for his wounded army. Today aloe is used to soothe skin complaints and treat burns, and is a common ingredient in many cosmetic products.

OTHER NAMES

Aloes, Barbados aloe, Curacao aloe

BOTANICAL NAME/FAMILY

Aloe vera (L.)/*Aloe barbadensis* (Mill.) (family Aloeaceae)

PLANT PARTS USED

The plant leaves are used, from which several different products are made; namely the exudate, gel, extract and juice. The exudate ('aloes' in older pharmacy texts) is a thick residue, yellow in colour and bitter in taste that comes from the latex that oozes out when the leaf is cut. The 'gel' refers to the clear gel or mucilage produced by the inner parenchymal cells in the central part of the leaf. Diluted aloe gel is commonly known as 'aloe vera extract' or 'aloe juice'.

CHEMICAL COMPONENTS

Aloe vera extract, or diluted aloe gel, is made of mostly water (99%) and mono- and polysaccharides, the most important of which are the monosaccharide mannose-6-phosphate and the polysaccharide gluco-mannans, which are long-chain sugars containing glucose and mannose. Gluco-mannan has been named acemannan and is marketed as Carrisyn. A glycoprotein with antiallergic properties has also been isolated, and has been named alprogen. Recently, C-glucosyl chromone, an anti-inflammatory compound, has also been identified.

Aloe gel also contains lignans, saponins, salicylic acid, sterols and triterpenoids, vitamins A, C, E, B_{12}, thiamine, niacin and folic acid, and the minerals sodium, calcium, potassium, manganese, magnesium, copper, chromium, zinc and iron (Shelton 1991, Yamaguchi et al 1993).

The fresh gel contains glutathione peroxidase, isozymes of superoxide dismutase and the proteolytic enzyme carboxypeptidase (Klein & Penneys 1988, Sabeh et al 1993). In vitro bioassays identified three malic acid-acylated carbohydrates from the gel, veracylglucan A, B and C, and determined that veracylglucan B exhibited potent anti-inflammatory and antiproliferative effects; veracylglucan C exhibited significant cell proliferative and anti-inflammatory activities; and the third carbohydrate, veracylglucan A, was highly unstable and provided no biological effects. Of interest is that veracylglucan B and C proved to be highly competitive in their effects on cell proliferation (Esua & Rauwald 2006).

Ultimately, the types and levels of components present in aloe gel vary according to geographic origin, variety and processing method.

There are significant constituent differences between aloe vera gel, juice and total leaf extracts. The exudate (latex layer) contains the pharmacologically active anthraquinone glycosides aloin, aloe-emodin, barbaloin, emodin and aloectic acid (Choi & Chung 2003, Rodriguez-Fragoso et al 2008), while aloe vera gel contains no anthraquinones (Vogler & Ernst 1999). It must be noted that, due to these central differences, evidence for a particular preparation of aloe may not necessarily be translatable across all types of aloe vera preparations.

MAIN ACTIONS

The active ingredients, whether acting alone or in concert, include glycoproteins, anthraquinones, polysaccharides, and low-molecular-weight species such as beta-sitosterol (Choi & Chung 2003).

Assists in wound healing

Wound healing is associated with various mechanisms and constituents. Thromboxane inhibits wound healing and aloe has been shown to inhibit thromboxane in vitro (Zachary et al 1987). Enzymes in aloe have also been shown to break down damaged tissue, which can then be removed by phagocytosis (Bunyapraphatsara et al 1996). A glycoprotein fraction was found to increase proliferation of human keratinocytes and increase the expression of receptors for epidermal growth factor and fibronectin in vitro (Choi et al 2001). The same research team then demonstrated that this glycoprotein enhanced wound healing by increasing cell proliferation in vivo. Beta-sitosterol appears to improve wound healing by stimulating angiogenesis and neovascularisation in vivo (Moon et al 1999). Aloe polysaccharides have been shown to ameliorate ultraviolet (UV)–induced immunosuppression (Strickland et al 1994).

In vitro and in vivo research generally shows that aloe vera application has beneficial effects in wound healing caused by thermal burns or frostbite. However few studies report on the levels of active constituents present in the test application or even the treatment regimen, making firm conclusions difficult. Not surprisingly, a 2012 Cochrane Review concluded that there is currently insufficient clinical trial evidence available to support the use of aloe vera topical agents or impregnated dressings as a treatment for acute and chronic wounds (Dat et al 2012). In future, better reporting of aloe vera preparations tested, their levels of active constituents and administration regimens, is necessary to better understand its effects.

Tests in animal models

Several animal studies support the application of aloe gel to skin damaged by frostbite as a means of maintaining circulation and reducing the vasoconstrictive effects of thromboxane in the affected dermis (Heggers et al 1987, Klein & Penneys 1988, McCauley et al 1990, Miller & Koltai 1995). In combination with pentoxifylline, it will act synergistically to further increase tissue survival (Miller & Koltai 1995).

A study to test the effectiveness of topical application versus oral administration in rats with full-thickness wounds showed topical use of aloe gel to be slightly more effective than internal use. The collagen content in granulation tissue was measured to be 89% in the topical group compared with 83% in the oral group (Chithra et al 1998). Oral administration of lyophilised *A. vera* powder was also found to increase wound contraction in rats with acute radiation-delayed wound healing, which was associated with increased transforming growth factor-β_1 (TGF-β_1) and basic fibroblast growth factor (Atiba et al 2011).

Other studies have found that aloe gel not only increases collagen content, but also changes collagen composition, in addition to increasing collagen cross-linking, which in turn increases the breaking strength of scar tissue, making the seal stronger (Chithra et al 1998, Heggers et al 1996). Conversely, a study using a porcine model of partial-thickness burns found that the application of aloe vera did not improve the re-epithelialisation of the wound, the scar size or visual appearance of the scar compared to control (no intervention) (Cuttle et al 2008). The study used leaves of a mature, well-established plant which were skinned and enough of the inner pulp and gel was collected and applied directly to the wound to cover it.

Full-thickness hot-plate burns (3% total surface area) in test animals healed more quickly with the application of aloe gel compared to silver sulfadiazine (SSD) or salicylic acid cream (aspirin) (Rodriguez-Bigas et al 1988). Guinea pigs treated with aloe recovered in 30 days as compared to 50 days for control animals (dressing only) and wound bacterial counts were effectively decreased. *A. vera* was also found to promote healing and decrease inflammation in second-degree burns in vivo (Somboonwong et al 2000). A significant reduction in vasodilation and postcapillary venular permeability was recorded on day 7 in the aloe group. At day 14 arteriolar diameter had returned to normal and the size of the wound was greatly reduced as compared to controls. More recently, a study found that treatment with aloe vera powdered gel (0.5%) 24 hours after a burn injury induced by hot water and then applied regularly over the next 25 days resulted in a significantly smaller wound size compared with SSD (Khorasani et al 2009). Additionally, a histological comparison showed aloe to increase re-epithelialisation in burn wounds significantly as compared with other cream-treated wounds which included SSD.

Aloe gel prevented delayed hypersensitivity of UV-irritated skin as well as contact hypersensitivity in animal models with allergic reactions (Strickland et al 1994). Acemannan gel (beta-(1,4)-acetylated mannan) has demonstrably improved radiation burns in mice. Best results were obtained when the gel was applied during the first week after injury (Roberts & Travis 1995).

Use with pharmaceutical agents

Several topical pharmaceutical antimicrobial agents, such as SSD, inhibit wound contraction, thereby slowing the rate of wound healing. An experimental model was used to investigate whether co-administration of aloe could reverse this effect and improve the wound-healing rate (Muller et al 2003). Full-thickness excised wounds were treated with placebo (aqueous cream or saline), SSD cream 0.5%, 1% or 1% with *A. vera* three times daily for 14 days, then observed until healed. *A. vera* was found to reverse the delayed wound healing produced by SSD, resulting in the shortest wound half-life and healing time.

A. vera (100 and 300 mg/kg daily for 4 days) blocked the ability of hydrocortisone acetate to suppress wound healing by up to 100% (Davis et al 1994a). Growth factors in *A. vera* were thought to mask sterols and certain amino acids that prevent wound healing. Another study identified the sugar mannose-6-phosphate to be one of the chief constituents responsible for wound healing (Davis et al 1994b).

Antioxidant

Studies have found that several compounds present in aloe gel protect tissues against oxidative damage caused by free radicals; however the clinical impact of this is yet to be determined (Singh et al 2000, 't Hart et al 1990, Wu et al 2006, Yagi et al 2002, Zhang et al 2006). This is achieved by direct antioxidant activity and indirect activity through stimulation of endogenous antioxidant systems. Two aloe dihydroisocoumarins have been identified and have demonstrated free radical scavenging properties (Zhang et al 2006, 2008).

Treatment with aloe gel extract decreased lipid peroxidation and hydroperoxides in diabetic rats to near-normal levels (Rajasekaran et al 2005). The extract also significantly increased superoxide dismutase, catalase, glutathione peroxidase and glutathione-*S*-transferase in the liver and kidney. In another study, data obtained 3, 7 and 10 days after exposure to radiation showed that aloe gel significantly reduced oxidative damage in the liver, lungs and kidney tissues of irradiated rats (Saada et al 2003). The oral administration of aloe vera to rats prior to 8 Gy gamma radiation exposure decreased serum lipid peroxidation and increased the reduced glutathione level and vitamin C levels (Saini & Saini 2011). This correlated with higher percentage survival after 30 days compared to untreated controls (93.3% vs 20% respectively).

A study by Jain et al (2010) identified that *A. vera* 30% gel increased thiobarbituric acid reactive substance, superoxide dismutase and catalase levels back to baseline levels in a model of induced diabetes in rats.

Three-year-old aloe plants appear to have the highest amounts of flavonoids and polysaccharides and hence the best free radical scavenging capacity, as compared to 2- and 4-year-old plants (Hu et al 2003). Interestingly, the 3-year-old plant demonstrated antioxidant activity of 72.19%, compared to alpha-tocopherol at 65.20%.

Immunostimulant

It has been suggested that aloe may have immune-stimulating capabilities. Much of the available research has been performed on mice or in vitro and aloe shows antiviral, antitumour and non-specific immunostimulant activity. An experiment in 1980 demonstrated that mice given aloe extract 2 days before exposure to pathogens were protected against a variety of fungi and bacteria (Brossat et al 1981).

Later, the isolated compound acemannan (beta-(1,4)-acetylated mannan) was shown to increase the response of lymphocytes to antigens in vitro (Womble & Helderman 1988). In mice, acemannan stimulated cytokines, bringing about an immune attack on implanted sarcoma cells, leading to necrosis and regression of cancer cells (Peng et al 1991). A later trial investigated the effects of acemannan on mouse macrophages (Zhang & Tizard 1996). Acemannan stimulated macrophage cytokine production (interleukin-6 (IL-6) and tumour necrosis factor-alpha (TNF-alpha), nitric oxide release, surface molecule expression and cellular morphological changes. Similarly, a polysaccharide fraction isolated from *A. vera* promoted human keratinocytes to secrete TGF-alpha, TGF-beta$_1$, IL-1beta, IL-6, IL-8 and TNF, and inhibited the release of nitric oxide as compared to control (Chen et al 2005). The immune-enhancing effects of acemannan may be due in part to the compound's ability to promote differentiation of immature dendritic cells (Lee et al 2001). These cells are crucial for the initiation of primary immune responses.

Multiple studies have highlighted the diverse immunomodulatory activities of aloe polysaccharides. Some studies have identified that immunomodulatory activity varies with the size of the polysaccharide entity. It appears that aloe polysaccharides that are of smaller molecular weight (specifically between 5 and 400 kDa) have the greatest immunological effects, possibly because they are better absorbed than larger-molecular-weight entities (Im et al 2005).

Three purified polysaccharide fractions (PAC-I, PAC-II and PAC-III) from *A. vera* stimulated peritoneal macrophages, and splenic T and B cells, and increased the ability of these cells to secrete TNF-alpha, IL-1beta, interferon-gamma, IL-2 and IL-6 (Leung et al 2004). The compound with the highest mannose content, and therefore the highest molecular weight (PAC-I), demonstrated the most potential. This finding was again repeated by Liu et al (2006), whereby PAC-I exhibited potent stimulation of murine macrophages and produced tumoricidal properties of activated macrophages in vitro, thus providing evidence in support of its antitumour properties.

A 99% pure carbohydrate compound (purified acemannan) isolated from aloe demonstrated potent haematopoietic and haematological activity in myelosuppressed mice (Talmadge et al 2004).

Specific manufacturing methods can be applied to enhance the extracts. For example, 1 g of extract obtained from leaves subjected to cold and dark treatment contained 400 mg of neutral polysaccharide compared with 30 mg in leaves not specially treated (Shida et al 1985).

> ***Clinical note — Wound-healing models***
>
> Acute wound healing occurs in four stages that tend to overlap: haemostasis, inflammation, proliferation and remodelling. Underlying metabolic disturbances and/or disease may disrupt the regenerative process, causing delayed healing. Much investigation is conducted with in vitro assays based on cell culture models of the various phases of healing, which provide information about possible mechanisms of action. Experimental models using animals are undertaken to determine the reduction of wound size (usually in terms of area) and hence the rate of healing. Histological examination of granulation and epidermal tissues provides a concurrent analysis at the molecular level. Human models of wound healing provide an opportunity to observe a variety of healing disorders that are less predictable than their cell or animal-based counterparts. *Aloe vera* is one of the very few traditional wound-healing herbal medicines that has been subjected to a variety of cell culture-based, animal and human-based studies (Krishnan 2006).

Anti-inflammatory

A number of in vitro and in vivo studies confirm the anti-inflammatory activity of *A. vera*.

The gel reduces oxidation of arachidonic acid, thereby reducing prostaglandin (PG) synthesis and inflammation (Davis et al 1987). It inhibits the production of PGE_2 by 30% and IL-8 by 20%, but has no effect on thromboxane B_2 production in vitro (Langmead et al 2004). Following burn injury in vivo, *A. vera* was also found to inhibit inflammation by reducing leucocyte adhesion and decreasing the proinflammatory cytokines TNF-alpha and IL-6 (Duansak et al 2003). Similarly, significant reductions in proinflammatory cytokines IL-1beta, IL-6 and TNF-alpha have been shown in in vitro models of monocyte-derived macrophages (Budai et al 2013) and human corneal cells (Woźniak and Paduch 2012).

An in vivo study of induced ulcerative colitis in rats found that dietary supplemention with aloe components aloin, aloesin and aloe gel resulted in significantly reduced plasma leukotriene B_4 and TNF-alpha concentrations, as well as colonic mucosal TNF-alpha and IL-1beta concentrations compared to controls (Park et al 2011). Similarly, IL-1beta, IL-6 and TNF-alpha were reduced following aloe vera treatment in a murine model of sepsis, which correlated with reduced bacterial count and increased survival (Yun et al 2009).

One study conducted on rats with croton oil-induced oedema reported a 47% reduction in swelling after the application of topical aloe gel (Davis et al 1989). Another study found aloe gel reduced vascularity and swelling by 50% in the inflamed synovial pouch in rats, along with a 48% reduction in the number of mast cells in the synovial fluid within the pouch. When aloe gel was applied topically there was also an increase in fibroblast cell numbers (Davis et al 1992). C-glucosyl chromone, isolated from aloe gel extracts, is chiefly responsible for the anti-inflammatory effect, with activity comparable to hydrocortisone in experimental models (Hutter et al 1996). A study of streptozotocin-induced diabetic mice further confirmed the anti-inflammatory activity of *A. vera* and identified the isolated constituent gibberellin as also effective (Davis & Maro 1989). Both compounds inhibited inflammation in a dose-dependent manner. A recent in vitro assessment using human immune cells displayed aloe's potential to reduce bacteria-induced proinflammatory cytokine production, specifically TNF-alpha and IL-1-beta, by peripheral blood leucocytes stimulated with *Shigella flexneri* or lipopolysaccharide (Habeeb et al 2007).

A number of studies have identified a possible role for aloe vera in the treatment of oral lichen planus (OLP), a chronic inflammation of the oral mucosal membranes. However, a 2011 Cochrane Review concluded that there was only weak evidence to support the use of *A. vera* to reduce pain and clinical signs of OLP compared to placebo (Thongprasom et al 2011).

Laxative

The aloe latex contains anthraquinones, which have a stimulant laxative activity. Studies in rats have shown that aloe latex increases intestinal water content, stimulates mucus secretion and induces intestinal peristalsis (Ishii et al 1994). However, aloe as a laxative is more irritating than other herbs (Reynolds & Dweck 1999) and long-term use can cause an electrolyte imbalance through depletion of potassium salts. Alternatives are recommended if long-term treatment is required.

Antiulcer

The antiulcer activity of *A. vera* has been proposed to be due to anti-inflammatory, cytoprotective, healing and mucus stimulatory effects. According to an in vivo study, *A. vera* promotes gastric ulcer healing (Eamlamnam et al 2006). In contrast to these results, in another study a stabilised fresh aloe gel preparation prolonged the effect of histamine-stimulated acid secretion but inhibited pepsin (Suvitayavat et al 2004).

Hypoglycaemic

Glucomannan slows carbohydrate absorption and slows the postprandial insulin response by up to 50% (McCarty 2002).

A. vera leaf gel has been investigated as a possible hepatoprotective and kidney-protective agent in diabetes type 2 using animal models. In one study, the leaf gel and glibenclamide both decreased degenerative kidney changes, serum urea levels and creatinine levels, but only aloe further reduced kidney lipid peroxidation (Bolkent et al 2004). Can et al (2004) tested aloe pulp, aloe gel extract and glibenclamide, finding that all treatments decreased liver tissue damage compared to control animals. Aloe gel extract also increased glutathione levels and decreased non-enzymatic glycosylation, lipid peroxidation, serum alkaline phosphatase and alanine transaminase. In a mouse model of type 2 diabetes mellitus, administration of aloe gel to diabetic mice over 8 weeks resulted in lowered blood glucose levels, which correlated with a reduced insulin resistance (Kim et al 2009).

Chemotherapeutic

Recent preclinical research has identified that aloe-emodin (an anthraquinone compound) present in the leaves of *A. vera* shows promising anticancer effects in human gastric carcinoma cell lines AGS and NCI-N87. Aloe-emodin induced cell death in a dose-dependent and time-dependent manner and caused the release of apoptosis-inducing factor and cytochrome c from mitochondria, followed by the activation of caspase-3, leading to nuclear shrinkage and apoptosis (AGS was more sensitive than NCI-N87 cells). In addition, casein kinase II activity was suppressed (time-dependent) and was accompanied by a reduced phosphorylation of Bid, a downstream substrate of casein kinase II and a proapoptotic molecule (Chen et al 2007).

Another study investigated the anticancer effect of aloe-emodin in T24 human bladder cancer cells and found that it induced apoptosis in T24 cells mediated through the activation of p53, p21, Fas/APO-1, Bax and caspase-3 (Lin et al 2006).

In mouse B16 melanoma and human A375 melanoma cell lines, aloe-emodin reduced cell viability in a dose-dependent manner through mechanisms of terminal differentiation and caspase-dependent apoptosis respectively (Radovic et al 2012).

Antimicrobial

A. vera is active against a wide variety of bacteria in vitro, such as *Pseudomonas aeruginosa*, *Klebsiella pneumoniae*, *Streptococcus pyogenes*, *Staphylococcus aureus* and *Escherichia coli* (Heck et al 1981, Shelton 1991). More recent research indicates antimicrobial activity against *Shigella flexneri*, methicillin-resistant *Staphylococcus aureus*, *Enterobacter cloacae* and *Enterococcus bovis* (Habeeb et al 2007).

Antiviral

In vitro studies suggest that *Aloe vera* has antiviral activity due to its interference with DNA synthesis (Saoo et al 1996). The polysaccharide fractions of aloe gel inhibit the binding of benzopyrene to primary rat hepatocytes and thus prevent the formation of potentially cancer-initiating benzopyrene-DNA adducts in vitro. This was later confirmed by in vivo studies (Kim & Lee 1997). Moreover, in vitro experiments have shown the anthraquinones in aloe to be virucidal against herpes simplex virus types 1 and 2, vaccinia virus, parainfluenza virus and vesicular stomatitis virus (Anderson 2003).

Investigation with the acemannan component has identified antiviral activity, particularly against feline AIDS, HIV type 1, influenza virus, measles virus and herpes simplex (Kahlon et al 1991a, 1991b, Sydiskis et al 1991).

Antifungal

An in vivo study using mice showed that the administration of processed *A. vera* gel reduced clearance of *Candida albicans* in both spleen and kidneys in a dose-dependent manner (Im et al 2010).

CLINICAL USE

Although *A. vera* products are used for many indications, the chief use is treating skin conditions. Various test preparations have been used, including fresh aloe vera mucilage, aloe vera gel, powdered aloe vera and aloe vera used with various gauzes. Commercial aloe vera preparations vary considerably in their quality and polysaccharide content, such as acemannan, which is considered an important functional component. Ideally, aloe vera preparations should have adequate amounts of the polysaccharide acemannan (at least 10% w/w) (Bozzi et al 2007). Unfortunately, researchers do not appear to test their preparations for adequate levels of polysaccharides or report on the polysaccharide content of their aloe vera preparation, which makes it difficult to interpret study results or make meaningful comparisons.

Skin conditions

Aloe is used in the treatment of wounds, burns, radiation burns, ulcers, frostbite, psoriasis and genital herpes, and is the only traditional wound-healing herbal medicine which has been subjected to a variety of cell culture-based, animal and human-based studies (Krishnan 2006). The healing properties may be attributed to antimicrobial, immune-stimulating, anti-inflammatory and antithromboxane activities. Allantoin has also been shown to stimulate epithelialisation, and acemannan has been shown to stimulate macrophage production of IL-1 and TNF, which are associated with wound healing (Liptak 1997).

Most human studies have found that topical application of aloe vera gel increases wound-healing rate and effectively reduces microbial counts; however, there are some negative studies, most likely related to the fact that the composition of aloe vera gel varies, even within the same species. Chemical composition depends on source, climate, region and the processing method used (Choi & Chung 2003).

Dry-coated aloe vera gloves were tested by 30 women suffering from dry, cracked hands, with or without contact dermatitis due to occupational exposure, in an open contralateral comparison study (West & Zhu 2003). Women wore a glove on one hand for 8 hours daily for 30 days followed by a rest period for 30 days and then 10 more days of treatment. Results indicated that the aloe vera glove significantly reduced dry skin, irritation, wrinkling, dermatitis and redness and improved skin integrity. It would be interesting to see this study repeated using a standard non-aloe-fortified glove on the opposing hand.

The effects of aloe gel applied to skin following dermabrasion in humans are more controversial, with some patients experiencing severe adverse reactions, including burning sensations and dermatitis (Hunter & Frumkin 1991). One study found that topical aloe vera gel actually slowed healing after caesarean delivery (Schmidt & Greenspoon 1991).

Burns

A systematic review of the efficacy of *A. vera* for healing of burns considered four controlled clinical trials involving 371 patients. Meta-analysis concluded that topical treatment with *A. vera* decreased healing time and was specifically more effective for first- and second-degree burns rather than third-degree burns. In particular, based on a meta-analysis using duration of wound healing as an outcome measure, the summary weighted-mean difference in healing time of the aloe vera group was 8.79 days shorter than those in the control group ($P = 0.006$). It was noted that, due to variations in the aloe preparations and outcome measures used in the studies, more specific conclusions cannot be drawn (Maenthalsong et al 2007). The types of aloe vera preparations studied include fresh aloe vera mucilage, gauze impregnated with 85% gel, aloe vera cream and gauze with 1% aloe vera powder. Importantly, none of the studies reported on the amount of key active constituents in their test preparations.

Comparisons to silver sulfadiazine (SSD)

Several studies have compared aloe vera to SSD. The most recent study found that treatment with aloe vera cream twice daily in patients with second-degree burns on two different body sites (n = 30) resulted in faster rates of re-epithelialisation (15.90 ± 2.00 vs 18.73 ± 2.65 days) compared to SSD and were considered fully healed faster than SSD (16 days vs 19 days) (Khorasani et al 2009). An older study comparing SSD with *A. vera* mucilage or a combination of both found that the success rate in the aloe vera group and the SSD group was 95% and 83%, respectively in the treatment of first- or second-degree burns (n = 38) (Thamlikitkul 1991).

Psoriasis

A 2010 double-blind, randomised trial found that topically applied *A. vera* significantly improved psoriasis area and severity index [PASI] scores compared to 0.1% triamcinolone acetonide cream (Choonhakarn et al 2010). After 8 weeks of treatment, *A. vera* treatment resulted in a mean reduction in PASI of 7.7 ± 2.3 compared to triamcinolone acetonide, which reduced PASI by 6.6 ± 2.1 (95% confidence interval: 1.1 (–2.13, –0.16), P = 0.0237).

A double-blind placebo-controlled study found topical aloe vera extract 0.5% in a hydrophilic cream to be beneficial in the treatment of psoriasis. Sixty patients aged 18–50 years with slight to moderate chronic psoriasis and PASI scores between 4.8 and 16.7 (mean 9.3) participated in the study, which was scheduled for 16 weeks with 12 months of follow-up. Patients were examined weekly and those showing a progressive reduction of lesions, desquamation followed by decreased erythema, infiltration and lowered PASI score were considered healed. By the end of the study, the *A. vera* extract cream had cured 83.3% of patients compared with the placebo cure rate of 6.6% ($P < 0.001$). Psoriatic plaques decreased in 82.8% of patients versus only 7.7% in the placebo group ($P < 0.001$). PASI scores decreased to a mean of 2.2 (Syed et al 1996a). In contrast, a randomised, double-blind, placebo-controlled trial found no significant benefits with a commercial aloe vera gel in 41 patients with stable plaque psoriasis (Paulsen et al 2005). Following a 2-week washout period patients applied either the aloe gel or the placebo twice daily for 1 month. Redness and desquamation decreased by 72.5% in the active treatment group as compared to 82.5% in the placebo group. It should be pointed out that 82.5% is an extremely high placebo responder rate. Fifty-five per cent of patients reported local side effects, mainly drying of the skin on test areas.

Genital herpes

Two clinical studies have investigated the effects of *Aloe vera* 0.5% topical preparations in genital herpes, producing good results.

A double-blind, placebo-controlled study has demonstrated that *A. vera* extract 0.5% in a hydrophilic cream is more efficacious than placebo in the treatment of initial episodes of genital herpes in men (n = 60, aged 18–40 years). Each patient was provided with a 40 g tube containing placebo or active preparation, with instructions on self-application of the trial medication to their lesions three times daily for 5 consecutive days (maximum 15 topical applications per week). The treatment was well tolerated by all patients (Syed et al 1997).

The other study involving 120 subjects used a preparation containing 0.5% of whole aloe leaf extract in a hydrophilic castor and mineral oil cream base, which was applied three times daily for 5 days per week for 2 weeks. Treatment resulted in a shorter mean duration of healing compared with placebo. Aloe cream also increased the overall percentage of healed patients and there were no significant adverse reactions reported (Syed et al 1996b).

Another study involving 18 outpatients with moderate to deep second-degree burns ranging from 2 to 12% of total body surface area showed that a commercial aloe vera ointment was as effective as SSD in regard to protection against bacterial colonisation and healing time. More specifically, the mean healing time with aloe vera treatment was 13 days compared with 16.15 days for SSD (Heck et al 1981).

Results are less encouraging for sunburn protection and healing. A randomised double-blind trial in 20 healthy volunteers evaluated the effect of aloe vera cream for both prevention and treatment of sunburn (Puvabanditsin & Vongtongsri 2005). The cream (70% aloe) was applied 30 minutes before, immediately after, or both before and after UV irradiation. The cream was then continually applied daily for 3 weeks. The results showed that the aloe vera cream did not protect against sunburn and was not an effective treatment.

Frostbite

In combination with other treatments, topical *A. vera* significantly enhances healing and has a beneficial effect in frostbite. One clinical study compared the effects of topical aloe vera cream in combination with standard treatment, such as rapidly rewarming the affected areas, analgesics, antibiotics and debridement (n = 56) with another group of 98 patients who did not receive *A. vera* treatment. Of those receiving *A. vera* in addition to usual treatment, 67% healed without tissue loss compared with 32.7% in the control group. Additionally, 7.1% of the total group of 56 required amputation compared with 32.7% in the control group. Although encouraging, this study is difficult to interpret because the groups were not well matched and combination therapies differed (Heggers et al 1987).

Radiation-induced dermatitis

There have been several studies which have focused on the effects of aloe on radiation-induced dermatitis. A 2005 review concluded that aloe gel was as effective as mild steroid creams, such as 1% hydrocortisone, in reducing the severity of radiation burn, without the side effects associated with steroid creams (Maddocks-Jennings et al 2005).

In contrast, another review concluded that aloe was ineffective for the prevention or reduction of side effects to radiation therapy in cancer patients (Richardson et al 2005). That review analysed one past review, five published randomised controlled trials (RCTs) and two unpublished RCTs. It is important to note that various preparations, such as creams, juices, gels and fresh aloe, had been tested, which makes it difficult to assess the evidence.

More recently, a study with good methodology was conducted, involving 60 patients with chiefly breast, pelvic or head or neck cancers. Volunteers were asked to apply an aloe vera cream to half the irradiated area twice daily, continuing for 2 weeks after radiation treatment ended (Haddad et al 2013). Significant benefits were not apparent until the end of the third week of radiotherapy, when the mean grade of dermatitis was lower on the aloe-treated half, with a statistically significant difference for weeks 4 ($P < 0.000$), 5 ($P < 0.000$) and 6 ($P = 0.006$) of radiotherapy, and weeks 2 ($P = 0.003$) and 4 ($P = 0.002$) afterwards. In particular, the effect was more evident in patients undergoing radiotherapy with larger treatment fields and higher doses of radiation. The aloe vera was in a lotion base consisting of lanolin oil, glyceryl stearate, diluted collagen, tocopherol, allantoin and paraben; however the concentration of aloe vera was not stated.

Leg ulcers

A number of case reports tell of a positive effect on leg ulcers with topical use of aloe gel, including cases that did not respond to standard medical interventions (Zawahry et al 1973). Application of water-based aloe gel saline soaks, broad-spectrum antibiotics and antifungals allowed a wound, caused by necrotising fasciitis, to heal in 45 days in a 72-year-old woman. Aloe gel and saline-soaked sponges were also used to treat two large seroma cavities caused by deep-vein thrombosis in a 48-year-old man (Ardire 1997).

A small study of 6 patients with chronic leg ulcers found that the ingestion of 60 mL aloe juice daily in addition to applying aloe gel directly to the ulcer and surrounding area resulted in less exudate, odour and seepage through the bandaging (Atherton 1998).

Acne

A double-blind RCT ($n = 60$) found that the combination of *A. vera* gel and the topical retinoid tretinoin leaf gel significantly reduced the presence of inflammatory lesions after 8 weeks' treatment by 78.4% compared to a reduction of 41.1% in patients receiving tretinoin alone (Hajheydari et al 2014). Similarly, comedone scores were significantly reduced in the tretinoin and *A. vera* group compared to tretinoin alone, with respective reductions of 88.2% compared to 60.1%.

Diabetes

Glycaemic control

Three systemic reviews of herbal medicines for glycaemic control in diabetes found that *A. vera* can lower blood glucose levels in diabetic patients (Grover et al 2002, Vogler & Ernst 1999, Yeh et al 2003). A recent double-blind RCT which investigated the effects of an orally ingested aloe vera gel complex on 136 patients with prediabetes or early diabetes determined that the aloe complex reduced body weight, body fat mass and insulin resistance after 8 weeks (Choi et al 2013). The aloe vera capsule contained 147 mg/cap of aloe vera and aloesin powder (95% aloesin) 3 mg/cap, yeast chromone 125 mg/cap and excipients (soy bean oil, yellow beeswax and lecithin) 425 mg/cap taken at a dose of two capsules after breakfast and two after dinner.

In another trial aloe juice consisting of 80% gel or placebo was given in a trial of 40 patients who were recently diagnosed with type 1 diabetes in a dose of 1 tablespoon twice daily. From day 14 the blood sugar levels in the aloe group began to fall significantly compared with the control group and continued to drop steadily during the study period ($P < 0.01$). Blood triglyceride levels were also substantially reduced but cholesterol levels remained the same (Yongchaiyudha et al 1996). A single-blind, placebo-controlled trial found that glibenclamide when combined with oral aloe gel was more effective in reducing blood sugar levels than glibenclamide alone in 72 patients with type 2 diabetes. Patients took 5 mg of glibenclamide twice daily and 1 tablespoon aloe gel. Fasting blood glucose levels dropped appreciably after just 2 weeks of treatment, and were still falling after 42 days (Bunyapraphatsara et al 1996).

Cancer

There are some epidemiological studies suggesting that aloe may reduce the risk of certain cancers; however, further research is required to clarify its place in practice (Sakai et al 1989, Siegers et al 1993).

Chemotherapy-induced oral and gastrointestinal mucositis

Earlier research reported that aloe gel may ameliorate chemotherapy-induced oral and gastrointestinal mucositis (Stargrove et al 2008); however, a 2011 Cochrane Review determined that, overall, there was currently insufficient evidence to support a role for aloe vera in the prevention of moderate to severe mucositis (Worthington et al 2011). Problems in determining the strength and quality of aloe vera preparations hamper interpretation of results.

Oral submucous fibrosis

A double-blind, placebo-controlled, parallel-group RCT ($n = 60$) identified that patients receiving adjuvant *Aloe vera* in addition to routine treatment (surgical or pharmacological) had significant improvement in most symptoms, including mouth burning sensation and mouth opening, compared to treatment alone (Alam et al 2013). In patients receiving medicinal treatment, after 6 months those who had received *A. vera* returned a pain score of 0.26 ± 0.40 on a 0–10 rating scale, whereas those without *A. vera* had a pain score of 2.96 ± 1.96.

HIV

The acemannan component of *Aloe vera* has been used as adjunctive therapy to antiretroviral therapy in HIV infection. A preliminary clinical trial found that acemannan may enhance the activity of the anti-HIV drug AZT. A dose of 800 mg acemannan daily significantly increased circulating monocytes (macrophages) in 14 HIV patients. Aloe increased the number and activity of the monocytes (McDaniel et al 1990). Subsequently, a randomised, double-blind placebo-controlled study of 63 male subjects with advanced HIV, taking zidovudine and didanosine, investigated the effects of 400 mg of acemannan taken four times daily for 48 weeks. Results showed a decrease in CD4 cell numbers in the acemannan group compared with placebo (Montaner et al 1996).

Gastrointestinal conditions

Oral *A. vera* is a popular treatment for a variety of gastrointestinal disorders. It has been shown to improve different parameters of gastrointestinal function in normal subjects, such as colonic bacterial activity, gastrointestinal pH, stool specific gravity and gastrointestinal motility (Bland 1986). Due to its anthraquinone content, the latex is used as a stimulant laxative.

Besides this indication, there is still a need for scientific validation to establish which gastrointestinal conditions are most receptive to treatment with aloe.

Irritable bowel syndrome

There is conflicting evidence surrounding the use of *A. vera* in irritable bowel syndrome (IBS). An RCT (n = 58) found that *A. vera* may be effective for patients with diarrhoea-predominant IBS (Davis et al 2006). In this study, both treatments were administered for 1 month with a follow-up period of 3 months. Within the first month, 35% of the patients receiving *A. vera* responded compared to 22% receiving placebo. Overall, diarrhoea-predominant IBS patients had a more statistically significant responder rate than placebo (43% vs 22%). Conversely, a multicentre, randomised, placebo-controlled, crossover study (n = 110) found *A. vera* to be no better than placebo in improving any aspect of quality of life for IBS patients (Hutchings et al 2011).

Ulcerative colitis

A double-blind, randomised, placebo-controlled trial evaluated the efficacy and safety of *A. vera* gel (100 mL twice daily for 4 weeks) in ulcerative colitis (Davis et al 2006). Aloe induced clinical remission in 30% of subjects compared to 7% for placebo and symptom improvement in 37% compared to 7% for placebo. The Simple Clinical Colitis Activity Index and histological scores also decreased significantly for patients on the aloe treatment, but not for those receiving placebo.

Practice points/Patient counselling

- Different parts of the *Aloe vera* plant are used therapeutically. The gel is used internally and topically and the latex is used internally. Differences in constituents between the different aloe extracts mean that evidence for a particular preparation may not be relevant for all aloe preparations.
- Some oral aloe preparations contain high sugar content to reduce bitterness, although this varies between brands. Be mindful of this if using aloe in diabetic patients.
- The gel may be beneficial in the treatment of skin conditions (wounds, burns, radiation burns, ulcers, frostbite, psoriasis and genital herpes). There is good scientific evidence for these indications.
- Traditionally, aloe latex is also used internally for gastrointestinal ulcers, dyspepsia and what is known today as IBS. Aloe is also used in conditions such as food allergies and disturbed bowel flora.
- Aloe may be a useful adjunct in the treatment of chronic poor immunity, HIV, cancer and chronic fatigue. There is preliminary scientific support for these indications.

DOSAGE RANGE

- Aloe vera gel: fresh from a living plant or as stabilised juice 25 mL (4.5 : 1) up to four times daily.
- Extracts standardised to acemannan: preparation containing up to 800 mg/day.
- Topical application: gel, cream or ointment as needed.
- 1.5–4.5 mL daily of 1 : 10 tincture of resin (latex).

According to clinical trials:

- Type 1 diabetes: 1 tablespoon of aloe juice consisting of 80% gel taken twice daily.
- Genital herpes: *Aloe vera* 0.5% topical applied three times a day.

HIV and AZT use: 800 mg acemannan daily

- Pre-diabetes: 147 mg/capsule of aloe vera (in combination) taken as 2 capsules twice daily.
- Psoriasis: aloe extract 0.5% cream applied three times daily.
- Second degree burns: Aloe cream containing aloe vera gel powder 0.5% applied twice daily.
- Ulcerative colitis: 100 mL twice daily for 4 weeks.

ADVERSE REACTIONS

Although adverse reactions are rare, hypersensitivities and contact dermatitis to aloe have been reported (Morrow et al 1980, Nakamura & Kotajima 1984). Hypersensitivity manifested by generalised nummular eczematous and papular dermatitis, and presumably by contact urticaria, developed in a 47-year-old man after 4 years of using oral and topical aloe. Patch tests for aloe were positive in this patient (Morrow et al 1980). Transient stinging and a mild itching sensation at oral lichen planus lesions have also been reported (Choonhakarn et al 2008).

SIGNIFICANT INTERACTIONS

A. vera juice was found to inhibit both CYP3A4 and CYP2D6 by both CYP and non-CYP mechanisms (Djuv & Nilsen 2012). The estimated IC50 inhibition values were suggestive of no major interference in humans; however some degree of caution and acknowledgement should be exercised.

Hypoglycaemic agents

Oral *A. vera* may have hypoglycaemic activity, therefore additive effects are theoretically possible — observe patients taking this combination.

Digoxin

Excessive or long-term use of oral *A. vera* may result in lowered potassium levels, which can alter the mechanism of action of digoxin on the heart. Avoid combination.

Laxatives

Additive effects are theoretically possible with oral aloe latex inducing griping pains. Use with caution.

Topical cortisone preparations

In addition to its own anti-inflammatory effects, animal studies have shown that *A. vera* increases the absorption of hydrocortisone by hydrating the stratum corneum, inhibits hydrocortisone's suppressive effects on wound healing and increases wound tensile strength — possible beneficial interaction (Davis et al 1994a).

Vitamins C and E

Concurrent prescription of oral *A. vera* (both gel and latex) with vitamins C and E shows improved absorption and increased plasma life of vitamin concentration for both vitamins when taken together (Vinson et al 2005).

Paclitaxel and doxorubicin

In vitro evidence suggests that aloe-emodin antagonises the cytotoxic effects on both paclitaxel and doxorubicin (Radovic et al 2012). While the clinical relevance of this remains unknown, caution should be observed in patients concurrently taking aloe with either of these chemotherapeutic agents.

CONTRAINDICATIONS AND PRECAUTIONS

Strong laxatives such as aloe latex are contraindicated in children. Avoid in patients with known hypersensitivity to aloe or with nausea, vomiting or signs and symptoms of gastrointestinal obstruction. Avoid excessive use and long-term use (more than 2 weeks), as potassium losses may occur, which may alter cardiac electrophysiology.

Use with caution in people with thyrotoxicosis.

A case study of depression of thyroid hormones in a woman taking *A. vera* juice has been reported (Pigatto & Guzzi 2005). The patient consumed 10 mL daily for 11 months and laboratory testing showed reduced levels of thyroxine (T_4) and triiodothyronine (T_3). Levels returned to normal progressively after discontinuing the aloe juice and the patient achieved full clinical remission after 16 months. Reduced serum levels of the thyroid hormones T_3 and T_4 have been reported for *A. vera* in vivo (Kar et al 2002).

Caution is suggested with topical applications that contain *A. vera* as they may enhance sensitivity to ultraviolet light (Xia et al 2007).

PREGNANCY USE

Strong laxatives such as aloe latex are not advised in pregnancy. Scientific evidence is unavailable to support conclusively the safe use of orally administered aloe.

PATIENTS' FAQs

What will this herb do for me?

Aloe gel is traditionally used for burns, wounds and inflammatory skin disorders. There is good scientific evidence that aloe may be of benefit in these conditions; however, the chemical composition of *A. vera* products will vary depending on geographical and processing factors. Traditionally, aloe is also used internally for dyspepsia, gastrointestinal ulcers and IBS.

When will it start to work?

Aloe can have an immediate soothing effect on burns and inflammatory skin diseases. Improvement in wound healing can occur within several weeks, with the condition continuing to improve with use. Chronic conditions may require long-term use. Internal use of *A. vera* as a laxative can produce results within 12–24 hours.

Are there any safety issues?

Aloe gel is considered safe and non-toxic when used topically. Avoid chronic use of laxative preparations that contain highly irritant compounds, known as anthraquinone glycosides, in the latex.

REFERENCES

Alam S et al. Efficacy of aloe vera as an adjuvant treatment of oral submucous fibrosis. Oral Surg Oral Med Oral Pathol Oral Radiol 116.6 (2013): 717–724.

Anderson D. Wound dressings unravelled. In Practice 25.2 (2003): 70–83.

Ardire L. Necrotizing fasciitis: case study of a nursing dilemma. Ostomy Wound Manage 43.5 (1997): 30–40.

Atherton P. Aloe vera: magic or medicine? Nurs Stand 12.41 (1998): 49–52, 54.

Atiba A et al. Aloe vera oral administration accelerates acute radiation-delayed wound healing by stimulating transforming growth factor β and fibroblast growth factor production. Am J Surg 201.6 (2011): 809–818.

Bland J. Aloe vera juice: an important role in gastrointestinal disorders? Altern Med 1 (1986): 280.
Bolkent S et al. Effect of *Aloe vera* (L.) Burm. fil. leaf gel and pulp extracts on kidney in type-II diabetic rat models. Indian J Exp Biol 42.1 (2004): 48–52.
Bozzi A et al. Quality and authenticity of commercial aloe vera gel powders. Food Chem 103.1 (2007): 22–30.
Brossat JY et al. Immunostimulating properties of an extract isolated from *Aloe vahombe*. 2. Protection in mice by fraction F1 against infections by *Listeria monocytogenes, Yersinia pestis, Candida albicans* and *Plasmodium berghei*. Arch Inst Pasteur Madagascar 48.1 (1981): 11–34.
Budai MM et al. Aloe vera downregulates LPS-induced inflammatory cytokine production and expression of NLRP3 inflammasome in human macrophages. Mol Immunol 56.4 (2013): 471–479.
Bunyapraphatsara N et al. Antidiabetic activity of *Aloe vera* juice, II: clinical trial in diabetes mellitus patients in combination with glibenclamide. Phytomedicine 3 (1996): 245–248.
Can A et al. Effect of *Aloe vera* leaf gel and pulp extracts on the liver in type-II diabetic rat models. Biol Pharm Bull 27.5 (2004): 694–698.
Chen XD et al. Effect of aloe vera polysaccharide on the release of cytokines and nitric oxide in cultured human keratinocytes. Zhongguo Wei Zhong Bing Ji Jiu Yi Xue 17.5 (2005): 296–298.
Chen SH et al. Aloe-emodin-induced apoptosis in human gastric carcinoma cell. Food Chem Tox 45.11 (2007): 2296–2303.
Chithra P, et al. Influence of *Aloe vera* on collagen characteristics in healing dermal wounds in rats. Mol Cell Biochem 181.1–2 (1998): 71–76.
Choi S, Chung MH. A review on the relationship between aloe vera components and their biologic effects. Semin Integr Med 1.1 (2003): 53–62.
Choi SW et al. The wound-healing effect of a glycoprotein fraction isolated from aloe vera. Br J Dermatol 145.4 (2001): 535–545.
Choi HC et al. Metabolic effects of aloe vera gel complex in obese prediabetes and early non-treated diabetic patients: Randomized controlled trial. Nutrition 29.9 (2013): 1110–1114.
Choonhakarn C et al. The efficacy of aloe vera gel in the treatment of oral lichen planus: a randomised controlled trial. Br J Dermatol 158.3 (2008): 573–577.
Choonhakarn C et al. A prospective, randomised clinical trial comparing topical aloe vera with 0.1% triamcinolone acetonide in mild to moderate plaque psoriasis. J Eur Acad Dermatol Venereol 24.2 (2010): 168–172.
Cuttle L et al. The efficacy of *Aloe vera*, tea tree oil and saliva as first aid treatment for partial thickness burns. Burns. 34.8 (2008):1176–1182.
Dat AD et al. Aloe vera for treating acute and chronic wounds. Cochrane Database of Systematic Reviews 2 (2012): Art No: CD008762.
Davis RH, Maro NP. Aloe vera and gibberellin: Anti-inflammatory activity in diabetes. J Am Podiatr Med Assoc 79.1 (1989): 24–26.
Davis RH et al. Biological activity of *Aloe vera*. Med Sci Res 15.5 (1987): 235.
Davis RH et al. Processed Aloe vera administered topically inhibits inflammation. J Am Podiatr Med Assoc 79.8 (1989): 395–397.
Davis RH et al. Aloe vera and the inflamed synovial pouch model. J Am Podiatr Med Assoc 82.3 (1992): 140–148.
Davis RH et al. Aloe vera, hydrocortisone, and sterol influence on wound tensile strength and anti-inflammation. J Am Podiatr Med Assoc 84.12 (1994a): 614–21.
Davis RH et al. Anti-inflammatory and wound healing activity of a growth substance in *Aloe vera*. J Am Podiatr Med Assoc 84.2 (1994b): 77–81.
Davis K et al. Randomised double-blind placebo-controlled trial of aloe vera for irritable bowel syndrome. Int J Clin Pract 60.9 (2006): 1080–1086.
Djuv A and Nilsen OG. Aloe vera juice: IC50 and Dual Mechanistic Inhibition of CYP3A4 and CYP2D6. Phytother Res 26.3 (2012): 445–451.
Duansak D, et al. Effects of *Aloe vera* on leukocyte adhesion and TNF-alpha and IL-6 levels in burn wounded rats. Clin Hemorheol Microcirc 29.3–4 (2003): 239–246.
Eamlamnam K et al. Effects of *Aloe vera* and sucralfate on gastric microcirculatory changes, cytokine levels and gastric ulcer healing in rats. World J Gastroenterol 12.13 (2006): 2034–2039.
Esua MF, Rauwald J-W. Novel bioactive maloyl glucans from *Aloe vera* gel: isolation, structure elucidation and in vitro bioassays. Carb Res 341.3 (2006): 355–364.
Grover JK, et al. Medicinal plants of India with anti-diabetic potential. J Ethnopharmacol 81.1 (2002): 81–100.
Habeeb F et al. The inner gel component of *Aloe vera* suppresses bacterial-induced pro-inflammatory cytokines from human immune-cells. Methods 42.4 (2007a): 388–393.
Haddad P et al. Aloe vera for prevention of radiation-induced dermatitis: a self-controlled clinical trial. Curr Oncol 20.4 (2013): e345–e348.
Hajheydari Z et al. Effect of *Aloe vera* topical gel combined with tretinoin in treatment of mild and moderate acne vulgaris: a randomized, double-blind, prospective trial. J Dermatol Treat 25.2 (2014): 123–129.
Heck E, et al. Aloe vera (gel) cream as a topical treatment for outpatient burns: Burns 7.4 (1981):291–4.
Heggers JP et al. Experimental and clinical observations on frostbite. Ann Emerg Med 16.9 (1987): 1056–1062.
Heggers JP et al. Beneficial effect of Aloe on wound healing in an excisional wound model. J Altern Complement Med 2.2 (1996): 271–277.
Hu Y, et al. Evaluation of antioxidant potential of aloe vera (*Aloe barbadensis* miller extracts). J Agric Food Chem 51.26 (2003): 7788–7791.
Hunter D, Frumkin A. Adverse reactions to vitamin E and aloe vera preparations after dermabrasion and chemical peel. Cutis 47.3 (1991): 193–196.
Hutchings HA et al. A randomised, cross-over, placebo-controlled study of aloe vera in patients with irritable bowel syndrome: effects on patient quality of life. ISRN Gastroenterol 2011 (2011): 206103.
Hutter JA et al. Antiinflammatory C-glucosyl chromone from *Aloe barbadensis*. J Nat Prod 59.5 (1996): 541–543.
Im SA et al. Identification of optimal molecular size of modified Aloe polysaccharides with maximum immunomodulatory activity. Int Immunopharm 5.2 (2005): 271–279.
Im SA et al. In vivo evidence of the immunomodulatory activity of orally administered aloe vera gel. Arch Pharm Res 33.3 (2010): 451–456.
Ishii Y, et al. Studies of aloe. V: Mechanism of cathartic effect. (4). Biol Pharm Bull 17.5 (1994): 651–3.
Jain N et al. Aloe vera gel alleviates cardiotoxicity in streptozocin-induced diabetes in rats. J Pharm Pharmacol 62.1 (2010): 115–123.
Kahlon JB et al. Inhibition of AIDS virus replication by acemannan in vitro. Mol Biother 3.3 (1991a): 127–35.
Kahlon JB et al. In vitro evaluation of the synergistic antiviral effects of acemannan in combination with azidothymidine and acyclovir. Mol Biother 3.4 (1991b): 214–23.
Kar A, et al. Relative efficacy of three medicinal plant extracts in the alteration of thyroid hormone concentrations in male mice. J Ethnopharmacol 81.2 (2002): 281–285.
Khorasani G et al. Aloe versus silver sulfadiazine creams for second-degree burns: a randomized controlled study. Surg Today 39.7 (2009): 587–591.
Kim HS, Lee BM. Inhibition of benzo[a]pyrene-DNA adduct formation by *Aloe barbadensis* Miller. Carcinogenesis 18.4 (1997): 771–776.
Kim K et al. Hypoglycaemic and hypolipidaemic effects of processed *Aloe vera* gel in a mouse model of non-insulin dependent diabetes mellitus. Phytomedicine 16.7 (2009): 856–863.
Klein AD, Penneys NS. Aloe vera. J Am Acad Dermatol 18 (4 Pt 1) (1988): 714–720.
Krishnan P. The scientific study of herbal wound healing therapies: Current state of play. Curr Anaes Crit Care 17.1–2 (2006): 21–27.
Langmead L, et al. Anti-inflammatory effects of aloe vera gel in human colorectal mucosa in vitro. Aliment Pharmacol Ther 19.5 (2004): 521–527.
Lee JK et al. Acemannan purified from *Aloe vera* induces phenotypic and functional maturation of immature dendritic cells. Int Immunopharmacol 1.7 (2001): 1275–1284.
Leung MY et al. Chemical and biological characterization of a polysaccharide biological response modifier from *Aloe vera* L. var. chinensis (Haw. Berg). Glycobiology 14.6 (2004): 501–510.
Lin JG et al. Aloe-Emodin induced apoptosis in T24 human bladder cancer cells through the p53 dependant apoptotic pathway, J Urol, 175.1 (2006): 343–347.
Liptak JM. An overview of the topical management of wounds. Aust Vet J 75.6 (1997): 408–413.
Liu C et al. Macrophage activation by polysaccharide biological response modifier isolated from *Aloe vera* L. Var. chinensis (Haw.) Berg. Int Immunopharm 6.11 (2006): 1634–1641.
Maddocks-Jennings W, et al. Novel approaches to radiotherapy-induced skin reactions: a literature review. Complement Ther Clin Pract 11.4 (2005): 224–231.
Maenthalsong R et al. The efficacy of aloe vera used for burn wound healing: A systematic review. Burns 33.6 (2007): 713–18.
McCarty MF. Glucomannan minimizes the postprandial insulin surge: a potential adjuvant for hepatothermic therapy. Med Hypotheses 58.6 (2002): 487–490.
McCauley RL, et al. Frostbite: Methods to minimize tissue loss. Postgrad Med 88.8 (1990): 67.
McDaniel HR et al. Extended survival and prognostic criteria for acemannan (ACE-M) treated HIV-1 patients. Antiviral Res Suppl 1 (1990): 117.
Miller MB, Koltai PJ. Treatment of experimental frostbite with pentoxifylline and aloe vera cream. Arch Otolaryngol Head Neck Surg 121.6 (1995): 678–680.
Montaner JS et al. Double-blind placebo-controlled pilot trial of acemannan in advanced human immunodeficiency virus disease.

J Acquir Immune Defic Syndr Hum Retrovirol 12.2 (1996): 153–157.

Moon EJ et al. A novel angiogenic factor derived from Aloe vera gel: beta-sitosterol, a plant sterol. Angiogenesis 3.2 (1999): 117–123.

Morrow DM, et al. Hypersensitivity to aloe. Arch Dermatol 116.9 (1980): 1064–1065.

Muller MJ et al. Retardation of wound healing by silver sulfadiazine is reversed by *Aloe vera* and nystatin. Burns 29.88 (2003): 34–6.

Nakamura T, Kotajima S. Contact dermatitis from aloe arborescens. Contact Dermatitis 11.1 (1984): 51.

Park MY et al. Dietary aloin, aloesin and aloe-gel exerts anti-inflammatory activity in a rat colitis model. Life Sciences 88.11–12 (2011): 486–492.

Paulsen E, et al. A double-blind, placebo-controlled study of a commercial *Aloe vera* gel in the treatment of slight to moderate psoriasis vulgaris. J Eur Acad Dermatol Venereol 19.3 (2005): 326–331.

Peng SY et al. Decreased mortality of Norman murine sarcoma in mice treated with the immunomodulator, Acemannan. Mol Biother 3.2 (1991): 79–87.

Pigatto PD, Guzzi G. Aloe linked to thyroid dysfunction. Arch Med Res 36.5 (2005): 608.

Puvabanditsin P, Vongtongsri R. Efficacy of aloe vera cream in prevention and treatment of sunburn and suntan. J Med Assoc Thai 88 (Suppl 4) (2005): S173–S176.

Radovic J et al. Cell-type dependent response of melanoma cells to aloe emodin. Food Chem Toxicol 50.9 (2012): 3181–3189.

Rajasekaran S, et al. Antioxidant effect of *Aloe vera* gel extract in streptozotocin-induced diabetes in rats. Pharmacol Rep 57.1 (2005): 90–96.

Reynolds T, Dweck AC. Aloe vera leaf gel: A review update. J Ethnopharmacol 68.1–3 (1999): 3–37.

Richardson J et al. Aloe vera for preventing radiation-induced skin reactions: a systematic literature review. Clin Oncol (R Coll Radiol) 17.6 (2005): 478–484.

Roberts DB, Travis EL. Acemannan-containing wound dressing gel reduces radiation-induced skin reactions in C3H mice. Int J Radiat Oncol Biol Phys 32.4 (1995): 1047–1052.

Rodriguez-Bigas M, et al. Comparative evaluation of aloe vera in the management of burn wounds in guinea pigs. Plast Reconstr Surg 81.3 (1988): 386–389.

Rodriguez-Fragoso L et al. Risks and benefits of commonly used herbal medicines in Mexico. Tox App Pharmacol 227.1 (2008): 125–135.

Saada HN, et al. Effectiveness of *Aloe vera* on the antioxidant status of different tissues in irradiated rats. Pharmazie 58.12 (2003): 929–931.

Sabeh F, et al. Purification and characterization of a glutathione peroxidase from the *Aloe vera* plant. Enzyme Protein 47.2 (1993): 92–98.

Saini DK, Saini MR. Evaluation of radioprotective efficacy and possible mechanism of action of Aloe gel. Environ Toxicol Pharmacol 31.3 (2011): 427–435.

Sakai K et al. Effect of water extracts of aloe and some herbs in decreasing blood ethanol concentration in rats. Tokyo: II. Chem Pharm Bull 37.1 (1989): 55–9.

Saoo K et al. Antiviral activity of aloe extracts against cytomegalovirus. Phytother Res 10.4 (1996): 348–350.

Schmidt JM, Greenspoon JS. Aloe vera dermal wound gel is associated with a delay in wound healing. Obstet Gynecol 78.1 (1991): 115–117.

Shelton RM. Aloe vera. Its chemical and therapeutic properties. Int J Dermatol 30.10 (1991): 679–683.

Shida T et al. Effect of Aloe extract on peripheral phagocytosis in adult bronchial asthma. Planta Med 3 (1985): 273–5.

Siegers CP, et al. Sennosides and aloin do not promote dimethylhydrazine-induced colorectal tumors in mice. Pharmacology 47 (Suppl 1) (1993): 205–208.

Singh RP, et al. Chemomodulatory action of *Aloe vera* on the profiles of enzymes associated with carcinogen metabolism and antioxidant status regulation in mice. Phytomedicine 7.3 (2000): 209–219.

Somboonwong J et al. Therapeutic effects of *Aloe vera* on cutaneous microcirculation and wound healing in second degree burn model in rats. J Med Assoc Thai 83.4 (2000): 417–425.

Stargrove MB, et al. Herb, nutrient and drug interactions — clinical applications and therapeutic strategies. St Louis: Mosby, Elsevier, 2008.

Strickland FM, et al. Prevention of ultraviolet radiation-induced suppression of contact and delayed hypersensitivity by *Aloe barbadensis* gel extract. J Invest Dermatol 102.2 (1994): 197–204.

Suvitayavat W et al. Effects of Aloe preparation on the histamine-induced gastric secretion in rats. J Ethnopharmacol 90.2–3 (2004): 239–247.

Sydiskis RJ et al. Inactivation of enveloped viruses by anthraquinones extracted from plants. Antimicrob Agents Chemother 35.12 (1991): 2463–2466.

Syed TA et al. Management of psoriasis with *Aloe vera* extract in a hydrophilic cream: A placebo-controlled, double-blind study. Trop Med Int Health 1.4 (1996a): 505–509.

Syed TA et al. *Aloe vera* extract 0.5% in hydrophilic cream versus *Aloe vera* gel for the management of genital herpes in males: A placebo-controlled, double-blind, comparative study [3]. J Eur Acad Dermatol Venereol 7.3 (1996b): 294–295.

Syed TA et al. Management of genital herpes in men with 0.5% *Aloe vera* extract in a hydrophilic cream: A placebo-controlled double-blind study. J Dermatol Treat 8.2 (1997): 99–102.

Talmadge J et al. Fractionation of *Aloe vera* L. inner gel, purification and molecular profiling of activity. Int Immunopharmacol 4.14 (2004): 1757–1773.

Thamlikitkul V et al. Controlled trial of Aloe vera Linn. for treatment of minor burns. Siriraj Hosp Gaz. 43 (1991): 313–316.

Thongprasom K et al. Interventions for treating oral lichen planus. Cochrane Database of Systematic Review 7 (2011): Art No CD001168.

't Hart LA et al. Effects of low molecular constituents from *Aloe vera* gel on oxidative metabolism and cytotoxic and bactericidal activities of human neutrophils. Int J Immunopharmacol 12.4 (1990): 427–434.

Vinson JA, et al. Effect of *Aloe vera* preparations on the human bioavailability of vitamins C and E. Phytomedicine 12.10 (2005): 760–65.

Vogler BK, Ernst E. Aloe vera: a systematic review of its clinical effectiveness. Br J Gen Pract 49.447 (1999): 823–828.

West DP, Zhu YF. Evaluation of aloe vera gel gloves in the treatment of dry skin associated with occupational exposure. Am J Infect Control 31.1 (2003): 40–42.

Womble D, Helderman JH. Enhancement of allo-responsiveness of human lymphocytes by acemannan (Carrisyn(TM)). Int J Immunopharmacol 10.8 (1988): 967–974.

Worthington HV et al. Interventions for preventing oral mucositis for patients with cancer receiving treatment. Cochrane Database of Systematic Reviews 4 (2011): Art No: CD000978.

Woźniak A and Paduch R. Aloe vera extract activity on human corneal cells. Pharmaceut Biol 50.2 (2012): 147–154.

Wu JH et al. Antioxidant properties and PC12 cell protective effects of APS-1, a polysaccharide from *Aloe vera* var. chinensis. Life Sci 78.6 (2006): 622–630.

Xia Q et al. Photo-irradiation of *Aloe vera* by UVA — Formation of free radicals, singlet oxygen, superoxide and induction of lipid peroxidation. Toxicol Lett 168.2 (2007): 165–175.

Yagi A et al. Antioxidant, free radical scavenging and anti-inflammatory effects of aloesin derivatives in *Aloe vera*. Planta Med 68.11 (2002): 957–960.

Yamaguchi I, et al. Components of the gel of *Aloe vera* (L.) burm. f. Biosci Biotechnol Biochem 57.8 (1993): 1350–1352.

Yeh GY et al. Systematic review of herbs and dietary supplements for glycemic control in diabetes. Diabetes Care 26.4 (2003): 1277–1294.

Yongchaiyudha S et al. Antidiabetic activity of *Aloe vera* L. juice: clinical trial in new cases of diabetes mellitus. Phytomedicine 3.3 (1996): 241–243.

Yun N et al. Protective effect of *Aloe vera* on polymicrobial sepsis in mice. Food Chem Toxicol 47.6 (2009):1341–1348.

Zachary LS, et al. The role of thromboxane in experimental inadvertent intra-arterial drug injections. J Hand Surg 12.2 (1987): 240–245.

Zawahry ME, et al. Use of aloe in treating leg ulcers and dermatoses. Int J Dermatol 12.1 (1973): 68–73.

Zhang L, Tizard IR. Activation of a mouse macrophage cell line by acemannan: the major carbohydrate fraction from *Aloe vera* gel. Immunopharmacology 35.2 (1996): 119–128.

Zhang XF et al. Isolation, structure elucidation, antioxidative and immunomodulatory properties of two novel dihydrocoumarins from *Aloe vera*. Bioorg Med Chem Lett 16.4 (2006): 949–953.

Zhang XF et al. Binding of the bioactive component Aloe dihydroisocoumarin with human serum albumin. J Mol Struct 891.1–2 (2008): 87–92.

Alpha lipoic acid

HISTORICAL NOTE Lipoic acid was first identified in bacteria in 1937 (Lodge & Packer 1999). In 1951, its isolation and chemical structure characterisation by Reed saw lipoic acid tentatively classified as a vitamin (Wang et al 2011). It was subsequently found to be endogenously produced in humans from octanoic acid and the sulfur residue of cysteine. By the early 1950s, lipoic acid was understood as an essential cofactor in oxidative metabolism, involved in acyl-group transfer and as a mitochondrial coenzyme in the Krebs cycle (Patel & Packer 2008). Currently used as a medicine in the treatment of diabetic neuropathies in Europe, research has focused on its unique antioxidant properties and their application, mainly in diabetes management, but also in various neuropathologies, as well as in immune and inflammation modulation (Shay et al 2009).

OTHER NAMES

Alpha lipoic acid (ALA), lipoic acid (LA), R-lipoic acid, S-lipoic acid, racemic lipoic acid, rhioctic acid, 6,8-thioctic acid, 1,2-dithiolane-3-valeric acid, dehydrolipoic acid (DHLA), 1,2-dithiolane-3-pentanoic acid.

BACKGROUND AND RELEVANT PHARMACOKINETICS

Chemical structure

ALA is a cyclic disulfide compound endogenously synthetised in the mitochondria from octanoic acid (caprylic acid) using cysteine as a source of sulfur. LA is manufactured in both R- and S-enantiomeric forms, but only the naturally produced R-form conjugates to lysine residues and attaches to a lipoyl protein carrier to act as an essential cofactor in physiolological systems (Wang et al 2011); free LA is only present in very small amounts in the body (Patel & Packer 2008, Shay et al 2009), and is usually found in free form after therapeutic supplementation (Teichert et al 1998).

LA is insoluble in water, but soluble in organic solvents. At physiological pH, LA is anionic and in this form it is commonly called lipoate.

Pharmocokinetics and bioavailability of LA

Most of the research for the bioavailability of ALA comes from studies using oral supplementation, usually made from manufactured racemic ALA.

Although not fully understood, the bioavailability of exogenous LA seems dependent on multiple carrier proteins. In vitro studies show that LA is absorbed through the cell membrane in a pH-dependent manner, through the monocarboxylate and Na^+-dependent multivitamin transporter (Keith et al 2012, Shay et al 2009).

The gastrointestinal uptake of ALA is rapid but variable. A pharmacokinetic study by Teichert et al (1998) showed that humans absorb 20–40% of oral racemic ALA. Additionally, preferential uptake of the R-enantiomer has been established, as plasma concentrations were 40–60% more than those of the L-enantiomer. However it is yet to be established if the S-form prevents polymerisation of ALA, thus increasing overall bioavailability (Breithaupt-Grogler et al 1999, Shay et al 2009).

Bioavailability fluctuates with concomitant absorption of food, suggesting nutrient interaction (Teichert et al 1998). Furthermore, it appears that the salt form has better bioavailability (Carlson et al 2007).

After rapid gastrointestinal uptake, ALA appears quickly in the plasma and generally peaks within 1 hour of administration and then declines rapidly, mainly via renal excretion (Harrison & McCormick 1974, Shay et al 2009). R-LA administered as a salt showed high plasma maximum concentrations and high area under the concentration versus time curve values (Carlson et al 2007). Ninety-eight per cent of radiolabelled LA is excreted within 24 hours (Schupke et al 2001).

Erythrocytes and a number of other cells take up ALA by glucose metabolism (GLUT 4), after which it reduces to DHLA, which is subsequently released in the extracellular environment (Packer & Cadenas 2010). However in adipocytes, it is poorly reduced and shows prooxidant activities (Cho et al 2003, Moini et al 2002a, 2002b, Packer & Cadenas 2010).

Supplemental LA has been shown to accumulate transiently in the liver, heart and skeletal muscles. Bioaccumulation in the brain has been debated (Chng et al 2009); however, in view of the large number of studies demonstrating a therapeutic effect on the brain, DHLA and other ALA metabolites should also be measured to establish their potential therapeutic benefits after oral ingestion of ALA (Shay et al 2009), as in vitro studies suggests that it is rapidly reduced to its DHLA form; catabolism of ALA, which occurs via β-oxidation, produces at least 12 major metabolites (Jones et al 2002).

FOOD SOURCES

ALA is found in various natural sources in the form lipoyllysine, which is protein-bound ALA. While it is ubiquitous in most food and especially in organ meats (liver, kidney) and spinach, with lesser amounts in broccoli floral buds, tomato, garden peas and Brussels sprouts, rice bran and yeast extract, it is only present in very low amounts and poorly bioavailable, thus it is not likely that it is consumed in appreciable amounts (Lodge & Packer 1999, Shay et al 2009, Sen & Packer 2000). Dietary supplements provide the main source of exogenous LA (Shay et al 2009).

DEFICIENCY SIGNS AND SYMPTOMS

ALA is endogenously synthesised, primarily in the liver but also in other tissues. Animal studies have established that it is essential to life. To determine deficiency signs and symptoms, animal models of decreased ALA production have been studied.

No recommended daily intake has been established.

As an endogenous nutrient, little is known about the effects of genetic alteration that modify lipoic acid synthase (LIAS) expression and the reduction in endogenous LA production on disease pathogenesis. A rodent study in which the LIAS gene (homozygous mutation) has been switched off demonstrated that absence of LA is incompatible with life and ends in the early demise of all embryos in early implantation, presumably due to the inability of cells to produce oxidative metabolism. Supplementation of the mother did not alter the outcome (Yi & Maeda 2005). Interestingly, the intraperitoneal (IP) injection of ALA to diabetic pregnant rats did improve fetal and placental outcome, suggesting it can travel through the placenta (Al Ghafli et al 2004).

Heterozygous mutation, impairing synthesis of ALA, showed an important decrease in erythrocyte glutathione levels and abnormal cellular antioxidant capacity (Yi & Maeda 2005).

Other animal models showed that LIAS deficiency resulted in overall cellular abnormality in antioxidant defence, increased inflammation and inflammatory cytokine expression, insulin resistance, mitochondrial dysfunction (Padmalayam et al 2009), and enhanced atherosclerosis formation, especially in males (Yi et al 2010). One case report of a newborn baby homozygous for LIAS deficiency manifested in mitochondrial encephalopathy with neonatal-onset epilepsy, muscular hypotonia, lactic acidosis and increased glycine in urine and plasma (Mayr et al 2011).

MAIN ACTIONS

While de novo endogenous synthesis is considered sufficient for metabolic function, less is understood of ALA's role as an oral nutritional supplement. The growing body of evidence suggests it is bioavailable, safe in moderate doses and displays a range of metabolic and clinical effects (Shay et al 2009).

Mitochondrial energy metabolism

De novo R-LA serves as an essential cofactor for the reduction of NAD to NADH in α-keto acid dehydrogenases (a multienzyme complex which includes pyruvate dehydrogenase) in the Krebs cycle, by catalysing the oxidative carboxylation of α-keto acids (Booker 2004, Rüdiger et al 1972, Shay et al 2009).

Antioxidant

Lipoate has the unique ability of being able to act as an antioxidant in fat and water-soluble tissues and also act as a 'metabolic antioxidant'. Enzymes in human cells accept it as a substrate for reduction. It is promptly taken up by cells and reduced to dihydrolipoate at the expense of cellular-reducing equivalents such as NADH and NADPH. As more of these reducing equivalents are used, the rate of cellular metabolism is sped up to cater for the enhanced demand (Sen & Packer 2000).

Both ALA (oxidised) and DHLA (reduced) act as a potent redox pair and scavenge a number of reactive oxygen species (ROS: hydroxyl radicals and hypochlorous acid). DHLA has been demonstrated to regenerate vitamin C and E in vitro (Bast & Haenen 2008, Biewenga et al 1997). R-LA feeding to rats has also been demonstrated to increase ascorbate levels in hepatocytes and cardiomyocytes subjected to normal aged-related loss (Lykkesfeldt et al 1999, Michels et al 2003, Suh et al 2001). Mechanisms of action appear indirect, by inducing the uptake from blood plasma, or promoting the synthesis of intracellular antioxidants via signal transduction (Shay et al 2009). DHLA increases intracellular glutathione by reducing cystine to cysteine (Han et al 1997, Suh et al 2001) and by enhancing cellular cysteine uptake (Suh et al 2004a).

Its role as an antioxidant and involvement in the broader antioxidant network underlie many of its observed actions in preclinical models.

Glucose uptake and metabolism

Lipoate is known to promote the efficiency of glucose uptake by cultured skeletal muscle cells at a magnitude comparable to that of insulin and has also been shown to retain its ability to stimulate glucose uptake even where L6 myotubes were insulin-resistant (Sen & Packer 2000). In a rat model, Streeper et al (1997) demonstrated that a 10-day administration of R-LA improved significantly glucose uptake, decreased insulin resistance and increased glycogen synthesis and glucose oxidation compared to S-LA; it is important to note that GLUT 4 was slightly decreased by S-LA at doses of 30 mg/kg of body weight in the same study.

A SDZ rat study had demonstrated that 10 days' ALA treatment (30 mg/kg IP) enhanced muscle glucose metabolism and increased gastrocnemius GLUT 4 translocation (Khamaisi et al 1997). R-LA enhanced glucose uptake more rapidly and in larger amounts than S-LA or rac-LA (Estrada et al 1996). In the presence of insulin, ALA's effects were increased by 33% (Henriksen et al 1997). Similar results were observed in rat heart cells (Strödter et al 1995).

Estrada et al (1996) and Moini et al (2002b) demonstrated in vitro PI3K involvement. In vivo studies, while supporting the finding of GLUT4 upregulation, indicated a mechanism independent of PI3K as well (Henriksen et al 1997, Packer & Cadenas 2010). It is important to note a great disparity in in vitro and in vivo study dosage administration, which could explain this difference.

Endothelial function

A number of clinical studies have demonstrated that treatment with ALA significantly improves endothelial function, increases nitric oxide (NO) synthesis and prevents loss in endothelial NO synthase phosphorylation, thus restoring vasodilation in diabetic and impaired-glycaemia patients. Although mechanisms are yet to be explained, it is thought to be acting through the PI3K/Akt signalling pathway (Heinisch et al 2010, Heitzer et al 2001, Sena et al 2008, Sola et al 2005, Xiang et al 2011).

Hypotensive

Oral ALA supplementation tested in a number of hypertensive rat models was shown to normalise systolic blood pressure and aortic superoxide production (Vasdev et al 2000a, 2000b, 2003, 2005). In addition to improving endothelial NO synthesis, ALA is thought to reduce sulfhydryl group denaturation of Ca^{2+} channels in vascular smooth muscles through the regeneration of reduced glutathione and by inhibition of renal and vascular overproduction of endothelin-1, an endothelial vasoconstrictor (Takaoka et al 2001). In vivo research further suggests that long-term treatment with ALA improves baroreflex sensitivity in rats with renovascular hypertension (Queiroz et al 2012).

ALA also appears to prevent the development of glucocorticoid-induced hypertension according to in vivo research, an effect not mediated by mitochondrial superoxide reduction (Ong et al 2013).

Anti-inflammatory

Numerous preclinical studies have demonstrated that LA affects several important inflammatory pathways in vivo, such as inducing a significant increase in cyclic adenosine monophosphate (cAMP) concentration and affecting the cAMP/protein kinase A signalling cascade (Salinthone et al 2010). These effects have also been demonstrated in humans.

In particular, LA, in either racemic or individual S- or R-forms, but not DHLA, is able to stimulate cAMP production in natural killer and T cells (Salinthone et al 2011, Schillace et al 2007), thus having an effect on inflammation, immunomodulation and autoimmunity.

It appears that LA stimulates cAMP production by activating G-protein coupled receptors, such as adenosine, likely to be responsible for the anti-inflammatory action of LA; curiously, LA also activated histamine, but not β-adrenergic receptors. The histamine activation pathway findings have an implication in the safety of long-term intake of LA and warrant further studies, especially in the development of allergies and cancers (Salinthone et al 2011).

LA, but not DHLA, downregulates $CD4^+$ expression in a concentration-dependent manner, potentially inhibiting T-cell activation to antigens, especially in the central nervous system environment, showing potential benefits in the management of multiple sclerosis (MS), and autoimmune pathologies (Marracci et al 2006).

In a small clinical study, ALA demonstrated an effect on exercise-induced inflammatory response in physically active males. Twenty minutes after a 90-minute exercise trial, ALA intake increased serum interleukin-6 (IL-6) and IL-10 (anti-inflammatory cytokines) and decreased IL-1β (proinflammatory). It also improved muscle regeneration (Zembron-Lacny et al 2013). In MS patients (n = 20), LA was shown to stimulate cAMP by 43%, reduce IL-6 and IL-17 (cytokines involved in MS pathogenesis) and inhibit T-cell proliferation by 90% and activation by 40%, demonstrating anti-inflammatory effects (Salinthone et al 2010).

Neuroprotective

ALA demonstrates neuroprotective effects in various test models. This is accomplished via several different mechanisms. As a result, ALA has a potential role in a number of neurodegenerative disorders, including diabetic neuropathies, Alzheimer's dementia, burning-mouth syndrome, amyotrophic lateral sclerosis, seizures, brain injuries and MS (Yamada et al 2011).

Peroxynitrite involvement has been demonstrated in the pathogenesis of various neurodegenerative diseases through DNA strand break; an in vitro study by Jia et al (2009) demonstrated the inhibition of peroxynitrite-mediated DNA damage by ALA, suggesting it may be partly responsible for the neuroprotective action. ALA's ability to promote the expression of antioxidative genes via the PI3K/Akt pathway that upregulates glutathione has also been demonstrated in SH-SY5Y brain cells in vitro (Yamada et al 2011).

In a cryo-injured rat brain model, ALA was shown to stimulate the synthesis of glutathione, decrease cell death, promote angiogenesis and decrease glial cell scar formation (Rocamonde et al 2012). ALA also appears to reduce monocyte migration across the blood–brain barrier effectively, protect its integrity and inhibit cerebral inflammation in a dose-dependent manner (Schreibelt et al 2006).

A number of experimental models demonstrate protective mechanisms in cerebral ischaemic-reperfusion injury when subjects are pretreated before occlusion (Connell et al 2011, Richard et al 2011). ALA was also shown to significantly prevent neuronal oxidative stress induced by a number a pharmacological drugs and environmental poisons in animal models: haloperidol (Perera et al 2011),

L-dopa (Abdin & Sarhan 2011), cyanide-induced seizures (Abdel-Zaher et al 2011), dimethoate, glyphosate and zineb (Astiz et al 2012) and morphine-induced tolerance and dependence (Abdel-Zaher et al 2011).

Hepatoprotective

Hepatoprotective activity has been demonstrated in different animal studies, indicating a potential role in chronic liver disease and damage.

A hepatoprotective effect was observed after ALA treatment in lipid peroxidation-induced liver injury, and thioacetamide-induced fibrosis. Treament with ALA resulted in a decrease in serum aspartate transaminase (AST) and alanine transaminase (ALT), decrease in lipid peroxidation, maintenance of antioxidant capacity, and reduction in histomorphological damage to hepatocytes (Kaya-Dagistanli et al 2013, Ning-Ping et al 2011).

Protection from paracetamol- and methotrexate-induced mitochondrial toxicity was demonstrated in rodent experimental models, again with maintenance of antioxidant capacity, inhibition of oxidative stress and protection of hepatocyte morphology (Abdel-Zaher et al 2008, Tabassum et al 2010).

Antiatherosclerotic

Animal models of LA synthase deficiency in apolipoprotein E-deficient animals show they have an increased propensity to develop atherosclerotic plaque, especially male subjects (Yi et al 2010, 2012b). In animal models fed high-fat, hypercholesterolaemic diets, ALA was shown to attenuate and decrease plaque formation, decrease inflammation, decrease T-cell content in plaque, decrease vascular smooth-muscle proliferation and improve lipid profile (Lee et al 2012, Xu et al 2012, Ying et al 2010).

Cardioprotective

Pretreatment of rats with LA reduced infarct size and preserved cardiac function in a study of myocardial ischaemia-reperfusion injury (Deng et al 2013).

OTHER ACTIONS

Metal chelation

ALA chelates transition metals by forming stable complexes with Mn^{2+}, Cu^{2+} and Zn^{2+} (Sigel et al 1978). DHLA, but not ALA, significantly inhibited ascorbate oxidation by Fe(III) and Cu(II) in a concentration-dependent manner through chelation, without removing copper or iron from the active sites of enzymes or altering the activity of copper- and iron-dependent enzymes (Suh et al 2004b).

While administration of ALA in lead-poisoned animal models or in vitro cellular models demonstrated a reduction in lead oxidation of the brain (Pande & Flora 2002), the kidney (Sivaprasad et al 2004), erythrocytes (Caylak et al 2008) and ovarian tissue (Gurer et al 1999), especially in combination with dimercaptosuccinic acid (DMSA, a pharmacological molecule commonly used as an antidote to heavy metal poisoning), it showed no chelation properties in decreasing the lead burden. Other studies showed a similar effect, alone or with DMSA, in cadmium-induced oxidation of rat heart, brain, testis and liver (Sumathi et al 1996), in arsenic-induced oxidation of rat brain (Shila et al 2005) and in in vitro human glial cells (Cheng et al 2007).

Signal transduction

ALA is involved in the reduction and oxidation of the thiol/disulfide bonds in transcription factors, and as such has been demonstrated to modulate cell signalling via NF-κB, AMPK and PI3K/Akt signalling (Packer & Cadenas 2010).

Cataract protection

ALA inhibited the development and progression of naphthalene and proton-induced cataract in healthy and diabetic rats (Chen et al 2010, Davis et al 2010, Kojima et al 2007). It also showed the ability to penetrate the human aqueous after topical application, showing a potential use of LA's antioxidant capacity in ophthalmology (Cagini et al 2010).

Cancer

Prevention

ALA has exhibited antimutagenic and anticlastogenic activities in tumorigenic animal and human cell models, including breast, melanoma, ovarian epithelial and colon cancers, through the inhibition of inflammatory mediators, the inhibition of NF-κB activity and DNA fragmentation and inhibition of metastasis (Goraca et al 2011).

Treatment

Four cases of pancreatic cancer patients undergoing a long-term treatment of 300–600 mg intravenous (IV) ALA twice a week, oral naltrexone (4.5 g/day) in addition to dietary modification, selenium (200 mcg bd) and silymarin (300 mg qd) were reported to have improved survival outcomes. These results warrant further investigation given the general poor prognosis of pancreatic cancer patients (Berkson et al 2009).

ALA also demonstrated neuroprotection from chemotherapy side effects (paclitaxel, cisplatin, frataxin and methotrexate) in human cell models of cancer and in vivo animal models (Dadhania et al 2010, Melli et al 2009, Tabassum et al 2010). Current clinical trials are underway.

Neuromodulation

LA improved the status of dopamine, serotonin and adrenaline in rodent's aged brain (Arivazhagan & Panneerselvan 2002).

Radioprotection

Report of a Russian open trial of the treatment of children exposed to radiation from the Chernobyl disaster is often stated as the basis of the radioprotective effects of ALA.

A small number of recent published in vitro and in vivo studies seem to support the potential role of ALA in radioprotection. These studies report protection of cerebellar structure and cognitive function in γ-irradiated rodents (Manda et al 2008), increased protection in cell membrane and DNA stability, as well as increased survival time in lethally radiated mice (Ramachandran & Nair 2011) and maintenance of haemogloblin integrity and rheology in irradiated blood bags for transfusion (Desouky et al 2011).

CLINICAL USE

Most clinical research has been conducted in diabetic populations and people with disease states where an antioxidant, neuroprotective and/or anti-inflammatory mechanism of action may have benefits.

Diabetes

Oral and injectable forms of LA have been investigated in diabetes as a means of enhancing insulin sensitivity and either preventing or treating chronic complications which occur years after the onset of disease, such as polyneuropathy, nephropathy and retinopathy. Many of these complications are the result of an overabundance of ROS produced by the mitochondrial transport chain as a result of a sustained hyperglycaemic state.

ALA was approved in Germany several years ago in the treatment of diabetic neuropathy and as a dietary supplement for patients affected by diabetic retinopathy (Nebbioso et al 2013). It is covered by medical insurance (Mijnhout et al 2012).

Insulin resistance

Increase in insulin sensitivity is primarily achieved through diet, exercise, weight loss and improvement of lean:fat body mass ratio and, lastly, pharmacological intervention if glycaemic control cannot be achieved and maintained.

Several clinical trials have investigated the effect of parenterally-administered LA to diabetic subjects. A study by Jacob et al (cited in Evans & Goldfine 2000) showed insulin-mediated metabolic clearance rates (MCR) of glucose improved by at least 30% in subjects with type 2 diabetes (well controlled with diet alone or with glibenclamide) at doses of 500 mg ALA/500 mL NaCl/day infusion for 10 days. A second study by the same group (Jacob et al 1996), using a dose of 1000 mg ALA/500 mL NaCl for 10 days, reported improvement in glucose infusion rates of 47%, MCR by 55% and insulin sensitivity by 57%. No effects were observed on fasting glucose and insulin levels.

More recently, a study by Zhang et al (2011) investigated 22 obese subjects with impaired glucose tolerance (IGT) (obese-IGT), 13 of whom underwent 2-week ALA treatment, 600 mg intravenously once daily. This short-term treatment significantly improved insulin sensitivity and plasma lipid profile. More specifically, the insulin sensitivity index was impressively enhanced by 41% and significant reductions were seen for plasma levels of free fatty acids, triglyceride, total cholesterol, low-density lipoprotein cholesterol, small dense lipoprotein cholesterol, oxidised lipoprotein cholesterol, and very-low-density lipoprotein cholesterol ($P < 0.01$). At the same time, both plasma oxidative products (malondialdehyde, 8-iso-prostaglandin) and inflammatory markers (tumour necrosis factor-alpha, IL-6) were remarkably decreased ($P < 0.01$), while adiponectin was increased ($P < 0.01$) (Zhang et al 2011).

Oral ALA supplementation has also been investigated in several studies and produced inconsistent results regarding effects on insulin sensitivity (de Oliveira et al 2011, Jacob et al 1999, Yan et al 2013).

Four weeks' treatment with oral ALA was found to improve insulin sensitivity in patients with type 2 diabetes according to this early randomised, placebo-controlled study involving 74 volunteers with type 2 diabetes (Jacob et al 1999). Patients were randomised to either placebo or active treatment in various doses of 600 mg once daily, twice daily (1200 mg) or three times daily (1800 mg); however no dose effect was observed. In contrast, no change in insulin sensitivity was reported in this double-blind randomised controlled trial (RCT) of 102 patients with type 2 diabetes which compared 4 months of treatment with 600 mg/day LA ($n = 26$); 800 mg/day α-tocopherol ($n = 25$); 800 mg/day α-tocopherol + 600 mg/day LA ($n = 25$) and placebo ($n = 26$). In this study, no treatment arm resulted in a significant change to the lipid profile or insulin sensitivity of patients (de Oliveira et al 2011).

Yan et al (2013) performed a double-blinded, randomised, cross-over trial involving 103 patients without cardiovascular disease, hypertension, diabetes or any other inflammatory diseases, to investigate whether oral ALA administration lowers the risk of cardiovascular disease by decreasing the level of oxidative stress markers or improving insulin sensitivity (Homeostatic Model Assessment of Insulin Resistance [HOMA-IR] levels, a method used to assess insulin resistance and beta-cell function). Treatment with oral ALA (1200 mg/day) over 8 weeks produced no significant difference in HOMA or oxidative biomarkers between the two groups. Interestingly, at this treatment dose, ALA was associated with significantly lower body mass index (BMI), weight and waist circumference after 8 weeks. There were no significant differences in the incidence of side effects between ALA and placebo.

Overall, it appears that oral supplementation of ALA may not be as effective as intravenous intake, possibly due to the short plasma half-life and limitations on maximal plasma levels achieved with oral dose forms (Evans & Goldfine 2000, Yan et al 2013). Enteric coating, sustained-release forms, timing of administration and form of LA used are also considerations that may influence future results.

Diabetic polyneuropathy

Diabetic polyneuropathy represents a considerable morbidity of long-term uncontrolled diabetes and occurs in about one-third of people. Symptoms of pain have been reported to occur in 13–34% of patients with diabetes, with the risk of painful neuropathic symptoms considerably higher in type 2 diabetes than in type 1 diabetes (Boulton et al 2013). Persistent hyperglycaemia leading to increased synthesis of ROS in the mitochondria and subsequent oxidative damage to endothelium and neuronal cells are part of the aetiology.

The use of ALA as a treatment for diabetic neuropathies has been studied since the 1950s, with numerous clinical trials of variable quality published (McIllduff & Rutkove 2011). In the last decade, several meta-analyses have been published, with results most consistent for injectable forms of ALA (300–600 mg daily) as a method of reducing symptoms; however the use of high oral doses (600–1200 mg/day) also appears to provide symptomatic relief and, possibly, slow disease progression.

An early meta-analysis from 2004 which analysed four RCTs concluded that 3 weeks of parenterally administered ALA (600 mg/day) provided a significant decrease in pain scores (Ziegler et al 2004). A similar conclusion was reached in a meta-analyis by McIllduff and Rutkove (2011), which included the ALADIN, SYDNEY, ORPIL, SYDNEY II and ALADIN III trials (n = 1160; level 2b evidence). Once again, authors reported that parenterally-administered ALA was associated with a clinically meaningful improvement on symptom scores compared to placebo, at IV doses of 600 mg/day for at least 3 weeks. Oral supplementation also produced a significant improvement in symptoms and impairment at doses of 600 mg, 1200 mg and 1800 mg/day over periods ranging from 3 weeks to 2 years. Side effects were described as dose-dependent, as an oral dose of 600 mg/day over 2 years was well tolerated; however the higher dose of 1200 mg/day was associated with an increase in side effects (nausea, vomiting and vertigo). This was particularly notable in the ALADIN study, whereby rates of adverse events were 32.6% for ALA 1200 mg/day, 18.2% for ALA 600 mg/day, 13.6% for ALA 100 mg/day and 20.7% for placebo. It is important to note that some of the studies selected did not exclude diet control, hypoglycaemic medication, insulin or recent antioxidant use, or the inclusion of some type 1 diabetes patients, which may have influenced the results.

In 2012, a new meta-analysis evaluated four level 1b RCTs (n = 653) with combined results for both oral and IV effects of LA for symptomatic control of neuropathies (pain, burning, paraesthesiae, numbness). All studies reported a reduction in total symptom scores; however, equivocal results were reported in trials using oral dose forms (Mijnhout et al 2012). Another 2012 meta-analysis, this time evaluating intravenous treatment only, concluded that treatment with 300–600 mg daily for 2–4 weeks was safe, and improved both nerve conduction velocity and neuropathic symptoms (Han et al 2012).

The NATHAN study, not reported in earlier meta-analyses, was a large multicentre, double-blind, RCT that evaluated the efficacy of oral ALA (600 mg/day) taken over 4 years by volunteers with mild to moderate diabetic distal symmetric sensorimotor polyneuropathy. The primary end point was a composite score (Neuropathy Impairment Score-Lower Limbs [NIS-LL] and seven neurophysiological tests), which was not significantly different for ALA compared to placebo after 4 years. However, change from baseline was significantly better with ALA than placebo for NIS (P = 0.028), NIS-LL (P = 0.05) and NIS-LL muscular weakness subscore (P = 0.045). Importantly, more patients showed a clinically meaningful improvement and fewer showed progression of NIS (P = 0.013) and NIS-LL (P = 0.025) with ALA than with placebo. Treatment was well tolerated, although the rates of serious adverse events were higher on ALA (38.1%) than on placebo (28.0%).

The most recent meta-analysis (Xu et al 2013) considered results from a larger cohort of 1106 patients with diabetic neuropathy in a series of 15 China-based trials, which demonstrated significant efficacy of a combined therapy of LA (300–600 mg IV) and methylcobalamin (500–1000 mg IV or intramuscularly) once a day for 2–4 weeks. The combination was shown to be more effective than monotherapy of LA or methylcobalamin. However, the authors recognised methodological quality issues and the small size sample, emphasising the need for larger, well-designed, multicentre RCTs.

Diabetic nephropathy

Administration of LA reduces diabetic nephropathy in animal models through mitonchondrial protection, glomerular histological changes and decrease in ROS generation (Wang et al 2013, Yi et al 2011). Protection of β cells, decrease in cholesterol levels, decrease in albuminuria, serum urea and creatinine, and amelioration of proteinuria have also been noted in these models (Obrosova et al 2003, Wang et al 2013, Winiarska et al 2008, Yi et al 2011). A rodent model of LIAS deficiency was shown to accelerate the development of nephropathy and treatment with ALA improved kidney metabolic regulation and antioxidant capacity (Yi et al 2012a).

In a small clinical study, oral ALA administration (600 mg/day) to diabetic patients (type 1 diabetes n = 20; type 2 diabetes n = 15) over a period of 18 months has shown a significant decrease in thrombomodulin and unchanged urea/creatinine ratio compared to a control group, demonstrating a slowing of kidney damage (Morcos et al 2001). Larger and better-designed studies are needed to confirm these findings.

Diabetic retinopathy

ALA is used as a dietary supplement to slow down the progression of diabetic retinopathy. ALA prevents microvascular damage and preserves pericyte coverage of retinal capillaries in addition to improving insulin sensitivity, thereby providing a theoretical basis for its use (Nebbioso et al 2013).

IN COMBINATION

One randomised study of 32 diabetic volunteers with pre-retinopathy and good metabolic control found that oral treatment with ALA at 400 mg/day (in association with genistein and vitamins) resulted in an increase in plasma antioxidant capacity after 30 days and significant increases in the electrophysiological response, as measured by electroretinography, suggesting a protective effect on retinal cells by strengthening the plasma antioxidant barrier (Nebbioso et al 2012).

In contrast, a randomised study examining the effects of ALA on macular oedema in patients with type 2 diabetes found an oral dose of 600 mg daily taken over 2 years did not produce a significant improvement in blood levels of glycated haemoglobin, visual acuity or any reduction in retinal thickness compared to placebo (Haritoglou et al 2011). Further clinical research is required, ideally with larger doses taken in divided daily doses. Alternatively, a combination of substances with antioxidant effects, such as the one used in the study by Nebbioso et al (2012), might have more promise.

Age-related macular degeneration (AMD)

A randomised study of 62 patients (50–75 years old) with early and intermediate dry form of AMD showed that treatment with ALA produced a significant increase in serum superoxide dismutase activity, suggesting that ALA may have a possible preventive effect in the development of AMD through an antioxidant mechanism (Sun et al 2012).

Peripheral neuropathic pain (sciatic nerve pain)

A double-blind RCT compared acetyl-L-carnitine (ALC: 1180 mg/day) to ALA (600 mg/day) over a 60-day treatment period in 64 consecutive patients (mean age 61 years; range 29–85 years) with acute backache and moderate sciatica associated with a herniated disc (Memeo & Loiero 2008). Treatment with ALA produced significantly greater mean improvement than ALC from baseline for NIS-LL, Neuropathy Symptoms and Change in the Lower Limbs and Total Symptom Score scores ($P < 0.05$ for all comparisons). Additionally, a significant reduction in analgesic requirements was reported for more patients taking ALA than ALC (71.0% vs 45.5%, respectively; $P < 0.05$).

Cardiac autonomic neuropathy and platelet reactivity

Cardiac neuropathy and platelet reactivity are complications in diabetes which increase the risk of cardiovascular events (Mollo et al 2012). One in vitro study investigating the mechanisms of LA's antiplatelet activity found it significantly inhibited platelet aggregation in a dose-dependent manner and suggested the mechanisms were linked to an increase in cAMP formation, followed by thromboxane A_2 inhibition, Ca^{2+} mobilisation and protein kinase C activation (Lai et al 2010).

One small clinical study looked at platelet reactivity in type 1 diabetes patients ($n = 56$) who were randomly assigned a 600 mg oral LA dose daily or a placebo for 5 weeks and found LA significantly reduced platelet activation. Mechanisms remain unclear, as markers of oxidative stress (8-iso-prostaglandin $F_{2\alpha}$) and inflammation (C-reactive protein) were unchanged (Mollo et al 2012).

In the Deutsche Kardiale Autonome Neuropathie (DEKAN), ALA supplementation (oral ALA, 800 mg daily for 4 months) in 73 type 2 diabetic patients showed modest improvement in heart rate variability, a validated tool in the assessment of cardiac neuropathy (Coleman et al 2001).

HIV/AIDS

Supplementation with ALA (300 mg three times daily) may positively impact patients with HIV and AIDS by restoring blood total glutathione level and improving functional reactivity of lymphocytes to T-cell mitogens, according to a placebo-controlled RCT (Jariwalla et al 2008). The mean blood total glutathione level in ALA-supplemented subjects was significantly elevated and the lymphocyte proliferation response was significantly enhanced or stabilised after 6 months compared to progressive decline in the placebo group (ALA vs placebo: $P < 0.001$ with phytohaemagglutinin; $P = 0.02$ with anti-CD3 monoclonal antibody). A positive correlation was seen between blood total glutathione level and lymphocyte response to anti-CD3 stimulation. There was no change in CD4 count over 6 months.

One study showed that antioxidant supplementation (with ALA + *N*-acetyl cysteine) may have a protective role on mitochondrial function, with limited effects on the reversal of clinical lipodystrophic abnormalities in HIV-1-infected patients (Milazzo et al 2010).

Multiple sclerosis

MS is a chronic inflammatory disease of the central nervous system, characterised mainly as an autoimmune neurodegenerative disorder. Excessive oxidative stress or a loss of the antioxidant/oxidant balance may contribute to its development or be a consequence of disease (Ferreira et al 2013). Additionally, transmigration of activated immune cells across the blood–brain barrier plays a significant role in MS pathogenesis as it leads to the development of new inflammatory lesions in MS. As such, it is not surprising that ALA has been investigated as a potential treatment in this disease.

ALA has been proven to be an effective treatment in the management of MS in experimental autoimmune encephalomyelitis (EAE) rats, the accepted model for MS. In these models, ALA was shown to decrease the migration of encephalitogenic T cells to the spinal cord through the inhibition of intercellular adhesion molecule 1 and vascular cell adhesion molecule-1. In vitro, ALA has been shown to activate cAMP-activated protein kinase A (an enzyme involved in immunomodulation and neuroprotection); this pathway is believed to be central in the pathogenesis of MS (Chaudhari et al 2006, Marracci et al 2002, Morini et al 2004, Salinthone et al 2010, Schreibelt et al 2006). Oral ALA supplementation (1200 mg/day) taken by MS volunteers resulted in increased cAMP levels in peripheral blood mononuclear cells 4 hours after ingestion and, on average, cAMP levels in 20 subjects were 43% higher than baseline (Salinthone et al 2010).

A small, double-blind, placebo-controlled, dose-finding trial (n = 37) found a significant dose relationship between ALA plasma levels and inhibition of metalloprotein 9 and intracellular adhesion molecules also involved in MS pathogenesis. Effects were noted after 2 weeks at doses of oral 1200 mg/day and were significantly better than a 600 mg/day dose; however, there was a significant individual variability in ALA peak serum — potentially an effect of the administration of ALA with food in this study (Yadav et al 2005). A more recent double-blind randomised controlled study testing the effect of oral ALA (1200 mg/day) in 52 MS patients (relapsing-remitting) over 12 weeks showed a significant increase in total antioxidant capacity ($P = 0.004$) compared to placebo but no change in malondialdehyde levels or the activities of superoxide dismutase or glutathione peroxidase (Khalili et al 2014).

MS is a common aetiology of optic neuritis and is often a presenting sign. A small animal study (n = 14) demonstrated protection against axonal loss and degeneration with ALA (100 mg/kg) reducing $CD4^+$ and $CD11b^+$ T cell, inflammation and demyelination in an EAE mice model (Chaudhari et al 2011).

A study by Yadav et al (2010) compared the pharmacokinetics of a 1200 mg single dose of three different formulations of racemic LA in 24 MS patients (formula A: 1200 mg tablet, excipients unknown; formula B: 300 mg gelatine capsule, cellulose and ascorbyl palmitate and silica; formula C: 600 mg capsule, pine cellulose and ascorbyl acid) against three different doses in rats (20 mg, 50 mg, 100 mg). The MS patients taking the capsule formulas B and C achieved C_{max} and area under the concentration curve (AUC) equivalent to subcutaneous 50 mg/kg in mice, the therapeutic dose in experimental MS mice models. As a result, the authors suggest 1200 mg as a therapeutic dose for further clinical trials. The tablet formulation showed the lowest AUC and clearance, and widest patient intervariability. The authors recognised that the postprandial administration, chosen to decrease potential gastric side effects, rather than the manufacturer-recommended fasting intake, may have influenced the pharmacokinetics of the tablet.

A placebo-controlled study is currently underway in the United States to determine whether oral ALA 1200 mg/day can slow the progression of MS over time.

Weight loss

According to a randomised, double-blind study involving 360 obese participants (BMI $\geq$ 30 kg/m^2 or 27–30 kg/m^2 plus hypertension, diabetes mellitus or hypercholesterolaemia), active treatment with 1800 mg/day of racemic ALA over 20 weeks led to significantly more weight loss than placebo. Weight loss was significantly greater with 1800 mg/day of ALA compared to placebo from week 4. Additionally, there was a significant difference between the groups with regard to percentage of subjects who achieved a ≥5% reduction in baseline body weight (21.6% vs 10.0%, $P < 0.01$). No significant changes were observed in triglyceride concentrations and triglyceride/high-density lipoprotein cholesterol ratios. The significant difference in weight loss was also reported for the group with BMI 27–30 kg/m^2 plus additional risk factors. Subjects with diabetes receiving 1800 mg/day ALA showed a mean 0.38% reduction from baseline in haemoglobin A_{1C} level ($P < 0.05$) but there was no change in blood pressure or fasting plasma glucose and cholesterol concentrations. Mild and transient urticaria and itching were experienced in ALA groups; however, overall incidence of side effects was similar to the placebo group (Koh et al 2011).

Oral ALA (1200 mg/day) was associated with significantly lower BMI, weight and waist circumference after 8 weeks in another double-blinded, randomised trial, conducted by Yan et al (2013), involving 103 patients without cardiovascular disease, hypertension, diabetes or any other inflammatory disease. There were no significant differences in incidence of side effects between ALA treatment and placebo.

Weight loss in schizophrenia

A case series of a 12-week ALA trial in 5 schizophrenia patients treated with atypical antipsychotic drugs found that treatment resulted in a mean weight loss of 3.16 kg ($P = 0.043$) and, on average, BMI showed a significant reduction ($P = 0.028$) over the 12 weeks (Kim et al 2008). No change was seen to the Brief Psychiatric Rating Scale and the Montgomery-Asberg Depression Rating Scale.

A small open study was more recently published, whereby ALA (1200 mg/day) taken for 10 weeks by 12 non-diabetic schizophrenic patients produced a significant weight loss during the intervention (–2.2 kg ± 2.5 kg). Treatment with ALA was well tolerated and particularly effective for individuals taking strongly antihistaminic antipsychotics (–2.9 kg ± 2.6 kg vs –0.5 kg ± 1.0 kg) (Ratliff et al 2013).

Migraine prophylaxis

An RCT using ALA in migraine prophylaxis was steered by the Belgian Headache Society and included five Belgian centres, which recruited 54 migraineurs (43 migraine without aura, 11 with aura; mean age 38 ± 8 years; 7 males) (Magis et al 2007). ALA (600 mg/day) was taken for 3 months and was found to reduce migraine attack frequency compared to placebo (P = 0.06). Within-group analyses showed a significant reduction of attack frequency (P = 0.005), headache days (P = 0.009) and headache severity (P = 0.03) in patients treated with ALA whereas these outcome measures remained unchanged in the placebo group. The treatment was well tolerated with no adverse effects reported.

Before any firm conclusion can be drawn, a larger clinical trial is now necessary.

OTHER USES

Alzheimer's disease (AD)

ALA, with its proven antioxidant, anti-inflammatory, neuroprotective, metal-chelating and glycaemic regulation activities, is showing potential in the treatment of AD and worthy of further investigation.

AD is characterised by neurofibrillary tangles and amyloid plaques leading to neuronal loss. Its pathophysiology is thought to involve progressive cholinergic deficit, a chronic inflammatory oxidative process leading to mitochondrial dysfunction. Recent preliminary studies are showing insulin abnormality and resistance in AD patients, including impaired cerebral glucose metabolism, leading to neuron toxicity (Maczureck et al 2008).

The first indication that ALA may be beneficial in AD and related dementias came from a serendipitous case of a 74-year-old woman with signs of cognitive impairment and diabetic polyneuropathy treated with an anticholinesterase inhibitor drug and 600 mg LA daily for her neuropathy. Since 1997, when treatment first began, several tests have been performed which show no substantial decline in cognitive function and neurological tests show unusually slow progress of her cognitive impairment (Maczureck et al 2008).

Since then, studies in rodents have shown a protective effect of cognitive deficits (Wang & Chen 2007) and chronic feeding of ALA in conjunction with *N*-acetyl cysteine showed improvement in cognition in aged subjects (Farr et al 2003).

A small open pilot trial (n = 9) of patients with AD were given 600 mg oral ALA daily, 30 minutes before breakfast in conjunction with standard treatment of acetylcholinesterase inhibitors over a period of 371 days. The treatment provided stabilisation in cognition compared to pretreatment decline in cognition. The size of this pilot study increased to 48 patients for up to 48 months, providing similar results. The need for well-designed RCTs is warranted to confirm these findings (Maczureck et al 2008).

Polycystic ovary syndrome (PCOS)

Although generally associated with high BMI, about 20% of women presenting with PCOS are of normal weight. Some studies have suggested that insulin resistance in PCOS is a result of genetic predisposition to a defective insulin-signalling pathway (and resulting compensatory hyperinsulinaemia), rather than dependent on BMI. In normoinsulaemic lean PCOS women, the use of insulin-reducing and sensitising drugs was shown to improve free testosterone and androstenedione serum values, suggesting insulin-related hyperandrogenism (Baptiste et al 2010); improving this resistance has been recognised as essential to improve metabolic and reproductive outcomes (Marshall & Dunaif 2012).

A pilot trial administering controlled-release lipoic acid 600 mg twice daily to 6 non-obese PCOS patients with no other comorbidity, including insulin resistance, and ingesting an isocaloric diet showed improvement in their insulin sensitivity, a decrease in their triglyceride and increase in low-density lipoprotein molecular size (Masharani et al 2010).

Hepatoprotection

A small trial (n = 24) of patients undergoing liver resection showed decreased serum AST and ALT (used in combination in the diagnosis of liver damage) and histomorphological damage to hepatocytes when 600 mg of IV ALA was administered 15 minutes before resection compared to the group administered IV NaCl (Dünschede et al 2006).

ALA (300 mg/day) has been investigated in alcoholic liver disease in a 6-month RCT (n = 40), which found that only those participants abstaining from alcohol showed significant improvement in AST and gamma-glutamyl transaminase (which is raised in chronic alcohol toxicity) values and histological biopsy with use (Marshall et al 1982). These results are problematic as the number of abstainers was not even in both groups, and the dose used was low. Hepatoprotective effects have been shown in animal studies in recent studies (Kaya-Dagistanli et al 2013, Foo et al 2011).

Hypertension

A cross-over double-blind study tested whether adding oral ALA to the angiotensin-converting enzyme inhibitor quinapril would potentiate regulation of blood pressure, endothelial function and proteinuria in obese diabetic patients with stage 1 hypertension. Patients were randomised to receive either quinapril (40 mg/day) alone or quinapril (40 mg/day) and LA (600 mg/day) for 6 weeks. Biomarkers of obesity and endothelial-dependent flow-mediated dilation were improved in the group of combination quinapril and ALA (Khan et al 2010). Another study noted a reduction in blood pressure, proteinuria and endothelial function (Rahman et al 2012).

Kwashiorkor

A small longitudinal clinical pilot study comparing the standard World Health Organization treatment protocol to one of three groups supplemented with reduced glutathione, LA or *N*-acetyl cysteine to a healthy control group showed that reduced glutathione and LA both positively increased recovery and survival, and correlated with erythrocyte glutathione concentration — a predictive value of survival (Becker et al 2005).

Burning-mouth syndrome

Three small clinical trials showed significant results in decreasing symptoms of burning-mouth syndrome with dosages of 600 mg daily for 1–2 months. However, the placebo groups in these studies also reported high levels, although non-significant, of symptomatic improvements, especially in the double-blind trial, compared to the open-label trials (Zakrzewska et al 2009); Crow and Gonzalez (2013) report three subsequent studies with similar dosage in which LA does not yield statistical significance over placebo, possibly due to the large variation in pain response in both groups.

Carpal tunnel syndrome — in combination

A study compared the efficacy of LA (600 mg/day) in combination with γ-linolenic acid 360 mg/day to a vitamin B complex (B6 150 mg; B1 100 mg; B12 500 mcg/1 daily) for 90 days in 112 subjects with moderate to severe carpal tunnel syndrome. The LA/γ-linolenic group scored significant improvement in symptoms, confirmed by electromyography, compared to the B vitamin group (Di Geronimo et al 2009).

Erectile dysfunction

With the classical causes of erectile dysfunction including diabetes mellitus, hypertension, obesity, hyperlipidaemia and cardiovascular conditions, and the pathophysiological mechanisms understood to involve oxidative stress, especially due to advanced glycosylated end products, and alteration of vascular and endothelial function through dysregulation of NO synthase (Shamloul & Ghanem 2012), a theoretical basis exists for the use of LA for this condition.

An animal study also demonstrated that the neurectomy associated with prostatectomy resulted in a loss of NO synthase-containing nerve fibres and in significant oxidative stress; treatment with LA (65 mg/kg/day IP) showed improvement in cavernous tissue regeneration (Alan et al 2010). No clinical trials are available at this time.

Wound healing

Human trials show that hyperbaric oxygen therapy increases IL-6 and ROS production. In a small double-blind randomised study, supplementation with LA (600 mg/day) in patients undergoing hyperbaric oxygen therapy for various conditions, with the inclusion criterion of leg ulcers older than 30 days, showed an 80% reduction or remission of the lesions at 40 days of treatment compared to the placebo group (Alleva et al 2005).

Glaucoma

Glaucoma is a progressive neurodegenerative condition in which the retinal ganglia and optic nerve are damaged due to increased intraocular pressure, leading to loss of vision. ALA has demonstrated a protective effect on retinal neurons in vitro and in animal models (Koriyama et al 2013). A small Russian study reported an improvement in visual function after 4 weeks of treatment with 150 mg/day of ALA in patients with glaucoma (Cotlier & Weinreb 2008).

Photoageing of skin

The low molecular weight of ALA, combined with its solubility characteristics, suggests the possibility of LA being absorbed by the skin and having pharmacological activities. Swift penetration through the epidermis has been demonstrated in a hairless mouse model and, after 4 hours, distribution to the dermis and subcutaneous tissue underneath. This was further explored in a 12-week RCT (n = 33) with a 5% ALA cream, which was applied twice daily to half the face and placebo cream to the other. Self-assessment, clinician assessment, standardised photography and laser profilometry before and after the period of treatment were used to evaluate effects. The ALA-enriched cream significantly improved profilometry in photoageing of facial skin.

According to photographic evaluations, ALA cream was shown to improve the appearance of fine lines ($P < 0.031$), decrease pigmentation ($P < 0.007$), decrease under-eye bags and puffiness ($P < 0.09$) and decrease pore size ($P < 0.08$). The clinical evaluation also reported a significant improvement in fine lines ($P = 0.01$). Additionally, self-assessment showed that 78% of subjects claimed the active side showed improvement, compared to 31% who claimed the placebo treatment was better ($P < 0.002$).

Amanita spp. mushroom poisoning

The use of thioctic acid in *Amanita* spp. has been a treatment of choice in Europe since the 1960s, often alongside silymarin or silibin. Intravenous doses of 300 mg/24 h with 10% glucose in saline for up to 6 days have been used (Becker et al 1976). However, usage of ALA remains controversial, with some reports of inefficacy (Enjalbert et al 2002, Tong et al 2007), mostly because of the inability to carry out blinded RCTs in mushroom poisoning ethically (Klein et al 1989). ALA is not currently used as an *Amanita* spp. antidote in Australia (Roberts et al 2013).

DOSAGE RANGE

As LA absorption decreases with food intake, it is recommended that LA be ingested 30–60 minutes before meals or 120 minutes after; however, side effects are more likely on an empty stomach (Gleiter et al 1996, McIllduff & Rutkove 2011, Shay et al 2009).

According to clinical studies, oral doses for ALA are:

- Diabetes and peripheral neuropathies: 600–1200 mg/day.
- Cardiac autonomic neuropathy in type 2 diabetes patients: 800 mg/day.
- MS: 1200 mg/day.
- AD: 600 mg/day in conjunction with *N*-acetyl cysteine.
- PCOS: 600 mg twice daily.
- Hypertension: 600 mg/day.
- Burning-mouth syndrome: 200–600 mg/day — efficacy uncertain.
- Carpal tunnel syndrome: 600 mg/day.
- Wound healing: 300 mg twice daily.
- Weight loss: 1800 mg/day.
- Migraine prevention: 600 mg/day.
- Sciatic nerve pain: 600 mg/day.
- Glaucoma: 150 mg/day.

Safety and dosage have not been studied in children.

TOXICITY

The maximum tolerated dose of ALA in human subjects has not been well defined; however, based on the observation that the oral lethal dose (LD_{50}) for rats and mice is 1130 and 502 mg/kg, respectively, it is assumed that human beings can tolerate several grams of ALA daily. The IP LD_{50} is 200 and 160 mg/kg for rats and mice, respectively (Biewenga et al 1997).

ADVERSE REACTIONS

Clinical trials testing oral ALA, at concentrations as high as 1800 mg/day for 6 months and as high as 1200 mg/day for 2 years, have not identified any serious adverse effects. Similarly, a clinical trial of obese volunteers found a daily dose of 1200 mg/day or 1800 mg/day over 20 weeks was well tolerated, with the most common side effects reported as itchiness and urticaria, although the overall incidence of side effects was no different from the placebo group (Koh et al 2011).

Overall, the most common side effects of oral supplementation tend to appear when used at doses of 1200 mg and above and include nausea, vomiting, rashes, tingling and itching sensations and headaches.

Topically, ALA has been used safely for up to 12 weeks at 5% concentration. Side effects can include mild rash and local irritation, stinging and burning sensations.

Intravenously, ALA has been used at doses of 600 mg and 1200 mg daily, with side effects reported at 1200 mg. Local irritations have been reported at the injection site.

A case was reported of a 63-year-old man with multiple pathologies and taking multiple medications who was administrated 600 mg/day of LA to treat diabetic neuropathy. He developed low-grade fever, nausea and fatigue and elevated serum transaminase. Discontinuation resulted in elimination of symptoms and return to normal of liver enzymes. A second attempt at treatment led to the return of symptoms and abnormal transaminase. The report investigated other potential aetiologies of liver injuries. While the authors recognise the case as unique and ALA as generally safe, they recommended liver enzyme monitoring in conjunction with ALA treatment (Ridruejo et al 2011). However the case report does not examine potential LA contamination or a drug–LA interaction as a potential aetiology for the liver enzyme abnormalities.

SIGNIFICANT INTERACTIONS

When controlled studies are not available, interactions are based on evidence of pharmacological activity, case reports and other evidence and are largely theoretical.

Copper

ALA is a metal chelator and binds to copper in vivo — separate doses by 3 h.

Manganese

ALA is a metal chelator and binds to manganese in vivo — separate doses by 3 h.

Zinc

ALA is a metal chelator and binds to zinc in vivo — separate doses by 3 h.

Hypoglycaemic agents

Theoretically, concomitant use may affect glucose control and require medication dosage changes — observe.

Vitamin E, vitamin C, coenzyme Q10 and glutathione

ALA reconstitutes these antioxidants from their oxidised form to their unoxidised form as part of the antioxidant cycle in humans — beneficial interaction.

Warfarin

ALA reduces platelet reactivity in vitro (Lai et al 2010). It is uncertain whether the effect is clinically significant — observe patients taking these agents together.

Levothyroxine

Uncertain interaction exists. When co-administered, ALA may suppress the conversion of thyroxine to triiodothyronine — decrease total cholesterol, triglycerides, albumin and total protein (Segermann et al 1991).

CONTRAINDICATIONS AND PRECAUTIONS

Age is believed to affect bioavailability markedly, with older age associated with reduced bioavailability of oral supplements (Keith et al 2012).

Insulin autoimmune syndrome is a condition that develops in individuals not previously injected with pharmacological insulin; it appears to be drug-induced in about 50% of cases, especially drugs from the sulfhydryl group. In East Asians, especially Japanese, and Native Americans, there is a high expression of a human leucocyte antigen genotype that confers susceptibility to this syndrome. A number of cases have been reported in Japan after intake of ALA. Anti-insulin antibody titres reduce after ALA discontinuation (Ishida et al 2007). The case of an Italian Caucasian woman was also reported in 2011 (Bresciani et al 2011).

ALA supplementation in pigeons and mice has caused fatal toxicity in thiamine-deficient subjects (20 mg/kg, a high dose). A theoretical basis exists for caution in prescribing LA to alcoholics, Wernicke–Korsakoff patients and other thiamine-depleting conditions. ALA does not, however, deplete thiamine in healthy or deficient individuals (Gal & Razevska 1960).

PREGNANCY USE

A study of diabetic rats injected intraperitoneally with ALA improved survival of their embryos, showing that is likely that ALA can cross the placenta. It also showed a decreased rate of neural tube defects (Al Ghafli et al 2004).

While ALA appears essential to fetal rat formation as an essential mitochondrial enzyme (Yi & Maeda 2005), no clinical trials of supplementation exist in human pregnancy or lactation.

Practice points/Patient counselling

- ALA is endogenously synthesised in the human body and is essential for cellular metabolism. It acts as an antioxidant, regenerates vitamins C and E and glutathione in the body, chelates metal ions and repairs oxidised proteins.
- ALA can be safely used in supplementary form at doses under 1200 mg for up to 2 years for a wide range of diseases.
- Meta-analysis supports its use in type 2 diabetes and diabetic neuropathy.
- There is preliminary clinical evidence suggesting a role in PCOS, MS, AD, hypertension, carpal tunnel syndrome, wound healing and glaucoma, although further research is required. Effects are uncertain in burning-mouth syndrome.
- Supplemental forms are often manufactured in a racemic form, but some trials show a greater efficacy with L-enantiomer.

PATIENTS' FAQs

What will this nutrient do for me?

LA supplementation is used in type 2 diabetes, diabetic neuropathy, hypertension, carpal tunnel syndrome, PCOS, MS and AD. ALA confers antioxidant and neuroprotective effects as well as improving glycaemia.

When will it start to work?

It depends on the dose and indication for use.

Are there any safety issues?

LA should be used with caution in people of East Asian and Native American origin; thiamine deficiency and alcoholics; patients with cancer, high homocysteine, liver impairment, thyroid disorders; people treated for diabetes or glycaemic impairment. There are also several drug interactions that should be considered before use.

REFERENCES

Abdel-Zaher A et al. The potential protective role of alpha-lipoic acid against acetaminophen-induced hepatic and renal damage. Toxicology 243 (2008): 261–270.

Abdel-Zaher A et al. Alpha-lipoic acid protect against potassium cyanide-induced seizures and mortality. Experimental and Toxicologic Pathology 23 (2011): 161–165.

Abdin A, Sarhan N. Intervention of mitonchondrial dysfunction-oxidative stress-dependent apoptosis as a possible neuroprotective mechanism od α-lipoic acid against rotenone induce parkinsonism and L-dopa toxicity. Neuroscience research 71 (2011): 387–395.

Alan C et al. Biochemical changes in cavernosal tissue caused by single sided cavernosal nerve resection and the effect of alpha-lipoic acid on these changes. Actas Urológicas Españolas 34.10 (2010): 874–881.

Alleva R et al. α-lipoic acide supplementation inhibits oxidative damage, accelerating chronic wound healing in patients undergoing hyperbaric oxygen therapy. Biochem Biophys Res Commun 333 (2005): 404–410.

Al Ghafli MH et al. Effect of alpha-lipoic acid supplementation on maternal diabetes-induced growth retardation and congenital abnormality in rat fetuses. Mol Cell Biochem 261.1/2 (2004): 123–35.

Arivazhagan P. et al. Effect of DL-alpha-lipoic acid on the status of lipid peroxidation and anti-oxidant enzymes in various brain regions of aged rats. Exp Gerontology 37.6 (2002): 803–11.

Astiz M et al. The oxidative damage and inflammation casued by pesticides are reverted in rat brains. Neurochemistry International 61 (2012): 1231–1242.

Baptiste CG et al. Insulin and hyperandrogenism in women with polycystic ovarian syndrome. The Journal of Steroid Biochemistry and Molecular Biology 122.1–3 (2010): 42–52.

Bast A, Haenen GR. Lipoic acid: a multifunctional antioxidant. BioFactors 17.1–4 (2008): 207–213.

Becker CE et al. Diagnosis and treatment of *Amanita phalloides*-type mushroom poisoning — Use of thioctic acid. West J Med 125 (1976): 100–109.

Becker K et al. Effects of antioxidants on glutathione levels and clinical recovery from the malnutrition syndrome kwashiorkor-a pilot study. Redox Rep 10.4 (2005): 215–26.

Berkson BM et al. Revisiting the ALA/N (α-lipoic acid/ low dose naltrexone) protocol for people with metastatic and non-metastatic pancreatic cancer: a report of 3 new cases. Integrative Cancer Therapies 8.4 (2009): 416–422.

Biewenga GP et al. The pharmacology of the antioxidant lipoic acid. Gen Pharmac. 29.3 (1997): 315–331.

Booker SJ. Uncovering the pathway of lipoic acid biosynthesis. Chemistry and Biology 11 (2004): 10–12.

Boulton, A.J., et al. 2013. Whither pathogenetic treatments for diabetic polyneuropathy? Diabetes Metab Res. Rev., 29, (5) 327–333.

Breithaupt-Grogler K et al. Dose-proportionality of oral thioctic acid — coincidence of assessments via pooled plasma and individual data. Eur J Pharm Sci 8 (1999):57–65.

Bresciani E et al. Insulin autoimmune syndrome induced by α-lipoic acid in a Caucasian woman: case report. Diabetes Care 34.9 (2011): e146.

Cagini C et al. Study of alpha-lipoic acid penetrationin the human aqueous after topical administration. Clin Experiment Opthalmol 38.6 (2010): 572–576.

Carlson DA et al. The plasma pharmacokinetics of R-(+)-lipoic acid deministered as sodium R-(+) lipoate to healthy human subjects. Alter Med Rev 12 (2007) 343–51.

Caylak E et al. Antioxidant effect of methionine, α-lipoic acid, *N*-acetylcysteine and homocysteine on lead-induced oxidative stress to erythrocytes in rats. Experimental and toxicologic pharmacology 60 (2008): 208–294.

Chaudhari P et al. Lipoic aicd inhibits expression of ICAM-1 and VCAM-1 by CNS endothelial cells and T cells migration into the spinal cordin experiemental autoimmune encephalomyelitis. Journal of Neuroimmunology 175 (2006): 87–96.

Chaudhari P et al. Lipoic acid decreases inflammation and confers neuroprotection in experimental autoimmune optic neuritis. J Neuroimmunology 233 (2011): 90–96.

Chen Y et al. Alpha-lipoic acid alters post-translational modificationand protects the chaperone activity of lens alpha-crystallin in naphthaline-induced cataract. Curr Eye Res 35.7 (2010): 620–630.

Cheng et al. Protection against arsenic trioxide-induced autophagic cell death in U118 human gliama cells by use of lipoic acid. Food and chemical toxicology 45 (2007): 1027–1038.

Chng HT et al. Distribution study of orally administrated lipoic acid in rat brain tissues. Brain research 1251 (2009): 80–86.

Cho KJ et al. Alpha-lipoic acid decreases thiol reactivity of the insulin receptor and protein tyrosine phosphatase 1B in 3T3-L1 adipocytes. Biochem Pharmacol 66 (2003): 849–858.

Coleman MD et al. The therapeutic use of lipoic acid in diabetes: a current perspective. Environ Toxicol Pharmacol 10 (2001): 167–172.

Connell BJ et al. Lipoic acid protects against reperfusion injury in the early stages of cerebral ischemia. Brain Res 1375 (2011): 128–136.

Cotlier E, Weinreb R. The potential value of natural antioxidative treatment in glaucoma. Survey of Ophthalmology 53.5 (2008): 479–505.

Crow HC, Gonzalez Y. Burning mouth syndrome. Oral Maxillofacial Surg Clin N Am. 25 (2013): 67–76.

Dadhania VP et al. Intervention of alpha-lipoic acidameliorates methotrexate-induced oxidative stress and genotoxicity; a study in rat intestine. Chemico-Biological Interactions 183.1 (2010): 85–97.

Davis JG et al. Dietary supplements reduce the caractogenic potential of proton and HZE — particle radiation in rats. Radiat Res (2010) 173(3): 353–361.

Deng C et al. α-lipoic acid reduces infarct size and preserve cardiac functions in rat myocardial ischemia/reperfusion injury through activation of PI3K/Akt/Nrf2 pathway. PLoSone 8.3 (2013): e58371.

de Oliveira, A.M., et al. 2011. The effects of lipoic acid and α-tocopherol supplementation on the lipid profile and insulin sensitivity of patients with type 2 diabetes mellitus: A randomized, double-blind, placebo-controlled trial. *Diabetes Research and Clinical Practice*, 92, (2) 253–260.

Desouky OS et al. Impact evaluation of α-lipoic acid in gamma-irradiated erythrocytes. Radiation physics and chemistry 80(2011): 446–452.

Di Geronimo G et al. Treatment of Tunnel carpal syndrome with alpha-lipoic acid. European Review for Medical and Pharcological Sciences 13 (2009): 133–139.

Dünschede F et al. Reduction of ischemia reperfusion injury after liver resection and hepatic inflow occlusion by alpha-lipoic acid in humans. World J Gastroenterol 12.42 (2006): 6812–7.

Enjalbert F et al. Treatment of amatoxin poisoning: 20 retrospective analyis. J Toxicol Clin Toxicol 40.6 (2002): 715–57.

Estrada et al. Stimulation of glucose uptake by the natural enzyme alpha-lipoic acid/thioctic acid: participation of elements of the insulin signaling pathway. Diabetes 45 (1996): 1798–804.

Evans JL Goldfine ID. α-lipoic acid: A multifunctional antioxidant that improve insulin sensitivity in patient with type 2 diabetes. Diabetes Technology and Research 2.3 (2000): 401–413.

Farr SA et al. The antioxidants α-lipoic acid and N-acetylcysteine reverse memory impairement and brain oxidative stress in aged SAMP8 mice. Journal of Neurochemistry 84 (2003): 1173–1183.

Ferreira, B., et al. 2013. Glutathione in multiple sclerosis. Br J Biomed. Sci., 70, (2) 75–79.

Foo NP et al. α-lipoic acid inhibits liver fibrosis through the attenuation of ROS-triggered signaling in hepatic stellate cells activated by PDGF and TGF-β. Toxicology 182.1/2 (2011): 39–46.

Gal E, Razevska DE. Studies on the in-vivo metabolism of lipoic acid. The fate of DL lipoic acid S- in normal and thiamine deficient rats. Archives of Biochemistry and Biophysics 89 (1960): 253–261.

Gleiter CH et al. Influence of food on the bioavailability of thioctic acid eniantomers. Eu J Clin Pharmacol. 50 (1996): 513–514.

Goraca A et al. Lipoic acid — biological activity and therapeutic potential. Pharmacological Report 63 (2011): 849–858.

Gurer et al. Antioxidant effects of α-lipoic acid in lead toxicity. Free radical toxicity and medicine 27.1/2 (1999): 75–81.

Han D et al. Lipic acid increases de novo synthesis of glutathione by improving cytine utilazation. Biofactors. 6 (1997): 321–38.

Han T et al. A systematic reiew and meta analysis of α-lipoic acid in the treatment of diabetic neuropathy. Eur J Endocrinil 167.4 (2012): 465–71.

Haritoglou, C., et al. 2011. Alpha-lipoic acid for the prevention of diabetic macular edema. Ophthalmologica, 226, (3) 127–137.

Harrison EH, McCormick DB. The metabolism of dl-(1,6–14C) lipoic acid in the rat. Arch Biochem Biophys 160 (1974): 514–522.

Heinisch BB et al. Alpha-lipoic acid improves vascular endothelial functions in patients with type 2 diabetes: a placebo-controlled randomized trial. Eur J Clin Invest 40.2 (2010): 148–54.

Heitzer T et al. Beneficial effecs of alpha-lipoic acid and ascorbic acid on endothelium-dependent, nitric oxide-mediated vasodialtion in diabetic patients: relation to parameters of oxidative stress. Free Radic Bio Med 31 (2001): 53–61.

Henriksen et al. Stimulation by alpha-lipoic acid of glucose transport activity in skeletal muscle of lean and obese Zucker rats. Life sci 61 (1997): 805–12.

Ishida Y et al. α-lipoic acid and insulin autoimmune syndrome. Diabetes care. 30.9 (2007): 2240–2241.

Jacob S et al. Improvement of insulin-stimulated glucose-disposal in type 2 diabetes after repeated parenteral administration of thioctic acid. Experimental and Clinical Endocrinology and Diabetes. 104 (1996): 284–288.

Jacob S et al. Oral adminstration of rac-α-lipoic acid modulates insulin sensitivity in patients with type-2 diabetes mellitus: a placebo-controlled pilot trial. Free radical Biology and Medicine 27.3/4 (1999): 309–314.

Jariwalla, R.J., et al. 2008. Restoration of blood total glutathione status and lymphocyte function following alpha-lipoic acid supplementation in patients with HIV infection. J Altern. Complement Med, 14, (2) 139–146.

Jia Z et al. Alpha-lipoic acid potently inhibits peroxynitrite-mediated DNA strand breakage and hydroxyl radical formation: implications for the neuroprotective effects of alpha-lipoic acid. Mol cell Biochem 323.2 (2009): 131–138.

Jones W et al. Uptake, recycling and antioxidant action of α-lipoic acid in endothelial cells. Free radical medicine and biology 33.1 (2002): 83–93.

Kaya-Dagistanli F et al. The effects of alpha lipoic acid on liver cell damages and apoptosis induced by polyunsaturated fatty acids. Food and Chemical Toxicology 53 (2013): 84–93.

Keith et al. Age and gender dependant bioavailability of R- and R/S-α-lipoic acid: a pilot study. Pharmacological Research 66 (2012): 199–206.

Khalili M et al. Effect of lipoic acid consumption on oxidative stress among multiple sclerosis patients: A randomized controlled clinical trial. Nutr. Neurosci 17 (1) 2014: 16–20.

Khamaisi M et al. Lipoic acid reduces glycemia and increases GLUT4 content in streptozotocin-diabetic rats. Metabolism 47.6 (1997): 763–768.

Khan BV et al. Quinapril and lipoic acid improve endothelial function and reduce markers of inflammation: Results of Quinapril and lipoic acid in the metabolic syndrome (QUALITY) study. Journal of the American College of Cardiology. 55.10 (2010): A54-E510.

Kim, E., et al. 2008. A preliminary investigation of alpha-lipoic acid treatment of antipsychotic drug-induced weight gain in patients with schizophrenia. J Clin. Psychopharmacol., 28, (2) 138–146.

Klein AS et al. *Amanita* poisoning: Treatment and the role of transplantation. The American Journal of Medicine 86 (1989): 187–193.

Koh EH et al. Effect of alpha-lipoic acid on body weight in obese subjects. The American Journal of Medicine 124.1 (2011): 85.e1–85.e8.

Kojima M et al. Efficacy of alpha-lipoic acid against diabetic cataract in rats. Jpn J Ophthalmol 51.1 (2007): 10–13.

Koriyama Y et al. Protective effect of lipoic acid against oxidative stress is mediated by Keap1/Nrf2 dependant heme oxigenase-1 induction in the RGC-5 cell line. Brain Research 1499 (2013): 145–157.

Lai YS et al. Antiplatelet activity of alpha-lipoic acid. J Agric Food Chem 58.15 (2010): 8596–608.

Lee WR et al. Alpha-lipoic acid attenuates athesclerotic lesions and inhibits proliferation of vascular smooth muscles through targeting the Ras/MEK/ERK signaling pathway. Mol Biol Rep 39.6 (2012): 6857–66.

Lodge JK, Packer L. Natural sources of lipoic acid in plant and animal tissues. in Packer L et al (eds) Antioxidant food supplements in human health. San Diego, CA: Academic Press (1999): 121–134.

Lykkesfeldt J et al. Age-associated decline in ascorbic acid concentration, recycling, and biosynthesis in rat hepatocytes — reversal with (R)-alpha-lipoic acid supplementation. Faseb J. 13.2 (1999): 411–418.

Maczureck A et al. Lipoic acid as an anti-inflammatory and neuroprotective treatment for Alzheimer's disease. Advanced Drug Delivery Review 60 (2008): 1463–1470.

Magis, D., et al. 2007. A randomized double-blind placebo-controlled trial of thioctic acid in migraine prophylaxis. Headache, 47, (1) 52–57.

Manda K et al. Memory impairment, oxidative stress and apoptosis induced by space radiation: ameliorative potential of α-lipoic acid. Behavioural Brain Research 187.2 (2008): 387–395.

Marracci GH et al. α lipoic acid inhibits T cell migration in the spinal cord and suppresses and treats experimental autoimmune encephalomyelitis. J Neuroimmunol. 131 (2002): 104–114.

Marracci GH et al. Lipoic acid downmodulates CD4 from human T lymphocytes by dissociation of p56lck. Biochemical and Biophysical Research Communications 344 (2006): 963–971.

Marshall AW et al. Treatment of liver-related disease with thioctic acid: a six-month randomized controlled trial. Gut 23.12 (1982): 1088–1093.

Marshall JC, Dunaif A. All women with PCOS should be treated for insulin resistance. Fertil Steril 97.1 (2012): 18–22.

Masharani U et al. Effects of controlled-release alpha lipoic acid in lean, non-diabetic patients with polycystic ovary syndrome. J diabetis Sci Technol 4.2 (2010) 359–364.

Mayr J et al. Lipoic acid synthase deficiency causes neonatal-onset epilepsy, defective mitochondrial energy metabolism, and glycine elevation. Am J Hum Genet 89.6 (2011): 792–797.

McIlldufF CE Rutkove SB Critical appraisal of the use of alpha lipoic acid (thioctic acid) in the treatment of symptomatic diabetic neuropathy. Therapeutics and clinical risk management 7 (2011): 377–385.

Melli G et al. Alpha-lipoic acid prevents mitochondrial damage and neurotoxicity in experimental chemotherapy neuropathy. Exp Neurol 214.2 (2009): 276–284.

Memeo, A. & Loiero, M. 2008. Thioctic acid and acetyl-L-carnitine in the treatment of sciatic pain caused by a herniated disc: a randomized, double-blind, comparative study. Clin. Drug Investig., 28, (8) 495–500.

Michels AJ et al. Age-related decline of sodium-dependant ascorbic acid transport in isolated rat hepatocytes. Arch Biochem Biophys 410 (2003): 112–120.

Mijnhout GS et al. Alpha-lipoic acid for symptomatic peripheral neuropathy in patients with diabetes : a meta-analysis of randomized controlled trials. International Journal of Endocrinology 2012 (2012) 456279.

Milazzo, L., et al. 2010. Effect of antioxidants on mitochondrial function in HIV-1-related lipoatrophy: a pilot study. AIDS Res. Hum. Retroviruses, 26, (11) 1207–1214.

Moini H et al. Antioxidant and proxidant activity of α-lipoic acid and dihydrolipoic acid. Toxicology and applied pharmacology 182 (2002a): 84–90.

Moini H et al. R-alpha lipoic acid action on cell redox status, the insulin receptor, and glucose uptake in 3T3-L1 adipocytes. Arch Biochem Biophys 397 (2002b): 384–391.

Mollo R et al. Effect of alpha-lipoic acid on platelet reactivity in type I diabetic patients. Diabetes Care 35.2 (2012): 196–197.

Morcos M et al. Effect of α-lipoic acid on the progression of endothelial cell damage and albuminuria in patients with diabetes mellitus: an exploratory study. Diabetic Research and Clinical Practice. 52.3 (2001): 175–183.

Morini M et al. Alpha lipoic acid is effective in prevention and treatment of experimental autoimmune encephalomyelitis. J. Neuroimmunology. 148.1/2 (2004): 146–153.

Nebbioso M et al. Oxidative stress in preretinopathic diabetes subjects and antioxidants. Diabetic Technology and Therapeutics. 14–3 (2012): 1–7.

Nebbioso, M., et al. 2013. Lipoic acid in animal models and clinical use in diabetic retinopathy. Expert. Opin. Pharmacother 14–13: 1829–38.

Ning-Ping F et al. α-lipoic acid inhibits liver fibrosis through the attenuation of ROS- triggered signaling in hepatic stellate cells activated by PDGF and TGF-β. Toxicology 182.1/2 (2011): 39–46.

Obrosova IG et al. Early oxidative stress in the diabetic kidney effect of DL-α-lipoic acid. Free Radical Biology and Medicine 34.2 (2003): 186–195.

Ong SLH et al. The effect of alpha lipoic acid on mitondrial superoxide and glucocorticoid-induced hypertension. Oxidative medicine and cellular longevity 2013 (2013): 517045.

Packer L, Cadenas E. Lipoic acid metabolism and redox regulation of transcription and cell signaling. J Clin Biochem Nutr. 48.1 (2010): 26–32.

Padmalayam E et al. Lipoic acid synthase (LASY): a novel role in inflammation, mitochondrial function and insulin resistance. Diabetes 58.3 (2009): 600–608.

Pande M Flora SJS. Lead induced oxidative damage and its response of combined administration of α-lipoic acid and succimers in rats. Toxicology 177 (2002): 187–196.

Patel M, Packer L. "Discovery and molecular structure" in Packer L, Cadenas E (eds) Lipoic acid: Energy production, antioxidant activity and health effects. CRC Press. Boca Raton, Florida (2008): 3–11.

Perera J et al. Neuroprotective effects of alpha lipoic acid on haloperidol-induced oxidative stress in the rat brain. Cell Biosci 1 (2011): 12.

Queiroz, T.M., et al. 2012. Alpha-lipoic acid reduces hypertension and increases baroreflex sensitivity in renovascular hypertensive rats. Molecules., 17, (11) 13357–13367.

Rahman ST et al. The impact of lipoic acid on endothelial function and proteinuria in quinapril-treated diabetic patient with stage I hypertension: results form the QUALITY study. J Cardiovasc Pharmacol Ther 17.2 (2012): 139–45.

Ramachandran L, Nair CK. Protection against genotoxic damages following total body exposure in mice by lipoic acid. Mutation Research 724 (2011): 52–58.

Ratliff, J.C., et al. 2013. An open-label pilot trial of alpha-lipoic acid for weight loss in patients with schizophrenia without diabetes. Clin Schizophr Relat Psychoses 1–13.

Richard M et al. Cellular mechanisms by which lipoic acid confers protection during the early stages of cerebral ischemia: a possible role for calcium. Neuroscience Research 69 (2011): 299–307.

Ridruejo E, et al. Thioctic acid-induced cholestatic hepatitis. Ann Pharmacother 45.7 (2011): 7–8.

Roberts DM et al. Amanita phalloides poisoning and treatment with silibin in the Australian Capital Territory and New South Wales. Med J Aust 198.1 (2013): 43–47.

Rocamonde B et al. Neuroprotection of lipoic acid treatment promotes angiogenesis and reduces the glial scar formation after brain injury. Neuroscience 224 (2012): 102–115.

Rüdiger HW et al. Lipoic acid dependency of human branched chain α-ketoacid oxidase. Biochim Biophys Acta 264 (1972): 220–223.

Salinthone S et al. Lipoic acid attenuates inflammation via camp ad protein kinase A signaling. PLoS ONE 5.9 (2010): e13058.

Salinthone S et al. Lipoic acid stimulates camp production via G-coupled receptor-dependent and independent mechanisms. Journal of nutritional biochemistry 22 (2011): 681–690.

Schillace RV et al. Lipoic acid stimulate camp production in T lymphocytes and NK cells. Biochemical and Biophysical Research Communication. 354 (2007): 259–264.

Schreibelt G et al. Lipoic acid affects cellular migration into the central nervous system and stabilizes blood-brain barrier integrity. The Journal of Immunology 177.4 (2006): 2630–2637.

Schupke H et al. New metabolic pathways of alpha lipoic acid. Drug Metab Dispos 29 (2001): 855–862.

Segermann J et al. Effect of alpha-lipoic acid on the peripheral conversion of thyroxine to triiodothyronine and on serum lipid-, protein- and glucose levels. Arzneimittleforschung 41.12 (1991): 1294–98.

Sen C.K. & Packer, L. 2000. Thiol homeostasis and supplements in physical exercise. Am J Clin. Nutr., 72, (2 Suppl) 653S-669S.

Sena CM et al. Effect of alpha-lipoic acid on endothelial function in aged diabetic and high-fat fed rats. Br J Pharmacol 153 (2008): 894–906.

Shamloul R Ghanem H. Erectile dysfunction. The Lancet 381 (2012): 153–165.

Shay KP et al. Lipoic acid as a dietary supplement: molecular mechanisms and therapeutic potential. Biochem Biophys Acta 1790.10 (2009): 1149–1160.

Shila S et al. Brain regional response in antioxidant systems to α-lipoic acid in arsenic intoxicated rats. Toxicology 210 (2005): 25–36.

Sigel H et al. Stability and structure of binary and ternary complexes of α-lipoate and lipoate derivatives in Mn2+, Cu2+ and Zn2+ in solution. Archives of biochemistry and biophysics 187.1 (1978): 208–214.

Sivaprasad TR et al. Therapeutic efficacy of lipoic acid in combination with dimercaptosuccinic acid against lead-induced renal tubular defects and on isolated brush-border enzyme activities. Chemico-biological interactions 147 (2004): 259–271.

Sola S et al. Irbesartan and lipoic acid improve endothelial function and reduce markers of inflammation in the metabolic syndrome: results of the ISLAND study. Molecular cardiology 111 (2005): 343–348.

Streeper RS et al. Differential effects of lipoic acid stereoisomers on glucose metabolism in insulin-resistant skeletal muscle. Am J physiolol 273 (1997): E185–91.

Strödter D et al. The influence of thioctic acid on metabolism and function of the diabetic heart. Diabetic Res Clin Prac. 29 (1995): 19–26.

Suh JH et al. Oxidative stress in the ageing rat heart is reversed by dietary supplementation with (R)-(alpha)-lipoic acid. Faseb J 15.3 (2001): 700–706.

Suh JH et al. (R)-alpha-lipoic acid reverses the age-related loss in GHS redox status in post-mitotic tissues: evidence for increased cysteine requirement for GSH redox status in post-mitotic tissues: evidence for increased cysteine requirement for GSH synthesis. Arch Biochem Biophys 423 (2004a): 126–135.

Suh JH et al. Dehydrolipoic acid lowers the redox activity of transition metal ions but does not remove them from the active sites of enzymes. Redox rep 9.1 (2004b) 57–61.

Sumathi L et al. Effect of DL α-lipoic acid on tissue redox state in acute cadmium-challenged tissues. Nutritional biochemistry 7 (1996): 85–92.

Sun YD et al. 2012. Effect of (R)-alpha-lipoic acid supplementation on serum lipids and antioxidative ability in patients with age-related macular degeneration. Ann. Nutr. Metab, 60, (4) 293–297.

Tabassum H et al. Protective effect of lipoic acid against methotrexate-induced oxidative stress in liver mitochondria. Food and Chemical toxicology 48 (2010): 1973–1979.

Takaoka M et al. Effects of alpha-lipoic acid on deoxycorticosterone acete-salt-induced hypertension in rats. Eur J Pharmacol 424 (2001): 121–129.

Teichert J et al. Investigations on the pharmacokinetics of alpha-lipoic acid in healthy volunteers. Int J Clin Pharmacol Ther 36 (1998): 625–628.

Tong et al. Comparative treatment of α-amanitin poisoning with N-acetyl-cysteine, benzylpenicillin, Cimetidine, thioctic acid, and sylibin in a murine model. Annals of Emmergency Medicine 50.3 (2007): 282–288.

Vasdev S et al. Dietary lipoic acid supplementation prevents fructose-induces hypertension in rats. Nutr Metab Cardiovasc Dis 10 (2000a): 339–46.

Vasdev S et al. Dietary alpha-lipoic acid supplementation lowers blood pressure in spontaneously hypertensive rats. J Hypers 18 (2000b): 567–573.

Vasdev S et al. Salt-induced hypertension in WKY rats: prevention by alpha-lipoic acid supplementation. Mol Cell Biochem 254 (2003): 319–326.

Vasdev S et al. Dietary lipoic acid supplementation attenuates hypertension in Dahl salt sensitive rats. Moll Cell Biochem 275 (2005): 135–141.

Wang L et al. The protective effect of α-lipoic acid on mitochondria in the kidney of diabetic rats. Int J Clin Exp Med 6.2 (2013): 90–97.

Wang MY et al. Activity assay of lipoamidase, an expected modulator of metabolic fate of externally administered lipoic acid. Inflammation and Regeneration 31.1 (2011): 88–94.

Wang SJ, Chen HH. Pre-synaptic mechanisms underlying the alpha-lipoic acid facilitation of glutamate exocytosis in rat cerebral cortex nerve terminals. Neurochem Int 50–1 (2007): 51–60.

Winiarska K et al. Lipoic acid ameliorates oxidative stress and renal injury in alloxan diabetic rabbits. Biochimie 90.3 (2008): 450–459.

Xiang et al. α-lipoic acid can improve endothelial dysfunction in subjects with impaired fasting glucose. Metabolism clinical and experimental 60 (2011): 480–485.

Xu J et al. Flaxseed oil and alpha-lipoic acid combination reduces atherosclerotis risk factors in rats fed a high-fat diet. Lipids Health Dis 11 (2012): 148.

Xu Q et al. Meta-analysis of methylcobalamin alone and in combination with lipoic acid in patients with diabetic peripheral neuropathy. Diabetes Res Clin Pract 101–2 (2013): 99–105.

Yadav V et al. Lipoic acid in multiple sclerosis: a pilot study. Multiple Sclerosis 11 (2005): 159–165.

Yadav V et al. Pharmacokinetics study of lipoic acid in multiple sclerosis: Comparing mice and human pharmacokinetic parameters. Mult Scler 16.4 (2010): 387–397.

Yamada T et al. α-lipoic acid (LA) enantiomers protect SH-SY5Y cells against glutathione depletion. Neurochemistry International 59 (2011): 1003–1009.

Yan W et al. Effect of oral ALA supplementation on oxidative stress and insulin sensitivity among overweight/obese adults: A double-blinded randomized, controlled cross over intervention trial. International Journal of cardiology 167 (2013): 602–3.

Yi X et al. Genetic reduction of lipoic acid synthase expression moderately increases atherosclerosis in male, but not female, apolipoprotein E-deficient mice. Atherosclerosis 211.2 (2010): 424–30.

Yi X et al. α-lipoic acid protects diabetic apolipoprotein E deficient mice from nephropathy. Journal of Diabetes and Its Complications 25 (2011): 193–201.

Yi X et al. Reduced expression of α-lipoic acid synthase accelerates diabetic nephropathy. J AM Soc Nephrol 23.1 (2012a): 103–111.

Yi X et al. Reduced alpha-lipoic acid synthase gene expression exacerbates atherosclerosis in diabetic apolipoprotein E-deficient mice. Atherosclerosis 223.1 (2012b): 17–143.

Yi X, Meada N. Endogenous production of lipoic acid is essential for mouse development. Molecular and cellular biology 25.18 (2005): 8387–92.

Ying Z et al. Lipoic acid effects on established atherosclerosis. Life Sci 86.3/4 (2010): 95–102.

Zakrzewska JM et al. Intervention for the treatment of burning mouth syndrome. Cochrane Oral Health Group. Cochrane Database of Systematic Reviews 1 (2009).

Zembron-Lacny A et al. Physical activity and lipoic acid modulate inflammatory response through changes in thiol redox status. J Physiol Biochem 69–3 (2013): 397–404.

Zhang, Y., et al. 2011. Amelioration of lipid abnormalities by alpha-lipoic acid through antioxidative and anti-inflammatory effects. Obesity. (Silver. Spring), 19, (8) 1647–1653.

Ziegler D et al. Treatment of symptomatic polyneuropathy with the antioxidant α-lipoic acid: a meta-analysis. Diabet Med 21.2 (2004): 114–121.

Andrographis

HISTORICAL NOTE Andrographis has long been used in traditional medicine systems in numerous countries. It has been included in the pharmacopoeias of India, Korea and China, possibly because it grows abundantly in India, Pakistan and various parts of Southeast Asia. In traditional Chinese medicine, andrographis is considered a 'cold' herb and is used to rid the body of heat, as in fevers and acute infections, and to dispel toxins from the body. In Ayurvedic medicine it is used as a bitter tonic, to stimulate digestion and as a treatment for a wide range of conditions such as diabetes and hepatitis. It is still a common household remedy and found in more than half the combination tonics used to treat liver conditions in India. In recent years, andrographis has gained popularity in Western countries as a treatment for upper respiratory tract infections and influenza.

COMMON NAMES

Andrographis, chirayata, chiretta, green chiretta, Indian echinacea, kalmegh, king of bitters

BOTANICAL NAME/FAMILY

Andrographis paniculata (family Acanthaceae)

PLANT PARTS USED

Leaves, aerial parts

CHEMICAL COMPONENTS

The main active constituent group is considered to be the bitter diterpenoid lactones known as andrographolides. This group includes andrographolide (AP1), 14-deoxy-11,12-didehydroandrographolide (AP3) and neoandrographolide (AP4) (Lim et al 2012). Other constituents found in the plant roots include flavonoids, diterpenoids, phenylpropanoids, oleanolic acid, beta-sitosterol and beta-daucosterol (Xu & Wang 2011). Constituents identified in the aerial parts include flavonoids, alkanes, ketones, aldehydes, lactones, diterpene glucosides, ditriterpenoids and diterpene dimers (Akbar 2011).

Clinical studies show that andrographis is well absorbed, with peak plasma concentrations reached after 1.5–2 hours and a half-life of 6.6 hours (Panossian et al 2000).

MAIN ACTIONS

The mechanism of action of andrographis has not been significantly investigated in clinical studies, so results from in vitro and animal tests provide most of the evidence for this herbal medicine.

Immunomodulation

A number of immunomodulatory actions have been identified with andrographis and its derivatives (Jayakumar et al 2013). One of the main constituents responsible for the immunostimulant activity is andrographolide, which has an effect on the stimulation and proliferation of immunocompetent cells and the production of key cytokines and immune markers in vitro (Panossian et al 2002).

In vitro and in vivo research demonstrates that andrographolide has the ability to interfere with T-cell proliferation, cytokine release and maturation of dendritic cells, as well as to substantially decrease the antibody response in delayed-type hypersensitivity (Iruretagoyena et al 2005). Additionally, andrographolide demonstrated a capacity to inhibit T-cell and antibody responses in experimental autoimmune encephalomyelitis in mice, and to protect against myelin sheath damage (Iruretagoyena et al 2005).

Andrographolide has been demonstrated to inhibit production of interleukin-12 (IL-12) and tumour necrosis factor-alpha (TNF-alpha) in lipopolysaccaride-stimulated mice macrophages, which appeared to relate to suppression of the ERK1/2 signalling pathway (Qin et al 2006). It has also been found to decrease interferon-gamma (IFN-gamma) and IL-2 production and therefore display an immunosuppressive effect. As a result, Burgos et al (2005) concluded that andrographis may be useful for autoimmune disease, especially where high levels of IFN-gamma are present, for example in multiple sclerosis and rheumatoid arthritis. Interestingly, andrographolide exerted antigrowth and proapoptotic effects in a study utilising rheumatoid arthritis fibroblast-like synoviocytes (Yan et al 2012).

Immunostimulatory activity of andrographolide in phytohaemagglutinin-stimulated human peripheral blood lymphocytes has been reported with laboratory studies (Kumar et al 2004).

Other pharmacologically active constituents are also present, as demonstrated by a study that found that the immunostimulant activity of the whole extract is greater than that of the isolated andrographolide constituent alone. Investigation with a combination of the whole extract and *Eleutherococcus senticosus* in the formula Kan Jang demonstrated a more profound effect (Panossian et al 2002).

Anticancer activity

In vivo and in vitro experiments have demonstrated the possible benefits of andrographolide and its derivatives on various cancer cells via multiple mechanisms. According to a recent review, Lim et al (2012) identified anticancer mechanisms, including inhibition of Janus tyrosine kinases-signal transducers, inhibition of activators of phosphatidylinositol 3-kinase, transcription and NF-κB signalling pathways, suppression of growth factors, cyclins, cyclin-dependent kinases, heat shock protein 90 and metalloproteins. Andrographolide has also been shown to induce tumour-suppressor proteins p53 and p21, leading to inhibition of cancer cell proliferation, survival, metastasis and angiogenesis (Lim et al 2012). Andrographolide increases apoptosis of prostate cancer cells and human leukaemic cells and increases cell cycle arrest (Cheung et al 2005, Geethangili et al 2008, Kim et al 2005, Zhao et al 2008, Zhou et al 2006). It also inhibits the proliferation of human cancer cells and increases IL-2 induction in human peripheral blood lymphocytes in vitro (Kumar et al 2004, Rajagopal et al 2003). A cytotoxic effect of andrographolide on HepG1 human hepatoma cells was observed in a laboratory study which was attributed primarily to the induction of cell cycle arrest via alteration of cellular redox status (Li et al 2007).

In vivo results show that andrographolide increases IL-2, IFN-gamma and T-cell activity (Sheeja et al 2007). In certain circumstances, andrographolide has been found to decrease IFN-gamma and IL-2 and may have an immunosuppressive effect (see Immunomodulation, above).

Andrographis and andrographolide may also inhibit angiogenesis and cancer cell adhesion (Jiang et al 2007, Sheeja et al 2007). Antiangiogenesis and chemotherapeutic potential of andrographolide have been shown in a lung tumour mouse model. In this study, andrographolide significantly reduced expression of hVEGF-A165 compared with a control group and also decreased tumour formation (Tung et al 2013).

Halogenated di-spiropyrrolizidino oxindole derivatives of andrographolide were more cytotoxic than andrographolide in some cancer cells, according to a recent study conducted in human cancer cell lines. One of the derivatives (CY2) induced death of a number of different types of cancer cells, involving cell rounding, nuclear fragmentation and an increase in percentage of apoptotic cells, cell cycle arrest at G1 phase, reactive oxygen species (ROS) generation and involvement of the ROS-dependent mitochondrial pathway (Dey et al 2013).

Antimicrobial

Aqueous extract of *Andrographis paniculata* has demonstrated antibacterial and antifungal activity in vitro. In various laboratory studies, activity was shown against *Bacillus subtilis, Escherichia coli, Pseudomonas aeruginosa, Staphylococcus aureus* and *Candida albicans* (Singha et al 2003, Voravuthikunchai & Limsuwan 2006). An ethanolic extract of *A. paniculata* demonstrated potent inhibitory activity against both Gram-positive and Gram-negative bacteria according to an in vitro study (Mishra et al 2009).

The andrographolides from andrographis have displayed antiviral activity against herpes simplex virus type 1 in vitro (Wiart et al 2005). Inhibitory activity against the dengue virus serotype 1 has also been demonstrated in a laboratory study using a methanolic extract of andrographis (Tang et al 2012).

Cardiovascular effects

Several in vivo studies have suggested a potential role for andrographis in cardiovascular disease. Antihypertensive effects have been demonstrated in animal models, which appear to be related to relaxation of vascular smooth muscle and a decrease in heart rate (Jayakumar et al 2013, Yoopan et al 2007). According to a recent review, early animal studies have shown that andrographis may reduce restenosis after angioplasty and may prevent myocardial reperfusion injury (Jayakumar et al 2013). In a study using rat hearts, a dichloromethane extract of andrographis significantly reduced coronary perfusion pressure by up to 24.5 ± 3.0 mmHg at a 3 mg dose and heart rate was also significantly decreased at this dose (Awang et al 2012). Andrographis has demonstrated hypolipidaemic action in an experimental rat model: a significant reduction ($P < 0.05$) in triglycerides, low-density lipoprotein cholesterol and blood glucose levels was observed after administration of a purified andrographolide extract (Nugroho et al 2012).

Hypoglycaemic

Andrographis has demonstrated significant hypoglycaemic activity in vitro and in various diabetic animal models.

In vitro tests reveal that andrographis has a strong dose-dependent action on insulin production in vitro (Wibudi et al 2008) and inhibits alpha-glucosidase (Subramanian et al 2008) and increases glucose uptake via the phospholipase C/protein kinase C pathway (Hsu et al 2004), all of which may contribute to the hypoglycaemic effect.

Hypoglycaemic and lipid lowering have also been observed in vivo in a model of type 2 diabetes. Administration of either andrographis or andrographolide extracts for 5 days significantly reduced preprandial and postprandial blood glucose levels in a dose-dependent manner. The effect was similar to that observed for metformin (90 mg/kg body weight) (Nugroho et al 2012). Similarly, oral administration of aqueous extract of andrographis to streptozotocin-induced diabetic rats resulted in a significant decrease in blood glucose levels at a dose of 400 mg/kg. This was accompanied by an antioxidant effect with an increase in superoxide dismutase and catalase activity (Dandu & Inamdar 2009). One in vivo study in alloxan-induced diabetic rats demonstrated significantly reduced blood glucose levels as compared to placebo (Reyes et al 2006). The authors commented that andrographis may restore impaired oestrous cycle in this model. A previous animal trial concluded that andrographolide (1.5 mg/kg) lowers plasma glucose by enhancing glucose utilisation in diabetic rats (Yu et al 2003).

Hepatoprotective

Hepatoprotective activity of andrographis has been identified in vitro and in vivo using various toxic liver insults and is mainly attributed to the andrographolide constituent. A significant dose-dependent protective action has been shown against paracetamol-induced hepatotoxicity in rats. Experimental rat models have also identified a protective action for andrographis and its constituents against liver toxicity induced by galactosamine, carbon tetrachloride and tertbutylhydroperoxide. Several mechanisms have been identified (Ghosh et al 2011, Jayakumar et al 2013). Pretreatment of mice for 7 days with andrographolide and another andrographis metabolite, arabinogalactan proteins, produced a protective effect against ethanol-induced toxicity to liver and kidney tissue. In this study, at doses of 500 mg/kg body weight andrographolide and 125 mg/kg body weight arabinogalactan proteins respectively, the results were comparable to that seen with silymarin 500 mg/kg body weight. Silymarin is an established heptoprotective agent and was used as a comparator substance in this animal study (Singha et al 2007).

Antipyretic and anti-inflammatory

Antipyretic activity with andrographis has been demonstrated in animal models (Mandal et al 2001, Suebsasana et al 2009).

Anti-inflammatory activity has also been observed in vitro and in vivo with andrographis, which is primarily associated with andrographolide (Jayakumar et al 2013).

Andrographolide has been shown to reduce production of cytokines, chemokines, adhesion molecules, nitric oxide and lipid mediators (Lim et al 2012) as well as IL-1beta, IL-6, prostaglandin E_2 and thromboxane B_2, and the allergic mediator leukotriene B_4 (Chandrasekaran et al 2010). A decreased induction of nitric oxide synthetase and cyclooxygenase-2 has been observed in laboratory studies, probably via inhibition of the NF-κB signalling pathway (Lee et al 2011, Lim et al 2012).

A. paniculata extract completely inhibited inflammation induced by carageenan in mice, compared to controls (Sheeja et al 2006). In vitro data from the same study showed that andrographis inhibited superoxide (32%), hydroxyl radicals (80%), lipid peroxidation (80%) and nitric oxide (42.8%). These antioxidant mechanisms are likely to contribute to the herb's anti-inflammatory effect.

Antiplatelet activity

Research has demonstrated that andrographis inhibits platelet-activating factor (PAF)-induced human platelet aggregation and also appears to confer additional antiplatelet activity, for which several mechanisms may be involved (Jayakumar et al 2013, Lu et al 2011, 2012, Thisoda et al 2006). A number of compounds appear to be involved in these actions. Thisoda et al (2006) identified andrographolide (AP1) and 14-deoxy-11,12 didehydroandrographolide (AP3) as key antiplatelet constituents. More recently, an additional four flavonoids were isolated that inhibit thrombin and PAF-induced platelet aggregation (Wu et al 2008).

OTHER ACTIONS

Anti-HIV activity

Andrographolide derivatives have been shown to possess anti-HIV activity in vitro. Inhibition of gp120-mediated cell fusion of HL2/3 cells with TZM-bl cells was observed. There is potential for future research in this area (Uttekar et al 2012).

Snake antivenom activity

Andrographis ethanolic extracts have been shown to exhibit neutralising effects on cobra venom. Andrographis was shown to prolong survival time in an animal study, but did not prevent death (Premendran et al 2011).

CLINICAL USE

Andrographis is most commonly used for its effects on immune function and inflammation, such as the treatment and prevention of upper respiratory tract infections (URTIs), while use in non-infective conditions such as ulcerative colitis and rheumatoid arthritis has also been investigated.

Upper respiratory tract infections and the common cold

A. paniculata has become popular as a treatment for URTIs. It is most often used in combination with other herbal medicines, in particular Siberian ginseng and sometimes echinacea. The fixed combination known as Kan Jang contains a standardised extract from *Andrographis paniculata* SHA-10 and *Eleutherococcus senticosus* and has been used for more than 20 years in Scandinavia as a herbal medicinal product in uncomplicated URTI (Gabrielian et al 2002). Clinical studies confirm that treatment with andrographis either by itself or in combination with Siberian ginseng (as in Kan Jang) is beneficial in cases of uncomplicated acute URTIs, providing some symptom relief within several days; however maximal effects appear by day 5.

Clinical evidence indicates that treatment with andrographis reduces the severity of cough, expectoration, nasal discharge, headache, fever, sore throat, malaise/fatigue, sinus pain and sleep disturbances. The dose of andrographis used in various studies has differed, but the majority have used a dose standardised to 60 mg andrographolide/day (Coon & Ernst 2004, Kligler et al 2006, Poolsup et al 2004, Saxena 2010).

A systematic review (Kligler et al 2006) of seven clinical trials (n = 879) concluded that evidence for the effectiveness of andrographis in the treatment of URTI is encouraging. At the time, the authors also made the comment that most of the studies have been done in conjunction with a major manufacturer of the product and further independent testing was required (Kligler et al 2006). Similar positive conclusions were drawn in two earlier systematic reviews. Coon and Ernst (2004) conducted a review that included seven double-blind randomised controlled trials (RCTs) and concluded that, collectively, the data suggest that andrographis is superior to placebo in alleviating symptoms of uncomplicated URTI, and has only mild, infrequent adverse effects. In five of the seven trials, the daily dose was equivalent to 60 mg of andrographolide, which was administered for 3–8 days. Another review of four RCTs confirmed that *A. paniculata*, either by itself or in combination with *E. senticosus* (Kan Jang), is effective for the treatment of uncomplicated acute URTI (Poolsup et al 2004).

More recently, the efficacy of a standardised extract of andrographis (KalmCold) was confirmed in a multicentre, double-blind RCT involving 223 adults with uncomplicated URTIs (Saxena 2010). Treatment with KalmCold (100 mg andrographis/capsule, standardised to 31.3% andrographolide), taken twice daily for a period of 5 days, resulted in a significant decrease in symptoms by day 5 compared to the placebo group for cough, expectoration, nasal discharge, headache, fever, sore throat, malaise/fatigue and sleep disturbances ($P \leq 0.05$); however no improvement in the symptom of earache was observed in either group. The overall efficacy of andrographis 200 mg/day (equivalent to approximately 60 mg andrographolide/day) as KalmCold was 2.1 times higher than placebo in reducing symptoms of URTIs (Saxena 2010).

Andrographis (as Kan Jang) may also reduce the incidence of the common cold according to the available evidence. A double-blind RCT of 107 healthy school children found that treatment with Kan Jan tablets (100 mg standardised to 5.6 mg andrographolide/tablet) taken twice daily for 5 days a week for a period of 3 months reduced the risk of developing a cold by approximately 50% after 2 months when compared to placebo. In the third month, the percentage occurrence of the common cold was 30% in the andrographis-treated group, compared to an occurrence of 62% in the placebo group. This represented a 2.1 times lower risk of the common cold in the group taking Kan Jang ($P < 0.05$) (Caceres et al 1997).

Comparisons between andrographis and echinacea in the treatment of the common cold in children

One study has compared andrographis to echinacea. However this was in the form of Kan Jang which also included Siberian ginseng, making a direct comparison difficult. An RCT involving 133 children with uncomplicated common cold compared the effectiveness of Kan Jang to Immunal (containing *Echinacea purpurea* [L.] extract), when both were used as adjuncts to standard treatment (Spasov et al 2004). The children were randomised to one of three groups. Group 1 received Kan Jang (2 tablets three times daily for 10 days) plus standard care; group 2 received Immunal (10 drops three times daily for 10 days) plus standard care; and group 3 received standard care only, including gargles and paracetamol as required. Adjuvant treatment with Kan Jang was shown to be significantly more effective than adjuvant treatment with Immunal or standard treatment alone. The group taking Kan Jang experienced less severe symptoms, in particular nasal congestion and volume of nasal secretion. Recovery time was also faster in the Kan Jang group than in the Immunal group as well as there being less need for additional standard treatment. Additionally, Kan Jang treatment was well tolerated and no side effects or adverse reactions were reported.

Pharyngotonsillitis

A clinical benefit of andrographis in the treatment of pharyngotonsillitis was reported in one early RCT involving 152 volunteers (Thamlikitkul et al 1991). Symptoms of sore throat and fever were reduced at a dose of 6 g/day of a non-standardised andrographis preparation after 3 days. No subsequent research appears to have been conducted for this indication to confirm these results.

Ulcerative colitis

Two RCTs have found benefits for andrographis treatment in mild to moderate ulcerative colitis.

The efficacy of *Andrographis paniculata* (HMPL-004) in the treatment of mild to moderate ulcerative colitis was assessed in a double-blind RCT ($n = 224$) (Sandborn et al 2013). Two different strengths of andrographis (1200 mg, or 1800 mg per day) were compared to placebo over 8 weeks. By the end of the treatment period, a clinical response was achieved in 60% of patients receiving andrographis 1800 mg/day ($P = 0.02$), compared to 45% taking the 1200 mg dose and 40% of those taking placebo ($P = 0.6$ andrographis 1200 mg vs placebo) (Sandborn et al 2013). Therefore, only the higher strength was significantly superior to placebo whereas the lower dose of andrographis was not effective. Interestingly, the lower dose of andrographis 1200 mg (HMPL-004) daily was as effective as slow-release mesalazine (4500 mg/day) after 8 weeks in another multicentre RCT involving 120 patients with mild to moderate ulcerative colitis (Tang et al 2011).

Rheumatoid arthritis

Anti-inflammatory and immunomodulating effects have been observed in laboratory and animal studies providing the basis of investigation into the effects of andrographis in rheumatoid arthritis. To date, only one clinical study has been published, producing promising results.

Treatment with andrographis tablets (standardised to 30 mg andrographolide/tablet) three times a day for 14 weeks significantly reduced joint tenderness, number of swollen or tender joints and total grade of swollen or tender joints compared to placebo in a double-blind RCT involving 60 patients with active rheumatoid arthritis (Burgos et al 2009). A reduction in rheumatoid factor IgA and C4 was also observed. Of note, participants were not permitted to take non-steroidal anti-inflammatory drugs during the study and paracetamol was only used in cases of severe pain. Joint pain intensity decreased in the andrographis treatment group compared to the placebo group, but the difference was not statistically significant (Burgos et al 2009).

OTHER USES

Familial Mediterranean fever — in combination

A standardised fixed combination (ImmunoGuard) of *Andrographis paniculata*, *Eleutherococcus senticosus*, *Schisandra chinensis* and *Glycyrriza glabra* was shown to be effective for the treatment of familial Mediterranean fever (FMF) in children (3–15 years), according to a small double-blind, randomised, placebo-controlled study (Amaryan et al 2003).

The herbal combination treatment significantly reduced the frequency, severity and duration of attacks compared to placebo. The treatment formulation included andrographis 50 mg/tablet (equivalent to 4 mg standardised andrographolide), which was given as four tablets three times a day for 1 month (Amaryan et al 2003). This herbal combination product, ImmunoGuard, has been shown to raise serum nitric oxide levels in FMF patients during attack-free periods and to have a normalising effect on blood levels of both nitric oxide and IL-6 during FMF attack periods (Panossian et al 2003).

HIV infection

A phase I clinical trial involving non-medicated HIV-positive patients and healthy controls found that oral andrographolides taken for 6 weeks at increasing doses produced no significant benefits and a high incidence of adverse effects, causing the trial to be stopped prematurely (Calabrese et al 2000). A recent in vitro study concluded that andrographolide derivatives may still hold promise as a potential agent in the prevention of HIV (Uttekar et al 2012).

Cancer (in combination)

An integrative treatment approach was investigated in 20 patients with various end-stage cancers. The patients were given a daily combination of six different immunoactive nutraceutical products plus *Andrographis paniculata* (500 mg twice daily) for 6 months. After 6 months, 16 of the 20 patients were still alive, with a statistically significant increase in both natural killer function and TNF-alpha levels. Haemoglobin, haematocrit and glutathione levels were all greatly increased (See et al 2002). Although these results are interesting, it is difficult to examine the direct effect of *A. paniculata*, as so many other nutritional supplements were given concurrently.

Spermatogenesis

Early studies with andrographis have reported antifertility effects in animal models at high doses (Jayakumar et al 2013). The only clinical studies investigating this further have used the herbal combination Kan Jang which contains andrographis and Siberian ginseng, making it difficult to ascertain the effect of andrographis alone.

A phase I clinical study investigated the effects of three different strengths of Kan Jang (combination of *Andrographis paniculata* and *Eleutherococcus senticosus*) on spermatogenesis and fertility in 14 healthy men aged between 18 and 35 years (Mkrtchyan et al 2005). The men were randomised into one of five groups to receive one of the following: (1) Kan Jang equivalent to 60 mg andrographolide; (2) Kan Jang equivalent to 120 mg andrographolide; (3) Kan Jang equivalent to 180 mg andrographolide; (4) a ginseng mixture; or (5) a valerian extract. The study confirmed no significant negative effects of Kan Jang on male sperm or fertility even at doses corresponding to three times the standard daily dose and only a positive trend towards the number of active spermatozoids in the whole ejaculate (Mkrtchyan et al 2005).

Traditional uses

The herb is traditionally given as a restorative and tonic in convalescence and used as a choleretic to stimulate bile production and flow, which improves appetite and digestion. It is often used in combination with aromatic herbs, such as peppermint, for stronger digestive effects and to prevent gastrointestinal discomfort at higher doses. It has also been used in traditional cultures for protection against snake bites, to treat fever, dysentery, cholera, gonorrhoea, diabetes, influenza and dyspepsia.

DOSAGE RANGE

The majority of clinical trials have been conducted using products standardised to the andrographolide fraction.

Upper respiratory tract infection

- Symptomatic treatment: 100 mg twice daily of a standardised andrographis extract providing 60 mg andrographolide per day — maximal effects by day 5.
- Prevention: Kan Jang 200 mg (equivalent to standardised extract of 11.2 mg/day of andrographolide) taken daily for 2 months has been used to prevent incidence of the common cold.
- Ulcerative colitis (mild to moderate): 1200–1800 mg/daily of andrographis (HMPL-004) — maximal effects reported by week 8.
- Rheumatoid arthritis: andrographis tablets (standardised to 30 mg andrographolide/tablet) taken three times daily for at least 3 months.

Toxicity

Animal tests suggest low toxicity (Mills & Bone 2000). Dose-related toxicity leading to termination of a study occurred at doses of 5–10 mg/kg/day of andrographolide (Calabrese et al 2000). This dose was 6–12 times higher than the standard dosage range used in all other studies.

ADVERSE REACTIONS

Generally well tolerated with adverse effects infrequent and mild at usual recommended doses. Unpleasant chest sensation, headache, fatigue, urticaria, gastrointestinal discomfort, nausea, vomiting and metallic taste have been reported at high doses (Coon & Ernst 2004).

SIGNIFICANT INTERACTIONS

No specific drug–herb interactions have been reported, therefore interactions are theoretical and based on evidence of pharmacological activity with uncertain clinical significance.

Anticoagulants

Increased risk of bruising and bleeding is theoretically possible, because andrographolide and other constituents in andrographis inhibit PAF-induced platelet aggregation. However andrographis used together with warfarin did not produce any significant effects on the pharmacokinetics of warfarin, and had even less effect on its pharmacodynamics in vivo (Hovhannisyan et al 2006). Caution should still be exercised until further research is available.

Antiplatelet drugs

Additive effects are theoretically possible, as andrographis has been shown to inhibit platelet aggregation in animal and laboratory research — patients should be observed for increased bruising or bleeding.

Barbiturates

Additive effects are theoretically possible, according to an animal study (Mandal et al 2001).

Hypoglycaemic agents

A hypoglycaemic effect has been observed in animal studies (Nugroho et al 2012, Wibudi et al 2008). Additive effects are theoretically possible.

Cytochrome p450 enzyme metabolism

Andrographolide was shown to induce the CYP1A1 enzyme pathway in laboratory studies; however, the clinical significance of this is unknown (Chatuphonprasert et al 2011, Jaruchotikamol et al 2007). Another in vitro study has demonstrated an inhibitive effect of andrographis extract and andrographolide on CYP3A and 2C9 pathways (Pekthong et al 2008). Further research is required before clinical relevance can be determined.

Immunosuppressants

Immunomodulatory activity has been observed with andrographis in vitro and in vivo (Jayakumar et al 2013). Clinical significance of use in combination with immunosuppressive drugs is not clear, but caution is advised.

CONTRAINDICATIONS AND PRECAUTIONS

Inhibition of platelet aggregation has been observed in vitro (Thisoda et al 2006). While it is uncertain whether the effect is clinically relevant, it is advised to suspend use 1 week prior to high-risk surgery, such as neurosurgery, where a small bleed can have serious consequences.

Doses equivalent to or higher than 5 mg/kg/day of the constituent andrographolide should be avoided due to a risk of significant adverse effects (Calabrese et al 2000).

PREGNANCY USE

There is insufficient reliable evidence available to determine safety.

PATIENTS' FAQs

What will this herb do for me?

Human studies confirm that it is effective in reducing symptoms of the common cold and uncomplicated URTIs. New research also suggests it can reduce symptoms in ulcerative colitis and possibly rheumatoid arthritis. It reduces the risk of developing the common cold when taken with Siberian ginseng for at least 2 months.

When will it start to work?

During an acute infection, effects may be seen within 3–4 days of starting the correct dose and maximal symptom-relieving effects are seen by day 5. Used together with Siberian ginseng, it can reduce the risk of developing a cold when used for at least 2 months. Symptom relief in ulcerative colitis develops within 8 weeks and a minimum of 3 months is required to achieve benefits in rheumatoid arthritis.

Are there any safety issues?

Andrographis is not recommended in pregnancy or lactation. This herb is well tolerated but may interact with certain medications.

Practice points/Patient counselling

- Several clinical studies suggest that andrographis, both as a stand-alone treatment and in combination with Siberian ginseng, is a useful symptomatic treatment in cases of common cold and uncomplicated URTIs, with significant symptom relief experienced after 3 days' use.
- It may also reduce the risk of the common cold when used daily for several months.
- New clinical research shows it can reduce symptoms in mild to moderate ulcerative colitis within 8 weeks and may also improve symptoms in rheumatoid arthritis when taken for at least 3 months.
- Preclinical experiments suggest that andrographis may be useful in cases of hepatotoxicity (paracetamol, alcohol), to reduce myocardial reperfusion injury, improve blood glucose management in diabetes, and in hypertension.
- Traditionally, the herb is used to increase bile production and relieve symptoms of dyspepsia and flatulence, loss of appetite and general debility.
- Because of the extreme bitterness of the herb, solid-dose forms may be better tolerated than liquid preparations.

REFERENCES

Akbar S. *Andrographis paniculata*: A review of pharmacological activities and clinical effects. Alternative Medicine Review. 16.1 (2011):66–77.

Amaryan G et al. Double-blind, placebo-controlled, randomized, pilot clinical trial of ImmunoGuard: a standardized fixed combination of *Andrographis paniculata* Nees, with *Eleutherococcus senticosus* Maxim, *Schizandra chinensis* Bail. and *Glycyrrhiza glabra* L. extracts in patients with familial Mediterranean fever. Phytomedicine 10.4 (2003): 271–285.

Awang K et al. Cardiovascular activity of labdane diterpenes from *Andrographis paniculata* in isolated rat hearts. Journal of Biomedicine and Biotechnogy. (2012): 2012;ID 876458.

Burgos RA et al. Andrographolide inhibits IFN-gamma and IL-2 cytokine production and protects against cell apoptosis. Planta Med 71.5 (2005): 429–434.

Burgos RA et al. Efficacy of an *Andrographis paniculata* composition for the relief of rheumatoid arthritis symptoms: a prospective randomized placebo-controlled trial. Clin Rheumatol 28.8 (2009): 931–46.

Caceres DD et al Prevention of common colds with *Andrographis paniculata* dried extract. A pilot double blind trial. Phytomedicine 4.2 (1997):101–104.

Calabrese C et al. A phase I trial of andrographolide in HIV positive patients and normal volunteers. Phytother Res 14.5 (2000): 333–338.

Chandrasekaran CV, et al. Effect of an extract of *Andrographis paniculata* leaves on inflammatory and allergic mediators in vitro. J Ethnopharmacol. 129.2 (2010):203–7.

Chatuphonprasert W et al. Different AhR binding sites of diterpenoid ligands from *Andrographis paniculata* caused differential CYP1A1 induction in primary culture in mouse hepatocytes. Toxicology in Vitro. 25.8 (2011):1757–63.

Cheung HY et al. Andrographolide isolated from *Andrographis paniculata* induces cell cycle arrest and mitochondrial-mediated apoptosis in human leukemic HL-60 cells. Planta Med 71.12 (2005): 1106–1111.

Coon JT, Ernst E. *Andrographis paniculata* in the treatment of upper respiratory tract infections: a systematic review of safety and efficacy. Planta Med 70.4 (2004): 293–298.

Dandu AM, Inamdar NM. Evaluation of beneficial effects of antioxidant properties of aqueous leaf extract of *Andrographis paniculata* in STZ-induced diabetes. Pakistan Journal of Pharmaceutical Sciences. 22.1 (2009):49–52.

Dey SK et al. Cytotoxic activity and apoptosis-inducing potential of di-spiropyrrolidino and di-spiropyrrolizino oxindole andrographolide derivatives. PLoS One 8.3 (2013).

Gabrielian, E.S.,et al. 2002. A double blind, placebo-controlled study of *Andrographis paniculata* fixed combination Kan Jang in the treatment of acute upper respiratory tract infections including sinusitis. Phytomedicine, 9, (7) 589–597.

Geethangili M et al. Cytotoxic constituents from *Andrographis paniculata* induce cell cycle arrest in jurkat cells. Phytother Res 22.10 (2008): 1336–1341.

Ghosh N et al. Recent advances in herbal medicine for treatment of liver diseases. Pharmaceutical Biology 19.9 (2011):970–988.

Hovhannisyan AS et al. The effect of Kan Jang extract on the pharmacokinetics and pharmacodynamics of warfarin in rats. Phytomedicine 13.5 (2006): 318–323.

Hsu JH et al. Activation of alpha1A-adrenoceptor by andrographolide to increase glucose uptake in cultured myoblast C2C12 cells. Planta Med 70.12 (2004): 1230–1233.

Iruretagoyena MI et al. Andrographolide interferes with T cell activation and reduces experimental autoimmune encephalomyelitis in the mouse. J Pharmacol Exp Ther 312.1 (2005): 366–372.

Jaruchotikamol A et al. Strong synergistic induction of CYP1A1 expression by andrographolide plus typical CYP1A inducers in mouse hepatocytes. Toxicol Appl Pharmacol 224.2 (2007): 156–162.

Jayakumar T et al. Experimental and clinical pharmacology of *Andrographis paniculata* and its major bioactive phytoconstituent andrographolide. Evidence-based Complementary and Alternative Medicine. (2013); 2013: 846740.

Jiang CG et al. Andrographolide inhibits the adhesion of gastric cancer cells to endothelial cells by blocking E-selectin expression. Anticancer Res 27 (4B) (2007): 2439–2447.

Kim TG, et al. Morphological and biochemical changes of andrographolide-induced cell death in human prostatic adenocarcinoma PC-3 cells. In Vivo 19.3 (2005): 551–557.

Kligler B et al. *Andrographis paniculata* for the treatment of upper respiratory infection: a systematic review by the natural standard research collaboration. Explore (NY) 2.1 (2006): 25–29.

Kumar RA et al. Anticancer and immunostimulatory compounds from *Andrographis paniculata*. J Ethnopharmacol 92.23 (2004): 291–295.

Lee KC et al. Andrographolide acts as an anti-inflammatory agent in LPS-stimulated RAW264.7 macrophages by inhibiting STAT3-mediated suppression of the NF-kB pathway. J Ethnopharmacol (2011) 135: 678–684.

Li J et al. Andrographolide induces cell cycle arrest at G2/M phase and cell death in HepG2 cells via alteration of reactive oxygen species. Eur J Pharmacol 568.1–3 (2007):31–44.

Lim JC et al. Andrographolide and its analogues: versatile bioactive molecules for combating inflammation and cancer. Clin Exp Pharmacol Physiol 39 (3) (2012):300–10.

Lu WJ et al. A novel role of andrographolide, an NK-kB inhibitor, on inhibition of platelet activation: the pivotal mechanisms of endothelial nitric oxide synthase/cyclic GMP. Journal of Molecular Medicine. 89.12 (2011):1263–1271.

Lu J et al. Suppression of NF-kB signaling by andrographolide with a novel mechanism in human platelets: regulatory roles of the p38 MAPK-hydroxyl radical0-ERK2 cascade. Biochemical Pharmacology 84 (2012):914–924.

Mandal SC, et al. Studies on psychopharmacological activity of *Andrographis paniculata* extract. Phytother Res 15.3 (2001): 253–256.

Mills S, Bone K. Principles and practice of phytotherapy. London: Churchill Livingstone, 2000.

Mishra U et al. Antibacterial activity of ethanol extract of *Andrographis paniculata*. Indian Journal of Pharmaceutical Sciences. 74.4 (2009):436–438.

Mkrtchyan AV et al. A phase I clinical study of *Andrographis paniculata* fixed combination Kan Jang versus ginseng and valerian on the semen quality of healthy male subjects. Phytomedicine 12.6–7 (2005): 403–409.

Nugroho AE et al. Antidiabetic and antihiperlipidemic effect of *Andrographis paniculata* (Burm. f) Nees and andrographolide in high-fructose-fat-fed rats. Indian J Pharmacol 44.3 (2012):377–81.

Panossian A et al. Pharmacokinetic and oral bioavailability of andrographolide from *Andrographis paniculata* fixed combination Kan Jang in rats and human. Phytomedicine 7.5 (2000): 351–364.

Panossian A et al. Effect of andrographolide and Kan Jang (fixed combination of extract SHA-10 and extract SHE-3) on proliferation of human lymphocytes, production of cytokines and immune activation markers in the whole blood cells culture. Phytomedicine 9.7 (2002): 598–605.

Panossian A et al. Plasma nitric oxide level in functional Mediterranean fever and its modulations by ImmunoGuard. Nitric Oxide 9 (2003): 103–110.

Pekthong DH et al. Differential inhibition of rat and human hepatic cytochrome P450 by *Andrographis paniculata* extract and andrographolide. J Ethnopharmacol 115.3 (2008): 432–440.

Poolsup N et al. *Andrographis paniculata* in the symptomatic treatment of uncomplicated upper respiratory tract infection: systematic review of randomized controlled trials. J Clin Pharm Ther 29.1 (2004): 37–45.

Premendran SJ et al. Anti-cobra venom activity of plant *Andrographis paniculata* and its comparison with polyvalent anti-snake venom. Journal of Natural Science, Biology, and Medicine 2.2 (2011):198–204.

Qin LH et al. Andrographolide inhibits the production of TNF-alpha and interleukin-12 in lipopolysaccharide-stimulated macrophages: role of mitogen-activated protein kinases. Biological & Pharmaceutical Bulletin 29.2 (2006):220–4.

Rajagopal S et al. Andrographolide, a potential cancer therapeutic agent isolated from *Andrographis paniculata*. J Exp Ther Oncol 3.3 (2003): 147–158.

Reyes BA et al. Anti-diabetic potentials of *Momordica charantia* and *Andrographis paniculata* and their effects on estrous cyclicity of alloxan-induced diabetic rats. J Ethnopharmacol 105.1–2 (2006): 196–200.

Sandborn WJ et al. *Andrographis paniculata* extract (HMPL-004) for active ulcerative colitis. Am J Gastroenterol 108.1 (2013):90–8.

Saxena RC. A randomized double blind placebo controlled clinical evaluation of extract of *Andrographis paniculata* (KalmCold) in patients with uncomplicated upper respiratory tract infection. Phytomedicine. 17(3–4) (2010):178–185.

See D, et al. Increased tumor necrosis factor alpha (TNF-alpha) and natural killer cell (NK) function using an integrative approach in late stage cancers. Immunol Invest 31.2 (2002): 137–153.

Sheeja K, et al. Antioxidant and anti-inflammatory activities of the plant *Andrographis paniculata* Nees. Immunopharmacol Immunotoxicol 28.1 (2006): 129–140.

Sheeja K, et al. Antiangiogenic activity of *Andrographis paniculata* extract and andrographolide. Int Immunopharmacol 7.2 (2007): 211–221.

Singha PK, et al. Antimicrobial activity of *Andrographis paniculata*. Fitoterapia 74.78 (2003): 692–694.

Singha PK, et al. Protective activity of andrographolide and arabinogalactan proteins from *Andrographis paniculata* Nees. against ethanol-induced toxicity in mice. J Ethnopharmacol 111.1 (2007): 13–21.

Spasov AA et al. Comparative controlled study of *Andrographis paniculata* fixed combination, Kan Jang and an Echinacea preparation as adjuvant, in the treatment of uncomplicated respiratory disease in children. Phytother Res 18.1 (2004): 47–53.

Subramanian R, et al. In vitro alpha-glucosidase and alpha-amylase enzyme inhibitory effects of *Andrographis paniculata* extract and andrographolide. Acta Biochim Pol 55.2 (2008): 391–398.

Suebsasana S et al. Analgesic, antipyretic, anti-inflammatory and toxic effects of andrographolide derivatives in experimental animals. Archives of Pharmacal Research 32.9 (2009):1191–1200.

Tang T et al. Randomised clinical trial: herbal extract HMPL-004 in active ulcerative colitis – a double-blind comparison with sustained release mesalazine. Aliment Pharmacol Ther 33.2 (2011):194–202.

Tang LI et al. Screening of anti-dengue activity in methanolic extracts of medicinal plants. BMC Complementary and Alternative Medicine. 12.3 (2012).

Thamlikitkul V et al. Efficacy of *Andrographis paniculata* nees for pharyngotonsillitis in adults. J Med Assoc Thai 74.10 (1991): 437–442.

Thisoda P et al. Inhibitory effect of *Andrographis paniculata* extract and its active diterpenoids on platelet aggregation. Eur J Pharmacol 553.1–3 (2006): 39–45.

Tung YT et al. Therapeutic potential of andrographolide isolated from the leaves of *Andrographis paniculata* Nees for treating lung adenocarcinoma. Evid Based Complement Alternat Med. (2013): 305898

Uttekar MM et al. Anti-HIV activity of semisynthetic derivatives of andrographolide and computational study of HIV-1 gp120 protein binding. European Journal of Medicinal Chemistry. 56 (2012) :368–74.

Voravuthikunchai SP; Limsuwan S. Medicinal plant extracts as anti-*Escherichia coli* 0157:H7 agents and their effects on bacterial cell aggregation. Journal of Food protection 69.10 (2006):2336–2341.

Wiart CK et al. Antiviral properties of ent-labdene diterpenes of *Andrographis paniculata* nees, inhibitors of herpes simplex virus type 1. Phytother Res 19 (12) (2005): 1069–1070.

Wibudi A et al. The traditional plant, *Andrographis paniculata* (Sambiloto), exhibits insulin-releasing actions in vitro. Acta Med Indones 40.2 (2008): 63–68.

Wu TS et al. Flavonoids and ent-labdane diterpenoids from *Andrographis paniculata* and their antiplatelet aggregatory and vasorelaxing effects. J Asian Nat Prod Res 10.1–2 (2008): 17–24.

Xu C, Wang ZT. [Chemical constituents from roots of *Andrographis paniculata*.] Yao Xue Xue Bao 46 (3) (2011):317–21

Yan J et al. Andrographolide induces cell cycle arrest and apoptosis in human rheumatoid arthritis fibroblast-like synoviocytes. Cell Biol Toxicol. 28.1 (2012):47–56.

Yoopan NP et al. Cardiovascular effects of 14-deoxy-11, 12-didehydroandrographolide and *Andrographis paniculata* extracts. Planta Med 73.6 (2007): 503–511.

Yu BC et al. Antihyperglycemic effect of andrographolide in streptozotocin-induced diabetic rats. Planta Med 69.12 (2003): 1075–1079.

Zhao F et al. Anti-tumor activities of andrographolide, a diterpene from *Andrographis paniculata*, by inducing apoptosis and inhibiting VEGF level. J Asian Nat Prod Res 10.5 (2008): 473–479.

Zhou J et al. Critical role of pro-apoptotic Bcl-2 family members in andrographolide-induced apoptosis in human cancer cells. Biochem Pharmacol 72.2 (2006): 132–144.

Astragalus

HISTORICAL NOTE Astragalus was first recorded in *Shen Nong's Materia Medica* about two thousand years ago and was believed to stimulate immune function and have antioxidant effects and other benefits in the treatment of viral infections and cardiovascular disease (Zhang et al 2007). The roots of astragalus are still considered among the most important and popular Chinese herbs for invigorating vital energy, health promotion and strengthening Qi. Western herbalists began using astragalus in the 1800s in various tonics and the gummy sap (tragacanth) is still used as an emulsifier, food thickener and antidiarrhoeal agent. Today, Western herbalists use astragalus as an immunomodulating agent, adaptogen and in the management of cardiovascular disease.

Clinical note — Polysaccharides and immunity

Plant polysaccharides are known for their ability to enhance host defence responses. Several types of immunomodulators have been identified, most recently botanically sourced polysaccharides isolated from mushrooms, algae, lichens and higher plants. These polysaccharides tend to have a broad spectrum of therapeutic properties and relatively low toxicity. One of the primary mechanisms responsible for immunomodulation involves non-specific induction of the immune system, which is thought to occur via macrophage stimulation and modulation of the complement system. According to one report, polysaccharides isolated from 35 plant species among 20 different families have been shown to increase macrophage cytotoxic activity against tumour cells and microorganisms, activate phagocytic activity, increase reactive oxygen species and nitric oxide production, and enhance secretion of cytokines and chemokines, such as tumour necrosis factor-alpha (TNF-alpha), inteleukin-1beta (IL-1beta), IL-6, IL-8, IL-12, interferfon-gamma (IFN-gamma) and IFN-beta2 (Schepetkin & Quinn 2006). These effects have a major influence on the body's ability to respond rapidly and potently to a diverse array of pathogens, giving the polysaccharides wide clinical application.

COMMON NAME

Astragalus

OTHER NAMES

Astragali, beg kei, bei qi, hwanggi, huang-qi, milk vetch, goat's horn, green dragon, Mongolian milk, ogi, Syrian tragacanth

BOTANICAL NAME/FAMILY

Astragalus membranaceus (family Fabaceae)

PLANT PART USED

Root

CHEMICAL COMPONENTS

Astragalus is a chemically complex herb and contains over 60 components, including beta-sitosterol, glycosides (astragalosides I–VII, soyasaponin, daucosterin), polysaccharides (astroglucans A–C), saponins such as cycloastragenol, astragalosides, isoflavones and other flavonoids, plant acid, choline, betaine, rumatakenin, formonetin, amino acids (including gamma-aminobutyric acid), monomeric lectin and various microelements (Duke 2003, Li & Wang 2005, Mills & Bone 2000, Yan et al 2010).

MAIN ACTIONS

Evidence about mechanisms of action is mainly derived from in vitro and animal studies.

Immune modulation

Studies using various experimental models indicate that astragalus and its saponins, polysaccharides and flavonoids have immune-modulating activity by stimulating macrophage activity and enhancing B- and T-cell activity (Chu et al 1988, Jin et al 1994, Kuo et al 2009, Lonkova 2010, Shen et al 2008, Sugiura et al 1993, Sun et al 2008). Astragalus enhances lymphocyte blastogenesis in vitro (Sun et al 1983). Immunostimulant effects have also been observed in the presence of immunosuppressive therapy in vivo (Jin et al 1999).

Although usually administered in the oral form, research has also been undertaken with injectable forms. A study conducted with both normal and immunosuppressed mice found that astragalus administration increased antibody responses and T-helper cell activity (Zhao et al 1990). A flavonoid identified in the stem and leaves of astragalus is believed to be one of the main constituents responsible for immune modulation (Jiao et al 1999) and, more recently, several studies have identified that astragalus polysaccharide also exerts significant biological effects, including increasing cellular and humoral immune responses in vivo (Guo et al 2004).

Other in vitro and animal studies reveal that astragalus polysaccharides increase beneficial gut flora and decrease harmful gut bacteria, suggesting beneficial immune effects within the gastrointestinal tract (Guo et al 2003).

A 2009 animal model observed a switch to Th-1-dominant immune regulation along with increased exercise tolerance in chronic fatigue rats (Kuo et al 2009), which suggests potential benefit for the use of astragalus in postviral syndrome and chronic fatigue.

Hypotensive and positive inotrope

Several constituents from *Astragalus* spp. have demonstrated effects on heart contractility, heart rate and blood pressure. In particular, 3-nitropropionic acid has been shown to decrease blood pressure and induce bradycardia when administered as an intravenous (IV) preparation in normotensive rats or renal hypertensive dogs (Castillo et al 1993). Another compound, astragaloside IV, demonstrated positive inotropic activity in patients with congestive heart failure (Luo et al 1995).

Recent research indicates that astragalus improves endothelial function by increasing the bioavailability of nitric oxide and decreasing reactive oxygen species production (Zhang et al 2007).

Antioxidant

In vivo studies have found that astragalus raises superoxide dismutase activity in the brain and liver, thus demonstrating an indirect antioxidant activity (Jin et al 1999). The constituent astragaloside IV (20 and 40 mg/kg) prevented the formation of cerebral infarction after induced focal ischaemia in an animal model, most likely due to its antioxidant and anti-inflammatory actions (Luo et al 2004). Recent in vitro experiments with astragalus polysaccharides also suggest they are potent free radical scavengers of hydroxyl radicals as well as hydrogen peroxide (Niu 2011).

Anticarcinogenic effects

Both in vitro and animal studies indicate that astragalus may have a role as adjunctive therapy in the treatment of some cancers. In vivo studies have shown that astragalus extract exerts anticarcinogenic effects in carcinogen-treated mice, mediated through activation of cytotoxic activity and the production of cytokines (Kurashige et al 1999). An extract of the root (90 and 180 mg/kg) prevented the development of preneoplastic lesions and delayed hepatic cancer in chemically-induced hepatocarcinogenesis in a rat model (Cui et al 2003). The saponin, astragaloside IV, can increase the fibrinolytic potential of cultured human umbilical vein endothelial cells by downregulating the expression of plasminogen activator inhibitor type 1 (Zhang et al 1997).

Another constituent (astragalan) increased the secretion of TNF-alpha and TNF-beta (Zhao & Kong 1993). More recent research attributes some of the antiproliferative effects of astragalus to lectins which inhibit the growth of tumour cells and induce apoptosis (L Huang et al 2012).

An animal study using a combination of *Astragalus membranaceus* and *Ligustrum lucidum* demonstrated antitumour effects by augmenting phagocyte and lymphokine-activated killer cell activities (Lau et al 1994). Via gene suppression, the saponin, astragaloside II, exerted antitumour effects, in both in vivo and in vitro experimental models on multi-drug-resistant hepatocellular carcinoma cell lines (C Huang et al 2012).

Hypoglycaemic

There is a growing body of experimental evidence demonstrating activities of relevance in insulin resistance and its comorbidities.

A meta-analysis of nine in vivo studies on rats published from 2005 to 2007 found that astragalus significantly lowers fasting blood glucose levels (Zhang et al 2009). In vivo and in vitro experimentation of polysaccharides of astragalus corroborates these findings and hypothesises that this effect is achieved via downregulation of gene expression and gene splicing for enzymes that regulate insulin signalling at a subcellular level (Mao et al 2009). These findings are significant within the context of emerging models of pathological understanding of non-insulin-dependent diabetes, which suggest that stress created at a subcellular level by hyperglycaemia perpetuates dysregulated insulin signalling and sensitivity.

Other rodent models demonstrate lowered blood glucose, and preservation of pancreatic beta cells when compared with controls (C Li et al 2011); improved insulin sensitivity in skeletal muscle (Liu 2010, Zou et al 2009); and restoration of defective hypoglycaemia (Zou et al 2010) with astragalus treatment.

In a diabetic hamster model with concomitant cardiomyopathy, astragalus polysaccharides reduced serum glucose, glycosylated serum protein and myocardial enzymes and lipid levels increased genetic expression for GLUT-4 transporters, suggesting that astragalus may have a significant role in diabetes and comorbid cardiomyopathy (W Chen et al 2012).

Hepatoprotective actions

Astragalus has hepatoprotective qualities against paracetamol, carbon tetrachloride and D-galactosamine poisoning (Zhang et al 1990). Increases in liver glutathione levels observed as a result of the herbal treatment may be partly responsible. Studies have identified the constituent betaine as an important contributor to this activity.

Renal protective

Alone and in combination, astragalus demonstrated reno-protective effects in animal models by reducing proteinuria and by protecting the microstructure of the kidney architecture (Li & Zhang 2009, Song et al 2009, Wojcikowski et al 2009).

Neuroprotective

A decoction of astragalus produced neuroprotective effects in rats with experimentally induced cerebral ischaemia, and memory enhancement has been observed in vivo (Jin et al 1999).

OTHER ACTIONS

Astragalus is also thought to have adaptogenic activity. It has shown weak oestrogenic activity in vitro when compared with other Chinese herbs and controls (17-beta-oestradiol). This could partially explain its traditional use in menopause.

Traditional action

Of note is a recent in vivo study (in rats) exploring the basis for meridian tropism theory in traditional Chinese medicine (TCM), the premise of which is that particular principles in plants have an affinity for specific tissues, organs and meridians, thus influencing the therapeutic application of herbal medicines in TCM. The results produced by Chang et al (2012) confirmed that astragaloside IV was mainly distributed to the liver, kidney, lung, spleen and heart, which reflects the traditional use of astragalus and may provide experimental validity for the application of meridian tropism.

Hypocholesterolaemic

A specific astragalus polysaccharide, extracted from *Astragalus membranaceus*, possessed hydroxyl radicals and hydrogen peroxide scavenging activities, and showed a chelating effect on ferrous ions in vitro (Niu 2011). This suggests that astragalus may have a cholesterol-lowering effect and reduces the risk of cardiovascular diseases.

Digestive effects

Astragalus strengthens the movement and muscle tone of the small intestine (especially the jejunum) in animal tests, which may account for its clinical application in a variety of common digestive symptoms (Yang 1993).

Improved sperm motility

An aqueous extract of *Astragalus membranaceus* was tested in vitro and found to have a significant stimulatory effect on sperm motility (Hong et al 1992). Astragalus has shown a significant effect on human sperm motility in vitro when compared with controls (Liu et al 2004).

Cytochrome 1A2 inhibition

An experimental model found astragaloside IV inhibited the activity of the cytochrome enzyme CYP1A2 in a rat model, suggesting that astragalus may affect the pharmacokinetics of co-administered medicines and that caution should be exercised, especially in medicines with a narrow therapeutic window (Zhang et al 2013).

CLINICAL USE

Astragalus is a popular Chinese herbal medicine and has been the subject of many clinical trials, mainly published in foreign-language peer-reviewed journals. To provide a more complete description of the evidence available, secondary sources have been used when necessary. As a reflection of clinical practice, astragalus is sometimes tested in combination with other herbal medicines, and also administered by injection in some countries. In these instances the preparation or route of administration is stated in this review.

Viral infection

Owing to its immunomodulatary actions, astragalus is widely used for preventing and treating various viral infections. A popular use is as a preventive treatment against common colds and influenza. To date, scientific evidence is scant to confirm effectiveness, although one review stated that astragalus has been tested in clinical trials in China, reducing the incidence and shortening the duration of the common cold (Murray 1995).

A 2013 systematic review found that astragalus reduced the incidence of upper respiratory tract infections in children with nephrotic syndrome, a very common complication in this patient group (Zhou et al 2013).

Viral myocarditis

The effect of astragalus on heart function has been the subject of several investigations and, most recently, a Cochrane systematic review, which analysed studies of Chinese herbs used in viral myocarditis. It concluded that astragalus significantly improves cardiac function, arrhythmia and creatinine kinase levels (Liu et al 2012). The review assessed data from 20 randomised controlled trials (RCTs) that used a variety of single preparations of astragalus as well as combination therapy across a range of dosage forms from decoction to injection. Where possible, comparable studies were included in a meta-analysis which revealed that astragalus injection had a significant positive effect on patients with abnormal electrocardiograms, especially the S-T segment. The authors concluded that the studies which met the inclusion criteria for the review were overall of poor quality in terms of design, reporting and methodology.

Cardiovascular disease

Congestive heart failure

Some of the clinical signs and symptoms recognised as indicators for this medicine by TCM practitioners suggest that the herb may be useful for congestive heart failure. Recent positive results obtained in clinical studies have reinforced this possibility.

Two clinical trials investigated continuous IV administration of astragalus. One study, involving 19 patients, found that after 2 weeks' continuous administration of astragaloside IV, major symptoms were alleviated in 15 patients. Treatment produced a positive inotropic effect and improved left ventricular modelling and ejection function (Luo et al 1995). The second study, involving 38 patients with congestive heart failure who were administered astragalus 24 g IV for 2 weeks, found that 13.6% had significantly shortened ventricular late potentials (Shi et al 1991).

IN COMBINATION

Huang-qi, a traditional Chinese medicine combination of astragalus root, licorice root and zizyphus fruit, has historically and prolifically been used and studied for the treatment of congestive heart failure. However a systematic review of 62 RCTs and quasi-RCT human trials found that, while the results seem promising for huang-qi injections, the overall methodological quality of the studies was poorly described (Fu et al 2011).

Angina pectoris

Two clinical studies have suggested that astragalus may be an effective treatment for angina pectoris. One study used Doppler echocardiography to study the action of astragalus on left ventricular function in 20 patients with angina pectoris. Treatment resulted in increased cardiac output after 2 weeks, but no improvement in left ventricular diastolic function (Lei et al 1994). One Chinese study reported 92 patients with ischaemic heart disease who were successfully treated with astragalus as measured by electrocardiogram readings. Results obtained with the herb were considered superior to those obtained with nifedipine (Li et al 1995).

Stroke

Astragalus membranaceus has an established history of use in China to assist recovery after stroke. Several clinical trials have been undertaken in China to explore the mechanism of action and to measure the effect; however they have not met the standards of the International Conference on Harmonization and Good Clinical Practice guidelines, and they used positive controls (C Chen et al 2012). A more robust trial with a sample size of 68 subjects has demonstrated that, when stroke patients are administered astragalus within 24 hours of the stroke, their functional independent outcome measures, such as dressing, eating and bladder control, were significantly improved when compared to controls at 4 and 12 weeks after the event. The researchers speculate that this may be due to the anti-inflammatory and antioxidant actions of astragalus, therefore reducing oedema (C Chen et al 2012). However inflammatory biomarkers such as erythrocyte sedimentation rate and C-reactive protein were not consistently measured after 7 days.

Cancer

Astragalus is used in cancer patients to enhance the effectiveness of chemotherapy and reduce associated side effects. It is additionally used to enhance immune function.

Few details are available of clinical studies looking at the potential for astragalus to alter patient survival outcomes, as most information has been published in non-English journals. However, two clinical studies are worth mentioning: they suggest that intravenously administered astragalus may have potential benefit as adjunctive therapy when given with chemotherapy. In one randomised study of 120 cancer patients receiving chemotherapy, IV astragalus extract was administered daily (20 mL in 250 mL normal saline), and tumour growth was slowed compared to controls (Duan & Wang 2002). Four treatment cycles were administered lasting 21 days each. Unfortunately, no further details are available about this study.

Another randomised study investigated IV astragalus in 60 patients with advanced non-small-cell lung cancer (Zou & Liu 2003). This time 2–3 treatment cycles were given of 21–18 days each. The mean remission rate was 5.4 months in the herbal-treated group vs 3.3 months in the untreated group, and the 1-year survival rate was 46.75% with herbal treatment vs 30.0% without. All differences were considered statistically significant. Once again, further details are not available in English.

Colorectal cancer

According to a 2005 Cochrane systematic review, astragalus may be a useful adjunct to chemotherapy in colorectal cancer as it reduces treatment side effects. The review assessed various Chinese herbal medicines taken in combination with chemotherapy for colorectal cancer for their ability to reduce common side effects of chemotherapy, such as nausea, vomiting, sore mouth, diarrhoea, hepatotoxicity, myelosuppression and immunosuppression (Taixiang et al 2005). Four trials were analysed: adjunctive treatment with astragalus was compared with chemotherapy alone in three trials, and with two other Chinese herbal treatments in the fourth trial. Overall, herbal treatment resulted in a significant reduction in the proportion of patients who experienced nausea and vomiting when decoctions of huang-qi (astragalus) compounds were given in addition to chemotherapy. There was also a decrease in the rate of leucopenia (white blood cell count $< 3 \times 10^9$/L) and increased proportions of T-lymphocyte subsets: CD3, CD4 and CD8 with no significant effects on immunoglobulins G, A or M. The authors concluded that astragalus may stimulate immunocompetent cells and decrease chemotherapy side effects; however a definitive conclusion could not be made because of the studies' methodological limitations. Additionally, no evidence of harm was identified with use of the Chinese herbal treatment in these studies.

Prostate cancer (in combination)

Although no human studies could be located, encouraging results were obtained from an in vitro study investigating the effects of a proprietary product known as Equiguard on prostate cancer cells. It is prepared according to TCM principles and contains standardised extracts of nine herbs: herb *Epimedium brevicornum maxim* (stem and leaves), *Radix Morindae officinalis* (root), *Fructus rosae laevigatae* Michx (fruit), *Rubus chingii* Hu (fruit), *Schisandra chinensis* (Turz.) Baill (fruit), *Ligustrum lucidum* Ait (fruit), *Cuscuta chinensis* Lam (seed), *Psoralea corylifolia* L. (fruit) and *Astragalus membranaceus* (root). It is used in TCM to restore Qi in the urogenital region. The product was shown to significantly reduce cancer cell growth, induce apoptosis, suppress expression of the androgen receptor and lower intracellular and secreted prostate-specific antigen (Hsieh et al 2002).

Chronic kidney disease

Astragalus is one of the most commonly prescribed Chinese herbs in chronic kidney disease. Pharmacological studies have confirmed that different constituents in the herb have effects which could be valuable in chronic kidney disease such as antioxidant, diuretic and anti-inflammatory effects, and studies in rat models indicate that astragalus decreases glomerular hyperperfusion and improves kidney function (Li & Wang 2005).

A meta-analysis of 14 RCTs involving 524 Chinese patients with primary nephrotic syndrome showed that treatment with astragalus for 1–3 months could increase the therapeutic effect of prednisone and immunosuppressants (reported in Li & Wang 2005). Herbal treatment decreased proteinuria and increased levels of total cholesterol and albumin. Although further details are unavailable, these results are encouraging.

A 2011 meta-analysis measuring the clinical effect of astragalus injection in diabetic nephropathy corroborated these results (M Li et al 2011). The pooled results from 25 clinical studies that included 945 patients and 859 control subjects demonstrated that astragalus injection, when compared with controls, provided greater renal protection and systemic improvement by reducing serum urea nitrogen, serum creatinine, urine protein and urine microalbumin; and increasing serum albumin in patients with diabetic nephropathy compared with controls (Okuda et al 2012).

A Cochrane systematic review compared the efficacy of pharmaceutical treatments and TCM for preventing infections in nephrotic syndrome in adults (Wu et al 2012). While the authors concluded that huang-qi granules (astragalus) may have positive effects on the prevention of infection in children with nephrotic syndrome, the methodological quality of all studies was poor, and there was no compelling evidence on the effectiveness of the intervention.

The efficacy of astragalus injection for hypertensive-induced renal damage was examined by systematic review of five RCTs comparing astragalus to placebo and antihypertensives (Sun et al 2012). Although the individual studies were considered to have poor methodological quality, the pooled data indicate that astragalus has protective effects for this patient group.

Glucose regulation

In a randomised trial of pregnant women with gestational diabetes ($n = 84$), the treatment group, who received insulin plus astragalus, had better outcomes for malondialdehyde, superoxide dismutase, renal function and blood lipids compared to the control group who received insulin alone (Liang et al 2009).

Adaptogenic tonic – traditional use

Within traditional Chinese herbal medicine, astragalus is used to invigorate and tonify Qi and the blood, as an adaptogen, for severe blood loss, fatigue, anorexia, organ prolapse, chronic diarrhoea, shortness of breath, sweating and to enhance recuperation (Mills & Bone 2000).

Clinical note — The concept of an adaptogen is foreign to Western medicine but often used in traditional medicine

The term 'adaptogen' was first coined by N. Lazarev in the Soviet Union in the mid 20th century, although the concept has been used for centuries in traditional herbal systems. Adaptogens are considered natural bioregulators that increase the ability of the organism to adapt to environmental factors and to avoid damage from such factors. Herbal medicines with adaptogenic activity are used when extremes of physical or emotional activity are present, environmental influences are severe or allostatic load has developed over time. The aim of treatment is to improve the patient's endurance and ability to deal with these changes in a healthy way, and for abnormal parameters to shift towards normal. The best-known example of a plant adaptogen is ginseng (*Panax ginseng*), but others are also well established, such as *Schisandra chinensis*, *Eleutherococcus senticosus* (Siberian ginseng), *Astragalus membranaceus* and *Withania somnifera* (see Siberian ginseng and Glossary).

Cholesterol reduction (in combination with other herbs)

A randomised, double-blind clinical trial compared the effects of a traditional Chinese herbal medicine combination known as jian yan ling (which includes astragalus as a main ingredient) to a placebo in 128 hyperlipidaemic patients. After 3 months' treatment it was found that total cholesterol, triglyceride, apoproteins and lipoprotein-a levels were significantly reduced in the treatment group compared with placebo.

Asthma (in combination with other herbs and minerals)

A herbal combination of *Astragalus membranaceus, Codonopsis pilulosa* and *Glycyrrhiza uralensis* was investigated in an open study for effects on airway responsiveness. Twenty-eight patients with asthma were treated with the herbal combination for 6 weeks, after which values for forced vital capacity, forced expiratory volume and peak expiratory flow were all higher than at baseline (Wang et al 1998).

In a 6-week randomised, double-blinded placebo-controlled trial of a proprietary preparation of astragalus and zinc, the intensity of rhinorrhoea was significantly improved in seasonal allergic rhinitis in 48 patients (Matkovic 2010).

Memory deficits (in combination with other herbs)

In TCM, invigorating Qi and warming Yang are believed to have a beneficial therapeutic effect on some brain diseases, such as senile dementia. Some studies have been conducted to determine the outcome of following this ancient principle.

DOSAGE RANGE

- Dried root: 2–30 g/day.
- Liquid extract (1:2) or solid-dose equivalent: 4.5–8.5 mL/day.
- Decoction: 8–12 g divided into two doses daily on an empty stomach.

TOXICITY

Animal studies have shown that the herb has a wide safety margin.

ADVERSE REACTIONS

None known.

SIGNIFICANT INTERACTIONS

Interactions are theoretical and based on the herb's pharmacodynamic effects; therefore clinical significance is unclear and remains to be confirmed. There is some evidence that a component in astragalus inhbits CYP 1A2 in vivo but no human studies have tested whether the effect is clinically significant for astragalus extract. Meanwhile, clinicians should supervise patients taking drugs with a narrow therapeutic index chiefly metabolised by CYP1A2 to avoid drug interactions.

Aciclovir

Possibly enhances antiviral activity against herpes simplex type 1 (Stargrove et al 2008) — adjunctive use may be beneficial.

Immunosuppressant medication

Reduced drug activity is theoretically possible, as immunostimulant activity has been demonstrated — use caution.

Positive inotropic drugs

Additive effects are theoretically possible with intravenous administration of astragalus, based on positive inotropic activity identified in clinical studies. The clinical significance of these findings for oral dose forms is unknown — observe patients using high-dose astragalus preparations.

Cyclophosphamide

Adjunctive treatment with astragalus may have beneficial effects in regard to improving patient wellbeing and reducing adverse effects associated with treatment, such as nausea and vomiting — only use combination under professional supervision.

Practice points/Patient counselling

- Astragalus is widely used as an immunostimulant medicine to reduce the incidence of the common cold and influenza and is sometimes used to improve immune responses to other viral infections, such as herpes simplex type 1.
- It is also used to enhance recuperation and reduce fatigue, and reduce the side effects of chemotherapy while improving immune function.
- Astragalus is a commonly prescribed Chinese herb in chronic kidney disease.
- According to TCM practice it is widely used to invigorate and tonify Qi and the blood, and as an important adaptogen.
- Some evidence suggests it enhances digestion, improves heart function in viral myocarditis, lowers cholesterol and fasting blood sugar and has hepatoprotective activity.
- Under the TCM system, astragalus is not used during periods of acute infection.
- In clinical practice it is often used in combination with other herbs, such as *Bupleurum chinense, Scutellaria baicalensis* and *Codonopsis pilulosa.* As such, most clinical trials have tested combination formulas.
- Astragalus injections are protective against chronic kidney conditions such as diabetic nephropathy and renal hypertenstion.
- Astragalus may improve the contractility of the heart muscle and prolong the S-T segment in patients with viral myocarditis.
- Astragalus root by oral and nasopharyngeal administration improves functional outcomes in stroke patients, when administered within 24 h of the stroke.

CONTRAINDICATIONS AND PRECAUTIONS

According to the principles of TCM, astragalus should not be used during the acute stages of an infection.

PREGNANCY USE

Safety is unknown, although no evidence of fetal damage has been reported in animal studies (Mills & Bone 2005). There were no reported safety concerns in the trial by Liang et al (2009) of pregnant women with gestational diabetes.

PATIENTS' FAQs

What will this herb do for me?

Astragalus appears to have numerous biological effects, such as digestive and immune system modulation, as a hypoglycaemic agent and cardiac tonic. Research suggests that it may have a role to play in recovery from viral infection, in chronic kidney disease and as an adjunct to chemotherapy treatment for cancer.

When will it start working?

This will depend on the indication and dose; some studies have shown that effects can begin within 2 weeks.

Are there any safety issues?

Overall the herb appears to be safe, although it has the potential to interact with some medicines. Professional supervision is advised for people receiving chemotherapy and considering using this herb.

REFERENCES

Castillo C et al. An analysis of the antihypertensive properties of 3-nitropropionic acid, a compound from plants in the genus *Astragalus*. Arch Inst Cardiol Mex 63.1 (1993): 11–6.

Chang Y et al. The experimental study of *Astragalus membranaceus* on meridian tropsim: The distribution study of astragaloside IV in rat tissues. J of Chromat 911 (2012): 71–75.

Chen CC, et al. Chinese Herb *Astragalus membranaceus* Enhances Recovery of Hemorrhagic Stroke: Double-Blind, Placebo-Controlled, Randomized Study. Evid Based Complement Alternat Med. 2012;2012:708452.

Chen W et al. Improvement of myocardial glycolipid metabolic disorder in diabetic hamster with *Astragalus* polysaccharides treatment. Mol Biol Rep. 2012 Jul;39(7):7609–15.

Chu DT, et al. Immunotherapy with Chinese medicinal herbs. I. Immune restoration of local xenogeneic graft-versus-host reaction in cancer patients by fractionated *Astragalus membranaceus* in vitro. J Clin Lab Immunol 25.3 (1988): 119–23.

Cui R et al. Suppressive effect of *Astragalus membranaceus* Bunge on chemical hepatocarcinogenesis in rats. Cancer Chemother. Pharmacol 51.1 (2003): 75–80.

Duan P, Wang ZM. Clinical study on effect of Astragalus in efficacy enhancing and toxicity reducing of chemotherapy in patients of malignant tumor. Zhongguo Zhong Xi Yi Jie He Za Zhi 22.7 (2002): 515–17.

Duke JA. Dr Duke's phytochemical and ethnobotanical databases. US Department of Agriculture, Agricultural Research Service, National Germplasm Resources Laboratory. Beltsville Agricultural Research Center, Beltsville, MD Online. Available www.ars-grin.gov/duke March 2003.

Fu S, et al. (2011) Huangqi injection (a traditional Chinese patent medicine) for chronic heart failure: a systematic review. PLoS ONE 6(5): e19604.

Guo FC et al. In vitro fermentation characteristics of two mushroom species, an herb, and their polysaccharide fractions, using chicken cecal contents as inoculum. Poult Sci 82.10 (2003): 1608–15.

Guo FC et al. Effects of mushroom and herb polysaccharides on cellular and humoral immune responses of *Eimeria tenella*-infected chickens. Poult Sci 83.7 (2004): 1124–32.

Hong CY, et al. *Astragalus membranaceus* stimulates human sperm motility in vitro. Am J Chin Med 20.3–4 (1992): 289–94.

Hsieh TC et al. Effects of herbal preparation Equiguard™ on hormone-responsive and hormone-refractory prostate carcinoma cells: mechanistic studies. Int J Oncol 20.4 (2002): 681–9.

Huang C, et al. Reversal of P-glycoprotein-mediated multidrug resistance of human hepatic cancer cells by Astragaloside II. J Pharm Pharmacol. 2012 Dec;64(12):1741–50.

Huang L et al. *Astragalus membranaceus* lectin (AML) induces caspase-dependent apoptosis in human leukemia cells. Cell Proliferation 45.1 (2012):15–21.

Jiao Y, et al. Influence of flavonoid of *Astragalus membranaceus*'s stem and leaves on the function of cell mediated immunity in mice. Zhongguo Zhong Xi Yi Jie He Za Zhi 19.6 (1999): 356–8.

Jin R et al. Effect of shi-ka-ron and Chinese herbs on cytokine production of macrophage in immunocompromised mice. Am J Chin Med 22.3–4 (1994): 255–66.

Jin R et al. Studies on pharmacological junctions of hairy root of *Astragalus membranaceus*. Zhongguo Zhong Yao Za Zhi 24.10 (1999): 619–21, 639.

Kurashige S, et al. Effects of astragali radix extract on carcinogenesis, cytokine production, and cytotoxicity in mice treated with a carcinogen, N-butyl-N-butanolnitrosoamine. Cancer Invest 17.1 (1999): 30–5.

Kuo Y, et al. . *Astragalus membranaceus* flavonoids (AMF) ameliorate chronic fatigue syndrome induced by food intake restriction plus forced swimming. J of Ethnopharm 122.1 (2009): 28–34.

Lau BH et al. Chinese medicinal herbs inhibit growth of murine renal cell carcinoma. Cancer Biother 9.2 (1994): 153–61.

Lei ZY, et al. Action of *Astragalus membranaceus* on left ventricular function of angina pectoris. Zhongguo Zhong Xi Yi Jie He Za Zhi 14.4 (1994): 195, 199–202.

Li SQ, et al. Clinical observation on the treatment of ischemic heart disease with *Astragalus membranaceus*. Zhongguo Zhong Xi Yi Jie He Za Zhi 15.2 (1995): 77–80.

Li X, Wang H. Chinese Herbal Medicine in the Treatment of Chronic Kidney Disease. Advances in Chronic Kidney Disease 12 (3) (2005): 276–81.

Li S, Zhang Y. Characterization and renal protective effect of a polysaccharide from *Astragalus membranaceus*. Carbo Polymers 78.2 (2009): 343–348.

Li C et al. Inhibitory effect of Astragalus polysaccharides on apoptosis of pancreatic beta-cells mediated by Fas in diabetes mellitus rats. Zhong Yao Cai. 2011; Oct;34(10):1579–82.

Li M, et al. Meta-analysis of the clinical value of *Astragalus membranaceus* in diabetic nephropathy. J Ethnopharmacol. 2011;133(2):412–9.

Liang HY et al. Clinical evaluation of the antioxidant activity of astragalus in women with gestational diabetes. Nan Fang Yi Ke Da Xue Xue Bao. 2009 Jul;29(7):1402–4.

Liu J et al. Effects of several Chinese herbal aqueous extracts on human sperm motility in vitro. Andrologia 36.2 (2004): 78–83.

Liu M, et al. Astragalus polysaccharide improves insulin sensitivity in KKAy mice: Regulation of PKB/GLUT4 signaling in skeletal muscle. Journal of Ethnopharmacology. 127.8 (2010): 32–37.

Liu JP, et al. Herbal medicines for viral myocarditis. Cochrane Database of Syst Rev 11. (2012): CD003711.

Lonkova, I. Biotechnological production of valuable plant pharmaceuticals: anticancer agents. Advances in Bulgarian Science (2010) 1: 5.

Luo HM, et al. Nuclear cardiology study on effective ingredients of *Astragalus membranaceus* in treating heart failure. Zhongguo Zhong Xi Yi Jie He Za Zhi 15.12 (1995): 707–9.

Luo Y et al. Astragaloside IV protects against ischemic brain injury in a murine model of transient focal ischemia. Neurosci Lett 363.3 (2004): 218–23.

Mao XX, et al. Hypoglycemic effect of polysaccharide enriched extract of Astragalus membranaceus in diet induced insulin resistant C57BL/6J mice and its potential mechanism. Phytomedicine 2009: 16, 416–425.

Matkovic Z. Efficacy and safety of *Astragalus membranaceus* in the treatment of patients with seasonal allergic rhinitis. Phyto Research 24.2(2010): 175–181.

Mills S, Bone K. Principles and practice of phytotherapy. London: Churchill Livingstone, 2000.

Mills S, Bone K. The essential guide to herbal safety. Edinburgh: Churchill Livingstone, 2005.

Murray M. The healing power of herbs. Rocklin CA: Prima Health, 1995.

Niu Y. Structural analysis and bioactivity of a polysaccharide from the roots of *Astragalus membranaceus* (Fisch) Bge. var. mongolicus (Bge.) Hsiao. Food Chemistry 128.3 (2011): 620–626.

Okuda M et al. Beneficial effect of *Astragalus membranaceus* on estimated glomerular filtration rate in patients with progressive chronic kidney disease. HK J of Neph 14.1(2012): 17–23.

Schepetkin IA, Quinn MT. Botanical polysaccharides: Macrophage immunomodulation and therapeutic potential. Int Immunopharmacol 6 (2006): 317–33.

Shen H, et al. *Astragalus membranaceus* prevents airway hyperreactivity in mice related to Th2 response inhibition. J of Ethnopharm 116.2 (2008): 363–369.

Shi HM, et al. Primary research on the clinical significance of ventricular late potentials (VLPs), and the impact of mexiletine, lidocaine and *Astragalus membranaceus* on VLPs. Zhong Xi Yi Jie He Za Zhi 11.5 (1991): 259, 265–7.

Song J et al. A combination of Chinese herbs, *Astragalus membranaceus* var. mongholicus and *Angelica sinensis*, improved renal microvascular insufficiency in 5/6 nephrectomized rats. Vasc Pharm 50.5 (2009): 185–193.

Stargrove M, et al. Herb, nutrient and drug interactions. St Louis: Mosby, 2008.

Sugiura H et al. Effects of exercise in the growing stage in mice and of *Astragalus membranaceus* on immune functions. Nippon Eiseigaku Zasshi 47.6 (1993): 1021–31.

Sun Y et al. Preliminary observations on the effects of the Chinese medicinal herbs *Astragalus membranaceus* and *Ligustrum lucidum* on lymphocyte blastogenic responses. J Biol Response Mod 2.3 (1983): 227–37.

Sun Y et al. Polysaccharides from *Astragalus membranaceus* promote phagocytosis and superoxide anion (O2–) production by coelomocytes from sea cucumber *Apostichopus japonicus* in vitro. Comp Biochem and Phys Part C: 147.3 (2008): 293–298.

Sun T, et al. *Astragalus* injection for hypertensive renal damage: a systematic review. Evid Based Complement Alternat Med. 2012;2012: 929025.

Taixiang W, et al. Chinese medical herbs for chemotherapy side effects in colorectal cancer patients. Cochrane Database Syst Rev 1 (2005): CD004540.

Wang H, et al. The effect of herbal medicine including *Astragalus membranaceus* (fisch) bge, Codonopsis pilulosa and Glycyrrhiza uralensis fisch on airway responsiveness. Zhonghua Jie He He Hu Xi Za Zhi 21.5 (1998): 287–8.

Wojcikowski K, et al. Beneficial effect of *Astragalus membranaceus* on estimated glomerular filtration rate in patients with progressive chronic kidney disease. Phyto Research 24.6 (2009): 875–884.

Wu HM, et al. Interventions for preventing infection in nephrotic syndrome. Cochrane Database Syst Rev. 2012 Apr 18;4:CD003964.

Yan Q, et al. Characterisation of a novel monomeric lectin (AML) from *Astragalus membranaceus* with anti-proliferative activity. Food Chemistry 122.3 (2010): 589–595.

Yang DZ [Effect of Astragalus membranaceus on myoelectric activity of small intestine.] Zhongguo Zhong Xi Yi Jie He Za Zhi. 1993;13: 582, 616–7.

Zhang ZL, et al. Hepatoprotective effects of astraglus root. J Ethnopharmacol 30.2 (1990): 145–9.

Zhang WJ, et al. Regulation of the fibrinolytic potential of cultured human umbilical vein endothelial cells: astragaloside IV downregulates plasminogen activator inhibitor-1 and upregulates tissue-type plasminogen activator expression. J Vasc Res 34.4 (1997): 273–80.

Zhang BQ et al. Effects of *Astragalus membranaceus* and its main components on the acute phase endothelial dysfunction induced by homocysteine. Vascular Pharmacology 46.4 (2007): 278–85.

Zhang J et al. Systematic review of the renal protective effect of *Astragalus membranaceus* (root) on diabetic nephropathy in animal models. Journal of Ethnopharmacology. 2009, 126(2):189–196.

Zhang YH et al, Astragaloside IV inhibited the activity of CYP1A2 in liver microsomes and influenced theophylline pharmokinetics in rats. J Pharm Pharmacol 65.1(2013): 149–55.

Zhao K S et al. Enhancement of the immuneresponse in mice by *Astragalus membranaceus* extracts. Immunopharmacology 20.3 (1990): 225–33.

Zhao KW, Kong HY. Effect of Astragalan on secretion of tumor necrosis factors in human peripheral blood mononuclear cells. Zhongguo Zhong Xi Yi Jie He Za Zhi 13.5 (1993): 259, 263–5.

Zhou C et al. Astragalus in the Prevention of Upper Respiratory Tract Infection in Children with Nephrotic Syndrome: Evidence-Based Clinical Practice (Review). Evidence-Based Comp and Alt Med 2013 (2013): 352130.

Zou YH, Liu XM. Effect of astragalus injection combined with chemotherapy on quality of life in patients with advanced non-small cell lung cancer. Zhongguo Zhong Xi Yi Jie He Za Zhi 23.10 (2003): 733–5.

Zou F et al 2009. Astragalus polysaccharides alleviates glucose toxicity and restores glucose homeostasis in diabetic states via activation of AMPK. Acta Pharmacol Sin. 2009 Dec;30(12):1607–15.

Zou F et al. *Radix astragali* (huangqi) as a treatment for defective hypoglycemia counterregulation in diabetes. Am J Chin Med. 2010; 38(6):1027–38.

Baical skullcap

HISTORICAL NOTE Baical skullcap is a herb used in Chinese medicine to clear 'heat and dry dampness'. Diseases with heat are associated with symptoms such as fever, irritability, thirst, cough and expectoration of thick, yellow sputum. Damp diseases may be associated with diarrhoea, a feeling of heaviness of the chest and painful urination (Bensky & Gamble 1986). From a modern perspective this suggests that baical may be useful for infection and inflammation of the respiratory, digestive and urinary systems. The experimental investigations described in this monograph demonstrate that baical skullcap's constituents have antibacterial, antiviral, anti-inflammatory, hepatoprotective, anxiolytic, hypocholesterolaemic, neuroprotective and antimetastatic actions.

OTHER NAMES

Baical skullcap, Chinese skullcap, huang qin (Mandarin), ogon (Japanese), scute

BOTANICAL NAME/FAMILY

Scutellaria baicalensis Georgi (family Lamiaceae)

PLANT PART USED

Root

In a notification for definition of pharmaceuticals from the Food Safety Bureau, Ministry of Health, Labour and Welfare of Japan, the roots of *Scutellaria baicalensis* were classified as raw materials used as pharmaceuticals (Makino et al 2008).

While it is typically and traditionally the root of *S. baicalensis* that is used therapeutically, experimentation is also being conducted on the aerial parts (Luo et al 2009).

CHEMICAL COMPONENTS

Baical skullcap contains resin, tannins, numerous flavonoids and their glycosides. Makino et al (2008) maintain that the flavone content in the root stock is significantly greater than that found in the aerial parts.

Baical also contains melatonin. It has been shown that dietary melatonin contributes directly to the circulating level of the hormone. The clinical effects of plant-derived melatonin remain to be investigated (Hardeland & Poeggeler 2003). Baicalin itself is poorly absorbed from the gut, but is hydrolysed to its aglycone, baicalein, by intestinal bacteria and then restored to its original form from the absorbed baicalein in the body (Akao et al 2000).

MAIN ACTIONS

The actions of baical skullcap, some of its individual constituents and combination formulations have been studied in various models.

Anti-inflammatory

The anti-inflammatory activity of baical skullcap has been well documented by in vitro and in vivo studies. The main constituents responsible are baicalein and wogonin (Chang et al 2001, Chi et al 2001, Chung et al 1995, Huang et al 2006, Krakauer et al 2001, Li et al 2000a, Park et al 2001, Wakabayashi 1999). Li and Lin (2011) identified six major biologically active flavones existing in the form of aglycones (baicalein, wogonin, oroxylin-A) and glycosides (baicalin, wogonoside, oroxylin A-7-glucuronide).

In an in vitro model, Yoon et al (2009) demonstrated that a water extract of baical skullcap exerted broad anti-inflammatory effects. It significantly inhibited the activation of macrophages by lipopolysaccharides (derived from Gram-negative bacteria cell walls), the production of nitric oxide, interleukin (IL)-3, IL-6, IL-10, IL-2p40 and IL-17, interferon-inducible protein-10, keratinocyte-derived chemokine and vascular endothelial growth factor.

These results are corroborated in a mouse model where baical skullcap was a potent inhibitor of multiple inflammatory markers and mediators, including inducible nitric oxide synthase (iNOS), cyclooxygenase-2 (COX-2), prostaglandin E_2 (PGE_2), IL-1β, IL-2, IL-6, IL-12 and tumour necrosis factor-α expression (Kim et al 2009).

In a study using mice, baicalein 50 mg/kg has been shown to ameliorate the inflammatory symptoms of induced colitis, including body weight loss, blood haemoglobin content, rectal bleeding and other histological and biochemical parameters (Hong et al 2002). Pretreatment with wogonin also significantly reduced ethanol-induced gastric damage in vivo (Park et al 2004) and reduced immunoglobulin E (IgE), IL-4, IL-5 and IL-10 secretion in a colitis-induced mouse model (Lim 2004). The methanolic extract of the baical skullcap root and its flavonoids wogonin, baicalein and baicalin have been shown to inhibit lipopolysaccharide-induced inflammation of the gingivae (gums) in vivo. The three flavonoids exerted an anti-inflammatory effect similar to prednisolone. In addition, the flavonoids exerted a moderate inhibition (33–36%) of collagenolytic activity, comparable to the 40% inhibition by tetracycline. Meanwhile, the cellular activity of fibroblasts was augmented remarkably (40%) by baicalein and slightly by baicalin and wogonin. Consistent with the cellular activation, the flavonoids enhanced the synthesis of both collagen and total protein in fibroblasts in vitro (Chung et al 1995).

The anti-inflammatory mechanisms are varied and summarised below.

Chemokine binding

In vivo and in vitro data suggest that *Scutellaria baicalensis* may prove to be a useful anti-inflammatory agent through its downregulation of the expression of various inflammatory mediators by limiting the biological function of chemokines (Jung et al 2012).

Excessive release of proinflammatory cytokines mediates the toxic effect of superantigenic staphylococcal exotoxins. In vitro data suggest that baicalin may be therapeutically useful for mitigating the pathogenic effects of staphylococcal exotoxins by inhibiting the signalling pathways activated by superantigens (Krakauer et al 2001).

Baicalin inhibited the binding of a number of chemokines to human leucocytes or cells expressing specific chemokine receptors, with an associated reduced capacity of the chemokines to induce cell migration. Based on these results, it is possible that the anti-inflammatory mechanism of baicalin is to bind a variety of chemokines and limit their biological function (Bao et al 2000, Li et al 2000a).

Four major flavonoids from baical skullcap have been shown in vitro to suppress eotaxin. Eotaxin is an eosinophil-specific chemokine associated with the recruitment of eosinophils to sites of allergic inflammation. Eotaxin is produced by IL-4 plus tumour necrosis factor (TNF)-alpha-stimulated human fibroblasts. This may explain why it has been used traditionally in the treatment of bronchial asthma (Nakajima et al 2001). In a rat model, baicalin inhibited induced eosinophilia and associated airway restriction by lowering IL-4 and IL-17A levels (Ma et al 2014).

COX-2 inhibition

Wogonin is a direct COX-2 inhibitor. Wogonin inhibits both iNOS and COX-2 induction (Chen et al 2001, 2008, Chi et al 2001, Wakabayashi & Yasui 2000). Wogonin has been shown to inhibit inducible PGE_2 production in macrophages by inhibiting COX-2 (Wakabayashi & Yasui 2000). Additionally baicalein, but not baicalin, has been shown to inhibit COX-2 expression in lipopolysaccharide-induced RAW 264.7 cells (a murine leukaemic macrophage-like cell line) (Woo et al 2006). Both compounds also suppressed iNOS protein expression, iNOS mRNA expression and NO production in a dose-dependent manner.

Wogonin may be beneficial for COX-2-related skin disorders. When applied topically to the dorsal skin of mice, it inhibited COX-2 expression and PGE_2 production (Byoung et al 2001, Chi et al 2003, Park et al 2001).

Lipoxygenase inhibition

The inhibition of the 5-lipoxygenase pathway of arachidonic acid metabolism may be one of the mechanisms of baicalein's anti-inflammatory activity, according to an in vivo study (Butenko et al 1993).

Antioxidant activity

The anti-inflammatory activity of baicalein may be associated with inhibition of leucocyte adhesion by the scavenging of reactive oxygen intermediates (Shen et al 2003).

Nuclear factor-kappa B (NF-κB) inhibition

Baicalin has been shown to inhibit NF-κB in vitro (Cheng et al 2007, Hsieh et al 2007, Kim et al 2006, Wang et al 2006), and microglial cells treated with wogonin indicated that the anti-inflammatory activity is exerted at least in part by suppressing microglial cell motility via inhibition of NF-κB activity (Piao et al 2008).

Antifibrotic

A methanolic extract of baical skullcap has been shown to inhibit fibrosis and lipid peroxidation induced by bile duct ligation or carbon tetrachloride in rat liver. Bile duct ligation in rodents is an experimental model for extrahepatic cholestasis caused by, for example, cholelithiasis (gallstones). Liver fibrosis was assessed by histological observation and by measuring levels of liver hydroxyproline, lipid peroxidation based on malondialdehyde production and serum enzyme activities. Treatment with baical skullcap significantly reduced the levels of liver hydroxyproline and malondialdehyde, with improved histological findings (Nan et al 2002).

In a 12-week study hypertensive rats treated with baicalein (flavone) had decreased heart to body weight ratio (a measure of left ventricular hypertrophy), decreased systolic blood pressure, decreased intraventricular thickness and a reduced expression of collagen and 12-lipoxygenase in cardiac tissue (antifibrotic), with the effect being more pronounced at the higher dose of 200 mg/kg/day (Kong 2011).

In an in vitro model, an ethanolic extract of baical skullcap (of unknown concentration) reduced markers associated with liver fibrogenesis such as collagen content and smooth-muscle actin, and also induced apoptosis of hepatic stellate cells, which are known to be implicated in the pathogenesis of liver fibrosis (Pan 2011).

Hepatoprotective

Baicalein, baicalin and wogonin have been shown to have hepatoprotective effects in vivo. The flavonoids decrease the toxicity produced by a variety of chemicals. Significant protective effects were seen by comparing the serum levels of aspartate transaminase (AST) and alanine aminotransferase (ALT) and by histopathological examination (Lin & Shieh 1996). Two different dried root preparations of baical skullcap (1% of total feed) were added to the diet of animals that were subsequently exposed to aflatoxin-B_1 (de Boer et al 2005). Mix A contained 3.13 mcg/g baicalin, 1.5 mcg/g baicalein, 0.021 mcg/g wogonin and 65.3 nmol/g melatonin compared to 0.94 mcg/g baicalin, 0.41 mcg/g baicalein, 0.003 mcg/g wogonin and 1176 nmol/g melatonin in mix B. The addition of mix A and B reduced hepatic damage by approximately 60% and 77%, respectively. The feed mixtures also increased the expression of the gene for glutathione-*S*-transferase A_5 by 2.5–3.0-fold. Interestingly, the mix with the lower concentration of flavonoids was the more protective. The authors explain this by stating that it was probably due to the much higher (18-fold) amount of melatonin which has been shown to enhance aflatoxin detoxification pathways in animals.

Baicalein, baicalin and wogonin have also been shown to inhibit haemin-nitrite-H_2O_2-induced liver injury in a dose-dependent manner by inhibiting oxidation and nitration (Zhao et al 2006). In other in vitro and in vivo studies baicalin reduced *tert*-butyl hydroperoxide hepatic damage, attenuated glutathione depletion, ALT and AST levels and reduced oxidative stress (Huang et al 2005). Additionally, further histopathological examination showed a significant reduction in the incidence of hepatic lesions and swelling. More recently it was found that baicalein significantly elevated the serum level of TNF-α and IL-6 in mice, in the early phase after liver injury was induced by carbon tetrachloride, suggesting that it may have a part to play in liver regeneration (Huang et al 2011).

IN COMBINATION

The combination Sho-saiko-to (a Japanese herbal supplement containing baical skullcap, also known as Minor Bupleurum Combination, and Xiao Chai Hu Tang in Mandarin) has been shown to inhibit chemical hepatocarcinogenesis in animals, act as a biological response modifier and suppress the proliferation of hepatoma cells by inducing apoptosis and arresting the cell cycle. These effects may be due to baicalin, baicalein and saikosaponins (from *Bupleurum falcatum*), which have the ability to inhibit cell proliferation (Shimizu 2000). Further testing is required to determine the role of baical skullcap in achieving these effects.

Antioxidant

Several studies have shown that baical skullcap constituents exert antioxidant activity in vitro and in vivo. Flavones produced a concentration-dependent protection of liposome membrane against ultraviolet-induced oxidation. The ability to scavenge free radicals and protect against the effects of lipid peroxidation (in this case, caused by sunlight irradiation) may in part account for the herb's underlying mechanism of action (Gabrielska et al 1997).

Fourteen flavonoids and flavone glycosides demonstrate good free radical-scavenging properties in vitro (Gao et al 1999, Lin & Shieh 1996). Baicalin has been found to have the most potent antioxidant effect (Bochorakova et al 2003).

Baicalin's antioxidant effect is based on scavenging superoxide radicals, whereas baicalein is a good xanthine oxidase inhibitor. Xanthine oxidase inhibitors are known to be therapeutically useful for the treatment of hepatitis and brain tumours (Gao et al 2001). Baicalin was also an efficient antioxidant in reducing hyperglycaemia-induced oxidative stress through the increased expression of antioxidant enzyme activities in rats (Waisundara et al 2011).

Oxidative stress plays an important role in the pathological process of neurodegenerative diseases, including Alzheimer's disease. The protective effects of baical flavonoids on the oxidative injury of neuronal cells have been demonstrated in vitro (Choi et al 2002, Gao et al 2001).

Antiallergic

Various flavonoids from baical skullcap, including wogonin and baicalein, have been shown to inhibit chemically induced histamine release from rat mast cells in vitro (Kubo et al 1984). *Scutellaria baicalensis* inhibited passive cutaneous anaphylaxis reaction and decreased histamine release in rat peritoneal mast cells. In human mast cells *S. baicalensis* moderated the allergic response by restoring IL-8 and TNF-α expression and inhibiting MAP kinase expression (Jung et al 2012).

Luteolin and baicalein have been shown to inhibit IgE antibody-mediated immediate and late-phase allergic reactions in mice. In an in vitro study, luteolin and baicalein inhibited IgE-mediated histamine release from mast cells. Wogonin, wogonoside and 3,5,7,2',6'-pentahydroxyl flavanone isolated from baical skullcap decrease histamine, leukotriene B_4 and IgE in vitro (Lim 2004).

In rats and in human mast cells baical skullcap inhibits IgE-mediated allergic reactions by decreasing histamine, and suppresssing IL-8 and TNF-alpha expression in human mast cells (Jung et al 2012, Kimata et al 2000).

Baicalein is 5–10-fold more potent than the antiallergic drug azelastine. Baicalein significantly suppressed leukotriene C_4 release by polymorphonuclear leucocytes obtained from asthmatic patients compared with healthy subjects (Niitsuma et al 2001).

Neuroprotective

Many in vitro and in vivo trials have demonstrated the neuroprotective effects of flavonoids derived from baical skullcap (Cho & Lee 2004, Heo et al 2004, Piao et al 2004, Shang et al 2006a, Son et al 2004). Gasiorowski et al (2011) suggest that the flavones of baical skullcap prevent neural injury through a strong antioxidant effect, by moderating inflammation and by increasing GABAergic signalling (anxiolytic and anticonvulsant effect) and that wogonin exerts neurogenerative action, based on in vitro and in vivo evidence.

Cerebral ischaemia can cause a significant elevation in the concentrations of amino acid neurotransmitters in the cerebral cortex. Baicalin administration can attenuate the elevations of glutamic acid and aspartic acid induced by cerebral ischaemia. This research demonstrates that baicalin may act as a neuroprotectant during cerebral ischaemia. Wogonin has been shown to exert a neuroprotective effect by inhibiting microglial activation, which is a critical component of pathogenic inflammatory responses in neurodegenerative diseases.

Baicalin (200 mg/kg) intraperitoneally injected into gerbils immediately after cerebral ischemia significantly improved neural dysfunction by reducing the damage to the gamma-aminobutyric acid (GABA)-inhibitory system, together with a protective effect observed at a protein-folding level (Dai et al 2013). In another gerbil model, baicalin injection immediately after induced ischaemia significantly reduced hippocampal neuronal damage at 100 and 200 mg/kg (Cao et al 2011). The investigators suspect the neuroprotective action is exerted via antioxidant (decreasing markers for lipid peroxidation), and antiapoptotic properties, increasing brain-derived neurotrophic factor, which inhibits caspase-3. These findings are significant as they suggest viable alternatives or adjuncts to the current treatment with thrombolytics. Comparatively, in a rat model of induced intracerebral haemorrhage, baicalin, injected intracerebrally, attenuated brain oedema and inhibited cell in a dose- and time-dependent manner, suggesting that baicalin has protective effects on intracerebral haemorrhage-induced brain injury (Zhou et al 2012).

An in vivo study in rats induced with permanent global ischaemia demonstrated that daily oral doses of baical skullcap flavonoids (35 mg/kg) for 19–20 days significantly increased learning and memory ability and attenuated neural injury (Shang et al 2005). A follow-up in vivo study demonstrated that the flavonoid fraction also reduced neural damage and memory deficits after permanent cerebral ischaemia (Shang et al 2006b). Huang lian jie du tang (HLJT) from China or oren gedoku to (Japan) is an important Asian multiherb combination remedy, containing *Scutellaria baicalensis*, which is clinically used to treat cerebral ischaemia (Zhu et al 2012).

It also appear that baical skullcap may have a role in neurogenerative disorders such as Parkinson's disease and Alzheimer's dementia. In induced memory loss model in rats treated with 30 mg/kg baical skullcap, increased numbers of cholinergic neurons (associated with memory and learning) were observed, along with and protected by *N*-methyl-D-aspartic receptors, which are associated with neuroplasticity (Heo et al 2009).

Mu et al (2009) also observed an antiapoptotic effect in a rat model of Parkinson's disease, as well as reduced tremor. In test tube and in vivo mouse model, Zhang et al (2013) noted that intraperitoneal injections of baicalin for 8 weeks retarded plaque formation and disease pathogenesis.

Another in vivo study investigated the neuroprotective effects of baicalein in a parkinsonian experimental model and demonstrated improved motor coordination and a reduction in spontaneous motor activity (Cheng et al 2008). This was thought to be the result of increased dopamine and serotonin levels in the striatum, leading to increased dopaminergic neurons and an inhibition of oxidative stress. Baical skullcap is used in traditional Chinese medicine (TCM) for the treatment of stroke. Methanol extracts from the dried roots (0.1–10 mg/kg intraperitoneally [IP]) significantly protected neurons against 10 minute transient forebrain ischaemia. The extract inhibited microglial TNF-alpha and NO production, and protected cells from hydrogen peroxide-induced toxicity in vitro (Kim et al 2001).

Hypotensive

Treatment with baicalein lowered blood pressure in hypertensive but not in normotensive rats according to one study (Takizawa et al 1998). Baical extract and baicalein have also been shown to lower blood pressure in rats and cats (Kaye et al 1997, Takizawa et al 1998). The exact mechanisms underlying the hypotensive action are unclear. One in vivo study has shown that *Scutellaria baicalensis* extract produces peripheral vasodilation (Lin et al 1980). A 2005 review concluded that baical skullcap is effective for renin-dependent hypertension and that in vivo effects may be due to the inhibition of lipoxygenase, reducing the production and release of arachidonic acid-derived vasoconstrictor substances (Huang et al 2005).

Vascular activity

Monocyte chemotactic protein-1 (MCP-1), a potent chemoattractant for monocytes, plays a crucial role in cases of early inflammatory responses, including atherosclerosis. Wogonin has been shown to inhibit MCP-1 induction by endothelial cells in a dose-dependent manner. Wogonin and baical skullcap may be potentially beneficial in inflammatory and vascular disorders (Chang et al 2001). Baicalein significantly suppressed intimal hyperplasia and cell proliferation in a vascular injury study in vivo (Peng et al 2008).

Antiplatelet

Baical flavonoids have been shown to inhibit platelet aggregation in vitro (Kubo et al 1985). Baicalein inhibited the elevation of calcium induced by thrombin and thrombin receptor agonist peptide. These findings suggest a potential benefit of baicalein in the treatment of arteriosclerosis and thrombosis (Kimura et al 1997).

Cholesterol reduction

Flavonoids are known to reduce cholesterol. A 30-day study of induced hyperlipidaemia in rats found that baicalein, quercetin, rutin and naringin reduced cholesterol, with baicalein the most potent. Baicalein was also the most effective flavonoid in reducing triglyceride levels (De Oliveira et al 2002). In another in vivo study, rats were fed a cholesterol-laden diet and half were also given *S. baicalensis* radix extract (Regulska-Ilow et al 2004). The treatment rats displayed a significant reduction in plasma triglycerides and total cholesterol compared with control animals. The mechanism may be due to the increased activity of lecithin cholesterol acyltransferase (You et al 2008).

Mice treated with 10 mg/kg of wogonin for 2 weeks had significantly decreased insulin, cholesterol, fat and glycogen accumulation in the liver and slowed weight gain, when compared with the control group (Bak et al 2013). Similarly, in an obese mouse model baical skullcap at 200 mg/kg for 4 weeks improved weight, hypertriglyceridaemia and hyperinsulinaemia, reduced ALT levels (a marker of liver damage) and restored metabolic process and insulin signalling pathways (Song et al 2013).

Anxiolytic

Wogonin, baicalein, scutellarein and baicalin (in reducing order of potency), which all contain a certain flavonoid phenyl benzopyrone nucleus, have been shown in vitro to bind with the benzodiazepine site of the GABA-A receptor (Hui et al 2000).

Oral administration of wogonin (7.5–30 mg/kg) has been shown to interact with GABA-A receptors and produce an anxiolytic response that was similar to diazepam in the elevated plus maze. Unlike benzodiazepines, wogonin was able to reduce anxiety without causing sedation or myorelaxation (Hui et al 2002, Kwok et al 2002).

Baicalin (10 mg/kg IP) and baicalin (20 mg/kg IP) have also been shown in vivo to produce an anxiolytic effect, mediated through activation of the benzodiazepine-binding sites of GABA-A receptors (Liao et al 2003).

Two other flavones, 5,7-dihydroxy-6-methoxyflavone (oroxylin A) and 5,7,2'-trihydroxy-6, 8-dimethoxyflavone (K36), also act as antagonists at the GABA-A recognition site and have demonstrated anxiolytic activity in vivo (Huen et al 2003a, 2003b).

A water extract of baical skullcap demonstrated anticonvulsant activity against electroshock-induced tonic seizures in vivo. Interestingly, the authors suggest that the effect might not be via the activation of the benzodiazepine-binding site of GABA-A receptors, but probably via the prevention of seizure spread (Liao et al 2003, Wang et al 2000). A more recent study has shown that wogonin has anticonvulsive effects mediated by GABA (Park et al 2007).

Hypnotic

In a rodent model baicalin exerted a biphasic effect on the sleep-wake cycle and exerted a delayed somnogenic effect by acting as a selective agonist of GABA receptors subtype A (Chang et al 2011). The authors speculate that the 8-hour delay to exert this effect may be due to low affinity for the receptor and also observe that another flavonoid, wogonin, has an antagonistic action on the same receptors, perhaps explaining why the whole plant is not traditionally noted for its hypnotic effect. An anxiolytic effect, via the GABA subtype A pathway and independently of a serotonergic effect, was also observed in a rodent model (de Carvalho et al 2011).

Antimicrobial

Numerous studies have found that baical extract and flavonoids exert antibacterial, antiviral and antifungal actions. The antimicrobial effect of baical extract is mild and the clinical efficacy of baical in infectious diseases may be more associated with its anti-inflammatory rather than its antimicrobial activities.

Antibacterial

Baical skullcap and its components have demonstrated antibacterial and bacteriostatic effects in vitro.

The addition of baicalein to standard antibiotic therapy for multiresistant *Staphylococcus aureus* (MRSA) prevents growth of the bacteria by increasing its susceptibility to the antibiotic ciprofloxacin, possibly by inhibiting the NorA efflux pump, which is known to pump the antibiotic out of the bacteria (Chan et al 2011). This finding provides optimism for the treatment of antibiotic-resistant bacterial strains.

Baical skullcap decoction was investigated for bacteriostatic and bactericidal activity against a selection of oral bacteria, including suspected periodontopathogens. At a concentration of 2%, the decoction was bacteriostatic for 8 of 11 bacteria tested, but a concentration of 3.13% or greater was required for bactericidal effect (Tsao et al 1982).

Baical aqueous extract, but not its flavonoids, baicalin and baicalein, demonstrated antibacterial effects against the enteric pathogen *Salmonella typhimurium*. The effect was compatible with commercial antibiotics, including ampicillin, chloramphenicol and streptomycin. In contrast, the growth of a non-pathogenic *Escherichia coli* strain was unaffected by baical (Hahm et al 2001). One study demonstrated that the addition of baical skullcap in vitro improved the responsiveness of antibiotics for the treatment of MRSA (Yang et al 2005). Baicalin has been shown to reduce the pathogenic effects of superantigenic staphylococcal exotoxins by inhibiting the signalling pathways activated by superantigens (Krakauer et al 2001).

Baicalin and *Scutellaria baicalensis* have been shown to be bactericidal against *Helicobacter pylori*, with the activity of the flavonoid baicalin greater than that of baical skullcap in assays (Wu et al 2008).

Antiviral

Antiviral effects have been demonstrated for baical in numerous in vitro and in vivo tests. Baical extract significantly inhibits hepatitis C RNA replication in vivo (Tang et al 2003) and in vitro studies have found that:

- Chloroform and ethyl acetate extracts of baical skullcap inhibited replication of influenza A virus subtypes in vitro, including pandemic 2009 H1N1, seasonal H1N1 and H3N2, via inhibition of neuraminidase by baicalin (Hour 2013). These findings are valuable in the development of antiviral agents; however, it must be noted that the solvent preparations used in this study do not reflect the traditional preparations of herbal medicines from Chinese or Western traditions.
- Intraperitoneal and intranasal administration of baical flavonoids significantly inhibits influenza virus in vivo and in vitro (Nagai et al 1989, 1992a, 1992b, 1995a, 1995b).
- Baicalein inhibits HIV-1 infection at the level of viral entry (a process known to involve interaction between HIV-1 envelope proteins and the cellular CD4 and chemokine receptors) (Li et al 2000b).
- Baicalin inhibits human T-cell leukaemia virus type I (Baylor et al 1992).
- Aqueous extract inhibits HIV-1 protease (Lam et al 2000).
- Baicalin inhibits HIV-1 infection and replication (Li et al 1993).
- Baical flavonoids inhibit Epstein-Barr virus early antigen activation (Konoshima et al 1992).
- Wogonin suppresses hepatitis B virus surface antigen production without evidence of cytotoxicity (Huang et al 2000).
- 5,7,4'-trihydroxy-8-methoxyflavone inhibits the fusion of influenza virus with endosome/lysosome membrane (Nagai et al 1995a).
- Virus replication is suppressed, partly by inhibiting the fusion of viral envelopes with the endosome/lysosome membrane, which occurs at the early stage of the virus infection cycle (Nagai et al 1995b).
- The flavones in baical have potent influenza virus sialidase-inhibitory activity and anti-influenza virus activity in vivo (Nagai et al 1992b).
- Baicalin may selectively induce apoptosis of HIV-infected human T-leukaemia (CEM-HIV) cells, which have a high virus-releasing capacity, and stimulate proliferation of CEM-HIV cells, which have a relatively lower capacity of HIV production (Wu et al 1995).
- In cell cultures and in mice, combinations of baicalein and ribavirin provided better protection against H1N1 influenza infection than each compound used alone and could potentially be clinically useful (Chen et al 2011).

Antifungal

Antifungal activity has been demonstrated by several studies (Blaszczyk et al 2000, Yang et al 1995). *Chlamydia trachomatis* was inhibited at doses of 0.12 and 0.48 mg/mL in vitro, by reducing CPAF expression, a protein which protects the infection was host immune defences (Hao et al 2009). Baical extract showed clear fungistatic activities in vitro against some cutaneous and unusual pathogenic fungi, and particularly against strains of *Candida albicans*, *Cryptococcus neoformans* and *Pityrosporum ovale*. The antifungal substance was isolated and found to be baicalein (Yang et al 1995). Of 56 Chinese antimicrobial plants, baical root extract had the highest activity against *Candida albicans* (Blaszczyk et al 2000).

Antiulcerogenic

Extracts prepared from grass and roots of *S. baicalensis* showed high antiulcerogenic activity in vivo (Amosova et al 1998). Pretreatment for 1 h with the flavonoid wogonin attenuated the rodent gastric mucosal damage in a dose-dependent fashion (3, 10, 30 mg/kg), with the protective effect being superior to the indicated medication rebamipide (Park 2004). This protective effect is exerted by inhibiting COX and lipoxygenase enzymes in the arachadonic acid pathway and the early induction of the anti-inflammatory PGE_2 as well as preventive apoptosis induction.

Antidiabetic

5-alpha-aldose inhibition

Diabetic patients may accumulate intracellular quantities of the sugars sorbitol and dulcitol, because of an increase in the polyol pathway involving the enzyme 5-alpha-aldose. Oral baicalin and liquid extract of licorice (also rich in flavonoids) reduced the sorbitol levels in the red blood cells of diabetic rats (Lin et al 1980, Zhou & Zhang 1989). *Scutellaria baicalensis* enhanced the antidiabetic effect of metformin in streptozocin-induced diabetic rats by improving the antioxidant status. It also increased pancreatic insulin content as well as improved the lipid profile in these rats (Waisundara et al 2008). And in healthy mice, administration of 10 mg/kg of wogonin produced improved glucose tolerance, reduced cholesterol and insulin, and reduced hepatic liver droplets when compared with controls (Bak et al 2013).

Alpha-glucosidase inhibition

Alpha-glucosidase inhibitors (e.g. acarbose) are a class of oral medicine for type 2 diabetes, which blocks the enzymes that digest starches in food. The result is a slower and lower rise in blood glucose throughout the day, especially immediately after meals. Methanol extracts of *S. baicalensis*, *Rheum officinale* and *Paeonia suffruticosa* showed potent inhibitory activity against rat intestinal sucrase. The active principles were identified as baicalein and methyl gallate (from the latter two plants). In addition to its activity against the rat enzyme, baicalein inhibited human intestinal sucrase in vitro (Nishioka et al 1998).

Antiemetic

Pretreatment with baical root extract has been shown to decrease cisplatin-induced pica in rats (animal models use the level of kaolin [type of clay] intake as a measure of the intensity of nausea). This suggests that baical may help to reduce cisplatin-induced nausea and emesis during cancer therapy (Aung et al 2003, Mehendale et al 2004, Wu et al 1995), although clinical testing is required to confirm significance.

Two in vivo trials found that *S. baicalensis* significantly attenuated ritonavir-induced pica, and demonstrated possible efficacy for the management of ritonavir-induced nausea in HIV treatment (Aung et al 2005, Mehendale et al 2007).

Renal–urinary tract activity

Baicalein inhibited angiotensin II-induced increases in the cellular protein content of aortic smooth-muscle cells in vitro (Natarajan et al 1994). In another in vitro study, baicalein prevented the angiotensin II-induced increase in renal vascular resistance by 50% and promoted glomerular filtration rate (Bell-Quilley et al 1993). Pretreatment with baicalein significantly inhibited a decrease in nephrotoxin-induced glomerular filtration rate and renal blood flow in vivo (Wu et al 1993). Oral intake of baical flavonoids and extract has been shown to produce a diuretic effect.

Anticancer

Immunostimulation (in combination)

Sho-saiko-to has been shown to stimulate granulocyte colony-stimulating factor (G-CSF), which may explain its use in infectious diseases and cancer (Yamashiki et al 1992). Like growth hormone, IL-2 and IL-4 and interferon, G-CSF is a signalling ligand that stimulates immune function. G-CSF, a glycoprotein produced mainly by macrophages, induces proliferation of neutrophil colonies and differentiation of precursor cells to neutrophils. It also stimulates the activity of mature neutrophils (Hill et al 1993).

Sho-saiko-to is known to significantly suppress cancer development in the liver. Moderate regulation of the cytokine production system in patients with hepatitis C with Sho-saiko-to may be useful in the prevention of disease progression (Yamashiki et al 1997). One possible mechanism for the beneficial effects of this formula in patients with liver cirrhosis may be the improvement in production of IL-12, which is an important cytokine for maintenance of normal systemic defence and bioregulation. This effect of Sho-saiko-to is attributed to two of its seven herb components, baical and licorice root (Yamashiki et al 1999).

Patients who were given baical skullcap showed a tendency towards an increase in the relative number of T lymphocytes and their theophylline-resistant population during antitumour chemotherapy. The immunoregulation index in this case was approximately twice the background value during the period of investigation. The inclusion of baical skullcap in the therapeutic complex promoted an increase in the number of IgA at a stable level of IgG (Smolianinov et al 1997).

Apoptosis induction

Baicalein, baicalin and wogonin have been shown to induce apoptosis, disrupt the mitochondria and inhibit proliferation in various human hepatoma cell lines (Chang et al 2002, Chen et al 2000). The platelet-type 12-lipoxygenase (12-LOX) pathway is a critical regulator of prostate cancer progression and apoptosis by affecting various proteins regulating these processes. Baicalein inhibits 12-LOX and may be a potential therapeutic agent in the treatment of prostate cancer (Pidgeon et al 2002) as well as breast cancer (Tong et al 2002) and lung cancer (Leung et al 2007). Crude ethanolic extracts of baical skullcap and its components baicalin, baicalein and wogonin are cytotoxic to lung cancer cell lines by inducing cell death, interfering with cell life cycles and regulating the expression of cyclin proteins (Gao 2010, Gao et al 2011).

Antiproliferative

Baicalein, baicalin and wogonin have been shown to induce apoptosis and inhibit proliferation in various human hepatoma cell lines (Chang et al 2002).

Baicalin has been shown to inhibit the proliferation of prostate cancer cells in vitro. However, the response to baicalin differed among different cell lines (Chan et al 2000). Whereas a baicalin-deprived fraction of baical skullcap arrested the growth of, and induced apoptosis of, breast cancer cell lines in an in vitro model, a whole extract of baical skullcap actually promoted cell growth (Wang et al 2010). Similar outcomes were observed on multiple myeloma cells exposed to wogonin in vitro (Zhang et al 2013).

COX-2, which converts arachidonic acid to PGE_2, is highly expressed in head and neck squamous cell carcinoma (HNSCC). *S. baicalensis*, but not baicalein, suppressed proliferation, cell nuclear antigen expression and PGE_2 synthesis. A 66% reduction in tumour mass was observed in the mice with HNSCC. Baical selectively and effectively inhibits cancer cell growth in vitro and in vivo and can be an effective chemotherapeutic agent for HNSCC (Zhang et al 2003).

In a study designed to determine the ability of baical skullcap to inhibit various human cancer cells in vitro, *S. baicalensis* demonstrated a significant dose-dependent growth inhibition on squamous cell carcinoma, breast cancer, hepatocellular carcinoma, prostate carcinoma and colon cancer cell lines (Ye et al 2002). Prostate and breast cancer cells were particularly sensitive. Baical skullcap has also been shown to arrest mouse leukaemia cell proliferation in vivo (Ciesielska et al 2002, 2004). Inhibition of PGE_2 synthesis via suppression of COX-2 expression may be responsible for its anticancer activity (Ye et al 2002). Differences in the biological effects of baical compared with baicalein suggest synergistic effects among components in baical (Zhang et al 2003). Another study has shown complete inhibition of acute lymphatic leukaemia, myeloma and lymphoma cell lines in vitro (Kumagai et al 2007). Baicalein, baicalin and wogonin have been shown to reduce proliferation of human bladder cancer cell lines in a dose-dependent manner, but baicalin exhibited the greatest antiproliferative activity. In an in vivo study baical skullcap extract had a significant inhibition of tumour growth ($P < 0.05$) (Ikemoto et al 2000).

Baical skullcap significantly inhibited prostate-specific antigen production and reduced PGE_2 synthesis via direct inhibition of COX-2 activity in vitro (Ye et al 2007). The extract also reduced cyclin D1, resulting in a G1 phase arrest, and inhibited cyclin-dependent kinase 1 (cdk1) expression and kinase activity, leading to a G2/M cell cycle arrest. An animal study reported a 50% reduction in tumour volume after 7 weeks (Ye et al 2007). Another study found that baicalein, wogonin, neobaicalein and skullcap flavone inhibited prostate cancer cell proliferation in vitro (Bonham et al 2005). Additionally, the in vivo phase of the study found that baicalein (20 mg/kg/day) reduced the growth of prostate cancer xenografts in mice by 55% after 2 weeks.

Wogonin inhibited phorbol 12-myristate 13-acetate-induced COX-2 protein and mRNA levels in human lung epithelial cancer cells (Chen et al 2008). It appears that this was due to activator protein 1 inhibition. *Scutellaria baicalensis* stem leaf total flavonoid inhibited the proliferation of vascular smooth-muscle cells directly by blocking cell cycle progression, and the ERK signal transduction way possibly participated in the cytoprotection of the flavonoid (Luo et al 2009).

Adjunct to chemotherapy

Baical skullcap shows promise as an adjunct to cancer therapy. In a cardiomyocyte in vivo model, baical skullcap attenuated the production of reactive oxygen species, cell death and cardiotoxicity typically associated with the chemotherapy drug doxorubicin (Chang et al 2011). Similarly, wogonin selectively inhibited apoptosis induced by the chemotherapy drug etoposide in normal cells, while potentiating it in tumour cells (Enomoto et al 2011). These studies suggest that components of baical skullcap show promise as adjunctive therapy in cancer treatment.

In a mouse model the combination of *S. baicalensis* and Qing-Shu-Yi-Qi-Tang alongside chemotherapy drugs minimises drug-induced cachexia, is actively anti-inflammatory, selectively cytotoxic to tumour cells and suppresses tumour growth (Wang et al 2012).

In experiments with murine and rat transplantable tumours, baical skullcap extract treatment improved cyclophosphamide and 5-fluorouracil-induced myelotoxicity and decreased tumour cell viability (Razina et al 1987). Wogonin has also demonstrated the ability to hasten etoposide-induced apoptotic cell death (Lee et al 2007). Another in vitro study found that wogonin increased apoptosis and induced cell cycle arrest at the G2/M phase (Himeji et al 2007).

Prevention of metastases

The advancement of Pliss' lymphosarcoma in rats is associated with disorders of platelet-mediated haemostasis, presenting with either lowered or increased aggregation activity of platelets. Extract of baical was shown to produce a normalising effect on platelet-mediated haemostasis whatever the pattern of alteration. This activity is thought to be important for antitumour and, particularly, metastasis-preventing effects (Razina et al 1989).

Experiments in mice inoculated with metastasising Lewis lung carcinoma showed that the antitumour and antimetastatic effects of cyclophosphamide are potentiated by baical, rose root (*Rhodiola rosea*), licorice (*Glycyrrhiza glabra*) and their principal acting components, baicalin, paratyrosol and glycyrrhizin (Razina et al 2000).

Chemoprevention

Baicalein prevents chemically induced DNA damage in a cell culture model (Chan et al 2002).

Antiangiogenesis

Baicalein, wogonin and baicalin have demonstrated anticancer activity against several cancers in vitro. The flavonoids have also been shown to be potent inhibitors of angiogenesis in vitro and in vivo. Baicalein was found to be more potent than baicalin (Liu et al 2003). Wogonin also exerts a potent anti-angiogenesis action on breast cancer cells lines, both in vivo and in vitro (Song 2013). Baical flavonoids inhibit hepatic cytochromes CYP1A2 and CYP3A2 in vitro and in vivo (de Boer et al 2005, Kim et al 2002).

Noise-induced hearing loss

A controlled mouse model was used by Kang et al (2010) to observe the effect of baical skullcap, baicalein and baicalin fractions on noise-induced hearing loss (NIHL), by exposing the mice to various noise intensities over 35 days. The results indicated the baical skullcap is protective in mild NIHL rather than severe NIHL, and that the flavonoid baicalein is largely responsible for this action.

CLINICAL USE

Baical skullcap is an ingredient in the very popular traditional Chinese/Japanese formulation, Minor Bupleurum Combination, also known as Xiao Chai Hu Tang (Chinese) and Sho-saiko-to (Japanese). Minor Bupleurum Combination has been used in China for about 3000 years for the treatment of pyretic diseases.

Minor Bupleurum Combination (Sho-saiko-to) is now a prescription drug approved by the Ministry of Health and Welfare of Japan and widely used in the treatment of chronic viral liver diseases. Since 1999, Sho-saiko-to has been administered to 1.5 million patients with chronic liver diseases, because it can significantly suppress cancer development in the liver (Yamashiki et al 1999). Sho-saiko-to is also used for the treatment of bronchial asthma in Japan (Nakajima et al 2001). As such, many studies have been conducted with the herbal combination, making it difficult to determine the role of baical skullcap as a stand-alone treatment.

Respiratory infection

Sixty patients with respiratory infection (mainly hospital-acquired pneumonia) were treated by injection of either baical compound or piperacillin sodium (intravenously). The total efficacy was evaluated after treatment for 1 week, after which it was found that total effective treatment rates were 73.3% for baical compared with 76.7% in the antibiotic treatment group. Body temperature was decreased similarly and symptoms disappeared or were relieved in 11.67 ± 6.75 days with the herb and 11.53 ± 7.30 days with the antibiotic. In the piperacillin sodium group, fungal infections occurred in 4 of 30 patients, but there were none in the baical treatment group (Lu 1990).

Bone marrow stimulation during chemotherapy

Haemopoiesis was studied in 88 patients with lung cancer during combination treatment with chemotherapy and a *S. baicalensis* extract. Administration of the plant preparation was associated with haemopoiesis stimulation, intensification of bone marrow erythrocytopoiesis and granulocytopoiesis, and increased numbers of circulating precursors of erythroid and granulomonocytic colony-forming units (Goldberg et al 1997).

Epilepsy (in combination with other herbs)

Saiko-keishi-to, a spray-dried decoction of bupleurum (cinnamon, peony, ginger, licorice, ginseng, pinellia, zizyphus and baical) was administered to 24 people with epilepsy who had frequent uncontrollable seizures (3–5 seizures per day in the most severe case and 5 seizures per month in the mildest case) of various types, despite treatment with pharmaceutical anticonvulsants. Of them, six were well controlled with Saiko-keishi-to, whereas thirteen experienced improvement and three showed no effect. No patients experienced worsening of their condition. Two patients dropped out during treatment (Narita et al 1982).

Chronic active hepatitis (in combination with other herbs)

In a double-blind, multicentre clinical study of 222 patients with chronic active hepatitis, Sho-saiko-to was found to significantly decrease AST and ALT values compared with placebo. The difference between the treatment and placebo groups in the mean value was significant after 12 weeks. In patients with chronic active hepatitis type B (HB), a tendency towards a decrease of HBe antigen and an increase of anti-HBe antibodies was also observed. No remarkable side effects were noticed (Hirayama et al 1989).

Liver fibrosis (in combination with other herbs)

Minor Bupleurum Combination (Sho-saiko-to) has been shown to play a chemopreventive role in the development of hepatocellular carcinoma in cirrhotic patients in a prospective study, and several studies have demonstrated the preventive and therapeutic effects of Sho-saiko-to on experimental hepatic fibrosis (Shimizu 2000). Sho-saiko-to has been shown to inhibit the activation of hepatic stellate cells, the major collagen-producing cells. Sho-saiko-to has a potent antifibrotic effect by inhibiting oxidative stress in hepatocytes and hepatic stellate cells. It is proposed that the active components are baicalin and baicalein, because they both have chemical structures very similar to silybinin, the active compound in *Silybum marianum* (St Mary's thistle), which exhibits antifibrotic activities. Sho-saiko-to combined with silymarin in 90 patients with hepatitis B-related liver fibrosis due to chronic hepatitis B virus improved indexes of liver function and serum liver fibrosis in the therapy group, while clearance of hepatitis B virus was comparable to control group (Bing et al 2010).

Gingivitis

In a randomised, controlled and blinded clinical gingivitis model, a topical preparation of 0.5% baical skullcap extract plus fluoride significantly reduced the severity of gingivitis and plaque development when compared with the control group, fluoride alone, which is an established therapy (Arweiler et al 2011). The participants rinsed with either preparation twice daily for 21 days, with the treatment group experiencing dramatic improvements. While the methods, including randomisation and blinding, are well described, a description of the type of extract, such as solvent, is not detailed.

OTHER USES

Because of its wide range of pharmacological effects, baical skullcap is used for many different indications. Although controlled trials are not yet available to determine its effectiveness, evidence from in vitro and animal studies provides a theoretical basis for the following uses:

- chronic inflammatory conditions such as asthma, arthritis and allergies (antiallergic and anti-inflammatory effects)
- hepatitis (as a hepatoprotective agent)
- common infections such as the common cold (antimicrobial and immunostimulant effects)
- nausea and vomiting (antiemetic effect).
- In practice, baical skullcap is used in combination with other herbs for these conditions.

DOSAGE RANGE

- Dried herb: 6–15 g/day (Bensky & Gamble 1986).
- Liquid extract (1:2): 30–60 mL/week or 4.5–8.5 mL/day in divided doses.

ADVERSE REACTIONS

There have been several case reports of interstitial pneumonia and acute respiratory failure associated with Japanese kampo medicines, specifically the formula Sho-saiko-to, and the content of baicalin is thought to be responsible for the reactions (Makino et al 2008). The incidence is increased by co-administration of interferon, duration of medication use, with the risk being greater in elderly populations (Lee et al 2011). One case of Sho-saiko-to-induced pneumonia in a patient with autoimmune hepatitis was reported (Katou & Mori 1999); however, direct toxicity is very low. Makino et al (2008) suggest that it is the high amount of baicalin (319 mg/day) in Oren-ge-doku-to and Sho-saiko-to which is responsible for the adverse drug reactions, and that the small amount derived from a tea, 12–27 mg, is safe.

Toxicity studies of three different traditional Chinese/Japanese formulations containing baical suggest a very low acute or subchronic toxicity for the herbs in them. The studies found no herb-related abnormalities such as changes in body weight or food consumption, abnormalities on ophthalmological and haematological examination, urinalysis and gross pathological examination, changes in organ weight or optical microscopic examination (Iijima et al 1995, Kanitani et al 1995, Kobayashi et al 1995, Minematsu et al 1992, 1995). The acute lethal activity of wogonin is low, with an LD_{50} of 3.9 g/kg (Kwok et al 2002).

SIGNIFICANT INTERACTIONS

There are reports of baical flavonoids interacting with P450 enzymes. Baical flavonoids inhibit hepatic CYP1A2 (Kim et al 2002) and CYP2E1 expression (Jang et al 2003). Theoretically, inhibition of CYP1A2 and CYP2E1 may affect certain medical drugs metabolised by these P450 enzymes. There are, however, no clinical reports of such herb–drug interactions.

A theoretical interaction may occur in the co-administration of ciprofloxacin, whereby baical skullcap makes more of the drug available to the bacteria (Ben 2011). Similarly, wogonin could theoretically interact and reduce drug-resistant breast cancer lines to the chemotherapeutic agent, doxorubicin (Zhong et al 2012).

Sho-saiko-to during interferon therapy

Sho-saiko-to, as well as interferon, is used for the treatment of chronic hepatitis. There have been reports of acute pneumonitis due to a possible interferon–herb interaction. Pneumonitis, also called extrinsic allergic alveolitis, is a complex syndrome caused by sensitisation to an allergen. The mechanism of the Sho-saiko-to–interferon interaction seems to be due to an allergic–immunological mechanism rather than direct toxicity (Ishizaki et al 1996) — contraindicated.

Cyclosporin

A decoction of *Scutellaria baicalensis* has been reported to significantly decrease plasma levels of cyclosporin in rats. The co-administration of these two substances should be avoided until further research is available (Lai et al 2004).

Warfarin/anticoagulants

Increased risk of bleeding is theoretically possible — use with caution.

CONTRAINDICATIONS AND PRECAUTIONS

Baical skullcap and the formulation Sho-saiko-to (Minor Bupleurum Combination, Xiao Chai Hu Tang) are contraindicated during interferon therapy. Baical is contraindicated in cold conditions in TCM.

PREGNANCY USE

Baical is used in TCM for restless fetus (threatened abortion) and toxaemia of pregnancy. A recent animal study found that baical skullcap combined with *Atractylodes macrocephala* had an antiabortive effect through inhibition of maternal–fetal interface immunity. The herbs prevented lipopolysaccharide-induced abortion by reducing natural killer cells and IL-2 activity (Zhong et al 2002). Although this is encouraging, safety in pregnancy is still unknown.

Practice points/Patient counselling

- Baical skullcap is a traditional Chinese herb used to treat fever, cough with thick yellow sputum, thirst and irritability, nausea, jaundice and diarrhoea.
- Baical skullcap extract, many of its constituents, and as part of herbal combination treatments, has been studied in many different experimental models. However, few clinical trials have been conducted using baical as a stand-alone treatment.
- It is used to treat chronic inflammatory conditions such as asthma, arthritis and allergy, because of its anti-inflammatory and antiallergic effects.
- It is used as a hepatoprotective agent in the treatment of hepatitis.
- Because of its antimicrobial and immunostimulant effects, baical is used to treat infections such as the common cold and bronchitis.
- Antiemetic effects suggest a role in nausea and vomiting.
- Hypotensive activity demonstrated in various animal models provides a basis for its use in hypertension.
- In practice, it is combined with other herbal medicines for a more targeted approach.
- Anti-inflamatory, antiallergic, antidiabetic, neuroprotective, antifibrotic and hepatoprotective effects of baical skullcap have been demonstrated repeatedly in in vitro and in vivo models.

PATIENTS' FAQs

What can this herb do for me?

Baical skullcap may be useful as an adjunctive therapy during cancer treatment to reduce nausea and immune suppression. Baical skullcap may also be beneficial in the treatment of vascular disorders, allergies, liver disease and infections, hypertension and arthritis; however, effectiveness is largely unknown.

When will it start to work?

For acute allergic and infectious conditions, the beneficial effects of baical skullcap should be noticeable within a few days. For chronic diseases, long-term use is recommended.

Are there any safety issues?

Baical skullcap is a safe and non-toxic herb which is used in both acute and chronic conditions. It should only be used during pregnancy on the recommendation of a healthcare practitioner. Baical and the formulation Sho-saiko-to (Minor Bupleurum Combination, known as Xiao Chai Hu Tang in Mandarin) are contraindicated during interferon therapy.

REFERENCES

Akao T et al. Baicalin, the predominant flavone glucuronide of *Scutellariae radix*, is absorbed from the rat gastrointestinal tract as the aglycone and restored to its original form. J Pharm Pharmacol 52.12 (2000): 1563–8.

Amosova EN et al. The search for new anti-ulcer agents from plants in Siberia and the Far East. Eksp Klin Farmakol 61.6 (1998): 31–5.

Arweiler NB et al. Clinical and antibacterial effect of an anti-inflammatory toothpaste formulation with *Scutellaria baicalensis* extract on experimental gingivitis. Clin Oral Investig (2011) 15(6):909–13.

Aung HH et al. *Scutellaria baicalensis* extract decreases cisplatin-induced pica in rats. Cancer Chemother Pharmacol 52.6 (2003): 453–8.

Aung HH et al. *Scutellaria baicalensis* decreases ritonavir-induced nausea. AIDS Res Ther 2.1 (2005): 12.

Bak EJ et al. Wogonin ameliorates hyperglycemia and dyslipidemia via PPARα activation in db/db mice. Clin Nutr (2013) S0261-5614(13)00091-5.

Bao QL et al. The flavonoid baicalin exhibits anti-inflammatory activity by binding to chemokines. Immunopharmacology 49.3 (2000): 295–306.

Baylor NW et al. Inhibition of human T cell leukemia virus by the plant flavonoid baicalin (7-glucuronic acid, 5,6-dihydroxyflavone). J Infect Dis 16.3 (1992): 433–7.

B

Bell-Quilley CP et al. Renovascular actions of angiotensin II in the isolated kidney of the rat: Relationship to lipoxygenases. J Pharmacol Exper Ther 267.2 (1993): 676–82.
Bensky D, Gamble A. Chinese herbal medicine: Materia Medica. Seattle: Eastland Press, 1986.
Bing QUI et al. Analysis of the clinical effect of sha-saiko-to combined with silymarin on liver fibrosis due to chronic hepatitis B. Chinese Journal Of Primary Medicine And Pharmacy (2010) 17(1): 1008–6706.
Blaszczyk T, et al. Screening for antimycotic properties of 56 traditional Chinese drugs. Phytother Res 14.3 (2000): 210–12.
Bochorakova H et al. Main flavonoids in the root of *Scutellaria baicalensis* cultivated in Europe and their comparative antiradical properties. Phytother Res 17.6 (2003): 640–4.
Bonham M et al. Characterization of chemical constituents in *Scutellaria baicalensis* with antiandrogenic and growth-inhibitory activities toward prostate carcinoma. Clin Cancer Res 11.10 (2005): 3905–14.
Butenko IG, et al. Anti-inflammatory properties and inhibition of leukotriene C4 biosynthesis in vitro by flavonoid baicalein from *Scutellaria baicalensis* georgi roots. Agents Actions 39 (Spec. No.) (1993): C49–51.
Byoung KP et al. Inhibition of TPA-induced cyclooxygenase-2 expression and skin inflammation in mice by wogonin, a plant flavone from *Scutellaria radix*. Eur J Pharmacol 425.2 (2001): 153–7.
Cao Y et al. Baicalin attenuates global cerebral ischemia/reperfusion injury in gerbils via anti-oxidative and anti-apoptotic pathways. Brain Research Bulletin 85 (2011) 396–402.
Chan FL et al. Induction of apoptosis in prostate cancer cell lines by a flavonoid, baicalin. Cancer Lett 160.2 (2000): 219–28.
Chan HY et al. Baicalein inhibits DMBA-DNA adduct formation by modulating CYP1A1 and CYP1B1 activities. Biomed Pharmacother 56.6 (2002): 269–75.
Chan BCL et al. Synergistic effects of baicalein with ciprofloxacin against NorA over-expressed methicillin-resistant *Staphylococcus aureus* (MRSA) and inhibition of MRSA pyruvate kinase. J Ethnopharmacol 137 (2011) 767–773.
Chang YL et al. Chinese herbal remedy wogonin inhibits monocyte chemotactic protein-1 gene expression in human endothelial cells. Mol Pharmacol 60.3 (2001): 507–13.
Chang W-H, et al. Different effects of baicalein, baicalin and wogonin on mitochondrial function, glutathione content and cell cycle progression in human hepatoma cell lines. Planta Med 68.2 (2002): 128–32.
Chang WT et al. Baicalein protects against doxorubicin-induced cardiotoxicity by attenuation of mitochondrial oxidant injury and JNK activation. J Cell Biochem (2011) 112(10):2873–81.
Chen L et al. Synergistic activity of baicalein with ribavirin against influenza A (H1N1) virus infections in cell culture and in mice. Antiviral Research 91(3) (2011); 314–320.
Chen C-H et al. Baicalein, a novel apoptotic agent for hepatoma cell lines: A potential medicine for hepatoma. Nutr Cancer 38.2 (2000): 287–95.
Chen YC et al. Wogonin, baicalin, and baicalein inhibition of inducible nitric oxide synthase and cyclooxygenase-2 gene expressions induced by nitric oxide synthase inhibitors and lipopolysaccharide. Biochem Pharmacol 61.11 (2001): 1417–27.
Chen LG et al. Wogonin, a bioactive flavonoid in herbal tea, inhibits inflammatory cyclooxygenase-2 gene expression in human lung epithelial cancer cells. Mol Nutr Food Res 52.11 (2008): 1349–57.
Chen Y et al. Wogonoside inhibits lipopolysaccharide-induced angiogenesis in vitro and in vivo via toll-like receptor 4 signal transduction. Toxicology (2009) 259(1–2):10-7.
Cheng PY et al. Protective effect of baicalein against endotoxic shock in rats in vivo and in vitro. Biochem Pharmacol 73.6 (2007): 793–804.
Cheng Y et al. Neuroprotective effect of baicalein against MPTP neurotoxicity: Behavioral, biochemical and immunohistochemical profile. Neurosci Lett 441.1 (2008): 16–20.
Chi YS, et al. Effect of wogonin, a plant flavone from *Scutellaria radix*, on the suppression of cyclooxygenase-2 and the induction of inducible nitric oxide synthase in lipopolysaccharide-treated RAW 264.7 cells. Biochem Pharmacol 61.10 (2001): 1195–203.
Chi YS et al. Effects of wogonin, a plant flavone from *Scutellaria radix*, on skin inflammation: in vivo regulation of inflammation-associated gene expression. Biochem Pharmacol 66.7 (2003): 1271–8.
Cho J, Lee HK. Wogonin inhibits ischemic brain injury in a rat model of permanent middle cerebral artery occlusion. Biol Pharm Bull 27.10 (2004): 1561–4.
Choi J et al. Flavones from *Scutellaria baicalensis* Georgi attenuate apoptosis and protein oxidation in neuronal cell lines. Biochim Biophys Acta Gen Subj 1571.3 (2002): 201–10.
Chung CP, et al. Pharmacological effects of methanolic extract from the root of *Scutellaria baicalensis* and its flavonoids on human gingival fibroblast. Planta Med 61.2 (1995):150–3.
Ciesielska E, et al. Anticancer, antiradical and antioxidative actions of novel Antoksyd S and its major components, baicalin and baicalein. Anticancer Res 22.5 (2002): 2885–91.
Ciesielska E et al. In vitro antileukemic, antioxidant and prooxidant activities of Antoksyd S (C/E/XXI): a comparison with baicalin and baicalein. In Vivo 18.4 (2004): 497–503.
Dai J et al. Activations of GABAergic signaling, HSP70 and MAPK cascades are involved in baicalin's neuroprotection against gerbil global ischemia/reperfusion injury. Brain Res Bull (2013) 90:1–9.
de Boer JG et al. Protection against aflatoxin-B1-induced liver mutagenesis by *Scutellaria baicalensis*. Mutat Res 578.1–2 (2005): 15–22.
De Carvalho RS et al. Involvement of GABAergic non-benzodiazepine sites in the anxiolytic-like and sedative effects of the flavonoid baicalein in mice. Behavioural Brain Research 221 (2011) 75–82.
De Oliveira TT et al. Effect of different doses of flavonoids on hyperlipidemic rats. Rev Nutr 15.1 (2002): 45–51 [in Portuguese].
Enomoto R et al. Wogonin potentiates the antitumor action of etoposide and ameliorates its adverse effects. Cancer Chemother Pharmacol (2011) 67(5):1063–72.
Gabrielska J et al. Antioxidant activity of flavones from *Scutellaria baicalensis* in lecithin liposomes. Z Naturforsch [C] 52.11–12 (1997): 817–23.
Gao J. Secondary metabolite mapping identifies *Scutellaria* inhibitors of human lung cancer cells. Journal of Pharmaceutical and Biomedical Analysis 53 (2010) 723–728.
Gao Z et al. Free radical scavenging and antioxidant activities of flavonoids extracted from the radix of *Scutellaria baicalensis* Georgi. Biochim Biophys Acta 1472.3 (1999): 643–50.
Gao Z, et al. Protective effects of flavonoids in the roots of *Scutellaria baicalensis* Georgi against hydrogen peroxide-induced oxidative stress in HS-SY5Y cells. Pharmacol Res 43.2 (2001): 173–8.
Gao J et al. The ethanol extract of *Scutellaria baicalensis* and the active compounds induce cell cycle arrest and apoptosis including upregulation of p53 and Bax in human lung cancer cells. Toxicol and App Pharmacol 254(3) (2011): 221–228.
Gasiorowski K et al. Flavones from the root of *Scutellaria baicalensis* Georgi: drugs of the future im neurogengeration. CNS & Neur Disorders and Drug Targers. (2011) 10(2): 184–191.
Goldberg VE et al. Dry extract of *Scutellaria baicalensis* as a hemostimulant in antineoplastic chemotherapy in patients with lung cancer. Eksp Klin Farmakol 60.6 (1997): 28–30.
Hahm D-H et al. Effect of *Scutellariae radix* as a novel antibacterial herb on the ppk (polyphosphate kinase) mutant of *Salmonella typhimurium*. J Microbiol Biotechnol 11.6 (2001): 1061–5.
Hardeland R, Poeggeler B. Non-vertebrate melatonin. J Pineal Res 34.4 (2003): 233–41.
Hao H et al. Baicalin suppresses expression of *Chlamydia* protease-like activity factor in Hep-2 cells infected by *Chlamydia trachomatis*. Fitoterapia 80(7) (2009): 448–452.
Heo HJ et al. Potent inhibitory effect of flavonoids in *Scutellaria baicalensis* on amyloid beta protein-induced neurotoxicity. J Agric Food Chem 52.13 (2004): 4128–32.
Heo H et al. Memory improvement in ibotenic acid induced model rats by extracts of *Scutellaria baicalensis*. J Ethnopharmacol (2009) 122(1):20–7.
Hill CP, et al. The structure of granulocyte-colony-stimulating factor and its relationship to other growth factors. Proc Natl Acad Sci USA 90.11 (1993): 5167–71.
Himeji M et al. Difference of growth-inhibitory effect of *Scutellaria baicalensis*-producing flavonoid wogonin among human cancer cells and normal diploid cell. Cancer Lett 245.1–2. (2007): 269–74.
Hirayama C et al. A multicenter randomized controlled clinical trial of Sho-saiko-to in chronic active hepatitis. Gastroenterol Jpn 24.6 (1989): 715–19.
Hong T et al. Evaluation of the anti-inflammatory effect of baicalein on dextran sulfate sodium-induced colitis in mice. Planta Med 68.3 (2002): 268–71.
Hour MJ. Baicalein, Ethyl Acetate, and Chloroform Extracts of *Scutellaria baicalensis* Inhibit the Neuraminidase Activity of Pandemic 2009 H1N1 and Seasonal Influenza A Viruses. Evidence-Based Complementary and Alternative Medicine. Volume 2013, Article ID 750803,
Hsieh CJ et al. Baicalein inhibits IL-1beta- and TNF-alpha-induced inflammatory cytokine production from human mast cells via regulation of the NF-kappaB pathway. Clin Mol Allergy 5 (2007): 5.
Huang RL et al. Anti-hepatitis B virus effects of wogonin isolated from *Scutellaria baicalensis*. Planta Med 66.8 (2000): 694–8.
Huang Y et al. Biological properties of baicalein in cardiovascular system. Curr Drug Targets Cardiovasc Haematol Disord 5.2 (2005): 177–84.
Huang WH, et al. Antioxidative and anti-inflammatory activities of polyhydroxyflavonoids of *Scutellaria baicalensis* Georgi. Biosci Biotechnol Biochem 70.10 (2006): 2371–80.
Huang HL et al. Hepatoprotective effects of baicalein against CCl_4-induced acute liver injury in mice. World J Gastroenterol 18(45) (2011): 6605–13.
Huen MS et al. Naturally occurring 2'-hydroxyl-substituted flavonoids as high-affinity benzodiazepine site ligands. Biochem Pharmacol 66.12 (2003a): 2397–407.

Huen MS et al. 5,7-Dihydroxy-6-methoxyflavone, a benzodiazepine site ligand isolated from *Scutellaria baicalensis* Georgi, with selective antagonistic properties. Biochem Pharmacol 66.1 (2003b): 125–32.

Hui KM, et al. Interaction of flavones from the roots of *Scutellaria baicalensis* with the benzodiazepine site. Planta Med 66.1 (2000): 91–3.

Hui KM et al. Anxiolytic effect of wogonin, a benzodiazepine receptor ligand isolated from *Scutellaria baicalensis* Georgi. Biochem Pharmacol 64.9 (2002): 1415–24.

Iijima OT et al. A single oral dose toxicity study and a 13-week repeated dose study with a 4-week recovery period of Tsumura Saiko-ka-ryukotsu-borei to (TJ-12) in rats. Jpn Pharmacol Ther 23 (Suppl. 7) (1995): 53–67 [in Japanese].

Ikemoto S et al. Antitumor effects of *Scutellariae radix* and its components baicalein, baicalin and wogonin on bladder cancer cell lines. Urology 55.6 (2000): 951–5.

Ishizaki T et al. Pneumonitis during interferon and/or herbal drug therapy in patients with chronic active hepatitis. Eur Respir J 9.12 (1996): 2691–6.

Jang SI et al. Hepatoprotective effect of baicalin, a major flavone from *Scutellaria radix*, on acetaminophen-induced liver injury in mice. Immunopharmacol Immunotoxicol 25.4 (2003): 585–94.

Jung HS et al. Antiallergic effects of *Scutellaria baicalensis* on inflammation in vivo and in vitro. J Ethnopharmacol (2012) 141(1):345–9.

Kang TH et al. Effect of baicalein from *Scutellaria baicalensis* on prevention of noise-induced hearing loss. Neurosci Lett 2010 469(3): 298–302.

Kanitani M et al. A single oral dose toxicity study and a 13-week repeated dose study with a 4-week recovery period of Tsumura Sairei-to (TJ-114) in rats. Jpn Pharmacol Ther 23 (Suppl. 7) (1995): 371–87 [in Japanese].

Katou K, Mori K. Autoimmune hepatitis with drug-induced pneumonia due to Sho-saiko-to. Nippon Kokyuki Gakkai Zasshi 37.8 (1999): 641–6.

Kaye AD et al. Effects of phospholipase A2, 12-lipoxygenase, and cyclooxygenase inhibitors in the feline pulmonary bed. Am J Physiol 272.4 (1997): L573–9.

Kim YO et al. Cytoprotective effect of *Scutellaria baicalensis* in CA1 hippocampal neurons of rats after global cerebral ischemia. J Ethnopharmacol 77.2–3 (2001): 183–8.

Kim J-Y et al. Effects of flavonoids isolated from *Scutellariae radix* on cytochrome P-450 activities in human liver microsomes. J Toxicol Environ Health 65.5–6 (2002): 373–81.

Kim DH et al. Short-term feeding of baicalin inhibits age-associated NF-kappaB activation. Mech Ageing Dev 127.9 (2006): 719–25.

Kim EH et al. Anti-inflammatory effects of *Scutellaria baicalensis* extract via suppression of immune modulators and MAP kinase signaling molecules. J Ethnopharmacol 126 (2009) 320–331.

Kimata M et al. Effects of luteolin and other flavonoids on IgE-mediated allergic reactions. Planta Med 66.1 (2000): 25–29.

Kimura Y et al. Effects of flavonoids isolated from *Scutellariae radix* on the production of tissue-type plasminogen activator and plasminogen activator inhibitor-1 induced by thrombin and thrombin receptor agonist peptide in cultured human umbilical vein endothelial cells. J Pharm Pharmacol 49.8 (1997): 816–22.

Kobayashi Y et al. A single oral dose toxicity study and a 13-week repeated dose study with a 4-week recovery period of Tsumura Oren-gedoku-to (TJ-15) in rats. Jpn Pharmacol Ther 23 (Suppl. 7) (1995): 69–89 [in Japanese].

Kong EKC. Novel anti-fibrotic agent, baicalein, for the treatment of myocardial fibrosis in spontaneously hypertensive rats. (2–3) 658 (2011) 175–181.

Konoshima T et al. Studies on inhibitors of skin tumor promotion. XI. Inhibitory effects of flavonoids from *Scutellaria baicalensis* on Epstein-Barr virus activation and their anti-tumor-promoting activities. Tokyo: Chem Pharm Bull 40.2 (1992): 531–3.

Krakauer T, et al. The flavonoid baicalin inhibits superantigen-induced inflammatory cytokines and chemokines. FEBS Lett 500.1–2 (2001): 52–5.

Kubo M, et al. *Scutellariae radix*. X: Inhibitory effects of various flavonoids on histamine release from rat peritoneal mast cells in vitro. Chem Pharm Bull 32.12 (1984): 5051–4.

Kubo M, et al. Studies on *Scutellariae radix*. XII: Anti-thrombic actions of various flavonoids from *Scutellariae radix*. Chem Pharm Bull 33.6 (1985): 2411–5.

Kumagai T et al. *Scutellaria baicalensis*, a herbal medicine: anti-proliferative and apoptotic activity against acute lymphocytic leukemia, lymphoma and myeloma cell lines. Leuk Res 31.4 (2007): 523–30.

Kwok MH et al. Anxiolytic effect of wogonin, a benzodiazepine receptor ligand isolated from *Scutellaria baicalensis* Georgi. Biochem Pharmacol 64.9 (2002): 1415–24.

Lai MY et al. Significant decrease of cyclosporine bioavailability in rats caused by a decoction of the roots of *Scutellaria baicalensis*. Planta Med 70.2 (2004): 132–7.

Lam TL et al. A comparison of human immunodeficiency virus type-1 protease inhibition activities by the aqueous and methanol extracts of Chinese medicinal herbs. Life Sci 67.23 (2000): 2889–96.

Lee E et al. Wogonin, a plant flavone, potentiates etoposide-induced apoptosis in cancer cells. Ann N Y Acad Sci 1095 (2007): 521–6.

Lee JK et al. Therapeutic effects of the oriental herbal medicine Sho-saiko-to on liver cirrhosis and carcinoma. Hepatol Res. (2011) Sep;41(9):825–37.

Leung HW et al. Inhibition of 12-lipoxygenase during baicalein-induced human lung nonsmall carcinoma H460 cell apoptosis. Food Chem Toxicol 45.3 (2007): 403–11.

Li C, Lin GZZ. Pharmacological effects and pharmacokinetics properties of Radix Scutellariae and its bioactive flavones. Biopharm. Drug Dispos (2011) 32: 427–445.

Li BQ et al. Inhibition of HIV infection by baicalin: a flavonoid compound purified from Chinese herbal medicine. Cell Mol Biol Res 39.2 (1993): 119–24.

Li BQ et al. The flavonoid baicalin exhibits anti-inflammatory activity by binding to chemokines. Immunopharmacology 49.3 (2000a): 295–306.

Li BQ et al. Flavonoid baicalin inhibits HIV-1 infection at the level of viral entry. Biochem Biophys Res Commun 276.2 (2000b): 534–8.

Liao J-F, et al. Anxiolytic-like effects of baicalein and baicalin in the Vogel conflict test in mice. Eur J Pharmacol 464.2–3 (2003): 141–6.

Lim BO. Efficacy of wogonin in the production of immunoglobulins and cytokines by mesenteric lymph node lymphocytes in mouse colitis induced with dextran sulfate sodium. Biosci Biotechnol Biochem 68.12 (2004): 2505–11.

Lin C-C, Shieh D-E. In vivo hepatoprotective effect of baicalein, baicalin and wogonin from *Scutellaria rivularis*. Phytother Res 10.8 (1996): 651–64.

Lin MT et al. Effects of Chinese herb, Huang Chin (*Scutellaria baicalensis* Georgi) on thermoregulation in rats. Jpn J Pharmacol 30.1 (1980): 59–64.

Liu JJ et al. Baicalein and baicalin are potent inhibitors of angiogenesis: inhibition of endothelial cell proliferation, migration and differentiation. Int J Cancer 106.4 (2003): 559–65.

Luo X et al. Effects of *Scutellaria baicalensis* stem-leaf total flavonoid on proliferation of vassel smooth muscle cells stimulated by high triglyceride blood serum. Zhongguo Zhong Yao Za Zhi (2009) 34(21):2803–7.

Lu Z. Clinical comparative study of intravenous piperacillin sodium or injection of scutellaria compound in patients with pulmonary infection. Zhong Xi Yi Jie He Za Zhi 10.7 389 (1990): 413–15.

Ma C et al. Anti-asthmatic Effects of Baicalin in a Mouse Model of Allergic Asthma. Phytother Res 2014; 28: 231–237.

Makino T et al. Comparison of the major flavonoid content of *S. baicalensis, S. lateriflora*, and their commercial products. J Nat Med. (2008) 62(3):294–9.

Mehendale SR et al. Effects of antioxidant herbs on chemotherapy-induced nausea and vomiting in a rat-pica model. Am J Chin Med 32.6 (2004): 897–905.

Mehendale SR et al. *Scutellaria baicalensis* and a constituent flavonoid, baicalein, attenuate ritonavir-induced gastrointestinal side-effects. J Pharm Pharmacol 59.11 (2007): 1567–72.

Minematsu S et al. A subchronic (3-month) oral toxicity study of Tsumura Sho-saiko-to (TJ-9) in the rat via oral gavage administration with a 4-week recovery period. Pharmacometrics 43.1 (1992): 19–42 [in Japanese].

Minematsu S et al. A single oral dose toxicity study of Tsumura Sho-saiko-to (TJ-9) in rats. Jpn Pharmacol Ther 23 (Suppl. 7) (1995): 29–32 [in Japanese].

Mu X et al. Baicalein exerts neuroprotective effects in 6-hydroxydopamine-induced experimental parkinsonism in vivo and in vitro. Pharmacology, Biochemistry and Behavior 92 (2009) 642–648.

Nagai T, et al. Inhibition of mouse liver sialidase by the root of *Scutellaria baicalensis*. Planta Med 55.1 (1989): 27–9.

Nagai T et al. In vivo anti-influenza virus activity of plant flavonoids possessing inhibitory activity for influenza virus sialidase. Antiviral Res 19.3 (1992a): 207–17.

Nagai T et al. Anti-influenza virus activity of plant flavonoids having inhibitory activity against influenza virus sialidase. J Pharmacobio-Dynamics 15.1 (1992b): S-1.

Nagai T et al. Mode of action of the anti-influenza virus activity of plant flavonoid, 5,7,4'-trihydroxy-8-methoxyflavone, from the roots of *Scutellaria baicalensis*. Antiviral Res 26.1 (1995a): 11–25.

Nagai T et al. Antiviral activity of plant flavonoid, 5,7, 4'-trihydroxy-8-methoxyflavone, from the roots of *Scutellaria baicalensis* against influenza A (H3N2) and B viruses. Biol Pharm Bull 18.2 (1995b): 295–9.

Nakajima T et al. Inhibitory effect of baicalein, a flavonoid in scutellaria root, on eotaxin production by human dermal fibroblasts. Planta Med 67.2 (2001): 132–5.

Nan J-X et al. *Scutellaria baicalensis* inhibits liver fibrosis induced by bile duct ligation or carbon tetrachloride in rats. J Pharm Pharmacol 54.4 (2002): 555–63.

Narita Y et al. Treatment of epileptic patients with the Chinese herbal medicine 'Saiko-Keishi-To' (SK). IRCS Med Sci 10.2 (1982): 88–9.
Natarajan R et al. Role of the lipoxygenase pathway in angiotensin II-induced vascular smooth muscle cell hypertrophy. Hypertension 23 (1 Suppl.) (1994): I142–7.
Niitsuma T et al. Effects of absorbed components of Saiboku-to on the release of leukotrienes from polymorphonuclear leukocytes of patients with bronchial asthma. Methods Find Exp Clin Pharmacol 23.2 (2001): 99–104.
Nishioka T, et al. Baicalein, an alpha-glucosidase inhibitor from *Scutellaria baicalensis*. J Natural Products 61.11 (1998): 1413–15.
Park S. Preventive Effect of the Flavonoid, Wogonin, Against Ethanol-Induced Gastric Mucosal Damage in Rats. Digestive Diseases and Sciences, Vol. 49(3)(2004): 384–394.
Park BK et al. Inhibition of TPA-induced cyclooxygenase-2 expression and skin inflammation in mice by wogonin, a plant flavone from *Scutellaria radix*. Eur J Pharmacol 425.2 (2001): 153–7.
Park S et al. Preventive effect of the flavonoid, wogonin, against ethanol-induced gastric mucosal damage in rats. Dig Dis Sci 49.3 (2004): 384–394.
Park HG et al. Anticonvulsant effect of wogonin isolated from *Scutellaria baicalensis*. Eur J Pharmacol 574.2–3 (2007): 112–19.
Peng CY et al. Baicalein attenuates intimal hyperplasia after rat carotid balloon injury through arresting cell-cycle progression and inhibiting ERK, Akt, and NF-kappaB activity in vascular smooth-muscle cells. Naunyn Schmiedebergs. Arch Pharmacol 378.6 (2008): 579–88.
Piao HZ et al. Neuroprotective effect of wogonin: potential roles of inflammatory cytokines. Arch Pharm Res 27.9 (2004): 930–6.
Piao HZ et al. Wogonin inhibits microglial cell migration via suppression of nuclear factor-kappa B activity. Int Immunopharmacol 8(12) (2008): 1658–1662.
Pidgeon GP et al. Mechanisms controlling cell cycle arrest and induction of apoptosis after 12-lipoxygenase inhibition in prostate cancer cells. Cancer Res 62.9 (2002): 2721–7.
Razina TG et al. Enhancement of the selectivity of the action of the cytostatics cyclophosphane and 5-fluorouracil by using an extract of the Baikal skullcap in an experiment. Vopr Onkol 33.2 (1987): 80–4.
Razina TG et al. The role of thrombocyte aggregation function in the mechanism of the antimetastatic action of an extract of Baikal skullcap. Vopr Onkol 35.3 (1989): 331–5.
Razina TG et al. Medicinal plant preparations used as adjuvant therapeutics in experimental oncology. Eksp Klin Farmakol 63.5 (2000): 59–61.
Regulska-Ilow B et al. Influence of bioflavonoids from the radix extract of *Scutellaria baicalensis* on the level of serum lipids, and the development of laboratory rats fed with fresh and oxidized fats. Nahrung 48.2 (2004): 123–8.
Shang Y et al. Scutellaria flavonoid reduced memory dysfunction and neuronal injury caused by permanent global ischemia in rats. Pharmacol Biochem Behav 82(1) (2005): 67–73.
Shang YZ et al. Prevention of oxidative injury by flavonoids from stems and leaves of *Scutellaria baicalensis* georgi in PC12 cells. Phytother Res 20.1 (2006a): 53–7.
Shang YZ et al. Effects of amelioration of total flavonoids from stems and leaves of *Scutellaria baicalensis* Georgi on cognitive deficits, neuronal damage and free radicals disorder induced by cerebral ischemia in rats. Biol Pharm Bull 29.4 (2006b): 805–10.
Shen Y-C et al. Mechanisms in mediating the anti-inflammatory effects of baicalin and baicalein in human leukocytes. Eur J Pharmacol 465.1–2 (2003): 171–81.
Shimizu I. Sho-saiko-to: Japanese herbal medicine for protection against hepatic fibrosis and carcinoma. J Gastroenterol Hepatol 15 (Suppl) (2000): D84–90.
Smolianinov ES et al. Effect of *Scutellaria baicalensis* extract on the immunologic status of patients with lung cancer receiving antineoplastic chemotherapy. Eksp Klin Farmakol 60.6 (1997): 49–51.
Son D et al. Neuroprotective effect of wogonin in hippocampal slice culture exposed to oxygen and glucose deprivation. Eur J Pharmacol 493.1–3 (2004): 99–102.
Song X. Wogonin inhibits tumor angiogenesis via degradation of HIF-1α protein. Toxicology and Applied Pharmacology 271 (2013) 144–155.
Song KH et al. Extracts of *Scutellaria baicalensis* reduced body weight and blood triglyceride in db/db Mice. Phytother Res (2013) 27(2):244–50.
Takizawa H, et al. Prostaglandin I2 contributes to the vasodepressor effect of baicalein in hypertensive rats. Hypertension 31.3 (1998): 866–71.
Tang ZM, et al. Screening 20 Chinese herbs often used for clearing heat and dissipating toxin with nude mice model of hepatitis C viral infection. Zhongguo Zhong Xi Yi Jie He Za Zhi 23.6 (2003): 447–8.
Tong WG, et al. The mechanisms of lipoxygenase inhibitor-induced apoptosis in human breast cancer cells. Biochem Biophys Res Commun 296.4 (2002): 942–8.
Tsao TF et al. Effect of Chinese and western antimicrobial agents on selected oral bacteria. J Dent Res 61.9 (1982): 1103–6.
Waisundara VY et al. Baicalin upregulates the genetic expression of antioxidant enzymes in Type-2 diabetic Goto-Kakizaki rats. Life Sci. Jun 6.88 (2011): 1016–1625.
Waisundara VY et al. *Scutellaria baicalensis* enhances the anti-diabetic activity of metformin in streptozotocin-induced diabetic Wistar rats. Am J Chin Med 36(3) (2008): 517–40.
Wakabayashi I. Inhibitory effects of baicalein and wogonin on lipopolysaccharide-induced nitric oxide production in macrophages. Pharmacol Toxicol 84.6 (1999): 288–91.
Wakabayashi I, Yasui K. Wogonin inhibits inducible prostaglandin E2 production in macrophages. Eur J Pharmacol 406.3 (2000): 477–81.
Wang H-H, et al. Anticonvulsant effect of water extract of *Scutellariae radix* in mice. J Ethnopharmacol 73.1–2 (2000): 185–90.
Wang GF et al. Influence of baicalin on the expression of receptor activator of nuclear factor-kappaB ligand in cultured human periodontal ligament cells. Pharmacology 77.2 (2006): 71–7.
Wang CZ et al. Improving cachectic symptoms and immune strength of tumour-bearing mice in chemotherapy by a combination of *Scutellaria baicalensis* and Qing-Shu-Yi-Qi-Tang. European J Can 48(7) (2012); 1074–1084.
Woo KJ et al. Differential inhibitory effects of baicalein and baicalin on LPS-induced cyclooxygenase-2 expression through inhibition of C/EBPbeta DNA-binding activity. Immunobiology 211.5 (2006): 359–68.
Wu S-H, et al. Hemodynamic role of arachidonate 12- and 5-lipoxygenases in nephrotoxic serum nephritis. Kidney Int 43.6 (1993): 1280–5.
Wu X, et al. Apoptosis of HIV-infected cells following treatment with Sho-saiko-to and its components. Jpn J Med Sci Biol 48.2 (1995): 79–87.
Wu J et al. Study of *Scutellaria baicalensis* and Baicalin against antimicrobial susceptibility of *Helicobacter pylori* strains in vitro. Zhong Yao Cai 31(5) (2008):707–10.
Yamashiki M et al. Herbal medicine sho-saiko-to induces in vitro granulocyte colony-stimulating factor production on peripheral blood mononuclear cells. J Clin Lab Immunol 37.2 (1992): 83–90.
Yamashiki M et al. Effects of the Japanese herbal medicine 'Sho-saiko-to' (TJ-9) on in vitro interleukin-10 production by peripheral blood mononuclear cells of patients with chronic hepatitis C. Hepatology 25.6 (1997): 1390–7.
Yamashiki M et al. Effects of the Japanese herbal medicine Sho-saiko-to (TJ-9) on interleukin-12 production in patients with HCV-positive liver cirrhosis. Dev Immunol 7.1 (1999): 17–22.
Yang D et al. Antifungal activity in vitro of *Scutellaria baicalensis* Georgi upon cutaneous and ungual pathogenic fungi. Ann Pharm Fr 53(3) (1995): 138–41.
Yang ZC et al. The synergistic activity of antibiotics combined with eight traditional Chinese medicines against two different strains of *Staphylococcus aureus*. Colloids Surf B Biointerfaces 41.2–3 (2005): 79–81.
Ye F et al. Anticancer activity of *Scutellaria baicalensis* and its potential mechanism. J Altern Complement Med 8.5 (2002): 567–72.
Ye F et al. Molecular mechanism of anti-prostate cancer activity of *Scutellaria baicalensis* extract. Nutr Cancer 57.1 (2007): 100–10.
Yoon S et al. Anti-inflammatory effects of *Scutellaria baicalensis* water extract on LPS-activated RAW264.7 macrophages. J Ethnopharmacol 125(2009); 286–290.
You CL, et al. Study on effect and mechanism of *Scutellaria baicalensis* stem-leaf total flavonoid in regulating lipid metabolism. Zhongguo Zhong Yao Za Zhi 33.9 (2008): 1064–6.
Zhang DY et al. Inhibition of cancer cell proliferation and prostaglandin E2 synthesis by *Scutellaria baicalensis*. Cancer Res 63.14 (2003): 4037–43.
Zhang SQ et al. Baicalein reduces β-amyloid and promotes nonamyloidogenic amyloid precursor protein processing in an Alzheimer's disease transgenic mouse model. Journal of Neuroscience Research (2013) 91:1239–1246.
Zhao Y et al. Effects of flavonoids extracted from *Scutellaria baicalensis* Georgi on hemin-nitrite-H_2O_2 induced liver injury. Eur J Pharmacol 536.1–2 (2006): 192–9.
Zhong XH et al. Anti-abortive effect of *Radix scutellariae* and *Rhizoma atractylodis* in mice. Am J Chin Med 30.1 (2002): 109–17.
Zhong Y et al. Drug resistance associates with activation of Nrf2 in MCF-7/DOX cells, and wogonin reverses it by down-regulating Nrf2-mediated cellular defense response. Mol Carcinog (2012) 10.1002/mc.21921.
Zhou Y, Zhang J. Oral baicalin and liquid extract of licorice reduce sorbitol levels in red blood cells of diabetic rats. Chin Med J 102.3 (1989): 203–6.
Zhou QB et al. Effects of baicalin on protease-activated receptor-1 expression and brain injury in a rat model of intracerebral hemorrhage. Chin J Physiol (2012) 55(3):202–9.
Zhu H et al. Integrated pharmacokinetics of major bioactive components in MCAO rats after oral administration of Huang-Lian-Jie-Du-Tang. J Ethnopharmacol 141 (2012) 158–169.

Bergamot

Bergamot is a common Italian citrus fruit and chiefly cultivated to produce essential oils. It is a natural hybrid fruit derived from bitter orange and lemon and produced almost exclusively on the south-eastern coast of Italy in the Reggio Calabria region, with an annual production of 25,000 tonnes (Pernice et al 2009). For centuries the essential oil obtained from the peel of *Citrus bergamia* was mainly used for its fragrant properties in perfumes, as an antiseptic, to facilitate wound healing, as an anthelminthic and also for heart disease (Bagetta et al 2010, Pernice et al 2009). It also provides the citrus aroma associated with Earl Grey tea.

LATIN BINOMIAL/CLASS

Citrus bergamia, Risso/Rutacee genus; subfamily Esperidea

OTHER NAMES

Aceite de bergamota, bergamot orange, bergamota, bergamotier, bergamoto, bergamotte, bergamotto, bigarade orange, huile de bergamote, oleum bergamotte, oranger bergamotte, sweet orange

PLANT PART USED

Bergamot is used mostly for production of the essential oil, obtained from the peel by wash-scraping the fruit. Until recently, bergamot juice (BJ) was considered a waste byproduct of this process; however, new research is finding potential uses for it.

CHEMICAL COMPONENTS

Bergamot juice

Present in the juice (BJ) are flavonoid and flavonoid glycosides and albedo, such as neoeriocitrin, neohesperidin, naringin, rutin, neodesmin, rhoifolin and poncirin. It is also rich in neohesperidosides of hesperetin and naringenin, such as melitidine and brutieridine (Mollace et al 2008).

Neoeriocitrin is one of the main flavonoids in BJ, accounting for 15%, whereas narirutin and naringin together represent only 14% of the total flavonoids (Pernice et al 2009).

The specific polyphenolic compounds in BJ include narirutin, naringin, isorhoifolin and rhoifolin and, to a lesser extent, rutin and other compounds: neoeriocitrin, neoponcirin, hesperidin and neodiosmin. Rhoifolin and isorhoifolin have been detected in substantial concentrations in BJ but are only present in very small amounts in orange, tangerine and grapefruit, and are completely absent in lemon (Pernice et al 2009).

Bergamot essential oil (BEO)

According to the Farmacopea Ufficiale Italiana (1991), BEO is obtained by cold pressing of the epicarp and, partly, of the mesocarp of the fresh fruit. BEO has poor water solubility, low stability and limited bioavailability (Celia et al 2013).

BEO consists of a volatile fraction (93–96%) and a non-volatile fraction (4–7%). The volatile fraction contains the monoterpene and sesquiterpene hydrocarbons and oxygenated derivatives such as limonene, γ-terpinene and β-pinene, the monoterpene alcohol, linalool and the monoterpene ester, linalyl acetate which, altogether, constitute more than 90% of the whole oil (Sakurada et al 2011). The non-volatile fraction contains waxes, polymethoxylated flavones, coumarins and psoralens such as bergamottin and bergapten (Bagetta et al 2010, Sakurada et al 2011). This hydrocarbon fraction does not have a fundamental role in determining the olfactory character of BEO.

MAIN ACTIONS

Antioxidant

BJ has an extraordinary high antioxidant activity, with values about 2800 and 1300 times greater than data obtained for apple and apricot juices respectively when measured using the *N,N*-dimethyl-*p*-phenylenediamine method (Pernice et al 2009). This method of determining antioxidant activity is widely used in food science. The bergamot polyphenols and, possibly, bergamot flavanones are the most important contributors to the antioxidant activity.

Lipid lowering

Experimental evidence obtained in animal models of diet-induced hypercholesterolaemia and renal damage as well as in the rat model of mechanical stress-induced vascular injury supports the hypolipaemic and vasoprotective effects of bergamot constituents (Mollace et al 2011).

Long-term administration of BJ (1 mL/day) induced a significant reduction in serum cholesterol, triglycerides and low-density lipoprotein (LDL) levels and an increase in high-density lipoprotein (HDL) levels in vivo (Miceli et al 2007). The hypocholesterolaemic effect of BJ may be mediated by the increase in faecal neutral sterols and total bile acid excretion, as observed after treatment.

The main constituents thought to be responsible for lipid-lowering activity are the flavanone glycosides brutieridin and melitidin, which both contain a 3-hydroxy-3-methylglutaric acid (HMG) moiety (Di et al 2009). As such, they have been described as structural analogues of statin drugs and it has been suggested that these compounds may interfere with the synthesis of mevalonate by mimicking endogenous HMG-CoA substrate (Leopoldini et al 2010).

Brutieridin and melitidin are present in bergamot fruit in concentrations of approximately 300–500 and 150–300 ppm respectively, as a function of the ripening stage (Di et al 2009).

Antimicrobial

Bergamot peel is a potential source of natural antimicrobial agents that are active against Gram-negative bacteria. In vitro tests demonstrate that bergamot ethanolic fractions were effective against the Gram-negative bacteria *Escherichia coli, Pseudomonas putida* and *Salmonella enterica* (Mandalari et al 2007).

Anxiolytic

BEO exhibits anxiolytic activity in vivo (Russo et al 2013). It has been shown to significantly increase gamma-aminobutyric acid levels in rat hippocampus. Rats exposed to bergamot aromatherapy also had a decrease in corticosterone levels; the combined effects provided a biological basis for an anxiolytic activity (Saiyudthong & Marsden 2011). Additionally, in vivo and in vitro results suggest that BEO induces release of glutamate, i.e. low concentrations stimulate exocytosis of the excitatory amino acid, possibly by activation of presynaptic receptors located on glutamate-releasing nerve endings; higher concentrations cause glutamate release via a Ca^{2+}-independent, carrier-mediated process (Bagetta et al 2010).

Anti-inflammatory

Bergapten and citropten from bergamot are strong inhibitors of interleukin-8 expression (Borgatti et al 2011). They have been investigated as possible treatment candidates to reduce lung inflammation in patients with cystic fibrosis.

Antinociceptive

In vivo research confirms antinociceptive activity for BEO (Russo et al 2013). Injected BEO has an antinociceptic effect and the isolated constituents linalool and linalyl acetate are even more potent. This suggests that the nociceptive effect of BEO may be dependent on the concentrations of linalool and linalyl acetate present. Interestingly, the effect of BEO and linalool appears to be opioid-mediated as naloxone abolishes activity (Sakurada et al 2011). Furthermore, an in vivo study identified that, when a combination of morphine (intraperitoneal and intrathecal) and intraplantar BEO or linalool was administered, a synergistic antinociceptive effect was seen for morphine. Of note, the morphine was administered at a subtherapeutic dose (Sakurada et al 2009).

Neuroprotection

BEO reduced neuronal damage caused by excitotoxic stimuli in vitro (Corasaniti et al 2007). Results obtained by using specific fractions of BEO suggested that monoterpene hydrocarbons were responsible for the neuroprotection afforded by BEO. Neuroprotection was also demonstrated in vivo as intraperitoneal injection of BEO reduced, in a dose-dependent manner, the brain damage caused by focal cerebral ischaemia in rats (Amantea et al 2009). It has been proposed that neuroprotection action may stem from its ability to enhance phosphorylation of Akt (Bagetta et al 2010).

Antitumour

In one study, BJ exhibited an antiproliferative effect but not a cytotoxic effect (Delle et al 2013). BEO also exhibits antitumour activity. BEO demonstrated antiproliferative activity against SH-SY5Y human neuroblastoma cells in vitro and BEO-derived compounds, such as limonene, limonene-related monoterpenes, perillyl alcohol and perillic acid have also been shown to inhibit cell proliferation of breast cancer cells and provide a chemopreventive and chemotherapeutic effect in mammary tumour models (Celia et al 2013).

Russo et al (2013) investigated several individual constituents in BEO for cytotoxic activity in human SH-SY5Y neuroblastoma cultures. They found significant cytotoxicity when cells were co-treated with limonene and linalyl acetate, whereas single exposure to limonene or linalyl acetate did not have the same effect. Based on current research, it appears likely that the combination of monoterpenes in BEO is responsible for the observed effects, which include caspase-3 activation, poly (ADP-ribose) polymerase cleavage, DNA fragmentation, cell shrinkage, cytoskeletal alterations, together with necrotic and apoptotic cell death (Russo et al 2013).

As a means of improving BEO and BEO-bergapten-free (BEO-BF) solubility, a liposomal formulation was developed by Celia et al (2013) which reduced the viability of SH-SY5Y cells at far lower concentrations than their free drug counterparts. The BEO-BF proved to be more efficacious than BEO when either administered as a free compound or encapsulated within a liposome.

OTHER ACTIONS

BEO contains several different constituents which can cause phototoxic reactions, such as bergapten, citropten, bergamoten and other furocoumarins (Kejlova et al 2007). Bergapten is one of the key constituents responsible for the phototoxicity of BEO, therefore, a bergapten-free extract of the essence (BEO-BF), together with a natural essence deprived of the hydrocarbon fraction and of bergapten (BEO-HF/BF) is prepared by extractive industries for perfumery and cosmetic uses (Bagetta et al 2010).

CLINICAL USAGE

Bergamot is traditionally used as an essential oil in aromatherapy or topical preparations, although recent research has suggested possible benefits for the juice or its isolated polyphenolic fraction when ingested orally.

Hypercholesterolaemia

Many naturally derived polyphenol compounds show potential benefits as therapeutic agents in cardiovascular disease and have been tested as a means of reducing blood lipids and addressing other underlying factors which may contribute to disease, such as inflammation and oxidative stress.

Recently, orally administered bergamot-derived polyphenols have been investigated in both animal models of diet-induced hyperlipidaemia and in patients with metabolic syndrome, where it was observed to significantly reduce serum cholesterol, triglycerides and glycaemia (Mollace et al 2011). A significant improvement in vascular reactivity was also seen in patients with both hyperlipidaemia and raised serum glucose, suggesting a possible role in metabolic syndrome.

A double-blind randomised controlled trial involving 237 participants tested three different dosages of bergamot fruit extract (500 mg/day, 1000 mg/day and 1500 mg/day) against placebo (Mollace et al 2011). The active treatment consisted of a bergamot preparation containing 26–28% of five main flavonoids: neoeriocitrin (7.7% ± 0.4%), naringin (6.3% ± 0.33%), neohesperidin (7.2% ± 0.35%), melitidin (1.56% ± 0.11%) and brutieridin (3.32% ± 0.17%). Patients were divided into subgroups: people with elevated cholesterol, hyperlipidaemia (elevated cholesterol and triglycerides) and those with mixed lipidaemia and glycaemia over 110 mg/dL who received either 500 or 1000 mg/day. A fourth group was comprised of 32 people who stopped statin therapy due to muscle pain and elevated serum creatine phosphokinase, and they received the highest dose (1500 mg/day) after a 60-day washout.

Bergamot treatment (500 and 1000 mg/day) resulted in a significant reduction in total cholesterol and LDL-cholesterol and a significant increase in HDL-cholesterol in most subjects in the first three subgroups. In particular, the group with metabolic syndrome experienced substantial effects on lipids and a highly significant ($P < 0.0001$) reduction in blood glucose levels (mean value of −18.9% with 500 mg/day and −22.4% with 1000 mg/day).

Both doses significantly lowered total cholesterol; however the higher dose of 1000 mg/day was significantly more effective at raising HDL-cholesterol.

For patients ($n = 32$) considered statin-intolerant, bergamot extract (1500 mg/day) produced a mean reduction in total cholesterol of 25% and 27.6% for LDL in 30 patients. Importantly, there was no reappearance of the side effects experienced with statin therapy.

More recently, a prospective, open-label study was conducted to determine whether natural bergamot-derived polyphenolic fraction (BPF) reduced total cholesterol when used as stand-alone therapy and also whether it could be used as an adjunct to statin therapy, allowing for a dose reduction in statin medication in patients with mixed hyperlipidaemia (Gliozzi et al 2013, Walker et al 2012).

The placebo-controlled study of 77 volunteers with LDL-cholesterol levels of >4.1 mmol/L and triglyceride levels >2.54 mmol/L were divided into five groups and received one of placebo, BPF 1000 mg/day, rosuvastatin 10 mg/day, rosuvastatin 20 mg/day or BPF (1000 mg/day) + rosuvastatin (10 mg/day) for 30 days. In addition, all groups were to follow a low-fat diet during the study duration.

Oral administration of BPF (1000 mg/daily for 30 consecutive days; $n = 15$) in patients with mixed hyperlipidaemia led to a significant reduction in total cholesterol, LDL-cholesterol, triglyceride and enhanced HDL-cholesterol levels, whereas no significant change was observed in the placebo group. The groups receiving rosuvastatin (10 and 20 mg/daily; $n = 16$ for each group) also experienced a significant reduction of total cholesterol and LDL-cholesterol compared to placebo; however, insignificant changes were seen for triglycerides at both doses and an elevation of HDL-cholesterol was found (Gliozzi et al 2013).

When BFG was combined with rosuvastatin (10 mg/day), a significant decrease in total cholesterol and LDL-cholesterol serum levels was seen when compared to rosuvastatin alone. Furthermore, the combination of low-dose rosuvastatin and BPF produced an effect which was nearly the same as that produced by 20 mg/day of rosuvastatin.

Changes to urinary mevalonate indicated that adding BPF to rosuvastatin further inhibited HMG-CoA reductase. A decrease in malondialdehyde levels for the combination treatment also confirms that BFG enhanced the antioxidant effect of rosuvastatin and changes in a range of other biomarkers indicate that vasoprotective effects were further enhanced.

Stress and anxiety

An open-label study of 54 elementary school teachers evaluated two 10-min sprays with bergamot oil aromatherapy for effects on stress. The BEO used was 100% pure and diluted to 2%. Exposure to BEO resulted in a significant decrease in blood pressure and heart rate when measured 5 min after exposure compared to 5 min before. Subgroup analysis revealed that aromatherapy was effective for high-anxiety and moderate-anxiety groups but not for people with mild anxiety (Chang & Shen 2011). While this was an open study measuring before and after effects to aromatherapy, there was strict control of the experimental environment, including subject's posture, measurement location and time, adding more rigour to the design.

A double-blind randomised controlled trial evaluating the effect of the respiratory administration of BEO or placebo on the anxiety, nausea and pain of 37 paediatric patients undergoing stem cell infusion and their parents found the treatment groups experienced greater anxiety ($P = 0.05$) and nausea ($P = 0.03$) 1 h postinfusion. There was no significant change to pain or parental anxiety, which reduced for both groups but did not reach statistical significance (Ndao et al 2012). Clearly the treatment was ineffective when given this way and poorly tolerated.

OTHER USES

Bergamot oil has been used for its fragrance properties in perfumes for generations; however these properties are quickly destroyed by exposure to sunlight.

Traditionally, BEO has been used in folk medicine as an antiseptic, to facilitate wound healing and as an anthelminthic agent. Today, it is still used for its antiseptic and antibacterial proprieties and by the cosmetic industries (e.g. in perfumes, body lotions, soaps and aromatherapy) (Bagetta et al 2010). It is also used in the food industries as aroma for the preparation of sweets, liquors and tea such as in Earl Grey tea.

DOSAGE RANGE

According to clinical studies

Hyperlipidaemia — oral bergamot fruit extract: 500–1500 mg/day.
Oral BPF: 1000 mg/day.
Anxiety — used as aromatherapy: 100% pure BEO and diluted to 2%.

ADVERSE REACTIONS

Phototoxic side effects can occur with bergamot application directly on the skin followed by exposure to sunlight (ultraviolet [UV]-A). This can result in oedema, long-lasting erythema and significant skin pigmentation. If a sunscreen-absorbing UV-A radiation is applied, the phototoxic reaction does not occur (Dubertret et al 1990).

BEO contains several different constituents which can cause phototoxic effects, such as bergapten, citropten, bergamoten and other furocoumarins (Kejlova et al 2007). Bergapten is one of the key constituents responsible for the phototoxicity of BEO; therefore, a bergapten-free extract of the essence together with a natural essence deprived of the hydrocarbon fraction and of bergapten are prepared by extractive industries for perfumery and cosmetic uses (Bagetta et al 2010).

The International Fragrance Association recommends a maximum of 0.4% of bergamot oil in the final leave-on products for application to areas of skin exposed to sunshine to avoid phototoxic and photocarcinogenic hazard. In order to guarantee safety, it is suggested to remove bergapten and other phototoxic components by distillation, the resulting oil being known as bergamot FCF (furocoumarin-free) (Kejlova et al 2007).

SIGNIFICANT INTERACTIONS

No significant drug interactions are known for oral bergamot preparations.

There is a theoretical concern about possible interactions due to the presence of naringin in bergamot (Pernice et al 2009). This constituent is also found in grapefruit juice and, while it does not have any appreciable effect on cytochromes, it may inhibit OATP1A2 according to clinical research (Bailey et al 2007). Whether the concentration of naringin present in commercial bergamot preparations is sufficient to cause such an effect is unlikely. Until this can be confirmed, people taking drugs with a narrow therapeutic index which are also OATP1A2 substrates should use caution.

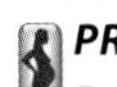

CONTRAINDICATIONS AND PRECAUTIONS

Bergamot oil should not be applied directly to the skin, especially by people with fair skin, as phototoxic side effects can occur. Use a sunscreen absorbing UV-A radiation at the same time to reduce the risk (Dubertret et al 1990).

PREGNANCY USE

Insufficient reliable information available to confirm safety in pregnancy.

Practice points/Patient counseling

- Bergamot fruit extract is an effective treatment for reducing total and LDL-cholesterol and raising HDL-cholesterol according to randomised studies. It can be used together with statin drugs to enable a dose reduction to occur. The available research suggests it can also be used by people intolerant of statins.
- BEO is used in aromatherapy and may reduce anxiety in highly stressed individuals.
- Bergamot has a range of activities, including antioxidant, anti-inflammatory, antimicrobial, neuroprotective, antinociceptive (probably opiate-mediated) and antitumour.
- BEO can be phototoxic and should not be applied directly to the skin, particularly by fair individuals before sun exposure.

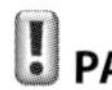

PATIENTS' FAQs

What will this herb do for me?

Bergamot fruit extract taken orally can effectively reduce total and LDL-cholesterol and raise HDL-cholesterol.

BEO, diluted and used as aromatherapy, may induce relaxation in highly stressed individuals.

When will it start to work?

The cholesterol-lowering effects develop within 1 month of use.

The relaxation effect should occur within 5–10 min of aromatherapy exposure.

Are there any safety issues?

Don't apply the BEO directly to the skin as it can make it highly sensitive to sunlight.

REFERENCES

Amantea, D., et al. 2009. Prevention of glutamate accumulation and upregulation of phospho-akt may account for neuroprotection afforded by bergamot essential oil against brain injury induced by focal cerebral ischemia in rat. Int. Rev. Neurobiol., 85, 389–405.

Bagetta, G., et al. 2010. Neuropharmacology of the essential oil of bergamot. Fitoterapia, 81, (6) 453–461.

Bailey, D.G., et al. 2007. Naringin is a major and selective clinical inhibitor of organic anion-transporting polypeptide 1A2 (OATP1A2) in grapefruit juice. Clin Pharmacol Ther., 81, (4) 495–502.

Borgatti, M., et al. 2011. Bergamot (*Citrus bergamia Risso*) fruit extracts and identified components alter expression of interleukin 8 gene in cystic fibrosis bronchial epithelial cell lines. BMC. Biochem., 12, 15.

Celia, C., et al. (2013). Anticancer activity of liposomal bergamot essential oil (BEO) on human neuroblastoma cells. Colloids Surf. B Biointerfaces., 112, 548–553.

Chang, K.M. & Shen, C.W. 2011. Aromatherapy benefits autonomic nervous system regulation for elementary school faculty in taiwan. Evid. Based. Complement Alternat. Med, 2011, 946537.

Corasaniti, M.T., et al. 2007. Cell signaling pathways in the mechanisms of neuroprotection afforded by bergamot essential oil against NMDA-induced cell death in vitro. Br J Pharmacol., 151, (4) 518–529.

Delle, M.S., et al. 2013. Mechanisms underlying the anti-tumoral effects of *Citrus bergamia* juice. PLoS.One., 8, (4) e61484.

Di, D.L., et al. 2009. Statin-like principles of bergamot fruit (*Citrus bergamia*): isolation of 3-hydroxymethylglutaryl flavonoid glycosides. J Nat. Prod., 72, (7) 1352–1354.

Dubertret, L., et al. 1990. Phototoxic properties of perfumes containing bergamot oil on human skin: photoprotective effect of UVA and UVB sunscreens. J Photochem.Photobiol. B, 7, (2–4) 251–259.

Gliozzi, M., et al. (2013) Bergamot polyphenolic fraction enhances rosuvastatin-induced effect on LDL-cholesterol, LOX-1 expression and protein kinase B phosphorylation in patients with hyperlipidemia. International Journal of Cardiology 170: 140–143.

Kejlova, K., et al. 2007. Phototoxicity of bergamot oil assessed by in vitro techniques in combination with human patch tests. Toxicol. In Vitro, 21, (7) 1298–1303.

Leopoldini, M., et al. 2010. On the inhibitor effects of bergamot juice flavonoids binding to the 3-hydroxy-3-methylglutaryl-CoA reductase (HMGR) enzyme. J Agric. Food Chem., 58, (19) 10768–10773.

Mandalari, G., et al. 2007. Antimicrobial activity of flavonoids extracted from bergamot (*Citrus bergamia Risso*) peel, a byproduct of the essential oil industry. J Appl. Microbiol., 103, (6) 2056–2064.

Miceli, N., et al. 2007. Hypolipidemic effects of *Citrus bergamia Risso* et Poiteau juice in rats fed a hypercholesterolemic diet. J Agric. Food Chem., 55, (26) 10671–10677.

Mollace, V., et al. 2008. The protective effect of bergamot oil extract on lecitine-like oxyLDL receptor-1 expression in balloon injury-related neointima formation. J Cardiovasc. Pharmacol. Ther., 13, (2) 120–129.

Mollace, V., et al. 2011. Hypolipemic and hypoglycaemic activity of bergamot polyphenols: from animal models to human studies. Fitoterapia, 82, (3) 309–316.

Ndao, D.H., et al 2012. Inhalation aromatherapy in children and adolescents undergoing stem cell infusion: results of a placebo-controlled double-blind trial. Psychooncology., 21, (3) 247–254.

Pernice, R., et al. 2009. Bergamot: A source of natural antioxidants for functionalized fruit juices. Food Chemistry, 112, (3) 545–550.

Russo, R., et al. 2013. Implication of limonene and linalyl acetate in cytotoxicity induced by bergamot essential oil in human neuroblastoma cells. Fitoterapia 89: 48–57.

Saiyudthong, S. & Marsden, C.A. 2011. Acute effects of bergamot oil on anxiety-related behaviour and corticosterone level in rats. Phytother. Res., 25, (6) 858–862.

Sakurada, T., et al. 2009. Intraplantar injection of bergamot essential oil into the mouse hindpaw: effects on capsaicin-induced nociceptive behaviors. Int. Rev. Neurobiol., 85, 237–248.

Sakurada, T., et al. 2011. Intraplantar injection of bergamot essential oil induces peripheral antinociception mediated by opioid mechanism. Pharmacol. Biochem. Behav., 97, (3) 436–443.

Walker, R., et al. 2012. Bergamot polyphenolic fraction potentiates rosuvastatin-induced effect on LDL-cholesterol, triglycerides and HDL cholesterol. Heart, Lung and Circulation, 21 (Suppl. 1), (0) S67.

Beta-Carotene

BACKGROUND AND RELEVANT PHARMACOKINETICS

Carotenoids

The carotenoids are a family of bright yellow, orange and red compounds found in fruit, vegetables and some animal products, such as salmon, lobster and egg yolk. Carotenoids can be divided into the provitamin A group, such as beta-carotene, and xanthophylls such as lutein, zeaxanthin and lycopene, which are important fat-soluble antioxidants. Of the 600 or so carotenoids known to exist in nature, approximately 20 are found in humans. In plants, carotenoids play a vital role in photosynthesis and participate in the energy-transfer process, as well as protecting plants from oxidative damage. The red, orange and yellow colours of these compounds is due to their preferential absorption of blue light, which is the most energetic and hence the most biologically damaging part of the visible spectrum.

In animals, carotenoids have many functions. In addition to providing direct photoprotection via absorption of blue light, carotenoids act as powerful fat-soluble antioxidants linked to oxidation prevention. They also play a role in cellular communication, including stimulation of gap-junction communication, which is important for cancer prevention, by regulating cell growth, differentiation, apoptosis and angiogenesis. Carotenoids may also be involved in detoxification of carcinogens, DNA repair and immunosurveillance. These properties are believed to contribute to their antioxidant, immune-enhancing, anticarcinogenic and photoprotective activity.

Beta-carotene was the first of the carotenoids to be discovered, being initially isolated from carrots. The bioavailability of beta-carotene is dependent on its source. In raw foods such as carrots it forms part of a protein-polysaccharide matrix, and absorption is only about 20% of that from supplemental forms. Although beta-carotene is lipid soluble, its absorption requires only a limited amount of fat (Roodenburg et al 2000); however, there is a wide individual variation in serum response to beta-carotene administration (Bowen et al 1993, Pryor et al 2000).

Although it has been suggested that different carotenoids compete for absorption, this was not confirmed by a postprandial study (Tyssandier et al 2002). Beta-carotene is absorbed in the intestine and released into the lymphatic circulation within chylomicrons. It is then taken up by hepatocytes and released into the blood, and transported predominantly within LDLs. It is distributed to adipose tissue and the skin and excreted in the faeces (Micromedex 2003). The time to reach peak concentration is up to 4–6 weeks with oral dosing (Mathews-Roth 1990a).

Animal feeding studies suggest that a natural algae-derived beta-carotene isomer mixture is more readily absorbed than synthetic all-*trans* beta-carotene, and that this higher bioavailability can be enhanced by increasing dietary lipid levels (Mokady & Ben-Amotz 1991). Studies on isomerisation that occurred following cooking further suggest that the food matrix may play a role in the effects of cooking on beta-carotene isomerisation (O'Sullivan et al 2010). Natural algal beta-carotene has also been shown to have higher accumulation in rat liver than synthetic all-*trans* beta-carotene (Ben-Amotz et al 1989, Takenaka et al 1993) with at least a 10-fold higher accumulation having been observed in chick and rat liver (Ben-Amotz et al 1989).

Animal studies suggest that there is some bioconversion within the body between different stereoisomers of beta-carotene (Ben-Amotz et al 2005). Further studies in humans suggest that, regardless of the isomer mix, there is preferential absorption or transport of the all-*trans* isomer in comparison with the 9-*cis* isomer, with plasma levels of the all-*trans* isomer being around 10 times that of the 9-*cis* form (Gaziano et al 1995b, Jensen et al 1987, Morinobu et al 1994, Stahl & Sies 1993, Tamai et al 1993).

It is suggested that *Helicobacter pylori* infection may impair the protective role of alpha-tocopherol and beta-carotene in the stomach, because infected people have been found to have reduced beta-carotene concentrations in gastric juice, and the presence of gastric atrophy and intestinal metaplasia is associated with reduced mucosal alpha-tocopherol and beta-carotene concentrations (Zhang et al 2000).

Chemical components

Beta-carotene comes in natural and synthetic forms. The natural form is derived mainly from algal sources and consists of roughly equal amount of 9-*cis* and all-*trans* isomers, with small amounts of the 13-*cis* isomer. Synthetic beta-carotene is primarily composed of the all-*trans* isomer, with small residues of the 13-*cis* isomer (PDRHealth 2005). Although all-*trans* beta-carotene is converted into vitamin A, which plays an essential role in vision, growth, reproduction, immune function and maintenance of the skin and mucous membranes (see *Vitamin A* monograph), the 9-*cis* isomer is not converted into vitamin A, but does act as a powerful antioxidant (Ben-Amotz & Levy 1996).

Food sources

Carrots are the major contributors of beta-carotene in the diet, but it is also found in rockmelon, broccoli and spinach. Carotenoids have emerged as the best single tissue marker for a diet rich in fruits and vegetables, and measurements of plasma and tissue carotenoids have an important role in defining the optimal diets for humans (Handelman 2001).

Natural beta-carotene for use in supplements is generally obtained from palm oil or the micromarine algae (phytoplankton) *Dunaliella salina* (also known as *D. bardawil*), which is the richest natural source of beta-carotene. Whole dried *D. salina* is also available in a supplemental form that contains between 1% and 2% beta-carotene. The typical Western diet is estimated to provide approximately 2–4 mg/day of beta-carotene (Pryor et al 2000).

Deficiency signs and symptoms

Beta-carotene is considered a conditionally essential nutrient and becomes an essential nutrient when the dietary intake of retinol (vitamin A) is inadequate.

Low serum beta-carotene levels have been associated with male gender, younger age, lower non-HDL-cholesterol, greater ethanol consumption and higher BMI (Brady et al 1996), insulin resistance (Arnlöv et al 2009), increased lipoprotein density and the presence of inflammation (Kritchevsky 1999), high C-reactive protein (Erlinger et al 2001, Wang et al 2008), high blood glucose (Abahusain et al 1999), hypertension (Coudray et al 1997), exposure to environmental tobacco smoke (Farchi et al 2001), as well as all measures of obesity (Wallstrom et al 2001), including obesity in children (Strauss 1999).

Low serum beta-carotene and/or low beta-carotene intake has also been associated with a number of clinical conditions, such as breast cancer (Hacisevki et al 2003), non-melanoma and melanoma skin cancer (Gollnick & Siebenwirth 2002), rheumatoid arthritis (Kacsur et al 2002), Alzheimer's dementia (Jimenez-Jimenez et al 1999), age-related macular degeneration (Cooper et al 1999a), metabolic syndrome (Revett 2008, Sugiura et al 2008), poor glycaemic control and type 2 diabetes (Abahusain et al 1999, Arnlöv et al 2009, Coudray et al 1997). It has been further shown that the inverse association between serum carotenoid and metabolic syndrome is more evident in current smokers (Revett 2008, Sugiura et al 2008).

Low serum beta-carotene has been independently associated with an increased all-cause mortality risk in older men. Apparently, a synergistic effect occurs between low beta-carotene and high inflammation burden in predicting higher mortality rates (Hu et al 2004). In another study of 668 hospitalised patients aged 70 years or over and 104 healthy controls, the diseased elderly people had reduced plasma levels of retinol, beta-carotene and alpha-tocopherol (Tebi et al 2000). It is unclear whether these observed low levels of beta-carotene seen in disease states are a cause or a result of disease processes.

MAIN ACTIONS

Pro-vitamin A

Beta-carotene is converted to retinoic acid (vitamin A — see *Vitamin A* monograph) by an enzyme found in the intestinal mucosa and liver, with 2 mcg of all-*trans* carotene being equal to 1 mcg of all-*trans* retinol (vitamin A) or 3.33 IU (PDRHealth 2005). This conversion is regulated by vitamin A status and may be enhanced by alpha-tocopherol (Wang & Krinsky 1998). Zinc may also be important for bio-conversion, as indicated by a double-blind, placebo-controlled trial of 170 pregnant women which found that supplementation zinc improved the post-partum vitamin A status of both mothers and infants (Dijkhuizen et al 2004).

Immunomodulation

The mechanisms by which beta-carotene influences immune function are not well understood, and both direct and indirect effects on immune function, via its pro-vitamin A activity, have been demonstrated (Watson et al 1991). Beta-carotene directly influences immune function by reducing oxidative damage to cell membranes and their receptors, by influencing the activity of redox-sensitive transcription factors and the production of cytokines and prostaglandins, and by enhancing cell-to-cell communication (Hughes 2001).

These actions are influenced by several factors, such as dose and timing of supplementation, age and health status of the individual. A double-blind, placebo-controlled, randomised crossover study in 25 healthy adult-male non-smokers found that 15 mg/day of beta-carotene enhanced cell-mediated immune responses, with significant increases in the percentages of monocytes expressing the major histocompatibility complex class II molecule HLA-DR and adhesion molecules, as well as increased ex vivo tumour necrosis factor alpha (TNF-alpha) secretion by blood monocytes (Hughes et al 1997). Beta-carotene has also been shown to increase plasma levels of TNF-alpha in patients given 30 mg/day for the treatment of oral leucoplakia (Prabhala et al 1993).

In controlled trials, supplementation with 30 mg beta-carotene was shown to protect against UV-induced photosuppression of immune function in young men (Fuller et al 1992), as well as in older men, with serum beta-carotene levels being significantly associated with maintenance of the delayed-type hypersensitivity response (Herraiz et al 1998). Another controlled trial found that 60 mg/day beta-carotene for 44 weeks increased the CD4–CD8 ratio after 9 months without affecting NK cells, virgin T-cells, memory T-cells or cytotoxic T-cells in healthy male non-smokers; supplementation with 60 mg/day beta-carotene for 4 weeks was shown to significantly increase lymphocyte counts and $CD4^+$ in a pilot study of seven patients with AIDS (Murata et al 1994).

Natural killer-cell activity was also found to increase in older adults in a dose-finding study in which 30 mg/day beta-carotene for 2 months significantly increased in a dose-dependent manner the percentage of lymphoid cells with surface markers for T-helper and NK cells, and cells with IL-2 and transferrin receptors (Watson et al 1991). In a further study of 59 men participating in the Physicians Health Study, 10–12 years of supplementation with 50 mg beta-carotene on alternate days was found to increase NK cell activity without increasing the percentage of NK cells, IL-2 production or receptor expression in elderly but not middle-aged men (Santos et al 1996).

Although beta-carotene supplementation has been shown to enhance NK cell responses, there are a number of randomised controlled trials (RCTs) that suggest it does not influence other aspects of immune activity in healthy individuals. In separate RCTs, supplementation with 90 mg beta-carotene for 3 weeks or 50 mg on alternate days for more than 10 years was not found to influence T-cell-mediated immunity of healthy elderly people (Santos et al 1997), and supplementation with 30 mg beta-carotene was not found to affect the T-lymphocyte proliferative response to phytohaemagglutinin in healthy lactating and non-lactating women (Gossage et al 2000). Another study found that supplementation with 8.2 mg/day of beta-carotene for 12 weeks did not influence several markers of T-cell-mediated immunity in well-nourished, healthy elderly individuals (Corridan et al 2001).

Antioxidant

Beta-carotene has consistently demonstrated antioxidant activity in vitro, although the mechanism of action is poorly understood. At low partial pressures of oxygen, such as those found in most tissues under physiological conditions, it exhibits good radical-trapping antioxidant behaviour; this capacity is lost at high oxygen pressures in vitro with autocatalytic, pro-oxidant effects observed (Burton & Ingold 1984).

Beta-carotene has been shown to quench singlet oxygen, scavenge peroxyl radicals and inhibit lipid peroxidation in vitro; however, there is ongoing debate about its ability to act as an antioxidant in vivo, with some evidence suggesting this varies from system to system for reasons that are poorly understood (Pryor et al 2000).

Beta-carotene acts synergistically with other antioxidants, such as vitamins E and C, or other dietary components as part of the antioxidant network (see *Vitamin E* monograph). A combination of beta-carotene and alpha-tocopherol has been shown to inhibit lipid peroxidation significantly more than the sum of the individual inhibitions in a membrane model (Palozza & Krinsky 1992), and a synergistic effect has also been demonstrated in vitro and in vivo with vitamins E and C (Bohm et al 1997, 1998a).

In vivo studies

A number of studies have demonstrated that beta-carotene has antioxidant activity in vivo. Supplementation with 180 mg of beta-carotene for 2 weeks was found to increase the beta-carotene content of LDL and significantly reduce plasma lipid peroxidation and LDL susceptibility to oxidation, as analysed by malondialdehyde generation (Levy et al 1996). Similarly, lipid peroxidation, as measured by breath pentane output, was found to be significantly reduced in healthy subjects by 4 weeks of daily supplementation with 120 mg of beta-carotene (Gottlieb et al 1993). In a case-controlled trial involving 20 patients with long-standing type 1 diabetes mellitus, as well as age- and sex-matched controls, supplementation with 60 mg/day of natural algae-derived beta-carotene for 3 weeks was found to significantly reduce malondialdehyde and lipid peroxide production and the increased susceptibility towards LDL oxidation seen in the diabetic subjects (Levy et al 2000). Beta-carotene supplementation was also found to significantly reduce serum lipid peroxidation in a dose-dependent manner in a number of double-blind, placebo-controlled trials (Greul et al 2002, Lee et al 2000). Beta-carotene supplementation has also been demonstrated to significantly reduce lipid peroxidation of erythrocytes membranes in people with beta-thalassaemia (Mahjoub et al 2007).

These results contrast with those from a number of studies that failed to demonstrate any in vivo antioxidant activity. A study of 79 healthy volunteers found that normal concentrations of carotenoids in plasma and tissues did not correlate with total antioxidant capacity of the plasma or breath pentane measurements (Borel et al 1998). In other studies supplementation was seen to increase LDL beta-carotene without changing LDL susceptibility to oxidation (Princen et al 1992, Reaven et al 1993).

It is possible that beta-carotene is more likely to demonstrate antioxidant activity in conditions of increased oxidative stress. This is suggested by the results of a randomised, double-blind controlled trial that involved 42 non-smokers and 28 smokers who received either 20 mg of beta-carotene or a placebo; this trial showed that beta-carotene reduced lipid peroxidation as indicated by breath pentane output in smokers, but not in non-smokers (Allard et al 1994). This is further supported by a study of whole-body irradiation in rats that found supplementation with natural algae-derived beta-carotene protected against the reduction in growth rate and the selective decline in 9-*cis* beta-carotene and retinol seen in irradiated animals, as well as partially reversing the effect of irradiation when given after the irradiation (Ben-Amotz et al 1996). Algae-derived beta-carotene was also found to protect against CNS oxygen toxicity in rats, as indicated by a significant increase in the latent period preceding oxygen seizures in supplemented animals (Bitterman et al 1994).

Isomer difference

Individual isomers and isomer mixtures demonstrate different antioxidant properties in vivo. The 9-*cis* isomer, which is present in greater amounts in natural beta-carotene, exhibits higher antioxidant potency than the all-*trans* isomer in vitro (Levin & Mokady 1994). Natural beta-carotene, such as that obtained from algal sources, also exhibits greater antioxidant activity than synthetic beta-carotene in vivo (Takenaka et al 1993).

In humans, supplementation with natural algal beta-carotene containing a 50:50 mix of all-*trans* and 9-*cis* isomers has been shown to be a more effective lipophilic antioxidant than all-*trans* beta-carotene (Ben-Amotz & Levy 1996). Human supplementation with natural algal and synthetic beta-carotene has also been shown to produce similar reductions in LDL oxidation, despite the fact that synthetic beta-carotene produced double the rise in LDL beta-carotene content (Levy et al 1995).

These studies contrasted with in vitro studies that suggest that 9-*cis* beta-carotene and all-*trans* beta-carotene have equal antioxidant activities (Liu et al 2000), and that synthetic beta-carotene is twice as effective as algal beta-carotene in inhibiting LDL lipid peroxidation following LDL incubation with copper ions (Lavy et al 1993).

Photoprotection

Beta-carotene, together with other carotenoids, is present in all photosynthetic organisms where it serves an important photoprotective function, either by dissipating excess excitation energy as heat or by scavenging reactive oxygen species and suppressing lipid peroxidation (Penuelas & Munne-Bosch 2005). Studies in bacteria, animals and humans have demonstrated that carotenoids can prevent or lessen photosensitivity by endogenous and exogenous photosensitisers (Mathews-Roth 1993). High doses of beta-carotene (from 180 mg/day up to 300 mg/day) have been used to treat the photosensitivity associated with erythropoietic protoporphyria (Mathews-Roth 1987). There is also consistent evidence from animal and human studies that beta-carotene has photoprotective effects.

Beta-carotene is present at the target sites of light-induced damage in the dermis, epidermis and stratum corneum, with levels varying in skin areas with higher concentration in the forehead and palms (Alaluf et al 2002). Skin levels are related to the levels found in the plasma (Sies & Stahl 2004). Beta-carotene and other endogenous antioxidants are reduced in both skin and blood by UV exposure (Gollnick et al 1996).

Although it is presumed that beta-carotene exerts a light-protective function by quenching excited species such as singlet oxygen and free radicals (Mathews-Roth 1987), there are a number of other ways that beta-carotene may contribute to photoprotection (i.e. protection against the absorption of UV light). These include the protection of target molecules through its antioxidant activity, enhancement of the repair of UV damage, modulation of enzyme activity and gene expression, enhancement of cell-to-cell communication and suppression of cellular responses and inflammation (Sies & Stahl 2004). It is also suggested that the UVA protection provided by beta-carotene is due to the siting of beta-carotene deep inside membranes in proximity to the UVA chromophores that initiate the cell damage (Bohm et al 1998b).

As a strong natural pigment, beta-carotene produces a yellow-orange colouration in the skin that adds to the red colouration from haemoglobin and the brown colouration from melanin to create the normal human skin colour (Alaluf et al 2002). Beta-carotene acts as a blue light filter by absorbing light in the range of 360–550 nanometers (Pathak 1982), with the *cis* isomers having been found to exhibit an additional absorption maximum in the UV range (Sies & Stahl 2004), thus suggesting a possible advantage for natural beta-carotene over synthetic all-*trans* beta-carotene in providing photoprotection.

As with titanium dioxide, the beta-carotene in the skin takes the form of finely dispersed particles that can increase the natural pigment action. This was observed in a human trial involving 20 subjects which found that supplementation with 50 mg of natural algal beta-carotene for 6 weeks increased the reflection capacity of the skin 2.3-fold, irrespective of the wavelength (Heinrich et al 1998). A study on whole albino hairless mouse skin and epidermis, however, suggests that although beta-carotene did impart a visible change in skin colour its absorbance was insufficient to impart significant photoprotection, which indicates that its photoprotective action is mediated through processes in addition to blue light absorption (Sayre & Black 1992).

In a controlled study injection of phytoene, the colourless triene precursor of beta-carotene was found to significantly reduce radiation-induced erythema in guinea pigs (Mathews-Roth & Pathak 1975); however, a further study on albino hairless mice found that 10 g/kg feed of beta-carotene and 200 mg/kg feed of 13-*cis* retinoic acid for 12 weeks did not prevent UVB-induced dermal damage (Kligman & Mathews-Roth 1990).

An in vitro study on human keratinocytes suggests that beta-carotene dose-dependently suppressed UVA-induction of matrix metalloproteases through quenching of singlet oxygen and that this action was not enhanced by vitamin E (Wertz et al 2004). Further studies suggest that beta-carotene also interferes with UVA-induced gene expression by multiple pathways, including inhibition of UVA-induced extracellular matrix degradation, enhanced UVA induction of tanning-associated protease-activated receptor-2, promotion of keratinocyte differentiation and synergistic induction of cell cycle arrest and apoptosis (Wertz et al 2005).

Beta-carotene has also been observed to have synergistic effects with other antioxidants in protecting cultured human fibroblasts from UVA, although only additive effects were observed for UVB (Bohm et al 1998b). The interaction between different antioxidants and/or other as yet unidentified phytochemicals has been used to explain the finding that UV carcinogenesis was enhanced with a beta-carotene-supplemented semi-defined diet in mice (Black 2004, Black & Gerguis 2003, Black et al 2000).

Enhanced intercellular communication

In addition to its antioxidant activity, beta-carotene enhances gap junction intercellular communication by upregulation of the gap junction protein connexin 43. This action may be important in its control of tumour growth (Yeh & Hu 2003), and is likely to be independent of its ability to quench singlet molecular oxygen (Stahl et al 1997).

Animal studies have indicated that a beta-carotene dose of 50 mg/kg/day for 5 days inhibits, whereas a lower dose (5 mg/kg/day) increases gap junction intercellular communication in rat liver. Further in vitro studies suggest that the observed inhibition is due, at least in part, to oxidised beta-carotene (Yeh & Hu 2003).

Anticarcinogenic activity

Observational epidemiological studies have consistently shown a relationship between dietary beta-carotene intake and low risk of various cancers (Cooper et al 1999b, Pryor et al 2000). In animal studies beta-carotene has been found to be chemoprotective, with inhibition of spontaneous mammary tumours (Fujii et al 1993, Nagasawa et al 1991), as well as prevention of skin carcinoma formation (Ponnamperuma et al 2000), UV-induced carcinogenesis in mice (Epstein 1977, Mathews-Roth 1982) and oral cancer in laboratory and animal models (Garewal 1995). Studies in ferrets suggest that the beta-carotene molecule becomes unstable in smoke-exposed lungs and that when given with alpha-tocopherol and ascorbic acid to stabilise the beta-carotene molecule, there is a protective effect against smoke-induced lung squamous metaplasia (Russell 2002).

A review of carotenoid research by the International Agency for Research on Cancer suggests there is sufficient evidence that beta-carotene has cancer-preventive activity in experimental animals, based on models of skin carcinogenesis in mice and buccal pouch carcinogenesis in hamsters (Vainio & Rautalahti 1998), despite a review suggesting that beta-carotene does not protect against lung cancer in animals (De Luca & Ross 1996).

Whether beta-carotene has anticancer properties in humans is unclear. It has been suggested any such effects could be mediated through multiple mechanisms that may include: antioxidant activity preventing oxidative damage to DNA and inhibition of lipid peroxidation; stimulation of gap junction communication; effects on cell transformation and differentiation; inhibition of cell proliferation and oncogene expression; effects on immune function; and inhibition of endogenous formation of carcinogens (Cooper et al 1999a). Additional mechanisms may include the metabolic conversion of beta-carotene to retinoids, which may in turn modulate the gene expression of factors linked to differentiation and cell proliferation. The modulation of enzymes that metabolise xenobiotics and inhibition of endogenous cholesterol synthesis by modulation of HMG-CoA reductase expression may also lead to a possible inhibition of cell proliferation and malignant transformation (PDRHealth 2005).

None of these mechanisms has been conclusively found to contribute to the prevention of cancer in vivo, and there is ongoing debate about the role of beta-carotene in cancer prevention (Cooper et al 1999a, Patrick 2000). This debate has been further fuelled by the findings of two large intervention studies: the Alpha-Tocopherol Beta-Carotene (ATBC) Cancer Prevention Study (the 'Finnish study': Heinonen et al 1994) and the Carotene and Retinol Efficacy Trial (CARET: Omenn et al 1996b), which found a significantly increased risk of lung cancer in high-risk individuals supplemented with synthetic beta-carotene (see *Clinical use* for more details).

The mixed findings from beta-carotene intervention trials have produced much controversy in the scientific literature and although it has been suggested there is no known biologically plausible explanation for the findings, a number of hypotheses have been put forward (Bendich 2004). It has been suggested that the dose, duration of study and/or choice of synthetic all-*trans*-beta-carotene may have been inappropriate in the intervention trials (Cooper et al 1999b), and that supplementation with monotherapy using synthetic beta-carotene may have inhibited the absorption of other carotenoids (Woodall et al 1996). It is also suggested that, although beta-carotene may be effective in the prevention of lung cancer before or during the phases of initiation and early promotion of cancer, the intervention studies that involved heavy smokers and asbestos workers probably included individuals in whom these processes were already initiated (Bendich 2004).

Additional possible explanations for the observed increase in lung cancer risk with beta-carotene supplementation include possible pro-oxidant activity of beta-carotene or its oxidative metabolites in the high-oxygen environment of smokers' lungs, with oxidised beta-carotene metabolites inducing carcinogen-bioactivating enzymes, facilitating the binding of metabolites to DNA, enhancing retinoic acid metabolism by P450 enzyme induction and acting as pro-oxidants, causing damage to DNA (Russell 2002), as well as inhibition of retinoid signalling (Wang et al 1999). It is further suggested that the beta-carotene molecule may become unstable due to the presence of a lower level of antioxidants, such as ascorbic acid, in smokers than in non-smokers (Bohm et al 1997), together with the presence of significant oxidative stress in smokers who consume high amounts of alcohol (PDRHealth 2005).

It has further been suggested that beta-carotene may increase lung cancer risk in smokers because of its ability to improve lung function. Thus smokers supplemented with beta-carotene may have increased lung capacity, resulting in deeper breathing of carcinogens and other oxidants. It is also suggested that beta-carotene may improve smokers' immune responses and thus reduce the number of days they suffer from upper respiratory tract infections, which enables them to smoke more (Bendich 2004).

The suggestion that beta-carotene may have pro-oxidant effects is supported by an in vitro study showing that although cell viability and DNA integrity were not affected by beta-carotene, they were significantly and dose-dependently decreased by oxidised beta-carotene (Yeh & Hu 2001). There was a dose-dependent increase of beta-carotene cleavage products, together with increasing genotoxicity in vitro when beta-carotene was supplemented during oxidative stress induced by hypoxia/reoxygenation (Alija et al 2004, 2005). Carotenoid cleavage products have also been found to impair mitochondrial function and increase oxidative stress in vitro (Siems et al 2002, 2005), as well as produce a booster effect on phase I carcinogen-bioactivating enzymes in the rat lung (Paolini et al 1999). Beta-carotene has also been shown to be degraded by stimulated polymorphonuclear leucocytes in vitro, producing highly reactive and potentially toxic cleavage products (Sommerburg et al 2003). These pro-oxidant effects have not been conclusively demonstrated in vivo, and beta-carotene at a dose of 50 mg/day for several years was not found to have pro-oxidant effects in either smokers or non-smokers, as measured by urinary excretion of F_2-isoprostanes (Mayne et al 2004).

Cardiovascular protection

There are a number of ways in which beta-carotene may act to protect against cardiovascular disease. Free-radical scavenging may prevent cellular transformations leading to atherosclerosis, and protection of LDL oxidation may further act to protect against atheroma formation (Halliwell 1993). Other mechanisms proposed for the possible favourable effect of antioxidants include an increase of HDL cholesterol and the preservation of endothelial functions (Tavani & La Vecchia 1999). Patients with acute myocardial infarction (AMI) have also been shown to have reduced plasma antioxidant vitamins and enhanced lipid peroxidation upon thrombolysis, suggesting that antioxidants may reduce free-radical generation processes in reperfusion injury in AMI (Levy et al 1998).

In an animal study, atherosclerosis was inhibited in rabbits fed a high-cholesterol diet supplemented with all-*trans* beta-carotene. In that study all-*trans* beta-carotene was undetectable in LDL, although tissue levels of retinyl palmitate were increased, suggesting that any anti-atherogenic effect is separate from the resistance of LDL to oxidation and that metabolites of beta-carotene may inhibit atherosclerosis in hypercholesterolaemic rabbits, possibly via stereospecific interactions with retinoic acid receptors in the artery wall (Shaish et al 1995). A randomised, placebo-controlled trial in 149 male smokers taking 20 mg/day of beta-carotene for 14 weeks, however, found no influence on haemostatic measures, suggesting that it is unlikely that cardiovascular protection from beta-carotene is via an effect on haemostasis (Van Poppel et al 1995).

OTHER ACTIONS

An animal study found that rats supplemented with beta-carotene-rich algae had improved reproduction and body growth, with a markedly lower stillbirth rate, a higher litter size or rearing rate, and enhanced body growth in male offspring (Nagasawa et al 1989).

CLINICAL USE

Vitamin A deficiency

In a series of large, double-blind, cluster-randomised, placebo-controlled field trials involving as many as 44,000 Nepalese women, weekly supplementation with 42 mg of *trans*-beta-carotene was found to reduce the prevalence of selected illness symptoms such as loose stools, night blindness and symptoms of high fever during late pregnancy, at the time of birth and during 6 months post-partum (Christian et al 2000b). Beta-carotene was further found to reduce maternal, but not infant, mortality among smokers and non-smokers by approximately 50%, with a protective effect becoming evident after 18 months of supplementation (Christian et al 2004, West et al 1999). Beta-carotene supplementation has also been found to reduce the five-fold increased risk of infection-related mortality in women who were night-blind because of vitamin A deficiency (Christian et al 2000a). In a randomised-controlled trial of children in rural China it was found that beta-carotene supplementation had a similar effect on correcting childhood vitamin A deficiency to retinol supplementation, with reduced morbidity and increased weight. The authors concluded that, considering the health risk of vitamin A supplementation and the easier acquisition and antioxidant value of dietary beta-carotene, dietary beta-carotene supplementation should be recommended for addressing vitamin A deficiency in this population (Lin et al 2009).

These studies contrast with one that found an association between self-reports of poor night vision and beta-carotene consumption in women involved in the Blue Mountain Eye Study, in which the authors concluded that perceived poor night vision caused an increase in carrot consumption in women (Smith et al 1999).

Cancer prevention

There are at least 35 observational epidemiological studies, including prospective cohort and case-controlled studies, involving smoking and non-smoking men and women from diverse regions of the world, that have found a positive association between dietary or serum beta-carotene levels and reduced risk of cancer (Cooper et al 1999a). This association, however, does not necessarily imply a causal link, because it may be an association between beta-carotene ingestion and other dietary or lifestyle factors (Peto et al 1981). Beta-carotene intake is linked to a variety of healthy dietary and lifestyle factors, as well as being highly correlated with the intake of many other protective dietary phytochemicals and nutrients (Cooper et al 1999a). Furthermore, these results have not always been consistent with a 6-year study of 137,001 European men, which found no link between plasma carotenoids and prostate cancer risk (Key et al 2007), and with a pooled analysis of 11 cohort studies suggesting no link with colorectal cancer risk (Männistö et al 2007). Similarly a pooled analysis of 10 cohort studies involving 521,911 women found no association between dietary carotenoids and the risk of ovarian cancer (Koushik et al 2006).

While the protective effect of dietary carotenoids on cancer risk is still being debated, findings of two large intervention trials have reported an increased lung cancer risk with synthetic beta-carotene supplementation (Heinonen et al 1994, Omenn et al 1996a).

The ATBC Cancer Prevention Study (Finnish study) was the first large intervention trial to test the hypothesis that beta-carotene reduces the risk of lung cancer. This double-blind, placebo-controlled primary-prevention trial involved 29,133 male smokers, 50–69 years of age, who were randomly selected to receive daily supplementation with alpha-tocopherol (50 mg/day) alone, synthetic (all-*trans*) beta-carotene (20 mg/day) alone, or both. After a follow-up period of 5–8 years, the results suggested that there was an unexpected 18% increase in the incidence of lung cancer with an associated 8% higher mortality among those who received beta-carotene (Heinonen et al 1994). Subgroup analysis revealed that the increased risk with beta-carotene supplementation was only greater for those who smoked at least 20 cigarettes per day, with the risk of those who smoked 5–19 cigarettes/day being no greater than that of the placebo group. An increased risk was also observed for those who consumed more than 11 g/day alcohol compared with those with a lower alcohol intake (Albanes et al 1996). Further analysis found no effect of beta-carotene supplementation on the risk of pancreatic cancer (Rautalahti et al 1999), colorectal cancer (Albanes et al 2000), urothelial or renal cell cancer (Virtamo et al 2000), or gastric cancer (Malila et al 2002).

The CARET trial tested the effect of synthetic, all-*trans* beta-carotene (30 mg) and retinyl palmitate (25,000 IU) on the incidence of lung cancer, other cancers and death in 18,314 participants who were at high risk of lung cancer because of a history of heavy smoking or asbestos exposure. CARET was stopped ahead of schedule in January 1996 because participants who were randomly assigned to receive the active intervention were unexpectedly found to have a 28% increase in incidence of lung cancer, a 17% increase in incidence of death and a higher rate of cardiovascular disease mortality compared with participants in the placebo group (Omenn et al 1996b). Further analysis revealed results similar to the ATBC study, with the increased risk of lung cancer being greatest for heavy smokers and those with the highest alcohol intake, while former smokers were found to have a similar risk to that of those taking the placebo (Omenn et al 1996b).

The finding of an increased risk of lung cancer in smokers taking beta-carotene in the ATBC and CARET studies is consistent with a number of other studies. A prospective cohort study of 59,910 French women found that self-reported supplemental use of beta-carotene was directly associated with double the risk of cancers among smokers, yet dietary beta-carotene intake was associated with less than half the risk of tobacco-related cancers among non-smokers in a statistically significant dose-dependent relationship (Touvier et al 2005). Similarly, the results of a case-control study of 362 adenoma cases and 427 polyp-free controls suggest a protective effect for colon cancer with beta-carotene in non-smokers and an adverse effect in smokers (Senesse et al 2005). Alcohol intake and cigarette smoking were also observed to modify the effect of beta-carotene supplementation on the risk of colorectal adenoma recurrence in another double-blind, placebo-controlled clinical trial involving 864 patients randomised to receive either beta-carotene (25 mg), vitamin C (1000 mg) or vitamin E (400 mg), beta-carotene with vitamins C and E, or a placebo. After 4 years this trial found no evidence that supplementation reduced the incidence of adenomas (Greenberg et al 1994). Subgroup analysis from this study, however, found that beta-carotene supplementation was associated with a marked decrease in the risk of one or more recurrent adenomas among subjects who neither smoked cigarettes nor drank alcohol, but conferred a modest increase in the risk of recurrence among those who either smoked or drank alcohol and doubled the risk for those who both smoked and drank (Baron et al 2003).

The results of these studies are contrasted with those from the Physicians' Health Study, which found that beta-carotene supplementation had no effect on cancer risk in smokers or non-smokers. This RCT of 50 mg of synthetic beta-carotene given on alternate days involved 22,071 US male doctors, 11% of whom were smokers. After more than 12 years of follow-up, no overall effect on cancer incidence was evident with beta-carotene supplementation (Hennekens et al 1996) and no benefit or harm was observed for lung, prostate or colon cancer (Cook et al 2000), or for squamous cell carcinoma (Frieling et al 2000). Subgroup analysis of this study population revealed that total cancer was modestly reduced with supplementation among those aged more than 70 years, and total cancers and colon cancer was reduced in those who drank alcohol daily (Cook et al 2000). Total cancers and prostate cancer were also reduced in those in the highest BMI quartile (Cook et al 2000) and those with low baseline beta-carotene levels (Cook et al 1999), while those with high baseline levels had a non-significant increased risk of prostate cancer with beta-carotene supplementation (Cook et al 1999).

Similar to the results of the Physicians' Health Study the results of the Women's Health Study, which involved 39,876 women supplemented with 50 mg of beta-carotene on alternate days for 2 years, found no benefit or harm from beta-carotene supplementation on the incidence of cancer or cardiovascular disease in apparently healthy women, and no benefit or harm observed for the 13% of women who were smokers at baseline (Lee et al 1999).

In contrast to these results, an RCT performed on a poorly nourished population found a lower cancer incidence with beta-carotene supplementation. This study involved 29,584 adults aged between 40 and 69 years from Linxian County, China, which has one of the world's highest rates of oesophageal/gastric cardia cancer and a persistently low intake of several micronutrients. In this study people were randomised to receive retinol and zinc, riboflavin and niacin, vitamin C and molybdenum, or beta-carotene, vitamin E and selenium, at doses that ranged from one- to two-fold the US RDI for a period of 6 years. Results revealed a significantly lower total mortality rate among those receiving supplementation with beta-carotene, vitamin E and selenium, mainly attributable to lower cancer rates, especially stomach cancer (Blot et al 1993).

Possible reasons for the mixed results

The mixed results from the beta-carotene intervention studies have created significant debate. The results of a review of carotenoid research by the International Agency for Research on Cancer suggest there is a lack of cancer-preventive activity for beta-carotene when it is used as a supplement at high doses (Vainio & Rautalahti 1998). This is supported by a more recent study that examined the relationship between dietary beta-carotene and lung cancer, using pooled data from seven cohort studies that involved 399,765 participants and 3155 lung cancer cases. This study found that dietary beta-carotene intake was not associated with increased or decreased lung cancer risk in those who had never smoked, past or current smokers (Männistö et al 2004). Similarly, a more recent systematic review and meta-analysis of six randomised clinical trials examining the efficacy of beta-carotene supplements and 25 prospective observational studies assessing the associations between carotenoids and lung cancer suggests that beta-carotene supplementation is not associated with a significant altered risk of developing lung cancer (Gallicchio et al 2008).

The mixed results from beta-carotene intervention studies may also be a reflection of a difference between natural and synthetic beta-carotene, as the negative intervention studies have all used synthetic rather than natural beta-carotene. These studies, however, do provide consistent evidence for a link between dietary and serum beta-carotene levels and reduced cancer risk. Even in the studies that found an adverse effect of beta-carotene supplementation, study participants with the highest intake and serum concentrations of beta-carotene at baseline developed fewer subsequent lung cancers, regardless of their intervention assignment (Albanes 1999, Holick et al 2002). Therefore, although monotherapy with synthetic beta-carotene is no longer generally recommended, there continues to be a consistent call for an increased consumption of beta-carotene-containing foods to assist in the prevention of cancer (Mayne 1996, Pryor et al 2000).

Oral leucoplakia

Beta-carotene consumption has been found to be inversely associated with precancerous lesions of the oral cavity in tobacco users (Gupta et al 1999), and it is suggested that there is a significant role for antioxidant nutrients in preventing oral cancer (Garewal & Schantz 1995). This is supported by the findings of multiple clinical trials in which beta-carotene and vitamin E have been shown to produce regression of oral leucoplakia, a premalignant lesion for oral cancer (Garewal 1994, Wright et al 2007).

In a more recent, double-blind RCT involving 160 people, 360 mg/week of beta-carotene for 12 months was found to induce regression in oral precancerous lesions, with half of the responders relapsing after ceasing supplementation. Similarly, another multicentre, double-blind, placebo-controlled trial found improvement in dysplasia with 60 mg/day of beta-carotene for 6 months (Garewal et al 1999).

These studies are contrasted with a subgroup analysis involving 409 white male cigarette smokers from the ATBC study, which suggested that beta-carotene supplementation does not play an essential role in preventing oral mucosal changes in smokers (Liede et al 1998).

Cardiovascular disease

Epidemiological studies support the idea that a diet rich in high-carotenoid-containing foods is associated with a reduced risk of heart disease (Kritchevsky 1999). A review of observational and intervention studies on beta-carotene and the risk of coronary heart disease found that seven cohort studies (Gaziano et al 1995a, Gey et al 1993, Knekt et al 1994, Manson et al 1991, Morris et al 1994, Rimm et al 1993, Street et al 1994) reported relative risks between 0.27 and 0.78 for high serum beta-carotene levels or high dietary intake; the review found this was supported by case-control studies (Bobak et al 1998, Bolton-Smith et al 1992, Kardinaal et al 1993, Torun et al 1994, Tavani et al 1997) which reported odds ratios between 0.37 and 0.71, with a possible stronger protection for current smokers (Tavani & La Vecchia 1999). More recently, a 16-year cohort study of 1031 Finnish men aged 46–65 years from the Kuopio Ischemic Heart Disease Risk Factor (KIHD) cohort, found that after controlling for other factors, low serum beta-carotene concentrations increased the risk of cardiovascular disease and total mortality in men and that men in the lowest tertile of serum concentrations of beta-carotene had a two-fold increased risk of sudden cardiac death compared to those in the highest tertile and men with the lowest quartile of beta-carotene had almost three-fold increased risk of congestive cardiac failure (Karppi et al 2013a, Karppi et al 2013b). This study further reported that the strongest risk of CVD mortality was observed among smokers with lowest levels of beta-carotene (Karppi et al 2012). These results contrast with those of four more recent cohort studies (Knekt et al 1994, Kushi et al 1996, Pandey et al 1995, Todd et al 1995) and five large RCTs (Hennekens et al 1996, Lee et al 1999, Redlich et al 1999, Vlot et al 1995) which have not reported any significant prevention of cardiovascular disease with beta-carotene supplementation.

The final results of the Physicians' Health Study (see *Cancer prevention* above) indicated that beta-carotene supplementation exerted no significant benefit or harm on cancer or cardiovascular disease during more than 12 years of treatment (Hennekens et al 1996). Similarly, the results of the Women's Health Study, involving 39,876 women aged 45 years or older, found that beta-carotene supplementation of 50 mg on alternate days did not influence cardiovascular disease after 2 years of supplementation and 2 years of further follow-up. Subgroup analysis revealed that beta-carotene supplementation had an apparent benefit on subsequent vascular events among 333 men with prior angina or revascularisation (Christen et al 2000c).

In contrast, analysis of the data from the ATBC cancer prevention study, which involved 23,144 male smokers, found that beta-carotene supplementation slightly increased the risk of angina (Rapola et al 1996) and intracerebral haemorrhage, while having no overall effect on the risk of stroke

(Leppala et al 2000a, 2000b), abdominal aortic aneurysm (Tornwall et al 2001), or symptoms and progression of intermittent claudication (Tornwall et al 1999). Beta-carotene, however, was found to decrease the risk of cerebral infarction modestly among a subgroup with greater alcohol consumption (Leppala et al 2000a, 2000b). In a 6-year post-intervention follow-up study, beta-carotene was found to increase the risk of first-ever myocardial infarction, while continuing to have no overall effect on the incidence of stroke (Tornwall et al 2004). An analysis of 52 men from the CARET study concluded that there was no significant effect on total, HDL or LDL cholesterol levels, which could account for the increase risk of cardiovascular disease observed in this study (Redlich et al 1999).

A pooled analysis of four randomised trials of beta-carotene therapy, ranging from 20 mg to 50 mg, involving 90,054 patients, found beta-carotene supplementation to be associated with a significant increase in all-cause mortality and cardiovascular death in patients at risk of coronary disease, with the increased risk being greatest in smokers. A further meta-analysis of eight randomised trials involving 138,113 patients found that supplementation with 15–50 mg of beta-carotene was associated with a small but significant increase in all-cause mortality and a slight increase in cardiovascular death (Vivekananthan et al 2003).

The apparent discrepancy between the findings of observational and intervention studies may be due to several factors, including the length and nature of the intervention (Tavani & La Vecchia 1999). For example, the intervention trials involved supplementation with synthetic beta-carotene in isolation or with other single nutrients, whereas the observational studies involved the consumption of beta-carotene-rich foods containing a range of additional antioxidant vitamins, phytonutrients and micronutrients.

Photoprotection

Excessive exposure to solar radiation, especially UVA (320–400 nm) and UVB (290–320 nm), may induce UV-carcinogenesis and erythema in the skin (Lee et al 2000). There have been a number of controlled clinical trials that have demonstrated that supplementation with beta-carotene alone, or in combination with other antioxidants, can reduce UV-induced erythema (Gollnick et al 1996, Heinrich et al 1998, Heinrich et al 2003, Lee et al 2000, Mathews-Roth et al 1972, Sies & Stahl 2004, Stahl et al 2000). These studies suggest that at least 8–10 weeks of supplementation required before protection against erythema becomes evident and that doses of at least 24 mg/day of beta-carotene are required (Sies & Stahl 2004).

In uncontrolled studies, a protective effect against UV-induced erythema was observed after supplementation with 180 mg of beta-carotene for 10 weeks (Mathews-Roth et al 1972) and with 50 mg for 6 weeks (Heinrich et al 1998). These results are supported by more rigorous studies that have shown photoprotective activity with smaller doses of beta-carotene. An RCT involving supplementation with 30 mg of natural beta-carotene for 8 weeks, with the dose increasing to 60 mg for a further 8 weeks and then to 90 mg for another 8 weeks, found a dose-dependent reduction in UVA- and UVB-induced erythema (Lee et al 2000). In another RCT, supplementation for 12 weeks with 24 mg/day of natural beta-carotene or a natural carotenoid mix supplying similar amounts of beta-carotene, lutein and lycopene also significantly reduced UV-induced erythema (Heinrich et al 2003). Similarly, a randomised trial found that supplementation with 25 mg of natural algal beta-carotene for 12 weeks significantly reduced UV-induced erythema, with the effect enhanced by the addition of alpha-tocopherol (Stahl et al 2000). Yet another trial suggests that the photoprotective action of beta-carotene enhances the action of topical sunscreens. In this randomised, placebo-controlled, double-blind study of 20 healthy young females, 30 mg/day beta-carotene for 10 weeks reduced UV-induced erythema and protected against UV-induced drop in serum beta-carotene levels and UV-induced reduction in Langerhans cells; beta-carotene combined with topical sunscreens was more effective than sunscreen cream alone (Gollnick et al 1996). A protective effect against photo-immunosuppression was demonstrated in another study in which 30 mg/day of beta-carotene for 4 weeks protected against UV-induced suppression of delayed-type hypersensitivity in young men (Fuller et al 1992).

It has been suggested that the duration of supplementation may be more important than the dose, as the studies that have not demonstrated significant reduction in UV-induced erythema have all involved supplementation of relatively short duration (Lee et al 2000). No photoprotective effects were observed with supplementation of 90 mg beta-carotene for 3 weeks (Garmyn et al 1995), 150 mg/day for 4 weeks (Wolf et al 1988) or 15 mg/day for 8 weeks (McArdle et al 2004).

It has also been suggested that a combination of antioxidants may be more effective than the sum of the separate components because the skin's antioxidant defence system appears to involve an intricate connection between individual antioxidants (Steenvoorden & Beijersbergen van Henegouwen 1997). This is supported by a randomised, double-blind, placebo-controlled study that found that short-term (2-week) supplementation with an antioxidative combination containing beta-carotene and lycopene, as well as vitamins C and E, selenium and proanthocyanidins, significantly decreases the UV-induced expression of matrix metalloproteinases, with a non-statistically significant trend towards reduced minimal erythema dose (Greul et al 2002).

Although beta-carotene supplementation may provide some degree of protection against sunburn, the effect is modest and there is still some debate about its use for routine photoprotection (Biesalski & Obermueller-Jevic 2001, Fuchs 1998). However, beta-carotene is likely to be clinically useful in providing photoprotection for people with specific photosensitivity. High doses (180 mg/day, up to 300 mg/day) have been shown to reduce photosensitivity in people with the genetic condition erythropoietic protoporphyria in a number of case series (Mathews-Roth et al 1970, 1974, Thomsen et al 1979), and the results of a double-blind RCT suggest that beta-carotene may be useful in conjunction with canthaxanthin in preventing polymorphous light eruptions (Suhonen & Plosila 1981).

The ability of beta-carotene to protect against UV-induced erythema and photosensitivity does not appear to extend to protecting against non-melanotic skin cancer. In a randomised placebo-controlled trial involving 1805 subjects with recent non-melanotic skin cancer, daily supplementation with 50 mg beta-carotene for 5 years had no effect on the incidence of new or recurring non-melanotic skin cancers, with similar results for those with low-baseline beta-carotene levels and smokers (Greenberg et al 1990). Similarly, in another randomised, placebo-controlled trial of 1621 adults aged between 25 and 74 years, daily supplementation with 30 mg beta-carotene did not reduce the development of solar keratoses over the 3-year study period (Darlington et al 2003, Green et al 1999). These results are supported by an analysis of data from the Physicians' Health Study which found that 12 years of beta-carotene supplementation had no effect on the incidence of non-melanotic skin cancer (Frieling et al 2000); a subgroup analysis from this study also found no effect on non-melanotic skin cancer in men with low-baseline plasma beta-carotene levels (Schaumberg et al 2004). In a further randomised, placebo-controlled study of 62 patients with numerous atypical naevi, 25 mg of beta-carotene given twice daily for 36 months resulted in a non-significant reduction in newly developed naevi, with a significant reduction observed for the lower arm and feet, but not for 10 other body sites (Bayerl et al 2003).

Oxidative stress

There are a number of human studies that suggest supplementation with beta-carotene can reduce the oxidative stress associated with different pathological conditions or stressors such as intense exercise or radiation. Supplementation with beta-carotene (30 mg/day) and vitamin E (500 mg/day) for 90 days has been found to enhance the antioxidant enzyme activity of superoxide dismutase and catalase in the neutrophils of sportsmen (Tauler et al 2002). Similarly, in a study of 13 professional basketball players, 35 days of antioxidant supplementation with 600 mg alpha-tocopherol, 1000 mg ascorbic acid and 32 mg beta-carotene led to a significant decrease in plasma lipid peroxides, with a significant decrease of lactate dehydrogenase serum activity and a non-significant increase in the anabolic/catabolic balance being observed during a 24-hour recuperation time after exercise (Schroder et al 2001).

The results of an Israeli study of 709 children exposed to radiation from the Chernobyl accident suggest that natural algae-derived beta-carotene may act as an in vivo lipophilic antioxidant or radioprotector. This study found that exposed children had increased susceptibility to lipid oxidation and that supplementation with 40 mg of natural 9-*cis* and all-*trans* equal isomer mixture beta-carotene twice daily for a period of 3 months reduced plasma markers of lipid oxidation (Ben-Amotz et al 1998).

A double-blind study has also found that beta-carotene supplementation reduced the severity, but not the incidence, of post-endoscopy pancreatitis, which is thought to be mediated by oxidative stress (Lavy et al 2004). A further small, controlled trial involving 15 patients with rheumatoid arthritis found that 3 weeks of supplementation with natural beta-carotene resulted in a significant increase in plasma antioxidants, but did not change indicators of disease (Kacsur et al 2002).

There is also evidence that beta-carotene may protect against the oxidative stress caused by chemotherapy and radiotherapy. A study on conditioning therapy found antioxidant protection after supplementation with 45 mg beta-carotene, 825 mg alpha-tocopherol and 450 mg ascorbic acid daily for 3 weeks preceding bone marrow transplantation. The conditioning therapy, which consists of high-dose chemotherapy and total body irradiation, has acute and delayed toxic effects that are considered to be due to peroxidation processes and exhaustion of antioxidants. Supplementation, however, was found to increase serum antioxidant levels and reduce the post-conditioning rise in plasma lipid hydroperoxides in patients receiving the conditioning therapy before transplantation (Clemens et al 1997). A higher than usual dietary intake of beta-carotene has also been found to reduce the occurrence of severe adverse effects of radiation therapy and decrease local cancer recurrence in people with head and neck cancer (Meyer et al 2007).

Contrasting with the above studies are two small studies showing no change in oxidative stress in healthy subjects after beta-carotene supplementation. Normal concentrations of carotenoids in plasma and tissues were not correlated with clinical markers of antioxidant and oxidative stress in a study of 79 healthy volunteers (Borel et al 1998), and a placebo-controlled, single-blind study found that daily supplementation with 15 mg of beta-carotene for 3 months did not significantly improve biomarkers of oxidative stress in healthy males (Hininger et al 2001).

Immune function

Beta-carotene supplementation of 15 mg/day has been shown to significantly reduce IgE and respiratory rate and improve recovery of pneumonia among children aged 6–36 months (Mohamed et al 2008). In a study of 652 non-institutionalised elderly people, the incidence of acute respiratory infections was reduced for those with the highest plasma levels, suggesting that beta-carotene may improve the immune response and result in decreased risk of infectious diseases (van der Horst-Graat et al 2004).

In contrast to these findings, analyses of male smokers who participated in the ATBC study found that supplementation with synthetic beta-carotene had no overall effect on the risk of hospital-treated pneumonia or the incidence of the common cold (Hemila et al 2002, 2004), but instead increased the risk of colds in subjects carrying out heavy exercise at leisure but not at work (Hemila et al 2003).

Asthma and chronic obstructive pulmonary disease

Studies have shown increased oxidative stress in patients with chronic airflow limitation (Ochs-Balcom et al 2005) and accumulating evidence suggests that dietary antioxidant vitamins are positively associated with lung function (Schunemann et al 2001), with serum beta-carotene levels being associated with improved forced expiratory volume in the first second (FEV_1) (Grievink et al 2000). Thus it has been suggested that antioxidant protection is important for protecting the lungs against high oxygen levels and that oxidative stress may contribute to respiratory pathology such as asthma (Rahman et al 2006, Wood et al 2003). This is supported by the finding of a significant association between serum vitamin C, vitamin E, beta-cryptoxanthin, lutein/zeaxanthin, beta-carotene and retinol with FEV_1 (Schunemann et al 2001), together with a study involving a subset from the CARET study of 816 asbestos-exposed men with a high rate of current and former cigarette smoking, which found that serum beta-carotene was associated with a significant improvement in forced expiratory volume in 1 second (FEV_1) and forced vital capacity (FVC) (Chuwers et al 1997).

Studies on the correlation between serum beta-carotene levels and asthma, however, have produced mixed results. A recent meta-analysis of 10 studies on the incidence of dietary antioxidant intake and the risk of asthma found no positive association between intakes of beta-carotene or vitamin E and asthma risk (Gao et al 2008). One small study of 15 asthmatic subjects and 16 healthy controls found that despite similar dietary intake, whole blood levels of total carotenoids — including beta-carotene, lycopene, lutein, beta-cryptoxanthin and alpha-carotene — were significantly lower in the asthmatics, with no differences in plasma or sputum carotenoid levels (Wood et al 2005). Another small study found that beta-carotene, alpha-tocopherol and ascorbic acid were significantly lower in asthmatics at remission compared to controls, and that beta-carotene was significantly lower and lipid peroxidation products significantly higher during attacks than in periods of remission (Kalayci et al 2000). A further small study found that increased dietary consumption of beta-carotene was associated with better quality of life (Moreira et al 2004).

These results are supported by an analysis of 7505 youths (4–16 years) from the Third National Health and Nutrition Examination Survey, which found that increased serum beta-carotene was associated with reduced asthma prevalence (Rubin et al 2004). Another analysis involving 4093 children from the same study, 9.7% of whom reported a diagnosis of asthma, found that asthma diagnosis was associated with lower levels of serum beta-carotene, vitamin C, alpha-carotene and beta-cryptoxanthin (Harik-Khan et al 2004).

In contrast to these findings, a much larger study involving 771 people with self-reported asthma, 352 people with former asthma and 15,418 people without asthma found that asthma status was not significantly associated with serum antioxidant concentrations (Ford et al 2004). Similarly, in a study of 15 mild asthmatics and 15 age- and sex-matched controls, oxidative stress was found to be increased in the asthmatics, with no difference in plasma dietary antioxidant vitamins (Wood et al 2000).

Although the role of antioxidant vitamins in prevention and/or treatment of asthma remains to be determined (Kalayci et al 2000), the results of one intervention study suggest that there may be a role for beta-carotene in exercise-induced asthma. This randomised, double-blind, placebo-controlled trial involved 38 subjects with proven exercise-induced asthma and found that supplementation with 64 mg/day of natural algal beta-carotene for 1 week protected against post-exercise reduction in FEV_1 (Neuman et al 1999).

Cystic fibrosis

Cystic fibrosis (CF) is characterised by exocrine pancreatic insufficiency and reduced absorption of fat-soluble vitamins, as well as by chronic lung inflammation and an associated increased oxygen free-radical generation. Patients with CF have been found to have lower levels of beta-carotene, and it has been suggested that they would benefit from beta-carotene supplementation (Cobanoglu et al 2002, Walkowiak et al 2004). This suggestion is supported by a study of 52 patients with CF, which found a statistically significant correlation between serum beta-carotene and the clinical course of the disease as indicated by faecal elastase-1 and FEV_1 (Walkowiak et al 2004), together with a study showing that the plasma levels of beta-carotene and vitamin E increased and the plasma levels of TNF-alpha and malondialdehyde decreased after 6 months of beta-carotene supplementation (Cobanoglu et al 2002). This is further supported by a RCT of 24 CF patients who were supplemented with up to 50 mg/day beta-carotene for 12 weeks and 10 mg/day beta-carotene for a further 12 weeks; a significant decrease in oxidative stress, correction of total antioxidative capacity and improved pulmonary response to treatment were found in the supplemented group (Rust et al 2000).

Cataracts

Although a high intake of foods containing beta-carotene has been associated with the prevention of cataracts, the role of supplementation is uncertain. An assessment of dietary beta-carotene intake in a subgroup of 472 non-diabetic female participants aged 53–73 years in the Nurses' Health Study found that the odds of posterior subcapsular cataracts were 72% lower in those with the highest intakes of beta-carotene who had never smoked, whereas beta-carotene intake and cataract risk were not associated in current or past smokers (Taylor et al 2002). In contrast to this finding, intervention studies have shown that beta-carotene may help prevent cataracts in smokers (Christen et al 2003, 2004a). Two years of beta-carotene treatment was found to have no significant beneficial or harmful effect on the development of cataract in a randomised, double-masked, placebo-controlled trial of 39,876 female health professionals aged 45 years or older who participated in the Women's Health Study, although a subgroup analysis suggests a possible beneficial effect in smokers (Christen et al 2004a). Similarly, the Physicians' Study (see above) found that 12 years of supplementation did not reduce the overall incidence of cataracts or cataract extraction; however, in a subgroup of smokers the risk of cataract was reduced by approximately 25% (Christen et al 2003).

In two randomised, double-masked trials that involved 5390 nutritionally deprived subjects in Linxian, China, supplementation with selenium, alpha-tocopherol and beta-carotene for 5–6 years was found to significantly reduce the prevalence of nuclear, but not cortical, cataracts in older subjects (Sperduto et al 1993). This contrasts with the finding that 500 mg of vitamin C, 400 IU of vitamin E and 15 mg of beta-carotene had no apparent effect on the 7-year risk of development or progression of age-related lens opacities or visual acuity loss in a relatively well-nourished older adult cohort of 4629 people, aged from 55 to 80 years, who participated in the Age-Related Eye Disease (ARED) study (Kassoff et al 2001).

Age-related macula degeneration

Although beta-carotene and other nutrients may have been found to be beneficial for preventing age-related macula degeneration (ARMD), the carotenoids lutein and zeaxanthin appear to provide the most protection (see monograph *Lutein and zeaxanthin*).

A high intake of beta-carotene-containing foods has been associated with the prevention of ARMD, and observational and experimental data suggest that carotenoid supplements may delay progression of both ARMD and vision loss. This is supported by the findings from the ARED study, in which an 11-centre, double-masked clinical trial involving 3640 participants with ARMD found that supplementation with vitamin C 500 mg, vitamin E 400 IU, beta-carotene 15 mg and zinc 80 mg for 6 years significantly reduced the development of advanced ARMD and moderate visual acuity loss (Kassoff et al 2001). A 5-year follow-up of 3549 participants from the ARED study found that the beneficial effects of the AREDS formulation persisted for development of neurovascular age, but not central geographic atrophy NV age-related macular degeneration, and not for CGA (Chew et al 2013). This result contrasts with findings from the Physicians' Study (see above), which found no beneficial or harmful effects of beta-carotene supplementation on the incidence of ARMD (Christen et al 2007).

Erythropoietic protoporphyria and photosensitivity

Studies in bacteria, animals and humans have demonstrated that carotenoid pigments can prevent or lessen photosensitivity to endogenous photosensitisers, such as chlorophyll or porphyrins, as well as to exogenous photosensitisers (Mathews-Roth 1993). High doses of beta-carotene (between 180 and 300 mg/day) have been used to effectively prevent or lessen photosensitivity in most patients with erythropoietic protoporphyria and in some patients with other photosensitivity diseases such as solar urticaria, hydroa aestivale, porphyria cutanea tarda and actinic reticuloid (Mathews-Roth 1986, 1987, Mathews-Roth et al 1977).

Cognitive function

A study of cognitive function in high-functioning older people found that beta-carotene may offer protection from cognitive decline in people with a greater genetic susceptibility, as evidenced by the presence of the apolipoprotein E4 allele (Hu et al 2006). There is also evidence to suggest that long-term supplementation with beta-carotene may provide cognitive benefits, whereas short-term supplementation does not. A study examining cognitive function in 5956 participants older than 65 years in the Physicians' Health Study found significant higher cognitive function in the beta-carotene group when 4052 continuing participants who had been receiving either beta-carotene supplementation or a placebo for an average of 18 years were examined, but no difference was found between the beta-carotene and placebo groups in 1904 newly recruited subjects after 1 year of intervention (Grodstein et al 2007).

DOSAGE RANGE

Consumption of the recommended five or more servings of fruits and vegetables per day provides 3–6 mg of beta-carotene. Supplemental intake of beta-carotene ranges from 3 to 30 mg/day, although medicinal doses to treat erythropoietic protoporphyria or prevent a reaction to sun in patients with polymorphous light eruption range from 30 to 300 mg/day (PDRHealth 2005). The dose required to provide photoprotection is greater than 24 mg/day for more than 2 months (Sies & Stahl 2004).

B

To enhance absorption, supplementation should be taken with meals.

TOXICITY

Beta-carotene is readily converted into vitamin A when required by the body and is considered to be non-toxic, even when given in doses as high as 300 mg/day (Mathews-Roth 1990b, 1993).

A review of the literature on adverse effects of carotenoids on human and animal development suggests that beta-carotene does not have any genotoxic affects (Mathews-Roth 1988), and a toxicity study performed on rats suggests a no-observed-adverse-effect-level (NOAEL) is at a dietary level of at least 5%, or more than 3000 mg/kg/day (Nabae et al 2005). Beta-carotene overdose is not reported in the literature.

Practice points/Patient counselling

- Beta-carotene is an antioxidant found in carrots, other vegetables and fruits, as well as in seaweed and algae. Together with other carotenoids, it is an effective marker for a diet rich in fruits and vegetables.
- Beta-carotene is fat soluble and should be consumed with meals.
- Although beta-carotene is converted into vitamin A in the body, unlike vitamin A it is considered non-toxic, even in large doses.
- When supplementing with beta-carotene, it is preferable to use supplements containing natural beta-carotene from the algae *Dunaliella salina* or palm oil, rather than synthetic beta-carotene.
- Beta-carotene is a powerful pigment that contributes to the normal yellow component of skin, and increased beta-carotene intake may protect from the effects of excessive exposure to sunlight and the symptoms of sunburn.
- Consumption of beta-carotene-rich food is associated with reduced risk of cancers, heart disease and eye disease; however, these benefits have not been found in large studies that have used synthetic beta-carotene, with two studies finding an increase in lung cancer in heavy smokers and asbestos workers taking large doses of synthetic beta-carotene.

ADVERSE REACTIONS

At doses greater than 30 mg/day, beta-carotene may cause an orange-yellow colouration of the skin (carotenodermia), which is usually seen first as yellowness of the palms and soles. This condition is harmless and reversible when intake ceases (Micozzi et al 1988). Carotenodermia is distinguished from jaundice by the absence of yellowed ocular sclerae. For some people, this skin colouration is actually considered desirable (Mathews-Roth 1990a) and is utilised in tanning tablets to produce a natural-looking skin tan (DerMarderosian & Beutler 2002).

At present it is unclear if there is a true link between increased lung cancer risk and long-term beta-carotene supplementation in smokers, because supplementation studies with synthetic beta-carotene have produced mixed results: two studies demonstrated an increased lung cancer risk in heavy smokers or those with high asbestos exposure (Group 1994, Heinonen et al 1994, Omenn et al 1996a), while other studies found either no effect (Hennekens et al 1996, Lee et al 1999) or a protective effect (Blot et al 1993).

The association between increased lung cancer risk and beta-carotene has not been found with natural beta-carotene, and there is no suggestion that heavy smokers should reduce their intake of beta-carotene-rich foods. A review suggests that there is no evidence at present that consuming small amounts of supplemental beta-carotene in a multivitamin tablet at amounts that exist in foods (< 6 mg) is unwise for any population (Pryor et al 2000).

SIGNIFICANT INTERACTIONS

Drugs reducing fat absorption

Drugs that reduce fat absorption, such as cholestyramine, colestipol and orlistat, may also reduce absorption of beta-carotene (PDRHealth 2005). This can be avoided by spacing the administration of these substances by at least 2 hours. Plant sterols have been found to reduce beta-carotene bioavailability by approximately 50% in normocholesterolaemic men (Richelle et al 2004).

Fibrates

There may be a positive interaction between fibrate and natural beta-carotene, which has been found to significantly increase HDL cholesterol levels in fibrate-treated mice and humans (Shaish et al 2006).

CONTRAINDICATIONS AND PRECAUTIONS

Heavy smokers should be advised not to take synthetic beta-carotene supplements for long periods of time.

PREGNANCY USE

Beta-carotene crosses the placenta. Adequate and well-controlled studies in humans have not been documented. No problems with pregnancy have been documented in women taking up to 30 mg beta-carotene daily (Micromedex 2003). As vitamin A is vital for the development of the fetus and the newborn baby, it has been recommended that pregnant women increase their vitamin A intake by 40% and breastfeeding women by 90%. It is further suggested that increasing dietary beta-carotene is an effective way for women to maintain their vitamin A levels (Strobel et al 2007).

Valproate

Epileptic patients who gain weight with valproate therapy have been found to have reduced plasma concentrations of beta-carotene and other fat-soluble antioxidant vitamins; this is reversible after valproate withdrawal (Verrotti et al 2004).

PATIENTS' FAQs

What will this supplement do for me?

Beta-carotene supplementation will ensure you maintain adequate vitamin A levels. It may possibly assist in preventing cancer and cardiovascular disease, help maintain a healthy immune system, prevent sunburn and photoageing of the skin, assist with asthma, and deal with oxidative stress.

When will it start to work?

It may take up to 2–3 months to see a benefit with UV protection, whereas other benefits may be observable only over many years.

Are there any safety issues?

Beta-carotene is considered non-toxic. Large doses may cause a yellowing of the skin, but this is harmless and reversible.

REFERENCES

Abahusain MA et al. Retinol, a-tocopherol and carotenoids in diabetes. Eur J Clin Nutr 53.8 (1999): 630–635.

Alaluf S et al. Dietary carotenoids contribute to normal human skin color and UV photosensitivity. J Nutr 132.3 (2002): 399–403.

Albanes D. Beta-carotene and lung cancer: a case study. Am J Clin Nutr 69.6 (1999): 1345–1350S.

Albanes D et al. Alpha-tocopherol and beta-carotene supplements and lung cancer incidence in the alpha-tocopherol, beta-carotene cancer prevention study: effects of base-line characteristics and study compliance. J Natl Cancer Inst 88.21 (1996): 1560–1570.

Albanes D et al. Effects of supplemental alpha-tocopherol and beta-carotene on colorectal cancer: results from a controlled trial (Finland). Cancer Causes Control 1.3 (2000): 197–205.

Alija AJ et al. Cytotoxic and genotoxic effects of beta-carotene breakdown products on primary rat hepatocytes. Carcinogenesis 25.5 (2004): 827–831.

Alija AJ et al. Cyto- and genotoxic potential of beta-carotene and cleavage products under oxidative stress. BioFactors 24.1–4 (2005): 159–163.

Allard JP et al. Effects of beta-carotene supplementation on lipid peroxidation in humans. Am J Clin Nutr 59.4 (1994): 884–890.

Arnlöv J et al. Serum and dietary beta-carotene and alpha-tocopherol and incidence of type 2 diabetes mellitus in a community-based study of Swedish men: Report from the Uppsala Longitudinal Study of Adult Men (ULSAM) study. Diabetologia 52.1 (2009): 97–105.

Baron JA et al. Neoplastic and antineoplastic effects of beta-carotene on colorectal adenoma recurrence: Results of a randomized trial. J Natl Cancer Inst 95.10 (2003): 717–722.

Bayerl C et al. A three-year randomized trial in patients with dysplastic naevi treated with oral beta-carotene. Acta Dermato-Venereol 834 (2003): 277–281.

Ben-Amotz A, Levy Y. Bioavailability of a natural isomer mixture compared with synthetic all-trans beta-carotene in human serum. Am J Clin Nutr 63.5 (1996): 729–734.

Ben-Amotz A et al. Bioavailability of a natural isomer mixture as compared with synthetic all-trans-[beta]-carotene in rats and chicks. J Nutr 119.7 (1989): 1013–1019.

Ben-Amotz A et al. Natural beta-carotene and whole body irradiation in rats. Radiat Environ Biophys 35.4 (1996): 285–288.

Ben-Amotz A et al. Effect of natural beta-carotene supplementation in children exposed to radiation from the Chernobyl accident. Radiat Environ Biophys 37.3 (1998): 187–193.

Ben-Amotz A et al. Selective distribution of beta-carotene stereoisomers in rat tissues. Nutr Res 25.11 (2005): 1005–1012.

Bendich A. From 1989 to 2001: What have we learned about the biological actions of beta-carotene? J Nutr 134.1 (2004): 225–30S.

Biesalski HK, Obermueller-Jevic UC. UV light, beta-carotene and human skin: beneficial and potentially harmful effects. Arch Biochem Biophys 389.1 (2001): 1–6.

Bitterman N et al. Beta-carotene and CNS oxygen toxicity in rats. J Appl Physiol 76.3 (1994): 1073–1076.

Black HS. Pro-carcinogenic activity of beta-carotene, a putative systemic photoprotectant. Photochem Photobiol Sci 3.8 (2004): 753–758.

Black HS, Gerguis J. Modulation of dietary vitamins E and C fails to ameliorate beta-carotene exacerbation of UV carcinogenesis in mice. Nutr Cancer 45.1 (2003): 36–45.

Black HS et al. Diet potentiates the UV-carcinogenic response to beta-carotene. Nutr Cancer 37.2 (2000): 173–178.

Blot WJ et al. Nutrition intervention trials in Linxian, China: supplementation with specific vitamin/mineral combinations, cancer incidence, and disease-specific mortality in the general population. J Natl Cancer Inst 85.18 (1993): 1483–1492.

Bobak M et al. Could antioxidants play a role in high rates of coronary heart disease in the Czech Republic? Eur J Clin Nutr 52 (1998a): 632.

Bohm F et al. Carotenoids enhance vitamin E antioxidant efficiency. J Am Chem Soc 119.3 (1997): 621–622.

Bohm F et al. [beta]-Carotene with vitamins E and C offers synergistic cell protection against NOx. FEBS Lett 436.3 (1998a): 387–389.

Bohm F et al. Enhanced protection of human cells against ultraviolet light by antioxidant combinations involving dietary carotenoids. J Photochem Photobiol B Biol 44.3 (1998b): 211–2115.

Bolton-Smith C et al. Dietary intake by food frequency questionnaire and odds ratios of coronary heart disease risk. II: The antioxidants vitamins and fibre. Eur J Clin Nutr 46 (1992): 85.

Borel P et al. Oxidative stress status and antioxidant status are apparently not related to carotenoid status in healthy subjects. J Lab Clin Med 132.1 (1998): 61–66.

Bowen PE et al. Carotenoid absorption in humans. Methods Enzymol 214 (1993): 3–17.

Brady WE et al. Human serum carotenoid concentrations are related to physiologic and lifestyle factors. J Nutr 126.1 (1996): 129–137.

Burton GW, Ingold KU. Beta-carotene: An unusual type of lipid antioxidant. Science 224.4649 (1984): 569–573.

Chew EY, Clemons TE et al. Long-term effects of vitamins C and E, beta-carotene, and zinc on age-related macular degeneration: AREDS Report No. 35. Ophthalmology (2013).

Christen WG et al. Design of Physicians' Health Study II: a randomized trial of beta-carotene, vitamins E and C, and multivitamins, in prevention of cancer, cardiovascular disease, and eye disease, and review of results of completed trials. Ann Epidemiol 10.2 (2000c): 125–134.

Christen WG et al. A randomized trial of beta carotene and age-related cataract in US physicians. Arch Ophthalmol 121.3 (2003): 372–378.

Christen WG et al. Age-related cataract in a randomized trial of beta-carotene in women. Ophthalmic Epidemiology 11.5 (2004a): 401–412.

Christen WG et al. Beta carotene supplementation and age-related maculopathy in a randomized trial of US physicians. Arch Ophthalmol 125.3 (2007): 333–339.

Christian P et al. Night blindness during pregnancy and subsequent mortality among women in Nepal: effects of vitamin A and beta-carotene supplementation. Am J Epidemiol 152.6 (2000a): 542–547.

Christian P et al. Vitamin A or beta-carotene supplementation reduces symptoms of illness in pregnant and lactating Nepali women. J Nutr 130.1 (2000b): 2675–2682.

Christian P et al. Cigarette smoking during pregnancy in rural Nepal: Risk factors and effects of beta-carotene and vitamin A. supplementation. Eur J Clin Nutr 58.2 (2004b): 204–211.

Chuwers P et al. The protective effect of [beta]-carotene and retinol on ventilatory function in an asbestos-exposed cohort. Am J Resp Crit Care Med 155.3 (1997): 1066–1071.

Clemens MR et al. Supplementation with antioxidants prior to bone marrow transplantation. Wiener Klin Wochensch 109.1 (1997): 771–776.

Cobanoglu N et al. Antioxidant effect of beta-carotene in cystic fibrosis and bronchiectasis: Clinical and laboratory parameters of a pilot study. Int J Paediatr 91.7 (2002): 793–798.

Cook NR et al. Beta-carotene supplementation for patients with low baseline levels and decreased risks of total and prostate carcinoma. Cancer 86.9 (1999): 1783–1792.

Cook NR et al. Effects of beta-carotene supplementation on cancer incidence by baseline characteristics in the Physicians' Health Study (United States). Cancer Causes Control 11.7 (2000): 617–626.

Cooper DA et al. Dietary carotenoids and certain cancers, heart disease, and age-related macular degeneration: a review of recent research. Nutr Rev 57(7) (1999a): 201–214.

Cooper DA et al. Dietary carotenoids and lung cancer: a review of recent research. Nutr Rev 57.5 (1999b): 133–145.

Corridan BM et al. Low-dose supplementation with lycopene or beta-carotene does not enhance cell-mediated immunity in healthy free-living elderly humans. Eur J Clin Nutr 55.8 (2001): 627–635.

Coudray C et al. Lipid peroxidation level and antioxidant micronutrient status in a pre-aging population; correlation with chronic disease

prevalence in a French epidemiological study (Nantes, France). J Am Coll Nutr 16.6 (1997): 584–591.
Darlington S et al. A randomized controlled trial to assess sunscreen application and beta carotene supplementation in the prevention of solar keratoses. Arch Dermatol 139.4 (2003): 451–455.
De Luca LM, Ross SA. Beta-carotene increases lung cancer incidence in cigarette smokers. Nutr Rev 54.6 (1996): 178–180.
DerMarderosian A, Beutler JA (eds), The review of natural products, St Louis: Facts and Comparisons, 2002.
Dijkhuizen MA et al. Zinc plus beta-carotene supplementation of pregnant women is superior to beta-carotene supplementation alone in improving vitamin A status in both mothers and infants. Am J Clin Nutr 80.5 (2004): 1299–1307.
Epstein JH. Effects of beta-carotene on ultraviolet induced cancer formation in the hairless mouse skin. Photochem Photobiol 25.2 (1977): 211–213.
Erlinger TP et al. Relationship between systemic markers of inflammation and serum [beta]-carotene levels. Arch Intern Med 161.15 (2001): 1903–1908.
Farchi S et al. Exposure to environmental tobacco smoke is associated with lower plasma [beta]-carotene levels among nonsmoking women married to a smoker. Cancer Epidemiol Biomarkers Prev 10.8 (2001): 907–909.
Ford ES et al. Serum antioxidant concentrations among U.S. adults with self-reported asthma. J Asthma 41.2 (2004): 179–187.
Frieling UM et al. A randomized, 12-year primary-prevention trial of beta carotene supplementation for nonmelanoma skin cancer in the Physician's Health Study. Arch Dermatol 136.2 (2000): 179–184.
Fuchs J. Potentials and limitations of the natural antioxidants RRR-alpha-tocopherol, L-ascorbic acid and beta-carotene in cutaneous photoprotection. Free Radic Biol Med 25.7 (1998): 848–873.
Fujii Y et al. Effects of beta-carotene-rich algae Dunaliella bardawil on the dynamic changes of normal and neoplastic mammary cells and general metabolism in mice. Anticancer Res 13.2 (1993): 389–393.
Fuller CJ et al. Effect of beta-carotene supplementation on photosuppression of delayed-type hypersensitivity in normal young men. Am J Clin Nutr 56.4 (1992): 684–690.
Gallicchio L et al. Carotenoids and the risk of developing lung cancer: A systematic review. American J Clin Nutr 88.2 (2008): 372–383.
Gao J et al. Observational studies on the effect of dietary antioxidants on asthma: A meta-analysis. Respirology 13.4 (2008): 528–536.
Garewal H. Chemoprevention of oral cancer: Beta-carotene and vitamin E in leukoplakia. Eur J Cancer Prev 3.2 (1994): 101–107.
Garewal HS. Antioxidants in oral cancer prevention. Am J Clin Nutr 62.(6 Suppl) (1995): 1410–1416S.
Garewal HS, Schantz S. Emerging role of beta-carotene and antioxidant nutrients in prevention of oral cancer. Arch Otolaryngol Head Neck Surg 121.2 (1995): 141–144.
Garewal HS et al. Beta-carotene produces sustained remissions in patients with oral leukoplakia: results of a multicenter prospective trial. Arch Otolaryngol Head Neck Surg 125.1 (1999): 1305–1310.
Garmyn M et al. Effect of beta-carotene supplementation on the human sunburn reaction. Exp Dermatol 4.2 (1995): 104–111.
Gaziano JM et al. A prospective study of consumption of carotenoids in fruits and vegetables and decreased cardiovascular mortality in the elderly. Ann Epidemiol 5 (1995a): 255.
Gaziano JM et al. Discrimination in absorption or transport of beta-carotene isomers after oral supplementation with either all-trans- or 9-cis-beta-carotene. Am J Clin Nutr 61.6 (1995b): 1248–1252.
Gey KF et al. Poor plasma status of carotene and vitamin C is associated with higher mortality from ischaemic heart diease and stroke: Basel Prospective Study. Clin Invest 71 (1993): 3.
Gollnick HP, Siebenwirth C. Beta-carotene plasma levels and content in oral mucosal epithelium is skin type associated. Skin Pharmacol Appl Skin Physiol 15.5 (2002): 360–366.
Gollnick HPM et al. Systemic beta carotene plus topical UV-sunscreen are an optimal protection against harmful effects of natural UV-sunlight: Results of the Berlin-Eilath study. Eur J Dermatol 6.3 (1996): 200–205.
Gossage C et al. Effect of [beta]-carotene supplementation and lactation on carotenoid metabolism and mitogenic T lymphocyte proliferation. Am J Clin Nutr 71.4 (2000): 950–955.
Gottlieb K et al. Beta-carotene decreases markers of lipid peroxidation in healthy volunteers. Nutr Cancer 19.2 (1993): 207–212.
Green A et al. Daily sunscreen application and betacarotene supplementation in prevention of basal-cell and squamous-cell carcinomas of the skin: a randomised controlled trial. Lancet 354.9180 (1999): 723–729.
Greenberg ER et al. A clinical trial of beta carotene to prevent basal-cell and squamous-cell cancers of the skin. The Skin Cancer Prevention Study Group. N Engl J Med 323.12 (1990): 789–795.
Greenberg ER et al. A clinical trial of antioxidant vitamins to prevent colorectal adenoma. New England J Med 331.3 (1994): 141–147.
Greul AK et al. Photoprotection of UV-irradiated human skin: an antioxidative combination of vitamins E and C, carotenoids, selenium and proanthocyanidins. Skin Pharmacol Appl Skin Physiol 15.5 (2002): 307–315.
Grievink L et al. Serum carotenoids, alpha-tocopherol, and lung function among Dutch elderly. Am J Resp Crit Care Med 161.3 (2000): 790–795.
Grodstein F et al. A randomized trial of beta carotene supplementation and cognitive function in men: The physicians' health study II. Arch Intern Med 167.20 (2007): 2184–2190.
Group AT. The effect of vitamin E and beta carotene on the incidence of lung cancer and other cancers in male smokers. N Engl J Med 330 (1994): 1029–1035.
Gupta PC et al. Influence of dietary factors on oral precancerous lesions in a population-based case-control study in Kerala. India. Cancer 85.9 (1999): 1885–1893.
Hacisevki AY et al. An evaluation of serum retinol and beta-carotene levels and the risk of breast cancer. Gazi Univ Eczacilik Fakult Dergisi 20.2 (2003): 87–94.
Halliwell B. Free radicals and vascular disease: how much do we know? BMJ 1093.307 (1993): 885.
Handelman GJ. The evolving role of carotenoids in human biochemistry. Nutrition 17.10 (2001): 818–822.
Harik-Khan RI et al. Serum vitamin levels and the risk of asthma in children. Am J Epidemiol 159.4 (2004): 351–357.
Heinonen OP et al. The effect of vitamin E and beta carotene on the incidence of lung cancer and other cancers in male smokers. N Engl J Med 330.15 (1994): 1029–1035.
Heinrich U et al. Photoprotection for ingested carotenoids. Cosmetics Toiletries 113 (1998): 61.
Heinrich U et al. Supplementation with beta-carotene or a similar amount of mixed carotenoids protects humans from UV-induced erythema. J Nutr 133.1 (2003): 98–101.
Hemila H et al. Vitamin C, vitamin E, and beta-carotene in relation to common cold incidence in male smokers. Epidemiology 13.1 (2002): 32–37.
Hemila H et al. Physical activity and the common cold in men administered vitamin E and beta-carotene. Med Sci Sports Exercise 35.11 (2003): 1815–1820.
Hemila H et al. Vitamin E and beta-carotene supplementation and hospital-treated pneumonia incidence in male smokers. Chest 125.2 (2004): 557–565.
Hennekens CH et al. Lack of effect of long-term supplementation with beta carotene on the incidence of malignant neoplasms and cardiovascular disease. N Engl J Med 334.18 (1996): 1145–1149.
Herraiz LA et al. Effect of UV exposure and [beta]-carotene supplementation on delayed-type hypersensitivity response in healthy older men. J Am Coll Nutr 17.6 (1998): 617–624.
Hininger IA et al. No significant effects of lutein, lycopene or beta-carotene supplementation on biological markers of oxidative stress and LDL oxidizability in healthy adult subjects. J Am Coll Nutr 20.3 (2001): 232–238.
Holick CN et al. Dietary carotenoids, serum beta-carotene, and retinol and risk of lung cancer in the alpha-tocopherol: beta-carotene cohort study. Am J Epidemiol 156.6 (2002): 536–547.
Hu P et al. The effects of serum beta-carotene concentration and burden of inflammation on all-cause mortality risk in high-functioning older persons: MacArthur studies of successful aging. J Gerontol Series A Biol Sci Med Sci 59.8 (2004): 849–854.
Hu P et al. Association between serum beta-carotene levels and decline of cognitive function in high-functioning older persons with or without apolipoprotein E 4 alleles: MacArthur studies of successful aging. J Geront A Biol Sci Med Sci 61.6 (2006): 616–620.
Hughes DA. Dietary carotenoids and human immune function. Nutrition 17.10 (2001): 823–827.
Hughes DA et al. The effect of [beta]-carotene supplementation on the immune function of blood monocytes from healthy male nonsmokers. J Lab Clin Med 129.3 (1997): 309–317.
Jensen CD et al. Observations on the effects of ingesting cis- and trans-beta-carotene isomers on human serum concentrations. Nutr Rep Int 35 (1987): 413–422.
Jimenez-Jimenez FJ et al. Serum levels of beta-carotene, alpha-carotene and vitamin A in patients with Alzheimer's disease. Eur J Neurol 6.4 (1999): 495–497.
Kacsur C et al. Plasma antioxidants and rheumatoid arthritis. Harefuah 141.2 (2002): 148–150.
Kalayci O et al. Serum levels of antioxidant vitamins (alpha tocopherol, beta carotene, and ascorbic acid) in children with bronchial asthma. Turk J Pediatr 42.1 (2000): 17–21.
Kardinaal AFM et al. Antioxidants in adipose tissue and risk of myocardial infarction: the EURAMIC study. Lancet 342 (1993): 1379.
Karppi J et al. Low β-carotene concentrations increase the risk of cardiovascular disease mortality among Finnish men with risk factors. Nutrition, Metabolism and Cardiovascular Diseases 22.10 (2012): 921–928.

Karppi J, Laukkanen JA et al. Serum β-carotene and the risk of sudden cardiac death in men: A population-based follow-up study. Atherosclerosis 226.1 (2013): 172–177.

Karppi J, Kurl S et al. Serum beta-carotene concentrations and the risk of congestive heart failure in men: A population-based study. Int J Cardiol (0) (2013).

Kassoff A et al. A randomized, placebo-controlled, clinical trial of high-dose supplementation with vitamins C and E, beta carotene, and zinc for age-related macular degeneration and vision loss: AREDS report no. 8. Arch Ophthalmol 119.10 (2001): 1417–1436.

Key TJ et al. Plasma carotenoids, retinol, and tocopherols and the risk of prostate cancer in the European Prospective Investigation into Cancer and Nutrition study. Am J Clin Nutr 86.3 (2007): 672–681.

Kligman LH, Mathews-Roth MM. Dietary beta-carotene and 13-cis-retinoic acid are not effective in preventing some features of UVB-induced dermal damage in hairless mice. Photochem Photobiol 51.6 (1990): 733–735.

Knekt P et al. Antioxidant vitamin intake and coronary mortality in a longitudinal population study. Am J Epidemiol 139 (1994): 1180.

Koushik A et al. Intake of the major carotenoids and the risk of epithelial ovarian cancer in a pooled analysis of 10 cohort studies. Int J Cancer 119.9 (2006): 2148–2154.

Kritchevsky SB. BETA-carotene, carotenoids and the prevention of coronary heart disease. J Nutr 129.1 (1999): 5–8.

Kushi LH et al. Dietary antioxidant vitamins and death from coronary heart disease in postmenopausal women. N Engl J Med 334 (1996): 1156.

Lavy A et al. Preferential inhibition of LDL oxidation by the all-trans isomer of beta-carotene in comparison with 9-cis beta-carotene. Eur J Clin Chem Clin Biochem 31.2 (1993): 83–90.

Lavy A et al. Natural beta-carotene for the prevention of post-ERCP pancreatitis. Pancreas 29.2 (2004): e45–e50.

Lee IM et al. Beta-carotene supplementation and incidence of cancer and cardiovascular disease: the Women's Health Study. J Natl Cancer Inst 91.24 (1999): 2102–2106.

Lee J et al. Carotenoid supplementation reduces erythema in human skin after simulated solar radiation exposure. Proc Soc Exp Biol Med 223.2 (2000): 170–174.

Leppala JM et al. Controlled trial of alpha-tocopherol and beta-carotene supplements on stroke incidence and mortality in male smokers. Arterioscler Thromb Vasc Biol 20.1 (2000a): 230–5.

Leppala JM et al. Vitamin E and beta carotene supplementation in high risk for stroke: a subgroup analysis of the Alpha-Tocopherol, Beta-Carotene Cancer Prevention Study. Arch Neurol 57.10 (2000b): 1503–9.

Levin G, Mokady S. Antioxidant activity of 9-cis compared to all-trans [beta]-carotene in vitro. Free Radic Biol Med 17.1 (1994): 77–82.

Levy Y et al. Effect of dietary supplementation of different [beta]-carotene isomers on lipoprotein oxidative modification. J Nutr Environ Med 5.1 (1995): 13–22.

Levy Y et al. Effect of dietary supplementation of beta-carotene on human monocyte-macrophage-mediated oxidation of low density lipoprotein. Israel J Med Sci 32.6 (1996): 473–478.

Levy Y et al. Plasma antioxidants and lipid peroxidation in acute myocardial infarction and thrombolysis. J Am Coll Nutr 17.4 (1998): 337–341.

Levy Y et al. Dietary supplementation of a natural isomer mixture of beta-carotene inhibits oxidation of LDL derived from patients with diabetes mellitus. Ann Nutr Metab 44.2 (2000): 54–60.

Liede K et al. Long-term supplementation with alpha-tocopherol and beta-carotene and prevalence of oral mucosal lesions in smokers. Oral Dis 4.2 (1998): 78–83.

Lin J et al. Effect of beta-carotene supplementation on health and growth of vitamin A deficient children in China rural villages: A randomized controlled trial. European e-Journal of Clinical Nutrition and Metabolism 4.1 (2009): e17–21.

Liu Q et al. Antioxidant activities of natural 9-cis and synthetic all-trans [beta]-carotene assessed by human neutrophil chemiluminescence. Nutr Res 20.1 (2000): 5–14.

Mahjoub S et al. The effects of beta-carotene and vitamin E on erythrocytes lipid peroxidation in beta-thalassemia patients. Journal of Research in Medical Sciences 12.6 (2007): 301–307.

Malila N et al. Effects of alpha-tocopherol and beta-carotene supplementation on gastric cancer incidence in male smokers (ATBC Study Finland). Cancer Causes Control 13.7 (2002): 617–623.

Männistö S et al. Dietary carotenoids and risk of lung cancer in a pooled analysis of seven cohort studies. Cancer Epidemiol Biomarkers Prev 13.1 (2004): 40–48.

Männistö S et al. Dietary carotenoids and risk of colorectal cancer in a pooled analysis of 11 cohort studies. Am J Epidemiol 165.3 (2007): 246–255.

Manson JE et al. A prospective study of antioxidant vitamins and incidence of coronary heart disease in women. Circulation 84 (1991): 546.

Mathews-Roth MM. Antitumor activity of beta-carotene, canthaxanthin and phytoene. Oncology 39.1 (1982): 33–37.

Mathews-Roth MM. Systemic photoprotection. Dermatol Clin 4.2 (1986): 335–339.

Mathews-Roth MM. Photoprotection by carotenoids. Fed Proc 46.5 (1987): 1890–1893.

Mathews-Roth MM. Lack of genotoxicity with beta-carotene. Toxicol Lett 41.3 (1988): 185–191.

Mathews-Roth MM. Carotenoid functions in photoprotection and cancer prevention. J Environ Pathol Toxicol Oncol 10.4–5 (1990a): 181–92.

Mathews-Roth MM. Plasma concentrations of carotenoids after large doses of [beta]-carotene. Am J Clin Nutr 52.3 (1990b): 500–1.

Mathews-Roth MM. Carotenoids in erythropoietic protoporphyria and other photosensitivity diseases. Ann NY Acad Sci 691 (1993): 127–138.

Mathews-Roth MM, Pathak MA. Phytoene as a protective agent against sunburn (>280 nm) radiation in guinea pigs. Photochem Photobiol. 21.4 (1975): 261–263.

Mathews-Roth MM et al. Beta-carotene as a photoprotective agent in erythropoietic protoporphyria. N Engl J Med 282.22 (1970): 1231–1234.

Mathews-Roth MM et al. A clinical trial of the effects of oral beta-carotene on the responses of human skin to solar radiation. J Invest Dermatol 59.4 (1972): 349–353.

Mathews-Roth MM et al. Beta-carotene as an oral photoprotective agent in erythropoietic protoporphyria. JAMA 228.8 (1974): 1004–1008.

Mathews-Roth MM et al. Beta carotene therapy for erythropoietic protoporphyria and other photosensitivity diseases. Arch Dermatol 113.9 (1977): 1229–1232.

Mayne ST. Beta-carotene, carotenoids, and disease prevention in humans. FASEB J 10(7) (1996): 690–701.

Mayne ST et al. Supplemental beta-carotene, smoking, and urinary F2-isoprostane excretion in patients with prior early stage head and neck cancer. Nutr Cancer 49.1 (2004): 1–6.

McArdle F et al. Effects of oral vitamin E and beta-carotene supplementation on ultraviolet radiation-induced oxidative stress in human skin. Am J Clin Nutr 80.5 (2004): 1270–1275.

Meyer F et al. Acute adverse effects of radiation therapy and local recurrence in relation to dietary and plasma beta carotene and alpha tocopherol in head and neck cancer patients. Nutr Cancer 59.1 (2007): 29–35.

Micozzi MS et al. Carotenodermia in men with elevated carotenoid intake from foods and beta-carotene. Am J Clin Nutr 48 (1988): 1061–1064.

Micromedex. Beta-carotene. Thomson, 2003. Available: www.micromedex.com June 2014.

Mohamed MS et al. Administration of lycopene and beta-carotene decreased risks of pneumonia among children. Pak J Nutr 7.2 (2008): 2713–2717.

Mokady S, Ben-Amotz A. Dietary lipid level and the availability of beta-carotene of Dunaliella-bardawil in rats. Nutr Cancer 15.1 (1991): 47–52.

Moreira A et al. Increased dietary beta-carotene intake associated with better asthma quality of life. Alergol Inmunol Clin 19.3 (2004): 1110–1112.

Morinobu T et al. Changes in beta-carotene levels by long-term administration of natural beta-carotene derived from Dunaliella bardawil in humans. J Nutr Sci Vitaminol 40.5 (1994): 421–430.

Morris DL et al. Serum carotenoids and coronary heart disease. The Lipid Research Clinics Coronary Primary Prevention Trial and Follow-up Study. JAMA 272 (1994): 1439.

Murata T et al. Effect of long-term administration of beta-carotene on lymphocyte subsets in humans. Am J Clin Nutr 60.4 (1994): 597–602.

Nabae K et al. A 90-day oral toxicity study of beta-carotene derived from Blakeslea trispora, a natural food colorant, in F344 rats. Food Chem Toxicol 43.7 (2005): 1127–1133.

Nagasawa H et al. Effects of beta-carotene-rich algae Dunaliella on reproduction and body growth in mice. Vivo 3.2 (1989): 79–81.

Nagasawa H et al. Suppression by beta-carotene-rich algae Dunaliella bardawil of the progression, but not the development, of spontaneous mammary tumours in SHN virgin mice. Anticancer Res 11.2 (1991): 713–7117.

Neuman I et al. Prevention of exercise-induced asthma by a natural isomer mixture of beta-carotene. Ann Allergy Asthma Immunol 82.6 (1999): 549–553.

O'Sullivan, L., K. Galvin, et al. Effects of cooking on the profile and micellarization of 9-cis, 13-cis- and all-trans-β-carotene in green vegetables. Food Research International 43.4 (2010): 1130–1135.

Ochs-Balcom HM et al. Oxidative stress and pulmonary function in the general population. Am J Epidemiol 162.1 (2005): 1137–1145.

Omenn GS et al. Effects of a combination of beta carotene and vitamin A on lung cancer and cardiovascular disease. N Engl J Med 334.18 (1996a): 1150–1155.

B

Omenn GS et al. Risk factors for lung cancer and for intervention effects in CARET, the beta-carotene and retinol efficacy trial. J Natl Cancer Inst 88.21 (1996b): 1550–1559.

Palozza PN, Krinsky I. [beta]-Carotene and [alpha]-tocopherol are synergistic antioxidants. Arch Biochem Biophys 297.1 (1992): 184–187.

Pandey DK et al. Dietary vitamin C and beta carotene and risk of death in middle aged men: The Western Electric Study. Am J Epidemiol 142 (1995): 1269.

Paolini M et al. Co-carcinogenic effect of beta-carotene. Nature 398.6730 (1999): 760–761.

Pathak MA. Sunscreens: topical and systemic approaches for protection of human skin against harmful effects of solar radiation. J Am Acad Dermatol 7.3 (1982): 285–312.

Patrick L. Beta carotene: The controversy continues. Altern Med Rev 5.6 (2000): 530–545.

PDRHealth. Beta carotene. Thomson Healthcare, 2005. Available: http://www.pdrhealth 16 June 2014.

Penuelas J, Munne-Bosch S. Isoprenoids: an evolutionary pool for photoprotection. Trends Plant Sci 10.4 (2005): 166–169.

Peto R et al. Can dietary betacarotene materially reduce human cancer rates? Nature 290 (1981): 201–208.

Ponnamperuma RM et al. [beta]-Carotene fails to act as a tumor promoter, induces RAR expression, and prevents carcinoma formation in a two-stage model of skin carcinogenesis in male sencar mice. Nutr Cancer 37.1 (2000): 82–88.

Prabhala RH et al. Influence of beta-carotene on immune functions. Ann NY Acad Sci 691 (1993): 262–263.

Princen HM et al. Supplementation with vitamin E but not beta-carotene in vivo protects low density lipoprotein from lipid peroxidation in vitro: Effect of cigarette smoking. Arterioscler Thromb 12.5 (1992): 554–562.

Pryor WA et al. Beta carotene: From biochemistry to clinical trials. Nutr Rev 58 (2000): 39–53.

Rahman I et al. Oxidant and antioxidant balance in the airways and airway diseases. Eur J Pharmacol 533.1–3 (2006): 222–229.

Rapola JM et al. Effect of vitamin E and beta carotene on the incidence of angina pectoris: A randomized, double-blind, controlled trial. JAMA 275.9 (1996): 693–698.

Rautalahti MT et al. The effects of supplementation with alpha-tocopherol and beta-carotene on the incidence and mortality of carcinoma of the pancreas in a randomized, controlled trial. Cancer 86.1 (1999): 37–42.

Reaven PD et al. Effect of dietary antioxidant combinations in humans: Protection of LDL by vitamin E but not by [beta]-carotene. Arterioscler Thromb 13.4 (1993): 590–600.

Redlich C et al. Effect of long-term beta-carotene and vitamin A on serum cholesterol and triglyceride levels among participants in the Carotene and Retinol Efficacy Trial (CARET). Atherosclerosis 145.2 (1999): 425–432.

Revett K. A machine learning investigation of a beta-carotenoid dataset. Studies in Fuzziness and Soft Computing 224 (2008): 211–227.

Richelle M et al. Both free and esterified plant sterols reduce cholesterol absorption and the bioavailability of beta-carotene and alpha-tocopherol in normocholesterolemic humans. Am J Clin Nutr 80.1 (2004): 171–177.

Rimm TV et al. Vitamin E consumption and the risk of coronary heart disease in men. N Engl J Med 328 (1993): 1450.

Roodenburg AJ et al. Amount of fat in the diet affects bioavailability of lutein esters but not of alpha-carotene, beta-carotene, and vitamin E in humans. Am J Clin Nutr 71.5 (2000): 1187–1193.

Rubin RN et al. Relationship of serum antioxidants to asthma prevalence in youth. Am J Resp Crit Care Med 169.3 (2004): 393–398.

Russell RM. Beta-carotene and lung cancer. Pure Appl Chem 74.8 (2002): 1461–1467.

Rust P et al. Long-term oral beta-carotene supplementation in patients with cystic fibrosis: effects on antioxidative status and pulmonary function. Ann Nutr Metab 44.1 (2000): 30–37.

Santos MS et al. Natural killer cell activity in elderly men is enhanced by [beta]-carotene supplementation. Am J Clin Nutr 64.5 (1996): 772–777.

Santos MS et al. Short- and long-term beta-carotene supplementation do not influence T cell-mediated immunity in healthy elderly persons. Am J Clin Nutr 66.4 (1997): 917–924.

Sayre RM, Black HS. Beta-carotene does not act as an optical filter in skin. J Photochem Photobiol B Biol 12.1 (1992): 83–90.

Schaumberg DA et al. No effect of beta-carotene supplementation on risk of nonmelanoma skin cancer among men with low baseline plasma beta-carotene. Cancer Epidemiol Biomarkers Prev 13.6 (2004): 1079–1080.

Schroder H et al. Effects of alpha-tocopherol, beta-carotene and ascorbic acid on oxidative, hormonal and enzymatic exercise stress markers in habitual training activity of professional basketball players. Eur J Nutr 40.4 (2001): 178–184.

Schunemann HJ et al. The relation of serum levels of antioxidant vitamins C and E, retinol and carotenoids with pulmonary function in the general population. Am J Resp Crit Care Med 163.5 (2001): 1246–1255.

Senesse P et al. Tobacco use and associations of beta-carotene and vitamin intakes with colorectal adenoma risk. J Nutr 135.10 (2005): 2468–2472.

Shaish A et al. Beta-carotene inhibits atherosclerosis in hypercholesterolemic rabbits. J Clin Invest 96.4 (1995): 2075–2082.

Shaish A et al. 9-cis [beta]-carotene-rich powder of the alga Dunaliella bardawil increases plasma HDL-cholesterol in fibrate-treated patients. Atherosclerosis 189.1 (2006): 215–221.

Siems W et al. Beta-carotene cleavage products induce oxidative stress in vitro by impairing mitochondrial respiration. FASEB J 16.10 (2002): 1289–1291.

Siems W et al. [beta]-Carotene breakdown products may impair mitochondrial functions — potential side effects of high-dose [beta]-carotene supplementation. J Nutr Biochem 16.7 (2005): 385–397.

Sies H, Stahl W. Nutritional protection against skin damage from sunlight. Annu Rev Nutr 24 (2004): 173–200.

Smith W et al. Carrots, carotene and seeing in the dark. Aust NZ J Ophthalmol 27.3–4 (1999): 200–203.

Sommerburg O et al. beta-carotene cleavage products after oxidation mediated by hypochlorous acid: A model for neutrophil-derived degradation. Free Radic Biol Med 35.11 (2003): 1480–1490.

Sperduto RD et al. The Linxian cataract studies: Two nutrition intervention trials. Arch Ophthalmol 111.9 (1993): 1246–1253.

Stahl WS, Sies H. Human serum concentrations of all-trans beta- and alpha-carotene but not 9-cis beta-carotene increase upon ingestion of a natural isomer mixture obtained from Dunaliella salina (Betatene). J Nutr 123 (1993): 847–851.

Stahl W et al. Biological activities of natural and synthetic carotenoids: induction of gap junctional communication and singlet oxygen quenching. Carcinogenesis 18.1 (1997): 89–92.

Stahl W et al. Carotenoids and carotenoids plus vitamin E protect against ultraviolet light-induced erythema in humans. Am J Clin Nutr 71.3 (2000): 795–798.

Steenvoorden DPT, Beijersbergen van Henegouwen GMJ. The use of endogenous antioxidants to improve photoprotection. J Photochem Photobiol B Biol 41.1–2 (1997): 1–110.

Strauss RS. Comparison of serum concentrations of alpha-tocopherol and beta-carotene in a cross-sectional sample of obese and nonobese children (NHANES III): National Health and Nutrition Examination Survey. J Pediatr 134.2 (1999): 160–165.

Street DA et al. Are low levels of carotenoids and alpha tocopherol risk factors for myocardial infarction? Circulation 90 (1994): 1154.

Strobel M et al. The importance of [beta]-carotene as a source of vitamin A with special regard to pregnant and breastfeeding women. Eur J Nutr 46 (Suppl 1) (2007): I/1–I/20.

Sugiura M et al. Associations of serum carotenoid concentrations with the metabolic syndrome: Interaction with smoking. Br J of Nutr 100.6 (2008): 1297–1306.

Suhonen R, Plosila M. The effect of beta-carotene in combination with canthaxanthin, Ro 8-8427 (Phenoro), in treatment of polymorphous light eruptions. Dermatologica 163.2 (1981): 172–176.

Takenaka H et al. Protective effect of Dunaliella bardawil on water-immersion-induced stress in rats. Planta Med 59.5 (1993): 421–424.

Tamai H et al. Bioavailability of beta-carotene in a carotenoid preparation derived from Dunaliella bardawil in human male adults. Ann NY Acad Sci 691 (1993): 238–240.

Tauler P et al. Diet supplementation with vitamin E, vitamin C and beta-carotene cocktail enhances basal neutrophil antioxidant enzymes in athletes. Pflugers Archiv Eur J Physiol 443.5–6 (2002): 791–797.

Tavani A, La Vecchia C. [beta]-Carotene and risk of coronary heart disease: A review of observational and intervention studies. Biomed Pharmacother 53.9 (1999): 409–416.

Tavani A et al. Beta Carotene intake and risk of nonfatal acute myocardial infarction in women. Eur J Epidemiol 13 (1997): 631.

Taylor A et al. Long-term intake of vitamins and carotenoids and odds of early age-related cortical and posterior subcapsular lens opacities. Am J Clin Nutr 75.3 (2002): 540–549.

Tebi A et al. Plasma vitamin, [beta]-carotene, and [alpha]-tocopherol status according to age and disease in hospitalized elderly. Nutr Res 20.10 (2000): 1395–1408.

Thomsen K et al. Beta-carotene in erythropoietic protoporphyria: 5 years' experience. Dermatologica 159.1 (1979): 82–86.

Todd S et al. An investigation of the relationship between antioxidant vitamin intake and coronary heart disease in men and women using logistic regression analysis. J Clin Epidemiol 48 (1995): 307.

Tornwall ME et al. The effect of alpha-tocopherol and beta-carotene supplementation on symptoms and progression of intermittent claudication in a controlled trial. Atherosclerosis 147.1 (1999): 193–197.

Tornwall ME et al. Alpha-tocopherol (vitamin E) and beta-carotene supplementation does not affect the risk for large abdominal aortic aneurysm in a controlled trial. Atherosclerosis 157.1 (2001): 167–173.

Tornwall ME et al. Postintervention effect of alpha tocopherol and beta carotene on different strokes: A 6-year follow-up of the alpha tocopherol, beta carotene cancer prevention study. Stroke 35.8 (2004): 1908–1913.

Torun M et al. Evaluation of serum beta carotene levels in patients with cardiovascular diseases. J Clin Pharm Ther 19 (1994): 61.

Touvier M et al. Dual association of beta-carotene with risk of tobacco-related cancers in a cohort of French women. J Natl Cancer Inst 97.18 (2005): 1338–1344.

Tyssandier V et al. Vegetable-borne lutein, lycopene, and beta-carotene compete for incorporation into chylomicrons, with no adverse effect on the medium-term (3-wk) plasma status of carotenoids in humans. Am J Clin Nutr 75.3 (2002): 526–534.

Vainio H, Rautalahti M. An international evaluation of the cancer preventive potential of carotenoids. Cancer Epidemiol Biomarkers Prev 7.8 (1998): 725–728.

Van der Horst-Graat JM et al. Plasma carotenoid concentrations in relation to acute respiratory infections in elderly people. Br J Nutr 92.1 (2004): 113–1118.

Van Poppel G et al. No influence of beta-carotene on haemostatic balance in healthy male smokers. Blood Coagul Fibrinolysis 6.1 (1995): 55–59.

Verrotti A et al. Obesity and plasma concentrations of alpha-tocopherol and beta-carotene in epileptic girls treated with valproate. Neuroendocrinology 79.3 (2004): 157–162.

Virtamo J et al. Effects of supplemental alpha-tocopherol and beta-carotene on urinary tract cancer: incidence and mortality in a controlled trial (Finland). Cancer Causes Control 11.10 (2000): 933–939.

Vivekananthan DP et al. Use of antioxidant vitamins for the prevention of cardiovascular disease: meta-analysis of randomised trials. Lancet 361.9374 (2003): 2017–2023.

Vlot WJ et al. The Lixian trials: mortality rates by vitamin-mineral intervention group. Am J Clin Nutr 62 (Suppl) (1995): 1424.

Walkowiak J et al. The deficiency of beta-carotene in cystic fibrosis patients is related to the clinical course of the disease. Pediatr Polska 79.7 (2004): 534–537.

Wallstrom P et al. Serum concentrations of beta-carotene and alpha-tocopherol are associated with diet, smoking, and general and central adiposity. Am J Clin Nutr 73.4 (2001): 777–785.

Wang XD, Krinsky NI. The bioconversion of beta-carotene into retinoids. SubCell Biochem 30 (1998): 159–180.

Wang XD et al. Retinoid signaling and activator protein-1 expression in ferrets given [beta]-carotene supplements and exposed to tobacco smoke. J Natl Cancer Inst 91.1 (1999): 60–66.

Wang L et al. Associations of plasma carotenoids with risk factors and biomarkers related to cardiovascular disease in middle-aged and older women. Am J Clin Nutr 88.3 (2008): 747–754.

Watson RR et al. Effect of beta-carotene on lymphocyte subpopulations in elderly humans: evidence for a dose-response relationship. Am J Clin Nutr 53.1 (1991): 90–94.

Wertz K et al. Beta-carotene inhibits UVA-induced matrix metalloprotease 1 and 10 expression in keratinocytes by a singlet oxygen-dependent mechanism. Free Radic Biol Med 37.5 (2004): 654–670.

Wertz K et al. Beta-carotene interferes with ultraviolet light A-induced gene expression by multiple pathways. J Invest Dermatol 124.2 (2005): 428–434.

West KP Jr. et al. Double blind, cluster randomised trial of low dose supplementation with vitamin A or beta carotene on mortality related to pregnancy in Nepal: The NNIPS-2 Study Group. BMJ (Clin Res Ed) 318.7183 (1999): 570–575.

Wolf C et al. Do oral carotenoids protect human skin against ultraviolet erythema, psoralen phototoxicity, and ultraviolet-induced DNA damage? J Invest Dermatol 90.1 (1988): 55–57.

Wood LG et al. Lipid peroxidation as determined by plasma isoprostanes is related to disease severity in mild asthma. Lipids 35.9 (2000): 967–974.

Wood LG et al. Biomarkers of lipid peroxidation, airway inflammation and asthma. Eur Resp J 21.1 (2003): 177–186.

Wood LG et al. Airway and circulating levels of carotenoids in asthma and healthy controls. J Am Coll Nutr 24.6 (2005): 448–455.

Woodall A et al. Caution with beta-carotene supplements. Lancet 347.9006 (1996): 967–968.

Wright EM et al. Effects of [alpha]-tocopherol and [beta]-carotene supplementation on upper aerodigestive tract cancers in a large, randomized controlled trial. Cancer 109.5 (2007): 891–898.

Yeh SL, Hu ML. Induction of oxidative DNA damage in human foreskin fibroblast Hs68 cells by oxidized beta-carotene and lycopene. Free Radic Res 35.2 (2001): 203–213.

Yeh SL, Hu ML. Oxidized [beta]-carotene inhibits gap junction intercellular communication in the human lung adenocarcinoma cell line A549. Food Chem Toxicol 41.12 (2003): 1677–1684.

Zhang ZW et al. Gastric [alpha]-tocopherol and [beta]-carotene concentrations in association with Helicobacter pylori infection. Eur J Gastroenterol Hepatology 12.5 (2000): 497–503.

Bilberry

HISTORICAL NOTE Bilberries have been used as a food for many centuries and are valued for their taste and high nutritional content. They are still commonly used to make jams, pies, syrups and beverages. Medicinally, the berries have been used internally to treat diarrhoea and haemorrhoids and externally for inflammation of the mouth and mucous membranes as they have significant astringent activity. According to folklore, World War II British Royal Air Force pilots noticed that their night vision seemed to improve after consuming bilberries or bilberry preserves, sparking a renewed interest in the medicinal properties of the fruits.

COMMON NAME

Bilberry

OTHER NAMES

Baies de myrtille, Blaubeeren, dwarf bilberry, European bilberry, European blueberries, huckleberry, hurtleberry, heidelbeeren, petit myrtle, whortleberry, wine berry

BOTANICAL NAME/FAMILY

Vaccinium myrtillus (family Ericaceae)

> ***Clinical note — Tannins***
> Tannins are polyphenolic compounds that have an affinity for proteins. They also complex with alkaloids and therefore should not be mixed with alkaloid-containing herbs.
> Anthocyanosides are condensed tannins. When they come into contact with mucous membranes they have an astringent action, making the mucosa less permeable. This activity has been used therapeutically in a variety of ways.
> Taken internally, herbs with a high tannin content such as bilberry have been used to treat diarrhoea; applied externally, a styptic action occurs that reduces blood loss.

> ***Clinical note — Cataract***
> Growing evidence suggests that senile cataract development may in part be linked to the endogenous generation of free radical molecules, such as superoxide derived from oxygen and light in the aqueous humour and lens (Varma & Richards 1988, Varma et al 1982, 1994). As such, substances with significant antioxidant activity such as anthocyanins, vitamin C and vitamin E have been investigated as potential prophylactic treatments.

PLANT PARTS USED

Dried ripe fruit or fresh fruit (berries)

CHEMICAL COMPONENTS

The fruit contains catechin tannins (up to 10%), invert sugar, fruit acids, flavonol glycosides including astragalin, hyperoside, isoquercitrin and quercitrin, phenolic acids, pectins, triterpenes, and polyphenols such as anthocyanosides. The volatile oil includes methyl salicylate, farnesol, vanillin, myristicin and citronellol. Bilberry also contains vitamin C and chromium, which are suspected of playing a role in its pharmacological activities.

Some of the anthocyanosides are responsible for the deep blue pigment of the fruit (Kahkonen et al 2001). As the fruit ripens the anthocyanoside content increases. Some commercially available extracts are standardised to anthocyanoside content. Recent research indicates that the anthocyanidin content is particularly high in the pulp of the fruit; however, all parts of the fruit are potential sources of phenolic compounds (Riihinen et al 2008). Anthocyanin (the aglycone and sugar moieties delphinidin, cyanidin, petunidin, peonidin and malvidin) concentration in the fresh fruit is approximately 0.1–0.5%, while concentrated bilberry extracts (BEs) are usually standardised to 25% anthocyanins (Ichiyanagi et al 2004, Yue & Xu 2008, Zhang et al 2004).

MAIN ACTIONS

The pharmacological actions of bilberry have not been significantly investigated in clinical studies, so information is generally derived from in vitro and animal studies or based on known information about key constituents found within the herb. Most of the research undertaken to understand the pharmacology of the herb has focused on the anthocyanin and anthocyanoside content.

Antioxidant

Many of the clinical effects attributed to bilberry are thought to be due, in some part, to the herb's antioxidant activity.

Anthocyanosides are the main phenolic constituents in bilberry and have well-established antioxidant activity (Bao et al 2010, Kahkonen et al 2001, Roy et al 2002). This activity is believed to be primarily due to their chemical structure (Mozaffarieh et al 2008, Yao & Vieira 2007). Anthocyanosides have exhibited direct superoxide radical scavenging properties, indirect antioxidant activity by amplifying endogenous antioxidant systems and cytoprotective activity against oxidative damage in animal models (Valentová et al 2007).

The observation that anthocyanosides induce clinical antioxidant effects has long puzzled researchers as these constituents have relatively poor bioavailability when orally ingested. A study examining the effect of both crude and standardised extracts of bilberry and blueberry on four different cell lines concluded that the small amount of bioavailable anthocyanosides that occurs after ingestion of a normal dietary serve is enough to promote a significant antioxidant response, particularly in vascular and hepatic cells (Bornsek et al 2012). It is thought that anthocyanosides enter the cell via active transport across the cell membrane, enabling small concentrations to promote an intracellular amplification of endogenous antioxidant systems.

Hepatoprotective

Several studies have focused on the protective effect of BE on hepatic mitochondrial response to stress (Bao et al 2008, 2010). These animal models have shown that bilberry protects mice mitochondria from stress-induced changes in cytochrome function and electron transport chain activity, and cellular membrane potential reduction. Bilberry also restored alanine aminotransferase and reactive oxygen species to normal levels. In another study (Domitrović & Jakovac 2011), mice with liver fibrosis induced by carbon tetrachloride were treated with 10 mg/kg BE, which reduced oxidative stress (measured by glutathione activity), decreased cytokines associated with fibrosis and resolved hepatic collagen deposits.

Cardioprotective

Two animal studies have shown BE may be protective against doxorubicin-induced cardiotoxicity, a dose-limiting side effect of this chemotherapy drug

(Ashour et al 2011, Choi et al 2010). Cardioprotection is most likely to be due to an antioxidant mechanism. While these results are promising, more studies are required to ensure that BE does not also reduce the therapeutic effects of doxorubicin.

In vitro studies show anthocyanins have antioxidant effects in cardiac mitochondria of rats (Trumbeckaitė et al 2013), which may reduce cytochrome c and protect against apoptosis of cardiac tissue during ischaemia (Skemiene et al 2013).

Antiatherogenic

A study involving apolipoprotein E-deficient mice confirmed that BE reduces atherosclerotic lesion development via the modulation of gene expression in the aorta. Treatment with BE resulted in over 1200 genes being modified; many were involved in atherogenic processes, including those known to influence oxidative stress, inflammation, angiogenesis and transendothelial migration. Additionally, total cholesterol was reduced by 20% whereas triglycerides and body weight remained unchanged (Mauray et al 2010).

Reduces ischaemic reperfusion injury

Bilberry anthocyanosides have been shown to improve ischaemic damage, preserve capillary perfusion, inhibit increased permeability of reperfusion and save arteriolar tone in an animal model of ischaemic reperfusion injury (Bertuglia et al 1995, Ziberna et al 2013).

Anti-inflammatory and antioedema activity

These effects have been demonstrated in both experimental studies and human trials.

Biochemical and histochemical data show that the anthocyanins in bilberry decrease vascular permeability and alter capillary wall dynamics. This is mainly due to an increase in the endothelial barrier effect as a result of stabilising membrane phospholipids and increasing the synthesis of the mucopolysaccharides in the connective ground substance, thereby restoring the altered pericapillary sheath (Mian et al 1977). These effects have been demonstrated in animal models for both oral administration and topical application of bilberry anthocyanins (1% alcohol solution) and were seen to be stronger and longer-lasting than those of rutin (Lietti et al 1976).

Bilberry (dried) and anthocyanins reduced inflammatory cytokines and decreased histological severity in experimental colitis in mice (Piberger et al 2011).

Anti-inflammatory activity has also been demonstrated in human studies. A small randomised controlled trial (RCT) of 27 people with metabolic syndrome looked at the effect of a diet enriched with bilberries (400 g/daily) on inflammatory markers. The special diet resulted in small decreases in a variety of inflammatory markers (C-reactive protein [CRP], interleukin-6 [IL-6], IL-12 and lipopolysaccharide) and an overall lower inflammatory score ($P = 0.024$) (Kolehmainen et al 2012). Similar results were achieved in an RCT of 62 people with cardiovascular disease with the treatment group receiving bilberry juice (not described further). The treated group experienced significant reductions in CRP, IL-6, IL-12 and interferon-gamma (Karlsen et al 2012).

Astringent

The astringent properties of bilberry are well established and attributed to its significant tannin content.

Improves visual function

Epidemiological investigations have indicated that moderate consumption of anthocyanin-containing herbs such as BE is associated with an improvement in visual function (Hou 2003). Several animal studies suggest a positive effect on dark adaptation (Canter & Ernst 2004). More specifically, bilberry enhances regeneration of rhodopsin in the retina, which is essential for optimal functioning of the rods and therefore light adaptation and night vision (Blumenthal et al 2000). Other possible mechanisms of action in the eye include accelerated modulation of retinal enzyme activity and improved microcirculation (Canter & Ernst 2004).

Jang et al (2005) demonstrated that two anthocyanins from bilberry were potent antioxidants that suppressed photo-oxidative processes initiated in retinal pigment epithelial cells by A2E, a component of retinal epithelial cells which is associated with ageing and some inherited forms of retinal degeneration (Kim et al 2008). Matsunaga et al (2009) also demonstrated in vitro and in vivo that anthocyanins from bilberry protected against chemically induced damage to retinal ganglion cells through mainly antioxidant processes. Other animal models found significant protection of bilberry in endotoxin-induced uveitis in mice (Miyake et al 2012, Yao et al 2010).

Gastroprotective activity

In vitro tests have found that a specific anthocyanin found in bilberry causes an increase in the efficiency of the gastric mucosal barrier (Cristoni et al 1989). When administered orally in an animal model it retarded the development of gastric ulcers induced by stress, non-steroidal anti-inflammatory drugs, ethanol, reserpine and histamine (Magistretti et al 1988).

Hypoglycaemic activity

This activity has been demonstrated in animal models and at least one human study.

A dried hydroalcoholic extract of bilberry leaf administered orally to streptozotocin-induced diabetic rats for 4 days decreased plasma glucose levels by 26% (Cignarella et al 1996).

Takikawa et al (2010) studied the effects of an anthocyanin-rich bilberry diet on type 2 diabetic mice, resulting in a reduction in hyperglycaemia and insulin sensitivity via AMP-activated protein kinase (AMPK), activated in white adipose tissue, skeletal muscle and liver tissue. AMPK is the target of drugs like metformin. Another effect of bilberry on the insulin pathway includes the inhibition of adipocyte differentiation (Suzuki et al 2011).

One clinical study tested the effects of two different strengths of bilberry beverage (10% and 47%) on the insulin index (II) in young healthy adults and compared them to two other beverages, a fermented oat-based drink and a 10% rosehip drink. The 10% bilberry beverage, 10% rosehip beverage and fermented oat drink had a similar glycaemic index of 95, but the bilberry 10% drink had a significantly lower II of 65 ($P < 0.05$). The II dropped to 49 with the higher-strength 47% bilberry beverage, which also had a lower (non-significant) glycaemic index of 79 compared to the other drinks (Granfeldt & Bjorck 2011).

Neuroprotective

The anthocyanoside content is chiefly responsible for reversing the course of neurodegeneration in animals by affecting calcium homeostasis and improving motor performance (Kolosova et al 2006, Landfield & Eldridge 1994).

Anticarcinogenic activity

Preliminary research has found that components of the hexane/chloroform fraction of bilberry exhibit anticarcinogenic activity (Bomser et al 1996). Anti-angiogenic activity has also been identified (Matsunaga et al 2010, Roy et al 2002), as well as anticarcinogenic activity via inhibition of the nuclear factor-kappa B activation pathway (Aggarwal & Shishodia 2006). One animal study demonstrated significant reduction in colon cancer in animals fed an anthocyanidin mixture derived from bilberry (Cooke et al 2006), while growth and invasiveness were suppressed in human non-small-cell lung cancer cells by bilberry-derived anthocyanins in animal models (Kauser et al 2012).

OTHER ACTIONS

BE inhibits platelet aggregation according to ex vivo tests (Pulliero et al 1989). There is also some early in vitro research investigating whether it provides ultraviolet protection of skin (Svobodová et al 2009), ameliorates pruritus in allergic dermatitis (Yamaura et al 2011), modifies amyloid in Alzheimer's disease (Vepsäläinen et al 2013) and reduces stress-induced depression mediated by the nitric oxide pathway (Kumar et al 2012).

According to an animal study, anthocyanins from bilberry induce vasorelaxation via a complex cascade of actions that start in the cell membrane and result in nitrous oxide release from the vascular endothelium (Ziberna et al 2013).

CLINICAL USE

BEs are popular in Europe and have been investigated in numerous clinical trials, primarily in non-English-speaking European countries. As a result, many research papers have been published in other languages. To provide a more complete description of the evidence available, secondary sources have been used when necessary. While many clinical trials are of a preliminary nature, several larger RCTs have been published in recent years.

Ulcerative colitis

Positive results were obtained for bilberry supplementation in a small open pilot study of 13 people with well-characterised mild to moderate ulcerative colitis on stable conventional medicine (Biedermann et al 2013). A preparation equivalent to 600 g of fresh fruit per day was taken in four divided doses over a 6-week period, delivering a mean anthocyanin concentration of 210 mg per dose. Remission was achieved in 63.4% of patients with a clinical activity index (CAI) <4, while 90.9% had a response (CAI value drop ≥3 points). Other endpoints such as the complete Mayo Score showed at least a 2-point drop in 100% of patients and a ≥3-point drop in 54%; however the endoscopic Mayo Score was not as significant, with mean at baseline of 1.5 dropping to 1.2 after treatment.

There was a highly significant reduction in faecal calprotectin, with mean levels dropping from 778 mcg/g of stool to 134 mcg/g. After treatment ceased in week 7, calprotectin levels rose in some patients, while 4 maintained undetectable levels (Biedermann et al 2013).

Non-specific acute diarrhoea

The considerable astringent activity of bilberry provides a theoretical basis for its use in non-specific acute diarrhoea. Commission E approved crude fruit preparations for this indication (Blumenthal et al 2000).

Mild inflammation of the mouth and throat

The considerable astringent, anti-inflammatory and antioedema activity of bilberry provides a theoretical basis for its use as a topical application in these indications. Commission E approved this indication (Blumenthal et al 2000).

Haemorrhoids, varicose veins, venous insufficiency

The considerable astringent, anti-inflammatory and antioedema activity of bilberry provides a theoretical basis for its use in these conditions. Several human case series and a single-blind trial report significant improvements in lower-extremity discomfort and oedema related to chronic venous insufficiency; however, further research is required to confirm these findings (Ulbricht & Basch 2005).

Pregnancy

A bilberry product (Myrtocyan) was taken at a dose of 320 mg daily in the last trimester by women aged 24–37 years with pregnancy-induced lower-extremity oedema and found to significantly improve symptoms of burning and itching, heaviness, pain, diurnal and nocturnal leg cramps, oedema and capillary fragility (Ghiringhelli et al 1978, as reported in Blumenthal 2003).

Ophthalmic conditions

Bilberry preparations have been used to improve poor night vision, light adaptation and photophobia and myopia and to prevent or retard diabetic retinopathy, macular degeneration and cataracts. Primarily the collagen-enhancing and antioxidant activities of bilberry provide a theoretical basis for these indications.

Visual acuity and light adaptation

Whether bilberry preparations have a significant effect on visual acuity and light adaptation is difficult to ascertain from the current available evidence. The safety of bilberry and lack of other safe and effective treatments for improving night vision should compel researchers to continue investigating this treatment and clinicians to consider recommending a trial to patients.

A systematic review of 12 placebo-controlled trials (five RCTs and seven placebo-controlled non-randomised trials) concluded that the anthocyanosides from *Vaccinium myrtillus* were not effective for improving night vision; however, the authors point out that the potential therapeutic role of these constituents should not yet be dismissed because confounding factors and supportive auxiliary evidence exist (Canter & Ernst 2004). Four of the RCTs showed no positive effects for *V. myrtillus* anthocyanosides on outcome measures relevant to vision in reduced light, whereas the fifth RCT and all seven non-randomised trials reported positive effects on outcome measures relevant to night vision. Seventeen other studies were located by Canter and Ernst, but not included in the analysis because they did not contain a placebo group. Sixteen of those studies produced positive results on measures relevant to night vision in either healthy subjects or patients with a range of visual disorders and only one was negative.

The authors point out several confounding factors, in particular the wide range of doses, possible geographical variations in extract composition, choice of subject (generally healthy) and methods used to obtain and interpret electroretinograms, which varied between older and newer studies. For example, two of the negative RCTs tested the lowest dose levels of any of the trials: 36 mg daily for acute treatment and ≤48 mg for short-term treatment.

A significant improvement in visual performance has been demonstrated for BE in people with retinitis pigmentosa and haemeralopia (inability to see distinctly in bright light), suggesting that effects may be more pronounced in cases of impaired visual acuity (Gloria & Peria 1966, Junemann 1967).

Glaucoma

Available research suggests bilberry anthocyanosides may be beneficial in glaucoma.

In one small study of 8 patients, a single oral dose of 200 mg bilberry anthocyanosides was shown to improve glaucoma, as assessed by electroretinography (Caselli 1985).

The largest study to date involved 332 subjects diagnosed with normal-tension glaucoma and compared treatment with bilberry anthocyanins (120 mg twice daily), *Ginkgo biloba* extract (80 mg twice daily) or no treatment. Humphrey visual field (HVF) test and logarithm of the minimal angle of resolution best-corrected visual acuity (BCVA) were performed at baseline and after treatment. A chart review follow-up was performed at a mean time of 24 months, with improvement shown in the bilberry anthocyanin group in BCVA ($P = 0.008$) and HVF ($P = 0.001$) (Shim et al 2012).

IN COMBINATION

A controlled but non-blinded trial testing of 38 volunteers testing the effects of Mirtogenol, a bilberry and marine pine bark supplement, on intraocular pressure found that treatment resulted in a significant mean drop from 25.2 mm to 22.2 mm after 3 months (Steigerwalt et al 2008).

Retinopathy

In Europe, bilberry anthocyanoside extracts are recognised as highly effective in preventing or treating diabetic retinopathy, with clinical research supporting its use (Lietti et al 1976, Orsucci et al 1983, Perossini et al 1987, Scharrer & Ober 1981).

One double-blind study involving 40 patients with diabetic and/or hypertensive retinopathy showed that a dose of BE (Tegens) equivalent to 160 mg anthocyanosides taken twice daily for 1 month significantly improved ophthalmoscopic parameters and angiographic parameters (Perossini et al 1987). Another study of 31 subjects with different forms of retinopathy (diabetic retinopathy, retinitis pigmentosa, macular degeneration or haemorrhage due to anticoagulant use) found that treatment with BE (Difrarel 100) reduced vascular permeability and the tendency to haemorrhage in all patients (Scharrer & Ober 1981). A small open study by Orsucci et al of 10 subjects with diabetic retinopathy found that 6 months of treatment with BE (Tegens) equivalent to 240 mg anthocyanosides daily resulted in reduction or disappearance of haemorrhages and improvement in the retinal picture (Orsucci et al 1983, and reported in Blumenthal 2003).

Myopia

Uncontrolled trials report a beneficial effect of the extract on patients with myopia (Canter & Ernst 2004).

Additional studies using purified anthocyanoside oligomers highlight significant improvements in subjective symptoms and objective contrast sensitivity in myopia patients with poor night vision (Lee et al 2005). However, as specificity of source is not provided, this information can only be used in conjunction with the additional supportive evidence listed above.

Cataract

In practice, bilberry has been recommended to delay cataract progression. A case series of 50 elderly subjects with early-stage cataract found that a combination of anthocyanosides extracted from bilberry and vitamin E slowed progression of lens opacities by 97% (Ulbricht & Basch 2005). Placebo-controlled trials are now required to confirm these results.

Dry eye

A placebo-controlled study of 22 subjects with dry eye found that treatment with bilberry (160 mg twice daily) for 30 days produced a statistically significant improvement ($P < 0.01$) compared to the placebo group (Anderson et al 2011).

Asthenopia

Asthenopia is a condition characterised by tired, red, painful eyes, headaches, shoulder stiffness, low-back pain and frustration. It has been attributed in some part to refractory problems in the eye. A randomised, double-blinded parallel study compared the effects of omega-3-rich fish oil 1000 mg, bilberry anthocyanins 59 mg and lutein 75 mg per day taken for 4 weeks to placebo. Symptoms were catalogued via questionnaire, which was completed three times a week and included a visual analogue scale for fatigue. While there was a response to placebo for many symptoms, shoulder stiffness, low-back pain and frustration were significantly improved in the treatment group (Kawabata & Tsuji 2011).

Hypercholesterolaemia

Treatment with a purified anthocyanin supplement 160 mg twice a day produced a significant increase in high-density lipoprotein and decrease in low-density lipoprotein in this randomised, double-blind, placebo-controlled study. The 24-week study of 150 people with hypercholesterolaemia also demonstrated that active treatment had a significant effect on inflammatory markers high sensitive CRP (hsCRP), soluble vascular cell adhesion molecule (sVCAM), IL-1β and tumour necrosis factor-alpha (TNF-α), which were measured at 12 and 14 weeks, with hsCRP ($P = 0.007$ and $P < 0.001$) and sVCAM ($P = 0.03$ and $P = 014$) and IL-1β ($P = 0.02$ and $P = 0.02$) being significantly decreased in the treatment group compared to the placebo group, but no change in TNF-α in either group (Zhu et al 2013).

OTHER USES

Traditionally, bilberry has been used to treat dysentery, diabetes, gastrointestinal inflammatory conditions, vaginal discharges and haemorrhoids, and to stop lactation. Externally, bilberry preparations have been used to treat wounds, ulcers and skin infections. More recently, other uses include treatment for bleeding gums, nose bleeds, spider veins, capillary fragility, peptic ulcers, Raynaud's syndrome and venous insufficiency (such as claudication).

Additionally, a double-blind placebo-controlled study confirmed that bilberry improves peripheral vascular disorders by improving subjective symptoms after 30 days' treatment (Mills & Bone 2000).

DOSAGE RANGE

Internal

- Fluid extract (1 : 1) standardised to provide 60–120 mg daily of anthocyanins: 6–12 mL/day taken in three divided doses.
- Oral dose forms: BEs providing 240–480 mg of anthocyanins daily.
- Decoction of dried herb: 5–10 g of crushed, dried fruit in 150 mL of cold water, which is then boiled for up to 10 minutes and strained while hot. For symptomatic treatment of diarrhoea, drink the cold decoction several times daily.
- Gargle: a 10% decoction of the above preparation.
- Fresh berries: 165–400 g daily.

TOXICITY

Rats administered high doses of up to 400 mg/kg showed no adverse effects (Murray 1995).

ADVERSE REACTIONS

No adverse effects were reported in a systematic review of 12 placebo-controlled trials of *V. myrtillus* anthocyanosides (Canter & Ernst 2004). According to the same authors, a postmarketing surveillance study of 2295 people identified that 4% experienced side effects related to the skin, nervous system or gastrointestinal tract.

SIGNIFICANT INTERACTIONS

Controlled studies are not available; therefore interactions are theoretical and based on evidence of pharmacological activity with uncertain clinical significance.

Anticoagulant and antiplatelet drugs

A theoretical risk exists that high doses (>170 mg anthocyanidins) may increase bleeding risk; however, this remains uncertain as there is inadequate clinical evidence (Aktaş et al 2011, Stargrove et al 2008).

Iron

Reduced absorption is theoretically possible if taken at the same time because of the tannin content of the herb — separate doses by 2 hours.

Hypoglycaemic agents

Additive effects are theoretically possible with leaf preparations — observe patient.

Topoisomerase chemotherapy drugs

An in vitro study using human colon cancer cells showed that anthocyanin-rich berry extracts may be protective of DNA damage caused by topoisomerase drugs and therefore may reduce chemotherapy effectiveness. As the concentration required (>50 mcg/mL) to cause this effect is likely to be greater than could be achieved through oral ingestion, it remains theoretical.

Practice points/Patient counselling

- Bilberry has antioxidant, anti-inflammatory and astringent actions and has considerable polyphenol content, and may therefore be of greatest benefit in the prevention of disorders where inflammation is a known precursor.
- BE is a popular treatment in Europe for preventing and treating retinopathy. It is also used to treat several other ophthalmic conditions, such as poor night vision, poor light adaptation and sensitivity to glare, photophobia, glaucoma, myopia, dry eye, asthenopia and cataract. Some clinical research suggests a possible role in glaucoma, retinopathy and dry eye, whereas the evidence for use in improving night vision is unclear.
- Some research also suggests that it is useful in venous insufficiency, peripheral vascular disorders (such as Raynaud's syndrome) and capillary fragility.
- There is new clinical research suggesting that BE has significant hypoglycaemic activity and lipid-lowering activity and that it may be beneficial in ulcerative colitis.
- Bilberry is approved by Commission E for the treatment of non-specific, acute diarrhoea and mild inflammatory conditions of the mouth and throat.
- Preliminary evidence suggests it may prevent peptic ulcer formation due to non-steroidal anti-inflammatory drugs or stress; however, clinical research is still required to confirm these effects.

CONTRAINDICATIONS AND PRECAUTIONS

High doses (>170 mg anthocyanidins) should be used with caution by people with haemorrhagic disorders. Avoid use with topoisomerase chemotherapy drugs until safety can be established.

PREGNANCY USE

A study investigating BE for pregnancy-induced lower-extremity oedema reported no adverse effects (Ulbricht & Basch 2005) — likely to be safe when berry is consumed in dietary amounts.

PATIENTS' FAQs

What will this herb do for me?

Bilberry is used to relieve the symptoms of mild diarrhoea and improve poor night vision, sensitivity to glare, photophobia, peptic ulcers, varicose veins, venous insufficiency and haemorrhoids when taken internally. It is also used as a mouthwash, gargle or paint for mild inflammation of the mouth or throat, such as gingivitis or pharyngitis. Clinical research also shows it may be useful for some ophthalmic conditions and as a treatment in ulcerative colitis, glaucoma and reducing low-density lipoprotein cholesterol while raising high-density lipoprotein cholesterol.

When will it start to work?

This depends on the indication. Improvements in night vision, photophobia and glare sensitivity have been reported within 2–4 weeks of use in some people whereas preventive effects are likely to require long-term use. In peripheral vascular disease, 30 days' treatment may be required before effects are noticed. In ulcerative colitis progressive symptom relief may occur over 6 weeks.

Are there any safety issues?

Bilberry is considered a safe herb which is well tolerated. Theoretically, it may reduce blood glucose levels so should be used carefully in diabetics on hypoglycaemic medication. Theoretically, it may increase the risk of bleeding when used at very high doses, and should be avoided with certain chemotherapy drugs. Due to its high tannin content, bilberry will reduce the absorption of iron if taken at the same time as iron-containing substances, so a 2-hour separation of doses is recommended.

REFERENCES

Aggarwal BB, Shishodia S. Molecular targets of dietary agents for prevention and therapy of cancer. Biochem Pharmacol 71.10 (2006): 1397–1421.

Aktaş, C et al. Bilberry potentiates Warfarin effect? Turk geratri Dergisi 14.1 (2011): 79–81.

Anderson, KG, et al. Potential use of bilberry for dry eye relief. Optometry 82.6 (2011): 380.

Ashour, O.M., et al. Protective effect of bilberry (*Vaccinium myrtillus*) against doxorubicin-induced oxidative cardiotoxicity in rats. Medical Science Monitor 17.4 (2011): 110–115.

Bao, L., et al. Protective effects of bilberry (*Vaccinium myrtillus* L.) extract on Kbro3-induced kidney damage in mice. J. Ag and Food Chem. 56.2 (2008): 420–25.

Bao. L., et al. Bilberry extract protein restraint stress-induced liver damage through attenuating mitochondrial dysfunction. Fitoterapia 81.8 (2010): 1094–101.

Bertuglia S, et al. Effect of *Vaccinium myrtillus* anthocyanosides on ischaemia reperfusion injury in hamster cheek pouch microcirculation. Pharmacol Res 31.3–4 (1995): 183–7.

Biedermann, L., et al. Bilberry ingestion improves disease activity in mild to moderate ulcerative colitis — an open pilot study. J. Crohn's and Colitis 7.4 (2013): 271–279.

Blumenthal M. The ABC clinical guide to herbs. New York: American Botanical Council and Thieme, 2003.

Blumenthal M, et al (eds). Herbal medicine: expanded Commission E monographs. Austin, TX: Integrative Medicine Communications, 2000.

Bomser J et al. In vitro anticancer activity of fruit extracts from *Vaccinium* species. Planta Med 62.3 (1996): 212–16.

Bornsek, S. M., et al. Bilberry and Blueberry Anthocyanins Act as Powerful Intracellular Antioxidants in Mammalian Cells. Food Chem. 134.4 (2012): 1878–84.

Canter PH, Ernst E. Anthocyanosides of *Vaccinium myrtillus* (bilberry) for night vision: a systematic review of placebo-controlled trials. Surv Opthalmol 49.1 (2004): 38–50.

Caselli L. Clinical and electroretinographic study on activity of anthocyanosides. Arch Med Int 37 (1985): 29–35.

Choi, E. H., et al. Alleviation of doxorubicin-induced toxicities by anthocyanin-rich bilberry (*Vaccinium myrtillus* L.) extract in rats and mice. BioFactors 36.4 (2010): 319–27.

Cignarella A et al. Novel lipid-lowering properties of *Vaccinium myrtillus* L. leaves, a traditional antidiabetic treatment, in several models of rat

dyslipidaemia: a comparison with ciprofibrate. Thromb Res 84.5 (1996): 311–22.
Cooke D et al. Effect of cyanidin-3-glucoside and an anthocyanin mixture from bilberry on adenoma development in the ApcMin mouse model of intestinal carcinogenesis-relationship with tissue anthocyanidin levels. Int J Cancer 119 (2006): 2213–20.
Cristoni A, et al. Effect of a natural flavonoid on gastric mucosal barrier. Arzneimittelforschung 39.5 (1989): 590–2.
Domitrović, R. and Jakovac, H. Effects of standardized bilberry fruit extract (Mirtoselectâ®) on resolution of ccl4-induced liver fibrosis in mice. Food and Chemical Toxicology 49.4 (2011): 848–54.
Ghiringhelli C, et al. Capillarotropic action of anthocyanosides in high dosage in phlebopathic stasis. Minerva Cardioangiol 24.4 (1978): 255–76.
Gloria E, Peria A. Effect of anthocyanosides on the absolute visual threshold. Ann Ottalmol Clin Ocul 92 (1966): 595–607 [in Italian].
Granfeldt, Y.E., and Bjorck, I.M.E. A bilberry drink with fermented oatmeal decreases postprandial insulin demand in young healthy adults. Nutrition Journal 10.1 (2011) 57.
Hou DX. Potential mechanisms of cancer chemoprevention by anthocyanins. Curr Mol Med 3.2 (2003): 149–59.
Ichiyanagi T et al. Complete assignment of bilberry (*Vaccinium myrtillus* L.) anthocyanins separated by capillary zone electrophoresis. Tokyo: Chemical & Pharmaceutical Bulletin 52.2 (2004): 226–9.
Jang YP et al. Anthocyanins protect against A2E photooxidation and membrane permeabilization in retinal pigment epithelial cells. Photochemistry and Photobiology 81.3 (2005): 529–36.
Junemann G. On the effect of anthocyanosides on hemeralopia following quinine poisoning. Klin Monatsbl Augenheilkd 151 (1967): 891–6 [in German].
Kahkonen MP, et al. Berry phenolics and their antioxidant activity. J Agric Food Chem 49.8 (2001): 4076–82.
Karlsen, A., et al. Bilberry juice modulates plasma concentration of NF-kappa B related inflammatory markers in subjects at increased risk of CVD. European Journal of Nutrition 46.6 (2012); 345–55.
Kauser, H., et al. Berry anthocyanidins synergistically suppress growth and invasive potential of human non-small-cell lung cancer cells. Cancer Letters 325.1 (2012): 54–62.
Kawabata, F., and Tsuji, T. Effects of dietary supplementation with a combination of fish oil, bilberry extract, and lutein on subjective symptoms of asthenopia in humans. Biomedical Research 32.6 (2011): 387–93.
Kim SR et al. Mechanisms involved in A2E oxidation. Experim Eye Res 86.6 (2008): 975–82.
Kolehmainen, M., et al. Bilberries reduce low-grade inflammation in individuals with features of metabolic syndrome. Mol. Nut and Food Research 56.10 (2012): 1501–10.
Kolosova NG, et al. Long-term antioxidant supplementation attenuates oxidative stress markers and cognitive deficits in senescent-accelerated OXYS rats. Neurobiol Aging 27 (2006): 1289–97.
Kumar, B., et al. *Vaccinium myrtillus* ameliorates unpredictable chronic mild stress induced depression: possible involvement of nitric oxide pathway. Phytotherapy Research 26.4 (2012): 488–97.
Landfield PW, Eldridge JC. The glucocorticoid hypothesis of age-related hippocampal neurodegeneration: role of dysregulated intraneuronal calcium. Ann NY Acad Sci 746 (1994): 308–321: discussion 321–6.
Lee J et al. Purified high-dose anthocyanoside oligomer administration improves nocturnal vision and clinical symptoms in myopia subjects. Br J Nutr 93.6 (2005): 895–9.
Lietti A, et al. Studies on *Vaccinium myrtillus* anthocyanosides. I. Vasoprotective and antiinflammatory activity. Arzneimittelforschung 26.5 (1976): 829–32.
Magistretti MJ, et al. Antiulcer activity of an anthocyanidin from *Vaccinium myrtillus*. Arzneimittelforschung 38.5 (1988): 686–90.
Matsunaga, N., et al. Bilberry and its main constituents have neuroprotective effects against retinal damage in vitro and in vivo. Molecular Nutrition and Food Research 53.7 (2009): 869–77.
Matsunaga, N., et al. *Vaccinium myrtillus* (bilberry) extracts reduce angiogenesis in vitro and in vivo. Evidence- based Complementary and Alternative Medicine 7.1 (2010): 47–56.
Mauray, A et al. Nutrigenomic analysis of the protective effects of bilberry anthocyanin-rich extract in apo E-deficient mice. Genes & nutrition 5.4 (2010): 343–353.
Mian E et al. Anthocyanosides and the walls of the microvessels: further aspects of the mechanism of action of their protective effect in syndromes due to abnormal capillary fragility. Minerva Med 68.52 (1977): 3565–81.
Mills S, Bone K. Principles and practice of phytotherapy. London: Churchill Livingstone, 2000.
Miyake, S et al. Vision preservation during retinal inflammation by anthocyanin-rich bilberry extract: cellular and molecular mechanism. Laboratory Investigation 92.1 (2012): 102–109.
Mozaffarieh M et al. The potential value of natural antioxidative treatment in glaucoma. Survey of Ophthalmology 53.5 (2008): 479–505.
Murray M. The healing power of herbs. Rocklin, CA: Prima Health, 1995.
Orsucci P et al. Treatment of diabetic retinopathy with anthocyanosides: a preliminary report. Clin Ocul 4 (1983): 377.
Perossini M et al. Diabetic and hypertensive retinopathy therapy with *Vaccinium myrtillus* anthocyanosides (Tegens™): Double-blind placebo controlled clinical trial. Ann Ottalmol Clin Ocul 113 (1987): 1173 [in Italian].
Piberger, H., et al. Bilberries and their anthocyanins ameliorate experimental colitis. Molecular Nutrition and Food Research 55.11 (2011): 1724–29.
Pulliero G et al. Ex vivo study of the inhibitory effects of *Vaccinium myrtillus* anthocyanosides on human platelet aggregation. Fitoterapia LX.I (1989): 69–75.
Riihinen K, et al. Organ-specific disribution of phenolic compounds in bilberry (*Vaccinium myrtillus*) and 'nrothblue' blueberry (*Vaccinium corymbosum* xV. *angustofolium*). Food Chem 110.1 (2008): 156–60.
Roy S et al. Anti-angiogenic property of edible berries. Free Radic Res 36.9 (2002): 1023–31.
Scharrer A, Ober M. Anthocyanosides in the treatment of retinopathies (author's transl.). Klin Monatsbl Augenheilkd 178.5 (1981): 386–9.
Shim, S.H., et al. Ginkgo biloba extract and bilberry anthocyanins improve visual function in patients with normal tension glaucoma. J. Med. Food 15.9 (2012) 818–23.
Skemiene, K., et al. Anthocyanins block ischemia-induces apoptosisin the perfused heart and support mitochondrial respiration potentially by reducing cytosolic cytochrome c. Internation Journal of Biochemistry and Cell Biology 45.1 (2013) 23–29.
Stargrove MB, et al. Herb, nutrient and drug interactions — clinical applications and therapeutic strategies. St Louis, MO: Mosby Elsevier, 2008.
Steigerwalt, R.D., et al. Effects of Mirtogenol® on ocular blood flow and intraocular hypertension in asymptomatic subjects. Molecular Vision 14 (2008):1288–92.
Suzuki, R., et al. Anthocyanidins-enriched bilberry extracts inhibit 3T3-L1 adipocyte differentiation via the insulin pathway. Nutrition and Metabolism 8 (2011):14.
Svobodová, A, et al. *Lonicera caerulea* and *Vaccinium myrtillus* fruit polyphenols protect HaCaT keratinocytes against UVB-induced phototoxic stress and DNA damage. Journal of dermatological science 56.3 (2009): 196–204.
Takikawa, M., et al. Dietary anthocyanin-rich bilberry extract ameliorates hyperglycemia and insulin sensitivity via activation of AMP-activated protein kinase in diabetic mice. J. of Nutrition 140.3 (2010): 527–33.
Trumbeckaitė, S et al. Direct effects of Vaccinium myrtillus L. fruit extracts on rat heart mitochondrial functions. Phytotherapy Research 27.4 (2013): 499–506.
Ulbricht CE, Basch EM. Natural standard herb and supplement reference. St Louis, MO: Mosby Inc., 2005.
Valentová K, et al. Cytoprotective effect of a bilberry extract against oxidative damage of rat heptocytes. Food Chem 101.3 (2007): 912–17.
Varma SD, Richards RD. Ascorbic acid and the eye lens. Ophthalmic Res 20.3 (1988): 164–73.
Varma SD, et al. Photoperoxidation in lens and cataract formation: preventive role of superoxide dismutase, catalase and vitamin C. Ophthalmic Res 14.3 (1982): 167–75.
Varma SD et al. Studies on Emory mouse cataracts: oxidative factors. Ophthalmic Res 26.3 (1994): 141–8.
Vepsäläinen, S et al. Anthocyanin-enriched bilberry and blackcurrant extracts modulate amyloid precursor protein processing and alleviate behavioral abnormalities in the APP/PS1 mouse model of Alzheimer's disease. The Journal of nutritional biochemistry 24.1 (2013): 360–370.
Yamaura, K., et al. Anthocyanins from bilberry (*Vaccinium myrtillus* L.) alleviate pruritus in mouse model of chronic allergic contact dermatitis. Pharacognosy Research 3.3 (2011): 173–77.
Yao Y, Vieira A. Protective activities of *Vaccinium* antioxidants with potential relevance to mitochondrial dysfunction and neurotoxicity. NeuroToxicity 28.1 (2007): 93–100.
Yao, N., et al. Protective effects of bilberry (*Vaccinium myrtillus* L.) extract against endotoxin –induced uveitis in mice. J. Ag and Food Chem. 58.8 (2010): 4731–36.
Yue, X. and Xu, Z. Changes of anthocyanins, anthocyanidins, and antioxidant activity in bilberry extract during dry heating. Journal of Food Science 73.6 (2008): c494–499.
Zhang Z et al. Comparison of HPLC methods for determination of anthocyanins and anthocyanidins in bilberry extracts. Journal of Agricultural and Food Chemistry 52.4 (2004): 688–91.
Zhu, Y., et al. Anti-inflammatory effect of purified dietary anthocyanin in adults with hypercholesterolemia: A randomized controlled trial. Nutrition, Metabolism and Cardiovascular Diseases 23.9 (2013): 843–849.
Ziberna, L., et al. The Endothelial plasma membrane transporter bilitranslocase mediates rat aortic vasoldilation induced by anthocyanins. Nutrition Metabolism, and Cardiovascular Diseases 23.1 (2013): 68–74.

Bitter melon

HISTORICAL NOTE Bitter melon is used as a traditional medicine wherever it is found. It has a long history of use in Asia, Africa and Latin America and has been widely acclaimed as an important remedy for diabetes mellitus since ancient times. The genus name *momordica* means 'to bite' and refers to the jagged edges of the leaf, which appear as if bitten. Bitter melon has been used to treat fevers, viral infections and as an emmenagogue in reproductive health. It has also been used to treat gastrointestinal complaints, worms, constipation, headaches, skin conditions and diabetes. The fruit is used topically for wound healing. The plant has also been used in traditional ceremonies and considered a powerful charm, which is worn as a necklace, wrist or ankle bracelet or crown (Beloin et al 2005). The ritual ceremonial importance of the plant is accompanied by its considerable reputation as a medicinal plant for the treatment of disease.

OTHER NAMES

African cucumber, balsam pear, bitter gourd, kakara, karela, ku gua, sushavi, wild cucumber

BOTANICAL NAME/FAMILY

Momordica charantia (family Curcubitaceae)

PLANT PARTS USED

Fruit, leaves

CHEMICAL COMPONENTS

It contains several biologically active constituents that include glycosides (e.g. momordicins I and II, 25ξ-isopropenylchole-5 [Liu et al 2012], taiwacin A(1),23,24,25,26,27-pentanorcucurbitane [Lin et al 2011]), steroidal saponins (e.g. charantins, Kuguacin J [Pitchakarn et al 2012]), alkaloids, fixed oils and proteins (e.g. MAP 30: *Momordica* anti-HIV protein; molecular weight, 30 kDa). The immature fruits are a good source of vitamin C and also provide vitamin A, phosphorus and iron (Grover & Yadav 2004).

MAIN ACTIONS

Bitter melon has been the subject of countless studies and has demonstrated significant pharmacological activity in a variety of experimental models.

Antidiabetic

The antidiabetic potential of bitter melon has been the subject of intense investigation, with over 140 studies having investigated the hypoglycaemic activity of various constituents of *Momordica charantia* in animal models and human studies.

The hypoglycaemic activity of bitter gourd is well established in normal, streptozocin- or alloxan-induced diabetic animals and in genetic models of diabetes (Ahmed et al 2004, Bailey et al 1985, Chaturvedi 2005, Day et al 1990, Harinantenaina et al 2006, Jayasooriya et al 2000, Kar et al 2003, Kumar et al 2008, Mamun 2011, Miura et al 2001, 2004, Ojewole et al 2006, Reyes et al 2006, Sarkar et al 1996, Shibib et al 1993, Shetty et al 2005). All parts of the plant (fruit pulp, seeds, leaves and whole plant) have shown activity. Superfine powdered bitter melon showed a higher antidiabetic effect than hot air-dried powder in vivo (Ying et al 2012). Whether the effect is sufficient to have a significant clinical effect in people with type 2 diabetes is uncertain, according to a recent systematic review of four clinical trials (Ooi et al 2012).

A systematic study comparing the hypoglycaemic activity of three extracts in vivo found that the methanolic extract of dried whole fruits and seeds reduced blood glucose by 49% at the end of the first week, which became 39% by week 5. The aqueous extract of fresh, unripe, whole fruits reduced fasting blood glucose by 50%, which was consistent until the study ended, and the chloroform extract of dried whole fruits and seeds showed almost no hypoglycaemic activity (Virdi et al 2003). These observations have special significance when one considers that the whole bitter gourd is cooked in water and consumed in many cultures, particularly in India.

Multiple mechanisms of action have been identified for bitter gourd. It also suggests that consideration should be made of the extraction used when interpreting human studies. In general, it appears to stimulate pancreatic insulin secretion (Fernandes et al 2007, Welihinda et al 1982), improve peripheral glucose uptake (Fernandes et al 2007, Welihinda & Karunanayake 1986) and improve insulin sensitivity and signalling (Sridhar et al 2008).

It has been demonstrated that *Momordica charantia* has a protective effect on pancreatic β-cells via downregulation of mitogen-activated protein kinases and nuclear factor kappa-light-chain enhancer of activated B cells (Kim & Kim 2011). Aqueous and alcohol extracts of *M. charantia* have been shown to stimulate glucose-6-phosphatase dehydrogenase and inhibit fructose 1,6-diphosphatase, glucose-6-phosphatase activities (Shetty et al 2005). Also, other biochemical and physiological processes such as glucose utilisation in skeletal muscles, intestinal glucose uptake inhibition and suppression of gluconeogenic enzymes have been inferred through in vivo and in vitro studies (Ahmed et al 2004). A study of streptozocin-induced diabetic animals further reveals a beneficial role for bitter gourd in controlling glycoconjugate- and heparan sulfate-related kidney complications in diabetes, thus prolonging late complications of diabetes (Kumar et al 2008).

The hypoglycaemic activity is attributed to a mixture of steroidal saponins known as charantins, insulin-like peptides and alkaloids that are concentrated in the fruit (Grover & Yadav 2004), whereas several different fractions of *M. charantia* extract may make different contributions to its cell-repairing activity and its ability to stimulate insulin secretion (Xiang et al 2007).

Lipid lowering

Lipid-lowering activity has been reported in studies of normal and diabetic animals for the fruit extract, flavonoids extracted from bitter melon or a methanolic fraction of the plant (Ahmed et al 2001, Anila & Vijayalakshmi 2000, Chaturvedi 2005, Chaturvedi et al 2004, Senanayake et al 2004, Singh et al 1989). Typically, decreases in triglyceride and low-density lipoprotein levels and increases in high-density lipoprotein levels are seen.

Antiviral

Several constituents found in bitter melon (e.g. alpha- and beta-momorcharin, lectin and MAP 30) have demonstrated in vitro antiviral activity against Epstein–Barr, herpes simplex virus type 1 (HSV-1), HIV, coxsackievirus B3 and polioviruses (Beloin et al 2005, Bourinbaiar & Lee-Huang 1996, Foa-Tomasi et al 1982, Grover & Yadav 2004, Sun et al 2001).

A study using a lyophilised extract of *Momordica charantia* against HSV-1 suggests that the presence of light may be important for antiviral activity (Beloin et al 2005). The active antiviral constituents are not the main bitter principles momordicins I and II, as these have not shown activity against HSV-1 (Beloin et al 2005). One constituent, referred to as MAP 30, has received special attention, as it exhibits potent inhibition of HIV-1 and HSV (Schreiber et al 1999).

Antibacterial and antiprotozoal

Broad-spectrum antibacterial activity has been demonstrated for the leaf extracts (aqueous, ethanol and methanol) (Grover & Yadav 2004). In vitro antimicrobial activity has been demonstrated against *Escherichia coli*, *Salmonella paratyphi*, *Shigella dysenterae* and *Streptomyces griseus* (Grover & Yadav 2004, Ogata et al 1991, Omoregbe et al 1996). A recent study found that both the aqueous and the ethanol extracts of bitter melon leaf inhibited the growth of *Staphylococcus aureus*, *Bacillus subtilis*, *Escherichia coli* and *Pseudomonas aeruginosa* (Mada et al 2013). In a phase II study, the leaf extracts inhibited the growth of *Mycobacterium tuberculosis* in vitro, using the BACTEC 460 susceptibility test method (Frame et al 1998).

Tests with an extract of the entire plant demonstrated antiprotozoal activity against *Entamoeba histolytica* (Grover & Yadav 2004) and a fruit extract exhibited activity against *Helicobacter pylori* (Yesilada et al 1999).

Anti-inflammatory

Bitter gourd extract has been found to suppress lipopolysaccharide-induced tumour necrosis factor-alpha production in vitro and, more recently, the butanol-soluble fraction was also found to strongly suppress lipopolysaccharide-induced tumour necrosis factor-alpha production (Kobori et al 2008).

Anthelminthic

The anthelminthic activity of the leaves of *Momordica charantia* against *Caenorhabditis elegans* was identified and described as high in one study (Beloin et al 2005). Triterpene glycosides of bitter melon (momordicins I and II) were found to be very active nematicides. A preparation of *M. charantia* exhibited stronger anthelminthic activity in vitro than piperazine hexahydrate against *Ascaridia galli* (Lal et al 1976). A recent in vitro study reported significant anthelminthic activity of ethanol extract of bitter melon leaf against *Ascaris suum* (Tjokropranoto et al 2011).

Abortifacient

Experimental studies with mice have demonstrated that bitter melon has abortifacient activity (Chan et al 1984, Tam et al 1984). According to an in vivo study, the glycoproteins alpha- and beta-momorcharin isolated from the seeds are effective in inducing early and midterm abortions (Chan et al 1986) and the momorcharins were teratogenic in cultured mouse embryos (Chan et al 1986).

Antifertility

A study on rats using bitter melon seed and pulp extract showed significant spermicidal activity in male rats and prolonged oestrous cycle in female rats, suggesting that bitter melon fruit may have antifertility activity (Sheeja et al 2012).

OTHER ACTIONS

Anticancer

Various preliminary studies (in vitro and in vivo) with crude bitter melon extract and its various constituents (e.g. MAP 30, momordin I, alpha-momorcharin) have shown anticancer activity (Basch et al 2003). An in vitro study on cucurbitane triterpenoids demonstrated antiproliferative activity on human breast adenocarcinoma, human medulloblastoma, human laryngeal carcinoma and human colon adenocarcinoma tumour cell lines (Hsiao et al 2013).

Analgesic

An in vivo study identified a dose-dependent analgesic effect for a methanolic extract of bitter melon seeds (Biswas et al 1991). The dose that produced a 50% response was 5 mg/kg subcutaneously. Analgesic activity was rapid and short-lived. The opiate pathway was not involved, as naloxone pretreatment did not modify the analgesic response.

Lipid lowering

A study on human preadipocytes treated with bitter melon juice demonstrated inhibition of lipogenesis and stimulation of lipolysis (Nerurkar et al 2010).

Wound healing

Momordica charantia Linn. fruit powder, in the form of an ointment (10% w/w dried powder in simple ointment base), was evaluated for wound-healing potential in an excision, incision and dead-space wound model in rats (Prasad et al 2006). The *Momordica* ointment produced a statistically significant response ($P < 0.01$), in terms of wound-contracting ability, wound closure time, period of epithelialisation, tensile strength of the wound and regeneration of tissues at wound site when compared with the control group. These results were comparable to those of the reference drug used, which was povidone-iodine ointment. In an experimental study on wounds in streptozotocin-induced diabetic rats, topical application of a bitter melon extract resulted in enhanced wound closure and an increase in protein content, suggesting faster cellular proliferation and healing (Teoh et al 2009).

CLINICAL USE

The clinical use of bitter melon is largely based on traditional evidence with mechanistic studies further providing a rationale for its use. Most clinical investigation has focused on its potential role in diabetes management.

Diabetes

Bitter melon has shown promising effects in prevention as well as delay in progression of diabetic complications (e.g. nephropathy, neuropathy, cataract and insulin resistance) in experimental animals (Grover & Yadav 2004).

Various bitter melon preparations, such as bitter melon fruit juice, dried fruit, seeds and tea, have been investigated for hypoglycaemic activity. Some preparations have demonstrated hypoglycaemic activity in clinical studies and experimental models; however, sample sizes are consistently small and statistical analyses are vaguely described (Dans et al 2007).

A Cochrane systematic review included four randomised controlled trials (RCTs) (n = 479) that assessed the effects of bitter melon for type 2 diabetes (Ooi et al 2012). Study duration varied from 4 weeks to 3 months and study preparations also varied. Two of the RCTs compared preparations from different parts of the bitter melon plant (tablets prepared from shade-dried whole fruit equivalent to 1 g three times a day and capsules prepared from the plant fruits and seeds) but found no statistically significant improvement in glycaemic control for bitter melon over the placebo. In a study comparing three doses of capsules prepared from oven-dried fruit pulp (500 mg/day, 1000 mg/day, 2000 mg/day) against metformin there was a significant reduction in mean fructosamine levels from baseline for both bitter melon 2000 mg/day (−10.2 micromol/L; 95% confidence interval [CI] −19.1 to −1.3 micromol/L) and metformin 1000 mg/day (−16.8 micromol/L; 95% CI −31.2 to −2.4 micromol/L), and the difference between the two treatments was and statistically significant ($P = 0.43$). The largest study that included 260 participants taking tablets prepared from the leaves showed statistically significant reductions in fasting blood glucose and HbA_{1C} that were comparable to low-dose glibenclamide (2.5 mg twice daily). There were also comparable improvements in polyuria, polyphagia, polydipsia, weight loss and nocturia. The four included trials used preparations from different parts of the plant and all were assessed as having a high risk of bias. Due to the supportive evidence of hypoglycemic activity and other mechanisms that would benefit diabetics, further research is warranted to identify the most effective extract, dose and plant part in humans.

Cancer

Controlled studies are not available to determine the clinical significance of the encouraging experimental findings. Bitter melon juice extracts have shown anticancer effects both in vivo and in vitro, especially against pancreatic carcinoma. Bitter melon juice extract resulted in strong apoptotic death of human pancreatic carcinoma cells and apoptosis is linked to the activation of the biomarker adenosine monophosphate-activated protein kinase (AMPK). Bitter melon juice extract displayed similar effects of inhibition of cancer cell proliferation, induction of apoptosis and activation of AMPK in mice, therefore suggesting possible clinical usefulness of bitter melon in pancreatic cancer (Kaur et al 2013).

HIV

Nine case reports of people with HIV taking bitter melon, sometimes in combination with other herbal medicines, suggest that it may normalise the CD4:CD8 ratio; however, further investigation is required (Zhang & Khanyile 1992). An in vitro study demonstrated that juice of bitter melon had a significant lipid-lowering effect on HIV-1 protease inhibitor-treated HepG2 cells, suggesting bitter melon's potential for decreasing hyperlipidaemia in HIV-infected patients with protease inhibitor-associated hyperlipidaemia (Nerurkar et al 2006).

OTHER USES

Traditionally, bitter melon has been used as a treatment for a variety of conditions, such as diabetes, gastrointestinal complaints, worms, constipation, headaches, skin conditions, viral infections and as an emmenagogue in reproductive health. Experimental studies support its use in some of these indications; however, controlled studies are still required to determine its role in practice.

DOSAGE RANGE

General guide

- Capsule of powdered bitter melon: 500–1000 mg/day.
- Juice: 50–100 mL/day.

B

According to clinical studies

- Diabetes: aqueous extract of bitter melon fruit juice containing 100 g of fruit in 100 mL of extract taken daily or oven-dried fruit pulp 2000 mg/day

ADVERSE REACTIONS

Gastrointestinal symptoms are the most common adverse effects seen. Clinically, this occurs as epigastric discomfort, pain and diarrhoea, which cease once treatment is stopped.

There are two case reports of bitter melon tea inducing hypoglycaemic coma and convulsions in children (Basch et al 2003). Headaches have been reported with ingestion of the seeds (Ulbricht & Basch 2005).

Practice points/Patient counselling

- Bitter melon is used as a traditional remedy for diabetes mellitus. Evidence from experimental studies and case reports supports moderate hypoglycaemic activity; however, evidence from clinical studies using a leaf extract or freeze-dried fruit pulp show better results.
- Traditionally, bitter melon has also been used as a treatment for gastrointestinal complaints, worms, constipation, headaches, skin conditions, viral infections and as an emmenagogue.
- According to experimental studies, bitter melon and/or its various constituents exert lipid-lowering, antibacterial, anthelminthic, abortifacient, antifertility, antineoplastic and analgesic activities.
- Bitter melon is contraindicated in pregnancy and people with glucose-6-phosphate dehydrogenase deficiency.
- Avoid bitter melon seed and the outer rind, which have toxic lectins.

CONTRAINDICATIONS AND PRECAUTIONS

Avoid bitter melon seed and the outer rind due to the presence of toxic lectins and avoid use of bitter melon in people with glucose-6-phosphate dehydrogenase deficiency (Ulbricht & Basch 2005).

When low doses of bitter melon extract were ingested for up to 2 months in experimental models, no signs of nephrotoxicity, hepatotoxicity or adverse effects on food intake, growth organ weights and haematological parameters were observed. However, toxicity and even death in laboratory animals have been reported when extracts in high doses were administered intravenously or intraperitoneally (Kusamran et al 1998).

SIGNIFICANT INTERACTIONS

Controlled studies are not available; therefore, interactions are based on evidence of activity and are largely theoretical and speculative.

Hypoglycaemic agents

Theoretically an additive effect is possible, resulting in increased hypoglycaemic effects — caution. Possible beneficial interaction when used under professional supervision.

PREGNANCY USE

Based on experimental studies in animal models and traditional use, bitter melon is contraindicated in pregnancy until safety is established. It should also not be used by men attempting to father a child.

PATIENTS' FAQs

What will this herb do for me?

According to preliminary research, bitter melon may lower blood glucose levels and aid in the management of diabetes.

When will it start to work?

This is difficult to predict. Diabetics should monitor their blood glucose readings when taking bitter melon, as they may require medication modification.

Are there any safety issues?

Bitter melon is contraindicated in pregnancy and people with glucose-6-phosphate dehydrogenase deficiency. The seeds and outer rind should be avoided because they contain toxic lectins. Diabetic patients should monitor their blood glucose when taking bitter melon to prevent hypoglycaemia.

REFERENCES

Ahmed I et al. Hypotriglyceridemic and hypocholesterolemic effects of anti-diabetic *Momordica charantia* (karela) fruit extract in streptozotocin-induced diabetic rats. Diabetes Res Clin Pract 51 (2001): 155–161.

Ahmed I et al. Beneficial effects and mechanism of action of *Momordica charantia* juice in the treatment of streptozotocin-induced diabetes mellitus in rat. Mol Cell Biochem 261 (2004): 63–70.

Anila L, Vijayalakshmi NR. Beneficial effects of flavonoids from *Sesamum indicum*, *Emblica officinalis* and *Momordica charantia*. Phytother Res 14 (2000): 592–595.

Bailey CJ et al. Cerasee, a traditional treatment for diabetes: studies in normal and streptozotocin diabetic mice. Diabetes Res 2 (1985): 81–84.

Basch E, et al. Bitter melon (*Momordica charantia*): a review of efficacy and safety. Am J Health Syst Pharm 60 (2003): 356–359.

Beloin N et al. Ethnomedicinal uses of *Momordica charantia* (Cucurbitaceae) in Togo and relation to its phytochemistry and biological activity. J Ethnopharmacol 96 (2005): 49–55.

Biswas AR, et al. Analgesic effect of *Momordica charantia* seed extract in mice and rats. J Ethnopharmacol 31 (1991): 115–118.

Bourinbaiar AS, Lee-Huang S. The activity of plant-derived antiretroviral proteins MAP30 and GAP31 against herpes simplex virus in vitro. Biochem Biophys Res Commun 219 (1996): 923–929.

Chan WY et al. The termination of early pregnancy in the mouse by beta-momorcharin. Contraception 29 (1984): 91–100.

Chan WY et al. Effects of momorcharins on the mouse embryo at the early organogenesis stage. Contraception 34 (1986): 537–544.

Chaturvedi P. Role of *Momordica charantia* in maintaining the normal levels of lipids and glucose in diabetic rats fed a high-fat and low-carbohydrate diet. Br J Biomed Sci 62.3 (2005): 124–126.

Chaturvedi P et al. Effect of *Momordica charantia* on lipid profile and oral glucose tolerance in diabetic rats. Phytother Res 18 (2004): 954–956.

Dans AM et al. The effect of *Momordica charantia* capsule preparation on glycemic control in type 2 diabetes mellitus needs further studies. J Clin Epidemiol 60.6 (2007): 554–559.

Day C et al. Hypoglycaemic effect of *Momordica charantia* extracts. Planta Med 56 (1990): 426–429.

Fernandes NP et al. An experimental evaluation of the antidiabetic and antilipidemic properties of a standardized *Momordica charantia* fruit extract. BMC Complement Altern Med 7 (2007): 29.

Foa-Tomasi L et al. Effect of ribosome-inactivating proteins on virus-infected cells. Inhibition of virus multiplication and of protein synthesis. Arch Virol 71 (1982): 323–332.

Frame AD et al. Plants from Puerto Rico with anti-*Mycobacterium tuberculosis* properties. P R Health Sci J 17 (1998): 243–252.

Grover JK, Yadav SP. Pharmacological actions and potential uses of *Momordica charantia*: a review. J Ethnopharmacol 93 (2004): 123–132.

Harinantenaina L et al. *Momordica charantia* constituents and antidiabetic screening of the isolated major compounds. Chem Pharm Bull (Tokyo) 54.7 (2006): 1017–1021.

Hsiao C et al. Anti-proliferative and hypoglycemic cucurbitane-type glycosides from the fruits of *Momordica charantia*. J Agric Food Chem 61.12(2013): 2979–2986.

Jayasooriya AP et al. Effects of *Momordica charantia* powder on serum glucose levels and various lipid parameters in rats fed with cholesterol-free and cholesterol-enriched diets. J Ethnopharmacol 72 (2000): 331–336.

Kar A et al. Comparative evaluation of hypoglycaemic activity of some Indian medicinal plants in alloxan diabetic rats. J Ethnopharmacol 84 (2003): 105–108.

Kaur M et al. Bitter melon juice activates cellular energy sensor AMP-activated protein kinase causing apoptotic death of human pancreatic carcinoma cells. Carcinogenesis 34.7 (2013): 1585–1592.

Kim K, Kim HY. Bitter melon (*Momordica charantia*) extract suppresses cytokineinduced activation of MAPK and NF-κB in pancreatic β-Cells. Food Sci. Biotechnol 20.2 (2011): 531–5.

Kobori M et al. Bitter gourd suppresses lipopolysaccharide-induced inflammatory responses. J Agric Food Chem 56.22 (2008): 10515–10520.

Kumar GS, et al. Modulatory effect of bitter gourd (*Momordica charantia* Linn.) on alterations in kidney heparan sulfate in streptozotocin-induced diabetic rats. J Ethnopharmacol 115.2 (2008): 276–283.

Kusamran WR et al. Effects of neem flowers, Thai and Chinese bitter gourd fruits and sweet basil leaves on hepatic monooxygenases and glutathione S-transferase activities, and in vitro metabolic activation of chemical carcinogens in rats. Food Chem Toxicol 36 (1998): 475–484.

Lal J et al. In vitro anthelmintic action of some indigenous medicinal plants on *Ascardia galli* worms. Indian J Physiol Pharmacol 20 (1976): 64–68.

Lin K-W et al. Antioxidant constituents from the stems and fruits of *Momordica charantia*. Food Chem 127.2 (2011): 609–14.

Liu P et al. A new C30 sterol glycoside from the fresh fruits of *Momordica charantia*. Chi. J. Nat. Med 10.2 (2012):88–91.

Mada SB et al. Antimicrobial activity and phytochemical screening of aqueous and ethnol extracts of *Momordica charantia* L. leaves. J Med Plant Res 7.10(2013): 579–586.

Mamun MD. A study on hypoglycemic effects of *Momordica charantia* (wild variety) in alloxan induced type 2 diabetic Long-Evans rats. Clin Biochem 44.13(2011): S116.

Miura T et al. Hypoglycemic activity of the fruit of the *Momordica charantia* in type 2 diabetic mice. J Nutr Sci Vitaminol (Tokyo) 47 (2001): 340–344.

Miura T et al. Suppressive activity of the fruit of *Momordica charantia* with exercise on blood glucose in type 2 diabetic mice. Biol Pharm Bull 27 (2004): 248–250.

Nerurkar PV et al. Lipid lowering effects of *Momordica charantia* (bitter melon) in HIV-1-protease inhibitor-treated human hepatoma cells, HepG2. Br J Pharmacol 148.8 (2006): 1156–64.

Nerurkar PV et al. *Momordica charantia* (bitter melon) inhibits primary human adipocyte differentiation by modulating adipogenic genes. BMC Complement Altern Med 10.1(2010): 34.

Ogata F et al. Purification and amino acid sequence of a bitter gourd inhibitor against an acidic amino acid-specific endopeptidase of Streptomyces griseus. J Biol Chem 266 (1991): 16715–16721.

Ooi CP et al. *Momordica charantia* for type 2 diabetes mellitus. Cochrane Database Syst Rev 8(2012): CD007845.

Ojewole JA, et al. Hypoglycaemic and hypotensive effects of *Momordica charantia* Linn (Cucurbitaceae) whole-plant aqueous extract in rats. Cardiovasc J S Afr 17.5 (2006): 227–232.

Omoregbe RE, et al. Antimicrobial activity of some medicinal plants extracts on *Escherichia coli, Salmonella paratyphi* and *Shigella dysenteriae*. Afr J Med Med Sci 25 (1996): 373–375.

Papiya Seeja EJ et al. Antifertility activity of *Momordica charantia* descourt pulp and seed hydroalcoholic extract. J App Pharm 03.04(2012): 682–696.

Pitchakarn P et al. Kuguacin J, a triterpenoid from *Momordica charantia* leaf, modulates the progression of androgen-independent human prostate cancer cell line, PC3. Food Chem Toxicol 50(2012): 840–47.

Prasad V et al. Wound-healing property of *Momordica charantia* L. fruit powder. J Herb Pharmacother 6.3–4 (2006): 105–115.

Reyes BA et al. Anti-diabetic potentials of *Momordica charantia* and *Andrographis paniculata* and their effects on estrous cyclicity of alloxan-induced diabetic rats. J Ethnopharmacol 105 (2006): 196–200.

Sarkar S, et al. Demonstration of the hypoglycemic action of *Momordica charantia* in a validated animal model of diabetes. Pharmacol Res 33 (1996): 1–4.

Schreiber CA et al. The antiviral agents, MAP30 and GAP31, are not toxic to human spermatozoa and may be useful in preventing the sexual transmission of human immunodeficiency virus type 1. Fertil Steril 72 (1999): 686–690.

Senanayake GV et al. The effects of bitter melon (*Momordica charantia*) extracts on serum and liver lipid parameters in hamsters fed cholesterol-free and cholesterol-enriched diets. J Nutr Sci Vitaminol (Tokyo) 50 (2004): 253–257.

Shetty AK et al. Effect of bitter gourd (*Momordica charantia*) on glycaemic status in streptozotocin induced diabetic rats. Plant Foods Hum Nutr 60.3 (2005): 109–112.

Shibib BA et al. Hypoglycaemic activity of *Coccinia indica* and *Momordica charantia* in diabetic rats: depression of the hepatic gluconeogenic enzymes glucose-6-phosphatase and fructose-1,6-bisphosphatase and elevation of both liver and red-cell shunt enzyme glucose-6-phosphate dehydrogenase. Biochem J 292 (1993): 267–270.

Singh N et al. Effects of long term feeding of acetone extract of *Momordica charantia* (whole fruit powder) on alloxan diabetic albino rats. Indian J Physiol Pharmacol 33 (1989): 97–100.

Sridhar MG et al. Bitter gourd (*Momordica charantia*) improves insulin sensitivity by increasing skeletal muscle insulin-stimulated IRS-1 tyrosine phosphorylation in high-fat-fed rats. Br J Nutr 99.4 (2008): 806–812.

Sun Y et al. Anti-HIV agent MAP30 modulates the expression profile of viral and cellular genes for proliferation and apoptosis in AIDS-related lymphoma cells infected with Kaposi's sarcoma-associated virus. Biochem Biophys Res Commun 287 (2001): 983–994.

Tam PP et al. Effects of alpha-momorcharin on preimplantation development in the mouse. J Reprod Fertil 71 (1984): 33–38.

Teoh S et al. The effect of topical extract of *Momordica charantia* (bitter gourd) on wound healing in nondiabetic rats and in rats with diabetes induced by streptozotocin. Clin Exp Dermatol 34.7(2009): 815–22.

Tjokropranoto R et al.Anthelmintic effect of ethanol extract of pare leaf (*Momordica charantia* L.) against female *Ascaris suum* worm in vitro. Jurnal Medica Planta 1.4(2011): 33–39.

Ulbricht C, Basch E. Bitter melon. Natural standard herb and supplement reference. St Louis: Mosby, 2005, pp 76–80.

Virdi J et al. Antihyperglycemic effects of three extracts from *Momordica charantia*. J Ethnopharmacol 88 (2003): 107–111.

Welihinda J, Karunanayake EH. Extra-pancreatic effects of *Momordica charantia* in rats. J Ethnopharmacol 17 (1986): 247–255.

Welihinda J et al. The insulin-releasing activity of the tropical plant *Momordica charantia*. Acta Biol Med Ger 41 (1982): 1229–1240.

Xiang L et al. The reparative effects of *Momordica charantia* Linn. extract on HIT-T15 pancreatic beta-cells. Asia Pac J Clin Nutr 16 (Suppl 1) (2007): 249–252.

Yesilada E et al. Screening of Turkish anti-ulcerogenic folk remedies for anti-*Helicobacter pylori* activity. J Ethnopharmacol 66 (1999): 289–293.

Ying Z et al. Effect of superfine grinding on antidiabetic activity of bitter melon powder. Int J Mol Sci 13.11 (2012): 14203–14218.

Zhang QC, Khanyile C. Primary report on the use of Chinese herbal extract of *Momordica charantia* (bitter melon) in HIV infected patients [abstract]. In: Proceedings of the VIII International Conference on AIDS/III STD World Congress, Vol. 3. Amsterdam, The Netherlands, July 19–24, 1992; as cited in Micromedex. Thomson 2003. Available at: www.micromedex.com (accessed 17-03-06).

Bitter orange

B

HISTORICAL NOTE The root word for orange is the Arabic, *narandj* (Sellar 1992). The orange is a symbol of innocence and fertility. Some scholars believe the 'golden apple' Paris presented to Venus was actually an orange. In return, Venus bestowed Helen on Paris as a reward for selecting her in a beauty contest, which eventually caused the Trojan War. The orange tree is indigenous to eastern Africa, Arabia and Syria and it is believed that the crusaders may have introduced the orange to Europe when they returned from the crusades. Unripe dried fruits and the fruit peel are incorporated into various products, including foods such as marmalade, alcoholic beverages, such as Curaçao, and medicinal products including weight-loss products. The essential oil is used in perfumes, cosmetics and aromatherapy (Leung & Foster 1996), as food flavouring and to disguise the unpleasant taste of medicines. Orange blossom water has been used for centuries in Mediterranean countries to flavour cakes and beverages (Jeannot et al 2005). Orange oil is used in various alcoholic beverages such as Grand Marnier, Curaçao, Triple Sec and Chinotto (*Citrus aurantium myrtifolia*), and in Chinese medicine (*Citrus aurantium daidai*). *Citrus aurantium* extract is also used in Chinese medicine.

COMMON NAME

Orange

OTHER NAMES

Bitter orange, *Citrus sinensis*, green orange, Seville orange, Zhi Shi

BOTANICIAL NAME/FAMILY

Citrus aurantium var. *dulcis* (sweet orange) and *Citrus aurantium* var. *amara* (bitter orange or neroli) (family Rutaceae).

PLANT PARTS USED

Dried outer peel of the ripe fruit (expressed essential oil), flowers (Neroli oil). Floral water is obtained during the extraction of essential oils from orange flowers (orange blossom water) and petitgrain essential oil from the leaves. Neroli and petitgrain are obtained by stream distillation or carbon dioxide extraction.

CHEMICAL COMPONENTS

Bitter orange peel

Essential oil (0.2–0.5%), monoterpenes linalyl acetate, pinene, limonene, linalool, nerol, geraniol, bitter substances, flavonoids and methyl anthranilate, the alkaloid synephrine and *N*-methyltyramine (Blumenthal et al 2000, Pellati et al 2002). Synephrine is also known as oxedrine in Australia.

Synephrine is considered the most biologically active component of the peel in regards to oral use. Synephrine levels are higher in unripe fruit, possibly because synephrine levels decrease as the fruit matures (Rossato et al 2011).

Essential oils

Terpeneless/deterpenated or concentrated orange oil is sometimes available. Although the terpenes are removed, terpeneless orange oils retain all their other chemical components, including the furanocoumarins, which are in larger amounts, increasing their

Essential oil species	Major components	Minor components
Citrus aurantium var. *dulcis*	Limonene 89%	Linalool
	Myrcene 1.7%	Neral
	Beta-bisabolene 1.29%	Geranial, neral, citronellal, sabinene, myracene
Citrus aurantium var. *amara*	*d*-limonene 89–96%	Nerol, geraniol, linalyl acetate
		Bergaptene 0.069–0.073%
		Furanocoumarins (in cold pressed but not in steam distilled oils)

(From Price and Price 1995, Sellar 1992, Verzera et al 2004)

phototoxic potential. Therefore, the safe concentration in blends containing terpeneless oils is less than 0.2% (Tisserand & Balacs 1995). Methyl anthranilate is an important compound that may give orange flowers their aroma (Jeannot et al 2005). The composition of orange essential oils is described by the International Standards Organisation (ISO) under the following standard numbers 1340: 2005

9844: 1991	Bitter orange *C. aurantium* var. *amara*
8901: 2003	*C. aurantium* (petitgrain)
3517: 2002	*C. aurantium* var. *amara* (neroli)
4735: 2002	Oils of citrus

MAIN ACTIONS

Sympathomimetic

C. aurantium (CA) contains biologically active adrenergic amines, and may exert sympathomimetic

Clinical note — Three different essential oils are obtained from the orange tree

C. aurantium var. *dulcis* (sweet orange) and *C. aurantium* var. *amara* (bitter orange or neroli) are obtained from the peel and are usually expressed oils.

Neroli essential oil is obtained from the flowers of *C. aurantium* var. *amara* by steam distillation or carbon dioxide extraction and very occasionally enfleurage and is known as Neroli Bigarade, which is said to be the best Neroli essential oil available. Neroli essential oil obtained from *C. aurantium* var. *dulcis* is known as Neroli of Portugal.

Petitgrain is obtained from the leaves of *C. aurantium* var. *amara* by steam distillation.

Each of these oils has a different chemical profile and, therefore, different uses. Basically, distilled essential oils are used in food flavourings and expressed and steam distilled essential oils in aromatherapy and perfumes because of their stronger fragrance (Tisserand & Balacs 1995). This monograph concentrates on expressed sweet orange and bitter orange essential oils, together with oral extracts of the plant.

activity. One of the most studied is *p*-synephrine, the primary protoalkaloid in *Citrus aurantium* (Kaats et al 2013), also known as oxedrine. It is also present in many other *Citrus* species and found in Seville oranges, nova tangerines, grapefruit, clementines and other orange-related species. Due to the structural similarity of *p*-synephrine found in bitter orange and ephedrine and phenylephrine (m-synephrine), it is assumed that *p*-synephrine exhibits somewhat similar pharmacological activities to these other amines and have a significant sympathomimetic action. However, there are several, small structural differences between *p*-synephrine and ephedrine and phenylephrine that result in markedly different binding characteristics, possibly accounting for the relative lack of sympathomimetic activity associated with oral bitter orange preparations and *p*-synephrine.

To clarify, *p*-synephrine has a hydroxyl group in the *para* position on the benzene ring of the molecule, whereas phenylephrine has a hydroxyl group in the *meta*-position on the benzene ring and is not found in plants in general (Kaats et al 2013). Additionally, ephedrine does not contain a para-substituted hydroxy group and *p*-synephrine lacks the methyl group on the side chain found in ephedrine. As a result of these structural differences, *p*-synephrine has different characteristics to ephedrine, such as being far less lipid soluble and less able to enter the CNS compared to ephedrine and able to be broken down by monoamine oxidase. Additionally, *p*-synephrine has very poor oral bioavailability.

Receptor binding studies further indicate that *p*-synephrine binds much more poorly to α, β-1 and β-2 adrenergic receptors than ephedrine and phenylephrine (*m*-synephrine) (Stohs et al 2011). To provide further perspective, in 1988 Brown et al identified that *p*-synephrine was 1000-fold less active binding to α-1 and α-2 adrenergic receptors than noradrenaline, and in 2010, Ma et al suggested that *p*-synephrine was in fact acting as an antagonist to human α-2a- and α-2c adrenergic receptors.

Whether CA has significant effects on blood pressure and heart function is unclear as inconsistent results have been obtained in various studies.

An in vivo study found no significant effects on blood pressure when two concentrations of *C. aurantium* tincture (standardised to 4% synephrine or 6% synephrine) were administered (Calapai et al 1999). However, analysis of myocardial electrical activity detected ECG alterations such as ventricular arrhythmias with enlarged QRS complex. The effect was present after 5 days of treatment and became significant at day 10 and was still evident after 15 days. This suggests a possible association between synephrine consumption and the occurrence of ventricular arrhythmias and increased cardiac output.

In 2008, a prospective, randomised, double-blind study of healthy adults with a BMI < 30 found that consumption of a single dose containing 900 mg of CA extract standardised to 6% of synephrine produced a significant increase in systolic pressure between 1 and 5 hours after the treatment (Bui et al 2006). More recently, a double-blind, placebo-controlled study found no significant changes to systolic or diastolic blood pressure for patients taking oral CA capsules providing a daily dose of 98 mg *p*-synephrine per day for 60 days alone and in combination with naringin and hesperidin. In relation to heart rate, a small, statistically significant difference was observed between the *p*-synephrine plus naringin and hesperidin treated group and the group receiving *p*-synephrine alone for 60 days as well as the placebo control group (Kaats et al 2013). Both differences were about 3 beats/min, a clinically insignificant finding, which was also observed for the placebo group, further casting doubt on the relevance of this finding.

Effects on blood pressure have been exhibited with the administration of intravenous synephrine where it is used to treat hypotension (Fugh-Berman & Myers 2004). The inconsistent effects on BP with oral use, but obvious effect when administered intravenously, may be due to the very poor oral bioavailability of *p*-synephrine.

Appetite suppressant and thermogenic

P-synephrine affects the human metabolism by stimulating lipolysis, raising metabolic rate and enhancing fat oxidation through increased thermogenesis (Pellati et al 2002). The thermogenic activity of bitter orange and synephrine appears to be dose-dependent with higher doses effectively promoting thermogenesis in humans, hamsters and guinea pigs (Carpene et al 1999). The dose-dependent effect is suggested because a later study found neither a single administration of 300 mg/kg of *p*-synephrine orally nor bitter orange extracts (5000 and 10,000 mg/kg standardised to contain 2.5% of *p*-synephrine) significantly altered body temperature in mice (Arbo et al 2008).

A controlled in vivo study of *C. aurantium* fruit hydro-alcoholic extracts standardised to synephrine 4% (Ci. au. 4%) and 6% (Ci. au. 6%) found that repeated administration of the extract significantly and dose-dependently reduced food intake and body weight (Calapai et al 1999). More recently, a reduction in body weight gain was seen in an animal study for *p*-synephrine 30 or 300 mg/kg given by oral gavage over 28 consecutive days (Arbo et al 2009).

Due to these combined actions, it appears to have potential benefits for use in obesity and weight management.

Antibacterial

Seville orange has strong in vitro antibacterial activity against *Escherichia coli* and *Staphylococcus aureus* (Melendez & Capriles 2006).

Antiviral

The fruit of *C. aurantium* has a potent inhibitory activity on rotavirus infection (Kim et al 2000). The active components are neohesperidin and hesperidin.

Antifungal

Bitter orange essential oil has been shown to be effective against resistant fungal skin conditions (Ramadan et al 1996).

Digestive effects

The essential oil of *C. aurantium* var. *dulcis* is believed to aid digestion by stimulating the flow of gastric juice and has antispasmodic and carminative actions. The essential oil of *C. aurantium* var. *amara* is considered to be a liver stimulant, reduces gastric spasm and relieves symptoms of indigestion (Price & Price 1995, Wichtl & Bisset 1994). It is also thought to lower cholesterol.

Aromatherapy effects

The essential oil of *C. aurantium* var. *dulcis* is considered to convey warmth and happiness and improve mood (Battaglia 1997), reduce stress, aid sleep by reducing stress (Miyake et al 1991) and aid concentration. The essential oil of *Citrus aurantium* var. *amara* is considered to have a calming anxiolytic effect (Faturi et al 2010) and is considered one of the most effective sedative essential oils (Battaglia 1997, Price & Price 1995, Wichtl & Bisset 1994). Anecdotally, many aromatherapists regard orange as the 'oil of joy and communication'.

OTHER ACTIONS

Antioxidant

Natural antioxidants obtained from 'citrus oils' have been shown to inhibit oxidation of LDL cholesterol in in vitro studies (Lv et al 2012, Takahashi et al 2003), possibly due to the gamma-terpinene content. Terpinolene and alpha-terpinene also have antioxidant properties. Takahashi et al suggested gamma-terpinene could be added to foods and beverages to prevent oxidation. Sellar (1992) suggested that sweet orange oil aids the absorption of vitamin C. Certain types of tissue damage are mediated by reactive oxygen species (free radicals) such as superoxide. Research suggests reactive oxygen metabolites (ROMS) are associated with inflammatory tissue injury and some antioxidants attenuate the inflammatory process by reducing ROMs, thereby attenuating the tissue injury (Lv et al 2012). Lv et al suggested a diet containing *C. aurantium* might improve oxidative injury and improve immunity in acute otitis media in rats. They showed essential oils obtained from orange peel reduced serum and cochlear malondialdehyde (MDA), immunoglobulins A (IgA), G (IgA) and immunoglobulin M (IgM) and increased the activity of antioxidant enzymes in rats. The clinical application requires further study.

CLINICAL USE

Bitter orange extract and the isolated constituent *p*-synephrine (oxedrine) are used in oral weight-loss and weight management supplements, cholesterol-lowering herbal mixtures, and in sports supplements.

Orange essential oil is available in tablets, capsules and liquid oil.

Heartburn and dyspeptic symptoms

A key indication for bitter orange tincture or extract is heartburn (Blumenthal et al 2000). The dried peel is officially listed in the British Pharmacopoeia (British Herbal Medicine Association Scientific Committee 1983) as a bitter tonic, and empirical evidence suggests that it acts as a carminative agent. Commission E approved the use of cut peel for loss of appetite and dyspeptic symptoms (Blumenthal et al 2000).

Weight loss

Citrus aurantium extract is growing increasingly popular as an ingredient in weight loss products, and is being substituted for the banned herbal product ephedra in the United States. The main active ingredient, *p*-synephrine, produces effects on human metabolism that could theoretically reduce fat mass in obese humans because it stimulates lipolysis, raises metabolic rate and increases fat oxidation through increased thermogenesis. Interestingly, m-synephrine is a more potent adrenergic stimulant than *p*-synephrine and although not thought to be found in nature, may be present in North American weight-loss products in order to achieve better results (Fugh-Berman & Myers 2004).

As a reflection of clinical use, most research has been conducted with bitter orange extract in combination with other ingredients, making it difficult to determine the effects of bitter orange on weight loss.

A randomised, pilot study of eight healthy subjects with body mass indexes of 25–40 kg/m^2 compared *Citrus aurantium* to placebo over 8 weeks for effects on body weight (Greenway et al 2006). The *Citrus aurantium* group gained 1.13 ± 0.27 (mean ± SEM) kg compared with 0.09 ± 0.28 kg in the placebo group (P < 0.04). Interestingly, resting metabolic rate at baseline rose more in the *Citrus aurantium* group, 144.5 ± 15.7 kcal/24 hours, than the placebo group, 23.8 ± 28.3 kcal/24 hours (P < 0.002) at 2 weeks, but not at 8 weeks.

Previously, two small clinical studies have been published and both suggest possible weight reduction (Preuss et al 2002); however, more research is required to confirm the effectiveness and safety of orange oil as an adjunct to weight loss.

Ergogenic aid — used in sports

IN COMBINATION

A nutritionally enriched JavaFrit (JF) coffee (450 mg of caffeine, 1200 mg of garcinia cambogia, 360 mg of citrus aurantium extract, and 225 mcg of chromium polynicotinate) was tested for effects on resting oxygen uptake (VO^2), respiratory exchange ratio (RER), heart rate (HR) and blood pressure (BP) in 10 healthy and physically active individuals using a randomised, double-blind methodology (Hoffman et al 2006). During each session, subjects reported to the Human Performance Laboratory after at least 3 hours post-absorptive state and were provided either 354 mL (1.5 cups) of freshly brewed JF or commercially available caffeinated coffee (P). The nutritionally-enriched coffee beverage increased resting energy expenditure in individuals that were shown to be sensitive to the caffeine and other herbal ingredients in addition to elevating their systolic blood pressure.

Superficial dermatophyte infection

The oil of bitter orange (*C. aurantium* var. *amara*) was an effective topical treatment in treatment-resistant, superficial dermatophyte infection in a study involving 60 patients (Ramadan et al 1996). Patients with tinea corporis, cruris or pedis were treated with one of three treatments based on oil of bitter orange and cure was assessed by clinical and mycological examinations. One group used a 25% emulsion of oil three times per day, the second group used 20% oil in alcohol three times per day and the third group applied pure oil once per day. Treatment with the 25% oil emulsion was the most successful and resulted in 80% of patients being cured after 1–2 weeks and 20% in 2–3 weeks. The group using the 20% oil in alcohol preparation also experienced substantial cure rates, but took longer to achieve. Application of the undiluted oil successfully cured 33% of subjects within the first week, 60% within 1–2 weeks and 7% in 2–3 weeks. The only side effect reported was mild irritation when the undiluted oil was used.

Aromatherapy

Citrus sinensis administered in massage or via inhalation has been shown to improve mood and reduce anxiety in a range of health care settings. Lehrner et al (2000) demonstrated reduced anxiety and more positive mood compared to placebo, particularly for women, using 0.25 mL essential oil added to a diffuser in a dental waiting room (n = 72). Fitzgerald et al (2007) also showed a greater effect on mood in girls than boys in a multicultural paediatric integrative medicine clinic. Interestingly, the girls reported feeling more energetic after inhaling spearmint, whereas males felt more energetic after inhaling ginger. Overall, ginger and lavender were the least liked oils. The self-reported reductions in anxiety were supported by objective measures of autonomous function: blood pressure, respiratory and pulse rates and skin temperature (Hongratanaworakit & Buchbauer 2007). These subjects also rated themselves as being more cheerful. Likewise Fewell et al (2007) reported sedative effects of sweet orange oil administered in a massage.

Faturi et al (2010) suggested the anxiolytic effects were most likely to be de to limonene in *C sinensis*, but anxiolytic activity may depend on the administration route.

Citrus aurantium var. *dulcis*

The essential oil is used to convey warmth and happiness and improve mood (Battaglia 1997), reduce stress and promote sleep (Miyake et al 1991). It is traditionally known as 'the oil of communication and happiness'. It is also used to improve digestion and as a carminative to relieve gastric cramping and discomfort.

Citrus aurantium var. *amara*

The essential oil is used to reduce anxiety, muscle tension and promote relaxation, and best used in the bath before bedtime when treating insomnia (Battaglia 1997). It is used in cosmetics to repair broken capillaries, stimulate cell regeneration and to manage acne-prone skin.

OTHER USES

Distilled orange oil is often added to foods and beverages to enhance their flavour and to medicines to reduce the unpleasant taste.

Orange blossom water or hydrosol contains small proportions of essential oils and is used on the skin as an astringent and orally as a gastrointestinal carminative (Jeannot et al 2005). There are no terpenes in orange hydrosol, so the likelihood of causing skin irritation is significantly reduced. It is also used topically as an astringent for acne-prone skin and to calm babies and induce sleep (Bellakhdar 1997, Hmamouchi 2000).

The essential oil of *C. aurantium* var. *amara* is used as an ingredient in perfumes.

DOSAGE RANGE

Bitter orange peel products

- General dose information: 4–6 g daily of cut peel for teas or other galenical preparations used for oral administration.
- Infusion: 2 g of cut peel in 150 mL boiling water taken three times daily.
- Weight loss: bitter orange 975 mg (used with caffeine 528 mg and St John's wort 900 mg in a small double-blind study) — efficacy uncertain

Essential oils

- Oral LD_{50} dose: 5 g/kg (rat).
- Dermal LD_{50} dose: >5 g/kg (rabbit) (Citrus and Allied Essences 2004).
- Oral LD_{50} dose for a 15-kg child: 83 g/kg.
- Oral LD_{50} dose for a 70-kg adult: 389 g/kg.
- Oral doses in teas and other preparations: 4–6 g/day or 2 g in 150 mL of boiled water as an infusion (American Botanical Council 1999). The inhalation LD_{50} dose has not been established.
- Topical application dose of bitter orange to skin exposed to UV rays: 1.4% of a blend. However, even when topical application is combined with inhalation, blood concentrations of *d*-limonene, a component of most citrus oils, during 20 minutes of massage is low (≤0.008 microgram/mL). It is detectable in the blood within 10 minutes, which represents an uptake of more than 1% of the dose administered (Fewell et al 2007).

ADVERSE REACTIONS

Skin sensitisation

The oils of both *C. sinensis* and *C. amara* are mild skin irritants, but are considered to be low risk. Skin reactions are more likely if undiluted oils are applied directly to the skin or when used on broken or inflamed skin, or when other skin pathology is present. Skin reactions are idiosyncratic and can be difficult to predict. Skin sensitisation with topically applied orange oil is largely due to the components citral and cinnamic acid and *d*-limonene and is dose dependent (Tisserand & Balacs 1995). It often occurs after long-term exposure (Verzera et al 2004).

Photosensitisation

Expressed *C. sinensis* essential oil is not normally phototoxic (Tisserand & Balacs 1995), whereas *C. amara* oil is moderately phototoxic due to its furanocoumarin content, although the risk is considered low unless higher than recommended concentrations are used or more than one potentially phototoxic oil is combined in a blend. The risk may be increased in fair-skinned individuals. Other phototoxic essential oils include *Citrus bergamia* (bergamot) and *Citrus limon* (lemon). Sensitivity to sunlight or UVB light after topical application increases in the first hour after application and declines over the following 8 hours. A general caution is to avoid UV exposure for at least 12 hours after topical application and use a sunscreen during this period. An early study (Zaynoun 1977) ($n = 63$) showed no significant differences in phototoxic reactions to bergamot oil for eye colour, age, gender or tanning, but smaller amounts of oil produced an effect in light-skinned people. It is not clear whether this also applies to orange essential oil.

Gastrointestinal symptoms

Abdominal pain, nausea, vomiting, diarrhoea and dizziness have been reported with oral use of the oil (Citrus and Allied Essences 2004).

Cardiotoxicity

Bitter orange, standardised to 4–6% synephrine, demonstrated cardiovascular toxicity (ventricular arrhythmias with enlargement of QRS complex) and mortality in rats (Calapai et al 1999). However, a more recent double-blind, placebo-controlled trial found that bitter extract treatment delivering 98 mg *p*-synephrine daily over 60 days produced no effects to systolic or diastolic blood pressure and no adverse effects with respect to the cardiovascular, hepatic, renal or haemopoietic systems (Kaats et al 2013). Intravenous administration of synephrine raises blood pressure (Fugh-Berman & Myers 2004) and is likely to have a different safety profile to the oral use of bitter orange extract preparations as *p*-synephrine has very poor oral bioavailability.

Many commercial products contain synephrine or *Citrus aurantium* (CA) in combination with other ingredients such as caffeine which makes it difficult to interpret case reports. In Canada, between January 1998 and February 2004, 16 cases of severe cardiovascular symptoms associated with weight-loss products containing CA or synephrine were reported and of these, only one contained CA as a sole ingredient. There is also some suspicion that ephedrine, which continues to be detected in adulterated dietary supplements found in North America, may be responsible for some cardiac adverse effects and that safety issues really increase when synephrine is taken as part of a combination with other sympathomimetic ingredients (Rossato et al 2011).

In 2010, Health Canada published new guidelines for the use of synephrine in natural products, establishing a daily limit of 30 mg as the maximum allowable dose for synephrine in these products and prohibiting caffeine in synephrine-containing products unless clinical evidence of its safe use in humans was demonstrated (Health-Canada 2010).

SIGNIFICANT INTERACTIONS

There are no known interactions between the essential oils and conventional medicines; however, interactions may occur with the fruit and fruit products.

Theoretically, an interaction exists for CYP3A and P-gp substrates, as human studies indicate that the juice made from *C. aurantium* (Seville orange) inhibits CYP3A and possibly P-glycoprotein (Di Marco et al 2002, Malhotra et al 2001) — use with caution.

More specifically, clinical research shows bergamottin and 6′,7′-dihydroxybergamottin found in Seville oranges inactivate intestinal CYP3A4. Other furanocoumarins, including bergapten, could also be involved (Malhotra et al 2001).

CONTRAINDICATIONS AND PRECAUTIONS

With aromatherapy use

Do not apply essential oils to eyes or undiluted to mucous membranes. Orange essential oil is flammable and should not be vapourised near sources of heat or open flames. Therefore, candle vapourisers are not recommended. Skin sensitisation and phototoxicity are possible with the essential oils, so exposure to UV light sources should be avoided for at least 12 hours after dermal application. The risk is increased in fair-skinned individuals and when a blend that also contains other phototoxic essential oils is used.

With internal use of CA preparations containing synephrine

Supplements are generally considered safe if they contain 3 mg or less of synephrine in a daily dose, based on a long tradition of safe use (Health Canada 2010). Doses above this should be used with caution by people with hypertension or known cardiac disease and not consumed with high doses of caffeine or other CNS stimulants.

In 2009, synephrine was added to the Monitoring Program in Competitions of the World Anti-Doping Agency (WADA). This program includes substances which WADA wishes to monitor in order to avoid misuse in sport such as caffeine, nicotine, phenylephrine stimulants (WADA 2013). However, synephrine is not a banned substance under WADA.

PREGNANCY

Bitter orange peel and associated products are not recommended for use in pregnancy (Blumenthal et al 2000).

Orange essential oil used in recommended doses is generally safe in pregnancy, but general safety precautions apply.

PATIENTS' FAQs

What will this herb do for me?

Orange essential oil can be used in a vapouriser or massage to aid focus and concentration and facilitate communication. Neroli oil is mostly used to reduce stress and promote sleep and relaxation. In teas and tinctures, cut peel may aid digestion and relieve dyspeptic symptoms. There is some evidence that orange oil may be an effective treatment for treatment-resistant fungal skin infections.

Taking bitter orange preparations containing synephrine may aid in weight loss or weight maintenance; however, this remains uncertain as more clinical research is required to confirm effects.

When will it start to work?

When used in aromatherapy, it usually acts soon after inhalation. When the oil or oil products are applied topically to fungal infections, results may be seen within 1–2 weeks; however, 3–4 weeks of treatment may be required. Used internally in capsules, tablets or lozenges, bitter orange peel products should provide symptom relief quickly. Used in the bath before bedtime to promote sleep, neroli oil should produce relaxing effects within half an hour.

Are there any safety issues?

Skin irritation and phototoxicity (chemical burn) are possible after topical application of the oil if the skin is exposed to UV light such as sunlight. Use in recommended doses and do not use more than 15% of orange essential oil in a blend. Oral use of bitter orange peel products is not recommended in pregnancy and Seville orange juice can induce multiple drug interactions. Oral bitter orange preparations containing more than 3 mg of *p*-synephrine should be used with caution by people with high blood pressure or heart conditions and not used with other stimulants.

Practice points/Patient counselling

- Bitter orange peel and associated products are used to improve digestion, relieve dyspeptic symptoms and improve appetite, according to traditional use.
- *Citrus aurantium* extract is growing increasingly popular as an ingredient in weight-loss products; however inconsistent research results means it is unclear whether it is effective.
- The oil of bitter orange (*Citrus aurantium* var. *amara*) is an effective topical treatment in treatment-resistant, superficial dermatophyte infection according to one study.
- Topical application of orange oil and bitter orange oil can induce skin sensitisation, which is more likely to occur if old orange essential oil is used because of its tendency to oxidise. Appropriate storage reduces oxidation. A patch test is recommended for atopic people or those who have a tendency to skin reactions to fragrance compounds, cosmetics or essential oils.
- Topical application of orange oil and bitter orange oil can induce photosensitivity in some individuals. After topical application, exposure to sunlight or UVB light should be avoided for at least 12 hours. The risk of phototoxicity increases if high concentrations of phototoxic essential oils are used or a blend contains several phototoxic essential oils or if used by fair-skinned people.

B

REFERENCES

American Botanical Council. Complete German E Commission Monographs: therapeutic guide to herbal medicines. Austin, TX: American Botanical Council, 1999.

Arbo MD et al. Concentrations of p-synephrine in fruits and leaves of Citrus species (Rutaceae) and the acute toxicity testing of Citrus aurantium extract and p-synephrine. Food Chem.Toxicol 46.8 (2008): 2770–2775.

Arbo MD et al. Subchronic toxicity of Citrus aurantium L. (Rutaceae) extract and p-synephrine in mice. Regul.Toxicol.Pharmacol 54.2 (2009)114–117.

Battaglia S. The complete guide to aromatherapy. Brisbane: The Perfect Potion Publishing, 1997.

Bellakhdar J. La Pharmacopee Marocaine Traditionnele. Casablanca: Le Fennec, 1997.

Blumenthal M, Goldberg A, Brinckmann J (eds). Herbal medicine: expanded Commission E monographs, Austin, TX: Integrative Medicine Communications, 2000, pp. 287–289.

British Herbal Medicine Association Scientific Committee. British Herbal Pharmacopoeia. Cowling: BHMA, 1983.

Bui LT, Nguyen DT, Ambrose, PJ. Blood pressure and heart rate effects following a single dose of bitter orange. Ann.Pharmacother 40.1 (2006): 53–57.

Calapai G et al. Antiobesity and cardiovascular toxic effects of Citrus aurantium extracts in the rat: a preliminary report. Fitoterapia 70 (1999): 586–592.

Carpene C et al. Selective activation of beta3-adrenoceptors by octopamine: comparative studies in mammalian fat cells. Naunyn Schmiedebergs Arch Pharmacol 359.4 (1999): 310–321.

Citrus and Allied Essences. Material Safety Data Sheet IOIIII. Lake Success. NY: Citrus and Allied Essences, 2004.

Di Marco MP et al. The effect of grapefruit juice and seville orange juice on the pharmacokinetics of dextromethorphan: the role of gut CYP3A and P-glycoprotein. Life Sci 71 (2002): 1149–1160.

Faturi C et al. Anxiolytic-like effect of sweet orange aroma in Wistar rats. Progress in Neuro-Psychopharmacology and Biological Psychiatry 34 (2010): 605–609.

Fewell F et al. Blood concentration and uptake of d-limonene during aromatherapy massage with sweet orange oil. A pilot study. International Journal of Essential Oil Therapeutics 1 (2007): 97–102.

Fitzgerald M et al. The effect of gender and ethnicity on children's attitudes and preferences for essential oils: a pilot study. Explore NY 3.4 (2007): 378–385.

Fugh-Berman A, Myers A. Citrus aurantium, an ingredient of dietary supplements marketed for weight loss: current status of clinical and basic research. Exp Biol Med (Maywood), 229.8 (2004): 698–704.

Greenway F et al. Dietary herbal supplements with phenylephrine for weight loss. J Med Food 9.4 (2006): 572–578.

Health Canada 2010 — website. Available: http://www.hc-sc.gc.ca/dhp-mps/prodnatur/legislation/docs/notice-avis-synephrine-eng.php 21 June 2014.

Hmamouchi M. Les plantes medicinales et aromatiques marocaines. Imprimerie de Fedala Mohammedia, 2000.

Hoffman JR et al. Thermogenic effect from nutritionally enriched coffee consumption. J Int Soc Sports Nutr 3 (2006): 35–41.

Hongratanaworakit T, Buchbauer G. Autonomic and emotional responses after transdermal absorption of sweet orange oil in humans: a placebo controlled trial. International Journal of Essential Oil Therapeutics 1 (2007): 29–34.

Jeannot V et al. Quantification and determination of chemical composition of the essential oil extracted from natural orange blossom water (*Citrus aurantium L. ssp. Aurantium*). International Journal of Aromatherapy 15.2 (2005): 94–97.

Kaats, G.R et al. A 60-day double-blind, placebo-controlled safety study involving Citrus aurantium (bitter orange) extract. Food and Chemical Toxicology, 55.0 (2013): 358–362.

Kim DH et al. Inhibitory effect of herbal medicines on rotavirus infectivity. Biol Pharm Bull 23 (2000): 356–358.

Lehrner J et al. Ambient odour of orange in a dental office reduces anxiety and improves mood in female patients. Physiol Behav 71 (2000): 83–86.

Leung A, Foster S. Encyclopaedia of common natural products used in food, drugs and cosmetics. New York: John Wiley, 1996.

Lv Y-X. Effect of orange peel essential oil on oxidative stress in AOM animals. International Journal of Biological Macromolecules 50 (2012):1144–1150.

Ma, G et al. Effects of synephrine and beta-phenethylamine on human alpha-adrenoceptor subtypes. Planta Med 76.10 (2010): 981–986.

Malhotra S et al. Seville orange juice-felodipine interaction: comparison with dilute grapefruit juice and involvement of furanocoumarins. Clin Pharmacol Ther 69 (2001): 14–23.

Melendez PA, Capriles VA. Antibacterial properties of tropical plants from Puerto Rico. Phytomedicine 13 (2006): 272–276.

Miyake Y, Nakagawa M, Asakura Y. Effects of odours on humans (1): effects on sleep latency. Chem Senses 16 (1991): 183.

Pellati F et al Determination of adrenergic agonists from extracts and herbal products of Citrus aurantium L. var. amara by LC. J Pharm Biomed Anal 29 (2002): 1113–11119.

Preuss HG et al Citrus aurantium as a thermogenic, weight-reduction replacement for ephedra: an overview. J Med 33 (2002): 247–264.

Price S, Price L. Aromatherapy for health professionals. Edinburgh: Churchill Livingstone, 1995.

Ramadan W et al. Oil of bitter orange: new topical antifungal agent. Int J Dermatol 35.6 (1996): 448–449.

Rossato LG et al. Synephrine: from trace concentrations to massive consumption in weight-loss. Food Chem Toxicol 49.1 (2011): 8–16.

Sellar W. The directory of essential oils. Essex, UK: Saffron Walden, 1992.

Stohs SJ, Preuss HG, Shara M. A review of the receptor-binding properties of p-synephrine as related to its pharmacological effects. Oxid Med Cell Longev 2011 (2011).

Takahashi Y et al. Antioxidant effect of citrus essential oil components on human low-density lipoprotein in vitro. Biosci Biotechnol Biochem 67 (2003): 195–197.

Tisserand R, Balacs T. Essential oil safety: a guide for health professionals. Edinburgh: Churchill Livingstone, 1995.

Verzera A et al. Biological lemon and sweet orange essential oil composition. Flavour and Fragrance Journal 19.6 (2004): 544–548.

WADA 2013 website. Available: http://www.wada-ama.org/Documents/World_Anti-Doping_Program/WADP-Prohibited-list/2013/WADA-Prohibited-List-2013-EN.pdf 20 June 2014.

Wichtl M, Bisset W (eds). Herbal drugs and phytopharmaceuticals, Stuttgart: Medpharm Scientific Publishers, 1994.

Zaynoun S. A study of bergamot and its importance as a phototoxic agent. Contact Dermatitis 3 (1977): 225–239.

Black cohosh

HISTORICAL NOTE Native Americans first used black cohosh many centuries ago, mainly as a treatment for female reproductive problems, including pain during childbirth, uterine colic and dysmenorrhoea, and also for fatigue, snakebite and arthritis. It was widely adopted by European settlers, eventually becoming a very popular treatment in Europe for gynaecological conditions. It was also a favourite of the Eclectic physicians in North America, who also used it for female reproductive conditions, myalgia, neuralgia and rheumatic conditions.

COMMON NAME

Black cohosh

OTHER NAMES

Baneberry, black snakeroot, bugbane, rattle-root, rattle-top, rattleweed, squawroot, traubensilberkerze, wanzenkraut

BOTANICAL NAME/FAMILY

Cimicifuga racemosa now known as *Actaea racemosa* Linnaeus (family Ranunculaceae)

PLANT PARTS USED

Rhizome and root

> ***Clinical note — Selective oestrogen receptor modulators (SERMs)***
> These are compounds that, in contrast to pure oestrogen agonists or antagonists, have a mixed and selective pattern of oestrogen agonist–antagonist activity, which largely depends on the tissue targeted. The therapeutic aim of using these substances is to produce oestrogenic actions in those tissues in which it would be beneficial (e.g. bone, brain, liver), and have either no activity or antagonistic activity in tissues, such as breast and endometrium, where oestrogenic actions (like cellular proliferation) might be deleterious. They are a relatively new class of pharmacologically active agents and are being used by women who cannot tolerate pharmaceutical HRT or are unwilling to use it. The most actively studied SERMs are tamoxifen and raloxifen (Hernandez & Pluchino 2003).

CHEMICAL COMPONENTS

Black cohosh contains numerous triterpene glycosides, including cimicifugoside, actein and 27-deoxyactein, *N*-methylcytosine and other quinolizidine alkaloids, phenolic acids, including isoferulic and fukinolic acid, salicylic acids, resins, fatty acids and tannins.

Until recently, the isoflavone formononetin was believed to be a pharmacologically important constituent of the herb; however, testing of numerous samples has failed to detect it in any sample, including the commercial products Remifemin (Schaper & Brummer GmbH & Co. KG, Salzgitter, Germany) and CimiPure (Kennelly et al 2002).

MAIN ACTIONS

Hormone modulation

The hormonal effects of black cohosh are believed to be the result of complex synergistic actions of several components, particularly the triterpene glycosides. Experimental and clinical evidence confirms that black cohosh does not contain natural oestrogens and does not exert significant oestrogenic activity, although some components may exert selective oestrogen receptor modulation. This has been confirmed in studies involving women where no oestrogenic effects on mammary glands or the endometrium were observed (Wuttke et al 2014).

Preclinical studies to determine how black cohosh works have yielded conflicting results, but several hypotheses have been proposed. It acts either (1) as a selective oestrogen receptor modulator (SERM); (2) through serotonergic pathways; (3) as an antioxidant; or (4) on inflammatory pathways (Ruhlen et al 2008). There is evidence to support all these actions.

One study suggests that black cohosh works as a SERM, augmented by central nervous effects (Viereck et al 2005). Results from studies found that it has SERM activity with a lower potency but comparable efficacy to that of 17 beta-oestradiol (Bolle et al 2007). It has no action in the uterus, but beneficial effects in the hypothalamopituitary unit and in bone (Seidlova-Wuttke et al 2003). This has been confirmed in a double-blind, randomised, multicentre study (Wuttke et al 2003). In that study, the standardised black cohosh extract BNO 1055 was equipotent with conjugated oestrogens in reducing menopausal symptoms, had beneficial effects on bone metabolism and significantly increased vaginal superficial cells; however, it did not exert uterotrophic activity. Most recently, a 2013 systematic review concluded that black cohosh does not appear to influence circulating levels of oestradiol, FSH or LH, nor to exert oestrogenic effects on breast, endometrial or vaginal tissues. However, it does appear to display oestrogenic activity on bone by stimulating bone formation and inhibiting bone breakdown (Fritz et al 2013). This validates the understanding of black cohosh as a SERM.

Overall, it is generally agreed that black cohosh reduces LH secretion in menopausal women. This has been confirmed in a human study and is believed to be the result of at least three different active constituents acting synergistically (Duker et al 1991). Reductions in LH have also been demonstrated in PCOS patients experiencing infertility (Kamel 2013).

Anti-inflammatory

Animal studies have identified some anti-inflammatory activity (Hirabayashi et al 1995). More recently, black cohosh extracts have demonstrated *in vitro* anti-inflammatory activity by inhibiting IL-6 and TNF-α, IFN-γ (Schmid et al 2009a) and nitric oxide (Schmid et al 2009b).

Serotonergic

In vitro tests identified compounds in a black cohosh methanol extract that were capable of strong binding to the 5-HT_{1A}, 5-HT_{1D}, and 5-HT_7 receptor subtypes (Burdette et al 2003). Further investigation by these authors found that the components functioned as a partial agonist of the 5-HT_7 receptor. Further investigation has identified triterpenoids and phenolic acids which bind weakly to the 5-HT_7 receptor and a new constituent, *N*ω-methylserotonin, which demonstrates strong 5-HT_7 receptor binding affinity, together with induction of cAMP and inhibition of serotonin re-uptake (Powell et al 2008). As 5-HT$_7$ receptors are present in the hypothalamus, it has been speculated that serotonergic activity in the hypothalamic thermoregulatory centres may be responsible for the reduction of hot flushes, although the precise mechanism of action remains unclear.

Dopaminergic

It is suggested that the effects of *A. racemosa* may be due to dopaminergic activity, because black cohosh extract BNO 1055 displayed dopaminergic activity with a D$_2$-receptor assay (Jarry et al 2003). Considering that dopaminergic drugs reduce some symptoms (e.g. hot flushes) associated with menopause, this theory is feasible; however, further studies are required to explain why black cohosh is devoid of the typical side effects associated with dopaminergic drugs (Borrelli & Ernst 2008).

Cytochromes and P-glycoprotein

Clinical studies have found no indication that Black cohosh affects CYP 3A, 1A2, 2E1 or 2D6 (Gurley et al 2005, 2006a, 2006b, 2008, 2012, Izzo 2012, Pang et al 2011).

Extremely high doses of black cohosh (1090 mg equivalent to 0.2% triterpene glycosides, twice daily for 28 days) demonstrated a minor inhibitory effect on CYP2D6; however, these results are unlikely to be clinically significant due to the high doses and negligible effect. Other studies have demonstrated that recommended doses (40 mg and 80 mg) did not modulate P-gp or CYP3A activity (Borrelli & Ernst 2008, Gurley et al 2006b, Shord et al 2009).

OTHER ACTIONS

Black cohosh serves as an agonist and competitive ligand for the mu-opioid receptor (Rhyu et al 2006), which provides some rationale for the herb's traditional reputation as a treatment for painful conditions such as dysmenorrhoea and arthritis.

A dose-dependent antihypertensive effect was identified for a triterpene found in black cohosh (actein) in animal tests. The clinical significance of this finding for humans using black cohosh root is unknown (Genazzani & Sorrentino 1962). *In vitro* research has demonstrated endothelium-independent vasorelaxation probably due to calcium channel activity (Kim et al 2011), suggesting possible benefit for vascular conditions.

Black cohosh is traditionally thought to act as a tonic and nervous system restorative medicine and to exert antispasmodic and anti-inflammatory activity.

CLINICAL USE

Most clinical research has investigated the use of various black cohosh preparations as either standalone treatments or in combination with other herbal medicines, notably St John's wort in the treatment of menopausal symptoms. More recently, investigation has begun to determine whether black cohosh has a role in female infertility.

Menopausal symptoms

Most clinical research on black cohosh has focused on its potential to prevent or decrease the severity of various menopausal symptoms. It can be described as the non-oestrogenic alternative treatment used for menopausal symptoms. Most trials test the commercial preparation of black cohosh known as Remifemin, which is standardised to contain triterpene glycosides (0.8–1.2 mg/tablet), and the extract BNO 1055, an aqueous ethanolic extract (58% vol/vol), sold as Klimadynon and Menofem (Bionorica AG, Neumarkt, Germany). There has also been some investigation with other black cohosh preparations, mainly in the United States. Overall, results from clinical studies have been positive for reducing the frequency of hot flushes, most consistently with the German/Swiss preparations and less consistently with US American black cohosh products. This is likely to be due to great variations in test dose, with lower doses appearing more effective, and differences in herbal extract quality and chemical profile. It may also be because the identity of many American black cohosh preparations is often unknown and they are on the market as food supplements. It was previously shown that many of them contain Asian *Cimicifuga* species, for which no clinical data are available. Importantly, the HPLC profiles of these Asian species look quite different from those of the species that grew originally in America, whereas the German/Swiss products contain extracts of original black cohosh rhizomes that stem from field-planted crops grown under rigidly controlled conditions (Wuttke et al 2014). Unlike hormone replacement therapy, the effect on menopausal symptoms is due to the presence of dopaminergic, adrenergic and serotonergic compounds and not oestrogen.

Systematic reviews and meta-analyses

Given the number of clinical trials conducted with black cohosh in alleviating menopausal symptoms, there have been a number of systematic reviews and meta-analyses of the evidence.

One of the early reviews was published in 1998 which discussed eight clinical trials and concluded that black cohosh (Remifemin) was a safe and effective alternative to HRT for menopausal patients in whom HRT is contraindicated (Lieberman 1998). Symptoms responding to treatment with black cohosh included hot flushes, vaginal thinning and drying, night sweats, sleep disturbances, anxiety and depression. In 2005, a systematic review, including randomised, controlled trials, open trials and comparison group studies, found that the evidence to date suggests that black cohosh is safe and effective for reducing menopausal symptoms, primarily hot flushes and possibly mood disorders (Geller & Studee 2005). Later reviews by the same research team showed that black cohosh significantly reduced depression and anxiety in all studies reviewed (Geller & Studee 2007). Another more recent systematic review identified seven randomised controlled trials of black cohosh and concluded that it may be beneficial in the treatment of menopausal vasomotor symptoms in some women (Cheema et al 2007).

A 2008 update of a previous systematic review evaluated the clinical evidence for or against the efficacy of black cohosh in alleviating menopausal symptoms. Seventy-two clinical trials were identified, but only six of these, with a total of 1163 peri- and postmenopausal women, met the inclusion criteria. With one exception, the results for each of these trials were positive; yet the authors concluded that the efficacy of black cohosh in reducing menopause symptoms is currently not supported by full conclusive evidence, citing small sample size as a limitation in establishing statistical significance (Borrelli & Ernst 2008). Similarly, a review of 16 eligible studies suggested that there were methodological flaws in many studies making a definitive conclusion difficult. Methodological issues included: lack of uniformity of the drug preparation used, variable outcome measures and lack of a placebo group (Palacio et al 2009).

A 2010 systematic review examined nine RCTs and compared black cohosh preparations to placebo in perimenopausal and postmenopausal women (excluding those with a history of breast cancer) for the frequency of vasomotor symptoms. Seven of these trials demonstrated a significant decrease in frequency of vasomotor symptoms in the treatment group and the combined improvement in these symptoms was 24% (95% CI) in the black cohosh group compared to placebo. Again, this review noted the significant heterogeneity of the trials. Black cohosh was found to be more efficacious in treating menopausal symptoms when given in combination with other botanicals such as St John's wort compared with black cohosh alone (Shams et al 2010). In contrast, a 2012 Cochrane review concluded that stand alone treatment with black cohosh was not superior to placebo for reducing the frequency of hot flushes in peri- and postmenopausal women. The authors analysed results of 16 RCTs involving 2027 women, but cautioned that a definitive conclusion could not be made due to the high level of heterogeneity between the studies. Additionally, due to insufficient data they were unable to pool the results for other menopause-related conditions, such as night sweats, bone health, vulvovaginal symptoms, quality of life and sexuality (Leach & Moore 2012).

A review by Wuttke et al (2014) makes the point that most placebo-controlled clinical trials have demonstrated amelioration of climacteric complaints, particularly hot flushes, and these positive effects have been seen mainly with German/Swiss preparations, whereas three out of four placebo controlled trials using US supplements have produced negative results (Geller et al 2009, Newton et al 2006, Pockaj et al 2006). A difference in dosage is one likely reason as the German/Swiss medications contained 2 × 20 mg CR (*Cimicifuga racemosa*) drug (4–8 mg extract), whereas two negative US American studies administered 15–25-fold the amounts used in the European trials and the third, a more moderate over-dosage. In contrast, the positive American trial used a preparation with a standardised amount of triterpenes (2.5%) which yielded a significant reduction of menopausal symptoms not seen when a triterpene-free extract was given.

There is also concern about the quality and herbal authenticity of US CR products as it has previously been shown that many contain Asian Cimicifuga species which have quite different constituent profiles (based on HPLC comparisons) compared to the CR species that originally grew in America. This is particularly of concern when products are not manufactured in countries that enforce strict GMP conditions.

Interestingly, since then another positive study has been published which used a European black cohosh extract (Ze450) in 442 unselected ambulatory female outpatients with menopausal complaints under daily practice conditions (Drewe et al 2013). For the first 3 months, doctors were advised to treat patients with 13 mg/day (high dose, HD) and to continue over additional 6 months either with this treatment or to switch to 6.5 mg/day CR (low dose, LD). The choice of treatment and its dose, however, was fully at the discretion of the doctor. After 3 months treatment with HD, symptom severity (Kupperman Menopause Index, KMI) decreased significantly ($p < 0.001$) from baseline values. Continuation of treatment with HD or LD decreased total KMI and its sub-item scores further (HD, LD: $p < 0.001$). However, more patients (84.9%) responded to HD than to LD (78.4%) and showed an improvement of symptoms ($p = 0.011$).

IN COMBINATION

A number of studies have been conducted investigating the combination of black cohosh and St John's wort for the treatment of symptoms of menopause with mood symptoms. One double-blind, randomised study of 301 women found that 16 weeks of herbal treatment produced a significant 50% reduction in the Menopause Rating Scale score compared with 20% for placebo and a significant 42% reduction in the Hamilton Depression Rating Scale compared with only 13% in the placebo group (Uebelhack et al 2006). Another large-scale (n = 6141), prospective, controlled open-label observational study supports the effectiveness and tolerability of black cohosh combined with St John's wort for alleviating menopausal mood symptoms (Briese et al 2007). In another double-blind, randomised, placebo-controlled, multicentre study, 89 peri- or postmenopausal women experiencing menopause symptoms were treated with a combination of St John's wort and black cohosh extract (Gynoplus) or a matched placebo. Hot flushes were significantly lower and HDL levels increased in the Gynoplus group (Chung et al 2007).

It is therefore no surprise that two systematic reviews have concluded that black cohosh is more efficacious in treating menopausal symptoms when given in combination with St John's wort, compared to black cohosh alone (Shams et al 2010, Laakmann et al 2012).

Comparison studies

Numerous comparison studies have been conducted utilising various pharmaceutical agents. One pilot study demonstrated that BNO 1055 is able to reduce oestrogen deficiency symptoms to the same degree as conjugated oestrogens (Wuttke et al 2006b). A randomised, double-blind, controlled 3-month study to investigate the efficacy–safety balance of black cohosh (Remifemin) in comparison with tibolone in 244 symptomatic menopausal Chinese women gave remarkable results. The efficacy of both treatments was similar and statistically significant. The safety for both groups was also good. However, the tolerability profile was greatly in favour of the herbal treatment with a significantly lower incidence of adverse events (Bai et al 2007).

An RCT of 120 healthy women with menopausal symptoms found, when compared with fluoxetine, black cohosh was more effective for treating hot flushes and night sweats by the third month, whereas fluoxetine was more effective for reducing mood change according to the Beck's Depression Scale (Beck et al 2003). Monthly scores for hot flushes and night sweats decreased significantly in both groups; however, black cohosh reduced monthly scores for hot flushes and night sweats to a greater extent than did fluoxetine. At the end of the sixth month of treatment, black cohosh reduced the hot flush score by 85%, compared with a 62% result for fluoxetine (Oktem et al 2007).

Wuttke et al (2003) conducted a double-blind, randomised, multicentre study which compared the effects of BNO 1055 (40 mg/day) to conjugated oestrogens (0.6 mg/day) and placebo on climacteric complaints, bone metabolism and endometrium (Wuttke et al 2003). The study involved 62 postmenopausal women who took their allocated treatment for 3 months. BNO 1055 proved to be equipotent to conjugated oestrogens and superior to a placebo in reducing climacteric symptoms, and both active treatments produced beneficial effects on bone metabolism. Vaginal superficial cells increased with both active treatments; however, BNO 1055 had no effect on endometrial thickness, which was significantly increased by conjugated oestrogens.

Commission E has approved the use of this herb as a treatment for menopausal symptoms (Blumenthal et al 2000). Similarly, the World Health Organization (WHO) recognises its use for the 'treatment of climacteric symptoms such as hot flushes, profuse sweating, sleeping disorders and nervous irritability'. The North American Menopause Society recommends black cohosh, in conjunction with lifestyle approaches, as a treatment option for women with mild menopause-related symptoms (North American Menopause Society 2004). In herbal practice generally, menopausal symptoms are usually addressed using a combination of herbs, supplements and dietary and lifestyle advice.

Weight gain

Rat models demonstrate that BNO 1055 black cohosh extract decreases enhanced pituitary LH secretion, attenuates body weight gain and intra-abdominal fat accumulation, lowers fasting plasma insulin and has no effects on uterine mass. The effects on plasma lipids are complex and are characterised by an increase of LDL cholesterol and decrease of triglyceride levels, which is in contrast to the effects of oestrogen (Rachon et al 2008). There has been no investigation of these effects in human trials.

Osteoporosis prevention

Black cohosh demonstrates osteoprotective effects comparable to oestrogen, although through a different mechanism of increasing osteoblast activity (Wuttke et al 2006a), mediated via an oestrogen receptor-dependent mechanism (Chan et al 2008). One experimental study has shown that a triterpenoid glycoside isolated from black cohosh (25-acetyl-cimigenol xylopyranoside) both blocks the osteoclastogenesis enhanced by cytokines in vitro and attenuates TNF-alpha-induced bone loss in vivo (Qiu et al 2007). These results demonstrate that black cohosh can offer effective prevention of postmenopausal bone loss.

Breast cancer protection

A number of in vitro studies on black cohosh show that it is cytotoxic to human breast cancer cells and inhibits the conversion of oestrone sulphate to active oestradiol in breast cancer cells (Rice et al 2007), and suppresses tumour cell invasion without affecting cell viability (Hostanska et al 2007). One in vitro study found that black cohosh enhances the action of some chemotherapy agents, most notably tamoxifen (Al-Akoum et al 2007). The triterpene glycoside, actein, induced a stress response and apoptosis in human breast cancer cells (Einbond et al 2006, 2007, 2008). A recent in vitro study suggests that a herbal combination, Avlimil (which includes black cohosh, licorice, red raspberry, red clover and kudzu), exhibits both stimulatory and inhibitory effects on the growth of oestrogen-dependent breast tumour (MCF-7) cells. This casts doubt on the safety of Avlimil for women with oestrogen-dependent breast cancer (Ju et al 2008).

A randomised study (Hernandez & Pluchino 2003) was performed with 136 young premenopausal breast cancer survivors experiencing hot flushes as a result of tamoxifen therapy. When BNO 1055 (Menofem/Klimadynon, corresponding to 20 mg of herbal drug) was used together with tamoxifen for 12 months, the number and severity of hot flushes were reduced, with almost 50% of subjects becoming free of hot flushes, and severe hot flushes were reported by only 24% compared with 74% for those using tamoxifen alone.

In contrast, a previous double-blind, placebo-controlled study (n = 85) failed to detect significant improvements with black cohosh for hot flush frequency or severity when used by patients with breast cancer for 2 months who were also taking tamoxifen (Jacobson et al 2001). Unfortunately, the authors of that study did not specify which black cohosh product was used or the dosage, making a comparison with the previous study difficult.

A 2013 systematic review on the efficacy of black cohosh in breast cancer found that black cohosh does not appear to influence circulating levels of oestradiol, FSH or LH, nor to exert oestrogenic effects on breast, endometrial or vaginal tissues. However, it does appear to display oestrogenic activity on bone by stimulating bone formation and inhibiting bone breakdown (Fritz et al 2013).

Premenstrual syndrome and dysmenorrhoea

Commission E has approved the use of black cohosh as a treatment in these conditions (Blumenthal et al 2000). Randomised clinical studies are still required to confirm efficacy in these conditions.

Menstrual migraine

IN COMBINATION

An RCT of 49 women with menstrual migraines tested placebo against a herbal combination consisting of 60 mg soy isoflavones, 100 mg dong quai and 50 mg black cohosh, with each component standardised to its primary alkaloid (Burke et al 2002). Over the course of the study, the average frequency of menstrually associated migraine episodes was significantly reduced in the active treatment group.

Primary and secondary infertility

Several RCTs have been conducted in the last few years investigating the use of a commercial black cohosh preparation (Klimadynon) as an adjunctive treatment for women with unexplained infertility, both producing promising results (Shahin et al 2008, 2009). One RCT has also been conducted with women diagnosed with polycystic ovarian syndrome (PCOS) and primary or secondary infertility.

Cimicifuga racemosa in conjunction with clomiphene citrate was investigated in a 2008 RCT (n = 119) in women under 35 years with primary or secondary unexplained infertility who were previously unsuccessful in achieving pregnancy after clomiphene citrate cycles. Both groups received clomiphene citrate (150 mg/day from days 3 to 7) and the treatment group also received *Cimicifuga racemosa* (Klimadynon 120 mg/day from days 1 to 12). In the treatment group, there were higher levels of oestradiol (274.5 ± 48.5 vs. 254.6 ± 20.6, NS) and LH concentrations, although these were considered non-significant. There was however a statistically significant increase in endometrial thickness (8.9 ± 1.4 mm vs. 7.5 ± 1.3 mm, $P < 0.001$), serum progesterone (13.3 ± 3.1 ng/mL vs. 9.3 ± 2.0 ng/mL, $P < 0.01$) and clinical pregnancy rate (36.7% vs. 13.6%, $P < 0.01$) (Shahin et al 2008).

A follow-up trial in the same population group (n = 134) compared *Cimicifuga racemosa* (CR) (Klimadynon 120 mg/day from days 1 to 12) to ethinyl oestradiol (EO) (100 mcg/day from days 1 to 12) in conjunction with clomiphene citrate (150 mg/day from day 3 to 7) (Shahin et al 2009). Although changes to clinical pregnancy rates did not reach statistical significance, these were higher in the black cohosh group (21.1% CR vs. 14.0% EO). The treatment group needed significantly fewer days for follicular maturation (13.55 ± 0.99 vs. 11.65 ± 0.98, $P < 0.001$), had a thicker endometrium (7.66 ± 0.68 vs. 8.08 ± 0.59, $P < 0.001$), higher luteal-phase serum progesterone (10.52 ± 0.89 vs. 12.15 ± 1.99, $P < 0.001$) and higher oestradiol concentration at the time of human chorionic gonadotrophin injection (245.10 ± 15.24 vs. 277.0 ± 27.73, $P < 0.001$).

A 2012 prospective RCT compared *Cimicifuga racemosa* as a stand-alone treatment to clomiphene citrate in 100 women aged 21–27 with polycystic ovarian syndrome (PCOS) and primary or secondary infertility (Kamel 2013). Both groups received black cohosh (Klimadynon 20 mg/day for 10 days) or clomiphene citrate (100 mg/day for 5 days) from the second day of the cycle for three consecutive cycles. Again, although the change in pregnancy rate was not statistically significant, more women taking *Cimicifuga racemosa* became pregnant (7 vs. 4 pregnancies; $P = 0.1$). Remarkable hormonal differences were noted in the black cohosh group, particularly in LH level and FSH/LH ratio, with a marked reduction in the LH level (first cycle 8.5 ± 0.28 vs. 8.9 ± 0.55; $P = 0.0001$) which was significant in all three treatment cycles. This confirms the understanding of black cohosh as a hypothalamic-pituitary-ovarian axis modulator. Progesterone was also statistically higher in the Klimadynon group, especially in the first cycle (10.12 ± 0.14 vs. 9.54 ± 0.15 ng/mL, $P = 0.0001$) along with endometrial thickness (first cycle: 8.34 vs. 6.89 mm; second cycle: 9.67 vs. 6.34 mm; third cycle: 9.11 vs. 7.32 mm; $P = 0.0004$). This study suggests that black cohosh has potential as an alternative to clomiphene citrate for ovulation induction in women with PCOS-related infertility.

Prostate cancer

Two in vitro studies suggest that black cohosh may have theoretical usefulness in the treatment of prostate cancer (Hostanska et al 2005, Jarry et al 2005, Seidlova-Wuttke et al 2006). Further research is now required to determine whether black cohosh may play a role in the prevention or treatment of prostate cancer.

OTHER USES

Black cohosh has been used traditionally to treat a variety of other female reproductive disorders and inflammatory disorders, especially menopausal arthritis and diarrhoea. It has also been used to promote menstruation. The British Herbal

Pharmacopoeia states it is indicated in ovarian dysfunction and ovarian insufficiency.

SAFETY

Evidence now confirms that black cohosh does not pose a risk in women with breast cancer, nor increase its incidence or recurrence. Four hundred postmenopausal women with symptoms related to oestrogen deficiency were enrolled into a prospective, open-label, multinational, multicentre study to investigate endometrial safety and the tolerability and efficacy of the black cohosh extract, BNO 1055. Low dose treatment (40 mg) for 52 weeks showed no case of hyperplasia or more serious adverse endometrial outcome occurred (Raus et al 2006). This finding is supported by the HALT study (Reed et al 2008).

A population-based case-control study consisting of 949 breast cancer cases and 1524 controls was used to evaluate the relationship between phyto-oestrogens and breast cancer risk. Use of black cohosh was found to have a significant breast cancer protective effect. This association was similar among women who reported use of either black cohosh or Remifemin (Rebbeck et al 2007). Another smaller trial demonstrated that Remifemin does not cause adverse effects on breast tissue. A total of 65 healthy, naturally postmenopausal women completed a trial with 40 mg black cohosh daily. Mammograms were performed, and breast cells were collected by percutaneous fine needle aspiration biopsies at baseline and after 6 months (Hirschberg et al 2007). A systematic review was conducted about the safety and efficacy of black cohosh in patients with cancer. There is laboratory evidence of antiproliferative properties but no confirmation from clinical studies for a protective role in cancer prevention. Black cohosh appears to be safe in breast cancer patients (Walji et al 2007).

A pharmacoepidemiological, observational, retrospective cohort study examined breast cancer patients to investigate the influence of Remifemin on recurrence-free survival after breast cancer, including oestrogen-dependent tumours. Remifemin was not found to be associated with an increase in the risk of recurrence but was associated with prolonged disease-free survival. After 2 years following initial diagnosis, 14% of the control group had developed a recurrence, while the Remifemin group reached this proportion after 6.5 years, demonstrating a protractive effect of black cohosh on the rate of recurrence of breast cancer for women with a history of breast cancer who had used Remifemin, compared to women who had not (Zepelin et al 2007).

In regards to safety, a 2013 systematic review of black cohosh in breast cancer found that the current evidence does not demonstrate an increased risk or recurrence of breast cancer in women with or without a history. Of the four studies investigating risk, two found no significant association with the use of black cohosh and two reported reduced risk, including a study that combined black cohosh with tamoxifen. When considering hormones, black cohosh does not appear to influence circulating levels of oestradiol, FSH or LH, nor to exert oestrogenic effects on breast, endometrial or vaginal tissues (Fritz et al 2013).

DOSAGE RANGE

- Decoction or powdered root: 0.3–2 g three times daily.
- Tincture (1:10): 2–4 mL three times daily.
- Fluid extract (1:1) (g/mL): 0.3–2 mL three times daily.
- Perimenopausal symptoms: 40–160 mg per day.
- Infertility: 20–120 mg per day.

Many practitioners have used black cohosh long term without safety concerns.

TOXICITY

Overdose has produced nausea and vomiting, vertigo and visual disturbances.

Idiosyncratic hepatic reactions

Rare, spontaneous hepatotoxicity has been reported in at least 42 case reports worldwide with treatment by *Cimicifugae racemosae rhizoma* (Levitsky et al 2005, Nisbet & O'Connor 2007, Teschke & Schwarzenboeck 2009, Whiting et al 2002). As a result, several safety reviews have been conducted to evaluate the available data and determine what risk exists with the use of this herb. A 2008 safety review of black cohosh products was conducted by the Dietary Supplement Information Expert Committee of the US Pharmacopeia's Council of Experts. All the reports of liver damage were assigned possible causality, and none were probable or certain causality. The clinical pharmacokinetic and animal toxicological information did not reveal unfavourable information about black cohosh. The Expert Committee determined that in the United States black cohosh products should be labelled to include a cautionary statement, a change from their decision of 2002, which required no such statement (Mahady et al 2008).

Assessment of the 42 cases by European Medicines Agency (EMEA) has shown a possible or probable causality in only four out of 42 patients. A diagnostic algorithm has been applied in the four patients with suspected BC (black cohosh) hepatotoxicity using several methods to allow objective assessment, scoring and scaling of the probability in each case. Due to incomplete data, the case of one patient was not assessable. For the remaining three patients, quantitative evaluation showed no causality for BC in any patient regarding the observed severe liver disease (Teschke & Schwarzenboeck 2009).

In Australia in February 2006, the TGA announced that based on the appraisal of case reports, a causal association between black cohosh and serious hepatitis exists; however, the incidence is very low considering its widespread use. As a result, products available in Australia containing black cohosh have to carry label warnings informing consumers of the risk. The conclusion made by the TGA is considered controversial by some experts because numerous confounding factors were present in many of the case reports, such as the use of multiple ingredient preparations, concurrent use of at least one pharmaceutical medicine and the presence of other medical conditions.

A 2008 study evaluated the effects of black cohosh extract on liver morphology and on levels of various hepatic function indices in an experimental model finding that at high doses, well above the recommended dosage, black cohosh appears quite safe (Mazzanti et al 2008).

More recently, Teschke (2010) investigated data from 69 spontaneous or published case reports of suspected black cohosh-induced hepatotoxicity and found confounding variables such as uncertainty about the quality and authenticity of the black cohosh product, dose or insufficient adverse event description, missing or inadequate evaluation of a clear temporal association, the possible presence of other medications or comorbidities and lack of de-challenge or re-exposure. A clear causal relationship between black cohosh and hepatotoxicity was not found.

A 2011 meta-analysis investigated the potential hepatotoxicity of black cohosh (Remifemin) from published RCTs in peri- and postmenopausal women. Liver function data (AST, ALT and γ-GT) from 1020 women was compared at baseline and after taking black cohosh (40–128 mg/day) for 3 to 6 months. No significant difference between the treatment and reference groups was found (Naser et al 2011).

ADVERSE REACTIONS

Black cohosh is a well tolerated treatment. A 2012 Cochrane systematic review of 16 RCTs involving 2027 women found no significant difference in incidence of adverse effects between black cohosh and placebo groups (Leach & Moore 2012). The adverse effects associated with black cohosh tend to be rare, mild and reversible. The most common adverse effects reported are gastrointestinal symptoms, musculoskeletal and connective tissue disorders such as rashes (Borrelli & Ernst 2008). According to data from clinical studies and spontaneous reporting programs, large doses can cause headache, tremors or giddiness in some people (Huntley & Ernst 2003).

A few rare but serious adverse events, including hepatic and circulatory conditions, have been reported, but without a clear causality relationship in most instances (see above).

SIGNIFICANT INTERACTIONS

Cisplatin

Black cohosh decreased the cytotoxicity of cisplatin in an experimental breast cancer model — while the clinical significance of this finding is unknown, it is recommended that patients taking cisplatin should avoid black cohosh until safety can be confirmed.

Clomiphene citrate

RCTs in women with infertility have demonstrated improved pregnancy rates, hormone profiles, follicular maturation and endometrial thickness when taking black cohosh in conjunction with clomid treatment when used during the follicular phase (Shahin et al 2008, Shahin et al 2009). Beneficial interaction possible under professional supervision.

Doxorubicin

Black cohosh increased the cytotoxicity of doxorubicin in an experimental breast cancer model — while the clinical significance of this finding is unknown, it is recommended patients taking doxorubicin avoid black cohosh until safety can be confirmed.

Docetaxel

A trial used mouse breast cancer cell line to test whether black cohosh altered the response of cancer cells to radiation and to four drugs commonly used in cancer therapy. The black cohosh extracts increased the cytotoxicity of doxorubicin and docetaxel and decreased the cytotoxicity of cisplatin, but did not alter the effects of radiation or 4-hydroperoxycyclophosphamide (4-HC), an analogue of cyclophosphamide which is active in cell culture. This evidence may be applicable to humans, so it is advisable that patients undergoing cancer therapy should be made aware that use of black cohosh could alter their response to the agents commonly used to treat breast cancer (Rockwell et al 2005).

? CONTRAINDICATIONS AND PRECAUTIONS

There is some controversy over the use of black cohosh in women with a history of breast cancer. Results from a 2002 study testing the safety of black cohosh in an in vitro model for oestrogen-dependent breast tumours found that the herbal extract significantly inhibited tumour cell proliferation, oestrogen-induced proliferation and enhanced the antiproliferative effects of tamoxifen (Bodinet & Freudenstein 2002). This finding is supported in a more recent in vitro study that showed black cohosh having a cytotoxic effect on both oestrogen-sensitive and oestrogen-insensitive breast cancer cells and a synergism with tamoxifen for inhibition of cancerous cell growth (Al-Akoum et al 2007). A 2013 systematic review of black cohosh in breast cancer found that the current evidence does not demonstrate an increased risk or recurrence of breast cancer in women with or without a history (Fritz et al 2013). As with all medicines, a risk-versus-benefit conversation should take place with patients.

B

Practice points/Patient counselling

- In general, clinical trials support the use of black cohosh for relieving menopausal symptoms, with most consistent benefits reported for the European extracts.
- It appears that 4–12 weeks continuous treatment are required for adequate menopausal symptom relief and it can be used successfully with St John's wort.
- Black cohosh is also used in the treatment of premenstrual syndrome and dysmenorrhoea and is Commission E-approved for these uses; however, controlled studies are not available to confirm its efficacy.
- Black cohosh has many different actions, including selective oestrogen receptor modulator activity, serotonergic, dopaminergic, anti-inflammatory and analgesic activity.
- Black cohosh should be used only under professional supervision by people with oestrogen-dependent tumours, or during pregnancy.
- Black cohosh is well tolerated with few side effects; however, rare case reports of idiosyncratic hepatic reactions have been described. Until safety can be confirmed, avoid prescribing black cohosh in conjunction with medications that are potentially hepatotoxic or in patients with liver disease.

PREGNANCY USE

Although it has been used to assist in childbirth, black cohosh is not traditionally recommended in pregnancy, particularly during the first trimester although it has been used in the final weeks of pregnancy to aid in delivery. Safety in lactation remains to be confirmed; however, it is usually avoided because of its hormonal effects (Dugoua et al 2006).

PATIENTS' FAQs

What will this herb do for me?

Black cohosh may be an effective treatment for menopausal symptoms in most women, especially those with mild to moderate symptoms. The European extracts give the most consistently positive results for reducing the frequency of hot flushes. Effects are also good when combined with the herb St John's wort. It may also be useful in the treatment of premenstrual syndrome and prevention of period cramping. Black cohosh can also be considered in women with unexplained or PCOS-related infertility.

When will it start to work?

Studies suggest that benefits are seen within 4–12 weeks for the treatment of menopausal symptoms.

Are there any safety issues?

Black cohosh is well tolerated with few side effects. It should only be used under professional supervision by people undergoing chemotherapy, receiving treatment for oestrogen-dependent tumours or during pregnancy.

Due to rare case reports of idiosyncratic hepatic reactions, avoid prescribing black cohosh in conjunction with medications that are potentially hepatotoxic or in patients with liver disease, until safety can be confirmed.

REFERENCES

Al-Akoum M, Dodin S, Akoum A. Synergistic cytotoxic effects of tamoxifen and black cohosh on MCF-7 and MDA-MB-231 human breast cancer cells: an in vitro study. Can J Physiol Pharmacol 85.11 (2007): 1153–1159.

Bai W et al. Efficacy and tolerability of a medicinal product containing an isopropanolic black cohosh extract in Chinese women with menopausal symptoms: a randomized, double blind, parallel-controlled study versus tibolone. Maturitas 58.1 (2007): 31–41.

Beck V et al. Comparison of hormonal activity (estrogen, androgen and progestin) of standardized plant extracts for large scale use in hormone replacement therapy. J Steroid Biochem Mol Biol 84.2–3 (2003): 259–68.

Blumenthal M, Goldberg A, Brinckmann J (eds). Herbal medicine: expanded Commission E monographs. Austin, TX: Integrative Medicine Communications, 2000.

Bodinet C, Freudenstein J. Influence of Cimicifuga racemosa on the proliferation of estrogen receptor-positive human breast cancer cells. Breast Cancer Res Treat 76.1 (2002): 1–10.

Bolle P et al. Estrogen-like effect of a Cimicifuga racemosa extract sub-fraction as assessed by in vivo, ex vivo and in vitro assays. J Steroid Biochem Mol Biol 107.3–5 (2007): 262–269.

Borrelli F, Ernst E. Black cohosh (Cimicifuga racemosa) for menopausal symptoms: a systematic review of its efficacy. Pharmacol Res 58.1 (2008): 8–14.

Briese V et al. Black cohosh with or without St. John's wort for symptom-specific climacteric treatment — results of a large-scale, controlled, observational study. Maturitas 57.4 (2007): 405–414.

Burdette JE et al. Black cohosh acts as a mixed competitive ligand and partial agonist of the serotonin receptor. J Agric Food Chem 51.19 (2003): 5661–5670.

Burke BE, Olson RD, Cusack BJ. Randomized, controlled trial of phytoestrogen in the prophylactic treatment of menstrual migraine. Biomed Pharmacother 56.6 (2002): 283–288.

Chan BY et al. Ethanolic extract of Actaea racemosa (black cohosh) potentiates bone nodule formation in MC3T3-E1 preosteoblast cells. Bone 43.3 (2008): 567–573.

Cheema D, Coomarasamy A, El-Toukhy T. Non-hormonal therapy of post-menopausal vasomotor symptoms: a structured evidence-based review. Arch Gynecol Obstet 276.5 (2007): 463–469.

Chung DJ et al. Black cohosh and St. John's wort (GYNO-Plus) for climacteric symptoms. Yonsei Med J 48.2 (2007): 289–294.

Drewe J, Zimmermann C, Zahner C. The effect of a Cimicifuga racemosa extracts Ze 450 in the treatment of climacteric complaints — an observational study. Phytomedicine, 20.8–9 (2013): 659–666.

Dugoua JJ et al. Safety and efficacy of black cohosh (Cimicifuga racemosa) during pregnancy and lactation. Can J Clin Pharmacol 13.3 (2006): e257–261.

Duker EM et al. Effects of extracts from Cimicifuga racemosa on gonadotropin release in menopausal women and ovariectomized rats. Planta Med 57.5 (1991): 420–424.

Einbond LS et al. Actein and a fraction of black cohosh potentiate antiproliferative effects of chemotherapy agents on human breast cancer cells. Planta Med 72.13 (2006): 1200–1206.

Einbond LS et al. The growth inhibitory effect of actein on human breast cancer cells is associated with activation of stress response pathways. Int J Cancer 121.9 (2007): 2073–2083.

Einbond LS et al. Growth inhibitory activity of extracts and compounds from Cimicifuga species on human breast cancer cells. Phytomedicine 15.6–7 (2008): 504–511.

Fritz H et al. Black Cohosh and Breast Cancer: A Systematic Review. Integr Cancer Ther. 2013 Mar 25 [Epub ahead of print]

Geller SE, Studee L. Botanical and dietary supplements for menopausal symptoms: what works, what does not. J Womens Health (Larchmt) 14.7 (2005): 634–649.

Geller SE, Studee L. Botanical and dietary supplements for mood and anxiety in menopausal women. Menopause 14.3 (Pt 1) (2007): 541–549.

Geller SE et al. Safety and efficacy of black cohosh and red clover for the management of vasomotor symptoms: a randomized controlled trial. Menopause 16.6 (2009): 1156–1166.

Genazzani E, Sorrentino L. Vascular action of actein: active constituent of Actaea racemosa L. Nature 194 (1962): 544–5 (as cited in Micromedex Thomsen 2003. www.micromedex.com).

Gurley BJ et al. In vivo effects of goldenseal, kava kava, black cohosh, and valerian on human cytochrome P450 1A2, 2D6, 2E1, and 3A4/5 phenotypes. Clin. Pharmacol. Ther., 77.5 (2005): 415–426.

Gurley B et al. Assessing the clinical significance of botanical supplementation on human cytochrome P450 3A activity: comparison of a milk thistle and black cohosh product to rifampin and clarithromycin. J Clin Pharmacol 46 (2006a): 201–213.

Gurley BJ et al. Effect of milk thistle (Silybum marianum) and black cohosh (Cimicifuga racemosa) supplementation on digoxin pharmacokinetics in humans. Drug Metab Dispos 34.1 (2006b): 69–74.

Gurley BJ et al. Clinical assessment of CYP2D6-mediated herb-drug interactions in humans: effects of milk thistle, black cohosh, goldenseal, kava kava, St. John's wort, and Echinacea. Mol Nutr Food Res 52.7 (2008) 755–763.

Gurley BJ, Fifer EK, Gardner Z. Pharmacokinetic herb -drug interactions (part 2): drug interactions involving popular botanical dietary ssupplements and their clinical relevance. Planta Med 78.13 (2012): 1490–1514.

Hernandez MG, Pluchino S. Cimicifuga racemosa for the treatment of hot flushes in women surviving breast cancer. Maturitas 44 (Suppl 1) (2003): S59–65.

Hirabayashi T et al. Inhibitory effect of ferulic acid and isoferulic acid on murine interleukin-8 production in response to influenza virus infections in vitro and in vivo. Planta Med 61.3 (1995): 221–6 (as cited in Micromedex Thomsen 2003. www.micromedex.com).

Hirschberg AL et al. An isopropanolic extract of black cohosh does not increase mammographic breast density or breast cell proliferation in postmenopausal women. Menopause 14.1 (2007): 89–96.

Hostanska K et al. Apoptosis of human prostate androgen-dependent and -independent carcinoma cells induced by an isopropanolic extract of black cohosh involves degradation of cytokeratin (CK) 18. Anticancer Res 25.1A (2005): 139–147.

Hostanska K et al. Inhibitory effect of an isopropanolic extract of black cohosh on the invasiveness of MDA-mB 231 human breast cancer cells. In Vivo 21.2 (2007): 349–355.

Huntley A, Ernst E. A systematic review of the safety of black cohosh. Menopause 10.1 (2003): 58–64.

Izzo AA. Interactions between herbs and conventional drugs: overview of the clinical data. Med Princ Pract 21.5 (2012): 404–428.

Jacobson JS et al. Randomized trial of black cohosh for the treatment of hot flashes among women with a history of breast cancer. J Clin Oncol 19.10 (2001): 2739–2745.

Jarry H et al. In vitro effects of the Cimicifuga racemosa extract BNO 1055. Maturitas 44 (Suppl 1) (2003): S31–38.

Jarry H et al. Cimicifuga racemosa extract BNO 1055 inhibits proliferation of the human prostate cancer cell line LNCaP. Phytomedicine 12.3 (2005): 178–182.

Ju YH, Doerge DR, Helferich WG. A dietary supplement for female sexual dysfunction, Avlimil, stimulates the growth of estrogen-dependent breast tumors (MCF-7) implanted in ovariectomized athymic nude mice. Food Chem Toxicol 46.1 (2008): 310–320.

Kamel HH. Role of phyto-oestrogens in ovulation induction in women with polycystic ovarian syndrome. Eur J Obstet Gynecol Reprod Biol 168.1 (2013): 60–63.

Kennelly EJ et al. Analysis of thirteen populations of black cohosh for formononetin. Phytomedicine 9.5 (2002): 461–467.

Kim EY, Lee YJ, Rhyu MR. Black cohosh (*Cimicifuga racemosa*) relaxes the isolated rat thoracic aorta through endothelium-dependentand -independent mechanisms. J Ethnopharmacol 138.2 (2011): 537–542.

Laakmann E et al. Efficacy of Cimicifuga racemosa, Hypericum perforatum and Agnus castus in the treatment of climacteric complaints: a systematic review. Gynecol Endocrinol 28.9 (2012):703–9.

Leach MJ, Moore V. Black cohosh (Cimicifuga spp.) for menopausal symptoms. Cochrane Database Syst Rev 12.9 (2012): CD007244.

Levitsky J et al. Fulminant liver failure associated with the use of black cohosh. Dig Dis Sci 50.3 (2005): 538–539.

Lieberman S. A review of the effectiveness of Cimicifuga racemosa (black cohosh) for the symptoms of menopause. J Womens Health 7.5 (1998): 525–529.

Mahady GB et al. United States Pharmacopeia review of the black cohosh case reports of hepatotoxicity. Menopause 15.4 Pt 1 (2008): 628–638.

Mazzanti G et al. Effects of Cimicifuga racemosa extract on liver morphology and hepatic function indices. Phytomedicine 15.11 (2008): 1021–1024.

Naser B et al. Suspected black cohosh hepatotoxicity: no evidence by meta-analysis of randomized controlled clinical trials for isopropanolic black cohosh extract. Menopause 18.4 (2011): 366–375.

Newton KM et al. Treatment of vasomotor symptoms of menopause with black cohosh, multibotanicals, soy, hormone therapy, or placebo: a randomized trial. Ann Intern Med 145.12 (2006): 869–879.

Nisbet BC, O'Connor RE. Black cohosh-induced hepatitis. Del Med J 79.11 (2007): 441–444.

North American Menopause Society. Treatment of menopause-associated vasomotor symptoms: position statement of The North American Menopause Society. Menopause 11 (2004): 11–33.

Oktem M et al. Black cohosh and fluoxetine in the treatment of postmenopausal symptoms: a prospective, randomized trial. Adv Ther 24.2 (2007): 448–461.

Palacio C, Masri G, Mooradian AD. Black cohosh for the management of menopausal symptoms: a systematic review of clinical trials. Drugs Aging 26.1 (2009): 23–26.

Pang X et al. Pregnane X receptor-mediated induction of Cyp3a by black cohosh. Xenobiotica 41.2 (2011): 112–123.

Pockaj BA et al. Phase III double-blind, randomized, placebo-controlled crossover trial of black cohosh in the management of hot flashes: NCCTG Trial N01CC1. J Clin Oncol 24.18 (2006): 2836–2841.

Powell SL et al. In vitro serotonergic activity of black cohosh and identification of N(omega)-methylserotonin as a potential active constituent. J Agric Food Chem 56.24 (2008):11718–11726.

Qiu SX et al. A triterpene glycoside from black cohosh that inhibits osteoclastogenesis by modulating RANKL and TNFalpha signaling pathways. Chem Biol 14.7 (2007): 860–869.

Rachon D et al. Effects of black cohosh extract on body weight gain, intra-abdominal fat accumulation, plasma lipids and glucose tolerance in ovariectomized Sprague-Dawley rats. Maturitas 60.3–4 (2008): 209–215.

Raus K et al. First-time proof of endometrial safety of the special black cohosh extract (Actaea or Cimicifuga racemosa extract) CR BNO 1055. Menopause 13.4 (2006): 678–691.

Rebbeck TR et al. A retrospective case-control study of the use of hormone-related supplements and association with breast cancer. Int J Cancer 120.7 (2007): 1523–1528.

Reed SD et al. Vaginal, endometrial, and reproductive hormone findings: randomized, placebo-controlled trial of black cohosh, multibotanical herbs, and dietary soy for vasomotor symptoms: the Herbal Alternatives for Menopause (HALT) Study. Menopause 15.1 (2008): 51–58.

Rhyu MR et al. Black cohosh (Actaea racemosa, Cimicifuga racemosa) behaves as a mixed competitive ligand and partial agonist at the human mu opiate receptor. J Agric Food Chem 54.26 (2006): 9852–9857.

Rice S, Amon A, Whitehead SA. Ethanolic extracts of black cohosh (Actaea racemosa) inhibit growth and oestradiol synthesis from oestrone sulphate in breast cancer cells. Maturitas 56.4 (2007): 359–367.

Rockwell S, Liu Y, Higgins SA. Alteration of the effects of cancer therapy agents on breast cancer cells by the herbal medicine black cohosh. Breast Cancer Res Treat 90.3 (2005): 233–239.

Ruhlen RL, Sun GY, Sauter ER. Black cohosh: insights into its mechanism/s of action. Integrative Medicine Insights 3 (2008): 21–32.

Schmid D et al. Aqueous extracts of Cimicifugas racemosa and phenolcarboxylic constituents inhibit production ofproinflammatory cytokines in LPS-stimulated human whole blood. Can J Physiol Pharmacol 87.11 (2009a): 963–972.

Schmid D et al. Inhibition of inducible nitric oxide synthesis by Cimicifuga racemosa (Actaea racemosa, black cohosh) extractsin LPS-stimulated RAW 264.7 macrophages. J Pharm Pharmacol 61.8 (2009b): 1089–1096.

Seidlova-Wuttke D et al. Evidence for selective estrogen receptor modulator activity in a black cohosh (Cimicifuga racemosa) extract: comparison with estradiol-17beta. Eur J Endocrinol 149 (2003): 351–362.

Seidlova-Wuttke D, Thelen P, Wuttke W. Inhibitory effects of a black cohosh (Cimicifuga racemosa) extract on prostate cancer. Planta Med 72.6 (2006): 521–526.

Shahin AY et al. Adding phytoestrogens to clomiphene induction in unexplained infertility patients — a randomized trial. Reprod Biomed Online 16.4 (2008): 580–588.

Shahin AY, Ismail AM, Shaaban OM. Supplementation of clomiphene citrate cycles with *Cimicifuga racemosa* or ethinyl oestradiol — a randomized trial. Reprod Biomed Online 19.4 (2009): 501–507.

Shams T et al. Efficacy of black cohosh-containing preparations on menopausal symptoms: a meta-analysis. Altern Ther Health Med 16.1 (2010): 36–44.

Shord SS, Shah K, Lukose A. Drug-botanical interactions: a review of the laboratory, animal, and human data for 8 common botanicals. Integr Cancer Ther 8.3 (2009): 208–227.

Teschke R. Black cohosh and suspected hepatotoxicity: inconsistencies, confounding variables, and prospective use of a diagnostic causality algorithm. A critical review. Menopause 17.2(2010): 426–440.

Teschke R, Schwarzenboeck A. Suspected hepatotoxicity by Cimicifugae racemosae rhizoma (black cohosh, root): critical analysis and structured causality assessment. Phytomedicine 16.1 (2009): 72–84.

Uebelhack R et al. Black cohosh and St John's wort for climacteric complaints: a randomized trial. Obstet Gynecol 107 (2006): 247–255.

Verhoeven MO et al. Effect of a combination of isoflavones and Actaea racemosa Linnaeus on climacteric symptoms in healthy symptomatic

perimenopausal women: a 12-week randomized, placebo-controlled, double-blind study. Menopause 12 (2005): 412–420.
Viereck V, Emons G, Wuttke W. Black cohosh: just another phytoestrogen? Trends Endocrinol Metab 16.5 (2005): 214–221.
Walji R et al. Black cohosh (Cimicifuga racemosa [L.] Nutt.): safety and efficacy for cancer patients. Support Care Cancer 15.8 (2007): 913–921.
Whiting PW, Clouston A, Kerlin P. Black cohosh and other herbal remedies associated with acute hepatitis. Med J Aust 177 (2002): 440–443.
Wuttke W, Seidlova-Wuttke D, Gorkow C. The Cimicifuga preparation BNO 1055 vs conjugated estrogens in a double-blind placebo-controlled study: effects on menopause symptoms and bone markers. Maturitas 44 (Suppl 1) (2003): S67–77.
Wuttke W, Gorkow C, Seidlova-Wuttke D. Effects of black cohosh (Cimicifuga racemosa) on bone turnover, vaginal mucosa, and various blood parameters in postmenopausal women: a double-blind, placebo-controlled, and conjugated estrogens-controlled study. Menopause 13.2 (2006a): 185–196.
Wuttke W, Raus K, Gorkow C. Efficacy and tolerability of the Black cohosh (Actaea racemosa) ethanolic extract BNO 1055 on climacteric complaints: a double-blind, placebo- and conjugated estrogens-controlled study. Maturitas 55(Supplement 1) (2006b): S83–91.
Wuttke W et al. The non-estrogenic alternative for the treatment of climacteric complaints: Black cohosh (Cimicifuga or Actaea racemosa). J Steroid Biochem Mol Biol 139 (2014): 302–310.
Zepelin HH et al. Isopropanolic black cohosh extract and recurrence-free survival after breast cancer. Int J Clin Pharmacol Ther 45.3 (2007): 143–154.

Brahmi

HISTORICAL NOTE Brahmi is the Sanskrit name for the herb *Bacopa monniera* and has been used in Ayurvedic medicine as a nerve tonic since time immemorial. Under this system, *B. monniera* is classified under 'Medhya rasayana', that is, medicinal plants rejuvenating intellect and memory, and has been used in India for almost 3000 years. The ancient classical Ayurvedic treatises recommend it for the promotion of memory, intelligence and general performance. Over time, it has earned a reputation as an important brain tonic (Williamson 2002).

COMMON NAME

Brahmi

OTHER NAMES

Bacopa, herb of grace, herpestis herb, Indian pennywort, jalanimba, jalnaveri, sambrani chettu, thyme-leave gratiola, keenmind, Nira-Brahmi, Sambrani Chettu

Centella asiatica (gotu kola) and *Merremia gangetica* have also been referred to by the name brahmi, but most authorities associate brahmi with *Bacopa monniera*. The name brahmi is derived from the word 'Brama', the mythical 'creator' in the Hindu pantheon. Because the brain is the centre for creative activity, any compound that improves brain health is called brahmi (Russo & Borrelli 2005).

BOTANICAL NAME/FAMILY

Bacopa monniera (family Scrophulariaceae)

PLANT PARTS USED

Dried whole plant or herb, mainly leaves and stems (aerial parts)

CHEMICAL COMPONENTS

Dammarene-type saponins (bacosides [A, B, C] and bacosaponines [D, E, F], based on the bacogenins A1–A5, are considered the most important) and alkaloids (brahmine, herpestine), flavonoids (luteolin-7-glucoside, glucuronyl-7-apigenin and glucuronyl-7-luteolin), phytosterols (Chakravarty et al 2003) and luteolin, phenylethanoid glycosides, monnierasides I–III and plantainoside B have been isolated (Adams et al 2007).

Standardised extract BacoMind has been shown to contain bacoside A_3, bacopaside I, bacopaside II, jujubogenin isomer of bacopasaponin C, bacosine, luteolin, apigenin and β-sitosterol D-glucoside (Dutta et al 2008).

The commercial extract KeenMind is standardised for bacosides A and B (no less than 55% of combined bacosides). Each capsule contains 150 mg *B. monniera* extract (20 : 1), equivalent to 3 g dried herb.

MAIN ACTIONS

Information about the mechanisms of action of brahmi chiefly comes from in vitro and animal tests using various experimental models, although an increasing number of clinical trials are now available. Some studies have investigated the effects of an Ayurvedic herbal combination known as brahmi rasayan, which consists of 10 parts bacopa, two parts cloves, one part cardamom, one part *Piper longum* and 40 parts sucrose.

Antioxidant

Brahmi has potent antioxidant activity, which appears to be a result of both direct free radical scavenging activity and increasing the activity of endogenous antioxidant systems (Bhattacharya et al 2000, Tripathi et al 1996). Administration of bacoside A reduced the effects of cigarette smoke in an animal model by increasing lactate dehydrogenase and its isoenzymes (Anbarasi et al 2005a). Bacoside A has also been shown to reduce creatine kinase in brain and cardiac tissue (Anbarasi et al 2005b), and prevent expression of hsp70 and neuronal apoptosis (Anbarasi et al 2006), thus preventing smoke-induced damage. An extract of brahmi provided protection against DNA damage in both animal cells (Russo et al 2003a) and human cells (Russo et al 2003b) in vitro. Dose-related increases in superoxide dismutase, catalase and glutathione peroxidase activities in several important regions of the brain have been demonstrated in animal models (Bhattacharya et al 2000) and it has been shown to induce the activity of superoxide dismutase and catalase in the liver (Kar et al 2002). Additionally, brahmi enhances antioxidant activity to protect against reactive oxygen species-induced damage in diabetic rats (Kapoor et al 2009).

Neuroprotective

Bacopa has demonstrated neuroprotective activity in a number of animal models, chiefly mediated by an antioxidant mechanism (Saini et al 2012). In particular, antioxidant effects have been observed for bacopa in areas of the brain that are key memory areas, such as hippocampus, frontal cortex and striatum (Bhattacharya et al 2000).

In one study, bacopa significantly protected lipids and proteins from oxidative stress-induced damage caused by aluminium. The protective antioxidant effect was described as similar to L-deprenyl (Jyoti et al 2007). In another experiment, bacopa improved memory functions in hypobaric conditions which induce hypoxia, most likely due to neuroprotective activity, antioxidant and mitochondria-stabilising effects (Hota et al 2009). Antioxidant activity and attenuation of oxidative damage were further confirmed for an oral bacopa extract in a study using a colchicine-induced dementia model (Saini et al 2012).

Administration of bacoside A prevented the structural and functional impairment of mitochondria upon exposure to cigarette smoke in vivo (Anbarasi et al 2005c). From the results, it was suggested that chronic cigarette smoke exposure induces damage to the mitochondria and that bacoside A protects the brain from this damage by maintaining the structural and functional integrity of the mitochondrial membrane.

In an Alzheimer's dementia model, bacopa extract significantly reduced beta-amyloid levels when administered prior to beta-amyloid deposition (Dhanasekaran et al 2004). The neuroprotective effect was specific for beta amyloid-induced cell death but not glutamate-induced excitotoxicity (Limpeanchob et al 2008). Bacopa extracts contain polyphenols and sulfhydryl compounds that demonstrate dose-dependent antioxidant activity, which reduces divalent metals, decreases the formation of lipid peroxides and inhibits lipoxygenase activity (Dhanasekaran et al 2007).

Cognitive or nootropic effects — multiple mechanisms

Cognitive and nootropic effects are not merely due to antioxidant activity and neuroprotection, as demonstrated in an experimental model of Alzheimer's dementia whereby the cognitive-enhancing effect of *Bacopa monniera* was not well correlated with its neuroprotection (Uabundit et al 2010).

Evidence shows that cognitive activation is due to a combination of mechanisms, which include serotonergic and cholinergic systems together with antioxidant and mitochondrial stabilisation activities. Further research with experimental models indicates that bacopa enhances synaptic plasticity (Preethi et al 2012). The saponins bacoside A and B are considered to be the most important active constituents responsible for enhancing cognitive function (Russo & Borelli 2005, Singh & Dhawan 1982).

Effects on the cholinergic system include the modulation of acetylcholine release, choline acetylase activity and muscarinic cholinergic receptor binding (Das et al 2002). Results from a double-blind, placebo-controlled trial using brahmi (300 mg/day) support this view, as one of the major effects seen was on speed of early information processing, a function predominantly modulated by the cholinergic system (Stough et al 2001). *Bacopa monniera* (120 mg/kg oral) significantly reversed diazepam-induced (1.75 mg/kg intraperitoneal) amnesia in an animal study (Saraf et al 2008), thereby confirming previous reports of cholinergic activity (Dhanasekaran et al 2007).

Research in animal models provides evidence of activation of the serotonergic system (Charles et al 2011). In one study, the level of serotonin (5-HT) increased in rat brains while dopamine decreased significantly. Based on this observation, the learning and memory enhancement effects are likely to be due to upregulation of serotonin-synthesising enzyme tryptophan hydroxylase-2 expression which could enhance 5-HT synthesis and also upregulated SERT (serotonin transporter) expression, which would enhance transportation of 5-HT and subsequent activation of the 5-HT_{3A} receptor during hippocampus-dependent learning. The characterised *Bacopa monniera* leaf extract used in this study contained 31.27% bacosides, i.e. bacopaside I (0.9%), bacoside A3 (9.47%), bacopaside II (17.15%), jujubogenin of bacopasaponin C (0.38%) and bacopasaponin C (3.37%). High-performance liquid chromatography analysis confirmed the presence of bioactive compounds in the serum of treated rats.

Antidepressant activity

A rodent model of depression found that an extract of brahmi produced significant antidepressant activity comparable to that of imipramine after 5 days of oral administration (Sairam et al 2002).

Serotonergic activity identified in animal models provides a mechanistic basis for the antidepressant activity.

> ***Clinical note — what is a nootropic agent?***
> Giurgen first coined the phrase when describing a proposed class of pharmacologically active substances that improve cognition or intelligence without side effects and which should protect the brain from damage (Stough et al 2011). This is in contrast to pharmaceutical cognitive activators such as amphetamine or modafinil that only improve cognition and are accompanied by side effects and therefore cannot be described as true nootropic agents. Bacopa is a good example of a nootropic agent due to its cognitive-enhancing and neuroprotective activities and excellent safety profile.

Antiulcer effects

Significant antiulcer activity for the fresh juice from the whole plant of *Bacopa monniera* has been demonstrated in an animal model of aspirin-induced gastric ulceration (Rao et al 2000). The study found that brahmi had a beneficial influence on the natural mucosal defensive factors, such as enhanced mucin secretion, mucosal glycoprotein production and decreased cell shedding, thereby reducing ulceration (Rao et al 2000). A follow-up in vivo study in various gastric ulcer models further confirmed brahmi's ability to increase the body's natural defence factors and showed that *B. monniera* is effective for both the prophylaxis and the treatment of gastric ulcers (Sairam et al 2001). In addition, brahmi was shown to reduce lipid peroxidation. An in vitro study demonstrated that *B. monniera* significantly inhibited *Helicobacter pylori*, and the effect was comparable to that of bismuth subcitrate, a known *H. pylori* growth inhibitor (Goel et al 2003).

Anti-inflammatory effects

Several different mechanisms are responsible for the observed anti-inflammatory activity of brahmi. Inhibition of cyclooxygenase-2, 5-lipoxygenase (5-LOX) and 15-LOX and downregulation of tumour necrosis factor-alpha were demonstrated in one study testing a methanolic extract of *B. monniera*. The activity was found for both ethyl acetate and bacoside fractions (Viji & Helen 2008). Channa et al (2006) also identified anti-inflammatory activity but reported that this was mediated by prostaglandin E_2 inhibition, inhibition of histamine, serotonin and bradykinin release (Channa et al 2006).

The anti-inflammatory activity of bacopa was found to be comparable to indomethacin without causing an associated gastric irritation (Jain et al 1994). Several constituents are thought to be responsible for the anti-inflammatory action, chiefly the triterpene, betulinic acid, saponins and flavonoids.

OTHER ACTIONS

Adaptogen

A standardised extract of *B. monniera* possesses adaptogenic effects in an animal model, which were found to be comparable to *Panax quinquefolium* (Rai et al 2003). The neuropharmacological adaptogenic activity of brahmi was identified by significant normalisation of stress-induced changes in plasma corticosterone, and monoamine levels and dopamine in cortex and hippocampus regions of the brain (Sheikh et al 2007).

Antinociceptive activity

Previously, brahmi rasayan (an Ayurvedic herbal combination containing brahmi) demonstrated antinociceptive activity in animal experiments (Shukia et al 1987). An interaction with the GABAergic system is believed to be involved. More recent research confirms antinociceptive activity specifically for *Bacopa monniera* (Bhaskar & Jagtap 2011). Research using an aqueous extract in an experimental model indicates that the endogenous adrenergic, serotonergic and opioidergic systems are involved in the analgesic mechanism of action of the herb.

Mast cell stabilisation

The methanolic fraction of brahmi exhibits potent mast cell-stabilising activity in vitro, which was found to be comparable to that of disodium cromoglycate (Samiulla et al 2001).

Increased thyroid hormone levels

Results from animal experiments have found that brahmi increases thyroxine concentrations by 41% without enhancing hepatic lipid peroxidation (Kar et al 2002).

Antispasmodic effect on smooth muscle

A spasmolytic effect on smooth muscle has been demonstrated in vivo, and is predominantly due to inhibition of calcium influx into the cell (Dar & Channa 1999). Bronchodilatory effects have also been demonstrated, most likely due to the same mechanism (Channa et al 2003).

Anticlastogenic effect

An in vitro study identified significant anticlastogenic effects of the standardised extract of BacoMind on human lymphocytes due to the herb's antioxidant activity (Dutta et al 2008).

Hepatoprotective

Bacoside A was hepatoprotective against D-galactosamine-induced liver injury in rat studies. Researchers found that bacoside A reduced alanine transaminase, aspartate transaminase, alkaline phosphatase, gamma-glutamyl transpeptidase, lactate dehydrogenase and 5'ND enzyme levels and restored the decreased levels of vitamins C and E reduced by D-galactosamine in both liver and plasma (Sumathi & Nongbri 2008).

Cholesterol-lowering activity

According to a study using an experimental model of hypercholesterolaemia, feeding test animals an ethanolic extract of whole plant material (*Bacopa monniera*) for 45 days resulted in a significant reduction in levels of total cholesterol (TC), triglycerides, low-density lipoproteins (LDL), very-low-density lipoprotein (VLDL), atherogenic index, LDL: high-density lipoprotein (HDL) ratio and TC: HDL ratio and significantly increased the level of HDL (Kamesh & Sumathi 2012).

Anticonvulsant activity

Using an experimental epileptic model, Matthew et al (2012) demonstrated that *Bacopa monniera* and bacoside A treatment reverses epilepsy-associated changes to near controls. The effect appears to be mediated via GABA-A receptors and attributed to the bacoside A constituent (Mathew et al 2010, 2011).

> ***Clinical note — Scientific investigation of Ayurvedic medicines in India***
>
> Modern-day interest in many Ayurvedic herbs, such as brahmi, really started in 1951 when the then Prime Minister of India set up the Central Drug Research centre in Lucknow. The goal of this initiative was to encourage scientists to investigate many of the traditional Ayurvedic herbs in a scientific way, and to determine their potential as contemporary drugs or as potential sources for newer drugs.

CLINICAL USE

Brahmi has been subject to many in vitro and animal studies, which indicate that the herb and several of its key constituents have significant pharmacological activity. Increasingly, clinical studies are being published which provide a scientific basis for its use in practice. Most clinical research has been conducted with standardised bacopa extracts and focused on its effects on memory and learning, overall supporting its traditional reputation as a 'brain tonic'.

Improving cognitive function — learning, memory, intelligence

In Ayurvedic medicine, bacopa is used to improve cognitive function and increase intelligence. Over time, it has developed an excellent reputation, prompting scientific researchers to investigate the activity of bacopa more closely.

The evidence available from clinical studies indicates a significant effect on various aspects of memory and learning when bacopa extract is taken long-term. Less is known about the acute neurocognitive effects as there is less research to draw on and the two available clinical trials have produced inconsistent results (Downey et al 2013, Nathan et al 2001).

The bacopa extract known as KeenMind has been the subject of most studies, although there is evidence that other extracts, including BacoMind, also have significant effects.

Healthy adults

A double-blind, placebo-controlled trial using a dose of 300 mg bacopa (KeenMind) over 12 weeks in 46 healthy volunteers aged between 18 and 60 years found that it significantly improved the speed of visual information processing, learning rate and memory consolidation and that it has a significant anxiolytic effect (Stough et al 2001).

Another study of the same design tested brahmi (KeenMind) in 76 adults aged 45–60 years taken for over 3 months (Roodenrys et al 2002); significant improvements in a test for new information retention was observed, but there were no changes in the rate of learning.

More recently, a 90-day double-blind placebo-controlled study demonstrated that bacopa (300 mg/day: KeenMind) produced significantly improved performance on the 'working memory' factor, more specifically spatial working memory accuracy and accuracy in the rapid visual information processing task compared to placebo (Stough et al 2008). Additionally, those receiving active treatment reported significantly greater incidence of increased energy. The only significant increase in side effects was for incidence of diarrhoea and reduction in the number of dreams. While 107 people were originally enrolled in the study, there were 45 withdrawals, a similar amount from both groups (23 and 22), so only 62 people were considered sufficiently compliant with treatment and included in the final analysis.

Older adults

In 2008, Calabrese et al demonstrated that whole-plant standardised dry extract of *Bacopa monniera* (300 mg/day) safely enhanced cognitive performance in the aged in a double-blind, randomised, placebo-controlled study. The trial involved 54 volunteers aged 65 years or older, without clinical signs of dementia, who received placebo or herbal treatment for 12 weeks. The group receiving active herbal treatment also experienced a reduction in anxiety, whereas anxiety increased in the placebo group.

A double-blind, placebo-controlled randomised study was conducted in India involving 40 volunteers aged over 55 years and complaining of memory impairment (Ranghav et al 2008). The subjects received either 125 mg of an ethanolic standardised bacopa extract (containing 55% bacosides) or placebo twice a day for a period of 12 weeks followed by a placebo period of another 4 weeks (total duration of the trial 16 weeks). Active treatment produced a significant improvement in calculating ability, logical memory and paired associate learning compared to the placebo group.

Calculating ability was significantly improved by the end of week 8 and became highly significant at the end of week 12 and was maintained for a further 4 weeks after treatment withdrawal. Logical memory and recall of story improved by the end of week 4 onwards with active treatment and, once again, remained for 4 weeks after treatment ceased. Paired associate learning improved by week 8.

In 2010, results from a 12-week, randomised, double-blind, placebo-controlled trial using a brahmi extract known as BacoMind (300 mg/day: Natural Remedies) were published (Morgan & Stevens 2010). The study involved 81 healthy participants aged over 55 years of age. This comprehensive study measured audioverbal and visual memory performance together with subjective memory performance using a battery of validated measures. Treatment with bacopa significantly improved memory acquisition and retention in healthy older people — specifically verbal learning, memory acquisition and delayed recall — when compared to controls.

Acute effects in healthy people

Whether bacopa has acute effects is uncertain as current clinical trials have produced inconsistent results. Nathan et al (2001) found no significant change in cognitive function 2 hours after ingesting 300 mg of a bacopa extract (standardised to 55% combined bacosides A and B). The double-blind, placebo-controlled trial of 38 healthy volunteers (ages 18–60) found no effects on working and short-term memory, memory consolidation, information processing, executive processes, problem solving or motor responsiveness.

In contrast, acute neurocognitive effects were identified in a double-blind, placebo-controlled, crossover study utilising bacopa extract (KeenMind) and involving 24 healthy participants (Downey et al 2013). Two doses of bacopa (320 mg and 640 mg) were compared to each other and placebo for effects on participants' performance on six repetitions of the Cognitive Demand Battery (CDB). The standard treatment dose of 320 mg improved performance on the first, second and fourth repetition of the CDB but had no effects on cardiovascular parameters, task-induced rating of stress or fatigue.

Children

Less research has been conducted with children; however the available evidence is promising. A single-blind open clinical study reported memory- and learning-enhancing effects and improved reaction time in children after 12 weeks of treatment (Sharma et al 1987). In this study children were given bacopa syrup three times daily (350 mg/dose) over 3 months. A small, randomised, double-blind trial of 36 children diagnosed with attention-deficit hyperactivity disorder (ADHD) showed that 12 weeks' treatment with fresh whole-plant extract of bacopa (50 mg twice daily) improved logical memory impairment (Negi et al 2000).

An Israeli study utilising a patented herbal and nutritional combination produced significant improvements to attention, cognition and impulse control in a larger double-blind, placebo-controlled study of 120 children with newly diagnosed ADHD (Katz et al 2010). After 4 months of treatment, the group showed substantial, statistically significant improvement in the four subscales and overall test of variables of attention scores, compared with no improvement in the control group, which persisted in an intention-to-treat analysis. The treatment being evaluated consisted of a patented blend of nutritive, food-grade herbs, prepared as a highly stable, dilute ethanol extract called Nurture & Clarity. Bacopa was one of the main herbal ingredients, but not the sole ingredient. Others in the treatment included *Paeoniae alba, Withania somnifera, Centella asiatica, Spirulina platensis* and *Mellissa officinalis,* together with a range of vitamins.

Anxiety

Bacopa has traditionally been used in Ayurvedic medicine to treat anxiety, and preliminary evidence is promising.

A placebo-controlled, randomised study of healthy subjects found that 300 mg of brahmi (KeenMind) daily reduced the anxiety compared with placebo, an effect most pronounced after 12 weeks compared to 5 weeks of treatment (Stough et al 2001). A reduction in anxiety was also reported by Calabrese et al (2008) in a double-blind, randomised, placebo-controlled study which tested whole-plant standardised dry extract of *Bacopa monniera* (300 mg/day) over 12 weeks. The trial of 54 volunteers aged 65 years or older, without clinical signs of dementia, found that active treatment reduced anxiety whereas anxiety increased in the placebo group.

OTHER USES

Traditional uses

Bacopa has been traditionally used as a brain tonic and is commonly recommended to improve memory and heighten learning capacity. It is also used as a nerve tonic to treat anxiety, nervous exhaustion or debility and is prescribed to enhance rehabilitation after any injury causing nervous deficit, such as stroke. Other traditional uses include promoting longevity, and treating diarrhoea and asthma. It is used as an anti-inflammatory, analgesic, anxiolytic and antiepileptic agent, with some support for these uses provided by in vitro and in vivo studies.

Irritable bowel syndrome

An Ayurvedic herbal combination consisting of *Aegle marmelos correa* and *Bacopa monniera* successfully treated 65% of patients with irritable bowel syndrome under double-blind, randomised conditions (Yadav et al 1989). Herbal treatment was particularly useful in the diarrhoea-predominant form of irritable bowel syndrome, compared with the placebo. Follow-up reviews 6 months after the trial found that relapse rates were the same among all test subjects. Although encouraging, it is not certain to what extent brahmi was responsible for these results.

DOSAGE RANGE

- Dried aerial parts of herb: 5–10 g/day.
- Fluid extract (1:2) or equivalent oral dose form: 5–13 mL/day in divided doses.
- Standardised extract (BacoMind or KeenMind) 300 mg/day.

For children aged 6 years and older: 350 mg of dried plant extract in a syrup form was administered three times daily.

According to clinical studies

- Cognitive activator effects: 300 mg/day.

Positive results obtained in one controlled study have found that 5–12 weeks' use is required before clinical effects are observed (Stough et al 2001).

TOXICITY

The LD_{50} data for an ethanolic extract of bacopa is 17 g/kg (oral) (Mills & Bone 2005).

Animal studies indicate that LD_{50} of standardised extract (BacoMind) is 2400 mg/kg body weight with no observed adverse effect limit of 500 mg/kg body weight after 90 days (Allan et al 2007).

ADVERSE REACTIONS

The most common side effects are minor gastrointestinal disturbances, nausea, abdominal cramps, increased stool frequency and diarrhoea (Morgan & Stevens 2010, Pravina et al 2007). Less frequent side effects include sleepiness, headache, palpitations, dry mouth, thirst and fatigue, insomnia and vivid dreams or lack of dreams.

SIGNIFICANT INTERACTIONS

Controlled studies are not available, so interactions are based on evidence of activity and are largely theoretical and speculative.

Cholinergic drugs

Cholinergic activity has been identified for brahmi, therefore increased drug activity is theoretically possible — observe patient, although a beneficial interaction is possible under professional supervision.

Serotonergic drugs

Serotonergic activity has been identified for bacopa extracts, therefore there is a theoretical increased risk of serotonin syndrome when bacopa is used together with selective serotonin reuptake inhibitor and serotonin-noradrenaline reuptake inhibitor medicines — the clinical significance of the interaction is unclear. Caution until further investigation can confirm.

Practice points/Patient counselling

- Brahmi is an Ayurvedic herb that has been used for several thousand years as a brain tonic, to enhance intellect, treat psychiatric illness, epilepsy and insomnia and as a mild sedative.
- There is now good evidence that bacopa exerts cognitive and nootropic activity via multiple mechanisms, including activation of the serotonergic and cholinergic systems, antioxidant and mitochondrial stabilisation activities and enhancement of synaptic plasticity.
- Human studies have shown that brahmi (KeenMind, BacoMind, whole-plant extract) has a significant effect on various aspects of learning and memory when used long-term; effects with short-term use or single doses are less well investigated. There is also evidence of anxiolytic activity according to clinical studies.
- Brahmi has potent antioxidant activity, which appears to be a result of both direct free radical scavenging activity and increasing endogenous antioxidant systems in the brain and liver.
- Anticholinesterase, antidepressant, antiulcer, antispasmodic, anti-inflammatory, antihistamine, neuroprotective, antinociceptive activities and lipid-lowering actions have been demonstrated in animal studies. Elevated thyroxine levels have also been observed.

CONTRAINDICATIONS AND PRECAUTIONS

Caution is advised in hyperthyroidism, as bacopa has been shown to significantly elevate thyroxine levels in vivo. The clinical significance of this finding is unknown.

Brahmi may cause gastrointestinal symptoms in people with coeliac disease, fat malabsorption syndrome, vitamins A, D, E or K deficiency, dyspepsia or pre-existing cholestasis due to the high saponins content of the herb (Mills & Bone 2005).

PREGNANCY USE

Brahmi is recommended as a tonic for anxiety in pregnancy according to traditional Ayurvedic medicine; however, insufficient information is available to confirm safety during pregnancy.

PATIENTS' FAQs

What will this herb do for me?

Brahmi has a long history of use as a brain tonic. Results from scientific studies demonstrate that it will enhance aspects of learning, memory and cognitive function with long-term use and is also likely to reduce anxiety,

B

When will it start to work?

Studies indicate that 5–12 weeks' continual use is required for benefits on cognitive function to become apparent. Acute effects may also be possible, but there is less evidence to be certain.

Are there any safety issues?

Information from traditional sources suggests that brahmi is well tolerated at the usual therapeutic doses and the most common side effects relate to gastrointestinal disturbances which are mild and reversible, such as nausea, frequent bowel motions and abdominal cramping. Clinical studies have not confirmed drug interactions so cautions are theoretical.

REFERENCES

Adams M, et al. Plants traditionally used in age-related brain disorders. A survey of ethnobotanical literature. J Ethnopharmacol 113.3 (2007): 363–81.

Allan JJ et al. Safety evaluation of a standardized phytochemical composition extracted from *Bacopa monnieri* in Sprague-Dawley rats. Food Chem Toxicol 45.10 (2007): 1928–1937.

Anbarasi K, et al. Protective effect of bacoside A on cigarette smoking-induced brain mitochondrial dysfunction in rats. J Environ Pathol Toxicol Oncol 24.3 (2005a): 225–34.

Anbarasi K, et al. Lactate dehydrogenase isoenzyme patterns upon chronic exposure to cigarette smoke: protective effects of bacoside A. Environmental Toxicology and Pharmacology 20 (2005b): 345–350.

Anbarasi K et al. Creatine kinase isoenzyme patterns upon chronic exposure to cigarette smoke: protective effect of bacoside A. Vascul Pharmacol 42.2 (2005c): 57–61.

Anbarasi K et al. Cigarette smoking induces heat shock protein 70 kDa expression and apoptosis in rat brain: modulation by bacoside A. Neuroscience 138.4 (2006): 1127–1135.

Bhaskar, M. & Jagtap, A.G. 2011. Exploring the possible mechanisms of action behind the antinociceptive activity of *Bacopa monniera*. Int. J Ayurveda.Res., 2, (1) 2–7.

Bhattacharya SK et al. Antioxidant activity of *Bacopa monniera* in rat frontal cortex, striatum and hippocampus. Phytother Res 14.3 (2000): 174–179.

Calabrese C et al. Effects of a standardized *Bacopa monnieri* extract on cognitive performance, anxiety, and depression in the elderly: a randomized, double-blind, placebo-controlled trial. J Altern Complement Med 14.6 (2008): 707–713.

Chakravarty AK, et al. Bacopasides III-V: three new triterpenoid glycosides from *Bacopa monniera*. Chem Pharm Bull (Tokyo) 51 (2003): 215–2117.

Channa S et al. Broncho-vasodilatory activity of fractions and pure constituents isolated from *Bacopa monniera*. J Ethnopharmacol 86.1 (2003): 27–35.

Channa S et al. Anti-inflammatory activity of *Bacopa monniera* in rodents. J Ethnopharmacol 104 (2006): 296–289.

Charles, P.D., et al. 2011. *Bacopa monniera* leaf extract up-regulates tryptophan hydroxylase (TPH2) and serotonin transporter (SERT) expression: implications in memory formation. J Ethnopharmacol., 134, (1) 55–61

Dar A, Channa S. Calcium antagonistic activity of *Bacopa monniera* on vascular and intestinal smooth muscles of rabbit and guinea-pig. J Ethnopharmacol 66.2 (1999): 167–174.

Das A et al. A comparative study in rodents of standardized extracts of *Bacopa monniera* and Ginkgo biloba. Anticholinesterase and cognitive enhancing activities. Pharmacol Biochem Behav 73.4 (2002): 893–900.

Dhanasekaran M et al. *Bacopa monniera* extract reduces beta-amyloid deposition in doubly transgenic PSAPP Alzheimer's disease mouse model. Neurology 63.8 (2004): 1545–8.

Dhanasekaran M et al. Neuroprotective mechanisms of ayurvedic antidementia botanical *Bacopa monniera*. Phytother Res 21.10 (2007): 965–969.

Downey, L.A., et al. 2013. An Acute, double-blind, placebo-controlled crossover study of 320 mg and 640 mg doses of a special extract of *Bacopa monnieri* (CDRI 08) on sustained cognitive performance. Phytother. Res. 27: 1407–1413.

Dutta D et al. In vitro safety evaluation and anticlastogenic effect of BacoMind™ on human lymphocytes. Biomed Environ Sci 21.1 (2008): 7–23.

Goel RK et al. In vitro evaluation of *Bacopa monniera* on anti-*Helicobacter pylori* activity and accumulation of prostaglandins. Phytomedicine 10.6–7 (2003): 523–527.

Hota SK et al. *Bacopa monniera* leaf extract ameliorates hypobaric hypoxia induced spatial memory impairment. Neurobiol Dis 34.1 (2009): 23–39.

Jain P et al. Anti-inflammatory effects of an Ayurvedic preparation, Brahmi Rasayan, in rodents. Indian J Exp Biol 32 (1994): 633–636.

Jyoti A, et al. *Bacopa monniera* prevents from aluminium neurotoxicity in the cerebral cortex of rat brain. J Ethnopharmacol 111.1 (2007): 56–62.

Kamesh, V. & Sumathi, T. 2012. Antihypercholesterolemic effect of *Bacopa monniera* Linn. on high cholesterol diet induced hypercholesterolemia in rats. Asian Pac. J Trop. Med, 5 (12) 949–955.

Kapoor R, et al. *Bacopa monnieri* modulates antioxidant responses in brain and kidney of diabetic rats. Environmental Toxicology and Pharmacology 27.1 (2009): 62–69.

Kar A, et al. Relative efficacy of three medicinal plant extracts in the alteration of thyroid hormone concentrations in male mice. J Ethnopharmacol 81.2 (2002): 281–285.

Katz, M., et al. 2010. A compound herbal preparation (CHP) in the treatment of children with ADHD: a randomized controlled trial. J Atten. Disord., 14, (3) 281–291.

Limpeanchob N et al. Neuroprotective effect of *Bacopa monnieri* on beta-amyloid-induced cell death in primary cortical culture. J Ethnopharmacol 120.1 (2008): 112–1117.

Mathew, J., et al. 2010. Behavioral deficit and decreased GABA receptor functional regulation in the cerebellum of epileptic rats: effect of *Bacopa monnieri* and bacoside A. Epilepsy Behav., 17, (4) 441–447.

Mathew, J., et al. 2011. Behavioral deficit and decreased GABA receptor functional regulation in the hippocampus of epileptic rats: effect of *Bacopa monnieri*. Neurochem.Res., 36, (1) 7–16.

Mathew, J., et al. 2012. Decreased GABA receptor in the cerebral cortex of epileptic rats: effect of *Bacopa monnieri* and Bacoside-A. J Biomed. Sci., 19, 25.

Mills S, Bone K. The essential guide to herbal safety. Edinburgh: Churchill Livingstone, 2005.

Morgan A, Stevens J. Does *Bacopa monnieri* improve memory performance in older persons? Results of a randomized, placebo-controlled, double-blind trial. J Altern Complement Med 2010;16:753–9.

Nathan PJ et al. The acute effects of an extract of *Bacopa monniera* (Brahmi) on cognitive function in healthy normal subjects. Hum Psychopharmacol 16.4 (2001): 345–351.

Negi, K.S., et al. 2000. Clinical evaluation of memory enhancing properties of Memory Plus in children with attention deficit hyperactivity disorder. Indian J Psychiatry, 42, (SUPPL.) 42–50

Pravina K et al. Safety evaluation of BacoMind™ in healthy volunteers: a phase 1 study. Phytomedicine 14.5 (2007): 301–308.

Preethi, J., et al. 2012. Participation of microRNA 124-CREB pathway: a parallel memory enhancing mechanism of standardised extract of *Bacopa monniera* (BESEB CDRI-08). Neurochem. Res., 37, (10) 2167–2177.

Rai D et al. Adaptogenic effect of *Bacopa monniera* (Brahmi). Pharmacol Biochem Behav 75.4 (2003): 823–830.

Ranghav, S., et al. Randomized controlled trial of standardized *Bacopa monniera* extract in age-associated memory impairment. Indian J Psychiatry. 48[4], 238–242. 2008.

Rao CV, et al. Experimental evaluation of *Bacopa monnieri* on rat gastric ulceration and secretion. Indian J Physiol Pharmacol 44.4 (2000): 435–441.

Roodenrys S et al. Chronic effects of Brahmi (*Bacopa monnieri*) on human memory. Neuropsychopharmacology 27.2 (2002): 279–281.

Russo A, Borrelli F. *Bacopa monniera*, a reputed nootropic plant: an overview. Phytomedicine 12 (2005): 305–317.

Russo A et al. Nitric oxide-related toxicity in cultured astrocytes: effect of *Bacopa monniera*. Life Sci 73.12 (2003a): 1517–26.

Russo A et al. Free radical scavenging capacity and protective effect of *Bacopa monniera* L. on DNA damage. Phytother Res 17.8 (2003b): 870–5.

Saini, N., et al. 2012. Neuroprotective effects of *Bacopa monnieri* in experimental model of dementia. Neurochem. Res., 37, (9) 1928–1937.

Sairam K et al. Prophylactic and curative effects of *Bacopa monniera* in gastric ulcer models. Phytomedicine 8.6 (2001): 423–430.

Sairam K et al. Antidepressant activity of standardized extract of *Bacopa monniera* in experimental models of depression in rats. Phytomedicine 9.3 (2002): 207–211.

Samiulla DS, et al. Mast cell stabilising activity of *Bacopa monnieri*. Fitoterapia 72.3 (2001): 284–285.

Saraf MK et al. *Bacopa monniera* ameliorates amnesic effects of diazepam qualifying behavioral-molecular partitioning. Neuroscience 155.2 (2008): 476–484.

Sharma R, et al. Efficacy of *Bacopa monniera* in revitalizing intellectual functions in children. J Res Edu Indian Med. 1987;1:12

Sheikh N et al. Effect of *Bacopa monniera* on stress induced changes in plasma corticosterone and brain monoamines in rats. J Ethnopharmacol 111.3 (2007): 671–6776.

Shukia B, et al. Effect of Brahmi Rasayan on the central nervous system. J Ethnopharmacol 21.1 (1987): 65–74.

Singh HK, Dhawan BN. Effect of *Bacopa monniera* Linn. (brahmi) extract on avoidance responses in rat. J Ethnopharmacol 5.2 (1982): 205–214.
Stough C et al. The chronic effects of an extract of *Bacopa monniera* (Brahmi) on cognitive function in healthy human subjects. Psychopharmacology (Berl) 156.4 (2001): 481–484.
Stough C, et al. Examining the nootropic effects of a special extract of *Bacopa monniera* on human cognitive functioning: 90 day double-blind placebo-controlled randomized trial. Phytother Res 2008;22:1629–34.
Stough, C., et al. 2011. Improving general intelligence with a nutrient-based pharmacological intervention. Intelligence, 39, (2–3) 100–107.
Sumathi T, Nongbri A. Hepatoprotective effect of bacoside-A, a major constituent of *Bacopa monniera*. Phytomedicine 15.10 (2008): 901–9005.
Tripathi YB et al. *Bacopa monniera* Linn. as an antioxidant: mechanism of action. Indian J Exp Biol 34.6 (1996): 523–526.
Uabundit, N., et al. 2010. Cognitive enhancement and neuroprotective effects of *Bacopa monnieri* in Alzheimer's disease model. J Ethnopharmacol., 127, (1) 26–31.
Viji V, Helen A. Inhibition of lipoxygenases and cycloxygenase-2 enzymes by extracts isolated from *Bacopa monniera*. J Ethnopharmacol 118.2 (2008): 305–311.
Williamson EM. Major herbs of Ayurveda. Dabur Research Foundation and Dabur Ayurvet Ltd. London: Churchill Livingstone, 2002.
Yadav SK et al. Irritable bowel syndrome: therapeutic evaluation of indigenous drugs. Indian J Med Res 90 (1989): 496–503.

Calcium

BACKGROUND AND RELEVANT PHARMACOKINETICS

In the context of both biosphere and biology (plant and animal) calcium plays a leading role. Its abundance in the environment (e.g. limestone, marble, coral) is reflected, in part, in the human body, with calcium being the most abundant mineral in the body. Calcium homeostasis reflects a balancing act between requirements for proper function and the organism's need to protect against excess cellular calcium levels and associated toxicity. This balance has ramifications not only for our own physiology, but also in terms of levels and bioavailability of dietary calcium.

Three hormones regulate calcium status in the body — calcitriol (active vitamin D), parathyroid hormone (PTH) and calcitonin. Calcitriol increases intestinal absorption of dietary calcium when blood levels are low. In addition, PTH signals the kidneys to reduce calcium loss, produce more calcitriol and also activate osteoclasts that release bone calcium. Calcitonin is secreted by the thyroid gland when calcium levels become too high and opposes the action of PTH, thereby returning calcium levels back to normal.

Calcium, found in the diet or supplements, exists in salt form, from which it must be released for absorption to occur. Adequate hydrochloric acid levels are required to solubilise the majority of these calcium ions, failing which calcium salts entering the higher pH environment of the small intestine are more likely to precipitate and be rendered insoluble (Wahlqvist 2002). Low or moderate calcium intakes (≤400 mg/day) are absorbed via active transport mechanisms that are influenced by vitamin D. When intake is high, active transport mechanisms become saturated, leading to greater passive absorption. Although most absorption occurs in the small intestine, the large intestine may also be responsible for up to 4% of absorption and provides compensatory mechanisms for those individuals with compromised small intestine absorption (Groff & Gropper 2009).

Calcium's bioavailability from both food and supplements shows substantial variation, and may be influenced by other foods present in the gastrointestinal tract. Phytates (in wholegrains, nuts and seeds), oxalates, all types of fibres, unabsorbed dietary fatty acids and other divalent minerals all potentially compromise its absorption, while lactose (especially in children) and other sugars, as well as protein and the presence of vitamin D, all enhance uptake (Groff & Gropper 2009).

Calcium salts differ in the amount of elemental calcium, which may have clinical implications and affect dose selection. Calcium carbonate contains the highest amount of elemental calcium by weight (40%), calcium citrate (21%), calcium lactate (14%) and calcium gluconate (9%) (Kopic & Geibel 2013). In addition to having variable calcium fractions, the different calcium salts have widely divergent water solubility, which may also affect absorption and bioavailability. For example, calcium citrate dissolves 17 times more readily than calcium carbonate in water. However, 86% of calcium carbonate will still dissolve in a slightly more acidic environment (pH 5.5), which is higher than a normal maximum stomach pH of 4.5. Researchers in this area have not reached consensus as to whether the difference in water solubility is clinically relevant, provided the stomach pH is sufficiently acidic to dissolve the calcium supplement and allow for absorption (Kopic & Geibel 2013).

Besides the variation in absorption due to gastric pH, other dietary components and type of calcium salt, there are differences between individuals in their calcium absorption efficiency which can be up to 60% variance; the underlying mechanisms, although unclear, may be linked to vitamin D receptor (VDR) polymorphisms (Heaney & Weaver 2003). Consistent with this, our understanding of the magnitude of vitamin D's influence upon calcium absorption continues to broaden, including the life-stage-dependent bioavailability of this mineral. The age-associated decline in calcium absorption (children absorb ≈75% compared with ≤30% in adults) (Groff & Gropper 2009) has now been linked to vitamin D via reduced available calcitriol and decreased intestinal VDR levels, producing vitamin D resistance (Groff & Gropper 2009, Pattanaungkul et al 2000). Similarly, the decreasing bioavailability associated with (peri)menopause and the increased absorption evident early in pregnancy (Prentice 2003) are attributed largely to vitamin D-mediated effects. Calcium absorption, however, is described as being generally inefficient, with a substantial amount of calcium remaining unabsorbed in the lumen (Heaney & Weaver 2003).

Distribution results in 99% of absorbed calcium being deposited in bones. The remainder of the absorbed calcium is present in teeth and the intracellular or extracellular fluids. Calcium is excreted in faeces, sweat and urine.

FOOD SOURCES

Good dietary sources of calcium include dairy products, fortified soy products, fish with bones (especially salmon and sardines), tofu, broccoli, collard greens, mustard greens, bok choy, clams and black strap molasses. Certain brands of soy milk, fruit juice, breakfast cereal and bread are also fortified with calcium, which provides an alternative for people who don't eat dairy products. People with limited dairy intake may still need to consider supplementation to ensure they meet RDI levels.

DEFICIENCY SIGNS AND SYMPTOMS

Optimal calcium intake is essential during every stage of life and insufficient intake in childhood years can have ramifications later in life.

While there is little information available about the prevalence of deficiency across the general Australian population, a Melbourne study of 1045 women aged 20–92 years in 2000 revealed that approximately 76% of women consumed calcium at levels less than the recommended daily intake (RDI), and an additional 14% demonstrated a grossly inadequate intake of less than 300 mg/day (Pasco et al 2000). Dietary calcium intake has been found to be inadequate and below Estimated Average Requirement (EAR) in the majority of elderly Australian women (Meng et al 2010). These figures are similar to those obtained by larger studies in the United States (Groff & Gropper 2009). Calculating the prevalence of calcium deficiency is partly hampered by physiological preservation of 'non-osseous' calcium for critical roles in exchange for the 'expendable' reserves in bone and, therefore, the slow development of overt deficiency features. Consequently, calcium deficiency is insidious in its early stages and potentially irreversible in the latter, making preventive optimisation the only successful pathway in all patients perceived to be at an increased risk. In addition to this, long-term suboptimal calcium has been linked to an increased risk of a range of other morbidities, including preeclampsia and colorectal cancer.

Deficiency signs and symptoms include:

- tetany: muscle pain, spasms and paraesthesias
- rickets
- osteomalacia
- increased neuromuscular irritability
- altered heart rate
- ambulatory developmental delays in children
- osteoporosis and increased risk of fractures
- bone pain and deformity
- tooth discolouration and increased decay
- hypertension
- increased risk of preeclampsia
- increased risk of colon cancer (controversial).

There are many situations and conditions in which the risk of hypocalcaemia may be increased.

Primary deficiency

Primary deficiency occurs as a result of inadequate dietary intake, with greatest risk seen in populations with increased calcium requirements e.g. children, adolescents, pregnant and lactating women, postmenopausal women (particularly those taking hormone replacement therapy [HRT] [Wahlqvist 2002]), people experiencing rapid weight loss or patients receiving total parenteral nutrition (TPN).

Secondary deficiency

Calcium absorption is impaired in achlorhydria (more common in the elderly), intestinal inflammation and any malabsorptive disorder accompanied by steatorrhoea (Wilson et al 1991). Increased faecal calcium loss occurs with higher intakes of fibre and in fat malabsorption, while renal excretion has been shown in some studies to be increased in those patients ingesting a high protein diet (Kerstetter et al 1998).

Factors that compromise vitamin D status or activity will also affect calcium status), e.g. oral and inhaled corticosteroids (Beers & Berkow 2003, Pattanaungkul et al 2000, Prince et al 1997, Rossi et al 2005).

Other conditions that can predispose to hypocalcaemia include hypoparathyroidism (a deficiency or absence of PTH), idiopathic hypoparathyroidism (an uncommon condition in which the parathyroid glands are absent or atrophied), pseudohypoparathyroidism (characterised not by deficiency of PTH, but by target organ resistance to its action), magnesium depletion, renal tubular disease, renal failure, acute pancreatitis, hypoproteinaemia, septic shock or the use of certain medicines such as anticonvulsants (phenytoin, phenobarbitone) and rifampicin, and corticosteroids (Beers & Berkow 2003, Rossi et al 2005).

MAIN ACTIONS

Calcium is an essential mineral required for the proper functioning of numerous intracellular and extracellular processes, including muscle contraction, nerve conduction, beating of the heart, hormone release, blood coagulation, energy production and maintenance of immune function. It also plays a role in intracellular signalling and is involved in the regulation of many enzymes.

Bone and teeth mineralisation

Calcium is found in bone where it is mainly complexed with other ions in the form of hydroxyapatite crystals. Approximately 1% of calcium in bone can be freely exchanged into the extracellular fluid in order to buffer changes in calcium balance.

Muscle contraction

Calcium plays a major role in muscle contraction. Ionised serum calcium helps to initiate both smooth and skeletal muscle contraction and in particular, the regulation of rhythmic contraction of the heart muscle in combination with sodium and potassium. During exercise, one cause of muscle fatigue is the impaired activity of calcium in muscle cells (Insel et al 2013).

Blood clotting

Calcium is required in order for blood to clot. It is involved in several steps of the blood clotting cascade and is required for the production of fibrin, the protein that gives structure to blood clots (Insel et al 2013).

Nerve conduction

Calcium is required for nerve cells to transmit signals. The strength of the signal is proportional to the number of calcium ions crossing the nerve cell membrane (Insel et al 2013).

Altered membrane functions

Calcium fluxes across membranes, both within the cell and across the plasma membrane, and acts as a vehicle for the signal transduction necessary for neurotransmitter and hormone function. It also selectively alters cell wall permeability to regulate passage of fluids in and out of cells.

OTHER ACTIONS

Regulates various enzyme systems responsible for muscle contraction, fat digestion and protein metabolism.

CLINICAL USE

Many of the indications for calcium supplements are conditions thought to arise from a gross or marginal deficiency; however, some are based on the concept of 'beyond-repletion' calcium therapy.

Calcium deficiency

Traditionally, calcium supplementation has been used to treat deficiency or prevent deficiency in high-risk conditions or people with increased calcium requirements such as pregnant and lactating women. Acute severe hypocalcaemic states are treated initially with intravenous infusion of calcium salts. In chronic cases, oral calcium supplements are often combined with vitamin D supplements to improve absorption and utilisation.

Rickets and osteomalacia

A deficiency of either calcium or vitamin D can produce these bone disorders. (See *Vitamin D* monograph for further information.)

Infants

The percentage and type of fats within an infant formula and their ability to bind calcium salts and increase excretion has been shown to influence the bone mineral content (BMC) of infants. One hundred 8-week-old infants given formulas considered to be more similar to breastmilk and less likely to form calcium soaps in the gut showed increased BMC after only 1 month's treatment compared with those infants on standard formula (Kennedy et al 1999).

Bone mineral density (BMD), osteoporosis prophylaxis and reducing fracture risk

Calcium supplements are prescribed widely to promote bone health, including the treatment and prevention of osteoporosis, a major cause of morbidity and mortality in older people (Hennekens & Barice 2011). RCTs assessing BMD generally show a beneficial effect of calcium treatment in both men and women (typically a 1%–2% absolute difference between the treatment and control groups over 2–3 years), which results in a sustained reduction in bone loss of 50%–60%. The effect appears to be greatest for people whose baseline dietary calcium intake is low (Sanders et al 2009).

Adequate calcium intake is particularly important to consider in at-risk populations because osteoporosis-related fractures can lead to early disability and death. Ensuring adequate calcium intake alone is not sufficient and vitamin D status is also important as both contribute to bone density and associated protective effects. Sufficient trace minerals such as manganese, zinc and copper and weight-bearing exercise is also suggested and the use of anti-resorptive drugs together with mineral supplementation may be required in high risk groups or those with preexisting osteoporosis.

The lifetime risk of fracture is highest in white women, and decreases successively among Hispanic, Asian and African-American people. For white women, it occurs 20% for the spine, 15% for the wrist and 18% for the hip, with an exponential increase in risk beyond the age of 50 years. Within 12 months after a hip fracture, approximately 13% of people die, with most survivors losing their previous independence. Calcium supplementation, together with vitamin D, may reduce vertebral and non-vertebral fractures (Vestergaard et al 2011). This is supported by a 2010 meta-analysis of seven randomised studies of vitamin D or calcium and vitamin D which included 68,517 participants (mean age 69.9 years, range 47–107 years, 14.7% men) (Abrahamsen 2010). The study found that calcium and vitamin D given together significantly reduced hip fractures and total fractures, and probably vertebral fractures, irrespective of age, sex or previous fractures. The protective effect is modest for combined therapy, whereas no significant effects were seen for vitamin D alone in doses of 10–20 microg/day for preventing fractures. Recently, a question has arisen as to whether calcium supplementation may in fact increase hip fracture risk; however, the issue has not been resolved and deserves further investigation.

Based on these findings, calcium could be considered a low potency anti-resorptive agent which should be taken in sufficient doses together with adequate vitamin D to produce any benefits.

The position statement from Osteoporosis Australia, the Endocrine Society of Australia and the Australian and New Zealand Bone and Mineral Society states that the balance of evidence remains in favour of combined calcium and vitamin D supplementation in elderly men and women for the prevention of fractures and calcium is regarded as an integral component of anti-resorptive regimens (Sanders et al 2009).

Children and adolescents

Most, but not all, RCTs involving children and adolescents using either dairy-supplemented foods or calcium supplementation have demonstrated some benefit at one or more of the BMD sites measured (Sanders et al 2009). However, a meta-analysis of 19 RCTs showed that there was no effect on BMD in children at the femoral neck or lumbar spine, and only a small benefit on total body BMD and upper limb BMD that was unlikely to substantially reduce adult fracture risk (Winzenberg et al 2006). The upper limb was the only site where a sustained BMD benefit was demonstrated after cessation of calcium supplementation. More studies are required in children with low calcium intakes and in peripubertal children.

The benefits of long-term supplementation may be greatest in children with pre-existing deficiency according to a meta-analysis of 21 RCTs (Huncharek et al 2008b). This study found no effect for calcium supplementation in individuals with (near) adequate calcium intake at baseline but found a significantly increased BMC (35–49 g) in individuals with a preexisting deficiency taking long-term treatment.

The same year, Lambert et al (2008) undertook an 18-month study of calcium-deficient adolescent girls (average age 12 years), increasing their mean daily intake by 555 mg in the treatment group which yielded a significantly increased BMC and BMD and reduced bone turnover markers in the treatment group compared with a placebo (Lambert et al 2008).

A more recent meta-analysis investigating whether weight-bearing exercises done by prepubertal children improves BMC found that the effect was strongest when done alongside a high calcium intake and only weak otherwise (Behringer et al 2014). Numerous studies, including one by Stear et al in 2003 of 144 pubertal girls, have confirmed a synergistic relationship between mechanical load through physical activity, calcium status and bone calcium accumulation; however, it is important to note that physical activity has a positive effect on BMD only at high calcium intakes, with no effect at calcium intakes of less than 1000 mg/day (Harkness & Bonny 2005).

The results of one long-term study has suggested that skeletal stature may be a determinant in whether long-term benefits are more likely with supplementation during puberty. The placebo-controlled study ($n = 354$ pubertal girls) used calcium supplements (670 mg/day) over a 7-year period and reported significant increases in BMD during growth spurts in the supplemented group; however, these gains did not uniformly persist into late adolescence and only girls of tall stature received long-lasting benefits. Interestingly, the placebo group exhibited a 'catch-up' in bone mineral accretion subsequent to the pubertal growth spurt (Matkovic et al 2005).

A second study introduces other issues regarding the impact of variable calcium status in adolescents. This RCT of 144 prepubertal girls used 850 mg/day of calcium over 1 year. After follow-up some 7 years later, in addition to positive effects on BMD outcomes, an inverse relationship became apparent between calcium supplementation and age of menarche. The authors speculate that higher calcium intake prior to menarche may favourably impact on long-term BMD through this dual mechanism (Chevalley et al 2005).

Postmenopausal women

Bone mass remains relatively stable during early adulthood but changes dramatically after menopause. For about the first 5 years after menopause, women lose bone at the rate of about 2%–3% per year and then continue to lose about 1% of bone mass per year to the end of life. During this time, there is a decline in intestinal calcium absorption and an increase in urinary calcium excretion (Sanders et al 2009).

Numerous studies have confirmed a role for calcium in bolstering BMD in late postmenopausal women where results are more consistent than for perimenopausal women (Sanders et al 2009). Clinical studies have assessed its efficacy as a sole agent against placebo, in comparison with steroid hormones, antiresorptive drugs and as part of combination therapy. While increased calcium intake provides some benefits it should be accompanied by sufficient vitamin D status for optimal results. In addition, a protein rich-diet together with weight-bearing exercise are considered the key pillars for osteoporosis prevention among postmenopausal women (Bischoff-Ferrari 2012). Adequate levels of trace minerals such as zinc, copper and manganese are also recommended (Strause et al 1994).

The efficacy of supplementation with calcium is not only dependent on vitamin D status but also baseline calcium levels as women with poor dietary intakes tend to achieve significant improvements over placebo, with more modest or no effect evident in groups with higher intakes at baseline (Daniele et al 2004, Fardellone et al 1998).

In a recent RCT trial of 159 postmenopausal women, calcium 1200 mg daily was shown to reduce the parathyroid hormone and bone turnover markers (cross-linked C-telopeptide and procollagen type 1 N-terminal propeptide) after 6 months (Aloia et al 2013). This provides some rationale for the long-term use of calcium supplements for osteoporosis prevention.

Men

While bone mineral density remains stable throughout adulthood, men start to lose bone density about the age of 50 years, although at a slower rate than women. By the age of 60 years, the rate of bone loss is similar for men and women as calcium absorption decreases over time (Sanders et al 2009).

The overwhelming majority of calcium studies for bone health have been conducted in postmenopausal women and often their results have simply been extrapolated to produce clinical protocols for men regarding osteoporosis prevention and management. The few studies conducted in male populations have produced inconsistent results, possibly due to differences in dosage and also vitamin D status of participants. For example, one study showed no benefit at 600 mg/day, while yielding BMD improvements secondary to higher doses (1200 mg/day) comparable with postmenopausal women (Reid et al 2008).

The elderly

A number of large studies have investigated the preventive effect of calcium alone or in combination with vitamin D in the elderly. Studies by Chapuy et al (1992, 1994, 2002), Dawson-Hughes et al (1997) and Larsen et al (2004) demonstrate a significant reduction in fracture risk (≤16%), while a meta-analysis of 29 RCTs conducted in 63,897 individuals 50 years of age or older over an average of 3.5 years also concluded that calcium alone (≥1200 mg/day) or in combination with vitamin D (≥800 IU/day) reduced the risk of fracture by 12–24% and reduced bone loss by 0.54% at the hip and 1.19% at the spine (Tang et al 2007).

More recently, a meta-analysis of over 68,000 participants (mean age 69.9 years) concluded that calcium combined with vitamin D significantly but modestly reduced hip fractures and total fractures, and probably vertebral fractures, irrespective of age, sex or previous fractures (2010).

In general, the greatest improvements are noted specifically in the elderly, institutionalised, underweight and calcium deficient.

Glucocorticoid (GC)-induced osteoporosis

Glucocorticoid-induced osteoporosis is the leading cause of osteoporosis in young adults and the most common cause of secondary osteoporosis. GCs induce rapid bone loss and increase the risk of fracture; however, the fracture risk is higher than expected based on bone mineral density values suggesting excess bone fragility is multifactorial (Soen 2013). GCs have a negative impact on bone through direct effects on bone cells and indirect effects on calcium absorption (Warriner & Saag 2013).

The use of GCs is widespread in medicine as they are used in almost all medical specialties. They are also used long-term by various patient groups such as those with severe asthma or rheumatological disease. In regards to rheumatological disease, morbidity secondary to the use of GCs represents an important aspect of the management as the incidences of vertebral and non-vertebral fractures are elevated, ranging from 30% to 50% of the individuals on GC for over 3 months (Pereira et al 2012). The risk or fracture is also elevated among asthmatics receiving inhaled and/or systemic glucocorticoids, with one report indicating approximately one in six people with asthma developed fractures over 5 years. The interaction with calcium plays a small role in this process, with GCs directly inhibiting vitamin D-mediated intestinal absorption of calcium. High vitamin D doses (50,000 IU twice weekly) in combination with 1.5 g calcium daily can overcome this interference (Wilson et al 1991), whereas treatment with calcium alone or in combination with etidronate may not be effective (Campbell et al 2004).

Supplementation during pregnancy and lactation

The NHMRC nutrient reference value recommendations for calcium intakes for pregnant women (ages 14–18 years) are 1300 mg/day and 1000 mg/day for older women (19–50 years). If the woman avoids dairy in her usual diet (e.g. lactose intolerant) and does not consume alternative high calcium food (e.g. calcium enriched soya milk), calcium supplementation is recommended at 1000 mg/day. Sufficient calcium intake is important as deficiency is associated with preeclampsia and intrauterine growth restriction. Supplementation may reduce both the risk of low birth weight and the severity of preeclampsia (Hovdenak & Haram 2012).

Evidence from 1997 found that approximately 40% of primiparous Australian women failed to meet the RDI for calcium. Considered a critical nutrient during pregnancy with at least a two-fold increase in requirements observed, its metabolism during gestation significantly changes from as early as 12 weeks, with doubling of both absorption and excretion, followed by additional losses through lactation, which can account for reductions in maternal bone mineral content of 3–10% (Prentice 2003).

Prevention of hypertension and preeclampsia

Gestational hypertensive disorders are the second leading cause of maternal deaths worldwide. Both epidemiological and clinical studies have shown that an inverse relationship exists between calcium intake and development of hypertension in pregnancy (Imdad & Bhutta 2012).

A 2012 systematic review analysing results from 15 RCTs confirmed that calcium supplementation during pregnancy is associated with a significant reduction in risk of gestational hypertensive disorders and pre-term birth and an increase in birthweight (85 gm) without any associated increased risk of kidney stones. Pooled analysis showed that calcium supplementation during pregnancy reduced risk of preeclampsia by 52% and that of severe preeclampsia by 25%. There was no effect on incidence of eclampsia. Importantly, there was a significant reduction for risk of maternal mortality/severe morbidity by 20% and a 24% reduction in risk of preterm birth with calcium supplementation during pregnancy (Imdad & Bhutta 2012).

Trials that included a 1996 meta-analysis of studies involving calcium and hypertension in pregnancy have shown a substantial mean reduction in both systolic blood pressure (SBP) and diastolic blood pressure (DBP), which was also confirmed by more recent reviews (Atallah et al 2002, Bucher et al 1996).

Further reviews of studies involving over 15,000 women, however, have supported calcium's preventive role with researchers demonstrating significant risk reduction in both low-risk (RR 0.48) and high-risk women (RR 0.22), hence concluding calcium supplementation should be recommended for those women with a low calcium intake who are at risk of developing gestational hypertension (Crowther et al 1999, Hofmeyr et al 2003, 2006, 2007).

There is currently no unanimous explanation for calcium's protective effect (Villar et al 2003). While the antagonistic relationship between calcium and lead has been previously hypothesised to be involved (Sowers et al 2002), recent evidence of calcium's lack of effect on platelet count, plasma urate and proteinuria, in spite of reducing preeclamptic incidence, implies that high-dose calcium effectively lowers blood pressure without influencing the condition's underlying pathology (Hofmeyr et al 2008).

A small number of studies have investigated the effects of calcium in combination with other nutrients, including antioxidant and omega-3 oils in this population. One randomised, placebo-controlled, double-blind study involving a sample of 48 primigravidas, using a combination of 600 mg/day calcium and 450 mg/day of conjugated linoleic acid (CLA) from weeks 18–22 until delivery, resulted in a significantly reduced incidence of pregnancy-induced hypertension (8% vs 42% of the control group) (Herrera et al 2005). Further studies are warranted to elicit the individual impact of both nutrients and to determine the superiority of sole or combination treatment.

Leg cramps

Calcium supplements are commonly prescribed in pregnancy when leg cramps are a problem. A Cochrane review of five trials involving 352 women taking various supplements for the treatment of leg cramps in pregnancy included only one placebo-controlled trial of calcium. From this, researchers concluded that any improvement in cramps in those groups treated solely with calcium was likely to be due to a placebo effect, with significant findings limited to the groups taking other nutrients (Young & Jewell 2013).

Lead toxicity

Increased blood lead levels may occur during pregnancy and lactation as a result of bone resorption to accommodate the calcium needs of the developing fetus or nursing infant. Lead exposure is considered a potential risk to fetal and infant health and may affect fetal neurodevelopment and growth. Ninety-five per cent of lead is stored in the bone and, if mobilised, can be transferred to the fetus and infant via cord blood and breast milk (Ettinger et al 2007). Several studies suggest a low placental barrier to lead, with 79% of the mobilised lead from maternal bone passed to the infant (Dorea & Donangelo 2005). While a number of studies have indicated lead levels in the breast milk of Australian women appear to be well within a safe range, recent data from a study conducted by Ettinger et al (2004) revealed that even low lead content in human milk appears to be highly influential on the lead levels of infants in their first month of life. A separate review published in 2005 discussed additional related trends, such as increased lead concentrations in cord blood during winter months, because of lower vitamin D status (Dorea 2004).

Dietary calcium supplementation of 1200 mg/day commencing in the first trimester was associated with modest reductions in blood lead during pregnancy and may reduce risk of fetal exposure, according to the findings of a RCT of 670 pregnant women (Ettinger et al 2009).

A RCT of 617 lactating women supplemented with high-dose calcium carbonate found that the women in the calcium group showed significant reductions in blood lead levels. Those subjects who showed improved compliance and also had baseline higher bone lead content produced an overall reduction of 16.4% (Hernandez-Avila et al 2003). Similar positive findings came from a study in Mexico of 367 lactating women; however, the maximal reduction in lead concentrations reached only 10% (Ettinger et al 2006). When considered together, these results suggest that calcium supplementation may represent an important interventional strategy, albeit with a modest effect, for reducing infant lead exposure.

Neonatal benefits

Calcium supplementation during pregnancy has been postulated to have prolonged benefits in the offspring, as indicated in a study of nearly 600 children aged 5–9 years whose mothers had previously participated in a calcium trial during their pregnancy. The children demonstrated reduced SBP, compared with the children whose mothers had taken placebo, with significance reached particularly for those in the upper BMI bracket (Belizan et al 1997). More recent reviews, while still demonstrating some association between gestational calcium supplementation and reduced blood pressure and incidence of hypertension in the offspring (particularly older children e.g. 7 years), highlight the weakness of the evidence to date, including small sample sizes, methodological issues and the fact that most of the studies have been conducted in developed countries where calcium intake is more likely to be adequate (Bergel & Barros 2007, Hiller et al 2007).

Dyspepsia

A first-line over-the-counter (OTC) treatment for heartburn, indigestion and dyspepsia has often been an antacid, based on calcium carbonate in combination with magnesium and aluminium salts. Calcium, alone or in combination with the other ingredients, neutralises stomach acid allowing for immediate short-term symptomatic relief (Kopic & Giebel 2013, Sulz et al 2007). There have been case-reports of milk-alkali syndrome associated with excessive prolonged use of calcium carbonate products, especially for dyspepsia, however the incidence appears rare (Kopic & Giebel 2013, Bailey et al 2008, Picolos et al 2004, Nabhan et al 2004, Beall & Scofield 1995). Long-term use of calcium carbonate as an antacid has largely been superseded by use of H_2-antagonists or proton pump inhibitors, thus the milk-alkali risk is possibly also of less clinical relevance than it was several years ago.

Prevention of cancer

Interest in a relationship between dairy consumption and cancer incidence continues to grow, with evidence of both protective and contributory effects dependent upon both cancer type and timing of exposure. The consumption of dairy products, however, represents a mix of numerous variables and biological pathways that potentially convey these underlying actions, from which calcium's role is difficult to extricate (van der Pols et al 2007). An interventional study of calcium (1400–1500 mg/day), alone or with vitamin D_3 (1100 IU/day) compared to placebo over 4 years, offers more specific information regarding calcium's role in cancer (Lappe et al 2007). The study, conducted in 1179 women of more than 55 years, was primarily designed to assess effects on fracture incidence; however, upon further analysis also demonstrated significant risk reduction (RR 0.40) for all cancer incidence among the calcium and vitamin D group. When the analysis was restricted to only those cancers diagnosed after the first year of treatment, the RR became 0.23. While the group receiving calcium alone also demonstrated a reduced risk, the researchers speculate that this may not be robust and conclude that vitamin D is the key variable in reduced incidence of all cancer.

Prevention of colorectal cancer and recurrence of adenomatous polyps

Currently, the gold standard for measuring risk reduction by an intervention in colorectal cancer investigates the incidence of recurrence of adenomatous polyps following removal of all colonic polyps by polypectomy; further analyses evaluate reduction of total adenomatous polyps and reduction of advanced polyps as defined by size and the presence of severe dysplasia.

Low calcium intake has been associated with a higher risk of colorectal cancer (Kim et al 2013). A meta-analysis of 10 cohort studies showed a reduction in risk of colorectal cancer in those with a higher calcium intake (Cho et al 2004). Reasonably consistent evidence suggests that calcium supplementation of 1200 mg/day reduces total adenomas by approximately 20% and advanced adenomas by about 45% (Holt 2008). Calcium supplementation may also significantly prevent risk of recurrence of adenomas 3–4 years after initial removal, according to findings of a meta-analysis of three trials (n = 1485) (Shaukat et al 2005). Further to this, a 2008 Cochrane review examining the effect of supplementary calcium on the incidence of colorectal cancer and the incidence or recurrence of adenomatous polyps included two double-blind, placebo-controlled trials with a pooled population of 1346 subjects. Doses of supplementary elemental calcium used were 1200–2000 mg/day for 3–4 years. Reviewers concluded that, while the evidence to date appears promising and suggests a moderate degree of prevention against colorectal adenomatous polyps, more research with similar findings is required before this can be translated into any preventive protocol (Weingarten et al 2008).

Interestingly, some studies show that calcium's protective effect against recurrent adenomas is largely restricted to individuals with baseline serum 25-hydroxy vitamin D above the median (≈ 29 ng/mL). These data, together with other research findings, strongly point to the importance of both calcium and vitamin D for reducing colorectal cancer risk and altering adenoma recurrence (Mizoue et al 2008, Grau et al 2003, Holt 2008, Oh et al 2007).

Interactions between calcium and other variables in colorectal carcinogenesis have also been explored, revealing gender-specific results; protective in males but not in females in most (Ishihara et al 2008, Jacobs et al 2007, Ryan-Harshman & Aldoori 2007), but not all, studies. Further research, including re-analysis of the Women's Health Initiative (WHI) findings pertaining to colorectal cancer incidence, has elucidated oestrogen's critical modifying effect upon calcium, whereby the higher oestrogen levels of both menstruating and postmenopausal women taking HRT negate calcium's otherwise protective effect (Ding et al 2008). Explanations for this phenomenon include oestrogen's influence upon calcium distribution: removing it from circulation for bone deposition and competition for binding evident between vitamin D and oestrogen (Ding et al 2008, Oh et al 2007).

Early hypotheses regarding calcium's general protective effects focused on its ability to bind bowel-irritating substances secreted into bile. This notion is further supported by a number of studies demonstrating enhanced chemoprotection when high doses of calcium have been combined with dietary factors such as reduced fat and increased carbohydrate, fibre and fluid intakes (Hyman et al 1998, Rozen et al 2001, Schatzkin & Peters 2004).

One significant development in our understanding has been the discovery of human parathyroid calcium-sensing receptors in the human colon epithelium, which function to regulate epithelial proliferation and differentiation. New in vitro studies suggest that expression of these receptors may be induced by the presence of extracellular calcium and vitamin D, therefore promoting greater differentiation of the epithelial cells (Chakrabarty et al 2005, Holt 2008) and inducing apoptosis (Miller et al 2005). The effect of the calcium-sensing receptor (CASR) gene on development of colorectal cancer has also been investigated, with in vitro studies suggesting that CASR may mediate the pro-cell proliferative effects of low intestinal calcium concentration. Results from a recent case-controlled study involving 1235 participants showed that low calcium intake was associated with an increase in colorectal cancer risk; however, this did not appear to relate directly to CASR polymorphism (Kim et al 2013).

Clear parameters for dosing are not yet available, with some studies showing no further benefit above 700–800 mg/day of total calcium, while other studies suggest an ongoing inverse dose-dependent relationship without cutoff (Schatzkin & Peters 2004). Current evidence for a combined protective role of calcium, either dietary or supplemental, and vitamin D, particularly in men and postmenopausal women not taking HRT, is strong and further elucidation of the independent and combined effects of these nutrients will assist in the development of preventive protocols.

Other cancers

Ongoing research regarding calcium's potential role in a range of other cancers suggests a possible protective effect against breast and ovarian cancers (Genkinger et al 2006, McCullough et al 2005, 2008); however, the research remains preliminary and largely of epidemiological design. A greater body of evidence has developed regarding the interplay between calcium and prostate cancer, with initial findings touting a positive association between dairy product consumption, total dietary calcium intake (especially >1500 mg/day) and risk. The results of ongoing extensive, prospective epidemiological research involving hundreds of thousands of men, however, have been conflicting, both confirming (Ahn et al 2008, Gao et al 2005) and negating (Huncharek et al 2008a, Park et al 2007a, 2007b) earlier evidence. Two important details have recently emerged regarding the potential interaction between calcium and prostate cancer risk with several studies consistently demonstrating that calcium derived from supplements does not convey a greater risk (Ahn et al 2008, Baron et al 2005, Park et al 2007a) and limiting calcium as a risk factor only when consumed as dairy products, while greater non-dairy calcium intake appears to lower the risk (Allen et al 2008, Park et al 2007b). A prospective study of serum calcium adds to the riddle, revealing that results in the highest tertile typically more than 9 years prior to diagnosis were strongly associated with increased risk of fatal prostate cancer (Skinner & Schwartz 2008); however, such results may be indicative of calcium dysregulation rather than high intakes.

Hypertension

Ongoing broad-scale international epidemiological data, including prospective studies, link low dietary calcium intake with a slightly increased risk of hypertension (Alonso et al 2005, Elliott et al 2008, Geleijnse et al 2005, Wang et al 2008), in particular raised systolic blood pressure. Conversely, increased dietary calcium, typically in the form of low-fat dairy products, has been shown to be independently protective (RR 0.87 for highest quintile of calcium intake) (Alonso et al 2005, Wang et al 2008). One study identified that high dietary calcium was associated with SBP/DBP reductions of −2.42/−1.48 mmHg, after controlling for other known risk factors (Elliott et al 2008). This effect was more pronounced when accompanied by increased magnesium and phosphorus consumption. Interestingly, neither high-fat dairy products nor calcium supplements convey protection (Wang et al 2008).

Additional findings attracting attention include epidemiological links between markers of low calcium status or calcium metabolism abnormalities, hypertension and insulin resistance. Supporting the possible link between these phenomena are the results of a Japanese study of 34 non-diabetic hypertensive and 34 non-diabetic normotensive women. Multiple group assessments revealed statistically significant increased urinary calcium, lower BMD, depressed serum calcium and elevated circulating PTH in the hypertensive sample (Gotoh et al 2005).

Underlying mechanisms for calcium's protective effect are speculated to involve reduced calcium influx into cells, inhibiting vascular smooth muscle cell constriction, reduced activity of the renin–angiotensin system and improved Na/K balance (Wang et al 2008).

A 2006 Cochrane review of 13 RCTs involving 485 volunteers found that calcium supplementation significantly reduced SBP (mean difference: −2.5 mmHg), but not DBP (mean difference: −0.8 mmHg) compared with controls (Dickinson et al 2006). The authors temper their conclusion, stating that the quality of included trials was poor and the heterogeneity between trials means there is a tendency to overestimate treatment effects. Earlier, an extensive systematic review, updated in 1999 to include 42 randomised comparative trials, showed modest reductions in both SBP and DBP (−2 mmHg and −1 mmHg, respectively) with 1–2 g/day calcium over a 4–14-week intervention (Griffith et al 1999). Dietary calcium appeared to have a larger effect than supplementation, a finding reiterated in more recent studies (Wang et al 2008). The clinical significance of these small effects has been questioned and the recommendation of calcium as a therapy for all types of hypertension appears premature (Kawano et al 1998), particularly in light of more recent negative findings from the WHI, which investigated the effects of 1 g of calcium together with 400 IU of vitamin D over a median follow-up period of 7 years in postmenopausal women (Margolis et al 2008). Some studies have proposed that it is only a particular hypertensive subset that is calcium responsive. A number of researchers, for example, have hypothesised a physiological correlation between 'salt sensitive' hypertension and responsiveness to calcium treatment (Coruzzi & Mossini 1997, Resnick 1999). The link may be that sodium excess encourages calcium losses. This theory is further supported by an epidemiological study demonstrating that, while blood pressure was inversely correlated with dietary calcium, further analysis revealed sodium intake to be the primary influence, increasing pressures while concomitantly reducing BMD (Woo et al 2008).

Premenstrual syndrome

Of all the vitamins and minerals used in the treatment of premenstrual syndrome (PMS), calcium supplements show overwhelmingly positive results.

One of the earliest trials to show that calcium supplementation can alleviate symptoms in PMS was conducted in 1989 (Thys-Jacobs et al 1989). A randomised, double-blind, crossover trial involving 33 women with confirmed PMS compared the effects of daily 1000 mg calcium carbonate with placebo over 6 months. Results showed that 73% of women reported improved symptoms while taking calcium supplementation, whereas 15% preferred placebo. The premenstrual symptoms responding significantly to calcium supplementation were mood changes, water retention and premenstrual pain. Menstrual pain was also significantly alleviated.

In 1993, the *American Journal of Obstetrics and Gynecology* published a study that compared the effects of calcium (587 mg or 1336 mg) and manganese (1.0 mg or 5.6 mg) on menstrual symptoms. Ten women with normal menstrual cycles were observed over four 39-day periods during the trial (Penland & Johnson 1993). The researchers found that increasing calcium intake reduced mood, concentration and behavioural symptoms generally and reduced water retention during the premenstrual phase. Additionally, menstrual pain was reduced.

A more recent large, double-blind, placebo-controlled, randomised parallel-group study was conducted in the United States and supports the previous findings (Thys-Jacobs et al 1998). Four hundred and sixty-six premenopausal women with confirmed moderate to severe PMS were randomly assigned to receive either 1200 mg elemental calcium (from calcium carbonate) or placebo for three menstrual cycles. Symptoms were documented daily by the subjects based on 17 core symptoms and four symptom factors (negative affect, water retention, food cravings and pain). Additionally, adverse effects and compliance were monitored daily. During the luteal phases of both the second and the third treatment cycles, a significantly lower mean symptom score was observed in the calcium group. By the third treatment cycle, calcium treatment resulted in a 48% reduction in total symptom score compared with baseline, whereas placebo achieved a 30% reduction. Furthermore, all four symptom factors responded in the calcium-treated group.

A 1999 review of multiple trials investigating calcium supplementation as an effective therapy for PMS has found overwhelming positive results (Ward & Holimon 1999).

The only RCT to be conducted in recent years was published in 2009 and once again produced positive results. The double-blind RCT compared 500 mg of calcium carbonate twice daily to placebo taken for 3 months by young female college students (mean age 21.4 ± 3.6 years) with diagnosed PMS. Active treatment resulted in significant improvements to early tiredness, appetite changes and depressive symptoms compared to placebo (Ghanbari et al 2009).

Some researchers in this area have hypothesised that part of the PMS aetiology lies in calcium dysregulation in the luteal phase and have highlighted the dramatic similarities between symptoms of PMS and hypocalcaemia (Thys-Jacobs 2000). Recent data from the Nurses' Health Study II support this theory, with evidence of low calcium and vitamin D levels in PMS populations when compared to controls (Bertone-Johnson et al 2005).

Weight loss

Evidence suggests that higher calcium intake may be associated with a lower body weight. This has been seen in several epidemiological studies and also some, but not all, studies using calcium supplementation (Onakpoya et al 2011, Tremblay & Gilbert 2011, Christensen et al 2009, Barba & Russo 2006, Garcia-Lorad et al 2007, Bueno et al 2008, Zhu et al 2013).

A relationship between low calcium intake and obesity was observed in an epidemiological study involving 1459 adults in Brazil, where the prevalence of participants that were overweight was higher in those with a low calcium intake, especially when less than 398.5 mg/day (Bueno et al 2008). Similarly, a negative relationship between calcium intake and BMI was reported in a study of 647 Spanish men and women (Garcia-Lorad et al 2007).

A meta-analysis of seven RCTs reported that calcium supplementation in overweight and obese individuals results in a small, but significant reduction in body weight (0.74 kg) and body fat (0.93 kg) compared to placebo. This review excluded studies that had been conducted for less than 6 months or that included subjects that were of a normal weight (Onakpoya et al 2011).

A prolific researcher in this area is Zemel (2004, Zemel et al 2004, 2005a, 2005b), having published three small trials investigating the effects of dietary and supplemental calcium in patients for weight maintenance or weight loss. These trials have consistently yielded positive results, demonstrating that in addition to enhanced weight loss on isocaloric and identical macronutrient profiles, with or without energy restriction, a diet providing high calcium levels of 1100–1200 mg/day results in central fat loss and corresponding improvements in blood pressure, insulin sensitivity and retention of lean tissue. Australian researchers Bowen and colleagues have also demonstrated similar results (Bowen et al 2004). Zemel et al conclude that dietary calcium and, in particular, dairy-based foods are the most effective form of calcium for weight loss and that results are significant within 12 weeks.An early review by Teegarden (2003), bringing together trials dating back 10 years to the first rat studies and updated in 2005, while acknowledging the promising data in relation to increased consumption of dairy products and weight management which had emerged over the intervening 2 years, noted the limitations of the current body of evidence that required addressing to elucidate the full extent of calcium's effect on weight. A more recent meta-analysis of 13 RCTs investigating calcium interventions ranging between 610 mg and 2400 mg/day over a period of 12 weeks–36 months failed to demonstrate a positive effect on weight loss for either calcium supplements or dairy products; however, once again methodological concerns were raised (Trowman et al 2006). In particular, this meta-analysis included RCTs designed to investigate the effects of calcium on bone health and only one of the included RCTs was specifically designed and powered to see if calcium supplementation altered fat loss. As Astrup (2008) notes in an editorial piece, this point is highly relevant, because a body fat loss of ≈1 kg/year may be extremely important in the prevention of weight gain and obesity, but large study groups are required in a randomised trial to obtain the statistical power necessary to detect such an effect (Astrup 2008).

In spite of this, studies have continued to emerge yielding positive findings in postmenopausal women as part of the WHI study (calcium and vitamin D treatment reducing risk of weight gain by 11%) (Caan et al 2007) and in overweight and obese type 2 diabetic patients (>8% more weight loss in those consuming calcium in the highest compared with the lowest tertile) (Shahar et al 2007). Additionally, one small study demonstrated an augmenting effect of calcium (1200 mg together with 400 IU vitamin D/day) over 15 weeks on weight loss-induced beneficial changes to blood lipids and lipoproteins (Major et al 2007). Most recently, an RCT involving 53 subjects showed that calcium (600 mg elemental/day) plus vitamin D_3 (125 IU/day) supplementation for 12 weeks promoted loss of body fat and visceral fat (Zhu et al 2013).

Although the underlying mechanism of action remains unclear, there is general acceptance that high calcium intake, particularly in the form of dairy products, and more recently calcium-fortified soy (Lukaszuk et al 2007), depresses PTH levels and $1,25(OH)_2D$, which in turn decreases intracellular calcium, thereby potentially inhibiting lipogenesis and stimulating lipolysis (Major et al 2007, McCarty & Thomas 2003, Schrager 2005, Zemel et al 2004). Additional proposed actions include promoting faecal fat loss and fat oxidation (Christensen et al 2009, Gonzalez et al 2012, Tremblay & Gilbert 2011), as well as by decreasing energy intake and facilitating appetite control (Tremblay & Gilbert 2011) and promoting satiety (Kabrnova-Hlavata et al 2008).

Christensen et al (2009) performed a meta-analysis of 15 RCTs that assessed the effect of calcium on faecal fat loss, The authors concluded that an increase in dietary calcium by about 1240 mg/day has the potential to increase faecal fat excretion by about 5.2 g/day, which is enough to be relevant for prevention of weight gain, or re-gain (Christensen et al 2009). Another meta-analysis investigating mechanisms by which calcium intake may affect weight reported that a high calcium intake appears to increase rate of fat oxidation, however the magnitude of effect appears relatively weak (Gonzalez et al 2012).

Nephrolithiasis

In spite of previous concerns regarding a causal relationship between dietary or supplemental calcium intake and the recurrence of oxalate stones, recent studies demonstrate that this fear appears unfounded. Collectively, the evidence points more towards a protective effect for increased dietary calcium, in relation to both urinary oxalate concentrations (Taylor & Curhan 2004) and reduced stone formation (Goldfarb 2009). The current view is that, rather than being a contributing factor for oxalate stones, dietary calcium, through its binding of oxalate in the gut, can minimise recurrence, as substantiated by other studies (Curhan et al 1997, Liebman & Chai 1997).

One study comprised 120 men with recurrent calcium oxalate stones due to idiopathic hypercalciuria and who were randomly assigned to either a low-calcium diet or low-animal protein, low-salt normal-calcium diet and assessed for changes in frequency of stone formation. Results clearly showed reduced oxalate excretion in those on a normal calcium intake, as well as a greater decrease in calcium oxalate saturation (Borghi et al 2002). In another study of 14 healthy men, assessment of the influence of dietary calcium on the given amount of oxalate demonstrated that with the inclusion of additional calcium (1121 mg) urinary oxalate levels increased in the control but not in the treatment group (Hess et al 1998).

OTHER USES

Hyperlipidaemia

Only a very few studies investigating calcium intake and serum lipids in postmenopausal women have been described and these showed significant increases in high-density lipoprotein and high-density lipoprotein to low-density lipoprotein ratio (Challoumas et al 2013).

For example, a randomised, placebo-controlled crossover trial of 56 patients with mild–moderate hypercholesterolaemia on a controlled low-cholesterol diet, calcium carbonate supplementation was shown to significantly reduce LDL levels by 4.4%, with additional 4.1% increases in HDL levels. No other effects on other blood lipids or blood pressure were observed (Bell et al 1992). Another small study demonstrated an augmenting effect of calcium (1200 mg together with 400 IU vitamin D/day) over 15 weeks on weight loss-induced beneficial changes to blood lipids and lipoproteins, with significantly greater reductions in total HDL, LDL:HDL and LDL levels (Major et al 2007).

Dry eye

A controlled double-masked study of petrolatum ointment containing 10% w/w calcium carbonate applied on the lower lid twice daily for 3 months resulted in significant improvements in all criteria assessed. However, significance over placebo was only found in ocular surface staining, therefore determination of the action of petrolatum needs to be established and controlled in future studies to identify the therapeutic value of calcium (Tsubota et al 1999).

Fluorosis

Calcium has been shown to reduce the clinical manifestations of fluorosis in children exposed to contaminated water (Gupta et al 1996).

DOSAGE RANGE

Australian RDIs

- Infants
  1–3 years: 500 mg/day.
  4–8 years: 700 mg/day.
- Children
  9–11 years: 1000 mg/day.
  12–18 years: 1300 mg/day.
- Adults
  <70 years: 1000 mg/day.
  >70 years: 1300 mg/day.
- Pregnancy: 1000–1300 mg/day.
- Lactation: 1000–1300 mg/day.

According to clinical studies

- Osteoporosis prophylaxis: 1500 mg/day in combination with vitamin D and accessory nutrients (e.g. zinc, manganese, copper and fluoride) and/or antiresorptive agents
- Premenstrual syndrome: 1200–1600 mg/day; however, 500 mg calcium carbonate twice daily for 3 months is also effective
- Prevention of preeclampsia: 2000 mg/day.
- Increased BMD in children with low intake: 100 mg/day.
- Supplementation during pregnancy to increase mineral accretion in fetus: 2000 mg/day for last trimester.
- Allergic rhinitis: 100 mg/day.
- Hyperacidity: 500–1500 mg/day as required.
- Hyperlipidaemia: 400 mg three times daily.
- Hypertension: 1000–2000 mg/day.
- Dry eye: 10% w/w calcium carbonate in petrolatum base applied twice daily.
- Fluorosis in children: 250 mg/day.
- Prevention of colorectal cancer: 1200 mg/day.
- Weight loss: 1000–1200 mg/day long term.

ADVERSE REACTIONS

Oral administration of calcium supplements may cause gastrointestinal discomfort, nausea, constipation and flatulence.

Hypercalcaemia

Increased serum calcium may be associated with anorexia, nausea and vomiting, constipation, hypotonia, depression and occasionally lethargy and coma. Prolonged hypercalcaemic states, especially if associated with normal or elevated serum phosphate, can precipitate ectopic calcification of blood vessels, connective tissues around joints, gastric mucosa, cornea and renal tissue (Wilson et al 1991).

SIGNIFICANT INTERACTIONS

Calcium carbonate when taken as an antacid alters the absorption and excretion of a wide range of drugs. Please refer to a drug interaction guide for specific concerns. Only those interactions encountered with oral administration of calcium supplements will be included in this section.

Antacids, including H_2 antagonists and proton pump inhibitors

Use of drugs that raise gastric pH may reduce calcium absorption, especially that of calcium carbonate or calcium phosphate as these salts require an acidic environment for solubilisation before

C

Clinical note — Is calcium supplementation a risk for increased vascular events?

Recently, concern has emerged regarding a potential increase in cardiovascular events associated with long-term high-dose calcium supplementation. This was largely triggered by the results of a New Zealand RCT investigating the effect of calcium supplements (1000 mg/day elemental calcium as calcium citrate) administered to 1471 postmenopausal women, with an average age 74 years, over 5 years. Concomitant vitamin D supplements were not given to participants in this trial (Bolland et al 2008). The primary outcome of this study was bone density; however, the researchers also hypothesised that a secondary effect of the treatment would be a reduction in cardiovascular (CV) events, based on existing observational studies highlighting calcium's positive effect on blood lipids and blood pressure (Nainggolan 2008). However, secondary analysis of the data revealed that the women taking calcium supplements experienced an increase in CV events rather than the expected decrease in CV event. In the calcium-treated group, there was a statistically significant higher rate of verified myocardial infarction (MI) ($P = 0.05$), and a non-significant increase in all vascular events ($P = 0.08$) and stroke ($P = 0.21$), compared to those taking placebo. While the authors concluded that their study does not unequivocally demonstrate causality, it did suggest that high calcium intakes may have an adverse effect on vascular health (Bolland et al 2008).

The same authors subsequently conducted a meta-analysis of 15 RCT of calcium ≥500 mg vs placebo, concluding that in the absence of vitamin D, calcium supplements were associated with a significant increase in MI ($P = 0.035$) and non-significant increase in composite end point of MI, stroke or sudden death ($P = 0.057$) or death ($P = 0.18$) (Bolland et al 2010). In addition, this research group conducted a re-analysis of data from a sub-group in the Women's Health Initiative Calcium Vitamin D study (WHI CaD) and concluded that calcium, with or without vitamin D, modestly increased risk of CV events, especially for MI (Bolland et al 2011).

While these findings have caused substantial alarm and led to much speculation, the evidence suggesting cardiovascular harm needs to be balanced against the body of opposing evidence that reports that calcium does not significantly increase cardiovascular event risk.

Daily supplementation with calcium carbonate 1000 mg plus vitamin D 400 IU for 7 years showed neither an increase nor a decrease in coronary or cerebrovascular events in a large-scale study (WHI CaD) involving 36,282 postmenopausal women aged 50–79 years (Hsia et al 2007). Another prospective study (EPIC-Heidelberg) that involved almost 24000 participants with an 11-year follow-up found no significant association between calcium intake and risk of stroke or cardiovascular mortality. Interestingly, a trend towards a decrease in MI risk was observed in those with a moderately high dairy calcium intake (mean = 820 mg/day), especially in women. By contrast, a statistically significant increase in MI was found in the group taking supplemental calcium in the absence of vitamin D; however, this may not be clinically meaningful as it translated to only 20 cases of MI in the calcium users, out of 24,000 participants (Li et al 2012). Results from the NHANES III study ($n = 20,024$) reported that there was no clear association for CVD death and intake of dietary or supplemental calcium (van Hemelrijk et al 2013). Another large prospective study involving 388,229 men and women aged 50–71 years, with a 12-year follow-up, reported that supplemental calcium intake was not associated with increased CVD or cerebrovascular death in women, although an increase CV risk was observed in men taking supplemental calcium (>1000 mg/day), who were also smokers (Xiao et al 2013).

Further to this, a 5-year study of 1460 older women suggested that supplementation with calcium carbonate (1200 mg/day) may reduce risk of hospitalisation and mortality in patients with pre-existing atherosclerotic CVD (Lewis et al 2011). It has been proposed that high calcium intake may increase risk of vascular calcification, or carotid atherosclerosis, although this effect was not demonstrated in recent studies (Lewis et al 2013, Kim et al 2012). In addition, there is some evidence that calcium may have a beneficial role in terms of cardiovascular disease by modestly reducing blood pressure and improving serum lipid profiles (Guessous et al 2011). In addition, a review of studies involving over 70,000 people concluded that mortality was reduced with vitamin D plus calcium (odds ratio, 0.94; 95% CI, 0.88–0.99), but not with vitamin D alone (odds ratio, 0.98; 95% CI, 0.91–1.06) (Rejnmark et al 2012).

While it is difficult at this stage to either confirm or refute the association between calcium supplementation and cardiovascular disease, there are a few factors for consideration:

- No RCTs have been conducted to specifically examine the effects of calcium supplementation on CVD morbidity and mortality; concerns have been raised due to secondary data analysis
- Current data does not support an association between dietary or supplemental calcium intake and an increased risk of stroke, cerebrovascular disease, cardiovascular disease or cardiovascular death
- Increased dietary intake of calcium has not been associated with an increase in risk of myocardial infarction
- Supplemental calcium may possibly be associated with an increased risk of myocardial infarction, but this appears to be limited to calcium given alone, without vitamin D.
- Known benefits of combined calcium and vitamin D therapy for reducing risk of osteoporotic fractures needs to be balanced against unproven risk of MI when making treatment decisions for an individual patient, and research now indicates that calcium and vitamin D reduce mortality in the elderly.

calcium can be absorbed. Aluminium- and magnesium-containing antacids may increase urinary excretion of calcium.

Bisphosphonates

Bisphosphonates (e.g. alendronate) are indicated for the treatment of osteoporosis; however, they commonly cause hypocalcaemia as an adverse effect, which reduces drug effectiveness in maintaining bone mineral density. Adequate intake of both calcium and vitamin D is essential for those taking bisphosphonates, however the drug must be taken on an empty stomach, at least 30 minutes before calcium supplementation.

Caffeine

Caffeine increases urinary excretion of calcium and may affect calcium absorption — ensure adequate calcium intake and monitor for signs and symptoms of deficiency in those with high caffeine intake.

Calcium channel blockers

Calcium supplements can have an antagonistic effect on the desired action of calcium channel blockers that could precipitate the re-emergence of arrhythmias — avoid high-dose supplements unless under professional supervision.

Cardiac glycosides (e.g. digoxin)

Administered concurrently, high-dose calcium may potentiate digoxin toxicity — use this combination with caution unless under medical supervision.

Corticosteroids

Long-term use of corticosteroids, especially oral formulations, may lead to reduced intestinal calcium absorption, increased calcium excretion and inhibition of osteoblasts, leading to drug-induced osteoporosis — ensure adequate calcium intake and monitor for signs and symptoms of deficiency. Consider supplementation with long-term drug therapy.

Excess dietary fat

This increases urinary excretion of calcium — ensure adequate calcium intake and monitor for signs and symptoms of deficiency.

Excess fibre, including guar gum

May simply delay or decrease absorption of calcium — separate doses by at least 2 hours.

Iron

Concurrent administration of calcium with iron may reduce absorption of both minerals. Separate supplemental or dietary intake of minerals by at least 2 hours.

Levothyroxine

Calcium administered concurrently may reduce drug absorption, while levothyroxine may block absorption of calcium, e.g. calcium carbonate — separate doses by at least 4 hours.

Lysine

Additive effects may occur as lysine enhances intestinal absorption and reduces renal excretion of calcium — potentially beneficial interaction.

Magnesium

Magnesium decreases calcium absorption as they compete for the same absorption pathway, however it is unclear if this mineral interaction is clinically significant — it is advisable to separate doses by at least 2 hours.

Oestrogen and progesterone

Calcium supplementation in combination with these hormones will have an additive effect on minimising bone resorption in postmenopausal women — potential beneficial interaction, so consider increasing intake.

Phosphorus

Excess intake (soft drinks, meat consumption) can increase urinary excretion of calcium — ensure adequate calcium intake and monitor for signs and symptoms of deficiency.

Quinolone antibiotics

Drug bioavailability may be reduced by concurrent administration with calcium supplements, reducing drug efficacy and increasing risk of developing bacterial resistance — quinolones should be taken either 2 hours before or 4–6 hours after calcium.

Tetracyclines

Calcium supplements form complexes with these antibiotics and render 50% or more insoluble, therefore reducing the efficacy of the drug and absorption of calcium — separate doses by at least 2 hours.

Thiazide diuretics

These diuretics decrease urinary excretion of calcium. Monitor serum calcium and look for signs of hypercalcaemia, such as anorexia, polydipsia, polyuria, constipation and muscle hypertonia when using high-dose calcium supplements. Contributing risk factors are the presence of hyperparathyroidism or concurrent use of vitamin D.

Zinc

Concurrent administration of calcium and zinc may reduce absorption of both minerals, however it is unclear if this is clinically significant. Calcium supplementation has been shown in some studies to increase faecal losses of zinc (McKenna et al 1997) — ensure adequate zinc intake and monitor for signs and symptoms of deficiency.

C

CONTRAINDICATIONS AND PRECAUTIONS

People with hyperparathyroidism, chronic renal impairment or kidney disease, sarcoidosis or other granulomatous diseases should only take calcium supplements under medical supervision. Calcium supplementation is contraindicated in hypercalcaemia.

PREGNANCY USE

The safety of calcium supplementation during pregnancy in doses up to 2000 mg elemental calcium per day is well established in clinical trials.

Practice points/Patient counselling

- Calcium is an essential mineral required for the proper functioning of numerous intracellular and extracellular processes, including muscle contraction, nerve conduction, beating of the heart, hormone release, blood coagulation, energy production and maintenance of immune function.
- Low-calcium states are associated with several serious diseases such as colorectal cancer, osteoporosis types I and II, hypertension, preeclampsia and eclampsia.
- Although supplementation is traditionally used to correct or avoid deficiency states, research has also shown a role in the prevention of osteoporosis, preeclampsia and management of numerous disease states and research now indicates that calcium and vitamin D reduces mortality in the elderly.
- Clinical studies show that calcium supplementation has benefits in symptomatic relief in premenstrual syndrome, reducing the risk of fracture (when combined with vitamin D), reducing the risk of preeclampsia and improving birthweight, weight loss and reducing incidence of some cancers.
- Calcium can interact with numerous drugs and should be used with caution by people with renal disease or hyperparathyroid conditions.

PATIENTS' FAQs

What will this supplement do for me?

Calcium is essential for health and wellbeing. Although used to prevent or treat deficiency states, and primarily associated with BMD, it is also beneficial in a wide range of conditions such as prevention of preeclampsia, premenstrual syndrome, reducing the risk of bone fractures (with vitamin D), aiding in weight loss, maintenance of fetal growth, treatment of lead toxicity. It is considered to be a critical nutrient in pregnancy, and may actually reduce mortality in the elderly when taken with vitamin D.

When will it start to work?

This will depend on the indication it is being used to treat; however, in most instances long-term administration is required (i.e. months to years).

Are there any safety issues?

In very high doses, calcium supplements can cause some side effects, including constipation, but generally calcium is considered safe and has a wide therapeutic range. High-dose supplements should not be used by people taking some medications. Caution should also be exercised with high doses in individuals with preexisting cardiovascular disease. (See *Significant interactions* above for specific information.)

REFERENCES

Abrahamsen B et al. Patient level pooled analysis of 68 500 patients from seven major vitamin D fracture trials in US and Europe. BMJ 340 (2010).

Ahn J et al. Serum vitamin D concentration and prostate cancer risk: a nested case-control study. J Natl Cancer Inst 100.11 (2008): 796–804.

Allen NE et al. Animal foods, protein, calcium and prostate cancer risk: the European Prospective Investigation into Cancer and Nutrition. Br J Cancer 98.9 (2008): 1574–1581.

Aloia JF et al. Calcium and vitamin D supplementationa in postmenopausal women. Journal of Clinical Endocrinology and Metabolism 98.11 (2013).

Alonso A et al. Low-fat dairy consumption and reduced risk of hypertension: the Seguimiento Universidad de Navarra (SUN) cohort. Am J Clin Nutr 82.5 (2005): 972–979.

Astrup A. The role of calcium in energy balance and obesity: the search for mechanisms. Am J Clin Nutr 88.4 (2008) 873–874.

Atallah AN et al. Calcium supplementation during pregnancy for preventing hypertensive disorders and related problems. Cochrane Database Syst Rev 1 (2002): CD001059.

Bailey CS et al. Excessive calcium ingestion leading to milk-alkali syndrome. Annals of Clinical Biochemistry. 45 (Pt 5) (2008): 527–529.

Barba G, Russo P. Dairy foods, dietary calcium and obesity: a short review of the evidence. Nutrition, Metabolism & Cardiovascular Diseases. 16 (2006): 445–451.

Baron JA et al. Risk of prostate cancer in a randomized clinical trial of calcium supplementation. Cancer Epidemiol Biomarkers Prev 14.3 (2005): 586–589.

Beall DP, Scofield RH. Milk-alkali syndrome associated with calcium carbonate consumption. Report of 7 patients with parathyroid hormone levels and an estimate of prevalence among patients hospitalized with hypercalcemia. Medicine. 74.2 (1995): 89–96.

Beers MH, Berkow R (eds). The Merck Manual of Diagnosis and Therapy, 17th edn. Rahway, NJ: Merck, 2003.

Behringer M et al. Effects of weight-bearing activities on bone mineral content and density in children and adolescents: a meta-analysis. J Bone Miner Res, 29.2 (2014) 467–478.

Belizan JM et al. Long-term effect of calcium supplementation during pregnancy on the blood pressure of offspring: follow up of a randomised controlled trial. BMJ 315.7103 (1997): 281–285.

Bell L et al. Cholesterol-lowering effects of calcium carbonate in patients with mild to moderate hypercholesterolemia. Arch Intern Med 152.12 (1992): 2441–2444.

Bergel E, Barros AJ. Effect of maternal calcium intake during pregnancy on children's blood pressure: a systematic review of the literature. BMC Pediatr 7 (2007): 15.

Bertone-Johnson ER et al. Calcium and vitamin D intake and risk of incident premenstrual syndrome. Arch Intern Med 165.11 (2005): 1246–1252.

Bischoff-Ferrari HA Which vitamin D oral supplement is best for postmenopausal women? Curr Osteoporos Rep 10.4 (2012): 251–257.

Bolland MJ et al. Calcium supplements with or without vitamin D and risk of cardiovascular events: reanalysis of the Women's Health Initiative limited access dataset and meta-analysis. BMJ 2011 doi 10.1136/bmj.d2040

Bolland MJ et al. Effect of calcium on risk of myocardial infarction and cardiovascular events:meta-analysis. BMJ 341 (2010): c3691.

Bolland MJ et al. Vascular events in healthy older women receiving calcium supplementation: randomised controlled trial. BMJ 336.7638 (2008): 262–266.

Borghi L et al. Comparison of two diets for the prevention of recurrent stones in idiopathic hypercalciuria. N Engl J Med 346.2 (2002): 77–84.

Bowen J, Noakes M, Clifton P. A high dairy protein, high-calcium diet minimizes bone turnover in overweight adults during weight loss. J Nutr 134 (2004): 568–573.

Bucher HC et al. Effect of calcium supplementation on pregnancy-induced hypertension and preeclampsia. JAMA 275 (1996): 1113–11117.

Bueno MB et al. Dietary calcium intake and overweight: An epidemiologic view. Nutrition 24 (2008):1110–1115.

Caan B et al. Calcium plus vitamin D supplementation and the risk of postmenopausal weight gain. Arch Intern Med 167.9 (2007): 893–902.

Campbell IA et al. Five year study of etidronate and/or calcium as prevention and treatment for osteoporosis and fractures in patients with asthma receiving long term oral and/or inhaled glucocorticoids. Thorax 59 (2004): 761–768.

Chakrabarty S et al. Calcium sensing receptor in human colon carcinoma: interaction with Ca(2+) and 1,25-dihydroxyvitamin D(3). Cancer Res 65.2 (2005): 493–498.

Challoumas D et al. Effects of calcium intake on the cardiovascular system in postmenopausal women. Atherosclerosis 231.1 (2013): 1–7

Chapuy MC et al. Combined calcium and vitamin D3 supplementation in elderly women: confirmation of reversal of secondary hyperparathyroidism and hip fracture risk: the Decalyos II study. Osteoporosis Int 13 (2002): 257–264.

Chapuy MC et al. Effect of calcium and cholecalciferol treatment for 3 years on hip fractures in elderly women. BMJ 308 (1994): 1081–1082.

Chapuy MC et al. Vitamin D3 and calcium to prevent hip fractures in elderly women. N Engl J Med 327 (1992): 1637–1642.

Chevalley T et al. Interaction between calcium intake and menarcheal age on bone mass gain: an eight-year follow-up study from prepuberty to postmenarche. J Clin Endocrinol Metab 90.1 (2005): 44–51.

Cho E et al. Dairy foods, calcium, and colorectal cancer: a pooled analysis of 10 cohort studies. J Natl Cancer Institute. 96.13 (2004):1015–1022.

Christensen R et al. Effects of calcium from dairy and dietary supplements on faecal fat excretion: a meta-analysis of randomized controlled trials. Obesity Review. 10 (2009):475–486.

Coruzzi P, Mossini G. Central hypervolemia does not invariably modulate calcium excretion in essential hypertension. Nephron 75 (1997): 368–369.

Crowther CA et al. Calcium supplementation in nulliparous women for the prevention of pregnancy-induced hypertension, preeclampsia and preterm birth: an Australian randomized trial: FRACOG and the ACT Study Group. Aust N Z J Obstet Gynaecol 39.1 (1999): 12–118.

Curhan GC et al. Comparison of dietary calcium with supplemental calcium and other nutrients as factors affecting the risk for kidney stones in women. Ann Intern Med 126 (1997): 497–504.

Daniele ND et al. Effect of supplementation of calcium and vitamin D on bone mineral density and bone mineral content in peri- and post-menopause women A double-blind, randomized, controlled trial. Pharmacol Res 50.6 (2004): 637–641.

Dawson-Hughes B et al. Effect of calcium and vitamin D supplementation on bone density in men and women 65 years of age or older. N Engl J Med 337 (1997): 670–676.

Dickinson HO et al. Calcium supplementation for the management of primary hypertension in adults. Cochrane Database Syst Rev 2 (2006): CD004639.alendula

Ding EL et al. Interaction of estrogen therapy with calcium and vitamin D supplementation on colorectal cancer risk: reanalysis of Women's Health Initiative randomized trial. Int J Cancer 122.8 (2008): 1690–1694.

Dorea JG, Donangelo CM. Early (in uterus and infant) exposure to mercury and lead. Clin Nutr (2005): [Epub ahead of print].

Dorea JG. Mercury and lead during breast-feeding. Br J Nutr 92 (2004): 21–40.

Elliott P et al. Dietary phosphorus and blood pressure: international study of macro- and micro-nutrients and blood pressure. Hypertension 51.3 (2008): 669–675.

Ettinger AS et al. Effect of breast milk lead on infant blood lead levels at 1 month of age. Environ Health Perspect 112.14 (2004): 1381–1385.

Ettinger AS et al. Effects of calcium supplementation on blood levels in pregnancy: a randomised placebo-controlled trial. Environ Health Perspect 117.1 (2009): 26–31.

Ettinger AS et al. Influence of maternal bone lead burden and calcium intake on levels of lead in breast milk over the course of lactation. Am J Epidemiol 163.1 (2006): 48–56.

Ettinger AS. Hu H, Avila MH. Dietary calcium supplementation to lower blood lead levels in pregnancy and lactation. J Nutr Biochem 18.3 (2007) :172–178.

Fardellone P et al. Biochemical effects of calcium supplementation in postmenopausal women: influence of dietary calcium intake. Am J Clin Nutr 67 (1998): 1273–1278.

Gao X, LaValley MP, Tucker KL. Prospective studies of dairy product and calcium intakes and prostate cancer risk: a meta-analysis. J Natl Cancer Inst 97.23 (2005): 1768–1777.

Garcia-Lorda P et al. Dietary calcium and body mass index in a Mediterranean population. In J Vitam Nutri Res. 77.1 (2007): 34–40.

Geleijnse JM, Grobbee DE, Kok FJ. Impact of dietary and lifestyle factors on the prevalence of hypertension in Western populations. J Hum Hypertens 19 (Suppl 3) (2005): S1–S4.

Genkinger JM et al. Dairy products and ovarian cancer: a pooled analysis of 12 cohort studies. Cancer Epidemiol Biomarkers Prev 15.2 (2006): 364–372.

Ghanbari Z et al. Effects of calcium supplement therapy in women with premenstrual syndrome. Taiwan J Obstet Gynecol 48.2 (2009): 124–129.

Goldfarb DS. Prospects for dietary therapy of recurrent nephrolithiasis. Adv Chronic Kidney Dis 16.1 (2009): 21–29.

Gonzalez JT, Rumbold PL, Stevenson EJ. Effect of calcium intake on fat oxidation in adults: a meta-analysis of randomized, controlled trials. Obes Rev. 13.10 (2012): 848–887.

Gotoh M et al. High blood pressure, bone-mineral loss and insulin resistance in women. Hypertens Res 28.7 (2005): 565–570.

Grau MV et al. Vitamin D, calcium supplementation, and colorectal adenomas: results of a randomized trial. J Natl Cancer Inst 95.23 (2003): 1765–1771.

Griffith LE et al. The influence of dietary and nondietary calcium supplementation on blood pressure: an updated metaanalysis of randomised controlled trials. Am J Hypertens 1291 (1999): 84–92.

Groff JL, Gropper SS. Advanced nutrition and human metabolism. Wadsworth, Belmont, CA, 2009.

Guessous I et al. Calcium, vitamin D and cardiovascular disease. Kidney Bloo Pres Res. 34 (2011): 404–417.

Gupta SK et al. Reversal of fluorosis in children. Acta Paediatr Jpn 38.5 (1996): 5113–5119.

Harkness LS, Bonny AE. Calcium and vitamin D status in the adolescent: key roles for bone, body weight, glucose tolerance, and estrogen biosynthesis. J Pediatr Adolesc Gynecol 18.5 (2005): 305–311.

Heaney RP, Weaver CM. Calcium and vitamin D. Endocrinol Metab Clin North Am 32.1 (2003): 181–188.

Hennekens CH, Barice EJ. Calcium supplements and risk of myocardial infarction: a hypothesis formulated but not yet adequately tested. Am J Med, 124.12 (2011): 1097–1098.

Hernandez-Avila M et al. Dietary calcium supplements to lower blood lead levels in lactating women: a randomized placebo-controlled trial. Epidemiology 14.2 (2003): 206–212.

Herrera JA et al. Calcium plus linoleic acid therapy for pregnancy-induced hypertension. Int J Gynecol Obstet 91.3 (2005): 221–227.

Hess B et al. High-calcium intake abolishes hyperoxaluria and reduces urinary crystallization during a 20-fold normal oxalate load in humans. Nephrol Dial Transplant 13 (1998): 2241–2247.

Hiller JE et al. Calcium supplementation in pregnancy and its impact on blood pressure in children and women: follow up of a randomised controlled trial. Aust N Z J Obstet Gynaecol 47.2 (2007): 115–121.

Hofmeyr GJ et al. Calcium supplementation during pregnancy for preventing hypertensive disorders is not associated with changes in platelet count, urate, and urinary protein: a randomized control trial. Hypertens Pregnancy 27.3 (2008): 299–304.

Hofmeyr GJ et al. Calcium supplementation to prevent pre-eclampsia: a systematic review. S Afr Med J 93.3 (2003): 224–228.

Hofmeyr GJ, Atallah AN, Duley L. Calcium supplementation during pregnancy for preventing hypertensive disorders and related problems. Cochrane Database Syst Rev 3 (2006): CD001059.

Hofmeyr GJ, Duley L, Atallah A. Dietary calcium supplementation for prevention of pre-eclampsia and related problems: a systematic review and commentary. BJOG 114.8 (2007): 933–943.

Holt PR. New insights into calcium, dairy and colon cancer. World J Gastroenterol 14.28 (2008): 4429–4433.

Hovdenak N, Haram K. Influence of mineral and vitamin supplements on pregnancy outcome. Eur J Obstet Gyneco Reprod Biol, 164.2 (2012): 127–132.

Hsia J et al. Calcium/vitamin D supplementation and cardiovascular events. Circulation. 115 (2007): 846–854.

Huncharek M et al. Dairy products, dietary calcium and vitamin D intake as risk factors for prostate cancer: a meta-analysis of 26,769 cases from 45 observational studies. Nutr Cancer 60.4 (2008a): 421–441.

Huncharek M et al Impact of dairy products and dietary calcium on bone-mineral content in children: results of a meta-analysis. Bone 43.2 (2008b): 312–321.

Hyman J et al. Dietary and supplemental calcium and the recurrence of colorectal adenomas. Cancer Epidemiol Biomarkers Prev 7.4 (1998): 291–295.

Imdad A, Bhutta ZA Effects of calcium supplementation during pregnancy on maternal, fetal and birth outcomes. Paediatr Perinat Epidemiol 26 (Suppl 1) (2012): 138–152.

Insel P et al. Discovering Nutrition; Jones and Burlington MA: Bartlett Learning, 2013.

Ishihara J et al. Dietary calcium, vitamin D, and the risk of colorectal cancer. Am J Clin Nutr 88.6 (2008): 1576–1583.

Jacobs ET, Thompson PA, Martínez ME. Diet, gender, and colorectal neoplasia. J Clin Gastroenterol 41.8 (2007): 731–746.

Kabrnova-Hlavata K et al. Calcium intake and the outcome of short-term weight management. Physiol Res 57.2 (2008): 237–45.

C

Kawano Y et al. Calcium supplementation in patients with essential hypertension assessment by office, home and ambulatory blood pressure. J Hypertens 16.11 (1998): 1693–1699.

Kennedy K et al. Double-blind, randomized trial of a synthetic triacylglycerol in formula-fed term infants: effects on stool biochemistry, stool characteristics, and bone mineralization. Am J Clin Nutr 70.5 (1999): 920–927.

Kerstetter JE et al. Dietary protein affects intestinal calcium absorption. Am J Clin Nutr 68 (1998): 859–865.

Kim JH et al. Increased dietary calcium intake is not associated with coronary artery calcification. International Journal of Cardiology. 157.3 (2012):429–431

Kim K-Z et al. Association between CASR polymorphisms, calcium intake, and colorectal cancer risk. PLoS ONE 8.3 (2013): e59628.

Kopic S, Geibel JP. Gastric acid, calcium absorption, and their impact on bone health. Physiol Rev 93 (2013): 189–268.

Lambert HL et al. Calcium supplementation and bone mineral accretion in adolescent girls: an 18-mo randomized controlled trial with 2-y follow-up. Am J Clin Nutr 87.2 (2008): 455–462.

Lappe JM et al. Vitamin D and calcium supplementation reduces cancer risk: results of a randomized trial. Am J Clin Nutr 85.6 (2007): 1586–1591.

Larsen ER, Mosekilde L, Foldspang A. Vitamin D and calcium supplementation prevents osteoporotic fractures in elderly community dwelling residents: a pragmatic population-based 3-year intervention study. J Bone Miner Res 19 (2004): 370–378.

Lewis JR et al. Calcium supplementation and the risks of atherosclerotic vascular disease in older women: results of a 5-year RCT and a 4.5-year follow-up. J Bone Miner Res. 26.1 (2011): 35–41.

Lewis JR et al. The effects of 3 years of calcium supplementation on common carotid artery intimal medial thickness and carotid atherosclerosis in older women: an ancillary study of the CAIFOS randomized controlled trial. J Bone Miner Res (2013).

Li K et al. Associations of dietary calcium intake and calcium supplementation with myocardial infarction and overall cardiovascular mortality in the Heidelberg cohort of the European Prospective Investigation into Cancer and Nutrition study (Epic-Heidelberg). Heart. 98 (2012): 920–925.

Liebman M, Chai W. Effect of dietary calcium on urinary oxalate excretion after oxalate loads. Am J Clin Nutr 65 (1997): 1453–1459.

Lukaszuk JM et al. Preliminary study: soy milk as effective as skim milk in promoting weight loss. J Am Diet Assoc 107.10 (2007): 1811–18114.

Major GC et al. Supplementation with calcium + vitamin D enhances the beneficial effect of weight loss on plasma lipid and lipoprotein concentrations. Am J Clin Nutr 85.1 (2007): 54–59.

Margolis KL et al. Effect of calcium and vitamin D supplementation on blood pressure: the Women's Health Initiative Randomized Trial. Hypertension 52.5 (2008): 847–855.

Matkovic V et al. Calcium supplementation and bone mineral density in females from childhood to young adulthood: a randomized controlled trial. Am J Clin Nutr 81.1 (2005): 175–188.

McCarty MF, Thomas CA. PTH excess may promote weight gain by impeding catecholamine-induced lipolysis-implications for the impact of calcium, vitamin D, and alcohol on body weight. Med Hypotheses 61.5–6 (2003): 535–542.

McCullough ML et al. Dairy, calcium, and vitamin D intake and postmenopausal breast cancer risk in the Cancer Prevention Study II Nutrition Cohort. Cancer Epidemiol Biomarkers Prev 14.12 (2005): 2898–2904.

McCullough ML et al. Vitamin D and calcium intake in relation to risk of endometrial cancer: a systematic review of the literature. Prev Med 46.4 (2008): 298–302.

McKenna AA et al. Zinc balance in adolescent females consuming a low- or high-calcium diet. Am J Clin Nutr 65 (1997): 1460–1464.

Meng X et al. Calcium intake in elderly Australian women is inadequate. Nutrients. 2 (2010):1036–1043.

Miller EA et al. Calcium, vitamin D, and apoptosis in the rectal epithelium. Cancer Epidemiol Biomarkers Prev 14.2 (2005): 525–528.

Mizoue T et al. Calcium, dairy foods, vitamin D, and colorectal cancer risk: the Fukuoka Colorectal Cancer Study. Cancer Epidemiol Biomarkers Prev 17.10 (2008): 2800–2807.

Nabhan FA et al. Milk-alkali syndrome from ingestion of calcium carbonate in a patient with hypoparathyroidism. Endocr Pract. 10.4 (2004): 372–375.

Nainggolan L. Calcium supplements increase vascular events? Medscape web MD Available: www.theheart.org.

Oh K et al. Calcium and vitamin D intakes in relation to risk of distal colorectal adenoma in women. Am J Epidemiol 165.10 (2007): 1178–1186.

Onakpoya IJ et al. Efficacy of calcium supplementation for management of overweight and obesity: systematic review of randomized clinical trials. Nutri Rev 69.6 (2011): 335–343.

Park SY et al. Calcium, vitamin D, and dairy product intake and prostate cancer risk: the Multiethnic Cohort Study. Am J Epidemiol 166.11 (2007a): 1259–1269.

Park Y et al. Calcium, dairy foods, and risk of incident and fatal prostate cancer: the NIH-AARP Diet and Health Study. Am J Epidemiol 166.11 (2007b): 1270–1279.

Pasco JA et al. Calcium intakes among Australian women: Geelong Osteoporosis Study. Aust N Z J Med 30.1 (2000): 21–27.

Pattanaungkul S et al. Relationship of intestinal calcium absorption to 1,25-dihydroxyvitamin D [1,25(OH)2D] levels in young versus elderly women: evidence for age-related intestinal resistance to 1,25(OH)2D action. J Clin Endocrinol Metab 85.11 (2000): 4023–4027.

Penland JG, Johnson PE. Dietary calcium and manganese effects on menstrual cycle symptoms. Am J Obstet Gynecol 168 (1993): 1417–1423.

Pereira RM et al. Guidelines for the prevention and treatment of glucocorticoid-induced osteoporosis. Rev Bras Reumatol 52.4 (2012): 580–593.

Picolos M et al. Milk-alkali syndrome in pregnancy. Obstet & Gynecology. 104.5 (pt2) (2004):1201–1204.

Prentice A. Micronutrients and the bone mineral content of the mother, fetus and newborn. J Nutr 133 (2003): 1693–1699.

Prince RL et al. The pathogenesis of age-related osteoporotic fracture: effects of dietary calcium deprivation. J Clin Endocrinol Metab 82.1 (1997): 260–264.

Reid IR et al. Randomized controlled trial of calcium supplementation in healthy, nonosteoporotic, older men. Arch Intern Med 168.20 (2008): 2276–2282.

Rejnmark L et al. Vitamin D with calcium reduces mortality: Patient level pooled analysis of 70,528 patients from eight major vitamin D trials. J Clin Endocrinol Metabol 97.8 (2012): 2670–2681.

Resnick LM. The role of dietary calcium in hypertension: a hierarchal overview (Review). Am J Hypertens 12 (1999): 99–112.

Rossi GA, Cerasoli F, Cazzola M. Safety of inhaled corticosteroids: room for improvement. Pulm Pharmacol Ther (2005) [Epub ahead of print].

Rozen P et al. Calcium supplements interact significantly with long-term diet while suppressing rectal epithelial proliferation of adenoma patients. Cancer 91.4 (2001): 833–840.

Ryan-Harshman M, Aldoori W. Diet and colorectal cancer: review of the evidence. Can Fam Physician 53.11 (2007): 1913–1920.

Sanders KM et al. Calcium and bone health: position statement for the Australian and New Zealand Bone and Mineral Society, Osteoporosis Australia and the Endocrine Society of Australia. Med J Aust 190.6 (2009): 316–320.

Schatzkin A, Peters U. Advancing the calcium–colorectal cancer hypothesis (Editorial). J Natl Cancer Inst 96.12 (2004): 893–894.

Schrager S. Dietary calcium intake and obesity evidence-based clinical practice. J Am Board Fam Pract 18 (2005): 205–210.

Shahar DR et al. Does dairy calcium intake enhance weight loss among overweight diabetic patients? Diabetes Care 30.3 (2007): 485–489.

Shaukat A, Scouras N, Schunemann HJ. Role of supplemental calcium in the recurrence of colorectal adenomas: a metaanalysis of randomized controlled trials. Am J Gastroenterol. 100.2 (2005): 390–394.

Skinner HG, Schwartz GG. Serum calcium and incident and fatal prostate cancer in the National Health and Nutrition Examination Survey. Cancer Epidemiol Biomarkers Prev 17.9 (2008): 2302–2305.

Soen, S. [The effects of glucocorticoid on bone architecture and strength]. Clin Calcium 23.7 (2013): 993–999.

Sowers M et al. Blood lead concentrations and pregnancy outcomes. Arch Environ Health 57.5 (2002): 489–495.

Stear SJ et al. Effect of a calcium and exercise intervention on the bone mineral status of 16–18-year-old adolescent girls. Am J Clin Nutr 77.4 (2003): 985–992.

Strause L et al. Spinal bone loss in postmenopausal women supplemented with calcium and trace minerals. J Nutr 124 (1994): 1060–1064.

Sulz MC et al. Comparison of two antacid preparations on intragastric acidity-a two-centre open randomised cross-over placebo-controlled trial. Digestion 75 (2007): 69–73.a

Tang BM et al. Use of calcium or calcium in combination with vitamin D supplementation to prevent fractures and bone loss in people aged 50 years and older: a meta-analysis. Lancet 370.9588 (2007): 657–666.

Taylor EN, Curhan GC. Role of nutrition in the formation of calcium-containing kidney stones. Nephron Physiol 98.2 (2004): 55–63.

Teegarden D. Calcium intake and reduction in weight or fat mass. J Nutr 133 (2003): 249–51S.

Thys-Jacobs S et al. Calcium carbonate and the premenstrual syndrome: effects on premenstrual and menstrual symptoms. Premenstrual Syndrome Study Group. Am J Obstet Gynecol 179.2 (1998): 444–452.

Thys-Jacobs S et al. Calcium supplementation in premenstrual syndrome: a randomized crossover trial. J Gen Intern Med 4 (1989): 183–189.

Thys-Jacobs S. Micronutrients and the premenstrual syndrome: the case for calcium. J Am Coll Nutr 19.2 (2000): 220–227.

Tremblay A, Gilbert JA. Human obesity: is sufficient calcium/dairy intake part of the problem? J Am Coll Nutri 20 (5 Suppl 1)(2011):449S–53S.
Trowman R et al. A systematic review of the effects of calcium supplementation on body weight. Br J Nutr 95.6 (2006): 1033–1038.
Tsubota K et al. New treatment of dry eye: the effect of calcium ointment through eyelid skin delivery. Br J Ophthalmol 83.7 (1999): 767–770.
van der Pols JC et al. Childhood dairy intake and adult cancer risk: 65-y follow-up of the Boyd Orr cohort. Am J Clin Nutr 86.6 (2007): 1722–1729.
Van Hemelrijck M et al. Calcium intake and serum concentration in relation to risk of cardiovascular death in NHANES III. PLoS One 10.8 (2013).
Vestergaard P et al. Fracture prevention in postmenopausal women. Clin Evid 2011.
Villar J et al. Nutritional interventions during pregnancy for the prevention or treatment of maternal morbidity and preterm delivery: an overview of randomized controlled trials. J Nutr 133 (Suppl) (2003): 1606–25.
Wahlqvist ML (ed). Food and nutrition: Australasia, Asia and the Pacific 2nd edn. Sydney: Allen & Unwin, 2002.
Wang L et al. Dietary intake of dairy products, calcium, and vitamin D and the risk of hypertension in middle-aged and older women. Hypertension 51.4 (2008): 1073–1079.
Ward MW, Holimon TD. Calcium treatment for premenstrual syndrome. Ann Pharmacother 33.12 (1999): 1356–1358.
Warriner AH, Saag KG. Glucocorticoid-related bone changes from endogenous or exogenous glucocorticoids. Curr Opin Endocrinol Diabetes Obes 20.6 (2013): 510–516.
Weingarten MA et al. Dietary calcium supplementation for preventing colorectal cancer and adenomatous polyps (Review). Cochrane Database Syst Rev 4 (2008): CD003548.
Wilson JD et al. Harrison's principles of internal medicine, 12th edn. New York: McGraw-Hill, 1991.
Winzenberg TM et al. Calcium supplementation for improving bone mineral density in children. Cochrane Database Syst Rev 2 (2006): CD005119.
Winzenberg T et al. Effects of calcium supplementation on bone density in healthy children: meta-analysis of randomised controlled trials. BMJ 333.7572 (2006): 775.
Woo J et al. Dietary intake, blood pressure and osteoporosis. J Hum Hypertens (2008 Dec 18) [Epub ahead of print].
Xiao Q et al. Dietary and Supplemental Calcium Intake and Cardiovascular Disease Mortality: The National Institutes of Health–AARP Diet and Health Study. JAMA Intern Med 173.8 (2013): 639–646.
Young GL, Jewell D. Interventions for leg cramps in pregnancy. Cochrane Database Syst Rev 1 (2013): CD000121.
Zemel MB et al. Calcium and dairy acceleration of weight and fat loss during energy restriction in obese adults. Obes Res 12 (2004): 582–590.
Zemel MB et al. Dairy augmentation of total and central fat loss in obese subjects. Int J Obes (Lond) 29.4 (2005a): 391–397.
Zemel MB et al. Effects of calcium and dairy on body composition and weight loss in African-American adults. Obes Res 13.7 (2005b): 218–225.
Zemel MB. Role of calcium and dairy products in energy partitioning and weight management. Am J Clin Nutr 79.5 (2004): 907S–912S.
Zhu W et al. Calcium plus vitamin D3 supplementation facilitated fat loss in overweight and obese college students with very low calcium consumption: a randomized controlled trial. Nutrition Journal 12.8 (2013).

Calendula

HISTORICAL NOTE Calendula is indigenous to Eastern Europe and the Mediterranean, where its medicinal value has been respected since ancient times. Calendula was popular in Ancient Greece and in earlier Indian and Arabic cultures. It has been a common garden plant since the 12th century and it is mentioned in several older herbals. The name calendula comes from the Latin *calends*, meaning the first day of the month, referring to the plant's near-continual flowering habit.

COMMON NAME

Marigold

OTHER NAMES

Pot or garden marigold, gold-bloom, holligold.

Field marigold (*Calendula arvensis*) is also used medicinally for the same indications because it has similar constituents. Take care not to confuse with *Tagetes erecta* (Mexican marigold).

BOTANICAL NAME/FAMILY

Calendula officinalis (family Asteraceae [Compositae or Daisy])

PLANT PARTS USED

The flowers are primarily used, but the stems, younger leaves, seeds and roots all have medicinal properties.

CHEMICAL COMPONENTS

The major constituents are triterpene saponins (2–10%) based on oleanolic acid and flavonols, including astragalin, hyperoside, isoquercitrin and rutin, as well as the carotenoids flavoxanthin and auroxanthin (Bako et al 2002). The triterpendiol esters faradiol laurate, faradiol myristate and faradiol palmitate have been identified as the major active compounds, which are also used as marker compounds for standardisation of calendula extracts (Hamburger et al 2003, Zitterl-Eglseer et al 2001).

Additional constituents include other phenolic compounds, steroids and other terpenoids, tocopherols, quinines, carotenes and resins (Re et al 2009), polysaccharides (WHO 2003), as well as minerals such as calcium, sodium, potassium, magnesium, iron, copper and manganese (Ahmed et al 2003).

MAIN ACTIONS

Antimicrobial and antiparasitic

Hydroalcoholic extracts have been shown to have antibacterial, antiparasitic, antiviral and antifungal activities.

The in vitro antibacterial activity of a hydroethanolic extract of calendula flower has been demonstrated against *Campylobacter jejenum* (Cwikla et al 2010) and an isolated oleanolic acid (triterpene) aglycone from calendula demonstrated the ability to affect morphology of Gram-positive bacteria in vitro (Szakiel et al 2008).

Glycosidic fractions of oleanolic acid isolated from calendula demonstrated antiparasitic activity against *Heligmosomoides bakeri* (Doligalska et al 2011) and a flower extract has been shown to inhibit the parasite *Trichomonas*. The oxygenated terpenes are thought to be the main active compounds (Gracza & Szasz 1968, Samochowiec et al 1979).

The in vitro antifungal activity of calendula flower extracts has been investigated against *Aspergillus niger, Rhizopus japonicum, Candida albicans, C. tropicalis* and *Rhodotorula glutinis, C. krusei, C. glabrata, C. parapsilosis, Aspergillus flavus, A. fumigatus* and *Exophiala dermatitidis*. Calendula extract showed a high degree of activity against all fungi and the inhibitory effect was comparable to that of standard antifungals (Efstratiou et al 2012, Kasiram et al 2000).

A 70% hydroalcoholic extract demonstrated virucidal activity against influenza virus and suppressed the growth of herpes simplex virus (Bogdanova et al 1970). Calendula flower extract has also been shown to possess anti-HIV and anti-Epstein–Barr virus activity in vitro (Kalvatchev et al 1997, Ukiya et al 2006).

Promotes wound healing

An ointment containing 5% calendula flower extract, as well as an ointment containing two different fractions of calendula extract combined with allantoin, has been shown to stimulate physiological regeneration and epithelialisation in experimentally-induced surgical wounds. The effect is thought to be due to more intensive metabolism of glycoproteins, nucleoproteins and collagen proteins during regeneration of the tissues (Klouchek-Popova et al 1982). A similar finding was reported in vivo for skin puncture wound healing, where collagen production was increased by application of a hydroethanolic extract of calendula flowers. The same study demonstrated increased angiogenic activity, suggesting that an increased blood supply may be involved (Parente et al 2012). Both a 5% and a 10% calendula gel showed accelerated healing in 5-fluorouracil-induced oral mucositis in vivo (Tanideh et al 2013). Hexane and ethanolic extracts of calendula stimulated both proliferation and migration of fibroblasts in an in vitro scratch assay. The triterpene esters faradiol myristate and palmitate contributed partially to this effect (Fronza et al 2009).

Anti-inflammatory

Anti-inflammatory activity has been demonstrated in several animal models for multiple chemical constituents found in calendula. Pretreatment with an 80% hydroalcoholic extract reduced carrageenan-induced rat paw oedema at a dose of 100 mg extract/kg. Indomethacin 5 mg/kg was shown to be fourfold more potent in the same experiment (Mascolo et al 1987). Application of a hydroethanolic extract to wounds decreased the presence of fibrin and hyperaemia in vivo, thus directly altering the inflammatory process (Parente et al 2012). Both a 70% hydroalcoholic extract and a CO_2 extract have been shown to inhibit experimentally induced inflammation and oedema. The triterpenoids faradiol, amidiol and calenduladiol demonstrate anti-inflammatory activity (Neukirch et al 2005), with the faradiol monoester appearing to be the most relevant compound due to its quantitative prevalence (Della et al 1994). A freeze-dried extract of calendula was found to suppress both the inflammatory effect and leucocyte infiltration in an inflammatory model induced by the simultaneous injection of carrageenan and prostaglandin E_1 (Shipochliev et al 1981).

Ten triterpenoid glycosides (including four new compounds) were isolated from calendula and tested for anti-inflammatory activity. Of these, nine were found to be effective against 12-*O*-tetradecanoylphorbol-13-acetate-induced inflammation in mice (Ukiya et al 2006).

OTHER ACTIONS

Reduces oedema

Oral administration of a triterpene-containing fraction prevented the development of ascites and increased survival time compared with controls in mice inoculated with a carcinoma (Boucaud-Maitre et al 1988). The main triterpendiol esters of calendula, the faradiol esters, have been shown to possess antioedema activity by inhibiting croton oil-induced oedema of the mouse ear (Zitterl-Eglseer et al 1997).

Immunomodulation

Isolated polysaccharides have been shown to stimulate phagocytosis of human granulocytes (Varljen et al 1989, Wagner et al 1985). A 70% ethanol extract of calendula was shown to completely inhibit the proliferation of lymphocytes in the presence of phytohaemagglutinin in vitro (Amirghofran et al 2000).

Antioxidant

Calendula has free radical scavenging and antioxidant activity, with aqueous extracts having greater activity than methanolic extracts. Antioxidant activity is related to the total phenolic and flavonoid content (Cetkovic et al 2004, Matic et al 2012).

The butanolic fraction of a calendula extract reduces superoxide and hydroxyl radicals, suggesting a free radical scavenging effect. Lipid peroxidation in liver microsomes is also reduced (Cordova et al 2002). Isorhamnetin glycosides isolated from calendula have been shown to inhibit the activity of lipo-oxygenase (Bezakova et al 1996).

Research with animal models also shows various antioxidant effects. A propylene glycol extract of calendula petals administered orally to rats on a high-polyunsaturated fatty acid diet protected lymphocyte DNA from oxidative damage and was comparable with vitamin E supplementation in preventing lipid peroxidation (Frankič et al 2009). Similarly, a dose-dependent protective effect against ultraviolet B-induced glutathione depletion was seen with an oral solution of a hydroethanolic extract of calendula in vivo (Fonseca et al 2010).

Antispasmodic activity

Calendula has demonstrated antispasmodic activity in isolated gut preparations (Bashir et al 2006). These effects appeared to be due to calcium channel blocking and cholinergic activity.

Hypoglycaemic activity

A methanolic extract and its butanol-soluble fraction have been found to have hypoglycaemic and gastroprotective effects and to slow gastric emptying. From the butanol-soluble fraction, four new triterpene oligoglycosides, calendasaponins A, B, C and D, were isolated, together with eight known saponins, seven known flavonol glycosides and a known sesquiterpene glucoside. Their structures were elucidated on the basis of chemical and physicochemical evidence. The principal saponin constituents, glycosides A, B, C, D and F, exhibited potent inhibitory effects on an increase in serum glucose levels in glucose-loaded rats, gastric emptying in mice and ethanol- and indomethacin-induced gastric lesions in rats (Yoshikawa et al 2001).

Hypolipidaemic activity

Oral administration of an isolated saponin fraction has been shown to reduce serum lipid levels in hyperlipidaemic rats (ESCOP 1996).

Hepatoprotective

Calendula extracts have been shown to have hepatoprotective effects on rat hepatocytes both in vitro and in vivo (Barajas-Farias et al 2006, Rusu et al 2005), with cytotoxic and genotoxic effects being evident at very high doses (Barajas-Farias et al 2006, Perez-Carreon et al 2002).

CLINICAL USE

Calendula is generally used in the treatment of inflammatory skin disorders or inflammation of the mucosa and as an aid to wound healing (Blumenthal et al 2000, ESCOP 1996). It is used both internally and topically for a variety of indications.

Wounds and burns

Historically, calendula flower preparations have been used to accelerate the healing of wounds, burns, bruises, grazes and minor skin infections. In recent times, it has been investigated for its effects on wound healing and burns in a variety of experimental models and clinical studies as either a stand-alone topical treatment or in combination with other ingredients. Generally, studies investigate various topical preparations; however, an oral mouthwash has also been tested for effects.

Calendula ointment (8%, 1:10 tincture in 70% alcohol) is a useful adjuvant treatment during cosmetic surgery, according to a study of 19 cleft-lip patients with discoloured scar tissue. Pretreatment with the calendula ointment under a gauze dressing every evening for 1 month improved the results of dermatography, a refined tattooing technique used to improve the appearance of scars (Van der Velden & Van der Dussen 1995).

In another controlled trial involving 34 patients with venous leg ulcers, a calendula extract applied twice daily for 3 weeks was found to produce a significant acceleration in healing compared to a saline solution (Duran et al 2005). Another clinical study used a mixture of chlorhexidine acetate and a 2% calendula extract as a haemostatic aerosol, producing good results (Garg & Sharma 1992).

A larger, open, randomised parallel study of 156 patients in four burn centres in France compared the effects of three different topical ointments (calendula, a proteolytic ointment and Vaseline) on the management of second- and third-degree burns. A thick layer of the test ointment was applied daily under a closed dressing until grafting or spontaneous healing occurred and effectiveness was evaluated between the eighth and 12th day of treatment. Failure was defined as the presence of an eschar, local infection, premature treatment discontinuation or failure to complete the study. A marginally significant difference in favour of calendula over Vaseline was observed and calendula was significantly better tolerated than the other treatments (Lievre et al 1992).

Prophylactic treatment with calendula ointment has also been used successfully to reduce the incidence and severity of bedsores in an open multicentre study. In other studies, positive results have been demonstrated in the treatment of poor venous return associated with ulcers, thrombophlebitis and other cutaneous changes, such as inflammation, cracks and eczema (Issac 1992).

Adjunct to radiation therapy

In a randomised controlled trial (RCT) involving 254 patients treated with adjuvant radiotherapy for breast cancer, topical treatment with calendula to the irradiated skin was found to be significantly more effective than trolamine in reducing acute dermatitis, with patients receiving calendula having less frequent interruption of radiotherapy and significantly reduced radiation-induced pain (Pommier et al 2004).

A 2012 RCT compared calendula cream to a standard aqueous cream to determine whether application would reduce the risk of severe acute radiation skin reactions in 411 patients undergoing radiation therapy for breast cancer. The study found no significant statistical difference between the two groups. The calendula application was reported as being more poorly absorbed than placebo, which may have been a factor; however, this remains to be tested further (Sharp et al 2012).

In contrast, a 2% calendula mouthwash decreased the intensity of radiation-induced oropharyngeal mucositis compared to placebo mouthwash in an RCT involving 40 patients with head and neck cancers. Patients were instructed to use 5 mL of mouthwash twice daily (placebo or calendula) over a period of 7 weeks during concurrent radiotherapy treatment. The severity of oropharyngeal mucositis was assessed by two doctors using the Oral Mucositis Assessment Scale (Babaee et al 2013).

IN COMBINATION

In practice, calendula is often combined with other herbs, such as St John's wort, to provide stronger effects. The combination of *Calendula arvensis* (field marigold) and *Hypericum perforatum* oils has been shown to improve the epithelial reconstruction of surgical wounds in childbirth with caesarean section (Lavagna et al 2001).

In a prospective, non-randomised study, 25 patients with venous ulcers were treated with an ointment containing calendula oil, *Hypericum perforatum* and *Allium sativa*. There was an average 99.1% improvement in epithelialisation by the end of the 7 weeks without any adverse effects (Kundakovic et al 2012).

A combination of calendula, *Arctium lappa* and *Geranium robertianum* has also been shown to improve healing of ulceration in 52 patients suffering herpetic keratitis compared with treatment with aciclovir alone (Corina et al 1999).

Commission E approves the external use of calendula for poorly healing wounds and leg ulcers (Blumenthal et al 2000).

Gastrointestinal inflammatory disorders

In practice, calendula is often combined with other herbs to provide stronger effects, a fact often reflected in the research.

IN COMBINATION

An oral mixture of *Symphytum officinalis* (comfrey) and calendula was beneficial in the treatment of duodenal ulcers and gastroduodenitis according to a study involving 170 patients. Of these, 137 were treated with the herbal combination and 33 also received an antacid. A dramatic 90% of treated patients became painfree and 85% had a reduction in dyspeptic complaints. Gastric acidity showed a statistically insignificant tendency to decrease in both groups. Gastroscopy later revealed that the ulcers had healed in 90% of patients (Chakurski et al 1981). Interestingly, a smaller study conducted by the same researchers involving only 32 patients with the same condition failed to detect a beneficial effect (Matev et al 1981).

A further study by the same authors found another mixture containing calendula to be beneficial in the treatment of chronic colitis. A combination of *Taraxacum officinale, Hypericum perforatum, Melissa officinalis, Calendula officinalis* and *Foeniculum vulgare* was shown to relieve the spontaneous and palpable pains along the large intestine in over 95% of the patients (n = 24) by day 15 of treatment. Defecation was normalised in patients with diarrhoea and constipated patients were successfully treated with the addition of *Rhamnus frangula, Citrus aurantium* and *Carum carvi*. The pathological admixtures in faeces disappeared (Chakurski et al 1981).

Although encouraging, the role of calendula as a stand-alone treatment is difficult to determine from these studies. Additionally, the oral ingestion of comfrey is not recommended due to potential hepatotoxic effects.

Gingivitis

Calendula has been shown in an open clinical study to be beneficial in the treatment of chronic catarrhal gingivitis (Krazhan & Garazha 2001). Interestingly, calendula extract failed to show any significant activity in vitro against common oral microorganisms in a second study that tested it against the saliva and dental plaque from 20 infants (Modesto et al 2000); however, a homeopathic preparation of calendula has been found to inhibit *Streptococcus mutans* (Giorgi et al 2004).

Commission E approves the internal and topical use of calendula flowers for inflammation of the oral and pharyngeal mucosa (Blumenthal et al 2000).

Nappy rash

In a postmarketing surveillance study (Guala et al 2007), 82 infants aged between 3 days and 48 months were randomised to receive either calendula cream (Weleda) or Babygella for treatment of their nappy rash. Both preparations were judged by doctors and mothers as useful; however mothers tended to describe the calendula cream more frequently than Babygella as very good rather than satisfactory. The calendula cream also contained other anti-inflammatory and healing ingredients, such as chamomile and zinc, making the contribution of calendula hard to judge.

In a double-blind RCT, 66 children suffering from diaper dermatitis ('nappy rash') were treated with either *Aloe vera* (syn. *Aloe barbadensis*) cream or calendula ointment. The treatment was applied three times a day over a period of 10 days and, while an improvement was observed in both treatment groups, there was a significantly greater reduction in rash severity with calendula treatment (Panahi et al 2012).

OTHER USES

The British Herbal Pharmacopoeia recommends calendula for gastric and duodenal ulcers, amenorrhoea, dysmenorrhoea and epistaxis (BHMA 1983). Topically it is recommended for leg ulcers, varicose veins, haemorrhoids, eczema and proctitis. The specific indications are for enlarged or inflamed lymphatic nodes, sebaceous cysts, duodenal ulcers and acute and chronic inflammatory skin conditions. Its styptic activity makes it a popular topical treatment for bleeding.

Practice points/Patient counselling

- Calendula has antimicrobial and anti-inflammatory activity and promotes wound healing.
- European textbooks recommend calendula for inflammation of the skin, poorly healing wounds, bruises, boils, rashes, bed sores, dermatitis resulting from chilblains, wound healing after amputations, cracked nipples during pregnancy and lactation, acne, sunburns, burns and nappy rashes. Calendula is also indicated for pharyngitis and tonsillitis (Bisset 1994, Bruneton 1999, Evans 2002, Issac 1992).
- There is some evidence from clinical trials that calendula may be beneficial in the treatment of burns, wounds and gastrointestinal inflammation and ulceration.
- People who are sensitive or allergic to foods or plants from the Asteraceae (previously Compositae) family should use calendula with caution.

DOSAGE RANGE

- Dried herb: 1–2 g as an infusion daily in divided doses.
- Liquid extract (1 : 2): 15–30 mL/week for internal use or 1.5–4.5 mL/day in divided doses. Dilute 1 : 3 for external application.
- Tincture (1 : 5): 0.3–1.2 mL three times daily.
- Calendula oil can be produced by steeping fresh flowers in vegetable oil for 1 week. Strain before use.

TOXICITY

Calendula has low toxicity. No symptoms of toxicity were found after long-term administration of a calendula extract in animal studies (Elias et al 1990, ESCOP 1996). A study evaluating an excessive dose (5 g/kg) in rats found no toxicity; however signs of liver and kidney burden were noted (Silva et al 2007). Similarly, changes to biochemical (alanine aminotransferase, aspartate aminotransferase and alkaline phosphatase) and haematological (haemoglobin, erythrocytes and leucocytes) parameters as well as slight changes to hepatic parenchyma were seen in male rats after subchronic daily administration (250 mg/kg/day and 1000 mg/kg/day) over 90 days (Lagarto et al 2011). Calendula has been found to be neither mutagenic nor carcinogenic (Elias et al 1990).

ADVERSE REACTIONS

Irritant dermatitis from calendula has been reported (Paulsen 2002, Reider et al 2001) but is rare. Sesquiterpene lactones are the most important allergens present in Compositae species, but there are also a few cases of sensitisation from a coumarin, a sesquiterpene alcohol and a thiophene (Paulsen 2002).

A study of over 1000 patients randomly chosen from several different patch test clinics identified only one who reacted to calendula (Bruynzeel et al 1992). Patch test results need to be carefully interpreted because false positives can occur, as the following case shows. A 35-year-old woman with recalcitrant atopic dermatitis, with a positive patch test reaction to Compositae mix, was told she was allergic to calendula. However, it turned out that she followed a self-devised diet consisting largely of food products of the Asteraceae (previously Compositae) family (which includes lettuces and artichoke). On excluding these foods her skin condition improved quickly. This case report underscores the difficulty in determining the relevance of positive patch tests, and shows that thorough analysis of positive patch tests, by both patient and doctor, may reveal unexpected or less common sources of contact allergens (Wintzen et al 2003).

SIGNIFICANT INTERACTIONS

Controlled studies are not available to assess the interaction potential of calendula.

CONTRAINDICATIONS AND PRECAUTIONS

Use with caution in patients with confirmed allergy to herbs or foods from the Compositae family.

PREGNANCY USE

Insufficient reliable information available to assess safety.

PATIENTS' FAQs

What will this herb do for me?

Calendula is used for inflammatory skin conditions, including poor wound healing, burns and ulcers, due to its non-irritant, antiseptic and healing properties. Internally it is used for inflammation and ulceration of the digestive tract.

When will it start to work?

Topical effects are quickly established and should improve with continuous use. Internal use may take longer.

Are there any safety issues?

Although there have been some reports of allergic reactions to calendula, these are very rare. Calendula is generally well tolerated by children and adults.

REFERENCES

Ahmed S et al. Elemental analysis of *Calendula officinalis* plant and its probable therapeutic role in health. Pakistan J Sci Ind Res 46.4 (2003): 283–287.

Amirghofran Z, et al. Evaluation of the immunomodulatory effects of five herbal plants. J Ethnopharmacol 72.1–2 (2000): 167–172.

Babaee, N. et al. Antioxidant capacity of *Calendula officinalis* flowers extract and prevention of radiation induced oropharyngeal mucositis in patients with head and neck cancers: a randomized controlled clinical study. DARU Journal of Pharmaceutical sciences 21.1 (2013): 18

Bako E, et al. HPLC study on the carotenoid composition of *Calendula* products. J Biochem Biophys Meth 53.1–3 (2002): 241–250.

C

Barajas-Farias LM et al. A dual and opposite effect of *Calendula officinalis* flower extract: Chemoprotector and promoter in a rat hepatocarcinogenesis model. Planta Med 72.3 (2006): 217–221.

Bashir S et al. Studies on spasmogenic and spasmolytic activities of *Calendula officinalis* flowers. Phytother Res 20.10 (2006): 906–910.

Bezakova L et al. Inhibitory activity of isorhamnetin glycosides from *Calendula officinalis* L. on the activity of lipoxygenase. Pharmazie 51.2 (1996): 126–127.

BHMA (British Herbal Medicine Association Scientific Committee). British herbal pharmacopoeia. Cowling, UK: BHMA, 1983.

Bisset NG. Herbal drugs and phytopharmaceuticals. Boca Raton: CRC Press, 1994.

Blumenthal M, et al. (eds). Herbal medicine: expanded Commission E monographs. Austin, TX: Integrative Medicine Communications, 2000.

Bogdanova NS et al. Study of antiviral properties of *Calendula officinalis*. Farmakol Toksikol 33.3 (1970): 349–355.

Boucaud-Maitre Y, et al. Cytotoxic and antitumoral activity of *Calendula officinalis* extracts. Pharmazie 43.3 (1988): 220–221.

Bruneton J. Pharmcognosy, Phytochemistry, medicinal plants. Paris: Lavoisier, 1999.

Bruynzeel DP et al. Contact sensitization by alternative topical medicaments containing plant extracts. Contact Dermatitis 27.4 (1992): 278–279.

Cetkovic GS et al. Antioxidant properties of marigold extracts. Food Res Int 37.7 (2004): 643–650.

Chakurski I et al. Treatment of chronic colitis with an herbal combination of *Taraxacum officinale, Hypericum perforatum, Melissa officinalis, Calendula officinalis* and *Foeniculum vulgare*. Vutr Boles 20.6 (1981): 51–54.

Cordova CA et al. Protective properties of butanolic extract of the *Calendula officinalis* L. (marigold) against lipid peroxidation of rat liver microsomes and action as free radical scavenger. Redox Rep 7.2 (2002): 95–102.

Corina P et al. Treatment with acyclovir combined with a new Romanian product from plants. Oftalmologia 46.1 (1999): 55–57.

Cwikla, C., et al. Investigations into the antibacterial activities of phytotherapeutics against *Helicobacter pylori* and *Campylobacter jejuni*. Phytother Res 24 (2010): 649–56.

Della LR et al. The role of triterpenoids in the topical anti-inflammatory activity of *Calendula officinalis* flowers. Planta Med 60.6 (1994): 516–520.

Doligalska, M., et al. 2011. Triterpenoid saponins affect the function of P-glycoprotein and reduce the survival of the free-living stages of *Heligmosomoides bakeri*. Veterinary Parasitology 179 (2011): 144–151.

Duran V et al. Results of the clinical examination of an ointment with marigold (*Calendula officinalis*) extract in the treatment of venous leg ulcers. Int J Tissue React 27.3 (2005): 101–106.

Efstratiou, E., et al. 2012. Antimicrobial activity of *Calendula officinalis* petal extracts against fungi, as well as Gram-negative and Gram-positive clinical pathogens. Complementary Therapies in Clinical Practice 18 (2012): 4.

Elias R et al. Antimutagenic activity of some saponins isolated from *Calendula officinalis* L., *C. arvensis* L. and *Hedera helix* L. Mutagenesis 5.4 (1990): 327–331.

ESCOP (European Scientific Co-operative on Phytomedicine). Calendulae flos — Calendula flower monograph. Stuttgart: Thieme, 1996.

Evans W. Trease and Evans: pharmacognosy, 15th edn. Edinburgh: WS Saunders, 2002.

Fonseca, Y. M., et al. Protective effect of *Calendula officinalis* extract against UVB-induced oxidative stress in skin: Evaluation of reduced glutathione levels and matrix metalloproteinase secretion. Journal of Ethnopharmacology, 127 (2010): 6.

Frankič, T., et al. The comparison of in vivo antigenotoxic and antioxidative capacity of two propylene glycol extracts of *Calendula officinalis* (marigold) and vitamin E in young growing pigs. Journal of Animal Physiology and Animal Nutrition 93 (2009): 688–694.

Fronza, M., et al. Determination of the wound healing effect of *Calendula* extracts using the scratch assay with 3T3 fibroblasts. Journal of Ethnopharmacology 126 (2009): 463–467.

Garg S, Sharma SN. Development of medicated aerosol dressings of chlorhexidine acetate with hemostatics. Pharmazie 47.12 (1992): 924–926.

Giorgi JSJ et al. In vitro study of *Calendula officinalis, Echinacea angustifolia* and *Streptococcus mutans*. Arztezeitschr Naturheilverfahr 45.4 (2004): 205–213.

Gracza L, Szasz K. Examination of active agents of petals of marigold (*Calendula officinalis* L). Acta Pharm Hung 38.2 (1968): 118–125.

Guala A, et al. Efficacy and safety of two baby creams in children with diaper dermatitis: results of a postmarketing surveillance study. J Altern Complement Med 13.1 (2007): 16–118.

Hamburger M et al. Preparative purification of the major anti-inflammatory triterpenoid esters from Marigold (*Calendula officinalis*). Fitoterapia 74.4 (2003): 328–338.

Issac O. Die Ringelblume: Botanik, Chemie, Pharmakologie, Toxikologie, Pharmazie und therapeutische Verwendung Wiss. Stuttgart: Verl Ges, 1992.

Kalvatchev Z, et al. Anti-HIV activity of extracts from *Calendula officinalis* flowers. Biomed Pharmacother 51.4 (1997): 176–180.

Kasiram K, et al. Antifungal activity of *Calendula officinalis*. Indian J Pharm Sci 62.6 (2000): 464–466.

Klouchek-Popova E et al. Influence of the physiological regeneration and epithelialization using fractions isolated from *Calendula officinalis*. Acta Physiol Pharmacol Bulg 8.4 (1982): 63–67.

Krazhan IA, Garazha NN. Treatment of chronic catarrhal gingivitis with polysorb-immobilized calendula. Stomatologiia (Mosk) 80.5 (2001): 11–113.

Kundakovic, T., et al. Treatment of venous ulcers with the herbal-based ointment Herbadermal(R): a prospective non-randomized pilot study. Forsch Komplementmed, 19 (2012): 26–30.

Lagarto, A., et al. Acute and subchronic oral toxicities of *Calendula officinalis* extract in Wistar rats. Experimental and Toxicologic Pathology 63 (2011): 387–391.

Lavagna SM et al. Efficacy of *Hypericum* and *Calendula* oils in the epithelial reconstruction of surgical wounds in childbirth with caesarean section. Farmaco 56.5–7 (2001): 451–453.

Lievre M et al. Controlled study of three ointments for the local management of 2nd and 3rd degree burns. Clin Trials Meta-Analysis 28.1 (1992): 9–12.

Mascolo N, et al. Biological screening of Italian medicinal plants for anti-inflammatory activity. Phytother Res 1.1 (1987): 28–31.

Matev M et al. Use of an herbal combination with laxative action on duodenal peptic ulcer and gastroduodenitis patients with a concomitant obstipation syndrome. Vutr Boles 20.6 (1981): 48–51.

Matic, I. Z., et al. Chamomile and Marigold Tea: Chemical Characterization and Evaluation of Anticancer Activity. Phytother Res.(2012)

Modesto A, et al. Effects of three different infant dentifrices on biofilms and oral microorganisms. J Clin Pediatr Dent 24.3 (2000): 237–243.

Neukirch H et al. Improved anti-inflammatory activity of three new terpenoids derived, by systematic chemical modifications, from the abundant triterpenes of the flowery plant *Calendula officinalis*. Chem Biodiversity 2.5 (2005): 657–671.

Panahi, Y., et al. A randomized comparative trial on the therapeutic efficacy of topical aloe vera and *Calendula officinalis* on diaper dermatitis in children. Scientific World Journal, (2012) 2012: 810234.

Parente, L. M., et al. Wound Healing and Anti-Inflammatory Effect in Animal Models of *Calendula officinalis* L. Growing in Brazil. Evid Based Complement Alternat Med (2012) 2012: 375671.

Paulsen E. Contact sensitization from Compositae-containing herbal remedies and cosmetics. Contact Dermatitis 47.4 (2002): 189–198.

Perez-Carreon JI et al. Genotoxic and anti-genotoxic properties of *Calendula officinalis* extracts in rat liver cell cultures treated with diethylnitrosamine. Toxicol in Vitro 16.3 (2002): 253–258.

Pommier P et al. Phase III randomized trial of *Calendula officinalis* compared with trolamine for the prevention of acute dermatitis during irradiation for breast cancer. J Clin Oncol 22.8 (2004): 1447–1453.

Re, T. A., et al. 2009. Application of the threshold of toxicological concern approach for the safety evaluation of calendula flower (*Calendula officinalis*) petals and extracts used in cosmetic and personal care products. Food and Chemical Toxicology 47 (2009): 1246–1254.

Reider N et al. The seamy side of natural medicines: Contact sensitization to arnica (*Arnica montana* L.) and marigold (*Calendula officinalis* L.). Contact Dermatitis 45.5 (2001): 269–272.

Rusu MA et al. The hepatoprotective action of ten herbal extracts in CCl4 intoxicated liver. Phytother Res 19.9 (2005): 744–749.

Samochowiec E et al. Evaluation of the effect of *Calendula officinalis* and *Echinacea angustifolia* extracts of *Trichomonas vaginalis* in vitro. Wiad Parazytol 25.1 (1979): 77–81.

Sharp, L., et al. No differences between *Calendula* cream and aqueous cream in the prevention of acute radiation skin reactions, Results from a randomised blinded trial. European Journal of Oncology Nursing (2012):1–7

Shipochliev T, et al. Anti-inflammatory action of a group of plant extracts. Vet Med Nauki 18.6 (1981): 87–94.

Silva EJ et al. Toxicological studies on hydroalcohol extract of *Calendula officinalis* L. Phytother Res 21.4 (2007): 332–336.

Szakiel, A., et al. Antibacterial and Antiparasitic Activity of Oleanolic Acid and its Glycosides isolated from Marigold (*Calendula officinalis*). Planta Medica 74(2008): 1709–1715.

Tanideh, N., et al. Healing acceleration in hamsters of oral mucositis induced by 5-fluorouracil with topical *Calendula officinalis*. Oral Surgery, Oral Medicine, Oral Pathology and Oral Radiology 115(2013): 332–338.

Ukiya M et al. Anti-inflammatory, anti-tumor-promoting, and cytotoxic activities of constituents of marigold (*Calendula officinalis*) flowers. J Nat Prod 69.12 (2006): 1692–1696.

Van der Velden EM, Van der Dussen MFN. Dermatography as an adjunctive treatment for cleft lip and palate patients. J Oral Maxillofac Surg 53.1 (1995): 9–12.
Varljen J, et al. Structural analysis of a rhamnoarabinogalactan and arabinogalactans with immuno-stimulating activity from *Calendula officinalis*. Phytochemistry 28 (1989): 2379–2383.
Wagner H et al. Immunostimulating action of polysaccharides (heteroglycans) from higher plants. Arzneimittelforschung 35.7 (1985): 1069–1075.
WHO (World Health Organization). Flos Calendulae. Online. Available: http://www.who.int/medicines/library/trm/medicinalplants/vol2/035to044.pdf 2003.
Wintzen M, et al. Recalcitrant atopic dermatitis due to allergy to Compositae. Contact Dermatitis 48.2 (2003): 87–88.
Yoshikawa M et al. Medicinal flowers. III. Marigold. (1): Hypoglycemic, gastric emptying inhibitory, and gastroprotective principles and new oleanane-type triterpene oligoglycosides, calendasaponins A, B, C, and D, from Egyptian *Calendula officinalis*. Chem Pharm Bull 49.7 (2001): 863–870.
Zitterl-Eglseer K et al. Anti-oedematous activities of the main triterpendiol esters of marigold (*Calendula officinalis* L.). J Ethnopharmacol 57.2 (1997): 139–144.
Zitterl-Eglseer K et al. Morphogenetic variability of faradiol monoesters in marigold *Calendula officinalis* L. Phytochem Anal 12.3 (2001): 199–201.

Carnitine

BACKGROUND AND RELEVANT PHARMACOKINETICS

Carnitine was discovered in 1905, although its role in metabolism was only described in the mid-1950s and deficiency symptoms outlined in 1972. It is a trimethylated amino acid, roughly similar in structure to choline, that is ingested in the diet and also synthesised from lysine and methionine in the body. To do this, a large number of cofactors are required, such as *S*-adenosyl methionine, methionine, magnesium, vitamins C, B_6, B_2, B_3, iron, alpha-ketoglutarate and oxygen (Kelly 1998). Dietary carnitine is absorbed in the intestine via a combination of active transport and passive diffusion (Li et al 1992). Mucosal absorption is saturated at around 2 g carnitine (Harper et al 1988). The bioavailability of carnitine is difficult to establish as reports vary widely, from 16% to 87% (Harper et al 1988, Rebouche & Chenard 1991). Peak blood levels occur 3.5 hours after digestion and excretion is primarily via the kidneys (Bach et al 1983).

CHEMICAL COMPONENTS

L-Carnitine is the form most commonly used. As the D form is not biologically active, there is concern that it might interfere with the use of the L isomer by competitive inhibition and thus cause L-carnitine deficiency (Tsoko et al 1995).

FOOD SOURCES

Red meat is the richest dietary source. Vegetarian sources include avocado and tempeh (Hendler & Rorvik 2001). Human colostrum also contains carnitine (Wahlqvist 2002).

DEFICIENCY SIGNS AND SYMPTOMS

L-Carnitine deficiency leads to an accumulation of free fatty acids in the cell cytoplasm and of acyl-coenzyme A (CoA) in the mitochondria. This produces a toxic effect and disturbs fatty acid use for

Clinical note — Acetyl-L-carnitine shows promise as a strong therapeutic agent

Acetyl-L-carnitine, an ester form of L-carnitine, has also been investigated for its use in the treatment of Alzheimer's disease (Brooks et al 1998, Pettegrew et al 1995, Sano et al 1992, Thal et al 1996); depression (Garzya 1990), physical and mental fatigue, cognitive status and physical function in the elderly (Malaguarnera et al 2008); diabetic (De Grandis & Minardi 2002), peripheral (Onofrj et al 1995) and antiretroviral toxic neuropathy (Youle & Osio 2007) as well as prevention of neuropathy in chemotherapy (Bianchi et al 2005, Maestri et al 2005). It has also been researched for fatigue in multiple sclerosis (Tomassini et al 2004), fibromyalgia syndrome (Rossini et al 2007), Peyronie's disease (Biagiotti & Cavallini 2001), degenerative cerebellar ataxia (Sorbi et al 2000) and cognitive disturbances in chronic alcoholics (Tempesta et al 1990).

Clinical note — Primary carnitine deficiency: an uncommon inherited disorder

Primary carnitine deficiency is an uncommon inherited disorder, related to a functional defect in plasma membrane carnitine transport in muscle and in the kidneys. These conditions have been classified as either systemic or myopathic (Evangeliou & Vlassopoulos 2003, Matera et al 2003). Systemic carnitine deficiency is reflected by low levels of carnitine in plasma and muscle and may result in cardiomyopathy, skeletal myopathy, hypoglycaemia and hyperammonaemia (Hendler & Rorvik 2001). Myopathic deficiency presents with normal plasma but low muscle carnitine levels and is a defect of carnitine transport across the muscle cell membrane (Winter et al 1987).

energy production (Kletzmayr et al 1999). Elevation of triglycerides may also occur due to the role of carnitine in fatty acid metabolism.

Deficiency symptoms (Kelly 1998) include the following:

- hypoglycaemia
- progressive myasthenia
- hypotonia
- fatigue
- cardiomyopathy
- congestive heart failure
- encephalopathy
- hepatomegaly
- neuromuscular disorders
- failure to thrive in infants
- muscle fatigue and cramps
- myoglobinaemia following exercise.

Elevation of triglycerides may also occur due to the role of carnitine in fatty acid metabolism.

Primary deficiency

People at risk of primary deficiency are vegetarians, preterm infants and infants receiving a carnitine-free formula, and those with an inherited functional defect.

Secondary deficiency

Secondary carnitine deficiency is associated with several inborn errors of metabolism and acquired medical or iatrogenic conditions, such as the following (Evangeliou & Vlassopoulos 2003):

- genetic defects of metabolism, including methylmalonic aciduria, cytochrome C oxidase deficiency, fatty acyl-CoA dehydrogenase deficiency
- medications (patients taking valproate and the anti-HIV drug azidothymidine are at risk)
- dialysis (carnitine depletion in haemodialysis patients is caused by insufficient carnitine synthesis and particularly by loss through the dialytic membranes. Many studies have shown that L-carnitine supplementation leads to improvements in several complications seen in uraemic patients, including cardiac complications, impaired exercise and functional capacities, muscle symptoms, increased symptomatic intradialytic hypotension and erythropoietin-resistant anaemia, normalising the reduced carnitine palmitoyl transferase activity in red cells [Matera et al 2003])
- liver disease, which impairs the last stage of carnitine synthesis, resulting in deficiencies in cardiac and skeletal muscle
- chronic renal failure and renal tubular disorders, in which excretion of carnitine may be excessive
- intestinal resection
- coeliac disease (a case report exists of a 48-year-old man developing encephalopathy due to carnitine deficiency as a result of coeliac disease [Karakoc et al 2006]. In patients with idiopathic dilated cardiomyopathy associated with coeliac disease, a gluten-free diet has been shown to increase serum carnitine levels [Curione et al 2005])
- preterm neonates (develop carnitine deficiency due to impaired proximal renal tubule carnitine reabsorption and immature carnitine biosynthesis)
- hypopituitarism (Martindale 1999)
- adrenal insufficiency (Hendler & Rorvik 2001)
- advanced AIDS (Hendler & Rorvik 2001)
- vitamin C deficiency (Hendler & Rorvik 2001)
- other chronic conditions — diabetes mellitus, heart failure, Alzheimer's disease.

C

MAIN ACTIONS

Carnitine is involved in a myriad of biochemical processes important for health and wellbeing.

Cellular energy production

Carnitine assists the transport of fat across cell membranes in muscle tissue for use as an energy source (Wahlqvist 2002). It is essential for mitochondrial fatty acid oxidation, which is the primary fuel source for the heart and skeletal muscles and therefore required for proper functioning (Evangeliou & Vlassopoulos 2003, Kelly 1998). This process is also required in order to maintain CoA levels. The combination of exercise training and L-carnitine (4 g/day) supplementation does not appear to augment fatty acid-binding protein (FABPc) expression and beta-hydroxyacyl CoA dehydrogenase (beta-HAD) activity in human skeletal muscle, indicating that combined treatment does not exert an additive effect in fat metabolism and would thus be unlikely to enhance exercise performance (Lee et al 2007).

Improved blood sugar control

Administration of L-carnitine reduces insulin secretion and improves peripheral glucose use (Grandi et al 1997) and tissue insulin sensitivity (Negro et al 1994).

Cellular function and integrity

Carnitine is involved in the protection of membrane structures, stabilising a physiological CoA-sulfate hydrate/acetyl-CoA ratio, and reduction of lactate production (Matera et al 2003).

Antioxidant

Carnitine acts as an antioxidant in the cell membrane, preventing protein oxidation and pyruvate and lactate oxidative damage (Peluso et al 2000). In vitro studies suggest a dose-dependent inhibition of lipid peroxidation of linoleic acid emulsion superior to alpha-tocopherol. In addition, L-carnitine may have an effect on superoxide anion radical scavenging, hydrogen peroxide scavenging, total reducing power and metal chelating on ferrous ions (Gulcin 2006).

OTHER ACTIONS

Increases male fertility

Based on the high concentrations of L-carnitine in the epididymis, it has been proposed that spermatozoa, which require beta oxidation for energy, may require L-carnitine for proper maturation (Lenzi et al 1992). Human trials have found carnitine therapy (2–3 g/day) to be effective in increasing semen quality, sperm concentration and total and forward sperm motility, especially in groups with lower baseline levels (Lenzi et al 2003). One trial also reported that improvements in sperm motility were only observed in the presence of normal mitochondrial function, determined by phospholipid hydroperoxide glutathione peroxidase levels (Garolla et al 2005).

Prevents apoptosis

In vitro and animal studies show that L-carnitine can prevent apoptosis of skeletal muscle cells (Vescovo et al 2002). In patients with HIV it decreases numbers of $CD4^+$ and $CD8^+$ cells undergoing apoptosis, and significantly increases $CD4^+$ counts (Moretti et al 2002).

Neuroprotective

Animal studies have demonstrated a reduction in mortality and neuronal degeneration in experimentally-induced neurotoxicity (Binienda et al 2004) and a reduction in hypoglycaemia-induced neuronal damage (Hino et al 2005) in rats that were pretreated with carnitine. In vitro studies suggest that the antiapoptotic and antioxidant actions of L-carnitine contribute to the neuroprotective effect (Ishii et al 2000, Tastekin et al 2005).

Lipid lowering

The role of carnitine in fatty acid metabolism suggests a potential role in hyperlipidaemia. Several studies have indicated that oral L-carnitine significantly reduces lipoprotein-a levels; however, effects on other lipids are inconsistent. According to human trials the addition of L-carnitine (2 g/day) to simvastatin therapy (20 mg/day) appears to lower lipoprotein-a serum levels in patients with type 2 diabetes mellitus (Solfrizzi et al 2006). In a separate placebo-controlled, double-blind randomised study L-carnitine (2 g/day) significantly reduced serum lipoprotein-a levels in 77.8% of subjects receiving active treatment after 12 weeks. No significant change was observed in other lipid parameters (Sirtori et al 2000). L-Carnitine (2 g/day) was also shown to significantly lower lipoprotein-a levels at 3 and 6 months in a double-blind placebo-controlled trial of 94 hypercholesterolaemic patients with newly diagnosed type 2 diabetes (Derosa et al 2003). In a trial of children with hyperlipidaemia, lipoprotein-a levels were only reduced in those with type II homozygotes and other lipid parameters worsened (Gunes et al 2005).

L-Carnitine has also been shown to decrease apolipoprotein B levels in paediatric peritoneal dialysis patients (Kosan et al 2003). A study of elderly people taking L-carnitine (2 g twice daily) demonstrated improvements in total serum cholesterol, low-density lipoprotein (LDL)-cholesterol, low-density lipoprotein (HDL)-cholesterol, triglycerides and apoproteins A1 and B at 30 days (Pistone et al 2003). Animal studies have also suggested the potential for carnitine to lower triglyceride levels (Eskandari et al 2004); however, clinical trials using oral doses in type 2 diabetes have indicated an increase in triglycerides (Rahbar et al 2005). Further human trials are required to confirm which population groups may benefit from carnitine supplementation.

CLINICAL USE

Carnitine supplementation may be administered as intravenous (IV) or oral doses. This review will only focus on oral supplementation as this is the form generally used by the public and available over the counter.

Treatment of deficiency

L-Carnitine supplementation is traditionally used to treat or prevent deficiency. It is indicated in primary L-carnitine deficiency and secondary deficiency due to inborn errors of metabolism or haemodialysis. L-Carnitine 50–200 mg/kg/day has been shown to normalise plasma carnitine levels within 10 days (Campos et al 1993).

Apnoea of prematurity

Preterm neonates develop carnitine deficiency due to impaired proximal renal tubule carnitine reabsorption and immature carnitine biosynthesis (Evangeliou & Vlassopoulos 2003) and are at risk of developing apnoea of prematurity. Despite a promising preliminary study, a blinded, randomised, placebo-controlled study found that infants who received supplemental carnitine did not demonstrate any reduction in apnoea of prematurity, days requiring ventilator or nasal continuous positive airway pressure, or the need for supplemental oxygen therapy (O'Donnell et al 2002). In a randomised controlled trial (RCT) premature neonates supplemented with carnitine (20 mg/kg/day) gained weight more rapidly and showed improvement in periodic breathing compared to placebo, although other respiratory markers were unaffected (Crill et al 2006). A 2004 Cochrane review was unable to locate studies of significant quality to confirm any effects (Kumar et al 2004a). Further studies are needed to determine the role of this treatment in clinical practice as present evidence does not support its use (Kumar et al 2004b).

Cardiovascular disease

L-Carnitine supplementation in doses ranging from 2 g to 4 g/day has been investigated in a number of controlled studies involving subjects with angina, heart failure, cardiogenic shock, cardiomyopathy and post myocardial infarction (MI). Overall, positive results have been obtained and reduced mortality reported for some populations.

In a small study investigating endothelial function in 31 patients receiving haemodialysis, 20 patients received 1500 mg oral L-carnitine (3 × 500 mg/day) on alternate days and 11 patients served as a control group, receiving placebo for 1 month. At completion of the study there were no significant differences in flow-mediated dilation or in carotid intima media thickness in either group of patients (Sabri et al 2012).

Chronic stable angina

Controlled studies indicate that L-carnitine supplements increase exercise tolerance and reduce frequency of angina attacks, enabling some patients to reduce nitrate requirements.

One RCT of 47 patients with chronic stable angina found that 2 g L-carnitine taken daily for 3 months moderately improved the duration of exercise and the time taken for ST changes to recover to baseline (Iyer et al 2000). This study confirmed the results of an earlier multicentre, double-blind, randomised, placebo-controlled crossover trial that examined the effects of L-carnitine 1 g twice daily for 4 weeks in 44 men with stable chronic angina (Cherchi et al 1985). This study showed that active treatment resulted in increased exercise tolerance and reduced electrocardiographic indices of ischaemia in stable effort-induced angina. A meta-analysis also highlighted a significant reduction in the number of angina attacks and nitrate requirements with doses of 2 g/day (Fernandez & Proto 1992).

Post myocardial infarction

L-carnitine supplementation may lead to a reduction in early mortality (assessed at day 5) without affecting the risk of death and heart failure at 6 months in patients with anterior acute MI (Tarantini et al 2006). A dose of 4 g/day L-carnitine over 12 months improved quality of life and increased life expectancy in patients who had suffered an MI, according to a controlled study (Davini et al 1992). This included an improvement in heart rate, systolic arterial pressure, a decrease in anginal attacks and improvement in the lipid profile. Changes were also accompanied by lower mortality in the treated group (1.2% vs 12.5% in the control group).

In a randomised, double-blind placebo-controlled trial, the effects of oral L-carnitine (2 g/day) for 28 days were assessed in patients with suspected acute MI. Total cardiac events, including cardiac deaths and non-fatal infarction, were 15.6% in the carnitine group and 26.0% in the placebo group. Angina pectoris (17.6% vs 36.0%), New York Heart Association class III or IV heart failure plus left ventricular enlargement (23.4% vs 36.0%) and total arrhythmias (13.7% vs 28.0%) were significantly less in the carnitine group compared with placebo (Singh et al 1996).

Cardiomyopathy

Cardiomyopathy appears to cause leakage of carnitine from heart stores, which may make cardiac tissue vulnerable to damage; however, it is unclear whether carnitine leakage is a cause or effect of cardiomyopathy (Baker et al 2005). Long-term placebo-controlled studies (10–54 months) using an oral dose of 2 g/day L-carnitine for treatment of heart failure caused by cardiomyopathy found a statistically significant advantage in survival rates with carnitine treatment (Rizos 2000). In patients with idiopathic dilated cardiomyopathy associated with coeliac disease, a gluten-free diet has been shown to increase serum carnitine levels (Curione et al 2005).

C

Cardiogenic shock

Several studies confirm the role of L-carnitine in the reversible phase of cardiogenic shock in terms of enzymic protection in the course of cellular oxidative damage. This has been reflected in improved survival rates (Corbucci & Lettieri 1991, Corbucci & Loche 1993).

Congestive heart failure

In congestive heart failure a specific myopathy secondary to myocyte apoptosis triggered by high levels of circulating tumour necrosis factor-alpha (TNF-alpha) has been described. The role of carnitine in preventing apoptosis in skeletal muscle and reducing TNF-alpha provides a theoretical basis for its use in the treatment of myopathy associated with congestive heart failure (Vescovo et al 2002).

Myocarditis resulting from diphtheria

Two studies using D,L-carnitine (100 mg/kg/day in two divided doses orally for 4 days) found a reduction in the incidence of, and mortality from, myocarditis in diphtheria (Ramos et al 1984, 1992).

Non-ST elevation acute coronary syndrome (NSTEMI)

In an RCT 96 patients with NSTEMI were randomised to treatment or control group. All patients received percutanenous coronary intervention within 24 hours from the onset of chest pain. The treatment group also received L-carnitine (5 g IV bolus followed by 10 g/day IV infusion for 3 days) and demonstrated significantly lower levels of cardiac markers (creatine kinase-MB and troponin-I) (Xue et al 2007).

Peripheral vascular disease

Due to its anti-ischaemic activity, L-carnitine supplements have also been used in peripheral vascular disease. A double-blind crossover study supports this use, finding L-carnitine supplements (2 g/day) taken for 3 weeks increased walking time in people with peripheral vascular disease (Brevetti et al 1988). A derivative of L-carnitine, known as propionyl-L-carnitine (PLC), taken for 6 months (2 g/day orally) has also demonstrated significant improvements in walking distance and speed in patients with claudication (Hiatt et al 2001).

A recent systematic review evaluating the effect of L-carnitine or PLC supplementation on walking performance in patients with intermittent claudication concluded that the majority of included studies

(17 articles, with 18 studies of varying duration [4–365 days]; five pretest/posttest studies in which 300–2000 mg PLC was administered orally or intravenously; eight parallel RCT in which PLC was administered orally [600–3000 mg in seven studies and 600 mg/day PLC, intravenously in one study]; five crossover RCTs in which 300–6000 mg L-carnitine or PLC was administered orally in two studies and intravenously in three studies) demonstrated a significant improvement in walking performance, particularly among patients with severe claudication, and also that oral administration was less effective compared to IV administration (Delaney et al 2013).

Likewise, in another recent systematic review and meta-analysis, the effect of PLC administration (daily dose range of 1.0–3.0 g among the included studies) was investigated regarding exercise performance in patients with claudication and it was concluded that oral PLC supplementation resulted in a statistically significant increase in peak walking distance (Brass et al 2013).

Hypertension

In a small open pilot study the effect of oral acetyl-L-carnitine (2 g/day given as 2 × 1 g/day) supplementation was investigated regarding components of the metabolic syndrome over the course of 24 weeks in non-diabetic subjects who were categorised in one of two groups (glucose disposal rate ≤7.9 [n = 16] or >7.9 [n = 16] mg/kg/min) who completed the study. Supplementation of acetyl-L-carnitine significantly reduced the arterial blood pressure and increased plasma adiponectin levels. Acetyl-L-carnitine was also effective in ameliorating insulin resistance and impaired glucose tolerance in patients who were insulin-resistant at the start of the study compared to those with normal or near-normal insulin sensitivity (Ruggenenti et al 2009).

However the role of L-carnitine and acylcarnitine derivatives remains to be determined, as a recent study of African (n = 101) and Caucasian (n = 101) men reported that, independently of ethnicity, higher levels of serum free L-carnitine were significantly associated with elevated blood pressure (Mels et al 2013). The authors of this study considered that increased carnitine biosynthesis may be due to reduced tissue uptake or reduced renal excretion or increased oxidative stress or higher cardiac energy demands due to increases in blood pressure.

Hyperthyroidism

Considering that this condition is associated with reduced body stores of carnitine and that L-carnitine is a peripheral antagonist of thyroid hormone action in some tissues according to in vivo studies, carnitine treatment has been investigated in hyperthyroidism.

One 6-month, randomised, double-blind placebo-controlled trial involving 50 women with induced suppression of thyroid-stimulating hormone showed that doses of 2 g or 4 g/day oral L-carnitine both reversed and prevented symptoms of the disease and had a beneficial effect on bone mineralisation (Benvenega et al 2001).

Male fertility

Some studies suggest that a combination of L-carnitine and acetyl-L-carnitine may provide benefit for the treatment of idiopathic asthenospermia and improve semen quality (Cheng & Chen 2008). A placebo-controlled, double-blind crossover trial of 100 infertile males (aged 20–40 years) found that L-carnitine therapy (2 g/day) was effective in increasing semen quality, sperm concentration and total and forward sperm motility, especially in groups with lower baseline levels (Lenzi et al 2003). The positive effects on sperm motility have also been shown in previous trials using L-carnitine 3 g/day (Costa et al 1994, Vitali et al 1995). In a later trial, improvements in sperm motility were only observed in the presence of normal mitochondrial function, determined by phospholipid hydroperoxide glutathione peroxidase levels (Garolla et al 2005). A meta-analysis comparing L-carnitine and/or acetyl-L-carnitine therapy to placebo found significant improvements in pregnancy rate ($P < 0.0001$), total sperm motility ($P = 0.04$), forward sperm motility ($P = 0.04$) and atypical sperm cells ($P < 0.00001$), but not sperm concentration or semen volume (Zhou et al 2007). One small RCT of 21 men (12 in the treatment group, 9 in the placebo group) with idiopathic asthenospermia showed that a combination of L-carnitine (2000 mg) and L-acetyl-carnitine (1000 mg) taken daily over 24 weeks failed to demonstrate improvements in sperm motility or total motile sperm counts (Sigman et al 2006).

In a 3-month study of patients (aged 22–35 years) with idiopathic infertility, 20 men were randomised to receive L-carnitine (25 mg/day) and 32 men received an antioestrogen clomiphene citrate (2 g/day). There was a significant increase in serum volume in the carnitine group ($P > 0.001$) and clomiphene citrate was reported to result in improved sperm motility and morphology (Moradi et al 2010).

Supplementary carnitine may have a role in assisted reproductive medicine because sperm quality can be adversely affected by cryopreservation. A recent study investigating the cryoprotective effect of L-carnitine on motility, vitality and DNA oxidation on human spermatozoa reported that semen samples from 22 infertile patients, when treated with L-carnitine at a ratio of 1:1 (v/v) (final carnitine concentration per cryovial of 0.5 mg/mL per 5 × 10^6 cell/mL) resulted in improved sperm motility and vitality ($P > 0.05$) compared to control semen samples that were cryopreserved without the addition of L-carnitine. However L-carnitine did not have any effect on sperm DNA oxidation after cryopreservation (Banihani et al 2013).

Decreased carnitine levels as well as low levels of testosterone in male patients on haemodialysis compared to healthy controls have been reported (Sakai et al 2013) and the role of supplementary carnitine remains to be determined in uraemic men on haemodialysis who are at risk of hypogonadism.

Ergogenic aid

L-Carnitine is a popular supplement amongst athletes in the belief that it will increase performance and recovery. This concept is largely based on the fact that carnitine assists in the transport of fat across cell membranes in muscle tissue and is involved in cellular energy production. However, the combination of exercise training and L-carnitine (4 g/day) supplementation does not appear to augment FABPc expression and beta-HAD activity in human skeletal muscle, suggesting that combined treatment does not exert an additive effect in fat metabolism and would thus be unlikely to enhance exercise performance (Lee et al 2007).

Carnitine reduces insulin secretion and significantly improves peripheral glucose use, when administered with glucose, according to human research (Grandi et al 1997). There is evidence that L-carnitine supplementation may increase maximal oxygen consumption, stimulate lipid metabolism and reduce postexercise plasma lactate (Karlic & Lohninger 2004). One trial reported that acute intake of L-carnitine (2 g) 1 hour prior to exercise did not appear to affect metabolic or blood lactate values of badminton players, although there was a significant difference in exercise maximum heart rate in male participants ($P < 0.05$) (Eroglu et al 2008).

In a placebo-controlled crossover trial using an L-carnitine–L-tartrate (LCLT) supplement (2 g L-carnitine/day) for 3 weeks, researchers suggested that LCLT supplementation was effective in assisting recovery from high-repetition squat exercise (Volek et al 2002). A similar trial of the same dose and duration suggested that recovery from postresistance exercise may be mediated by upregulation of androgen receptor content (Kraemer et al 2006). However, other clinical trials using 2 g L-carnitine twice daily for 3 months found no significant increase in muscle carnitine content, mitochondrial proliferation or physical performance (Wachter et al 2002). Similarly, a study using glycine PLC (1–3 g/day) for 8 weeks in conjunction with aerobic exercise training failed to demonstrate improvement in muscle carnitine content, aerobic or anaerobic exercise performance (Smith et al 2008).

Ergogenic aid in cardiovascular disease

Trials in subjects with cardiovascular disorders have been more promising. This is supported by the clinical trial discussed earlier involving patients with chronic stable angina (Iyer et al 2000). In addition, a clinical trial using 1 g L-carnitine or placebo three times daily for 120 days has indicated a potential for improved performance and effort tolerance in patients with cardiac insufficiency (Loster et al 1999).

Ergogenic aid in chronic obstructive pulmonary disease (COPD)

Compared to placebo, L-carnitine (2 g/day) for 6 weeks can significantly improve inspiratory muscle strength (14 ± 5 vs 40 ± 14 cm H_2O) and exercise tolerance (walking test: 34 ± 29 vs 87 ± 30 m, $P < 0.05$) in COPD patients, as well as reducing lactate production (2.3 ± 0.7 vs 1.6 ± 0.7 mM, $P < 0.05$) (Borghi-Silva et al 2006).

OTHER USES

Cancer

Animal studies have reported that L-carnitine can modulate the inflammatory mechanisms via regulation of carnitine palmityl transferase (Liu et al 2011) and human cell line studies have demonstrated inhibition of apoptosis and DNA damage as a result of L-carnitine supplementation (Zaugg et al 2011). As L-carnitine is well known for its role in energy generation by mitochondrial β-oxidation, the utility of supplementary L-carnitine in patients with advanced cancer has been investigated because of L-carnitine deficiency in cancer cachexia and cancer-related fatigue.

In a recent prospective, multicentre, placebo-controlled, randomised and double-blinded study, 72 patients with advanced pancreatic cancer received either 4 g oral L-carnitine or placebo for 12 weeks. At enrolment there were 38 patients in the carnitine-supplemented group and 34 in the control group, and 14 and 12 patients completed the study, respectively and the drop-outs were related to medical issues, not the intervention. The patients in the carnitine-supplemented group were reported to have increased their body mass index by 3.4 ± 1.4% compared to the control group, whose body mass index decreased by 1.5 ± 1.4% ($P < 0.05$) (Kraft et al 2012). In addition the carnitine-supplemented group was reported to have an improvement in some quality-of-life measures, as determined by European Organisation for Research and Treatment of Cancer (EORTC)-Quality of Life Questionnaire (QLQ)-C30, with a pancreatic cancer-specific module. In addition there was a trend in increased overall survival (median 519 ± 50 days vs 399 ± 43 days) and also reduced hospital stay (36 ± 4 days vs 41 ± 9 days), although these results were not statistically significant (Kraft et al 2012).

Neuropathy

The role of acetyl-L-carnitine as a potential neural protective agent has been investigated in cancer treatment-related neuropathy. In a large 24-week placebo-controlled double-blind randomised study of breast cancer, women undergoing adjuvant taxane-based chemotherapy who received acetyl-L-carnitine ($n = 208$, 3000 mg/day) were reported to have a significant increase in chemotherapy-induced peripheral neuropathy by 24 weeks, although there were no differences between the groups at 12 weeks and fatigue levels did not differ either. The study reported that the supplemented group was more likely to have a >5-point decrease in the neurotoxicity component of the FACT-NXT scores (38% vs 28%; $P = 0.05$) (Hershman et al 2013).

In contrast, in a placebo-controlled double-blind RCT of ovarian cancer (OC: $n = 98$) and castration-resistant prostate cancer ($n = 52$) patients receiving sagopilone (16 mg/m^2 intravenously over 3 hours every 3 weeks), the group ($n = 75$) given supplementation of acetyl-L-carnitine (1000 mg every 3 days) reported significantly lower incidence of grade 3 or 4 peripheral neuropathy in the OC group compared to the OC group receiving placebo. However there was no significant difference in duration of neuropathy or overall incidence of peripheral neuropathy (Campone et al 2013).

Fatigue

Chronic fatigue syndrome (CFS)

Studies investigating whether people with CFS have lower levels of free L-carnitine have shown contradictory results (Jones et al 2005), and trials using L-carnitine supplementation in CFS have generally produced mixed results (Plioplys & Plioplys 1995, 1997, Soetekouw et al 2000). One RCT did find that 1 g L-carnitine (three times daily) produced a significant clinical improvement, especially between the fourth and eighth week of treatment (Plioplys & Plioplys 1997).

Fatigue in cancer patients

A number of studies have reported the benefits of oral L-carnitine in patients with chemotherapy-related side effects such as fatigue. In a trial of advanced cancer patients, 76% were found to be carnitine-deficient. In a subset of patients (those whose carnitine levels increase with supplementation) doses up to 3 g/day are deemed to be safe and may reduce fatigue (Cruciani et al 2006).

In a large double-blind, placebo-controlled trial of 376 patients with cancer and fatigue, the change in fatigue was determined in 189 patients who were randomly assigned to 2 g/day of L-carnitine oral supplementation and 187 received a placebo for 4 weeks. The supplemented group resulted in a significant increase in plasma carnitine levels but did not produce a significant change in fatigue levels beyond placebo (L-carnitine: −0.96, 95% confidence interval [CI] −1.32 to −0.60; placebo: −1.11, 95% CI −1.44 to −0.78; $P = 0.57$) (Cruciani et al 2012).

Fatigue in coeliac disease patients

L-Carnitine blood levels are low in coeliac disease patients most likely due to reduced OCTN2 levels (the specific carnitine transporter). In 60 coeliac disease patients, L-carnitine supplementation (2 g/day) for 180 days has been shown to be safe and effective in ameliorating fatigue measured by the Scott-Huskisson Visual Analogue Scale for Asthenia compared with placebo ($P = 0.0021$) (Ciacci et al 2007).

Fatigue in multiple sclerosis

A recent systematic review evaluated the effect of carnitine supplementation on quality of life and symptoms of fatigue in patients with multiple sclerosis-related fatigue; the review included a currently ongoing randomised, placebo-controlled, crossover trial and one completed study which was randomised, active-comparator, crossover in design and conducted over 12 months. In the completed study, 30 patients were exposed to both acetyl-L-carnitine 2 g/day (as two divided doses) and amantadine 200 mg/day (divided as two doses). The effect of carnitine was not clear and therefore it was concluded that at present there is a lack of evidence to support the use of supplemental carnitine for multiple sclerosis-related fatigue (Tejani et al 2012). It is expected that results from ongoing and future studies will provide more data regarding the effects of carnitine supplementation on multiple sclerosis-related symptoms.

Attention deficit-hyperactivity disorder (ADHD)

In a randomised, double-blind, placebo-controlled double-crossover trial, treatment with L-carnitine (100 mg/kg twice daily, maximum 4 g/day) over 24 weeks significantly decreased attention problems, delinquency and aggressive behaviour in boys with ADHD (Van-Oudheusden & Scholte 2002). At 6-month follow-up 19 of 24 boys had responded to treatment as judged by parents and teachers.

In a 12-month multicentre randomised, double-blind placebo-controlled, parallel study of fragile X syndrome, young boys aged 6–13 years ($n = 51$) with ADHD who were given either L-acetylcarnitine (500 mg twice daily) or a placebo (L-acetylcarnitine supplemented $n = 24$; placebo $n = 27$), improved behaviour was reported in both groups and reduction of hyperactivity. However, improvement of social behaviour was more pronounced in patients treated with L-acetylcarnitine compared with the placebo group (Torrioli et al 2008).

Diabetes

Only high circulating serum insulin concentrations (90 mU/L) are capable of stimulating skeletal muscle carnitine accumulation (Stephens et al 2007). Carnitine is essential for lipid and carbohydrate metabolism, and correct metabolic control. It has been suggested that some people with diabetes may have reduced levels of total and free carnitine (Mamoulakis et al 2004). Administration of L-carnitine reduces insulin secretion and improves peripheral glucose use (Grandi et al 1997) and tissue insulin sensitivity (Negro et al 1994). Additionally, in type 2 diabetes, L-carnitine (1 g three times daily) significantly lowers fasting plasma glucose, but may increase fasting triglycerides (Rahbar et al 2005).

In a large 1-year study of obese patients with uncontrolled type 2 diabetes, 258 patients were randomised to receive either orlistat (120 mg, 3 × day) or orlistat (120 mg, 3 × day) with L-carnitine (2 g daily) and the latter group was reported to have improvements in their body weight, blood lipid, inflammatory biomarkers and glycaemic control compared to the group that did not receive L-carnitine (Derosa et al 2011).

In a recent systematic review and meta-analysis evaluating the metabolic effects of L-carnitine supplementation in type 2 diabetes, four trials with 284 patients were included. Oral L-carnitine supplementation was reported to result in improved glycaemia and plasma lipids, although there were no significant changes in triglycerides, lipoprotein-a or HbA_{1C} (Vidal-Casariego et al 2013).

Type 1 diabetes

L-Carnitine (2 g/m^2/day) in the early stage (stage 1a) of type 1 diabetes may improve nerve conduction velocity, suggesting benefits for the treatment of subclinical neuropathy (Uzun et al 2005).

Haemodialysis

Carnitine depletion in haemodialysis patients is caused by insufficient carnitine synthesis and excessive loss through the dialytic membranes (Matera et al 2003). Carnitine supplementation has been approved by the US Food and Drug Administration for the treatment and prevention of carnitine depletion in dialysis patients. Supplementation in such patients is said to improve lipid metabolism, protein nutrition, antioxidant status and anaemia, and may reduce the incidence of intradialytic muscle cramps, hypotension, asthenia, muscle weakness and cardiomyopathy (Bellinghieri et al 2003).

In maintenance haemodialysis patients, L-carnitine supplementation (20 mg/kg) has been associated with protein-sparing effects during hyperinsulinaemia (Biolo et al 2008). L-carnitine supplementation (10 mg/kg orally) immediately after haemodialysis sessions three times a week for 12 months induced regression of left ventricular hypertrophy in patients with normal cardiac systolic function undergoing haemodialysis (Sakurabayashi et al 2008).

However, the routine use of L-carnitine in dialysis patients to manage anaemia and refractory dialysis-associated hypotension is contentious and some authors believe that there is insufficient evidence to support this indication (Steinman et al 2003).

In a randomised study of maintenance haemodialysis patients, the effect of L-carnitine supplementation was evaluated in 35 patients regarding lipid parameters, apoproteins (apoprotein A1 and B) and inflammatory (highly sensitive C-reactive protein: hsCRP), and nutritional markers (total protein, albumin). Twenty patients received 1 g/day of L-carnitine supplementation intravenously three times a week after each session of haemodialysis and 15 patients served as a control group for 6 months. At completion of the study, the carnitine-supplemented group was reported to have a significant decrease in hsCRP levels, with no other significant differences being noted (Suchitra et al 2011).

In a recent study of 30 patients on maintenance haemodialysis, the effect of oral L-carnitine supplementation (750 mg/day; 250 mg tablets three times a day for 8 weeks) was investigated regarding lipid profile and compared with 30 matched patients who served as the control group. At completion of the study period, the carnitine-supplemented group had a significant decrease in total cholesterol (190 ± 36.8 vs 177 ± 31.2 mg/dL), triglyceride (210 ± 64.7 vs 190 ± 54.1 mg/dL) and LDL-cholesterol (117 ± 30.1 vs 106 ± 26.3 mg/dL), although there was no significant change in HDL-cholesterol levels (Naini et al 2012).

A recent systematic review and meta-analysis of 49 RCTs that included 1734 participants investigated the effectiveness of L-carnitine supplementation in adults with end-stage renal disease who required maintenance haemodialysis. This study confirmed the role of carnitine in reducing serum LDL (mean difference: −5.82 mg/dL; 95% CI −11.61 to −0.04 mg/dL) and C-reactive protein (−3.65 mg/L; −6.19 to −1.12 mg/L) levels, but there was no significant change in the required erythropoietin dose or triglyceride, cholesterol and HDL levels. The authors reported the reductions in C-reactive protein and LDL levels to be clinically relevant (Chen et al 2014).

Hepatitis

A prospective, randomised, open-label study of 69 patients with chronic hepatitis C investigated the effect of supplemental L-carnitine regarding alleviation of anaemia, thrombocytopenia and leucopenia in patients in treatment with interferon-alpha (IFN-α) plus ribavirin. One group of patients (n = 35; 30 completed the study) received Peg-IFN-α2b plus ribavirin plus L-carnitine, and the control group (n = 34; 27 completed study) received Peg-IFN-α and ribavirin for 12 months. At study completion the L-carnitine-supplemented group demonstrated a significant improvement of sustained virological response in 50% of patients vs 25% of the control group. The study reported a significantly greater decrease in platelets and red and white cells in the Peg-IFN-α plus ribavirin group compared to the Peg-IFN-α plus ribavirin plus L-carnitine group (Malaguarnera et al 2011d).

Hepatic encephalopathy

Hepatic encephalopathy is a major complication of cirrhosis. A 2008 systematic review suggested that L-acetyl-carnitine is promising as a safe and effective treatment for hepatic encephalopathy (Shores & Keeffe 2008). Human trials have demonstrated a protective effect of L-carnitine (2 g twice daily) in ammonia-precipitated hepatic encephalopathy in cirrhotic patients at 30 days and, more significantly, at 60 days (Malaguarnera et al 2003).

In a randomised, double-blind, placebo-controlled study the effect of supplementary acetyl-L-carnitine was evaluated in 121 patients with mild (*n* = 61 total; 31 received 2 g acetyl-L-carnitine and 30 received placebo twice a day for 90 days) and moderate hepatoencephalopathy (*n* = 60 total; 30 received 2 g acetyl-L-carnitine and 30 received placebo twice a day for 90 days) regarding physical and mental fatigue, fatigue severity and physical activity. The acetyl-L-carnitine-supplemented groups had a significant decrease in mental and physical fatigue, while physical activity levels were also increased (Malaguarnera et al 2011a).

The same authors also reported that acetyl-L-carnitine improves cognitive functions in severe hepatic encephalopathy in a randomised, double-blind, placebo-controlled study of 61 patients with severe hepatic encephalopathy: 31 patients received 2 g acetyl-L-carnitine twice a day for 90 days and 30 patients received a placebo. At completion of the study there was an improvement in electroencephalograms for both patient groups (88% of acetyl-L-carnitine group vs 72% of placebo group), and patients treated with acetyl-L-carnitine were also reported to have significant improvements in cognitive deficits, and a reduction of ammonia compared to the control group (Malaguarnera et al 2011b).

Similarly, in another randomised, double-blind, placebo-controlled study of 67 patients with minimal hepatic encephalopathy, of which 33 were randomly assigned to receive 2 g acetyl-L-carnitine twice a day and 34 patients to receive a placebo for 90 days, the acetyl-L-carnitine group was reported to have a significant improvement in quality-of-life parameters (physical function, role physical, general health, social function, role emotional, mental health), and to be associated with reduction of anxiety and depression (Malaguarnera et al 2011c).

Inflammatory bowel disease

Short-chain fatty acids (SCFAs) are a major energy source for colonocytes and in ulcerative colitis there is some evidence to indicate that a deficiency of SCFAs may lead to an energy deficit due to impaired beta-oxidation of SCFAs. Studies have reported lower levels of plasma PLC in patients with ulcerative colitis compared to healthy matched controls but similar levels of plasma L-carnitine. It has been proposed that PLC may be serving as a source of L-carnitine and propionyl-coenzyme-A and therefore supplementary PLC may improve cellular energy levels due to the role of L-carnitine in releasing energy as a result of beta-oxidation of fatty acids and propionyl-coenzyme-A as an energy source via the citric acid cycle (Mikhailova et al 2011).

In a recent multicentre, phase II, double-blind, parallel-group study of patients with mild to moderate ulcerative colitis who were receiving stable oral aminosalicylate or thiopurine therapy, the efficacy of colon release PLC was investigated. Patients (*n* = 121) with disease activity index score 3–10 inclusive were randomised to receive PLC 1 g/day, PLC 2 g/day or placebo. Overall, the majority of patients (57 of 79: 72%) receiving PLC (combined 1 g and 2 g cohort) had a clinical/endoscopic response compared to 50% of patients receiving the placebo (20 of 40) ($P = 0.02$). The PLC doses were similar in their effects, although the 1 g/day dose was the more effective (clinical/endoscopic response in PLC 1 g/day: 30 of 40 [75%]: $P = 0.02$ vs placebo and clinical/endoscopic response in PLC 2 g/day: 27 of 39 [69%]: $P = 0.08$ vs placebo). The rates of remission were greater in the supplemented groups (PLC 1 g/day: 22/40 [55%], PLC 2 g/day: 19/39 [49%], placebo: 14/40 [35%:]) (Mikhailova et al 2011).

Narcolepsy

Narcolepsy patients have been reported to have altered fatty acid beta-oxidation and it has been suggested that supplementary L-carnitine may improve fatty acid oxidation and potentially alleviate symptoms of narcolepsy (Miyagawa et al 2011).

In a randomised, double-blind, crossover, placebo-controlled trial of 16 weeks' duration, 28 narcolepsy patients received 510 mg/day supplemental L-carnitine (as three doses of 170 mg each; two doses were administered in the morning and one dose in the evening) for two 8-week periods; carnitine supplementation resulted in a reduction in excessive daytime sleepiness (Miyagawa et al 2013).

Rett syndrome

A case is reported of a 17-year-old girl with Rett syndrome whose condition improved while using L-carnitine (50 mg/kg/day). Upon cessation, she relapsed, whereas re-establishing the treatment saw improvements after 1 week. More specifically, alertness increased; she started reaching for objects with both hands, and answered simple questions with one or two words. Interestingly, serum carnitine levels (free and total) were within normal limits before and after L-carnitine treatment (Plioplys & Kasnicka 1993). An 8-week randomised, placebo-controlled, double-blind crossover trial of L-carnitine has since been completed detecting improvements on the Hand Apraxia Scale and in subjects' general wellbeing (Ellaway et al 1999).

Beta-thalassaemia major

In a small study of regularly transfused and chelated beta-thalassaemia patients (*n* = 40; mean age 17.5 ± 5.0 years) and 10 age-matched controls, L-carnitine levels were assessed. The thalassaemic patients had significantly lower L-carnitine levels (23.71 ± 7.3 microM) as compared to the control group (29.26 ± 2.37 microM) ($P < 0.0001$). Vegetarians also had lower levels compared to non-vegetarians (22.34 ± 6.55 microM vs 26.91 ± 8.4 microM) but the difference was not statistically significant ($P = 0.072$) (Merchant et al 2010).

L-Carnitine appears to be a safe and effective adjunctive therapy in thalassaemia patients, especially younger patients. L-Carnitine therapy (50 mg/kg/day) for 6 months resulted in a significant increase in oxygen consumption, cardiac output and oxygen pulse at maximal exercise ($P < 0.001$, $P = 0.002$ and $P < 0.001$, respectively). There was also a significant increase in the blood transfusion intervals after L-carnitine administration ($P = 0.008$) (El-Beshlawy et al 2007). Additionally L-carnitine (100 mg/kg/day) for 1 month may prevent red blood cell deterioration in beta-thalassaemia major patients (Toptas et al 2006).

Ageing

In a randomised, double-blind, placebo-controlled trial of 84 elderly subjects (aged 70–92 years) who experienced onset of fatigue after slight physical activity, L-carnitine (2 g twice daily) for 30 days resulted in significant improvements in total fat mass, total muscle mass and lipid profiles, as well as overall improvements in physical and mental fatigue (Pistone et al 2003). Similarly, in a placebo-controlled, randomised, double-blind, two-phase study of 66 centenarians with onset of fatigue even after slight physical activity, L-carnitine (2 g/day)-treated centenarians showed significant improvements compared with the placebo group. Improvements included total fat mass (–1.80 vs 0.6 kg; $P < 0.01$), total muscle mass (3.80 vs 0.8 kg; $P < 0.01$), plasma concentrations of total carnitine (12.60 vs –1.70 micromol; $P < 0.05$), plasma long-chain acylcarnitine (1.50 vs –0.1 micromol; $P < 0.001$), and plasma short-chain acylcarnitine (6.0 vs –1.50 micromol; $P < 0.001$). Significant differences were also found in physical fatigue (–4.10 vs –1.10; $P < 0.01$), mental fatigue (–2.70 vs 0.30; $P < 0.001$), fatigue severity (–23.60 vs 1.90; $P < 0.001$), and Mini-Mental State Examination (4.1 vs 0.6; $P < 0.001$) (Malaguarnera et al 2007).

Animal studies have demonstrated that supplementation of carnitine (300 mg/kg/day) and lipoic acid (100 mg/kg/day) for 30 days protects mitochondria from ageing by raising mitochondrial energy production and reversing the age-associated decline in mitochondrial enzyme activity (Savitha et al 2005). Studies using standard oral doses of L-carnitine in humans are required to confirm these effects.

Weight loss

Carnitine is a popular supplement for weight loss when combined with an exercise programme. This is based on its biochemical role in the production of energy from fatty acids. Carnitine deficiency impairs fatty acid beta-oxidation and may partly explain weight gain in valproate-treated patients. However, L-carnitine (15 mg/kg/day) for 26 weeks failed to improve weight loss outcomes in valproate-treated bipolar patients consuming an energy-restricted, low-fat diet (Elmslie et al 2006). Currently, one clinical trial that has investigated carnitine supplementation together with an aerobic training programme failed to detect a significant effect on weight loss (Villani et al 2000).

DOSAGE RANGE

- Deficiency: L-carnitine 50–200 mg/kg/day.
- Most conditions: L-carnitine 2–4 g/day in divided dose.

Note: Maximum plasma concentration may be achieved at 500 mg. Therefore individual doses exceeding this level may not provide any additional benefits (Bain et al 2006). Larger doses should be divided.

According to clinical studies

- Cardiovascular disorders: 2 g/day for at least 3 months may improve exercise tolerance and recovery in people with conditions such as chronic stable angina and cardiac insufficiency, and may also reduce lipoprotein-a levels and improve peripheral vascular disease.
- Hyperthyroidism: 2–4 g/day in divided doses.
- Chronic fatigue syndrome: 1 g three times daily.
- Ergogenic aid: 2 g/day.
- Fertility: 2–3 g/day may be useful to increase sperm motility and concentration.
- Peripheral vascular disease: 2 g/day.
- COPD: 2 g/day.
- Thalassaemia (as adjunct): 50 mg/kg/day.
- Ageing (to reduce fatigue): 2 g daily or twice daily.

ADVERSE REACTIONS

Carnitine is well tolerated at recommended doses. Mild gastrointestinal symptoms including abdominal cramps, diarrhoea, nausea and vomiting, heartburn or gastritis may occur. Mild myasthenia has been reported in uraemic patients using the D,L form (Hendler & Rorvik 2001). Changes in body odour have also been noted (Sigma-Tau Pharmaceuticals 1999, Van-Oudheusden & Scholte 2002).

SIGNIFICANT INTERACTIONS

Anticoagulants

According to one case report, L-carnitine 1 g/day may potentiate the anticoagulant effects of acenocoumarol (also known as nicoumalone or acenocoumarin) (Martinez et al 1993). Use this combination with caution. Monitor bleeding time and signs and symptoms of excessive bleeding.

Anticonvulsants (including valproate, phenobarbitone, phenytoin, carbamazepine)

Trials with children and adults have shown a reduction in carnitine levels during anticonvulsant therapy (Hug et al 1991, Rodriguez-Segade et al 1989). A study evaluating carnitine deficiency in children and adolescents with epilepsy found 27.3% taking valproic acid and 14.3% taking carbamazepine showed low free carnitine levels. Polytherapy, female sex, psychomotor or mental retardation and abnormal neurological examination appeared to increase the risk of hypocarnitinaemia. Patients taking topiramate or lamotrigine or on a ketogenic diet did not appear to be affected (Coppola et al 2006). L-Carnitine deficiency may cause or potentiate valproate toxicity and supplementation is known to reduce the toxicity of valproate, as well as symptoms of fatigue. In a trial using L-carnitine for acute valproate poisoning, no adverse events were noted (LoVecchio et al 2005). Increased carnitine intake may be required with long-term therapy — potentially beneficial interaction under professional supervision.

Betamethasone

An RCT has shown that a combination of low-dose betamethasone (2 mg/day) and L-carnitine (4 g/5 days) was more effective in the prevention of respiratory distress syndrome (7.3% vs 14.5%) and death (1.8% vs 7.3%) in preterm infants than high-dose betamethasone given alone (8 mg/2 days) (Kurz et al 1993) — beneficial interaction possible under professional supervision.

Chemotherapy

Adriamycin (doxorubicin)

Animal studies suggest long-term carnitine administration may reduce the cardiotoxic side effects of Adriamycin (Kawasaki et al 1996). A small randomised placebo-controlled trial attempted to determine these effects in humans, administering 3 g L-carnitine before each chemotherapy cycle, followed by 1 g L-carnitine/day during the following 21 days to the treatment group. The trial reported no cardiotoxicity in either group and was able to demonstrate stimulation of oxidative metabolism in white blood cells through carnitine uptake (Waldner et al 2006). Increased carnitine intake may be required with long-term therapy — potentially beneficial interaction, only under professional supervision.

Carboplatin

Treatment with carboplatin appears to result in marked urinary losses of L-carnitine and acetyl-L-carnitine, most likely due to inhibition of carnitine reabsorption in the kidney (Mancinelli et al 2007).

Cisplatin

Research into the use of L-carnitine 4 g/day for 7 days showed a reduction in fatigue resulting from treatment with cisplatin (Graziano et al 2002) — beneficial interaction is possible under professional supervision.

HIV drugs (zidovudine)

In vitro studies indicate prevention of muscle damage due to carnitine depletion (Dalakas et al 1994, Moretti et al 2002, Semino-Mora et al 1994). Patients with HIV infection undergoing highly active antiretroviral therapy can be carnitine-deficient and supplementation of L-carnitine has been proposed to 'increase the number of CD4 cells and reduce lymphocyte apoptosis; improve symptoms of polyneuropathy; prevent cardiovascular damage from wasting and diarrhoea syndromes; decrease serum levels of triglycerides and TNF(alpha)' (Ilias et al 2004). Beneficial interaction is possible. Increased carnitine intake may be required with long-term therapy — use under professional supervision.

HMG CoA-reductase inhibitors (statins)

According to human trials the addition of L-carnitine (2 g/day) to simvastatin therapy (20 mg/day) appears to lower lipoprotein-a serum levels in patients with type 2 diabetes mellitus (Solfrizzi et al 2006). Beneficial interaction possible.

Interferon-alpha

Clinical trials with patients being treated with IFN-alpha for hepatitis C observed reduced fatigue when carnitine 2 g/day was co-administered (Neri et al 2003). L-Carnitine may reduce hepatic steatosis associated with IFN-alpha and ribavirin treatment in patients with hepatitis C (Romano et al 2008). Increased carnitine intake may be required with long-term therapy — potentially beneficial interaction under professional supervision.

Interleukin-2 immunotherapy

Clinical trials using L-carnitine (1 g/day orally) found that it may be used successfully to prevent

? CONTRAINDICATIONS AND PRECAUTIONS

- Chronic liver disease — may impair metabolism or increase biosynthesis of L-carnitine (Krahenbuhl 1996).
- Seizures — may increase incidence of seizures in those with a pre-existing condition (Sigma-Tau Pharmaceuticals 1999).

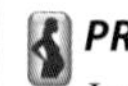

PREGNANCY USE

Insufficient reliable information is available. However, animal studies have revealed no evidence of decreased fertility or harm to the fetus (Hendler & Rorvik 2001). In fact, some research suggests a role for carnitine.

Requirements for carnitine may increase during pregnancy and a small trial found a positive effect in women diagnosed with placental insufficiency taking 1 g L-carnitine twice daily (Genger et al 1988). Due to the role of L-carnitine in the synthesis of surfactant, trials have also been conducted using L-carnitine in combination with low-dose betamethasone in women with imminent premature delivery, with an improvement in respiratory distress syndrome and mortality rates (Kurz et al 1993).

cardiac complications during IL-2 immunotherapy in cancer patients with clinically relevant cardiac disorders (Lissoni et al 1993). Thus a beneficial interaction is possible under professional supervision.

Practice points/Patient counselling

- Carnitine is an amino acid that is ingested through the diet and also synthesised from lysine and methionine in the body.
- It is involved in numerous biochemical processes and is essential for energy production in the mitochondria of every cell.
- Vegetarians, and preterm infants or those on a carnitine-free formula, are at risk of deficiency. Secondary risk factors include genetic defects of metabolism, liver and renal disease, dialysis, certain medicines and hypopituitarism.
- L-Carnitine 2 g/day for 3 months has been shown to improve exercise tolerance and recovery, especially in people with cardiovascular disorders such as chronic stable angina and cardiac insufficiency. Preliminary evidence also suggests a possible role in hyperthyroidism, male infertility and peripheral vascular diseases such as intermittent claudication.
- Carnitine supplements are also used to promote weight loss and as an ergogenic aid, although large controlled studies are unavailable to assess their effectiveness.

PATIENTS' FAQs

What will this supplement do for me?

L-Carnitine supplements improve clinical outcomes in people with cardiovascular disorders by reducing the frequency of angina attacks, and improving outcomes after heart attack, cardiogenic shock and in cardiomyopathy. It may also reduce symptoms in hyperthyroidism, increase male fertility, increase walking distance in people with peripheral vascular disease and reduce the side effects of some medicines.

When will it start to work?

People with cardiovascular disorders such as chronic stable angina and cardiac insufficiency should experience benefits within 1–3 months.

Are there any safety issues?

Carnitine is well tolerated, but people with chronic liver disease or epilepsy should use it with caution.

REFERENCES

Bach AC et al. Free and total carnitine in human serum after oral ingestion of L-carnitine. Diabet Metab 9 (1983): 121–124.

Bain MA, et al. Disposition and metabolite kinetics of oral L-carnitine in humans. J Clin Pharmacol 46.10 (2006): 1163–1170.

Baker H et al. Cardiac carnitine leakage is promoted by cardiomyopathy. Nutrition 21.3 (2005): 348–350.

Banihani S, et al. Cryoprotective effect of L-carnitine on motility, vitality and DNA oxidation of human spermatozoa. Andrologia. 2013 Jul 3. doi: 10.1111/and.12130.

Bellinghieri G et al. Carnitine and hemodialysis. Am J Kidney Dis 41.3 (Suppl 1) (2003): S116–S122.

Benvenega S et al. Usefulness of L-carnitine, a naturally occurring peripheral antagonist of thyroid hormone action, in iatrogenic hyperthyroidism: a randomized, double-blind, placebo-controlled clinical trial. J Clin Endocrinol Metab 86.8 (2001): 3579–3594.

Biagiotti G, Cavallini G. Acetyl-L-carnitine vs tamoxifen in the oral therapy of Peyronie's disease: a preliminary report. BJU Int 88.1 (2001): 63–67.

Bianchi G et al. Symptomatic and neurophysiological responses of paclitaxel- or cisplatin-induced neuropathy to oral acetyl-L-carnitine. Eur J Cancer 41.12 (2005): 1746–1750.

Binienda Z et al. Neuroprotective effect of carnitine in the 3-nitropropionic acid (3-NPA)-evoked neurotoxicity in rats. Neurosci Lett 367.2 (2004): 264–267.

Biolo G et al. Insulin action on glucose and protein metabolism during L-carnitine supplementation in maintenance haemodialysis patients. Nephrol Dial Transplant 23.3 (2008): 991–997.

Borghi-Silva A et al. L-Carnitine as an ergogenic aid for patients with chronic obstructive pulmonary disease submitted to whole-body and respiratory muscle training programs. Braz J Med Biol Res 39.4 (2006): 465–474.

Brass EP, et al. A systematic review and meta-analysis of propionyl-L-carnitine effects on exercise performance in patients with claudication. Vasc Med. 2013 Feb;18(1):3–12.

Brevetti G et al. Increases in walking distance in patients with peripheral vascular disease treated with L-carnitine: a double-blind, crossover study. Circulation 77.4 (1988): 767–773.

Brooks JO et al. Acetyl L-Carnitine slows decline in younger patients with Alzheimer's disease: a reanalysis of a double-blind, placebo-controlled study using the trilinear approach. Int Psychogeriatr 10.2 (1998): 193–203.

Campone M, et al. A double-blind, randomized phase II study to evaluate the safety and efficacy of acetyl-L-carnitine in the prevention of sagopilone-induced peripheral neuropathy. Oncologist. 2013;18(11):1190–1.

Campos Y et al. Plasma carnitine insufficiency and effectiveness of L-carnitine therapy in patients with mitochondrial myopathy. Muscle Nerve 16.2 (1993): 150–153.

Chen Y, et al. L-Carnitine supplementation for adults with end-stage kidney disease requiring maintenance hemodialysis: a systematic review and meta-analysis. Am J Clin Nutr. 2014;99(2):408–22.

Cheng HJ, Chen T. Clinical efficacy of combined L-carnitine and acetyl-L-carnitine on idiopathic asthenospermia. Zhonghua Nan Ke Xue 14.2 (2008): 149–151.

Cherchi A et al. Effects of L-carnitine on exercise tolerance in chronic stable angina: a multicenter, double-blind, randomized, placebo controlled crossover study. Int J Clin Pharmacol Ther Toxicol 23.10 (1985): 569–572.

Ciacci C et al. L-Carnitine in the treatment of fatigue in adult celiac disease patients: a pilot study. Dig Liver Dis 39.10 (2007): 922–928.

Coppola G et al. Plasma free carnitine in epilepsy children, adolescents and young adults treated with old and new antiepileptic drugs with or without ketogenic diet. Brain Dev 28.6 (2006): 358–365.

Corbucci GG, Lettieri B. Cardiogenic shock and L-carnitine: clinical data and therapeutic perspectives. Int J Clin Pharmacol Res 11.6 (1991): 283–293.

Corbucci GG, Loche F. L-Carnitine in cardiogenic shock therapy: pharmacodynamic aspects and clinical data. Int J Clin Pharmacol Res 13.2 (1993): 87–91.

Costa M et al. L-Carnitine in idiopathic asthenozoospermia: a multicentre study. Andrologia 26 (1994): 155–159.

Crill CM et al. Carnitine supplementation in premature neonates: effect on plasma and red blood cell total carnitine concentrations, nutrition parameters and morbidity. Clin Nutr 25.6 (2006): 886.

Cruciani RA et al. Safety, tolerability and symptom outcomes associated with L-carnitine supplementation in patients with cancer, fatigue, and carnitine deficiency: a phase I/II study. J Pain Symptom Manage 32.6 (2006): 551–559.

Cruciani RA, et al. L-carnitine supplementation for the management of fatigue in patients with cancer: an eastern cooperative oncology group phase III, randomized, double-blind, placebo-controlled trial. J Clin Oncol. 2012 Nov 1;30(31):3864–9.

Curione M et al. Carnitine deficiency in patients with coeliac disease and idiopathic dilated cardiomyopathy. Nutr Metab Cardiovasc Dis 15.4 (2005): 279–283.

Dalakas MC et al. Zidovudine-induced mitochondrial myopathy is associated with muscle carnitine deficiency and lipid storage. Ann Neurol 35 (1994): 482–487.

Davini P et al. Controlled study on L-carnitine therapeutic efficacy in post-infarction. Drugs Exp Clin Res 18.8 (1992): 355–365.
De Grandis D, Minardi C. Acetyl-L-carnitine (levacecarnine) in the treatment of diabetic neuropathy. A long-term, randomised, double-blind, placebo-controlled study. Drugs R D 3.4 (2002): 223–231.
Delaney CL, et al. A systematic review to evaluate the effectiveness of carnitine supplementation in improving walking performance among individuals with intermittent claudication. Atherosclerosis. 2013 Mar 15. pii: S0021-9150(13)00179-2.
Derosa G et al. The effect of L-carnitine on plasma lipoprotein(a) levels in hypercholesterolemic patients with type 2 diabetes mellitus. Clin Ther 25.5 (2003): 1429–1439.
Derosa G, et al. Comparison between orlistat plus L-carnitine and orlistat alone on inflammation parameters in obese diabetic patients. Fundam Clin Pharmacol. 2011 Oct;25(5):642–51
El-Beshlawy A et al. Effect of L-carnitine on the physical fitness of thalassemic patients. Ann Hematol 86.1 (2007): 31–34.
Ellaway C et al. Rett syndrome: randomized controlled trial of L-carnitine. J Child Neurol 14.3 (1999): 162–167.
Elmslie JL et al. Carnitine does not improve weight loss outcomes in valproate-treated bipolar patients consuming an energy-restricted, low-fat diet. Bipolar Disord 8.5 Pt 1 (2006): 503–507.
Eroglu H, et al. Effects of acute L-carnitine intake on metabolic and blood lactate levels of elite badminton players. Neuro Endocrinol Lett 29.2 (2008): 261–266.
Eskandari HG et al. Short term effects of L-carnitine on serum lipids in STZ-induced diabetic rats. Diabetes Res Clin Pract 66.2 (2004): 129–132.
Evangeliou A, Vlassopoulos D. Carnitine metabolism and deficit: When is supplementation necessary? Curr Pharm Biotechnol 4.3 (2003): 211–2119.
Fernandez C, Proto C. L-Carnitine in the treatment of chronic myocardial ischemia: An analysis of 3 multicenter studies and a bibliographic review. Clin Ther 140.4 (1992): 353–377 [in Italian].
Garolla A et al. Oral carnitine supplementation increases sperm motility in asthenozoospermic men with normal sperm phospholipid hydroperoxide glutathione peroxidase levels. Fertil Steril 83.2 (2005): 355–361.
Garzya G. Evaluation of the effects of L-acetylcarnitine on senile patients suffering from depression. Drugs Exp Clin Res 16.2 (1990): 101–106.
Genger H, et al. Carnitine in therapy of placental insufficiency: initial experiences. Z Geburtshilfe Perinatol 192 (1988): 155–157.
Grandi M, et al. Effect of acute carnitine administration on glucose insulin metabolism in healthy subjects. Int J Clin Pharm Res 17.4 (1997): 143–147.
Graziano F et al. Potential role of levocarnitine supplementation for the treatment of chemotherapy-induced fatigue in non-anaemic cancer patients. Br J Cancer 86.12 (2002): 1854–1857.
Gulcin I. Antioxidant and antiradical activities of L-carnitine. Life Sci 78.8 (2006): 803–811.
Gunes B et al. The effect of oral L-carnitine supplementation on the lipid profiles of hyperlipidaemic children. Acta Paediatr 94.6 (2005): 711–7116.
Harper P, et al. Pharmacokinetics of intravenous and oral bolus doses of L-carnitine in healthy subjects. Eur J Clin Pharmacol 35 (1988): 555–562.
Hendler SS, Rorvik D (eds). PDR for Nutritional Supplements, Montvale, NJ: Medical Economics Co., 2001.
Hershman DL, et al. Randomized double-blind placebo-controlled trial of acetyl-L-carnitine for the prevention of taxane-induced neuropathy in women undergoing adjuvant breast cancer therapy. J Clin Oncol. 2013, 10;31(20):2627–33.
Hiatt WR et al. Propionyl-L-carnitine improves exercise performance and functional status in patients with claudication. Am J Med 110.8 (2001): 616–622.
Hino K, et al. L-Carnitine inhibits hypoglycemia-induced brain damage in the rat. Brain Res 1053.1–2 (2005): 77–87.
Hug G et al. Reduction of serum carnitine concentrations during anticonvulsant therapy with phenobarbital, valproic acid, phenytoin and carmazepine in children. J Pediatr 119 (1991): 799–802.
Ilias I et al. L-Carnitine and acetyl-L-carnitine in the treatment of complications associated with HIV infection and antiretroviral therapy. Mitochondrion 4.2–3 (2004): 163–168.
Ishii T et al. Anti-apoptotic effect of acetyl-L-carnitine and L-carnitine in primary cultured neurons. Jpn J Pharmacol 83.2 (2000): 119–124.
Iyer RN et al. L-carnitine moderately improves the exercise tolerance in chronic stable angina. J Assoc Physicians India 48.11 (2000): 1050–1052.
Jones MG et al. Plasma and urinary carnitine and acylcarnitines in chronic fatigue syndrome. Clin Chim Acta 360.1–2 (2005): 173–177.
Karakoc E et al. Encephalopathy due to carnitine deficiency in an adult patient with gluten enteropathy. Clin Neurol Neurosurg 108.8 (2006): 794–797.
Karlic H, Lohninger A. Supplementation of L-carnitine in athletes: does it make sense? Nutrition 20.7–8 (2004): 709–715.
Kawasaki N et al. Long-term L-carnitine treatment prolongs the survival in rats with andiamycin induced heart failure. J Card Fail 2 (1996): 293–299.
Kelly GS. L-Carnitine: Therapeutic applications of a conditionally-essential amino acid. Altern Med Rev 3.5 (1998): 345–360.
Kletzmayr J et al. Anemia and carnitine supplementation in hemodialyzed patients. Kidney Int 55.69 (1999): S93–106.
Kosan C et al. Carnitine supplementation improves apolipoprotein B levels in pediatric peritoneal dialysis patients. Pediatr Nephrol 18.11 (2003): 1184–1188.
Kraemer WJ et al. Androgenic responses to resistance exercise: effects of feeding and L-carnitine. Med Sci Sports Exerc 38.7 (2006): 1288–1296.
Kraft M, et al. L-Carnitine-supplementation in advanced pancreatic cancer (CARPAN)—a randomized multicentre trial. Nutr J. 2012 Jul 23;11:52.
Krahenbuhl S. Carnitine metabolism in chronic liver disease. Life Sci 59.19 (1996): 1579–1599.
Kumar M, et al. Carnitine supplementation for preterm infants with recurrent apnea. Cochrane Database Syst Rev 4 (2004a): CD004497.
Kumar M, et al. Role of carnitine supplementation in apnea of prematurity: a systematic review. J Perinatol 24.3 (2004b): 158–163.
Kurz C et al. L-Carnitine-betamethasone combination therapy versus betamethasone therapy alone in prevention of respiratory distress syndrome. Z Geburtshilfe Perinatol 197.5 (1993): 215–2119 [in German].
Lee JK et al. Effect of L-carnitine supplementation and aerobic training on FABPc content and beta-HAD activity in human skeletal muscle. Eur J Appl Physiol 99.2 (2007): 193–199.
Lenzi A et al. Metabolism and action of L-carnitine: its possible role in sperm tail function. Arch Ital Urol Nephrol Androl 64 (1992): 187–196.
Lenzi A et al. Use of carnitine therapy in selected cases of male factor infertility: a double-blind crossover trial. Fertil Steril 79.2 (2003): 292–300.
Li B et al. The effect of enteral carnitine administration in humans. Am J Clin Nutr 55 (1992): 838–845.
Lissoni P et al. Prevention by L-carnitine of interleukin-2 related cardiac toxicity during cancer immunotherapy. Tumori 79 (1993): 202–204.
Liu S, et al L-Carnitine ameliorates cancer cachexia in mice by regulating the expression and activity of carnitine palmityl transferase. Cancer Biol Ther 2011, 12:125–30.
Loster H et al. Prolonged oral L-carnitine substitution increases bicycle ergometer performance in patients with severe, ischemically induced cardiac insufficiency. Cardiovasc Drugs Ther 13.6 (1999): 537–546.
LoVecchio F, et al. L-Carnitine was safely administered in the setting of valproate toxicity. Am J Emerg Med 23.3 (2005): 321–322.
Maestri A et al. A pilot study on the effect of acetyl-L-carnitine in paclitaxel- and cisplatin-induced peripheral neuropathy. Tumori 91.2 (2005): 135–138.
Malaguarnera M et al. L-Carnitine in the treatment of mild or moderate hepatic encephalopathy. Dig Dis 21.3 (2003): 271–275.
Malaguarnera M et al. L-Carnitine treatment reduces severity of physical and mental fatigue and increases cognitive functions in centenarians: a randomized and controlled clinical trial. Am J Clin Nutr 86.6 (2007): 1738–1744.
Malaguarnera M et al. Acetyl L-Carnitine (ALC) treatment in elderly patients with fatigue. Arch Gerontol Geriatr 46.2 (2008): 181–190.
Malaguarnera M, et al. Oral acetyl-L-carnitine therapy reduces fatigue in overt hepatic encephalopathy: a randomized, double-blind, placebo-controlled study. Am J Clin Nutr. 2011(a) Apr;93(4):799–808
Malaguarnera M, et al. Acetyl-L-carnitine improves cognitive functions in severe hepatic encephalopathy: a randomized and controlled clinical trial. Metab Brain Dis. 2011(b) Dec;26(4):281–9.
Malaguarnera M, et al. Acetyl-L-carnitine reduces depression and improves quality of life in patients with minimal hepatic encephalopathy. Scand J Gastroenterol. 2011(c) Jun;46(6):750–9.
Malaguarnera M, et al. L-carnitine supplementation improves hematological pattern in patients affected by HCV treated with Peg interferon-α 2b plus ribavirin. World J Gastroenterol. 2011(d) Oct 21;17(39):4414–20.
Mamoulakis D et al. Carnitine deficiency in children and adolescents with type 1 diabetes. J Diabetes Complic 18.5 (2004): 271–274.
Mancinelli A et al. Urinary excretion of L-carnitine and its short-chain acetyl-L-carnitine in patients undergoing carboplatin treatment. Cancer Chemother Pharmacol 60.1 (2007): 19–26.
Martindale W. Extra pharmacopoeia. London: Pharmaceutical Press, 1999.
Martinez E, et al. Potentiation of acenocoumarol action by L-carnitine (Letter). J Intern Med 233 (1993): 94.
Matera M et al. History of L-carnitine: implications for renal disease. J Renal Nutr 13.1 (2003): 2–14.

Mels CM, et al. L-carnitine and long-chain acylcarnitines are positively correlated with ambulatory blood pressure in humans: the SABPA study. Lipids. 2013 Jan;48(1):63–73.

Merchant R, et al. L-carnitine in beta thalassemia. Indian Pediatr. 2010 Feb;47(2):165–7.

Mikhailova TL, et al. Randomised clinical trial: the efficacy and safety of propionyl-L-carnitine therapy in patients with ulcerative colitis receiving stable oral treatment. Aliment Pharmacol Ther. 2011 Nov;34(9):1088–97.

Miyagawa T, et al. Abnormally low serum acylcarnitine levels in narcolepsy patients. Sleep (2011); 34: 349–353A.

Miyagawa T, et al. Effects of oral L-carnitine administration in narcolepsy patients: a randomized, double-blind, cross-over and placebo-controlled trial. PLoS One. 2013;8(1):e53707.

Moradi M, et al. Safety and Efficacy of Clomiphene Citrate and L-Carnitine in Idiopathic Male Infertility. A Comparative Study. Urol J. 2010;7:188–93.

Moretti S et al. L-Carnitine reduces lymphocyte apoptosis and oxidant stress in HIV-1-infected subjects treated with zidovudine and didanosine. Antioxid Redox Signal 4.3 (2002): 391–403.

Naini AE, et al. Oral carnitine supplementation for dyslipidemia in chronic hemodialysis patients. Saudi J Kidney Dis Transpl. 2012 May;23(3):484–8.

Negro P et al. The effect of L-carnitine, administered through intravenous infusion of glucose, on both glucose and insulin levels in healthy subjects. Drugs Exp Clin Res 20.6 (1994): 257–262.

Neri S et al. L-Carnitine decreases severity and type of fatigue induced by interferon-alpha in the treatment of patients with hepatitis C. Neuropsychobiology 47.2 (2003): 94–97.

O'Donnell J, et al. Role of L-carnitine in apnea of prematurity: a randomized, controlled trial. Pediatrics 109.4 (2002): 622–626.

Onofrj M et al. L-Acetylcarnitine as a new therapeutic approach for peripheral neuropathies with pain. Int J Clin Pharmacol Res 15.1 (1995): 9–15.

Peluso G et al. Cancer and anticancer therapy-induced modifications on metabolism mediated by carnitine system. J Cell Physiol 182 (2000): 339–350.

Pettegrew JW et al. Clinical and neurochemical effects of acetyl-L-carnitine in Alzheimer's disease. Neurobiol Aging 16.1 (1995): 1–4.

Pistone G et al. Levocarnitine administration in elderly subjects with rapid muscle fatigue: effect on body composition, lipid profile and fatigue. Drugs Aging 20.10 (2003): 761–767.

Plioplys AV, Kasnicka I. L-Carnitine as a treatment for Rett syndrome. South Med J 86.12 (1993): 1411–1412.

Plioplys AV, Plioplys S. Serum levels of carnitine in chronic fatigue syndrome: clinical correlates. Neuropsychobiology 32.3 (1995): 132–138.

Plioplys AV, Plioplys S. Amantadine and L-carnitine treatment of chronic fatigue syndrome. Neuropsychobiology 35.1 (1997): 16–23.

Rahbar AR et al. Effect of L-carnitine on plasma glycemic and lipidemic profile in patients with type II diabetes mellitus. Eur J Clin Nutr 59.4 (2005): 592–596.

Ramos AC et al. The protective effect of carnitine in human diphtheric myocarditis. Pediatr Res 18.9 (1984): 815–819.

Ramos AC et al. Carnitine supplementation in diphtheria. Indian Pediatr 29.12 (1992): 1501–1505.

Rebouche CJ, Chenard CA. Metabolic fate of dietary carnitine in human adults: identification and quantification of urinary and fecal metabolites. J Nutr 121 (1991): 539–545.

Rizos I. Three-year survival of patients with heart failure caused by dilated cardiomyopathy and L-carnitine administration. Am Heart J 139.2 (2000): S120–S123.

Rodriguez-Segade S et al. Carnitine deficiency associated with anticonvulsant therapy. Clin Chim Acta 181.2 (1989): 175–181.

Romano M et al. L-Carnitine treatment reduces steatosis in patients with chronic hepatitis C treated with alpha-interferon and ribavirin. Dig Dis Sci 53.4 (2008): 1114–1121.

Rossini M et al. Double-blind, multicenter trial comparing acetyl l-carnitine with placebo in the treatment of fibromyalgia patients. Clin Exp Rheumatol 25.2 (2007): 182–188.

Ruggenenti P, et al. Ameliorating hypertension and insulin resistance in subjects at increased cardiovascular risk: effects of acetyl-L-carnitine therapy. Hypertension. 2009 Sep;54(3):567–74.

Sabri MR, et al. Does L-carnitine improve endothelial function in hemodialysis patients? J Res Med Sci. 2012 May;17(5):417–21.

Sakai K, et al. Evidence for a positive association between serum carnitine and free testosterone levels in uremic men with hemodialysis. Rejuvenation Res. 2013 Jun;16(3):200–5.

Sakurabayashi T et al. L-Carnitine supplementation decreases the left ventricular mass in patients undergoing hemodialysis. Circ J 72.6 (2008): 926–931.

Sano M et al. Double-blind parallel design pilot study of acetyl levocarnitine in patients with Alzheimer's disease. Arch Neurol 49.11 (1992): 1137–1141.

Savitha S et al. C. Efficacy of levo carnitine and alpha lipoic acid in ameliorating the decline in mitochondrial enzymes during aging. Clin Nutr 24.5 (2005): 794–800.

Semino-Mora MC et al. Effect of L-carnitine on the zidovudine-induced destruction of human myotubes: Part 1: L-carnitine prevents the myotoxicity of AZT in vitro. Lab Invest 71 (1994): 102–112.

Shores NJ, Keeffe EB. Is oral L-acyl-carnitine an effective therapy for hepatic encephalopathy? Review of the literature. Dig Dis Sci 53.9 (2008): 2330–2333.

Sigman M et al. Carnitine for the treatment of idiopathic asthenospermia: a randomized, double-blind, placebo-controlled trial. Fertil Steril 85.5 (2006): 1409–1414.

Sigma-Tau Pharmaceuticals. Carnitor [levocarnitine] package insert. Gaithersberg, MD: Sigma-Tau Pharmaceuticals Inc, Dec. 1999.

Singh RB et al. A randomised, double-blind, placebo-controlled trial of L-carnitine in suspected acute myocardial infarction. Postgrad Med J 72.843 (1996): 45–50.

Sirtori CR et al. L-Carnitine reduces plasma lipoprotein(a) levels in patients with hyperLp(a). Nutr Metab Cardiovasc Dis 10.5 (2000): 247–251.

Smith WA et al. Effect of glycine propionyl-L-carnitine on aerobic and anaerobic exercise performance. Int J Sport Nutr Exerc Metab 18.1 (2008): 19–36.

Soetekouw PM et al. Normal carnitine levels in patients with chronic fatigue syndrome. Neth J Med 57.1 (2000): 20–24.

Solfrizzi V et al. Efficacy and tolerability of combined treatment with L-carnitine and simvastatin in lowering lipoprotein(a) serum levels in patients with type 2 diabetes mellitus. Atherosclerosis 188.2 (2006): 455–461.

Sorbi S et al. Double-blind, crossover, placebo-controlled clinical trial with L-acetylcarnitine in patients with degenerative cerebellar ataxia. Clin Neuropharmacol 23.2 (2000): 114–118.

Steinman TI et al. L-Carnitine use in dialysis patients: is national coverage for supplementation justified? What were CMS regulators thinking: or were they? Nephrol News Issues 17.5 (2003): 28–30: 32–4, 36.

Stephens FB et al. A threshold exists for the stimulatory effect of insulin on plasma L-carnitine clearance in humans. Am J Physiol Endocrinol Metab 292.2 (2007): E637–E641.

Suchitra MM, et al. The effect of L-carnitine supplementation on lipid parameters, inflammatory and nutritional markers in maintenance hemodialysis patients. Saudi J Kidney Dis Transpl. 2011 Nov;22(6):1155–9

Tarantini G et al. Metabolic treatment with L-carnitine in acute anterior ST segment elevation myocardial infarction. A randomized controlled trial. Cardiology 106.4 (2006): 215–223.

Tastekin A et al. L-Carnitine protects against glutamate- and kainic acid-induced neurotoxicity in cerebellar granular cell culture of rats. Brain Dev 27.8 (2005): 570–573.

Tejani AM, et al. Carnitine for fatigue in multiple sclerosis. Cochrane Database Syst Rev. 2012 May 16;5:CD007280.

Tempesta E et al. Role of acetyl-L-carnitine in the treatment of cognitive deficit in chronic alcoholism. Int J Clin Pharmacol Res 10.1–2 (1990): 101–107.

Thal LJ et al. A 1-year multicenter placebo-controlled study of acetyl-L-carnitine in patients with Alzheimer's disease. Neurology 47.3 (1996): 705–711.

Tomassini V et al. Comparison of the effects of acetyl L-carnitine and amantadine for the treatment of fatigue in multiple sclerosis: results of a pilot, randomised, double-blind, crossover trial. J Neurol Sci 218.1–2 (2004): 103–108.

Toptas B et al. L-Carnitine deficiency and red blood cell mechanical impairment in beta-thalassemia major. Clin Hemorheol Microcirc 35.3 (2006): 349–357.

Torrioli MG, et al. A double-blind, parallel, multicenter comparison of L-acetylcarnitine with placebo on the attention deficit hyperactivity disorder in fragile X syndrome boys. Am J Med Genet A. 2008 Apr 1;146(7): 803–812

Tsoko M et al. Enhancement of activities relative to fatty acid oxidation in the liver of rats depleted of L-carnitine by D-carnitine and gammabutyrobetaine hydroxylase inhibitor. Biochem Pharmacol 49.10 (1995): 1403–1410.

Uzun N et al. Peripheric and automatic neuropathy in children with type 1 diabetes mellitus: the effect of L-carnitine treatment on the peripheral and autonomic nervous system. Electromyogr Clin Neurophysiol 45.6 (2005): 343–351.

Van-Oudheusden LJ, Scholte HR. Efficacy of carnitine in the treatment of children with attention-deficit hyperactivity disorder. Prostaglandins Leukot Essent Fatty Acids 67.1 (2002): 33–38.

Vescovo G et al. L-Carnitine: a potential treatment for blocking apoptosis and preventing skeletal muscle myopathy in heart failure. Am J Physiol Cell Physiol 283.3 (2002): C802–C810.

Vidal-Casariego A, et al. Metabolic Effects of L-carnitine on Type 2 Diabetes Mellitus: Systematic Review and Meta-analysis. Exp Clin Endocrinol Diabetes. 2013; 121(4):234–8
Villani RG et al. L-Carnitine supplementation combined with aerobic training does not promote weight loss in moderately obese women. Int J Sport Nutr Exerc Metab 10.2 (2000): 199–207.
Vitali G, et al. Carnitine supplementation in human idiopathic asthenospermia: clinical results. Drugs Exp Clin Res 21 (1995): 157–159.
Volek JS et al. L-Carnitine L-tartrate supplementation favorably affects markers of recovery from exercise stress. Am J Physiol Endocrinol Metab 282.2 (2002): E474–E482.
Wachter S et al. Long-term administration of L-Carnitine to humans: effect on skeletal muscle carnitine content and physical performance. Clin Chim Acta 318.1–2 (2002): 51–61.
Wahlqvist ML (ed). Food and nutrition, 2nd edn. Sydney: Allen & Unwin, 2002.
Waldner R et al. Effects of doxorubicin-containing chemotherapy and a combination with L-Carnitine on oxidative metabolism in patients with non-Hodgkin lymphoma. J Cancer Res Clin Oncol 132.2 (2006): 121–128.
Winter S et al. Plasma carnitine deficiency. Am J Dis Child 141.6 (1987): 660–665.
Xue YZ et al. L-Carnitine as an adjunct therapy to percutaneous coronary intervention for non-ST elevation myocardial infarction. Cardiovasc Drugs Ther 21.6 (2007): 445–448.
Youle M, Osio M. A double-blind, parallel-group, placebo-controlled, multicentre study of acetyl L-Carnitine in the symptomatic treatment of antiretroviral toxic neuropathy in patients with HIV-1 infection. HIV Med 8.4 (2007): 241–250.
Zaugg K, et al: Carnitine palmitoyltransferase 1 C promotes cell survival and tumor growth under conditions of metabolic stress. Genes Dev 2011, 25:1041–51.
Zhou X, et al. Effect of L-carnitine and/or L-acetyl-carnitine in nutrition treatment for male infertility: a systematic review. Asia Pac J Clin Nutr 16 (Suppl 1) (2007): 383–390.

Celery

HISTORICAL NOTE Celery is widely used as a food. The ancient Greeks used celery to make a wine called selinites, which was served as an award at athletic games. Dioscorides described celery as an effective remedy for 'heated stomach' and breast lumps and used it as a diuretic for urinary retention and dropsy.

OTHER NAMES

Smallage, marsh parsley, wild celery

BOTANICAL NAME/FAMILY

Apium graveolens (family Umbelliferae [Apiaceae])

PLANT PART USED

Fruit (seed)

CHEMICAL COMPONENTS

Celery is high in minerals, including sodium (Murphy et al 1978), and contains furocoumarins such as psoralen and bergapten (Beier et al 1983). The major constituents of celery seed oil include pinene and D-limonene (Saleh et al 1985). Celery also contains flavonoids, such as apigenin, luteolin and isoquercitrin, and phenolic acids and alkaloids (Fisher & Painter 1996).

MAIN ACTIONS

Anti-inflammatory activity

An ethanol extract of aerial celery parts has been found to have anti-inflammatory activity, with suppression of carrageenan-induced paw oedema observed in rats (Al-Hindawi et al 1989). Several constituents show anti-inflammatory activity, such as apigenin, eugenol, ferulic acid, luteolin, bergapten and apiin (Duke 2003, Mencherini et al 2007, Ovodova et al 2009, Ziyan et al 2007). Studies in rats suggest that some celery seed extracts are highly effective in suppressing experimental arthritis without exhibiting any gastrotoxicity (Whitehouse et al 1999). Further in vivo studies suggest that celery seed extracts were gastroprotective for non-steroidal anti-inflammatory drug (NSAID) gastropathy and that this effect is mediated through non-prostaglandin mechanisms (Whitehouse et al 2001). Luteolin may also be useful for mitigating neuroinflammation (Jang et al 2008).

Cholagogue

Aqueous celery extract has also been found to increase bile acid excretion and lower total serum cholesterol levels in genetically hypercholesterolaemic rats (Tsi & Tan 2000).

Chemoprotective

Human in vivo trials imply that apiaceous vegetable intake may be chemopreventive by inhibiting cytochrome P450-mediated carcinogen activation (Peterson et al 2006). Based on in vivo studies in mice, it has been suggested that the phthalide components of celery may be effective chemoprotective agents (Zheng et al 1993). Other studies show that celery consumption, in particular due to its flavones luteolin and apigenin (Lim do et al 2007, Meeran & Katiyar 2008), has been linked to a reduced risk of developing colon cancer (Slattery et al 2000), stomach cancer (Haenszel et al 1976), liver cancer (Sultana et al 2005) and lung cancer (Galeone et al 2007).

Antioxidant

There are a number of studies providing evidence of the antioxidative effects of some constituents in celery (Popovic et al 2006, Yeh & Yen 2005, Zidorn et al 2005).

Lipid-lowering activity

One study of vegetables, including celery, showed that cooking enhanced the amount of phytosterols which are known to decrease plasma cholesterol, mainly the atherogenic low-density lipoprotein cholesterol (Kaloustian et al 2008). In vivo studies of aqueous celery extract on rats showed a significant reduction in total serum cholesterol (Tsi et al 1995, 1996). A significant reduction in total serum cholesterol has been observed in several in vivo studies in rats, which used either aqueous celery extract or diets supplemented with celery leaf (El-Mageed 2011, Tsi et al 1995, 1996).

Hepatoprotective

An in vivo study using *Pangasuis sutchi* freshwater fish found that celery leaf powder reduced hepatotoxic markers aspartate transaminase, alanine aminotransferase and alkaline phosphatase and abnormal liver histology following paracetamol-induced liver damage (Shivashri et al 2013).

Protection against plasticiser toxicities

In animal studies, a 6-week treatment with celery seed oil extract was found to ameliorate the toxic effects of di (2-ethylhexyl) phthalate, which included normalising of lipid profiles and liver function, reduction of peroxisome proliferator-activated receptor-alpha expression, and reduced vascular oxidative stress (El-Shinnawy 2013). Another in vivo study showed celery oil pretreatment partially prevented changes to testicular weight, sperm parameters and sperm hormone levels induced by di (2-ethylhexyl) phthalate (Madkour 2012).

Testicular protection

Pretreatment of rats with celery oil prevented sodium valproate-induced reductions in testes weight, sperm count and sperm motility (Hala 2011). As previously mentioned, celery oil pretreatment partially prevented di (2-ethylhexyl) phthalate-induced testicular toxicities, including changes in weight and sperm parameters (Madkour 2012).

OTHER ACTIONS

Celery is said to have antirheumatic, carminative, antispasmodic, diuretic, antihypertensive and urinary antiseptic activity. An in vivo study in rats identified that celery seed extracts had antihypertensive properties, which correlated with *n*-butylphthalide content (Moghadam et al 2013). Celery extracts have also been found to have significant activity as a mosquito repellent (Pitasawat et al 2007, Tuetun et al 2004, 2005, 2008). Research has shown that the flavones and coumarins, as well as the nutritional compounds, of vegetables, including celery, have immunomodulatory functions (Cherng et al 2008). Some antimicrobial activity is also reported from in vitro studies of the essential oil component (Misic et al 2008), while other studies show celery extracts to be ineffective against Gram-negative bacteria (Watt et al 2007). In vitro tests reveal the flavone apigenin has multiple effects on osteoblasts, suggesting that it could prevent bone loss in vivo (Bandyopadhyay et al 2006) and be a useful pharmacological tool for the treatment of osteoporosis (Choi 2007).

CLINICAL USE

Celery has not been significantly investigated under clinical trial conditions, so evidence is mainly derived from in vitro and animal studies and is largely speculative.

Osteoarthritis

Evidence of anti-inflammatory activity in experimental models provides a theoretical basis for its use; however, controlled trials are not available to determine effectiveness.

A small uncontrolled trial of 15 patients with chronic arthritis found that treatment with celery seed extract significantly reduced pain symptoms after 3 weeks (Bone 2003).

Urinary tract infection

Celery is used in combination with other herbal medicines for the treatment of this condition. Although it is not certain that the herb has antibacterial activity against microorganisms implicated in urinary tract infection, it is used for its diuretic effect.

OTHER USES

Traditional

Celery has been traditionally used as a diuretic, to improve appetite and digestion, and as a treatment for nervousness and hysteria. The British Herbal Pharmacopoeia gives the specific indication of celery for rheumatoid arthritis and depression (Fisher & Painter 1996).

Oriental medicine uses the seeds to treat headaches and as a digestive aid and emmenagogue.

In Trinidad and Tobago, celery is used as a heart tonic and for low blood pressure (Lans 2006); while in some parts of Indonesia it is one of a number of kitchen plants used in saunas for postpartum recuperation (Zumsteg & Weckerle 2007).

Animal studies on isolated constituents from celery have been found to be valuable in the treatment of acute ischaemic stroke via multiple mechanisms, such as strong antioedema activity (Deng et al 1997) as well as antioxidation, antiapoptosis and anti-inflammatory actions (Chang & Wang 2003). Animal studies also demonstrate that the phthalide components improve cognitive impairment induced by chronic cerebral hypoperfusion, indicating its therapeutic potential for the treatment of dementia caused by decreased cerebral blood flow (Peng et al 2007).

DOSAGE RANGE

- Fluid extract (1:2): 4.5–8.5 mL/day in divided doses.
- Decoction of dried fruit: 0.5–2 g three times daily.

TOXICITY/ADVERSE REACTIONS

Celery can cause food allergy (Luttkopf et al 2000), with cross-reactivity to a number of other foods (Moneret-Vautrin et al 2002, Vieths et al 2002). One incidence of severe anaphylaxis following celery ingestion has been reported (Palgan et al 2012). Topical exposure to celery may cause contact dermatitis, angio-oedema and urticaria (Kauppinen et al 1980). Photodermatitis has been recorded with occupational exposure (Seligman et al 1987) and celery has been suggested to cause ocular phototoxicity (Fraunfelder 2004).

SIGNIFICANT INTERACTIONS

Controlled studies are not available, so interactions are based on evidence of activity and are largely theoretical and speculative.

NSAIDs

Celery seed extract may reduce gastrointestinal symptoms associated with NSAIDs — beneficial interaction possible.

Pentobarbitone

Celery juice has been found to prolong the action of pentobarbitone in rats (Jakovljevic et al 2002) — use with caution.

Thyroxine

Celery seed might decrease the effects of levothyroxine replacement therapy according to one case report — observe patient.

Sodium valproate

In animal studies celery was found to have a protective effect against sodium valproate's well-established toxicity to the testes and sperm production (Hamza & Amin 2007).

Psoralen–UVA (PUVA) therapy

Although celery has been found to contain psoralens, celery extract does not seem to be photosensitising, even after ingestion of large amounts; however, it may increase the risk of phototoxicity with concurrent PUVA therapy (Gral et al 1993) — use with caution.

Practice points/Patient counselling

- Celery has been traditionally used as a diuretic. It is used to treat osteoarthritis and demonstrates anti-inflammatory activity in experimental models. Celery is likely to be safe when used in quantities commonly used in foods; however, there is the possibility for allergy and contact sensitivity.
- It is prudent to avoid using celery seed essential oil in amounts greater than those ingested when used as a food.

CONTRAINDICATIONS AND PRECAUTIONS

Usual dietary intakes are likely to be safe.

PREGNANCY USE

Safe when consumed in dietary amounts; however.

REFERENCES

Al-Hindawi MK et al. Anti-inflammatory activity of some Iraqi plants using intact rats. J Ethnopharmacol 26.2 (1989): 163–168.

Bandyopadhyay S et al. Attenuation of osteoclastogenesis and osteoclast function by apigenin. Biochem Pharmacol 72.2 (2006): 184–197.

Beier RC et al. HPLC analysis of linear furocoumarins (psoralens) in healthy celery (*Apium graveolens*). Food Chem Toxicol 21.2 (1983): 163–165.

Bone K. A clinical guide to blending liquid herbs. Edinburgh: Churchill Livingstone, 2003.

Chang Q, Wang XL. Effects of chiral 3-n-butylphthalide on apoptosis induced by transient focal cerebral ischemia in rats. Acta Pharmacol Sin 24.8 (2003): 796–804.

Cherng J-M, et al. Immunomodulatory activities of common vegetables and spices of Umbelliferae and its related coumarins and flavonoids. Food Chemistry 106.3 (2008): 944–950.

Choi EM. Apigenin increases osteoblastic differentiation and inhibits tumor necrosis factor-alpha-induced production of interleukin-6 and nitric oxide in osteoblastic MC3T3-E1 cells. Pharmazie 62.3 (2007): 216–220.

Deng W et al. Effect of di-3-n-butylphthalide on brain edema in rats subjected to focal cerebral ischemia. Chin Med Sci J 12.2 (1997): 102–107.

Duke JA. Dr Duke's Phytochemical and Ethnobotanical Databases. US Department of Agriculture–Agricultural Research Service–National Germplasm Resources Laboratory. Beltsville Agricultural Research Center, Beltsville, MD. Online. Available www.ars-grin.gov/duke March 2003.

El-Mageed NMA. Hepatoprotective effects of feeding celery leaves mixed with chicory leaves and barley grains to hypercholesterolemic rats. Pharmacogn Mag 7.26 (2011): 151–156

El-Shinnawy NA. The therapeutic applications of celery oil seed extract on the plasticizer di(2-ethylhexyl)phthalate toxicity. Toxicol Ind Health [ePub ahead of print] (2013)

Fisher C, Painter G. Materia Medica for the Southern Hemisphere. Auckland: Fisher-Painter Publishers, 1996.

Fraunfelder F. Ocular side effects from herbal medicines and nutritional supplements. Am J Opthalmol 138.4 (2004): 639–648.

Galeone C et al. Dietary intake of fruit and vegetable and lung cancer risk: a case-control study in Harbin, northeast China. Ann Oncol 18.2 (2007): 388–392.

Gral N et al. Plasma levels of psoralens after celery ingestion. Ann Dermatol Venereol 120.9 (1993): 599–603.

Haenszel W et al. Stomach cancer in Japan. J Ntl Cancer Inst 56.2 (1976): 265–274.

Hala MA. Protective effects of *Nigella sativa*, linseed and celery oils against testicular toxicity induced by sodium valproate in male rats. J Am Sci 7.5 (2011):687–693

Hamza AA, Amin A. Apium graveolens modulates sodium valproate-induced reproductive toxicity in rats. J Exp Zool Part A Ecol Genet Physiol 307.4 (2007): 199–206.
Jakovljevic V et al. The effect of celery and parsley juices on pharmacodynamic activity of drugs involving cytochrome P450 in their metabolism. Eur J Drug Metab Pharmacokinet 27.3 (2002): 153–156.
Jang S, Kelley KW, Johnson RW. Luteolin reduces IL-6 production in microglia by inhibiting JNK phosphorylation and activation of AP-1. Proc Natl Acad Sci USA 105.21 (2008): 7534–7539.
Kaloustian J et al. Effect of water cooking on free phytosterol levels in beans and vegetables. Food Chemistry 107.4 (2008): 1379–1386.
Kauppinen K et al. Aromatic plants: a cause of severe attacks of angio-edema and urticaria. Contact Dermatitis 6.4 (1980): 251–254.
Lans CA. Ethnomedicines used in Trinidad and Tobago for urinary problems and diabetes mellitus. J Ethnobiol Ethnomed 2 (2006): 45.
Lim do Y et al. Induction of cell cycle arrest and apoptosis in HT-29 human colon cancer cells by the dietary compound luteolin. Am J Physiol Gastrointest Liver Physiol 292.1 (2007): G66–G75.
Luttkopf D et al. Celery allergens in patients with positive double-blind placebo-controlled food challenge. J Allergy Clin Immunol 106.2 (2000): 390–399.
Madkour NK. The beneficial role of celery oil in lowering of di(2-ethylhexyl) phthalate-induced testicular damage. Toxicol Ind Health (2012) [epub ahead of print]
Meeran SM, Katiyar SK. Cell cycle control as a basis for cancer chemoprevention through dietary agents. Front Biosci 13 (2008): 2191–2202.
Mencherini T et al. An extract of *Apium graveolens* var. *dulce* leaves: structure of the major constituent, apiin, and its anti-inflammatory properties. J Pharm Pharmacol 59.6 (2007): 891–897.
Misic D et al. Antimicrobial activity of celery fruit isolates and SFE process modeling. Biochemical Engineering Journal 42.2 (2008): 148–152.
Moghadam MH, et al. Antihypertensive effect of celery seed on rat blood pressure in chronic administration. J Med Food 16.6 (2013): 558–563
Moneret-Vautrin DA et al. Food allergy and IgE sensitization caused by spices: CICBAA data (based on 589 cases of food allergy). Allerg Immunol 34.4 (2002): 135–140.
Murphy EW et al. Nutrient content of spices and herbs. J Am Diet Assoc 72.2 (1978): 174–176.
Ovodova RG et al. Chemical composition and anti-inflammatory activity of pectic polysaccharide isolated from celery stalks. Food Chem 114.2 (2009): 610–615
Palgan K et al. Celery –cause of severe anaphylactic shock. Postepy Hig Med Dosw 66 (2012): 132–134
Peng Y et al. l-3-n-butylphthalide improves cognitive impairment induced by chronic cerebral hypoperfusion in rats. J Pharmacol Exp Ther 321.3 (2007): 902–910.
Peterson S et al. Apiaceous vegetable constituents inhibit human cytochrome P-450 1A2 (hCYP1A2) activity and hCYP1A2-mediated mutagenicity of aflatoxin B1. Food Chem Toxicol 44.9 (2006): 1474–1484.
Pitasawat B et al. Aromatic plant-derived essential oil: An alternative larvicide for mosquito control. Fitoterapia 78.3 (2007): 205–210.
Popovic M et al. Effect of celery (*Apium graveolens*) extracts on some biochemical parameters of oxidative stress in mice treated with carbon tetrachloride. Phytother Res 20.7 (2006): 531–537.
Saleh MM et al. The essential oil of *Apium graveolens* var. *secalinum* and its cercaricidal activity. Pharmaceut Weekblad (Scientific Edn) 7.6 (1985): 277–279.
Seligman PJ et al. Phytophotodermatitis from celery among grocery store workers. Arch Dermatol 123.11 (1987): 1478–1482.
Shivashri C, et al. Hepatoprotective action of celery (*Apium graveolens*) leaves in acetaminophen-fed freshwater fish (*Pangasius sutchi*). Fish Physiol Biochem. 39.5 (2013): 1057–1069
Slattery ML et al. Carotenoids and colon cancer. Am J Clin Nutr 71.2 (2000): 575–582.
Sultana S et al. Inhibitory effect of celery seed extract on chemically induced hepatocarcinogenesis: modulation of cell proliferation, metabolism and altered hepatic foci development. Cancer Lett 221 (1) (2005): 11–20.
Tsi D, Tan BK. The mechanism underlying the hypocholesterolaemic activity of aqueous celery extract, its butanol and aqueous fractions in genetically hypercholesterolaemic RICO rats. Life Sci 66.8 (2000): 755–767.
Tsi D et al. Effects of aqueous celery (*Apium graveolens*) extract on lipid parameters of rats fed a high fat diet. Planta Medica 61.1 (1995): 18–21.
Tsi D et al. Effects of celery extract and 3-N-butylphthalide on lipid levels in genetically hypercholesterolaemic (RICO) rats. Clin Exp Pharmacol Physiol 23.3 (1996): 214–2117.
Tuetun B et al. Mosquito repellency of the seeds of celery (*Apium graveolens* L.). Ann Trop Med Parasitol 98.4 (2004): 407–417.
Tuetun B et al. Repellent properties of celery, *Apium graveolens* L., compared with commercial repellents, against mosquitoes under laboratory and field conditions. Trop Med Intern Health 10.11 (2005): 1190–1198.
Tuetun B et al. Celery-based topical repellents as a potential natural alternative for personal protection against mosquitoes. Parasitol Res 104.1 (2008): 107–11915.
Vieths S et al. Current understanding of cross-reactivity of food allergens and pollen. Ann NY Acad Sci 964 (2002): 47–68.
Watt K, et al. The detection of antibacterial actions of whole herb tinctures using luminescent *Escherichia coli*. Phytother Res 21.12 (2007): 1193–1199.
Whitehouse MW et al. Over the counter (OTC) oral remedies for arthritis and rheumatism: How effective are they? Inflammopharmacology 7.2 (1999): 89–105.
Whitehouse MW et al. NSAID gastropathy: Prevention by celery seed extracts in disease-stressed rats. Inflammopharmacology 9.1–2 (2001): 201–209.
Yeh CT, Yen GC. Effect of vegetables on human phenolsulfotransferases in relation to their antioxidant activity and total phenolics. Free Radic Res 39.8 (2005): 893–904.
Zheng GQ et al. Chemoprevention of benzo[a]pyrene-induced forestomach cancer in mice by natural phthalides from celery seed oil. Nutr Cancer 19.1 (1993): 77–86.
Zidorn C et al. Polyacetylenes from the Apiaceae vegetables carrot, celery, fennel, parsley, and parsnip and their cytotoxic activities. J Agric Food Chem 53.7 (2005): 2518–2523.
Ziyan L et al. Evaluation of the anti-inflammatory activity of luteolin in experimental animal models. Planta Med 73.3 (2007): 221–226.
Zumsteg IS, Weckerle CS. Bakera, a herbal steam bath for postnatal care in Minahasa (Indonesia): Documentation of the plants used and assessment of the method. J Ethnopharmacol 111.3 (2007): 641–650.

Chaste tree

HISTORICAL NOTE Chaste tree fruits and leaves were a popular remedy in ancient Greece and Rome to promote celibacy. Leaves of the chaste tree were worn by vestal virgins in ancient Rome as a symbol of chastity. In the 17th century it was written that the chaste tree is a 'remedy for such as would willingly live chaste' (Gerard 1975). The dried fruits of the chaste tree have a peppery taste and smell and were used in place of pepper in monasteries to 'check violent sexual desires', hence one of its common names, monk's pepper. The berries have also been used to reduce fever and headaches, stimulate perspiration and dispel wind. However, since ancient times the chaste tree has primarily been used for a variety of gynaecological purposes, primarily to treat menstrual abnormalities and mastalgia, to aid in expulsion of the placenta after birth, to facilitate lactation and to promote menstruation. A commercial preparation of chaste tree has been available in Germany for over 50 years and it is still commonly used for menstrual irregularities.

OTHER NAMES

Vitex agnus castus, chasteberry, monk's pepper, gattilier, hemp tree, Keusch-Lamm-Fruechte, wild pepper.

BOTANICAL NAME/FAMILY

Vitex agnus-castus (family Labiatae)

PLANT PART USED

Dried, ripened or fresh ripe fruits (berries)

CHEMICAL COMPONENTS

Vitex agnus-castus contains many different chemical constituents: 10 flavonoids (including luteolin-like flavonoids casticin, orientin, isovitexin), five terpenoids (viteagnusins A–E), three neolignans and four phenolic compounds, as well as one glyceride, essential fatty acids (linoleic acid) and the essential oils cineole, limonene and sabinene. The phenolic and flavonoid compounds confer antioxidant and antimicrobial activity. Apigenin, 3-methylkaempferol, luteolin and casticin are weak ligands of delta and mu-opioid receptors, exhibiting dose-dependent receptor binding (Chen et al 2011, Ono et al 2008, Sarikurkcu et al 2009, Stojkovic et al 2011). Casticin is a potent immunomodulatory and cytotoxic compound (Mesaik et al 2009). Several secondary metabolites exhibit significant anti-inflammatory and lipo-oxygenase inhibition activity (Choudhary et al 2009).

MAIN ACTIONS

Vitex displays multiple mechanisms of action identified through in vitro and experimental model research.

One major area of activity is the pituitary–hypothalamic axis.

Decreases prolactin release

The most thoroughly studied mechanism for vitex is its interaction with dopamine receptors in the anterior pituitary. Several studies have indicated that vitex acts on dopamine D_2 receptors and decreases prolactin levels (Berger et al 2000, Halaska et al 1998, Jarry et al 1994, Meier & Hoberg 1999, Meier et al 2000, Milewicz et al 1993, Sliutz et al 1993, Wuttke et al 2003). It is likely that this mechanism is responsible for the symptom-relieving effects seen with vitex in mastodynia and hyperprolactinaemia (Meier & Hoberg 1999, Milewicz et al 1993, Wuttke et al 1997) and provides some rationale for its use by herbalists in disorders complicated by hyperprolactinaemia, such as amenorrhoea, mastalgia or polycystic ovarian syndrome.

Results from one study involving healthy males propose that this effect is dose-dependent, as lower doses (120 mg) were found to increase secretion and higher doses (204–480 mg) were found to decrease secretion (Merz et al 1996).

A study using the vitex extract BNO 1095 (70% ethanol, 30% H_2O extract, Bionorica, Neumarkt, Germany) identified that the major dopaminergic compounds are the clerodadienols, which act as potent inhibitors of prolactin release; however, other active compounds of lesser activity were also identified (Wuttke et al 2003). Dopaminergic bicyclic diterpenes have also been isolated that inhibit cAMP formation and prolactin release in rat pituitary cell cultures (Jarry et al 2006).

Oestrogen receptor binding

Vitex contains oestrogenic compounds, the flavonoids penduletin and apigenin. There are inconsistent results on whether vitex competitively binds to oestrogen receptors alpha and beta in vitro (Cavieres & Castillo 2011, Jarry et al 2003, Liu et al 2001, Wuttke et al 2003).

Increases progesterone levels

In vitro research has found that vitex stimulates progesterone receptor expression (Liu et al 2001), significantly increases plasma progesterone and total oestrogen levels and significantly reduces luteinising hormone (LH) and plasma prolactin (Ibrahim et al 2008). A randomised controlled trial of women with hyperprolactinaemia showed that vitex extract (20 mg daily) normalises progesterone levels after 3 months' treatment (Milewicz et al 1993).

Opioid receptors

Recent research reported that a methanol extract of vitex had affinity to the mu-opioid and delta-opioid (but not kappa-opioid) receptors (Webster et al 2011). Of note, the mu-opiate receptor is the primary action site for beta-endorphin in vivo, a peptide which assists in regulating the menstrual cycle through inhibition of the hypothalamus–pituitary–adrenal axis.

Cytotoxic activity

Cytotoxic activity has been reported for an ethanolic extract of the dried ripe fruit of vitex against various human cancer cell lines (Imai et al 2009, Ohyama et al 2003, 2005, Weisskopf et al 2005). The extract increased intracellular oxidative stress and mitochondrial damage, leading to apoptosis. In vitro studies demonstrate that vitex extract inhibits the proliferation of human prostate epithelial cell lines via apoptosis (Weisskopf et al 2005) and induces apoptosis in human colon carcinoma cell lines (Imai et al 2009).

OTHER ACTIONS

Conflicting results have been obtained in studies with regard to the effect on follicle-stimulating hormone (FSH), LH and testosterone levels. In vivo research suggests that vitex significantly decreases LH and testosterone levels (Nasri et al 2007). However, one clinical study found that vitex extract did not alter FSH or LH levels, whereas another showed that it increased LH release (Lauritzen et al 1997, Milewicz et al 1993). Inconsistent clinical results may be due to variations in chemical constituent levels present in the different test herbal products.

In vivo research on male rats demonstrated osteoprotective effects (Sehmisch et al 2009).

CLINICAL USE

Although double-blind studies have recently been conducted with chasteberry, uncontrolled trials go back to the 1940s, when a product known as Agnolyt was tested. The product was developed and patented by Dr Gerhard Madaus in Germany and contained *Vitex agnus-castus*. Several different vitex products have been investigated to date, including: Agnolyt (standardised to 3.5–4.2 mg of dried chasteberry extract), *Vitex agnus-castus* L. extract Ze440 (each 20 mg tablet standardised for casticin and agnuside), Femicur (contains 1.6–3.0 mg of dried extract per capsule) and Mastodynon (53% v/v ethanol), a homeopathic preparation. The BNO 1095 extract contains 4.0 mg of dried ethanolic (70%) extract of vitex (corresponding to 40 mg of herbal drug) and is found in Agnucaston/Cyclodynon (Bionorica, Neumarkt, Germany).

Premenstrual syndrome

Vitex is an effective and well-tolerated treatment for mild, moderate and severe premenstrual syndrome (PMS) according to numerous clinical trials (Atmaca et al 2003, Berger et al 2000, Dittmar 1992, He et al 2009, Lauritzen et al 1997, Loch et al 2000, Schellenberg 2001, Schellenberg et al 2012, Zamani et al 2012). According to these studies, the PMS symptoms that respond best to treatment are breast tenderness, irritability, depressed mood, anger, mood changes, headache and constipation. The most studied extract investigated in PMS is Ze440 and, more recently, BNO 1095 extract (see Clinical note).

A recent systematic review evaluated the evidence for the efficacy and safety of vitex extracts from randomised controlled trials investigating women's health. Of the 12 trials included in this review, eight investigated PMS. Seven of the eight trials found vitex extracts to be superior to placebo (five of six studies), pyridoxine (one study) and magnesium oxide (one study). Additionally, adverse events with vitex were mild and generally infrequent (van Die et al 2013). A Cochrane review investigating the use of *Vitex agnus-castus* for the treatment of PMS symptoms is currently underway (Shaw et al 2011).

The most recent double blind study was conducted with 162 women and tested three different doses : Ze 440 (8, 20 and 30 mg) over three menstrual cycles. Improvement in the total symptom score (TSS) in the 20 mg group was significantly higher than in the placebo and 8 mg treatment group. The highest dose of 30 mg did not significantly decrease symptom severity compared to the 20 mg treatment, providing a rationale for the usage of 20 mg daily as the effective dose (Schellenberg et al 2012).

Two prospective randomised double-blind placebo-controlled studies investigating efficacy of vitex extract (BNO 1095) in the treatment of Chinese women suffering moderate to severe PMS ($n = 67$ and $n = 217$, respectively) found that vitex significantly ameliorated all symptoms except abdominal cramping, and especially improved negative affect (depressed mood) and fluid retention. In the treatment arm, there was a significantly greater decrease in depressive symptoms in the luteal phase and PMS self-assessment compared to placebo after two menstrual cycles, with the differences between placebo and active treatment groups becoming even more significant after 3 months' treatment. This further supports the use of vitex in PMS and indicates that full benefit requires at least three menstrual cycles to become established. Of note, these studies found a placebo effect of 50%, but still a significantly greater effect of vitex (He et al 2009, Ma et al 2010).

A multicentre, randomised, controlled, double-blind study investigating the effects of vitex (Ze440) for PMS involved 170 women and was published in the *British Medical Journal* (Schellenberg 2001). Of the group, 13% were also taking oral contraceptive pills (OCP). Treatment with a 20-mg tablet of dry extract of chasteberry taken daily resulted in a significant improvement of PMS symptoms, particularly headache, breast fullness, irritability, anger and mood changes. Over 50% of women in the active treatment group achieved at least a 50% reduction in symptoms. Similar results were obtained in a 2006 prospective, open, non-comparative study of 121 women with moderate to severe PMS who took vitex (BNO 1095) over three menstrual cycles. Assessment using the validated PMS diary and the premenstrual tension syndrome score showed that the severity of PMS symptoms consistently decreased during treatment (Prilepskaya et al 2006).

Another three-arm double-blind study of women with premenstrual dysphoric disorder ($n = 108$), compared 20–40 mg fluoxetine, 20 mg vitex or multivitamin placebo for 6 months. Women in both treatment arms showed significant improvement on the Hamilton Depression Rating Scale ($P < 0.001$ and $P < 0.05$ respectively) compared with placebo, and the vitex group demonstrated no side effects (Ciotta et al 2012).

Previously, a number of open studies had generally produced positive results for vitex as a symptomatic treatment in PMS. One multicentre, open-label study showed that daily treatment with a 20-mg tablet of vitex (Ze440) over three menstrual cycles significantly reduced the Moor menstrual distress self-assessment questionnaire (MMDQ), with 46% of women experiencing a 50% reduction in the MMDQ. Treatment also reduced the duration of PMS symptoms from 7.5 days to 6 days and was as effective for women taking OCP as for those who were not (Berger et al 2000). Once treatment was stopped, PMS symptoms gradually returned to baseline within three further cycles.

The largest multicentre trial was an open study of 1634 women with PMS, which found that treatment with vitex (Femicur) for three menstrual cycles decreased the number of PMS symptoms in 93% of subjects (Loch et al 2000). Symptoms completely resolved in 40% of subjects and 94% overall rated vitex treatment as well tolerated. An early study using vitex (Agnolyt) in 1542 women with PMS reported an improvement in symptoms with an average dose of 42 drops daily taken for an average of 25 days (Dittmar 1992, as reported in

Ulbricht & Basch 2005). According to Ulbricht and Basch (2005), three earlier uncontrolled studies produced inconclusive results.

An open-label clinical trial of 100 women with PMS and migraine headaches was conducted using 40 mg/day vitex extract over a 3-month period. Sixty-six women reported a dramatic reduction of PMS symptoms, 26 a mild reduction, with no effect in eight of the trial participants. Forty-two women experienced greater than 50% reduction in frequency of premenstrual migraine. No patients reported side effects. While this was not a placebo-controlled trial, it points to vitex being a safe and effective treatment for women with premenstrual migraine headaches: the frequency and duration of migraine attacks were reduced (Ambrosini et al 2013).

Clinical note — The opiate system and PMS

The opiate system consists of mu, delta and kappa opiate receptors and endogenous opiate peptides such as beta-endorphin (Webster et al 2006). The opiate system plays an essential role in regulating tonic pain perception, mood, appetite and other functions. PMS is characterised by a reduction of opiate activity and the severity of symptoms such as anxiety, food cravings and physical discomfort is inversely proportional to the amount of decline in beta-endorphin levels in the luteal phase. Based on recent research, the symptom-relieving effects of vitex in PMS may be due to direct activation of analgesic and mood-regulatory pathways via opiate receptor activation and/or reversal of the loss of opiate inhibition in the luteal phase.

Clinical note — Ze440 extract

The naming of the Ze440 extract (Premular in Australia) is derived from the name Zeller, the 150-year-old Swiss company manufacturing it, combined with a unique number ascribed during the initial studies. In order to ensure that products deliver consistent results, Ze440 is measured by both composition and consistency from batch to batch. To promote product uniformity, every batch is grown, harvested and manufactured into tablets under controlled conditions and is extracted in a standardised method that ensures consistent and high levels of the important lipophilic compound casticin and an established marker compound, the iridoid glycoside, named agnuside. A daily dose of 20 mg (equivalent to one tablet) has demonstrated effectiveness (Schellenberg et al 2012).

IN COMBINATION

A 2008 Australian study investigated the effects of a combination of *Vitex agnus-castus* (equivalent to 1000 mg dry fruit) and *Hypericum perforatum* (St John's wort) on PMS-like symptoms in a small subpopulation of late perimenopausal women participating in a double-blind, placebo-controlled, randomised trial on menopausal symptoms. Of 100 volunteers recruited to the larger study, 14 late perimenopausal women who had menstruated at least once within the last 12 weeks of the treatment phase provided data for PMS-like symptoms. This herbal combination was found to be superior to placebo for total PMS-like symptoms and the subclusters, PMS-D (depression) and PMS-C (cravings) (van Die et al 2009a).

Comparison to SSRI drugs

A systematic review of herbal treatments for alleviating premenstrual symptoms looked at four clinical trials of vitex and found it had significant efficacy for relieving physical symptoms of PMS, but lesser effectiveness compared with fluoxetine for treating the psychological symptoms of premenstrual dysphoric disorder and a similar incidence to placebo of self-limiting minor adverse reactions (nausea, headaches) (Dante & Facchinetti 2011). In 2003, a randomised 8-week study involving 42 women compared the effects of 20–40 mg daily of fluoxetine, a selective serotonin reuptake inhibitor (SSRI), and 20–40 mg of vitex extract and found no statistically significant difference between the groups with respect to the rate of responders (Atmaca et al 2003). More specifically, patients with premenstrual dysphoric disorder responded well to both treatments; however, fluoxetine was more effective for psychological symptoms such as depression and irritability, whereas the herbal extract was more effective for diminishing physical symptoms such as breast tenderness, cramps, food cravings and swelling. Unfortunately, the authors did not report the type of vitex extract used in the study.

Comparison to vitamin B_6

Although vitamin B_6 (pyroxidine) is a popular treatment for PMS symptoms, the results from a double-blind comparative study have found that vitex (Agnolyt) is as effective, and possibly more so (Lauritzen et al 1997). The randomised, double-blind study of 175 women compared vitex, pyridoxine and placebo. In the study, 77% of women receiving vitex reported symptom alleviation compared with 61% with pyridoxine (200 mg/day), which was considered a small but significant difference. Additionally, doctors' assessments were more likely to rate treatment with vitex as 'excellent' compared with pyridoxine.

Commission E approves the use of vitex for PMS.

Mastalgia

Mastalgia is considered to relate to latent and increased basal prolactin levels; therefore, agents that reduce prolactin levels are anticipated to reduce symptoms. Vitex is a popular treatment for cyclical mastalgia as it interacts with dopamine D_2 receptors to reduce prolactin levels.

In two randomised, double-blind studies, vitex (Mastodynon) effectively reduced premenstrual mastalgia (Halaska et al 1998, Wuttke et al 1997, Wuttke et al 2003). Subjects completed a visual analogue scale and rated their breast pain from 0 (lowest breast pain) to 10 (extremely strong breast pain). Active treatment reduced the mastalgia score by 35–40%, an effect significantly stronger than that of placebo (25%). One of these studies also demonstrated that treatment with vitex reduced serum prolactin levels (Wuttke et al 1997, as reported in Wuttke et al 2003). According to Halaska et al (1998), symptom relief was experienced after the first month of treatment, with continued improvements experienced after the second and third months.

Commission E approves the use of vitex for this indication.

Irregularities of the menstrual cycle

Vitex is used to normalise menstruation in women with shortened, lengthened or infrequent menstruation, particularly when low progesterone and luteal-phase defects are suspected. In practice, vitex has also been used traditionally to treat both amenorrhoea and menorrhagia. Herbalists speculate that beneficial effects obtained in practice may be due to the herb's ability to reduce elevated prolactin levels in these conditions. This is particularly indicated where chronic stress is also present, as this has an effect on the hypothalamus–pituitary axis, resulting in elevated prolactin levels (Mills 2000, Trickey 1998). While the use of vitex in all these indications has not yet been tested under double-blind conditions, one randomised controlled trial of women with luteal-phase defect due to latent hyperprolactinaemia demonstrated that vitex extract (20 mg daily) effectively reduced prolactin levels and normalised luteal-phase length and progesterone levels after treatment for 3 months (Milewicz et al 1993).

Commission E approves the use of vitex for this indication.

Menopause

Vitex has only recently been utilised for menopause-related complaints. Based on pharmacological studies and clinical research, there is emerging support for its role in the alleviation of menopausal symptoms (van Die et al 2009c). While evidence from rigorous randomised controlled trials is lacking for the use of vitex as an individual herb in this context, further investigation is warranted.

IN COMBINATION

Vitex has been studied as part of several different polyherbal treatments for effectiveness in treating menopausal symptoms. The use of herbal combinations reflects real-world practice but makes it difficult to assess the value of vitex as a stand-alone treatment for this indication. To date, these studies using combination herbal therapy, including vitex, have produced mixed results.

A systematic review assessed the effectiveness of a combination of vitex and St John's wort versus placebo and found no significant differences in measured end points, including vasomotor symptoms, somatic complaints, sleep disorders, sexual disorders or mental disorders, with side effects comparable between the two (Laakmann et al 2012). It has been suggested, however, that some of the symptoms typically attributed to menopause may be more related to PMS in some women and, in these cases, the vitex and St John's wort combination could provide some relief (van Die et al 2009b).

Vitex (200 mg daily), in combination with other herbs, notably black cohosh, produced a significantly superior mean reduction in menopausal symptoms compared to placebo according to a 2007 randomised controlled study (Rotem & Kaplan 2007). The study of 50 healthy pre- and postmenopausal women found herbal treatment improved menopausal symptoms gradually and, after 3 months of treatment, there was a 73% decrease in hot flushes and a 69% reduction in frequency of night sweats, accompanied by a decrease in their intensity and a significant benefit in terms of sleep quality. Importantly, hot flushes ceased completely in 47% of women in the study group, compared with only 19% in the placebo group. No changes were detected for vaginal epithelium or levels of relevant hormones (oestradiol, FSH), liver enzymes or thyroid-stimulating hormone in either group.

Poor lactation

Vitex has been used since ancient times as a galactagogue to promote milk production, especially in the first 10 days after delivery.

Currently, there are no double-blind studies to confirm its efficacy; however, an early uncontrolled study provides some support for the use of vitex in lactation, finding a favourable effect on milk production in 80% of women (Noack 1943). Results from a small study of males suggest that increases in prolactin may be possible with low-dose vitex (120 mg daily), whereas higher doses (480 mg daily) result in decreased levels (Merz et al 1996).

Fertility disorders

Vitex is used in practice with other herbal medicines to enhance fertility in women with progesterone deficiency or luteal-phase defects. Currently, no large studies have been published to evaluate the effectiveness of this approach; however, a double-blind, randomised, placebo-controlled study of 96 women with fertility disorders (38 with secondary amenorrhoea, 31 with luteal insufficiency and 27 with idiopathic infertility) used the vitex product Mastodynon, with encouraging results (Gerhard et al 1998). Treatment of 30 drops was administered twice daily for 3 months and resulted in women with amenorrhoea or luteal insufficiency achieving pregnancy more than twice as often as the placebo group, with 15 women conceiving during the study period (n = 7 with amenorrhoea, n = 4 with idiopathic infertility, n = 4 with luteal insufficiency). Although promising, this study has been criticised for pooling of diverse conditions, unclear reporting of results and variable significance (Ulbricht & Basch 2005).

Acne vulgaris

An open study of 117 subjects (male and female) with different forms of acne found that, after 6 weeks' treatment with a 0.2% dried extract of *Vitex agnus-castus* and a topical disinfectant, 70% of cases experienced total resolution, with the highest success rates reported for acne vulgaris, follicularis and excoriated acne (Amann 1975). A group that was not treated with the herb took 30–50% longer to achieve similar results. Although encouraging, it is difficult to determine the contribution of vitex treatment to these results. Until controlled studies using vitex as a stand-alone treatment are conducted, the herb's role in this condition is still uncertain.

OTHER USES

Vitex is used to aid the expulsion of the placenta after birth. It is also used to treat fibroids, to normalise hormones following the use of OCP and in cases of premature ovarian failure. Studies on rats suggest that the dopaminergic agonist action of vitex may be useful to reduce or control epileptic seizures (Saberi et al 2008).

Practice points/Patient counselling

- Clinical trials support the use of vitex in mild, moderate and severe PMS. It is particularly suited to treating common PMS symptoms, such as mood changes and irritability, breast tenderness, headaches and constipation. According to the available evidence, it is more effective than pyridoxine treatment and has a similar response rate to fluoxetine.
- It may also be effective in the treatment of menstrual irregularities and mastalgia.
- Vitex is also used to relieve perimenopausal symptoms, enhance fertility in women with progesterone deficiency or luteal-phase defects, aid the expulsion of the placenta after birth, reduce fibroids and normalise hormones following the use of oral contraceptives.
- Traditionally, it is described as a galactagogue (i.e. a medicine able to increase milk production in lactation) and is used in low doses for this indication.
- A mechanism of action has not been conclusively identified, but it appears to inhibit prolactin release by selective stimulation of pituitary dopamine D_2 receptors, to increase progesterone levels and works via the opiate system.

DOSAGE RANGE

General guide

- Liquid extract (1 : 2): 1–2.5 mL in the morning.
- Dried fruit: 1.5–3 g in the morning.
- Dry fruit flesh (solid-dose form): 1000–1800 mg/day.
- Manufacturers have recommended vitex preparations be taken daily as a single dose upon rising, before breakfast, throughout the menstrual cycle.

According to clinical studies

PMS

- Ze440 extract (Premular) 20 mg daily.
- Femicur 40 mg daily.

Cyclic mastalgia

- Mastodynon 60 drops daily or one tablet daily.

Menstrual irregularities

- 20 mg daily (extract unknown).

Infertility

- Mastodynon 30 drops twice daily.

ADVERSE REACTIONS

A systematic review of the herb's safety, published in 2005, analysed data from six electronic databases, postmarketing surveillance studies, spontaneous reporting schemes (including the World Health Organization), herbalist organisations and manufacturers (Daniele et al 2005). The review concluded that vitex is a safe herbal medicine and any adverse effects associated with its use tend to be mild and reversible. The most common adverse effects are nausea, headache, dizziness, tiredness, mild gastrointestinal disturbances, dry mouth, menstrual disorders, acne, pruritus and erythematous rash. Additionally, no drug interactions have been reported. More recently, a 2009 placebo-controlled study of 202 women with moderate to severe PMS found no significant difference between incidence of adverse effects in the placebo- or vitex-treated groups (He et al 2009). Headache was reported as one of the more common side effects experienced by both groups, but was attributed to the PMS itself and not treatment.

SIGNIFICANT INTERACTIONS

Controlled studies are not available, so interactions are based on evidence of activity and are largely theoretical and speculative.

Dopamine antagonists

An antagonistic interaction is theoretically possible — observe patients.

Oral contraceptives

There has been speculation about the effectiveness of vitex when OCP are being taken. Several clinical studies involving women taking oral contraceptives have confirmed the herb still reduces PMS symptoms and does not affect OCP.

C

CONTRAINDICATIONS AND PRECAUTIONS

People with tumours sensitive to oestrogen or progesterone should avoid using this herb until safety can be established. It has been suggested that the ability of vitex to reduce prolactin levels may inhibit medical investigations and may mask diagnosis and proper treatment of prolactinoma (Gallagher et al 2008).

PREGNANCY USE

Vitex is not traditionally recommended in pregnancy. In practice, some herbalists use it during the first 10 weeks of pregnancy in cases of difficult conception.

PATIENTS' FAQs

What will this herb do for me?
Vitex is used to relieve common symptoms of PMS, such as irritability, mood swings, breast tenderness, headache and constipation. It is also used in combination with other herbal medicines to enhance fertility, relieve menopausal symptoms, regulate irregular menstruation, improve acne and promote milk production in new mothers.

When does it start to work?
Most trials show that treatment for at least three menstrual cycles may be required before symptom relief is experienced in PMS.

Are there any safety issues?
In cases of irregular menstruation, investigation for serious pathology should be undertaken before use of this herb.

REFERENCES

Amann W. Acne vulgaris and *Agnus castus* (Agnolyt). Z Allgemeinmed 51.35 (1975): 1645–1648.

Ambrosini, A., et al. (2013). Use of *Vitex agnus-castus* in migrainous women with premenstrual syndrome: an open-label clinical observation. Acta Neurol Belg, 113(1), 25-29.

Atmaca M, et al. Fluoxetine versus *Vitex agnus castus* extract in the treatment of premenstrual dysphoric disorder. Hum Psychopharmacol 18.3 (2003): 191–195.

Berger D et al. Efficacy of *Vitex agnus castus* L. extract Ze 440 in patients with pre-menstrual syndrome (PMS). Arch Gynecol Obstet 264.3 (2000): 150–153.

Cavieres, M., & Castillo, R. (2011). Evaluation of the estrogenicity of *Vitex agnus castus*. Toxicology Letters, 205 Supplement, S250.

Chen, S.-N., et al. (2011). Phytoconstituents from *Vitex agnus-castus* fruits. Fitoterapia, 82, 528-533.

Choudhary, M., et al. (2009). Antiinflammatory and lipoxygenase inhibitory compounds from *Vitex agnus-castus*. Phytotherapy Research, 23(9), 1336-1339.

Ciotta, L., et al. (2012). Long-term treatment with *Vitex agnus castus* (VAC) in premenstrual dysphoric disorders (PMDD). International Journal of Gynecology & Obstetrics, 119(Supplement 3), S605.

Daniele C et al. *Vitex agnus castus*: a systematic review of adverse events. Drug Saf 28.4 (2005): 319–332.

Dante, G., & Facchinetti, F. (2011). Herbal treatments for alleviating premenstrual symptoms: a systematic review. Journal of Psychosomatic Obstetrics & Gynecology, 32(1), 42-51.

Dittmar FW. Premenstrual syndrome: treatment with a phytopharmaceutical. TW Gynakologie 5.1(1992): 60–68.

Gallagher, J., et al. (2008). A prolactinoma masked by a herbal remedy. European Journal of Obstetrics, Gynecology and Reproductive Biology, 137(2), 257-258.

Gerard J. The herbal, or general history of plants. The complete 1633 edition as revised and enlarged by Thomas Johnson. New York: Dover Publications, 1975.

Gerhard II et al. Mastodynon(R) bei weiblicher Sterilitat. Forsch Komplementarmed 5.6 (1998): 272–278.

Halaska M et al. [Treatment of cyclical mastodynia using an extract of *Vitex agnus castus*: results of a double-blind comparison with a placebo.] Ceska Gynekol 63.5 (1998): 388–392.

He Z et al. Treatment for premenstrual syndrome with *Vitex agnus castus*: a prospective, randomized, multi-center placebo controlled study in China. Maturitas 63.1 (2009): 99–103.

Ibrahim, N., et al. (2008). Gynecological efficacy and chemical investigation of *Vitex agnus-castus* L. fruits growing in Egypt. Natural Product Research, 22(6), 537-546.

Imai, M., et al. (2009). Cytotoxic effects of flavonoids against a human colon cancer derived cell line, COLO 201: A potential natural anti-cancer substance. Cancer Letters, 276(1), 74-80.

Jarry H et al. In vitro prolactin but not LH and FSH release is inhibited by compounds in extracts of *Agnus castus*: direct evidence for a dopaminergic principle by the dopamine receptor assay. Exp Clin Endocrinol 102.6 (1994): 448–454.

Jarry H et al. Evidence for estrogen receptor beta-selective activity of *Vitex agnus-castus* and isolated flavones. Planta Med 69.10 (2003): 945–947.

Jarry H et al. In vitro assays for bioactivity-guided isolation of endocrine active compounds in *Vitex agnus-castu*. Maturitas 55 (Supplement 1) (2006): S26–S36.

Laakmann, E., et al. (2012). Efficacy of *Cimicifuga racemosa, Hypericum perforatum* and *Agnus castus* in the treatment of climacteric complaints: a systematic review. Gynecological Endocrinology, 28(9), 703-709.

Lauritzen C et al. Treatment of premenstrual tension syndrome with *Vitex agnus castus*: controlled, double-blind study versus pyridoxin. Phytomedicine 4 (1997): 183–189.

Liu J et al. Evaluation of estrogenic activity of plant extracts for the potential treatment of menopausal symptoms. J Agric Food Chem 49.5 (2001): 2472–2479.

Loch EG, et al. Treatment of premenstrual syndrome with a phytopharmaceutical formulation containing *Vitex agnus castus*. J Womens Health Gend Based Med 9.3 (2000): 315–320.

Ma, L., et al. (2010). Treatment of moderate to severe premenstrual syndrome with *Vitex agnus castus* (BNO 1095) in Chinese women. Gynecological Endocrinolfog, 26(8), 612-616.

Meier B, Hoberg E. Agni-casti fructus: an overview of new findings in phytochemistry, pharmacology and biological activity. Zeitschr Phytother 20.3 (1999): 140–158.

Meier B et al. Pharmacological activities of *Vitex agnus-castus* extracts in vitro. Phytomedicine 7.5 (2000): 373–381.

Merz PG et al. The effects of a special *Agnus castus* extract (BP1095E1) on prolactin secretion in healthy male subjects. Exp Clin Endocrinol Diabetes 104.6 (1996): 447–453.

Mesaik, M., et al. (2009). Isolation and immunomodulatory properties of a flavonoid, casticin from *Vitex agnus-castus*. Phytotherapy Research, 23(11), 1516-1520.

Milewicz A et al. *Vitex agnus castus* extract in the treatment of luteal phase defects due to latent hyperprolactinemia: results of a randomized placebo-controlled double-blind study. Arzneimittelforschung 43.7 (1993): 752–756.

Mills SB. Principles and practice of phytotherapy: modern herbal medicine. Sydney: Churchill Livingstone, 2000.

Nasri, S., et al. (2007). The effects of *Vitex agnus castus* extract and its interaction with dopaminergic system on LH and testosterone in male mice. Pakistan Journal of Biological Sciences, 10(14), 2300-2307.

Noack M. Dtsch Med Wochenschr (1943): 204. Available at: www.phytotherapies.org.

Ohyama K et al. Cytotoxicity and apoptotic inducibility of *Vitex agnus-castus* fruit extract in cultured human normal and cancer cells and effect on growth. Biol Pharm Bull 26.1 (2003): 10–1118.

Ohyama K et al. Human gastric signet ring carcinoma (KATO-III) cell apoptosis induced by *Vitex agnus-castus* fruit extract through intracellular oxidative stress. Int J Biochem Cell Biol 37.7 (2005): 1496–1510.

Ono, M., et al. (2008). Five new diterpenoids, viteagnusians A-Z, from the fruit of *Vitex angus-castus*. Chemical & Pharmaceutical Bulletin, 56(11), 1621-1624.

Prilepskaya VN et al. *Vitex agnus castus*: successful treatment of moderate to severe premenstrual syndrome. Maturitas 55 (Supplement 1) (2006): S55–S63.

Rotem C, Kaplan B. Phyto-female complex for the relief of hot flushes, night sweats and quality of sleep: randomized, controlled, double-blind pilot study. Gynecol Endocrinol 23.2 (2007): 117–122.

Saberi M, et al. The antiepileptic activity of *Vitex agnus castus* extract on amygdala kindled seizures in male rats. Neurosci Lett 441.2 (2008): 193–196.

Sarikurkcu, C., et al. (2009). Studies on the antioxidant activity of essential oil and different solvent extracts of *Vitex agnus castus* L. fruits from Turkey. Food and Chemical Toxicology, 47, 2479-2483.
Schellenberg R. Treatment for the premenstrual syndrome with agnus castus fruit extract: prospective, randomised, placebo controlled study. BMJ 322.7279 (2001): 134–137.
Schellenberg, R., et al. (2012). Dose-dependent efficacy of the *Vitex agnus castus* extract Ze 440 in patients suffering from premenstrual syndrom. Phytomedicine, 19(14), 1325-1331.
Sehmisch, S., et al. (2009). *Vitex agnus castus* as prophylaxis for osteopenia after orchidectomy in rats compared with estradiol and testosterone supplementation. Phytotherapy Research, 23(6), 851-858.
Shaw, S., et al. (2011). *Vitex agnus castus* for premenstrual syndrome (Protocol). Cochrane Database of Systematic Reviews.
Sliutz G et al. Agnus castus extracts inhibit prolactin secretion of rat pituitary cells. Horm Metab Res 25.5 (1993): 253–255.
Splitt G et al. Behandlung zyklusabhangiger Brustschmerzen mit einem Agnus castus-haltigen Arzneimittel: Ergebnisse einer randomisierten, plazebokontrollierten Doppelblindstudie. Geburtsh u Frauenheilk 57 (1997): 569–574.
Stojkovic, C., Sokovic, M., Glamoclija, J., et al. (2011). Chemical composition and antimicrobial activity of *Vitex agnus-castus* L. fruits and leaves essential oils. Food Chemistry, 128, 1017-1022.
Trickey R. Women, hormones & the menstrual cycle. St Leonards, NSW. Australia: Allen & Unwin, 1998.
Ulbricht C, Basch E. Chasteberry. Missouri: Mosby, 2005:136–43.
van Die, M., et al. (2009a). Effects of a Combination of *Hypericum perforatum* and *Vitex agnus-castus* on PMS-Like Symptoms in Late-Perimenopausal Women: Findings from a Subpopulation Analysis. The Journal of Alternative and Complementary Medicine, 15(9), 1045-1048.
van Die, M., et al. (2009b). Effects of a combination of *Hypericum perforatum* and *Vitex agnus-castus* on PMS-like symptoms in late-perimenopausal women: findings from a subpopulation analysis. Journal of Alternative & Complementary Medicine, 15(9), 1045-1048.
van Die, M., et al. (2009c). *Vitex agnus-castus* (Chaste-Tree = Berry) in the Treatment of Menopause-Related Complaints. The Journal of Alternative and Complementary Medicine, 15(8), 853-862.
van Die, M. D., Burger, H. G., Teede, H. J., et al. (2013). *Vitex agnus-castus* Extracts for Female Reproductive Disorders: A Systematic Review of Clinical Trials. Planta Med, 79(8), 562-575.
Webster DE et al. Activation of the mu-opiate receptor by *Vitex agnus-castus* methanol extracts: implication for its use in PMS. J Ethnopharmacol (2006): 106: 216-221.
Webster, D., et al. (2011). Opiodergic mechanisms underlying the actions of *Vitex agnus-castus* L. Biochemical Pharmacology, 81(1), 170-177.
Weisskopf M et al. A *Vitex agnus-castus* extract inhibits cell growth and induces apoptosis in prostate epithelial cell lines. Planta Med 71.10 (2005): 910–916.
Wuttke W et al. Chaste tree (*Vitex agnus-castus*): pharmacology and clinical indications. Phytomedicine 10.4 (2003): 348–357.
Zamani, M., et al. (2012). Therapeutic Effect of *Vitex agnus castus* in Patients with Premenstrual Syndrome. Acta Medica Iranica, 50(2), 101-106.

Chickweed

HISTORICAL NOTE Chickweed is one of the most common weeds worldwide. It has been used since ancient times to treat external inflammatory conditions and is also consumed as a tasty and nutritious vegetable, as well as poultry fodder to improve egg production. Other medicinal claims include its use as an astringent, carminative, antiasthmatic, demulcent, depurative, diuretic, emmenagogue, expectorant, galactagogue, useful in kidney complications, rheumatic joints, wounds and ulcers (Chidrawar et al 2011). Its water is an old wives remedy for obesity (Rani et al 2012). Modern herbalists mainly prescribe chickweed for skin diseases but also bronchitis, rheumatic pains, arthritis and period pain (Ma et al 2012).

COMMON NAME

Chickweed

OTHER NAMES

Mouse-ear, star chickweed, starweed, satinflower, starwort, stellaria, winterweed

BOTANICAL NAME/FAMILY

Stellaria media (family Caryophyllaceae)

PLANT PARTS USED

Aerial parts — leaves, stems and flowers

CHEMICAL COMPONENTS

Chickweed is commonly used as a food and is rich in essential vitamins A, B-complex and C, and minerals including calcium and iron. It is also a dietary source of carotenoids, including beta-carotene and gamma-linolenic acid (Fisher 2009, Rani et al 2012).

Other chemical constituents which may contribute to the pharmacological action of chickweed include: saponins, coumarins, flavonoids, triterpenoids, pentasaccharide, polysaccharides and sitosterols (Ma et al 2012, Rani et al 2012, Vanhaecke et al 2008).

Chromatography isolates include apigenin 6-C-beta-D-galactopyranosyl-8-C-alpha-L-arabinopyranoside, apigenin 6-C-alpha-L-arabinopyranosyl-8-C-beta-D-galactopyranoside, apigenin 6-C-beta-D-galactopyranosyl-8-C-beta-L-arabinopyranoside, apigenin 6-C-beta-D -glucopyranosyl-8-C-beta-D-galactopyranoside, and apigenin 6,8-di-C-alpha-L-arabinopyranoside (Dong et al 2007).

Chickweed essential oil has been found to contain several well-known contact allergens: borneol, menthol, linalool, 1,8-cineole, and other terpenes such as epoxy-dehydro-caryophyllene, monoterpene alcohol-ester and caryophyllene (Jovanović et al 2003).

MAIN ACTIONS

The pharmacological actions of chickweed have not been significantly investigated, so traditional use and an understanding of the actions of individual constituents is used.

Internal use

Antitussive, expectorant and demulcent effects

Herbal saponins are well known to irritate mucous membranes and are successfully used as expectorants (e.g. senega). Herbs such as chickweed that contain saponins are also suspected to have a degree of expectorant activity when used internally; however, this has not been investigated in controlled studies.

Antimicrobial

Defensins are a family of peptides that exhibit antimicrobial activity and play an important role in resistance against pathogens in the plant kingdom. Two defensins have been successfully isolated from chickweed that display strong antifungal activity. Their amino acid sequence was identified. The understanding of sequence coding of these peptides may lead to further understanding of their antimicrobial action and development of new extractions and applications of chickweed (Slavokhotova 2011).

Antiviral effects

An in vitro study investigated chickweed against Hepatitis B virus (HBV). The extract was shown to suppress the secretion of Hepatitis B surface antigen (HBsAg) and hepatitis B e antigen (HBeAg) in a cell culture medium — 27.92% and 25.35% after 6 days of treatment, respectively. The chickweed fraction also reduced the level of HBV DNA in a dose-dependent manner. Characterisation of the chemical constituents of the extract found the presence of flavonoid C-glycosides, polysaccharides and protein exhibited antiviral activities (Ma et al 2012).

Hepatoprotective

A water-soluble polysaccharide extracted from chickweed was administered to rats with induced hepatitis, at a dose of 100 mg/kg. The extract was shown to reduce liver enzymes ALT, AST and AP by 41%, 37% and 56% respectively. The concentration of total and conjugated bilirubin decreased by 63% and 87% respectively. Histological results revealed a three-fold reduction in the number of necrotic and degenerative hepatocytes; and a significant increase in the regeneration of hepatic tissue with a proliferation of hepatocytes. These results are suggestive of a promising action for the novel constituent of chickweed in promoting liver regeneration and protecting against hepatocyte necrosis associated with liver disease (Gorina et al 2013).

External use

Soothing irritated skin and enhancing wound healing

Chickweed is traditionally thought to have soothing properties when applied to the skin in an appropriate vehicle, although controlled studies are not available to confirm these effects. The saponin content may account for the herb's ability to help reduce itchiness.

OTHER ACTIONS

An in vitro study identified that a chickweed decoction had activity against human hepatoma cell lines (Lin et al 2002). An ethanolic extract of chickweed has been found to strongly inhibit xanthine oxidase in vitro, suggesting that it may have a use against hyperuricaemia and gout (Pieroni et al 2002).

CLINICAL USE

Chickweed has not been significantly investigated under clinical trial conditions, so evidence is derived from traditional, in vitro and animal studies.

Urticaria, eczema, rashes, burns

Chickweed is most commonly used in external preparations for inflamed and itchy skin conditions such as urticaria, eczema, insect bites and stings, as well as minor wounds and cuts. Anecdotal evidence suggests that it may have some effects; however, controlled studies are not available to confirm effectiveness.

Bronchial phlegm and bronchitis

Taken orally, chickweed is often combined with other herbs for treating conditions characterised by fever and bronchial phlegm; however, controlled studies are not available to confirm effectiveness.

Obesity/Weight loss

Traditional Indian medicine claims chickweed has anti-obesity activity. Recent investigations using animal models have shown promising results. The effect of methanolic and alcoholic extracts of chickweed on food consumption pattern, change in body weight, thermogenesis, lipid metabolism and histology of fat pad was examined in progesterone-induced obese female mice. Food consumption behaviours, adiposity index, white adipose tissue and liver and body weight increases were significantly decreased in a dose-dependent manner (100 mg, 200 mg, 400 mg per kg body weight). There was no significant change in body temperature. The possible weight loss properties are believed to be due to saponins, flavonols and partly by β-sitosterol, which has a chemical structure similar to dietary fat and thereby competitively inhibits dietary fat absorption (Chidrawar et al 2011).

Moreover, another study investigated a lyophilised juice extract of chickweed and its anti-obesity action at two doses, 400 mg/kg and 900 mg/kg body weight, in mice fed a high-fat-diet for 6 weeks. In addition, pancreatic lipase activity was evaluated by measurement of plasma triacylglycerol levels. The lyophilised juice extract of chickweed significantly suppressed the increase in body weight, retroperitoneal adipose tissue, liver weights and serum parameters of total cholesterol, total triglyceride and LDL-cholesterol levels at the dose of 900 mg/kg body weight. The results indicate that chickweed might confer an anti-obesity action by delaying the intestinal absorption of dietary fat and carbohydrate by inhibiting digestive enzymes (Rani et al 2012).

Further investigations including clinical trials are required to verify the clinical use of chickweed in obesity.

OTHER USES

Chickweed can be eaten raw in salads, served as cooked greens, juiced or infused as a tea. It has also been used as a mild laxative and diuretic substance.

DOSAGE RANGE

- Tincture (1:5): 2–10 mL three times daily.
- Infusion of dried herb: 1–5 g three times daily.
- Chickweed is commonly incorporated into a topical ointment or cream base for external use (1 part chickweed to 5 parts base) and applied as required.

TOXICITY

Allergic skin reactions can occur with topical use.

ADVERSE REACTIONS

There is insufficient reliable information available about the safety of chickweed when used internally or externally. Allergy to chickweed causing contact erythema multiforme has been reported (Jovanović et al 2003), and it is advised to apply a test patch to a small area before applying more widely.

SIGNIFICANT INTERACTIONS

Not known.

CONTRAINDICATIONS AND PRECAUTIONS

Allergic skin reactions can occur with topical use.

PREGNANCY USE

Likely to be safe when consumed in dietary amounts; however, safety is not known when used in larger quantities.

Practice points/Patient counselling

- Chickweed has been traditionally used as an ingredient in herbal creams and ointments to soothe inflamed, itchy skin and promote wound healing. Although controlled studies are unavailable, the pharmacological actions of several constituents within the herb suggest that it may be useful.
- Although it is likely to be safe, it is prudent to avoid using chickweed in pregnancy in amounts greater than those ingested when used as a food.

PATIENTS' FAQs

What will this herb do for me?

When chickweed is applied topically it may soothe inflamed and itchy skin. It is taken orally as a cough suppressant and expectorant. Large doses in animal models have shown it may reduce fat absorption in the gastrointestinal tract.

How quickly will it work?

In practice, topical preparations are reported to produce symptom relief within 30 minutes; however, there are no controlled trials to confirm this.

Are there any safety issues?

Chickweed can be consumed as a food in salads, cooked as greens or prepared as a juice; however, the safety of larger intakes is unknown. Used as part of a herbal cream, it is likely to be safe, although it would be wise to do a test patch in a small area before applying to large areas. The safety of large doses in pregnancy is unknown.

REFERENCES

Chidrawar VR et al. Antiobesity effect of Stellaria media against drug induced obesity in Swiss albino mice. Ayu 32.4 (2011): 576–584.

Dong Q, Huang Y, Qiao SY. [Studies on chemical constituents from stellaria media. I]. Zhongguo Zhong Yao Za Zhi 32.11 (2007): 1048–1051.

Fisher C, Materia medica of Western Herbs. Vitex Medica (2009).

Gorina YV et al. Evaluation of hepatoprotective activity of water-soluble polysaccharide fraction of stellaria media L. Bulletin of experimental biology and medicine 154.5 (2013): 645–648.

Jovanović M et al. Erythema multiforme due to contact with weeds: a recurrence after patch testing. Contact Dermatitis 48.1 (2003): 17–25.

Lin L-T et al. In vitro anti-hepatoma activity of fifteen natural medicines from Canada. Phytother Res 16.5 (2002): 440–444.

Ma L et al. Anti-hepatitis B virus activity of chickweed [Stellaria media (L.) Vill.] extracts in HepG2.2.15 cells. Molecules (Basel, Switzerland) 17.7 (2012): 8633–8646.

Pieroni A et al. In vitro antioxidant activity of non-cultivated vegetables of ethnic Albanians in southern Italy. Phytother Res 16.5 (2002): 467–473.

Rani N, Vasudeva N, Sharma SK. Quality assessment and anti-obesity activity of Stellaria media (Linn.) Vill. BMC Complementary and Alternative Medicine 12 (2012): 145.

Slavokhotova AA Isolation, molecular cloning and antimicrobial activity of novel defensins from common chickweed (Stellaria media L.) seeds. Biochimie 93.3 (2011): 450–456.

Vanhaecke M et al. Isolation and characterization of a pentasaccharide from Stellaria media. Journal of natural products 71.11 (2008): 1833–1836.

Chitosan

C

HISTORICAL NOTE With the exception of cellulose, chitin is the most abundant natural polysaccharide on Earth. The most useful chitin derivative is chitosan. It is produced by different crustaceans, molluscs, insects, algae, fungi and yeasts. Recently, the commercial value of chitin has increased because of the beneficial properties of its soluble derivatives, which are used in chemistry, biotechnology, agriculture, food processing, cosmetics, veterinary science, medicine, dentistry, environmental protection and paper or textile production.

BACKGROUND AND RELEVANT PHARMACOKINETICS

Chitosan is a form of poorly soluble fibre, chemically derived from chitin through deactylation, which is extracted from the exoskeletons of crustaceans or squid. It is a cationic polysaccharide composed of β-1,4–linked D-glucosamine and *N*-acetyl-D-glucosamine. Similar to other forms of fibre, such as oat bran, chitosan is thought to bind bile acids and dietary lipids. The solubility, biocompatibility and immunological activity and physicochemical properties of chitosan are altered by its molecular weight and degree of N-acetylation. The most useful chitosan is one that has the highest degree of acylation and lowest molecular weight, for example, 8kD (Synowiecki & Al-Khateeb 2003).

The solubility of chitosan increases in the acidic environment of the stomach, but at a pH above 6.3 (for example, in the intestines) the amino groups of chitosan, together with dietary fatty acids, bile acids, cholesterol and lipids, form a complex (Ylitalo et al 2002). The decreased availability of bile acids limits intestinal emulsification and the absorption of lipids, which are then excreted in the faeces.

CHEMICAL COMPONENTS

Chitosan is a cationic polysaccharide prepared by N-deacetylation of chitin.

DEFICIENCY SIGNS AND SYMPTOMS

Chitosan is not an essential nutrient, so deficiencies do not occur.

MAIN ACTIONS

Binds to fat

Chitosan displays unique cationic properties which enables it to bind fatty acids via electrostatic forces. As it passes through the digestive tract, positively-charged chitosan binds to negatively-charged fat, bile acids and cholesterol, preventing their absorption. The complexes that form between chitosan and various fats are then excreted in the faeces.

A human study investigating whether this effect is clinically significant found that a dose of 4.5 g/day, taken in divided doses 30 minutes before meals, trapped only negligible amounts of fat as measured by fat excretion in stools (Gades & Stern 2003). A subsequent study by the same authors investigated 2.5 g chitosan/day in 12 men and 12 women, and found faecal excretion of fat increased by 1.8 g/day in men and was negligible in women (Gades & Stern 2005). However, another trial using a larger dose of chitosan (6.3 g/day) found a mean increase of 3.63 g/day faecal fat excretion (Barroso Aranda et al 2002).

These trials suggest the ability for chitosan to bind fats is clinically insignificant unless taken in doses >6 g/day; however, chitosan's binding of fatty acids appears to be selective, determined by chain length and degree of fatty acid saturation. Animal models suggest chitosan binds strongly with lauric and myristic acid, both highly artherogenic fats, but it has a lower affinity for stearic acid. Chitosan also binds more strongly to omega-6 isomers than omega-3, suggesting that in addition to reducing fat absorption generally, it may ultimately have a positive effect on balancing this ratio in the Western diet (Santas et al 2012).

Antibacterial and antifungal activity

Animal studies have identified antibacterial activity against *Bifidobacterium* and *Lactobacillus*, which are part of the normal flora of the intestinal tract (Tanaka et al 1997). Clinical trials with a chitosan mouthwash and chewing gum have shown antibacterial activity against *Streptococcus mutans* (Sano et al 2003). Chitosan also inhibits the adhesion of *Candida albicans* to human buccal cells and has antifungal activity (Senel et al 2000). The mechanism of its antimicrobial action is believed to be due to its cationic properties. The positively charged anions of chitosan bind to the cell wall of bacteria causing damage and leakage of cytoplasmic content, leading to cell lysis (Hayashi et al 2007a, 2007b). Due to differences in cell wall characteristics, chitosan is more effective against Gram-positive than Gram-negative bacteria. In vitro studies against *Candida albicans* demonstrated the cell wall was still identifiable; however, intracellular structure had either disappeared or changed, suggesting a different mechanism of action.

Wound healing

Chitosan exhibits a wound-healing action. When applied topically it is considered a haemostatic agent by binding with blood cells, assisting to form a clot (Dai et al 2011). It has been reported to enhance inflammatory cells involved in wound healing, including leucocytes, macrophages and fibroblasts. As a result, chitosan leads to acceleration of granulation and organisation of the healing process (Ueno et al 2001). Because infection can significantly impair healing time, the antimicrobial actions mentioned previously also contribute to chitosan's attributes as a wound healer.

OTHER ACTIONS

Chitosan can also absorb urea and ammonia and generally displays similar actions to other dietary fibres (Hendler & Rorvik 2001).

CLINICAL USE

The most biologically effective products contain a chitosan fraction having a low molecular weight, for example, 8kD. The smaller the chitosan fraction, the stronger the positive charge. Unfortunately, not every clinical study indicates whether low-molecular-weight chitosan has been used. Therefore, aside from the usual variables, discrepant results may be due to differences in the type of chitosan used. Some applications of chitosan also use chemically modified chitosan derivatives, in particular, for wound-healing applications, but this remains unknown. The process aims to favourably change the physical properties such as solubility, for use in film- or gel-forming capabilities (Chang et al 2013).

Weight loss

Chitosan is sometimes marketed as a weight-loss aid, primarily due to its ability to bind to fats and reduce their absorption in the digestive tract.

A Cochrane systematic review published in 2005 analysed the results of 14 randomised studies involving 1131 subjects and concluded that use of chitosan resulted in a significantly greater weight loss, decrease in total cholesterol and decrease in systolic and diastolic blood pressure than placebo (Ni et al 2005). The studies were a minimum of 4 weeks duration and were conducted in overweight or obese subjects. With regard to the frequency of adverse events or faecal fat excretion, no clear differences were observed between the placebo and chitosan groups. Although encouraging, the authors noted that the quality of the studies were suboptimal and, overall, results were variable. A look at the studies of highest quality suggests that the effects are minimal. The mean trial duration was 8.3 weeks (range 4–24 weeks) and eight of the 14 studies combined the use of chitosan or placebo with a low-calorie or weight-reducing diet. Interpretation of the data is not straightforward because the dose of chitosan used in studies varied considerably, from 0.24 g/day to 15 g/day (mean 3.7 g/day), and six of the studies used treatment preparations that contained other active ingredients in addition to chitosan. Additionally, the review excluded some potentially important trials because they did not meet criteria for inclusion (for example, subjects were not enrolled for being overweight but selected for other reasons).

In 2008, an updated Cochrane systematic review was published which evaluated 15 clinical studies (n = 1219) (Jull et al 2008). Analyses indicated that chitosan preparations result in a significantly greater weight loss (weighted mean difference −1.7 kg; $P <$ 0.00001), decrease in total cholesterol (−0.2 mmol/L; $P < 0.00001$), and a decrease in systolic and diastolic blood pressure compared with placebo. Chitosan treatment was well tolerated, as there were no clear differences between intervention and control groups in terms of frequency of adverse events or in faecal fat excretion. While these results appear more positive than the initial Cochrane review, their clinical significance is unclear, and reviewers once again reported that the quality of many studies was suboptimal and analysis of only high-quality trials yielded less convincing evidence.

Since the 2008 Cochrane review, a double-blind study was conducted in 60 hyperlipidaemia patients treated with low molecular chitosan (2 g/day) or placebo. Both the supplement and the placebo were administered in conjunction with a physical activity program for 4 months duration. Caloric intake was similar in both groups. In comparison to the placebo, chitosan significantly reduced body weight (respectively 6.9 ± 1.87 vs 3.0 ± 1.61 kg), waist circumference (7.3 ± 2.49 vs 3.1 ± 4.21 cm), LDL cholesterol (44 ± 14.7 vs 12.5 ± 12.6 mg/dL), and triacylglycerol (52 ± 29.3 vs 39 ± 15.2 mg/dL); HDL increase was also higher (6 ± 3.6 vs 3 ± 4.2 mg/dL). Metabolic syndrome was reduced in 12 cases of the chitosan group, compared with three cases in the placebo (Cornelli et al 2008).

Further well-reported research is required, using longer time frames and clearly stating the complete characteristics of the chitosan preparations.

Hyperlipidaemia

The ability of chitosan to form complexes with various fats, including cholesterol, provides a theoretical basis for its use in hyperlipidaemia. Dietary chitosan has been tested and found to be effective in reducing serum cholesterol levels and atherosclerosis in normal and diabetic mice, and, therefore, has been investigated in the treatment of hypercholesterolaemia in humans (Muzzarelli 1999).

A 2002 review stated that in humans, dietary chitosan reduces serum total cholesterol levels by 5.8–42.6% and LDL levels by 15.1–35.1% (Ylitalo et al 2002). Reduction in LDL cholesterol was evident after 4 weeks' treatment with chitosan (1.2 g twice daily) according to one double-blind study (Wuolijoki et al 1999) and after 8 weeks treatment using a low dose of 1.2 g/day of chitosan in another randomised double-blind study (Bokura & Kobayashi 2003).

These results, however, are not a reflection of more recent investigations. One randomised double-blind study found no effect with 1.5 g chitosan tablets taken three times daily (Zahorska-Markiewicz et al 2002). In a randomised placebo-controlled study, no significant effect on total cholesterol, LDL cholesterol or triglycerides was seen, which tested chitosan capsules (1 g twice daily) (Guha et al 2005). The group receiving chitosan did report a significant reduction in mean body weight (3.14% versus 1.29% of body weight, $P < 0.05$) and a significant rise in HDL cholesterol value (3.8% versus 1.07%, $P = 0.02$). At higher doses which reflect those used in weight-loss studies, a more recent 2008 study found no significant effects on total cholesterol levels or LDL cholesterol concentration for chitosan (4.5 or 6.75 g/day) after 8 weeks of treatment (Tapola et al 2008).

The 2008 Cochrane review concluded that based on the current evidence, chitosan supplementation significantly reduced total cholesterol (Jull et al 2008). A second meta-analysis published in 2008 concurred that chitosan supplementation lowers total cholesterol but not LDL cholesterol or triglycerides, nor did it significantly increase HDL cholesterol (Baker et al 2009). The electrically neutral nature of triglycerides may mean that chitosan is unable to form complexes with it, and, therefore, is unable to influence its absorption.

Insulin sensitivity

Both preliminary animal and human studies have investigated chitosan and its derivatives for hypoglycaemic potential. A randomised, double blind trial involving 12 obese men treated with chitosan (750 mg, 3 times daily) or placebo for 3 months found a significant increase in insulin sensitivity (2.4 ± 1.4 vs 3.6 ± 1.4 mg kg^{-1} min^{-1}; $P = 0.43$) in those taking chitosan. This group also had a significant decrease in weight, BMI, waist circumference and TG. As there was no significant change in actual glucose levels, the authors concluded that the change in insulin sensitivity may be secondary to the decrease in weight and lipid profile (Hernandez-Gonzalez et al 2010). However, oral treatment with chitosan for 12 weeks was shown to decrease fasting plasma glucose, plasma insulin and leptin levels in rats (Liu et al 2012). Larger human trials, specifying the molecular weight of chitosan used, are required to clarify its effects on insulin sensitivity.

Hypertension

A patented NaCl salt containing 3% chitosan has been clinically trialled in a randomised, double-blind crossover trial involving 40 patients with mild hypertension. The chitosan salt was compared with standard sea salt to determine if this substitute was effective at lowering salt intake and BP. In addition to lifestyle advice, patients were ordered to consume no more than 3 g total salt per day. Patients were given saltshakers of either NaCl with chitosan 3% or NaCl alone for a period of 8 weeks. Following a 2-week washout period the patients crossed over and were given the other salt for a further 8-weeks. The results found a significantly greater reduction in BP using the patented chitosan salt compared with standard sea salt; 8.7 ± 10 mmHg vs 3.2 ± 8.5 mmHg ($P = 0.0156$) for systolic BP and 7.2 ± 8.00 mmHg vs 3.7 ± 7.4 mmHg ($P = 0.0285$) for diastolic BP. The exact mechanism for this effect is still unclear (Allaert 2013).

Dental plaque prevention

Because of chitosan's antibacterial activity against *Streptococcus mutans* and antifungal action against *Candida albicans*, it has been added to mouthwashes and dental gels. One randomised, crossover clinical trial involving 24 volunteers found that rinsing with a mouthwash containing 0.5% chitosan for 14 days was significantly more effective in reducing plaque formation than a placebo (Sano et al 2003). Several clinical studies have investigated the effect of chitosan-containing chewing gum. One clinical study reported that chewing the gum significantly decreased oral bacterial counts and significantly increased salivary secretion (Hayashi et al 2007a). Another confirmed antibacterial activity for the gum, especially reducing total streptococci, streptococci mutans in saliva (Hayashi et al 2007b). Hayashi et al suggested that chewing chitosan-containing gum could be an effective method for controlling the number of cariogenic bacteria in situations where it is difficult for a person to brush their teeth. The gum used in the study was xylitol-based and supplemented with chitosan so it dissolved in saliva at a rate of about 2% (w/v).

Periodontal disease

Chitosan was tested both as a carrier in gel form for the antibiotic metronidazole and as an active agent in the treatment of chronic periodontitis (CP) (Akncbay et al 2007). The chitosan gel (1% w/w) incorporated with or without 15% metronidazole was prepared and applied adjunctive to scaling and root planing (SRP) and compared to SRP alone in CP patients. All groups experienced significant improvements for clinical parameters between baseline and week 24 ($P < 0.05$). Chitosan was found to be effective in itself, as well as in combination with metronidazole in CP treatment due to its antimicrobial properties.

A small pilot trial involving 20 patients with periodontitis investigated three applications of chitosan after initial periodontal surgery: chitosan gel 1% w/v; chitosan gel plus demineralised bone matrix; and chitosan gel plus collagenous membrane. The control group received a flap only that contained no chitosan. Clinical and radiographic evaluation found no significant differences between the chitosan treatment groups; however, radiographic results indicated that compared with the control, all three chitosan groups showed statistically significant bone fills indicative of periodontal regeneration (Boynuegri et al 2009).

> ***Clinical note — Periodontal disease***
> Periodontal disease is a collective term used to describe several pathological conditions characterised by degeneration and inflammation of gums, periodontal ligaments, alveolar bone and dental cementum. It is a localised inflammatory response caused by bacterial infection of a periodontal pocket associated with subgingival plaque. Periodontal disease has been considered as a possible risk factor for other systemic diseases such as cardiovascular diseases and preterm, low-birth-weight infants. Increasingly, chitosan is being used as a polymeric matrix in the form of film enriched with taurine (antioxidant agent). Taurine enhances the wound-healing ability of chitosan and is considered beneficial in tissue repair in destructive diseases like periodontitis (Jain et al 2008).

Kidney failure

One open study of 80 patients with renal failure undergoing haemodialysis found that 1350 mg of chitosan taken three times daily effectively reduced total serum cholesterol levels (from 10.14 ± 4.40 mmol/L to 5.82 ± 2.19 mmol/L) and increased serum haemoglobin levels (from 58.2 ± 12.1 g/L to 68 ± 9.0 g/L) (Jing et al 1997). After 4 weeks, significant reductions in serum urea and creatinine levels were observed. After 12 weeks, patients reported subjective improvements, such as feeling physically stronger, with increased appetite and improved sleep, which were also significantly greater than the placebo group. Importantly, during the treatment period, no clinically problematic symptoms were observed.

Hyperphosphataemia is a common complication of chronic renal failure and is a risk factor for cardiovascular calcification in these patients. Chitosan strongly binds to salivary phosphate and lower serum levels in haemodialysis patients. In 13 haemodialysis patients with elevated serum phosphate levels, 20 mg of chewing gum containing a highly de-acetylised chitosan, was administered twice daily for 2 weeks in addition to their prescribed regimen. At the end of the 2 weeks, salivary phosphate had decreased by 55% from baseline (73.21 ± 19.19 to 33.19 ± 6.53; P = 0.00001), and serum phosphate decreased 31% from baseline (7.60 ± 0.91 to 5.25 ± 0.89 mg/dL; P = 0.00001). Serum phosphate took 30 days to return to baseline after the trial (Savica et al 2009). Interestingly, in a separate publication, the authors later analysed the CRP values from the blood samples of the patients, and found the chitosan chewing gum significantly lowered CRP values (from 1.38 ± 0.61 mg/L before the gum use to 0.39 ± 0.16 after the gum, P = <0.0003). The reduction was parallel with the reduced phosphate levels and is an important biomarker for cardiovascular health risk.

Wound healing — topical use

Chitosan is applied to burns and wound dressings in the form of films, bandages, cotton-like materials and non-woven napkins. Chitosan dressings have good hydroscopicity, show high bacteriostatic effect and are completely biodegradable in the human body. Another significant advantage is that repeated dressings are not usually needed (Synowiecki & Al-Khateeb 2003). Topical application of chitosan enhances wound healing and has been used to promote donor-site tissue regeneration in plastic surgery. Its use is supported by findings that indicate chitosan accelerates the reformation of connective tissue (Ueno et al 2001).

Chitosan was compared alongside conventional wound dressings in 20 patients undergoing skin grafts. These related to either skin malignancy, limb trauma or burn wounds. Compared with silicone net gauze, healing time was significantly shorter in the chitosan group; however, compared with alginates there was no significant benefit. However, three patients agreed to punch biopsy at the newly-healed time point. Histology results compared to the alginates showed chitosan biopsies had a marked looser connective tissue stroma, which was richer in both glycosaminoglycan matrix and capillaries. Small dermal nerve fibres were also more numerous. In addition, digital images of the scars demonstrated an earlier return to normal skin colour at the chitosan-treated areas (Stone et al 2000).

In a randomised controlled trial of 40 patients undergoing endoscopic sinus surgery for the treatment of chronic rhinosinusitis, chitosan was applied in the form of a gel and compared to control (no treatment). Chitosan achieved rapid haemostasis compared to the control group; 2–4 minutes compared with 10 minutes ($P < 0.001$). There was also significantly less adhesions at all follow-up time points (2, 6 and 12 weeks post-surgery). There was no change with respect to crusting, mucosal oedema, infection or granulation tissue formation (Valentine et al 2010).

OTHER USES

Drug delivery systems

Chitosan is considered a good carrier for the controlled release of drugs over an extended period of time (Synowiecki & Al-Khateeb 2003). Additionally, it has been shown to excel in transcellular transport.

Chitosan is also used as a component of different cosmetics, toothpaste, hand and body creams and hair-care products (Synowiecki & Al-Khateeb 2003).

DOSAGE RANGE

- The standard dose of chitosan is 3–6 g/day, taken with food.

According to clinical studies

- Weight loss: 3.0–4.5 g taken daily in divided doses, 30 minutes before meals.

- Hyperlipidaemia: 1.2–4.5 g/day in divided doses.
- Insulin sensitivity: 750 mg 3 times daily.
- Hypertension: NaCl with chitosan 3% used as a salt replacement.
- Dental plaque prevention: rinse daily with mouthwash containing 0.5%.
- Periodontal disease: chitosan gel (1% w/w) applied as an adjunct to scaling and root planing.
- Renal failure: 1.35 g taken three times daily.
- Hyperphosphataemia: 20 mg chewing gum loaded with highly deacetylated chitosan; twice daily for 1 hour.

ADVERSE REACTIONS

A systematic review of 14 randomised studies found that the most common side effects reported were constipation, nausea, bloating, indigestion and abdominal pain (Ni et al 2005). Increased water consumption may reduce some of these side effects.

Overall, chitosan is considered very safe and well tolerated according to safety studies in experimental models (Kim et al 2001).

SIGNIFICANT INTERACTIONS

Fat-soluble nutrients

Given chitosan's capacity to bind dietary fats and reduce their absorption, chitosan can also affect the absorption of fat-soluble vitamins. However, the effect may be dose-dependent as one study using a dose of 2 g/day found no changes to the levels of vitamins A, D, E and beta-carotene after 4 weeks use (Pittler et al 1999). A more recent study confirmed that there were no significant effects on serum vitamins (vitamin A, vitamin E, 25-hydroxyvitamin D) and carotenes (alpha- and beta-carotene) with oral chitosan after 8 weeks, even at a dose of 6.75 g daily (Tapola et al 2008).

Lipophilic drugs

Considering chitosan binds to dietary fats and reduces their absorption, it can also affect the absorption of lipophilic drugs, such as those that require passage across the blood–brain barrier, for example, some antihistamines, sleep aids and other psychiatric medications. Separate doses by at least 2 hours.

Vitamin C

According to a preliminary study in rats, taking vitamin C together with chitosan might provide additional benefit in lowering cholesterol.

B-group vitamins

In vitro studies using fluorescence and ultraviolet-visible absorption measurements have shown vitamin B_2 and B_{12} interact with chitosan in an acid-aqueous environment replicating the stomach. These studies suggest chitosan may inhibit the absorption of these nutrients; however, the degree of clinical significance is unknown (Rodrigues et al 2011, 2012).

Warfarin

Chitosan may potentiate warfarin by inhibiting absorption of fat-soluble vitamin K. A case report details an 83-year-old patient on a regimen of 2.5 mg warfarin/day. After 6 months supplementation of 1.2 g chitosan twice daily, the patient's INR levels had risen significantly. The patient was administered vitamin K intravenously and INR levels returned to normal. Against medical advice, the patient restarted chitosan supplementation and INR levels increased over the following 3 months. Once discontinued, the levels returned to within target range (Huang et al 2007).

CONTRAINDICATIONS AND PRECAUTIONS

Chitosan is contraindicated in people with allergies to shellfish.

> ***PREGNANCY USE***
>
> Pregnant women should avoid avoid taking chitosan at mealtimes as it may reduce absorption of essential dietary nutrients.

> ***Practice points/Patient counselling***
>
> - Chitosan is a form of poorly soluble fibre, chemically derived from chitin, which is extracted from the exoskeletons of crustaceans or squid. The most biologically active forms have a low molecular weight.
> - It forms insoluble complexes with dietary fats, fatty acids, bile acids, cholesterol and other lipids in the digestive tract and has antibacterial and antifungal activity that is useful in dental hygiene and topically for wound healing.
> - Chitosan is a popular weight-loss supplement. Clinical studies have produced mixed results; however, best effects occur when chitosan is used over several months and combined with dietary and lifestyle modifications.
> - Chitosan has been shown to significantly lower total cholesterol in hypercholesterolaemic patients, but not LDL cholesterol, HDL cholesterol or triglycerides. Clinical studies suggest chitosan is most beneficial in individuals consuming high cholesterol diets.
> - Chitosan is contraindicated in people with allergies to shellfish and should be recommended together with a multivitamin supplement with long-term use.

PATIENTS' FAQs

What will this supplement do for me?

Taken orally, chitosan may aid in weight loss when combined with dietary and lifestyle modifications and may reduce total cholesterol levels.

When will it start to work?

Effects in weight loss require at least 8 weeks continual use before effects are seen, according to research, whereas cholesterol-lowering requires 4–8 weeks.

Are there any safety issues?

Chitosan is contraindicated in people with allergies to shellfish and must not be used in patients taking warfarin.

REFERENCES

Akncbay H, Senel S, Ay ZY. Application of chitosan gel in the treatment of chronic periodontitis. J Biomed Mater Res B Appl Biomater 80.2 (2007): 290–296.

Allaert F. Double-blind, randomized, crossover, controlled clinical trial of NaCl + Chitosan 3% versus NaCl on mild or moderate high blood pressure during the diet and lifestyle improvement period before possible prescription of an antihypertensive treatment. International Angiology, 32 (2013): 94–101.

Baker W et al. A meta-analysis evaluating the impact of chitosan on serum lipids in hypercholesterolemic patients. Annals of Nutrition and Metabolism, 55 (2009): 368–374.

Barroso Aranda J et al. Efficacy of a novel chitosan formulation on fecal fat excretion: A double-blind, crossover, placebo-controlled study. Journal of Medicine, 33 (2002): 209–225.

Bokura H, Kobayashi S. Chitosan decreases total cholesterol in women: a randomized, double-blind, placebo-controlled trial. Eur J Clin Nutr 57.5 (2003): 721–725.

Boynuegri D et al. Clinical and radiographic evaluations of chitosan gel in periodontal intraosseous defects: a pilot study. Journal of Biomedical Materials Research. Part B: Applied Biomaterials (2009): 461–466.

Chang J et al. Investigation of the skin repair and healing mechanism of N-carboxymethyl chitosan in second-degree burn wounds. Wound Repair and Regeneration, 21 (2013) 113–121.

Cornelli U et al. Use of polyglucosamine and physical activity to reduce body weight and dyslipidemia in moderately overweight subjects. Minerva Cardioangiol 56 (2008): 71–78.

Dai T et al. Chitosan preparations for wounds and burns: antimicrobial and wound healing effects. Expert Review of Anti-Infective Therapy, 9 (2011): 857–879.

Gades M, Stern J. Chitosan supplementation and fat absorption in men and women. Journal of the American Dietetic Association, 105 (2005): 72–77.

Gades MD, Stern JS. Chitosan supplementation and fecal fat excretion in men. Obes Res 11.5 (2003): 683–688.

Guha S et al. Effect of chitosan on lipid levels when administered concurrently with atorvastatin—a placebo controlled study. J Indian Med Assoc 103.8 (2005): 418, 420.

Hayashi Y et al. Chitosan-containing gum chewing accelerates antibacterial effect with an increase in salivary secretion. J Dent 35(11) (2007a): 871–874.

Hayashi Y et al. Chewing chitosan-containing gum effectively inhibits the growth of cariogenic bacteria. Arch Oral Biol 52.3 (2007b): 290–294.

Hendler SS, Rorvik D (eds). PDR for nutritional supplements. Montvale, NJ: Medical Economics, 2001.

Hernandez-Gonzalez S et al. Chitosan improves insulin sensitivity as determined by the euglycemic-hyperinsulinemic clamp technique in obese subjects. Nutrition Research, 30 (2010).

Huang S, Sung S, Chiang C. Chitosan potentiation of warfarin effect. The annals of pharmacotherapy, 41 (2007): 1912–1914.

Jain N et al. Recent approaches for the treatment of periodontitis. Drug Discov Today 13.21–22 (2008): 932–943.

Jing SB et al. Effect of chitosan on renal function in patients with chronic renal failure. J Pharm Pharmacol 49.7 (1997): 721–723.

Jull AB et al. Chitosan for overweight or obesity. Cochrane Database Syst Rev 3 (2008): CD003892.

Kim SK et al. Subacute toxicity of chitosan oligosaccharide in Sprague-Dawley rats. Arzneimittelforschung 51.9 (2001): 769–774.

Liu X et al. Effect of chitosan, O-carboxymethyl chitosan and N-[(2-hydroxy-3-N,N-dimethylhexadecyl ammonium)propyl] chitosan chloride on overweight and insulin resistance in a murine diet-induced obesity. Journal of Agricultural and Food Chemistry, 60 (2012): 3471–3476.

Muzzarelli RA. Clinical and biochemical evaluation of chitosan for hypercholesterolemia and overweight control. EXS 87 (1999): 293–304.

Ni MC et al. Chitosan for overweight or obesity. Cochrane Database Syst Rev 3 (2005): CD003892.

Pittler MH et al. Randomized, double-blind trial of chitosan for body weight reduction. Eur J Clin Nutr 53.5 (1999): 379–381.

Rodrigues M, de Oliveira H, Lacerda F. Use of chitosan in the treatment of obesity: evaluation of interaction with vitamin B2. International journal of food sciences and nutrition, 63 (2011) 195–199.

Rodrigues M, de Oliveira H. Use of chitosan in the treatment of obesity: evaluation of interaction with vitamin B12. International Journal of Food Sciences and Nutrition, 63 (2012): 548–552.

Sano H et al. Effect of chitosan rinsing on reduction of dental plaque formation. Bull Tokyo Dent Coll 44.1 (2003): 9–16.

Santas J et al. Selective in vivo effect of chitosan on fatty acid, netural sterol and bile acid excretion: a longitudinal study. Food Chemistry, 134 (2012): 940–947.

Savica V et al. Salivary phosphate-binding chewing gum reduces hyperphosphatemia in dialysis patients. Journal of the American Society of Nephrology, 20 (2009): 639–644.

Senel S et al. Chitosan films and hydrogels of chlorhexidine gluconate for oral mucosal delivery. Int J Pharm 193.2 (2000): 197–203.

Stone C et al. Healing at skin graft donor sites dressed with chitosan. British journal of plastic surgery, 53 (2000): 601–606.

Synowiecki J, Al-Khateeb NA. Production and properties and some new applications of chitin and its derivatives. Crit Rev Food Sci Nutr 43.2 (2003): 145.

Tanaka Y et al. Effects of chitin and chitosan particles on BALB/c mice by oral and parenteral administration. Biomaterials 18.8 (1997): 591–595.

Tapola NS et al. Safety aspects and cholesterol-lowering efficacy of chitosan tablets. J Am Coll Nutr 27.1 (2008): 22–30.

Ueno H et al. Evaluation effects of chitosan for the extracellular matrix production by fibroblasts and the growth factors production by macrophages. Biomaterials 22.15 (2001): 2125–2130.

Valentine R et al. The efficacy of a novel chitosan gel on hemostasis and wound healing after endoscopic sinus surgery. American Journal of Rhinology and Allergy, 24 (2010): 70–75.

Wuolijoki E, Hirvela T, Ylitalo P. Decrease in serum LDL cholesterol with microcrystalline chitosan. Methods Find Exp Clin Pharmacol 21.5 (1999): 357–361.

Ylitalo R et al. Cholesterol-lowering properties and safety of chitosan. Arzneimittelforschung 52.1 (2002): 1–7.

Zahorska-Markiewicz B et al. Effect of chitosan in complex management of obesity. Pol Merkur Lekarski 13.74 (2002): 129–132.

Chondroitin

OTHER NAMES

Chondroitin sulfate, chondroitin sulfuric acid, chondroitin 4-sulfate, chondroitin 4- and 6-sulfate

BACKGROUND AND RELEVANT PHARMACOKINETICS

Chondroitin sulfate is an amino sugar polymer, made up of glucuronic acid and galactosamine, that is in the class of large polymers known as glucosaminoglycans or mucopolysaccharides. These compounds act as the flexible connecting matrix between the protein filaments in cartilage and connective tissue (Liesegang 1990) as well as being a major component of the extracellular matrix in the brain (Kwok et al 2012). It has been found that serum levels of chondroitin sulfate are increased in patients with both rheumatoid arthritis and osteoarthritis (OA) and this may provide the basis for systemic detection of OA (Pothacharoen et al 2006).

Chondroitin sulfate molecules represent a heterogeneous population, the structure of which varies with source, manufacturing processes, presence of contaminants and other factors (Lauder 2009). There are also differences in the absorption and bioavailability of chondroitin formulations due to differences in molecular mass, charge density and cluster of disulfated disaccharides of the parental molecules (Volpi 2003). This has led to a call for reference standards with high specificity, purity and well-known physicochemical properties for use in accurate and reproducible quantitative analyses (Volpi 2007).

Chondroitin is generally manufactured from natural sources, such as shark and bovine (usually tracheal) cartilage and may have a molecular weight that varies from 10 to 50 kDa, depending on the product's source or preparation (Ross 2000). Low-molecular-weight chondroitin appears to be absorbed orally in both animals and humans (Adebowale et al 2002, Du et al 2004) and displays accumulation after multiple dosing (Adebowale et al 2002). Chondroitin is concentrated in the intestine, liver, kidneys, synovial fluid and cartilage (Conte et al 1995) and the elimination half-life is about 5–6 hours, with 40–50% being excreted in the urine (Conte et al 1991, Ronca & Conte 1993). Oral chondroitin is absorbed as several metabolites, and as the active moiety has not yet been identified it is difficult to establish bioequivalence between different products (Volpi 2003).

CHEMICAL COMPONENTS

Chondroitin sulfate is a linear polymer of two alternating sugars, alpha-D-*N*-acetylgalactosamine and beta-D-glucuronic acid, with the sulfate moiety being a covalent part of the molecule and not a counter ion, as is the case with glucosamine sulfate (Ross 2000).

FOOD SOURCES

Chondroitin is naturally present in the gristle in meat. As a supplement it is generally produced from natural sources, such as shark or bovine (usually tracheal) cartilage and it can also be manufactured in the laboratory using various methods. The purity and content of products have been questioned in the United States, where it is regarded as a nutritional supplement and its quality is unregulated (Consumer-lab 2009).

MAIN ACTIONS

Chondroprotective effect

A review of chondroitin sulfate in the pathophysiology of OA suggests that chondroitin exerts its anti-arthritic effects via the stimulation of proteoglycan synthesis and reduction of chondrocyte catabolic activity. It does this by inhibiting the synthesis of proteolytic enzymes as well as via anti-inflammatory activity and actions on osteoblasts in subchondral bone, with modulation of osteoprotegerin/receptor activator of NF-κB ligand ratio in favour of reduced bone resorption (Martel-Pelletier et al 2010). Chondroitin appears to protect cartilage by providing it with the raw material required for repair, as well as inhibiting the enzymes in synovial fluid, such as elastase and hyaluronidase, that damage joint cartilage. It improves chondrocyte nutrition by increasing hyaluronic acid production in articular cells (Raoudi et al 2005) and hence, the fluid content of the extracellular matrix (Sasada et al 2005), which not only acts as a shock absorber but also brings nutrients into the cartilage (Krane & Goldring 1990).

In vitro studies have shown that low-dose combinations of glucosamine hydrochloride and chondroitin sulfate stimulate collagen and non-collagenous protein synthesis by ligament cells, tenocytes and chondrocytes (Lippiello 2007). An overall chondroprotective effect of chondroitin has also been demonstrated in different animal models. In a rabbit model oral or intramuscular chondroitin sulfate was shown to protect articular cartilage from experimental chymopapain injury (Uebelhart et al 1998a) and inhibit the destruction of the cartilage extracellular matrix (Sumino et al 2005). In a dog model, chondroitin sulfate was seen to stimulate articular cartilage and decrease or delay the alterations of degenerative joint disease (Melo et al 2008). In other animal models, co-administration with glucosamine was shown to prevent both biochemical and histological alterations and provide pain reduction (Silva et al 2009).

It has been suggested that at least some of the chondroprotective action of chondroitin sulfate is due to the provision of a source of additional inorganic sulfur which is essential for glycosaminoglycan synthesis, as well as being a structural component of glutathione and other key enzymes, coenzymes and metabolites that play fundamental roles in cellular homeostasis and control of inflammation (Nimni et al 2006). This is supported by the finding that the chondroprotective action of chondroitin is potentiated by high-sulfur mineral water (Caraglia et al 2005).

Urinary chondroitin sulfate and keratan sulfate excretion is reported to reflect the turnover rates of cartilage matrix proteoglycans, leading to the suggestion that the measurement of these compounds could provide an objective means of evaluating and monitoring joint diseases (Baccarin et al 2012). Furthermore, it has been found that technetium-99m-chondroitin sulfate accumulates in cartilage tissue, either by acting as a substrate for proteoglycan synthesis or by adsorption to cartilage, suggesting that this compound could serve to target and radioimage OA (Sobal et al 2009).

Anti-inflammatory

Chondroitin exerts an anti-inflammatory action with an inhibitory effect over complement (Pipitone 1991). In an in vitro study of bovine cartilage, chondroitin alone, and in combination with glucosamine, was found to regulate gene expression and synthesis of nitric oxide and prostaglandin E_2, suggesting a basis for its anti-inflammatory properties (Chan et al 2005). Chondroitin sulfate has been found to increase the levels of antioxidant enzymes and reduce inflammation and cirrhosis of liver tissue in an ovariectomised rat model, suggesting that it enhances antioxidant activity (Ha 2004). It has been suggested that chondroitin's multiple anti-inflammatory effects in chondrocytes and synoviocytes are primarily due to a common mechanism, through the inhibition of NF-κB nuclear translocation (Iovu et al 2008). Chondroitin sulfate has also been shown to inhibit the production of prostaglandin E_2 and matrix metalloproteinases in osteoblasts, leading to the suggestion that chondroitin's action in OA is not only due to effects on cartilage but may also be due to effects on subchondral bone (Pecchi et al 2012).

Based on in vitro and in vivo evidence, it is suggested that the antioxidant and anti-inflammatory effects of chondroitin contribute to neuro-protective properties (Egea et al 2010). A recent review further suggests that chondroitin improves moderate to severe psoriasis and experimental and clinical data suggest chondroitin might be a useful therapeutic agent in inflammatory diseases such as inflammatory bowel disease, atherosclerosis, Parkinson's and Alzheimer's disease, multiple sclerosis, amyotrophic lateral sclerosis, rheumatoid arthritis and systemic lupus erythematosus (Vallieres & du Souich 2010).

Viscoelastic agent

Chondroitin sulfate is a viscoelastic agent and, together with similar substances such as sodium hyaluronate and hydroxypropyl methylcellulose, is used in ophthalmic surgery to protect and lubricate cells and tissues (Larson et al 1989, Liesegang 1990).

OTHER ACTIONS

There are suggestions from laboratory studies and uncontrolled human trials that chondroitin may have potential antiatherogenic properties (Morrison 1969, 1971, Morrison & Enrick 1973).

A review of the potential therapeutic applications of chondroitin sulfate/dermatan sulfate suggest that chondroitin sulfate may have potential applications in parasitic and viral infections, regenerative medicine and development of antitumour therapies (Yamada & Sugahara 2008).

CLINICAL USE

Osteoarthritis: symptom control and retarding disease progression

There are now a number of reviews and meta-analyses of clinical data (Bruyere & Reginster 2007, Hochberg 2010, Monfort et al 2008, Uebelhart 2008, Vangsness et al 2009), including a critical appraisal of five separate meta-analyses (Monfort et al 2008), which indicate that oral chondroitin sulfate is a valuable and safe symptomatic treatment for OA disease (Kubo et al 2009). Chondroitin sulfate appears to produce a slow but gradual reduction of the clinical symptoms of OA. Multiple human clinical trials lasting from a few weeks to 3 years have shown that chondroitin sulfate can significantly alleviate symptoms of pain and improve function in patients with OA of the knee, finger and hip (Bourgeois et al 1998, Bucsi & Poor 1998, Fioravanti et al 1991, Lazebnik & Drozdov 2005, Mazieres et al 2001, Morreale et al 1996, Oliviero et al 1991, Rovetta 1991, Uebelhart 2008, Zegels et al 2013) and that these effects last months after the cessation of treatment (Mazieres et al 2005), as well as being evident with intermittent treatment (Uebelhart et al 2004).

There is also evidence from double-blind clinical trials that chondroitin can reverse, retard or stabilise the pathology of OA (Volpi 2005), as evidenced by stabilisation of the joint space (Uebelhart et al 1998b), less progression of erosions (Rovetta et al 2002, Verbruggen et al 1998) and improved articular cartilage thickness (Pipitone et al 1992, Raynauld et al 2012) and interarticular space, as observed by X-rays (Conrozier 1998, Michel et al 2005, Uebelhart et al 2004). A subanalysis of patients involved in the Glucosamine/Chondroitin Arthritis Intervention Trial (GAIT) study (see below and Glucosamine monograph) further suggests that chondroitin sulfate may have differential effects on OA symptoms depending on the degree of radiographic involvement, and that chondroitin may provide improvements in knee pain in patients with relatively early radiographic disease (Clegg et al 2005). These results are supported by a more recent controlled trial that found that chondroitin sulfate, but not paracetamol, reduced synovitis and clinical symptoms of OA with a carry-over effect and high safety profile (Monfort et al 2012). In contrast to the above findings, a 24-month, double-blind, placebo-controlled study of 572 patients conducted as part of the GAIT study did not demonstrate reductions in joint space narrowing, although there was a trend for improvement in knees with Kellgren/Lawrence grade 2 radiographic OA. The authors state, however, that power of this study was diminished by the limited sample size, variance of joint

> ***Clinical Note***
>
> In 2014 the European Society for Clinical and Economic Aspects of Osteoporosis and Osteoarthritis (ESCEO) gathered an international task force of 13 members to determine clinical management of patients with OA. They concluded that the first step in patients with OA and pain is to use either glucosamine sulfate ± chondroitin sulphate or paracetamol on a regular basis, while NSAIDS should only be used as an advanced step, if response is not adequate. They recommended that the safer, more sensible approach is not to use paracetamol due to its side effects and questionable efficacy on pain with chronic use, but to recommend chronic symptomatic, slow-acting dugs for osteoarthritis such as chondroitin sulphate. For chondroitin, the effect size on pain is clinically significant and there are benefits on joint structure changes in patients with mild-to-moderate disease using prescription chondroitin 4&6 sulfate. (Bruyere et al 2014). Interestingly, they noted that US groups are reluctant to recommend dietary supplements due to quality issues, whereas there is less concern in Europe as pharmaceutical grade preparations are used.

space width measurement and a smaller than expected loss in joint space (Sawitzke et al 2008).

Comparisons with NSAIDs

Although chondroitin appears to be at least as effective as non-steroidal anti-inflammatory drugs (NSAIDs) in treating the symptoms of OA (Fioravanti et al 1991, Morreale et al 1996), it has a slower onset of action, taking 2–4 months to establish an effect (Leeb et al 2000, Morreale et al 1996). Chondroitin may, however, provide benefits that persist after treatment is stopped (Mazieres et al 2001, Morreale et al 1996). A cost-effectiveness analysis suggests that chondroitin sulfate in the treatment for OA has less cost and better gastrointestinal tolerability compared than NSAIDs and that, for every 10,000 cases treated, 2666 cases of gastrointestinal adverse events (including 90 serious adverse events) will have been avoided (Rubio-Terres & Grupo del estudio 2010).

Combined use of chondroitin sulfate and glucosamine sulfate

Chondroitin and glucosamine are frequently marketed together in combination products and some studies suggest that this combination is effective in treating symptoms (Das & Hammad 2000, Leffler et al 1999, McAlindon et al 2000, Miller & Clegg 2011, Nguyen et al 2001) or reducing joint space narrowing (Rai et al 2004, Fransen et al 2014). These findings are supported by an in vitro study on horse cartilage that found that a combination of glucosamine and chondroitin was more effective than either product alone in preventing articular cartilage glycosaminoglycan degradation (Dechant et al 2005), as well as an in vivo study on rats that found that the combined treatment prevented the development of cartilage damage and was associated with a reduction in interleukin-1-beta and matrix metalloprotease-9 synthesis (Chou et al 2005). The GAIT trial (see above and Glucosamine monograph) provides evidence that glucosamine hydrochloride and chondroitin are more effective when given in combination than when either substance is given alone, with the combined treatment being more effective than the cyclooxygenase-2 inhibitor, celecoxib, for treating moderate to severe arthritis compared with chondroitin alone (Clegg et al 2006). A substudy of the GAIT trial on the pharmacokinetics of glucosamine and chondroitin sulfate when taken separately or in combination suggests that pain relief following ingestion of chondroitin probably does not depend on simultaneous or prior intake of glucosamine and that any effect on joint pain probably does not result from ingested chondroitin reaching the joint space but rather from changes in cellular activities in the gut lining or in the liver, where concentrations of ingested chondroitin, or its breakdown products, could be substantially elevated following oral ingestion (Jackson et al 2010). More recently, a large double-blind, placebo-controlled, randomised study (n = 605) conducted in Australia concluded that 2 years of treatment with glucosamine sulfate 1500 mg/day, taken together with chondroitin sulfate 800 mg/day, resulted in significant and clinically relevant joint structure modification (Fransen et al 2014). The same effect was not seen for stand-alone chondroitin sulfate or glucosamine sulfate.

A small randomised controlled trial has suggested that the addition of high-molecular-weight hyaluronate to glucosamine and chondroitin may provide additional benefits to the use of glucosamine and chondroitin alone (Bucci et al 2005).

Topical preparations

A topical preparation containing chondroitin with glucosamine and camphor has been shown to reduce pain from OA of the knee in one randomised controlled trial (Cohen et al 2003).

OTHER USES

Heart disease

There are suggestions that chondroitin in doses of up to 10 g/day may have antiatherogenic actions and beneficial effects on serum lipid levels and may be useful for reducing the risk of myocardial infarction (Morrison 1969, 1971, Morrison & Enrick 1973, Morrison et al 1969).

Snoring

The results of a pilot crossover study of seven subjects suggest that chondroitin sulfate instilled into the nostril at bedtime may reduce snoring (Lenclud et al 1998).

Ophthalmic surgery and dry eyes

Chondroitin sulfate is used as a viscoelastic substance to protect and lubricate cells and tissues during ophthalmic surgery, as well as to preserve corneas before transplantation (Larson et al 1989, Liesegang 1990). In a double-blind, crossover study of 20 subjects, 1% chondroitin sulfate was found to be as effective as polyvinyl alcohol artificial tear formulation and 0.1% hyaluronic acid in reducing itching, burning and foreign-body sensation in people with keratoconjunctivitis sicca (Limberg et al 1987).

Psoriasis

It has been found that some patients with psoriasis experience a significant clinical and histological improvement in their psoriatic lesions after taking chondroitin to treat their OA (Verges et al 2004, 2005), and this has been confirmed in a clinical trial which suggests that chondroitin could represent a special benefit in patients with both pathologies, since NSAIDs have been reported to induce or exacerbate psoriasis (Moller et al 2010).

Interstitial cystitis

Evidence from community-based clinical practice studies along with small randomised controlled trials suggests that intravesical chondroitin sulfate may play a role in the treatment of interstitial cystitis

(Berger 2011, Gentile et al 2011, Nickel et al 2009, 2010, 2012).

DOSAGE RANGE

- Oral doses of chondroitin range from 800 to 1200 mg/day in either single or divided doses. Intramuscular, intravenous and topical forms are also available.
- A 4–5-month trial is generally used in order to determine whether it is effective for an individual patient.
- A dose-finding study in patients with knee OA suggests that administration of 800 mg of chondroitin sulfate orally had nearly the same effect as 1200 mg/day, while the use of a sequential 3-month administration mode, twice a year, was also shown to provide the same results as continuous treatment (Uebelhart 2008). More recently a double-blind randomised placebo-controlled trial found no significant difference in efficacy, security or tolerability between a single oral daily dose of 1200 mg and three divided doses of 400 mg (Zegels et al 2013).

ADVERSE REACTIONS

Chondroitin is generally deemed to be extremely safe, with the incidence of adverse reactions being comparable to placebo in studies lasting from 2 months to 6 years (Bourgeois et al 1998, Bucsi & Poor 1998, Hathcock & Shao 2007, Leeb et al 2000, McAlindon et al 2000, Uebelhart et al 1998b, Vangsness et al 2009).

Oral chondroitin may cause mild gastrointestinal disturbance. While there is a theoretical risk of anticoagulant activity, this has not been demonstrated in clinical trials (Chavez 1997) and chondroitin has been assessed as having a complete absence of adverse effects and an observed safe level at doses of up to 1200 mg/day (Hathcock & Shao 2007).

SIGNIFICANT INTERACTIONS

Controlled studies are not available; therefore, interactions are based on evidence of activity and are largely theoretical and speculative.

Anticoagulants

Additive effect theoretically possible — observe patient.

Non-steroidal anti-inflammatory drugs

Chondroitin may enhance drug effectiveness, suggesting a beneficial interaction is possible — drug dosage may require modification.

CONTRAINDICATIONS AND PRECAUTIONS

Due to theoretical anticoagulant activity, chondroitin should be used with caution in people with clotting disorders.

Some forms of chondroitin are produced from bovine (usually tracheal) cartilage, so it is theoretically possible that it may be a source of transmission of bovine spongiform encephalopathy (mad-cow disease) and other diseases. This transmission has not been demonstrated and is deemed unlikely.

PREGNANCY USE

Insufficient reliable information is available to advise on safety in pregnancy.

Practice points/Patient counselling

- Chondroitin is a naturally-occurring building block of joint tissue and cartilage. Supplements are made from shark cartilage or bovine tracheal cartilage.
- Chondroitin is an effective symptomatic treatment in OA and considered to improve the disability associated with the condition. It appears to slow disease progression when used long-term with positive results most consistently reported when it is used with glucosamine sulphate together. Its symptom-relieving effects occur after several weeks as it is a slow-acting substance.
- It is considered extremely safe and may reduce the need for NSAIDs, which can have serious side effects. In 2014, the European Society for Clinical and Economic Aspects of Osteoporosis and Osteoarthritis (ESCEO) recommended that chondroitin sulfate, glucosamine sulfate or paracetamol be used before NSAIDS in OA.
- Taking chondroitin in conjunction with glucosamine for treating arthritis provides the best results when being used long-term for delaying disease progression.
- Patients undergoing anticoagulant therapy or with clotting disorders should have their blood clotting monitored while taking chondroitin.

PATIENTS' FAQs

What will this supplement do for me?

Multiple scientific studies have shown that chondroitin sulfate reduces the symptoms of OA and may also slow down further progression of the condition. When used long term for slowing the progression of OA, it should be used together with glucosamine. Some people find that they do not require NSAIDs as often when taking chondroitin sulfate.

When will it start to work?

Symptom relief takes 2–4 months to reach maximal effect, but protection effects on the joints occur only with long-term use of several years.

Are there any safety issues?

Generally considered a very safe treatment and far safer than pharmaceutical anti-inflammatory drugs; however, it should be used with caution by people with clotting disorders or taking anticoagulants.

REFERENCES

Adebowale A et al. The bioavailability and pharmacokinetic of glucosamine hydrochloride and low molecular weight chondroitin sulfate after single and multiple doses to beagle dogs. Biopharm Drug Dispos 23.6 (2002): 217–225.

Baccarin, R. Y., et al. (2012). Urinary glycosaminoglycans in horse osteoarthritis. Effects of chondroitin sulfate and glucosamine. Res Vet Sci, 93(1), 88–96.

C

Berger, R E. (2011). Re: Prevention of Recurrent Urinary Tract Infections by Intravesical Administration of Hyaluronic Acid and Chondroitin Sulphate: A Placebo-Controlled Randomised Trial. The Journal of Urology, 186(1), 132.
Bourgeois P et al. Efficacy and tolerability of chondroitin sulfate 1200 mg/day vs chondroitin sulfate 3 × 400 mg/day vs placebo. Osteoarthritis Cartilage 6 (Suppl A) (1998): 25–30.
Bruyere O, Reginster JY. Glucosamine and chondroitin sulfate as therapeutic agents for knee and hip osteoarthritis. Drugs and Aging 24.7 (2007): 573–580.
Bucci LR et al. P196 Comparison between glucosamine with chondroitin sulfate and glucosamine with chondroitin sulfate and hyaluronate for symptoms of knee osteoarthritis. Osteoarthritis Cartilage 13 (Suppl 1) (2005): S99.
Bucsi L, Poor G. Efficacy and tolerability of oral chondroitin sulfate as a symptomatic slow-acting drug for osteoarthritis (SYSADOA) in the treatment of knee osteoarthritis. Osteoarthritis Cartilage 6 (Suppl A) (1998): 31–36.
Caraglia M et al. Alternative therapy of earth elements increases the chondroprotective effects of chondroitin sulfate in mice. Exp Mol Med 37.5 (2005): 476–481.
Chan PS et al. Glucosamine and chondroitin sulfate regulate gene expression and synthesis of nitric oxide and prostaglandin E2 in articular cartilage explants. Osteoarthritis Cartilage 13.5 (2005): 387–394.
Chavez ML. Glucosamine sulfate and chondroitin sulfates. Hosp Pharm 32.9 (1997): 1275–1285.
Chou MM et al. Effects of chondroitin and glucosamine sulfate in a dietary bar formulation on inflammation, interleukin-1-beta, matrix metalloprotease-9, and cartilage damage in arthritis. Exp Biol Med (Maywood) 230.4 (2005): 255–262.
Clegg DO et al. P145 Chondroitin sulfate may have differential effects on OA symptoms related to degree of radiographic involvement. Osteoarthritis Cartilage 13 (Suppl 1) (2005): S76–S77.
Clegg DO et al. Glucosamine, chondroitin sulfate, and the two in combination for painful knee osteoarthritis. N Engl J Med 354.8 (2006): 795–808.
Cohen M et al. A randomized double blind, placebo controlled trial of a topical cream containing glucosamine sulfate, chondroitin sulfate, and camphor for osteoarthritis of the knee. J Rheumatol 30 (2003): 523–528.
Conrozier T. Anti-arthrosis treatments: efficacy and tolerance of chondroitin sulfates (CS 4&6). Presse Med 27.36 (1998): 1862–1865.
Consumer-lab. Product review: glucosamine and chondroitin. Available online: www.consumerlab.com/reviews/Joint_Supplements_Glucosamine_Chondroitin_and_MSM/jointsupplements February 2009.
Conte A et al. Metabolic fate of exogenous chondroitin sulfate in man. Arzneimittelforschung 41.7 (1991): 768–772.
Conte A et al. Biochemical and pharmacokinetic aspects of oral treatment with chondroitin sulfate. Arzneimittelforschung 45.8 (1995): 918–925.
Das A Jr, Hammad TA. Efficacy of a combination of FCHG49 glucosamine hydrochloride, TRH122 low molecular weight sodium chondroitin sulfate and manganese ascorbate in the management of knee osteoarthritis. Osteoarthritis Cartilage 8.5 (2000): 343–350.
Dechant JE et al. Effects of glucosamine hydrochloride and chondroitin sulphate, alone and in combination, on normal and interleukin-1 conditioned equine articular cartilage explant metabolism. Equine Vet J 37.3 (2005): 227–231.
Du J, et al. The bioavailability and pharmacokinetics of glucosamine hydrochloride and chondroitin sulfate after oral and intravenous single dose administration in the horse. Biopharm Drug Dispos 25.3 (2004): 109–116.
Egea, J., et al. (2010). Antioxidant, antiinflammatory and neuroprotective actions of chondroitin sulfate and proteoglycans. Osteoarthritis Cartilage, 18 Suppl 1(0), S24–27.
Fioravanti A et al. Clinical efficacy and tolerance of galactosoaminoglucuronoglycan sulfate in the treatment of osteoarthritis. Drugs Exp Clin Res 17.1 (1991): 41–44.
Fransen M et al. Glucosamine and chondroitin for knee osteoarthritis: a double-blind randomised placebo-controlled clinical trial evaluating single and combination regimens. Ann Rheum Dis (2014) [Epub ahead of print].
Gentile, B., et al. (2011). UP-01.074 Recurrent Bacterial Cystitis, Bladder Instillation with a Combined Solution of Sodium Halurate and Chondroitin Sulfate (IALURIL): One Year of Follow-Up. Urology, 78(3), S209.
Ha BJ. Oxidative stress in ovariectomy menopause and role of chondroitin sulfate. Arch Pharm Res 27.8 (2004): 867–872.
Hathcock JN, Shao A. Risk assessment for glucosamine and chondroitin sulfate. Regul Toxicol Pharmacol 47.1 (2007): 78–83.
Hochberg, M. C. (2010). Structure-modifying effects of chondroitin sulfate in knee osteoarthritis: an updated meta-analysis of randomized placebo-controlled trials of 2-year duration. Osteoarthritis Cartilage, 18 Suppl 1(0), S28–31.
Iovu M, et al. Anti-inflammatory activity of chondroitin sulfate. Osteoarthritis Cartilage 16 (Suppl 3) (2008): S14–S118.
Jackson, C. G., et al. (2010). The human pharmacokinetics of oral ingestion of glucosamine and chondroitin sulfate taken separately or in combination. Osteoarthritis Cartilage, 18(3), 297–302.
Krane SM, Goldring MB. Clinical implications of cartilage metabolism in arthritis. Eur J Rheumatol Inflamm 10.1 (1990): 4–9.
Kubo, M., et al. (2009). Chondroitin sulfate for the treatment of hip and knee osteoarthritis: current status and future trends. Life Sci, 85(13-14), 477–483.
Kwok, J. C., et al. (2012). Chondroitin sulfate: a key molecule in the brain matrix. Int J Biochem Cell Biol, 44(4), 582–586.
Larson RS et al. Viscoelastic agents. Contact Lens Assoc Ophthalmol J 15.2 (1989): 151–160.
Lauder RM. Chondroitin sulphate: a complex molecule with potential impacts on a wide range of biological systems. Complement Ther Med 17.1 (2009): 56–62.
Lazebnik LB, Drozdov VN. Efficacy of chondroitin sulphate in the treatment of elderly patients with gonarthrosis and coxarthrosis. Ter Arkh 77.8 (2005): 64–69.
Leeb BF et al. A metaanalysis of chondroitin sulfate in the treatment of osteoarthritis. J Rheumatol 27.1 (2000): 205–211.
Leffler CT et al. Glucosamine, chondroitin, and manganese ascorbate for degenerative joint disease of the knee or low back: a randomized, double-blind, placebo-controlled pilot study. Mil Med 164.2 (1999): 85–91.
Lenclud CCP et al. Effects of chondroitin sulfate on snoring characteristics: a pilot study. Curr Ther Res 59.4 (1998): 234–243.
Liesegang TJ. Viscoelastic substances in ophthalmology. Surv Ophthalmol 34.4 (1990): 268–293.
Limberg MB et al. Topical application of hyaluronic acid and chondroitin sulfate in the treatment of dry eyes. Am J Ophthalmol 103.2 (1987): 194–197.
Lippiello L. Collagen synthesis in tenocytes, ligament cells and chondrocytes exposed to a combination of glucosamine HCl and chondroitin sulfate. Evid Based Complement Alternat Med 4.2 (2007): 219–224.
Martel-Pelletier, J., et al. (2010). Effects of chondroitin sulfate in the pathophysiology of the osteoarthritic joint: a narrative review. Osteoarthritis Cartilage, 18 Suppl 1(0), S7–11.
Mazieres B et al. Chondroitin sulfate in osteoarthritis of the knee: a prospective, double blind, placebo controlled multicenter clinical study. J Rheumatol 28.1 (2001): 173–181.
Mazieres B, et al. P140 Chondroitin sulfate in the treatment for knee osteoarthritis: a randomized, double blind, multicenter, placebo-controlled trial. Osteoarthritis Cartilage 13 (Suppl 1) (2005): S74.
McAlindon TE et al. Glucosamine and chondroitin for treatment of osteoarthritis: a systematic quality assessment and meta-analysis. JAMA 283.11 (2000): 1469–1475.
Melo EG et al. [Chondroitin sulfate and sodium hyaluronate in the treatment of the degenerative joint disease in dogs. Histological features of articular cartilage and synovium.] Arq Bras Med Vet Zootec 60.1 (2008): 83–92.
Michel BA et al. Chondroitins 4 and 6 sulfate in osteoarthritis of the knee: a randomized, controlled trial. Arthritis Rheum 52.3 (2005): 779–786.
Miller, K. L., & Clegg, D. O. (2011). Glucosamine and chondroitin sulfate. Rheum Dis Clin North Am, 37(1), 103–118.
Moller, I., et al. (2010). Effectiveness of chondroitin sulphate in patients with concomitant knee osteoarthritis and psoriasis: a randomized, double-blind, placebo-controlled study. Osteoarthritis Cartilage, 18 Suppl 1(0), S32–40.
Monfort J, et al. Chondroitin sulphate for symptomatic osteoarthritis: critical appraisal of meta-analyses. Curr Med Res Opin 24.5 (2008): 1303–1308.
Monfort, J., et al. (2012). Chondroitin sulfate and not acetaminophen effectively reduces synovitis in patients with knee osteoarthritis: results from a pilot study. Osteoarthritis and Cartilage, 20(0), S283–S284.
Morreale P et al. Comparison of the antiinflammatory efficacy of chondroitin sulfate and diclofenac sodium in patients with knee osteoarthritis. J Rheumatol 23.8 (1996): 1385–1391.
Morrison LM. Response of ischemic heart disease to chondroitin sulfate-A. J Am Geriatr Soc 17.10 (1969): 913–923.
Morrison LM. Reduction of ischemic coronary heart disease by chondroitin sulfate A. Angiology 22.3 (1971): 165–174.
Morrison LM, Enrick NL. Coronary heart disease: reduction of death rate by chondroitin sulfate-A. Angiology 24.5 (1973): 269–287.
Morrison LM et al. The prevention of coronary arteriosclerotic heart disease with chondroitin sulfate A: preliminary report. Exp Med Surg 27.3 (1969): 278–289.
Nguyen P et al. A randomized double-blind clinical trial of the effect of chondroitin sulfate and glucosamine hydrochloride on temporomandibular joint disorders: a pilot study. Cranio 19.2 (2001): 130–139.
Nickel JC et al. A real-life multicentre clinical practice study to evaluate the efficacy and safety of intravesical chondroitin sulphate for the treatment of interstitial cystitis. BJU Int 103.1 (2009): 56–60.
Nickel, J. C., et al. (2010). A multicenter, randomized, double-blind, parallel group pilot evaluation of the efficacy and safety of intravesical sodium chondroitin sulfate versus vehicle control in patients with interstitial cystitis/painful bladder syndrome. Urology, 76(4), 804–809.
Nickel, J. C., et al. (2012). Second multicenter, randomized, double-blind, parallel-group evaluation of effectiveness and safety of intravesical

sodium chondroitin sulfate compared with inactive vehicle control in subjects with interstitial cystitis/bladder pain syndrome. Urology, 79(6), 1220–1224.
Nimni ME, et al. Chondroitin sulfate and sulfur containing chondroprotective agents: is there a basis for their pharmacological action? Curr Rheum Rev 2.2 (2006): 137–149.
Oliviero U et al. Effects of the treatment with matrix on elderly people with chronic articular degeneration. Drugs Exp Clin Res 17.1 (1991): 45–51.
Pecchi, E., et al. (2012). A potential role of chondroitin sulfate on bone in osteoarthritis: inhibition of prostaglandin E(2) and matrix metalloproteinases synthesis in interleukin-1beta-stimulated osteoblasts. Osteoarthritis Cartilage, 20(2), 127–135.
Pipitone V. Chondroprotection with chondroitin sulfate. Drugs Exp Clin Res 17.1 (1991): 3–7.
Pipitone V et al. A multicenter, triple-blind study to evaluate galactosaminoglucuronoglycan sulfate versus placebo in patients with femorotibial gonarthritis. Curr Ther Res 52.4 (1992): 608–638.
Pothacharoen P et al. Raised chondroitin sulfate epitopes and hyaluronan in serum from rheumatoid arthritis and osteoarthritis patients. Osteoarthritis Cartilage 14.3 (2006): 299–301.
Rai J et al. Efficacy of chondroitin sulfate and glucosamine sulfate in the progression of symptomatic knee osteoarthritis: a randomized, placebo-controlled, double blind study. Bull Postgrad Inst Med Educ Res Chandigarh 38.1 (2004): 18–22.
Raoudi M et al. P152 Effect of chondroitin sulfate on hyaluronan synthesis and expression of udp-glucose dehydrogenase and hyaluronan synthases in synoviocytes and articular chondrocytes. Osteoarthritis Cartilage 13 (Suppl 1) (2005): S79–S80.
Raynauld, J. P., et al. (2012). Prediction of Total Knee Replacement in a 6-Month Multicentre Clinical Trial with Chondroitin Sulfate in Knee Osteoarthritis: Results from a 4-Year Observation. Osteoarthritis and Cartilage, 20(0), S175–S175.
Ronca G, Conte A. Metabolic fate of partially depolymerized shark chondroitin sulfate in man. Int J Clin Pharmacol Res 13 (Suppl) (1993): 27–34.
Ross I. A submission to the Complementary Medicines Evaluation Committee concerning chondroitin sulfate. Canberra: Complementary Healthcare Council of Australia, 2000.
Rovetta G. Galactosaminoglycuronoglycan sulfate (matrix) in therapy of tibiofibular osteoarthritis of the knee. Drugs Exp Clin Res 17.1 (1991): 53–57.
Rovetta G et al. Chondroitin sulfate in erosive osteoarthritis of the hands. Int J Tissue React 24.1 (2002): 29–32.
Rubio-Terres, C., & Grupo del estudio, Vectra. (2010). [An economic evaluation of chondroitin sulfate and non-steroidal anti-inflammatory drugs for the treatment of osteoarthritis. Data from the VECTRA study.] Reumatol Clin, 6(4), 187–195.
Sasada T et al. Role of chondroitin sulfate on mechanical behavior of articular cartilage. Report of Chiba Institute of Technology 52 (2005): 91–97.
Sawitzke AD et al. The effect of glucosamine and/or chondroitin sulfate on the progression of knee osteoarthritis: a report from the glucosamine/chondroitin arthritis intervention trial. Arthritis Rheum 58.10 (2008): 3183–3191.
Silva FS Jr et al. Combined glucosamine and chondroitin sulfate provides functional and structural benefit in the anterior cruciate ligament transection model. Clin Rheumatol 28.2 (2009): 109–117.
Sobal, G., et al. (2009). Uptake of 99mTc-labeled chondroitin sulfate by chondrocytes and cartilage: a promising agent for imaging of cartilage degeneration? Nucl Med Biol, 36(1), 65–71.
Sumino T et al. P163 Effect of long term oral administration of glucosamine hydrochloride and chondroitin sulfate on the progression of cartilage degeneration in a guinea pig model of spontaneous osteoarthritis. Osteoarthritis Cartilage 13 (Suppl 1) (2005): S84.
Uebelhart D. Clinical review of chondroitin sulfate in osteoarthritis. Osteoarthritis Cartilage 16 (Suppl 3) (2008): S19–S21.
Uebelhart D et al. Protective effect of exogenous chondroitin 4,6-sulfate in the acute degradation of articular cartilage in the rabbit. Osteoarthritis Cartilage 6 (Suppl A) (1998a): 6–13.
Uebelhart D et al. Effects of oral chondroitin sulfate on the progression of knee osteoarthritis: a pilot study. Osteoarthritis Cartilage 6 (Suppl A) (1998b): 39–46.
Uebelhart D et al. Intermittent treatment of knee osteoarthritis with oral chondroitin sulfate: a one-year, randomized, double-blind, multicenter study versus placebo. Osteoarthritis Cartilage 12.4 (2004): 269–276.
Vallieres, M., & du Souich, P. (2010). Modulation of inflammation by chondroitin sulfate. Osteoarthritis Cartilage, 18 Suppl 1(0), S1–6.
Vangsness CT Jr, et al. A review of evidence-based medicine for glucosamine and chondroitin sulfate use in knee osteoarthritis. Arthroscopy 25.1 (2009): 86–94.
Verbruggen G, et al. Chondroitin sulfate: S/DMOAD (structure/disease modifying anti-osteoarthritis drug) in the treatment of finger joint OA. Osteoarthritis Cartilage 6 (Suppl A) (1998): 37–38.
Verges J et al. Clinical and histopathological improvement of psoriasis in patients with osteoarthritis treated with chondroitin sulfate: report of 3 cases. Med Clin (Barc) 123.19 (2004): 739–742.
Verges J et al. P156 Chondroitin sulfate: a novel symptomatic treatment for psoriasis. Report of eleven cases. Osteoarthritis Cartilage 13 (Suppl 1) (2005): S81.
Volpi N. Oral absorption and bioavailability of ichthyic origin chondroitin sulfate in healthy male volunteers. Osteoarthritis Cartilage 11.6 (2003): 433–441.
Volpi N. Chondroitin sulphate for the treatment of osteoarthritis. Curr Med Chem Anti-Inflamm Anti-Allergy Agents 4.3 (2005): 221–234.
Volpi N. Analytical aspects of pharmaceutical grade chondroitin sulfates. J Pharm Sci 96.12 (2007): 3168–3180.
Yamada S, Sugahara K. Potential therapeutic application of chondroitin sulfate/dermatan sulfate. Curr Drug Discov Technol 5.4 (2008): 289–301.
Zegels, B., et al. (2013). Equivalence of a single dose (1200 mg) compared to a three-time a day dose (400 mg) of chondroitin 4&6 sulfate in patients with knee osteoarthritis. Results of a randomized double blind placebo controlled study. Osteoarthritis Cartilage, 21(1), 22–27.

Chromium

HISTORICAL NOTE Shortly after its discovery in 1959, chromium's importance and role in insulin sensitivity and glucose control was observed in vitro (Schwarz & Mertz 1959). Its importance was confirmed in 1977 when a woman on long-term total parenteral nurtrition (TPN), without chromium, developed symptoms of diabetes that could not be controlled by insulin. After further investigation it was noted that she was deficient in chromium and when < 50 mcg was added to her TPN solution, symptoms resolved. This led to the US FDA listing chromium as an essential trace nutrient. However, problems in elucidating the effects of chromium supplementation persist, due to a lack of practical methods for diagnosing deficiency (Mertz 1998). Over the years researchers have focused on investigating the effects of chromium supplementation on insulin sensitivity and management and prevention of type 2 diabetes (and to a lesser extent PCOS and other presentations) and cardiovascular disease (Hummel et al 2007), and more recently, mental health and atypical depression (Arthur 2008).

BACKGROUND AND RELEVANT PHARMACOKINETICS

Absorption of chromium occurs by passive diffusion and is inversely related to dietary intake (e.g. from a dose of 10 mcg, 2% is absorbed; from a dose of 40 mcg, 0.5% is absorbed) (Anderson & Kozlovsky 1985). Absorption may be inhibited by zinc (Hahn & Evans 1975) and phytates, and enhanced by oxalate (Bryson & Goodall 1983) and ascorbic acid (Offenbacher 1994). Unfortunately, much of the current information is based on chromium chloride, which is an inorganic and poorly absorbed form, so effects may vary for different forms (Arthur 2008). For example, the complexation of picolinic acid with chromium increases its bioavailability (Press et al 1990). Nicotinic acid is a metabolite of tryptophan that also improves the absorption of chromium (Arthur 2008).

Chromium is transported around the systemic circulation primarily by transferrin (Campbell et al 1997), therefore potentially competing with iron and other microminerals that use this transport mechanism, and accumulates in kidney, muscle and liver (Hepburn & Vincent 2003). It is excreted primarily in urine, but small amounts are lost in hair, perspiration and faeces.

CHEMICAL COMPONENTS

Chromium exists mostly in two valence states in nature: hexavalent chromium (chromium (VI)) and trivalent chromium (chromium (III)). The hexavalent form is toxic and poses a significant risk mainly via occupational exposure. It is recognised as a potent carcinogen to animals and humans, orally, often as a result of water contamination from industry (Kirman et al 2013, Sedman et al 2006) or when inhaled (Haney 2012). Trivalent chromium is an essential trace element in the human body and approved as a supplement.

Supplemental forms used in trials include organic chromium complexes, such as chromium picolinate and chromium nicotinate/polynicotinate (niacin-bound chromium [NBC]), and inorganic salts such as chromium chloride. While a number of different commercial trivalent chromium supplements exist the best evidence is for the picolinate and polynicotinate forms (Preuss et al 2008).

The picolinate form has been plagued by some controversy over the years — relating to both questions over its effects on iron levels and DNA damage (see below).

FOOD SOURCES

The chromium content of food is geochemically dependent and Australian soils appear to vary widely in chromium content, thus dietary sources are likely to vary in chromium content due to growing location together with processing methods. In particular, Australian soils appear to be low in chromium, unlike some other locations such as USA (Thor et al 2011). Recommended dietary sources of chromium in Australia include Brewer's yeast, wholegrain breads and cereals, processed meat products and chocolate products (Ashton et al 2003). Other sources documented in the international literature include organ meat, cheese, green beans, broccoli, egg yolk, nuts, poultry, spices, tea, beer, wine (Arthur 2008).

Clinical note — Problems testing for chromium deficiency

Currently, testing for chromium deficiency is a serum assay. This is problematic as it is unclear whether serum levels correlate with tissue levels. Previous studies have shown that subjects with widely varying serum chromium levels respond favourably to chromium supplementation, suggesting that this marker is misleading (Bahijri 2000). As a consequence, serum tests should not be solely relied upon, leaving the diagnosis of deficiency up to a practitioner's clinical judgement. Other tests have been proposed, such as toenail chromium concentration (Ayodele & Ajala 2009, Guallar et al 2005) and urinary chromium response to glucose load (Bahijri & Mufti 2002), as conditions that increase circulating glucose and insulin concentrations increase urinary chromium output (Vincent 2004); however, further research is required to confirm the validity of these tests. The recent development and change towards a more sensitive and accurate whole blood test (Cieslak et al 2013) may be better than serum testing; however, there still remains some uncertainty as to whether this newer test provides an accurate reflection of tissue levels.

DEFICIENCY SIGNS AND SYMPTOMS

Primary deficiency

Symptoms of weight loss, glucose intolerance and neuropathy have been noted in patients on TPN deficient in chromium (Verhage et al 1996). Deficiency may also be a precursor to the development of insulin resistance, and thus associated with hyperglycaemia, hypoglycaemia and obesity. Up to 90% of US diets have been found to be below the minimum suggested adequate daily intake for chromium of 50 mcg/day (Anderson & Kozlovsky 1985); as previously mentioned, Australian foods have been found to contain lower levels of this mineral (Ashton 2003), suggesting that the average Australian diet is likely to be lower.

Animal studies suggest that maternal chromium deficiency prior to and during gestation may also have detrimental effects in the offspring such as increased body weight, central obesity and overall percentage of body fat, together with impaired glycaemia (Padmavathi et al 2011). It remains to be tested whether the same results occur in humans.

Secondary deficiency

Factors that may exacerbate deficiency, generally by increasing requirements for or urinary excretion of chromium, include pregnancy, excessive exercise, infection, physical trauma and stress (Anderson 1986). Diets high in simple sugars have been found to increase urinary chromium excretion up to 30-fold, thereby increasing the risk of deficiency

(Kozlovsky et al 1986). Corticosteroids also increase urinary losses of chromium (Kim et al 2002).

MAIN ACTIONS

Most of chromium's main actions are ultimately related to its role in glycaemic control and regulation and secondary benefits for antioxidant systems.

Important cofactor

Chromium is an essential trace mineral required for carbohydrate, lipid, protein and corticosteroid metabolism (Kim et al 2002).

Improves blood sugar control

Trivalent chromium is an essential trace element for normal carbohydrate metabolism and insulin sensitivity (Wilson & Gondy 1995), aiding the ability of insulin to transport glucose into cells. In particular, chromium improves the ability of insulin to bind to cells by enhancing skeletal muscle Glut4 translocation; enhancing beta-cell sensitivity; increasing the number of insulin receptors; and activating insulin receptor kinase, thus increasing insulin sensitivity; it also appears to reduce the cholesterol ratio in plasma membrane, improving insulin sensitivity (Anderson 1997, Hua 2012, Penumathsa 2009, Wang 2009). Additionally, in vitro studies have shown that chromium inhibits the secretion of TNF-alpha, a cytokine known to reduce the sensitivity and action of insulin, and that this appears to be mediated by its antioxidant effects (Jain & Kannan 2001). In vitro studies also show that chromium chloride prevents the increase in protein glycosylation and oxidative stress caused by high levels of glucose in erythrocytes (Jain et al 2006).

Lipid-lowering activity

Although the mechanism of action is yet to be fully explained, studies show that chromium supplementation may decrease triglyceride levels, total and LDL-cholesterol and modestly increase HDL-cholesterol (Bahijri 2000, Lee & Reasner 1994, Press et al 1990, Preuss et al 2000, Sundaram 2013b). In a study by Cefalu (2010), chromium decreased and modulated peripheral tissue lipids in insulin-resistant subjects with improved insulin response post-chromium supplementation. Another in vitro study suggested chromium may have a role in modulating cellular cholesterol accumulation induced by hyperinsulinaemia; mechanisms are thought to involve the upregulation of HDL-C (Sealls et al 2011).

Antihypertensive, cardioprotective

In rats with sugar-induced hypertension, niacin-bound chromium lowers systolic blood pressure, at least in part due to its effects on the renin-angiotensin system (Perricone et al 2008). Niacin-bound chromium and chromium phenylalanine also demonstrated improvement in cardiac contractile function and protection in ischaemic-reperfusion injury in a diabetic rat model (Hua 2012).

Antidepressant/neurotransmitter effects

According to McCarty (1994), a large proportion of unipolar depressive patients may also have insulin resistance, indicating that people with diabetes may have an increased risk of depression. Increased brain insulin levels, secondary to elevated cortisol or insulin resistance, influences the normal functioning of catecholaminergic neurons, contributing to a depressive state (McCarty 1994). The reputed antidepressant effects of chromium may be explained by improvements in insulin sensitivity (Davidson et al 2003) and related increases in tryptophan availability and/or noradrenaline release (McLeod & Golden 2000). Chromium has also been shown to lower the cortisol response to challenge with 5-hydroxy-L-tryptophan (5-HTP) and decrease the sensitivity of 5-HT_{2A} receptors (Attenburrow et al 2002). Influences on serotonergic pathways have also been reported in animal studies using chromium picolinate (Khanam & Pillai 2006) and potassium channels are thought to be involved. Chromium chloride in a rodent model of depression showed antagonistic activities to glutamanergic NMDA and AMPA receptors, as well as a 5-HT_{1A} agonistic effect, resulting in antidepressant effects (Piotrowska 2008).

OTHER ACTIONS

Immunomodulation

A review detailing the effects of chromium on the immune system found that chromium has both immunostimulatory and immunosuppressive effects, as shown by its effects on T- and B-lymphocytes, macrophages and cytokine production (Shrivastava et al 2002).

Bone density protection

It has been suggested that modulation of insulin by chromium may have positive effects on bone density, reducing bone resorption and promoting collagen production by osteoblasts (McCarty 1995). One placebo-controlled study using chromium picolinate (equivalent to 200 mcg chromium/day for 60 days) has shown a 47% reduction in the urinary hydroxyproline : creatinine ratio, indicating a decrease in calcium excretion and a potential role in the prevention of osteoporosis (Evans et al 1995).

Antioxidant

A placebo-controlled trial using 1000 mcg/day of chromium (in yeast form) for 6 months found chromium to be an effective treatment in reducing oxidative stress in people with type 2 diabetes (T2DM) and severe hyperglycaemia ($HbA_{1C} > 8.5\%$); however, the authors noted that it may act as a pro-oxidant in euglycaemic people (Cheng et al 2004).

A similar randomised study confirmed chromium's antioxidant capacity in a similar cohort; chromium (1000 mcg in yeast form), alone or in combination with vitamin C (1000 mg) and vitamin E

(800 IU), reduced oxidation markers after 6 months in 30 T2DM subjects with similar Cr and oxidation markers plasma baseline values (Lai 2008).

The histadinate form of chromium may be superior to picolinate for antioxidant activity according to in vivo research with a diabetic model, notably by decreasing cerebral levels of NF-κB and 4-HNE, two inflammatory markers found in diabetic subjects (Sahin et al 2012).

Anti-inflammatory

In diabetic rats, chromium supplementation can lower the risk of vascular inflammation. Chromium niacinate appears to be more effective than the picolinate form in lowering blood levels of pro-inflammatory cytokines (TNF-alpha, IL-6) and C-reactive protein, and in reducing oxidative stress and lipid levels (Jain et al 2007).

Increases dehydroepiandrosterone (DHEA)

In a placebo-controlled trial, chromium picolinate (equivalent to 200 mcg chromium/day for 60 days) increased DHEA by 24% in postmenopausal women (Evans et al 1995).

Hepatoprotection

In alloxan-induced diabetic rats with mild chronic hepatic injury, supplementation with chromium picolinate prevented and ameliorated histopathological damage, elevation in AST and ALT, as well as LFABP, a biomarker of hepatic injury (Fan 2013).

CLINICAL USE

Supplemental forms used in trials include organic chromium complexes, such as chromium picolinate and chromium nicotinate, and inorganic salts such as chromium chloride. Chromium is known to improve insulin sensitivity and metabolic markers, and as such its clinical applications reflect this central action; it is used in conditions associated with insulin resistance such as T2DM, gestational diabetes (GDM), polycystic ovarian syndrome (PCOS), obesity and syndrome X. It is also used in practice to curb sugar cravings and stabilise blood sugar levels. More recently, it is attracting interest as a potential treatment in mental health disorders, depression in particular.

Deficiency states: prevention and treatment

Although frank demonstrable chromium deficiency is uncommon (Vincent 2004) and is mostly described in relation to the use of TPN with inadequate chromium levels, subclinical deficiency states in the USA and Australia are thought to be more prevalent (Anderson & Kozlovsky 1985, Ashton 2003); however, it is difficult to detect chromium deficiency via pathology testing so true estimates remain unknown. Chromium supplementation is used in cases ***at risk*** of deficiency, such as long-term corticosteroid use (Kim et al 2002), patients with evidence of impaired insulin sensitivity, people with a high sugar intake (Kozlovsky et al 1986) or those suspected to be deficient after a thorough clinical history has been taken.

Diabetes

Subjects with diabetes (both T1DM & T2DM) appear to have lower tissue levels of chromium and a correlation exists between low circulating levels of chromium and incidence of T2DM (Hummel et al 2007). Additionally, insulin resistance has been associated with higher rates of chromium excretion (Bahijri & Alyssa 2011) and a study of people with T2DM of less than 2 years' duration found they had lower chromium plasma levels (33%) and increased chromium excretion (100%) compared with healthy controls (Morris et al 1999). While still controversial, a number of studies and reviews suggest that chromium supplementation may facilitate insulin signalling and therefore improve systemic insulin sensitivity. A review of 15 clinical studies involving a total of 1690 subjects (1505 of which received chromium picolinate) reported significant improvement in at least one outcome of glycaemic control. The pooled data showed substantial reductions in both hyperglycaemia and hyperinsulinaemia (Broadhurst & Domenico 2006).

Type 2 diabetes mellitus (T2DM)

Results have shown that chromium supplementation appears to be more effective in patients with T2DM than in those with T1DM (Ravina & Slezack 1993, Wang & Cefalu 2010).

In 2013, a meta-analysis of seven RCTs comparing chromium supplementation (>250 mcg/day for at least 3 months) to placebo on glucose and lipid profiles in patients with T2DM concluded that chromium significantly reduced fasting blood sugar compared to the placebo ($P < 0.0001$), but had no significant effects on glycated haemoglobin, total cholesterol (TC), high-density lipoprotein cholesterol (HDL-C), low-density lipoprotein cholesterol (LDL-C), very low-density lipoprotein cholesterol (VLDL-C), triglyceride (TG) or body mass index (BMI) (Abdollahi et al 2013).

Despite this conclusion, not all studies have produced positive results and several researchers have sought to identify the best responders. It is accepted that chromium supplementation given to human subjects in documented deficiency states experience improved glucose levels. However, it also appears that a clinical response to chromium (i.e. decreased glucose and improved insulin sensitivity) may be more likely in insulin-resistant individuals with T2DM who have more elevated fasting glucose and haemoglobin A(1C) levels (Wang & Cefalu 2010).

In support of this, a more recent study seeking to evaluate the metabolic and physiological differences in responders and non-responders found that a clinical response to a dose of 1000 mcg was correlated to baseline values of poorer insulin sensitivity, high glycosylated haemoglobin (HbA_{1C}) and high fasting blood glucose (Cefalu 2010).

Furthermore, in a double-blind RCT of 31 non-obese, normo-glycaemic subjects, those with the highest serum chromium at the start experienced a worsening of their insulin sensitivity after treatment with chromium (500 mcg twice daily for 16 weeks) compared to placebo (Marashani et al 2012).

Some study findings suggest that improvements are dose-related but may also be affected by treatment duration, initial chromium status (Ghosh et al 2002, Amato et al 2000, Masharani et al 2012) and age. A controlled trial of elderly T2DM patients (average age 73 years) reported that supplementation with chromium (200 mcg twice daily) for 3 weeks improved fasting blood glucose, HbA_{1C}, and total cholesterol levels (Rabinovitz et al 2004), suggesting lower doses may be effective in older patients. Another study (single blind prospective) in 40 newly diagnosed T2DM subjects (ages 35–67 years) supplemented with 9 g of a chromium-containing brewer's yeast for 3 months also yielded improvements of glycaemia, reducing glycosylated haemoglobin and fasting blood glucose values as well as improving their lipid profile (Sharma 2011).

The most promising RCT to date tested chromium picolinate at doses of 200 and 1000 mcg/day in subjects with T2DM who were instructed to maintain their current medications, diet and lifestyle habits. HbA_{1C} values improved significantly in the higher treatment group after 2 months and in both groups after 4 months' treatment. Fasting glucose was lower in the 1000 mcg group after 2 and 4 months (4-month values: 7.1 ± 0.2 mmol/L vs placebo 8.8 ± 0.3 mmol/L). Two-hour glucose values were also significantly lower in the 1000 mcg group after both 2 and 4 months (4-month values: 10.5 ± 0.2 mmol/L vs placebo 12.3 ± 0.4 mmol/L). Fasting and 2-hour insulin values decreased significantly in both groups receiving supplemental chromium after 2 and 4 months. Plasma total cholesterol also decreased in the subjects receiving 1000 mcg chromium after 4 months (Anderson et al 1997). In another study T2DM patients taking sulfonylurea agents, chromium picolinate supplementation (equivalent to 1000 mcg chromium) for 6 months significantly improved insulin sensitivity and glucose control; and attenuated bodyweight gain and visceral fat accumulation compared with the placebo (Martin et al 2006).

Studies using chromium nicotinic acid have proven more promising with higher doses of nicotinic acid (100 mg/day) (Urberg & Zemel 1987) than those with low-dose nicotinic acid (1.8 mg) (Thomas & Gropper 1996), demonstrating a synergistic effect with chromium (200 mcg/day).

It appears the picolinate form of chromium is crucial in obtaining improvements of glycaemic parameters.

Type 1 diabetes mellitus (T1DM)

As chromium appears to improve insulin sensitivity rather than secretion its therapeutic potential in T1DM is limited (Edmondson 2002). One study did show reduced requirements for insulin in 33.6% of patients with T1DM taking 200 mcg chromium/day (Ravina & Slezack 1993), and another showed a 30% reduction in insulin requirements in 71% of subjects at the same dose (Ravina et al 1995), but it is unclear which patients might respond to treatment. No further studies have been done on this population.

Gestational diabetes mellitus (GDM)

Pregnancy can be described as an increased insulin resistant state, which may result in GDM if the pancreas is unable to increase insulin levels to maintain blood glucose balance (Jovanovic & Peterson 1996). While chromium serum measurement in pregnancy yielded inconclusive results (Sundararaman 2012, Wood 2008), it appears that chromium excretion is elevated in normal pregnancy, potentially contributing to the insulin resistance (Morris et al 2000). The beneficial effect of chromium on insulin sensitivity provides a theoretical basis for its use in this condition. A small placebo-controlled trial using 4 or 8 mcg/kg of chromium daily in GDM found a significant dose-dependent improvement in fasting insulin, 1-hour insulin and glucose, and postprandial glucose levels after 8 weeks supplementation (Jovanovic et al 1999).

Corticosteroid-induced diabetes mellitus

Human trials have shown that corticosteroid use significantly increases urinary chromium excretion. Supplementation with chromium picolinate (equivalent to 600 mcg chromium/day) in patients experiencing steroid-induced diabetes resulted in decreased fasting blood glucose values (from >13.9 mmol/L to <8.3 mmol/L). Furthermore, hypoglycaemic medications were also reduced by 50% in all patients within 1 week (Ravina et al 1999).

Antiretroviral medication-induced dysglycaemia

In a study of people with HIV (n = 56) and evidence of elevated glucose, altered lipids or body-fat redistribution secondary to antiretroviral medication, supplementation with chromium nicotinate (400 mcg daily) for 16 weeks significantly decreased insulin, triglycerides and total body fat mass; however, blood glucose, HbA_{1C}, HDL and LDL values remained unchanged (Aghdassi 2010).

Prevention of long-term diabetic complications

Both QTc interval prolongation and chronic hyperinsulinaemia have been associated with atherosclerosis progression and increased cardiovascular morbidity in patients with T2DM. In a crossover trial of 60 subjects, chromium picolinate (1000 mcg/day) for 3 months was shown to reduce both QTc interval duration and plasma insulin levels (Vrtovec et al 2005), probably by reducing the adrenergic activation of the sympathetic nervous system due to hyperinsulinaemia. Benefits were most significant in obese patients with higher peripheral insulin resistance (Vrtovec et al 2005).

In a retrospective study of patients hospitalised with uncontrolled acute hyperglycaemia non-responsive to intravenous insulin, treatment with intravenous chromium chloride at 20 mcg/hour for 10 to 15 hours decreased insulin needs and improved glucose control at 12 and 24 hours post-treatment (Drake 2012).

Animal studies have found that chromium supplementation in mice with T2DM reduces the symptoms of hyperglycaemia and improves the renal function by recovering renal chromium concentration (Mita et al 2005, Mozaffari et al 2005, 2012, Selcuk 2012), which may hold promise for human trials investigating the potential role of chromium in reducing the incidence of diabetic nephropathy.

Hypoglycaemia

Eight patients with reactive hypoglycaemia were given chromium chloride (equivalent to 200 mcg chromium) for 3 months in a double-blind crossover study. Chromium supplementation significantly improved blood sugar regulation, insulin binding to receptors and red blood cells, and alleviated symptoms of hypoglycaemia (Anderson et al 1987).

A double-blind crossover study using chromium chloride (equivalent to 200 mcg/day elemental chromium) for 8 weeks found a significant improvement in glycaemic control in subgroups where the 2-hour glucose level was >10% above or below the fasting level (Bahijri 2000). In these subgroups chromium supplementation resulted in a 2-hour mean not significantly different to the fasting mean, suggesting an amphoteric effect on glycaemic control.

Hyperlipidaemia

It has been suggested that some of the potential benefits of HRT on total and LDL-cholesterol and total:HDL-cholesterol ratio may be related to its ability to improve chromium status (Bureau et al 2002, Roussel et al 2002), and trials yielding both positive and negative results for supplemental chromium in hyperlipidaemia have been reported. In a systematic review of 41 trials, 18 studies, with a total 655 participants, reported lipid data for participants with either T2DM or glucose intolerance (Balk 2007). Overall, chromium supplementation was not found to exert a statistically significant effect on lipid levels in either group, although brewer's yeast supplementation did result in a statistically significant increase in HDL cholesterol (+0.21 mmol/L) compared to chromium picolinate.

Currently, it is unclear what circumstances or conditions and type of subjects are most likely to respond to treatment, so in practice a treatment trial period is often used to establish usefulness in individual patients.

A placebo-controlled trial using chromium tripicolinate (equivalent to 200 mcg chromium/day) for 42 days found a reduction in total cholesterol, LDL and apolipoprotein B (the major protein of the LDL fraction) with a slight increase in HDL and a significant increase in apolipoprotein A1 (the major protein of the HDL fraction) (Press et al 1990). Another RCT of 40 hypercholesterolaemic subjects found that chromium polynicotinate (equivalent to 200 mcg elemental chromium) twice daily for 2 months decreased total (10%) cholesterol and LDL-cholesterol (14%) (Preuss et al 2000).

Another double-blind RCT of young, non-obese adults taking chromium nicotinate (equivalent to 220 mcg elemental chromium) for 90 days found no statistically significant differences in lipid levels (total cholesterol, HDL-cholesterol, LDL-cholesterol, triglycerides) at this dose compared to the placebo; however, this dose is lower than used in most successful studies (Wilson & Gondy 1995).

Lipid-lowering activity does not appear to be significant in people with T2DM according to a meta-analysis of seven RCTs that tested chromium supplementation (>250 mcg/day) taken for at least 3 months (Abdollahi et al 2013).

Obesity

As chromium has a role in maintaining carbohydrate and lipid metabolism, it has been suggested that chromium supplementation may positively impact body composition, including reducing fat mass and increasing lean body mass (Vincent 2003).

A meta-analysis of RCTs concluded that chromium picolinate elicited a relatively small effect compared with placebo for reducing body weight (Pittler et al 2003). One study, however, did show promising results using 200 mcg niacin-bound chromium TIDS (600 mcg/day) with moderate exercise. At these high doses, while overall reduction in body weight was similar for both the chromium and the placebo groups, total fat loss was more significant in the chromium group, suggesting a muscle-sparing effect (Crawford et al 1999). More recent RCTs using chromium picolinate (equivalent to 200 mcg and 1000 mcg/day) were unable to reproduce these effects (Lukaski et al 2007).

A more recent meta analysis of 20 RCTs concurred with Pittler's findings, and found a small but significant difference in weight loss (1 kg) over placebo for studies lasting at least 16 weeks, but not in studies of shorter duration (Onakpoya et al 2013).

Atypical depression

The anti-depressant activity of chromium has been noted in a small number of rodent and human studies (Khanam & Pillai 2006, Komorowski et al 2012), however mechanisms are poorly understood (Iovieno et al 2011). Preclinical studies provide a biological basis for its use in depression, chiefly relating to neurotransmitter synthesis and release (McCarty 1994, Liu & Lin 1997) with decreases seen for serotonergic 5-HT_{2A} receptor expression and increased receptor sensitivity (Attenburrow et al 2002, Piotrowska et al 2008), antagonistic effects on NMDA and AMPA glutamanergic receptors (Piotrowska et al 2008) and antagonist effects on the dopamine and noradrenergic pathway (Piotrowska et al 2013).

In humans, a case series and a single blind trial conducted by McLeod and colleagues (1999, 2000) have shown that supplementation with chromium 400–600 mcg/day alone or in conjunction with sertraline or nortriptyline antidepressant led to the improvement of symptoms of patients with various treatment-resistant mood disorders.

A small placebo-controlled double-blind study of chromium picolinate (600 mcg/day) for 8 weeks was conducted in 15 patients with DSM-IV major depressive disorder, atypical type. Seven (70%) of 10 patients receiving chromium picolinate and none of the placebo group responded to treatment. Six subjects in the chromium group also experienced remission compared with none in the placebo group. However, only a moderate difference was detected in the Hamilton Depression Scale at the end of treatment for a small number of patients (Davidson et al 2003). A replication of the Davidson study by Docherty and colleagues (2005) with a larger cohort (n = 113) demonstrated similar significant improvements compared to the placebo. The study highlighted that patients with carbohydrate cravings, increased appetite and hyperphagia and diurnal mood variation responded particularly well. While these studies have limitations because they include patients with varied depressive pathologies, they provide encouraging evidence for further studies (Iovieno et al 2011).

OTHER USES

Chromium is also used in the following conditions, based on a theoretical understanding of its pharmacological actions.

Exercise aid – not effective

Chromium has demonstrated an ability to enhance insulin-mediated glucose uptake in cultured cells; however, human supplementation does not appear to exert such benefits. In a small RCT, 16 overweight men were randomised to receive chromium picolinate (equivalent to 600 mcg chromium/day) for 4 weeks before being subjected to supramaximal cycling exercises to deplete glycogen stores, followed by high glycaemic index carbohydrate feedings. At this dose, supplementation did not appear to improve glycogen synthesis during the recovery phase (Volek et al 2006).

In addition, studies in female athletes have shown no effect on body composition or muscle strength following supplementation with 500 mcg chromium picolinate daily during 6 weeks of resistance training (Livolsi et al 2001). In a clinical trial of older women a high-dose chromium picolinate supplement did not affect body composition, skeletal muscle size or maximal strength above that of resistance training alone (Campbell et al 2002). A meta-analysis of trials of dietary supplements for enhancing lean muscle mass and strength during resistance training did not support the use of chromium for this purpose (Nissen & Sharp 2003).

POLYCYSTIC OVARIAN SYNDROME (PCOS)

The relationship between PCOS and insulin resistance provides a theoretical basis for the use of chromium in this condition. A small study has found that chromium picolinate (200 mcg/day) appears to improve glucose tolerance but not ovulatory frequency in women with polycystic ovary syndrome (Lucidi et al 2005). Larger studies are required to investigate the potential benefits of chromium supplementation in this population.

Critical care

It is reported that up to 67% of critical care patients present on admission to intensive care with acute insulin resistance and blood sugar control may have better outcomes with intra-venous (IV) chromium (Surani et al 2012). Surani reports a case study of a 62-year-old diabetic, hypercholesterolaemic woman presenting to ICU with cardiac arrest and respiratory failure secondary to aspiration pneumonia and septic shock presenting with acute insulin resistance and requiring 7000 units of insulin over 12 hours, successfully stabilised with an IV infusion of chromium chloride at the rate of 3 mcg/hr (100 mcg in 1 L of saline infused at 30 mL/hr) and leading to the cessation of the insulin infusion.

Osteoporosis

Effects on bone resorption, calcium excretion and collagen production suggest a role in the prevention of osteoporosis (Evans et al 1995, McCarty 1995); however, there are no controlled trials to determine clinical effectiveness.

DOSAGE RANGE

The ESADDI is 50–200 mcg/day. The most common doses studied include 200, 400, 600 and 1000 mcg daily. Doses in the upper range appear to produce more convincing trial results.

- Glycaemic control – 200–1000 mcg for at least 1 to 3 months.

Australian adequate intake

- Women: 25 mcg/day.
- Men: 35 mcg/day.

Chromium picolinate is the best absorbed form (Press et al 1990); chromium nicotinate, which also improves absorption (Arthur 2008), may have a better safety profile and the synergistic effects with nicotinic acid (providing a minimum of 100 mg) may have further benefits in some conditions, especially with regard to lipid profiles and anti-inflammatory effects (Jain et al 2007).

ADVERSE REACTIONS

It is important to differentiate between hexavalent chromium (Cr IV) and trivalent chromium (Cr III) when discussing the potential toxicity of chromium. Cr IV is used in industry and is highly toxic, whereas Cr III is approved for use as a supplement and does not attract the same concerns. Recent in vitro

> ***Clinical note — Does chromium picolinate cause cancer?***
> There has been some concern in the past arising from in vitro studies suggesting chromium picolinate exerts clastogenic effects in hamster ovarian cells (Stearns et al 1995a, 2002) and possible DNA damage (Levina & Lay 2008, Speetjens et al 1999). While some recent reviews seem to maintain the controversy (Jana 2009, Wise 2012, Golubnitschaja 2012), this genotoxicity has been refuted by a number of authors, suggesting the doses tested were several thousand times higher than equivalent human doses (McCarty 1997, Salmon 1996) and that chromium has a relatively short half-life so that the accumulated doses suggested by researchers (Stearns et al 1995a) were not clinically relevant (Hepburn & Vincent 2003). Furthermore, in vivo evidence from animals and humans suggests that under normal circumstances trivalent chromium (Cr III) has only restricted access to cells, which would limit or prevent genotoxic effects. A recent rodent study by Komorowski (2008) showed no DNA deletions, chromosome gaps or breaks after a single megadose of 7,500 mg/kg. A 2-year study in rats and mice fed CrPic daily at doses three to five times higher than those commonly recommended showed a general lack of toxicity, except in male rats which developed preputial gland adenomas at the highest doses. The reasons for this remain unclear (Stout 2009). Another study showed no histopathological changes or DNA damage in the kidney of male rats supplemented chromium picolinate (100 mg/kg diet), despite accumulation in the kidney (Mozaffari 2012). Therefore, supplementation at low to moderate doses is not currently considered to be detrimental (Eastmond et al 2008). It should also be noted that picolinic acid appears to be the source of the concern and other forms of chromium have not been implicated (Bagchi et al 2002, Stearns et al 1995b).

studies suggest a possibility that Cr III may oxidise to Cr V, a potential carcinogen (Shrivastava et al 2005); however, this requires confirmation from in vivo studies.

Irritability and insomnia have been reported with chromium yeast supplementation (Schrauzer et al 1992).

A follow-up survey found no side effects for doses up to 1000 mcg/day of chromium picolinate at 1 year (Cheng et al 1999).

Of five anecdotal adverse reports attributed to chromium picolinate and reviewed by Lamson and Plaza (2002), only one reporting transient and vague symptoms was considered to be a possible adverse reaction (Huszonek 1993). Three could not be validated by the reviewers due to concurrent medications (Cerulli et al 1998, Martin & Fuller 1998, Wasser et al 1997), and another involved the inappropriate use of potassium dichromate, a strong oxidising agent known to elicit reactions in a majority of people (Fowler 2000). A case report exists of toxic hepatitis and greatly elevated hepatic chromium levels (>10-fold normal) after 5 months' ingestion of chromium polynicotinate in combination with vegetable extracts (Lanca et al 2002). Whether chromium supplementation was responsible for this incident is currently unclear.

No adverse effects on iron status

As chromium competes with iron for binding to transferrin it has been suggested that high-dose chromium supplementation may adversely affect iron status. While some studies support this (Ani & Moshtaghie 1992), others show that serum iron concentrations and serum ferritin concentrations are unaffected by chromium picolinate supplementation (Campbell et al 1997, Lukaski et al 2007). Iron does not use all available transferrin binding sites and therefore this situation is unlikely under normal conditions.

SIGNIFICANT INTERACTIONS

Corticosteroids

Corticosteroids increase urinary losses of chromium, and chromium supplementation has been shown to aid in recovery from steroid-induced diabetes mellitus. Therefore a beneficial interaction may be possible (Kim et al 2002).

Hypoglycaemic medicines

Chromium may reduce requirements for hypoglycaemic agents (Ravina & Slezack 1993, Ravina et al 1995). While a beneficial interaction is possible, this combination should be used with caution and drug requirements monitored and adjusted if necessary by a healthcare professional.

Hormone replacement therapy

Women receiving HRT appear to have improved chromium status (Bureau et al 2002, Roussel et al 2002) and the addition of trivalent chromium to 17-beta-oestradiol may enhance IL-6 inhibition in experimental models (Jain et al 2004). Whether this alters chromium requirements is unknown.

Lipid-lowering medicines

Additive effects are theoretically possible as some clinical studies have indicated lipid-lowering effects. Observe patients taking this combination and monitor drug requirements.

 ***CONTRAINDICATIONS AND PRECAUTIONS***

Hypersensitivity to chromium.

PREGNANCY USE

Oral ingestion of doses typically found in the diet are likely to be safe. Taken under professional supervision, supplements are also likely to be safe and may be beneficial in the prevention and treatment of gestational diabetes (Jovanovic & Peterson 1996, Jovanovic et al 1999).

Practice points/Patient counselling

- Chromium is an essential trace mineral required for carbohydrate, lipid, protein and corticosteroid metabolism.
- Dietary intakes are generally below the minimum suggested safe and adequate levels, and factors such as high-sugar diets, corticosteroid use, excessive exercise, infection, physical trauma and psychological stress further increase the risk of deficiency.
- Chromium supplements are used in the management of T2DM, hypoglycaemia, gestational diabetes and hyperlipidaemia. It appears chromium supplementation taken by people with T2DM for at least 3 months can reduce fasting glucose levels, but have no significant effect on lipids.
- It is also used in the treatment of obesity, atypical depression, polycystic ovary syndrome, to curb sugar cravings and improve osteoporosis.
- Supplemental forms used in trials include organic chromium complexes, such as chromium picolinate and chromium nicotinate, and inorganic salts such as chromium chloride.

PATIENTS' FAQs

What will this supplement do for me?

Chromium is essential for health and wellbeing. It reduces fasting glucose levels in people with T2DM when taken as a supplement for at least 3 months. It may also have benefits in gestational diabetes, hypoglycaemia and elevated cholesterol and triglyceride levels in some people, although scientific research has produced mixed results. In practice, it is also used to curb sugar cravings.

When will it start to work?

Effects in T2DM take at least 3 months.

Are there any safety issues?

Used under professional supervision, chromium supplements are considered safe.

REFERENCES

Abdollahi M et al. Effect of chromium on glucose and lipid profiles in patients with type 2 diabetes; a meta-analysis review of randomized trials. J Pharm Pharmaceut Sci 16.1 (2013): 99–114.

Aghdassi E et al. In patients with HIV-infection, chromium supplementation improves insulin resistance and other metabolic abnormalities: a randomized, double-blind, placebo controlled trial. Curr HIV Res 8.2(2010): 113–120.

Amato P et al. Effects of chromium picolinate supplementation on insulin sensitivity, serum lipids, and body composition in healthy, nonobese, older men and women. J Gerontol A Biol Sci Med Sci 55.5 (2000): M260–M263.

Anderson RA et al. Effects of supplemental chromium on patients with symptoms of reactive hypoglycemia. Metabolism 36.4 (1987): 351–355.

Anderson RA et al. Elevated intakes of supplemental chromium improve glucose and insulin variables in individuals with type 2 diabetes. Diabetes 46.11 (1997): 1786–1791.

Anderson RA, Kozlovsky AS. Chromium intake, absorption and excretion of subjects consuming self-selected diets. Am J Clin Nutr 41.6 (1985): 1177–1183.

Anderson RA. Chromium metabolism and its role in disease processes in man. Clin Physiol Biochem 4 (1986): 31–41 [cited in Salmon B. The truth about chromium. What science knows won't kill you. Let's Live Apr 1996].

Anderson RA. Nutritional factors influencing the glucose/insulin system: chromium. J Am Coll Nutr 16.5 (1997): 404–410.

Ani M, Moshtaghie AA. The effect of chromium on parameters related to iron metabolism. Biol Trace Elem Res Jan–Mar 32 (1992): 57–64.

Arthur R. Chromium. J Compl Med 7.4 (2008): 33–42.

Ashton, J.F. (2003) The Chromium content of some Australian foods. Food Australia 55.5 (2003): 201–204.

Attenburrow MJ et al. Chromium treatment decreases the sensitivity of 5-HT2A receptors. Psychopharmacology (Berl) 159.4 (2002): 432–436.

Ayodele JT, Ajala IC. Chromium and copper in toenails of some Kano inhabitants. Journal of Public Health and Epidemiology 1.2 (2009): 46–52.

Bagchi D et al. Cytotoxicity and oxidative mechanisms of different forms of chromium. Toxicology 180.1 (2002): 5–22.

Bahijri SM, Alyssa EM. Increased insulin resistance is associated with increased urinary excretion of chromium in non-diabetic, normotensive Saudi adults. J Clin Biochem Nutr 49.3 (2011): 164–168.

Bahijri SM, Mufti AM. Beneficial effects of chromium in people with type 2 diabetes, and urinary chromium response to glucose load as a possible indicator of status. Biol Trace Elem Res 85.2 (2002): 97–109.

Bahijri SM. Effect of chromium supplementation on glucose tolerance and lipid profile. Saudi Med J 21.1 (2000): 45–50.

Balk EM et al. Effect of chromium supplementation on glucose metabolism and lipids: a systematic review of randomized controlled trials. Diabetes Care 30.8 (2007): 2154–2163.

Broadhurst CL, Domenico P. Clinical studies on chromium picolinate supplementation in diabetes mellitus–a review. Diabetes Technol Ther 8.6 (2006): 677–687.

Bryson WG, Goodall CM. Differential toxicity and clearance kinetics of chromium III or IV in mice. Carcinogenesis 4 (1983): 1535–1539.

Bureau I et al. Trace mineral status in post menopausal women: impact of hormonal replacement therapy. J Trace Elem Med Biol 16.1 (2002): 9–13.

Campbell WW et al. Chromium picolinate supplementation and resistive training by older men: effects on iron-status and hematologic indexes. Am J Clin Nutr 66.4 (1997): 944–949.

Campbell WW et al. Effects of resistive training and chromium picolinate on body composition and skeletal muscle size in older women. Int J Sport Nutr Exerc Metab 12.2 (2002): 125–135.

Cefalu SD et al. Characterization of the metabolic and physiologic response to chromium supplementation in subjects with type 2 diabetes mellitus. Metabolism 59.5 (2010): 755–762.

Cerulli J et al. Chromium picolinate toxicity. Ann Pharmacother 32 (1998): 428–431.

Cheng HH et al. Antioxidant effects of chromium supplementation with type 2 diabetes mellitus and euglycemic subjects. J Agric Food Chem 52.5 (2004): 1385–1389.

Cheng N et al. Follow-up survey of people in China with type-II diabetes mellitus consuming supplemental chromium. J Trace Elem Exper Med 12 (1999): 55–60.

Cieslak W et al. Highly sensitive measurement of whole blood chromium by inductively coupled plasma mass spectrometry. Clinical Biochemistry 46 (2013): 266–270.

Crawford V, Scheckenbach R, Preuss HG. Effects of niacin-bound chromium supplementation on body composition in overweight African-American women. Diabetes Obes Metab 1.6 (1999): 331–337.

Davidson JR et al. Effectiveness of chromium in atypical depression: a placebo-controlled trial. Biol Psychiatry 53.3 (2003): 261–264.

Docherty JP et al. A double-blind, placebo-controlled, exploratory trial of chromium picolinate in atypical depression: effect on carbohydrate cravings. J. Psychiatr. Pract. 11 (2005): 302–314.

Drake TC. Chromium infusion in hospitalized patients with severe insulin resistance: a retrospective analysis. Endocr Prat 18.3 (2012): 394–398.

Eastmond DA et al. Trivalent chromium: assessing the genotoxic risk of an essential trace element and widely used human and animal nutritional supplement. Crit Rev Toxicol 38.3 (2008): 173–190.

Edmondson C. Can chromium be used for diabetes? Drug Utilization Rev 18.11 (2002): 5.

Evans GW, Swensen G, Walters K. Chromium picolinate decreases calcium excretion and increases dehydroepiandrosterone [DHEA] in postmenopausal women. FASEB J 9 (1995): A449.

Fan W et al. Role of liver fatty acid binding protein in hepatocellular injury: effect of CrPic treatment. Journal of inorganic chemistry 124 (2013): 46–53.

Fowler JF Jr. Systemic contact dermatitis caused by oral chromium picolinate. Cutis 65 (2000): 116.

Ghosh D et al. Role of chromium supplementation in Indians with type 2 diabetes mellitus. J Nutr Biochem 13.11 (2002): 690–697.

Golubnitschaja O, Yeghiazaryan K. Opinion controversy to chromium picolinate therapy's safety and therapy: ignoring 'anectodes" of case reports or recognizing individual risks and new guidelines urgency to introduce innovation by predictive diagnosis. EPMA J 3.1 (2012): 11.

Guallar E et al. Low toenail chromium concentration and increased risk of nonfatal myocardial infarction. Am J Epidemiol 162.2 (2005): 157–164.

Hahn CJ, Evans GW. Absorption of trace minerals in zinc-deficient rats. Am J Physiol 228 (1975): 1020–1023.

Haney JT et al. Development of a cancer-based chronic inhalation reference value for hexavalent chromium based on a nonlinear-threshold carcinogenic assessment. Regul Toxicol Pharmacol 64.3(2012): 466–480.

Hepburn DD, Vincent JB. Tissue and subcellular distribution of chromium picolinate with time after entering the bloodstream. J Inorg Biochem 94.1–2 (2003): 86–93.

Hua Y et al. Molecular mechanisms of chromium in alleviating insulin resistance. J Nutr Biochem 23.4 (2012): 313–319.

Hummel M et al. Chromium in metabolic and cardiovascular disease. Horm Metab Res 39.10 (2007): 743–751.

Huszonek J. Over-the-counter chromium picolinate. Am J Psychiatry 150 (1993): 1560–1561.

Iovieno N et al. Second-tier natural antidepressants: Review and critique. Journal of Affective Disorders 130 (2011): 343–357.

Jain SK et al. Effect of chromium niacinate and chromium picolinate supplementation on lipid peroxidation, TNF-alpha, IL-6, CRP, glycated hemoglobin, triglycerides, and cholesterol levels in blood of streptozotocin-treated diabetic rats. Free Radic Biol Med 43.8 (2007): 1124–1131.

Jain SK et al. Protective effects of 17beta-estradiol and trivalent chromium on interleukin-6 secretion, oxidative stress, and adhesion of monocytes: relevance to heart disease in postmenopausal women. Free Radic Biol Med 37.11 (2004): 1730–1735.

Jain SK et al. Trivalent chromium inhibits protein glycosylation and lipid peroxidation in high glucose-treated erythrocytes. Antioxid Redox Signal 8.1–2 (2006): 238–241.

Jain SK, Kannan K. Chromium chloride inhibits oxidative stress and TNF-alpha secretion caused by exposure to high glucose in cultured U937 monocytes. Biochem Biophys Res Commun 289.3 (2001): 687–691.

Jana M et al. Chromium picolinate induced apoptosis of lymphocytes and the signalling mechanisms thereof. Toxicology and applied pharmacology 237.3 (2009): 331–344.

Jovanovic L, Gutierrez M, Peterson CM. Chromium supplementation for women with gestational Diabetes mellitus. J Trace Elem Exp Med 12 (1999): 91–97.

Jovanovic L, Peterson CM. Vitamin and mineral deficiencies which may predispose to glucose intolerance of pregnancy. J Am Coll Nutr 15.1 (1996): 14–20.

Khanam R, Pillai KK. Effect of chromium picolinate on modified forced swimming test in diabetic rats: involvement of serotonergic pathways and potassium channels. Basic Clin Pharmacol Toxicol 98.2 (2006): 155–159.

Kim DS et al. Effects of chromium picolinate supplementation on insulin sensitivity, serum lipids, and body weight in dexamethasone-treated rats. Metabolism 51.5 (2002): 589–594.

Kirman CR et al. Physiologically based pharmacokinetics for humans orally exposed to chromium. Chemico-Biological Interactions 204.1 (2013): 13–27.

Komorowski JR et al. Chromium picolinate does not produce chromosome damage. Toxicology in vitro 22 (2008): 819–826.

Komorowski JR et al. Chromium picolinate modulates serotonergic properties and carbohydrate metabolism in a rat model of diabetes. Biol Trace Elem Res 149.1 (2012): 50–56.

Kozlovsky AS et al. Effects of diets high in simple sugars on urinary chromium losses. Metabolism 35.6 (1986): 515–5118.

Lai MH. Antioxidant effects and insulin resistance improvement of chromium combined with vitamin C and E supplementation for type 2 daibetes mellitus. J Clin Biochem Nutr 43 (2008): 191–198.

Lamson DW, Plaza SM. The safety and efficacy of high-dose chromium. Alt Med Rev 7.3 (2002): 218–235.

Lanca S et al. Chromium-induced toxic hepatitis. Eur J Int Med 13.8 (2002): 518–520.

Lee NA, Reasner CA. Beneficial effect of chromium supplementation on serum triglyceride levels in type 2 diabetes. Diabetes Care 17.12 (1994): 1449–1452.

Levina A, Lay PA. Chemical properties and toxicity of chromium(III) nutritional supplements. Chem Res Toxicol 21.3 (2008): 563–571.

Liu, P.S., Lin, M.K. Biphasic effects of chromium compounds oncatecholamine secretion from bovine adrenal medullary cells. Toxicology 117 (1997) 45–53.

Livolsi JM, Adams GM, Laguna PL. The effect of chromium picolinate on muscular strength and body composition in women athletes. J Strength Cond Res 15.2 (2001): 161–166.

Lucidi RS et al. The effect of chromium supplementation on insulin resistance and ovarian/menstrual cyclicity in women with polycystic ovary syndrome. Fertil Steril 84 (Suppl 1) (2005): S427–S428.

Lukaski HC et al. Chromium picolinate supplementation in women: effects on body weight, composition, and iron status. Nutrition 23.3 (2007): 187–195.

Marashani U et al. Chromium supplementation in non-obese non-diabetic subjects is associated with a decline in insulin sensitivity. BMC Endocr Disord 12.31 (2012).

Martin J et al. Chromium picolinate supplementation attenuates body weight gain and increases insulin sensitivity in subjects with type 2 diabetes. Diabetes Care 29.8 (2006): 1826–1832.

Martin WR, Fuller RE. Suspected chromium picolinate-induced rhabdomyolysis. Pharmacotherapy 18 (1998): 860–862.

Masharani U et al. Chromium supplementation in non-obese non-diabetic subjects is associated with a decline in insulin sensitivity. BMC Endocrine Disorders 12.31 (2012).

McCarty MF. Anabolic effects of insulin on bone suggest a role for chromium picolinate in preservation of bone density. Med Hypotheses 45.3 (1995): 241–246.

McCarty MF. Enhancing central and peripheral insulin activity as a strategy for the treatment of endogenous depression: an adjuvant role for chromium picolinate? Med Hypotheses 43.4 (1994): 247–252.

McCarty MF. Subtoxic intracellular trivalent chromium is not mutagenic: implications for safety of chromium supplementation. Med Hypotheses 49.3 (1997): 263–269.

McLeod MN, Golden RN. Chromium treatment of depression. Int J Neuropsychopharmacol 3.4 (2000): 311–14.

McLeod MN, Gaynes BN, Golden RN. Chromium potentiation of antidepressant pharmacotherapy for dysthymic disorder in 5 patients. J. Clin. Psychiatry 60 (1999) 237–240.

Mertz W. Chromium research from a distance: from 1959 to 1980. J Am Coll Nutr 17.6 (1998): 544–547.

Mita Y et al. Supplementation with chromium picolinate recovers renal Cr concentration and improves carbohydrate metabolism and renal function in type 2 diabetic mice. Biol Trace Elem Res 105.1–3 (2005): 229–248.

Morris BW et al. Chromium homeostasis in patients with type II (NIDDM) diabetes. J Trace Elem Med Biol 13.1–2 (1999): 57–61.

Morris BW et al. Increased chromium excretion in pregnancy is associated with insulin resistance. J Trace Elem Exp Med 13 (2000): 389–396.

Mozafarri M S et al. Renal and glycemic effects of high dose chromium picolinate in *db/db* mice: assessment of DNA damage. J Nutrit Biochem 23.8 (2012): 977–985.

Mozaffari MS et al. Effects of chronic chromium picolinate treatment in uninephrectomized rat. Metabolism 54.9 (2005): 1243–1249.

Nissen SL, Sharp RL. Effect of dietary supplements on lean mass and strength gains with resistance exercise: a meta-analysis. J Appl Physiol 94.2 (2003): 651–659.

Offenbacher EG. Promotion of chromium absorption by asccorbic acid. Trace Elem Electrolytes 11 (1994): 178.

Onakpoya I et al. Chromium supplementation in overweight and obesity: a systematic review and meta-analysis of randomized clinical trials. Obesity Reviews 14 (2013): 496–507.

Padmavathi IJN et al. Impact of maternal chromium restriction on glucose tolerance, plasma insulin and oxidative stress in WNIN rat offspring. Journal of molecular endocrinology 47 (2011): 261–271.

Penumathsa SV et al. Niacin bound chromium treatment induces myocardial glut4 translocation and caveolar interaction via Akt, AMPK and eNOS phosphorylation in streptozotocin induced diabetic rats after ischemia-reperfusion injury. BBA 1792.1 (2009): 39–48.

Perricone NV et al. Blood pressure lowering effects of niacin-bound chromium(III) (NBC) in sucrose-fed rats: renin-angiotensin system. J Inorg Biochem 102.7 (2008): 1541–1548.

Piotrowska A et al. Antidepressant-like effect of chromium chloride in the mouse forced swim test: involvement of glutamatergic and serotonergic receptors. Pharmacological Report 60 (2008): 991–995.

Piotrowska A et al. involvement of the monoaminergic system in the antidepressant-like activity of chromium chloride in the force swim test. Journal of Physiology and Pharmacology 64(2013): 493–498.

Pittler MH, Stevinson C, Ernst E. Chromium picolinate for reducing body weight: meta-analysis of randomized trials. Int J Obes Relat Metab Disord 27.4 (2003): 522–529.

Press RI, Geller J, Evans GW. The effect of chromium picolinate on serum cholesterol and apolipoprotein fractions in human subjects. West J Med 152.1 (1990): 41–45.

Preuss HG et al. Comparing metabolic effects of six different commercial trivalent chromium compounds. J Inorg Biochem 102.11 (2008): 1986–90.

Preuss HG et al. Effects of niacin-bound chromium and grape seed proanthocyanidin extract on the lipid profile of hypercholesterolemic subjects: a pilot study. J Med 31.5–6 (2000): 227–246.

Rabinovitz H et al. Effect of chromium supplementation on blood glucose and lipid levels in type 2 diabetes mellitus elderly patients. Int J Vitam Nutr Res 74.3 (2004): 178–182.

Ravina A et al. Clinical use of the trace element chromium III in the treatment of diabetes mellitus. J Trace Elem Exp Med 8 (1995): 183–190.

Ravina A et al. Reversal of corticosteroid-induced diabetes mellitus with supplemental chromium. Diabet Med 16.2 (1999): 164–167.

Ravina A, Slezack L. Chromium in the treatment of clinical diabetes mellitus. Harefuah 125.5–6 (1993): 142–45, 191 [in Hebrew].

Roussel AM et al. Beneficial effects of hormonal replacement therapy on chromium status and glucose and lipid metabolism in postmenopausal women. Maturitas 42.1 (2002): 63–69.

Sahin K et al. The effects of chromium picolinate and chromium histidinate administration on NF-κB and Nrf2/HO-1 pathway in the brain of diabetic rats. Bio Trace Elem Res 150.3 (2012): 291–96.

Salmon B. The truth about chromium: What science knows won't kill you. Let's Live (Apr 1996).

Schrauzer GN, Shrestha KP, Arce MF. Somatopsychological effects of chromium supplementation. J Nutr Med 3.1 (1992): 43–48.

Schwarz K, Mertz W. Chromium(III) and the glucose tolerance factor. Arch Biochem Biophys 85 (1959): 292–295.

Sealls W Penque BA Elmendorf JS. Evidence that chromium modulates cellular cholesterol homeostasis and ABCA1 functionality impaired by hyperinsulinemia. Arterioscler Thromb Vasc Biol 31.5 (2011): 1139–1140.

Sedman RM et al. Review of the evidence regardingthe carcinogenicity of hexavalent chromium in drinking water. J Environ Sci Health C Environ Carcinog Ecotoxicol Rev 24.1 (2006): 155–82.

Selcuk M et al. chromium picolinate and chromium histidinate protect against renal dysfunction by modulation of NF-κB pathway in high-fat diet fed rats and streptozotocin-induced diabetic rats. Nutrition and Metabolism 9 (2012): 30.

Sharma S et al. Beneficial effects of chromium supplementation on glucose, HbA1C, and lipid variables in individuals with newly onset type-2 diabetes. Journal of Trace Elements in Medicine and Biology 25 (2011): 149–153.

Shrivastava HY et al. Cytotoxicity studies of chromium(III) complexes on human dermal fibroblasts. Free Rad Biol Med 38.1 (2005): 58–69.

Shrivastava R et al. Effects of chromium on the immune system. FEMS Immunol Med Microbiol 34.1 (2002): 1–7.

Speetjens JK et al. The nutritional supplement chromium(III) tris(picolinate) cleaves DNA. Chem Res Toxicol 12.6 (1999): 483–487.

Stearns DM et al. Chromium(III) picolinate produces chromosome damage in Chinese hamster ovary cells. FASEB J 9.15 (1995a): 1643–1648.

Stearns DM et al. Chromium(III) tris(picolinate) is mutagenic at the hypoxanthine (guanine) phosphoribosyltransferase locus in Chinese hamster ovary cells. Mutat Res 513.1–2 (2002): 135–142.

Stearns DM, Belbruno JJ, Wetterhahn KE. A prediction of chromium (III) accumulation in humans from chromium dietary supplements. FASEB J 9.15 (1995b): 1650–1657.

Stout MD et al. Chronic toxicity and carcinogenicity studies of chromium picolinate monohydrate administered in feed to F344N rats and B6C3F1 mice for 2 years. Food Chem Toxicol 47.4 (2009): 729–733.

Sundaram B et al. Anti-atherogenic effects of chromium picolinate in streptozotocin-induced experimental diabetes. J Diabetes 5.1 (2013b): 43–50.

Sundararaman PG et al. Serum chromium levels in gestational diabetes. Indian J Endocrinol Metab 16.1 (2012): S70–73.

Surani SR et al. Severe insulin resistance treatment with intravenous chromium in septic shock patient. World J Diabetes 3.9 (2012): 170–173.

Thomas VL, Gropper SS. Effect of chromium nicotinic acid supplementation on selected cardiovascular disease risk factors. Biol Trace Elem Res 55.3 (1996): 297–305.

Thor MY et al. Evaluation of the comprehensiveness and reliability of the chromium composition of foods in the literature. J Food Compost Anal. 24.8 (2011): 1147–1152 [pubmed]

Urberg M, Zemel MB. Evidence for synergism between chromium and nicotinic acid in the control of glucose tolerance in elderly humans. Metabolism 36.9 (1987): 896–899.

Verhage AH, Cheong WK, Jeejeebhoy KN. Neurologic symptoms due to possible chromium deficiency in long-term parenteral nutrition that closely mimic metronidazole-induced syndromes. J Parenter Enteral Nutr 20.2 (1996): 123–127.

Vincent J. The potential value and toxicity of chromium picolinate as a nutritional supplement, weight loss agent and muscle development agent. Sports Med 33.3 (2003): 213–230.

Vincent JB. Recent advances in the nutritional biochemistry of trivalent chromium. Proc Nutr Soc 63.1 (2004): 41–47.

Volek JS et al. Effects of chromium supplementation on glycogen synthesis after high-intensity exercise. Med Sci Sports Exerc 38.12 (2006): 2102–2109.

Vrtovec M et al. Chromium supplementation shortens QTc interval duration in patients with type 2 diabetes mellitus. Am Heart J 149.4 (2005): 632–636.

Wang, Y, Yao M, Effects of chromium picolinate on glucose uptake in insulin-resistant 3T3-L1 adipocytes involve activation of p38 MAPK, J Nutritional Biochemistry 20 (2009): 982–991.

Wang ZQ, Cefalu WT. Current concepts about chromium supplementation in type 2 diabetes and insulin resistance. Curr Diab Rep, 10.2 (2010): 145–151.

Wasser WG, Feldman NS, Agnati VD. Chronic renal failure after ingestion of over-the-counter chromium picolinate. Ann Intern Med 126 (1997): 410.

Wilson BE, Gondy A. Effects of chromium supplementation on fasting insulin levels and lipid parameters in healthy, non-obese young subjects. Diabetes Res Clin Pract 28.3 (1995): 179–184.

Wise SS, Wise SP. Chromium and genomic stability. Mutation Research 733 (2012): 78–82.

Woods SE et al. Serum chromium and gestational diabetes. J Am Board Fam Med 21.2 (2008): 153–157.

Cinnamon

HISTORICAL NOTE Since ancient times cinnamon has been used for a variety of purposes and was valued as a precious commodity. In ancient Egypt it was used as a flavouring for beverages, in combination with other spices for embalming, and as a medicinal agent. Ancient Chinese herbals document it as a medicinal treatment as early as 2700 BC (Castleman 1991), and it has a long history of use as a remedy for diabetes in China, Korea, Russia and India. In medieval Europe, cinnamon was a common ingredient in cooking, often used together with ginger. Due to the high demand for cinnamon, discovering lands where it grew was a primary motive for a number of explorers in the 15th and 16th centuries. There are more than 250 evergreen shrubs and trees in the genus *Cinnamomum*. Today, two main species of cinnamon are cultivated, *Cinnamomum verum*, also known as Ceylon cinnamon, and *Cinnamomum cassia*, also known as Chinese cinnamon.

OTHER NAMES

Cinnamomum verum (also known as *C. zeylanicum*): cannelle de ceylan, Ceylon celonzimi cinnamon, Ceylon cinnamon, cinnamon bark, cortex cinnamomi ceylanici, dalchini, ecorce de cannelier de Ceylan, echter, gujerati-dalchini, kannel, kuei-pi, kurundu, kulit kayumanis, ob choei, tamalpatra, wild cinnamon.

Cinnamomum cassia Blume: cassia, Chinese cinnamon, dalchini, guipi, kannan keihi, keishi, lavanga-pattai, lurundu, macrophyllos cassia bark tree, rou gui, Saigon cinnamon, saleekha, taj, toko keihi, Viet Nam cinnamon.

BOTANICAL NAME/FAMILY

Cinnamomum verum J.S. Presl (also known as *C. zeylanicum* Nees) and *C. cassia* Blume (family Lauraceae).

PLANT PARTS USED

Dried inner bark of the shoots grown on cut stock of *C. verum* or of the trunk bark, freed from the underlying parenchyma; outer cork of *C. cassia* Blume.

CHEMICAL COMPONENTS

Both forms of cinnamon contain an essential oil that consists primarily of cinnamaldehyde (up to 80% in *C. verum* and 90% in *C. cassia*) and differ primarily in their eugenol and coumarin content. The volatile oil from *C. verum* contains 10% eugenol, whereas the oil from *C. cassia* contains only trace amounts. Also, *C. cassia* contains coumarin, which is not found substantially in *C. verum*. The bark of *C. verum* contains caryophyllene, cinnamyl acetate and linalool, whereas the bark of *C. cassia* contains catechin and 1,8 cineole. A- and B-type procyanidin oligomers are recognised as bioactive in a number of species, including *C. parthenoxylon*, *C. cassia*, *C. japonica* and *C. burmannii* (Lu et al 2011).

MAIN ACTIONS

Cinnamon has diverse mechanisms of action. The cinnamaldehyde constituent in cinnamon is attributed with producing most of the herb's biological activity. This component is found in large amounts in both forms of cinnamon. More recently, several other constituents have also been tested in isolation and found to exert significant pharmacological effects.

Antibacterial and fungicidal effects

Several in vitro studies have identified broad-spectrum antibacterial and fungicidal effects for both forms of cinnamon. This has been chiefly attributed to cinnamaldehyde although other constituents such as eugenol, caryophyllene and 1,8 cineole also exhibit antimicrobial properties.

C. verum demonstrated activity against a wide range of bacteria and fungi, including *Bacillus subtilis*, *Escherichia coli*, *Saccharomyces cerevisiae*, *Candida albicans*, *Listeria monocytogenes* and *Salmonella enterica* (De et al 1999, Friedman et al 2002, Matan et al 2006, Simic et al 2004, Tampieri et al 2005). Cinnamon and thyme extracts were found to be superior to two other botanical antifungals (garlic and marigold) in an in vitro study, and recommended as an effective herbal treatment for candidiasis (Moghim & Shahabi 2011).

C

C. cassia extracts significantly inhibited *Helicobacter pylori* in vitro and produced zones of inhibition greater than or equal to commonly used antibiotics (Tabak et al 1999). The essential oil of *C. cassia* also exhibited strong antifungal properties in vitro (Giordani et al 2006). When tested with amphotericin, a reduced amount of drug was required for adequate antifungal effects.

Antibacterial activity for the oil has also been demonstrated against antibiotic-resistant *E. coli* and *Staphylococcus aureus* (Friedman et al 2004).

Fungi in bakery products

Antifungal activity against the more common fungi causing spoilage of bakery products, *Eurotium amstelodami*, *E. herbariorum*, *E. repens*, *E. rubrum*, *Aspergillus flavus*, *A. niger* and *Penicillium corylophilum*, was demonstrated for cinnamon oil in vitro (Guynot et al 2003).

Respiratory tract pathogens

An in vitro study of the antibacterial activity of essential oils and their major components against the major bacteria-causing respiratory tract infection indicated that cinnamon bark oil was effective against *Haemophilus influenzae*, *Streptococcus pneumoniae* and *S. pyogenes* (Inouye et al 2001).

Oral pathogens

According to in vitro research, cinnamon bark oil is an effective inhibitor of bacteria-causing dental caries and periodontal disease (Saeki et al 1989).

Carminative

The essential oil exhibits carminative activity and decreases smooth muscle contractions in guinea-pig trachea and ileum, and in dog ileum, colon and stomach (WHO 2004). The oil has also demonstrated antifoaming activity in a foam generator model for flatulence (ESCOP 2003). The active antispasmodic constituent is considered to be cinnamaldehyde.

Hypoglycaemic activity

Using an experimental model of diabetes, Kim et al (2006) observed that cinnamon extract significantly reduced blood glucose levels after two weeks of treatment. Both A- and B-type procyanidin oligomers in different *Cinnamon cassia* extracts have been identified as having hypoglycaemic activity and may improve insulin sensitivity in the treatment of rats with induced type 2 diabetes (Lu et al 2011). In vitro studies on related species of cinnamon, with the same polyphenols as *C. cassia,* have also demonstrated potential for hypoglycaemic effects (Cao et al 2010).

Enhanced insulin sensitivity

Water-soluble compounds extracted from *C. cassia* potentiate insulin activity, as measured by glucose oxidation in the rat epididymal fat-cell assay. The most active compound, methylhydroxy chalcone polymer (MHCP), increased glucose metabolism approximately 20-fold and was an effective mimetic of insulin according to an in vitro study. When combined with insulin, the responses were greater than additive, indicating synergism between the two compounds (Jarvill-Taylor et al 2001). According to Anderson et al (2004), MHCP is actually a water-soluble polyphenolic type-A polymer that increases insulin sensitivity by activating the key enzymes that stimulate insulin receptors, while inhibiting the enzymes that deactivate them. More specifically, extracts of cinnamon activate insulin receptor kinase and inhibit dephosphorylation of the insulin receptor, leading to maximal phosphorylation of the insulin receptor.

The United States Agricultural Research Service has filed a patent application on the active substances.

Anti-atherosclerotic activity

Data from animal experiments suggest that cinnamon may be of benefit in controlling lipid metabolism (Jin et al 2010, Qin et al 2008). In an in-vivo and ex-vivo animal study, rats and hamsters were fed a high-fructose diet and given an olive oil loading and a water soluble cinnamon extract, called Cinnulin PF (10 or 50 mg/kg body weight). Cinnulin PF is a 20 : 1 extract of whole cinnamon powder, standardised to contain at least 3% of the active type A polyphenols. The treatment induced an acute inhibition of elevated postprandial serum triglycerides and an overproduction of intestinal apoB48-lipoproteins. The observed intestinal effects of the cinnamon extract were partly mediated by regulating both abnormal mRNA expression of intestinal insulin signalling and the key proteins involved in intestinal lipoprotein metabolism. The cinnamon extract improved insulin sensitivity in the rats' intestinal enterocytes (Qin et al 2008).

In vitro studies have demonstrated that cinnamon hydrophilic extracts exhibit strong anti-glycation activity; inhibit copper-mediated LDL oxidation and LDL phagocytosis by macrophages; display some ferric ion removal ability; and also exhibit hypolipidaemic activity in vivo. These activities indicate potential in the treatment of chronic metabolic diseases (Jin et al 2010).

Antitumour activity

Cinnamon extract displayed antitumour activity when administered orally or by intra-tumour injection (Kwon et al 2009). It strongly inhibited the expression of pro-angiogenic factors and master regulators of tumour progression. The effects were seen not only in melanoma cell lines but also in an experimental melanoma model. In addition, cinnamon extract treatment increased the anti-tumour activities of $CD8^+$ T cells by increasing the levels of cytolytic molecules and their cytotoxic activity. These findings are important as tumour cells recruit new blood vessels by excessive production of pro-angiogenic factors that play a pivotal role in tumour progression and tumour survival.

According to a study in mice grafted with human melanoma cells, cinnamon effectively impaired human metastatic melanoma cell proliferation and tumour growth. The equivalent dose in humans is 120 mg/kg daily, which is large. This chemopreventive and chemotherapeutic anti-cancer activity occurs via different intracellular mechanisms, namely G1 cell-cycle arrest, elevated intracellular ROS and impairing invasiveness (Cabello et al 2009). Aqueous extract of cinnamon has also been shown to disrupt the G2/M phase of leukaemic cells in vitro affecting cell proliferation (Schoene et al 2009).

Anti-allergy and anti-asthmatic effects

Cinnamon extract mediates anti-allergy activities in vitro, by reducing degranulation, reducing cysteinyl leukotriene production and reducing the expression of proinflammatory cytokines and proteases in human intestinal mast cells (Hagenlocher et al 2012).

Animal studies using type-A procyanidine polyphenols from *Cinnamomum zeylanicum* bark showed anti-asthmatic effects, and may have potential as a therapeutic agent in asthma management. This study demonstrated histological reductions in lung inflammation, increased oxygen supply to the cells, reduction in goblet cell hyperplasia, reduced mucous secretion, reduced inflammatory cell infiltrates (eosinophils) and mast cell stabilisation. Overall an anti-inflammatory, bronchoprotective and mucolytic potential was suggested; however, additional studies are needed to fully elucidate the exact mechanism (Kandhare et al 2013).

OTHER ACTIONS

A myriad of other effects have been demonstrated in various in vitro and animal models.

Cinnamon extract may have anti-depressant activity, according to research with a preclinical model. An evaluation of rat behaviours in a forced swimming test showed that *C. zeylanicum* at both 150 and 300 mg/kg had similar effects to imipramine (Emamghoreishi & Ghasemi 2011).

In vitro studies suggest that type A cinnamon polyphenols may exhibit neuroprotective effects by upregulating prosurvival proteins, activating mitogen-activated protein kinase pathways and decreasing proinflammatory cytokines (Qin et al 2013).

Potent antioxidant and anti-inflammatory activity for cinnamon bark oil has been demonstrated in vitro and for the dry ethanolic extract in vivo (ESCOP 2003, Jarvill-Taylor et al 2001, Lee et al 2003, Mathew & Abraham 2006).

A dose-dependent antinociceptive activity has been demonstrated for *Cinnamomum zeylanicum* when administered orally to mice in the hot plate and acetic acid writhing induced tests (Atta & Alkofahi 1998).

C. cassia also possesses antipyretic activity (Kurokawa et al 1998) and reduced the occurrence of ulcers in rats in a dose-dependent manner in a study that administered an aqueous extract (Tanaka et al 1989).

Besides antispasmodic and broad-spectrum antibacterial and fungicidal activities, cinnamaldehyde exhibits antitumour effects (Kwon et al 1998) and cytotoxicity (Moon & Pack 1983).

C. zeylanicum exhibits strong inhibitory effects on osteoclast-like cell formation without affecting cell viability (Tsuji-Naito 2008). This finding presents a novel approach in the treatment of osteopenic disease and warrants further investigation.

CLINICAL USE

Cinnamon has been used as a medicinal agent in several traditional healing systems. In the last two decades, scientific investigation has been undertaken to investigate its clinical effects. Evidence to support its clinical use is predominantly derived from in vitro and in vivo research, and from traditional usage; however, an increasing number of clinical trials are now being published.

Dyspepsia and related symptoms

Cinnamon bark oil and crushed cinnamon bark is used in the treatment of dyspeptic conditions, such as mild spastic conditions of the gastrointestinal tract, fullness and flatulence, loss of appetite and diarrhoea. Although controlled studies are unavailable, evidence of antispasmodic and antifoaming activity in animal models and a long tradition of use provide some support for its use in these indications.

Cinnamon bark and Chinese cinnamon are approved by the German Commission E for the treatment of loss of appetite and dyspeptic complaints such as mild gastrointestinal spasms, bloating and flatulence (Blumenthal et al 1998).

Helicobacter pylori infection

A placebo-controlled study of 15 volunteers, 11 women and 4 men aged 16–79 years, with documented *H. pylori* infection, demonstrated that an ethanolic extract of cinnamon was ineffective at eradicating the infection, when used at a dose of 40 mg twice daily for 4 weeks (Nir et al 2000). Considering this is an extremely low dose, and *C. cassia* extracts significantly inhibit *Helicobacter pylori* in vitro to a greater or equal extent than commonly used antibiotics (Tabak et al 1999), further research may be warranted.

Diabetes and blood glucose regulation

Cinnamon has a long history of use for diabetes in China, India, Korea and Russia. Additionally, a plethora of studies have shown the beneficial metabolic effects of cinnamon and its components in vitro and in animal models. To date, clinical investigations into the effects of cinnamon on blood glucose regulation have produced mixed results. There are several possible explanations for this, which should be addressed in future studies.

Theories proposed to explain inconsistent clinical results

It appears that duration of use, dosage and baseline glycaemic levels may be important factors influencing results and worthy of further investigation. Additionally, effects on type 2 diabetes (T2DM) are more promising than type 1 diabetes (T1DM), which could be expected as T1DM is primarily a disease of insulin secretion and not insulin resistance. Another factor is the type of cinnamon used as many different species are available in commercial products and they may differ in chemical composition and resultant activities. For example, some studies have used the water-soluble extract of cinnamon, rather than the whole spice. Unfortunately, some studies do not specify which cinnamon has been used, making interpretation of the evidence difficult. Finally, the concomitant diabetic drugs used may also be a factor. An initial and very successful study, showing that oral cinnamon had significant effects on fasting glucose levels involved patients also taking sulfonylurea drugs, which increase insulin secretion; increased secretion coupled with the role of cinnamon in reducing insulin resistance may have led to improved outcomes (Rafehi et al 2012).

The first major study suggesting oral cinnamon may be useful in T2DM was reported in 2003 (Khan et al 2003). The randomised, placebo-controlled study of 60 people demonstrated that cinnamon extracts at all test doses (1, 3 or 6 g daily) produced a clinically significant glucose- and lipid-lowering effect. The volunteers were not using insulin therapy and had a fasting blood glucose reading between 140 and 400 mg/dL. After 40 days of treatment, all three doses of cinnamon reduced mean fasting serum glucose by 18 to 29%, triglycerides by 23 to 30%, LDL-cholesterol by 7 to 27% and total cholesterol by 12 to 26%. No significant changes were observed in the placebo groups. The effect on glucose and lipid levels was sustained 20 days after treatment had ceased, suggesting that cinnamon would not need to be consumed every day. The cinnamon used was *C. cassia*, which was finely ground and put into capsules.

Since then, numerous other interventional studies have been performed, allowing for systematic reviews and meta-analyses to be conducted, producing inconsistent conclusions.

A 2013 systematic review and meta-analysis of ten RCTs (n = 543) reported that cinnamon in doses of 120 mg to 6 g per day for 4 to 18 weeks was associated with a significant decrease in levels of fasting plasma glucose, total cholesterol, LDL-C and triglyceride levels. Cinnamon also significantly increased levels of HDL-C but had no significant effect on HbA_{1C} (Allen et al 2013).

In 2012 several systematic reviews and meta-analyses were also published.

A 2012 Cochrane review reported that cinnamon did not significantly affected HbA_{1C} levels, serum insulin or postprandial glucose when administered at a mean dose of 2 g daily, for a period of 4 to 16 weeks (Leach & Kumar 2012). Importantly, they combined studies involving people with either type 1 or type 2 diabetes and analysed results from 10 prospective, parallel-group design, randomised controlled trials, involving a total of 577 participants. The authors concluded there is insufficient evidence to support the use of cinnamon for type 1 or type 2 diabetes and stated that poor trial reporting standards was a major problem.

Rafehi et al (2012) reviewed 16 clinical studies of which only five found no significant effect on the parameters studied, while all of the other studies found significant beneficial changes caused by cinnamon. Of the studies conducted, five investigated the effects of cinnamon consumption in healthy individuals and six studies investigated effects in individuals with T2DM. The remaining studies have investigated the effects of cinnamon in people with T1DM, metabolic syndrome, impaired fasting glucose, postmenopausal women and women with polycystic ovarian syndrome. Of the five studies performed in healthy individuals, four showed some beneficial effects of cinnamon, whereas only one did not. The authors concluded that positive results were most often seen in studies of at least 12 weeks duration and less likely in short-term studies. Since cinnamon is believed to promote insulin sensitivity, it may be expected that the effectiveness would be greater in those whose disease state was more progressed such as in T2DM, rather than those with milder insulin resistance or minimal insulin resistance.

Another 2012 systematic review and meta-analysis was conducted using results from six clinical trials (n = 435). Test doses ranged from 1–6 g cinnamon per day, with follow-up periods from 40 days to 4 months. The review also concluded that the majority of studies did not demonstrate therapeutic efficacy for people with T2DM but acknowledged that cinnamon may be a viable addition to conventional diabetes management in patients with an HbA_{1C} exceeding 7%. The meta-analysis demonstrated that the short-term effects of cinnamon on glycaemic control were promising (Akilen et al 2012). The HbA_{1C} cut-off had been demonstrated previously in a randomised study by Akilen et al (2012), which showed that 2 g daily of encapsulated cinnamon powder (*C. cassia*) over 12 weeks significantly decreased HbA_{1C} ($P < 0.005$) compared to placebo in volunteers with T2DM, $HbA_{1C} > 7\%$ and treated with hypoglycaemic agents that remained unchanged during the study.

Since these reviews and meta-analyses were published, three more clinical trials have been published, demonstrating positive results.

One small 2012 clinical study of 15 young adults, testing apple cider vinegar and cinnamon, alone and combined, showed that cinnamon may mitigate postprandial blood glucose in healthy adults, but has no impact on satiety (Chezem et al 2012). Another trial (n = 30) using 6 g of ground cinnamon indicated that the postprandial glucose response in both obese and normal weight adults may be moderated by cinnamon (Magistrelli & Chezem 2012). In addition, a trial of 66 Chinese subjects with T2DM taking only gliclazide showed that a water-extracted Chinese cinnamon supplementation (at 120 and 360 mg/day) for 3 months was able to significantly improve blood glucose in this cohort. The low dose cinnamon group also demonstrated reduced blood triglycerides (Lu et al 2012).

Gestational diabetes

A randomised, double-blind placebo-controlled study of 51 women with gestational diabetes found that 6 weeks of treatment with 1 g of cinnamon daily produced a trend towards decreased insulin requirements (53.85% cinnamon vs 44% placebo, $P = 0.58$); however, this did not reach significance (Graham et al 2005). The cinnamon used was *C. cassia*. The researchers suggested that a longer duration of treatment may be required to produce better results.

Hypertension

In 2010, Akilen et al demonstrated that a dose of 2 g daily of encapsulated cinnamon powder (*C. cassia*) over 12 weeks significantly decreased systolic and diastolic blood pressure compared to placebo (systolic blood pressure 129 vs 135, P = 0.011; diastolic blood pressure 81 vs. 86, P = 0.008) in volunteers with T2DM, $HbA_{1C} > 7\%$ and treated with hypoglycaemic and antihyperlipidaemic agents that remained unchanged during the study. Salt, carbohydrate and protein intake was similar for the two groups during the test period.

A systematic review and meta-analysis of three studies evaluated the short-term effect of cinnamon on blood pressure regulation in patients with prediabetes and type 2 diabetes. Cinnamon significantly decreased SBP and DBP by 5.39 mmHg (95% CI, −6.89 to −3.89) and 2.6 mmHg (95% CI, −4.53 to −0.66) respectively (Akilen et al 2013).

Metabolic syndrome

A water-soluble extract of cinnamon (Cinnulin PF 500 mg/day) significantly reduced fasting blood glucose, systolic blood pressure and increased lean body mass according to a placebo-controlled trial of 22 subjects with prediabetes and metabolic syndrome (Ziegenfuss et al 2006). The study was conducted over 12 weeks and also detected small but statistically significant decreases in body fat in the cinnamon-treated group when within-group analyses were performed.

Polycystic ovarian syndrome

A pilot study involving 15 non-diabetic women with oligomenorrhoea or amenorrhoea and polycystic ovaries compared cinnamon (333 mg cinnamon extract taken three times a day) to placebo (Wang et al 2007). The randomised study found oral cinnamon extract resulted in a significant reduction in fasting glucose as well as insulin resistance, as measured by various indices of insulin sensitivity from fasting and oral glucose tolerance test (OGTT) values. Specifically, fasting glucose was reduced by 17% during the 8-week treatment period. The reduction in insulin resistance appears to be mediated through an increase in glucose utilisation, as there were no significant alterations in hyperinsulinaemia measured by fasting insulin or mean insulin levels during OGTT. These preliminary findings are consistent with prior in vivo animal and human studies.

OTHER USES

Administration of 3 g cinnamon for 6 weeks in 60 athletic women resulted in a reduction in muscle soreness but no significant effect on IL-6 levels (Mashhadi et al 2013a), body composition or exercise performance (Mashhadi et al 2013b).

Traditional uses

Cinnamon has been used traditionally by ancient healers from many backgrounds for stomach cramps, flatulence, nausea, vomiting, diarrhoea, infant colic, common infections and also female reproductive problems such as dysmenorrhoea, menorrhagia, lactation and pain in childbirth. It has also been used as an ingredient in topical preparations for pain and inflammation. Cinnamon is often used in combination with other herbs and spices for most of these indications. In TCM it is considered to warm the kidneys and fortify yang, so is used for impotence, among other indications. In Ayurvedic medicine and in China, Korea and Russia, it has long been used as a treatment for diabetes.

Practice points/Patient counselling

- Cinnamon has been used since ancient times as a flavouring and medicinal agent.
- It is a natural food preservative with antioxidant and wide-ranging antimicrobial and antifungal properties.
- It has been used traditionally to treat dyspepsia, nausea, flatulence, poor appetite, stomach cramps and diarrhoea. Some evidence suggests it may be effective for some of these indications.
- Whether ground cinnamon (*C. cassia*) reduces blood glucose and lipid levels and can be useful for people with type 2 diabetes is uncertain as clinical studies have produced mixed results — individuals wanting to try cinnamon should try a 12-week trial to determine whether they respond.
- Cinnamon oil can cause allergic contact dermatitis when used topically and should be avoided by people with allergies to cinnamon or Peru balsam, pregnant women or those with active gastrointestinal ulcers.

Natural food preservative

Spices such as cinnamon have been used traditionally to preserve food products. The considerable antimicrobial, fungicidal and antioxidant properties of cinnamon provide a theoretical basis for its use.

DOSAGE RANGE

General guide

- Dried bark (crushed cinnamon): 1.5–4 g taken up to four times daily.
- Fluid extract 1 : 1: 0.5–1.0 mL taken up to three times daily.
- Tea: half to three-quarters teaspoon of powdered cinnamon in a cup of boiling water taken 2–3 times daily with meals.
- Essential oil: 0.05–0.2 mL diluted in carrier oil.

According to clinical studies

Diabetes Type 2

- 1–6 g daily of powdered cinnamon (*C. cassia*) — a 12-week trial will determine whether an individual responds

Loss of appetite or digestive complaints

- Essential oil: 0.05–0.2 g daily.
- Fluid extract (1 : 1 g/mL): 0.7–1.3 mL three times daily.
- Infusion or decoction: 0.7–1.3 g in 150 mL water three times daily.
- Tea: 1–4.5 g daily using *C. cassia* bark.

TOXICITY

The oral LD_{50} for cinnamon bark oil in rats is 4.16 g/kg and 3.4 mL/kg body weight.

ADVERSE REACTIONS

When the powdered herb is ingested orally, it is generally well tolerated; however, when cinnamon oil is applied topically, allergic reactions are possible as cinnamaldehyde may cause allergic contact dermatitis (Cheung et al 2003).

SIGNIFICANT INTERACTIONS

Controlled studies are not available, therefore interactions are based on pharmacological activity and are largely theoretical and speculative.

Hypoglycaemic agents

Oral ingestion of cinnamon capsules may reduce blood glucose levels, therefore theoretically, an additive effect is possible with concurrent use — observe; potential beneficial interaction under professional supervision.

CONTRAINDICATIONS AND PRECAUTIONS

Cinnamon is contraindicated in people with an allergy to cinnamon or Peru balsam, in cases of fever of unknown origin or active stomach or duodenal ulcers (WHO 2004).

PREGNANCY USE

C. cassia or *C. zeylanicum/verum* should not be used in pregnancy; however, usual dietary intakes are likely to be safe. Currently, evidence of teratogenicity from animal studies is contradictory.

PATIENTS' FAQs

What will this herb do for me?
Cinnamon is a natural food preservative with wide-ranging antimicrobial and antifungal properties. It may improve digestion and ease symptoms of dyspepsia, flatulence and nausea. It may also lower blood glucose, total cholesterol and triglyceride levels, however more research is required to confirm these effects and the best dose and form.

When will it start to work?
The effects on digestion should start rapidly; however, effects on blood glucose and lipid levels may take 1 month or more.

Are there any safety issues?
Cinnamon oil can cause allergic contact dermatitis when used topically and should be avoided by people with allergies to cinnamon or Peru balsam, pregnant women or those with active gastrointestinal ulcers.

REFERENCES

Akilen R et al. Cinnamon in glycaemic control: Systematic review and metaanalysis, Clinical Nutrition 31 (2012): 609–615.

Akilen R et al. Effect of short-term administration of cinnamon on blood pressure in patients with prediabetes and type 2 diabetes, Nutrition, 29.10 (2013): 1192–1196.

Allen RW et al. Cinnamon use in type 2 diabetes: an updated systematic review and meta-analysis. Ann Fam Med 11.5 (2013): 452–459.

Anderson RA et al. Isolation and characterization of polyphenol type-A polymers from cinnamon with insulin-like biological activity. J Agric Food Chem 52 (2004): 65–70.

Atta AH, Alkofahi A. Anti-nociceptive and anti-inflammatory effects of some Jordanian medicinal plant extracts. J Ethnopharmacol 60.2 (1998): 117–124.

Blumenthal M et al. The complete German Commission E monographs: therapeutic guide to herbal medicines. Austin, TX: American Botanical Council, 1998.

Cabello CM et al. The cinnamon-derived Michael acceptor cinnamic aldehyde impairs melanoma cell proliferation, invasiveness, and tumor growth, Free Rad Biol Med 46.2 (2009): 220–231.

Castleman M. Cinnamon. In: The healing herbs. Schwartz Books, Melbourne (1991), pp. 115–118.

Cheung C, Hotchkiss SA, Pease CK. Cinnamic compound metabolism in human skin and the role metabolism may play in determining relative sensitisation potency. J Dermatol Sci 31.1 (2003): 9–19.

Chezem J et al. Effects of Ground Cinnamon and Apple Cider Vinegar on Postprandial Blood Glucose Levels in Healthy Adults, Journal of the Academy of Nutrition and Dietetics, 112.9 (2012): A43.

Cao H, Graves DJ, Anderson RA. Cinnamon extract regulates glucose transporter and insulin-signaling gene expression in mouse adipocytes, Phytomedicien 17.13 (2010): 1027–1032.

De M, Krishna DA, Banerjee AB. Antimicrobial screening of some Indian spices. Phytother Res 13.7 (1999): 616–618.

Emamghoreishi M, Ghasemi F. Antidepressant Effect of Aqueous and Hydroalcoholic Extracts of Cinnamon zeylanicum in the Forced Swimming Test, Asian Journal of Psychiatry 4 Sup 1 (2011): S44.

European Scientific Co-operative On Phytomedicine (ESCOP). Cinnamomi cortex. In: ESCOP Monographs, 2nd edn. Stuttgart: Thieme (2003): 92–97.

Friedman M, Buick R, Elliott CT. Antibacterial activities of naturally occurring compounds against antibiotic-resistant Bacillus cereus vegetative cells and spores, Escherichia coli, and Staphylococcus aureus. J Food Prot 67.8 (2004): 1774–1778.

Friedman M, Henika PR, Mandrell RE. Bactericidal activities of plant essential oils and some of their isolated constituents against Campylobacter jejuni, Escherichia coli, Listeria monocytogenes, and Salmonella enterica. J Food Prot 65.10 (2002): 1545–1560.

Giordani R et al. Potentiation of antifungal activity of amphotericin B by essential oil from Cinnamomum cassia. Phytother Res 20.1 (2006): 58–61.

Graham F et al. Cinnamon for glycemic control in gestational diabetes: A randomized double-blind placebo controlled pilot study. Am J Obst Gynecol 193.6 (Suppl 1) (2005): S91.

Guynot ME et al. Antifungal activity of volatile compounds generated by essential oils against fungi commonly causing deterioration of bakery products. J Appl Microbiol 94.5 (2003): 893–899.

Hagenlocher Y et al. Cinnamon extract strongly reduces IgE-Dependent activation of Mast Cells, Clinical Nutrition Supplements 7.1 (2012): 91.

Inouye S, Yamaguchi H, Takizawa T. Screening of the antibacterial effects of a variety of essential oils on respiratory tract pathogens, using a modified dilution assay method. J Infect Chemother 7.4 (2001): 251–254.

Jarvill-Taylor KJ, Anderson RA, Graves DJ. A hydroxychalcone derived from cinnamon functions as a mimetic for insulin in 3T3-L1 adipocytes. J Am Coll Nutr 20.4 (2001): 327–336.

Jin SR et al. Water extracts of cinnamon and clove exhibits potent inhibition of protein clycation and anti-atherosclerotic activity in vitro and in vivo, Atherosclerosis Supplements 11.2 (2010): 109–222.

Kandhare AD et al. Anti-asthmatic effects of type-A procyanidine polyphenols from cinnamon bark in ovalbumin-induced airway hyperresponsiveness in laboratory animals. Biomedicine & Aging Pathology 3(2013): 23–30.

Khan A et al. Cinnamon improves glucose and lipids of people with type 2 diabetes. Diabetes Care 26.1 (2003): 3215–32118.

Kim SH et al. Anti-diabetic effect of cinnamon extract on blood glucose in db/db mice. J Ethnopharmacol 104.1–2 (2006): 119–123.

Kurokawa M et al. Antipyretic activity of cinnamyl derivatives and related compounds in influenza virus-infected mice. Eur J Pharmacol 348.1 (1998): 45–51.

Kwon BM et al. Synthesis and in vitro cytotoxicity of cinnamaldehydes to human solid tumor cells. Arch Pharm Res 21.2 (1998): 147–152.

Kwon HK et al. Cinnamon extract suppresses tumor progression by modulating angiogenesis and the effector function of CD8+ T cells. Cancer Lett 278.2 (2009): 174–182.

Leach, MJ, Kumar, S Cinnamon for diabetes mellitus, Cochrane Database Syst Rev, 9 (2012).

Lee SE et al. Screening of medicinal plant extracts for antioxidant activity. Life Sci 73.2 (2003): 167–179.

Lu T et al. Cinnamon extract improves fasting blood glucose and glycosylated hemoglobin levels in Chinese patients with type 2 diabetes, Nutirtion Research 32 (2012): 408–412.

Lu Z et al. Hypoglycemic activities of A- and B-type procyanidin oligomer-rich extracts from different Cinnamon barks, Phytomedicine 18.4 (2011): 298–302.

Magistrelli A, Chezem JC. Effect of Ground Cinnamon on Postprandial Blood Glucose Concentreationin Normal-Weight and Obese Adults, J Acad Nutr Diet 112 (2012): 1806–1809.

Mashhadi NS et al. Influence of ginger and cinnamon intake on inflammation and muscle soreness endued by exercise in Iranian female athletes, Int J Prev Med 4.1 (2013a): S11–15.

Mashhadi, NS et al. Effect of ginger and cinnamon intake on oxidative stress and exercise performance and body composition in Iranian female athletes, Int J Prev Med 4.1 (2013b): S31–35.

Matan N et al. Antimicrobial activity of cinnamon and clove oils under modified atmosphere conditions. Int J Food Microbiol 107.2 (2006): 180–185.

Mathew S, Abraham TE. Studies on the antioxidant activities of cinnamon (Cinnamomum verum) bark extracts, through various in vitro models. Food Chem 94.4 (2006): 520–528.

Moghim, H, Shahabi GA. Comparison of antifungal effects of extracts of marigold, cinnamon, garlic and thyme on candida albicans, Clinical Biochemistry 44. 13 (2011): S339.

Moon KH, Pack MY. Cytotoxicity of cinnamic aldehyde on leukemia L1210 cells. Drug Chem Toxicol 6.6 (1983): 521–535.

Nir Y et al. Controlled trial of the effect of cinnamon extract on Helicobacter pylori. Helicobacter 5.2 (2000): 94–97.

Qin B et al. Cinnamon extract inhibits the postprandial overproduction of apolipoprotein B48-containing lipoproteins in fructose-fed animals, J. Nut Bio 20.11 (2008): 901–908.

Qin, B, Panickar, KS, Anderson, RA, Cinnamon polyphenols regulate S100beta, sirtuins, and neuroactive proteins in rat C6 glioma cells, Nutrition. Nov 12. (2013) pii: S0899-9007(13)00333-X. doi: 10.1016/j.nut.2013.07.001.

Rafehi H, Ververis K, Karagiannis TC. Diabetes, Obesity and Metabolism 14 (2012): 493–499.

Saeki Y et al. Antimicrobial action of natural substances on oral bacteria. Bull Tokyo Dent Coll 30.3 (1989): 129–135.

Schoene NW et al. A polyphenol mixture from cinnamon targets p38 MAP kinase-regulated signaling pathways to produce G2/M arrest, Journal of Nutritional Biochemistry 20 (2009): 614–620.
Simic A et al. The chemical composition of some Lauraceae essential oils and their antifungal activities. Phytother Res 18.9 (2004): 713–717.
Tabak M, Armon R, Neeman I. Cinnamon extract's inhibitory effect on Helicobacter pylori. J Ethnopharmacol 67.3 (1999): 269–277.
Tampieri MP et al. The inhibition of Candida albicans by selected essential oils and their major components. Mycopathologia 159.3 (2005): 339–345.
Tanaka S et al. Antiulcerogenic compounds isolated from Chinese cinnamon. Planta Med 55.3 (1989): 245–248.
Tsuji-Naito K. Aldehydic components of Cinnamon bark extract suppresses RANKL-induced osteoclastogensis through NFATc1 downregulation, Bioorganic & Medicinal Chemistry 16 (2008) 9176–9183
Wang JG et al. The effect of cinnamon extract on insulin resistance parameters in polycystic ovary syndrome: a pilot study. Fertility and Sterility 88.1 (2007): 240–243.
WHO (World Health Organization). Cortex Cinnamomi. In: WHO Monographs on Selected Medicinal Plants, Geneva: WHO, 2004.
Ziegenfuss TN et al. Effects of a water-soluble cinnamon extract on body composition and features of the metabolic syndrome in pre-diabetic men and women. J Int Soc Sports Nutr 3 (2006): 45–53.

C

Cloves

HISTORICAL NOTE Spices such as cloves have been used as food preservatives, disinfectants and antiseptics for centuries (De et al 1999). Modern research has confirmed that cloves are an effective preservative that inhibits the growth of many food-poisoning and food-spoiling bacteria.

COMMON NAME

Cloves

OTHER NAMES

Oil of cloves, Oleum caryophylli, *Eugenia carylophyllata*, *Eugenia aromatica*, *Caryophyllus aromaticus*, Myrtaceae

SCIENTIFIC NAME

Syzygium aromaticum (family Myrtaceae)

PLANT PART USED

Dried flower buds (clove oil is distilled from this plant part)

CHEMICAL COMPONENTS

The main constituent of clove oil is eugenol. Other components include beta-caryophyllene, acetyl eugenol, isoeugenol, eugenine, kaemferol, tannins, gallic acid, vitamin C, minerals (boron, calcium, chromium, iron, manganese, magnesium, potassium, phosphorus) and flavonoids (Nassar 2006).

MAIN ACTIONS

Because of cloves' significant eugenol content, most pharmacological activity is based on studies involving eugenol.

Local analgesic, local anaesthetic and anti-inflammatory

The analgesic action of clove oil and aqueous extract of clove has been established in animal models. It is mainly due to the eugenol component, although other active constituents also exist. Recently, an aqueous extract of clove demonstrated significant analgesic activity that is reversible by naloxone, indicating it is mediated by an opiate pathway (Kamkar et al 2012). Eugenol acts on contact to depress nociceptors, the sensory receptors involved in pain perception (Brodin & Roed 1984). Eugenol also inhibits prostaglandin biosynthesis through potent cyclooxygenase-1 (COX-1) and COX-2 inhibitory activity (Huss et al 2002, Kelm et al 2000) and modulates inflammatory pathways by inhibiting the release of leukotrienes (Kamatou et al 2012, Raghavenra et al 2006). According to experiments with an animal model, daily doses of eugenol produce a cumulative effect after 5 days of continuous administration, producing a statistically significant reduction in neuropathic pain (Guénette et al 2007). Although eugenol is chiefly responsible for much of the pharmacological activity of cloves, other constituents are also involved (Ghelardini et al 2001a). Eugenol is thought to activate vanilloid 1 receptors, resulting in the modulation of pain (Kamatou et al 2012). In an induced osteoarthritis rat model, daily oral administration of eugenol (40 mg/kg) resulted in improved gait parameters, decreased levels of spinal substance P and calcitonin gene-related peptide and increased dynorphin (Ferland et al 2012).

Inhibitory 15-lipo-oxygenase (LOX) and 5-LOX (involved in asthma and allergic rhinitis) activity of clove has also been demonstrated (Kamatou et al 2012).

Beta-caryophyllene is another key component of clove oil, which exhibits significant anti-inflammatory and rapid local anaesthetic activity in several animal models (Ghelardini et al 2001b, Muruganandan et al 2001). Local anaesthetic effects develop within 5 minutes of application and diminish after about 15 minutes.

Fungicidal

Clove oil has an inhibitory effect against yeasts and fungi in vitro (Arora & Kaur 1999). Cloves are effective against species belonging to the *Eurotium*, *Aspergillus* and *Penicillium* genera in vitro (Guynot et al 2003) and clove essential oil has exhibited strong antifungal activity against *Aspergillus* and aflatoxigenic strains (Bluma et al 2008, Viuda-Martos et al 2007), as well as various other fungal and dermatophyte species (Park et al 2007, Pinto et al 2009), including fluconazole-resistant strains of *Candida* spp. and *Aspergillus* spp. (Kamatou et al 2012, Pinto et al 2009).

Experiments with animal models have identified significant activity against *Candida albicans*. Vaginal candidiasis responded to treatment of topical application of clove oil in animal models, suggesting that further investigation is warranted to determine clinical relevance (Ahmad et al 2005). Another animal experiment found that oral intake of cloves reduced *Candida albicans* growth in the alimentary tract (Taguchi et al 2005). The eugenol component is important for such effects, as in vitro experiments identified that eugenol displays anticandidal activity by affecting the envelope of the organism (Braga et al 2007, Fu et al 2007), specifically through the disruption of the cell membrane sterol pathway (thus decreasing ergosterol, a fungi-specific cell membrane component), leading to cell demise (Kamatou et al 2012, Pinto et al 2009).

Antibacterial

Antibacterial activity has also been demonstrated for cloves and several of its key constituents. Cloves has activity against Gram-negative, anaerobic, periodontal oral pathogens, including *Porphyromonas gingivalis* and *Prevotella intermedia* (Cai & Wu 1996), *Streptoccocus mutans* strains and *Streptoccocus salivarius* and 15 other strains of pathogenic bacteria frequently involved in tooth decay and other oral pathologies (Koba et al 2011). In vitro experiments demonstrated a synergistic effect of clove oil and gentamicin against 11 strains of cariogenic bacteria. Eugenol also demonstrated a synergistic effect, except for *S. mutans* and *S. ratti*. A synergistic effect was also demonstrated for both clove oil and eugenol and ampicillin against all 11 strains tested (Moon et al 2011).

Hydroethanolic extract of clove showed significant antimicrobial activity against nosocomial strain isolates of *Klebsiella pneumoniae, Escherichia coli* and *C. albicans* (Khan et al 2009). Clove oil also produced a significant decrease in *K. pneumoniae* colonies in the lung of mice induced with acute pneumonia (Saini et al 2009).

Activity has also been demonstrated against *Bacillus subtilis*, *Listeria monocytogenes*, *Salmonella enterica*, *E. coli* and *Saccharomyces cerevisiae* (Burt & Reinders 2003, Chami et al 2005, De et al 1999, Dorman & Deans 2000, Friedman et al 2002, Fu et al 2007) and *Staphylococcus epidermidis* (Fu et al 2007). Ethanolic extract of clove showed superior activity to a garlic extract against a variety of Gram-negative and Gram-positive food-associated bacteria and moulds, including *Staphyloccocus aureus* and *E. coli* (Pundir et al 2010). Aqueous extract of cloves demonstrated a strong inhibitory action against six *Helicobacter pylori* strains in vitro (Yang et al 2005).

Eugenol is thought to act through disruption and destruction of the cytoplasmic membrane via rapid ATPase inhibition and release (Devi et al 2010, Gill & Holley 2006a, 2006b). Hemaiswarya and Doble (2009) demonstrated a 50% membrane integrity loss after a 10-minute exposure to eugenol in vitro. Furthermore, a synergistic interaction of eugenol with hydrophilic antibiotics (vancomycin, β-lactam, ampicillin, gentamicin) against Gram-negative bacteria has been demonstrated, with no cytotoxic effects to erythrocytes (effects to erythrocytes is a measurement of substance toxicity) (Hemaiswarya & Doble 2009, Kamatou et al 2012). Further pharmacodynamic studies are needed to establish an effective dosage and potential as treatment strategy to reduce antibiotic resistance and toxicity in clinical trials (Hemaiswarya & Doble 2009).

Antiviral

In vitro assays have identified inhibitory effects on hepatitis C virus protease (Hussein et al 2000) and human cytomegalovirus (Shiraki et al 1998, Yukawa et al 1996). An animal model confirmed significant activity against herpes simplex virus type 1 (Kurokawa et al 1998). An inhibitory effect against parasitic growth has been demonstrated in vitro for clove oil (Santoro et al 2007).

Acaricidal

Clove essential oil and eugenol demonstrated potential for further in vivo and clinical trials for acaricidal properties against permethrin-resistant and permethrin-sensitive scabies mites (*Sarcoptes scabiei*). In vitro bioassays against live populations of scabies mites showed clove oil and eugenol to be of toxicity levels equivalent or superior to the positive control benzyl benzoate (a topical acaricide). The acaricidal effect was more rapid in sensitive specimens than non-sensitive ones.

Antiprotozoan

The essential oil of clove and eugenol inhibited the adhesion of *Giardia lamblia* to bovine epithelial cells in vitro by altering viability, adherence and incubation time. The essential oil, but not eugenol, induced death by lysis, suggesting another constituent is responsible. No cytotoxic effect on the bovine epithelial cells was noted (Machado et al 2011).

Antioxidant

Several constituents within the flower have antioxidant activity, especially eugenol, which has been the focus of most antioxidant research (Duke 2002). Studies with cloves and eugenol have demonstrated protective effects against several agents, which cause damage to cells and tissues via an oxidative stress mechanism.

Cloves illustrated a protective effect against a cytotoxic agent (peroxynitrite) that causes damage to proteins, lipids and DNA (Ho et al 2008) and significantly reversed isoprenaline-induced cardiac hypertrophy in rats (Choudhary et al 2006). In other studies, eugenol was shown to reduce radiation-induced membrane damage (Pandey et al 2006), and to demonstrate a 97.3% inhibition of lipid peroxidation (Gülçin et al 2012, Kabuto et al 2007) and increase glutathione (Kabuto et al 2007). Further activities against a number of reactive oxygen species were demonstrated (DPPH, ABTS, superoxide anion radical, hydrogen peroxide-scavenging and ferric ion [Fe^{3+}]-reducing and ferrous ion [Fe^{2+}]-chelating activities) (Gülçin et al 2012).

Anticarcinogenic

Eugenol essential oil showed anticancer apoptosis activity on HL-60 human promyelocytic leukaemia cells in vitro (Yoo et al 2005). Further chemopreventive potential was explored in mice with induced lung carcinogenesis. A clove infusion, administered orally, was found to significantly reduce proliferating cells and increase apoptosis. The cloves down-regulated some growth-promoting proteins, while at the same time upregulating the expression of some proapoptotic proteins (Banerjee et al 2006). Later in vitro studies confirmed apoptosis induction of eugenol (and its analogues) as well as anti-inflammatory action through downregulation of Bcl-2, COX-2 and interleukin-1β (IL-1β) (Hussein et al 2011), suggesting that it may have a chemotherapeutic role (Carrasco et al 2008). An aqueous infusion of cloves, administered orally, in a mouse experiment delayed the formation and reduced skin papilloma (Banerjee & Das 2005).

A comparative in vitro study showed indiscriminate cytotoxicity of gemcitabine (a chemotherapeutic agent used in cervical cancer) to both healthy and cancerous cell lines, whereas a crude clove extract diluted in 2% Dubecco's modified Eagle medium was found to preferentially be more cytotoxic to cancer cell lines. A low-dose gemcitabine and crude clove extract was synergistically more cytotoxic towards cervical cell lines than individual preparations (Hussein et al 2009).

Clove essential oil and eugenol showed a 40–80% inhibition of melanin production in B16 melanoma cells in vitro at a concentration of 100–200 mcg/mL; however, the essential oil showed cytotoxicity at higher concentration, a strong consideration in establishing safe therapeutic dose in the development of further studies (Arung et al 2011).

A 2012 review (Jaganathan & Supriyanto 2012) established the antiproliferative, apoptotic and chemopreventive activities as well as the molecular mechanisms of eugenol and some of its dimers against melanomas, skin tumours, osteosarcoma, leukaemia, androgen-insensitive prostate, hepG2 hepatoma, lymphoma and gastric in vitro cancer cell lines and in animal models (Jaganathan & Supriyanto 2012, Kamatou et al 2012).

Antigenotoxic and antimutagenic activity of eugenol was non-significant in vitro. A small human study of 10 healthy non-smoking males administered a dose of 150 mg of eugenol/day did not demonstrate any antigenotoxic activity (Kamatou et al 2012).

OTHER ACTIONS

C

Improvement of cognition — memory

An animal study found that intraperitoneally-administered clove extract (200 mg/kg) improved short-term memory recall but caused some impairment in learning ability (Morshedi et al 2006). A 3-week treatment with clove oil (0.05 mL/kg) has been shown to reverse memory acquisition latency and memory deficit in a rodent model of scopolamine-induced memory impairment. Malondialdehyde and glutathione brain levels in the clove mice were increased; the reversal of short-term and long-term memory deficit is thought to be due to antioxidant activity on clove (Halder et al 2011).

Antihistamine

Clove bud extracts inhibit histamine release from mast cells in vivo and in vitro (Kim et al 1997, 1998, Shakila et al 1996).

Immunomodulatory

An in vitro study found that clove inhibited murine macrophage production of cytokines IL-1β, IL-6 and IL-10 and eugenol inhibited IL-6 and counteracted significantly lipopolysaccharide (endotoxins produced by Gram-negative bacteria) (Bachiega et al 2012).

A previous study found no significant influence in Th1/Th2 modulation in mice fed a water extract of clove (Bachiega et al 2009).

Antispasmodic

Both beta-caryophyllene and eugenol have antispasmodic activity (Duke 2002).

Anticholinesterase

Clove extract, its oil and eugenol showed inhibition of AChE in vitro (Dalai et al 2014).

Antiplatelet

Eugenol inhibits platelet aggregation in vitro (Srivastava 1993, Srivastava & Malhotra 1991). It was more potent than aspirin in several experimental models and equivalent to indomethacin in one (Srivastava 1993).

Antidiabetic

In vitro tests have identified hypoglycaemic activity for cloves. It appears that a phenolic compound in cloves may be the key constituent responsible and acts by repressing the expression of genes which control hepatic gluconeogenesis (Prasad et al 2005). Commercially sold culinary cloves were also shown to be potent inhibitors of fructose-mediated protein glycation and so may have antidiabetic potential (Dearlove et al 2008). Further research is required with in vivo models of diabetes to determine whether these effects may have clinical significance.

Gastroprotective and antiulcerogenic

Prophylactic use of both *Syzygium aromaticum* steamed distilled essential oil and eugenol displayed antiulcer and gastroprotective activity through increased quantification of free gastric mucus production in indomethacin and ethanol-HCl-induced rat models (Santin et al 2011).

CLINICAL USE

The clinical effects of cloves and clove oil have not been significantly investigated; however, an understanding of the herb's pharmacological activity suggests a role in the treatment of several conditions.

Toothache and relief of dry-socket pain

Clove oil and dried clove buds are used in dentistry to relieve dental pain and reduce infection. The anaesthetic effects of eugenol, the main component of clove, as well as its analgesic and anti-inflammatory effects have been well documented in vivo. Based on the evidence available, Commission E has approved cloves for use as a local anaesthetic and antiseptic (Blumenthal et al 2000). In one study, 2 g of a 2:3 clove:glycerin gel was found to be as effective as 2 g of a 20% benzocaine gel as a topical anaesthetic before needle insertion in dentistry (Alqareer et al 2006).

Oral hygiene

Used as an antiseptic and antibacterial agent for the oral mucosa, clove is used as an ingredient in mouth rinses and gargles. Its established antiseptic activity provides a theoretical basis for efficacy. Aqueous extract of cloves has also demonstrated significant analgesic activity mediated by an opiate pathway, according to in vivo research (Kamkar et al 2012).

Anal fissures

A small (n = 55) single-blind randomised trial comparing topical application of 1% clove oil cream or a 5% lignocaine cream and stool softeners in the treatment of anal fissure showed statistically significant healing of fissures and reduction in anal pressure with the clove cream (60%) compared to the lignocaine treatment (12%) (Elwakeet 2006, Nelson et al 2012).

Herpes simplex virus type 1

One study using a combination of aciclovir and cloves administered orally found this to be superior to aciclovir alone in the treatment of herpes simplex virus type 1 infection (Kurokawa et al 1995). The combination significantly reduced the development of skin lesions and/or prolonged survival times of infected mice and reduced viral loads.

Headache (as part of a combination)

Tiger balm is a popular over-the-counter preparation that contains clove oil, menthol, cassia oil, camphor, cajuput oil and sometimes peppermint oil. It is generally used to relieve the symptoms of sore muscles, but a randomised, double-blind study found that it is also as effective as paracetamol in reducing headache severity (Schattner & Randerson 1996). Although encouraging, the role of cloves in this combination is difficult to assess from the study.

Type 2 diabetes

In a small study, 36 people with type 2 diabetes were given 0, 1, 2 or 3 g capsules of cloves for 30 days. All the groups administered with cloves had significantly lowered serum glucose, triglycerides, total and low-density lipoprotein cholesterol and there was no change in high-density lipoprotein cholesterol. After a 10-day washout period all these parameters were still significantly lower than at the start of the trial (Khan et al 2006). Further research is warranted to confirm clinical use in type 2 diabetes and to assess any side effects with oral ingestion of cloves.

OTHER USES

Cloves have been investigated as an agent to protect harvests from fungal contamination (Ranasinghe et al 2002).

Practice points/Patient counselling

- Clove flower buds and clove oil have antiseptic, analgesic, anti-inflammatory and local anaesthetic properties.
- As a gel, it is directly applied to relieve the symptoms of toothache, dry socket and anal fissures.
- Clove oil is also used in mouth rinses and gargles to improve oral hygiene.
- Massaging one drop of oil into the temples has been used to treat headache.
- This herb and its essential oil should not be taken internally.

DOSAGE RANGE

- Powder: 120–300 mg as a single dose.
- Oil: 0.05–0.2 mL as a single dose.
- Toothache or gum inflammation: oil of clove is applied directly to the site.
- Dry socket: the area is packed with dried flower buds steeped in oil.
- Anal fissure: 1% clove essential oil in base cream.
- Headache: one drop of oil massaged into each temple or area of pain.

ADVERSE REACTIONS

According to one review, contact dermatitis and several adverse reactions to eugenol used in dentistry have been reported, and local application may cause irritation to mucous membranes in sensitive individuals (Kamatou et al 2012). Used neat, clove oil is considered hazardous, and dermal irritation is reported with topical ointment at concentrations above 20% (Lis-Balchin 2006). Oral use of the oil can cause nervous system depression, seizures, hepatic dysfunction and irritation and necrosis to mucosal tissues. Five cases of fulminant hepatic failure were reported by the European Medicine Agency (2011). All were associated with the ingestion of 5–10 mL of clove oil by children under 2 years.

SIGNIFICANT INTERACTIONS

Cloves have been found in vitro to strongly inhibit metabolism mediated by CYP3A4 and CYP2D6, but clinical relevance has yet to be established (Usia et al 2006). If cloves are only used topically, these interactions are unlikely to be relevant.

CONTRAINDICATIONS AND PRECAUTIONS

None known.

PREGNANCY USE

Safety unknown.

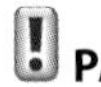

PATIENTS' FAQs

What will this herb do for me?

Clove flower buds and clove oil have antiseptic, anti-inflammatory properties. As a gel, its analgesic and local anaesthetic properties are useful in the treatment of toothache, dry socket and common mouth infections. It has applications with anal fissure as a 1% cream. Massaging one drop of the oil into the temples may relieve the symptoms of headache.

When will it start to work?

Research suggests that effects are almost immediate, although short-lasting.

Are there any safety issues?

Clove buds and clove oil should not be taken internally, and only applied externally in diluted form, as pure essential oil is reportedly hazardous. Using cloves as a spice in cooking may give you some of the antioxidant benefits.

REFERENCES

Ahmad N et al. Antimicrobial activity of clove oil and its potential in the treatment of vaginal candidiasis. J Drug Target 13.10 (2005): 555–561.

Alqareer A, et al. The effect of clove and benzocaine versus placebo as topical anesthetics. J Dent 34.10 (2006): 747–750.

Arora DS, Kaur J. Antimicrobial activity of spices. Int J Antimicrob Agents 12.3 (1999): 257–262.

Arung ET et al. Inhibitory components from the buds of clove (*Syzygium aromaticum*) on melanin formation in B16 melanoma cells. Fitoterapa 82-2 (2011): 198–202.

Bachiega TF et al. Th1/Th2 cytokine production by clove treated mice. Nat Prod Res 23.16 (2009): 1552–8

Bachiega TF et al. Clove and eugenol in noncytotoxic concentrations exert immunomodulatory/anti-inflammatory action on cytokine production by murine macrophages. J Pharm Pharmacol 264.4 (2012):610–6.

Banerjee S, Das S. Anticarcinogenic effects of an aqueous infusion of cloves on skin carcinogenesis. Asian Pac J Cancer Prev 6.3 (2005): 304–308.

Banerjee S, et al. Clove (*Syzygium aromaticum* L.), a potential chemopreventive agent for lung cancer. Carcinogenesis 27.8 (2006): 1645–1654.

Bluma R, et al. Screening of Argentine plant extracts: impact on growth parameters and aflatoxin B1 accumulation by *Aspergillus* section Flavi. Int J Food Microbiol 122.1–2 (2008): 114–25.

Blumenthal M et al. Herbal medicine: expanded Commission E monographs. Austin, TX: American Botanical Council, 2000.

Braga PC et al. Eugenol and thymol, alone or in combination, induce morphological alterations in the envelope of *Candida albicans*. Fitoterapia 78.6 (2007): 396–400.

Brodin P, Roed A. Effects of eugenol on rat phrenic nerve and phrenic nerve-diaphragm preparations. Arch Oral Biol 29.8 (1984): 611–6115.

Burt SA, Reinders RD. Antibacterial activity of selected plant essential oils against *Escherichia coli* O157:H7. Lett Appl Microbiol 36.3 (2003): 162–167.

Cai L, Wu CD. Compounds from *Syzygium aromaticum* possessing growth inhibitory activity against oral pathogens. J Nat Prod 59.10 (1996): 987–990.

Carrasco HL et al. Eugenol and its synthetic analogues inhibit cell growth of human cancer cells (Part 1). Journal of the Brazilian Chemical Society 19.3 (2008): S1–13.

Chami F et al. Oregano and clove essential oils induce surface alteration of *Saccharomyces cerevisiae*. Phytother Res 19.5 (2005): 405–408.

Choudhary R, et al. Prevention of isoproterenol-induced cardiac hypertrophy by eugenol, an antioxidant. Indian Journal of Clinical Biochemistry 21.2 (2006): 107–113.

Dalai MK et al. Anti-cholinesterase activity of the standardized extract of Syzygium aromaticum L. Pharmacogn Mag 10 (Suppl 2) (2014): S276–S282.

De M, et al. Antimicrobial screening of some Indian spices. Phytother Res 13.7 (1999): 616–6118.

Dearlove RP et al. Inhibition of protein glycation by extracts of culinary herbs and spices. J Med Food 11.2 (2008): 275–281.

Devi KP et al. Eugenol (an essential oil of clove) acts as an antibacterial agent against *Salmonella typhi* by disrupting the cellular membrane. Journal of Ethnophamacology 130 (2010): 107–115.

Dorman HJ, Deans SG. Antimicrobial agents from plants: antibacterial activity of plant volatile oils. J Appl Microbiol 88.2 (2000): 308–316.

Duke JA. Dr Duke's Phytochemical and Ethnobotanical Databases. US Department of Agriculture–Agricultural Research Service–National Germplasm Resources Laboratory. Beltsville, MD: Beltsville Agricultural Research Center. Available at: www.ars-grin.gov/duke (accessed 11-10-02)

Elwakeel HA et al. Clove oil cream: a new effective treatment for chronic anal fissure. Colorectal Dis 9.6 (2007): 549–552.

European Medicines Agency. Assessment report on *Syzygium aromaticum* (L.) Merill et L.M. Perry, flos and *Syzygium aromaticum* (L.) Merill et L.M. Perry, *Floris aetheroleum*. Committee on Herbal Medicinal Products. (2011) EMA/HMPC/534946/2010. Viewed online 28/02/2013 [http://www.ema.europa.eu/docs/en_GB/document_library/Herbal_-_HMPC_assessment_report/2011/12/WC500119923.pdf]

Ferland CE, et al. Antinociceptive effects of eugenol in a monoiodoacetate-induced osteoarthritis rat model. Phytotherapy Research, 26 (2012): 1278–1285.

Friedman M, et al. Bactericidal activities of plant essential oils and some of their isolated constituents against *Campylobacter jejuni, Escherichia coli, Listeria monocytogenes*, and *Salmonella enterica*. J Food Prot 65.10 (2002): 1545–1560.

Fu Y et al. Antimicrobial activity of clove and rosemary essential oils alone and in combination. Phytother Res 21.10 (2007): 989–994.

Ghelardini C, et al. Local anaesthetic activity of monoterpenes and phenylpropanes of essential oils. Planta Med 67.6 (2001a): 564–6.

Ghelardini C et al. Local anaesthetic activity of beta-caryophyllene. Farmaco 56.5–7 (2001b): 387–9.

Gill, A.O., Holley, R.A. Disruption of *Escherichia coli, Listeria monocytogenes* and *Lactobacillus sakei* cellular membrane by plant oil aromatics. Int. J. Food Microbiol. 108 (2006a): 1–9.

Gill, A.O., Holley, R.A. Inhibition of membrane bound ATPases of *Escherichia coli* and *Listeria monocytogenes* by plant oil aromatics. Int. J. Food Microbiol. 111 (2006b): 170–174.

Guénette SA et al. Pharmacokinetics of eugenol and its effects on thermal hypersensitivity in rats. Eur J Pharmacol 562.1–2 (2007): 60–67.

Gülçin I et al. Antioxidant activity of clove oil – a powerful antioxidant source. Arabian Journal of Chemistry 5.4 (2012): 489–499.

Guynot ME et al. Antifungal activity of volatile compounds generated by essential oils against fungi commonly causing deterioration of bakery products. J Appl Microbiol 94.5 (2003): 893–899.

Halder S, et al. Clove oil reverses learning and memory deficits in scopolamine-treated mice. Planta Medica 77.8 (2011):830–4.

Hemaiswarya S, Doble M Synergistic interaction of eugenol with antibiotics against Gram negative bacteria. Phytomedicine 16.11 (2009): 997–1005.

Ho S-C et al. Protective capacities of certain spices against peroxynitrite-mediated biomolecular damage. Food Chem Toxicol 46.3 (2008): 920–928.

Huss U et al. Screening of ubiquitous plant constituents for COX-2 inhibition with a scintillation proximity based assay. J Nat Prod 65.11 (2002): 1517–1521.

Hussein G et al. Inhibitory effects of Sudanese medicinal plant extracts on hepatitis C virus (HCV) protease. Phytother Res 14.7 (2000): 510–5116.

Hussein A et al. Clove (*Syzygium aromaticum*) extract potentiates gemcitabine cytotoxic effect on human cervical cancer cell line. Intl J Cancer Res 5.3 (2009): 95–104.

Hussein A et al. Eugenol enhances the chemotherapeutic potential of Gemcitabine and induces anticarcinogenic and anti-inflammatory activity in human cervical cancer cells. Cancer Biother Radiopharm 26.5 (2011): 519–527.

Jaganathan SK, Supriyanto E. Antiproliferative and molecular mechanism of eugenol-induced apoptosis in cancer cells. Molecules. 6.17 (2012): 6290–6304.
Kabuto H et al. Eugenol [2methoxy4(2propenyl)phenol] prevents 6hydroxydopamineinduced dopamine depression and lipid peroxidation inductivity in mouse striatum. Biol Pharm Bull 30.3
Kamatou GP et al. Eugenol – From the remote Maluku Island to the international market place: a review of a remarkable molecule. Molecule 6.17 (2012): 6953–6981.
Kamkar AM et al. Analgesic effect of the aqueous and ethanolic extracts of clove. Avicenna J Phytomed 3.2 (2013):186–192.
Kelm MA et al. Antioxidant and cyclooxygenase inhibitory phenolic compounds from *Ocimum sanctum* Linn. Phytomedicine 7.1 (2000): 7–13.
Khan A et al. Cloves improve glucose, cholesterol, and triglycerides of people with type 2 diabetes mellitus [abstract]. Journal of Federation of American Societies Experimental Biology 20.5 (2006): A990: 640.3.
Khan R et al. Antimicrobial activity of five herbal extracts against multi drug resistant (MDR) strains of bacteria and fungus of clinical origin. 4.14.2 Molecules (2009): 586–97.
Kim HM et al. Antianaphylactic properties of eugenol. Pharmacol Res 36.6 (1997): 475–480.
Kim HM et al. Effect of *Syzygium aromaticum* extract on immediate hypersensitivity in rats. J Ethnopharmacol 60.2 (1998): 125–131.
Koba K et al. Antibacterial activities of the buds essential oil of *Syzygium aromaticum* (L.) Merr. & Perry from Togo. Journal of Biologically Active Products from Nature 1.1 (2011):42–57
Kurokawa M et al. Efficacy of traditional herbal medicines in combination with acyclovir against herpes simplex virus type 1 infection in vitro and in vivo. Antiviral Res 27.1–2 (1995): 19–37.
Kurokawa M et al. Purification and characterization of eugeniin as an anti-herpesvirus compound from *Geum japonicum* and *Syzygium aromaticum*. J Pharmacol Exp Ther 284.2 (1998): 728–735.
Lis-Balchin M, Aromatherapy Science: A Guide for Healthcare Professionals. London: Pharmaceutical Press, 2006: p171
Machado M et al. Anti-*Giardia* activity of *Syzygium aromaticum* essential oil and eugenol effects on growth, viability, adherence and ultrastructure. Experimental Parasitology 4.11, (2011): 732–739.
Moon SE, et al, Synergistic effect between clove oil and its major compounds and antibiotics against oral bacteria. Archives of oral biology 56.9 (2011): 907–916
Morshedi A et al. P19.4 The effect of *Syzygium aromaticum* (clove) and vitamin C on learning and memory in rats. Clin Neurophysiol 117 (Suppl 1) (2006): 211–2112.
Muruganandan S et al. Anti-inflammatory activity of *Syzygium cumini* bark. Fitoterapia (2001) 72.4
Nassar MI. Flavonoid triglycosides from the seeds of *Syzygium aromaticum*. Carbohydr Res 341.1 (2006): 160–163.
Nelson RL, et al. Non surgical therapy for anal fissure. Çochrane Database of Systematic Reviews 2012, Issue 2. Art. No.: CD003431.
Pandey BN, et al. Modification of radiation-induced oxidative damage in liposomal and microsomal membrane by eugenol. Radiat Phys Chem 75.3 (2006): 384–391.
Park MJ et al. Antifungal activities of the essential oils in *Syzygium aromaticum* (L.) Merr. Et Perry and Leptospermum petersonii Bailey and their constituents against various dermatophytes. J Microbiol 45.5 (2007): 460–465.
Pinto E et al. Antifungal activity of the clove essential oil from *Syzygium aromaticum* on *Candida*, *Aspergillus* and dermatophyte species. J of Medical Microbiology 58 (2009):1454–1462
Prasad RC et al. An extract of *Syzygium aromaticum* represses genes encoding hepatic gluconeogenic enzymes. J Ethnopharmacol 96.1–2 (2005): 295–301.
Pundir, RK et al. Antimicrobial activity of ethanolic extracts of *Syzygium aromaticum* and *Allium sativum* against food associated bacteria and fungi. Ethnobotanical Leaflets (2010):3–11.
Raghavenra H et al. Eugenol—the active principle from cloves inhibits 5-lipoxygenase activity and leukotriene-C4 in human PMNL cells. Prostaglandins Leukot Essent Fatty Acids 74.1 (2006): 23–27.
Ranasinghe L, et al. Fungicidal activity of essential oils of *Cinnamomum zeylanicum* (L.) and *Syzygium aromaticum* (L.) against crown rot and anthracnose pathogens isolated from banana. Lett Appl Microbiol 35.3 (2002): 208–211.
Saini A, et al. Induction of resistance to respiratory tract infection with *Klebsiella pneumoniae* in mice fed on a diet supplemented with tulsi (*Ocimum sanctum*) and clove (*Syzgium aromaticum*) oils. J Microbiol Immunol Infect. 42 (2009):107–113
Santin JR et al. Gastroprotective activity of the essential oil of *Sygyzium aromaticum* and its major component eugenol in different animal models. Naunyn-Schmied Arch Pharmacol 383 (2011):149–158.
Santoro GF et al. *Trypanosoma cruzi*: activity of essential oils from *Achillea millefolium* L., *Syzygium aromaticum* L. and *Ocimum basilicum* L. on epimastigotes and trypomastigotes. Exp Parasitol 116.3 (2007): 283–290.
Schattner P, Randerson D. Tiger Balm as a treatment of tension headache: a clinical trial in general practice. Aust Fam Physician 25.2 (1996): 216, 218, 220.
Shakila RJ, et al. Inhibitory effect of spices on in vitro histamine production and histidine decarboxylase activity of *Morganella morganii* and on the biogenic amine formation in mackerel stored at 30 degrees C. Z Lebensm Unters Forsch 203.1 (1996): 71–76.
Shiraki K et al. Cytomegalovirus infection and its possible treatment with herbal medicines. Nippon Rinsho 56.1 (1998): 156–160.
Srivastava KC. Antiplatelet principles from a food spice clove (*Syzygium aromaticum* L) [corrected]. Prostaglandins Leukot Essent Fatty Acids 48.5 (1993): 363–372.
Srivastava KC, Malhotra N. Acetyl eugenol, a component of oil of cloves (*Syzygium aromaticum* L.) inhibits aggregation and alters arachidonic acid metabolism in human blood platelets. Prostaglandins Leukot Essent Fatty Acids 42.1 (1991): 73–81.
Taguchi Y et al. Protection of oral or intestinal candidiasis in mice by oral or intragastric administration of herbal food, clove (*Syzygium aromaticum*). Nippon Ishinkin Gakkai Zasshi 46.1 (2005): 27–33.
Usia T et al. CYP3A4 and CYP2D6 inhibitory activities of Indonesian medicinal plants. Phytomedicine 13.1–2 (2006): 67–73.
Viuda-Martos M et al. Antifungal activities of thyme, clove and oregano essential oils. J Food Saf 27.1 (2007): 91–101.
Yang L et al. In vitro anti-*Helicobacter pylori* action of 30 Chinese herbal medicines used to treat ulcer diseases. J Ethnopharmacol 98.3 (2005): 329–333.
Yoo C et al. Eugenol isolated from the essential oil of *Eugenia caryophyllata* induces a reactive oxygen species-mediated apoptosis in HL-60 human promyelocytic leukemia cells. Cancer Lett 225.1 (2005): 41–52.
Yukawa TA et al. Prophylactic treatment of cytomegalovirus infection with traditional herbs. Antiviral Res 32.2 (1996): 63–70.

Cocoa

HISTORICAL NOTE Cocoa originates from Mexico, where the Mayas, Incas and Aztecs considered it the food of the gods. Chocolate, mixed with vanilla and sugar, was first introduced as a beverage in Europe by Columbus and was considered an aphrodisiac and a symbol of wealth and power. The phenolics in chocolate prevent the fat becoming rancid, decreasing the need for added preservatives. This quality was exploited during World War II when at times US troops were rationed three chocolate bars per day during heavy combat as their sole source of nourishment (Waterhouse et al 1996). While an amusing association between countries' annual chocolate consumption and the number of Nobel laureates per capita has been described, direct correlation between past Nobel prize winners' chocolate intake and their academic success hasn't been established (Maurage et al 2013, Messerli 2012).

COMMON NAME

Chocolate, cocoa, cocoa liquor, cocoa mass, baking chocolate, Cocoapro, Acticoa

BOTANICAL NAME/FAMILY

Theobroma cacao (family Sterculiaceae)

C

PLANT PARTS USED

Cocoa is produced through a process of fermenting the seeds from the pods of the cacao tree, *Theobroma cacao*. The beans are dried, roasted and crushed to produce high-fat, unsweetened chocolate, which is also called baking chocolate. This intermediate is pressed and alkalised to form cocoa powder, which is then homogenised with sugar and cocoa butter, and sometimes milk, to ultimately form chocolate. Dark chocolate generally contains more than 50% cocoa, whereas mass-produced milk chocolate contains only around 10% cocoa. White chocolate is based on cocoa butter (or theobroma oil) without the cocoa solids.

Although many different types of cocoa beans grow throughout the world, three varieties of cocoa beans are mainly used to make chocolate products: (1) criollo (meaning 'native'), distributed to the north and west of the Andes; (2) forastero (meaning 'foreign'), found mainly in the Amazon basin; and (3) trinitario (meaning 'sent from heaven') (Bruinsma & Taren 1999).

Cocoa beans from different countries along with postharvesting and processing procedures can have a striking influence on the flavanol content of chocolate and cocoa (Hollenberg et al 2004). As flavanols impart a bitter, astringent flavour, chocolate often undergoes extensive processing, dilution and the addition of flavour modifiers to improve its palatability, despite these processes having the potential to negatively impact on cocoa's nutritional and clinical value (McShea et al 2008). While a study that examined the total phenolic content of chocolate found that the antioxidant properties of the artisan-made chocolate were significantly better than those of the factory-produced chocolate (Cervellati et al 2008), recent attention to flavonoid content has led to the development of commercial processes that protect and preserve the naturally occurring flavonoids, with Cocoapro being developed by Mars and Acticoa by the Swiss-based Barry Callebaut.

CHEMICAL COMPONENTS

Cocoa is among the most concentrated sources of the flavanols, catechin and epicatechin, with four times the catechin content of tea (Arts et al 1999). Chocolate also contains additional flavonoids not found in tea, with high concentrations of oligomeric procyanidins (Lazarus et al 1999). Dark chocolate has the highest total catechin content, with approximately 53.5 mg/100 g, whereas milk chocolate contains approximately 15.9 mg/100 g (Arts et al 1999). White chocolate primarily contains cocoa butter with minimal levels of polyphenols. The bioavailability of cocoa flavanols may change depending on the type of sugar used in the chocolate formulation, with maltitol-containing chocolate being associated with reduced flavanol absorption compared to its sucrose-containing equivalent (Rodriguez-Mateos et al 2012).

In addition to flavanols, cocoa also contains the methylxanthines caffeine and theobromine, the biogenic amines phenylethylamine, phenylalanine and tyrosine (Bruinsma & Taren 1999) and the cannabinoid-like fatty acid anandanine analogues, *N*-oleoylethanolamine and *N*-linoleoylethanolamine (Di Tomaso et al 1996). Chocolate is also a rich source of minerals, including magnesium, calcium, iron, copper, phosphorus, potassium and zinc (Steinberg et al 2003) and it is suggested that the presence of methylxanthines, peptides and minerals could synergistically enhance or reduce cocoa's antioxidant properties (Jalil & Ismail 2008).

Food source

Cocoa and chocolate are nutritious foods that contribute to caloric as well as trace mineral intake (Steinberg et al 2003). Milk chocolate has a relatively low glycaemic index of approximately 40 (Foster-Powell et al 2002) and this is attributed to the fat in chocolate slowing gastric emptying and thus the rate of subsequent digestion and absorption. The glycaemic effect of milk chocolate can be further reduced by replacing the sucrose with fructose or isomalt (Gee et al 1991).

MAIN ACTIONS

Antioxidant

Cocoa has been found to have much higher levels of total phenolics and flavonoids, with a correspondingly higher antioxidant capacity per serving, than black tea, green tea or red wine (Lee et al 2003). It has been suggested that the antioxidant capacity of cocoa polyphenols is greater than synthetic antioxidants and that they have the potential to complement or replace synthetic antioxidants in aqueous and oil-based food applications (Osman et al 2004). There is, however, tremendous variability in cocoa processing, flavonoid content and measurement of flavonoids,

Cocoa has been consistently shown to confer significant protection against oxidation both in vitro (Martin et al 2008, Sies et al 2005, Waterhouse et al 1996) and in vivo (Kondo et al 1996). In addition to reducing lipid oxidation, consumption of a flavanol-rich cocoa beverage has been shown to reduce susceptibility of erythrocytes to haemolysis and to increase their ability to buffer free radicals (Zhu et al 2005).

While the antioxidant activity of cocoa is well established, questions remain around best forms for maximal bioavailability and dosing frequency (Fisher & Hollenberg 2006).

Cocoa powder dissolved in milk as one of the most common ways of cocoa powder consumption seems to have a negative effect on the absorption of polyphenols; however, statistical analyses have shown that milk does not impair the bioavailability of flavonoids (Keogh et al 2007, Roura et al 2007). High-flavonoid cocoa products may lead to greatly enhanced flavonoid bioavailability in humans (Tomas-Barberan et al 2007).

A feeding study demonstrated that procyanidins were remarkably stable in the stomach environment and thus most ingested procyanidins reach the small intestine intact and are available for absorption or metabolism (Rios et al 2002). Epicatechin and its metabolites reach maximal levels 2 hours after either chocolate or cocoa intake, with rapid excretion in the urine (Baba et al 2000) and dimeric procyanidins have been detected in human plasma as early as 30–60 minutes after the consumption of flavanol-rich beverages providing 0.25–0.50 g/kg cocoa/kg body weight (Holt et al 2002, Zhu et al 2005). Human studies have confirmed that the polyphenols in chocolate are indeed bioavailable and able to increase the antioxidant capacity of plasma, with one study reporting that ingestion of 80 g of procyanidin-rich chocolate increased plasma epicatechin concentrations 12-fold, significantly increased plasma total antioxidant capacity by 31% and significantly decreased 2-thiobarbituric acid-reactive substances by 40% after 2 hours, with levels returning to normal within 6 hours (Rein et al 2000a). Similarly, a 2012 study identified that both dark chocolate and high-antioxidant dark chocolate had a peak total antioxidant capacity 2 hours postingestion, with the high-antioxidant dark chocolate showing raised levels for over 5 hours postingestion (Lettieri-Barbato et al 2012).

There is evidence that the polyphenols are not the only antioxidants in chocolate, as suggested by a study that found that consumption of chocolate containing 200 mg of polyphenols, as well as chocolate with less than 10 mg of polyphenols, reduced faecal free-radical production (Record et al 2003). Furthermore, similar reductions in markers of lipid peroxidation have been observed after daily consumption of 75 g of dark chocolate and dark chocolate enriched with cocoa polyphenols, as well as with white chocolate, which contains very little polyphenols (Mursu et al 2004).

In a crossover study in 23 healthy subjects, cocoa powder and dark chocolate were seen to modestly reduce low-density lipoprotein (LDL) oxidation susceptibility while increasing serum total antioxidant capacity and high-density lipoprotein (HDL) cholesterol concentrations (Wan et al 2001), and another crossover trial of 25 healthy subjects found that supplementation with 36.9 g of dark chocolate (30 g of cocoa powder drink) for 6 weeks reduced LDL oxidisability (Mathur et al 2002). Similar results were seen in a randomised, double-blind crossover trial that found that a high-flavanol cocoa drink providing 187 mg flavan-3-ols/100 mL significantly reduced lipid peroxidation, compared with a low-flavanol cocoa drink providing only 14 mg/100 mL (Wiswedel et al 2004).

In contrast to these studies a further randomised, double-blind, placebo-controlled study of 21 healthy adults, however, found that intake of high-flavonoid (213 mg procyanidins, 46 mg epicatechin) dark chocolate bars for 2 weeks did not alter resistance to LDL oxidation, total antioxidant capacity, 8-isoprostanes, blood pressure, lipid parameters, body weight or body mass index (BMI), despite increasing plasma epicatechin concentrations and improving endothelium-dependent flow-mediated dilation of the brachial artery (Engler et al 2004).

Lipid-modifying

A 3-week clinical supplementation trial of 45 non-smoking, healthy volunteers consuming high-polyphenol chocolate found a significant increase in serum HDL cholesterol with dark and high-polyphenol chocolate (11.4% and 13.7%, respectively), whereas white chocolate consumption resulted in a small decrease in HDL. Markers of lipid peroxidation decreased 11.9% in all three study groups, suggesting that, while cocoa polyphenols may increase the concentration of HDL cholesterol, chocolate fatty acids may modify the fatty acid composition of LDL, making it more resistant to oxidative damage (Mursu et al 2004).

A new soluble cocoa fibre product rich in soluble dietary fibre and antioxidant polyphenols diminished the negative impact of the cholesterol-rich diet in an animal model of dietary-induced hypercholesterolaemia (Ramos et al 2008). Similarly, in an animal model of hypercholesterolaemia a cholesterol- and triglyceride-lowering effect along with a reduction of biomarkers of oxidative stress and increasing faecal bulking was seen after 3 weeks of consuming a fibre-rich cocoa product (Bravo et al 2008).

It appears that chronic intake of cocoa-based products is required for effects, as an acute dosing study using 100 g of either dark chocolate (55% dry cocoa solids) or high-antioxidant dark chocolate (66% dry cocoa solids) did not significantly affect total cholesterol levels 5 hours afterwards, although triacylglycerol was significantly increased in both products after 1 hour (Lettieri-Barbato et al 2012).

Effects on microcirculation and nitric oxide

Flavanols have been shown in several in vitro or ex vivo studies to modify the production of proinflammatory cytokines, the synthesis of eicosanoids, the activation of platelets and nitric oxide (NO)-mediated mechanisms (Selmi et al 2008). A double-blind, dose-finding study found that flavanol-rich cocoa increased circulating NO species in the plasma of male smokers, with maximal effects seen with ingestion of 176–185 mg flavanols (Heiss et al 2005). Another double-blind trial found that ingestion of a high-flavanol cocoa drink, but not a low-flavanol one, enhanced NO bioactivity and increased plasma concentrations of nitroso compounds and flow-mediated dilation of the brachial artery (Sies et al 2005). Similarly, ingestion of flavanol-rich cocoa is associated with acute elevations in levels of circulating NO species, enhanced flow-mediated dilation response of conduit arteries and an augmented microcirculation, with these effects being mimicked by ingestion of chemically pure epicatechin. Moreover, chronic consumption of a cocoa–flavanol-rich diet has been associated with augmented urinary excretion of NO metabolites (Schroeter et al 2006).

Double-blind, crossover intervention studies in both humans and rats suggest that an increase in the circulating NO pool following flavanol consumption is correlated with decreased arginase activity as the availability of L-arginine can be a rate-limiting factor for cellular NO production by nitric oxide synthase (NOS) (Schnorr et al 2008).

Cardioprotection

A significant reduction in experimentally induced myocardial infarct size was observed following treatment with the cocoa-derived flavanol (–)-epicatechin in vivo. Test animals who were 48 hours and 3 weeks post permanent coronary occlusion experienced a 52% and 33% reduction in myocardial infarct size respectively (Yamazaki et al 2010). The left ventricular scar area strain was improved following (–)-epicatechin treatment, suggesting possible cardioprotective mechanisms (Arranz et al 2013).

Inhibits platelet activation

Numerous dietary intervention studies in humans and animals indicate that flavanol-rich foods and beverages might exert cardioprotective effects with respect to vascular function and platelet reactivity (Keen et al 2005). Acute doses of flavanols and oligomeric procyanidins from cocoa have been observed to inhibit platelet activation (Pearson et al 2002, Rein et al 2000b) and have an aspirin-like effect on primary haemostasis 2 and 6 hours after consumption (Hermann et al 2006, Pearson et al 2002, Rein et al 2000b), with the effects being similar to, but less profound than, aspirin (Pearson et al 2002). Similar results have been observed in longer studies with lower doses of cocoa flavanols, with a double-blind, controlled trial demonstrating significantly lower platelet aggregation and significantly higher plasma ascorbic acid concentrations after supplementation with cocoa flavanols (234 mg cocoa flavanols and procyanidins/day) over 28 days (Murphy et al 2003).

In a randomized controlled trial (RCT) of 30 healthy volunteers, 100 mg of dark chocolate, but not white or milk chocolate, was found to significantly inhibit collagen-induced platelet aggregation (Innes et al 2003). The alteration of eicosanoid synthesis has been suggested as a plausible mechanism by which procyanidins can decrease platelet activation, and this has been observed in an in vitro study of the effect of procyanidin on aortic endothelial cells, as well as in a randomised, blinded, crossover study of high-procyanidin chocolate (4.0 mg/g) (Schramm et al 2001).

Diabetes — glycaemic control

Pretreatment with a cocoa extract high in polyphenols was seen to normalise body weight, plasma glucose levels, total cholesterol, triglycerides and HDL levels in streptozotocin-diabetic rats (Ruzaidi et al 2008). The supplementation of 0.5% epicatechin in drinking water of non-obese diabetic mice reduced the incidence of hyperglycaemia (16.6% of treated vs 66.7% of control mice), significantly increased plasma insulin levels (0.392 mcg/L in treated vs 0.129 mcg/L in controls) and lowered glycosylated haemoglobin levels (5.2% in treated vs 7.4% in controls) (Fu et al 2013). In preadipocytes, cocoa polyphenol extract is able to inhibit insulin receptor activity, as well as prevent the development of obesity in mice given a high-fat diet (Min et al 2013).

In humans, short-term administration of flavonoid-rich dark chocolate significantly improved insulin sensitivity and endothelial function in healthy and hypertensive subjects (Grassi et al 2008b), while a double-blind, placebo-controlled crossover study found that flavanol-rich dark chocolate but not flavanol-free white chocolate ameliorated insulin sensitivity and beta-cell function, decreased blood pressure and increased flow-mediated dilation in hypertensive patients with impaired glucose tolerance (Grassi et al 2008a). Similar results were obtained from another small RCT that found that high-flavanol cocoa reversed vascular dysfunction in diabetic patients (Balzer et al 2008). In contrast to these findings, a double-blind, crossover study found that daily consumption of flavanol-rich cocoa for 2 weeks was not sufficient to reduce blood pressure or improve insulin resistance in human subjects with essential hypertension (Muniyappa et al 2008). Similarly, a randomised crossover study determined that the short-term (5-day) intake of cocoa flavanols (30–900 mg per day) did not have any effect on glucose metabolism in 20 obese participants at risk of insulin resistance; however markers of oxidative stress, inflammation and haemostasis were significantly reduced (Stote et al 2012).

Psychological effects

Chocolate is purported to have a range of psychological effects, including enhanced arousal and cognitive function, stimulation of feelings of wellbeing and euphoria, as well as initiating cravings. The orosensory aspects of chocolate, including its taste, smell and texture, certainly contribute to chocolate's positive appeal. Chocolate contains large amounts of fat in the form of cocoa butter, which melts at body temperature, producing a pleasurable melt-in-the-mouth experience. Chocolate also often contains large amounts of sugar and thus satisfies the seemingly innate preference for sweet, high-fat foods (Bruinsma & Taren 1999).

In addition to unique sensory properties, chocolate also contains many pharmacologically active substances. Several endogenous biogenic amines with sympathomimetic properties are found in chocolate, most notably tyramine and phenylethylamine (Hurst et al 1982). Phenylethylamine is an amphetamine analogue structurally related to methylenedioxy-methamphetamine that may act to potentiate dopaminergic and noradrenergic neurotransmission and modulate mood (Bruinsma & Taren 1999).

Cocoa is also known to contain methylxanthines, including caffeine and theobromine, both of which are stimulants. Although the stimulatory and sympathomimetic effects of caffeine are well documented, the psychological effects of theobromine are less certain.

A group of biologically active constituents, including *N*-oleoylethanolamine and *N*-linoleoylethanolamine, have been identified in chocolate and appear to be related to anandamide, the 'internal bliss' chemical, which is the endogenous lipoprotein that binds cannabinoid receptors within the brain (Di Tomaso et al 1996). Although it has been suggested that these compounds may elicit heightened sensitivity and euphoria by directly activating cannabinoid receptors or by increasing anandamide levels (Bruinsma & Taren 1999), measurements have suggested that their amount in cocoa is several orders of magnitude below those required to reach the blood and cause observable central effects (Di Marzo et al 1998).

Chocolate craving, which is reported to be the most common food craving (Weingarten & Elston 1991), is more common in women, with fluctuations occurring with hormonal changes just before and during the menses (Rozin et al 1991). The basis for chocolate craving, however, remains undetermined, but it is suggested that aroma, sweetness, texture and calorie content are likely to play a more important role in chocolate cravings than pharmacological factors (Bruinsma & Taren 1999, Michener & Rozin 1994, Rozin et al 1991, Smit et al 2004).

In 2013, a randomised, placebo-controlled trial (n = 72) identified that ingesting a cocoa treatment (500 mg polyphenols) daily for 30 days significantly improved self-rated calmness and contentedness compared to placebo (Pase et al 2013). This effect was not observed after acute treatment, and cognition was unaffected both acutely and after 30 days.

Modulation of immune function and inflammation

The procyanidin fraction from cocoa demonstrates immunomodulatory function in vitro, with stimulation of tumour necrosis factor-alpha (Mao et al 2002) and modulation of the secretion of the cytokine transforming growth factor (Mao et al 2003), as well as inhibiting induced nuclear transcription of human interleukin-1β (IL-1β) (Mao et al 2000a), phytohaemagglutinin-induced stimulation of IL-2 (Mao et al 1999) and mitogen-stimulated secretion of IL-4 (Mao et al 2000b) in peripheral blood mononuclear cells in vitro. In vivo cocoa intake has been shown to modulate intestinal immune responses in young rats (Ramiro-Puig et al 2008), while cocoa polyphenols have been shown to reduce leukotriene synthesis through inhibition of human 5-lipo-oxygenase in humans (Sies et al 2005).

In vivo rat studies have also shown that a diet supplemented with 10% (w/w) cocoa for 7 weeks resulted in significantly reduced serum immunoglobulin A (IgA), IgG2b and IgM levels compared to those fed an isocaloric unsupplemented diet (Pérez-Berezo et al 2012). Additionally gut IgA and IgM levels were significantly reduced to approximately 30% and 50% of control animals, respectively.

Anti-inflammatory

While flavanols are known to modify the production of proinflammatory cytokines, the synthesis of eicosanoids, the activation of platelets and NO-mediated mechanisms (Selmi et al 2008), evidence for any beneficial effects of cocoa flavanols in providing a meaningful anti-inflammatory action has been gathered predominantly from in vitro experiments and only more recently have in vivo studies been conducted.

An in vivo study of induced colon carcinogenesis found that a cocoa-rich diet reduced NF-κB levels and the expression of proinflammatory enzymes, including cyclooxygenase-2 and iNOS (Rodríguez-Ramiro et al 2013). A study which investigated the effects of cocoa supplementation on trigeminal nerve inflammation identified that 1% (w/w) and 10% (w/w) cocoa repressed MKP-1 and -3, as well as resulted in reduced MAPK proteins, all of which indicates a reduced inflammatory response (Cady & Durham 2010). This study was conducted using immunofluorescence as the main indicative biomarker.

More recently, a randomised, crossover study of 20 obese volunteers confirmed that beverages containing cocoa flavanols (30–900 mg flavanol per day) produced a dose-dependent effect on the inflammation marker C-reactive protein and also significantly reduced IL-6 concentrations (Stote et al 2012).

Altered cellular signalling

Flavonoids have been shown to modulate tumour pathology in vitro and in animal models, and the pentameric procyanidin fraction isolated from cocoa is reported to slow the growth of cultured human aortic endothelial cells (Kenny et al 2004a), as well as inhibit the proliferation of human dermal microvascular endothelial cells in vitro through inhibition of tyrosine kinase ErbB2 expression. This has led to the suggestion that polyphenols may influence endothelial growth signalling in vitro, with potential beneficial effects for specific neoplasias in which cells overexpress ErbB2 (Kenny et al 2004b).

Inhibition of dental caries

Cocoa contains substances that protect against dental caries (Palenik et al 1977, s'Gravenmade et al 1977) and in vitro experiments have shown that monomeric polyphenols and tannins from cocoa may interfere with glucosyltransferase activity of *Streptococcus mutans* and reduce plaque formation (Kashket et al 1985). Similar results were reported in hamsters, with a marked caries-inhibitive effect found with a water extract of cocoa (Stralfors 1966). Cocoa bean husk, while not used in cocoa or chocolate, demonstrates antibacterial properties attributed to its unsaturated fatty acids and antiglucosyltransferase activities attributed to epicatechin polymers, as well as being shown both in vitro and in vivo to possess significant antiplaque activity (Matsumoto et al 2004).

Antitussive

It has been suggested that theobromine, a methylxanthine derivative present in cocoa, may form the basis for a new class of antitussive drugs, as it has been shown to effectively inhibit citric acid-induced cough in guinea pigs in vivo, as well as suppress capsaicin-induced cough in a human double-blind trial (Usmani et al 2005). The observation that theobromine inhibits capsaicin-induced sensory nerve depolarisation of the guinea pig and human vagus nerve suggests that its antitussive action may be mediated peripherally through an inhibitory effect on afferent nerve activation.

Skin antiageing and photoprotection

Cocoa and, more specifically, cocoa-derived flavanols have multiple beneficial effects on skin integrity, according to several clinical trials.

Long-term cocoa ingestion appears to lead to an increased resistance to UV-induced erythema and a lowered transepidermal water loss. In a crossover design study in 10 healthy women, a single dose of cocoa rich in flavanols (329 mg) was found to enhance dermal blood flow by 1.7-fold and elevate oxygen saturation of haemoglobin at 1 mm skin depth 1.8-fold 2 hours after consumption, while there was no effect seen after consumption of low-flavanol cocoa (27 mg) (Neukam et al 2007).

In a study using a model of ex vivo human skin explants, cocoa polyphenols were seen to exhibit a positive action on several indicators of skin elasticity and skin tonus, and an enhancing effect of cocoa butter on activity of cocoa polyphenol was observed (Gasser et al 2008).

There is evidence to suggest that dietary flavanols from cocoa contribute to endogenous photoprotection, improve dermal blood circulation and affect cosmetically relevant skin surface and hydration variables in women. A 12-week RCT, comparing high-flavanol (326 mg/day containing epicatechin [61 mg/day] and catechin [20 mg/day]) and low-flavanol (27 mg/day containing 6.6 mg epicatechin and 1.6 mg catechin) cocoa consumption found that high-flavanol consumption led to significantly reduced ultraviolet-induced erythema (by 15% and 25%, after 6 and 12 weeks of treatment). The high-flavanol group also experienced increased skin density, skin hydration and skin thickness along with increased blood flow in cutaneous and subcutaneous tissues, and significantly decreased skin roughness and scaling, compared with no change in the low-flavanol group (Heinrich et al 2006).

Antineurodegenerative

The major flavonoids of cocoa, epicatechin and catechin, protected cellular membrane from amyloid beta-protein-induced neurotoxicity in vitro, suggesting that cocoa may have antineurodegenerative effects (Heo & Lee 2005). This is supported by a study that found that 1-year administration of a cocoa polyphenolic extract (Acticoa powder) affects the onset of age-related cognitive deficits, urinary free dopamine levels and lifespan in old Wistar-Unilever rats (Bisson et al 2008a, 2008b). Daily oral administration of Acticoa powder was also seen to protect rats from cognitive impairments after heat exposure by counteracting the overproduction of free radicals (Rozan et al 2007). A 2012 human study confirms that the effects are also seen clinically. The study of 90 elderly men and woman with mild cognitive impairment identified that the consumption of 520–990 mg cocoa flavanols daily for 8 weeks improved the outcome of cognitive function assessments, including verbal fluency test and the trail-making test compared to those taking low (45 mg daily) flavanols (Desideri et al 2012).

OTHER ACTIONS

Acticoa powder has been observed to protect rats from prostate carcinogenesis (Bisson et al 2008a) and prostate hyperplasia as well as improve established prostate hyperplasia in an animal model (Bisson et al 2007). The clinical significance of these findings is yet to be determined.

CLINICAL USE

Cocoa consumption is not only highly pleasurable for many people, it is also correlated with reduced health risks of cardiovascular diseases, hypertension, atherosclerosis and cancer (Kim et al 2014). These benefits are mainly mediated by a range of cocoa-derived phytochemicals.

Cardiovascular disease

There is evidence to support that the flavanols in cocoa can be absorbed, are bioactive and may be responsible for the cardiovascular benefits associated with regular cocoa consumption. Several mechanisms have been proposed to explain this positive influence, including metabolic, antihypertensive, anti-inflammatory and antioxidant effects, along with decreased platelet activation and function, effects on serum lipids, insulin sensitivity, immune function and vascular endothelial function (Ding et al 2006, Eo 2008, Lippi 2008).

A 2012 Cochrane review performed a meta-analysis of 20 studies involving 856 mainly healthy adults, and found that flavanol-enriched cocoa exhibited a small but statistically significant blood pressure-lowering effect compared to controls in short-term trials of 2–18 weeks' length (Reid et al 2012).

Additionally, two recent systematic reviews and meta-analyses on the effects of chocolate, cocoa and flavanols on major cardiovascular disease risk factors found benefits on markers of vascular function, insulin resistance and cholesterol (Hooper et al 2012, Shrime et al 2011). In addition to significant antihypertensive benefits, these reviews reported significant effects on LDL (−0.07 mmol/L; 95% confidence interval (CI) −0.13, 0.00 mmol/L) and HDL (+0.03 mmol/L; 95% CI 0.00, 0.06 mmol/L), cholesterol (Hooper et al 2012) and insulin resistance (−0.94 points; 95% CI −0.59, −1.29) (Shrime et al 2011).

The impact of other chocolate constituents must be considered when evaluating the effects of chocolate on cardiometabolic health. An animal study found that the chronic supplementation of two chocolate preparations with equivalent composition aside from fibre and polyphenol content resulted in significant differences in systemic inflammatory markers, liver weight and endothelial activation markers (Yakala et al 2013).

Of the epidemiological studies conducted thus far, inverse associations between dietary polyphenols and mortality from coronary heart disease have also been identified. Small, short-term intervention studies have indicated that cocoa-containing foods may provide many cardiovascular benefits, including reducing blood pressure, inhibiting platelet function, preventing lipid oxidation, reducing LDL, increasing HDL, improving endothelial function, increasing insulin sensitivity, reducing insulin resistance and reducing inflammation.

A meta-analysis of 133 trials on flavonoid-rich foods and cardiovascular risk found that chocolate increased flow-mediated dilation after acute (3.99%; 95% CI 2.86, 5.12; six studies) and chronic (1.45%; 0.62, 2.28; two studies) intake and reduced systolic (−5.88 mmHg; −9.55, −2.21; five studies) and diastolic (−3.30 mmHg; −5.77, −0.83; four studies) blood pressure (Hooper et al 2008, Innes et al 2003). A 2006 systematic review of 136 experimental, observational and clinical studies on cocoa products and the risk of cardiovascular disease concluded that stearic acid may be neutral, while flavonoids are likely to be protective against cardiovascular mortality. The review found that multiple short-term, randomised feeding trials suggest cocoa and chocolate may exert beneficial effects on cardiovascular risk, with a meta-analysis finding that flavonoids may lower risk of cardiovascular mortality (relative risk = 0.81; 95% CI 0.71–0.92), comparing highest and lowest tertiles (Ding et al 2006).

While there are no published long-term RCTs or prospective intervention studies of cocoa with hard clinical end points (Hooper et al 2008, Maron 2004), the cardiovascular benefits of cocoa are evident in a 15-year epidemiological study of 470 elderly men, which found that cocoa intake was inversely associated with blood pressure and 15-year cardiovascular and all-cause mortality. This study found a 50% reduction in cardiovascular-related death and all-cause mortality in men with the highest tertile of cocoa intake compared to the lowest tertile, suggesting that the pharmacological actions described for cocoa do, in fact, translate into reduced cardiovascular risk and other positive clinical outcomes (Buijsse et al 2006).

Hyperlipidaemia

While the lipid content of chocolate is relatively high, around one-third of the lipid in cocoa butter is composed of the fat, stearic acid, which exerts a neutral cholesterolaemic response in humans by an unknown mechanism (Kris-Etherton et al 1993, Steinberg et al 2003). Cocoa butter, however, is considered a high-calorie fat because it has a high digestibility with a digestible energy value of 37 kJ/g in humans (Shahkhalili et al 2000). The results of a randomised, double-blind, crossover design supplementation study suggest that the addition of calcium to chocolate can significantly reduce the absorption of cocoa butter, thus reducing the absorbable energy value of the chocolate by approximately 9% while at the same time reducing the plasma LDL cholesterol level and leaving the plasma HDL cholesterol level and taste of the chocolate unchanged (Shahkhalili et al 2001).

A systematic review and meta-analysis of 10 clinical trials (n = 320) found that dark chocolate significantly reduced serum LDL by 5.90 mg/dL (95% CI −10.47, −1.32 mg/dL) and total cholesterol levels by 0.35 mmol/L (95% CI −0.64, −0.05 mmol/L) compared to low or nil cocoa control (Tokedo et al 2011). No statistically significant effects on HDL or triglycerides were found (difference in means [95% CI] −0.04 mmol/L [−0.16, 0.08], and −0.28 mmol/L [−0.75, 0.18], respectively).

Since then, a double-blind RCT of 152 healthy adults (aged 40–70 years) reported that 850 mg theobromine, a non-flavonoid constituent of cocoa, independently increased serum HDL concentrations by 0.16 mmol/L compared to placebo (Neufingerl et al 2013). In this study, the use of cocoa in addition to theobromine supplementation (total 1000 mg theobromine) did not have a significant effect on HDL.

Cocoa bran may also have a use in hypercholesterolaemia, as well as constipation, because this low-fat, high-fibre material has been shown in a randomised, controlled, double-blind study to increase faecal bulk similarly to wheat bran and reduce the LDL/HDL cholesterol ratio, with no effect on LDL cholesterol oxidation (Jenkins et al 2000).

Blood pressure

A 2012 Cochrane review of 20 studies involving 856 mainly healthy adults found that flavanol-enriched chocolate supplementation over 2–18 weeks reduced mean systolic blood pressure by 2.77 mmHg (95% CI −4.72, −0.82) and mean diastolic blood pressure by 2.20 mmHg (95% CI −3.46, −0.93; n = 19) (Reid et al 2012). These modest effects for flavanol-containing dark chocolate have been observed in various populations, including normotensive people with mild hypercholesterolaemia (Erdman et al 2008), overweight adults (Davison et al 2008, Faridi et al 2008), patients with newly diagnosed essential hypertension (Grassi et al 2005b), patients with untreated upper-range prehypertension and stage 1 hypertension without concomitant risk factors (Taubert et al 2007a) and healthy people (Grassi et al 2005a, Vlachopoulos et al 2007), including male soccer players (Fraga et al 2005).

While cocoa appears to have mild antihypertensive actions, this is complemented by positive effects on other cardiovascular risk factors, such as serum lipids, blood glucose and vascular function. These benefits are evident from the results of various clinical trials. For example, an RCT using 100 g of dark chocolate containing approximately 500 mg of polyphenol consumed daily for 15 days found reductions in diastolic blood pressure by −11.9 ± 7.7 mmHg, decreases in serum LDL cholesterol from 3.4 to 3.0 mmol/L, improvements in flow-mediated dilation and reductions in insulin resistance and increased insulin sensitivity in patients with newly diagnosed essential hypertension (Grassi et al 2005b). An 8-week double-blind, placebo-controlled crossover study found that consumption of a cocoa flavanol-containing dark chocolate bar with added plant sterols lowered serum lipids and blood pressure in a normotensive population with elevated cholesterol (Allen et al 2008). Yet another study found that 12 weeks of supplementation with high-flavanol cocoa led to reduced insulin resistance, diastolic blood pressure and mean arterial blood pressure and improved endothelial function independently of exercise in overweight and obese subjects (Davison et al 2008).

Use in children

In children, 7 g dark chocolate once daily for 7 weeks (n = 124) did not significantly affect blood pressure compared to controls (n = 70), with mean systolic pressure differing by 1.7 mmHg (95% CI −0.6 to 4.1) and mean diastolic pressure differing by −1.2 mmHg (95% CI −3.6 to 1.3) (Chan et al 2012). This study did conclude that, while providing dark chocolate appeared feasible and acceptable in a school setting, further studies would be required to clarify possible cardiovascular benefits of dark chocolate supplementation in children.

Vascular function

In a 2008 meta-analysis it was found that acute and chronic intake of chocolate increases flow-mediated dilation (Hooper et al 2008). A 30-day double-blind RCT in 41 medicated diabetic patients which compared thrice-daily dosing of flavanol-rich cocoa with a nutrient-matched control found that vascular function was significantly improved in the cocoa-treated group, as measured by flow-mediated dilation of the brachial artery (Balzer et al 2008). More recently, a randomised, placebo-controlled crossover study found that women, but not men, also experienced significant reductions in arterial stiffness (augmentation index (AI) reduced by 83% and AI at 75 beats per minute reduced by 129%) following 4-weeks of high-flavanol cocoa and dark chocolate treatment (West et al 2014). Given that the women in this study had higher AI at baseline, the clinical relevance of this finding is unclear.

A review of evidence from both animal and human studies suggests that human ingestion of the flavanol epicatechin is, at least in part, causally linked to the reported beneficial effects on vascular function (Schroeter et al 2006), while results from a controlled trial suggest that formation of vasodilative NO contributes to beneficial vascular effects (Taubert et al 2007b).

Improved vascular function after cocoa consumption has been demonstrated in a number of clinical trials involving congestive heart failure patients (Flammer et al 2012), hypercholesterolaemic postmenopausal women (Wang-Polagruto et al 2006), heart transplant recipients (Flammer et al 2007), diabetics (Balzer et al 2008), healthy subjects (Faridi et al 2008, Grassi et al 2012, Vlachopoulos et al 2007) and people with coronary artery disease (Horn et al 2013).

It has also been found that flavanol-rich cocoa enhanced several measures of endothelial function to a greater degree among older than younger healthy subjects, leading to the suggestion that the vascular effects of flavanol-rich cocoa may be greater among older people in whom endothelial function is more disturbed (Fisher & Hollenberg 2006).

There is evidence to suggest that the improved vascular function with flavanol-rich cocoa occurs acutely and in a sustained and dose-dependent manner, with a maximal flow-mediated dilation at 2 hours after a single-dose ingestion of flavanol-rich cocoa seen in a trial involving individuals with smoking-related endothelial dysfunction (Heiss et al 2007). Similar acute results were seen in a double-blind RCT involving 22 heart transplant recipients in which flavonoid-rich dark chocolate was seen to induce coronary vasodilation, improve coronary vascular function, decrease platelet adhesion and reduce serum oxidative stress 2 hours after consumption compared to cocoa-free control chocolate (Flammer et al 2007). Further evidence for acute effects comes from a study in which dark chocolate, but not white chocolate, was observed to significantly improve endothelial and platelet function in healthy smokers, with increased flow-mediated dilation, increased total antioxidant status and reduced shear stress-dependent platelet function seen 2–8 hours after ingestion (Hermann et al 2006).

The above findings are contrasted by a 6-week double-blind, placebo-controlled, fixed-dose, parallel-group clinical trial of 101 healthy older adults that compared consumption of a 37 g dark chocolate bar or 237 mL of artificially sweetened cocoa beverage with placebo. This study failed to demonstrate the predicted beneficial effects of short-term dark chocolate and cocoa consumption on neuropsychological or cardiovascular health-related variables (Crews et al 2008).

Whether sugar-free cocoa products have different effects to those containing sugar has also been investigated. A single-blind, crossover RCT of 45 healthy adults suggested that endothelial function improved significantly more with sugar-free than with regular cocoa (Faridi et al 2008). Despite this, Njike et al (2011) found that both sugar-free and sugar-sweetened cocoa beverages improved endothelial function compared to sugar-sweetened placebo, in a double-blind crossover RCT of 44 healthy, overweight (BMI 25–35 kg/m^2) adults. The same study found no significant changes for blood pressure, BMI, lipids or blood glucose levels for these cocoa beverages compared to placebo (Njike et al 2011).

Cardiac ischaemia

A prospective analysis of the self-reported chocolate consumption habits of 33,372 Swedish women over a mean follow-up of 10.4 years suggested that high chocolate consumption may be associated with a lower risk of stroke (Larsson & Virtamo 2011). There is evidence suggesting that cocoa flavanols may help in reducing cardiac ischaemia, with an animal study finding that epicatechin pretreatment confers cardioprotection in the setting of ischaemia-reperfusion injury and that the effects are independent of changes in haemodynamics, sustained over time, and accompanied by reduced levels of indicators of tissue injury (Yamazaki et al 2008). Human studies suggest that cocoa consumption may have clinical benefits for cerebrovascular ischaemic syndromes, including dementias and stroke with dietary intake of flavanol-rich cocoa being associated with a significant increase in cerebral blood flow velocity in 34 healthy elderly humans (Sorond et al 2008). It is further suggested that the prospect of increasing cerebral perfusion with cocoa flavanols is extremely promising, with implications for stroke and dementia (Fisher et al 2006).

Premenstrual syndrome

Magnesium deficiency may contribute to premenstrual syndrome symptoms, which may be improved by chocolate or cocoa powder, which contain a high concentration of magnesium (≈100 mg/100 g in chocolate and 520 mg/100 g in cocoa powder). There is also some evidence to suggest that serotonin levels are low premenstrually, and it is possible that premenstrual chocolate cravings are the body's attempt to raise central nervous system (CNS) concentrations of serotonin (Bruinsma & Taren 1999).

Enhanced cognitive function

A recent systematic review of RCTs on the neurocognitive effects of chocolate or cocoa concluded that neither cocoa nor chocolate exerted cognitive effects in chronic or subchronic administration (Scholey & Owen 2013). Despite this, the review acknowledged that some specific physiological functions underlying cognition did appear affected, including cerebral blood flow and region-specific brain activity (Crews et al 2008, Francis et al 2006).

Previously, a double-blind study suggested that improvements in cognitive function following chocolate consumption are due to the methylxanthine content of chocolate, with 11.6 g of cocoa powder producing identical improvements in cognitive function and the mood construct 'energetic arousal' as a mixture of caffeine (19 mg) and theobromine (250 mg) (Smit et al 2004).

A randomised, single-blinded, cross-over study determined that consuming 35 g dark chocolate (720 mg cocoa flavanols) improved visual contrast sensitivity and spatial memory and reduced time required to detect motion compared to 35 g white chocolate (trace flavanols) in a group of 30 healthy young adults (Field et al 2011).

Consumption of a 65-g chocolate bar was shown to significantly increase driving accuracy and reduce collisions compared to an equicaloric snack of cheese and biscuits or no snack in a small controlled trial of 12 volunteers (Smith & Rich 1998).

Motor function in Parkinson's disease

A 2012 crossover study compared the effects of a single dose of dark chocolate (200 g) containing 80% cocoa with the equivalent cocoa-free white chocolate in 26 adults diagnosed with moderate non-fluctuating Parkinson's disease (Wolz et al 2012). The study found that the single dose of dark chocolate did not result in any significant improvement in Parkinson's disease motor function. As a number of cocoa components, such as xanthine derivatives, are thought to have anti-Parkinson activity, quantifying plasma concentration of these compounds in this population may help to explain the observed effects from this study.

Colonic health and constipation

Cocoa mass has been suggested to have beneficial effects on metabolism of colonic microbiota (Mäkivuokko et al 2007) and cocoa husk rich in dietary fibre may assist paediatric patients with idiopathic chronic constipation. This is supported by an RCT that found that benefits seem to be more evident in paediatric constipated patients with slow colonic transit time (Castillejo et al 2006). Similarly, a double-blind, crossover RCT (n = 22) found that daily intake of high-flavanol cocoa over 4 weeks resulted in significant increases in faecal bifidobacterial and lactobacilli microflora and reduced clostridia compared to low-flavanol cocoa (Tzounis et al 2011).

OTHER USES

Chocolate consumption 15 minutes before exercise has been shown to enhance exercise capacity, spare glycogen stores, delay fatigue and contribute to the recovery of glycogen repletion in healthy subjects (Chen et al 1996).

Milk chocolate has also been shown to be a cheap, effective and palatable form of fatty meal for producing gallbladder contraction prior to cholecystography (Harvey 1977).

Cocoa may also be of use in lactose intolerance, with a feeding study of 35 subjects finding that the addition of cocoa significantly reduced breath hydrogen levels, as well as bloating and cramping, with the result being independent of the presence of sucrose and carrageenan (Lee & Hardy 1989).

Cocoa butter is used in the formation of suppositories and pessaries, as well as preparations for rough or chafed skin, chapped lips, sore nipples and various cosmetics (Raintree Nutrition 1996).

There is empiric evidence indicating successful treatment of copper deficiency by adding copper-rich cocoa powder to tube-feeding formulas. It is suggested that, although there are other high-copper-containing foods such as seaweed, oyster and beans, cocoa powder is advantageous due to the ease of adding it to feeding formulas (Tokuda et al 2006, Tokuda 2007).

DOSAGE RANGE

There is enormous variability in the polyphenol content of cocoa and chocolate and the flavanols in cocoa exist in a multitude of different stereochemical configurations, thus giving rise to a unique and complex mixture of compounds. Given this complexity, the quantitative analysis of cocoa flavanols can be challenging. It is only through the use of methods that can accurately quantify these flavanols that it will be possible to make meaningful dietary recommendations regarding the consumption of cocoa flavanol-containing foods (Kwik-Uribe & Bektash 2008).

Trials suggest that effective doses are approximately 40–100 g dark chocolate or 15–30 g cocoa powder, providing approximately 200–500 mg polyphenols. Beneficial effects are more likely to result from the use of cocoa powder or dark chocolate containing more than 50–60% cocoa mass.

TOXICITY

Cocoa contains caffeine, which is a mild CNS stimulant that can be profoundly toxic in large doses, resulting in arrhythmia, tachycardia, vomiting, convulsions, coma and death. The caffeine content of cocoa is variable, being approximately 0.009% by weight (Kondo et al 1996), with a typical milk chocolate bar containing approximately 10 mg of caffeine, compared to a cup of coffee, which contains approximately 100 mg (Bruinsma & Taren 1999). Fatal caffeine overdoses in adults have been reported, but are rare and typically require ingestion of more than 5 g of caffeine, which would require consumption of more than 50 kg of chocolate (Kerrigan & Lindsey 2005).

ADVERSE REACTIONS

It is believed that chocolate is a trigger for migraine, yet there is inconsistent support for this. In one small double-blind, parallel-group study of 12 patients who believed that chocolate could provoke their attacks, chocolate ingestion was more likely than placebo to trigger a typical migraine episode, with the median time until the onset of the attack of 22 hours (Gibb et al 1991). Three other double-blind, placebo-controlled trials suggest that chocolate on its own rarely precipitates migraine (Marcus et al 1997, Moffett et al 1974), with the results of one trial suggesting that chocolate was no more likely to provoke headache than was carob in typical migraine, tension-type or combined headache sufferers (Marcus et al 1997).

One case of paroxysmal supraventricular tachycardia in a healthy 53-year-old female following the consumption of 'a large amount' of chocolate has been reported (Parasramka & Dufresne 2012).

Allergy to cocoa has been documented (Taibjee et al 2004) and it has been suggested that workers employed in the processing of cocoa and flour may be at high risk for the development of allergic sensitisation and respiratory impairment (Zuskin et al 1998). One case report of cocoa aspiration causing severe aspiration pneumonitis in a 4-year-old has been documented (Lopatka et al 2004).

There is insufficient evidence to determine whether cocoa contributes to acne (Goh et al 2011, Ravenscroft 2005, Smith et al 2007). This may be due to other ingredients, such as fat and sugar content, which are known contributors to acne development and were not adequately controlled for as contributing variables (Smith et al 2007). Further studies which control for these additional factors in chocolate are required to fully evaluate the effects of cocoa on acne. The arginine content of most chocolate formulations may theoretically increase the susceptibility of consumers to cold sores (herpes simplex labialis virus). And sleep may also be adversely affected by high chocolate consumption due to its caffeine content (Lodato et al 2013).

Practice points/Patient counselling

- Cocoa consumption is associated with reduced health risks of cardiovascular diseases, hypertension, atherosclerosis and cancer.
- Cocoa has many potential benefits for the cardiovascular system and may reduce blood pressure, improve vascular function, inhibit platelet function and improve the serum cholesterol profile, as well as having beneficial effects on insulin sensitivity. However, further research is required to confirm the benefits.
- Cocoa may act to enhance cognitive function in a similar way to coffee, albeit with one-tenth the caffeine content.
- The most active agents in cocoa are the polyphenols, which are present in high amounts in dark chocolate, with lesser amounts in milk chocolate and minimal amounts in white chocolate.
- Cocoa powder contains minimal fat while dark chocolate contains less fat and sugar than milk or white chocolate. Beneficial effects are more likely to result from the use of cocoa powder or dark chocolate containing more than 50–60% cocoa mass.

SIGNIFICANT INTERACTIONS

Polyphenols may reduce iron absorption, with a cocoa beverage containing 100–400 mg total polyphenols per serving having been shown to reduce iron absorption by approximately 70% (Hurrell et al 1999).

PREGNANCY USE

Cocoa and chocolate can be considered safe to use in pregnancy.

PATIENTS' FAQs

What will this herb do for me?

Cocoa is a nutritious food that appears to have beneficial effects on blood pressure, cholesterol, blood clotting and psychological wellbeing.

When will it start to work?

Psychological effects of dark chocolate consumption may be evident immediately, whereas beneficial effects on blood pressure and cholesterol may be evident after 2–4 weeks.

Are there any safety issues?

Cocoa powder and dark chocolate are extremely safe and are unlikely to precipitate migraine, acne or dental caries or produce adverse effects from the caffeine content.

REFERENCES

Allen RR et al. Daily consumption of a dark chocolate containing flavanols and added sterol esters affects cardiovascular risk factors in a normotensive population with elevated cholesterol. J Nutr 138.4 (2008): 725–731.

Arranz S et al. Cardioprotective effects of cocoa: Clinical evidence from randomized clinical intervention trials in humans. Mol Nutr Food Res 57.6 (2013): 936–947

Arts CI et al. Chocolate as a source of tea flavonoids. Lancet 354.9177 (1999): 488.

Baba S et al. Bioavailability of (–)-epicatechin upon intake of chocolate and cocoa in human volunteers. Free Radic Res 33.5 (2000): 635–641.

Balzer J et al. Sustained benefits in vascular function through flavanol-containing cocoa in medicated diabetic patients. A double-masked, randomized, controlled trial. J Am Coll Cardiol 51.22 (2008): 2141–2149.

Bisson JF et al. Therapeutic effect of ACTICOA powder, a cocoa polyphenolic extract, on experimentally induced prostate hyperplasia in Wistar-Unilever rats. J Med Food 10.4 (2007): 628–635.

Bisson JF et al. Protective effect of Acticoa powder, a cocoa polyphenolic extract, on prostate carcinogenesis in Wistar-Unilever rats. Eur J Cancer Prev 17.1 (2008a): 54–61.

Bisson JF et al. Effects of long-term administration of a cocoa polyphenolic extract (Acticoa powder) on cognitive performances in aged rats. Br J Nutr 100.1 (2008b): 94–101.

Bravo L et al. A diet rich in dietary fibre from cocoa improves lipid profile. Agro Food Industry Hi-Tech 19.5 (Suppl) (2008): 10–112.

Bruinsma K, Taren DL. Chocolate: food or drug? J Am Diet Assoc 99.10 (1999): 1249–1256.

Buijsse B et al. Cocoa intake, blood pressure, and cardiovascular mortality: The Zutphen Elderly Study. Arch Intern Med 166.4 (2006): 411–417.

Cady RJ and Durham PL. Cocoa-enriched diets enhance expression of phosphatases and decrease expression of inflammatory molecules in trigeminal ganglion neurons. Brain Res 1323 (2010): 18–32

Castillejo G et al. A controlled, randomized, double-blind trial to evaluate the effect of a supplement of cocoa husk that is rich in dietary fiber on colonic transit in constipated pediatric patients. Pediatrics 118.3 (2006): e641–68.

Cervellati R et al. A comparison of antioxidant properties between artisan-made and factory-produced chocolate. Int J Food Sci Technol 43.10 (2008): 1866–1870.

Chan EK et al. Dark chocolate for children's blood pressure: randomised trial. Arch Dis Child 97.7 (2012): 637–640

Chen J et al. The effect of a chocolate bar supplementation on moderate exercise recovery of recreational runners. Biomed Environ Sci 9.2–3 (1996): 247–255.

Crews WD Jr et al. A double-blind, placebo-controlled, randomized trial of the effects of dark chocolate and cocoa on variables associated with neuropsychological functioning and cardiovascular health: clinical findings from a sample of healthy, cognitively intact older adults. Am J Clin Nutr 87.4 (2008): 872–880.

Davison K et al. Effect of cocoa flavanols and exercise on cardiometabolic risk factors in overweight and obese subjects. Int J Obes 32.8 (2008): 1289–1296.

Desideri G et al. Benefits in cognitive function, blood pressure, and insulin resistance through cocoa flavanol consumption in elderly subjects with mild cognitive impairment: the Cocoa, Cognition, and Aging (CoCoA) study. Hypertension 60.3 (2012): 794–801

Di Marzo V et al. Trick or treat from food endocannabinoids? Nature 396.6712 (1998): 636–637.

Di Tomaso E, et al. Brain cannabinoids in chocolate. Nature 382.6593 (1996): 677–678.

Ding EL et al. Chocolate and prevention of cardiovascular disease: a systematic review. Nutr Metab 3 (2006): 2.

Engler MB et al. Flavonoid-rich dark chocolate improves endothelial function and increases plasma epicatechin concentrations in healthy adults. J Am Coll Nutr 23.3 (2004): 197–204.

Eo A. Cocoa and chocolate consumption - are there aphrodisiac and other benefits for human health? South African J Clin Nutr 21.3 (2008): 107–113.

Erdman JW Jr et al. Effects of cocoa flavanols on risk factors for cardiovascular disease. Asia Pac J Clin Nutr 17 (Suppl 1) (2008): 284–287.

Faridi Z et al. Acute dark chocolate and cocoa ingestion and endothelial function: a randomized controlled crossover trial. Am J Clin Nutr 88.1 (2008): 58–63.

Field DT et al. Consumption of cocoa flavanols results in an acute improvement in visual and cognitive functions. Physiol & Behav 103.3–4 (2011): 255–260

Fisher ND, Hollenberg NK. Aging and vascular responses to flavanol-rich cocoa. J Hypertens 24.8 (2006): 1575–1580.

Fisher NDL et al. Cocoa flavanols and brain perfusion. J Cardiovasc Pharmacol 47.Suppl 2 (2006): S221–153.

Flammer AJ et al. Dark chocolate improves coronary vasomotion and reduces platelet reactivity. Circulation 116.21 (2007): 2376–2382.

Flammer AJ et al. Cardiovascular effects of flavanol-rich chocolate in patients with heart failure. Eur Heart J 33.17 (2012): 2172–2180

Foster-Powell K, et al. International table of glycemic index and glycemic load values. Am J Clin Nutr 76 (2002): 5–56.

Fraga CG et al. Regular consumption of a flavanol-rich chocolate can improve oxidant stress in young soccer players. Clin Dev Immunol 12.1 (2005): 11–117.

Francis S et al. The effect of flavanol-rich cocoa on the fMRI response to a cognitive task in healthy young people. J Cardiovasc Pharmacol 47.Suppl 2 (2006): S215–220

Fu Z et al. Dietary Flavonol Epicatechin Prevents the Onset of Type 1 Diabetes in Nonobese Diabetic Mice. J Agric Food Chem 61.18 (2013):4303–4309

Gasser P et al. Cocoa polyphenols and their influence on parameters involved in ex vivo skin restructuring. Int J Cosmet Sci 30.5 (2008): 339–345.

Gee JM et al. Effects of conventional sucrose-based, fructose-based and isomalt-based chocolates on postprandial metabolism in non-insulin-dependent diabetics. Eur J Clin Nutr 45.11 (1991): 561–566.

Gibb CM et al. Chocolate is a migraine-provoking agent. Cephalalgia 11.2 (1991): 93–95.

Goh W et al. Chocolate and acne: how valid was the original study? Clin Dermatol 29.4 (2011): 459–460.

Grassi D et al. Short-term administration of dark chocolate is followed by a significant increase in insulin sensitivity and a decrease in blood pressure in healthy persons. Am J Clin Nutr 81.3 (2005a): 611–14.

Grassi D et al. Cocoa reduces blood pressure and insulin resistance and improves endothelium-dependent vasodilation in hypertensives. Hypertension 46.2 (2005b): 398–405.

Grassi D et al. Blood pressure is reduced and insulin sensitivity increased in glucose-intolerant, hypertensive subjects after 15 days of consuming high-polyphenol dark chocolate. J Nutr 138.9 (2008a): 1671–1676.

Grassi D et al. Chocolate, endothelium and insulin resistance. Agro Food Industry Hi-Tech 19.3 (Suppl) (2008b): 8–12.

Grassi D et al. Protective effects of flavanol-rich dark chocolate on endothelial function and wave reflection during acute hyperglycemia. Hypertension 60.3 (2012): 827–832

Harvey IC. Milk chocolate as the fatty meal in oral cholecystography. Clin Radiol 28.6 (1977): 635–636.

Heinrich U et al. Long-term ingestion of high flavanol cocoa provides photoprotection against UV-induced erythema and improves skin condition in women. J Nutr 136.6 (2006): 1565–1569.

Heiss C et al. Acute consumption of flavanol-rich cocoa and the reversal of endothelial dysfunction in smokers. J Am Coll Cardiol 46.7 (2005): 1276–1283.

Heiss C et al. Sustained increase in flow-mediated dilation after daily intake of high-flavanol cocoa drink over 1 week. J Cardiovasc Pharmacol 49.2 (2007): 74–80.

Heo HJ, Lee CY. Epicatechin and catechin in cocoa inhibit amyloid beta protein induced apoptosis. J Agric Food Chem 53.5 (2005): 1445–1448.

Hermann FL et al. Dark chocolate improves endothelial and platelet function. Heart 92.1 (2006): 119–120.

Hollenberg NK et al. Cocoa, flavanols and cardiovascular risk. Br J Cardiol 11.5 (2004): 379–386.

Holt RR et al. Procyanidin dimer B2 [epicatechin-(4-Beta-8)-epicatechin] in human plasma after the consumption of a flavanol-rich cocoa. Am J Clin Nutr 76.4 (2002): 798–804.

Hooper L et al. Flavonoids, flavonoid-rich foods, and cardiovascular risk: a meta-analysis of randomized controlled trials. Am J Clin Nutr 88.1 (2008): 38–50.

Hooper L et al. Effects of chocolate, cocoa, and flavan-3-ols on cardiovascular health: a systemiatic review and meta-analysis of randomized trials. Am J Clin Nutr 95.3 (2012): 740–751

Hurrell RF et al. Inhibition of non-haem iron absorption in man by polyphenolic-containing beverages. Br J Nutr 81.4 (1999): 289–295.

Hurst WJ et al. Biogenic amines in chocolate: a review. Nutr Rep Int 26 (1982): 1081–1086.

Innes AJ et al. Dark chocolate inhibits platelet aggregation in healthy volunteers. Platelets 14.5 (2003): 325–327.

Jalil AMM, Ismail A. Polyphenols in cocoa and cocoa products: is there a link between antioxidant properties and health? Molecules 13.9 (2008): 2190–219.

Jenkins DJ et al. Effect of cocoa bran on low-density lipoprotein oxidation and fecal bulking. Arch Intern Med 160.15 (2000): 2374–2379.

Kashket S et al. In-vitro inhibition of glucosyltransferase from the dental plaque bacterium *Streptococcus mutans* by common beverages and food extracts. Arch Oral Biol 30.11–12 (1985): 821–826.

Keen CL et al. Cocoa antioxidants and cardiovascular health. Am J Clin Nutr 81.1 (2005): 298–303S.

Kenny TP et al. Cocoa procyanidins inhibit proliferation and angiogenic signals in human dermal microvascular endothelial cells following stimulation by low-level H_2O_2. Exp Biol Med 229.8 (2004a): 765–71.

Kenny TP et al. Pentameric procyanidins isolated from *Theobroma cacao* seeds selectively downregulate erbb2 in human aortic endothelial cells. Exp Biol Med 229.3 (2004b): 255–63.

Keogh JB, et al. The effect of milk protein on the bioavailability of cocoa polyphenols. J Food Sci 72.3 (2007): S230–3.

Kerrigan S, Lindsey T. Fatal caffeine overdose: two case reports. Forensic Sci Int 153.1 (2005): 67–69.

Kim J et al. Cocoa phytochemicals: recent advances in molecular mechanisms on health. Crit Rev Food Sci Nutr 54.11 (2011): 1458–1472.

Kondo K et al. Inhibition of LDL oxidation by cocoa. Lancet 348.9040 (1996): 1514.

Kris-Etherton P et al. The role of fatty acid saturation on plasma lipids, lipoproteins, and apolipoproteins: I. Effects of whole food diets high in cocoa butter, olive oil, soybean oil, dairy butter, and milk chocolate on the plasma lipids of young men. Metab Clin Exp 42.1 (1993): 121–129.

Kwik-Uribe C, Bektash RM. Cocoa flavanols: measurement, bioavailability and bioactivity. Asia Pac J Clin Nutr 17 (Suppl 1) (2008): 280–283.

Larsson SC and Virtamo J. Chocolate consumption and Risk of Stroke in Women. J Am Coll Cardiol 58.17 (2011): 1828–1829

Lazarus SA et al. Chocolate contains additional flavonoids not found in tea. Lancet 354.9192 (1999): 1825.

Lee CM, Hardy CM. Cocoa feeding and human lactose intolerance. Am J Clin Nutr 49.5 (1989): 840–844.

Lee KW et al. Cocoa has more phenolic phytochemicals and a higher antioxidant capacity than teas and red wine. J Agric Food Chem 51.25 (2003): 7292–7295.

Lettieri-Barbato D et al. Effect of ingestion of dark chocolate with similar lipid composition and different cocoa content on antioxidant and lipid status in healthy humans. Food Chem 132.3 (2012): 1305–1310

Lippi GM. Dark chocolate: consumption for pleasure or therapy? J Thromb Thrombolysis (2008): 1–7.

Lodato F et al (2013). Caffeine intake reduces sleep duration in adolescents. Nutr Res 33.9 (2013): 726–732

Lopatka J et al. Cocoa powder aspiration. Clin Pediatr 43.1 (2004): 111–1114.

Mäkivuokko H et al. The effect of cocoa and polydextrose on bacterial fermentation in gastrointestinal tract simulations. Biosci Biotechnol Biochem 71.8 (2007): 1834–1843.

Mao TK et al. Influence of cocoa procyanidins on the transcription of interleukin-2 in peripheral blood mononuclear cells. Int J Immunother 15.1 (1999): 23–29.

Mao T et al. Cocoa procyanidins and human cytokine transcription and secretion. J Nutr 130.8 (2000a): 2093–9S.

Mao TK et al. Effect of cocoa procyanidins on the secretion of interleukin-4 in peripheral blood mononuclear cells. J Med Food 3.2 (2000b): 107–14.

Mao TK et al. Modulation of TNF-alpha; secretion in peripheral blood mononuclear cells by cocoa flavanols and procyanidins. Dev Immunol 9.3 (2002): 135–141.

Mao TK et al. Cocoa flavonols and procyanidins promote transforming growth factor-beta1 homeostasis in peripheral blood mononuclear cells. Exp Biol Med 228.1 (2003): 93–99.

Marcus DA et al. A double-blind provocative study of chocolate as a trigger of headache. Cephalalgia 17.8 (1997): 855–862: discussion 800.

Maron DJ. Flavonoids for reduction of atherosclerotic risk. Curr Atheroscler Rep 6.1 (2004): 73–78.

Martin MA et al. Protection of human HepG2 cells against oxidative stress by cocoa phenolic extract. J Agric Food Chem 56.17 (2008): 7765–7772.

Mathur S et al. Cocoa products decrease low density lipoprotein oxidative susceptibility but do not affect biomarkers of inflammation in humans. J Nutr 132.12 (2002): 3663–3667.

Matsumoto M et al. Inhibitory effects of cacao bean husk extract on plaque formation in vitro and in vivo. Eur J Oral Sci 112.3 (2004): 249–252.

Maurage P et al. Does chocolate consumption really boost nobel award chances? The peril of over-interpreting correlations in health studies. J Nutr 143 (2013): 931–933

McShea A et al. Clinical benefit and preservation of flavonols in dark chocolate manufacturing. Nutr Rev 66.11 (2008): 630–641.

Messerli FH (2012). Chocolate consumption, cognitive function, and Nobel laureates. N Engl J Med 367.16 (2012): 1562–1564

Michener W, Rozin P. Pharmacological versus sensory factors in the satiation of chocolate craving. Physiol Behav 56.3 (1994): 419–422.

Min SY et al. Cocoa polyphenols suppress adipogenesis in vitro and obesity in vivo by targeting insulin receptor. Int J Obes (Lond) 37.4 (2013): 584–92

Moffett AM et al. Effect of chocolate in migraine: a double blind study. J Neurol Neurosurg Psychiatr 37.4 (1974): 445–448.

Muniyappa R et al. Cocoa consumption for 2 wk enhances insulin-mediated vasodilatation without improving blood pressure or insulin resistance in essential hypertension. Am J Clin Nutr 88.6 (2008): 1685–1696.

Murphy KJ et al. Dietary flavanols and procyanidin oligomers from cocoa (*Theobroma cacao*) inhibit platelet function. Am J Clin Nutr 77.6 (2003): 1466–1473.

Mursu J et al. Dark chocolate consumption increases HDL cholesterol concentration and chocolate fatty acids may inhibit lipid peroxidation in healthy humans. Free Radic Biol Med 37.9 (2004): 1351–1359.

Neufingerl N et al. Effect of cocoa and theobromine consumption on serum HDL-cholesterol concentrations: a randomised controlled trial. Am J Clin Nutr 97.6 (2013): 1201–1209

Neukam K et al. Consumption of flavanol-rich cocoa acutely increases microcirculation in human skin. Eur J Nutr 46.1 (2007): 53–56.

Njike VY et al. Effects of sugar-sweetened and sugar-free cocoa on endothelial function in overweight adults. Int J Cardiol 149.1 (2011): 83–88

Osman H et al. Extracts of cocoa (*Theobroma cacao* L.) leaves and their antioxidation potential. Food Chem 86.1 (2004): 41–46.

Palenik CJ et al. Studies of antiplaque substances derived from cocoa. J Dent Res 56 Spec. B (1977): 272.

Parasramka S and Dufresne A. Supraventricular tachycardia induced by chocolate: is chocolate too sweet for the heart? Am J Emerg Med 30.7 (2012): 1325e5–1325e7

Pase MP et al. Cocoa polyphenols enhance positive mood states but not cognitive performance: a randomized, placebo-controlled trial. J Psychopharm 27.5 (2013):451–458

Pearson DA et al. The effects of flavanol-rich cocoa and aspirin on ex vivo platelet function. Thromb Res 106.4–5 (2002): 191–197.

Pérez-Berezo T et al. Mechanisms involved in down-regulation of intestinal IgA in rats by high cocoa intake. J Nutr Biochem 23.7 (2012): 838–844

Raintree Nutrition. Tropical plant database: database file for chocolate (Theobroma cacao). Carson City: Raintree Nutrition, 1996.

Ramiro-Puig E et al. Intestinal immune system of young rats influenced by cocoa-enriched diet. J Nutr Biochem 19.8 (2008): 555–565.

Ramos S et al. Hypolipidemic effect in cholesterol-fed rats of a soluble fiber-rich product obtained from cocoa husks. J Agric Food Chem 56.16 (2008): 6985–6993.

Ravenscroft J. Evidence based update on the management of acne. Arch Dis Child Educ Pract 90 (2005): 98–101.

Record IR et al. Chocolate consumption, fecal water antioxidant activity, and hydroxyl radical production. Nutr Cancer 47.2 (2003): 131–135.

Reid K et al. Effect of cocoa on blood pressure. Cochrane Database of Systematic Reviews 2012. 8 (2012): Art. No. CD008893

Rein D et al. Epicatechin in human plasma: in vivo determination and effect of chocolate consumption on plasma oxidation status. J Nutr 130.8 (2000a): 2109–14S.

Rein D et al. Cocoa inhibits platelet activation and function. Am J Clin Nutr 72.1 (2000b): 30–5.

Rios LY et al. Cocoa procyanidins are stable during gastric transit in humans. Am J Clin Nutr 76.5 (2002): 1106–1110.

Rodriguez-Mateos A et al. Influence of sugar type on the bioavailability of cocoa flavanols. Br J Nutr 108.12 (2012): 2243–2250

Rodríguez-Ramiro I et al. Cocoa polyphenols prevent inflammation in the colon of azoxymethane-treated rats and in TNF-α-stimulated Caco-2 cells. Br J Nutr 110.2 (2013): 206–215

Roura E et al. Milk does not affect the bioavailability of cocoa powder flavonoid in healthy human. Ann Nutr Metab 51.6 (2007): 493–498.

Rozan P et al. Preventive antioxidant effects of cocoa polyphenolic extract on free radical production and cognitive performances after heat exposure in Wistar rats. J Food Sci 72.3 (2007): S203–496.

Rozin P et al. Chocolate craving and liking. Appetite 17.3 (1991): 199–212.

Ruzaidi AMM et al. Protective effect of polyphenol-rich extract prepared from Malaysian cocoa (*Theobroma cacao*) on glucose levels and lipid profiles in streptozotocin-induced diabetic rats. J Sci Food Agric 88.8 (2008): 1442–1447.

Scholey A, Owen L. The effects of chocolate on mood and cognitive function: a systematic review. Nutrition Reviews 71 (2013): 665–681.

Schnorr O et al. Cocoa flavanols lower vascular arginase activity in human endothelial cells in vitro and in erythrocytes in vivo. Arch Biochem Biophys 476.2 (2008): 211–2115.

Schramm DD et al. Chocolate procyanidins decrease the leukotriene-prostacyclin ratio in humans and human aortic endothelial cells. Am J Clin Nutr 73.1 (2001): 36–40.

Schroeter H et al. (–)-Epicatechin mediates beneficial effects of flavanol-rich cocoa on vascular function in humans. Proc Natl Acad Sci U S A 103.4 (2006): 1024–1029.

Selmi C et al. Chocolate at heart: the anti-inflammatory impact of cocoa flavanols. Mol Nutr Food Res 52.11 (2008): 1340–1348.

s'Gravenmade EJ et al. A potential cariostatic factor in cocoa beans. Caries Res 11.2 (1977): 138.

Shahkhalili Y et al. Digestibility of cocoa butter from chocolate in humans: a comparison with corn-oil. Eur J Clin Nutr 54.2 (2000): 120–125.

Shahkhalili Y et al. Calcium supplementation of chocolate: effect on cocoa butter digestibility and blood lipids in humans. Am J Clin Nutr 73.2 (2001): 246–252.

Shrime MG et al. Flavonoid-rich cocoa consumption affects multiple cardiovascular risk factors in a meta-analysis of short-term studies. J Nutr 141.11 (2011): 1982–1988

Sies H et al. Cocoa polyphenols and inflammatory mediators. Am J Clin Nutr 81.1 (2005): 304–12S.

Smit HJ et al. Methylxanthines are the psycho-pharmacologically active constituents of chocolate. Psychopharmacologia 176.3–4 (2004): 412–4119.

Smith AP, Rich N. Effects of consumption of snacks on simulated driving. Percept Motor Skills 87.3 Pt 1 (1998): 817–818.

Smith NR et al. A low glycemic load diet improved symptoms in acne vulgaris patients: a randomized controlled trial. Am J Clin Nutr 86.1 (2007): 107–115

Sorond FA et al. Cerebral blood flow response to flavanol-rich cocoa in healthy elderly humans. Neuropsychiatr Dis Treat 4.2 (2008): 433–440.

Steinberg FM et al. Cocoa and chocolate flavonoids: implications for cardiovascular health. J Am Diet Assoc 103.2 (2003): 215–223.

Stote KS et al. Effect of cocoa and green tea on biomarkers of glucose regulation, oxidative stress, inflammation and hemostasis in obese adults at risk for insulin resistance. Eur J Clin Nutr 66.10 (2012): 1153–1159

Stralfors A. Effect on hamster caries by dialysed, detanned or carbon-treated water-extract of cocoa. Arch Oral Biol 11.6 (1966): 609–615.

Taibjee SM et al. Orofacial granulomatosis worsened by chocolate: results of patch testing to ingredients of Cadbury's chocolate. Br J Dermatol 150.3 (2004): 595.

Taubert D, et al. Effect of cocoa and tea intake on blood pressure: a meta-analysis. Arch Intern Med 167.7 (2007a): 626–634.

Taubert D et al. Effects of low habitual cocoa intake on blood pressure and bioactive nitric oxide: a randomized controlled trial. JAMA 298.1 (2007b): 49–60.

Tokedo OA et al. Effects of cocoa products / dark chocolate on serum lipids: a meta-analysis. Eur J Clin Nutr 65.8 (2011): 879–886

Tokuda Y. Cocoa supplementation for copper deficiency. Agro Food Industry Hi-Tech 18.3 (2007): 11–4913.

Tokuda Y et al. Cocoa supplementation for copper deficiency associated with tube feeding nutrition. Intern Med 45.19 (2006): 1079–85.

Tomas-Barberan FA et al. A new process to develop a cocoa powder with higher flavonoid monomer content and enhanced bioavailability in healthy humans. J Agric Food Chem 55.10 (2007): 3926–3935.

Tzounis X et al. Prebiotic evaluation of cocoa-derived flavanols in healthy humans by using a randomized, controlled, double-blind, crossover intervention study. Am J Clin Nutr 93.1 (2011): 62–72

Usmani OS et al. Theobromine inhibits sensory nerve activation and cough. FASEB J 19.2 (2005): 231–233.

Vlachopoulos CV et al. Relation of habitual cocoa consumption to aortic stiffness and wave reflections, and to central hemodynamics in healthy individuals. Am J Cardiol 99.10 (2007): 1473–1475.

Wan Y et al. Effects of cocoa powder and dark chocolate on LDL oxidative susceptibility and prostaglandin concentrations in humans. Am J Clin Nutr 74.5 (2001): 596–602.

Wang-Polagruto JF et al. Chronic consumption of flavanol-rich cocoa improves endothelial function and decreases vascular cell adhesion molecule in hypercholesterolemic postmenopausal women. J Cardiovasc Pharmacol 47 (Suppl 2) (2006): S177–4986.

Waterhouse AL et al. Antioxidants in chocolate. Lancet 348.9030 (1996): 834.

Weingarten HP, Elston D. Food cravings in a college population. Appetite 17 (1991): 167–175.

West SG et al. Effects of dark chocolate and cocoa consumption on endothelial function and arterial stiffness in overweight adults. Br J Nutr [published online ahead of print] (2014) 111: 653–661.

Wiswedel I et al. Flavanol-rich cocoa drink lowers plasma F(2)-isoprostane concentrations in humans. Free Radic Biol Med 37.3 (2004): 411–421.

Wolz M et al. Comparison of chocolate to cacao-free white chocolate in Parkinson's disease: a single-dose, investigator-blinded, placebo-controlled, crossover trial. J Neurol 259.11 (2012): 2447–2451

Yakala GK et al. Effects of chocolate supplementation on metabolic and cardiovascular parameters in ApoE3L mice fed a high-cholesterol atherogenic diet. Mol Nutr Food Res 57.11 (2013): 2039–2048

Yamazaki KG et al. Short- and long-term effects of (–)-epicatechin on myocardial ischemia-reperfusion injury. Am J Physiol Heart Circ Physiol 295.2 (2008): H761–497.

Yamazaki KG et al. Effects of (–)-epicatechin on myocardial infarct size and left ventricular remodeling after permanent coronary occlusion. J Am Coll Cardiol 55.25 (2010): 2869–2876

Zhu QY et al. Influence of cocoa flavanols and procyanidins on free Radic-induced human erythrocyte hemolysis. Clin Dev Immunol 12.1 (2005): 27–34.

Zuskin E et al. Respiratory function and immunological status in cocoa and flour processing workers. Am J Indust Med 33.1 (1998): 24–32.

Coenzyme Q10

OTHER NAMES

Ubiquinone, ubidecarenone, ubiquinol

BACKGROUND AND RELEVANT PHARMACOKINETICS

Coenzyme Q10 (CoQ10) is an endogenous enzyme cofactor produced in humans from tyrosine through a cascade of reactions that itself requires eight vitamin coenzymes: tetrahydrobiopterin, vitamins B_6, C, B_2, B_{12}, folic acid, niacin and pantothenic acid (Folkers et al 1990). CoQ10 is also a fat-soluble antioxidant vitamin that plays an indispensable role in intracellular energy production.

Absorption occurs in the small intestine and tends to be poor, and is influenced by the presence of food and drink. CoQ10 is better absorbed in the presence of a fatty meal and is primarily bound to

VLDL and LDL cholesterol and transported to the systemic circulation via the lymphatic system. As such, serum levels of CoQ10 depend mostly on the amount of CoQ10-containing lipoproteins in circulation.

After incorporation into lipoproteins in the liver, CoQ10 is subsequently concentrated in various tissues, including the adrenal glands, spleen, kidneys, lungs and myocardium. Physical activity markedly reduces muscle tissue levels of CoQ10, which do not correlate to serum levels, suggesting that they are independently regulated (Laaksonen et al 1995, Overvad et al 1999).

CHEMICAL COMPONENTS

The basic structure of ubiquinones is a benzoquinone head and terpinoid tail. The number of isoprenoid units in the tail portion varies among coenzymes. CoQ10 contains one quinine group and 10 isoprenyl units (Overvad et al 1999). Ubiquinones have been found in microorganisms, plants and animals but the CoQ10 form is the most common type found in mammals and humans.

FOOD SOURCES

Meat and fish products are the most concentrated sources of CoQ10, although lesser quantities are found in boiled broccoli, cauliflower, nuts, spinach and soy. Dietary intake of CoQ10 is approximately 3–5 mg per day (Potgieter et al 2013).

DEFICIENCY SIGNS AND SYMPTOMS

No recommended daily intake (RDI) levels have been established, but there has been some speculation as to possible deficiency signs and symptoms. These include fatigue, muscle aches and pains and chronic gum disease.

Based on biopsy and/or serum samples, it has been observed that relative CoQ10 deficiency is associated with:

- congestive heart failure (Sole & Jeejeebhoy 2002, Spigset 1994a, Molyneux et al 2008)
- cardiomyopathy (Mortensen et al 1990, Senes et al 2008)
- hypertension (Karlsson et al 1991)
- ischaemic heart disease (Karlsson et al 1991, Lee et al 2012a, 2012b, 2012c)
- hyperthyroidism (Bianchi et al 1999)
- breast cancer (Folkers et al 1997)
- cystic fibrosis (Laguna et al 2008)
- pancreatic insufficiency (Laguna et al 2008)
- depression (Maes et al 2009)
- fibromyalgia (Cordero et al 2012, Miyamae et al 2013)
- septic shock (Dupic et al 2011, Donnino et al 2011)
- chronic fatigue syndrome (Maes et al 2009)
- mitochondrial myopathy (Sacconi et al 2010).

At this stage, it is still unclear whether an observation of relative deficiency in a particular disease state can be interpreted as part of the aetiology of that disease, or whether lowered levels are a consequence of disease.

A deficiency state may result from:

- impaired or reduced synthesis due to nutritional deficiencies, advancing age or medication use.
- interactions with drugs — there is clinical evidence that lovastatin, pravastatin and simvastatin reduce CoQ10 status in humans, which may, in part, explain the incidence of side effects, particularly myopathy, associated with their use (Bargossi et al 1994a, 1994b, Folkers et al 1990, Mortensen et al 1997). Clinical evidence also suggests that use of gemfibrozil and other fibric acid derivatives reduce CoQ10 levels (Aberg et al 1998). The clinical significance and long-term consequences of decreased CoQ10 synthesis due to chronic use of lipid-lowering drugs remains to be tested.

  In vitro evidence suggests that other drugs, such as clonidine, hydralazine, hydrochlorothiazide, methyldopa, metoprolol and propranolol, may also decrease endogenous production of CoQ10 (Kishi et al 1975). Other sources cite tricyclic antidepressants as further medicines that can reduce CoQ10 status (Pelton et al 1999). Whether this evidence translates to significant clinical outcomes, remains to be seen.
- inadequate intake or biosynthesis to meet increased requirements resulting from illness or excess physical exertion.
- genetic defects — deficiencies of CoQ10 have been associated with four major clinical phenotypes: (1) encephalomyopathy characterised by a triad of recurrent myoglobinuria, brain involvement and ragged-red fibres; (2) infantile multisystemic disease, typically with prominent nephropathy and encephalopathy; (3) cerebellar ataxia with marked cerebellar atrophy; and (4) pure myopathy (Quinzii et al 2008).

MAIN ACTIONS

Antioxidant

CoQ10 is a powerful antioxidant that buffers the potential adverse consequences of free radicals produced during oxidative phosphorylation in the inner mitochondrial membrane (Young et al 2007). It also binds to a site in the inner mitochondrial membrane that inhibits the mitochondrial permeability transition pore (MPTP).

Being a vital electron and proton carrier, CoQ10 supports adenosine triphosphate (ATP) synthesis in the mitochondrial inner membrane and stabilises cell membranes, preserving cellular integrity and function. It also reconstitutes vitamin E into its antioxidant form by transforming vitamin E radicals to their reduced (active) form (Kaikkonen et al 2002).

Cardioprotective

CoQ10 supplementation offers myocardial protection during cardiac surgery, as indicated by clinical trials that observed improved postoperative cardiac function and reduced myocardial structural damage with presurgery administration of CoQ10. Studies with animal models have found that CoQ10

Clinical note — Improving bioavailability

Absorption of compounds from the gastrointestinal tract is one of the important determinants of oral bioavailability. The absorption of oral CoQ10 is slow and limited due to its hydrophobicity and large molecular weight (Ochiai et al 2007). Research indicates that intestinal absorption of CoQ10 is enhanced when taken with food. To further improve bioavailability, specialty formulations have been produced by various manufacturers. Ochiai et al (2007) report that an emulsified form of CoQ10 had superior intestinal absorption and achieved a higher peak concentration than for a suspension formulation. Zmitek et al (2008) found that the water solubility and bioavailability of CoQ10 was increased significantly with the use of an inclusion complex with beta-cyclodextrin. This complex is widely used as Q10Vital in the food industry. PureSorb-Q40 (water-soluble type CoQ10 powder) is reported in single-dose human and rat studies to have a greater absorption rate and absorbed volume of CoQ10, even taken postprandially, than those of regular CoQ10, which is lipid-soluble and generally taken in the form of soft gel capsules (Nuku et al 2007). Ullmann et al (2005) tested the bioavailability of DSM Nutritional Products Ltd (Kaiseraugst, Switzerland). CoQ10 10% TG/P (all-Q), a new tablet-grade formulation, with CoQ10 Q-Gel Softsules based on the Bio-Solv technology (Tishcon Corp., Salisbury, MD; marketed by Epic4Health, Smithtown, NY) and Q-SorB (Nature's Bounty, Bohemia, NY). They conducted a crossover study, which showed a bioequivalence between Q-Gel and all-Q, and both preparations were found to have better bioavailability properties than Q-SorB.

Recently, CoQ10 producers in Kaneka, Japan, have synthesised ubiquinol (the reduced form of CoQ10) in an attempt to achieve better bioavailability and higher plasma concentrations with lower oral doses. This form is now available in Australia for over-the-counter use. Single-blind, placebo-controlled studies with healthy subjects testing single oral doses of 150 or 300 mg/day and longer term (4 weeks) oral administration of 90, 150 or 300 mg/day confirmed significant absorption of ubiquinol from the gastrointestinal tract (Hosoe et al 2007). Additionally, no safety concerns were noted on standard laboratory tests for safety or on assessment of adverse events for doses of up to 300 mg for up to 2 weeks after treatment completion.

improves preservation of mitochondrial ATP-generating capacity after ischaemia and reperfusion (Pepe et al 2007). Treated animals demonstrate improved myocardial contractile function, increased coronary flow, reduced release of creatine kinase and malondialdehyde in the cardiac effluent. Recent RCTs have found supplementation of 150 mg daily of CoQ10 reduced the inflammatory marker interleukin-6 by 14% (Lee et al 2012a), reduced lipid peroxidation (plasma malondialdehyde) and increased endogenous antioxidant activity (superoxide dismutase and catalase) in patients with coronary heart disease (Lee et al 2012a, 2012b). However, it did not have any effect on homocysteine or highly sensitive C-reactive protein (Lee et al 2012c). Recently, in vitro evidence has suggested CoQ10 protects LDL cholesterol from oxidation, which may have benefits in atherosclerosis (Ahmadvand et al 2013).

Doxorubicin — induced cardiotoxicity

Irreversible oxidative damage to cardiac mitochondria is believed to account for the dose-related cardiomyopathy induced by anthracyclines. Tests in animal models have demonstrated that CoQ10 protects against doxorubicin cardiotoxicity, possibly via antioxidant activity and protection of mitochondrial function (Combs et al 1977, Folkers et al 1978). Clinical studies provide some support for the use of oral CoQ10 and indicate that adjunctive treatment provides protection against cardiotoxicity or liver toxicity during cancer therapy; however, further studies are required to prove this association conclusively and confirm safety (Roffe et al 2004).

Antihypertensive

In the 1970s, Yamagami et al (1975, 1976) observed a deficiency in CoQ10 in patients with hypertension and suggested that correction of the deficiency could result in hypotensive effects. Small studies were initially conducted with hypertensive patients identified as CoQ10-deficient.

Since then, numerous studies have been conducted. In 2007, a meta-analysis was published which evaluated 12 clinical trials (n = 362) and found that oral CoQ10 has the potential in hypertensive patients to lower systolic blood pressure by up to 17 mmHg and diastolic blood pressure by up to 10 mmHg without significant side effects (Rosenfeldt et al 2007). Interestingly, most trials fail to identify the subjects' baseline CoQ10 plasma levels and determine whether oral administration restored levels to within the normal range. It has been suggested that CoQ10 supplementation is associated with a decrease in total peripheral resistance, possibly because of action as an antagonist of vascular superoxide, either scavenging or suppressing its synthesis (McCarty 1999).

More specifically, suspected mechanisms of action include: increased antioxidant activity reducing free-radical damage to the endothelial lining and increasing nitric oxide bioavailability (Graham et al 2009); increasing superoxide dismutase-1 which scavenges superoxide anion, which reacts with nitric oxide impairing endothelium-derived relaxation (Kedziora-Kornatowska et al 2010), reduced aldosterone secretion (Louis et al 1965), improved angiotensin II-induced oxidative stress and endothelial dysfunction and reduced angiotensin II-induced upregulation of intercellular adhesion molecule 1 (ICAM-1) and vascular cell adhesion molecule 1 (VCAM-1) (Tsuneki et al 2013).

Immunostimulant activity

Several models of immune function have demonstrated the immunostimulant activity of CoQ10 (Folkers & Wolaniuk 1985), and immunomodulating activity of CoQ10 (Bessler et al 2010).

Endothelial function

The vascular endothelium is the interface between the blood and vascular smooth muscle in arteries and is easily damaged by oxidative stress, resulting in impaired endothelial function. Substances with antioxidant and anti-inflammatory activity, such as CoQ10, have been studied for beneficial effects on endothelial function. A recent meta-analysis ($n = 194$) found CoQ10 supplementation (150–300 mg/daily) taken for 4 to 12 weeks was associated with a significant improvement in endothelial function compared to placebo, as assessed peripherally by flow-mediated dilation (FMD) of the brachial artery (Gao et al 2012). The improvement measured by FMB was a clinically significant 1.7%, which may translate to 10–25% reduction in residual cardiovascular risk for these patients. FMD is designated as an endothelium-dependent process that reflects vasorelaxation. CoQ10 supplementation was not found to improve nitrate-mediated dilation, suggesting no effect on endothelium-independent vasorelaxation. Of the study participants, 33% were women, 44% had diabetes, 34.5% had hypertension and 28% had established coronary artery disease, indicating activity in patients with and without overt cardiovascular disease. The studies included in this meta-analysis were Watts et al 2002, Tiano et al 2008, Hamilton et al 2009 and Dai et al 2011.

Recently, several in vitro studies have examined the mechanisms of CoQ10 on endothelial function using human umbilical vein endothelial cells. CoQ10 was found to prevent the oxidative stress and subsequent endothelial dysfunction induced by angiotensin II (Tsuneki et al 2013) and by the expression of oxidised low-density lipoprotein receptor (via suppressing NADPH oxidase activation) (Tsai et al 2011). In another study examining CoQ10 on the effects of oxidised LDL cholesterol on endothelial dysfunction, it was found to suppress inflammation and oxidative damage by protecting the activity of superoxide dismutase and catalase, reducing the increase in intracellular calcium and attenuating changes to nitric oxide synthase (Tsai et al 2012).

Neuroprotective

Oxidative stress, resulting in glutathione loss and oxidative DNA and protein damage, has been implicated in many neurodegenerative disorders, including Alzheimer's disease, Parkinson's disease and Huntington's disease (Young et al 2007). Of relevance in Alzheimer's disease, CoQ10 inhibits the formation of beta-amyloid protein in vitro (Ono et al 2005) and clinically, lower levels of CoQ10 have been found in the cortex of the brain in Parkinson's patients (Hargreaves et al 2008). Experimental studies in animal models suggest that CoQ10 may protect against neuronal damage that is produced by ischaemia, atherosclerosis and toxic injury. Though most have tended to be pilot studies, there are published preliminary clinical trials showing that CoQ10 may offer promise in many brain disorders.

Regulates genomic expression

CoQ10 targets the expression of multiple genes, especially those involved in cell signalling, intermediary metabolism and transport (Groneberg et al 2005, Pepe et al 2007) and inflammation (Schmelzer et al 2008, Sohet et al 2009). These mechanisms may account for some of the pharmacological effects observed with CoQ10 supplementation.

OTHER ACTIONS

Tissue protection

A protective effect of coenzyme Q10 against acute paracetamol hepatotoxicity, mostly via antioxidant, anti-inflammatory and antiapoptotic effects, has been demonstrated in vivo (Fouad & Jresat 2012). Additionally, pretreatment of test animals with coenzyme CoQ10 for 6 days protected against acute cisplatin nephrotoxicity, reducing the induced adverse effects on antioxidant defences, lipid peroxidation, tumour necrosis factor-alpha and nitric oxide concentration (Fouad et al 2010).

CoQ10 affects the transport activity of P-gp according to an in vitro test, although the clinical significance of this remains to be established (Itagaki et al 2008).

Recently, a possible antidepressant activity was identified for CoQ10 in vivo. Test animals treated with CoQ10 (25, 50, 100 and 150 mg/kg/day, for 3 weeks) found CoQ10 reduced the hippocampal DNA damage induced by chronic restraint stress in an experimental model of depression, possibly via antioxidant mechanisms and activity within the mitochondria (Aboul-Fotouh 2013).

CLINICAL USE

Cardiovascular diseases

In 1972, Folkers and Littaru from Italy documented a deficiency of CoQ10 in human heart disease (Ernster & Dallner 1995). Since those early reports, a steady stream of research articles has been published and clinical experience in its use as an adjunct to conventional treatment in various forms of heart disease has accumulated. Data from laboratory studies have also accumulated and generally provide a supportive basis for its use.

A review by Langsjoen and Langsjoen of over 34 controlled studies and additional open studies concluded that CoQ10 supplementation goes beyond the correction of a simple deficiency state with strong evidence to show that it has the potential to reduce the risk of cardiovascular disease by the maintenance of optimal cellular and mitochondrial function in cardiomyocytes.

Although investigation into specific cardiovascular diseases has been undertaken, the results of an open study of 424 patients suggested that CoQ10 may have widespread benefits. The study found that CoQ10 supplementation produced clinically significant improvements in cardiac function and reduced medication requirements in patients with a range of cardiovascular disorders, including ischaemic cardiomyopathy, dilated cardiomyopathy, primary diastolic dysfunction, hypertension, mitral valve prolapse and valvular heart disease (Langsjoen et al 1994).

A review by Langsjoen & Langsjoen (1999) of more than 34 controlled studies and additional open studies concluded that CoQ10 supplementation goes beyond the correction of a simple deficiency state, with strong evidence to show that it has the potential to reduce the risk of cardiovascular disease by the maintenance of optimal cellular and mitochondrial function in cardiomyocytes. Furthermore, a recent meta-analysis confirms that CoQ10 supplementation is associated with a significant improvement in endothelial function as measured by FMD, which may translate to 10–25% reduction in residual cardiovascular risk in people both with and without established cardiovascular disease (Gao et al 2012).

Congestive heart failure (CHF)

The potential of CoQ10 as a therapeutic agent is of great interest because it is a safe and well tolerated supplement and CHF causes significant morbidity and mortality and currently has no known cure. CoQ10 has been reported to improve symptoms of congestive heart failure (CHF) and quality of life (QOL), and to reduce hospitalisation, and is used as standard therapy for CHF in some parts of Europe, Russia and Japan.

At the cellular level, oxidative stress, mitochondrial dysfunction and energy starvation are believed to play important roles in the aetiology of CHF (Overvad et al 1999). As such, it has been suggested that low CoQ10 levels identified in patients with CHF may play a role in disease development (Jeejeebhoy et al 2002), and that restoring myocyte nutrition with vitamin supplementation, including CoQ10, produces significant improvement (Sole & Jeejeebhoy 2002). Furthermore, an inverse relationship has been found between the severity of CHF and CoQ10 levels in blood from endocardial biopsies. Some evidence suggests that decreased myocardial function is associated with decreased CoQ10 myocardial tissue concentrations and observational studies have reported that the plasma CoQ10 concentration was an independent predictor of mortality in patients with CHF (Fotino et al 2013).

Recently, the CORONA study by McMurray et al (2010) showed that while low coenzyme Q10 was a marker of greater disease severity, it is very unlikely to have utility as a clinically important prognostic biomarker in heart failure. They observed that people with lower baseline serum coenzyme Q10 levels were found to have risk factors associated with more advanced disease and poorer prognosis such as being older, more severe heart failure (higher NYHA functional class), lower EF and lower estimated glomerular filtration rate; however, multivariate analysis did not find serum coenzyme Q10 to be an independent prognostic variable (McMurray et al 2010). These results are in contrast to those published by Molyneux et al (2008), who had previously identified that plasma CoQ10 concentration in people with CHF was an independent predictor of mortality.

Clinical studies

A meta-analysis of studies published prior to 2012 examined whether CoQ10 supplementation could improve the ejection fraction (EF) and/or New York Heart Association (NYHA) classification of people with congestive heart failure (Fotino et al 2013). The analysis included 13 placebo-controlled clinical trials (seven crossover and six parallel-arm) involving a total of 395 subjects, with several additional studies not included in an earlier meta-analysis (Berman et al 2004). The included studies had a duration of 4–28 weeks, testing a dose of CoQ10 from 60–300 mg daily. Importantly, baseline EF ranged from 22% to 46% and the baseline NYHA functional class ranged from 2.3 to 3.4.

From the limited number of studies available, the changes in EF for CoQ10 compared with placebo ranged from −3.0% to 17.8% (mean 3.67%) and the pooled mean net change in NYHA classification was −0.30, which meant a slight, but non-significant improvement in NYHA heart failure classification. Additional post hoc analysis by a subgroup found positive effects in crossover trials, study duration less than 12 weeks, conducted prior to 1994 (which tended to include less sick patients) using doses less than 100 mg daily, and in those with a milder stage of CHF (baseline EF ≥ 30%). The authors stated that due to the small number of studies with NYHA classification, use of various different CoQ10 formulations and doses and lack of information about adjunctive medications used and comorbidities, results should be viewed cautiously and the study may have been under-powered to detect a true effect.

The finding regarding changes to EF largely supports the conclusion made in an earlier meta-analysis (Sander et al 2006). The primary outcome measure was EF and secondary outcome measures were cardiac output (CO), cardiac index (CI), stroke volume (SV) and stroke index (SI). The analyses used data from 11 eligible trials (randomised, double-blind, placebo-controlled) and CoQ10 doses ranging from 60 to 200 mg/day with treatment periods ranging from 1 to 6 months. Overall, there was a significant 3.7% net improvement in EF ($P <$ 0.00001). Interestingly, more profound effects on EF were observed for patients not receiving angiotensin-converting enzyme inhibitors (6.74% net improvement). To put the degree of EF improvement into perspective, the beta-blocker drug, metoprolol, is associated with an average increase in EF of 7.4% (range 3–16%), whereas carvedilol is associated with an increase of 5% (3–11%). CoQ10 also significantly increased the cardiac output by an average of 0.28 L/min. When a less conservative meta-analysis model was used, cardiac index, stroke volume and stroke index were also significantly improved. Sander et al (2006) used data from clinical trials by Hofman-Bang et al 1995, Judy et al 1986, Keogh et al 2003, Khatta et al 2000, Langsjoen et al 1985, Morisco et al 1994, Munkholm et al 1999, Permanetter et al 1992, Pogessi et al 1991, Serra et al 1991 and Watson et al 1999.

The largest controlled trial in adult cardiomyopathy and CHF was reported in 1993 and not included in the 2013 meta-analysis (Morisco et al 1993). It involved 641 patients with CHF New York Heart Association (NYHA) classes III and IV. The double-blind, placebo-controlled study used a dose of 2 mg CoQ10 per kg daily over 1 year and found that active treatment significantly improved arrhythmias and episodes of pulmonary oedema, as well as reducing the number of hospitalisations and overall mortality rate. The same researchers conducted a smaller double-blind, crossover study that again produced positive results. Oral CoQ10 (150 mg/day) taken for 4 weeks significantly improved EF, stroke volume and cardiac output in chronic heart failure patients (Morisco et al 1994).

Although CoQ10 is generally studied in heart failure patients (NYHA class II and III), a double-blind, placebo-controlled, randomised study published in 2004 (Berman et al) describes its effects in end-stage heart failure among patients awaiting heart transplantation. The study of 32 subjects compared Ultrasome CoQ10 (60 mg/day) to placebo over 3 months as an adjunct to conventional therapy. Significant improvements in functional status, clinical symptoms and QOL were reported for CoQ10; however, no significant changes in the echocardiography parameters (dimensions and contractility of cardiac chambers) or atrial natriuretic factor and tumour necrosis factor (ANF and TNF) blood levels were observed.

While the overall body of evidence generally supports the use of CoQ10 in mild heart failure, not every trial has produced positive results. One theory proposes that the most profound effects on myocardial function occur when supplementation is given shortly after the diagnosis of CHF and before the development of irreversible myocyte loss and fibrosis. Some commentators have suggested that the sample sizes, severity and duration of disease, treatment dose and duration of treatment may have contributed to the inconsistent results observed (Langsjoen 2000). An important issue that often fails to be considered is the measurement of plasma and myocyte CoQ10 concentrations and whether supplementation has achieved levels that are within the range likely to produce clinical results.

Langsjoen and Langsjoen (2008) reported that patients with CHF, NYHA class IV, often fail to achieve adequate plasma CoQ10 levels on supplemental ubiquinone at dosages up to 900 mg/day. These patients often have plasma total CoQ10 levels of less than 2.5 microgram/mL and limited clinical improvement. Interestingly, the 2013 meta-analysis reported that CHF patients had a baseline blood CoQ10 concentration ranging from 0.61 to 1.01 mcg/mL and those receiving CoQ10 supplementation had a pooled mean net increase in blood CoQ10 concentration of 1.4 mcg/mL, suggesting some may have had plasma levels at less than the optimal range (Fotino et al 2013).

One theory proposed to explain this discrepancy is that critically ill patients have intestinal oedema, which reduces oral CoQ10 absorption. To test this hypothesis, seven patients with advanced CHF were identified (mean EF 22%) with subtherapeutic plasma CoQ10 levels with mean level of 1.6 microgram/mL on an average dose of 450 mg of ubiquinone daily (150–600 mg/day) (Langsjoen & Langsjoen 2008). The doses of all patients were increased by an average of 580 mg/day of ubiquinol (450–900 mg/day) with follow-up plasma CoQ10 levels, clinical status and EF measurements by echocardiography. At these higher doses, mean plasma CoQ10 levels increased from 1.6 microgram/mL (0.9–2.0 microgram/mL) up to 6.5 microgram/mL (2.6–9.3 microgram/mL) with a subsequent mean improvement in EF from 22% (10–35%) to 39% (10–60%). Substantial clinical improvements were also reported with higher dosing as patients' NYHA class improving from a mean of IV to a mean of II (I–III).

Stocker and Macdonald make the observation that a major change in the treatment of CHF in the mid-1990s with the increase in prescription of β-blockers may account for the less impressive results obtained in CoQ10 studies conducted after this period compared to earlier ones (as reported by Fotino et al 2013). They suggest it is possible that there is an incremental benefit of CoQ10 when added to treatment that includes angiotensin-converting enzyme inhibitors but no or less incremental benefit of CoQ10 in addition to angiotensin-converting enzyme inhibitors plus β-blockers (Stocker & Macdonald 2013). To test the theory, a future study utilising CoQ10 with adjunctive beta-blockade would be necessary, but as they point out, funding such an expensive study without patent protection for CoQ10 will be near impossible.

Mortality and CHF

Ultimately, whether CoQ10 has a significant effect on EF or NYHA classifications is relatively less important than whether it affects mortality. To this end, the Q-SYMBIO trial has been conducted, a randomised, double-blind, multicentre trial with CoQ10 as adjunctive treatment of CHF, with focus on SYMptoms, BIOmarker status and long-term outcome (hospitalisations/mortality) (Stocker & Macdonald 2013). Most recently, the preliminary results were presented at the 7th International Coenzyme Q10 Association Meeting in Seville,

Spain (SA Mortensen, unpublished data, 2012 reported by Stocker and Macdonald). At completion, 422 patients with CHF were recruited and those receiving CoQ10 (2 mg/kg/day) experienced a significantly reduced all-cause mortality at 2 years compared with placebo. This important trial makes a major addition to the evidence base supporting a role of CoQ10 in the management of CHF.

Paediatric myopathy

The potential role of CoQ10 in paediatric idiopathic dilated cardiomyopathy has been investigated in a small double blind RCT. Thirty-eight subjects (<18 years) using standard treatment were given additional placebo or 2 mg/kg/daily of CoQ10 in divided doses which were increased to the maximum dose of 10 mg/kg/daily or until side effects occurred. After 6 months of treatment, those receiving CoQ10 supplementation had improved cardiac performance with t-ejection fraction, heart rate and grading of diastolic dysfunction (measured by electrocardiogram) reaching statistical significance. Additionally, the cardiac failure index score was reduced in those receiving treatment compared to the controls and CoQ10 was well tolerated (Kocharian et al 2009).

Haemodialysis

In a prospective, double-blind, placebo-controlled, crossover study, haemodialysis patients were given CoQ10 200 mg/day during 8 weeks, with a 4-week washout period. There was no significant improvement in left ventricle diastolic functions compared with placebo; however, it did improve left ventricle hypertrophy (Turk et al 2013).

IN COMBINATION

A randomised, double-blind, placebo-controlled trial the addition of a supplement containing water-soluble CoQ10 (320 mg) terclatrate and creatine (340 mg) on exercise tolerance and health-related quality of life in 67 patients with stable chronic heart failure was examined. After 8 weeks, exercise tolerance measured by peak oxygen consumption and health-related quality of life (physical component) were significantly improved compared to placebo (Fumagalli et al 2011).

Hypertension

CoQ10 has been studied both as stand-alone and adjunctive treatment in hypertension. In 2007, a meta-analysis was published which evaluated 12 clinical trials (n = 362) consisting of three randomised controlled trials, one crossover study and eight open label studies (Rosenfeldt et al 2007). In the randomised controlled trials (n = 120), systolic blood pressure in the treatment group decreased by 16.6 mmHg (12.6–20.6, $P < 0.001$), with no significant change in the placebo group. Diastolic blood pressure in the treatment group was also significantly reduced after treatment by 8.2 mmHg (6.2–10.2, $P < 0.001$), with no significant change in the placebo group. In the crossover study (n = 18), systolic blood pressure decreased by 11 mmHg and diastolic blood pressure by 8 mmHg with no significant change in the placebo group. In the open label studies (n = 214), mean systolic blood pressure decreased by 13.5 mmHg (9.8–17.1, $P < 0.001$) with active treatment and mean diastolic blood pressure significantly decreased by 10.3 mmHg (8.4–12.3, $P < 0.001$). Previously, a review of eight studies concluded that supplemental CoQ10 results in a mean decrease in systolic blood pressure of 16 mmHg and in diastolic blood pressure of 10 mmHg (Rosenfeldt et al 2003). The effect on blood pressure has been reported within 10 weeks of treatment at doses usually starting at 100 mg daily.

A 2009 Cochrane review of CoQ10 in the treatment of essential hypertension reported that despite a clinically significant greater reduction in blood pressure in the treatment group receiving 100–120 mg daily for 4–12 weeks (systolic by 11 mmHg and diastolic by 7 mmHg) compared to the placebo group, caution is needed in interpreting the findings due to the limited available data and the possibility of bias (Ho et al 2009). The review analysed results from one crossover study and two RCTs which met the inclusion criteria (n = 96) (Digiesi 1994, Singh 1999, Yamagami 1976) and were also included in the earlier meta-analysis by Rosenfeldt et al 2007).

In conjunction

The effect of CoQ10 in patients with metabolic syndrome and inadequately controlled hypertension (n = 30) was examined in a randomised, double blind, placebo-controlled, crossover trial. Subjects received either 100 mg CoQ10 twice daily or placebo for 12 weeks in addition to their antihypertensive medication, and were then changed over to the alternative treatment following a 4-week washout period. Plasma levels of CoQ10 increased 3.7 fold following treatment, however, there was no significant reduction in clinic or 24-hour ambulatory blood pressure compared to placebo, though there was a non-statistically significant trend towards reduction in 24-hour blood pressure, and a reduction in daytime diastolic blood pressure loads (the proportion of 24-hour blood pressure readings increased above 90 mmHg and ≥ 85 mmHg in diabetics) (Young et al 2012).

Cardiac surgery

The use of CoQ10 supplementation before cardiac surgery has been studied since the early 1980s. Since that time, growing evidence has suggested that CoQ10 can reduce reperfusion injury after coronary artery bypass surgery, reduce surgical complications, accelerate recovery times and, possibly, shorten hospital stays (Chello et al 1996, Chen et al 1994, Judy et al 1993, Rosenfeldt et al 2002, Taggart et al 1996, Tanaka et al 1982, Zhou et al 1999). In general, the studies that achieved positive results had provided supplements for 1–2 weeks prior to surgery. One study observed that continuing to administer CoQ10 for 30 days after surgery hastened the recovery course to 3–5 days without complications, compared with a 15–30-day recovery period for a control group, which did experience complications (Judy et al 1993, Rosenfeldt et al 2002).

A randomised, double-blind trial investigated the effects of preoperative high-dose CoQ10 therapy (300 mg/day) in patients undergoing elective cardiac surgery (mainly coronary artery bypass graft surgery (CABG) or valve replacement) (Rosenfeldt et al 2005). Approximately 2 weeks of active treatment resulted in significantly increased CoQ10 levels in the serum, atrial myocardium and mitochondria compared with placebo, but no significant change in the duration of hospital stay. Active treatment also improved subjective assessment of physical QOL (+13%) compared with placebo; however, the authors point out that physical QOL does not necessarily indicate improved cardiac pump function and further studies are required with larger sample sizes to clarify the role of CoQ10 in QOL.

More recently, a prospective, randomised trial involving patients undergoing CABG compared coenzyme Q10 supplementation (150–180 mg/day) taken for 7 to 10 days prior to surgery as an adjunct to standard care to a cohort receiving standard care only. Compared to the control group, those receiving CoQ10 experienced shorter hospital stays (7.1 vs 10.3 days) and better clinical outcomes, such as fewer reperfusion arrhythmias, greater spontaneous return of heartbeat and normal sinus rhythm after clamping, lower total inotropic medication requirements (dopamine and adrenaline). Interestingly, no significant difference in plasma levels of total antioxidants was observed between the groups until 24 hours after aortic clamp release, where it was significantly higher than baseline ($P < 0.05$) for CoQ10 treatment (Makhija et al 2008).

The use of CoQ10 as preoperative treatment may hold special significance for older patients, who generally experience poorer recovery of cardiac function after cardiac surgery than their younger counterparts. One explanation gaining support is that the aged myocardium has less homeostatic reserve and so is more sensitive to both aerobic and physical stress and less well equipped to deal with cardiac surgery. Two studies have confirmed this theory, demonstrating an age-related deficit in myocardial performance after aerobic and ischaemic stress and the capacity of CoQ10 treatment to correct age-specific diminished recovery of function (Rosenfeldt et al 1999).

Besides improving cardiac resilience, CoQ10 has been found to reduce skeletal muscle reperfusion injury after clamping and declamping by reducing the degree of peroxidative damage (Chello et al 1996).

IN COMBINATION

CoQ10 supplementation has been utilised as part of a multi-component metabolic treatment in a double-blind, randomised, placebo-controlled trial of 117 elective CABG and valve surgery patients at The Alfred Hospital (Melbourne, Australia) (Leong et al 2010). Treatment was commenced while on the waiting list for surgery (approximately 2 months) and continued for 1 month after surgery. Active treatment consisted of CoQ10 (Blackmore's CoQ10; 300 mg/day), magnesium orotate, alpha lipoic acid, omega-3 EFAs and selenium which was taken for a mean of 76 ± 7.5 days and resulted in increased antioxidant levels preoperatively so that the adverse effect of surgery on redox status was attenuated. Active treatment also reduced plasma troponin I, 24 hours postoperatively from 1.5 (1.2–1.8) mcg/L, to 2.1 (1.8–2.6) mcg/L ($P = 0.003$) and shortened the mean length of postoperative hospital stay by 1.2 days from 8.1 (7.5–8.7) to 6.9 (6.4–7.4) days ($P = 0.004$) and reduced associated hospital costs.

As a result of these positive findings, the Integrative Cardiac Wellness Program was established at The Alfred Hospital in 2008, whereby metabolic therapy is provided to all elective cardiothoracic patients prior to surgery. Metabolic therapy consists of: CoQ10 225 mg/day; R,S alpha-lipoic acid 225 mg/day; magnesium orotate 1500 mg/day (as FIT Bioceutical's Cardionutrients) and omega-3 EFAs 3000 mg/day (as FIT Bioceuticals UltraClean). Supplements are commenced after visiting the surgery pre-admission clinic, continued until the day before surgery and resumed on the ward, once solids are recommenced. A clinical audit of 337 elective cardiothoracic surgical patients in the program was recently undertaken, which found that coronary artery bypass patients had a relative reduction of 42% for positive inotropic requirements post-surgery compared to controls ($P < 0.001$) and valve repair/replacement patients, a 40% relative reduction ($P = 0.02$). Multivariate analysis was used to compare them to a historical control group receiving standard care only in the previous 3 years at the same hospital (Braun et al 2013).

Angina pectoris

Based on the observation of relative CoQ10 deficiency in patients with ischaemic heart disease, and in animal models showing that it prevents reperfusion injury, several randomised clinical trials have been performed in angina pectoris. The doses used have varied from 60 mg to 600 mg daily, and the time frames for use varied from 4 days to 4 weeks. Overall, CoQ10 appears to delay signs of oxygen deficiency in the myocardium, increases patients' stamina on a treadmill or during exercise and delays the onset of angina (Overvad et al 1999), as well as reducing glyceryl trinitrate consumption (Kamikawa et al 1985).

Statin drug use

The mechanism of action of the statin group of drugs is inhibition of 3-hydroxy-3-methylglutaryl-coenzyme A (HMG-CoA) reductase, an enzyme involved in the biosynthesis of cholesterol from acetyl-CoA. Inhibition of this enzyme also adversely affects the intrinsic biosynthesis of CoQ10, as demonstrated in laboratory animals and humans and reduces plasma and myocardial levels of CoQ10 (Bargossi et al 1994b, Folkers et al 1990, Rosenfeldt et al 2005).

This fact, plus the role of CoQ10 in mitochondrial energy production, which is required in muscle function, has prompted the hypothesis that statin-induced CoQ10 deficiency is involved in the pathogenesis of statin myopathy and long-term statin use may actually impair cardiac function.

At least nine observational studies and six RCTs have demonstrated that statins reduce plasma/serum levels of CoQ10 by 16–54% (Marcoff & Thompson 2007). This could be related to the fact that statins lower plasma LDL levels, and CoQ10 is mainly transported in LDL; however, a decrease is also found in platelets and in lymphocytes of statin-treated patients and, therefore, it could truly depend on inhibition of CoQ10 synthesis (Littarru & Langsjoen 2007). Additionally, studies have also demonstrated that co-administration of oral CoQ10 can still effectively raise serum levels when taken together with statin drugs (Bargossi et al 1994, Silver et al 2004).

Reduced muscle CoQ10 concentrations are of greater concern because they may be associated with impaired cardiac function and, theoretically, increased risk of myopathy and possibly side effects such as physical fatigue. The results obtained by Folkers et al (1990), Silver et al (2004) and Paiva et al (2005) provide support for an association between statin use and reduced intramuscular CoQ10 levels, whereas other studies find no change to intramuscular CoQ10 concentrations (Laaksonen et al 1994, 1995, 1996), increased risk of cardiovascular disease or impaired left ventricular systolic or diastolic function in hypercholesterolaemic subjects (Colquhoun et al 2005, Stocker et al 2006). Further investigation is required to determine whether long-term reductions of CoQ10 as a result of chronic statin therapy increases the risk of myopathy and whether subpopulations at risk, such as patients with familial hypercholesterolaemia, heart failure or who are over 65 years of age, may benefit from CoQ10 supplementation (Levy & Kohlhaas 2006).

Statin-induced myalgia

The decreased formation of coenzyme Q10 (CoQ10) within the body due to statin use is suspected of contributing to the incidence of statin-associated muscle pain (myalgia), one of the possible side effects of statins. The question of whether supplemental CoQ10 can help prevent or treat statin myopathy is regularly asked by clinicians.

In recent years, several intervention studies have been performed whereby CoQ10 supplementation has been tested in volunteers also taking statin medication and experiencing myalgia.

A 2012 study examined the effect of CoQ10 supplementation (Q max 30 mg twice daily) on statin-associated myopathy in 28 patients. After 6 months, serum CoQ10 levels had substantially increased (194%), subjective muscle pain reduced by almost 54% and muscle weakness by 44% (Zlatohlavek et al 2012). Similarly, positive results were obtained in a controlled double-blind randomised trial, which demonstrated 100 mg CoQ10 daily produced a 40% reduction in pain severity and 38% in pain interference with daily activities compared to a control group receiving 400 IU of vitamin E (Caso et al 2007).

In contrast, a 3-month placebo-controlled, randomised trial found no difference in the reduction of muscle pain between CoQ10 (60 mg twice daily) or placebo in patients who had developed myalgia within 2 months of starting or increasing statins. Interestingly, both the groups demonstrated significant reduction in pain after one month, suggesting a substantial placebo effect. The endpoints measured in this trial were the 10 cm visual analogue scale and the McGill pain questionnaire (Bookstaver et al 2012). Additionally, Young et al (2007) found no change in the myalgia score compared to placebo in a group receiving 200 mg CoQ10 for 12 weeks (Caso et al 2007).

It is difficult to explain the reasons for these inconsistent results; however some of the following factors should be considered. As there was no measurement of CoQ10 levels (serum or muscle) at baseline or at the end of treatment it is not possible to know if there were any differences between the study groups at baseline, if there was any change in levels by the end of the study, and therefore if the bioavailability or dose of CoQ10 used may have been factors.

There is another placebo controlled study currently being conducted in the USA to test whether CoQ10 supplementation is beneficial for reducing pain intensity in statin-induced myalgic patients (Parker et al 2013). In practice, a 3-month trial of supplemental CoQ10 can be safely considered for patients with fatigue, mild muscle soreness or slightly impaired concentration while taking long-term statins and with other risk factors for low CoQ10, such as advanced age, low meat intake or multi-system diseases.

Statin-induced cognitive impairment

Cognitive problems are also identified among some patients reporting statin adverse events. Brain tissue shares with muscle tissue a high mitochondrial vulnerability and both are the dominant organs clinically affected in CoQ10-deficiency mitochondrial syndromes (Golomb & Evans 2008). Whether the cognitive side effects reported by statin users are due to CoQ10 depletion or responds to CoQ10 treatment is not well explored. To date, a study with aged dogs that had undergone long-term statin use demonstrated significant cognitive deficits with statin use compared to age-matched controls. In addition, poorer cognition was associated with lower parietal cortex CoQ10, and statin use was associated with a significant reduction in serum

CoQ10 (Martin et al 2011). Human trials are now warranted to determine whether CoQ10 supplementation improves cognitive function in long-term statin users.

Statin use and CoQ10 supplementation

Overall, whether supplementation is effective as a treatment in statin-associated myalgia remains unclear because test results are inconsistent. Due to the low risk nature of CoQ10, a 3-month trial is worth considering in people presenting with statin-associated myalgia or generalised muscle pain and who cannot be satisfactorily treated with other agents.

It is also worth considering for people reporting fatigue, poor concentration and headaches in association with long-term statin use. Particularly consider it for those with a family history of heart failure, elevated cholesterol levels, and who are over 65 years of age and taking statin drugs long-term (Levy & Kohlhaas 2006). A trial of therapy may also be worthwhile in patients reporting fatigue, malaise, cognitive impairment and headaches as possible side effects to statin treatment.

Arrhythmias

A small open study of 27 volunteers showed that CoQ10 exerts antiarrhythmic effects in some individuals (Fujioka et al 1983).

Hypercholesterolemia

Oral CoQ10 reduces cholesterol levels, according to two clinical trials. One small 10-week open study of 26 subjects with essential hypertension study found that an oral dose of 50 mg CoQ10 taken twice daily also reduced total serum cholesterol levels with a modest increase in serum HDL cholesterol (Digiesi et al 1994). A reduction in total cholesterol was also seen in a 2013 randomised, double-blind, placebo-controlled study of 64 people with type 2 diabetes. A dose of CoQ10 (200 mg/day) significantly reduced total cholesterol, LDL-cholesterol and improved glycaemic control compared to placebo in the 12-week trial (Kolahdouz et al 2013).

Sports supplement/ergogenic aid

Because CoQ10 is essential for energy metabolism and reduces oxidative stress, researchers have speculated that it may improve athletic performance. Clinical studies investigating the effects of CoQ10 supplementation on physical capacity generally show negative results. One theory as to the differences in study results is due to great variations in serum CoQ10 levels resulting from differences in dosage and also individual responses to treatment. Nine earlier studies used test doses of CoQ10 which varied from 60 mg to 150 mg daily over time periods of 28 days to 8 weeks. Of these eight studies, only two produced positive results. One was a double-blind, crossover trial which produced positive results on both objective and subjective parameters of physical performance (Ylikoski et al 1997). In that study 94% of athletes felt that CoQ10 had improved their performance and recovery times, compared with the 33% receiving placebo. Most recently, another double-blind, placebo-controlled, crossover study of healthy people found that oral CoQ10 (300 mg/day) taken for 8 days improved subjective fatigue sensation and physical performance during fatigue-inducing workload trials (Mizuno et al 2008).

Of the others, one study found that 150 mg CoQ10 taken over 2 months had no effect on maximal oxygen consumption, lactate thresholds or forearm blood flow, although it did improve the subjective perceived level of vigour (Porter et al 1995). Another study demonstrated that CoQ10 did not alter physiological or metabolic parameters measured as part of cardiopulmonary exercise testing; however, it did extend the time and the workload required to reach muscular exhaustion (Bonetti et al 2000). Five further clinical trials produced negative results.

One retrospective study found that muscle CoQ10 levels were positively related to exercise capacity and/or marathon performance, suggesting that runners with the highest levels performed better than those with lower levels (Karlsson et al 1996).

More recent studies also demonstrate mixed results, though the majority of studies are negative. Whether negative results are due to insufficient dose or treatment time frames or differences in baseline CoQ10 levels remains to be clarified.

In another double-blind RCT of trained and untrained subjects, a single dose of CoQ10 (200 mg) resulted in raised plasma levels and significantly correlated with higher muscle CoQ10 levels, maximal oxygen consumption and treadmill time to exhaustion. After supplementation for 2 weeks, there was an increase in plasma CoQ10 levels and a non-significant trend towards increased time to exhaustion (Cooke et al 2008). In a study where 18 elite kendo athletes were given either 300 mg CoQ10 or placebo for 20 days, the active treatment group had reduced exercise-induced muscular injury with lower levels of creatine kinase, myoglobin and lipid peroxides compared with the corresponding values in the placebo group (Kon et al 2008). Similarly, the increase in lipid peroxidation induced by repeated bouts of supramaximal exercises was partially prevented following 8 weeks of CoQ10 supplementation (100 mg) in a randomised, double-blind, crossover study involving 15 sedentary men (Gul et al 2011). Recently, a small, randomised, double-blind, crossover study involving 15 healthy sedentary men found supplementation with 100 mg CoQ10 increased mean power during repeated bouts of supramaximal exercises, suggesting possible benefits in performance; however, while fatigue indexes decreased, they did not significantly differ from placebo (Gokbel et al 2010). A study by Ostman et al (2012) also failed to show any benefit from 8 weeks of supplemental CoQ10 (90 mg) daily on exercise capacity, muscle damage or oxidative stress in a small randomised, double-blind, controlled study involving moderately trained healthy men.

Postpolio syndrome

One randomised, double-blind study tested whether adding oral CoQ10 to resistance training would further improve muscle strength and endurance as well as functional capacity and health-related quality of life (Skough et al 2008). All 14 patients (8 women and 6 men) with postpolio syndrome in the 12-week study undertook muscular resistance training 3 days/week and were randomised to receive either CoQ10 200 mg/day or placebo. For all patients, muscle strength, muscle endurance and quality of life regarding mental health increased statistically significantly, but there was no significant difference between the CoQ10 and placebo groups.

Chronic obstructive pulmonary disease (COPD)

Patients with COPD have increased oxidative stress, which increases further during periods of exacerbation, so the investigation of supplements with antioxidant activity has been of interest in this cohort (Tanrikulu et al 2011). At least two clinical trials have investigated the use of CoQ10 supplementation in COPD (Fujimoto et al 1993, Satta et al 1991). In one study, 20 patients with COPD were randomly assigned CoQ10 (50 mg) or placebo as part of their pulmonary rehabilitation program (Satta et al 1991). Treatment resulted in a 13% increase in maximum oxygen consumption and a 10% increase in maximum expired volume — both significant improvements. A dose of CoQ10 (90 mg) daily over 8 weeks was studied in a smaller trial of patients with COPD (Fujimoto et al 1993 Significantly elevated serum CoQ10 levels were associated with improved hypoxaemia at rest, but pulmonary function was unchanged.

IN COMBINATION

A double-blind, placebo-controlled study found that supplementation of CoQ10 (Q-Ter) and creatine in COPD patients with chronic respiratory failure (in long term O_2 therapy) during the stable phase of the disease significantly increased lean body mass, exercise tolerance as measured by the 6-minute walk test, reduced severity of dyspnoea, improved quality of life and decreased exacerbations. Treatment consisted of Creatine 340 mg + 320 mg Coenzyme Q-Ter (Eufortyn), Scharper Therapeutics SRL taken for 2 months while diet and lifestyle remained unchanged and the study involved 55 volunteers (Marinari et al 2013).).

Cystic fibrosis

Pancreatic insufficiency and a diminished bile acid pool cause malabsorption of important essential nutrients and other dietary components in cystic fibrosis (CF) (Papas et al 2008). Of particular significance is the malabsorption of fat-soluble antioxidants such as carotenoids, tocopherols and CoQ10. Despite supplementation, CF patients are often deficient in these compounds, resulting in increased oxidative stress, which may contribute to adverse health effects. Papas et al (2008) conducted a pilot study to evaluate the safety of a novel micellar formulation (CF-1) of fat-soluble nutrients and antioxidants, which included CoQ10 (30 mg/10 mL), alpha-tocopherol (200 IU), beta-carotene (30 mg), gamma tocopherol (94 mg), vitamin D_3 (400 IU) and other tocopherols (31 mg). Ten CF subjects aged 8–45 years were given 10 mL of the formulation orally daily for 56 days after a 21-day washout period in which subjects stopped supplemental vitamin use, except for a standard multivitamin. No serious adverse effects, laboratory abnormalities or elevated nutrient levels (above normal) were identified for the treatment. Supplementation with CF-1 significantly increased CoQ10, beta-carotene and gamma tocopherol from baseline in all subjects and improvements in antioxidant plasma levels were associated with reductions in airway inflammation in CF patients.

Periodontal disease

Dry mouth is associated with ageing and may also contribute to diseases such as periodontal disease. CoQ10 is used both topically and internally for the treatment of chronic periodontal disease. Topical application has been shown to improve adult periodontitis (Hanioka et al 1994) and a small open study has shown that oral CoQ10 supplementation can produce dramatic results within 5–7 days, making location of baseline biopsy sites impossible (Wilkinson et al 1975).

Supplemental CoQ10 (100 mg ubiquinol or ubiquinone) taken for 1 month was found to significantly increase salivary secretion and salivary CoQ10 concentration in patients with dry mouth compared to placebo. The authors suggest the effects were due to improving the decreased energy production and reducing oxidative stress in salivary glands (Ryo et al 2011).

Parkinson's disease

Parkinson's disease (PD) is a neurodegenerative disorder characterised by progressive loss of dopaminergic neurons within the substantia nigra pars compacta. The pathogenesis of PD remains obscure, but there is increasing experimental and clinical data that points to a defect of the mitochondrial respiratory chain, oxidative damage and inflammation as major pathogenetic factors in PD, inducing degeneration of nigrostriatal dopaminergic neurons (Beal 2003, Ebadi et al 2001, Gotz et al 2000, Storch 2007).

It has been theorised that restoration of mitochondrial respiration and reduction of oxidative stress by CoQ10 could induce neuroprotective effects against the dopaminergic cell death in PD and could also enhance dopaminergic dysfunction (Storch 2007). As a result, CoQ10 might exert both neuroprotective and symptomatic effects in PD.

Current data from controlled clinical trials are not sufficient to answer conclusively whether CoQ10 is neuroprotective in PD or has significant symptomatic effects, as results are inconsistent. The data are presented here.

A number of preclinical studies using in vitro and in vivo models of PD have demonstrated that CoQ10 can protect the nigrostriatal dopaminergic system, and levels of CoQ10 have been reported to be decreased in blood and platelet mitochondria from subjects with PD (Shults 2005, Mischley et al 2012), as well as reduced brain CoQ10 status (Hargreaves 2008).

As a result, several clinical intervention studies have been conducted to determine whether CoQ10 supplementation can provide benefits for people with PD. An early randomised, placebo-controlled, double-blind study compared three different doses of CoQ10 (300 mg, 600 mg or 1200 mg) with placebo in 80 subjects with early PD. After 9 months of treatment, subjects taking 1200 mg CoQ10 daily experienced significant improvements in disability compared with the placebo group. CoQ10 was also well tolerated at the dosages studied (Shults et al 2002). In 2003, results were published of a double-blind, placebo-controlled study, which showed that even a relatively low dose of CoQ10 (360 mg/day) taken for a short period (4 weeks) produced a significant mild benefit on PD symptoms and significantly improved visual function compared with placebo (Muller et al 2003).

The safety and tolerability of high-dose CoQ10 in subjects with PD was investigated in an open study of 17 patients (Shults et al 2004). The study used an escalating dosage of 1200, 1800, 2400 and 3000 mg/day administered together with vitamin E (alpha-tocopherol) 1200 IU/day and failed to identify any serious adverse effects with CoQ10 administration. It also identified that plasma CoQ10 levels reached a plateau at 2400 mg/day, suggesting that higher treatment doses are not required.

In 2007, a multicentre, randomised, double-blind, placebo-controlled, stratified, parallel-group, single-dose trial was conducted which used nanoparticular CoQ10, as it has been shown to provide symptomatic effects in patients with mid-stage PD without motor fluctuations (Storch et al 2007). The study of 131 volunteers with PD without motor fluctuations and a stable anti-parkinsonian treatment were randomly assigned to receive placebo or nanoparticular CoQ10 (100 mg three times a day) for a treatment period of 3 months. This form and dose of CoQ10 led to plasma levels similar to 1200 mg/day of standard formulations; however, no significant changes to the Unified Parkinson's Disease Rating Scale (UPDRS) were observed with CoQ10 after stratification for L-dopa dosing in this group of people with mid-stage PD.

More recently, a 2011 Cochrane review examined the efficacy and safety of coenzyme Q10 in patients with early and midstage Parkinson's disease. Four randomised, double-blind, placebo-controlled trials (Muller 2003, Shults 2002, Storch 2007, The NINDS NET-PD 2007) involved a total of 452 patients, with CoQ10 doses ranging from 300 mg to 2400 mg/day. Positive effects were identified in activities of daily life in Unified Parkinson's Disease Rating Scale and the Schwab and England scale for Q10 at 1200 mg/day for 16 months versus placebo. There were no differences in the withdrawals from adverse effects between treatment and placebo groups, although there was a mildly increased relative risk ratio for pharyngitis and diarrhoea (Liu et al 2011).

A large phase III trial comparing placebo and 1200 and 2400 mg of CoQ10 daily was recently published that found no effect for oral CoQ10 supplementation on slowing the progression of disease (Beal et al 2014).

Another form of parkinsonism is progressive supranuclear palsy. A short-term double-blind, randomised, placebo-controlled, phase II trial was conducted in patients with progressive supranuclear palsy, a disease which causes down-gaze palsy with progressive rigidity and imbalance. Impairment of mitochondrial ETC complex I activity is thought to play a role in its pathogenesis suggesting a possible role for CoQ10 in its treatment. Twenty-one patients received either CoQ10 at a dose of 5 mg/kg/day or placebo. After 6 weeks, magnetic resonance spectroscopy showed a statistically significant increase in oxidative phosphorylation in the occipital cortex with an increase in the ratio of high-energy to low-energy phosphates, and an increase in motor and neuropsychological dysfunction measured by the PSP rating scale and the Frontal Assessment Battery (Stamelou et al 2008).

Alzheimer's dementia

Similar to Parkinson's disease, mitochondrial dysfunction and oxidative damage appear to play a role in the pathogenesis of Alzheimer's dementia and, therefore, CoQ10 supplementation has been investigated as a possible treatment. Currently, evidence is limited to test tube and animal studies and is far from definitive.

CoQ10 was shown to inhibit beta-amyloid formation in vitro (Ono et al 2005) and in an animal model of AD (Dumont et al 2011, Choi et al 2012, Yang et al 2008, Yang et al 2010), activate the phosphatidylinositol 3-kinase pathway involved in neuronal cell survival and adult neurogenesis (Choi et al 2013), and protect against brain mitochondrial dysfunction induced by a neurotoxic beta-peptide in a study using brain mitochondria isolated from diabetic rats (Moreira et al 2005). McDonald et al (2005) conducted two studies with test animals and found that supplemental CoQ10 (123 mg/kg/day) taken with alpha-tocopherol acetate (200 mg/kg/day) improved age-related learning deficits; however, supplementation of CoQ10 alone at this dose, or higher doses of 250 or 500 mg/kg/day, failed to produce comparable effects.

Haemodialysis

Increased oxidative stress is associated with various complications in haemodialysis (HD) patients (Sakata et al 2008). Due to its antioxidant activity, CoQ10 was administered for 6 months to 36 HD patients. Treatment was found to partially reduce oxidative stress as measured by a decrease of oxygen radical absorbing capacity (ORAC) and Trolox equivalent antioxidant capacity (TEAC).

Migraine

There is now good supportive evidence to recommend the use of CoQ10 supplementation as a preventive treatment for migraine headache. Due to its relatively good safety profile when compared to pharmaceutical migraine treatments, a 3-month trial can be considered for prevention.

Research began over a decade ago to determine whether CoQ10 could affect the course of migraine attacks and reduce their frequency, largely because migraine was starting to become known as a disorder with an underlying mitochondrial dysfunction component.

An open-labelled trial investigated the effects of oral CoQ10 supplementation (150 mg/day) over 3 months in 32 volunteers with a history of episodic migraine with or without aura. CoQ10 significantly reduced both the frequency of attacks and the number of days with migraine after 3 months' treatment (Rozen et al 2002). In 2005, Sandor et al investigated the effects of CoQ10 (300 mg/day) taken over 3 months in 42 migraine subjects in a double-blind, randomised, placebo-controlled study; 47.6% of CoQ10-treated patients responded to treatment compared with 14.4% for placebo, experiencing a (50% or less) reduction in migraine frequency (number needed to treat, 3). Active treatment was superior to placebo for reducing attack frequency, headache days and days with nausea in the third treatment month and was well tolerated.

In 2007, Hershey et al assessed 1550 paediatric patients (mean age 13.3 ± 3.5, range 3–22 yrs) attending a tertiary care centre with frequent headaches for CoQ10 deficiency (Hershey et al 2007). Of these patients, 32.9% were below the reference range. Patients with low CoQ10 were recommended to start 1 to 3 mg/kg/day of CoQ10 in liquid gel capsule formulation as part of their multidisciplinary treatment plan. Those patients who returned for follow-up (mean, 97 days) demonstrated significantly increased total CoQ10 levels and significant improvements for headache disability and headache frequency (19.2 ± 10.0 to 12.5 ± 10.8). In a subsequent, placebo-controlled, double-blind, crossover, add-on trial, 120 paediatric and adolescent migraine patients were given either CoQ10 (100 mg/day) or placebo for 32 weeks. Migraine frequency, severity and duration improved in both groups by the end of the study; however, the treatment group had significant early improvement in frequency in the first 4 weeks (Slater et al 2011).

In 2012, the Canadian Headache Society made a strong recommendation for the use of CoQ10 supplementation as a preventive treatment in migraine (Pringsheim et al 2012). This was based on a comprehensive search strategy to identify randomised, double-blind, controlled trials of drug treatments for migraine prophylaxis and relevant Cochrane reviews and then grading the evidence according to criteria developed by the US Preventive Services Task Force.

Fibromyalgia

Fibromyalgia presents with a range of symptoms including chronic pain, allodynia, fatigue, joint stiffness and migraines. Oxidative stress and mitochondrial dysfunction are thought to play a role in its pathogenesis, with some academics suggesting CoQ10 deficiency as part of the pathophysiology of fibromyalgia (Alcocer-Gomez et al 2013). This theory has gained momentum as a result of the observation that, compared to healthy controls, several studies have identified lower levels of CoQ10 in fibromyalgia patients (Cordero et al 2009, 2012, Miyamae et al 2013), as well as increased levels of oxidative stress and decreased ATP production (Cordero et al 2009, 2012). Cordero et al identified a significant correlation between high oxidative stress (measured as low CoQ10 or catalase levels, and high levels of lipid peroxidation) with headache symptoms experienced by fibromyalgia subjects.

Futhermore, in fibromyalgia subjects given CoQ10 (300 mg/day for 12 weeks), the level of oxidative stress decreased to similar levels to the controls, and the levels of CoQ10, ATP and catalase significantly increased, although they were still lower than controls. Supplementation also improved clinical symptoms and headaches measured by tender points, Fibromyalgia Impact Questionnaire, visual analogue scales and the Headache Impact Test scores (Cordero et al 2012). A small case series involving four patients who met the American College of Rheumatology (ACR) Diagnostic Criteria of 1990 and 2010 for FM found that all were CoQ10-deficient. Treatment with CoQ10 resulted in an improvement in clinical symptoms as assessed by three different methods (Alcocer-Gomez et al 2013).

In a study involving young patients with fibromyalgia (14.7 ± 2.9 years), CoQ10 100 mg/day for 12 weeks similarly increased CoQ10 levels and decreased the ratio of ubiquinone-10 to total coenzyme Q10. Cholesterol metabolism was also improved with treatment (decreased free cholesterol and cholesterol esters) as well as fatigue (measured by the Chalder Fatigue Scale); however, subjective pain intensity (assessed by VAS) and health-related QOL did not change (Miyamae et al 2013).

Further investigation with doubled-blind, placebo-controlled clinical trials is warranted.

Male infertility

Several studies have recently examined the role of coenzyme Q10 in the treatment of male infertility, with most reporting positive results. Potentially beneficial mechanisms include its role as an antioxidant, improving mitochondrial activity and energy production, all of which influence spermatogenesis and motility.

The level of seminal plasma coenzyme Q10 and oxidative stress was examined in patients with different types of male infertility in a case-controlled study. Compared to the age-matched healthy controls, those with infertility had lower seminal levels of CoQ10 and lower CoQ10 was associated with higher levels of oxidative stress (measured by malondialdehyde (MDA) (Abdul-Rasheed et al 2010). A randomised, placebo-controlled study examined the seminal levels and antioxidants effects of CoQ10 in infertile men with idiopathic oligoasthenoteratozoospermia. After 3 months of 200 mg CoQ10 supplementation daily, the levels of CoQ10 increased in the treatment group, as did the activity of seminal antioxidants catalase and superoxide dismutase while the marker of oxidative stress, seminal plasma 8-isoprostane, decreased. There was significant correlation found between the reduction in seminal oxidative stress and improved sperm morphology (Nadjarzadeh et al 2013).

Several clinical trials have suggested treatment with CoQ10 improves sperm parameters and may increase the pregnancy rate in those with male infertility. In a placebo-controlled, double-blind, randomised trial, men with idiopathic infertility receiving 200 mg/day of CoQ10 for 6 months had significantly increased seminal plasma and sperm levels of CoQ10 and increased sperm motility. The greatest response was seen in those with the lowest baseline CoQ10 and sperm motility levels (Balercia et al 2009). Similarly, in a study by Safarinejad et al (2009) involving 212 infertile men (aged 21–42 years) with idiopathic oligoasthenoteratospermia, 300 mg/day of CoQ10 for 26 weeks led to a significant increase in sperm density (increase of 21.5% versus 1.3%) and motility (increase of 30.7% versus 2%), as well as a decrease in serum follicle-stimulating hormone (suggesting better spermatogenesis) and increase in inhibin B (reflecting better Sertoli's cell function); however, there was no difference in the pregnancy rate compared to placebo. Interestingly, at the 56 week follow-up (30 weeks post-treatment) sperm count, motility and morphology were still higher in the CoQ10 treated group compared to placebo, although it was not statistically significant. More recently, Safarinejad has conducted two additional studies. Using the same study design as above, 200 mg ubiquinol/day was given to 114 infertile men with idiopathic oligoasthenoteratozoospermia for 26 weeks. Compared to the placebo group (n = 114), active treatment improved several sperm parameters including sperm density, sperm motility (35.8% versus 25.4%) and sperm morphology (17.6% versus 14.8%). As in the 2009 study, serum follicle-stimulating hormone decreased while inhibin B levels increased. Sperm parameters had decreased again at the 12-week follow-up post-treatment; however, there was still a statistically significant improvement from the placebo group for sperm density and motility (Safarinejad et al 2012b). An open label prospective study was conducted with 287 infertile men with idiopathic oligoasthenoteratospermia who had previously undergone at least two failed infertility treatments. They received CoQ10 300 mg (Nutri Q10) twice daily for 12 months. Compared to baseline, blood and seminal CoQ10 levels increased at 3 months and remained steady for the remainder of the study. Sperm parameters significantly increased concentration by 114%, progressive motility by 105%, and morphology by 79%. There was also a pregnancy rate of 34.1% achieved within a 8.4 ± 4.7 months (Safarinejad 2012).

In contrast, a double-blind, placebo-controlled clinical trial (n = 47) found 200 mg CoQ10 for 3 months did not significantly change sperm concentration, motility and morphology in infertile men with idiopathic oligoasthenoteratozoospermia, although total antioxidant capacity of seminal plasma significantly increased (Nadjarzadeh et al 2011). As this study was shorter than those reporting positive results, the shorter treatment timeframe may have been a factor.

OTHER USES

Cancer

Currently, controlled studies are not available to determine the clinical effectiveness of CoQ10 in cancer; however, there have been several case reports of CoQ10 (390 mg/day) successfully reducing metastases or eliminating tumours entirely (Lockwood et al 1994, 1995). This supports numerous recent in vitro and animal studies that also suggest a protective role for CoQ10 against cancer development (Bahar et al 2010, Fouad et al 2012, Kim & Park 2010, Mizushina et al 2008). An in vivo study found that CoQ10 enhances the effects of immunochemotherapy (Kokawa et al 1983).

Studies investigating the plasma level of CoQ10 in those with cancer have reported variable correlation. In postmenopausal women, higher CoQ10 levels were found to be associated with an increased risk of breast cancer (Chai et al 2010), while a moderate amount was associated with reduced risk of prostate cancer in men (Chai et al 2011). Furthermore, compared to placebo, supplementation with CoQ10 for 12 weeks significantly lowered PSA levels from baseline in men with PSA levels below 2.5 ng/L, and there was a strong correlation between serum CoQ10 and PSA (Safarinejad et al 2012a).

Reducing cardiotoxic effects of anthracyclines

There is some evidence that CoQ10 supplementation protects the mitochondria of the heart from anthracycline-induced damage. A systematic review of six studies (three randomised), in which patients in five of the six studies received anthracyclines, concluded that CoQ10 provides some protection against cardiotoxicity or liver toxicity during cancer treatment; however, weaknesses in design and reporting made it difficult to reach a definitive conclusion (Roffe et al 2004). Despite the high level of heterogeneity, it appeared that CoQ10 had a stabilising effect on the heart. Importantly, CoQ10 was not shown to interfere with standard treatments in the clinical trials reviewed and no adverse effects were reported in any single study for CoQ10 administration.

Sample sizes in the studies ranged from 19 to 88 patients and one study included children. The methods researchers used to measure patient tolerance to anthracyclines and other cancer treatments were heart function and toxicity in five studies, and hair loss and liver enzymes in one study. The dose of CoQ10 investigated in the trials ranged from 90 mg/day to 240 mg/day. The lack of adverse effect by CoQ10 on cytotoxicity of doxorubicin was also supported by a recent in vitro study using breast cancer cell lines treated with doxorubicin at a range of CoQ10 concentrations (Greenlee et al 2012).

Reducing side effects of tamoxifen

Tamoxifen is a common treatment used by those with breast cancer and is associated with some adverse effects, such as increasing oxidative stress and causing hypertriglyceridaemia. A study examining the effects of Coenzyme Q10 (100 mg) supplementation in addition to tamoxifen in breast cancer patients found it counteracted the effects of tamoxifen on raising triglycerides and increasing angiogenesis (increasing potential tumour metastasis) (Sachdanandam 2008). Similarly, in a study examining postmenopausal women with breast cancer treated with tamoxifen, the addition of CoQ10 combined with niacin and riboflavin for 90 days reduced oxidative stress and improved antioxidant status.

Several animal and in vitro studies have suggested a protective effect of CoQ10 from chemotherapy-induced organ toxicity (Celebi et al 2013, da Silva Machado et al 2013, El-Sheikh et al 2012, Sato et al 2013).

Mitochondrial myopathy

An open multicentre study involving 44 volunteers with mitochondrial myopathies showed that treatment with CoQ10 (2 mg/kg daily) over 6 months decreased post-exercise lactate levels by at least 25% in 16 patients. Of those responding, a further 3 months' treatment with either CoQ10 or placebo produced no significant differences (Bresolin et al 1990). A more recent randomised, double-blind, crossover trial involving 30 patients with mitochondrial disease (mostly due to MELAS, chronic external progressive encephalopathy and mitochondrial DNA deletions) tested a high dose of oral CoQ10 (1200 mg/day). After 60 days of treatment, plasma CoQ10 levels were increased 5.5-fold, the post-exercise rise in lactate was reduced and the cycle aerobic capacity (measured by oxygen consumption in lean body mass) was increased, There was no effect on other measurements including grip strength, or resting lactate production during a non-ischaemic isometric forearm exercise protocol (Glover et al 2010).

Age-related macular degeneration (in combination)

Mitochondrial dysfunction is likely to play a role in the pathophysiology of age-related macular degeneration (Littarru & Tiano 2005). The level of CoQ10 in the retina has been shown to decrease with age by approximately 40% and the reduction in antioxidant protection and ATP synthesis may contribute to age-associated eye diseases, such as macular degeneration (Qu et al 2009). Further potential benefits of CoQ10 for eye health include in vitro evidence of its ability to protect lens epithelial cells from light-induced damage (Kernt et al 2010) and retinal cells from radiation-induced apoptosis (Lulli et al 2012a, Lulli et al 2012b). As a result, researchers are investigating therapeutic agents, such as CoQ10, which affect mitochondrial function.

Metabolic therapy consisting of a combination of omega-3 fatty acids, CoQ10 and acetyl-L-carnitine may have potential benefits as a treatment for early age-related macular degeneration by improving mitochondrial dysfunction, specifically improving lipid metabolism and ATP production in the retinal pigment epithelium, improving photoreceptor turnover and reducing generation of reactive oxygen species (Feher et al 2007). According to a pilot study and a randomised, placebo-controlled, double-blind clinical trial, both central visual field and visual acuity slightly improved after 3–6 months of treatment with the metabolic combination; however, the difference was not statistically significant when compared to the baseline or to controls. Treatment produced an improvement in fundus alterations as the drusen-covered area decreased significantly compared to baseline readings or controls, and was most marked in the less-affected eyes. Interestingly, a prospective case study on long-term treatment confirmed these observations. Visual function remained stable and, generally, drusen regression continued for years and for some intermediate and advanced cases, significant regression of drusen was found with treatment.

Friedreich's ataxia

Decreased mitochondrial respiratory chain function and increased oxidative stress and iron accumulation play significant roles in the disease mechanism of Friedreich's ataxia (FRDA), raising the possibility that energy enhancement and antioxidant therapies may be an effective treatment (Cooper & Schapira 2007). Therapeutic avenues for patients with FRDA are beginning to be explored; in particular, targeting antioxidant protection, enhancement of mitochondrial oxidative phosphorylation and iron chelation. The use of quinone therapy (ubiquinone and idebenone) has been the most extensively studied to date, with clear benefits demonstrated using evaluations of both disease biomarkers and clinical symptoms (Mariotti et al 2003).

A 4-year follow-up on 10 Friedreich's ataxia patients treated with CoQ10 (400 mg/day) and vitamin E (2100 IU/day) showed a substantial improvement in cardiac and skeletal muscle bioenergetics and heart function, which was maintained over the test period and some clinical feature of disease (Hart et al 2005). Comparison with cross-sectional data from 77 patients with FRDA indicated the changes in total International Cooperative Ataxia Rating Scale and kinetic scores over the trial period were better than predicted for seven patients, but the posture and gait and hand dexterity scores progressed as predicted.

In a more recent pilot study involving 50 subjects, the potential for high dose CoQ10 and vitamin E to modify the clinical progression of Friedreich's ataxia was investigated. Patients were randomly assigned to either high- or low-dose CoQ10 and vitamin E. At baseline, both groups had low serum CoQ10 and vitamin E, which significantly increased in both groups over the course of the 2-year trial. There was improvement in the International Cooperative Ataxia Rating Scale (ICARS) in 49% of patients when compared to cross-sectional data, but the response did not differ between the high- and low-dose groups. Serum CoQ10 levels were the best predictor of positive clinical response to treatment with CoQ10/vitamin E (Cooper et al 2008).

Tinnitus and hearing loss

CoQ10 has been considered in hearing impairment due to its ability to act as an antioxidant and inhibit oxidative stress in the inner ear and reduce damage induced by noise (Hirose et al 2008).

In patients with a low plasma CoQ10 concentration, CoQ10 supply may decrease the tinnitus expression in chronic tinnitus aurium according to a 16-week prospective, non-randomised clinical trial (n = 20) (Khan et al 2007). CoQ10 was tested in this population because of its antioxidant activity.

IN COMBINATION

A controlled prospective study (n = 120) examined the effects of CoQ10 in addition to steroid treatment in patients diagnosed with sudden sensorineural hearing loss. The CoQ10 was administered at a dose of 200 mg three times daily for 5 days and then 100 mg three times daily for another 10 days. After 3 months, the CoQ10 group had a non-statistically-significant additional benefit in hearing improvement compared to the steroid treatment alone (78.3% compared to 71.7%), but had a significantly better improvement in speech discrimination (Ahn et al 2010). This was supported by a more recent study in patients with presbycusis, a disorder with progressive bilateral symmetrical age-related sensorineural hearing loss. Patients (n = 60) were given either a water-soluble form of CoQ10 (Q-TER, 160 mg), vitamin E (50 mg) or placebo for 30 days. All patients receiving the CoQ10 had improvement in hearing, which was significant at most frequencies compared to the vitamin E group. No differences were found in those receiving the placebo treatment (Salami et al 2010).

Myelodysplastic syndromes

The myelodysplastic syndromes (MDS) are a collection of haematopoietic disorders with varying degrees of mono- to trilineage cytopenias and bone marrow dysplasia. In recent years, much progress has been made in the treatment of MDS and there are now several therapeutic compounds used with varying levels of success; however, side effects make them unattractive for patients (Galili et al 2007).

Galili et al tested CoQ10 supplementation in MDS patients with low- to intermediate-2-risk disease. A variety of responses were observed in 7 of 29 patients. Sequencing mitochondrial DNA (mtDNA) from pretreatment bone marrows showed multiple mutations, some resulting in amino acid changes, in 3 in 5 non-responders, 1 in 4 responders and in two control samples. Based on these observations, it appears that CoQ10 may be of clinical benefit in a subset of MDS patients, but responders cannot be easily preselected on the basis of either the conventional clinical and pathological characteristics or mtDNA mutations.

Huntington's chorea

A randomised, double-blind study involving 347 patients with early Huntington's chorea showed that a dose of CoQ10 (600 mg/day) taken over 30 months produced a trend towards slow decline as well as beneficial trends in some secondary measures; however, changes were not significant at this dosage level (Huntington's Study Group, 2001).

In a more recent 20-week open-label study by the same group, the effect on blood levels and safety of high dose CoQ10 supplementation was tested. Subjects (8 healthy and 20 with Huntington's disease) were supplemented with 1200 mg CoQ10 for 4 weeks, with the dose increasing by 1200 mg every 4 weeks to the maximum of 3600 mg/day. Blood levels of CoQ10 increased steadily from baseline 1.26 ± 1.27 mcg/mL to a peak of 7.49 ± 4.09 mcg/mL at a dose of 3600 mg at 12 weeks, and then declined again to 6.78 ± 3.36 mcg/mL at the same dose at week 20. The most common adverse effects reported were gastrointestinal symptoms. Most symptoms developed at the initial dosage of 1200 mg/day, with no new symptoms occurring at the 2400 mg dose although two new cases occurred at the 3600 mg dose. It is possible that a smaller initial dose may reduce initial symptoms. The authors suggest that 2400 mg provides the best balance between increased blood levels and tolerability (Huntington Study Group, 2010).

C

Preeclampsia

Teran et al (2009) conducted a randomised, double-blind, placebo-controlled trial involving 235 pregnant women at increased risk of preeclampsia. Women who received 100 mg of CoQ10 twice daily from week 20 until delivery had significantly reduced risk of developing preeclampsia compared to the placebo group (14.4% versus 25.6%). Possible mechanisms of action include reducing oxidative stress and improving endothelial function, but further research is required to clarify the outcomes.

Diabetes

In 2009, the observation was made that plasma CoQ10 was significantly lower in a cohort of 28 people with type 2 diabetes compared to healthy controls and there was a negative correlation between plasma CoQ10 and glycosylated haemoglobin (El-ghoroury et al 2009). Soon after, a small open-label study found that volunteers with type 2 diabetes given 200 mg ubiquinol daily for 12 weeks, in addition to their existing hypoglycaemic medication, improved their glycosylated haemoglobin readings. No significant differences were seen for blood pressure, lipid profile, oxidative stress or inflammatory markers. Furthermore, five healthy volunteers who received 200 mg ubiquinol daily for 4 weeks had improved insulinogenic index and ratio of proinsulin to insulin, suggesting that CoQ10 may improve glucose control via increasing insulin secretion (Mezawa et al 2012). In 2013, a randomised, double-blind, placebo-controlled study of 64 people with type 2 diabetes, CoQ10 (200 mg/day) significantly reduced total cholesterol, LDL-cholesterol and improved glycaemic control compared to placebo (Kolahdouz et al 2013). Treatment was taken for 12 weeks, resulting in serum HbA_{1C} concentration decreasing in the CoQ10-treated group (8 ± 2.28% vs 8.61 ± 2.47%) with no significant changes seen for placebo.

Peyronie's disease

Peyronie's disease is an acquired idiopathic localised fibrosis of the penis which causes the penis to curve and associated sexual dysfunction. Safarinejad et al investigated the effects of CoQ10 supplementation in the treatment of early chronic Peyronie's disease in 186 patients. Treatment with CoQ10 300 mg/day for 24 weeks significantly reduced plaque size and penile curvature, improved erectile function (International Index of Erectile Function increasing by 117.1 versus 8.6%) and slowed disease progression compared to the placebo group (Safarinejad 2010).

DOSAGE RANGE

According to clinical studies

- Generally 100–150 mg/day has been used for conditions such as congestive cardiac failure (Mortensen et al 1990), hypertension, neurological disease, performance enhancement, periodontal disease (Wilkinson et al 1975).
- As preparation for cardiac surgery: 100–300 mg/day for 2 weeks before surgery followed by 100–225 mg/day for 1 month after surgery has been used (Judy et al 1993, Rosenfeldt et al 2002, 2005, Braun et al 2013).
- Adjunct to chemotherapy (anthracyclines) 90–240 mg/day, but evidence is not definitive.
- Angina pectoris: 60–600 mg daily.
- Chronic obstructive pulmonary disease: 50–90 mg daily.
- Cholesterol lowering: 200 mg daily (in type 2 diabetes).
- Congestive heart failure: 60–200 mg/day or 2 mg/kg/day for reducing mortality.
- Dry mouth: 100 mg/day.
- Fibromyalgia: 100–300 mg/day.
- Huntington's chorea: 600 mg daily.
- Hypertension: 100–120 mg/day.
- Male infertility: 200–600 mg/day.
- Migraine: 150–300 mg daily.
- Parkinson's disease: 1200 mg/day.
- Peyronie disease: 300 mg/day.
- Type 2 diabetes: 200 mg daily ubiquinol for improved glycosylated Hb levels.
- Sports supplement: 60–300 mg/day — inconsistent results.
- Statin-associated myalgia: 60–200 mg/day — inconsistent results.

ADVERSE REACTIONS

CoQ10 appears relatively safe and non-toxic and is extremely well tolerated. Dizziness, nausea, epigastric discomfort, anorexia, diarrhoea, photophobia, irritability and skin rash occur in less than 1% of patients. This tends to occur with higher doses (> 200 mg/day).

SIGNIFICANT INTERACTIONS

When controlled studies are not available, interactions are based on evidence of pharmacological activity, case reports and other evidence and are largely theoretical.

Beta-adrenergic antagonists

Induces CoQ10 depletion — beneficial interaction with co-administration (Stargrove et al 2008).

Doxorubicin

Tests in animal models have demonstrated that CoQ10 protects against doxorubicin cardiotoxicity (Combs et al 1977, Folkers et al 1978) and clinical studies provide some support for the use of oral CoQ10, and indicate that adjunctive treatment provides some protection against cardiotoxicity or liver toxicity during cancer therapy; however, further studies are required to prove this association conclusively (Roffe et al 2004). Furthermore, in vivo results indicate that CoQ10 has no significant effect on the pharmacokinetics of doxorubicin and the formation of the cytotoxic metabolite, doxorubicinol (Combs et al 1977, Zhou & Chowbay 2002) — potentially beneficial interaction with co-administration under professional supervision.

Phenothiazines

CoQ10 reduces adverse effect this drug class has on CoQ10-related enzymes, NADH oxidase and succinoxidase — beneficial interaction with co-administration (Stargrove et al 2008).

Statin drugs

Currently, it is still not clear whether CoQ10 supplementation should be considered a necessary adjunct to all patients taking statin drugs; however, there are no known risks to this supplement and there is some anecdotal and clinical trial evidence of its effectiveness (Marcoff & Thompson 2007). Consequently, CoQ10 can be tested in patients requiring statin treatment, who develop statin myalgia, headache, fatigue or malaise as statin-induced side effects. It may also prove useful for patients considered at risk of deficiency, in particular, patients with a family history of heart failure, elevated cholesterol levels and who are older than 65 years and taking statin drugs long term (Levy & Kohlhaas 2006) — possible beneficial interaction with co-administration, particularly with the antioxidant effects of superoxide dismutase (Okello et al 2009).

Sulfonylureas

CoQ10 reduces adverse effect this drug class has on CoQ10-related enzymes, NADH oxidase and low CoQ10 levels have been observed in people with diabetes — beneficial interaction with co-administration (Stargrove et al 2008).

Tamoxifen

Concomitant use of CoQ10 reduced triglyceride levels in one study — potentially beneficial.

Theophylline

An animal study suggests significant changes to the pharmacokinetics of theophylline, such as time to peak concentration, half-life and distribution following treatment with CoQ10. While there is very limited research, there may be possible interactions (Baskaran et al 2008).

Timolol

Eye drops — oral CoQ10 reduced the vascular side effects of timolol without affecting eye pressure (Takahashi 1989) — beneficial interaction with co-administration.

Tricyclic antidepressants

CoQ10 reduces adverse effect this drug class has on CoQ10-related enzymes, NADH-oxidase and succinoxidase — beneficial interaction with co-administration (Stargrove et al 2008).

Warfarin

There are three case reports suggesting that CoQ10 may decrease the international normalised ratio (INR) in patients previously stabilised on anticoagulants (Spigset 1994b). However, a double-blind crossover study involving 24 outpatients on stable long-term warfarin found that oral CoQ10 (100 mg) daily had no significant effect on INR or warfarin levels (Engelson et al 2003). One observational study suggested an increase in minor bleeding events but not INR (Shalansky et al 2007). Observe patients using high CoQ10 doses and taking warfarin.

Vitamin E

Reconstitutes oxidised vitamin E to its unoxidised form — beneficial interaction with co-administration.

CONTRAINDICATIONS AND PRECAUTIONS

Insufficient reliable evidence — unknown.

PREGNANCY USE

Since this is an endogenously produced substance that has been tested in preeclampsia without serious negative outcomes, it is likely to be safe in this population during the final trimester.

Practice points/Patient counselling

- CoQ10 is a safe antioxidant vitamin used in supplement form for a wide range of diseases.
- Meta-analyses provide support for its use in congestive heart failure and hypertension.
- Clinical evidence further supports the use of presurgical supplementation in cardiac surgery, as it improves recovery and has cardioprotective activity.
- Clinical evidence supports its use in the prevention of migraine headache.
- There is also some clinical evidence suggesting a role in fibromyalgia, dry mouth, type 2 diabetes, Huntington's chorea, mitochondrial myopathy, COPD, periodontal disease, haemodialysis, Friedreich's ataxia, tinnitus, age-related macular degeneration, cystic fibrosis, male infertility and reducing cardiotoxicity and liver toxicity associated with anthracyclines, although further research is required.
- Whether CoQ10 may slow the progression of PD is unclear.
- Several common medicines, such as statins, have been found to reduce serum CoQ10 status. It is still unclear whether CoQ10 should be considered a necessary adjunct to statin drugs; however, there are no known risks to this supplement and there is some anecdotal and clinical trial evidence of its effectiveness. In particular, it may be useful in patients who develop statin myalgia, headache, fatigue or malaise and those considered at risk of deficiency, such as people of advanced age and vegetarians..

PATIENTS' FAQs

What will this vitamin do for me?

CoQ10 is an antioxidant vitamin used in every cell of the body. It is necessary for healthy function and can improve heart function, lower blood pressure and reduce angina. Taken before cardiac surgery, it has been shown to reduce complications and hasten recovery in some studies. It may also provide benefits in preventing migraine headache, Huntington's chorea, mitochondrial myopathy, COPD, type 2 diabetes, chronic obstructive airways disease, periodontal disease, haemodialysis, Friedreich's ataxia, tinnitus, age-related macular degeneration, cystic fibrosis and reducing cardiotoxicity and liver toxicity associated with anthracyclines, although further research is required to definitively confirm effect. Whether it is helpful in Parkinson's disease is not clear. People taking statin drugs long term and experiencing mild side effects could safely take a 3-month trial of CoQ10 and see whether it helps them.

When will it start to work?

This depends on the indication. For heart conditions and to reduce migraine, 10–12 weeks may be required. To delay the progression of PD, one study found that effects started after 9 months' use.

Are there any safety issues?

Medical monitoring is required in patients taking warfarin and starting high-dose CoQ10 supplements; however, even high-dose supplements are well tolerated and considered safe.

REFERENCES

Abdul-Rasheed OF et al. Coenzyme Q10 and oxidative stress markers in seminal plasma of Iraqi patients with male infertility. Saudi Med J 31.5 (2010): 501–506.

Aberg F et al. Gemfibrozil-induced decrease in serum ubiquinone and alpha- and gamma-tocopherol levels in men with combined hyperlipidaemia. Eur J Clin Invest 28.3 (1998): 235–242.

Aboul-Fotouh S. Coenzyme Q10 displays antidepressant-like activity with reduction of hippocampal oxidative/nitrosative DNA damage in chronically stressed rats. Pharmacol Biochem Behav 104 (2013): 105–112.

Ahmadvand H et al. Effects of coenzyme Q10 on LDL oxidation in vitro. Acta Med Iran 51.1 (2013): 12–18.

Ahn JH et al. Coenzyme Q10 in combination with steroid therapy for treatment of sudden sensorineural hearing loss: a controlled prospective study. Clin Otolaryngol 35.6 (2010): 486–489.

Alcocer-Gomez E et al. Effect of coenzyme Q10 evaluated by 1990 and 2010 ACR Diagnostic Criteria for Fibromyalgia and SCL-90-R: Four case reports and literature review. Nutrition 29.11–12 (2013): 1422–1425.

Bahar M et al. Exogenous coenzyme Q10 modulates MMP-2 activity in MCF-7 cell line as a breast cancer cellular model. Nutr J 9 (2010): 62.

Balercia G et al. Coenzyme Q10 treatment in infertile men with idiopathic asthenozoospermia: a placebo-controlled, double-blind randomized trial. Fertil Steril 91.5 (2009): 1785–1792.

Bargossi AM et al. Exogenous CoQ10 preserves plasma ubiquinone levels in patients treated with 3-hydroxy-3-methylglutaryl coenzyme A reductase inhibitors. Int J Clin Lab Res 24.3 (1994a): 171–176.

Bargossi AM et al. Exogenous CoQ10 supplementation prevents plasma ubiquinone reduction induced by HMG-CoA reductase inhibitors. Mol Aspects Med 15 (Suppl) (1994b): S187–193.

Baskaran R et al. The effect of coenzyme Q10 on the pharmacokinetic parameters of theophylline. Arch Pharm Res 31(7) (2008): 938–944.

Beal MF et al. A randomized clinical trial of high-dosage coenzyme Q10 in early Parkinson disease: no evidence of benefit. JAMA Neurol 71.5 (2014): 543–552.

Beal MF. Mitochondria, oxidative damage, and inflammation in Parkinson's disease. Ann N Y Acad Sci 991 (2003): 120–131.

Berman M et al. Coenzyme Q10 in patients with end-stage heart failure awaiting cardiac transplantation: a randomized, placebo-controlled study. Clin Cardiol 27 (2004): 295–299.

Bessler, H., Bergman, M., et al. Coenzyme Q10 decreases TNF-alpha and IL-2 secretion by human peripheral blood mononuclear cells. J Nutr Sci Vitaminol (Tokyo) 1 (2010): 77–81.

Bianchi G et al. Oxidative stress and anti-oxidant metabolites in patients with hyperthyroidism: effect of treatment. Horm Metab Res 31.11 (1999): 620–624.

Bonetti A et al. Effect of ubidecarenone oral treatment on aerobic power in middle-aged trained subjects. J Sports Med Phys Fitness 40.1 (2000): 51–57.

Bookstaver DA et al. Effect of coenzyme Q10 supplementation on statin-induced myalgias. Am J Cardiol 110.4 (2012): 526–529.

Braun L et al. A wellness program for cardiac surgery improves clinical outcomes. Advances in Integrative Medicine 1.1 (2013): 32–37.

Bresolin N et al. Ubidecarenone in the treatment of mitochondrial myopathies: a multi-center double-blind trial. J Neurol Sci 100.1–2 (1990): 70–78.

Caso G et al. Effect of coenzyme q10 on myopathic symptoms in patients treated with statins. Am J Cardiol 99.10 (2007): 1409–1412.

Celebi N et al. Protective effect of coenzyme Q10 in paclitaxel-induced peripheral neuropathy in rats. Neurosciences (Riyadh) 18(2) (2013): 133–137.

Chai W et al. Plasma coenzyme Q10 levels and postmenopausal breast cancer risk: the multiethnic cohort study. Cancer Epidem Biomar 19.9 (2010): 2351–2356.

Chai W et al. Plasma coenzyme Q10 levels and prostate cancer risk: the multiethnic cohort study. Cancer Epidem Biomar 20.4 (2011): 708–710.

Chello M et al. Protection by coenzyme Q10 of tissue reperfusion injury during abdominal aortic cross-clamping. J Cardiovasc Surg (Torino) 37.3 (1996): 229–235.

Chen YF et al. Effectiveness of coenzyme Q10 on myocardial preservation during hypothermic cardioplegic arrest. J Thorac Cardiovasc Surg 107 (1994): 242–247.

Choi H et al. Coenzyme Q10 protects against amyloid beta-induced neuronal cell death by inhibiting oxidative stress and activating the P13K pathway. Neurotoxicology 33.1 (2012): 85–90.

Choi, H et al. Coenzyme Q10 restores amyloid beta-inhibited proliferation of neural stem cells by activating the PI3K Pathway. Stem Cells Dev. 1.22 (2013): 2112–2120.

Colquhoun DM et al. Effects of simvastatin on blood lipids, vitamin E, coenzyme Q10 levels and left ventricular function in humans. Eur J Clin Invest 35 (2005): 251–258.

Combs AB et al. Reduction by coenzyme Q10 of the acute toxicity of adriamycin in mice. Res Commun Chem Pathol Pharmacol 18.3 (1977): 565–568.

Cooke M et al. Effects of acute and 14-day coenzyme Q10 supplementation on exercise performance in both trained and untrained individuals. J Int Soc Sports Nutr 5 (2008): 8.

Cooper JM et al. Coenzyme Q10 and vitamin E deficiency in Friedreich's ataxia: predictor of efficacy of vitamin E and coenzyme Q10 therapy. Eur J Neurol 15.12 (2008): 1371–1379.

Cooper JM, Schapira AH. Friedreich's ataxia: coenzyme Q10 and vitamin E therapy. Mitochondrion 7 (Suppl) (2007): S127–S135.

Cordero MD et al. Oxidative stress correlates with headache symptoms in fibromyalgia: coenzyme Q(1)(0) effect on clinical improvement. PLoS One 7(4) (2012): e35677.

da Silva Machado C et al. Coenzyme Q10 protects Pc12 cells from cisplatin-induced DNA damage and neurotoxicity. Neurotoxicology 36C (2013): 10–16.

Dai Y-L et al. Reversal of mitochondrial dysfunction by coenzyme Q10 supplement improves endothelial function in patients with ischaemic left ventricular systolic dysfunction: a randomized controlled trial. Atherosclerosis 216.2 (2011): 395–401.

Digiesi V et al. Coenzyme Q10 in essential hypertension. Mol Aspects Med 15 (Suppl) (1994): S257–S263.

Donnino MW et al. Coenzyme Q10 levels are low and may be associated with the inflammatory cascade in septic shock. Crit Care. Aug 9 15.4 (2011): R189.

Dumont, M et al. Coenzyme Q10 decreases amyloid pathology and improves behavior in a transgenic mouse model of Alzheimer's disease. J Alzheimer's Disease 27.1 (2011): 211–223.

Dupic, L et al. Coenzyme Q!0 deficiency in septic shock patients. Critical Care. 15 (2011):194.

Ebadi M et al. Ubiquinone (coenzyme q10) and mitochondria in oxidative stress of parkinson's disease. Biol Signals Recept 10.3–4 (2001): 224–253.

El-ghoroury EA et al. Malondialdehyde and coenzyme Q10 in platelets and serum in type 2 diabetes mellitus: correlation with glycemic control. Blood Coagul Fibrinolysis, 20.4 (2009): 248–251.

El-Sheikh AA et al. Effect of coenzyme-q10 on Doxorubicin-induced nephrotoxicity in rats. Adv Pharmacol Sci 2012 (2012): 981461.

Engelson J et al. Effect of coenzyme Q10 and Ginkgo biloba on warfarin dosage in patients on long-term warfarin treatment: a randomized, double-blind, placebo-controlled cross-over trial. Ugeskr Laeger 165.18 (2003): 1868–1871.
Ernster L, Dallner G. Biochemical, physiological and medical aspects of ubiquinone function. Biochim Biophys Acta 1271.1 (1995): 195–204.
Feher J et al. [Metabolic therapy for early treatment of age-related macular degeneration]. Orv Hetil 148.48 (2007): 2259–2268.
Folkers K et al. Activities of vitamin Q10 in animal models and a serious deficiency in patients with cancer. Biochem Biophys Res Commun 234.2 (1997): 296–299.
Folkers K et al. Lovastatin decreases coenzyme Q levels in humans. Proc Natl Acad Sci U S A 87.22 (1990): 8931–8934.
Folkers K, Choe JY, Combs AB. Rescue by coenzyme Q10 from electrocardiographic abnormalities caused by the toxicity of adriamycin in the rat. Proc Natl Acad Sci U S A 75.10 (1978): 5178–5180.
Folkers K, Wolaniuk A. Research on coenzyme Q10 in clinical medicine and in immunomodulation. Drugs Exp Clin Res 11.8 (1985): 539–545.
Fotino AD et al. Effect of coenzyme Q(1)(0) supplementation on heart failure: a meta-analysis. Am J Clin Nutr 97.2 (2013): 268–275.
Fouad AA et al. Coenzyme Q10 treatment ameliorates acute cisplatin nephrotoxicity in mice. Toxicology 274(1–3) (2010): 49–56.
Fouad AA, Jresat I. Hepatoprotective effect of coenzyme Q10 in rats with acetaminophen toxicity. Environ Toxicol Pharmacol 33.2 (2012): 158–167.
Fujimoto S et al. Effects of coenzyme Q10 administration on pulmonary function and exercise performance in patients with chronic lung diseases. Clin Invest 71.8 (Suppl) (1993): S162–S166.
Fujioka T et al. Clinical study of cardiac arrhythmias using a 24-hour continuous electrocardiographic recorder (5th report): antiarrhythmic action of coenzyme Q10 in diabetics. Tohoku J Exp Med 141 (Suppl) (1983): 453–463.
Fumagalli S et al. Coenzyme Q10 terclatrate and creatine in chronic heart failure: a randomized, placebo-controlled, double-blind study. Clin Cardiol 34(4) (2011): 211–217.
Galili N et al. Clinical response of myelodysplastic syndromes patients to treatment with coenzyme Q10. Leuk Res 31.1 (2007): 19–26.
Gao L et al. Effects of coenzyme Q10 on vascular endothelial function in humans: a meta-analysis of randomized controlled trials. Atherosclerosis, 221.2 (2012): 311–316.
Glover EI et al. A randomized trial of coenzyme Q10 in mitochondrial disorders. Muscle Nerve 42.5 (2010): 739–748.
Gokbel H et al. The effects of coenzyme Q10 supplementation on performance during repeated bouts of supramaximal exercise in sedentary men. J Strength Cond Res 24.1 (2010): 97–102.
Golomb BA, Evans MA. Statin adverse effects: a review of the literature and evidence for a mitochondrial mechanism. Am J Cardiovasc Drugs 8.6 (2008): 373–418.
Gotz ME et al. Altered redox state of platelet coenzyme Q10 in Parkinson's disease. J Neural Transm 107.1 (2000): 41–48.
Graham D et al. Mitochondria-targeted antioxidant MitoQ10 improves endothelial function and attenuates cardiac hypertrophy. Hypertension 54(2) (2009): 322–328.
Greenlee H et al. Lack of effect of coenzyme q10 on doxorubicin cytotoxicity in breast cancer cell cultures. Integr Cancer Ther 11(3) (2012): 243–250.
Groneberg DA et al. Coenzyme Q10 affects expression of genes involved in cell signalling, metabolism and transport in human CaCo-2 cells. Int J Biochem Cell Biol 37 (2005): 1208–1218.
Gul I et al. Oxidative stress and antioxidant defense in plasma after repeated bouts of supramaximal exercise: the effect of coenzyme Q10. J Sports Med Phys Fitness 51.2 (2011): 305–312.
Hamilton SJ et al. Coenzyme Q10 improves endothelial dysfunction in statin-treated type 2 diabetic patients. Diabetes Care. 32.5 (2009): 810–812.
Hanioka T et al. Effect of topical application of coenzyme Q10 on adult periodontitis. Mol Aspects Med 15 (Suppl) (1994): S241–S248.
Hargreaves IP et al. The coenzyme Q10 status of the brain regions of Parkinson's disease patients. Neurosci Lett 447.1 (2008): 17–19.
Hart PE et al. Antioxidant treatment of patients with Friedreich ataxia: four-year follow-up. Arch Neurol 62.4 (2005): 621–626.
Hershey AD et al. Coenzyme Q10 deficiency and response to supplementation in pediatric and adolescent migraine. Headache 47.1 (2007): 73–80.
Hirose Y et al. Effect of water-soluble coenzyme Q10 on noise-induced hearing loss in guinea pigs. Acta Otolaryngol 128(10) (2008): 1071–1076.
Ho MJ et al. Blood pressure lowering efficacy of coenzyme Q10 for primary hypertension. Cochrane Database Syst Rev(4) (2009): CD007435.
Hofman-Bang C et al. Coenzyme Q10 as an adjunctive in the treatment of chronic congestive heart failure. The Q10 Study Group. J Card Fail 1.2 (1995): 101–107.
Hosoe K et al. Study on safety and bioavailability of ubiquinol (Kaneka QH) after single and 4-week multiple oral administration to healthy volunteers. Regul Toxicol Pharmacol 47.1 (2007): 19–28.
Huntington Study Group Pre et al. Safety and tolerability of high-dosage coenzyme Q10 in Huntington's disease and healthy subjects. Mov Disord 25.12 (2010): 1924–1928.
Huntington's Study Group. A randomized, placebo-controlled trial of coenzyme Q10 and remacemide in Huntington's disease. Neurology 57.3 (2001): 397–404.
Itagaki S et al. Interaction of coenzyme Q10 with the intestinal drug transporter P-glycoprotein. J Agric Food Chem 56.16 (2008): 6923–6927.
Jeejeebhoy F et al. Nutritional supplementation with MyoVive repletes essential cardiac myocyte nutrients and reduces left ventricular size in patients with left ventricular dysfunction. Am Heart J 143.6 (2002): 1092–1100.
Judy WV et al. Double-blind-double crossover study of coenzyme Q10 in heart failure. In: Folkers K, Yamamura Y (eds). Biomedical and Clinical Aspects of Coenzyme Q. Vol 5, Amsterdam: Elsevier, 1986: 315–323.
Judy WV et al. Myocardial preservation by therapy with coenzyme Q10 during heart surgery. Clin Invest 71.8 (Suppl) (1993): S155–S161.
Kaikkonen J et al. Coenzyme Q10: absorption, antioxidative properties, determinants, and plasma levels. Free Radic Res 36.4 (2002): 389–397.
Kamikawa T et al. Effects of coenzyme Q10 on exercise tolerance in chronic stable angina pectoris. Am J Cardiol 56.4 (1985): 247–251.
Karlsson J et al. Muscle fibre types, ubiquinone content and exercise capacity in hypertension and effort angina. Ann Med 23.3 (1991): 339–344.
Karlsson J et al. Muscle ubiquinone in healthy physically active males. Mol Cell Biochem 156.2 (1996): 169–172.
Kedziora-Kornatowska K et al. Effects of coenzyme Q10 supplementation on activities of selected antioxidative enzymes and lipid peroxidation in hypertensive patients treated with indapamide. A pilot study. Arch Med Sci 6.4 (2010): 513–518.
Keogh A et al. Randomised double-blind, placebo-controlled trial of coenzyme Q10 therapy in class II and III systolic heart failure. Heart Lung Circ 12 (2003): 135–141.
Kernt M et al. Coenzyme Q10 prevents human lens epithelial cells from light-induced apoptotic cell death by reducing oxidative stress and stabilizing BAX / Bcl-2 ratio. Acta Ophthalmol 88.3 (2010): e78–86.
Khan M et al. A pilot clinical trial of the effects of coenzyme Q10 on chronic tinnitus aurium. Otolaryngol Head Neck Surg 136.1 (2007): 72–77.
Khatta M et al. The effect of coenzyme Q10 in patients with congestive heart failure. Ann Intern Med 132 (2000): 636–640.
Kim JM, Park E. Coenzyme Q10 attenuated DMH-induced precancerous lesions in SD rats. J Nutrit Sci Vitaminology, 56.2 (2010): 139–144.
Kishi H et al. Bioenergetics in clinical medicine. III. Inhibition of coenzyme Q10-enzymes by clinically used anti-hypertensive drugs. Res Commun Chem Pathol Pharmacol 12.3 (1975): 533–540.
Kocharian A et al. Coenzyme Q10 improves diastolic function in children with idiopathic dilated cardiomyopathy. Cardiol Young 19.5 (2009): 501–506.
Kokawa T et al. Coenzyme Q10 in cancer chemotherapy: experimental studies on augmentation of the effects of masked compounds, especially in the combined chemotherapy with immunopotentiators. Gan To Kagaku Ryoho 10.3 (1983): 768–774.
Kolahdouz MR et al. The effect of coenzyme Q10 supplementation on metabolic status of type 2 diabetic patients. Minerva Gastroenterol Dietol 59.2 (2013): 231–236.
Kon M et al. Reducing exercise-induced muscular injury in kendo athletes with supplementation of coenzyme Q10. Br J Nutr 100.4 (2008): 903–909.
Laaksonen R et al. Decreases in serum ubiquinone concentrations do not result in reduced levels in muscle tissue during short-term simvastatin treatment in humans. Clin Pharmacol Ther 57.1 (1995): 62–66.
Laaksonen R et al. Serum ubiquinone concentrations after short- and long-term treatment with HMG-CoA reductase inhibitors. Eur J Clin Pharmacol 46.4 (1994): 313–317.
Laaksonen R et al. The effect of simvastatin treatment on natural antioxidants in low-density lipoproteins and high-energy phosphates and ubiquinone in skeletal muscle. Am J Cardiol 77.10 (1996): 851–854.
Laguna TA et al. Decreased total serum coenzyme-Q10 concentrations: a longitudinal study in children with cystic fibrosis. J Pediatr 153.3 (2008): 402–407.
Langsjoen PH et al. Usefulness of coenzyme Q10 in clinical cardiology: a long-term study. Mol Aspects Med 15 (Suppl) (1994a): S165–S175.
Langsjoen PH, Langsjoen AM. Overview of the use of CoQ10 in cardiovascular disease. Biofactors 9 (1999): 273–284.
Langsjoen PH, Langsjoen AM. Supplemental ubiquinol in patients with advanced congestive heart failure. Biofactors 32.1–4 (2008): 119–128.

Langsjoen PH, Vadhanavikit S, Folkers K. Effective treatment with coenzyme Q10 of patients with chronic myocardial disease. Drugs Exp Clin Res 11.8 (1985): 577–579.

Langsjoen PH. Lack of effect of coenzyme Q on left ventricular function in patients with congestive heart failure. J Am Coll Cardiol 35.3 (2000): 816–8117.

Lee BJ et al. Coenzyme Q10 supplementation reduces oxidative stress and increases antioxidant enzyme activity in patients with coronary artery disease. Nutrition 28.3 (2012b): 250–255.

Lee BJ et al. Effects of coenzyme Q10 supplementation on inflammatory markers (high-sensitivity C-reactive protein, interleukin-6, and homocysteine) in patients with coronary artery disease. Nutrition 28.7–8 (2012a): 767–772.

Lee BJ et al. The relationship between coenzyme Q10, oxidative stress, and antioxidant enzymes activities and coronary artery disease. Sci World J 2012 (2012c): 792756.

Leong JY et al. Perioperative metabolic therapy improves redox status and outcomes in cardiac surgery patients: a randomised trial. Heart Lung Circ 19.10 (2010): 584–591.

Levy HB, Kohlhaas HK. Considerations for supplementing with coenzyme Q10 during statin therapy. Ann Pharmacother 40.2 (2006): 290–294.

Littarru GP, Langsjoen P. Coenzyme Q10 and statins: biochemical and clinical implications. Mitochondrion 7 (Suppl) (2007): S168–S174.

Littarru GP, Tiano L. Clinical aspects of coenzyme Q10: an update. Curr Opin Clin Nutr Metab Care 8.6 (2005): 641–646.

Liu J et al. Coenzyme Q10 for Parkinson's disease. Cochrane Database Syst Rev (12) (2011): CD008150.

Lockwood K et al. Partial and complete regression of breast cancer in patients in relation to dosage of coenzyme Q10. Biochem Biophys Res Commun 199.3 (1994): 1504–1508.

Lockwood K et al. Progress on therapy of breast cancer with vitamin Q10 and the regression of metastases. Biochem Biophys Res Commun 212.1 (1995): 172–177.

Louis F et al. Effects of ubiquinone and related substances on secretion of aldosterone and cortisol. Am J Physiol 208 (1965): 1275–1280.

Lulli M et al. Coenzyme Q10 instilled as eye drops on the cornea reaches the retina and protects retinal layers from apoptosis in a mouse model of kainate-induced retinal damage. Invest Ophthalmol Vis Sci 53.13 (2012b): 8295–8302.

Lulli M et al. Coenzyme Q10 protects retinal cells from apoptosis induced by radiation in vitro and in vivo. J Radiat Res 53.5 (2012a): 695–703.

Maes M et al. Coenzyme Q10 deficiency in myalgic encephalomyelitis/chronic fatigue syndrome (ME/CFS) is related to fatigue, autonomic and neurocognitive symptoms and is another risk factor explaining the early mortality in ME/CFS due to cardiovascular disorder. Neuro Endocrinol Lett 30.4 (2009): 470–476.

Makhija N et al. The role of oral coenzyme Q10 in patients undergoing coronary artery bypass graft surgery. J Cardiothorac Vasc Anesth 22.6 (2008): 832–839.

Marcoff L, Thompson PD. The role of coenzyme Q10 in statin-associated myopathy: a systematic review. J Am Coll Cardiol 49.23 (2007): 2231–2237.

Marinari S et al. Effects of nutraceutical diet integration, with coenzyme Q10 (Q-Ter multicomposite) and creatine, on dyspnea, exercise tolerance, and quality of life in COPD patients with chronic respiratory failure. Multidiscip Respir Med 8.1 (2013): 40.

Mariotti C et al. Idebenone treatment in Friedreich patients: one-year-long randomized placebo-controlled trial. Neurology 60.10 (2003): 1676–1679.

Martin SB et al. Coenzyme Q10 and cognition in atorvastatin treated dogs. Neurosci Lett 501.2 (2011): 92–95.

McCarty MF. Coenzyme Q versus hypertension: does CoQ decrease endothelial superoxide generation? Med Hypotheses 53.4 (1999): 300–304.

McDonald SR et al. Concurrent administration of coenzyme Q10 and alpha-tocopherol improves learning in aged mice. Free Radic Biol Med 38 (2005): 729–736.

McMurray JJ et al. (2010). Coenzyme Q10, rosuvastatin, and clinical outcomes in heart failure: a pre-specified substudy of CORONA (controlled rosuvastatin multinational study in heart failure). J Am Coll Cardiol 56(15): 1196–1204.

Mezawa M et al. The reduced form of coenzyme Q10 improves glycemic control in patients with type 2 diabetes: an open label pilot study. Biofactors 38.6 (2012): 416–421.

Mischley LK et al. Coenzyme Q10 deficiency in patients with Parkinson's disease. J Neurol Sci 318(1–2) (2012): 72–75.

Miyamae T et al. Increased oxidative stress and coenzyme Q10 deficiency in juvenile fibromyalgia: amelioration of hypercholesterolemia and fatigue by ubiquinol-10 supplementation. Redox Rep 18.1 (2013): 12–19.

Mizuno K et al. Antifatigue effects of coenzyme Q10 during physical fatigue. Nutrition 24.4 (2008): 293–299.

Mizushina Y et al. Coenzyme Q10 as a potent compound that inhibits Cdt1–geminin interaction. Biochimica et Biophysica Acta (BBA)-General Subjects, 1780.2 (2008): 203–213.

Molyneux SL et al. Coenzyme Q10: an independent predictor of mortality in chronic heart failure. J Am Coll Cardiol 52.18 (2008): 1435–1441.

Moreira PI et al. CoQ10 therapy attenuates amyloid beta-peptide toxicity in brain mitochondria isolated from aged diabetic rats. Exp Neurol 196 (2005): 112–119.

Morisco C et al. Noninvasive evaluation of cardiac hemodynamics during exercise in patients with chronic heart failure. Effects of short-term coenzyme Q10 treatment. Mol Aspects Med 15 (Suppl) (1994): S155–S163.

Morisco C, Trimarco B, Condorelli M. Effect of coenzyme Q10 therapy in patients with congestive heart failure: a long-term multicenter randomized study. Clin Invest 71 (1993): S134–S136.

Mortensen SA et al. Coenzyme Q10: clinical benefits with biochemical correlates suggesting a scientific breakthrough in the management of chronic heart failure. Int J Tissue React 12.3 (1990): 155–162.

Mortensen SA et al. Dose-related decrease of serum coenzyme Q10 during treatment with HMG-CoA reductase inhibitors. Mol Aspects Med 18 (Suppl) (1997): S137–S144.

Muller T et al. Coenzyme Q10 supplementation provides mild symptomatic benefit in patients with Parkinson's disease. Neurosci Lett 341 (2003): 201–204.

Munkholm H, Hansen HH, Rasmussen K. Coenzyme Q10 treatment in serious heart failure. Biofactors 9.2–4 (1999): 285–289.

Nadjarzadeh A et al. Effect of Coenzyme Q10 supplementation on antioxidant enzymes activity and oxidative stress of seminal plasma: a double-blind randomised clinical trial. Andrologia 46.2 (2013): 177–183.

Nadjarzadeh, A., Sadeghi, M. R., et al. (2011). Coenzyme Q10 improves seminal oxidative defense but does not affect on semen parameters in idiopathic oligoasthenoteratozoospermia: a randomized double-blind, placebo controlled trial. J Endocrinol Invest 34(8): e224–228.

Nuku K et al. Safety assessment of PureSorb-Q40 in healthy subjects and serum coenzyme Q10 level in excessive dosing. J Nutr Sci Vitaminol (Tokyo) 53.3 (2007): 198–206.

Ochiai A et al. Improvement in intestinal coenzyme q10 absorption by food intake. Yakugaku Zasshi 127.8 (2007): 1251–1254.

Okello E et al. Combined statin/coenzyme Q10 as adjunctive treatment of chronic heart failure. Med Hypoth 73.3 (2009): 306–308.

Ono K et al. Preformed beta-amyloid fibrils are destabilized by coenzyme Q10 in vitro. Biochem Biophys Res Commun 330 (2005): 111–116.

Ostman B et al. Coenzyme Q10 supplementation and exercise-induced oxidative stress in humans. Nutrition 28.4 (2012): 403–417.

Overvad K et al. Coenzyme Q10 in health and disease. Eur J Clin Nutr 53.10 (1999): 764–770.

Paiva H et al. High-dose statins and skeletal muscle metabolism in humans: a randomized, controlled trial. Clin Pharmacol Ther 78.1 (2005): 60–68.

Papas KA et al. A pilot study on the safety and efficacy of a novel antioxidant rich formulation in patients with cystic fibrosis. J Cyst Fibros 7.1 (2008): 60–67.

Parker BA et al. A randomized trial of coenzyme Q10 in patients with statin myopathy: rationale and study design. J Clin Lipidol 7.3 (2013): 187–193.

Pelton R et al. Drug-induced nutrient depletion handbook 1999–2000. Lexi-Comp (1999).

Pepe S et al. Coenzyme Q10 in cardiovascular disease. Mitochondrion 7 (Suppl) (2007): S154–S167.

Permanetter B et al. Ubiquinone (coenzyme Q10) in the long-term treatment of idiopathic dilated cardiomyopathy. Eur Heart J 13.11 (1992): 1528–1533.

Pogessi L et al. Effect of coenzyme Q10 on left ventricular function in patients with dilative cardiomyopathy. Curr Ther Res 49 (1991): 878–886.

Porter DA et al. The effect of oral coenzyme Q10 on the exercise tolerance of middle-aged, untrained men. Int J Sports Med 16.7 (1995): 421–427.

Potgieter M et al. Primary and secondary coenzyme Q10 deficiency: the role of therapeutic supplementation. Nutrition Reviews 71.3 (2013): 180–188.

Pringsheim T et al. Canadian Headache Society guideline for migraine prophylaxis. Can J Neurol Sci 39 (2 Suppl 2) (2012): S1–S59.

Qu J et al. Coenzyme Q10 in the human retina. Invest Ophthalmol Vis Sci 50.4 (2009): 1814–1818.

Quinzii CM et al. Human CoQ10 deficiencies. Biofactors 32.1–4 (2008): 113–118.

Roffe L et al. Efficacy of coenzyme Q10 for improved tolerability of cancer treatments: a systematic review. J Clin Oncol 22.21 (2004): 4418–4424.

Rosenfeldt F et al. Coenzyme Q10 improves the tolerance of the senescent myocardium to aerobic and ischemic stress: studies in rats and in human atrial tissue. Biofactors 9.2–4 (1999): 291–299.

Rosenfeldt F et al. Coenzyme Q10 therapy before cardiac surgery improves mitochondrial function and in vitro contractility of myocardial tissue. J Thorac Cardiovasc Surg 129 (2005): 25–32.

Rosenfeldt F et al. Systematic review of effect of coenzyme Q10 in physical exercise, hypertension and heart failure. Biofactors 18 (2003): 91–100.

Rosenfeldt F et al. The effects of ageing on the response to cardiac surgery: protective strategies for the ageing myocardium. Biogerontology 3 (2002): 37–40.

Rosenfeldt FL et al. Coenzyme Q10 in the treatment of hypertension: a meta-analysis of the clinical trials. J Hum Hypertens 21.4 (2007): 297–306.

Rozen TD et al. Open label trial of coenzyme Q10 as a migraine preventive. Cephalalgia 22.2 (2002): 137–141.

Ryo, K., Ito, A., et al. (2011). Effects of coenzyme Q10 on salivary secretion. Clin Biochem 44(8–9): 669–74.

Sacconi S et al. Coenzyme Q10 is frequently reduced in muscle of patients with mitochondrial myopathy. Neuromuscul Disord 20.1 (2010): 44–48.

Sachdanandam P. Antiangiogenic and hypolipidemic activity of coenzyme Q10 supplementation to breast cancer patients undergoing Tamoxifen therapy. Biofactors 32.1–4 (2008):151–159.

Safarinejad MR et al. Effects of EPA, gamma-linolenic acid or coenzyme Q10 on serum prostate-specific antigen levels: a randomised, double-blind trial. Br J Nutr (2012): 1–8.

Safarinejad MR et al. Effects of the reduced form of coenzyme Q10 (ubiquinol) on semen parameters in men with idiopathic infertility: a double-blind, placebo controlled, randomized study. J Urol 188(2) (2012b): 526–531.

Safarinejad MR. Efficacy of coenzyme Q10 on semen parameters, sperm function and reproductive hormones in infertile men. J Urol 182.1 (2009): 237–248.

Safarinejad MR. Safety and efficacy of coenzyme Q10 supplementation in early chronic Peyronie's disease: a double-blind, placebo-controlled randomized study. Int J Impot Res 22.5 (2010): 298–309.

Safarinejad MR. The effect of coenzyme Q(1)(0) supplementation on partner pregnancy rate in infertile men with idiopathic oligoasthenoteratozoospermia: an open-label prospective study. Int Urol Nephrol 44(3) (2012): 689–700.

Sakata T et al. Coenzyme Q10 administration suppresses both oxidative and antioxidative markers in hemodialysis patients. Blood Purif 26.4 (2008): 371–378.

Salami A et al. Water-soluble coenzyme Q10 formulation (Q-TER((R))) in the treatment of presbycusis. Acta Otolaryngol 130.10 (2010): 1154–1162.

Sander S et al. The impact of coenzyme Q10 on systolic function in patients with chronic heart failure. J Card Fail 12.6 (2006): 464–472.

Sandor PS et al. Efficacy of coenzyme Q10 in migraine prophylaxis. a randomized controlled trial. Neurology 64 (2005): 713–715.

Sato Y et al. Emulsification Using Highly Hydrophilic Surfactants Improves the Absorption of Orally Administered Coenzyme Q10. Biolog and Pharmaceut Bulletin 36.12 (2013): 2012–2017.

Satta A et al. Effects of ubidecarenone in an exercise training program for patients with chronic obstructive pulmonary diseases. Clin Ther 13.6 (1991): 754–757.

Schmelzer C et al. Functions of coenzyme Q10 in inflammation and gene expression. Biofactors 32.1–4 (2008): 179–183.

Senes M et al. Coenzyme Q10 and high-sensitivity C-reactive protein in ischemic and idiopathic dilated cardiomyopathy. Clin Chem Lab Med 46.3 (2008): 382–386.

Serra G et al. Evaluation of coenzyme Q10 in patients with moderate heart failure and chronic stable effort angina. In: Folkers K, Yamamura Y (eds). Biomedical and Clinical Aspects of Coenzyme Q. Vol 6, Amsterdam: Elsevier, 1991: 327–338.

Shalansky S et al. Risk of warfarin-related bleeding events and supratherapeutic international normalized ratios associated with complementary and alternative medicine: a longitudinal analysis. Pharmacotherapy, 27.9 (2007): 1237–1247.

Shults CW et al. Effects of coenzyme Q10 in early Parkinson disease: evidence of slowing of the functional decline. Arch Neurol 59.10 (2002): 1541–1550.

Shults CW et al. Pilot trial of high dosages of coenzyme Q10 in patients with Parkinson's disease. Exp Neurol 188 (2004): 491–494.

Shults CW. Therapeutic role of coenzyme Q(10) in Parkinson's disease. Pharmacol Ther 107 (2005): 120–130.

Silver MA et al. Effect of atorvastatin on left ventricular diastolic function and ability of coenzyme Q10 to reverse that dysfunction. Am J Cardiol 94 (2004): 1306–1310.

Singh RB et al. Effect of hydrosoluble coenzyme Q10 on blood pressure and insulin resistance in hypertensive patients with coronary artery disease. J Hum Hypertens 13 (1999): 203–208.

Skough K et al. Effects of resistance training in combination with coenzyme Q10 supplementation in patients with post-polio: a pilot study. J Rehabil Med 40.9 (2008): 773–775.

Slater SK et al. c. Cephalalgia 31.8 (2011): 897–905.

Sohet FM et al. Coenzyme Q10 supplementation lowers hepatic oxidative stress and inflammation associated with diet-induced obesity in mice. Biochem Pharmacol 78.11 (2009): 1391–400.

Sole MJ, Jeejeebhoy KN. Conditioned nutritional requirements: therapeutic relevance to heart failure. Herz 27.2 (2002): 174–178.

Spigset O. Coenzyme Q10 (ubiquinone) in the treatment of heart failure. Are any positive effects documented? Tidsskr Nor Laegeforen 114.8 (1994a): 939–942.

Spigset O. Reduced effect of warfarin caused by ubidecarenone. Lancet 344 (1994b): 1372–1373.

Stamelou M et al. Short-term effects of coenzyme Q10 in progressive supranuclear palsy: a randomized, placebo-controlled trial. Mov Disord 23(7) (2008): 942–949.

Stargrove M et al. Herb, nutrient and drug interactions. St Louis: Mosby, 2008.

Stocker R et al. Neither plasma coenzyme Q10 concentration, nor its decline during pravastatin therapy, is linked to recurrent cardiovascular disease events: a prospective case-control study from the LIPID study. Atherosclerosis 187.1 (2006): 198–204.

Stocker R, Macdonald P. The benefit of coenzyme Q10 supplements in the management of chronic heart failure: a long tale of promise in the continued absence of clear evidence. Am J Clin Nutr 97.2 (2013): 233–234.

Storch A et al. Randomized, double-blind, placebo-controlled trial on symptomatic effects of coenzyme Q(10) in Parkinson disease. Arch Neurol 64.7 (2007): 938–944.

Storch A. [Coenzyme Q10 in Parkinson's disease. Symptomatic or neuroprotective effects?]. Nervenarzt 78.12 (2007): 1378–1382.

Taggart DP et al. Effects of short-term supplementation with coenzyme Q10 on myocardial protection during cardiac operations. Ann Thorac Surg 61 (1996): 829–833.

Takahashi N et al. Effect of coenzyme Q10 on hemodynamic response to ocular timolol. J Cardiovasc Pharmacol 14.3 (1989): 462–468.

Tanaka J et al. Coenzyme Q10: the prophylactic effect on low cardiac output following cardiac valve replacement. Ann Thorac Surg 33.2 (1982): 145–151.

Tanrikulu AC et al. Coenzyme Q10, copper, zinc, and lipid peroxidation levels in serum of patients with chronic obstructive pulmonary disease. Bio Trace Elem Res 143.2 (2011): 659–667.

Teran E et al. Coenzyme Q10 supplementation during pregnancy reduces the risk of pre-eclampsia. Int J Gynaecol Obstet 105.1 (2009): 43–45.

Tiano L et al. Coenzyme Q10 and oxidative imbalance in Down syndrome: biochemical and clinical aspects. Biofactors 32(1–4) (2008): 161–167.

Tsai KL et al. A novel mechanism of coenzyme Q10 protects against human endothelial cells from oxidative stress-induced injury by modulating NO-related pathways. J Nutr Biochem 23.5 (2012): 458–468.

Tsai, K. L., Chen, L. H., et al. (2011). Coenzyme Q10 suppresses oxLDL-induced endothelial oxidative injuries by the modulation of LOX-1-mediated ROS generation via the AMPK/PKC/NADPH oxidase signaling pathway. Mol Nutr Food Res 55 Suppl 2: S227–40.

Tsuneki H et al. Protective effects of coenzyme Q10 against angiotensin II-induced oxidative stress in human umbilical vein endothelial cells. European J Pharmacol 701.1 (2013): 218–227.

Turk S et al. Coenzyme Q10 supplementation and diastolic heart functions in hemodialysis patients: A randomized double-blind placebo-controlled trial.Hemodialysis International, 17.3 (2013): 374–381.

Ullmann U et al. A new Coenzyme Q10 tablet-grade formulation (all-Q) is bioequivalent to Q-Gel and both have better bioavailability properties than Q-SorB. J Med Food 8.3 (2005): 397–399.

Watson PS et al. Lack of effect of coenzyme Q on left ventricular function in patients with congestive heart failure. J Am Coll Cardiol 33.6 (1999): 1549–1552.

Watts GF et al. Coenzyme Q(10) improves endothelial dysfunction of the brachial artery in type II diabetes mellitus. Diabetologia 45 (2002): 420–426.

Wilkinson EG et al. Bioenergetics in clinical medicine. II. Adjunctive treatment with coenzyme Q in periodontal therapy. Res Commun Chem Pathol Pharmacol 12.1 (1975): 111–123.

Yamagami T, Shibata N, Folkers K. Bioenergetics in clinical medicine: studies on coenzyme Q10 and essential hypertension. Res Commun Chem Pathol Pharmacol 11 (1975): 273–288.

Yamagami T, Shibata N, Folkers K. Bioenergetics in clinical medicine. VIII. Adminstration of coenzyme Q10 to patients with essential hypertension. Res Commun Chem Pathol Pharmacol 14 (1976): 721–727.

Yang X et al. Coenzyme Q10 reduces β-amyloid plaque in an APP/PS1 transgenic mouse model of Alzheimer's disease. J Mol Neurosci 41.1 (2010): 110–113.
Yang, X et al. Coenzyme Q10 attenuates β-amyloid pathology in the aged transgenic mice with Alzheimer Presenilin 1 mutation. J Mol Neurosci 34.2 (2008): 165–171.
Ylikoski T et al. The effect of coenzyme Q10 on the exercise performance of cross-country skiers. Mol Aspects Med 18 (Suppl) (1997): S283–S290.
Young AJ et al. Coenzyme Q10: a review of its promise as a neuroprotectant. CNS Spectr 12.1 (2007): 62–68.
Young JM et al. A randomized, double-blind, placebo-controlled crossover study of coenzyme Q10 therapy in hypertensive patients with the metabolic syndrome. Am J Hypertens 25.2 (2012): 261–270.
Zhou M et al. Effects of coenzyme Q10 on myocardial protection during cardiac valve replacement and scavenging free radical activity in vitro. J Cardiovasc Surg (Torino) 40 (1999): 355–361.
Zhou Q, Chowbay B. Effect of coenzyme Q10 on the disposition of doxorubicin in rats. Eur J Drug Metab Pharmacokinet 27.3 (2002): 185–192.
Zlatohlavek L et al. The effect of coenzyme Q10 in statin myopathy. Neuro Endocrinol Lett 33 (2012): 98–101.
Zmitek J et al. Relative bioavailability of two forms of a novel water-soluble coenzyme Q10. Ann Nutr Metab 52.4 (2008): 281–287.

Colostrum

Clinical note — Hyperimmune bovine colostrum

Bovine colostrum contains a variety of Ig, but the specific Ig present varies and is influenced by previous immune system challenges. Hyperimmune BC, in which the concentration of specific antibodies is raised, can be produced by immunising cows with either specific pathogens or their antigens. For example, BC from cows exposed to rotavirus might contain a relatively high neutralising Ig titre against the virus (as well as many other pathogenic microorganisms), whereas BC collected from cows never exposed to rotavirus is less likely to have specific neutralising Ig against rotavirus. This is an important distinction, because much of the research on BC as prophylaxis or treatment for infectious disease has focused on products that are, as a consequence of specific immune provocation, immunologically unique (Kelly 2003).

BACKGROUND AND RELEVANT PHARMACOKINETICS

Colostrum is the milk produced by female mammals towards the end of pregnancy and secreted from the mammary gland in the first 2 days after giving birth. It is a very complex fluid, rich in nutrients, antibodies, growth factors, vitamins and minerals (Uruakpa et al 2002). The antibodies provide passive immunity to the newborn, and the growth factors stimulate development of the gastrointestinal tract. In contrast to humans, where immonoglobulins are transferred in utero via the placenta, newborn calves are wholly dependent on colostrum to provide passive immunity via intestinal absorption of immunoglobulins, which do not cross the placenta in cattle. This provides a highly concentrated immunoglobulin-rich substance (Rathe et al 2014).

CHEMICAL COMPONENTS

Colostrum contains macronutrients, such as protein and carbohydrate, micronutrients, such as vitamins and minerals, together with cytokines, including IL-1-beta, IL-6, trypsin inhibitors, protease inhibitors and oligosaccharides. It also contains growth factors, such as insulin-like growth factor (IGF)-1 and -2, transforming growth factor-alpha and -beta, lactoferrin, epidermal growth factor and others. High amounts of insulin-like growth factors (IGF-1 and IGF-2) are present and are heat and acid stable, able to withstand dairy processing, and the acid conditions of the GIT (Rathe et al 2014). Several different antimicrobial factors are also present, such as immunoglobulin (Ig) A, secretory IgA, IgG-1, IgG-2 and IgM, lactoferrin, lactoperoxidase and lysozyme, which produce both specific and non-specific bacteriostatic and bacteriocidal effects on many pathological microorganisms, including bacteria, viruses and fungi. IgG-1 is the principal immunoglobulin type in colostrums, and IgM, IgA and IgG-2 are present in lower amounts (Mach & Pahud 1971). Colostrum is the only natural source of two major growth factors: transforming growth factors alpha and beta, and high amounts of insulin-like growth factors 1 and 2. These growth factors have significant muscle and cartilage repair characteristics (Uruakpa et al 2002). The presence of fibroblast growth factors and platelet-derived growth factor is thought to be instrumental in tissue repair and wound healing. Transforming growth factor-β has anti-inflammatory effects and is implicated in tissue proliferation and repair, while transforming growth factor-α has a role in maintenance of epithelial function and integrity (Rathe et al 2014).

Evidence for stability of bioactive substances in GIT transit has been documented for bovine immunoglobulin; however, other constituents such as cytokines may be less resilient to changes in conditions related to collection and administration, which may account for variable effects (Rathe et al 2014).

FOOD SOURCES

Bovine colostrums (BC) are derived from cows, and hyperimmune BC is derived from cows that have been exposed to organisms that can cause disease in humans.

MAIN ACTIONS

In a recent systematic review, Rathe et al (2014) suggest that while methodological quality of clinical trials has been generally less than robust, the main benefits of bovine colostrums are provided in gastrointestinal and immunological effects. Further, more robust studies are required to confirm findings to date in humans, and animal model studies may help to elucidate the biological mechanisms underlying any observed effect and the best methods for dosage and administration.

Imparts passive immunity and stimulates growth of the neonatal gastrointestinal tract

Just as the immunoglobulins of human colostrum impart passive immunity to the newborn child, so too BC provides protection against microbial infections and confers passive immunity to the newborn calf until its own immune system matures (Korhonen et al 2000). Studies with targeted hyperimmune BC suggest that passive immunity may prevent or treat infectious diseases that affect the entire length of the gastrointestinal tract (Pacyna et al 2001).

In contrast, two studies examining the effects of BC on short bowel syndrome in both children (Aunsholt et al 2014) and adults (Lund et al 2012) found that the inclusion of BC to the diet did not improve intestinal function in either population.

Rathe et al (2014) reviewed research that suggests that the antimicrobial effect of bovine colostrum lies in its constituent elements that contain numerous proteins and peptides that are attributable to both the innate and the acquired immune systems (Stelwagen et al 2009).

Immunomodulatory activity

An animal study found that BC has a Th1-promoting activity, which may be helpful in treating various infectious diseases, including influenza (Biswas et al 2007, Yoshioka et al 2005). When BC was administered to weaned piglets, this intervention increased total serum IgA levels, stimulated ileal Peyer's patch (PP) and both Th1 and Th2 cytokine production (Boudry et al 2007). Further research would be needed to assess if BC increases Th1 in already high Th1 profiles or simply modulates the immune function where there is dysfunction.

Uchida et al (2012) demonstrated in their study that skimmed and concentrated bovine late colostrum (SCBLC) activates the immune system and protects against the influenza (flu) virus infection. Activity of natural killer (NK) cells of PP cells significantly increased following oral administration of SCBLC to mice. This was seen in splenocytes and lung cells, indicating that oral administration of SCBLC activates systemic cellular immunity and also local cellular immunity, such as in the respiratory tract, and that activation of cellular immunity is one of the mechanisms of amelioration of flu infection.

In an analysis of human colostrum and breast milk, Marcuzzi et al (2013) confirmed the presence of high levels of cytokines, cytokine receptors and chemokines. The concentrations of these were significantly higher in colostrum, including the presence of IL-9, which was first described by these researchers. Of the cytokines investigated, IL-1β, IL-2, IL-4, IL-5, IL-7 and MIP-1α were present in colostrum only. The presence of these substances is indicative of the influence on the development of the immune system of the newborn.

For children aged 1–10 years, with non-organic failure to thrive, Panahi et al (2010) found that daily supplementation with 40 mg oral BC significantly improved the Gomez index for weight status after 3 months. One hundred and twenty children with mild to moderate non-organic failure to thrive were randomised to routine treatment or to 40 mg oral BC plus routine treatment. The mean Gomez index significantly improved in the oral BC group, but height status, as measured by the Waterlow I index, was no different between the groups.

In contrast, a clinical study found no significant effect on immune parameters for healthy volunteers aged 40–80 years who received BC concentrate 1.2 g/day. The researchers suggested that improving immune function in people with healthy immune responses is difficult, thereby explaining why no significant effect was observed (Wolvers et al 2006).

Jensen et al (2012), however, investigated the effects of bovine colostrum low-molecular weight fraction (CLMWF) on aspects of innate immune function in healthy adults. In a double-blind, placebo-controlled, randomised crossover study, a single dose of CLMWF resulted in a rapid increase in phagocytic activity of monocytes at 1 hour and polymophonuclear cells at 1 hour and 2 hours. The relative increase of NK cells suggested that new NK cells were mobilised into action following the interaction of CLMWF with immune cells in the gut mucosa. Local immune events in the gut are triggered acutely, with systemic consequences. This is reiterated by Rathe et al (2014), suggesting that BC constituents may contribute to systemic immunological events following contact with gut mucosa, as well as localised direct antimicrobial and endotoxin-neutralising effects throughout the GIT. Further, the authors suggested other growth-stimulating factors may be at work, indicated by suppression of gut inflammation and the promotion of mucosal integrity and tissue repair in the context of injury (Rathe et al 2014).

Antibacterial and antiviral effects

Targeted hyperimmune BCs have proven effective in prophylaxis against various human infectious diseases caused by organisms such as rotavirus, *Shigella flexneri*, *Escherichia coli*, *Clostridium difficile*, *Streptococcus mutans*, *Cryptosporidium parvum* and *Helicobacter pylori* (Korhonen et al 2000). Hyperimmune BC from cows previously immunised with a vaccine of 17 strains of pathogenic diarrhoea bacteria was shown to inhibit in vitro growth of the same pathogens by destroying cell walls and agglutinating with bacteria (Xu et al 2006).

It is suspected that colostrum may modulate the interaction of *H. pylori* and other adhesin-expressing

Clinical note — Ovine colostrum and colostrum proline-rich polypeptides

There is new research appearing in the literature regarding colostrum from ewes, mostly using a product called Colostrinin, which is a proline-rich, polypeptide complex from mammalian colostrum. In vitro, in vivo and clinical trials using this product have gained attention as having possible therapeutic benefit in the treatment of mild or moderate Alzheimer's disease (AD) by improving cognitive symptoms and delaying the disease process. Two mechanisms have been proposed to explain these benefits — an antioxidant mechanism which reduces oxidative stress and prevention of beta-amyloid aggregation (Bilikiewicz & Gaus 2004, Boldogh & Kruzel 2008, Stewart 2008). The anti-inflammatory action of this substance may also have an effect on decreasing IgE/IgG-1 production, which could prevent or reduce allergic responses (Boldogh et al 2008). It seems that bovine colostrum proline-rich polypeptides have also displayed some potential in this anti-allergenic arena. Ovine colostrum, Colostrinin and colostrum proline-rich polypeptides are products to watch and would benefit from broader clinical trials to confirm their potential therapeutic uses.

pathogens with their target tissues, chiefly due to phosphatidylethanolamine and its derivatives, rather than to an antibody response (Bitzan et al 1998).

Benson et al (2012) evaluated the effects on the innate immune system in the mouse model after exposure to a low-molecular weight fraction (CLMWF) of immunoglobulin-depleted bovine colostrum whey. Reduced bacterial (Streptococcus) and viral (influenza) loads were observed in lungs within 24 hours when product is introduced across mucosal membranes. The results are confirmed by Jensen et al (2012), with a follow-up human study linking a rapid and immediate increase in phagocytic activity of monocytes with a subsequent triggering of new natural killer cells into systemic circulation.

Improves gut permeability

Studies with agents known to disrupt gut permeability indicate that BC has a preventive effect that is likely to be a result of more than one growth factor present in the colostrum (Mir et al 2010, Playford et al 1999, 2000, Rathe et al 2014).

Reduces NSAID-induced intestinal damage

Defatted BC had major beneficial effects in preventing non-steroidal anti-inflammatory drug (NSAID)-induced gut injury in a variety of well-validated in vivo and in vitro models (Kim et al 2005a, 2005b, Playford et al 1999, 2001). BC improves the integrity of intestinal villi and prevents NSAID-induced increases in small intestine permeability. More specifically, the studies indicate that it stimulates both cell migration and proliferation, thereby enhancing the natural repair mechanisms that occur during acute mucosal injury. One of the studies, by Kim et al (2005a), identified that when BC is administered together with glutamine, gastrointestinal protection is greater than when either agent is used alone. Further, the other study found that the overgrowth of enteric aerobic bacteria seen with NSAID administration did not occur to the same extent with BC (Kim et al 2005b).

OTHER ACTIONS

The high nutritional content of BC makes it an excellent source of many macro- and micronutrients.

Antioxidant activity

BC given to intestinal ischaemia/reperfusion-injured rats experienced reduced oxidative stress and reduced nitric oxide (NO) overproduction in the lungs, which reduced lung injury. Superoxide dismutase and glutathione peroxidase levels were significantly increased and myeloperoxidase and malondialdehyde were significantly reduced in lung tissue, indicating an overall reduction in oxidative stress (Choi et al 2007). The same research team went on to show that BC may reduce damage in brain ischaemia/reperfusion-injured rats (Choi & Ko 2008). Following this, the same research team (Choi et al 2009) demonstrated that BC may have beneficial effects in treating and preventing intestinal barrier damage, bacterial translocation and the related systemic inflammatory response syndrome (SIRS) and multiple organ dysfunction syndrome (MODS) in an intestinal ischaemia/reperfusion (I/R)-injured rat model.

CLINICAL USE

The use of BC as a dietary supplement has increased substantially over the past two decades. Unlike other dietary supplements, the composition of BC is not precisely defined and varies greatly according to the breed and health status of the donor animal feeding practices, previous exposure to infectious organisms and time collected postparturition (Kelly 2003).

Prevention and treatment of infection

Targeted hyperimmune BC products have proven effective in prophylaxis against various infectious diseases in humans, such as URTI, influenza and shigella (Rathe et al 2014, Tacket et al 1992).

Infectious diarrhoea

Rotavirus infection

The clinical evidence available suggests that hyperimmune BC is a promising agent in the prophylaxis and treatment of infectious diarrhoea caused by rotavirus. One Australian study using BC containing high titres of antibody to all four human rotavirus serotypes found that administration successfully prevented symptomatic infection in 100% of children treated with the preparation (Davidson et al 1989). It also reduced the duration of rotavirus excretion, which may have implications for preventing cross-infection. A double-blind study of 75 boys aged 6–24 months with rotavirus diarrhoea compared ordinary BC to hyperimmune BC (100 mL three times daily for 3 days) from cows immunised with four serotypes of human rotavirus (Mitra et al 1995). Diarrhoea ceased within 48 hours in 50% of children receiving hyperimmune BC, whereas 100% of children receiving ordinary BC continued to have diarrhoea. Total stool output (g/kg) between admission and cessation of diarrhoea was also reduced in the group receiving hyperimmune BC compared with ordinary BC. Another double-blind study also found that treatment with antirotavirus immunoglobulin of BC origin is effective in the management of children with acute rotavirus diarrhoea (Sarker et al 1998).

A double-blind study of children aged 6–30 months found that treatment with hyperimmune BC (100 mL solution four times daily for 4 days) leads to improved weight gain, decreased duration of diarrhoea and resulted in fewer stools, although the differences were not statistically significant compared to ordinary colostrum or placebo (Ylitalo et al 1998).

Studies using hyperimmune BC in young children have identified rotavirus antibodies as early as 8 hours after ingestion and up to 72 hours after consumption has ceased, with a strong relation between the titre of rotavirus antibody administered and the level of antibody activity detected in the faeces (Pacyna et al 2001). This suggests that passive immunity is imparted to the entire length of the gastrointestinal tract.

Shigella infection

According to one small study, hyperimmune BC with a high titre of anti-*Shigella flexneri* 2a lipopolysaccharide prevented the incidence of shigella infection in 10 of 10 volunteers, whereas 5 of 11 volunteers administered a control substance went on to develop the infection (Tacket et al 1992).

HIV-induced diarrhoea

BC has also been investigated as a potential treatment in HIV-induced diarrhoea, a symptom that occurs in most patients infected with AIDS. A BC product (Lactobin, Biotest, Dreieich, Germany) containing high titres of antibodies against a wide range of bacterial, viral and protozoal pathogens, as well as against various bacterial toxins, was tested in a multicentre pilot study involving 29 HIV-infected patients (Rump et al 1992). An oral dose of 10 g/day produced a transient (10 days) or long-lasting (>4 weeks) normalisation of the stool frequency in 21 patients. Mean daily stool frequency decreased from 7.4 to 2.2 at the end of the treatment. Some success was also obtained 1 year later in a prospective, open, uncontrolled study of 25 HIV patients with chronic refractory diarrhoea and either confirmed cryptosporidiosis ($n = 7$) or absence of demonstrable pathogenic organisms ($n = 18$) (Plettenberg et al 1993). An oral dose of 10 g/day of an immunoglobulin preparation from BC over a period of 10 days led to complete remission of cryptosporidiosis infection in three of seven subjects and two had partial remission. Complete remission was also seen in seven of 18 patients with diarrhoea and negative stool culture and a further four had partial remission. Of those subjects not responding to treatment, doubling of the dose to 20 g/day led to partial remission in four more patients and complete remission in one.

A BC product designed for slow passage through the gastrointestinal tract (ColoPlus) was tested over 4 weeks in an open-label study of 30 people with HIV-associated diarrhoea (Floren et al 2006). Treatment resulted in a dramatic decrease in daily stool evacuations (from 7.0 ± 2.7 to 1.3 ± 0.5), a mean increase of 7.3 kg of body weight, a 125% increase in $CD4^+$ count and a substantial decrease in self-estimated fatigue. However, in a 2011 study by Byakwaga et al researchers found that the administration of neither raltegravir nor hyperimmune bovine colostrum (HIBC) for 24 weeks resulted in any significant change to $CD4^+$ count.

Reducing incidence of upper respiratory tract infections (URTIs)

There is good evidence that daily supplementation with bovine colostrum for a number of weeks (and preliminary evidence for acute effects after a single dose) can maintain intestinal barrier integrity, immune function and reduce the chances of suffering URTI or URT symptoms in athletes or those undertaking heavy training (Davison 2012). IgA is found in saliva and acts as a major barrier preventing pathogens entering the body via the oral route. As such, the level of secretory IgA has been found to correlate with resistance to some viral infections. According to two clinical studies, BC (20 g/day) increases salivary IgA levels, a factor that could feasibly increase the host's resistance to infection (Crooks et al 2006, Mero et al 2002). In the study by Crooks et al, secretory IgA levels were elevated by 79% after 12 weeks of BC administration in athletes. The presence of numerous immune factors in BC further provides a theoretical basis for its use; however, little clinical investigation has been conducted to confirm its preventive effects.

In 2003, results of a randomised, double-blind, placebo-controlled trial were published, providing some support for its use as a prophylactic agent (Brinkworth & Buckley 2003). The study of 174 physically active young males compared colostrum powder (60 g/day; intact, Numico Research Australia Pty Ltd) to concentrated whey powder over 8 weeks. During the test period, a significantly smaller proportion of subjects taking BC reported URTI symptoms than the control group; however, BC did not alter the duration of URTI once infection was established. Due to the self-reporting method used in this study, results should be viewed as preliminary and require further confirmation. An open study with 605 children in India achieved exceptional results as a prophylactic in preventing recurrent episodes of upper respiratory tract infections and diarrhoea. The children received a BC (Pedimune) for 12 weeks, which reduced the incidence of URTI by 91% and diarrhoea by 86% (Patel & Rana 2006). This was an open study, and more rigorous clinical trials are needed to confirm these findings.

Influenza prophylactic

Colostrum may reduce the incidence of influenza according to a trail which compared a colostrum supplement, given over 2 months, with an influenza vaccination and a combination of the two, for the prevention of flu. Over the next 3 months, the group receiving colostrum treatment only had the lowest number of flu episodes (13), with the next highest in the colostrum and vaccination group (14), then the vaccination only (41), highest in non-treated subjects (57). The study was repeated with 65 high-risk cardiovascular patients, which once again produced positive results, as the incidence of hospital admissions and complications was higher in those who received only the vaccination compared to people receiving colostrum. Overall, colostrum supplementation was considered at least three times more effective than vaccination for flu prevention (Cesarone et al 2007). Benson et al's (2012) mouse model study, followed by the Jensen et al (2012) human study, suggests reduced bacterial (Streptococcus) and viral (influenza) load observed in the lungs within 24 hours of administration of a consumable low-molecular weight fraction (CLMWF) bovine colostrum whey is the result of a rapid immediate increase in phagocytic activity of monocytes with a subsequent triggering of new natural killer cells into systemic circulation.

Improved physical performance and preservation of muscle mass

BC has been used by athletes mainly as a natural source of IGF-1 because it has an anabolic effect and is involved in the regulatory feedback of growth hormone. It is taken with the belief that protein catabolism will be reduced during intense training periods and physical performance will improve.

A double-blind, crossover study of nine male athletes confirmed that ingestion of BC (125 mL/day; Bioenervie, Viable Bioproducts) resulted in elevated concentrations of IGF-1; however, no significant effects were reported for serum IgG or saliva IgA concentrations (Mero et al 1997). Several years later in a larger study of athletes, under double-blind study conditions, researchers confirmed that BC ingestion produced significant increases in serum IGF-1 (Mero et al 2002). The dose of 20 g/day of BC (dynamic supplement) was used during a 2-week training period in this study, which further found that saliva IgA levels increased with this particular treatment.

In a more recent trial, 29 cyclists were randomly assigned to take either 10 g/day of a BC protein concentrate or a placebo consisting of 10 g/day of whey protein during normal training over 5 weeks. Performance tests showed that BC treatment improved results in a 40-km time trial during a high-intensity training regimen and also maintained ventilatory threshold (Shing et al 2006). The same researchers also found that the supplement modulated immunity before and after training and prevented postexercise reductions in serum IgG2 at the end of the high-intensity training period. A trend towards fewer upper respiratory tract illnesses was also detected (Shing et al 2007). In 2013, these same researchers undertook a pilot study (n = 10) to examine the effects of bovine colostrum protein concentrate (CPC) (10 g per day) supplementation on salivary hormones, salivary IgA and heart rate variability (HRV) over consecutive days of competitive cycling, compared with a control group receiving whey protein concentrate (10 g per day). They found that bovine CPC supplementation was associated with maintained salivary testosterone concentration and modulated autonomic activity (HRV) over consecutive days of competitive cycling. No differences were found in salivary IgA between groups. Implications for improved recovery is implied for endurance athletes in this pilot study, and further research is warranted (Shing et al 2013).

Conversely, in a study by Carol et al (2011), BC was investigated for its effect in post exercise immune modulation after short-term intense exercise in nine male athletes. No significant effect was found for BC in preventing post-exercise immune suppression. Similarly, a study by Crooks et al (2010) on the effect of BC on mucosal defence in the respiratory tracts of athletes and a non-exercising control group found no measurable effect on either saliva or plasma immunoglobulin levels in the BC group or the control group.

However, a trial by Davison and Diment (2010), designed to model stress-induced immunodepression by examining exercise-induced immunodepression, found that while previous research had focused primarily on salivary IgA levels, a more useful measure may be to examine the exercise-induced changes in innate immunity as measured by neutrophil function and salivary lysozyme, in addition to salivary IgA. They found that there were significant increases in these stress markers in both groups, but that over time there were observed differences in neutrophil function and salivary lysozyme concentration and release. Significant exercise-induced decreases were observed in these parameters, but the BC group had a more speedy recovery of the neutrophil function and prevention of the decrease in salivary lysozyme, as measures of innate immunity. Therefore, the authors suggest that BC supplementation limits the immunodepressive effects induced by an acute prolonged physical stressor.

Appukutty et al (2011) found in a 6-week intervention of bovine colostrum in active adolescent boys that supplementation resulted in modulated interferon-γ activity.

The review by Rathe et al (2014) suggest that collectively, results from studies of athletes, and GIT re-activity to BC, confirm systemic effects, which follow immunological events triggered by contact with gut mucosa.

Gastrointestinal protection against NSAID-induced damage

BC has also been investigated in a small, randomised, crossover study as prophylaxis against NSAID-induced gastrointestinal damage (Playford et al 2001). A spray-dried, defatted colostrum (125 mL three times daily) was co-administered with indomethacin (50 mg three times daily) for 5 days in the first phase, then the effect of 7 days treatment with the colostral solution on gut permeability was determined in subjects taking NSAID long-term. Indomethacin (150 mg/day) caused a threefold increase in gut permeability after 5 days, whereas no change was observed when colostrum was co-administered, suggesting a protective effect. In contrast, no protective effect was seen in subjects who had been using NSAIDs long-term and then administered colostrum for 1 week. Various animal and human studies suggest the protective effect of BC on the gut aginst NSAID exposure (Rathe et al 2014).

Antidiabetic

It has been suggested that BC may have an effect on blood glucose levels. A small, randomised study of 16 patients with type 2 diabetes tested the effects of BC (10 g/day) over 4 weeks. Total cholesterol and triglyceride levels decreased significantly with active treatment, and a reduction in blood glucose levels and ketones were observed, which suggests a potential role for BC in diabetes management (Kim et al 2009). Larger clinical studies are warranted to confirm this finding.

Hammon et al (2013) state that BC affects intestinal growth and function and is likely to enhance the absorptive capacity of the GIT, and therefore improve the glucose status in neonatal calves by increasing glucose absorption and elevating postprandial plasma glucose concentrations. This is thought to occur by improved glucose absorption and therefore storage in the liver, enhancing availability in the postprandial state (Hammon et al 2013). In a study by Tozier (2013), neonatal admissions to the intensive care unit (NICU) for glucose stabilisation decreased following the initiation of routine colostrum feeds for newborns of diabetic mothers, replacing routine formula supplementation for this population. Rates of exclusive breastfeeding were also increased, in line with best practice recommendations from the WHO. Marinelli et al (2012) note that the high protein content of colostrum helps with glucose stabilisation and promotion of ketogenesis.

Wound healing

In a small study by Doillon et al (2011), a complex compound (immune ('IM') fraction) from colostrum-derived whey was investigated for potential wound-healing capabilities. In vitro, the compound was able to significantly inhibit the contraction of collagen gel while fibroblast density remained similar to control gels, and did not exhibit evidence of stress fibres. This effect was dose-dependent. In vivo studies of guinea pig models demonstrated significantly delayed wound closure by contraction, resulting in minimised residual scarring, and the wound covered a significantly larger surface area, with unchanged collagen deposition. The mechanism of action may reflect a contraction rate modulation and wound remodelling.

OTHER USES

Due to its effects on gut permeability, BC is used in a variety of other conditions, such as inflammatory bowel disease, coeliac disease, food allergies, intestinal infection and inflammatory joint diseases. It has also been used to restore normal gut permeability in people using chemotherapy. In some instances, it is used with glutamine for these indications (Kim et al 2005a).

DOSAGE RANGE

According to clinical studies

- Diarrhoea due to rotavirus: 100 mL three times daily for 3 days of BC from cows immunised with the four serotypes of human rotavirus.
- HIV-induced diarrhoea: 10 g/day (Lactobin, Biotest, Dreieich, Germany).
- Prevention of URTI: 60 g/day (intact, Numico Research Australia Pty Ltd).
- Increasing serum IGF-1 levels: 125 mL/day (Bioenervie, Viable Bioproducts) or 20 g/day (Dynamic supplement).
- Prevention of NSAID-induced gastrointestinal damage: 125 mL three times daily of spray-dried, defatted BC.
- For improving performance in high-intensity training and reducing exercise-induced URTI: 10 g/day.

TOXICITY

Not known.

ADVERSE REACTIONS

Not known.

SIGNIFICANT INTERACTIONS

Not known.

CONTRAINDICATIONS AND PRECAUTIONS

Only BC products produced under strict quality control guidelines should be used. They typically contain lactose, so should be avoided by people with lactose intolerance.

PREGNANCY USE

Likely to be safe.

Practice points/Patient counselling

- Colostrum is a very complex fluid that is rich in nutrients, antibodies, growth factors, vitamins and minerals.
- Targeted hyperimmune BC products have proven effective in prophylaxis against various infectious diseases in humans, notably infectious diarrhoea.
- BC is a popular supplement among athletes and used mainly as a natural source of IGF-1 because it has an anabolic effect and is involved in the regulatory feedback of growth hormone.
- Preliminary evidence suggests that BC may prevent NSAID-induced gastrointestinal damage and improve gut permeability.
- Most studies use hyperimmune BC in which the concentration of specific antibodies is raised.
- Preliminary evidence shows some potential for BC in flu prevention and upper respiratory tract infections.

PATIENTS' FAQs

What will this supplement do for me?

Bovine colostrum contains nutrients, antibodies, growth factors, vitamins and minerals, and has a variety of effects on the gastrointestinal tract, immune function and the ability to fight some infections, and may possibly reduce muscle catabolism. It also may reduce the risk of developing an upper respiratory tract infection.

When will it start to work?

Studies with infectious diarrhoea have reported benefits within 3–4 days, and improvement in gut permeability within 5 days.

Are there any safety issues?

Bovine colostrum produced under quality control guidelines is a safe substance; however, it should be avoided by people with lactose intolerance.

REFERENCES

Appukutty M, et al. Modulation of interferon gamma response through orally administered bovine colostrums in active adolescent boys. Biomed Res 22 (2011): 135–145.

Aunsholt L et al. Bovine colostrum to children with short bowel syndrome: A randomised, double-blind, crossover pilot study. J Parenteral and Enteral Nutrition. 38.1 (2014): 99–106.

Benson K et al. A novel extract from bovinge colostrum whey supports anti-bacterial and anti-viral innate immune functions in vitro and in vivo I. Enhanced immunce activity in vitro translates to improved microbial clearance in animal infection models. Prev Med 54 (2012): S116–S123.

Bilikiewicz A, Gaus W. Colostrinin (a naturally occurring, proline-rich, polypeptide mixture) in the treatment of Alzheimer's disease. J Alzheimers Dis 6.1 (2004): 17–26.

Biswas P et al. Immunomodulatory effects of bovine colostrum in human peripheral blood mononuclear cells. New Microbiol 30.4 (2007): 447–454.

Bitzan MM et al. Inhibition of Helicobacter pylori and Helicobacter mustelae binding to lipid receptors by bovine colostrum. J Infect Dis 177 (1998): 955–961.

Boldogh I et al. Colostrinin decreases hypersensitivity and allergic responses to common allergens. Int Arch Allergy Immunol 146.4 (2008): 298–306.

Boldogh I, Kruzel ML. Colostrinin: an oxidative stress modulator for prevention and treatment of age-related disorders. J Alzheimers Dis 13.3 (2008): 303–321.

Boudry C et al. Effects of oral supplementation with bovine colostrum on the immune system of weaned piglets. Res Vet Sci 83.1 (2007): 91–101.

Brinkworth GD, Buckley JD. Concentrated bovine colostrum protein supplementation reduces the incidence of self-reported symptoms of upper respiratory tract infection in adult males. Eur J Nutr 42 (2003): 228–232.

Byakwaga H et al. Intensification of antiretroviral therapy with raltegravir or addition of hyperimmune bovine colostrum in HIV-infected patients with suboptimal CD4⁺ T-cell response: A randomised controlled trial. J Infectious Dis 204 (2011): 1532–40.

Carol A et al. Bovine colostrum supplementation's lack of effect on immune variables during short-term intense exercise in well-trained athletes. Int J Sp Nutr & Ex Metab 21.2 (2011): 135–145.

Cesarone MR et al. Prevention of influenza episodes with colostrum compared with vaccination in healthy and high-risk cardiovascular subjects: the epidemiologic study in San Valentino. Clin Appl Thromb Hemost 13.2 (2007): 130–136.

Choi H, et al. Bovine colostrum prevents bacterial translocation in an intestinal ischemia/reperfusion-injured rat model. J Medicinal Food. 12.1 (2009): 37–49.

Choi H, Ko Y. P032 protective effects of bovine colostrum on brain ischemia/reperfusion injury in rat. Clin Nut Supp 3 (Suppl 1) (2008): 42.

Choi H, Ko Y, Hong H. Antioxidant activity of a bovine colostrum in intestinal ischemia/reperfusion injured rat model. J Emerg Med 33.3 (2007): 337–338.

Choi HS, et al. Bovine colostrum prevents bacterial translocation in an intestinal ischemia/reperfusion-injured rat model. J Med Food 12.1 (2009): 37.

Crooks C et al. Effect of bovine colostrum supplementation on respiratory tract mucosal defenses in swimmers. Int J Sp Nutr & Ex Metab 20.3 (2010): 224–235.

Crooks CV et al. The effect of bovine colostrum supplementation on salivary IgA in distance runners. Int J Sport Nutr Exerc Metab 16 (2006): 47–64.

Davidson GP et al. Passive immunisation of children with bovine colostrum containing antibodies to human rotavirus. Lancet 2 (1989): 709–712.

Davison G. Bovine colostrum and immune function after exercise. Med Sport Sci 59 (2012): 62–69.

Doillon, CJ et al. Modulatory effect of a complex fraction derived from colostrum on fibroblast contractibility and consequences on repair tissue. Int Wound J 8 (2011): 280–290.

Floren CH et al. ColoPlus, a new product based on bovine colostrum, alleviates HIV-associated diarrhoea. Scand J Gastroenterol 41 (2006): 682–686.

Hammon HM et al. Lactation biology symposium: Role of colostrum and colostrum components on glucose metabolism in neonatal calves. J Anim Sci 91 (2013): 685–695.

Jensen GS, Patel D, Benson KF. A novel extract from bovine colostrum whey supports innate immune functions. II. Rapid changes in cellular immune function in humans. Pev Med 54 (2012): S124–S129.

Kelly GS. Bovine colostrums: a review of clinical uses. Altern Med Rev 8 (2003): 378–394.

Kim JH et al. Health-promoting effects of bovine colostrum in type 2 diabetic patients can reduce blood glucose, cholesterol, triglyceride and ketones. J Nutr Biochem 20 (2009): 298–303.

Kim JH et al. Health-promoting effects of bovine colostrum in type 2 diabetic patients can reduce blood glucose, cholesterol, triglyceride and ketones. J Nutr Biochem 20.4 (2009): 298–303.

Kim JW et al. Protective effects of bovine colostrum on non-steroidal anti-inflammatory drug induced intestinal damage in rats. Asia Pac J Clin Nutr 14 (2005b): 103–107.

Kim JW, Jeon WK, Kim EJ. Combined effects of bovine colostrum and glutamine in diclofenac-induced bacterial translocation in rat. Clin Nutr 24 (2005a): 785–793.

Korhonen H, Marnila P, Gill HS. Bovine milk antibodies for health. Br J Nutr 84 (Suppl 1) (2000): S135–S146.

Lund P et al. Randomised controlled trial of colostrum to improve intestinal function in patients with short bowel syndrome. European J Clinical Nutrition 66.9 (2012): 1059–1065.

Mach JP, Pahud JJ. Secretory IgA, a major immunoglobulin in most bovine external secretions. J Immunol 106 (1971): 552–563.

Marcuzzi A et al. Presence of IL-9 in paired samples of human colostrum and transitional milk. J Hum Lact 29.1 (2013): 26–31.

Mero A et al. Effects of bovine colostrum supplementation on serum IGF-I, IgG, hormone, and saliva IgA during training. J Appl Physiol 83 (1997): 1144–1151.

Mero A et al. IGF-I, IgA, and IgG responses to bovine colostrum supplementation during training. J Appl Physiol 93 (2002): 732–739.

Mir R et al. Structural and binding studies of C-terminal half (C-lobe) of lactoferrin protein with COX-2-specific non-steroidal anti-inflammatory drugs (NSAIDs). Arch Biochem Biophys. 500 (2010): 196–202.
Mitra AK et al. Hyperimmune cow colostrum reduces diarrhoea due to rotavirus: a double-blind, controlled clinical trial. Acta Paediatr 84 (1995): 996–1001.
Pacyna J et al. Survival of rotavirus antibody activity derived from bovine colostrum after passage through the human gastrointestinal tract. J Pediatr Gastroenterol Nutr 32 (2001): 162–167.
Panahi Y et al. Bovine colostrum in the management of nonorganic failure to thrive: A randomized clinical trial. J Ped Gastro & Nutr 50.5 (2010): 551–554.
Patel K, Rana R. Pedimune in recurrent respiratory infection and diarrhoea — the Indian experience — the pride study. Indian J Pediatr 73.7 (2006): 585–591.
Playford RJ et al. Bovine colostrum is a health food supplement which prevents NSAID induced gut damage. Gut 44 (1999): 653–658.
Playford RJ et al. Co-administration of the health food supplement, bovine colostrum, reduces the acute non-steroidal anti-inflammatory drug-induced increase in intestinal permeability. Clin Sci (Lond) 100 (2001): 627–633.
Playford RJ et al. Colostrum and mild-derived peptide growth factors for the treatment of gastrointestinal disorders. Am J Clin Nutr 72.5 (2000): 5–14.
Plettenberg A et al. A preparation from bovine colostrum in the treatment of HIV-positive patients with chronic diarrhoea. Clin Invest 71 (1993): 42–45.
Rathe M et al. Clinical applications of bovine colostrums therapy: a systematic review. Nutr Rev 72.4 (2014): 237–254.
Rump JA et al. Treatment of diarrhoea in human immunodeficiency virus-infected patients with immunoglobulins from bovine colostrum. Clin Investig 70 (1992): 588–594.
Sarker SA et al. Successful treatment of rotavirus diarrhoea in children with immunoglobulin from immunized bovine colostrum. Pediatr Infect Dis J 17 (1998): 1149–1154.
Shing CM et al. A pilot study: bovine colostrum supplementation and hormonal and autonomic responses to competitive cycling. J Sp Med & Phys Fit 53.5 (2013): 490.
Shing CM et al. Effects of bovine colostrum supplementation on immune variables in highly trained cyclists. J Appl Physiol 102.3 (2007): 1113–1122.
Shing CM et al. The influence of bovine colostrum supplementation on exercise performance in highly trained cyclists. Br J Sports Med 40.9 (2006): 797–801.
Stelwagen K et al. Immune components of bovine colostrums and milk. J amin Sci 87 Suppl 1 (2009): 3–9.
Stewart MG. Colostrinin: a naturally occurring compound derived from mammalian colostrum with efficacy in treatment of neurodegenerative diseases, including Alzheimer's. Expert Opin Pharmacother 9.14 (2008): 2553–2559.
Tacket CO et al. Efficacy of bovine milk immunoglobulin concentrate in preventing illness after Shigella flexneri challenge. Am J Trop Med Hyg 47 (1992): 276–283.
Tozier PK. Colostrum versus formula supplementation for glucose stabilization in newborns of diabetic mothers. JOGNN 42.6 (2013): 619–628.
Uchida K et al. Augmentation of cellular immunity and protection against influenza virus infection by bovine late colostrum in mice. Nutr 28 (2012): 442–446.
Uruakpa FO et al. Colostrum and its benefits: a review. Nutr Res 22 (2002): 755–767.
Wolvers DA et al. Effect of a mixture of micronutrients, but not of bovine colostrum concentrate, on immune function parameters in healthy volunteers: a randomized placebo-controlled study. Nutr J 5 (2006): 28.
Xu LB et al. Bovine immune colostrum against 17 strains of diarrhea bacteria and in vitro and in vivo effects of its specific IgG. Vaccine 24.12 (2006): 2131–2140.
Ylitalo S et al. Rotaviral antibodies in the treatment of acute rotaviral gastroenteritis. Acta Paediatr 87 (1998): 264–267.
Yoshioka Y et al. Oral administration of bovine colostrum stimulates intestinal intraepithelial lymphocytes to polarize Th1-type in mice. Int Immunopharmacol 5.3 (2005): 581–590.

C

Coriolus versicolor

HISTORICAL NOTE In traditional medical practices of China and Japan, *Coriolus versicolor* or Yun Zhi mushroom was harvested, dried, ground and made into tea. It has an established history of use in these cultures and is included in the Chinese Materia Medica, being widely prescribed for cancer and infection. Not surprisingly, the healing properties of coriolus has been further investigated in clinical trials, mainly by Chinese and Japanese scientists. The dose of the active polymers in the traditional tea was similar to that used in modern clinical practice. Of the mushroom-derived therapeutics, polysaccharopeptides (PSP) obtained from *Coriolus versicolor* are commercially available and are of most interest. In addition to its medical applications, *C. versicolor* is widely used to degrade recalcitrant organic pollutants such as pentachlorophenol (Cui et al 2003).

COMMON NAME

Coriolus, Yun Zhi

OTHER NAMES

Agaricus versicolor, Boletus versicolor, champignon coriolus, Krestin, *Polyporus versicolor, Polystictus versicolor, Poria versicolor, Trametes versicolor*, Yun Zhi (Chinese), Kawaratake (Japanese), polysaccharide-K, polysaccharide Krestin, PSK

In North America, *C. versicolor* is commonly known as 'turkey tail' mushroom.

BOTANICAL NAME/FAMILY

Coriolus versicolor (family Agamidae)

PLANT PART USED

Fruiting body

CHEMICAL COMPONENTS

Coriolus versicolor consists of saccharide, protein, polyphenol and triterpenoid components, with PSP and polysaccharide-K (PSK, krestin) being the most noteworthy fractions (Cui & Chisti 2003, Hsu et al 2013), The protein-bound polysaccharides and their polypeptide moieties are rich in aspartic acid and glutamic acid and also contain the amino acids: alanine, tyrosine, threonine, cysteine, phenylalanine, serine, valine, tryptophan, methionine, lysine, praline, isoleucine and histadine, glycine, leucine and arginine (Yeung & Or 2012). The polysaccharide component contains the sugars mannose, xylose, galactose, arabinose, glucose and rhamnose (Yeung & Or 2011).

MAIN ACTIONS

Studies exploring the mechanisms of action for coriolus have utilised various different extracts and also isolated constituents, but mainly focused on PSK (krestin) and PSP, which are chemically similar and display similar activities. In vitro and in vivo tests reveal an extremely broad range of pharmacological activity and physiological effects for coriolus, PSK and PSP.

Immunomodulatory activity

The ability to influence immune regulation via anti-inflammatory and cell-signalling pathways is well documented in experimental literature. Overall, polysaccharides from coriolus have been shown to activate various types of immune effector cells, such as B lymphocytes, T lymphocytes, cytotoxic T cells, macrophages, polymorphonuclear cells, natural killer cells, lymphokine-activated killer cells and tumour-infiltrating lymphocytes (Wong et al 2004).

PSP from Coriolus has also been shown to regulate gene expression and cytokine secretion related to Toll-like receptor signalling pathway in human peripheral blood mononuclear cells (PBMCs) (Li et al 2010).

Anticancer

Research into the anticancer properties of coriolus has largely focused on the effects of the mushroom to strengthen the immune response of cancer patients. Additionally, direct anticancer activity has been demonstrated for both PSK and PSP in vitro and in vivo for several cancers.

A dose-dependent cytotoxic activity was demonstrated in vitro for a standardised aqueous ethanolis extract of coriolus. The extract was shown to suppress the proliferation of Raji, NB-4 and HL-60 cells by more than 90%, with ascending order of IC50 values. It was also found that it did not exert any significant cytotoxic effect on normal liver cell line WRL when compared with a chemotherapeutic anticancer drug, mitomycin C, confirming the tumour-selective cytotoxicity (Lau et al 2004). In a rat model PSP enhanced the cytotoxic effect of cyclophosphamide on a cancer cell line in vitro and altered the pharmacokinetics of cyclophosphamide (Chan et al 2006b). A methanol extract exerted pronounced antimelanoma activity, both directly through antiproliferative and cytotoxic effects on tumour cells and indirectly through promotion of macrophage antitumour activity in vitro. The methanol extract treatment was also shown to inhibit tumour growth in C57BL/6 mice inoculated with syngeneic B16 tumour cells. Moreover, peritoneal macrophages collected 21 days after tumour implantation from methanol extract-treated animals exerted stronger tumoristatic activity ex vivo than macrophages from control melanoma-bearing mice (Harhaji et al 2008).

Coriolus versicolor polysaccharide-B was also shown to inhibit proliferation and enhance apoptosis of oesophageal cancer cell lines (Wang et al 2012), and, in a double-blind, pilot randomised controlled trial (RCT), high-dose PSP significantly delayed the progression of metastases and afforded the longest survival times reported in canine haemangiosarcoma (Brown et al 2012). Other studies show that coriolus extract dose-dependently suppressed the proliferation of HL-60 cells, with increased nucleosome production from apoptotic cells. Expression of pro-apoptotic protein Bcl-2-associated X protein was significantly upregulated in HL-60 cells treated with the coriolus extract, especially after 16 and 24 hours, and expression of antiapoptotic protein Bcl-2 was concomitantly downregulated, as reflected by the increased Bcl-2-associated X protein : Bcl-2 protien ratio and markedly, but transiently, promoted the release of cytochrome c from mitochondria to cytosol after 24-hour incubation and may be useful in the treatment of some forms of human leukaemia (Ho et al 2006).

Analgesic activity

Analgesic activity has been demonstrated in several animal models and found to be dose-dependent for polysaccharopeptide (Ng et al 1997, Chan et al 2006a). The activity appears to be partly mediated by interleukin-2 (IL-2), which is activated by polysaccharopeptide and interacts with IL-2 receptors in the mediobasal hypothalamus, as demonstrated in mice (Gong et al 1998).

Antioxidant

A direct antioxidant effect of Yun Zhi against oxidant challenge on the DNA of lymphocytes was evidenced in vitro and the active component in Yun Zhi is thought likely to be membrane-permeable (Szeto et al 2013).

OTHER ACTIONS

Anti-inflammatory

The anti-inflammatory effects of *Coriolus versicolor* can be explained by its ability to inhibit certain proinflammatory cytokines, as was seen in a study of male mice with experimentally-induced ulcerative colitis. There was a significant reduction in the expression of STAT1 and STAT6 molecules, thereby leading to lower interferon-γ and IL-4 expression (Lim et al 2011).

Anti-HIV

The inhibitory effect of polysaccharopeptide from *Coriolus versicolor* on HIV-1 reverse transcriptase and alpha-glucosidase was enhanced after chemical modification with chlorosulfonic acid (Wang et al 2001). In a series of in vitro assays it demonstrated inhibition of the interaction between HIV-1 gp 120 and immobilised CD4 receptor (IC50 150 mcg/mL) and potent inhibition of recombinant HIV-1 reverse transcriptase (IC50 6.25 mcg/mL) and it inhibited a glycohydrolase enzyme associated with viral glycosylation (Collins et al 1997).

Hepatoprotection

PSP dose-dependently decreased the binding of [^{14}C]-paracetamol to microsomal proteins in vitro. When PSP was given to rats subchronically for 7 days, the subsequent microsomes obtained also showed a 25% decrease in covalent binding to [^{14}C]-paracetamol, suggesting that PSP interacted with the microsomal proteins rather than the chemically reactive metabolite of paracetamol (Yeung et al 1994).

CLINICAL USE

Preparations containing coriolus and PSK and PSP have been extensively used in Japan and China in the last 30 years, mainly as adjuvant treatment in various cancers to improve patient survival.

Cancer

Both PSP and PSK are considered a new type of biological response modifier which appears to counter the immunosuppressive effect of standard cancer treatments, improve appetite and liver function, enhance the pain threshold and, according to a 2012 meta-analysis, provide a significant survival advantage when used together with standard anticancer treatments compared with standard conventional anticancer treatments alone (Cui & Chisti 2003, Eliza et al 2012, Wong et al 2004). PSK is a Japanese product, while PSP is a Chinese product, and both are approved as adjuvant agents of cancer treatment in Japan and China (Eliza et al 2012).

The 2012 meta-analysis was conducted on 13 RCTs in which coriolus or its extracts (PSP or PSK) were compared to placebo or standard therapy in cancer patients (n = 2587) (Eliza et al 2012). Importantly, no language restrictions limited access to RCTs and trials using coriolus in combination with other herbs were excluded. The overall 5-year survival rate compared was defined as the common end point and was used to assess the differences between the Yun Zhi and standard conventional anticancer treatment groups. The authors identified 22 RCTs that met inclusion criteria; however data were only available from 13 RCTs in a form that could be used for meta-analysis. All RCTs compared Yun Zhi or its extracts (PSK or PSP) with conventional anticancer treatment with or without placebo, using a dose range of 1–3.6 g daily, and the duration of therapy was 1–36 months.

Coriolus treatment or its extracts produced a highly significant difference in overall survival at 5 years when compared to patients solely receiving standard oncology treatment ($P < 0.00001$; relative risk = 1.14; 95% confidence interval = 1.09, 1.20). More specifically, in the patients randomised to receive coriolus preparations, there was a 9% absolute reduction in 5-year mortality, resulting in one additional patient alive for every 11 patients treated. The increase in 5-year survival was most evident for people with breast cancer, gastric cancer or colorectal cancer who were also treated with chemotherapy, according to the RCTs that were assessed.

This is not to assume that coriolus is ineffective in other cancers. Eliza et al (2012) stated they could not be sure whether people with oesophageal cancer were responders from the data available.

The possibility that PSK and PSP could be effective adjuvant treatments in people with cancer is not new. In Japanese trials since 1970, PSK significantly extended survival at 5 years or beyond in cancers of the stomach, colon/rectum, oesophagus, nasopharynx and lung (non-small-cell types), and in an HLA B40-positive breast cancer subset. PSP was subjected to phase II and III trials in China. In double-blind trials, PSP significantly extended 5-year survival in oesophageal cancer. PSP significantly improved quality of life, provided substantial pain relief and enhanced immune status in 70–97% of patients with cancers of the stomach, oesophagus, lung, ovary and cervix. PSK and PSP boosted immune cell production, ameliorated chemotherapy symptoms and enhanced tumour infiltration by dendritic and cytotoxic T cells. Their extremely high tolerability, proven benefits to survival and quality of life and compatibility with chemotherapy and radiation therapy make them well suited for cancer management regimens (Kidd et al 2000). A study to evaluate the effects of 28-day administration of PSP in 34 patients with non-small-cell lung carcinoma showed a significant improvement in blood leucocyte and neutrophil counts, serum immunoglobulin G (IgG) and IgM, and percentage of body fat among the PSP, but not the control, patients. Although the evaluable PSP patients did not improve in non-small-cell lung carcinoma-related symptoms, there were significantly fewer PSP patients withdrawn due to disease progression than their control counterparts. There was no reported adverse reaction attributable to the trial medications (Tsang et al 2003).

> ***Clinical note — PSP and PSK successful development of traditional medicine***
>
> PSK was the first polysaccharide to be commercialised from coriolus. It was tested extensively in clinical trials and approved for use in Japan in 1977. Within a decade it was ranked 19th in the world's most commercially successful drug list and annual sales grew to $357 million in Japan in 1987. About 10 years after the development of PSK, PSP was commercialised by the Chinese (Cui & Chisti 2003).

OTHER USES

Immunomodulatory

IN COMBINATION

The regular oral consumption of Yun Zhi together with a Chinese herb known as Danshen is able to promote immunological function in the posttreatment period of breast cancer patients, according to a study in 82 patients. Results showed that the absolute counts of T-helper lymphocytes ($CD4^+$), the ratio of T-helper ($CD4^+$):T suppressor and cytotoxic lymphocytes ($CD8^+$) and the percentage and absolute counts of B lymphocytes were significantly elevated in patients with breast cancer after taking Yun Zhi-Danshen capsules, while plasma-soluble receptors for IL-2 concentration were significantly decreased (Wong et al 2005). Similarly, multiple effects on immune function were reported in a study of healthy subjects, where oral consumption of Yun Zhi-Danshen capsules significantly elevated PBMC gene expression of IL-2 receptor, increased the percentage and absolute counts of T-helper cell and ratio of $CD4^+$ (T-helper):$CD8^+$ (T-suppressor and cytotoxic T) cell, and significantly enhanced the ex vivo production of typical Th1 cytokine interferon-gamma from PBMCs activated by a lectin found in plants, called phytohaemagglutinin and lipopolysaccharide. Such consumption had no adverse effects on liver or renal function (Wong et al 2004).

DOSAGE RANGE

2–6 g daily

TOXICITY

The oral lethal dose of *Coriolus versicolor* water extract is more than 5000 mg/kg and no observed adverse effect level of the extract for both male and female rats is 5000 mg/kg per day for 28 days (Hor et al 2011).

ADVERSE REACTIONS

The use of *Coriolus versicolor*, PSK and PSP has not been associated with any serious adverse reactions. No toxicity has been observed and serious adverse effects have not been reported in clinical trials. Doses of the extract up to 15 g daily over a long period have not been linked with any side effects (Kidd et al 2000).

SIGNIFICANT INTERACTIONS

In sarcoma-bearing mice, PSK, a protein-bound polysaccharide from *Coriolus versicolor*, was not found to affect microsomal enzymatic activities and, when administered concomitantly, is predicted to not cause changes in the pharmacokinetics of drugs (Fujita et al 1988).

Immunosuppressant medication

The use of *C. versicolor* polysaccharopeptides is contraindicated when immune suppression is desired. Polysaccharopeptides reduce the potency of immunosuppressants such as cyclosporin — avoid.

CONTRAINDICATIONS AND PRECAUTIONS

People with cancer choosing to use coriolus treatment or its polysaccharides should seek professional guidance when doing so, to ensure safety and monitor for response.

Given its immune-stimulating action *Coriolus versicolor* should be used with caution by people with autoimmune diseases as well as people who are organ transplant recipients, particularly in the case of bone marrow transplant (Chu et al 2002).

PREGNANCY USE

PSP did not produce adverse effects on female reproductive or embryonic development in mice treated intraperitoneally, suggesting safety in pregnancy (Ng et al 1997).

Practice points/Patient counselling

- Coriolus is a medicinal mushroom which is used extensively in China and Japan as adjuvant treatment in cancer
- Clinical trials show that coriolus and the derived polysaccharides PSK and PSP increase the chances of 5-year survival when used as adjuvant treatment with chemotherapy in several cancers — current evidence supports its use in breast, gastric and colorectal cancer, but it may also have benefits in other cancers.
- It improves immune function, has direct anticancer effects, reduces liver toxicity, decreases pain and stimulates appetite.
- Coriolus, PSK and PSP may counteract immunosuppression therapy and should be used with caution by people with autoimmune disease.
- The treatment is well tolerated and can be used long-term.

PATIENTS' FAQs

What will this supplement do for me?

Clinical studies show that coriolus and the derived polysaccharides PSK and PSP increase the chances of 5-year survival when used as adjuvant treatment with chemotherapy in several cancers. To date the evidence most strongly supports use in breast, gastric and colorectal cancer, but it may also have benefits in other cancers.

When will it start to work?

It is usually used long-term by people with cancer and studies use frames lasting from 1 month to 36 months; there do not appear to be any safety issues associated with long-term use.

Are there any safety issues?

Coriolus, PSP and PSK are well tolerated and safe. They should not be used by people taking immunosuppressive medicines or organ transplant recipients due to their immunostimulating effects. People with autoimmune disease should use this treatment with caution.

REFERENCES

Brown DC et al. Single agent polysaccharopeptide delays metastases and improves survival in naturally occurring hemangiosarcoma. Evid Based Complement Alternat Med (2012):384301

Chan S et al. Polysaccharide peptides from COV-1 strain of *Coriolus versicolor* induce hyperalgesia via inflammatory mediator release in the mouse. Life Sci (2006a); 78(21): 2463–2470.

Chan S et al. Effects of polysaccharide peptide (PSP) from *Coriolus versicolor* on the pharmacokinetics of cyclophosphamide in the rat and cytotoxicity in HepG2 cells. Food and Chemical Toxicology (2006b) 44(5):689–694

Chu KK et al. *Coriolus versicolor*: a medicinal mushroom with promising immunotherapeutic values. J Clin Pharmacol (2002) 42(9):976–84

Collins RA et al. Polysaccharopeptide from *Coriolus versicolor* has potential for use against human immunodeficiency virus type 1 infection. Life Sci (1997) 60(25):PL383–7

Cui J et al. Polysaccharopeptides of *Coriolus versicolor*: physiological activity, uses, and production. Biotechnol Adv (2003) 21(2):109–122

Eliza WLY et al. Efficacy of Yun Zhi (*Coriolus versicolor*) on survival in cancer patients: systematic review and meta-analysis. Centre for Reviews and Dissemination (2012):78–87

Fujita H et al, Effect of PSK, a protein-bound polysaccharide from *Coriolus versicolor*, on drug-metabolizing enzymes in sarcoma-180 bearing and normal mice. Int J Immunopharm (1988) 10(4): 445–450

Gong S et al. Involvement of interleukin-2 in analgesia produced by *Coriolus versicolor* polysaccharide peptides. Zhongguo Yao Li Xue Bao (1998) 19(1):67–70

Harhaji L et al. Anti-tumor effect of *Coriolus versicolor* methanol extract against mouse B16 melanoma cells: In vitro and in vivo study. Food and Chemical Toxicology (2008) 46(5):1825–1833

Ho CY et al. *Coriolus versicolor* (Yunzhi) extract attenuates growth of human leukemia xenografts and induces apoptosis through the mitochondrial pathway. Oncol Rep. (2006) 16(3):609–16

Hor S et al. Acute and subchronic oral toxicity of *Coriolus versicolor* standardized water extract in Sprague-Dawley rats. J Ethnopharmacol (2011) 13(3):1067–1076

Hsu W et al. Separation, purification, and — glucosidase inhibition of polysaccharides from *Coriolus versicolor* LH1 mycelia. Carbohydrate Polymers. 92 (2013) 297–306

Kidd PM et al. The use of mushroom glucans and proteoglycans in cancer treatment. Altern Med Rev (2000) 5(1):4–27

Lau CBS et al. Cytotoxic activities of *Coriolus versicolor* (Yunzhi) extract on human leukemia and lymphoma cells by induction of apoptosis. Life Sciences (2004) 75(7):797–808

Li W et al. Immunomodulatory effects of polysaccharopeptide (PSP) in human PBMC through regulation of TRAF6/TLR immunosignal-transduction pathways. Immunopharmacol Immunotoxicol (2010) 32(4):576–84

Lim BO et al. oriolus versicolor suppresses inflammatory bowel disease by Inhibiting the expression of STAT1 and STAT6 associated with IFN-γ and IL-4 expression. Phytother Res (2011) 25(8):1257–61

Ng TG et al. Polysaccharopeptide from the mushroom *Coriolus versicolor* possesses analgesic activity but does not produce adverse effects on female reproductive or embryonic development in mice. Gen Pharmacol (1997) 29(2):269–273

Szeto YT et al. Direct human DNA protection by *Coriolus versicolor* (Yunzhi) extract. Pharm Biol (2013) 51(7):851–5

Tsang KW et al. *Coriolus versicolor* polysaccharide peptide slows progression of advanced non-small cell lung cancer. Respiratory Medicine (2003) 97(6):618–624

Wang HX et al. Examination of lectins, polysaccharopeptide, polysaccharide, alkaloid, coumarin and trypsin inhibitors for inhibitory activity against human immunodeficiency virus reverse transcriptase and glycohydrolases. Planta Med (2001) 67(7):669–72

Wang DF et al. Effect of *Coriolus versicolor* polysaccharide-B on the biological characteristics of human esophageal carcinoma cell line eca109. Cancer Biol Med (2012) 9(3):164–7

Wong CK et al. Immunomodulatory effects of yun zhi and danshen capsules in health subjects — a randomized, double-blind, placebo-controlled, crossover study. Int Immunopharmacol (2004) 4(2):201–11.

Wong CK et al. Immunomodulatory activities of Yunzhi and Danshen in post-treatment breast cancer patients. Am J Chin Med (2005) 33(3):381–95

Yeung JH and Or P. Polysaccharide peptides from *Coriolus versicolor* competitively inhibit tolbutamide 4-hydroxylation in specific human CYP2C9 isoform and pooled human liver microsomes. Phytomedicine 18 (2011) 1170–1175.

Yeung JH and Or P. Polysaccharide peptides from *Coriolus versicolor* competitively inhibit modelcytochrome P450 enzyme probe substrates metabolism in human liver microsomes. Phytomedicine 19 (2012) 457–463

Yeung JH et al. Effect of polysaccharide peptide (PSP) on glutathione and protection against paracetamol-induced hepatotoxicity in the rat. Methods Find Exp Clin Pharmacol (1994) 16(10):723–9

C

Cranberry

HISTORICAL NOTE Native American Indians used cranberries as both a food and a treatment for bladder and kidney diseases. In the mid-1800s, German scientists suggested that cranberry juice had antibacterial activity, supporting its use as a treatment for bladder infections. Recent investigation has confirmed its usefulness in the prevention of urinary tract infections.

OTHER NAMES

Kronsbeere, marsh apple, moosbeere, preisselbeere

BOTANICAL NAME/FAMILY

Vaccinium oxycoccus, *Vaccinium macrocarpon* (family Ericaceae)

PLANT PART USED

Fruit

CHEMICAL COMPONENTS

Catechin, flavone glycosides, fructose, organic acids, proanthocyanidins, vitamin C. Cranberry has a high flavonol content (100–263 mg/kg) (Hakkinen et al 1999) — higher than commonly consumed fruits and vegetables.

MAIN ACTIONS

Bacteriostatic and antiadhesive activity

The adhesion of pathogenic organisms to a tissue surface is required to initiate most infectious diseases (Sharon & Ofek 2002). Various in vitro and in vivo studies have identified that cranberry has antiadhesion properties relevant to several different strains of bacteria, including *Escherichia coli*, *Staphylococcus aureus*, *Helicobacter pylori*, *Streptococcus pneumoniae* and *Streptococcus mutans*.

The proanthocyanidins in cranberry are potent inhibitors of *E. coli* adhesion, thereby influencing the initiation of disease without exerting bactericidal activity. One in vitro study found that cranberry juice inhibited adhesion of 46 different *E. coli* isolates by 75% (Sobota 1984): when administered to mice for 14 days, adherence of *E. coli* to uroepithelial cells was inhibited by 80%. Significant inhibition of adherence was also observed in samples of human urine 1–3 hours after subjects drank a cranberry drink. A water-soluble extract was found to be most effective in its antimicrobial inhibition of seven bacterial strains, including *E. coli, Listeria monocytogenes* and *Salmonella typhimurium* (Côté et al 2011).

The morphology of *E. coli* is changed when grown in the presence of cranberry juice or extract (Johnson et al 2008). It appears that the antiadhesion effects are a result of irreversible inhibition of the expression of P-fimbriae of *E. coli* (Ahuja et al 1998). Electron micrographic evidence suggests that cranberry juice acts either on the cell wall, preventing proper attachment of the fimbrial subunits, or as a genetic control, preventing the expression of normal fimbrial subunits, or both (Gupta et al 2007). Of the cranberry constituents, it appears that the sugars in conjunction with organic acids cause osmotic stress and the anthocyanins and phenolics lead to the disintegration of the outer membrane when tested against *E. coli* (Lacombe et al 2010). Furthermore, cranberry juice has been shown to disrupt bacterial ligand-uroepithelial cell receptor binding (Liu et al 2008). This inhibitory effect has been seen with *Staphylococcus aureus* (Magarinos et al 2008, Su et al 2012), *E. coli* and uroepithelial tissues, but also in the adhesion of *Helicobacter pylori* to human gastrointestinal cells (Burger et al 2002) and in the co-aggregation of oral bacteria and *Streptococcus mutans* counts in saliva (Sharon & Ofek 2002, Weiss et al 1998).

New research on human bronchial cells found a 90% adhesion inhibition for *Streptococcus pneumoniae* (a common cause of pneumonia, meningitis and otitis media) with cranberry juice (Huttunen et al 2011). Two studies have looked at the effect of cranberry extracts on biofilm production, which can cause infections with catheter use and corneal infections caused by contact lens use. Both studies found a reduction in growth of biofilm with Gram-positive bacteria, specifically *Staphylococcus* spp. (LaPlante et al 2012, Leshem et al 2011).

Antioxidant

Cranberries consistently rank highly among common fruits with antioxidant activity. In particular, the polyphenolic compounds in cranberry display substantial antioxidant capacity. In vitro tests with whole fruit and isolated flavonol glycosides found in cranberry showed free radical scavenging activity comparable or superior to that of vitamin E (Yan et al 2002). In vivo studies demonstrate that cranberry juice increases plasma antioxidant status (Villarreal et al 2007). A small human trial demonstrated that a single 240-mL serving of cranberry juice increased plasma antioxidant capacity significantly greater than controls receiving an equivalent amount of vitamin C in solution (Vinson et al 2008).

Increases excretion of oxalic acid and uric acid

According to an open study, a dose of 330 mL cranberry juice can increase the excretion of oxalic acid and uric acid (Kessler et al 2002).

Alterations to urinary pH

Earlier hypotheses that cranberry juice prevents urinary tract infection (UTI) by acidification of urine or by its hippuric acid content have not been substantiated. Results from human studies are contradictory, but overall suggest no significant change in urinary pH at doses less than 330 mL daily. A crossover study of 27 patients with indwelling urinary catheters and chronic bacteriuria showed no change in urinary pH (Nahata et al 1982); the results of a double-blind study of 153 women were the same (Avorn et al 1994). One small, open study involving 12 healthy subjects found that 330 mL of cranberry juice reduced the urinary pH (Kessler et al 2002).

Chemoprotective

Studies employing mainly in vitro tumour models show that cranberry extracts and compounds inhibit the growth and proliferation of several types of tumour, including lymphoma, bladder, breast, colon, prostate, ovaries, oesophageal, lung, oral squamous cell carcinoma and gastric cancer cells (Chatelain et al 2008, Ferguson et al 2006, Hochman et al 2008, Kim et al 2012, Kresty et al 2008, Liu et al 2009, MacLean et al 2011, Prasain et al 2008, Singh et al 2009, Sun & Hai Liu 2006, Vu et al 2012). The flavonoid components may act in a complementary fashion to limit carcinogenesis by inducing apoptosis in tumour cells (Neto et al 2008).

Cytochromes

Although some studies with animal models have suggested effects on various cytochromes, human studies have found that cranberry juice has no significant effect on CYP 2C9, 1A2 or 3A4 (Greenblatt et al 2006, Grenier et al 2006, Lilja et al 2007, Mohammed Abdul et al 2008, Ushijima et al 2009).

Before we can definitively conclude that cranberry juice has no effect on CYP3A4, it must be noted that a human study testing five commercial cranberry juices has identified substantial interbrand variations in ability to inhibit intestinal (but not hepatic) CYP3A, ranging from 34% to abolishment (Ngo et al 2009). Further testing indicates that three triterpenes are able to inhibit CYP3A in humans, suggesting it may be the natural variation in concentration of these constituents between products which is responsible for the inconsistent results seen between in vivo and clinical trials to date (Kim et al 2011a).

OTHER ACTIONS

Preliminary research with in vitro tests and those using animal models are identifying many different actions which are worthy of further exploration.

Antiviral activity

A non-specific antiviral effect has been demonstrated in vitro for a commercially produced cranberry fruit juice drink (Lipson et al 2007).

Antifungal activity

A recent in vitro study of cranberry proanthocyanidin fractions on human fungi, *Candida* spp. and *Cryptococcus neoformans* reported antifungal activity (Patel et al 2011).

ACE inhibitor

Cranberry powders have been shown in vitro to have a limited inhibitory activity on alpha-amylase and to significantly impact angiotensin 1-converting enzyme (ACE) (Pinto Mda et al 2010).

Lipid lowering and anti-inflammatory

According to a rat study, cranberry powder may modify serum lipids and reduce inflammatory markers (Kim et al 2011b).

CLINICAL USE

Prevention of UTI

A number of controlled clinical trials support the use of cranberry products (solid-dose form and juice) in the prevention of UTIs in women experiencing recurrent infections; however, the heterogeneity of studies makes a clear interpretation difficult. There is emerging evidence to suggest that cranberry juice with high concentrations of Type A proanthocyanidin may be more effective than other forms; however further studies are required to assess this (Afshar et al 2012).

A significant preventive effect was concluded in a 2012 systematic review and meta-analysis of 10 randomised controlled trials (RCTs) which included 1494 subjects (Wang et al 2012). Wang et al reported that, on subgroup analysis, cranberry-containing products seemed to be more effective in several subgroups, including women with recurrent UTIs (relative risk [RR] 0.53), female populations (RR 0.49), children (RR 0.33), cranberry juice drinkers (RR 0.47) and subjects using cranberry-containing products more than twice daily (RR 0.58). While the conclusion was positive, authors cautioned that the results should be interpreted in the context of substantial heterogeneity across the studies.

In contrast, a 2012 Cochrane review evaluated data from RCTs and also quasi-RCTs of cranberry products for the prevention of UTIs in all populations (n = 4473) and concluded that there is no statistically significant difference between cranberry and placebo for the prevention of UTIs (Jepson et al 2012). The effects of cranberry/cranberry-lingonberry juice versus placebo, juice, lactobacillus, antibiotics or water were evaluated in 13 studies (with amounts ranging from 30 mL to 1000 mL), and cranberry tablets versus placebo in nine studies (daily dose range from 400 mg to 2000 mg); one study evaluated both juice and tablets. Overall, cranberry products did not significantly reduce the incidence of UTIs at 12 months compared with placebo/control. Cranberry products showed a small benefit in some of the smaller studies for women with recurrent UTIs; however no significant benefit was seen in the elderly, pregnant women, children with recurrent UTIs, cancer patients, those with neuropathic bladder or spinal injury or people requiring catheterisation. Only one study reported a significant result for the outcome of symptomatic UTIs. One study (McMurdo et al 2009) showed that cranberry treatment was as effective as an antibiotic. Beerepoot et al (2011) did not get the same result. Gurley (2011) suggests the negative result with Beerepoot was because he used a cranberry treatment whereby the quantity of type-A proanthocyanidins used amounted to only 9 mg/g, making the amount of free proanthocyanidins reaching the urinary tract of study participants less than 1 mg/day. Side effects were common in all studies, and dropouts/withdrawals in several of the studies were high (Jepson et al 2012).

Why the conflicting conclusions?

The systematic review and meta-analysis completed by Wang et al, also in 2012, reported conflicting results, possibly due to the significant heterogeneity of the trials, making the literature difficult to evaluate in a meaningful way. The Wang review confirmed the findings of the earlier 2008 Cochrane review, concluding that cranberry products were effective especially for women with recurrent UTIs. It excluded the Barbosa-Cesnik RCT of women with recurrent UTIs (Barbosa-Cesnik et al 2011), as they inadvertently used ascorbic acid in the placebo. As this in itself may reduce UTIs, it may have masked the effects of cranberry, especially as the authors expected the placebo arm to have 30% recurrence of UTIs and the rate was only 14%. The study also used the lowest threshold of bacteria in the urine to determine a UTI (Wang et al 2012). Gurley (2011) reports that the amount of type A procyanidin present in the test extracts needs to be of a sufficient quantity to have an effect, as they tend to have very poor bioavailability and some studies, such as Beerepoot et al (2011), use extracts with insufficient amounts.

Since these two reviews were published, further RCTs have also been published.

A clear protective effect and significant decrease in the rate of relapse were seen amongst women aged aged over 50 years taking cranberry juice in a double-blind RCT by Takahashi et al (2013). The study involved 118 women aged 20–79, given 125 mL of cranberry juice to drink daily before going to sleep over a 24-week period. In a subgroup analysis of women aged over 50 years, relapse of UTI was observed in 16 of 55 (29.1%) patients drinking cranberry juice compared with 31 of 63 (49.2%) in the placebo group.

In 2012, an RCT of 176 premenopausal women with a history of UTIs found cranberry juice (120–240 mL/day) demonstrated a potentially protective effect with a hazard ratio for UTI of 0.68 compared with placebo, but it was not statistically significant. In addition, researchers found that the group ingesting cranberry juice had reduced infection with P-fimbriated *E. coli* strains, which suggests benefits from cranberry juice therapy are possible and confirms the antiadhesion mechanism clinically. One major limitation of this study was that it was underpowered to show a significant effect of cranberry on the cumulative rate of UTI, as they did not achieve the necessary sample size (Stapleton et al 2012).

A concentrated cranberry liquid blend (UTI-Stat with Proantinox) was tested for safety, tolerability and maximal tolerated dose in 28 women with a history of recurrent UTI and an average age of 46 years. A secondary outcome was UTI recurrence. The secondary end points demonstrated that 2 (9.1%) of 23 women reported a recurrent UTI, a rate considered superior to their historical data. At 12 weeks, there was a significant reduction in worry about recurrent infection and increased quality of life in regard to the physical functioning domain and role limitations from physical health domain, as measured by the Medical Outcomes Study short-form 36-item questionnaire ($P = 0.0097$). A lower American Urological Association Symptom Index indicating greater quality of life was also significant ($P = 0.045$) (Efros et al 2010).

Another RCT with 137 women aged 45 years or older, who had experienced cystitis at least twice in the past year and been treated with antibiotics, were given a 500 mg cranberry capsule (Cran-Max, Buckton Scott Health Products, UK) at bedtime for a period of 6 months or 100 mg of the antibiotic trimethoprim. Overall, 28% of women experienced a UTI during the study (25 in the cranberry group and 14 in the trimethoprim group), with median time to recurrence of 84.5 days for the cranberry group and 91 days for the trimethoprim group. Trimethoprim was more effective at reducing UTIs in older women in this study but it was not statistically significant and compared with cranberry the trimethoprim conferred only 7 extra UTI-free days. Cranberry may be a cheaper, better-tolerated option for recurrent UTI treatment in older women and does not carry the risk of antimicrobial antibiotic resistance (McMurdo et al 2009).

Renal transplant patients

A small retrospective trial of 82 renal transplant patients receiving cranberry juice (2 × 50 mL/day) found the annual number of UTI episodes was reduced by 63.9% (Pagonas et al 2012).

Spinal cord injuries

Patients with spinal cord injuries are a high-risk group for catheter-associated UTIs, so cranberry products are popular in this group. One double-blind, factorial-design, RCT of 305 people with spinal cord injuries showed no significant UTI-free period compared to placebo when taking 800 mg of cranberry tablets twice daily (Lee et al 2007), while another randomised, double-blind, placebo-controlled, crossover trial in 47 patients with spinal cord injury demonstrated a significant reduction in the frequency of UTIs (Hess et al 2008). An open pilot study involving 15 volunteers with spinal cord injuries showed that three glasses of cranberry juice daily significantly reduced the adhesion of Gram-negative and Gram-positive bacteria to uroepithelial cells (Reid 2002). Treatment using catheter device with proanthocyanidin solutions has also been shown to inhibit adhesion of bacteria to non-biological particles such as PVC (Eydelnant & Tufenkji 2008). While these results are promising, a 2010 review of five studies of spinal cord injury patients reported that there is limited evidence that cranberry may be helpful in preventing or treating UTIs and suggests that more rigorous research is required (Opperman 2010).

Radiotherapy and UTI prevention

Bladder infections are a common side effect of radiotherapy for prostate cancer. This controlled trial of 370 patients who were receiving radiotherapy for prostate cancer in an Italian hospital were given a 200 mg enteric-coated tablet (VO370 or Monoselect Macrocarpon) containing standardised cranberry extract titrated as 30% proanthocyanidins. This trial took place over 6–7 weeks and a significant reduction was found in the number of UTIs and recurrent UTIs in the treatment group vs controls. Good compliance and only two gastric complaints were reported. It was also found to help reduce urinary symptoms of dysuria, nocturia, urinary frequency and urgency (Bonetta & Di Pierro 2012).

Gynaecological surgery and UTI prevention

The short-term use of cranberry capsules produced no statistically significant difference in UTI incidence in a cohort of 286 women undergoing gynaecological surgery. The treatment group received cranberry capsules for 4 days prior to surgery and 5 days postoperatively (Cadkova et al 2009).

Children

Catheterisation and renal disease

Cranberry use is popular for children with renal disease. An anonymous survey of 117 parents of children seen in a hospital paediatric nephrology clinic identified that 29% gave cranberry products to their children to treat as well as prevent diverse renal problems (Super et al 2005). Most parents felt that it was beneficial and only one reported an adverse reaction (nausea).

Two studies conducted in children managed by clean intermittent catheterisation found no clinical or statistical difference in the number of symptomatic UTIs observed in either the cranberry or the placebo group (Foda et al 1995, Schlager et al 1999). Foda et al used a dose of 5 mL/kg/day of cranberry cocktail for 6 months and the dose used by Schlager et al was 2 oz (≈55 g) of cranberry concentrate.

Recurrent UTIs in children

There has been a recent Cochrane systematic review and a meta-analysis by Wang et al, both published in 2012 and both reporting different conclusions. The Cochrane review found no significant difference of cranberry compared to placebo in children with recurrent UTIs (RR 0.48, 95% confidence interval [CI] 0.19–1.22); whereas the Wang meta-analysis concluded benefit for children (RR 0.33; 95% CI 0.16–0.69). The Cochrane review included three studies, one RCT (Ferrara et al 2009) of 84 girls randomised to cranberry (50 mL daily), *Lactobacillus* or control for 6 months, and reported that daily cranberry drink significantly reduced recurrent UTIs in children. Also in the Cochrane review was a study by Salo et al (2012) which was a randomised placebo-controlled trial with 263 children recruited in seven hospitals in Finland reported no significant difference in the number of children with recurrent UTIs, although there was a non-significant reduction, with 20 children (16%) in the cranberry group and 28 (22%) in the placebo group experiencing a recurrent UTI (difference −6%; 95% CI −16 to 4%; $P = 0.21$). The cranberry juice dose was 5 mL/kg up to 300 mL per day. Although cranberry did not significantly reduce the number of children with a UTI, the authors reported a significant reduction in the number of times a child got a UTI and also the number of days the child needed to take antibiotics.

The third study (Uberos et al 2010) mentioned in the Cochrane review was dismissed as it was unclear about whether they were testing for a UTI or just a positive culture. Uberos et al did report that cranberry syrup was equally effective to trimethoprim for recurrent UTIs in their population of 192 children.

The Wang meta-analysis included only the Ferrara study for children with recurrent UTIs and report that the current data support the use of cranberry products in children with UTIs, although suggest that more trials are needed. Overall the differences in the two meta-analyses appear to be that Wang did not include either the Salo et al (2012) or the Uberos et al (2010) trials. The difference in the individual trial results may be explained by the variety of cranberry products used and the dosage levels (for children, dosage may need to be adjusted by body weight), although in general the trend on all the trials is towards benefit for children with recurrent UTIs.

A later RCT looked at a cranberry juice with high concentrations of proanthocyanidin and compared that to regular cranberry juice for 1 year. There were 40 children in the study and the incidence of infection in the treatment group of high proanthocyanidins was 0.4 per patient per year and 1.15 in the placebo group, showing a 65% reduction in the risk of UTIs in non-febrile children (Afshar et al 2012). This high-proanthocyanidin-containing cranberry juice shows promise and further investigation is warranted.

Treatment of UTI

Although cranberry may be a viable adjunctive treatment in UTI when antibiotic resistance is encountered, there is no reliable evidence that it is an effective sole treatment in diagnosed UTI (Ulbricht & Basch 2005). One study of pregnant women demonstrated comparable effects of daily cranberry juice mixture to those of placebo for asymptomatic bacteriuria and symptomatic UTIs; however, the results were not statistically significant and more than one-third of participants withdrew from the study because of gastrointestinal upset (Wing et al 2008). In another study, cranberry exhibited only weak antimicrobial activity in urine specimens of symptom-free subjects after ingestion of a single dose (Lee et al 2010).

Nephroprotection

Cranberries have an antioxidant function and may prevent infection-induced oxidative renal damage. Animal studies suggest that cranberries might be used clinically as a beneficial adjuvant treatment to prevent damage due to pyelonephritis in children with vesicoureteric reflux (Han et al 2007).

OTHER USES

Gout

Cranberry juice has been used to treat gout. Evidence of increased uric acid excretion in humans provides a theoretical basis for the indication, although studies in patients with gout are not available to confirm effectiveness (Kessler et al 2002).

Oral hygiene

The antiadhesion effect of cranberry on oral microbial flora has been demonstrated in vitro (Bodet et al 2008, Koo et al 2006, Polak et al 2013, Yamanaka et al 2007). More specifically, cranberry polyphenol fraction significantly decreased the hydrophobicity of oral streptococci in a dose-dependent manner, suggesting that it may reduce bacterial adherence to the tooth surface (Yamanaka-Okada et al 2008). It has been shown in vitro to prevent biofilm formation and reduce adherence of *Candida albicans* and so may have a role in the prevention or treatment of oral candidiasis (Feldman et al 2012). The same research group also found the synergy of cranberry proanthocyanidins and licochalcone A inhibited *Porphyromonas gingivalis* growth and biofilm formation, offering potential in the treatment and prevention of periodontal disease (Feldman & Grenier 2012).

Prevention and treatment of *Helicobacter* infection

Cranberry inhibits the adhesion of *H. pylori* to human gastrointestinal cells in vitro (Matsushima et al 2008); however, very little clinical evidence is available to confirm significance in humans (Burger et al 2002). A multicentre, randomised controlled, double-blind trial found that regular intake of cranberry juice or a probiotic inhibited *H. pylori* in a trial of 295 children (Gotteland et al 2008). Another double-blind, randomised clinical study was carried out in 177 patients with *H. pylori* infection to investigate the possible additive effect of cranberry juice to triple therapy with omeprazole, amoxicillin and clarithromycin. Overall, there was no statistically significant difference; however, analysis by gender showed that the eradication rate was higher in females taking cranberry, but not in males (Shmuely et al 2007).

Cardioprotection

Consumption of 250 mL cranberry juice daily is associated with decreasing markers of oxidative stress (Ruel et al 2008) and a significant increase in plasma high-density lipoprotein (HDL) cholesterol concentration (Ruel et al 2006). A small study of 30 abdominally obese, healthy, middle-aged men who consumed increasing doses of cranberry juice, up to 500 mL/day over 12 weeks, found a significant reduction in plasma matrix metalloproteinase-9, a substance which can accelerate atherosclerotic progression (Ruel et al 2009). The same authors recruited 35 overweight men in an RCT using an intervention of 500 mL/day of low-calorie cranberry juice or placebo juice. In a 4-week trial there was no significant difference in the cardiometabolic parameters but some benefit was noted in the augmentation index measuring arterial stiffness (Ruel et al 2013). These potential cardioprotective effects (which may be useful in reducing hypertension and atherosclerotic plaque vulnerability) need larger studies to confirm the findings. In addition, cranberry extract increases cholesterol uptake and the synthesis of low-density lipoprotein (LDL) receptors (Chu & Liu 2005), suggesting that accelerated cholesterol excretion may occur in vivo (McKay & Blumberg 2007). An oestrogen-deficient animal model found improvements in cholesterol parameters and endothelial function and suggested that cranberry juice consumption may be a useful food for postmenopausal women (Yung et al 2013).

Type 2 diabetes

Some studies have suggested that consumption of a low-calorie cranberry juice is associated with a favourable glycaemic response (Wilson et al 2008a, 2008b). In a double-blind RCT, 60 males with type 2 diabetes, some of whom were taking oral hypoglycaemic drugs, were asked to drink one cup of cranberry juice daily for 12 weeks or placebo. A significant decrease in serum glucose and apolipoprotein B and a significant increase in serum apolipoprotein A-1 and paraoxonase 1 activity in the cranberry juice group resulted. The authors concluded that cranberry juice may assist in the management of type 2 diabetic males to reduce cardiovascular disease risk factors (Shidfar et al 2012). However, a randomised, placebo-controlled, double-blind study of 16 males and 14 females demonstrated that a 500 mg capsule of cranberry extract had a neutral effect on glycaemic control in type 2 diabetics who were on oral glucose-lowering medication. This same study found, however, that cranberry supplements are effective in reducing atherosclerotic cholesterol profiles, including LDL cholesterol and total cholesterol levels, as well as total:HDL cholesterol ratio in people with type 2 diabetes (Lee et al 2008). A study of 13 participants with type 2 diabetes, attempting to find palatable options for food choices, found that raw cranberries and sweetened dried cranberries containing less sugar and with polydextrose added as a bulking agent significantly improved glycaemic control when compared to sweetened dried cranberries alone or white bread (Wilson et al 2010).

Prostate health

A trial of 42 men at risk of prostate disease (with negative prostate biopsy) with UTIs, elevated prostate-specific antigen (PSA) and chronic non-bacterial prostatitis were prescribed cranberry powder (1500 mg) for 6 months, with the control group receiving no treatment. The treatment group showed benefits with statistically significant improvement in International Prostate Symptom Score, quality of life, urination parameters and lower total PSA levels (Vidlar et al 2009, 2010). More research is required to confirm these promising findings.

Urinary deodorising activity

Cranberry juice and solid-dose forms are popular in nursing homes as urinary deodorising agents in older adults with incontinence. Although no clinical study is available to confirm efficacy, numerous anecdotal reports suggest that it is useful when used on a regular basis.

DOSAGE RANGE

Preventing UTI

According to clinical studies

- Adults: 120–400 mL daily or 400–500 mg capsule 1–3 times daily.
- Children: 15 mL/kg or up to 300 mL daily.

In practice, much higher doses are being used in an attempt to achieve quicker results (e.g. cranberry capsules or tablets 10,000 mg/day for prevention).

Recent studies reveal that cranberry extract regimens containing 72 mg of type-A proanthocyanidins produced significant bacterial anti-adhesion activity in human urine, therefore the dose of bioavailable type-A proanthocyanidins is important to consider (Gurley 2011).

ADVERSE REACTIONS

At high doses (3 L or greater), gastrointestinal discomfort and diarrhoea can occur (Ulbricht & Basch 2005).

SIGNIFICANT INTERACTIONS

The composition of bioactive components of cranberry juice can vary substantially and there is potential for drug interaction (Ngo et al 2009).

CYP3 A substrates

Whether cranberry juice inhibits the metabolism of drugs chiefly metabolised by CYP3A isoenzymes appears to be dependent on the concentration of three triterpenes (maslinic acid, corosolic acid and ursolic acid) in the juice (Kim et al 2011a). These have been identified as the important constituents responsible for inhibiting intestinal CYP3A and most likely explain the interbrand differences seen in various clinical and preclinical trials.

Caution — monitor patients taking high-strength cranberry preparations and medicines chiefly metabolised by CYP3A. Special care should be taken if the medicines have a narrow therapeutic index.

Proton pump inhibitors

Cranberry juice increases the absorption of vitamin B_{12} when used concurrently with proton pump inhibitor medicines (Saltzman et al 1994) — beneficial interaction.

Warfarin

There are a small number of case reports suggesting that cranberry juice may increase the international normalised ratio (INR) in patients taking warfarin; however, clinical pharmacokinetic studies have found no clinically relevant interaction between cranberry and warfarin (Ansell et al 2008, Pham & Pham 2007), changes to the anticoagulant activity of warfarin or a significant effect on the activities of CYP2C9, CYP1A2 or CYP3A4 (Lilja et al 2007). Other clinical studies have found a daily glass of cranberry juice has no significant effect on INR compared to placebo (Ansell et al 2009) and two glasses of cranberry juice daily do not change prothrombin times (Mellen et al 2010). Ansell et al (2009) conducted an RCT with 30 patients on stable warfarin anticoagulation (international normalised ratio [INR], 1.7–3.3) and found 240 mL of CJ had no effect on plasma S- or R-warfarin plasma levels, thereby excluding a pharmacokinetic interaction.

An earlier study suggests that a pharmacodynamic interaction is more likely (Mohammed Abdul et al 2008).

CONTRAINDICATIONS AND PRECAUTIONS

People with diabetes should take care when using commercially prepared cranberry juices because of the high sugar content.

If symptoms of UTI become more severe while cranberry is being administered, other treatments may be required and medical advice is recommended.

Cranberries contain oxalates and theoretically this could encourage kidney stone formation. People with a history of oxalate kidney stones should therefore limit their intake of cranberry juice.

PREGNANCY USE

Women experience UTIs with greater frequency during pregnancy. A systematic review of the literature for evidence on the use, safety and pharmacology of cranberry, focusing on issues pertaining to pregnancy and lactation, found that there is no direct evidence of safety or harm to the mother or fetus as a result of consuming cranberry during pregnancy. A survey of 400 pregnant women did not uncover any adverse events when cranberry was regularly consumed. In lactation, the safety or harm of cranberry is unknown (Dugoua et al 2008). Recent trials have not shown evidence for benefit of cranberry juice in preventing UTIs in pregnant women so, although it has a good safety profile, its benefit may be limited.

Practice points/Patient counselling

- Cranberry preparations are widely used to prevent minor UTIs.
- Overall, clinical testing suggests that cranberry products, particularly the juice, with high concentrations of type-A proanthocyanidin may have some benefits for UTI prevention in certain populations.
- It may be more effective to take the cranberry products more than twice daily.
- Cranberry exerts bacteriostatic effects by reducing bacterial adhesion to host tissues.
- Overall, evidence suggests no significant alteration to urinary pH at doses less than 330 mL daily.
- Cranberry products have also been used to treat gout and to deodorise urine in people with incontinence.
- Preliminary research suggests a possible role in preventing conditions such as *Helicobacter pylori* infection, dental plaque formation and periodontal disease, managing glucose control in type 2 diabetes, prostate health and reducing cardiovascular risk among type 2 diabetics.
- Patients taking warfarin and regular cranberry intake should have their INR monitored.

In regard to the case reports, a systematic review concluded that the suggested drug interactions were questionable and that moderate consumption of cranberry juice was unlikely to affect coagulation (Zikria et al 2010).

Until the interaction can be better understood, patients taking warfarin with cranberry juice should continue to monitor their INR changes and signs and symptoms of bleeding.

PATIENTS' FAQS

What will this herb do for me?

Cranberry products, in particular the juice, with high concentrations of proanthocyanidin, may reduce the risk of developing UTI in some populations.

When will it start to work?

Studies using 1–2 glasses of cranberry juice suggest that 4–8 weeks' continual use is required.

Are there any safety issues?

If fever or pain exists or symptoms of UTI become more severe, seek medical advice. People taking warfarin together with cranberry should monitor their INR for changes. People taking concentrated cranberry juice should also check with their healthcare provider if also taking medication to avoid drug interactions.

REFERENCES

Afshar, K et al. 2012. Cranberry juice for the prevention of pediatric urinary tract infection: a randomized controlled trial. J Urol, 188, 1584–7.

Ahuja S, et al. Loss of fimbrial adhesion with the addition of *Vaccinium macrocarpon* to the growth medium of P-fimbriated *Escherichia coli*. J Urol 159.2 (1998): 559–562.

Ansell, J., et al. 2008. A randomized, double-blind trial of the interaction between cranberry juice and warfarin. Journal of Thrombosis and Thrombolysis, 25, 112–112.

Avorn J et al. Reduction of bacteriuria and pyuria after ingestion of cranberry juice. JAMA 271.10 (1994): 751–754.

Barbosa-Cesnik, C, et al. 2011. Cranberry juice fails to prevent recurrent urinary tract infection: results from a randomized placebo-controlled trial. Clin Infect Dis, 52, 23–30.

Beerepoot MA, ter RG, Nys S, van der Wal WM, de Borgie CA, de Reijke TM, et al. Cranberries vs antibiotics to prevent urinary tract infections: a randomized double-blind noninferiority trial in premenopausal women. Arch Intern Med 171(14) (2011): 1270–1278.

Bodet C et al. Potential oral health benefits of cranberry. Crit Rev Food Sci Nutr 48.7 (2008): 672–680.

Bonetta, A. & Di Pierro, F. 2012. Enteric-coated, highly standardized cranberry extract reduces risk of UTIs and urinary symptoms during radiotherapy for prostate carcinoma. Cancer Manag Res, 4, 281–6.

Burger O et al. Inhibition of *Helicobacter pylori* adhesion to human gastric mucus by a high-molecular-weight constituent of cranberry juice. Crit Rev Food Sci Nutr 42.3 (Suppl) (2002): 279–284.

Cadkova, I., et al. 2009. [Effect of cranberry extract capsules taken during the perioperative period upon the post-surgical urinary infection in gynecology.] Ceska Gynekol, 74, 454–8.

Chatelain K et al. Cranberry and grape seed extracts inhibit the proliferative phenotype of oral squamous cell carcinomas. Evid Based Complement Altern Med (2008); 2011: 467691.

Chu YF, Liu RH. Cranberries inhibit LDL oxidation and induce LDL receptor expression in hepatocytes. Life Sci 77 (2005): 1892–1901.

Côté, J., et al. 2011. Antimicrobial effect of cranberry juice and extracts. Food Control, 22, 1413–1418.

Dugoua JJ et al. Safety and efficacy of cranberry (*Vaccinium macrocarpon*) during pregnancy and lactation. Can J Clin Pharmacol 15.1 (2008): e80–e86.

Efros, M., et al. 2010. Novel Concentrated Cranberry Liquid Blend, UTI-STAT With Proantinox, Might Help Prevent Recurrent Urinary Tract Infections in Women. Urology, 76, 841–845.

Eydelnant IA, Tufenkji N. Cranberry derived proanthocyanidins reduce bacterial adhesion to selected biomaterials. Langmuir 24.18 (2008): 10273–10281.

Feldman, M. & Grenier, D. 2012. Cranberry proanthocyanidins act in synergy with licochalcone A to reduce *Porphyromonas gingivalis* growth and virulence properties, and to suppress cytokine secretion by macrophages. J Appl Microbiol, 113, 438–47.

Feldman, M., et al. 2012. Cranberry proanthocyanidins inhibit the adherence properties of *Candida albicans* and cytokine secretion by oral epithelial cells. BMC Complement Altern Med, 12, 6.

Ferrara P et al. Cranberry juice for the prevention of recurrent urinary tract infections: a randomized controlled trial in children. Scand J Urol Nephrol 43.5 (2009): 369–372.

Ferguson PJ et al. In vivo inhibition of growth of human tumor lines by flavonoid fractions from cranberry extract. Nutr Cancer 56.1 (2006): 86–94.

Foda MM et al. Efficacy of cranberry in prevention of urinary tract infection in a susceptible pediatric population. Can J Urol 2.1 (1995): 98–102.

Gotteland M et al. Modulation of *Helicobacter pylori* colonization with cranberry juice and *Lactobacillus johnsonii* La1 in children. Nutrition 24.5 (2008): 421–426.

Greenblatt, D.J., et al. 2006. Interaction of flurbiprofen with cranberry juice, grape juice, tea, and fluconazole: in vitro and clinical studies. Clin.Pharmacol.Ther., 79, (1) 125–133.

Grenier, J., et al. 2006. Pomelo juice, but not cranberry juice, affects the pharmacokinetics of cyclosporine in humans. Clin.Pharmacol.Ther., 79, (3) 255–262.

Gupta K et al. Cranberry products inhibit adherence of P-fimbriated *Escherichia coli* to primary cultured bladder and vaginal epithelial cells. J Urol 177.6 (2007): 2357–2360.

Gurley B. Cranberries as Antibiotics? Comment on 'Cranberries vs Antibiotics to Prevent Urinary Tract Infections: A Randomized Double-Blind Noninferiority Trial in Premenopausal Women' Arch Intern Med 171.14 (2011): 1279–1280.

Hakkinen SH et al. Content of the flavonols quercetin, myricetin, and kaempferol in 25 edible berries. J Agric Food Chem 47.6 (1999): 2274–2279.

Han CH et al. Protective effects of cranberries on infection-induced oxidative renal damage in a rabbit model of vesico-ureteric reflux. BJU Int 100.5 (2007): 1172–1175.

Hess MJ et al. Evaluation of cranberry tablets for the prevention of urinary tract infections in spinal cord injured patients with neurogenic bladder. Spinal Cord 46.9 (2008): 622–626.

Hochman N et al. Cranberry juice constituents impair lymphoma growth and augment the generation of antilymphoma antibodies in syngeneic mice. Nutr Cancer 60.4 (2008): 511–517.

Huttunen, S., et al. 2011. Inhibition activity of wild berry juice fractions against *Streptococcus pneumoniae* binding to human bronchial cells. Phytother Res, 25, 122–7.

Jepson, R. G., et al. 2012. Cranberries for preventing urinary tract infections. Cochrane Database Syst Rev, 10, CD001321.

Johnson BJ et al. Impact of cranberry on *Escherichia coli* cellular surface characteristics. Biochem Biophys Res Commun 377.3 (2008): 992–994.

Kessler T, et al. Effect of blackcurrant-, cranberry- and plum juice consumption on risk factors associated with kidney stone formation. Eur J Clin Nutr 56.10 (2002): 1020–1023.

Kim, E., et al. 2011a. Isolation and identification of intestinal CYP3A inhibitors from cranberry (*Vaccinium macrocarpon*) using human intestinal microsomes. Planta Med, 77, 265–70.

Kim, M. J., et al. 2011b. Effects of freeze-dried cranberry powder on serum lipids and inflammatory markers in lipopolysaccharide treated rats fed an atherogenic diet. Nutr Res Pract, 5, 404–11.

Kim, K. K., et al. 2012. Anti-angiogenic activity of cranberry proanthocyanidins and cytotoxic properties in ovarian cancer cells. Int J Oncol, 40, 227–35.

Koo H et al. Influence of cranberry juice on glucan-mediated processes involved in *Streptococcus mutans* biofilm development. Caries Res 40.1 (2006): 20–27.

Kresty LA, et al. Cranberry proanthocyanidins induce apoptosis and inhibit acid-induced proliferation of human esophageal adenocarcinoma cells. J Agric Food Chem 56.3 (2008): 676–680.

Lacombe, A., et al. 2010. Antimicrobial action of the American cranberry constituents; phenolics, anthocyanins, and organic acids, against *Escherichia coli* O157:H7. Int J Food Microbiol, 139, 102–7.

Laplante, K. L., et al. 2012. Effects of cranberry extracts on growth and biofilm production of *Escherichia coli* and *Staphylococcus* species. Phytother Res, 26, 1371–4.

Lee BB et al. Spinal-injured neuropathic bladder antisepsis (SINBA) trial. Spinal Cord 45.8 (2007): 542–550.

Lee IT et al. Effect of cranberry extracts on lipid profiles in subjects with type 2 diabetes. Diabet Med 25.12 (2008): 1473–7.

Lee YL et al. Anti-microbial activity of urine after ingestion of cranberry: a pilot study. Evid Based Complement Alternat Med (2010); 7: 227–232.

Leshem, R., et al. 2011. The effect of nondialyzable material (NDM) cranberry extract on formation of contact lens biofilm by *Staphylococcus epidermidis*. Invest Ophthalmol Vis Sci, 52, 4929–34.

Lilja JJ, et al. Effects of daily ingestion of cranberry juice on the pharmacokinetics of warfarin, tizanidine, and midazolam—probes of CYP2C9, CYP1A2, and CYP3A4. Clin Pharmacol Ther 81.6 (2007): 833–839.
Lipson SM et al. Antiviral effects on bacteriophages and rotavirus by cranberry juice. Phytomedicine 14.1 (2007): 23–30.
Liu Y et al. Cranberry changes the physicochemical surface properties of *E. coli* and adhesion with uroepithelial cells. Colloids Surf B Biointerfaces 65.1 (2008): 35–42.
Liu, M., et al. 2009. Cranberry phytochemical extract inhibits SGC-7901 cell growth and human tumor xenografts in Balb/c nu/nu mice. J Agric Food Chem, 57, 762–8.
MacLean, M. A., et al. 2011. North American cranberry (*Vaccinium macrocarpon*) stimulates apoptotic pathways in DU145 human prostate cancer cells in vitro. Nutr Cancer, 63, 109–20.
Magarinos HL et al. In vitro inhibitory effect of cranberry (*Vaccinium macrocarpon* Ait.) juice on pathogenic microorganisms. Prikl Biokhim Mikrobiol 44.3 (2008): 333–336.
Matsushima M et al. Growth inhibitory action of cranberry on *Helicobacter pylori*. J Gastroenterol Hepatol 23 (Suppl 2) (2008): S175–S180.
McKay DL, Blumberg JB. Cranberries (*Vaccinium macrocarpon*) and cardiovascular disease risk factors. Nutr Rev 65.11 (2007): 490–502.
McMurdo, M. E. T., et al. 2009. Cranberry or trimethoprim for the prevention of recurrent urinary tract infections? A randomized controlled trial in older women. Journal of Antimicrobial Chemotherapy, 63, 389–395.
Mellen, C. K., et al. 2010. Effect of high-dose cranberry juice on the pharmacodynamics of warfarin in patients. Br J Clin Pharmacol, 70, 139–42.
Mohammed Abdul MI et al. Pharmacodynamic interaction of warfarin with cranberry but not with garlic in healthy subjects. Br J Pharmacol 154.8 (2008): 1691–1700.
Nahata MC et al. Effect of urinary acidifiers on formaldehyde concentration and efficacy with methenamine therapy. Eur J Clin Pharmacol 22.3 (1982): 281–284.
Neto CC, et al. Anticancer activities of cranberry phytochemicals: an update. Mol Nutr Food Res 52 (Suppl 1) (2008): S18–S27.
Ngo N et al. Identification of a cranberry juice product that inhibits enteric CYP3A-mediated first-pass metabolism in humans. Drug Metab Dispos 37.3 (2009): 514–522.
Opperman, E. A. 2010. Cranberry is not effective for the prevention or treatment of urinary tract infections in individuals with spinal cord injury. Spinal Cord, 48, 451–6.
Pagonas, N., et al. 2012. Prophylaxis of Recurrent Urinary Tract Infection After Renal Transplantation by Cranberry Juice and L-Methionine. Transplantation Proceedings, 44, 3017–3021.
Patel, K. D., et al. 2011. Proanthocyanidin-rich extracts from cranberry fruit (*Vaccinium macrocarpon* Ait.) selectively inhibit the growth of human pathogenic fungi *Candida* spp. and *Cryptococcus neoformans*. J Agric Food Chem, 59, 12864–73.
Pham DQ, Pham AQ. Interaction potential between cranberry juice and warfarin. Am J Health Syst Pharm 64.5 (2007): 490–494.
Pinto Mda, S., et al. 2010. Potential of cranberry powder for management of hyperglycemia using in vitro models. J Med Food, 13, 1036–44.
Polak, D., et al. 2013. The Protective Potential of Non-Dialysable Material Fraction of Cranberry Juice on the Virulence of P. Gingivalis and F. Nucleatum Mixed Infection. J Periodontol 84: 1019–1025.
Prasain JK et al. Effect of cranberry juice concentrate on chemically-induced urinary bladder cancers. Oncol Rep 19.6 (2008): 1565–1570.
Reid G. The role of cranberry and probiotics in intestinal and urogenital tract health. Crit Rev Food Sci Nutr 42.3 (Suppl) (2002): 293–300.
Ruel G et al. Favourable impact of low-calorie cranberry juice consumption on plasma HDL-cholesterol concentrations in men. Br J Nutr 96.2 (2006): 357–364.
Ruel G et al. Low-calorie cranberry juice supplementation reduces plasma oxidized LDL and cell adhesion molecule concentrations in men. Br J Nutr 99.2 (2008): 352–359.
Ruel, G., et al. 2009. Plasma matrix metalloproteinase (MMP)-9 levels are reduced following low-calorie cranberry juice supplementation in men. J Am Coll Nutr, 28, 694–701.
Ruel, G., et al. 2013. Evidence that cranberry juice may improve augmentation index in overweight men. Nutrition Research, 33, 41–49.
Salo J et al. Cranberry juice for the prevention of recurrences of urinary tract infections in children: a randomized placebo-controlled trial. Clin Infect Dis 54.3 (2012): 340–346.
Saltzman JR et al. Effect of hypochlorhydria due to omeprazole treatment or atrophic gastritis on protein-bound vitamin B12 absorption. J Am Coll Nutr 13.6 (1994): 584–591.
Schlager TA et al. Effect of cranberry juice on bacteriuria in children with neurogenic bladder receiving intermittent catheterization. J Pediatr 135.6 (1999): 698–702.
Sharon N, Ofek I. Fighting infectious diseases with inhibitors of microbial adhesion to host tissues. Crit Rev Food Sci Nutr 42.3 (Suppl) (2002): 267–272.
Shidfar, F., et al. 2012. The effects of cranberry juice on serum glucose, apoB, apoA-I, Lp(a), and Paraoxonase-1 activity in type 2 diabetic male patients. J Res Med Sci, 17, 355–60.
Shmuely H et al. Effect of cranberry juice on eradication of *Helicobacter pylori* in patients treated with antibiotics and a proton pump inhibitor. Mol Nutr Food Res 51.6 (2007): 746–751.
Singh AP et al. Cranberry proanthocyanidins are cytotoxic to human cancer cells and sensitize platinum-resistant ovarian cancer cells to paraplatin. Phytother Res 23.8 (2009): 1066–1074.
Sobota AE. Inhibition of bacterial adherence by cranberry juice: potential use for the treatment of urinary tract infections. J Urol 131.5 (1984): 1013–10116.
Stapleton, A. E., et al. 2012. Recurrent urinary tract infection and urinary *Escherichia coli* in women ingesting cranberry juice daily: a randomized controlled trial. Mayo Clin Proc, 87, 143–50.
Su, X., et al. 2012. Antibacterial effects of plant-derived extracts on methicillin-resistant *Staphylococcus aureus*. Foodborne Pathog Dis, 9, 573–8.
Sun J, Hai Liu R. Cranberry phytochemical extracts induce cell cycle arrest and apoptosis in human MCF-7 breast cancer cells. Cancer Lett 241.1 (2006): 124–134.
Super EA et al. Cranberry use among pediatric nephrology patients. Ambul Pediatr 5.4 (2005): 249–252.
Takahashi, S., et al. 2013. A randomized clinical trial to evaluate the preventive effect of cranberry juice (UR65) for patients with recurrent urinary tract infection. J Infect Chemother 19: 112–117.
Uberos J et al. Urinary excretion of phenolic acids by infants and children: a randomised double-blind clinical assay. Clin Med Insights Pediatr 6 (2012): 67–74.
Ulbricht CE, Basch EM. Natural standard herb and supplement reference. St Louis: Mosby, 2005.
Ushijima, K., et al. 2009. Cranberry juice suppressed the diclofenac metabolism by human liver microsomes, but not in healthy human subjects. Br J Clin.Pharmacol., 68, (2) 194–200.
Vidlar, A., et al. 2009. C10 Beneficial effects of cranberries on prostate health: Evidence from a randomized controlled trial. European Urology Supplements, 8, 660.
Vidlar, A., et al. 2010. The effectiveness of dried cranberries (*Vaccinium macrocarpon*) in men with lower urinary tract symptoms. Br J Nutr, 104, 1181–9.
Villarreal A et al. Cranberry juice improved antioxidant status without affecting bone quality in orchidectomized male rats. Phytomedicine 14.12 (2007): 815–820.
Vinson JA et al. Cranberries and cranberry products: powerful in vitro, ex vivo, and in vivo sources of antioxidants. J Agric Food Chem 56.14 (2008): 5884–5891.
Vu, K. D., et al. 2012. Effect of different cranberry extracts and juices during cranberry juice processing on the antiproliferative activity against two colon cancer cell lines. Food Chemistry, 132, 959–967.
Wang, C. H., et al. 2012. Cranberry-containing products for prevention of urinary tract infections in susceptible populations: a systematic review and meta-analysis of randomized controlled trials. Arch Intern Med, 172, 988–96.
Weiss EI et al. Inhibiting interspecies coaggregation of plaque bacteria with a cranberry juice constituent. J Am Dent Assoc 129.12 (1998): 1719–1723: [published erratum J Am Dent Assoc 130.1(1999): 36 and 130.3 (1999): 332].
Wilson T et al. Favorable glycemic response of type 2 diabetics to low-calorie cranberry juice. J Food Sci 73.9 (2008a): H241–5.
Wilson T et al. Human glycemic response and phenolic content of unsweetened cranberry juice. J Med Food 11.1 (2008b): 46–54.
Wilson, T., et al. 2010. Glycemic responses to sweetened dried and raw cranberries in humans with type 2 diabetes. J Food Sci, 75, H218–23.
Wing DA et al. Daily cranberry juice for the prevention of asymptomatic bacteriuria in pregnancy: a randomized, controlled pilot study. J Urol 180.4 (2008): 1367–1372.
Yamanaka A et al. Inhibitory effect of cranberry polyphenol on biofilm formation and cysteine proteases of *Porphyromonas gingivalis*. J Periodontal Res 42.6 (2007): 589–592.
Yamanaka-Okada A et al. Inhibitory effect of cranberry polyphenol on cariogenic bacteria. Bull Tokyo Dent Coll 49.3 (2008): 107–112.
Yan X et al. Antioxidant activities and antitumor screening of extracts from cranberry fruit (*Vaccinium macrocarpon*). J Agric Food Chem 50.21 (2002): 5844–5849.
Yung, L. M., et al. 2013. Chronic cranberry juice consumption restores cholesterol profiles and improves endothelial function in ovariectomized rats. Eur J Nutr 52: 1145–1155.
Zikria, J., et al. 2010. Cranberry juice and warfarin: when bad publicity trumps science. Am J Med, 123, 384–92.

Creatine

HISTORICAL NOTE Creatine was first discovered in 1832 when it was identified in meat. The word creatine is derived from the Greek *kreas* for flesh, similar to the word 'creature'. About 15 years after its discovery, the meat from foxes killed in the wild was found to have 10-fold more creatine than meat from domesticated ones, suggesting that physical exercise must influence the amount of creatine that accumulates in muscles. Early last century, orally consumed creatine was shown to be partly retained in the body and able to increase creatine content in muscles, leading some to suspect this could influence the performance of muscles. Nowadays, creatine supplementation enjoys enormous popularity as a sports supplement and is being recommended to elite athletes by respected sporting bodies such as the Australian Institute of Sport (AIS) (AIS 2009). There is also new research investigating its potential role in other areas such as central nervous system and metabolic disturbances, cancer, muscle wasting and low bone density.

BACKGROUND AND RELEVANT PHARMACOKINETICS

Creatine is a naturally occurring nitrogenous compound produced in the human liver, pancreas and kidneys at a rate of 1–2 g daily. The amino acids glycine, arginine and methionine and the three enzymes L-arginine-glycine amidinotransferase, guanidinoacetate methyltransferase and methionine adenosyltransferase are required for its synthesis. Any drain on glycine metabolism from creatine synthesis is minimal; however the demand is more appreciable for methionine (via S-adenosylmethionine) and arginine (Brosnan et al 2011). Cellular creatine uptake is controlled by the specific transporter protein Creat-T, which moves creatine into the cell against a concentration gradient which is sodium- and chloride-dependent (Gualano et al 2012). It is stored primarily in skeletal muscle, where it is in dynamic equilibrium with phosphocreatine and is a precursor to adenosine triphosphate (ATP), the main source of energy for muscle activity and many other biological functions. Orally ingested creatine is absorbed from the small intestine, then distributed via creatine transporters around the body to muscles and nerves (Persky et al 2003). These transporters also serve as a clearance mechanism because of creatine 'trapping' by skeletal muscle. Creatine monohydrate is not degraded during normal digestion and nearly 99% of orally ingested creatine monohydrate is either taken up by muscle or excreted in urine after being converted to creatinine.

CHEMICAL COMPONENTS

Creatine is chemically known as *N*-(aminoiminomethyl)-*N*-methyl glycine.

FOOD SOURCES

Animal protein and fish. It has been estimated that approximately 1–5 g is ingested daily from the diet by omnivores (Gualano et al 2012).

DEFICIENCY SIGNS AND SYMPTOMS

Several rare inborn errors of synthesis (L-arginine-glycine amidinotransferase deficiency and guanidinoacetate methyltransferase deficiency) or in the creatine transporter result in a lack of creatine and phosphorylcreatine in the brain and severe mental retardation. Other symptoms and signs of milder deficiencies include involuntary extrapyramidal movements, speech disability, epilepsy, muscular hypotonia and weakness; in older patients, autism with self-injurious behaviour has also been reported (Beard & Braissant 2010, Wyss & Schulze 2002). While supplementation has been found to be beneficial in those with impaired creatine synthesis (Longo et al 2011, Ndika et al 2012), it does not improve cerebral symptoms in those with defective transport (Valayannopoulos et al 2012, van de Kamp et al 2012).

People involved in intense physical activity, vegetarians and those with muscle diseases may have lower residual muscle creatine levels than others.

MAIN ACTIONS

Energy production

Although the exact mechanism is unclear, much is known about the biochemistry of endogenous creatine. In skeletal muscle tissue, it is used for the production of phosphocreatine, an important form of high-energy phosphate. Phosphocreatine is broken down into phosphate and creatine during high-intensity exercise lasting 15–30 s, in a reaction catalysed by creatine kinase. During the process, energy is released and is used to regenerate ATP, the primary source of energy. Creatine is involved in an energy transport system (the creatine-phosphocreatine shuttle), transferring energy from the mitochondria to the cytosol, linking sites of ATP generation to those of consumption (Sahlin & Harris 2011).

Supplemental creatine

Oral supplementation with creatine has been shown to increase phosphocreatine levels in muscles and, as such, has been described as 'fuelling up' natural energy stores. Increased phosphocreatine creatine stores lead to faster regeneration of ATP, thereby making more energy immediately available to muscles. This is particularly important during high-intensity physical activity where rapid energy production is required. Theoretically, increased free creatine allows depleted stores to replenish more quickly, thus shortening recovery times during repeated bouts of intense exercise. Increased muscle creatine may also buffer the lactic acid produced during exercise, delaying muscle fatigue and soreness. Another possible benefit of creatine supplementation is muscle glycogen-sparing during high-intensity intermittent exercise (Roschel et al 2010) and increased muscle glycogen accumulation (Hickner et al 2010), although not all evidence supports this theory (Rico-Sanz et al 2008). It has been estimated that short-term supplementation over 5–7 days with a daily dose of 20 g creatine increases total creatine content by 10–30% and phosphocreatine stores by 10–40% (Kreider 2003).

Overall, the response to creatine supplementation is highly variable and may be influenced by an individual's pretreatment levels, so that people with low levels, such as vegetarians, may respond to a greater extent than those with higher starting levels (AIS 2009).

Neuroprotective

Creatine supplementation has displayed neuroprotective effects in several animal models of neurological diseases, such as Huntington's disease, Parkinson's disease (PD) or motor neuron disease (also known as amyotrophic lateral sclerosis or ALS) (Andreassen et al 2001, Dedeoglu et al 2003, Ferrante et al 2000, Wyss & Schulze 2002). The National Institute of Neurological Disorders and Stroke (NINDS) is currently conducting a large double-blind, placebo-controlled, phase III study involving 1720 people with early-stage PD to evaluate the effects of long-term creatine supplementation.

Creatine may exhibit antiageing benefits according to an in vivo study, where creatine-fed mice lived longer and exhibited improvements in neurobehavioural tests. Further, creatine significantly lowered the amounts of ageing pigment, lipofuscin, and upregulated various genes involved in neuroprotection and learning (Bender et al 2008). Preliminary data from a randomised, comparative, open study have shown a neuroprotective effect in cases of children with traumatic brain injury. Treatment with creatine improved a number of parameters, including duration of posttraumatic amnesia, length of recovery time, social/behaviour and cognitive function (Sakellaris et al 2006).

A number of theories of a possible mechanism for neuroprotection have been put forward. One theory proposes that creatine exerts antioxidant activity and mitochondrial stabilising effects, two mechanisms of benefit in neurodegenerative diseases, which are characterised by mitochondrial dysfunction and oxidative damage (Shefner et al 2004). Other protective actions suggested by in vitro and in vivo studies include attenuation of energy depletion (Shen & Goldberg 2012), reducing damage to the brain induced by ischaemia, apoptosis, excitotoxicity (Genius et al 2012, Klopstock et al 2011, Perasso et al 2013) and ammonia toxicity (Braissant 2010). Oral doses of creatine have been shown to pass the blood–brain barrier (Andres et al 2008); however this occurs in relatively small amounts, with most creatine supplied by endogenous synthesis within the central nervous system (Braissant 2012). Interestingly, results from a recent in vivo study suggest that creatine supplementation may also play a protective role in neurodevelopment (Sartini et al 2012).

Glycaemic control

The exact mechanisms of action for creatine on blood glucose regulation have not been well elucidated (Rocic et al 2011); however, it appears to modulate the expression of proteins and genes involved in insulin sensitivity and glycaemic control. These include protein kinase B, myocyte enhancer factor-2, insulin-like growth factor-1 (Safdar et al 2008) and AMPK-alpha protein (Alves et al 2012), which increases GLUT-4 translocation. In vitro and in vivo results also suggest the possibility that creatine increases insulin release (Roci et al 2007, 2011).

Mood

Antidepressant activity has been demonstrated in vivo using several different animal models (Allen et al 2010, 2012, Cunha et al 2012). Creatine appears to interact with several neurotransmitter receptors, including dopamine (D_1 and D_2) (Cunha et al 2012), serotonin (Cunha et al 2013) and N-methyl-D-aspartate (Royes et al 2008). Interestingly, this action was observed only in females (Allen et al 2012).

Anticancer

The anticancer effect of creatine had been demonstrated in experimental models and recent literature has reported low creatine content in several types of malignant cells. There are several reports of the anticancer effect of creatine and cyclocreatine and different theories, such as inhibition of glycolysis, generation of acidosis, had been put forward, together with an apoptosis-independent pathway. More recently, research with animal models suggests that tumour tissue supplemented with creatine might sequester significant amounts of ATP necessary for any growth-oriented cells such as malignant cells, thereby essentially starving the cells of fuel (Patra et al 2012).

OTHER ACTIONS

Creatine has a direct and indirect antioxidant effect in the cell (Gualano et al 2012). It has been shown to reduce infarct volume after stroke by 40% in vivo. By using magnetic resonance imaging, the study found augmented cerebral blood flow after stroke in mice treated with creatine (Prass et al

2006). Creatine monohydrate exhibited a positive influence on bone mineral density in vivo (Antolic et al 2007) and affected bone mineral resorption clinically.

CLINICAL USE

Creatine supplementation has been primarily used in sports where it is an extremely popular supplement. In the United States alone, creatine-containing dietary supplements make up a large portion of the estimated $2.7 billion in annual sales of sports nutrition supplements (Jager et al 2011). Beyond its use in sports, there is growing investigation of its potential use in a variety of conditions such as myopathies, neurodegenerative, neuromuscular, neurometabolic and inflammatory diseases, diabetes and cancer.

Creatine monohydrate is the form generally used and tested in clinical trials; however it has very poor solubility. In practice, this is available in different forms, which differ according to particle size (granular, powder and micronised), with the belief that smaller particles are more fully absorbed and cause less gastric distress. Other forms of creatine are appearing and include creatine anhydrous, buffered creatine monohydrate, various creatine salts — pyruvate, citrate, malate, phosphate and oratate — as well as creatine ethyl esters and creatine gluconate. An effervescent form has also been produced (Jager et al 2011). The newer forms claim to have increased solubility and bioavailability, which may reduce some adverse effects (Gufford et al 2010); however, not all studies have shown this to be the case (Jagim et al 2012). Some manufacturers have started putting several different creatine forms together in the one supplement in an attempt to ensure sufficient creatine enters the target tissues and, possibly, as a means of extending the release of creatine into the system over a longer period of time.

According to in vivo research, creatine monohydrate bioavailability can be improved when taken together with insulin-stimulating ingredients such as high amounts of glucose or protein (Jager et al 2011). It is suspected that creatine uptake could be mediated in part by glucose and insulin.

Ergogenic aid

Creatine supplementation has become one of the most widely used supplements taken by athletes and is touted by some as the only truly effective ergogenic aid, besides carbohydrate loading. It is used by athletes engaged in sprint disciplines (e.g. 100-m run or 50-m swim), strength disciplines (e.g. weight lifting) or high-intensity, repetitive-burst exercise (e.g. tennis, hockey, football, soccer) separated by short bouts of recovery.

Several hundred published studies have been conducted over the last few decades involving a variety of different athletes doing different physical tasks to clarify what types of physical activity may be improved, how and to what extent with oral creatine supplementation. In general, the majority of studies with exercise performance outcomes support an ergogenic effect of creatine (Gualano et al 2012). Overall, studies indicate that creatine supplementation (about 20 g/day for 5 days or about 2 g/day for 30 days) results in increased skeletal muscle creatine and phosphocreatine concentrations by approximately 15–40%, enhances anaerobic exercise capacity and increases training volume, leading to potentially greater gains in strength, power and muscle mass (Jager et al 2011, Rawson & Venezia 2011). Studies have also been conducted with older adults in an attempt to determine whether creatine has benefits in this population and the available evidence appears to support a potential additive or synergistic effect of combining creatine supplementation with resistance training for improving lean mass and muscle strength (Buford et al 2013).

Creatine supplementation increases muscle fibre hypertrophy, myosin heavy-chain expression and swelling of myocytes, which may in turn affect carbohydrate and protein metabolism. Supplementation also increases acute weight-lifting performance and training volume, which may allow for greater overload and adaptation to training. Creatine significantly increases phosphocreatine resynthesis after intense muscle contractions and it is this improvement in resynthesis rates which is thought to contribute to positive improvements in body composition, muscle strength and exercise performance reported when combining creatine supplementation with exercise training (Buford et al 2013).

According to a double-blind, placebo study, creatine in combination with physical training increases fibre growth by increasing satellite cell number and myonuclei concentration. Researchers took muscle biopsies at various intervals during 16 weeks of heavy resistance training, where participants were given 6 g of creatine monohydrate four times a day for the loading phase of 7 days and then once a day (Olsen et al 2006). More recently identified effects of creatine on skeletal muscle hypertrophy include increased myogenic transcription factors (Saremi et al 2010), increased insulin-like growth factor-1 (Burke et al 2008), increased gene expression for collegen and glucose 4 transporter (Deldicque et al 2008) and increased neuromuscular function. In a double-blind randomised controlled trial (RCT), 16 men receiving 20 g of creatine for 5 days demonstrated enhanced neuromuscular function of the elbow flexors in both electrically induced and voluntary contractions during short-duration intermittent exercises, but not in endurance performance (Bazzucch et al 2009).

Cycling creatine loading

Due to the fact that human muscle appears to have an upper limit of creatine storage of 150–160 mmol/kg of dry muscle, which, once achieved with diet or supplementation, cannot be exceeded, creatine supplementation is likely to produce larger effects in subjects who ingest lower creatine in diet (e.g.

vegetarians) and consequently display lower tissue creatine than people on long-term high dietary creatine intakes (Gualano et al 2012). The fact that muscle storage is finite provides some rationale for undertaking creatine loading in cycles, thereby enabling muscle levels to reach maximal storage after a number of weeks, followed by a period of withdrawal when creatine supplementation stops, followed by another reloading phase after several weeks. When combined with a continuous training program, this could theoretically lead to even greater performance gains.

Who will respond?

The observation that not every athlete responds to creatine supplementation with improved strength, performance and recovery has prompted investigation to identify the key features of responders. One study identified that responders had the lowest initial levels of muscle creatine, greatest percentage of type 2 fibres and greatest preload muscle fibre cross-sectional area and fat-free mass in comparison to non-responders (Syrotuik & Bell 2004). Other factors that are likely to influence an individual's response to creatine include training status, diet, age and the bioavailability of the creatine supplement being used. One review on the use of creatine in the elderly suggested that timing of creatine intake may be important, and if creatine is taken closely before or after the resistance training session it is likely to be more effective (Candow & Chilibeck 2008). Benefits would therefore be expected to be greater in those with the lower creatine levels at baseline, such as vegetarians. Not taking these factors into account may partly explain the inconsistent results obtained in RCTs.

Short-duration, high-intensity exercise

Studies have been conducted in a variety of athletes, such as sprint cyclists, soccer players and sprint swimmers, and generally have used a dose of 20 g daily taken for at least 5 days. Most, but not all, controlled studies have shown that supplementation improves performance and delays muscle fatigue (Balsom et al 1995, Becque et al 2000, Burke et al 1996, Cox et al 2002, Finn et al 2001, Gilliam et al 2000, Kreider et al 1998, Maganaris & Maughan 1998, Mujika & Padilla 1997, Mujika et al 2000, Rawson et al 2011, Tarnopolsky & MacLennan 2000, Williams & Branch 1998).

A meta-analysis of placebo-controlled RCTs investigating the effects of creatine on swim performance concluded that the majority of studies report an ergogenic effect, particularly in those activities lasting less than 30 s (Branch 2003). A later 2006 review reported that evidence did not suggest benefits for single bouts of swimming (distance 25–400 m) but did show improved performance for repeated bouts (2–15 bouts) and distances 25–100 m (Hopwood et al 2006). In regard to cycling, creatine supplementation appears most effective at improving exercise performance during repeated bouts of brief (30 s) high-intensity exercise (Branch 2003). The few studies conducted in athletic sprint running suggest positive ergogenic effects (Gualano et al 2012).

Since the Hopwood et al (2006) and Branch reviews (2003), many other RCTs have been published, generally supporting the use of creatine supplementation in physical activity requiring sprint-like exertion.

For example, Juhasz et al (2009) reported creatine supplementation (20 g/day for 5 days) in elite young swimmers (n = 16 males) reduced their swim time by approximately 1.8 s in two successive 100-m swims. This small change could make the difference between winning a medal at a major competition or not. In a study examining gender differences in response to creatine citrate (20 g/day), males (but not females) receiving 20 g creatine citrate for 4 days had a 23% greater anaerobic energy reserve during running sprints (Fukuda et al 2010). One small study with 10 cyclists found improved sprint cycling in the heat with a dose of 5 g given four times a day for 6 days (Wright et al 2007). In another study, 42 college-aged men undergoing high-intensity interval training (five 2-minute exercise bouts on a cycle ergometer) and receiving creatine (10 g/day) had greater endurance performance compared to those receiving the placebo (Kendall et al 2009). Similarly, Oliver et al (2013) found 5 g creatine (plus 15 g glucose) daily improved time to fatigue and reduced lactate during incremental cycling exercise following 6 days of supplementation.

The effects of creatine on jump height performance have recently been examined in two studies. In a study on 12 elite volleyball players receiving 4 weeks of creatine or placebo supplementation (loading dose of 20 g/day for 4 days, then 10 g/day on days 5–6, followed by 5 g/day for the remainder of the trial) in a double-blind RCT, the treatment group demonstrated improved repeated jump height capability but did not influence muscular fatigue and the decline in repeated performance (Lamontagne-Lacasse et al 2011). The effect of creatine compared to carbohydrate in maintaining performance during repeated bouts of high-intensity jumping exercises was investigated in another RCT. Active males (n = 60) performed two sets of jump height tests (10 jumps over 60 s) separated by 5 days. The high-dose carbohydrate (containing 250 kcal carbohydrate drink) and the creatine group (creatine monohydrate 25 g supplement) had similar effects on increasing jump height compared to the placebo and low-carbohydrate groups (250 kcal carbohydrate drink). As the creatine group increased weight (1.52 ± 0.89 kg), the authors suggested that high-dose carbohydrates may be preferred by weight-conscious athletes (Koenig et al 2008).

While low-dose creatine supplementation does not usually have an ergogenic activity, a recent double-blind RCT in healthy young adult subjects found low-dose creatine (0.03 g/kg — approximately

2.3 g) for 6 weeks was beneficial in reducing resistance to fatigue during repeated bouts of high-intensity contractions compared to placebo (Rawson et al 2011). Similarly, a trial involving 18 rugby players during an 8-week rugby season of Rugby Union football found that creatine, at a relatively low dose (0.1 g/kg/day), increased muscular endurance without detrimentally affecting body composition or aerobic endurance (Chilibeck et al 2007).

While many studies show benefits with creatine supplementation, there are several that have not, such as a placebo-controlled RCT with 17 ice hockey players given 0.3 g/kg/day of creatine for 5 days (Cornish et al 2006). Also a double-blind study found no significant improvement on multiple sprint performance, fatigue or blood lactate concentration when testing creatine use with 42 physically active men who were given 5 g four times a day for 5 days (Glaister et al 2006). An RCT found lower-dose creatine monohydrate supplementation (3 g/day for 28 days) failed to improve sprint cycling performance in 12 subjects at the end of a 2-hour endurance cycle; however submaximal oxygen consumption near the end of the 2-hour ride was decreased by approximately 10% by creatine supplementation ($P < 0.05$) (Hickner et al 2010). Another study examining the effects in sprint cycling performance failed to demonstrate a significant improvement on fatigue threshold in college men after receiving creatine loading for 5 days (four doses of 5 g dicreatine citrate plus 10 g fructose powder) (Walter et al 2008). A study with 36 tennis players found no significant benefits of creatine supplementation for 6 days on repetitive sprint power or strength of the upper and lower extremities (Pluim et al 2006). Similarly, a small recent study in males competing in judo failed to find significant benefit in anaerobic capacity or aerobic power (Sterkowicz et al 2012).

A review by Gualano et al (2012) provides further reading for those wanting greater details about creatine supplementation in specific sports.

Lean body mass

Creatine increases exercise-related gains in lean body mass (Aguiar 2013, Chrusch et al 2001, Jowko et al 2001, Stone et al 1999). In 2009, a double-blind RCT examining the effects of creatine in men with HIV undergoing three weekly training sessions demonstrated a greater increase in lean muscle mass, but no difference in muscle strength compared to the placebo group. The dose used in this study was 20 g creatine monohydrate capsules daily for 5 days followed by 4.8 g daily for the remainder of the 14-week trial (Sakkas et al 2009).

Enhanced power and/or strength

Many studies show that creatine supplementation in conjunction with resistance training augments muscle strength and size, although the effect is not consistent for everybody (Gualano et al 2012, Spriet & Gibala 2004, Volek & Rawson 2004, Zungia et al 2012). A 2003 review of 22 studies estimated that the average increase in muscle strength following creatine supplementation as an adjunct to resistance training was 8% greater than the placebo (20% vs 12%) (Rawson & Volek 2003). Similarly, the average increase in weight-lifting performance (maximal repetitions at a given percentage of maximal strength) following creatine supplementation plus resistance training was 14% greater than the placebo (26% vs 12%).

Numerous recent studies have further investigated the effects of different types of creatine on various aspects of muscle performance, which have added to the understanding of its potential benefits. It appears that effects take at least 5 days to develop, often in combination with resistance training, different forms of creatine may have different effects and combining creatine with other substances may also change an individual's response.

Law et al (2009) examined the effect of 20 g creatine supplementation versus placebo in 17 trained men undergoing resistance training. Muscle performance was tested prior to supplementation and again after 2 and 5 days of supplementation. While creatine increased muscle strength and power compared to training alone, benefits were only seen after the 5 days of supplementation. Candow et al studied the effects of the timing and frequency of creatine supplement on muscle mass and muscle strength in a 6-week RCT of university students (21–28 years). The treatment groups received either creatine 0.15 g/kg creatine twice a week or 0.10 g/kg creatine three times a week on days they underwent resistance training. Compared to the control groups receiving the same dose and frequency of placebo, muscle thickness of the elbow flexors increased, and muscle strength increased in the men but not the women. There was no difference in effects between the frequency of supplementation (Candow et al 2011).

In a double-blind RCT, the effects of two different types of creatine were compared on performance of high-intensity intermittent hand grip exercises. Compared to placebo, both creatine citrate and creatine pyruvate (5 g/day for 28 days) increased mean power initially; however after numerous repetitions only creatine pyruvate was effective (Jager et al 2008), suggesting a superior effect on endurance.

Creatine monohydrate was compared with creatine ethyl ester in an RCT of 30 young men undergoing resistance training. A loading dose of approximately 20 g/day for 5 days followed by 5 g/day for 42 days of creatine ethyl ester, creatine monohydrate or placebo were compared. Neither creatine group was found to significantly improve muscle strength or performance compared to placebo, and furthermore the creatine ethyl ester supplementation significantly increased serum creatinine levels while not increasing serum or total muscle creatine content, suggesting it may be degraded within the gastrointestinal tract after ingestion (Spillane et al 2009).

While many studies show some positive results, not all studies have shown benefits of adding creatine supplementation to a training protocol on either strength or lean body mass. It appears that some of these studies suffer from using insufficient doses or not using the correct dosage for an appropriate period of time (Carter et al 2005, Eckerson et al 2008, Ferguson & Syrotuik 2006).

IN COMBINATION

Combining creatine and sodium bicarbonate supplementation increased peak and mean power and had the greatest attenuation of decline in relative peak power over six repeated sprints. These data suggest that combining these two supplements may be advantageous for athletes participating in high-intensity, intermittent exercise. This crossover study utilised supplementation for 2 days followed by a 3-week washout and involved 13 trained men assessed during six 10-s repeated Wingate sprint tests on a cycle ergometer with a 60-s rest period between each sprint (Barber 2013).

One study examined the effect of creatine combined with glycerol on running economy in endurance. The supplement, taken for 7 days, was beneficial in attenuating the cardiovascular strain and thermal effects of a 30-min run in hot conditions (35°C), and, while it did increase body mass, it did not negatively affect running economy (Beis 2011).

The combined effects of supplementation with creatine, conjugated linoleic acid and whey protein for 5 weeks in addition to strength training resulted in a greater increase in muscle strength and lean mass compared to either creatine plus placebo or placebo alone (Cornish et al 2009). Another study examined the additive effects of creatine combined with other nutrients on muscle strength and body composition. This randomised double-blind study in 24 resistance-trained men aged 18–35 years compared the effects of creatine monohydrate (loading dose of 18 g/day for 5 days followed by 4.5 g/day for 23 days) combined with either 2 g/day of corn starch or D-pinitol for 5 days followed by 0.5 g/day for the remaining 23 days. While both groups increased upper- and lower-body strength and body composition, the creatine-only group had greater improvement in increases in lean mass and fat-free mass, suggesting that the addition of pinitol may negate some of the benefits of creatine on body composition (Kirksick et al 2009).

Creatine without resistance training

The effects of creatine on muscle strength in untrained young adults without resistance training have recently been studied in a double-blind RCT. The treatment group received 5 g polyethylene glycosylated creatine daily for 28 days. There was a significant increase in upper-body strength (measured by one-repetition maximum bench press) but not lower-body strength or muscular power in the treatment group (n = 10) compared to the placebo group (n = 12) (Camic et al 2010), suggesting some benefit to muscle strength may occur even without exercise. Furthermore, the effect of creatine on muscle mass and strength on immobilised limbs has been investigated. In a single-blind crossover study, 7 men aged 18–25 years received placebo on days 1–7 and creatine 20 g/day on days 15–21. An upper limb was immobilised in a cast during the placebo supplementation period, removed between days 8–14 and then the opposite limb was immobilised during creatine treatment. Compared to the placebo, the creatine supplementation better maintained lean muscle mass and muscle strength during immobilisation (Johnston et al 2009).

Physical performance benefits in the elderly

Ageing accompanied by reduced physical activity results in decreased muscle creatine, muscle mass, bone density and strength, which may be addressed by increasing creatine intake (Rawson & Venezia 2011). Short-term creatine supplementation in older adults, independently of physical exercise training, has shown increased muscle strength and performance of activities of daily living, and enhanced fatigue resistance and body mass in the majority of studies. When supplementation is combined with resistance training these benefits are amplified.

Several RCTs show benefits in both male and female older adults (Aguiar 2013, Brose et al 2003, Candow & Chilibeck 2008, Chrusch et al 2001, Gotshalk et al 2008, Kreider et al 1998, Stout et al 2007). Study volunteers have included people aged over 70 years, and demonstrated benefits in lean tissue mass, leg strength, endurance and average power greater than placebo (Chrusch et al 2001), increase in total and fat-free mass, and gains in several indices of isometric muscle strength (Brose et al 2003), increases in grip strength, muscle endurance and physical working capacity at fatigue threshold (Stout et al 2007), muscle strength and function compared to placebo (Aguiar 2013, Gotshalk et al 2008). Doses used have ranged from 5 g to 20 g daily for at least 5 days.

In contrast, a 7-day study of elderly women produced mixed results, as creatine supplementation (dosage 0.3 g/kg/day) did not show any benefits for endurance but did help volunteers to perform lower-body function exercises that involved quick movements (Canete et al 2006). No additional benefits were found in two studies in which creatine was given either alone or combined with protein powder (given on training days three times a week) on muscle strength or muscle mass in men aged 48–72 undergoing resistance training (Bemden et al 2010, Eliot et al 2008).

Improve recovery from exercise damage

Several studies have recently found positive effects in creatine in attenuating exercise-induced muscle injury, suggesting a therapeutic role in injured athletes. A small study of triathletes (n = 8) receiving creatine (20 g/day plus 50 g maltodextrin in two doses) for 5 days prior to competition had decreased markers of muscle damage (creatine kinase, lactate dehydrogenase and aldolase, glutamic oxaloacetic acid transaminase and glutamic pyruvic acid transaminase) following the IronMan competition, compared to the placebo group (Bassit 2010). In the second study, creatine loading in young males for 5 days prior to an eccentric resistance training session (0.3 g/day kg body weight) and postmaintenance for 14 days (0.1 g/day kg body weight) attenuated the loss of strength and muscle damage (measured by creatine kinase activity) compared to the placebo group (Cooke et al 2009). Positive results were also observed in a study in which 20 g/day creatine monohydrate for 6 days given to young men reduced markers of muscle damage, muscle soreness and a smaller reduction in range of movement after repeated bouts of resistance exercise compared to placebo (Veggi et al 2013). Possible reasons for these effects are the pre-exercise creatine enhancing the calcium-buffering capacity of the muscle, and postexercise creatine enhancing the regenerative response of the muscle (Cooke et al 2009).

Another mechanism of creatine which may protect muscles is its role as an antioxidant (Barros et al 2012, Coco & Perciavalle 2012, Deminice & Jordao 2012, Sestili et al 2011). In a study by Rahimi (2011) in resistance-trained males (n = 27), 7 days of creatine supplementation (5 g four times daily) reduced the oxidation of DNA and lipid peroxidation following a single bout of strenuous resistance training. Creatine has direct and indirect antioxidant activity in the cell; however this has not always been observed clinically (Percario et al 2012, Silva et al 2013).

Clinical note — The Australian Institute of Sport Supplement Program

The AIS is world-renowned for its professionalism and high-quality training programs. In 2000, a project called the AIS Sports Supplement Program (AIS 2009) was developed to ensure that athletes use supplements correctly and confidently, and receive 'cutting-edge' advice on nutritional practices. In order to streamline the information available, a panel of experts categorised some of the most popular sports supplements into various classes to clarify which are approved or recommended and which are directly banned by international doping rules. Some of the approved supplements recommended for use include creatine, antioxidants (vitamins C and E), multivitamins, iron, calcium supplements and sports drinks.

Heart failure

Muscle fatigue due to loss of skeletal muscle mass and strength, decreased oxidative capacity and other abnormalities of muscle metabolism have been associated with heart failure.

As a result, creatine supplementation has been suggested as a possible therapeutic agent in this condition and current RCT evidence suggests possible improvements in dyspnoea and reducing dysrhythmia but no change in ejection fraction.

This was most recently reported in a 2012 Cochrane systematic review which analysed the results of RCTs (n = 1474) which examined the effectiveness of creatine supplementation and its analogues (creatine phosphate — orally, intravenously or intramuscularly; and phosphocreatinine) in adults with heart failure (six RCTs, n = 1226), acute myocardial infarction (four RCTs, n = 220) and one RCT in ischaemic heart disease (n = 28). The duration of treatment ranged from acute 2-hour intravenous to 6 months. In regard to heart failure, no improvement was reported for ejection fraction; however there was improvement in reducing dysrhythmia and dyspnoea. There was insufficient evidence to determine which form of creatine, dose, route of administration and duration of therapy is most effective (Horjus et al 2011).

Other studies have sought to identify whether creatine has any other benefits in people with congestive heart failure (CHF). Three double-blind RCTs involving people with CHF have found improvements in muscle strength compared to placebo when creatine was taken for at least 5 days (Andrews et al 1998, Gordon et al 1995, Kuethe et al 2006). More recently, low-dose creatine (5 g/day) taken for 6 months by volunteers (n = 33) with CHF showed no significant improvement in functional capacity over placebo, as assessed by cardiopulmonary exercise test and the six-minute walk test in a double-blind study (Carvalho et al 2012).

Fibromyalgia

Theoretically, creatine supplementation may have value in fibromyalgia as a means of reducing muscle fatigue and/or improving strength. Two studies suggest it may be worth considering in this population.

An 8-week open-label study testing creatine monohydrate (3 g/day for 3 weeks then 5 g/day until 8 weeks) showed improvements in the symptoms of fibromyalgia measured by the Fibromyalgia Impact Questionnaire, sleep quality and pain levels. In addition, patients' impression of disease burden had reduced at 8 weeks and again at the 4-week posttreatment mark (Leader et al 2009).

More recently, a 16-week, double-blind RCT involving 28 women showed that creatine monohydrate (20 g for 5 days in four equal doses, followed by 5 g/day for the remainder of the study) increased phosphoryl creatine muscle content and improved lower- and upper-body muscle function and strength (measured by leg-press and chest-press exercises) compared to placebo. However, no differences were seen in other outcomes measured, including aerobic conditioning, cognitive function, quality of sleep and quality of life (Alves et al 2012).

Neurological degenerative diseases

Over the past few years, a considerable body of scientific evidence has given support to the idea that creatine supplementation may alleviate some of the clinical symptoms of neurological disease and delay disease progression (Wyss & Schulze 2002). Unfortunately, neuroprotective effects demonstrated in animal models have not been consistently demonstrated in clinical trials. This may be not only because the pathophysiological processes of neurodegenerative disease are different in humans, but also due to differences in dosage and timing of creatine supplementation relative to disease onset (Klopstock et al 2011). Traditionally, the existing studies may also have been underpowered and limited the detection of statistically significant effects (Klopstock et al 2011) and used insufficient doses, as some animal studies have used doses 10 times higher than in clinical trials (Andres et al 2008).

Theoretically, a combination of creatine and CoQ10 may have added benefits in neurological diseases as they both work in the mitochondria and are involved in ATP production, together with exerting antioxidant effects. Although thus far only studied in animal models of PD and Huntington's disease, several measurements of neuroprotection were enhanced, and motor performance and survival were improved (Yang et al 2009).

Huntington's disease

A number of studies conducted with experimental animal models of Huntington's disease have identified a possible role for creatine supplementation (Andreassen et al 2001, Dedeoglu et al 2003, Ferrante et al 2000). Creatine was shown to increase survival, delay onset of symptoms and exert neuroprotective effects in vivo. A double-blind, placebo RCT with 64 Huntington's disease patients given creatine at a dose of 8 g/day for 16 weeks found that creatine concentrations in the brain and serum increased with supplementation and reduced oxidative injury to DNA (Hersch et al 2006).

Parkinson's disease

Decreased muscle mass and strength are features of PD. Creatine monohydrate combined with resistance training showed improved muscular endurance and improvements in upper-body strength. This double-blind, placebo RCT had 20 patients given 20 g/day of creatine for 5 days and then 5 g/day for 12 weeks (Hass et al 2007). Another placebo RCT followed 60 patients for a 2-year period and found that creatine had no overall effect on Unified Parkinson's Disease Rating Scale scores (covering behaviour and mood, daily living activities, motor skills and complications of therapy; patients taking creatine did experience elevated mood and required smaller increases in dopamine medication) (Bender et al 2006). In a randomised, blinded phase II clinical trial, creatine showed a delay in the progression of PD by 50% compared to the placebo group (NINDS NET-PD Investigators 2006). In a follow-up study 18 months later, the safety of creatine supplementation (10 g/day) was confirmed, as it did not cause any safety concerns or interactions with the PD therapy (minocycline 200 mg/day) in subjects with early PD (NINDS NET-PD Investigators 2008). It is currently in phase III trials (Elm et al 2012).

Interestingly, the effects of creatine on L-dopa-induced dyskinesia, which occurs with long-term treatment in PD patients, were investigated in an animal model. Rats which had a 6-hydroxydopamine lesion were fed creatine for 1 month prior to receiving 21 days of L-dopa medication. Treated rats had significantly fewer abnormal involuntary movements without any worsening of the disease, suggesting that creatine may attenuate the motor complications associated with L-dopa treatment (Valastro et al 2009).

Amyotrophic lateral sclerosis/motor neuron disease (MND)

Despite the positive results from animal model MND, human trials have produced mixed results (Groeneveld et al 2003, Mazzini et al 2001, Rosenfeld et al 2008, Shefner et al 2004). A systematic review of three RCTs conducted in MND patients (n = 386) found that low-dose creatine supplementation of 5–10 g/day did not improve disease survival or MND progression. There was a slight trend towards creatine worsening breathing ability (measured by forced vital capacity); however the authors suggested this may have been a misleading statistical variability (Pastula & Bedlack 2010). One possible explanation for this finding is the dose used. In a phase I open-label study on the pharmacokinetics of creatine in 6 patients with MND, the effects of escalating doses of 5 g, 10 g and 15 g twice daily (taken for 1 week at each dose) were evaluated via changes in blood levels of creatine and brain metabolites measured by proton magnetic resonance spectroscopy. Plasma levels of creatine increased in a dose-dependent manner, with the magnetic resonance spectroscopy results suggesting it crosses the blood–brain barrier at the highest dose, increasing brain creatine levels. The highest dose was also found to reduce brain glutamate concentrations by 17%, which may be of significance as glutamate-mediated injury to motor neurons is thought to occur in MND (Atassi et al 2010).

Charcot-Marie-Tooth disease (CMT)

Muscle function improved when creatine and resistance training were undertaken by people with CMT, according to a randomised, placebo-controlled trial of 18 people. Over the 12-week period, combined treatment also resulted in improved muscle myosin heavy-chain composition (Smith et al 2006).

Multiple sclerosis (MS)

In a small double-blind, crossover trial, with a 3-week wash-out period, in multiple sclerosis subjects (n = 11) given either creatine (5 g four times a day for a week: 2.5 g twice a day for the second week) or placebo for two 14-day periods, creatine did not improve muscle capacity or habitual fatigue (Malin et al 2008).

Cervical-level spinal cord injury

According to a randomised, double-blind, placebo-controlled crossover trial, creatine supplementation enhances upper-extremity work capacity in subjects with complete cervical-level spinal cord injury (Jacobs et al 2002).

Bone mineral density

The combination of high energy requirement for bone and cartilage repair and development and the positive role muscle plays on bone mass makes creatine a possible therapy for bone disorders such as osteoporosis and osteoarthritis.

According to a double-blind, placebo-controlled study with 29 older men, creatine (0.3 g/kg for 5 days and 0.07 g/kg thereafter) administered for 12 weeks while undergoing resistance training significantly increased bone density. Creatine supplementation had an additional benefit for regionalised bone mineral content where there was a change in lean tissue mass. It was suggested that the effect may be due to greater tension on the bone due to an increase in muscle mass in the creatine participants (Chilibeck et al 2005). Additionally, creatine supplementation 0.1 g/kg for 3 days/week (for 10 weeks) in healthy older males undergoing supervised resistance training was found to reduce bone resorption (measured by cross-linked *N*-telopeptides of type I collagen) by 27% (Candow & Chilibeck 2008).

Osteoarthritis

Creatine supplementation (20 g/day for 1 week and then 5 g daily thereafter) in addition to strengthening exercises for 3 months improved quality of life, physical function, stiffness and lower-limb lean mass compared to placebo in a double-blind RCT of 24 postmenopausal women with knee osteoarthritis. The authors attributed the positive outcomes to creatine's effect on strength training and possibly increased cartilage metabolism, as a direct role in cartilage repair is unlikely to occur within 3 months (Neves et al 2011a).

Muscular dystrophy

A number of muscle diseases are associated with a decrease in intracellular creatine concentration, which could theoretically contribute to muscle weakness and degeneration of muscle tissue (Wyss et al 1998).

An updated 2011 systematic review of literature looking at creatine supplementation in muscle diseases evaluated 14 RCTs (n = 364) and found that both short- and medium-term creatine supplementation improved muscular strength activities of daily living in those with muscular dystrophies and idiopathic inflammatory myopathy but there was no significant improvement in metabolic myopathies. However, people with glycogen storage disease type V should avoid high-dose creatine supplementation, as it caused a significant increase in pain in one study (Kley et al 2011).

It appears the potential positive or negative effects of creatine supplementation depend on the type of myopathy and creatine transport system disorder (Tarnopolsky 2011).

Reduces mental fatigue and improves cognitive function

Creatine supplementation improves cognitive performance, with generally positive effects being reported in both young (Benton & Donohoe 2011, Ling et al 2009, Watanabe et al 2002) and older individuals (McMorris et al 2007). Supplementation has been found to increase brain creatine and phosphocreatine levels and is associated with improved cognitive performance (Rawson & Venezia 2011).

Hammett et al (2010) showed that creatine (20 g/day for 5 days then 5 g for 2 days) given to healthy adults (n = 22) improved short-term memory and abstract reasoning compared to placebo. Treatment with 5 g/day creatine ethyl ester improved tasks associated with memory and attention span (assessed by memory scanning, arrow flankers and Raven's matrices) compared to placebo in another study of 14 young adults (Ling et al 2009). Similarly, creatine (8 g/day for 5 days) reduced mental fatigue when examined under double-blind, placebo-controlled conditions in 24 healthy volunteers (Watanabe et al 2002). A study of 45 healthy vegetarians showed that creatine significantly improved tasks requiring speed of processing, both working memory and intelligence (Raven's advanced progressive matrices) (Rae et al 2003). This is further supported by a recent double-blind RCT (n = 128) in which creatine supplementation (20 g/day for 5 days) was found to have a greater effect on memory in young healthy vegetarians compared to omnivores (Benton & Donohoe 2011).

A placebo RCT demonstrated that creatine improved cognitive function in elderly patients, with various cognitive performance tasks showing significant improvement on baseline, apart from backward number recall, where no improvement was found (McMorris et al 2007). Alternatively, a negative double-blind, placebo-controlled study of 22 individuals given low-dose creatine (0.03 g/kg of body weight) daily for 6 weeks found no significant difference in cognitive function (Rawson et al 2008).

Depression

A potential role for the use of creatine in psychiatric disorders is beginning to be explored, with magnetic resonance spectroscopy finding changes to brain creatine metabolism in a number of psychiatric illnesses, including depression; reduced creatine metabolism has been associated with a worse disease course and outcome (Allen et al 2012).

Three clinical trials of different designs have also found a beneficial effect of augmenting antidepressant medication with creatine (4–5 g/day) in those with major depression disorder (Kondo et al 2011, Lyoo et al 2012, Roitman et al 2007). Current evidence suggests it may be best suited to unipolar depression; however, further research is required to confirm the role of creatine in depression.

In a recent double-blind placebo-controlled trial, 52 women with major depression were given either 5 g creatine monohydrate or placebo in addition to the selective serotonin reuptake inhibitor (SSRI) escitalopram for 8 weeks. Significant improvements in symptoms, as measured by the Hamilton Depression Rating Scale score, were seen in the treatment group commencing after 2 weeks of treatment. There was no difference in adverse effects reported (Lyoo et al 2012). This supports the findings of two earlier preliminary studies. An open-label, add-on study involving 5 treatment-resistant female adolescents receiving fluoxetine reported that 4 g of creatine daily for 8 weeks had increased brain phosphocreatine concentrations compared to healthy controls and there was a 56% reduction in the depressive symptom score (measured by Children's Depression Rating Scale-Revised) (Kondo et al 2011). In contrast, a shorter pilot study involving 18 treatment-resistant patients (4 men and 14 women) with major depression treated with SSRI/serotonin-noradrenaline reuptake inhibitor or noradrenergic specific serotonin antidepressant for 3 weeks, who received either 5 or 10 g/day creatine or placebo for 4 weeks in addition to their antidepressant, reported no difference in symptoms measured by the Hamilton Depression Rating Scale and the Clinical Global Impression Severity Scale compared to placebo (Nemets & Levine 2013). The lack of effect reported in this trial may be due to the shorter timeframe — only 4 weeks compared to 8 weeks in previous positive studies. However this should be explored further for confirmation.

An open-label study suggests that creatine supplementation may be better suited to unipolar depression. In this trial, people with treatment-resistant depression were given creatine 3–5 g/day for 4 weeks. This treatment resulted in symptom improvement in patients with unipolar depression. However, in two patients with bipolar, hypomania/mania was experienced, suggesting the need for caution (Roitman et al 2007).

Diabetes

Creatine supplementation (10 g/day) for 3 months improved glucose tolerance but not insulin sensitivity when combined with aerobic training in a double-blind, randomised, placebo-controlled trial with 22 healthy sedentary males (Gualano et al 2008). A 12-week randomised, double-blind, placebo-controlled trial of 25 subjects with type 2 diabetes undergoing exercise training found creatine 5 g/day resulted in improved glycaemic control (HbA_{1C}), postprandial glycaemia and GLUT-4 translocation compared to placebo. No changes were seen in the surrogate measures of insulin sensitivity such as insulin and C-peptide concentrations, physical capacity or lipid profile. The underlying mechanism in increased glucose disposal is thought to be further enhancement of GLUT-4 recruitment to the sarcolemma compared to exercise alone (Gualano et al 2011).

The effectiveness of short-term creatine on glycaemic control in type 2 diabetics has been examined in two crossover RCTs.

The first randomised crossover study (n = 30 unmedicated subjects) found that creatine (2 × 3 g/day) was as effective as metformin (2 × 500 mg/day) in reducing fasting and postprandial blood glucose levels measured at 60, 90, 120, 180 and 240 minutes post-meal consumption; however creatine had a greater effect at 120 minutes. Neither treatment resulted in changes in blood insulin, C-peptide or HbA_{1C} (Rocic et al 2009). Soon after, Rocic et al (2011) reported that creatine (3 g/day) was as effective as glibenclamide (3.5 g/day) in lowering blood glucose levels from baseline, measured before and postprandially. The study of 31 people with type 2 diabetes also showed both treatments increased plasma insulin and C-peptide (Rocic et al 2011).

OTHER USES

Gyrate atrophy

Doses of 1.5 g/day for 1 year resulted in improvement of the skeletal muscle abnormality that accompanies gyrate atrophy, a genetically acquired form of blindness (Feldman 1999).

DOSAGE RANGE

There are two common dosing regimens.

Loading

Creatine loading protocols have been well studied.

- Rapid loading: a dose of 5 g is taken four times daily for 5–7 days as a loading phase, followed by 2–10 g daily as maintenance for 1 week to 6 months (Bemben & Lamont 2005). This is followed by a 4-week break and then restarted, in a process known as 'cycling'.
- Slower loading: a similar effect can be achieved by taking 3 g daily over 28 days.

Concurrent ingestion of carbohydrate (50–100 g) may improve creatine uptake.

Once muscles have become saturated, it takes approximately 4 weeks to return to baseline levels.

Non-loading

- Daily dose of 3 g.

In practice, creatine is often taken with simple carbohydrates, such as glucose or fruit juice, in order to increase creatine accumulation within muscle.

Clinical note — Interview with Steve Brown, former Mr Australia National Powerlifting Champion, world record holder and personal trainer

In practice, micronised creatine supplements have changed enormously since their introduction to the mainstream market 10 years ago. The greater majority of creatine supplements have no negative impact or side effects on the gastrointestinal tract and, typically, most creatine supplements are now available as hybrids. This means they are presented as a combination of different forms all blended together and are very easily assimilated into the body with water. Good hydration is very important when using a creatine supplement in order to ensure minimal fluid retention within the layers of skin, according to Steve Brown (personal communication, 2014). The loading regimen typically increases the ability to lift heavier weights for greater repetitions within a week and occurs quite suddenly. Also, creatine increases alertness and mental sharpness, effects that are obvious after the first week. Although there can be a very slight weight gain due to water retention, lean body mass also increases, because the body is able to work harder and for longer with creatine. Once supplementation stops, the physical effects on performance quickly reduce and are noticeable after the first week.

Dosing range according to clinical studies

- Short-duration, high-intensity exercise: 20 g/day for 5 days.
- Lean muscle mass: 20 g/day for 5 days followed by 4.8 g daily.
- Muscle strength with training: 0.15 g/kg body weight twice a week; 0.10 g/kg three times a week; 5 g/day creatine pyruvate.
- Muscle strength without training: 5 g polyethylene glycosylated creatine daily for 28 days.
- Maintaining muscle mass with limb immobilisation: 20 g/day for 1 week.
- Muscle strength and function in the elderly: 5–20 g/day for at least 5 days.
- Muscle recovery from exercise: 20 g/day plus 50 g maltodextrin for 5 days prior to competition/training; 0.3 g/kg body weight for 5 days prior to training and 0.1 g/kg body weight posttraining.
- Fibromyalgia: 3 g/day for 3 weeks followed by 5 g/day; 20 g/day for 5 days followed by 5 g/day.
- Bone mineral density: 0.3 g/kg body weight for 5 days followed by 0.07 g/kg combined with resistance training.
- Osteoarthritis: 20 g/day for 1 week followed by 5 g daily combined with resistance training.
- Huntington's disease: 8 g/day.
- PD: 20 g/day for 5 days followed by 5 g/day.
- Mental fatigue and brain function: 5–20 g for 5 days.
- Depression: 4–5 g/day for 4–8 weeks as an add-on therapy to antidepressant medication.
- Diabetes / glucose intolerance: 5–10 g/day.
- Gyrate atrophy: 1.5 g/day.
- Reducing effects of sleep deficit: 50–100 mg/kg body weight.
- Rett's syndrome: 200 mg/kg body weight.

ADVERSE REACTIONS

Side effects can include gastrointestinal distress with nausea and vomiting, diarrhoea, muscle fatigue, pain and cramping, dehydration and heat intolerance. The effects may be reduced when micronised forms of creatine are taken together with glucose or simple carbohydrates. A systematic review and meta-analysis however found creatine supplementation did not increase symptoms, adversely affect hydration or thermoregulation in athletes exercising in the heat (Lopez et al 2009) and, interestingly, may even reduce perceived exertion when exercising in the heat (Hadjicharalambous et al 2008). Recent reviews of creatine safety found no negative effects on kidney function in healthy individuals (Gualano et al 2012, Kim et al 2011); however in those with a pre-existing kidney disease or dysfunction, supplementation greater than 3–5 g/day should be avoided (Kim et al 2011). Splitting the daily dose or using a slow-release formulation may assist in reducing the accumulation of potential toxic metabolites (Gualano et al 2012).

CONTRAINDICATIONS AND PRECAUTIONS

Use of high-dose creatine is contraindicated in individuals with renal failure, although it appears to be relatively safe in people at risk of kidney dysfunction. This was seen in several studies examining the effect of creatine in those at risk of kidney dysfunction, including type 2 (Gualano et al 2011b), older individuals (postmenopausal women) (Neves et al 2011), elderly Parkinson's patients (Bender et al 2008) or those with a single kidney (Gualano et al 2010b): no negative effects on renal function were found.

Caution in people with bipolar depression based on a report of increased mania in an open study (Roitman et al 2007).

A risk assessment report using data from clinical trials concluded that, overall, creatine has a good safety profile in healthy individuals, with the main side effect being gastrointestinal upset when taken in large doses. Doses up to 5 g/day are generally considered safe but the long-term safety of larger doses is yet to be established (Shao & Hathcock 2006). Creatine supplementation for up to 8 weeks has not been associated with major health risks, but the safety of long-term creatine supplementation has not been established (Gualano et al 2012, Williams & Branch 1998).

Gastrointestinal disturbance may further be reduced if doses are divided (e.g. two doses of 5 g/day may be better tolerated than a single 10-g dose) (Ostojic & Ahmetovic 2008).

Fluid retention is commonly observed during the loading phase of supplementation and it can result in early weight gain of 1.6–2.4 kg.

SIGNIFICANT INTERACTIONS

Controlled studies are not available and there is insufficient reliable evidence to determine interaction potential.

PREGNANCY USE

Insufficient reliable data are available, but it is generally not recommended in pregnancy.

Practice points/Patient counselling

- Creatine is a very popular sports supplement and is not a substance banned by the International Olympic Committee. Although scientific evidence supports its use in high-intensity, repetitive-burst exercise, not every individual will respond. It appears that vegetarians and those with low starting creatine levels in muscle are most likely to respond.
- Creatine is also used in the treatment of numerous conditions involving fatigue or muscle weakness.
- Creatine is used in the production of ATP, the main source of energy for muscle activity and many other biological functions.
- Clinical studies suggest that creatine supplementation may improve cognitive function and mood, glycaemic control in type 2 diabetes and possibly also have benefits in fibromyalgia, PD and osteoarthritis when combined with exercise and improving bone mineral density.
- Neuroprotective effects observed in animal studies and some clinical studies suggest a possible role in neurodegenerative diseases; however, further research is still required to clarify its role.
- In practice, creatine is often taken in high doses for 5–7 days, followed by lower maintenance doses for up to 8 weeks. This is called 'loading'. Stopping creatine after this time and then starting the treatment regimen again is common among athletes and is supported by the fact that muscles have a finite storage capacity for creatine.
- High-dose creatine is contraindicated in renal failure.

PATIENTS' FAQs

What will this supplement do for me?

Creatine enhances physical power and recovery in most cases and appears most effective when combined with resistance training. It may also reduce mental fatigue, enhance mood and memory and have a protective effect on nerves. Research shows a possible role in neurodegenerative diseases, glycaemic control in type 2 diabetes, fibromyalgia, PD and osteoarthritis when combined with exercise and improving bone mineral density.

When will it start to work?

The physical effects generally develop within 1–4 weeks of use. The effects on mood and concentration take longer — 4–8 weeks.

Are there any safety issues?

Creatine should not be taken in high doses by people with kidney disease and its long-term safety has not been established.

REFERENCES

AIS 2009 http://www.ausport.gov.au/__data/assets/pdf_file/0019/466030/Creatine_11-_website_fact_sheet.pdf

Alves, CR, et al 2012, 'Creatine-induced glucose uptake in type 2 diabetes: a role for AMPK-alpha?', Amino Acids, vol. 43, no. 4, pp. 1803–7.

Andreassen OA et al. Creatine increases survival and delays motor symptoms in a transgenic animal model of Huntington's disease. Neurobiol Dis 8.3 (2001): 479–491.

Andres RH et al. Functions and effects of creatine in the central nervous system. Brain Res Bull 76.4 (2008): 329–343.

Andrews R et al. The effect of dietary creatine supplementation on skeletal muscle metabolism in congestive heart failure. Eur Heart J 19.4 (1998): 617–622.

Antolic A et al. Creatine monohydrate increases bone mineral density in young Sprague-Dawley rats. Med Sci Sports Exerc 39.5 (2007): 816–820.

Balsom PD et al. Skeletal muscle metabolism during short duration high-intensity exercise: influence of creatine supplementation. Acta Physiol Scand 154.3 (1995): 303–310.

Beard, E & Braissant, O 2010, 'Synthesis and transport of creatine in the CNS: importance for cerebral functions', J Neurochem, vol. 115, no. 2, pp. 297–313.

Becque MD, et al. Effects of oral creatine supplementation on muscular strength and body composition. Med Sci Sports Exerc 32.3 (2000): 654–658.

Bemben MG, Lamont HS. Creatine supplementation and exercise performance: recent findings. Sports Med 35.2 (2005): 107–125.

Bender A et al. Creatine supplementation in Parkinson disease: a placebo-controlled randomized pilot trial. Neurology 67.7 (2006): 1262–1264.

Bender A et al. Creatine improves health and survival of mice. Neurobiol Aging 29.9 (2008): 1404–1411.

Braissant, O 2010, 'Ammonia toxicity to the brain: effects on creatine metabolism and transport and protective roles of creatine', Mol Genet Metab, vol. 100 Suppl 1, pp. S53–8.

Braissant O 2012 Creatine and guanidinoacetate transport at blood-brain and blood-cerebrospinal fluid barriers. J Inherit Metab Dis 35, 655–664.

Branch, J.D. 2003. Effect of creatine supplementation on body composition and performance: a meta-analysis. Int. J Sport Nutr. Exerc. Metab, 13, (2) 198–226.

Brose A et al. Creatine supplementation enhances isometric strength and body composition improvements following strength exercise training in older adults. J Gerontol A Biol Sci Med Sci 58.1 (2003): B11–B119.

Brosnan, JT, et al 2011, 'The metabolic burden of creatine synthesis', Amino Acids, vol. 40, no. 5, pp. 1325–31.

Buford, T.W., et al. (2013) Optimizing the Benefits of Exercise on Physical Function in Older Adults. PM&R (0) available from: http://www.sciencedirect.com/science/article/pii/S1934148213011878

Burke LM, et al. Effect of oral creatine supplementation on single-effort sprint performance in elite swimmers. Int J Sport Nutr 6.3 (1996): 222–233.

Candow DG, Chilibeck PD. Timing of creatine or protein supplementation and resistance training in the elderly. Appl Physiol Nutr Metab 33.1 (2008): 184–190.

Canete S et al. Does creatine supplementation improve functional capacity in elderly women? J Strength Cond Res 20.1 (2006): 22–28.

Carter JM et al. Does nutritional supplementation influence adaptability of muscle to resistance training in men aged 48 to 72 years. J Geriatr Phys Ther 28.2 (2005): 40–47.

Chilibeck PD et al. Creatine monohydrate and resistance training increase bone mineral content and density in older men. J Nutr Health Aging 9.5 (2005): 352–353.

Chilibeck PD, et al. Effect of in-season creatine supplementation on body composition and performance in rugby union football players. Appl Physiol Nutr Metab 32.6 (2007): 1052–1057.

Chrusch MJ et al. Creatine supplementation combined with resistance training in older men. Med Sci Sports Exerc 33.12 (2001): 2111–2117.

Cornish SM, et al. The effect of creatine monohydrate supplementation on sprint skating in ice-hockey players. J Sports Med Phys Fitness 46.1 (2006): 90–98.

Cox G et al. Acute creatine supplementation and performance during a field test simulating match play in elite female soccer players. Int J Sport Nutr Exerc Metab 12.1 (2002): 33–46.

Cunha, MP, et al 2012, 'Antidepressant-like effect of creatine in mice involves dopaminergic activation', J Psychopharmacol, vol. 26, no. 11, pp. 1489–501.

Cunha, MP, et al 2013, 'Evidence for the involvement of 5-HT(1A) receptor in the acute antidepressant-like effect of creatine in mice', Brain Res Bull. 2013; 95: 61–69.

Dedeoglu A et al. Creatine therapy provides neuroprotection after onset of clinical symptoms in Huntington's disease transgenic mice. J Neurochem 85.6 (2003): 1359–1367.

Deldicque, L, et al 2008, 'Effects of resistance exercise with and without creatine supplementation on gene expression and cell signaling in human skeletal muscle', J Appl Physiol, vol. 104, no. 2, pp. 371–8.

Deminice, R & Jordao, AA 2012, 'Creatine supplementation reduces oxidative stress biomarkers after acute exercise in rats', Amino Acids, vol. 43, no. 2, pp. 709–15.

Eckerson, JM, et al 2008, 'Effect of thirty days of creatine supplementation with phosphate salts on anaerobic working capacity and body weight in men', J Strength Cond Res, vol. 22, no. 3, pp. 826–32.

Eliot, KA, et al 2008, 'The effects of creatine and whey protein supplementation on body composition in men aged 48 to 72 years during resistance training', J Nutr Health Aging, vol. 12, no. 3, pp. 208–12.

Elm, JJ & Investigators, NN-P 2012, 'Design innovations and baseline findings in a long-term Parkinson's trial: the National Institute of Neurological Disorders and Stroke Exploratory Trials in Parkinson's Disease Long-Term Study-1', Mov Disord, vol. 27, no. 12, pp. 1513–21.

Feldman EB. Creatine: a dietary supplement and ergogenic aid. Nutr Rev 57.2 (1999): 45–50.

Ferguson TB, Syrotuik DG. Effects of creatine monohydrate supplementation on body composition and strength indices in experienced resistance trained women. J Strength Cond Res 20.4 (2006): 939–946.

Ferrante RJ et al. Neuroprotective effects of creatine in a transgenic mouse model of Huntington's disease. J Neurosci 20.12 (2000): 4389–4397.

Finn JP et al. Effect of creatine supplementation on metabolism and performance in humans during intermittent sprint cycling. Eur J Appl Physiol 84.3 (2001): 238–243.

Fukuda, DH, et al 2010, 'The effects of creatine loading and gender on anaerobic running capacity', J Strength Cond Res, vol. 24, no. 7, pp. 1826–33.

Genius, J, et al 2012, 'Creatine protects against excitoxicity in an in vitro model of neurodegeneration', PLoS One, vol. 7, no. 2, p. e30554.

Gilliam JD et al. Effect of oral creatine supplementation on isokinetic torque production. Med Sci Sports Exerc 32.5 (2000): 993–996.

Glaister M et al. Creatine supplementation and multiple sprint running performance. J Strength Cond Res 20.2 (2006): 273–277.

Gordon A et al. Creatine supplementation in chronic heart failure increases skeletal muscle creatine phosphate and muscle performance. Cardiovasc Res 30.3 (1995): 413–418.

Groeneveld JG et al. A randomized sequential trial of creatine in amyotrophic lateral sclerosis. Ann Neurol 53.4 (2003): 437–445.

Gualano B et al. Effects of creatine supplementation on glucose tolerance and insulin sensitivity in sedentary healthy males undergoing aerobic training. Amino Acids 34.2 (2008): 245–250.

Gualano, B., et al 2012. In sickness and in health: the widespread application of creatine supplementation. Amino Acids, 43, (2) 519–529.

Hass CJ, et al. Resistance training with creatine monohydrate improves upper-body strength in patients with Parkinson disease: a randomized trial. Neurorehabil Neural Repair 21.2 (2007): 107–115.

Hersch SM et al. Creatine in Huntington disease is safe, tolerable, bioavailable in brain and reduces serum 8OH2'dG". Neurology 66.2 (2006): 250–252.

Hickner, RC, et al 2010, 'Effect of 28 days of creatine ingestion on muscle metabolism and performance of a simulated cycling road race', J Int Soc Sports Nutr, vol. 7, p. 26.

Hopwood, M.J., et al. 2006. Creatine Supplementation and Swim Performance: A Brief Review. J Sports Sci.Med, 5, (1) 10–24.

Jacobs PL et al. Oral creatine supplementation enhances upper extremity work capacity in persons with cervical-level spinal cord injury. Arch Phys Med Rehabil 83.1 (2002): 19–23.

Jager, R, et al 2008, 'The effects of creatine pyruvate and creatine citrate on performance during high intensity exercise', J Int Soc Sports Nutr, vol. 5, p. 4.

Jager, R, et al 2011, 'Analysis of the efficacy, safety, and regulatory status of novel forms of creatine', Amino Acids, vol. 40, no. 5, pp. 1369–83.

Jagim, AR, et al 2012, 'A buffered form of creatine does not promote greater changes in muscle creatine content, body composition, or training adaptations than creatine monohydrate', J Int Soc Sports Nutr, vol. 9, no. 1, p. 43.

Johnston, AP, et al 2009, 'Effect of creatine supplementation during cast-induced immobilization on the preservation of muscle mass, strength, and endurance', J Strength Cond Res, vol. 23, no. 1, pp. 116–20.

Jowko E et al. Creatine and beta-hydroxy-beta-methylbutyrate (HMB) additively increase lean body mass and muscle strength during a weight-training program. Nutrition 17.7–8 (2001): 558–566.

Juhasz, I, et al 2009, 'Creatine supplementation improves the anaerobic performance of elite junior fin swimmers', Acta Physiol Hung, vol. 96, no. 3, pp. 325–36.

Kendall, KL, et al 2009, 'Effects of four weeks of high-intensity interval training and creatine supplementation on critical power and anaerobic working capacity in college-aged men', J Strength Cond Res, vol. 23, no. 6, pp. 1663–9.

Kim, HJ, et al 2011, 'Studies on the safety of creatine supplementation', Amino Acids, vol. 40, no. 5, pp. 1409–18.

Kley, RA, et al 2011, 'Creatine for treating muscle disorders', Cochrane Database Syst Rev, no. 2, p. CD004760.

Klopstock, T, et al 2011, 'Creatine in mouse models of neurodegeneration and aging', Amino Acids, vol. 40, no. 5, pp. 1297–303.

Kreider RB. Effects of creatine supplementation on performance and training adaptations. Mol Cell Biochem 244.1–2 (2003): 89–94.

Kreider RB et al. Effects of creatine supplementation on body composition, strength, and sprint performance. Med Sci Sports Exerc 30.1 (1998): 73–82.

Kuethe F et al. Creatine supplementation improves muscle strength in patients with congestive heart failure. Pharmazie 61.3 (2006): 218–222.

Lamontagne-Lacasse, M, et al 2011, 'Effect of creatine supplementation on jumping performance in elite volleyball players', Int J Sports Physiol Perform, vol. 6, no. 4, pp. 525–33.

Law, YL, et al 2009, 'Effects of two and five days of creatine loading on muscular strength and anaerobic power in trained athletes', J Strength Cond Res, vol. 23, no. 3, pp. 906–14.

Leader, A, et al 2009, 'An open-label study adding creatine monohydrate to ongoing medical regimens in patients with the fibromyalgia syndrome', Ann N Y Acad Sci, vol. 1173, pp. 829–36.

Ling, J, et al 2009, 'Cognitive effects of creatine ethyl ester supplementation', Behav Pharmacol, vol. 20, no. 8, pp. 673–9.

Longo, N, et al 2011, 'Disorders of creatine transport and metabolism', Am J Med Genet C Semin Med Genet, vol. 157, no. 1, pp. 72–8.

Lopez, RM, et al 2009, 'Does creatine supplementation hinder exercise heat tolerance or hydration status? A systematic review with meta-analyses', J Athl Train, vol. 44, no. 2, pp. 215–23.

Lyoo, IK, et al 2012, 'A randomized, double-blind placebo-controlled trial of oral creatine monohydrate augmentation for enhanced response to a selective serotonin reuptake inhibitor in women with major depressive disorder', Am J Psychiatry, vol. 169, no. 9, pp. 937–45.

Maganaris CN, Maughan RJ. Creatine supplementation enhances maximum voluntary isometric force and endurance capacity in resistance trained men. Acta Physiol Scand 163.3 (1998): 279–287.

Malin, SK, et al 2008, 'Effect of creatine supplementation on muscle capacity in individuals with multiple sclerosis', J Diet Suppl, vol. 5, no. 1, pp. 20–32.

Mazzini L et al. Effects of creatine supplementation on exercise performance and muscular strength in amyotrophic lateral sclerosis: preliminary results. J Neurol Sci 191.1–2 (2001): 139–144.

McMorris T et al. Creatine supplementation and cognitive performance in elderly individuals. Neuropsychol Dev Cogn B Aging Neuropsychol Cogn 14.5 (2007): 517–528.

Mujika I, Padilla S. Creatine supplementation as an ergogenic acid for sports performance in highly trained athletes: a critical review. Int J Sports Med 18.7 (1997): 491–496.

Mujika I et al. Creatine supplementation and sprint performance in soccer players. Med Sci Sports Exerc 32.2 (2000): 518–525.

Ndika, JD, et al 2012, 'Developmental progress and creatine restoration upon long-term creatine supplementation of a patient with arginine:glycine amidinotransferase deficiency', Mol Genet Metab, vol. 106, no. 1, pp. 48–54.

Nemets, B & Levine, J 2013, 'A pilot dose-finding clinical trial of creatine monohydrate augmentation to SSRIs/SNRIs/NASA antidepressant treatment in major depression', Int Clin Psychopharmacol, vol. 28, no. 3, pp. 127–33.

Neves, M, Jr., et al 2011a, 'Beneficial effect of creatine supplementation in knee osteoarthritis', Med Sci Sports Exerc, vol. 43, no. 8, pp. 1538–43.

C

Neves, M, Jr., et al 2011b, 'Effect of creatine supplementation on measured glomerular filtration rate in postmenopausal women', Appl Physiol Nutr Metab, vol. 36, no. 3, pp. 419–22.

Oliver, JM, et al 2013, 'Oral Creatine Supplementation Decreases Blood Lactate during Exhaustive, Incremental Cycling', Int J Sports Physiol Perform. 23: 252–259.

Olsen S et al. Creatine supplementation augments the increase in satellite cell and myonuclei number in human skeletal muscle induced by strength training. J Physiol 573 (Pt 2) (2006): 525–534.

Ostojic SM, Ahmetovic Z. Gastrointestinal distress after creatine supplementation in athletes: are side effects dose dependent? Res Sports Med 16.1 (2008): 15–22.

Patra, S., et al. 2012. A short review on creatine-creatine kinase system in relation to cancer and some experimental results on creatine as adjuvant in cancer therapy. Amino Acids, 42, (6) 2319–2330.

Perasso, L, et al 2013, 'Therapeutic use of creatine in brain or heart ischemia: available data and future perspectives', Med Res Rev, vol. 33, no. 2, pp. 336–63.

Percario, S, et al 2012, 'Effects of creatine supplementation on oxidative stress profile of athletes', J Int Soc Sports Nutr, vol. 9, no. 1, p. 56.

Persky AM, et al. Pharmacokinetics of the dietary supplement creatine. Clin Pharmacokinet 42.6 (2003): 557–574.

Pluim BM et al. The effects of creatine supplementation on selected factors of tennis specific training. Br J Sports Med 40.6 (2006): 507–511; discussion 511–12.

Prass K et al. Improved reperfusion and neuroprotection by creatine in a mouse model of stroke. J Cereb Blood Flow Metab 27.3 (2006): 452–459.

Rae C et al. Oral creatine monohydrate supplementation improves brain performance: a double-blind, placebo-controlled, cross-over trial. Proc Biol Sci 270.1529 (2003): 2147–2150.

Rahimi, R 2011, 'Creatine supplementation decreases oxidative DNA damage and lipid peroxidation induced by a single bout of resistance exercise', J Strength Cond Res, vol. 25, no. 12, pp. 3448–55.

Rawson ES, Volek JS. Effects of creatine supplementation and resistance training on muscle strength and weightlifting performance. J Strength Cond Res 17.4 (2003): 822–831.

Rawson, E.S. & Venezia, A.C. 2011. Use of creatine in the elderly and evidence for effects on cognitive function in young and old. Amino. Acids, 40, (5) 1349–1362.

Rawson, ES & Venezia, AC 2011b, 'Use of creatine in the elderly and evidence for effects on cognitive function in young and old', Amino Acids, vol. 40, no. 5, pp. 1349–62.

Rawson ES et al. Creatine supplementation does not improve cognitive function in young adults. Physiol Behav 95.1–2 (2008): 130–134.

Rawson, ES, et al 2011, 'Low-dose creatine supplementation enhances fatigue resistance in the absence of weight gain', Nutrition, vol. 27, no. 4, pp. 451–5.

Rico-Sanz, J, et al 2008, 'Creatine feeding does not enhance intramyocellular glycogen concentration during carbohydrate loading: an in vivo study by 31P- and 13C-MRS', J Physiol Biochem, vol. 64, no. 3, pp. 189–96.

Rocic, B, et al 2011, 'Comparison of antihyperglycemic effects of creatine and glibenclamide in type II diabetic patients', Wien Med Wochenschr, vol. 161, no. 21–22, pp. 519–23.

Roitman S et al. Creatine monohydrate in resistant depression: a preliminary study. Bipolar Disord 9.7 (2007): 754–758.

Roschel, H, et al. 2010, 'Creatine supplementation spares muscle glycogen during high intensity intermittent exercise in rats', J Int Soc Sports Nutr, vol. 7, no. 1, p. 6.

Rosenfeld, J, et al 2008, 'Creatine monohydrate in ALS: effects on strength, fatigue, respiratory status and ALSFRS', Amyotroph Lateral Scler, vol. 9, no. 5, pp. 266–72.

Royes, LF, et al 2008, 'Neuromodulatory effect of creatine on extracellular action potentials in rat hippocampus: role of NMDA receptors', Neurochem Int, vol. 53, no. 1–2, pp. 33–7.

Safdar, A, et al 2008, 'Global and targeted gene expression and protein content in skeletal muscle of young men following short-term creatine monohydrate supplementation', Physiol Genomics, vol. 32, no. 2, pp. 219–28.

Sahlin, K & Harris, RC 2011, 'The creatine kinase reaction: a simple reaction with functional complexity', Amino Acids, vol. 40, no. 5, pp. 1363–7.

Sakellaris G et al. Prevention of complications related to traumatic brain injury in children and adolescents with creatine administration: an open label randomized pilot study. J Trauma 61.2 (2006): 322–329.

Sakkas, GK, et al 2009, 'Creatine fails to augment the benefits from resistance training in patients with HIV infection: a randomized, double-blind, placebo-controlled study', PLoS One, vol. 4, no. 2, p. e4605.

Saremi, A, et al 2010, 'Effects of oral creatine and resistance training on serum myostatin and GASP-1', Mol Cell Endocrinol, vol. 317, no. 1–2, pp. 25–30.

Sartini, S, et al 2012, 'Creatine affects in vitro electrophysiological maturation of neuroblasts and protects them from oxidative stress', J Neurosci Res, vol. 90, no. 2, pp. 435–46.

Sestili, P, et al 2011, 'Creatine as an antioxidant', Amino Acids, vol. 40, no. 5, pp. 1385–96.

Shao A, Hathcock JN. Risk assessment for creatine monohydrate. Regul Toxicol Pharmacol 45.3 (2006): 242–251.

Shefner JM et al. A clinical trial of creatine in ALS. Neurology 63.9 (2004): 1656–1661.

Shen, H & Goldberg, MP 2012, 'Creatine pretreatment protects cortical axons from energy depletion in vitro', Neurobiol Dis, vol. 47, no. 2, pp. 184–93.

Silva, LA, et al 2013, 'Creatine supplementation does not decrease oxidative stress and inflammation in skeletal muscle after eccentric exercise', J Sports Sci. 31: 1164–1176.

Smith CA et al. Effects of exercise and creatine on myosin heavy chain isoform composition in patients with Charcot-Marie-Tooth disease. Muscle Nerve 34.5 (2006): 586–594.

Spillane, M, et al 2009, 'The effects of creatine ethyl ester supplementation combined with heavy resistance training on body composition, muscle performance, and serum and muscle creatine levels', J Int Soc Sports Nutr, vol. 6, p. 6.

Spriet LL, Gibala MJ. Nutritional strategies to influence adaptations to training. J Sports Sci 22.1 (2004): 127–141.

Sterkowicz, S, et al 2012, 'The effects of training and creatine malate supplementation during preparation period on physical capacity and special fitness in judo contestants', J Int Soc Sports Nutr, vol. 9, no. 1, p. 41.

Stone MH et al. Effects of in-season (5 weeks) creatine and pyruvate supplementation on anaerobic performance and body composition in American football players. Int J Sport Nutr 9.2 (1999): 146–165.

Stout JR et al. Effects of creatine supplementation on the onset of neuromuscular fatigue threshold and muscle strength in elderly men and women (64–86 years). J Nutr Health Aging 11.6 (2007): 459–464.

Syrotuik DG, Bell GJ. Acute creatine monohydrate supplementation: a descriptive physiological profile of responders vs nonresponders. J Strength Cond Res 18.3 (2004): 610–6117.

Tarnopolsky, MA 2011, 'Creatine as a therapeutic strategy for myopathies', Amino Acids, vol. 40, no. 5, pp. 1397–407.

Tarnopolsky MA, MacLennan DP. Creatine monohydrate supplementation enhances high-intensity exercise performance in males and females. Int J Sport Nutr Exerc Metab 10.4 (2000): 452–463.

Valastro, B, et al 2009, 'Oral creatine supplementation attenuates L-DOPA-induced dyskinesia in 6-hydroxydopamine-lesioned rats', Behav Brain Res, vol. 197, no. 1, pp. 90–6.

Valayannopoulos, V, et al 2012, 'Treatment by oral creatine, L-arginine and L-glycine in six severely affected patients with creatine transporter defect', J Inherit Metab Dis, vol. 35, no. 1, pp. 151–7.

van de Kamp, JM, et al 2012, 'Long-term follow-up and treatment in nine boys with X-linked creatine transporter defect', J Inherit Metab Dis, vol. 35, no. 1, pp. 141–9.

Veggi, KF, et al 2013, 'Oral Creatine Supplementation Augments the Repeated Bout Effect', Int J Sport Nutr Exerc Metab. 23: 378–387.

Volek JS, Rawson ES. Scientific basis and practical aspects of creatine supplementation for athletes. Nutrition 20.7–8 (2004): 609–614.

Walter, AA, et al 2008, 'Effects of creatine loading on electromyographic fatigue threshold in cycle ergometry in college-age men', Int J Sport Nutr Exerc Metab, vol. 18, no. 2, pp. 142–51.

Watanabe A, et al. Effects of creatine on mental fatigue and cerebral hemoglobin oxygenation. Neurosci Res 42.4 (2002): 279–285.

Williams MH, Branch JD. Creatine supplementation and exercise performance: an update. J Am Coll Nutr 17.3 (1998): 216–234.

Wright GA, et al. The effects of creatine loading on thermoregulation and intermittent sprint exercise performance in a hot humid environment. J Strength Cond Res 21.3 (2007): 655–660.

Wyss M, Schulze A. Health implications of creatine: can oral creatine supplementation protect against neurological and atherosclerotic disease? Neuroscience 112.2 (2002): 243–260.

Wyss M et al. The therapeutic potential of oral creatine supplementation in muscle disease. Med Hypotheses 51.4 (1998): 333–336.

Yang, L, et al 2009, 'Combination therapy with coenzyme Q10 and creatine produces additive neuroprotective effects in models of Parkinson's and Huntington's diseases', J Neurochem, vol. 109, no. 5, pp. 1427–39.

Damiana

HISTORICAL NOTE Damiana is a wild deciduous shrub found in the arid and semiarid regions of South America, Mexico, the United States and West Indies. It is believed that Mayan Indians used damiana to prevent giddiness, falling and loss of balance, and as an aphrodisiac. It has also been used during childbirth, and to treat colic, stop bedwetting and bring on suppressed menses. Today its leaves are used for flavouring in food and beverages, and infusions and other preparations are used for a variety of medicinal purposes.

COMMON NAME

Damiana

OTHER NAMES

Herba de la pastora, Mexican damiana, miziboc, old woman's broom, shepherd's herb, stag's herb

BOTANICAL NAME/FAMILY

Turnera diffusa, *Damiana aphrodisiaca*, *Turnera aphrodisiaca* (family Turneraceae)

PLANT PARTS USED

Dried leaves and stems

CHEMICAL COMPONENTS

Alkaloids, flavonoids, arbutin (a glycosylated hydroquinone), essential oils containing caryophyllene, delta-cadinene, beta-elemene and 1,8-cineole and other lesser constituents, tetraphylin B (a cyanogenic glycoside, 0.26%), resin, tannins, gum, mucilage, starch, a bitter element and possibly caffeine (Piacente et al 2002, Zhao et al 2007).

MAIN ACTIONS

Hormonal effects

One study that investigated the effects of over 150 herbs for their relative capacity to compete with oestradiol and progesterone binding to intracellular receptors identified damiana as a herb that binds to intracellular progesterone receptors, exerting a neutral effect and also exerting weak oestrogen agonist activity (Zava et al 1998). It has been reported that delta-cadinene is a testosterone inducer and 1,8-cineole is a testosterone hydroxylase inducer (Duke 2006).

A study analysing the constituents of the essential oils found in various damiana samples identified that fresh and dry samples contained both compounds, but wild plants contained more delta-cadinene than cultivated plants (Alcaraz-Melendez et al 2004). The action of these constituents may support the common belief that damiana is useful as an aphrodisiac. An in vitro study assaying the antiaromatase activity of a methanolic extract of damiana found a dose-dependent inhibitory effect on aromatase enzyme. The isolates pinocembrin and acacetin (flavonoids) were the most potent inhibitors of 24 compounds isolated from the methanolic extract. Further studies are required to verify if these findings can be replicated in vivo (Zhao et al 2008).

Hypoglycaemic agent

A decoction of dried damiana leaves caused a significant reduction of the hyperglycaemic peak, exerting a hypoglycaemic effect comparable to that of tolbutamide in an experimental model (Alarcon-Aguilara et al 1998).

OTHER ACTIONS

Anxiolytic activity

An animal model investigated the antianxiety effects of damiana in mice exposed to the elevated pulse maze. A methanolic extract was found to exhibit anxiolytic activity at a dose of 25 mg/kg (Kumar & Shumar 2005). A further preclinical study using an apigenin (flavone) fraction derived from damiana demonstrated anxiolytic effects in mice exposed to various animal models of anxiety (Kumar et al 2008).

CLINICAL USE

Damiana has not been significantly investigated under clinical trial conditions; therefore, evidence is derived from traditional use, in vitro and animal studies, and its clinical significance is unknown.

Sexual dysfunction or decreased libido

Damiana has been used traditionally for sexual dysfunction or as an aphrodisiac to enhance sexual activity. Scientific studies in experimental models provide preliminary support for its use in these conditions, but controlled trials testing damiana as a stand-alone treatment are lacking. One in vivo study established that damiana fluid extract significantly improves the copulatory performance of sexually sluggish animals, but has no effect on normally functioning ones (Arletti et al 1999). The effect appears to be dose-dependent, as positive results were obtained only when the highest dose was administered.

A study investigating the effects of damiana on sexually exhausted male rats showed a significant increase in proportion of copulating animals following a single oral dose of damiana aqueous extract (80 mg/kg), with a significantly reduced postejaculatory interval (Estrada-Reyes et al 2009). It is thought the prosexual effects are exerted via the nitric oxide pathway and anxiolytic-like effects (Estrada-Reyes et al 2013).

IN COMBINATION

In an randomised controlled trial involving 78 men suffering from mild to moderate erectile dysfunction, oral treatment with a multi-herb preparation containing *Turnera diffusa, Panax ginseng, Serenoa repens, Crataegus rivularis, Ginkgo biloba, Tribulus terrestris, Erythroxylum catuaba, Cuscuta chinensis, Epimedium sagittatum* and bioperine resulted in significantly improved erectile function scores after 12 weeks of treatment (Shah et al 2012).

Another clinical study of unknown design compared a herbal combination product consisting of ginseng, ginkgo, damiana, l-arginine and a variety of vitamins and minerals with placebo in 77 female volunteers. After 4 weeks, 73.5% of the women in the treatment group reported an increase in sexual satisfaction compared with 37.2% receiving placebo (Ito et al 2001). Although promising, the role of damiana in achieving this result is unknown.

Diabetes

Although in vivo studies suggest significant hypoglycaemic activity, no clinical studies are available to determine whether the effects are clinically significant.

Weight loss

No controlled studies are available to determine the effectiveness of damiana as a stand-alone treatment in weight loss; however, one study that used a combination of herbs that included damiana has produced positive results. The randomised, double-blind study involving 47 overweight subjects tested a herbal combination product known as YGD (*Yerba mate, Paullinia cupana* and damiana) for weight loss activity. Treatment resulted in a prolonged gastric emptying time and a body weight reduction of 5.1 ± 0.5 kg compared with 0.3 ± 0.08 kg after placebo over 45 days. A 12-month follow-up revealed that weight loss was maintained in the active treatment group (Andersen & Fogh 2001). A further double-blind, placebo-controlled crossover study on the YGD formulation revealed a decrease in food intake and energy intake in female subjects, suggesting an effect on in-meal satiation. The same study showed an increased amount of satiation following administration of YGD and a soluble fermentable fibre together (Harrold et al 2013). Until studies using damiana as sole therapy are conducted, the effectiveness of this herb in weight loss is still unknown.

OTHER USES

In practice, damiana is sometimes used to treat anxiety and depression associated with hormonal changes (e.g. menopause) or where there is a sexual factor involved. It is also used as a mild stimulant and aphrodisiac, to enhance stamina generally and for nervous dyspepsia and constipation.

DOSAGE RANGE

- Dried leaf: 2–4 g taken three times daily.
- Infusion: pour a cup of boiling water on to one teaspoonful of the dried leaves and let infuse for 10–15 min. Drink three cups daily.
- Liquid extract (1 : 2) or solid-dose equivalent: 20–40 mL/week or 3–6 mL/day.

D

ADVERSE REACTIONS

There is insufficient reliable information available.

SIGNIFICANT INTERACTIONS

Controlled studies are not available; therefore, interactions are based on evidence of activity and are largely theoretical and speculative.

Hypoglycaemic agents

Additive effects are theoretically possible, with unknown clinical significance — observe patients.

CONTRAINDICATIONS AND PRECAUTIONS

Traditionally, the herb is not recommended for people with overactive sympathetic nervous system activity.

PREGNANCY USE

Safety in pregnancy has not been scientifically evaluated; however, no increase in fetal abnormalities has been observed from limited use in women (Mills & Bone 2005).

Practice points/Patient counselling

- Damiana is a herb with a traditional reputation as being an aphrodisiac, stimulant, mood enhancer and general tonic.
- Currently, evidence to support its use as an aphrodisiac is limited to research in animals, which has produced some positive results.
- In vivo studies have identified significant anti-inflammatory and hypoglycaemic activity, although human studies are still required to determine clinical significance.
- It is also suspected that the herb exerts some degree of hormonal activity.

PATIENTS' FAQs

What will this herb do for me?

Damiana has not been significantly tested in human studies, so much information is taken from traditional sources or preliminary research in animals. According to these sources, it may increase sexual function and libido in some cases of dysfunction, lower blood glucose levels and exert anti-inflammatory actions.

When will it start to work?

There is insufficient evidence to predict when effects may develop.

Are there any safety issues?

A long history of use suggests it is generally safe. However, scientific testing has not been conducted.

REFERENCES

Alarcon-Aguilara FJ et al. Study of the anti-hyperglycemic effect of plants used as antidiabetics. J Ethnopharmacol 61.2 (1998): 101–110.

Alcaraz-Melendez L, et al. Analysis of essential oils from wild and micropropagated plants of damiana (*Turnera diffusa*). Fitoterapia 75 (2004): 696–701.

Andersen T, Fogh J. Weight loss and delayed gastric emptying following a South American herbal preparation in overweight patients. J Hum Nutr Diet 14.3 (2001): 243–250.

Arletti R et al. Stimulating property of *Turnera diffusa* and *Pfaffia paniculata* extracts on the sexual behavior of male rats. Psychopharmacology (Berl) 143.1 (1999): 15–119.

Duke JA. Dr Duke's Phytochemical and Ethnobotanical Databases. Beltsville, MD: US Department of Agriculture–Agricultural Research Service–National Germplasm Resources Laboratory, Beltsville Agricultural Research Center. www.ars-grin.gov/duke/ (accessed January 2006).

Estrada-Reyes R et al. *Turnera diffusa* Wild (Tunreraceae) recovers sexual behavior in sexually exhausted males. Journal of Ethnopharmacology 123 (2009): 423–429.

Estrada Reyes R, et al. Pro-sexual effects of *Turnera diffusa* Wild (Turneraceae) in male rats involves the nitric oxide pathway. Journal of Ethnopharmacology 146 (2013): 164–172.

Harrold et al. Acute effects of a herb extract formulation and inulin fibre on appetite, energy intake and food choice. Appetite 62 (2013): 84–90.

Ito TY, et al. A double-blind placebo-controlled study of ArginMax, a nutritional supplement for enhancement of female sexual function. J Sex Marital Ther 27.5 (2001): 541–549.

Kumar S & Sharma A. Anti-anxiety activity studies of various extracts of *Turnera aphrodisiaca* Ward. Journal of Herbal Pharmacotherapy 5.4 (2005):13–21.

Kumar S, et al. Pharmacological evaluation of bioactive principle of *Turnera aphrodisiaca*. Indian Journal of Pharmaceutical Sciences 70.6 (2008):740–744.

Mills S, Bone K. The essential guide to herbal safety. St Louis, MO: Churchill Livingstone, 2005.

Piacente S et al. Flavonoids and arbutin from *Turnera diffusa*. Z Naturforsch [C] 57.11–12 (2002): 983–985.

Shah et al. Evaluation of a multi-herb supplement for erectile dysfunction: a randomized double-blind, placebo-controlled study. BMC Complementary & Alternative Medicine 12 (2012); 155–163.

Zava DT, et al. Estrogen and progestin bioactivity of foods, herbs, and spices. Proc Soc Exp Biol Med 217.3 (1998): 369–378.

Zhao J et al. Phytochemical investigation of *Turnera diffusa*. J. Nat. Prod. 70 (2007): 289–292.

Zhao J et al. Anti-aromatase activity of the constituents from damiana (*Turnera diffusa*). Journal of Ethnopharmacology 120 (2008): 387–393.

Dandelion

HISTORICAL NOTE Dandelion grows as a perennial native herb throughout the Northern Hemisphere and as a weed in other temperate zones. It has a long history of medicinal and culinary use. Dandelion is an entirely edible plant (Gonzales-Castejon et al 2012). Its leaves are added to salads, providing a good source of minerals, and the roasted root is used as a coffee substitute. In Europe, dandelion flowers were used for the preparation of drinks and salads (Mlcek & Rop 2011), and particular extracts used as flavourings in various dairy desserts, baked goods, candy gelatins, puddings and cheese (Gonzales-Castejon et al 2012). Traditionally, dandelion leaves are used as a diuretic, and the root as a liver tonic. This use has no doubt led to its trivial names *pissenlit* (French) and *piscialetto* (Italian) both hinting at its property of enuresis provocation (Gonzales-Castejon et al 2012).

OTHER NAMES

Blowball, cankerwort, common dandelion, lion's tooth, priest's crown, puffball, swine snout, taraxacum, wild endive, white endive

BOTANICAL NAME/FAMILY

Taraxacum officinale Weber; synonyms: *Leontodon taraxacum*, *Taraxacum vulgare* (family Compositae [Asteraceae])

PLANT PARTS USED

Leaf, root and flowers (used less commonly)

CHEMICAL COMPONENTS

Nutritionally, dandelion is a particularly rich source of potassium (Hook et al 1993, Gonzales-Castejon et al 2012), as well as iron, magnesium, zinc, manganese, copper, choline, selenium, calcium, boron and silicon (Queralt et al 2005), and a rich source of vitamins A, C, D and B complex (US Department of Agriculture 2003). It is one of the richest green-vegetable sources of β-carotene (Gonzales-Castejon et al 2012). The relatively high protein, fibre and linoleic acid content of dandelion leaves has led to suggestions that dandelion is a nutritious and underutilised food source (Escudero et al 2003). Dandelion's constituents also include sugars and mucilage (Blumenthal et al 2000).

Seasonal variations, soil composition, growing location, companion plants, fungi and insects may result in phytochemical variations in dandelion (Romm et al 2010b).

The major phytochemical groups identified in dandelion are terpenes, phenolic compounds and storage carbohydrates. Some phytochemicals are found in all parts of the planet (i.e. the phenolic caffeic acid); however, some are unique to a single plant part. The root contains at least nine different sesquiterpene lactones (anti-inflammatory and anti-microbial properties), nine different triterpenes and phytosterols (promote reduced cholesterol absorption), at least twelve different phenolic acids (immunostimulatory properties), three different coumarins (cardiovascular system actions) and the prebiotic-acting, oligosaccharide soluble fibre inulin (Gonzales-Castejon et al 2012). The levels of inulin in dandelion root range from 2% to 40% from spring to autumn (Romm et al 2010b). Dandelion leaves and stems contain two sesquiterpene lactones, three triterpenes, five phenolic acids, five different flavonoids with antioxidant properties and two coumarins. There are numerous xanthophylls within dandelion leaf, with particularly high levels of lutein (Znidarcic 2011). Dandelion flowers contain three different phenolic acids and four flavonoids (Gonzales-Castejon et al 2012).

MAIN ACTIONS

Diuretic

Dandelion leaf has been found to have a greater diuretic effect than the roots, with activity comparable to that of frusemide, without causing potassium loss because of the leaves' high potassium content (Newell et al 1996). A small clinical trial confirmed oral intake of dandelion leaf extract significantly increases urinary output (Clare et al 2009). Dandelion root does not appear to have the same diuretic effect according to research with animal models using an infusion of the root (Grases et al 1994), and no secondary metabolites showing major diuretic activity were found (Hook et al 1993).

Choleretic

The bitter constituents in dandelion root are believed to be responsible for increasing bile production and flow, as well as contributing to the root's mild laxative effects.

Hepatic enzyme induction

In vivo studies have demonstrated decreased activity of CYP1A2 and CYP2E enzymes and dramatic increases in levels of the phase II detoxifying enzyme UDP-glucuronosyltransferase in liver microsomes of rats receiving dandelion tea (Maliakal & Wanwimolruk 2001). The same study found that dandelion tea had no effect on the activities of CYP2D and CYP3A.

Anti-inflammatory

Dandelion extract exhibited a mild analgesic and anti-inflammatory effect in vivo (Tito et al 1993). Dandelion influences inflammatory mediators (TNF-alpha, COX-2, IL-1, iNOS) in leucocytes (root methanol extract), astrocytes (leaf extract) and macrophages (isolated polyphenols) in vitro. Dandelion ethanolic, aqueous and methanolic extracts have been found to inhibit inflammatory cytokines in vivo. (Gonzales-Castejon et al 2012).

Antioxidant activity

Dandelion flower, root, stems and leaf extracts demonstrate antioxidant activity in a number of preclinical models (Cho et al 2002, Colle 2012, Kaurinovic et al 2003, Liu et al 2010, Yanghee 2010).

Dandelion flower extract demonstrated marked antioxidant activity that has been attributed to its phenolic content, with suppression of reactive oxygen species and nitric oxide (Hu & Kitts 2003, 2005, Kery et al 2004). Dandelion aqueous extract demonstrated antioxidant activity in a diabetic rat model, preventing diabetic complications due to lipid peroxidation and excessive free radicals (Cho et al 2002), and in a model of acute lung injury (Liu et al 2010). Aqueous extract of dandelion root provided protection against the development of alcoholic liver disease by increasing antioxidant capacity (Yanghee 2010). The leaf extract also protected against paracetamol-induced hepatoxicity via an antioxidant mechanism (Colle 2012).

Anti-Cancer Activity

Traditional medicines of China, Arabia and Native America all use the plants of the genus *Taraxacum* (dandelions) to treat a variety of diseases, including cancer. An extract of dandelion leaf (but not root or flowers) has been demonstrated to decrease the growth of MCF-7/AZ breast cancer cells in vitro, suggesting that it may be of value as an anticancer agent. There is preliminary scientific evidence from animal and in vitro studies that suggest the roots of *Taraxacum japonicum* (Japanese dandelion) may have a cancer-preventive effect. The extract has been shown to induce cytotoxicity through TNF-alpha and IL-1-alpha secretion in vitro. The ethanol extract of dried, arial *Taraxacum officinalis* (n-butanol fraction (BuOH)) exhibited potent anti-angiogenic activity. The flavonoid luteolin is one of the key constituents responsible for the activity (Jeon et al 2008), and is particularly potent in inhibiting hepatocellular carcinoma cells (Stagos et al 2012). Furthermore, aqueous extract of dandelion root contains compounds which selectively induce apoptosis in human leukaemia cells in vitro (Ovadje et al 2011).

OTHER ACTIONS

Traditionally, dandelion root is understood to have laxative activity and to stimulate digestion, whereas dandelion leaf has antirheumatic effects. Dandelion root infusion, which contains oligofructans, has been found to stimulate the growth of multiple strains of bifidobacteria, suggesting its use as a prebiotic (Trojanova et al 2004). Possible hypolipidaemic effects were suggested in a cholesterol study of rabbits fed dandelion leaf and roots (Ung-Kyu 2010).

Dandelion may have antidiabetic actions because ethanolic extracts of whole dandelion exhibited insulin secretagogue activity (Hussain et al 2004).

Three peptides purified from *Taraxacum officinalis* flowers have been discovered which display strong antifungal and antibacterial properties. The peptides are cationic and cysteine-rich, and represent two novel families of plant antimicrobial peptides, evidently evolved to protect the plant from fungal and microbial invasion (Astafieva 2012).

Dose-dependent activity was observed against the replication of a pseudotyped HIV-1 in test tube studies using an aqueous extract of the entire dandelion plant (Han et al 2011).

CLINICAL USE

The therapeutic effectiveness of dandelion has not been significantly investigated under clinical trial conditions, so evidence is derived from traditional, in vitro and animal studies.

Diuretic

Dandelion has a long history of use as a diuretic in well-established systems of traditional medicines; however, the scientific and clinical evidence to support this use is limited to animal studies (see above). The high potassium content of dandelion is considered to be partly responsible for any diuretic activity (Hook et al 1993). A significant increase in the frequency of urination ($P < 0.05$) has been confirmed in a small study ($n = 17$) which gave volunteers 8 mL TDS of 1:1 high quality hydroethanolic dandelion leaf extract in a single day and compared urinary output to the previous 2 days. The effect was apparent within the 5-hour period immediately after the first dose, indicating relatively quick-acting effects. There was also a significant ($P < 0.001$) increase in the volume of urine within the 5-hour period after the second dose of extract.

IN COMBINATION

A double-blind RCT of 57 women with recurrent cystitis found that a commercial preparation known as Uva-E (a combination of bearberry leaves and dandelion root) significantly reduced the frequency of recurrence of cystitis compared with placebo. At the end of 12 months, none of the patients taking Uva-E had a recurrence of cystitis, compared with 23% recurrence in the control group ($P < 0.05$) (Larsson et al 1993). The role of dandelion in achieving this result is unknown; however, the researchers suggested that its diuretic effect was likely to have contributed to the positive results.

Liver tonic

Dandelion root has a long history of use as a liver tonic (Macia et al 2005); however, the scientific and clinical evidence to support this use is limited. Preliminary studies suggest that dandelion root stimulates the flow of bile.

Commission E approves the use of dandelion root and herb for disturbances in bile flow, loss of appetite and dyspepsia (Blumenthal et al 2000).

European Scientific Co-Operative on Phytotherapy (ESCOP 2003) recommends dandelion root for 'restoration of hepatic and biliary function, dyspepsia, and loss of appetite'.

OTHER USES

Dandelion has been used traditionally as a source of minerals and for treating diabetes, rheumatic conditions, heartburn, bruises and for recurrent hives, urticaria and eczema. It has also been used to treat various digestive complaints, such as dyspepsia, lack of appetite and constipation (Newell et al 1996), as well as for breast and uterine cancers (Koo et al 2004). The sap has been used topically on warts (Guarrera 2005).

DOSAGE RANGE

Leaf

- Infusion of dried herb: 4–10 g three times daily.
- Fluid extract (25%): 4–10 mL three times daily.
- Fresh juice: 10–20 mL three times daily.

Root

- Decoction of dried root: 2–8 g three times daily.
- Tincture (1:5): 5–10 mL three times daily.
- Fluid extract (30%): 2–8 mL three times daily.
- Juice of fresh root: 4–8 mL three times daily.

According to clinical studies

Diuresis: 8 mL three times daily for a 1:1 hydroethanolic extract of dandelion leaf.

ADVERSE REACTIONS

Dandelion is generally considered safe when consumed in amounts commonly found in foods. Side effects are rare, and the likelihood of dandelion leaf preparations causing a contact allergy is low. However, cross-reactivity may exist between dandelion and other members of the Compositae (Asteraceae) family, such as ragweed, mugwort, sunflower, daisy and chamomile (Cohen et al 1979, Fernandez et al 1993, Jovanovic et al 2004). The most common type of allergy to dandelion is dermatitis following direct skin contact. Contact allergy to herbal teas derived from the plant family was investigated in patients allergic to sesquiterpene lactones (SLs). Ninety per cent had positive test reactions to the Compositae teas, mainly to those based on dandelion, German chamomile and wormwood. Children with a family or personal history of atopy, summer-related or -exacerbated dermatitis of any kind may be more sensitive to exposure to Compositae weeds, especially dandelions.

Avoid in patients with hypersensitivity/allergy to dandelion or other member of the Asteraceae family.

SIGNIFICANT INTERACTIONS

Controlled studies are not available; therefore, interactions are based on evidence of activity and are largely theoretical and speculative.

Diuretic agents

Dandelion leaf may theoretically potentiate the diuretic effect of pharmaceutical diuretics—observe.

D

Quinolone antibiotics

The high mineral content of dandelion may result in the formation of chelate complexes with quinolone antibiotics and reduce their absorption and bioavailability. This has been demonstrated in rats with *Taraxacum mongolicum* (Chinese dandelion) (Zhu et al 1999). While the clinical significance of this is unknown, it is recommended to avoid concomitant use of these substances or to separate their dosing.

Practice points/Patient counselling

- Dandelion leaf and root have a long tradition of culinary and medicinal use.
- Dandelion has been traditionally used as a diuretic and liver tonic. It has also been used to treat various digestive complaints such as dyspepsia, lack of appetite and constipation.
- The therapeutic effectiveness of dandelion has not been significantly investigated under clinical trial conditions, so evidence is derived from traditional, in vitro and animal studies.
- Dandelion is generally considered to be safe and non-toxic, but may cause allergy in people allergic to ragweed and daisies.

CONTRAINDICATIONS AND PRECAUTIONS

It is recommended that dandelion not be used by people with obstruction of the bile ducts or other serious diseases of the gall bladder (Blumenthal et al 2000).

PREGNANCY USE

Based on a long history of use in traditional medicine, dandelion is generally considered safe in pregnancy and lactation (Blumenthal et al 2000, McGuffin et al 1997). Dandelion root and leaf is used for various complaints, such as digestive issues, diuretics and iron support during pregnancy (Romm et al 2010a).

PATIENTS' FAQs

What will this do for me?

In practice, dandelion is used to improve digestion and detoxification, as a diuretic and laxative and to treat diabetes, rheumatic conditions, heartburn, bruises and for recurrent hives, urticaria and eczema. Controlled studies are not available to determine its effectiveness in these conditions.

When will it work?

Stimulation of digestive processes is thought to occur rapidly after one dose.

Are there any safety issues?

Dandelion is generally considered to be safe and non-toxic but may cause allergy in people allergic to ragweed and daisies.

Does the roasted dandelion root drink have the same properties?

Heating will affect some constituents in the root, however as no studies have been performed on the roasted dandelion root, it is not possible to comment on its therapeutic effect.

REFERENCES

Astafieva A et al Discovery of novel antimicrobial peptides with unusual cysteine motifs in dandelion Taraxacum officinale Wigg. Flowers. Peptides 36 (2012): 266–271.

Blumenthal M et al (eds) Herbal medicine: expanded commission E monographs. Austin, TX: Integrative Medicine Communications, 2000.

Cho SY et al. Alternation of hepatic antioxidant enzyme activities and lipid profile in streptozotocin-induced diabetic rats by supplementation of dandelion water extract. Clin Chim Acta 317.1–2 (2002): 109–117.

Clare BA et al. The diuretic effect in human sujects of an extract of Taraxacum officinale folium over a single day, J Alt Comp Med 15.8 (2009): 929–34.

Cohen SH et al. Acute allergic reaction after composite pollen ingestion. J Allergy Clin Immunol 64.4 (1979): 270–274.

Colle D et al. Antioxidant properties of Taraxacum officinale leaf extract are involved in the protective effect against hepatoxicity induced by acetaminophen in mice. J Med Food. 15.6 (2012): 549–56.

ESCOP. European Scientific Co-operative on Phytomedicine, 2nd edn. Stuttgart: Thieme, 2003.

Escudero NL et al. Taraxacum officinale as a food source. Plant Foods Hum Nutr 58.3 (2003): 1–110.

Fernandez Martin-Esteban CM et al. Analysis of cross-reactivity between sunflower pollen and other pollens of the Compositae family. J Allergy Clin Immunol 92.5 (1993): 660–667.

González-Castejón M et al. Diverse biological activities of dandelion. Nutrition Reviews 70.9 (2012): 534–547.

Grases F et al. Urolithiasis and phytotherapy. Int Urol Nephrol 26.5 (1994): 507–511.

Guarrera PM. Traditional phytotherapy in Central Italy (Marche, Abruzzo, and Latium). Fitoterapia 76.1 (2005): 1–25.

Han H et al. Inhibitory effect of aqueous Dandelion extract on HIV-1 replication and reverse transcriptase activity, BMC Complement Altern Med. Nov 14.11 (2011): 112.

Hook I et al. Evaluation of dandelion for diuretic activity and variation in potassium content. Int J Pharmacog 31.1 (1993): 29–34.

Hu C, Kitts DD. Antioxidant, prooxidant, and cytotoxic activities of solvent-fractionated dandelion (Taraxacum officinale) flower extracts in vitro. J Agric Food Chem 51.1 (2003): 301–310.

Hu C, Kitts DD. Dandelion (Taraxacum officinale) flower extract suppresses both reactive oxygen species and nitric oxide and prevents lipid oxidation in vitro. Phytomedicine 12.8 (2005): 588–597.

Hussain ZA et al. The effect of medicinal plants of Islamabad and Murree region of Pakistan on insulin secretion from INS-1 cells. Phytother Res 18.1 (2004): 73–77.

Jeon Hye-Jin et al. Anti-inflammatory activity of Taraxacum officinale. Journal of Ethnopharmacology 115 (2008): 82–88.

Jovanovic MA et al. Sesquiterpene lactone mix patch testing supplemented with dandelion extract in patients with allergic contact dermatitis, atopic dermatitis and non-allergic chronic inflammatory skin diseases. Contact Dermatitis 51.3 (2004): 101–110.

Kaurinovic B et al. Effects of Calendula officinalis L. and Taraxacum officinale Weber (Asteraceae) extracts on the production of OH radicals. Fresenius Environ Bull 12.2 (2003): 250–253.

Kery A et al. Free radical scavenger and lipid peroxidation inhibiting effects of medicinal plants used in phytotherapy. Acta Pharm Hung 74.3 (2004): 158–165.

Koo H-N et al. Taraxacum officinale induces cytotoxicity through TNF-[alpha] and IL-1[alpha] secretion in Hep G2 cells. Life Sci 74.9 (2004): 1149–1157.

Larsson B et al. Prophylactic effect of Uva-E in women with recurrent cystitis: a preliminary report. Curr Ther Res 53.4 (1993): 441–443.

Liu L et al. Taraxacum officinale protects against lipopolysaccharide-induced injury in mice. J Ethnopharmacology 130 (2010): 392–397.

Macia MJ et al. An ethnobotanical survey of medicinal plants commercialized in the markets of La Paz and El Alto, Bolivia. J Ethnopharmacol 97.2 (2005): 337–350.

Maliakal PP, Wanwimolruk S. Effect of herbal teas on hepatic drug metabolizing enzymes in rats. J Pharm Pharmacol 53.10 (2001): 1323–9.

McGuffin M (ed). American Herbal Products Association's botanical safety handbook. Boca Raton, FL: CRC Press, 1997, p. 114.

Mlcek J, Rop O. Fresh edible flowers of ornamental plants – A new source of nutraceutical foods, Trends in Food Science & Technology 22 (2011): 561–569.

Newell CA, Anderson LA, Phillipson JD. Herbal medicines: a guide for health care professionals. London, UK: The Pharmaceutical Press, 1996.
Ovadje P et al. Selective induction of apoptosis through activation of caspase-8 in human leukemia cells (Jurkat) by dandelion root extract. Journal of Ethnopharmacology 133 (2011): s86–91.
Queralt I et al. Quantitative determination of essential and trace element content of medicinal plants and their infusions by XRF and ICF techniques. X-Ray Spectrometry 34.3 (2005): 213–217.
Romm A et al. Botanical Medicine for Women's Health, Churchill Livingstone (2010).
Romm A et al. Fundamental Principles of Herbal Medicine, Botanical Medicine for Women's Health, Churchill Livingstone (2010).
Stagos D et al. Chemoprevention of liver cancer by plant polyphenols, Food and Chemical Toxicology, 50.6 (2012): 2155–2170.
Tito B et al. Taraxacum officinale W: pharmacological effect of ethanol extract. Pharmacol Res 27 (Supp 1) (1993): 23–24.
Trojanova I et al. The bifidogenic effect of Taraxacum officinale root. Fitoterapia 75.7–8 (2004): 760–763.
Ung-Kyu Choi et al. Hypolipidemic and Antioxidant Effects of Dandelion (Taraxacum officinale) Root and Leaf on Cholesterol-Fed Rabbits, Int J Mol Sci. 2010 January; 11(1): 67–78.
US Department of Agriculture. Phytochemical Database. Agricultural Research Service–National Germplasm Resources Laboratory. Beltsville, MD: Beltsville Agricultural Research Center, 2003.
Yanghee You et al, In vitro and in vivo hepatoprotective effects of the aqueous extract from Taraxacum officinale (dandelion) root against alcohol-induced oxidative stress. Food and Chemical Toxicology 48 (2010): 1632–1637.
Zhu M, Wong PY, Li RC. Effects of taraxacum mongolicum on the bioavailability and disposition of ciprofloxacin in rats. J Pharm Sci 88.6 (1999): 632–634.
Znidarcic D, Ban D, Sircelj H, Carotenoid and chlorophyll composition of commonly consumed leafy vegetables in Mediterranean countries. Food Chemistry 129 (2011): 1164–1168.

Devil's claw

HISTORICAL NOTE The botanical name *Harpagophytum* means 'hook plant' in Greek, after the hook-covered fruits of the plant. Devil's claw is native to southern Africa and has been used traditionally as a bitter tonic for digestive disturbances, febrile illnesses and allergic reactions, and to relieve pain (Mills & Bone 2000). It has been used in Europe for the treatment of rheumatic conditions for over 50 years, and was first cited in the literature by Zorn at the University of Jena, Germany, who described his observations on the antiphlogistic and anti-arthritic effects after administration of oral aqueous extracts prepared from the secondary roots of *H. procumbens* in patients suffering from arthritides (Chrubasik et al 2006).

COMMON NAMES

Devil's claw root, grapple plant, harpagophytum, wood spider

BOTANICAL NAME/FAMILY

Harpagophytum procumbens (family Pedaliaceae)

The closely related *H. zeyheri* and *H. procumbens* are collectively known as devil's claw and have been used interchangeably. However, *H. zeyheri* has a lower concentration of the biologically active constituents. Sometimes it is included in raw materials and products as an adulterant of *H. procumbens*, the preferred species of commerce (Mncgwangi et al 2014).

Plant Part Used

Dried tuber/roots. Forms used include dried raw materials, aqueous and ethanol extracts, aqueous-ethanol extracts standardised for harpagocide content, and powdered dry herb tablets (Mncgwangi et al 2012).

Chemical Components

The major active constituent is considered to be the bitter iridoid glycoside, harpagoside (8-cinnamoyl harpagide), which should constitute not less than 1.2% of the dried herb (Georgiev et al 2013). Other iridoid glycosides include harpagide, procumbide, 8-O-(p-coumaroyl)-harpagide and verbascoside, and a newly discovered minor constituent, tentatively identified as methoxypagoside (Karioti et al 2011).

About 50% of the herb consists of sugars. There are also triterpenes, phytosterols, plant phenolic acids, flavonol glycosides and phenolic glycosides. *Harpagophytum zeyheri*, which has a lower level of active compounds, may be partially substituted for *H. procumbens* in some commercial preparations (Stewart & Cole 2005). The extraction solvent (e.g. water, ethanol) has a major impact on the active principle of the products (Chrubasik 2004a), and a concentrated aqueous maceration blended with methanol was found to be most efficient for optimal extraction of harpagoside (El Babili et al 2012). When administering *H. procumbens* extract topically it was found that higher penetration of all compounds occurred from an ethanol/water preparation (Abdelouahab & Heard 2008b), and the hydro-alcoholic tincture of devil's claw is very stable when tested over a 6 month period, with levels of marker iridoids not falling below 90% of their initial concentration (Karioti et al 2011).

MAIN ACTIONS

Anti-inflammatory/analgesic

There is good in vitro and in vivo pharmacological evidence of the anti-inflammatory and analgesic properties of devil's claw, although some negative findings have also been reported (McGregor et al 2005). Overall, greatest activity appears to be in semi-chronic rather than acute conditions.

Devil's claw exerted significant analgesic effects against thermally and chemically-induced nociceptive pain stimuli in mice and significant dose-related reduction of experimentally-induced acute inflammation in rats (Mahomed & Ojewole 2004), as well as reducing pain and inflammation in Freund's adjuvant-induced arthritis in rats (Andersen et al 2004). Results from a study in mice suggest that the opioid system is involved in the antinociceptive effects of *H. procumbens* extract (Uchida et al 2008).

The iridoids, particularly harpagoside, are thought to be the main active constituents responsible for the anti-inflammatory activity; however, in vitro evidence suggests that the anti-inflammatory effect may in part be due to antioxidant activity (Denner 2007, Grant et al 2009, Langmead et al 2002), and it is particularly rich in water-soluble antioxidants (Betancor-Fernandez et al 2003). A study administering *H. procumbens* extract intraperitoneally to rats found that the anti-inflammatory response does not depend on the release of adrenal corticosteroids (Catelan et al 2006).

Contradictory evidence exists as to whether devil's claw affects prostaglandin (PG) synthesis. Early in vitro and in vivo and clinical studies suggest that it does not inhibit PG synthesis (Whitehouse et al 1983, Moussard et al 1992); however, more recent investigations have suggested that its anti-inflammatory and analgesic activities are due to suppression of PGE_2 synthesis and nitric oxide production and that the herb may suppress expressions of COX-2 and iNOS (Jang et al 2003). Harpagoside alone has been shown to suppress COX-2 and iNOS at both the mRNA and the protein level in vitro due to a suppression of NF-kappaB activation, although no influence on COX-1 was noted (Huang et al 2006). In vitro research shows that harpagoside and 8-O-(p-coumaroyl)-harpagide exhibit a greater reduction in COX-2 expression than verbascoside and that harpagide on the other hand causes a significant increase in COX-2 expression (Abdelouahab & Heard 2008a). Methanolic extracts of devil's claw have been shown to inhibit COX-2 in vivo (Kundu et al 2005, Na et al 2004), and more recently an ethanol extract of devil's claw was found to inhibit the expression of COX-2 and PGE_2 when applied to freshly excised porcine skin, although no significant effect on 5-LOX or iNOS was noted (Quitas & Heard 2009).

Inhibition of leukotriene synthesis has been observed in vitro, which appears to relate to the amount of harpagoside present (Loew et al 2001, Anauate et al 2010). A study using subcritical and supercritical CO_2 extracts (15 to 30% harpagoside) showed almost total inhibition of 5-lipoxygenase biosynthesis at 51.8 mg/mL of extract, whereas the conventional extract (2.3% harpagoside) did not inhibit the enzyme significantly (Gunther et al 2006).

In vivo experiments have determined that the method of administration of devil's claw affects its anti-inflammatory properties. Intraperitoneal and intraduodenal administration was shown to reduce carrageenan-induced oedema, whereas oral administration had no effect, suggesting that exposure to stomach acid may reduce its anti-inflammatory activity (Soulimani et al 1994). This is supported by a study that found a loss of anti-inflammatory activity after acid treatment (Bone & Walker 1997). In addition, harpagoside inhibits release of the inflammatory mediator RANTES (Regulated on Activation, Normal T cell Expressed and Secreted) by stimulated human bronchial epithelial (BEAS-2B) cells, indicating that it has potential utility for treating respiratory disorders (Boeckenholt et al 2012). It also ameliorates dopaminergic neurodegeneration and movement disorder in a mouse model of Parkinson's disease by elevating the glial cell line-derived neurotrophic factor (Sun et al 2012).

In vitro studies on rat mesangial cells suggest that devil's claw may be used as an anti-inflammatory agent in the treatment of glomerular inflammatory diseases (Kaszkin et al 2004a). Devil's claw extract produced a concentration-dependent suppression of nitrite formation in rat mesangial cells in vitro due to an inhibition of iNOS expression through interference with the transcriptional activation of iNOS. It was found that this activity was due to harpagoside, together with other constituents that possibly have strong anti-oxidant activity (Kaszkin et al 2004b).

It has been suggested that the suppression of inflammatory cytokine synthesis, demonstrated in vitro and vivo (Fiebich et al 2001, Spelman et al 2006), could explain its therapeutic effect in arthritic inflammation (Kundu et al 2005). Fiebich and co-workers found that a 60% ethanolic extract decreases the expression of IL-1-beta, IL-6 and TNF-alpha (Fiebich et al 2001). A follow up study by the same authors found a dose-dependent inhibition of release of TNF-α, interleukin (IL)-6, IL-1-beta and prostaglandin E_2 (PGE_2) in addition to inhibiting the induction of pro-inflammatory gene expression in human monocytes (Fiebich et al 2012). Another study showed that devil's claw extract inhibits inflammation in the chronic stage of adjuvant-induced arthritis, and the same study showed that devil's claw extract displays potent inhibitory activity against IL-1β, IL-6, and TNF-α production in mouse macrophages. Harpagoside also inhibited production of these inflammatory cytokines without cytotoxicity (Inaba et al 2010).

Chondroprotective

In vitro data suggest that the active principles of *H. procumbens* inhibit not only inflammatory mediators but also mediators of cartilage destruction, such as matrix metalloproteinases, NO and elastase (Boje et al 2003, Schulze-Tanzil et al 2004). A study using an animal model confirmed a chondroprotective effect in which the tissue inhibitor of metalloproteinase-2 is involved (Chrubasik et al 2006).

Hypoglycaemic

Devil's claw extract produced a dose-dependent, significant reduction in the blood glucose concentrations of both fasted normal and fasted diabetic rats (Mahomed & Ojewole 2004).

OTHER ACTIONS

Traditional uses include dyspepsia, fever, blood diseases, urinary tract infections, postpartum pain, sprains, sores, ulcers and boils (Mncwangi et al 2012). Recent research with animal models indicates an analgesic effect on acute postoperative and chronic neuropathic pain (Lim et al 2014). In vitro and in vivo evidence suggests that harpagoside may exhibit cardiac affects and lower blood pressure, heart rate and reduce arrhythmias (Fetrow & Avila 1999). As an extremely bitter herb, devil's claw is thought to increase appetite and bile production. Diterpenes extracted from the roots and seeds of devil's claw exhibited selective antiplasmodial (Clarkson et al 2003) and antibacterial activity (Weckesser et al 2007) in vitro, which may have future relevance in view of the increasing resistance to conventional antimalarials and antibiotics. One study showed that aqueous devil's claw extract can markedly delay the onset, as well as reduce the average duration, of convulsion in mice. Although not conclusive, it seems that the extract produces its anticonvulsant activity by enhancing GABAergic neurotransmission and/or facilitating GABAergic action in the brain (Mahomed & Ojewole 2006).

CLINICAL USE

Arthritis

Devil's claw is mainly used to reduce pain and inflammation in practice, with a focus on musculoskeletal conditions. Overall, evidence from clinical trials suggests that devil's claw is effective in the treatment of arthritis; however, additional well-designed, long term studies are required in order to determine effects of its long-term administration in chronic models of joint inflammation and the minimum effective doses, safety and optimal administration routes must be thoroughly determined (Georgiev et al 2013, DiLorenzo et al 2013).

An observational study of 6 months' use of 3–9 g/day of an aqueous extract of devil's claw root reported significant benefit in 42–85% of the 630 people suffering from various arthritic complaints (Bone & Walker 1997). In a 12-week uncontrolled multicentre study of 75 patients with arthrosis of the hip or knee, a strong reduction in pain and the symptoms of osteoarthritis were observed in patients taking 2400 mg of devil's claw extract daily, corresponding to 50 mg harpagoside (Wegener & Lupke 2003). Similar results were reported in a 2-month observational study of 227 people with osteoarthritic knee and hip pain and non-specific low back pain, where both the generic and the disease-specific outcome measures improved by week 4 and further by week 8 (Chrubasik et al 2002). A double-blind study of 89 subjects with rheumatic complaints used powdered devil's claw root (2 g/day) for 2 months, which also provided significant pain relief, whereas another double-blind study of 100 people reported benefit after 1 month (Bone & Walker 1997). A case report suggests that devil's claw relieved strong joint pain in a patient with Crohn's disease (Kaszkin et al 2004b). A single group open study of 8 weeks duration involving 259 patients showed statistically significant improvements in patient assessment of global pain, stiffness and function, and significant reductions in mean pain scores for hand, wrist, elbow, shoulder, hip, knee and back pain. Moreover, quality of life scores significantly increased and 60% of patients either reduced or stopped concomitant pain medication (Warnock et al 2007).

Comparison studies

Comparisons with standard treatment have also been investigated. In 2000, encouraging results of a randomised double-blind study comparing the effects of treatment with devil's claw 2610 mg/day with diacerein 100 mg/day were published (Leblan et al 2000). The study involved 122 people with osteoarthritis of the hip and/or knee and was conducted over 4 months. It found that both treatment groups showed similar considerable improvements in symptoms of osteoarthritis; however, those receiving devil's claw required fewer rescue analgesics.

One double-blind, randomised, multicentre clinical study of 122 patients with osteoarthritis of the knee and hip found that treatment with Harpadol (6 capsules/day, each containing 435 mg of cryoground powder of *H. procumbens*) given over 4 months was as effective as diacerein (an analgesic) 100 mg/day (Chantre et al 2000). However, at the end of the study, patients taking Harpadol were using significantly fewer NSAIDs and had a significantly lower frequency of adverse events. In a 6-week study of only 13 subjects, similar benefits for devil's claw and indomethacin were reported (Newall et al 1996). A preliminary study comparing the proprietary extract Doloteffin with the COX-2 inhibitor rofecoxib reported a benefit with the herbal treatment but suggested that larger studies are still required (Chrubasik et al 2003b).

Previously reviews have concluded that there is moderate evidence of the effectiveness of *H. procumbens* in the treatment of osteoarthritis of the spine, hip and knee; however it is suggested, as with many herbal medicines, that evidence of effectiveness is not transferable from product to product and that the evidence is more robust for products that contain at least 50 mg of harpagoside in the daily dosage (Chrubasik et al 2003a, Gagnier et al 2004, Long et al 2001, Lopez 2012). Two reviews have concluded that 'data from higher quality studies suggest that devil's claw appeared effective in the reduction of the main clinical symptom of pain' (Brien et al 2006) and that the evidence of effectiveness was 'strong' for at least 50 mg of harpagoside as the daily dose, with extracts of devil's claw resulting in pain relief for 60% of patients with an osteoarthritic hip or knee, or nonspecific lower back pain (Chrubasik JE et al 2007). Nevertheless, two other reviews concluded that there was only 'limited evidence' (Ameye & Chee 2006) and 'insufficient reliable evidence' regarding the long term effectiveness of devil's claw (Gregory et al 2008), however this may be as the result of lack of continuity in clinical testing and the definition of 'physical impairment'. Different measures of physical impairment have been used in the clinical trials (including the Arhus low back pain index, the Schober test and the Waddell scale), and this may be a reason for varied results rather than a lack of effectiveness of the extracts (Chrubasik 2008).

The herb is Commission E approved as supportive therapy for degenerative musculoskeletal disorders (Blumenthal et al 2000) and approved for painful osteoarthritis by the European Scientific Cooperative on Phytotherapy (ESCOP 2003).

Back pain

Three reviews looking at the treatment of low back pain concluded that there is strong evidence for short-term improvements in pain and reduction in rescue medication for devil's claw treatment, standardised to 50 and 100 mg harpagoside as daily doses (Chrubasik et al 2007, Gagnier 2008, Gagnier et al 2006, 2007). The reliability and quality of some of these clinical trials have been investigated in detail by different research groups (Brien et al 2006, Chrubasik et al 2003a, Gagnier et al 2004, 2007). All reviews of clinical studies conclude that Harpagophytum extracts show strong evidence of efficacy and reliability in the treatment of lower back pain.

Eight weeks treatment with devil's claw extract LI 174, known commercially as Rivoltan, significantly decreased back pain and improved mobility in a double-blind RCT of 117 people (Laudahn & Walper 2001) although another double blind RCT using the same product found that pain relief was established more quickly, after 4 weeks amongst subjects with muscle stiffness (Gobel et al 2001). Similar results were reported in two double-blind studies of 118 people (Chrubasik et al 1996) and 197 people (Chrubasik et al 1999) with chronic lower back pain.

Devil's claw appears to compare favourably to conventional treatments. A 6-week double-blind study of 88 subjects comparing devil's claw to rofecoxib found equal improvements in both groups (Chrubasik et al 2003b). A follow-up of the subjects from that study who were all given devil's claw for 1 year found that it was well tolerated and improvements were sustained (Chrubasik et al 2005). In an open, prospective study, an unspecific lower back pain treatment with *Harpagophytum* extract and conventional therapy were found to be equally effective (Schmidt et al 2005).

Dyspepsia

Traditionally, devil's claw has also been used to treat dyspepsia and to stimulate appetite (Fisher & Painter 1996). The bitter principles in the herb provide a theoretical basis for its use in these conditions, although controlled studies are not available to determine effectiveness. The herb is Commission E (Blumenthal et al 2000) and ESCOP (2003) approved for dyspepsia and loss of appetite.

OTHER USES

Use in oncology

There is a case report that two Stage IIIA follicular lymphoma patients demonstrated objective tumour regression after taking 500 mg daily doses of devil's claw without cytotoxic therapy, which was confirmed by computed tomography (CT) scans. This result was presumably as a result of COX-2 inhibition, which has been implicated in lymphomagenesis. Although this case report introduces a possible use of the herb, it is unknown as to whether the regression was spontaneous (as has been observed in up to 16% of lymphoma patients) or due to devil's claw, and further studies are warranted (Wilson 2009).

Traditional use

Traditionally, the herb is also used internally to treat febrile illnesses, allergic reactions and to induce sedation, and topically for wounds, ulcers, boils and pain relief (Fisher & Painter 1996, Mills & Bone 2000), as well as for diabetes, hypertension, indigestion and anorexia (Van Wyk 2000).

DOSAGE RANGE

Musculoskeletal conditions

- Dried root or equivalent aqueous or hydroalcoholic extracts: 2–6 g daily for painful arthritis; 4.5–9 g daily for lower back pain.
- Liquid extract (1 : 2): 6–12 mL/day.
- Tincture (1 : 5): 2–4 mL three times daily.

It is suggested that devil's claw extracts with at least 50 mg harpagoside in the daily dosage should be recommended for the treatment of pain, and dosages corresponding to 30–100 mg harpagosides have been used in clinical trials (Chrubasik 2004a, 2004b, Street & Prinsloo 2012).

Digestive conditions (e.g. dyspepsia)

- Dosages equivalent to 1.5 g/day dried herb are used (Blumenthal et al 2000). It is suggested that devil's claw preparations be administered between meals, when gastric activity is reduced.

TOXICITY

The acute LD_{50} of devil's claw was more than 13.5 g/kg according to one study (Bone & Walker 1997). In a recent review of 28 clinical trials only a few reports on acute toxicity were found, whereas no reports on chronic toxicity had been reported. The review concluded that more studies for long-term treatment are needed (Vlachojannis et al 2008). An earlier review looking at 14 clinical trials had come to the same conclusion (Brien et al 2006).

ADVERSE REACTIONS

Devil's claw is a well tolerated treatment. In a recent review of 28 clinical trials it was found that only minor adverse events, mainly mild gastrointestinal symptoms (e.g. diarrhoea), occur in 3% of the patients. The incidence of adverse effects in the treatment groups was never higher than in the placebo groups for all 28 trials (Vlachojannis et al 2008).

SIGNIFICANT INTERACTIONS

Devil's claw was previously found to moderately inhibit cytochrome P450 enzymes (CYP2C9, 2C19, 3A4) in vitro (Unger & Frank 2004); however a subsequent study found no significant interactions when testing 10 different commercial devil's claw preparations (Modari et al 2011). An in vitro study found commercial preparations of devil's claw and pure harpagoside upregulated P-glycoprotein in a dose-dependent manner (Romiti et al 2009); however the effect has not been tested in vivo. In contrast to NSAIDs, devil's claw does not affect platelet function (Izzo et al 2005).

Warfarin

Rare case reports suggest that devil's claw may potentiate the effects of warfarin, but the reports are mostly inconclusive (Argento et al 2000, Heck et al 2000, Izzo et al 2005). Clinical testing would be required to confirm a possible interaction.

Anti-arrhythmic drugs

Theoretical interaction exists when the herb is used in high doses; however, clinical testing is required to determine significance — observe patients taking concurrent antiarrhythmics (Fetrow & Avila 1999).

Practice points/Patient counselling

- Devil's claw reduces pain and inflammation and is a useful treatment in arthritis and back pain, according to controlled studies.
- The anti-inflammatory action appears to be different to that of NSAIDs and has not been fully elucidated. There is also preliminary evidence of a chondroprotective effect.
- Preliminary research suggests that it is best to take devil's claw between meals, on an empty stomach.
- Devil's claw appears to be relatively safe but should not be used in pregnancy and should be used with caution in people with ulcers or gallstones or in those taking warfarin.

CONTRAINDICATIONS AND PRECAUTIONS

Use cautiously in patients with gastric and duodenal ulcers, gallstones or acute diarrhoea, as devil's claw may cause gastric irritation (Blumenthal et al 2000).

PREGNANCY USE

Devil's claw is not recommended in pregnancy, as it has exhibited oxytocic activity in animals.

PATIENTS' FAQs

What will this herb do for me?
Devil's claw is a useful treatment for arthritis and back pain. It may also increase appetite and improve digestion and dyspepsia.

When will it start to work?
Results from studies suggest that pain-relieving effects will start within 4–12 weeks reaching maximum pain relief after 3–4 months (Chrubasik S et al 2007, Thanner et al 2008).

Are there any safety issues?
Devil's claw should be used cautiously by people with gallstones, diarrhoea, stomach ulcers and those taking the drug warfarin. It is also not recommended in pregnancy.

REFERENCES

Abdelouahab N, Heard C. Effect of the major glycosides of Harpagophytum procumbens (Devil's Claw) on epidermal cyclooxygenase-2 (COX-2) in vitro. J Nat Prod 71.5 (2008a): 746–749.

Abdelouahab N, Heard CM. Dermal and transcutaneous delivery of the major glycoside constituents of Harpagophytum procumbens (Devil's Claw) in vitro. Planta Med 74.5 (2008b): 527–531.

Ameye LG, Chee WS. Osteoarthritis and nutrition. From nutraceuticals to functional foods: a systematic review of the scientific evidence. Arthritis Res Ther 8.4 (2006): R127.

Andersen ML et al. Evaluation of acute and chronic treatments with Harpagophytum procumbens on Freund's adjuvant-induced arthritis in rats. J Ethnopharmacol 91.2–3 (2004): 325–330.

Anauate, MC et al. Effect of Isolated Fractions of Harpagophytum Procumbens D.C. (devil's Claw) on COX-1, COX-2 Activity and Nitric Oxide Production on Whole-blood Assay. Phyto Res 24.9 (2010): 1365–369.

Argento AE et al. Oral anticoagulants and medicinal plants: An emerging interaction. Ann Ital Med Intern 15.2 (2000): 139–143.

Betancor-Fernandez A et al. Screening pharmaceutical preparations containing extracts of turmeric rhizome, artichoke leaf, devil's claw root and garlic or salmon oil for antioxidant capacity. J Pharm Pharmacol 55.7 (2003): 981–986.

Blumenthal M, Goldberg A, Brinckmann J (eds). Herbal medicine: expanded Commission E monographs. Austin, TX: Integrative Medicine Communications, 2000.

Boeckenholt, C et al. Effect of silymarin and harpagoside on inflammation reaction of BEAS-2B cells, on ciliary beat frequency (CBF) of trachea explants and on mucociliary clearance (MCC). Planta Med. 78 (2012): 761–766.

Boje K, Lechtenberg M, Nahrstedt A. New and known iridoid- and phenylethanoid glycosides from Harpagophytum procumbens and their in vitro inhibition of human leukocyte elastase. Planta Med 69 (2003): 820–825.

Bone K, Walker M. Devil's claw. MediHerb Professional Review. Australia: Mediherb Pty Ltd (February 1997).

Brien S, Lewith GT, McGregor G. Devil's Claw (Harpagophytum procumbens) as a treatment for osteoarthritis: a review of efficacy and safety. J Altern Complement Med 12.10 (2006): 981–993.

Catelan SC et al. The role of adrenal corticosteroids in the anti-inflammatory effect of the whole extract of Harpagophytum procumbens in rats. Phytomedicine 13.6 (2006): 446–451.

Chantre P et al. Efficacy and tolerance of Harpagophytum procumbens versus diacerhein in treatment of osteoarthritis. Phytomedicine 7.3 (2000): 177–183.

Chrubasik JE et al. Potential molecular basis of the chondroprotective effect of Harpagophytum procumbens. Phytomedicine 13.8 (2006): 598–600.

Chrubasik JE, Roufogalis BD, Chrubasik S. Evidence of effectiveness of herbal antiinflammatory drugs in the treatment of painful osteoarthritis and chronic low back pain. Phytother Res 21.7 (2007): 675–683.

Chrubasik S. Devil's claw extract as an example of the effectiveness of herbal analgesics. Der Orthopade 33.7 (2004a): 804–808.

Chrubasik S. Salix and Harpagophytum for chronic joint and low back pain: From evidence-based view herbal medicinal products are recommended. Schweiz Z Ganzheits Med 16.6 (2004b): 355–359.

Chrubasik S et al. Effectiveness of Harpagophytum procumbens in treatment of acute low back pain. Phytomedicine 3.1 (1996): 1–110.

Chrubasik S et al. Effectiveness of Harpagophytum extract WS 1531 in the treatment of exacerbation of low back pain: a randomized, placebo-controlled, double-blind study. Eur J Anaesthesiol 16.2 (1999): 118–129.

Chrubasik S et al. Comparison of outcome measures during treatment with the proprietary Harpagophytum extract doloteffin in patients with pain in the lower back, knee or hip. Phytomedicine 9.3 (2002): 181–194.

Chrubasik S et al. The quality of clinical trials with Harpagophytum procumbens. Phytomedicine 10.6–7 (2003a): 613–623.

Chrubasik S et al. A randomized double-blind pilot study comparing Doloteffin(R) and Vioxx(R) in the treatment of low back pain. Rheumatology 42.1 (2003b): 141–148.

Chrubasik S et al. A 1-year follow-up after a pilot study with Doloteffin(R) for low back pain. Phytomedicine 12.1–2 (2005): 1–9.

Chrubasik S et al. Patient-perceived benefit during one year of treatment with Doloteffin. Phytomedicine 14.6 (2007): 371–376.

Chrubasik C et al. Impact of herbal medicines on physical impairment. Phytomedicine 15 (2008): 536–539.

Clarkson C et al. In vitro antiplasmodial activity of abietane and totarane diterpenes isolated from Harpagophytum procumbens (Devil's Claw). Planta Med 69.8 (2003): 720–724.

Denner SS. A review of the efficacy and safety of devil's claw for pain associated with degenerative musculoskeletal diseases, rheumatoid, and osteoarthritis. Holist Nurs Pract 21.4 (2007): 203–207.

Di Lorenzo C et al. Plant food supplements with anti-inflammatory properties: A Systematic Review (II). Crit Rev in Food Sc Nutr 53:5 (2013): 507–516.

ESCOP. European Scientific Co-operative on Phytomedicine, 2nd edn. Stuttgart: Thieme, 2003.

El Babili F et al. Anatomical study of secondary tuberized roots of *Harpagophytum procumbens* DC and quantification of harpagoside by highperformance liquid chromatography method. Pharmacogn Mag. 8.30 (2012): 175–180.

Fetrow CW, Avila JR. Professionals' handbook of complementary and alternative medicines. Springhouse, PA: Springhouse Publishing, 1999.

Fiebich BL et al. Inhibition of TNF-alpha synthesis in LPS-stimulated primary human monocytes by Harpagophytum extract SteiHap 69. Phytomedicine 8.1 (2001): 28–30.

Fiebich BL et al. Molecular targets of the anti-inflammatory Harpagophytum procumbens (devil's claw): inhibition of TNFa and COX-2 gene expression by preventing activation of AP-1. Phytother Res 26.6 (2012): 806–11.

Fisher C, Painter G. Materia Medica for the Southern hemisphere. Auckland: Fisher-Painter Publishers, 1996.

Gagnier JJ et al. Harpgophytum procumbens for osteoarthritis and low back pain: a systematic review. BMC Complement Altern Med 4 (2004): 13.

Gagnier JJ et al. Herbal medicine for low back pain. Cochrane Database Syst Rev 2 (2006): CD004504.

Gagnier JJ et al. Herbal medicine for low back pain: a Cochrane review. Spine 32.1 (2007): 82–92.

Gagnier JJ Evidence-informed management of chronic low back pain with herbal, vitamin, mineral, and homeopathic supplements. The Spine Journal 8 (2008): 70–79.

Georgiev MI et al Harpagoside: from Kalahari Desert to pharmacy shelf. Phytochemistry Aug (2013): 8–15.

Gobel HA et al. Effects of Harpagophytum procumbens LI 174 (devil's claw) on sensory, motor and vascular muscle reagibility in the treatment of unspecific back pain. Schmerz 15.1 (2001): 10–118.

Grant L et al. The inhibition of free radical generation by preparations of Harpagophytum procumbens in vitro. Phytother Res 23.1 (2009): 104–110.

Gregory PJ, Sperry M, Wilson AF. Dietary supplements for osteoarthritis. Am Fam Physician 77.2 (2008): 177–184.

Gunther M, Laufer S, Schmidt PC. High anti-inflammatory activity of harpagoside-enriched extracts obtained from solvent-modified super- and subcritical carbon dioxide extractions of the roots of Harpagophytum procumbens. Phytochem Anal 17.1 (2006): 1–7.

Heck AM et al. Potential interactions between alternative therapies and warfarin. Am J Health-System Pharm 57.13 (2000): 1221–1227: quiz 1228–30.

Huang TH et al. Harpagoside suppresses lipopolysaccharide-induced iNOS and COX-2 expression through inhibition of NF-kappaB activation. J Ethnopharmacol 104 (2006): 149–155.

Inaba K et al. Inhibitory effects of devil's claw (secondary root of Harpagophytum procumbens) extract and harpagoside on cytokine production in mouse macrophages. J Nat Med 64 (2010): 219–222.

Izzo AA et al. Cardiovascular pharmacotherapy and herbal medicines: the risk of drug interaction. Int J Cardiol 98.1 (2005): 1–114.

Jang MH et al. Harpagophytum procumbens suppresses lipopolysaccharide-stimulated expressions of cyclooxygenase-2 and inducible nitric oxide synthase in fibroblast cell line L929. J Pharmacol Sci 93.3 (2003): 367–371.

Karioti A et al. Analysis and stability of the constituents of Curcuma longa and Harpagophytum procumbens tinctures by HPLC-DAD and HPLC-ESI-MS. J Pharma Biomed Anal 55 (2011): 479–486.

Kaszkin M et al. Downregulation of iNOS expression in rat mesangial cells by special extracts of Harpagophytum procumbens derives from harpagoside-dependent and independent effects. Phytomedicine 11.7–8 (2004a): 585–595.

Kaszkin M et al. High dosed Harpagophytum special extract for maintenance of remission in patients with Crohn's disease: A case report. Arztezeitschr Naturheilverfahr 45.2 (2004b): 102–106.

Kundu JK et al. Inhibitory effects of the extracts of Sutherlandia frutescens (L.) R. Br. and Harpagophytum procumbens DC. on phorbol ester-induced COX-2 expression in mouse skin: AP-1 and CREB as potential upstream targets. Cancer Lett 218.1 (2005): 21–31.

Langmead L et al. Antioxidant effects of herbal therapies used by patients with inflammatory bowel disease: an in vitro study. Aliment Pharmacol Ther 16.2 (2002): 197–205.

Laudahn D, Walper A. Efficacy and tolerance of Harpagophytum extract LI 174 in patients with chronic non-radicular back pain. Phytother Res 15.7 (2001): 621–624.

Leblan D, Chantre P, Fournie B. Harpagophytum procumbens in the treatment of knee and hip osteoarthritis: Four-month results of a prospective, multicenter, double-blind trial versus diacerhein. Joint Bone Spine 67.5 (2000): 462–467.

Lim DW et al. Analgesic effect of Harpagophytum procumbens on postoperative and neuropathic pain in rats. Molecules 19.1 (2014): 1060–1068.

Loew D et al. Investigations on the pharmacokinetic properties of Harpagophytum extracts and their effects on eicosanoid biosynthesis in vitro and ex vivo. Clin Pharmacol Ther 69.5 (2001): 356–364.

Long L, Soeken K, Ernst E. Herbal medicines for the treatment of osteoarthritis: a systematic review. Rheumatology 40 (2001): 779–4693.

Lopez H. Nutritional Interventions to Prevent and Treat Osteoarthritis. Part II: Focus on Micronutrients and Supportive Nutraceuticals. Phys Med Rehab 4 (2012) S:155–68.

Mahomed IM, Ojewole JAO. Analgesic, antiinflammatory and antidiabetic properties of Harpagophytum procumbens DC (Pedaliaceae) secondary root aqueous extract. Phytother Res 18.12 (2004): 982–989.

Mahomed IM, Ojewole JA. Anticonvulsant activity of Harpagophytum procumbens DC [Pedaliaceae] secondary root aqueous extract in mice. Brain Res Bull 69.1 (2006): 57–62.

McGregor GB et al. Devil's claw (Harpagophytum procumbens): An anti-inflammatory herb with therapeutic potential. Phytochem Rev 4.1 (2005): 47–53.

Mills S, Bone K. Principles and practice of phytotherapy. London: Churchill Livingstone, 2000.

Moussard CD et al. A drug used in traditional medicine, Harpagophytum procumbens: no evidence for NSAID-like effect on whole blood eicosanoid production in human. Prostaglandins Leukot Essent Fatty Acids 46.4 (1992): 283–286.

Mncwangi N et al. Devil's Claw—A review of the ethnobotany, phytochemistry and biological activity of Harpagophytum procumbens. J Ethnopharmacology 143 (2012): 755–771.

Mncgwangi N et al. Mid-infrared spectroscopy and short wave infrared hyperspectral imaging—A novel approach in the qualitative assessment of Harpagophytum procumbens and H. zeyheri (Devil's Claw). Phytochemistry Letters 7 (2014):143–149.

Modari M et al. The interaction potential of herbal medicinal products: a luminescence-based screening platform assessing effects on cytochrome P450 and its use with devil's claw (*Harpagophyti radix*) preparations. J Pharm Pharmacol 63 (2011) 429–438.

Na HK et al. Inhibition of phorbol ester-induced COX-2 expression by some edible African plants. Oxford: BioFactors 21.1–4 (2004): 149–353.

Newell CA, Anderson LA, Phillipson JD. Herbal medicines: A guide for health care professionals. London, UK: The Pharmaceutical Press, 1996.

Quitas NA, Heard CM A novel ex vivo skin model for the assessment of the potential transcutaneous anti-inflammatory effect of topically applied Harpagophytum procumbens extract. Int J Pharm. 376.1–2 (2009):63–8.

Romiti, N et al Effects of Devil's Claw (Harpagophytum procumbens) on the multidrug transporter ABCB1/P-glycoprotein. Phytomedicine 16.12 (2009): 1095–100.

Schmidt A et al. Effectiveness of Harpagophytum procumbens in treatment of unspecific low back pain. Physikal Med Rehabilitationsmed Kurortmed 15.5 (2005): 317–321.

Schulze-Tanzil G, Hansen C, Shakibaei M. Effect of a Harpagophytum procumbens DC extract on matrix metalloproteinases in human chondrocytes in vitro. Arzneimittelforschung 54 (2004): 213–220.

Soulimani R et al. The role of stomachal digestion on the pharmacological activity of plant extracts, using as an example extracts of Harpagophytum procumbens. Can J Physiol Pharmacol 72.12 (1994): 1532–1536.
Spelman K et al. Modulation of cytokine expression by traditional medicines: a review of herbal immunomodulators. Altern Med Rev 11.2 (2006): 128–150.
Stewart KM, Cole D. The commercial harvest of devil's claw (Harpagophytum spp.) in southern Africa: The devil's in the details. J Ethnopharmacol 100.3 (2005): 225–236.
Street RA, Prinsloo G. Commercially important medicinal plants of South Africa: A Review. J Chemistry (2013) Article ID 205048.
Sun, X et al. Harpagoside attenuates MPTP/MPP(+) induced dopaminergic neurodegeneration and movement disorder via elevating glial cell line derived neurotrophic factor. J. Neurochem. 120 (2012):1072–1083.
Thanner J et al. Retrospective evaluation of biopsychosocial determinants and treatment response in patients receiving devil's claw extract (doloteffin(R)). Phytother Res 23.5 (2008): 742–744.
Uchida S et al. Antinociceptive effects of St. John's wort, Harpagophytum procumbens extract and Grape seed proanthocyanidins extract in mice. Biol Pharm Bull 31.2 (2008): 240–245.
Unger M, Frank A. Simultaneous determination of the inhibitory potency of herbal extracts on the activity of six major cytochrome P450 enzymes using liquid chromatography/mass spectrometry and automated online extraction. Rapid Commun in Mass Spectrometry 18.19 (2004): 2273–2281.
Van Wyk BE, Gericke N. People's plants: a guide to useful plants of Southern Africa. Pretoria: Briza Publications, 2000.
Vlachojannis J, Roufogalis BD, Chrubasik S. Systematic review on the safety of Harpagophytum preparations for osteoarthritic and low back pain. Phytother Res 22.2 (2008): 149–152.
Warnock M et al. Effectiveness and safety of Devil's Claw tablets in patients with general rheumatic disorders. Phytother Res 21.12 (2007): 1228–1233.
Weckesser S et al. Screening of plant extracts for antimicrobial activity against bacteria and yeasts with dermatological relevance. Phytomedicine 14.7–8 (2007): 508–516.
Wegener T, Lupke N-P. Treatment of patients with arthrosis of hip or knee with an aqueous extract of devil's claw (Harpagophytum procumbens DC). Phytother Res 17.10 (2003): 1165–1172.
Whitehouse LW et al. Devil's claw (Harpagophytum procumbens): no evidence for anti-inflammatory activity in the treatment of arthritic disease. Can Med Assoc J 129.3 (1983): 249–251.
Wilson KS. Regression of follicular lymphoma with Devil's Claw: coincidence or causation? Curr Onc 16.4 (2009): 67–70.

Dunaliella salina

HISTORICAL NOTE Microalgae are nutrient-dense natural foods and medicines that have been used for thousands of years by the Aztecs, some African and Asian peoples and South Pacific islanders. It has been suggested that gram for gram, microalgae are the most nutrient-dense food on earth (Passwater & Solomon 1997) with minimal indigestible structures, in contrast to higher plants or animals, which typically have less than half their dry weight being nutritionally useful (Bruno 2001). Examples of edible algae include *Spirulina*, *Chlorella* and *Dunaliella salina*. The last may be the most nutrient dense of the three, primarily due to its extremely high concentration of carotenoid antioxidants. The high carotenoid content imparts a pink colouring to salt lakes where the microalgae flourish. This colour is amplified through the food chain to give the pink colour to brine shrimp and flamingos (Skinner & Tomkins 2008).

COMMON NAME

Dunaliella salina

BOTANICAL NAME/FAMILY

Dunaliella salina and *Dunaliella bardawil* are considered to be the same species (Borowitzka & Borowitzka 1988).

OTHER NAMES

Red marine phytoplankton (microalgae)

PLANT PARTS USED

Dunaliella salina is a marine phytoplankton that is a unicellular, biflagellate, soft-walled, green alga that lives in salt-water lakes and coastal waters. As a phytoplankton, *D. salina* can be considered a whole plant; yet, it has a soft cell membrane that makes it easily digestible, compared with other microalgae that have hard cell walls (Ben-Amotz & Avron 1983). *D. salina* is one of the most salt-tolerant life forms known and is found in hypersaline waters generally >20% (salt lakes and evaporation ponds of salt works). It has a wide tolerance to environmental extremes, especially salinity, pH (pH 1–11), temperature (>45°C) and high ultraviolet (UV) exposure (Borowitzka & Borowitzka 1988). To cope with these extreme environments, *D. salina* produces very high levels of carotenoids in the chloroplast (organelles that conduct photosynthesis) as well as maintaining a high mineral content.

CHEMICAL COMPONENTS

D. salina contains a range of macro- and micronutrients, including amino acids, lipids and fatty acids, carbohydrates, chlorophyll, vitamins and minerals, along with very high levels of carotenoids. As a phytoplankton that grows in seawater, *D. salina* is rich in many trace minerals. *D. salina* is also extremely high in carotenoids and, while it contains over 500 different carotenoids, including alpha-carotene, lutein, zeaxanthin and cryptoxanthum, it is the richest known natural source of beta-carotene (USDA 2005), which can make up to 8% of its dry weight (Ben-Amotz & Avron 1983). *D. salina* is therefore commonly used as a source of natural beta-carotene or mixed carotenoids in nutritional supplements (see *Beta-carotene* monograph).

Unlike synthetic (all-*trans*) beta-carotene, the beta-carotene from *D. salina* is composed of near-equal amounts of the all-*trans* and 9-*cis* stereoisomers, which differ in their physicochemical features and antioxidative activity. The 9-*cis* isomer is considered to be one of nature's most powerful antioxidants and provides much greater bioavailability and antioxidant activity than synthetic beta-carotene supplements (Ben-Amotz & Levy 1996, Ben-Amotz et al 1989, Stahl et al 1993) (see *Beta-carotene* monograph).

D. salina is the richest natural source known of the 9-*cis* isomer (Ye et al 2008) and it is believed that exposure to reactive oxygen species triggers extensive carotenoid accumulation in *D. salina* (Ye et al 2008). There are a number of biotechnology processes aimed at extracting its natural beta-carotene content (Lamers et al 2008, Raja et al 2007a). As a supplement, *D. salina* can be produced in either the whole dried (unwashed) form that contains high levels of minerals or a washed (desalinated) form that has higher carotenoid levels and lower mineral levels. Recently, advances in production technology have allowed the whole dried *D. salina* biomass with its full range of nutrients and minerals to become commercially available in supplement form (Tracton & Bobrov 2005).

MAIN ACTIONS

Antioxidant and anti-inflammatory

Animal studies suggest that natural beta-carotene from *D. salina* can protect rats against central nervous system oxygen toxicity (Bitterman et al 1994), whole-body irradiation (Ben-Amotz et al 1996) and gastrointestinal inflammation (Lavy et al 2003, Takenaka et al 1993). It is suggested that the gastric cytoprotective effect may depend on the amount of beta-carotene accumulated. A study that fed rats with diets containing up to 0.1% beta-carotene for 2 weeks using dry *D. salina*, purified natural beta-carotene from *D. salina* or synthetic beta-carotene found that the rats showed higher accumulations of the algal beta-carotene than of the synthetic all-*trans* beta-carotene and that the *D. salina* and algal beta-carotene supplementation both significantly decreased the gastric mucosal lesions after water immersion stress, while synthetic beta-carotene did not (Takenaka et al 1993).

Cytoprotection

Animal studies suggest that supplementation with *D. salina* has hepatoprotective effects and can protect rats against laboratory models of liver toxicity to a significantly greater degree than synthetic beta-carotene. This is most likely due to the presence of various isomeric forms of carotene and other oxygenated carotenoids (Chidambara Murthy et al 2005, Vanitha et al 2007). *D. salina* supplementation has also been found to protect rats against laboratory-induced fibrosarcoma (Raja et al 2007b). Further studies have shown that prefeeding rats with *D. salina* ameliorated acid-induced enteritis (Lavy et al 2003). A double-blind trial in humans found that a single dose of natural beta-carotene from *D. salina* reduced the severity, but not the incidence, of postprocedural pancreatitis after endoscopic retrograde cholangiopancreatography (Lavy et al 2004).

Anti-atherogenic

Supplementation with *D. salina* powder inhibited atherogenesis in animal models using high-fat diet-fed low-density lipoprotein (LDL) receptor knockout mice. Reductions of plasma cholesterol of 40–63% and atherosclerotic lesions of 60–83%, along with reduced liver fat accumulation, liver inflammation and mRNA levels of inflammatory genes, were also observed. By administrating *D. salina* powder containing different levels of 9-*cis* and all-*trans* beta-carotene isomers, these effects were shown to be 9-*cis*-dependent (Harari et al 2008).

D

Photoprotection

The red, orange and yellow colours of *D. salina* preferentially absorb UV light; therefore, ingestion of the microalgae adds pigmentation to the skin which helps to absorb UV light and reduce the effects of UV-induced erythema (sunburn) (Heinrich et al 2003). The beta-carotene in *D. salina* demonstrates photoprotective activity in plant cells and human skin (Heinrich et al 2003, Stahl et al 2000) and supplementation with *D. salina* was found to exhibit potent protective effects on UVB radiation-induced corneal oxidative damage in mice (Tsai et al 2012).

OTHER ACTIONS

Detoxification

D. salina contains chlorophyll, along with other vitamins and minerals such as selenium and magnesium that are believed to aid in detoxification (Murray 1997). A small cohort study found that 14 weeks of supplementation with 3 g/day of *D. salina* powder produced marked reduction in hair tissue levels of various heavy metals. These findings await further confirmation in controlled trials (Bobrov et al 2008).

Antibacterial

A study on the antimicrobial activity of different pressurised liquid extracts obtained from *D. salina* found that 15 different volatile compounds as well as several fatty acids (mainly palmitic, alpha-linolenic and oleic acids) may be responsible for the observed antibacterial activity (Herrero et al 2006).

Antiproliferative

An ethanol extract of *D. salina* has been found to have antiproliferative effects and induce cell cycle G0/G1 arrest and apoptosis of human lung cancer (Sheu et al 2008) and prostate cancer cells (Jayappriyan et al 2013). An ethanolic extract of *D. salina* has also been found to inhibit proliferation of rat and human smooth-muscle cells, suggesting a possible role in preventing restenosis following balloon angioplasty (Sheu et al 2010).

Chemoprevention

There has been considerable research into carotenoids and chemoprevention. Many studies have shown the correlation between high intakes of natural beta-carotene from food and a decreased risk in the carcinogenesis of stomach, prostate and breast cancers (see *Beta-carotene* monograph). It is likely that natural beta-carotene from *D. salina* has different biological activity from synthetic beta-carotene — while synthetic beta-carotene has been shown to increase the risk of lung cancer in some populations, this has not been demonstrated with natural beta-carotene. As such, it is possible that long-term usage of *D. salina* may also decrease the risk of various cancers; however, this has yet to be investigated.

CLINICAL USE

D. salina is nature's richest source of natural beta-carotene and as such has similar uses to beta-carotene. To date, most of the clinical research on *D. salina* has been conducted with beta-carotene-containing extracts rather than the whole organism. This research suggests that potential benefits of supplementation with *D. salina* include prevention of cancer and cardiovascular disease, protection against sun damage and photosensitivity, supporting healthy eye, skin and immune function, providing benefits in asthma, macular degeneration and promotion of overall health and wellbeing (see *Beta-carotene* monograph). Human studies on *D. salina* extracts suggest many positive clinical effects, mainly due to its antioxidant activity.

Diabetes

A reduction in oxidative injury (Levy et al 1999) along with normalisation of LDL oxidation (Levy et al 2000) was reported in two studies involving supplementation with a *D. salina* extract containing 60 mg/day of beta-carotene given for 3 weeks in patients with non-insulin-dependent diabetes mellitus.

Radiation exposure

A study of 709 children with long-term exposure to radiation during and after the Chernobyl accident found that 3-month supplementation with 40 mg of beta-carotene powder from *D. salina* reduced serum markers for oxidisation and acted as a lipophilic antioxidant and radioprotector (Ben-Amotz et al 1998).

Photoprotection

D. salina extracts protect the skin from sunburn and sun damage due to increased protective pigmentation of the skin along with reduced susceptibility to sunburn, according to a clinical study (Heinrich & Tronnier 1998, Stahl et al 1993). The placebo-controlled ($n = 24$) trial found 12 weeks of supplementation with 24 mg/day of *Dunaliella*-derived carotenoids significantly increased protection from sunburn (Heinrich et al 2003).

Exercise-induced asthma

A double-blind, placebo-controlled trial involving 38 subjects found that 1-week supplementation with *D. salina* provided a protective effect for patients with exercise-induced asthma (Neuman et al 1999).

Practice points/Patient counselling

- *D. salina* is a marine phytoplankton that grows in extreme environments and is nature's richest source of natural beta-carotene.
- Dunaliella is a 'whole-food' supplement that provides a range of trace minerals and other nutrients that provide antioxidant, anti-inflammatory and photoprotection activity.
- Supplementation with *D. salina* may assist in the prevention of a range of conditions, including cardiovascular disease, some cancers and exercise-induced asthma.
- The antioxidants in *D. salina* may provide some protection against exposure to the sun and other sources of radiation.

DOSAGE RANGE

1–3 g of whole dried *D. salina* powder (which contains around 1–2% beta-carotene) when taken as a supplement.

ADVERSE REACTIONS

D. salina is classified as an edible species of microalgae. While no human toxicology studies have been carried out, there are no reported adverse effects from consumption of the whole microalgae or beta-carotene extract from *D. salina* in human clinical studies. An orange or yellow skin colouration (carotenodermia) may become evident after a few months of consumption but this is harmless and reversible on discontinuation (see *Beta-carotene* monograph).

SIGNIFICANT INTERACTIONS

No known interactions at this time.

PREGNANCY USE

While *D. salina* is considered safe, there is insufficient information to guide its use in pregnancy.

PATIENTS' FAQs

What will it do for me?

D. salina provides a source of natural beta-carotene and minerals that may promote energy and vitality, enhance skin health and appearance and assist in healthy ageing. As a rich source of beta-carotene, *D. salina* acts to supplement vitamin A levels without the risk of vitamin A toxicity. It may be used to assist in maintaining healthy skin, eyes and immune function, preventing cancer and cardiovascular disease and reducing oxidative stress. *D. salina* may also provide photoprotection, detoxification of heavy metals and protective effect for patients with exercise-induced asthma.

When will it start to work?

Effects may be observable within 1 week but may take up to 3 months to obtain full benefits, while benefits of long-term supplementation on disease prevention may take many years to become evident. *D. salina* should be taken with meals or other dietary fats to increase the bioavailability of carotenoids.

Are there any safety issues?

D. salina is considered non-toxic. Large doses over long periods of time may produce carotenodermia, which is a harmless and reversible yellow-orange discolouration of the skin.

STORAGE

D. salina should be stored in airtight containers or capsules away from direct sunlight, as carotenoids will oxidise on exposure to air and light.

REFERENCES

Ben-Amotz A, Avron M. Accumulation of metabolites by halotolerant algae and its industrial potential. Annu Rev Microbiol 37.1 (1983): 95–119.

Ben-Amotz A, Levy Y. Bioavailability of a natural isomer mixture compared with synthetic all-trans beta-carotene in human serum. Am J Clin Nutr 63.5 (1996): 729–734.

Ben-Amotz A et al. Bioavailability of a natural isomer mixture as compared with synthetic all-trans-[beta]-carotene in rats and chicks. J Nutr 119.7 (1989): 1013–10119.

Ben-Amotz A et al. Natural beta-carotene and whole body irradiation in rats. Radiat Environ Biophys 35.4 (1996): 285–288.

Ben-Amotz A et al. Effect of natural beta-carotene supplementation in children exposed to radiation from the Chernobyl accident. Radiat Environ Biophys 37.3 (1998): 187–193.

Bitterman N, et al. Beta-carotene and CNS oxygen toxicity in rats. J Appl Physiol 76.3 (1994): 1073–1076.

Bobrov Z et al. Effectiveness of whole dried *Dunaliella salina* marine microalgae in the chelating and detoxification of toxic minerals and heavy metals. J Altern Complement Med 14.1 (2008): S8–S9.

Borowitzka MA, Borowitzka LJ. Micro-algal biotechnology. Cambridge: Cambridge University Press, 1988.

Bruno JJ. Edible microalgae: a review of the health research. Pacifica: Center of Nutritional Psychology Press, 2001.

Chidambara Murthy KN et al. Protective effect of *Dunaliella salina* — A marine micro alga, against carbon tetrachloride-induced hepatotoxicity in rats. Hepatol Res 33.4 (2005): 313–3119.

Harari A et al. A 9-cis β-carotene-enriched diet inhibits atherogenesis and fatty liver formation in LDL receptor knockout mice. J Nutr 138.10 (2008): 1923–1930.

Heinrich U, Tronnier H. Systemic photoprotection: dream and reality. Aktuelle Dermatologie 24.10 (1998): 298–302.

Heinrich U et al. Supplementation with carotene or a similar amount of mixed carotenoids protects humans from UV-induced erythema. J Nutr 133.1 (2003): 98–101.

Herrero M et al. *Dunaliella salina* microalga pressurized liquid extracts as potential antimicrobials. J Food Prot 69.10 (2006): 2471–2477.

Jayappriyan, K. R., et al. (2013). In vitro anticancer activity of natural β-carotene from *Dunaliella salina* EU5891199 in PC-3 cells. Biomedicine and Preventive Nutrition. 3: 99–105.

Lamers PP et al. Exploring and exploiting carotenoid accumulation in *Dunaliella salina* for cell-factory applications. Trends Biotechnol 26.11 (2008): 631–638.

Lavy A et al. Dietary *Dunaliella bardawil*, a beta-carotene-rich alga, protects against acetic acid-induced small bowel inflammation in rats. Inflamm Bowel Dis 9.6 (2003): 372–379.

Lavy A et al. Natural beta-carotene for the prevention of post-ERCP pancreatitis. Pancreas 29.2 (2004): e45–e50.

Levy Y et al. Beta-carotene affects antioxidant status in non-insulin-dependent diabetes mellitus. Pathophysiology 6.3 (1999): 157–161.

Levy Y et al. Dietary supplementation of a natural isomer mixture of beta-carotene inhibits oxidation of LDL derived from patients with diabetes mellitus. Ann Nutr Metab 44.2 (2000): 54–60.

Murray MT. Encyclopaedia of nutritional supplements. Roseville, California: Prima Publishing, 1997.

Neuman I, et al. Prevention of exercise-induced asthma by a natural isomer mixture of beta-carotene. Ann Allergy Asthma Immunol 82.6 (1999): 549–553.

Passwater R, Solomon N. Algae: the next generation of superfoods. The Experts' Optimal Health Journal 1 (1997): 2.

Raja R, et al. Exploitation of *Dunaliella* for beta-carotene production. Appl Microbiol Biotechnol 74.3 (2007a): 517–23.

Raja R et al. Protective effect of *Dunaliella salina* (*Volvocales, Chlorophyta*) against experimentally induced fibrosarcoma on wistar rats. Microbiol Res 162.2 (2007b): 177–84.

Sheu M-J et al. Ethanol extract of *Dunaliella salina* induces cell cycle arrest and apoptosis in A549 human non-small cell lung cancer cells. In Vivo 22.3 (2008): 369–378.

Sheu, M. J., et al. (2010). Molecular mechanism of green microalgae, *Dunaliella salina*, involved in attenuating balloon injury-induced neointimal formation. British Journal of Nutrition, 104(3), 326–335.

Skinner G, Tomkins S. In the pink: colour from carotenes. Catalyst 29.2 (2008): 1–3.

Stahl W, et al. Human serum concentrations of all-trans beta- and alpha-carotene but not 9-cis beta-carotene increase upon ingestion of a natural isomer mixture obtained from *Dunaliella salina* (Betatene). J Nutr 123.5 (1993): 847–851.

Stahl W et al. Carotenoids and carotenoids plus vitamin E protect against ultraviolet light-induced erythema in humans. Am J Clin Nutr 71.3 (2000): 795–798.

Takenaka H et al. Protective effect of *Dunaliella bardawil* on water-immersion-induced stress in rats. Planta Med 59.5 (1993): 421–422.

Tracton I, Bobrov Z. Media release: world's first organic, super-anti-oxidant, wholefood to be released. NutriMed Group (2005).

Tsai, C. F., et al. (2012). Protective effects of *Dunaliella salina* — a carotenoids-rich alga — against ultraviolet B-induced corneal oxidative damage in mice. Molecular Vision, 18, 1540–1547.

USDA (2005). US Department of Agriculture National nutrient database for standard references. Release 18. Available online at: http://ndb.nal.usda.gov/.

Vanitha A et al. Effect of the carotenoid-producing alga, *Dunaliella bardawil*, on CCl4-induced toxicity in rats. Int J Toxicol 26.2 (2007): 159–167.

Ye ZW, et al. Biosynthesis and regulation of carotenoids in *Dunaliella*: progresses and prospects. Biotechnol Adv 26.4 (2008a): 352–360.

Ye, Z-W, et al. (2008b). Biosynthesis and regulation of carotenoids in *Dunaliella*: Progresses and prospects. Biotechnology Advances, 26(4), 352–360.

E

Echinacea

HISTORICAL NOTE Echinacea was first used by Native American Sioux Indians centuries ago as a treatment for snakebite, colic, infection and external wounds, among other things. It was introduced into standard medical practice in the United States during the 1800s as a popular anti-infective medication, which was prescribed by eclectic and traditional doctors until the 20th century. Remaining on the national list of official plant drugs in the United States until the 1940s, it was produced by pharmaceutical companies during this period. With the arrival of antibiotics, echinacea fell out of favour and was no longer considered a 'real' medicine for infection. Its use has re-emerged, probably because we are now in a better position to understand the limitations of antibiotic therapy and because there is growing public interest in self-care. The dozens of clinical trials conducted overseas have also played a role in its renaissance.

COMMON NAME

Echinacea

OTHER NAMES

Echinacea angustifolia — American coneflower, black sampson, black susans, coneflower, echinaceawurzel, Indian head, kansas snakeroot, purple coneflower, purpursonnenhutkraut, racine d'echinacea, *Rudbeckia angustifolia* L., scurvy root, snakeroot

E. purpurea — *Brauneria purpurea* (L.) Britt., combflower, purple coneflower, red sunflower

Rudbeckia purpurea L. — *E. pallida*, *Brauneria pallida* (Nutt.) Britt., pale coneflower, *Rudbeckia pallida* Nutt.

BOTANICAL NAME/FAMILY

Echinacea species (family Asteraceae [Compositae])

The name 'echinacea' generally refers to several different plants within the genus — *E. purpurea*, *E. pallida* and *E. angustifolia.*

PLANT PARTS USED

Root, leaf and aerial parts

CHEMICAL COMPONENTS

The most important constituents with regard to pharmacological activity are the polysaccharides, caffeic acid derivatives, alkylamides, essential oils and polyacetylenes, although there are other potentially active constituents, as well as a range of vitamins, minerals, fatty acids, resins, glycoproteins and sterols (Pizzorno & Murray 2006). Cynarin, a potential immunosuppressant and CD28 ligand, was also identified in *E. purpurea* (Dong et al 2006). Constituent concentrations vary depending on the species, plant part and growing conditions. With regard to the final chemical composition of an echinacea-containing product, the drying and extraction processes further alter chemical composition. Therefore, the pharmacological effects of an echinacea product depend very much on which constituents are present and their relative ratios. This is outlined further in the following sections.

Pharmacokinetics

The absorption of *E. purpurea* alkylamides from lozenges is rapid and linear (Guiotto et al 2008).

A clinical study with healthy volunteers showed that, following ingestion of tablets containing ethanolic echinacea extract, alkylamides were detectable in plasma 20 minutes after ingestion, whereas caffeic acid derivatives were not detectable in the plasma at any time after tablet ingestion (Matthias et al 2005a). A further study by the same authors showed that there was no significant difference in the bioavailability of alkylamides from a liquid and solid oral dosage form of an echinacea product (mixture of *E. purpurea* and *E. angustifolia*), with T_{max} reached at 20 and 30 minutes, respectively (Matthias et al 2007b). Two other studies reported that, 30–45 minutes following administration of *E. purpurea* products (Echinaforce tincture, tablets, spray) containing milligram amounts of alkylamides, plasma concentrations of alkylamides of about 0.07–0.40 ng/mL were recorded (Woelkart et al 2006, 2008b), and effects on the immune markers were observed 23 hours after oral administration (Woelkart et al 2006).

Furthermore, tetraene alkylamides, present in *E. angustifolia* and *E. purpurea*, are metabolised by CYP450 enzymes (Matthias et al 2005b). In addition, the metabolism of tetraene alkylamides can be significantly decreased by monoene alkylamides that are only found in *E. angustifolia* (Matthias et al 2005b). A recent study found that the human CYP450 enzymes involved in the metabolism of one of the most abundant alkylamides, *N*-isobutyldodeca-2E,4E,8Z,10Z-tetraenamide, are CYP2E1, CYP2C9 and CYP1A2 (Toselli et al 2010).

MAIN ACTIONS

Due to the wide assortment of chemical constituents found in echinacea, it has varied pharmacological effects.

Immunomodulator

Experimental results suggest that echinacea functions more as a modulator of the immune response rather than as a straightforward immune stimulant. This is well illustrated by a recent study conducted by Ritchie et al (2011), which showed that the response to treatment with the product Echinaforce was dependent on subjects' baseline constitution. For example, echinacea treatment induced an additional formation of antiviral interferon-gamma, chemotactic molecules (interleukin-8 [IL-8]) or monocyte chemoattractant protein-1 in subjects with a low initial production at baseline (from +18 to +49%). In contrast, subjects with higher levels of these factors at baseline experienced no further increase after treatment (Ritchie et al 2011). Similarly, volunteers reporting higher stress levels or higher susceptibility to cold infections have reacted to echinacea treatment with improved immune responses (Schapowal 2013).

The immunomodulator activity of echinacea has been the subject of countless studies and appears to be the result of multiple mechanisms.

Overall, the fresh-pressed leaf juice of *E. purpurea* and alcoholic extracts of the roots of *E. pallida*, *E. angustifolia* and *E. purpurea* have been shown to act mainly on non-specific cellular immunity (Blumenthal et al 2000). It was reported that no one single constituent is responsible for the herb's immunomodulating action, with the most important elements being polysaccharides, glycoproteins, alkamides and flavonoids (Ernst 2002). More recent research indicates that the water-soluble compounds (such as polysaccharides) rather than lipophilic constituents are chiefly responsible for the immunostimulatory activity (Pillai et al 2007).

Macrophage activation has been well demonstrated, as has stimulation of phagocytosis (Barrett 2003, Bauer et al 1988, Groom et al 2007, Pugh et al 2008, Zhai et al 2009a). Orally administered root extracts of echinacea have produced stronger effects on phagocytosis than aerial parts, with *E. purpurea* roots producing the greatest effect, followed by that of *E. angustifolia* and *E. pallida* (Pizzorno & Murray 2006).

The activation of polymorphonuclear leucocytes and natural killer (NK) cells and increased numbers of T-cell and B-cell leucocytes have also been reported for echinacea (Groom et al 2007, Zhai et al 2007a).

Echinacea stimulates cytokine (Altamirano-Dimas et al 2007, Brush et al 2006, Dong et al 2006, 2008, Farinacci et al 2009, Sharma et al 2006, Zhai et al 2007a, Zwickey et al 2007) and chemokine production (Wang et al 2006, 2008).

Moreover, various echinacea species stimulate nitric oxide (NO) production in vitro (Classen et al 2006, Sullivan et al 2008).

Contradictory results were obtained for tumour necrosis factor-alpha (TNF-alpha) production, possibly due to the different preparations used producing different effects. In one study, echinacea significantly increased TNF-alpha production (Senchina et al 2006), whereas no effects on TNF-alpha were observed for all echinacea species in another study (McCann et al 2007), and in a third study, NF-κB expression and TNF-alpha levels decreased in non-stimulated macrophages following echinacea treatment (Matthias et al 2007a).

In lipopolysaccharide-stimulated (endotoxin) cells, echinacea inhibited NF-κB, TNF-alpha, NO and cytokine production, with different alkylamides exerting different effects (Matthias et al 2007a, 2008, Raduner et al 2006, Sasagawa et al 2006, Stevenson et al 2005, Woelkart et al 2006, Zhai et al 2007a). Another study found that the *E. purpurea* root extract (polysaccharide-rich) increased specific surface biomarkers whereas the leaf extract (alkylamide-rich) inhibited their expression. Moreover, IL-6 and TNF-alpha production was increased due to the root extract, but unchanged following exposure to the leaf extract (Benson et al 2010).

Similarly, a more recent study found that different alkylamides either suppressed or stimulated influenza A-induced secretion of cytokines, chemokines and prostaglandin E_2 from RAW264.7 macrophage-like cells (Cech et al 2010). Unidentified constituents from echinacea have been shown to stimulate inositol-1,4,5-trisphosphate receptor and phospholipase C mediation of cytosolic Ca^{2+} levels in non-immune mammalian cells (Wu et al 2010).

Anti-inflammatory

Studies indicate that alcohol extracts of all three echinacea species (*E. angustifolia*, *E. purpurea* and *E. pallida*) exert significant anti-inflammatory activity (Raso et al 2002, Zhai et al 2009a). The result is due to multiple constituents acting with multiple mechanisms. The alkylamide fraction inhibits inducible nitric oxide synthase (iNOS) and the caffeic acid fraction enhances arginase activity (Zhai et al 2009a). In vivo tests further identify anti-inflammatory effects also for *E. angustifolia* and *E. pallida* when applied topically (Speroni et al 2002, Tragni et al 1985, Tubaro et al 1987).

A recent study reports on the selective induction of pro- and anti-inflammatory cytokines by low-dose *E. purpurea* (Kapai et al 2011). Similarly, anti-inflammatory effects have been identified for the essential oils of *E. purpurea* extract, with proinflammatory cytokines such as IL-2, IL-6 and TNF-alpha being reduced in the blood of treated mice (Yu et al 2013).

COX-1/COX-2

Alkylamides from the roots of *E. purpurea* partially inhibit both cyclooxygenase-1 (COX-1) and COX-2 isoenzymes, thus decreasing prostaglandin E_2 levels (Clifford et al 2002, LaLone et al 2007, Raman et al 2008). Several alkylamides isolated from a CO_2 extract of the roots of *E. angustifolia* have been shown to inhibit COX-2-dependent prostaglandin E_2 formation, although COX-2 mRNA and protein expression were not inhibited, but rather increased (Hinz et al 2007). A 2009 study further confirmed that certain alkylamides and ketones present in various *Echinacea* species were the key anti-inflammatory contributors inhibiting prostaglandin E_2 production (LaLone et al 2009).

Cannabinoid and TRPV1 receptor interaction

The alkamides from echinacea also modulate TNF-alpha mRNA expression in human monocytes/macrophages via the cannabinoid type 2 (CB2) receptor, thus identifying a possible mode of action for its immunomodulatory activity (Raduner et al 2006, Woelkart & Bauer 2007). Two alkylamides, which bind to the CB2 receptor more strongly than endogenous cannabinoids and activate it, have been classified as a new class of cannabinomimetics (Gertsch et al 2006). It was found that some of the alkylamides in echinacea self-assemble into micelles in aqueous solution, which then determines their binding to the CB2 receptor (Raduner et al 2007). In a subsequent study, Chicca et al (2009) showed that ethanolic *E. purpurea* root and herb extracts and specific *N*-alkylamides within produce synergistic pharmacological effects on the endocannabinoid system in vitro by simultaneously targeting the CB2 receptor, endocannabinoid transport and degradation. In contrast, ketoalkenes from *E. pallida* did not interact with cannabinoid receptors (Egger et al 2008).

Ethanol extracts from echinacea roots showed potent agonist activity on TRPV1, a mammalian pain receptor. The compounds involved in the TRPV1 receptor activation differ from those involved in the inhibition of prostaglandin E_2 production (Birt et al 2008).

Antiviral activity

Four different *Echinacea* species (*E. angustifolia, E. purpurea, E. tennesseensis* and *E. pallida)* increase the amount of iNOS protein, but to varying degrees. The results suggest that any potential antiviral activities of *Echinacea* spp. extracts are not likely to be mediated through large inductions of type 1 interferon, but may involve iNOS (Senchina et al 2010). *E. purpurea* extract Echinaforce inhibited the induction of multiple proinflammatory cytokines by respiratory viruses (Sharma et al 2009). The same authors showed in a three-dimensional tissue model of normal human airway epithelium that this specific *E. purpurea* extract, Echinaforce, reversed rhinovirus type 1A (RV1A)-stimulated mucopolysaccharide inclusion in goblet cells, RV1A-induced mucin secretion and the RV1A-stimulated secretion of proinflammatory cytokines (Sharma et al 2010).

Herpes simplex virus

Extracts of eight taxa of the genus *Echinacea* were found to have antiviral activity against herpes simplex virus type 1 (HSV-1) in vitro when exposed to visible and ultraviolet A light (Binns et al 2002). Antiviral activity was confirmed for *E. purpurea* extracts in 2008, with evidence suggesting that polyphenolic compounds other than the known HIV inhibitor, cichoric acid, may also be involved (Birt et al 2008). A 2010 study found that hydroalcoholic *E. pallida* extracts interfere with free HSV-1 or HSV-2 and pressed juice is able to interact with HSV-1 or HSV-2 inside and outside the cell, as well as to protect cells against viral infection, probably by interfering with virus attachment (Schneider et al 2010). Another study in mice showed that *E. purpurea* polysaccharide reduces the latency rate in HSV-1 infections when supplied prior to infection (Ghaemi et al 2009).

Antibacterial activity

An in vitro study showed that Echinaforce inhibits the proliferation of *Propionibacterium acnes* and decreases bacterial-induced inflammation (Sharma et al 2011). Antiadhesive activity against *Campylobacter jejuni* was found for two different *Echinacea* species, with *E. purpurea* extract displaying a higher activity than *E. angustifolia.* The extracts used were of the MediHerb brand (Bensch et al 2011). The standardised extract of *E. purpurea* (Echinaforce) readily inactivated *Streptococcus pyogenes*, *Haemophilus influenzae* and *Legionella pneumophila* and also reversed their proinflammatory responses. *Staphylococcus aureus* (methicillin-resistant and sensitive strains) and *Mycobacterium smegmatis* were less sensitive to the bactericidal effects of *Echinacea*; however, their proinflammatory responses were still completely reversed. In contrast, some other pathogens tested, including *Candida albicans*, were relatively resistant (Sharma et al 2010).

Cytochromes and P-glycoprotein

Earlier research suggested caution when using echinacea with anticancer and antiretroviral agents (Meijerman et al 2006, van den Bout-van den Beukel et al 2006), due to possible effects on drug-metabolising and transporting enzymes. However, most of the warnings were based on in vitro studies, which now appear to have little or no clinical relevance in vivo (Heinrich et al 2008, Huntimer et al 2006, Izzo 2012, Unger 2010). Moreover, recent research found no pharmacokinetic interactions between echinacea and different antiretrovirals and warfarin (Abdul et al 2010, Hermann & von Richter 2012).

In fact, clinical studies found that echinacea has no clinically significant effect on CYP1A2, CYP2D6, CYP2E1 or CYP3A4 activity (Gurley et al 2004). This was demonstrated for the *E. purpurea* extract Echinaforce (Modarai et al 2011) and 400 mg of powdered dried root of *E. purpurea* taken four times daily for 8 days (Gorski et al 2004). Moreover, studies by Gurley et al found no effects on CYP2D6 in healthy volunteers after echinacea (*E. purpurea)* use for 14 days (Gurley et al 2008a).

To further confirm no clinically significant effects of *E. purpurea* on CYP3A4, two more recent studies using a dose of 500 mg three times daily found no change to the pharmacokinetics of lopinavir-ritonavir (CYP3A4 substrates) in healthy people (Penzak et al 2010) and darunavir-ritonavir in HIV patients (Moltó et al 2011).

In another study investigating echinacea 1275 mg, four times daily (capsules containing a mixture of 600 mg of *E. angustifolia* roots and 675 mg of *E. purpurea* root; standardised to contain 5.75 mg of total alkylamides per tablet) with warfarin in 12 healthy male subjects (single oral dose of 25 mg warfarin or received this dose after 14 days of pretreatment with echinacea) significantly reduced plasma concentrations of S-warfarin and no change for R-warfarin were reported. Warfarin pharmacodynamics, platelet aggregation and baseline were not significantly affected by echinacea (Abdul et al 2010).

Differences between in vitro and clinical results were also found among studies investigating effects on P-glycoprotein, indicating that the effect on P-glycoprotein is not clinically significant (Hellum & Nilsen 2008). A 14-day clinical trial of 18 healthy volunteers detected no significant alteration to digoxin pharmacokinetics for *E. purpurea* extract consisting of 195 mg aerial, root and seed parts, and 72 mg *E. angustifolia* root parts which were standardised to contain 2.2 mg isobutylamides per capsule (Gurley et al 2008b).

> ***Clinical note — Echinacea and cannabinoid receptors***
> Alkylamides found in echinacea show a structural similarity with anandamide, an endogenous ligand of cannabinoid receptors. CB1 and CB2 receptors belong to G-protein-coupled receptors. CB2 receptors are believed to play an important role in various processes, including metabolic dysregulation, inflammation, pain and bone loss. Compounds such as cannabinoids, which act on these receptors, are becoming more and more popular as they represent new targets for drug discovery. A well-known plant cannabinoid is delta-9-tetrahydrocannabinol, a constituent of *Cannabis sativa*.

OTHER ACTIONS

Antioxidant

Free radical scavenging activity can be attributed to numerous antioxidant constituents found in echinacea, such as vitamin C, beta-carotene, flavonoids, selenium and zinc. One in vitro study reported that the antioxidant activity exerted by echinacea tincture was significantly greater than that observed for *Ginkgo biloba* (Masteikova et al 2007).

Anaesthetic

The alkylamides exert a mild anaesthetic activity, which is typically experienced as a tingling sensation on the tongue (Pizzorno & Murray 2006).

Apoptosis

Apoptosis, or programmed cell death, is a physiological, active cellular suicide process that can be modulated by various stimuli, including hormones, cytokines, growth factors and some chemotherapeutic agents. Research has been undertaken with the three clinically used *Echinacea* spp., several key constituents and different herbal fractions to investigate mechanisms of action, strength of activity and specificity of effect.

The *n*-hexane extracts of all three *Echinacea* spp. exert cytotoxic effects on human pancreatic and colon cancer cells in a concentration- and time-dependent manner, with *E. pallida* being the most active species (Aherne et al 2007). The effects were partially due to apoptosis by significantly increasing caspase-3/7 activity (Chicca et al 2007, 2008). Cytotoxic effects of the *n*-hexane extract of *E. angustifolia* on lung cancer cells have also been reported (Ramirez-Erosa et al 2007). However, in comparison to other herbal medicines such as wild yam and dichora root, echinacea exhibits only weak tumoricidal effects (Mazzio & Soliman 2009).

Isolated hydroxylated polyacetylenes and polyenes (more hydrophilic) from *E. pallida* are less cytotoxic than the more hydrophobic compounds (Pellati et al 2006).

It has been shown that the effects of isolated constituents on cell proliferation vary. In cervical and breast cancer cells treated with doxorubicin and *E. purpurea* extract or isolated echinacea constituents (i.e. cynarin, chicoric acid), the ethyl acetate fraction of echinacea extract and chicoric acid increased breast cancer cell growth and cynarin enhanced the growth of cervical cancer cells. However, cynarin showed antiproliferative effects on breast cancer cells (Huntimer et al 2006).

Chemoprevention

Several experimental studies with mice have found that treatment with echinacea reduces the incidence of tumour development (Brousseau & Miller 2005, Hayashi et al 2001, Miller 2005). Most research has been conducted with *E. purpurea*. In a study with gamma-irradiated mice, *E. purpurea* was able to show radioprotection (use before radiation) as well as radio-recovery effectiveness (Abouelella et al 2007). One study reported that *E. angustifolia* can stimulate mammary epithelial cell differentiation (Starvaggi Cucuzza et al 2008).

An animal study showed that the administration of *E. purpurea* extract to rats with hyperplasia for 4 and 8 weeks gradually and significantly reduced the prostate mass and reversed the degenerative changes in the structure of the prostate gland (Skaudickas et al 2009).

Immunological adjuvants

In vitro studies in human lymphocytes activated with different lectins showed that using *E. purpurea* root extract in addition to individual lectins increased lymphoproliferation, which would suggest adjuvant activity (Chaves et al 2007). In mice, no adjuvant activity was detected for lipophilic, neutral and acidic extracts of echinacea (Gaia Herbs) (Ragupathi et al 2008).

Antifungal activity

Hexane extracts of echinacea have phototoxic antimicrobial activity against fungi (Binns et al 2000). The extracts inhibited growth of yeast strains of *Saccharomyces cerevisiae*, *Candida shehata*, *C. kefyr*, *C. albicans*, *C. steatulytica* and *C. tropicalis*. A recent study reports on antifungal activities of echinacea against *S. cerevisiae* and *Cryptococcus neoformans* by disrupting the fungal cell wall structure (Mir-Rashed et al 2010).

Antiparasitic

Aqueous extracts of echinacea showed activity against gastrointestinal nematodes in goats and pigs (Lans et al 2007). Four preparations of echinacea, with distinct chemical compositions, inhibited the proliferation of *Leishmania donovani*, *Leishmania major* and *Trypanosoma brucei* and at least one extract seems to reverse the proinflammatory activity of *L. donovani* (Canlas et al 2010).

Anxiolytic

The anxiolytic potential of five different echinacea preparations (*E. purpurea*: two different root and one herb extract; *E. angustifolia:* two different root extracts) were tested in a rat model. Three of these decreased anxiety but two of them had a very narrow effective dose range. One extract, *E. purpurea* root extract (70% ethanol v/v), decreased anxiety within a wide dose range (3–8 mg/kg) in three different tests of anxiety. These findings suggest for the first time that certain preparations have a considerable anxiolytic potential (Haller et al 2010).

Hypoglycaemic

Alkylamides and fatty acids isolated from an *n*-hexane extract of the flowers of *E. purpurea* were found to activate peroxisome proliferator-activated receptor gamma without stimulating adipocyte differentiation. This suggests that these compounds have the potential to manage insulin resistance and type 2 diabetes (Christensen et al 2009).

CLINICAL USE

Clinical trials using echinacea have used various preparations, such as topical applications, homeopathic preparations, injectable forms and oral dose forms, characteristics that should be noted when reviewing the data available. Overall, the majority of clinical studies performed in Europe have involved a commercial product known as Echinacin (Madaus, Germany), which is a hydrophilic product prepared from the stabilised juice of fresh *E. purpurea* tops (aerial parts). However, other preparations have also been tested, such as the fresh plant tincture of the whole plant of *E. purpurea* and several preparations manufactured by an Australian company, Mediherb. Due to the different species, plant parts and extraction processes used, the chemical constituent profiles of the different preparations will vary, which may partly account for the differences in test results.

Upper respiratory tract infections

Clinical studies investigating the use of various echinacea preparations in the treatment of upper respiratory tract infections (URTIs) have produced inconsistent results due to the use of different extracts and plant parts, *Echinacea* species, populations and study designs, making interpretation difficult. Overall, the most consistently positive results are obtained from preparations containing *E. purpurea* and *E. angustifolia* for reducing symptoms and possibly the duration of infection, when used as soon as symptoms arise. However, supportive evidence has also accumulated for the use of echinacea as a preventive approach.

In 2000, a Cochrane review was published that had assessed the evidence available from 16 clinical trials (eight treatment and eight prevention) involving a total of 3396 subjects (Melchart et al 2000), and it concluded that some echinacea preparations may be better than placebo, with a majority of studies reporting favourable effects.

Certain facets of quality of life improve with echinacea treatment during an URTI, according to a 2006 review, suggesting that treatment provides symptom relief and improved wellbeing (Gillespie & Coleman 2006). A more recent Cochrane systematic review (Linde et al 2009) evaluated data from 16 trials (up to October 2007). While reviewers reported that evaluation was difficult because of the heterogeneity of preparations tested and variability of trial approaches, it was concluded that preparations based on the aerial parts of *E. purpurea* might be effective for the early treatment of colds in adults, although results are not completely consistent. Also, beneficial effects of other echinacea preparations (i.e. from *E. angustifolia* and *E. pallida*) may exist, but independently replicated rigorous randomised controlled trials (RCTs) are lacking (Linde et al 2009) and further research is needed (Woelkart et al 2008b).

A review including evidence until August 2009 concluded that there is moderate evidence to support the use of *E. purpurea* for treatment of the common cold (Nahas & Balla 2011). Treatment should be commenced at the first signs of infection (Schoop et al 2006a, Woelkart et al 2008a).

Since then a large placebo-controlled trial (n = 719) testing an echinacea preparation made from the roots of *E. purpurea* and *E. angustifolia* (tablets containing the equivalent of 675 mg *E. purpurea* root standardised to 2.1 mg alkamides and 600 mg *E. angustifolia* root standardised to 2.1 mg alkamides: MediHerb brand) failed to find that treatment decreased the severity and duration of the common cold compared to placebo (Barrett et al 2010). Frequency of adverse effects did not differ between the placebo and echinacea group.

Commission E approves the use of *E. purpurea* herb as an immune system support in cases of respiratory and lower urinary tract infection, and *E. pallida* root as supportive treatment in influenza-like infections (Blumenthal et al 2000).

Prevention

According to a 2009 Cochrane systematic review, the beneficial effects of echinacea preparations for the prevention of URTIs may also exist, but require further investigation (Linde et al 2009). Since then, two new RCTs have been published confirming *E. purpurea* preparations are effective at reducing the incidence of the common cold (Jawad et al 2012, Tiralongo et al 2012).

An Australian study published by Tiralongo et al (2012) used a standardised echinacea tablet, known as Echinacea Premium, by MediHerb, which contained 112.5 mg *Echinacea purpurea* 6:1 extract (equivalent to 675 mg dry root) and 150 mg *Echinacea angustifolia* 4:1 extract (equivalent to 600 mg dry root), standardised to 4.4 mg alkylamides. The prevention study did not use artificial rhinovirus inoculation, unlike previous studies, choosing to test the treatment effectiveness in preventing respiratory symptoms in air travellers. The RCT included 175 adults travelling overseas on a long-haul, economy flight for a period of 1–5 weeks. Treatment with the echinacea preparation before and during travel reduced the incidence of respiratory symptoms during travel compared to placebo (Tiralongo et al 2012).

A much larger RCT (n = 755 healthy adults) found that compliant prophylactic use of *E. purpurea* (Echinaforce, produced by Bioforce, Switzerland, containing an alcoholic extract of *E. purpurea*, 95% herb and 5% roots) over a 4-month period reduced the total number of cold episodes, cumulated episode days and painkiller-medicated episodes, inhibited virally confirmed colds and especially prevented enveloped virus infections ($P < 0.05$). Preventive effects increased with therapy compliance and adherence to the protocol (Jawad et al 2012).

Additionally, the treatment was considered well tolerated, with adverse event incidence similar to placebo and no induction of allergic reactions, leucopenia or autoimmune diseases (Schapowal 2013).

Previously, a 2006 meta-analysis by Schoop et al concluded that the odds of experiencing a clinical cold were 55% higher with placebo than with pressed *Echinacea purpurea* juice or hydroethanolic *E. angustifolia* extract following inoculation with rhinovirus. Schoop et al concluded that *E. purpurea* (pressed juice) and *E. angustifolia* (alcoholic extract) show the most promise as preventive treatment, although further investigation is still required to confirm this (Schoop et al 2006b). A 2007 meta-analysis published in *Lancet Infectious Diseases* was also positive and concluded that echinacea products from all species were beneficial in significantly decreasing the incidence (by 58%) and duration (by 1.4 days) of the common cold (Shah et al 2007b).

Athletes

Echinacea has been used to prevent exercise-induced immunosuppression (Gleeson et al 2001). Standardised *E. purpurea* extract (Echinaforce Forte) was effective in the prophylaxis, as well as treatment, of athletes in an open-label study (n = 80) (Ross 2010, Schoop et al 2006a). It is believed that echinacea attenuates mucosal immune suppression known to occur with intensive exercise and can reduce the duration of URTIs that exercising people incur (Hall et al 2007).

Interestingly, a double-blind study of 24 healthy men (20–28 years of age) showed that oral echinacea supplementation resulted in significant increases in erythropoietin, VO_{2max} and running economy (Whitehead 2012).

Paediatric studies

Four randomised studies published after 2000 were conducted with children and generally produced disappointing results (Cohen et al 2004, Spasov et al 2004, Taylor et al 2003, Weber et al 2005). A short review by Koenig and Roehr (2006) has also concluded that there is currently no evidence for the efficacy of *E. purpurea* in the treatment of URTI in children (Koenig & Roehr 2006). A 2008 clinical study with 60 children aged 12–60 months suggests that treating cold with *E. purpurea* in otitis-prone young children does not decrease the risk of acute otitis media, but is associated with a borderline increased risk of having at least one episode of acute otitis media during a 6-month follow-up compared to placebo (Wahl et al 2008).

No clear evidence of benefit in children was also reported in the most recent Cochrane reviews (Fashner et al 2012, Linde et al 2009).

> ***Clinical note — Common cold symptoms: What is usual?***
>
> The pathogenesis of the common cold involves a complex interplay between replicating viruses and the host's inflammatory response (Heikkinen & Jarvinen 2003). The onset of cold symptoms after viral incubation varies considerably and depends on the causative virus. In experimental rhinovirus infections, the onset of symptoms has been reported to occur as soon as 10–12 hours after intranasal inoculation. Generally, the severity of the symptoms increases rapidly, peaks within 2–3 days of infection and decreases soon after. The mean duration of the common cold is 7–10 days, but in a proportion of patients some symptoms can still be present after 3 weeks. Symptoms typically start with a sore throat, which is soon accompanied by nasal stuffiness and discharge, sneezing and cough. The soreness of the throat usually disappears quickly, whereas the initial watery rhinorrhoea becomes thicker and more purulent over time and can be accompanied by fever, most usually in children. Other symptoms associated with the cold syndrome include hoarseness, headache, malaise and lethargy.

Acute sore throat

A multicentre, randomised, double-blind, double-dummy-controlled trial (n = 154) found that an echinacea/sage preparation is as efficacious and well tolerated as a chlorhexidine/lignocaine spray in the treatment of acute sore throat (Schapowal et al 2009).

Wound healing

Several uncontrolled clinical studies support the topical use of echinacea to enhance wound healing. A trial involving 4598 people investigated the effects of a preparation consisting of the juice of the aerial parts of *E. purpurea* on various wounds, burns, skin infections and inflammatory skin conditions (Kinkel et al 1984). Topical application of echinacea produced an 85% overall success rate, and the key constituent responsible for enhancing wound healing appears to be echinacoside (Speroni et al 2002).

Preclinical research with a mice model provides some support for its role. An alcoholic extract of *E. pallida* reversed stress-delayed wound healing in mice, but had no apparent wound-healing effect for the non-stressed mice when compared to controls (Zhai et al 2009b).

Commission E approves the external use of *E. purpurea* herb for poorly healing wounds and chronic ulcerations (Blumenthal et al 2000).

Genital herpes *(Condyloma acuminata)*

Human papillomavirus is the most common cause of sexually transmitted disease. It is associated with immunosuppression and shows a marked tendency to recur.

A prospective, double-blind, placebo-controlled, crossover trial conducted over 1 year investigated the effects of an extract of the plant and root of *E. purpurea* (Echinaforce 800 mg twice daily) on the incidence and severity of genital herpes outbreaks in 50 patients (Vonau et al 2001). Treatment was taken for 6 months, then crossed over to the alternative treatment for an additional 6 months. The entry criteria specified a minimum of four recurrences during the previous 12 months or prior to suppressive aciclovir. The study found no statistically significant benefit compared with placebo after 6 months of therapy. It is important to note that, during the study, 15 people dropped out, thereby reducing the sample size, which was considered insufficient by the authors.

IN COMBINATION

A preventive effect against recurrence was found in a more recent RCT for a herbal combination consisting of echinacea, uncaria, tabebuja, papaya, grapefruit and andrographis (*Andrographis paniculata*). In this study, 261 patients allocated to surgical excision were divided into two groups, with one receiving additional treatment with the herbal combination in a dose of three tablets per day for 1 month postoperatively or no additional treatment after surgery. Over a 6-month follow-up period, the group receiving the herbal combination experienced a significantly reduced incidence of recurrence of anal condylomata (7.2% [10/139] compared to 27.1% [33/122] in the control group which received no additional treatment: $P < 0.0001$) (Mistrangelo et al 2010).

Reducing chemotherapy side effects

Results from a small, open, prospective study of subjects with advanced gastric cancer suggest that intravenous administration of a polysaccharide fraction isolated from *E. purpurea* may be effective in reducing chemotherapy-induced leucopenia (Melchart et al 2002). Test subjects had advanced gastric cancer and were undergoing palliative chemotherapy with etoposide, leucovorin and 5-fluorouracil. The median number of leucocytes 14–16 days after chemotherapy was 3630/mcL (range 1470–5770 mcL) in the patients receiving herbal treatment compared with 2370/mcL (870–3950 mcL) in the patients of the historical control group ($P = 0.015$).

Radiation-associated leucopenia

Equivocal evidence exists for the use of echinacea in radiation-induced leucopenia, according to a small number of randomised studies (Ulbricht & Basch 2005). The product tested was Esberitox, which contains ethanolic extracts of three herbs, including root of echinacea. A study investigated the radioprotective properties of *E. purpurea* tablets (two 275 mg echinacea tablets twice daily) in a group of radiation workers who were identified as carrying dicentric chromosomes in their lymphocytes. After the 2-week treatment, lymphocyte chromosome aberration frequency dropped significantly, and the number of apoptotic cells increased, indicating that echinacea treatment may be beneficial for the prevention of adverse health effects in workers exposed to ionising radiation (Joksić et al 2009).

Halitosis

A study with healthy volunteers suggests that a palatal adhesive tablet containing echinacea may serve as an effective means of treatment for patients complaining of oral malodour, because it resulted in a significant reduction in both oral malodour scores and volatile sulfide compound levels. The reduction in volatile sulfide compound levels was significantly higher than with zinc and chlorhexidine (Sterer et al 2008).

Recurrent candidiasis

The herb is used to treat recurrent candidiasis, chiefly because of its antifungal and immunostimulant properties. Controlled studies are unavailable to determine effectiveness in this condition.

OTHER USES

Echinacea has also been used to treat urinary tract infections, allergies, acne and abscesses, and as adjunctive therapy in cancer (Mills & Bone 2000). Based on the herb's antiviral activity against HSV-1 in vitro, it is also used in the treatment of herpes infections. In practice, it is prescribed with other herbs to treat common infections and to prevent infections generally.

A recent study reported on preliminary results suggesting that Polinacea could be used to improve the immune response to influenza vaccine (Di Pierro et al 2012). The extract is made from the roots of *E. angustifolia* standardised to the complex polysaccharide IDN5405, the phenylethanoid echinacoside and substantial lack of alkamide. This follows a previous study showing that this preparation modulates bovine peripheral blood mononuclear cell proliferation (Wu et al 2009).

It may have potential as a topical cream for improving skin hydration and reducing wrinkles, according to a small study with 10 healthy people aged 25–40 years; however it showed low storage stability (Yotsawimonwat et al 2010).

DOSAGE RANGE

General guide

- Dried herb: 3 g/day of either *E. angustifolia* or *E. purpurea*.
- Liquid extract (1:2): 3–6 mL/day of either *E. angustifolia* or *E. purpurea*.

This dose may be increased to 10–20 mL/day in acute conditions.

Treatment is usually started at the first sign of URTI and continued for 7–14 days.

Specific guide

- *E. angustifolia* dried root: 1–3 g/day.
- *E. purpurea* dried root: 1.5–4.5 g/day.
- *E. purpurea* dried aerial parts: 2.5–6.0 g/day.
- *E. purpurea* expressed juice of fresh plant: 6–9 mL/day.

It appears that the cold-pressed juice and ethanolic extract of the aerial parts of *E. purpurea* and the hydroethanolic extracts from the roots of *E. angustifolia* are the most studied preparation for URTIs.

Doses according to clinical trials

URTI: Treatment

- 10.2 g of dried echinacea root during the first 24 hours and 5.1 g during each of the next 4 days. One tablet contained: 675 mg *E. purpurea* root and 600 mg *E. angustifolia* root standardised to 2.1 mg alkamides (MediHerb brand, produced by Integria Healthcare).
- 4000 mg of extract/day taken as 0.9 mL five times a day, Echinaforce, produced by Bioforce, Switzerland (alcoholic extract of *E. purpurea*, 95% herb and 5% roots, 5 mg/100 g, standardised to contain 5 mg/100 g of dodecatetraenoic acid isobutylamide)

Prevention

- 3825 mg dry root equivalent/day, taken as one tablet three times a day for 6 weeks. One tablet contained: 675 mg *E. purpurea* root and 600 mg *E. angustifolia* root standardised to 2.1 mg alkamides (MediHerb brand, produced by Integria Healthcare).
- 2400 mg of extract/day taken as 0.9 mL three times a day for 1 month, Echinaforce, produced by Bioforce, Switzerland (alcoholic extract of *E. purpurea*, 95% herb and 5% roots, 5 mg/100 g, standardised to contain 5 mg/100 g of dodecatetraenoic acid isobutylamide).
- Two tablets per day, over 8 weeks; each 750-mg tablet contained 1200 mg of tincture mass of Echinaforce, which corresponded to 18.6 mg dry mass of *E purpurea* (drug extract ratio of the 95% herb = 1:12; ratio of the 5% root = 1:11).

Protection from radiation

- Two 275 mg *E. purpurea* tablets twice daily for 2 weeks (brand not specified).

Genital herpes

- Echinaforce 800 mg twice daily for 1 year.

ADVERSE REACTIONS

E

Echinacea is well tolerated. A recent analysis of systematic reviews noted only minor adverse effects for *Echinacea* spp. (Posadzki 2013). Short-term use of echinacea is associated with a good safety profile, with a slight risk of transient, reversible and self-limiting gastrointestinal symptoms and rashes (Huntley et al 2005). However, cases of allergic reactions have been reported, resulting in pruritus, urticaria, angio-oedema and anaphylaxis (Mullins 1998, Mullins & Heddle 2002), especially in people with known plant allergies (Tiralongo et al 2012). Hypereosinophilia has been reported, and various authors suggest that the allergic reaction observed is an IgE-mediated hypersensitivity reaction (Maskatia & Baker 2010, Mullins & Heddle 2002).

Overall, echinacea is safe for asthmatics and only in rare instances has been associated with allergic reactions or disease exacerbation (Huntley et al 2005).

It is unclear whether children are more prone to rashes with *E. purpurea* than adults. One study found that rash occurred in 7.1% of children using echinacea compared with 2.7% taking placebo (Taylor et al 2003), whereas a more recent study failed to identify allergic responses or adverse reactions in children with echinacea use (Saunders et al 2007).

There is no clear evidence from basic science or human studies to show that echinacea causes liver toxicity (Ulbricht & Basch 2005). Echinacea (8000 mg/day) taken over 28 days resulted in an increase in serum erythropoietin levels at days 7, 14 and 21, but did not significantly alter red blood cell, haemoglobin and haematocrit levels (Whitehead et al 2007). A single 350-mg dose of *E. purpurea* had no effect on electrocardiographic and blood pressure measurements (Shah et al 2007a).

One clinical study has reported that 1 g *E. purpurea* administered over 10 days altered the gastrointestinal microflora by significantly increasing total aerobic bacteria and bacteria belonging to the *Bacteroides* genus, but not significantly changing the number of enteric bacteria, enterococci, lactobacilli, bifidobacteria or total anaerobic bacteria (Hill et al 2006). Moreover, a review reported several ocular adverse effects due to *E. purpurea* (Santaella & Fraunfelder 2007). A recent review states that echinacea contributes to dry eye (Askeroglu et al 2013). One case report exists where it is believed that an ethanolic extract of *E. pallida*, taken 10–20 days before, may have induced or exacerbated severe thrombotic thrombocytopenic purpura in a healthy 32-year-old man (Liatsos et al 2006).

SIGNIFICANT INTERACTIONS

Cyclophosphamide

Echinacea appears to increase the immunostimulatory effect of low-dose cyclophosphamide, which may be detrimental in autoimmune disease where low doses are used (Stargrove et al 2008) — the clinical significance of this observation is unknown — avoid until safety can be assured.

Immunosuppression agents (e.g. cyclosporine)

Theoretically, there may be an antagonistic pharmacodynamic interaction with immunosuppressive medication, but the clinical relevance is unclear. Exercise caution when using immunosuppressive agents and echinacea concurrently.

Myelosuppressive chemotherapeutic agents

Use of echinacea between treatment cycles may theoretically improve white cell counts, reduce dose-limiting toxicities on myelopoeisis and improve patient's quality of life — potentially beneficial interaction under professional supervision.

Etoposide

One recent case study of a 61-year-old man undergoing chemoradiation with cisplatin and etoposide reports on a probable interaction with echinacea resulting in profound thrombocytopenia requiring platelet transfusion. The authors postulated an interaction via the CYP3A4 enzyme, with echinacea being an inhibitor of CYP3A4 in vitro and etoposide being a substrate of CYP3A4 (Bossaer & Odle 2012). However clinical research casts doubt on this given that various echinacea extracts had no effect on CYP3A4 in human studies (see section on cytochromes and P-glycoprotein, above).

Duration of use

Based on evidence that parenterally administered echinacea reversibly depresses immune parameters, Commission E has recommended that echinacea should not be used for more than 8 weeks. However, in a study in which it was taken orally for up to 6 months, no changes in immune parameters were detected (Vonau et al 2001). As such, no conclusive evidence demonstrates that long-term use is detrimental.

PREGNANCY USE

Oral use of echinacea has generally been considered safe in pregnancy when used in recommended doses (Mills & Bone 2005). This was substantiated by preliminary results from a prospective study of 206 women who had inadvertently taken echinacea during their pregnancy; the study found that gestational use was not associated with an increased risk for major malformations (Gallo et al 2000). Moreover, a review concluded that echinacea is non-teratogenic when used during pregnancy, but that caution should prevail when using echinacea during lactation until further high-quality human studies can determine its safety (Perri et al 2006).

Studies in animal models have reported that echinacea preparations derived from *E. purpurea* produce unwanted effects in pregnant animals, such as interference with embryonal angiogenesis (Barcz et al 2007), alteration of maternal haemopoiesis, fetal growth and a reduction in number of viable fetuses (Chow et al 2006). Due to the high rate of false positives obtained in such animal studies and problems with extrapolating data to humans from these models, the clinical significance of these findings remains unknown.

CONTRAINDICATIONS AND PRECAUTIONS

Contraindicated in people with allergies to the Asteraceae (Compositae) family of plants (e.g. chamomile, ragweed).

Commission E warns against using echinacea in cases of autoimmune disorders, such as multiple sclerosis, systemic lupus erythematosus and rheumatoid arthritis, as well as tuberculosis or leucocytosis (Blumenthal et al 2000). A recent review identifies echinacea as one of the herbs with the largest number of documented contraindications, adding multiple sclerosis, tuberculosis and HIV infection to the above list. However, most references used in this review to support this claim were older than 2004 and were not critically evaluated (Tsai et al 2012). As highlighted by Lee and Werth (2004), most contraindications are based on theoretical considerations and case reports with a questionable causal relationship; however, this warning does not appear to be warranted. For example, Boullata and Nace (2000) recommended the avoidance of echinacea use in patients with autoimmune disease, but this recommendation was only seen as the 'extrapolation from experimental observations of echinacea's effects on the immune system' by other authors (Logan & Ahmed 2003).

Moreover, no adverse effects were reported when echinacea was consumed by mice afflicted with autoimmune (type 1) diabetes for up to 18 weeks. Instead, a consistent, long-lasting immunostimulation of only NK cells was observed, thus warranting further research (Delorme & Miller 2005). In addition, recent human studies reported safe and effective systemic echinacea treatment of low-grade autoimmune idiopathic uveitis, resulting in longer steroid-free treatment periods for patients on echinacea treatment (Neri et al 2006).

In practice, echinacea has been successfully used by herbalists in autoimmune disease without mishap (Mills & Bone 2005).

Practice points/Patient counselling

- Different types of echinacea have demonstrated immunomodulating, anti-inflammatory, antifungal, antiviral and antioxidant activity.
- Overall, clinical studies support the use of echinacea in URTIs, such as bacterial sinusitis, common cold, influenza-like viral infections and streptococcal throat. Current evidence supports its use as acute treatment in URTIs, with some evidence supporting its use as prophylactic treatment.
- Several uncontrolled clinical studies support the topical use of echinacea to enhance wound healing.
- Echinacea is also used to treat urinary tract infections, allergies, acne and abscesses, as adjunctive therapy in cancer, herpesvirus infections and candidiasis.
- Although controversy still exists over which part of the plant and which particular plant has the strongest pharmacological activity, it appears that the cold-pressed juice and ethanolic extracts of the *E. purpurea* plant and *E. angustifolia* root are the most-studied preparations for URTIs.

PATIENTS' FAQs

What will this herb do for me?

Echinacea stimulates immune function and also has antifungal (candida), antiviral (herpes) and anti-inflammatory activity. Human studies support its use as an acute treatment and preventive medicine for URTIs in adults. It may also be useful as an adjunct to reduce chemotherapy and radiation-associated side effects. Topically it seems to be useful for chronic wounds and sore throats.

When will it start to work?

As an acute treatment for URTI, echinacea should be started when the first signs and symptoms of infection appear.

Are there any safety issues?

Echinacea is well tolerated, although allergic reactions are possible in rare cases. Patients being treated for autoimmune diseases should be cautious due to echinacea's immune-stimulating effects. Interactions with some immunosuppressant medicines may occur.

REFERENCES

Abdul MI, et al. Pharmacokinetic and pharmacodynamic interactions of echinacea and policosanol with warfarin in healthy subjects. Br J Clin Pharmacol. 2010 May;69(5):508–15.

Abouelella AM et al. Phytotherapeutic effects of *Echinacea purpurea* in gamma-irradiated mice. J Vet Sci 8.4 (2007): 341–51.

Aherne SA, et al. Effects of plant extracts on antioxidant status and oxidant-induced stress in Caco-2 cells. Br J Nutr 97.2 (2007): 321–8.

Altamirano-Dimas M et al. Modulation of immune response gene expression by echinacea extracts: results of a gene array analysis. Can J Physiol Pharmacol 85.11 (2007): 1091–8.

Askeroglu U, et al. Pharmaceutical and herbal products that may contribute to dry eyes. Plast Reconstr Surg. 2013 Jan;131(1):159–67.

Barcz E et al. Influence of *Echinacea purpurea* intake during pregnancy on fetal growth and tissue angiogenic activity. Folia Histochem Cytobiol 45 (Suppl 1) (2007): S35–9.

Barrett B. Medicinal properties of *Echinacea*: a critical review. Phytomedicine 10.1 (2003): 66–86.

Barrett B, et al. Echinacea for treating the common cold: a randomized trial. Ann Intern Med. 2010 Dec 21;153(12):769–77

Bauer VR et al. Immunologic in vivo and in vitro studies on Echinacea extracts. Arzneimittelforschung 38.2 (1988): 276–81.

Bensch K et al. Investigations into the anti-adhesive activity of herbal extracts against *Campylobacter jejuni*. Phytotherapy Research 2011;25(8): 1125–32

Benson JM, et al. *Echinacea purpurea* extracts modulate murine dendritic cell fate and function. Food Chem Toxicol. 2010 May;48(5):1170–7.

Binns SE et al. Light-mediated antifungal activity of Echinacea extracts. Planta Med 66.3 (2000): 241–4.

Binns SE et al. Antiviral activity of characterized extracts from *Echinacea* spp. (Heliantheae: Asteraceae) against herpes simplex virus (HSV-1). Planta Med 68.9 (2002): 780–3.

Birt DF et al. Echinacea in infection. Am J Clin Nutr 87.2 (2008): 488S–92S.

Blumenthal M, et al. (eds). Herbal medicine: expanded commission E monographs. Austin, TX: Integrative Medicine Communications, 2000.

Bossaer JB, Odle BL. Probable etoposide interaction with Echinacea. J Diet Suppl. 2012 Jun;9(2):90–5.

Boullata JI, Nace AM. Safety issues with herbal medicine. Pharmacotherapy 20.3 (2000): 257–69.

Brousseau M, Miller SC. Enhancement of natural killer cells and increased survival of aging mice fed daily Echinacea root extract from youth. Biogerontology 6.3 (2005): 157–63.

Brush J et al. The effect of *Echinacea purpurea, Astragalus membranaceus* and *Glycyrrhiza glabra* on CD69 expression and immune cell activation in humans. Phytother Res 20.8 (2006): 687–95.

Canlas J, et al. Echinacea and trypanasomatid parasite interactions: growth-inhibitory and anti-inflammatory effects of Echinacea. Pharm Biol. 2010 Sep;48(9):1047–52.

Cech NB, et al. Echinacea and its alkylamides: effects on the influenza A-induced secretion of cytokines, chemokines, and PGE_2 from RAW 264.7 macrophage-like cells. Int Immunopharmacol. 2010 Oct; 10(10):1268–78.

Chaves F et al. Effect of *Echinacea purpurea* (Asteraceae) aqueous extract on antibody response to Bothrops asper venom and immune cell response. Rev Biol Trop 55.1 (2007): 113–19.

Chicca A et al. Cytotoxic effects of Echinacea root hexanic extracts on human cancer cell lines. J Ethnopharmacol 110.1 (2007): 148–53.

Chicca A et al. Cytotoxic activity of polyacetylenes and polyenes isolated from roots of *Echinacea pallida*. Br J Pharmacol 153.5 (2008): 879–85.

Chicca A, et al. Synergistic immunomopharmacological effects of N-alkylamides in *Echinacea purpurea* herbal extracts. Int Immunopharmacol. 2009 Jul;9(7–8):850–8.

Chow G, et al. Dietary *Echinacea purpurea* during murine pregnancy: effect on maternal hemopoiesis and fetal growth. Biol Neonate 89.2 (2006): 133.

Christensen KB, et al. Activation of PPARgamma by metabolites from the flowers of purple coneflower (*Echinacea purpurea*). J Nat Prod. 2009 May 22;72(5):933–7.

Classen B et al. Immunomodulatory effects of arabinogalactan-proteins from Baptisia and Echinacea. Phytomedicine 13.9–10 (2006): 688–94.

Clifford LJ et al. Bioactivity of alkamides isolated from *Echinacea purpurea* (L.) Moench. Phytomedicine 9.3 (2002): 249–53.

Cohen HA et al. Effectiveness of an herbal preparation containing echinacea, propolis, and vitamin C in preventing respiratory tract infections in children: a randomized, double-blind, placebo-controlled, multicenter study. Arch Pediatr Adolesc Med 158.3 (2004): 217–21.

Delorme D, Miller SC. Dietary consumption of Echinacea by mice afflicted with autoimmune (type I) diabetes: effect of consuming the herb on hemopoietic and immune cell dynamics. Autoimmunity 38.6 (2005): 453–61.

Di Pierro F, et al. Use of a standardized extract from *Echinacea angustifolia* (Polinacea) for the prevention of respiratory tract infections. Altern Med Rev. 2012 Mar;17(1):36–41.

Dong GC et al. Immuno-suppressive effect of blocking the CD28 signaling pathway in T-cells by an active component of Echinacea found by a novel pharmaceutical screening method. J Med Chem 49.6 (2006): 1845–54.

Dong GC et al. Blocking effect of an immuno-suppressive agent, cynarin, on CD28 of T-cell receptor. Pharm Res 26.2 (2008): 375–81.

Egger M et al. Synthesis and cannabinoid receptor activity of ketoalkenes from Echinacea pallida and nonnatural analogues. Chemistry 14.35 (2008): 10978–84.

Ernst E. The risk-benefit profile of commonly used herbal therapies: Ginkgo, St. John's Wort, Ginseng, Echinacea, Saw Palmetto, and Kava. Ann Intern Med 136.1 (2002): 42–53.

Farinacci M, et al. Modulation of ovine neutrophil function and apoptosis by standardized extracts of *Echinacea angustifolia*, *Butea frondosa* and *Curcuma longa*. Vet Immunol Immunopathol 128.4 (2009): 366–73.

Fashner J, et al., Treatment of the common cold in children and adults., Am Fam Physician. 2012 Jul 15;86(2):153–9.

Gallo M et al. Pregnancy outcome following gestational exposure to echinacea: a prospective controlled study. Arch Intern Med 160.20 (2000): 3141–3.

Gertsch J, et al. New natural noncannabinoid ligands for cannabinoid type-2 (CB2) receptors. J Recept Signal Transduct Res 26.5–6 (2006): 709–30.

Ghaemi A, et al. *Echinacea purpurea* polysaccharide reduces the latency rate in herpes simplex virus type-1 infections. Intervirology. 2009;52(1):29–34.

Gillespie EL, Coleman CI. The effect of Echinacea on upper respiratory infection symptom severity and quality of life. Conn Med 70.2 (2006): 93–7.

Gleeson M, et al. Nutritional strategies to minimise exercise-induced immunosuppression in athletes. Can J Appl Physiol 26 (Suppl) (2001): S23–35.

Gorski JC et al. The effect of echinacea (*Echinacea purpurea* root) on cytochrome P450 activity in vivo. Clin Pharmacol Ther. 2004 Jan;75(1):89–100.

Groom SN, et al. The potency of immunomodulatory herbs may be primarily dependent upon macrophage activation. J Med Food 10.1 (2007): 73–9.

Guiotto P et al. Pharmacokinetics and immunomodulatory effects of phytotherapeutic lozenges (bonbons) with *Echinacea purpurea* extract. Phytomedicine 15.8 (2008): 547–54.

Gurley BJ et al. In vivo assessment of botanical supplementation on human cytochrome P450 phenotypes: *Citrus aurantium*, *Echinacea purpurea*, milk thistle, and saw palmetto. Clin Pharmacol Ther 76.5 (2004): 428–40.

Gurley BJ et al. Clinical assessment of CYP2D6-mediated herb–drug interactions in humans: effects of milk thistle, black cohosh, goldenseal, kava kava, St. John's wort, and Echinacea. Mol Nutr Food Res 52.7 (2008a): 755–63.

Gurley BJ, et al. Gauging the clinical significance of P-glycoprotein-mediated herb–drug interactions: comparative effects of St. John's wort, Echinacea, clarithromycin, and rifampin on digoxin pharmacokinetics. Mol Nutr Food Res. (2008b) Jul;52(7):772–9.

Hall H, et al. *Echinacea purpurea* and mucosal immunity. Int J Sports Med 28.9 (2007): 792–7.

Haller J. et al. The Effect of Echinacea Preparations in Three Laboratory Tests of Anxiety: Comparison with Chlordiazepoxide. Phytother. Res. 24: 1605–1613 (2010).

Hayashi I et al. Effects of oral administration of *Echinacea purpurea* (American herb) on incidence of spontaneous leukemia caused by recombinant leukemia viruses in AKR/J mice. Nihon Rinsho Meneki Gakkai Kaishi 24.1 (2001): 10–20.

Heikkinen T, Jarvinen A. The common cold. Lancet 361.9351 (2003): 51–9.

Heinrich M, et al. Herbal extracts used for upper respiratory tract infections: are there clinically relevant interactions with the cytochrome P450 enzyme system? Planta Med 74.6 (2008): 657–60.

Hellum BH, Nilsen OG. In vitro inhibition of CYP3A4 metabolism and P-glycoprotein-mediated transport by trade herbal products. Basic Clin Pharmacol Toxicol 102.5 (2008): 466–75.

Hermann R, von Richter O. Clinical evidence of herbal drugs as perpetrators of pharmacokinetic drug interactions. Planta Med. 2012 Sep;78(13):1458–77.

Hill LL et al. *Echinacea purpurea* supplementation stimulates select groups of human gastrointestinal tract microbiota. J Clin Pharm Ther 31.6 (2006): 599–604.

Hinz B, et al. Alkamides from Echinacea inhibit cyclooxygenase-2 activity in human neuroglioma cells. Biochem Biophys Res Commun 360.2 (2007): 441–6.

Huntimer ED, et al. Proliferative activity of *Echinacea angustifolia* root extracts on cancer cells: Interference with doxorubicin cytotoxicity. Chem Biodivers 3.6 (2006): 695–703.

Huntley AL, et al. The safety of herbal medicinal products derived from *Echinacea* species: a systematic review. Drug Saf 28.5 (2005): 387–400.

Izzo AA. Interactions between herbs and conventional drugs: overview of the clinical data. Med Princ Pract. 2012;21(5):404–28.

Jawad M, et al. Safety and efficacy profile of *Echinacea purpurea* to prevent common cold episodes: a randomized, double-blind, placebo-controlled trial. Evid Based Complement Alternat Med. 2012:841315.

Joksić G, et al. Biological effects of *Echinacea purpurea* on human blood cells. Arh Hig Rada Toksikol. 2009 Jun;60(2):165–72.

Kapai NA, et al. Selective cytokine-inducing effects of low dose Echinacea. Bull Exp Biol Med. 2011 Apr;150(6):711–3.

Kinkel HJ, et al. Effect of Echinacin ointment in healing of skin lesions. Med Klin 1984; 79: 580–4; as cited in Micromedex Thomson 2003. www.micromedex.com.

Koenig K, Roehr CC. Does treatment with *Echinacea purpurea* effectively shorten the course of upper respiratory tract infections in children? Arch Dis Child 91.6 (2006): 535–7.

LaLone CA et al. Echinacea species and alkamides inhibit prostaglandin E(2) production in RAW264.7 mouse macrophage cells. J Agric Food Chem 55.18 (2007): 7314–22.

LaLone CA, et al. Endogenous levels of Echinacea alkylamides and ketones are important contributors to the inhibition of prostaglandin E2 and nitric oxide production in cultured macrophages. J Agric Food Chem. 2009 Oct 14;57(19):8820–30.

Lans C et al. Ethnoveterinary medicines used to treat endoparasites and stomach problems in pigs and pets in British Columbia, Canada. Vet Parasitol 148.3–4 (2007): 325–40.

Lee AN, Werth VP. Activation of autoimmunity following use of immunostimulatory herbal supplements. Arch Dermatol 140.6 (2004): 723–7.

Liatsos G et al. Severe thrombotic thrombocytopenic purpura (TTP) induced or exacerbated by the immunostimulatory herb Echinacea. Am J Hematol 81.3 (2006): 224.

Linde K et al. Echinacea for preventing and treating the common cold. Cochrane Database Syst Rev 1 (2009): CD000530.

Logan JL, Ahmed J. Critical hypokalemic renal tubular acidosis due to Sjogren's syndrome: association with the purported immune stimulant echinacea. Clin Rheumatol 22.2 (2003): 158–9.

Maskatia ZK, Baker K. Hypereosinophilia associated with echinacea use. South Med J. 2010 Nov;103(11):1173–4.

Masteikova R et al. Antioxidative activity of Ginkgo, Echinacea, and Ginseng tinctures. Medicina (Kaunas) 43.4 (2007): 306–9.

Matthias A et al. Bioavailability of Echinacea constituents: Caco-2 monolayers and pharmacokinetics of the alkylamides and caffeic acid conjugates. Molecules 10.10 (2005a): 1242–51.

Matthias A et al. Cytochrome P450 enzyme-mediated degradation of Echinacea alkylamides in human liver microsomes. Chem Biol Interact 155 (2005b): 62–70: 1–2.

Matthias A et al. Alkylamides from echinacea modulate induced immune responses in macrophages. Immunol Invest 36.2 (2007a): 117–30.

Matthias A et al. Comparison of Echinacea alkylamide pharmacokinetics between liquid and tablet preparations. Phytomedicine 14.9 (2007b): 587–90.

Matthias A et al. Echinacea alkylamides modulate induced immune responses in T-cells. Fitoterapia 79.1 (2008): 53–8.

Mazzio EA, Soliman KF. In vitro screening for the tumoricidal properties of international medicinal herbs. Phytother Res 23.3 (2009): 385–98.

McCann DA et al. Cytokine- and interferon-modulating properties of *Echinacea* spp. root tinctures stored at −20 degrees C for 2 years. J Interferon Cytokine Res 27.5 (2007): 425–36.

Meijerman I, et al. Herb–drug interactions in oncology: focus on mechanisms of induction. Oncologist 11.7 (2006): 742–52.

Melchart D et al. Echinacea for preventing and treating the common cold. Cochrane Database Syst Rev 2 (2000): CD000530.

Melchart D et al. Polysaccharides isolated from *Echinacea purpurea* herba cell cultures to counteract undesired effects of chemotherapy: a pilot study. Phytother Res 16.2 (2002): 138–42.

Miller SC. Echinacea: a miracle herb against aging and cancer? Evidence in vivo in mice. Evid Based Complement Altern Med 2.3 (2005): 309–14.

Mills S, Bone K. Principles and practice of phytotherapy. London: Churchill Livingstone, 2000.

Mills S, Bone K. The essential guide to herbal safety. St Louis, MO: Churchill Livingstone, 2005.

Mir-Rashed N, et al. Disruption of fungal cell wall by antifungal Echinacea extracts. Med Mycol. 2010 Nov;48(7):949–58.

Mistrangelo M, et al. Immunostimulation to reduce recurrence after surgery for anal condyloma acuminata: a prospective randomized controlled trial. Colorectal Dis. 2010 Aug;12(8):799–803.

Modarai M, et al. Safety of herbal medicinal products: echinacea and selected alkylamides do not induce CYP3A4 mRNA expression. Evid Based Complement Alternat Med. 2011;2011:213021.

Moltó J, et al. Herb–drug interaction between *Echinacea purpurea* and darunavir-ritonavir in HIV-infected patients. Antimicrob Agents Chemother. 2011 Jan;55(1):326–30.

Mullins RJ. Echinacea-associated anaphylaxis. Med J Aust 168.4 (1998): 170–171.

Mullins RJ, Heddle R. Adverse reactions associated with echinacea: the Australian experience. Ann Allergy Asthma Immunol 88.1 (2002): 42–51.

Nahas R, Balla A. Complementary and alternative medicine for prevention and treatment of the common cold. Can Fam Physician. 2011 Jan;57(1):31–6.

Neri PG et al. Oral *Echinacea purpurea* extract in low-grade, steroid-dependent, autoimmune idiopathic uveitis: a pilot study. J Ocul Pharmacol Ther 22.6 (2006): 431–6.

Pellati F et al. Isolation and structure elucidation of cytotoxic polyacetylenes and polyenes from Echinacea pallida. Phytochemistry 67.13 (2006): 1359–64.

Penzak SR, et al. *Echinacea purpurea* significantly induces cytochrome P450 3A activity but does not alter lopinavir-ritonavir exposure in healthy subjects. Pharmacotherapy. 2010 Aug;30(8):797–805.

Perri D et al. Safety and efficacy of echinacea (*Echinacea angustafolia, E. purpurea* and *E. pallida*) during pregnancy and lactation. Can J Clin Pharmacol 13.3 (2006): e262–7.

Pillai S et al. Use of quantitative flow cytometry to measure ex vivo immunostimulant activity of echinacea: the case for polysaccharides. J Altern Complement Med 13.6 (2007): 625–34.

Pizzorno J, Murray M. Textbook of natural medicine. St Louis: Elsevier, 2006.

Posadzki P, (2013) "http://www.ncbi.nlm.nih.gov/pubmed?term=Posadzki%20P%5BAuthor%5D&cauthor=true&cauthor_uid=23472485"

Pugh ND et al. The majority of in vitro macrophage activation exhibited by extracts of some immune enhancing botanicals is due to bacterial lipoproteins and lipopolysaccharides. Int Immunopharmacol 8.7 (2008): 1023–32.

Raduner S et al. Alkylamides from *Echinacea* are a new class of cannabinomimetics: Cannabinoid type 2 receptor-dependent and -independent immunomodulatory effects. J Biol Chem 281.20 (2006): 14192–206.

Raduner S et al. Self-assembling cannabinomimetics: supramolecular structures of N-alkyl amides. J Nat Prod 70.6 (2007): 1010–15.

Ragupathi G et al. Evaluation of widely consumed botanicals as immunological adjuvants. Vaccine 26.37 (2008): 4860–5.

Raman P, et al. Lipid peroxidation and cyclooxygenase enzyme inhibitory activities of acidic aqueous extracts of some dietary supplements. Phytother Res 22.2 (2008): 204–12.

Ramirez-Erosa I et al. Xanthatin and xanthinosin from the burrs of *Xanthium strumarium* L. as potential anticancer agents. Can J Physiol Pharmacol 85.11 (2007): 1160–72.

Raso GM et al. In-vivo and in-vitro anti-inflammatory effect of *Echinacea purpurea* and *Hypericum perforatum*. J Pharm Pharmacol 54.10 (2002): 1379–83.

Ritchie, M.R., et al. 2011. Effects of Echinaforce(R) treatment on ex vivo-stimulated blood cells. Phytomedicine, 18, (10) 826–831 available from: PM:21726792

Ross SM. A standardized Echinacea extract demonstrates efficacy in the prevention and treatment of colds in athletes. Holist Nurs Pract. 2010 Mar-Apr;24(2):107–9.

Santaella RM, Fraunfelder FW. Ocular adverse effects associated with systemic medications: recognition and management. Drugs 67.1 (2007): 75–93.

Sasagawa M et al. Echinacea alkylamides inhibit interleukin-2 production by Jurkat T cells. Int Immunopharmacol 6.7 (2006): 1214–21.

Saunders PR, et al. *Echinacea purpurea* L. in children: safety, tolerability, compliance, and clinical effectiveness in upper respiratory tract infections. Can J Physiol Pharmacol 85.11 (2007): 1195–9.

Schapowal, A. 2013. Efficacy and safety of Echinaforce(R) in respiratory tract infections. Wien.Med Wochenschr., 163, (3–4) 102–105.

Schapowal A, et al. Echinacea/sage or chlorhexidine/lidocaine for treating acute sore throats: a randomized double-blind trial. Eur J Med Res. 2009 Sep 1;14(9):406–12.

Schneider S, et al Anti-herpetic properties of hydroalcoholic extracts and pressed juice from *Echinacea pallida*. Planta Med. 2010 Feb;76(3):265–72

Schoop R, et al. Open, multicenter study to evaluate the tolerability and efficacy of Echinaforce Forte tablets in athletes. Adv Ther 23.5 (2006a): 823–33.

Schoop R et al. Echinacea in the prevention of induced rhinovirus colds: a meta-analysis. Clin Ther 28.2 (2006b): 174–83.

Senchina DS et al. Phenetic comparison of seven Echinacea species based on immunomodulatory characteristics. Econ Bot 60.3 (2006): 205–11.

Senchina DS, et al. Effects of Echinacea extracts on macrophage antiviral activities. Phytother Res. 2010 Jun;24(6):810–6.

Shah SA et al. Effects of echinacea on electrocardiographic and blood pressure measurements. Am J Health Syst Pharm 64.15 (2007a): 1615–18.

Shah SA et al. Evaluation of echinacea for the prevention and treatment of the common cold: a meta-analysis. Lancet Infect Dis 7.7 (2007b): 473–80.

Sharma M et al. Echinacea extracts modulate the pattern of chemokine and cytokine secretion in rhinovirus-infected and uninfected epithelial cells. Phytother Res 20.2 (2006): 147–52.

Sharma M, et al. Induction of multiple pro-inflammatory cytokines by respiratory viruses and reversal by standardized Echinacea, a potent antiviral herbal extract. Antiviral Res. 2009 Aug;83(2):165–70.

Sharma SM, et al Bactericidal and anti-inflammatory properties of a standardized Echinacea extract (Echinaforce): dual actions against respiratory bacteria. Phytomedicine. 2010 Jul;17(8–9):563–8

Sharma M, et al. The potential use of Echinacea in acne: control of *Propionibacterium acnes* growth and inflammation. Phytother Res. 2011 Apr;25(4):517–21.

Skaudickas D, et al. The effect of *Echinacea purpurea* (L.) Moench extract on experimental prostate hyperplasia. Phytother Res. 2009 Oct;23(10): 1474–8.

Spasov AA et al. Comparative controlled study of *Andrographis paniculata* fixed combination, Kan Jang and an Echinacea preparation as adjuvant, in the treatment of uncomplicated respiratory disease in children. Phytother Res 18.1 (2004): 47–53.

Speroni E et al. Anti-inflammatory and cicatrizing activity of *Echinacea pallida* Nutt. root extract. J Ethnopharmacol 79.2 (2002): 265–72.

Stargrove M, et al. Herb, nutrient and drug interactions. St Louis: Mosby, Elsevier, 2008.

Starvaggi Cucuzza L et al. Effect of *Echinacea augustifolia* extract on cell viability and differentiation in mammary epithelial cells. Phytomedicine 15.8 (2008): 555–62.

Sterer N et al. Oral malodor reduction by a palatal mucoadhesive tablet containing herbal formulation. J Dent 36.7 (2008): 535–9.

Stevenson LM et al. Modulation of macrophage immune responses by Echinacea. Molecules 10.10 (2005): 1279–85.

Sullivan AM et al. Echinacea-induced macrophage activation. Immunopharmacol Immunotoxicol 30.3 (2008): 553–74.

Taylor JA et al. Efficacy and safety of echinacea in treating upper respiratory tract infections in children: a randomized controlled trial. JAMA 290.21 (2003): 2824–30.

Tiralongo, E., et al. Randomised, double blind, placebo controlled trial of *Echinacea* supplementation in air-travellers, eCAM, 2012;2012: 417267.

Toselli F, et al. Metabolism of the major Echinacea alkylamide N-isobutyldodeca-2E,4E,8Z,10Z-tetraenamide by human recombinant cytochrome P450 enzymes and human liver microsomes. Phytother Res. 2010 Aug;24(8):1195–201.

Tragni E et al. Evidence from two classic irritation tests for an anti-inflammatory action of a natural extract, Echinacina B. Food Chem Toxicol 23.2 (1985): 317–19.

Tsai HH et al Evaluation of documented drug interactions and contraindications associated with herbs and dietary supplements: a systematic literature review. Int J Clin Pract. 2012 Nov;66(11): 1056–78.

Tubaro A et al. Anti-inflammatory activity of a polysaccharidic fraction of *Echinacea angustifolia*. J Pharm Pharmacol 39.7 (1987): 567–9.

Ulbricht CE, Basch EM. Natural standard herb and supplement reference. St Louis: Mosby, 2005.

Unger M. Pharmacokinetic drug interactions by herbal drugs: Critical evaluation and clinical relevance. Wien Med Wochenschr. 2010 Dec;160(21–22):571–7.

Van den Bout-van den Beukel CJ et al. Possible drug-metabolism interactions of medicinal herbs with antiretroviral agents. Drug Metab Rev 38.3 (2006): 477–514.

Vonau B et al. Does the extract of the plant *Echinacea purpurea* influence the clinical course of recurrent genital herpes? Int J STD AIDS 12.3 (2001): 154–8.

Wahl RA et al. *Echinacea purpurea* and osteopathic manipulative treatment in children with recurrent otitis media: a randomized controlled trial. BMC Complement Altern Med 8 (2008): 56.

Wang CY et al. Modulatory effects of *Echinacea purpurea* extracts on human dendritic cells: a cell- and gene-based study. Genomics 88.6 (2006): 801–8.

Wang CY et al. Genomics and proteomics of immune modulatory effects of a butanol fraction of *Echinacea purpurea* in human dendritic cells. BMC Genomics 9 (2008): 479.

Weber W et al. *Echinacea purpurea* for prevention of upper respiratory tract infections in children. J Altern Complement Med 11.6 (2005): 1021–6.

Whitehead MT Running economy and maximal oxygen consumption after 4 weeks of oral echinacea supplementation. J Strength Cond Res. 2012 Jul;26(7):1928–33.

Whitehead MT et al. The effect of 4 wk of oral echinacea supplementation on serum erythropoietin and indices of erythropoietic status. Int J Sport Nutr Exerc Metab 17.4 (2007): 378–90.

Woelkart K, Bauer R. The role of alkamides as an active principle of echinacea. Planta Med 73.7 (2007): 615–23.

Woelkart K et al. Bioavailability and pharmacokinetics of *Echinacea purpurea* preparations and their interaction with the immune system. Int J Clin Pharmacol Ther 44.9 (2006): 401–8.

Woelkart K, et al. Echinacea for preventing and treating the common cold. Planta Med 74.6 (2008a): 633–7.

Woelkart K et al. Pharmacokinetics of the main alkamides after administration of three different *Echinacea purpurea* preparations in humans. Planta Med 74.6 (2008b): 651–6.

Wu H, et al. Effects of a standardized purified dry extract from *Echinacea angustifolia* on proliferation and interferon gamma secretion of peripheral blood mononuclear cells in dairy heifers. Res Vet Sci. 2009 Dec;87(3):396–8.
Wu L, Rowe EW, Jeftinija K, et al. Echinacea-induced cytosolic Ca^{2+} elevation in HEK293. BMC Complement Altern Med. 2010 Nov 23;10:72.
Yotsawimonwat S, et al. Skin improvement and stability of *Echinacea purpurea* dermatological formulations. Int J Cosmet Sci. 2010 Apr 1 (epub ahead of print).
Yu D, et al. Anti-inflammatory effects of essential oil in *Echinacea purpurea* L. Pak J Pharm Sci. 2013 Mar;26(2):403–8.
Zhai Z et al. Alcohol extracts of Echinacea inhibit production of nitric oxide and tumor necrosis factor-alpha by macrophages in vitro. Food Agric Immunol 18.3–4 (2007a): 221–36.
Zhai Z et al. Echinacea increases arginase activity and has anti-inflammatory properties in RAW 264.7 macrophage cells, indicative of alternative macrophage activation. J Ethnopharmacol 122.1 (2009a): 976–85.
Zhai Z, et al. Alcohol extract of *Echinacea pallida* reverses stress-delayed wound healing in mice. Phytomedicine. 2009b Jun;16(6–7):669–78.
Zwickey H et al. The effect of *Echinacea purpurea*, *Astragalus membranaceus* and *Glycyrrhiza glabra* on CD25 expression in humans: a pilot study. Phytother Res 21.11 (2007): 1109–12.

Elder

HISTORICAL NOTE The elder tree has enjoyed much popularity throughout the ages. Ancient Egyptians used elderflowers to heal burns and improve their complexion. Throughout England elder was termed 'the medicine chest of the country people', and Native Americans used elder for coughs, colds, infections and skin conditions. Elderflowers are a favorite ingredient in herb teas, cordials and some wines.

COMMON NAME

Elder

OTHER NAMES

Black elder, common elder

BOTANICAL NAME/FAMILY

Sambucus nigra/Caprifoliaceae

PLANT PART USED

Flower or ripe berry

CHEMICAL COMPONENTS

Flowers

Flavonoids, primarily quercertin, isoquercertin, rutin and astragaline (Dawidowicz et al 2006, Wach et al 2007), as well as alpha-linolenic acid and linoleic acid and the predominant flavanone in grapefruit, naringenin, has been reported to be present in elderflowers (Christensen et al 2010). Elderflowers also contain essential oils.

Berries

Anthocyanins are abundant in the berries, including cyanidin 3-sambubioside-5-glucoside, cyanidin 3,5-diglucoside, cyanidin 3-sambubioside, cyanidin 3-glucoside and cyanidin 3-rutinoside. Cyanidin 3-sambubioside is the most abundant anthrocyanin and accounts for more than 50% of all anthocyanins found in the berries (Veberic et al 2009, Murkovic et al 2000). The berries also contain flavonoids, including quercertin, quercertin 3-rutinoside and quercetin 3-glucoside, organic acids and sugars (Veberic et al 2009). The unripe berries contain cyanogenic glycosides (Dellagreca et al 2003).

MAIN ACTIONS

There is more research evaluating the actions of elderberries than elderflowers; however, most research has been conducted in vitro or with animal models with relatively few human clinical trials available.

Antioxidant

Elderflowers contain flavonoids such as quercertin, isoquercertin and rutin which all possess potent antioxidant properties (Dawidowicz et al 2006). The berries also contain these flavonoids and additionally have appreciable amounts of anthocyanins, chiefly cyanidin 3-sambubioside and cyanidin 3-glucoside (Veberic et al 2009, Murkovic et al 2000).

The effects of dietary cyanidin-3-O-glucoside (2 g/kg) and a concentrate of elderberry (2 g/kg) on the plasma and tissue concentrations of tocopherol and cholesterol were investigated for a period of 4 weeks in vivo (Frank et al 2002). Cyanidin-3-O-glucoside increased the levels of vitamin E in the liver and lungs and appeared to have a sparing effect. Cholesterol levels were not affected, but both cyanidin-3-O-glucoside and elderberry reduced the amount of saturated fatty acid in the liver. Higher temperatures (100 degrees C) during aqueous extraction appear to yield a higher flavonoid content (Dawidowicz et al 2006).

Antiviral/Antimicrobial

In vitro studies have shown that a proprietary product known as Sambucol, whose chief ingredient is elderberry extract (1.9 g per 5 mL) is effective against ten strains of influenza virus (Zakay-Rones et al 1995). Other ingredients in the product include raspberry extract, sucrose, citric acid and honey.

Interestingly, recent research suggests that the in vitro anti-influenza activity of concentration elderberry juice is relatively weak, while the in vivo activity is relatively strong (Kinoshita et al 2012).

Research investigating the activity of several flavonoids from the elderberry extract (5,7,3', 4'-tetra-O-methylquercetin and 5,7-dihydroxy-4-oxo-2-(3,4,5-trihydroxyphenylchroman-3-yl-3,4,5-trihydroxycyclohexanecarboxylate), as well as the synthetic analogue dihydromyricetin have demonstrated an ability to bind to H1N1 virions, thus blocking the ability of the viruses to infect host cells (Roschek et al 2009).

These combined findings warrant further investigation to determine whether the effects of oral elderberry extracts have a role as a treatment in pandemic influenza infections (Kong 2009).

'Rubini' (BerryPharma AG), a standardised elderberry extract, was investigated for its antimicrobial and antiviral activity in the treatment of respiratory tract infections (e.g. pneumonia). This standardised elderberry liquid extract displayed an inhibitory effect on the propagation of human pathogenic influenza viruses. It also showed antimicrobial activity against both Gram-positive bacteria of *Streptococcus pyogenes* group C and G, streptococci and the Gram-negative bacterium *Branhamella catarrhalis* in liquid cultures (Krawitz et al 2011).

Immunostimulating

The standardised black elderberry product Sambucol has been shown to increase the production of certain inflammatory cytokines (IL-1 beta, TNF-alpha, IL-6, IL-8) in human monocytes (Barak et al 2001). It is proposed that this may be one of the mechanisms via which elderberry improves immune system activity. Another study confirmed these results and, in addition, showed that elderberry also increases the anti-inflammatory cytokine IL-10 (Barak et al 2002). An in vitro study using a lectin isolated from elderflower (*Sambucus nigra* agglutinin) found the extract increased the release of IL-4 from basophils (Haas et al 1999). In vivo evidence confirms that concentrated elderberry juice suppresses viral replication and stimulates the immune response (Kinoshita et al 2012).

Chemo-preventative

Elderberry extract exhibited a dose-dependent inhibitory effect on the growth of human colorectal adenocarcinoma HT29 cells in vitro (Jing et al 2008).

Anti-inflammatory

An extract of elderflower was found to reduce inflammatory mediators in monocytes, macrophages and neutrophils incubated with whole cells of the periodontal pathogens *Porphyromonas gingivalis* and *Actinobacillus actinomycetemcomitans* (Harokopakis et al 2006). The extract appeared to inhibit the activation of nuclear factor kappa B and phosphatidylinositol 3-kinase. Human trials are required to determine whether the effect occurs clinically and the potential of elderflower extract as a treatment for reducing inflammation in periodontitis.

Diuretic

Elderflower has traditionally been used as a diuretic agent. An in vivo study found that the extract possessed diuretic properties comparable to the reference product hydrochlorothiazide (Beaux et al 1999). The extract also increased sodium excretion. However, *Sambucus nigra L.* has no impact on urinary pH and therefore does not affect the solubility of stone-inducing ions (Walz & Chrubasik 2008).

Antidiabetic

An aqueous extract of elderflowers has been shown to increase insulin secretion and enhance muscle glucose uptake (70%), glucose oxidation (50%) and glycogenesis (70%) in pancreatic beta cells in vitro (Gray et al 2000). Extracts of elderflowers have been found to activate human PPAR (peroxisome proliferator-activated receptor) gamma and to stimulate insulin-dependent glucose uptake, suggesting a potential role in the prevention and/or treatment of insulin resistance (Christensen et al 2010). The insulinotropic effects of elder were slightly stronger with a hot preparation. An aqueous extract of elder failed to increase glucose diffusion in another in vitro study (Gallagher et al 2003). The authors theorise that the anti-diabetic effects of elder may not be related to intestinal absorption.

Preliminary in vivo evidence suggests that the natural polyphenols extracted from elder berries may positively influence bone mineral density in diabetic rats (Badescu et al 2012).

Cardioprotective

It has been proposed that *Sambucus nigra* polyphenols have cardioprotective effects that may be useful in practice. These cardioprotective effects are believed to be due to antioxidant, hypolipidaemic and hypocholesterolaemic properties of the polyphenols (Ciocoiu et al 2009). In vivo evidence suggests elderberry has the potential to improve endothelial function (Morosanu et al 2011). Polyphenols extracted from elderberries have been shown to lower oxidative stress in rats with hypertension, resulting in a biostatistically significant ($P < 0.05$) blood pressure drop between the control group (who received no polyphenols) and the intervention group (Ciocoiu et al 2012).

Whether these in vivo observations have clinical relevance in humans remains uncertain, based on current clinical research. For example, a placebo-controlled RCT of 52 healthy postmenopausal women found treatment with 500 mg/day anthocyanins as cyanidin glycosides (from elderberry) taken for 12 weeks (2 capsules twice daily) did not significantly alter biomarkers of CVD risk (inflammatory biomarkers, platelet reactivity, lipids and glucose) (Curtis et al 2009). Similarly, another placebo-controlled

RCT of 34 healthy volunteers failed to find any evidence of lipid-lowering activity with oral capsules of freeze-dried elderberry juice (400 mg containing 10% anthocyanins) when taken three times daily for 2 weeks (Murkovic et al 2004).

OTHER ACTIONS

Elderflower preparations are traditionally believed to have expectorant, decongestant and diaphoretic activity.

CLINICAL USE

Most human research has been conducted exploring the use of elderberry preparations for treating infections. Some studies have investigated commercial elder preparations that also contain ingredients such as echinacea, vitamin C and zinc.

Influenza

Three clinical trials investigating elderberry oral mixture (Sambucol) or oral lozenges demonstrate that it reduces symptom severity more rapidly than placebo and may shorten the duration of infection.

In regards to clinical use, the elderberry extract Sambucol (contains 1.9 g of elderberry extract per 5 mL; other ingredients include raspberry extract, sucrose, citric acid and honey) was evaluated in a multi-centre, randomised, placebo-controlled clinical trial to investigate its efficacy in decreasing the severity and duration of influenza A and B infections (Zakay-Rones et al 2004). Sixty patients aged between 18 and 54 years were enrolled in the study when they had three or more symptoms of influenza (fever, malaise, nasal discharge, etc). Patients were given 15 mL four times daily with meals for 4 days. The first dose was given within 48 hours of the onset of symptoms. The global evaluation scores for the elderberry group using visual analogue scales showed a significant improvement after an average of 3.1 days (± 1.3) as compared to 7.1 (± 2.5) days for the placebo group ($P < 0.001$).

The same extract was investigated in a placebo-controlled study of 27 children and adults during an outbreak of influenza B Panama (Zakay-Rones et al 1995). Children were given 2 tablespoons of mixture for 3 days, while adults received 4 tablespoons for the same duration. Patients were followed for 6 days and their symptoms were monitored. A significant improvement in symptoms was seen in 93.3% of people in the treatment group within 2 days whereas it was not until after 6 days that 91.7% of the patients in the placebo group were feeling better ($P < 0.001$).

A randomized, double-blind clinical trial involving 64 participants (aged 16–60 years) evaluated the efficacy of a standardised, proprietary elderberry extract in reducing influenza symptoms ($n = 32$) compared to placebo ($n = 32$) (Kong 2009). The elderberry extract was administered in the form of slowly dissolving lozenges taken 4 times daily for 2 days. Both the proprietary elderberry extract and placebo lozenges were supplied by HerbalScience Singapore Pte. Ltd. After 24 hours, the group receiving active treatment showed significant improvements in most of the symptoms, whereas the placebo group showed no such improvements. By 48 hours, 9 patients (28%) in the active treatment group were void of all symptoms, and 19 patients (60%) showed relief from some symptoms. In comparison, no patient in the placebo group achieved complete recovery, and only 5 patients (16%) showed improvement in one or two symptoms at the same time point.

Hyperlipidaemia—not effective

Negative results have been obtained to date showing no significant lipid-lowering activity in humans with the tested preparations.

One randomised, double-blind, placebo-controlled study investigated the effect of elderberry juice on serum cholesterol and triglyceride levels (Murkovic et al 2004). The study began with 34 healthy volunteers who took capsules containing either spray-dried elderberry juice (400 mg containing 10% anthocyanins) or placebo three times a day for two weeks. A subgroup of 14 participants continued for another week to further evaluate the resistance of LDL-cholesterol to copper-induced oxidation. In the next phase, six subjects took a single dose of elderberry juice 50 mL together with a fat-laden breakfast to test the short-term effects of elderberry on serum lipid levels.

Results from the main study found that a small but not statistically significant change was noted in cholesterol concentrations in the elderberry group (from 199 to 190 mg/dL) compared to the placebo group (from 192 to 196 mg/dL). Additionally, elder did not improve LDL-cholesterol oxidation and failed to significantly reduce postprandial triglyceride concentrations after a high-fat meal.

More recently, a randomised, placebo-controlled trial of 52 healthy postmenopausal women found treatment with 500 mg/day anthocyanins as cyanidin glycosides (from elderberry) was ineffective when taken for 12 weeks (2 capsules twice daily). Treatment did not alter biomarkers of CVD risk (inflammatory biomarkers, platelet reactivity, lipids and glucose) (Curtis et al 2009).

Chronic constipation—*in combination*

No studies were located that evaluated the effects of elder preparations on constipation however, one study did produce supportive evidence when it was used as part of a herbal combination treatment.

A phytotherapic combination containing *Sambucus nigra L.*, *Pimpinella anisum L.*, *Foeniculum vulgare* Miller, and *Cassia angustifolia* was assessed for efficacy in 20 subjects with chronic constipation. This randomised, crossover, placebo-controlled, single-blind study revealed that active herbal treatment produced a laxative effect and was a safe treatment option for the treatment of constipation (Picon et al 2010). The contribution of elder to producing this effect is unknown.

Other uses

Elder preparations have also been used traditionally to treat colds, influenza, scarlet fever, bronchitis, sinusitis, hayfever, wounds and skin disorders. They have also been used as diaphoretic agents to increase sweating during temperatures or fevers. It is believed that the action is greatly improved by the use of a hot infusion. German Commission E approves the use of elderflowers as a diaphoretic and expectorant treatment (Blumenthal et al 1998).

DOSAGE RANGE

General guide

Flowers

- Tea: 10–15 g flowers/day.
- Liquid extract: 2–6 mL of 1:2 extract/day.

Berries

- Elderberry syrup: usually contains 30–38% elderberry; dose at 15 mL, 3 times daily (Sambucus nigra (elderberry) 2005).
- Powdered extracts: often available in 500 mg capsules, dose 2–3 times daily (Sambucus nigra (elderberry) 2005).

According to clinical studies

Influenza

- 15 mL of the elderberry syrup (Sambucol) taken 4 times daily.
- 1 slow-release lozenge, four times daily, for 2 days. Each lozenge must contain 175 mg of elderberry extract.

ADVERSE REACTIONS

Elderberries have been generally well tolerated in clinical trials (Zakay-Rones et al 1995, 2004). Although there are no clinical studies using elderflowers, it is generally thought that they are most likely to also be very safe. In large doses elder may produce nausea, diarrhoea and polyuria (Mills & Bone 2005).

SIGNIFICANT INTERACTIONS

'Sambucus Force', a commercially manufactured capsulated formulation containing *E. purpurea* and *S. nigra*, has been shown in vitro to be a relatively weak inhibitor of CYP3A4 (Schrøder-Aasen et al 2012). Whether this is clinically relevant remains to be tested.

Diuretic drugs

Elderflower has diuretic activity. Increased diuresis is possible with concomitant use — observe (Beaux et al 1999).

Hypoglycaemic drugs

Elderflower has demonstrated hypoglycaemic effects in vitro; the clinical significance of this observation remains unknown, and further research is required (Gray et al 2000, Gallagher et al 2003).

CONTRAINDICATIONS AND PRECAUTIONS

A small number of people in the general population may experience allergy to elderflowers as shown by skin prick and RAST tests (Forster-Waldl et al 2003). Avoid in sensitive patients.

Never consume unripe or uncooked berries. They contain cyanogenic glycosides and can be dangerous.

PREGNANCY USE

Elder is likely to be safe when consumed in dietary amounts; however, safety is not known when used in larger quantities.

Practice points/Patient counselling

- Elder is a popular herbal medicine and both the fruit and the berry are used medicinally.
- Elderflower exhibits antiviral, anti-inflammatory, antioxidant, antibacterial, antiproliferative, diaphoretic, diuretic and anti-diabetic properties. The berry also possesses antioxidant and antiviral properties.
- Commission E approves the use of elderflowers as a diaphoretic and to increase bronchial secretion.
- Elderflower has been used traditionally to treat colds, influenza, scarlet fever, bronchitis, sinusitis, hay fever and skin disorders.
- Three clinical trials investigating elderberry oral mixture (Sambucol) or oral lozenges demonstrate that it reduces symptom severity more rapidly than placebo and may shorten the duration of infection.
- The unripe and uncooked berries should never be consumed as they contain cyanide.

PATIENTS' FAQs

What will this herb do for me?

Elderberry preparations appear to reduce the severity and duration of flu symptoms, according to clinical trials. They may also be useful in the treatment of colds, sinusitis and bronchitis; however, less research has been conducted to date to confirm this.

When will it start to work?

Clinical trials of elderberry in influenza have shown that symptom relief may be experienced within 24–48 hours and that the duration of illness may be reduced by up to 3 days. Elder, when taken as a hot infusion, appears to work immediately as a diaphoretic.

Are there any safety issues?

Elderflowers and berries (when cooked) appear to be very safe. No serious adverse events have been reported with the proprietary elderberry extract (Sambucol) in trials with adults and children suggesting it may be suitable for children and elderly influenza patients, who can develop complications more readily (Kong 2009). The unripe and uncooked berries however should never be consumed as they contain cyanide.

REFERENCES

Badescu L et al. Mechanism by Sambucus nigra Extract Improves Bone Mineral Density in Experimental Diabetes. Evid Based Complement Alternat Med. 2012: 848269.
Barak V et al. The effect of Sambucol, a black elderberry-based, natural product, on the production of human cytokines: I. Inflammatory cytokines. Eur Cytokine Netw 12.2 (2001): 290–6.
Barak V et al. The effect of herbal remedies on the production of human inflammatory and anti-inflammatory cytokines. Isr Med Assoc J 4.11 (Suppl) (2002): 919–922.
Beaux D et al. Effect of extracts of Orthosiphon stamineus Benth, Hieracium pilosella L., Sambucus nigra L. and Arctostaphylos uva-ursi (L.) Spreng. in rats. Phytother Res 13.3 (1999): 222–225.
Blumenthal M et al. The complete German Commission E monographs: therapeutic guide to herbal medicines. Austin, TX: American Botanical Council, 1998.
Christensen KB et al. Identification of bioactive compounds from flowers of black elder (Sambucus Nigra L.) that activate the human peroxisome proliferator-activated receptor (ppar) gamma. Phytother Res 24 (Suppl 2) (2010): S129–132.
Ciocoiu M et al. The effects of Sambucus nigra polyphenols on oxidative stress and metabolic disorders in experimental diabetes mellitus. J Physiol Biochem. 65.3 (2009): 297–304.
Ciocoiu M et al. Intervention of Sambucus Nigra Polyphenolic Extract in Experimental Arterial Hypertension. World Academy of Science, Engineering and Technology. 64 (2012): 244–247.
Curtis PJ et al. Cardiovascular disease risk biomarkers and liver and kidney function are not altered in postmenopausal women after ingesting an elderberry extract rich in anthocyanins for 12 weeks. J Nutr 139.12 (2009): 2266–2271.
Dawidowicz AL et al. The antioxidant properties of alcoholic extracts from Sambucus nigra L. (antioxidant properties of extracts). LWT — Food Science and Technology 39.3 (2006): 308–315.
Dellagreca M et al. Synthesis of degraded cyanogenic glycosides from Sambucus nigra. Nat Prod Res 17.3 (2003): 177–181.
Forster-Waldl E et al. Type I allergy to elderberry (Sambucus nigra) is elicited by a 33.2 kDa allergen with significant homology to ribosomal inactivating proteins. Clin Exp Allergy 33.12 (2003): 1703–1710.
Frank J et al. Effects of dietary anthocyanins on tocopherols and lipids in rats. J Agric Food Chem 50.25 (2002): 7226–7230.
Gallagher AM et al. The effects of traditional antidiabetic plants on in vitro glucose diffusion. Nutrition Research 23.3 (2003): 413–424.
Gray AM et al. The traditional plant treatment, Sambucus nigra (elder), exhibits insulin-like and insulin-releasing actions in vitro. J Nutr 130.1 (2000): 15–20.
Haas H et al. Dietary lectins can induce in vitro release of IL-4 and IL-13 from human basophils. Eur J Immunol 29.3 (1999): 918–927.
Harokopakis E et al. Inhibition of proinflammatory activities of major periodontal pathogens by aqueous extracts from elder flower (Sambucus nigra). J Periodontol 77.2 (2006): 271–279.
Jing P et al. Structure-function relationships of anthocyanins from various anthocyanin-rich extracts on the inhibition of coloncancer cell growth. J Agric Food Chem. 56.20 (2008): 9391–9398.
Kinoshita E et al. Anti-influenza virus effects of elderberry juice and its fractions. Biosci Biotechnol Biochem. 76.9(2012): 1633–1638.
Kong F. Pilot clinical study on a proprietary elderberry extract: efficacy in addressing influenza symptoms. Onl J Pharmacol Pharmacokinetics 5 (2009): 32–43.
Krawitz C et al. Inhibitory activity of a standardized elderberry liquid extract against clinically-relevant human respiratory bacterial pathogens and influenza A and B viruses. BMC Complement Altern Med. 11.16 (2011).
Mills S, Bone K. The essential guide to herbal safety. St Louis: Elsevier, 2005.
Moronsanu AJ et al. Antioxidant effect of Aronia versus Sambucus on murine model with or without arterial hypertension. Annals of the Romanian Society for Cell Biology. 16.1 (2011): 222.
Murkovic M et al. Analysis of anthocyanins in plasma for determination of their bioavailability. J Food Comp Analysis 13.4 (2000): 291–296.
Murkovic M et al. Effects of elderberry juice on fasting and postprandial serum lipids and low-density lipoprotein oxidation in healthy volunteers: a randomized, double-blind, placebo-controlled study. Eur J Clin Nutr 58.2 (2004): 244–249.
Picon PD et al. Randomized clinical trial of a phytotherapic compound containing Pimpinella anisum, Foeniculum vulgare,Sambucus nigra, and Cassia augustifolia for chronic constipation. BMC Complement Altern Med. 10:17 (2010).
Roschek, B et al. Elderberry Flavonoids Bind to and Prevent H1n1 Infection in Vitro. Phytochemistry 70.10 (2009): 1255–1261.
Sambucus nigra (elderberry). Altern Med Rev 10.1 (2005): 51–54.
Schrøder-Aasen T et al. In vitro inhibition of CYP3A4 by the Multiherbal commercial product sambucus force and its main constituents Echinacea purpurea and Sambucus nigra. Phytother Res. 26.11 (2012): 1606–1613.
Veberic R et al. European elderberry (Sambucus nigra L.) rich in sugars, organic acids, anthocyanins and selected polyphenols. Food Chemistry 114.2 (2009): 511–515.
Wach A et al. Quercetin content in some food and herbal samples. Food Chemistry 100.2 (2007): 699–704.
Walz B, Chrubasik S. Impact of a proprietary concentrate of Sambucus nigra L. on urinary pH. Phytother Res. 22 (2008): 977–978.
Zakay-Rones Z et al. Inhibition of several strains of influenza virus in vitro and reduction of symptoms by an elderberry extract (Sambucus nigra L.) during an outbreak of influenza B Panama. J Altern Complement Med 1.4 (1995): 361–369.
Zakay-Rones Z et al. Randomized study of the efficacy and safety of oral elderberry extract in the treatment of influenza A and B virus infections. J Int Med Res 32.2 (2004): 132–140.

Eucalyptus

HISTORICAL NOTE Indigenous Australians traditionally used eucalyptus to treat wounds, fungal infections, fevers and respiratory infections, accounting for its name 'fevertree' (Chevallier 2001). European settlers also recognised the medicinal qualities of eucalyptus and surgeon Considen is credited with producing the first essential oil sample in 1788. Bosisto investigated oils from several Australian plants and in 1854 eventually produced essential oils, including Eucalyptus, commercially in association with Müeller, a pharmacist. Bosisto and Müeller concentrated on oils rich in 1,8-cineole, which includes *Eucalyptus* species. In the late 1800s, articles about its medicinal use appeared in medical journals such as *The Lancet*, focusing on its potential use in scarlet fever and diphtheria.

COMMON NAME

Eucalyptus

OTHER NAMES

The term 'Eucalyptus' encompasses a large genus of more than 900 species and subspecies of trees and shrubs native to Australia, but many species are cultivated in other parts of the world.

OTHER NAMES

Aetheroleum Eucalypti, cineole, *Oleum Eucalypti*, *Essence of eucalyptus rectifiee*
Common names include Australian fevertree leaf, blue gum, eucalyptol, fevertree, gum tree, red gum, stringy bark tree.

BOTANICAL NAME/FAMILY

Eucalyptus species (family Myrtaceae)

The species most commonly used in healthcare are:

- *Eucalyptus globulus* (blue gum)
- *Eucalyptus citriodora* (lemon scented gum)
- *Eucalyptus dives* (broad leaf peppermint)
- *Eucalyptus polybractea*
- *Eucalyptus olida*
- *Eucalyptus staigeriana*
- *Eucalyptus sideroxylon*

PLANT PARTS USED

The essential oil is primarily extracted by steam distillation from fresh twigs and leaves. Once the oil is extracted it is analysed to determine the chemical composition using gas chromatography and mass spectrograph analysis. Modern eucalyptus essential oils are primarily extracted from *E. polybractea*, *E. dives*, *E. leucoxylon*, *E. sideroxylon*, *E citriodora* and *E. radiata* in Australia, but other species are used in other countries (Gilles et al 2010, Lassak & McCarthy 2001).

CHEMICAL COMPONENTS

The major chemical constituents of many eucalyptus species are oxides and hydroterpenes, primarily 1,8-cineole, which is the most significant constituent and ranges from 54–95% depending on the species. The 1,8-cineole component is particularly high in *E. globulus* and *E. radiata*. However, the chemical make-up of essential oils extracted from the same species depends on the parts of the plant used; for example oil extracted from the fruit of *E. globulus* contains ~31% aromadendrene in addition to cineole and other constituents (Mulyaningsih et al 2011). The dominant constituents in *E. dives* are piperitone, α-phellandrene, p-cymene and terpin-4-ol. *E. staigeriana* contains 1,8-cineole, neral, geranial, α-phellandrene and methyl geranate. In contrast, *E. olida* contains one major constituent, (E)-methyl cinnamate, although over 20 constituents are present in the oil (Gilles et al 2010).

Eucalyptus oils also contain citronellal, camphone, fenchone, limonene, α-phellandrene, geranial, methyl geranate, (E)-methyl cinnamate and pinene depending on the species (Clarke 2002, Gilles et al 2010, Mulyaningsih et al 2011).

The exact chemical composition of an essential oil depends on the particular species from which it is extracted and to some extent the extraction process and, as indicated, the part of the plant used; most eucalyptus species contain over 20 chemical constitutes. Small amounts of alpha-pinene (2.6%), alpha-cymene (2.7%), aromadendrene, ciminaldehyde, globulol and pinocarveol and *d*-limonene, alpha-phellandrene, camphene and alpha-terpinene are often present (Bisset 1994, Bruneton 1995, Serafino et al 2008).

Other essential oils high in 1,8-cineole include *Rosmarinus officinalis* ct. cineole, *Laurus nobilis*, *Cinnamomum camphora* ct. cineole and *Melaleuca cajuputi*.

MAIN ACTIONS

The main reported actions are expectorant, antitussive (Misawa & Kizawa 1990), nasal decongestant (Burrows 1983, FDA 1994), analgesic (Gobel 1995), antimicrobial (Gilles et al 2010, Raho 2012), antioxidant (Shahwar et al 2012) and anti-inflammatory and antispasmodic properties have been reported in animal and human studies.

Antitussive

Antitussive effects were compared with codeine in guinea pigs in which cough was mechanically stimulated. Essential oil 5% in normal saline was administered by inhalation and had a significant antitussive effect relative to codeine ($P < 0.05$) (Misawa & Kizawa 1990). The antitussive effects of 1,8-cineole were demonstrated in humans in 1980 in a single-blind crossover study in healthy volunteers using a commercially available chest rub where eucalyptus was the active ingredient in the blend (Packman & London 1980). It appears that 1,8-cineole interacts with the M8 (TRPM8) receptor potential channel, the cool-sensitive thermoreceptor primarily affected by menthol, which produces a cooling sensation (Behrendt et al 2004). However, the antitussive effect may also be due to an effect on pulmonary C-fibres, which also contain TRPM8 receptors. Likewise, topically applied vapour rubs (containing camphor, menthol and eucalyptus oil) applied on two consecutive days might be effective in improving nocturnal cough, congestion and sleep in children with coughs due to upper respiratory tract infections (URTI) (Paul 2012).

Nasal decongestant

Two clinical studies have demonstrated that inhalation of eucalyptus oil reduces nasal congestion (Burrows 1983, FDA 1994). Likewise, Cohen and Dressler (1982) showed statistically significant differences in patients with acute coryza inhaling a volatile mixture of menthol 56% and eucalyptus oil 9% for 20 minutes compared to a control group on 14 of the 22 indices of respiratory function, measured from baseline to 60 minutes after inhalation. In contrast, Burrows et al (1983) showed no decongestant effect of inhaling camphor, eucalyptus or menthol for 5-minute periods via a face mask (n = 31), although cold receptors in the nose were stimulated, creating a sensation of increased airflow and improved comfort.

Oral doses or inhaling eucalyptus oil is an effective treatment for purulent and non-purulent respiratory infections such as bronchitis, asthma and chronic obstructive pulmonary airways disease (COPD), possibly due to eucalyptus' broad spectrum antimicrobial action (Sadlon & Lamson 2010).

Antimicrobial

Previous studies indicate eucalyptus has antimicrobial activity in vitro against *Pseudomonas aeruginosa, Bacillus subtilis, Enterococcus faecalis* and *Escherichia coli* (Kurrerath & Mundulaldo 1954), herpes simplex (Schnitzler et al 2001) and oral pathogens (Takarada et al 2004). A clinical observational study involving 30 patients with head and neck cancer and necrotic malodorous ulcers demonstrated improved quality of life and social interaction with the addition of a twice-daily cleansing of the ulcers with an essential oil mix whose main component was eucalyptus (Warnke et al 2006). In addition, the researchers reported evidence of re-epithelialisation and anti-inflammatory effects. Raho and Benali (2012) showed antimicrobial activity of *E. globulus* oil obtained from the leaves against *Escherichia coli* (Gram negative) and *Staphyloccus aureus* (Gram positive) in an in vitro assay. Gilles et al (2010) reported on varying degrees of antimicrobial activity of oils from *E. staigeriana, E. dives* and *E. olida*: *E. staigeriana* had the highest activity in general. Gram-positive bacteria were more sensitive to the essential oils than Gram-negative organisms. *Staphyloccus aureus* was the most sensitive organism and *Pseudomonas aeruginosa* the most resistant organism. The authors stated the antimicrobial activity of the three essential oils, especially *E. staigeriana* and *E. dives*, 'compared favourably with that of the standard antibiotics tested', but did not describe the comparison process or list the 'standard antibiotics' in the method. From the results these appear to be chloramphenicol and nystatin. The clinical utility of these findings requires further study.

Ceremelli et al (2008) evaluated the antimicrobial activity of *E. globulus* against isolates of a range of bacteria such as *Streptococcus pyrogenes, S. pneumoniae, Stapholcoccus aureus, Haemophilus influenzae* and *Klebsiella pneumoniae* and two viruses, *adenovirus* and a mumps virus strain. *Haemophilus influenzae* and *S. pneumoniae* were the most susceptible bacteria and there was a mild inhibitory effect on the mumps virus. As indicated earlier, oil extracted from the fruit of *E. globulus* is effective against methicillin-resistant *Stapholcoccus aureus* (Mulyaningsih et al 2011).

Anti-inflammatory

Eucalyptus inhibits prostaglandin synthesis in vitro (Wagner 1986) at a concentration of 37 micromol/L. Anti-inflammatory and antinociceptive effects have been demonstrated in animal models (Ulbricht & Basch 2005). Alternatively, a study in which 1,8-cineole was injected into the rat hind-paw demonstrated that eucalyptus induced oedema, most likely due to the release of mast cell mediators (Santos & Rao 1997). The clinical implications of this finding for topically-applied eucalyptus oil require further investigation. Anti-inflammatory activity of *E. radiata* has been demonstrated in patients with dry and weeping dermatitis, most probably due to inhibition of inflammatory markers such as TNF-alpha, COX enzymes, 5-lipoxygenase and other leukotrienes, and it could be an alternative to topical steroid medicines (Hadji-Minglou & Bolcato 2005, Santos & Rao 2000). Juergens et al (2003) demonstrated 1,8-cineole maintained lung function four times better than controls in a double blind clinical trial of patients (n = 32) with severe steroid-dependent bronchial asthma. Patients were randomly assigned to 1,8-cineole 200 mg three times daily for 3 weeks or placebo. Steroid doses were reduced by 2.5 mg every 3 weeks. Twelve of the 16 receiving 1,8-cineole remained stable despite reduced steroid doses.

Analgesic

Analgesic properties are attributed to the monoterpene components of eucalyptus oil. The monoterpenoid profile differs among eucalypt species and may account for variations in therapeutic effect. *E. globulus* has a high 1,8-cineole content (60–90%) (Juergens et al 1998, Shahwar et al 2012, Wei & Shibamoto 2010). Silva et al (2003) investigated the analgesic and anti-inflammatory effects of *E. tereticornis, E. citriodora* and *E. globulus* in rats. The results showed central and peripheral analgesic effects of the three oils. Santos and Rao (2000) also demonstrated 1,8-cineole had anti-inflammatory properties and reduced granuloma in rat studies.

OTHER ACTIONS

Eucalyptus oil is metabolised in the liver; however, evidence is contradictory as to whether it induces the cytochrome P450 enzyme system. One study conducted with an animal model demonstrated a slight increase in CYP4A expression (Ngo et al 2003), whereas 1,8-cineole has demonstrated CYP450 induction in vitro and in animal studies (Ulbricht & Basch 2005). *E. globulus* induces a cell-mediated immune response, and morphological and functional activation in human macrophages stimulates the phagocytic response (Serafino et al 2008). Some eucalyptus species, such as *E. sideroxylon*, have antioxidant properties, but the clinical application is unknown. Some essential oils have chemopreventive properties, thus inducing enzymes to detoxify the carcinogen (Wei & Shibamoto 2010). In addition, they have chemotherapeutic properties by inhibiting tumour proliferation and enhancing tumour death. The inhibitory actions may be due to dietary isoprenoids, especially monoterpenes, in essential oils (Wei & Shibamoto 2010).

Umezu (2012) compared the effects of 20 essential oils, including eucalyptus, with conventional medicines that act on the central nervous system (CNS) to determine whether the essential oils had stimulant, depressive or neither of these effects in mice. They found that essential oils from eucalyptus and rose reduced the avoidance rate (number of avoidance responses/number of avoidance trials) without affecting the response rate, which suggests that these essential oils may have some effect on the CNS.

CLINICAL USE

Eucalyptus oil has been investigated in numerous forms; however, there is a lack of controlled, clinical studies.

It is mainly used in topical preparations or as an inhalant and not generally used internally.

Respiratory conditions

As indicated in other sections, eucalyptus oil is used as symptomatic treatment in obstructive respiratory conditions such as bronchitis, asthma, the common cold and other conditions associated with catarrh of the upper respiratory tract. Although it is used internally and externally in Europe for these indications, in Australia the oil is generally used externally in vaporisers, chest rubs and nasal inhalations.

Nasal decongestant properties were assessed in 31 healthy volunteers using inhalations of 10 mL of essential oil for 5 minutes. There was no effect on nasal resistance to air flow, but there was a stimulant effect on the cold receptors in the nose and the majority of subjects reported being able to breathe more easily (FDA 1994). A single-blind, parallel clinical trial (n = 234) was conducted to assess whether vaporised essential oil reduced nasal congestion compared with steam. The essential oil was significantly more effective ($P < 0.02$), but only in the first hour after inhalation. Other researchers found no significant differences in nasal decongestion compared with placebo (Burrows 1983). There was no significant difference between placebo and topically applied *E. piperita* to the forehead and temples to treat headache in a randomised, double crossover trial (n = 32); however, cognitive performance and muscle and mental relaxation were greater in the essential oil group (Gobel 1995).

Eucalyptus oil has mucolytic, bronchodilating and anti-inflammatory properties largely due to 1,8-cineole and is known to reduce exacerbations of COPD (Sadlon & Lamson 2010, Worth & Dethlesen 2012). A double-blind placebo trial involving 247 people with a confirmed diagnosis of asthma were randomly assigned to 200 mg cineole or placebo three times per day as concomitant therapy for 6 months (Worth & Dethlesen 2012). The cineole group showed statistically significant improvements in forced expiratory volume and asthma symptoms and quality of life using the Asthma Quality of Life Questionnaire.

Aromatherapy

Eucalyptus, as it is traditionally used in aromatherapy, has not been systematically investigated under clinical trial conditions. Therefore, most evidence is derived from traditional sources.

Aromatherapists use eucalyptus for its mentally uplifting and stimulating effects and to aid concentration. It is also used in massage and vaporisers to relieve respiratory symptoms, treat minor skin infections and acne and relieve headache and muscular aches and pain. Usually eucalyptus oil is included in a blend of 3–5 essential oils for a massage, but may be used alone for an inhalation. One study investigating the effects of topical application of eucalyptus oil to the forehead and temples found it was an ineffective treatment for headache (Gobel 1995).

E

OTHER USES

Eucalyptus oil is often included in OTC and other medicines in various formulations such as rubs, mouthwashes, 'cold and 'flu' preparations, cleansing products, inhalers, soaps and insect repellents in which the 1,8-cineole content is standardised to 80–90%. Bosisto's Eucalyptus Oil is commonly sold in supermarkets and has an Aust R label (10908). It is not used in aromatherapy and is dispensed in a ribbed poison bottle with a childproof cap.

Dust mite removal

Eucalyptus oil can be formulated with a kitchen detergent concentrate to form an inexpensive acaricidal wash that reduces the number of live mites found in blankets during normal machine washing (Tovey & McDonald 1997). When compared with detergent concentrate alone, a 30-minute pre-wash soak of woollen blankets with the eucalyptus oil/detergent formula reduced the number of live mites that could be recovered by 97%. This eliminates the need for very hot water and may maintain low allergen levels in bedding for longer than normal laundering alone because mites are adversely affected by low concentrations of eucalyptus oil vapour, which lingers for 2–3 days. In this study, the dishwashing liquid detergent concentrate (Kit, L&K, Rexona, Sydney, Australia) was used to form an emulsion in water because the essential oil is not soluble in water.

Cleaning agent

Washing in diluted eucalyptus oil is also used as a method of removing stains from fabric; however, it does leave a faint characteristic odour for 2–3 days despite rinsing and drying, and some people may find this irritating.

Malodorous necrotic ulcers

These ulcers are a major concern for cancer patients and can lead to social isolation and reduced QOL because current treatments inadequately reduce the foul smell to acceptable levels. A paper published in 2006 reported that rinsing the ulcers twice a day with an antibacterial essential oil mixture (mainly eucalyptus oil) resulted in complete disappearance of odour by day 3 or 4 in all patients (n = 30) (Warnke et al 2006). The eucalyptus was used in combination with a standard course of antibiotics. A number of beneficial secondary findings were anti-inflammatory activity, promotion of healing and complete re-epithelialisation and emotional relief on resolution of the condition.

DOSE RANGE

Dose recommendations vary, but generally low doses are used. Internal formulations may take longer to show an effect than conventional medicines.

- Inhalation: 12 drops in 150 mL of boiling water or 5 drops in a nebuliser, which delivers approximately 35 mg (unpubl. data: Harris & Harris—Aromatic Medicine: The Interfaces of Absorption, seminar course notes, Melbourne, 2003). High doses are not recommended because they can irritate the eyes and mucous membranes and may trigger an asthma-like attack.
- Mouth wash: 20 mL (0.91 mg/mL) solution gargled twice daily.
- Massage: traditionally aromatherapists use essential oils as 3.5–5% in a carrier substance but doses between 5 and 20% are used for adults and much lower doses for children and older people.
- Ointments, creams, gels and poultices: 5–10% in a carrier substance such as beeswax.
- Internal use: 0.3–0.6 mL/day essential oil 1–4 times daily; capsules 100–200 mg; lozenges 0.2–15.0 mg dissolved slowly in the mouth every 30–60 minutes.

Most Australian aromatherapists do not currently administer essential oils via the internal route (oral, vaginal and rectal), but they are administered via these routes in other countries, especially France. The safety risk is great with internal use.

TOXICITY

Toxicity is influenced by the purity of the essential oil, the administration mode and the knowledge and competence of the individuals using the oil. Toxicity symptoms occur rapidly, but may be delayed for hours and include altered consciousness state, drowsiness and unconsciousness, which are dose-dependent. Symptoms reported in other studies include epigastric burning, nausea, vomiting, dizziness, muscular weakness, delirium and convulsions, especially with oral ingestion.

The acute oral LD_{50} dose of 1,8-cineole in rats is 2.48 g/kg and the dermal LD_{50} dose in rabbits is > 5 g/kg.

Fatal poisoning has occurred in children after accidental ingestion of whole or diluted eucalyptus oil in amounts ranging from 2 to 10 mL. Tibballs (1995) reported 109 children who were admitted to hospital for eucalyptus oil poisoning in an 11-year period; 27 had been accidentally poisoned when an adult administered the oil orally by mistake and most of the remaining 82 children had ingested the oil from a vaporiser. Another review of 41 cases of eucalyptus oil poisoning (Webb & Pitt 1993) indicated that 80% were asymptomatic. There was no relationship between the amount of oil ingested and the presence and severity of symptoms. A recent case reports shows dermal application of eucalyptus oil can induce seizures. A healthy 4-year-old girl was treated with eucalyptus for head lice. Her symptoms included vomiting, ataxia, lethargy and tonic-clonic seizure, which resolved spontaneously when the skin was washed (Waldman 2011). Oral ingestion of eucalyptus is known to induce neurological symptoms and seizures. Waldman's case report suggests dermal application might also induce seizures in susceptible individuals.

Another case study demonstrated severe poisoning following a low oral dose of eucalyptus in a

Practice points/Patient counselling

- It is essential to buy eucalyptus essential oils from reputable sources and to ensure the products have appropriate labels that contain enough information to use the oils safely. That is, the product should comply with safety and manufacturing and labelling requirements.
- Eucalyptus essential oils are steam-distilled from a number of *Eucalyptus* species, and have different chemical compositions depending on the species. Many contain a large proportion of 1,8-cineole, which appears to be responsible for the action on the respiratory system.
- Eucalyptus is primarily used in aromatherapy as an inhalation to relieve nasal congestion and in massage to relieve muscular aches and pain, as well as in ointments, gels and compresses, and via a vaporiser for mental stimulation and to aid concentration.
- Eucalyptus leaf extract is an approved food additive in Australia and is used in lozenges, lollies, teas, tinctures and conventional medicines.
- When used topically in an appropriate manner and appropriate doses, eucalyptus oil is considered to be safe; however, several cautions should be considered when determining the risk of adverse reactions and toxicity. People using eucalyptus essential oil should be monitored for allergies and the oil should not be applied to the face of children. Eucalyptus should not be used internally unless it is diluted and used in the recommended doses and dose intervals on the advice of appropriately qualified practitioners.
- Signs of poisoning usually occur rapidly and include confusion, irritability, respiratory distress, hypotension, nausea and vomiting. If poisoning is suspected medical care should be sought urgently. Do not induce vomiting. Use oral charcoal and monitor consciousness.
- Several medicine-essential oil interactions are theoretically possible; however, their clinical significance is unknown.

58-year-old chemist suffering from acute delusions who drank 4–5 drops of undiluted eucalyptus oil. He developed complications, including compromised respiratory and cardiac function and hypertension, which resolved after treatment (Waldman et al 2011). This case history highlights the importance of storing essential oils and vaporisors out of reach of children and cognitively impaired adults.

The Victorian Poisons Information Centre (see Appendix 3) recommends that all people who ingest ≥ 1 mL of eucalyptus oil be assessed in an emergency department. The centre attributes the toxicity to the 1,8-cineole, terpene and α-phellandrene content and indicates that, although hydrocyanic acid is only present in small amounts, it may be responsible for most of the toxicity.

ADVERSE REACTIONS

Eucalyptus oil is generally safe when used externally in an appropriate manner.

A number of adverse reactions are reported for topical application, including systemic toxicity in a 6-year-old girl, and urticaria, contact dermatitis and skin irritation in other cases (Darben 1988). Likewise, there is a low risk of skin sensitivity to *E. staigeriana* because of the citral content in geranial acetate (Tisserand & Balacs 1995). However, when considering the risks of topical application of eucalyptus oil the state of the skin must be considered as well as the individual's susceptibility to atopic conditions such as eczema and asthma.

Allergic reactions to lozenges have also been reported anecdotally.

Inhalations may irritate the eyes and mucous membranes.

SIGNIFICANT INTERACTIONS

Due to the lack of clinical evidence, interactions are theoretical and speculative.

CNS depressants

Oral ingestion of eucalyptus has been associated with CNS depression, therefore additive effects are theoretically possible — use with caution.

Medicines metabolised by CYP 450

Some evidence suggests CYP induction is possible; however, it is not known which CYP enzymes are affected, thus making recommendations difficult. Interactions are unlikely when used topically or inhaled, but could theoretically occur when used internally (Springhouse Corporation 2001).

Hypoglycaemic agents

If used in combination with oral glucose-lowering conventional or complementary medicines by people with diabetes, doses of eucalyptus might contribute to hypoglycaemia. Blood glucose levels should be monitored to detect hypoglycaemia (Springhouse Corporation 2001).

CONTRAINDICATIONS AND PRECAUTIONS

Essential oils are not recommended in the first 3 months of life because the barrier function of the skin is not fully developed. In addition, inhaling menthol can induce transient apnoea in premature infants due to its effects on the TRPM8 receptor (Javorka et al 1980); thus, essential oils containing 1,8-cineole should not be applied on or near the face of babies and small children. *E. globulus* may cause skin allergy in susceptible individuals such as people prone to asthma and allergies, and those who had a previous reaction to eucalyptus. Skin testing might be indicated in these people.

Eucalyptus oil should not be administered internally to children or people with inflammatory gastrointestinal tract disease or impaired liver function, or during pregnancy.

Eucalyptus oil should not be applied to the face, especially of infants and young children because of the risk of bronchospasm and irritation.

The oil should be stored out of the reach of children and confused people. This precaution includes eucalyptus essential oil in vaporisers, which should also be placed out of reach. Poisoning has occurred following essential oil ingestion from vaporisers.

Oily carrier fluids should not be used for nasal sprays because they inhibit protective nasal ciliary movement and could cause lipid pneumonia.

The essential oil is highly flammable and represents a fire risk when used in candle vaporisers.

PREGNANCY USE

No studies have been undertaken. The essential oil is not teratogenic in animal studies, but doses of 500 mg/kg cross the placenta in large enough amounts to stimulate hepatic activity in rodents (Jori & Briatico 1973). Aromatherapists do not recommend using eucalyptus essential oil during pregnancy, especially in the first trimester.

PATIENTS' FAQs

What will this essential oil do for me?

Eucalyptus essential oil can be used in a vaporiser or on tissues to help clear the nose and make breathing easier if you have an upper respiratory tract infection (URTI). It can also increase mental alertness. In a massage blend eucalyptus can help relieve muscular and arthritic pain.

Eucalyptus oil can be added to the washing machine to help kill dust mites in human clothes and animal bedding. Dust mites are responsible for many respiratory conditions such as asthma.

When will it start to work?

Inhaled eucalyptus oil usually acts quickly and provides symptomatic relief quickly. Oral doses and massage blends usually take longer to have an effect.

Are there any safety issues?

Ingested eucalyptus oil has caused poisoning especially in children and therefore any source of the oil, including from vaporisers, should be placed out of reach of children and confused people.

Eucalyptus can irritate the eyes and mucous membranes. It should be kept away from the face, especially of infants and children.

Ingested eucalyptus oil could affect the action of some medicines such as antidepressants, sedatives and anaesthetic agents. It increases absorption of nicotine.

REFERENCES

Behrendt H-J et al. Characterisation of the mouse cold-menthol receptor TRPM8 and vallinoid receptor type-1 VRI using a fluorometric imaging plate reader (FLIPR) assay. Br J Pharmacology 141 (2004): 733–737.

Bisset N. Herbal drugs and pharmaceuticals. Boca Raton, CA: CRC Press, 1994.

Bruneton J. Pharmacognosy, phytochemistry, medicinal plants. Paris: Lavoisier, 1995.

Burrows A. The effects of camphor, eucalyptus and menthol vapour on nasal resistance to airflow and nasal sensation. Acta Otolaryngol 96 (1983): 157–161.

Cermelli C et al. Effect of Eucalyptus essential oil on respiratory bacteria viruses. Current Microbiology 56.1 (2008): 88–92.

Chevallier A. Encyclopedia of Medicinal Plants. St Leonards NSW: Dorling Kimberley (2001).

Clarke S. Essential oil chemistry for safe aromatherapy. Edinburgh: Churchill Livingstone, 2002.

Cohen BM, Dressler WE. Acute aromatics inhalation modifies the airways. Effects of the common cold. Respiration 43.4 (1982): 285–293.

Darben T. Topical Eucalyptus oil poisoning. Aust J Dermatol 39 (1988): 265–267.

Food and Drug Administration (FDA). Over the counter drugs: monograph for OTC nasal decongestant drug products. Fed Reg 41 (1994): 38408–38409.

Gilles M, Zhao J, An M, Agboola S. Chemical composition and antimicrobail properties of essential oils of three Australain Eucalyptus species. Food Chemistry. (2010): 731–737.

Gobel H. Essential plant oils and headache mechanisms. Phytomedicine 2 (1995): 93–102.

Hadji-Minaglou A, Bolcato O. The potential role of specific essential oils in replacement of dermocorticoid drugs (strong, medium, weak) in the treatment of acute dry or weeping dermatitis. Int J Aromather 15.2 (2005): 66–73.

Javorka K, Tomori Z, Zavarska L. Protective and defensive airway reflexes in premature infants. Physiol Bohemoslov 29.1 (1980): 29–35.

Jori A, Briatico G. Effects of eucalyptol on microsomal enzyme activity of foetal and newborn rats. Biochem Pharmacol 22 (1973): 543–544.

Juergens U et al. Antiinflammatory effects of eucalyptol (1,8-cineole) in bronchial asthma: inhibition of arachidonic acid metabolism in human blood monocytes ex vivo. Eur J Med Res 3.9 (1998): 407–412.

Juergens U et al. Anti-inflammatory activity of 1,8-cineole (eucalyptol) in bronchial asthma: a double-blind placebo-controlled trial. Eur J Med Res 97 (2003): 250–256.

Kurrerath F, Mundulaldo G. The activity of some preparations containing essential oils in tuberculosis. Fitoterpia 25 (1954): 483–485.

Lassak E, McCarthy T. Australian medicinal plants. Sydney: Reed New Holland, 2001.

Misawa M, Kizawa M. Antitussive effects of several volatile oils especially cedar leaf oil in guinea pigs. Pharmacometrics 39 (1990): 81–87.

Mulyaningsih S, Spor F, Reichling J, Wink M. Antibacterial activity of essential oils from eucalyptus and of selected components against multidrug-resistant bacterial pathogens. Pharmacological Biology 49.9 (2011): 893–899.

Ngo SNT et al. The effects of Eucalyptus terpenes on hepatic cytochrome P450 CYP4A, peroxisomal Acyl CoA oxidase (AOX) and peroxisome proliferator activated receptor alpha (PPAR[alpha]) in the common brush tail possum (Trichosurus vulpecula). Comp Biochem Physiol C Toxicol Pharmacol 136.2 (2003): 165–173.

Packman F, London S. The utility of artificially induced cough as a clinical model for evaluating the antitussive effects of aromatics delivered by inunction. Eur J Resp Dis 61 (Suppl) (1980): 101–109.

Paul I. Therapeutic options for acute cough due to upper respiratory infections in children. Lung 190.1 (2012): 41–44.

Raho B, Benali M. Antibacterial activity of the essential oils from the leaves of *Eucalyptus globulus* against *Escherichia coli* and *Staphylococcus aureus*. Asian Pacific Journal of Tropical Biomedicine. (2012): 739–742.

Sadlon A, Lamson D. Immune-modifying and antimicrobial effects of eucalyptus and simple inhalation devices. Alternative Medicine Review 15.1 (2010): 33–47.

Santos FA, Rao VSN. Mast cell involvement in the rat paw oedema response to 1,8-cineole, the main constituent of eucalyptus and rosemary oils. Eur J Pharmacol 331.2–3 (1997): 253–258.

Santos F, Rao V. Antiinflammatory and antinocieptive effects of 1,8-cineole, a terpenoid oxide present in many plant essential oils. Phytotheraphy Reseaech (2000):14: 240–244.

Santos F, Raos V. Antiinflammatory and antinociceptive effects of 1,8-cineole and terpenoid oxide present in many plant essential oils. Phytother Res 14 (2000): 240–244.

Schnitzler P et al. Antiviral activity of Australian tea tree oil and eucalyptus oil against herpes simplex virus. Pharmazie 56 (2001): 343–347.

Serafino A et al. Stimulatory effect of Eucalyptus essential oil on innate cell-mediated immune response. BMC Immunology 9 (2008).

Shahwar D, Raza M, Bukhan S, Bukhan G. Ferric reducing antioxidant power of essential oils extracted from *Eucalyptus* and *Curcuma* species. Asian Pacific Journal of Tropical Biomedicine. (2012): S1633–S1636.

Silva J et al. Analgesic and anti-inflammatory effects of essential oils of Eucalyptus. J Ethnopharmacology 89.2–3 (2003): 277–283.

Springhouse Corporation. Nursing drug handbook series: herbal medicine. Springhouse, PA: Springhouse Corporation, 2001.

Takarada K et al. A comparison of the effects of essential oils against oral pathogens. Oral Microbiol Immunol 19 (2004): 61–64.

Tibballs J. Clinical effects and management of eucalyptus oil ingestion in infants and young children. Med J Aust 163 (1995): 177–180.

Tisserand R, Balacs T. Essential oil safety: a guide for health professionals, Edinburgh: Churchill Livingstone 1995.

Tovey ER, McDonald LG. A simple washing procedure with eucalyptus oil for controlling house dust mites and their allergens in clothing and bedding. J Allergy Clin Immunol 100.4 (1997): 464–466.

Ulbricht CE, Basch EM. Natural standard herb and supplement reference. St Louis: Mosby, 2005.

Umezu T. Evaluation of the effects of plant-derived essential oils on central nervous system function using discrete shuttle-type conditioned avoidance response in mice. Phytotherapy Research 26.6 (2012): 884–891.

Wagner H. In vitro inhibition of prostaglandin biosynthesis by essential oils and phenolic compounds. Planta Med 3 (1986): 184–187.

Waldman N. Seizure caused by dermal application of over-the-counter eucalyptus oil head lice preparation. Clinical Toxicology 49.8 (2011): 750–751.

Waldman W, Barwina M, Sein J. Accidental intoxication with eucalyptus oil—a case report. Przegl Lek (Polish) 68.8 (2011): 555–556.

Warnke P et al. Antibacterial essential oils in malodorous cancer patients: clinical observations of 30 patients. Phytomedicine 13.7 (2006): 463–467.

Webb N, Pitt W. Eucalyptus and poisoning in childhood: 41 cases in South East Queensland. J Paediatr Child Health 29 (1993): 368–371.

Wei A, Shibamoto T. Medicinal activities of essential oils: role in disease prevention. Chapter 4 in Bioactive Foods in Promoting Health Elsevier (2010).

Worth H, Dethlefsen U. Patients with asthma benefit from concomitant therapy with cineole: a placebo controlled, double blind trial. Journal of Asthma 49.8 (2012): 849–853.

Fenugreek

HISTORICAL NOTE Fenugreek's seeds and leaves are used as food, and as traditional medicine throughout the world. It is indigenous to Western Asia and Southern Europe and now mainly cultivated in India, Pakistan, France, Argentina and North African countries. In ancient Egypt it was used as an aphrodisiac and, together with honey, for the treatment of rickets, diabetes, dyspepsia, rheumatism, anaemia and constipation. It has also been described in early Greek and Latin pharmacopoeias for hyperglycaemia and was used by Yemenite Jews for type 2 diabetes (Yeh et al 2003). In India, China and the Middle East, it is still widely used as a therapeutic agent and as an ingredient in traditional Indian chutney and spice blends and in Egyptian confectionery (Basu & Srichamroen 2010). In the United States, it has been used therapeutically since the 19th century for postmenopausal vaginal dryness and dysmenorrhoea (Ulbricht & Basch 2005), and commercially is a principal flavouring ingredient of simulated maple syrup, flavouring agent of tobacco and of hydrolysed vegetable protein powder (Basu & Srichamroen 2010). It is a herb still used today as part of traditional herbal treatment for type 2 diabetes in Tunisia and Palestine (Ali-Shtayeh et al 2012, Othman et al 2013).

F

COMMON NAME

Fenugreek

OTHER NAMES

Trigonella seeds, bird's foot, Greek hay, hu lu ba, methi, trigonella

BOTANICAL NAME/FAMILY

Trigonella foenum-graecum (family Leguminosae)

PLANT PARTS USED

Dried mature seed. Leaves are used less commonly.

CHEMICAL COMPONENTS

The main chemical constituents are fibre, tannic acid, fixed and volatile oils and a bitter extractive, steroidal saponins, flavonoids, polysaccharides, alkaloids, trigonelline, trigocoumarin, trigomethyl coumarin, mucilage (up to 30%), seven essential amino acids and vitamins A, C, D, B_1, B_2 and B_3 (Bin-Hafeez et al 2003, Fisher & Painter 1996, Shang et al 1998, Zia et al 2001). Leaves contain 25% protein and 25.9% starch and are a rich source of calcium, iron and beta-carotene. The seeds contain 6–10% lipids (mostly unsaturated), 44–59% carbohydrates (mostly galactomannans) and 20–30% protein (rich in arginine, alanine and glycine and low in lysine and methionine) (Basu & Srichamroen 2010).

MAIN ACTIONS

Hypoglycaemic and antidiabetic

The hypoglycaemic effect of fenugreek seeds has been demonstrated in numerous studies involving experimentally-induced diabetes (both type 1 and type 2) in rats, dogs, mice and rabbits as well as diabetic humans (Alarcon-Aguilara et al 1998, Eidi et al 2007, Madar et al 1988, Mohammad et al 2006, Raju et al 2001, Ribes et al 1984, 1986, Riyad et al 1988, Sharma et al 1990, Vats et al 2002), and the effect has been described as slow but sustained (Puri et al 2002). Interestingly, however, no reduction in fasting or postprandial blood sugar levels was observed in a placebo-controlled study in non-diabetic people who used a dose of 5 g/day over 3 months (Bordia et al 1997).

It is recognised that there is a synergistic effect from a range of compounds, resulting in both glucose absorption inhibition and the promotion of pancreatic function to effect lower blood glucose and enhance other metabolic indicators (Basu & Srichamroen 2010). The mechanism for the hypoglycaemic effect of fenugreek has been explored in many in vivo trials. The viscous fibre, galactomannan, reduces intestinal absorption of glucose and thus postprandial blood glucose (Kaur et al 2011, Srichamroen et al 2009). Fenugreek also has an insulinomimetic effect and may increase the sensitivity of tissues to available insulin (Puri et al 2002), and enhance utilisation of glucose (Al Habori et al 2001). Extracts of fenugreek stimulated insulin secretion of INS-1 cells in vitro (Kaur et al 2011). Biguanides (metformin) are the widely used pharmaceutical treatment for type 2 diabetes. Significant levels of biguanide-related compounds were found in analyses of fenugreek seeds (Perla & Jayanty 2013). Another mouse study revealed that an extract of fenugreek opposed the development of diabetes in mice fed a high-fat diet and had an antidiabetic effect in mice with established diabetes (Hamza et al 2012).

Antiulcerogenic activity

Both an aqueous extract and a gel fraction isolated from the seeds demonstrated significant ulcer-protective effects in vivo (Pandian et al 2002). The seed fractions given orally to test animals provided dose-dependent gastric protection against the effects of ethanol, which was as potent as that of omeprazole. Furthermore, histological studies found that the soluble gel fraction was significantly more protective than omeprazole. Preliminary research suggests that the polysaccharide composition and/or flavonoid components of the mucilaginous gel are responsible for the gastroprotective and antisecretory activities of the seeds.

Hypocholesterolaemic effect

Significant cholesterol-lowering activity has been demonstrated in numerous animal studies and human studies with diabetic volunteers (Belguith-Hadriche et al 2013, Boban et al 2008, Gupta et al 2001, Petit et al 1995, Rao et al 1996, Sharma et al 1990, Sowmya & Rajyalakshmi 1999, Stark & Madar 1993).

One mechanism of action, although unclear, appears to be the fibre and steroidal saponins interacting with bile salts in the digestive tract (Stark & Madar 1993). In one study, an unusual amino acid, 4-hydroxyisoleucine 5, was isolated and tested in dyslipidaemic hamsters and was found to significantly decrease plasma triglyceride levels by 33%, total cholesterol by 22% and free fatty acids by 14%, accompanied by an increase in high-density lipoprotein (HDL) cholesterol: total cholesterol ratio by 39% (Narender et al 2006). A thermostable extract of fenugreek seeds (TEFS) upregulated low-density lipoprotein receptors, resulting in enhanced low-density lipoprotein (LDL) uptake in vitro. Studies of fat-supplemented mice showed that TEFS decreased serum triglycerides, LDL and body weight in a time-dependent manner, indicating inhibition of fat accumulation and upregulation of LDL receptors (Vijayakumar et al 2010). Another in vivo study showed that ethyl acetate extracts of fenugreek seeds had significant hypocholesterolaemic and antioxidant effects in cholesterol-fed rats when other extracts did not. There was speculation that this was due to the flavonoid content of the extract (Belguith-Hadriche et al 2013).

Immunostimulant activity

Enhanced humoral immunity, significant increases in macrophage activity and a stimulatory effect on lymphoproliferation have been demonstrated in vivo (Bin-Hafeez et al 2003). Stimulatory effects were observed at 100 mg/kg and in some cases at 250 mg/kg.

Anti-inflammatory and antipyretic activity

Potent anti-inflammatory activity was demonstrated in an animal model for both single-dose and chronic-dose applications of a dried-leaf decoction of fenugreek (Ahmadiani et al 2001). The effectiveness of the 1000 mg/kg dose of the extract was relatively equal to 300 mg/kg sodium salicylate for single dosing; however, chronic administration was more effective than sodium salicylate. Additionally, the fenugreek decoction exhibited stronger antipyretic activity than that of sodium salicylate. These findings have been supported in an in vivo study of a water-soluble fraction of fenugreek seed that was shown to have significant analgesic and anti-inflammatory actions (Vyas et al 2008).

Antinociceptive effects

Two studies in animal models have identified antinociceptive activity for fenugreek (Ahmadiani et al 2001, Javan et al 1997). This seems to be mediated through central and peripheral mechanisms. According to Javan et al (1997), the antinociceptive effects of 2000 mg/kg of the extract were more potent than those of 300 mg/kg sodium salicylate. One animal study concluded that the anti-inflammatory effects of fenugreek reduced pain in peripheral neuropathy (Morani et al 2012).

Effect on thyroid hormones

Administration of fenugreek seed extract for 15 days to both mice and rats significantly decreased serum triiodothyronine (T_3), suggesting that thyroxine (T_4)-to-T_3 conversion is inhibited and leads to increases in T_4 levels (Panda et al 1999).

Stimulates digestion

Traditionally, fenugreek is used to improve digestion. In vivo studies have identified that it enhances the activities of pancreatic and intestinal lipases, and sucrase and maltase, thereby providing support for this traditional use (Platel & Srinivasan 1996, 2000).

Effect on neurotransmitters

A range of constituents extracted from fenugreek seeds exhibited potential anticholinesterase activity and therefore should be explored for potential benefits in the treatment of memory disorders (Satheesh Kumar et al 2010, Sharififar et al 2012). An amino acid constituent of fenugreek, 4-hydrosyisoleucine, exhibited antidepressant-like effects by enhancing brain serotonin turnover in preclinical studies (Gaur et al 2012).

OTHER ACTIONS

Fenugreek has been studied for a wide range of actions. Positive findings for other properties of fenugreek have been found in vitro and in vivo, including antioxidant, antihypertensive, hepatoprotective, chemoprotective and renoprotective actions (Amin et al 2005, Annida & Stanely Mainzen Prince 2005, Balaraman et al 2006, Bhatia et al 2006, Dixit et al 2005, 2008, Liu et al 2012, Shetty & Salimath 2009). The polyphenolic compounds of fenugreek seeds confer antioxidant and hepatoprotective properties comparable to silymarin in trials on rats (Kaviarasan & Anuradha 2007, Kaviarasan et al 2004, 2006, 2008). Analysis of fenugreek ethyl acetate extract showed it to be a good source of flavonoids and flavonoid glycosides, possibly responsible for the majority of its antioxidant properties (Kenny et al 2013). The fenugreek mucilage, in rat studies, demonstrated potential beneficial effect on induced arthritis in rats (Sindhu et al 2012).

Antineoplastic activity has been observed for fenugreek in the Ehrlich ascites carcinoma model in mice (Sur et al 2001). Protodioscin, purified from fenugreek, has also exhibited antineoplastic activity on human leukaemia cell lines in vitro (Hibasami et al 2003). Fenugreek extract induces apoptosis in vitro to breast, pancreatic and prostate cancer cell lines, but not normal cells (Sebastian & Thampan 2007, Shabbeer et al 2009).

Ethanol extract (50%) seemed to possess profound antiplasmodial activity in vitro (Palaniswamy et al 2010), but no in vivo trials have yet been undertaken. Although fenugreek contains coumarin constituents, a placebo-controlled study found that it does not affect platelet aggregation, fibrinolytic activity or fibrinogen (Bordia et al 1997).

Traditionally, it is thought to promote lactation in nursing mothers and act as a general tonic; however there is conflicting scientific evidence to support its efficacy. The mechanism as a galactogogue is also unclear. Fenugreek is thought to exert oestrogenic activity through its phyto-oestrogen and diosgenin content (Mortel & Mehta 2013).

CLINICAL USE

Fenugreek is both a food and medicine that has demonstrated significant pharmacological effects beyond its nutrient value. It is one of the more validated herbal medicines for blood glucose lowering and has multiple mechanisms of relevance to the diabetic patient.

Dyspepsia and loss of appetite

Although controlled studies are unavailable, the increased activities of pancreatic and intestinal lipases seen in animal studies provide a theoretical basis for its use in dyspepsia.

Commission E approved the internal use of fenugreek seed for loss of appetite (Blumenthal et al 2000).

Elevated lipid levels

Several clinical studies conducted in people with and without diabetes have identified significant lipid-lowering activity with different fenugreek preparations, such as defatted fenugreek, germinated seed and hydroalcoholic extracts (Bordia et al 1997, Gupta et al 2001, Sharma et al 1990, Sowmya & Rajyalakshmi 1999). As can be expected, the dose used and type of preparation tested have an influence on the results.

An open study using a daily dose of 18 g germinated fenugreek seed in healthy volunteers demonstrated significant reductions in total cholesterol and LDL cholesterol levels. A placebo-controlled study found no effect after 3 months with a lower dose of 5 g seed daily (Bordia et al 1997, Sowmya & Rajyalakshmi 1999), suggesting that higher intakes may be required for lipid-lowering activity to become significant.

Diabetes

Fenugreek is a popular natural treatment used to aid blood sugar regulation in diabetes in numerous cultures, particularly Asia. A meta-analysis of various herbal medicines affecting HbA_{1C} levels concluded that fenugreek supplements are effective in controlling glycaemic levels in people with type 2 diabetes (Suksomboon et al 2011).

This was further confirmed in a 2014 meta-analysis which reviewed results from 10 clinical trials ($n = 278$). The meta-analysis concluded that ingestion of fenugreek seeds (1–100 g/day; median 25 g) for at least 1 week significantly changed fasting blood glucose by −0.96 mmol/L (95% confidence interval [CI] −1.52, −0.40; I2 = 80%; 10 trials), 2-h post-load glucose by −2.19 mmol/L (95% CI −3.19, −1.19; I2 = 71%; seven trials) and HbA_{1C} by −0.85% (95% CI −1.49%, −0.22%; I2 = 0%; three trials) compared with control interventions (Neelakantan et al 2014). Significant effects on fasting and 2-h glucose levels were only found for studies that administered medium or high doses of fenugreek seed powder (≥5 g) to people with diabetes and not in overweight people without established diabetes. The effect on fasting blood glucose appears to be dose-dependent, as no effects were seen for low doses (<5 g/day) and greater effects were seen with higher doses.

The mean age of study participants in the 10 clinical studies reviewed by Neelakantan et al (2014) ranged from 22.0 to 54.4 years (median: 43.1 years) and most trials included participants with type 2 diabetes treated with diet or oral antidiabetic medication. A variety of different fenugreek preparations have been studied, including powdered fenugreek seeds, debitterised powdered fenugreek seeds (25–50 g twice daily) or hydroalcoholic seed extract (1 g/day) either in the form of capsules or as an ingredient of unleavened bread. These were provided in equal doses 2–3 times daily.

The effect is quite quick, as demonstrated in a study of people with type 2 diabetes ($n = 166$), which showed that 2-h post prandial plasma glucose levels were positively affected by fenugreek seed consumption (Bawadi et al 2009).

Fenugreek is also being incorporated into other foods as a means of improving glycaemic control. Bread baked with 5% fenugreek significantly reduced insulin levels in a pilot double-blind study of 8 diet-controlled diabetic subjects (Losso et al 2009).

Trigonelline, a major alkaloid component of fenugreek, is one of the key constituents responsible for the effects seen in diabetes and has been shown to affect beta-cell regeneration, insulin secretion, activities of various enzymes related to glucose metabolism, reactive oxygen species, axonal extension and neuron excitability (Zhou et al 2012).

With sulfonylureas

The efficacy and safety of fenugreek in the treatment of patients with type 2 diabetes mellitus were investigated in 69 patients whose blood glucose levels were not well controlled by oral sulfonylureas (Lu et al 2008). This 12-week trial demonstrated that combined treatment of fenugreek with sulfonylureas improved glycaemic control, further reduced blood glucose levels and ameliorated clinical symptoms in the treatment of type 2 diabetes. Fenugreek treatment was also found to be safe.

Lipid lowering in diabetes

Studies investigating the effects of fenugreek seed and seed powder have demonstrated significant lipid-lowering activity in this population. Oral doses of 25 g fenugreek seed powder taken twice daily significantly reduced serum total cholesterol, triacylglyceride and LDL cholesterol in hypercholesteraemia according to a study of hypercholesterolaemic type 2 diabetic patients. Results were recorded at 3 weeks and 6 weeks (Moosa et al 2006). A placebo-controlled study using a lower dose of 2.5 g unaltered fenugreek seed twice daily over 3 months found that this was ineffective in type 1 diabetes but did have a lipid-lowering effect in patients with diabetes and coronary artery disease (Bordia et al 1997). In this population, total cholesterol and triglyceride levels were significantly reduced.

Studies with defatted fenugreek seed (100 g/day) in patients with type 1 diabetes also identified significant reductions in total cholesterol, LDL and very-low-density lipoprotein cholesterol and triglyceride levels, but no changes to HDL cholesterol under randomised conditions (Sharma et al 1990).

Ethanolic extracts of fenugreek have also demonstrated good results. A 2001 double-blind, placebo-controlled study found that a dose of 1 g ethanolic extract of fenugreek was able to significantly decrease serum triglyceride levels and increase HDL cholesterol in mild to moderate type 2 diabetes mellitus (Gupta et al 2001). Previously, similar results were obtained with an ethanolic extract of defatted fenugreek seeds in vivo, which produced an 18–26% reduction in plasma cholesterol level (Stark & Madar 1993).

IN COMBINATION

A combination powdered mixture of three traditional Indian medicinal plants — fenugreek seeds, bitter gourd and jamun seeds — in raw and cooked form produced benefits in a study of 60 non-insulin-dependent people with diabetes. Daily supplementation of 1 g of this mixture for a 1.5-month period and then a further increase to 2 g for another 1.5 months significantly reduced the fasting and postprandial glucose levels in this population. A significant decrease in oral hypoglycaemic drug requirements was observed and, for some subjects, cessation of drug therapy could be achieved after the 3-month feeding trial (Kochhar & Nagi 2005).

Promoting lactation

Although fenugreek has been used traditionally for centuries as a galactogogue, to increase milk production and improve lactation, and is the most commonly used herbal galactogogue in published literature, there is only one valid clinical trial supporting its use. A double-blind randomised controlled trial involving 66 mother–infant pairs demonstrated that three cups of fenugreek herb tea per day were able to enhance breast milk production (measured on day 3 post-birth) and facilitate infant birth weight regain in the early postnatal days in exclusively breast-fed infants compared to placebo (Turkyilmaz et al 2011). In contrast, another placebo-controlled study of mothers of premature newborns suggested that fenugreek had no effect on prolactin levels or on volume of breast milk (Rowe et al 2013).

While little scientific research has been conducted to truly explore the effects of fenugreek in lactation, contemporary lactation consultants in the United States and Europe, midwives, herbalists and the general public continue to use it to increase milk supply when milk supply is low, with few side effects for mother or baby. Fenugreek is often mixed with other herbs such as blessed thistle (*Carduus marianum*) and taken up to 3 g a day (Humphrey & Romm 2010).

Due to the safety of fenugreek, a trial is worthwhile considering before any pharmaceutical options are used (Forinash et al 2012).

Externally — to reduce local inflammation

Although controlled studies are not available, evidence of anti-inflammatory and antinociceptive activity provides a theoretical basis for this indication.

Commission E approves the external use of fenugreek as a poultice for local inflammation (Blumenthal et al 2000).

OTHER USES

In Ayurvedic and Unani systems of medicine, fenugreek is used to treat fever, epilepsy, paralysis, gout, dropsy, chronic cough and piles. In Morocco, fenugreek is used as a preventive treatment against the development of kidney stones. There are some tests in experimental models which provide support for this use (Laroubi et al 2007).

In Ayurveda the seeds are reported to have nutritive properties and to stimulate digestive processes, and have been used to treat a range of gastrointestinal disorders. It is also used as a general tonic, mixed with milk and sugar, to promote lactation and to lower lipid and glucose levels.

Parkinson's disease

A double-blind study of 50 people with Parkinson's disease (diagnosis of over 6 months), showed that a fenugreek standardised extract (IBHB) reduced deterioration as measured by the Unified Parkinson's Disease Rating Scale. All participants were stabilised and taking L-dopa therapy together with IBHB 300 mg twice daily. IBHB had an excellent safety and tolerability profile and offers a novel use for fenugreek as integrative treatment with Parkinson's sufferers (Nathan et al 2013).

DOSAGE RANGE

Internal use

According to clinical studies

- General dose range: liquid extract (1:2): 2–6 mL/day.

- Diabetes: 50–100 g seed daily taken in divided doses with meals, or >1 g/day ethanolic seed extract.
- Lipid-lowering activity: according to the above studies, 18.0 g germinated fenugreek or 100 g defatted seeds daily taken in divided doses with meals.

External use

- As a poultice: 50 g powdered seed in 0.5–1 L hot water applied topically to affected area.

TOXICITY

Safety studies indicate that fenugreek is extremely safe. When consumed as 20% of the diet, it did not produce toxic effects in animal tests.

ADVERSE REACTIONS

One clinical study found that a dose of 50 g taken twice daily produced mild gastrointestinal symptoms, such as diarrhoea and flatulence, which subsided after 3–4 days. Allergic reactions have been reported, more usually as a consequence of cross-reactivity in patients with peanut allergy. Primary fenugreek allergy is rare (Faeste et al 2009). The Norwegian Food Allergy Register identified two legumes, lupine and fenugreek, as 'new' allergens in processed foods. Mandatory labeling of lupine, but not fenugreek, has since been established (Namork et al 2011). A 'maple-syrup' odour can appear after fenugreek ingestion. Rats fed a diet of 30% fenugreek seeds exhibited antifertility effects to the point of toxicity (Kassem et al 2006). Doses of 500 and 1000 mg/kg/day aqueous extracts of fenugreek resulted in increase in fetal death rates, decreased litter sizes, reduction in fetal body weight and increased incidence of morphological abnormalities (Khalki et al 2010). Proportional doses in humans would be near-impossible to administer.

Practice points/Patient counselling

- Fenugreek seeds and leaves are used as a functional food and as an ingredient in traditional medicine systems.
- Clinical studies have identified significant hypoglycaemic and potential for lipid-lowering activity.
- In animal studies, fenugreek has been shown to exert immunostimulant, anti-inflammatory and antinociceptive activity, stimulate digestive enzyme production and provide significant antiulcerogenic effects.
- In practice, it is used to manage blood sugar levels in patients with diabetes, to lower cholesterol levels, to provide symptom relief in dyspepsia and to promote lactation.
- Externally it is made into a poultice with hot water and used as an anti-inflammatory application.

SIGNIFICANT INTERACTIONS

Where controlled studies are not available, interactions are speculative and based on evidence of pharmacological activity and case reports.

Hypoglycaemic agents

Additive effects are theoretically possible in diabetes and drug dose reductions may be required in some patients — monitor serum glucose levels closely — potentially beneficial interaction.

Iron

Frequent use of fenugreek can inhibit iron absorption — separate doses by 2 h.

Warfarin

A placebo-controlled study found that fenugreek does not affect platelet aggregation, fibrinolytic activity or fibrinogen (Bordia et al 1997) so it should be considered safe.

CONTRAINDICATIONS AND PRECAUTIONS

Fenugreek is contraindicated in people with allergy to the herb, which has been observed in several case reports (Patil et al 1997), or those with allergy to chickpeas, because of possible cross-reactivity (Ulbricht & Basch 2005). Monitor patients with thyrotoxicosis when using this herb at doses above usual dietary intake.

PREGNANCY USE

When taken in usual dietary amounts, fenugreek is likely to be safe; however, the safety of larger doses has not been scientifically evaluated.

PATIENTS' FAQs

What will this herb do for me?
Fenugreek lowers blood sugar levels in patients with diabetes, reduce cholesterol levels and stimulate digestion. It may also protect the gastrointestinal tract from ulcers, stimulate immune function and provide anti-inflammatory and antipyretic effects. Traditionally, it has also been used to promote lactation.

When will it start to work?
Studies suggest that blood sugar effects can be seen within 10 days in type 1 diabetes, whereas lipid-lowering effects can take up to 3 months to establish. Traditionally, digestive effects are thought to occur soon after ingestion of the seeds.

Are there any safety issues?
Used as a food, fenugreek appears extremely safe but may interact with blood-thinning medicines. When used in high doses as a medicine, it may cause flatulence, diarrhoea and mild stomach discomfort. Allergies to fenugreek are possible. When

used with diabetic medicine, it may increase sugar-lowering activity and safety should be monitored.

REFERENCES

Ahmadiani A et al. Anti-inflammatory and antipyretic effects of *Trigonella foenum-graecum* leaves extract in the rat. J Ethnopharmacol 75.2–3 (2001): 283–286.

Alarcon-Aguilara FJ et al. Study of the anti-hyperglycemic effect of plants used as antidiabetics. J Ethnopharmacol 61.2 (1998): 101–110.

Al Habori M et al. In vitro effect of fenugreek extracts on intestinal sodium-dependent glucose uptake and hepatic glycogen phosphorylase A. Int J Exp Diabetes Res 2.2 (2001): 91–99.

Ali-Shtayeh M, et al. Complementary and alternative medicine use amongst Palestinian diabetic patients, Complementary Therapies in Clinical Practice 18 (2012) 16–21.

Amin A et al. Chemopreventive activities of *Trigonella foenum graecum* (Fenugreek) against breast cancer. Cell Biol Int 29.8 (2005): 687–694.

Annida B, Stanely Mainzen Prince P. Supplementation of fenugreek leaves reduces oxidative stress in streptozotocin-induced diabetic rats. J Med Food 8.3 (2005): 382–385.

Balaraman RDS, et al. Antihypertensive effect of *Trigonella foenum-graecum* seeds in experimentally induced hypertension in rats. Pharm Biol 44.8 (2006): 568–575.

Basu TK & Srichamroen A. "Health benefits of Fenugreek" in Bioactive Foods in Promoting Health: Fruits and Vegetables, Edmonton, AB Canada: Department of Agriculture, Food and Nutritional Science, Faculty of Agricultural, Environmental and Life Sciences, University of Alberta/Elsevier (2010) pp425–435,

Bawadi H, et al. The post prandial hypoglycemic activity of fenugreek seed and seeds' extract in type 2 diabetics: a pilot study, Pharmacognosy Magazine (2009) 5.18;134–8.

Belguith-Hadriche O, et al. Comparative study on hypocholesterolemic and antioxidant activities of various extracts of fenugreek seeds, Food Chemistry 138 (2013) 1448–1453.

Bhatia K et al. Aqueous extract of *Trigonella foenum-graecum* L. ameliorates additive urotoxicity of buthionine sulfoximine and cyclophosphamide in mice. Food Chem Toxicol 44.10 (2006): 1744–1750.

Bin-Hafeez B et al. Immunomodulatory effects of fenugreek (*Trigonella foenum graecum* L.) extract in mice. Int Immunopharmacol 3.2 (2003): 257–265.

Blumenthal M, et al. (eds). Herbal medicine: expanded commission E monographs. Austin, TX: Integrative Medicine Communications, 2000.

Boban PT, et al. Dietary mucilage promotes regression of atheromatous lesions in hypercholesterolemic rabbits. Phytother Res 23.5 (2008): 725–730.

Bordia A, et al. Effect of ginger (*Zingiber officinale* Rosc.) and fenugreek (*Trigonella foenum-graecum* L.) on blood lipids, blood sugar and platelet aggregation in patients with coronary artery disease. Prostaglandins Leukot Essent Fatty Acids 56.5 (1997): 379–384.

Dixit P et al. Antioxidant properties of germinated fenugreek seeds. Phytother Res 19.11 (2005): 977–983.

Dixit PP, et al. Formulated antidiabetic preparation Syndrex has a strong antioxidant activity. Eur J Pharmacol 581.1–2 (2008): 216–225.

Eidi A, et al. Effect of fenugreek (*Trigonella foenum-graecum* L.) seeds on serum parameters in normal and streptozotocin-induced diabetic rats. Nutr Res 27.11 (2007): 728–733.

Faeste CK, et al. Allergenicity and antigenicity of fenugreek (*Trigonella foenum-graecum*) proteins in foods. J Allergy Clin Immunol 123.1 (2009): 187–194.

Fisher C, Painter G (eds). Materia medica for the southern hemisphere. Auckland: Fisher-Painter Publishers, 1996.

Forinash AB, et al. The use of galactogues in the breastfeeding mother, Ann Pharmacother 46.10.(2012):1392–404.

Gaur V, et al. Antidepressant-like effect of 4-hydroxyisoleucine from *Trigonella foenum graecum* L. seeds in mice, Biomedicine & Aging Pathology 2 (2012) 121–125.

Gupta A, et al. Effect of *Trigonella foenum-graecum* (fenugreek) seeds on glycaemic control and insulin resistance in type 2 diabetes mellitus: a double blind placebo controlled study. J Assoc Physicians India 49 (2001): 1057–1061.

Hamza N, et al. Preventive and curative effect of *Trigonella foenum-graecum* L. seeds in C57BL/6J models of type 2 diabetes induced by high-fat diet, Journal of Ethnopharmacology 142 (2012) 516–522.

Hibasami H et al. Protodioscin isolated from fenugreek (*Trigonella foenum-graecum* L.) induces cell death and morphological change indicative of apoptosis in leukemic cell line H-60, but not in gastric cancer cell line KATO III. Int J Mol Med 11.1 (2003): 23–26.

Humphrey S, Romm A "Breastfeeding and Botanical Medicine". Botanical Medicine for Women's Health, (2010) St Louis, MO: Churchill Livingstone

Javan M et al. Antinociceptive effects of *Trigonella foenum-graecum* leaves extract. J Ethnopharmacol 58.2 (1997): 125–129.

Kassem A et al. Evaluation of the potential antifertility effect of fenugreek seeds in male and female rabbits. Contraception 73.3 (2006): 301–306.

Kaur L, et al. Indian culinary plants enhance glucose-induced insulin secretion and glucose consumption in INS-1 B-cells and 3T3-L1 adipocytes, Food Chemistry 129 (2011) 1120–1125.

Kaviarasan S, Anuradha CV. Fenugreek (*Trigonella foenum graecum*) seed polyphenols protect liver from alcohol toxicity: a role on hepatic detoxification system and apoptosis. Pharmazie 62.4 (2007): 299–304.

Kaviarasan S, et al. Polyphenol-rich extract of fenugreek seeds protect erythrocytes from oxidative damage. Plant Foods Hum Nutr 59.4 (2004): 143–147.

Kaviarasan S et al. Fenugreek (*Trigonella foenum-graecum*) seed extract prevents ethanol-induced toxicity and apoptosis in Chang liver cells. Alcohol Alcohol 41.3 (2006): 267–273.

Kaviarasan S, et al. Protective action of fenugreek (*Trigonella foenum-graecum*) seed polyphenols against alcohol-induced protein and lipid damage in rat liver. Cell Biol Toxicol 24.5 (2008): 391–400.

Kenny, O., et al. (2013). Antioxidant properties and quantitative UPLC-MS analysis of phenolic compounds from extracts of fenugreek (*Trigonella foenum-graecum*) seeds and bitter melon (*Momordica charantia*) fruit. Food Chemistry, 141(4), 4295.

Khalki L, et al. Evaluation of the developmental toxicity of the aqueous extract from *Trigonella foenum-graecum* (L.) in mice, Journal of Ethnopharmacology 131 (2010) 321–325.

Kochhar A, Nagi M. Effect of supplementation of traditional medicinal plants on blood glucose in non-insulin-dependent diabetics: a pilot study. J Med Food 8.4 (2005): 545–549.

Laroubi A et al. Prophylaxis effect of *Trigonella foenum graecum* L. seeds on renal stone formation in rats. Phytother Res 21.10 (2007): 921–925.

Liu Y, et al. Compounds in functional food fenugreek spice exhibit anti-inflammatory antioxidant activities, Food Chemistry 131 (2012) 1187–1192.

Losso, JN., et al. Fenugreek bread: a treatment for diabetes mellitus, J Med Food 2009 12(5): 1046–9.

Lu F et al (2008) Clinical observations on *Trigonella foenum-gracum* L. total saponins in combination with sulfonylureas in the treatment of type 2 diabetes mellitus. Chin J Integr Med 2008, 14:56–60.

Madar Z et al. Glucose-lowering effect of fenugreek in non-insulin dependent diabetics. Eur J Clin Nutr 42.1 (1988): 51–54.

Mohammad S et al. In vivo effect of *Trigonella foenum graecum* on the expression of pyruvate kinase, phosphoenolpyruvate carboxykinase, and distribution of glucose transporter (GLUT4) in alloxan-diabetic rats. Can J Physiol Pharmacol 84.6 (2006): 647–654.

Moosa ASM et al. Hypolipidemic effects of fenugreek seed powder. Bangladesh J Pharmacol 1 (2006): 64–67.

Morani A, et al. Ameliorative effects of standardized extract from *Trigonella foenum-graecum* L. seeds on painful peripheral neuropathy in rats, Asian Pacific Journal of Tropical Medicine (2012) 385–390.

Mortel M & Mehta SD Systematic review of the efficacy of herbal galactogogues, J Human Lact (2013) 29.2:154–162.

Namork E, et al. Severe allergic reactions to food in Norway: A ten year survey of cases reported to the Food Allergy Register, Int J Environ Res Public Health (2011), 8, 3144–3155.

Narender T et al. 4-hydroxyisoleucine an unusual amino acid as antidyslipidemic and antihyperglycemic agent. Bioorg Med Chem Lett 16.2 (2006): 293–296.

Nathan J, et al. Efficacy and safety of standardized extract of *Trigonella foenum-graecum* L seeds as an adjuvant to L-dopa in the management of patients with Parkinson's disease. Phytother Res 2013 28(2): 172–8.

Neelakantan, N., et al. 2014. Effect of fenugreek (*Trigonella foenum-graecum* L.) intake on glycemia: a meta-analysis of clinical trials. Nutr.J, 13, (1) 7 available from: PM:24438170.

Othman RB, et al. Use of hypoglycemic plants by Tunisian diabetic patients, Alexandria Journal of Medicine (2013) 49:261–264.

Palaniswamy M et al. In vitro anti-plasmodial activity of *Trigonella foenum-graecum* L. Evid Based Complement Alternat Med (2010). 7(4); 441–445.

Panda S, et al. Inhibition of triiodothyronine production by fenugreek seed extract in mice and rats. Pharmacol Res 40.5 (1999): 405–409.

Pandian RS, et al. Gastroprotective effect of fenugreek seeds (*Trigonella foenum-graecum*) on experimental gastric ulcer in rats. J Ethnopharmacol 81.3 (2002): 393–397.

Patil SP, et al. Allergy to fenugreek (*Trigonella foenum-graecum*). Ann Allergy Asthma Immunol 78.3 (1997): 297–300.

Perla V & Jayanty SS. Biguanide related compounds in traditional antidiabetic functional foods, Food Chemistry, 138 (2013) 1574–1580.

Petit PR et al. Steroid saponins from fenugreek seeds: extraction, purification, and pharmacological investigation on feeding behavior and plasma cholesterol. Steroids 60.10 (1995): 674–680.

Platel K, Srinivasan K. Influence of dietary spices or their active principles on digestive enzymes of small intestinal mucosa in rats. Int J Food Sci Nutr 47.1 (1996): 55–59.

Platel K, Srinivasan K. Influence of dietary spices and their active principles on pancreatic digestive enzymes in albino rats. Nahrung 44.1 (2000): 42–46.

Puri D, et al. Mechanism of action of a hypoglycemic principle isolated from fenugreek seeds. Indian J Physiol Pharmacol 46.4 (2002): 457–462.

Raju J et al. *Trigonella foenum graecum* (fenugreek) seed powder improves glucose homeostasis in alloxan diabetic rat tissues by reversing the altered glycolytic, gluconeogenic and lipogenic enzymes. Mol Cell Biochem 224.1–2 (2001): 45–51.

Rao P et al. Short term nutritional and safety evaluation of fenugreek. Nutr Res 16.9 (1996): 1495–1505.

Ribes G et al. Effects of fenugreek seeds on endocrine pancreatic secretions in dogs. Ann Nutr Metab 28.1 (1984): 37–43.

Ribes G et al. Antidiabetic effects of subfractions from fenugreek seeds in diabetic dogs. Proc Soc Exp Biol Med 182.2 (1986): 159–166.

Riyad MA, et al. Effect of fenugreek and lupine seeds on the development of experimental diabetes in rats. Planta Med 54.4 (1988): 286–290.

Rowe H, et al. Maternal Medication, Drug Use and Breast feeding, Pediatri Clin N Am 60 (2013) 275–294.

SatheeshKumar N, et al. Acetylcholinesterase enzyme inhibitory potential of standardized extract of *Trigonella foenum graecum* L and its constiuents, Phytomedicine 17 (2010) 292–295.

Sebastian KS, Thampan RV. Differential effects of soybean and fenugreek extracts on the growth of MCF-7 cells. Chem Biol Interact 170.2 (2007): 135–143.

Shabbeer S et al. Fenugreek: a naturally occurring edible spice as an anticancer agent. Cancer Biol Ther 8.3 (2009) 8:272–8.

Shang M, et al. Analysis of amino acids in *Trigonella foenum-graecum* seeds. Zhong Yao Cai 21.4 (1998): 188–190.

Sharififar, F., Moshafi, MH., Shafazand, E., et al. Acetyl cholinesterase inhibitory, antioxidant and cytotoxic activity of three dietary medicinal plants, Food Chemistry, 130 (2012) 20–23.

Sharma RD, et al. Effect of fenugreek seeds on blood glucose and serum lipids in type I diabetes. Eur J Clin Nutr 44.4 (1990): 301–306.

Shetty AK., Salimath, PV., Renoprotective effects of fenugreek (*Trigonella foenum graecum*) during experimental diabetes. e-SPEN, the European e-journal of Clinical Nutrition and Metabolism 4 (2009) e137–142.

Sindhu G, et al. Anti-inflammatory and antioxidative effects of mucilage of *Trigonella foenum graecum* (Fenugreek) on adjuvant induced arthritic rats, International Immunopharmacology 12 (2012) 205–211.

Sowmya P, Rajyalakshmi P. Hypocholesterolemic effect of germinated fenugreek seeds in human subjects. Plant Foods Hum Nutr 53.4 (1999): 359–365.

Srichamroen A et al. In vitro intestinal glucose uptake is inhibited by galactomannan from Canadian fenugreek seed (*Trigonella foenum-graecum* L.) in genetically lean and obese rats. Nutr Res 29.1 (2009): 49–54.

Stark A, Madar Z. The effect of an ethanol extract derived from fenugreek (*Trigonella foenum-graecum*) on bile acid absorption and cholesterol levels in rats. Br J Nutr 69.1 (1993): 277–287.

Suksomboon N, et al. Meta-analysis of the effect of herbal supplement on glycemic control in type 2 diabetes, Journal of Ethnopharmacology 137 (2011) 1328–1333.

Sur P et al. *Trigonella foenum-graecum* (fenugreek) seed extract as an antineoplastic agent. Phytother Res 15.3 (2001): 257–259.

Turkyilmaz C, et al. The effect of galactagogue herbal tea on breast milk production and short-term catch-up of birth weight in the first week of life, The journal of Alt and Comp med, (2011), 17(2):139–142.

Ulbricht CE, Basch EM. Natural standard herb and supplement reference. St Louis: Mosby, 2005.

Vats V, et al. Evaluation of anti-hyperglycemic and hypoglycemic effect of *Trigonella foenum-graecum* Linn, *Ocimum sanctum* Linn and *Pterocarpus marsupium* Linn in normal and alloxanized diabetic rats. J Ethnopharmacol 79.1 (2002): 95–100.

Vijayakumar MV, et al. Hypolipidemic effect of fenugreek seeds is mediated through inhibition of fat accumulation and upregulation of LDL receptor, Obesity 2010, 18 (4): 667–674.

Vyas S et al. Analgesic and anti-inflammatory activities of *Trigonella foenum-graecum* (seed) extract. Acta Pol Pharm 65.4 (2008): 473–476.

Yeh GY et al. Systematic review of herbs and dietary supplements for glycemic control in diabetes. Diabetes Care 26.4 (2003): 1277–1294.

Zhou, J., et al. 2012. Trigonelline: a plant alkaloid with therapeutic potential for diabetes and central nervous system disease. Curr.Med Chem., 19, (21) 3523–3531.

Zia T, et al. Evaluation of the oral hypoglycaemic effect of *Trigonella foenum-graecum* L. (methi) in normal mice. J Ethnopharmacol 75.2–3 (2001): 191–195.

Feverfew

HISTORICAL NOTE Feverfew has been used traditionally to treat migraine (Shrivastava et al 2006). Feverfew has been used for centuries as a febrifuge, with the common plant name being derived from the Latin term 'febrifugia' which means to 'drive out fevers' (Knight 1995). Feverfew has been used for centuries in Europe to treat headaches, arthritis, coughs and colds, atonic dyspepsia, worm infestation and menstrual disorders, and used as an emmenagogue and anthelmintic agent. In the 1970s it was 'rediscovered' by the medical establishment and subjected to clinical studies, which produced encouraging results that suggested feverfew was an effective prophylactic medicine for migraine headache. The ancient Greeks called it parthenium because legend has it that it was used to save the life of a worker who had fallen from the Parthenon during its construction (Setty & Sigal 2005).

Clinical note — Natural variations in parthenolide content

The amount of parthenolide present in commercial preparations of feverfew leaves varies significantly, with some exhibiting levels as high as 1.7% dry weight and others as low as 0.01% to non-detectable (Cutlan et al 2000). The study by Cutlan et al measured the parthenolide content in plants produced from seeds taken from over 30 different sources and germinated under identical conditions. According to this study, feverfew collected from the wild and distributed by botanical gardens or US Department of Agriculture seed banks yielded plants with the highest mean parthenolide value, and plants with yellow leaves also had significantly higher parthenolide levels than those with green leaves.

OTHER NAMES

Altamisa, bachelor's button, camomilegrande, featherfew, featherfoil, chrysanthemum parthenium, mutterkraut, matrem, midsummer daisy, tanaceti parthenii herba/folium

BOTANICAL NAME/FAMILY

Tanacetum parthenium (family [Asteraceae] Compositae)

PLANT PART USED

Leaf

CHEMICAL COMPONENTS

The leaves and flowering tops contain many monoterpenes and sesquiterpenes as well as sesquiterpene lactones (chrysanthemolide, chrysanthemonin, 10-epi-canin, magnoliolide and parthenolide), reynosin, santamarin, tanaparthins and other compounds. Until recently, the sesquiterpene lactone parthenolide was thought to be the major biologically active constituent. However, in vitro and in vivo research suggests that others are also present (Brown et al 1997, Pugh & Sambo 1988). A study from the early 1990s (Heptinstall et al 1992) found that feverfew grown in the United Kingdom contained a high level of parthenolide in leaves, flowering tops and seeds but had lower levels in stalks and roots. The level of parthenolide in powdered-leaf material fell during storage. Melatonin has been detected in leaf samples of feverfew (1.37–2.45 mcg/g) and in a commercially available product (0.57 mcg/g) (Murch et al 1997).

MAIN ACTIONS

Anti-inflammatory and analgesic

Parthenolide has been shown to have multiple effects on target cells, ranging from phosphorylation to transcriptional inhibition activities (Mathema et al 2012). Several in vivo studies have identified anti-inflammatory and antinociceptive activity for feverfew extracts and parthenolide. When feverfew extracts were orally administered, or pure parthenolide was injected intraperitoneally, significant dose-dependent, anti-inflammatory and antinociceptive effects were observed in animal models (Jain & Kulkarni 1999). Similarly, when feverfew extracts and parthenolide from *Tanacetum vulgare* were administered orally in a rat model, gastric ulcer index was significantly reduced (Tournier et al 1999).

The mechanisms responsible for these effects are not well elucidated. Jain and Kulkarni (1999) demonstrated that the antinociceptive effect was not mediated through the opiate pathway and was not associated with sedation. With regard to the anti-inflammatory effect, several mechanisms appear to be responsible.

In vitro studies have found evidence of cyclooxygenase (COX) and lipoxygenase (LOX) inhibition (Capasso 1986, Pugh & Sambo 1988, Sumner et al 1992), while other tests reveal no effect on COX (Collier et al 1980, Makheja & Bailey 1982). Preincubation of intact rat and human leucocytes for 10 minutes with crude chloroform extracts of fresh feverfew leaves caused a dose-dependent and potent inhibition of their capacity to generate COX and LOX pathways (Sumner et al 1992).

Inhibition of phospholipase A_2 has also been suggested (Heptinstall 1988, Sumner et al 1992). Direct binding and inhibition of I-kappa B kinase beta, an important subunit involved in cytokine-mediated signalling, has been demonstrated for parthenolide in in vitro studies (Kwok et al 2001). Parthenolide also inhibits nitric oxide production, an important regulator and inducer of various inflammatory states (Wong & Menendez 1999). More recently, results from an in vivo study confirm that parthenolide inhibits proinflammatory cytokine responses, although the authors propose that proinflammatory mediators, including chemokines (MIP-2), plasma enzyme mediators (complement, kinin and clotting systems) and lipid mediators (COX, prostaglandins, platelet-activating factor), are also likely to be involved (Smolinski & Pestka 2003). Parthenolide acts as inhibitor of inflammasomes. Inflammasomes engage and activate caspase-1, which in turn processes the inactive pro-IL-18 and pro-IL-1β into their corresponding active forms of proinflammatory cytokines, IL-18 and IL-1β, respectively (Mathema et al 2012). In an in vitro study, synovial fibroblasts were cultured with and without feverfew extract and subsequently stimulated with interleukin-1 (IL-1), interferon (IFN) and tumour necrosis factor (TNF) to induce expression of intercellular adhesion molecule-1 (ICAM-1). The most potent inhibition of ICAM-1 was seen in cultures stimulated with IL-1 and TNF (46–95% suppression) and less so in cultures stimulated with IFN-gamma (17–39% suppression). One of the major proinflammatory functions of ICAM-1 in vivo is as a cellular ligand for T cells. Feverfew inhibition of ICAM-1 was associated with a decrease in functional T-cell adhesion. Feverfew inhibition of IL-1-induced ICAM-1 was dose-dependent (Piela-Smith & Liu 2001).

Parthenolide suppresses inflammation by inhibiting activity of NF-κB (Mathema et al 2012). The majority of NF-κB activities are related to TNF-alpha and oxidative stress.

In vitro testing has identified that parthenolide-induced reduction in IL-6 secretion is dose-dependent: 29% by 200 nm ($P < 0.001$); 45% by 1 mcm ($P < 0.001$); 98% by 5 mcm ($P < 0.001$). At the highest concentration tested, at 5 mcm, it reduced the secretion of TNF-alpha by 54% ($P < 0.001$) (Magni et al 2012). These combined actions, inhibiting proinflammatory agents and reducing microglial activation, provide a theoretical rationale behind the proposed clinical effects of feverfew in reducing the frequency and severity of acute migraine attacks.

The essential oil constituent of feverfew, chrysanthenyl acetate, inhibits prostaglandin synthetase in vitro and also seems to possess analgesic properties (Pugh & Sambo 1988).

Antispasmodic

The results from several in vitro studies generally indicate that feverfew decreases vascular smooth-muscle spasm (Barsby et al 1992, 1993a, 1993b, Collier et al 1980).

Inhibits serotonin release and binding

Parthenolide and several other sesquiterpene lactone constituents inhibit serotonin release but do not bind to 5-HT_1 receptors, according to in vivo data (Groenewegen & Heptinstall 1990, Marles et al 1992, Weber et al 1997a). Some tests with 5-HT_{2A} receptors show that parthenolide is a low-affinity antagonist (Weber et al 1997b), whereas other tests found no effect on 5-HT_{2A} or 5-HT_{2B} receptors. Feverfew extract potently and directly blocked 5-HT_{2A} and 5-HT_{2B} receptors and neuronally released 5-HT, suggesting that feverfew powder or extracts are more effective than isolated parthenolide (Mittra et al 2000).

Anticancer activity

In the last decade, there has been increasing investigation into the parthenolide constituent from feverfew as an anticancer agent. It displays multiple mechanisms, such as its selectivity to biological and/or epigenetic targets, tumours and cancer stem cells (Ghantous et al 2013), which make it an attractive candidate for further cancer research.

Parthenolide has been shown to withdraw cells from cell cycle or to promote cell differentiation, and finally to induce programmed cell death (Pajak et al 2008). It has an ability to induce apoptosis in a variety of cancer lines, has chemosensitising properties and is non-toxic to normal cells. The potent anticancer activity of parthenolide is in part due to its ability to inhibit transcription factor NF-κB, thereby reducing survival potential in a number of cancer cells (Anderson & Bejcek 2008, Pajak et al 2008, Zunino et al 2007). The effect is specific to tumour cells. Parthenolide-induced generation of reactive oxygen species (ROS) in cancer cells has also been shown to play a role in promoting apoptotic cell death. Interestingly, experiments in animal models indicate that, in non-cancerous cells, parthenolide acts as an antioxidant molecule by increasing levels of intracellular glutathione, resulting in a decrease in ROS. In contrast, an increase in ROS generation in response to parthenolide appears to increase apoptotic cell death in cancer cells. Recently, parthenolide was found to induce apoptosis in cancer cells, through mitochondrial dysfunction. Through this mechanism, it was shown to significantly inhibit tumour growth and angiogenesis in a xenograft model, exhibiting anticancer activity in human colorectal cancer in vitro and in vivo (Kim SL et al 2012). This proapoptotic action is suggested to occur through the activation of p53 and the increased production of ROS (Mathema et al 2012).

Signal transducer and activator of transcription (STAT) proteins are transcriptional factors responding to extracellular ligands that mediate diverse biological functions, such as cell proliferation, differentiation and apoptosis. Parthenolide shows strong NF-κB and STAT inhibition-mediated transcriptional suppression of proapoptotic genes. Parthenolide induced ROS exclusively in tumour cells. Parthenolide was found to have the unique ability to induce sensitisation to extrinsic as well as intrinsic apoptosis signalling in cancer cells. The proapoptotic activity is not observed in normal cells (Mathema et al 2012). A comparison of parthenolide treatment with that of the standard chemotherapy drug cytosine arabinoside (Ara-C) found it was much more specific to leukaemia cells (Guzman et al 2005), whereas Ara-C killed both leukaemia cells and normal cells to an equivalent extent; parthenolide showed significantly less toxicity to normal haematopoietic cells from bone marrow and cord blood.

Parthenolide is cytotoxic to several breast cancer cell lines, one human cervical cancer cell line (SiHa), prostate tumour-initiating cells isolated from prostate cancer cell lines, as well as primary prostate tumour-initiating cells, glioblastoma cells and pre-B acute lymphoblastic leukaemia lines (Anderson & Bejcek 2008, Kawasaki et al 2009, Wu et al 2006, Zunino et al 2007).

An in vitro and in vivo study of parthenolide in breast cancer found that parthenolide has significant in vivo chemosensitising properties in the metastatic breast cancer setting (Sweeney et al 2005). Parthenolide was effective either alone or in combination with docetaxel in reducing colony formation, inducing apoptosis and reducing the expression of prometastatic genes IL-8 and the antiapoptotic gene GADD45beta1 in vitro. In an adjuvant setting, animals treated with parthenolide and docetaxel combination showed significantly enhanced survival compared with untreated animals or animals treated with either drug. The enhanced survival in the combination arm was associated with reduced lung metastases. In addition, nuclear NF-κB levels were lower in residual tumours and lung metastasis of animals treated with parthenolide, docetaxel or both.

Studies are being conducted with a series of aminoparthenolide analogues, which have been synthesised by a conjugate addition of several primary and secondary amines to the alpha-methylene-gamma-butyrolactone function of the sesquiterpene lactone, parthenolide (Nasim & Crooks 2008).

Metastatic melanoma is a highly life-threatening disease. Parthenolide has been found to inhibit the proliferation of various cancer cells, mainly by inducing apoptosis (Lesiak et al 2010). In this in vitro study, parthenolide reduced the number of viable adherent cells in melanoma cultures. Half maximal inhibitory concentration values were around 4 mcmol/L. Cell death accompanied by mitochondrial membrane depolarisation and caspase-3 activation was observed as the result of parthenolide application (Lesiak et al 2010). In breast cancer cell lines, parthenolide reduced the number of viable MCF-7 and MDA-MB-231 cells, with half maximal inhibitory concentration values between 6 and 9 mcmol/L (Wyrębska et al 2013).

In colorectal cancer cell line COLO205, parthenolide depletes intracellular thiols and increases ROS and cytosolic calcium levels, resulting in cellular stress, which consequently leads to cell apoptosis. Similar effects of parthenolide mediate mitochondrial damage and cell death in human gastric cancer cell line SGC7901, suggesting that parthenolide-induced ROS-mediated apoptosis may be common to many types of cancer cells (Mathema et al 2012).

Parthenolide has been found to selectively affect gene regulation or activity and consequently controls of target cells (Mathema et al 2012).

OTHER ACTIONS

Platelet aggregation inhibition

Evidence is contradictory as to whether feverfew inhibits platelet aggregation. Several in vitro studies and animal models have observed inhibition of platelet aggregation (Heptinstall et al 1988, Jain & Kulkarni 1999, Makheja & Bailey 1982). However, no significant effects were seen in a clinical study of 10 patients receiving feverfew (Biggs et al 1982). Feverfew was found to inhibit secretory activity in platelets. Release of serotonin from platelets induced by various aggregating agents (adenosine diphosphate, adrenaline, arachidonic acid, collagen and U46619) was inhibited. Platelet aggregation was consistently inhibited. It is interesting to note that parthenolide stimulated functional platelet production from human megakaryocyte cell lines as well as from primary mouse and human megakaryocytes in vitro. Parthenolide enhanced platelet production via inhibition of NF-κB signalling in megakaryocytes. Parthenolide significantly reduced the basal NF-κB activity at 6 h. This effect was found to be independent of the parthenolide-induced oxidative stress response. Additionally, parthenolide treatment of human peripheral blood platelets attenuated activation of stimulated platelets (Sahler et al 2011).

Mast cell stabilisation

Tests with rat mast cells indicate that feverfew extract inhibits histamine release, but the mechanism of action is different from cromoglycate and quercetin (Hayes & Foreman 1987). In vivo tests confirm that parthenolide significantly inhibits IgE antigen-induced mast cell degranulation in a dose-dependent manner (Miyata et al 2008). The formation of microtubules is well known to be crucial for IgE antigen-induced degranulation in mast cells, and parthenolide exhibits tubulin/microtubule-interfering activity. The mast cell stabilisation effect is rapid in vivo, as an immediate-type allergic response was induced in test animals and strongly inhibited by parthenolide administration.

Hepatoprotective effects

Parthenolide exhibits potent antifibrotic activity both in vitro and in vivo. The apoptotic and antifibrotic effects of parthenolide have been investigated for its apoptotic effects in test tube studies on hepatic stellate cells and for antifibrotic action on hepatic fibrosis in an in vivo rat model (Kim IH et al 2012). Parthenolide inhibited cell growth and induced apoptotic cell death in a dose-dependent manner in hepatic stellate cells. Parthenolide (at 2 and 4 mg/kg) significantly reduced hepatic fibrosis in thioacetamide-treated rats and decreased expression of transforming growth factor-beta-1.

Bone regulation effects

Parthenolide shows potential in bone-destructive disorders associated with osteoclast-mediated bone resorption (Kim SL et al 2012).

Osteoclasts, which are bone-resorbing multinucleated giant cells differentiated from haematopoietic stem cells upon stimulation by two essential cytokines, receptor activator of NF-κB ligand (RANKL) and macrophage colony-stimulating factor (M-CSF), play a central role in bone-destructive disorders. RANKL promotes osteoclast formation from osteoclast precursors while M-CSF supports proliferation and survival of precursor cells during osteoclast differentiation. In a mouse model, parthenolide suppressed RANKL-mediated osteoclast differentiation in bone marrow macrophages. In addition, parthenolide inhibited mRNA expression of osteoclast-associated receptor, tartrate-resistant acid phosphatase, dendritic cell-specific transmembrane protein and cathepsin K by RANKL, suggesting that parthenolide inhibits the bone-resorbing activity of mature osteoclasts. Parthenolide inhibits differentiation and bone-resolving activity of osteoclast by RANKL.

CLINICAL USE

Migraine headache

Currently available research investigating the use of feverfew for migraine prophylaxis is promising, especially with the dried feverfew leaf formulations, whereas ethanolic extracts have produced inconsistent results.

Ideally, more research into the most effective formulation and dosage regimen is required to provide more consistent results. In particular, further work is needed to determine which other constituents, beside parthenolide, are important for producing the desired clinical effect, whether by pharmacodynamic or pharmacokinetic interaction with parthenolide or as stand-alone active constituents (Saranitzky et al 2009).

Traditionally, feverfew has been used in the treatment and prevention of headaches. Its growing popularity in the United Kingdom, in the 1970s and 1980s, prompted researchers to investigate its usefulness under controlled trial conditions. The first double-blind study investigating feverfew in

> ***Clinical note — Migraine***
>
> Migraine is a common episodic familial headache disorder characterised by a combination of headache and neurological, gastrointestinal and autonomic symptoms. It has a 1-year prevalence of approximately 18% in women, 6% in men and 4% in children before puberty (Silberstein 2004). Several underlying mechanisms are considered responsible for the onset of migraine.
>
> One of the genes linked to migraine is associated with dysfunction in P-type neuronal calcium channels, which mediate 5-HT and excitatory neurotransmitter release. This dysfunction can impair release of 5-HT and predispose patients to migraine attacks or impair their self-aborting mechanism (Silberstein 2004). Additionally, nitric oxide may be involved in the initiation and maintenance of migraine headache (Ferrari 1998). Migraine aura is now thought to be caused by neuronal dysfunction, not ischaemia, and headache begins while cortical blood flow is reduced.
>
> In clinical practice, the three goals of migraine-preventive therapy are to reduce attack frequency, severity and duration, improve responsiveness to treatment of acute attacks, improve function and reduce disability. Ultimately, choice of treatment should be based on efficacy, adverse effects and coexisting conditions, with a full therapeutic trial taking 2–6 months.

migraine prophylaxis was published in 1985 and involved 17 patients who had been chewing fresh feverfew leaves on a daily basis (Johnson et al 1985). Therapeutic effect was maintained when capsules containing freeze-dried feverfew powder were continued, whereas those allocated placebo capsules experienced a significant increase in the frequency and severity of headache, nausea and vomiting during the early months of withdrawal.

Since then, numerous clinical studies have been conducted to determine the role of feverfew in the prevention of migraine headache.

In 2000, Ernst and Pittler published a systematic review of six randomised, placebo-controlled, double-blind trials of feverfew as a prophylactic treatment and concluded that the evidence favours feverfew as an effective preventive treatment against migraine headache, and is generally well tolerated. One of the studies in the systematic review noted a 24% reduction in the number of attacks during feverfew treatment but found no significant alteration in the duration of individual attacks. There was a non-significant tendency ($P = 0.06$) towards milder headaches with feverfew and a significant reduction ($P < 0.02$) in nausea and vomiting accompanying the attacks (Murphy et al 1988).

A Cochrane systematic review of five placebo-controlled, randomised, double-blind trials ($n = 343$) concluded that there was insufficient evidence to determine whether feverfew was superior to placebo in reducing migraine frequency or incidence, severity of nausea or severity of migraines (Pittler & Ernst 2004). A closer look at the studies reveals that results were mixed, methodological quality varied and various dosage regimens, administration forms and extracts were used. One study used three different dosing regimens for a CO_2 extract, two studies used an alcoholic and CO_2 extract, three studies used dried feverfew leaves for 8–24 weeks and one study used an alcoholic extract for 8 weeks. Interpretation of test results is made even more difficult when one considers the naturally occurring chemical variations among the preparations.

The authors have offered several explanations for the inconsistent clinical findings and point out that previous negative studies used extracts standardised for parthenolide concentration; however, it is possible that other compounds found in whole-leaf preparations may also be important for pharmacological activity. In vivo studies support this view (Mittra et al 2000). Others have also suggested that the alcoholic extracts may not contain the same amount of adjunctive compounds necessary for action or, conversely, the alcoholic extract may contain greater concentrations of compounds which reduce the action of parthenolide (Saranitzky et al 2009). It is also possible that the negative results obtained by some studies may be due to underdosing.

Since then, positive results were obtained for a CO_2 extract of feverfew (with enriched parthenolide) in a randomised, double-blind, placebo-controlled, multicentre study of 170 patients with frequent migraine headache (Diener et al 2005). Active treatment with feverfew (MIG-99) at a dose of 6.25 mg, three times daily, significantly reduced the frequency of migraine headache episodes, the number of migraine headache days and migraine duration over a 16-week period. More specifically, migraine frequency decreased from 4.8 to 2.9 attacks per month in the MIG-99 group and to 3.5 attacks for placebo ($P = 0.046$). The prophylactic effect was most pronounced in the first 2 months and then appeared to stabilise. The treatment was very well tolerated. Participants included in this study needed to have experienced migraine headaches for at least 1 year, have an average of 4–6 migraine attacks in the month before commencing treatment and a duration of attack between 4 and 72 hours. All prophylactic migraine treatment was ceased at least 4 weeks prior to study commencement.

IN COMBINATION

A number of trials have tested feverfew in combination with other herbs and nutritional supplements. Shrivastava et al (2006) tested a combination of feverfew (600 mg/day) and willow bark (600 mg/day), known as Mig-RL, in a 12-week prospective study for the prophylaxis of migraine and the combination was shown to significantly reduce attack frequency and severity. The combination was selected because previous in vitro studies identified that feverfew and willow bark inhibit binding to 5-$HT_{2A/2C}$ receptors and the combination of willow bark with feverfew further inhibited 5-HT_{1D} receptors, whereas feverfew on its own did not. Combination herbal treatment significantly reduced migraine attack frequency by 57.2% at 6 weeks ($P < 0.029$) and by 61.7% at 12 weeks ($P < 0.025$) in nine of 10 patients, with 70% of patients having a reduction of at least 50%. Attack intensity was reduced by 38.7% at 6 weeks ($P < 0.005$) and by 62.6% at 12 weeks ($P < 0.004$) in all of the 10 patients, with 70% of patients having a reduction of at least 50%. Attack duration decreased by 67.2% at 6 weeks ($P < 0.001$) and by 76.2% at 12 weeks ($P < 0.001$) in all of the 10 patients. Two patients were excluded for reasons unrelated to treatment. Self-assessed general health, physical performance, memory and anxiety also improved by the end of the study. The treatment was well tolerated and no adverse events occurred (Shrivastava et al 2006).

The combination of feverfew with ginger (GelStat Migraine) in a sublingually administered fluid was evaluated as an acute treatment in an open-label study involving 29 patients with 1-year history of migraine meeting International Headache Society diagnostic criteria of 2–8 migraines per month and ≤15 headache days per month, with or without aura. People ingested the test substance during the early mild headache phase of an oncoming migraine. Herbal treatment was found to totally relieve pain in 48% of people within 2 hours and a further 34% reported pain had remained mild and not worsened. Of the group, 59% were satisfied with their response to GelStat Migraine therapy (Cady et al 2005). Of note, the product is marketed as a homeopathic product and contains extremely small amounts of both herbs.

In 2011, a randomised, multicentre study of 60 patients found that 2 hours after acute treatment with sublingual feverfew/ginger, 32% of subjects receiving active medication and 16% of subjects receiving placebo were pain-free ($P = 0.02$). At 2 hours, 63% of subjects receiving feverfew/ginger found pain relief (pain-free or mild headache) vs 39% for placebo ($P = 0.002$) and pain severity was significantly less with the feverfew/ginger combination (Cady et al 2011). All subjects in this study had <15 headache days per month and were not experiencing medication overuse headache.

Feverfew (100 mg) combined with riboflavin (400 mg) and magnesium (300 mg) was compared to stand-alone riboflavin (25 mg) treatment in a randomised, double-blind study of migraine sufferers (Maizels et al 2004). Both treatments showed a significant reduction in number of migraines, migraine days and migraine index in the 3-month trial, which was greater than responses for placebo in other trials of migraine prophylaxis. When treatment responses were compared, no significant differences were seen between the groups, indicating that feverfew at this low dose is ineffective.

Women patients ($n = 22$) with headache who were treated with acupuncture for 10 weeks showed significant improvements in symptoms, migraine disability assessment score (MIDAS; quantifies headache-related disability over a 3-month period) and overall health-related quality of life (Ferro et al 2012). When feverfew (150 mg/day taken at bedtime) was combined with acupuncture ($n = 23$), the results were better than in patients who received acupuncture ($n = 22$) or feverfew alone ($n = 23$). There was a substantial mean reduction from baseline in the visual analogue scale (rated from 0 [pain-free] to 10 [unbearable pain]) outcome measure in both treatment groups. However, the combination of acupuncture and feverfew was statistically significantly more effective than acupuncture or feverfew alone in reducing the mean of score of pain on the visual analogue scale.

Arthritic conditions

Although traditionally used as a treatment for inflammatory joint conditions, the results of a randomised, double-blind study involving 41 patients with symptoms of rheumatoid arthritis found no difference between chopped dried feverfew (70–86 mg) or placebo after 6 weeks' treatment (Pattrick et al 1989).

OTHER USES

Dermatology

Feverfew may protect the skin from the numerous external aggressions encountered daily by the skin as well as reduce the damage to oxidatively challenged skin (Martin et al 2008). Parthenolide-free feverfew extract is being investigated in various dermatological conditions. It has been found to protect the skin against inflammation and ultraviolet (UV)-induced damage (Finkey et al 2005). When the parthenolide-free feverfew extract was topically applied, it significantly reduced loss of cell viability, increase in proinflammatory mediator release and induction of DNA damage induced by solar-simulated UV radiation in a human epidermal model. It also exhibited potent antioxidant activity in vitro and has been shown to dismutate superoxide, thereby protecting cells from the pro-oxidant depletion of endogenous skin antioxidants.

In the next phase of testing, a clinical study was conducted with an emollient containing the parthenolide-free feverfew extract, which confirmed that treatment significantly reduced the erythema effects of acute UVB exposure by up to 60% compared to placebo. Assessment was done by a blinded clinical grader and a chroma meter. These results suggest that topical application of parthenolide-depleted feverfew extract (PD-feverfew) can protect skin from UV-induced damage and from oxidative damage and help to repair damaged DNA.

In another study, PD-feverfew extract was found to possess free radical scavenging activity against a wide range of ROS and with greater activity than vitamin C (Martin et al 2008). In vitro, PD-feverfew attenuated the formation of UV-induced hydrogen peroxide and reduced proinflammatory cytokine release. It also restored cigarette smoke-mediated depletion of cellular thiols. In vivo, topical PD-feverfew reduced UV-induced epidermal hyperplasia, DNA damage and apoptosis. This suggests that feverfew has the ability to scavenge free radicals, preserve endogenous antioxidant levels, reduce DNA damage and induce DNA repair enzymes, which can help repair damaged DNA.

Oncology

Parthenolide has demonstrated potent antitumour activity in a variety of experimental models (in vitro and in vivo), and its mechanisms of action are becoming better elucidated. The positive results obtained in these preliminary studies indicate that it may have potential in the treatment of cancer; however, no clinical studies have been published to date to determine its efficacy in humans.

DOSAGE RANGE

- Dried leaf: 50–200 mg daily.
- Fresh plant tincture (1 : 1): 0.7–2.0 mL/day.
- Dried plant tincture (1 : 5): 1–3 mL/day.
- Prevention of migraine headaches (based on clinical studies): 125–600 mg/day of powder, standardised to contain a minimum parthenolide content of 0.2%, or 400 mcg, which should be taken for at least 4 months. It is still controversial as to whether ethanolic standardised extracts are best for migraine prophylaxis or not.
- According to a large 2005 randomised controlled trial: a commercial CO_2 extract of *Tanacetum parthenium* (MIG-99) 6.25 mg taken three times daily

TOXICITY

Unknown, although no major safety issues have been identified (Ernst & Pittler 2000).

ADVERSE REACTIONS

According to a Cochrane systematic review of five studies (Pittler & Ernst 2004), feverfew is well tolerated and adverse events are generally mild and reversible. Symptoms were most frequently reported by long-term users and were predominantly mouth ulceration and gastrointestinal symptoms. Contact dermatitis, mouth soreness and lip swelling have also been reported when leaves are chewed. People allergic to the Asteraceae (Compositae) family of plant, or feverfew in particular, should avoid feverfew products that contain parthenolide, as it is this component which is thought to be the main inducer of the allergic response (Sharma & Sethuraman 2007).

SIGNIFICANT INTERACTIONS

Controlled studies are not available; therefore, interactions are based on evidence of activity and are largely theoretical and speculative.

Anticoagulants

Theoretically, feverfew may increase bruising and bleeding; however, although feverfew inhibits platelet aggregation in vitro and in vivo, no effects were seen in a clinical study (Biggs et al 1982) — observe patients taking this combination.

CONTRAINDICATIONS AND PRECAUTIONS

Hypersensitivity to plants in the daisy (Asteraceae/Compositae) family (e.g. chamomile, ragweed).

PREGNANCY USE

Feverfew is contraindicated in pregnancy. An in vitro and in vivo preliminary screen using a rat model suggested that feverfew consumption may have detrimental effects in pregnancy, a finding which needs to be more fully explored in larger studies (Yao et al 2006). Feverfew-treated animals had reduced litter sizes, a greater proportion of smaller fetuses than the control group and increased pre-implantation loss, indicating maternal and embryonic effects. However, it should be noted that the doses used were 59 times the accepted human dose, and therefore the clinical relevance of the findings are unclear. A full reproductive toxicity study is warranted to determine whether the observed effects are clinically significant.

Practice points/Patient counselling

- Currently available research investigating the use of feverfew for migraine prophylaxis is promising, especially with the dried feverfew-leaf formulations, whereas ethanolic extracts have produced inconsistent results.
- A study with a commercial CO_2 extract of *Tanacetum parthenium* (MIG-99) showed it reduced the frequency, severity and duration of migraine headache in chronic sufferers.
- Tincture or solid-dose preparations may be better tolerated than chewing the fresh leaves, which have been associated with mouth ulcers and lip swelling in some individuals.
- Traditionally, feverfew has also been used to treat coughs and colds, fevers, atonic dyspepsia, worm infestation, menstrual disorders, nervous debility, joint pain and headaches.
- Parthenolide-free feverfew shows promise as a dermatological and UV-protective agent when used topically.
- Many preliminary studies with parthenolide confirm that it has potent antitumour activity; however, it has not yet been tested in humans.
- Use is contraindicated in pregnancy until safety can be better established.

PATIENTS' FAQs

What will this herb do for me?

Evidence suggests that feverfew may reduce the frequency and severity of migraine headaches when dried-leaf preparations are used, whereas results with ethanolic extracts are inconsistent. Topical application with parthenolide-free feverfew cream shows promise as a dermatological preparation to reduce redness after sun exposure and help heal damaged skin.

When will it start to work?

Of those studies producing positive results, it appears that benefits in migraine occur within 2 months of use; however, in practice, some patients experience benefits within the first 4 weeks.

Are there any safety issues?

Feverfew should not be used in pregnancy or by people with Asteraceae (Compositae) allergy.

REFERENCES

Anderson KN, Bejcek BE. Parthenolide induces apoptosis in glioblastomas without affecting NF-kappaB. J Pharmacol Sci 106.2 (2008): 318–20.

Barsby RW et al. Feverfew extracts and parthenolide irreversibly inhibit vascular responses of the rabbit aorta. J Pharm Pharmacol 44.9 (1992): 737–40.

Barsby RW, et al. A chloroform extract of the herb feverfew blocks voltage-dependent potassium currents recorded from single smooth muscle cells. J Pharm Pharmacol 45.7 (1993a): 641–5.

Barsby RW et al. Feverfew and vascular smooth muscle: extracts from fresh and dried plants show opposing pharmacological profiles, dependent upon sesquiterpene lactone content. Planta Med 59.1 (1993b): 20–5.

Biggs MJ et al. Platelet aggregation in patients using feverfew for migraine. Lancet 2.8301 (1982): 776.

Brown AM et al. Pharmacological activity of feverfew (*Tanacetum parthenium* (L.) Schultz-Bip.): assessment by inhibition of human polymorphonuclear leukocyte chemiluminescence in-vitro. J Pharm Pharmacol 49.5 (1997): 558–61.

Cady RK et al. Gelstat Migraine (sublingually administered feverfew and ginger compound) for acute treatment of migraine when administered during the mild pain phase. Med Sci Monit 11.9 (2005): I65–9.

Cady, R.K., et al. 2011. A double-blind placebo-controlled pilot study of sublingual feverfew and ginger (LipiGesic M) in the treatment of migraine. Headache, 51, (7) 1078–1086.

Capasso F. The effect of an aqueous extract of *Tanacetum parthenium* L. on arachidonic acid metabolism by rat peritoneal leucocytes. J Pharm Pharmacol 38.1 (1986): 71–2.

Collier HO et al. Extract of feverfew inhibits prostaglandin biosynthesis. Lancet 2.8200 (1980): 922–3.

Cutlan AR et al. Intra-specific variability of feverfew: correlations between parthenolide, morphological traits and seed origin. Planta Med 66.7 (2000): 612–17.

Diener HC et al. Efficacy and safety of 6.25 mg t.i.d. feverfew CO2-extract (MIG-99) in migraine prevention: a randomized, double-blind, multicentre, placebo-controlled study. Cephalalgia 25.11 (2005): 1031–41.

Ernst E, Pittler MH. The efficacy and safety of feverfew (*Tanacetum parthenium* L.): an update of a systematic review. Public Health Nutr 3.4A (2000): 509–14.

Ferrari MD. Migraine. Lancet 351.9108 (1998): 1043–51.

Ferro EC et al. The combined effect of acupuncture and *Tanacetum parthenium* on quality of life in women with headache: randomised study. Acupunct Med 30.4 (2012): 252–7.

Finkey MB et al. Parthenolide-free feverfew extract protects the skin against UV damage and inflammation. J Am Acad Dermatol 52.3 (2005): 93.

Ghantous A et al. Parthenolide: from plant shoots to cancer roots. Drug Discov Today (2013) May 17. S1359-6446.

Groenewegen WA, Heptinstall S. A comparison of the effects of an extract of feverfew and parthenolide, a component of feverfew, on human platelet activity in-vitro. J Pharm Pharmacol 42.8 (1990): 553–7.

Guzman ML et al. The sesquiterpene lactone parthenolide induces apoptosis of human acute myelogenous leukemia stem and progenitor cells. Blood 105.11 (2005): 4163–9.

Hayes NA, Foreman JC. The activity of compounds extracted from feverfew on histamine release from rat mast cells. J Pharm Pharmacol 39.6 (1987): 466–70.

Heptinstall S. Feverfew: an ancient remedy for modern times? J R Soc Med 81.7 (1988): 373–4.

Heptinstall S et al. Inhibition of platelet behaviour by feverfew: a mechanism of action involving sulphydryl groups. Folia Haematol Int Mag KlinMorpholBlutforsch 115.4 (1988): 447–9.

Heptinstall S et al. Parthenolide content and bioactivity of feverfew (*Tanacetum parthenium* (L.) Schultz-Bip.). Estimation of commercial and authenticated feverfew products. J Pharm Pharmacol 44.5 (1992): 391–5.

Jain NK, Kulkarni SK. Antinociceptive and anti-inflammatory effects of *Tanacetum parthenium* L. extract in mice and rats. J Ethnopharmacol 68.1–3 (1999): 251–9.

Johnson ES et al. Efficacy of feverfew as prophylactic treatment of migraine. BMJ (Clin Res Ed) 291.6495 (1985): 569–73.

Kawasaki BT et al. Effects of the sesquiterpene lactone parthenolide on prostate tumor-initiating cells: an integrated molecular profiling approach. Prostate 69.8 (2009): 827–37.

Kim IH et al. Parthenolide-induced apoptosis of hepatic stellate cells and anti-fibrotic effects in an in vivo rat model. Exp Mol Med 44.7 (2012): 448–56.

Kim SL et al. Parthenolide suppresses tumor growth in a xenograft model of colorectal cancer cells by inducing mitochondrial dysfunction and apoptosis. Int.J Oncol 41.4 (2012): 1547–1553.

Knight DW. Feverfew: chemistry and biological activity. Nat. Prod. Rep 12.3 (1995): 271–276.

Kwok BH et al. The anti-inflammatory natural product parthenolide from the medicinal herb Feverfew directly binds to and inhibits IkappaB kinase. Chem Biol 8.8 (2001): 759–66.

Lesiak K et al. Parthenolide, a sesquiterpene lactone from the medical herb feverfew, shows anticancer activity against human melanoma cells in vitro. Melanoma Res 20.1 (2010):21–34.

Magni P et al. Parthenolide inhibits the LPS-induced secretion of IL-6 and TNF-alpha and NF-kappaB nuclear translocation in BV-2 microglia. Phytother Res 26.9 (2012) 1405–1409.

Maizels M, et al. A combination of riboflavin, magnesium, and feverfew for migraine prophylaxis: a randomized trial. Headache 44.9 (2004): 885–90.

Makheja AN, Bailey JM. A platelet phospholipase inhibitor from the medicinal herb feverfew (*Tanacetum parthenium*).Prostaglandins Leukot Med 8.6 (1982): 653–60.

Marles RJ et al. A bioassay for inhibition of serotonin release from bovine platelets. J Nat Prod 55.8 (1992): 1044–56.

Martin K et al. Parthenolide-depleted Feverfew (*Tanacetum parthenium*) protects skin from UV irradiation and external aggression. Arch Dermatol Res 300.2 (2008): 69–80.

Mathema VB et al. Parthenolide, a sesquiterpene lactone, expresses multiple anti-cancer and anti-inflammatory activities. Inflammation 35.2 (2012): 560–5.

Mittra S et al. 5-hydroxytryptamine-inhibiting property of feverfew: role of parthenolide content. Acta Pharmacol Sin 21.12 (2000): 1106–14.

Miyata N et al. Inhibitory effects of parthenolide on antigen-induced microtubule formation and degranulation in mast cells. Int Immunopharmacol 8.6 (2008): 874–80.

Murch SJ et al. Melatonin in feverfew and other medicinal plants. Lancet 350.9091 (1997):1598–9.

Murphy JJ et al. Randomised double-blind placebo-controlled trial of feverfew in migraine prevention. Lancet 2.8604 (1988): 189–92.

Nasim S, Crooks PA. Antileukemic activity of aminoparthenolide analogs. Bioorg Med ChemLett 18.14 (2008): 3870–3.

Pajak B, et al. Molecular basis of parthenolide-dependent proapoptotic activity in cancer cells. Folia HistochemCytobiol 46.2 (2008): 129–35.

Pattrick M, et al. Feverfew in rheumatoid arthritis: a double blind, placebo controlled study. Ann Rheum Dis 48.7 (1989): 547–9.

Piela-Smith T, Liu X. Feverfew extracts and sesquiterpene lactone parthenolide inhibit intercellular adhesion molecule-1 expression in human synovial fibroblasts. Cell Immunol, 209 (2001), 89–96.

Pittler M, Ernst E. Feverfew for preventing migraine. Cochrane Database Syst Rev 1 (2004): CD 002286.

Pugh WJ, Sambo K. Prostaglandin synthetase inhibitors in feverfew. J Pharm Pharmacol 40.10 (1988): 743–5.

Sahler J et al. The Feverfew plant-derived compound, parthenolide enhances platelet production and attenuates platelet activation through NF-κB inhibition. Thromb Res 127.5 (2011):426–34.

Saranitzky E et al. Feverfew for migraine prophylaxis: a systematic review. J Diet Suppl 6.2 (2009): 91–103.

Setty AR, Sigal LH. Herbal medications commonly used in the practice of rheumatology: mechanisms of action, efficacy, and side effects. Semin Arthritis Rheum 34.6 (2005):773–84.

Sharma VK, Sethuraman G. Parthenium dermatitis. Dermatitis 18.4 (2007): 183–90.

Shrivastava R, et al. *Tanacetum parthenium* and *Salix alba* (Mig-RL) combination in migraine prophylaxis: a prospective, open-label study. Clin Drug Investig 26.5 (2006): 287–96.

Silberstein SD. Migraine. Lancet 363.9406 (2004): 381–91.

Smolinski AT, Pestka JJ. Modulation of lipopolysaccharide-induced proinflammatory cytokine production in vitro and in vivo by the herbal constituents apigenin (chamomile), ginsenoside Rb1 (ginseng) and parthenolide (feverfew). Food ChemToxicol 41.10 (2003): 1381–90.

Sumner H et al. Inhibition of 5-lipoxygenase and cyclo-oxygenase in leukocytes by feverfew. Involvement of sesquiterpene lactones and other components. Biochem Pharmacol, 43.11 (1992), 2313–2320.

Sweeney CJ et al. The sesquiterpene lactone parthenolide in combination with docetaxel reduces metastasis and improves survival in a xenograft model of breast cancer. Mol Cancer Ther 4.6 (2005): 1004–12.
Tournier H et al. Effect of the chloroform extract of *Tanacetum vulgare* and one of its active principles, parthenolide, on experimental gastric ulcer in rats. J Pharm Pharmacol 51.2 (1999): 215–19.
Weber JT et al. Rabbit cerebral cortex 5HT1a receptors. Comp Biochem Physiol C Pharmacol Toxicol Endocrinol 117.1 (1997a): 19–24.
Weber JT et al. Activity of Parthenolide at 5HT2A receptors. J Nat Prod 60.6 (1997b): 651–3.
Wong HR, Menendez IY. Sesquiterpene lactones inhibit inducible nitric oxide synthase gene expression in cultured rat aortic smooth muscle cells. BiochemBiophys Res Commun 262.2 (1999): 375–80.
Wu C et al. Antiproliferative activities of parthenolide and golden feverfew extract against three human cancer cell lines. J Med Food 9.1 (2006): 55–61.
Wyrębska A et al. Apoptosis-mediated cytotoxic effects of parthenolide and the new synthetic analog MZ-6 on two breast cancer cell lines. Mol Biol Rep 40.2 (2013):1655–63.
Yao M, et al. A reproductive screening test of feverfew: is a full reproductive study warranted? Reprod Toxicol 22.4 (2006): 688–93.
Zunino SJ, et al. Parthenolide induces significant apoptosis and production of reactive oxygen species in high-risk pre-B leukemia cells. Cancer Lett 254.1 (2007): 119–27.

Fish oils

BACKGROUND AND RELEVANT PHARMACOKINETICS

One of the two human essential fatty acids (EFAs) EFAs is alpha-linolenic acid (ALA or 18:3ω-3), which, due to the position of its first double bond, is classified as an omega-3 (ω-3) EFA. Although mammals have the ability to introduce double bonds into most positions of the fatty-acid chain in fat metabolism, therefore producing various unsaturated metabolites, they lack the capacity to insert double bonds at the ω-3 and ω-6 positions. Consequently, linoleic acid (LA) and ALA, which already have the double bond at the ω-3 or ω-6 position, respectively, are considered essential and must be consumed in the diet. When the EFAs are consumed in this precursor state they follow a pathway of further elongation and desaturation via the action of delta-6- and delta-5-desaturase until they form the 'active' fatty acids: eicosapentaenoic acid (20:5ω-3) (EPA) and docosahexaenoic acid (DHA) (22:6ω-3), also referred to as the ω-3 long-chain polyunsaturated fats (ω-3 LCPUFAs).

Fish oils, also known as marine oils, are rapidly absorbed from the gastrointestinal tract and compete with arachidonic acid (AA) for incorporation into phospholipids, particularly of platelets, erythrocytes, neutrophils, monocytes and liver cells (Simopoulos 1999). When stimulated, the cell membranes release polyunsaturated fatty acids (PUFAs), which are then converted into 20-carbon eicosanoids, which have profound and extensive physiological effects. The most active of these metabolites are prostaglandins, prostacyclins and thromboxanes, which affect blood chemistry, muscle contraction, immune function and inflammation. Dietary fats not used in this way are stored in adipose tissue and ultimately oxidised to produce energy. The fatty-acid cell membrane profile of different tissues will have varying ratios of EPA and DHA, but generally DHA is considered the major component of phospholipids in the retina, brain, male reproductive tissue and myocardium (Groff & Gropper 2004).

Supplements based on fish liver oils, such as cod and halibut, contain EPA and DHA together with high levels of vitamins A and D. As such, they have additional actions and safety issues besides those found with traditional marine lipid supplements. This review will focus on the research surrounding those fish oils that are not liver extractions.

CHEMICAL COMPONENTS

Dietary fish contains a number of nutrients important for health, such as several B vitamins, vitamin E, calcium, magnesium and potassium, and are an excellent source of protein with a low saturated fat content. Importantly, they also contain the two PUFAs: EPA and DHA. EPA has 20 carbon atoms and five double bonds, and DHA has 22 carbon atoms and six double bonds. Both are derived from ALA and are considered conditionally essential. The EPA and DHA found in whole fish are predominantly esterified in the *sn*-2 position of triacylglycerols and glyercophospholipids; however, when found in supplements, most commonly exist as ethyl esters (Visioli et al 2003). This minor chemical distinction may explain the speculated superior bioavailability of these fats when derived from the diet as opposed to supplements.

FOOD SOURCES

Most dietary EPA and DHA are consumed in the form of fish or seafood. Deep-sea cold-water fish, such as salmon, mackerel, halibut and herring, provide the most concentrated sources. Current Australian estimates of intake indicate inadequate consumption according to World Health Organization (WHO) standards (Meyer et al 2003).

DEFICIENCY SIGNS AND SYMPTOMS

Based on epidemiological studies, low levels of ω-3 LCPUFAs are associated with:

- fetal alcohol syndrome (DHA) (Horrocks & Yeo 1999)
- attention-deficit hyperactivity disorder (ADHD) (DHA) (Horrocks & Yeo 1999)

- learning deficits (DHA) (Horrocks & Yeo 1999)
- cystic fibrosis (DHA) (Horrocks & Yeo 1999)
- phenylketonuria (DHA) (Horrocks & Yeo 1999)
- cardiovascular disease (CVD), including an increased risk of sudden death due to heart disease (Siscovick et al 2003)
- inflammatory disorders
- rheumatoid arthritis (RA) (Navarro et al 2000)
- unipolar depression (DHA) (Horrocks & Yeo 1999)
- senile dementia.

In addition to these symptoms, lack of dietary EFAs has been implicated in the development or aggravation of numerous diseases such as breast cancer, prostate cancer, RA, asthma, pre-eclampsia, depression and schizophrenia (Yehuda et al 2005).

Clinical note — Are ALA-rich oils a worthy substitute for fish oils?

Both EPA and DHA are derived from ALA, so food sources containing ALA are seen as indirect dietary sources. ALA is commonly found in non-hydrogenated canola oil, linseed oil, soybean oil, flaxseed, pumpkin and walnuts. Studies investigating the effects of ALA supplementation have not consistently produced the same positive results as for fish oils, most likely due to inefficient conversion of ALA into EPA and DHA. This is reportedly poor in healthy individuals, with only 5–10% of ALA converted to EPA and 2–5% of ALA converted to DHA (Davis & Kris-Etherton 2003). Consequently, the few foods that contain both EPA and DHA in their preformed state offer a significant advantage over other sources. The most concentrated dietary source of both EPA and DHA is deepsea oily fish (See Flaxseed monograph for further information.)

Primary deficiency

Full-term babies fed a skim-milk formula low in ALA are at risk of primary deficiency. In the past, patients fed long-term with fat-free total parenteral nutrition solutions were at risk, but fat emulsions are now in general use and prevent deficiency. Studies have demonstrated lower plasma levels of EPA and DHA in vegetarians and vegans, suggesting they may be at risk of deficiency; however, the findings of a cross-sectional study comparing the dietary intakes and plasma levels of 196 meat-eating, 231 vegetarian and 232 vegan men in the United Kingdom did not suggest that there is cause for alarm (Rosell et al 2005). Vegans and vegetarians had significantly lower levels of these fatty acids; however, they remained steady and there is evidence of some conversion of ALA into EPA and DHA.

There is much discussion regarding the inadequate intake of EPA and DHA generally in the Western diet. Australian data, based on dietary intake records from the 1995 National Nutrition Survey, have estimated the average daily intake of EPA and DHA to be 0.008 g and 0.015 g, respectively. If correct, this indicates that the majority of Australians are failing to meet recommended amounts (Meyer et al 2003).

Secondary deficiency

People with fat malabsorption syndromes, serious trauma or burns are at risk of reduced PUFA levels (Beers & Berkow 2003). A secondary deficiency may also manifest as a result of abnormal or compromised activity of the delta-6 and delta-5 desaturase enzymes, for example in diabetics, patients with a variety of metabolic disorders and individuals with increased dietary saturated fats and *trans* fatty acids, alcoholics and the elderly (Davis & Kris-Etherton 2003, Houston 2005).

MAIN ACTIONS

As precursors of eicosanoids, PUFAs found in fish oils exert a wide influence over many important physiological processes.

Cardiovascular effects

Fish oils exert myriad different effects on the heart and vessels, demonstrated in both experimental models and human studies. It is speculated that the clinical effects attributed to ω-3 PUFAs are due to the summation of many small pharmacological effects, adding up to a larger protective effect on mortality and/or cardiovascular events.

Prevent malignant cardiac arrhythmias

Dietary fish or fish oil intake has been shown to prevent cardiac arrhythmias and associated sudden death in numerous animal studies (Billman et al 1997, 1999, Kang & Leaf 1996, 2000, McLennan et al 1988, 1990), in vitro and more recently in human clinical trials (Jung et al 2008). This has been achieved using intakes below those required to alter plasma lipids or blood pressure. It appears that the myocardial membrane phospholipid content increases in DHA but not always EPA, with fish intake. The preferential accumulation of DHA affords protection against ventricular fibrillation induced under a variety of conditions, such as ischaemia and reperfusion (McLennan 2001).

Inadequate DHA in myocyte membranes has been reported to be associated with altered sodium, calcium and potassium ion channel functions, mitochondrial function and increased arrhythmia susceptibility with an increased prevalence of sudden cardiac death (Jung et al 2008, Siscovick et al 2003). One in vivo study suggests that fish oils electrically stabilise myocytes, increasing the electrical impulse required to produce an action potential by approximately 50% and prolonging the refractory time by 150% (Kang & Leaf 2000).

Triglyceride (TG)-lowering activity

Fish oil supplements effectively reduce TG levels, as demonstrated in human studies. This is of particular interest, given only moderate elevations in TG levels have been associated with a progressively increased risk of ischaemic heart disease, independently of other major risk factors, including high-density lipoprotein (HDL) cholesterol (Jeppesen et al 1998). A significant plasma TG-lowering activity has also been demonstrated for a highly potent form of ω-3 fatty acids, available as Lovaza in the United States (previously Omacor) (Kar 2014).

Lipoprotein effects

Both ω-6 and ω-3 LCPUFAs can inhibit the expression of genes involved in fatty-acid and TG synthesis (Jung et al 2008). Dietary ω-3 LCPUFAs, in particular, and their metabolites, through this mechanism are reported to increase beta-oxidation and inhibit adipogenesis. Ultimately, this may result in reduced substrate for TG synthesis and thus explain ω-3 PUFAs' profound TG-lowering effects.

Concerns raised previously about increased LCPUFAs in lipoproteins increasing the susceptibility to oxidation of the low-density lipoproteins (LDLs) have recently been moderated, with a demonstrable difference between EPA and DHA. While increased levels of EPA (4.8 g/day) did increase the LDL susceptibility to damage, DHA supplementation (4.9 g/day) had no effect on the oxidation process (Mesa et al 2004). Concurrent supplementation with antioxidants however appears prudent with high doses of ω-3 PUFAs.

Improved endothelial function

Studies have indicated that fish oils can improve endothelial relaxation by enhancing nitric oxide-(NO) and non-NO-induced vasodilation (Holub 2002).

A double-blind study conducted by Mori et al (2000) showed that, relative to placebo, DHA, but not EPA, enhances vasodilator mechanisms and attenuates constrictor responses in forearm microcirculation.

Reducing resting heart rate

Regular ω-3 LCPUFA intake can lower resting heart rate by up to 5 beats/min in patient and healthy populations, in healthy individuals during exercise without compromising maximum heart rate and during exercise recovery in post myocardial infarction (MI) patients (McLennan 2014).

Reduce blood pressure

Three meta-analyses have concluded that fish oils exert a significant blood pressure-lowering effect in hypertensive people; however, the effects can only be described as modest, between 2 and 5 mmHg (Geleijnse et al 2002, Miller et al 2014, Morris et al 1993). Hypotensive activity appears to be dose-dependent and DHA may have greater effect than EPA. Alternatively, a 2006 Cochrane review found no significant changes to systolic or diastolic blood pressure with ω-3 LCPUFA consumption (Hooper et al 2006). The review assessed studies that used both plant- and fish-based ω-3 fatty acids, dietary sources and supplements.

While the mechanism is unknown, current theories include EPA stimulation of prostacyclin synthesis and increased NO production — both vasodilators. An additional action may be improved autonomic nervous system function, and inhibition of adrenal activation (Din et al 2004, Ross 2005); however, these are inconsistent with the attribution of action to DHA. In addition to the actions improving endothelial function generally, other posited mechanisms for a hypotensive effect include: blunting of the renin–angiotensin–aldosterone system via reduced adrenal aldosterone synthesis, altered AA metabolism, modulation of calcium release and influx into vascular smooth-muscle cells and activation of vascular adenosine triphosphate-sensitive potassium channels (Jung et al 2008).

F

Reduce and possibly reverse atherogenesis

Ω-3 fatty acids alter eicosanoid synthesis and inhibit smooth-muscle cell proliferation, suggesting a role in reducing atherosclerotic development (Holub 2002). One controlled study demonstrated that fish oil ingestion had a clinically significant influence on atherosclerosis (von Schacky et al 2001). This randomised, double-blind study of 223 patients found that a dose of 1.5 g ω-3 fatty acids reduced progression and increased regression of established coronary artery disease as assessed by coronary angiography. The content of diets and relevant risk factors were examined through a health survey on the inhabitants in a fishing village ($n = 261$) and in a farming village ($n = 209$) in Japan (Yamada et al 2000). Pulse wave velocity of the aorta, intima media thickness (IMT) of the carotid artery and atherosclerotic plaques as obtained by ultrasonography were used as measures of atherosclerosis. The fish consumption of both males and females in the fishing village was about 1.8 and 1.6 times higher, respectively, than that reported in the farming village ($P < 0.0001$). Dietary consumption of EPA and DHA was significantly higher in the fishing village versus the farming village ($P < 0.001$). Pulse wave velocity and IMT were significantly lower in the fishing village than in the farming village in males ($P < 0.01$ and $P < 0.001$, respectively). IMT was significantly lower in females ($P < 0.001$). There was an eightfold difference in the average number of plaques in the common carotid arteries in males ($P < 0.0001$) and a fivefold difference in females between the villages ($P < 0.0001$).

Antithrombotic and antiplatelet

Dietary ω-3 PUFAs enhance antiaggregatory and antiadhesive platelet activity by inducing increased production of prostacyclin I_3 and suppressing synthesis of the chemotactic platelet adhesion-promoting substances, leukotriene B_4 and thromboxane A_2 (Jung et al 2008, Kinsella 1987). A meta-analysis of randomised controlled trials (RCTs) ($n = 15$) with 409 participants found daily supplementation with ω-3 PUFA significantly reduced adenosine diphosphate (ADP)-induced platelet aggregation compared with placebo ($P = 0.02$) (Gao et al 2013). Independently of this, ω-3 LCPUFAs reduce levels of several coagulating factors (e.g. VII and X, and fibrinogen) (Jung et al 2008).

Clinical interest — Do fish oil supplements pose a significant bleeding risk?

A search through Medline reveals several case reports where bleeding episodes are attributed to fish oil ingestion (Buckley et al 2004, Jalili & Dehpour 2007, McClaskey & Michalets 2007). In each case, the person affected was elderly and also taking warfarin. One was a report of an elderly man taking high-dose ω-3 fatty acids (6 g/day) with both aspirin and warfarin who developed a subdural haematoma after a minor fall (McClaskey & Michalets 2007). Another case is reported of a 67-year-old woman taking warfarin for 1.5 years who doubled the fish oil dose from 1000 to 2000 mg/day, causing an associated elevation in international normalised ratio (INR) from 2.8 to 4.3 within 1 month (Buckley et al 2004). A third case was of a 65-year-old male who had been taking warfarin for 6 months and then was recommended trazodone and fish oils, causing his INR to rise to 8.06 (Jalili & Dehpour 2007).

Although these case reports would lead us to believe that ω-3 fatty acids interact with warfarin and increase the risk of bleeding, several intervention studies have come to a different conclusion. One randomised study of 511 patients taking either aspirin (300 mg/day) or warfarin (INR aimed at 2.5–4.2) found that a dose of 4 g/day of fish oils did not increase the number of bleeding episodes, bleeding time or any parameters of coagulation and fibrinolysis (Eritsland et al 1995). A smaller placebo-controlled study by Bender et al (1998) of patients receiving chronic warfarin therapy found that fish oil doses of 3–6 g/day produced no statistically significant difference in INR between the placebo lead-in and treatment period within each group. There was also no difference in INR between groups.

More recently, Harris (2007) examined 19 clinical studies which used doses of fish oils varying from 1 g/day to 21 g/day in patients undergoing major vascular surgery (coronary artery bypass grafting, endarterectomy) or femoral artery puncture for either diagnostic cardiac catheterisation or percutaneous transluminal coronary angioplasty. Of note, in 16 studies patients were taking aspirin and in three studies patients were taking heparin. The review concluded that the risk for bleeding was virtually non-existent. Frequent comments accompanying the studies were 'no difference in clinically significant bleeding noted' or 'no patient suffered from bleeding complications'. The same conclusion was reached in a 2008 review which stated that no published studies have reported clinically significant bleeding episodes amongst patients treated with antiplatelet drugs and fish oils (3–7 g/day) (Harris et al 2008). In 2014, a clinical audit of over 900 cardiac surgery patients at the Alfred Hospital found that those taking 3 g of fish oils daily in the week before surgery did not have a significantly increased risk of major haemorrhage or re-admission due to bleeding, once again demonstrating the lack of risk for fish oil supplements in this population (Braun et al 2014).

Overall, when we consider the body of evidence available regarding ω-3 fatty acid supplementation, it is clear that the benefits for cardioprotection far outweigh the risk of bleeding. This not only applies to patients taking aspirin but also those patients about to undergo coronary artery bypass surgery or percutaneous transluminal coronary angioplasty. While the evidence suggests that fish oils in low to moderate doses do not increase bleeding risk with warfarin, a general caution should still apply to patients taking high doses with antiplatelet or anticoagulant medication.

Platelet aggregation studies and flow cytometric analyses of platelet activation and platelet–leucocyte aggregates were determined at baseline and after 4 weeks of a moderate dose of ω-3 (DHA 520 mg and EPA 120 mg) supplementation in 40 healthy subjects and 16 patients with a history of CVD. In healthy subjects, ω-3 PUFA significantly reduced ADP-induced platelet aggregation, as measured by maximum amplitude of platelet aggregation ($P = 0.036$) and velocity of aggregation ($P = 0.014$), as well as adrenaline-induced platelet aggregation (maximum slope, $P = 0.013$; lag time to platelet aggregation, $P = 0.002$). ω-3 PUFA also reduced P-selectin expression ($P = 0.049$) on platelets and platelet–monocyte aggregates ($P = 0.022$). There were fewer changes in platelet aggregation and activation found in subjects with CVD. Nevertheless, there was a reduction in the velocity of AA-induced platelet aggregation ($P = 0.009$) and increased lag time to platelet aggregation for U46619-induced platelet aggregation. ω-3 PUFA had a greater effect on platelet aggregation and activation in healthy subjects and the findings of this study support the recommendation of a higher dose of ω-3 PUFA in patients with CVD who are already receiving antiplatelet medication than in healthy people with CVD ($P = 0.018$) (McEwen et al 2013).

In animal models of arterial thrombosis, fish oil-enriched diets have been shown to have an antithrombotic effect; however, there is evidence suggesting that this is most likely to occur when associated with reduced saturated fat intake (Hornstra 1989).

Clinical observations of Eskimos have found lowered platelet counts, inhibition of platelet aggregation and prolonged bleeding times compared with age- and sex-matched Danes. However, intervention studies using fish oil supplements have produced conflicting results (Hellsten et al 1993, Kristensen et al 1989, Radack et al 1990) and, more recently, a review of clinical studies concluded that there was no clinically significant effect on bleeding with usual therapeutic doses (Harris 2007).

Anti-inflammatory

Fish oils induce a series of chemical changes in the body that ultimately exert an anti-inflammatory action. They partially replace AA in inflammatory cell membranes, and compete with it for the enzymes cyclo-oxygenase and lipoxygenase, leading to reduced production of proinflammatory metabolites such as 2-series prostaglandins and 4-series leukotrienes (Calder 2002, 2003, Cleland et al 2003). Resolvins are compounds that reduce cellular inflammation by inhibiting the production and transportation of inflammatory cells and chemicals. EPA-derived lipid mediator resolvin E1 has potent anti-inflammatory and pro-resolution actions both in vitro and in vivo. In addition, EPA-derived and DHA-derived products such as resolvin D1 and protectin D1 have potent anti-inflammatory and pro-resolution properties (Seki et al 2009).

Besides this, ω-3 PUFAs suppress the production of proinflammatory cytokines, and reduce the expression of cell adhesion molecules, critical in recruiting circulating leucocytes to the vascular endothelium (Calder 2002, Din et al 2004). According to new research, it appears that anti-inflammatory activity may vary among different sources of fish oils due to variations in EPA/DHA content (Bhattacharya et al 2007).

Neurological effects

Fatty acids are major components of the brain and are found in high concentrations in two structural components: the neuronal membrane and the myelin sheath. About 50% of the neuronal membrane is composed of fatty acids (one-third from ω-3 LCPUFAs), while in the myelin sheath lipids constitute about 70% (Yehuda et al 2005). The lipid component has a relatively high turnover, in contrast to the protein component, which is fundamentally stable. The de novo synthesis of PUFA is very low within the brain (Chen & Bazinet 2014). The supply of PUFA to the brain is via the blood, either from exogenous PUFA obtained through diet or from endogenous liver synthesis of PUFA from dietary precursors. Brain DHA levels are 250–300-fold higher than EPA compared to about four-, five-, 14- and 86-fold higher levels of DHA versus EPA in plasma, erythrocyte, liver and heart, respectively. EPA enters the brain at a broadly similar rate to DHA and is rapidly and extensively β-oxidised upon entry into the brain (Chen & Bazinet 2014).

ω-3 fatty acids play an active role in neuronal membrane function, fluidity and control of neuronal growth factors. They also potentially influence each step in biogenic amine function, including neurotransmitter synthesis, degradation, release, reuptake and binding (Bruinsma & Taren 2000). Studies indicate that dietary PUFAs may influence noradrenergic and serotonergic neurotransmission and receptor function in the nervous system and, thereby, have a direct effect on function, mood and behaviour. Other actions at the neuronal cell membrane include suppression of the phosphatidyl-associated signal transduction pathways, blocking of the calcium ion influx through L-calcium channels and direct inhibition of protein kinase C, which are similar actions to those exhibited by some pharmaceutical mood stabilisers.

Prenatal and postnatal neurological development

DHA plays an important, if not critical, role in the growth and functional development of the brain during the third trimester and the early postnatal period when maximal growth occurs (Horrocks & Yeo 1999). Given that 15% of brain growth occurs during infancy, much attention has been paid to the consequences of variable ω-3 levels during late pregnancy and early infancy. It also plays an important role in retinal development, where DHA constitutes 60% of total PUFAs.

Chemopreventive effects

Marine fatty acids, particularly EPA and DHA, have been consistently shown to inhibit the proliferation of breast and prostate cancer cell lines in vitro and to reduce the risk and progression of these tumours in animal experiments (Bagga et al 2002, Terry et al 2003). Similar effects have also been observed for colorectal and prostate cancers (Calder et al 1998, Llor et al 2003, Stoll 2002).

Chemopreventive actions demonstrated by ω-3 LCPUFAs include suppression of neoplastic transformation, cell growth inhibition and enhanced apoptosis and antiangiogenicity (Rose & Connolly 1999). The proposed mechanisms for these are extensive, including the suppression of ω-6 eicosanoid synthesis; influences on transcription factor activity, gene expression and signal transduction pathways; effects on oestrogen metabolism; increased or decreased production of free radicals and reactive oxygen species, and influences on both insulin sensitivity and membrane fluidity (Larsson et al 2004). Ongoing research is attempting to elucidate the specific chemopreventive mechanisms of fish oils with the individual cancer cell lines.

CLINICAL USE

Thousands of studies have been conducted in various populations to determine the clinical consequences of regular fish consumption and fish oil supplementation. Initially, interest was focused on CVD but in recent years this has extended to other areas such as neurological conditions, neonatal and childhood health and development and mental health. While the plethora of studies published have begun to clarify the potential benefits of increasing intakes of ω-3 EFAs and fish on a regular basis, some are inconsistent with the general body of evidence, an issue which needs to be resolved.

There are multiple factors which could account for the sometimes inconsistent results that are seen.

Some studies have focused on ω-3 fatty acids intake as a whole and included both vegetable and marine-based sources; however, in light of the lack of bio-equivalence and clinical efficacy between the ω-3 precursors (e.g. ALA) and their long-chain derivatives (e.g. EPA/DHA), the results of these studies are likely to be confounded. Similarly, prospective studies investigating the effects of ω-3 PUFAs may be producing inconsistent results due to improper placebo selection (e.g. olive oil) (Pizzorno & Murray 2006). This was most recently seen in a large RCT comparing ω-3 EFAs to olive oil (placebo) and both groups experiencing a reduction in cardiovascular risk factors (Roncaglioni et al 2013). It is also important to note that few studies or reviews have considered the effect of variations in ω-3 : ω-6 ratio, which may be important, and the ratio of EPA : DHA being administered. McLennan (2014) suggests that dietary fish tends to have a greater amount of DHA than EPA whereas many studies use supplements containing EPA > DHA, which means they don't replicate the usual dietary sources which tend to show multiple health benefits. In regard to cardiovascular benefits, this could be important, as the human myocardium selectively incorporates DHA over EPA. De (2011) further suggests that the great variation in dietary fish intakes between populations could be another influence, as people with low baseline levels of ω-3 EFAs are more likely to experience a range of benefits with supplementation compared to those who already have high dietary intakes. Finally, the role of mercury in fish needs to be taken into account as research suggests it counteracts the benefits of ω-3 PUFAS on sudden cardiac death and MI and possibly other outcomes. Unfortunately, few studies consider participants' mercury levels when analysing results (see Clinical note p. 330).

Prevention of morbidity and mortality of cardiovascular disease

Consuming fatty fish at least twice per week reduces the risk of developing cardiovascular disease. In addition, a reduced risk of all-cause mortality, cardiovascular death, sudden death, and myocardial infarction is often reported in population studies. This is largely based on research conducted over the last three decades, which has linked fish and fish oils to CV health. Benefits have also been reported in people with pre-existing CV disease. This association was first recognised when significantly lower death rates from acute MI were found among Greenland's Inuit population, despite only moderate differences between the Inuits' blood cholesterol levels and those of other populations (Holub 2002). A high dietary ω-3 LCPUFA intake in the form of marine mammals (seal, whale) and various fish was thought to be responsible for the protective effect (Bang et al 1980).

In 1989, results from the first large, randomised, clinical trial investigating the effects of fatty fish consumption on survival and risk of secondary MI confirmed a link to cardiovascular health (Burr et al 1989). The Diet and Reinfarction Trial (DART) found that a modest intake of two to three portions weekly of fatty fish reduced mortality in men who had previously experienced an MI and produced a relative reduction in total mortality of 29% during the 2-year follow-up, attributed mainly to a reduction in deaths from coronary heart disease (CHD). Increased consumption of fish (relative risk [RR] = 0.66 for five or more times per week) was further confirmed in the Nurses Study as significantly reducing risk in both CHD and CHD-related mortality independent of the cardiovascular status (Hu et al 2002).

Since then, 25 studies involving a total of 280,000 participants have identified an inverse association between fish consumption and morbidity or mortality from CHD. Blood levels of ω-3 fatty acids also appear to correlate inversely with death from cardiovascular causes and total mortality (De 2011). Similar findings were reached in another 2011 review which concluded that prospective observational studies and adequately powered RCTs provide strong concordant evidence of the benefits of ω-3 PUFA, most consistently for CHD mortality and sudden cardiac death (Mozaffarian & Wu 2011). More specifically, both epidemiological and interventional approaches have clearly demonstrated that individuals with a diet rich in fish (30–35 g/day) or supplemented with EPA and DHA (up to 665 mg/day) show a 30–50% reduction in CHD and CHD-related mortality compared to individuals who did not eat fish (Russo 2009). It appears that, while some level of primary CVD prevention occurs, secondary prevention effects are more notable.

These protective effects are achieved via multiple mechanisms which include lowering plasma TGs, resting heart rate and blood pressure and possibly also improvements to myocardial filling and efficiency and lowering inflammation. There is also evidence that ω-3-PUFAs have the ability to protect vascular endothelial cells by decreasing oxidative stress, halting atherosclerotic events and preventing vascular inflammatory and adhesion cascades (Balakumar & Taneja 2012). The effects have been succinctly described as both intrinsic and extrinsic. Intrinsic effects refer to effects on cardiac function dependent upon membrane incorporation at <1 g/day; extrinsic effects are indirect cardiac effects through vascular disease which require EPA + DHA doses >3 g/day (McLennan 2014).

Not surprisingly, in 2004, the US Food and Drug Administration (FDA) reported that it would allow products containing ω-3 fatty acids to claim that eating the product may reduce the risk of heart disease. The FDA based its decision on the wealth of scientific evidence that suggests a correlation between ω-3 fatty acids such as EPA and DHA and a reduced risk of coronary artery disease. The FDA subsequently approved ω-3 fatty acids as a treatment to reduce plasma TGs (Frishman et al 2009).

The largest study is known as the GISSI trial, which involved 11,324 survivors of MI, demonstrating that a low-dose fish oil supplement (1 g/

day) significantly reduced the risk of all-cause death, non-fatal MI and non-fatal stroke compared to vitamin E (300 mg/day) (Stone 2000). The group receiving ω-3 EFAs experienced a 15% reduction in the composite primary end point of death, non-fatal MI or non-fatal stroke ($P < 0.02$), with a 20% reduction in the rate of death from any cause ($P < 0.01$) and a 45% reduction in the rate of sudden death, an end point adjudicated by a committee whose members were unaware of the group assignments ($P < 0.001$), whereas the incidence of MI was not significantly reduced. Vitamin E provided no additional benefit. The effect on significantly reducing total mortality was evident early on, within 3 months (RR 0.59), and the rate of sudden death after only 4 months (RR 0.47) (De 2011). The effect was highly significant at 3.5 years, the end of the study, when it accounted for 59% of the ω-3 PUFA advantage in mortality. The reduction observed in all-cause mortality and in cardiovascular mortality resulted mainly from the prevention of sudden cardiac death by the ω-3 LCPUFAs. (Marchioli et al 2002).

The Japan Eicosapentaenoic Acid Lipid Intervention (JELIS) study followed afterwards and was a very large open-label study testing the long-term use of isolated EPA (1800 mg/day) in addition to statin therapy for the prevention of major coronary events in Japanese patients with hypercholesterolaemia. At a mean follow-up of 4.6 years a 19% relative reduction in major coronary events ($P = 0.01$) was observed with the combination therapy compared to statins alone and there was also a significant reduction in stroke (Tanaka et al 2008, Yokoyama 2009). Non-fatal coronary events were also significantly reduced in the EPA group, but sudden death from cardiac causes and death from coronary causes were not. Importantly, the reduction in events associated with EPA was similar in patients with and those without a history of coronary artery disease, but it was significant only in the former group, with a very low number needed to treat (De 2011). The JELIS study involved a total of 18,645 patients with total cholesterol levels ≥6.5 mmol/L who were randomly assigned to 1800 mg of EPA per day with statins or statins alone. A later analysis comparing people with good adherence (>80% of dose) to others found that, in good adherers with previous coronary artery disease, EPA substantially reduced the risk compared with statin alone (hazard ratio 0.55, $P < 0.014$). Furthermore, the clinical benefit of EPA + statin was significantly larger in patients with good adherence than in those with poor adherence ($P = 0.041$) (Origasa et al 2010). De Caterina (2011) suggests that the high dietary intake of fish amongst the Japanese population may account for the lack of effect on death from cardiac causes in this trial as a result of high baseline levels.

More recently, a 2013 double-blind study which compared fish oils (1 g/day) to placebo (olive oil) in people with multiple cardiovascular risk factors or atherosclerotic vascular disease but not MI found no change to the end points of cumulative rate of death, non-fatal MI and non-fatal stroke. Interestingly, at 1 year the event rate was found to be lower than anticipated so the researchers revised the primary end point to death from cardiovascular causes or admission to hospital for cardiovascular causes. They concluded that daily treatment with ω-3 fatty acids did not reduce cardiovascular mortality and morbidity as compared to the placebo group (Roncaglioni et al 2013). Unlike the GISSI trial, which used vitamin E as a comparator, this study used olive oil, a choice which must be questioned as it was obviously active because both groups experienced lower event rates than expected and, by the end of the trial, the overall cardiovascular risk profile had improved in both groups.

Unfortunately, the authors of these three studies did not report on the ratio of EPA:DHA used in their ω-3 EFA capsules or baseline EPA + DHA measures, thereby limiting further comparisons and interpretation.

Meta-analyses

In 2002, a high-quality systematic review of 11 RCTs on the effect of fish-based dietary or supplemental ω-3 fatty acids on cardiovascular morbidity and mortality in people with CHD found a strongly significant benefit (Bucher et al 2002); however, a 2006 Cochrane review came to a different conclusion (Hooper et al 2006). The review assessed 48 studies that compared at least 6 months of ω-3 fats (vegetable- and fish-based) with placebo or control and used data involving 36,913 participants. Meta-analysis of the studies assessing the effects of increased ω-3 fats on total mortality or combined cardiovascular events found strongly significant statistical heterogeneity. When randomised studies considered to be at medium or high risk of bias were removed, there was no significant effect of ω-3 fats on total mortality (RR 0.87; 95% confidence interval [CI] 0.73–1.03, with significant heterogeneity), whereas the cohort studies suggested significant protection (RR 0.65; 95% CI 0.48–0.88, no significant heterogeneity).

It is important to note that, until the publication of the DART-2 trial in 2003 (Burr et al 2003), the evidence showed that ω-3 from oily fish or supplements reduced the risks of fatal MI, sudden death and overall mortality among people with existing disease. Inclusion of the DART-2 trial in the Cochrane review had a major influence on the conclusion, as removing it produced RRs similar to those in the Bucher review (fatal MI: RR 0.70, 95% CI 0.54–0.91; sudden death: RR 0.68, 95% CI 0.42–1.10; overall mortality: RR 0.83, 95% CI 0.75–0.91). The DART-2 trial included 3114 men with stable angina and tested the hypothesis that the main benefit of ω-3 fat is derived from its antiarrhythmic action in the presence of chronic disease. Surprisingly, it did not confirm this, showing an excess of sudden and total cardiac deaths most clearly in participants taking fish oil capsules rather than eating oily fish. Authors of the Cochrane review report that something about the DART-2 study is different from the other included studies; however, further investigation has failed to clarify the issue. It is possible that, based on this latest review, the effect of ω-3 fats on CVD is smaller than previously thought or that effects in people who have had an MI are protective, but the effects in men with angina and no MI are not.

More recently, a 2013 meta-analysis of 11 double-blind RCTs for investigating the cardiovascular-preventive effects of ω-3 EFA supplementation (at least 1 g/day) for at least 1 year in patients with existing CVD concluded that there were significant protective effects observed for cardiac death (RR 0.68; 95% CI 0.56–0.83), sudden death (RR 0.67; 95% CI 0.52–0.87) and MI (RR 0.75; 95% CI 0.63–0.88) (Casula et al 2013). The review, involving 15,348 patients with a history of CVD, also found no statistically significant association for all-cause mortality (RR 0.89; 95% CI 0.78–1.02) and stroke (RR 1.31; 95% CI 0.90–1.90).

Congestive heart failure

The current body of evidence indicates modest benefits for fish oils in patients with chronic heart failure. One of the first major studies was published in 2005: this was a large epidemiology study of 4738 adults aged over 65 years that showed 20% reduced incidence of heart failure associated with the consumption of tuna or other broiled or baked fish (but not fried), delivering estimated intakes of ω-3 LC-PUFA as low as 260 mg/day (Mozaffarian et al 2005). In 2008, a large, double-blind, placebo-controlled trial involving 6975 patients with CHF New York Heart Association class II–IV (GISSI-HF) demonstrated that the use of 1 g of ω-3 EFAs was associated with a statistically significant 9% reduction in all-cause mortality and cardiac-cause hospitalisations, with specific improvement in the proportion of subjects with low (<40%) ejection fraction (Tavazzi et al 2008).

More recently, a large cohort trial which recruited 12,500 patients with multiple CVD risk factors reported a 35% reduction in hospitalisations from heart failure as the only physiologically and clinically meaningful outcome from treatment with 850 mg/day EPA + DHA over 5 years (Risk and Prevention Study Collaborative Group 2013). These outcomes reflect improved myocardial function in clinical populations.

EPA levels appear to be more important than DHA levels in patients with CHF, according to a 2013 study which tested baseline levels of ω-3 EFAs in patients with CHF enrolled in the GISSI-HF study. An average difference of 43% was seen between patients with the lowest and highest consumptions of dietary fish ($P < 0.0001$). Baseline EPA but not DHA was inversely related to C-reactive protein, pentraxin-3, adiponectin, natriuretic peptide and troponin levels and 3 months of supplementation raised their levels of PUFA by 43%, independently of dietary fish consumption. Additionally, increases in EPA levels were associated with decreased pentraxin-3. Importantly, low EPA levels were inversely related to total mortality in patients with chronic heart failure (Masson et al 2013).

Patients with implantable cardioverter defibrillators (ICDs)

At least three double-blind RCTs have been conducted in patients with ICDs exploring whether ω-3 EFAs can reduce ventricular tachycardia. In one study, a dose of 2.6 g/day of combined EPA and DHA demonstrated significantly increased 'time to first ICD event' for ventricular tachycardia, fibrillation or death (Jung et al 2008). However, not all studies have produced such positive results, with some suggesting that the ω-3 LCPUFAs are ineffective in this patient group (Jenkins et al 2008, Nair & Connolly 2008).

Clinical note — The ω-3 : ω-6 balance: implications in cardiovascular disease and cancer

In recent years, attention has been drawn to the importance of not only ω-3 fatty acid intake but also its relation to concurrent ω-6 fatty acid intake (Simopoulos 2008). When there is increased ω-3 LCPUFAs in the diet and in our bodies, a shift in AA metabolism occurs, which results in the production of metabolites that have beneficial effects on cardiovascular physiology and cancer incidence and promotion (Leaf 2002). For example, when EPA is available to compete with AA, production of thromboxane A_2 (a potent vasoconstrictor and platelet activator) is reduced and production of thromboxane B_3 results, which is only weakly active. Additionally, several forms of research implicate ω-6 PUFAs as stimulating processes that promote human cancer development and progression, whereas ω-3 LCPUFAs have the opposite effect (Weisburger 1997). Once again, competition with AA is thought to be involved, although several other protective mechanisms have also been identified. Overall, it seems that, in order to obtain maximal cardiovascular and chemopreventive benefits, intake of ω-3 LCPUFAs should be increased and intake of ω-6 PUFAs must be reduced.

It has been estimated that the ratio of ω-6 to ω-3 EFAs in the Western diet is some 15 : 1 to 20 : 1 or higher, whereas the optimal ratio appears to be closer to 2 : 1 or 1 : 1 (Leaf 2002, Simopoulos 1999, 2008).

Elevated triglyceride levels

DHA and EPA supplementation significantly reduces TG levels in both normo- and hyperlipidaemic individuals and is used as sole therapy in cases of elevation or as adjunctive therapy with cholesterol-lowering medication when indicated. ω-3 LCPUFAs reduce TG concentrations in a dose-dependent manner, with intakes approximating 4 g/day lowering serum TGs by 25–30% in hyperlipidaemic patients at baseline (Balk et al 2006, Din et al 2004, Jung et al 2008). Studies have emerged using ω-3 LCPUFA in combination with statins for the treatment of hyperlipidaemia (Barter & Ginsberg 2008). While LDL reduction is the primary target of statins, fish oil co-supplementation both enhances this action and produces additional beneficial changes in other lipid parameters (e.g. HDL, TGs and lipoprotein particle size).

Overall, it appears that the smallest amount of ω-3 LCPUFAs required to lower serum TG levels significantly is approximately 1 g/day, as provided by a fish diet (Weber & Raederstorff 2000).

In the United States in 2004, the FDA approved Omacor as an ω-3 fatty acid prescription for adults with severe hypertriglyceridaemia (>5.65 mmol/L). Each 1 g capsule contains 465 mg (46%) EPA ethyl esters, 375 mg (38%) DHA ethyl esters and approximately 60 mg (6%) other ω-3 fatty acid ethyl esters. The remaining part is mainly composed of ω-6 fatty acids along with 4 mg α-tocopherol (Nicholson et al 2013). In 2007 the name was changed to Lovaza. Evidence to support its use as an effective therapy for elevated TGs is derived from clinical trials involving patients suffering from dyslipidaemia, familial combined hyperlipidaemia and CHD and studies examining its effects in combination with statin therapy (atorvastatin, simvastatin). A dose of 4 g daily was used in all studies, taken as a single dose or as two capsules twice daily. The reduction in TGs ranged from 19.1% to 45%; however, changes in LDL and HDL cholesterol were inconsistent and often insignificant (Nicholson et al 2013).

Hypertension

According to three meta-analyses, fish oils have a significant but modest dose-dependent effect on blood pressure in hypertension (Geleijnse et al 2002, Miller et al 2014, Morris et al 1993). The DHA component is likely to have stronger effects than EPA.

The most recent meta-analysis analysed results from 70 RCTs and confirmed that fish oils significantly reduce blood pressure, most notably amongst hypertensive patients but also to a modest extent amongst normotensive people (Miller et al 2014). More specifically, compared with placebo, EPA + DHA reduced systolic blood pressure (−1.52 mmHg; 95% CI −2.25 to −0.79) and diastolic blood pressure (−0.99 mmHg; 95% CI −1.54 to −0.44). The strongest effects of EPA + DHA were observed amongst untreated hypertensive subjects (systolic blood pressure = −4.51 mmHg, 95% CI −6.12 to −2.83; diastolic blood pressure = −3.05 mmHg, 95% CI −4.35 to −1.74), although blood pressure also was lowered among normotensive subjects but to a very modest extent only (systolic blood pressure = −1.25 mmHg, 95% CI −2.05 to −0.46; diastolic blood pressure = −0.62 mmHg, 95% CI −1.22 to −0.02). Doses of at least 2 g/day are required to achieve the effect.

Prior to cardiac surgery

While many secondary CHD prevention trials require months of treatment before the benefits of ω-3 fatty acid supplementation are detected, a clinical study with cardiothoracic surgical patients suggests acute benefits within weeks. Calo et al (2005) conducted a randomised, placebo-controlled study which found that patients taking 2 g/day of fish oils for at least 5 days prior to coronary artery bypass grafting and until discharge had a significantly reduced incidence of postoperative atrial fibrillation. Specifically, 15.2% of patients receiving fish oils experienced postoperative atrial fibrillation compared with 33.3% of patients who were not taking the supplement. In addition, hospital length of stay was significantly reduced by 1 day. Except for a single case of allergy, no adverse effects were observed.

A meta-analysis of 21 high-quality RCTs and subgroup analysis of trials using intravenously administered fish oil-enhanced lipid emulsions found that active treatment was associated with a significant reduction in the length of hospital stay (mean = −2.14 days, 95% CI = −3.02 to −1.27), infections (odds ratio [OR] = 0.53, 95% CI = 0.35–0.81), alanine aminotransferase (mean = −6.35 U/L, 95% CI = −11.75 to −0.94), gamma-glutamyl transferase (mean = −11.01 U/L, 95% CI = −20.77 to −1.25) and total bilirubin (mean = −2.06 micromol/L, 95% CI = −3.6 to −0.52), as well as a non-significant change in mortality and postoperative medical cost (Li et al 2014).

Intermittent claudication

A 2007 Cochrane review of six studies involving 313 subjects suffering from intermittent claudication and treated with ω-3 LCPUFAs (typical dose 1.8 g EPA and 1.2 g DHA per day) over weeks to years found that, in spite of some haematological improvements (e.g. reduced viscosity), there were no demonstrable improvements in clinical outcomes (Sommerfield et al 2007). A more recent 2013 Cochrane systematic review came to a similar conclusion, stating that ω-3 fatty acids appear to have little benefit in this condition (Campbell et al 2013). A closer look at the studies reveals there is relatively little research looking at long-term use of fish oils as a stand-alone treatment for this indication and further research is required to better explore this potential treatment option.

Neurological effects

There is evidence that alterations to ω-3 fatty acid metabolism and the composition of the phospholipids in serum and membranes are involved in the pathogenesis of some neurological disorders (Ulbricht & Basch 2005). Also, several epidemiological studies have reported low-plasma DHA status in individuals with schizophrenia, ADHD, dyslexia, personality disorder, depression and bipolar disorder

Clinical note — Would you like methylmercury (MeHg) or organohalogen pollutants (OHPs) with that?

In aquatic environments, inorganic mercury, either naturally occurring or as an industrial byproduct (e.g. coal-fired power plants, waste incinerators), is converted into MeHg by microorganisms present in sediment or within the intestine of fish themselves (Dórea 2006). The MeHg, which is the most hazardous dietary form, then accumulates in the aquatic food chain, making fish the primary source of exposure for most individuals (FSANZ 2004). There has been increasing public awareness and concern regarding MeHg exposure secondary to fish consumption. This has been partly in response to the health warnings issued by Food Standards Australia and New Zealand (FSANZ) in March 2004 regarding maximal intake of selected fish species during pregnancy and childhood (Bambrick & Kjellstrom 2004). Interestingly, while the main public concern relates to neurodevelopmental toxicity, some data show a relationship between increasing MeHg exposure and CVD, in particular MI (Stern 2005). Postulated mechanisms include the oxidative stress and reactive oxygen species observed with in vitro exposures to MeHg, as well as impaired calcium homeostasis and kidney function.

MeHg concentrations in fish and shellfish species, which represent 80–90% of the mercury present, range from <0.1 ppm for shellfish, such as oysters and mussels, to multiple parts per million in large predatory fish such as tuna, marlin, swordfish and shark. Consequently, MeHg intake depends on the species and age of fish consumed, as well as the quantity eaten. Previous American data determined that adults consumed an average of 18 mcg MeHg/day, with 80–90% coming from fish and shellfish (Mahaffey et al 2004).

Inorganic mercury is readily excreted in the urine, whereas MeHg accumulates in erythrocytes across a wide range of exposures (Mahaffey et al 2004). Multiple international studies assessing MeHg exposure levels have revealed that approximately 10% of blood samples were high. American studies have identified populations at greater risk, among them a subpopulation consuming a substantial amount of fish in pursuit of health benefits. Blood MeHg analysis revealed blood mercury levels up to 90 mcg/L (Hightower & Moore 2003). This is concerning, given levels >5 mcg/L have been reported as potentially detrimental in women of child-bearing age.

Some researchers propose that the potentially cardiotoxic effects of MeHg are countered by the presence of the ω-3 oils also found within fish, and interestingly, there is some overlap between those species with the highest concentrations of both (Bambrick & Kjellstrom 2004). However, there is also concern that the converse is true and MeHg could counteract the health-giving benefits of fish.

While fish oil supplements are not a major source of mercury and as such there is no need to restrict their intake (Bays 2007, FSANZ 2004, Levine et al 2005, Schaller 2001), OHPs such as polychlorinated biphenyls, dioxins and organochlorine pesticides, widely used in flame retardants, pesticides, paints and electrical equipment prior to their ban in the 1980s in most countries (Bays 2007), may be present in these products. OHPs also accumulate in the aquatic food chain and are lipophilic carcinogens as well as being associated with other health risks (Dórea 2006). Data across the board confirm significantly higher OHPs in farmed fish and the supplements produced from these (Jacobs et al 1998, 2004) compared with wild harvested samples. These higher levels are attributed most consistently with use of contaminated feed (Domingo & Bocio 2007, Dórea 2006, Easton et al 2002, Jacobs et al 2002, Melanson et al 2005).

A UK study analysing the OHP content of 21 commercially available fish (both whole-body fish and cod liver oil) and vegetable oil dietary supplements in 2004 found that levels in all fish oil products had increased dramatically in brands tested 8 years previously (Jacobs et al 1998, 2004). For example, OHP levels in cod liver oils, which originally ranged from 0 to 13 ng/g, were found to contain 15–34 ng/g in the most recent analysis. The findings of an American study contrast with this, however, with OHP levels below the level of detection in five over-the-counter fish oil products (Melanson et al 2005). There are no published data on Australian products.

There remains little doubt that the discriminating inclusion of fish is an important part of a healthy diet. Recent research suggests that high exposure to mercury may reduce the benefits of long-chain ω-3 PUFA on sudden cardiac death (Virtanen et al 2012). It also reduces the benefits of fish oils on preventing MI, according to a Scandinavian study involving over 500 volunteers. It was identified that a small increase in fish consumption (increasing serum PUFA by 1%) would prevent 7% of MI, despite a small increase in mercury (Wennberg et al 2012). However, the higher the hair–mercury, the more the benefits on preventing MI were counteracted. Thus, MI risk may be reduced by the consumption of fish high in PUFAs and low in methylmercury.

(BD) (Riediger et al 2009). As a result, there has been much interest in understanding the effects of supplemental ω-3 fatty acids in neurological development, cognitive function, behavioural problems and other neurological conditions.

Cognitive function

Low-serum DHA level is considered a significant risk factor for the development of Alzheimer's dementia (Conquer et al 2000). Additionally, both DHA and total ω-3 LCPUFAs are significantly lower in cognitively impaired but non-demented people and people with other dementias. One of the first interventional studies was a small RCT of 4.3 g/day DHA in 20 elderly nursing-home residents, assessing the efficacy of fish oil in the treatment of vascular dementia. DHA supplementation resulted in a small improvement in dementia-rating scores within 3 months of treatment (Terano et al 1994).

Dietary factors influence the association between physical activity and cognitive performance. Executive and memory functions were investigated in 344 participants. High levels of DHA relative to AA mitigated the effects of lower levels of physical activity on cognitive performance. The combination of higher AA:DHA ratios with lower physical activity was associated with markedly decreased performance. In contrast, there were no significant associations between serum AA:DHA ratio levels and cognitive function (Leckie et al 2014).

The results from numerous animal studies, demonstrating neuroprotection and slowing of neurodegeneration from the ω-3 LCPUFAs, appear promising (Hashimoto et al 2005, Mucke & Pitas 2004); however, more clinical trials are required to determine the clinical implications of these positive findings.

Alzheimer's dementia

Epidemiological studies have shown that dementia and CVD may share several common risk factors, including high intakes of dietary total fat, high saturated fat, high ω-6:ω-3 fatty acid ratio and low fish intake (Riediger et al 2009). Considering ω-3 fatty acids possess anti-inflammatory properties and inflammatory markers have been located in the brain of patients with Alzheimer's disease, it seems reasonable to suggest that ω-3 fatty acids may delay the onset of Alzheimer's disease by reducing brain inflammatory state. This may be one of the reasons behind prevention of Alzheimer's disease/dementia by adequate DHA/EPA intake suggested by the Framingham heart study (Kalmijn 2000, Kalmijn et al 2004), the Rotterdam study (Kalmijn et al 1997) and the 2003 prospective study by Morris et al (2003), although later follow-up of the Rotterdam study found no association (Engelhart et al 2002).

In 2005, a review of the evidence prepared for the US Department of Health and Human Services concluded that there is a significant correlation between fish consumption and reduced incidence of Alzheimer's disease. Total ω-3 LCPUFA and DHA consumption correlated with this risk reduction; however, ALA and EPA did not (MacLean et al 2004). A Cochrane review came to a similar conclusion, reporting that there is a growing body of evidence from biological, observational and epidemiological studies to suggest a protective effect of ω-3 LCPUFAs against dementia; however, further research is required before firm conclusions can be made (Lim et al 2006). A study investigating supplementation with 1.8 g/day of fish oils over 24 weeks in subjects with either mild to moderate Alzheimer's disease or mild cognitive impairment yielded greatest benefits in individuals suffering only mild cognitive impairment (Chiu et al 2008). Further studies using higher doses, larger sample sizes and only subjects mildly affected by the condition are recommended.

Brain trauma injury

Brain trauma injury is characterised by significant neuroinflammation. Acute administration of ω-3 PUFA after injury and dietary exposure before or after injury have the potential to improve neurological outcomes in traumatic brain injury and spinal cord injury. The mechanisms include decreased neuroinflammation and oxidative stress, neurotrophic support and activation of cell survival pathways (Michael-Titus & Priestley 2014). A paper by Sears et al (2013) reported a case where ω-3 supplementation was given (10.8 g of EPA and 5.4 g of DHA) in two divided doses on a daily basis. The patient was a 26-year-old male exposed to a carbon monoxide and methane gas atmosphere for 41 hours following an explosion at a coal mine. When rescued, his breathing was laboured, and he had significant neurological, cardiovascular and renal dysfunction (being the classic symptoms of carbon monoxide poisoning), dehydration and rhabdomyolysis. Magnetic resonance imaging scans indicated significant cytotoxic cell injury and demyelination. He emerged from the coma after 3 weeks. He spent the next 2 months in a rehabilitation facility, at which time the ω-3 fatty acid supplementation was continued for another 2 months. He steadily improved over time. He was released into home care nearly 3 months after the explosion. Six years after the explosion he was functionally normal and had fathered two young children (Sears et al 2013). Although this is a single case report, ω-3 PUFAs show potential in brain trauma injury and are worthy of further investigation.

Autism spectrum disorder (ASD)

Two studies have found evidence of low levels of EPA and DHA in autistic patients (Curtis & Patel 2008). A moderately sized epidemiological study of women with children with ASD (n = 317) revealed that pregnant mothers with the lowest ω-3 intake had a significant increase in offspring ASD risk as compared with the remaining distribution (n = 17,728; RR = 1.53). The data obtained from online survey research from 861 parents of autistic children also suggest that consumption of a formula devoid in DHA and AA during infancy is associated with an OR of 4.41 for autism generally and 12.96 for regressive autism, compared with breastfed infants (Schultz et al 2006). However, the heavy reliance upon self-reporting in addition to the non-random sample leaves these results open to scrutiny. Given all this epidemiological evidence, surprisingly few studies have investigated the effects of ω-3 LCPUFAs in autistic individuals. One study conducted in a sample of 12 children, employing 5 g/day of ω-3

LCPUFAs over 6 weeks, produced significant remission of hyperactivity (Amminger et al 2007); however another using comparable doses in adults failed to demonstrate efficacy on any behavioural parameter (Politi et al 2008). The paucity of ω-3 studies in ASD is striking and has been commented on by reviewers (Frye et al 2013), including the Cochrane review which failed to find a single study that met their inclusion criteria in this area (Tan et al 2012).

While theories abound about the potential role of aberrant LCPUFA metabolism in ASD (Das 2013) as an explanation for the higher incidence in boys, secondary to hormonal differences in fat metabolism (Field 2014), other reviewers argue there isn't a plausible biological mechanism by which ω-3 could be implicated (Prior & Galduroz 2012).

Pregnancy, breastfeeding and infants

The three big focus points in ω-3 research for improved offspring health are in the areas of reduced adulthood obesity, prevention of atopy in at-risk individuals (≥1 atopic primary family member) and improved cognitive outcomes.

Animal studies suggest that changes in peri- and early postnatal ω-3 intake can affect the development of adulthood obesity (Bagley et al 2013); however, attempts to replicate these findings in humans have so far produced negative findings in both early infancy and even adolescence (Hauner et al 2013, Rytter et al 2011).

Prevention of atopy in at-risk infants

Cross-sectional studies measuring breast milk ω-3 content in new mothers found an inverse relationship between LCPUFA levels and positive skin prick test responses in infants at 12 months (Soto-Ramirez et al 2012), while maternal and infant phospholipid ω-3 were inversely correlated with non-atopic persistent infant wheezing and positive skin prick test at 6 years old (Pike et al 2012). These later cross-sectional studies suggest ≤50% reduced incidence.

Pregnancy ω-3 interventions in high-risk mothers for allergic offspring have demonstrated a protective effect against immunoglobulin E (IgE) sensitisation; however, an absolute reduction in atopic incidence is less certain (Dunstan et al 2008, Furuhjelm et al 2011, Noakes et al 2012, Storro et al 2010). There have been several RCTs with positive findings, such as a significantly reduced incidence of food allergy (2% vs 15%) and atopic eczema (8% vs 24%) in 1-year-old infants whose mothers consumed high-dose ω-3 (1.6 g/day EPA and 1.1 g/day DHA) from week 25 to 3–4 months postpartum compared with those receiving placebo (Furuhjelm et al 2008). A follow-up study of this original cohort found the decreased incidence was sustained at 2-years-old and higher maternal and infant ω-3 levels were associated with less IgE-associated disease and reduced severity of the allergic phenotype (Furuhjelm et al 2011). One of the strengths of this study was the comprehensive diagnosis of food allergy — a combination of clinical picture assessment, IgE antibody assays and skin prick test.

A large Mexican RCT of 869 pregnant women administered 400 mg/day DHA from the third trimester to delivery observed a significant protective effect of DHA treatment on respiratory symptoms (phlegm and nasal discharge) following adjustment for potential confounders, among infants of atopic mothers (Escamilla-Nunez et al 2014). Interestingly, however, there was no significant difference in cord blood IgE levels between the treatment and placebo groups (Hernandez et al 2013). A large Norwegian study adopted a multipronged approach to reducing asthma in offspring, advising pregnant women in the treatment group to increase their ω-3 intake, stop parental smoking and reduce exposure to damp environments during the first 2 years of life (Dotterud et al 2013). The combined effect was a significantly reduced incidence of asthma compared with controls but only in girls (OR 0.41).

One of the longest longitudinal studies in this area to date is a 16-year follow-up investigation of offspring born to women supplemented with 2.7 g/day fish oils from week 30 until delivery as part of an RCT (Olsen et al 2008). Children born to mothers in the fish oil group demonstrated a 63% reduction in asthma diagnoses and 87% reduction in the prevalence of allergic asthma. In line with these findings, it has been suggested that longer follow-up may be necessary to accurately ascertain the impact of ω-3 interventions on offspring allergy incidence (Almqvist et al 2007, Marks et al 2006).

In regard to infants' diets, the results of a prospective, longitudinal study from Sweden of 4921 infants' diets, exposure patterns and eczema diagnoses have found a protective effect for early introduction of fish (Alm et al 2009). Infants introduced to fish prior to 9 months of age demonstrated reduced rates of eczema at 1 year (OR 0.76). This finding flies in the face of previous primary prevention strategies whereby many child health authorities have encouraged delaying the introduction of fish in order to reduce allergy.

Cognitive development

Although numerous studies of mothers and infants have demonstrated that consuming greater amounts of EFAs had a positive effect on the subsequent cognitive development and IQ of their young offspring (Cohen et al 2005, Helland et al 2003, Williams et al 2001), the Evidence Report/Technology Assessment prepared for the Agency of Healthcare Research and Quality of the US Department of Health and Human Services concludes that, based on the small number of current well-designed studies, there is no conclusive evidence of any benefit (Moher 2005). The report observes that studies demonstrating a positive relationship between ω-3 LCPUFAs and cognition are those that assessed children under 1 year of age, whereas in studies of older children a significant statistical relationship is not sustained. Despite the conclusions of this report, several studies with longer follow-up periods have demonstrated both improved eye and hand coordination (Dunstan et al 2008) and IQ at 4 years old (Helland et al 2003), but not at 7 years old (Helland et al 2008). The latter is an Australian study, following up on 98 women who were supplemented with 2.2 g DHA and 0.1 g EPA per day or placebo from 20 weeks' gestation. Children's eye and hand coordination scores correlated with ω-3 LCPUFA levels in cord blood red blood cells (RBC) and inversely correlated with ω-6 LCPUFA at 2½ years of age.

Other studies investigating fish oil supplementation during lactation have produced mixed findings, including possible negative outcomes only in male offspring (impaired working memory and inhibitory control, increased diastolic blood pressure at 7 years old). However, these figures all come from the same small study (n = 122) of Danish mothers administered either 1.5 g/day of fish or olive oil for 4 months during lactation and these conclusions were based on only 36 children in the treatment group who were assessed at 7 years old (Asserhoj et al 2009, Cheatham et al 2011). Therefore, additional research is necessary before any firm conclusions can be drawn.

According to the WHO and Food and Agriculture Organization (FAO), pregnant women should take at least 2.6 g of ω-3 EFAs, incorporating 100–300 mg of DHA, daily to look after the needs of the fetus (Bambrick & Kjellstrom 2004). Postnatal deficiencies have been associated with reduced visual acuity, poor neurodevelopment and ill effects on behaviour. Breastfed infants generally receive sufficient DHA if the maternal diet is adequate, but it is not known whether formula-fed infants receive adequate amounts if their formula does not contain PUFAs.

Prevention and treatment of postpartum depression (PPD)

The rationale for considering ω-3 EFAs as potential risk reducers in PPD relates to consistent evidence of maternal DHA depletion and increasing inflammation throughout pregnancy. However, in spite of evidence of decreased DHA in the frontal cortex correlated with lower serotonin in pregnant animals (Chen et al 2012) and several international cross-sectional epidemiological studies suggesting that higher seafood intake (reflected especially in higher breast milk DHA content) is protective against PPD (Jans et al 2010, Kendall-Tackett 2010), interventional studies in humans have not produced consistently positive findings.

A large Australian study of 2399 pregnant women randomised to DHA-rich fish oil (800 mg DHA and 100 mg EPA/day) or placebo found a non-significant reduction in the percentage of women with high levels of depressive symptoms overall and in the subgroup of women with previously diagnosed depression (Makrides et al 2010). Criticisms of this study include the lack of dietary ω-3 assessment, the inclusion of individuals with depression at baseline, the use of self-rated depression scales only and the reliance on high-dose DHA with nominal EPA. A systematic review published the same year, which didn't include the trial by Makrides, examined seven studies of EPA/DHA administration in pregnancy for the prevention of

Clinical note — What determines infants' ω-3 inheritance?

Many expectant mothers are aware that one 'breast is best' argument relates to an improved fatty-acid profile in breast milk compared with formula milk. Adding to this is a study by Meldrum et al (2012), investigating the efficacy of direct high-dose fish oil supplementation of infants from birth to 6 months, which found that even in supplemented infants, the ω-3 content of the breast milk was the stronger determinant of infant RBC DHA, in spite of total daily exposure being approximately a third of that provided by the supplement. While this result may be the consequence of methodological error, there is speculation that this underscores the superior bioavailability of LCPUFAs in breast milk.

Consistent evidence points to a correlation between ω-3 intake during pregnancy (dietary or supplements) and breast milk ω-3 concentrations (Urwin et al 2012), but what else influences the infant's ω-3 inheritance? Breast milk DHA levels are at their highest in the early postpartum period and progressively decline over the first month of lactation (Weiss et al 2013). However, other variables that dictate how much is available to begin with include birth order (levels decline with each subsequent pregnancy) and multiple versus single pregnancies (Al et al 2000). Additionally, there is growing interest in genetic variations with the FADS1/2 gene clusters which code for the desaturases and how this impacts on ω-3 status of mother and infant. Molto Puigment (2010) found that, while plasma DHA levels rose in mothers regardless of genotype, their breast milk DHA changed. Women homozygous for a mutation, with reduced efficacy of these enzymes, demonstrated limited incorporation into breast milk. The results of another interesting but very small study suggest that women with atopic eczema had lower ω-3 breast milk levels compared with non-atopic mothers and even atopic mothers who were free from eczema, in spite of comparable intake (Johansson et al 2011). The key take-home message currently seems to be that, while good ω-3 intake during pregnancy and lactation is sensible, intake and breast milk concentrations will not perfectly correlate due to a range of other variables we are just starting to identify.

PPD (four studies sampled healthy individuals and in three studies individuals were depressed at baseline) and found the pooled mean effect size was non-significant and indicated no or a small pre- to posttreatment decrease in perinatal depression.

More recently, 126 women in early pregnancy at high risk of depression were randomised in a trial to receive EPA-rich or DHA-rich fish oil or placebo throughout pregnancy. While fatty-acid analyses revealed increased ω-3 levels in the DHA-rich group particularly, demonstrating an inverse relationship between DHA levels and depression-rating scores evident at 34–36 weeks, overall there were no statistically significant differences in the mean depression scores among the groups at entry or at any of the study visits and no statistically significant differences among the groups in the proportion of women who started antidepressant medications (Mozurkewich et al 2013). In summary, these findings have led researchers, and the latest Cochrane review on nutritional prevention of PPD, to currently conclude that fish oil is not effective (Miller et al 2013). In spite of these findings, Goren and Tewksbury (2011) reiterate the numerous benefits of adequate DHA during pregnancy (e.g. fetal neurocognitive development, reduced cardiovascular risks) and encourage pregnant women to continue supplementing high-dose DHA during the third trimester.

Preventing depression

After adjusting for several confounding factors, Kamphuis et al (2006) reported that every 50 mg/day increase in ω-3 fatty acid intake was correlated with a 7% risk reduction of depressive symptoms in elderly men. It has been suggested that the balance between ω-6 and ω-3 EFA influences the metabolism of biogenic amines, an interaction that may be relevant to changes in mood and behaviour (Bruinsma & Taren 2000). In several observational studies, low concentrations of ω-3 LCPUFAs predicted impulsive behaviours and greater severity of depression. Additionally, early research by Horrobin and Bennett (1999) revealed that almost all studies on depression have found increased prostaglandin G_2 series or related thromboxanes and there is evidence that the older antidepressants (monoamine oxidase inhibitors and tricyclic antidepressants) either inhibit prostaglandin synthesis or are powerful antagonists of their actions. The findings of a number of studies showing a correlation between low erythrocyte ω-3 EFAs and suicide attempts go one step further. One demonstrated an eightfold difference in suicide attempt risk between the lowest and highest RBC EPA quartiles (Huan et al 2004). Belgian researchers have also speculated about seasonal variations in EFA status that correlate with seasonal patterns of suicide (De Vriese et al 2004); however, studies on larger populations of depressed people are required to confirm this link.

Several international cross-sectional studies have found a correlation between ω-3 intake and rates of depression, including that depression rates are 10 times higher in countries with limited seafood intake and PPD 10–50 times higher (Kendall-Tackett 2010). In countries with traditionally high seafood consumption, such as Finland, individuals who consume smaller amounts were found to have a 31% higher chance of developing depression, even when other risk factors were controlled for. Noaghiul and Hibbeln (2003) postulated that countries where individuals consumed less than ≈ 450–680 g of seafood per person per week demonstrated the highest rates of affective disorders.

Superior epidemiological evidence comes from longitudinal rather than cross-sectional studies of ω-3 intake in healthy individuals and subsequent depression diagnoses. Four such trials were included in a recent review (Sanhueza et al 2013). While two of these did not find any association between fish consumption and depression incidence, the other two found that an inverse relationship was only seen with intermediate intake which equated to ≈0.16% of the total energy intake or 1.17 g/day (energy-adjusted) and produced a significant risk reduction of 35–40% in depression. The loss of apparent protection with the highest fish intake remains unexplained, possibly an issue of excess exposure to the contaminants found in certain fish (see Would you like methylmercury (MeHg) or organohalogen pollutants (OHPs) with that?). However, it is noteworthy that a similar phenomenon was evident with ω-3 supplementation (Peet & Horrobin 2002).

Treating depression

In spite of widespread epidemiological data correlating ω-3 status with a range of depressive disorders, including major depression, PPD and seasonal affective disorder, and extensive evidence of the role of inflammation in depression (Kendall-Tackett 2010), there are relatively few interventional studies and those published are typically compromised by small sample size and possess heterogeneous designs, particularly with regard to the composition and dose of the intervention itself (Grenyer et al 2007). More recent reviews have focused on eliminating the confounding issue of variable ω-3 forms and dose. These reviews (Martins 2009, Ross et al 2007, Sublette et al 2011) appear to have reached a consensus regarding the superiority of EPA over DHA in depressed individuals. Sublette et al (2011) in particular postulate that interventions providing >60% EPA and a minimum of 200–2200 mg EPA in excess of DHA were significantly more effective. Although DHA is more prevalent in the brain and possesses actions that would suggest it would be helpful in depression, several theories are proposed why this doesn't translate into clinical findings, including that oral DHA supplementation has not conclusively been shown to increase brain DHA levels. Secondly, it is EPA that directly competes with AA for conversion to eicosanoids and therefore may have the most relevant anti-inflammatory action.

Trials published since these reviews include a small, double-blind randomised study (n = 66) of mildly depressed elderly individuals (mean age 80 years) administered low-dose EPA and DHA (180 mg and 120 mg/day, respectively) over 6 months to Iranian nursing-home patients with extremely low dietary ω-3, e.g. three fish meals over 6 months. Using self-assessment via the Geriatric Depression Scale-15, 40.7% of subjects in the treatment group demonstrated improved mood compared with only 27.6% of placebo, which was a significant difference (Tajalizadekhoob et al 2011). In young healthy adults (aged 18–35 years) also with low baseline ω-3 intake, EPA-rich (EPA 300 mg and DHA 200 mg/day) and DHA-rich (450 mg and EPA 90 mg/day) supplements were compared with placebo for improving cognition and, as a secondary assessment, mood, via the Depression Anxiety Stress Scale and Bond-Lager visual analogue (Jackson et al 2012). Treatment with fish oils at these doses failed to produce any mood or cognitive benefits, which the authors argue may be illustrative that baseline ω-3 levels need to be lower and functional impairment evident in order to benefit from fish oil supplementation. However, the results could also be explained by inadequate unopposed EPA according to the work of Sublette et al (2011). Most recently, a randomised double-blind placebo-controlled study of 152 patients preparing for interferon treatment revealed that those treated with EPA 2 weeks before interferon treatment started reported significantly lower rates of depression (10%) compared with both DHA-supplemented individuals (28%) and subjects taking placebo (30%) (Su et al 2014).

Bipolar disorder

Interest in the role and therapeutic potential of ω-3 in BD is substantial and has moved beyond the epidemiological associations to more sophisticated investigations, i.e. fatty-acid levels present in specific brain regions of BD sufferers, genetic variations in expression of LCPUFA metabolic enzymes (Igarashi et al 2010). Proposed mechanisms of action include their capacity to increase cell membrane fluidity (altering receptor numbers and dampening signal transduction pathways), reduce brain inflammation, antagonise phosphoinositide protein kinase C and, to a small extent, inhibit reuptake of serotonin and dopamine, which would all be beneficial in BD depression (Sarris et al 2011). Additionally, some researchers have found a correlation between individuals' LCPUFA levels and BD severity (DHA and depression; EPA and mania) (Clayton et al 2009). It is also noteworthy that many of the medications prescribed in BD (e.g. lithium, valproate) reduce turnover of AA and therefore are postulated to be anti-inflammatory (Goren & Tewksbury 2011).

Poor methodological quality as well as heterogeneous design have plagued ω-3 interventional studies, however, as illustrated by the Cochrane review which based their negative conclusion on the results of one study (Frangou et al 2006), while >23 others failed to meet their inclusion criteria (Montgomery & Richardson 2008).

A broader review by Sarris et al (2011) notes that, of nine adjunctive ω-3 trials in BD, seven were randomised, double-blind and placebo-controlled and four of these demonstrated a statistically significant positive effect on reducing depression. While generally ω-3 oils have not demonstrated significantly superior results to placebo in the management of mania, Sarris et al comment that all studies are in favour of fish oils over placebo in this respect; however, small sample sizes could explain the lack of statistically significant findings. Again, particular note is made of the differences in ω-3 preparations, which range from high-dose EPA alone, EPA : DHA blends, to flaxseed oil and with dosage variations, e.g. up to 3400 mg DHA and 6000 mg ethyl-EPA. One of the open-label studies also included by Sarris is a small Australian study (n = 18) of juvenile BD, in which subjects stable on pharmaceutical medications then took ω-3 (360 mg/day EPA 1560 mg/day DHA) for 6 weeks, producing a 50% reduction in depression ratings, and again a non-significant improvement in mania (Clayton et al 2009).

Addiction/abstinence

A study in polysubstance abusers (Buydens-Branchey et al 2008), using 2.25 g EPA and 500 mg DHA administered over 3 months to 24 individuals, resulted in decreased anger and anxiety scores, corresponding with plasma increases in both EPA and DHA. A randomised double-blind placebo-controlled study of abstinent alcoholics revealed that 3 weeks of supplementation with fish oil (60 mg/day EPA and 252 mg/day DHA) produced lower basal salivary cortisol levels compared with placebo, accompanied by lower depression and anxiety ratings. At the end of intervention, amplitude and duration of stress-evoked cortisol response did not differ between groups; however, the peak of cortisol response was temporally anticipated in supplemented subjects (Barbadoro et al 2013).

An animal study which injected rats with amphetamine and fed subgroups different dietary fats (soybean, hydrogenated vegetable fats or fish oil) found that fish oils largely attenuated the detrimental effects on brain structure, mitochondrial activity and vitamin C levels typically seen with chronic amphetamine exposure. The researchers hypothesise that this action could be similar to the protective effects of ω-3 oils in other forms of mania (Trevizol et al 2001).

Aggressive and impulsive behaviour

Animal studies demonstrate increased aggression test scores in rats and other species deprived of ω-3 LCPUFAs during either gestation or early life. This has been linked to deficits in neuronal arborisation and multiple indices of synaptic pathology, including deficits in serotonin and mesocorticolimbic dopamine neurotransmission (Hibbeln et al 2006, Liu & Raine 2006). Human data also support this proposition, whereby preterm delivery is associated with deficits in fetal cortical DHA accrual, and children/adolescents born preterm exhibit deficits in

F

cortical grey-matter maturation, neurocognitive deficits, particularly in the realm of attention, impulsivity and increased risk of ADHD and schizophrenia (Hibbeln et al 2006, McNamara & Carlson 2006). While there is strong support for the biological basis for a relationship between ω-3 LCPUFAs and aggressive and impulsive behaviour (Garland & Hallahan 2006), the results of interventional studies have been somewhat mixed.

DHA has been used to reduce aggressive behaviour in children and adolescents. One placebo-controlled study of 42 college students showed that DHA supplementation (1.5–1.8 g/day) prevented an increase in aggression towards others at times of mental stress (Hamazaki et al 1996); however, there was no effect on aggressive behaviour under non-stressful conditions (Hamazaki et al 1998). A 2005 randomised, placebo-controlled clinical trial looked at 166 Japanese children aged 9–12 years administered 3.6 g DHA and 840 mg per week via both supplements and fortified foods over a period of 3 months (Itomura et al 2005). While reducing aggression in girls, concomitant with improved EPA:AA RBC ratios, the same effect was not evident in boys. Impulsivity amongst female subjects was also significantly reduced in the treatment group.

Other small successful studies for anger reduction have been conducted in abstaining polysubstance abusers (2.25 g EPA, 500 mg DHA administered over 3 months) (Buydens-Branchey et al 2008), borderline personality disorder (1 g/day ethyl EPA over 8 weeks) (Zanarini et al 2003) and borderline personality disorder in adolescents at high risk of psychosis (1.2 g/day ω-3 over 12 weeks) (Amminger et al 2013). In a separate study, however, individuals exhibiting recurrent self-harm, scores for impulsivity, aggression and hostility remained unchanged, in spite of decreased depression and suicidality scores, when treated with 1.2 g EPA and 900 mg DHA per day over 12 weeks (Hallahan et al 2007). New research has found a relationship between AA/EPA + DHA RBC ratios and individuals' vulnerability to anger with interferon treatment. Marked anger and irritability are common adverse effects of interferon that can compromise compliance and success of the treatment, therefore co-administration of ω-3 LCPUFA may represent an effective way to reduce the likelihood of this occurrence (Lotrich et al 2013).

Anxiety

In spite of consistent animal evidence that decreased ω-3 LCPUFA leads to chronic mild stress-induced anxiety (Vinot et al 2011), limited well-designed studies have been conducted in patients with anxiety disorders as a stand-alone diagnosis rather than a comorbidity, e.g. BD, substance abuse (Goren & Tewksbury 2011).

Animal studies of both supplemental ω-3 during the perinatal period and, more recently, adulthood confirm a moderate anxiolytic action (Vinot et al 2011) and new mechanisms such as improved neural plasticity and endocannibinoid activity have been elucidated (Larrieu et al 2011). A placebo-controlled, double-blind 12-week RCT compared ω-3 (2085 mg EPA and 348 mg DHA) supplementation with placebo on proinflammatory cytokine production and anxiety symptoms in medical students (n = 68) for 12 weeks. ω-3 supplementation produced a 20% reduction in anxiety symptoms (P = 0.04), as measured by the Beck Anxiety Inventory, and a 14% decrease in stimulated interleukin-6 production (P = 0.04). ω-3 PUFA also had a borderline effect on serum tumour necrosis factor-alpha (TNF-α) (7% decrease, P = 0.06). At the completion of the study, plasma levels of EPA and DHA were approximately sixfold and ½-fold higher compared to levels prior to supplementation. The levels of EPA and DHA in peripheral blood mononucleated cells (PBMCs) also increased but were not as dramatic in increase: threefold and 1/3-fold, respectively, for EPA and DHA. Supplementation with the placebo oil resulted in no changes of either plasma or PBMC EPA and DHA. There was no significant change in depressive symptoms (Kiecolt-Glaser et al 2011). Further human studies of anxiety disorders are needed to confirm these findings.

Attention-deficit hyperactivity disorder

It has been reported that many children with ADHD have EFA deficiency (mainly ω-3 fatty acid), with a high correlation between severity of symptoms and severity of deficiency (Yehuda et al 2005). Deficiency may be due to insufficient dietary intake or inefficient conversion of EFA to LCPUFAs. Several studies have investigated the effects of supplemental fatty acids in ADHD with mixed results; however, interpretation of findings is difficult because of the use of different treatments, measurements and subject selection (Richardson & Puri 2000). Although the evidence is hampered by small samples and other methodological issues, at this time ω-3 LCPUFAs do not appear to be effective in ADHD (Goren & Tewksbury 2011).

Schizophrenia

Schizophrenic patients have been frequently found to have low LCPUFAs (Peet 2003, 2006). Some studies have found higher saturated and monounsaturated fat in red cells at the expense of LCPUFAs of both the ω-3 and ω-6 families (Kemperman et al 2006). The evidence linking LCPUFAs with this condition was so persuasive it generated the 'membrane phospholipid theory of schizophrenia'; however, while most evidence points to increased LCPUFA turnover, a consensus on the exact nature of this disturbance is still pending (Atker et al 2012). Interestingly, an in vitro study of cells exposed to H_2O_2 as a model of the high oxidative stress seen in schizophrenia found that respiridone and fish oils together reduced lipid peroxidation and free Ca^{2+} while simultaneously increasing glutathione, glutathione peroxidase and vitamin C levels (Altinkilic 2010).

A key researcher in the area of EFAs and psychiatry also points to the significant overlap between core features of the metabolic syndrome and established physiological aberrations evident in schizophrenia, including visceral adiposity, insulin resistance, dyslipidaemias, increased inflammatory markers and reduced ω-3 LCPUFAs in cell membranes (Peet 2006). Importantly, these similarities predate the introduction of the novel antipsychotics, which are known to be diabesogenic. Schizophrenic patients demonstrate a two- to fourfold increased risk of type 2 diabetes mellitus (T2DM) and two to three times greater risk of coronary artery disease mortality, which cannot be entirely related to secondary lifestyle behaviours.

In a 2003 review, four out of five placebo-controlled, double-blind trials of EPA in the adjunctive treatment of schizophrenia have produced positive results with a typical effective dose of 2 g/day of EPA for a minimum of 3 months (Peet 2003). An updated Cochrane review of six studies, involving 353 subjects, has similarly concluded that ethyl-EPA may exert positive effects when added to standard medication; however, more large well-designed, conducted and reported studies are needed (Joy et al 2006). Since this time another systematic review has reached similar conclusions (Akter et al 2012), with small sample sizes (n = 16–122), short intervention duration (6–16 weeks) and heterogeneous LCPUFA interventions hampering more robust findings. The authors note, however, with suggestive positive effects in this cohort and an excellent safety profile, many clinicians may opt to add ω-3 into their schizophrenic patient management.

A new area of research opening up is psychosis prevention in high-risk individuals. One randomised double-blind placebo-controlled study of 81 adolescents classified as being at ultra-high risk of psychosis, treated with either fish oils (480 mg/day DHA, 700 mg/day EPA, 7.6 mg vitamin E) or placebo over 12 weeks, found that, while 27.5% of the control group transitioned to their first psychotic episode, only 4.9% of those taking fish oil did (Amminger et al 2010). Impressively, these benefits were sustained following cessation of the intervention throughout the year of follow-up. Early treatment of psychosis is considered to be a major determinant of overall outcomes and, compared to the risks associated with long-term antipsychotic medications, ω-3 supplements are an appealing alternative.

Cancer

It is well established that dietary fat has an influence on human cancer development and progression. Several forms of research implicate ω-6 PUFAs as catalysts, whereas ω-3 LCPUFAs have the opposite effect and have been shown to inhibit development and progression (Leitzmann et al 2004, Weisburger 1997). Therefore, it is the ratio of ω-3 to ω-6 PUFAs intake that appears to be an important factor influencing cancer incidence and progression.

This observation is supported by both animal and epidemiological studies. The largest to date involved 24 European countries and identified a significant inverse correlation with fish and fish oil consumption, when expressed as a proportion of total or animal fat, for both male and female colorectal cancer and for female breast cancer (Caygill et al 1996). Importantly, the protective effects were only detected in countries with a high animal fat intake, suggesting that fish oil protects against the promotional effects of animal fat in carcinogenesis.

Breast and prostate cancers

Increased intake of ω-3 fatty acids associated with decreased ω-6, resulting in a higher ω-3/ω-6 ratio compared with the western diet, are inversely associated with breast cancer risk, as shown by Yang et al in their meta-analysis (de Lorgeril and Salen 2014). A 2003 review found that overall it remains unclear as to whether dietary fish or fish oil consumption exerts a protective effect against the development of breast and prostate cancers (Terry et al 2003). The assessment of EPA and DHA intake and their relation to ω-6 fatty acid intake and cancer incidence still requires further examination before conclusions can be confidently made. An updated review conducted by the same researchers in 2004 (Terry et al 2004) reached a similar conclusion; however, they also observed that those studies that assess ω-3 intake concomitant with the ω-6 consumption were most likely to yield a statistically significant inverse relationship between fish oils and breast and prostate cancers. Once again this reinforces the understanding that due to interrelated metabolism and actions the fats should not be viewed independently.

A prospective cohort study in the United States of 47,866 men aged 40–75 years with no cancer history were assessed using a 131-item semiquantitative food frequency questionnaire administered annually over 14 years, as part of the Health Professionals Follow-Up study. Nutrient intake data from this trial suggest an association between ALA and advanced prostate cancer, but an inverse relationship with the ALA metabolites, EPA and DHA. Earlier studies investigating the relationship between ALA and prostate cancer have had mixed results while the inverse relationship with EPA/DHA appears to be largely supported. Again the authors demonstrate that ratios of ω-3 : ω-6 appear to be highly influential in conveyed risk (Leitzmann et al 2004).

More recently, an association was confirmed between consuming salted or smoked fish and an increased risk of advanced prostate cancer, whereas fish oil consumption may be protective against progression of prostate cancer in elderly men (Torfadottir et al 2013). Interestingly, serum PSA concentrations from 6018 men (from the 2003–2010 National Health and Nutrition Examination Survey), matched with dietary intake of fish, found little evidence for ω-3PUFA consumption in influencing PSA levels (Patel et al 2014). Emerging data further suggest ω-3 PUFAs may slow the growth of many tumours, including prostate (Masko et al 2013).

Colorectal cancer

Epidemiological evidence investigating associations between fish intake and colorectal cancer have produced mixed findings (Caygill et al 1996, Daniel et al 2009), with the most recent prospective cohort study (Cancer Prevention Study-II Nutrition Cohort) involving over 99,000 individuals failing to demonstrate a protective effect of increased ω-3 intake. In fact, increased consumption of ALA was associated with increased risk in women. Contrastingly, higher marine ω-3 intake did appear protective. The latter finding is consistent with the results of other large prospective studies on this issue (Hall et al 2008).

Other sources of evidence attribute both EPA and DHA and their main dietary source, fish oil, with antineoplastic effects in colorectal cancer (Llor et al 2003). Fish oil supplementation, in one study, providing 4.1 g EPA and 3.6 g DHA per day in patients with sporadic adenomatous colorectal polyps, was reported to reduce the percentage of cells in the S-phase in the upper crypt of the rectal mucosa (Anti et al 1992). The evidence to date, as reviewed in 2004 by Roynette et al, suggests a primary preventive effect with some residual ambiguity over the safety of ω-3 LCPUFA with respect to secondary tumour formation.

One study has investigated the effects of ω-3 LCPUFA parenteral supplementation postoperatively on clinical outcomes and immunomodulation in colorectal cancer patients using a randomised, double-blind design (Liang et al 2008). Treatment effect comparisons revealed that those treated with ω-3 LCPUFAs had significantly lower serum interleukin, TNF-alpha and increased ratios of $CD4^+$/$CD8^+$. These patients also tended towards shorter postoperative hospital stays. Consequently, the authors conclude that such a treatment regimen may have beneficial effects on lowering the magnitude of inflammatory responses and modulating the immune response in this patient group.

The results of an in vitro study have demonstrated synergistic inhibition of proliferating colon cancer cells using a combination of lycopene and EPA (Tang et al 2009). The results of other in vitro studies attribute the protective effects of ω-3 LCPUFAs with DHA rather than EPA (Kato et al 2007). Both animal studies and RCTs are now required to clarify the 'active' fatty acid and confirm these findings.

Diabetes

Increasing the intake of ω-3 LCPUFA has been shown to be both preventive in a healthy population and beneficial in people with diabetes (Montori et al 2000, Nettleton et al 2005, Sirtori & Galli 2002, Sirtori et al 1997). A recent systematic review and meta-analysis revising results from 24 studies, including 24,509 type 2 diabetes patients and 545,275 participants overall, found marine ω-3 PUFA to have beneficial effects on the prevention of type 2 diabetes in Asian populations (Zheng et al 2012). Alternately, no clear association was found between ω-3 EFAS and type 2 diabetes in a review of 16 studies comprising 540,184 individuals (Wu et al 2012). In addition, no major harms or benefits of fish/seafood or EPA+DHA on development of DM were observed, but there was suggestion of modestly lower risk with ALA.

While the preventative effect of ω-3 EFAS on diabetes is still being investigated, ω-3EFAs do provide other benefits for people with established diabetes. Diets higher in fish and ω-3 PUFA may reduce cardiovascular risk in diabetes by inhibiting platelet aggregation, improving lipid profiles and reducing cardiovascular mortality (McEwen et al 2010). Two meta-analyses found that fish oil supplementation lowers plasma TG levels in type 2 diabetic subjects; however, a possible rise in plasma LDL cholesterol may occur (Balk et al 2006, Montori et al 2000). Although an increase in LDL cholesterol was noted after ω-3 supplementation, the levels of LDL were not significantly increased in subgroup analyses of hypertriglyceridaemic patients, high (greater than 2 g of EPA and DHA daily) or low ω-3 PUFA doses and in trials lasting longer than 2 months (Hartweg et al 2008). The rise in plasma LDL cholesterol has been speculated to be the result of enhanced conversion of very LDLs and studies in primates suggest that ω-3 LCPUFA-enriched LDLs do not convey the same atherogenic potential (Jung et al 2008). Additionally, no significant effect occurs on glycaemic control, total cholesterol or HDL cholesterol. In addition, studies reveal an average of 7.4% increase in HDL levels concomitant with a 25% reduction in TGs in response to 1020 mg EPA and 700 mg DHA supplementation over 6 months (Sirtori et al 1998). Such findings are supported by the results of other trials in patients with diabetes (Nettleton et al 2005).

In a randomised study, serum phospholipid ω-3 PUFA levels were found to be significantly decreased in patients with type 2 diabetes and non-alcoholic fatty liver disease ($n = 51$; $P < 0.05$). In addition, serum ω-3 levels were negatively related with insulin resistance. Homeostasis model assessment method (HOMA-IR) levels were higher in patients with type 2 diabetes and non-alcoholic fatty liver disease than in the type 2 diabetes ($n = 50$), non-alcoholic fatty liver disease ($n = 45$) and healthy control groups ($n = 42$; $P < 0.05$). Furthermore, Pearson analysis showed that the ω-3 PUFA level was negatively correlated with HOMA-IR ($r = -0.491$), total cholesterol ($r = -0.376$), TGs ($r = -0.462$) and LDL cholesterol ($r = -0.408$), all $P < 0.05$ (Lou et al 2014).

The effect of fish on endothelial function was investigated in 23 postmenopausal women with type 2 diabetes. Participants were assigned to two 4-week periods of either a fish-based diet (ω-3 PUFAs ≥ 3.0 g/day) or a control diet in a randomised cross-over design. Endothelial function was measured with reactive hyperaemia using strain-gauge plethysmography and peak forearm blood flow, duration of reactive hyperaemia and flow debt repayment (FDR). This was then compared with the serum levels of fatty acids and their metabolites. In the fish-first group, the peak forearm blood flow response and FDR increased markedly after the fish-based diet period (4 weeks), and these effects were sustained after the control diet period (8 weeks). In addition, the durations of reactive hyperaemia and FDR increased significantly, and the peak forearm blood flow showed improvement. Conversely, in the control diet-first group, the peak forearm blood flow response, duration of reactive hyperaemia and FDR were unchanged after the control diet period (4 weeks) (Kondo 2014).

Furthermore, the anti-inflammatory properties of ω-3 PUFA, such as the reduction of prostaglandin E_2, leukotrienes (B_4 and E_4), thromboxane B_2 and C-reactive protein, may be of beneficial use in patients with diabetes and CVD. Large trials are suggested to assess the therapeutic potential of ω-3 PUFA as an anti-inflammatory agent in patients with diabetes and CVD (McEwen et al 2010). Despite the potential benefits associated with ω-3 LCPUFAs, a 2008 Cochrane review of 23 RCTs involving 1075 individuals concluded there is currently insufficient evidence to recommend high-dose fish oils to T2DM patients for cardiovascular benefits (Hartweg et al 2008).

Weight reduction

Animal studies illustrate the potential for ω-3 as disease modifiers in obesity via anti-inflammatory mechanisms such as activation of peroxisome proliferator-activated receptors, lowering levels of TNF-α produced by adipocytes and therefore attenuating secondary insulin resistance (Pedersen et al 2011), and that ω-3 interventions consistently reduce body weight and fat mass (Munro & Garg 2013). The results of ω-3 interventions in humans, however, are very mixed. Some positive findings include attenuating negative PUFA changes associated with weight loss regimes (Hlavatý et al 2008) and improving insulin resistance in overweight subjects (Ramel et al 2008), and possible reduced incidence of obesity, increased ease of weight loss and maintenance of body weight in this population (Nettleton et al 2005). One study found that overweight and obese subjects consuming >1300 mg/day ω-3 LCPUFAs compared with those consuming <240 mg/day demonstrated significantly increased satiety 2 hours postprandially, which correlated with increased ω-3 : ω-6 (Parra et al 2008). In contrast there are numerous interventional studies which have failed to produce these anticipated outcomes, including a recent small Australian trial (n = 33) conducted over 12 weeks (Munro & Garg 2013). Speculation regarding such inconsistent results includes the heterogeneous nature of the supplements, with highly variable DHA and EPA ratios and dose, the possible need for longer treatment periods and the perennial issue of human dietary compliance. A new finding in animal research may shed some light on this, with evidence that background diet exerts a crucial influence on the ability of fish oil to protect against obesity development and adipose tissue inflammation (Hao et al 2012). In fact, in this study of mice the beneficial effects of ω-3 intake in mice were significantly diminished or completely abrogated by a simultaneous intake of high-glycaemic index carbohydrates. Another Australian study posits the question of whether other nutrients in fish beyond LCPUFAs contribute to positive weight- and insulin-lowering effects, with a small human trial showing statistically greater adiponectin increases with high dietary ω-3 versus comparable EPA/DHA from supplements (Neale et al 2012). Finally, preliminary research investigating ω-3's effect on lowering endocannibinoid levels in obese rats and humans suggests that krill oil may be superior for this application (Banni et al 2011). Further human studies investigating these issues are necessary.

F

Polycystic ovarian syndrome (PCOS)

Evidence of fish oil's ability to improve insulin sensitivity has led to several small investigations in PCOS populations. One study of 45 non-obese PCOS sufferers administered 1.5 g of ω-3 for 6 months found that body mass index, insulin and HOMA levels decreased significantly, in addition to hormonal improvements e.g. lower serum LH, testosterone and higher SHBG. Glucose levels themselves however didn't change and TNF-α levels showed a significant increase (Oner & Muderris 2013). Similar results were obtained in another study of 61 PCOS patients administered 720 mg/day EPA and 480 mg/DHA or placebo over 8 weeks. Again statistically significant improvements were evident on multiple parameters (TGs, HDLs, HOMA) but the inflammatory marker, this time CRP, was unchanged (Mohammadi et al 2012). Interestingly, in a study of PCOS patients which included those with healthy body mass index, favourable lipid changes were lessened. Several of these studies illustrate the androgen-lowering effect of high-dose ω-3 (Oner & Muderris 2013, Phelan et al 2011) which is hypothesised to be the result of reduced ω-6 : ω-3 rather than a direct effect of ω-3 (Phelan et al 2011).

Inflammatory diseases

Numerous clinical trials have investigated the effects of fish oil supplementation in several inflammatory and autoimmune diseases, such as RA, Crohn's disease, ulcerative colitis, lupus erythematosus and migraine headaches (Belluzzi 2002, Belluzzi et al 1996, Miura et al 1998, Simopoulos 2002). Although not all trials have produced positive results, many of the placebo-controlled trials reveal significant benefit in chronic disease, including decreased disease activity and sometimes reduced requirement for anti-inflammatory medicines (Adam et al 2003).

Rheumatoid arthritis

Of the inflammatory diseases, the use of fish oil supplementation is most widely seen and supported in RA. RCTs, meta- and mega-analysis of RCTs indicate reduction in tender joint counts, pain intensity, morning stiffness and decreased use of non-steroidal anti-inflammatory drugs with fish oil supplementation in long-standing RA (Adam et al 2003, Cleland et al 2003, Goldberg & Katz 2007, James et al 2010, Kremer 2000, Miles & Calder 2012, Ulbricht & Basch 2005, Volker et al 2000). Since non-steroidal anti-inflammatory drugs confer cardiovascular risk and there is increased cardiovascular mortality in RA, an additional benefit of fish oil in RA may be reduced cardiovascular risk via direct mechanisms and decreased non-steroidal anti-inflammatory drug use. Interestingly, fish oil has been shown to slow the development of RA in animal models and to reduce disease severity (Miles & Calder 2012).

Generally, supplements are taken daily as adjuncts to standard therapy, with clinical effects appearing after 12 weeks. A dose ranging from 30 mg to 40 mg/kg of EPA and DHA daily has been used successfully, although some studies have found a minimum of 3 g/day is required. Results from a double-blind, crossover study suggest that the beneficial effects obtained from fish oil capsules are further enhanced when combined with an anti-inflammatory diet providing less than 90 mg/day of AA (Adam et al 2003).

Symptomatic relief with ω-3 LCPUFAs in RA was more recently confirmed in a meta-analysis of 17 RCTs assessing the pain-relieving effects in RA patients or joint pain secondary to inflammatory bowel disease and dysmenorrhoea (Goldberg & Katz 2007). Supplementation for 3–4 months significantly reduced patient-reported joint pain intensity, minutes of morning stiffness, number of painful and/or tender joints and non-steroidal anti-inflammatory drug consumption. Significant effects were not detected, however, for doctor-assessed pain or Ritchie articular index. These papers, together with other authoritative reviews, conclude that, based on high-level evidence, ω-3 LCPUFAs are an attractive adjunctive treatment for joint pain associated with RA and have a beneficial follow-on effect on cardiovascular morbidity and mortality pertinent to this population (Proudman et al 2008).

Although the anti-inflammatory activity of fish oil supplementation is thought to be chiefly responsible for symptom-relieving effects, there is also evidence that ω-3 LCPUFAs can modulate expression and activity of degradative factors that cause cartilage destruction (Curtis et al 2000). A 2005 randomised study found that fish oil supplements (3 g/day), whether taken alone or in combination with olive oil (9.6 mL), produced a statistically significant improvement ($P < 0.05$) compared to placebo on several clinical parameters (Berbert et al 2005). Significant improvements were observed for joint pain intensity, right and left handgrip strength after 12 and 24 weeks, duration of morning stiffness, onset of fatigue, Ritchie's articular index for pain joints after 24 weeks, ability to bend down to pick up clothing from the floor and getting in and out of a car after 24 weeks. The group using a combination of oils showed additional improvements with respect to duration of morning stiffness after 12 weeks, patient global assessment after 12 and 24 weeks, ability to turn taps on and off after 24 weeks and rheumatoid factor after 24 weeks. In addition, this group showed a significant improvement in patient global assessment compared with fish oils alone after 12 weeks.

Based on these results, it appears that, while fish oils will not improve all parameters of RA, overall they have demonstrated symptomatic relief in the majority and result in significantly reduced use of anti-inflammatory and corticosteroid use, a fact that MacLean et al (2004) acknowledge and which is confirmed by a 2005 review by Stamp et al and meta-analysis by Goldberg and Katz (2007). There appears to be little evidence of sustained improvements following cessation of the supplements.

A 2008 paper from the Joint Nutrition Society notes that, in addition to modifying the lipid mediator profile, ω-3 LCPUFAs exert effects on other aspects of immunity relevant to RA, such as antigen presentation, T-cell reactivity and inflammatory cytokine production (Calder 2008).

Reducing incidence of RA

A large prospective cohort study ($n = 57{,}053$) investigating the association between dietary factors and risk of RA found that each increase in intake of 30 g fatty fish (≥8 g fat/100 g fish) per day was associated with 49% reduction in the risk of RA ($P = 0.06$); however, a medium intake of fatty fish (3–7 g fat/100 g fish) was associated with significantly increased risk of RA (Pedersen et al 2005). No associations were found between risk of RA and intake of a range of other dietary factors, including long-chain fatty acids, olive oil, vitamins A, C, D and E, zinc, selenium, iron and meat. The authors caution that, due to the limited number of patients who developed RA during follow-up, it is not yet possible to make firm conclusions.

Asthma

Ω-3 LCPUFAs exhibit anti-inflammatory activity and epidemiological evidence has demonstrated an inverse relationship between fish intake, asthma risk and improved lung function (Wong 2005). Evidence suggests this protective effect may extend back as far as adequate fetal ω-3 LCPUFA exposure (Salam et al 2005).

A 2002 Cochrane review of nine RCTs conducted between 1986 and 2001 concluded that ω-3 LCPUFA supplementation demonstrated no consistent effect on any of the analysable outcomes: forced expiratory volume in 1 s, peak flow rate, asthma symptoms, asthma medication use or bronchial hyperreactivity (Woods et al 2002). However, one of the RCTs involving children showed that, when fish oil supplementation was combined with dietary changes, positive results were obtained, as evidenced by improved peak flow and reduced asthma medication use.

An interesting crossover study of 72 asthmatic children aged 7–10 years involved five randomised phases of treatment each lasting 6 weeks: placebo; ω-3 (300 mg/day combined EPA and DHA); zinc (15 mg/day); vitamin C (200 mg/day); combination of all nutrients (Biltagi et al 2009). While the ω-3 LCPUFA supplementation was associated with improved lung function and a reduction in both sputum production and markers of airway inflammation, these positive effects were significantly augmented when combined with zinc and vitamin C, suggesting that a broader nutritional approach to inflammation and oxidation control results in greatest clinical outcomes.

The equivocal nature of ω-3 LCPUFAs interventions, as documented by a 2005 review (Wong 2005), may be clarified in future with the identification of a subtype of asthma more likely to respond to EFA manipulation.

Another interesting paper reports on three patients with disabling salicylate intolerance producing urticaria, asthma and anaphylactic reactions who, following administration of 10 g/day fish oils for 6–8 weeks, experienced complete or virtually complete resolution of symptoms (Healy et al 2008). Treatment response was so effective corticosteroids could be discontinued; however, symptoms reappeared following fish oil dose reduction.

The focus for fish oils in asthma has broadened to include other populations such as athletes. One randomised, double-blind, crossover study of 16 non-atopic asthmatic patients with documented exercise-induced broncoconstriction compared the effects of 3.2 g of EPA and 2.0 g DHA per day and placebo capsules for 3 weeks. During treatment with fish oils, subjects demonstrated improved pulmonary function to below the diagnostic exercise-induced broncoconstriction threshold, which was associated with a concurrent reduction in bronchodilator use. Measurement of leukotriene B_4 and B_5 levels also confirmed a significant reversal of the inflammatory picture (Mickleborough et al 2006).

Clinical note — Oils ain't oils

Arguably the biggest ongoing methodological sticking point in ω-3 research is the heterogeneous nature of the interventions used, which has hindered comparisons, meta-analyses and consensus about their therapeutic actions. While the inferiority of plant-based ω-3 EFAs has now been established (see Are ALA-rich oils a worthy substitute for fish oils?), new questions over different forms — e.g. fish versus supplements, supplemental forms, e.g. TGs, ethyl esters, ratios of EPA to DHA and sources, e.g. krill, algal — have arisen and there is a focused effort to clarify differences in the behaviour and bioavailability of each, such that researchers can better understand disparate outcomes of RCTs and, most importantly, identify superior ways of improving ω-3.

Fish versus fish oil supplements

Underpinning interest and excitement about ω-3s, particularly in the context of CVD prevention, stemmed from epidemiological studies of high fish-consuming populations. Early on an assumption was made that these benefits were entirely attributable to the ω-3 fatty acids. More recently, however, this has been questioned, with increasing speculation that EPA/DHA may interact with other nutrients, e.g. taurine, selenium, astaxanthin, within fish and/or that dietary fish may displace other unhealthy food choices and therefore may be superior to supplementation with fish oils (Brazionis et al 2012, Deckelbaum & Torrejon 2012, Harvard Heart Letter 2011, He 2009). Some researchers reason that this explains the disparate and somewhat disappointing results of fish oil interventions in some RCTs compared with studies of increasing fish intake in the prevention of CVD, especially fatal CHD (He 2009). An interesting small crossover Australian study found that fish consumption (150 g of Atlantic salmon twice a week) significantly reduced blood pressure and waist circumference when compared with fish oil (1.2 g/day 6 days/week) in spite of comparable changes in ω-3 index (Brazionis et al 2012). The current consensus is: eat low mercury-containing fish where possible and if not possible, take supplements; however, more research in other conditions is necessary.

Triglycerides versus ethyl esters

Several studies confirm improved bioavailability from fish oils presented as TGs (either natural or re-esterified) over ethyl esters, including a long-term study (6 months) of moderate intake (1.01 g EPA and 0.67 g DHA) and its effects on RBC levels in healthy individuals (Neubronner et al 2011). Another debate is the impact of the position of the LCPUFAs along the glycerol backbone in these TGs; this differs between natural TGs and chemically re-esterified TGs. However, a small study found that EPA bioavailability at least was significantly greater from the re-esterified TGs than the NTGs (Wakil et al 2010). Other similar studies reviewing DHA uptake, however, are inconsistent.

Atopic dermatitis and eczema

In a sample of adult patients (n = 53), randomised to 5.4 g/day DHA or isoenergetic saturated fats for 20 weeks, active fish oil treatment produced significant clinical improvements which correlated with increases in plasma DHA (Koch et al 2008);

Comparing krill, algal and fish oil

Pressing issues of non-sustainability of both wild harvesting and aquaculture together with increasing contaminants in fish and their products have motivated researchers to search for alternative sources to meet our increasing ω-3 demand (Racine & Deckelbaum 2007, Robert 2006). Two key emerging areas are algal and krill oil (*Euphausia superba*). Microalgae, such as *Cryptheco-dinium cohnii* and *Schizochytrium* spp., represent part of the coastal food chain as a primary food source for shellfish, contain no contaminants (Arterburn et al 2000, Doughman et al 2007) and are currently commercially developed as sustainable crops (Doughman et al 2007, Whelan & Rust 2006). Krill is by far the most dominant member of the Antarctic zooplankton in terms of biomass, which also makes it attractive as a more sustainable crop (Ulven et al 2011); however, both algal and krill oil are produced at significantly higher production costs (Deckelbaum & Torrejon 2012) and differ chemically and behaviourally from fish oil, e.g. both algal and krill oil contain the astaxanthin not found in fish oil. Also, algal oil predominates in DHA and initial human studies have confirmed both bioequivalence and comparable clinical efficacy with other DHA sources such as salmon (Arterburn et al 2000, Doughman et al 2007). However, some conditions respond preferentially to higher EPA levels (see Depression), which would limit the application of these products. Attempts to produce high EPA forms have been unsuccessful to date (Deckelbaum & Torrejon 2012).

In contrast, krill oil has a lower yield per gram of LCPUFAs compared with fish oil but its ratio of EPA : DHA is greater. Additionally, LCPUFAs in fish oils are presented as either TGs or ethyl esters; however, 30–65% found in krill oil are incorporated into phospholipids. This phospholipid form appears to favour increased bioavailability and several studies have found that krill oil can produce comparable or superior improvements in ω-3 levels in spite of lower actual EPA and DHA content (approximately 68% of that used in fish oil comparator studies) (Banni et al 2011, Ramprasath et al 2013, Schuchardt et al 2011, Ulven et al 2011). Preliminary evidence suggests that krill oil may offer a therapeutic advantage over fish oil in the treatment of metabolic syndrome and weight loss (Banni et al 2011, Vigerust et al 2013); however the vast majority of RCTs performed to date with PUFAs have used fish oils.

however, due to the small sample size, larger studies are required to confirm these preliminary results.

Previously, a double-blind multicentre study involving 145 patients with moderate to severe atopic dermatitis showed that ω-3 LCPUFAs (6 g/day) improved clinical symptom scores by 30% after 4 months' treatment (Soyland et al 1994). The results were confirmed by patients' subjective scoring. An earlier, 12-week, prospective, double-blind study produced similar results, with a dose of 10 g/day (fish oil) improving overall severity of atopic dermatitis and reducing scaling (Bjorneboe et al 1989). A 2012 Cochrane review that included all four studies concluded that two trials suggest a moderate effect on reducing severity in adults; however, further research is needed (Bath-Hextall et al 2012).

OTHER USES

Fish oil supplements are also used in the management of acute respiratory distress syndrome, psoriasis, multiple sclerosis, osteoporosis and dysmenorrhoea and in children with dyslexia.

DOSAGE RANGE

- Fish should be considered part of a healthy diet for everybody and be consumed at least twice a week. Care should be taken to avoid intake of fish known or suspected to contain higher levels of mercury.
- Additional administration of ω-3 LCPUFA supplements should be considered in specific groups.
- Fish meals should consist of deep-sea oily fish, whereas fried or processed fish containing partially hydrogenated fats and salted or pickled fish should be avoided.

Cardiovascular disease

Secondary prevention trials after MI indicate that consumption of 0.5–1.8 g/day of EPA and DHA from fish or fish oil supplements may be beneficial. Intake of marine-derived ω-3 fatty acids can be increased through diet or with fish oil supplements.

- An expert US panel of nutrition scientists has recommended an intake of 0.65 g/day, whereas the British Nutrition Foundation's recommendation is 1.2 g/day (Din et al 2004).
- National Heart Foundation/Cardiac Society of Australia and New Zealand: >2 servings/week.
- Patients who have experienced coronary artery bypass surgery with venous grafts: 4 g/day of ω-3 LCPUFAs.
- Moderate hypertension: 4 g/day of fish oils.
- Elevated TG levels: 1–4.6 g/day of fish oils; Lovaza 4 g/day.

Other conditions

- Aggression induced by mental stress: DHA supplementation, 1.5–1.8 g/day.
- Anger and anxiety reduction in polysubstance abuse withdrawers: 2.25 g EPA, 500 mg DHA and 250 mg other ω-3 per day.
- Asthma prevention in pregnancy: 2.7 g/day from week 20 gestation until delivery.
- Asthma treatment in children: 300 mg combined EPA and DHA with 15 mg zinc and 200 mg vitamin C per day.
- Atopic dermatitis: 6 g/day fish oils or 5.4 g/day DHA.
- Autism: 5 g/day (limited evidence to support).
- BD: 1 g/day EPA.

- Colorectal cancer: 4.1 g EPA + 3.6 g DHA daily.
- Dementia: DHA supplementation, 4.32 g/day.
- Depression: 1 g/day EPA or a combined supplement with ≥60% EPA.
- Exercise-induced asthma in non-atopic individuals: 3.2 g EPA + 2.0 g DHA daily.
- High blood pressure: 3–5.6 g/day.
- Intermittent claudication: 1.8 g EPA and 1.2 g DHA per day (limited evidence to support).
- Pregnancy: According to the WHO and FAO, the pregnant woman should take at least 2.6 g of ω-3 EFAs, incorporating 100–300 mg of DHA daily to look after the needs of the fetus.
- Psychosis prevention in high-risk individuals: 480 mg/day DHA, 700 mg/day EPA for 12 weeks.
- RA: 30–40 mg/kg body weight of EPA and DHA daily.
- Schizophrenia: 2 g/day EPA for a minimum of 3 months.
- Weight reduction and improved insulin sensitivity: 660 mg EPA and 440 mg DHA/day.

ADVERSE REACTIONS

Fish oil supplementation is generally safe and well tolerated. The few side effects reported are usually mild and can include gastrointestinal discomfort and loose bowels, halitosis and a fishy odour of the skin and urine.

Studies using Lovaza (previously Omacor) report the main side effects as belching, indigestion, taste aversions, fishy taste, infection and flu-like symptoms. Reports have also shown that it may increase levels of alanine aminotransferase; in addition ratio of LDL:apolipoprotein B may increase after pharmacological doses of ω-3 (Nicholson et al 2013).

SIGNIFICANT INTERACTIONS

Antiplatelet agents

Theoretically, concomitant use with antiplatelet agents may increase the risk of bleeding; however, multiple clinical studies have found no clinically significant effect on bleeding and one study has suggested that the combined effects may be beneficial (Engstrom et al 2001) — no clinically significant interaction expected at therapeutic doses.

Anticoagulants

Clinical studies of surgical patients taking warfarin have not found a clinically significant increase in bleeding. According to one clinical study, bleeding time is increased at very high doses of 12 g/day. Usual therapeutic doses, which tend to fall below this dosage, appear safe in this population, although care should still be taken. Very high doses >12 g should be used only under professional supervision to ensure no adverse outcomes.

Non-steroidal anti-inflammatory drugs

Additional anti-inflammatory effects are theoretically possible with concurrent use of fish oil supplements, suggesting a beneficial interaction. Drug dosage may require modification.

CONTRAINDICATIONS AND PRECAUTIONS

One area of concern is the growing problem of heavy-metal contamination found in fish, specifically mercury. In areas where contamination is possible, fish oil supplements may represent a safer option. According to the *Australia New Zealand Food Standards Code*, fish with higher levels of mercury include: marlin, swordfish, southern bluefin tuna, barramundi, ling, orange roughy, rays and shark. Fish considered to have lower levels of mercury include: mackerel, silver wahoo, Atlantic salmon, canned salmon and canned tuna in oil, herrings and sardines.

People with bleeding disorders should take fish oil supplements under medical supervision.

PREGNANCY USE

Fish oils appear to be safe during pregnancy at dietary doses and are likely to have benefits.

Practice points/Patient counselling

- As precursors of eicosanoids, PUFAs found in fish oils exert a wide influence over many important physiological processes.
- They have demonstrated anti-inflammatory, immunological, neurological, antiplatelet and chemopreventive effects, and a range of beneficial actions within the cardiovascular system.
- Daily ingestion of at least 1 g EPA and DHA (equivalent to fish eaten at least twice weekly) may result in a reduction in total mortality, cardiovascular mortality and morbidity and incidence of dementia and depression.
- Trials generally support the use of supplements in a range of inflammatory and autoimmune diseases such as RA and atopic dermatitis, elevated TGs, hypertension and other cardiovascular conditions, poor cognitive function and diabetes. Preliminary research suggests a possible role in depression.
- People with bleeding disorders should take fish oil supplements under medical supervision.

Pravastatin

Low-dose pravastatin combined with fish oil supplementation is more effective than pravastatin alone for changing the lipid profile after renal transplantation, according to one clinical study — potential beneficial interaction.

PATIENTS' FAQs

What will this supplement do for me?

Regular consumption of fish oils may reduce total mortality, cardiovascular mortality and morbidity, dementia, depression and possibly diabetes and various cancers. Additionally, beneficial effects have been demonstrated in a wide variety of conditions.

When will it start to work?

This will depend on the dosage taken and indication for use.

Are there any safety issues?

People with bleeding disorders should take fish oil supplements under medical supervision.

REFERENCES

Adam O et al. Anti-inflammatory effects of a low arachidonic acid diet and fish oil in patients with rheumatoid arthritis. Rheumatol Int 23.1 (2003): 27–36.

Alm B et al. Early introduction of fish decreases the risk of eczema in infants. Arch Dis Child 94.1 (2009): 11–15.

Almqvist C et al. CAPS team. Omega-3 and omega-6 fatty acid exposure from early life does not affect atopy and asthma at age 5 years. J Allergy Clin Immunol 119.6 (2007): 1438–1444.

Amminger GP et al. Omega-3 fatty acids supplementation in children with autism: a double-blind randomized, placebo-controlled pilot study. Biol Psychiatry 61.4 (2007): 551–553.

Anti M et al. Effect of omega-3 fatty acids on rectal mucosal cell proliferation in subjects at risk for colon cancer. Gastroenterology 103 (1992): 883–891.

Arterburn LM et al. A combined subchronic (90-day) toxicity and neurotoxicity study of a single-cell source of docosahexaenoic acid triglyceride (DHASCO oil). Food Chem Toxicol 38.1 (2000): 35–49.

Bagga D et al. Long-chain n-3 to n-6 polyunsaturated fatty acid ratios in breast adipose tissue from women with and without breast cancer. Nutr Cancer 42.2 (2002): 180–185.

Balakumar, P. & Taneja, G. 2012. Fish oil and vascular endothelial protection: bench to bedside. Free Radic.Biol.Med, 53, (2) 271–279.

Balk EM et al. Effects of omega-3 fatty acids on serum markers of cardiovascular disease risk: a systematic review. Atherosclerosis 189.1 (2006): 19–30.

Bambrick HJ, Kjellstrom TE. Good for your heart but bad for your baby? Revised guidelines for fish consumption in pregnancy. Med J Aust 181.2 (2004): 61–62.

Bang HO, et al. The composition of the Eskimo food in north western Greenland. Am J Clin Nutr 33.12 (1980): 2657–2661.

Barter P, Ginsberg HN. Effectiveness of combined statin plus omega-3 fatty acid therapy for mixed dyslipidemia. Am J Cardiol 102.8 (2008): 1040–1045.

Bays HE. Safety considerations with omega-3 fatty acid therapy. Am J Cardiol 99.6A (2007): 35C–43C.

Beers MH, Berkow R (eds), The Merck manual of diagnosis and therapy, 17th edn. Rahway, NJ: Merck, 2003.

Belluzzi A et al. Effect of an enteric-coated fish-oil preparation on relapses in Crohn's disease. N Engl J Med 334.24 (1996): 1557–1560.

Belluzzi A. N-3 fatty acids for the treatment of inflammatory bowel diseases. Proc Nutr Soc 61.3 (2002): 391–395.

Bender NK et al. Effects of marine fish oils on the anticoagulation status of patients receiving chronic warfarin therapy. J Thromb Thrombolysis 5.3 (1998): 257–261.

Berbert AA et al. Supplementation of fish oil and olive oil in patients with rheumatoid arthritis. Nutrition 21.2 (2005): 131–136.

Bhattacharya A et al. Different ratios of eicosapentaenoic and docosahexaenoic omega-3 fatty acids in commercial fish oils differentially alter pro-inflammatory cytokines in peritoneal macrophages from C57BL/6 female mice. J Nutr Biochem (2007); 18: 23–30.

Billman GE, et al. Prevention of ischemia-induced cardiac sudden death by n-3 polyunsaturated fatty acids in dogs. Lipids 32.11 (1997): 1161–1168.

Billman GE, et al. Prevention of sudden cardiac death by dietary pure omega-3 polyunsaturated fatty acids in dogs. Circulation 99.18 (1999): 2452–2457.

Biltagi MA et al. Omega-3 fatty acids, vitamin C and Zn supplementation in asthmatic children: a randomized self-controlled study. Acta Paediatr 2009; 98: 737–742.

Bjorneboe A et al. Effect of n-3 fatty acid supplement to patients with atopic dermatitis. J Intern Med Suppl 225.731 (1989): 233–236.

Braun L et al. A wellness program for cardiac surgery improves clinical outcomes. Adv in Integrat Med 1.1 (2014): 32–37.

Bruinsma KA, Taren DL. Dieting, essential fatty acid intake, and depression. Nutr Rev 58.4 (2000): 98–108.

Bucher HC et al. N-3 polyunsaturated fatty acids in coronary heart disease: a meta-analysis of randomized controlled trials. Am J Med 112.4 (2002): 298–304.

Buckley MS, et al. Fish oil interaction with warfarin. Ann Pharmacother 38.1 (2004): 50–52.

Burr ML et al. Effects of changes in fat, fish, and fibre intakes on death and myocardial reinfarction: diet and reinfarction trial (DART). Lancet 2.8666 (1989): 757–761.

Burr ML et al. Lack of benefit of dietary advice to men with angina: results of a controlled trial. Eur J Clin Nutr 57.2 (2003): 193–200.

Buydens-Branchey L, et al. Associations between increases in plasma n-3 polyunsaturated fatty acids following supplementation and decreases in anger and anxiety in substance abusers. Prog Neuropsychopharmacol Biol Psychiatry 32.2 (2008): 568–575.

Calder PC. Dietary modification of inflammation with lipids. Proc Nutr Soc 61.3 (2002): 345–358.

Calder PC. N-3 polyunsaturated fatty acids and inflammation: from molecular biology to the clinic. Lipids 38.4 (2003): 343–352.

Calder PC. Session 3: Joint Nutrition Society and Irish Nutrition and Dietetic Institute Symposium on 'Nutrition and autoimmune disease' PUFA, inflammatory processes and rheumatoid arthritis. Proc Nutr Soc 67.4 (2008): 409–418.

Calder PC et al. Dietary fish oil suppresses human colon tumour growth in athymic mice. Clin Sci (Lond) 94.3 (1998): 303–311.

Calo L et al. N-3 Fatty acids for the prevention of atrial fibrillation after coronary artery bypass surgery: a randomized, controlled trial. J Am Coll Cardiol 45.10 (2005): 1723–1728.

Campbell, A., et al. 2013. Omega-3 fatty acids for intermittent claudication. Cochrane Database Syst Rev., 7, CD003833.

Casula, M., et al. 2013. Long-term effect of high dose omega-3 fatty acid supplementation for secondary prevention of cardiovascular outcomes: A meta-analysis of randomized, placebo controlled trials [corrected]. Atheroscler. Suppl, 14, (2) 243–251.

Caygill CP et al. Fat, fish, fish oil and cancer. Br J Cancer 74.1 (1996): 159–164.

Chen CT and Bazinet RP. β-Oxidation and rapid metabolism, but not uptake regulate brain eicosapentaenoic acid levels. Prostaglandins, Leukotrienes and Essential Fatty Acids (PLEFA) (in press).

Chiu CC et al. The effects of omega-3 fatty acids monotherapy in Alzheimer's disease and mild cognitive impairment: a preliminary randomized double-blind placebo-controlled study. Prog Neuropsychopharmacol Biol Psychiatry 32.6 (2008): 1538–1544.

Cleland LG et al. The role of fish oils in the treatment of rheumatoid arthritis. Drugs 63.9 (2003): 845–853.

Cohen JT et al. A quantitative analysis of prenatal intake of n-3 polyunsaturated fatty acids and cognitive development. Am J Prev Med 29.4 (2005): 366: e1–e12.

Conquer JA et al. Fatty acid analysis of blood plasma of patients with Alzheimer's disease, other types of dementia, and cognitive impairment. Lipids 35.12 (2000): 1305–1312.

Curtis CL et al. N-3 fatty acids specifically modulate catabolic factors involved in articular cartilage degradation. J Biol Chem 275.2 (2000): 721–724.

Curtis LT, Patel K. Nutritional and environmental approaches to preventing and treating autism and attention deficit hyperactivity disorder (ADHD): a review. J Altern Complement Med 14.1 (2008): 79–85.

Daniel CR et al. Dietary intake of omega-6 and omega-3 fatty acids and risk of colorectal cancer in a prospective cohort of U.S. men and women. Cancer Epidemiol Biomarkers Prev 18.2 (2009): 516–525.

Davis BC, Kris-Etherton PM. Achieving optimal essential fatty acid status in vegetarians: current knowledge and practical implications. Am J Clin Nutr 78.3 (2003): 640–6S.

De, C.R. 2011. N-3 fatty acids in cardiovascular disease. N. Engl. J Med, 364, (25) 2439–2450.

de Lorgeril M, Salen P. Helping women to good health: breast cancer, omega-3/omega-6 lipids, and related lifestyle factors. BMC Med 12.54 (2014): PM:24669767.

De Vriese SR, et al. In humans, the seasonal variation in poly-unsaturated fatty acids is related to the seasonal variation in violent suicide and serotonergic markers of violent suicide. Prostaglandins Leukot Essent Fatty Acids 71.1 (2004): 13–18.

Din JN, et al. Omega 3 fatty acids and cardiovascular disease: fishing for a natural treatment. BMJ 328 (2004): 30–35.

Domingo J. Omega-3 fatty acids and the benefits of fish consumption: is all that glitters gold? Environ Int 33.7 (2007): 993–998.

Domingo J, Bocio A. Levels of PCDD/PCDFS and PCBS in edible marine species and human intake: a literature review. Environ Int 33.3 (2007): 397–405.

Dórea J. Fish meal in animal feed and human exposure to persistent bioaccumulative and toxic substances. J Food Prot 69.11 (2006): 2777–2785.

Doughman S, et al. Omega-3 fatty acids for nutrition and medicine: considering microalgae oil as a vegetarian source of EPA and DHA. Curr Diabetes Rev 3.3 (2007): 198–203.

Dunstan JA et al. Cognitive assessment of children at age 2½ years after maternal fish oil supplementation in pregnancy: a randomised controlled trial. Arch Dis Child Fetal Neonatal Ed 93.1 (2008): F45–F50.

Easton M, et al. Preliminary examination of contaminant loadings in farmed salmon, wild salmon and commercial salmon feed. Chemosphere 46.7 (2002): 1053–1074.

Engelhart MJ et al. Diet and risk of dementia: Does fat matter? The Rotterdam Study. Neurology 59.12 (2002): 1915–1921.

Engstrom K, et al. Effect of low-dose aspirin in combination with stable fish oil on whole blood production of eicosanoids. Prostaglandins Leukot Essent Fatty Acids 64.6 (2001): 291–297.

Eritsland J et al. Long-term effects of n-3 polyunsaturated fatty acids on haemostatic variables and bleeding episodes in patients with coronary artery disease. Blood Coagul Fibrinolysis 6.1 (1995): 17–22.

Food Standards Australia New Zealand (FSANZ). www.foodstandards.gov.au (accessed 18-03-04).

Foran J et al. Quantitative analysis of the benefits and risks of consuming farmed and wild salmon. J Nutr 135.11 (2005): 2639–2643.

Frangou S, et al. Efficacy of ethyl-eicosapentaenoic acid in bipolar depression: randomised double-blind placebo-controlled study. Br J Psychiatry 188 (2006): 46–50.

Frishman WH, et al. Alternative and complementary medicine for preventing and treating cardiovascular disease. Dis Mon 55.3 (2009): 121–192.

FSANZ. Mercury in Fish. Canberra: FSANZ, 2004.

Gao L et al. Influence of omega-3 polyunsaturated fatty acid-supplementation on platelet aggregation in humans: A meta-analysis of randomized controlled trials. Atherosclerosis. 226.2 (2013): 328–334.

Garland MR, Hallahan B. Essential fatty acids and their role in conditions characterised by impulsivity. Int Rev Psychiatry 18.2 (2006): 99–105.

Geleijnse JM et al. Blood pressure response to fish oil supplementation: metaregression analysis of randomized trials. J Hypertens 20.8 (2002): 1493–1499.

Goldberg RJ, Katz J. A meta-analysis of the analgesic effects of omega-3 polyunsaturated fatty acid supplementation for inflammatory joint pain. Pain 129.1–2 (2007): 210–223.

Grenyer BF et al. Fish oil supplementation in the treatment of major depression: a randomised double-blind placebo-controlled trial. Prog Neuropsychopharmacol Biol Psychiatry 31.7 (2007): 1393–1396.

Groff J, Gropper S. Advanced nutrition and human metabolism. Belmont USA: Wadsonworth Thomsen Learning, 2004.

Hall MN et al. A 22-year prospective study of fish, n-3 fatty acid intake, and colorectal cancer risk in men. Cancer Epidemiol Biomarkers Prev 17.5 (2008): 1136–1143.

Hallahan B et al. Omega-3 fatty acid supplementation in patients with recurrent self-harm. Single-centre double-blind randomised controlled trial. Br J Psychiatry 190 (2007): 118–122.

Hamazaki T et al. The effect of docosahexaenoic acid on aggression in young adults: A placebo-controlled double-blind study. J Clin Invest 97.4 (1996): 1129–1133.

Hamazaki T et al. Docosahexaenoic acid does not affect aggression of normal volunteers under nonstressful conditions: a randomized, placebo-controlled, double-blind study. Lipids 33.7 (1998): 663–667.

Harris WS. Expert opinion: omega-3 fatty acids and bleeding — cause for concern? Am J Cardiol 99.6A (2007): 44C–46C.

Harris WS et al. Omega-3 fatty acids and coronary heart disease risk: clinical and mechanistic perspectives. Atherosclerosis 197.1 (2008): 12–24.

Hartweg J et al. Omega-3 polyunsaturated fatty acids (PUFA) for type 2 diabetes mellitus. Cochrane Database Syst Rev 23; (1) (2008): CD003205.

Hashimoto M et al. Chronic administration of docosahexaenoic acid ameliorates the impairment of spatial cognition learning ability in amyloid beta-infused rats. J Nutr 135.3 (2005): 549–555.

Healy E et al. Control of salicylate intolerance with fish oils. Br J Dermatol 159.6 (2008): 1368–1369.

Helland IB et al. Maternal supplementation with very-long chain n-3 fatty acids during pregnancy and lactation augments children's IQ at 4 years of age. Pediatrics 111.1 (2003): e39–e44.

Helland IB et al. Effect of supplementing pregnant and lactating mothers with n-3 very-long-chain fatty acids on children's IQ and body mass index at 7 years of age. Pediatrics 122.2 (2008): e472–e479.

Hellsten G et al. Effects on fibrinolytic activity of corn oil and a fish oil preparation enriched with omega-3-polyunsaturated fatty acids in a long-term study. Curr Med Res Opin 13.3 (1993): 133–139.

Hibbeln JR, et al. Omega-3 fatty acid deficiencies in neurodevelopment, aggression and autonomic dysregulation: opportunities for intervention. Int Rev Psychiatry 18.2 (2006): 107–118.

Hightower JM, Moore D. Mercury levels in high-end consumers of fish. Environ Health Perspect 111 (2003): 604–608.

Hlavatý P et al. Change in fatty acid composition of serum lipids in obese females after short-term weight-reducing regimen with the addition of n-3 long chain polyunsaturated fatty acids in comparison to controls. Physiol Res 57 (Suppl 1) (2008): S57–S65.

Holub BJ. Clinical nutrition: 4. Omega-3 fatty acids in cardiovascular care. Can Med Assoc J 166.5 (2002): 608–615.

Hooper L et al. Risks and benefits of omega 3 fats for mortality, cardiovascular disease, and cancer: systematic review. BMJ 332.7544 (2006): 752–760.

Hornstra G. Influence of dietary fish oil on arterial thrombosis and atherosclerosis in animal models and in man. J Intern Med (Suppl) 225.731 (1989): 53–59.

Horrobin DF, Bennett CN. Depression and bipolar disorder: relationships to impaired fatty acid and phospholipid metabolism and to diabetes, cardiovascular disease, immunological abnormalities, cancer, ageing and osteoporosis. Possible candidate genes. Prostaglandins Leukot Essent Fatty Acids 60.4 (1999): 217–234.

Horrocks LA, Yeo YK. Health benefits of docosahexaenoic acid (DHA). Pharmacol Res 40.3 (1999): 211–225.

Houston MC. Nutraceuticals, vitamins, antioxidants, and minerals in the prevention and treatment of hypertension. Progr Cardiovasc Dis 47.6 (2005): 396–449.

Hu FB et al. Fish and omega-3 fatty acid intake and risk of coronary heart disease in women. JAMA 287 (2002): 1815–1821.

Huan M et al. Suicide attempt and n-3 fatty acid levels in red blood cells: A case control study in China. Biol Psychiatry 56.7 (2004): 490–496.

Itomura M et al. The effect of fish oil on physical aggression in schoolchildren — a randomized, double-blind, placebo-controlled trial. J Nutr Biochem 16.3 (2005): 163–171.

Jackson, P. A., et al. (2012). No effect of 12 weeks' supplementation with 1 g DHA-rich or EPA-rich fish oil on cognitive function or mood in healthy young adults aged 18–35 years. British Journal Of Nutrition, 107(8), 1232–1243.

Jacobs M et al. Organochlorine residues in fish oil dietary supplements: comparison with industrial grade oils. Chemosphere 37.9–12 (1998): 1709–1721.

Jacobs M, et al. Investigation of selected persistent organic pollutants in farmed Atlantic salmon (*Salmo salar*), salmon aquaculture feed, and fish oil components of the feed. Environ Sci Technol 36.13 (2002): 2797–2805.

Jacobs M et al. Time Trend Investigation of PCBs, PBDEs, and organochlorine pesticides in selected n-3 polyunsaturated fatty acid rich dietary fish oil and vegetable oil supplements; nutritional relevance for human essential n-3 fatty acid requirements. J Agric Food Chem 52.6 (2004): 1780–1788.

Jalili M, Dehpour AR. Extremely prolonged INR associated with warfarin in combination with both trazodone and omega-3 fatty acids. Arch Med Res 38.8 (2007): 901–904.

James, M., et al. 2010. Fish oil and rheumatoid arthritis: past, present and future. Proc.Nutr.Soc., 69, (3) 316–323.

Jans, L. A., et al. (2010). The efficacy of n-3 fatty acids DHA and EPA (fish oil) for pernatal depression. British Journal of Nutrition, 104(11), 1577–1585.

Jenkins DJ et al. Fish-oil supplementation in patients with implantable cardioverter defibrillators: a meta-analysis. CMAJ 178.2 (2008): 157–164.

Jeppesen J et al. Triglyceride concentration and ischemic heart disease: an eight-year follow-up in the Copenhagen Male Study. Circulation 97.11 (1998): 1029–1036.

Joy CB, et al. Polyunsaturated fatty acid supplementation for schizophrenia. Cochrane Database Syst Rev 3 (2006): CD001257.

Jung UJ et al. N-3 Fatty acids and cardiovascular disease: mechanisms underlying beneficial effects. Am J Clin Nutr 87.6 (2008): 2003S–2009S.

Kalmijn S. Fatty acid intake and the risk of dementia and cognitive decline: a review of clinical and epidemiological studies. J Nutr Health Aging 4.4 (2000): 202–207.

Kalmijn S et al. Dietary fat intake and the risk of incident dementia in the Rotterdam Study. Ann Neurol 42.5 (1997): 776–782.

Kalmijn S et al. Dietary intake of fatty acids and fish in relation to cognitive performance at middle age. Neurology 62.2 (2004): 275–280.

Kamphuis MH et al. Depression and cardiovascular mortality: a role for n-3 fatty acids? Am J Clin Nutr 84.6 (2006): 1513–1517.

Kang JX, Leaf A. The cardiac antiarrhythmic effects of polyunsaturated fatty acid. Lipids 31 (Suppl) (1996): S41–S44.

Kang JX, Leaf A. Prevention of fatal cardiac arrhythmias by polyunsaturated fatty acids. Am J Clin Nutr 71. (1 Suppl) (2000): 202–27S.

Kar, S. 2014. Omacor and omega-3 fatty acids for treatment of coronary artery disease and the pleiotropic effects. Am J Ther., 21, (1) 56–66.

Kato T, et al. Docosahexaenoic acid (DHA), a primary tumor suppressive omega-3 fatty acid, inhibits growth of colorectal cancer independent of p53 mutational status. Nutr Cancer 58.2 (2007): 178–187.

Kemperman RF et al. Low essential fatty acid and B-vitamin status in a subgroup of patients with schizophrenia and its response to dietary supplementation. Prostaglandins Leukot Essent Fatty Acids 74.2 (2006): 75–85.

Kendall-Tackett, K. (2010). Long-chain omega-3 fatty acids and women's mental health in the perinatal period and beyond. Journal of Midwifery & Women's Health, 55(6), 561–567.

Kiecolt-Glaser JK et al. Omega-3 supplementation lowers inflammation and anxiety in medical students: A randomized controlled trial. Brain, Behavior, and Immunity. 25.8 (2011): 1725–1734.

Kinsella JE. Effects of polyunsaturated fatty acids on factors related to cardiovascular disease. Am J Cardiol 60.12 (1987): 23G–32G.

Koch C et al. Docosahexaenoic acid (DHA) supplementation in atopic eczema: a randomized, double-blind, controlled trial. Br J Dermatol 158.4 (2008): 786–792.

Kondo K. A fish-based diet intervention improves endothelial function in postmenopausal women with type 2 diabetes mellitus: A randomized crossover trial. Metabolism. 63.7 (2014): 930–940.

Kremer JM. N-3 fatty acid supplements in rheumatoid arthritis. Am J Clin Nutr 71.(1 Suppl) (2000): 349S–351S.

Kristensen SD, et al. Dietary supplementation with n-3 polyunsaturated fatty acids and human platelet function: a review with particular emphasis on implications for cardiovascular disease. J Intern Med (Suppl) 225.731 (1989): 141–150.

Larsson SC et al. Dietary long-chain n-3 fatty acids for the prevention of cancer: a review of potential mechanisms. Am J Clin Nutr 79.6 (2004): 935–945.

Leaf A. On the reanalysis of the GISSI-Prevenzione. Circulation 105.16 (2002): 1874–1875.

Leckie RL et al. Omega-3 fatty acids moderate effects of physical activity on cognitive function. Neuropsychologia. 59 (2014): 103–111.

Leitzmann MF et al. Dietary intake of n-3 and n-6 fatty acids and the risk of prostate cancer. Am J Clin Nutr 80.1 (2004): 204–216.

Levine KE et al. Determination of mercury in an assortment of dietary supplements using an inexpensive combustion atomic absorption spectrometry technique. J Autom Methods Manag Chem 2005 (2005): 211–216.

Li, N.N., et al. 2014. Does intravenous fish oil benefit patients post-surgery? A meta-analysis of randomised controlled trials. Clin Nutr., 33, (2) 226–239.

Liang B et al. Impact of postoperative omega-3 fatty acid-supplemented parenteral nutrition on clinical outcomes and immunomodulations in colorectal cancer patients. World J Gastroenterol 14.15 (2008): 2434–2439.

Lim WS et al. Omega 3 fatty acid for the prevention of dementia. Cochrane Database Syst Rev 1 (2006): CD005379.

Liu J, Raine A. The effect of childhood malnutrition on externalizing behavior. Curr Opin Pediatr 18.5 (2006): 565–570.

Llor X et al. The effects of fish oil, olive oil, oleic acid and linoleic acid on colorectal neoplastic processes. Clin Nutr 22.1 (2003): 71–79.

Lou DJ et al. Serum phospholipid omega-3 polyunsaturated fatty acids and insulin resistance in type 2 diabetes mellitus and non-alcoholic fatty liver disease. J Diabetes Complications. 2014 (epub ahead of print).

MacLean CH et al. Effects of omega-3 fatty acids on lipids and glycemic control in type II diabetes and the metabolic syndrome and on inflammatory bowel disease, rheumatoid arthritis, renal disease, systemic lupus erythematosus, and osteoporosis. Evid Rep Technol Assess (Summ) 89 (2004): 1–4.

Mahaffey KR, et al. Blood organic mercury and dietary mercury intake: National Health and Nutrition Examination Survey, 1999 and 2000. Environ Health Perspect 112.5 (2004): 562–570.

Makrides, M., et al. (2010). Effect of DHA supplementation during pregnancy on maternal depression and neurodevelopment of young children: a randomized controlled trial. JAMA 304(15), 1675–1683.

Marchioli R et al. Early protection against sudden death by n-3 polyunsaturated fatty acids after myocardial infarction: time-course analysis of the results of the Gruppo Italiano per lo Studio della Sopravvivenza nell'Infarto Miocardico (GISSI)-Prevenzione. Circulation 105 (2002): 1897–1903.

Marks GB et al. Prevention of asthma during the first 5 years of life: a randomized controlled trial. J Allergy Clin Immunol 118.1 (2006): 53–61.

Masko EM et al. The Relationship Between Nutrition and Prostate Cancer: Is More Always Better? Eur Urol 63.5 (2013): 810–820.

Masson, S., et al. 2013. Plasma n-3 polyunsaturated fatty acids in chronic heart failure in the GISSI-Heart Failure Trial: relation with fish intake, circulating biomarkers, and mortality. Am Heart J, 165, (2) 208–215.

McClaskey EM, Michalets EL. Subdural hematoma after a fall in an elderly patient taking high-dose omega-3 fatty acids with warfarin and aspirin: case report and review of the literature. Pharmacotherapy 27.1 (2007): 152–160.

McEwen B et al. Effect of omega-3 fish oil on cardiovascular risk in diabetes. Diabetes Educ. 36.4 (2010): 565–84.

McEwen BJ et al. Effects of omega-3 polyunsaturated fatty acids on platelet function in healthy subjects and subjects with cardiovascular disease. Semin Thromb Hemost. 39.1 (2013): 25–32.

McLennan PL. Myocardial membrane fatty acids and the antiarrhythmic actions of dietary fish oil in animal models. Lipids 36 (Suppl) (2001): S111–S114.

McLennan, P.L. 2014a. Cardiac physiology and clinical efficacy of dietary fish oil clarified through cellular mechanisms of omega-3 polyunsaturated fatty acids. Eur J Appl. Physiol, 114, (7) 1333–1356.699892.

McLennan, P.L. 2014b. Cardiac physiology and clinical efficacy of dietary fish oil clarified through cellular mechanisms of omega-3 polyunsaturated fatty acids. Eur J Appl. Physiol, 114, (7) 1333–1356.

McLennan PL, et al. Dietary fish oil prevents ventricular fibrillation following coronary artery occlusion and reperfusion. Am Heart J 116.3 (1988): 709–717.

McLennan PL, et al. Reversal of the arrhythmogenic effects of long-term saturated fatty acid intake by dietary n-3 and n-6 polyunsaturated fatty acids. Am J Clin Nutr 51.1 (1990): 53–58.

McNamara RK, Carlson SE. Role of omega-3 fatty acids in brain development and function: potential implications for the pathogenesis and prevention of psychopathology. Prostaglandins Leukot Essent Fatty Acids 75.4–5 (2006): 329–349.

Melanson S et al. Measurement of organochlorines in commercial over-the-counter fish oil preparations: implications for dietary and therapeutic recommendations for omega-3 fatty acids and a review of the literature. Arch Pathol Lab Med 129.1 (2005): 74–77.

Mesa MD et al. Effects of oils rich in eicosapentaenoic and docosahexaenoic acids on the oxidizability and thrombogenicity of low-density lipoprotein. Atherosclerosis 175.2 (2004): 333–343.

Meyer BJ et al. Dietary intakes and food sources of omega-6 and omega-3 polyunsaturated fatty acids. Lipids 38.4 (2003): 391–398.

Michael-Titus AT and Priestley JV. Omega-3 fatty acids and traumatic neurological injury: from neuroprotection to neuroplasticity? Trends in Neurosciences. 37.1 (2014): 30–38.

Mickleborough TD et al. Protective effect of fish oil supplementation on exercise-induced bronchoconstriction in asthma. Chest 129.1 (2006): 39–49.

Miles, E.A. & Calder, P.C. 2012. Influence of marine n-3 polyunsaturated fatty acids on immune function and a systematic review of their effects on clinical outcomes in rheumatoid arthritis. Br J Nutr., 107 Suppl 2, S171–S184.

Miller, B. J., et al. (2013). Dietary supplements for preventing postnatal depression. Cochrane Database Syst Rev, 10, CD009104.

Miller PE et al. Long-chain omega-3 fatty acids eicosapentaenoic acid and docosahexaenoic acid and blood pressure: a meta-analysis of randomized controlled trials. Am J Hypertens. 27.7 (2014): 885–96.

Miura S et al. Modulation of intestinal immune system by dietary fat intake: relevance to Crohn's disease. J Gastroenterol Hepatol 13.12 (1998): 1183–1190.

Moher D. Effects of omega-3 fatty acids on child and maternal health. Rockville, MD: US Department of Health and Human Services, 2005.

Montgomery P, Richardson AJ. Omega-3 fatty acids for bipolar disorder. Cochrane Database Syst Rev 2 (2008): CD005169.

Montori VM et al. Fish oil supplementation in type 2 diabetes: a quantitative systematic review. Diabetes Care 23.9 (2000): 1407–1415.

Mori TA et al. Differential effects of eicosapentaenoic acid and docosahexaenoic acid on vascular reactivity of the forearm microcirculation in hyperlipidemic, overweight men. Circulation 102.11 (2000): 1264–1269.

Morris MC, et al. Does fish oil lower blood pressure? A meta-analysis of controlled trials. Circulation 88.2 (1993): 523–533.

Morris MC et al. Consumption of fish and n-3 fatty acids and risk of incident Alzheimer disease. Arch Neurol 60.7 (2003): 940–946.

Mozaffarian D et al. Fish intake and risk of incident heart failure. J Am Coll Cardiol 45.12 (2005): 2015–2021.

Mozaffarian D, Rimm E. Fish intake, contaminants, and human health: evaluating the risks and the benefits. JAMA 296.15 (2006): 1885–1899.

Mozaffarian, D. & Wu, J.H. 2011. Omega-3 fatty acids and cardiovascular disease: effects on risk factors, molecular pathways, and clinical events. J Am Coll. Cardiol., 58, (20) 2047–2067.

Mozurkewich, E. L., et al. (2013). The Mothers, Omega-3, and Mental Health Study: a double-blind, randomized controlled trial. American Journal of Obstetrics & Gynecology, 208(4), 313.e311–319.

Mucke L, Pitas RE. Food for thought: essential fatty acid protects against neuronal deficits in transgenic mouse model of AD. Neuron 43.5 (2004): 596–599.

Nair GM, Connolly SJ. Should patients with cardiovascular disease take fish oil? CMAJ 178.2 (2008): 181–182.

Navarro E et al. Abnormal fatty acid pattern in rheumatoid arthritis. A rationale for treatment with marine and botanical lipids. J Rheumatol 27.2 (2000): 298–303.

Nettleton JA, et al. N-3 long-chain polyunsaturated fatty acids in type 2 diabetes: a review. J Am Diet Assoc 105.3 (2005): 428–440.

Nicholson, T., et al. 2013. The role of marine n-3 fatty acids in improving cardiovascular health: a review. Food Funct., 4, (3) 357–365.

Noaghiul, S., & Hibbeln, J. R. (2003). Cross-national comparisons of seafood consumption and rates of bipolar disorders. Am J Psychiatry, 160(12), 2222–2227.

Olsen SF et al. Fish oil intake compared with olive oil intake in late pregnancy and asthma in the offspring: 16 y of registry-based follow-up from a randomized controlled trial. Am J Clin Nutr 88.1 (2008): 167–175.

Origasa, H., et al. 2010. Clinical importance of adherence to treatment with eicosapentaenoic acid by patients with hypercholesterolemia. Circ.J, 74, (3) 510–517.

Parra D et al. A diet rich in long chain omega-3 fatty acids modulates satiety in overweight and obese volunteers during weight loss. Appetite 51.3 (2008): 676–680.

Patel D et al. Omega-3 polyunsaturated fatty acid intake through fish consumption and prostate specific antigen level: Results from the 2003 to 2010 national health and examination survey. Prostaglandins, Leukotrienes and Essential Fatty Acids (PLEFA) 91.4 (2014): 155–160.

Pedersen M et al. Diet and risk of rheumatoid arthritis in a prospective cohort. J Rheumatol 32.7 (2005): 1249–1252.

Peet, M., & Horrobin, D. F. (2002). A dose-ranging study of the effects of ethyl-eicosapentaenoate in patients with ongoing depression despite apparently adequate treatment with standard drugs. Arch Gen Psychiatry, 59(10), 913–919.

Peet M. Eicosapentaenoic acid in the treatment of schizophrenia and depression: rationale and preliminary double-blind clinical trial results. Prostaglandins Leukot Essent Fatty Acids 69.6 (2003): 477–485.

Peet M. The metabolic syndrome, omega-3 fatty acids and inflammatory processes in relation to schizophrenia. Prostaglandins Leukot Essent Fatty Acids 75.4–5 (2006): 323–327.

Pizzorno J, Murray M. Textbook of natural medicine. St Louis: Elsevier, 2006.

Politi P et al. Behavioral effects of omega-3 fatty acid supplementation in young adults with severe autism: an open label study. Arch Med Res 39.7 (2008): 682–685.

Proudman SM, et al. Dietary omega-3 fats for treatment of inflammatory joint disease: efficacy and utility. Rheum Dis Clin North Am 34.2 (2008): 469–479.

Racine R, Deckelbaum R. Sources of the very-long-chain unsaturated omega-3 fatty acids: eicosapentaenoic acid and docosahexaenoic acid. Curr Opin Clin Nutr Metab Care 10.2 (2007): 123–128.

Radack K, et al. The comparative effects of n-3 and n-6 polyunsaturated fatty acids on plasma fibrinogen levels: a controlled clinical trial in hypertriglyceridemic subjects. J Am Coll Nutr 9.4 (1990): 352–357.

Ramel A et al. Beneficial effects of long-chain n-3 fatty acids included in an energy-restricted diet on insulin resistance in overweight and obese European young adults. Diabetologia 51.7 (2008): 1261–1268.

Richardson AJ, Puri BK. The potential role of fatty acids in attention-deficit/hyperactivity disorder. Prostaglandins Leukot Essent Fatty Acids 63.1–2 (2000): 79–87.

Riediger ND et al. A systemic review of the roles of n-3 fatty acids in health and disease. J Am Diet Assoc 109.4 (2009): 668–679.

Risk and Prevention Study Collaborative Group (2013) n-3 Fatty acids in patients with multiple cardiovascular risk factors. N Engl J Med 368(19):1800–1808.

Robert SS. Production of eicosapentaenoic and docosahexaenoic acid-containing oils in transgenic land plants for human and aquaculture nutrition. Mar Biotechnol (NY) 8.2 (2006): 103–109.

Roncaglioni, M.C., et al. 2013. N-3 fatty acids in patients with multiple cardiovascular risk factors. N. Engl. J Med, 368, (19) 1800–1808.

Rose DP, Connolly JM. Omega-3 fatty acids as cancer chemopreventive agents. Pharmacol Ther 83.3 (1999): 217–244.

Rosell MS et al. Long-chain n-3 polyunsaturated fatty acids in plasma in British meat-eating, vegetarian, and vegan men. Am J Clin Nutr 82.2 (2005): 327–334.

Ross CM. Fish oil, adrenal activation, and cardiovascular health [Letter]. Thromb Res 116.3 (2005): 273.

Roynette CE et al. N-3 polyunsaturated fatty acids and colon cancer prevention. Clin Nutr 23.2 (2004): 139–151.

Russo GL. Dietary n-6 and n-3 polyunsaturated fatty acids: from biochemistry to clinical implications in cardiovascular prevention. Biochem Pharmacol 77.6 (2009): 937–946.

Salam MT et al. Maternal fish consumption during pregnancy and risk of early childhood asthma. J Asthma 42.6 (2005): 513–518.

Sanhueza, C., et al. (2013). Diet and the risk of unipolar depression in adults: systematic review of cohort studies. Journal of Human Nutrition & Dietetics, 26(1), 56–70.

Schaller JL. Mercury and fish oil supplements. Med Gen Med 3.2 (2001): 20.

Schultz ST et al. Breastfeeding, infant formula supplementation, and autistic disorder: the results of a parent survey. Int Breastfeed J 1 (2006): 16.

Sears B et al. Therapeutic uses of high-dose omega-3 fatty acids to treat comatose patients with severe brain injury. PharmaNutrition. 1.3 (2013): 86–89.

Seki H et al. Omega-3 PUFA derived anti-inflammatory lipid mediator resolvin E1. Prostaglandins & Other Lipid Mediators. 89.3–4 (2009): 126–130.

Simopoulos AP. Essential fatty acids in health and chronic disease. Am J Clin Nutr 70.(3 Suppl) (1999): 56–9S.

Simopoulos AP. Omega-3 fatty acids in inflammation and autoimmune diseases. J Am Coll Nutr 21.6 (2002): 495–505.

Simopoulos AP. The importance of the omega-6/omega-3 fatty acid ratio in cardiovascular disease and other chronic diseases. Exp Biol Med (Maywood) 233.6 (2008): 674–688.

Sirtori CR et al. N-3 fatty acids do not lead to an increased diabetic risk in patients with hyperlipidemia and abnormal glucose tolerance: Italian Fish Oil Multicenter Study. Am J Clin Nutr 65.6 (1997): 1874–1881.

Sirtori CR et al. One-year treatment with ethyl esters of n-3 fatty acids in patients with hypertriglyceridemia and glucose intolerance: reduced triglyceridemia, total cholesterol and increased HDL-C without glycemic alterations. Atherosclerosis 137.2 (1998): 419–427.

Sirtori CR, Galli C. N-3 fatty acids and diabetes. Biomed Pharmacother 56.8 (2002): 397–406.

Siscovick DS, et al. The fish story: a diet-heart hypothesis with clinical implications: n-3 polyunsaturated fatty acids, myocardial vulnerability, and sudden death. Circulation 107.21 (2003): 2632–2634.

Sommerfield T, et al. Omega-3 fatty acids for intermittent claudication. Cochrane Database Syst Rev 4 (2007): CD003833.

Soyland E et al. Dietary supplementation with very long-chain n-3 fatty acids in patients with atopic dermatitis: A double-blind, multicentre study. Br J Dermatol 130.6 (1994): 757–764.

Stamp LK, et al. Diet and rheumatoid arthritis: A review of the literature. Semin Arthritis Rheum 35.2 (2005): 77–94.

Stern AH. A review of the studies of the cardiovascular health effects of methylmercury with consideration of their suitability for risk assessment. Environ Res 98.1 (2005): 133–142.

Stoll BA. N-3 fatty acids and lipid peroxidation in breast cancer inhibition. Br J Nutr 87.3 (2002): 193–198.

Stone NJ. The Gruppo Italiano per lo Studio della Sopravvivenza nell' Infarto Miocardio (GISSI)-Prevenzione Trial on fish oil and vitamin E supplementation in myocardial infarction survivors. Curr Cardiol Rep 2.5 (2000): 445–451.

Tacon A, Metian M. Aquaculture feed and food safety. Ann N Y Acad Sci 1140 (2008): 50–59.

Tajalizadekhoob, Y. et al. (2011). The effect of low-dose omega 3 fatty acids on the treatment of mild to moderate depression in the elderly: a double-blind, randomized, placebo-controlled study. European Archives of Psychiatry & Clinical Neuroscience, 261(8), 539–549.

Tanaka, K., et al. 2008. Reduction in the recurrence of stroke by eicosapentaenoic acid for hypercholesterolemic patients: subanalysis of the JELIS trial. Stroke, 39, (7) 2052–2058.

Tang FY et al. Concomitant supplementation of lycopene and eicosapentaenoic acid inhibits the proliferation of human colon cancer cells. J Nutr Biochem (2009); 20: 426–434.

Tavazzi L et al. Effect of n-3 polyunsaturated fatty acids in patients with chronic heart failure (the GISSI-HF trial): a randomised, double-blind, placebo-controlled trial. Lancet 372.9645 (2008): 1223–1230.

Terano T et al. Docosahexanoic acid supplementation improves the moderately severe dementia from thrombotic cerebrovascular disease. Lipids 34 (Suppl) (1994): S345–S346.

Terry PD, et al. Intakes of fish and marine fatty acids and the risks of cancers of the breast and prostate and of other hormone-related cancers: a review of the epidemiologic evidence. Am J Clin Nutr 77.3 (2003): 532–543.

Terry PD, et al. Long-chain (n-3) fatty acid intake and risk of cancers of the breast and the prostate: recent epidemiological studies, biological mechanisms, and directions for future research. J Nutr 134 (2004): 3412–320S.

Torfadottir JE et al. Consumption of fish products across the lifespan and prostate cancer risk. PLoS.One 8.4 (2013): e59799.

Ulbricht CE, Basch EM. Natural standard herb and supplement reference. St Louis: Mosby, 2005.

Visioli F et al. Dietary intake of fish vs. formulations leads to higher plasma concentrations of n-3 fatty acids. Lipids 38.4 (2003): 415–418.

Virtanen JK et al. Serum long-chain n-3 polyunsaturated fatty acids, mercury, and risk of sudden cardiac death in men: a prospective population-based study. PLoS.One 7.7 (2012): e41046.

Volker D et al. Efficacy of fish oil concentrate in the treatment of rheumatoid arthritis. J Rheumatol 27.10 (2000): 2343–2346.

von Schacky C, et al. The effect of n-3 fatty acids on coronary atherosclerosis: results from SCIMO, an angiographic study, background and implications. Lipids 36 (Suppl) (2001): S99–102.

Weber P, Raederstorff D. Triglyceride-lowering effect of omega-3 LC-polyunsaturated fatty acids: a review. Nutr Metab Cardiovasc Dis 10.1 (2000): 28–37.

Weisburger JH. Dietary fat and risk of chronic disease: mechanistic insights from experimental studies. J Am Diet Assoc 97.(7 Suppl) (1997): S16–S23.

Wennberg M et al. Myocardial infarction in relation to mercury and fatty acids from fish: a risk-benefit analysis based on pooled Finnish and Swedish data in men. Am J Clin Nutr 96.4 (2012): 706–713.

Whelan J, Rust C. Innovative dietary sources of n-3 fatty acids. Annu Rev Nutr 26 (2006): 75–103.

Williams C et al. Stereo acuity at age 3–5 years in children born full term is associated with pre-natal and post-natal dietary factors: a report from a population-based cohort study. Am J Clin Nutr 73 (2001): 316–322.

Wong KW. Clinical efficacy of n-3 fatty acid supplementation in patients with asthma. J Am Diet Assoc 105.1 (2005): 98–105.

Woods RK, et al. Dietary marine fatty acids (fish oil) for asthma in adults and children. Cochrane Database Syst Rev 3 (2002): CD001283.

Wu JH et al. Omega-3 fatty acids and incident type 2 diabetes: a systematic review and meta-analysis. Br J Nutr 107(Suppl 2) (2012): S214–S227.

Yamada T et al. Atherosclerosis and ω-3 fatty acids in the populations of a fishing village and a farming village in Japan. Atherosclerosis. 153.2 (2000): 469–481.

Yehuda S, et al. Essential fatty acids and the brain: from infancy to aging. Neurobiol Aging 26.(Suppl 1) (2005): 98–102.

Yokoyama, M. 2009. [Japan EPA Lipid Intervention Study (JELIS). Randomized clinical trial involving primary and secondary prevention of cardiovascular events with EPA in hypercholesterolemia.] Nihon Ronen Igakkai Zasshi, 46, (1) 22–25.

Zheng JS et al. Marine N-3 polyunsaturated fatty acids are inversely associated with risk of type 2 diabetes in Asians: a systematic review and meta-analysis. PLoS.One 7.9 (2012): e44525.

Flaxseed oil

HISTORICAL NOTE For over 5000 years, flaxseed in its various forms has been a part of the diet of people in Asia, Africa and Europe. It has a long history of use as both a food and a medicine, with the seed being most commonly used. The oil was also popular and has been a traditional food of the Egyptians from the time of the Pharaohs to the present day. The oil is also consumed by the Chinese, who documented its medicinal properties in the Pen-T's AO, the Great Chinese Pharmacopeia (Judd 1995). Its Latin name *usitatissimum* means 'most useful', suggesting its various uses have been recognised for centuries (Kolodziejczyk & Fedec 1995). Interestingly, research into its nutritional properties and effects on human health were not studied in earnest until the 1980s (Cunnane & Thompson 1995). In Australia in 1981, cultivation of a low alpha-linolenic acid (ALA) variety, now known as Linola, was pioneered in an attempt to improve the stability of the oil and increase its commercial viability as a cooking oil. Such modifications were successful and resulted in ALA content <3.0% and a higher concentration of linoleic acid than the naturally occurring form (Bhatty 1995, Hall et al 2006). These modified oils are not used for medicinal purposes.

OTHER NAMES

Flax oil and linseed oil.

Internationally, it is accepted that 'flaxseed' refers to products for human consumption, whereas 'linseed oil' refers to products that have been denatured, made unfit for human consumption and used in commercial products, such as paints and varnishes.

BOTANICAL NAME/FAMILY

Linium usitatissimum (family Linaceae)

PLANT PART USED

Fixed oil is derived from the seeds of the plant. Due to the highly polyunsaturated nature of the oil (≈ 73%), extracts are obtained by cold-pressing rather than heat extraction. Flaxseed oil (FSO) is highly susceptible to photo-oxygenation, so it is packaged in opaque bottles. It is also susceptible to auto-oxidation, resulting in the production of hydroperoxides and aldehydes that can give a rancid flavour. Encapsulated FSO is considered more stable, particularly when antioxidants are added (Kolodziejczyk & Fedec 1995).

Eating the seeds versus defatted flour or taking the oil

With the growth of flaxseed-based bakery goods that have arrived on the market in recent years, it is valuable to review the bioavailability and therapeutic potential of such products. A study compared the effect of consuming flaxseeds (30 g/day) versus both milled flaxseed (30 g/day) and FSO (6 g/day) over a 3-month period on corresponding blood lipid profiles (Austria et al 2008). These results revealed that while the milled preparation and oil extract produced significant physiological increases in ALA levels (with the FSO producing the largest effect), consumption of the whole seeds did not (Austria et al 2008). Effects in individuals consuming the whole seeds also demonstrated the greatest inter-individual variability, probably related to the degree of chewing each subject performed. Consequently, while the consumption of whole flaxseeds can boost dietary fibre and phyto-oestrogen content, they do not appear to be a reliable means to supplying ALA. In a study comparing the energy and macronutrient balance between flaxseed (FS), defatted flaxseed flour (FF) and flaxseed oil (FO), investigators found a higher energy excretion in the FF and FS groups, and higher total lipid and PUFA (ALA) excretion in the FS group, with a maintenance of body weight despite a higher energy intake (Gonçalves de Oliveira et al 2012). Further, in a study of flaxseed oil bioavailability, emulsified versus non-emulsified FO was examined in rats. ALA bioavailability was improved in rats who ingested FO in the emulsified state.

CHEMICAL COMPONENTS

Flaxseed oil contains several types of fatty acids (FAs). It contains a high concentration of ALA, ranging from 40% to 60%, and is the most concentrated plant source of omega-3 FA identified to date.

FSO also contains unsaturated FAs, such as linolenic acid, linoleic acid and oleic acid. Linoleic acid (LA or C18:2 ω-6) and oleic acid each contribute 15% to the total FA content of the oil. Due to the range of FA present, it contains precursors for the omega-3, -6 and -9 families. Environmental factors can profoundly influence the unsaturated FA composition and ratios (Hall et al 2006). FSO may also contain varying amounts of the lignan, secoisolariciresinol diglycoside (SDG), which is a precursor to enterodiol and enterolactone.

Flax seeds contain 41% fat, 28% dietary fibre, 21% protein and significantly higher amounts of lignans, which behave as phyto-oestrogens (Morris 2001). This review, however, focuses on FSO.

Clinical note — Is FSO equivalent to the fish oils?

FSO has been commercially promoted as the vegetarian or vegan alternative to fish oils, with many of the health benefits ascribed to fish oils also being attributed to FSO. A review of the literature suggests that FSO is unlikely to be equipotent with fish oils in the treatment of a variety of conditions.

The ALA present in FSO can theoretically undergo desaturation and elongation to synthesise eicosapentaenoic acid (EPA) and docosahexaenoic (DHA), which are found in fish oil; however, most studies using oral FSO intake demonstrate only moderate increases in EPA and DHA remains unchanged (Allman et al 1995, Arterburn et al 2006, Barcelo-Coblijn et al 2008, Kelley et al 1993, Mantzioris et al 1994, Nestel et al 1997). Although results from one early study suggest that increases in DHA levels may be achieved with long-term supplementation (Cunnane et al 1993), more recent studies fail to confirm this result (Barcelo-Coblijn et al 2008, Harper et al 2006a, Hussein et al 2005).

Conversion rates of ALA to EPA and docosapentaenoic acid (DPA) are reported to be <10% and approximately 8%, respectively, whereas the DHA yield ranges from 0% to 0.5%. One explanation for this is that DHA synthesis is under separate regulatory control, a hypothesis supported by enzymatic studies (Burdge 2004). Theoretically, therefore, a 20 mL serve of FSO, providing 11.1 g of ALA, would result in a maximum of 880 mg DPA and 5 mg of DHA. A recent study investigating optimal minimal dosing of FSO, however, reported that increased red blood cell omega-3 concentrations are evident at a minimum of 2.4 g/day taken over 2 weeks, with the largest effect seen at the 6–8-week timeframe (Barcelo-Coblijn et al 2008). These authors also report that 1.2 g/day of fish oil produced comparable changes, concluding that FSO or other plant-based ALA sources represent a realistic alternative source of omega-3s, and at doses much lower than previously studied.

However, there is marked inter-individual variation in conversion efficacy, even in the face of comparable background diets and some notable gender differences, with resultant DHA typically undetectable in males consuming high-dose ALA (Arterburn et al 2006). Adding to this puzzle is a wide range of other variables that can inhibit the conversion of ALA into its metabolites. For instance, high dietary intake of linoleic acid (LA), common in Western cultures (Arterburn et al 2006, Breslow 2006, Faintuch et al 2011), inhibits both the uptake of ALA and its conversion to long-chain metabolites due to competition for shared enzymes. An interesting study conducted in 1998, which used radioactively labelled ALA, showed that a diet high in omega-6 fats reduced conversion by 40–50% (Gerster 1998), resulting in 70% net reduction of long chain omega-3 end products (Arterburn et al 2006). This adds weight to the argument that the ratios of FAs may have the primary influence on their resultant health benefits. The authors of this study suggest that the ratio of omega-6:omega-3 should not exceed 4. In contrast, the typical American diet demonstrates an LA:ALA ratio of ≥11.5 (Arterburn et al 2006, Breslow 2006). However, there are authors who refute that the ratios are a major determinant (Goyens et al 2006).

Other studies have reported abnormal or compromised activity of the delta-6 and delta-5 desaturase enzymes in the elderly, diabetics and patients with a variety of metabolic disorders, as well as those individuals with increased dietary intake of saturated fats, *trans*-fatty acids and alcohol (David & Kris-Etherton 2003). Studies using radioisotopes of ALA have revealed significant gender differences in conversion capability, with women demonstrating higher levels of FA metabolites. It is believed that this is due to their higher oestrogen levels, a theory supported by the increased conversion capacity evident in women taking synthetic oestrogens and speculated as representing a physiological adaptation that ensures adequate essential fatty acid (EFA) delivery to the fetus in pregnancy (Burdge 2004).

Finally, it appears that ALA conversion to long chain omega-3 FA is also self-limiting, with high intakes producing significantly increased oxidation and impairing conversion into EPA and DHA (Arterburn et al 2006, Schwab et al 2006). Based on the available evidence, it appears that ALA conversion is relatively inefficient in humans, making ALA a poor means of increasing omega-3 levels (Arterburn et al 2006).

MAIN ACTIONS

The main actions of FSO have been attributed to its high ALA content. ALA is subject to three different metabolic fates: (a) incorporation into structural, transport or storage pools, (b) beta-oxidation as an energy source, and (c) elongation and further desaturation to form EPA, DPA and DHA. It appears that all three contribute to the biological effects of this oil.

ALA's direct role in cell membrane structure is likely to be minor, with ALA representing less than 0.5% of the total FA in cell membranes and blood lipids in healthy adults and possessing a limited distribution (e.g. adipose, rectal epithelium, cheek, heart) (Arterburn et al 2006). However, its limited propensity to generate the ω-3 metabolites, EPA and DHA, the major FAs in cell membranes, could represent an indirect effect via this mechanism

(Burdge 2004). Studies exploring the metabolism of ALA have revealed that 22% of ALA undergoes beta-oxidation in women and 33% in men. Once broken down, the carbon chain can be used as fuel or in the synthesis of cholesterol and other fatty acids such as palmitic, palmitoleic, stearic and oleic acids de novo (Burdge 2004). FSO also influences the eicosanoid production cascade via conversion of the ω-3 and ω-6 parent FAs in FSO to their respective metabolites.

It is also thought that some of the actions of FSO may be independent of its FA content and can be attributed to the lignan SDG. This has been supported by research conducted by Prasad et al in 1998 and again in 1999. The SDG has been confirmed as the main lignin present in flaxseed, and that this lignin is converted to the mammalian lignans enterodiol (ED) and enterolactone (EL) by gastrointestinal microbiota (Bassett et al 2009, Dukes et al 2012, Gagnon et al 2009, Park & Velasquez 2012, Rhee and Brunt 2008). In a study of ruminal metabolism of flaxseed in dairy cows, researchers identified that concentrations of SDG were higher in urine, plasma and milk when placed in the rumen of the cows and that ruminal microbiota are important in the metabolism of flaxseed lignans.

Anti-inflammatory

Metabolites of ALA and LA act as substrates for the formation of the anti-inflammatory eicosanoids, comprising prostaglandins, thromboxanes and leukotrienes (Gerster 1998). ALA suppresses AA production by interfering with the conversion of LA to AA, and reduces the biosynthesis of inflammatory eicosanoids, although not to the same extent as EPA and DHA (Morris 2001). Cytokines, another important group of inflammatory mediators, are generated in response to these eicosanoids and are influenced by changes in the ω-3 : ω-6 ratios in cell membranes (James et al 2000). In one study, ingestion of FSO (equivalent to 13.7 g/day ALA) for 4 weeks by healthy male subjects resulted in a 30% reduction in TNF-alpha, 31% reduction in IL-1-beta, 29% reduction in eicosanoids thromboxane B(2) and 30% reduction in PGE_2 (Caughey et al 1996). In contrast, more recent studies have failed to demonstrate anti-inflammatory effects (Barcelo-Coblijn et al 2008, Paschos et al 2007, Sturgeon et al 2011, Zong et al 2013).

In animal models, ALA has consistently demonstrated eicosanoid-mediated anti-inflammatory effects; however, the magnitude of the effect has been dependent on the levels of both ALA and LA in the diet, duration of use and type of tissue studied (Cunnane & Thompson 1995).

Immune effects

Evidence of ALA deficiency has been reported in patients on prolonged total parenteral nutrition (TPN), which resulted in reduced T-helper cells to below the normal range and impaired proliferation of peripheral blood mononuclear cells. Although supplementation with small doses of ALA corrected these abnormalities, the effect of ALA on human immune cells appears to be paradoxical, with evidence of immune function inhibition at higher doses (≥40 mL/day FSO) (Kelley 1992).

More recently, animal models have suggested some beneficial effects of chronic flaxseed intake on haematological and immunological function in the development of Wistar rats. Female rats were fed 25% flaxseed during gestation, and continuing in the male newborn pups through to adult life (250 days old). A significant increase in haemoglobin and albumin, and a smaller percentage of segmented lymphocytes was observed, as well as a significant reduction in body mass (Ferreira Medeiros de Franca Cardozo et al 2011). In human studies, researchers have not found convincing evidence of increased immune function as a result of effects of flaxseed lignan, secoisolariciresinol diglucoside (SDG) (Rhee & Brunt 2008). More research is required.

Cardiovascular effects

Because ALA can be converted to long-chain (ω-3) PUFA in humans and may potentially reproduce the beneficial effects of fish oils, FSO and ALA have been studied as possible preventive or treatment agents for cardiovascular disease. Epidemiological evidence of secondary coronary event prevention from ALA, in the context of a modified Mediterranean diet, support this premise (Schwab et al 2006). While numerous studies have suggested that FSO and ALA exert a myriad of different mechanisms in the body, which can be beneficial in cardiovascular disease, inconsistent results have been reported. In secondary prevention trials, such as the Lyon Diet Heart Study (1999), reporting on the effects of the Mediterranean Diet, it was shown that dietary ALA has a significant cardioprotective effect, with a decreased risk of recurrent fatal and nonfatal myocardial infarction and a significant reduction in risk (73%) in primary end points of cardiac mortality and morbidity (Rodriguez-Leyva et al 2010).

In a symposium paper, researchers suggest that the ω-3 ALA component in FXO contributes to the antiatherogenic effect via anti-inflammatory and antiproliferative mechanisms. They suggest that dietary flaxseed may also protect against ischaemic heart disease by improving vascular relaxation responses and inhibiting the incidence of ventricular fibrillation (Bassett et al 2009).

Antithrombotic and antiplatelet activities

The question of whether supplementation with ALA affects platelet aggregation appears to now suggest that this is not part of flaxseed's main profile (Kaul et al 2008; Finnegan et al 2003; Austria et al 2008)). A major determinant appears to be the degree of conversion to EPA (Garg et al 1989), and the ratio of ω-3 PUFAs to ω-6 PUFAs in modulating haemostatic function (Rodriguez-Leyva et al 2010). When there is an increase in total EPA and reduced AA, due to ALA inhibition of LA conversion, the result is EPA replacing AA in the cell membrane and a decrease in thromboxane synthesis. In addition, SDG, another component of FSO, is metabolised to enterolactone and enterodiol, and these substances may have antiplatelet-activating factor activity, although studies suggest the results are isolated and modest at best. Due to the variable lignan content of FSO, it is difficult to determine the clinical significance of this (Prasad 1999). Studies assessing the actual antiaggregatory effect of FSO in humans have produced mixed results.

Reduced endothelial inflammation

A number of studies have confirmed that consumption of high-dose FSO reduces endothelium inflammation. One study assessing the cardiovascular effects of a diet in which 6.5% of total kilocalorie intake was contributed by ALA and compared with the Standard American Diet (SAD) showed that the ALA-enriched diet produced a 75% reduction in C-reactive protein, a 19% reduction in cellular adhesion molecule and a 15.6% reduction in vascular cellular adhesion molecule (VCAM) (Zhao et al 2004). An earlier study had reported these findings, demonstrating a 28% reduction in VCAM with additional reductions in soluble E-selectin (17%) (Thies et al 2001). ALA levels examined as part of a plasma cholesterol fraction have been found to be negatively correlated with CRP concentrations (Klein-Platat et al 2005). Research in the mouse model demonstrated that flaxseed (0.4 g/day) inhibits the expression of inflammatory markers like interleukin (IL)-6, mac-3 and vascular cell adhesion molecule-1 (VCAM-1) in aortic atherosclerotic tissue (Dupasquier et al 2007).

Lipid-lowering effect

Whole flaxseed is the form most commonly investigated in lipid-lowering studies, because the high fibre content and ALA have been speculated to act synergistically, therefore there are relatively few studies using FSO. Those that have been conducted with FSO have produced conflicting results with an almost 50/50 weighting of research showing no effect (Austria et al 2008, Harper et al 2006, Kaul et al 2008, Schwab et al 2006) or a positive one. At worst, FSO has produced increased fasting triacylglycerol concentrations and lower HDL cholesterol (Bemelmans et al 2002, Finnegan et al 2003, Wilkinson et al 2005). At best, it has been described in earlier studies as having comparable effects with bioequivalent doses of fish oils (Harris 1997, Singer et al 1986). The reality probably lies somewhere in between; however, further investigation is required. The results of a small study of 57 men by Wilkinson et al (2005), who substituted 45 g of fat per day with 15 g/day ALA derived from FSO over 12 weeks, adds to the puzzle. While confirming the mixed cardiovascular effects noted above, this treatment group also demonstrated a reduction of total cholesterol by 12.3% in comparison to a reduction of 7.3% in the group receiving equivalent LA. While another study comparing the effects of an ALA-rich (6.8 g/day) versus EPA/DHA-rich (1.6 g/day) diet in mildly hypercholesterolaemic elderly subjects over 6 weeks revealed improved lipid responses in the ALA than the EPA/DHA group (Goyens & Mensink 2006).

The same equivocal trend is evident from studies assessing the effects of FSO on lipoproteins. Zhao's trial (2004) using an ALA-enriched diet produced a reduction in apolipoproteins A1 and B, the latter by almost 10%, however, more recent studies administering ≥3 g/day of ALA from FSO over 6–26 weeks failed to demonstrate any effect on lipoprotein particle or size concentrations (Goyens & Mensink 2006, Harper et al 2006b). In spite of these seemingly disappointing findings, some researchers note a preventive effect against cardiovascular morbidity associated with increased ALA consumption in the substantial Lyon diet study was not accompanied by cholesterol changes and therefore may point to an alternative mechanism (Kaul et al 2008). Additionally, the context of diet may be important. In a rat model, rats fed a high-fat, high-fructose diet supplemented with lignan-enriched flaxseed powder (LEFP) showed an improvement in lipid profile, as well as reduced bodyweight and fat accumulation and blood pressure control, compared to the high-fat, high-fructose diet, the normal control diet and the normal diet supplemented with LEFP (Park and Velasquez 2012). In a healthy rat model, supplementation with 20% FS raised HDL-cholesterol, and reduced LDL-cholesterol, glucose and uric acid indicating preventive potential of FS for CVD (Tomaz Pacheco et al 2011).

Antiarrhythmic

Four studies have identified an antiarrhythmic effect mediated by ALA (Albert et al 2005, Ander et al 2004, Christensen et al 2005, Djoussé et al 2005), although one meta-analysis concluded otherwise (Matthan et al 2005). Although the majority of research has been conducted in animals, one of the most interesting human trials involved 106 women with a mean age of 59.5 years referred for coronary angiography due to suspected coronary artery disease. Following adipose sampling for ALA levels and monitoring of 24-hour heart rate variability (HRV), it was concluded that a positive and independent association was present between ALA in adipose tissue and HRV, which was even stronger in smokers (Christensen et al 2005).

Antiatherogenic

Earlier positive findings and promising epidemiological data have been substantially challenged by RCTs of FSO in atherosclerosis. Following earlier positive outcomes in cardiovascular disease trials with whole flaxseed, a 1999 study showed that a low-ALA variety could produce comparable results with the earlier trials, suggesting that the antiatherogenic properties of flaxseed are independent of its ALA content (Prasad 1999).

More recent large-scale epidemiological studies continue to suggest a relationship between higher ALA intake and reduced coronary artery calcification (Djousse et al 2005); however, there is ongoing criticism that important variables have not been sufficiently accounted for, such as corresponding reductions in *trans*-FAs (Harris 2005, Wilkinson et al 2005).

Antiproliferative

ALA has demonstrated the capacity to inhibit tumour progression in animal models of mammary tumour (Chen et al 2002, Cognault et al 2000); however, the clinical significance of these findings needs to be examined further. An immunostimulant action, which is both eicosanoid and non-eicosanoid mediated, has been suggested as one possible mechanism of action. Another theory suggests that through ALA's competitive inhibition of LA, tumour cells may not receive sufficient LA, which would inhibit further cell growth (Johnston 1995). It is interesting to observe that higher dietary ALA intake is associated with a reduction in cancer deaths; however, this is not seen with higher EPA/DHA intakes, suggesting that the protective effect is not reliant on the conversion of ALA to EPA/DHA (Cunnane 1995). In addition, results from epidemiological studies show an association between low ALA consumption in humans and increased cancer deaths in general (Dolecek 1992).

Animal studies testing SDG and its metabolites from the seeds have produced promising results and suggest that they may act as selective oestrogen receptor modulating agents and therefore play a protective role against oestrogen-dependent cancers (Kitts et al 1999, Wang et al 2005).

Hypotensive

The mechanism for ALA's potential hypotensive action remains to be elucidated and in light of the bulk of negative findings, more research to support these current results is necessary (Paschos et al 2007). Research investigating the effects of FS on inflammation and carotid diameter in morbidly obese patients may point to a possible mechanism. Researchers found that after 12 weeks of flaxseed supplementation, large artery diameter and inflammatory markers deteriorated less compared with controls whose clinical course continued to deteriorate (Faintuch et al 2011). In a review of flaxseed on cardiovascular effects, flaxseed was proposed to protect against the loss of endothelial-dependent vascular function, which is induced by hypertensive or cholesterolaemic conditions (Bassett et al 2009). The effects of flaxseed on the preservation of arterial relaxation requires further investigation.

Insulin sensitising

Preliminary animal studies suggested a protective role for ALA against the development of insulin resistance and an ability to counter the associated oxidative stress (Ghafoorunissa & Natarajan 2005, Suresh & Das 2003). However, a series of clinical trials examining high-dose FSO in patients with type 2 diabetes failed to demonstrate any positive effect on glycaemic control (Barre et al 2008, Schwab et al 2006). Nor was any effect demonstrated in post-menopausal women in circulating levels of insulin and IGF-1 or C-peptide (Sturgeon et al 2011).

CNS development

Animal studies present some evidence for FSO in the fetal and early development of the central nervous system (CNS) in rats. The importance of essential fatty acids (EFA), especially omega-3 FAs, in the CNS development of newborns is known. It was found that there were significant increases in the brain weight of newborn pups from mothers fed with FSO, and that ω-3 FAs were found to be incorporated into the brain tissue of the pups (Almeida et al 2011). In a further study, body growth was shown to be adequate and brain development, incorporating omega-3 FA into the tissue, was increased up to 52 days post-birth, representing equivalent childhood and adolescence of rats (Ferreira et al 2011). In a study of behavioural development and habituation to environment, brain weight was superior in the FSO rats, as was aggregation of omega-3 FA in the brain tissue. Habituation and behavioural management in this group was superior demonstrating lower levels of stress (de Meneses et al 2011).

Antioxidant

The health benefits and preventative capacity of antioxidants for chronic diseases and ageing is well documented; however, in recent years, peptides with antioxidant capacity have gained interest. These peptides are reported to be released from the parent protein by gastrointestinal enzymes and/or microflora or in vitro by stimulated digestion using isolated enzymes (Silva et al 2013). The preliminary research suggest that Flaxseed protein hydrolysate (FPH) and Flaxseed protein isolate (FPI) may have some antioxidant capacity, and that hydrolysis produced by gastric conversion to produce peptides in vitro may have an optimal range. However, in this study, FPI or FPH did not produce a protective effect on U937 human cell lines. Interestingly, there have been reports of a converse effect where flaxseed supplementation produced an increase in oxidative stress (Bassett et al 2009). Further research is required to understand the potential of flaxseed's antioxidant capacity (Silva et al 2013).

CLINICAL USE

Reduced mortality in coronary heart disease

The most likely mechanism by which ALA may prevent coronary heart disease (CHD) mortality is by reducing cardiac arrhythmia (Rodriguez-Leyva et al 2010). In Western populations, almost 50% of all deaths from cardiovascular disease can be attributed to sudden cardiac death and the majority of sudden deaths are directly caused by acute ventricular arrhythmia (Brouwer et al 2004). A review in 2001 (Lanzmann-Petithory 2001) and a meta-analysis of three studies in 2004 (Brouwer et al) both found in favour of a protective effect from increased ALA consumption against fatal CHD (RR 0.24). The dose associated with this trend was small; only 1–3 g/day ALA higher than controls (Brouwer et al 2004). A study published in 2005, which derived data from the Nurses' Health Study (Albert et al 2005), found that women consuming ALA in the highest two quintiles had a 38–40% lower risk of sudden cardiac death than women in the lowest quintile; however, the protective effect did not extend to other fatal forms of CHD or non-fatal myocardial infarction. A cross-sectional study found that in both men and women high levels of dietary ALA were associated with a shorter QT interval, and suggests a protective effect against abnormally long repolarisation, and therefore risk of ventricular filbrillation (Djoussé et al 2005). Animal data also demonstrated shorter QT intervals and a marked reduction in ventricular fibrillation, and suggest alterations in the calcium/sodium exchange (Ander et al 2004).

Much criticism has been directed at those researchers wanting to extrapolate prescriptive advice from these findings. An editorial by Harris (2005) notes that an early primary prevention study with ALA in CHD has been conducted and that was in the 1960s. The 1-year trial involved 13,578 Norwegian men and compared 10 g of FSO (providing 5.5/day ALA) with a sunflower seed placebo. In the analysis, there was no demonstrable difference in end points between the two groups. Recent attempts to explain this lack of effect, such as high baseline ω-3 consumption by this population, appear to be well founded (Mozaffarian et al 2005).

The research regarding ALA found in flaxseed and its effects on CAD is not as mature as the marine ω-3 PUFAs, EPA and DHA data, and the role of ALA in human nutrition is still being debated. In a review by Rodriguez-Leyva et al (2010) on the effects of flaxseed, it was reported that results from nine major studies suggest that ALA levels are inversely correlated with primary cardiovascular events. The studies used large sample sizes and extended over a relatively long follow-up time. In animal studies, researchers found that atherosclerosis was significantly prevented by flaxseed supplementation in the hypercholesterolaemic rabbit (Dupasquier et al 2006) and in the cholesterol-fed, low-density lipoprotein (LDL) receptor-deficient mouse; however, the review speculates that because there was relatively poor correlation with cholesterol-lowering effect of flaxseed, the hypolipidaemic effect is likely to be only one of the contributing factors to its antiatherogenic potential (Rodriguez-Leyva et al 2010).

In secondary prevention trials, as stated above, ALA was associated with a decreased risk of recurrent fatal and nonfatal myocardial infarction and cardiac mortality and morbidity (Lyon Diet Heart Study — de Lorgeril et al 1999).

Anticlotting

There have been a surprising number of studies investigating the influence of ALA from FSO on coagulation and fibrinolysis, and enormous variation in results. Methodological issues have plagued the overall quality of evidence, with small sample sizes, inconsistent methodologies and diverse sample characteristics making interpretation difficult.

One early study compared different dietary ratios of ω-6 and ω-3 EFAs in relation to prostanoid production in a group of normolipidaemic men (Kelley et al 1993). The high ALA dietary intervention constituted an overall ω-6 : ω-3 ratio of 2.7 versus control ratio of up to 27.4. Following the 18 days of the intervention, groups showed significant differences in measured outcomes, notably, that 6-keto-$PGF_{1\alpha}$ was significantly higher following the high ALA diet, but no evidence of significant effect on bleeding time or thromboxane B_2 production. A second study published in the same year also failed to show an effect on clotting; however, the dose of FSO used was only 4.3 g/day (Kelley et al 1993). In contrast, the results of a study using a much larger dose of 40 g/day of FSO over 23 days in 11 healthy men showed that FSO significantly reduced collagen-induced aggregation response when compared to 40 g/day sunflower seed oil (Allman et al 1995).

A follow-up study of 29 healthy males that was conducted over 6 weeks investigated the effects of a diet in which approximately 7% of the total kilocalories from polyunsaturated fat was made up of either an ALA-rich (ω-3 : ω-6 = 1 : 1.2) or LA-rich diet (ω-3 : ω-6 = 1 : 21). The ALA-enriched diet resulted in triple the EPA phospholipid levels compared to the LA-enriched diet, but had no demonstrable effect on coagulation or fibrinolysis, other than an increase in the ratio of activated protein C. The authors speculated that the latter finding may still prove significant, but suggest that future studies should be conducted in patients with vascular pathology, as healthy clotting profiles may have obscured the true effects of FSO (Allman-Farinelli et al 1999).

In the same year, another group of Australian researchers published the results of their study of 17 vegetarian men who were assigned to either a low- or a high-ALA diet (derived from FSO) for 28 days following a run-in baseline diet for 14 days. Again there were no significant differences in prothrombin time, activated partial thromboplastin time or plasminogen activities with the different ALA diets, despite increases in EPA and DPA levels (Li et al 1999).

Since 1994, Mutanen and Freese have conducted many studies assessing the effect of ALA and

LA:ALA ratios on haemostatic factors (Freese et al 1994, Freese & Mutanen 1997, Mutanen & Freese 2001). Their 1997 study was the largest and involved a sample of 46 subjects who were given FSO to provide 5.9 g/day ALA or a fish/sunflower oil combination equal to 5.2 g/day EPA/DHA over 4 weeks. Extensive analysis of the sample throughout the intervention, as well as at the 12-week follow-up, revealed no difference in collagen-induced platelet aggregation, thromboxane production or bleeding time between the two groups, suggesting equivalent anticoagulant effects for FSO and fish oil when consumed in comparable quantities. This was despite smaller increases in EPA levels in the platelets of the subjects taking FSO.

The largest and most recent trial (Finnegan et al 2003) compared the effects of small increases in ALA (4.5 or 9.5 g/day) and EPA and DHA (0.8 or 1.7 g/day EPA + DHA) intake on blood coagulation and fibrinolytic factors over 6 months. The randomised, placebo-controlled, parallel study of 150 moderately hyperlipidaemic subjects found no significant differences in coagulation or fibrinolysis for any intervention.

The most recent review of flaxseed by Rodriguez-Leyva et al (2010) report that although anticoagulant effects of flaxseed have been noted in diabetic patients (Tohgi et al 2004), flaxseed ingestion does not influence platelet function in healthy individuals.

Currently, the evidence is equivocal, but may indicate a minor antiaggregatory role for FSO in high doses. Further research, with more heterogeneous designs, is required to form any valid conclusion.

Endothelial function

In one 12-week study of healthy subjects aged 55–75 years, low levels of ALA (equivalent to approximately 5 mL/day of FSO) were shown to decrease some markers of endothelial activation (Thies et al 2001). More specifically, ALA decreased the plasma concentrations of soluble VCAM-1 by 16% and soluble E-selectin by 23%.

High blood pressure

In spite of a large number of studies which failed to demonstrate a relationship between ALA intake and blood pressure, a prospective trial, administering 8 g/day of ALA from FSO to middle-aged dyslipidaemic men over 12 weeks, produced a small but significant reduction in median blood pressure readings of 3–6% (≈5 mmHg) when compared to a similarly high intake of LA from safflower oil (Paschos et al 2007). The clinical significance of this result is questionable.

Lipid-lowering

The largest trial involved over 150 moderately hyperlipidaemic patients in a double-blind, placebo-controlled, 5-arm parallel design conducted over 6 months. Two groups received FSO at different doses (equivalent to 4.5 g/day and 9.5 g/day of ALA), two groups received bioequivalent levels of EPA/DHA, and one group received LA and served as a control group. Although the higher ALA dose induced comparable changes in serum and cell membrane EPA levels to the fish oil group, ALA failed to significantly lower lipid levels, whereas EPA and DHA reduced triacylglycerides (Finnegan et al 2003).

Alternatively, a shorter study of only 2 weeks supplementing with much higher doses of FSO (60 mL/day) or sunflower oil or 130 g/day of mackerel in hypertensive males produced positive results. Subjects taking either FSO or consuming fish experienced an equal decrease in serum triglycerides, total cholesterol and LDL cholesterol (Singer et al 1986). Interestingly, FSO intake resulted in only marginal increases in EPA levels, suggesting that lipid-lowering activity is not reliant on conversion to EPA.

One possible explanation for this comes from the results of a number of trials conducted by Prasad (Prasad 1997, 1999, Prasad et al 1998), who investigated low-ALA FSO and later isolated extracts of the lignan SDG and found significant lipid-lowering effects in animal models. In rabbits, administration of the lignan at high doses produced significant changes to blood lipids, including a 33% reduction in total cholesterol, 35% reduction in LDL cholesterol and an astonishing increase of over 140% in HDL cholesterol by week 8 (Prasad 1999). As exciting as these results are, it is difficult to determine the clinical significance of these findings because the lignan content of FSO is variable. It is possible that the high dose of FSO (60 mL/day used by Singer et al 1986) contained a substantial amount of SDG, which could explain the effects seen; however, this is speculation. Results from a rat study confirmed these effects of lignin SDG on lowering serum total and LDL-cholesterol levels and hepatic lipid accumulation. There was also a reduction in body weight gain (Felmlee et al 2009).

In research investigating the effects of supplementation in healthy volunteers with fish oil, flaxseed oil and hempseed oil, compared with placebo, none of the groups showed any differences in lipid parameters, although the flaxseed group showed a transient increase in ALA levels (Kaul et al 2008). Choice of subjects may be a factor in interpreting the effects of PUFA supplementation in healthy individuals. Prospective studies in at-risk populations may be required to elucidate the effectiveness of PUFAs on cardiovascular health.

Fukumitsu et al (2010) have also reported on the effects of the lignan SDG intake on hypercholesterolaemia and liver disease risk factors in moderately hypercholesterolaemic men. They found that 100 mg SDG significantly reduced the ratio of LDL/HDL cholesterol at 12 weeks. The participants also had a significant decrease in hepatic biomarkers, indicating a protective effect for hepatic disease risk in moderately hypercholesterolaemic men.

In a recent study, high-lignan flaxseed (FLX) decreased total cholesterol, LDL and oxidised-LDL in 36 healthy men and women. The difference in effect between high-lignan FLX and regular lignin FLX on oxidised-LDL was highly significant. The potential for decreasing oxidised-LDL is important, as it is an independent risk factor for CVD (Almario et al 2013).

Interestingly, Akpolat et al (2011) report a significant decrease in the serum cholesterol and lipid levels in hyper-lipidaemic rats fed a high cholesterol diet treated with FXO. This was accompanied by a decreased deposition of neutral lipid, and prevented renal injuries associated with hypercholesterolaemia in these rats.

In an animal study, a rise in serum cholesterol was induced by overiectomy in five groups of hamsters. Results found that both FLX and FXO more than doubled the hepatic protein levels, and researchers suggest that increased bile acid synthesis is only one of the major cholesterol-lowering mechanisms of FLX and FXO (Lucas et al 2011).

In an RCT crossover trial of 36 hypercholesterolaemic men and women, researchers found that FXO consumption significantly reduced total cholesterol by 11%, LDL:HDL ratio by 7.5% and significantly decreased E-selectin concentration, which is an inflammatory biomarker. The cardioprotective potential of FXO may be through lipid-lowering effects, and the mechanism of action may include anti-inflammatory effects (Gillingham et al 2011).

In a review by Bassett et al (2009), researchers report on multiple clinical dietary interventions, stating that daily flaxseed consumption can modestly reduce circulating total cholesterol (TC) by 6–11%, and low-density lipoprotein (LDL) by 9–18% in normolipaemic humans, and by 5–17% for TC and 4–10% for LDL cholesterol in hypercholesterolaemic patients, as well as lowering various markers associated with atherosclerotic CVD in humans. The review suggests that the dietary fibre and lignan content provides the hypocholesterolaemic action, and that flaxseed oil fractions may, in fact, increase circulating lipid levels (Bassett et al 2009).

Anti-inflammatory effects

Inflammation from a variety of causes, such as infectious disease or hyperlipidaemia, has a deleterious effect on vascular function and is a major contributor to atherosclerosis (Bassett et al 2009). There have been inconsistent results of studies of flaxseed and its anti-inflammatory effects. Many studies that have been mentioned in this monograph report little or no change to serum levels of IL-6, TNF-α, CRP and soluble adhesion molecules (Dodin et al 2008, Hallund et al 2008, Kaul et al 2008). However some studies have reported an anti-inflammatory action. Faintuch et al (2007), in an investigation of obese adults, had significantly lower inflammatory markers (CRP, SAA, fibronectin) after 2 weeks of flaxseed supplementation. Three further studies reported beneficial effects on inflammation markers (Caughey et al 1996, Hallund et al 2008, Thies et al 2001). These inconsistencies require further clarification in future studies, but it is possible that the anti-inflammatory benefits are more pronounced in compromised individuals.

Menopausal symptoms

A recent RCT of 38 post-menopausal women examined the effectiveness of partially defatted ground flaxseed in bread on number of daily hot flushes, a menopausal index (Kupperman Menopausal Index (KMI)) and endometrial thickness. Plasma lipid profile (total cholesterol and HDL, LDL and VLDL cholesterol fractions and triglycerides) and the hormones oestradiol, FSH, TSH and free thyroxin were also measured. Both the flaxseed and the placebo group had significant, but similar, reductions in hot flushes and the menopausal index following 12 weeks of treatment. There were lower levels of triglycerides in the flaxseed group, and HDL, but higher LDL concentrations. Both groups had unaffected endometrial thickness. The authors acknowledge that urine tests to confirm levels of enterodiol and enterolactone were not performed (Simbalista et al 2010). However, the outcomes from a randomised study in Brazil showed lower frequency scores for hot flushes and a tendency for lower KMI scores in the flaxseed extract and the SDG groups as compared with placebo. Consistently with the previous studies there were no changes in biomarkers of oestrogenic effects to endometrial thickness, or on the vaginal epithelium (Constantino Colli et al 2012).

More recently in an RCT of healthy menopausal women, flaxseed was not found to be effective in reducing either the severity or the frequency of hot flushes (Carlson et al 2011). Additionally, in a RCT of menopausal women with or without breast cancer, flaxseed bars with 410 mg of lignans versus placebo for 6 weeks found both groups had a reduction in hot flushes, but this was not significantly different, and both experienced mild gastrointestinal effects likely to be due to the fibre content of the bars (Pruthi et al 2012).

In a large, well-controlled RCT of 179 menopausal women, flaxseed supplementation versus wheatgerm placebo for 12 months was investigated for its effect on markers of CVD risk. FS was found to increase ω-3 FA (total, docosapentaenoic and ALA), but demonstrated a limited effect on apolipoprotein metabolism (Dodin et al 2008). Similarly, in a placebo crossover study, 22 healthy menopausal women consumed a low-fat muffin with or without the flaxseed lignin SDG, daily. Levels of C-reactive protein (CRP) were significantly reduced in the SDG group, with CRP being a biomarker of inflammation. CRP levels increased in the placebo group over the course of the trial. However, there were no differences in concentrations of other inflammation biomarkers (IL-6, TNF-α, soluble intracellular adhesion molecule-1, soluble vascular cell adhesion molecule-1 and monocyte chemoattractant protein-1) (Hallund et al 2008).

Lung disease

A group of researchers has been investigating the effects of flaxseed on various forms of lung disease and genetic changes seen. Their results suggest that flaxseed has a protective role in the mouse model on acute and chronic lung injury (Christofidou-Solomidou et al 2011, Kinniry et al 2006, Lee et al 2008, Lee et al 2009). They have confirmed that it takes 3 weeks of supplementation in the mouse model for the flaxseed lignans to reach steady state, and in their latest research looked at specific gene groups shown to be relevant to acute lung injury. The results showed that a significant proportion of the genes were differently expressed following exposure to flaxseed supplementation, including genes in protective pathways. They provide valuable insight into modulation of gene expression in lung tissue and how they might be related to protective mechanisms, confirming therapeutic applications of flaxseed on lung disease (Dukes et al 2012). These exciting results need to be followed up with human trials.

Appetite suppression and weight maintenence

In a study investigating the impact of dietary flaxseed on appetite and post-meal lipaemia in young men, an inhibitory effect was seen on the hunger-signalling hormone ghrelin on the day consumption, combined with a delay in gastric emptying observed when FS was in a high mucilage form. However, subsequent energy intake was not affected (Kristensen et al 2013). This same group of researchers previously demonstrated an increased sensation in satiety and fullness, and subsequent energy intake when flaxseed was taken in a tablet or a drink form, compared with controls (Ibrügger et al 2012). In animal models a significant reduction in body mass following FS supplementation has been observed (Ferreira Medeiros de Franca Cardozo et al 2011, Felmlee et al 2009); however, this should be viewed with caution as an increase in lipid cell size and redistributed accumulation around internal organs rather than subcutaneous distribution may be responsible for the observed effect.

Increased excretion has been noted for flaxseed supplementation above, and further research notes that partially defatted flaxseed meal (PDFM) in constipated mice significantly increased stool frequency and weight in both the normal and the constipated mice (Xu et al 2012).

Insulin sensitivity/metabolic syndrome

It has been proposed that FSO may be of benefit in insulin resistance (IR) based on its possible cardioprotective activities; however, direct evidence of improved insulin sensitivity remains elusive. One small study published in 1997 demonstrated improved systemic arterial compliance in 12 subjects with suspected IR, fed a high dose of ALA over 12

Clinical note — Are vegetarians at risk of omega-3 deficiency?

Omnivores can obtain ω-3 long-chain PUFAs in two ways: from the partial conversion of dietary ALA or directly through the consumption of fish, eggs or animal products (Li et al 1999). Lacto-ovovegetarians obtain ω-3 EFAs from the conversion of plant-based ALA and a limited amount of preformed EPA and DHA from milk, dairy products and eggs; however, their EFA content is highly dependent upon animal diets. In contrast, strict vegetarians and vegans are at risk of inadequate ω-3 EFA, DHA and EPA intake because they are solely reliant on plant-based ALA, which has poor conversion to ω-3 EFA metabolites in the body and they have no dietary intake of preformed DHA or EPA.

This has been demonstrated in studies in which lower plasma and platelet levels of ω-3 EFAs have been identified in vegetarians compared with omnivores, together with lower EPA and DHA levels (Arterburn et al 2006). For vegetarians and vegans, increased consumption and conversion of ALA has been proposed as a strategy to ensure omega-3 adequacy; however, the evidence to date suggests that this is not effective (Burdge 2004, Phinney et al 1990).

Average daily intake of ALA has been estimated at 1.3–1.5 g in the general population and may be lower in vegetarians and vegans. Based on current conversion calculations, general consumption levels already fall short of EPA and DHA requirements. Studies investigating increased ALA consumption at 9.5 g/day, the equivalent of approximately 17 mL FSO, found this increased EPA and DPA, yet failed to improve DHA concentrations, which further proves that ALA is not an effective substitute for animal-derived omega-3 EFAs (Burdge 2004).

To complicate matters, there is evidence suggesting that high intakes of ALA downregulate the delta-6-desaturase enzyme, therefore inhibiting its own conversion (Arterburn et al 2006, Gerster 1998). Vegetarian diets are also notoriously rich in the ω-6 EFA, LA, which if consumed in significantly higher quantities than omega-3 will further retard conversion of ALA (Kris-Etherton & Skulas 2005). Alternatively, background omega-3 deficiency has been speculated to improve conversion efficacy, making vegetarians and vegans potentially superior converters (Arterburn et al 2006).

Vegans and vegetarians are recommended to consume additional sources of ALA, such as algae, that may contain some preformed EPA and DHA in an attempt to reduce risk of deficiency (Kris-Etherton & Skulas 2005, Li et al 1999).

weeks, although an additional finding in this study was evidence of slight deterioration in insulin sensitivity (Nestel et al 1997). Another study using relatively low-dose FSO (1.7 g/day ALA) in normoglycaemic adults found no changes in glycaemic response (Curran et al 2002). A series of clinical trials examining high-dose FSO in patients with type 2 diabetes failed to demonstrate any positive effect on glycaemic control (Barre et al 2008). Similarly, a study examining milled flaxseed (FS) or flaxseed oil (FXO) in bakery products did not affect glycaemic control in adults with well-controlled type 2 diabetes. However compared with the control group, who experienced a 4% weight gain, the FXS and FXO group gained no weight, suggesting possible prevention of weight gain by flax (Noto et al 2010).

In a study of 25 overweight or obese men and post-menopausal women with pre-diabetes it was found that when participants consumed 0, 13 or 26 g ground flaxseed for 12 weeks, glucose decreased, insulin decreased and homeostatic model assessment decreased on the 13 g intervention, but not the 26 g intervention compared with 0 g. Fructosamine, high sensitivity C-reactive protein, adiponectin and high-sensitivity interleukin-6 had no significant differences (Hutchins et al 2013). Similarly, in a study of 173 Chinese with risk factors of metabolic syndrome, it was found that participants receiving lifestyle counselling (LC) plus 30 g/day faxseed supplementation (LCF groups), compared with LC alone, had a significant increase in total erythrocyte ω-3 PUFAs, ALA, eicosapentaenoic acid and docosapentaenoic acid, and a decrease in total ω-6 PUFAs and ω-6, ω-3 ratio. Arachidonic acid increased significantly in the LC group, presumably due to low levels of ALA. However, there were no additional benefits seen on biomarkers of inflammation, endothelial dysfunction, thrombosis and oxidative stress (Zong et al 2013).

The beneficial effect of FS may be in prevention of complications of diabetes. Tao et al (2008) found that high dietary intake of ALA was associated with lower odds of peripheral neuropathy. Velasquez et al (2003) found in an animal model that FS consumption ameliorated nephropathy in type 2 diabetes mellitus.

Anticancer effects

Breast and colon cancer

Bougnoux et al (1994) made an important observation when they demonstrated an inverse relationship between ALA levels in breast tissue and risk of lymph node involvement and visceral metastases in breast cancer. This has been followed up with larger studies of similar design (Klein et al 2000, Maillard et al 2002) and one meta-analysis, all yielding comparable results (Saadatian-Elahi et al 2004).

FS contains two main bioactive anti-cancer components, FS oil (FXO) and plant lignans (a class of phyto-oestrogens). FXO represents 40% of FS, but has more than 50% as the ω-3 fatty acid, ALA. The predominant plant lignan is secoisolariciresinol diglucoside (SDG) which can be converted into the 'mammalian lignans' enterodiol and enterolactone by intestinal bacteria, and has been reported to possess the oestrogenic properties of lignans (Chen et al 2011). The data indicate that those women with the highest breast tissue concentrations of ALA have a relative risk of breast cancer between 0.36 and 0.39, while other FA levels fail to exhibit a statistically significant relationship. Interestingly, an epidemiological study has identified an association between low consumption of ALA in humans and increased cancer deaths in general (Dolecek 1992).

In an in vitro study, SDG and two other lignan isolates from FSO, secoisolariciresinol and anhydrosecoisolariciresinol, were shown to modulate the growth of human breast cells, with the most significant decrease of cell growth at 50–100 microM (Attoumbre et al 2010).

In athymic mouse models, with low-circulating oestrogen concentrations, SDG, FS and the lignin-rich fraction FS hull (FH) were compared for the effect of breast tumour growth. All treatments significantly inhibited cell proliferation, FS and SDG induced significantly higher apoptosis and FS and SDG significantly decreased expressions of various tumour biomarkers, including downregulating ER- and growth factor-mediated cell signalling, but the lesser effects of FH may indicate a need for higher doses (Chen et al 2009). In a further study by these researchers, the ω-3 FA-rich cotyledon fraction of FS (FC), alone or in combination with tamoxifen, was examined for effect on breast cancer cells in athymic mice. FC was found to reduce the growth of oestrogen-receptor (ER) positive (ER+) breast tumours alone and in combination with tamoxifen, partly through modulating ER and growth factor-mediated signalling pathways (Chen et al 2011). In a study of ovariectomised (OVX) athymic mice, SDG and FXO were compared alone and in combination on established ER+ human breast tumours. All treatments reduced the tumour growth; however, SDG had the greatest effect, mainly through reduction of cell proliferation as opposed to increasing apoptosis. SDG alone lowered biomarkers indicating an effect involving modulation of the ER- and growth factor receptor-mediated signalling pathways confirming previous studies (Saggar et al 2010).

Abrahamsson et al's (2012) study demonstrated a significant positive correlation between oestradiol and in vivo levels of the pro-inflammatory cytokine IL-1β in breast tissue and abdominal subcutaneous fat, and a significant negative correlation with IL-1Ra and oestradiol, which exerts an inhibitory effect on IL-1β. Tamoxifen or a dietary supplement of FS produced significant increases in levels of IL-1Ra, suggesting a potential therapeutic target.

In a large prospective analysis of the Ontario Women's Diet and Health Study (2002–03), researchers investigated associations between consumption of flaxseed and flax breads and breast cancer risk, with confounding factors accounted for. A significant association with breast cancer risk reduction was observed for flaxseed (OR = 0.82 [95% CI, 0.69–0.97]) and flax bread (OR = 0.77 [95% CI, 0.67–0.89]) (Lowcock et al 2013).

In a recent study in athymic mice, the potential for dietary FS to enhance the effectiveness of trastuzumab (TRAS), which is a first line therapy for the treatment on HER2 (human epidermal growth factor receptor 2) overexpressing breast cancer, was conducted. HER2 is overexpressed in about a quarter of breast cancers and results in often highly metastatic, aggressive tumours, and provides a relatively poor prognosis. FS was found to not further improve TRAS in tumour reduction; however, a significant improvement was seen in overall survival of the mice (Mason et al 2013). In a mechanistic study, researchers examined the link between flaxseed supplementation and urinary levels of oestrogen metabolites that may be involved in the development of breast cancer. They found no evidence to support shifts in oestrogen metabolism pathways from flaxseed supplementation for postmenopausal women (Sturgeon et al 2010).

In a commentary by Patterson (2011), the evidence for flaxseed and breast cancer is discussed. In a large RCT of 1140 postmenopausal patients with breast cancer, those who had the highest levels of serum enterolactone concentrations (highest quartile) had a reduced risk of overall mortality by 42%, and a distant disease risk reduction of 38% (Buck et al 2011). The biological plausibility of this is supported by a meta-analysis indicating that enterolactone biomarkers are indeed associated with a breast cancer risk reduction of 28% (Zaineddin et al 2012). However, Patterson is clear that naturally occurring biomarkers, signifying perhaps not more than a healthy lifestyle with well balanced dietary intake, does not necessarily equate to continued health benefits and disease risk reduction with further supplementation with flaxseed lignans.

Therefore, until prospective human trials are completed, the evidence for flaxseed supplementation for breast cancer treatment or risk reduction is uncertain, but may be promising.

SDG is reported to have a broad range of biological effects as a chemopreventive agent against the development of breast, prostate and colon cancers, and has potential antioxidant activity (Attoumbre et al 2010).

Currently, the only evidence from interventional studies using FSO as a chemoprotective agent is provided by animal trials, which demonstrate that dietary FSO is effective in preventing colon tumour development (Dwivedi et al 2005). In a recent study of Sprague Dawley rats, both flaxseed and its total non-digestible fraction (TNDF) exhibited a preventive effect against colon cancer. Two tablespoons (human daily dose) were administered daily. The treatments induced cell cycle arrest, and in an analysis of the expressed genes, an association with the presence of dietary antioxidants linked to the cell wall of flaxseed was demonstrated (Hernández-Salazar et al 2013).

Prostate cancer

There is much debate surrounding research into the hypothesised link between ALA and the risk of prostate cancer. Giovannucci, a prolific prostate cancer researcher, has contributed to numerous papers on this topic, deriving data from large epidemiological or prospective cohort studies, including The Health Professionals Follow-Up, The Physician's Health Study and the Alpha-Tocopherol, Beta-Carotene Cancer Prevention Study (Gann et al 1994, Giovannucci et al 1993, Leitzmann et al 2004, Mannisto et al 2003). The conclusions oscillate between a positive independent association between increased ALA intake and prostate cancer risk (Gann et al 1994, Giovannucci et al 1993, Leitzmann et al 2004) to no significant association (Mannisto et al 2003). Further support of ALA as a risk factor has come from a large Norwegian epidemiological study (Harvei et al 1997), a review by Astorg (2004) and a meta-analysis by Brouwer et al in 2004. Although the majority of published data appear to implicate ALA as a prostate cancer risk factor, it is worthy of note that none of the trials were interventional and many relied exclusively on food frequency questionnaires rather than independent biochemical indices of ALA. Other researchers have also presented sound arguments against this theory, such as those articulated by de Lorgeril and Salen (2004), which query the quality of evidence being considered, the exclusion of trials that demonstrated minor risk reduction with increased ALA intake (Schuurman et al 1999) and other weaknesses of the study designs. Additional criticisms include the lack of distinction in the sources of dietary ALA, with red meat an independent risk factor for prostate cancer, being a major dietary source of ALA in some studies (Brouwer et al 2004).

In a study of 147 patients with prostate cancer, a presurgical trial of flaxseed supplementation (30 g/day) for approximately 30 days was examined for effects on prostatic tumour expression of NFκB, VEGF and Ki67. A significant correlation between intake of plant lignan and urinary concentrations of total enterolignans, enterolactone and enterodiol (main lignans of FS) was observed. The results showed an inverse association between urinary concentrations of total enterolignans and enterolactone with Ki67, and a near-significant inverse association with enterodiol. A near statistical significance was observed for NFκB and enterolactone. The authors concluded that FS enterolignans may hinder cancer cell proliferation via VEGF-associated pathways (Azrad et al 2013). However, further studies are required to elucidate the effects of FS on prostate cancer.

DOSAGE RANGE

- Anticlotting: 5.9 g/day ALA.
- Improved endothelial function: 2 g/day ALA.

- Lipid-lowering: 60 mL/day FSO.
- Reduced CHD mortality: 1–3 g/day ALA.
- Reduced cancer (esp breast) risk: 2 tsp/day.

A key consideration with FSO supplementation is product quality. Due to the high potential for FSO to become oxidised, ingestion of inadequately manufactured or preserved FSO could result in higher intakes of peroxides. It is recommended that only refrigerated FSO packaged in opaque containers be used. Once opened, the product should be consumed within a few weeks of opening and kept stored in the fridge.

ADVERSE REACTIONS

FSO may cause loose stools and gastrointestinal distress in some individuals (Austria et al 2008). There is a report of an allergic reaction to FSO, with a 40-year-old woman experiencing ocular pruritis and weeping followed by generalised urticaria and nausea, and vomiting within 10 minutes of taking a spoonful of linseed oil. A subsequent skin prick test produced a positive response to linseed. It remains unclear, however, whether this patient consumed FSO or linseed oil, which is denatured and unfit for human consumption (Alonso et al 1996).

SIGNIFICANT INTERACTIONS

None known.

CONTRAINDICATIONS AND PRECAUTIONS

- Hypersensitivity to flaxseed/linseed.
- Prostate cancer.
- Pregnancy and lactation.

There are a number of studies that link increased ALA intake with a higher risk of prostate or aggressive prostate cancer. Although the evidence is preliminary and widely debated, it is recommended that at-risk individuals avoid high-dose consumption of FSO and only consume FSO that is packaged in opaque containers and refrigerated.

PATIENTS' FAQs

What will this supplement do for me?

Regular consumption of flaxseed oil, in the presence of balanced linoleic acid (omega-6) intake, may reduce cardiovascular mortality and possibly the risk of some cancers; however, this remains speculative.

When will it start to work?

This will depend on the dosage taken and indication for use.

Are there any safety issues?

Long-term high doses may compromise immune function in susceptible individuals.

Preliminary evidence suggests a possible link between high ALA intake and increased risk of prostate cancer; however, this is controversial.

PREGNANCY USE AND USE DURING LACTATION

There is some animal evidence to suggest safety concerns when using flaxseed during gestation and lactation. In female Wistar rats, flaxseed use during the perinatal and post-weaning periods improved the offsprings' spatial ability, but did so to the detriment of growth (Fernandes et al 2011). However the research suggests that consumption during lactation does not interfere with reproductive/sexual maturation of female rat offspring (Leal Soares et al 2010).

In the most recent animal research, evidence suggests that extensive use of flaxseed during lactation is not desirable, as maternal supplementation produces a decrease in adiposity of offspring and an increase in pituitary leptin signalling, and higher thyroid leptin receptor in adulthood, indicating induction of insulin resistance in adult offspring. These offspring also demonstrated a higher adult subcutaneous and visceral adipocyte areas, with no change in body fat mass (Sarto Figueiredo et al 2013).

F

Practice points/Patient counselling

- Good quality, cold-pressed FSO is a good source of the essential fatty acid ALA, which is often deficient in the Western diet. Capsules are more stable than the bottled oil which must be stored in a dark bottle, refrigerated after opening and consumed within a few weeks.
- The polyunsaturated fatty acids found in FSO, particularly ALA, are precursors of eicosanoids and influence many important physiological processes. Additional actions may be attributed to the variable amount of lignan present in FSO, but which is found in higher concentrations in the actual seed.
- FSO has demonstrated anti-inflammatory, immunological, minor antiplatelet and chemopreventive effects and a range of beneficial actions within the cardiovascular system; however, large RCTs are still required to determine the role of FSO in clinical practice.
- FSO is not an adequate substitute for animal sources of ω-3 EFAs. Most studies of oral FSO demonstrate only moderate increases in EPA, while DHA remains unchanged. Strict vegetarians and vegans using FSO as ω-3 EFA substitute may be at risk of EPA and DHA deficiency.
- There is some evidence to suggest that daily ingestion of an additional 1–3 g of ALA (equivalent to 5 mL FSO) may reduce the incidence of some cancers and coronary heart disease mortality; however, this remains speculative.

REFERENCES

Abrahamsson A et al. Estradiol, Tamoxifen, and flaxseed Alter IL-1β and IL-1Ra levels in normal human breast tissue *in vivo*. J Clin Endocrinol Metab 97.11 (2012): E2044–E2054.

Akpolat M et al. Protective effect of flaxseed oil on renal injury in hyperlipidaemic rats: The effect of flaxseed oil on hyperlipidaemia. Phytother Res 25 (2011): 796–802.

Albert CM et al. Dietary alpha-linolenic acid intake and risk of sudden cardiac death and coronary heart disease. Circulation 112.21 (2005): 3232–3238.

Allman-Farinelli MA et al. Comparison of the effects of two low fat diets with different alpha-linolenic: linoleic acid ratios on coagulation and fibrinolysis. Atherosclerosis 3 (1999): 159–168.

Allman MA, Pena MM, Pang D. Supplementation with flaxseed oil versus sunflowerseed oil in healthy young men consuming a low fat diet: effects on platelet composition and function. Eur J Clin Nutr 49.3 (1995): 169–178.

Almario RU, Karakas SE. Lignan content of the flaxseed influences its biological effects in health men and women. J Am Coll Nutr 32.3 (2013): 194–199.

Almeida KC et al. Influence of omega-3 fatty acids from the flaxseed (Linum usitatissimum) on the brain development of newborn rats. Nutr Hosp. 26.5 (2011): 991–996.

Alonso L et al. Anaphylaxis caused by linseed (flaxseed) intake. J Allergy Clin Immunol 98.2 (1996): 469–470.

Ander BP et al. Dietary flaxseed protects against ventricular fibrillation induced by ischemia-reperfusion in normal and hypercholesterolemic rabbits. J Nutr 134.12 (2004): 3250–3256.

Arterburn LM, Hall EB, Oken H. Distribution, interconversion, and dose response of ω-3 fatty acids in humans. Am J Clin Nutr 83 (6 Suppl) (2006): 1467S–1476S.

Astorg P. Dietary Ω-6 and Ω-3 polyunsaturated fatty acids and prostate cancer risk: a review of epidemiological and experimental evidence. Cancer Causes Control 15 (2004): 367–386.

Attoumbre J et al. Extraction of lignans from flaxseed and evaluation of their biological effects on breast cancer MCF-7 and MDA-MB-231 cell lines. J Med Food 13.4 (2010): 834–844.

Austria JA et al. Bioavailability of alpha-linolenic acid in subjects after ingestion of three different forms of flaxseed. J Am Coll Nutr 27.2 (2008): 214–221.

Azrad M et al. Flaxseed-derived enterolactone is inversely associated with tumor cell proliferation in men with localized prostate cancer. J Med Food 16.4 (2013): 357–360.

Barceló-Coblijn G et al. Flaxseed oil and fish-oil capsule consumption alters human red blood cell ω-3 fatty acid composition: a multiple-dosing trial comparing 2 sources of ω-3 fatty acid. Am J Clin Nutr 88.3 (2008): 801–809.

Barre DE et al. High dose flaxseed oil supplementation may affect fasting blood serum glucose management in human type 2 diabetics. J Oleo Sci 57.5 (2008): 269–273.

Bassett C, Rodriguez-Leyva D, Pierce G. Experimental and clinical research findings on the cardiovascular benefits of consuming flaxseed. Appl. Physiol. Nutr. Metab. 34 (2009): 965–974.

Bemelmans WJE et al. Effect of an increased intake of alpha-linolenic acid and group nutritional education on cardiovascular risk factors: the Mediterranean Alpha-linolenic Enriched Groningen Dietary Intervention (MARGARIN) study. Am J Clin Nutr 75.2 (2002): 221–227.

Bhatty RS. Nutrient composition of whole flaxseed and flaxseed meal. In: Cunnane SC, Thompson LU (eds), Flaxseed in human nutrition, Illinois, ACOS Press, 1995: pp 22–42.

Bougnoux P et al. alpha-Linolenic acid content of adipose breast tissue: a host determinant of the risk of early metastasis in breast cancer. Br J Cancer 70.2 (1994): 330–334.

Breslow JL. ω-3 fatty acids and cardiovascular disease. Am J Clin Nutr 83 (6 Suppl) (2006 Jun): 1477S–1482S.

Brouwer IA, Katan MB, Zock PL. Dietary alpha-linolenic acid is associated with reduced risk of fatal coronary heart disease, but increased prostate cancer risk: a meta-analysis. J Nutr 134.4 (2004): 919–922.

Buck K, et al. Serum enterolactone and prognosis of postmenopausal breast cancer. J Clin Oncol 29 (2011): 3730–3738.

Burdge G. Alpha-linolenic acid metabolism in men and women: nutritional and biological implications. Curr Opin Clin Nutr Metab Care 7.2 (2004): 137–144.

Carlson, R et al. Hot Flashes: Flaxseed Not Effective in Reducing Either Frequency or Severity. Oncol Times 33.18 (2011): 34–35.

Caughey GE et al. The effect on human tumor necrosis factor alpha and interleukin 1-beta production of diets enriched in ω-3 fatty acids from vegetable oil or fish oil. Am J Clin Nutr 63.1 (1996): 116–122.

Chen J et al. Dietary flaxseed inhibits human breast cancer growth and metastasis and downregulates expression of insulin-like growth factor and epidermal growth factor receptor. Nutr Cancer 43.2 (2002): 187–92.

Chen J et al. Flaxseed and pure secoisolariciresinol diglucoside, but not flaxseed hull, reduce human breast tumor growth (MCF-7) in athymic mice. J Nutr 139.11 (2009): 2061–2065.

Chen J et al. Flaxseed cotyledon fraction reduces tumour growth and sensitizes tamoxifen treatment of human breast cancer xenograft (MCF-7) in athymic mice. Br J Nutr 105 (2011): 339–347.

Christensen JH et al. Alpha-linolenic acid and heart rate variability in women examined for coronary artery disease. Nutr Metab Cardiovasc Dis 15.5 (2005): 345–351.

Christofidou-Solomidou M et al. Dietary flaxseed administered post thoracic radiation treatment improves survival and mitigates radiation-induced pneumonopathy in mice. BMC Cancer 11.1 (2011): 269.

Cognault S et al. Effect of an alpha-linolenic acid-rich diet on rat mammary tumor growth depends on the dietary oxidative status. Nutr Cancer 36.1 (2000): 33–41.

Constantino Colli M et al. Evaluation of the efficacy of flaxseed meal and flaxseed extract in recuing menopausal syptoms. J Med Food 15.9 (2012): 840–845.

Cunnane SC et al. High alpha-linolenic acid flaxseed (Linum usitatissimum): some nutritional properties in humans. Br J Nutr 69.2 (1993): 443–453.

Cunnane SC, Thompson LU (eds), Flaxseed in human nutrition. Illinois, ACOS Press, 1995.

Curran RRD et al. Influence of flaxseed oil administration on glycemic response in active, healthy adults. Top Clin Nutr 17.5 (2002): 28–35.

David BC, Kris-Etherton PM. Achieving optimal essential fatty acid status in vegetarians: current knowledge and practical implications (Review). Am J Clin Nutr 78 (3 Suppl) (2003): 640–646S.

de Lorgeril M. et al. Mediterranean diet, traditional risk factors, and the rate of cardiovascular complications after myocardial infarction. Heart failure 11 (1999): 6.

de Lorgeril M, Salen P. Alpha-Linolenic acid, coronary heart disease, and prostate cancer. J Nutr 134 (2004): 3385.

de Meneses MJ et al. Behavioral analysis of Wistar rats fed with a flaxseed based eiet added to an environmental enrichment. Nutr Hosp 26.4 (2011): 716–721.

Djousse L et al. Dietary linolenic acid is inversely associated with calcified atherosclerotic plaque in the coronary arteries: the National Heart, Lung, and Blood Institute Family Heart Study. Circulation 111 (2005): 2921–2926.

Dodin S et al. Flaxseed on cardiovascular disease markers in healthy menopausal women: a randomized, double-blind, placebo-controlled trial. Nutrition 24.1 (2008): 23–30.

Dolecek TA. Epidemiological evidence of relationships between dietary polyunsaturated fatty acids and mortality in the multiple risk factor intervention trial. Proc Soc Exp Biol Med 200.2 (1992): 177–182.

Dukes F et al. Gene expression profiling of flaxseed in mouse lung tissues-modulation of toxicologically relevant genes. BMC CAM 12.1 (2012): 47–58.

Dupasquier CMC, et al. Dietary flaxseed inhibits atherosclerosis in the LDL receptor-deficient mouse in part through antiproliferative and anti-inflammatory actions. Am J Physiol Heart Circ Physiol 293.4 (2007): H2394–H2402.

Dupasquier CMC, et al. The effects of dietary flaxseed on vascular contractile function and atherosclerosis in rabbits during prolonged hypercholesterolemia. Am J Physiol Heart Circ Physiol 291 (2006): H2987–H2996.

Dwivedi C, Natarajan K, Matthees DP. Chemopreventive effects of dietary flaxseed oil on colon tumor development. Nutr Cancer 51.1 (2005): 52–58.

Faintuch J et al. Systemic inflammation and carotid diameter in obese patients: pilot comparative study with flaxseed powder and cassava powder. Nutr Hosp 26.1 (2011): 208–213.

Faintuch J et al. Systemic inflammation in morbidly obese subjects: Response to oral supplementation with alpha-linolenic acid. Obes Surg 17 (2007): 341–347.

Felmlee M et al. Effects of the flaxseed lignans secoisolariciresinol diglucoside and its aglycone on serum and hepatic lipids in hyperlipidaemic rats. Br J Nutr 102 (2009): 361–369.

Fernandes FS, et al. Maternal intake of flaxseed-based diet (Linum usitatissimum) on hippocampus fatty acid profile: Implications for growth, locomotor activity and spatial memory. Nutr 27 (2011): 1040–1047.

Ferreira Costa Leite, CD et al. Flaxseed and its contribution to body growth and brain of Wistar rats during childhood and adolescence. Nutr Hosp 26.2 (2011): 415–420.

Ferreira Medeiros de França Cardozo L et al. Hematologic and immunological indicators are altered by chronic intake of flaxseed in Wistar rats. Nutr Hosp 26.5 (2011): 1091–1096.

Finnegan YE et al. Plant- and marine-derived ω-3 polyunsaturated fatty acids have differential effects on fasting and postprandial blood lipid concentrations and on the susceptibility of LDL to oxidative modification in moderately hyperlipidemic subjects. Am J Clin Nutr 77.4 (2003): 783–795.

Freese R, Mutanen M. Alpha-linolenic acid and marine long-chain ω-3 fatty acids differ only slightly in their effects on hemostatic factors in healthy subjects. Am J Clin Nutr 66.3 (1997): 591–598.

Freese R et al. Comparison of the effects of two diets rich in monounsaturated fatty acids differing in their linoleic/alpha-linolenic acid ratio on platelet aggregation. Thromb Haemost 71.1 (1994): 73–77.

Fukumitsu S et al. Flaxseed lignan lowers blood cholesterol and decreases liver disease risk factors in moderately hypercholesterolemic men. Nutr Res 30 (2010): 441–446.

Gagnon N et al. Ruminal metabolism of flaxseed (Linum usitatissimum) lignans to the mammalian lignin enterolactone and its concentration in ruminal fluid, plasma, urine nd mild of dairy cows. Br J Nutr 102 (2009): 1015–1023.

Gann PH et al. Prospective study of plasma fatty acids and risk of prostate cancer. J Natl Cancer Inst 86.4 (1994): 281–286.

Garg ML et al. Dietary saturated fat level alters the competition between alpha-linolenic and linoleic acid. Lipids 24.4 (1989): 334–339.

Gerster H. Can adults adequately convert alpha-linolenic acid (18: 3ω-3) to eicosapentaenoic acid (20: 5ω-3) and docosahexaenoic acid (22: 6ω-3)? Int J Vitam Nutr Res 68.3 (1998): 159–173.

Ghafoorunissa Ibrahim A, Natarajan S. Substituting dietary linoleic acid with alpha-linolenic acid improves insulin sensitivity in sucrose fed rats. Biochim Biophys Acta 1733.1 (2005): 67–75.

Gillingham, LG et al. High-oleic rapeseed (canola) and flaxseed oils modulate serum lipids and inflammatory biomarkers in hypercholesterolaemic subjects. Br J Nutr 105 (2011): 417–427.

Giovannucci E et al. A prospective study of dietary fat and risk of prostate cancer. J Natl Cancer Inst 85.19 (1993): 1571–1579.

Gonçalves de Oliveira C et al. Flaxseed energy and macronutrients balance. Nutr Hosp 27.5 (2012): 1598–1604.

Goyens PL et al. Conversion of alpha-linolenic acid in humans is influenced by the absolute amounts of alpha-linolenic acid and linoleic acid in the diet and not by their ratio. Am J Clin Nutr 84.1 (2006): 44–53.

Goyens PL, Mensink RP. Effects of alpha-linolenic acid versus those of EPA/DHA on cardiovascular risk markers in healthy elderly subjects. Eur J Clin Nutr 60.8 (2006): 978–984.

Hall C 3rd, Tulbek MC, Xu Y. Flaxseed. Adv Food Nutr Res 51 (2006): 1–97.

Hallund J et al. The effect of a lignin complex isolated from flaxseed on inflammation markers in health postmenopausal women. Nut. Metab and CV Diseases 18.7 (2008): 497–502.

Harper CR, Edwards MC, Jacobson TA. Flaxseed oil supplementation does not affect plasma lipoprotein concentration or particle size in human subjects. J Nutr 136.11 (2006a): 2844–2848.

Harper CR et al. Flaxseed oil increases the plasma concentrations of cardioprotective (ω-3) fatty acids in humans. J Nutr 136.1 (2006b): 83–87.

Harris WS et al. ω-3 fatty acids and serum lipoproteins: human studies. Am J Clin Nutr 65 (5 Suppl) (1997): 1645–1654S.

Harris WS. Alpha-linolenic acid: a gift from the land?. (Editorial) Circulation 111.22 (2005): 2872–2874.

Harvei S et al. Prediagnostic level of fatty acids in serum phospholipids: omega-3 and omega-6 fatty acids and the risk of prostate cancer. Int J Cancer 71 (1997): 545–551.

Hernández-Salazar M et al. Flaxseed (Linum usitatissimum L.) and its total non-digestible fraction influence the expression of genes involved in azoxymethane-induced colon cancer in rats. Plant Foods Hum Nutr 68 (2013): 259–267.

Hutchins A et al. Daily flaxseed consumption improves glycemic control in obese men and women with pre-diabetes: a randomized study. Nutr Res 33 (2013): 367–375.

Hussein N et al. Long-chain conversion of [13C]linoleic acid and alpha-linolenic acid in response to marked changes in their dietary intake in men. J Lipid Res 46.2 (2005): 269–280.

Ibrügger S, et al. Flaxseed dietary fiber supplements for suppression of appetite and food intake. Appetite 58 (2012): 490–495.

James MJ, Gibson RA, Cleland LG. Dietary polyunsaturated fatty acids and inflammatory mediator production. Am J Clin Nutr 71.1 (2000): 343–348s.

Johnston PV. Alpha-Linolenic acid and carcinogenesis. In: Cunnane SC, Thompson LU (eds), Flaxseed in human nutrition, ACOS Press, 1995, pp 207–218.

Judd A. Flax: some historical considerations. In: Cunnane SC, Thompson LU (eds), Flaxseed in human nutrition, ACOS Press, 1995, pp 1–10.

Kaul N et al. A comparison of fish oil, flaxseed oil and hempseed oil supplementation on selected parameters of cardiovascular health in healthy volunteers. J Am Coll Nutr 27.1 (2008): 51–58.

Kelley DS. Alpha-linolenic acid and immune response. Nutrition 8.3 (1992): 215–217.

Kelley DS et al. Dietary alpha-linolenic acid alters tissue fatty acid composition, but not blood lipids, lipoproteins or coagulation status in humans. Lipids 28.6 (1993): 533–537.

Kitts DD et al. Antioxidant activity of the flaxseed lignan secoisolariciresinol diglycoside and its mammalian lignan metabolites enterodiol and enterolactone. Mol Cell Biochem 202.1–2 (1999): 91–100.

Kinniry P et al. Dietary flaxseed supplementation ameliorates inflammation and osidative tissue damage in experimental models of acute lung injury in mice. J Nutr 136.6 (2006): 1545–1551.

Klein V et al. Low alpha-linolenic acid content of adipose breast tissue is associated with an increased risk of breast cancer. Eur J Cancer 36.3 (2000): 335–340.

Klein-Platat, C et al. Plasma fatty acid composition is associated with the metabolic syndrome and low-grade inflammation in overweight adolescents. Am J of Clin Nutr 82 (2005): 1178–1184.

Kolodziejczyk PP, Fedec P. Processing flaxseed for human consumption. In: Cunnane SC, Thompson LU (eds), Flaxseed in human nutrition, ACOS Press, 1995, pp 261–80.

Kris-Etherton P, Skulas A. Essential fatty acids and vegetarians: the missing link in long-chain omega-3 fatty acid recommendations. Nutr MD 31.8 (2005): 1–4.

Kristensen M et al. Flaxseed dietary fibers suppress postprandial lipemia and appetite sensation in young men. Nut. Metab. CVD 23 (2013): 136–143.

Lanzmann-Petithory D. Alpha-linolenic acid and cardiovascular diseases (Review). J Nutr Health Aging 5.3 (2001): 179–183.

Leal Soares L et al. Influence of flaxseed during lactation on the reproductive system of female Wistar rats. Nutr Hosp 25.3 (2010): 437–442.

Lee JC et al. Dietary flaxseed enhances antioxidant defenses and is protective in a mouse model of lung ischemia-reperfusion injury. Am J Physiol Lung Cell Mol Physiol 294.2 (2008): L255–256.

Lee JC et al. Dietary flaxseed prevents radiation-induced oxidative lung damage, inflammation and fibrosis in a mouse model of thoracic radiation injury. Cancer Biol Ther 8.1 (2009): 47–53.

Leitzmann MF et al. Dietary intake of n–3 and n–6 fatty acids and the risk of prostate cancer. Am J Clin Nutr 80.1 (2004): 204–216.

Li D et al. Effect of dietary alpha-linolenic acid on thrombotic risk factors in vegetarian men. Am J Clin Nutr 69.5 (1999): 872–882.

Lowcock E, Cotterchio M. Consumption of flaxseed, a rich source of lignans, is associated with reduced breast cancer risk. Cancer Causes Control 24 (2013): 813–816.

Lucas EA et al. Flaxseed but not flaxseed oil prevented the rise in serum cholesterol due to overiectomy in the Golden Syrian Hamsters. J Med Food 14.3 (2011): 261–267.

Maillard V et al. Ω-3 and Ω-6 fatty acids in breast adipose tissue and relative risk of breast cancer in a case-control study in Tours, France. Int J Cancer 98.1 (2002): 78–83.

Mannisto S et al. Fatty acids and risk of prostate cancer in a nested case-control study in male smokers. Cancer Epidemiol Biomarkers Prev 12.12 (2003): 1422–1428.

Mantzioris E et al. Dietary substitution with an alpha-linolenic acid-rich vegetable oil increases eicosapentaenoic acid concentrations in tissues. Am J Clin Nutr 59.6 (1994): 1304–1309.

Mason JK et al. Dietary flaxseed-Trastuzumab interactive effects on the growth of HER2-Overexpressing human breast tumors (BT-474). Nutr & Cancer 65.3 (2013): 451–459.

Matthan NR et al. A systematic review and meta-analysis of the impact of omega-3 fatty acids on selected arrhythmia outcomes in animal models. Metabolism 54.12 (2005): 1557–1565.

Morris D. Essential nutrients and other functional compounds in flaxseed. Nutr Today 36.3 (2001): 159–62.

Mozaffarian D et al. Interplay between different polyunsaturated fatty acids and risk of coronary heart disease in men. Circulation 111 (2005): 157–164.

Mutanen M, Freese R. Fats, lipids and blood coagulation. Curr Opin Lipidol 12.1 (2001): 25–29.

Nestel PJ et al. Arterial compliance in obese subjects is improved with dietary plant ω-3 fatty acid from flaxseed oil despite increased LDL oxidizability. Arterioscler Thromb Vasc Biol 17.6 (1997): 1163–1170.

Noto AD, Stringer DM, Taylor CG. Dietary milled flaxseed and flaxseed oil improve *n*-3 fatty acid status and do not affect glycemic control in individuals with well-controlled type 2 diabetes. J Am Coll Nutr 15.3 (2010): 288.

Park JB, Velasquez MT. Potential effects of lignan-enriched flaxseed powder on bodyweight, visceral fat, lipid profile, and blood pressure in rats. Fitoterapia 83 (2012): 941–946.

Paschos GK et al. Dietary supplementation with flaxseed oil lowers blood pressure in dyslipidaemic patients. Eur J Clin Nutr 61.10 (2007): 1201–1206.

Patterson R. Flaxseed and breast cancer: What should we tell our patients? J Clin Onc 29.18 (2011): 3723–3724.

Phinney SD et al. Reduced arachidonate in serum phospholipids and cholesteryl esters associated with vegetarian diets in humans. Am J Clin Nutr 51.3 (1990): 385–392.

Prasad K. Dietary flaxseed in prevention of hypercholesterolemic atherosclerosis. Atherosclerosis 132 (1997): 69–76.

Prasad K. Reduction of serum cholesterol and hypercholesterolemic atherosclerosis in rabbits by secoisolariciresinol diglucoside isolated from flaxseed. Circulation 99.10 (1999): 1355–1362.

Prasad K et al. Reduction of hypercholesterolemic atherosclerosis by CDC-flaxseed with very low alpha-linolenic acid. Atherosclerosis 136 (1998): 367–75.

Pruthi, S et al. A phase III, randomized, placebo-controlled, double-blind trial of flaxseed for the treatment of hot flashes: North Central Cancer Treatment Group N08C7. Menopause 19.1 (2012): 48.

Rhee Y Brunt A. Effects of flaxseed lignan on *in vitro* mitogen-stimulated T cell proliferation. J App Res 8.32 (2008): 208–214.

Rodriguez-Leyva D, et al. The cardiovascular effects of flaxseed and its omega-3 fatty acid, alpha-linolenic acid. Can J Cardiol 26.9 (2010) 489–496.

Saadatian-Elahi M et al. Biomarkers of dietary fatty acid intake and the risk of breast cancer: a meta-analysis. Int J Cancer 111.4 (2004): 584–91.

Saggar, K et al. The effect of secoisolariciresinol diglucoside and flaxseed oil, alone and in combination, on MCF-7 tumor growth and signaling pathways. J Nutr & Cancer 62.4 (2010): 533–542.

Schuurman AG et al. Association of energy and fat intake with prostate carcinoma risk: results from The Netherlands Cohort Study. Cancer 86 (1999): 1019–1027.

Schwab US et al. Effects of hempseed and flaxseed oils on the profile of serum lipids, serum total and lipoprotein lipid concentrations and haemostatic factors. Eur J Nutr 45.8 (2006): 470–7.

Simbalista R et al. Consumption of a flaxseed-rich food is not more effective than a placebo in alleviating the climacteric symptoms of postmenopausal women. J Nutr 40.2 (2010): 293–297.

Singer P et al. Slow desaturation and elongation of linoleic and alpha-linolenic acids as a rationale of eicosapentaenoic acid-rich diet to lower blood pressure and serum lipids in normal, hypertensive and hyperlipemic subjects. Prostaglandins Leukot Med 24.2–3 (1986): 173–193.

Silva FGD et al. Antioxidant capacity of flaxseed products: The effect of *in vitro* digestion. Plant Foods Hum Nutr 68 (2013): 24–30.

Sturgeon S et al. Effect of flaxseed consumption on urinary levels of estrogen metabolites in postmenopausal women. Nutr & Cancer 62.2 (2010): 175–180.

Sturgeon S et al. Dietary intervention of flaxseed: Effect on serum levels of IGF-1, IGF-BP3, and C-Peptide. Nutr & Cancer 63.3 (2011): 376–380.

Suresh Y, Das UN. Long-chain polyunsaturated fatty acids and chemically induced diabetes mellitus: Effect of omega-3 fatty acids. Nutrition 19.3 (2003): 213–228.

Tao M, et al. Relationship of polyunsaturated fatty acid intake to peripheral neuropathy among adults with diabetes int eh National Health and Nutrition Examination Survey (NHANES) 1999–2004. Diab Care 31 (2008): 93–95.

Thies F et al. Influence of dietary supplementation with long-chain ω-3 or ω-6 polyunsaturated fatty acids on blood inflammatory cell populations and functions and on plasma soluble adhesion molecules in healthy adults. Lipids 36.11 (2001): 1183–1193.

Tohgi N et al. Effect of alpha-linolenic acid-containing linseed oil on coagulation in type 2 diabetes. Diab Care 27 (2004): 2563–2564.

Tomaz Pacheco J et al. Impact of dietary flaxseed (linum usitatissumum) supplementation on biochemical profile in healthy rats. Nutr Hosp 26.4 (2011): 798–802.

Velasquez MT, et al. Dietary flaxseed meal reduces proteinuria and ameliorates nephropathy in an animal model of type II diabetes mellitus. Kidney Int 64 (2003): 2100–2107.

Wang L, Chen J, Thompson LU. The inhibitory effect of flaxseed on the growth and metastasis of estrogen receptor negative human breast cancer xenografts is attributed to both its lignan and oil components. Int J Cancer 116.5 (2005): 793–798.

Wilkinson P et al. Influence of alpha-linolenic acid and fish oil on cardiovascular risk with an atherogenic lipoprotein phenotype. Atherosclerosis 181.1 (2005): 115–124.

Xu J et al. Laxative effects of partially defatted flaxseed meal on normal and experimental constipated mice. BMC CAM 12 (2012): 14–19.

Zaineddin AK, et al. Serum enterolactone and postmenopausal breast cancer risk by estrogen, progesterone and herceptin 2 receptor status. Int J Cancer, (2012): 1401–1410.

Zhao G et al. Dietary alpha-linolenic acid reduces inflammatory and lipid cardiovascular risk factors in hypercholesterolemic men and women. J Nutr 134 (2004): 2991–2997.

Zong G et al. Effects of flaxseed supplementation on erythrocyte fatty acids and multiple cariometabolic biomarkers among Chinese with risk factors of metabolic syndrome. Eur J Nutr 52 (2013): 1547–1551.

Folate

HISTORICAL NOTE Folic acid was isolated from spinach leaves in 1941 and synthesised in 1946; hence, its name comes from the Latin *folium*, which means leaf.

OTHER NAMES

Folacin, vitamin B_9, folic acid, pteroylmonoglutamic acid (PGA)

BACKGROUND AND RELEVANT PHARMACOKINETICS AND CHEMICAL COMPONENTS

Folate is the generic term for a large family of chemically similar trace compounds that fall within the vitamin B group. Folic acid is the most oxidised and stable form and the one characteristically used in supplements and food fortification. Folate found in animal sources is present in a 'free form' and is readily absorbed; however, aside from the organ meats, animal products are notoriously poor sources. Folate found in plant foods exists in conjugated forms, which require deconjugation by zinc-dependent enzymes in the gut prior to absorption. (Kelly 1998). This step is inhibited by chronic alcohol ingestion and some foods, including oranges and legumes (Gropper et al 2009). Secondary to this difference, the average bioavailability of natural folate is half that of the synthetic form (e.g. 55–66% versus ≈ 100% (Carmel et al 2006, Kelly 1998). Small amounts of folate are endogenously produced by bacteria in the intestines, but this appears to be predominantly lost via the faeces (Gropper et al 2009).

Dietary folate and synthetic folic acid alike then undergo complex conversion into folate's active forms, e.g. tetrahydrofolate (THF). This occurs via a multistep pathway now proposed to occur solely within the liver (Wright et al 2007). In contrast, a less common supplemental form of folate — folinic acid (5-formyltetrahydrofolate or 5-formylTHF), as an intermediate folate metabolite — bypasses some of these steps to readily form 5,10-methylenetetrohydrofolate (5,10-formylTHF) (Kelly 1998, McGuire et al 1987, Priest et al 1991).

Secretion into the bile of the THF derivatives and their subsequent reabsorption through the enterohepatic circulation enable redistribution throughout the body. Distribution of folate appears to be regulated via an unknown mechanism, ensuring increased availability to those tissues demonstrating rapid cell division (Gropper et al 2009). Although many of the biochemical pathways in which folate is involved act to regenerate the nutrient, there is still a significant amount that is broken down and eliminated, chiefly in the urine.

Clinical note — Food fortification with folate: still not enough for pregnant women?

In 1997, voluntary folic acid fortification of foods was introduced in Australia and New Zealand to improve the folate status, particularly of pregnant women. Following this, a study evaluating mean serum folate levels in over 20,000 Australian women aged 14–45 years found that although concentrations had increased by 19%, the prevalence of poor folate status in this age group had only reduced from 8.5% to 4.1% (Metz et al 2002). Several state-based studies since 1997 have shown a variety of improvements in a range of measures, including haematological markers, folate awareness and supplementation rates among Australian women (Brown et al 2011, Chan et al 2008, du Plessis et al 2008, Hickling et al 2005) and corresponding reductions in NTD births have varied from 17% to 40%; however, some researchers suggest that this decrease occurred in the first 2 years following fortification and the launch of awareness campaigns, and that there has been no further reduction since this time (du Plessis et al 2008). Unsurprisingly, an economic evaluation of the Australian mandatory fortification determined that while it was a cost-effective approach offering substantial long-term benefits with respect to life years gained and quality-adjusted life years, mandatory supplementation alone would be insufficient to achieve folate status required for NTD prevention (Rabovskaja et al 2013). Although fortification programs, including mandatory fortification of bread flour in Australia and New Zealand (FSANZ 2007), provide some measure of protection for women of reproductive age, supplementation is still required. Unfortunately, widespread public health campaigns have had limited success and many women remain unaware of the need to take supplements prior to pregnancy, or are aware but still fail to use supplements (du Plessis et al 2008, Metz et al 2002). In Australia, only 36% and 46% of new mothers in Victoria and New South Wales, respectively, took folate supplements in 2006, with even lower rates reported for women of low socio-economic or non-English speaking backgrounds (Watson et al 2006) and women aged 20–24 years. The last group also experiences the highest rate of NTD births (du Plessis et al 2008).

Clinical note — A challenge to the perceived safety and superiority of synthetic folic acid?

Given its relative stability in processing and enhanced bioavailability, synthetic folic acid in food fortificants and supplements has long been regarded as more reliable than natural dietary sources for ensuring folate adequacy (Kelly 1998). This, in turn, has led to widening implementation of mandatory folate fortification programs aimed at the prevention of neural tube defects (NTDs). Recently, however, the safety of increased exposure to synthetic folic acid has been thrown into question. Individuals who consume high doses (≥400 mcg/day) exhibit unmetabolised folic acid in their blood, a form that does not naturally occur in human physiology (Kelly 1998, Lucock 2004, 2006, Sauer et al 2009, Smith et al 2008, Sweeney et al 2007, Troen et al 2006, Wright et al 2007). While this will eventually be hepatically converted into a natural folate derivative, there is speculation regarding the interim effects, with evidence of competition between the unmetabolised folic acid and the main active folate form methyl-THF at receptors and their subsequent down-regulation on cell surfaces (Sauer et al 2009, Smith et al 2008). Particular at-risk groups identified by researchers include those individuals taking anti-folate medications, folate-replete cancer patients and elderly patients with B_{12} deficiency (Smith et al 2008, Wright et al 2007), while others question the long-term safety for the unborn fetus (Kelly 1998). Until further research is conducted in this area, the implications remain unclear.

F

FOOD SOURCES

Good dietary sources of folate are fresh green leafy vegetables, such as cabbage and spinach, asparagus, broccoli, sprouts, mushrooms, legumes, nuts and fortified cereals and organ meats.

Food preparation and processing can destroy up to 100% of the naturally occurring folate, as it is sensitive to light and air but especially heat; therefore, raw foods, as well as fortified foods, are considered superior sources, which in Australia provide 100 mcg per serve (Gropper et al 2009, Hickling et al 2005).

DEFICIENCY

Folate deficiency is not uncommon and can develop within just 4 months of an inadequate diet (Carmel et al 2006, Gropper et al 2009, Wilson et al 1991).

In light of folate's fundamental role in DNA synthesis, deficiency of this nutrient will predictably impact most on those cells and tissues that exhibit a high turnover (e.g. blood and the cells in the gastrointestinal tract), which also applies to those stages of development with increased rates of growth, such as pregnancy and fetal tissue development.

Signs and symptoms of deficiency

- Macrocytic/megaloblastic anaemia
- Fatigue
- Psychological symptoms such as irritability and depression (Reynolds 2002)
- Headache
- Hair loss
- Nausea
- Insomnia (Pelton et al 2000)
- Peripheral neuropathy
- Myelopathy (Okada et al 2014)
- Tendon hyperreflexivity
- Diarrhoea
- Weight loss
- Cerebral disturbances (Botez 1976), cerebral cortex atrophy and cognitive decline
- Increased blood levels of homocysteine

Primary deficiency

This develops in response to inadequate dietary intake and can be caused by a diet generally lacking in fresh, lightly cooked vegetables. Risk is increased in patients with *MTHFR* gene polymorphisms, in people receiving total parenteral nutrition (TPN), chronic alcoholics, phenylketonuria patients on restricted diets, patients with sickle cell anaemia and the institutionalised elderly (Carmel et al 2006, Wahlqvist 2002).

Folate enzyme polymorphisms

Single allele substitution in the gene encoding for the *N*5,10-methylenetetrahydrofolate reductase enzyme, responsible for converting folate into its methylated 'active' form, results in several possible polymorphisms. Individuals who are homozygous for the *MTHFR* C677T polymorphism (2–16% white populations) convert the active folate form at only 30% of the normal capacity, while the *MTHFR* A1298C genotype produces an enzyme with 60% of the unaffected enzyme activity (Gilbody et al 2007). Homozygotes for either polymorphism are at a significantly increased risk of folate deficiency and cannot maintain adequacy with recommended dietary intake levels (NHMRC 2006).

Secondary deficiency

Secondary deficiency is caused by compromised absorption, increased excretion or increased demands or losses. Inadequate absorption can occur in malabsorption syndromes such as coeliac and Crohn's disease, with long-term use of certain medications such as phenytoin, sulfasalazine, cimetidine, antacids and oral contraceptive pill (OCP), in congenital malabsorption states and in blind loop syndrome (Beers & Berkow 2003), especially when combined with suboptimal dietary intake (Carmel et al 2006). In chronic kidney disease, down-regulation of folate transporters in the intestine, heart, liver and brain can lead to reduced intestinal absorption of folate (Bukhari et al 2011). Significantly impaired absorption has also been observed in HIV patients (Revell et al 1991).

Besides impaired absorption, inadequate use can occur with concurrent vitamin B_{12} or C deficiency, smoking (Gabriel et al 2006, Okumura & Tsukamoto 2011) or acute or chronic alcoholism (Hamid & Kaur 2007). A genetic variation in folate requirement has also been identified, as a congenital enzyme deficiency exists in approximately 13% of the Western population (Ma et al 1996). In these cases, total or partial absence of the enzyme responsible for the final step in converting folate to its major active metabolite (methylenetetrahydrofolate reductase) results in decreased plasma levels (Kumar & Clarke 2002). Therefore, these individuals have a higher folate requirement than others without this congenital enzyme deficiency and display increased susceptibility to folate deficiency.

A number of pharmaceutical drugs, such as folic acid antagonists (e.g. methotrexate), can affect status by interfering with absorption, use and conversion to its active forms. In such cases, oral folic acid supplements are sometimes given to reduce side effects, although it may marginally reduce drug efficacy (Kumar & Clarke 2002, Strober & Menon 2005). Oral isotretinoin treatment may induce folic acid deficiency, although the mechanisms underlying this observation remain unclear (Karadag et al 2011).

Additionally, there are several subpopulations with increased demands for folic acid, such as pregnant and lactating women, the elderly and patients with malignancies, haemolytic anaemias such as sickle cell disease, chronic exfoliative skin disorders or achlorhydria (Gropper et al 2009). Extra losses have also been reported in haemodialysis patients.

The chronic use of alcohol during pregnancy may be associated with reduced folate transport to the fetus (Hutson et al 2012). The ratio of serum folate in maternal blood compared to umbilical cord blood at time of delivery was significantly lower in pregnancies with chronic and heavy alcohol exposure ($P = 0.014$), further emphasising the need for abstinence from alcohol during pregnancy.

Excess folic acid

Adults and children with phenylketonuria may be at risk of receiving folic acid at higher doses than daily recommendations as a result of high folic acid content in protein substitutes (Stølen et al 2013). These patients should be individually monitored for nutrient status, as the effects of very high doses, in particular in children, is uncertain.

MAIN ACTIONS

Folate's actions are all secondary to its ability to donate methyl groups and its central role, therefore, in one-carbon metabolism.

Coenzyme

As a key methyl donor, folate is involved in a variety of reactions important for the metabolism of amino acids and nucleic acids.

DNA and RNA synthesis

Folate plays an essential part in the production of purines and pyrimidines that make up DNA, making it a critical nutrient in relation to cell division and repair of genetic material, and is generally required for genomic stability. Subsequently, folate plays an indirect role in the synthesis of transfer RNA.

Production of the active form of B_{12}

Folate and B_{12} are intrinsically linked; for example, the conversion of B_{12} into methylcobalamin is dependent upon the presence of a THF derivative.

Reduction of homocysteine levels

Folate, via B_{12} activation, donates a methyl group to homocysteine facilitating its recycling back to methionine. Together with vitamin B_6, necessary for homocysteine catabolism, folate effectively lowers homocysteine levels.

Synthesis of S-adenosyl-l-methionine (SAMe)

Following regeneration of methionine from homocysteine, the methyl group donated by folate is then taken up by SAMe, enabling it to become a carbon donor in multiple transmethylation reactions throughout the body, including neurotransmitter synthesis (Hendler & Rorvik 2001).

Amino acid metabolism

Folate is involved in the synthesis of some of the non-essential amino acids such as serine and glycine. It is also required for the conversion of histidine into glutamate (Gropper et al 2009).

CLINICAL USE

The conditions for which folate is indicated as a potential treatment are primarily due to an existing deficiency, through either primary or secondary pathways. Research has focused particularly on those conditions in which folate deficiency is a consequence of medication use and the benefits of improved folate status.

Prevention and treatment of deficiency

Commonly, folic acid supplements are used to correct identifiable deficiency states, such as macrocytic anaemia, or given as preventive treatment to those patients at risk of deficiency, such as in malabsorption syndromes or taking long-term folate antagonist medication. Increased oral intake of folate has been found to be effective, even in cases of malabsorption due to the passive diffusion evident with pharmacological doses (Carmel et al 2006).

Preconception and during pregnancy

Neural tube defects

Poor folate status either 1 month before conception or during the first trimester of pregnancy is an independent risk factor for NTD in the newborn. One study has suggested that the increased risk could be as high as 10-fold (Daly et al 1995). Despite a wealth of scientific evidence and global health promotion campaigns, it would appear many pregnant women still fail to meet folate intake requirements (Manniën et al 2013, Timmermans et al 2008). It is estimated that, worldwide, only 25% of folic acid-preventable spina bifida and anencephaly are currently being prevented through folic acid fortification (Youngblood et al 2013). Interestingly, a study from Northern Ireland found that women who had been pregnant previously were less likely to follow folate intake recommendations compared to women in their first pregnancy ($P = 0.001$), highlighting the need to emphasise supplementation irrespective of previous pregnancy experience (McNulty et al 2011).

The continued supplementation of 400 mcg folic acid daily in the second and third trimester of pregnancy has been found to increase maternal and placental cord blood folate status, and prevent the increase in homocysteine concentration that otherwise occurs in late pregnancy (McNulty et al 2013). The clinical implication on pregnancy outcomes or early childhood development requires further investigation.

Intervention trials for pregnancy have routinely used 400 mcg folic acid/day; however, there is some suggestion that routine ingestion of only 100 mcg folate from fortified food would prevent the majority of NTDs. Studies have also been conducted on women with a previous NTD birth, with benefits demonstrated at doses of 4 mg/day. There is a general consensus among researchers and health authorities that due to the inconsistent nature of natural food sources, taking a supplement or incorporating fortified foods is the most reliable way to increase levels sufficiently (Cuskelly et al 1996). A maternal red blood cell folate concentration >906 nmol/L is thought to be optimal for lowering risk (Pietrzik et al 2007).

The prevalence of NTD-affected pregnancies has been reported as up to 75% higher in obese women and up to threefold higher for women who are severely obese (Rasmussen et al 2008, Stothard et al 2009). An observational study found obese women to have lower serum folate levels but increased red blood cell folate concentrations, which may be due to body mass index and tissue type affecting the distribution of folate (Tinker et al 2012).

Other neonatal outcomes

While a number of other birth defects besides NTD have been attributed to folate deficiency in recent times, including Down syndrome (Eskes 2006) and cleft lip and/or palate (CL/P), a 2010 Cochrane review concluded that there was no statistically significant evidence of any effects of folate supplementation on prevention of cleft palate, cleft lip, congenital cardiovascular defects, miscarriage or other birth defects (De-Regil et al 2010).

A more recent case-control study from the Netherlands found that regular folic acid supplementation during 0–12 weeks after conception was associated with increased risk of cleft formation in the offspring (OR 1.72, 95% CI 1.19–2.49) (Rozendaal et al 2013). Despite this, available evidence surrounding the role of folic acid in non-NTD birth defects is still contradictory (Bean et al 2011, Hollis et al 2013); as such, the role that supplementation has in the aetiology of these conditions still remains unclear.

Data from numerous studies have suggested that supplementation with folic acid prior to conception and during early pregnancy may reduce autism spectrum disorder (ASD) risk (Berry 2013, Schmidt et al 2012). Analysis of the Norwegian Mother and Child Cohort Study (n = 85,176) found that the maternal supplementation from 4 weeks before to 8 weeks after the start of pregnancy was associated with a lower risk of autistic disorder, the most severe form of ASD, in children (adjusted OR 0.61, 95% CI 0.41–0.90) (Surén et al 2013). Using the same data, another study identified that folic acid supplementation or dietary folate did not protect against spontaneous pre-term delivery; pre-conceptional folic acid supplementation starting more than 8 weeks before conception was associated with an increased risk of pre-term delivery (hazard ratio 1.19, 95% CI 1.05–1.34) (Sengpiel et al 2013).

Higher folate levels are linked to the prevention of miscarriages, decreased risk of intrauterine growth retardation, increased birth weight in the offspring of smoking mothers (Sram et al 2005) and increased rates of twin pregnancies, from both natural and in vitro fertilisation (IVF) conception (Haggarty et al 2006). Folic acid supplementation may modify some of the adverse effects of maternal smoking on neonatal outcomes and fetal growth, particularly during the first trimester, although no effect on risk of preterm birth or on risk of 'small size for gestational age' at birth (Bakker et al 2011).

A recent Cochrane review concluded that folic acid supplementation was associated with an improved mean birth weight (mean difference (MD) 135.75, 95% CI: 47.85–223.68) and with a reduction in megaloblastic anaemia incidence (RR 0.21, 95% CI 0.11–0.38) (Lassi et al 2013). Conversely, this review also found that folic acid supplementation had no conclusive benefit on pregnancy outcomes such as preterm birth (RR 1.33, 95% CI 0.73–1.38), stillbirths/neonatal deaths (RR 1.33, 95% CI 0.96–1.85) or some haematological parameters including pre-delivery anaemia (RR 0.62, 95% CI 0.35–1.10), mean pre-delivery haemoglobin level (MD −0.03, 95% CI −0.25–0.19), mean pre-delivery serum folate levels (standardised mean difference 2.03, 95% CI 0.80–3.27) and mean pre-delivery red cell folate levels (SMD 1.59, 95% CI −0.07–3.26).

A large population-based cohort study (n = 193,554) found that daily supplementation with 400 mcg folic acid did not prevent preeclampsia or gestational hypertension in Chinese women (Li et al 2013). Periconception folate supplementation was found to be associated with lower uteroplacental vascular resistance and higher blood pressures during pregnancy in a population-based cohort study (n = 5993) (Timmermans et al 2011). These observed effects were small and remained within normal physiological ranges, and did not correlate with risk of preeclampsia or gestational hypertension.

A case-control study in Chinese mothers found that folic acid supplementation was associated with significantly reduced risk of congenital heart defects (Li et al 2013). Supplementing with folic acid for a longer period of time appeared to be more effective in reducing the risk of heart defects. Similarly, a prelimary study found that mothers with the *MDR1* 3435T allele who did not use folic acid during the 4 weeks prior to conception until 10 weeks post-conception were at an increased risk of congenital heart defects in their offspring (OR 2.8, 95% CI 1.2–6.4) (Obermann-Borst et al 2011). Further studies are suggested to clarify this finding. Interestingly, several studies have failed to demonstrate a significant relationship between the *MTHFR* C677T genotype and CL/P (Boyles et al 2008, Butali et al 2013, Chevrier et al 2007); however, this may be confounded by concurrent folic acid supplementation in some individuals.

Childhood diseases

There is a small amount of evidence suggesting folic acid supplementation during early pregnancy may increase the risk of asthma and allergic diseases (Håberg et al 2009, Hollingsworth et al 2008). Despite this, a 2013 systematic review and meta-analysis concluded that there was no evidence of an association between maternal folic acid supplementation and increased risk of asthma in children (RR 1.01, 95% CI 0.78–1.30) (Crider et al 2013). Due to limitations of current studies, further high-quality studies may be of benefit (Ownby et al 2009).

OCP-induced folate deficiency

Long-term use of the oral contraceptive pill (OCP) (>5 years) has historically been associated with a progressive decrease in serum folate levels, of up to 40%, which could feasibly result in changes to cognition and mood, increased risk of macrocytic anaemia and increased risk of NTD in newborns once use has ceased. Results from some studies suggest this last concern may be unfounded (Lussanaa et al 2003, Sütterlin et al 2003).

There are a number of proposed mechanisms for folate depletion with OCP use, including concurrent depletion of B_{12}, which is involved in the regeneration pathway of THF (Bielenberg 1991), and impaired folate resorption (Sütterlin et al 2003).

Hyperhomocysteinaemia

Together with vitamins B_{12} and B_6, folic acid has been shown to reduce high plasma levels of homocysteine (Hcy). Of the three, folate appears to have the strongest effect (Voutilainen et al 2001). A randomised dose-response clinical trial found that for adults with existing folate deficiencies, there was a trend towards reduced homocysteine levels with increasing folic acid dose (Anderson et al 2010). Supplementation in healthy adults with adequate folate status did not appear to reduce homocysteine.

Although elevated Hcy has been implicated as a risk for cardiovascular disease (including atherosclerosis and coronary artery disease), cerebrovascular disease, peripheral vascular disease and venous thromboembolism (Clarke et al 1991, den Heijer et al 1996, Malinow et al 1989, Selhub et al 1995), exudative age-related macular degeneration (Nowak et al 2005), noise-related hearing loss (Gok et al 2004), cognitive dysfunction, posttraumatic stress disorder (Jendricko et al 2008), breast cancer incidence in postmenopausal women (Gatt et al 2007) and adverse pregnancy outcomes (Bjorke Monsen & Ueland 2003) including postnatal depression (Behzadi et al 2008), clinical trials are ongoing to determine the clinical relevance of these associations.

Bone health and fracture risk

Elevated Hcy has been identified as a strong risk factor for osteoporotic fractures (Abrahamsen et al 2006, Green et al 2007, McLean et al 2008, Rejnmark et al 2008). While a significant association between the *MTHFR* C677T polymorphism and fractures has also been demonstrated, this is only significant when coupled with low reported intake of folate, B_{12}, B_2 and B_6 (Abrahamsen et al 2006). This has led some researchers to conclude that the response rate to folate treatment among an osteoporotic population is likely to be as little as 2% (Abrahamsen et al 2006). This may explain the lack of positive effect on bone turnover seen in an RCT of hyperhomocysteinaemic (>5 mmol/L) older patients treated with 1 mg folate, 500 mcg B_{12} and 10 mg B_6 treated for 2 years, in spite of significant Hcy lowering (Green et al 2007). Similarly, 800 mcg daily folic acid supplemented for 4 months in 31 women with Hcy > 10 micromol/L failed to identify any significant effect on bone turnover markers compared to placebo despite lowering of Hcy ($P = 0.007$) (Keser et al 2013).

Cardiovascular protection and treatment

In spite of two early meta-analyses which concluded that risk of ischaemic heart disease could be reduced by 16% following a decrease in Hcy of 3 mmol/L (Homocysteine Study Collaboration 2002, Wald et al 2002), there are few folate interventional studies in established hyperhomocysteinaemic cardiovascular populations and recent studies have produced mixed findings.

In patients with kidney disease, two recent meta-analyses have yielded conflicting conclusions concerning the effect of folic acid supplementation on cardiovascular disease. A 2013 meta-analysis (9 RCTs, $n = 8234$) determined that folic acid supplementation reduced the risk of cardiovascular disease in patients with kidney disease, in patients with folate deficiency, diabetes or advanced and end-stage renal disease (RR 0.85, 95% CI 0.77–0.94) (Qin et al 2013a). Conversely, a 2012 systematic review and meta-analysis (11 RCTs, $n = 10{,}951$) determined that folic acid-based homocysteine lowering does not reduce cardiovascular events in patients with kidney disease (RR 0.97, 95% CI 0.92–1.03) and thus should not be used solely for CVD prevention in this population (Jardine et al 2012).

An interesting trial investigating the benefits of combined B vitamins (5 mg folic acid and high-dose B complex, both administered twice weekly) to patients with a history of cardiovascular events has revealed that those participants whose Hcy decreased within the first 3 months demonstrated significantly reduced cardiovascular risk over the next 5 years; however, no protection was conveyed for slower responders (Siragusa et al 2007). While another small study of B vitamins in hyperhomocysteinaemic elderly subjects failed to improve blood pressure (McMahon et al 2007), elevated Hcy secondary to impaired kidney function in this population group cannot be excluded as a confounding variable.

Alzheimer's dementia and impaired cognitive function in the elderly

Findings such as the prevalence of folate deficiency in the elderly, increasing Hcy levels with age, evidence of an inverse relationship between total plasma Hcy levels and cognitive function and preliminary evidence of correlation between Hcy and plasma amyloid peptide levels in Alzheimer patients (Aisen et al 2008) have attracted attempts to link the phenomena, providing an explanation for neurodegenerative disorders.

In spite of this, and a large number of investigations of B vitamins, very few have restricted participation to only hyperhomocysteinaemic individuals, which may partly explain their negative findings. The Folic Acid and Carotid Intima-Media Thickness (FACIT) trial, however, administered 800 mcg/day over 3 years to participants with elevated baseline Hcy (≥ 13 mmol/L), producing a mean increase in serum folate of 576% and 26% reduction in plasma Hcy (Durga et al 2007). Treated subjects demonstrated significant improvements in three of the six cognitive testing domains (memory, information processing speed and sensorimotor speed), leading the authors to conclude that folic acid is an effective agent for improving cognitive function that tends to decline with age.

In patients with organic brain disease including Alzheimer's and vascular dementia, again only one

F

study has restricted participation to hyperhomocysteinaemic individuals, administering 5 mg folic acid together with 1 mg B_{12} daily over 2 months (Nilsson et al 2001). As this stands alone in its positive findings, it is suggestive that Hcy is a key indicator of likelihood for response to B vitamin supplementation (Nilsson et al 2001).

It is important to note that hyperhomocysteinaemic patients suffering dementia do not typically co-present with macrocytic anaemia, as might be expected (McCaddon et al 2004). Therefore, the neurological and haematological features of B_{12} and folate deficiency are often unrelated in these patients.

Diabetes mellitus

An RCT (n = 48) of overweight and obese men with type 2 diabetes mellitus found that folic acid supplementation (5 mg daily for 8 weeks) significantly reduced HbA_{1C} by 8% (P = 0.005), reduced serum insulin by 16.2% (P = 0.02), reduced insulin resistance by 20.5% (P = 0.04) and reduced plasma homocysteine by 21.2% (P = 0.000) (Gargari et al 2011).

More recently, a systematic review and meta-analysis of 4 studies (n = 183) also found that daily supplementation of 5 mg folic acid in patients with type II diabetes mellitus significantly reduced plasma total homocysteine levels (Sudchada et al 2012). However, the meta-analysis concluded that the effect of folic acid on HbA_{1C} levels was not found to be significant and that further large-scale studies with larger sample sizes would be required to accuracy determine any effect of folic acid in type 2 diabetes mellitus.

Renal transplant recipients

Combination vitamin B treatment (folate, B_{12} and B_6) may be of benefit in renal transplant patients, according to an RCT of 56 renal transplant patients, which found that vitamin supplementation with folic acid (5 mg/day), vitamin B_6 (50 mg/day) and vitamin B_{12} (400 mcg/day) for 6 months reduced the progression of atherosclerosis, as evidenced by a significant decrease in carotid intima-media thickness. Additionally, a significant decrease in homocysteine levels was observed (Marcucci et al 2003).

Restenosis after percutaneous coronary intervention

An RCT found that treatment with vitamin B_{12} (cyanocobalamin 400 mcg/day), folic acid (1 mg/day) and vitamin B_6 (pyridoxine hydrochloride 10 mg/day) for 6 months significantly decreased the incidence of major adverse events, including restenosis, after percutaneous coronary intervention (Schnyder et al 2002). By contrast, one trial demonstrated an increased risk of in-stent restenosis in those patients intravenously administered 1 mg of folic acid, 5 mg of vitamin B_6 and 1 mg of vitamin B_{12} followed by daily oral doses of 1.2 mg of folic acid, 48 mg of vitamin B_6 and 60 mcg of vitamin B_{12} for 6 months (Lange et al 2004). Further research with more consistent study designs is required to elucidate the true effects.

Idiopathic recurrent miscarriage (IRM)

Maternal hyperhomocysteinaemia and poor folate status are risk factors for recurrent embryo loss and for first early embryo loss (George et al 2002). There has also been conflicting evidence in relation to the role of *MTHFR* polymorphisms and pregnancy, although many studies point towards increased risk of recurrent spontaneous abortion. One explanation for the discrepant results may be that the numbers of study participants have been relatively small (Zetterberg 2004). Although researchers encourage the periconceptional use of both folate and B_{12} to reduce these risks, there is a lack of interventional studies in this area other than one investigation of combined aspirin (100 mg/day) and folic acid (5 mg/alternate days) throughout gestation, on top of initial (12 weeks) prednisone and progesterone treatment (Tempfer et al 2006). This treatment yielded higher live birth rate compared with no treatment in women with IRM.

Cardiovascular disease protection and treatment independent of homocysteine status

In the absence of a causal relationship between Hcy and cardiovascular disease, what remains most promising for folate are studies illustrating its protective effects, mediated through other mechanisms. This has led some researchers to suggest that folate deficiency may be the primary cause of an increased vascular risk and that elevated Hcy levels should principally be considered an indicator of low folate status rather than a pathogenetic marker (Verhaar et al 2002). Demonstrations of in vitro antioxidant activity, effects on co-factor availability and direct and indirect interactions with the endothelial NO synthase enzyme have been proposed as plausible mechanisms, through which folate may prevent endothelial dysfunction (Antoniades et al 2007, Das 2003, Verhaar et al 2002).

Several meta-analyses have been conducted that assess the impact of folate alone or in combination on cardiovascular and all-cause mortality, including in individuals with preexisting cardiovascular or kidney disease, and have concluded that the treatments conveyed no significant benefits (Bazzano et al 2002, Bleys et al 2006, Leung et al 2010, Yang et al 2012). This was confirmed in a recent meta-analysis (n = 27,418) which concluded that folic acid supplementation had no significant effect on coronary revascularisation, coronary artery bypass grafting, percutaneous coronary intervention, coronary restenosis or total revascularisation (Qin et al 2014).

Combined B vitamins failed to reduce cardiovascular risk in high-risk women (Albert et al 2008), improve mortality and cardiovascular event frequency in patients with coronary artery disease (Ebbing et al 2008), failed to protect against cardiovascular events over 40 months (Bønaa et al 2006) and failed to prevent vascular events in patients with a stroke history after 3.9 years (Potter et al 2008).

On a more promising note, 51 heart transplant recipients who took 15 mg/day of methyltetrahydrofolate for 1 year following transplantation were found at their 7-year follow-up to have reduced all-cause mortality with a relative risk (RR) 0.53 when compared to the placebo group (Potena et al 2008).

Stroke

Several studies show the cardiovascular protective effects of folic acid, including the predictive value of low folate status on stroke risk (Bazzano et al 2002, Verhaar et al 2002).

Primary prevention with folic acid was found to effectively reduce the risk of stroke in a large-scale meta-analysis (n = 16,841; RR 0.82) (Wang et al 2007). The greatest beneficial effect was seen in subjects who received folic acid for longer than 3 years. A more recent 2012 meta-analysis of 26 RCTs similarly suggested there may be a modest benefit of folic acid supplementation in stroke prevention (Yang et al 2012).

Carotid intima-media thickness

Several studies have observed a beneficial effect of folic acid supplementation on markers of atherosclerosis, such as carotid intima-media thickness (Ntaios et al 2010, Vianna et al 2007).

A 2012 meta-analysis of 10 RCTs (n = 2052) found that folic acid supplementation was effective in reducing the progression of carotid intima-media thickness, a measure of atherosclerosis progression ($P < 0.001$) (Qin et al 2012). In particular, subjects with chronic kidney disease or high cardiovascular risk appeared to benefit from folic acid supplementation.

Hypertension and glucose control

In a multi-centre RCT, the combination of folic acid (400 mcg or 800 mcg) with enalapril (10 mg), an ACE inhibitor, was no more effective than enalapril alone in reducing blood pressure over 8 weeks (Mao et al 2008). The same study found that in subjects with hyperglycaemia, the combination of enalapril and 800 mcg folic acid significantly reduced fasting plasma glucose compared to enalapril alone and enalapril with 400 mcg ($P < 0.015$). Conversely, 8-week folic acid supplementation (400 mcg/day) in elderly women (n = 122) resulted in increased overnight fasting blood glucose concentrations (baseline: 84.8 ± 1.0 mg/dL; at 8 weeks: 98.2 ± 5.2 mg/dL, $P < 0.01$) (Chmurzynska et al 2013). When this cohort was stratified by *MTHFR* genotype, significant differences in HDL-cholesterol before and after supplementation were observed, with levels almost 10% lower in T-allele carriers than in CC homozygous subjects ($P < 0.05$).

Another small study, employing high-dose folate (10 mg/day) in patients with a recent history of acute myocardial infarction, demonstrated improved endothelial function (Moens et al 2007). These positive findings were independent of Hcy levels at baseline or changes to Hcy throughout the trial.

Cognitive decline, dementia and Alzheimer's disease prevention or treatment independent of homocysteine status

Independent of Hcy, folate is implicated in cognition and neurodegeneration due to its ability to improve nitric oxide levels in the brain and facilitate synthesis of neurotransmitters (Malouf & Grimley Evans 2008). Additionally, atrophy of the cerebral cortex results from folate deficiency. Despite an abundance of epidemiological evidence and a limited number of studies showing a positive correlation between folate status and dementia, the role of folic acid supplementation in cognition remains unclear.

A 2008 Cochrane review examining the effects of folic acid supplementation, with or without vitamin B_{12}, concluded that there was no consistent evidence that folate had any beneficial effect on cognitive function of healthy or cognitively impaired subjects (Malouf & Grimley Evans 2008). This was corroborated by a 2010 meta-analysis which found no effect of folic acid, with or without other B vitamins, on cognitive function within 3 years of the start of treatment.

Of the evidence available, including trials examined by the Cochrane review, a 2002 review has estimated that 71% of acute hospital admissions with severe folate deficiency have organic brain syndrome, compared with 31% of controls (Reynolds 2002). Low baseline serum folate also predicted dementia in a sample of 625 individuals followed over 2.4 years (Kim et al 2008), with onset of dementia significantly associated with exaggerated declines in folate and B_{12} and increases in Hcy, which may, however, have been the result of concomitant weight loss. In spite of this knowledge, the results of studies investigating supplemental folic acid have been equivocal and warrant closer examination of the disparate methodologies.

A review by Balk et al in 2007, which sub-analysed folic-acid-only treatments (three RCTs, using 750 mcg to 15 mg/day over 5–10 weeks) in elderly patients who were either healthy or cognitively impaired, found that while folic acid was not universally effective, there was evidence to suggest that patients with low baseline folate (<3 ng/mL) may significantly benefit.

Several studies investigating folic acid, either alone or in combination with other B vitamins, for slowing cognitive decline in Alzheimer's disease have failed to demonstrate an effect, independent of the hyperhomocysteinaemic population (Aisen et al 2008). One small study using 1 mg folic acid/day in conjunction with cholinesterase inhibitors over 6 months did, however, point towards an additive effect on patients' function (rather than cognition per se) regardless of Hcy (Connelly et al 2008); however, a similar study using higher doses of combined B vitamins failed to produce any statistically significant benefits (Sun et al 2007).

Anticonvulsant-induced folate deficiency

Anticonvulsant medications such as phenytoin, carbamazepine and valproate reduce serum folate status. Individual studies have estimated an incidence of 15% folate deficiency in this group, compared with 2% for control groups (Froscher et al 1995). However, the figure may be as high as 97% with long-term phenytoin therapy (Rivey et al 1984). This may be due to increased use of folate in drug metabolism and/or decreased mucosal absorption (Berg et al 1992, Pelton et al 2000). Often, folic acid supplements are recommended to avoid deficiency, but this requires close supervision to ensure drug efficacy is not substantially reduced (Rivey et al 1984). A series of published case reports documenting NTD births to women supplemented with folic acid 5 mg/day while on anticonvulsants has thrown into question whether this commonly recommended dose is sufficient or whether concomitant administration of other B vitamins, especially B_6, may be necessary (Candito et al 2007).

Psychiatric illness

Over the past three decades, a vast number of case reports, open studies and, to a lesser extent, case-control studies have been published on the topic of psychopathology and folate deficiency. Many report a high incidence of serum folate deficiency in patients with symptoms of depression and various psychiatric disorders, particularly in geriatric populations (Reynolds 2002). For instance, one review identified that rates of deficiency varied between 8% and 50% in patients with various psychiatric disorders, including depression and schizophrenia (Young & Ghadirian 1989). Two large studies, involving over 350 patients diagnosed with acute psychiatric presentations, identified low folate levels or frank deficiency (31% and 12% respectively). The patients with the most marked deficiency were also the group with the highest percentage of inpatients (Carney et al 1990). Another study of similar design found that 30% of 224 newly admitted psychiatric patients had low serum folate (<3.5 ng/mL) compared to just 2.4% of controls, and that patients with low folate were 3.5-fold more likely to present with depressive features (Lerner et al 2006). Disturbingly, the researchers also identified a significant trend between folate deficiency and hospital readmissions.

Depression

Aetiological role

It has been estimated that 15–38% of depressed people are folate deficient (Alpert & Fava 1997, Lerner et al 2006). Studies have also demonstrated that low dietary folate consumption (<256 mcg/day) (Tolmunen et al 2004), low serum folate (<3.5 ng/mL) (typically co-occurring with B_{12} deficiency) (Gilbody et al 2007, Lerner et al 2006) and an *MTHFR* C677T genotype (OR 1.36) are all independently associated with an increased risk of depression (Gilbody et al 2007, Kelly et al 2004). One study found that while folic acid supplementation did not reduce the risk of depression during and up to 8 months after pregnancy, it appeared to protect against depression for up to 21 months postpartum (Lewis et al 2012). This effect was more pronounced in those with the MTHFR C677T TT genotype ($P = 0.01$). The lesser-studied *MTHFR* A1298C genotype (although more active than the C677T genotype, but still 40% underactive) also demonstrates a weak positive relationship with depression incidence; however, more studies are required (Gilbody et al 2007). Following on from these findings, serum folate has also been negatively correlated with depression severity and duration in some, but not all, studies (Kim et al 2008). One proposed explanation for these inconsistencies is that low folate and elevated Hcy are only found in a sub-group of depressed patients; in particular, those who experience increased anger and hostility as part of their depression (Fraguas et al 2006).

Additional studies also highlight an association between antenatal and postnatal depression and elevated Hcy or low folate levels but not serum B_{12} nor dietary intake of these two nutrients (Abou-Saleh et al 1999, Miyake et al 2006) and depression in antenatal and postnatal patients, with Hcy naturally peaking in the third trimester (Abou-Saleh et al 1999, Behzadi et al 2008). The link between folate and B_{12} and depression has been hypothesised to be via Hcy and independent of this, due to its methylation role generally (Bottiglieri 2005, Coppen & Bolander-Gouaille 2005, Das 2008, Gilbody et al 2007, Lerner et al 2006, Roberts et al 2007, Tiemeier et al 2002).

Therapeutic role

Given the volume of evidence linking folate with depression, it is surprising that so few clinical trials have been conducted. A Cochrane systematic review of three RCTs involving 247 depressed people suggested that, on the limited evidence available, folate shows potential as an augmenting agent, but speculated that its effectiveness might be restricted to folate-deficient patients (Taylor et al 2003). The studies included in this review used 500 mcg folic acid, 15 mg or 50 mg of methyltetrahydrofolate once daily and lasted from 8 weeks to 6 months.

More recent studies, particularly in the elderly, who exhibit high rates of both folate deficiency and depression, have investigated the effects of broad-scale nutritional supplementation (meeting recommended daily intakes (RDIs) for all essential micronutrients) over a 6-month period with promising results. Red cell folate and serum B_{12} values rose in supplemented individuals in accordance with significantly reduced scores on depression scales (Gariballa & Forster 2007). Prophylactic treatment of non-depressed elderly men with 2 mg folic acid, 25 mg B_6 and 400 mcg B_{12}, in another study, however, failed to reduce depression incidence over 2 years (Ford et al 2008).

Improves response to standard antidepressants

Research investigating folate's adjunctive role in depression treatment has escalated in recent years and there is now evidence of an impaired fluoxetine response in patients with low folate levels, with response rates dropping from 44.7% in subjects with normal serum folate to only 7.1% of deficient patients (<2.5 ng/mL) (Papakostas et al 2004a, 2004b), as well as a potentiating effect when only 500 mcg/day of folic acid is added to fluoxetine (Coppen & Bailey 2000). Reduced folate levels have also been associated with reduced response to sertraline (Alpert et al 2003). Poor folate status negatively impacts response time (+1.5 weeks) (Papakostas et al 2005) and relapse rates during continuation of fluoxetine (42.9% relapse in patients with low folate levels versus 3.2%) (Papakostas et al 2004a, 2004b), independent of B_{12} and Hcy levels.

Schizophrenia

Folate has been implicated in schizophrenic aetiology since the 1950s with one-carbon metabolism abnormalities proposed as a distinct hypothesis at a similar time (Regland 2005). With current knowledge linking the two, there has been renewed interest in the role of folate in this disorder. In particular, folate deficiency fits with the neurodevelopmental theory, implicating malnutrition amongst other environmental stressors during gestation in the subsequent susceptibility to neurological disorders of offspring (Applebaum et al 2004, Gilbody et al 2007, Haidemenos et al 2007, Muntjewerff & Blom 2005). Specifically, elevated Hcy in the third trimester has been associated with significantly elevated risk. This theory is supported in part by the parallel increases in NTD births and schizophrenia incidence in populations affected by famine (Muntjewerff & Blom 2005). Further evidence of folate's role comes from elevated Hcy and a high incidence of the *MTHFR* C677T genotype which are frequently, but not consistently, found in this patient group (Kemperman et al 2006, Regland 2005). A meta-analysis of links between this folate polymorphism and schizophrenia found an odds ratio of 1.44 (Gilbody et al 2007).

Several studies in adult schizophrenic patients have reported increased rates of active folate deficiency. One, in addition to this, demonstrated an inverse relationship between serum folate and degree of negative symptoms and a positive association between Hcy and extra-pyramidal symptoms (Goff et al 2004). There have been several case reports of successful treatment using 15–30 mg folate together with B_{12} injections (1 mg every 10 days) and *N*-acetylcysteine (200 mg twice daily) (Regland 2005), as well as a study which administered a combination of 2 mg folic acid, 25 mg B_6 and 400 mcg B_{12} to schizophrenic patients with baseline Hcy > 15 mmol, which produced improvements in both clinical features and neuropsychological test performance (Levine et al 2006).

Other neurological and psychiatric presentations

Significantly decreased red cell folate (not serum) has been documented in both phases of bipolar disorder (Hasanah et al 1997), as well as frequently found in patients chronically treated with lithium (Coppen & Bolander-Gouaille 2005). There is also preliminary evidence of mildly elevated Hcy in post-traumatic stress disorder (PTSD) sufferers; however, more thorough investigation is required to confirm this tentative association (Jendricko et al 2008).

A 2011 Cochrane review determined that there are insufficient high-quality data to determine the effect of folic acid on fragile X-syndrome patients (Rueda & Ballesteros 2011).

Chemopreventative role

Epidemiological, animal and human studies all suggest that folate status may affect the risk of developing cancers in selected tissues; however, the exact nature of this relationship continues to elude researchers (Bollheimer et al 2005, Powers 2005). One current theory points to the negative synergism between ageing and folate inadequacy, producing aberrations in one-carbon transfer such as gene hypomethylation, implicated in potentially carcinogenic genomic changes (Jang et al 2005). Despite the wealth of studies available concerning folate and cancer risk, recent meta-analyses of over 50,000 subjects concluded that folic acid supplementation did not substantially increase or decrease incidence of site-specific cancer during the first five years of treatment (RR 1.06, $P = 0.10$) (Vollset et al 2013). This large-scale study also found no significant effect of folic acid supplementation on the incidence of cancer within the breast, prostate, lung, large intestine or any other specific site. Conversely, a meta-analysis by Qin and colleagues (2013) found that folic acid supplementation was associated with a significantly reduced risk of melanoma (RR 0.47) although no significant effect was observed with total cancer incidence, colorectal cancer, prostate cancer, lung cancer, breast cancer or haematological malignancy (Qin et al 2013b).

Previously, high folate intake was purported to have an almost universally protective effect. An extensive review of the role of the *MTHFR* C677T polymorphism in cancer risk concluded that, in spite of the poor folate status associated with this polymorphism, however, many studies identify it as protective against a range of cancers (Sharp & Little 2004). In addition to this, a group of Swedish researchers have demonstrated that the relationship between serum folate and colorectal cancer follows a bell-shaped curve distribution (Van Guelpen et al 2006). Speculation regarding the role of additional co-factors involved in folate activity has also emerged (Powers 2005).

Folate's actions, however, still constitute a plausible cancer risk modulator, due to its critical role in the production, methylation and repair of DNA, regulation of cell turnover and suppression of excessive proliferation (Choi & Mason 2000, 2002).

Colon cancer

The link between folate status and colorectal cancer was first suggested as a result of 1990s epidemiological findings. Subsequent rodent studies further strengthened the theory, when chemically induced colorectal carcinogenesis was shown to be enhanced under dietary folate deprivation and reduced with folate administration (Cravo et al 1992, Kim et al 1996). The *MTHFR* C677T genotype has been identified as a risk factor (OR 1.34), compounded by dietary folate below median intakes (Murphy et al 2008). Based on a recent systematic review and meta-analysis, folate may be associated with a protective effective against colorectal cancer (Kennedy et al 2011); however, this is not yet definitive as some studies show no effects. A 2013 meta-analysis of RCTs concluded that long-term folic acid use (3.5 years) did not increase or decrease the occurrence of new colorectal adenomas in patients with history of adenoma (RR any adenoma 0.98; RR advanced adenoma 1.06) (Figueiredo et al 2013). Similarly, in subjects with a history of colorectal cancer, a 2008 multicentre RCT found 0.5 mg/day folate did not reduce the risk of colorectal adenoma recurrence (RR any adenoma 1.07; RR advanced adenoma 0.98) (Logan et al 2008). Additionally, a large placebo-controlled RCT ($n = 5442$) of women at high risk of cardiovascular disease found that use of B-vitamins, including folate, was not associated with the prevention of colorectal adenoma, with no apparent benefit or harm being identified (Song et al 2012).

Breast cancer

While the epidemiological evidence with respect to dietary folate and breast cancer risk has produced equivocal results, more consistent evidence points to low folate intake as a risk factor only when combined with increased alcohol consumption (Larsson et al 2007, Mahoney et al 2007). This negative synergy is further supported by evidence that maintaining adequate folate intake, usually via supplementation, can reduce or eliminate the excess risk due to increased alcohol consumption (Mahoney et al 2007). A comparable detrimental additive effect has been demonstrated between the *MTHFR* genotype and low folate intake (OR 2.80) (Suzuki et al 2008).

Cervical cancer

Folate deficiency may increase the risk of cervical cancer in individuals infected with high risk human papiloma virus (HR-HPV) (Piyathilake et al 2004). Evidence suggests a diet rich in fruit and vegetables generally (OR 0.52), and folate independently (OR 0.55), reduces the risk of developing cervical cancer (Ghosh et al 2008); however, much of the other evidence pertaining to a protective relationship has been ambiguous and results from intervention studies on cervical cancer have been inconsistent (Henao et al 2005, Kwanbunjan et al 2005, Sedjo et al 2003). The most surprising finding is that the *MTHFR* genotype appears protective against cervical cancer (Shekari et al 2008), enhanced further by a concomitant low intake of B_2 (Piyathilake et al 2007).

The most promising RCT involved 47 patients taking an OCP who demonstrated mild to moderate intraepithelial dysplasia. A dose of 10 mg folic acid daily over 3 months resulted in significantly lower biopsy scores in the treatment group and a significant reduction in cytology scores from baseline (Butterworth et al 1982). Other studies have shown that folic acid treatment does not alter the course of disease in patients with pre-established cervical dysplasia (Childers et al 1995).

Other cancers

A protective role for folate in the prevention of a growing number of other cancers, e.g. prostate (Marchal et al 2008), lung (Suzuki et al 2007), pancreas (Suzuki et al 2008) and nervous system cancers (Milne et al 2012, Sirachainan et al 2008), has been tentatively made. Due to the limited or, in some cases, conflicting evidence that is available, more research is required to validate these preliminary findings (Rycyna et al 2013).

In a case-control study, maternal folic acid supplementation before and during pregnancy may reduce the risk of childhood acute leukaemia (OR 0.4) (Amigou et al 2012). This study also suggested that genotypes homozygous for any of the MTHFR polymorphisms or carrying both MTRR variant alleles may also be a risk factor for developing acute leukaemia; however, this study had some limitations thus further research is recommended.

Periodontal disease

A series of RCTs have shown that rinsing with a solution of folate (5 mg/dose) twice daily alleviates gingival inflammation in all age groups and in pregnant and non-pregnant women (Pack 1984, Thomson & Pack 1982). Treatment results in a significant reduction in inflammation without altering plaque levels or folate serum status and appears to be more successful than oral supplements (Vogel et al 1976).

Preliminary evidence suggests that topical folate may also have a role in controlling gingival hyperplasia associated with long-term phenytoin use (Drew et al 1987).

Methotrexate toxicity

Methotrexate is a cytotoxic drug with folate antagonist properties. In part, its efficacy is dependent on this effect, but severe deficiency symptoms such as macrocytic anaemia are sometimes induced (Lambie & Johnson 1985). Co-administration of folic acid or folinic acid has been investigated as preventive treatment, with both forms capable of reducing drug side effects (Ortiz et al 1998, Strober & Menon 2005). A 2013 Cochrane review found a statistically significant and clinically important reduction in the incidence of GI adverse effects, hepatic dysfunction and methotrexate discontinuation in methotrexate patients with rheumatoid arthritis receiving folic or folinic acid (Shea et al 2013). A trend towards a reduction in stomatitis was observed; however, this did not reach statistical significance.

Sickle cell anaemia

In the past, folate supplements were recommended to patients with sickle cell anaemia, but more recent studies show that clinically significant folate deficiency occurs in a very small percentage of these patients and other nutrients may be indicated (Reed et al 1987).

Vitiligo

Although a number of uncontrolled studies testing combination treatments have been promising, folate has never been assessed as a sole treatment. As such, it is difficult to determine its role in the treatment of this condition. In previous studies, a combination of oral folic acid and vitamin B_{12}, together with increased sun exposure, has produced response rates in the vicinity of 50% (Juhlin & Olsson 1997). A controlled study by a different group of researchers found that exposure to a specific band width of UV radiation produced repigmentation in 92% of subjects, irrespective of vitamin supplementation (Tjioe et al 2002).

Erectile dysfunction

The combination of folic acid (5 mg daily) with tadalafil (10 mg every other day) was found to be more effective in improving sexual function than tadalafil alone (10 mg every other day) in an RCT of 83 patients with type 2 diabetes mellitus (Hamidi Madani et al 2013). Due to limitations in study design, including failure to obtain baseline serum folate levels or serum testosterone levels, more research into the clinical implication of this finding is recommended.

DOSAGE RANGE

Australian RDI (NHMRC 2006)

- 400 mcg/day for adults; up to 1 mg/day in deficiency states.
- Up to 600 mcg/day is recommended as the Suggested Dietary Target to reduce chronic disease risk in adults.
- 600 mcg/day in pregnancy.
- 500 mcg/day during lactation.

According to clinical studies

- Preconception care or early pregnancy supplementation: 400–600 mcg/day.
- Preconception and pregnancy supplementation in women with a previous NTD birth: 4 mg/day.
- Idiopathic recurring miscarriage: aspirin (100 mg/day) and folic acid (5 mg/alternate days) throughout gestation plus prednisone and progesterone treatment for first 12 weeks.
- Anticonvulsant-induced deficiency: 15 mg/day (under supervision).
- Prevention of cervical cancer: 800–10,000 mcg/day.
- Prevention of breast cancer in high alcohol consumers: 400 mcg/day.
- Alzheimer's dementia in the presence of elevated Hcy: 800 mcg/day.
- Alzheimer's dementia with normal Hcy: 1 mg/day in combination with cholinesterase inhibitors.
- Cognitive decline in elderly with folate deficiency: 750 mcg/day.
- Depression: minimum of 2 mg or sufficient dose to reduce elevated homocysteine as stand-alone treatment.
- Depression as an augmenting agent with standard antidepressants: 500 mcg/day.
- Acute psychiatric presentation: 15–30 mg methylfolate daily in combination with standard psychotropic treatment.
- Hyperhomocysteinaemia: 500–5000 mcg/day.
- Cardiovascular protection in patients with elevated Hcy: 5 mg/day with high-dose B complex.
- Cardiovascular protection in heart transplant recipients or patients with recent history of MI: 10–15 mg/day.
- Methotrexate toxicity: 5 mg/week.
- OCP-induced folate deficiency: 2 mg/day.
- Periodontal disease: rinse mouth with a solution of folate (5 mg/dose) twice daily.
- Prevention of restenosis after percutaneous coronary intervention: 1 mg in combination with vitamin B_{12} (400 mcg) and vitamin B_6 (10 mg) daily.
- Schizophrenia with marked negative symptoms: 2 mg/day in combination with 25 mg/day B_6 and 400 mcg/day B_{12}.
- Sickle cell anaemia: 1 mg/day.
- Ulcerative colitis: 15 mg/day.
- Vitiligo: 2–10 mg/day.

ADVERSE REACTIONS

Adverse reactions appear to be limited to oral doses greater than 5 mg/day. Reactions include a generalised urticaria associated with an allergic response, nausea, flatulence and bitter taste in the mouth, irritability and excitability.

One study found high-dose folic acid supplementation in children aged 6–30 months was associated with an increased risk of persistent diarrhoea (Taneja et al 2013).

SIGNIFICANT INTERACTIONS

Antacids

Reduce folic acid absorption — separate doses by 2–3 hours.

Anticonvulsants (phenytoin)

Reduced folate levels frequently develop with long-term use, but macrocytic anaemia is rare (Lambie & Johnson 1985). Supplementation can reduce toxicity, which is a beneficial interaction, although medical supervision is advised.

Cholestyramine (e.g. Questran)

Reduced folate absorption — observe patient for signs and symptoms of folate deficiency and separate doses by at least 4 hours.

Gastric acid inhibitors (proton-pump inhibitors)

Reduced folic acid absorption — separate doses by 2–3 hours.

Methotrexate

Methotrexate is a folate antagonist drug. Folate supplementation can reduce toxicity, which is a beneficial interaction; however, it may reduce the efficacy of methotrexate (Al-Dabagh et al 2013) — medical supervision advised.

Oral contraceptives

Folate levels are reduced with long-term use of the OCP, particularly those with high oestrogen content; therefore, increased intakes may be required for women undertaking long-term use.

Pancreatin

Reduced folate absorption (Kelly 1998) — separate doses by 2–3 hours.

Pyrimethamine (e.g. maloprim)

Impairs the use of folate and, as such, supplementation with folinic acid may be beneficial.

Sulfasalazine

Folic acid can reduce drug absorption — separate doses by 2–3 hours.

Trimethoprim

Trimethoprim is a folate antagonist drug. Supplementation can reduce toxicity, which is a beneficial interaction — medical supervision advised.

Zinc

At high doses (>15 mg/day), minor zinc depletion may develop (Carmel et al 2006, Kelly 1998) — observe patients for signs and symptoms of zinc deficiency.

Practice points/Patient counselling

- Folate is involved in a number of important biochemical pathways required for health and wellbeing, in particular development and cell growth.
- Folate supplements are often given to correct deficiencies or prevent deficiency in people at risk, such as those with malabsorption syndromes (e.g. coeliac disease and Crohn's disease), long-term use of certain medications such as phenytoin, sulfasalazine, cimetidine, antacids and the OCP, in congenital malabsorption states and blind loop syndrome, chronic alcoholism, HIV infection, the institutionalised elderly, pregnant and lactating women.
- It is considered to be the most important supplement to be taken by women in the weeks leading up to conception and during the first 12 weeks of pregnancy, in order to significantly reduce the risk of NTD in newborns. Food fortification is not considered sufficient.
- Both tablet and multivitamin softgel capsules have similar bioavailability profiles, with both peak level and total serum folate similar between each dosage form. Time to peak concentration appears slower in softgel capsules compared to tablets (Maki et al 2012).
- Other uses for folic acid supplements include reducing homocysteine levels (often in combination with vitamins B_{12} and B_6), reducing primary cardiovascular disease risk and cancer risk in general, periodontal disease (as a topical application), depression, schizophrenia and other psychiatric presentations and vitiligo.

CONTRAINDICATIONS AND PRECAUTIONS

Use of folate supplements may mask a B_{12} deficiency state by correcting an apparent macrocytic anaemia without altering progression of neurological damage. It is recommended that patients be screened for vitamin B_{12} deficiency.

PREGNANCY USE

According to the Australian Drug Evaluation Committee (1999), folate is considered to be safe to take during both pregnancy and lactation. Retrospective analysis of a trial of folate in pregnancy in the 1960s has suggested a possible increase in all-cause mortality and breast cancer in pregnant women taking 5 mg/day folate; however, this finding could be due to a number of factors unrelated to folate (Bland 2005, Charles et al 2004). The only context requiring special consideration is those pregnant women taking anticonvulsant medication (see Significant interactions).

PATIENTS' FAQs

What will this supplement do for me?

Folic acid is essential for health and wellbeing. Supplements have a critical role in preventing NTD in newborns and may also reduce the risk of primary cardiovascular disease and improve brain function in Alzheimer's dementia and non-Alzheimer's dementia and depression. It can also reduce the toxic effects of some medicines and may reduce the risk of developing some forms of cancer.

When will it start to work?

This depends on the indication.

Are there any safety issues?

The major concern with high doses of folate is that they may mask an underlying vitamin B_{12} deficiency and allow it to progress unnoticed, which means that a vitamin B_{12} deficiency should be excluded. It also interacts with some drugs in both a potentially harmful and a beneficial way. High doses should not be used in patients with a history of bowel polyps or adenomas.

REFERENCES

Abou-Saleh MT et al. The role of pterins and related factors in the biology of early postpartum depression. Eur Neuropsychopharmacol 9.4 (1999): 295–300.

Abrahamsen B et al. MTHFR c.677C > T polymorphism as an independent predictor of peak bone mass in Danish men–results from the Odense Androgen Study. Bone 38.2 (2006): 215–2119.

Aisen PS et al. High-dose B vitamin supplementation and cognitive decline in Alzheimer disease: a randomized controlled trial. JAMA 300.15 (2008): 1774–1783.

Albert CM et al. Effect of folic acid and B vitamins on risk of cardiovascular events and total mortality among women at high risk for cardiovascular disease: a randomized trial. JAMA 299.17 (2008): 2027–2036.

Al-Dabagh A et al. The effect of folate supplementation on methotrexate efficacy and toxicity in psoriasis patients and folic acid use by dermatologists in the USA. Am J Clin Dermatol 14.3 (2013): 155–161.

Alpert JE, Fava M. Nutrition and depression: the role of folate. Nutr Rev 55.5 (1997): 145–149.

Alpert M. et al. Prediction of treatment response in geriatric depression from baseline folate level: interaction with an SSRI or a tricyclic antidepressant. J Clin Psychopharmacol 23 (2003): 309–313.

Amigou A et al. Folic acid supplementation, MTHFR and MTRR polymorphisms, and the risk of childhood leukemia: the ESCALE study (SFCE). Cancer Causes Control 23.8 (2012): 1265–1277.

Anderson CA et al. Effects of folic acid supplementation on serum folate and plasma homocysteine concentrations in older adults: a dose-response trial. Am J Epidemiol 172.8 (2010): 932–941.

Antoniades C et al. Homocysteine lowering: any use in atherosclerosis? Hellenic J Cardiol 48.5 (2007): 249–251.

Applebaum J et al. Homocysteine levels in newly admitted schizophrenic patients. J Psychiatr Res 38.4 (2004): 413–4116.

Australian Drug Evaluation Committee. Prescribing medicines in pregnancy, 4th edn. Canberra: TGA Publications, 1999.

Bakker R et al. Folic acid supplements modify the adverse effects of maternal smoking on fetal growth and neonatal complications. J Nutr 141.12 (2011): 2171–2179.

Balk EM et al. Vitamin B6, B12, and folic acid supplementation and cognitive function: A systematic review of randomized trials. Arch Intern Med 167.1 (2007): 21–30.

Bazzano LA et al. Dietary intake of folate and risk of stroke in US men and women: NHANES1 epidemiological follow-up study. Stroke 33 (2002): 1183–1189.

Bean LJ et al. Lack of maternal folic acid supplementation is associated with heart defects in Down syndrome: a report from the National Down Syndrome Project. Birth Defects Res A Clin Mol Teratol 91.10 (2011): 885–893.

Beers MH, Berkow R (eds), The Merck manual of diagnosis and therapy, 17th edn. Whitehouse, NJ: Merck, 2003.

Behzadi AH, Behbahani AS, Ostovar N. Therapeutic effects of folic acid on ante partum and postpartum depression. Med Hypotheses 71.2 (2008): 313–14.

Berg MJ et al. Phenytoin pharmacokinetics: before and after folic acid administration. Epilepsia 33.4 (1992): 712–720.

Berry RJ. Maternal prenatal folic acid supplementation is associated with a reduction in development of autistic disorder. J Pediatr 163.1 (2013): 302–306.

Bielenberg J. Folic acid and vitamin deficiency caused by oral contraceptives. Med Monatsschr Pharm 14.8 (1991): 244–247.

Bjorke Monsen AL, Ueland PM. Homocysteine and methylmalonic acid in diagnosis and risk assessment from infancy to adolescence. Am J Clin Nutr 78.1 (2003): 7–21.

Bland JM. Taking folate in pregnancy and risk of maternal breast cancer. What's in a name? BMJ 330 (2005): 600.

Bleys J et al. Vitamin-mineral supplementation and the progression of atherosclerosis: a meta-analysis of randomized controlled trials. Am J Clin Nutr 84.4 (2006): 880–887.

Bollheimer LC et al. Folate and its preventative potential in colorectal carcinogenesis. How strong is the biological and epidemiological evidence? Crit Rev Oncol Hematol 55 (2005): 13–36.

Bønaa K et al. Homocysteine lowering and cardiovascular events after acute myocardial infarction. N Engl J Med 354 (2006): 1578–1588.

Botez MI. Folate deficiency and neurological disorders in adults. Med Hypotheses 2 (1976): 135–240.

Bottiglieri T. Homocysteine and folate metabolism in depression. Progr Neuro-psychopharmacol Biol Psychiatry 29 (2005): 1103–1112.

Boyles AL et al. Folate and one-carbon metabolism gene polymorphisms and their associations with oral facial clefts. Am J Med Genet A 146A.4 (2008): 440–449.

Brown RD et al. The impact of mandatory fortification of flour with folic acid on the blood folate levels of an Australian population. Med J Aust 194.2 (2011): 65–67.

Bukhari FJ et al. Effect of chronic kidney disease on the expression of thiamin and folic acid transporters. Nephrol Dial Transplant 26.7 (2011): 2137–2144.

Butali A et al. Folic acid supplementation use and the MTHFR C677T polymorphism in orofacial clefts etiology: An individual participant data pooled-analysis. Birth Defects Res A Clin Mol Teratol. 97.8 (2013): 509–514.

Butterworth CE Jr. et al. Improvement in cervical dysplasia associated with folic acid therapy in users of oral contraceptives. Am J Clin Nutr 35.1 (1982): 73–82.

Candito M et al. Plasma vitamin values and antiepileptic therapy: case reports of pregnancy outcomes affected by a neural tube defect. Birth Defects Res A Clin Mol Teratol 79.1 (2007): 62–64.

Carmel R et al. Folic acid. in: Shils M (ed), Modern nutrition in health and disease. Baltimore: Lippincott Williams & Wilkins, 2006, pp 470–481.

Carney MW et al. Red cell folate concentrations in psychiatric patients. J Affect Disord 19.3 (1990): 207–213.

Chan AC et al. Folate awareness and the prevalence of neural tube defects in South Australia, 1966–2007. Med J Aust 189.10 (2008): 566–569.

Charles D et al. Taking folate in pregnancy and risk of maternal breast cancer. BMJ 329 (2004): 1375–1376.

Chevrier C et al. Fetal and maternal MTHFR C677T genotype, maternal folate intake and the risk of nonsyndromic oral clefts. Am J Med Genet A 143.3 (2007): 248–257.

Childers JM et al. Chemoprevention of cervical cancer with folic acid: phase III Southwest Oncology Group Intergroup study. Cancer Epidemiol Biomarkers Prev 4.2 (1995): 155–159.

Chmurzynska A et al. Elderly women: Homocysteine reduction by short-term folic acid supplementation resulting in increased glucose concentrations and affecting lipid metabolism (C677T *MTHFR* polymorphism). Nutrition 29.6 (2013): 841–844.

Choi SW, Mason JB. Folate and carcinogenesis: an integrated scheme. J Nutr 130 (2000): 129–132.

Choi SW, Mason JB. Folate status: effects on pathways of colorectal carcinogensis. J Nutr 132 (2002): 2413–18S.

Clarke R et al. Hyperhomocysteinemia: an independent risk factor for vascular disease. N Engl J Med 324 (1991): 1149–1155.

Connelly PJ et al. A randomised double-blind placebo-controlled trial of folic acid supplementation of cholinesterase inhibitors in Alzheimer's disease. Int J Geriatr Psychiatry 23.2 (2008): 155–160.

Coppen A, Bailey J. Enhancement of the antidepressant action of fluoxetine by folic acid: A randomised, placebo controlled trial. J Affect Disord 60.2 (2000): 121–130.

Coppen A, Bolander-Gouaille C. Treatment of depression: time to consider folic acid and vitamin B12. J Psychopharmacol 19.1 (2005): 59–65.

Cravo ML et al. Folate deficiency enhances the development of colonic neoplasia in dimethylhydrazine-treated rats. Cancer Res 52.18 (1992): 5002–5006.

Crider KS et al. Prenatal folic acid and risk of asthma in children: a systematic review and meta-analysis. Am J Clin Nutr 98.5 (2013): 1272–1281.

Cuskelly GJ, McNulty H, Scott JM. Effect of increased dietary folate on red-cell folate: implications for the prevention of neural tube defects. Lancet 47.9002 (1996): 657–659.

Daly LE et al. Folate levels and neural tube defects. Implications for prevention. JAMA 274 (1995): 1698–1702.

Das U. Folic acid says NO to vascular diseases. Nutrition 19.7–8 (2003): 686–692.

Das UN. Folic acid and polyunsaturated fatty acids improve cognitive function and prevent depression, dementia, and Alzheimer's disease–but how and why? Prostaglandins Leukot Essent Fatty Acids 78.1 (2008): 11–119.

De-Regil LM et al. Effects and safety of periconceptional folate supplementation for preventing birth defects. Cochrane DB Syst Rev 10 (2010): CD007950.

den Heijer M et al. Hyperhomocysteinemia as a risk factor for deep-vein thrombosis. N Engl J Med 334 (1996): 759–762.

Drew HJ et al. Effect of folate on phenytoin hyperplasia. J Clin Periodontal 14.6 (1987): 350–356.

du Plessis L et al. What has happened with neural tube defects and women's understanding of folate in Victoria since 1998? Med J Aust 189.10 (2008): 570–574.

Durga J et al. Effect of 3-year folic acid supplementation on cognitive function in older adults in the FACIT trial: a randomised, double blind, controlled trial. Lancet 369.9557 (2007): 208–216.

Ebbing M et al. Mortality and cardiovascular events in patients treated with homocysteine-lowering B vitamins after coronary angiography: a randomized controlled trial. JAMA 300.7 (2008): 795–804.

Eskes T. Abnormal folate metabolism in mothers with Down syndrome offspring: review of the literature. Eur J Obstet Gynecol Reprod Biol 124 (2006): 130–133.

Figueiredo JC et al. Folic acid and prevention of colorectal adenomas: a combined analysis of randomized clinical trials. Int J Cancer 129.1 (2013): 192–203.

Ford AH et al. Vitamins B12, B6, and folic acid for onset of depressive symptoms in older men: results from a 2-year placebo-controlled randomized trial. J Clin Psychiatry 69.8 (2008): 1203–1209.

Fraguas R Jr. et al. Anger attacks in major depressive disorder and serum levels of homocysteine. Biol Psychiatry 60.3 (2006): 270–274.

Froscher W et al. Folate deficiency, anticonvulsant drugs, and psychiatric morbidity. Clin Neuropharmacol 18.2 (1995): 165–182.

FSANZ. Consideration of mandatory fortification with folic acid. Canberra: Food Standards Australia New Zealand, 2007.

Gabriel HE et al. Chronic cigarette smoking is associated with diminished folate status, altered folate form distribution, and increased genetic damage in the buccal mucosa of healthy adults. Am J Clin Nutr 83.4 (2006): 835–841.

Gargari BP et al. Effect of folic acid supplementation on biochemical indices in overweight and obese men with type 2 diabetes. Diabetes Res Clin Pract 94.1 (2011): 33–38.

Gariballa S, Forster S. Effects of dietary supplements on depressive symptoms in older patients: a randomised double-blind placebo-controlled trial. Clin Nutr26.5 (2007): 545–551.

Gatt A et al. Hyperhomocysteinemia in women with advanced breast cancer. Int J Lab Hematol 29.6 (2007): 421–425.

George L et al. Plasma folate levels and risk of spontaneous abortion. JAMA 288.15 (2002): 1867–1873.

Ghosh C et al. Dietary intakes of selected nutrients and food groups and risk of cervical cancer. Nutr Cancer 60.3 (2008): 331–341.

Gilbody S, Lewis S, Lightfoot T. Methylenetetrahydrofolate reductase (MTHFR) genetic polymorphisms and psychiatric disorders: a HuGE review. Am J Epidemiol 165.1 (2007): 1–13.

Goff DC et al. Folate, homocysteine, and negative symptoms in schizophrenia. Am J Psychiatry 161.9 (2004): 1705–1708.

Gok U et al. Comparative analysis of serum homocysteine, folic acid and vitamin B12 levels in patients with noise-induced hearing loss. Auris Nasus Larynx 31.1 (2004): 19–22.

Green TJ et al. Lowering homocysteine with B vitamins has no effect on biomarkers of bone turnover in older persons: a 2-y randomized controlled trial. Am J Clin Nutr 85.2 (2007): 460–464.

Gropper S, Smith J, Groff J. Advanced nutrition and human metabolism, 4th edn. Belmont, CA: Wadsworth Thomson Learning, 2009.

Håberg SE et al. Folic acid supplements in pregnancy and early childhood respiratory health. Arch Dis Child 94.3 (2009): 180–184.

Haggarty P et al. Effect of B vitamins and genetics on success of in-vitro fertilisation: prospective cohort study. Lancet 367 (2006): 1513–15119.

Haidemenos A et al. Plasma homocysteine, folate and B12 in chronic schizophrenia. Prog Neuropsychopharmacol Biol Psychiatry 31.6 (2007): 1289–1296.

Hamid A, Kaur J. Long-term alcohol ingestion alters the folate-binding kinetics in intestinal brush border membrane in experimental alcoholism. Alcohol 41.6 (2007): 441–446.

Hamidi Madani A et al. Assessment of the efficacy of combination therapy with folic acid and tadalafil for the management of erectile dysfunction in men with type 2 diabetes mellitus. J Sex Med 10.4 (2013): 1146–1150.

Hasanah CI et al. Reduced red-cell folate in mania. J Affect Disord 46.2 (1997): 95–99.

Henao O et al. Women with polymorphisms of methylenetetrahydrofolate reductase (MTHFR) and methionine synthase (MS) are less likely to have cervical intraepithelial neoplasia (CIN) 2 or 3. Int J Cancer 113.6 (2005): 991–997.

Hendler SS, Rorvik D (eds), PDR for nutritional supplements. Montvale, NJ: Medical Economics, 2001.

Hickling S et al. Impact of voluntary folate fortification on plasma homocysteine and serum folate in Australia from 1995 to 2001: a population based cohort study. J Epidemiol Community Health 59 (2005): 371–376.

Hollingsworth JW et al. In utero supplementation with methyl donors enhances allergic airway disease in mice. J Clin Invest 118.10 (2008): 3462–3469.

Hollis ND et al. Preconception folic acid supplementation and risk for chromosome 21 nondisjunction: a report from the National Down Syndrome Project. Am J Med Genet A 161A.3 (2013): 438–444.

Homocysteine Study Collaboration. Homocysteine and risk of ischemic heart disease and stroke: a meta-analysis. JAMA 288.16 (2002): 2015–2022.

Hutson JR et al. Folic acid transport to the human fetus is decreased in pregnancies with chronic alcohol exposure. PLoS One 7.5 (2012): e38057.

Jang H, Mason JB, Choi SW. Genetic and epigenetic interactions between folate and aging in carcinogenesis. J Nutr 135 (12 Suppl) (2005): 2967S–2971S.

Jardine MJ et al. The effect of folic acid based homocysteine lowering on cardiovascular events in people with kidney disease: systematic review and meta-analysis. BMJ 344 (2012): e3533.

Jendricko T et al. Homocysteine and serum lipids concentration in male war veterans with posttraumatic stress disorder. Prog Neuropsychopharmacol Biol Psychiatry (2008 Nov 14): [Epub ahead of print].

Juhlin L, Olsson MJ. Improvement of vitiligo after oral treatment with vitamin B12 and folic acid and the importance of sun exposure. Acta Derm Venereol 77.6 (1997): 460–462.

Karadag AS et al. Effect of isotretinoin treatment on plasma holotranscobalamin, vitamin B12, folic acid, and homocysteine levels: non-controlled study. Int J Dermatol 50.12 (2011): 1564–1569.

Kelly C et al. The MTHFR C677T polymorphism is associated with depressive episodes in patients from Northern Ireland. J Psychopharmacol 18.4 (2004): 567–571.

Kelly GS. Folate supplemental forms and therapeutic applications. Altern Med Rev 3 (1998): 208–220.

Kemperman R et al. Low essential fatty acids and B-vitamin status in a subgroup of patients with schizophrenia and its response to dietary supplementation. Prostaglandins Leukot Essent Fatty Acids 74 (2006): 75–85.

Kennedy DA et al. Folate intake and the risk of colorectal cancer: A systematic review and meta-analysis. Cancer Epidemiol 35.1 (2011): 2–10.

Keser I et al. Folic acid and vitamin B_{12} supplementation lowers plasma homocysteine but has no effect on serum bone turnover markers in elderly women: a randomized, double-blind, placebo-controlled trial. Nutr Res 33.3 (2013): 211–219.

Kim JM et al. Changes in folate, vitamin B12 and homocysteine associated with incident dementia. J Neurol Neurosurg Psychiatry 79.8 (2008): 864–868.

Kim YI et al. Dietary folate protects against the development of macroscopic colonic neoplasia in a dose responsive manner in rats. Gut 39.5 (1996): 732–740.

Kumar P, Clarke M. Clinical medicine, 5th edn. London: WB Saunders, 2002.

Kwanbunjan K et al. Low folate status as a risk factor for cervical dysplasia in Thai women. Nutr Res 25 (2005): 641–654.

Lambie DG, Johnson RH. Drugs and folate metabolism. Drugs 30.2 (1985): 145–155.

Lange H et al. Folate therapy and in-stent restenosis after coronary stenting. N Engl J Med 350 (2004): 2673–2681.

Larsson SC, Giovannucci E, Wolk A. Folate and risk of breast cancer: a meta-analysis. J Natl Cancer Inst 99.1 (2007): 64–76.

Lassi ZS et al. Folic acid supplementation during pregnancy for maternal health and pregnancy outcomes. Cochrane DB Syst Rev (2013) Issue 3 Art:CD006896.

Lerner V et al. Vitamin B12 and folate serum levels in newly admitted psychiatric patients. Clin Nutr 25 (2006): 60–67.

Leung J et al. Folic Acid Supplementation and Cardiac and Stroke Mortality among Hemodialysis Patients. J Ren Nutr 20.5 (2010): 293–302.

Levine J et al. Homocysteine-reducing strategies improve symptoms in chronic schizophrenic patients with hyperhomocysteinemia. Biol Psychiatry 60.3 (2006): 265–269.

Lewis SJ et al. Folic acid supplementation during pregnancy may protect against depression 21 months after pregnancy, an effect modified by MTHFR C677T genotype. Eur J Clin Nutr 66.1 (2012): 97–103.
Li X et al. The association between periconceptional folic acid supplementation and congenital heart defects: A case–control study in China. Prev Med 56.6 (2013): 385–389.
Li Z et al. Folic acid supplementation during early pregnancy and the risk of gestational hypertension and preeclampsia. Hypertension 61.4 (2013): 873–879.
Logan RFA et al. Aspirin and folic acid for the prevention of recurrent colorectal adenomas. Gastroenterol 134.1 (2008): 29–38.
Lucock M. Is folic acid the ultimate functional food component for disease prevention? BMJ 328.7433 (2004): 211–214.
Lucock MD. Synergy of genes and nutrients: the case of homocysteine. Curr Opin Clin Nutr Metab Care 9.6 (2006): 748–756.
Lussanaa F et al. Blood levels of homocysteine, folate, vitamin B6 and B12 in women using oral contraceptives compared to non-users. Thromb Res 112.1–2 (2003): 37–41.
Ma J et al. Methylenetertahydrofolate reductase polymorphism, plasma folate, homocysteine, and risk of myocardial infarction in US physicians. Circulation 94.10 (1996): 2410–24116.
Mahoney MC. et al. Breast cancer risk reduction and counseling: lifestyle, chemoprevention, and surgery. J Natl Compr Canc Netw 5.8 (2007): 702–710.
Maki KC et al. Absorption of Folic Acid from a Softgel Capsule Compared to a Standard Tablet. J Acad Nutr Diet 112.7 (2012):1062–1067.
Malinow MR et al. Prevalence of hyperhomocyst(e)inemia in patients with peripheral arterial occlusive disease. Circulation 79 (1989): 1180–1188.
Malouf R, Grimley Evans J. Folic acid with or without vitamin B12 for the prevention and treatment of healthy elderly and demented people. Cochrane Database Syst Rev 8.4 (2008): CD004514.
Manniën J et al. Factors associated with not using folic acid supplements preconceptionally. Public Health Nutr (2013) [Epub ahead of print].
Mao G et al. Efficacy of folic acid and enalapril combined therapy on reduction of blood pressure and plasma glucose: A multicenter, randomized, double-blind, parallel-controlled, clinical trial. Nutrition 24.11–12 (2008): 1088–1096.
Marchal C et al. Association between polymorphisms of folate-metabolizing enzymes and risk of prostate cancer. Eur J Surg Oncol 34.7 (2008): 805–810.
Marcucci R et al. Vitamin supplementation reduces the progression of atherosclerosis in hyperhomocysteinemic renal-transplant recipients. Transplantation 75.9 (2003): 1551–1555.
McCaddon A et al. Absence of macrocytic anaemia in Alzheimer's disease. Clin Lab Haematol 26.4 (2004): 259–263.
McGuire BW et al. Absorption kinetics of orally administered leucovorin calcium. NCI Monogr 5 (1987): 47–56.
McLean RR et al. Plasma B vitamins, homocysteine, and their relation with bone loss and hip fracture in elderly men and women. J Clin Endocrinol Metab 93.6 (2008): 2206–2212.
McMahon JA et al. Lowering homocysteine with B vitamins has no effect on blood pressure in older adults. J Nutr 137.5 (2007): 1183–1187.
McNulty B et al. Impact of continuing folic acid after the first trimester of pregnancy: findings of a randomized trial of Folic Acid Supplementation in the Second and Third Trimesters. Am J Clin Nutr 98.1 (2013): 92–98.
McNulty B et al. Women's compliance with current folic acid recommendations and achievement of optimal vitamin status for preventing neural tube defects. Hum Reprod 26.6 (2011): 1530–1536.
Metz J et al. Changes in serum folate concentrations following voluntary food fortification in Australia. Med J Aust 176.2 (2002): 90–91.
Milne E et al. Maternal use of folic acid and other supplements and risk of childhood brain tumors. Cancer Epidemiol Biomarkers Prev 21.11 (2012): 1933–1941.
Miyake Y et al. Dietary folate and vitamins B12, B6, and B2 intake and the risk of postpartum depression in Japan: the Osaka Maternal and Child Health Study. J Affect Disord 96.1–2 (2006): 133–138.
Moens AL et al. Effect of folic acid on endothelial function following acute myocardial infarction. Am J Cardiol 99.4 (2007): 476–481.
Muntjewerff J-W, Blom H. Aberrant folate status in schizophrenic patients: what is the evidence? Prog Neuro-psychopharmacol Biol Psychiatry 29.7 (2005): 1133–1139.
Murphy G et al. Folate and MTHFR: risk of adenoma recurrence in the Polyp Prevention Trial. Cancer Causes Control 19.7 (2008): 751–758.
NHMRC (National Health and Medical Research Council). Nutrient reference values for Australia and New Zealand. Canberra: Department of Health and Ageing, 2006.
Nilsson K, Gustafson L, Hultberg B. Improvement of cognitive functions after cobalamin/folate supplementation in elderly patients with dementia and elevated plasma homocysteine. Int J Geriatr Psychiatry 16.6 (2001): 609–614.
Nowak M et al. Homocysteine, vitamin B12, and folic acid in age-related macular degeneration. Eur J Ophthalmol 15.6 (2005): 764–767.
Ntaios G et al. The effect of folic acid supplementation on carotid intima-media thickness in patients with cardiovascular risk: A randomized, placebo-controlled trial. Int J Cardiol 143.1 (2010): 16–19.
Obermann-Borst SA et al. General maternal medication use, folic acid, the *MDR1*C3435T polymorphism, and the risk of a child with a congenital heart defect. Am J Obstet Gynecol 204.3 (2011): 236. e1–236.e8.
Okada A et al. Slowly progressive folate-deficiency myelopathy: Report of a case. J Neurol Sci 336.1–2 (2014): 273–275.
Okumura K & Tsukamoto H. Folate in smokers. Clin Chim Acta 412.7–8 (2011): 521–526.
Ortiz Z et al. The efficacy of folic acid and folinic acid in reducing methotrexate gastrointestinal toxicity in rheumatoid arthritis. A meta-analysis of randomized controlled trials. J Rheumatol 25.1 (1998): 36–43.
Ownby DR. et al. Has mandatory folic acid supplementation of foods increased the risk of asthma and allergic disease? J All Clin Immunol 123.6 (2009): 1260–1261.
Pack ARC. Folate mouthwash: effects on established gingivitis in odontal patients. J Clin Periodontol 11.9 (1984): 619–628.
Papakostas G et al. Serum folate, vitamin B12, and homocysteine in major depressive disorder. Part 1: predictors of clinical response in fluoxetine-resistant depression. J Clin Psychiatry 65.8 (2004a): 1090–5.
Papakostas G et al. Serum folate, vitamin B12, and homocysteine in major depressive disorder. Part 2: predictors of relapse during the continuation phase of pharmacotherapy. J Clin Psychiatry 65.8 (2004b): 1096–8.
Papakostas G et al. The relationship between serum folate, vitamin B12, and homocysteine levels in major depressive disorder and the timing of improvement with fluoxetine. Int J Neuro-psychopharmacol 8.4 (2005): 523–528.
Pelton R et al. Drug-induced nutrient depletion handbook 1999–2000. Hudson, OH: Lexi-Comp, 2000.
Pietrzik K et al. Calculation of red blood cell folate steady state conditions and elimination kinetics after daily supplementation with various folate forms and doses in women of childbearing age. Am J Clin Nutr 86.5 (2007): 1414–14119.
Piyathilake C et al. Folate is associated with the natural history of high-risk human papillomaviruses. Cancer Res 64 (2004): 8788–8793.
Piyathilake CJ et al. Protective association of MTHFR polymorphism on cervical intraepithelial neoplasia is modified by riboflavin status. Nutrition 23.3 (2007): 229–235.
Potena L et al. Long-term effect of folic acid therapy in heart transplant recipients: follow-up analysis of a randomized study. Transplantation 85.8 (2008): 1146–1150.
Potter K et al. The effect of long-term homocysteine-lowering on carotid intima-media thickness and flow-mediated vasodilation in stroke patients: a randomized controlled trial and meta-analysis. BMC Cardiovasc Disord 8 (2008): 24.
Powers HJ. Interaction among folate, riboflavin, genotype, and cancer, with reference to colorectal and cervical cancer. J Nutr 135 (2005): 2960–6S.
Priest DG et al. Pharmacokinetics of leucovorin metabolites in human plasma as a function of dose administered orally and intravenously. J Natl Cancer Inst 83.24 (1991): 1806–1812.
Qin X et al. Effect of folic acid supplementation on the progression of carotid intima-media thickness: A meta-analysis of randomized controlled trials. Atherosclerosis 222.2 (2012): 307–313.
Qin X et al. Homocysteine-lowering therapy with folic acid is effective in cardiovascular disease prevention in patients with kidney disease: A meta-analysis of randomized controlled trials. Clin Nutr 32.5 (2013a): 722–727.
Qin X et al. Folic acid supplementation and cancer risk: a meta-analysis of randomized controlled trials. Int J Cancer 133.5 (2013b): 1033–1041.
Qin X et al. Folic acid supplementation with and without vitamin B6 and revascularization risk: A meta-analysis of randomized controlled trials. Clin Nutr (2014) http://dx.doi.org/10.1016/j.clnu.2014.01.006.
Rabovskaja V et al. The Cost-Effectiveness of Mandatory Folic Acid Fortification in Australia. J Nutr 143.1 (2013): 59–66.
Rasmussen SA et al. Maternal obesity and risk of neural tube defects: a metaanalysis. Am J Obstet Gynecol 198.6 (2008): 611–619.
Reed JD et al. Nutrition and sickle cell disease. Am J Hematol 24.4 (1987): 441–455.
Regland B. Schizophrenia and single-carbon metabolism. Prog Neuro-psychopharmacol Biol Psychiatry 29 (2005): 1124–1132.
Rejnmark L et al. Dietary intake of folate, but not vitamin B2 or B12, is associated with increased bone mineral density 5 years after the menopause: results from a 10-year follow-up study in early postmenopausal women. Calcif Tissue Int 82.1 (2008): 1–111.
Revell P et al. Folic acid absorption in patients infected with human immunodeficiency virus. J Intern Med 230 (1991): 227–231.

Reynolds EH. Folic acid, ageing, depression and dementia. BMJ 324 (2002): 1512–15115.

Rivey MP, Schottelius DD, Berg MJ. Phenytoin-folic acid: a review. Drug Intell Clin Pharm 18.4 (1984): 292–301.

Roberts SH et al. Folate augmentation of treatment — evaluation for depression (FolATED): protocol of a randomised controlled trial. BMC Psychiatry 7 (2007): 65.

Rozendaal AM et al. Periconceptional folic acid associated with an increased risk of oral clefts relative to non-folate related malformations in the Northern Netherlands: a population based case-control study. Eur J Epidemiol 28.11 (2013): 875–887.

Rueda J-R & Ballesteros J. Folic acid for fragile X syndrome. Coch DB Syst Rev 5 (2011): CD008476.

Rycyna KJ et al. Opposing Roles of Folate in Prostate Cancer. Urology 82.6 (2013): 1197–1203.

Sauer J, Mason JB, Choi SW. Too much folate: a risk factor for cancer and cardiovascular disease? Curr Opin Clin Nutr Metab Care12 (2009): 30–6.

Schmidt RJ et al. Maternal periconceptional folic acid intake and risk of autism spectrum disorders and developmental delay in the CHARGE (CHildhood Autism Risks from Genetics and Environment) case-control study. Am J Clin Nutr 96.1 (2012): 80–89.

Schnyder G et al. Effect of homocysteine-lowering therapy with folic acid, vitamin B12, and vitamin B6 on clinical outcome after percutaneous coronary intervention: the Swiss Heart study: a randomized controlled trial. JAMA 288.8 (2002): 973–979.

Sedjo R et al. Folate, vitamin B12, and homocysteine status. findings of no relation between human papillomavirus persistence and cervical dysplasia. Nutrition 19.6 (2003): 497–502.

Selhub J et al. Association between plasma homocysteine concentrations and extracranial carotid-artery stenosis. N Engl J Med 332 (1995): 286–291.

Sengpiel V et al. Folic acid supplementation, dietary folate intake during pregnancy and risk for spontaneous preterm delivery: a prospective observational cohort study. BMC Pregnancy Childbirth 13.160 (2013). doi 10.1186/1471-2393-13-160.

Sharp L, Little J. Polymorphisms in genes involved in folate metabolism and colorectal neoplasia: a HuGE review. Am J Clin Epidemiol 159.5 (2004): 423–443.

Shea B et al. Folic acid and folinic acid for reducing side effects in patients receiving methotrexate for rheumatoid arthritis. Cochrane DB Syst Rev (2013) Issue 5 Art CD000951.

Shekari M et al. Impact of methylenetetrahydrofolate reductase (MTHFR) codon (677) and methionine synthase (MS) codon (2756) on risk of cervical carcinogenesis in North Indian population. Arch Gynecol Obstet 278.6 (2008): 517–524.

Sirachainan N et al. Folate pathway genetic polymorphisms and susceptibility of central nervous system tumors in Thai children. Cancer Detect Prev 32.1 (2008): 72–78.

Siragusa S et al. The risk of recurrent cardiovascular events in patients with increased plasma homocysteine levels is reduced by short but not long-term therapy with folate and B vitamins. Thromb Res 121.1 (2007): 51–53.

Smith AD, Kim YI, Refsum H. Is folic acid good for everyone? Am J Clin Nutr 87.3 (2008): 517–533.

Song Y et al. Effect of combined folic acid, vitamin B(6), and vitamin B(12) on colorectal adenoma. J Natl Cancer Inst 104.20 (2012): 1562–1575.

Sram R et al. The impact of plasma folate levels of mothers and newborns on intrauterine growth retardation and birth weight. Mutat Res 591 (2005): 302–310.

Stølen LH et al. High Dietary Folic Acid and High Plasma Folate in Children and Adults with Phenylketonuria. JIMD Rep (2013) [epub ahead of print] doi: 10.1007/8904_2013_260.

Stothard KJ et al. Maternal overweight and obesity and the risk of congenital anomalies. A systematic review and meta-analysis. JAMA 301.6 (2009): 636–650.

Strober B, Menon K. Folate supplementation during methotrexate therapy for patients with psoriasis. J Am Acad Dermatol 53 (2005): 652–659.

Sudchada P et al. Effect of folic acid supplementation on plasma total homocysteine levels and glycemic control in patients with type 2 diabetes: A systematic review and meta-analysis. Diabetes Res Clin Pr 98.1 (2012): 151–158.

Sun Y et al. Efficacy of multivitamin supplementation containing vitamins B6 and B12 and folic acid as adjunctive treatment with a cholinesterase inhibitor in Alzheimer's disease: a 26-week, randomized, double-blind, placebo-controlled study in Taiwanese patients. Clin Ther 29.10 (2007): 2204–2214.

Surén P et al. Association between maternal use of folic acid supplements and risk of autism in children. JAMA 309.6 (2013): 570–577.

Sütterlin M et al. Serum folate and vitamin B12 levels in women using modern oral contraceptives (OC) containing 20 μg ethinyl estradiol. Eur J Obstet Gynecol Reprod Biol 107.1 (2003): 57–61.

Suzuki T et al. Alcohol drinking and one-carbon metabolism-related gene polymorphisms on pancreatic cancer risk. Cancer Epidemiol Biomarkers Prev 17.10 (2008): 2742–2747.

Suzuki T et al. Impact of one-carbon metabolism-related gene polymorphisms on risk of lung cancer in Japan: a case control study. Carcinogenesis 28.8 (2007): 1718–1725.

Sweeney MR, McPartlin J, Scott J. Folic acid fortification and public health: report on threshold doses above which unmetabolised folic acid appear in serum. BMC Public Health 22.7 (2007): 41.

Taneja S et al. Folic acid and vitamin B-12 supplementation and common infections in 6–30-mo-old children in India: a randomized placebo-controlled trial. Am J Clin Nutr 98.3 (2013): 731–737.

Taylor MJ et al. Folate for depressive disorders. Cochrane Database Syst Rev 2 (2003).

Tempfer CB et al. A combination treatment of prednisone, aspirin, folate, and progesterone in women with idiopathic recurrent miscarriage: a matched-pair study. Fertil Steril 86.1 (2006): 145–148.

Thomson ME, Pack ARC. Effects of extended systemic and topical folate supplementation on gingivitis of pregnancy. J Clin Periodontol 9.3 (1982): 275–280.

Tiemeier H et al. Vitamin B12, folate, and homocysteine in depression: the Rotterdam Study. Am J Psychiatry 159.12 (2002): 2099–2101.

Timmermans S et al. Determinants of folic acid use in early pregnancy in a multi-ethnic urban population in The Netherlands: The Generation R study. Prev Med 47.4 (2008): 427–432.

Timmermans S et al. Folic acid is positively associated with uteroplacental vascular resistance: The Generation R Study. Nutr Metab Cardiovas 21.1 (2011): 54–61.

Tinker SC et al. Does obesity modify the association of supplemental folic acid with folate status among nonpregnant women of childbearing age in the United States? Birth Defects Res Part A Clin Mol Teratol 94.10 (2012): 749–755.

Tjioe M et al. Treatment of vitiligo with narrow band UVB (311 nm) for one year and the effect of addition of folic acid and vitamin B12. Acta Derm Venereol 82.5 (2002): 369–372.

Tolmunen T et al. Dietary folate and the risk of depression in Finnish middle-aged men: a prospective follow-up study. Psychother Psychosom 73.6 (2004): 334–339.

Troen AM et al. Unmetabolized folic acid in plasma is associated with reduced natural killer cell cytotoxicity among postmenopausal women. J Nutr 136.1 (2006): 189–194.

Van Guelpen B et al. Low folate levels may protect against colorectal cancer. Gut 55.10 (2006): 1461–1466.

Verhaar MC, Stroes E, Rabelink TJ. Folates and cardiovascular disease. Arterioscler Thromb Vasc Biol 22 (2002): 6.

Vianna AC et al. Uremic hyperhomocysteinemia: a randomized trial of folate treatment for the prevention of cardiovascular events. Hemodial Int 11.2 (2007): 210–216.

Vogel RI et al. The effect of folic acid on gingival health. J Periodontol 47.11 (1976): 667–668.

Vollset SE et al. Effects of folic acid supplementation on overall and site-specific cancer incidence during the randomised trials: meta-analyses of data on 50,000 individuals. Lancet 381.9871 (2013): 1029–1036.

Voutilainen S et al. Low dietary folate intake is associated with an excess incidence of acute coronary events. Circulation 103 (2001): 2674–2680.

Wahlqvist ML (ed), Food and nutrition, 2nd edn. Sydney: Allen & Unwin, 2002.

Wald DS, Law M, Morris JK. Homocysteine and cardiovascular disease: evidence on causality from a meta-analysis. BMJ 325.7374 (2002): 1202.

Wang X et al. Efficacy of folic acid supplementation in stroke prevention: a meta-analysis. Lancet 369.9576 (2007): 1876–1882.

Watson L, Brown S, Davey M. Use of periconceptional folic acid supplements in Victoria and New South Wales. Australia. Aust NZ J Public Health 30.1 (2006): 42–49.

Wilson JD et al. Harrison's principles of internal medicine, 12th edn. New York: McGraw-Hill, 1991.

Wright AJ, Dainty JR, Finglas PM. Folic acid metabolism in human subjects revisited: potential implications for proposed mandatory folic acid fortification in the UK. Br J Nutr 98.4 (2007): 667–675.

Yang H-T et al. Efficacy of folic acid supplementation in cardiovascular disease prevention: An updated meta-analysis of randomized controlled trials. Eur J Int Med 23.8 (2012): 745–754.

Young SN, Ghadirian AM. Folic acid and psychopathology. Prog Neuro-psychopharmacol Biol Psychiatry 13.6 (1989): 841–863.

Youngblood ME et al. 2012 Update on global prevention of folic acid–preventable spina bifida and anencephaly. Birth Defects Res A Clin Mol Teratol 97.10 (2013): 658–663.

Zetterberg H. Methylenetetrahydrofolate reductase and transcobalamin genetic polymorphisms in human spontaneous abortion: biological and clinical implications. Reprod Biol Endocrinol 2.7 (2004): 1–8.

Garlic

HISTORICAL NOTE Garlic has been used as both a food and a medicine since antiquity. Legend has it that garlic was used in ancient Egypt to increase workers' resistance to infection and later used externally to prevent wound infection. Other ancient civilisations have also used it medicinally. Sanskrit records document the use of garlic approximately 5000 years ago and the Chinese have been using it for over 3000 years. One of the uses of garlic was as a treatment for tumours, a use that extends back to the Egyptian Codex Ebers of 1550 BC (Hassan 2004). Louis Pasteur was one of the first scientists to confirm that garlic had antimicrobial properties. Garlic was used to prevent gangrene and treat infection in both world wars. Traditionally, garlic has been used as a warming and blood-cleansing herb to prevent and treat colds, flu, coughs and menstrual pain and to expel worms and other parasites.

COMMON NAME

Garlic

OTHER NAMES

Ail, ajo, allium, camphor of the poor, da-suan, knoblauch, la-juan, poor man's treacle, rustic treacle, stinking rose

BOTANICAL NAME/FAMILY

Allium sativum (family Liliaceae)

PLANT PART USED

Bulb, and oil from the bulb

CHEMICAL COMPONENTS

Garlic bulbs contain organosulfur compounds (OSCs), protein (mainly alliinase), amino acids (such as arginine, lysine, threonine and tryptophan), fibre, lipids, phytic acid, saponins, beta-sitosterol and small quantities of vitamins and minerals, such as vitamin C, vitamin E, beta-carotene, chromium, iron and selenium (Duke 2003). Of the numerous constituents present, it is the alliin component and resultant degradation products, such as allicin and ajoene, that produce much of the herb's pharmacological activity. These are formed when garlic is crushed or chewed and alliin is exposed to the enzyme alliinase. According to Commission E, 1 mg of alliin produces 0.458 mg of allicin (Blumenthal 2000). Allicin is unstable and degrades to various sulfides depending on the conditions. Steam distillation converts water-soluble thiosulfanates to lipid-soluble diallyl sulfides (DAS), whereas oil maceration results in the production of ajoenes and vinyldithines (Stargrove et al 2008).

The pharmacological actions of the herb are due to its organosulfur components: alliin, allyl cysteine, allyl disulfide and allicin (Chung 2006). In garlic oil, there are three major OSCs: diallyl trisulfide (DATS), DAS and diallyl disulfide (DADS) (Liu et al 2006). In aged garlic the sulfur compounds are metabolites of γ-glutamylcysteine; including water-soluble S-allylcysteine (SAC) and its metabolites S-allylmercaptocysteine (SAMC) and S-methylcysteine (Tsai et al 2012).

MAIN ACTIONS

Antioxidant

Garlic and many of its constituents have strong antioxidant activity and is capable of directly scavenging free radicals, and indirectly enhancing endogenous antioxidant systems such as glutathione, superoxide dismutase (SOD), catalase and glutathione peroxidase (Arhan et al 2009). This has been demonstrated in vitro and in vivo (Arhan et al 2009, Hassan et al 2010).

When tested individually, the four main chemical classes of garlic, allyl disulfide, alliin, allicin and allyl cysteine, have been shown to exhibit different patterns of antioxidant activity. Alliin scavenges superoxide via the oxanthine oxidase system; alliin, allyl cysteine and allyl disulfide act as hydroxyl scavengers; and allyl disulfide prevents lipid peroxidation (Chung 2006). SAC has also been shown to scavenge reactive oxygen and nitrogen species, including superoxide anion, hydrogen peroxide, hydroxyl radical and peroxynitrite anion (Medina-Campos et al 2007).

According to in vitro tests, garlic prevents cadmium- and arsenic-induced oxidative damage by inducing endogenous antioxidant defence mechanisms (Chowdhury et al 2008, Ola-Mudathir et al 2008, Suru 2008). A later study demonstrated the protective effects of DADS from garlic on human osteoblasts exposed to cigarette smoke (Ehnert et al 2012).

In vivo studies suggest protection from radiofrequency electromagnetic radiation associated with mobile phone use via the reduction of protein oxidation (Avci et al 2012), and cardioprotection with aged garlic on doxorubicin-induced cardiotoxicity (Alkreathy et al 2010, 2012). Large doses of garlic (500 mg/kg) improved sperm viability and partially preserved seminiferous tubule histological organisation after 28 days when compared to controls, most likely due to an antioxidant mechanism (Asadpour et al 2013).

Antioxidant activity and lower levels of oxidative stress have further been demonstrated in several clinical studies for garlic supplementation. One study used a dose of garlic 0.1 g/kg/day for 1 month; this was shown to induce a significant reduction in erythrocyte malondialdehyde (an indicator of oxidative stress) and significantly increase levels of SOD and glutathione peroxidase (Avci et al 2008). Similarly, oral garlic (250 mg/day) taken for 2 months caused a significant reduction in markers of lipid peroxidation in people with essential hypertension compared to normotensive controls (Dhawan & Jain 2005).

Protection against ischaemic and reperfusion injury

Prophylactic administration of garlic protects against renal and hepatic ischaemia/reperfusion injury in vitro and in a rat model (Kabasakal et al 2005, Sener et al 2005) prevents ischaemic and perfusion injuries after testicular torsion and detorsion in rats (Unsal et al 2006). More recently, pre-feeding mice with garlic attenuated oxidative damage in isoproterenol-induced myocardial infarction (MI) via the nitric oxide (NO) signalling pathway (Khatua et al 2012).

Anti-inflammatory activity

Fresh garlic extracts and garlic oil exert anti-inflammatory action in various models. Mechanisms of action identified include a direct action upon Toll-like receptor-mediated signalling pathway, inhibiting NF-kappa activation (Youn et al 2008), modification of the expression of cyclooxygenase (COX) activity (Thomson et al 2000) and suppression of inducible nitric oxide synthase (iNOS) and NO production (Liu et al 2006). The sulfur compounds Z- and E-aejones and their sulfonyl analogues have been shown to suppress lipopolysaccharide-promoted NO and prostaglandin E_2-mediated NF-κB-induced expression of iNOS/COX-2 genes (D Lee et al 2012). Lee et al investigated the anti-inflammatory action of DAS in articular chondrocytes and synovial fibroblasts harvested from patients undergoing joint replacement for osteoarthritis. Incubation with DAS inhibited the upregulation of COX-2 expression in synovial cells and chondrocytes and ameliorated crystal-induced synovitis through the inhibition of NF-κB (Lee et al 2009). Mice infected with malaria (*Plasmodium yoelli* 17XL) then treated with allicin 3 mg or 9 mg/kg had increased inflammatory mediators tumour necrosis factor, interferon-gamma, interleukin-12 (IL-12), p70, and NO; and immune cells, $CD4^+$ T cells, dendritic cells and macrophages were significantly higher in the treatment group, resulting in longer survival in a dose-dependent manner (Feng et al 2012).

Inhibits platelet aggregation and antithrombotic effects

In vitro studies indicate that garlic inhibits platelet aggregation through multiple mechanisms, including inhibition of COX activity and thromboxane A_2 formation, via the suppression of intraplatelet Ca^{2+} mobilisation and by increasing cAMP and cGMP levels. The antioxidant action of garlic also increased platelet-derived NO, and interaction with glycoprotein IIb/IIIa receptors reduces platelets' ability to bind to fibrinogen (Allison et al 2006, Chan et al 2007, Rahman 2007).

Importantly, the method of garlic preparation can influence its antiplatelet activity in humans (Lawson et al 1992, Rahman & Billington 2000), yet microwaving, oven heating at 200°C or submersion in boiling water for 3 min has shown no reduction in inhibition of platelet aggregation as compared to raw garlic (Cavagnaro et al 2007).

The clinical significance of the in vitro findings is hard to determine, as a double-blind, placebo-controlled crossover study of 14 volunteers concluded that solvent-extracted garlic oil had minimal or no effect on platelet aggregation. Researchers found that administration of garlic 9.9 g over 4 h exerted little or no effect on both collagen and adenosine 5'-diphosphate (ADP)-induced aggregation. Adrenaline-induced aggregation did, however, exert a slight but significant ($P < 0.05$; 12) reduction (Wojcikowski et al 2007).

Stimulates fibrinolysis

A significant increase in fibrinolysis has been observed in several clinical tests for both raw and fried garlic, which appears to be dose-dependent (Bordia et al 1998, Chutani & Bordia 1981, Gadkari & Joshi 1991). A recent controlled animal study found a statistically significant decrease in plasma fibrinogen and increase in clotting time in treatment groups receiving doses of raw garlic 750 and 1000 mg/kg, respectively, in comparison to that of 500 mg/kg (Gorinstein et al 2006). Odourless garlic has been shown to stimulate fibrinolytic activity via accelerated tissue plasminogen activator-mediated plasminogen activation and to inhibit the formation of thrombin, leading to suppression of coagulation (Fukao et al 2007).

Antiatherosclerotic activity

Evidence from in vitro, animal and human research has shown that garlic supplementation significantly reduces the atherosclerotic process (Campbell et al 2001, Durak et al 2002, Ferri et al 2003, Koscielny et al 1999, Kwon et al 2003, Orekhov et al 1995, Tsai et al 2012). Early research demonstrated that garlic significantly decreases accumulation of aortic tissue cholesterol, fatty-streak formation and the size of atherosclerotic plaque in vivo (Campbell et al 2001).

The adherence of leucocytes/monocytes to endothelium is also implicated in early-stage atherogenesis. In vitro studies have shown that incubation with garlic compounds significantly inhibits the oxidation of low-density lipoprotein (LDL) (Lau 2006), prevents adhesion of monocytes to IL-1alpha-stimulated endothelial cells (Rassoul et al 2006), suppresses oxidised LDL-mediated leucocyte adhesion to human endothelial cells (Lei et al 2008) and inhibits the uptake of oxidised LDL and CD36 expression (homocysteine-induced) by human macrophages (Morihara et al 2011).

A critical review conducted on in vitro studies established that garlic inhibits enzymes involved in lipid synthesis, platelet aggregation and oxidisation of LDL, while increasing antioxidant status (Rahman & Lowe 2006). Results from several published animal studies further exhibit antiatherogenic effects and have investigated the mechanisms responsible (Durak et al 2002, Ferri et al 2003, Kwon et al 2003). One in vivo study found that garlic activated antioxidant systems and decreased peroxidation in aortic tissue (Durak et al 2002), whereas ajoene inhibited smooth-muscle cell proliferation in another (Ferri et al 2003). The administration of 9 mg/kg of pure allicin in an animal model was found to reduce atherosclerotic plaque, Cu^{2+} binding to LDL, macrophages and the inhibition of LDL and oxidised LDL degradation. Allicin was also found to directly bind to lipoproteins, suggesting a further mechanism of action (Gonen et al 2005).

Similar results have been obtained using ultrasound techniques. Koscielny et al (1999) conducted a long-term randomised, double-blind, placebo-controlled trial involving 152 volunteers to determine whether garlic powder supplements (Kwai 900 mg daily) directly alter plaque volumes in carotid and/or femoral arteries. After 4 years' treatment, garlic intake significantly reduced the expected increase in arteriosclerotic plaque volume by 5–18%, with a slight regression also observed. A subsequent re-evaluation of the results found that significant effects were limited to women (Siegel & Klussendorf 2000).

In a multifactor prognostic evaluation of high-risk patients assessing risk of coronary heart disease (CHD), MI and sudden death, prolonged administration of Allicor containing 150 mg of dehydrated garlic powder in a slow-release form significantly reduced multifactor risk of CHD in both genders. However, reduced risk of MI and sudden death was achieved significantly in men, but not in women. A pilot study suggests that incremental benefits were identified when evaluating the role of garlic therapy in coronary artery calcification with patients also on concomitant statin therapy (Budoff 2006).

A published review suggested that the antiatherosclerotic action of garlic, while dose-dependent, is a valuable component in an atherosclerosis-preventing diet (Gorinstein et al 2007). A need for the standardisation of garlic products has been called for, to enable the opportunity to evaluate and draw conclusions from research findings (El-Sabban & Abouazra 2008).

A possible role for garlic in the prevention of cerebrovascular damage has been postulated through a reduction in levels of beta-amyloid and apoptosis, associated with the pathogenesis of Alzheimer's disease (Borek 2006). S-allyl-L-cysteine, an OSC purified from aged garlic extract (AGE), exerted an antiamyloidogenic activity in vitro, protecting against amyloid-beta-induced neuronal cell death, inhibiting amyloid-beta fibril formation and defibrillating amyloid-beta preformed fibrils (Gupta & Rao 2007, Gupta et al 2009, Imai et al 2007, Ishige et al 2007).

Reduces serum cholesterol levels

Two recent meta-analyses confirm that long-term garlic treatment modestly reduces total cholesterol levels (Ried et al 2013, Zeng et al 2012). Garlic powder capsules (mainly Kwai) are the most studied preparation; however the AGE preparations appear to have slightly stronger cholesterol-lowering activity than other forms.

A critical review published in 2006 suggests that garlic and its constituents exert a capacity to inhibit the enzymes involved in cholesterol and fatty acid synthesis, particularly mono-oxygenase and 3-hydroxy-3-methyl-glutaryl-CoA reductase (Rahman & Lowe 2006).

A 75% inhibition of cholesterol synthesis was achieved in garlic-treated human hepatoma cells without any evidence of cytotoxicity. Results indicated that compounds containing allyl-disulfide or allyl-sulfhydryl have the strongest inhibitory effect, likely to be through mediation of sterol 4-alpha-methyl oxidase (Singh & Porter 2006). Administration of high-dose (500 mg/kg) raw garlic extract to rats showed a significant (38%) reduction in triglycerides and cholesterol (Thomson et al 2006).

The capacity for modulating lipids may be attributed to the release of allicin through enzyme activation. A clinical crossover study involving 50 renal transplant patients involved the ingestion of one garlic clove daily for 2 months, either by swallowing or chewing. The swallowing route achieved a significant reduction in systolic blood pressure (SBP) and malondialdehyde (MDA) but no change in lipid parameters. However, chewing garlic achieved a reduction in cholesterol and a significant reduction in triglycerides, MDA and systolic and diastolic blood pressures, but no changes in high-density lipoprotein (HDL) or LDL (Jabbari et al 2005).

The metabolic activity of garlic has been studied in an obese rat model which compared three interventions to controls (garlic, exercise, garlic plus exercise). While all groups showed positive effects on cholesterol lowering, obesity and inflammation, the combination of garlic plus exercise group showed the greatest effects ($P < 0.001$) (Seo et al 2012).

Garlic's beneficial effects on serum lipids have been shown to decline following cessation of treatment, suggesting that long-term supplementation is required. A reduction in cholesterol and triglycerides and an increase in HDL were achieved in 30 participants with elevated blood cholesterol ingesting 5 g of raw garlic twice daily for 42 days. However, following a 42-day washout period, cholesterol and triglycerides increased and HDL decreased (Mahmoodi et al 2006). This study was repeated in 30 participants with blood cholesterol >245 mg/dL, with decreases in total blood

G

cholesterol ($P < 0.001$) and triglycerides ($P < 0.01$), while HDL-C was increased ($P < 0.01$); these results were again reversed after a 42-day washout period (Hosseini et al 2013). Earlier clinical evidence also supports these results (Bordia et al 1998, Sobenin et al 2005).

Hypoglycaemic activity

Animal studies have shown that garlic and its constituents exhibit a hypoglycaemic action (Hattori et al 2005, Jelodar et al 2005) and produce significant changes in glucose tolerance and insulin secretion (Liu et al 2005, Padiya et al 2011). An antioxidant isolated from garlic, S-allyl cysteine sulfoxide, was found to stimulate insulin secretion from beta cells in rats (Augusti & Sheela 1996). Oral administration of garlic extract for 14 days significantly decreased serum glucose in streptozotocin-induced diabetic rats but not in normal rats. The garlic extract was also compared to that of glibenclamide, a known antidiabetic drug, and was found to be more effective (Eidi et al 2006). A similar study using garlic oil found no effect on oral glucose tolerance acutely, but did report significantly improved oral glucose tolerance at 4, 8, 12 and 16 weeks (Liu et al 2006). A study in a diabetic animal model showed garlic 100 mg/kg significantly reduced blood glucose levels and increased serum insulin levels in dogs when compared to controls. The effect was comparable to metformin (Mosallanejad et al 2013). A similar study in rabbits testing several doses of garlic extract in both normal and diabetic test animals found that the highest dose (350 mg/kg) had the strongest effect and significantly lowered blood glucose compared to controls in both cohorts. Levels of triglycerides and cholesterol also significantly reduced in both groups compared to controls, 4 h after administration. When compared to metformin, garlic had greater lipid-lowering activity whereas metformin was superior for hypoglycaemic activity (Sher et al 2012).

Antihypertensive activity

Numerous clinical studies have identified mild to moderate antihypertensive activity with various garlic preparations when used for at least 12 weeks (Andrianova et al 2002, Dhawan & Jain 2005, Ried et al 2013, Silagy & Neil 1994, Stabler et al 2012, Tsai et al 2012). Although the mechanism of action has not been fully elucidated, evidence from in vivo research suggests that both the renin–angiotensin system and the NO system are responsible for this activity (Al-Qattan et al 2006, Mohamadi et al 2000). A controlled animal study found that both raw and aged garlic produced a reduction in induced elevated SBP compared to control. A reduction in pulse pressure was also achieved in the aged garlic-treated group (Harauma & Moriguchi 2006). Rats receiving a conjugate of allicin and captopril (allylmercaptocaptopril) showed a greater reduction in blood pressure and improved cardiac hypertrophy than those receiving captopril alone. Allylmercaptocaptopril improved, whereas captopril impaired, fasting glucose tolerance (Ernsberger et al 2007). A similar study compared the effect of a fresh garlic homogenate (125–250 mg/kg) and its bioactive sulfur compound S-allylcysteine sulfoxide (SACS) in potentiating antihypertensive and cardioprotective activities of captopril (30 mg/kg) in rats. The combined treatment of garlic plus captopril was more effective than either alone and significantly reduced SBP, cholesterol, triglycerides and glucose in a dose-dependent manner (Asdaq & Inamdar 2010). In particular, a synergistic effect was seen for the blood pressure-lowering activity.

Enhances microcirculation

Jung et al (1991) found that, 5 hours after the administration of garlic powder (Kwai: total dose 900 mg garlic powder), a significant increase in capillary skin perfusion (55%) occurred in healthy volunteers, whereas Kiesewetter et al (1993a) showed a 48% increase with a dose of 800 mg garlic.

Antimicrobial and immune-enhancing activities

Garlic and its components have been demonstrated in vitro to exert a direct and indirect activity against various pathogens, including bacteria (both Gram-negative and Gram-positive), fungi and parasites. Antimicrobial sensitivity tests conducted on *Escherichia coli*, *Shigella* spp., *Salmonella* spp. and *Proteus mirabilis* found that no isolates were resistant to garlic; moreover, Gram-negative isolates were found to be highly sensitive to garlic in comparison to ciprofloxacin and ampicillin (Eja et al 2007).

Multiple chemical components in garlic demonstrate immunomodulating activity, including garlic sulfur compounds, lectins ASA I and II, agglutinins, proteins and fructans (Chandrashekar & Venkatesh 2009, Clement & Venkatesh 2010, Clement et al 2010, Chandrashekar et al 2011).

Allicin was initially believed to be chiefly responsible for the antimicrobial activity of garlic. Research found it to exert antibacterial activity against a wide range of Gram-negative and Gram-positive bacteria, including multidrug-resistant enterotoxicogenic strains of *Escherichia coli*, *Staphylococcus aureus*, *Mycobacterium tuberculosis*, *Proteus* spp., *Streptococcus faecalis* and *Pseudomonas aeruginosa*; antifungal activity, particularly against *Candida albicans*; antiparasitic activity against some of the major human protozoan parasites such as *Cryptosporidium parvum*, *Trichomonas vaginalis*, *Entamoeba histolytica* and *Giardia lamblia* and antiviral activity (Ankri & Mirelman 1999, Davis 2005, Gaafar et al 2012, Ibrahim 2013, Tessema et al 2006). Allicin has been found to exert an antimalarial action in vitro and in vivo (Coppi et al 2006, Feng et al 2012) and to significantly enhance the effect of amphotericin B against *Candida albicans* in vitro and in vivo, mediated through oxidative damage to *C. albicans* (An et al 2008, 2009). Additionally, in vitro investigations have identified the capacity of allicin to activate macrophage activity

(Dong et al 2011, Ghazanfari et al 2006) and inhibit macrophage apoptosis (Cho et al 2006).

Ajoene, another important antimicrobial constituent, has been attributed to more biological activities in vitro and in vivo, including antifungal and antiparasitic actions (Ledezma & Apitz-Castro 2006), with greater antiviral activity than that of allicin, according to one in vitro test (Weber et al 1992), plus an interesting anti-leech effect (Eftekhari et al 2012).

The role of garlic in oral hygiene and the pathogenesis of dental disease has been investigated. All isolates of *Streptococcus mutans* identified in human carious teeth were sensitive to garlic extract, suggesting a role for garlic in mouthwashes for the prevention of dental caries (Fani et al 2007). This antimicrobial effect against streptococci was found to continue for 2 weeks posttreatment (Groppo et al 2007). Garlic extract was also found to significantly kill *Porphyromonas gingivalis* and its protease enzymes, indicating a role in the treatment of periodontitis (Bakri & Douglas 2005). A randomised trial of 56 patients found garlic paste to be as effective as that of clotrimazole solution in suppressing signs of oral candidiasis (Sabitha et al 2005).

Helicobacter pylori infection

Several in vitro and in vivo tests have shown that garlic has activity against *H. pylori* (Chung et al 1998, Jonkers et al 1999, O'Gara et al 2000); however, results from clinical studies are equivocal. Two studies found that a combination of garlic and omeprazole produced synergistic effects against *H. pylori* (Cellini et al 1996, Jonkers et al 1999). A rapid anti-*H. pylori* action of garlic oil was observed in artificial gastric juice, suggesting it as a useful treatment (O'Gara et al 2008).

Antineoplastic and chemopreventive effects

Garlic was first used over 3500 years ago in Egypt for the treatment of cancer. Garlic, and, in particular, its OSCs, including allicin, DAS, DADS, DATS and ajoene, have been investigated for their chemoprotective actions (Shukla & Kalra 2007). Many review articles have identified the multiple mechanisms by which garlic's compounds exert anticarcinogenic properties.

Garlic OSCs demonstrate a capacity to modulate detoxification enzyme systems often responsible for the activation of carcinogens (Yang et al 2001); for example, DAS and its metabolites have been found to competitively inhibit the metabolism of cytochrome P450 2E1 substrates in vitro (Brady et al 1991). This inhibitory activity has been shown in rat nasal mucosa (Hong et al 1991) and hepatocytes (Brady et al 1991). In addition, garlic OSCs increase the expression of phase II enzymes by enhancement of detoxification of activated carcinogenic intermediates such as quinine reductase and glutathione transferases (Bianchini & Vainio 2001, Rose et al 2005). Phase II enzyme modulation by OSCs has been reported in forestomach and lung cancer in mice (Singh et al 1998), and hepatoma cells (Chen et al 2004). Further investigations have established garlic OSCs' capacity to upregulate gene expression of glutathione S-transferase.

Garlic OSCs have been shown to suppress neoplastic cell formation by inhibition of cell cycle progression, leading to cellular accumulation in the G2/M phase (Frantz et al 2000, Zheng et al 1997). Human colon cancer cells treated with DADS have not only been seen to arrest the G2/M phase: concomitant alterations were also seen to DNA repair and cellular adhesion factors (Knowles & Milner 2003), with increases in cyclin B1 expression and p53 expression leading to cellular apoptosis (Jo et al 2008, Song et al 2009). DATS also induced apoptosis in primary colorectal cancer cells via mitochondrial-signalling pathways (Yu et al 2012), while treatment with DATS was reported to be more effective in arresting the G2/M phase of the cell cycle than DADS or DAS in human prostate cells (Xiao et al 2005). However DADS induced apoptosis in prostate cancer cells through modulation of the insulin growth factor pathway and the resulting inhibition of Akt phosphorylation, which resulted in reduced expression of antiapoptotic molecules and increased expression of proapoptotic signalling molecules (Arunkumar et al 2012). In human cervical cell cancer lines (Ski) DAS caused apoptosis via p53-induced cell cycle arrest and mitochondrial disruption (Chiu et al 2013).

Treatment with garlic and its compounds has been shown to display characteristics of mitotic arrest, exhibiting alterations to tubulin network and chromatin condensation (Herman-Antosiewicz & Singh 2005). Treatment of human colon cells with garlic-derived compound SAMC resulted in depolymerisation of microtubules and cytoskeleton disruption (Xiao et al 2005). Similarly, DATS treatment induced rapid microtubule disassembly and cell cycle arrest in human colon cancer cells (Hosono et al 2008).

Garlic and its constituents have demonstrated actions that modify apoptopic pathways mostly through regulation of antiapoptotic Bcl-2 and proapoptotic Bax and Bac proteins (Herman-Antosiewicz et al 2007). For example, modification to transcription ratios of Bax/Bcl-2 proteins following treatment with OSCs has induced apoptosis in neuroblastoma and lung cancer cells (Hong et al 2000), breast cancer cell lines (Nakagawa et al 2001) and prostate cancer cells (Arunkumar et al 2012, Xiao et al 2004). Another mechanism shown to induce cellular apoptosis following treatment with OSCs is the induction of reactive oxygen species (ROS) generation (Song et al 2009, Sriram et al 2008). DATS has been shown to induce ROS, reduce cell viability, increase apoptosis and inhibit cell migration in human breast cancer cells, but not in normal breast tissue cells (Chandra-Kuntal et al 2013). It has also been shown to induce ROS-related mitochondrial membrane disruption in hepatic cancer cells (Kim et al 2012). Additionally regulation of Akt-Bad (protein kinase B) pathway (Arunkumar et al 2012, Xiao & Singh 2006) and increased free intracellular calcium (Lin et al 2006) have been demonstrated. Malignant cells appear to be more sensitive to OSC-mediated apoptosis than normal cells (Chandra-Kuntal et al 2013, Powolny & Singh 2008). Garlic OSCs' protective qualities include increased histone acetylation by the inhibition of histone deacetylase, leading to cancer cell growth inhibition; for example, treatment of rodent erythroleukaemia and human leukaemia cells with DADS increases H4 and H3 histone acetylations (Lea & Randolph 2001). Increased acetylation has also been reported with treatment of OSCs in human colon cancer cells (Druesne et al 2004), breast cancer cells (Altonsy et al 2012) and prostate cancer cells (Arunkumar et al 2007). Similar research has been repeated in many different human cancer cell lines (Tsai et al 2012).

Finally, in vitro studies in human and animal cell lines indicate garlic and/or its constituents' ability to inhibit angiogenesis and metastasis. In human colon cancer cells, AGE was shown to inhibit angiogenesis by reducing endothelial cell motility, inhibiting tube formation, proliferation and invasion (Matsuura et al 2006). Administration of alliin exerted a dose-dependent inhibition of fibroblast growth factor-2-induced human endothelial cell tube formation and angiogenesis (Mousa & Mousa 2005). Similarly, treatments with DATS, DADS and DAS have been shown to inhibit capillary-like tube formation, cellular proliferation and migration (Thejass & Kuttan 2007). DADS was also found to inhibit angiogenesis by inhibiting the activation of matrix metalloproteinase (Thejass & Kuttan 2007). In human breast tumour cells, SAC reduced cell adhesion and invasion through expression of E-cadherin and reduced expression of matrix metalloproteinase-2 (Gapter et al 2008). In animal studies, intravenous administration of ajoene significantly inhibited lung metastasis of melanoma cells (Taylor et al 2006) and AGE inhibited sarcoma cell migration (Hu et al 2002). A mouse model of inserted fibrosarcoma showed treatment with AGE reduced tumour progression and significantly improved survival with $CD4^+/CD8^+$ T-cell modulation (Fallah-Rostami et al 2013).

There are many published reviews confirming garlic and its constituents' chemoprotective capacity in various human cancer cell lines (Herman-Antosiewicz et al 2007, Moriarty et al 2007, Nagini 2008, Powolny & Singh 2008, Seki et al 2008, Shukla & Kalra 2007). It is suggested that future research should focus on pharmacokinetics and pharmacodynamics in humans (Powolny & Singh 2008).

OTHER ACTIONS

Hepatoprotective effects

AGE has a glutathione-sparing effect in the liver and specifically elevates reduced glutathione content, thereby enhancing endogenous protective mechanisms, according to in vitro tests (Wang et al 1999). The protective effects of a single simultaneous dose of garlic oil have been demonstrated on acute ethanol-induced fatty liver in mice, by significantly inhibiting elevation of MDA levels, restoring glutathione levels and enhancing SOD, glutathione reductase and glutathione S-tranferase activities (Zeng et al 2008). More recent studies with organosulfur components from garlic have also demonstrated hepatoprotective effects in vivo (D'Argenio et al 2013, Xiao et al 2013) and a small clinical trial demonstrated a dose-dependent protective effect of a garlic oil and diphenyl-dimethyldicarboxylate (DDM) supplement, as measured by aspartate aminotransferase and alanine aminotransferase levels in patients with chronic hepatitis, with the greatest benefit seen in doses of 75–100 mg of DDB and 100–150 mg of garlic oil (M Lee et al 2012).

Homocysteine-lowering action

AGE exhibits homocysteine-lowering action that indicates its potential for the treatment of cardiovascular disease (Yeh & Yeh 2006). A pilot study conducted in patients with cardiovascular disease showed that pretreatment for 6 weeks with AGE significantly reduced the effects of acute hyperhomocysteinaemia (Weiss et al 2006). It is postulated that the homocysteine-lowering action of AGE is due to its ability to inhibit CD36 expression and OxLDL uptake in macrophages involved in the formation of atherosclerotic lesions (Ide et al 2006).

Inhibits CYP 2E1 and induces P-glycoprotein

According to in vitro and animal studies, garlic and some of its components may affect various cytochromes (Engdal et al 2009, Fisher et al 2007, Greenblatt et al 2006); however, human research has not produced the same findings (Cox et al 2006, Dalvi 1992, Foster et al 2001, Gurley et al 2002, 2005) and now confirmed that it is only clinically relevant for cytochrome 2E1 and P-glycoprotein with no effects on CYP3A4.

Researchers using human volunteers found that garlic oil reduced CYP2E1 activity by 39%, but had no effect on CYP1A2, CYP2D6 or CYP3A4 activity (Gurley et al 2002). The lack of a clinically significant effect on CYP1A2, CYP2D6 and CYP3A4 activity was confirmed in a later study of 12 elderly healthy volunteers receiving garlic oil for 28 days, followed by a 30-day washout period. Garlic oil had a mild inhibitory effect on CYP2E1 activity (by approximately 22%) (Gurley et al 2005). Additionally, tests with allicin found no effect on CYP3A4 in women receiving docetaxel treatment (Cox et al 2006).

More recently, a clinical study further confirmed no significant effect on CYP3A4 for oral ingestion of garlic extract by human volunteers but a significant induction of P-glycoprotein (Hajda et al 2010). Specifically, the ingestion of garlic extract increased expression of duodenal P-glycoprotein to 131% (95% confidence interval [CI] 105–163%)

and negatively correlated with changes to the average area under the plasma concentration curve of saquinavir, which decreased to 85% (95% CI 66–109%).

Another clinical study identified that co-administration of garlic did not significantly alter warfarin pharmacokinetics or pharmacodynamics in healthy volunteers who had taken a single dose of 25 mg warfarin administered after 2 weeks of pre-treatment with garlic (Mohammed Abdul et al 2008).

Quality of life

A small open-label study observed the effect of a Japanese garlic extract supplement (Aomori) 500 mg daily on 17 active workers with significant improvements in self-assessed stress, sleep quality, fatigue, dehydroepiandrosterone sulfate and cortisol awakening response, as measurements of improved quality of life (Ohiro et al 2013).

CLINICAL USE

The use of garlic to treat a variety of conditions is supported by several authorities. Treatment of atherosclerosis, arterial vascular disease, blood lipids, respiratory tract infections and catarrhal conditions has been indicated by the European Scientific Cooperative on Phytotherapy (ESCOP). Treatment of hyperlipidaemia and age-related vascular changes with garlic is supported by the expert German panel, the Commission E, while the World Health Organization (WHO) also reports that there are sufficient clinical data to indicate the use of garlic in hyperlipidaemia, age-dependent atherosclerosis and mild hypertension. Many different dietary forms and commercial preparations of garlic have been tested in clinical trials and several meta-analyses have been published to further aid our understanding of its role in practice.

Cardiovascular disease

Epidemiological studies show an inverse correlation between garlic consumption and progression of CVD in general (Rahman & Lowe 2006). Several intervention studies have also been published producing promising results for various forms of garlic treatment.

A double-blind, placebo-controlled study of 167 patients with hyperlipidaemia demonstrated that Allicor was effective in reducing the 10-year absolute multifactorial risk of cardiovascular diseases (Sobenin et al 2005). Garlic was also found to reduce the 10-year risk of acute MI and sudden death in a double-blind, placebo-controlled study of 51 patients with coronary artery disease receiving Allicor for a 12-month period (Sobenin et al 2007).

Previously, Koscielny et al (1999) conducted a long-term randomised, double-blind, placebo-controlled trial involving 152 volunteers to determine whether garlic powder supplements (Kwai 900 mg daily) directly alter plaque volumes in carotid and/or femoral arteries. After 4 years' treatment, garlic intake significantly reduced the expected increase in arteriosclerotic plaque volume by 5–18%, with a slight regression also observed. A subsequent re-evaluation of the results found that significant effects were limited to women (Siegel & Klussendorf 2000).

In a multifactor prognostic evaluation of high-risk patients assessing risk of CHD, MI and sudden death, prolonged administration of Allicor significantly reduced multifactor risk of CHD in both genders. However, reduced risk of MI and sudden death was achieved significantly in men, but not in women (Sobenin et al 2005).

G

Long-term use of AGE (1200 mg/day) appears to retard calcification of coronary arteries according to a placebo-controlled, double-blind, randomised pilot study involving high-risk patients while on a stable course of statin and aspirin therapy (Budoff 2006). Active treatment slowed down progression of disease, as the study showed that patients on placebo (with statin baseline therapy) progressed at a rate of 22.2% per year compared to those also taking AGE, who had a reduced progression to 7.5%.

IN COMBINATION

In 2009 Budoff et al reported on a well-designed double-blind randomised controlled trial (RCT) of 65 intermediate-risk patients taking statin medication and presenting with subclinical atherosclerosis coronary artery disease. Subjects were treated with a capsule containing 250 mg of AGE, B_{12} 100 mcg, folic acid 300 mcg, B_6 12.5 mg and l-arginine 100 mg or placebo daily for 1 year. The treatment group achieved significantly favourable changes in oxidative biomarkers, vascular factors and reduced progression of atherosclerosis. In 2012, results of an RCT once again found that coronary artery calcification could be significantly decreased with AGE (1200 mg/day), this time used together with coenzyme Q10 (120 mg/day) for 1 year. The placebo-controlled study involved 65 intermediate-risk firemen and found both coronary artery calcium and C-reactive protein significantly decreased with active treatment compared to placebo ($P = 0.01$). Interestingly, only 24.4% of participants were on statin drugs (Zeb et al 2012).

Hypertension

The current clinical evidence indicates that garlic treatment has a slow-onset blood pressure-reducing effect when taken for approximately 12 weeks; however, it is difficult to quantify the size of effect. It has been tested as a stand-alone treatment or used together with standard antihypertensive medication to produce further reductions in blood pressure. Based on current clinical and preclinical research, the effectiveness of treatment is primarily determined by its content of SAC and ability to yield allicin, although other compounds may also be important.

An early meta-analysis reported in 1994 analysing results from seven trials using Kwai 600–900 mg daily showed a mean reduction of 7.7 mmHg for

SBP and 5 mmHg for diastolic blood pressure (DBP) (Silagy & Neil 1994). Isolating the results of the two placebo-controlled trials involving hypertensive patients, the reduction in SBP was 11.1 mmHg and 6.5 mmHg reduction in DBP with garlic treatment.

In 2000, the Agency for Health Care Research and Quality analysed results from 27 randomised, placebo-controlled trials and reported that results were mixed, with occasional small reductions reported (Mulrow et al 2000).

In contrast, in 2008 Reinhart et al analysed 10 clinical trials, reporting that garlic reduced blood pressure in patients with an elevated SBP, but not in those with normal SBP. The same year, Ried et al (2008) conducted a meta-analysis of 11 randomised placebo-controlled trials (n = 1298) and concluded that garlic preparations are superior to placebo in reducing SBP and DBP in normotensive people and those with hypertension (Ried et al 2008).

In 2012, a Cochrane systematic review confirmed that garlic treatment reduces blood pressure when compared to placebo; however, the magnitude of this effect cannot be accurately quantified. The review analysed the results of two studies (n = 87) which met the entry criteria of being randomised, blinded, controlled to treatment, including intention-to-treat data and involving only participants with primary hypertension. One of the included studies reported that 12 weeks of treatment with 200 mg garlic powder (Kwai) three times daily reduced supine SBP by 10–12 mmHg and DBP by 5–9 mmHg and significantly reduced standing SBP by 21 mmHg (from 171 to 150 mmHg) and DBP by 11 mmHg (from 101 to 90 mmHg) (Auer et al 1990). The other study found that 12 weeks' treatment with two capsules of 100 mg high-potency garlic powder taken three times daily produced a statistically significant mean reduction in supine SBP of 16 mmHg (from 178 to 162 mmHg) and supine DBP of 15 mmHg (from 100 to 85 mmHg). Treatment also produced a statistically significant mean reduction in standing SBP of 16 mmHg (from 174 to 158 mmHg) and standing DBP of 16 mmHg (from 99 to 83 mmHg) (Stabler et al 2012).

Due to the limited data available, the Cochrane systematic review was unable to determine whether garlic treatment reduced all-cause mortality, cardiovascular events or cerebrovascular events in hypertensive patients (Stabler et al 2012).

Since then, three further randomised trials have been published. An RCT of 50 participants with uncontrolled hypertension taking standard treatment were given additional AGE 960 mg (standardised to 2.4 mg SAC) or placebo and found active treatment produced a significant reduction in SBP after 12 weeks for people with baseline SBP > 140 mmHg ($P = 0.036$). There was no significant reduction seen across the whole treatment group, which also consisted of people with SBP < 140 mmHg (Ried et al 2010).

In 2013 the same authors published results of a double-blind, randomised trial comparing three different dosages (240/480/960 mg containing 0.6/1.2/2.4 mg SAC) of AGE (Kyolic aged garlic; extract: High Potency Everyday Formula 112; Wakunaga/Wagner) plus regular treatment in 79 subjects with uncontrolled systolic hypertension. Similar to previous studies, SBP was significantly lowered after 12 weeks of treatment by 11.8 ± 5.4 mmHg compared with placebo ($P = 0.006$). The effect was only seen in the groups taking at least 480 mg daily. Interestingly, the hypotensive effect did not occur in all patients and ranged from −40 mmHg to +5 mmHg across all groups; however this study was unable to predict responder characteristics. Mild gastrointestinal side effects were reported, mainly in the highest-dose group (Ried et al 2013).

A traditional Japanese garlic homogenate (300 mg/day)-supplemented diet was compared to placebo in a randomised, double-blind study involving 81 participants with prehypertension or mild hypertension. Once again, treatment for 12 weeks induced significant reductions in SBP (−6.6 mmHg to −7.5 mmHg) and DBP (−4.6 mmHg to −5.2 mmHg) compared to placebo with no major side effects. Importantly, the effect was only clinically relevant in subjects with hypertension (Nakasone et al 2013).

Hyperlipidaemia

The most recent meta-analyses confirm that long-term garlic treatment modestly reduces total cholesterol levels. Garlic powder capsules (mainly Kwai) are the most-studied preparation; however the AGE preparations appear to have slightly stronger cholesterol-lowering activity than the powder forms.

In 2000, a meta-analysis of 13 clinical trials concluded that garlic reduces total cholesterol levels significantly more than placebo; however, the effects can only be described as modest (Stevinson et al 2001). The same year, a systematic review and meta-analysis were published by the Agency for Health Care Research and Quality, which analysed results from 44 studies with lipid outcomes (Mulrow et al 2000). Most studies involved fewer than 100 volunteers and randomisation techniques were unclear in 82% of the studies. Pooled data from the placebo-controlled trials reporting changes in total cholesterol levels found a significant average reduction in total cholesterol levels of 7.2 mg/dL after 4–6 weeks, using any form of garlic, and a reduction of 17.1 mg/dL at 8–12 weeks. Results at 20–24 weeks were not significant and thought to be due to low statistical power, fewer long-term studies or a time-dependent effect of garlic.

Two meta-analyses have been published more recently. The first, in 2012, analysed results from 26 RCTs and did not discriminate between preparation or dose, finding that total cholesterol and triglycerides were significantly reduced ($P = 0.001$), with the most marked outcomes seen in people with higher triglyceride levels and long-term interventions. The most-studied preparation was garlic powder, mainly Kwai brand, with doses ranging from 600 to 900 mg, whereas four studies used garlic oil and three studies used AGE. The duration of treatment ranged from 2 weeks to 1 year and no other lipid parameters were affected. Further, the review surmises that total cholesterol is most affected by aged garlic and powdered garlic, while triglycerides were most affected by powdered preparations (Zeng et al 2012).

In 2013, Ried et al published a meta-analysis of 37 RCTs (n = 2,298) which produced similar results: a significant cholesterol-lowering effect of garlic preparations compared with placebo and that the cholesterol-lowering treatment effect was more pronounced in trials of longer duration. The best effects were obtained when the intervention was used for longer than 12 weeks. More specifically, interventions >2 months in those with total cholesterol >200 mg/dL (~5.2 mmol/L) had significant reductions in total cholesterol by 17 ± 6 mg, reduction in LDL cholesterol by 9 ± 6 mg/dL, only marginal improvements in HDL cholesterol (1.5 ± 1.3 mg/dL) and no significant improvement in triglycerides. Subgroup analysis by single type of garlic preparation suggested a greater cholesterol-lowering effect for AGE than for garlic powder, and a borderline effect for garlic oil, The effect of garlic on HDL cholesterol levels was significant but small and most pronounced for garlic oil and the effect on triglycerides was non-significant overall (Ried et al 2013).

Clinical note — Not all garlic preparations are the same

One of the difficulties encountered when interpreting the research available for garlic is comparing the effects of different preparations, which often have not been tested for the presence of important constituents or allicin-releasing potential. It is known that fresh garlic and dried garlic powder contain alliin. When cut, crushed, chewed or dehydrated, the enzyme allinase is rapidly released, which allows the biotransformation of alliin to active organo-sulfur compounds. Some other forms may only contain alliin, and not the necessary alliinase component, thus compromising allicin-releasing potential. An example of the manufacturing process affecting potency has been suggested for a commercial garlic product known as Kwai, which has often been used in cholesterol research (Lawson et al 2001). According to a 2001 experiment, substantial differences were found between tablets manufactured before 1993 (the years when all but one of the positive trials were conducted) and those manufactured after 1993 (the years when all of the negative trials were conducted). Kwai products manufactured after 1993 released only one-third as much allicin as older preparations. Those preparations from before 1993 disintegrated more slowly, protecting alliinase from acid exposure and inactivation.

Comparative studies

Two clinical studies have compared different garlic preparations with pharmaceutical cholesterol-lowering medicines. Garlic taken as 300 mg three times daily (Kwai) produced similar lipid-lowering effects to 200 mg Bezafibrate (a hypolipidaemic fibrate) three times daily in subjects with primary hyperlipidaemia (Holzgartner et al 1992), whereas Clofibrate 500 mg was more effective than an essential oil extract of 50 g raw garlic (Arora & Arora 1981). The administration of 600 mg of fish oil with 500 mg of garlic pearls (garlic oil) per day to 16 hypercholesterolaemic subjects with a total cholesterol above 220 mg/dL for 60 days was found to reduce total cholesterol, LDL, serum triglyceride and very-low-density lipoprotein (Jeyaraj et al 2005).

Commission E approves the use of garlic as an adjunct to dietary changes in the treatment of hyperlipidaemia (Blumenthal 2000).

Diabetes mellitus (plus hyperlipidaemia)

Garlic may be of benefit to people with diabetes, according to the available clinical research; however mixed results hamper the interpretation of results.

In the 1990s, one double-blind study reported that 800 mg garlic powder taken daily for a period of 4 weeks reduced blood glucose concentrations by 11.6% (Kiesewetter et al 1993b); however, another study using a higher dose of 3 g/day over 26 weeks found no effects (Ali & Thomson 1995).

Ten years later, a 12-week, placebo-controlled, single-blind, randomised study found that treatment with a garlic tablet (Garlex: Bosch Pharmaceuticals, 300 mg, containing 1.3% allicin) twice daily, together with a diet and exercise plan, resulted in a significant reduction in total cholesterol of 28 mg/dL (12.03%) compared to placebo (Ashraf et al 2005). The study involved 70 patients with type 2 diabetes and newly diagnosed dyslipidaemia.

The metabolic action of Allicor (INAT-Farma, Russia) was investigated in a 4-week, double-blind, placebo-controlled study of 60 type 2 diabetic patients taken off their hypoglycaemic medication. Active treatment resulted in better metabolic control compared to placebo as measured by several parameters. In particular, a significant decrease in serum triglyceride levels was observed after 3 weeks of treatment, and by the end of the study the difference from baseline levels accounted for 36% (P < 0.05). Additionally, fasting blood glucose levels decreased and were maintained at the mean levels below 7.0 mmol/L during the whole study period whereas they began to rise in the placebo group (Sobenin et al 2008). Allicor contains 150 mg of dehydrated garlic powder in a slow-release form and the dose used was 300 mg twice daily.

In contrast, a short-term double-blind placebo-controlled crossover trial of 26 people with type 2 diabetes found no change in endothelial function, vascular inflammation, insulin resistance or oxidative stress when 1200 mg of AGE was added to usual treatment for 4 weeks followed by a 4-week washout period (Atkin 2011).

In the past few years, several more clinical studies have been published, one comparing garlic to metformin and others adding garlic to metformin treatment to see if further benefits develop.

A single-blind placebo-controlled, escalating dose study was conducted with 210 people with type 2 diabetes comparing the effects of garlic 300, 600, 900, 1200, 1500 mg, metformin and placebo for 24 weeks. Results showed significant effects ($P < 0.005$) for both fasting blood sugar and HbA_{1C} with the higher garlic doses (1200 and 1500 mg) compared to placebo, both being comparable to metformin (Phil et al 2011).

Adjunctive therapy to metformin

An RCT involving 60 participants taking metformin 500 mg twice daily compared the addition of garlic 300 mg three times daily or placebo over a 24-week test period. Results showed that adding garlic to the treatment induced an improvement in both glycaemic control and cholesterol markers ($P < 0.005$) compared to placebo (Ashraf et al 2011). Most recently an open-label study of 60 obese patients with type 2 diabetes compared the effects of stand-alone metformin 500 mg twice daily to metformin and garlic 250 mg twice daily for 12 weeks. Combination treatment resulted in significantly improved postprandial blood glucose levels ($P < 0.001$), total cholesterol, triglycerides, LDL ($P < 0.05$), adenosine deaminase ($P < 0.01$) and C-reactive protein ($P < 0.05$); however changes in HbA_{1C} were not significantly different between the two groups (Kumar et al 2013).

Antiplatelet effects

Antiplatelet effects of garlic are well recognised, but the dose at which this becomes significant remains uncertain. Results from a 1996 double-blind study have identified a dose of 7.2 g/day of AGE as significantly inhibiting platelet aggregation and adhesion (Steiner et al 1996). In contrast, a double-blind, placebo-controlled crossover study of 14 volunteers concluded that solvent-extracted garlic oil had minimal or no effect on platelet aggregation. Researchers found that administration of garlic 9.9 g over 4 hours exerted little or no effect on both collagen and ADP-induced aggregation. Adrenaline-induced aggregation did, however, exert a slight but significant ($P < 0.05$; 12) reduction (Wojcikowski et al 2007).

Peripheral arterial occlusive disease

In 2000, Mulrow et al reported on two double-blind placebo-controlled trials in participants with atherosclerotic lower-extremity disease. One study of 64 participants showed that pain-free walking distance increased by approximately 40 m with standardised dehydrated garlic (Kwai 800 mg daily), compared with approximately 30 m with placebo over 12 weeks. The other study of 100 participants (Mulrow et al 2000) showed that a combination treatment of garlic oil macerate/soya lecithin/hawthorn oil/wheatgerm oil significantly increased the maximum walking distance (114%) compared to placebo (17%) ($P < 0.05$). A 2008 Cochrane review found only one study meeting quality criteria and having a diagnosis of peripheral vascular atherosclerosis. The study included 78 participants, with garlic powder coated tablets 200 mg twice a day being no better than placebo for measured outcomes of walking distance and subjective symptoms after 12 weeks (Jepson et al 2008).

Infection

Garlic oil is effective against numerous bacteria, viruses and fungi, including *Staphylococcus aureus*, methicillin-resistant *Staphylococcus aureus* and several species of *Candida*, *Aspergillus* and *Cryptococcus neoformans* in vitro (Davis et al 1994, Tsao & Yin 2001, Yoshida et al 1987). As such, it has been used both internally and externally to treat various infections and prevent wound infection.

Tinea pedis, tinea corporis, tinea cruris

A trial comparing the effects of three different strengths of ajoene cream (0.4%, 0.6% and 1%) with 1% terbinafine applied twice daily found the cure rate to be 72% for 0.6% ajoene, 100% for 1% ajoene and 94% for 1% terbinafine after 60 days (Ledezma et al 2000).

Vaginitis

Taken internally as a 'natural antibiotic' or applied topically in a cream base, garlic is used to treat vaginitis. The considerable antibacterial activity of garlic provides a theoretical basis for its use in this condition, but controlled studies are not available to determine its effectiveness.

Common cold prevention

A 12-week, double-blind, randomised study involving 146 people demonstrated that allicin-containing garlic preparations significantly reduce the incidence of colds and accelerate recovery compared with placebo (Josling 2001). More specifically, the number of symptom days in the placebo group was 5.01 compared with 1.52 days in the garlic-treated group. Additionally, garlic reduced the incidence of developing a second cold, whereas placebo did not. These results were similar to those reported in a randomised, double-blind, placebo-controlled parallel intervention study of 120 participants given AGE 2.56 g/day for 90 days. At day 45 $\gamma\delta$ T-cell and natural killer cell proliferation were significantly increased, and at day 90 there was no change in cold and flu incidence between the two groups; however the treatment group had fewer symptoms

(21%), fewer sick days (58%) and fewer days lost from school/work (58%) than placebo (Nantz et al 2012).

Helicobacter pylori infection

It has been suggested that gastrointestinal lesions, such as gastric ulcers, duodenal ulcers and gastric cancers, are strongly associated with *H. pylori* infection (Scheiman & Cutler 1999). Medical treatment consisting of 'triple therapy' has a high eradication rate, yet is associated with side effects and has started to give rise to antibiotic resistance. Since garlic intake has been associated with a lowered incidence of stomach cancer, researchers have started investigating whether garlic has activity against *H. pylori*. Several in vitro and in vivo tests have shown garlic to be effective against *H. pylori* (see section on Main actions, above). However, to date only a few small clinical trials have been conducted, with disappointing and controversial results (Aydin et al 2000, Graham et al 1999, McNulty et al 2001).

A small pilot study of dyspeptic patients with confirmed *H. pylori* infection found that treatment with 4 mg garlic oil capsules taken four times daily with meals for 14 days did not alter symptoms or lead to *H. pylori* eradication (McNulty et al 2001). Another small study using garlic oil 275 mg three times a day (allicin 800 mcg/capsule) either as stand-alone treatment or in combination with omeprazole (20 mg twice daily) found that both treatments produced similar results (Aydin et al 2000). These results were confirmed in another small clinical study (Graham et al 1999).

Protective effects against cancer

Whether long-term garlic consumption reduces the risk of cancer is uncertain. A 2001 critical review of the epidemiological evidence suggests a preventive effect for garlic consumption in stomach and colorectal cancers, but not other cancers (Fleischauer & Arab 2001). With regard to gastric cancer protection, case-control studies suggested a protective effect for raw and/or cooked garlic when eaten at least once a week, whereas protective effects against colorectal cancer seem to require at least two servings of garlic per week. A similar view was reported in a 2003 review by Ernst, which stated that the weight of evidence to support the use of allium vegetables, such as garlic, in cancer is clearly positive. However, a 2009 review of 19 human studies evaluated the evidence supporting a relationship between garlic intake and a reduction in risk of different cancers with respect to food labelling. No evidence was found to suggest that garlic consumption reduced the risk of gastric, breast, lung or endometrial cancer, with very limited evidence supporting a reduction in risk of colon, prostate, oesophageal, larynx, oral, ovary or renal cell cancers due to garlic consumption (Kim & Kwon 2009). This has been reinforced by a 2012 systematic review of RCTs that found no benefit in reducing risk of cancer (Ernst & Posadzki 2012). Additionally, a report on the Nurses' study and Health Professional follow-up study, which followed 76,208 women and 45,592 men for up to 24 years, found no benefit in either dietary garlic or garlic supplement use (Meng et al 2013). Data collected included those using up to one clove of garlic (or equivalent) per day and only 6% of participants used supplements, not enough to perform statistical analysis, and no information on dosage or preparation was collected.

In addition, the Cancer Prevention Study-II investigating colorectal cancer risk in the nutrition cohort of 42,824 men and 56,876 women, whose garlic use was tracked for 7 years, indicated at best a weak protective effect in women, and a slight increase in risk for men (McCullough et al 2012).

G

Intervention study in colorectal cancer

A preliminary double-blind, randomised clinical trial in patients with colorectal adenomas — precancerous lesions of the large bowel — produced promising results with the use of high-dose AGE 2.4 mL/day (Tanaka et al 2006). The study of 51 patients measured the number and size of adenomas at baseline and at 6 and 12 months and found that AGE significantly suppressed both the size and the number of colon adenomas in patients after 1 year of treatment ($P = 0.04$). In comparison, the number of adenomas increased linearly in the control group from the beginning.

A systematic review of scientific evidence from all studies conducted over the last decade that examined the effects of garlic on colorectal cancer was conducted. Five of eight case-control/cohort studies suggested that a high intake of raw/cooked garlic produced a chemoprotective effect. Review of 11 animal studies showed a significant anticarcinogenic effect of garlic. Overall, the authors concluded that there was consistent scientific evidence derived from RCT animal studies, despite heterogeneity of human epidemiological studies (Ngo et al 2007).

Endometrial cancer

Analysis of data from a multicentre, case-control study of 454 endometrial cancer cases and 908 controls found a moderately protective role for allium vegetables on the risk of endometrial cancer, with a significant inverse trend identified for high intakes of garlic (Galeone et al 2008). Topical application of garlic-derived ajoene to tumours of 21 patients with either nodular or superficial basal cell carcinoma resulted in reduction in tumour size in 17 patients. Chemical assays prior to and posttreatment showed a significant decrease in the expression of the apoptosis suppression protein Bcl-2 (Tilli et al 2003).

OTHER USES

Some early research suggests that garlic may prevent the incidence of altitude sickness (Fallon et al 1998, Kim-Park & Ku 2000) and reduce mosquito numbers (Jarial 2001).

A small Indian trial randomly assigned 41 patients with hepatopulmonary syndrome to receive garlic oil capsules (1–2 g/m^2/day) or placebo in divided doses over a period of 18 months, with monthly evaluations. After 9 months there was a 24.7% increase in baseline arterial oxygen levels ($P < 0.001$) compared to a 7.4% increase in placebo. There was a 28.4% decrease in the alveolar-arterial oxygen gradient ($P < 0.001$) and a 10.7% reduction in placebo, which was significantly better than placebo ($P < 0.001$). Hepatopulmonary syndrome was reversed in 66.7% of patients in the treatment group compared to 5% in placebo (intention to treat) and at 18-month follow-up two had died in the treatment group compared to seven in the placebo group (De Binay et al 2010). This is an interesting study looking at a condition widely believed to be associated with increased NO production in liver cirrhosis.

DOSAGE RANGE

General guide

- Fresh garlic: 2–5 g/day (ensure it is bruised, crushed or chewed).
- Dried powder: 0.4–1.2 g/day.
- AGEs have been studied in amounts ranging from 2.4 to 7.2 g/day.
- Oil: 2–5 mg/day.
- Garlic preparations that will provide 4–12 mg alliin daily.
- Fluid extract (1 : 1): 0.5–2 mL three times daily.

According to clinical studies

- Type 2 diabetes: Allicor 300 mg twice daily.
- Hypertension: AGE: 480–960 mg standardised to SAC 4.8 mg/day in divided doses and taken for at least 12 weeks to see maximal results.
- Hyperlipidaemia: 600–900 mg/day.
- Hyperglycaemia: 1200–1500 mg/day.
- Fungal infection: topical 0.4–0.6% ajoene cream applied twice daily.
- Occlusive arterial disease: 600–800 mg/day.

It is important to be aware of the thiosulfinate content, in particular the allicin-releasing ability, of any commercial product to ensure efficacy.

ADVERSE REACTIONS

Internal use

Side effects tend to be limited to mild gastrointestinal side effects such as bloating, reflux, flatulence, garlic odour and breath. A dose–response study with hypertensive subjects found 32% of people using AGE at a dose of 960 mg daily experienced mild gastrointestinal side effects compared to 15% taking 480 mg daily. These effects were minimised by taking the garlic treatment in the morning (Ried et al 2013). Others have reported garlic odour and breath, allergic reactions, nausea, abdominal discomfort and diarrhoea (Berthold & Sudhop 1998). These side effects are more common when garlic is taken on an empty stomach and at doses greater than 1 g.

Headache, myalgia and fatigue were reported in one study using a dose of 900 mg garlic powder (standardised to 1.3% alliin) (Holzgartner et al 1992).

A meta-analysis of 37 RCTs investigating garlic for lipid lowering found no changes in liver function, biochemistry or haematology with use (Ried et al 2013).

Topical use

An ajoene 0.6% gel produces a transient burning sensation after application, according to one study (Ledezma et al 1999). Garlic has been classified as a type 1 allergen with various reactions, including contact dermatitis, urticaria, asthma, pemphigus and anaphylaxis, being reported. DADS, allylpropyl disulfide and allylmercaptin have been identified as allergens (Tsai et al 2012).

SIGNIFICANT INTERACTIONS

Saquinavir, darunavir and ritonavir

Ritonavir toxicity has been reported in AIDS patients co-administering with garlic, most likely due to P-glycoprotein inhibition by allicin in garlic (Tsai et al 2012) — avoid using concurrently (Piscitelli et al 2002).

Anticoagulants

Theoretically, a pharmacodynamic interaction is possible when using garlic at high doses (>7 g), in excess of usual dietary amounts; however, results from clinical studies cast doubt on this proposition. Published clinical studies have identified no significant action of enteric-coated or aged garlic on warfarin pharmacodynamics or pharmacokinetics. A double-blind, randomised, placebo-controlled pilot study of 48 patients demonstrated that the concomitant use of garlic containing 14.7 mg/day of SAC and warfarin showed no adverse effects (Macan et al 2006). An open-label, three-treatment, randomised, crossover clinical trial involving 12 healthy males, investigating potential effects of garlic and cranberry on warfarin (25 mg single dose), found that two garlic tablets daily containing 2000 mg of fresh garlic bulb equivalent to 3.71 mg of allicin per tablet did not significantly alter warfarin's pharmacokinetics or pharmacodynamics (Mohammed Abdul et al 2008). Use caution with doses >7 g/day.

Antiplatelet drugs

Theoretically, a pharmacodynamic interaction is possible when using garlic at high doses in excess of usual dietary amounts, although a small clinical study involving 10 adult participants showed garlic had no effect on platelet function (Beckert et al 2007). Observe.

Antihypertensive agents

Theoretically, potentiation effects are possible when using garlic at high doses in excess of usual dietary amounts — this can be used as adjunctive therapy to produce beneficial results — observe.

Antihyperlipidaemic agents

Theoretically, potentiation effects are possible when using garlic at high doses in excess of usual dietary amounts — this can be used as adjunctive therapy to produce beneficial results — observe.

Helicobacter pylori triple therapy

Additive effects are theoretically possible. While it is prudent to observe the patient for adverse reactions, the interaction may be beneficial.

Hepatotoxic drugs

Garlic may exert hepatoprotective activity against liver damage induced by drugs, according to in vitro tests, which suggest a beneficial interaction.

Paracetamol

In vivo protection from garlic and ajoene on paracetamol-induced hepatotoxicity has been observed (Hsu et al 2006) — beneficial interaction.

Hydrochlorothiazide

Co-administration may require a reduction in the dose of hydrochlorothiazide due to a pharmacokinetic interaction raising drug serum levels (Asdaq & Inamdar 2009). Cautious use under medical supervision.

CONTRAINDICATIONS AND PRECAUTIONS

Patients with bleeding abnormalities should avoid high doses of garlic. Although usual dietary intakes are likely to be safe prior to major surgery, suspend the use of high-dose garlic supplements 1 week before, as there is a theoretical increased risk of bleeding.

Avoid if known allergy to sulfurous vegetables. If being used as part of a topical application, a test patch is advised before more widespread application.

PREGNANCY USE

Garlic is not recommended at doses greater than usual dietary intakes in the first trimester until safety can be confirmed. A small trial in 100 pre-eclamptic primigravida women prescribed 800 mg of a dried garlic powder supplement throughout the third trimester reported no side effects or unexpected birth outcomes (Ziaei et al 2001).

Practice points/Patient counselling

- Garlic is both a food and a therapeutic medicine capable of significant and varied pharmacological activity.
- It has antioxidant, antimicrobial, modest antiplatelet, antithrombotic, antiatherosclerotic and vasoprotective activities.
- Human research confirms that some garlic preparations lower total cholesterol levels and blood pressure and possibly blood glucose levels in people with type 2 diabetes.
- It also enhances microcirculation and may have anti-inflammatory and immunostimulant activities.
- Garlic is used as a treatment for many common infections, to reduce the incidence of colds, to improve peripheral circulation and to manage hyperlipidaemia and hypertension.
- Topical garlic preparations have been used to treat common fungal infections.
- Several important drug interactions are possible with garlic (see significant interactions, above).

PATIENTS' FAQs

What will this herb do for me?

Garlic has many different actions in the body and is used to treat conditions such as elevated blood pressure and cholesterol levels, poor peripheral circulation, higher than normal blood glucose levels and common infections such as the common cold, flu and athlete's foot. Research suggests that it may be effective in all of these conditions; however, in some cases, the effect is small.

When will it start to work?

This varies greatly, depending on the reason for use. For example, garlic has been shown to improve microcirculation within 5 hours of ingestion, whereas slowing down of the atherosclerotic process or cancer-protective effects are likely to require several years' continuous use.

Are there any safety issues?

When garlic is taken at doses above the usual dietary levels, it may interact with a number of medications. Also, it should not be taken by people with bleeding disorders.

REFERENCES

Ali M, Thomson M. Consumption of a garlic clove a day could be beneficial in preventing thrombosis. Prostaglandins Leukot Essent Fatty Acids 53.3 (1995): 211–212.

Alkreathy, H., et al. Aged garlic extract protects against doxorubicin-induced cardiotoxicity in rats. Food and chemical toxicology 48 (2010) 951–956.

Alkreathy, H.M., et al. Mechanisms of cardioprotective effect of aged garlic extract against doxorubicin induced cardiotoxicity. Integrative Cancer Therapies 11.4 (2012): 364–370.

Allison GL, Lowe GM, Rahman K. Aged garlic extract may inhibit aggregation in human platelets by suppressing calcium mobilization. J Nutr 136 (3 Suppl) (2006): 789S–792S.

Al-Qattan KK et al. Nitric oxide mediates the blood-pressure lowering effect of garlic in the rat two-kidney, one-clip model of hypertension. J Nutr 136 (3 Suppl) (2006): 774S–776S.

Altonsy, M. O., T. N. Habib, and S. C. Andrews. Diallyl Disulfide-Induced Apoptosis in a Breast-Cancer Cell Line (MCF-7) may be caused by Inhibition of Histone Deacetylation. Nutrition and cancer 64.8 (2012): 1251–60.

An M et al. Allicin enhances the oxidative damage effect of amphotericin B against *Candida albicans*. Int J Antimicrob Agents 33.3 (2008): 258–263

An, MM et al. Allicin enhances the oxidative damage effect of amphotericin B against *Candida albicans*. International journal of antimicrobial agents 33.3 (2009): 258–263.

Andrianova IV, Fomchenkov IV, Orekhov AN. [Hypotensive effect of long-acting garlic tablets allicor (a double-blind placebo-controlled trial)]. Ter Arkh 74.3 (2002): 76–78.

Ankri S, Mirelman D. Antimicrobial properties of allicin from garlic. Microbes Infect 1.2 (1999): 125–129.

Arhan M et al. Hepatic oxidant/antioxidant status in cholesterol-fed rabbits: effects of garlic extract. Hepatol Res 39.1 (2009): 70–77.

Arora RC, Arora S. Comparative effect of clofibrate, garlic and onion on alimentary hyperlipemia. Atherosclerosis 39.4 (1981): 447–452.

Arunkumar A et al. Induction of apoptosis and histone hyperacetylation by diallyl disulfide in prostate cancer cell line PC-3. Cancer Lett 251.1 (2007): 59–67.

Arunkumar, R., et al. Effect of Diallyl Disulfide on Insulin-Like Growth Factor Signaling Molecules Involved in Cell Survival and Proliferation of Human Prostate Cancer Cells in Vitro and in Silico Approach through Docking Analysis. Phytomedicine 19.10 (2012): 912–23.

Asadpour, R., et al. Comparison of the Protective Effects of Garlic (*Allium sativum* L) Extract, Vitamin E and N Acetyl Cystein on Testis Structure and Sperm Quality in Rats Treated with Lead Acetate. Revue de Medecine Veterinaire 164.1 (2013): 28–33.

Asdaq, S. M. B., and M. N. Inamdar. The potential for interaction of hydochlorothiazide with Garlic in Rats. Chemico-biological Interactions 181 (2009):472–79.

Asdaq, S. M. & Inamdar, M. N. Potential of garlic and its active constituent, S-allyl cysteine, as antihypertensive and cardioprotective in presence of captopril. Phytomed. 17 (2010) 1016–26.

Ashraf R et al. Effects of garlic on dyslipidemia in patients with type 2 diabetes mellitus. J Ayub Med Coll Abbottabad 17.3 (2005): 60–64.

Ashraf, R., et al. Garlic (*Allium sativum*) supplementation with standard antidiabetic agent provides better diabetic control in type 2 diabetes patients. Pak J Pharm Sci. 24.4 (2011): 565–70.

Atkin, M. The effects of garlic upon endothelial function, vascular inflammation, oxidative stress and insulin resistance in patients with type 2 diabetes at high cardiovascular risk: a double blind randomised placebo controlled trial. Dissertation. University of Portsmouth, 2011.

Auer, W., Eiber, A., Hertkorn, E., et al. 1990. Hypertension and hyperlipidaemia: garlic helps in mild cases. Br J Clin. Pract. Suppl, 69, 3–6.

Augusti KT, Sheela CG. Antiperoxide effect of S-allyl cysteine sulfoxide, an insulin secretagogue, in diabetic rats. Experientia 52.2 (1996): 115–120.

Avci A et al. Effects of garlic consumption on plasma and erythrocyte antioxidant parameters in elderly subjects. Gerontology 54.3 (2008): 173–176

Avci, B., et al. Oxidative Stress Induced by 1.8 GHz Radio Frequency Electromagnetic Radiation and Effects of Garlic Extract in Rats. International journal of radiation biology 88.11 (2012): 7

Aydin A et al. Garlic oil and *Helicobacter pylori* infection. Am J Gastroenterol 95.2 (2000): 563–564.

Bakri IM, Douglas CW. Inhibitory effect of garlic extract on oral bacteria. Arch Oral Biol 50.7 (2005): 645–651.

Beckert BW et al. The effect of herbal medicines on platelet function: an in vivo experiment and review of the literature. Plast Reconstr Surg 120.7 (2007): 2044–2050.

Berthold HK, Sudhop T. Garlic preparations for prevention of atherosclerosis. Curr Opin Lipidol 9.6 (1998): 565–569.

Bianchini F, Vainio H. Allium vegetables and organosulfur compounds: do they help prevent cancer? Environ Health Perspect 109.9 (2001): 893–902.

Blumenthal M. Herbal medicine — expanded Commission E monographs. Newton: American Botanical Council, 2000.

Bordia A, Verma SK, Srivastava KC. Effect of garlic (*Allium sativum*) on blood lipids, blood sugar, fibrinogen and fibrinolytic activity in patients with coronary artery disease. Prostaglandins Leukot Essent Fatty Acids 58.4 (1998): 257–263.

Borek C. Garlic reduces dementia and heart-disease risk. J Nutr 136 (3 Suppl) (2006): 810S–812S.

Brady JF et al. Inhibition of cytochrome P-450 2E1 by diallyl sulfide and its metabolites. Chem Res Toxicol 4.6 (1991): 642–647.

Budoff M. Aged garlic extract retards progression of coronary artery calcification. J Nutr 136 (3 Suppl) (2006): 741S–744S.

Budoff, M. J., et al. Aged garlic extract supplemented with B vitamins, folic acid and L-arginine retards the progression of subclinical atherosclerosis: a randomized clinical trial. Preventive Medicine, 49(2), (2009). 101–107.

Campbell JH et al. Molecular basis by which garlic suppresses atherosclerosis. J Nutr 131.3s (2001): 1006S–1009S.

Cavagnaro PF et al. Effect of cooking on garlic (*Allium sativum* L.) antiplatelet activity and thiosulfinates content. J Agric Food Chem 55.4 (2007): 1280–1288.

Cellini L et al. Inhibition of *Helicobacter pylori* by garlic extract (*Allium sativum*). FEMS Immunol Med Microbiol 13.4 (1996): 273–277.

Chan KC, Yin MC, Chao WJ. Effect of diallyl trisulfide-rich garlic oil on blood coagulation and plasma activity of anticoagulation factors in rats. Food Chem Toxicol 45.3 (2007): 502–507.

Chandra-Kuntal, K., J. Lee, and S. V. Singh. Critical Role for Reactive Oxygen Species in Apoptosis Induction and Cell Migration Inhibition by Diallyl Trisulfide, a Cancer Chemopreventive Component of Garlic. Breast cancer research and treatment 138.1 (2013): 69–79.

Chandrashekar, P.M. Venkatesh, Y. P. Identification of the protein components displaying immunomodulatory activity in aged garlic extract. Journal of ethnopharmacology 124.3 (2009): 384–390.

Chandrashekar, P. M., Prashanth, K. V. H., and Venkatesh, Y. P. Isolation, structural elucidation and immunomodulatory activity of fructans from aged garlic extract. Phytochemistry 72.2 (2011): 255–264.

Chen C et al. Induction of detoxifying enzymes by garlic organosulfur compounds through transcription factor Nrf2: effect of chemical structure and stress signals. Free Radic Biol Med 37.10 (2004): 1578–1590.

Chiu, T. -H, et al. Diallyl Sulfide Promotes Cell-Cycle Arrest through the p53 Expression and Triggers Induction of Apoptosis Via Caspase- and Mitochondria-Dependent Signaling Pathways in Human Cervical Cancer Ca Ski Cells. Nutrition and cancer 65.3 (2013): 505–14.

Cho SJ, Rhee DK, Pyo S. Allicin, a major component of garlic, inhibits apoptosis of macrophage in a depleted nutritional state. Nutrition 22.11–12 (2006): 1177–1184.

Chowdhury R et al. In vitro and in vivo reduction of sodium arsenite induced toxicity by aqueous garlic extract. Food Chem Toxicol 46.2 (2008): 740–751.

Chung LY. The antioxidant properties of garlic compounds: allyl cysteine, alliin, allicin, and allyl disulfide. J Med Food 9.2 (2006): 205–213.

Chung, J. G., et al. Effects of garlic compounds diallyl sulfide and diallyl disulfide on arylamine N-acetyltransferase activity in strains of *Helicobacter pylori* from peptic ulcer patients. The American journal of Chinese medicine 26.03–04 (1998): 353–364.

Chutani SK, Bordia A. The effect of fried versus raw garlic on fibrinolytic activity in man. Atherosclerosis 38.3–4 (1981): 417–421.

Clement, F, Venkatesh YP. Dietary garlic (*Allium sativum*) lectins, ASA I and ASA II, are highly stable and immunogenic. International immunopharmacology 10.10 (2010): 1161–1169.

Clement F, Pramod SN, Venkatesh YP. Identity of the immunomodulatory proteins from garlic (*Allium sativum*) with the major garlic lectins or agglutinins. International Immunopharmacology 10.3 (2010): 316–324.

Coppi A et al. Antimalarial activity of allicin, a biologically active compound from garlic cloves. Antimicrob Agents Chemother 50.5 (2006): 1731–1737.

Cox MC et al. Influence of garlic (*Allium sativum*) on the pharmacokinetics of docetaxel. Clin Cancer Res 12.15 (2006): 4636–4640.

Dalvi RR. Alterations in hepatic phase I and phase II biotransformation enzymes by garlic oil in rats. Toxicol Lett 60.3 (1992): 299–305.

D'Argenio, G., et al. Garlic Extract Attenuating Rat Liver Fibrosis by Inhibiting TGF-β1. Clinical Nutrition 32.2 (2013): 252–8.

Dae Yun Seo, et al. Aged garlic extract enhances exercise-mediated improvement of metabolic parameters in high fat diet induced obese rats. Nutr Res Pract 6.6 (2012): 513–519.

Davis SR. An overview of the antifungal properties of allicin and its breakdown products – the possibility of a safe and effective antifungal prophylactic. Mycoses 48.2 (2005): 95–100.

Davis LE, Shen J, Royer RE. In vitro synergism of concentrated *Allium sativum* extract and amphotericin B against *Cryptococcus neoformans*. Planta Med 60.6 (1994): 546–549.

De Binay K., et al. The role of garlic in hepatopulmonary syndrome: a randomized controlled trial. Canadian Journal of Gastroenterology 24.3 (2010): 183.

Dhawan V, Jain S. Garlic supplementation prevents oxidative DNA damage in essential hypertension. Mol Cell Biochem 275.1–2 (2005): 85–94.

Dong, Q., et al. Stimulation of IFN-γ Production by Garlic Lectin in Mouse Spleen Cells: Involvement of IL-12 via Activation of p38 MAPK and ERK in Macrophages. Phytomedicine 18.4 (2011): 309–16.

Druesne N et al. Diallyl disulfide (DADS) increases histone acetylation and p21(waf1/cip1) expression in human colon tumor cell lines. Carcinogenesis 25.7 (2004): 1227–1236.

Duke Dr. Dr Duke's phytochemical and ethnobotanical database. Available online at: http://www.ars-grin. gov/duke/ (accessed 2003).

Durak I et al. Effects of garlic extract on oxidant/antioxidant status and atherosclerotic plaque formation in rabbit aorta. Nutr Metab Cardiovasc Dis 12.3 (2002): 141–147.

Eftekhari, Z., et al. Evaluating the Anti-Leech (*Limnatis nilotica*) Activity of Methanolic Extract of *Allium sativum* L. Compared with Levamisole and Metronidazole. Comparative Clinical Pathology 21.6 (2012): 1219–22.

Ehnert, S., et al. Diallyl-disulphide is the effective ingredient of garlic oil that protects primary human osteoblasts from damage due to cigarette smoke. Food Chemistry 132.2 (2012): 724–729.

Eidi A, Eidi M, Esmaeili E. Antidiabetic effect of garlic (*Allium sativum* L.) in normal and streptozotocin-induced diabetic rats. Phytomedicine 13.9–10 (2006): 624–629.

Eja ME et al. A comparative assessment of the antimicrobial effects of garlic (*Allium sativum*) and antibiotics on diarrheagenic organisms. Southeast Asian J Trop Med Public Health 38.2 (2007): 343–348.

El-Sabban F, Abouazra H. Effect of garlic on atherosclerosis and its factors. East Mediterr Health J 14.1 (2008): 195–205.

Engdal S, Klepp O, Nilsen OG. Identification and exploration of herb-drug combinations used by cancer patients. Integr Cancer Ther 8.1 (2009): 29–36.

Ernsberger P et al. Therapeutic actions of allylmercaptocaptopril and captopril in a rat model of metabolic syndrome. Am J Hypertens 20.8 (2007): 866–874.

Ernst, E. The current position of complementary/alternative medicine in cancer. European Journal of Cancer 39.16 (2003): 2273–2277.

Ernst, E., and P. Posadzki. Can Garlic-Intake Reduce the Risk of Cancer? A Systematic Review of Randomised Controlled Trials. Focus on Alternative and Complementary Therapies 17.4 (2012): 192–6.

Fallah-Rostami, F., et al. "Immunomodulatory Activity of Aged Garlic Extract Against Implanted Fibrosarcoma Tumor in Mice." North American Journal of Medical Sciences 5.3 (2013): 207–12.

Fallon MB et al. Garlic prevents hypoxic pulmonary hypertension in rats. Am J Physiol 275.2 (Pt 1) (1998): L283–L287.

Fani MM, Kohanteb J, Dayaghi M. Inhibitory activity of garlic (*Allium sativum*) extract on multidrug-resistant *Streptococcus mutans*. J Indian Soc Pedod Prev Dent 25.4 (2007): 164–168.

Feng, Y., et al. Allicin Enhances Host Pro-Inflammatory Immune Responses and Protects Against Acute Murine Malaria Infection. Malaria Journal 11 (2012) 10–1186.

Ferri N et al. Ajoene, a garlic compound, inhibits protein prenylation and arterial smooth muscle cell proliferation. Br J Pharmacol 138.5 (2003): 811–8118.

Fisher CD et al. Induction of drug-metabolizing enzymes by garlic and allyl sulfide compounds via activation of constitutive androstane receptor and nuclear factor E2-related factor 2. Drug Metab Dispos 35.6 (2007): 995–1000.

Fleischauer AT, Arab L. Garlic and cancer: a critical review of the epidemiologic literature. J Nutr 131.3s (2001): 1032S–1040S.

Foster BC et al. An in vitro evaluation of human cytochrome P450 3A4 and P-glycoprotein inhibition by garlic. J Pharm Pharm Sci 4.2 (2001): 176–184.

Frantz DJ et al. Cell cycle arrest and differential gene expression in HT-29 cells exposed to an aqueous garlic extract. Nutr Cancer 38.2 (2000): 255–264.

Fukao H et al. Antithrombotic effects of odorless garlic powder both in vitro and in vivo. Biosci Biotechnol Biochem 71.1 (2007): 84–90.

Gaafar, MR. Efficacy of *Allium sativum* (garlic) against experimental cryptosporidiosis. Alexandria Journal of Medicine 48.1 (2012): 59–66.

Gadkari JV, Joshi VD. Effect of ingestion of raw garlic on serum cholesterol level, clotting time and fibrinolytic activity in normal subjects. J Postgrad Med 37.3 (1991): 128–131.

Galeone C et al. Allium vegetables intake and endometrial cancer risk. Public Health Nutr (2008): 1–4.

Gapter LA, Yuin OZ, Ng KY. S-Allylcysteine reduces breast tumor cell adhesion and invasion. Biochem Biophys Res Commun 367.2 (2008): 446–451.

Ghazanfari T, Hassan ZM, Khamesipour A. Enhancement of peritoneal macrophage phagocytic activity against *Leishmania major* by garlic (*Allium sativum*) treatment. J Ethnopharmacol 103.3 (2006): 333–337.

Gonen A et al. The antiatherogenic effect of allicin: possible mode of action. Pathobiology 72.6 (2005): 325–334.

Gorinstein S et al. Dose-dependent influence of commercial garlic (*Allium sativum*) on rats fed cholesterol-containing diet. J Agric Food Chem 54.11 (2006): 4022–4027.

Gorinstein S et al. The atherosclerotic heart disease and protecting properties of garlic: contemporary data. Mol Nutr Food Res 51.11 (2007): 1365–1381.

Graham DY, Anderson SY, Lang T. Garlic or jalapeno peppers for treatment of *Helicobacter pylori* infection. Am J Gastroenterol 94.5 (1999): 1200–1202.

Greenblatt DJ, Leigh-Pemberton RA, von Moltke LL. In vitro interactions of water-soluble garlic components with human cytochromes p450. J Nutr 136 (3 Suppl) (2006): 806S–809S.

Groppo FC et al. Antimicrobial activity of garlic against oral streptococci. Int J Dent Hyg 5.2 (2007): 109–115.

Gupta VB, Rao KS. Anti-amyloidogenic activity of S-allyl-L-cysteine and its activity to destabilize Alzheimer's beta-amyloid fibrils in vitro. Neurosci Lett 429.2–3 (2007): 75–80.

Gupta VB, Indi SS, Rao KS. Garlic extract exhibits antiamyloidogenic activity on amyloid-beta fibrillogenesis: relevance to Alzheimer's disease. Phytother Res 23.1 (2009): 111–115.

Gurley BJ et al. Cytochrome P450 phenotypic ratios for predicting herb–drug interactions in humans. Clin Pharmacol Ther 72.3 (2002): 276–287.

Gurley BJ et al. Clinical assessment of effects of botanical supplementation on cytochrome P450 phenotypes in the elderly: St John's wort, garlic oil, Panax ginseng and Ginkgo biloba. Drugs Aging 22.6 (2005): 525–539.

Hajda, J., Rentsch, K.M., Gubler, C., et al. 2010. Garlic extract induces intestinal P-glycoprotein, but exhibits no effect on intestinal and hepatic CYP3A4 in humans. Eur.J Pharm.Sci., 41, (5) 729–735.

Harauma A, Moriguchi T. Aged garlic extract improves blood pressure in spontaneously hypertensive rats more safely than raw garlic. J Nutr 136 (3 Suppl) (2006): 769S–73S.

Hassan HT. Ajoene (natural garlic compound): a new anti-leukaemia agent for AML therapy. Leuk Res 28.7 (2004): 667–671.

Hassan A., et al. Garlic oil as a modulating agent for oxidative stress and neurotoxicity induced by sodium nitrite in male albino rats. Food and Chemical Toxicology 48 (2010): 1980–1985.

Hattori A et al. Antidiabetic effects of ajoene in genetically diabetic KK-A(y) mice. Tokyo: J Nutr Sci Vitaminol, 51.5 (2005): 382–40.

Herman-Antosiewicz A, Singh SV. Checkpoint kinase 1 regulates diallyl trisulfide-induced mitotic arrest in human prostate cancer cells. J Biol Chem 280.31 (2005): 28519–28528.

Herman-Antosiewicz A, Powolny AA, Singh SV. Molecular targets of cancer chemoprevention by garlic-derived organosulfides. Acta Pharmacol Sin 28.9 (2007): 1355–1364.

Holzgartner H, Schmidt U, Kuhn U. Comparison of the efficacy and tolerance of a garlic preparation vs. bezafibrate. Arzneimittelforschung 42.12 (1992): 1473–1477.

Hong JY et al. Metabolism of carcinogenic nitrosamines by rat nasal mucosa and the effect of diallyl sulfide. Cancer Res 51.5 (1991): 1509–1514.

Hong YS et al. Effects of allyl sulfur compounds and garlic extract on the expression of Bcl-2, Bax, and p53 in non small cell lung cancer cell lines. Exp Mol Med 32.3 (2000): 127–134.

Hosono T et al. Alkenyl group is responsible for the disruption of microtubule network formation in human colon cancer cell line HT-29 cells. Carcinogenesis 29.7 (2008): 1400–1406.

Hosseini, E., Bahrami, A.M., Razmjo, M. Study of the effects of raw garlic consumption on lipids and some blood biochemical factors in hyperlipdemic individuals. Global Veterinaria 10.1 (2013): 9–12.

Hsu CC et al. Protective effect of s-allyl cysteine and s-propyl cysteine on acetaminophen-induced hepatotoxicity in mice. Food and Chemical Toxicology 44.3 (2006): 393–397.

Hu X et al. Attenuation of cell migration and induction of cell death by aged garlic extract in rat sarcoma cells. Int J Mol Med 9.6 (2002): 641–643.

Ibrahim, A. N. Comparison of in Vitro Activity of Metronidazole and Garlic-Based Product (Tomex®) on *Trichomonas vaginalis*. Parasitology research 112.5 (2013): 2063–7

Ide N, Keller C, Weiss N. Aged garlic extract inhibits homocysteine-induced CD36 expression and foam cell formation in human macrophages. J Nutr 136 (3 Suppl) (2006): 755S–758S.

Imai T et al. Amyloid beta-protein potentiates tunicamycin-induced neuronal death in organotypic hippocampal slice cultures. Neuroscience 147.3 (2007): 639–651.

Ishige K et al. Role of caspase-12 in amyloid beta-peptide-induced toxicity in organotypic hippocampal slices cultured for long periods. J Pharmacol Sci 104.1 (2007): 46–55.

Jabbari A et al. Comparison between swallowing and chewing of garlic on levels of serum lipids, cyclosporine, creatinine and lipid peroxidation in renal transplant recipients. Lipids Health Dis 4 (2005): 11.

Jarial MS. Toxic effect of garlic extracts on the eggs of *Aedes aegypti* (Diptera: Culicidae): A scanning electron microscopic study. J Med Entomol 38.3 (2001): 446–450.

Jelodar GA et al. Effect of fenugreek, onion and garlic on blood glucose and histopathology of pancreas of alloxan-induced diabetic rats. Indian J Med Sci 59.2 (2005): 64–69.

Jepson, R.G. et al. Garlic for peripheral arterial occlusive disease. John Wiley and Sons, The Cochrane Library Issue 3 (2008)

Jeyaraj S et al. Effect of combined supplementation of fish oil with garlic pearls on the serum lipid profile in hypercholesterolemic subjects. Indian Heart J 57.4 (2005): 327–331.

Jo HJ et al. Diallyl disulfide induces reversible G2/M phase arrest on a p53-independent mechanism in human colon cancer HCT-116 cells. Oncol Rep 19.1 (2008): 275–280.

Jonkers D et al. Antibacterial effect of garlic and omeprazole on *Helicobacter pylori*. J Antimicrob Chemother 43.6 (1999): 837–839.

Josling P. Preventing the common cold with a garlic supplement: a double-blind, placebo-controlled survey. Adv Ther 18.4 (2001): 189–193.

Jung EM et al. Influence of garlic powder on cutaneous microcirculation. A randomized placebo-controlled double-blind cross-over study in apparently healthy subjects. Arzneimittelforschung 41.6 (1991): 626–630.

Kabasakal L et al. Protective effect of aqueous garlic extract against renal ischemia/reperfusion injury in rats. J Med Food 8.3 (2005): 319–326.

Khatua, T. N., et al. Garlic provides protection to mice heart against isoproterenol-induced oxidative damage: Role of nitric oxide. Nitric Oxide 27 (2012):9–17.

Kiesewetter H et al. Effects of garlic coated tablets in peripheral arterial occlusive disease. Clin Investig 71.5 (1993a): 383–386.

Kiesewetter H, Jung F, Jung EM, et al. Effect of garlic on platelet aggregation in patients with increased risk of juvenile ischaemic attack. Eur J Clin Pharmacol 45.4 (1993b): 333–336.

Kim JY, Kwon O. Garlic intake and cancer risk: an analysis using the Food and Drug Administration's evidence-based review system for the scientific evaluation of health claims. Am J Clin Nutr 89.1 (2009): 257–264.

Kim, H. J., et al. Hexane Extracts of Garlic Cloves Induce Apoptosis through the Generation of Reactive Oxygen Species in Hep3B Human Hepatocarcinoma Cells. Oncology reports 28.5 (2012): 1757–63.

Kim-Park S, Ku DD. Garlic elicits a nitric oxide-dependent relaxation and inhibits hypoxic pulmonary vasoconstriction in rats. Clin Exp Pharmacol Physiol 27.10 (2000): 780–786.

Knowles LM, Milner JA. Diallyl disulfide induces ERK phosphorylation and alters gene expression profiles in human colon tumor cells. J Nutr 133.9 (2003): 2901–2906.

Koscielny J et al. The antiatherosclerotic effect of *Allium sativum*. Atherosclerosis 144.1 (1999): 237–249.

Kwon MJ et al. Cholesteryl ester transfer protein activity and atherogenic parameters in rabbits supplemented with cholesterol and garlic powder. Life Sci 72.26 (2003): 2953–2964.

Kumar, R., et al. Antihyperglycemic, antihyperlipidemic, anti-inflammatory and adenosine deaminase – lowering effects of garlic in patients with type 2 diabetes mellitus with obesity Diabetes, Metabolic Syndrome and Obesity: Targets and Therapy 6 (2013): 49–56.

Lau BH. Suppression of LDL oxidation by garlic compounds is a possible mechanism of cardiovascular health benefit. J Nutr 136 (3 Suppl) (2006): 765S–768S.

Lawson LD, Ransom DK, Hughes BG. Inhibition of whole blood platelet-aggregation by compounds in garlic clove extracts and commercial garlic products. Thromb Res 65.2 (1992): 141–156.

Lawson LD, Wang ZJ, Papadimitriou D. Allicin release under simulated gastrointestinal conditions from garlic powder tablets employed in clinical trials on serum cholesterol. Planta Med 67.1 (2001): 13–118.

Lea MA, Randolph VM. Induction of histone acetylation in rat liver and hepatoma by organosulfur compounds including diallyl disulfide. Anticancer Res 21.4A (2001): 2841–2845.

Ledezma E, Apitz-Castro R. [Ajoene the main active compound of garlic (*Allium sativum*): a new antifungal agent.] Rev Iberoam Micol 23.2 (2006): 75–80.

Ledezma, E et al. Ajoene in the topical short-term treatment of tinea cruris and tinea corporis in humans. Arzneimittelforschung 49.06 (1999): 544–547.

Ledezma E et al. Efficacy of ajoene in the treatment of tinea pedis: a double-blind and comparative study with terbinafine. J Am Acad Dermatol 43.5 Pt 1 (2000): 829–832.

Lee HS et al. Inhibition of cyclooxygenase 2 expression by diallyl sulfide on joint inflammation induced by urate crystal and IL-1beta. Osteoarthritis Cartilage 17.1 (2009): 91–99.

Lee, D. Y., et al. Anti-Inflammatory Activity of Sulfur-Containing Compounds from Garlic. Journal of Medicinal Food 15.11 (2012a): 992–9.

Lee, M. H., Y. M. Kim, and S. G. Kim. Efficacy and Tolerability of Diphenyl-Dimethyldicarboxylate Plus Garlic Oil in Patients with Chronic Hepatitis. International journal of clinical pharmacology and therapeutics 50.11 (2012b): 778–86.

Lei YP et al. Diallyl disulfide and diallyl trisulfide suppress oxidized LDL-induced vascular cell adhesion molecule and E-selectin expression through protein kinase A- and B-dependent signaling pathways. J Nutr 138.6 (2008): 996–1003.

Lin HL et al. The role of Ca2+ on the DADS-induced apoptosis in mouse-rat hybrid retina ganglion cells (N18). Neurochem Res 31.3 (2006): 383–393.

Liu CT et al. Effects of garlic oil and diallyl trisulfide on glycemic control in diabetic rats. Eur J Pharmacol 516.2 (2005): 165–173.

Liu KL et al. DATS reduces LPS-induced iNOS expression, NO production, oxidative stress, and NF-kappaB activation in RAW 264.7 macrophages. J Agric Food Chem 54.9 (2006): 3472–3478.

Macan H et al. Aged garlic extract may be safe for patients on warfarin therapy. J Nutr 136 (3 Suppl) (2006): 793S–795S.

Mahmoodi M et al. Study of the effects of raw garlic consumption on the level of lipids and other blood biochemical factors in hyperlipidemic individuals. Pak J Pharm Sci 19.4 (2006): 295–298.

Matsuura N et al. Aged garlic extract inhibits angiogenesis and proliferation of colorectal carcinoma cells. J Nutr 136 (3 Suppl) (2006): 842S–846S.

McCullough, M. L., et al. "Garlic Consumption and Colorectal Cancer Risk in the CPS-II Nutrition Cohort." Cancer Causes and Control 23.10 (2012): 1643–51.

McNulty CA et al. A pilot study to determine the effectiveness of garlic oil capsules in the treatment of dyspeptic patients with *Helicobacter pylori*. Helicobacter 6.3 (2001): 249–253.

Medina-Campos ON et al. S-allylcysteine scavenges singlet oxygen and hypochlorous acid and protects LLC-PK(1) cells of potassium dichromate-induced toxicity. Food Chem Toxicol 45.10 (2007): 2030–2039.

Meng, S., et al. No Association between Garlic Intake and Risk of Colorectal Cancer. Cancer Epidemiology 37.2 (2013): 152–5.

Mohamadi A et al. Effects of wild versus cultivated garlic on blood pressure and other parameters in hypertensive rats. Heart Dis 2.1 (2000): 3–9.

Mohammed Abdul MI, Jiang X, Williams, K.M., et al. Pharmacodynamic interaction of warfarin with cranberry but not with garlic in healthy subjects. Br J Pharmacol 154.8 (2008): 1691–1700.

Moriarty RM, Naithani R, Surve B. Organosulfur compounds in cancer chemoprevention. Mini Rev Med Chem 7.8 (2007): 827–838.

Morihara, N., Nagatoshi, I., Weiss, N. Aged garlic extract inhibits homocysteine-induced scavenger receptor CD36 expression and oxidized low-density lipoprotein cholesterol uptake in human macrophages in vitro. J of ethnopharm. 134 (2011): 711–716.

Mosallanejad, B., et al. A Comparison between Metformin and Garlic on Alloxan-Induced Diabetic Dogs. Comparative Clinical Pathology 22.2 (2013): 169–74.

Mousa AS, Mousa SA. Anti-angiogenesis efficacy of the garlic ingredient alliin and antioxidants: role of nitric oxide and p53. Nutr Cancer 53.1 (2005): 104–110.

Mulrow C et al. Garlic: effects on cardiovascular risks and disease, protective effects against cancer, and clinical adverse effects. Evid Rep Technol Assess (Summ) 20 (2000): 1–4.

Nagini S. Cancer chemoprevention by garlic and its organosulfur compounds-panacea or promise? Anticancer Agents Med 8.3 (2008): 313–321.

Nakagawa H et al. Growth inhibitory effects of diallyl disulfide on human breast cancer cell lines. Carcinogenesis 22.6 (2001): 891–897.

Nakasone, Y., et al. Effect of a Traditional Japanese Garlic Preparation on Blood Pressure in Prehypertensive and Mildly Hypertensive Adults. Experimental and Therapeutic Medicine 5.2 (2013): 399–405.

Nantz, M. P., et al. Supplementation with aged garlic extract improves both nk and γδ-t cell function and reduces the severity of cold and flu symptoms: a randomized, double-blind, placebo-controlled nutrition intervention. Clinical Nutrition 31.3 (2012): 337–44

Ngo SN et al. Does garlic reduce risk of colorectal cancer? A systematic review. J Nutr 137.10 (2007): 2264–2269.

O'Gara EA, Hill DJ, Maslin DJ. Activities of garlic oil, garlic powder, and their diallyl constituents against *Helicobacter pylori*. Appl Environ Microbiol 66.5 (2000): 2269–2273.

O'Gara EA et al. The effect of simulated gastric environments on the anti-*Helicobacter* activity of garlic oil. J Appl Microbiol 104.5 (2008): 1324–1331.

Ohiro, A., et al. Effects of the "Aomori Garlic Extract"-Containing Dietary Supplement on the Stress, Quality of Sleep, Fatigue, and Quality of Life in Active Workers. Japanese Pharmacology and Therapeutics 41.3 (2013): 281–7.

Ola-Mudathir KF et al. Protective roles of onion and garlic extracts on cadmium-induced changes in sperm characteristics and testicular oxidative damage in rats. Food Chem Toxicol 46.12 (2008): 3604–3611.

Orekhov AN et al. Direct anti-atherosclerosis-related effects of garlic. Ann Med 27.1 (1995): 63–65.

Padiya, R., et al. Garlic improves insulin sensitivity and associated metabolic syndromes in fructose fed rats. Nutrition and metabolism (2011); 8: 53.

Phil, R. A. M., et al. Effects of garlic on blood glucose levels and HbA1c in patients with type 2 diabetes mellitus. J. of Med. Plants Research 5.13 (2011): 2922–28.

Piscitelli SC et al. The effect of garlic supplements on the pharmacokinetics of saquinavir. Clin Infect Dis 34.2 (2002): 234–238.

Powolny AA, Singh SV. Multitargeted prevention and therapy of cancer by diallyl trisulfide and related *Allium* vegetable-derived organosulfur compounds. Cancer Lett 269.2 (2008): 305–314.

Rahman K. Effects of garlic on platelet biochemistry and physiology. Mol Nutr Food Res 51.11 (2007): 1335–1344.

Rahman K, Billington D. Dietary supplementation with aged garlic extract inhibits ADP-induced platelet aggregation in humans. J Nutr 130.11 (2000): 2662–2665.
Rahman K, Lowe GM. Garlic and cardiovascular disease: a critical review. J Nutr 136 (3 Suppl) (2006): 736S–740S.
Rassoul F et al. The influence of garlic (*Allium sativum*) extract on interleukin 1alpha-induced expression of endothelial intercellular adhesion molecule-1 and vascular cell adhesion molecule-1. Phytomedicine 13.4 (2006): 230–235.
Reinhart KM et al. Effects of garlic on blood pressure in patients with and without systolic hypertension: a meta-analysis. Ann Pharmacother 42.12 (2008): 1766–1771.
Ried K et al. Effect of garlic on blood pressure: a systematic review and meta-analysis. BMC Cardiovasc Disord 8 (2008): 13.
Ried, K., O. R. Frank, and N. P. Stocks. Aged Garlic Extract Lowers Blood Pressure in Patients with Treated but Uncontrolled Hypertension: A Randomised Controlled Trial. Maturitas 67.2 (2010): 144–50.
Ried, K., et al. Aged garlic extract reduces blood pressure in hypertensives: a dose-response trial. European journal of clinical nutrition 67.1 (2013): 64–70.
Ried, K., et al. Effect of garlic on serum lipids: an updated meta-analysis. Nutr Rev 71.5 (2013): 282–299
Rose P et al. Bioactive S-alk(en)yl cysteine sulfoxide metabolites in the genus Allium: the chemistry of potential therapeutic agents. Nat Prod Rep 22.3 (2005): 351–368.
Sabitha P et al. Efficacy of garlic paste in oral candidiasis. Trop Doct 35.2 (2005): 99–100.
Scheiman JM, Cutler AF. *Helicobacter pylori* and gastric cancer. Am J Med 106.2 (1999): 222–226.
Seki T et al. Anticancer effects of diallyl trisulfide derived from garlic. Asia Pac J Clin Nutr 17 (Suppl 1) (2008): 249–252.
Sener G et al. Chronic nicotine toxicity is prevented by aqueous garlic extract. Plant Foods Hum Nutr 60.2 (2005): 77–86.
Seo, D Y, et al. Aged garlic extract enhances exercise-mediated improvement of metabolic parameters in high fat diet-induced obese rats. Nutrition research and practice 6.6 (2012): 513–519.
Sher, A., et al. Effect of Garlic Extract on Blood Glucose Level and Lipid Profile in Normal and Alloxan Diabetic Rabbits. Advances in Clinical and Experimental Medicine 21.6 (2012): 705–11.
Shukla Y, Kalra N. Cancer chemoprevention with garlic and its constituents. Cancer Lett 247.2 (2007): 167–181.
Siegel G, Klussendorf D. The anti-atheroslerotic effect of *Allium sativum*: statistics re-evaluated. Atherosclerosis 150.2 (2000): 437–438.
Silagy CA, Neil HA. A meta-analysis of the effect of garlic on blood pressure. J Hypertens 12.4 (1994): 463–468.
Singh DK, Porter TD. Inhibition of sterol 4alpha-methyl oxidase is the principal mechanism by which garlic decreases cholesterol synthesis. J Nutr 136.(3 Suppl) (2006): 759S–764S.
Singh SV et al. Differential induction of NAD(P)H:quinone oxidoreductase by anti-carcinogenic organosulfides from garlic. Biochem Biophys Res Commun 244.3 (1998): 917–920.
Sobenin IA et al. [Allicor efficacy in lowering the risk of ischemic heart disease in primary prophylaxis.] Ter Arkh 77.12 (2005): 9–13.
Sobenin IA et al. [Use of allicor to lower the risk of myocardial infarction.] Klin Med (Mosk) 85.3 (2007): 25–28.
Sobenin IA et al. Lipid-lowering effects of time-released garlic powder tablets in double-blinded placebo-controlled randomized study. J Atheroscler Thromb 15.6 (2008): 334–338.
Song JD et al. Molecular mechanism of diallyl disulfide in cell cycle arrest and apoptosis in HCT-116 colon cancer cells. J Biochem Mol Toxicol 23.1 (2009): 71–79.
Sriram N et al. Diallyl sulfide induces apoptosis in Colo 320 DM human colon cancer cells: involvement of caspase-3, NF-kappaB, and ERK-2. Mol Cell Biochem 311.1–2 (2008): 157–165.
Stabler, S. N., et al. Garlic for the prevention of cardiovascular morbidity and mortality in hypertensive patients., Cochrane Database of Systematic Reviews, no. 8, Article ID CD007653, 2012
Stargrove M, Treasure J, McKee D. Herb, nutrient and drug interactions. St Louis: Mosby, Elsevier, 2008.
Steiner M et al. A double-blind crossover study in moderately hypercholesterolemic men that compared the effect of aged garlic extract and placebo administration on blood lipids. Am J Clin Nutr 64.6 (1996): 866–870.
Stevinson C, Pittler MH, Ernst E. Garlic for treating hypercholesterolemia. A meta-analysis of randomized clinical trials. Ann Intern Med 133.6 (2001): 420–429.
Suru SM. Onion and garlic extracts lessen cadmium-induced nephrotoxicity in rats. Biometals 21.6 (2008): 623–633.
Tanaka S et al. Aged garlic extract has potential suppressive effect on colorectal adenomas in humans. J Nutr 136. (3 Suppl) (2006): 821S–826S.
Taylor P et al. Ajoene inhibits both primary tumor growth and metastasis of B16/BL6 melanoma cells in C57BL/6 mice. Cancer Lett 239.2 (2006): 298–304.
Tessema B et al. An in vitro assessment of the antibacterial effect of garlic (*Allium sativum*) on bacterial isolates from wound infections. Ethiop Med J 44.4 (2006): 385–389.
Thejass P, Kuttan G. Inhibition of angiogenic differentiation of human umbilical vein endothelial cells by diallyl disulfide (DADS). Life Sci 80.6 (2007): 515–521.
Thomson M, Mustafa T, Ali M. Thromboxane-B(2) levels in serum of rabbits receiving a single intravenous dose of aqueous extract of garlic and onion. Prostaglandins Leukot Essent Fatty Acids 63.4 (2000): 217–221.
Thomson M et al. Including garlic in the diet may help lower blood glucose, cholesterol, and triglycerides. J Nutr 136 (3 Suppl) (2006): 800S–802S.
Tilli CM et al. The garlic-derived organosulfur component ajoene decreases basal cell carcinoma tumor size by inducing apoptosis. Arch Dermatol Res 295.3 (2003): 117–123.
Tsai, C-W., et al. Garlic: health benefits and actions. Biomedicine (2012) 17–29.
Tsao SM, Yin MC. In-vitro antimicrobial activity of four diallyl sulphides occurring naturally in garlic and Chinese leek oils. J Med Microbiol 50.7 (2001): 646–649.
Unsal A et al. Protective role of natural antioxidant supplementation on testicular tissue after testicular torsion and detorsion. Scand J Urol Nephrol 40.1 (2006): 17–22.
Wang BH et al. Treatment with aged garlic extract protects against bromobenzene toxicity to precision cut rat liver slices. Toxicology 132.2–3 (1999): 215–225.
Weber ND et al. In vitro virucidal effects of *Allium sativum* (garlic) extract and compounds. Planta Med 58.5 (1992): 417–423.
Weiss N et al. Aged garlic extract improves homocysteine-induced endothelial dysfunction in macro- and microcirculation. J Nutr 136 (3 Suppl) (2006): 750S–754S.
Wojcikowski K, Myers S, Brooks L. Effects of garlic oil on platelet aggregation: a double-blind placebo-controlled crossover study. Platelets 18.1 (2007): 29–34.
Xiao D, Singh SV. Diallyl trisulfide, a constituent of processed garlic, inactivates Akt to trigger mitochondrial translocation of BAD and caspase-mediated apoptosis in human prostate cancer cells. Carcinogenesis 27.3 (2006): 533–540.
Xiao D et al. Diallyl trisulfide-induced apoptosis in human prostate cancer cells involves c-Jun N-terminal kinase and extracellular-signal regulated kinase-mediated phosphorylation of Bcl-2. Oncogene 23.33 (2004): 5594–5606.
Xiao D et al. Diallyl trisulfide-induced G(2)-M phase cell cycle arrest in human prostate cancer cells is caused by reactive oxygen species-dependent destruction and hyperphosphorylation of Cdc 25 C. Oncogene 24.41 (2005): 6256–6268.
Xiao, J et al. Garlic-derived S-allylmercaptocysteine is a hepato-protective agent in non-alcoholic fatty liver disease in vivo animal model. European journal of nutrition 52.1 (2013): 179–191.
Yang CS et al. Mechanisms of inhibition of chemical toxicity and carcinogenesis by diallyl sulfide (DAS) and related compounds from garlic. J Nutr 131.3s (2001): 1041S–1045S.
Yeh YY, Yeh SM. Homocysteine-lowering action is another potential cardiovascular protective factor of aged garlic extract. J Nutr 136 (3 Suppl) (2006): 745S–749S.
Yoshida S et al. Antifungal activity of ajoene derived from garlic. Appl Environ Microbiol 53.3 (1987): 615–6117.
Youn HS et al. Garlic (*Allium sativum*) extract inhibits lipopolysaccharide-induced Toll-like receptor 4 dimerization. Biosci Biotechnol Biochem 72.2 (2008): 368–375.
Yu, C. -S, et al. Diallyl Trisulfide Induces Apoptosis in Human Primary Colorectal Cancer Cells. Oncology reports 28.3 (2012): 949–54.
Zeb, I., et al. Aged Garlic Extract and Coenzyme Q10 have Favorable Effect on Inflammatory Markers and Coronary Atherosclerosis Progression: A Randomized Clinical Trial. Journal of Cardiovascular Disease Research 3.3 (2012): 185–90.
Zeng T et al. The anti-fatty liver effects of garlic oil on acute ethanol-exposed mice. Chem Biol Interact 176.2–3 (2008): 234–242.
Zeng, T., et al. A Meta-Analysis of Randomized, Double-Blind, Placebo-Controlled Trials for the Effects of Garlic on Serum Lipid Profiles. Journal of the science of food and agriculture 92.9 (2012): 1892–902.
Zheng S et al. Initial study on naturally occurring products from traditional Chinese herbs and vegetables for chemoprevention. J Cell Biochem Suppl 27 (1997): 106–112.
Ziaei, S. et al. The effect of garlic tablet on plasma lipids and platelet aggregation in nulliparous pregnants at high risk of preeclampsia. European Journal of Obstetrics & Gynecology and Reproductive Biology 99.2 (2001): 201–206.

Gentian

HISTORICAL NOTE The genus *Gentiana* is derived from Gentius, king of ancient Illyria, who is attributed with the discovery of its therapeutic effects (Blumenthal 2000). In ancient Greece and Rome it was used to relieve common gastrointestinal symptoms, much as it is used today. It was first noted in the Chinese medical literature in 50 BC (Willard 1991).

OTHER NAMES

Gentiana, yellow gentian, wild gentian, bitter wort

BOTANICAL NAME/FAMILY

Gentiana lutea (family Gentianaceae)

PLANT PARTS USED

Root and rhizome

CHEMICAL COMPONENTS

Secoiridoid bitter glycosides (swertiamarin, gentiopicroside, amarogentin, sweroside), oligosaccharides, phenolic acids, phytosterols, polysaccharides (inulin and pectin), tannin, lupeol, beta-amyrin triterpenes, xanthones (genitsine, isogenitsine), xanthone glycosides (gentiosides) and essential oil.

Analysis of several commercially available *G. lutea* samples showed that gentiopicroside is the most prevalent bioactive compound (4.46–9.53%), followed by loganic acid (0.10–0.76%), swertiamarin (0.21–0.45%) and then the xanthone glycosides. The xanthones, gentisine, isogentisine and the secoiridoid bitter glycosides, amarogentin were found in concentrations of only 0.02%, 0.11% (Aberham et al 2007) and 0.025–0.4% respectively (European Medicines Agency 2010).

MAIN ACTIONS

The bitter taste of gentian root is due to the secoiridoid glycosides: gentiopicroside and amarogentin. (Aberham et al 2011, European Medicines Agency 2010) The bitterness values of gentiopicroside and amarogentin are 12,000 and 58 million respectively. Amarogentin is the most bitter natural substance known (Aberham et al 2011, European Medicines Agency 2010). It is through the stimulating effect of this bitter taste that most of the beneficial effects of *Gentiana lutea* are achieved.

Digestive stimulant

The bitter principles induce reflex excitation of taste receptors and increased saliva, gastric juice and bile secretion, thereby stimulating appetite and digestion according to in vivo experiments. A small human study confirmed that oral administration of gentian root extract increases gastric juice secretion and emptying of the gallbladder (ESCOP 2003). This was also confirmed by the European Medicines Agency report, which states that bitters stimulate the gustatory nerves in the mouth, leading to increased secretion of gastric fluid and bile (European Medicines Agency 2010).

Antioxidant

Antioxidant activity has been observed in vitro for the ethyl acetate and chloroform fractions of gentian (Calliste et al 2001). An orally administered crude extract of *Gentiana lutea* (1 g/kg body weight/day) prevented both the reproductive toxicity and oxidative damage induced in rat testes in response to a high, acute dose of ketoconazole (Amin 2008).

In vitro testing of *Gentiana lutea* confirmed antioxidant activity using both the free radical scavenging test, 2,2-diphenyl-1-picrylhydrazyl and cyclic voltammetry. The 50% ethanolic extract showed the highest antioxidant capacity with IC_{50} values of 20.6 mcg/mL. The ethanolic and water extracts contained the highest phenolic content (Nastasijevic et al 2012).

Promotes wound healing

The gentiopicroside, sweroside and swertiamarin constituents from *Gentiana lutea* demonstrate wound-healing properties in animal models, due to increased stimulation of collagen production and mitotic activity (Ozturk et al 2006).

Analgesic

An animal study has shown that gentiopicroside exerts its analgesic activity by down-regulation of the *N*-methyl-D-aspartate (NMDA) NR2B receptor expression in the anterior cingulate cortex; part of the forebrain responsible for pain transmission and modulation (Chen et al 2008). In this study gentiopicroside (50–200 mg/kg) caused a significant dose-related reduction of persistent inflammatory pain stimuli through the modulation of glutamatergic synaptic transmission in response to peripheral injury (Chen et al 2008).

Antiaddictive

Gentian significantly reversed overexpression of the GluN2B-containing NMDA receptors and dopamine D2 receptors in the nucleus accumbens (forebrain area involved in drug addiction) during the first week of morphine withdrawal, reducing morphine dependence (Liu et al 2012).

Anti-inflammatory

In vitro testing of *Gentiana lutea* extracts and its constituents found that gentiopricroside was the strongest inhibitor of myeloperoxidase, a peroxidase enzyme released during neutrophil and monocyte degranulation and inflammation. The inhibition of this enzyme has an anti-inflammatory effect (Nastasijevic et al 2012).

OTHER ACTIONS

Traditionally, gentian is considered to have stomachic, anthelminthic, antiseptic, anti-inflammatory and tonic activity (Willard 1991).

Antimicrobial

Gentiana lutea leaves and flowers extracts (not the traditional parts used) showed antimicrobial activity against an array of Gram-negative and Gram-positive bacteria and one human yeast pathogen. The minimum inhibitory concentration (MIC) values of the *G. lutea* leaf extract against *Pseudomonas aeruginosa, Bacillus subtilis, Proteus mirabilis, Staphylococcus epidermis* and *Candida albicans* ranged from 0.12 to 0.31 mg/mL, showing sensitivity to this extract. The most susceptible microorganism to the flower extract of *G. lutea* was *Salmonella enteritidis* (MIC 0.15 mg/mL) (Savikin et al 2009). A gentian root preparation inhibited *Helicobacter pylori* in vitro (Mahady et al 2005) and animal studies with amarogentin have identified antileishmanial properties (Medda et al 1999).

Antidiabetic

Gentiana lutea was tested in an in vitro study to evaluate its inhibitory activity on aldose reductase (ALR2) and thereby its ability to prevent the accumulation of intracellular sorbitol in dysglycaemia. Inhibitory activities against both rat lens and human recombinant ALR2 with IC_{50} values of 23–82 mcg/mL were measured. Amarogentin showed the greatest specificity for effective inhibition of ALR2, compared to the other *G. lutea* constituents. Further research in vivo is required to confirm these findings, and if confirmed, *G. lutea* has potential in the prevention or treatment of diabetic complications (Akileshwari et al 2012).

CLINICAL USE

Gentian root preparations have not been significantly investigated under clinical trial conditions, so evidence is mainly derived from traditional, in vitro and animal studies. It is a popular remedy amongst naturopaths and herbalists.

Dyspepsia and flatulence

The considerable bitter taste of gentian provides a theoretical basis for its use in dyspepsia and flatulence, for which increased saliva and gastric acid secretion would be beneficial. Commission E and the European Scientific Co-operative on Phytomedicine (ESCOP) approve its use for this indication (Blumenthal 2000, ESCOP 2003).

Loss of appetite

The considerable bitter taste of gentian provides a theoretical basis for its use in anorexia, when increased saliva and gastric acid secretions would be beneficial. Commission E and ESCOP approve its use for this indication (Blumenthal 2000, ESCOP 2003).

Radioprotective

In vitro and ex vivo testing of lymphocytes (peripheral blood mononuclear cells) and human cervix carcinoma (HeLa cell lines) in nine healthy persons given 15 g of *Gentiana lutea* extract and mangiferin (xanthone) showed it may reduce the cytotoxic effect of ionising radiation (6 and 8 Gy doses) without changing the efficacy of irradiation destroying malignant cells. This is significant as the protection of immunocompetent cells during tumour-destructive radiation therapy is clinically important (Menkovic et al 2010).

OTHER USES

Traditionally, gentian has also been used for gout, amenorrhoea, diarrhoea and worms in the stomach and bowel (Willard 1991). Gentian is also used in alcoholic drinks such as brandy, medicinal wines and vermouth.

Clinical note — Herbs in alcoholic drinks

The maceration of herbs and spices in wine was common practice in antiquity, and the invention of aromatised wine, the ancestor of vermouth, has been attributed to Hippocrates (Liddle & Boero 2003). Herbs are still commonly used in alcoholic drink production today, either as flavourings, or as both fermentation substrates and flavouring agents. The volatile components of a herb will provide its distinctive odour, whereas non-volatile constituents can affect some gustatory reactions and produce a physiological effect. Bitter herbs such as gentian are used for flavour, but also because they contain a significant amount of fermentable sugars that can be converted by strains of yeast into ethanol in an alcoholic fermentation process. Examples of other herbs that are used in brandies, flavoured spirits, liqueurs, medicinal wines and vermouth are anise, caraway, cardamom, coriander, dandelion, sage and yarrow (Veljkovic & Stankovic 2003).

DOSAGE RANGE

General guide

- Cut root or dried extract: 2–4 g/day.
- Fluid extract (1:1): 1–2 mL taken 1 hour before meals up to three times daily.
- Tincture (1:5): 3–12 mL/day.
- Infusion: 1–2 g in 150 mL boiled water taken 1 hour before meals and up to three times daily.

Practice points/Patient counselling

- Gentian root and its preparations are extremely bitter.
- Gentian preparations stimulate salivation, gastric juice and bile secretion.
- They are used to improve digestion, relieve flatulence and stimulate appetite.
- Gentian has shown potential in pain management, morphine withdrawal, reducing the cytotoxicity of ionising radiation without compromising its effectiveness, as well as the potential to reduce complications in diabetes.
- Little clinical investigation has been undertaken with the herb, so evidence of efficacy relies on traditional and animal studies. More research is needed.
- It should not be used in cases of gastric or duodenal ulcer or hyperacidity.

ADVERSE REACTIONS

Headaches have been reported (ESCOP 2003), as have nausea and vomiting with high doses.

SIGNIFICANT INTERACTIONS

Interactions are unknown.

CONTRAINDICATIONS AND PRECAUTIONS

Contraindicated in gastric or duodenal ulcers and hyperacidity according to Commission E (Blumenthal 2000, European Medicines Agency 2010).

PREGNANCY USE

There is insufficient reliable information available to make a recommendation.

PATIENTS' FAQs

What will this herb do for me?

Gentian preparations stimulate taste buds when taken orally, and increase gastric juice secretion, thereby improving digestion.

When will it start to work?

Effects are expected within several minutes of ingestion.

Are there any safety issues?

It should not be used by people with gastric or duodenal ulcers or with gastric hyperacidity.

REFERENCES

Aberham A et al. Quantitative analysis of iridoids, secoiridoids, xanthones and xanthone glycosides in *Gentiana lutea* L. roots by RP-HPLC and LC-MS. J Pharm Biomed Anal 45.3 (2007): 437–442.

Aberham, A., et al. 2011. Analysis of iridoids, secoiridoids and xanthones in *Centaurium erythraea, Frasera caroliniensis* and *Gentiana lutea* using LC-MS and RP-HPLC. J Pharm Biomed Anal, 54, 517–25.

Akileshwari, C., et al. 2012. Inhibition of aldose reductase by *Gentiana lutea* extracts. Exp Diabetes Res, 2012, 147965.

Amin A. Ketoconazole-induced testicular damage in rats reduced by Gentiana extract. Exp Toxicol Pathol 59.6 (2008): 377–384.

Blumenthal M (ed). Herbal medicine: expanded commission E monographs. Austin, TX: Integrative Medicine Communications, 2000.

Calliste CA et al. Free radical scavenging activities measured by electron spin resonance spectroscopy and B16 cell antiproliferative behaviors of seven plants. J Agric Food Chem 49 (2001): 3321–3327.

Chen, L., et al. 2008. Down-regulation of NR2B receptors partially contributes to analgesic effects of Gentiopicroside in persistent inflammatory pain. Neuropharmacology, 54, 1175–81.

ESCOP. Gentianae Radix. In: European scientific co-operative on phytomedicine (ESCOP), 2nd edn. Stuttgart: Thieme, 2003, pp 174–177.

European Medicines Agency 2010. Assessment Report on *Gentiana lutea* L., Radix. In: Committee on Herbal Medicinal Reports (HMPC) (ed.). London: European Medicines Agency.

Liddle P, Boero L. Vermouth. In: Benjamin C (ed). Encyclopedia of food sciences and nutrition. Oxford: Academic Press, 2003, pp 5980–5984.

Liu, S. B., et al. 2012. Gentiopicroside attenuates morphine rewarding effect through downregulation of GluN2B receptors in nucleus accumbens. CNS Neurosci Ther, 18, 652–8.

Mahady GB et al. In vitro susceptibility of *Helicobacter pylori* to botanical extracts used traditionally for the treatment of gastrointestinal disorders. Phytother Res 19 (2005): 988–991.

Medda S, et al. Evaluation of the in-vivo activity and toxicity of amarogentin, an antileishmanial agent, in both liposomal and niosomal forms. J Antimicrob Chemother 44 (1999): 791–794.

Menkovic, N., et al. 2010. Radioprotective activity of *Gentiana lutea* extract and mangiferin. Phytother Res, 24, 1693–6.

Nastasijevic, B., et al. 2012. Inhibition of myeloperoxidase and antioxidative activity of *Gentiana lutea* extracts. J Pharm Biomed Anal, 66, 191–6.

Ozturk N et al. Effects of gentiopicroside, sweroside and swertiamarine, secoiridoids from gentian (*Gentiana lutea* ssp. *symphyandra*), on cultured chicken embryonic fibroblasts. Planta Med 72.4 (2006): 289–294.

Savikin, K., et al. 2009. Antimicrobial activity of *Gentiana lutea* L. extracts. Z. Naturforsch, 64c, 339–342.

Veljkovic VB, Stankovic MZ. Herbs used in alcoholic drinks. In: Benjamin C (ed). Encyclopedia of food sciences and nutrition., Oxford: Academic Press, 2003, pp 3098–3107.

Willard T. Gentian. The wild rose scientific herbal. Calgary: Wild Rose College of Natural Healing, 1991, pp 135–7.

Ginger

HISTORICAL NOTE Ginger has been used as both a food and a medicine since ancient times. Confucius wrote about it in his Analects, the Greek physician Dioscorides listed ginger as an antidote to poisoning, as a digestive, and as being warming to the stomach in De Materia Medica, and the Koran, the Talmud and the Bible all mention ginger. Records suggest that ginger was highly valued as an article of trade and in 13th- and 14th-century England, one pound of ginger was worth the same as a sheep (Rosengarten 1969). Ginger is still extremely popular in the practice of phytotherapy, particularly in traditional Chinese medicine (TCM), which distinguishes between the dried and fresh roots. It is widely used to stimulate circulation, treat various gastrointestinal disorders and as a stimulant heating agent.

OTHER NAMES

African ginger, Indian ginger, Jamaica ginger, common ginger, rhizoma zingiberis, shokyo (Japanese).

BOTANICAL NAME/FAMILY

Zingiber officinale Roscoe (family Zingiberaceae)

PLANT PART USED

Rhizome

CHEMICAL COMPONENTS

The ginger rhizome contains an essential oil and resin known collectively as oleoresin. The composition of the essential oil varies according to the geographical origin, but the chief constituents, sesquiterpene hydrocarbons, which are responsible for the characteristic aroma, are fairly constant.

The oleoresin contains:

- Sesquiterpenes: zingiberene, ar-curcumene, beta-sesquiphellandrene and beta-bisabolene.
- Pungent phenolic compounds: gingerols and their corresponding degradation products, shogaols, zingerone and paradol. Zingerone and shogaols are found in small amounts in fresh ginger and in larger amounts in dried or extracted products (Govindarajan 1982).
- Other constituents: diarylheptanoids galanolactone (diterpenoid), 6-gingesulfonic acid, monoacyldigalactosylglycerols (Awang 1992, Bhattarai et al 2001, Charles et al 2000, Govindarajan 1982, Kikuzaki et al 1991, WHO 2003, Yamahara et al 1992, Yoshikawa et al 1992, 1993).

PHARMACOKINETICS

Metabolites of [6]-, [8]- and [10]-gingerol as well as [6]-shogaol have been detected as glucuronide and sulfate conjugates in the plasma of healthy human volunteers after oral ingestion of 100 mg–2 gram doses of ginger (Zick et al 2008). A clinical study estimated the half-life of [6]-, [8]- and [10]-gingerol as well as [6]-shogaol and their metabolites to be 1–3 hours in human plasma (Yu et al 2011).

MAIN ACTIONS

Anti-emetic

Ginger has demonstrated anti-emetic activity in both experimental models and human studies. It appears that several key constituents are responsible, which exert several different mechanisms. In vivo studies have demonstrated [6]-, [8]- and [10]-gingerol as well as [6]-shogaol exert anti-emetic activity (Abdel-Aziz et al 2006, Kawai et al 1994), most likely by acting on the 5-HT_3 receptor ion-channel complex, either by binding directly to a modulatory site distinct from the serotonin binding site or indirectly via underlying muscarinic receptors. Specific constituents of ginger volatile oil including terpinolene, beta-pinene and alpha-phellandrene were also found to induce an antispasmodic effect via interaction with the 5-HT_3 receptor channel system in rat ileum (Riyazi et al 2007). Galactone has also been identified as a serotonin-receptor antagonist (Huang et al 1991, Mustafa et al 1993, Yamahara et al 1990). Such mechanisms of action also explain the inhibitory effect of ginger on serotonin-induced diarrhoea and antispasmodic effect on visceral and vascular smooth muscle.

Ginger has been shown to blunt gastric dysrhythmias and nausea evoked by acute hyperglycaemia in humans. The anti-arrhythmic and anti-emetic effects are thought to be due to a blockade of prostaglandins rather than inhibition of their release (Gonlachanvit et al 2003). Ginger has also been shown to reduce radiation-induced gastrointestinal distress and emesis in rat models, which is thought to be due at least in part to its antioxidant properties and the ability to scavenge free radicals and inhibit lipid peroxidation (Sharma et al 2005). Ginger extract displayed comparable radioprotection against radiation-induced taste aversion (CTA) when compared to dexamethasone and ondansetron in male and female rats. The most effective concentration was 1000 microgram/mL of ginger extract, which exerted free radial scavenging of hydroxyl ions and nitric oxide and modulation of CTA (Haksar et al 2006).

G

Gastrointestinal activity

Ginger exerts several effects in the gastrointestinal tract, which lead to an improvement in gastrointestinal symptoms. It stimulates the flow of saliva, bile and gastric secretions (Platel & Srinivasan 1996, 2001; Yamahara et al 1985), and has been shown to increase gastrointestinal motility in several animal models and human studies (Gupta & Sharma 2001, Micklefield et al 1999, Phillips et al 1993). In a double-blind RCT involving 24 healthy volunteers, ginger was found to accelerate gastric emptying and stimulate antral contractions (Wu et al 2008), a result that was confirmed in a follow-up double blind RCT using 1.2 g ginger root (Hu et al 2011). Ginger has also been observed to have prokinetic activity in mice in vivo and antispasmodic activity in vitro (Ghayur & Gilani 2005). These findings appear to support the traditional use of ginger in the treatment of gastrointestinal discomfort, colic, diarrhoea and bloating, and its use as a carminative agent. New insight into the mechanisms of the antidiarrhoeal action of a decoction of ginger root indicates that it may modify bacterial as well as host cell metabolism, reducing colonisation of epithelial cells (Daswani et al 2010). In vitro studies confirm cholinergic agonistic activity on postsynaptic M3 receptors, as well as suggesting an inhibitory effect on presynaptic muscarinic autoreceptors; the [6]-gingerol constituent displayed the strongest antispasmodic activity (Ghayur et al 2008).

Anti-ulcer activity

A number of in vivo studies have identified anti-ulcer activity for ginger extract and several of its isolated constituents. The orally administered acetone extract of ginger at a dose of 1000 mg/kg and zingiberene, the main terpenoid in this extract, at 100 mg/kg significantly inhibited gastric lesions by 97.5% and 53.6%, respectively. Additionally, the pungent principle, [6]-gingerol at 100 mg/kg, significantly inhibited gastric lesions by 54.5%. These results suggest that both zingiberene and [6]-gingerol are important constituents responsible for ginger's anti-ulcer activity (Yamahara et al 1988). Other constituents demonstrating anti-ulcer properties in gastric ulcer models in rats include beta-sesquiphellandrene, beta-bisabolene, ar-curcumene and shogaol (Sertie et al 1992, Yoshikawa et al 1994). Furthermore, an animal study showed that ginger was able to protect against indomethacin-induced gastric ulceration when administered at 100, 200 and 400 mg/kg, and was comparable in efficacy to the study's reference drug, ranitidine (Anoiske et al 2009).

Helicobacter pylori has been identified as a major causative factor in gastric ulcers. In vitro studies have established ginger extract containing gingerols effectively inhibited the growth of 19 strains of *H. pylori* including CagA+ strains (Mahady et al 2003, 2005). While ginger is effective in inhibiting *H. pylori*, its ability to prevent bacterial adhesion to the stomach tissue is limited (O'Mahony et al 2005).

In addition to direct anti-ulcer activity, ginger exerts synergistic effects with the antibiotic clarithromycin in inhibiting different *H. pylori* isolates independent of the organisms' susceptibility to clarithromycin (Nostro et al 2006). Ginger-free phenolic and ginger hydrolysed phenolic fractions were found to be potent inhibitors of gastric cell proton potassium ATPase and *H. pylori*, exhibiting a six-to-eight-fold better potency over lansoprazole (Siddaraju & Dharmesh 2007).

Hypolipidaemic

Ginger demonstrates significant lipid lowering activity in several animal models and, more recently, a double-blind clinical trial.

High doses of an aqueous extract of ginger (500 mg/kg) significantly reduced serum cholesterol according to an animal study that used oral doses of a raw aqueous extract of ginger administered daily for a period of 4 weeks (Thomson et al 2002). Treatment with ginger methanol and ethyl acetate extracts (250 mg/kg) for 8 weeks also resulted in a significant reduction in lipid levels in vivo (Goyal & Kadnur 2006). Similarly, methanolic and ethyl acetate extracts of dried ginger rhizome significantly reduced fructose-elevated lipid levels and body weight in vivo (Kadnur & Goyal 2005). Reductions in lipid levels were further reported for ethanolic extract of ginger (200 mg/kg for 20 days) by using a streptozocin-induced diabetic rat model. In addition, herbal treatment effectively reduced serum glucose (Bhandari et al 2005).

Effects on triglyceride levels are more difficult to determine, as one study demonstrated that 250 microgram ginger extract/day reduced serum triglyceride levels by 27% in mice (Fuhrman et al 2000), whereas another study using a high dose of 500 mg/kg found no significant effects (Thomson et al 2002).

An ex vivo study found that 250 mcg/day of a standardised ginger extract significantly reduced plasma cholesterol, triglycerides and LDL cholesterol levels, the LDL basal oxidative state, as well as LDL cholesterol and serum cholesterol's susceptibility to oxidation and aggregation, compared with placebo. Ginger also reduced aortic atherosclerotic lesions by 44% in atherosclerotic mouse aorta (Fuhrman et al 2000).

According to a double-blind controlled clinical trial study of 85 volunteers, ginger (3 g/day) demonstrates clinically significant lipid lowering effects compared to controls. After 45 days of treatment, triglyceride and cholesterol levels were reduced, as well as a reduction in LDL levels and an increase in HDL levels (Alizadeh-Navaei et al 2008).

Glycaemic response

Ginger improves insulin sensitivity and reduces serum glucose levels in vivo (Al-Amin et al 2006, Goyal & Kandur 2006). The mechanisms underlying these actions are associated with the inhibition of key enzymes controlling carbohydrate metabolism, an insulinotropic effect rather than hypoglycaemic (Islam & Choi 2008), increased insulin release/sensitivity (Goyal & Kandur 2006), resulting in enhanced glucose uptake in peripheral adipose and skeletal muscle tissues. Significant lipid lowering activity further contributes to improving the insulin resistant condition (Li et al 2012).

Gingerols have been identified as the main constituent group responsible for improving insulin sensitivity. In an assay for aldose reductase inhibitors within ginger, five active compounds were isolated and two were found to be inhibitors of recombinant human aldose reductase (Kato et al 2006).

Anti-inflammatory and analgesic

The anti-inflammatory and analgesic effects reported for ginger are attributed to multiple constituents exerting several different mechanisms.

An acetone extract containing gingerols, shogaols and minor compounds like gingerenone A, [6]-gingerdiol, hexahydrocurcumin and zingerone has been shown synergistically to produce dose-dependent anti-inflammatory effects (Schuhbaum & Franz 2000). Other studies have identified the gingerols and diarylheptanoids and gingerdione as the key compounds responsible (Flynn et al 1986, Kiuchi et al 1992).

Investigations on macrophages in vitro found that [6]-shogaol and [6]-gingerol inhibit the expression of inflammatory iNOS and COX-2 proteins (Pan et al 2008). [6]-Gingerol has also been shown to inhibit catalytic activity of iNOS in murine macrophages via attenuation of NF-kappaB-mediated iNOS gene expression (Aktan et al 2006). [6]-Gingerol proved to be useful in treatment of inflammation by selectively inhibiting the production of inflammatory cytokines of murine peritoneal macrophages without interfering with the antigen-presenting function of the macrophages (Tripathi et al 2007). Ginger extract inhibited interleukin (IL)-12, tumour necrosis factor (TNF)-alpha, IL-1-beta in lipopolysaccharide-stimulated macrophages and significantly reduced T-cell proliferation (Tripathi et al 2008).

Ginger has been found to modulate the arachidonic acid cascade, as COX-1 and -2 and lipoxygenase inhibition has been shown in vitro (Kobayashi et al 1987) and high oral doses of an aqueous extract of ginger (500 mg/kg) significantly lowered serum PGE_2 and thromboxane B_2 levels in rats (Thomson et al 2002). A hydroalcoholic extract of ginger exerted anti-inflammatory and attenuated COX metabolites in rat trachea hyperactivity for 90 minutes and 48 hours after exposure to lipopolysaccharide (LPS). Ginger reduced serum levels of prostaglandin (PGE_2) and thromboxane (TXA_2) post LPS exposure (Aimbire et al 2007). Ginger also suppresses leukotriene biosynthesis by inhibiting 5-lipoxygenase, thus distinguishing ginger from non-steroidal anti-inflammatory drugs (NSAIDs). Additionally, ginger extract has been shown to inhibit thromboxane synthase (Langner et al 1998) and a ginger extract (EV.EXT 77) has been found to inhibit the induction of several genes involved in the inflammatory response. These include genes encoding cytokines, chemokines and the inducible enzyme COX-2, thus providing evidence that ginger modulates biochemical pathways activated in chronic inflammation (Grzanna et al 2005). A positive response to ginger administration was also demonstrated in an arthritic animal model whereby a significant reduction in inflammatory cytokines occurred that was superior to indomethacin (Ramadan et al 2011).

Gingerol and [8]-gingerol have been found to evoke capsaicin-like intracellular Ca^{2+} transients and ion currents in vitro and it has been suggested that gingerols represent a novel class of naturally occurring vanilloid receptor agonists that contribute to ginger's medicinal properties (Dedov et al 2002). This is supported by the finding that topical application of ginger creams or compresses produce an analgesic capsaicin-like effect on the release of the immunoreactive substance P from primary afferent neurons (Onogi et al 1992). In animal models of chemically induced inflammation, ginger extract reduced oedema that was partly caused by serotonin-receptor antagonism (Penna et al 2003) and has been shown to reduce inflammation in a non-dose dependent manner, and display equivalent efficacy to indomethacin (Anosike et al 2009). Additionally, ginger oil has shown anti-inflammatory activity, significantly suppressing both paw and joint swelling in severe adjuvant arthritis in rats (Sharma et al 1994).

In an animal model of rheumatoid arthritis, both crude ginger extract and gingerols were efficacious in preventing streptococcal cell wall-induced arthritis. However, the crude ginger extract, which also contained essential oils, was more effective in preventing both joint inflammation and attenuating cellular destruction (Funk et al 2009).

Antiplatelet

It has been suggested that gingerols and their derivatives represent a potential new class of platelet activation inhibitors, with synthetic gingerols being found to inhibit the arachidonic acid-induced platelet release reaction in vitro in a similar dose range as aspirin possibly due to an effect on COX activity in platelets (Koo et al 2001, Lu 2005, Nurtjahja-Tjendraputra et al 2003, Tjendraputra et al 2001).

Powdered ginger exerted an antiplatelet activity when taken in very high doses of at least 10 g, according to one human study (Bordia et al 1997). A randomised double-blind study found that doses up to 2 g of dried ginger had no effect on bleeding time, platelet aggregation or platelet count (Lumb 1994). This lack of effect has been demonstrated in healthy volunteers (Janssen et al 1996) and those with type 1 diabetes mellitus or coronary artery disease (Bordia et al 1997).

Antimicrobial and antiparasitic

Ginger extract, several of its main constituents and essential oil of ginger exhibit antimicrobial activity in vitro and in vivo. Ginger extract has been shown to have an antibacterial effect against *Staphylococcus aureus*, *Streptococcus pyogenes*, *Streptococcus pneumoniae* and *Haemophilus* collected from throat swabs of infected individuals. The minimum inhibitory concentration of ginger ranged from 0.0003 to 0.7 mcg/mL, and the minimum bactericidal concentration ranged from 0.135 to 2.04 mcg/mL (Akoachere et al 2002). Recent in vitro studies confirmed ginger compounds were effective against *Penicillium* spp., *Escherichia coli, Bacillus subtilis* and *Staphylococcus aureus*, with minimal inhibitory concentrations of the oleoresin and essential oil 2 mg/mL and 869.2 mg/mL, respectively (Bellik 2014). The anti-*H. pylori* effects of ginger have also been shown to inhibit *H. pylori* $CagA^+$ strains in vitro (Mahady et al 2003). Essential oils of ginger have also been shown to have antimicrobial activity against Gram-positive and Gram-negative bacteria in vitro (Martins et al 2001).

Various ginger extracts have demonstrated significant larvicidal potential against larvae of the dengue fever mosquito vector, *Aedes aegypti*. The application of ginger alcoholic and oil-based extracts resulted in complete mortality with no pupal or adult emergence (Kalaivani et al 2012, Kumar et al 2012).

Ginger constituents

[10]-Gingerol and [12]-gingerol successfully inhibited oral bacteria associated with periodontitis. Ethanol and *n*-hexane extracts of ginger have demonstrated antibacterial activities against the bacteria

Porphyromonas gingivalis, *Porphyromonas endodontalis* and *Prevotella intermedia*, associated with periodontal disease, effectively inhibited the growth of these anaerobic Gram-negative bacteria (Park et al 2008). Intraperitoneally administered ginger exerted a dose-dependent antimicrobial activity against *Pseudomonas aeruginosa*, *Salmonella typhimurium*, *Escherichia coli* and *Candida albicans* (Jagetia et al 2003).

Gingerols demonstrated antibacterial activity against *Bacillus subtilis* and *Escherichia coli* in vitro (Yamada et al 1992). [10]-Gingerol was found to potentiate the antibacterial actions of aminoglycosides in vancomycin-resistant enterococci, bacitracin and polymixin B suggesting [10]-gingerol increases membrane permeability of enterococcal cells promoting an enhanced influx of aminoglycosides (Nagoshi et al 2006).

Ginger has also shown antischistosomal activity. Gingerol (5.0 ppm) completely abolished the infectivity of *Schistosoma* spp (blood flukes) in animal studies (Adewunmi et al 1990). Gingerol and shogaol exhibited potent molluscicidal activity in vivo. Shogaol and gingerol have demonstrated anti-nematode activities; 6.25 mcg/mL 6-shogaol destroyed *Anisakis* larvae within 16 hours in vitro, whereas the anti-nematodal medication pyrantel pamoate had no lethal effect at 1 mg/mL (Goto et al 1990).

Antifungal and antiviral

Ginger constituents have demonstrated antifungal and antiviral activity. Shogaol and zingerone strongly inhibited *Salmonella typhi*, *Vibrio cholerae* and *Tricophyton violaceum*. Aqueous extracts have also been shown to be effective against *Trichomonas vaginalis* (Henry & Piggott 1987). Several sesquiterpenes, but especially beta-sesquiphellandrene, isolated from ginger have also been shown to have antirhinoviral activity in vitro (Denyer et al 1994).

Essential oils of ginger have been shown to have activity yeasts and filamentous fungi in vitro (Martins et al 2001). Such oils have exhibited virucidal activity against aciclovir-sensitive and resistant strains of herpes simplex-1 reducing plaque formation significantly (Schnitzler et al 2007). A further in vitro study has indicated a dose-dependent virucidal activity against herpes simplex-2 is possible by interaction with the viral envelope (Koch et al 2008).

Antioxidant

Various investigations have confirmed that ginger displays strong in vitro and in vivo antioxidant properties. Orally administered ginger significantly lowered levels of free radicals and raised the activities of endogenous antioxidants, superoxide dismutase and catalase and had a sparing effect on vitamins C and E (Jeyakumar et al 1999). Ginger has been found to protect against lipid peroxidation in the liver (Ahmed et al 2008) and kidney (Asnani & Verma 2007). Ginger root aqueous extract taken orally (500 mg/kg/day) reduced testicular toxicity, including the restoration of sperm function, testicular steroidogenesis and reproductive organo-somatic indices in an animal model, effects which were attributed to the antioxidant activity of ginger (Morakinyo et al 2010).

An in vivo and in vitro research has shown [6]-gingerol to be effective in reducing ultraviolet B (UVB)-induced intracellular reactive oxygen species (ROS), UVB-induced expression of COX-2 and inhibited the translocation of NF-kappaB from cytosol to cell nucleus. Moreover, topical application of [6]-gingerol prior to UVB exposure on hairless mice inhibited COX-2 mRNA, and protein and NF-kappaB translocation (Kim et al 2007).

Immunomodulation

In vitro and in vivo research suggests that ginger extract exerts some degree of immunomodulatory activity (Ahui et al 2008, Imanishi et al 2006, Tripathi et al 2008).

Ginger exerted an immunosuppressive in vitro lymphocyte proliferation analysis, an effect modulated through IL-2 production (Wilasrusmee et al 2002). Ginger oil has also been shown to have immunomodulatory activity in mice, with dose-dependent inhibition of T lymphocyte proliferation and IL-1-alpha secretion and reduced delayed type of hypersensitivity response in vivo (Zhou et al 2006).

Hepatoprotective

Experimental models of alcohol-induced liver damage previously showed that ginger has significant hepatoprotective effects comparable to those of silymarin (Bhandari et al 2003). The effect appears to be mediated by an antioxidative mechanism. Reversal of ethanol-induced liver damage was achieved following the treatment with 1% ginger for 4 weeks. The hepatoprotective action was mediated by preventing a decline in antioxidant status (Mallikarjuna et al 2008). Pretreatment with an ethanol extract of ginger exerted a protective effect against carbon tetrachloride and paracetamol-induced acute liver damage in rats, with attenuation of serum and liver marker enzymes (Yemitan & Izegbu 2006). In a similar study ginger exerted significant declines in the activities of serum transaminases and alkaline phosphatase and restoration of hepatic oxidative status post administration of a single dose (Ajith et al 2007). More recently, two animal studies comparing ginger to silymarin (an active constituent in St Mary's thistle), oral extracts of ginger were found to attenuate carbon tetrachloride-induced damage of the liver. The first study involved the use of methanolic extract, resulting in reductions of the inflammatory enzymes alkaline phosphatase (ALP) and gamma-glutamyl transpeptidase (GGT) and also showed no symptoms of morbidity or mortality in dosages of up to 5000 mg/kg in rats (Atta et al 2010). In the second, ethanolic extract of ginger significantly increased glutathione, superoxide dismutase and protein levels in addition to reduced aspartate and alanine amintransferases (AST and ALT), GGT and bilirubin levels and markedly reduced necrosis and collagen deposition fibrosis (Motawi et al 2011).

Nephroprotection

Ginger prevented the decline in renal antioxidant status by increasing glutathione-S-transferase activity in an experimental model of nephrotoxicity (Ajith et al 2008). Ginger exhibited a significant dose-dependent nephroprotective role in experimentally induced acute renal damage when administered as a stand-alone treatment (250 mg/kg) and when used in combination with vitamin E (Ajith et al 2007).

Chemoprotective

The inhibitory effects of ginger and its constituents in tumour development have previously been demonstrated in animal models and human cell lines with activity observed against human breast cancer (Lee et al 2008), ovarian cancer (Rhode et al 2007), gastric cancer (Ishiguro et al 2007) and pancreatic cancer (Park et al 2006).

Antitumour properties have been isolated to several key constituents of ginger including [6]-gingerol, [6]-paradol, shogaols, zerumbone and zingerone and are partly due to an antioxidative and anti-inflammatory mechanism (Kim et al 2005).

Application of ginger or its constituents achieved induction of apoptosis in cancerous cells resulting in suppression of proliferation (Lee & Surh 1998) and apoptosis resulting in cell transformation (Bode et al 2001). The apoptotic effect of ginger constituents was also demonstrated in human promyelocytic leukaemia cells (Wei et al 2005), and an ethanolic extract of ginger also demonstrated cytotoxic activity against cultured non-hormone-dependent cancer cell lines, arresting development in the sub-G1 phase (Sabli et al 2012) The modulation of proteins involved in apoptosis has also been demonstrated in in vivo and in vitro prostate cancer models (Shukla et al 2007). [6]-Gingerol administration exerted actions of cell cycle arrest and induction of apoptosis in suppression of hepatoma cells (Yagihashi et al 2008). [6]-Gingerol was also found to exert a direct suppressive effect on colon cancer cell growth and inhibit angiogenesis by reduction in tumour blood supply (Brown et al 2008). [6]-Shogaol has been found to effectively induce apoptotic cell death in human hepatoma p53 mutant cells by way of an intracellular oxidative stress mediated cascade which ultimately leads to cell death (Chen et al 2007), and the same constituent was shown to be a potent inhibitor of MDA-MB-231 breast cancer cell invasion, possibly by down-regulating transcription by targeting the NF-kappaB activation cascade (Ling et al 2010).

Reduction of lipid peroxidation and increased antioxidant activity was attributed to suppression of colon carcinogenesis by ginger in male Wistar rats (Manju & Nalini 2005). Differing types of tumours exhibit high NF-kappa B activity sustaining angiogenesis and cell proliferation gingerols were found to display properties inhibiting the activation of NF-kappaB (Kim et al 2009, Takada et al 2005).

The activity seen in test tube and animal models may have clinical significance according to a double blind RCT. The trial involved 33 participants with normal risk of colorectal cancer who were given ginger powder (2 g/day) for 28 days. Colon biopsy results showed that compared to placebo, ginger significantly reduced prostaglandin E_2 and the eicosanoid 5-hydroxyeicosatetraenoic normalised to arachidonic acid, indicating that ginger extract may have an inhibitory effect on colon tissue cyclooxygenase and lipoxygenase enzymes in humans (Zick et al 2011).

G

Clinical note — Ginger and moxibustion — a clinical perspective

Moxibustion as a part of acupuncture has been well noted in TCM and is widely accepted as a useful complementary and alternative medicine therapy (Okada & Kawakita 2009). Indirect moxibustion utilises ginger slices placed at specific acupuncture points to insulate the skin from burning moxa sticks and provides therapeutic effects via thermal stimulation and sympathetic vibration (Shen et al 2006).

A review of 587 acupuncture and moxibustion randomised controlled papers from 1978 to 2007 conducted by Du et al (2009) demonstrated the growing indications for, and applications of, the use of moxibustion and acupuncture. Clinical trials have shown ginger-partitioned moxibustion to be therapeutically effective in the treatment of child diarrhoea (Liu et al 2003), cervical vertigo (Xiaoxiang 2006), poststroke urination disorders (Liu & Wang 2006), leucopenia induced by chemotherapy (Zhao et al 2007) and rheumatoid arthritis (Xie & Lei 2008).

OTHER ACTIONS

Antihistamine

Shogaols and certain gingerols exhibit dose-dependent inhibition of drug-induced histamine release from rat peritoneal mast cells in vitro (Yamahara et al 1995).

Anxiolytic

A combination of ginger and *Ginkgo biloba* has been shown to reduce anxiety in an animal model (elevated plus-maze test). The effect was similar to diazepam (Hasenohrl et al 1996). A highly non-polar fraction of a ginger extract has been shown to possess anticonvulsant, anxiolytic and antiemetic activities in animals (Vishwakarma et al 2002).

Antifibrotic

Supplementation with 5 g ginger not only prevented a decrease, but also significantly increased

Clinical note — Morning sickness

Nausea and vomiting are the most common symptoms experienced in early pregnancy, with nausea affecting between 70% and 85% of women. About half of pregnant women experience vomiting (Jewell & Young 2002). Hyperemesis gravidarum is more severe and affects between 0.3% and 2% of all pregnant women. It is a multifactorial disease in which pregnancy-induced hormonal changes associated with concurrent gastrointestinal dysmotility and possible *Helicobacter pylori* infection function as contributing factors (Eliakim et al 2000).

fibrinolytic activity in 30 healthy adult volunteers who consumed 50 g fat in a meal in an open clinical study (Verma & Bordia 2001).

Positive inotrope

Gingerols and shogaols isolated from ginger have positive inotropic activity, as demonstrated on isolated heart muscle (Shoji et al 1982, Yamahara et al 1995). The effect of gingerol seems to be rather specific to SR Ca^{2+}–ATPase activity (Kobayashi et al 1987).

Thermogenic

Ginger helps to maintain body temperature and inhibit serotonin-induced hypothermia in vivo (Huang et al 1991, Kano et al 1991). However, the addition of a ginger-based sauce to a meal did not produce any significant effect on metabolic rate in humans (Henry & Piggott 1987).

Hypotensive

Aqueous ginger extract has been shown to lower blood pressure via stimulation of muscarinic receptors and blockade of Ca^{2+} channels in guinea pig atria (Ghayur et al 2005). The calcium channel blocking effect of ginger has been demonstrated in acetycholine (ACh)-induced airway constriction of mouse lung tissue. Pretreatment with a 70% aqueous methanolic crude extract of ginger 30 minutes prior to ACh administration achieved significant reduction in airway contraction and Ca^{2+}. Similar results were achieved with verapamil, indicating comparable modes of action. Concomitant use of both ginger extract and verapamil achieved the same outcome as when each was used alone (Ghayur et al 2008).

CLINICAL USE

Although ginger is used in many forms, including fresh ginger used in cooking or chai (Indian spicy tea), pickled or glazed ginger, ethanol extracts and concentrated powdered extracts, preparations made with the root are used medicinally. Depending on the specific solvent used, the resultant preparation will contain different concentrations of the active constituents and may differ markedly from crude ginger. The great majority of research refers specifically to the species *Zingiber officinale*; however, there is the potential for confusion with other species or even with other genera (Canter 2004). Furthermore, there are reported to be wide variations in the quality of commercial ginger supplements with concentrations of gingerols ranging from 0.0 to 9.43 mg/g. As such, the results of specific extracts cannot necessarily be extrapolated to different preparations (Schwertner et al 2006).

Prevention of nausea and vomiting

Many clinical studies have investigated the effects of ginger in the prevention and treatment of nausea and vomiting associated with different circumstances, including pregnancy (Fischer-Rasmussen et al 1990, Keating & Chez 2002, Portnoi et al 2003, Smith et al 2004, Sripramote & Lekhyananda 2003, Vutyavanich et al 2001, Willetts et al 2003), the postoperative period (Arfeen et al 1995, Bone et al 1990, Meyer et al 1995, Phillips et al 1993, Visalyaputra et al 1998), motion sickness (Grontved & Hentzer 1986, Lien et al 2003, Mowrey & Clayson 1982, Schmid et al 1994, Stewart et al 1991) and chemotherapy (Manusirivithaya et al 2004, Meyer et al 1995, Sontakke et al 2003, Ryan et al 2012).

A systematic review of 24 randomised controlled trials (RCTs) covering 1073 patients suggests that results for the treatment of nausea and vomiting in pregnancy are encouraging and generally supportive; however, results for postoperative nausea and vomiting and motion sickness are unclear and daily doses of up to 6 g of ginger seem to have few side effects (Betz et al 2005). More reviews provide further encouragement and suggest that ginger may indeed be effective in nausea associated with pregnancy (Boone & Shields 2005) and the postoperative period (Chaiyakunapruk et al 2006). Similarly a review of four well-controlled, double-blind, randomised clinical studies concluded there was convincing evidence for application of ginger in the treatment of nausea and vomiting of pregnancy (Bryer 2005).

Nausea and vomiting in pregnancy

There is supportive evidence from clinical studies that ginger preparations in pregnancy reduce the duration and severity of nausea and vomiting.

Nausea of pregnancy

There are many studies, including an observational study (Portnoi et al 2003) and at least seven RCTs (Fischer-Rasmussen et al 1990, Keating & Chez 2002, Portnoi et al 2003, Smith et al 2004, Sripramote & Lekhyananda 2003, Vutyavanich et al 2001, Willetts et al 2003), as well as multiple systematic reviews, including a Cochrane review (Matthews et al 2010), that suggest that ginger powder or extract may be safe and effective in treating nausea and vomiting of pregnancy (Boone & Shields 2005, Borrelli et al 2005, Bryer 2005, Dib & El-Saddik 2004, Ernst & Pittler 2000, Jewell 2003). A subsequent review, considering four double-blind RCTs including 504 subjects, suggests that ginger is superior to placebo and as effective as vitamin B_6 in reducing the frequency and intensity of pregnancy-related nausea and vomiting and that there is an absence of significant side effects and adverse pregnancy outcomes; however, the review does mention uncertainty regarding the maximum safe dosage and the need for further research (Ding et al 2013).

In three double-blind, placebo-controlled, randomised trials of ginger for pregnancy-related nausea and vomiting, including one trial on hyperemesis gravidarum, 1 g ginger in divided doses was significantly more effective than placebo in reducing nausea and vomiting (Fischer-Rasmussen et al 1990, Keating & Chez 2002, Vutyavanich et al 2001). In a further double-blind trial of 120 women, 25 mg of the ginger extract EV.EXT 35 (equivalent to 1.5 g of dried ginger) four times daily was useful in patients experiencing nausea and retching, although no significant result was seen for vomiting (Willetts et al 2003).

Comparative studies

A comparative double-blind randomised controlled trial of 170 pregnant women who attended an antenatal clinic with the symptoms of nausea and vomiting in pregnancy found one capsule of ginger (0.5 g ginger powder) twice daily was identical in efficacy to treatment with 50 mg dimenhydrinate twice daily. In addition, ginger treatment resulted in fewer side effects (Pongrojpaw et al 2007). Initial comparative randomised, double-blind controlled trials found ginger to be equivalent to vitamin B_6 in helping to reduce pregnancy-related nausea, dry retching and vomiting (Smith et al 2004, Sripramote & Lekhyananda 2003). However, ginger (650 mg qid) proved more effective than vitamin B_6 (25 mg qid) in a randomised double-blind controlled trial involving 126 pregnant women, with a gestational age of ≤16 weeks who had nausea and vomiting (Chittumma et al 2007). Investigations over a 3-month duration into the efficacy of ginger compared to vitamin B_6 of 70 pregnant women with nausea and a gestational age of ≤17 weeks were randomised to receive either ginger 1 g/day or vitamin B_6 40 mg/day for 4 days. Treatment with ginger (1 g/day) was found to be more effective than vitamin B_6 (40 mg/day) for relieving the severity of nausea, as well as equally effective in decreasing the episodes of vomiting (Ensiyeh & Sakineh 2008). Another clinical trial suggests that ginger at a dose of 250 mg taken four times per day is as effective as the higher dose of B_6 40 mg twice per day for reducing pregnancy-induced nausea (Haji Seid Javadi et al 2013).

Postoperative nausea

Ginger may be useful for the prevention of postoperative nausea; however, not all studies have produced positive results and as the ginger preparations used have not been standardised, it is difficult to directly compare studies. A meta-analysis of five randomised trials (n = 363) found that a fixed dose of at least 1 g of ginger was more effective than placebo for the prevention of postoperative nausea and vomiting (Chaiyakunapruk et al 2006).

Most of the studies on postoperative nausea and vomiting have been conducted on patients undergoing gynaecological surgery. Powdered ginger (2 g) was administered to 239 women undergoing elective caesarean section at term, in order to evaluate the effects on intra- and post-operative nausea and vomiting. Ginger reduced the number of episodes of intraoperative nausea compared to placebo, but had no effect on incidence of nausea, vomiting or pain during or after elective caesarean section (Kalava et al 2013). In two other double-blind RCTs, ginger significantly reduced the incidence of postoperative nausea and vomiting (Bone et al 1990, Phillips et al 1993), although two further studies failed to show any benefit with ginger (Arfeen et al 1995, Eberhart et al 2003). A fifth study of 80 women undergoing gynaecological laparoscopy found that 1 g of ginger taken 1 hour before surgery was significantly superior to placebo in reducing the incidence of nausea 2–4 hours afterwards; however, it failed to show statistical significance for an observed reduction in the incidence and frequency of vomiting (Pongrojpaw & Chiamchanya 2003).

A double-blind RCT of 120 patients who underwent major gynaecological surgery found that a pretreatment with ginger powder (0.5 g) as compared to placebo resulted in lower incidence and frequency of vomiting in the treatment group. Frequency of vomiting was evaluated at 0, 2, 6, 12 and 24 hours postoperatively with the most statistically significant differences between ginger and placebo occurring at the 2- and 6-hour time intervals (Nanthakomon & Pongrojpaw 2006). Similarly a randomised study of 60 inpatients who underwent laparoscopic operations for non-cancer gynaecological conditions found that pretreatment 1 hour prior to surgery with three capsules of ginger (0.5 g of ginger powder per capsule) when compared to placebo significantly prevented vomiting at 6 hours postoperation. The effect was not apparent at 2 hours postoperation (Apariman et al 2006).

Although other types of surgery have not been as extensively studied as gynaecological surgery, there is a report on 6 months of clinical anaesthetic experience that suggests that a nasocutaneously administered 5% solution of essential oil of ginger given pre-operatively, together with conventional therapies, to general anaesthesia patients at high risk for postoperative nausea and vomiting is a safe and cost-effective way of reducing nausea and vomiting post anaesthesia (Geiger 2005).

Another RCT recently showed that inhaled ginger essential oil produced significant benefits by reducing postoperative nausea. The study involving 303 subjects in an ambulatory post anaesthesia care unit were administered three deep inhalations of a gauze pad soaked with saline (placebo), alcohol, ginger essential oil (EO) or a combination of ginger, spearmint, peppermint and cardamom. The ginger EO and the ginger blend showed significant beneficial effects over placebo for nausea severity and a significant reduction in postoperative antiemetic medication was required (Hunt et al 2013).

In the only double-blind, placebo-controlled study of postoperative nausea and vomiting in patients undergoing middle ear surgery, ginger was ineffective and the use of 1 g of ginger 1 hour before surgery was associated with significantly more postoperative nausea and vomiting than the use of ondansetron or placebo (Gulhas et al 2003).

Motion sickness

Commission E approves the use of ginger root for the prevention of motion sickness (Blumenthal et al 2000) and several clinical studies have assessed its effects as either prophylaxis or treatment. An early double-blind, randomised, placebo-controlled study involving 80 naval cadets found that ginger was significantly superior to placebo in reducing symptoms of vomiting and cold sweats due to seasickness. Fewer symptoms of nausea and vertigo were also reported with ginger, but the difference was not statistically significant (Grontved & Hentzer 1986). In another randomised double-blind study of seasickness involving over 1700 tourists on a whale-watching safari 300 km north of the Arctic Circle, 500 mg ginger was found to be as effective for the treatment of motion sickness as several common antiemetic medications (cinnarizine, cyclizine, dimenhydrinate, domperidone, meclizine and scopolamine) with ginger preventing seasickness in 80% of the subjects during the 6-hour boat trip, although the incidence of severe vomiting did not differ significantly between treatment groups (Schmid et al 1994).

At least three studies have had mixed results from experimental models of motion sickness whereby subjects are seated in a rotating chair. The first study involving 28 volunteers found no significant protective effects for powdered ginger (500 mg or 1000 mg) or fresh ginger root (1000 mg) (Stewart et al 1991), whereas a second study involving 36 undergraduate men and women who reported very high susceptibility to motion sickness found that ginger was superior to dimenhydrinate (Mowrey & Clayson 1982). Another double-blind, randomised, placebo-controlled crossover study showed positive benefits with ginger pretreatment on prolonging time before nausea, shortening recovery time and effectively reducing nausea (Lien et al 2003). This study used pretreatment doses of 1000 mg and 2000 mg, which were also shown to reduce tachygastria and plasma vasopressin.

Chemotherapy-induced nausea and vomiting (CINV)

A review of seven RCTs and crossover trials concluded that ginger may be useful as an adjuvant therapy; however, interpretation is difficult because of mixed results due to methodological differences and the complex aetiology of chemotherapy-induced nausea and vomiting (CINV). Chemotherapy may affect both the central nervous system and the gastrointestinal tract which can influence their development of CINV. Patients may also be affected by sensory input (e.g. smell, sight) or 'anticipatory nausea' as a result of the individual's psychological condition (e.g. fear, anxiety) (Marx et al 2013).

One of the largest most recent placebo-controlled studies was conducted by Ryan et al (2012) which involved 576 cancer patients and showed that supplementation of 0.5, 1.0 and 1.5 g powdered ginger significantly reduced self-assessed acute nausea severity compared to placebo when administered for 3 days prior and 3 days after chemotherapy administration (Ryan et al 2012).

Comparative studies

Powdered ginger root effectively reduced cyclophosphamide-induced nausea and vomiting in a randomised, prospective, crossover double-blind study, with the antiemetic effect of ginger being equal to metoclopramide (Sontakke et al 2003). Ginger was found to have similar efficacy to metoclopramide in reducing cisplatin-induced emesis in a randomised, double-blinded, crossover study of 48 gynaecological cancer patients receiving chemotherapy (Manusirivithaya et al 2004); however, the current clinical significance of this result is questionable, due to the fact that metoclopramide is no longer used as a stand-alone antiemetic treatment (Marx et al 2013).

Use with other anti-nausea medication

A recent combination study found that 1.5 g/day ginger taken with granisetron plus dexamethasone was more effective at reducing CINV than granisetron plus dexamethasone alone. A significantly lower prevalence of nausea, vomiting and retching was observed in the 6–24 hour post-chemotherapy period (Panahi et al 2012). Another RCT compared ginger root powder capsules or placebo in addition to ondansetron and dexamethasone for chemotherapy-induced nausea and vomiting in children and young adults, undergoing 60 cycles of cisplatin/doxorubicin for bone sarcoma (Pillai et al 2011). Acute moderate to severe vomiting and delayed nausea were reduced by 37–47% in the ginger group compared to placebo, highlighting the potential for ginger to act as an effective add-on therapy.

Nausea and vomiting with antiretroviral treatment

Ginger (500 mg twice daily) was effective in ameliorating antiretroviral-induced nausea and vomiting in a placebo-controlled RCT involving 102 HIV-positive patients (Dabaghzadeh et al 2014).

Musculoskeletal disorders

Ginger is described in Ayurvedic (traditional Indian) and Tibb (traditional Arabian) systems of medicine to be useful in inflammation and rheumatism and this traditional use is supported by modern studies demonstrating ginger's anti-inflammatory activity.

A highly purified and standardised ginger extract (EV.EXT 77) moderately reduced the symptoms of osteoarthritis (OA) of the knee in a double-blind, placebo-controlled, multicentre, parallel-group 6-week study of 261 patients (Altman & Marcussen 2001). Similarly, 250 mg of the ginger extract (Zintona EC) taken four times daily for 6 months was significantly more effective than placebo in reducing pain and disability in 29 OA patients in a double-blind, placebo-controlled, crossover study (Wigler et al 2003).

These studies are supported by an open retrospective study involving 56 patients (28 with RA, 18 with OA, 10 with muscular discomfort) that revealed more than three-quarters experienced varying degrees of relief of pain and swelling from the long-term use of powdered ginger (Srivastava & Mustafa 1992). Further support comes from studies comparing ginger to NSAIDs.

In one double-blind RCT involving 120 patients, 30 mg of an ethanolic ginger extract equivalent to 1 g of ginger and prepared from fresh ginger purchased from a local market in India was found to be significantly more effective than placebo and was as effective as 1.2 g of ibuprofen in the symptomatic treatment of OA (Haghighi et al 2005). In another double-blind crossover study, 170 mg of the ginger extract EV.EXT 33 with a standardised content of hydroxy-methoxy-phenyl compounds given twice daily was found to be significantly more effective than placebo but not as effective as ibuprofen in reducing pain and disability in 75 patients with OA before the crossover period, whereas no statistical difference was seen between ginger and placebo in the analysis after the crossover period. The authors commented that the washout period may have been insufficient to prevent carry-over effects, and that ginger might need to be administered for longer than 3 weeks, and possibly in a higher dosage, to be clinically effective (Bliddal et al 2000).

Topical ginger preparation

In a small pilot study, 10 patients with osteoarthritis applied external ginger compresses over the kidneys for 7 days in a phenomenological approach and found benefits such as improved posture, more comfortable and flexible joint mobility and a positive shift in pain perception (Therkleson 2010).

Post-exercise muscle pain

In a double blind, placebo-controlled clinical trial of healthy volunteers, daily consumption of 2 g of raw or heated ginger for 11 days was found to reduce eccentric exercise-induced muscle pain when compared to placebo (Black et al 2010). In this study, dried powdered ginger was placed in a sealed bottle with deionised water and heated in a water bath for 3 hours and 15 minutes at 100 degrees Celsius. No significant difference in pain reduction effect was found with the heated versus raw ginger (Black et al 2010).

Dysmenorrhoea

Ginger has been used orally to treat dysmenorrhoea and appears to be effective based on available evidence. Due to its ability to inhibit thromboxane synthetase and activate endorphin receptors, the use of ginger has been suggested in treatment of dysmenorrhoea (Backon 1991). A double-blind comparative clinical trial involving 150 participants demonstrated that ginger (250 mg ginger rhizome powder qid for 3 days from the start of their menstrual period) was just as effective as 250 mg mefenamic acid or 400 mg ibuprofen capsules in relieving pain in women with primary dysmenorrhoea (Ozgoli et al 2009). Significant benefits were also seen in a RCT of 120 participants with mild-moderate dysmenorrhoea. Treatment with 500 mg powdered ginger given three times per day for 3–5 days produced a significant improvement in intensity and duration of menstrual pain (Rahnama et al 2012).

Dyspepsia

Ginger stimulates the flow of saliva, bile and gastric secretions and therefore is traditionally used to stimulate appetite, reduce flatulence and colic, gastrointestinal spasms and generally act as a digestive aid. Commission E approves the use of ginger root for the treatment of dyspepsia (Blumenthal et al 2000).

Hyperlipidaemia

A double-blind controlled clinical trial of 85 volunteers with hyperlipidaemia showed ginger treatment (3 g/day) produced a significant lipid-lowering effect compared to controls. Measurement of lipid concentrations before and after 45 days of treatment showed significantly higher mean changes in triglyceride and cholesterol levels for ginger compared to control ($P < 0.05$) as well as significant mean reduction in LDL level and increase in HDL levels compared to controls (Alizadeh-Navaei et al 2008). This initial study shows promising results; however, further controlled human trials are necessary to prove efficacy, a conclusion shared by a review of the pharmacological properties of ginger (Li et al 2012).

Migraine

Ginger is used to prevent and treat migraine headache. Its ability to inhibit thromboxane A_2 and exert antihistamine, anti-inflammatory and gastric actions makes it a theoretically attractive choice (Mustafa & Srivastava 1990). This use is supported by an open-label study of 30 migraine sufferers reporting that treatment with a sublingual ginger and feverfew preparation (GelStat MigraineO) in the initial phase of a migraine resulted in most patients being satisfied with the therapy and being pain-free or only having mild headache post-treatment (Cady et al 2005).

IN COMBINATION

In a follow-up randomised pilot study of 60 patients, 221 migraine episodes were treated with sublingual feverfew/ginger (LipiGesic) or placebo, resulting in significant reductions in migraine and headache pain when used as a first line suppressive treatment (Cady et al 2011). Due to the use of a combination product, it is difficult to determine which herb is clinically effective from this study.

Pain

A review of eight RCTs for the treatment of any type of pain raised methodological concerns regarding previous clinical trial designs. Specifically, it concluded that the form of ginger (powder or ethanolic extract) results in variation in active constituent profiles, and this in combination with different therapeutic dosages results in variable levels of efficacy. Administration of over 1 g ginger per day results in amelioration of pain in most trials, whereas less than 510 mg per day does not (Terry et al 2011).

OTHER USES

Ginger cream or compress is used externally for mastitis.

Cognitive function

As a follow-up trial to a successful animal study, a double-blind RCT was conducted which involved 60 healthy middle aged women who received 800 mg ginger per day for 1 month or placebo. When compared to placebo, active treatment resulted in statistically significant improvements in attention, cognitive processing and working memory, including speed of recall and quality of memory (Saenghong et al 2012).

Diabetes

A randomised, double-blind placebo-controlled trial of 88 diabetic participants recently found that 1 g ginger capsules taken three times daily for 8 weeks significantly improved fasting blood sugar, fasting insulin and insulin sensitivity (Mozaffari-Khosravi et al 2014). Animal studies have also shown that ginger may have potential benefits in the treatment of diabetes, indicating that ginger improves insulin sensitivity and reduces serum glucose levels. Further clinical trials are required to confirm the significance of these findings in humans.

Weight loss

Further investigations in animal models and mixed-herbal clinical trials suggest a potential role for ginger in weight loss (Hasani-Ranjbar et al 2009). A significant reduction in body weight and parametrial adipose tissue following oral administration of zingerone in ovariectomised rats indicated that by increasing noradrenaline-induced lipolysis in adipocytes, zingerone may prevent fat storage (Han et al 2008). The anti-obesity action of ginger may be a result of slowed intestinal absorption of dietary fat (Han et al 2008).

Asthma

A possible therapeutic role for gingerol in the treatment of asthma has been indicated through a recent animal model. An aqueous ginger extract enriched in *n*-gingerols was investigated in Th2-mediated pulmonary inflammation where gingerols were found to decrease recruitment of eosinophils to the lungs and suppress Th2 cell response to allergen. Serum IL-4, IL-5 and IgE titres were diminished in ginger-treated mice relative to controls (Ahui et al 2008).

Ulcerative colitis

Recent research has identified a potential role for ginger in attenuating inflammatory bowel disease. In an in vitro study involving ulcerated male Wistar rats, ginger extract was found to be comparable to sulfasalazine in attenuating colonic mucosal injury. The effect of ginger against acetic acid-induced ulcerative colitis has been attributed to its anti-inflammatory and antioxidant properties (El-Abhar et al 2008). Clinical trials are required to determine the significance of this effect in humans.

DOSAGE RANGE

The recommended dose ranges widely from 500 mg to 9 g/day dried root or equivalent; however, a safe maximal dose is 4 g/day. As there are wide variations in the gingerol concentrations in commercial ginger supplements (Schwertner et al 2006), the effective dosage will depend on the preparation and the indication for use.

- Liquid extract (1 : 2): 0.7–4.0 mL/day.
- Dried root: 1–3 g daily in divided doses.
- Infusion: 4–6 slices of fresh ginger steeped in boiling water for 30 minutes.

According to clinical studies

- Dysmenorrhoea: 250 mg ginger rhizome powder taken four times daily for 3 days from the start of the menstrual period.
- Hyperlipidaemia: 3 g/day.
- Nausea and vomiting of pregnancy: 1–2 g taken daily in divided doses.
- Motion sickness: powdered ginger (500 mg or 1000 mg) or fresh ginger root (1000 mg) up to 2000 mg.
- Osteoarthritis: 250 mg of the ginger extract (Zintona EC) four times daily.
- Prevention of postoperative nausea: 1 g 1 hour prior to surgery.
- Rheumatoid arthritis: 1–2 g/day of powdered ginger.

ADVERSE REACTIONS

Gastric irritation, heartburn and bloating have been reported in clinical trials (Arfeen et al 1995). Contact dermatitis of the fingertips has also been reported (Seetharam & Pasricha 1987) with topical use.

SIGNIFICANT INTERACTIONS

Controlled studies are not available for many interactions; therefore they are based on evidence of activity and are largely theoretical and speculative.

Antibiotics

According to a recent review, ginger may enhance the absorption of antibiotics such as azithromycin, erythromycin and cephalexin when used in doses of between 10 and 30 mg/kg due to the herb's modulating effect on the gastric mucosa; however, the clinical significance of this effect is untested (Kesarwani & Gupta 2013).

Warfarin

Due to the herb's antiplatelet effects there is a theoretical risk of increased bleeding at high doses (>10 g), although this is not evident clinically. There is no evidence of an interaction with warfarin at the usual dietary and therapeutic intakes (Jiang et al 2005, Stenton et al 2001, Vaes & Chyka 2000), and ginger has been shown not to alter prothrombin times in pooled human plasma collected from male volunteers between the ages of 18 and 57 years (Jones et al 2001). A standardised ginger extract, EV.EXT 33, has demonstrated no significant effect on coagulation parameters or on warfarin-induced changes in blood coagulation in rats (Weidner & Sigwart 2000) and three ginger capsules (each containing an extract equivalent to 400 mg of ginger rhizome powder) taken three times daily for 2 weeks had no effect on the pharmacokinetics or pharmacodynamics of a single 25-mg dose of warfarin taken on day 7. Moreover, ginger alone did not affect the International Normalised Ratio (INR), platelet aggregation or the pharmacokinetics or pharmacodynamics of warfarin in healthy human subjects (Jiang et al 2005).

Antiplatelet drugs

Theoretically, increased antiplatelet and anti-inflammatory effects may occur with high-dose ginger preparations, but the clinical significance of this is unknown. Caution should be exercised with doses > 10 g — possible beneficial effect.

PREGNANCY USE

Although Commission E suggests that ginger is contraindicated in pregnancy, more recent research suggests that ginger is not contraindicated in pregnancy — doses up to 2 g/day of dried ginger root have been used safely.

No adverse effects on pregnancy were observed in multiple studies of ginger for nausea and vomiting (Boone & Shields 2005, Borrelli et al 2005, Bryer 2005, Dib & El-Saddik 2004, Ernst & Pittler 2000, Jewell & Young 2002).

Cisplatin

Pretreatment has restored testicular antioxidant parameters and sperm motility in cisplatin-induced damage in an animal model (Amin & Hamza 2006). Clinical implications are uncertain; however, potential benefits may be found upon further testing.

CONTRAINDICATIONS AND PRECAUTIONS

Ginger in high doses is not recommended for children under 6 years of age due to the pungent nature of ginger. However, if the benefits of ginger treatment outweigh the potential for gastric irritation, then it can be used. Alternatively, ginger lollies or ginger ale is sometimes used and a dose of 250 mg every 4 hours for motion sickness is safe.

Commission E suggests that people with gallstones consult with their doctor before using ginger. People with gastric ulcers or reflux should use this herb with caution. Suspend use of high-dose supplements (>10 g) 1 week before major surgery.

Practice points/Patient counselling

- Ginger is most often used for its antiemetic, anti-inflammatory and gastrointestinal effects.
- There is good clinical support for the use of ginger in the treatment of nausea and vomiting associated with pregnancy and some evidence for its use in motion sickness, the postoperative period and chemotherapy although this is less consistent.
- Ginger is traditionally used for gastrointestinal disorders, including dyspepsia, poor appetite, flatulence, colic, vomiting, diarrhoea and spasms, as well as a diaphoretic in the treatment of the common cold and influenza.
- Ginger is also used as an anti-inflammatory agent for arthritis, although large controlled studies have yet to produce strong support for this use.
- Although antiplatelet effects have been reported, these require very large doses and are not likely to be significant in normal therapeutic doses or dietary intake levels.
- A study of 24 subjects found that ginger did not significantly affect clotting status or pharmacokinetics of warfarin in healthy subjects (Jiang et al 2006).
- Due to the potential seriousness of the proposed interaction, people taking warfarin should use high-dose supplements (>10 g/day) with caution.

PATIENTS' FAQs

What will this herb do for me?

Ginger is a useful treatment for nausea and vomiting associated with pregnancy and may also be of benefit in motion sickness, postoperative nausea and seasickness. It is also useful for treating symptoms of dyspepsia and may have symptom-relieving effects in arthritis, although this is less certain.

When will it start to work?

In the case of dyspepsia and motion sickness prevention, ginger will have an almost immediate effect, with improvement reported within 30 minutes. For motion sickness, 0.5–1.0 g ginger should be taken 30 minutes before travel and repeated 4-hourly. For nausea of pregnancy it should be taken for at least 4 days; however, symptoms should start to reduce within 1 hour of administration.

Are there any safety issues?

Ginger is well tolerated, although it should be used with caution by people with gallstones, gastric ulcers or reflux.

REFERENCES

Abdel-Aziz H et al. Mode of action of gingerols and shogaols on 5-HT3 receptors: binding studies, cation uptake by the receptor channel and contraction of isolated guinea-pig ileum. Eur J Pharmacol 530.1–2 (2006): 136–143.

Adewunmi CO, Oguntimein BO, Furu P. Molluscicidal and antischistosomal activities of Zingiber officinale. Planta Med 56.4 (1990): 374–376.

Ahmed RS et al. Protective effects of dietary ginger (Zingiber officinale Rosc.) on lindane-induced oxidative stress in rats. Phytother Res 22.7 (2008): 902–906.

Ahui ML et al. Ginger prevents Th2-mediated immune responses in a mouse model of airway inflammation. Int Immunopharmacol 8.12 (2008): 1626–1632.

Aimbire F et al. Effect of hydroalcoholic extract of Zingiber officinalis rhizomes on LPS-induced rat airway hyperreactivity and lung inflammation. Prostaglandins Leukot Essent Fatty Acids 77.3–4 (2007): 129–138.

Ajith TA, Hema U, Aswathy MS. Zingiber officinale Roscoe prevents acetaminophen-induced acute hepatotoxicity by enhancing hepatic antioxidant status. Food Chem Toxicol 45.11 (2007): 2267–2272.

Ajith TA et al. Protective effect of Zingiber officinale Roscoe against anticancer drug doxorubicin-induced acute nephrotoxicity. Food Chem Toxicol 46.9 (2008): 3178–3181.

Akoachere JF et al. Antibacterial effect of Zingiber officinale and Garcinia kola on respiratory tract pathogens. East Afr Med J 79.11 (2002): 588–592.

Aktan F et al. Gingerol metabolite and a synthetic analogue Capsarol inhibit macrophage NF-kappaB-mediated iNOS gene expression and enzyme activity. Planta Med 72.8 (2006): 727–734.

Al-Amin ZM et al. Anti-diabetic and hypolipidaemic properties of ginger (Zingiber officinale) in streptozotocin-induced diabetic rats. Br J Nutr 96.4 (2006): 660–666.

Alizadeh-Navaei R et al. Investigation of the effect of ginger on the lipid levels. A double blind controlled clinical trial. Saudi Med J 29.9 (2008): 1280–1284.

Altman RD, Marcussen KC. Effects of a ginger extract on knee pain in patients with osteoarthritis. Arthritis Rheum 44.11 (2001): 2531–2538.

Amin A, Hamza AA. Effects of Roselle and Ginger on cisplatin-induced reproductive toxicity in rats. Asian J Androl 8.5 (2006): 607–612.

Anoiske CA et al. Anti-inflammatory and anti-ulcerogenic activity of the ethanol extract of ginger (*Zingiber officinale*). Afr J of Biochem Res 3.12 (2009): 379–384.

Apariman S et al. Effectiveness of ginger for prevention of nausea and vomiting after gynecological laparoscopy. J Med Assoc Thai 89.12 (2006): 2003–2009.

Arfeen Z et al. A double-blind randomised controlled trial of ginger for the prevention of postoperative nausea and vomiting. Anaesth Intensive Care 23.4 (1995): 449–452.

Asnani V, Verma RJ. Antioxidative effect of rhizome of Zinziber officinale on paraben induced lipid peroxidation: an in vitro study. Acta Pol Pharm 64.1 (2007): 35–37.

Atta AH et al Hepatoprotective effect of methanol extracts of Zingiber officinale and Cichorium intybus Indian J of Pharm Sc 72.5 (2010): 564–70.

Awang DVC. Ginger. Can Pharm J 125.7 (1992): 309–311.

Backon J. Mechanism of analgesic effect of clonidine in the treatment of dysmenorrhea. Med Hypotheses 36.3 (1991): 223–224.

Bellik Y Total antioxidant activity and antimicrobial potency of the essential oil and oleoresin of Zingiber officinale Roscoe. Asian Pac J Trop Dis 4.1 (2014): 40–44.

Betz O et al. Is ginger a clinically relevant antiemetic? A systematic review of randomised controlled trials. Forsch Komplementarmed Klass Naturheilkd 12.1 (2005): 14–23.

Bhandari U et al. Antihepatotoxic activity of ginger ethanol extract in rats. Pharm Biol 41.1 (2003): 68–71.

Bhandari U, Kanojia R, Pillai KK. Effect of ethanolic extract of Zingiber officinale on dyslipidaemia in diabetic rats. J Ethnopharmacol 97.2 (2005): 227–230.

Bhattarai S, Tran VH, Duke CC. The stability of gingerol and shogaol in aqueous solutions. J Pharm Sci 90.10 (2001): 1658–1664.

Black CD et al. Ginger (Zingiber officinale) Reduces Muscle Pain Caused by Eccentric Exercise. Journal of Pain 11.9 (2010): 894–903.

Bliddal H et al. A randomised, placebo-controlled, cross-over study of ginger extracts and ibuprofen in osteoarthritis. Osteoarthritis Cartilage 8.1 (2000): 9–12.

Blumenthal M, Goldberg A, Brinckmann J (eds). Herbal medicine: expanded commission E monographs. Austin, TX: Integrative Medicine Communications, 2000.

Bode AM et al. Inhibition of epidermal growth factor-induced cell transformation and activator protein 1 activation by [6]-gingerol. Cancer Res 61.3 (2001): 850–853.

Bone ME et al. Ginger root: a new antiemetic: the effect of ginger root on postoperative nausea and vomiting after major gynaecological surgery. Anaesthesia 45.8 (1990): 669–671.

Boone SA, Shields KM. Treating pregnancy-related nausea and vomiting with ginger. Ann Pharmacother 39.10 (2005): 1710–1713.

Bordia A, Verma SK, Srivastava KC. Effect of ginger (Zingiber officinale Rosc.) and fenugreek (Trigonella foenum-graecum L.) on blood lipids, blood sugar and platelet aggregation in patients with coronary artery disease. Prostaglandins Leukot Essent Fatty Acids 56.5 (1997): 379–384.

Borrelli F et al. Effectiveness and safety of ginger in the treatment of pregnancy-induced nausea and vomiting. Obstet Gynecol 105.4 (2005): 849–856.

Brown AC et al. Ginger's (Zingiber officinale Roscoe) inhibition of rat colonic adenocarcinoma cells proliferation and angiogenesis in vitro. Phytother Res 23.5 (2008): 640–645.

Bryer E. A literature review of the effectiveness of ginger in alleviating mild-to-moderate nausea and vomiting of pregnancy. J Midwifery Womens Health 50.1 (2005): e1–e3.

Cady RK et al. Gelstat Migraine (sublingually administered feverfew and ginger compound) for acute treatment of migraine when administered during the mild pain phase. Med Sci Monitor Int Med J Exp Clin Res 11.9 (2005): PI65–PI69.

Cady RK et al A double-blind placebo-controlled pilot study of sublingual feverfew and ginger (LipiGesic M) in the treatment of migraine. Headache 51.7 (2011): 1078–86.

Canter PH. Ginger: do we know what we are talking about? Focus Altern Complement Ther 9.3 (2004): 184–185.

Chaiyakunapruk N et al. The efficacy of ginger for the prevention of postoperative nausea and vomiting: a meta-analysis. Am J Obstet Gynecol 194.1 (2006): 95–99.

Charles R et al. New gingerdione from the rhizomes of Zingiber officinale. Fitoterapia 71.6 (2000): 716–718.

Chen CY et al. 6-shogaol (alkanone from ginger) induces apoptotic cell death of human hepatoma p53 mutant Mahlavu subline via an oxidative stress-mediated caspase-dependent mechanism. J Agric Food Chem 55.3 (2007): 948–954.

Chittumma P et al. Comparison of the effectiveness of ginger and vitamin B6 for treatment of nausea and vomiting in early pregnancy: a randomized double-blind controlled trial. J Med Assoc Thai 90.1 (2007): 15–20.

Dabaghzadeh F et al. Ginger for prevention of antiretroviral-induced nausea and vomiting: a randomized clinical trial. Expert Opin Drug Saf 13.7 (2014): 859–866.

Daswani PG et al Antidiarrhoeal activity of Zingiber officinale (Rosc). Current Science 98.2 (2010): 222–229.

Dedov VN et al. Gingerols: a novel class of vanilloid receptor (VR1) agonists. Br J Pharmacol 137.6 (2002): 793–798.

Denyer CV et al. Isolation of antirhinoviral sesquiterpenes from ginger (Zingiber officinale). J Nat Prod 57.5 (1994): 658–662.

Dib JG, El-Saddik RA. Ginger for nausea and vomiting in pregnancy. J Pharm Pract Res 34.4 (2004): 305–307.

Ding M et al. The effectiveness and safety of ginger for pregnancy-induced nausea and vomiting:A systematic review. Women Birth 26.1 (2013): e26–30.

Du YH et al. [Preliminary study on disease menu of acupuncture and moxibustion abroad]. Zhongguo Zhen Jiu 29.1 (2009): 53–55.

Eberhart LHJ et al. Ginger does not prevent postoperative nausea and vomiting after laparoscopic surgery. Anesth Analg 96.4 (2003): 995–998.

El-Abhar HS et al. Modulating effect of ginger extract on rats with ulcerative colitis. J Ethnopharmacol 118.3 (2008): 367–372.

Eliakim R, Abulafia O, Sherer DM. Hyperemesis gravidarum: a current review. Am J Perinatol 17.4 (2000): 207–218.

Ensiyeh J, Sakineh MA. Comparing ginger and vitamin B6 for the treatment of nausea and vomiting in pregnancy: a randomised controlled trial. Midwifery (2008).

Ernst E, Pittler MH. Efficacy of ginger for nausea and vomiting: a systematic review of randomized clinical trials. Br J Anaesth 84.3 (2000): 367–371.

Fischer-Rasmussen W et al. Ginger treatment of hyperemesis gravidarum. Eur J Obstet Gynecol Reprod Biol 38.1 (1990): 19–24.

Flynn DL et al. Inhibition of human neutrophil 5-lipoxygenase activity by gingerdione, shogaol, capsaicin and related pungent compounds. Prostaglandins Leukot Med 24.2–3 (1986): 195–198.

Fuhrman B et al. Ginger extract consumption reduces plasma cholesterol, inhibits LDL oxidation and attenuates development of atherosclerosis in atherosclerotic, apolipoprotein E-deficient mice. J Nutr 130.5 (2000): 1124–1131.

Funk JL et al. Comparative effects of two gingerol-containing Zingiber officinale extracts on experimental rheumatoid arthritis (perpendicular). J Nat Prod (2009).

Geiger JL. The essential oil of ginger, Zingiber officinale, and anaesthesia. Int J Aromather 15.1 (2005): 7–14.

Ghayur MN, Gilani AH. Pharmacological basis for the medicinal use of ginger in gastrointestinal disorders. Dig Dis Sci 50.10 (2005): 1889–1897.

Ghayur MN et al. Muscarinic, Ca(++) antagonist and specific butyrylcholinesterase inhibitory activity of dried ginger extract might explain its use in dementia. J Pharm Pharmacol 60.10 (2008): 1375–1383.

Gonlachanvit S et al. Ginger reduces hyperglycemia-evoked gastric dysrhythmias in healthy humans: possible role of endogenous prostaglandins. J Pharmacol Exp Ther 307.3 (2003): 1098–1103.

Goto C et al. Lethal efficacy of extract from Zingiber officinale (traditional Chinese medicine) or [6]-shogaol and [6]-gingerol in Anisakis larvae in vitro. Parasitol Res 76.8 (1990): 653–656.

Govindarajan VS. Ginger: chemistry, technology, and quality evaluation: part 2. Crit Rev Food Sci Nutr 17 (1982): 189–258.

Goyal RK, Kadnur SV. Beneficial effects of Zingiber officinale on goldthioglucose induced obesity. Fitoterapia 77.3 (2006): 160–163.

Grontved A, Hentzer E. Vertigo-reducing effect of ginger root: a controlled clinical study. ORL J Otorhinolaryngol Relat Spec 48.5 (1986): 282–286.

Grzanna R et al. Ginger: an herbal medicinal product with broad anti-inflammatory actions. J Med Food 8.2 (2005): 125–132.

Gulhas N et al. The effect of ginger and ondansetron on nausea and vomiting after middle ear surgery. Anestezi Dergisi 11.4 (2003): 265–268.

Gupta YK, Sharma M. Reversal of pyrogallol-induced delay in gastric emptying in rats by ginger (Zingiber officinale). Methods Find Exp Clin Pharmacol 23.9 (2001): 501–503.

Haghighi M et al. Comparing the effects of ginger (Zingiber officinale) extract and ibuprofen on patients with osteoarthritis. Arch Iran Med 8.4 (2005): 267–271.

Haji Seid Javadi, E et al. Comparing the effectiveness of Vitamin B6 and Ginger in the treatment of pregnancy-induced nausea and vomiting. Obstet Gynecol Int (2013): Article ID 927834.

Haksar A et al. Zingiber officinale exhibits behavioral radioprotection against radiation-induced CTA in a gender-specific manner. Pharmacol Biochem Behav 84.2 (2006): 179–188.

Han LK et al. Effects of zingerone on fat storage in ovariectomized rats. Yakugaku Zasshi 128.8 (2008): 1195–1201.

Hasani-Ranjbar S et al. A systematic review of the efficacy and safety of herbal medicines used in the treatment of obesity. World J Gastroenterol 15.25 (2009): 3073–3085.

Hasenohrl RU et al. Anxiolytic-like effect of combined extracts of Zingiber officinale and ginkgo biloba in the elevated plus-maze. Pharmacol Biochem Behav 53.2 (1996): 271–275.

Henry CJ, Piggott SM. Effect of ginger on metabolic rate. Hum Nutr Clin Nutr 41.1 (1987): 89–92.

Hu ML et al. Effect of ginger on gastric motility and symptoms of functional dyspepsia. World J. Gastroenterol.17.1 (2011) 105–10.

Huang QR et al. Anti-5-hydroxytryptamine3 effect of galanolactone, diterpenoid isolated from ginger. Chem Pharm Bull 39.2 (1991): 397–399.

Hunt R et al. Aromatherapy as treatment for postoperative nausea: a randomized trial. Anaesth Analg 117.3 (2013): 597–604.

Imanishi N et al. Macrophage-mediated inhibitory effect of Zingiber officinale Rosc., a traditional oriental herbal medicine, on the growth of influenza A/Aichi/2/68 virus. Am J Chin Med 34.1 (2006): 157–169.

Ishiguro K et al. Ginger ingredients reduce viability of gastric cancer cells via distinct mechanisms. Biochem Biophys Res Commun 362.1 (2007): 218–223.

Islam MS, Choi H. Comparative effects of dietary ginger (Zingiber officinale) and garlic (Allium sativum) investigated in a type 2 diabetes model of rats. J Med Food 11.1 (2008): 152–159.

Jagetia GC et al. Influence of ginger rhizome (Zingiber officinale Rosc.) on survival, glutathione and lipid peroxidation in mice after whole-body exposure to gamma radiation. Radiat Res 160.5 (2003): 584–592.

Janssen PL et al. Consumption of ginger (Zingiber officinale Roscoe) does not affect ex vivo platelet thromboxane production in humans. Eur J Clin Nutr 50.11 (1996): 772–774.

Jewell D, Young G. Interventions for nausea and vomiting in early pregnancy. Cochrane Database Syst Rev 1 (2002): CD000145.

Jewell D. Nausea and vomiting in early pregnancy. Am Fam Physician 68.1 (2003): 143–144.

Jeyakumar SM et al. Antioxidant activity of ginger (Zingiber officinale Rosc.) in rats fed a high fat diet. Med Sci Res 27.5 (1999): 341–344.

Jiang X et al. Investigation of the effects of herbal medicines on warfarin response in healthy subjects: a population pharmacokinetic-pharmacodynamic modeling approach. J Clin Pharmacol 46.11 (2006): 1370–1378.

Jiang X et al. Effect of ginkgo and ginger on the pharmacokinetics and pharmacodynamics of warfarin in healthy subjects. Br J Clin Pharmacol 59.4 (2005): 425–432.

Jones SC et al. The development of a human tissue model to determine the effect of plant-derived dietary supplements on prothrombin time. J Herbal Pharmacother 1.1 (2001): 21–34.

Kadnur SV, Goyal RK. Beneficial effects of Zingiber officinale Roscoe on fructose induced hyperlipidemia and hyperinsulinemia in rats. Indian J Exp Biol 43.12 (2005): 1161–1164.

Kano Y et al. Pharmacological properties of galenical preparation. XIV. body temperature retaining effect of the Chinese traditional medicine, goshuyu-to and component crude drugs. Tokyo: Chem Pharm Bull 39.3 (1991): 690–692.

Kalaivani K et al. Biological activity of selected Lamiaceae and Zingiberaceae plant essential oils against the dengue vector Aedes aegypti L. (Diptera: Culicidae). Parasitol Res 110 (2012): 1261–1268.

Kalava A et al. Efficacy of ginger on intraoperative and postoperative nausea and vomiting in elective cesarean section patients. Euro J Obstet Gynecol Repro Biol 169.2 (2013): 184–188.

Kato A et al. Inhibitory effects of Zingiber officinale Roscoe derived components on aldose reductase activity in vitro and in vivo. J Agric Food Chem 54.18 (2006): 6640–6644.

Kawai T et al. Anti-emetic principles of Magnolia obovata bark and Zingiber officinale rhizome. Planta Med 60.1 (1994): 17–20.

Keating A, Chez RA. Ginger syrup as an antiemetic in early pregnancy. Altern Ther Health Med 8.5 (2002): 89–91.

Kesawarni K, Gupta R. Bioavailability enhancers of herbal origin. Asian Pac J Trop Biomed 3.4 (2013): 253–266.

Kikuzaki H et al. Constituents of Zingiberaceae. I. Diarylheptanoids from the rhizomes of ginger (Zingiber officinale Roscoe). Chem Pharm Bull 39.1 (1991): 120–122.

Kim JH et al. [6]-Gingerol suppresses interleukin-1 beta-induced MUC5AC gene expression in human airway epithelial cells. Am J Rhinol Allergy 23.4 (2009): 385–391.

Kim JK et al. [6]-Gingerol prevents UVB-induced ROS production and COX-2 expression in vitro and in vivo. Free Radic Res 41.5 (2007): 603–614.

Kim SO et al. [6]-Gingerol inhibits COX-2 expression by blocking the activation of p38 MAP kinase and NF-kappaB in phorbol ester-stimulated mouse skin. Oncogene 24.15 (2005): 2558–2567.

Kiuchi F et al. Inhibition of prostaglandin and leukotriene biosynthesis by gingerols and diarylheptanoids. Chem Pharm Bull 40.2 (1992): 387–391.

Kobayashi M, Shoji N, Ohizumi Y. Gingerol, a novel cardiotonic agent, activates the Ca^{2+}-pumping ATPase in skeletal and cardiac sarcoplasmic reticulum. Biochim Biophys Acta 903.1 (1987): 96–102.

Koch C et al. Inhibitory effect of essential oils against herpes simplex virus type 2. Phytomedicine 15.1–2 (2008): 71–78.

Koo KL et al. Gingerols and related analogues inhibit arachidonic acid-induced human platelet serotonin release and aggregation. Thromb Res 103.5 (2001): 387–397.

Kumar S et al. Evaluation of 15 local plant species as larvicidal agents against an Indian strain of dengue fever mosquito, *Aedes aegypti* L.(Diptera: Culicidae). Frontiers in Phys. 3 (2012) Art 104.

Langner E et al. Ginger: history and use. Adv Ther 15.1 (1998): 25–44.

Lee E, Surh YJ. Induction of apoptosis in HL-60 cells by pungent vanilloids, [6]-gingerol and [6]-paradol. Cancer Lett 134.2 (1998): 163–168.

Lee HS et al. [6]-Gingerol inhibits metastasis of MDA-MB-231 human breast cancer cells. J Nutr Biochem 19.5 (2008): 313–3119.

Li Y et al. Preventive and protective properties of Zingiber officinale (Ginger) in diabetes mellitus, diabetic complications, and associated lipid and other metabolic disorders: a brief review. Evidence-Based Complementary and Alternative Medicine Volume 2012 (2012): ID 516870.

Lien HC et al. Effects of ginger on motion sickness and gastric slow-wave dysrhythmias induced by circular vection. Am J Physiol Gastrointest Liver Physiol 284.3 (2003): G481–G489.

Ling H et al. 6-Shogaol, an active constituent of ginger, inhibits breast cancer cell invasion by reducing matrix metalloproteinase-9 expression via blockade of nuclear factor-kB activation. British J Pharma 161 (2010): 1763–1777.

Liu HL, Wang LP. [Randomized controlled study on ginger-salt-partitioned moxibustion at shenque (CV 8) on urination disorders poststroke]. Zhongguo Zhen Jiu 26.9 (2006): 621–624.

Liu N et al. [Effect of Zingiber Officinale Rosc on lipid peroxidation in hyperlipidemia rats]. Wei Sheng Yan Jiu 32.1 (2003): 22–23.

Lu CJ. Function of ginger on cerebrovascular disease and its gateway. Chin J Clin Rehab 9.45 (2005): 187–189.

Lumb AB. Effect of dried ginger on human platelet function. Thromb Haemost 71.1 (1994): 110–1111.

Mahady GB et al. Ginger (Zingiber officinale Roscoe) and the gingerols inhibit the growth of Cag A+ strains of Helicobacter pylori. Anticancer Res 23.5A (2003): 3699–3702.

Mahady GB et al. In vitro susceptibility of Helicobacter pylori to botanical extracts used traditionally for the treatment of gastrointestinal disorders. Phytother Res 19.11 (2005): 988–991.

Mallikarjuna K et al. Ethanol toxicity: rehabilitation of hepatic antioxidant defense system with dietary ginger. Fitoterapia 79.3 (2008): 174–178.

Manju V, Nalini N. Chemopreventive efficacy of ginger, a naturally occurring anticarcinogen during the initiation, post-initiation stages of 1,2 dimethylhydrazine-induced colon cancer. Clin Chim Acta 358.1–2 (2005): 60–67.

Manusirivithaya S et al. Antiemetic effect of ginger in gynecologic oncology patients receiving cisplatin. Int J Gynecol Cancer 14.6 (2004): 1063–1069.

Martins AP et al. Essential oil composition and antimicrobial activity of three Zingiberaceae from S.Tome e Principle. Planta Med 67.6 (2001): 580–584.

Marx WM et al. Ginger (Zingiber officinale) and chemotherapy-induced nausea and vomiting: a systematic literature review. Nutrition Reviews 71.4 (2013): 245–254.

Matthews A et al. Interventions for nausea and vomiting in early pregnancy. Cochrane Database Sys Rev 9 (2010):CD007575.

Meyer K et al. Zingiber officinale (ginger) used to prevent 8-Mop associated nausea. Dermatol Nurs 7.4 (1995): 242–244.

Micklefield GH et al. Effects of ginger on gastroduodenal motility. Int J Clin Pharmacol Ther 37.7 (1999): 341–346.

Morakinyo AO et al. Effect of Zingiber officinale (Ginger) on sodium arsenite-induced reproductive toxicity in male rats. Afr. J. Biomed. Res. 13 (2010): 39–45.

Motawi TK et al. *Zingiber officinale* acts as a nutraceutical agent against liver fibrosis. Nutr Metab (Lond). 8 (2011): 40.

Mowrey D, Clayson D. Motion sickness, ginger and psychosis. Lancet 319.8273 (1982): 655–657.

Mozaffari-Khosravi H et al. The effect of ginger powder supplementation on insulin resistance and glycemic indices in patients with Type 2 diabetes: a randomized, double-blind, placebo-controlled trial. Complementary Therapies in Medicine (2014): http://dx.doi.org/10.1016/j.ctim.2013.12.017 online ahead of print.

Mustafa T, Srivastava KC. Possible leads for arachidonic acid metabolism altering drugs from natural products. J Drug Develop 3.1 (1990): 47–60.

Mustafa T et al. Pharmacology of ginger. Zingiber officinale. J Drug Dev 6.11 (1993): 25–39.

Nagoshi C et al. Synergistic effect of [10]-gingerol and aminoglycosides against vancomycin-resistant enterococci (VRE). Biol Pharm Bull 29.3 (2006): 443–447.

Nanthakomon T, Pongrojpaw D. The efficacy of ginger in prevention of postoperative nausea and vomiting after major gynecologic surgery. J Med Assoc Thai 89 (Suppl 4) (2006): S130–S136.

Nostro A et al. Effects of combining extracts (from propolis or Zingiber officinale) with clarithromycin on Helicobacter pylori. Phytother Res 20.3 (2006): 187–190.

Nurtjahja-Tjendraputra E et al. Effective anti-platelet and COX-1 enzyme inhibitors from pungent constituents of ginger. Thromb Res 111.4–5 (2003): 259–265.

Okada K, Kawakita K. Analgesic action of acupuncture and moxibustion: a review of unique approaches in Japan. Evid Based Complement Alternat Med 6.1 (2009): 11–117.

O'Mahony R et al. Bactericidal and anti-adhesive properties of culinary and medicinal plants against Helicobacter pylori. World J Gastroenterol 11.47 (2005): 7499–7507.

Onogi T et al. Capsaicin-like effect of (6)-shogaol on substance P-containing primary afferents of rats: a possible mechanism of its analgesic action. Neuropharmacology 31.11 (1992): 1165–1169.

Ozgoli G et al. Comparison of effects of ginger, mefenamic acid, and ibuprofen on pain in women with primary dysmenorrhea. J Altern Complement Med 15.2 (2009): 129–32.

Pan MH et al. 6-Shogaol suppressed lipopolysaccharide-induced up-expression of iNOS and COX-2 in murine macrophages. Mol Nutr Food Res 52.12 (2008): 1467–1477.

Panahi Y et al. Effect of ginger on acute and delayed chemotherapy-induced nausea and vomiting: a pilot, randomized, open-label clinical trial. Integr Cancer Ther 11.3 (2012): 204–211.

Park YJ et al. [6]-Gingerol induces cell cycle arrest and cell death of mutant p53-expressing pancreatic cancer cells. Yonsei Med J 47.5 (2006): 688–697.

Park M et al. Antibacterial activity of [10]-gingerol and [12]-gingerol isolated from ginger rhizome against periodontal bacteria. Phytother Res 22.11 (2008): 1446–1449.

Penna SC et al. Anti-inflammatory effect of the hydralcoholic extract of Zingiber officinale rhizomes on rat paw and skin edema. Phytomedicine 10.5 (2003): 381–385.

Phillips S et al. Zingiber officinale (ginger): an antiemetic for day case surgery. Anaesthesia 48.8 (1993): 715–7117.

Pillai AK et al. Anti-emetic effect of ginger powder versus placebo as an add-on therapy in children and young adults receiving high emetogenic chemotherapy. Pediatr Blood Cancer 56.2 (2011): 234–8.

Platel K, Srinivasan K. Influence of dietary spices or their active principles on digestive enzymes of small intestinal mucosa in rats. Int J Food Sci Nutr 47.1 (1996): 55–59.

Platel K, Srinivasan K. Studies on the influence of dietary spices on food transit time in experimental rats. Nutr Res 21.9 (2001): 1309–1314.

Pongrojpaw D, Chiamchanya C. The efficacy of ginger in prevention of post-operative nausea and vomiting after outpatient gynecological laparoscopy. J Med Assoc Thailand 86.3 (2003): 244–250.

Pongrojpaw D et al. A randomized comparison of ginger and dimenhydrinate in the treatment of nausea and vomiting in pregnancy. J Med Assoc Thai 90.9 (2007): 1703–1709.

Portnoi G et al. Prospective comparative study of the safety and effectiveness of ginger for the treatment of nausea and vomiting in pregnancy. Am J Obstet Gynecol 189.5 (2003): 1374–1377.

Rahnama et al. Effect of Zingiber officinale R. rhizomes (ginger) on pain relief in primary dysmenorrhea: a placebo randomized trial. BMC Complementary and Alternative Medicine 12.92 (2012).

Ramadan G et al. anti-inflammatory and anti-oxidant properties of Curcuma longa (Turmeric) versus Zingiber officinale (Ginger) rhizomes in rat adjuvant-induced arthritis. Inflammation 34.4 (2011): 291–301.

Rhode J et al. Ginger inhibits cell growth and modulates angiogenic factors in ovarian cancer cells. BMC Complement Altern Med 7 (2007): 44.

Riyazi A et al. The effect of the volatile oil from ginger rhizomes (Zingiber officinale), its fractions and isolated compounds on the 5-HT3 receptor complex and the serotoninergic system of the rat ileum. Planta Med 73.4 (2007): 355–362.

Ryan JL et al. Ginger (Zingiber officinale) reduces acute chemotherapy-induced nausea: a URCC CCOP study of 576 patients. Support Care Cancer 20.7 (2012): 1479–489.

Rosengarten FJ. The book of spices. Wynnewood, PA: Livingston Publishing, 1969.

Sabli F et al Cytotoxic Properties of selected *Etlingera* spp. and *Zingiber* spp. (Zingiberaceae) endemic to Borneo. Pertanika J. Trop. Agric. Sci. 35.3 (2012): 663–671.

Saenghong N et al. Zingiber officinale improves cognitive function of the middle-aged healthy women. Evidence-Based Complementary and Alternative Medicine 2012 (2012): ID 383062.

Schmid R et al. Comparison of seven commonly used agents for prophylaxis of seasickness. J Travel Med 1.4 (1994): 203–206.

Schnitzler P et al. Susceptibility of drug-resistant clinical herpes simplex virus type 1 strains to essential oils of ginger, thyme, hyssop, and sandalwood. Antimicrob Agents Chemother 51.5 (2007): 1859–1862.

Schuhbaum H, Franz G. Ginger: spice and versatile medicinal plant. Z Phytother 21.4 (2000): 203–209 [in German].

Schwertner HA et al. Variation in concentration and labeling of ginger root dietary supplements. Obstet Gynecol 107.6 (2006): 1337–1343.

Seetharam KA, Pasricha JS. Condiments and contact dermatitis of the finger-tips. Indian J Dermatol Venereol Leprol 53.6 (1987): 325–328.

Sertie JAA et al. Preventive anti-ulcer activity of the rhizome extract of Zingiber officinale. Fitoterapia 63.1 (1992): 55–59.

Sharma JN et al. Suppressive effects of eugenol and ginger oil on arthritic rats. Pharmacology 49.5 (1994): 314–3118.

Sharma A et al. Zingiber officinale Rosc. modulates gamma radiation-induced conditioned taste aversion. Pharmacol Biochem Behav 81.4 (2005): 864–870.

Shen X et al. An infrared radiation study of the biophysical characteristics of traditional moxibustion. Complement Ther Med 14.3 (2006): 213–2119.

Shoji N et al. Cardiotonic principles of ginger (Zingiber officinale Roscoe). J Pharm Sci 71.10 (1982): 1174–1175.

Shukla Y et al. In vitro and in vivo modulation of testosterone mediated alterations in apoptosis related proteins by [6]-gingerol. Mol Nutr Food Res 51.12 (2007): 1492–1502.

Siddaraju MN, Dharmesh SM. Inhibition of gastric H^+, K^+-ATPase and Helicobacter pylori growth by phenolic antioxidants of Zingiber officinale. Mol Nutr Food Res 51.3 (2007): 324–332.
Smith C et al. A randomized controlled trial of ginger to treat nausea and vomiting in pregnancy. Obstet Gynecol 103.4 (2004): 639–645.
Sontakke S et al. Ginger as an antiemetic in nausea and vomiting induced by chemotherapy: a randomized, cross-over, double blind study. Indian J Pharmacol 35.1 (2003): 32–36.
Sripramote M, Lekhyananda N. A randomized comparison of ginger and vitamin B6 in the treatment of nausea and vomiting of pregnancy. J Med Assoc Thai 86.9 (2003): 846–853.
Srivastava KC, Mustafa T. Ginger (Zingiber officinale) in rheumatism and musculoskeletal disorders. Med Hypotheses 39.4 (1992): 342–348.
Stenton SB et al. Interactions between warfarin and herbal products, minerals, and vitamins: a pharmacist's guide. Can J Hospital Pharm 54.3 (2001): 184–190.
Stewart JJ et al. Effects of ginger on motion sickness susceptibility and gastric function. Pharmacology 42.2 (1991): 111–120.
Takada Y et al. Zerumbone abolishes NF-kappaB and IkappaBalpha kinase activation leading to suppression of antiapoptotic and metastatic gene expression, upregulation of apoptosis, and downregulation of invasion. Oncogene 24.46 (2005): 6957–6969.
Terry R. et al. The use of ginger (*Zingiber officinale*) for the treatment of pain: a systematic review of clinical trials. Pain Medicine 12 (2011) 1808–1818.
Therkleson T. Ginger compress therapy for adults with osteoarthritis. J Adv Nurs 66.10 (2010), 2225–2233.
Thomson M et al. The use of ginger (Zingiber officinale Rosc.) as a potential anti-inflammatory and antithrombotic agent. Prostaglandins Leukot Essent Fatty Acids 67.6 (2002): 475–478.
Tjendraputra E et al. Effect of ginger constituents and synthetic analogues on cyclooxygenase-2 enzyme in intact cells. Bioorgan Chem 29.3 (2001): 156–163.
Tripathi S et al. Ginger extract inhibits LPS-induced macrophage activation and function. BMC Complement Altern Med 8 (2008): 1.
Tripathi S et al. Effect of 6-gingerol on pro-inflammatory cytokine production and costimulatory molecule expression in murine peritoneal macrophages. J Surg Res 138.2 (2007): 209–213.
Vaes LP, Chyka PA. Interactions of warfarin with garlic, ginger, ginkgo, or ginseng: nature of the evidence. Ann Pharmacother 34.12 (2000): 1478–1482.
Verma SK, Bordia A. Ginger, fat and fibrinolysis. Indian J Med Sci 55.2 (2001): 83–86.
Visalyaputra S et al. The efficacy of ginger root in the prevention of postoperative nausea and vomiting after outpatient gynaecological laparoscopy. Anaesthesia 53.5 (1998): 506–510.
Vishwakarma SL et al. Anxiolytic and antiemetic activity of Zingiber officinale. Phytother Res 16.7 (2002): 621–626.
Vutyavanich T et al. Ginger for nausea and vomiting in pregnancy: Randomized, double-masked, placebo-controlled trial. Obstet Gynecol 97.4 (2001): 577–582.
Wei QY et al. Cytotoxic and apoptotic activities of diarylheptanoids and gingerol-related compounds from the rhizome of Chinese ginger. J Ethnopharmacol 102.2 (2005): 177–184.
Weidner MS, Sigwart K. The safety of a ginger extract in the rat. J Ethnopharmacol 73.3 (2000): 513–520.
WHO. Rhizoma Zingiberis. Geneva: World Health Organization. Available online at: www.who.int/medicines/library/trm/medicinalplants (accessed 15-12-03).
Wigler I et al. The effects of Zintona EC (a ginger extract) on symptomatic gonarthritis. Osteoarthritis Cartilage 11.11 (2003): 783–789.
Wilasrusmee C et al. In vitro immunomodulatory effects of herbal products. Am Surg 68.10 (2002): 860–864.
Willetts KE, Ekangaki A, Eden JA. Effect of a ginger extract on pregnancy-induced nausea: a randomised controlled trial. Aust NZ J Obstet Gynaecol 43.2 (2003): 139–144.
Wu KL et al. Effects of ginger on gastric emptying and motility in healthy humans. Eur J Gastroenterol Hepatol 20.5 (2008): 436–440.
Xiaoxiang Z. Jinger moxibustion for treatment of cervical vertigo — a report of 40 cases. J Tradit Chin Med 26.1 (2006): 17–118.
Xie XX, Lei QH. [Observation on therapeutic effect of the spreading moxibustion on rheumatoid arthritis]. Zhongguo Zhen Jiu 28.10 (2008): 730–732.
Yagihashi S et al. Inhibitory effect of gingerol on the proliferation and invasion of hepatoma cells in culture. Cytotechnology 57.2 (2008): 129–136.
Yamada Y et al. Identification of antimicrobial gingerols from ginger (Zingiber officinale Roscoe). J Antibact Antifungal Agents Jpn 20.6 (1992): 309–311.
Yamahara J et al. Cholagocic effect of ginger and its active constituents. J Ethnopharmacol 13.2 (1985): 217–225.
Yamahara J et al. The anti-ulcer effect in rats of ginger constituents. J Ethnopharmacol 23.2–3 (1988): 299–304.
Yamahara J et al. Gastrointestinal motility enhancing effect of ginger and its active constituents. Chem Pharm Bull 38.2 (1990): 430–431.
Yamahara J et al. Stomachic principles in ginger. II. Pungent and anti-ulcer effects of low polar constituents isolated from ginger, the dried rhizoma of Zingiber officinale Roscoe cultivated in Taiwan: the absolute stereostructure of a new diarylheptanoid. Yakugaku Zasshi 112.9 (1992): 645–655 [in Japanese].
Yamahara J et al. Pharmacological study on ginger processing. I. Antiallergic activity and cardiotonic action of gingerols and shogaols. Nat Med 49.1 (1995): 76–83: [in Japanese].
Yemitan OK, Izegbu MC. Protective effects of Zingiber officinale (Zingiberaceae) against carbon tetrachloride and acetaminophen-induced hepatotoxicity in rats. Phytother Res 20.11 (2006): 997–1002.
Yoshikawa M et al. 6-Gingesulfonic acid, a new anti-ulcer principle, and gingerglycolipids A, B and C, three new monoacyldigalactosylglycerols from Zingiberis rhizoma originating in Taiwan. Chem Pharm Bull 40.8 (1992): 2239–2241.
Yoshikawa M et al. Crude drug processing by far-infrared treatment. II. Chemical fluctuation of the constituents during the drying of Zingiberis Rhizoma. Yakugaku Zasshi 113.10 (1993): 712–7117.
Yoshikawa M et al. Stomachic principles in ginger. III: An anti-ulcer principle, 6-gingesulfonic acid, and three monoacyldigalactosylglycerols, gingerglycolipids A, B, and C, from Zingiberis Rhizoma originating in Taiwan. Chem Pharm Bull 42.6 (1994): 1226–1230.
Yu, Y et al Examination of the Pharmacokinetics of Active Ingredients of Ginger in Humans. The AAPS Journal 13.3 (2011) 417–26.
Zhao XX et al. [Multi-central clinical evaluation of ginger-partitioned moxibustion for treatment of leukopenia induced by chemotherapy]. Zhongguo Zhen Jiu 27.10 (2007): 715–720.
Zhou H-L, Deng YM, Xie QM. The modulatory effects of the volatile oil of ginger on the cellular immune response in vitro and in vivo in mice. J Ethnopharmacol 105.1–2 (2006): 301–305.
Zick SM et al. Pharmacokinetics of 6-gingerol, 8-gingerol, 10-gingerol, and 6-shogaol and conjugate metabolites in healthy human subjects. Cancer Epidemiol Biomarkers Prev 17 (2008): 1930–1936.
Zick SM et al Phase II study of the effects of ginger root extract on eicosanoids in colon mucosa in people at normal risk for colorectal cancer. Cancer Prev Res 4.11 (2011): 1929–1937.

Ginkgo biloba

HISTORICAL NOTE *Ginkgo biloba* is one of the world's oldest living tree species, earning it the name 'living fossil'. Its existence can be traced back more than 200 million years and it was commonly found in North America and Europe before the Ice Age. Its place of origin is believed to be remote mountainous valleys of Zhejiang province of eastern China and, up to 350 years ago, knowledge about this plant was restricted to China (Singh et al 2008). Ginkgo was first introduced into Europe in 1690 by the botanist Engelbert Kaempfer, who described it as the 'tree with duck feet'. Ginkgo has been used medicinally for decades and is now one of the most popular therapeutic agents prescribed in Europe by medical doctors. It has been estimated that, in Germany and France, prescriptions for ginkgo make up 1% and 1.3%, respectively, of total prescription sales (Pizzorno & Murray 2006). Also popular in the United States, it was the top-selling herbal medicine in 1999, with sales of US$148 million. Current estimates indicate that the use of *G. biloba* has been growing at a very rapid rate worldwide, at 25% per year in the open-world commercial market (Singh et al 2008). Germany, Switzerland and France have respectively 31%, 8% and 5% of the world commercial market. To meet the demand for ginkgo products, 50 million *G. biloba* trees are grown, especially in China, France and South Carolina, United States, producing 8000 tons of dried leaves each year.

COMMON NAME

Ginkgo

In England, it is known as 'maidenhair tree' based on its resemblance to the foliage of the 'maidenhair fern' (*Adiantum*). In Japan, it is known as 'ginkyo' and in France, 'l'arbre aux quarante écus' and 'noyer du Japon' (Singh et al 2008).

OTHER NAMES

Adiantifolia, arbre aux quarante écus, bai guo ye, duck foot tree, fossil tree, gin-nan, icho, Japanese silver apricot, kew tree, maidenhair tree, salisburia, silver apricot, tempeltrae, temple balm, yinhsing

BOTANICAL NAME/FAMILY

Ginkgo biloba (family Ginkgoaceae)

PLANT PARTS USED

In modern times only the leaf is used, but traditionally the nut was also used.

CHEMICAL COMPONENTS

Important constituents present in the leaves are the terpene trilactones (i.e. ginkgolides A, B, C and J and bilobalide), many flavonol glycosides (mostly derivatives of quercetin and kaempferol) (Hibatallah et al 1999), biflavones, proanthocyanidins, alkylphenols, simple phenolic acids, 6-hydroxykynurenic acid, 4-*O*-methylpyridoxine and polyprenols (van Beek 2002). *G. biloba* contains more than 30 genuine flavonoids, of which the flavonol glycosides are the most abundant (Singh et al 2008).

There has been some interest in ginkgo alkylphenols (ginkgolic acids) because of their allergenic properties, so most manufacturers limit the concentration of alkylphenols to 5 ppm.

> ***Clinical note — Ginkgo extract used in practice***
> The standardised ginkgo extract is made from dried ginkgo leaves extracted in 60% acetone. Only a fraction of the leaf matter is extracted; 98% is not extracted. Of the 2% extracted, the flavones account for 25%, the ginkgolides 3% and the bilobalide 3%. The remaining 69% is not specified. The drug ratio may vary from 35:1 to 67:1 (average ratio 50:1). This means that, on average, it takes 50 kg dried leaf to produce 1 kg of extract. Standardised ginkgo extract (e.g. EGb 761) must be standardised to 22–27% flavone glycosides, 5–7% terpene lactones (2.8–3.4% ginkgolides A, B and C, and 2.6–3.2% bilobalide). The content of ginkgolic acids must be less than 5 ppm (Blumenthal et al 2000). Although the standardisation is very specific, the compounds are considered to be marker compounds, as the active constituents of *G. biloba* have not been fully identified (unpublished data: Keller K, Chair of the Herbal Medicinal Products Working Group, European Medicines Evaluation Agency. Quality Assurance of Herbal Medicines, March 2001).

MAIN ACTIONS

The many and varied pharmacological actions of ginkgo preparations are related to the presence of several classes of active constituents. Research has mainly been conducted with a standardised ginkgo biloba extract (GBE) and also several of its key constituents, such as ginkgetin. Various preparations have also been tested, including oral, injectable and topical preparations.

Antioxidant

GBE and several of its individual constituents, such as quercetin and kaempferol, have demonstrated significant antioxidant properties in vitro (Hibatallah et al 1999, Sloley et al 2000). Antioxidant activity has further been demonstrated in several different animal models.

Experimental models investigating the effects of ginkgo on reducing ischaemic injury in various tissues have shown positive results, indicating that ginkgo reduces the damage caused by oxidative stress during reperfusion (Liu et al 2007, Schneider et al 2008).

Hepatoprotective effects, via an antioxidant action, have also been seen in an animal study in the treatment of non-alcoholic steatohepatitis (Zhou et al 2010).

A novel study has investigated the effect of *G. biloba* on mobile phone-induced oxidative damage in brain tissue of rats (Ilhan et al 2004). Rats were exposed to the same amount of mobile phone-induced radiation for 7 days, with some also pretreated with *G. biloba*. After exposure, oxidative damage was evident by the: (1) increase in malondialdehyde and nitric oxide (NO) levels in brain tissue; (2) decrease in brain superoxide dismutase and glutathione peroxidase activities; and (3) increase in brain xanthine oxidase and adenosine deaminase activities. *Ginkgo biloba* prevented these alterations and the mobile phone-induced cellular injury in brain tissue histopathologically.

Initial research on apoptosis of human lens epithelial cells when exposed to high glucose suggests that GBE has a protective effect inhibiting this oxidative stress (Wu et al 2008b).

G. biloba's antioxidant action and prevention of mitochondrial degeneration may have some effect on protecting Sertoli and spermatid cells in a rat model with testicular torsion (Kanter 2011).

Topical antioxidant effects have also been investigated. *G. biloba* has been shown to reduce the effects of ultraviolet radiation on skin (Aricioglu et al 2001, Hibatallah et al 1999, Kim 2001, Lin & Chang 1997). When applied topically, ginkgo increases the activity of superoxide dismutase within skin, thereby enhancing the skin's natural defences.

Cardioprotective

Ginkgo reduces the damage caused by oxidative stress during reperfusion according to research with various preclinical models.

One study using a model of myocardial infarction found that pretreatment with GBE EGb 761 reduced ischaemic myocardial injury compared to untreated controls (Schneider et al 2008) and another showed *G. biloba* may provide cardioprotection in preventing diabetic complications of cardiovascular autonomic neuropathy, as seen in diabetes-induced myocardial nervous damage (Schneider et al 2010). Another animal study demonstrated that *G. biloba* phytosomes conferred significant cardiac protection with antioxidant activity and decreased lipid peroxidation (Panda & N 2009).

EGb 761 may have a role in reducing cardiotoxic effects of the antineoplastic drug, Adriamycin, as pretreatment for 10 days prior to drug use resulted in normalisation of cardiac enzymes (having an effect on cardiac malondialdehyde, total antioxidant capacity, tumour necrosis factor-alpha [TNF-alpha] and NO levels) (El-Boghdady 2013b). A recent rat study revealed cardioprotective effects reducing ischaemic free radical damage to the heart mitochondria (Bernatoniene et al 2011). These cardiac benefits found in animal studies did not translate to show a clinical effect in the Ginkgo Evaluation of Memory study assessing *G. biloba*'s effect on cardiovascular disease. This enormous double-blind trial randomised 3069 participants over 75 years (120 mg of *G. biloba* EGb 761 twice daily) with follow-up over 6.1 years; no reduction was found in cardiovascular disease events or mortality (Kuller et al 2010).

Anti-inflammatory

The anti-inflammatory activity of ginkgo has been investigated for the whole extract and an isolated biflavonoid component known as ginkgetin, with both forms demonstrating significant anti-inflammatory activity.

Ginkgo extract

Intravenously administered ginkgo extract produced an anti-inflammatory effect that was as strong as the same dose of prednisolone (i.e. 1 mg GBE = 1 mg prednisolone) in an experimental model. Ginkgo extract was also found to significantly reduce the concentration of prostaglandin E_2, TNF-alpha and NO production in vitro (Ilieva et al 2004). Studies with subcutaneously administered GBE in experimental models have further confirmed significant anti-inflammatory activity, with the addition of antinociceptive effects (Abdel-Salam et al 2004).

Investigation with an animal model of colitis revealed that *G. biloba* (EGb 761) extract reduces markers of inflammation (inducible nitric oxide synthase [iNOS], cyclooxygenase-2 [COX-2] and TNF-alpha) and inflammatory stress (p53 and p53-phosphoserine 15) (Kotakadi et al 2008). In the case of ischaemia-reperfusion injury in a rat model, *G. biloba* was found to inhibit inflammatory cytokines (interleukin-6 [IL-6]) and promote anti-inflammatory cytokines (IL-4) (Bao et al 2010).

Ginkgetin

Ginkgetin showed a stronger anti-inflammatory activity than prednisolone when administered by intraperitoneal injection in an animal model of arthritis. Histological examination of the knee joints confirmed the effect (Kim et al 1999). When used topically in an animal model of chronic skin inflammation and proinflammatory gene expression, it was found to inhibit ear oedema by approximately 26% and prostaglandin E_2 production by 30% (Lim et al 2006). Histological comparisons revealed that ginkgetin reduced epidermal hyperplasia, inhibited phospholipase A_2 and suppressed COX-2 and iNOS expression (Lim et al 2006).

Vascular effects

Vasodilation

Ginkgo promotes vasodilation and improves blood flow through arteries, veins and capillaries. Increases in microcirculatory blood flow occur rapidly and have been confirmed under randomised crossover test conditions 1 h after administration (Jung et al 1990).

Several mechanisms of action are responsible. Currently, these are considered to be: inhibition of NO release, activation of Ca^{2+}-activated K^+ channels, increased prostacyclin release and an antioxidant and anti-inflammatory effect (Chen et al 1997, 2011a, Koltermann et al 2007, Nishida & Satoh 2003). In 2008, a clinical study by Wu et al investigated the effects of GBE on the distal left anterior descending coronary artery (LAD) blood flow and plasma NO and endothelin-1 (ET-1) levels (Wu et al 2008c). The randomised controlled trial (RCT) of 80 volunteers with coronary artery disease (CAD) used Doppler echocardiography to determine blood flow, which was measured at baseline and after 2 weeks of treatment. A significant improvement in maximal diastolic peak velocity, maximal systolic peak velocity and diastolic time velocity integral was observed for the group treated with GBE compared with controls ($P < 0.01$). Additionally, a significant increase in NO and decrease in ET-1 was observed, suggesting that the observed increase of LAD blood flow might be related to restoration of the delicate equilibrium between NO and ET-1.

Reduces oedema

Various flavonoids, including anthocyanosides and GBE, have been shown to be effective against experimentally induced capillary hyperfiltration (Cohen-Boulakia et al 2000).

Antiplatelet and anticoagulant — no significant effect

Standardised *G. biloba* therapy is not associated with a higher bleeding risk, according to a 2011 meta-analysis of 18 RCTs (Kellermann & Kloft 2011). This level 1 evidence overrides previous speculation based on several case reports suggesting ginkgo biloba can cause bleeding and some evidence that one of its components, ginkgolide B, is a platelet-activating factor antagonist (Smith et al 1996).

Controlled studies have included young healthy volunteers, older adults, people with multiple sclerosis (MS) and people using warfarin or aspirin at the same time as *G. biloba* (Aruna & Naidu 2007, Bal Dit et al 2003, Beckert et al 2007, Carlson et al 2007, Engelsen et al 2003, Gardner et al 2007, Jiang et al 2005, Kohler et al 2004, Lovera et al 2007, Wolf 2006). An escalating-dose study found that 120 mg, 240 mg or 480 mg given daily for 14 days did not alter platelet function or coagulation (Bal Dit et al 2003).

Only one study could be located which demonstrated that EGb 761 (80 mg/day) produced a significant reduction in blood viscosity after 30 days' treatment (Galduroz et al 2007). When measured again 90 days after commencement of EGb 761 treatment, a further reduction was observed which appeared to stabilise, as no further reduction was observed after 180 days of use.

Alters neurotransmitters

Monoamine oxidase (MAO) inhibition — not in vivo

In vitro tests in rat brains suggest that EGb 761 may exert MAO-A and MAO-B inhibitor activity (Wu & Zhu 1999). Tests with isolated constituents, kaempferol, apigenin and chrysin, have demonstrated these to be potent MAO inhibitors, with greater effect on MAO-A than MAO-B (Sloley et al 2000). A recent rat model showed MAO activity was not affected by EGb 761, suggesting the effect is not significant in vivo (Fehske et al 2009). The lack of significant in vivo MAO-inhibitory activity was confirmed in a human study using positron emission tomography, which found that treatment with *G. biloba* (EGb 761: 120 mg/day) for 1 month did not produce significant changes in brain MAO-A or MAO-B in the 10 participating volunteers (Fowler et al 2000).

Serotonin

An in vitro study found that oral EGb 761 significantly increases the uptake of serotonin, but not dopamine, in cerebral cortex samples from mice (Ramassamy et al 1992) and a later in vivo study identified an antiaggressive effect mediated by 5-HT_{2A} receptors (Shih et al 2000). In contrast, an animal study suggests no change in 5-HT uptake after 14 days of oral treatment with EGb 761 (Fehske et al 2009).

Cholinergic effects

Considering that *G. biloba* appears to be as effective as anticholinesterase drugs, several researchers have investigated whether it exerts cholinergic effects. Evidence from behavioural, in vitro and ex vivo tests with *G. biloba* has shown both direct and indirect cholinergic activities (Das et al 2002, Nathan 2000). The extract appears to increase the rate of acetylcholine turnover and stimulate the binding activity of ligands to muscarinic receptors in the hippocampus (Muller 1989).

Gamma-aminobutyric acid (GABA) receptors

Bilobalide in *G. biloba* is a competitive antagonist for GABA-A receptors according to in vitro tests (Huang et al 2003). The effect is almost as potent as bicuculline and pictrotoxin.

Corticosterone

In vivo tests have found that EGb 761 has stress-alleviating properties mediated through its moderation of corticosterone levels (Puebla-Perez et al 2003).

Dopamine

Chronic, but not acute, treatment with *G. biloba* (EGb 761) significantly increases extracellular dopamine in vivo, which may be one of the mechanisms in improving cognitive function (Yoshitake et al 2010). *G. biloba* (EGb 761) affects the dopaminergic system, which was observed as a reduction in serum prolactin levels in male rats (Yeh et al 2008) and an increase in dopamine and acetylcholine levels in the prefrontal cortex (Kehr et al 2012). *G. biloba*'s dopamine-enhancing effect may be explained by its ability to decrease the uptake of noradrenaline as dopamine clearance in the frontal cortex is mediated by noradrenaline (Fehske et al 2009).

Neuroprotection

G. biloba leaf extract (EGb 761) has demonstrated neuroprotective effects in a variety of studies ranging from molecular and cellular, to animal and human; however not all the cellular and molecular mechanisms have been elucidated (Ao et al 2006, Kaur et al 2013, Smith et al 2002). Of the constituents studied, it appears that the bilobalide constituent is chiefly responsible for this activity, although others are also involved (DeFeudis & Drieu 2000).

Until recently, it was believed that the antioxidant, membrane-stabilising and platelet-activating factor antagonist effects were chiefly responsible for neuroprotection, but effects at the mitochondria may also be important contributing mechanisms. Recent research suggests that *G. biloba* (EGb 761) exerts a multifunctional neuroprotective role associated with activation of the haem oxygenase 1 (HO1) and nuclear factor erythroid 2-related factor 2 (Nrf2), upregulation of vascular endothelial growth factor (VEGF) and downregulation of inflammatory mediators (Tulsulkar & Shah 2012). Another in vivo animal study suggests the neuroprotection may also be a result of antiapoptotic activity and effects on energy metabolism (Mahdy et al 2011).

Beta-amyloid

GBE EGb 761 protects cells against toxicity induced by beta-amyloid in a concentration-dependent manner, according to in vitro tests (Bastianetto & Quirion 2002a, 2002b, Bastianetto et al 2000). In vivo studies have confirmed that ginkgo extract has an antiamyloid aggregation effect (Luo 2006). It appears that ginkgo increases transthyretin RNA levels in mouse hippocampus, which is noteworthy because transthyretin is involved in the transport of beta-amyloid and may provide a mechanism to reduce amyloid deposition in brain (Watanabe et al 2001). There is also evidence that *G. biloba* modulates alpha-secretase, the enzyme that cuts the amyloid precursor protein and prevents amyloidogenic fragments from being produced (Colciaghi et al 2004).

Cerebral ischaemia

There is evidence from experimental and clinical studies that GBE protects cerebral tissues from ischaemia/reperfusion damage and, while the effect has been reported for prophylactic use (Janssens et al 2000, Kaur et al 2013, Peng et al 2003), some research also suggests *G. biloba* exerts significant neuroprotective effects after acute ischaemic stroke (Ma et al 2012, Nada & Shah 2012, Zhang et al 2012b). This was confirmed most recently in a 2013 placebo-controlled RCT of 102 consecutive patients with acute ischaemic stroke which found that treatment with GBE for 4 months produced a significant reduction in poststroke National Institutes of Health Stroke Scale (NIHSS) score compared to placebo, showing improved function (Oskouei et al 2013). The treatment used was *G. biloba* tablets (Gol-Darou, Isfahan, Iran) with a total dose of 120 mg/day (40 mg three times/day),

G. biloba crosses the blood–brain barrier and reaches extracellular concentrations in the brain, allowing efficient interaction with target molecules. The availability of ginkgo in cerebral tissue is high when given before ischaemia, but severely limited after the occurrence of ischaemia, which may explain the greater success seen in animal model research when used prophylactically and mean higher doses are required poststroke (Oskouei et al 2013).

Stabilisation and protection of mitochondrial function

Several in vitro tests have demonstrated that EGb 761 stabilises and protects mitochondrial function (Eckert et al 2005, Janssens et al 2000). These observations are gaining the attention of researchers interested in neurodegenerative diseases, as it is suspected that the mitochondria and the phenomenon of mitochondrial permeability transition play a key role in neuronal cell death and the development of such diseases (Beal 2003, Shevtsova et al 2005). Animal studies are confirming these in vitro findings and it may be that both the ginkgolides and the bilobalide compounds have this mitochondrial protective action on neural function (Eckert 2012).

Immunostimulant

Immunostimulatory activity has been demonstrated in several experimental models (Puebla-Perez et al 2003, Tian et al 2003, Villasenor-Garcia et al 2004).

The beneficial effects of EGb 761 on immune function are based on its antioxidant properties, as well as the cell proliferation-stimulating effect. An in vitro animal study has suggested that nebulised total ginkgo flavone glycosides have a therapeutic effect for asthmatic mice, perhaps through regulating Th1/Th2 imbalance (Chen et al 2008).

Anticancer

Studies conducted with various molecular, cellular and whole-animal models have revealed that leaf extracts of *G. biloba* may have anticancer (chemopreventive) properties that are related to its antioxidant, antiangiogenic and gene-regulatory actions (DeFeudis et al 2003). Both the flavonoid and terpenoid constituents are thought to be responsible for many of these mechanisms, meaning that the whole extract is required for activity. In vitro and in vivo studies have shown GBE inhibits the growth and proliferation of several types of tumour, including colon cancer cells (Chen et al 2011b), gastric precancerous lesions (Jiang et al 2009), pancreatic cancer cells (Zhang et al 2008), liver cancer cells (Hao et al 2009, Wang et al 2011), breast cancer cells (Jiang et al 2011, Park et al 2013) and ovarian cancer BRCA1 gene mutation cells (Jiang et al 2011) and provides protection from cigarette smoke in human lung cells (Hsu et al 2009). An in vitro study identified the kaempferol and quercetin constituents of *G. biloba* as key components inducing apoptosis in oral-cavity cancer cells (Kang et al 2010). Studies in humans have found that ginkgo extracts inhibit the formation of radiation-induced (chromosome-damaging) clastogenic factors and ultraviolet-induced oxidative stress, both effects that may contribute to the overall chemopreventive activity. As a result of these observations, there has been a call by some academics for ginkgo to be more widely investigated and used in the prevention and treatment of cancer (Eli & Fasciano 2006).

OTHER ACTIONS

Antiatherosclerotic

Animal models have found *G. biloba* to be effective against atherosclerosis (Chen et al 2011a, Lim et al 2011, Pierre et al 2008). An in vitro study suggests an antiatherosclerotic effect via downregulation of VEGF (Liu et al 2009) and an in vivo study suggests that *G. biloba* may have a cholesterol-lowering effect via HMG-CoA reductase activity and decreasing cholesterol influx (Xie et al 2009). Another animal model found *G. biloba*'s antiatherosclerotic action was through lipid modulation, reducing vascular lesions and modulation of connexin 43 protein (Wei et al 2013).

Antiviral

Ginkgolic acid inhibits HIV protease activity and HIV infection in vitro (Lu et al 2012). In vitro research also identified anti-influenza action with GBE, but only with pretreatment before cell exposure, suggesting it interferes with the interaction between the virus and erythrocytes (Haruyama & Nagata 2013).

Glycaemia

Some in vitro and animal research has suggested that *G. biloba* may have a beneficial effect on reducing insulin resistance (Cong et al 2011, Zhou et al 2011).

Antiosteoporotic

G. biloba treatment produced a significant reversal in bone loss of the mandible and femur in a glucocorticoid-induced osteoporosis model (Lucinda et al 2010).

Activity on cytochromes and P-glycoprotein

Several studies have investigated *G. biloba* for effects on different cytochromes in test tube and animal models and, more recently, human studies. While early in vitro tests demonstrated that *G. biloba* inhibits CYP 3A4, clinical studies have found no such effect (Budzinski et al 2000, Gurley et al 2002, 2005, 2012, Markowitz et al 2003). In vitro tests have suggested that the effect on cytochromes is biphasic, with low doses of ginkgo extract inducing CYP 1A2 and inhibiting 2D6 and higher doses exhibiting the opposite effect (Hellum et al 2007). Studies investigating ginkgo extract and its various constituents in animal models have identified induction of CYP 3A1, 1A1, 1A2, 2E1, 2B12 for ginkgo, which appears to be largely mediated by the bilobalide constituent, whereas no effect on CYP 2D6, 2C11 or 2C7 has been demonstrated (Deng et al 2008, Ribonnet et al 2011, Taki et al 2009, Tang et al 2007a, Zhao et al 2006).

The question arises of clinical significance and whether the effects observed in animal models also occur in humans to an appreciable degree. To this end, clinical studies have been conducted clarifying the issue (Duche et al 1989, Gurley et al 2002, 2005, Kim et al 2010, Markowitz et al 2003, Tang et al 2007a, Zadoyan et al 2012, Zuo et al 2010). Tests with human volunteers have found no significant effect on CYP 3A4, 2D6 or 1A2 with GBE. Gurley et al (2012) report that 29 drugs mediated by various cytochromes have been evaluated and conclude that there is little risk of herb–drug interactions with *G. biloba* at doses of 240 mg/day or less.

Less is known about the effects of ginkgo on the drug transporter molecule P-glycoprotein (P-gp, also known as ABCB1). In vitro studies have identified induction of P-gp with ginkgo (Hellum & Nilsen 2008, Yeung et al 2008). A human study found no effects on P-gp after a single ginkgo dose (120 mg); however use of 120 mg three times daily (360 mg/day) for 14 days did show significant P-gp inhibition for *G. biloba* (Fan et al 2009). The most common therapeutic dose used is 240 mg daily, suggesting some minor effects are possible clinically. More clinical trials are needed to confirm this finding.

Antiasthmatic

In an asthma mouse study ginkgolide B exhibited a significant effect on regulating the kinase/MAPK pathway and a significant decrease in eosinophil count in bronchoalveolar lavage fluid after treatment (Chu et al 2011). Emerging research demonstrates how GBE may be useful in asthma treatment and acute lung injury by its action of suppressing NF-κB gene expression (Huang et al 2013, Li et al 2008).

CLINICAL USE

G. biloba is a complex herb that contains many different active constituents and works by means of multiple mechanisms. In practice, its therapeutic effect is a result of interactions between constituents and mechanisms, giving it applications in many varied conditions. To date, most of the research conducted in Europe has used a standardised preparation known as EGb 761.

Dementia, memory impairment

G. biloba has been used and studied as a cognitive activator in a variety of populations, such as cognitively intact people and those with cerebral insufficiency, age-related memory impairment, Alzheimer's dementia or multi-infarct dementia and dementia with neuropsychiatric features. It has also been tested in healthy adults with poor memory and others with no cognitive deficits to determine whether treatment can further improve memory. Overall, the evidence suggests that oral ginkgo extract improves cognitive function in people with mild to moderate cognitive impairment when used long-term and it also provides benefits for people with dementia and neuropsychiatric symptoms when used long-term (approximately 6 months). Some benefits may also be possible for various aspects of cognitive function in older adults, such as retrieval of learned material, but results are inconsistent for cognitive function overall. In regard to younger healthy adults, acute dosing appears more successful than chronic use.

While ginkgo biloba demonstrates neuroprotective effects in experimental models, the current evidence indicates long-term use does not protect against the development of dementia.

Clinical note — What is cerebral insufficiency?
Cerebral insufficiency is a syndrome characterised by a collection of symptoms, although it is not associated with any clear pathological changes. The 12 symptoms associated with this condition are: (1) difficulties of memory; (2) difficulties of concentration; (3) being absent-minded; (4) confusion; (5) lack of energy; (6) tiredness; (7) decreased physical performance; (8) depressive mood; (9) anxiety; (10) dizziness; (11) tinnitus; and (12) headaches (Kleijnen & Knipschild 1992). Some of these symptoms are also described as early symptoms of dementia and appear to be associated with decreased cerebral blood flow, although frequently no explanation is found.

A 2013 systematic review and meta-analysis of eight RCTs involving people with dementia reported significant, although modest, improvements in both cognitive function and daily activities. All studies used the GBE EGb 761 and two of the studies compared the extract to the drug donepezil and found no significant difference between the two treatments when treating mild to moderate dementia (Brondino et al 2013). Two of the studies included in the Brondino review focused on outpatients (n = 410) with mild to moderate dementia and neuropsychiatric symptoms who were treated with *G. biloba* (240 mg daily EGb 761) for 24 weeks; a significant improvement was produced in apathy, sleep, irritability, depression and aberrant motor behaviour and improved wellbeing of their caregivers (Bachinskaya et al 2011, Herrschaft et al 2012). Another trial in the 2013 review was a double-blind RCT of 400 subjects with mild to moderate dementia (Alzheimer's disease or vascular dementia) with neuropsychiatric features testing EGb 761 extract over 22 weeks (Napryeyenko & Borzenko 2007). Active treatment produced a mean −3.2-point improvement in the Specialty Knowledge Test (SKT) with an average deterioration by +1.3 points on placebo ($P < 0.001$). EGb 761 was significantly superior to placebo on all secondary outcome measures, including the Neuropsychiatric Inventory (NPI), and an activities-of-daily-living scale. Treatment results were essentially similar for Alzheimer's disease or vascular dementia subgroups. The drug was well tolerated and adverse events were similar for ginkgo and placebo treatment. A secondary analysis of this Napryeyenko RCT found *G. biloba* (EGb 761 240 mg/day) to be effective for both Alzheimer's disease and vascular dementia for neuropsychiatric symptoms (Napryeyenko et al 2009).

A 2009 Cochrane systematic review of 36 RCTs for ginkgo (any dose) in the treatment of dementia and cognitive decline (any severity) concluded that the results were inconsistent and unreliable but explained that the studies were mainly small, often poorly designed and of less than 3 months' duration, which may explain the inconsistency. All but one study used the EGb 761 extract (dose ranging from 80 to 600 mg/day, with most less than 200 mg daily). The authors reported that, although earlier studies found significant benefits, later studies were inconsistent and they found no difference between the 120 mg and 240 mg standard dosing (Birks & Grimley Evans 2009). This inconsistency may be in part due to reviewers pooling all studies regardless of patient diagnoses, the myriad of different scales and measures used and the fact that some studies are over 20 years old and randomisation and blinding techniques have changed in recent years. As a result, the findings are not straightforward and deserve more detailed description to be better understood. A literature review in 2012 suggested that the evidence for the use of *G. biloba* for cognitive impairment and dementia was not convincing (Roland & Nergard 2012).

However, other meta-analyses, with well-defined parameters, have found *G. biloba* to be clinically effective. One review and meta-analysis included nine well-designed studies between 12 and 52 weeks (n = 2372), all using the standardised extract EGb 761 (once-a-day dose of 240 mg) and found *G. biloba* to be more effective than placebo; with the Alzheimer's disease subgroup experiencing a larger cognitive benefit (Weinmann et al 2010). Another meta-analysis of six RCTs took a bivariate random approach considering the influence of baseline risk and found *G. biloba* to be effective for cognitive function in dementia with 6 months of treatment (Wang et al 2010). Kaschel undertook a literature review in 2009, aiming to discover the differential effects in neuropsychological improvement with *G. biloba* use, hypothesising that there may be certain parts of our memory that improve with this herb. Results from 29 RCTs were analysed, giving psychometric scores in different cognitive domains and 14 cognitive subfunctions. This reviewer suggested there is consistent evidence for long-term use of *G. biloba* in providing benefits for selective attention, fluid intelligence and long-term memory for both verbal and non-verbal material. It does not seem to have much effect on pure speed or on the less age-sensitive area of short-term memory (Kaschel 2009). This selective testing has provided a credible explanation for why there may be inconsistent study results and is perhaps the best way forward for future studies.

Two trials were not included in the recent reviews: the first was a double-blind, parallel-group RCT of 176 subjects with mild to moderate dementia which used low-dose standardised extract of *G. biloba* (120 mg daily) over 6 months, finding no benefits beyond placebo (McCarney et al 2008). The second trial was a larger double-blind RCT of 400 patients with dementia associated with neuropsychiatric features, testing a higher dose of EGb 761 extract (240 mg/day) (Scripnikov et al 2007).

The study population included people with probable or possible Alzheimer's disease with cerebrovascular disease or vascular dementia. At this dose, EGb 761 was significantly superior to placebo with respect to the primary outcome (SKT battery) and all secondary outcome variables. While herbal treatment improved outcomes, the placebo group showed evidence of deterioration as measured by the mean composite score (frequency × severity) and the mean caregiver distress score ($P < 0.001$). The largest effects for EGb 761 were found for apathy/indifference, anxiety, irritability/lability, depression/dysphoria and sleep/nighttime behaviour.

Some smaller recent trials report benefit in treating mild cognitive impairment (Dong et al 2012) and one group found that episodic memory of patients with mild cognitive impairment improved (Zhao et al 2012).

Several recent reviews have focused on the role of ginkgo in Alzheimer's disease, producing inconsistent conclusions, which may be due to differences in exclusion criteria and the heterogeneity of the studies making data analysis difficult. A Cochrane systematic review in 2009 found 925 patients from nine Alzheimer's disease and ginkgo trials and suggested no consistent pattern of benefit (Birks & Grimley Evans 2009) and another systematic review suggested results were inconclusive (Fu & Li 2011). However, in 2010, a systematic review of the use of *G. biloba* in Alzheimer's disease found evidence of high-dose *G. biloba* (240 mg/day EGb 761) improving daily living, mood and cognition; the results were statistically significant in three of the four studies within the subgroup analysis. The complete meta-analysis included six quality studies of at least 16 weeks' duration and, although benefit for *G. biloba* was reported, the authors found that no potential effect size could be estimated because of the heterogeneous results and recommend future research focusing on subgroups of Alzheimer's disease. No evidence of harm was found in any of the studies (Janssen et al 2010).

Alzheimer's disease or vascular dementia with neuropsychiatric features

A 2013 review of four RCTs testing EGb 761 in elderly patients ($n = 1294$) with a total score of 9–23 in the SKT cognitive test battery (cognitive domain) and with a composite score of 6 and greater in the NPI (behavioural domain) concluded that active treatment with ginkgo was safe, effective and well tolerated (Ihl 2013). Patients treated with EGb 761 showed improvements of cognitive performance and behavioural symptoms that were associated with advances in activities of daily living and a reduced burden to caregivers, whereas the placebo groups showed only minimal improvements or signs of disease progression. EGb 761 was significantly superior to placebo groups in all mentioned domains ($P < 0.01$) and had similar effects to donepexil. The RCTs compared a dose of EGb 761 2 capsules of 120 mg/day or one capsule of 240 mg/day to placebo while one RCT used donepezil as an active control. The duration of treatment was 22 or 24 weeks.

Use in healthy subjects

Many double-blind studies have investigated the effects of *G. biloba* (120–600 mg/day) on cognitive function in younger and older healthy subjects. Some studies have evaluated the effects of a single dose, whereas others are long-term studies (2 days–13 weeks).

A 2012 meta-analysis of *G. biloba* as a cognitive enhancer in healthy individuals identified 10 RCTs (with 13 data sets) and concluded that, on measures of memory, executive function and attention, there was no significant effect on cognitive function. In the analysis the authors reported all effect sizes as non-significant and found no difference with age of participants, dose, time of trial or type of GBE. In the 13 studies assessing memory, not one of the studies found a significant effect (Laws et al 2012).

Previously, a systematic review of placebo-controlled trials, published in 2007, investigated whether *G. biloba* enhances cognitive function in healthy subjects aged under 60 years (Canter & Ernst 2007). A number of the acute studies included in the analysis used multiple outcomes and reported positive effects on one or more of these at particular time points with particular doses, but these findings were either not replicated or contradicted by other studies. The evidence from long-term studies is largely negative. Of those studies that measured subjective effects, only one of five acute studies and one of six long-term studies reported any significant positive results.

More recently, a benefit was found in 188 healthy middle-aged volunteers who were given placebo or ginkgo 240 mg once daily (EGb 761) for 6 weeks. There was significant improvement on the demanding standardised free-recall test but no benefit in another memory test on recalling a driving route. This confirms previous evidence suggesting a role for *G. biloba* in retrieval of learned material, which is known to be sensitive to ageing (Kaschel 2011).

Overall, tests with younger subjects taking *G. biloba* long-term have failed to show positive effects on memory; however, short-term benefits after acute dosing may be possible for some aspects of memory. Healthy older adults with poorer cognitive performance appear to experience greater benefit than those with higher cognitive function levels. This was confirmed in a 2011 RCT which found a more pronounced and consistent improvement in cognition in subjects with a lower memory function at baseline in mild cognitive impairment ($n = 300$) who were taking *G. biloba* (240 mg/daily EGb 761) for 12 weeks (Grass-Kapanke et al 2011).

Tests with younger (18–43 years) and older volunteers (55–79 years) produced different results in a 12-week, double-blind, placebo-controlled study

(Burns et al 2006). The effects of ginkgo (120 mg/day) were assessed for both groups on a wide range of cognitive abilities, executive function, attention and mood. The older group responded to treatment as long-term memory assessed by associational learning tasks showed significant improvement with ginkgo; however, no other significant differences were found on any other measure. The young adult group (n = 104) failed to respond on any measure, as no significant differences were observed for the treatment or placebo groups. Similarly, no significant effects on mood or any of the cognitive tests employed by Elsabagh et al (2005a) were found for ginkgo (120 mg/day) taken over 6 weeks in a placebo-controlled study of 52 young adults. In contrast, acute treatment of younger subjects with ginkgo (120 mg) significantly improved performance on the sustained-attention task and pattern recognition memory task according to a randomised, double-blind study (Elsabagh et al 2005a). The study of 52 students found no further effects for ginkgo on working memory, planning, mental flexibility or mood.

Kennedy et al (2007b) reported on a re-analysis of data from three methodologically identical, double-blind, crossover studies that each included a treatment of 120 mg ginkgo extract and matched placebo. The analysis found that 120 mg of ginkgo conferred a significant improvement on the 'quality of memory' factor and was most evident at 1 and 4 hours after single-dose treatment, but had a negative effect on performance on the 'speed of attention' factor, which was most evident at 1 and 6 hours after treatment.

Vascular cognitive impairment

One study of 80 patients diagnosed with vascular cognitive impairment compared conventional treatment with antiplatelet medication to treatment with adjunctive *G. biloba* and the antiplatelet medication. The 3-month trial found addition of ginkgo improved the therapeutic effect, with increases in cerebral blood flow and cognitive enhancement observed (Zhang & Xue 2012).

Ginkgo complexed with phospholipids

Some recent data suggest that the complexation of standardised GBE with soy-derived phospholipids may enhance the bioavailability of active components, thereby producing better results. Kennedy et al (2007a) tested two different ginkgo products complexed with either phosphatidylserine or phosphatidylcholine in a placebo-controlled study of younger volunteers. Test subjects were given an acute dose of ginkgo, one of the ginkgo combinations or placebo on separate days (7 days apart). Confirming earlier results, *G. biloba* (120 mg) as sole treatment was not associated with markedly improved performance on the primary outcomes in this younger population; however, administration of GBE complexed with phosphatidylserine resulted in improved secondary memory performance and significantly increased speed of memory task performance across all of the postdose testing sessions. Interestingly, all three herbal treatments were associated with improved calmness. Whether the superior effect obtained for this combination is due to the complexation of the extracts, their mere combination or the separate psychopharmacological actions of the two extracts remains to be tested.

Cognitive effects in postmenopausal women

A systematic review of herbal and dietary supplements and their use in menopause for cognitive function included two *G. biloba* studies, both using a low dose of 120 mg/day (Clement et al 2011). In one RCT, 57 postmenopausal women were given a combination of ginkgo at 120 mg and ginseng at 200 mg (Gincosan) over 12 weeks. No significant effects were found in any of the symptoms measured of anxiety and mood and cognitive measures of attention and memory (Hartley et al 2004). The second was a double-blind RCT of 87 postmenopausal women; it was found that 1 week's treatment with ginkgo (120 mg/day) significantly improved mental flexibility in older (mean age 61 years) postmenopausal women beyond placebo. However no significant benefits were seen for younger women with better cognitive performance at baseline and no benefit for any of the women for the cognitive function of memory and sustained attention (Elsabagh et al 2005b). The study tested ginkgo extract (LI 1370, Lichtwer Pharma, Marlow, UK) over 6 weeks (Elsabagh et al 2005b).

Comparisons with anticholinesterase drugs

The type of central nervous system effects produced by EGb 761 in elderly dementia patients is similar to those induced in tacrine responders and those seen after the administration of other 'cognitive activators', according to a small randomised study involving 18 elderly people diagnosed with mild to moderate dementia (possible or probable Alzheimer's disease) (Itil et al 1998). The results also demonstrated that 240 mg EGb produced typical cognitive activator electrocardiogram profiles (responders) in more subjects (8 of 18) than 40 mg tacrine (3 of 18 subjects). Later reviews concluded that ginkgo extract and second-generation cholinesterase inhibitors (donepezil, rivastigmine, metrifonate) should be considered equally effective in the treatment of mild to moderate Alzheimer's dementia (Kasper & Schubert 2009, Wettstein 2000). One double-blind exploratory RCT with 96 outpatients compared *G. biloba*, donepezil or combined treatment over 22 weeks and found no significant differences between them and only superior benefits when they were combined (Yancheva et al 2009).

Commission E approves the use of standardised ginkgo extract in dementia syndromes, including vascular, primary degenerative and mixed types (Blumenthal et al 2000).

Dementia prevention

The many mechanisms attributed to ginkgo make it an ideal candidate for the long-term prevention of many age-related diseases such as dementia. Two clinical trials were published in 2008, which investigated whether treatment with *G. biloba* could significantly reduce the incidence of dementia and, more recently, a large RCT released results in 2012. Overall, the current body of evidence indicates that ginkgo treatment does not protect against the development of dementia or Alzheimer's disease when taken by people over 70 years (DeKosky et al 2008, Dodge et al 2008, Vellas et al 2012).

DeKosky et al (2008) compared the effectiveness of *G. biloba* to placebo in reducing the incidence of all-cause dementia and Alzheimer's disease in elderly individuals with normal cognition and those with mild cognitive impairment. The large randomised, double-blind, placebo-controlled clinical trial involved 3069 community-dwelling subjects aged 75 years or older with normal cognition ($n = 2587$) or mild cognitive impairment ($n = 482$). It was conducted at five academic medical centres in the United States between 2000 and 2008, with a median follow-up of 6.1 years. Treatment consisted of a twice-daily dose of 120 mg extract of *G. biloba* and was not shown to reduce the overall incidence rate of either dementia or Alzheimer's disease incidence in elderly individuals. Treatment was well tolerated by this population, as the incidence of side effects was similar for both groups.

In the same year, Dodge et al (2008) published the results of a double-blind study involving 118 cognitively intact older subjects (85 years or older). In the intention-to-treat analysis, there was no reduced risk of progression to clinical dementia among the GBE group; however, in the secondary analysis, where medication adherence level was controlled, the GBE group had a significantly lower risk of progression and a smaller decline in memory scores. Importantly, more stroke and transient ischaemic attack cases were observed among the GBE group; further investigation is required to confirm this finding.

A 5-year double-blind RCT (GuidAge) released results in 2012. This large clinical trial recruited participants aged over 70 years who had consulted their primary care doctor for memory problems; 1404 patients were prescribed a dose of 120 mg twice daily (EGb 761) and 1414 were given placebo. The findings were negative and *G. biloba* did not reduce the incidence of Alzheimer's disease in elderly patients with memory complaints (Vellas et al 2012).

Acute ischaemic stroke

GBE is widely used in the treatment of acute ischaemic stroke in China.

A 2005 Cochrane systematic review identified 14 trials, of which 10 (792 patients) were included (Zeng et al 2005). In those 10 trials, follow-up was performed at 14–35 days after stroke and, in all studies, neurological outcome was assessed, but none of them reported on disability (activities of daily living function) or quality of life and only three trials reported adverse events. Nine of the trials were considered to be of inferior quality. Overall, results from the 10 studies found that GBE was associated with a significant increase in the number of improved patients. Of note, one placebo-controlled trial, assessed to be of good quality, failed to show an improvement in neurological deficit at the end of treatment. A recent review of *G. biloba* confirmed previous Cochrane reviews and concluded that there was no convincing evidence of ginkgo being effective for acute ischaemic stroke (Roland & Nergard 2012).

However, the story is not yet complete, as two more recent studies have shown benefits for ginkgo treatment in ischaemic stroke. A double-blind RCT of 31 patients after an acute ischaemic stroke or a cerebrovascular accident were administered standard pharmacotherapy or standard treatment with the addition of *G. biloba* (1500 mg/day) for 30 days. Blood samples before and after the treatment showed greater antioxidant status and lower inflammatory markers, such as C-reactive protein, which may assist in neuroprotection after a stroke (Thanoon et al 2012). Of more interest is a 2013 placebo-controlled RCT of 102 consecutive patients with acute ischaemic stroke which tested treatment with *G. biloba* tablets (Gol-Darou, Isfahan, Iran) with a total dose of 120 mg/day (40 mg three times/day) over 4 months (Oskouei et al 2013). The primary outcome was a 50% reduction in the 4-month NIHSS, which was used to measure functional outcome. Treatment with ginkgo was significantly superior to placebo and the risk ratio and number needed to treat were 3.16 and 2.50, respectively. In addition, multivariate regression adjusted for age and sex revealed a significant NIHSS decline in the *G. biloba* group compared to the placebo group ($P < 0.05$).

Depression

Although studies have investigated the effects of *G. biloba* in cerebral insufficiency, a syndrome that is often characterised by depression and dementia with neuropsychiatric features, no clinical studies are available that have specifically investigated its use in clinical depression.

One randomised, double-blind, placebo-controlled study has investigated its effects in seasonal affective disorder (SAD). GBE PN246, in tablet form (Bio-Biloba), was tested in 27 patients with SAD over 10 weeks or until they developed symptoms, starting in a symptom-free phase about 1 month before symptoms were expected. In this trial, *G. biloba* failed to prevent the development of SAD (Lingaerde et al 1999).

Cieza et al (2003) tested EGb 761 (240 mg/day) on the subjective emotional wellbeing of healthy older subjects (50–65 years) in a randomised, double-blind study. Ginkgo treatment produced a statistically significant difference for the visual analogue scale on mental health and for quality of life, as well as for the Subjective Intensity Scale: Mood score in week 2 compared with placebo. At the end of the study, statistically significant improvement in the EGb 761 group was observed for the variables of depression, fatigue and anger. Several more-recent studies investigating the effects of ginkgo on memory have also measured effects on mood. The double-blind studies found no significant effects for healthy older or younger volunteers (Burns et al 2006, Carlson et al 2007, Elsabagh et al 2005a). Whether ginkgo may have a mood-enhancing effect in a population with diagnosed depression remains to be tested.

Generalised anxiety disorder (GAD)

EGb 761 has demonstrated stress-alleviating and anxiolytic-like activity in preclinical studies, and in a randomised study of 107 patients with GAD (n = 82) or adjustment disorder with anxious mood (n = 25) (Woelk et al 2007). *G. biloba* was tested in two different doses (480 mg/day and 240 mg/day) against placebo over 4 weeks and found to be significantly superior, with a dose–response trend being identified. Beneficial effects were observed after 4 days of treatment. Additionally, ginkgo treatment was safe and well-tolerated. A review of controlled studies of the use of medicinal plants for GAD found only a small number of studies on *G. biloba* but in those studies ginkgo showed an effect similar to or better than anxiolytic drugs (Faustino et al 2010).

Peripheral vascular diseases

Ginkgo has been used in the treatment of intermittent claudication, Raynaud's syndrome and chilblains (Mouren et al 1994, Pittler & Ernst 2000). This is often based on the known pharmacological actions of ginkgo in improving peripheral circulation and exerting antioxidant and anti-inflammatory activities. While clinical trials have produced inconsistent results, the lack of non-surgical and safe pharmaceutical treatment options means ginkgo biloba is worthy of consideration in practice as a 3-month trial to determine individual response.

Intermittent claudication

A 2013 Cochrane database systematic review included 14 trials with 739 patients and found a non-significant increase of only 64.5 m on a flat treadmill being the absolute claudication distance (ACD) and concluded no significant benefit for patients with peripheral arterial disease. In the 24 weeks subgroup, authors found a significant improvement in ACD with an increase of 85.3 m. Nine trials compared 120–160 mg *G. biloba* daily with placebo and three of the trials used larger doses of 240 mg (Wang et al 2007), 300 mg (Gardner et al 2008) and 320 mg (Mouren et al 1994), with the majority of the trials lasting 12–24 weeks. The authors suggest that a publication bias and exclusion of some 'negative' trials in earlier reviews skewed the results and also suggested that exercise therapy alone has shown a 5–10 times greater benefit than GBE (Nicolai et al 2013).

The earlier trials referred to included a 2004 meta-analysis reporting that ginkgo was more effective than placebo in intermittent claudication (Horsch & Walther 2004). Nine double-blind studies of EGb 761 for intermittent claudication were assessed in a total of 619 patients. A sensitivity analysis of a homogeneous sample in terms of design, treatment duration, inclusion and exclusion criteria and methods of measurement confirms these findings. Most studies have used a dose of 120 mg/day taken in divided doses, although one trial found that 240 mg/day gave better results. It should be recommended as long-term therapy and as an adjunct to exercise for the best results. An earlier randomised study measuring transcutaneous partial pressure of oxygen during exercise showed that a dose of 320 mg/day EGb 761 taken for 4 weeks significantly decreased the amount of ischaemic area by 38%, compared with no change with placebo (Mouren et al 1994).

Commission E approved the use of standardised ginkgo extract for intermittent claudication (Blumenthal et al 2000).

Clinical note — Peripheral arterial disease

Peripheral arterial disease is the chronic obstruction of the arteries supplying the lower extremities. The most frequent symptom is intermittent claudication, which results from poor oxygenation of the muscles of the lower extremities and is experienced typically as an aching pain, cramping or numbness in the calf, buttock, hip, thigh or arch of the foot. Symptoms are induced by walking or exercise and are relieved by rest. Presently, medical treatment revolves around lifestyle changes, such as increased exercise, and surgery as a final option.

Raynaud's syndrome

Whether ginkgo is an effective treatment in Reynaud's syndrome is difficult to ascertain. A review and meta-analysis of complementary medicine and Raynaud's syndrome (Malenfant et al 2009) included only one study on *G. biloba* by Muir et al (2002), which found a non-significant change in duration and severity of symptoms (P = 0.75 and 0.23, respectively). This study used a standardised GBE (Seredrin 360 mg daily) taken over a 10-week period which significantly reduced the number of attacks per week (from 13.2 to 5.8) compared with placebo (Muir et al 2002).

Several later studies were published, including an RCT conducted over 8 weeks, with 93 patients, which compared the use of the calcium channel blocker nifedipine with *G. biloba* and found a 50% improvement in the drug group versus a 31%

improvement in the ginkgo group (Choi et al 2009). Another RCT conducted during the coldest part of the year involved 41 participants and found no significant differences between EGb 761 (240 mg/day) and placebo after 10 weeks (Bredie & Jong 2012). Whether participants in these last two studies had more severe symptoms than in the previous positive study is unknown

Vertigo, tinnitus, labyrinthitis and sudden deafness

Ginkgo is used to treat these and other symptoms of vestibulocochlear disorders.

Tinnitus

A recent Cochrane review included only four quality trials (n = 1543) and they found no evidence to suggest that *G. biloba* was effective in patients whose primary issue was tinnitus, although they did report a small, statistically significant reduction in tinnitus in patients with vascular dementia and Alzheimer's disease (Hilton et al 2013). Two double-blind studies included in the recent Cochrane review have shifted the evidence against the use of *G. biloba* in tinnitus. The first was a large, double-blind, placebo-controlled study involving 1121 people aged between 18 and 70 years with tinnitus and 978 matched controls, which found that 12 weeks of treatment with ginkgo extract, LI 1370 (Lichtwer Pharma, Berlin, Germany), 50 mg three times daily resulted in no significant differences when subjects assessed their tinnitus in terms of loudness and how troublesome it was (Drew & Davies 2001). The second RCT of 66 subjects with tinnitus failed to show benefits with active treatment using a dose of 120 mg extract daily over 12 weeks (Rejali et al 2004). The primary outcome measures used were the Tinnitus Handicap Inventory, the Glasgow Health Status Inventory and the average hearing threshold at 0.5, 1, 2 and 4 kHz. In 2004, Rejali et al conducted a meta-analysis of clinical trials and found that 21.6% of patients with tinnitus reported benefit from *G. biloba* versus 18.4% of patients who reported benefit from a placebo.

Importantly, a 2011 systematic review which looked at the quality of plant extract and dosage levels included results of eight trials (all with EGb 761 with 120–240 mg/day) and excluded trials such as the Rejali study that did not specify the ginkgo preparation and which had a large drop-out rate due to illness. This review found that GBE EGb 761 was superior to placebo and was an effective treatment option for tinnitus. The authors suggest that trials with other GBEs were often of poor methodological quality (von Boetticher 2011).

Salicylate-induced tinnitus

One in vivo study investigating the effects of ginkgo in salicylate-induced tinnitus found a statistically significant decrease in the behavioural manifestation of tinnitus for ginkgo in doses of 25, 50 and 100 mg/kg/day (Jastreboff et al 1997).

Vertigo

Despite being a common disease, there is no effective and side effect-free pharmaceutical agent that has shown efficacy for vertigo, creating interest in well-tolerated treatments such as ginkgo biloba, which displays mechanisms of action which may be relevant, such as antioxidant, neuroprotective, cognitive enhancing, improved perfusion and possibly vigilance enhancing. Research with animal models further indicates EGb 761 has an effect on the vestibular system and vestibular compensation (Hamann 2007).

In 2013, the REVERT registry collected data from 4294 patients with vertigo in 13 countries over 28 months and found that, in real-life medical practice, the most common treatments prescribed were betahistine followed by piracetam, ginkgo biloba and diuretics, and the greatest improvements were seen in the more severely ill, and those with benign paroxysmal positional vertigo or 'other vertigo of peripheral origin' (Agus et al 2013). Although the registry reported that 93% of patients had some improvement in the 6-month follow-up, there were no specific data on the ginkgo subsection.

A systematic review of preclinical studies and five double-blind RCTs investigating the effects of EGb 761 in vestibular and non-vestibular vertigo concluded that ginkgo has benefits in vertiginous syndromes (Hamann 2007). The RCTs used a daily dose between 120 and 160 mg which was taken for 3 months.

Labyrinthitis

A novel guinea pig model has shown that *G. biloba* can minimise cochlear damage on otitis media-induced labyrinthitis (Jang et al 2011). Clinical trials are needed to confirm if this has any clinical relevance.

Sudden deafness

Ginkgo extract was as effective as pentoxifylline in the treatment of sudden deafness, according to one randomised, double-blind study (Reisser & Weidauer 2001). Both treatments equally reduced associated symptoms of tinnitus and produced the same effects on the return to normal of speech discrimination. Subjective assessment suggested that GBE was more beneficial than pentoxifylline. EGb 761 (240 mg/day) has also been shown to accelerate and secure recovery of acute idiopathic sudden sensorineural hearing loss, observable within 1 week of treatment under randomised double-blind test conditions (Burschka et al 2001).

Commission E approves the use of standardised ginkgo extract in these conditions when of vascular origin (Blumenthal et al 2000).

Macular degeneration, glaucoma and retinopathy

With regard to these ophthalmological conditions, ginkgo has numerous properties that should theoretically make it a useful treatment, such as increasing ocular blood flow, antioxidant and platelet-activating factor inhibitor activity, NO inhibition, protecting retinal ganglion cells against apoptosis (Wang et al 2012) and neuroprotective abilities.

Macular degeneration

Although some positive evidence exists, a 2013 Cochrane review has suggested that, overall, there is insufficient evidence currently available to conclude that *G. biloba* treatment is effective in macular degeneration, with further testing required (Evans 2013). Based on its known mechanisms of action, it is a worthy candidate for further research.

Glaucoma

With regard to glaucoma, the little research conducted so far appears promising. Researchers using colour Doppler imaging have observed significantly increased end-diastolic velocity in the ophthalmic artery after treatment with EGb (120 mg/day) in a placebo-controlled, randomised, crossover study (Chung et al 1999).

A randomised, double-blind, crossover study found that EGb 761 (120 mg/day) taken for 4 weeks produces positive effects in normal-tension glaucoma (Quaranta et al 2003). Furthermore, ginkgo treatment did not significantly alter intraocular pressure, blood pressure or heart rate and was well tolerated.

Other more recent studies have confirmed a benefit for normal-tension glaucoma. One RCT of 30 patients, administered 80 mg GBE twice a day over 4 weeks, found that retinal blood flow increased significantly in these normal-tension glaucoma patients (Park et al 2011). A retrospective study of 42 patients with a mean follow-up time of 12.3 years showed that 80 mg GBE twice daily slowed visual field defect damage (Lee et al 2013). These findings were also confirmed in a retrospective study with 332 patients who were compared to controls (n = 97); of the cohort, 132 patients were given bilberry anthocyanins and 103 patients received *G. biloba* (ginkgo leaf extract from SK Chemicals, Gyeonggi-do, Korea) at a dose of one 80-mg tablet twice a day. Both treatments were found to improve visual function in some patients with normal-tension glaucoma (Shim et al 2012).

Chloroquine retinopathy

In vivo tests using electroretinography have identified protective effects against the development of chloroquine-induced retinopathy using *G. biloba* (Droy-Lefaix et al 1992). This has been observed in both acute and chronic chloroquine toxicity of the retina (Droy-Lefaix et al 1995).

Prevention of altitude sickness/acute mountain sickness

Acetazolamide and ginkgo biloba are the two most investigated drugs for the prevention of acute mountain sickness (AMS) (Ke et al 2013). In general, research indicates that ginkgo may be useful as a prophylactic treatment when started 4–5 days prior to ascent to reduce the incidence of AMS (van Patot et al 2009). Considering its excellent safety profile, it is a treatment worthy of consideration.

While many studies have shown that pretreatment with ginkgo extract reduces the incidence of developing AMS, not all studies are positive when compared to placebo. This was most clearly seen in a study which consisted of two RCTs, one of which showed significant results (standardised *Ginkgo biloba* produced by Spectrum Chemical and Laboratory Products, Gardena, CA, United States) and the other did not (*Ginkgo biloba* 24/6/5 from Technical Sourcing International, TSI, Missoula, MT, United States) (Leadbetter et al 2009). The positive study used a dose of 120 mg twice daily starting 4 days before ascent to 4300 m and the other used prophylaxis at the same dose for 3 days.

In the positive study, treatment with 120 mg GBE twice daily significantly reduced both the incidence and the severity of AMS in participants rapidly exposed to high altitude; 68% of participants had AMS in the placebo group, compared to 33% in the GBE group and the number needed to treat was 3. In contrast, no significant effects on AMS incidence or severity were seen with the other ginkgo treatment and AMS developed in 45% of the placebo group compared to 27% taking ginkgo. Of note, the incidence of AMS in both ginkgo groups was still lower than placebo; however, the higher rate of AMS in the placebo group in the positive study may have been responsible for the discrepant results. The authors noted that the studies were underpowered to confirm these suspicions; however, the rates of AMS observed with placebo reflected the rates reported in the literature (50–75%).

A 2012 systematic shortcut review of literature (Seupaul et al 2012) on prophylaxis for AMS suggested that *G. biloba* was not effective; however, this review only included one study with *G. biloba* which was negative and involved 487 healthy Western hikers (Gertsch et al 2004). While the study by Gertsch et al is considered to be the only adequately powered GBE and AMS study published, treatment was not administered until participants reached approximately 4300 m without evidence of AMS, thus skewing the population towards those who are less susceptible to the condition and not being a proper trial design to test prophylaxis (Leadbetter et al 2009).

Numerous other studies not reported in the 2012 systematic review by Seupaul et al have been conducted, with research commencing in the 1990s and generally showing some benefits with ginkgo biloba pretreatment. Roncin et al (1996) involved 44 subjects and found that a dose of 160 mg/day taken for 5 days as prophylactic treatment resulted in 0% of subjects developing the cerebral symptoms of AMS versus 41% of subjects in the placebo group, whereas only 3 subjects (13.6%) in the EGb 761 group developed respiratory symptoms of AMS; 18 (81.8%) in the placebo group developed these symptoms. Besides effectively preventing AMS for moderate altitude (5400 m), the treatment also decreased vasomotor disorders of the extremities. In 2001, Maakestad et al reported on a randomised, double-blind trial of *G. biloba* (120 mg twice daily starting 5 days before ascent) compared to placebo for the prevention of AMS in 40 college students who underwent rapid ascent from 1400 to 4300 m. Using the Lake Louise Symptoms score and Environmental Symptoms Questionnaire as outcomes, *G. biloba* was shown to significantly reduce the incidence of AMS compared to placebo.

In subsequent years, some researchers compared ginkgo to acetazolamide. In 2003, two studies produced conflicting results. The study by Moraga et al (2003) compared prophylaxis with *G. biloba* (80 mg twice daily) versus acetazolamide (250 mg twice daily) versus placebo, which was started 24 hours before rapid ascent to 3700 m. Of 32 subjects enrolled, none of those in the *G. biloba* group developed AMS, compared with 35% of those in the acetazolamide group and 54% of those receiving placebo. Alternatively, ginkgo (120 mg twice daily) started 3 days before ascent produced no significant effects when compared to placebo or acetazolamide in a randomised, double-blind study by Leadbetter and Hackett (2003). The study involved 59 subjects who experienced a rapid ascent to 4300 m. Negative results were also obtained by Chow et al (2005) in a small RCT, showing no benefits over placebo and superiority of acetazolamide.

A study published in 2007 tested a different type of treatment regimen that produced significant benefits. The placebo-controlled study of 36 people found that pretreatment followed by continued treatment with *G. biloba* prevented AMS and was significantly more effective than acetazolamide (Moraga et al 2007). Volunteers were given placebo, acetazolamide (250 mg per dose) or ginkgo (80 mg per dose) every 12 hours starting 24 hours before ascending and continuing throughout the 3-day stay at high altitude. Not a single person treated with ginkgo experienced AMS, compared with 36% taking acetazolamide and 54% taking placebo. While ginkgo did not alter arterial oxygen saturation compared to acetazolamide, a marked increased saturation in arterial oxygen was seen in comparison with the placebo group.

Premenstrual syndrome (PMS)

A double-blind RCT evaluating the effects of EGb 761 in treating congestive symptoms of PMS in a group of 165 women found that treatment over two menstrual cycles (from day 16 until day 5 of the next cycle) was successful. Treatment was particularly effective in reducing breast symptoms, although neuropsychological symptoms were also alleviated (Tamborini & Taurelle 1993). A more recent placebo-controlled RCT with 85 participants has confirmed that *G. biloba* can significantly reduce the severity of PMS symptoms when given at a dose of 40 mg ginkgo extract three times a day from day 16 of the menstrual cycle to day 5 of the next menstrual cycle (Ozgoli et al 2009).

Vitiligo

A dose of 120 mg/day ginkgo extract significantly stopped active progression of depigmentation in slow-spreading vitiligo and induced repigmentation in some treated patients under double-blind, placebo-controlled study conditions (Parsad et al 2003). Although the mechanism of action responsible is unknown, antioxidant activity is thought to be important. An open-label trial of just 12 participants also reported repigmentation with *G. biloba* 120 mg/day given over 12 weeks (Szczurko et al 2011).

Sexual dysfunction/sexual function

Due to its vasodilatory effects, ginkgo has been used in the management of sexual dysfunction in cases where compromised circulation is suspected. One open study has been conducted with subjects experiencing sexual dysfunction associated with antidepressant use (Cohen & Bartlik 1998). Ginkgo extract (average dose 209 mg/day) was found to be 84% effective in treating antidepressant-induced sexual dysfunction, predominantly caused by selective serotonin reuptake inhibitor, in a study of 63 subjects. A relative success rate of 91% was observed for women, compared with 76% for men, and a positive effect was reported on all four phases of the sexual response cycle: desire, excitement (erection and lubrication), orgasm and resolution. Although this was an open trial, the results are encouraging when one considers that the placebo effect is about 25% from past randomised trials of US Federal Drug Administration-approved medications for erectile dysfunction (Moyad 2002).

More recently, a small, triple-blind (investigator, patient, statistician), randomised, placebo-controlled trial of *G. biloba* (240 mg/day for 12 weeks) was undertaken with 24 subjects experiencing sexual impairment caused by antidepressant drugs (Wheatley 2004). The authors report some spectacular individual responses in both groups, but no statistically significant differences, and no differences in side effects.

Meston et al (2008) conducted two studies of women with sexual dysfunction. The first was a single-dose, placebo-controlled study using 300 mg ginkgo extract, which produced a small but significant facilitatory effect on physiological, but not subjective, sexual arousal in 99 sexually dysfunctional women. The second study investigated long-term use of ginkgo (300 mg/day) over 8 weeks, and found that herbal treatment combined with sex therapy significantly increased sexual desire and contentment compared to placebo or ginkgo as sole treatment. A newer study looking at the effect of *G. biloba* on menopausal women's sexual function reported significant improvement in sexual desire, sexual pleasure, orgasm and importance of sex in comparison to previous years. The triple-blind, randomised, placebo-controlled trial included 80 healthy women aged 50–60 years who were given a dose of 120–240 mg *G. biloba* daily (Taavoni et al 2012).

OTHER USES

G. biloba is used for many other indications, including improving connective tissue conditions such as haemorrhoids, common allergies, reducing the effects of exposure to radiation and to prevent some of the complications associated with diabetes. In the United Kingdom and other European countries, the cardioprotective effects of EGb 761 in myocardial ischaemia and reperfusion are currently being investigated in preclinical studies.

Attention-deficit hyperactivity disorder and autism — no effect

A clinical trial in children with attention-deficit hyperactivity disorder (ADHD) found *G. biloba* to be less effective than the drug methylphenidate (Salehi et al 2010). A systematic review of herbal and nutritional products for treating ADHD confirmed no evidence of benefit with ginkgo (Sarris et al 2011). Additionally, *G. biloba* provided no benefits when used as add-on therapy in autism, according to a double-blind clinical trial adding the herb to risperidone therapy (Hasanzadeh et al 2012).

Addiction — no effect

A pilot study for the treatment of cocaine dependence found no benefit to *G. biloba*. In the RCT 10-week trial 44 participants dependent on cocaine took piracetam (4.8 g/day) or ginkgo (120 mg/day) or placebo. The results found that piracetam was associated with more cocaine use and that ginkgo was not superior to placebo (Kampman et al 2003).

Allergic conjunctivitis

An RCT of 60 patients with symptomatic allergic conjunctivitis using a topical GBE with hyaluronic acid ophthalmic solution (Trium) or hyaluronic acid alone found that additional *G. biloba* produced a significant decrease in symptoms of conjunctival hyperaemia, conjunctival discharge and chemosis (Russo et al 2009).

Adjunct in cancer treatment

As a herb with significant antioxidant and neuroprotective activities, ginkgo has been used to reduce the toxic side effects of some chemotherapeutic drugs. Evidence from in vivo studies demonstrates protective effects against nephrotoxicity induced by cisplatin, cardiotoxicity induced by doxorubicin (El Boghdady 2013a, Naidu et al 2002, Ozturk et al 2004), cisplatin-induced ototoxicity (Huang et al 2007), Adriamycin-induced hyperlipidaemic nephrotoxicity (Abd-Ellah & Mariee 2007) and protective effects for testicular tissue after doxorubicin therapy (Yeh et al 2009). An in vitro study produced a protective effect against radiation of human peripheral blood lymphocytes (Esmekaya et al 2011) and another found *G. biloba* may be helpful with cisplatin therapy sensitising ovarian cancer cells to treatment (Jiang et al 2014).

Little clinical research has been conducted thus far to determine its potential use in practice. One recent open-label clinical study enrolled 34 irradiated brain tumour patients who were given *G. biloba* (120 mg/day) for 24 weeks and found some improvement in quality of life and cognitive function (Attia et al 2012). Another trial with low-dose *G. biloba* (60 mg/day EGb 761) found no benefit in reducing cognitive dysfunction, which can often be associated with treatment in women who are undergoing chemotherapy for breast cancer (Barton et al 2013).

G

Patients (n = 23) undergoing radioiodine therapy for differentiated thyroid cancer were assigned placebo or GBE before and after treatment (120 mg/day for a month). The treated group did not have a significant increase in lymphocytes and ginkgo was found to be protective from possible oxidative and genotoxic damage from the treatment (Dardano et al 2012).

Asthma

Ginkgo shows promise as a treatment for asthma, according to studies using a mouse model of asthma (Babayigit et al 2008) and two clinical studies (Li et al 1997, Tang et al 2007b). Ginkgo significantly reduced airway hyperreactivity and improved clinical symptoms and pulmonary function in asthmatic patients in a placebo-controlled study (Li et al 1997). Platelet-activating factor inhibitor, antioxidant and anti-inflammatory activities are likely to be involved.

Reduced airway inflammation was reported in another study of 75 asthma patients, which compared the effects of fluticasone propionate with fluticasone propionate plus ginkgo (Tang et al 2007b). The addition of ginkgo to treatment resulted in a significant decrease in the infiltration of inflammatory cells such as eosinophils and lymphocytes in the asthmatic airway and relieved airway inflammation.

Cancer prevention

A 2006 review proposes that *G. biloba* should be more widely used as a safe preventive agent for reducing cancer incidence. This recommendation is based on results from numerous in vitro and experimental studies showing that ginkgo affects many factors associated with the incidence and mortality of cancer (Eli & Fasciano 2006). However, a more recent secondary analysis of the Ginkgo Evaluation of Memory study, which is the largest placebo-controlled RCT of ginkgo, evaluated cancer hospitalisations during the 6.1-year follow-up and found no evidence of reduced incidence of cancer. The intervention of 120 mg twice daily of ginkgo extract (EGb 761) was chosen for cognition and not cancer prevention, and the authors also suggested that the follow-up may have been too short to detect benefits with regard to cancer prevention (Biggs et al 2010).

Cardiac surgery support

An RCT of 20 patients undergoing cardiac surgery found the GBE group (0.5 mg/kg Ginaton) increased the production of plasma VEGF, offering some myocardial protection in the perioperative period (Deng et al 2009). Another study with 80 CAD patients found that the GBE group caused an increase in coronary artery blood flow (Wu et al 2008a).

Diabetic nephropathy

Ginkgo had a beneficial effect on vascular endothelial function in patients with early-stage diabetic nephropathy, according to an RCT of 64 patients (Li et al 2009).The known pharmacological mechanisms of ginkgo provide some basis for this finding.

Migraine headache

Ginkgolide B demonstrates anti-inflammatory activity and a reduction of the excitatory effect of glutamate in the central nervous system, which may be of benefit in the treatment of migraine headache with and without aura. Initial studies have been undertaken, often with a combination of nutrients, showing promise in the prevention of migraine.

An open study of 50 women with a history of migraine with typical aura used a product (Migrasoll) containing ginkgolide B from *G. biloba* (60 mg) with coenzyme Q10 (11 mg) and vitamin B_2 (8.7 mg) for 4 months, whereby migraine frequency and duration were reduced, an effect seen after the first 2 months and further enhanced after taking the product for 4 months (D'Andrea et al 2009). Another open-label study with 119 school-aged volunteers with a history of migraine found that treatment with a combination product (ginkgolide B, coenzyme Q10, riboflavin and magnesium) taken twice daily as a prophylactic therapy for 3 months significantly reduced migraine frequency (Esposito & Carotenuto 2011). A similar combination of nutrients with ginkgolide B (80 mg), coenzyme Q10 (20 mg), vitamin B_2 (1.6 mg) and magnesium (300 mg) was given to 30 children twice a day for 3 months. In this open-label prospective trial the children were followed up over a year; combination treatment was shown to be an effective preventive treatment in significantly reducing migraine frequency and reducing analgesic medication after 3 months and at 1-year follow-up (Usai et al 2011).

Multiple sclerosis

MS is a chronic demyelinating neurological disease afflicting young and middle-aged adults, resulting in problems with coordination, strength, cognition, affect and sensation. Several clinical studies have investigated whether ginkgo treatment may help reduce some of these impairments, generally producing disappointing results.

Johnson et al (2006) conducted a randomised, double-blind study which compared the effects of ginkgo (EGb 761: 240 mg/day) to placebo on depression, anxiety, fatigue, symptom severity and functional performance using validated measures for each outcome. Twenty-two people with MS were enrolled in the study. Significantly, more people administered ginkgo showed improvement on four or more measures, with improvements associated with significantly larger effect sizes on measures of fatigue, symptom severity and functionality. The ginkgo group also exhibited less fatigue at follow-up compared with the placebo group and treatment was well tolerated, with no side effects or adverse effects reported.

The cognitive function of people with MS did not significantly improve after 12 weeks of treatment with GBE (120 mg twice a day), according to a randomised, double-blind, placebo-controlled trial (Lovera et al 2007). However, a treatment effect trend, limited to the Stroop test, indicated that ginkgo treatment may have an effect on cognitive domains assessed by this test, such as susceptibility to interference and mental flexibility. People with greater cognitive impairment at the start of the study experienced more improvement with treatment than higher-functioning people. No serious drug-related side effects occurred. A Cochrane systematic review of treatment for memory disorders in MS patients only found the 2007 Lovera study worthy of inclusion and confirmed *G. biloba* was not effective as an intervention in this group (He et al 2011). The same author, Lovera, repeated his earlier study with a RCT of 120 subjects with MS and *G. biloba* (120 mg twice daily) over 12 weeks and confirmed that there were no improvements in cognitive performance (Lovera et al 2012).

Parkinson's disease

There is great interest in the application of safe substances, such as *G. biloba*, in neurodegenerative diseases such as Parkinson's disease because of their neuroprotective and mitochondrial protective effects. Currently, investigation with ginkgo is limited to animal studies of experimentally induced Parkinson's disease, which have shown it to afford some protection against neuronal loss (Ahmad et al 2005, Kim et al 2004) and neuronal damage (Rojas et al 2012).

Schizophrenia — adjunctive treatment

G. biloba given as an adjunct to the atypical antipsychotic medicine clozapine in the treatment of refractory schizophrenia was shown to enhance drug effects on negative symptoms according to a placebo-controlled study involving 42 patients with chronic, treatment-resistant schizophrenia (Doruk et al 2008). Ginkgo was used at a dose of 120 mg/day for 12 weeks. This study has been further validated by a review and meta-analysis conducted in 2010 which included six studies of 466 patients taking ginkgo and 362 people taking placebo. When prescribed in combination with antipsychotic medication, *G. biloba* resulted in statistically significant positive effects with symptoms of chronic schizophrenia (Singh et al 2010). Since the publication of the meta-analysis a further randomised double-blind, placebo-controlled trial found benefit of using GBE (EGb 761) for reducing symptoms of tardive dyskinesia in schizophrenia patients. This trial recruited 157 in a psychiatric hospital in China and the treatment arm were given 240 mg/day of *G. biloba* or placebo for 12 weeks. The authors hypothesise that the improvement may be due to the antioxidant activity of this herb (Zhang et al 2011, 2012a).

Tardive syndromes — including tardive dyskinesias

The American Academy of Neurology in 2013 conducted a broad literature review to make evidence-based recommendations regarding management of tardive syndromes, including tardive dyskinesias (Bhidayasiri et al 2013). They came to the conclusion that clonazepam probably improves tardive dyskinesias and ginkgo biloba probably improves tardive syndromes (both level B) and both should be considered as treatment.

DOSAGE RANGE

The recommended dose varies, depending on indication and condition treated.

General guide

- Dried herb: 9–10 g/day.
- 120–240 mg of a 50 : 1 standardised extract daily in divided doses (40 mg extract is equivalent to 1.4–2.7 g leaves).
- Fluid extract (1 : 1): 0.5 mL three times daily.

According to clinical studies

- Asthma: 40 mg three times daily.
- Dementia and memory impairment: 120–240 mg standardised extract daily in divided doses.
- Generalised anxiety disorder: 240–480 mg daily.
- Intermittent claudication, vertigo: 120–320 mg standardised extract daily in divided doses.
- Normal-tension glaucoma: 120–160 mg standardised extract daily.
- MS — to improve energy levels, cognitive function and mood: 120 mg twice daily.
- PMS: 80 mg twice daily, starting on the 16th day of the menstrual cycle until the 5th day of the next cycle.
- Prevention of altitude sickness: 160 mg standardised extract daily, starting 5 days prior to ascent or ginkgo (80 mg per dose) every 12 hours, starting 24 hours before ascending and continuing throughout stay at high altitude.
- Schizophrenia: as an adjunct to clozapine in refractory cases: 120–240 mg daily.
- Raynaud's syndrome: 240–360 mg/day divided into three doses.
- Sexual dysfunction associated with antidepressant drugs: 200 mg standardised extract daily.
- Sexual dysfunction (women): 300 mg daily in conjunction with sex therapy.
- Vitiligo: 120 mg standardised extract daily.

Although some studies report positive effects after 4–6 weeks' continual use, a trial of at least 12 weeks is recommended in chronic conditions.

ADVERSE REACTIONS

In most placebo-controlled studies, there is no difference between the side effect incidence with ginkgo and placebo. Standardised ginkgo leaf extracts have been used safely in trials lasting from several weeks to up to 6 years. In a few cases (less than 0.001%), gastrointestinal upset, headaches and dizziness were reported. Ginkgo does not appear to alter heart rate and blood pressure, change cholesterol and triglyceride levels or increase intraocular pressure in clinical studies (Chung et al 1999).

A 2011 systematic review of bleeding associated with *G. biloba* therapy found no higher bleeding risk associated with standardised GBE in a meta-analysis of 18 RCTs (Kellermann & Kloft 2011); however, rare case reports of subarachnoid haemorrhage, subdural haematoma, intracerebral haemorrhage, subphrenic haematoma, vitreous haemorrhage and postoperative bleeding have been reported.

Crude ginkgo plant parts that may contain concentrations of 5 ppm of the toxic ginkgolic acid constituents should be avoided, as they can induce severe allergic reactions.

SIGNIFICANT INTERACTIONS

A small clinical study suggests that *G. biloba* inhibits P-gp, so caution is advised when taking GBE and P-gp substrates together, as drug doses may need to be adjusted. Various cytochromes have been evaluated, and drugs metabolised this way seem to have little risk of herb–drug interactions with *G. biloba* at doses of 240 mg/day or less (Gurley et al 2012).

Adriamycin

Studies with an animal model indicate that ginkgo extract EGb 761 reduces the hyperlipidaemia and proteinuria associated with Adriamycin-induced nephropathy, which might be beneficial to enhance the therapeutic index of Adriamycin (Abd-Ellah & Mariee 2007). Clinical trials have not been conducted to confirm the activity.

Antidepressant drugs

Ginkgo may reduce the sexual dysfunction side effects of these drugs and improve sleep continuity; however, results from clinical studies are mixed — possible beneficial interaction.

Clinical note — Does* Ginkgo biloba *cause significant bleeding and does it interact with warfarin?

The current body of evidence casts doubt on the clinical significance of the proposed interaction between warfarin and ginkgo, revealing that there is little evidence from controlled studies to demonstrate significant platelet inhibition, bleeding or changes to international normalised ratio (INR) with use of ginkgo (especially EGb 761 or phytochemically similar extracts).

Several clinical trials have been published in peer-reviewed journals which demonstrate that *G. biloba* does not have a significant effect on platelet function, two studies showing no interaction with warfarin, one study showing no interaction with aspirin and a further study showing no interaction with clopidogrel (Aruna & Naidu 2007, Bal Dit et al 2003, Beckert et al 2007, Carlson et al 2007, Engelsen et al 2003, Gardner et al 2007, Jiang et al 2005, Kohler et al 2004). Studies have included young healthy volunteers and older adults, using doses up to 480 mg/day of ginkgo and time frames up to 4 months.

The first controlled study was published in 2003. Bal Dit et al conducted a double-blind, randomised, placebo-controlled study of 32 young healthy volunteers to evaluate the effect of three doses of GBE (120, 240 and 480 mg/day for 14 days) on haemostasis, coagulation and fibrinolysis (Bal Dit et al 2003). This escalating dose study found no effect on platelet function or coagulation for any dose tested. A year later, results from a larger randomised, placebo-controlled, crossover study that produced similar results were published (Kohler et al 2004). The study by Kohler et al investigated the effects of ginkgo (2 × 120 mg/day EGb 761) on 29 different coagulation and bleeding parameters. Once again, no evidence of inhibition of blood coagulation and platelet aggregation was detected. In Australia, Jiang et al (2005) investigated the interaction between warfarin and *G. biloba* using a randomised, cross-over study design. The study of 12 healthy males found no evidence that INR or platelet aggregation was affected by *G. biloba*. Engelsen et al (2003) also found no evidence of an interaction between *G. biloba* and warfarin under double-blind, placebo-controlled trial conditions. The study involved patients stable on long-term warfarin and reported no changes to INR values.

In 2007, four more studies were published. Carlson et al (2007) conducted a study of 90 older adults (65–84 years) who were randomly assigned to placebo or a *G. biloba*-based supplement (160 mg/day) for 4 months. No evidence of alteration to platelet function was seen at this dose. Beckert et al (2007) conducted a smaller trial of 10 volunteers who were administered ginkgo for 2 weeks, after which in vivo platelet function was quantified using the PFA-100 assay. The study used aspirin as a control agent and found that platelet function was not affected by *G. biloba*, but was markedly inhibited by the administration of aspirin. No clinically or statistically significant differences were seen in a randomised, double-blind, placebo-controlled trial, which investigated the effects of *G. biloba* (EGb 761, 300 mg/day) on several measures of platelet aggregation among 55 older adults (age 69 ± 10 years) also consuming 325 mg/day aspirin (Gardner et al 2007). Reports of bleeding or bruising were infrequent and similar for both study groups. A study of 10 healthy volunteers investigated the effects of two different doses of *G. biloba* (120 mg and 240 mg) taken together with clopidogrel (75 mg) (Aruna & Naidu 2007). Platelet inhibition with the combination of *G. biloba* and clopidogrel was not statistically significant, compared with individual doses of drugs. Finally, a 2011 randomised, double-blind, placebo-controlled, two-way cross-over trial was conducted on 12 healthy volunteers for 5 weeks. It was found that there was no effect on clotting process alone and *G. biloba* had limited effects on the pharmacokinetics and no effect on the pharmacodynamics of single-dose warfarin in health volunteers (Zhou & Zeng 2011).

Bleomycin

Studies with an animal model indicate that ginkgo extract EGb 761 reduces oxidative stress induced by bleomycin. This may improve drug tolerance; however, clinical studies have not yet been conducted to test this further (Erdogan et al 2006).

Cholinergic drugs

Cholinergic activity has been identified for ginkgo; therefore, combined use may theoretically increase drug activity — observe patients using this combination, although the effects may be beneficial when used under supervision.

Cilostazol

Used for intermittent claudication with peripheral arterial disease. Adjunctive use with *G. biloba* may produce additional benefits based on in vivo studies (Jung et al 2012) — observe.

Cisplatin

As a herb with significant antioxidant activity, ginkgo has also been employed as a means of reducing the nephrotoxic effects of cisplatin, a use supported by two in vivo studies (Gulec et al 2006, Ozturk et al 2004). Other researchers using animal models have indicated that ginkgo may protect against cisplatin-induced ototoxicity (Huang et al

2007). Clinical trials are required to confirm significance — adjunctive use may be beneficial when used under professional supervision.

Clozapine

Ginkgo may enhance the effects of clozapine on negative affect in refractory schizophrenic patients, according to a placebo-controlled study (Doruk et al 2008) — beneficial interaction.

Doxorubicin

In vivo research suggests that ginkgo can prevent doxorubicin-induced cardiotoxicity, suggesting a potentially beneficial interaction, although no human studies are available to confirm clinical significance (Naidu et al 2002).

Haloperidol

In three clinical trials, the effectiveness of haloperidol was enhanced when co-administered with 360 mg of ginkgo daily (Chavez et al 2006) — beneficial interaction under supervision.

Platelet inhibitor drugs

Due to its platelet-activating factor antagonist activity, *G. biloba* may theoretically enhance the effects of these drugs and increase the risk of bruising or bleeding; however, evidence from recent clinical trials and a systematic review has cast doubt on the clinical significance of this activity (Diamond & Bailey 2013, Kim et al 2010, Ryu et al 2009) — observe.

Valproate, Dilantin, Depakote

There is a report of 2 patients using valproate who experienced seizures with ginkgo use (Chavez et al 2006). There is also a report of a patient taking Dilantin, Depakote and ginkgo, together with other herbal medicines, who suffered a fatal breakthrough seizure, with no evidence of non-compliance with anticonvulsant medications (Kupiec & Raj 2005). The autopsy report revealed subtherapeutic serum levels for both anticonvulsants, Depakote and Dilantin; however, it is uncertain whether effects can be attributed to ginkgo — observe patient taking ginkgo with these medicines.

Warfarin

Theoretically, ginkgo may increase bleeding risk when used together with warfarin; however, evidence from controlled clinical studies does not support this conclusion and has failed to identify any clinically significant pharmacodynamic or pharmacokinetic interaction. This conclusion is supported by a systematic review (Bone 2008) — observe.

Cerebral haemorrhage and epilepsy

Rare case reports have suggested that ginkgo should be used with caution in people with known risk factors for cerebral haemorrhage and epilepsy until further investigation can clarify its safety (Benjamin et al 2001, Granger 2001, Vale 1998).

CONTRAINDICATIONS AND PRECAUTIONS

If unusual bleeding or bruising occurs, stop use immediately. Although new clinical evidence suggests that *G. biloba* does not affect clotting times, it may be prudent to suspend use for 1 week prior to major surgery in at-risk populations.

PREGNANCY USE

Insufficient reliable evidence in humans to determine safety. In clinical usage there would be no adverse effects expected (Bone 2003).

Practice points/Patient counselling

- *G. biloba* is a complex herb that contains many different active constituents and works by means of multiple mechanisms. Therefore, it has applications in many varied conditions.
- Oral ginkgo extract improves cognitive function in people with mild to moderate cognitive impairment or those people with dementia with neuropsychiatric features, but it is less successful in people with normal cognitive function.
- Long-term use does not protect against the development of dementia.
- It may be an effective treatment in peripheral vascular diseases such as intermittent claudication; however, study findings are not always consistent. Due to the herb's inherent safety, a therapeutic trial may be useful in practice to determine an individual's response.
- Some positive evidence exists for PMS, sudden deafness, tardive syndromes, preventing altitude sickness, ischaemic stroke, SAD and vertigo.
- Largely based on the herb's physiological actions, ginkgo is also used to treat chilblains and haemorrhoids, and prevent macular degeneration, glaucoma, sexual dysfunction, impotence, allergies and asthma, and improve wellbeing.
- The form of ginkgo most often tested and used is a preparation known as EGb 761, which is standardised to 24% ginkgo flavonol glycosides and 6% terpene lactones.
- Overall, *G. biloba* is a very safe herb and is extremely well tolerated.

PATIENTS' FAQs

What will this herb do for me?

Ginkgo is a very popular herbal treatment that increases peripheral circulation, beneficially influences brain chemicals, protects nerve cells from damage and may stimulate immune function and reduce inflammation. Scientific evidence has shown that it may improve cognitive function in people with mild to moderate cognitive impairment when used long-term in sufficient dosage, but it is less successful in people with normal function. It may also improve some aspects of memory in younger people when used short-term. Ginkgo may improve symptoms of intermittent claudication and be useful in treating chilblains, PMS and vitiligo, preventing altitude sickness, vertigo and SAD and possibly sexual dysfunction such as impotence. If taken long-term, it does not protect against the development of dementia in the future.

When will it start to work?

This will depend on the condition treated and the dose used. Generally, *G. biloba* is a slow-acting herb that can take anywhere from 4 weeks to 6 months to exert maximal effects.

Are there any safety issues?

Ginkgo has been extensively studied and appears to be extremely safe with virtually no side effects in healthy people. Some contraindications and interactions are possible, so it is recommended that it should be taken under professional supervision.

REFERENCES

Abd-Ellah MF, Mariee AD. *Ginkgo biloba* leaf extract (EGb 761) diminishes adriamycin-induced hyperlipidaemic nephrotoxicity in rats: association with nitric oxide production. Biotechnol Appl Biochem 46 (2007): 35–40.

Abdel-Salam OM et al. Evaluation of the anti-inflammatory, anti-nociceptive and gastric effects of *Ginkgo biloba* in the rat. Pharmacol Res 49.2 (2004): 133–142.

Agus, S., et al. 2013. Clinical and Demographic Features of Vertigo: Findings from the REVERT Registry. Front Neurol., 4, 48 available from: PM:23675366.

Ahmad M et al. *Ginkgo biloba* affords dose-dependent protection against 6-hydroxydopamine-induced parkinsonism in rats: neurobehavioural, neurochemical and immunohistochemical evidences. J Neurochem 93.1 (2005): 94–104.

Ao Q et al. Protective effects of extract of *Ginkgo biloba* (EGb 761) on nerve cells after spinal cord injury in rats. Spinal Cord 44.11 (2006): 662–667.

Aricioglu A et al. Changes in zinc levels and superoxide dismutase activities in the skin of acute, ultraviolet-B-irradiated mice after treatment with *Ginkgo biloba* extract. Biol Trace Elem Res 80.2 (2001): 175–179.

Aruna D, Naidu MU. Pharmacodynamic interaction studies of *Ginkgo biloba* with cilostazol and clopidogrel in healthy human subjects. Br J Clin Pharmacol 63.3 (2007): 333–338.

Attia, A., et al. 2012. Phase II study of *Ginkgo biloba* in irradiated brain tumor patients: effect on cognitive function, quality of life, and mood. J Neurooncol, 109, 357–63.

Babayigit A et al. Effects of *Ginkgo biloba* on airway histology in a mouse model of chronic asthma. Allergy Asthma Proc 30.2 (2008): 186–2591.

Bachinskaya, N., et al. 2011. Alleviating neuropsychiatric symptoms in dementia: the effects of *Ginkgo biloba* extract EGb 761. Findings from a randomized controlled trial. Neuropsychiatr Dis Treat, 7, 209–15.

Bal Dit SC et al. No alteration in platelet function or coagulation induced by EGb 761 in a controlled study. Clin Lab Haematol 25.4 (2003): 251–253.

Bao, Y. M., et al. 2010. [Effects of *Ginkgo biloba* extract 50 preconditioning on contents of inflammation-related cytokines in myocardium of rats with ischemia-reperfusion injury.] Zhong Xi Yi Jie He Xue Bao, 8, 373–8.

Barton, D. L., et al. 2013. The use of *Ginkgo biloba* for the prevention of chemotherapy-related cognitive dysfunction in women receiving adjuvant treatment for breast cancer, N00C9. Support Care Cancer. 21: 1185–1192.

Bastianetto S, Quirion R. EGb 761 is a neuroprotective agent against beta-amyloid toxicity. Cell Mol Biol (Noisy-le-grand) 48.6 (2002a): 693–7.

Bastianetto S, Quirion R. Natural extracts as possible protective agents of brain aging. Neurobiol Aging 23.5 (2002b): 891–7.

Bastianetto S et al. The *Ginkgo biloba* extract (EGb 761) protects hippocampal neurons against cell death induced by beta-amyloid. Eur J Neurosci 12.6 (2000): 1882–1890.

Beal MF. Bioenergetic approaches for neuroprotection in Parkinson's disease. Ann Neurol 53 (Suppl 3) (2003): S39–S47.

Beckert BW et al. The effect of herbal medicines on platelet function: an in vivo experiment and review of the literature. Plast Reconstr Surg 120.7 (2007): 2044–2050.

Benjamin J et al. A case of cerebral haemorrhage: can *Ginkgo biloba* be implicated? Postgrad Med J 77.904 (2001): 112–1113.

Bernatoniene, J., et al. 2011. The effect of *Ginkgo biloba* extract on mitochondrial oxidative phosphorylation in the normal and ischemic rat heart. Phytother Res, 25, 1054–60.

Bhidayasiri, R., et al. 2013. Evidence-based guideline: treatment of tardive syndromes: report of the Guideline Development Subcommittee of the American Academy of Neurology. Neurology, 81, (5) 463–469 available from: PM:23897874.

Biggs, M. L., et al. 2010. *Ginkgo biloba* and risk of cancer: secondary analysis of the Ginkgo Evaluation of Memory (GEM) Study. Pharmacoepidemiol Drug Saf, 19, 694–8.

Birks, J. & Grimley Evans, J. 2009. *Ginkgo biloba* for cognitive impairment and dementia. Cochrane Database Syst Rev, CD003120.

Blumenthal M, et al. (eds). Herbal medicine expanded commission E monographs. Austin, TX: Integrative Medicine Communications, 2000.

Bone, K. 2003. A Clinical guide to blending liquid herbs, Qld, Australia, Churchill Livingstone.

Bone KM. Potential interaction of *Ginkgo biloba* leaf with antiplatelet or anticoagulant drugs: what is the evidence? Mol Nutr Food Res 52.7 (2008): 764–771.

Bredie, S. J. & Jong, M. C. 2012. No significant effect of ginkgo biloba special extract EGb 761 in the treatment of primary Raynaud phenomenon: a randomized controlled trial. J Cardiovasc Pharmacol, 59, 215–21.

Brondino, N., et al. 2013. A Systematic Review and Meta-Analysis of *Ginkgo biloba* in Neuropsychiatric Disorders: From Ancient Tradition to Modern-Day Medicine. Evid Based Complement Alternat Med, 2013, 915691.

Budzinski JW et al. An in vitro evaluation of human cytochrome P450 3A4 inhibition by selected commercial herbal extracts and tinctures. Phytomedicine 7.4 (2000): 273–282.

Burns NR, et al. *Ginkgo biloba*: no robust effect on cognitive abilities or mood in healthy young or older adults. Hum Psychopharmacol 21.1 (2006): 27–37.

Burschka MA et al. Effect of treatment with *Ginkgo biloba* extract EGb 761 (oral) on unilateral idiopathic sudden hearing loss in a prospective randomized double-blind study of 106 outpatients. Eur Arch Otorhinolaryngol 258.5 (2001): 213–2119.

Canter PH, Ernst E. *Ginkgo biloba* is not a smart drug: an updated systematic review of randomised clinical trials testing the nootropic effects of *G. biloba* extracts in healthy people. Hum Psychopharmacol 22.5 (2007): 265–278.

Carlson JJ et al. Safety and efficacy of a ginkgo biloba-containing dietary supplement on cognitive function, quality of life, and platelet function in healthy, cognitively intact older adults. J Am Diet Assoc 107.3 (2007): 422–432.

Chavez ML, et al. Evidence-based drug: herbal interactions. Life Sci 78.18 (2006): 2146–2157.

Chen X, et al. Extracts of *Ginkgo biloba* and ginsenosides exert cerebral vasorelaxation via a nitric oxide pathway. Clin Exp Pharmacol Physiol 24.12 (1997): 958–959.

Chen, L. L., et al. 2008. [Effect of nebulized TFG on Th1/Th2 imbalance in mouse model with asthma.] Zhongguo Zhong Yao Za Zhi, 33, 1865–8.

Chen, J. S., et al. 2011a. Nrf-2 mediated heme oxygenase-1 expression, an antioxidant-independent mechanism, contributes to anti-atherogenesis and vascular protective effects of *Ginkgo biloba* extract. Atherosclerosis, 214, 301–9.

Chen, X. H., et al. 2011b. Effects of *Ginkgo biloba* extract EGb761 on human colon adenocarcinoma cells. Cell Physiol Biochem, 27, 227–32.

Choi, W. S., et al. 2009. To compare the efficacy and safety of nifedipine sustained release with *Ginkgo biloba* extract to treat patients with primary Raynaud's phenomenon in South Korea; Korean Raynaud study (KOARA study). Clin Rheumatol, 28, 553–9.

Chow T et al. *Ginkgo biloba* and acetazolamide prophylaxis for acute mountain sickness: a randomized, placebo-controlled trial. Arch Intern Med 165.3 (2005): 296–301.

Chu, X., et al. 2011. A novel anti-inflammatory role for ginkgolide B in asthma via inhibition of the ERK/MAPK signaling pathway. Molecules, 16, 7634–48.

Chung HS et al. *Ginkgo biloba* extract increases ocular blood flow velocity. J Ocul Pharmacol Ther 15.3 (1999): 233–240.

Cieza A, et al. [The effect of ginkgo biloba on healthy elderly subjects.] Fortschr Med Orig 121.1 (2003): 5–10.

Clement, Y. N., et al. 2011. Effects of herbal and dietary supplements on cognition in menopause: a systematic review. Maturitas, 68, 256–63.

Cohen AJ, Bartlik B. *Ginkgo biloba* for antidepressant-induced sexual dysfunction. J Sex Marital Ther 24.2 (1998): 139–143.

Cohen-Boulakia F et al. In vivo sequential study of skeletal muscle capillary permeability in diabetic rats: effect of anthocyanosides. Metabolism 49.7 (2000): 880–885.

Colciaghi F et al. Amyloid precursor protein metabolism is regulated toward alpha-secretase pathway by *Ginkgo biloba* extracts. Neurobiol Dis 16.2 (2004): 454–460.

Cong, W.-N., et al. 2011. EGb761, an extract of *Ginkgo biloba* leaves, reduces insulin resistance in a high-fat-fed mouse model. Acta Pharmaceutica Sinica B, 1, 14–20.

D'Andrea, G., et al. 2009. Efficacy of Ginkgolide B in the prophylaxis of migraine with aura. Neurol Sci, 30 Suppl 1, S121–4.

Dardano, A., et al. 2012. The effect of *Ginkgo biloba* extract on genotoxic damage in patients with differentiated thyroid carcinoma receiving thyroid remnant ablation with iodine-131. Thyroid, 22, 318–24.

Das A et al. A comparative study in rodents of standardized extracts of *Bacopa monniera* and *Ginkgo biloba*: anticholinesterase and cognitive enhancing activities. Pharmacol Biochem Behav 73.4 (2002): 893.

DeFeudis FV, Drieu K. *Ginkgo biloba* extract (EGb 761) and CNS functions: basic studies and clinical applications. Curr Drug Targets 1.1 (2000): 25–58.

DeFeudis FV, et al. *Ginkgo biloba* extracts and cancer: a research area in its infancy. Fundam Clin Pharmacol 17.4 (2003): 405–417.

DeKosky ST et al. *Ginkgo biloba* for prevention of dementia: a randomized controlled trial. JAMA 300.19 (2008): 2253–2262.

Deng Y et al. Induction of cytochrome P450s by terpene trilactones and flavonoids of the *Ginkgo biloba* extract EGb 761 in rats. Xenobiotica 38.5 (2008): 465–481.

Deng, Y. K., et al. 2009. [Effect of ginkgo biloba extract on plasma vascular endothelial growth factor during peri-operative period of cardiac surgery.] Zhongguo Zhong Xi Yi Jie He Za Zhi, 29, 40–2.

Diamond, B. J. & Bailey, M. R. 2013. *Ginkgo biloba*: indications, mechanisms, and safety. Psychiatr Clin North Am, 36, 73–83.

Dodge HH et al. A randomized placebo-controlled trial of *Ginkgo biloba* for the prevention of cognitive decline. Neurology 70.19 (Pt 2) (2008): 1809–1817.

Dong, Z. H., et al. 2012. [Effects of ginkgo biloba tablet in treating mild cognitive impairment.] Zhongguo Zhong Xi Yi Jie He Za Zhi, 32, 1208–11.

Doruk A, et al. A placebo-controlled study of extract of ginkgo biloba added to clozapine in patients with treatment-resistant schizophrenia. Int Clin Psychopharmacol 23.4 (2008): 223–227.

Drew S, Davies E. Effectiveness of *Ginkgo biloba* in treating tinnitus: double blind, placebo controlled trial. BMJ 322.7278 (2001): 73.

Droy-Lefaix MT et al. Effect of *Gingko biloba* extract (EGb 761) on chloroquine induced retinal alterations. Lens Eye Toxic Res 9.3–4 (1992): 521–528.

Droy-Lefaix MT et al. Antioxidant effect of a *Ginkgo biloba* extract (EGb 761) on the retina. Int J Tissue React 17.3 (1995): 93–100.

Duche JC et al. Effect of *Ginkgo biloba* extract on microsomal enzyme induction. Int J Clin Pharmacol Res 9.3 (1989): 165–168.

Eckert, A. 2012. Mitochondrial effects of *Ginkgo biloba* extract. Int Psychogeriatr, 24 Suppl 1, S18–20.

Eckert A et al. Stabilization of mitochondrial membrane potential and improvement of neuronal energy metabolism by *Ginkgo biloba* extract EGb 761. Ann NY Acad Sci 1056 (2005): 474–485.

El Boghdady, N. A. 2013a. Antioxidant and antiapoptotic effects of proanthocyanidin and ginkgo biloba extract against doxorubicin-induced cardiac injury in rats. Cell Biochem Funct 13: 344–351.

El-Boghdady, N. A. 2013b. Increased cardiac endothelin-1 and nitric oxide in adriamycin-induced acute cardiotoxicity: protective effect of *Ginkgo biloba* extract. Indian J Biochem Biophys, 50, 202–9.

Eli R, Fasciano JA. An adjunctive preventive treatment for cancer: ultraviolet light and ginkgo biloba, together with other antioxidants, are a safe and powerful, but largely ignored, treatment option for the prevention of cancer. Med Hypotheses 66.6 (2006): 1152–1156.

Elsabagh S et al. Differential cognitive effects of *Ginkgo biloba* after acute and chronic treatment in healthy young volunteers. Psychopharmacology (Berl) 179.2 (2005a): 437–46.

Elsabagh S, et al. Limited cognitive benefits in Stage +2 postmenopausal women after 6 weeks of treatment with *Ginkgo biloba*. J Psychopharmacol 19.2 (2005b): 173–81.

Engelsen J, et al. Effect of coenzyme Q10 and *Ginkgo biloba* on warfarin dosage in patients on long-term warfarin treatment: a randomized, double-blind, placebo-controlled cross-over trial. Ugeskr Laeger 165.18 (2003): 1868–1871.

Erdogan H et al. Effects of *Ginkgo biloba* on plasma oxidant injury induced by bleomycin in rats. Toxicol Ind Health 22.1 (2006): 47–52.

Esmekaya, M. A., et al. 2011. Mutagenic and morphologic impacts of 1.8GHz radiofrequency radiation on human peripheral blood lymphocytes (hPBLs) and possible protective role of pre-treatment with *Ginkgo biloba* (EGb 761). Sci Total Environ, 410–411, 59–64.

Esposito, M. & Carotenuto, M. 2011. Ginkgolide B complex efficacy for brief prophylaxis of migraine in school-aged children: an open-label study. Neurol Sci, 32, 79–81.

Evans, J. R. 2013. *Ginkgo biloba* extract for age-related macular degeneration. Cochrane Database Syst Rev, 1, CD001775.

Fan, L., et al. 2009. Effects of *Ginkgo biloba* extract ingestion on the pharmacokinetics of talinolol in healthy Chinese volunteers. Ann Pharmacother, 43, 944–9.

Faustino, T. T., et al. 2010. [Medicinal plants for the treatment of generalized anxiety disorder: a review of controlled clinical studies.] Rev Bras Psiquiatr, 32, 429–36.

Fehske, C. J., et al. 2009. *Ginkgo biloba* extract (EGb761) influences monoaminergic neurotransmission via inhibition of NE uptake, but not MAO activity after chronic treatment. Pharmacol Res, 60, 68–73.

Fowler JS et al. Evidence that gingko biloba extract does not inhibit MAO A and B in living human brain. Life Sci 66.9 (2000): L141–L146.

Fu, L. M. & Li, J. T. 2011. A systematic review of single Chinese herbs for Alzheimer's disease treatment. Evid Based Complement Alternat Med, 2011, 640284.

Galduroz JC, et al. Gender- and age-related variations in blood viscosity in normal volunteers: a study of the effects of extract of *Allium sativum* and *Ginkgo biloba*. Phytomedicine 14.7–8 (2007): 447–451.

Gardner CD et al. Effect of *Ginkgo biloba* (EGb 761) and aspirin on platelet aggregation and platelet function analysis among older adults at risk of cardiovascular disease: a randomized clinical trial. Blood Coagul Fibrinolysis 18.8 (2007): 787–793.

Gardner CD et al. Effect of *Ginkgo biloba* (EGb 761) on treadmill walking time among adults with peripheral artery disease: a randomized clinical trial. J Cardiopulm Rehabil Prev 28.4 (2008): 258–65.

Gertsch JH et al. Randomised, double blind, placebo controlled comparison of ginkgo biloba and acetazolamide for prevention of acute mountain sickness among Himalayan trekkers: the prevention of high altitude illness trial (PHAIT). BMJ 328.7443 (2004): 797.

Granger AS. *Ginkgo biloba* precipitating epileptic seizures. Age Ageing 30.6 (2001): 523–525.

Grass-Kapanke, B., et al. 2011. Effects of Ginkgo Biloba Special Extract EGb 761® in Very Mild Cognitive Impairment (vMCI). Neuroscience and Medicine, 2, 48–56.

Gulec M et al. The effects of ginkgo biloba extract on tissue adenosine deaminase, xanthine oxidase, myeloperoxidase, malondialdehyde, and nitric oxide in cisplatin-induced nephrotoxicity. Toxicol Ind Health 22.3 (2006): 125–130.

Gurley BJ et al. Cytochrome P450 phenotypic ratios for predicting herb-drug interactions in humans. Clin Pharmacol Ther 72.3 (2002): 276–287.

Gurley BJ et al. Clinical assessment of effects of botanical supplementation on cytochrome P450 phenotypes in the elderly: St John's wort, garlic oil, *Panax ginseng* and *Ginkgo biloba*. Drugs Aging 22.6 (2005): 525–539.

Gurley, B., et al. 2012. Pharmacokinetic Herb-Drug Interactions (Part 2): Drug Interactions Involving Popular Botanical Dietary Supplements and Their Clinical Relevance. Planta Med 2012, 78, 1490–1514.

Hamann, K.F. 2007. [Special ginkgo extract in cases of vertigo: a systematic review of randomised, double-blind, placebo controlled clinical examinations.] HNO, 55, (4) 258–263.

Hao, Y. R., et al. 2009. [*Ginkgo biloba* extracts (EGb761) inhibits aflatoxin B1-induced hepatocarcinogenesis in Wistar rats.] Zhong Yao Cai, 32, 92–6.

Hartley, D. E., et al. 2004. Gincosan (a combination of *Ginkgo biloba* and *Panax ginseng*): the effects on mood and cognition of 6 and 12 weeks' treatment in post-menopausal women. Nutr Neurosci, 7, 325–33.

Haruyama, T. & Nagata, K. 2013. Anti-influenza virus activity of *Ginkgo biloba* leaf extracts. J Nat Med, 67, 636–42.

Hasanzadeh, E., et al. 2012. A double-blind placebo controlled trial of *Ginkgo biloba* added to risperidone in patients with autistic disorders. Child Psychiatry Hum Dev, 43, 674–82.

He, D., et al. 2011. Pharmacologic treatment for memory disorder in multiple sclerosis. Cochrane Database of Systematic Reviews [Online]. Available: http://onlinelibrary.wiley.com/doi/10.1002/14651858.CD008876.pub2/abstract.

Hellum BH, Nilsen OG. In vitro inhibition of CYP3A4 metabolism and P-glycoprotein-mediated transport by trade herbal products. Basic Clin Pharmacol Toxicol 102.5 (2008): 466–475.

Hellum BH, et al. The induction of CYP1A2, CYP2D6 and CYP3A4 by six trade herbal products in cultured primary human hepatocytes. Basic Clin Pharmacol Toxicol 100.1 (2007): 23–30.

Herrschaft, H., et al. 2012. *Ginkgo biloba* extract EGb 761(R) in dementia with neuropsychiatric features: a randomised, placebo-controlled trial to confirm the efficacy and safety of a daily dose of 240 mg. J Psychiatr Res, 46, 716–23.

Hibatallah J, et al. In-vivo and in-vitro assessment of the free-radical-scavenger activity of Ginkgo flavone glycosides at high concentration. J Pharm Pharmacol 51.12 (1999): 1435–1440.

Hilton, M. P., et al. 2013. *Ginkgo biloba* for tinnitus. Cochrane Database Syst Rev, 3, CD003852.

Horsch S, Walther C. *Ginkgo biloba* special extract EGb 761 in the treatment of peripheral arterial occlusive disease (PAOD): a review based on randomized, controlled studies. Int J Clin Pharmacol Ther 42.2 (2004): 63–72.

Hsu, C. L., et al. 2009. *Ginkgo biloba* extract confers protection from cigarette smoke extract-induced apoptosis in human lung endothelial cells: Role of heme oxygenase-1. Pulm Pharmacol Ther, 22, 286–96.

Huang SH et al. Bilobalide, a sesquiterpene trilactone from *Ginkgo biloba*, is an antagonist at recombinant alpha1beta2gamma2L GABA(A) receptors. Eur J Pharmacol 464.1 (2003): 1–8.

Huang X, et al. *Ginkgo biloba* extract (EGb 761) protects against cisplatin-induced ototoxicity in rats. Otol Neurotol 28.6 (2007): 828–833.

Huang, C. H., et al. 2013. *Ginkgo biloba* leaves extract (EGb 761) attenuates lipopolysaccharide-induced acute lung injury via inhibition of oxidative stress and NF-kappaB-dependent matrix metalloproteinase-9 pathway. Phytomedicine 20: 303–309.

Ihl, R. 2013. Effects of *Ginkgo biloba* extract EGb 761 (R) in dementia with neuropsychiatric features: review of recently completed randomised, controlled trials. Int.J Psychiatry Clin Pract., 17 Suppl 1, 8–14.

Ilhan A et al. *Ginkgo biloba* prevents mobile phone-induced oxidative stress in rat brain. Clin Chim Acta 340.1–2 (2004): 153–162.

Ilieva I et al. The effects of *Ginkgo biloba* extract on lipopolysaccharide-induced inflammation in vitro and in vivo. Exp Eye Res 79.2 (2004): 181–187.

Itil TM et al. The pharmacological effects of ginkgo biloba, a plant extract, on the brain of dementia patients in comparison with tacrine. Psychopharmacol Bull 34.3 (1998): 391–397.

Jang, C. H., et al. 2011. Effect of *Ginkgo biloba* extract on endotoxin-induced labyrinthitis. International Journal of Pediatric Otorhinolaryngology, 75, 905–909.

Janssen, I. M., et al. 2010. *Ginkgo biloba* in Alzheimer's disease: a systematic review. Wien Med Wochenschr, 160, 539–46.

Janssens D et al. Protection by bilobalide of the ischaemia-induced alterations of the mitochondrial respiratory activity. Fundam Clin Pharmacol 14.3 (2000): 193–201.

Jastreboff PJ et al. Attenuation of salicylate-induced tinnitus by *Ginkgo biloba* extract in rats. Audiol Neurootol 2.4 (1997): 197–212.

Jiang X et al. Effect of ginkgo and ginger on the pharmacokinetics and pharmacodynamics of warfarin in healthy subjects. Br J Clin Pharmacol 59.4 (2005): 425–432.

Jiang, X. Y., et al. 2009. Interventional effect of *Ginkgo biloba* extract on the progression of gastric precancerous lesions in rats. J Dig Dis, 10, 293–9.

Jiang, W., et al. 2011. Ginkgo may prevent genetic-associated ovarian cancer risk: multiple biomarkers and anticancer pathways induced by ginkgolide B in BRCA1-mutant ovarian epithelial cells. Eur J Cancer Prev, 20, 508–17.

Jiang, W., et al. 2014. Ginkgo may sensitize ovarian cancer cells to cisplatin: antiproliferative and apoptosis-inducing effects of ginkgolide B on ovarian cancer cells. Integr Cancer Ther 13: NP10–NP17.

Johnson SK et al. a pilot randomized controlled trial. The effect of *Ginkgo biloba* on functional measures in multiple sclerosis. NY: Explore 2.1 (2006): 19–24.

Jung F et al. Effect of *Ginkgo biloba* on fluidity of blood and peripheral microcirculation in volunteers. Arzneimittelforschung 40.5 (1990): 589–593.

Jung, I. H., et al. 2012. *Ginkgo biloba* extract (GbE) enhances the anti-atherogenic effect of cilostazol by inhibiting ROS generation. Exp Mol Med, 44, 311–8.

Kampman, K., et al. 2003. A pilot trial of piracetam and ginkgo biloba for the treatment of cocaine dependence. Addict Behav, 28, 437–48.

Kang, J. W., et al. 2010. Kaempferol and quercetin, components of *Ginkgo biloba* extract (EGb 761), induce caspase-3-dependent apoptosis in oral cavity cancer cells. Phytother Res, 24 Suppl 1, S77–82.

Kanter, M. 2011. Protective effects of *Ginkgo biloba* (EGb 761) on testicular torsion/detorsion-induced ischemia-reperfusion injury in rats. Exp Mol Pathol, 91, 708–13.

Kaschel, R. 2009. *Ginkgo biloba*: specificity of neuropsychological improvement — a selective review in search of differential effects. Hum Psychopharmacol, 24, 345–70.

Kaschel, R. 2011. Specific memory effects of *Ginkgo biloba* extract EGb 761 in middle-aged healthy volunteers. Phytomedicine, 18, 1202–7.

Kasper, S. & Schubert, H. 2009. [*Ginkgo biloba* extract EGb 761 in the treatment of dementia: evidence of efficacy and tolerability.] Fortschr Neurol Psychiatr, 77, 494–506.

Kaur, S., et al. 2013. *Ginkgo biloba* extract attenuates hippocampal neuronal loss and cognitive dysfunction resulting from trimethyltin in mice. Phytomedicine, 20, (2) 178–186.

Ke, T., et al. 2013. Effect of acetazolamide and gingko biloba on the human pulmonary vascular response to an acute altitude ascent. High Alt.Med Biol., 14, (2) 162–167.

Kehr, J., et al. 2012. *Ginkgo biloba* leaf extract (EGb 761(R)) and its specific acylated flavonol constituents increase dopamine and acetylcholine levels in the rat medial prefrontal cortex: possible implications for the cognitive enhancing properties of EGb 761(R). Int Psychogeriatr, 24 Suppl 1, S25–34.

Kellermann, A. J. & Kloft, C. 2011. Is there a risk of bleeding associated with standardized *Ginkgo biloba* extract therapy? A systematic review and meta-analysis. Pharmacotherapy, 31, 490–502.

Kennedy DO et al. Acute cognitive effects of standardised *Ginkgo biloba* extract complexed with phosphatidylserine. Hum Psychopharmacol 22.4 (2007a): 199–210.

Kennedy DO et al. Modulation of cognitive performance following single doses of 120 mg *Ginkgo biloba* extract administered to healthy young volunteers. Hum Psychopharmacol 22.8 (2007b): 559–66.

Kim SJ. Effect of biflavones of *Ginkgo biloba* against UVB-induced cytotoxicity in vitro. J Dermatol 28.4 (2001): 193–199.

Kim HK et al. Inhibition of rat adjuvant-induced arthritis by ginkgetin, a biflavone from ginkgo biloba leaves. Planta Med 65.5 (1999): 465–467.

Kim MS et al. Neuroprotective effect of *Ginkgo biloba* L. extract in a rat model of Parkinson's disease. Phytother Res 18.8 (2004): 663–666.

Kim, B. H., et al. 2010. Influence of *Ginkgo biloba* extract on the pharmacodynamic effects and pharmacokinetic properties of ticlopidine: an open-label, randomized, two-period, two-treatment, two-sequence, single-dose crossover study in healthy Korean male volunteers. Clin Ther, 32, 380–90.

Kleijnen J, Knipschild P. *Ginkgo biloba* for cerebral insufficiency. Br J Clin Pharmacol 34.4 (1992): 352–358.

Kohler S, et al. Influence of a 7-day treatment with *Ginkgo biloba* special extract EGb 761 on bleeding time and coagulation: a randomized, placebo-controlled, double-blind study in healthy volunteers. Blood Coagul Fibrinolysis 15.4 (2004): 303–309.

Koltermann A et al. *Ginkgo biloba* extract EGb 761 increases endothelial nitric oxide production in vitro and in vivo. Cell Mol Life Sci 64.13 (2007): 1715–1722.

Kotakadi VS et al. *Ginkgo biloba* extract EGb 761 has anti-inflammatory properties and ameliorates colitis in mice by driving effector T cell apoptosis. Carcinogenesis 29.9 (2008): 1799–1806.

Kuller, L. H., et al. 2010. Does *Ginkgo biloba* reduce the risk of cardiovascular events? Circ Cardiovasc Qual Outcomes, 3, 41–7.

Kupiec T, Raj V. Fatal seizures due to potential herb-drug interactions with *Ginkgo biloba*. J Anal Toxicol 29.7 (2005): 755–758.

Laws, K. R., et al. 2012. Is *Ginkgo biloba* a cognitive enhancer in healthy individuals? A meta-analysis. Hum Psychopharmacol, 27, 527–33.

Leadbetter GW, Hackett P. Comparison of *Ginkgo biloba*, acetazolamide, and placebo for prevention of acute mountain sickness. High Alt Med Biol 3 (2003): 455.

Leadbetter, G., et al. 2009. *Ginkgo biloba* does — and does not — prevent acute mountain sickness. Wilderness Environ Med, 20, 66–71.

Lee, J., et al. 2013. Effect of *Ginkgo biloba* Extract on Visual Field Progression in Normal Tension Glaucoma. J Glaucoma 22: 780–784.

Li MH, et al. Effects of ginkgo leaf concentrated oral liquor in treating asthma. Zhongguo Zhong Xi Yi Jie He Za Zhi 17.4 (1997): 216–2118.

Li, G. H., et al. 2008. [Studies on the effect of *Ginkgo biloba* extracts on NF-kappaB pathway.] Zhong Yao Cai, 31, 1357–60.

Li, X. S., et al. 2009. Effect of Ginkgo leaf extract on vascular endothelial function in patients with early stage diabetic nephropathy. Chin J Integr Med, 15, 26–9.

Lim H et al. Effects of anti-inflammatory biflavonoid, ginkgetin, on chronic skin inflammation. Biol Pharm Bull 29.5 (2006): 1046–1049.

Lim, S., et al. 2011. EGb761, a *Ginkgo biloba* extract, is effective against atherosclerosis in vitro, and in a rat model of type 2 diabetes. PLoS One, 6, e20301.

Lin SY, Chang HP. Induction of superoxide dismutase and catalase activity in different rat tissues and protection from UVB irradiation after topical application of *Ginkgo biloba* extracts. Methods Find Exp Clin Pharmacol 19.6 (1997): 367–371.

Lingaerde O, et al. Can winter depression be prevented by *Ginkgo biloba* extract? A placebo-controlled trial. Acta Psychiatr Scand 100.1 (1999): 62–66.

Liu KX et al. *Ginkgo biloba* extract (EGb 761) attenuates lung injury induced by intestinal ischemia/reperfusion in rats: roles of oxidative stress and nitric oxide. World J Gastroenterol 13.2 (2007): 299–305.

Liu, H. J., et al. 2009. Inhibitions of vascular endothelial growth factor expression and foam cell formation by EGb 761, a special extract of *Ginkgo biloba*, in oxidatively modified low-density lipoprotein-induced human THP-1 monocytes cells. Phytomedicine, 16, 138–45.

Lovera J et al. *Ginkgo biloba* for the improvement of cognitive performance in multiple sclerosis: a randomized, placebo-controlled trial. Mult Scler 13.3 (2007): 376–385.

Lovera, J. F., et al. 2012. *Ginkgo biloba* does not improve cognitive function in MS: a randomized placebo-controlled trial. Neurology, 79, 1278–84.

Lu, J. M., et al. 2012. Ginkgolic acid inhibits HIV protease activity and HIV infection in vitro. Med Sci Monit, 18, BR293–298.

Lucinda, L. M. F., et al. 2010. Evidences of osteoporosis improvement in Wistar rats treated with *Ginkgo biloba* extract: A histomorphometric study of mandible and femur. Fitoterapia, 81, 982–987.

Luo Y. Alzheimer's disease, the nematode Caenorhabditis elegans, and *Ginkgo biloba* leaf extract. Life Sci 78.18 (2006): 2066–2072.

Ma, S., et al. 2012. Neuroprotective effect of ginkgolide K against acute ischemic stroke on middle cerebral ischemia occlusion in rats. J Nat Med, 66, 25–31.

Maakestad K et al. *Ginkgo biloba* reduces incidence and severity of acute mountain sickness. Wilderness Environ Med 12 (2001): 51.

Mahdy, H. M., et al. 2011. The effect of *Ginkgo biloba* extract on 3-nitropropionic acid-induced neurotoxicity in rats. Neurochem Int, 59, 770–778.

Malenfant, D., et al. 2009. The efficacy of complementary and alternative medicine in the treatment of Raynaud's phenomenon: a literature review and meta-analysis. Rheumatology (Oxford), 48, 791–5.

Markowitz JS et al. Multiple-dose administration of *Ginkgo biloba* did not affect cytochrome P-450 2D6 or 3A4 activity in normal volunteers. J Clin Psychopharmacol 23.6 (2003): 576–581.

McCarney R et al. *Ginkgo biloba* for mild to moderate dementia in a community setting: a pragmatic, randomised, parallel-group, double-blind, placebo-controlled trial. Int J Geriatr Psychiatry 23.12 (2008): 1222–1230.

Meston CM, et al. Short- and long-term effects of *Ginkgo biloba* extract on sexual dysfunction in women. Arch Sex Behav 37.4 (2008): 530–547.

Moraga F et al. *Ginkgo biloba* decreases acute mountain sickness at 3700 m. High Alt Med Biol 3 (2003): 453.

Moraga FA et al. *Ginkgo biloba* decreases acute mountain sickness in people ascending to high altitude at Ollague (3696 m) in northern Chile. Wilderness Environ Med 18.4 (2007): 251–257.

Mouren X, et al. Study of the antiischemic action of EGb 761 in the treatment of peripheral arterial occlusive disease by TcPo2 determination. Angiology 45.6 (1994): 413–4117.

Moyad MA. Dietary supplements and other alternative medicines for erectile dysfunction. What do I tell my patients? Urol Clin North Am 29.1 (2002): 11–22: vii.

Muir AH et al. The use of *Ginkgo biloba* in Raynaud's disease: a double-blind placebo-controlled trial. Vasc Med 7.4 (2002): 265–267.

Muller WE. Nootropics, the therapy of dementia between aspiration and reality. Drug News Perspect 2 (1989): 295–300.

Nada, S. E. & Shah, Z. A. 2012. Preconditioning with *Ginkgo biloba* (EGb 761(R)) provides neuroprotection through HO1 and CRMP2. Neurobiol Dis, 46, 180–9.

Naidu MU et al. Protective effect of *Gingko biloba* extract against doxorubicin-induced cardiotoxicity in mice. Indian J Exp Biol 40.8 (2002): 894–900.

Napryeyenko O, Borzenko I. *Ginkgo biloba* special extract in dementia with neuropsychiatric features. A randomised, placebo-controlled, double-blind clinical trial. Arzneimittelforschung 57.1 (2007): 4–11.

Napryeyenko, O., et al. 2009. Efficacy and tolerability of *Ginkgo biloba* extract EGb 761 by type of dementia: analyses of a randomised controlled trial. J Neurol Sci, 283, 224–9.

Nathan P. Can the cognitive enhancing effects of ginkgo biloba be explained by its pharmacology? Med Hypotheses 55.6 (2000): 491–493.

Nicolai, S. P., Kruidenier, L. M., Bendermacher, B. L., et al. 2013. *Ginkgo biloba* for intermittent claudication. Cochrane Database Syst Rev, 6, CD006888.

Nishida S, Satoh H. Mechanisms for the vasodilations induced by *Ginkgo biloba* extract and its main constituent, bilobalide, in rat aorta. Life Sci 72.23 (2003): 2659–2667.

Oskouei, D.S., et al. 2013. The Effect of *Ginkgo biloba* on Functional Outcome of Patients with Acute Ischemic Stroke: A Double-blind, Placebo-controlled, Randomized Clinical Trial. Journal of Stroke and Cerebrovascular Diseases, 22, (8) e557–e563.

Ozgoli, G., et al. 2009. A randomized, placebo-controlled trial of *Ginkgo biloba* L. in treatment of premenstrual syndrome. J Altern Complement Med, 15, 845–51.

Ozturk G et al. The effect of Ginkgo extract EGb761 in cisplatin-induced peripheral neuropathy in mice. Toxicol Appl Pharmacol 196.1 (2004): 169–175.

Panda, V. S. & N, S. R. 2009. Evaluation of cardioprotective activity of *Ginkgo biloba* and *Ocimum sanctum* in rodents. Altern Med Rev, 14, 161–71.

Park, J. W., et al. 2011. Short-term effects of *Ginkgo biloba* extract on peripapillary retinal blood flow in normal tension glaucoma. Korean J Ophthalmol, 25, 323–8.

Park, Y. J., et al. 2013. Chemopreventive effects of *Ginkgo biloba* extract in estrogen-negative human breast cancer cells. Arch Pharm Res 36: 102–108.

Parsad D, et al. Effectiveness of oral *Ginkgo biloba* in treating limited, slowly spreading vitiligo. Clin Exp Dermatol 28.3 (2003): 285–287.

Peng H, et al. Effects of *Ginkgo biloba* extract on acute cerebral ischemia in rats analyzed by magnetic resonance spectroscopy. Acta Pharmacol Sin 24.5 (2003): 467–471.

Pierre, S. V., et al. 2008. The standardized *Ginkgo biloba* extract Egb-761 protects vascular endothelium exposed to oxidized low density lipoproteins. Cell Mol Biol (Noisy-le-grand), 54 Suppl, OL1032–42.

Pittler MH, Ernst E. *Ginkgo biloba* extract for the treatment of intermittent claudication: a meta-analysis of randomized trials. Am J Med 108.4 (2000): 276–281.

Pizzorno J, Murray M. Textbook of natural medicine. St Louis: Elsevier, 2006.

Puebla-Perez AM, et al. Effect of *Ginkgo biloba* extract, EGb 761, on the cellular immune response in a hypothalamic-pituitary-adrenal axis activation model in the rat. Int Immunopharmacol 3.1 (2003): 75–80.

Quaranta L et al. Effect of *Ginkgo biloba* extract on preexisting visual field damage in normal tension glaucoma. Ophthalmology 110.2 (2003): 359–362.

Ramassamy C et al. The *Ginkgo biloba* extract, EGb761, increases synaptosomal uptake of 5-hydroxytryptamine: in-vitro and ex-vivo studies. J Pharm Pharmacol 44.11 (1992): 943–945.

Reisser CH, Weidauer H. *Ginkgo biloba* extract EGb 761 or pentoxifylline for the treatment of sudden deafness: a randomized, reference-controlled, double-blind study. Acta Otolaryngol 121.5 (2001): 579–584.

Rejali D, et al. *Ginkgo biloba* does not benefit patients with tinnitus: a randomized placebo-controlled double-blind trial and meta-analysis of randomized trials. Clin Otolaryngol Allied Sci 29.3 (2004): 226–231.

Ribonnet, L., et al. 2011. Modulation of CYP1A1 activity by a *Ginkgo biloba* extract in the human intestinal Caco-2 cells. Toxicol Lett, 202, 193–202.

Rojas, P., et al. 2012. *Ginkgo biloba* extract (EGb 761) modulates the expression of dopamine-related genes in 1-methyl-4-phenyl-1,2,3,6-tetrahydropyridine-induced Parkinsonism in mice. Neuroscience, 223, 246–57.

Roland, P. D. & Nergard, C. S. 2012. [*Ginkgo biloba* — effect, adverse events and drug interaction.] Tidsskr Nor Laegeforen, 132, 956–9.

Roncin JP, et al. EGb 761 in control of acute mountain sickness and vascular reactivity to cold exposure. Aviat Space Environ Med 67.5 (1996): 445–452.

Russo, V., et al. 2009. Clinical efficacy of a *Ginkgo biloba* extract in the topical treatment of allergic conjunctivitis. Eur J Ophthalmol, 19, 331–6.

Ryu, K. H., et al. 2009. *Ginkgo biloba* extract enhances antiplatelet and antithrombotic effects of cilostazol without prolongation of bleeding time. Thromb Res, 124, 328–34.

Salehi, B., et al. 2010. *Ginkgo biloba* for attention-deficit/hyperactivity disorder in children and adolescents: a double blind, randomized controlled trial. Prog Neuropsychopharmacol Biol Psychiatry, 34, 76–80.

Sarris, J., et al. 2011. Complementary medicines (herbal and nutritional products) in the treatment of Attention Deficit Hyperactivity Disorder (ADHD): a systematic review of the evidence. Complement Ther Med, 19, 216–27.

Schneider R et al. Cardiac ischemia and reperfusion in spontaneously diabetic rats with and without application of EGb 761: I. Cardiomyocytes. Histol Histopathol 23.7 (2008): 807–817.

Schneider, R., et al. 2010. Cardiovascular autonomic neuropathy in spontaneously diabetic rats with and without application of EGb 761. Histol Histopathol, 25, 1581–90.

Scripnikov A, et al. Effects of *Ginkgo biloba* extract EGb 761 on neuropsychiatric symptoms of dementia: findings from a randomised controlled trial. Wien Med Wochenschr 157.13–14 (2007): 295–300.

Seupaul, R. A., et al. 2012. Pharmacologic prophylaxis for acute mountain sickness: a systematic shortcut review. Ann Emerg Med, 59, 307–317 e1.

Shevtsova EF, et al. [Mitochondria as the target for neuroprotectors.] Vestn Ross Akad Med Nauk 9 (2005): 13–117.

Shih JC et al. *Ginkgo biloba* abolishes aggression in mice lacking MAO A. Antioxid Redox Signal 2.3 (2000): 467–471.

Shim, S. H., et al. 2012. *Ginkgo biloba* extract and bilberry anthocyanins improve visual function in patients with normal tension glaucoma. J Med Food, 15, 818–23.

Singh B et al. Biology and chemistry of *Ginkgo biloba*. Fitoterapia 79.6 (2008): 401–418.

Singh, V., et al. 2010. Review and meta-analysis of usage of ginkgo as an adjunct therapy in chronic schizophrenia. Int J Neuropsychopharmacol, 13, 257–71.

Sloley BD et al. Identification of kaempferol as a monoamine oxidase inhibitor and potential Neuroprotectant in extracts of *Ginkgo biloba* leaves. J Pharm Pharmacol 52.4 (2000): 451–459.

Smith PF, et al. The neuroprotective properties of the *Ginkgo biloba* leaf: a review of the possible relationship to platelet-activating factor (PAF). J Ethnopharmacol 50.3 (1996): 131–139.

Smith JV et al. Anti-apoptotic properties of *Ginkgo biloba* extract EGb 761 in differentiated PC12 cells. Cell Mol Biol (Noisy-le-Grand) 48.6 (2002): 699–707.

Szczurko, O., et al. 2011. *Ginkgo biloba* for the treatment of vitilgo vulgaris: an open label pilot clinical trial. BMC Complement Altern Med, 11, 21.

Taavoni, S., et al. 2012. 160 Effect of *Ginkgo biloba* on menopausal women's sexual function: a randomized placebo controlled trial, Tehran, 2011. Maturitas, 71, Supplement 1, S65.

Taki, Y., et al. 2009. Time-dependent induction of hepatic cytochrome P450 enzyme activity and mRNA expression by bilobalide in rats. J Pharmacol Sci, 109, 459–62.

Tamborini A, Taurelle R. Value of standardized *Ginkgo biloba* extract (EGb 761) in the management of congestive symptoms of premenstrual syndrome. Rev Fr Gynecol Obstet 88.7–9 (1993): 447–457.

Tang J et al. Herb-drug interactions: effect of *Ginkgo biloba* extract on the pharmacokinetics of theophylline in rats. Food Chem Toxicol 45.12 (2007a): 2441–5.

Tang Y et al. The effect of *Ginkgo biloba* extract on the expression of PKCalpha in the inflammatory cells and the level of IL-5 in induced sputum of asthmatic patients. J Huazhong Univ Sci Technolog Med Sci 27.4 (2007b): 375–80.

Thanoon, I. A., et al. 2012. Oxidative Stress and C-Reactive Protein in Patients with Cerebrovascular Accident (Ischaemic Stroke): The role of *Ginkgo biloba* extract. Sultan Qaboos Univ Med J, 12, 197–205.

Tian YM et al. Effects of *Ginkgo biloba* extract (EGb 761) on hydroxyl radical-induced thymocyte apoptosis and on age-related thymic atrophy and peripheral immune dysfunctions in mice. Mech Ageing Dev 124.8–9 (2003): 977–983.

Tulsulkar, J. & Shah, Z. A. 2012. *Ginkgo biloba* prevents transient global ischemia-induced delayed hippocampal neuronal death through antioxidant and anti-inflammatory mechanism. Neurochem Int, 62, 189–197.

Usai, S., et al. 2011. Gingkolide B as migraine preventive treatment in young age: results at 1-year follow-up. Neurol Sci, 32 Suppl 1, S197–9.

Vale S. Subarachnoid haemorrhage associated with *Ginkgo biloba*. Lancet 352.9121 (1998): 36.

van Beek TA. Chemical analysis of *Ginkgo biloba* leaves and extracts. J Chromatogr A 967.1 (2002): 21–55.

Van Patot, M. C., et al. 2009. *Ginkgo biloba* for prevention of acute mountain sickness: does it work? High Alt Med Biol, 10, 33–43.

Vellas, B., et al. 2012. Long-term use of standardised *Ginkgo biloba* extract for the prevention of Alzheimer's disease (GuidAge): a randomised placebo-controlled trial. Lancet Neurol, 11, 851–9.

Villasenor-Garcia MM et al. Effect of *Ginkgo biloba* extract EGb 761 on the nonspecific and humoral immune responses in a hypothalamic-pituitary-adrenal axis activation model. Int Immunopharmacol 4.9 (2004): 1217–1222.

Von Boetticher, A. 2011. *Ginkgo biloba* extract in the treatment of tinnitus: a systematic review. Neuropsychiatr Dis Treat, 7, 441–7.

Wang J et al. Supervised exercise training combined with ginkgo biloba treatment for patients with peripheral arterial disease. Clin Rehabil 21.7 (2007): 579–586.

Wang, B. S., et al. 2010. Effectiveness of standardized ginkgo biloba extract on cognitive symptoms of dementia with a six-month treatment: a bivariate random effect meta-analysis. Pharmacopsychiatry, 43, 86–91.

Wang, W. W., et al. 2011. [The effect of extract of ginkgo biloba leaf during the formation of HBV-related hepatocellular carcinoma.] Zhonghua Shi Yan He Lin Chuang Bing Du Xue Za Zhi, 25, 325–7.

Wang, Z. Y., et al. 2012. [Ginkgolide B promotes axonal growth of retina ganglion cells by anti-apoptosis in vitro.] Sheng Li Xue Bao, 64, 417–24.

Watanabe CM et al. The in vivo neuromodulatory effects of the herbal medicine ginkgo biloba. Proc Natl Acad Sci U S A 98.12 (2001): 6577–6580.

Wei, J. M., et al. 2013. Ginkgo suppresses atherosclerosis through downregulating the expression of connexin 43 in rabbits. Arch Med Sci, 9, 340–6.

Weinmann, S., et al. 2010. Effects of *Ginkgo biloba* in dementia: systematic review and meta-analysis. BMC Geriatr, 10, 14.

Wettstein A. Cholinesterase inhibitors and Gingko extracts: are they comparable in the treatment of dementia? Comparison of published placebo-controlled efficacy studies of at least six months' duration. Phytomedicine 6.6 (2000): 393–401.

Wheatley D. Triple-blind, placebo-controlled trial of *Ginkgo biloba* in sexual dysfunction due to antidepressant drugs. Hum Psychopharmacol 19.8 (2004): 545–548.

Woelk H et al. *Ginkgo biloba* special extract EGb 761((R)) in generalized anxiety disorder and adjustment disorder with anxious mood: a randomized, double-blind, placebo-controlled trial. J Psychiatr Res (2007) 41: 472–480.

Wolf HR. Does *Ginkgo biloba* special extract EGb 761 provide additional effects on coagulation and bleeding when added to acetylsalicylic acid 500 mg daily? Drugs R D 7.3 (2006): 163–172.

Wu WR, Zhu XZ. Involvement of monoamine oxidase inhibition in neuroprotective and neurorestorative effects of *Ginkgo biloba* extract against MPTP-induced nigrostriatal dopaminergic toxicity in C57 mice. Life Sci 65.2 (1999): 157–164.

Wu, Y. Z., et al. 2008a. *Ginkgo biloba* extract improves coronary artery circulation in patients with coronary artery disease: contribution of plasma nitric oxide and endothelin-1. Phytother Res, 22, 734–9.

Wu, Z. M., et al. 2008b. *Ginkgo biloba* extract prevents against apoptosis induced by high glucose in human lens epithelial cells. Acta Pharmacol Sin, 29, 1042–50.

Wu YZ et al. *Ginkgo biloba* extract improves coronary artery circulation in patients with coronary artery disease: contribution of plasma nitric oxide and endothelin-1. Phytother Res 22.6 (2008c): 734–739.

Xie, Z. Q., et al. 2009. Molecular mechanisms underlying the cholesterol-lowering effect of *Ginkgo biloba* extract in hepatocytes: a comparative study with lovastatin. Acta Pharmacol Sin, 30, 1262–75.

Yancheva, S., et al. 2009. *Ginkgo biloba* extract EGb 761(R), donepezil or both combined in the treatment of Alzheimer's disease with neuropsychiatric features: a randomised, double-blind, exploratory trial. Aging Ment Health, 13, 183–90.

Yeh, K. Y., et al. 2008. *Ginkgo biloba* extract enhances male copulatory behavior and reduces serum prolactin levels in rats. Horm Behav, 53, 225–31.

Yeh, Y. C., et al. 2009. A standardized extract of *Ginkgo biloba* suppresses doxorubicin-induced oxidative stress and p53-mediated mitochondrial apoptosis in rat testes. Br J Pharmacol, 156, 48–61.

Yeung EY et al. Identification of *Ginkgo biloba* as a novel activator of pregnane X receptor. Drug Metab Dispos 36.11 (2008): 2270–2276.

Yoshitake, T., et al. 2010. The *Ginkgo biloba* extract EGb 761(R) and its main constituent flavonoids and ginkgolides increase extracellular dopamine levels in the rat prefrontal cortex. Br J Pharmacol, 159, 659–68.

Zadoyan, G., et al. 2012. Effect of *Ginkgo biloba* special extract EGb 761(R) on human cytochrome P450 activity: a cocktail interaction study in healthy volunteers. Eur J Clin Pharmacol, 68, 553–60.

Zeng X et al. *Ginkgo biloba* for acute ischaemic stroke. Cochrane Database Syst Rev 4 (2005): CD003691.

Zhang, S. J. & Xue, Z. Y. 2012. Effect of Western medicine therapy assisted by *Ginkgo biloba* tablet on vascular cognitive impairment of none dementia. Asian Pac J Trop Med, 5, 661–4.

Zhang, Y., et al. 2008. *Ginkgo biloba* Extract Kaempferol Inhibits Cell Proliferation and Induces Apoptosis in Pancreatic Cancer Cells. Journal of Surgical Research, 148, 17–23.

Zhang, W. F., et al. 2011. Extract of *Ginkgo biloba* treatment for tardive dyskinesia in schizophrenia: a randomized, double-blind, placebo-controlled trial. J Clin Psychiatry, 72, 615–21.

Zhang, X. Y., et al. 2012a. Brain-derived neurotrophic factor levels and its Val66Met gene polymorphism predict tardive dyskinesia treatment response to *Ginkgo biloba*. Biol Psychiatry, 72, 700–6.

Zhang, Z., et al. 2012b. Experimental evidence of *Ginkgo biloba* extract EGB as a neuroprotective agent in ischemia stroke rats. Brain Research Bulletin, 87, 193–198.

Zhao LZ et al. Induction of propranolol metabolism by *Ginkgo biloba* extract EGb 761 in rats. Curr Drug Metab 7.6 (2006): 577–587.

Zhao, M. X., et al. 2012. [Effects of *Ginkgo biloba* extract in improving episodic memory of patients with mild cognitive impairment: a randomized controlled trial.]. Zhong Xi Yi Jie He Xue Bao, 10, 628–34.

Zhou, Y. & Zeng, R. 2011. [Effects of *Ginkgo biloba* extract on anticoagulation and blood drug level of warfarin in healthy wolunteers]. Zhongguo Zhong Yao Za Zhi, 36, 2290–3.

Zhou, Z. Y., et al. 2010. Antioxidant and hepatoprotective effects of extract of ginkgo biloba in rats of non-alcoholic steatohepatitis. Saudi Med J, 31, 1114–8.

Zhou, L., et al. 2011. *Ginkgo biloba* extract enhances glucose tolerance in hyperinsulinism-induced hepatic cells. J Nat Med, 65, 50–6.

Zuo, X. C., et al. 2010. Effects of *Ginkgo biloba* extracts on diazepam metabolism: a pharmacokinetic study in healthy Chinese male subjects. Eur J Clin Pharmacol, 66, 503–9.

Ginseng — Korean

HISTORICAL NOTE *Gin* refers to man and *seng* to essence in Chinese, whereas *Panax* is derived from the Greek word *pan* (all) and *akos* (cure), referring to its use as a cure-all. Ginseng is a slow-growing perennial herb, with fleshy roots native to Korea and China, and has been used as a herbal remedy in eastern Asia for thousands of years. It is considered to be the most potent Qi or energy tonic in traditional Chinese medicine (TCM). Modern indications include low vitality, poor immunity, cancer, cholesterol and cardiovascular disease, metabolic dysfunction and enhancement of physical performance and sexual function (Nagappan et al 2012). However, a systematic review of randomised controlled trials (RCTs) found that the efficacy of ginseng root extract could not be established beyond doubt for any of these indications (Coon & Ernst 2002). While many more clinical trials have been conducted in the past decade, and understanding of the active constituents has progressed markedly, no update to this systematic review, or any other, has been performed.

COMMON NAME

Korean ginseng

OTHER NAMES

Ren shen (Mandarin), red ginseng, white ginseng

BOTANICAL NAME/FAMILY

Panax ginseng C.A. Meyer (family Araliaceae)

It should be differentiated from *P. aquifolium* (American ginseng), *P. notoginseng* (Tien chi, pseudoginseng), *Eleutherococcus senticosus* (Siberian ginseng), *Withania somnifera* (Indian Ginseng) and other ginsengs.

PLANT PART USED

Main and lateral roots. The smaller root hairs are considered an inferior source. There are two types of preparations produced from ginseng: white ginseng, which is prepared by drying the raw herb, and red ginseng, prepared by steaming before drying. Cultivated ginseng differs from wild ginseng, and plants from different countries or regions may also differ greatly. Processing of the crude herb to produce red ginseng appears to increase its potency. Steaming has been shown to alter the composition of the ginsenosides; for example, steaming produces the active 20(S)-ginsenoside-Rg(3) (Matsuda et al 2003) and makes certain ginsenosides more cytotoxic (Park IH et al 2002). Kim et al (2010) suggest that two rounds of heating is optimal for producing Korean red ginseng (KRG) with the highest amount of arginyl-fructose (AF) and arginyl-fructose-glucose (AFG), which contribute to some of the antioxidant effects of KRG. This effect was specific to the hydroxyl radical scavenging capacity of KRG. Hydroxyl radicals are one of the most harmful radical oxygen species (ROS) found in the body. This effect of hydroxyl-preventing capacity was attributed to the metal-chelating capacity of AF and AFG. On the other hand, after seven rounds of heating, thus reducing the concentration, Kim et al (2010) found that the KRG extract decreased the extent of intracellular oxidative stress due to peroxyl radicals. This peroxyl radical scavenging ability of KRG extract is thought to be due to total phenolic compound content providing the ability of bioactive substances to permeate the cell membrane. Studies have also found different therapeutic effects for different concentrations of ginsenosides in the rootlets versus body of the KRG. This indicates that elucidation from clinical trials as to dose range of therapeutics is required. De Souza et al (2011) found that extracts from the KRG body, although containing lower concentrations of ginsenosides, had a superior postprandial blood glucose lowering effect than the rootlets, which had no significant effect on glucose levels in diabetics.

The British Herbal Pharmacopoeia (1983) stipulates that ginseng should contain not less than 20% solids (70% ethanol). The German Pharmacopoeia requires not less than 1.5% total ginsenosides, calculated as ginsenoside Rg 1.

Chewing gums containing ginseng saponins have also been developed and demonstrate therapeutic effects in some trials (Ding et al 2004).

CHEMICAL COMPONENTS

The most characteristic compounds in the ginseng roots are the ginsenosides, and most biological effects have been ascribed to these compounds. The ginsenosides are dammarane saponins and can be divided into two classes: the protopanaxatriol class consisting primarily of Rg1, Rg2, Rf and Re and the protopanaxadiol class consisting primarily of Rc, Rd, Rb1 and Rb2 (Ho et al 2012). Ginseng also contains other saponins, polysaccharides, amino acids (in particular glutamine and arginine) (Kuo et al 2003), essential oils and other compounds. Three sesquiterpene hydrocarbons have been isolated from the essential oil: panaxene, panaginsene and ginsinsene (Richter et al 2005). The major component of *Panax ginseng* is ginsenoside Rb1, otherwise the major component of KRG is Rg3 (Park et al 2012).

Ginsenosides Rh1, Rh2 and Rg3 are obtained from red ginseng as artifacts produced during steaming and drying, which suggests the transformation of chemical and physiological properties and involves ginsenosides, peptides, polysaccharides, polyacetylenic alcohols and fatty acids (Park et al 2012). It is likely that ginsenoside is actually a prodrug that is converted in the body by intestinal bacterial deglycosylation and fatty acid esterification into an active metabolite (Hasegawa 2004). Rg3 has been shown to be metabolised to ginsenoside Rh2 by intestinal microflora. Jin et al (2012) have shown that the bioactive novel soponin metabolite, IH-901 (or compound K), is formed by intestinal flora, and fermentation by intestinal bacteria and enzymatic digestion of ginsensides in vivo and in vitro produces its pharmacological effects. The authors suggest that fermentation in vitro may enhance its pharmokinetic properties for medicinal purposes. Ho et al (2012) suggest that the metabolite compound K is then absorbed from the gastrointestinal tract, and has a variety of pharmacological activies, including antitumour, antidiabetic, anti-inflammatory and antiallergic effects.

Therefore, extrapolation from in vitro studies or studies in which ginseng or isolated constituents were given by injection must be made very cautiously.

Commercial ginseng preparations are variable in quality. An analysis of 50 products sold in 11 countries showed that there was a large variation in the concentration of ginsenosides (from 1.9 to 9.0%). Some products were even found to be void of any specific ginsenosides. Some ginseng products have also been discovered to be contaminated with ephedrine. Therefore, it is essential that only quality ginseng products be used (Cui et al 1994). Although the root hairs have a higher level of total ginsenosides than the main root, the main and lateral roots are the preferred medicinal parts. In all probability, it is the ratio of ginsenosides that is important and other important compounds are also active.

MAIN ACTIONS

Adaptogen

The pharmacological effects of ginseng are many and varied, contributing to its reputation as a potent adaptogen. The adrenal gland and the pituitary gland are both known to have an effect on the body's ability to respond to stress and alter work capacity (Filaretov et al 1988), and ginseng is thought to profoundly influence the hypothalamic–pituitary–adrenal axis (Kim DH et al 2003). The active metabolites of protopanaxadiol and protopanaxatriol saponins reduce acetylcholine-induced catecholamine secretion in animal models (Tachikawa & Kudo 2004, Tachikawa et al 2003), and this may help to explain the purported antistress effects of ginseng.

Ginseng has been shown in numerous animal experiments to increase resistance to a wide variety of chemical, physical and biological stressors. Ginseng extract or its isolated constituents have been shown to prevent immunosuppression induced by cold water swim stress (Luo et al 1993) and to counter stress-induced changes from heat stress (Yuan 1989), food deprivation (Lee et al 1990), electroshock (Banerjee & Izquierdo 1982) and radiation exposure (Takeda et al 1981). As there are more than 1500 studies on ginseng and its constituents, it is outside the scope of this monograph to include all studies, so we have attempted to include those studies most relevant to the oral use of ginseng.

Animal models suggest that ginseng is most useful for chronic rather than acute stress, significantly reducing elevated scores on ulcer index, adrenal gland weight, plasma glucose, triglycerides, creatine kinase activity and serum corticosterone during chronic stress (Rai et al 2003). Oxidative stress resulting from the excessive exposure to reactive oxygen species (ROS) is generated in many stressful situations and induces cell death by either apoptosis or necrosis. Ginsenosides, the main pharmacological constituents of ginseng, are reported to have antineoplastic, anti-stress, anti-inflammatory, antioxidant and hepatoprotective activities (Park et al 2012).

(Refer to the *Siberian ginseng* monograph for more information about adaptogens and allostasis.)

Cardiovascular effects

According to in vitro and animal studies, ginseng may benefit the cardiovascular system 'through diverse mechanisms, including antioxidant, modifying vasomotor function, reducing platelet adhesion, influencing ion channels, altering autonomic neurotransmitter release, improving lipid profiles' and glycaemic control (Zhou et al 2004).

Antihypertensive

Red ginseng has been used as an antihypertensive agent in Korea, but its clinical effect is unclear despite several in vivo and in vitro experimental studies. Data suggest that the antihypertensive effects may be partly attributed to an angiotensin-converting enzyme (ACE) inhibitory effect demonstrated by *P. ginseng* extract in vitro (Persson et al 2006). These effects were additive to the traditional ACE inhibitor enalapril.

A study of isolated muscle preparations of animal heart and aorta with an alcohol-based extract of ginseng suggested that the hypotensive effect of ginseng is associated with a direct inhibition of myocardial contractility due to a reduction of calcium ion influx into cardiac cells, as well as the inhibition of catecholamine-induced contractility of vascular smooth muscles (Hah et al 1978). Nagappan et al (2012) suggest that ginsenoside Rb1 releases nitric oxide and decreases intracellular-free calcium in cardiac myocytes.

In a prospective, randomised, double-blind, placebo-controlled study of 30 healthy adults, 200 mg ginseng extract given for 28 days was found to increase the QTc interval and decrease diastolic blood pressure 2 hours after ingestion on the first day of therapy. These changes, however, were not thought to be clinically significant (Caron et al 2002).

Further, in a randomised controlled trial of Korean red ginseng (KRG) versus placebo on arterial stiffness in subjects with hypertension and taking antihypertensive medication, no difference was found between the groups in terms of arterial stiffness after 3 months of treatment. Blood pressure readings for both groups were significantly reduced in the study period (Rhee et al 2011).

Conversely, a study by Chen et al (2012) suggests that the reported effect of increasing blood pressure may provide KRG with a haemodynamic stabilising capacity in patients undergoing haemodialysis who commonly experience intradialytic hypotension (IDH). They found that chewing 3.5 g KRG at each haemodialysis session over a 4-week period significantly reduced the degree of BP drop and the frequency of symptomatic IDH during haemodialysis. Activation of vasoconstrictors (endothelin-1 and angiotensis II) during haemodialysis was found, and the authors concluded that chewing KRG could be an effective adjunct treatment for IDH.

Antiplatelet

Although reports from in vitro and in vivo assays claim that *P. ginseng* is not one of the herbs that contributes to the antiplatelet effects of a Korean combination formula known as Dae-Jo-Hwan (Chang et al 2005), a number of studies have found that several ginsenosides inhibit platelet aggregation. Panaxynol has been shown to inhibit platelet aggregation induced by adenosine diphosphate, collagen and arachidonic acid. Panaxynol and ginsenosides Ro, Rg and Rg2 inhibit rabbit platelets, while panaxynol prevented platelet aggregation and thromboxane formation (Kuo et al 1990).

Antihyperlipidaemic

Ginsenoside Rb1 has been shown to lower triglyceride and cholesterol levels via cyclic adenosine monophosphate (cAMP) production in the rat liver (Park KH et al 2002). *P. ginseng* extract (6 g/day) for 8 weeks resulted in a reduction in serum total cholesterol, triglyceride, low density lipoprotein (LDL) and plasma malondialdehyde levels and an increase in high density lipoprotein (HDL) (Kim & Park 2003) in eight males. Ginseng has also been reported to decrease hepatic cholesterol and triglyceride levels in rats, indicating a potential use of ginseng in the treatment of fatty liver (Yamamoto et al 1983).

Other cardiovascular effects

Ginsenoside Rb2 has been shown to enhance the fibrinolytic activity of bovine aortic endothelial cells (Liu 2003). In animal studies, ginseng inhibits cardiomyocyte apoptosis induced by ischaemia and reperfusion injury (Zeng et al 2004) and the crude saponins have been shown to reduce body weight, food intake and fat content in rats fed a high-fat diet (Kim J et al 2005). In vitro studies report that an extract of ginseng fruit can promote vascular endothelial cell proliferation, migration, DNA synthesis and vascular endothelial growth factor mRNA expression, suggesting an effect on the genesis and development of new vessels in the ischaemic myocardium (Lei et al 2008).

Gastrointestinal

Hepatorestorative

Oral administration of Korean red ginseng (250 and 500 mg/kg) on liver regeneration has been investigated in 15 dogs with partial hepatectomy. All haematological values except leucocyte counts were within normal ranges for 3 days postoperatively. The levels of aspartate transaminase (AST) and alanine aminotransferase (ALT) in the ginseng groups were significantly decreased compared with those in the control group ($P < 0.05$). The numbers of degenerative cells and areas of connective tissue were significantly decreased in the livers of the dogs treated with ginseng ($P < 0.01$) (Kwon et al 2003).

In a recent study, Korean red ginseng (KRG) and its primary ginsenosides (Rg3 and Rh2) were examined for their effect on alcohol-induced oxidative injury to mouse hepatocytes (TIB-73). Hepatocytic injury was measured by: cell viability; lactate dehydrogenase (LDL); aspartate amino-transferase (AST); reactive oxygen species (ROS); and mitochondria membrane potential (MMP) in hepatocytes. The authors report that ROS can induce cell death, and induce 'MAPK' activation, by which hepatocytes mediate reaction to oxidative stress. This family of serine/threonine kinases is central to integrating signal transduction processes generating various cell responses. Chronic activation is reported to lead to cellular growth arrest (Park et al 2012).

Lee and Shukla (2007) found that an increase in ROS from alcohol exposure leads to injury and apoptosis in hepatocytes by mediating several signal transduction pathways. The study by Park et al (2012) found that KRG, Rg3 or Rh2 inhibited the alcohol-induced apoptotic changes. Alcohol was found to induce cell death in the mouse hepatocytes by an increase in membrane damage and intracellular ROS and by decreasing Mg^{2+}. Treatment with KRG, Rg3 or Rh2 significantly attenuated the alcohol-induced decrease in cell viability; recovered the decrease in cell numbers; and attenuated the increase in LDH release, AST protein and ROS. A decrease in cellular concentrations of magnesium (Mg^{2+}), indicating cytotoxicity, was also inhibited by exposure to KRG and its primary ginsenosides. Therefore, the authors concluded that KRG and its primary constituents exert a protective effect on alcohol-induced hepatocytic injury.

Anti-ulcerative

Ginseng has been shown in several studies to protect against ulceration. Among the hexane, chloroform, butanol and water fractions, the butanol fraction of a ginseng extract has been shown to be the most potent inhibitor of HCl-induced gastric lesions and ulcers induced by aspirin, acetic acid and Shay (ulcer induced by pylorus ligation). The butanol fraction showed significant increase in mucin secretion, and inhibited malondialdehyde and H^+/K^+ ATPase activity in the stomach. These results indicate that the effectiveness of ginseng on gastric damage might be related to inhibition of acid secretion, increased mucin secretion and antioxidant properties (Jeong 2002). Furthermore, inhibition of *Helicobacter pylori*-stimulated 5-lipoxygenase activity may have a beneficial effect on *H. pylori*-associated gastric inflammation (Park et al 2007). Results from a mouse-model study investigating the effects of Korean red ginseng (KRG) and Korean red ginseng containing drug (KRGCD) found that both KRG and KRGCD significantly decreased ethanol- and indomethacin-induced gastric ulcer, and increased gastric mucosal blood flow. These preparations were significantly protective against gastric ulcers in a dose-dependent manner (100 mg/kg and 300 mg/kg being significantly and relatively effective); however, only KRGCD demonstrated a significant reduction in the measures of oxidative stress, shown by attenuation of lipid peroxidation in the gastric lining. This study suggests that KRG's anti-ulcer properties may lie primarily in its capacity to increase basal gastric mucosal blood flow, rather than via anti-oxidant activities (Oyagi et al 2010). The authors note that in previous studies (Chen et al 1997) that saponin fraction of KRG increased levels of nitric oxide in endothelial cells, in an endothelium-dependent manner, stating that vaso-relaxation may be the vehicle for effect.

Effects on peristalsis

Ginseng root extract and its components, ginsenoside Rb1(4) and ginsenoside Rd(7), have been shown to significantly ameliorate chemically induced acceleration of small intestinal transit in vivo. The test results suggest that the protective mechanism involves both an inhibitory effect on the cholinergic nervous system and a direct suppressive effect on intestinal muscles (Hashimoto et al 2003).

Anti-inflammatory

Both a crude and a standardised extract (G115) of ginseng varying in saponin concentrations have been found to protect against muscle fibre injury and inflammation after eccentric muscle contractions in rats on a treadmill. The oral ginseng extracts significantly reduced plasma creatine kinase levels by about 25% and lipid peroxidation by 15%. Certain markers of inflammation were also significantly reduced (Cabral de Oliveira et al 2001). In a later study, pretreatment with ginseng extract (3, 10, 100 or 500 mg/kg) administered orally for 3 months to male Wistar rats resulted in a 74% decrease in lipid peroxidation caused by eccentric exercise (Voces et al 2004).

The many and varied effects of ginseng may be partly associated with the inhibition of transcription factor nuclear factor (NF)-kappaB, which is pivotal in the regulation of inflammatory genes. Inhibition of NF-kappaB may reduce inflammation and protect cells against damage.

Topical application of several ginsenosides (Rb1, Rc, Re, Rg1, Rg3) significantly attenuated chemically-induced ear oedema in mice. The ginsenosides also suppressed expression of cyclooxygenase-2 (COX-2) and activation of NF-kappaB in the skin. Of the ginsenosides tested, Rg3 was found to be most effective (Surh et al 2002).

Immunomodulation

The immunomodulatory effect of ginseng is based on the production of cytokines, activation of macrophages, stimulation of bone marrow cells and stimulation of inducible nitric oxide synthase (iNOS), which produces high levels of NO in response to activating signals from Th1-associated cytokines and plays an important role in cytotoxicity and cytostasis (growth inhibition) against many pathogenic microorganisms. In addition to its direct effector function, NO serves as a potent immunoregulatory factor.

Ginseng enhances interleukin (IL)-12 production and may therefore induce a stronger Th1 response, resulting in improved protection against infection from a variety of pathogens (Larsen et al 2004), including *Pseudomonas aeruginosa* lung infection in animal models (Song et al 2005). However, other studies suggest that it may also assist in the correction of Th1-dominant pathological disorders (Lee E-J et al 2004).

Ginseng polysaccharides have been shown to increase the cytotoxic activity of macrophages against melanoma cells, increase phagocytosis and induce the levels of cytokines, including tissue necrosis factor (TNF)-alpha, IL-1-beta, IL-6 and interferon-gamma in vitro (Shin et al 2002). Ginseng has been shown to be an immunomodulator and to enhance antitumour activity of macrophages in vitro (Song et al 2002). Ginseng has also been shown to significantly enhance natural killer (NK) function in an antibody-dependent cellular cytotoxicity of peripheral blood mononuclear cells in vitro (See et al 1997).

Incubation of macrophages with increasing amounts of an aqueous extract of ginseng showed a dose-dependent stimulation of iNOS. Polysaccharides isolated from ginseng showed strong stimulation of iNOS, whereas a triterpene-enriched fraction from an aqueous extract did not show any stimulation. As NO plays an important role in immune function, ginseng could modulate several aspects of host defence mechanisms due to stimulation of iNOS (Friedl et al 2001).

Ginseng promotes the production of granulocytes in the bone marrow (granulocytopoiesis). The ginseng saponins have been shown to directly and/or indirectly promote the stromal cells and lymphocytes to produce human granulocyte–macrophage colony-stimulating factor (GM-CSF) and other cytokines, and induce bone marrow haematopoietic cells to express GM-CSF receptors, leading to a proliferation of human colony-forming units for granulocytes and macrophages in vitro (Wang et al 2003).

Ginseng polysaccharides have been shown to have potent antisepticaemic activity by stimulating macrophages and helping modulate the reaction against sepsis induced by *Staphylococcus aureus*. Ginseng polysaccharides have been shown to reduce the intracellular concentration of *S. aureus* in macrophages in infected animals by 50% compared with controls. Combination of the ginseng polysaccharides with vancomycin resulted in 100% survival of the animals, whereas only 67 or 50% of the animals survived, respectively, when treated with the ginseng polysaccharides or vancomycin alone (Lim DS et al 2002).

According to animal studies, long-term oral administration of ginseng extract may potentiate humoral immune response, but suppress spleen cell functions (Liou et al 2005).

Anticancer

Oral intake of standardised *P. ginseng* extract demonstrates a dose-dependent (1, 3 or 10 mg/kg), chemoprotective and antimutagenic effect in animal studies (Panwar et al 2005), and ginsenoside Rg3 has recently been produced as an antiangiogenic anticarcinogenic drug in China (Shibata 2001).

Ho et al (2012) described the tumour-inhibitory activity of Rh2, which is reported to constrain cell growth in MCF-7 human breast cancer and SK-Hep1 hepatoma and can induce apoptosis in various cell lines (Oh et al 2005). Ginsenoside Rg3 has been reported to reduce the gelatinolytic activities of some matrix metalloproteinases (MMPs). MMPs degrade the extracellular matrix and are abundantly expressed in various malignant tumours and are critical in tumour metastasis. Inhibition of MMP activity is important in respect of preventing cell metastasis (Ho et al 2012). Other ginseng saponins with chemopreventive actions include Rb2, which may partly contribute to the inhibition of lung tumour metastasis by arresting tumour-associated angiogenesis (Yue et al 2006), and Rp1, derived from Rg5, whose anti-cancer effect is thought to be due to inhibition of tumour cell metastasis and viability, possibly through impeding adhesion and vessel formation (Kumar et al 2009).

Ho et al (2012) undertook a study to investigate the antimetastatic effect of KRG on human hepatoma as well as possible mechanisms of action. The authors found that the inhibitory effect of the water extract of KRG (WKRG), rather than ethanolic extract of KGR (EKRG), exerted a dose-dependent inhibitory effect on the invasion and motility, but not adhesion, of highly metastatic SK-Hep1 cells.

Jo et al (2013) demonstrated in their study that KRG extract alone was sufficient to induce growth inhibition in acute promyleocytic leukaemia (APL), and describe a sequential molecular mechanism by which KRG extract operates to arrest growth in human APL. In a study by Park et al (2009), KRG extract treatment to U937 human leukaemia cells showed significant growth inhibition and induction of apoptosis in a concentration-dependent manner. The authors observed that KRG extract markedly inhibited COX-2 mRNA and protein expression in leukaemia cells, suggesting that inhibition of growth and induced apoptosis is consistent with COX-2 inhibition. Additionally, KRG progressively down-regulated the expression of human telomerase-related genes in U937 human leukaemia cells, which appeared to account for its anti-proliferative activity. Loss of COX-2 and telomerase activity may be a strategy for assessing the anti-tumour effects of KRG extract.

Chemoprotection

Oral administration of red ginseng extracts (1% in diet for 40 weeks) significantly ($P < 0.05$) suppressed spontaneous liver tumour formation in male mice. Oral white ginseng was also shown to suppress tumour promotion in vitro and in vivo (Nishino et al 2001).

Dietary administration of red ginseng in combination with 1,2-dimethylhydrazine suppresses colon carcinogenesis in rats (rats were fed 1% ginseng for 5 weeks). It is thought that the inhibition may be partly associated with inhibition of cell proliferation in the colonic mucosa (Fukushima et al 2001).

Oral administration of 50 mg/kg/day for 4 weeks of a ginseng intestinal metabolite has been shown to partially protect against doxorubicin-induced testicular toxicity in mice. The metabolite significantly ($P < 0.01$) prevented decreases in body weight, spermatogenic activities, serum levels of lactate dehydrogenase and creatine phosphokinase induced by doxorubicin. It also significantly attenuated germ cell injuries (Kang et al 2002).

The methanol extract of red ginseng has been shown to attenuate the lipid peroxidation in rat brain and scavenge superoxides in differentiated human promyelocytic leukaemia (HL-60) cells. Topical application of the same extract, as well as purified ginsenoside Rg3, has been demonstrated to suppress skin tumour promotion in mice. Rg3 also suppresses COX, NF-kappaB and extracellular-regulated protein kinase, which are all involved in tumour promotion (Surh et al 2001).

Pretreatment with oral red ginseng extract significantly reduced the development of cancer from diethylnitrosamine-induced liver cancer nodules in rats (the developmental rate of liver cancer in the experimental group was 14.3% compared with 100% in the control group). When ginseng was given concomitantly with diethylnitrosamine, the hepatoma nodules were smaller than those of the control group, the structure of hepatic tissue was well preserved and the structure of hepatocytes was normal. Ginseng also prolonged the average life span. These findings suggest benefits of ginseng in the prevention and treatment of liver cancer (Wu et al 2001).

Irradiation protection

Ginsenosides and specifically panaxadiol have been shown to have radioprotective effects in mice irradiated with high-dose and low-dose gamma radiation. Jejunal crypts were protected by pretreatment with extract of whole ginseng (50 mg/kg body weight intraperitoneally at 12 and 36 hours before irradiation, $P < 0.005$). Extract of whole ginseng ($P < 0.005$), total saponin ($P < 0.01$) or panaxadiol ($P < 0.05$) administration before irradiation (50 mg/kg body weight IP at 12 and 36 hours before irradiation) resulted in an increase in the formation of the endogenous spleen colony. The frequency of radiation-induced apoptosis in the intestinal crypt cells was also reduced by pretreatment with extract of whole ginseng, total saponin and panaxadiol (Kim DH et al 2003).

These radioprotective effects are partly associated with the immunomodulatory effect of ginseng. Ginsan, a purified polysaccharide isolated from ginseng, has been shown to have a mitogenic activity, induce lymphokine-activated killer cells and increase levels of several cytokines. Ginsan reduced mutagenicity in a dose-dependent manner when applied to rats 30 minutes before or 15 minutes after 1.5 Gy of gamma irradiation. The radioprotective effect of ginsan has been partly attributed to a reduction in radiation-induced genotoxicity (Ivanova et al 2006). Ginsan has also been found to increase the number of bone marrow cells, spleen cells, granulocyte–macrophage colony-forming cells and circulating neutrophils, lymphocytes and platelets significantly in irradiated mice (Song et al 2003).

One of the causes of radiation damage is lipid peroxidation, which alters lysosomal membrane permeability, leading to the release of hydrolytic enzymes. Ginseng has been shown to markedly inhibit lipid peroxidation and protect against radiation damage in testes of mice (Kumar et al 2003).

Antitumour, antiproliferative, antimetastatic and apoptosis-inducing stimulation of the phagocytic activity of macrophages may play a role in the anticarcinogenic and antimetastatic activities demonstrated for ginseng in vivo (Shin M 2004), and research has continually found tumour-inhibitory effects, especially in the promotion and progression phases (Helms 2004).

Ginsenosides Rg3, Rg5, Rk1, Rs5 and Rs4 have been shown to be cytotoxic to Hep-1 hepatoma cancer cells in vitro. Their 50% growth inhibition concentration (GI50) values were 41, 11, 13, 37 and 13 micromol/L, respectively. Cisplatin had a GI50 of 84 micromol/L in the same assay conditions (Park IH et al 2002). Several triterpenoids found in the leaves have also demonstrated cytotoxic activity in vitro (Huang et al 2008).

Constituents in ginseng have also been shown to inhibit proliferation of cancer cells. Panaxytriol isolated from red ginseng was shown to have a significant dose-dependent cytotoxic activity and inhibit DNA synthesis in various tumour cells tested (Kim JY et al 2002). Ginsenoside Rg3 has displayed inhibitory activity against human prostate cancer cells in vitro (Liu et al 2000).

Ginsenosides, especially 20(R)-ginsenoside Rg3, have been shown to specifically inhibit cancer cell invasion and metastasis (Shibata 2001), and ginsenoside Rh2 has been shown to inhibit human ovarian cancer growth in mice (Nakata et al 1998). It is likely that the antitumour-promoting activity of Rg3 is mediated through down-regulation of NF-kappaB and other transcription factors (Keum et al 2003).

Oral administration of 20(S)-protopanaxatriol (M4), the main bacterial metabolite of protopanaxatriol-type ginsenosides, has been shown to inhibit melanoma growth in mice, and pretreatment was shown to reduce metastases to the lungs. This effect is thought to be due to stimulation of NK-mediated tumour lysis (Hasegawa et al 2002).

The antimetastatic effects of ginseng are related to inhibition of the adhesion and invasion of tumour cells and also to antiangiogenesis activity. Ginsenosides Rg3 and Rb2 have been shown to significantly inhibit adhesion of melanoma cells to fibronectin and laminin, as well as preventing invasion into the basement membrane in vitro. Other experiments have demonstrated that the saponins exert significant antiapoptotic activity, decreasing the number of blood vessels oriented towards the tumour mass (Mochizuki et al 1995, Sato et al 1994).

Ginseng saponins have also been found to promote apoptosis (programmed cell death) in cancer cells in vitro (Hwang et al 2002).

Neurological

Analgesia

Intraperitoneal administration of ginsenoside Rf has been shown to potentiate opioid-induced analgesia in mice. Furthermore, ginsenosides prevented tolerance to the opiate that was not associated with opioid or GABA receptors (Nemmani & Ramarao 2003).

Neuroprotection

Ginseng saponins have demonstrated dose-dependent neuroprotective activity in vitro and in vivo (Kim J-H et al 2005). Ginsenosides Rb1 and Rg1 have a partial neurotrophic and neuroprotective role in dopaminergic cell cultures (Radad et al 2004), and Rg3 has been shown to inhibit chemically-induced injuries in hippocampal neurons. Pretreatment with ginsenosides (50 or 100 mg/kg for 7 days) has been shown to be neuroprotective in vivo. An in vitro survival assay demonstrated that ginsenosides Rb1 and Rg1 protect spinal cord neurons against damage. The ginsenosides protect spinal neurons from excitotoxicity induced by glutamate and kainic acid, as well as oxidative stress induced by H_2O_2. The optimal doses are 20–40 micromol/L for ginsenosides Rb1 and Rg1 (Liao et al 2002). The lipophilic fraction of ginseng has been shown to induce differentiation of neurons and promote neuronal survival in the rat cortex. The effect is thought to be mediated via protein kinase-C-dependent pathways (Mizumaki et al 2002). In vitro studies have also suggested a benefit for ginseng in hypoxia-induced neuronal injury including ischaemia, trauma and degenerative diseases (Park et al 2007). Beneficial effects have yet to be demonstrated in clinical trials.

It has been suggested that the neuroprotective effects of ginseng against hypoperfusion/reperfusion-induced brain injury demonstrated in animal models suggest a potential for use in cardiovascular disease (CVD) (Shah et al 2005). In a study by Lee et al (2011), focal cerebral ischaemia/reperfusion injury rats were fed Korean red ginseng (KRG) extract (100 mg/kg/day) or saline after reperfusion. Infarct volume was significantly reduced in the KRG rats, and neurological deficits were rapidly improved. Serum levels of tumour necrosis factor-alpha (TNF-α), interleukin-1 beta (IL-1β) and IL-6 were significantly attenuated in the KRG rats after 7 days, and serum IL-10 levels were significantly increased. This suggests that KRG provides neuroprotection possibly due to raised IL-10 expression and a reduction in the serum levels of TNFα, IL-1β and IL-6.

Cognitive function

Following oral consumption, the active metabolites of protopanaxadiol saponins may reactivate neuronal function in Alzheimer's disease according to in vivo evidence (Komatsu et al 2005). Ginseng also enhances the survival of newly generated neurons in the hippocampus, which may contribute to the purported benefits of ginseng for improving learning tasks (Qiao et al 2005).

Anticonvulsant

Pretreatment (30 min) with 100 mg/kg ginseng significantly protected rats against pentylenetetrazole-induced seizures (Gupta et al 2001).

Hearing loss

Pretreatment with ginseng extract has been shown to significantly attenuate the effect on auditory cell lines from chemotherapy drug cisplatin-induced increases in reactive oxygen species (ROS). KRG was demonstrated to inhibit the expression of caspase-3 and poly-ADP-ribose polymerase related to cisplatin-induced apoptosis. The cisplatin-induced toxicity involves ROS production, indicating an anti-apoptotic and anti-oxidative role of KRG in cisplatin-induced ototoxicity in auditory cell lines (Im et al 2010). Use of animoglycosides, such as gentamicin (GM), has been noted for its ototoxicity, including hearing loss and vestibular dysfunction. In a study examining GM-induced ototoxicity, Choung et al (2011) found that co-treatment with KRG significantly limited stereocilia (hair cells) death and hearing loss in rats. KRG was thought to attenuate apoptosis, which is medicated by reactive oxygen species (ROS) and intracellular signalling pathways, highlighting its antioxidant and antiapoptotic effects. The saponin components Rb1 and/or Rb2 only were found to be effective as protective agents against GM-induced hearing loss.

Antidiabetic

Hypoglycaemic/antihyperglycaemic effects

G

While human and animal studies have found American ginseng to lower blood glucose level (Vuksan et al 2000a, 2000b, 2000c, 2001a, 2001b), results for Korean ginseng are less consistent (Sievenpiper et al 2003, 2004). Both ginseng root and berry (150 mg/kg) have been shown to significantly decrease fasting blood glucose levels in hyperglycaemic rats (Dey et al 2003). Intraperitoneal administration of glycans (polysaccharides known as panaxans) and other unidentified compounds has demonstrated hypoglycaemic activity in both normal and alloxan-induced hyperglycaemic mice (Waki et al 1982).

Oral administration of *P. ginseng* root (125.0 mg/kg) three times daily for 3 days reduced hyperglycaemia and improved insulin sensitivity in rats fed a high-fructose chow, suggesting a possible role in delaying or preventing insulin resistance (Liu et al 2005). However, these doses are very high, and human trials need to be conducted to confirm these results.

In more recent studies, when KRG-rootlet and KRG-body preparations were compared for their effect on postprandial glucose levels on healthy individuals, it was found that despite the KRG-rootlets having >6-fold higher total ginsenosides than KRG-body, the KRG-body preparations were more effective in lowering postprandial glucose levels at 45, 60, 90 and 120 min during the test ($P < 0.05$), giving an overall reduction of 27% in area under the curve (glucose) (de Souza et al 2011). This is important for potential dose range of therapeutics. Cho et al (2013) also found that a KRG-rootlet preparation for healthy overweight or obese adults without overt diabetes and hypertension had no significant effect on improving insulin sensitivity over time.

In a study investigating the prophylactic effects of KRG on type 1 diabetes (T1DM), which is a chronic autoimmune disease rather than a metabolic disorder characterised by insulin resistance as in type 2 diabetes (T2DM), Hong et al (2012) found that KRG extract significantly lowered glucose levels and improved glucose challenge testing. The histological findings report KRG extract protected against induced destruction of pancreatic tissue and restored insulin secretion. Importantly, this effect was accompanied by restoration of lymphocytes in secondary lymphoid organs, indicating a striking effect on immune homeostasis.

Diabetic complications

Aqueous extract of ginseng was shown to exert no significant effect on weight in normal rats, while it prevented weight loss in rats with streptozotocin-induced diabetes. Cell proliferation in the dentate gyrus of diabetic rats was increased by ginseng treatment, but it had no effect on cell proliferation in normal rats. These results suggest that ginseng may help reduce the long-term central nervous system complications of diabetes mellitus (Lim BV et al 2002).

According to experimental studies, ginseng may also inhibit the formation of glycated haemoglobin due to its antioxidative activity (Bae & Lee 2004).

Steroid receptor activity

Ginseng has been shown to increase the mounting behaviour of male rats and increase sperm counts in rabbit testes. The effect is not by a direct sex hormone-like function, but probably via a gonadotrophin-like action. Ginsenoside Rb1 has been shown to increase luteinising hormone (LH) secretion by acting directly on the anterior pituitary gland in male rats (Tsai et al 2003). Ginsenoside Rh1 failed to activate the glucocorticoid and androgen receptors, but did demonstrate an interaction with oestrogen receptors in vitro. The effect was much weaker than 17-beta-oestradiol. Ginseng is therefore considered to contain phyto-oestrogens (Lee et al 2003). However, there are conflicting reports about oestrogen-binding activity, which may in part be explained by the presence or absence of zearalenone, an oestrogenic mycotoxin contaminant (Gray et al 2004).

OTHER ACTIONS

Prevention of damage from toxins

Ginseng extract has been shown to be beneficial in the prevention and treatment of testicular damage induced by environmental pollutants. Dioxin is one of the most potent toxic environmental pollutants. Exposure to dioxin either in adulthood or during late fetal and early postnatal development causes a variety of adverse effects on the male reproductive system. The chemical decreases spermatogenesis and the ability to conceive and carry a pregnancy to full term. Pretreatment with 100 or 200 mg/kg ginseng aqueous extract intraperitoneally for 28 days prevented toxic effects of dioxin in guinea pigs. There was no loss in body weight, testicular weight or damage to spermatogenesis (Kim 1999). In guinea pigs, *P. ginseng* also improves the survival and quality of sperm exposed to dioxin (Hwang et al 2004).

Promoting haemopoiesis

Ginseng is traditionally used to treat anaemia. The total saponin fraction, and specifically Rg1 and Rb1, has been shown to promote haematopoiesis by stimulating proliferation of human granulocyte–macrophage progenitors (Niu et al 2001). The total saponins at a concentration of 50 mcg/mL most effectively promote CD34^{+} cells to proliferate and differentiate by cooperating with haematopoietic growth factors (Wang et al 2006).

Antioxidant

In vitro studies did not find various extracts of ginseng to be particularly potent antioxidants against several different free radicals (Kim YK et al 2002). However, animal models have demonstrated effects in type 2 diabetes (Ryu et al 2005), particularly for the leaf, which may suppress lipid peroxidation in diabetic rats (Jung et al 2005). Ginseng extract has also been shown to protect muscle from exercise-induced oxidative stress in animal studies (Voces et al 2004).

Whether these effects are directly due to the antioxidant activity of ginseng components or secondary to other mechanisms, such as blood glucose regulation, is unclear. Additionally, ginseng compounds may require in vivo conversion to active metabolites in order to exert their full effects.

Antiviral

Pretreatment with Korean red ginseng (KRG) extract, reported to have immunomodulatory effects, was shown to be effective in increasing survival rates of mice infected with the influenza H1N1 strain. This was a particularly virulent influenza virus responsible for the 2009 pandemic. Daily oral treatment with KRG extract provided increased protection against two distinct viruses: H1N1 and H3N2. Infected mice showed lower levels of lung viral titres and IL-6, but higher levels of interferon-γ, which is critical for innate and adaptive immunity against viral and intracellular bacterial infections and for tumour control (Yoo et al 2012). Additionally, KRG extract inhibited replication of the virus in vitro, demonstrating important antiviral properties in vivo and in vitro.

Hair growth

Red ginseng extract (more so than white ginseng), and especially ginsenoside Rb1 and 20(S)-ginsenoside Rg3, has been shown to promote hair growth in mouse hair follicles in vitro (Matsuda et al 2003).

Anti-allergic activity

Ginsenosides have been demonstrated to have anti-allergic activity in vitro. One of the metabolites, 20-O-beta-D-glucopyranosyl-20(S)-protopanaxadiol, was found to inhibit beta-hexosaminidase release from rat basophil leukaemia cells and potently reduce passive cutaneous anaphylaxis reaction. The inhibitory activity of protopanaxadiol was more potent than that of disodium cromoglycate, an anti-allergic drug. The compound stabilised membranes but had no effect on hyaluronidase and did not scavenge free radicals. These results suggest that the anti-allergic action of protopanaxadiol originates from its cell membrane-stabilising activity and that the ginsenosides are prodrugs with anti-allergic properties (Choo et al 2003).

Anxiolytic effects

Ginsenosides, and especially ginsenoside Rc, regulate GABA-A receptors in vitro (Choi SE et al 2003), and animal models have demonstrated an anxiolytic effect for ginseng saponins (Park J et al 2005).

Antidepressant effects

In a mouse model of depression, a 2-week administration of: hydrolysed red ginseng (HRG); acetate-fermented red ginseng (ARG); ginsenoside Rg3; red ginseng (RG); and fluoxetine (a classical antidepressant) were assessed for their effects using forced swimming test (FST) compared with a control group. HRG, ARG, Rg3, RG and fluoxetine all significantly improved serum glucose levels and total protein levels compared with the control group ($P < 0.05$), which indicated a beneficial effect in treating depressive-like behaviours (Kim & Kim 2011).

Wound healing

Ginsenoside Rb2 has been reported to improve wound healing. It is believed that ginsenoside Rb2 enhances epidermal cell proliferation by enhancing the expressions of protein factors related to cell proliferation, such as epidermal growth factor and fibronectin (and their receptors), keratin and collagenase (Choi 2002). Ginsenoside Re may also enhance tissue regeneration by inducing angiogenesis (Huang et al 2005). Topical application of ginseng root extract may also promote collagen production via type I procollagen synthesis, suggesting potential anti-wrinkle effects (Lee 2007).

Improves acne

In an animal model of acne, ginseng extracts reduced the size of comedones by altering keratinisation of the skin and desquamating horny cells in comedones. In a study of experimentally-induced hyperkeratosis, ginseng reduced the accumulation of lipids in the epidermis by regulating enzymes associated with epidermal metabolism (Kim et al 1990).

Male fertility

Ginseng-treated rats exhibit a significant increase in sperm count and motility due to activation of cAMP-responsive element modulator in the testes (Park et al 2007).

CLINICAL USE

In the scientific arena, ginseng and the various ginsenosides are used in many forms and administered via various routes. This review will focus primarily on those methods commonly used in clinical practice.

Cancer prevention

The various anticancer actions of *P. ginseng*, as demonstrated in animal and in vitro trials, support its use as an agent to prevent the development and progression of cancer. A 5-year prospective study of 4634 patients over 40 years of age found that ginseng reduced the relative risk of cancer by nearly 50% (Yun 1996).

A retrospective study of 905 case-controlled pairs taking ginseng showed that ginseng intake reduced the risk of cancer by 44% (odds ratio equal to 0.56). The powdered and extract forms of ginseng were more effective than fresh sliced ginseng, juice or tea. The preventive effect was highly significant ($P < 0.001$). There was a significant decline in cancer occurrence with increasing ginseng intake ($P < 0.05$) (Yun & Choi 1990).

Epidemiological studies in Korea strongly suggest that cultivated Korean ginseng is a non-organ-specific human cancer preventive agent. In case–control studies, odds ratios of cancer of the lip, oral cavity and pharynx, larynx, lung, oesophagus, stomach, liver, pancreas, ovary and colorectum were significantly reduced by ginseng use. The most active compounds are thought to be ginsenosides Rg3, Rg5 and Rh2 (Yun 2003).

Ginseng polysaccharide (18 mg/day) has also been shown to be effective in improving immunological function and quality of life (QOL) in elderly patients with non-small cell lung cancer (Zhang et al 2004).

In a randomised, double-blinded, placebo-controlled trial of 643 chronic atrophic gastritis patients in four hospitals in the Zhejiang Province, China, oral administration of KRG extract powder (1 g) per week for 3 years, with a follow-up period of 8 years, to determine the risk of all non-organ-specific cancers, showed a significant risk reduction of all cancers for male subjects of 65% (RR = 0.35; $P = 0.03$). However the risk reduction was non-significant for whole group analysis including both genders (RR = 0.54; $P = 0.13$). In the follow-up period 24 cancers of various organs were diagnosed, with 21 cases being male (Yun et al 2010).

Chemotherapy

Overexpression of P-glycoprotein or multidrug resistance-associated protein may lead to multidrug resistance of cancer cells. Protopanaxatriol ginsenosides have been shown to sensitise cancer cells to chemotherapeutic agents in vitro by increasing the intracellular accumulation of the drugs through direct interaction with P-glycoprotein (Choi CH et al 2003, Kim S-W et al 2003). The ginsenoside Rh2 possesses strong tumour-inhibiting properties and sensitises multidrug-resistant breast cancer cells to paclitaxel (Jia et al 2004), and animal models demonstrate a synergistic antitumour effect for ginseng acidic polysaccharides and paclitaxel (Shin H et al 2004).

Panax ginseng polysaccharide (12 mg IV daily) has also been trialled during treatment for ovarian cancer, and the authors suggest that it is 'effective, safe and reliable for reducing the toxic effects of chemotherapy' (Fu et al 2005).

In a cohort of 1455 patients with breast cancer recruited to the Shanghai Breast Cancer Study, ginseng use prior to diagnosis was associated with a significantly reduced risk of death (adjusted hazard ratios 0.71; 95% confidence interval: 0.52–0.98). Use of the following diagnosis resulted in a dose-dependent improvement in QOL scores (especially for psychological and social wellbeing) (Cui et al 2006).

Diabetes

The putative effects of Korean ginseng on blood glucose and lipid regulation, oxidative stress and protein glycation suggest a possible role as an adjunctive therapy in the management of diabetes and diabetic complications. Diabetes mellitus is characterised by excessive glucose production, which causes oxidative stress and the formation of advanced glycation end-products. These have been significantly linked to diabetic complications such as neuropathy, retinopathy and nephropathy (Kim HY et al 2008).

A double-blind, placebo-controlled study with 36 subjects found that 200 mg ginseng elevated mood, improved psychophysical performance and reduced fasting blood glucose and body weight in patients with newly-diagnosed type 2 diabetes (Sotaniemi et al 1995). A double-blind, randomised, dose-finding study reported that 2 g of Korean ginseng rootlets is sufficient to achieve reproducible reductions in postprandial glycaemia (Sievenpiper 2006), although studies using 200–400 mg have also demonstrated benefits for lowering fasting blood glucose levels (Reay et al 2006a).

In a clinical trial, 19 participants with well-controlled type 2 diabetes (sex: 11 M:8 F, age: 64 ± 2 years, body mass index (BMI): 28.9 ± 1.4 kg/m^2, HbA_{1C}: 6.5%) received 2 g Korean ginseng preparation (rootlets) 40 minutes prior to meals (total 6 g/day) for 12 weeks in addition to their usual antidiabetic therapy. While HbA_{1C} levels remained unchanged, improvements were noted for plasma glucose (75 g-oral glucose tolerance test-plasma glucose (OGTT-PG) reduced by 8–11%), plasma insulin (PI) (fasting PI and 75 g-OGTT-PI reduced by 33–38%) and insulin sensitivity index (ISI) (75 g-OGTT-ISI increased by 33%) compared with placebo ($P < 0.05$) (Vuksan et al 2008).

HY Kim et al (2008), in a study of KRG and heat-processed KRG (H-KRG) on diabetic renal damage, used streptazotocin-induced diabetic rats in a direct-comparison model. Protein expressions related to oxidative stress and advanced glycation end-products were significantly reduced in diabetic rats. Both formulations had a significant effect and may improve diabetic pathological conditions and prevent renal damage associated with diabetic nephropathy; however, H-KRG had a more pronounced effect than KRG.

In a study looking at KRG effects in obese insulin-resistant animal models, the KRG rats were fed 200 mg/kg, per oral and a high fat diet. Compared with a control group and a high-fat-diet-only group, the KRG rats had a significant reduction in weight, especially fat mass, and a significantly increased insulin sensitivity. The authors conclude that KRG may have antidiabetic and antiobesity effects due to partly-increased insulin sensitivity by increased adipokine and partly-enhanced insulin signalling (Lee et al 2012). Kim and Kim (2012) concluded from their study of diabetic rats that KRG may primarily target processes that increase insulin action and insulin secretion and decrease β-cell mass, which causes the normalisation in glucose homeostasis. Conversely, HJ Kim et al (2012) found that in a human study, a preparation of ginseng roots, mulberry leaf water extract and banaba leaf extract (1 : 1 : 1; 6 g/day for 24 weeks) had no impact on glucose homeostasis control measures, however, plasma intracellular adhesion molecule-1 (ICAM-1) concentration was decreased significantly between the groups, and vascular cell adhesion molecule-1 (VCAM-1) and the oxidised low-density lipoprotein (ox-LDL) concentration were decreased within the treatment group from baseline. The authors suggest that these markers indicate a suppression of the inflammatory responses in type 2 diabetes mellitus.

Bang and colleagues (2014) summarise four theories that could explain the anti-diabetic effect of KRG that have been supported by animal models: modulation of the way glucose is absorbed in the digestive system; increase of insulin secretion from the pancreatic islets and binding in the liver; modulation of glucose transport which is increased in various cell lines such as glucose transporter GLUT-1 protein expression; and lastly by an increase in enzymes related to glucose disposal, such as isomerase and lactate dehydrogenase. In their study, they suggest that results indicate a glucose transport mechanism coupled with insulin sensitisation, evidenced by the decreases in serum and whole blood glucose levels and decrease in insulin concentrations.

Different formulations of KGR and its constituents may demonstrate different mechanisms of action, or a combination of effect. Further studies are warranted, as KRG shows promise in the prevention and treatment of both type 1 and type 2 diabetes mellitus.

Cardiovascular disease

A 2006 systematic review concluded that there is currently a lack of well-designed, randomised, controlled trials to support the use of ginseng to treat cardiovascular risk factors despite some studies suggesting improvements in blood pressure, blood glucose and lipid profiles (Buettner et al 2006).

Although there are reports of ginseng causing hypertension, red ginseng is actually used as an antihypertensive agent in Korea.

Acute administration of an aqueous preparation of Korean ginseng (100 mg/kg body weight) to 12 healthy, non-smoking male volunteers resulted in an increase in NO levels and a concomitant reduction in mean blood pressure and heart rate (Han et al 2005).

Ginseng is often used in practice as an adjuvant to both conventional and complementary and alternative medicine (CAM) treatments. Trials have reported that 1.5 g three times daily of Korean red ginseng (4.5 g/day) is useful as an adjuvant to antihypertensive medication (Han et al 1995, 1998). It should be noted, however, that results in these trials, while statistically significant (e.g. systolic pressure −5.7 mmHg), may not be clinically significant. A combination of red ginseng and digoxin was found to be more beneficial than either drug alone in an open study of advanced congestive heart failure. There were no adverse reactions (Ding et al 1995). A combination of ginseng and ginkgo extracts has been found to improve circulation and lower blood pressure in a controlled single-dose study of 10 healthy young volunteers (Kiesewetter et al 1992).

Korean red ginseng has also been shown to improve vascular endothelial function in patients with hypertension. The effect is thought to be mediated through increasing the synthesis of nitric oxide (Sung et al 2000).

Hyperlipidaemia

In a small trial of eight males receiving 2 g Panax ginseng extract three times daily (total Panax ginseng extract (PGE) 6 g/day) for 8 weeks, serum total cholesterol, LDL and triglyceride concentrations were decreased by 12, 45 and 24%, respectively, and a 44% increase in HDL was reported (Kim & Park 2003).

Red ginseng, 1.5 g three times daily before meals for 7 days, reduced liver cholesterol, decreased the atherogenic index and elevated HDL cholesterol in 11 patients (5 normal subjects and 6 with hyperlipidaemia). Serum cholesterol was not significantly altered, but serum triglycerides were significantly decreased (Yamamoto & Kumagai 1982).

Immunomodulation

Ginseng has been shown to significantly enhance NK function in healthy subjects and in those suffering from chronic fatigue syndrome or AIDS ($P < 0.01$) (See et al 1997).

Ginseng polysaccharide injection has been shown, in a randomised study, to improve immunity in 130 patients with nasopharyngeal carcinoma and to reduce adverse reactions to radiotherapy compared with controls (Xie et al 2001).

Red ginseng powder has been shown to restore immunity after chemotherapy and reduce the recurrence of stage III gastric cancer. The 5-year disease-free survival and overall survival rates were significantly higher in patients taking the red ginseng powder during postoperative chemotherapy versus control (68.2 vs 33.3%, 76.4 vs 38.5%, respectively, $P < 0.05$). Despite the limitation of a small number of patients ($n = 42$), these findings suggest that red ginseng powder may help to improve postoperative survival in these patients. Additionally, red ginseng powder may have some immunomodulatory properties associated with CD3 and CD4 activity in patients with advanced gastric cancer during postoperative chemotherapy (Suh et al 2002).

Vaccine adjuvant activity

Ginseng extract (100 mg ginsan G115/day) improved the response to an influenza vaccine in a multicentre, randomised, double-blind, placebo-controlled, two-arm study of 227 subjects. Compared with vaccine without the ginseng, the addition of ginseng resulted in fewer cases of influenza and common cold. Ginseng increased NK activity and increased antibody production (Scaglione et al 1996).

The addition of 2 mg ginseng dry extract per vaccine dose has been shown to potentiate the antibody response of commercial vaccines without altering their safety. The enhancing effect of ginseng was demonstrated during the vaccination of pigs against porcine parvovirus and *Erysipelothrix rhusiopathiae* infections using commercially available vaccines (Rivera et al 2003).

G

Cognitive function

There is some contention about the benefits of ginseng for improving memory, concentration and learning (Persson et al 2004). Well-controlled clinical trials are lacking, and variations in dosage and standardisation may affect study results.

Some studies have demonstrated that ginseng improves the quality of memory and associated secondary memory (Kennedy et al 2001a). In a randomised, placebo-controlled, double-blind, balanced, crossover study of healthy, young adult volunteers, 400 mg ginseng was shown to improve secondary memory performance on a Cognitive Drug Research computerised assessment battery and two serial subtraction mental arithmetic tasks. Ginseng also improved attention and the speed of performing the memory tasks (Kennedy et al 2002). In a later double-blind, placebo-controlled, balanced, crossover study of 30 healthy young adults, acute administration of ginseng (400 mg) was again shown to improve speed of attention (Sunram-Lea et al 2005).

In a double-blind, placebo-controlled study of healthy young subjects, ginseng extract (G115) improved accuracy and slowed responses during one of two computerised serial subtraction tests (Serial Sevens) and it was also shown to improve mood during these tasks (Kennedy et al 2001b). In acute dosing trials, a single dose of ginseng (200 mg G115 extract, with or without 25 g glucose) and glucose has been shown to enhance cognitive performance in healthy young adults. Participants experienced enhanced performance on a mental arithmetic task and a reduction in subjective feelings of mental fatigue during the later stages of the sustained, cognitively demanding task (Reay et al 2006b).

In a double-blind, randomised, placebo-controlled 8–9-week trial, standardised ginseng extract 400 mg was found to significantly improve abstract thinking ($P < 0.005$) and reaction time (not significant) in 112 healthy subjects over 40 years of age. Ginseng was found not to affect concentration or memory (Sorensen & Sonne 1996).

In a controlled open-label study, 97 consecutive patients with Alzheimer's disease were randomly assigned to a treatment (n = 58) or control group (n = 39). The treatment group received Korean ginseng powder (4.5 g/day) for 12 weeks, which resulted in improvements in the cognitive subscale of Alzheimer's disease assessment scale (ADAS) and the mini-mental state examination (MMSE) ($P = 0.029$ and $P = 0.009$ vs baseline, respectively). After discontinuing ginseng, the improved ADAS and MMSE scores declined to the levels of the control group (Lee 2008). In addition, similar trials using 0, 4.5 or 9 g ginseng daily found that patients in the high-dose group showed significant improvement on the ADAS and Clinical Dementia Rating after 12 weeks of ginseng therapy ($P = 0.032$ and 0.006, respectively). Improvements in MMSE did not reach statistical significance (Heo et al 2008).

In clinical practice, Korean ginseng and *Ginkgo biloba* are frequently used in combination for cognitive benefits. Combining ginseng with ginkgo dramatically improves memory, concentration and speed of completing mental tasks (Kennedy et al 2001a, Scholey & Kennedy 2002). In clinical trials, ginseng directly modulates cerebral electrical activity on EEG recordings to a greater extent than *Ginkgo biloba* (Kennedy et al 2003).

In a double-blind, placebo-controlled study, postmenopausal women aged 51–66 years were randomly assigned to 12 weeks' treatment with a combination formula containing 120 mg *Ginkgo biloba* and 200 mg *Panax ginseng* (n = 30) or matched placebo (n = 27). The combination appeared to have no effect on mood or cognition after 6 and 12 weeks; however, these doses may be too low (Hartley et al 2004). According to other trials, it would appear that doses of 400–900 mg of ginseng are required for best results and 200 mg doses have been associated with 'cognitive costs', slowing performance on attention tasks (Kennedy & Scholey 2003).

Menopausal symptoms

Korean red ginseng is used to alleviate symptoms associated with menopause; 6 g ginseng for 30 days was shown in a small study of 20 women significantly ($P < 0.001$) to improve menopausal symptoms, in particular fatigue, insomnia and depression. The women treated had a significant decrease in cortisol and cortisol-to-dehydroepiandrosterone ratio ($P < 0.05$). No adverse effects were recorded (Tode et al 1999).

Erectile dysfunction

Korean red ginseng has been shown to alleviate erectile dysfunction and improve the ability to achieve and maintain erections even in patients with severe erectile dysfunction (Price & Gazewood 2003). Ginsenosides can facilitate penile erection by directly inducing the vasodilation and relaxation of the penile corpus cavernosum. Moreover, the effects of ginseng on the corpus cavernosum appear to be mediated by the release and/or modification of release of NO from endothelial cells and perivascular nerves (Murphy & Lee 2002). In men with type 2 diabetes, oxidative stress has been suggested as a contributing factor to erectile dysfunction and animal studies suggest that ginseng can preserve 'potency' via its antioxidant effect (Ryu et al 2005).

In a double-blind, placebo-controlled study, 60 patients presenting with mild or mild to moderate erectile dysfunction received 1 g (three times daily) of Korean ginseng or placebo. In the five-item International Index of Erectile Function (IIEF)-5, 66.6% (20 patients) reported improved erection, rigidity, penetration and maintenance ($P < 0.01$) after 12 weeks. Serum testosterone, prolactin and cholesterol were not significantly different (de Andrade et al 2007).

In a double-blind crossover study, 900 mg Korean red ginseng was found to significantly improve the Mean IIEF scores compared with placebo. Significant subjective improvements in penetration and maintenance were reported by participants, and penile tip rigidity on the RigiScan showed significant improvement for ginseng versus placebo (Hong et al 2002).

A significant improvement in erectile function, sexual desire and intercourse satisfaction was demonstrated in 45 subjects following 8 weeks' oral administration of Korean red ginseng (900 mg three times daily) in a double-blind, placebo-controlled, crossover trial. Subjects demonstrated significant improvement in mean IIEF scores compared with placebo (baseline, 28 ± 16.7; Korean red ginseng, 38.1 ± 16.6; placebo, 30.9 ± 15.7) (Hong et al 2003).

Quality of life

An 8-week, randomised, double-blind study found that 200 mg/day ginseng (n = 15, placebo: n = 15) improved aspects of mental health and social functioning after 4 weeks' therapy, but that these differences disappeared with continued use (Ellis & Reddy 2002). A review of eight clinical studies with ginseng found some improvement in QOL scores. However, the findings were equivocal. Despite some positive results, improvement in overall health-related QOL cannot, given the current research, be attributed to *P. ginseng*. However, the possibility that various facets of QOL may have improved and the potential of early transient effects cannot be discounted (Coleman et al 2003). A double-blind, placebo-controlled, randomised clinical trial of 83 subjects also did not find ginseng to enhance psychological wellbeing in healthy young adults (Cardinal & Engels 2001).

A double-blind, placebo-controlled, crossover study found that 1200 mg ginseng was only slightly more effective than placebo and not as effective as a good night's sleep in improving bodily feelings, mood and fatigue in 12 fatigued night nurses. Volunteers slept less and experienced less fatigue, but rated sleep quality worse after ginseng administration (Hallstrom et al 1982).

A recent double-blind, placebo-controlled, balanced, crossover design of 30 healthy young adults taking *P. ginseng* extract (200 or 400 mg) or placebo demonstrated improvements in performance and subjective feelings of mental fatigue during sustained mental activity. It has been hypothesised that this effect may be due in part to the ability of ginseng to regulate blood glucose levels (Reay et al 2005).

Adaptogenic and tonic effects

A randomised double-blind study involving 232 subjects between the ages of 25 and 60 years found that extract equivalent to about 400 mg ginseng root for 4 weeks significantly improved fatigue. Side effects were uncommon, with only two subjects withdrawing from the study (Le Gal & Cathebras 1996).

A randomised double-blind study of 83 subjects found that extract equivalent to 1 g ginseng root for 4 months decreased the risk of contracting a common cold or bronchitis and improved appetite, sleep, wellbeing and physical performance (Gianoli & Riebenfeld 1984).

Improved athletic performance

Ginseng is used by many athletes to improve stamina and to facilitate rapid recovery from injuries; however, supporting evidence from well-designed clinical trials is lacking. To examine the effects of ginseng supplements on hormonal status following acute resistance exercise, eight male college students were randomly given water (control group) or 20 g ginseng root extract treatment immediately after a standardised training exercise. Human growth hormone, testosterone, cortisol and insulin-like growth factor 1 levels were determined by radioimmunoassay. The responses of plasma hormones following ginseng consumption were not significant between the control and the ginseng groups during the 2-hour recovery period (Youl et al 2002).

Although ginseng is commonly used to improve endurance, a double-blind study of 19 healthy, active women found that 400 mg of a ginseng extract (G115) did not improve supramaximal exercise performance or short-term recovery. Analysis of variance using pretest to posttest change scores revealed no significant difference between the ginseng and placebo study groups for the following variables measured: peak anaerobic power output, mean anaerobic power output, rate of fatigue and immediate postexercise recovery heart rates (Engels et al 2001). A recent study by the same authors also failed to find any benefit from ginseng (400 mg/day G115; equivalent to 2 g *P. ginseng* C.A. Meyer root material for 8 weeks) on improving physical performance and heart rate recovery of individuals undergoing repeated bouts of exhausting exercise (Engels et al 2003). When 60 men from the Naval Medical Corps, Royal Thai Navy (aged 17–22 years), given 3 g/day of ginseng or placebo for an 8-week period, were measured for blood lactic acid levels for determination of lactate threshold (LT), no improvements were noted, nor was there any beneficial effect on physical performance (Kulaputana et al 2007).

A small study of seven healthy male subjects given 2 g ginseng (three times daily) for 8 weeks reported a significant increase in exercise duration until exhaustion (+1.5 min; $P < 0.05$), which was related to improvements in lipid peroxidation and scavenger enzymes (Kim et al 2005); however, this study is too small to make generalisations.

G

OTHER USES

Gastroprotection during heart surgery

In a trial of 24 children undergoing heart surgery for congenital heart defects, 12 children received 1.35 mg/kg ginsenoside compound or placebo intravenously before and throughout the course of cardiopulmonary bypass surgery. Ginseng administration resulted in attenuation of gastrointestinal injury and inflammation (Xia et al 2005).

Respiratory disease

Ginseng extract (G115) has been shown to significantly ($P < 0.05$) improve pulmonary function test, maximum voluntary ventilation, maximum inspiratory pressure and maximal oxygen consumption (VO_{2max}) in a study of 92 patients suffering moderately severe chronic obstructive pulmonary disease ($n = 49$, G115 100 mg twice daily for 3 months) (Gross et al 2002).

Helicobacter pylori

Helicobacter pylori can provoke gastric inflammation, ulceration and DNA damage, resulting in an increased risk of carcinogenesis. As preliminary evidence suggests that *P. ginseng* inhibits the growth of *H. pylori* (Kim J et al 2003) and can inhibit adhesion (Lee J et al 2004), it may be useful as a gastroprotective agent against *H. pylori*-associated gastric mucosal cell damage (Park S et al 2005).

HIV infection

Long-term intake of Korean ginseng slows the depletion of $CD4^+$ T cells and may delay disease progression in people with HIV type 1 (Sung et al 2005). Ginseng intake in HIV-1-infected patients may also be associated with the occurrence of grossly deleted nef genes (gDeltanef) (Cho et al 2006) and gross deletions (gDelta) in HIV-1 5'-LTR and gag regions (Cho & Jung 2008). Long-term intake (60 ± 15 months) has also been shown to delay the development of resistance mutation to zidovudine (Cho et al 2001).

DOSAGE RANGE

- Extract equivalent to 0.9–3 g crude ginseng root (Bensky & Gamble 1986).

- Standardised extract: 1.5–4.0% total ginsenosides calculated as ginsenoside Rg1.
- Liquid extract (1 : 2): 1–6 mL/day.
- Cognitive function: Clinical trials using 1.5–3 g three times daily have reported benefits. Lower doses may be associated with 'cognitive costs' and slowing performance on attention tasks (Kennedy & Scholey 2003).
- Cardiovascular use: 1.5–2 g three times daily.

Many of the clinical studies published in the scientific literature have used a proprietary extract of ginseng standardised to 4% total ginsenosides (G115 or Ginsana produced by Pharmaton, Lugano, Switzerland).

Ginseng is usually given in the earlier part of the day. It should not be given in the evening, unless it is used to promote wakefulness. Ginseng is usually not given to children.

ADVERSE REACTIONS

Ginseng abuse syndrome (hypertension, nervousness, insomnia, morning diarrhoea, inability to concentrate and skin reactions) has been reported, and there has been a report of a 28-year-old woman who had a severe headache after ingesting a large quantity of ethanol-extracted ginseng. Cerebral angiograms showed 'beading' appearance in the anterior and posterior cerebral and superior cerebellar arteries, consistent with cerebral arteritis (Ryu & Chien 1995). High doses (15 g/day) have been associated with confusion, depression and depersonalisation in four patients (Coon & Ernst 2002).

However, the majority of the scientific data suggest that ginseng is rarely associated with adverse events or drug interactions. A systematic review found that the most commonly experienced adverse events are headache, sleep and gastrointestinal disorders. Data from clinical trials suggest that the incidence of adverse events with ginseng monopreparations is similar to that of placebo. Any documented effects are usually mild and transient. Combined preparations are more often associated with adverse events, but causal attribution is usually not possible (Coon & Ernst 2002).

Allergic reactions to Korean ginseng, including occupation asthma, may occur via an IgE-mediated mechanism (Kim KM 2008). A case of suspected ginseng allergy has recently been reported in the scientific literature. The case involved a 20-year-old male who developed urticaria, dyspnoea and hypotension after ingesting ginseng syrup. The subject recovered fully and was discharged after 24 hours (Wiwanitkit & Taungjararuwinai 2004).

While ginseng use has been associated with the development of hypertension, it has actually been shown to reduce blood pressure in several studies (Coon & Ernst 2002).

Ginseng has very low toxicity. Subacute doses of 1.5–15 mg/kg of a 5 : 1 ginseng extract did not produce negative effect on body weight, food consumption, haematological or biochemical parameters or histological findings in dogs (Hess et al 1983), and no effects have been observed from the administration of similar doses in two generations of rat offspring (Hess et al 1982).

Traditionally, ginseng is not recommended with other stimulants such as caffeine and nicotine, and a case report exists of a 39-year-old female experiencing menometrorrhagia, arrhythmia and tachycardia after using oral and topical ginseng, along with coffee and cigarettes (Kabalak et al 2004).

SIGNIFICANT INTERACTIONS

Albendazole

Panax ginseng significantly accelerated the intestinal clearance of the anthelmintic albendazole sulfoxide, when coadministered to rats (Merino et al 2003).

Alcohol

Ginseng may increase the clearance of alcohol from the blood according to an open trial of 14 healthy volunteers (Coon & Ernst 2002) — beneficial interaction possible, but needs confirmation.

Chemotherapy, radiotherapy and general anaesthetics

Preliminary evidence suggests that *P. ginseng* saponins may reduce nausea and vomiting associated with chemotherapy, radiotherapy and general anaesthetics by antagonising serotonin (5-hydroxytryptamine) type 3A receptors (Min et al 2003). Ginseng may also help to sensitise cancer cells to chemotherapeutic agents according to preliminary evidence.

Digoxin

Ginseng contains glycosides with structural similarities to digoxin, which may modestly interfere with digoxin results (Dasgupta et al 2003). These naturally-occurring glycosides may cause false elevation of fluorescence polarisation and falsely low microparticle enzyme results, although Tina-quant results appear unaffected (Dasgupta & Reyes 2005). It should be noted that measuring free digoxin does not eliminate these modest interferences in serum digoxin measurement by the Digoxin III assay (Dasgupta et al 2008). There are no confirmed case reports of actual interaction (Chow et al 2003, Dasgupta et al 2003).

Drugs metabolised chiefly by CYP1A, CYP2D6 and CYP3A4

Mixed reports exist as to whether ginseng may act as an inhibitor of cytochrome CYP1A (Gurley et al 2005, Lee HC et al 2002, Yu et al 2005) or CYP2D6 (Gurley et al 2005). Ginsenosides F1 and Rh1 (but not ginseng extract) may inhibit CYP3A4 at 10 micromolar (Etheridge et al 2007). Whether these effects are likely to be clinically significant has not been established. Observe for increased drug bioavailability and clinical effects.

Nifedipine

Ginseng increased the mean plasma concentration of the calcium channel blocker nifedipine by 53% at 30 minutes in an open trial of 22 healthy subjects. Effects at other time points were not reported (Smith et al 2001).

Vancomycin

In animal studies, the combination of ginseng polysaccharides with vancomycin resulted in a 100% survival rate for animals treated for *Staphylococcus aureus* compared to only 67 or 50% survival in animals treated with ginseng polysaccharides or vancomycin alone (Lim BV et al 2002). A beneficial additive effect is possible, but clinical use in humans has not yet been established.

Warfarin

No effects on the pharmacokinetics or pharmacodynamics of either S-warfarin or R-warfarin were revealed in an open-label, crossover randomised trial of 12 healthy male subjects who received a single 25-mg dose of warfarin alone or after 7 days' pretreatment with ginseng (Jiang et al 2004). Whether these effects are consistent in less 'healthy' people likely to be taking warfarin or for prolonged concurrent use is unclear.

There have been two case reports of ginseng reducing the antithrombotic effects of warfarin (Janetzky & Morreale 1997, Rosado 2003). Additionally, it inhibits platelet aggregation according to both in vitro and animal studies. Avoid using this combination unless under medical supervision to monitor antithrombotic effects.

Zidovudine

Long-term intake (60 ± 15 months) of Korean red ginseng in HIV-1-infected patients has been shown to delay the development of resistance mutation to zidovudine (Cho et al 2001).

CONTRAINDICATIONS AND PRECAUTIONS

Korean ginseng is generally contraindicated in acute infections with fever and in persons who are very hot, tense and overly stimulated. Overuse may result in headache, insomnia and palpitation (Bensky & Gamble 1986). Ginseng should not be taken concurrently with other stimulants including caffeine and should be discontinued 1 week before major surgery. Use in hypertension should be supervised; however, it may prove beneficial for this indication.

PREGNANCY USE

Ginseng is traditionally used in Korea as a tonic during pregnancy. Commission E does not list any restrictions (Blumenthal 2001). There is in vitro evidence of teratogenicity based on exposure to isolated ginsenosides (especially Rb1) (Chan et al 2003) at much higher levels than achievable through normal consumption in humans and conflicting evidence as to its oestrogenic properties. In light of the lack of good clinical evidence, Korean ginseng should be used cautiously during pregnancy (especially the first trimester) and lactation until more data are available (Seely et al 2008).

In a two-generation rat study, a ginseng extract fed at doses as high as 15 mg/kg/day did not produce adverse effects on reproductive performance, including embryo development and lactation (Hess et al 1982).

Practice points/Patient counselling

Traditional use:

Ginseng is traditionally used for deficiency of Qi (energy/life force) manifested by shallow respiration, shortness of breath, cold limbs, profuse sweating and a weak pulse (such as may occur from severe blood loss). Ginseng is also used for wheezing, lethargy, lack of appetite, abdominal distension and chronic diarrhoea. Ginseng may also be used for palpitations, anxiety, insomnia, forgetfulness and restlessness associated with low energy and anaemia (Bensky & Gamble 1986).

Scientific evidence:

There is some scientific evidence for the beneficial effects of ginseng for the following conditions. In practice, it is mostly used as a supportive treatment and combined with other herbs to treat a specific condition.

- Prevention and supportive treatment of cancer
- Chronic immune deficiency
- Menopausal symptoms
- Erectile dysfunction
- Chronic respiratory disease
- Enhancement of psychomotor activity, memory and concentration
- Adaptogenic effects in any chronic condition and for the elderly and infirm
- Type 1 diabetes
- Cardiovascular disease (the effects on hypertension/hypotension remain to be fully investigated)
- QOL (equivocal scientific support)

Commission E recommends ginseng as a tonic for invigoration and fortification in times of fatigue, debility and convalescence or declining capacity for work and concentration. The World Health Organization suggests that ginseng can be used as a prophylactic and restorative agent for enhancement of mental and physical capacities, in cases of weakness, exhaustion, tiredness and loss of concentration and during convalescence (Blumenthal 2001).

G

PATIENTS' FAQs

What will this herb do for me?

Ginseng is a safe herb used to support the body during times of prolonged stress or chronic disease and to restore mental and physical functioning during the rehabilitative process. Numerous studies have identified a range of pharmacological activities that suggest that it may be useful in the treatment of many conditions.

When will it start to work?

In practice, it generally appears that ginseng has a quick onset of action with the condition continuing to improve with long-term use; however, this will vary depending on the individual and the indication.

Are there any safety issues?

Ginseng may interact with warfarin and other blood-thinning drugs and should not be used with these medications, unless under medical supervision. Avoid use in children or in hypertension, unless under supervision. Use with caution in pregnancy.

REFERENCES

Bae J, Lee M. Effect and putative mechanism of action of ginseng on the formation of glycated hemoglobin in vitro. J Ethnopharmacol 91.1 (2004): 137–140.

Banerjee U, Izquierdo JA. Antistress and antifatigue properties of Panax ginseng: comparison with piracetam. Acta Physiol Lat Am 32.4 (1982): 277–285.

Bang H et al. Korean red ginseng improves glucose control in subjects with impaired fasting glucose, impaired glucose tolerance, or newly diagnosed type 2 diabetes mellitus. J Med Food 17.1 (2014): 128–134.

Bensky D, Gamble A. Chinese herbal medicine: materia medica 1843. Seattle, WA: Eastland Press, 1986.

Blumenthal M. Asian ginseng: potential therapeutic uses. Adv Nurse Pract 9.2 (2001): 26–28, 33.

British Herbal Medicine Association Scientific Committee. British herbal pharmacopoeia. Lane House. Cowling, UK: BHMA, 1983.

Buettner C et al. Systematic review of the effects of ginseng on cardiovascular risk factors. Ann Pharmacother 40.1 (2006): 83–95.

Cabral de Oliveira AC et al. Protective effects of Panax ginseng on muscle injury and inflammation after eccentric exercise. Comp Biochem Physiol C Toxicol Pharmacol 130.3 (2001): 369–377.

Cardinal BJ, Engels HJ. Ginseng does not enhance psychological well-being in healthy, young adults: results of a double-blind, placebo-controlled, randomized clinical trial. J Am Diet Assoc 101.6 (2001): 655–660.

Caron MF et al. Electrocardiographic and hemodynamic effects of Panax ginseng. Ann Pharmacother 36.5 (2002): 758–763.

Chan L et al. An in vitro study of ginsenoside Rb1-induced teratogencity using a whole rat embryo culture model. Hum Reprod 18.10 (2003): 2166–2168.

Chang G-T et al. Inhibitory effect of the Korean herbal medicine, Dae-Jo-Whan, on platelet-activating factor-induced platelet aggregation. J Ethnopharmacol 102.3 (2005): 430–439.

Chen X et al. Extracts of *Ginkgo biloba* and ginsenosides exert cerebral vas orrelaxation via a nitric oxide pathway. Clin Exp Pharmal Physiol 24 (1997): 958–959.

Chen IJ et al. Korean red ginseng improves blood pressure stability in patients with intradialytic hypotension. Evid-Based CAM (eCAM) 2012 (2012): id 595271.

Cho YK, Jung YS. High frequency of gross deletions in the 5' LTR and gag regions in HIV type 1-infected long-term survivors treated with Korean red ginseng. AIDS Res Hum Retroviruses 24.2 (2008): 181–193.

Cho YK et al. Long-term intake of Korean red ginseng in HIV-1-infected patients: development of resistance mutation to zidovudine is delayed. Int Immunopharmacol 1.7 (2001): 1295–1305.

Cho YK et al. High frequency of grossly deleted nef genes in HIV-1 infected long-term slow progressors treated with Korean red ginseng. Curr HIV Res 4.4 (2006): 447–457.

Cho YH et al. Effect of Korean red ginseng on insulin sensitivity in non-diabetic healthy overweight and obese adults. Asia Pac J Clin Nutr 22.3 (2013): 365–371.

Choi S. Epidermis proliferative effect of the Panax ginseng ginsenoside Rb2. Arch Pharm Res 25.1 (2002): 71–76.

Choi SE et al. Effects of ginsenosides on GABA(A) receptor channels expressed in Xenopus oocytes. Arch Pharm Res 26.1 (2003): 28–33.

Choi CH et al. Reversal of P-glycoprotein-mediated multidrug resistance by protopanaxatriol ginsenosides from Korean red ginseng. Planta Med 69.3 (2003): 235–40.

Choo MK et al. Antiallergic activity of ginseng and its ginsenosides. Planta Med 69.6 (2003): 518–522.

Choung YH et al. Korean red ginseng prevents gentamicin-induced hearing loss in rats. Laryngoscope 121.6 (2011): 1294–1302.

Chow L et al. Effect of the traditional Chinese medicines Chan Su, Lu-Shen-Wan, Dan Shen, and Asian ginseng on serum digoxin measurement by Tina-quant (Roche) and Synchron LX system (Beckman) digoxin immunoassays. J Clin Lab Anal 17.1 (2003): 22–27.

Coleman CI, Hebert JH, Reddy P. The effects of Panax ginseng on quality of life. J Clin Pharm Ther 28.1 (2003): 5–15.

Coon JT, Ernst E. Panax ginseng: a systematic review of adverse drug reactions and interactions. Drug Safety 25.5 (2002): 323–344.

Cui J et al. What do commercial ginseng preparations contain? Lancet 344.8915 (1994): 134.

Cui Y et al. Association of ginseng use with survival and quality of life among breast cancer patients. Am J Epidemiol 163.7 (2006): 645–653.

Dasgupta A, Reyes M. Effect of Brazilian, Indian, Siberian, Asian, and North American ginseng on serum digoxin measurement by immunoassays and binding of digoxin-like immunoreactive components of ginseng with Fab fragment of antidigoxin antibody (Digibind). Am J Clin Pathol 124.2 (2005): 229–236.

Dasgupta A et al. Effect of Asian and Siberian ginseng on serum digoxin measurement by five digoxin immunoassays: significant variation in digoxin-like immunoreactivity among commercial ginsengs. Am J Clin Pathol 119.2 (2003): 298–303.

Dasgupta A et al. Effect of Asian ginseng, Siberian ginseng, and Indian ayurvedic medicine Ashwagandha on serum digoxin measurement by Digoxin III, a new digoxin immunoassay. J Clin Lab Anal 22.4 (2008): 295–301.

de Andrade E et al. Study of the efficacy of Korean Red Ginseng in the treatment of erectile dysfunction. Asian J Androl 9.2 (2007): 241–244.

de Souza L et al. Korean red ginseng (Panax ginseng C.A. Meyer) root fractions: Differential effects on postprandial glycemia in healthy individuals. J Ethnopharm 137 (2011): 245–250.

Dey L et al. Anti-hyperglycemic effects of ginseng: comparison between root and berry. Phytomedicine 10.6–7 (2003): 600–605.

Ding DZ et al. Effects of red ginseng on the congestive heart failure and its mechanism. Zhongguo Zhong Xi Yi Jie He Za Zhi 15.6 (1995): 325–327.

Ding Y et al. Preparation of ginseng saponin chewing gum and observation of improving intelligence and movement function. Chin J Clin Rehab 8.16 (2004): 3206–3207.

Ellis JM, Reddy P. Effects of Panax ginseng on quality of life. Ann Pharmacother 36.3 (2002): 375–379.

Engels HJ et al. Effects of ginseng supplementation on supramaximal exercise performance and short-term recovery. J Strength Cond Res 15.3 (2001): 290–295.

Engels HJ et al. Effects of ginseng on secretory IgA, performance, and recovery from interval exercise. Med Sci Sports Exerc 35.4 (2003): 690–696.

Etheridge AS et al. An in vitro evaluation of cytochrome P450 inhibition and P-glycoprotein interaction with goldenseal, Ginkgo biloba, grape seed, milk thistle, and ginseng extracts and their constituents. Planta Med 73.8 (2007): 731–741.

Filaretov AA et al. Role of pituitary-adrenocortical system in body adaptation abilities. Exp Clin Endocrinol 92.2 (1988): 129–136.

Friedl R et al. Stimulation of nitric oxide synthesis by the aqueous extract of Panax ginseng root in RAW 264.7 cells. Br J Pharmacol 134.8 (2001): 1663–1670.

Fu W et al. The role of Panax ginseng polysaccharide injection in chemotherapy of patients with ovarian cancer. Pharm Care Res 5.2 (2005): 169–171.

Fukushima S, Wanibuchi H, Li W. Inhibition by ginseng of colon carcinogenesis in rats. J Korean Med Sci 16 (Suppl) (2001): S75–S80.

Gianoli A, Riebenfeld D. Doppelblind-Studie zur Beurteilung der Verträglichkeit und Wirkung des standardisierten Ginseng-Extraktes G115®. Cytobiol Rev 8.3 (1984): 177–186.

Gray S et al. Mycotoxins in root extracts of American and Asian ginseng bind estrogen receptors alpha and beta. Exp Biol Med 229.6 (2004): 560–568.

Gross D et al. Ginseng improves pulmonary functions and exercise capacity in patients with COPD. Monaldi Arch Chest Dis 57.5–6 (2002): 242–246.

Gupta YK et al. Antiepileptic activity of Panax ginseng against pentylenetetrazole induced kindling in rats. Indian J Physiol Pharmacol 45.4 (2001): 502–506.

Gurley B et al. Clinical assessment of effects of botanical supplementation on cytochrome P450 phenotypes in the elderly: St John's Wort, garlic oil, Panax ginseng and Ginkgo biloba. Drugs Aging 22.6 (2005): 525–539.

Hah JS et al. Effect of Panax ginseng alcohol extract on cardiovascular system. Yonsei Med J 19.2 (1978): 11–118.
Hallstrom C et al. Effects of ginseng on performance of nurses on night duty. Comp Med East West 6.4 (1982): 277–282.
Han KH et al. Effect of red ginseng on blood pressure in patients with essential hypertension and white coat hypertension assessed by twenty-four-hour ambulatory blood pressure monitoring. J Korean Soc Clin Pharmacol Ther 3.2 (1995): 198–208 [Korean].
Han KH et al. Effect of red ginseng on blood pressure in patients with essential hypertension and white coat hypertension. Am J Chin Med 26.2 (1998): 199–209.
Han K et al. Korea red ginseng water extract increases nitric oxide concentrations in exhaled breath. Nitric Oxide Biol Chem 12.3 (2005): 159–162.
Hartley D et al. Gincosan (a combination of ginkgo biloba and panax ginseng): the effects on mood and cognition of 6 and 12 weeks' treatment in post-menopausal women. Nutr Neurosci 7.5–6 (2004): 325–333.
Hasegawa H. Proof of the mysterious efficacy of ginseng: basic and clinical trials: metabolic activation of ginsenoside: eglycosylation by intestinal bacteria and esterification with fatty acid. J Pharmacol Sci 95.2 (2004): 153–157.
Hasegawa H et al. Prevention of growth and metastasis of murine melanoma through enhanced natural-killer cytotoxicity by fatty acid-conjugate of protopanaxatriol. Biol Pharm Bull 25.7 (2002): 861–866.
Hashimoto K et al. Components of Panax ginseng that improve accelerated small intestinal transit. J Ethnopharmacol 84.1 (2003): 115–119.
Helms S. Cancer prevention and therapeutics: Panax ginseng. Altern Med Rev 9.3 (2004): 259–274.
Heo JH et al. An open-label trial of Korean red ginseng as an adjuvant treatment for cognitive impairment in patients with Alzheimer's disease. Eur J Neurol 15.8 (2008): 865–868.
Hess FG Jr et al. Reproduction study in rats or ginseng extract G115. Food Chem Toxicol 20.2 (1982): 189–192.
Hess FG Jr. et al. Effects of subchronic feeding of ginseng extract G115 in beagle dogs. Food Chem Toxicol 21.1 (1983): 95–97.
Ho YL et al. Korean red ginseng suppresses metastasis of human hepatoma SK-Hep1 cells by inhibiting matrix metalloproteinase-2/-9 and urokinase plasminogen activator. Evidence-Based CAM 2012 (2012): 1–8.
Hong B et al. A double-blind crossover study evaluating the efficacy of Korean red ginseng in patients with erectile dysfunction: a preliminary report. J Urol 168.5 (2002): 2070–2073.
Hong B et al. Korean red ginseng effective for treatment of erectile dysfunction. J Fam Pract 52.1 (2003): 20–21.
Hong YJ et al. Korean red ginseng (Panax ginseng) ameliorates type 1 diabetes and restores immune cell compartments. J Ethnopharm 144 (2012): 225–233.
Huang Y et al. A natural compound, Ginsenoside Re (isolated from Panax ginseng), as a novel angiogenic agent for tissue regeneration. Pharm Res 22.4 (2005): 636–646.
Huang J et al. A new triterpenoid from Panax ginseng exhibits cytotoxicity through p53 and the caspase signaling pathway in the HepG2 cell line. Arch Pharm Res 31.3 (2008): 323–329.
Hwang SJ et al. Diol- and triol-type ginseng saponins potentiate the apoptosis of NIH3T3 cells exposed to methyl methanesulfonate. Toxicol Appl Pharmacol 181.3 (2002): 192–202.
Hwang S et al. Panax ginseng improves survival and sperm quality in guinea pigs exposed to 2,3,7,8-tetrachlorodibenzo-p-dioxin. BJU Int 94.4 (2004): 663–668.
Im GJ et al. Protective effect of Korean red ginseng extract on cisplatin ototoxicity in HE1-OC1 auditory cells. Phytother Res 24 (2010): 614–621.
Ivanova T et al. Antimutagenic effect of polysaccharide ginsan extracted from Panax ginseng. Food Chem Toxicol 4.4 (2006): 517–521.
Janetzky K, Morreale AP. Probable interaction between warfarin and ginseng. Am J Health Syst Pharm 54.6 (1997): 692–693.
Jeong CS. Effect of butanol fraction of Panax ginseng head on gastric lesion and ulcer. Arch Pharm Res 25.1 (2002): 61–66.
Jia W et al. Rh2, a compound extracted from ginseng, hypersensitizes multidrug-resistant tumor cells to chemotherapy. Can J Physiol Pharmacol 82.7 (2004): 431–437.
Jiang X et al. Effect of St John's wort and ginseng on the pharmacokinetics and pharmacodynamics of warfarin in healthy subjects. Br J Clin Pharmacol 57.5 (2004): 592–599.
Jin H et al. Pharmacokinetic comparison of ginsenoside metabolite IH-901 from fermented and non-fermented ginseng in healthy Korean volunteers. J Ethnopharm 139 (2012): 664–667.
Jo S et al. Korean red ginseng extract induces proliferation to differentiation transition of human acute promyelocytic leukemia cells via MYC-SKP2-CDKN1B axis. J Ethnopharm 150 (2013): 700–707.
Jung C-H et al. Effects of wild ginseng (Panax ginseng C.A. Meyer) leaves on lipid peroxidation levels and antioxidant enzyme activities in streptozotocin diabetic rats. J Ethnopharmacol 98.3 (2005): 245–250.
Kabalak A et al. Menometrorrhagia and tachyarrhythmia after using oral and topical ginseng. J Womens Health 13.7 (2004): 830–833.
Kang J et al. Ginseng intestinal metabolite-I (GIM-I) reduces doxorubicin toxicity in the mouse testis. Reprod Toxicol 16.3 (2002): 291–298.
Kennedy DO, Scholey AB. Ginseng: potential for the enhancement of cognitive performance and mood. Pharmacol Biochem Behav 75 (2003): 687–700.
Kennedy DO et al. Differential, dose dependent changes in cognitive performance following acute administration of a Ginkgo biloba/Panax ginseng combination to healthy young volunteers. Nutr Neurosci 4.5 (2001a): 399–412.
Kennedy DO et al. Dose dependent changes in cognitive performance and mood following acute administration of Ginseng to healthy young volunteers. Nutr Neurosci 4.4 (2001b): 295–310.
Kennedy DO et al. Modulation of cognition and mood following administration of single doses of Ginkgo biloba, ginseng, and a ginkgo/ginseng combination to healthy young adults. Physiol Behav 75.5 (2002): 739–751.
Keum YS et al. Inhibitory effects of the ginsenoside Rg3 on phorbol ester-induced cyclooxygenase-2 expression, NF-kappaB activation and tumor promotion. Mutat Res 523–524 (2003): 75–85.
Kiesewetter H et al. Hemorrheological and circulatory effects of gincosan. Int J Clin Pharmacol Ther Toxicol 30.3 (1992): 97–102.
Kim W. Panax ginseng protects the testis against 2,3,7, 8-tetrachlorodibenzo-p-dioxin induced testicular damage in guinea pigs. BJU Int 83.7 (1999): 842–849.
Kim KM. Korean ginseng-induced occupational asthma and determination of IgE binding components. J Korean Med Sci 23.2 (2008): 232–235.
Kim HY, Kim K. Regulation of signaling molecules associated with insulin action, insulin secretion and pancreatic β-cell mass in the hypoglycemic effects of Korean red ginseng in Goto-Kakizaki rats. J Ethnopharm 142 (2012): 53–58.
Kim SH, Park KS. Effects of Panax ginseng extract on lipid metabolism in humans. Pharmacol Res 48.5 (2003): 511–513.
Kim H et al. Actions of Korean ginseng and benzoyl peroxide on inflammation relevant to acne. Korean J Ginseng Sci 14 (1990): 391–398.
Kim JY et al. Inhibitory effect of tumor cell proliferation and induction of G2/M cell cycle arrest by panaxytriol. Planta Med 68.2 (2002): 119–122.
Kim YK et al. Free radical scavenging activity of red ginseng aqueous extracts. Toxicology 172.2 (2002): 149–156.
Kim J et al. Inhibitory effect of ginseng polyacetylenes on infection and vacuolation of Helicobacter pylori. Nat Prod Sci 9.3 (2003): 158–160.
Kim DH et al. Effects of ginseng saponin administered intraperitoneally on the hypothalamo-pituitary-adrenal axis in mice. Neurosci Lett 343.1 (2003): 62–66.
Kim S-W et al. Reversal of P-glycoprotein-mediated multidrug resistance by ginsenoside Rg3. Biochem Pharmacol 65.1 (2003): 75–82.
Kim J et al. Effect of crude saponin of Korean red ginseng on high-fat diet-induced obesity in the rat. J Pharmacol Sci 97.1 (2005): 124–131.
Kim J-H et al. Protective effects of ginseng saponins on 3-nitropropionic acid-induced striatal degeneration in rats. Neuropharmacology 48.5 (2005): 743–756.
Kim SH et al. Effects of Panax ginseng extract on exercise-induced oxidative stress. J Sports Med Phys Fitness 45.2 (2005): 178–182.
Kim HY et al. Comparison of the effects of Korean ginseng and heat-processed Korean ginseng on diabetic oxidative stress. Am J Chin Med 36.5 (2008): 989–1004.
Kim GN et al. Heat processing decreases Amadori products and increases total phenolic content and antioxidant activity of Korean red ginseng. J Med Food 13.6 (2010): 1478–1484.
Kim HJ et al. A six-month supplementation of mulberry, Korean red ginseng, and banaba decreases biomarkers of systemic low-grade inflammation in subjects with impaired glucose tolerance and type 2 diabetes. Evid-based CAM 2012 (2012): 735191.
Kim NH et al. Antidepressant-like effect of altered Korean red ginseng in mice. Beh Med 37 (2011): 42–46.
Komatsu K et al. Ginseng drugs: molecular and chemical characteristics and possibility as antidementia drugs. Curr Top Nutraceut Res 3.1 (2005): 47–64.
Kulaputana O et al. Ginseng supplementation does not change lactate threshold and physical performances in physically active Thai men. J Med Assoc Thai 90.6 (2007): 1172–1179.
Kumar M et al. Radioprotective effect of Panax ginseng on the phosphatases and lipid peroxidation level in testes of Swiss albino mice. Biol Pharm Bull 26.3 (2003): 308–312.
Kumar A et al. Molecular mechanisms of ginsenoside Rp1-mediated growth arrest and apoptosis. Int J Molec Med 24.3 (2009): 381–386.
Kuo Y-H, Ikegami F, Lambein F. Neuroactive and other free amino acids in seed and young plants of Panax ginseng. Phytochemistry 62.7 (2003): 1087–1091.
Kuo SC et al. Antiplatelet components in Panax ginseng. Planta Med 56.2 (1990): 164–167.
Kwon YS et al. The effects of Korean red ginseng (ginseng radix rubra) on liver regeneration after partial hepatectomy in dogs. J Vet Sci 4.1 (2003): 83–92.

Larsen M et al. Ginseng modulates the immune response by induction of interleukin-12 production. APMIS 112.6 (2004): 369–373.

Le Gal M, Cathebras K. Pharmaton capsules in the treatment of functional fatigue: a double-blind study versus placebo evaluated by a new methodology. Phytother Res 10 (1996): 49–53.

Lee J. Panax ginseng induces human Type I collagen synthesis through activation of Smad signaling. J Ethnopharmacol 109.1 (2007): 29–34.

Lee ST. Panax ginseng enhances cognitive performance in Alzheimer disease. Alzheimer Dis Assoc Disord 22.3 (2008): 222–226.

Lee YJ, Shukla SD. Pro-and anti-apoptotic roles of c-Jun N-terminal kinase (JNK) in ethoanol and acetaldehyde exposed rat hepatocytes. European Journal of Pharmacology 508 (2007) 31–45.

Lee SP et al. Chronic intake of panax ginseng extract stabilizes sleep and wakefulness in food-deprived rats. Neurosci Lett 111.1–2 (1990): 217–221.

Lee HC et al. In vivo effects of Panax ginseng extracts on the cytochrome P450-dependent monooxygenase system in the liver of 2,3,7,8-tetrachlorodibenzo-p-dioxin-exposed guinea pig. Life Sci 71.7 (2002b): 759–769.

Lee Y et al. A ginsenoside-Rh1, a component of ginseng saponin, activates estrogen receptor in human breast carcinoma MCF-7 cells. J Steroid Biochem Mol Biol 84.4 (2003): 463–468.

Lee E-J et al. Ginsenoside Rg1 enhances CD4+T-cell activities and modulates Th1/Th2 differentiation. Int Immunopharmacol 4.2 (2004a): 235–244.

Lee J et al. Inhibition of Helicobacter pylori adhesion to human gastric adenocarcinoma epithelial cells by acidic polysaccharides from Artemisia capillaris and Panax ginseng. Planta Med 70.7 (2004b): 615–619.

Lee JS et al. Therapeutic effect of Korean red ginseng on inflammatory cytokines in rats with focal cerebral ischemia/reperfusion injury. Amer. J Chin Med. 39.1 (2011): 83–94.

Lee SH et al. Korean red ginseng (Panax ginseng) improves insulin sensitivity in high fat fed Sprague-Dawley rats. Phytother Res 26 (2012): 142–147.

Lei Y et al. Effects of extracts from Panax notoginseng and Panax ginseng fruit on vascular endothelial cell proliferation and migration in vitro. Chin J Integr Med 14.1 (2008): 37–41.

Liao B et al. Neuroprotective effects of ginseng total saponin and ginsenosides Rb1 and Rg1 on spinal cord neurons in vitro. Exp Neurol 173.2 (2002): 224–234.

Lim DS et al. Anti-septicaemic effect of polysaccharide from Panax ginseng by macrophage activation. J Infect 45.1 (2002a): 32–38.

Lim BV et al. Ginseng radix increases cell proliferation in dentate gyrus of rats with streptozotocin-induced diabetes. Biol Pharm Bull 25.12 (2002b): 1550–1554.

Liou C et al. Long-term oral administration of ginseng extract modulates humoral immune response and spleen cell functions. Am J Chin Med 33.4 (2005): 651–661.

Liu JW. Enhancement of fibrinolytic activity of bovine aortic endothelial cells by ginsenoside Rb2. Acta Pharmacol Sin 24.2 (2003): 102–108.

Liu W et al. Anti-proliferative effect of ginseng saponins on human prostate cancer cell line. Life Sci 67.11 (2000): 1297–1306.

Liu T et al. Improvement of insulin resistance by Panax ginseng in fructose-rich chow-fed rats. Horm Metab Res 37.3 (2005): 146–151.

Luo YM et al. Effects of ginseng root saponins and ginsenoside Rb1 on immunity in cold water swim stress mice and rats. Zhongguo Yao Li Xue Bao 14.5 (1993): 401–404.

Matsuda H et al. Promotion of hair growth by ginseng radix on cultured mouse vibrissal hair follicles. Phytother Res 17.7 (2003): 797–800.

Merino G et al. Ginseng increases intestinal elimination of albendazole sulfoxide in the rat. Comp Biochem Physiol C Toxicol Pharmacol 136.1 (2003): 9–15.

Min K et al. Effect of ginseng saponins on the recombinant serotonin type 3A receptor expressed in Xenopus oocytes: implication of possible application as an antiemetic. J Altern Complement Med 9.4 (2003): 505–510.

Mizumaki Y et al. Lipophilic fraction of Panax ginseng induces neuronal differentiation of PC12 cells and promotes neuronal survival of rat cortical neurons by protein kinase C dependent manner. Brain Res 950.1–2 (2002): 254–260.

Mochizuki M et al. Inhibitory effect of tumor metastasis in mice by saponins, ginsenoside-Rb2, 20(R)- and 20(S)-ginsenoside-Rg3, of red ginseng. Biol Pharm Bull 18.9 (1995): 1197–1202.

Murphy LL, Lee TJ. Ginseng, sex behavior, and nitric oxide. Ann N Y Acad Sci 962 (2002): 372–377.

Nagappan A et al. Comparative root protein profiles of Korean ginseng (Panax ginseng) and Indian ginseng (Withania somnifera). Am J Chin Med 40.1 (2012): 203–218.

Nakata H et al. Inhibitory effects of ginsenoside Rh2 on tumor growth in nude mice bearing human ovarian cancer cells. Jpn J Cancer Res 89.7 (1998): 733–740.

Nemmani KV, Ramarao P. Ginsenoside Rf potentiates U-50, 488H-induced analgesia and inhibits tolerance to its analgesia in mice. Life Sci 72.7 (2003): 759–768.

Nishino H et al. Cancer chemoprevention by ginseng in mouse liver and other organs. J Korean Med Sci 16 (Suppl) (2001): S66–S69.

Niu YP et al. Effects of ginsenosides Rg1 and Rb1 on proliferation of human marrow granulocyte-macrophage progenitor cells. Zhongguo Shi Yan Xue Ye Xue Za Zhi 9.2 (2001): 178–180.

Oh JI et al. Caspase-3-dependent protein kinase C delta activity is required for the progression of Ginsenoside-Rh2-induced apoptosis in SK-HEP-1 cells. Cancer Letters 230.2 (2005): 228–238.

Oyagi A et al. Protective effects of a gastrointestinal agent containing Korean red ginseng on gastric ulcer models in mice. BMC CAM 10 (2010): 45–54.

Panwar M et al. Evaluation of chemopreventive action and antimutagenic effect of the standardized Panax Ginseng extract, EFLA400 in Swiss albino mice. Phytother Res 19.1 (2005): 65–71.

Park IH et al. Cytotoxic dammarane glycosides from processed ginseng. Chem Pharm Bull (Tokyo) 50.4 (2002): 538–540.

Park KH et al. Possible role of ginsenoside Rb1 on regulation of rat liver triglycerides. Biol Pharm Bull 25.4 (2002): 457–460.

Park J et al. Anxiolytic-like effects of ginseng in the elevated plus-maze model: comparison of red ginseng and sun ginseng. Prog Neuropsychopharmacol Biol Psychiatry 29.6 (2005): 895–900.

Park S et al. Rescue of Helicobacter pylori-induced cytotoxicity by red ginseng. Dig Dis Sci 50.7 (2005): 1218–1227.

Park H et al. Panax ginseng increases hypoxia-induced down-regulated cellular response related genes in human neuroblastoma cells, SK-N-MC. Neurol Res 29 (Suppl 1) (2007): S78–S87.

Park ES et al. Korean red ginseng extract induces apoptosis and decreases telomerase activity in human leukemia cells. J Ethnopharm 121 (2009): 304–312.

Park HM et al. Korean red ginseng and its primary ginsenosides inhibit ethanol-induced oxidative injury by suppression of the MAPK pathway in TIB-73 cells. J Ethnopharm 141 (2012): 1071–1076.

Persson IA-L, Dong L, Persson K. Effect of Panax ginseng extract (G115) on angiotensin-converting enzyme (ACE) activity and nitric oxide (NO) production. J Ethnopharmacol 105.3 (2006): 321–325.

Persson J et al. The memory-enhancing effects of Ginseng and Ginkgo biloba in healthy volunteers. Psychopharmacology 172.4 (2004): 430–434.

Price A, Gazewood J. Korean red ginseng effective for treatment of erectile dysfunction. J Fam Pract 52.1 (2003): 20–21.

Qiao C et al. Ginseng enhances contextual fear conditioning and neurogenesis in rats. Neurosci Res 51.1 (2005): 31–38.

Radad K et al. Ginsenosides Rb1 and Rg1 effects on mesencephalic dopaminergic cells stressed with glutamate. Brain Res 1021.1 (2004): 41–53.

Rai D et al. Anti-stress effects of Ginkgo biloba and Panax ginseng: a comparative study. J Pharmacol Sci 93.4 (2003): 458–464.

Reay JL et al. The glycaemic effects of single doses of Panax ginseng in young healthy volunteers. Br J Nutr 96.4 (2006a): 639–642.

Reay JL et al. Effects of Panax ginseng, consumed with and without glucose, on blood glucose levels and cognitive performance during sustained 'mentally demanding' tasks. J Psychopharmacol 20.6 (2006b): 771–781.

Reay J et al. Single doses of Panax ginseng (G115) reduce blood glucose levels and improve cognitive performance during sustained mental activity. J Psychopharmacol 19.4 (2005): 357–365.

Rhee MY et al. Effect of Korean red ginseng on arterial stiffness in subjects with hypertension. J alt and comp med 17.1 (2011): 45–49.

Richter R et al. Three sesquiterpene hydrocarbons from the roots of Panax ginseng C.A. Meyer (Araliaceae). Phytochemistry 66.23 (2005): 2708–2713.

Rivera E et al. Ginseng extract in aluminium hydroxide adjuvanted vaccines improves the antibody response of pigs to porcine parvovirus and Erysipelothrix rhusiopathiae. Vet Immunol Immunopathol 91.1 (2003): 19–27.

Rosado MF. Thrombosis of a prosthetic aortic valve disclosing a hazardous interaction between warfarin and a commercial ginseng product. Cardiology 99.2 (2003): 111.

Ryu SJ, Chien YY. Ginseng-associated cerebral arteritis. Neurology 45.4 (1995): 829–830.

Ryu J et al. Free radical-scavenging activity of Korean red ginseng for erectile dysfunction in non-insulin-dependent diabetes mellitus rats. Urology 65.3 (2005): 611–615.

Sato K et al. Inhibition of tumor angiogenesis and metastasis by a saponin of Panax ginseng, ginsenoside-Rb2. Biol Pharm Bull 17.5 (1994): 635–639.

Scaglione F et al. Efficacy and safety of the standardised Ginseng extract G115 for potentiating vaccination against the influenza syndrome and protection against the common cold [corrected]. Drugs Exp Clin Res 22.2 (1996): 65–72.

Scholey AB, Kennedy DO. Acute, dose-dependent cognitive effects of Ginkgo biloba, Panax ginseng and their combination in healthy young volunteers: differential interactions with cognitive demand. Hum Psychopharmacol 17.1 (2002): 35–44.

See DM et al. In vitro effects of echinacea and ginseng on natural killer and antibody-dependent cell cytotoxicity in healthy subjects and chronic fatigue syndrome or acquired immunodeficiency syndrome patients. Immunopharmacology 35.3 (1997): 229–235.
Seely D et al. Safety and efficacy of panax ginseng during pregnancy and lactation. Can J Clin Pharmacol 15.1 (2008): e87–e94.
Shah ZA et al. Cerebroprotective effect of Korean ginseng tea against global and focal models of ischemia in rats. J Ethnopharmacol 101.1–3 (2005): 299–307.
Shibata S. Chemistry and cancer preventing activities of ginseng saponins and some related triterpenoid compounds. J Korean Med Sci 16 (Suppl) (2001): S28–S37.
Shin M. Enhancement of antitumor effects of paclitaxel (taxol) in combination with red ginseng acidic polysaccharide (RGAP). Planta Med 70.11 (2004): 1033–1038.
Shin JY et al. Immunostimulating effects of acidic polysaccharides extract of Panax ginseng on macrophage function. Immunopharmacol Immunotoxicol 24.3 (2002): 469–482.
Shin H et al. A further study on the inhibition of tumor growth and metastasis by red ginseng acidic polysaccharide (RGAP). Nat Prod Sci 10.6 (2004): 284–288.
Sievenpiper JL. Korean red ginseng rootlets decrease acute postprandial glycemia: results from sequential preparation- and dose-finding studies. J Am Coll Nutr 25.2 (2006): 100–107.
Sievenpiper J et al. Null and opposing effects of Asian ginseng (Panax ginseng C.A. Meyer) on acute glycemia: results of two acute dose escalation studies. J Am Coll Nutr 22.6 (2003): 524–532.
Sievenpiper J et al. Decreasing, null and increasing effects of eight popular types of ginseng on acute postprandial glycemic indices in healthy humans: the role of ginsenosides. J Am Coll Nutr 23.3 (2004): 248–258.
Smith M et al. An open trial of nifedipine-herb interactions: nifedipine with St. John's Wort, ginseng, or Ginkgo biloba. Clin Pharmacol Ther 69.2 (2001): 86.
Song JY et al. Induction of secretory and tumoricidal activities in peritoneal macrophages by ginsan. Int Immunopharmacol 2.7 (2002): 857–865.
Song JY et al. Radioprotective effects of ginsan, an immunomodulator. Radiat Res 159.6 (2003): 768–774.
Song Z et al. Ginseng modulates the immune response via its effect on cytokine production. Ugeskr Laeger 167.33 (2005): 3054–3056.
Sorensen H, Sonne J. A double-masked study of the effects of ginseng on cognitive functions. Curr Ther Res Clin Exp 57.12 (1996): 959–968.
Sotaniemi EA et al. Ginseng therapy in non-insulin-dependent diabetic patients: Effects of psychophysical performance, glucose homeostasis, serum lipids, serum aminoterminalpropeptide concentration, and body weight. Diabetes Care 18.10 (1995): 1373–1375.
Suh SO et al. Effects of red ginseng upon postoperative immunity and survival in patients with stage III gastric cancer. Am J Chin Med 30.4 (2002): 483–494.
Sung J et al. Effects of red ginseng upon vascular endothelial function in patients with essential hypertension. Am J Chin Med 28.2 (2000): 205–216.
Sung H et al. Korean red ginseng slows depletion of CD4 T cells in human immunodeficiency virus type 1-infected patients. Clin Diagn Lab Immunol 12.4 (2005): 497–501.
Sunram-Lea S et al. The effect of acute administration of 400 mg of Panax ginseng on cognitive performance and mood in healthy young volunteers. Curr Top Nutraceut Res 3.1 (2005): 65–74.
Surh YJ et al. Effects of selected ginsenosides on phorbol ester-induced expression of cyclooxygenase-2 and activation of NF-kappaB and ERK1/2 in mouse skin. Ann NY Acad Sci 973 (2002): 396–401.
Surh YJ et al. Molecular mechanisms underlying anti-tumor promoting activities of heat-processed Panax ginseng C.A. Meyer. J Korean Med Sci 16 (Suppl) (2001): S38–S41.
Tachikawa E, Kudo K. Proof of the mysterious efficacy of ginseng: basic and clinical trials: suppression of adrenal medullary function in vitro by ginseng. J Pharmacol Sci 95.2 (2004): 140–144.
Tachikawa E et al. In vitro inhibition of adrenal catecholamine secretion by steroidal metabolites of ginseng saponins. Biochem Pharmacol 66.11 (2003): 2213–2221.
Takeda A et al. Restoration of radiation injury by ginseng. I. Responses of X-irradiated mice to ginseng extract. J Radiat Res (Tokyo) 22.3 (1981): 323–335.
Tode T et al. Effect of Korean red ginseng on psychological functions in patients with severe climacteric syndromes. Int J Gynaecol Obstet 67.3 (1999): 169–174.
Tsai SC et al. Stimulation of the secretion of luteinizing hormone by ginsenoside-Rb1 in male rats. Chin J Physiol 46.1 (2003): 1–7.
Voces J et al. Ginseng administration protects skeletal msucle from oxidative stress induced by acute exercise in rats. Braz J Med Biol Res 37.12 (2004): 1863–1871.
Vuksan V et al. American ginseng (Panax quinquefolius L) reduces postprandial glycemia in nondiabetic subjects and subjects with type 2 diabetes mellitus. Arch Intern Med 160.7 (2000a): 1009–1013.
Vuksan V et al. American ginseng improves glycemia in individuals with normal glucose tolerance: effect of dose and time escalation. J Am Coll Nutr 19.6 (2000b): 738–744.
Vuksan V et al. Similar postprandial glycemic reductions with escalation of dose and administration time of American ginseng in type 2 diabetes. Diabetes Care 23.9 (2000c): 1221–1226.
Vuksan V et al. American ginseng (Panax quinquefolius L.) attenuates postprandial glycemia in a time-dependent but not dose-dependent manner in healthy individuals. Am J Clin Nutr 73.4 (2001a): 753–758.
Vuksan V et al. Konjac-Mannan and American ginsing: emerging alternative therapies for type 2 diabetes mellitus. J Am Coll Nutr 20.5 (Suppl) (2001b): 370S–380S.
Vuksan V et al. Korean red ginseng (Panax ginseng) improves glucose and insulin regulation in well-controlled, type 2 diabetes: results of a randomized, double-blind, placebo-controlled study of efficacy and safety. Nutr Metab Cardiovasc Dis 18.1 (2008): 46–56.
Waki I et al. Effects of a hypoglycemic component of ginseng radix on insulin biosynthesis in normal and diabetic animals. J Pharmacobiodyn 5.8 (1982): 547–554.
Wang SL et al. Modulation of expression of human GM-CSF and GM-CSFRalpha by total saponins of Panax ginseng. Sheng Li Xue Bao 55.4 (2003): 487–492.
Wang JW et al. [Synergistic effects of total saponins of panax ginseng in combination with hematopoietic growth factor on proliferation and differentiation of CD34(+) cells ex vivo]. Zhongguo Shi Yan Xue Ye Xue Za Zhi 14.5 (2006): 959–963.
Wiwanitkit V, Taungjararuwinai W. A case report of suspected ginseng allergy. Medscape Gen Med 6.3 (2004): 1–2.
Wu XG, Zhu DH, Li X. Anticarcinogenic effect of red ginseng on the development of liver cancer induced by diethylnitrosamine in rats. J Korean Med Sci 16 (Suppl) (2001): S61–S65.
Xia Z-Y et al. Ginsenosides compound (Shen-fu) attenuates gastrointestinal injury and inhibits inflammatory response after cardiopulmonary bypass in patients with congenital heart disease. J Thorac Cardiovasc Surg 130.2 (2005): 258–264.
Xie FY et al. Clinical observation on nasopharyngeal carcinoma treated with combined therapy of radiotherapy and ginseng polysaccharide injection. Zhongguo Zhong Xi Yi Jie He Za Zhi 21.5 (2001): 332–334.
Yamamoto M, Kumagai M. Anti-atherogenic action of Panax Ginseng in rats and in patients with hyperlipidemia. Planta Med 45 (1982): 149–166.
Yamamoto M et al. Serum HDL-cholesterol-increasing and fatty liver-improving actions of Panax ginseng in high cholesterol diet-fed rats with clinical effect on hyperlipidemia in man. Am J Chin Med 11.1–4 (1983): 96–101.
Yoo DG et al. Protective effect of Korean red ginseng extract on the infections by H1N1 and H3N2 influenza viruses in mice. J Med Food 15.10 (2012): 855–862.
Youl KH et al. Effects of ginseng ingestion on growth hormone, testosterone, cortisol, and insulin-like growth factor 1 responses to acute resistance exercise. J Strength Cond Res 16.2 (2002): 179–183.
Yu C et al. Lack of evidence for induction of CYP2B1, CYP3A23, and CYP1A2 gene expression by Panax ginseng and Panax quinquefolius extracts in adult rats and primary cultures of rat hepatocytes. Drug Metab Dispos 33.1 (2005): 19–22.
Yuan WX. Effects of ginseng root saponins on brain monoamines and serum corticosterone in heat-stressed mice. Zhongguo Yao Li Xue Bao 10.6 (1989): 492–496.
Yue PYK et al. The angio-suppressive effects of 20®- gensenoside Rg3. Biochem Pharm 72.4 (2006): 437–445.
Yun TK. Experimental and epidemiological evidence of the cancer-preventive effects of Panax ginseng C.A. Meyer. Nutr Rev 54.11 (Pt 2) (1996): S71–S81.
Yun TK. Experimental and epidemiological evidence on non-organ specific cancer preventive effect of Korean ginseng and identification of active compounds. Mutat Res 5234 (2003): 63–74.
Yun TK et al. Non-organ-specific preventative effect of long-term administration of Korean red ginseng extract on incidence of human cancers. J Med Food 13.3 (2010): 489–494.
Yun T-K, Choi SY. A case-control study of ginseng intake and cancer. Int J Epidemiol 19.4 (1990): 871–876.
Zeng H et al. Inhibitory effects of Radix ginseng rubra on cardiomyocyte apoptosis induce by ischemia and reperfusion in rats. Chin J Clin Rehab 8.9 (2004): 1784–1786.
Zhang L et al. Effect of ginseng polysaccharide compound on immunological function and quality of life in elder patients with advanced non-small cell lung cancer. Chin J Clin Rehab 8.5 (2004): 916–9117.
Zhou W et al. Molecular mechanisms and clinical applications of ginseng root for cardiovascular disease. Med Sci Monit 10.8 (2004): RA187–RA192.

Ginseng — Siberian

HISTORICAL NOTE Siberian ginseng has been used for over 2000 years, according to Chinese medical records, where it is referred to as ci wu jia. It was used to prevent colds and flu and to increase vitality and energy. In modern times, it has been used by Russian cosmonauts to improve alertness and energy and to aid in adaptation to the stresses of life in space. It also has been used as an ergogenic aid by Russian athletes before international competitions (Mills & Bone 2000) and after the Chernobyl accident to counteract the effects of radiation (Chevallier 1996).

Clinical note — Allostasis

Allostasis is the body's adaptation to stress. Allostatic (adaptive) systems are critical to survival and enable us to respond to changes in our physical (such as asleep, awake, standing, sitting, eating, exercising and infection) and psychological states (such as anticipation, fear, isolation, worry and lack of control). The consumption of tobacco, alcohol and our dietary choices also induces allostatic responses (McEwan 1998). These systems are complex and have broad boundaries, in contrast to the body's homeostatic systems (e.g. blood pH and body temperature), which are maintained within a narrow range.

Most commonly, allostatic responses involve the sympathetic nervous system and the hypothalamic-pituitary-adrenal (HPA) axis. Upon activation (e.g. when a challenge is perceived), catecholamines are released from nerves and the adrenal medulla, corticotrophin is secreted from the pituitary and cortisol is released from the adrenal cortex. Once the threat has passed (e.g. the environment is more comfortable or infection is controlled), the system is inactivated and levels of cortisol and catecholamine secretion return to baseline.

Chronic exposure to stress can lead to allostatic load, a situation resulting from chronic overactivity or underactivity of allostatic systems. The situation is characterised by maladaptive responses whereby systems become inefficient or do not turn off appropriately. Currently, there is much interest in understanding the association between numerous diseases such as cardiovascular disease and overwhelming allostatic load.

One measure that is used to gauge an individual's allostatic response is the cortisol response to a variety of stressors. As such, cortisol is seen as the classical 'stress' hormone.

OTHER NAMES

Ci wu jia, devil's bush, devil's shrub, eleuthero, eleutherococcus, eleuthero root, gokahi, ogap'I, russisk rod, taigawurzel, touch-me-not, wu jia pi

BOTANICAL NAME/FAMILY

Eleutherococcus senticosus (synonym: *Acanthopanax senticosus*) (family Araliaceae)

PLANT PART USED

Root, rhizome

CHEMICAL COMPONENTS

Glycosides (eleutherosides A–M, including saponins, coumarins, lignans, phenylpropanoids, oleanolic acids, triterpenes, betulinic acid and vitamins), steroid glycoside (eleutheroside A), lignans (syringin, sesamin, chlorigenic acid), glycans (eleutherans A–G), triterpenoid saponins (friedelin), saponin (protoprimulagenin A), hydroxycoumarin (isofraxidin), phenolics, polysaccharides, lignans, coumarins and resin.

Nutrients include magnesium 723 mcg/g, aluminium 188 mcg/g and manganese 37 mcg/g and vitamins A and E (*Eleutherococcus senticosus* 2006, Meacham et al 2002, Nissen 2003, Panossian et al 1999, Skidmore-Roth 2001).

MAIN ACTIONS

Adaptogenic (modulates stress response)

Siberian ginseng appears to alter the levels of different neurotransmitters and hormones involved in the stress response, chiefly at the HPA axis. Various mechanisms have been proposed, including inhibition of catechol-*O*-methyltransferase, which inactivates catecholamines (Gaffney et al 2001a). As a result, catecholamine levels are not depleted and release of new catecholamines from nerve synapses is decreased (Panossian et al 1999). In theory, this may reduce the risk of the organism's adaptive responses becoming depleted and moving into the exhaustion phase of the stress response. In addition, eleutherosides have been shown to improve carbohydrate metabolism and energy provision and increase the synthesis of protein and nucleic acids, although the direct molecular targets responsible for this adaptive response remain unknown (Panossian et al 1999). Eleutherosides have also been reported to bind to receptor sites for progestin, oestrogen, mineralocorticoids and glucocorticoids in vitro and therefore may theoretically exert numerous pharmacological actions important for the body's stress response (Pearce et al 1982).

Owing to such actions, herbalists and naturopaths describe the herb's overall action as 'adaptogenic'. The term 'adaptogen' describes substances that increase the ability of an organism to adapt to environmental factors and to avoid damage from such factors (Panossian et al 1999). The term 'allostasis' (see Clinical note) has been adopted in the medical arena to describe 'the ability to achieve stability through change'.

Although the mechanism of action responsible is still unclear, several theories have been proposed to explain the effect of Siberian ginseng on allostatic systems, largely based on the pharmacological actions observed in test tube and animal studies. Depending on the stage of the stress response, Siberian ginseng can act in different ways to support the 'stress system'. Research suggests that there is a threshold of stress below which the herb increases the stress response and above which it decreases the stress response (Gaffney et al 2001b). Therefore, for example, if allostatic load is such that responses have become inadequate, then the resulting increase in hormone levels would theoretically induce a more efficient response. Alternatively, situations of chronic overactivity, also due to allostatic load, would respond to Siberian ginseng in a different way, with negative-feedback systems being triggered to inactivate the stress response (Gaffney et al 2001a).

The dosing regimen may also be significant. While multidose administration in chronic stress engages the HPA axis, balancing the switch-on and switch-off responses, single doses (~4 mL) in acute stress trigger a rapid response from the sympatho-adrenal system, resulting in secretion of catecholamines, neuropeptides, adenosine triphosphate and nitric oxide (NO) (Panossian & Wagner 2005). Studies have demonstrated that maximal effects are achieved around 4 weeks but do not persist at the 8-week time point, which may help to explain the practice of giving Siberian ginseng for 6 weeks with a 2-week break before repeating.

Immunomodulation

Siberian ginseng appears to exert an immunomodulatory rather than just an immunosuppressive or stimulating action; however, evidence for the immune-enhancing effects of Siberian ginseng is contradictory. Clinical studies, in vitro and in vivo, have revealed stimulation of general non-specific resistance and an influence on T lymphocytes, natural killer (NK) cells and cytokines (Bohn et al 1987, Schmolz et al 2001), although other studies suggest that Siberian ginseng does not significantly stimulate the innate macrophage immune functions that influence cellular immune responses (Wang et al 2003). Alternatively, another in vitro study has demonstrated that activation of macrophages and NK cells does occur and may be responsible for inhibiting tumour metastasis both prophylactically and therapeutically (Yoon et al 2004).

The main constituents responsible appear to be lignans (sesamin, syringin) and polysaccharides, such as glycans, which demonstrate immunostimulant effects in vitro (Davydov & Krikorian 2000, Wagner et al 1984). Additionally, effects on the HPA axis will influence immune responses.

A liposoluble fraction from a crude extract of Siberian ginseng enhanced the forced swimming capacity of mice by decreasing muscle damage, effectively preventing the increase in blood urea nitrogen concentration and increasing fat utilisation (Huang et al 2010).

Antiviral

In vitro studies show a strong antiviral action, inhibiting the replication of ribonucleic acid-type viruses such as human rhinovirus, respiratory syncytial virus and influenza A virus (Glatthaar-Saalmuller et al 2001).

Anabolic activity

Syringin and other eleutherosides appear to improve carbohydrate metabolism and energy provision by increasing the formation of glucose-6-phosphate and activating glucogen transport (Panossian et al 1999), and Siberian ginseng extracts have been reported to improve the metabolism of lactic and pyruvic acids (Farnsworth et al 1985).

While initial animal studies showed promise for improving weight gain and increasing organ and muscle weight (Farnsworth et al 1985, Kaemmerer & Fink 1980), clinical studies confirming whether anabolic effects occur also in humans could not be located.

Anti-inflammatory

Excess production of NO is a characteristic of inflammation, and Siberian ginseng has been shown to significantly suppress NO production and inducible NO synthase (iNOS) gene expression in a dose-dependent manner (Lin et al 2008). The downregulation of iNOS expression may be the result of inhibition of intracellular peroxide production (Lin et al 2008) or through blocking c-Jun NH_2-terminal kinase (JNK) and Akt activation (Jung et al 2007). Cyanidin-3-*O*-(2″-xylosyl)-glucoside (C-3-*O*-(2″-xylosyl)-G), which was analysed as an active constituent from the fruit of Siberian ginseng, was shown to act by suppressing cyclooxygenase-2 expression and AP-1 and NF-κB transactivation and JNK, MAPKK3/6 and MEK/ERK1/2 phosphorylation (Jung et al 2013). *Acanthopanax senticosus* also exhibited significantly higher immunomodulatory activities against lymphocyte proliferation in vitro. It also demonstrated pronounced reductive power, strong hydroxyl radical-scavenging activity, moderate superoxide radicals and 2,2-diphenyl-1-picrylhydrazyl radical-scavenging activities. This however needs to be further explored for use in functional foods or medicine (Chen et al 2011).

Glycaemic control and insulin-sensitising effect

Animal studies have indicated a potential for hypoglycaemic effects when used intravenously. Syringin appears to enhance glucose utilisation (Niu et al 2008) and lower plasma glucose levels in animal experiments. The effect may be due to an increase in the release of acetylcholine from nerve terminals, stimulating muscarinic M_3 receptors in pancreatic cells to increase insulin release (Liu et al 2008). Syringin may also enhance the secretion of beta-endorphin from the adrenal medulla to stimulate peripheral micro-opioid receptors, resulting in a decrease of plasma glucose in insulin-depleted diabetic rats (Niu et al 2007).

Eleutherans A–G exert marked hypoglycaemic effects in normal and alloxan-induced hyperglycaemic mice (Hikino et al 1986), and eleutherosides show an insulin-like action in diabetic rats (Dardymov et al 1978). However, these effects have not been borne out in human studies (Farnsworth et al 1985). A glucose tolerance study in db/db mice orally administered *Acanthopanax senticosus* lowered plasma glucose levels more than the control group 30 minutes after sucrose loading, without affecting plasma insulin levels, and significantly inhibited α-glucosidase activity in the small-intestine mucosa (Watanabe et al 2010).

A small, double-blind, randomised, multiple, crossover study using 12 healthy participants actually showed an increase in postprandial plasma glucose at 90 and 120 minutes when 3 g Siberian ginseng was given orally 40 minutes before a 75-g oral glucose tolerance test (Sievenpiper et al 2004). More recently, oral administration of an aqueous extract of Siberian ginseng was shown to improve insulin sensitivity and delay the development of insulin resistance in rats (Liu et al 2005). As a result, further trials in people with impaired glucose tolerance and/or insulin resistance are warranted.

Hepatoprotective

Animal studies have demonstrated that an intravenous extract of Siberian ginseng decreased thioacetamide-induced liver toxicity when given before and after thioacetamide administration (Shen et al 1991). More recently, oral administration of aqueous extract and polysaccharide was found to attenuate fulminant hepatic failure induced by D-galactosamine/lipopolysaccharide in mice, reducing serum aspartate aminotransferase, alanine aminotransferase and tissue necrosis factor-alpha levels (Park et al 2004). The protective effect is thought to be due to the water-soluble polysaccharides. Coadministration of Siberian ginseng may also act to enhance the action of amtizole, improving the protective effect on hepatic antitoxic function and lipid metabolism (Kushnerova & Rakhmanin 2008). Diabetic rats treated with *Acanthopanax senticosus* plus metformin showed a more beneficial promotion for relieving the symptoms of diabetes and reversing liver and kidney damage to normal level than only metformin administration (Fu et al 2012).

Neuroprotective

Preliminary animal studies have suggested possible neuroprotective effects in transient middle cerebral artery occlusion in Sprague-Dawley rats. Infarct volume was reduced by 36.6% by inhibiting inflammation and microglial activation in brain ischaemia after intraperitoneal injection of a water extract of Siberian ginseng (Bu et al 2005). Similarly, intraperitoneal injection of Siberian ginseng was found to relieve damage to neurons following hippocampal ischaemia hypoxia and improve the learning and memory of rats with experimentally induced vascular dementia (Ge et al 2004). Siberian ginseng extract appears to protect against neuritic atrophy and cell death under amyloid beta treatment; the effect is thought to be due at least in part to eleutheroside B (Tohda et al 2008). The saponins present in Siberian ginseng have also been shown to protect against cortical neuron injury induced by anoxia/reoxygenation by inhibiting the release of NO and neuron apoptosis in vitro (Chen et al 2004).

Using a cerebral-ischaemic rat model, researchers demonstrated that an ethanolic extract of Siberian ginseng, given at the time of the ischaemic event and 90 minutes after, was protective against delayed neuronal cell death and also attenuated inflammatory markers, suggesting that some of the protective effect may be attributed to an anti-inflammatory effect (Lee et al 2012). In the Parkinson-induced mice model, oral administration of Siberian ginseng at low dose, 45 mg/kg, and high dose, 182 mg/kg, increased dopamine levels in the substantia nigra and enhanced coordination and motor function (Liu et al 2012). The researchers noted that more dopamine was present in the low-dose group (equivalent to 9 g/day for humans), suggesting that therapeutic effect is not necessarily a function of increasing dose.

In an in vitro depression model induced by stress hormone corticosterone, Siberian ginseng prolonged cell life and may account for the antidepressant effects reported in in vivo models (Wu et al 2013). And in sleep-deprived mice, treatment with eleutheroside E reduced the monoamines induced through sleep deprivation and restored their behaviour, suggesting that this component of Siberian ginseng could be valuable for the stress experienced from chronic sleeplessness (Huang et al 2011).

OTHER ACTIONS

Anticoagulant and antiplatelet effects

Animal studies have demonstrated prevention against thrombosis induced by immobilisation (Shakhmatov et al 2007), and the 3,4-dihydroxybenzoic acid constituent of Siberian ginseng has demonstrated antiplatelet activity in vivo (Yun-Choi et al 1987). A controlled trial using Siberian ginseng tincture for 20 days in 20 athletes detected a decrease in the blood coagulation potential and activity of the blood coagulation factors that are normally induced by intensive training of the athletes (Azizov 1997). Whether the effects also occur in non-athletes is unknown.

Antiallergic

In vitro studies demonstrate that Siberian ginseng has antiallergic properties in mast cell-mediated allergic reactions (Jeong et al 2001). The mechanism appears to involve inhibition of histamine, tumour necrosis factor-alpha and interleukin-6.

Antioxidant

Results using aqueous extracts of *Acanthopanax senticosus* indicated that it protects against oxidative stress which may be generated via the induction of Nrf2 and related antioxidant enzymes (Wang et al 2010). It was shown that *A. senticosus* orally administered to rats experienced significantly lower oxidative stress, as indicated by the expression of certain genes (Kim et al 2010).

Cardioprotective

Oral administration of Siberian ginseng (1 mL/kg) to rats for 8 days prevented stress-induced heart damage and chronic administration increased beta-endorphin levels and improved cardiac tolerance to D,L-isoproterenol and arrhythmia caused by adrenaline. The cardioprotective and antiarrhythmic effect may be related to an increase in endogenous opioid peptide levels (Maslov & Guzarova 2007). Benefits following a 45-minute coronary artery occlusion were not demonstrated in this study (Maslov & Guzarova 2007) but have been in studies using Siberian ginseng in a polypharmacy combination known as Tonizid (Lishmanov et al 2008).

Radioprotective

Animal studies have found that administration of Siberian ginseng prior to a lethal dose of radiation produced an 80% survival rate in mice (Miyanomae & Frindel 1988). Interestingly, α-difluoromethylornithine (DFMO), a chemotherapeutic drug which has a cytostatic effect, had a more pronounced effect than Siberian ginseng root tincture (SGRT) in radiation-induced carcinogenesis; however, in combination DFMO and SGRT increased survival rate and decreased frequency and multiplicity of malignant and benign tumours in irradiated rats (Bespalov et al 2013).

Vascular relaxant

In vitro studies have demonstrated vasorelaxant effects for Siberian ginseng. The effect is thought to be endothelium-dependent and mediated by NO and/or endothelium-derived hyperpolarising factor, depending on the size of the blood vessel. Other vasorelaxation pathways may also be involved (Kwan et al 2004).

CLINICAL USE

Due to its long history of use and myriad pharmacological actions, Siberian ginseng is used for many varied indications.

Stress

Siberian ginseng is widely used to treat individuals with nervous exhaustion or anxiety due to chronic exposure to stress or what is now termed 'allostatic load situations'. The biochemical effects on stress responses observed in experimental and human studies provide a theoretical basis for this indication (Abramova et al 1972, Gaffney et al 2001a).

G

One placebo-controlled study conducted over 6 weeks investigated the effects of an ethanolic extract of Siberian ginseng (8 mL/day, equivalent to 4 g/day dried root). In the study, active treatment resulted in increased cortisol levels, which may be consistent with animal research, suggesting a threshold of stress below which Siberian ginseng increases the stress response and above which it decreases the stress response (Gaffney et al 2001b). In a randomised, controlled study in 144 participants suffering from asthenia and reduced working capacity related to chronic stress, *Eleutherococcus senticosus* improved parameters over time and a significant difference was found in mental fatigue and restlessness, both in favour of *E. senticosus* versus 2-day professional stress management training (Schaffler et al 2013).

Fatigue

Siberian ginseng is used to improve physical and mental responses during convalescence or fatigue states. While traditional stimulants can produce a temporary increase in work capacity followed by a period of marked decrease, the initial increase in performance from adaptogens is followed by only a slight dip and performance remains above basal levels (Panossian et al 1999). The ability of Siberian ginseng to increase levels of noradrenaline, serotonin, adrenaline and cortisol provides a theoretical basis for its use in situations of fatigue. However, controlled studies are limited.

A randomised, double-blind, placebo-controlled trial of 300 mg/day (*E. senticosus* dry extract) for 8 weeks assessed health-related quality-of-life scores in 20 elderly people. Improvements were observed in social functioning after 4 weeks of therapy but did not persist to the 8-week time point. It would appear that improvements diminish with continued use (Cicero et al 2004), which may help to explain the practice of giving Siberian ginseng for 6 weeks with a 2-week break before repeating.

A randomised placebo-controlled trial evaluated the effectiveness of Siberian ginseng in chronic fatigue syndrome (CFS). No significant improvements were demonstrated overall; however, subgroup analysis showed improvements in fatigue severity and duration ($P < 0.05$) in CFS sufferers with less severe fatigue at 2-month follow-up (Hartz et al 2004). Further studies are required to determine whether Siberian ginseng may be a useful therapeutic option in cases of mild to moderate fatigue.

IN COMBINATION

A double-blind, placebo-controlled, randomised study of single-dose effects of a standardised fixed combination of *Rhodiola rosea, Schisandra chinensis* and *Eleutherococcus senticosus* extracts on mental performance, such as attention, speed and accuracy, in tired individuals performing stressful cognitive tasks showed that subjects gained improved attention and increased speed and accuracy during stressful cognitive tasks, in comparison to placebo (Aslanyan et al 2010).

Commission E approves the use of Siberian ginseng as a tonic in times of fatigue and debility, for declining capacity for work or concentration and during convalescence (Blumenthal et al 2000). In practice, it is often used in low doses in cases of fatigue due to chronic stress (Gaffney et al 2001a).

Cardioprotective

Due to its effects on vascular relaxation, stress response, anti-inflammatory and antioxidant activities, it is also believed to be a good tonic for the heart. Furthermore, a 2008 study shows that *Acanthopanax senticosus* significantly decreased serum low-density lipoprotein (LDL) (127.54 ± 29.79 mg/dL vs 110.33 ± 22.26 mg/dL) and the LDL/high-density lipoprotein ratio (2.40 ± 0.65 vs 2.11 ± 0.58) after supplementation in 40 postmenopausal women (Lee et al 2008).

Ergogenic aid

While initial animal studies showed promise for improving weight gain, increasing organ and muscle weight, improving the use of glycogen and metabolism of lactic and pyruvic acids (Farnsworth et al 1985, Wagner et al 1985), randomised controlled trials have produced inconsistent results in healthy individuals and athletes (Asano et al 1986, Dowling et al 1996, Eschbach et al 2000, Goulet & Dionne 2005, Kuo et al 2010, Mahady et al 2000). The evidence to date is inconsistent and further research is required to determine the potential role for Siberian ginseng in improving performance in sports.

In the mid-1980s, a Japanese controlled study conducted on six male athletes over 8 days showed that Siberian ginseng extract (2 mL twice daily) improved work capacity compared with a placebo (23.3 vs 7.5%) in male athletes, owing to increased oxygen uptake ($P < 0.01$). Time to exhaustion (stamina) also increased (16.3 vs 5.4%, $P < 0.005$) (Asano et al 1986). Other research however has failed to confirm these effects (Dowling et al 1996, Eschbach et al 2000).

A randomised, double-blind, crossover trial using a lower dose of 1200 mg/day Siberian ginseng for 7 days reported that treatment did not alter steady-state substrate use or 10-km cycling performance time (Eschbach et al 2000). Additionally, an 8-week, double-blind, placebo-controlled study involving 20 experienced distance runners failed to detect significant changes to heart rate, oxygen consumption, expired minute volume, respiratory exchange ratio, perceived exertion or serum lactate levels compared with placebo. Overall, both submaximal and maximal exercise performance were unchanged (Dowling et al 1996).

More recently, when recreationally trained males were treated for 8 weeks with *Eleutherococcus senticosus* supplementation there was marked enhancement in endurance time and elevated cardiovascular functions and this altered the metabolism of plasma free fatty acid and glucose after 8-week supplementation. This is the first well-controlled study that showed positive effects of Siberian ginseng on endurance exercise capacity in human clinical studies (Kuo et al 2010).

Siberian ginseng may however reduce blood coagulation factors induced by intensive training in athletes (Azizov 1997) and has been shown in combination with micronutrients to improve iron metabolism and immunological responsiveness in 39 high-grade unarmed self-defence sportsmen (Nasolodin et al 2006). Whether these effects also occur in other scenarios is yet to be established.

Siberian ginseng does not appear on the 2014 Prohibited List of the World Anti-doping Agency (WADA 2014).

Prevention of infection

Due to the herb's ability to directly and indirectly modulate immune responses, it is also used to increase resistance to infection. One double-blind study of 1000 Siberian factory workers supports this, reporting a 50% reduction in general illness and a 40% reduction in absenteeism over a 12-month period, following 30 days' administration of Siberian ginseng (Farnsworth et al 1985). More recently, a 6-month controlled trial in males and females with recurrent herpes infection found that Siberian ginseng (2 g/day) successfully reduced the frequency of infection by 50% (Williams 1995).

In practice, Siberian ginseng is generally used as a preventive medicine, as administration during acute infections is widely thought to increase the severity of the illness, although this has not been borne out in controlled studies using Siberian ginseng in combination with other herbs.

IN COMBINATION

A small randomised controlled trial demonstrated a significant reduction in the severity of familial Mediterranean fever in children using a combination of Siberian ginseng with licorice, andrographis and schisandra (Amaryan et al 2003), and a combination of Siberian ginseng with schisandra and rhodiola was found to expedite the recovery of patients with acute non-specific pneumonia (Narimanian et al 2005).

There is also clinical research conducted with an oral combination of Siberian ginseng and *Andrographis paniculata,* which is commonly known as Kan Jang, showing significant improvement of cold and flu symptoms (see Andrographis monograph for details).

Herpes simplex virus type 2 infection

Siberian ginseng (standardised to eleutheroside 0.3%) taken orally for 3 months reduced the severity, duration and frequency of genital herpes outbreaks; however more research is required before recommendations can be made about use (Ulbricht 2012).

Cancer therapy

A polypharmacy preparation known as AdMax, which contains *Eleutherococcus senticosus* in combination with *Leuzea carthamoides*, *Rhodiola rosea* and *Schizandra chinensis*, has been shown to boost suppressed immunity in patients with ovarian cancer who are subject to chemotherapy (Kormosh et al 2006). Which herb or combination of herbs is responsible for the effect is unclear.

OTHER USES

Given the herb's ability to increase levels of serotonin and noradrenaline in animal studies (Abramova et al 1972), a theoretical basis exists for the use of Siberian ginseng in depression.

In traditional Chinese medicine, Siberian ginseng is used to encourage the smooth flow of Qi and blood when obstructed, particularly in the elderly, and is viewed as a general tonic. It is therefore used for a myriad of indications, usually in combination with other herbal medicines. Numerous studies use Siberian ginseng in combination with other adaptogens, such as *Rhodiola rosea* and *Schisandra chinensis*, which may potentially act synergistically for improved effects.

Clinical note — Case reports of Siberian ginseng need careful consideration

Some adverse reactions attributed to Siberian ginseng have subsequently been found to be due to poor product quality, herbal substitution and/or interference with test results. For example, initial reports linking maternal ginseng use to neonatal androgenisation are now suspected to be due to substitution with another herb, *Periploca sepium* (called Wu jia or silk vine), as American herb companies importing Siberian ginseng from China have been known to be supplied with two or three species of *Periploca* (Awang 1991). Additionally, rat studies have failed to detect significant androgenic action (Awang 1991, Waller et al 1992) for Siberian ginseng.

Another example is the purported interaction between digoxin and Siberian ginseng, which was based on a single case report of a 74-year-old man found to have elevated digoxin levels for many years (McRae 1996). It was subsequently purported that the herbal product may have been adulterated with digitalis. Additionally, Siberian ginseng contains glycosides with structural similarities to digoxin that may modestly interfere with digoxin fluorescence polarisation (FPIA), microparticle enzyme (MEIA) results, falsely elevating digoxin values with FPIA and falsely lowering digoxin values with MEIA (Dasgupta & Reyes 2005). It should be noted that measuring free digoxin does not eliminate these modest interferences in serum digoxin measurement by the Digoxin III assay (Dasgupta et al 2008).

G

DOSAGE RANGE

- 1–4 g/day dried root or equivalent preparations.
- Fluid extract (1:2): 2–8 mL/day (15–55 mL/week).
- Tincture (1:5): 10–15 mL/day.
- Acute dosing: 4 mL in a single dose before activity.

Extracts with standardised levels of eleutheroside E (syringin) (>0.5 mg/mL) are recommended. Russian and Korean sources appear to have higher levels of this constituent. So, variations in therapeutic activity may be predicted (Wagner et al 1982). As there can be a significant product variability in the level of eleutherosides between capsules and liquids, standardisation may be necessary for quality assurance (Harkey et al 2001).

In practice, Siberian ginseng is often given for 6 weeks with a break of at least 2 weeks before resuming treatment.

ADVERSE REACTIONS

Clinical trials of 6 months' duration have shown no side effects from treatment (Bohn et al 1987). High doses may cause slight drowsiness, irritability, anxiety, mastalgia, palpitations or tachycardia, although these side effects may be more relevant to *Panax ginseng*.

SIGNIFICANT INTERACTIONS

As controlled studies are not available, interactions are currently speculative and based on evidence of pharmacological activity and case reports. Studies have reported that normal doses of Siberian ginseng are unlikely to affect drugs metabolised by CYP2D6 or CYP3A4 (Donovan et al 2003).

Anticoagulants

An in vivo study demonstrated that an isolated constituent in Siberian ginseng has anticoagulant activity (Yun-Choi et al 1987), and a clinical trial found a reduction in blood coagulation induced by intensive training in athletes (Azizov 1997). Whether these effects also occur in non-athletes is unknown. Given that a study looking at the concomitant application of Kan Jang (Siberian ginseng in combination with andrographis) and warfarin did not produce significant effects on the pharmacokinetics or pharmacodynamics of the drug (Hovhannisyan et al 2006), a negative clinical effect is unlikely.

Chemotherapy

An increased tolerance for chemotherapy and improved immune function has been demonstrated in women with breast (Kupin 1984, Kupin & Polevaia 1986) and ovarian (Kormosh et al 2006) cancer undergoing chemotherapy treatment. Caution — as coadministration may theoretically reduce drug effects. However, beneficial interaction may be possible under medical supervision.

> **CONTRAINDICATIONS AND PRECAUTIONS**
>
> Some authors suggest that high-dose Siberian ginseng should be avoided by those with cardiovascular disease or hypertension (blood pressure > 80/90 mmHg) (Mahady et al 2000). Others merely suggest a caution, as reports are largely unsubstantiated (Holford & Cass 2001). As such, it is recommended that people with hypertension should be monitored.

> ***Practice points/Patient counselling***
>
> - Siberian ginseng appears to alter the levels of different neurotransmitters and hormones involved in the stress response, chiefly at the HPA axis.
> - It is widely used to treat individuals with nervous exhaustion or anxiety due to chronic exposure to stress or what are now termed 'allostatic load situations'. It is also recommended during convalescence or fatigue to improve mental and physical responses.
> - Siberian ginseng may increase resistance to infection and has been shown to reduce frequency of genital herpes outbreaks with long-term use.
> - The herb is popular among athletes in the belief that endurance, performance and power may improve with its use, but clinical studies have produced inconsistent results.
> - It is not recommended for use in pregnancy, and people with hypertension should be monitored if using high doses.
> - In a study of elderly people with hypertension, 8 weeks of Siberian ginseng use did not affect blood pressure control (Cicero et al 2004).
> - Due to possible effects on glycaemic control (Sievenpiper et al 2004), care should be taken in people with diabetes until safety is established. Suspend use 1 week before major surgery.
> - Traditional contraindications include hormonal changes, excess energy states, fever, acute infection, concurrent use of other stimulants and prolonged use.

Diabetic medications

Claims that Siberian ginseng has hypoglycaemic effects are based on intravenous use in animal studies and not observed in humans, for whom oral intake may actually increase postprandial glycaemia (Sievenpiper et al 2004). Observe diabetic patients taking ginseng.

Influenza virus vaccine

Ginseng may reduce the risk of postvaccine reactions (Zykov & Protasova 1984), a possible beneficial interaction.

> 
>
> ***PREGNANCY USE***
>
> Insufficient reliable information is available, but the herb is not traditionally used in pregnancy.

PATIENTS' FAQs

What will this herb do for me?

Siberian ginseng affects many chemicals involved in switching on and off the body's stress responses. As such, it is used to improve wellbeing during times of chronic stress and enhance physical performance and recovery from exercise. The scientific research has yet to fully investigate its use in this regard; however, experimental findings suggest that the neuroprotective, anti-inflammatory and antioxidant properties of the herb may be responsible.

It may also boost immune function and reduce the frequency of genital herpes outbreaks. Evidence for improved performance in athletes is inconsistent so its role remains unclear.

When will it start to work?

Effects on stress levels should develop within 6 weeks, whereas immune responses develop within 30 days.

Are there any safety issues?

It should not be used in pregnancy, and high doses should be used with care by those with hypertension.

REFERENCES

Abramova ZI et al. Lek Sredstva Dal'nego Vostoka 11 (1972): 106–8. In: Mills S, Bone K. Principles and practices of phytotherapy. London: Churchill Livingstone, 2000.

Amaryan G et al. Double-blind, placebo-controlled, randomized, pilot clinical trial of ImmunoGuard(R): a standardized fixed combination of *Andrographis paniculata* Nees, with *Eleutherococcus senticosus* Maxim, *Schizandra chinensis* Bail. and *Glycyrrhiza glabra* L. extracts in patients with Familial Mediterranean Fever. Phytomedicine 10.4 (2003): 271–85.

Asano K et al. Planta Med 3 (1986): 175–7. In: Mills S, Bone K. Principles and practices of phytotherapy. London: Churchill Livingstone, 2000.

Aslanyan G et al. Double-blind, placebo-controlled, randomised study of single dose effects of ADAPT-232 on cognitive functions. Phytomedicine (2010) 17(7):494–9

Awang DVC. Maternal use of ginseng and neonatal androgenization (so-called Siberian ginseng is probably *Periploca sepium*, or silk vine) [Letter]. JAMA 266.3 (1991): 363.

Azizov AP. Effects of eleutherococcus, elton, leuzea, and leveton on the blood coagulation system during training in athletes. Eksp Klin Farmakol 60.5 (1997): 58–60 [in Russian].

Bespalov V.G et al. Comparative effects of difluoromethylornithine and Siberian ginseng root tincture on radiation-induced carcinogenesis in rats and their lifespan. Advances in Gerontology, Jan 2013, Volume 3, Issue 1, pp 70–76
Blumenthal M, et al (eds). Herbal medicine expanded commission E monographs. Austin, TX: Integrative Medicine Communications, 2000.
Bohn B, et al. Flow-cytometric studies with *Eleutherococcus senticosus* extract as an immunomodulatory agent. Arzneimittelforschung 37.10 (1987): 1193–6.
Bu Y et al. Siberian ginseng reduces infarct volume in transient focal cerebral ischaemia in Sprague-Dawley rats. Phytother Res 19.2 (2005): 167–9.
Chen Y, et al. Protective effect of *Acanthopanax senticosus* saponins on anoxia/reoxygenation injury of neuron. Chin J Clin Rehab 8.31 (2004): 6964–5.
Chen R et al. Antioxidant and immunobiological activity of water-soluble polysaccharide fractions purified from *Acanthopanax senticosus*. Food Chemistry (2011) 127(2):34–440
Chevallier A. The encyclopedia of medicinal plants. London: Dorling Kindersley, 1996.
Cicero AF et al. Effects of Siberian ginseng (*Eleutherococcus senticosus* Maxim.) on elderly quality of life: a randomized clinical trial. Arch Gerontol Geriatr 38 (Suppl 1) (2004): 69–73.
Dardymov IV, et al. Rastit Resur 14.1 (1978): 86–9. In: Mills S, Bone K. Principles and practices of phytotherapy. London: Churchill Livingstone, 2000.
Dasgupta A, Reyes MA. Effect of Brazilian, Indian, Siberian, Asian, and North American ginseng on serum digoxin measurement by immunoassays and binding of digoxin-like immunoreactive components of ginseng with Fab fragment of antidigoxin antibody (Digibind). Am J Clin Pathol 124.2 (2005): 229–236.
Dasgupta A, et al. Effect of Asian ginseng, Siberian ginseng, and Indian ayurvedic medicine Ashwagandha on serum digoxin measurement by Digoxin III, a new digoxin immunoassay. J Clin Lab Anal 22.4 (2008): 295–301.
Davydov M, Krikorian AD. *Eleutherococcus senticosus* Maxim as an adaptogen: a closer look. J Ethnopharmacol 72.3 (2000): 345–93.
Donovan JL et al. Siberian ginseng (*Eleutheroccus senticosus*) effects on CYP2D6 and CYP3A4 activity in normal volunteers. Drug Metab Dispos 31.5 (2003): 519–22.
Dowling EA et al. Effect of *Eleutherococcus senticosus* on submaximal and maximal exercise performance. Med Sci Sports Exerc 28.4 (1996): 482–9.
Eleutherococcus senticosus. Altern Med Rev 11.2 (2006): 151–155.
Eschbach LF et al. The effect of Siberian ginseng (*Eleutherococcus senticosus*) on substrate utilization and performance. Int J Sport Nutr Exerc Metab 10.4 (2000): 444–51.
Farnsworth NR et al. Siberian ginseng (Eleutherococcus senticosus): current status as an adaptogen. In: Farnsworth NR (ed). Economic and medicinal plant research, vol. 1. London: Academic Press, 1985, p 178.
Fu J et al 2012. Anti-diabetic activities of *Acanthopanax senticosus* polysaccharide (ASP) in combination with metformin. Int J Biological Macromolecules, Vol 50, Issue 3, 1 April 2012, Pages 619–623.
Gaffney BT, et al. *Panax ginseng* and *Eleutherococcus senticosus* may exaggerate an already existing biphasic response to stress via inhibition of enzymes which limit the binding of stress hormones to their receptors. Med Hypotheses 56.5 (2001a): 567–72.
Gaffney BT, et al. The effects of *Eleutherococcus senticosus* and *Panax ginseng* on steroidal hormone indices of stress and lymphocyte subset numbers in endurance athletes. Life Sci 70.4 (2001b): 431–2.
Ge X et al. Effects of *Acanthopanax senticosus* saponins against vascular dementia in rats. Chin J Clin Rehab 8.34 (2004): 7734–35.
Glatthaar-Saalmuller B, et al. Antiviral activity of an extract derived from roots of *Eleutherococcus senticosus*. Antiviral Res 50 (2001): 223–8.
Goulet ED, Dionne IJ. Assessment of the effects of *Eleutherococcus senticosus* on endurance performance. Int J Sport Nutr Exerc Metab 15.1 (2005): 75–83.
Harkey MR et al. Variability in commercial ginseng products: an analysis of 25 preparations. Am J Clin Nutr 73.6 (2001): 1101–6.
Hartz AJ et al. Randomized controlled trial of Siberian ginseng for chronic fatigue. Psychol Med 34.1 (2004): 51–61.
Hikino H et al. Isolation and hypoglycemic activity of eleutherans A, B, C, D, E, F, and G: glycans of *Eleutherococcus senticosus* roots. J Nat Prod 49.2 (1986): 293–7.
Holford P, Cass H. Natural highs. Piatkus (2001): 90.
Hovhannisyan AS et al. The effect of Kan Jang extract on the pharmacokinetics and pharmacodynamics of warfarin in rats. Phytomedicine 13.5 (2006): 318–23.
Huang LZ et al. (2010) Antifatigue activity of the liposoluble fraction from *Acanthopanax senticosus*. Phytother. Res., 25: 940–943.
Huang LZ et al. The effect of Eleutheroside E on behavioral alterations in murine sleep deprivation stress model. Eur J Pharmacol (2011) 658(2–3):150–5
Jeong HJ et al. Inhibitory effects of mast cell-mediated allergic reactions by cell cultured Siberian Ginseng. Immunopharmacol Immunotoxicol 23.1 (2001): 107–17.
Jung CH et al. *Eleutherococcus senticosus* extract attenuates LPS-induced iNOS expression through the inhibition of Akt and JNK pathways in murine macrophage. J Ethnopharmacol 113.1 (2007): 183–7.
Jung SK et al. Cyanidin-3-*O*-(2″-xylosyl)-glucoside, an anthocyanin from Siberian ginseng (*Acanthopanax senticosus*) fruits, inhibits UVB-induced COX-2 expression and AP-1 transactivation. Food Science and Biotechnology, April 2013, Volume 22, Issue 2, pp 507–513
Kaemmerer K, Fink J. Prakt Tierarzt 61.9 (1980): 748, 750–2, 754, 759–60. In: Mills S, Bone K (eds). Principles and practices of phytotherapy. London: Churchill Livingstone, 2000: 538.
Kim KJ et al. The effects of *Acanthopanax senticosus* on global hepatic gene expression in rats subjected to heat environmental stress. Toxicol (2010) 278 (2):217–223
Kormosh N, et al. Effect of a combination of extract from several plants on cell-mediated and humoral immunity of patients with advanced ovarian cancer. Phytother Res 20.5 (2006): 424–5.
Kuo J et al. The effect of eight weeks of supplementation with *Eleutherococcus senticosus* on endurance capacity and metabolism in human. Chinese Journal of Physiology 53(2): 105–111, 2010.
Kupin VJ. Eleutherococcus and other biologically active modifiers in oncology. Medexport, Moscow, 1984: 21. In: Lininger SW et al (eds). A-Z guide to drug-herb-vitamin interactions. Healthnotes, 1999.
Kupin VI, Polevaia EB. Stimulation of the immunological reactivity of cancer patients by Eleutherococcus extract. Vopr Onkol 32.7 (1986): 21–6 [in Russian].
Kushnerova NF, Rakhmanin Iu A. [The impact of nitric oxide intoxication on hepatic metabolic reactions and the prevention of lesions.] Gig Sanit 1 (2008): 70–3.
Kwan CY et al. Vascular effects of Siberian ginseng (*Eleutherococcus senticosus*): endothelium-dependent NO- and EDHF-mediated relaxation depending on vessel size. Naunyn Schmiedebergs Arch Pharmacol 369.5 (2004): 473–80.
Lee YJ et al. The effects of A. senticosus supplementation on serum lipid profiles, biomarkers of oxidative stress, and lymphocyte DNA damage in postmenopausal women. Biochem and Biophysical Res Comm (2008) 375(1):Pages 44–48
Lee D et al. Neuroprotective effects of *Eleutherococcus senticosus* bark on transient global cerebral ischemia in rats. J Ethnopharmacol (2012) 139(1):Pages 6–11
Lin QY et al. Inhibition of inducible nitric oxide synthase by *Acanthopanax senticosus* extract in RAW264.7 macrophages. J Ethnopharmacol 118.2 (2008): 231–6.
Lishmanov IuB et al. [Cardioprotective, inotropic, and anti-arrhythmia properties of a complex adaptogen "Tonizid"]. Eksp Klin Farmakol 71.3 (2008): 15–22.
Liu T et al. Improvement of insulin resistance by *Acanthopanax senticosus* root in fructose-rich chow-fed rats. Clin Exp Pharmacol Physiol 32.8 (2005): 649–54.
Liu KY et al. Release of acetylcholine by syringin, an active principle of *Eleutherococcus senticosus*, to raise insulin secretion in Wistar rats. Neurosci Lett 434.2 (2008): 195–9.
Liu SM et al. Protective effect of extract of *Acanthopanax senticosus* harms on dopaminergic neurons in Parkinson's disease mice. Phytomedicine (2012) 19(7):631–638
Mahady GB et al. Ginsengs: a review of safety and efficacy. Nutr Clin Care 3.2 (2000): 90.
Maslov LN, Guzarova NV. [Cardioprotective and antiarrhythmic properties of preparations from *Leuzea carthamoides*, *Aralia mandshurica*, and *Eleutherococcus senticosus*]. Eksp Klin Farmakol 70.6 (2007): 48–54.
McEwan BS. Seminars in medicine of the Beth Israel Deaconess Medical Center: protective and damaging effects of stress mediators. N Engl J Med 338.3 (1998): 171–9.
McRae S. Elevated serum digoxin levels in a patient taking digoxin and Siberian ginseng. CMAJ 155.3 (1996): 293–5.
Meacham S et al. Nutritional assessments for cancer patients can be improved when mineral concentrations in dietary supplements are considered during medical nutrition therapy consultations. J Nutr 132.11 (2002): 3547S.
Mills S, Bone K. Siberian ginseng, principles and practice of phytotherapy. UK: Churchill Livingstone, 2000, pp 534–41.
Miyanomae T, Frindel E. Radioprotection of hemopoiesis conferred by *Acanthopanax senticosus* Harms (Shigoka) administered before or after irradiation. Exp Hematol 16.9 (1988): 801–6.
Narimanian M et al. Impact of Chisan® (ADAPT-232) on the quality-of-life and its efficacy as an adjuvant in the treatment of acute non-specific pneumonia. Phytomedicine 12.10 (2005): 723–9.
Nasolodin VV et al. [Prevention of iron deficiencies in high-qualification athletes.] Gig Sanit 2 (2006): 44–7.
Nissen D (ed). Mosby's drug consult, St Louis: Mosby, 2003, pp. 17.
Niu HS et al. Increase of beta-endorphin secretion by syringin, an active principle of *Eleutherococcus senticosus*, to produce antihyperglycemic action in type 1-like diabetic rats. Horm Metab Res 39.12 (2007): 894–8.
Niu HS et al. Hypoglycemic effect of syringin from *Eleutherococcus senticosus* in streptozotocin-induced diabetic rats. Planta Med 74.2 (2008): 109–13.

Panossian A, Wagner H. Stimulating effect of adaptogens: an overview with particular reference to their efficacy following single dose administration. Phytother Res 19.10 (2005): 819–38.
Panossian A, et al. Plant adaptogens. III. Earlier and aspects and concepts on their mode of action. Phytomedicine 6.4 (1999): 287–300.
Park EJ et al. Water-soluble polysaccharide from *Eleutherococcus senticosus* stems attenuates fulminant hepatic failure induced by D-galactosamine and lipopolysaccharide in mice. Basic Clin Pharmacol Toxicol 94.6 (2004): 298–304.
Pearce PT et al. Panax ginseng and *Eleutherococcus senticosus* extracts: in vitro studies on binding to steroid receptors. Endocrinol Jpn 29.5 (1982): 567–73.
Schaffler K et al. 2013. No benefit adding *Eleutherococcus senticosus* to stress management training in stress-related fatigue/weakness, impaired work or concentration, a randomized controlled study. Pharmacopsychiatry. E-pub ahead of print Apr 2013.
Schmolz MW, et al. The synthesis of Rantes, G-CSF, IL-4, IL-5, IL-6, IL-12 and IL-13 in human whole-blood cultures is modulated by an extract from *Eleutherococcus senticosus* L. roots. Phytother Res 15.3 (2001): 268–70.
Shakhmatov II et al. [Effect of eleutherococcus on hemostasis in immobilized rats]. Eksp Klin Farmakol 70.2 (2007): 45–7.
Shen ML et al. Immunopharmacological effects of polysaccharides from *Acanthopanax senticosus* on experimental animals. Int J Immunopharmacol 13.5 (1991): 549–54.
Sievenpiper JL et al. Decreasing, null and increasing effects of eight popular types of ginseng on acute postprandial glycemic indices in healthy humans: the role of ginsenosides. J Am Coll Nutr 23.3 (2004): 248–58.
Skidmore-Roth L. Mosby's handbook of herbs and natural supplements. St Louis: Mosby, 2001.
Tohda C et al. Inhibitory effects of *Eleutherococcus senticosus* extracts on amyloid beta(25-35)-induced neuritic atrophy and synaptic loss. J Pharmacol Sci 107.3 (2008): 329–39.
Ulbricht C. Herpes: An Integrative Approach. Alternative and Complementary Therapies. October 2012, 18(5): 269–276
WADA. The World Anti-Doping Code. The 2014 prohibited list: international standard. World Anti Doping Agency (2014).
Wagner H et al. Die DC-and HPLC-analyse der Eleutherococcus Droge DC-and HPLC-analysis of Eleutherococcus. Planta Med 44.4 (1982): 193–8.
Wagner H et al. Immunostimulant action of polysaccharides (heteroglycans) from higher plants: preliminary communication. Arzneimittelforschung 34.6 (1984): 659–61 [in German].
Wagner H et al. Economic and medicinal plant research. London: Academic Press, 1985, pp 155–215.
Waller DP et al. Lack of androgenicity of Siberian ginseng (Siberian ginseng fails to cause sex differentiation disorder in rats) [Letter]. JAMA 267.17 (1992): 232.
Wang H et al. Asian and Siberian ginseng as a potential modulator of immune function: an in vitro cytokine study using mouse macrophages. Clin Chim Acta 327.1–2 (2003): 123–8.
Wang X et al. The protective effects of *Acanthopanax senticosus* Harms aqueous extracts against oxidative stress: Role of Nrf2 and antioxidant enzymes. J Ethanopharmacol Volume 127, Issue 2, 3 February 2010, Pages 424–432
Watanabe K et al. Fundamental studies on the inhibitory action of *Acanthopanax senticosus* Harms on glucose absorption. J Ethnopharmacology, Vol 132, Issue 1, 28 October 2010, Pages 193–199
Williams M. Immunoprotection against herpes simplex type II infection by eleutherococcus root extract. Int J Alt Complement Med 13 (1995): 9–12.
Wu F et al. Protective effects of aqueous extract from *Acanthopanax senticosus* against corticosterone-induced neurotoxicity in PC12. J Ethnopharmacol (2013) 148(3):861–868
Yoon T et al. Anti-metastatic activity of *Acanthopanax senticosus* extract and its possible immunological mechanism of action. J Ethnopharmacol 93.2–3 (2004): 247–53.
Yun-Choi HS et al. Potential inhibitors of platelet aggregation from plant sources, III (Part 3). J Nat Prod 50.6 (1987): 1059–64.
Zykov MP, Protasova SF. Prospects of immunostimulating vaccination against influenza including the use of Eleutherococcus and other preparations of plants. In: New data on Eleutherococcus: proceedings of the second international symposium on Eleutherococcus. Moscow, 1984: 164–9.

Globe artichoke

HISTORICAL NOTE Artichoke has a long history of use as a vegetable delicacy and medicinal agent, and its cultivation in Europe dates back to ancient Greece and Rome. It was domesticated in Roman times, possibly in Sicily, and spread by the Arabs during the early Middle Ages. Traditional use of artichoke has always pertained to the liver, where it is considered to increase bile flow and act as a protective agent against various toxins. As such, it has been used for jaundice, dyspepsia, nausea, gout, pruritus and urinary stones. It is still a popular medicine in Europe today.

COMMON NAME

Artichoke

OTHER NAMES

Alcachofa, artichaut, alcaucil, carciofo, cynara, cynarae folium (ESCOP 2009)

BOTANICAL NAME/FAMILY

Cynara cardunculus L., formerly *Cynara scolymus* L. (family Asteraceae) (WHO 2009)

PLANT PART USED

Leaf

CHEMICAL COMPONENTS

Key constituents of the leaf include phenolic acids, mainly caffeic acid derivatives (e.g. chlorogenic acid, cynarin), sesquiterpenes, lactones (e.g. cynaropicrin) and flavonoids (e.g. cynaroside, luteolin derivatives, anthocyanin), phytosterols, inulin and free luteolin.

MAIN ACTIONS

The main pharmacologically active constituents are thought to be the phenolic acids and flavonoids.

Antioxidant

Artichoke leaf extract (ALE) exerts antioxidant effects, according to in vitro and clinical studies (Juzyszyn et al 2010, Kusku-Kiraz et al 2010, Skarpanska-Stejnborn et al 2008, Speroni et al 2003). According to a double-blind trial, ALE (400 mg three times daily for 5 weeks) significantly elevates plasma total antioxidant capacity compared to placebo (Skarpanska-Stejnborn et al 2008). Even edible artichokes were able to protect hepatocytes from oxidative stress (Miccadei et al 2008). ALE significantly inhibited the oxidation of the mitochondrial respiratory chain complex I and II substrates (Juzyszyn et al 2010).

Hepatoprotective

The hepatoprotective action of *Cynara scolymus* is synonymous with its choleretic and antioxidant actions (Speroni et al 2003). As well as improving the synthesis and flow of bile (Saenz et al 2002, Speroni et al 2003) it can protect the bile canalicular membrane from chemically induced distortions (Gebhardt 2002b).

Tests with primary hepatocyte cultures and animal models support the suggestion that the hepatoprotective effect of globe artichoke may be due to its direct antioxidant action (Gebhardt 1997, Mehmetcik et al 2008, Miccadei et al 2008), as well as indirectly by increasing glutathione peroxidase by up to 39.5% in rat livers (Mehmetcik et al 2008).

Choleretic and cholagogue

Choleretic activity was reported in a randomised, double-blind, placebo-controlled study, with maximum effects on mean bile secretion observed 60 minutes after a single dose (Kirchhoff et al 1994). A significant increase in bile flow was also demonstrated in studies using isolated perfused rat liver in vivo after acute treatment, as well as after repeated administration (Saenz et al 2002).

A study that evaluated the choleretic and hepatoprotecive effects of four commercially available ALEs in terms of their cynarin, chlorogenic acid and caffeoyol derivatives content determined that the effect was dose-dependent: the extract with the highest concentration of phenolic derivatives exerted the strongest choleretic and antioxidant effects (Speroni et al 2003). However chlorogenic acid or cynarin alone did not exert a protective effect, suggesting a synergistic relationship between plant components and effects.

Lipid lowering

ALE inhibited cholesterol biosynthesis in primary cultured rat hepatocytes (Gebhardt 1998); indirect modulation of hydroxymethylglutaryl-CoA-reductase activity is the most likely inhibitory mechanism. When several known constituents were screened for activity, cynaroside, and particularly its aglycone, luteolin, were mainly responsible for the effect (Gebhardt 2002). Clinical studies have found that ALE compared to placebo causes a modest but statistically significant reduction in total cholesterol (Bundy et al 2008, Skarpanska-Stejnborn et al 2008, Wider et al 2009) and low-density lipoprotein (LDL) cholesterol (Wider et al 2009).

In addition, ALE lowered plasma cholesterol levels by a mechanism involving greater faecal excretion of neutral bile acids and sterols, an effect that was more pronounced in male compared to female hamsters (Qiang et al 2012).

OTHER ACTIONS

According to German Commission E, human studies have confirmed carminative, spasmolytic and antiemetic actions (Blumenthal et al 2000). The antispasmodic activity of some fractions and cynaropicrin, a sesquiterpene lactone from *Cynara* spp., has been confirmed in vivo (Emendorfer et al 2005).

Artichoke administration (500–1500 mg/kg) led to a significant decrease in postprandial glycaemia in normal and obese rats (Fantini et al 2011).

Studies with implications for atherosclerosis using artichoke leaf juice showed that it protected in vitro endothelial cells and improved brachial flow-mediated vasodilation, most likely by its antioxidant constituents (Juzyszyn et al 2008, Lupattelli et al 2004).

Fresh artichoke buds (115–125 g) were found to have an apoptotic effect in the human breast cancer cell line, oestrogen receptor-negative (MDA-MB231) (Mileo et al 2012). Previously, the artichoke buds were found to have an apoptotic effect in a human hepatoma cell line (HepG2) (Miccadei et al 2008).

Ten per cent fish oil and 1 g of artichoke leaves or heads administered for 25 days was protective against diethylnitrosamine-induced hepatocellular carcinoma in rats (Metwally et al 2011).

Pharmacokinetics

Studies further confirm the bioavailability of the metabolites of hydroxycinnamic acids after ingestion of cooked edible globe artichoke (Azzini et al 2007).

Cooked baby artichokes had higher total phenolics, caffeic acid, chlorogenic acid and cynarin content ($P < 0.05$) compared to cooked mature artichokes (Lutz et al 2011).

Clinical note — Inulin: a natural prebiotic

Inulin is a plant-derived carbohydrate that is not digested or absorbed in the small intestine, but is fermented in the colon by beneficial bacteria. It functions as a prebiotic, stimulating growth of bifidobacteria in the intestine, and has been associated with the enhanced function of the gastrointestinal system and immune system (Di Bartolomeo et al 2013, Lopez-Molina et al 2005). Increasing levels of beneficial bacteria, such as bifidobacteria, allow them to 'outcompete' potentially detrimental organisms and improve the health of the host. Inulin also increases calcium and magnesium absorption, influences blood glucose levels and reduces the levels of cholesterol and serum lipids. Globe artichoke contains 3% of fresh-weight inulin and smaller amounts are found in the leaves. According to animal studies, this concentration is sufficient to favourably affect the intestinal health (Goñi et al 2005).

CLINICAL USE

Treatment of digestive complaints (e.g. dyspepsia, feeling of fullness, flatulence, nausea, stomach ache and vomiting). Adjunct treatment of mild to moderate hypercholesterolaemia (WHO 2009).

Hyperlipidaemia

European Scientific Co-operative of Phytotherapy (ESCOP) approves the use of artichoke leaf as an adjunct to a low-fat diet in the treatment of mild to moderate hyperlipidaemia (ESCOP 2003, 2009).

Overall, evidence from five uncontrolled studies, case series and placebo-controlled trials suggests that ALE and cynarin have lipid-lowering effects and a possible role as adjunctive therapy in hyperlipidaemia (Ulbricht & Basch 2005).

Data are available from both controlled and uncontrolled studies that have investigated the effects of ALE in hyperlipidaemia. Most studies use Hepar SL forte (600 mg) or Valverde Artischocke bei Verdauungsbeschwerden (artichoke dry extract) containing 450 mg of herbal extract as a coated tablet.

A Cochrane systematic review that analysed the results of three studies concluded that ALE appears to have a modest positive effect on the levels of total cholesterol and LDL; however, the evidence is not compelling enough to recommend it as a treatment option for hypercholesterolaemia. The results from the two controlled studies suggest that patients with severely elevated total cholesterol levels at baseline might benefit more from ALE than those with moderately elevated levels (Wider et al 2009). One of the studies was a randomised, placebo-controlled, double-blind, multicentre trial involving 143 subjects with total cholesterol levels > 7.3 mmol/L (>280 g/dL) (Englisch et al 2000). A dose of 1800 mg ALE was administered daily for 6 weeks. Active treatment resulted in 18.5% decrease in serum cholesterol compared with 8.6% for placebo, a result that was significant. No differences were observed between the groups for blood levels of either high-density lipoprotein (HDL) or triglycerides. Although dietary habits were recorded, the food intake was not strictly controlled in the entire patient sample.

The second randomised, placebo-controlled, double-blind study involved 44 healthy volunteers and compared 1920 mg artichoke extract daily to placebo over a 12-week treatment period. No significant effects on serum cholesterol levels were observed in this study; however, subgroup analyses suggested that patients with higher initial total cholesterol levels experienced a significant reduction in total cholesterol levels compared to placebo (Petrowicz et al 1997, Wider et al 2009).

Two placebo-controlled clinical studies were published which further demonstrated modest but significant reductions in total cholesterol for ALE. Bundy et al (2008) conducted a 12-week, randomised study of 75 adults which found that treatment with artichoke leaf (1280 mg of a standardised extract, PE 4–6:1) significantly reduced plasma total cholesterol by an average of 4.2% (from 7.16 mmol/L [SD 0.62] to 6.86 mmol/L [SD 0.68]) compared with controls, although no significant differences were observed for LDL cholesterol, HDL cholesterol or triglyceride levels.

A smaller randomised, double-blind study of 22 volunteers found that oral ALE (400 mg three times daily) significantly reduced serum total cholesterol levels by the end of the 5-week study compared to placebo (Skarpanska-Stejnborn et al 2008).

In a randomised, double-blind, placebo-controlled clinical trial, 92 patients with mild hypercholesterolaemia (5.4–7.0 mmol/L) took two daily doses of 250 mg of standardised ALE for 8 weeks. The mean HDL cholesterol (HDL-C) significantly increased in the ALE group compared to the placebo group (primary outcome measure). The LDL:HDL ratio significantly improved in the supplemented group but not in the placebo group (Rondanelli et al 2013). It is postulated that chlorogenic acid in ALE may enhance the activity of paraxonase, an enzyme which prevents the oxidation of HDL-C.

Dyspepsia

The German Commission E approves artichoke leaf and preparations made from artichoke leaf as a choleretic agent for dyspeptic problems (Blumenthal et al 2000). ALE has been studied as a bile secretion stimulant and primarily recommended in this way for non-ulcer dyspepsia.

A double-blind, randomised, placebo-controlled trial of 247 patients with functional dyspepsia (persistent or recurrent pain or discomfort in the upper abdomen with one or more of the following symptoms: early satiety, postprandial fullness, bloating and nausea) found that treatment with two capsules of 320 mg ALE LI 220 (Hepar SL) taken three times daily significantly improved overall symptoms over the 6 weeks compared with placebo (Holtmann et al 2003). Additionally, active treatment significantly improved global quality of life (QOL) scores compared with the placebo.

A randomised, open study of 454 subjects investigated the efficacy of a low-dose ALE (320 mg or 640 mg daily) on amelioration of dyspeptic symptoms and improvement of QOL (Marakis et al 2002). Both doses achieved a significant reduction of all dyspeptic symptoms, with an average reduction of 40% in global dyspepsia score. Although no differences in primary outcome measures were reported between the two treatment groups, the higher dosage resulted in greater improvements in anxiety.

An uncontrolled study of 553 patients with nonspecific digestive disorders (dyspeptic discomfort, functional biliary colic and severe constipation) demonstrated a significant reduction of symptoms after 6 weeks of treatment with artichoke extract. Symptoms improved by an average of 70.5%, with strongest effects on vomiting (88.3%), nausea (82.4%), abdominal pain (76.2%), loss of appetite

(72.3%), constipation (71.0%), flatulence (68.2%) and fat intolerance (58.8%). In 85% of patients, the global therapeutic efficacy of artichoke extract was judged by the doctors as excellent or good (Fintelmann 1996).

Constipation

In a randomised, double-blind trial, 20 patients with constipation were given 180 g per day of artichoke alone or artichoke enriched with *Lactobacillus paracasei* (2×10^{10} colony-forming unit) for 15 days. The results showed that the Gastrointestinal Symptom Rating Scale for constipation was significantly lower in the probiotic-enriched artichoke group compared to the ordinary artichoke group (Riezzo et al 2012).

Appetite control and glycaemia reduction — in combination

A double-blind randomized controlled trial of 39 overweight patients compared placebo to 300 mg of standardised *Phaseolus vulgaris* (kidney bean) and 600 mg standardised *Cynara scolymus* flowering bud extract taken daily in three divided doses for 2 months. The participants were also placed on a concurrent hypocaloric diet. Active treatment resulted in a significant increase in the Haber's satiety scale in the treatment group compared to the placebo group (primary outcome measure). There was also a significant reduction in glycaemia (homeostasis model assessment [HOMA] and the quantitative insulin sensitivity check index [QUICKI]), indicating that *Phaseolus vulgaris* and *Cynara scolymus* may be useful in the treatment of overweight patients with dysglycaemia (Rondanelli et al 2011).

Hepatitis C

An open prospective study of 17 chronic hepatitis C patients administered 3200 mg of standardised ALE for 12 weeks found that no patients had alanine aminotransferase normalisation (primary outcome measure). Significant improvements in fatigue and joint pain occurred at week 4, but this improvement was lost at week 12. However, as the numbers in this study were small, the trial was of short duration and there was no control group, it is hard to draw meaningful clinical conclusions from this study (Huber et al 2009).

Irritable-bowel syndrome (IBS)

ALE appears to have substantial benefits in IBS, according to the available evidence; however, large controlled studies are required to confirm these observations. The antispasmodic and prebiotic activities of artichoke leaf are likely to contribute to the beneficial effects produced by this preparation.

A subgroup of patients with IBS symptoms was identified from a sample of subjects with dyspeptic syndrome who were being monitored for 6 weeks (Walker et al 2001). Analysis of the data revealed that 96% of patients rated ALE as better than or at least equal to previous therapies administered for their symptoms. Doctors also provided favourable reports on the effects of ALE in these patients.

In a study of 208 adults with IBS, changes in symptoms were observed before and after a 2-month intervention period (Bundy et al 2004). A significant reduction in the incidence of IBS by 26.4% and a significant shift in self-reported usual bowel pattern towards 'normal' were also reported after treatment. The Nepean Dyspepsia Index (NDI) total symptom score significantly decreased by 41% after treatment and there was a significant 20% improvement in the NDI total QOL score.

OTHER USES

Traditional uses include treatment for jaundice, dyspepsia, nausea, gout, pruritus and urinary stones. Due to its choleretic effect, it has also been used to improve fat digestion.

Wild artichoke significantly restores proper vasomotion after simulation of oxidative stress in rat models. This may have clinical significance for treatment in the elderly, where a progressive loss of vascular endothelial function and concurrent loss of vasomotor control are frequently seen (Rossoni et al 2005). The antioxidant activity of artichoke has been shown to offer a protective effect on gonads of cadmium-treated rats (Gurel et al 2007).

DOSAGE RANGE

- 1:2 liquid extract: 3–8 mL/day in divided doses.
- 6 g daily of dried cut leaves, pressed juice of the fresh plant or equivalent.

According to clinical studies

- Hyperlipidaemia: 4–9 g/day of dried leaves or 1800 mg/day of ALE.
- Dyspepsia: ALE 640 mg/day.
- IBS: ALE 640 mg/day.

ADVERSE REACTIONS

Studies with hyperlipidaemic subjects indicate that globe ALE is generally well tolerated. Mild symptoms of flatulence, hunger and weakness were reported in approximately 1% of subjects when the fresh plant was used (Fintelmann 1996). Contact dermatitis is possible with the fresh plant and urticaria–angio-oedema has been reported in one case of ingestion of raw and boiled herb (Mills & Bone 2005).

CONTRAINDICATIONS AND PRECAUTIONS

Not to be used by people with known allergy to globe artichoke or other members of the Asteraceae/Compositae family of plants.

Herbs with choleretic and cholagogue activities should be used with caution by people with bile duct obstruction (Blumenthal et al 2000), acute or severe hepatocellular disease (e.g. cirrhosis), septic cholecystitis, intestinal spasm or ileus, liver cancer or with unconjugated hyperbilirubinaemia (Mills & Bone 2005).

G

SIGNIFICANT INTERACTIONS

None known.

PREGNANCY USE

Safety has not been scientifically established for the leaf extract. Dietary intake is likely to be safe.

PATIENTS' FAQs

What will this herb do for me?

ALE effectively reduces symptoms in non-ulcer dyspepsia and possibly IBS. It also modestly reduces total cholesterol levels and improves digestion, flatulence and nausea.

When will it start to work?

Symptomatic relief in dyspepsia and IBS appears after 2–3 weeks of treatment; however, further improvements are possible with long-term use. A reduction in cholesterol may take 4–6 weeks and is best achieved when combined with a low-fat Mediterranean diet.

Are there any safety issues?

The extract is well tolerated with few side effects, but should not be used by people with known allergy to globe artichoke or other members of the Asteraceae/Compositae family of plants. It should be used with caution in bile duct obstruction, acute or severe hepatocellular disease (e.g. cirrhosis), septic cholecystitis, intestinal spasm or ileus, liver cancer or in people with unconjugated hyperbilirubinaemia.

Practice points/Patient counselling

- ALE has antioxidant, choleretic, apoptotic, diuretic, antispasmodic and lipid-lowering activity and hepatoprotective, hypoglycaemic, chemopreventive and antiemetic effects.
- According to controlled clinical trials, ALE has a modest but significant effect in lowering total cholesterol and LDL levels, and may increase HDL cholesterol levels. ESCOP recommends that a low-fat diet should also be undertaken when ALE is used for mild to moderate hyperlipidaemia.
- ALE is an effective symptomatic treatment for non-ulcer dyspepsia and shows promise for IBS.
- ALE may be beneficial in overweight patients with dysglycaemia.
- Include baby artichokes in your diet for optimal antioxidant activity and to improve beneficial bacteria in the gut.
- The extract is well tolerated, with few side effects, but should not be used by people with known allergy to globe artichoke or other members of the Asteraceae/Compositae family of plants. It should be used with caution in bile duct obstruction, acute or severe hepatocellular disease (e.g. cirrhosis), septic cholecystitis, intestinal spasm or ileus or liver cancer or in people with unconjugated hyperbilirubinaemia.

REFERENCES

Azzini E et al. Absorption and metabolism of bioactive molecules after oral consumption of cooked edible heads of *Cynara scolymus* L. (cultivar Violetto di Provenza) in human subjects: a pilot study. Br J Nutr 97.5 (2007): 963–969.

Blumenthal M, et al. (eds). Herbal medicine: expanded commission E monographs. Austin, TX: Integrative Medicine Communications, 2000, pp 10–113.

Bundy R et al. Artichoke leaf extract (*Cynara scolymus*) reduces plasma cholesterol in otherwise healthy hypercholesterolemic adults: a randomized, double blind placebo controlled trial. Phytomedicine 15.9 (2008): 668–675.

Di Bartolomeo, F., et al. 2013. Prebiotics to Fight Diseases: Reality or Fiction? Phytother Res. 27: 1457–1473.

Emendorfer F et al. Antispasmodic activity of fractions and cynaropicrin from *Cynara scolymus* on guinea-pig ileum. Biol Pharm Bull 28.5 (2005): 902–904.

Englisch W et al. Efficacy of Artichoke dry extract in patients with hyperlipoproteinemia. Arzneimittelforschung 50 (2000): 260–265.

European Scientific Co-operative On Phytomedicine (ESCOP). Cynarae folium. ESCOP Monographs, 2nd edn. Stuttgart: Thieme, 2003, pp. 118–126.

ESCOP 2009. ESCOP Monographs: The Scientific Foundation for Herbal Medicinal Products Supplement 2009, Stuttgart, Thieme.

Fantini, N., et al. 2011. Evidence of glycemia-lowering effect by a *Cynara scolymus* L. extract in normal and obese rats. Phytother Res, 25, 463–6.

Fintelmann V. Antidyspeptic and lipid-lowering effects of artichoke leaf extract: results of clinical studies into the efficacy and tolerance of Hepar-SL® forte involving 553 patients. J Gen Med 1996: 2: 3–19; as cited on Micromedex 27(Healthcare Series). Artichoke. Thomson 2006. Available at: www.micromedex.com (accessed 15-02-06).

Gebhardt R. Antioxidative and protective properties of extracts from leaves of the artichoke (*Cynara scolymus* L.) against hydroperoxide-induced oxidative stress in cultured rat hepatocytes. Toxicol Appl Pharmacol 144 (1997): 279–286.

Gebhardt R. Inhibition of cholesterol biosynthesis in primary cultured rat hepatocytes by artichoke (*Cynara scolymus* L.) extracts. J Pharmacol Exp Ther 286 (1998): 1122–1128.

Gebhardt R. Inhibition of cholesterol biosynthesis in HepG2 cells by artichoke extracts is reinforced by glucosidase pretreatment. Phytother Res 16 (2002): 368–372.

Goñi I et al. Artichoke (*Cynara scolymus* L.) modifies bacterial enzymatic activities and antioxidant status in rat cecum. Nutr Res 25.6 (2005): 607–615.

Gurel E et al. Effects of artichoke extract supplementation on gonads of cadmium-treated rats. Biol Trace Elem Res 119.1 (2007): 51–59.

Holtmann G et al. Efficacy of artichoke leaf extract in the treatment of patients with functional dyspepsia: a six-week placebo-controlled, double-blind, multicentre trial. Aliment Pharmacol Ther 18 (2003): 1099–1105.

Huber, R., et al. 2009. Artichoke leave extract for chronic hepatitis C — a pilot study. Phytomedicine, 16, 801–4.

Juzyszyn Z et al. The effect of artichoke (*Cynara scolymus* L.) extract on ROS generation in HUVEC cells. Phytother Res 22.9 (2008): 1159–1161.

Juzyszyn, Z., et al. 2010. The effect of artichoke (*Cynara scolymus* L.) extract on respiratory chain system activity in rat liver mitochondria. Phytother Res, 24 Suppl 2, S123–8.

Kirchhoff R et al. Increase in choleresis by means of artichoke extract. Phytomedicine 1994; 1: 107–15; as cited on Micromedex 27 (Healthcare Series). Artichoke. Thomson 2006, www.micromedex.com (accessed 15-02-06).

Kusku-Kiraz, Z., et al. 2010. Artichoke leaf extract reduces oxidative stress and lipoprotein dyshomeostasis in rats fed on high cholesterol diet. Phytother Res, 24, 565–70.

Lopez-Molina D et al. Molecular properties and prebiotic effect of inulin obtained from artichoke (*Cynara scolymus* L.). Phytochemistry 66 (2005): 1476–1484.

Lupattelli G et al. Artichoke juice improves endothelial function in hyperlipemia. Life Sci 76 (2004): 775–782.

Lutz, M., et al. 2011. Chemical composition and antioxidant properties of mature and baby artichokes (*Cynara scolymus* L.), raw and cooked. J Food Comp Anal, 24, 49–54.

Marakis G et al. Artichoke leaf extract reduces mild dyspepsia in an open study. Phytomedicine 9 (2002): 694–699.

Mehmetcik G et al. Effect of pretreatment with artichoke extract on carbon tetrachloride-induced liver injury and oxidative stress. Exp Toxicol Pathol 60.6 (2008): 475–480.
Metwally, N. S., et al. 2011. The protective effects of fish oil and artichoke on hepatocellular carcinoma in rats. Eur Rev Med Pharmacol Sci, 15, 1429–44.
Miccadei S et al. Antioxidative and apoptotic properties of polyphenolic extracts from edible part of artichoke (*Cynara scolymus* L.) on cultured rat hepatocytes and on human hepatoma cells. Nutr Cancer 60.2 (2008): 276–283.
Mileo, A. M., et al. 2012. Artichoke polyphenols induce apoptosis and decrease the invasive potential of the human breast cancer cell line MDA-MB231. J Cell Physiol, 227, 3301–9.
Mills S, Bone K. The essential guide to herbal safety. St Louis, MO: Churchill Livingstone, 2005, pp 437–9.
Petrowicz, O., et al. 1997. Efficacy of artichoke leaf extract (ALE) on lipoprotein metabolism in vitro and in vivo. Atherosclerosis, 129, 147.
Qiang, Z., et al. 2012. Artichoke extract lowered plasma cholesterol and increased fecal acids in Golden Syrian hamsters. Phytother Res, 26, 1048–52.
Riezzo, G., et al. 2012. Randomised clinical trial: efficacy of *Lactobacillus paracasei*-enriched artichokes in the treatment of patients with functional constipation — a double-blind, controlled, crossover study. Aliment Pharmacol Ther, 35, 441–50.
Rondanelli, M., et al. 2011. Appetite control and glycaemia reduction in overweight subjects treated with a combination of two highly standardized extracts from *Phaseolus vulgaris* and *Cynara scolymus*. Phytother Res, 25, 1275–1282.
Rondanelli, M., et al. 2013. Beneficial effects of artichoke leaf extract supplementation on increasing HDL-cholesterol in subjects with primary mild hypercholesterolaemia: a double-blind, randomized, placebo-controlled trial. Int J Food Sci Nutr, 64, 7–15.
Rossoni G et al. Wild artichoke prevents the age-associated loss of vasomotor function. J Agric Food Chem 53.26 (2005): 10291–10296.
Saenz RT et al. Choleretic activity and biliary elimination of lipids and bile acids induced by an artichoke leaf extract in rats. Phytomedicine 9 (2002): 687–693.
Skarpanska-Stejnborn A et al. The influence of supplementation with artichoke (*Cynara scolymus* L.) extract on selected redox parameters in rowers. Int J Sport Nutr Exerc Metab 18.3 (2008): 313–327.
Speroni E et al. Efficacy of different *Cynara scolymus* preparations on liver complaints. J Ethnopharmacol 86 (2003): 203–211.
Ulbricht CE, Basch EM. Natural standard herb and supplement reference. St Louis: Mosby, 2005, pp 29–33.
Walker AF, et al. Artichoke leaf extract reduces symptoms of irritable bowel syndrome in a post-marketing surveillance study. Phytother Res 15 (2001): 58–61.
WHO 2009. WHO monographs on selected medicinal plants. 2009 ed. Spain: World Health Organization.
Wider, B., et al. 2009. Artichoke leaf extract for treating hypercholesterolaemia. Cochrane Database Syst Rev, CD003335.

Glucosamine

OTHER NAMES

D-Glucosamine, amino monosaccharide, glucosamine sulfate, glucosamine hydrochloride, glucosamine hydroiodide, *N*-acetyl D-glucosamine, 2-amino-2-deoxy-beta-D-glucopyranose

BACKGROUND AND RELEVANT PHARMACOKINETICS

Glucosamine is a naturally occurring substance that is required for the production of proteoglycans, mucopolysaccharides and hyaluronic acid, which are substances that make up joint tissue, such as articular cartilage, tendons and synovial fluid. It is also a component of blood vessels, heart valves and mucus secretions (Kelly 1998).

Glucosamine sulfate is 90% absorbed after oral administration. The bioavailability is approximately 20% after first-pass metabolism (Aghazadeh-Habashi et al 2002). Unbound glucosamine is concentrated in the articular cartilage and the elimination half-life is 70 hours, with excretion as CO_2 in expired air, as well as by the kidneys and in faeces (Setnikar & Canali 1993). A study of the pharmacokinetics of glucosamine sulfate in humans found that it is rapidly absorbed after oral administration and its elimination half-life was tentatively estimated to average 15 hours, therefore supporting once-daily dosing (Persiani et al 2005). Twice-daily dosing with 500 mg of a time-release formula has also been shown to provide comparable serum levels after 24 hours as three divided doses of 500 mg (Basak et al 2004).

A further study suggests that glucosamine is bioavailable both systemically and at the joint, and that steady state concentrations in human plasma and synovial fluid were correlated and in line with levels deemed effective in in vitro studies (Persiani et al 2007). This is contrasted by the suggestion from a study of 18 people with osteoarthritis (OA) which found serum glucosamine levels were significantly less than those previously shown to have in vitro effects (Biggee et al 2006). Similar results were reported in an equine study that found levels attained in serum and synovial fluid were 500-fold lower than those reported to modify chondrocyte anabolic and catabolic activities in tissue and cell culture experiments (Laverty et al 2005).

It is interesting to note that co-adminstration of glucosamine and chondroitin has been observed to reduce plasma levels of glucosamine compared to administration of glucosamine alone (Jackson et al 2010). There is also some research being undertaken to improve the intestinal absorption of glucosamine, due to the large first pass effect. For example, one study found that glucosamine oral formulations containing chitosan (0.5% w/v) (QD-Glu solution and QD-Glu tablet) increased Cmax (2.8-fold) and AUC0-infinity (2.5-fold) of glucosamine (Qian et al 2013). Further pharmacokinetic studies in beagle dogs demonstrated that QD-Glu solution and QD-Glu tablets had higher relative bioavailabilities of 313% and 186%, compared to several other glucosamine products (Wellesse solution and Voltaflex tablet respectively).

CHEMICAL COMPONENTS

2-amino-2-deoxy-D-glucose

FOOD SOURCES

Glucosamine is present in chitin from the shells of prawns and other crustaceans. As a supplement, glucosamine is derived from marine exoskeletons or produced synthetically and is available in salt forms, including glucosamine sulfate, glucosamine hydrochloride, glucosamine hydroiodide and *N*-acetyl glucosamine. Glucosamine salts are likely to be completely ionised in the stomach, although clinical equivalence of the different salts has not been established. The purity and content of products has been questioned in the USA, where glucosamine is regarded as a food supplement and its quality was largely unregulated before GMP in 2010.

MAIN ACTIONS

Chondroprotective effect

Glucosamine is a primary substrate and stimulant of proteoglycan biosynthesis and inhibitor of proteoglycan degradation (Roman-Blas et al 2010). Glucosamine also stimulates synovial production of hyaluronic acid, a compound responsible for the lubricating and shock-absorbing properties of synovial fluid (McCarty 1998a, McCarty et al 2000) with the production of hyaluronic acid being higher in synovial cells than chondrocytes (Nagaoka et al 2012). Glucosamine also causes a statistically significant stimulation of proteoglycan production by chondrocytes from human osteoarthritic cartilage culture (Bassleer et al 1998) and modifies cultured OA chondrocyte metabolism by acting on protein kinase C, cellular phospholipase A_2, protein synthesis and possibly collagenase activation (Piperno et al 2000).

In animal models of OA, glucosamine has demonstrated limited site-specific, partial disease-modifying effects (Tiraloche et al 2005) which have been attributed to the inhibition of the cytokine intracellular signalling pathways and reversal of the proinflammatory and joint-degenerating effects of IL-1 (Roman-Blas et al 2010). In rabbits, *N*-acetyl glucosamine has been found to produce proliferation of matured cartilaginous tissues and matured cartilage substrate in experimentally produced cartilaginous injuries (Tamai et al 2003) and partially reverse structural effects of OA, restoring cartilage thickness to that of healthy joints and preventing superficial fibrillation (López et al 2013). In another animal model, co-administration with chondroitin was seen to prevent both biochemical and histological alterations and provide pain reduction (Silva et al 2009). Glucosamine is also reported to induce osteoblastic cell differentiation and suppress the osteoclastic cell differentiation, thereby increasing bone matrix deposition and decreasing bone resorption to modulate bone metabolism in OA (Nagaoka et al 2012).

An in vitro study using bovine chondrocytes suggested that the experimental effects of glucosamine were sensitive to the model, dose and length of treatment (de Mattei et al 2002). In another in vitro study, exogenous glucosamine was found not to stimulate chondroitin sulfate synthesis in human chondrocytes and the capacity to form glucosamine from glucose was estimated to be far in excess of the levels achievable through oral administration (Mroz & Silbert 2004). In human trials, glucosamine is suspected of reducing joint loading with decreased serum cartilage oligomeric matrix protein observed over a 12-week physical training period (Petersen et al 2010). Glucosamine, however, had no effect on type 2 collagen fragment levels in serum or urine in a 6-month RCT of 137 subjects with OA of the knee (Cibere et al 2005).

Part of the chondroprotective action of glucosamine sulfate is due to the provision of a source of additional inorganic sulfur, which is essential for glycosaminoglycan (GAG) synthesis as well as being a structural component of glutathione and other key enzymes, coenzymes and metabolites that play fundamental roles in cellular homeostasis and control of inflammation (Nimni & Cordoba 2006).

Anti-inflammatory

A number of in vitro and in vivo tests have identified anti-inflammatory activity for glucosamine (Nagaoka et al 2011). Anti-inflammatory and chondroprotective activities have been observed in human OA cartilage (Sumantran et al 2008). In vitro studies have found that glucosamine sulphate exerts anti-inflammatory effects by altering production of TNF-alpha, interleukins and prostaglandin E_2 in macrophage cells (Kim et al 2007), as well as suppression of mast cell activation (Sakai et al 2010).

Glucosamine restores proteoglycan synthesis and prevents the production of inflammatory mediators induced by the cytokine IL-1-beta in rat articular chondrocytes according to in vitro research (Gouze et al 2001). Glucosamine sulfate and *N*-acetyl glucosamine have also been found to inhibit IL-1-beta- and TNF-alpha-induced NO production in normal human articular chondrocytes (Shikhman et al 2001) and it is suggested that the anti-IL-1beta effect of glucosamine is accomplished by suppression of NF-κB activation. It is further suggested that glucosamine sulfate inhibits IL-1beta-stimulated gene expression of COX-2, inducible nitric oxide synthase, cytokines and metalloproteinases at concentrations found in human plasma and synovial fluid after administration of glucosamine sulfate standard oral doses (Roman-Blas 2010). It is further reported that glucosamine has epigenetic effects and can prevent cytokine-induced demethylation of a specific CpG site in the IL-1-beta promoter which is associated with decreased expression of IL-1-beta (Imagawa et al 2011).

Glucosamine demonstrates an ability to suppress PGE_2 production and partly suppress NO production in chondrocytes in vitro (Mello et al 2004, Nakamura et al 2004) and to suppress the production of matrix metalloproteases in normal chondrocytes and synoviocytes (Nakamura et al 2004). Glucosamine is further reported to exert an anti-inflammatory action through suppression of neutrophil function such as superoxide generation, phagocytosis, granule enzyme release and chemotaxis (Hua et al 2002).

Glucose metabolism

Exogenous glucosamine is actively taken up by cells. Its entry into cells is stimulated by insulin and involves the glucose transporter system (Pouwels et al 2001); however, the affinity of glucosamine for these transporters is substantially lower than that of glucose (Nelson et al 2000).

Early preliminary evidence suggested that glucosamine may cause changes in glucose metabolism and insulin secretion similar to those seen in type 2 diabetes in both rats (Balkan & Dunning 1994, Giaccari et al 1995, Lippiello et al 2000, Shankar et al 1998) and humans (Monauni et al 2000); however, these findings have been disputed (Echard et al 2001). In the 10 years following the original research, most clinical trial evidence has failed to find any significant effect on glucose metabolism in humans (Anderson et al 2005, Tannis et al 2004, Onigbinde et al 2011). It is suggested, however, that there could be some effect in people with impaired glucose tolerance or insulin resistance (Dostrovsky et al 2011).

Gastrointestinal protection

Glycoproteins are important in protecting the bowel mucosa from damage, and the breakdown of glycosaminoglycans is an important consequence of inflammation of mucosal surfaces (Salvatore et al 2000). Abnormalities in colonic glycoprotein synthesis have been implicated in the pathogenesis of ulcerative colitis and Crohn's disease (Burton & Anderson 1983, Winslet et al 1994).

OTHER ACTIONS

Glucosamine might have some activity against HIV. Preliminary evidence shows that it inhibits intracellular viral movement and blocks viral replication (Bagasra et al 1991). Other studies have found that glucosamine has immunosuppressive properties and can prolong graft survival in mice (Ma et al 2002). Oral, intraperitoneal and intravenously administered glucosamine significantly reduces CNS inflammation and demyelination in an animal model of multiple sclerosis (Zhang et al 2005).

CLINICAL USE

Osteoarthritis

There is very good evidence to suggest that glucosamine sulphate is effective in treating the symptoms of OA, in particular moderate severity OA, as well as slowing disease progression as per studies mainly investigating knee OA. This is further supported by studies with animal models that unequivocally confirm glucosamine has anti-inflammatory and disease modifying effects.

While there have been some inconsistencies in human studies, reviews of clinical trials generally confirm the efficacy of glucosamine sulphate in providing pain relief from OA whereas studies investigating glucosamine hydrochloride tend to produce inconsistent results (Black et al 2009, Bruyere & Reginster 2007, Chan and Ng 2011, Fox & Stephens 2009, Henrotin et al 2012, Kwoh et al 2013, Miller & Clegg 2011, Provenza et al 2014, Reginster et al 2007, 2012, Vangsness et al 2009, Wandel et al 2010, Wu et al 2013). Benefits appear most consistent when glucosamine sulfate is taken together with chondroitin sulfate long term.

> ***Clinical note***
>
> In 2014, the European Society for Clinical and Economic Aspects of Osteoporosis and Osteoarthritis (ESCEO) gathered an international task force of 13 members to determine clinical management of patients with OA. They concluded that the first step for patients with OA and pain is to use either glucosamine sulfate +/− chondroitin sulphate or paracetamol on a regular basis, while NSAIDS should only be used as an advanced step, if response is not adequate. They recommended that the safer, more sensible approach is not to use paracetamol due to its side effects and questionable efficacy on pain with chronic use, but to recommend chronic symptomatic slow-acting drugs for osteoarthritis such as glucosamine sulphate (Bruyere et al 2014). Interestingly, they noted that US groups are reluctant to recommend dietary supplements due to quality issues, whereas there is less concern in Europe as pharmaceutical grade preparations are used.

One explanation for the inconsistent results could relate to dosing. Pharmacokinetic studies have shown that glucosamine is easily absorbed, but the current treatment doses (1500 mg/day) barely reach the required therapeutic concentration in plasma and tissue. Therefore, it is likely that many patients, in particular obese patients, are being under-dosed at the current tested concentrations (Aghazadeh-Habashi & Jamali 2011, Henrotin et al 2012). Other reasons for some of the inconsistent results include: inconsistency in the chemical potency of some products used as well as variable and erratic bioavailability indices. Some support for a higher dose was recently obtained via a 12-week randomised study that showed 3000 mg/day of glucosamine sulphate provided effective symptom relief in knee OA. All outcome measures (WOMAC and Lequesne algofunctional indices) were significantly improved (Coulson et al 2013).

Compared to standard treatments

Several clinical studies indicate that glucosamine is at least as effective as NSAIDs in treating the symptoms of OA however the effect takes longer to be established (approximately 2–6 weeks) (Herrero-Beaumont et al 2007, Muller-Fassbender et al 1994, Reichelt et al 1994, Rovati 1992, Ruane & Griffiths 2002). In addition, a double-blind, random controlled trial (RCT) involving 318 people with moderately severe knee OA showed that more people responded to daily glucosamine sulphate (1500 mg/day) than paracetamol (3 gm/day) or placebo over

6 months, as seen by improvements to the Lequesne score (Herrero-Beaumont et al 2007).

The first Cochrane systematic review was published in 2003 and analysed results from 16 RCTs testing glucosamine for OA. It concluded that 'there is good evidence that glucosamine is both effective and safe in treating OA' and that 'glucosamine therapy may indeed represent a significant breakthrough in the pharmacological management of OA' (Towheed et al 2003). The most recent Cochrane review (updated in 2008) looked at 20 studies involving a total of 2570 patients and found that the Rottapharm glucosamine sulfate preparation was superior to placebo in the treatment of pain and functional impairment, whereas studies using non-Rottapharm glucosamine hydrochloride preparations failed to show benefit in pain and function (Towheed et al 2006).

The first placebo-controlled clinical trials investigating glucosamine in OA were published in the early 1980s. Drovanti et al (1980) showed that a dose of 1500 mg glucosamine sulfate significantly reduced symptoms of OA, almost twice as effectively and twice as fast as placebo. Perhaps the most exciting results were found when electron microscopy analysis of cartilage showed that those people taking glucosamine sulfate had cartilage more similar to healthy joints than the placebo group. Based on this finding, researchers suggested that glucosamine sulfate had not only provided symptom relief but also had the potential to induce rebuilding of the damaged cartilage.

Since that time, multiple human clinical trials lasting from a few weeks (Coulson et al 2013, Crolle & D'Este 1980, Drovanti et al 1980, Lopes Vaz 1982, McAlindon 2001, Pujalte et al 1980, Qiu et al 1998) to 3 years (Pavelka et al 2002, Reginster et al 2001), as well as systematic reviews (Poolsup et al 2005, Towheed et al 2003, 2006) and meta-analyses (McAlindon et al 2000, Richy et al 2003) have shown that glucosamine sulfate (1500 mg/day) can significantly improve symptoms of pain and functionality measures in patients with OA of the knee, with side effects comparable to those of placebo. This is not to say that all studies have produced positive results for symptom relief in OA.

Probably the most well-known study showing 'apparent' negative results was published in 2005 after the National Institutes of Health (NIH) spent US$14 million on a Glucosamine hydrochloride and Chondroitin Arthritis Intervention Trial (GAIT). The 24-week, placebo-controlled, parallel, double-blind, five-arm trial involving 1583 patients aimed to answer the question as to whether glucosamine hydrochloride and/or chondroitin was more effective than placebo or the COX-2 inhibitor celecoxib for symptom relief (Clegg et al 2006, NIH 2002). The results of this study provide evidence that glucosamine hydrochloride and chondroitin are more effective when given in combination than when either substance is given alone and that combined treatment with glucosamine hydrochloride and chondroitin is more effective than celecoxib for treating moderate-to-severe, but not mild, arthritis. Furthermore, the combined treatment was significantly better than placebo for patients with either mild or moderate-to-severe disease when the internationally accepted Outcome Measures in Rheumatology-Osteoarthritis Research Society International (OMERACT-OARSI) response criteria for judging clinical trials of OA was used (Clegg et al 2006). A 2-year sub-study however, found no clinically important differences in symptoms or function with any treatments compared to placebo (Sawitzke et al 2010) and no reductions in joint space narrowing, although there was a trend for improvement in knees with Kellgren and Lawrence (K/L) grade 2 radiographic OA. The authors acknowledge that the statistical power of this 2-year follow-up study was diminished by the limited sample size, variance of joint space width measurements and a smaller than expected loss in joint space (Sawitzke et al 2008).

The design and overall inconclusive results of the GAIT trial have been strongly criticised for the fact that the trial included a large number of people with very mild disease at baseline who were more likely to be susceptible to placebo (as evidenced by the very high (60%) placebo response) and who were given ready access to rescue medication. Furthermore, the unusually high 50% drop-out rate at 2 years meant that the structural study was underpowered. The use of intention-to-treat rather than an according-to-protocol analysis further compromised the ability to detect any significant differences (Pelletier et al 2010).

Long-term use

A meta-analysis of six studies involving 1052 cases suggests that daily administration of glucosamine sulfate delays radiological progression of OA of the knee after 3 years (Lee et al 2010). A small to moderate protective effect on minimum joint space narrowing ($P < 0.001$) was observed after long-term use, but not yet apparent after the first 12 months. This was further confirmed in a more recent 2013 meta-analysis of 19 RCTs ($n = 3159$) which identified that long-term use (over 6 months) of glucosamine sulphate exerts disease-modifying effects in OA (Wu et al 2013).

The first of these long term structural studies was performed by Reginster et al (2000) and compared the effects of 1500 mg glucosamine sulfate with placebo daily over 3 years in 212 patients aged over 50 years with primary knee OA. This was heralded as a landmark study at the time because it not only detected modest symptom-relieving effects, but also was the first to identify significant joint-preserving activity with long-term use. Two years later, Pavelka et al confirmed these results in another randomised, double-blind study that involved 202 patients with knee OA (Pavelka et al 2002) and once again observed that long-term treatment with glucosamine sulfate retarded disease progression. A post hoc analysis of these studies found that the disease-modifying effect was evident in 319 postmenopausal women (Bruyere et al 2004) and another sub-analysis found that patients with less severe radiographic knee OA, who are likely to experience the most dramatic disease progression, may be particularly responsive to treatment with glucosamine (Bruyere et al 2003). A 1-year trial involving 104 subjects with OA of the hands, hip and knee also found that treatment with both glucosamine and chondroitin reduced pain and significantly slowed disease progression as measured by radiographs and measures of urinary C-terminal cross-linking telopeptides of type I collagen (Scarpellini et al 2008).

A recent 2-year double blind RCT with 605 participants that compared glucosamine sulfate (1500 mg/day) with or without chondroitin sulfate (1200 mg/day) to placebo, found that while those in the combination group experienced significant reduction in joint space narrowing after 2 years, and all groups experienced a reduction in pain, none of the treatment groups demonstrated significant symptomatic benefit above placebo (Fransen et al 2014).

Furthermore, results confirming a disease-modifying effect using cartilage volume assessment were also obtained in the National Institutes of Health Osteoarthritis Initiative (OAI) (a longitudinal observational cohort study) which analysed a sub-group of 600 people with knee osteoarthritis, who were followed over a 2-year period (Martel-Pelletier et al 2013). The cohort had complete radiographic and MRI data for the most symptomatic knee enabling close observation of disease progression. Importantly, this was the first study to use fully automated MRI analysis and not rely on manual or semi-automated techniques. The protective effect of glucosamine plus chondroitin appears to mainly target the medial subregions in subjects with less severe damage and in the more early stages of knee OA. This is highly relevant as the MRI parameter of medial compartment cartilage volume/thickness loss seems to be able to predict progression to total knee replacement, according to a recent report by the European Society for Clinical and Economic Aspects of Osteoporosis and Osteoarthritis (ESCEO). While this was not a controlled study, over 85% of subjects that reported using glucosamine plus chondroitin stated they did this nearly every day or every day; however, no details were obtained about the forms or doses used.

It is therefore interesting to note the results of a pharmacoeconomic study which suggests that treatment with glucosamine sulfate for at least 12 months results in significant reduction in health resource utilisation even after treatment is discontinued. This study, which involved 275 subjects previously involved in 12-month glucosamine intervention trials, followed subjects for up to 5 years after treatment was discontinued (making up a total of 2178 patient-years of observation). The study showed that total knee replacement had occurred in over twice as many patients from the placebo group (19/131 or 14.5%), than in those formerly receiving glucosamine sulphate (9/144 or 6.3%) (Bruyere et al 2008).

Clinical note: Theories to explain inconsistencies across studies

Although many forms of glucosamine are used in practice, there is significantly more evidence supporting the use of the glucosamine sulfate than glucosamine hydrochloride. It has been suggested the inconsistent results may be due to the type of preparation, inadequate allocation concealment and industry bias as most clinical trials of glucosamine sulfate have used a specific patented oral formulation from Rottapharm, Italy, which is available as a prescription medicine in Europe (Vlad et al 2007). The greater efficacy seen with the Rottapharm glucosamine sulfate formulation may be due to the fact it uses vacuum sealed sachets to protect the physiologically active and highly hygroscopic, crystalline glucosamine sulfate from degradation in air, while the less hygroscopic 'stabilised' glucosamine hydrochloride preparations have been found to crystallise out of solution and therefore may contain less than the optimal amount of the physiologically active ingredient (Sahoo et al 2012). Pharmacokinetic studies have also suggested that the current treatment doses (500 mg three times daily) barely reach the required therapeutic concentration in plasma and tissue and it is likely that many patients are being underdosed at the current tested concentrations (Aghazadeh-Habashi & Jamali 2011, Henrotin et al 2012). This is most likely with obese patients who tend to require higher doses of many medications. Henrotin et al (2012) further suggest that inconsistent results are likely to be due to inconsistency in the chemical potency of some products used as well as variable and erratic bioavailability indices.

Combination therapy

With chondroitin sulfate (see Chondroitin monograph for more information)

Chondroitin sulfate and glucosamine are frequently marketed together in combination products and many studies suggest that this combination is effective in treating symptoms (Clegg et al 2006, Das & Hammad 2000, Leffler et al 1999, McAlindon et al 2000, Nguyen et al 2001, NIH 2002) and reducing joint space narrowing (Rai et al 2004). In a cluster-randomised, placebo-controlled trial in 251 patients, a combination of chondroitin sulfate and glucosamine hydrochloride but not glucosamine hydrochloride alone was found to be effective in alleviating symptoms and improving the dysfunction with Kashin-Beck disease (Yue et al 2012). This is supported by in vitro studies using horse cartilage, which report that a combination of glucosamine sulfate and chondroitin sulfate can partially mitigate the catabolic response to inflammatory stress and mechanical trauma (Harlan et al 2012) and that combination treatment is more effective than either product alone in preventing articular cartilage glycosaminoglycan degradation (Dechant et al 2005). Further support for combination therapy comes from an in vivo study of rats, which found that combined treatment with chondroitin and glucosamine sulfate prevented the development of cartilage damage and was associated with a reduction in IL-1-beta and matrix metalloprotease-9 synthesis (Chou et al 2005). While combination therapy with glucosamine and chondroitin is supported by clinical evidence, the mechanism of any synergistic action is unknown. Furthermore, research indicates that co-administration of chondroitin actually reduces the uptake of glucosamine sulphate resulting in reduced circulating plasma levels. Thus, it is suggested that any combined effect may be due to effects on the gut lining or liver rather than the joint space (Jackson et al 2010).

With omega-3 EFAs

Results from a recent study further suggest that glucosamine may be more effective in combination with omega-3 fatty acids. A recent RCT involving 177 patients with moderate to severe hip or knee osteoarthritis compared glucosamine sulfate (1500 mg/day) alone with glucosamine sulfate in combination with the omega-3 polyunsaturated fatty acids eicosapentaenoic acid (EPA) and docosahexaenoic acid (DHA). After 26 weeks the combination therapy group was significantly superior to glucosamine sulphate alone in reducing WOMAC by either 80% (P = 0.044) or 90% (P = 0.015). (Gruenwald et al 2009).

With MSM

In a 12-week, randomised, placebo-controlled trial of glucosamine and methylsulfonylmethane involving 118 patients, combined therapy was found to produce a greater and more rapid reduction in pain, swelling and loss of function than either agent alone (Usha & Naidu 2004).

Topical, with camphor

A topical preparation containing glucosamine along with chondroitin and camphor has been shown to reduce pain from OA of the knee in one randomised controlled trial (Cohen et al 2003).

With NSAIDs

Although glucosamine has not been shown to have direct analgesic activity, certain combinations with non-opioid analgesics have demonstrated synergistic (e.g. ibuprofen and ketoprofen), additive (e.g. diclofenac, indomethacin, naproxen and piroxicam) or sub-additive (e.g. aspirin and paracetamol) effects in animal pain models, suggesting that combinations of certain ratios of glucosamine and specific non-steroidal anti-inflammatory drugs (NSAIDs) might enhance pain relief or provide adequate pain relief with lower doses of NSAIDs (Tallarida et al 2003).

Comparisons with NSAIDs

There are many studies suggesting that glucosamine is at least as effective as NSAIDs in treating the symptoms of OA (Herrero-Beaumont et al 2007, Muller-Fassbender et al 1994, Reichelt et al 1994, Rovati 1992, Ruane & Griffiths 2002), although glucosamine has a slower onset of action, taking 2–6 weeks to establish an effect. The GAIT trial (see earlier) found that the combination of glucosamine hydrochloride and chondroitin was more effective than celecoxib in treating moderate to severe OA in the shorter term, whereas glucosamine alone was not (Clegg et al 2006).

Inflammatory bowel disease

In vitro and in vivo studies suggest that glucosamine may be useful in treating inflammatory bowel disease with in vitro studies demonstrating suppression of cytokine-induced activation of intestinal epithelial cells and in vivo studies finding that glucosamine improved clinical symptoms and suppressed colonic inflammation and tissue injury in a rat model of inflammatory bowel diseases (Yomogida et al 2008). The anti-inflammatory activity of glucosamine is partly mediated by an increased production of heparan sulfate proteoglycans by the vascular endothelium, thereby improving the endothelium's barrier function (McCarty 1998b). It is possible that the step in glycoprotein synthesis involving the amino sugar is relatively deficient in patients with inflammatory bowel disease and this could reduce the synthesis of the glycoprotein cover that protects the mucosa from damage by bowel contents (Burton & Anderson 1983, Winslet et al 1994). In a pilot study, *N*-acetyl glucosamine proved beneficial in children with chronic inflammatory bowel disease (Salvatore et al 2000).

Chronic lower back pain

A systematic review of 3 RCTs concluded that there was insufficient data to determine whether the use of glucosamine is useful for lower back pain (Sodha et al 2013). Wilkens et al (2012) conducted a double blind RCT over 6 months of 250 subjects with chronic lower back pain (>6 months) and MRI findings indicating degenerative lumbar disease, finding no significant pain relieving effects with glucosamine sulfate (1500 mg/day) (Wilkens et al 2012). Similarly, no pain relief was observed in a small double blind, placebo controlled, crossover study which tested a combination of glucosamine HCl (1500 mg/day), chondroitin sulfate (1200 mg/day) and manganese ascorbate (228 mg/day) over 16 weeks (Leffler et al 1999). In contrast, Tant et al (2005) conducted an open label, RCT of glucosamine taken over 12 weeks in combination with other ingredients such as MSM (methylsulfonylmethane) and found a clinically significant reduction in pain; however, the trial was an open study using a multiple ingredient combination treatment.

OTHER USES

There is the suggestion from one small RCT that glucosamine may provide symptomatic relief for people with rheumatoid arthritis (Nakamura et al 2007).

Veterinary use

Glucosamine demonstrates benefits in alleviating symptoms of degenerative joint disease in both horses (Forsyth et al 2006, Baccarin et al 2012) and dogs (McCarthy et al 2007).

Skincare use

It has been suggested that glucosamine may be a suitable cosmetic ingredient for use in skin care products. Because of its stimulation of hyaluronic acid synthesis, glucosamine has been shown to accelerate wound healing, improve skin hydration and decrease wrinkles. In addition, as an inhibitor of tyrosinase activation, it inhibits melanin production and is useful in treatment of disorders of hyperpigmentation (Bissett 2006). This is supported by an 8-week, double-blind, placebo-controlled trial, which found that hyperpigmentation was reduced with topical use of *N*-acetyl glucosamine with the effect being enhanced by niacinamide (Bissett et al 2007).

DOSAGE RANGE

- Typical dosing is 1500 mg glucosamine (either HCl or sulphate)/day (500 mg three times daily). This is based on preclinical animal models which used 20 mg/kg of body weight per day, which translates to 1500 mg/day for a 75 kg adult. Higher dosing may therefore be required in heavier individuals.
- A 2–3-month trial is generally used to determine whether it is effective for an individual patient. Use for 3+ years is required to slow down knee joint degeneration and potentially reduce the risk of knee replacement.
- Intramuscular glucosamine sulfate: 400 or 800 mg three times/week (Reichelt et al 1994) for 4–6 weeks or longer if required.
- Glucosamine sulfate, hydrochloride, hydroiodide and *N*-acetyl forms are available. Most research has been done on the sulfate forms. Topical, intravenous, intramuscular and intraarticular forms are also available in some countries.

ADVERSE REACTIONS

Glucosamine has been used safely in multiple clinical trials lasting from 4 weeks to 3 years with minimal or no adverse effects (Lopes Vaz 1982, Pavelka et al 2002, Pujalte et al 1980, Reginster et al 2001). A 2006 Cochrane systematic review concluded that glucosamine is as safe as placebo (Towheed et al 2006). Glucosamine has an observed safe level (OSL) of 2000 mg/day and while it is considered safe, some uncommon and minor adverse effects have been reported, including epigastric pain or tenderness (3.5%), heartburn (2.7%), diarrhoea (2.5%) and nausea (1%) (Sherman et al 2012).

Glucosamine sulphate has no significant effect on serum lipids (Albert et al 2007, Østergaard et al 2007). While it is unlikely that glucosamine has any significant effects on glucose tolerance, people with impaired glucose tolerance or insulin resistance should be monitored (Dostrovsky et al 2011).

There is one case report of asthma being exacerbated by glucosamine–chondroitin supplementation (Tallia & Cardone 2002).

SIGNIFICANT INTERACTIONS

Controlled studies are not available so interactions remain speculative and are based on evidence of pharmacological activity.

Non-steroidal anti-inflammatory drugs

Glucosamine reduces the requirements for NSAID use by people with knee OA according to a large French study (Bertin & Taieb 2013) — drug dosage may require modification after several weeks' glucosamine use — a potentially beneficial combination.

Warfarin

Case reports exist of glucosamine and glucosamine/chondroitin combinations increasing bruising, bleeding and INR amongst people taking warfarin (Knudsen & Sokol 2008). Until the interaction can be tested in a controlled study, caution is advised.

Practice points/Patient counselling

- Glucosamine is a naturally occurring building block of joint tissue and cartilage.
- Glucosamine sulphate is an effective symptomatic treatment for pain and disability associated with OA, with most research conducted with knee OA. When used long term (more than 6 months) it slows the progression of the disease, and appears to work best long-term with chondroitin sulfate.
- It is considered extremely safe and may reduce the need for NSAIDs (which can have serious side effects).
- People who are overweight or obese may require higher doses than the usual dose of 1500 mg/day.
- People with severe shellfish allergy should be advised to use a form that is not derived from shellfish.
- Patients with diabetes should monitor their blood glucose levels while taking glucosamine, although no significant changes are anticipated.

PATIENTS' FAQs

What will this supplement do for me?

Multiple scientific studies have shown that glucosamine sulfate reduces symptoms of OA and also slows progression of the condition when used

Clinical note — Should people with diabetes avoid glucosamine?

Clinicians' concern about the safety of glucosamine in diabetes were probably first fuelled by an article published in *Lancet* in 1999 (Adams 1999). The article entitled 'Hype about glucosamine' by Adams stated that glucosamine increases glucose resistance in normal and in experimentally diabetic animals (McClain & Crook 1996) and intravenous glucosamine in doses as low as 0.1 mg/kg/minute result in a 50% reduction in the rate of glucose uptake in skeletal muscle (Baron et al 1995). Adams concluded by suggesting that perhaps all people, but especially those who are overweight or have diabetes, should be urged to have caution when using glucosamine. In 2005, a critical review of 33 clinical studies involving 3063 human subjects concluded that glucosamine does not affect glucose metabolism, and that there are no adverse effects of oral glucosamine administration on blood, urine or faecal parameters (Anderson et al 2005). A more recent systematic review of 11 studies, however, suggests that glucosamine may have some effect on glucose metabolism in people with impaired glucose tolerance or insulin resistance and that more studies are required before definitive conclusion can be made (Dostrovsky et al 2011).

CONTRAINDICATIONS AND PRECAUTIONS

Diabetics using glucosamine should have their blood sugar levels checked regularly.

Glucosamine is made from shellfish and, although it is not extracted from the protein component and appears to pose no threat to shrimp-allergic individuals (Villacis et al 2006), it should be used with caution in patients with shellfish allergy.

Whether glucosamine poses a serious bleeding risk in major surgery is unclear. Multiple case reports suggesting an interaction between warfarin and glucosamine have been collected by the FDA and WHO however it is unknown whether the interaction is pharmacokinetic or pharmacodynamic (Knudsen & Sokol 2008). Of the 21 documented case reports indicating increased INR and held in the WHO adverse drug reaction database, 17 resolved when glucosamine was ceased. While this does not provide strong evidence that glucosamine used by itself will cause bleeding, caution is advised. Due to the fact that glucosamine is long term therapy, suspending use one week before major surgery and resuming use afterwards seems reasonable.

long-term. The sulfate form is superior to the hydrochloride form for improving symptoms. Some people find that they do not require NSAIDs as often when taking it.

PREGNANCY USE

Insufficient reliable information is available to advise on safety in pregnancy. Some limited data suggest no increased risk for major malformations or other adverse fetal effects with glucosamine use during pregnancy (Sivojelezova et al 2007).

When will it start to work?

Symptom relief generally takes 2–6 weeks to establish, but joint protection effects occur only with long-term use of at least 6 months to several years.

Are there any safety issues?

Although considered very safe for the general population, it should be used with caution in people with severe shellfish allergies.

REFERENCES

Adams ME. Hype about glucosamine. Lancet 354.9176 (1999): 353–354.

Aghazadeh-Habashi A et al. Single dose pharmacokinetics and bioavailability of glucosamine in the rat. J Pharmacy Pharm Sci 5.2 (2002): 181–184.

Aghazadeh-Habashi A, Jamali F. The glucosamine controversy; a pharmacokinetic issue. J Pharm Pharm Sci 14.2 (2011): 264–273.

Albert SG et al. The effect of glucosamine on serum HDL cholesterol and apolipoprotein AI levels in people with diabetes. Diabetes Care 30.11 (2007): 2800–2803.

Anderson JW et al. Glucosamine effects in humans: a review of effects on glucose metabolism, side effects, safety considerations and efficacy. Food Chem Toxicol 43.2 (2005): 187–201.

Baccarin RYA et al. Urinary glycosaminoglycans in horse osteoarthritis. Effects of chondroitin sulfate and glucosamine. Research in Veterinary Science 93.1 (2012): 88–96.

Bagasra O et al. Anti-human immunodeficiency virus type 1 activity of sulfated monosaccharides: comparison with sulfated polysaccharides and other polyions. J Infect Dis 164.6 (1991): 1082–1090.

Balkan B, Dunning BE. Glucosamine inhibits glucokinase in vitro and produces a glucose-specific impairment of in vivo insulin secretion in rats. Diabetes 43.10 (1994): 1173–1179.

Baron AD et al. Glucosamine induces insulin resistance in vivo by affecting GLUT 4 translocation in skeletal muscle. Implications for glucose toxicity. J Clin Invest 96.6 (1995): 2792–2801.

Basak M et al. Comparative bioavailability of a novel timed release and powder-filled glucosamine sulfate formulation: a multi-dose, randomized, crossover study. Int J Clin Pharmacol Ther 42.11 (2004): 597–601.

Bassleer C, Rovati L, Franchimont P. Stimulation of proteoglycan production by glucosamine sulfate in chondrocytes isolated from human osteoarthritic articular cartilage in vitro. Osteoarthritis Cartilage 6.6 (1998): 427–434.

Bertin P, Taieb C. NSAID-sparing effect of glucosamine hydrochloride in patients with knee osteoarthritis: an analysis of data from a French database. Curr Med Res Opin (2013).

Biggee BA et al. Low levels of human serum glucosamine after ingestion of glucosamine sulphate relative to capability for peripheral effectiveness. Ann Rheum Dis 65.2 (2006): 222–226.

Bissett DL et al. Reduction in the appearance of facial hyperpigmentation by topical N-acetyl glucosamine. J Cosmet Dermatol 6.1 (2007): 20–26.

Bissett DL. Glucosamine: an ingredient with skin and other benefits. J Cosmet Dermatol 5.4 (2006): 309–15.

Black C et al. The clinical effectiveness of glucosamine and chondroitin supplements in slowing or arresting progression of osteoarthritis of the knee: a systematic review and economic evaluation. Health Technology Assessment 13(52) (2009).

Bruyere O et al. Correlation between radiographic severity of knee osteoarthritis and future disease progression: results from a 3-year prospective, placebo-controlled study evaluating the effect of glucosamine sulfate. Osteoarthritis Cartilage 11.1 (2003): 1–5.

Bruyere O et al. Glucosamine sulfate reduces osteoarthritis progression in postmenopausal women with knee osteoarthritis: evidence from two 3-year studies. Menopause 11.2 (2004): 138–143.

Bruyere O et al. Total joint replacement after glucosamine sulphate treatment in knee osteoarthritis: results of a mean 8-year observation of patients from two previous 3-year, randomised, placebo-controlled trials. Osteoarthritis Cartilage 16.2 (2008): 254–260.

Bruyere O, Reginster JY. Glucosamine and chondroitin sulfate as therapeutic agents for knee and hip osteoarthritis. Drugs Aging 24.7 (2007): 573–80.

Burton AF, Anderson FH. Decreased incorporation of 14C-glucosamine relative to 3H-N-acetyl glucosamine in the intestinal mucosa of patients with inflammatory bowel disease. Am J Gastroenterol 78.1 (1983): 19–22.
Chan KOW, Ng GYF. A review on the effects of glucosamine for knee osteoarthritis based on human and animal studies. Hong Kong Physiotherapy Journal 29.2 (2011): 42–52.
Chou MM et al. Effects of chondroitin and glucosamine sulfate in a dietary bar formulation on inflammation, interleukin-1-beta, matrix metalloprotease-9, and cartilage damage in arthritis. Exp Biol Med 230.4 (2005): 255–262.
Cibere J et al. Glucosamine sulfate and cartilage type II collagen degradation in patients with knee osteoarthritis: randomized discontinuation trial results employing biomarkers. J Rheumatol 32.5 (2005): 896–902.
Clegg DO et al. Glucosamine, chondroitin sulfate, and the two in combination for painful knee osteoarthritis. N Engl J Med 354.8 (2006): 795–808.
Cohen M et al. A randomized double blind, placebo controlled trial of a topical cream containing glucosamine sulfate, chondroitin sulfate, and camphor for osteoarthritis of the knee. J Rheumatol 30 (2003): 523–528.
Consumer Lab 2; Product review: glucosamine and chondroitin. Available at www.consumerlab.com (accessed January 2006).
Coulson S et al. Green-lipped mussel extract (Perna canaliculus) and glucosamine sulphate in patients with knee osteoarthritis: therapeutic efficacy and effects on gastrointestinal microbiota profiles. Inflammopharmacology 21.1 (2013): 79–90.
Crolle G, D'Este E. Glucosamine sulphate for the management of arthrosis: a controlled clinical investigation. Curr Med Res Opin 7.2 (1980): 104–109.
Das A Jr, Hammad TA. Efficacy of a combination of FCHG49 glucosamine hydrochloride, TRH122 low molecular weight sodium chondroitin sulfate and manganese ascorbate in the management of knee osteoarthritis. Osteoarthritis Cartilage 8.5 (2000): 343–350.
de Mattei M et al. High doses of glucosamine-HCl have detrimental effects on bovine articular cartilage explants cultured in vitro. Osteoarthritis Cartilage 10.10 (2002): 816–825.
Dechant JE et al. Effects of glucosamine hydrochloride and chondroitin sulphate, alone and in combination, on normal and interleukin-1 conditioned equine articular cartilage explant metabolism. Equine Vet J 37.3 (2005): 227–231.
Dostrovsky NR et al. The effect of glucosamine on glucose metabolism in humans: a systematic review of the literature. Osteoarthritis and Cartilage 19.4 (2011): 375–380.
Drovanti A, Bignamini AA, Rovati AL. Therapeutic activity of oral glucosamine sulfate in osteoarthrosis: a placebo-controlled double-blind investigation. Clin Ther 3.4 (1980): 260–272.
Echard BW et al. Effects of oral glucosamine and chondroitin sulfate alone and in combination on the metabolism of SHR and SD rats. Mol Cell Biochem 225 (2001): 85–91.
Forsyth RK et al. Double blind investigation of the effects of oral supplementation of combined glucosamine hydrochloride (GHCL) and chondroitin sulphate (CS) on stride characteristics of veteran horses. Equine Vet J 36 (Suppl) (2006): 622–625.
Fox BA, Stephens, MM. Glucosamine/chondroitin/primorine combination therapy for osteoarthritis. Drugs Today (Barc.) 45.1 (2009): 21–31.
Fransen M et al. Glucosamine and chondroitin for knee osteoarthritis: a double-blind randomised placebo-controlled clinical trial evaluating single and combination regimens. Annals of Rheumatic Diseases 0 (2014): 1–8.
Giaccari A et al. In vivo effects of glucosamine on insulin secretion and insulin sensitivity in the rat: possible relevance to the maladaptive responses to chronic hyperglycaemia. Diabetologia 38.5 (1995): 518–524.
Gouze JN et al. Interleukin-1beta down-regulates the expression of glucuronosyltransferase I, a key enzyme priming glycosaminoglycan biosynthesis: influence of glucosamine on interleukin-1beta-mediated effects in rat chondrocytes. Arthritis Rheum 44.2 (2001): 351–360.
Gruenwald J et al. Effect of glucosamine sulfate with or without omega-3 fatty acids in patients with osteoarthritis. Adv Ther 26.9 (2009): 858–871.
Harlan RS et al. The Effect of Glucosamine and Chondroitin on Stressed Equine Cartilage Explants. Journal of Equine Veterinary Science 32.1 (2012): 12–14.
Henrotin, Y et al. Is there any scientific evidence for the use of glucosamine in the management of human osteoarthritis? Arthritis Res Ther 14.1(2012): 201.
Herrero-Beaumont G et al. Glucosamine sulfate in the treatment of knee osteoarthritis symptoms: a randomized, double-blind, placebo-controlled study using acetaminophen as a side comparator. Arthritis Rheum 56.2 (2007): 555–67.
Hua J, Sakamoto K, Nagaoka I. Inhibitory actions of glucosamine, a therapeutic agent for osteoarthritis, on the functions of neutrophils. J Leukocyte Biol 71.4 (2002): 632–640.
Imagawa K et al. The epigenetic effect of glucosamine and a nuclear factor-kappa B (NF-kB) inhibitor on primary human chondrocytes — Implications for osteoarthritis. Biochemical and Biophysical Research Communications 405.3 (2011): 362–367.
Jackson CG et al. The human pharmacokinetics of oral ingestion of glucosamine and chondroitin sulfate taken separately or in combination. Osteoarthritis and Cartilage 18(3) (2010): 297–302.
Kelly GS. The role of glucosamine sulfate and chondroitin sulfates in the treatment of degenerative joint disease. Altern Med Rev 3.1 (1998): 27–39.
Kim MM et al. Glucosamine sulfate promotes osteoblastic differentiation of MG-63 cells via anti-inflammatory effect. Bioorg Med Chem Lett 17.7 (2007): 1938–1942.
Knudsen JF, Sokol GH. Potential glucosamine-warfarin interaction resulting in increased international normalized ratio: case report and review of the literature and MedWatch database. Pharmacotherapy, 28.4 (2008): 540–548.
Laverty S et al. Synovial fluid levels and serum pharmacokinetics in a large animal model following treatment with oral glucosamine at clinically relevant doses. Arthritis Rheum 52.1 (2005): 181–191.
Lee YH et al. Effect of glucosamine or chondroitin sulfate on the osteoarthritis progression: a meta-analysis. Rheumatology International 30 (2010): 357–363.
Leffler CT et al. Glucosamine, chondroitin, and manganese ascorbate for degenerative joint disease of the knee or low back: a randomized, double-blind, placebo-controlled pilot study. Mil Med 164.2 (1999): 85–91.
Lippiello L et al. In vivo chondroprotection and metabolic synergy of glucosamine and chondroitin sulfate. Clin Orthopaed Rel Res 381 (2000): 229–240.
Lopes Vaz A. Double-blind clinical evaluation of the relative efficacy of ibuprofen and glucosamine sulphate in the management of osteoarthrosis of the knee in out-patients. Curr Med Res Opin 8.3 (1982): 145–149.
López M et al. Effects of Glucosamine Sulphate, Chondroitin Sulphate and Hyaluronic Acid on Articular Cartilage. Journal of Comparative Pathology 148.1 (2013): 97.
Ma L et al. Immunosuppressive effects of glucosamine. J Biol Chem 277.42 (2002): 39343–39349.
Martel-Pelletier J et al. First-line analysis of the effects of treatment on progression of structural changes in knee osteoarthritis over 24 months: data from the osteoarthritis initiative progression cohort. Ann.Rheum. Dis. (2013).
McAlindon T. Glucosamine and chondroitin for osteoarthritis? Bull Rheum Dis 50.7 (2001): 1–4.
McAlindon TE et al. Glucosamine and chondroitin for treatment of osteoarthritis: a systematic quality assessment and meta-analysis [Comment]. JAMA 283.11 (2000): 1469–1475.
McCarthy G et al. Randomised double-blind, positive-controlled trial to assess the efficacy of glucosamine/chondroitin sulfate for the treatment of dogs with osteoarthritis. Vet J 174.1 (2007): 54–61.
McCarty MF, Russell AL, Seed MP. Sulfated glycosaminoglycans and glucosamine may synergize in promoting synovial hyaluronic acid synthesis. Med Hypotheses 54.5 (2000): 798–802.
McCarty MF. Enhanced synovial production of hyaluronic acid may explain rapid clinical response to high-dose glucosamine in osteoarthritis. Med Hypotheses 50.6 (1998a): 507–10.
McCarty MF. Vascular heparan sulfates may limit the ability of leukocytes to penetrate the endothelial barrier: implications for use of glucosamine in inflammatory disorders. Med Hypotheses 51.1 (1998b): 11–15.
McClain DA, Crook ED. Hexosamines and insulin resistance. Diabetes 45.8 (1996): 1003–1009.
Mello DM et al. Comparison of inhibitory effects of glucosamine and mannosamine on bovine articular cartilage degradation in vitro. Am J Vet Res 65.10 (2004): 1440–1445.
Miller KL, Clegg DO. Glucosamine and chondroitin sulfate. Rheum Dis Clin North Am 37.1 (2011): 103–118.
Monauni T et al. Effects of glucosamine infusion on insulin secretion and insulin action in humans. Diabetes 49.6 (2000): 926–935.
Mroz PJ, Silbert JE. Use of 3H-glucosamine and 35S-sulfate with cultured human chondrocytes to determine the effect of glucosamine concentration on formation of chondroitin sulfate. Arthritis Rheum 50.11 (2004): 3574–3579.
Muller-Fassbender H et al. Glucosamine sulfate compared to ibuprofen in osteoarthritis of the knee. Osteoarthritis Cartilage 2.1 (1994): 61–69.
Nagaoka I et al. Chapter 22 — Biological Activities of Glucosamine and Its Related Substances. Advances in Food and Nutrition Research. K. Se-Kwon, Academic Press 65 (2012): 337–352.
Nagaoka I et al. Recent aspects of the anti-inflammatory actions of glucosamine. Carbohydrate Polymers 84.2 (2011): 825–830.
Nakamura H et al. Effects of glucosamine administration on patients with rheumatoid arthritis. Rheumatol Int 27.3 (2007): 213–2118.
Nakamura H et al. Effects of glucosamine hydrochloride on the production of prostaglandin E2, nitric oxide and metalloproteases by chondrocytes and synoviocytes in osteoarthritis. Clin Exp Rheumatol 22.3 (2004): 293–299.

G

National Institutes of Health NIH; National Centre for Complementary and Alternative Medicine GAIT Study, 2002. www.nih.com (accessed January 2008).

Nelson BA, Robinson KA, Buse MG. High glucose and glucosamine induce insulin resistance via different mechanisms in 3T3-L1 adipocytes. Diabetes 49.6 (2000): 981–991.

Nguyen P et al. A randomized double-blind clinical trial of the effect of chondroitin sulfate and glucosamine hydrochloride on temporomandibular joint disorders: a pilot study. Cranio 19.2 (2001): 130–139.

Nimni ME, Cordoba F. Chondroitin sulfate and sulfur containing chondroprotective agents: Is there a basis for their pharmacological action? Curr Rheum Rev 2.2 (2006): 137–149.

Onigbinde AT et al. Acute effects of combination of glucosamine sulphate lontophoresis with exercise on fasting plasma glucose of participants with knee osteoarthritis. Hong Kong Physiotherapy Journal 29.2 (2011): 79–85.

Ostergaard K et al. The effect of glucosamine sulphate on the blood levels of cholesterol or triglycerides — a clinical study. Ugeskr Laeger 169.5 (2007): 407–410.

Pavelka K et al. Glucosamine sulfate use and delay of progression of knee osteoarthritis: a 3-year, randomized, placebo-controlled, double-blind study. Arch Intern Med 162.18 (2002): 2113–2123.

Pelletier JP et al. Long term knee OA trial design: an ounce of prevention is worth a pound of cure. Annals of Rheumatic Diseases Letter to Editor (2010).

Persiani S et al. Glucosamine oral bioavailability and plasma pharmacokinetics after increasing doses of crystalline glucosamine sulfate in man. Osteoarthritis Cartilage 13.12 (2005): 1041–1049.

Persiani S et al. Synovial and plasma glucosamine concentrations in osteoarthritic patients following oral crystalline glucosamine sulphate at therapeutic dose. Osteoarthritis Cartilage 15.7 (2007): 764–772.

Petersen SG et al. Glucosamine but not ibuprofen alters cartilage turnover in osteoarthritis patients in response to physical training. Osteoarthritis and Cartilage 18.1 (2010): 34–40.

Piperno M et al. Glucosamine sulfate modulates dysregulated activities of human osteoarthritic chondrocytes in vitro. Osteoarthritis Cartilage 8.3 (2000): 207–212.

Poolsup N et al. Glucosamine long-term treatment and the progression of knee osteoarthritis: systematic review of randomized controlled trials. Ann Pharmacother 39.6 (2005): 1080–1087.

Pouwels MJ et al. Short-term glucosamine infusion does not affect insulin sensitivity in humans. J Clin Endocrinol Metab 86.5 (2001): 2099–2103.

Provenza JR et al. Combined glucosamine and chondroitin sulfate, once or three times daily, provides clinically relevant analgesia in knee osteoarthritis. Clin Rheumatol 2014 [Epub ahead of print].

Pujalte JM, Llavore EP, Ylescupidez FR. Double-blind clinical evaluation of oral glucosamine sulphate in the basic treatment of osteoarthrosis. Curr Med Res Opinion 7.2 (1980): 110–1114.

Qian, S et al. Bioavailability enhancement of glucosamine hydrochloride by chitosan. Int.J Pharm., 455.1–2 (2013): 365–373.

Qiu GX et al. Efficacy and safety of glucosamine sulfate versus ibuprofen in patients with knee osteoarthritis. Arzneimittelforschung 48.5 (1998): 469–474.

Rai J et al. Efficacy of chondroitin sulfate and glucosamine sulfate in the progression of symptomatic knee osteoarthritis: a randomized, placebo-controlled, double blind study. Bull Postgrad Inst Med Educ Res Chandigarh 38.1 (2004): 18–22.

Reginster JY et al. Evidence of nutriceutical effectiveness in the treatment of osteoarthritis. Curr Rheumatol Rep 2.6 (2000): 472–477.

Reginster JY et al. Long-term effects of glucosamine sulphate on osteoarthritis progression: a randomised, placebo-controlled clinical trial [Comment]. Lancet 357.9252 (2001): 251–256.

Reginster JY et al. Current role of glucosamine in the treatment of osteoarthritis. Rheumatology (Oxford) 46.5 (2007): 731–5.

Reginster J-YN et al. Role of glucosamine in the treatment for osteoarthritis. Rheumatology International 32 (2012): 2959–2967.

Reichelt A et al. Efficacy and safety of intramuscular glucosamine sulfate in osteoarthritis of the knee: a randomised, placebo-controlled, double-blind study. Arzneimittelforschung 44.1 (1994): 75–80.

Richy F et al. Structural and symptomatic efficacy of glucosamine and chondroitin in knee osteoarthritis: a comprehensive meta-analysis. Arch Intern Med 163.13 (2003): 1514–1522.

Roman-Blas J et al. Glucosamine sulfate for knee osteoarthritis: science and evidence-based use. Therapy 7.6 (2010): 591–604.

Rovati LC. Clinical research in osteoarthritis: design and results of short-term and long-term trials with disease-modifying drugs. Int J Tissue React 14.5 (1992): 243–251.

Ruane R, Griffiths P. Glucosamine therapy compared to ibuprofen for joint pain. Br J Community Nurs 7.3 (2002): 148–152.

Sahoo SC et al. Glucosamine Salts: Resolving Ambiguities over the Market-Based Compositions Crystal Growth and Design 12 (2012): 5148–5154.

Sakai S et al. Effect of glucosamine and related compounds on the degranulation of mast cells and ear swelling induced by dinitrofluorobenzene in mice. Life Sciences 86(9–10) (2010): 337–343.

Salvatore S et al. A pilot study of N-acetyl glucosamine, a nutritional substrate for glycosaminoglycan synthesis, in paediatric chronic inflammatory bowel disease. Aliment Pharmacol Ther 14.12 (2000): 1567–1579.

Sawitzke AD et al. The effect of glucosamine and/or chondroitin sulfate on the progression of knee osteoarthritis: a report from the glucosamine/chondroitin arthritis intervention trial. Arthritis Rheum 58.10 (2008): 3183–91.

Sawitzke AD et al Clinical efficacy and safety of glucosamine, chondroitin sulphate, their combination, celecoxib or placebo taken to treat osteoarthritis of the knee: 2-year results from GAIT. Annals of Rheumatic Diseases 69 (2010): 1459–1464.

Scarpellini M et al. Biomarkers, type II collagen, glucosamine and chondroitin sulfate in osteoarthritis follow-up: the Magenta osteoarthritis study. J Orthop Traumatol 9.2 (2008): 81–87.

Setnikar IP, Canali S. Pharmacokinetics of glucosamine in man. Arzneimittelforschung 43.10 (1993): 1109–1113.

Shankar RR et al. Glucosamine infusion in rats mimics the beta-cell dysfunction of non-insulin-dependent diabetes mellitus. Metabolism 47.5 (1998): 573–577.

Sherman AL et al Use of Glucosamine and Chondroitin in Persons With Osteoarthritis. PM&R 4(5, Supplement) (2012): S110–S116.

Shikhman AR et al. N-acetylglucosamine prevents IL-1 beta-mediated activation of human chondrocytes. J Immunol 166.8 (2001): 5155–5160.

Silva FS Jr et al. Combined glucosamine and chondroitin sulfate provides functional and structural benefit in the anterior cruciate ligament transection model. Clin Rheumatol 28.2 (2009): 109–117.

Sivojelezova A et al. Glucosamine use in pregnancy: an evaluation of pregnancy outcome. J Womens Health (Larchmt) 16.3 (2007): 345–348.

Sodha, R et al. The use of glucosamine for chronic low back pain: a systematic review of randomised control trials. BMJ Open 3.6 (2013).

Sumantran VN et al. The relationship between chondroprotective and antiinflammatory effects of Withania somnifera root and glucosamine sulphate on human osteoarthritic cartilage in vitro. Phytother Res 22.10 (2008): 1342–1348.

Tallarida RJ et al. Antinociceptive synergy, additivity, and subadditivity with combinations of oral glucosamine plus nonopioid analgesics in mice. J Pharmacol Exp Ther 307.2 (2003): 699–704.

Tallia AF, Cardone DA. Asthma exacerbation associated with glucosamine-chondroitin supplement. J Am Board Fam Pract 15.6 (2002): 481–484.

Tamai Y et al. Enhanced healing of cartilaginous injuries by N-acetyl-glucosamine and glucuronic acid. Carbohydr Polym 54.2 (2003): 251–262.

Tannis AJ et al. Effect of glucosamine supplementation on fasting and non-fasting plasma glucose and serum insulin concentrations in healthy individuals. Osteoarthritis Cartilage 2.6 (2004): 506–511.

Tant L et al. Open-label, randomized, controlled pilot study of the effects of a glucosamine complex on low back pain. Curr Ther Res 66 (2005): 511–21.

Tiraloche G et al. Effect of oral glucosamine on cartilage degradation in a rabbit model of osteoarthritis. Arthritis Rheum 52.4 (2005): 1118–1128.

Towheed TE et al. Glucosamine therapy for treating osteoarthritis. Cochrane Database Syst Rev 1 (2003).

Towheed TE et al. Glucosamine therapy for treating osteoarthritis. Cochrane Database Syst Rev 2 (2006).

Usha PR, Naidu MUR. Randomised, double-blind, parallel, placebo-controlled study of oral glucosamine, methylsulfonylmethane and their combination in osteoarthritis. Clin Drug Invest 24.6 (2004): 353–363.

Vangsness CT Jr et al. A review of evidence-based medicine for glucosamine and chondroitin sulfate use in knee osteoarthritis. Arthroscopy 25.1 (2009): 86–94.

Villacis J et al. Do shrimp-allergic individuals tolerate shrimp-derived glucosamine? Clin Exp Allergy 36.11 (2006): 1457–1461.

Vlad SC et al. Glucosamine for pain in osteoarthritis: why do trial results differ? Arthritis Rheum 56.7 (2007): 2267–2277.

Wandel S et al. Effects of glucosamine, chondroitin, or placebo in patients with osteoarthritis of hip or knee: network meta-analysis. BMJ 341 (2010): c4675.

Wilkens P et al. No effect of 6-month intake of glucosamine sulfate on Modic changes or high intensity zones in the lumbar spine: sub-group analysis of a randomized controlled trial. J Negat Results Biomed 11.13 (2012).

Winslet MC et al. Mucosal glucosamine synthetase activity in inflammatory bowel disease. Dig Dis Sci 39.3 (1994): 540–544.

Wu, D et al. Efficacies of different preparations of glucosamine for the treatment of osteoarthritis: a meta-analysis of randomised, double-blind, placebo-controlled trials. Int.J Clin Pract 67.6 (2013): 585–594.

Yomogida S et al. Glucosamine, a naturally occurring amino monosaccharide, suppresses dextran sulfate sodium-induced colitis in rats. Int J Mol Med 22.3 (2008): 317–323.

Yue J et al. Chondroitin sulfate and/or glucosamine hydrochloride for Kashin-Beck disease: a cluster-randomized, placebo-controlled study. Osteoarthritis and Cartilage 20.7 (2012): 622–629.

Zhang GX et al. Glucosamine abrogates the acute phase of experimental autoimmune encephalomyelitis by induction of Th2 response. J Immunol 175.11 (2005): 7202–7208.

Goji

HISTORICAL NOTE For thousands of years in traditional Chinese medicine, the fruit of the lycium shrub has been used as both a food and an important medicinal substance. In fact, the earliest known Chinese medicinal monograph documented the medicinal use of *Lycium barbarum* around 2300 years ago. According to this tradition, it is believed that the fruit has antiageing properties, nourishes the kidneys and liver by tonifying yin deficiency and brightens the eyes. It also has a long history of use as a traditional remedy for male infertility and is included in most fertility-promoting Chinese herbal remedies (Luo et al 2006). In China it is known by several names, such as Gou Qi Zi or Gouqizi, which probably led to the name it is known as here, goji.

G

COMMON NAME

Goji

OTHER NAMES

Gou Qi Zi, Gouqizi, Fructus lycii, Kei Tze, wolfberry

SCIENTIFIC NAME

Lycium barbarum (Solanaceae family)

PLANT PART USED

Fruit

Goji berry is a deep-red, dried fruit about the same size as a raisin, but with a different taste. The berries have a slight chewy consistency and taste like a mixture of cherries and cranberries, without the sweetness of raisins.

CHEMICAL COMPONENTS

The reddish orange colour of the fruit is derived from a group of carotenoids, which make up only 0.03–0.5% of the dried fruit. The predominant carotenoid is zeaxanthin, which comprises about one-third to one-half of the total carotenoids present (Inbaraj et al 2008). The fruit also contains various small molecules, such as betaine, cerebroside, beta-sitosterol, *p*-coumaric acid, various vitamins (e.g. B_1, B_2, vitamin C) and minerals (e.g. iron, selenium, zinc). Among these chemical constituents, the most valuable and pharmacologically active components are a group of unique, water-soluble glycoconjugates — collectively termed *Lycium barbarum* polysaccharides (LBPs). Nineteen different constituents of LBP have been isolated, and they are estimated to comprise 5–8% of the dried fruit (Amagase et al 2009a, Tang et al 2012).

MAIN ACTIONS

Antioxidant

LBPs have demonstrated high antioxidant activity in a number of in vitro and in vivo studies (Amagase et al 2009a, Guoliang et al 2011, Ke et al 2011, Lin et al 2009, Niu 2008, Zhang et al 2011a). Pretreatment with LBP increased endurance, decreased malondialdehyde and increased superoxide dismutase and glutathione peroxidase (GSH-Px) levels in rats subjected to exhaustive exercise (Shan et al 2011).

Pretreatment of pregnant rats with LBP prevented prenatal stress-induced cognitive dysfunction in offspring, possibly via prevention of oxidative damage to brain tissue mitochondria (Feng et al 2010).

A study of streptozocin-induced diabetic animals found that LBP restored abnormal oxidative indices to near-normal levels (Li 2007).

Goji stimulates endogenous antioxidant mechanisms and has been shown to significantly increase superoxide dismutase and GSH-Px, and reduce lipid peroxidation (indicated by decreased levels of malondialdehyde) in humans (Amagase et al 2009a, Liang et al 2011).

The zeaxanthin component found in whole goji berries is bioavailable in humans (Cheng et al 2005) and is likely to contribute the fruit's in vivo antioxidant effects. Bioavailability of zeaxanthin from freeze-dried wolfberries can be greatly enhanced when consumed in hot skimmed milk compared to hot water or warm milk (Benzie et al 2006).

Conversely, a hepatic ischaemia-reperfusion injury rat model found that LBP did not attenuate ischaemia-reperfusion-induced free radical production, and in fact resulted in an increased production of hydroxyl radicals. Explanations for these unexpected results include loss of antioxidant components during isolation of LBP, and mediation of hepatic injury via pathways other than free radical production. Since the results of this study are not in accord with other studies demonstrating antioxidant activity for LBP, further investigations are needed to expand upon the findings of this study (Wang et al 2009).

Antidiabetic

Goji exhibits a variety of mechanisms of relevance in diabetes.

A study by Zhao et al (2005b) demonstrated that diabetic animals treated with LBP for 3 weeks resulted in a significant decrease in the concentration of plasma triglyceride and weight in non-insulin-dependent diabetes mellitus (NIDDM) rats. Furthermore, LBP markedly decreased the plasma cholesterol levels, fasting plasma insulin levels and postprandial glucose levels at 30 minutes during oral glucose tolerance test and significantly increased the Insulin Sensitivity Index in NIDDM rats.

An acidic polysaccharide isolated from *L. barbarum* (LBP-I) has been shown to protect pancreatic islet cells from oxidative damage, significantly enhance cell survival and inhibit the development of insulin resistance in HepG2 cells in vitro (Zou et al 2010).

Furthermore, LBP prevented diabetic nephropathy in streptozotocin-induced diabetic mice via mediation of oxidative stress and inhibition of protein kinase C, which play a major role in oxidative stress-induced glomerular injury (Zhao et al 2009).

The fruit extract of goji has also shown hypoglycaemic and lipid-lowering activities in diabetic animals while not affecting healthy animals (Jing et al 2009, Luo et al 2004). It appears that the polysaccharides and vitamin antioxidants may be responsible for these particular effects.

Neuroprotective

Goji berry extract and LBP display neuroprotective activity in several different experimental models (Yao et al 2011).

An aqueous extract isolated from *L. barbarum* exhibited significant protection on cultured neurons against harmful chemical toxins (A beta and dithiothreitol) by reducing the activity of both caspase-3 and -2, but not caspase-8 and -9 (Yu et al 2007). A new arabinogalactan-protein (LBP-III) was isolated from LBP, which appeared to have the strongest effect.

The polysaccharide-containing extract (LBP) from LBP protects neurons against beta-amyloid peptide toxicity in neuronal cell cultures (Chang & So 2008) and demonstrates neuroprotective effects in the retina in several experimental models, including retinal ischaemia-reperfusion injury, glaucoma and diabetic retinopathy (Chan et al 2007, Chang & So 2008, Hu et al 2012, Li et al 2011, Miranda et al 2010, Song et al 2011, 2012, Yang et al 2011, Yu et al 2007) as well as ocular hypertension in animal models (Chiu et al 2010, Mi et al 2012, Yu et al 2007).

In vivo studies suggest that LBP may be used to protect neuronal brain cells from a range of insults. LBP attenuated neuronal damage in rat hippocampal neurons injured by oxygen glucose deprivation/reperfusion in a dose-dependent manner (Rui et al 2012). Prophylactic treatment with LBP improved neurological deficits and decreased infarct size in an experimental stroke model using mice (Yang et al 2012). LBP enhanced learning and memory capabilities of manganese-poisoned mice via promotion of neurogenesis in the hippocampus (Wen et al 2010).

Pretreatment with LBP has been found to prevent homocysteine- and glutamate-induced apoptosis in cortical neuronal cells (Ho et al 2009, 2010). Whether *L. barbarum* has a potential role in degenerative diseases such as Alzheimer's disease and Parkinson's disease, as homocysteine and glutamate neurotoxicity have been implicated in their pathophysiology, remains to be tested.

Anticancer

The antiproliferative activity of LBP has been demonstrated in several in vitro models. LBP demonstrated inhibition of proliferation of human cervical carcinoma cells (HeLa cells) via changing cell cycle distribution and inducing apoptosis (Zhu & Zhang 2012). Another study found that AA-2βG (a vitamin C analogue in *L. barbarum*) induced apoptosis and repressed the proliferation of HeLa cells via stabilisation of p53 protein (Zhang et al 2011b).

In vitro studies have also demonstrated that LBP inhibited the growth of breast cancer cells (MCF-7) by arresting the cell cycle in S phase and inducing apoptosis through the extracellular signal-regulated protein kinase (ERK) pathway, which is an important regulating pathway of cell proliferation (Shen & Du 2012).

Pretreatment of human epidermal keratinocyte cell lines and dermal fibroblasts with LBP attenuated the ultraviolet (UV) B radiation-induced expression of p1, p21 and p53 genes (Wang X et al 2011). Juice of the *L. barbarum* berry protected mouse epithelia cells from UV radiation-induced skin damage by preventing UV-induced lipid peroxidation and immunosuppression (Reeve et al 2010).

Furthermore, LBP has been shown to inhibit the growth of human colon cancer cells and human gastric cancer cells by inducing cell cycle arrest at G0/G1 and S phase (Bucheli et al 2011, Mao et al 2011, Miao 2010). It inhibits growth and induces apoptosis in human prostate cancer cells in vitro and prevents prostate tumour growth in vivo (Luo et al 2009). LBP has also been shown to inhibit the growth of oestrogen receptor-positive breast cancer cells in vitro by altering oestradiol metabolism (Li et al 2009).

Reduces chemotherapy- and radiotherapy-induced toxicity

LBP elicited a typical cardioprotective effect on doxorubicin-related oxidative stress in an experimental model (Xin et al 2007). Furthermore, an in vitro cytotoxic study showed the antitumour activity of doxorubicin was not compromised by LBP.

Interestingly, another animal study identified that LBP promotes the peripheral blood recovery of irradiation- or chemotherapy-induced myelosuppressive mice (Gong et al 2005). Compared to controls, 50 mg/kg LBP significantly ameliorated the decrease of peripheral white blood cells and peripheral red cells in irradiated myelosuppressive mice. Higher doses significantly enhanced peripheral platelet counts.

Ototoxicity is a major dose-limiting side effect of cisplatin. Uptake of cisplatin by hair cells in the organ of Corti results in increased local reactive oxygen species production and hair cell damage, leading to progressive and irreversible hearing loss. An animal study found that LBP attenuated cisplatin-induced damage to the organ of Corti via antioxidant activity (Liu et al 2011). Further research is required to determine whether using goji extracts and cisplatin at the same time affects the chemotherapeutic activity of cisplatin.

Immune modulation

LBPs have been known to have a variety of immunomodulatory functions, including activation of T cells, B cells, natural killer (NK) cells and macrophages (Chen et al 2008, Zhang et al 2011c, Zhu et al 2007).

A polysaccharide–protein complex isolated from *L. barbarum* (LBP) activated macrophages in vivo (Chen et al 2009). The mechanism may be through activation of transcription factors nuclear factor-kappaB and activator protein-1 to induce tumour necrosis factor-alpha production and upregulation of major histocompatibility complex class II costimulatory molecules. LBP also activates T cells.

A milk-based *L. barbarum* preparation attenuated symptoms and pathology of influenza virus A infection in mice via enhanced systemic T-cell function and reduced inflammatory cytokines (Ren et al 2012).

L. barbarum glycopeptide 3, a specific polysaccharide, was found to reverse apoptotic resistance of T cells in aged mice (Yuan et al 2008). Apoptotic resistance of T cells occurs as part of the ageing process. The ability of *L. barbarum* glycopeptides 3 to regulate T-cell apoptosis suggests that it may be of use to promote healthy ageing.

Sexual behaviour and male reproductive function

Studies with experimental models suggest the polysaccharides in goji berries may improve sexual behaviour and reproductive function (Luo et al 2006, 2011). LBP improved the copulatory performance and reproductive function of hemicastrated male rats, such as shortened penis erection latency and mount latency, regulated secretion of sexual hormones and increased hormone levels, raised accessory sexual organ weights and improved sperm quantity and quality (Luo et al 2006). Another study found that LBP improved the copulatory performance, including increase of copulatory efficiency, increase of ejaculation frequency and shortening of ejaculation latency in male rats. LBP prevented corticosterone-induced sexual inhibition and reversed corticosterone-induced suppression of neurogenesis in the subventricular zone and hippocampus. Prosexual effects were not seen in rats in which neurogenesis was blocked, suggesting the prosexual effect of LBP may be modulated via regulation of neurogenesis (Lau et al 2012).

Studies with LBP indicate a protective effect on testicular cells against a variety of insults. Pretreatment with LBP reversed a number of parameters of testicular oxidative stress and toxicity in doxorubicin-treated rats. LBP reversed the doxorubicin-induced increase in abnormal sperm rate and tissue oxidation, and the reduction in sperm concentration, percentage of motile sperm and testicular weight. LBP-treated rats also had significantly increased plasma testosterone levels compared to controls (Xin et al 2012).

Luo et al (2006) demonstrated a dose-dependent protective effect for LBP against DNA oxidative damage of mouse testicular cells in vivo. LBP also inhibits time- and hyperthermia-induced structural damage in murine seminiferous epithelium in vitro (Wang et al 2002). Moreover, LBP delays apoptosis in this system, both at normothermic and hyperthermic culture conditions. Considering the oxidative stress is suspected to be a major cause of structural degradation and apoptosis in hyperthermic testes, the protective effect of LBP may be mediated by an antioxidant mechanism of action.

G

Hepatoprotective

Animal studies have demonstrated the protective activity of *L. barbarum* against the hepatotoxic effects of alcohol and a high-fat diet (Cheng & Kong 2011, Cui et al 2011, Wu et al 2010).

Pretreatment with LBP effectively reduced oxidative stress, hepatic necrosis and serum alanine transaminase levels in mice with CCL4-induced acute hepatotoxicity (Xiao et al 2012). Similar results were found in a study using an aqueous extract of *L. barbarum* and *Rehmannia glutinosa*; however it is difficult to determine the individual efficacy of *L. barbarum* due to the use of the herbal combination (Wu et al 2011).

Cardioprotective

Pretreatment with LBP significantly reduced doxorubicin-induced cardiac conduction abnormalities, and alleviated doxorubicin-induced increases in serum creatine kinase and aspartate transaminase. The suggested mechanism for the cardioprotective effect of LBP is via mediation of oxidative stress (Xin et al 2011a, 2011b).

Supplementation with LBP attenuated myocardial cell apoptosis in rats with ischaemia-reperfusion injury (Lu & Zhao 2010).

OTHER ACTIONS

One of *L. barbarum*'s glycoconjugates promoted the survival of human fibroblasts cultured in suboptimal conditions and demonstrated important skin-protective properties (Zhao et al 2005a).

LBP reduced heat stress-induced apoptosis of germ cells in rats (Tan et al 2012).

Cationised LBP nanoparticles successfully facilitated nuclear uptake of DNA encoding for transforming growth factor-beta 1 by rat mesenchymal stem cells in vitro. That cationised LBP may have a role as a carrier for gene delivery is a promising result for the field of gene therapy, as research in this area is attempting to develop new therapies for genetically-based and infectious diseases, such as haemophilia and cystic fibrosis, by introducing nucleic acids into the cell nucleus (Wang, M et al 2011).

LBPs demonstrated antidepressant activity in an animal model, potentially by enhancing synaptic plasticity (Zhang et al 2012). Administration of LBP to mice fed a high-fat diet significantly decreased total cholesterol, low-density lipoprotein, triglycerides and blood glucose (Ming et al 2009).

Administration of LBP to ovariectomised rats resulted in increased bone gene expression, bone mineral density and bone mineral content (Zhu et al 2010).

CLINICAL USE

Goji has become more popular in the last few years due to its public acceptance as a 'functional food' with highly advantageous nutritive and antioxidant properties. It is touted as being able to improve wellbeing and protect against cancer and other serious diseases. Most investigation with goji has been conducted in China and there is little clinical research information available in English-language journals.

Improved wellbeing

A meta-analysis of four small, randomised, placebo-controlled trials (three double-blind and one single-blind) was conducted to examine the effects a standardised *L. barbarum* fruit juice (GoChi, FreeLife International, Phoenix, AZ) on perceived general wellbeing. All four studies involved oral consumption of 120 mL/day of the standardised juice. A total of 161 participants, aged 18–72 years, were given a questionnaire consisting of symptoms graded 0–5. Pre- and posttreatment symptom scores were compared. The treatment group (n = 81) showed significant improvements in a number of subjective measurements of overall feelings of health and wellbeing, including fatigue, depression, stress, calmness, weakness, mental acuity, focus on activity, sleep quality, ease of awakening, daydreaming and shortness of breath, compared to the control group (n = 80) (Hsu et al 2012).

A randomised, double-blind, placebo-controlled clinical trial examined the general effects of orally consumed goji berry, *L. barbarum*, as a standardised juice (GoChi; FreeLife International, Phoenix, AZ) in healthy adults for 14 days (Amagase & Nance 2008). The study was designed to measure multiple outcomes based on the traditionally understood properties of the product. Comparisons between day 1 and day 15 revealed that goji treatment significantly increased ratings for energy level, athletic performance, quality of sleep, ease of awakening, ability to focus on activities, mental acuity, calmness and subjective feelings of general wellbeing. Furthermore, goji significantly reduced fatigue and stress, and improved regularity of gastrointestinal function. In contrast, the placebo group (n = 18) showed only two significant changes: decreased heartburn and elevated mood.

Immunomodulating

A randomised, double-blind, placebo-controlled trial examined the immunomodulatory effects of a standardised *L. barbarum* fruit juice (GoChi, FreeLife International, Phoenix, AZ). Sixty participants aged 55–72 years consumed 120 mL/day (equivalent to 150 g of fresh fruit) or placebo for 30 days. The treatment group showed statistically significant increases in lymphocytes (27%), interleukin-2 (IL-2) (58%) and immunoglobulin G (IgG) (19%) compared to both the placebo group and pretreatment levels. Other outcomes measured include levels of CD4, CD8, NK cells, IL-4 and IgA; however no significant changes were seen in any of these outcomes. The treatment group also reported significant improvement in general wellbeing, energy, sleep, short-term memory and concentration compared to both the placebo group and pretreatment reports. No adverse reactions were reported (Amagase et al 2009b).

A randomised, double-blind, placebo-controlled trial evaluated the effect of a milk-based *L. barbarum* formulation (Lacto-Wolfberry; Nestlé R&D Centre Shanghai, Shanghai, China) on immune function in the elderly. A total of 150 healthy elderly Chinese people aged 65–70 years were given a milk-based *L. barbarum* formulation or placebo (13.7 g/day) for 90 days. The treatment group had significantly higher postvaccination serum influenza-specific IgG levels and seroconversion rate, between days 30 and 90, compared with the placebo group. There was no statistically significant difference in postvaccination positive rate, delayed-type hypersensitivity response or inflammatory markers between the treatment group and the placebo group. No serious adverse reactions were reported. This study suggests the milk-based *L. barbarum* formulation can enhance the immune response to an antigenic challenge in elderly subjects without adversely affecting immune function (Vidal et al 2012).

Weight loss

Amagase and Nance (2011) conducted two small, randomised, double-blind, placebo-controlled studies on *L. barbarum* standardised juice (GoChi; FreeLife International, Phoenix, AZ) and its effect on caloric expenditure and waist circumference. One was an acute dosing study and the other tested the effects of treatment after 14 days.

In the first study, after a 12-hour overnight fast, 8 healthy participants received a nutritional beverage containing 360 kcal and one of three doses of standardised juice (30, 60 or 120 mL) or placebo (a formulation designed to match the colour and flavour of the juice). Resting metabolic rate (RMR) was measured at baseline, 1, 2 and 4 hours postintervention. The RMR rose in all groups from baseline, and after 4 hours had returned to baseline levels in all groups except the 120 mL *L. barbarum* treatment group. This group had an RMR that was significantly higher than placebo and other doses of *L. barbarum*.

In the second study, 33 participants were administered 90 mL of standardised juice or placebo in the morning with food and 30 mL at bedtime for 14 days. Caloric intake was restricted to 1200 kcal/day, and 15 minutes of walking each day was implemented for all subjects. Waist circumference was measured as baseline, midintervention and postintervention. The treatment group showed significant reductions in waist circumference at both mid- and postintervention assessment, whereas no significant change in waist circumference was seen in the placebo group. The results of both studies are promising; however, larger-scale studies of longer duration are required to clarify these findings.

Aphrodisiac and increased male fertility

Traditional evidence and animal studies provide some support for its use; however, well-controlled clinical studies are not available to determine the effectiveness of goji in this capacity.

Age-related macular degeneration

A randomised, double-blind, placebo-controlled trial evaluated the effect of a milk-based goji berry formulation (Lacto-Wolfberry; Nestlé R&D Centre Shanghai, Shanghai, China) on the clinical risk factors for age-related macular degeneration. A total of 133 healthy volunteers aged 65–70 years were administered 13.7 g Laco-Wolfberry (LBW, containing 530 mg/g goji berry, 290 mg/g skim milk powder and 180 mg/g maltodextrin) or placebo (290 mg/g skim milk powder, 200 mg/g maltodextrin, 476 mg/g sucrose and 34 mg/g yellow/caramel colourants) once per day for 90 days as a freeze-dried powder consumed in 200 mL of soup or warm water at lunch. LBW provided 10 mg/day goji berry-derived zeaxanthin, and 68.5 mg/day goji berry-derived vitamin C precursor. After 90 days, the LBW group showed significantly less macular hypopigmentation and fewer soft macular drusen than the control group. Plasma zeaxanthin (the carotenoid that composes the pre-retinal pigment and is abundant in goji berries) and antioxidant activity were significantly increased in the LBW group versus control. These findings suggest that milk-based goji formulations may protect against age-related macular degeneration by preventing hypopigmentation and soft drusen formation. Interestingly, no relationship was found between change in plasma zeaxanthin levels and changes in macular characteristics, therefore the mechanism of protection remains unclear (Bucheli et al 2011). It is worth noting that three of the authors are employees of the company that manufactures the milk-based goji berry formulation used in this study.

OTHER USES

Goji is broadly marketed as a 'functional food' with significant health-promoting qualities. The high concentration of antioxidants, vitamins and minerals in the fruit makes it a nutritious substance; however, claims that it cures major diseases are not founded on sound clinical evidence.

The high concentration of zeaxanthin in the berries makes it a good dietary source of this carotenoid. As such, indications which respond to increased zeaxanthin intake may also respond to an equivalent dose from goji berries. (See Lutein and zeaxanthin monograph for further information.)

G

Clinical note — Pesticide residues

Levels of pesticides pyridaben and imidacloprid, for which there are zero-tolerance levels, were found in commercial goji juice samples. Methomyl, a carbamate insecticide whose use is restricted due to its high toxicity in humans, was also found. Other pesticides were also found but these levels were below tolerance levels (Tran et al 2012). Practitioners should be aware of the source and quality of goji products.

Practice points/Patient counselling

- Goji berries are a nutritious source of antioxidants, vitamins and minerals.
- The LBPs in the fruit that are considered to be the most important for pharmacological activity are attracting research interest.
- Preliminary studies in test tubes and with animal models indicate the berry and/or polysaccharides enhance immune function, exert neuroprotective effects, reduce lipid and blood glucose levels in diabetic models and improve male fertility; however, human tests are not available to determine whether these effects are significant in humans.
- Use with caution in people taking warfarin.

DOSAGE RANGE

Daily dose: 6–15 g daily.

Bioavailability of zeaxanthin from freeze-dried wolfberries can be greatly enhanced when consumed in hot skimmed milk compared to hot water or warm milk (Benzie et al 2006).

ADVERSE REACTIONS

Cases of allergic reactions, including anaphylaxis after goji berry consumption, have been reported. Sensitivities to nuts, tomato, peach and *Artemisia* appear to be common in people sensitive to goji berries. Non-specific lipid transfer proteins seem to be the major allergens involved in sensitisation and cross-reactivity (Ballarin et al 2011, Carnes et al 2013, Larramendi et al 2012). One case study suggests that individuals with latex sensitivity may also be sensitive to goji berries (Gomez et al 2013).

One case of *L. barbarum*-induced photosensitivity has been reported in a 53-year-old male who presented with pruriginous eruptions on sun-exposed areas of 2-week duration. The man had been taking *L. barbarum* berries and *Uncaria tomentosa* infusions for 5 and 3 months, respectively. Photoprovocation tests with *L. barbarum* berries and *U. tomentosa* revealed that photosensitivty was not increased with *U. tomentosa*, but was increased with *L. barbarum* berries (Gomez-Bernal et al 2011).

One case of hepatotoxicity related to the consumption of *L. barbarum* has been reported. A 60-year-old woman was admitted to the hospital with a 24-hour history of asthenia, arthralgias, non-bloody diarrhoea and abdominal pain. The patient presented with mild jaundice and a generalised rash. She had been consuming a tea of goji berries three times daily for the previous 10 days and no other medication. Liver enzymes were raised, but no other abnormalities were detected in laboratory tests or abdominal ultrasound. Consumption of the tea was stopped, and liver enzymes returned to normal after 1 month (Arroyo-Martinez et al 2011). As it is unknown whether the tea was tested for authenticity and presence of contaminants, the causality cannot be established.

SIGNIFICANT INTERACTIONS

Warfarin

Three case reports exist in the literature suggesting that an interaction between warfarin and goji is possible. However causality remains unclear as it is unknown whether the suspected products were tested for authenticity and presence of contaminants.

One case was of an 80-year-old Chinese woman on a chronic stable dose of warfarin, who experienced two episodes of an elevated international normalised ratio (INR) after drinking herbal tea containing goji (Leung et al 2008). Another case describes a 61-year-old Chinese woman, previously stabilised on anticoagulation therapy (INR 2–3) who had an elevated INR of 4.1 as a result of drinking a concentrated Chinese herbal tea made from *L. barbarum* L. fruits (3–4 glasses daily). No changes in her other medications, lifestyle or dietary habits were revealed (Lam et al 2001). A third case describes a 71-year-old Ecuadorean-American woman who had been on warfarin for 3 months following knee surgery. The woman presented with epistaxis, bruising and rectal bleeding, and was found to have a markedly elevated INR. No changes in dietary habits or lifestyle were reported other than drinking goji juice for 4 days prior to hospitalisation (Rivera et al 2012). Until confirmation from controlled trials is available, caution is advised.

CONTRAINDICATIONS AND PRECAUTIONS

Allergic reactions in sensitised individuals, especially those with sensitivities to nuts, tomato, peach, latex and *Artemisia*.

PREGNANCY USE/PATIENT COUNSELLING

The fruit is likely to be safe when taken in typical dietary doses; however, the safety of higher doses is unknown.

PATIENTS' FAQs

What will this herb do for me?
Goji fruits are a nutritious source of vitamins, minerals and antioxidants. Preliminary tests show that it has multiple health-promoting effects, but little human research is available to confirm activity.

When will it start to work?
As a concentrated source of nutrients, general benefits will start within several days.

Are there any safety issues?
Three case reports suggest a possible interaction between warfarin and goji berry, but this remains to be confirmed.

REFERENCES

Amagase H, Nance DM. A randomized, double-blind, placebo-controlled, clinical study of the general effects of a standardized *Lycium barbarum* (Goji) juice. GoChi, J Altern Complement Med 14.4 (2008): 403–412.

Amagase H, Nance DM. *Lycium barbarum* increases caloric expenditure and decreases waist circumference in healthy overweight men and women: pilot study. Journal Of The American College Of Nutrition 30.5 (2011): 304–9.

Amagase H et al. *Lycium barbarum* (goji) juice improves in vivo antioxidant biomarkers in serum of healthy adults. Nutr Res 29.1 (2009a): 19–25.

Amagase H et al. Immunomodulatory effects of a standardized *Lycium barbarum* fruit juice in Chinese older healthy human subjects. Journal Of Medicinal Food 12.5 (2009b): 1159–65.

Arroyo-Martinez Q et al. *Lycium barbarum*: a new hepatotoxic "natural" agent? Digestive And Liver Disease 43.9 (2011): 749.

Ballarin S et al. Anaphylaxis associated with the ingestion of Goji berries (*Lycium barbarum*). Journal Of Investigational Allergology & Clinical Immunology 21.7 (2011): 567–70.

Benzie IF et al. Enhanced bioavailability of zeaxanthin in a milk-based formulation of wolfberry (Gou Qi Zi; *Fructus barbarum* L.). Br J Nutr 96.1 (2006): 154–160.

Bucheli P et al. Goji berry effects on macular characteristics and plasma antioxidant levels. Optometry And Vision Science 88.2 (2011): 257–262.

Carnes J et al. Recently introduced foods as new allergenic sources: Sensitisation to Goji berries (*Lycium barbarum*). Food Chemistry 137.1 (2013): 130–5.

Chan HC et al. Neuroprotective effects of Lycium barbarum Lynn on protecting retinal ganglion cells in an ocular hypertension model of glaucoma. Exp Neurol 203.1 (2007): 269–273.

Chang RC, So KF. Use of anti-aging herbal medicine, Lycium barbarum, against aging-associated diseases. What do we know so far? Cell Mol Neurobiol 28.5 (2008): 643–652.

Chen Z, et al. Activation of T lymphocytes by polysaccharide-protein complex from Lycium barbarum L. Int Immunopharmacol 8.12 (2008): 1663–1671.

Chen Z et al. Activation of macrophages by polysaccharide-protein complex from Lycium barbarum L. Phytother Res 23.8 (2009): 1116–1122.

Cheng D, Kong H. The effect of *Lycium barbarum* polysaccharide on alcohol-induced oxidative stress in rats. Molecules 16.3 (2011): 2542–50.

Cheng CY et al. Fasting plasma zeaxanthin response to *Fructus barbarum* L. (wolfberry; Kei Tze) in a food-based human supplementation trial. Br J Nutr 93.1 (2005): 123–130.

Chiu K et al. Up-regulation of crystallins is involved in the neuroprotective effect of wolfberry on survival of retinal ganglion cells in rat ocular hypertension model. Journal Of Cellular Biochemistry 110.2 (2010): 311–20.

Cui B et al. Effects of *Lycium barbarum* aqueous and ethanol extracts on high-fat-diet induced oxidative stress in rat liver tissue. Molecules 16.11 (2011): 9116–28.

Feng Z et al. A milk-based wolfberry preparation prevents prenatal stress-induced cognitive impairment of offspring rats, and inhibits

oxidative damage and mitochondrial dysfunction in vitro. Neurochemical Research 35.5 (2010): 702–11.
Gomez C et al. Goji berry: A potential new player in latex-food syndrome. Annals of Allergy, Asthma & Immunology 110.3 (2013): 206–7.
Gomez-Bernal S et al. Systemic photosensitivity due to Goji berries. Photodermatology, Photoimmunology & Photomedicine 27.5 (2011): 245–7.
Gong H et al. Therapeutic effects of Lycium barbarum polysaccharide (LBP) on irradiation or chemotherapy-induced myelosuppressive mice. Cancer Biother Radiopharm 20.2 (2005): 155–162.
Guoliang L et al. Supercritical CO2 cell breaking extraction of *Lycium barbarum* seed oil and determination of its chemical composition by HPLC/APCI/MS and antioxidant activity. Food Science and Technology 44.4 (2011): 1172–78.
Ho YS et al. Polysaccharides from wolfberry antagonizes glutamate excitotoxicity in rat cortical neurons. Cellular And Molecular Neurobiology 29.8 (2009): 1233–44.
Ho YS et al. Neuroprotective effects of polysaccharides from wolfberry, the fruits of *Lycium barbarum*, against homocysteine-induced toxicity in rat cortical neurons. Journal Of Alzheimer's Disease 19.3 (2010): 813–27.
Hsu CH, et al. A meta-analysis of clinical improvements of general well-being by a standardized *Lycium barbarum*. Journal Of Medicinal Food 15.11 (2012): 1006–14.
Hu C et al. The protective effects of *Lycium barbarum* and *Chrysanthemum morifolum* on diabetic retinopathies in rats. Veterinary Ophthalmology 15.2 (2012): 65–71.
Inbaraj BS et al. Determination of carotenoids and their esters in fruits of Lycium barbarum Linnaeus by HPLC-DAD-APCI-MS. J Pharm Biomed Anal 47.4–5 (2008): 812–818.
Jing L et al. Evaluation of hypoglycemic activity of the polysaccharides extracted from *Lycium barbarum*. African Journal Of Traditional, Complementary, And Alternative Medicines 6.4 (2009): 579–84.
Ke M et al. Extraction, purification of *Lycium barbarum* polysaccharides and bioactivity of purified fraction. Carbohydrate Polymers 86.1 (2011): 136–41.
Lam AY, et al. Possible interaction between warfarin and Lycium barbarum L. Ann Pharmacother 35.10 (2001): 1199–1201.
Larramendi C et al. Goji berries (*Lycium barbarum*): risk of allergic reactions in individuals with food allergy. Journal Of Investigational Allergology & Clinical Immunology 22.5 (2012): 345–50.
Lau B et al. Polysaccharides from wolfberry prevents corticosterone-induced inhibition of sexual behavior and increases neurogenesis. Plos One 7.4 (2012): e33374.
Leung H et al. Warfarin overdose due to the possible effects of Lycium barbarum L. Food Chem Toxicol 46.5 (2008): 1860–1862.
Li XM. Protective effect of *Lycium barbarum* polysaccharides on streptozotocin-induced oxidative stress in rats. Int J Biol Macromol 40.5 (2007): 461–465.
Li G et al. *Lycium barbarum* inhibits growth of estrogen receptor positive human breast cancer cells by favorably altering estradiol metabolism. Nutrition And Cancer 61.3 (2009): 408–14.
Li SY et al. *Lycium barbarum* polysaccharides reduce neuronal damage, blood-retinal barrier disruption and oxidative stress in retinal ischemia/reperfusion injury. Plos One 6.1 (2011): e16380.
Liang B, et al. Water-soluble polysaccharide from dried *Lycium barbarum* fruits: Isolation, structural features and antioxidant activity. Carbohydrate Polymers 83.4 (2011): 1947–51.
Lin CL et al. Antioxidative activity of polysaccharide fractions isolated from *Lycium barbarum* Linnaeus. International Journal of Biological Macromolecules 45.2 (2009): 146–51.
Liu Q et al. *Lycium barbarum* polysaccharides attenuate cisplatin-induced hair cell loss in rat cochlear organotypic cultures. International journal of molecular sciences 12.12 (2011): 8982–92.
Lu SP, Zhao PT. Chemical characterization of *Lycium barbarum* polysaccharides and their reducing myocardial injury in ischemia/reperfusion of rat heart. International Journal of Biological Macromolecules 47.5 (2010): 681–84.
Luo Q et al. Hypoglycemic and hypolipidemic effects and antioxidant activity of fruit extracts from *Lycium barbarum*. Life Sci 76.2 (2004): 137–149.
Luo Q et al. *Lycium barbarum* polysaccharides: Protective effects against heat-induced damage of rat testes and H_2O_2-induced DNA damage in mouse testicular cells and beneficial effect on sexual behavior and reproductive function of hemicastrated rats. Life Sci 79.7 (2006): 613–21.
Luo Q et al. *Lycium barbarum* polysaccharides induce apoptosis in human prostate cancer cells and inhibits prostate cancer growth in a xenograft mouse model of human prostate cancer. Journal Of Medicinal Food 12.4 (2009): 695–703.
Luo Q et al. Antagonistic effects of *Lycium barbarum* polysaccharides on the impaired reproductive system of male rats induced by local subchronic exposure to ^{60}**Co-γ** irradiation. Phytotherapy Research 25.5 (2011): 694–701.
Mao F et al. Anticancer effect of *Lycium barbarum* polysaccharides on colon cancer cells involves G0/G1 phase arrest. Medical Oncology 28.1 (2011): 121–26.
Mi XS et al. Protection of retinal ganglion cells and retinal vasculature by *Lycium barbarum* polysaccharides in a mouse model of acute ocular hypertension. Plos One 7.10 (2012): e45469.
Miao Y. Growth inhibition and cell-cycle arrest of human gastric cancer cells by *Lycium barbarum* polysaccharide. Medical Oncology 27.3 (2010): 785–90.
Ming M et al. Effect of the *Lycium barbarum* polysaccharides administration on blood lipid metabolism and oxidative stress of mice fed high-fat diet in vivo. Food Chemistry 113.4 (2009): 872–77.
Miranda MA et al.. Antioxidants rescue photoreceptors in rd1 mice: Relationship with thiol metabolism. Free Radical Biology & Medicine 48.2 (2010): 216–22.
Niu AJ. Protective effect of *Lycium barbarum* polysaccharides on oxidative damage in skeletal muscle of exhaustive exercise rats. International Journal of Biological Macromolecules 425 (2008): 447–49.
Reeve VE et al. Mice drinking goji berry juice (*Lycium barbarum*) are protected from UV radiation-induced skin damage via antioxidant pathways. Photochemical & Photobiological Sciences 9.4 (2010): 601–7.
Ren Z et al. Dietary supplementation with lacto-wolfberry enhances the immune response and reduces pathogenesis to influenza infection in mice. The Journal Of Nutrition 142.8 (2012) 1596–1602.
Rivera CA et al. Probable interaction between *Lycium barbarum* (goji) and warfarin. Pharmacotherapy 32.3 (2012): e50–e53.
Rui C et al. Protective effects of *Lycium barbarum* polysaccharide on neonatal rat primary cultured hippocampal neurons injured by oxygen-glucose deprivation and reperfusion. Journal Of Molecular Histology 43.5 (2012): 535–42.
Shan X et al. *Lycium barbarum* polysaccharides reduce exercise-induced oxidative stress. International journal of molecular sciences 12.2 (2011): 1081–88.
Shen L, Du, G. *Lycium barbarum* polysaccharide stimulates proliferation of MCF-7 cells by the ERK pathway. Life Sciences 91 (2012): 353–57.
Song MK et al. *Lycium barbarum* (Goji berry) extracts and its taurine component inhibit PPAR-γ-dependent gene transcription in human retinal pigment epithelial cells: Possible implications for diabetic retinopathy treatment. Biochemical Pharmacology 82.9 (2011): 1209–18.
Song MK, et al. Reversal of the caspase-dependent apoptotic cytotoxicity pathway by taurine from *Lycium barbarum* (goji berry) in human retinal pigment epithelial cells: potential benefit in diabetic retinopathy. Evidence-Based Complementary And Alternative Medicine 1.0 (2012): e323784.
Tan QH et al. [Protective effect of *Lycium barbarum* polysaccharides against heat stress-induced germ cell apoptosis in rats and its mechanism.] Zhonghua Nan Ke Xue = National Journal Of Andrology 18.1 (2012): 88–92.
Tang W et al. A review of the anticancer and immunomodulatory effects of *Lycium barbarum* fruit. Inflammopharmacology 20.6 (2012): 307–14.
Tran K et al. Finding of pesticides in fashionable fruit juices by LC-MS/MS and GC-MS/MS. Food Chemistry 134.4 (2012): 2398–405.
Vidal K et al. Immunomodulatory effects of dietary supplementation with a milk-based wolfberry formulation in healthy elderly: a randomized, double-blind, placebo-controlled trial. Rejuvenation Research 15.1 (2012): 89–97.
Wang Y et al. Protective effect of *Fructus lycii* polysaccharides against time and hyperthermia-induced damage in cultured seminiferous epithelium. J Ethnopharmacol 82.2–3 (2002): 169–175.
Wang NT et al. Effects of the antioxidants *Lycium barbarum* and ascorbic acid on reperfusion liver injury in rats. Transplantation Proceedings 41.10 (2009): 4110–13.
Wang M et al. Efficient gene transfer into rat mesenchymal stem cells with cationized *Lycium barbarum* polysaccharides nanoparticles. Carbohydrate Polymers 86.4 (2011): 1509–18.
Wang X, et al. Ginsenoside Rb1, Rg1 and three extracts of traditional Chinese medicine attenuate ultraviolet B-induced G1 growth arrest in HaCaT cells and dermal fibroblasts involve down-regulating the expression of p16, p21 and p53. Photodermatology, Photoimmunology & Photomedicine 27.4 (2011): 203–12.
Wen J, et al. Effect of *Lycium barbarum* polysaccharides on neurogenesis and learning & memory in manganese poisoning mice. Chinese Journal Of Integrated Traditional And Western Medicine 30.3 (2010): 295–8.
Wu H et al. Chemical characterization of *Lycium barbarum* polysaccharides and its inhibition against liver oxidative injury of high-fat mice. International Journal of Biological Macromolecules 46.5 (2010): 540–3.
Wu P et al. Hot water extracted *Lycium barbarum* and *Rehmannia glutinosa* inhibit liver inflammation and fibrosis in rats. The American Journal Of Chinese Medicine 39.6 (2011): 1173–91.
Xiao J et al. *Lycium barbarum* polysaccharides protect mice liver from carbon tetrachloride-induced oxidative stress and necroinflammation. Journal Of Ethnopharmacology 139.2 (2012): 462–70.

Xin YF et al. Protective effect of Lycium barbarum on doxorubicin-induced cardiotoxicity. Phytother Res 21.11 (2007): 1020–1024.
Xin Y et al. Electrocardiographic and biochemical evidence for the cardioprotective effect of antioxidants in acute doxorubicin-induced cardiotoxicity in the beagle dogs. Biological & Pharmaceutical Bulletin 34.10 (2011a): 1523–26.
Xin Y et al. Alleviation of the acute doxorubicin-induced cardiotoxicity by *Lycium barbarum* polysaccharides through the suppression of oxidative stress. Food and Chemical Toxicology 49.1 (2011b): 259–64.
Xin Y et al. Protective effect of *Lycium barbarum* polysaccharides against doxorubicin-induced testicular toxicity in rats. Phytotherapy Research 26.5 (2012): 716–21.
Yang M et al. Protective effect of *Lycium barbarum* polysaccharide on retinal ganglion cells in vitro. International Journal Of Ophthalmology 4.4 (2011): 377–79.
Yang D et al. *Lycium barbarum* extracts protect the brain from blood-brain barrier disruption and cerebral edema in experimental stroke. Plos One 7.3 (2012): e33596.
Yao XL et al. Protective effects of *Lycium barbarum* extract against MPP(+) -induced neurotoxicity in *Caenorhabditis elegans* and PC12 cells. Journal Of Chinese Medicinal Materials 34.8 (2011): 1241–6.
Yu MS et al. Characterization of the effects of anti-aging medicine *Fructus lycii* on beta-amyloid peptide neurotoxicity. Int J Mol Med 20.2 (2007): 261–268.
Yuan LG et al. Reversal of apoptotic resistance by *Lycium barbarum* glycopeptide 3 in aged T cells. Biomedical and Environmental Sciences 21.3 (2008): 212–17.
Zhang Z et al. Comparative evaluation of the antioxidant effects of the natural vitamin C analog 2-O-β-*D*-glucopyranosyl-L-ascorbic acid isolated from Goji berry fruit. Archives Of Pharmacal Research 34.5 (2011a): 801–10.
Zhang Z et al. Selective suppression of cervical cancer Hela cells by 2-O-β-*D*-glucopyranosyl-L-ascorbic acid isolated from the fruit of *Lycium barbarum* L. Cell Biology And Toxicology 27.2 (2011b): 107–21.
Zhang XR et al. Macrophages, rather than T and B cells are principal immunostimulatory target cells of *Lycium barbarum* L. polysaccharide LBPF4-OL. Journal Of Ethnopharmacology 136.3 (2011c): 465–72.
Zhang E et al. Synaptic plasticity, but not hippocampal neurogenesis, mediated the counteractive effect of wolfberry on depression in rats. Cell Transplantation 21.12 (2012): 2635–49.
Zhao H et al. *Lycium barbarum* glycoconjugates: effect on human skin and cultured dermal fibroblasts. Phytomedicine 12.1–2 (2005a): 131–7.
Zhao R, et al. Effect of *Lycium barbarum* polysaccharide on the improvement of insulin resistance in NIDDM rats. Yakugaku Zasshi 125.12 (2005b): 981–8.
Zhao R et al. Protective effect of *Lycium barbarum* polysaccharide 4 on kidneys in streptozotocin-induced diabetic rats. Canadian Journal Of Physiology And Pharmacology 87.9 (2009): 711–19.
Zhu CP, Zhang SH. *Lycium barbarum* polysaccharide inhibits the proliferation of HeLa cells by inducing apoptosis. Journal Of The Science Of Food And Agriculture 93.0 (2012): 149–56.
Zhu J et al. *Lycium barbarum* polysaccharides regulate phenotypic and functional maturation of murine dendritic cells. Cell Biol Int 31.6 (2007): 615–619.
Zhu M et al. Extraction, characterization of polysaccharides from *Lycium barbarum* and its effect on bone gene expression in rats. Carbohydrate Polymers 80.3 (2010): 672–6.
Zou S et al. Structure characterization and hypoglycemic activity of a polysaccharide isolated from the fruit of *Lycium barbarum* L. Carbohydrate Polymers 80.4 (2010): 1161–7.

Goldenrod

HISTORICAL NOTE *Solidago virgaurea* (goldenrod) is a perennial herb that is common in Europe and found at lower altitudes (below 1500 m). It is recognisable by its elongated and branched golden yellow flower heads that bloom in summer (Laurençon et al 2013). Goldenrod has been used in European phytotherapy for over 700 years for the treatment of chronic nephritis, cystitis, urolithiasis, rheumatism (Apáti et al 2003) and wound healing. The name *Solidago* is from the Latin verb 'to make whole'. In 1934, reports from the US Department of Agriculture suggested that goldenrod was considered as a potential future source of commercially prepared rubber, although it was noted that domestication of the plant would be difficult as it is vulnerable to fungal infection and insect attack.

COMMON NAME

Goldenrod

OTHER NAMES

Aaron's rod, blue mountain tea, sweet goldenrod, woundwort

BOTANICAL NAME/FAMILY

Solidago canadensis (Canadian goldenrod), *Solidago virgaurea* (European goldenrod) (family Asteraceae [Compositae]). There are numerous species of goldenrod.

PLANT PARTS USED

Dried aerial parts — flowers and leaves.

CHEMICAL COMPONENTS

Flavonoids, sesquiterpenes, diterpenes, triterpenes, saponins, phenolic glycosides (Zhang et al 2007), diterpenes (Starks et al 2010, Zhang et al 2007), rutin, catechol tannins, phenolic acids, one essential oil, diterpene lactones and polysaccharides.

MAIN ACTIONS

The pharmacology of goldenrod has not been significantly investigated; therefore, evidence of activity derives from traditional, in vitro and animal studies.

Diuretic

Goldenrod is considered an aquaretic medicine, as it promotes fluid loss without an associated disruption to electrolytes. Two animal studies have confirmed diuretic activity (Chodera et al 1991, Leuschner 1995). According to one study, excretion of calcium increases whereas excretion of potassium and sodium decreases (Chodera et al 1991). A review of herbal medicines for the urinary tract concluded that goldenrod is a major diuretic herb (Yarnell 2002).

Antispasmodic and anti-inflammatory

High doses of a commercial preparation of *S. gigantea* extract have demonstrated anti-inflammatory activity in an animal model, comparable to those of the pharmaceutical anti-inflammatory medicine diclofenac (Leuschner 1995). Other tests with an extract of *S. virgaurea* have also produced similar results (el Ghazaly et al 1992).

The herbal combination consisting of *Populus tremula*, *S. virgaurea* and *Fraxinus excelsior* has demonstrated dose-dependent anti-inflammatory, analgesic and antipyretic effects comparable to those of non-steroidal anti-inflammatory drugs (NSAIDs) in several animal models (Okpanyi et al 1989). Although encouraging, the role of *Solidago* in this study is uncertain.

OTHER ACTIONS

Traditionally believed to have an effect on the microarchitecture of the kidney.

Antifungal

Inhibitory effects on human pathogenic yeasts such as *Candida* and *Cryptococcus* spp. have been demonstrated for triterpenoid glycosides isolated from *S. virgaurea* (Bader et al 1990). The saponins are considered chiefly responsible for the antimicrobial activity of *S. virgaurea* extract against *Candida albicans* hyphae formation. A study which isolated six triterpene saponins (virgaureasaponin 1–6) from the dried aerial parts of *S. virgaurea* found that four saponins showed an inhibition of *C. albicans* yeast–hyphal conversion, whereas fractions F1 and F2 were inactive. In contrast, fractions F3 and F4 showed significant inhibition of yeast–hyphal conversion (Laurençon et al 2013).

Antibacterial

A moderate antibacterial activity in vitro against certain strains of bacteria, including species of *Bacillus*, *Proteus* and *Staphylococcus*, has been demonstrated from an extract of *Solidago virgaurea* (Thiem & Goslinska 2002). Clerodane diterpenes isolated from *S. virgaurea* were observed to have moderate antibacterial activity against *Staphylococcus aureus* (Starks et al 2010).

Anticancer effects

An extract of *Solidago virgaurea* has demonstrated antineoplastic activity in vitro using a variety of cell lines, including prostate, breast, small-cell lung carcinoma and melanoma, and in vivo in a mouse model of prostate cancer (Gross et al 2002).

Antiplatelet effects

Polyphenolic–polysaccharide conjugates from *S. virgaurea*, even at a concentration of 50 mcg/mL, could markedly reduce the level in nitrotyrosine in platelet proteins treated with ONOO−. The results indicated that the tested conjugates may protect platelet proteins against oxidation, leading to changed haemostatic function of platelets caused by peroxynitrite or its intermediates (Saluk-Juszczak et al 2010). With this antiplatelet effect, goldenrod may have a potential use in cardiovascular disease, with further research expanding on the mechanism of action in the treatment of cardiovascular disease.

Cardioprotective effects

A significant cardioprotective effect was observed in vivo against isoproterenol-induced cardiotoxicity when test rats were pretreated with *Solidago virgaurea* extract at a dose of 250 mg/kg once daily for 5 weeks. Without pretreatment, subcutaneous injections of isoproterenol led to a significant increase in serum lactate dehydrogenase, creatine phosphokinase, alanine transaminase, aspartate transaminase, angiotensin-converting enzyme activities, total cholesterol, triglycerides, free serum fatty acids, cardiac tissue malondialdehyde and nitric oxide levels ($P < 0.05$). In addition, there was a significant decrease in levels of glutathione and superoxide dismutase in cardiac tissue as compared to the normal control group ($P < 0.05$) (El-Tantawy 2014).

G

CLINICAL USE

Goldenrod has not been significantly investigated under controlled study conditions, so most evidence is derived from traditional use, in vitro and animal studies.

Cystitis

The most common use of goldenrod is in the treatment of bladder infections. Both the Commission E (Blumenthal et al 1998) and European Scientific Co-operative On Phytomedicine (ESCOP) (2003) have approved its use for irrigation of the urinary tract, with ESCOP also indicating usefulness as adjunctive treatment for bacterial urinary tract infections (UTIs).

IN COMBINATION

Two clinical studies have been performed using a test combination which included *Solidago*, *Orthosiphon*, birch extract and cranberry (Cistimev Plus and Cistimev). One study involved people with indwelling catheters and the other women with recurrent UTIs; both produced encouraging results.

The first randomised study evaluated the efficacy of 1 × 600 mg Cistimev Plus tablet daily compared to no therapy in reducing microbial colonisation and biofilm development in patients with indwelling urinary catheters. After 30 days, a statistically significant reduction of microbial colonisation was found for the test group (10/43) vs the control group (16/30) ($P = 0.013$) (Cai et al 2013).

The second study investigated the use of 3 months of antibiotic prophylaxis (prulifloxacin 600 mg, one tablet/week or phosphomycin one cachet/week) with and without the addition of Cistimev (one capsule/day) in 164 patients with UTI. The group using stand-alone antibiotics experienced a significantly greater UTI relapse risk (2.5 times greater) compared to the group taking combination therapy ($P < 0.0001$). Of the group taking both antibiotic prophylaxis plus Cistimev, 25% had no recurrence at 1 year, whereas all the patients receiving stand-alone antibiotic therapy experienced at least one recurrence within 1 year. In addition, the time to UTI recurrence was longer in the combination-therapy group (10.4 months) compared to antibiotics only (3.6 months; $P < 0.0001$) (Frumenzio et al 2013).

Arthritis (in combination)

The product Phytodolor contains alcoholic extracts of *Populus tremula*, *Fraxinus excelsior* and *Solidago virgaurea* and is standardised to 0.14 mg/mL of isofraxidine, 1 mg/mL salicine and 0.07 mg/mL of total flavonoids. As part of this combination, goldenrod has been investigated in patients with rheumatoid arthritis, osteoarthritis and back pain. Pain was significantly reduced by treatment with Phytodolor in a placebo-controlled study of 47 patients (Weiner & Ernst 2004). Symptom relief was equally effective amongst patients receiving half-strength, normal (60 drops three times daily) or double-strength treatment. A shorter placebo-controlled study of 2 weeks' duration found that Phytodolor reduced the need for conventional drug doses in subjects with 'at least one rheumatological diagnosis' (Weiner & Ernst 2004). Similarly, Phytodolor reduced requirements of diclofenac compared to placebo in a smaller study of 30 patients (Weiner & Ernst 2004). A 2-week placebo-controlled study of 30 subjects with osteoarthritis demonstrated that treatment with Phytodolor significantly reduced pain and improved grip strength (Weiner & Ernst 2004). A review found that Phytodolor may be a suitable alternative to NSAIDs and cyclooxygenase-2 inhibitors for the treatment of rheumatic disease (Gundermann & Muller 2007). The role of goldenrod in achieving these results is unclear.

Inflammation of the nasopharynx with catarrh

Goldenrod is also used to relieve symptoms in this condition. The astringent activity of the tannin components provides a theoretical basis for its use.

OTHER USES

In many countries, goldenrod is used to prevent urolithiasis and eliminate renal calculi (Skidmore-Roth 2001). Although only at the level of in vitro studies, goldenrod may be beneficial in reducing *Candida* overgrowth and in conditions associated with dry-mouth problems, without affecting the biofilm (Laurençon et al 2013). It is also used in children with otitis media and nasal catarrh.

Traditional uses

Goldenrod is used both internally and externally for a variety of conditions. Internally it is used to treat upper respiratory tract catarrh, arthritis, menorrhagia and urological complaints, vomiting and dyspepsia, and externally it is used to support wound healing and as a mouth rinse for inflammatory conditions of the mouth and gums.

DOSAGE RANGE

- Infusion of dried herb: 0.5–2 g in 150 mL of boiled water for at least 10 min.
- Fluid extract (1:1) (g/mL): 0.5–2 mL taken 2–4 times daily between meals.

ADVERSE REACTIONS

Handling the plant has been associated with allergic reactions ranging from allergic rhinoconjunctivitis and asthma to urticaria. There is one study of a cohort predominantly comprising florists who had presented with complaints relating to the handling of plants; extensive cross-sensitisation to pollen of several members of the Asteraceae family (e.g. *Matricaria*, *Chrysanthemum* and *Solidago*) and to pollen of the Amaryllidaceae family (*Alstroemeria* and *Narcissus*) was found (de Jong et al 1998).

SIGNIFICANT INTERACTIONS

None known.

Practice points/Patient counselling

- Goldenrod has a long history of use, but has not been tested in humans to any significant extent.
- Traditionally, it has been used internally to reduce upper respiratory catarrh, arthritis, menorrhagia, urological complaints and dyspepsia, and externally to promote wound healing and as a mouth rinse for inflammatory conditions of the mouth and gums.
- In Europe, goldenrod is a popular herb for treating lower UTIs and preventing kidney stones.
- When used as part of the commercial preparation Phytodolor, it provides effective symptom relief in rheumatoid arthritis and osteoarthritis, according to several clinical studies.
- It is considered an aquaretic herb: it induces diuresis but not potassium and sodium loss.
- Preliminary studies in animal models suggest anti-inflammatory activity comparable to that of NSAIDs, but human studies are not available to confirm the clinical significance of these findings.

CONTRAINDICATIONS AND PRECAUTIONS

Commission E cautions against use as irrigation therapy when heart or kidney disease is also present (Blumenthal et al 1998).

People with known allergy to goldenrod or who are allergic to the Asteraceae (Compositae) family of plants should avoid this herb.

PREGNANCY USE

From limited use in pregnant women, it appears that no increase in frequency of malformation or other harmful effects has been reported, although animal studies are lacking (Mills & Bone 2005).

PATIENTS' FAQs

What will this herb do for me?
Goldenrod has diuretic and anti-inflammatory activity, which may be useful in cases of bladder inflammation, although clinical testing has not yet been conducted to confirm this.
When will it start to work?
This is unknown.
Are there any safety issues?
People who are allergic to goldenrod or the Asteraceae family of plants should avoid taking this herb.

REFERENCES

Apáti P et al. Herbal remedies of Solidago — correlation of phytochemical characteristics and antioxidative properties. J Pharm Biomed Anal. 32.4–5 (2003): 1045–1053.
Bader G, et al. The antifungal action of polygalactic acid glycosides. Pharmazie 45.8 (1990): 618–620.
Blumenthal M et al. The complete German commission E monographs: therapeutic guide to herbal medicines. Austin, TX: The American Botanical Council, 1998.
Cai T et al. Solidago, orthosiphon, birch and cranberry extracts can decrease microbial colonization and biofilm development in indwelling urinary catheter: a microbiologic and ultrastructural pilot study. World J Urol. 2013 Oct 4 (epub ahead of print).
Chodera A et al. Effect of flavonoid fractions of *Solidago virgaurea* L. on diuresis and levels of electrolytes. Acta Pol Pharm 48.5–6 (1991): 35–37.
de Jong NW et al. Occupational allergy caused by flowers. Allergy 53.2 (1998): 204–209.
el Ghazaly M et al. Study of the anti-inflammatory activity of *Populus tremula, Solidago virgaurea* and *Fraxinus excelsior*. Arzneimittelforschung 42.3 (1992): 333–336.
El-Tantawy WH. Biochemical effects of Solidago virgaurea extract on experimental cardiotoxicity. J Physiol Biochem 70.1 (2014): 33–42.
ESCOP. European Scientific Co-operative On Phytomedicine, 2nd edn. Stuttgart: Thieme, 2003.
Frumenzio E et al. Role of phytotherapy associated with antibiotic prophylaxis in female patients with recurrent urinary tract infections. Arch Ital Urol Androl. 85.4 (2013): 197–9.
Gross SC et al. Antineoplastic activity of *Solidago virgaurea* on prostatic tumor cells in a SCID mouse model. Nutr Cancer 43.1 (2002): 76–81.
Gundermann KJ, Muller J. Phytodolor — effects and efficacy of a herbal medicine. Wien Med Wochenschr 157.13–14 (2007): 343–347.
Laurençon L et al 2013. Triterpenoid saponins from the aerial parts of *Solidago virgaurea alpestris* with inhibiting activity of *Candida albicans* yeast-hyphal conversion. Phytochemistry. 86 (2013): 103–111.
Leuschner J. Anti-inflammatory, spasmolytic and diuretic effects of a commercially available *Solidago gigantea* herb extract. Arzneimittelforschung 45.2 (1995): 165–168.
Mills S, Bone K. The essential guide to herbal safety. St Louis, MO: Churchill Livingstone, 2005.
Okpanyi SN, et al. Anti-inflammatory, analgesic and antipyretic effect of various plant extracts and their combinations in an animal model. Arzneimittelforschung 39.6 (1989): 698–703.
Saluk-Juszczak J et al. The effect of polyphenolic-polysaccharide conjugates from selected medicinal plants of Asteraceae family on the peroxynitrite-induced changes in blood platelet proteins. International Journal of Biological Macromolecules. 47.5 (2010): 700–705.
Skidmore-Roth L. Mosby's handbook of herbs and natural supplements. St Louis, MO: Mosby, 2001.
Starks CM et al. Antibacterial clerodane diterpenes from Goldenrod (*Solidago virgaurea*). Phytochemistry. 71.1 (2010): 104–109.
Thiem B, Goslinska O. Antimicrobial activity of *Solidago virgaurea* L. from in vitro cultures. Fitoterapia 73.6 (2002): 514–5116.
Weiner DK, Ernst E. Complementary and alternative approaches to the treatment of persistent musculoskeletal pain. Clin J Pain 20 (2004): 244–255.
Yarnell E. Botanical medicines for the urinary tract. World J Urol 20.5 (2002): 285–293.
Zhang J et al. A new phenolic glycoside from the aerial parts of *Solidago canadensis*. Fitoterapia. 78.1 (2007): 69–71.

G

Goldenseal

HISTORICAL NOTE Goldenseal is indigenous to North America and was traditionally used by the Cherokees and then by early American pioneers. Preparations of the root and rhizome were used for gastritis, diarrhoea, vaginitis, dropsy, menstrual abnormalities, eye and mouth inflammation and general ulceration. In addition to this, the plant was used for dyeing fabric and weapons. Practitioners of the eclectic school created a high demand for goldenseal around 1847. This ensured the herb's ongoing popularity in Western herbal medicine, but unfortunately led to it being named a threatened species in 1997. Today, most high-quality goldenseal is from cultivated sources.

Clinical note — Isoquinoline alkaloids

Isoquinoline alkaloids are derived from phenylalanine or tyrosine and are most frequently found in the Ranunculaceae, Berberidaceae and Papaveraceae families (Pengelly 2004). This is a very large class of medicinally active compounds that include the morphinane alkaloids (morphine, thebaine and codeine), the ipecac alkaloids (emetine and cephaeline), the atropine alkaloid (boldine) and the protoberberines (berberine and hydrastine). Many other plants contain berberine, including *Berberis vulgaris* (barberry), *Mahonia aquifolium/Berberis aquifolium* (Oregon mountain grape), *Berberis aristata* (Indian barberry), *Coptis chinensis* (Chinese goldthread), *Coptis japonica* (Japanese goldthread) and *Thalictrum minus*.

COMMON NAME

Goldenseal

OTHER NAMES

Eye root, jaundice root, orange root, yellow root

BOTANICAL NAME/FAMILY

Hydrastis canadensis (family Ranunculaceae)

PLANT PARTS USED

Root and rhizome

CHEMICAL COMPONENTS

Isoquinoline alkaloids, including hydrastine (1.5–5%), berberine (0.5–6%) and canadine (tetrahydroberberine, 0.5–1.0%). Other related alkaloids include canadaline, hydrastidine, corypalmine and isohydrastidine.

There are significant seasonal variations in biomass yields and hydrastine contents of goldenseal roots, although rhizome yield are largely unaffected (Douglas et al 2010). Late summer or winter harvesting has been shown to provide the highest yield and alkaloid contents.

MAIN ACTIONS

A wealth of empirical data exists for the medicinal use of goldenseal; however, much of the research has been conducted using the chief constituent berberine. It is recommended that goldenseal products be standardised to contain at least 8 mg/mL of berberine and 8 mg/mL of hydrastine (Bone 2003).

Antimicrobial

In vitro testing has demonstrated antibacterial activity of both the whole extract of goldenseal and the major isolated alkaloids (berberine, beta-hydrastine, canadine and canadaline) against *Staphylococcus aureus*, *Streptococcus sanguis*, *Escherichia coli* and *Pseudomonas aeruginosa* (Scazzocchio et al 2001). In a study, two flavonoids isolated from goldenseal were shown to exhibit antibacterial activity against the oral pathogens *Streptococcus mutans* and *Fusobacterium nucleatum* (Hwang et al 2003). An added antimicrobial effect against *S. mutans* was noted with the addition of berberine. The synergistic effect of berberine with other goldenseal-derived alkaloids has been demonstrated against *Staphylococcus aureus*, whereby sideroxylin, 8-desmethyl-sideroxylin and 6-desmethyl-sideroxylin all enhanced the antimicrobial effect of berberine despite displaying no antimicrobial properties individually (Junio et al 2011). This effect was shown to be mediated through inhibition of the NorA multidrug-resistant pump.

Root and rhizome ethanolic extract of goldenseal has been shown to exhibit antibacterial activity against *Helicobacter pylori* and *Campylobacter jejeuni* (Cwikla et al 2010). The methanolic extract of the rhizome inhibited the growth of 15 strains of *H. pylori* in vitro (Mahady et al 2003). The authors identified berberine and beta-hydrastine as the main active constituents.

Berberine alone, and in combination with both ampicillin and oxacillin, has demonstrated strong antibacterial activity against all strains of methicillin-resistant *Staphylococcus aureus* (MRSA) in vitro (Yu et al 2005); 90% inhibition was demonstrated with 64 microgram/mL or less of berberine. Berberine was also found to enhance the effectiveness of ampicillin and oxacillin against MRSA in vitro.

Many of the *Berberis* spp. contain the flavonolignan 5′-methoxyhydnocarpin, which inhibits the expression of the multidrug-resistant efflux pumps (Musumeci et al 2003, Stermitz et al 2000a, 2000b); however, it is unknown whether goldenseal contains this compound.

Berberine inhibits the adherence of streptococci to host cells by aiding the release of an adhesin lipoteichoic acid (an acid that is responsible for the adhesion of the bacteria to the host tissue) from the streptococcal cell surface (Sun et al 1998). Berberine is also able to dissolve lipoteichoic acid–fibronectin complexes once they have been formed. Berberine displays well-defined antimicrobial properties against certain bacteria and such data suggest that it may also be able to prevent adherence and destroy already-formed complexes.

Berberine may also possess antifungal and antiviral properties. Antimycotic synergism between berberine and miconazole was observed against *Candida albicans* in both plantonic or biofilm growth phases (Wei et al 2011). When used alone, berberine was shown to destroy cell wall and sterol biosynthesis in *Candida* spp. in vitro (Park et al 1999).

The antiviral activities of goldenseal and its constituents have also been demonstrated in a number of studies. Ethanolic extracts of goldenseal, stardardised to contain 25 microM berberine, were found to inhibit the growth of influenza A and the subsequent production of pro-inflammatory mediators TNF-α and PGE_2 after 24 hours exposure in RAW 264.7 cells (Cecil et al 2011). A study demonstrated the antiviral activity of berberine to be as effective as the DNA polymerase inhibitor ganciclovir in human cytomegalovirus (Hayashi et al 2007). It appeared to work via a different mechanism and may prove useful if used in conjunction to prevent tolerance and reduce toxicity.

Antidiarrhoeal

Berberine decreases intestinal activity by activating alpha-2-adrenoceptors and reducing cyclic adenosine monophosphate (cAMP) (Hui et al 1991). Berberine also inhibits intestinal iron secretion and inhibits toxin formation from microbes (Birdsall & Kelly 1997).

Berberine has demonstrated efficacy in vitro for many bacteria that cause infective diarrhoea, including *E. coli*, *Shigella dysenteriae*, *Salmonella paratyphi*, *Clostridium perfringens* and *Bacillus subtilis* (Mahady & Chadwick 2001). It has also demonstrated activity in vitro against parasites that cause diarrhoea, including *Entamoeba histolytica*, *Giardia lamblia* and *Trichomonas vaginalis*. Berberine was effective against multiple strains of Shigella in vitro, with effects almost comparable to standard ciprofloxacin (Joshi et al 2011). An in vitro model of human intestinal epithelia found that berberine increased expression of the Na^+/H^+ exchanger 3 and aquaporin 4 proteins in a model of induced diarrhoea, suggesting its actions may be mediated through enhancing sodium and water absorption (Zhang et al 2012). Further, in vivo studies have shown that berberine treatment delayed the onset of experimentally induced diarrhoea and number of diarrhoeal episodes in a dose-dependent manner. The effects of berberine on cholera toxin-induced water and electrolyte secretion were investigated in an experimental in vivo model (Swabb et al 1981). Secretions of water, sodium and chlorine were reduced 60–80 minutes after exposure to berberine. Berberine did not alter ileal water or electrolyte transport in the control model. It produced a significant reduction in fluid accumulation caused by infection with *E. coli* in vivo (Khin-Maung & Nwe Nwe 1992). Oral doses of berberine before the toxin was introduced and intragastric injection after infection were both effective. Berberine was shown to inhibit by approximately 70% the secretory effects of *Vibrio cholerae* and *E. coli* in a rabbit ligated intestinal loop model (Sack & Froehlich 1982). As in the other study, the drug was effective when given either before or after enterotoxin binding. In an investigation using pig jejunum, berberine demonstrated a reduction in water and electrolyte secretion after intraluminal perfusion with *E. coli* (Zhu & Ahrens 1982).

Berberine significantly slowed small intestine transit time in an experimental in vivo model (Eaker & Sninsky 1989). Berberine inhibited myoelectric activity, which appears to be partially mediated by opioid and alpha-adrenergic receptors. The antidiarrhoeal properties of berberine may be partially due to the constituents' ability to delay small intestinal transit time.

Cardiovascular actions

Berberine may be effective for congestive heart failure and arrhythmia, as it has demonstrated positive inotropic, negative chronotropic, antiarrhythmic and vasodilator properties (Lau et al 2001).

In a 12-week rat model of hypercholesterolaemia and hyperglycaemia, berberine treatment (30 mg/kg/day) resulted in a 64% increase in cardiac output, 16% increase in left ventricular systolic pressure and a 121% decrease in left ventricular end diastolic pressure compared to no treatment (Dong et al 2011). Through analysis of cardiac biomarkers and protein expression, it was suggested these results were due to berberine's effects on alleviating cardiac lipid accumulation and promoting glucose transport.

In similar studies, after 8 weeks of treatment, oral doses of berberine (10 mg/kg) improved cardiac function and prevented development of left ventricular hypertrophy induced by pressure overload in rats (Hong et al 2002, 2003). Berberine was found to reduce left ventricular end-diastolic pressure, improve contraction and relaxation and decrease the amount of the atrophied heart muscle.

Berberine has also been found to increase cardiac output in dogs with left ventricular failure due to ischaemia (Huang et al 1992). Over 10 days, intravenous administration of berberine (1 mg/kg, within 3 minutes) followed by a constant infusion (0.2 mg/kg/min, 30 minutes) increased the cardiac output and decreased left ventricular end-diastolic pressure, diastolic blood pressure (DBP) and systemic vascular resistance, but did not affect heart rate. This study shows that berberine may be able to improve impaired left ventricular function by exerting positive inotropic effects and mild systemic vasodilatation. These results, although interesting, should be evaluated cautiously as the method of administration was intravenous. The hypotensive effects of the berberine derivative, 6-protoberberine (PTB-6), were studied in spontaneously hypertensive rats (Liu et al 1999). PTB-6 lowered systolic blood pressure (SBP) in a dose-dependent manner (5 mg/kg: -31.1 ± 1.6 mmHg; 10 mg/kg: -42.4 ± 3.1 mmHg). The berberine derivative also reduced cardiac output and heart rate. The authors conclude that the antihypertensive effect of PTB-6 is probably caused by a central sympatholytic effect.

Hypocholesterolaemic/anti-atherogenic

Berberine upregulates the LDL receptor (LDLR) by stabilising the LDLR mRNA (Abidi et al 2005, Kong et al 2004). A follow-up study confirmed this and went on to demonstrate that the whole root preparation of goldenseal was more effective in up-regulating liver LDLR expression and reducing plasma cholesterol and LDL cholesterol in hyperlipidaemic hamsters than the pure berberine compound (Abidi et al 2006). The authors also noted that canadine effectively upregulated LDLR expression and unlike berberine was not affected by MDR1-mediated efflux from liver cells. In another study, hamsters fed a high-fat diet for 2 weeks, followed by treatment with oral doses of berberine (100 mg/kg) for 10 days, demonstrated a 40% reduction of cholesterol, including a 42% reduction in LDL cholesterol (Kong et al 2004). No effect on HDL cholesterol was noted.

The synergistic effects of berberine with plant stanols has been described in a number of studies. One study found that the supplementation of hamster diet ($n = 17$) with 0.17% (100 mg/kg/day) berberine alone significantly reduced total cholesterol, HDL-cholesterol and non-HDL cholesterol compared to untreated control (Wang et al 2010). When co-administered with plant stanols, total cholesterol, non-HDL-cholesterol and triacylglycerols significantly decreased compared to untreated control, and both plant stanols and berberine alone. Conversely, the same research group found that in a rat model, berberine alone did not lower cholesterol, but when combined with plant stanols significantly reduced both total cholesterol and non-HDL cholesterol (Jia et al 2008). Rats being fed a high-sucrose, high-fat diet were given berberine (100 mg/kg), plant sterols (1% of total diet), a combination of both or a control mixture for 6 weeks. While berberine on its own made no appreciable difference, the combination reduced total cholesterol by 41% and non-HDL cholesterol by 59%. Berberine also reduced plasma triglycerides by 31%, which was of marginal statistical significance ($P = 0.054$).

In combination with mevastatin, a HMG-CoA reductase inhibitor, berberine increased LDL receptor mRNA and protein levels and suppressed mRNA levels of PCSK9, a gene which downregulated the LDL receptor (Cameron et al 2008). Further studies have been recommended to clarify the usefulness of berberine as an adjuvant therapy for patients receiving statins.

Berberine may have potential as an anti-atherosclerotic agent because of a demonstrated inhibition of lysophosphatidylcholine (lysoPC)-induced DNA synthesis and cell proliferation in vascular smooth muscle cells (VSMCs) in vivo (Cho et al 2005). Berberine also inhibited the migration of lysoPC-stimulated VSMCs and the activity of extracellular signal-regulated kinases, reduced transcription factor AP-1 and intracellular reactive oxygen species. An in vitro study found that in PMA-induced macrophages, berberine inhibits the up-regulated expression of MMP-9 and EMMPRIN, both of which have been shown to contribute to plaque instability and rupture (Huang et al 2011). This suggests that berberine may be useful for the prevention and stabilisation of atherosclerosis.

Antidiabetic

A glucose-lowering effect similar to metformin was observed in vitro for berberine; however, no effect was seen on insulin secretion (Yin et al 2002).

In high-fat diet-induced obese mice, the administration of 3 mg/kg/day berberine for 36 days resulted in significantly reduced food intake and blood glucose levels compared to untreated control (Hu & Davies 2010). A reduction in body weight and serum triglycerides was also seen at berberine concentrations of 0.75–3 mg/kg/day and a decrease in total serum cholesterol from 1.5–5 mg/kg/day. Results from this study suggest that berberine may be a useful adjunct in the prevention of obesity, although further tests are warranted.

Blood glucose, blood lipids, muscle triglycerides and insulin sensitivity were measured before and after the ingestion of berberine or metformin in rats fed a high-fat diet (Gao et al 1997). In this trial, berberine and metformin improved insulin resistance and liver glycogen levels, but had no effect on blood glucose, insulin, lipid and muscle triglyceride levels. The study was able to demonstrate that berberine was as effective as metformin for improving insulin sensitivity in the rats.

Similarly, fasting blood glucose, total cholesterol and triglyceride levels significantly decreased after 8 weeks of treatment with 187.5 or 562.5 mg/kg of berberine in an experimental model of glucose intolerance (Leng et al 2004). An additional in vitro study using insulin secreted from pancreatic cells, incubated with berberine for 12 hours, concluded that berberine increased insulin production. The relationship of these trials to oral doses in humans is unknown. In another in vivo test, diabetic rats were treated with berberine (100 or 200 mg/kg) via intragastric means for 21 days (Tang et al 2006). The researchers found that berberine demonstrated hypoglycaemic, hypolipidaemic and antioxidant effects.

Berberine inhibits alpha-glucosidase and therefore reduces the transport of glucose through the intestinal epithelium (Pan et al 2003). Berberine also appears to stimulate glucose uptake through the AMP-AMPK-p38 MAPK pathway, which may be at least partly responsible for its hypoglycaemic effects (Cheng et al 2006).

Berberine may be able to attenuate the renal complications of diabetes. Streptozotocin-induced diabetic rats were fed berberine (200 mg/kg) for 12 weeks in order to examine the effects on kidney function (Liu et al 2008). The results showed significant reductions in fasting blood glucose, blood urea nitrogen, protein and creatinine over 24 hours as compared to control animals.

Anti-inflammatory

Rats treated long-term with golden seal (25,000 ppm in feed) over 2 years exhibited reduced lung and sinus inflammation as well as reduced neutrophil, macrophage and lymphocyte infiltration within both regions, indicative of reduced inflammatory mediation (Dunnick et al 2011).

Supplementation of berberine (50–500 mg/kg) over 14 weeks in non-obese diabetic mice was found to reduce the ratio of pro-/anti-inflammatory cytokines in the liver and kidney, as well as reduced the Th1/Th2 ratios in the spleen, thereby protecting these organs from spontaneous chronic inflammation (Chueh & Lin 2012).

Both in vitro and in vivo studies have found that berberine inhibits cyclo-oxygenase 2 (COX-2) transcriptional activity (Feng et al 2012, Fukuda et al 1999, Kuo et al 2005) and reduces prostaglandin (PG) synthesis (Kuo et al 2004). Berberine also inhibits kappa B-alpha phosphorylation and degradation, therefore reducing certain inflammatory mediators such as induced tumour necrosis factor (TNF)-alpha and interleukin (IL)-1beta productions in human lung cells (Lee et al 2007). The compound has also been found to reduce proliferation of human lymphocytes in vitro by inhibiting DNA synthesis in activated cells (Ckless et al 1995).

Skin Ageing

Berberine inhibits basal and UV-induced matrix metalloproteinase (MMP)-1 activity, an interstitial collagenase, as well as increasing type I procollagen expression in primary human dermal fibroblasts (Kim & Chung 2008). The same group also demonstrated that berberine inhibited both basal and TPA-induced expression of MMP-9 and suppressed TPA-induced IL-6 expression in normal human keratinocytes (Kim et al 2008). These preliminary results suggest berberine may be of use in the prevention of skin damage associated with ageing and UV exposure, although further studies are recommended.

Immune activity

Intragastric administration of the crude extract of goldenseal for 6 weeks increased the production of IgM in vivo (Rehman et al 1999). Berberine has also been found to induce IL-12 p40, a large subunit of IL-12, through the activation of p38 mitogen-activated protein kinase in mouse macrophages (Kang et al 2002). Interleukin-12 is crucial for the development of the Th1 immune response and thus may also have a therapeutic effect in reducing Th2 allergic disorders. A follow-up study demonstrated that pretreatment with berberine induced IL-12 production in stimulated macrophages and dendritic cells (Kim et al 2003). Macrophages pretreated with berberine had an increased ability to induce interferon (IFN)-gamma and a reduced ability to induce IL-4 in antigen-primed CD4+ T-cells. Increased levels of IL-12 appear to deviate CD4+ T-cells from the Th2 to the Th1 pathway. This inhibition of type 2 cytokine responses indicates that berberine may be an effective anti-allergic compound.

The immunosuppressive effects of berberine were investigated in an induced autoimmune model in vivo (Marinova et al 2000). Berberine was administered daily (10 mg/kg) for 3 days before intravenous induction of tubulo-interstitial nephritis (TIN).

Significantly less damage and an increase in renal function were demonstrated in the animals pretreated with berberine as compared to controls after 2 months. Berberine decreased CD3, CD4 and CD8 lymphocytes in comparison with the non-treated animals. These results suggest that berberine may exert an immunosuppressive effect in a TIN model. Clinical trials in human kidney autoimmune diseases are warranted.

Carcinogenic vs anticancer properties

A 2-year study by the National Toxicology Program investigated the effect of long-term administration of goldenseal (0–25,000 ppm in feed) in male and female rats and mice (Dunnick et al 2011). In both male and female rats, an increased incidence of hepatocellular adenoma was observed at doses of 25,000 ppm goldenseal. In male and female mice, significantly increased incidence of multiple hepatocellular adenoma was also observed from 9000 ppm. Further in vivo studies are recommended to determine whether use of goldenseal is likely to be safe and effective in a clinical setting (Tang et al 2009).

In contrast to this, there are a number of laboratory studies that have identified anticancer effects of berberine in the absence of other constituents of goldenseal (Tang et al 2009). Berberine has demonstrated cytotoxic activity in vitro against many strains of human cancer cells (Chen et al 2013, Hwang et al 2006, Kettmann et al 2004, Kuo et al 2005, Meeran et al 2008, Piyanuch et al 2007, Serafim et al 2008, Wang et al 2008). This is due in part to the reduction of COX-2 enzymes (Kuo et al 2005, Tai & Luo 2003), damage to the cytoplasmic membrane, DNA fragmentation (Letasiova et al 2005) and inhibition of topoisomerase II (Chen et al 2013). Pro-apoptotic activity of berberine through modulation of the HER2/PI3K/AKT signalling pathway and the mitochondrial apoptotic pathway have also been described (Tillhon et al 2012).

In an animal model of induced hepatocarcinoma, the combination of berberine and S-allyl-cysteine (SAC) inhibited Akt-mediated cellular proliferation, restored liver function and prevented morphological alterations in treated mice compared to control (Sengupta et al 2014). This study identified the inhibition of Akt-mediated pathways, inhibition of JNK and activation of PP2A may play a role in the underlying mechanisms of berberine and SAC in the induced hepatocarcinoma model. Similarly, another in vivo study found the oral administration of berberine (50 mg/kg) reduced hepatocarcinogenesis through reductions in iNOS, hepatocyte proliferation and reduce cytochrome P450 activities (Zhao et al 2008).

The antitumour effects of berberine were investigated on malignant brain tumours in an in vitro and in vivo model (Zhang et al 1990). Berberine (150 mg/mL) demonstrated an ability to kill 91% of cells in six human malignant brain tumour cell lines and 10 mg/kg exhibited an 80.9% cell-kill rate against solid brain tumours in vivo. The addition of berberine to 1,3-bis(2-chloroethyl)-1-nitrosourea increased cytotoxicity.

G

Neuroprotective

An in vivo study was designed to investigate the neuroprotective effects of berberine in ischaemic brain injury (Zhou et al 2008). Berberine (20 mg/kg) was intragastrically administered 30 minutes before and 1 day after middle cerebral artery occlusion (MCAO) was performed. After 48 hours, infarct size and neurological deficits were significantly reduced in the treatment group as compared to control. The authors were interested in discovering the mechanisms of action and designed a follow-up in vitro study. They found that berberine inhibited reactive oxygen species and protected PC12 cells against glucose and oxygen deprivation.

Berberine may also be effective in Alzheimer's disease according to early in vitro data (Asai et al 2007). Berberine significantly reduced extracellular amyloid-beta peptide levels by modulating amyloid precursor proteins in human neuroglioma H4 cells.

Antidepressant

A number of in vivo studies have shown berberine to have antidepressant effects at doses up to 20 mg/kg (Kulkarni & Dhir 2008, Peng et al 2007). Within mouse models, berberine has been shown to inhibit both noradrenaline and serotonin uptake in mouse brain synaptosomes, an effect which may be mediated by human organic cation transporters hOCT2 and hOCT3 (Sun et al 2014).

Oral doses of berberine (10 and 20 mg/kg) were shown to possess antidepressant effects in both the forced swim and tail suspension tests (Peng et al 2007). It was found to be slightly weaker than the positive control desipramine, a tricyclic antidepressant. In the forced swim test, however, berberine was shown to have additive benefits when used with desipramine, fluoxetine (a selective 5-HT reuptake inhibitor) and moclobemide (a monoamine oxidase inhibitor). The authors also noted that noradrenaline and serotonin levels were increased in the frontal cortex and hippocampus of animals in the berberine group (20 mg/kg).

Another in vivo study used the same models and gave animals either 5, 10 or 20 mg/kg of berberine IP (Kulkarni & Dhir 2008). They also found that animals in the berberine group demonstrated a reduced immobility period. Berberine (5 mg/kg IP) also improved the efficacy of subeffective doses of standard antidepressant medications in the forced swim test. The acute administration of berberine (5 mg/kg IP) increased noradrenaline (31%), serotonin (47%) and dopamine (31%) in the brain. The authors add that the mechanism may at least in part involve the nitric oxide pathway and/or sigma receptors.

Antioxidant

It has been suggested that berberine's diverse range of biological activities may be a result of its antioxidant properties (Siow et al 2011). Berberine quenches superoxide radicals, peroxynitrite and nitric oxide (Choi et al 2001, Jung et al 2009, Shirwaikar et al 2006). The molecular mechanisms underlying these observations, as well as specific clinical links to disease states, remain unclear.

Hepatoprotective

An in vivo study investigating the effects of oral goldenseal (300 mg/kg and 1000 mg/kg) on paracetamol-induced hepatotoxicity found that 300 mg/kg treatment attenuated increases in serum ALT and AST (Yamaura et al 2011). It was hypothesised by the authors that the inhibition of CYP2EI, which metabolises paracetamol to the hepatotoxic metabolite NAPQI, may be responsible for both observed effects.

In mice treated with carbon tetrachloride, berberine (5–10 mg/kg) was found to suppress the increase in serum ALT, AST, ALP, lipid peroxidation and the decrease in superoxide dismutase activity association with induced hepatotoxicity (Domitrovíc et al 2011). This study also found that berberine treatment reduced the histopathological changes associated with CCl_4-induced hepatotoxicity, possibly through the attenuation of pro-inflammatory cytokines TNF-α and COX-2, and antioxidant activity.

Mitochondrial function

In an animal model of metabolic syndrome, rats fed high-fat diets who then received 100 mg/kg/day berberine treatment were found to have increased hepatic mitochondrial efficiency and back to levels seen in normal, untreated rats (Teodoro et al 2013). The recovery of mitochondrial function, including normalisation of mitochondrial membrane potential, by berberine was associated with an increased activity of the mitochondrial sirtuin 3 (SirT3).

Urolithiasis

In a murine model of urolithiasis, berberine (10 mg/kg) prevented calcium oxalate crystal deposition in renal tubules and subsequent associated physical manifestations, including weight loss, impaired renal function and oxidative stress (Bashir & Gilani 2011).

Periodontal disease

Data from in vitro and in vivo experimentation suggest that berberine may slow periodontal degradation through regulation of matrix-metalloproteinases (Tu et al 2013). Berberine (0–100 microM) was added to LPS-treated human gingival fibroblast cultures and U-937 cultures, and was found to significantly decrease MMP activity in a dose-dependent manner. In periodontitic rats, berberine (75 mg/kg daily for 8 days) reduced gingival tissue degradation as assessed through micro-CT, histology and immunohistology, suggesting a possible role for berberine in periodontal disease.

OTHER ACTIONS

Traditionally, goldenseal is described as having the following activities: anticatarrhal, astringent, bitter, choleretic, depurative, mucus membrane tonic, vulnerary and oxytocic.

CLINICAL USE

Goldenseal has not been significantly investigated under clinical trial conditions, so evidence is derived from traditional, in vitro and animal studies. Many of these studies have been conducted on the primary alkaloids, in particular the isolated compound berberine. Although this compound appears to have various demonstrable therapeutic effects, extrapolation of these results to crude extracts of goldenseal is premature. It should also be noted that equivalent doses of the whole extract of goldenseal are exceptionally high.

Diarrhoea

Diarrhoea and constipation are common clinical complaints that negatively affect quality of life. Unlike drugs that require systemic absorption to exert their effects, luminally acting agents improve diarrhoea by altering intestinal and/or colonic motility, as well as mucosal absorption and secretion, through a variety of mechanisms. Berberine is an example of a luminally acting agent for diarrhoea. Berberine from *Hydrastis canadensis* L., Chinese herb Huanglian, and also found in many other plants, is widely used in traditional Chinese medicine as an antimicrobial in the treatment of dysentery and infectious diarrhoea (Lau et al 2001).

In accordance with both in vitro and in vivo studies, human studies have shown that berberine treatment has antidiarrhoeal activity.

A double-blind, placebo-controlled, randomised trial examined the effect of berberine alone (100 mg four times daily) and in combination with tetracycline for acute watery diarrhoea in 400 patients (Khin-Maung et al 1985). Patients were divided into four groups and given tetracycline, tetracycline plus berberine, berberine or placebo; 185 patients tested positive for cholera and those in the tetracycline and tetracycline plus berberine groups achieved a significant reduction in diarrhoea after 16 hours and up to 24 hours. The group given berberine alone showed a significant reduction in diarrhoea volume (1 L) and a 77% reduction in cAMP in stools. Noticeably, fewer patients in the tetracycline and tetracycline plus berberine groups excreted vibrios in their stool after 24 hours and interestingly no statistically significant improvements for patients with non-cholera diarrhoea in the tetracycline or berberine group were shown. A later randomised, double-blind clinical trial compared 200 mg of berberine four times daily plus tetracycline with tetracycline alone in 74 patients with diarrhoea resulting from *V. cholerae* (Khin-Maung et al 1987). There were no statistically significant differences between the two groups.

An RCT evaluated the effect of berberine sulfate in 165 men with *E. coli-* or *V. cholerae*-induced diarrhoea as compared to tetracycline (Rabbani et al 1987). Patients with *E. coli* were given a single 400 mg dose and those with *V. cholerae* were given either a single 400 mg dose or 1200 mg (400 mg every 8 hours), combined with tetracycline. Berberine reduced mean stool volumes by 48% in the *E. coli* group as compared to control over 24 hours. Patients in the *V. cholerae* group who received 400 mg of berberine as a single dose also had a reduction in stool volume after 16 hours as compared to placebo. The combination of berberine and tetracycline did not show any statistical improvement over tetracycline alone in the *V. cholerae* group.

A follow-up randomised, placebo-controlled trial was designed to evaluate the antisecretory and antimicrobial potential of various antidiarrhoeal agents including berberine in patients with active diarrhoea due to *Vibrio cholerae* or enterotoxic *E. coli* (Rabbani 1996). Berberine at a lower dose of 200 mg resulted in a reduction in stool volume of between 30% and 50% without significant side effects. Berberine was again shown to be more effective in the treatment of diarrhoea resulting from *E. coli* than in cholera.

Small-intestinal transit time was evaluated in 30 healthy subjects in a controlled study (Yuan et al 1994). Transit time was significantly delayed from 71.10 ± 22.04 minutes to 98.25 ± 29.03 minutes after oral administration of 1.2 g of berberine. These results suggest that the antidiarrhoeal effect of berberine might be partially due to its ability to delay small-intestinal transit time.

Giardiasis

Berberine may also be effective in the treatment of giardiasis. A comparison-controlled study of 359 children aged between 4 months and 14 years compared berberine (10 mg/kg/day) with metronidazole (20 mg/kg/day) for up to 10 days (Gupte 1975). Negative stool samples were evident in 90% of children receiving berberine after 10 days with 83% remaining negative after 1 month's duration. The results were comparative with the metronidazole (Flagyl) group (95% after 10 days and 90% after 1 month), without side effects. In a similar study, 40 children aged 1–10 years with giardiasis were given berberine (5 mg/kg/day), metronidazole (10 mg/kg/day) or placebo (vitamin B syrup) for 6 days (Choudry et al 1972). In the berberine group, 48% of children were symptom-free after 6 days and 68% had no giardia cysts on stool analysis as compared to the metronidazole group who experienced a 33% reduction in symptoms and a 100% clearance rate for cysts. These results show that berberine may be more effective than Flagyl for symptom relief, but not as effective for clearing the organism from the gastrointestinal tract. The aforementioned study (Gupte 1975) used a higher dose of berberine (10 mg/kg/day), which produced better results; however, the equivalent amount of goldenseal for either dose would be exceedingly high based on an average berberine content of 5%, which would be inappropriate.

Radiation-induced acute intestinal symptoms (RIAISs)

RIAISs are the most relevant complication of abdominal or pelvic radiation and have a negative impact on patients' daily activities. A RCT found that pretreatment with oral berberine significantly decreased the incidence and severity of RIAIs in patients with abdominal/pelvic radiotherapy when compared with the patients of the control group ($P < 0.05$) (Li et al 2010, Menees et al 2010). Oral berberine also significantly postponed the occurrence of RIAIs in patients with abdominal or whole pelvic radiation. The study included 36 patients with seminoma or lymphomas who were randomised to receive berberine oral (n = 18) or not (n = 18) and an additional 42 patients with cervical cancer were randomised to a trial group (n = 21) and control group (n = 21). Active treatment consisted of 300-mg berberine taken orally three times daily. In addition, 8 patients with RIAIs were treated with 300-mg berberine three times daily from the third to the fifth week.

G

Eye infection

A controlled clinical trial of 51 patients with ocular trachoma infections investigated the effectiveness of berberine over 3 weeks with a 1-year follow-up (Babbar et al 1982). Subjects who used the 0.2% berberine either by itself or combined with sulfacetamide demonstrated significant symptom improvement and tested negative for *Chlamydia trachomatis*, with no relapse after 1 year.

A later comparison-controlled clinical study also evaluated the effectiveness of the topical treatment of berberine for trachoma in 32 microbiologically confirmed patients (Khosla et al 1992). A 0.2% berberine solution (2 drops in each eye, three times daily) was found to be more effective than sulfacetamide (20%) in reducing both the course of the trachoma and the serum antibody titres against *C. trachomatis*. Berberine eyedrops were compared to berberine plus neomycin ointment, sulfacetamide and placebo in a double-blind, controlled clinical trial in 96 primary school children (Mohan et al 1982). Patients in the berberine group were asked to use 2 drops (0.2% berberine) of the solution in each eye, three times daily and to additionally apply a berberine ointment (0.2%) at night for 3 months. Children treated with only the berberine had an 87% clinical response rate, compared to 58% in the berberine and neomycin group; however, only 50% tested negative in follow-up microbiological tests.

A study addressed safety concerns about berberine eye products (Chignell et al 2007). They concluded that caution should be taken when eyes are exposed to strong sunlight.

Hypercholesterolaemia

In an RCT, oral doses of 0.5 g of berberine, given twice daily for 3 months in 32 hypercholesterolaemic patients, resulted in a 29% reduction in serum cholesterol, a 35% reduction in triglycerides and a 25% reduction in LDL cholesterol (Kong et al 2004). HDL cholesterol levels remained unchanged. Berberine also significantly improved liver function, as noted by liver enzyme levels.

Use of berberine (500 mg three times daily) in newly diagnosed type 2 diabetics ($n = 26$) compared to standard metformin therapy (500 mg three times daily) for 13 weeks resulted in significantly reduced total cholesterol (reduced by 0.57 mmol/L) and triglycerides levels (reduced by 0.24 mmol/L) in patients taking berberine compared to the metformin group ($P = 0.05$) (Yin et al 2008). In the same study, the combination of standard metformin therapy with berberine treatment resulted in significantly lowered LDL cholesterol, total cholesterol and triglyceride levels compared to baseline after 13 weeks.

A 2008 trial compared berberine, simvastatin and a combination of both (Kong et al 2008). Patients ($n = 63$) diagnosed with hypercholesterolaemia (total cholesterol over 5.2 mmol/L) were randomised into three groups and given either berberine (1 g/day), simvastatin (20 mg/day) or both. After 2 months of oral treatment, the results were as follows: monopreparation of berberine reduced LDL cholesterol by 23.8% and triglycerides by 22.1%; simvastatin reduced LDL cholesterol by 14.3% and triglycerides by 11.4%; combination therapy reduced LDL cholesterol by 31.8% and triglycerides by 38.9%. Total cholesterol reductions were similar to LDL reductions and HDL cholesterol did not change significantly in any group. All preparations were found to be safe.

Chronic congestive heart failure

The efficacy and safety of berberine in chronic congestive heart failure were studied in a randomised, double-blind, controlled study in 156 patients with chronic heart failure (Zeng et al 2003). All patients received conventional treatment and 79 patients in the treatment group also received 1.2–2.0 g/day of berberine for 8 weeks. Quality of life was greatly improved in the berberine group in comparison to controls, as measured by a significant increase in left ventricular ejection fraction, less fatigue and a greater capacity to exercise. A significant reduction in mortality was also noted during the 24-month follow-up (7 in the treatment group as compared to 13).

The acute cardiovascular effects of intravenous berberine (0.02 and 0.2 mg/kg/minute for 30 minutes) were studied in 12 patients with refractory congestive heart failure (Marin-Neto et al 1988). At the lower dose, a 14% reduction in heart rate was noted, whereas 0.2 mg/kg resulted in a 48% decrease in systemic vascular resistance and a 41% decrease in pulmonary vascular resistance. Right atrium and left ventricular end-diastolic pressures were reduced by 28% and 32%, respectively. Cardiac index, stroke index and left ventricular ejection fraction were also significantly enhanced.

Diabetes

Despite a large amount of preclinical data, well designed clinical trials investigating the role of goldenseal or berberine in glucose metabolism are still lacking. Preliminary studies suggest that berberine may be effective in lowering fasting blood glucose and Haemoglobin A_{1C} (HbA_{1C}) in patients with type 2 diabetes, as well as patients with comorbidities such as chronic hepatitis (Zhang et al 2010).

A pilot study was designed to determine the safety and efficacy of berberine in patients with type 2 diabetes mellitus (Yin et al 2008). Eighty-four subjects were divided into two groups. Study A consisted of 36 newly-diagnosed type 2 diabetics who received either berberine (500 mg three times daily) or metformin (500 mg three times daily) for 13 weeks. The second group (study B) consisted of 48 diabetics who were poorly controlled on their current medication. They all stayed on their current regimen and half also received berberine (500 mg three times daily) for 13 weeks.

Results for study A: Participants in the berberine group had very similar results to the metformin group. HbA_{1C} reduced by 2%, fasting blood glucose reduced by 3.8 mmol/L and postprandial blood glucose reduced by 8.8 mmol/L. Fasting insulin levels and postprandial insulin were also the same as the metformin group.

Results for study B: Participants in the combination group had reductions in haemoglobin A_{1C} from 8.1% to 7.3% ($P = 0.001$). Fasting blood glucose and postprandial blood glucose also improved significantly ($P = 0.001$), and fasting insulin was also reduced by 29.0%.

Polycystic ovary syndrome (PCOS) and IVF

An RCT involving 150 infertile women with PCOS found that 3 months of berberine treatment before ovarian stimulation produced greater reductions in total testosterone, free androgen index, fasting glucose, fasting insulin and HOMA-IR, compared with placebo (An et al 2014). The same study confirmed that berberine and metformin treatments prior to IVF improved the pregnancy outcome by normalising the clinical, endocrine and metabolic parameters in PCOS women but that berberine had a more pronounced therapeutic effect and achieved more live births with fewer side effects than metformin. Furthermore, treatment with berberine, in comparison with metformin, was associated with decreases in BMI, lipid parameters and total FSH requirement.

> ***Clinical note — Berberine absorption***
> Berberine is poorly absorbed, with up to 5% bioavailability (Pan et al 2002). In vitro data have clearly demonstrated that berberine is a potent antibacterial; however, in vivo data have established low bioavailability. Berberine has been shown to upregulate the expression and function of the drug transporter P-glycoprotein (Pgp) (Lin et al 1999). Pgp belongs to the super family of ATP-binding cassette transporters that are responsible for the removal of unwanted toxins and metabolites from the cell (Glastonbury 2003). It appears that Pgp in normal intestinal epithelia greatly reduces the absorption of berberine in the gut. In vivo and in vitro methods have been used to determine the role of Pgp in berberine absorption by using the known Pgp inhibitor cyclosporin A (Pan et al 2002). Co-administration increased berberine absorption sixfold and clearly demonstrated the role of Pgp in absorption.
>
> Increased expression of Pgp can lead to cells displaying multidrug resistance (Glastonbury 2003). As previously reported, a certain flavonolignan in many *Berberis* spp. has the ability to inhibit the expression of multidrug-resistant efflux pumps (Stermitz et al 2000a, 2000b), allowing berberine and certain antibiotics to be more effective.

Radiation-induced lung injury (RILI)

A prospective, randomised, placebo-controlled, double-blind trial was designed to determine whether berberine might reduce RILI in patients receiving radiation treatment for non-small cell lung cancer (Liu et al 2008). Ninety patients were randomised to receive either 20 mg/kg/day of berberine or placebo for 6 weeks during three-dimensional conformal radiation therapy. At 6 weeks, 45.2% of patients in the treatment group developed RILI as compared to 72.1% in the placebo group. At 6 months, 35.7% of patients in the berberine group experienced RILI as compared to 65.1% in the control group. Significant improvements in lung function were also demonstrated.

Recurrent apthous stomatitis

A randomised, placebo-controlled trial ($n = 84$) found that the application of a gelatin containing berberine (5 mg/g) four times a day for 5 days significantly reduced ulcer pain, ulcer size, exudate level and erythema level in patients diagnosed with minor recurrent apthous stomatitis compared to gelatin vehicle alone (Jiang et al 2013). Despite this, it should be noted that reductions across all four end-points were also seen in the control group, suggesting that occlusion of the ulcer with gelatin alone exerted some beneficial action. The authors did not comment on the significance of this finding compared with normal progression of ulcer wound healing.

OTHER USES

Menorrhagia, dysmenorrhoea, peptic ulcer, gastritis, dyspepsia, skin disorders, sinusitis, chronic inflammation of mucous membranes and topically for ulceration and infection. Goldenseal is included in some remedies to treat allergic rhinitis, though evidence for this indication is lacking (Kushnir 2011).

Traditionally, it is used as a bitter digestive stimulant that improves bile flow and liver function.

DOSAGE RANGE

Internal

- Tincture (1:3): 2.0–4.5 mL/day or 15–30 mL/week (Bone 2003).
- Tincture (1:10): 6–12 mL/day (Mills & Bone 2005).
- Dried rhizome and root: 1.5–3 g/day by decoction (Mills & Bone 2005).

External

- Eyewash: 0.2% berberine solution, 2 drops in each eye, three times daily (Khosla et al 1992).

ADVERSE REACTIONS

Goldenseal is generally regarded as safe in recommended doses (Blumenthal 2003). Doses higher than 0.5 g of pure berberine may cause lethargy, dizziness, dyspnoea, skin and eye irritation, gastrointestinal irritation, nausea, vomiting, diarrhoea, nephritis and kidney irritation (Blumenthal et al 1998).

SIGNIFICANT INTERACTIONS

Because controlled studies are not available, interactions are currently speculative and based on evidence of pharmacological activity. Many studies have shown that extracts of goldenseal significantly inhibit cytochrome P450 enzymes (Budzinski et al 2000, 2007, Etheridge et al 2007, Gurley et al 2005, 2008a, 2008b, Raner et al 2007). Two studies in healthy volunteers demonstrated that CYP3A4 and CYP2D6 were significantly down-regulated following goldenseal treatment (Gurley et al 2008a, 2008b). The inhibitory effects of berberine on CYP1A1/2, CYP1B1, CYP2C8, CYP2D6, CYP2E1, CYP3A4/5/11 and CYP4A10/14 have been reported in vitro and in vivo with one study finding that CYP2D6 and CYP3A4/5 were each down-regulated by 40% (Chatuphonprasert et al 2012, Gurley et al 2005, 2008a, 2008b, Lo et al 2013). As such, a pharmacokinetic interaction is likely between drugs chiefly metabolised by CYP3A4 or CYP2D6 and goldenseal.

Cyclosporin A

Berberine increased the blood concentration of cyclosporin A in renal transplant patients in an RCT (Wu et al 2005): 52 patients received 0.2 g of berberine orally three times daily for 3 months. The final blood concentration in the berberine/cyclosporin A group was 29.3% higher than the group given cyclosporin A only. The relevance of this to oral ingestion of goldenseal is unknown — caution advised.

Digoxin

Twenty healthy volunteers took 3210 mg of goldenseal and 0.5 mg digoxin daily for 14 days (Gurley et al 2007). There was no change in the pharmacokinetics of digoxin suggesting that this dose of goldenseal is not a potent modulator of Pgp.

Practice points/Patient counselling

- Goldenseal has been used traditionally as an antidiarrhoeal agent and digestive stimulant.
- Most clinical evidence has been conducted using the chemical constituent berberine. These data have shown effectiveness against diarrhoea, congestive heart failure, infection, plasma glucose and cholesterol.
- It has been suggested that berberine may also possess immunosuppressive, antidepressant and hepatoprotective properties based on animal and in vitro studies, though studies in humans are yet to confirm this.
- Goldenseal inhibits two key cytochromes (3A4 and 2D6) and therefore caution should be exercised if co-administering drugs metabolised via these routes.
- Goldenseal is not to be used in pregnancy or during breastfeeding, or in patients with kidney disease.
- Use with caution in patients who have hypertension or taking cyclosporin.

CONTRAINDICATIONS AND PRECAUTIONS

Goldenseal is contraindicated in kidney disease because of inadequate excretion of the alkaloids (Blumenthal 2003). Berberine has been found to be a potent displacer of bilirubin (Chan 1993). A review published in 1996 stated that berberine can cause severe acute haemolysis and jaundice in babies with glucose-6-phosphate dehydrogenase deficiency (Ho 1996). Goldenseal is therefore not recommended in pregnancy, lactation or cases of neonatal jaundice. Goldenseal is also contraindicated in hypertension (BHMA 1983) as large amounts of hydrastine have been reported to restrict peripheral blood vessels and cause hypertension (Genest & Hughes 1969). The dose required to induce this effect is unknown and the ability to reach this threshold using the whole extract is unlikely; however, until this is clarified goldenseal is best avoided in hypertension.

PREGNANCY USE

Contraindicated in pregnancy and lactation.

In addition to the preceding concerns about bilirubin, berberine has caused uterine contractions in pregnant and non-pregnant experimental models (Mills & Bone 2005). An in vivo study using 65-fold the average human oral dose of goldenseal investigated effects on gestation and birth and found no increase in implantation loss or malformation (Yao et al 2005). The authors conclude that the low bioavailability of goldenseal from the gastrointestinal tract was likely to explain the differences between in vitro and in vivo effects in pregnancy. Hydrastine (0.5 g) has also been found to induce labour in pregnant women (Mills & Bone 2005). Until more pharmacokinetic studies are done, goldenseal is best avoided in pregnancy.

PATIENTS' FAQs

What will this herb do for me?

Goldenseal may be used in the treatment of diarrhoea, dyspepsia, infection, diabetes and cholesterol. Most of the available research has been done on the alkaloid berberine. More clinical trials of the whole extract are needed to determine if the same effect will be seen.

When will it start to work?

Antibacterial and antidiarrhoeal activities should be apparent quite quickly. The lipid-lowering effects of goldenseal have been reported within 12 weeks.

Are there any safety issues?

The herb should not be taken during pregnancy or lactation and may interact with some medications.

REFERENCES

Abidi P et al. Extracellular signal-regulated kinase-dependent stabilization of hepatic low-density lipoprotein receptor mRNA by herbal medicine berberine. Arterioscler Thromb Vasc Biol 25.10 (2005): 2170–2176.

Abidi P et al. The medicinal plant goldenseal is a natural LDL-lowering agent with multiple bioactive components and new action mechanisms. J Lipid Res 47.10 (2006): 2134–2147.

An Y et al. The use of berberine for women with polycystic ovary syndrome undergoing IVF treatment. Clin Endocrinol.(Oxf) 80.3 (2014): 425431.

Asai M et al. Berberine alters the processing of Alzheimer's amyloid precursor protein to decrease Abeta secretion. Biochem Biophys Res Commun 352.2 (2007): 498–502.

Babbar OP et al. Effect of berberine chloride eye drops on clinically positive trachoma patients. Indian J Med Res 76 (Suppl) (1982): 83–88.

Bashir S, Gilani AH. Antiurolithic effect of berberine is mediated through multiple pathways. Eur J Pharmacol 651.1–3 (2011): 168–175.

Birdsall T, Kelly G. Therapeutic potential of an alkaloid found in several medicinal plants. Altern Med Rev 2 (1997): 94–103.

Blumenthal M. The ABC clinical guide to herbs. New York: Thieme, 2003.

Blumenthal M et al. Therapeutic guide to herbal medicines. The complete German commission E monographs. Austin, TX: The American Botanical Council, 1998.

Bone K. A clinical guide to blending liquid herbs. St Louis: Churchill Livingstone, 2003.

British Herbal Medicine Association (BHMA) Scientific Committee. British Herbal Pharmacopoeia. Cowling, UK: BHMA: Lane House, 1983.

Budzinski JW et al. An in vitro evaluation of human cytochrome P450 3A4 inhibition by selected commercial herbal extracts and tinctures. Phytomedicine 7.4 (2000): 273–282.

Budzinski JW et al. Modulation of human cytochrome P450 3A4 (CYP3A4) and P-glycoprotein (P-gp) in Caco-2 cell monolayers by selected commercial-source milk thistle and goldenseal products. Can J Physiol Pharmacol 85.9 (2007): 966–978.

Cameron J et al. Berberine decreases PCSK9 expression in HepG2 cells. Atherosclerosis 201.2 (2008): 266–273

Cecil CE et al. Inhibition of H1N1 influenza A virus growth and induction of inflammatory mediators by the isoquinoline alkaloid berberine and extracts of goldenseal (Hydrastis canadensis). Int Immunopharmacol. 11.11 (2011): 1706–1714.

Chan E. Displacement of bilirubin from albumin by berberine. Biol Neonate 63 (1993): 201–208.

Chatuphonprasert W et al. Modulations of cytochrome P450 expression in diabetic mice by berberine. Chemico Biol Interact 196.1–2 (2012): 23–29.
Chen S et al. Mechanism study of goldenseal-associated DNA damage. Toxicol Letters 221.1 (2013): 64–72.
Cheng Z et al. Berberine-stimulated glucose uptake in L6 myotubes involves both AMPK and p38 MAPK. Biochim Biophys Acta 1760.11 (2006): 1682–1689.
Chignell CF et al. Photochemistry and photocytotoxicity of alkaloids from Goldenseal (Hydrastis canadensis L.) 3: effect on human lens and retinal pigment epithelial cells. Photochem Photobiol 83.4 (2007): 938–943.
Cho BJ et al. Berberine inhibits the production of lysophosphatidylcholine-induced reactive oxygen species and the ERK1/2 pathway in vascular smooth muscle cells. Mol Cells 20.3 (2005): 429–434.
Choi DS et al. Inhibitory activity of berberine on DNA strand cleavage induced by hydrogen peroxide and cytochrome C. Biosci, Biotechnol, Biochem 65.2 (2001): 452–455.
Choudry VP, Sabir M, Bhide VN. Berberine in giardiasis. Indian Pediatr 9.3 (1972): 143–166.
Chueh W-H & Lin J-Y. Protective effect of isoquinoline alkaloid berberine on spontaneous inflammation in the spleen, liver and kidney of non-obese diabetic mice through downregulating gene expression ratios of pro-/anti-inflammatory and Th1/Th2 cytokines. Food Chem 131.4 (2012): 1263–1271.
Ckless K et al. Inhibition of in-vitro lymphocyte transformation by the isoquinoline alkaloid berberine. J Pharm Pharmacol 47.12A (1995): 1029–1031.
Cwikla C et al. Investigations into the antibacterial activities of phytotherapeutics against Helicobacter pylori and Campylobacter jejuni. Phytother Res 24.5 (2010): 649–656.
Domitrović R et al 2011. Hepatoprotective activity of berberine is mediated by inhibition of TNF-α, COX-2, and iNOS expression in CCl_4-intoxicated mice. Toxicol 280.1–2 (2011): 33–43.
Dong S-F et al. Berberine attenuates cardiac dysfunction in hyperglyceamic and hypercholesterolaemic rats. Eur J Pharmacol 660.2–3 (2011): 368–374.
Douglas JA et al. Seasonal variation of biomass and bioactive alkaloid content of goldenseal, *Hydrastis canadensis*. Fitoterapia 81.7 (2010): 925–928.
Dunnick JK et al. Investigating the Potential for Toxicity from Long-Term Use of the Herbal Products, Goldenseal and Milk Thistle. Toxicol Pathol 39.2 (2011): 398–409.
Eaker EY, Sninsky CA. Effect of berberine on myoelectric activity and transit of the small intestine in rats. Gastroenterology 96.6 (1989): 1506–1513.
Etheridge AS et al. An in vitro evaluation of cytochrome P450 inhibition and P-glycoprotein interaction with goldenseal, Ginkgo biloba, grape seed, milk thistle, and ginseng extracts and their constituents. Planta Med 73.8 (2007): 731–741.
Feng A-W et al. Berberine ameliorates COX-2 expression in rat small intestinal mucosa partially through PPARγ pathway during acute endotoxemia. Int Immunopharmacol 12.1 (2012):182–188.
Fukuda K et al. Inhibition by berberine of cyclooxygenase-2 transcriptional activity in human colon cancer cells. J Ethnopharmacol 66.2 (1999): 227–233.
Gao CR, Zhang JQ, Huang QL. Experimental study on berberine raised insulin sensitivity in insulin resistance rat models. Zhongguo Zhong Xi Yi Jie He Za Zhi 17.3 (1997): 162–164.
Genest K, Hughs DW. Natural products in Canadian pharmaceuticals. II: Hydrastis canadensis. Can J Pharm Sci 4: 41; as cited in Mahady GB, Chadwick LR. 2001 Golden Seal (Hydrastis canadensis): Is there enough scientific evidence to support safety and efficacy? Nutr Clin Care 4.5 (1969): 243–249.
Glastonbury S. Scientific evaluation of the use of traditional herbal depuratives via modulation of ABC transporters. Aust J Med Herbalism 15.2 (2003): 34–38.
Gupte S. Use of berberine in treatment of giardiasis. Am J Dis Child 129.7 (1975): 866.
Gurley BJ et al. In vivo effects of goldenseal, kava kava, black cohosh, and valerian on human cytochrome P450 1A2, 2D6, 2E1, and 3A4/5 phenotypes. Clin Pharmacol Ther 77.5 (2005): 415–426.
Gurley BJ et al. Effect of goldenseal (Hydrastis canadensis) and kava kava (Piper methysticum) supplementation on digoxin pharmacokinetics in humans. Drug Metab Dispos 35.2 (2007): 240–245.
Gurley BJ et al. Clinical assessment of CYP2D6-mediated herb-drug interactions in humans: effects of milk thistle, black cohosh, goldenseal, kava kava, St. John's wort, and Echinacea. Mol Nutr Food Res 52.7 (2008a): 755–763.
Gurley BJ et al. Supplementation with goldenseal (Hydrastis canadensis), but not kava kava (Piper methysticum), inhibits human CYP3A activity in vivo. Clin Pharmacol Ther 83.1 (2008b): 61–69.
Hayashi K et al. Antiviral activity of berberine and related compounds against human cytomegalovirus. Bioorg Med Chem Lett 17.6 (2007): 1562–1564.
Ho NK. Traditional Chinese medicine and treatment of neonatal jaundice. Singapore Med J 37.6 (1996): 645–651.
Hong Y et al. Effect of berberine on regression of pressure-overload induced cardiac hypertrophy in rats. Am J Chin Med 30.4 (2002): 589–599.
Hong Y et al. Effect of berberine on catecholamine levels in rats with experimental cardiac hypertrophy. Life Sci 72.22 (2003): 2499–2507.
Hu Y and Davies GE. Berberine inhibits adipogenesis in high-fat diet-induced obesity mice. Fitoterapia 81.5 (2010): 358–366.
Huang WM et al. Beneficial effects of berberine on hemodynamics during acute ischemic left ventricular failure in dogs. Chin Med J (Engl) 105.12 (1992): 1014–1019.
Huang Z et al. Berberine reduces both MMP-9 and EMMPRIN expression through prevention of p38 pathway activation in PMA-induced macrophages. Int J Cardiol 146.2 (2011): 153–158.
Hui KK et al. Interaction of berberine with human platelet alpha 2 adrenoceptors. Life Sci 49.4 (1991): 315–324.
Hwang BY et al. Antimicrobial constituents from goldenseal (the rhizomes of Hydrastis canadensis) against selected oral pathogens. Planta Med 69.7 (2003): 623–627.
Hwang JM et al. Berberine induces apoptosis through a mitochondria/caspases pathway in human hepatoma cells. Arch Toxicol 80.2 (2006): 62–73.
Jia X et al. Co-administration of berberine and plant stanols synergistically reduces plasma cholesterol in rats. Atherosclerosis 201.1 (2008): 101–107.
Jiang X-W et al. Effects of berberine gelatin on recurrent aphthous stomatitis: a randomized, placebo-controlled, double-blind trial in a Chinese cohort. Oral Surg Oral Med Oral Pathol Oral Radiol 115.2 (2013): 212–217.
Joshi, P.V., et al. Antidiarrheal activity, chemical and toxicity profile of Berberis aristata. Pharm.Biol 29.1 (2011): 94–100.
Jung HA et al. Anti-Alzheimer and antioxidant activities of Coptidis Rhizoma alkaloids. Biol Pharm Bull 32.8 (2009): 1433–1438.
Junio HA et al. Synergy-directed fractionation of botanical medicines: a case study with goldenseal (Hydrastis canadensis). J Nat Prod 74.7 (2011): 1621–1629.
Kang BY et al. Involvement of p38 mitogen-activated protein kinase in the induction of interleukin-12 p40 production in mouse macrophages by berberine, a benzodioxoloquinolizine alkaloid. Biochem Pharmacol 63.10 (2002): 1901–1910.
Kettmann V et al. In vitro cytotoxicity of berberine against HeLa and L1210 cancer cell lines. Pharmazie 59.7 (2004): 548–551.
Khin-Maung U et al. Clinical trial of berberine in acute watery diarrhoea. Br Med J (Clin Res Ed) 291.6509 (1985): 1601–1605.
Khin-Maung U et al. Clinical trial of high-dose berberine and tetracycline in cholera. J Diarrhoeal Dis Res 5.3 (1987): 184–187.
Khin-Maung U, Nwe Nwe W. Effect of berberine on enterotoxin-induced intestinal fluid accumulation in rats. J Diarrhoeal Dis Res 10.4 (1992): 201–204.
Khosla PK et al. Berberine, a potential drug for trachoma. Rev Int Trach Pathol Ocul Trop Subtrop Sante Publique 69 (1992): 147–165.
Kim S & Chung JH. Berberine prevents UV-induced MMP-1 and reduction of type I procollagen expression in human dermal fibroblasts. Phytomedicine 15.9 (2008): 749–753.
Kim TS et al. Induction of interleukin-12 production in mouse macrophages by berberine, a benzodioxoloquinolizine alkaloid, deviates $CD4^+$ T cells from a Th2 to a Th1 response. Immunology 109.3 (2003): 407–414.
Kim S et al. Berberine inhibits TPA-induced MMP-9 and IL-6 expression in normal human keratinocytes. Phytomedicine 15.5 (2008): 340–347.
Kong W et al. Berberine is a novel cholesterol-lowering drug working through a unique mechanism distinct from statins. Nat Med 10.12 (2004): 1344–1351.
Kong WJ et al. Combination of simvastatin with berberine improves the lipid-lowering efficacy. Metabolism 57.8 (2008): 1029–1037.
Kulkarni SK, Dhir A. On the mechanism of antidepressant-like action of berberine chloride. Eur J Pharmacol 589.1–3 (2008): 163–172.
Kuo CL, Chi CW, Liu TY. The anti-inflammatory potential of berberine in vitro and in vivo. Cancer Lett 203.2 (2004): 127–137.
Kuo CL, Chi CW, Liu TY. Modulation of apoptosis by berberine through inhibition of cyclooxygenase-2 and Mcl-1 expression in oral cancer cells. In Vivo 19.1 (2005): 247–252.
Kushnir NM. The Role of Decongestants, Cromolyn, Guafenesin, Saline Washes, Capsaicin, Leukotriene Antagonists, and Other Treatments on Rhinitis. Immunol Allergy Clin North Am 31.3 (2011): 601–617.
Lau CW et al. Cardiovascular actions of berberine. Cardiovasc Drug Rev 19.3 (2001): 234–244.
Lee CH et al. Berberine suppresses inflammatory agents-induced interleukin-1beta and tumor necrosis factor-alpha productions via the inhibition of I[kappa]B degradation in human lung cells. Pharmacol Res 56.3 (2007): 193–201.
Leng SH, Lu FE, Xu LJ. Therapeutic effects of berberine in impaired glucose tolerance rats and its influence on insulin secretion. Acta Pharmacol Sin 25.4 (2004): 496–502.
Letasiova S et al. Antiproliferative activity of berberine in vitro and in vivo. Biomed Pap Med Fac Univ Palacky Olomouc Czech Repub 149.2 (2005): 461–463.

Li, G.H. et al. Berberine inhibits acute radiation intestinal syndrome in human with abdomen radiotherapy. Med Oncol 27.3 (2010): 919–925.

Lin HL et al. Up-regulation of multidrug resistance transporter expression by berberine in human and murine hepatoma cells. Cancer 85.9 (1999): 1937–1942.

Liu JC et al. The antihypertensive effect of the berberine derivative 6-protoberberine in spontaneously hypertensive rats. Pharmacology 59.6 (1999): 283–289.

Liu W et al. Berberine inhibits aldose reductase and oxidative stress in rat mesangial cells cultured under high glucose. Arch Biochem Biophys 475.2 (2008): 128–134.

Liu Y et al. Protective effects of berberine on radiation-induced lung injury via intercellular adhesion molecular-1 and transforming growth factor-beta-1 in patients with lung cancer. Eur J Cancer 44.16 (2008): 2425–2432.

Lo S-N et al. Inhibition of CYP1 by berberine, palmatine, and jatrorrhizine: Selectivity, kinetic characterization, and molecular modeling. Toxicol Appl Pharm 272 (2013): 671–680.

Mahady GB, Chadwick LR. Golden Seal (Hydrastis canadensis): is there enough scientific evidence to support safety and efficacy? Nutr Clin Care 4.5 (2001): 243–249.

Mahady GB et al. In vitro susceptibility of Helicobacter pylori to isoquinoline alkaloids from Sanguinaria canadensis and Hydrastis Canadensis. Phytother Res 17.3 (2003): 217–221.

Marin-Neto JA et al. Cardiovascular effects of berberine in patients with severe congestive heart failure. Clin Cardiol 11.4 (1988): 253–260.

Marinova EK et al. Suppression of experimental autoimmune tubulointerstitial nephritis in BALB/c mice by berberine. Immunopharmacology 48.1 (2000): 9–16.

Meeran SM, Katiyar S, Katiyar SK. Berberine-induced apoptosis in human prostate cancer cells is initiated by reactive oxygen species generation. Toxicol Appl Pharmacol 229.1 (2008): 33–43.

Menees, S. et al. Agents that act luminally to treat diarrhoea and constipation. Nat Rev Gastroentero Hepatol 9.11 (2010): 661–674.

Mills S, Bone K. The essential guide to herbal safety. St Louis: Churchill Livingstone, 2005.

Mohan M et al. Berberine in trachoma: A clinical trial. Indian J Ophthalmol 30.2: 69–75; as cited in Mahady GB, Chadwick LR. 2001, Golden Seal (Hydrastis canadensis): Is there enough scientific evidence to support safety and efficacy? Nutr Clin Care 4.5 (1982): 243–249.

Musumeci R et al. Berberis aetnensis C. Presl. extracts: antimicrobial properties and interaction with ciprofloxacin. Int J Antimicrob Agents 22.1 (2003): 48–53.

Pan GY et al. The involvement of P-glycoprotein in berberine absorption. Pharmacol Toxicol 91.4 (2002): 193–197.

Pan GY et al. The antihyperglycaemic activity of berberine arises from a decrease of glucose absorption. Planta Med 69.7 (2003): 632–636.

Park KS et al. Differential inhibitory effects of protoberberines on sterol and chitin biosyntheses in Candida albicans. J Antimicrob Chemother 43.5 (1999): 667–674.

Peng W-H et al. Berberine produces antidepressant-like effects in the forced swim test and in the tail suspension test in mice. Life Sci 81.11 (2007): 933–938.

Pengelly A. The constituents of medicinal plants. Sydney: Allen & Unwin, 2004.

Piyanuch R et al. Berberine, a natural isoquinoline alkaloid, induces NAG-1 and ATF3 expression in human colorectal cancer cells. Cancer Lett 258.2 (2007): 230–240.

Rabbani GH et al. Randomized controlled trial of berberine sulfate therapy for diarrhea due to enterotoxigenic Escherichia coli and Vibrio cholerae. J Infect Dis 155.5 (1987): 979–984.

Rabbani GH. Mechanism and treatment of diarrhoea due to Vibrio cholerae and Escherichia coli: roles of drugs and prostaglandins. Dan Med Bull 43.2 (1996): 173–185.

Raner GM et al. Effects of herbal products and their constituents on human cytochrome P450(2E1) activity. Food Chem Toxicol 45.12 (2007): 2359–2365.

Rehman J et al. Increased production of antigen-specific immunoglobulins G and M following in vivo treatment with the medicinal plants Echinacea angustifolia and Hydrastis Canadensis. Immunol Lett 68.2–3 (1999): 391–395.

Sack RB, Froehlich JL. Berberine inhibits intestinal secretory response of Vibrio cholerae and Escherichia coli enterotoxins. Infect Immun 35.2 (1982): 471–475.

Scazzocchio F et al. Antibacterial activity of Hydrastis canadensis extract and its major isolated alkaloids. Planta Med 67.6 (2001): 561–564.

Sengupta D et al. Berberine and S allyl cysteine mediated amelioration of DEN + CCl4 induced hepatocarcinoma. BBA-Gen Subjects 1840.1 (2014): 219–244.

Serafim TL et al. Different concentrations of berberine result in distinct cellular localization patterns and cell cycle effects in a melanoma cell line. Cancer Chemother Pharmacol 61.6 (2008): 1007–1018.

Shirwaikar A et al. In vitro antioxidant studies on the benzyl tetra isoquinoline alkaloid berberine. Biol Pharm Bull 29.9 (2006): 1906–1910.

Siow YL et al. Redox regulation in health and disease — Therapeutic potential of berberine. Food Res Int 44.8 (2011): 2409–2417.

Stermitz FR et al. Synergy in a medicinal plant: antimicrobial action of berberine potentiated by 5'-methoxyhydnocarpin, a multidrug pump inhibitor. Proc Natl Acad Sci USA 97.4 (2000a): 1433–1437.

Stermitz FR et al. 5'-Methoxyhydnocarpin-D and pheophorbide A: Berberis species components that potentiate berberine growth inhibition of resistant Staphylococcus aureus. J Nat Prod 63.8 (2000b): 1146–1149.

Sun D et al. Berberine sulfate blocks adherence of streptococcus pyogenes to epithelial cells, fibronectin, and hexadecane. Antimicrob Agents Chemother 32.9 (1998): 1370–1374.

Sun S et al. Inhibition of organic cation transporter 2 and 3 may be involved in the mechanism of the antidepressant-like action of berberine. Prog Neuropsychopharmacol Biol Psychiatry 49.3 (2014): 1–6.

Swabb EA, Tai YH, Jordan L. Reversal of cholera toxin-induced secretion in rat ileum by luminal berberine. Am J Physiol 241.3 (1981): G248–G252.

Tai WP, Luo HS. [The inhibit effect of berberine on human colon cell line cyclooxygenase-2]. Zhonghua Nei Ke Za Zhi 42.8 (2003): 558–560.

Tang LQ et al. Effects of berberine on diabetes induced by alloxan and a high-fat/high-cholesterol diet in rats. J Ethnopharmacol 108.1 (2006): 109–115.

Tang J et al. Berberine and Coptidis Rhizoma as novel antineoplastic agents: A review of traditional use and biomedical investigations. J Ethnopharmacol 126.1 (2009): 5–17.

Teodoro JS et al. Berberine reverts hepatic mitochondrial dysfunction in high-fat fed rats: A possible role for SirT3 activation. Mitochondrion 13.6 (2013): 637–646.

Tillhon M et al. Berberine: New perspectives for old remedies. Biochem Pharmacol 84.10 (2012): 1260–1267.

Tu HP et al. Berberine's effect on periodontal tissue degradation by matrix metalloproteinases: an in vitro and in vivo experiment. Phytomedicine 20.13 (2013): 1203–1210.

Wang XN et al. Enhancement of apoptosis of human hepatocellular carcinoma SMMC-7721 cells through synergy of berberine and evodiamine. Phytomedicine 15.12 (2008): 1062–1068.

Wang Y et al. Berberbine and plant stanols synergistically inhibit cholesterol absorption in hamsters. Atherosclerosis 209.1 (2010): 111–117.

Wei G-X et al. In vitro synergism between berberine and miconazole against planktonic and biofilm Candida cultures. Arch Oral Biol 56.6 (2011): 565–572.

Wu X et al. Effects of berberine on the blood concentration of cyclosporin A in renal transplanted recipients: clinical and pharmacokinetic study. Eur J Clin Pharmacol 61.8 (2005): 567–572.

Yamaura K et al. Protective effects of goldenseal (Hydrastis canadensis L.) on acetaminophen-induced hepatotoxicity through inhibition of CYP2E1 in rats. Pharmacognosy Res 3.4 (2011): 250–255.

Yao M, Ritchie HE, Brown-Woodman PD. A reproductive screening test of goldenseal. Birth Defects Res B Dev Reprod Toxicol 74.5 (2005): 399–404.

Yin J et al. Effects of berberine on glucose metabolism in vitro. Metabolism 51.11 (2002): 1439–1443.

Yin J, Xing H, Ye J. Efficacy of berberine in patients with type 2 diabetes mellitus. Metabolism 57.5 (2008): 712–7117.

Yu HH et al. Antimicrobial activity of berberine alone and in combination with ampicillin or oxacillin against methicillin-resistant Staphylococcus aureus. J Med Food 8.4 (2005): 454–461.

Yuan J, Shen XZ, Zhu XS. Effect of berberine on transit time of human small intestine. Zhongguo Zhong Xi Yi Jie He Za Zhi 14.12 (1994): 718–720.

Zeng XH, Zeng XJ, Li YY. Efficacy and safety of berberine for congestive heart failure secondary to ischemic or idiopathic dilated cardiomyopathy. Am J Cardiol 92.2 (2003): 173–176.

Zhang H et al. Berberine lowers blood glucose in type 2 diabetes mellitus patients through increasing insulin receptor expression. Metabolism 59.2 (2010): 285–292.

Zhang RX, Dougherty DV, Rosenblum ML. Laboratory studies of berberine used alone and in combination with 1,3-bis(2-chloroethyl)-1-nitrosourea to treat malignant brain tumors. Chin Med J (Engl) 103.8 (1990): 658–665.

Zhang Y et al. Berberine increases the expression of NHE3 and AQP4 in sennosideA-induced diarrhea model. Fitoterapia 83.6 (2012): 1014–1022.

Zhao X et al. Effect of berberine on hepatocyte proliferation, inducible nitric oxide synthase expression, cytochrome P450 2E1 and 1A2 activities in diethylnitrosamine- and phenobarbital-treated rats. Biomed Pharmacother 62.9 (2008): 567–572.

Zhou X et al. Neuroprotective effects of Berberine on stroke models in vitro, in vivo. Neuroscience Letters 447.1 (2008): 31–36.

Zhu B, Ahrens FA. Effect of berberine on intestinal secretion mediated by Escherichia coli heat-stable enterotoxin in jejunum of pigs. Am. J Vet Res 43.9 (1982): 1594–1598.

Grapeseed extract

HISTORICAL NOTE Since the time of Ancient Greece, grape leaves, fruit and sap have been used medicinally to treat a variety of ailments, such as skin and eye irritation, varicose veins, diarrhoea, bleeding and cancer. In the 1500s, a French expedition in North America found itself trapped in ice and forced to survive on salted meat and stale biscuits. After a time, the crew began to show signs of what we now recognise as scurvy. It is believed that the men survived because a Native American Indian showed them how to make a tea from the bark and needles of pine trees. The French explorer wrote of this encounter in a book that was subsequently read by researcher Jacques Masquelier, also a Frenchman, in the 20th century. Intrigued by the story, he began to investigate the chemistry and properties of pine bark and identified oligomeric proanthocyanidin complexes (OPCs). Several years later, he extracted OPCs from grapeseed extract, which is now considered the superior source of OPCs (Murray & Pizzorno 1999).

COMMON NAME

Grapeseed extract

BOTANICAL NAME/FAMILY

Vitis vinifera/Vitaceae

PLANT PARTS USED

Seeds, grape skins

CHEMICAL COMPONENTS

The skin of the grapeseed is a rich source of proanthocyanidins (PCs: also referred to as procyanidins). Mixtures of procyanidins are referred to as OPCs. Grapeseed extract contains OPCs made up of dimers or trimers of (+)-catechin and (−)-epicatechin (Fine 2000) and also trimers and polymers of PCs. *Vitis vinifera* also contains stilbenes (resveratrol and viniferins) (Bavaresco et al 1999); however, it is unclear whether significant amounts are present in the seeds.

MAIN ACTIONS

Most evidence of activity derives from in vitro and animal studies for OPCs or grapeseed extract; however, some clinical studies are also available. The stilbene resveratrol (3,4',5 trihydroxystilbene) has also been the focus of much investigation and exhibits anti-inflammatory, antithrombotic, anticarcinogenic and antibacterial activities, but it is not clear whether significant amounts are present in the seeds and grapeseed extract (Fremont 2000).

Antioxidant

Grapeseed PC extract has demonstrated excellent free radical-scavenging abilities, in both test tube and animal models, and provided significantly greater effects than vitamins C, E and beta-carotene (Bagchi et al 1997, 1998, 2000, 2001, Castillo et al 2000, Facino et al 1999, Fauconneau et al 1997, Maffei et al 1994, 1996). In vitro tests have further identified a vitamin E-sparing effect, in which PCs prevent vitamin E loss and cause alpha-tocopherol radicals to revert to their antioxidant form (Maffei et al 1998). Animal studies have also demonstrated that grapeseed extract exerts significant improvements in antioxidant enzyme activity in obesity- and diet-related oxidative stress (Castrillejo et al 2011, Choi et al 2012). A recent randomised controlled trial (RCT) found that 400 mg/day of catechin-rich grapeseed extract for a period of 1 month resulted in a positive effect on oxidative markers in obese adults — better than resveratrol alone, and on par

> ***Clinical note — Proanthocyanidins***
>
> PCs are a group of naturally occurring polyphenolic bioflavonoids that are present in many fruits (e.g. apples, pears, grapes and peaches), vegetables, nuts, beans (e.g. cocoa), seeds, flowers and bark (e.g. pine) (Bavaresco et al 1999). Grapeseeds are a particularly rich source of PCs, containing more than any other grape products, such as red, white or rosé wine or grape juice, and more than most commonly available foods (Rasmussen et al 2005). PCs are also found in many medicinal herbs, such as *Ginkgo biloba, Camellia sinensis, Hypericum perforatum* and *Crataegus monogyna*; however, grapeseed extract is considered the superior source. PCs demonstrate a wide range of biological actions according to various in vitro, in vivo and clinical studies. However, in recent years, bioavailability studies have demonstrated that not all orally ingested PCs are absorbed. In particular, PC polymers have negligible absorption from the gastrointestinal tract, whereas low-molecular-weight PCs (monomers, dimers and trimers) are absorbed (Rasmussen et al 2005). In addition, some PCs are degraded by microflora in the caecum and large intestine into low-molecular-weight phenolic acids, chiefly hydroxyphenylpropionic acid and 4-*O*-methylgallic acid (Ward et al 2004), which are likely to contribute to the biological effects. These findings have implications when interpreting in vitro data because this method of testing does not take into account the variations in bioavailability and metabolism in the body.

with resveratrol triphosphate (a more stable resveratrol derivative) (De Groote et al 2012).

Inhibits platelet aggregation

Grapeseed extract has been shown to inhibit platelet aggregation, and combining extracts of grapeseed and grape skin produces a far greater antiplatelet effect in test tube and ex vivo tests (Shanmuganayagam et al 2002). Inhibition of platelet function was confirmed more recently (Sano et al 2005, Vitseva et al 2005).

Stabilises capillary walls and enhances dermal wound healing

In vivo studies have found that PCs stabilise the capillary wall and prevent increases in capillary permeability when chemically induced in tests, such as carrageenan-induced hindpaw oedema (Zafirov et al 1990) and dextran-induced oedema (Robert et al 1990). Components in grapeseed extract have the ability to cross-link collagen fibres, thereby strengthening the collagen matrix (Tixier et al 1984). Clinical studies confirm that grapeseed extract improves capillary resistance when used at a dose of 150 mg daily (Lagrue et al 1981). Not unexpectedly, research has also identified wound-healing properties.

A 2002 study in mice found that topical application of grapeseed PCs considerably accelerated wound contraction and closure and provided additional support during the wound-healing process (Khanna et al 2002). It has been shown that a grapeseed extract preparation containing 5000 ppm resveratrol facilitates oxidant-induced vascular endothelial growth factor expression in keratinocytes in vitro, which may account for its beneficial effects in promoting dermal wound healing and resolution of related skin disorders (Khanna et al 2001).

Anticarcinogenic, antimutagenic

Most tests have been conducted with PCs from grapeseed extract and show significant activity.

A number of in vitro studies have demonstrated that PCs from *Vitis vinifera* strongly suppress tumour growth and have cytotoxic activity against a range of cancer cells, including breast, lung, prostate, colon and gastric adenoma cells (Bagchi et al 2000, Dinicola et al 2010, Engelbrecht et al 2007, Fernandez-Perez et al 2012, Joshi et al 2001, Kaur et al 2006, Tyagi et al 2003, Ye et al 1999). More specifically, PCs from grapeseeds exerted antitumour properties in several animal models (Kim et al 2004, Martinez Conesa et al 2005, Nomoto et al 2004, Raina et al 2007, Ray et al 2005, Tong et al 2011, Zhang et al 2005). One study also found that grapeseed PCs enhanced the growth and viability of human gastric mucosal cells at the same time (Ye et al 1999).

Tests with grapeseed extract showed that it induced apoptosis in acute myeloid leukaemic cells (Fernandez-Perez et al 2012, Hu & Qin 2006) and an in vitro study identified gallic acid within grapeseed extract to be effective against human prostate carcinoma cells (Agarwal et al 2006). In breast cancer cells, its mechanism of action is to inhibit aromatase activity and expression (Kijima et al 2006).

PCs from grape stems have also demonstrated inhibitory action against liver and cervical cancer cell growth in vitro, comparable to PCs from grapeseeds, preventing reactive oxygen species-induced DNA damage (Apostolou et al 2013).

Anti-inflammatory

In vitro evidence suggests that grapeseed extract has anti-inflammatory activity (Sen & Bagchi 2001). Two compounds isolated from *Vitis vinifera* exhibit non-specific inhibitory activity against cyclooxygenase-1 and -2 (Waffo-Teguo et al 2001). Inhibition of the proinflammatory 5-lipoxygenase is another mechanism identified recently for grapeseed extract (Leifert & Abeywardena 2008). Rats fed on a hyperlipidic diet and grapeseed extract had a reduction in pro-inflammatory markers such as C-reactive protein, interleukin-6 and tumour necrosis factor-alpha (Terra et al 2009). Mice subjected to immunological liver injury demonstrated a significant reduction in inflammatory cytokines when treated with grapeseed extract (Liu et al 2012).

Cardioprotective effects

Considering that grapeseed extract demonstrates antioxidant, antiplatelet and anti-inflammatory actions, it may have a role in the prevention of cardiovascular disease. A number of researchers have investigated this issue further, mainly using animal models. One series of studies was conducted by Bagchi et al (2003) using a natural, standardised, water–ethanol extract made from California red grapeseeds, which contained approximately 75–80% oligomeric PCs and 3–5% monomeric PCs. According to in vivo research, treatment with grapeseed extract provided resistance to myocardial ischaemia-reperfusion injury, better postischaemic ventricular recovery and reduced incidence of reperfusion-induced ventricular fibrillation and ventricular tachycardia, as compared with corresponding control animals. Another study using a hamster atherosclerosis model found that 50 and 100 mg grapeseed extract/kg body weight led to a 49% and 63% reduction in foam cells, respectively. Additionally, cholesterol- and triglyceride-lowering activity has been reported (Yu et al 2002). One animal study identified that grapeseed extract significantly reduced total cholesterol by 42%, low-density lipoproteins (LDLs) by 56% and elevated high-density lipoprotein (HDL) cholesterol by 56% (El-Adawi et al 2006). This lipid-lowering action has been attributed to enhanced bile acid secretion (Jiao et al 2010). A study with hyperlipidaemic rabbits showed that grapeseed extract administered over 15 weeks produced a significant reduction in aortic atherosclerosis in males, although no effect was observed in females (Frederiksen et al 2007).

A small RCT (n = 50) assessed the role of 1300 mg/day of oral grapeseed extract, for a period of 4 weeks, on vascular endothelial function in high-risk subjects. The study found that, while there was no improvement in endothelial function after 4 weeks' treatment, there was a significant increase in brachial diameter, demonstrating measurable vascular effect (Mellen et al 2010).

A more recent in vitro study demonstrated that PCs from grapeseed extract inhibited angiotensin-converting enzyme activity (Eriz et al 2011), a finding that should be confirmed in vivo.

Cognition enhancer/neuroprotective

Grapeseed PC extract demonstrated neuroprotective effects in vivo and an increase in superoxide dismutase with the highest test dose (Devi et al 2006). Some in vivo studies have identified that grapeseed extract reduces age-related oxidative DNA damage and improves memory performance and cognitive enhancement, most likely achieved via an antioxidant mechanism (Balu et al 2005, 2006, Sarkaki et al 2007, Sreemantula et al 2005). Interestingly, along with grapeseed extract's antioxidant action, one study demonstrated a neurorescue effect when grapeseed extract was given to rats 3 hours after neurotoxic injury (Feng et al 2005, 2007).

The ability of grapeseed extract to protect critical proteins in the brain that are most affected in Alzheimer's disease suggests a potential clinical application (Kim et al 2005, 2006).

Reducing drug-induced toxicity

Protection against chemically induced multiorgan toxicity has also been reported (Bagchi et al 2001). Hepatoprotection was demonstrated in studies where rats were exposed to a hepatotoxin. It is thought that this effect was due to inhibiting lipid peroxidation via antioxidant activity (Dulundu et al 2007, Jamshidzadeh et al 2008, Pan et al 2011). Grapeseed extract demonstrated potent antioxidant activity and protected kidneys from gentamicin-induced nephrotoxicity in an experimental model. The same study found that bone marrow chromosomes were also protected (El-Ashmawy et al 2006). Grapeseed extract was also protective in rats from toxicity due to radiation exposure (Enginar et al 2007, Saada et al 2009).

Grapeseed extract protected against the cardiotoxic side effects of the chemotherapy drug doxorubicin in vivo. It is thought that the antioxidant properties of grapeseed extract protecting cardiomyocytes was chiefly responsible (Du & Lou 2008). Protection against chemotherapy-induced small-intestine mucositis was observed in another animal study where rats were administered with 400 mg/kg of grapeseed extract before and during chemotherapy (Cheah et al 2008).

Modulating insulin response

Animal studies have shown that catechin-rich grapeseed extract significantly affected body weight development over 12 weeks, suppressing weight gain in mice fed a high-fat diet. Grapeseed extract supplementation also decreased blood glucose and plasma insulin, leptin, glutamic pyruvate transaminase and cholesterol, compared to control (Meeprom et al 2011, Ohyama et al 2011). PCs have also demonstrated a direct effect on insulin resistance in an animal model, lowering insulin response after 10 days' treatment of 25 mg/kg day. However, longer-term dosing of 30 days showed better maintenance of fasting glycaemia. This dose was also shown to reduce visceral adipose tissue (Montagut et al 2010).

A recent RCT involving 8 healthy adults showed that supplementation of between 100 mg and 300 mg grapeseed extract, ingested together with a high-carbohydrate meal, significantly reduced postprandial plasma glucose. This result was seen within 15 minutes of ingestion and lasted up to 2 hours (Sapwarobol et al 2012). Longer term, 4 weeks' treatment with 600 mg/day grapeseed extract significantly improved markers of inflammation and glycaemia in 32 obese adults with type 2 diabetes (Kar et al 2009).

G

OTHER ACTIONS

There is preliminary evidence from many other studies indicating a range of pharmacological effects. Results from a clinical study suggest that grapeseed extract increases the rhodopsin content of the retina or accelerates its regeneration after exposure to bright light (Boissin et al 1988). Reduced incidence of cataract development and cataract progression was also observed in an experimental model using grapeseed PC extract (Durukan et al 2006). Grapeseed extract shows evidence of antibacterial and antifungal actions, specifically against *Candida albicans* (Furiga et al 2009, Han 2007). Grapeseed extract has also been shown in vitro to have an antivenom action against the saw-scaled viper (Mahadeswaraswamy et al 2008). Antinociceptive effects demonstrated in vivo for grapeseed extract show a reduction in pain and a potentiating effect of morphine (Uchida et al 2008). An animal study demonstrated antiageing potential due to grapeseed extract maintaining the erythrocyte membrane integrity that is often impaired in the elderly (Sangeetha et al 2005). In vitro, grapeseed extract has demonstrated antiallergenic potential via the inhibition of mast cell degranulation (Chen et al 2012).

CLINICAL USE

Free radical damage has been strongly associated with virtually every chronic degenerative disease, including cardiovascular disease, arthritis and cancer. Due to the potent antioxidant activity of grapeseed and its myriad of other pharmacological effects, its therapeutic potential is quite broad. The majority of clinical studies have been conducted in Europe using a commercial product known as Endotelon. Due to the poor bioavailability of high-molecular-weight PCs, it is advised that products containing chiefly low-molecular-weight PCs be used in practice.

Fluid retention, peripheral venous insufficiency and capillary resistance

There is good supportive evidence from clinical studies that have investigated the use of grapeseed extract in fluid retention, capillary resistance or venous insufficiency (Amsellem et al 1987, Costantini et al 1999, Delacroix 1981, Henriet 1993, Lagrue et al 1981).

Hormone replacement therapy and fluctuations in hormone levels can produce symptoms of venous insufficiency in some women. One large study involving 4729 subjects with peripheral venous insufficiency due to hormone replacement therapy showed that grapeseed extract decreased the sensation of heaviness in the legs in just over half the subjects by day 45, whereas 89.4% of subjects experienced an improvement by day 90 (Henriet 1993). According to an open multicentre study of women aged 18–50 years with oedema due to premenstrual syndrome, grapeseed extract (Endotelon) administered from day 14 to 28 improved various symptoms of fluid retention, such as abdominal swelling, weight gain and pelvic pain and also venous insufficiency (Amsellem et al 1987). The treatment was taken for four cycles, with most women (60.8%) responding after two cycles and 78.8% responding after four cycles.

An open study involving 24 patients with non-complicated chronic venous insufficiency found that over 80% of subjects receiving OPCs (100 mg/day) reported lessened or no symptoms after 10 days. Symptoms of itching and pain responded best, completely disappearing during the course of treatment in 80% and 53% of the patients, respectively (Costantini et al 1999). A double-blind study of 50 patients with symptoms of venous insufficiency found that grapeseed extract (Endotelon 150 mg daily) improved both subjective and objective markers of peripheral venous insufficiency, such as pain (Delacroix 1981).

In some pathological conditions, such as inflammation or diabetes, vascular permeability can be abnormally increased (Robert et al 1990). Two studies investigated the effects of grapeseed extract on capillary resistance in hypertensive and diabetic patients under both open and double-blind, placebo-controlled conditions, with treatment producing significant improvements in both groups (Lagrue et al 1981). The studies used a daily dose of 150 mg (Endotelon).

Diabetes

Diabetic retinopathy

Grapeseed extract (Endotelon 150 mg) was found to stabilise diabetic retinopathy in 80% of subjects compared to 47% with placebo, under double-blind test conditions (Arne 1982). These results were obtained by measuring objective markers such as visual acuity, muscular tone and ocular tone.

Diabetic nephropathy

Preliminary in vitro research indicates that grapeseed polyphenols have a protective effect against cell damage, including renal cell damage, caused by high glucose levels (Fujii et al 2006). Other in vitro research also points to possible therapeutic benefits in preventing and treating vascular problems and diabetic complications (Zhang et al 2007).

A study with diabetic rats given grapeseed PC extracts identified nephroprotection, which might be related to the free radical-scavenging activity of grapeseed PC extracts (Liu et al 2006). Further research would be required to confirm a clinical application.

Metabolic syndrome and blood pressure reduction

A randomised trial in 27 adults with metabolic syndrome found that treatment with either 150 mg or 300 mg grapeseed extract/day resulted in a significant reduction of both systolic and diastolic blood pressures after 4 weeks' treatment. In the 300 mg/day group, there was also significant reduction of oxidative LDL and an increase of plasma catechin concentrations (Sivaprakasapillai et al 2009).

Eye strain

A double-blind study involving 75 patients with eye strain caused by viewing a computer screen found that a 300 mg dose of grapeseed extract daily significantly improved objective and subjective measures (Bombardelli & Morrazzoni 1995). Grapeseed extract (Endotelon) has also been shown to significantly improve visual adaptation to and from bright light in a dual-centre study involving 100 volunteers (Boissin et al 1988, Corbe et al 1988). A dose of 200 mg daily over 5 weeks was used. It has been proposed that grapeseed extract increases rhodopsin content of the retina or accelerates its regeneration after exposure to bright light.

Hyperlipidaemia/atherosclerosis

A single-blind, placebo-controlled study where 61 healthy subjects took 200 or 400 mg grapeseed extract over 12 weeks showed that active treatment significantly lowered oxidised LDL levels at the end of the test period. The group receiving the higher dose experienced results at the earlier 6-week point as well as at 12 weeks (Sano et al 2007). A randomised, double-blind study of 40 subjects with hypercholesterolaemia compared the effects of placebo, chromium polynicotinate (400 mcg/day), grapeseed extract (200 mg/day) or a combination of both. Over 2 months, the combination treatment decreased total cholesterol and LDL levels significantly but did not significantly alter homocysteine, HDL or blood pressure among the four groups (Preuss et al 2000). The role of grapeseed extract in achieving this result is unclear.

Enhances dermal wound healing

A 2002 study in mice found that topical application of grapeseed PCs considerably accelerated wound contraction and closure and provided additional support during the wound-healing process (Khanna et al 2002).

Chloasma

Chloasma is a condition characterised by hyperpigmentation and is generally considered recalcitrant to treatment. PC-rich grapeseed extract successfully reduced hyperpigmentation in women with chloasma after 6 months of oral treatment, according to an open study involving 12 subjects (Yamakoshi et al 2004). The study continued for another 6 months but failed to find any additional improvement with further use. The researchers suggested that a preventive effect may be possible with long-term oral grapeseed extract when used in the months prior to summer.

Pancreatitis

It is believed that the oxygen-derived free radicals mediate tissue damage in acute and chronic pancreatitis. Therefore, antioxidant treatment is being investigated. A small, open study of three patients with difficult-to-treat chronic pancreatitis found that a commercially available IH636 grapeseed extract produced a reduction in the frequency and intensity of abdominal pain, as well as resolution of vomiting in one patient.

Preventing reperfusion injury

Procyanidin administration reduced the adverse effects of myocardial ischaemia-reperfusion injury during cardiac surgery in several in vivo studies (Facino et al 1999, Maffei et al 1996). This appears to be positively associated with an increase in plasma antioxidant activity. An animal model also suggests that a PC-rich extract from grapeseed was protective against renal damage from ischaemia-reperfusion injury (Nakagawa et al 2005). Another animal model showed protection against hepatic ischaemia-reperfusion injury by regulating the release of inflammatory mediators and by its antioxidant action (Sehirli et al 2008).

Reduces sunburn

Topical application of grapeseed extract has been shown to enhance sun protection factor in human volunteers (Bagchi et al 2000). A study, with a grapeseed extract supplement, topical cream and a topical lotion (both Anthogenol products), assessed 42 individuals randomised into two groups, with one group taking the dietary supplement. Ultraviolet radiation-induced erythema was treated and it was found that both the topical applications decreased erythema formation, with slightly better results for those volunteers also taking the oral supplements. Application of the topical lotion produced the best results (53% reduction) and the lotion plus the grapeseed extract supplement added a further 13% reduction in skin inflammation, while all groups found improved skin hydration (Hughes-Formella et al 2007).

Practice points/Patient counselling

- Grapeseed extract has considerable antioxidant activity and appears to regenerate alpha-tocopherol radicals to their antioxidant form.
- Grapeseed extract also has anti-inflammatory actions, reduces capillary permeability, enhances dermal wound healing and reduces photodamage, inhibits platelet aggregation and may enhance rhodopsin regeneration or content in the retina.
- It is popular in Europe as a treatment for venous insufficiency and capillary fragility, both of which are supported by clinical evidence. It is also used to relieve eye strain and stabilise diabetic retinopathy and connective tissue disorders.
- Preliminary research has identified cardioprotective effects due to a variety of mechanisms. Possible benefits include pancreatitis and multi-organ protection against damage caused by several pharmaceutical drugs, including several chemotherapy drugs, and radiation. Anticarcinogenic activity has also been reported.
- It shows promise for neurodegenerative disorders in preliminary studies.
- Most clinical research has been conducted in Europe with a commercial grapeseed product known as Endotelon.
- Due to concerns with bioavailability, it is recommended that only preparations containing low-molecular-weight PCs be used.
- It provides protection against multiorgan drug and chemical toxicity.

The results from a number of in vivo studies have suggested that pre-exposure to grapeseed extract can provide multiorgan protection against damage caused by various drugs, such as paracetamol, amiodarone, doxorubicin, cadmium chloride and dimethylnitrosamine treatment (Bagchi et al 2000, 2001). This is most likely via an antioxidant mechanism.

OTHER USES

Some preliminary in vitro research suggests a potential use for periodontal diseases and oral hygiene for prevention of periodontitis. This is due to grapeseed extract's antimicrobial effect against specific oral bacteria and its strong antioxidant action (Furiga et al 2009, Houde et al 2006).

An in vitro study suggests a promising use for grapeseed extract as active against *Candida albicans* and a possible synergistic action with the drug amphotericin B, which would enable this strong drug dose to be reduced by 75% when given in conjunction with grapeseed extract. Clinical studies are needed to confirm this potential use (Han 2007).

DOSAGE RANGE

- Fluid extract 1:1 (g/mL): 20–40 mL per week.
- Solid-dose forms: 12,000 mg of grapeseed extract standardised to OPCs taken 2–3 times daily in order to provide 150–300 mg of OPCs daily. Due to the poor bioavailability of high-molecular-weight PCs, it is advised that products containing chiefly low-molecular-weight PCs be used in practice.

According to clinical studies:

- Chloasma: 162 mg/day grapeseed extract.
- Cardiovascular disease: 200–300 mg/day grapeseed extract.
- Hypercholesterolaemia: 200–400 mg/day grapeseed extract.
- Chronic pancreatitis: ActiVin 200–300 mg/day.
- Oedema due to premenstrual syndrome: grapeseed extract (Endotelon) 150–400 mg taken from day 14 to 28.
- Oedema due to injury or surgery: 200–400 mg/day grapeseed extract (Endotelon).
- Diabetic retinopathy: 150–400 mg/day grapeseed extract (Endotelon).
- Insulin resistance: 300 mg/day grapeseed extract.
- Vascular fragility: 150–400 mg/day grapeseed extract (Endotelon).
- Venous insufficiency and poor leg circulation: grapeseed extract (Endotelon) 150–300 mg/day.
- Vision problems: grapeseed extract (Endotelon) 200 mg/day.

TOXICITY

Tests in animal models have found grapeseed extract to be extremely safe (Bentivegna & Whitney 2002).

ADVERSE REACTIONS

Studies using doses of 150 mg/day have found it to be well tolerated. Side effects are generally limited to gastrointestinal disturbances, including nausea and indigestion.

SIGNIFICANT INTERACTIONS

Controlled studies are not available; therefore, interactions are theoretical and based on evidence of pharmacological activity.

Antiplatelet drugs

Additive effect theoretically possible — observe patient.

Anticoagulant drugs

Increased risk of bleeding theoretically possible — monitor patient for increased bruising or bleeding.

Iron and iron-containing preparations

Decreased iron absorption. Tannins can bind to iron, forming insoluble complexes — separate doses by 2 hours.

CONTRAINDICATIONS AND PRECAUTIONS

None known.

PREGNANCY USE

Safety has not been scientifically established.

PATIENTS' FAQs

What will this herb do for me?

There is evidence that grapeseed extract is a useful treatment for venous insufficiency, poor leg circulation and capillary fragility and has considerable antioxidant activity. It may also assist with blood sugar regulation and hyperlipidaemia in overweight and high-risk individuals. Grapeseed extract is used to treat eye strain and diabetic retinopathy and enhance wound healing when applied locally.

When will it start to work?

It appears to relieve symptoms of venous insufficiency within 10 days and eye strain within 5 weeks. Other uses may take longer before results are seen.

Are there any safety issues?

Research suggests that it is well tolerated and generally safe; however, people taking anticoagulant medicines should refer to their healthcare professional before taking this substance.

REFERENCES

Agarwal C, et al. Gallic acid, the major active constituent in grape seed extract, causes S phase arrest via activation of ATM-Chk1/2-Cdc25A/C-Cdc2 pathway, and leads to caspase-mediated apoptotic death of human prostate carcinoma DU145 cells. AACR Meeting Abstracts 2006 (1) (2006): 1318–b-.

Amsellem M et al. Endotelon in the treatment of venolymphatic problems in premenstrual syndrome: multicenter study on 165 patients. Tempo Med 282 (1987): 46–57.

Apostolou A et al. Assessment of polyphenolic content, antioxidant activity, protection against 3 ROS-induced DNA damage and anticancer activity of *Vitis vinifera* stem extracts. Food Chem Toxicol 61 (2013): 60–68.

Arne JL. Contribution to the study of procyanidolic oligomers: endotelon in diabetic retinopathy. Gaz Med France 89 (1982): 3610–36114.

Bagchi D et al. Oxygen free radical scavenging abilities of vitamins C and E, and a grape seed proanthocyanidin extract in vitro. Res Commun Mol Pathol Pharmacol 95 (1997): 179–189.

Bagchi D et al. Protective effects of grape seed proanthocyanidins and selected antioxidants against TPA-induced hepatic and brain lipid peroxidation and DNA fragmentation, and peritoneal macrophage activation in mice. Gen Pharmacol 30 (1998): 771–776.

Bagchi D et al. Free radicals and grape seed proanthocyanidin extract: importance in human health and disease prevention. Toxicology 148 (2000): 187–197.

Bagchi D et al. Protection against drug- and chemical-induced multiorgan toxicity by a novel IH636 grape seed proanthocyanidin extract. Drugs Exp Clin Res 27 (2001): 3–15.

Bagchi D et al. Molecular mechanisms of cardioprotection by a novel grape seed proanthocyanidin extract. Mutat Res 523–4 (2003): 87–97.

Balu M et al. Age-related oxidative protein damages in central nervous system of rats: modulatory role of grape seed extract. Int J Dev Neurosci 23.6 (2005): 501–507.

Balu M et al. Modulatory role of grape seed extract on age-related oxidative DNA damage in central nervous system of rats. Brain Res Bull 68.6 (2006): 469–473.

Bavaresco L et al. Stilbene compounds: from the grapevine to wine. Drugs Exp Clin Res 25 (1999): 57–63.

Castrillejo V et al. Antioxidant effects of a grapeseed procyanidin extract and oleoyl-estrone in obese Zucker rats. Nutrition 27 (2011): 1172–1176.

Choi S et al. Suppression of oxidative stress by grape seed supplementation in rats. Nutr Res Pract 6.1 (2012): 3–8.

Corbe C, et al. Light vision and chorioretinal circulation: Study of the effect of procyanidolic oligomers (Endotelon). J Fr Ophtalmol 11 (1988): 453–460.
Costantini A, et al. Clinical and capillaroscopic evaluation of chronic uncomplicated venous insufficiency with procyanidins extracted from *Vitis vinifera*. Minerva Cardioangiol 47 (1999): 39–46.
Bentivegna SS, Whitney KM. Subchronic 3-month oral toxicity study of grape seed and grape skin extracts. Food Chem Toxicol 40 (2002): 1731–1743.
Boissin JP, et al. Chorioretinal circulation and dazzling: use of procyanidol oligomers (Endotelon). Bull Soc Ophtalmol Fr 88 (1988): 173–179.
Bombardelli E, Morrazzoni P. *Vitis vinifera* L. Fitoterapia 66 (1995): 291–317.
Castillo J et al. Antioxidant activity and radioprotective effects against chromosomal damage induced in vivo by X-rays of flavan-3-ols (procyanidins): from grape seeds (*Vitis vinifera*): comparative study versus other phenolic and organic compounds. J Agric Food Chem 48 (2000): 1738–1745.
Cheah KY et al. T1321 An Extract from Grape Seed Protects IEC-6 Cells from Chemotherapy-Induced Cytotoxicity and Improves Parameters of Small Intestinal Mucositis in Rats with Experimentally-Induced Mucositis. Gastroenterology 134 (4 Suppl 1) (2008): A-530.
Chen B et al. Anti-allergic activity of grapeseed extract (GSE) on RBL-2H3 mast cells. Food Chem 132 (2012): 968–974.
De Groote D et al. Effect of the Intake of Resveratrol, Resveratrol Phosphate, and Catechin-Rich Grape Seed Extract on Markers of Oxidative Stress and Gene Expression in Adult Obese Subjects. Ann Nutr Metab 61.1 (2012): 15–24.
Delacroix P. Double-blind trial of endotelon in chronic venous insufficiency. Rev Med 27–8 (1981): 1793–1802.
Devi A, et al. Grape seed proanthocyanidin extract (GSPE) and antioxidant defense in the brain of adult rats. Med Sci Monit 12.4 (2006): BR124–BR129.
Dinicola S et al. Apoptosis-inducing factor and caspase-dependent apoptotic pathways triggered by different grape seed extracts on human colon cancer cell line Caco-2. Br Journ Nut 104 (2010): 824–832.
Du Y, Lou H. Catechin and proanthocyanidin B4 from grape seeds prevent doxorubicin-induced toxicity in cardiomyocytes. Eur J Pharmacol 591.1–3 (2008): 96–101.
Dulundu E et al. Grape seed extract reduces oxidative stress and fibrosis in experimental biliary obstruction. J Gastroenterol Hepatol 22.6 (2007): 885–892.
Durukan AH et al. Ingestion of IH636 grape seed proanthocyanidin extract to prevent selenite-induced oxidative stress in experimental cataract. J Cataract Refract Surg 32.6 (2006): 1041–1045.
El-Adawi H et al. Study on the effect of grape seed extract on hypercholesterolemia: prevention and treatment. Inter J of Pharmac 2.6 (2006): 593–600.
El-Ashmawy IM, et al. Grape seed extract prevents gentamicin-induced nephrotoxicity and genotoxicity in bone marrow cells of mice. Basic Clin Pharmacol Toxicol 99.3 (2006): 230–236.
Engelbrecht AM et al. Proanthocyanidin from grape seeds inactivates the PI3-kinase/PKB pathway and induces apoptosis in a colon cancer cell line. Cancer Lett 258.1 (2007): 144–153.
Enginar H et al. Effect of grape seed extract on lipid peroxidation, antioxidant activity and peripheral blood lymphocytes in rats exposed to x-radiation. Phytother Res 21.11 (2007): 1029–1035.
Eriz G et al. Inhibition of the angiotensin-converting enzyme by grape seed and skin proanthocyanidins extracted from Vitis vinífera L. cv. País. Food Science and Technology 44 (2011): 860–865.
Facino RM et al. Diet enriched with procyanidins enhances antioxidant activity and reduces myocardial post-ischaemic damage in rats. Life Sci 64 (1999): 627–642.
Fauconneau B et al. Comparative study of radical scavenger and antioxidant properties of phenolic compounds from *Vitis vinifera* cell cultures using in vitro tests. Life Sci 61 (1997): 2103–2110.
Feng Y et al. Grape seed extract suppresses lipid peroxidation and reduces hypoxic ischemic brain injury in neonatal rats. Brain Res Bull 66.2 (2005): 120–127.
Feng Y et al. Grape seed extract given three hours after injury suppresses lipid peroxidation and reduces hypoxic-ischemic brain injury in neonatal rats. Pediatr Res 61.3 (2007): 295–300.
Fernandez-Perez F et al. Cytotoxic Effect of Natural trans-Resveratrol Obtained from Elicited *Vitis vinifera* Cell Cultures on Three Cancer Cell Lines. Plant Foods Hum Nutr 67 (2012): 422–429.
Fine AM. Oligomeric proanthocyanidin complexes: history, structure, and phytopharmaceutical applications. Altern Med Rev 5 (2000): 144–151.
Frederiksen H et al. Effects of red grape skin and seed extract supplementation on atherosclerosis in Watanabe heritable hyperlipidemic rabbits. Mol Nutr Food Res 51.5 (2007): 564–571.
Fremont L. Biological effects of resveratrol. Life Sci 66 (2000): 663–673.
Fujii H et al. Protective effect of grape seed polyphenols against high glucose-induced oxidative stress. Biosci Biotechnol Biochem 70.9 (2006): 2104–2111.
Furiga A, et al. In vitro study of antioxidant capacity and antibacterial activity on oral anaerobes of a grape seed extract. Food Chem 113 (2009): 1037–1040.
Han Y. Synergic effect of grape seed extract with amphotericin B against disseminated candidiasis due to *Candida albicans*. Phytomedicine 14.11 (2007): 733–738.
Henriet JP. Veno-lymphatic insufficiency: 4,729 patients undergoing hormonal and procyanidol oligomer therapy. Phlebologie 46 (1993): 313–325.
Houde V, et al. Protective effects of grape seed proanthocyanidins against oxidative stress induced by lipopolysaccharides of periodontopathogens. J Periodontol 77.8 (2006): 1371–1379.
Hu H, Qin YM. Grape seed proanthocyanidin extract induced mitochondria-associated apoptosis in human acute myeloid leukaemia 14.3D10 cells. Chin Med J (Engl) 119.5 (2006): 417–421.
Hughes-Formella B, et al. Anti-inflammatory and skin-hydrating properties of a dietary supplement and topical formulations containing oligomeric proanthocyanidins. Skin Pharmacol Physiol 20.1 (2007): 43–49.
Jamshidzadeh A, et al. Hepatoprotective effect of grape seed extract on rat liver. Toxicology Letters 180 (Suppl 1) (2008): S50.
Jiao R et al. Hypocholesterolemic activity of grape seed proanthocyanidin is mediated by enhancement of bile acid excretion and up-regulation of CYP7A1. J Nutr Biochem 21.11 (2010): 1134–1139.
Joshi SS, et al. The cellular and molecular basis of health benefits of grape seed proanthocyanidin extract. Curr Pharm Biotechnol 2 (2001): 187–200.
Kar P et al. Effects of grape seed extract in Type 2 diabetic subjects at high cardiovascular risk: a double blind randomized placebo controlled trial examining metabolic markers, vascular tone, inflammation, oxidative stress and insulin sensitivity. Diabet Med 26.5 (2009): 526–31.
Kaur M et al. Grape seed extract inhibits in vitro and in vivo growth of human colorectal carcinoma cells. Clin Cancer Res 12.20 (Pt 1) (2006): 6194–6202.
Khanna S et al. Upregulation of oxidant-induced VEGF expression in cultured keratinocytes by a grape seed proanthocyanidin extract. Free Radic Biol Med 31 (2001): 38–42.
Khanna S et al. Dermal wound healing properties of redox-active grape seed proanthocyanidins. Free Radic Biol Med 33 (2002): 1089–1096.
Kijima I et al. Grape seed extract is an aromatase inhibitor and a suppressor of aromatase expression. Cancer Res 66.11 (2006): 5960–5967.
Kim H et al. Chemoprevention by grape seed extract and genistein in carcinogen-induced mammary cancer in rats is diet dependent. J Nutr 134 (2004): 3445–52S.
Kim H et al. Consideration of grape seed extract as a preventive against Alzheimer disease. Alzheimers Dement 1 (1 Suppl 1) (2005): S100–S101.
Kim H et al. Proteomics analysis of the actions of grape seed extract in rat brain: Technological and biological implications for the study of the actions of psychoactive compounds. Life Sci 78.18 (2006): 2060–2065.
Lagrue G, et al. A study of the effects of procyanidol oligomers on capillary resistance in hypertension and in certain nephropathies (author's transl). Sem Hop 57 (1981): 1399–1401.
Leifert WR, Abeywardena MY. Grape seed and red wine polyphenol extracts inhibit cellular cholesterol uptake, cell proliferation, 5-lipoxygenase activity. Nutr Res 28.11 (2008): 729–737.
Liu YN, et al. Effects of grape seed proanthocyanidins extracts on experimental diabetic nephropathy in rats. Wei Sheng Yan Jiu 35.6 (2006): 703–705.
Liu T et al. Hepatoprotective Effects of Total Triterpenoids and Total Flavonoids from *Vitis vinifera* L against Immunological Liver Injury in Mice. eCAM (2012): 1–8.
Maffei FR et al. Free radicals scavenging action and anti-enzyme activities of procyanidines from *Vitis vinifera*: a mechanism for their capillary protective action. Arzneimittelforschung 44 (1994): 592–601.
Maffei FR et al. Procyanidines from *Vitis vinifera* seeds protect rabbit heart from ischemia/reperfusion injury: antioxidant intervention and/or iron and copper sequestering ability. Planta Med 62 (1996): 495–502.
Maffei FR et al. Sparing effect of procyanidins from *Vitis vinifera* on vitamin E in vitro studies. Planta Med 64 (1998): 343–347.
Mahadeswaraswamy YH et al. Local tissue destruction and procoagulation properties of *Echis carinatus* venom: inhibition by *Vitis vinifera* seed methanol extract. Phytother Res 22.7 (2008): 963–969.
Martinez Conesa C et al. Experimental model for treating pulmonary metastatic melanoma using grape-seed extract, red wine and ethanol. Clin Transl Oncol 7.3 (2005): 115–121.
Meeprom A et al. Grape seed extract supplementation prevents high-fructose diet-induced insulin resistance in rats by improving insulin and adiponectin signaling pathways. Br J Nutr 106 (2011): 1173–1181.
Mellen P et al. Effect of Muscadine Grape Seed Supplementation on Vascular Function in Subjects with or at Risk for Cardiovascular Disease: A Randomized Crossover Trial. J Am Coll Nutr 29.5 (2010): 469–475.
Montagut G et al. Effects of a grapeseed procyanidin extract (GSPE) on insulin resistance. J Nutritional Biochem 21 (2010): 961–967.

Murray M, Pizzorno J. Procyanidolic oligomers. Textbook of natural medicine, 2nd edn. London: Churchill-Livingstone, 1999, pp 899–902.
Nakagawa T et al. Attenuation of renal ischemia-reperfusion injury by proanthocyanidin-rich extract from grape seeds. J Nutr Sci Vitaminol (Tokyo) 51.4 (2005): 283–6.
Nomoto H et al. Chemoprevention of colorectal cancer by grape seed proanthocyanidin is accompanied by a decrease in proliferation and increase in apoptosis. Nutr Cancer 49 (2004): 81–88.
Ohyama K et al. Catechin-Rich Grape Seed Extract Supplementation Attenuates Diet-Induced Obesity in C57BL/6J Mice. Ann Nutr Metab 58 (2011): 250–258.
Pan X et al. Inhibition of arsenic induced-rat liver injury by grape seed exact through suppression of NADPH oxidase and TGF-β/Smad activation. Toxicol Appl Pharmacol 254 (2011): 323–331.
Preuss HG et al. Effects of niacin-bound chromium and grape seed proanthocyanidin extract on the lipid profile of hypercholesterolemic subjects: a pilot study. J Med 31 (2000): 227–246.
Raina K et al. Oral grape seed extract inhibits prostate tumor growth and progression in TRAMP mice. Cancer Res 67.12 (2007): 5976–5982.
Rasmussen SE et al. Dietary proanthocyanidins: occurrence, dietary intake, bioavailability, and protection against cardiovascular disease. Mol Nutr Food Res 49 (2005): 159–174.
Ray SD, et al. Proanthocyanidin exposure to B6C3F1 mice significantly attenuates dimethylnitrosamine-induced liver tumor induction and mortality by differentially modulating programmed and unprogrammed cell deaths. Mutat Res 579 (2005): 81–106.
Robert L et al. The effect of procyanidolic oligomers on vascular permeability. a study using quantitative morphology. Pathol Biol (Paris) 38 (1990): 608–16.
Saada HN et al. Grape seed extract *Vitis vinifera* protects against radiation-induced oxidative damage and metabolic disorders in rats. Phytother Res 23.3 (2009): 434–438.
Sangeetha P et al. Age associated changes in erythrocyte membrane surface charge: Modulatory role of grape seed proanthocyanidins. Exp Gerontol 40.10 (2005): 820–828.
Sano T et al. Anti-thrombotic effect of proanthocyanidin, a purified ingredient of grape seed. Thromb Res 115.1–2 (2005): 115–121.
Sano A et al. Beneficial effects of grape seed extract on malondialdehyde-modified LDL. J Nutr Sci Vitaminol (Tokyo) 53.2 (2007): 174–82.
Sapwarobol S et al. Postprandial blood glucose response to grape seed extract in healthy participants: A pilot study. Pharmacogn Mag 8.31 (2012): 192–196.
Sarkaki A, et al. The effect of grape seed extract (GSE) on spatial memory in aged male rats. Pak J Med Sci 23.4 (2007): 561–5.
Sehirli O et al. Grape seed extract treatment reduces hepatic ischemia-reperfusion injury in rats. Phytother Res 22.1 (2008): 43–48.
Sen CK, Bagchi D. Regulation of inducible adhesion molecule expression in human endothelial cells by grape seed proanthocyanidin extract. Mol Cell Biochem 216 (2001): 1–7.
Shanmuganayagam D et al. Grape seed and grape skin extracts elicit a greater antiplatelet effect when used in combination than when used individually in dogs and humans. J Nutr 132 (2002): 3592–3598.
Sivaprakasapillai B et al. Effect of grape seed extract on blood pressure in subjects with the metabolic syndrome. Metabolism 58.12 (2009): 1743–1746.
Sreemantula S et al. Adaptogenic and nootropic activities of aqueous extract of *Vitis vinifera* (grape seed): an experimental study in rat model. BMC Complement Altern Med 5 (2005): 1.
Terra X et al. Grape-seed procyanidins prevent low-grade inflammation by modulating cytokine expression in rats fed a high-fat diet. J Nutr Biochem 20 (2009): 210–218.
Tixier JM et al. Evidence by in vivo and in vitro studies that binding of pycnogenols to elastin affects its rate of degradation by elastases. BioChem Pharmacol 33 (1984): 3933–3939.
Tong H et al. Immunomodulatory and Antitumor Activities of Grape Seed Proanthocyanidins. J Agric Food Chem 59 (2011): 11543–11547.
Tyagi A, et al. Grape seed extract inhibits EGF-induced and constitutively active mitogenic signaling but activates JNK in human prostate carcinoma DU145 cells: possible role in antiproliferation and apoptosis. Oncogene 22 (2003): 1302–1316.
Uchida S et al. Antinociceptive effects of St. John's wort, *Harpagophytum procumbens* extract and Grape seed proanthocyanidins extract in mice. Biol Pharm Bull 31.2 (2008): 240–245.
Vitseva O et al. Grape seed and skin extracts inhibit platelet function and release of reactive oxygen intermediates. J Cardiovasc Pharmacol 46 (2005): 445–451.
Waffo-Teguo P et al. Two new stilbene dimer glucosides from grape (*Vitis vinifera*) cell cultures. J Nat Prod 64 (2001): 136–138.
Ward NC et al. Supplementation with grape seed polyphenols results in increased urinary excretion of 3-hydroxyphenylpropionic acid, an important metabolite of proanthocyanidins in humans. J Agric Food Chem 52 (2004): 5545–5549.
Yamakoshi J et al. Oral intake of proanthocyanidin-rich extract from grape seeds improves chloasma. Phytother Res 18 (2004): 895–899.
Ye X et al. The cytotoxic effects of a novel IH636 grape seed proanthocyanidin extract on cultured human cancer cells. Mol Cell Biochem 196 (1999): 99–108.
Yu H et al. Effect of grape seed extracts on blood lipids in rabbits model with hyperlipidemia. Wei Sheng Yan Jiu 31 (2002): 114–1116.
Zafirov D et al. Antiexudative and capillaritonic effects of procyanidines isolated from grape seeds (*V. vinifera*). Acta Physiol Pharmacol Bulg 16 (1990): 50–54.
Zhang XY et al. Proanthocyanidin from grape seeds potentiates anti-tumor activity of doxorubicin via immunomodulatory mechanism. Int Immunopharmacol 5 (2005): 1247–1257.
Zhang FL, et al. Inhibitory effect of GSPE on RAGE expression induced by advanced glycation end products in endothelial cells. J Cardiovasc Pharmacol 50.4 (2007): 434–440.

Green tea

HISTORICAL NOTE Tea has been a popular beverage for thousands of years and was originally grown in China, dating back 5000 years, where it has been used as part of various ceremonies and to maintain alertness. Green tea and the partially fermented oolong tea have remained popular beverages in Asia since that time, whereas black tea is the preferred beverage in many English-speaking countries. Tea was introduced to the Western culture in the sixth century by Turkish traders (Ulbricht & Basch 2005). Second to water, tea is now considered to be the world's most popular beverage.

COMMON NAME

Green tea

OTHER NAMES

Chinese tea, camellia tea, gruner tea, Matsu-cha, green Sencha tea, Japanese tea, Yame tea

BOTANICAL NAME/FAMILY

Camellia sinensis (family Theaceae)

PLANT PART USED

Leaf

CHEMICAL COMPONENTS

The composition of green tea varies according to the growing and harvesting methods, but the most abundant components are polyphenols, which are predominantly flavonoids (e.g. catechin, epicatechin, epicatechin gallate, epigallocatechin gallate,

> ***Clinical note — The difference between teas***
> Black, green and oolong tea are produced from the same plant (*Camellia sinensis*) but differ in polyphenol content according to the way the leaves are processed. Black tea is made from oxidised leaves, whereas oolong tea is made from partially oxidised leaves and green tea leaves are not oxidised at all. Because the oxidising process converts many polyphenolic compounds into others with less activity, green tea is considered to have the strongest therapeutic effects and the highest polyphenol content (Lin et al 2003). Caffeine concentrations also vary between the different teas: black tea > oolong tea > green tea > fresh tea leaf (Lin et al 2003). Variation in caffeine content is further influenced by growing conditions, manufacturing processes and size of the tea leaves (Astill et al 2001). The highest-quality leaves are the first spring leaf buds, called the 'first flush'. The next set of leaf buds produced is called the 'second flush' and considered to be of poorer quality. Tea varieties also reflect the area they are grown in (e.g. Darjeeling in India), the form produced (e.g. pekoe is cut, gunpowder is rolled) and processing method (black, oolong or green) (Ulbricht & Basch 2005).

proanthocyanidins). Caffeine content in green tea varies but is estimated at about 3%, along with very small amounts of the other common methylxanthines, theobromine and theophylline (Graham 1992). It also contains many other constituents, such as tannin, diphenylamine, oxalic acid, trace elements and vitamins.

Epigallocatechin gallate is one of the most abundant polyphenols in tea and is regarded as the most important pharmacologically active component.

MAIN ACTIONS

It is suspected that the polyphenol content is chiefly responsible for the chemoprotective, antiproliferative, antimicrobial and antioxidant activity of green tea. The caffeine content is predominantly responsible for central nervous system (CNS) activity and an interaction between both appears necessary for increasing thermogenesis.

Antioxidant

Green tea has consistently demonstrated strong antioxidant activity. A recent systematic review of 31 controlled intervention studies concluded that green tea reduced lipid peroxidation and increased antioxidant capacity when the beverage was consumed regularly (0.6–1.5 litres a day) (Ellinger et al 2011). In a controlled human trial, 24 healthy women consumed two cups of green tea (250 mg catechins/day) for 42 days (Erba et al 2005). The results showed a significant increase in plasma antioxidant status, reduced plasma peroxides and reduced low-density lipoprotein (LDL) cholesterol when compared with controls. Several other in vitro animal and human studies have also demonstrated that green tea inhibits lipid peroxidation and scavenges hydroxyl and superoxide radicals (Leenen et al 2000, Rietveld & Wiseman 2003, Sung et al 2000).

Antibacterial activity

Green tea extract has moderate and wide-spectrum inhibitory effects on the growth of many types of pathogenic bacteria, according to in vitro tests, including seven strains of *Staphylococcus* spp., seven strains of *Streptococcus* spp., 26 strains of *Salmonella*, 19 strains of *Escherichia coli* spp. and one strain of *Corynebacterium suis* (Ishihara et al 2001). In one in vitro study green tea was effective against most of the 111 bacteria tested, including two genera of Gram-positive and seven genera of Gram-negative bacteria. It was also confirmed that in vivo it could protect against *Salmonella typhimurium* (Bandyopadhyay et al 2005).

Recent in vitro research is looking at a possible role for (–)(–)-epigallocatechin-3-gallate (EGCG) in fighting antibiotic-resistant bacteria. It has been shown to be effective against 21 clinical isolates of *Acinetobacter baumannii*, a common cause of infection in intensive-care units, and against the antibiotic resistant *Stenotrophomonas maltophilia* (Gordon & Wareham 2010, Osterburg et al 2009).

Green tea has also been found to inhibit *Helicobacter pylori* in animal models (Matsubara et al 2003, Stoicov et al 2009). According to one study, which compared the antibacterial activity of black, green and oolong tea, it seems that fermentation adversely affects antibacterial activity, as green tea exhibited the strongest effects, and black tea the weakest (Chou et al 1999). An in vitro study has demonstrated that green tea can significantly lower bacterial endotoxin-induced cytokine release and therefore may reduce mortality from sepsis. Part of the antibacterial activity may be a selective anti-adhesive effect, with green tea inhibiting pathogen adhesion to cells (Lee et al 2009).

Oral pathogens

In a recent randomised controlled trial (RCT), 66 healthy subjects rinsed with a green tea extract for 1 minute three times a week, and at the end of 4 and 7 days there was a significant reduction in *Streptococcus mutans* and lactobacilli in the green tea group (Ferrazzano et al 2011). Both in vitro and in vivo tests have identified strong antibacterial activity against a range of oral pathogens, such as *Streptococcus mutans*, *S. salivarius* and *E. coli* (Otake et al 1991, Rasheed & Haider 1998). The mechanism of action appears to involve antiadhesion effects, with the strongest activity associated with epigallocatechin gallate and epicatechin gallate. Green tea catechins (GTCs) have also showed an antibacterial effect against *Porphyromonas gingivalis* and *Prevotella* spp. in vitro (Araghizadeh et al 2013, Hirasawa et al 2002).

Furthermore, green tea polyphenols, especially epigallocatechin gallate, have been found to completely inhibit the growth and adherence of *Porphyromonas gingivalis* on buccal epithelial cells (Sakanaka et al 1996).

Antiviral activity

A number of in vitro studies have shown that epigallocatechin gallate strongly inhibits HIV replication (Chang et al 1994, Fassina et al 2002, Liu et al 2005, Tao 1992, Williamson et al 2006) and inhibits attachment of HIV virus to T cells (Nance et al 2009). The theaflavins from black tea have shown even stronger anti-HIV activity than catechins in vitro by inhibiting viral entry into target cells (Liu et al 2005). Antiviral activity has also been identified against Epstein–Barr virus, herpes simplex virus 1, influenza A and B, rotavirus and enterovirus (Chang et al 2003, de Oliveira et al 2013, Imanishi et al 2002, Isaacs et al 2008, Mukoyama et al 1991, Tao 1992, Weber et al 2003). EGCG and epicatechin gallate show antiviral activity inhibiting influenza virus replication in vitro with differences in the strength of the antiviral activity depending on the strain of influenza (Song et al 2005). In vitro research shows green tea extract and EGCG inhibit human papillomavirus in human cervical cancer cells (Tang et al 2008). Antiviral activity seems to be attributable to interference with virus adsorption (Mukoyama et al 1991).

Antimalarial

Antimalarial properties have been shown in vitro, with crude extract of green tea, EGCG and epicatechin gallate strongly inhibiting *Plasmodium falciparum* growth (Sannella et al 2007).

Anticarcinogenic

Several in vitro studies have shown a dose-dependent decreased proliferation and/or increased apoptosis in a variety of cancer cell lines (lung, prostate, colon, stomach, pancreatic, bladder, oral, leukaemia, breast, cervical and bone) (Garcia et al 2006, Gupta et al 2003, Han et al 2009, Honicke et al 2012, Kavanagh et al 2001, Khan et al 2009a, Kinjo et al 2002, Qanungo et al 2005, Qin et al 2007, Sen & Chatterjee 2011, Shimizu et al 2005, Siddiqui et al 2011, Srinivasan et al 2008, Valcic et al 1996, Wang & Bachrach 2002, Yamauchi et al 2009, Yoo et al 2002, Zhang et al 2002, Zou et al 2010). Additionally, photochemopreventive effects for green tea and epigallocatechin gallate have been demonstrated in vitro, in vivo and on human skin for the prevention of skin cancer (Afaq et al 2003, Katiyar 2011) and apoptosis of skin tumour cells (Mantena et al 2005).

The mechanism of action by which tea polyphenols exert antimutagenic and antitumorigenic effects is still largely speculative. A review of research suggests there is increasing experimental evidence of multiple signalling pathways and reducing cancer metastasis (Khan & Mukhtar 2010, Thakur et al 2012). A systematic review of in vitro and in vivo studies on epithelial ovarian cancer cells concluded green tea components had an impact on cell signalling, cell motility, angiogenesis, apoptosis and inflammation (Trudel et al 2012). The following has been observed: inhibition of the large multicatalytic protease and metalloproteinases, which are involved in tumour survival and metastasis, respectively, and inhibition of many tumour-associated protein kinases, while not affecting kinase activity in normal cells (Kazi et al 2002, Wang & Bachrach 2002). Tea polyphenols have also been found to inhibit some cancer-related proteins that regulate DNA replication and transformation. There is increasing evidence that catechins possess antiangiogenic properties (Sachinidis & Hescheler 2002). Inhibition of angiogenic factors and antitumour immune reactivity, including an increase in cytotoxic T-lymphocyte cells, was found to be the mechanism of action in preventing photocarcinogenesis (Mantena et al 2005). Recent work suggests tea polyphenols may inhibit microsomal aromatase and 5 alpha-reductase, so suppressing prostate carcinogenesis. Tea catechins may work to suppress proteasomal activities, thereby inhibiting breast cancer cell proliferation (Ho et al 2009). Modification of oestrogen metabolism was found with both premenopausal and menopausal women, which may modify the risk of breast cancer (Fuhrman et al 2013).

Adjunct in cancer treatment

There has been some exploratory in vitro research to study the combination of green tea and anticancer drugs, with findings suggesting that EGCG with cyclooxygenase-2 inhibitors increased apoptosis mediated through the MAPK signalling pathway and the combination of EGCG and tamoxifen increased the effectiveness in apoptosis more than tamoxifen alone (Suganuma et al 2011). In this cell culture research the issue of ovarian cancer cells developing resistance to chemotherapy was explored. They found EGCG and sulforaphane from cruciferous vegetables may offer a novel treatment in ovarian cancer. The combination of EGCG and sulforaphane increased apoptosis significantly after 6 days of treatment in cells that were resistant to paclitaxel and it may offer a solution for overcoming paclitaxel resistance in this disease (Chen et al 2013). This initial in vitro work may point the way to future research.

Antihypertensive

Recent human studies have found antihypertensive benefit, with a small RCT reporting significant reduction in both systolic and diastolic blood pressure in obese patients with hypertension (Bogdanski et al 2012) and other studies reporting blood pressure-lowering effects (Brown et al 2009, Nantz et al 2009). In vitro experiments using green tea extracts have identified angiotensin-converting enzyme inhibition (Persson et al 2006). Animal experiments have also shown that a green tea extract protected against arterial hypertension induced by angiotensin II (Antonello et al 2007).

Cardioprotective

Studies on animals and humans find that green tea has multiple mechanisms that have an impact on the cardiovascular system, including lipid lowering, hypocholesterolaemic, anti-inflammatory, antithrombogenic, antioxidant, antihypertensive and antiatherosclerotic (Babu & Liu 2008, Neves et al 2008) and shows a beneficial effect on endothelial function in healthy volunteers (Alexopoulos et al 2008). The catechins in the green tea also have the ability to prevent atherosclerosis, as well as inhibiting thrombogenesis through a platelet aggregation action (Bhardwaj & Khanna 2013).

Neuroprotective/neurorescue

Neuroprotective activity refers to the use of an agent before exposure to a neurotoxin which prevents toxicity. Neurorescue is a different term which refers to the use of an agent after exposure to a neurotoxin, which is able to reverse toxicity effects. In vitro and animal research indicates that EGCG found in green tea has the ability to act as both a neuroprotective and a neurorescue agent (Guo et al 2007, Hou et al 2008, Jeong et al 2007). In vitro tests reveal that EGCG reduces apoptosis of human neuroblastoma cells (Avramovich-Tirosh et al 2007). Additionally, in vivo studies have found a neuroprotective effect for EGCG on dopamine neurons, which is being further investigated as a potential preventive treatment in Parkinson's disease (Guo et al 2007, Jeong et al 2007). Animal research has found a number of neuroprotective benefits, such as reducing neuronal cell death, of EGCG in multiple sclerosis (Herges et al 2011), following a traumatic brain injury (Itoh et al 2011) and protecting the retina against neurodegeneration in a rat diabetic retinopathy model (Silva et al 2013). In vitro epicatechin and EGCG have been shown to have a neuroprotective effect which may be suitable for the neurological complications associated with HIV infection (Nath et al 2012).

Two animal studies found that EGCG reduced beta-amyloid deposition — one study reported 60% reduction in the frontal cortex and 52% in the hippocampus over the 3 months of the study (Li et al 2006, Rezai-Zadeh et al 2008). This may have implications in the development and progression of Alzheimer's dementia and is being further investigated in other models. Beta-amyloid deposition impacts on mitochondrial function and recent in vitro and in vivo research suggests EGCG can restore and protect brain mitochondrial function and integrity (Dragicevic et al 2011).

Numerous in vitro and animal models suggest several different mechanisms of action appear to be responsible for neuroprotective and neurorescue activity, including antioxidant, iron chelating, anti-inflammatory, cell apoptosis, signal transduction, gene regulation and an effect on amyloid precursor protein (Assuncao et al 2010, Biasibetti et al 2013, Mandel et al 2006, Ostrowska et al 2007). These actions taken together make green tea polyphenols a promising agent in reversing age-related neuronal decline (Andrade & Assuncao 2012). A rat model found improvement in spatial learning and memory over long-term treatment, with green tea protecting against oxidative damage in the rat hippocampal region (Assuncao et al 2011). In an aged rat model improved cognitive function after EGCG might be due to its impact on neurotransmitters, with a positive effect found for dopamine, acetylcholine and serotonin (Srividhya et al 2012).

Iron chelation

EGCG has been shown to chelate metals such as iron, zinc and copper (Guo et al 1996, Kumamoto et al 2001). Since the accumulation of iron has been implicated in the aetiology of both Alzheimer's dementia and Parkinson's disease and in vivo research shows EGCG's iron-chelating effect penetrates the brain barrier, it may offer neuroprotective and neurorescue effects in these diseases. EGCG has further been shown to reduce amyloid precursor protein and beta-amyloid peptide, most likely due to its iron-chelating activity (Reznichenko et al 2006). It is possible that iron chelation effects enabling iron to be removed from the brain may provide a novel therapy to prevent progression in neurodegenerative diseases (Mandel et al 2007).

Thermogenic activity

Although the thermogenic activity of green tea is often attributed to its caffeine content, an in vivo study has shown that stimulation of brown adipose tissue thermogenesis occurs to a greater extent than would be expected from the caffeine content alone (Dulloo et al 2000). The interaction between catechin polyphenols and caffeine on stimulating noradrenaline release and reducing noradrenaline catabolism may be responsible. Clinical investigation has produced similar results, with green tea consumption significantly increasing 24-hour energy expenditure and urinary noradrenaline excretion, whereas an equivalent concentration of caffeine had no effect on these measures (Dulloo et al 2000).

OTHER ACTIONS

Green tea exhibits a variety of other pharmacological actions, such as anti-inflammatory activity, CNS stimulation, inhibition of platelet aggregation, stimulation of gastric acid secretion and diuresis, increased mental alertness, relaxation of extracerebral vascular and bronchial smooth muscle, and reduced cholesterol, triglyceride and leptin levels (Fassina et al 2002, Sayama et al 2000). Recent in vitro and animal models suggest potential as a therapeutic agent for T-cell-mediated autoimmune conditions (Pae & Wu 2013). A significant genoprotective effect was found with an in vitro study and a small human trial using a biomarker of oxidative stress (Han et al 2011).

Some animal studies suggest that EGCG activates gamma-aminobutyric acid (GABA)-A receptors, causing sedative and hypnotic effects (Adachi et al 2006, Vignes et al 2006). A number of rat experiments have shown memory improvement in older animals. Improved spatial cognition learning ability in rats was demonstrated after the administration of long-term GTCs (Haque et al 2006). Significant improvement in memory and learning was found in older rats administered with green tea extract over 8 weeks (Kaur et al 2008).

Hepatoprotective

Preliminary evidence from in vitro experiments demonstrates hepatoprotective activity with GTCs improving insulin sensitivity, decreasing lipids and through their antioxidant and anti-inflammatory actions (Masterjohn & Bruno 2012, Ueno et al 2009).

Antithyroid

In vitro research and a recent rat model has found catechins have an antithyroid action, decreasing the activities of thyroid peroxidase and the synthesis of thyroid hormone (Chandra & De 2013). An action preventing autoimmune inflammation in an animal model suggests EGCG may delay or manage autoimmune disorders such as Sjögren's syndrome (Gillespie et al 2008). Another recent animal model of multiple sclerosis reported a protection against autoimmune expression by inhibiting immune cell infiltration and modulating proautoimmune cells and antiautoimmune cells (Meydani 2011). In vitro and in vivo studies and some preclinical research suggests an antiarthritic and antirheumatic activity for EGCG (Ahmed 2010).

CLINICAL USE

Evidence is largely based on epidemiological studies, with few clinical studies available.

Cancer prevention

It is still unclear whether green tea consumption reduces the incidence of all cancers or has any effect on mortality; however, studies of individual cancers show some protective effects. Supportive evidence is most consistent for breast, ovarian, endometrial and prostate cancers, with some supportive evidence for colerectal, pancreatic cancers and leukaemia and less consistent evidence for lung, liver, bladder, oesophageal and gastric cancers.

All cancers

A Cochrane review concluded that there was conflicting evidence regarding an inverse association between green tea drinking and cancer risk and suggests it remains unproven as a cancer intervention (Boehm et al 2009). Other systematic reviews and meta-analyses have suggested a trend towards protection in breast and prostate cancers and improved survival rates in epithelial ovarian cancer (Clement 2009, Johnson et al 2012). Another review concluded that green tea was associated with a reduced risk of upper gastrointestinal tract cancers and had a beneficial role in breast cancer. However they suggested results on overall cancer prevention were inconclusive (Yuan et al 2011). A 2003 study using 13-year follow-up data found increased green tea consumption was associated with an apparent delay of cancer onset and death, and all-cause deaths (Nakachi et al 2003).

The conflicting results from different studies and reviewers may be due to confounding factors in different populations, dosages and differences in the EGCG content of green teas.

Breast cancer

There appears to be a benefit of green tea drinking of three or more cups daily with reduction in the risk of breast cancer. Some recent studies are suggesting the aromatase-inhibiting action may be more effective for women drinking green tea premenopause, which may delay onset of breast cancer later in life. A meta-analysis of three cohort studies from Japan and one population case-control study from the United States concluded that green tea consumption reduced the risk of breast cancer (Sun et al 2006). Similar protective effects were observed in a case–control study in China, which found that regular drinking of green tea reduced breast cancer risk (Zhang et al 2007a). In a meta-analysis of nine studies — seven studies on the incidence and two on the recurrence of breast cancer — consumption of three or more cups of green tea daily was associated with reduced recurrence (pooled relative risk [RR] = 0.73, 95% confidence interval [CI]: 0.56–0.96). No association was found in the cohort studies for reduced incidence of breast cancer; however the case-control studies did find an inverse association with incidence (pooled RR 0.81, 95% CI: 0.75–0.88) (Ogunleye et al 2010). In this review it is suggested that the difference in numbers of pre- or postmenopausal women in the case-controlled or cohort studies may explain the conflicting results. One review examining data from the Shanghai Women's Health Study (n = 74,942 Chinese women) considered the hypothesis that, because of the difference in oestrogens pre- and postmenopause, and green tea's aromatase-inhibiting action, tea-drinking protection might depend on menopausal status. Their analysis found that regularly drinking green tea from 25 years of age may delay the onset of breast cancer, suggesting a largely beneficial effect in premenopausal women (Dai et al 2010). This hypothesis may explain in part some of the conflicting evidence from studies, but larger studies and RCTs are required to confirm findings.

Ovarian cancer

A recent meta-analysis included six case-control and cohort studies with a total of 9113 subjects (3842 cases and 5271 controls) reporting that green tea drinking can significantly decrease the risk of ovarian cancer (odds ratio [OR] 0.81; 95% CI: 0.73–0.89;

$P < 0.0001$). More research is suggested to assess different teas and dosages, and how different subgroups are affected (Gao et al 2013). The case-control Australian Ovarian Cancer Study conducted over 3.5 years (1368 patients and 1416 controls) reported a significant inverse association between green tea drinking (four or more cups) and ovarian cancer. They found no difference between green and black tea consumption and there was no dose-response effect. The same authors conducted a meta-analysis (which included 17 studies) and found a trend towards green tea drinking and ovarian cancer prevention (Nagle et al 2010). A 2011 review of the literature found only four case-control studies (Goodman 2003, Nagle et al 2010, Song et al 2008, Zhang et al 2002) of green tea and ovarian cancer and a meta-analysis of these studies found evidence of a combined inverse association (OR 0.66; 95% CI: 0.54–0.80) between green tea drinking and ovarian cancer, with a 32% reduction in risk for green tea drinkers. Both prospective and retrospective observational analysis found an inverse association; however the authors suggested caution in interpretation of the results, with very different levels of tea drunk in the studies and lack of prospective cohort results (Butler & Wu 2011). A systematic review of in vitro, in vivo and epidemiological studies on epithelial ovarian cancer included four case-control studies and concluded that it was difficult to extrapolate data as the catechins in the green tea varied, there were different cup sizes and various definitions of high tea intake. Despite these factors it did appear that green tea consumption was associated with a decreased ovarian cancer risk and better prognosis of the disease (Trudel et al 2012).

Endometrial cancer

Green tea drinking was found to be mildly protective against endometrial cancer risk in a population-based case–control study in China where 995 cases were interviewed. This protective effect might be limited to premenopausal women (Gao et al 2005). A total of two cohort and five case-control studies were included in a meta-analysis that reported a significant reduction in risk of endometrial cancer for green tea drinkers, with an increase of two cups a day associated with a reduction in risk of endometrial cancer by 25% (Tang et al 2009b). A more recent review and meta-analysis of six observational studies confirmed a dose-dependent protective role of green tea drinking and endometrial cancer risk, suggesting a 23% reduction in risk for regular green tea drinkers (OR 0.78; 95% CI: 0.62–0.98). However the authors suggest caution in interpreting the results because of the differences in green teas and the amount of tea consumed (Butler & Wu 2011).

Prostate cancer

Although evidence is inconclusive, there is a mounting body of research showing a preventive role for reducing the risk of prostate cancer with a therapeutic dose of five or more cups of green tea a day. A Cochrane review included five studies and reported that in the higher-quality observational studies and in the only RCT there was a decreased risk of prostate cancer with high consumption of green tea (Boehm et al 2009). A case-control study in China with 130 prostate cancer patients found that green tea was protective against prostate cancer, with lower risk associated with an increase in the frequency, duration and quantity of green tea consumed (Jian et al 2004). Drinking green tea was also associated with a reduction in the risk of advanced prostate cancer in 49,920 men aged 40–69 years who completed questionnaires over a 10-year period in the Japan Public Health Center-based Prospective Study. The effect was dose-dependent and strongest for men drinking five or more cups/day compared with less than 1 cup/day (Kurahashi et al 2008). The more recent evidence appears to be inconclusive, with mixed results from a number of clinical trials and population studies (Henning et al 2011, Khan et al 2009a, Lee & Pasalich 2013). A meta-analysis of observational studies included seven studies with green tea and reported a borderline significant decrease (38%) in prostate cancer risk for Asian populations with high green tea consumption (Zheng et al 2011a). One of the plausible reasons for the conflicting evidence is that some studies include low tea consumption, which may skew the results, as it appears that dosage is important in cancer protection.

Colorectal cancer

A recent meta-analysis of 13 case-control studies found a weak, non-statistically-significant reduction in colorectal cancer risk for those drinking high doses of green tea (Wang et al 2012c). This benefit did not seem to extend to US and European populations. More research would be required to confirm these findings. A meta-analysis of six prospective cohort studies (including 1675 cases of colorectal cancer) reported that in Shanghai populations there was an inverse risk between green tea consumption and the incidence of colon and colorectal cancers. The results overall were insufficient to suggest green tea may protect against colorectal cancer (Wang et al 2012e).

Pancreatic cancer

A recent Chinese population-based case-control study (908 patients with pancreatic cancer and 1067 healthy controls) found that women had a 32% less risk of pancreatic cancer with regular low-temperature green tea consumption, especially drinking higher amounts and with long-term use. Drinking more than 150 g of dry tea leaves per month (also lower-temperature tea) resulted in a reduction in risk by 43% (OR 0.56, 95% CI 0.32–0.98) for women compared with non-tea drinkers. With men there was only an association between pancreatic cancer risk and tea for regular tea drinkers consuming lukewarm and cool tea compared to hot tea (Wang et al 2012b).

Leukaemia

Leukaemia risk may be reduced with drinking sufficient amounts of green tea. The protective effect was significant in the 16–29-year age range with higher amounts of green tea consumption; there was no significant relationship to green tea drinking and leukaemia risk in younger people in the 0–15-year age range. These findings were from a population-based study in Taiwan (Kuo et al 2009). A hospital-based case-control study (107 patients) in China found that there was a reduction of risk in adult leukaemia with high green tea consumption (Zhang et al 2007b).

Lung cancer

A systematic review of epidemiological studies on the risk of lung cancer and tea drinking found a significant reduction in risk for the high-level tea drinkers in only four out of 20 studies. Overall the review found a small benefit for green tea drinking in reducing the risk of lung cancer, which was especially noticeable in those who had never smoked (Arts 2008). A meta-analysis including 22 studies (12 studies on green tea only) also reported a borderline significant association with a 22% reduction in the risk of developing lung cancer for the highest green tea drinkers. Increasing green tea by two cups a day was shown to reduce lung cancer risk by 18% (Tang et al 2009a). This was confirmed in a dose–response analysis of six studies where a significant non-linear relationship between green tea and risk of lung cancer was reported. This beneficial effect was especially strong in those drinking more than seven cups a day (Wang et al 2012d). It appears that green tea may have a small beneficial effect in reducing lung cancer risk but, as a recent systematic review suggests, more well-designed studies are needed (Fritz et al 2013).

Liver cancer

The protective effect of green tea drinking to reduce liver cancer risk appears to be stronger for high-risk patients with hepatitis B or C and also for long-term green tea drinkers. A recent meta-analysis included 13 epidemiological studies (six case-control and seven prospective cohort studies) and reported borderline significance showing green tea was preventive (for both men and women) in reducing the risk of developing primary liver cancer (Fon Sing et al 2011). Evidence is conflicting and one analysis of data from a Japanese Public Health Cohort study with 18,815 subjects found no association with green tea drinking and liver cancer risk (Inoue et al 2009a). However another larger Japanese cohort study (Ohsaki Cohort Study, following 41,761 subjects over 9 years) found a significant reduction in risk for liver cancer and green tea for men and women drinking five or more cups of green tea a day (Ui et al 2009). The differences in reporting data may be linked to quantity of tea drunk, number of years of green tea drinking and also whether the group had a high- or low-risk cohort. A recent case-control study of 204 hepatocellular carcinoma (HCC) patients and 415 healthy controls found that drinking high amounts of green tea for longer periods of time resulted in a protective effect, with those drinking green tea for over 30 years having the lowest risk. In the subgroup of patients with chronic hepatitis infection, the risk of HCC in non-green tea drinkers was twice that of those consuming green tea. Further research in this subgroup of people with a higher HCC risk may be warranted (Li et al 2011). According to a placebo-controlled, randomised study, green tea polyphenols may reduce the incidence of HCC in high-risk patients (Yu et al 2006). The study involved 1209 males, who tested positive for hepatitis B virus and then were allocated to the control group or active treatment with green tea polyphenols (two capsules daily of 500 mg). The trial lasted 3 years, with a further 2-year follow-up period. Ten cases of HCC were reported in the green tea group and 18 cases in the placebo group.

Bladder/kidney cancer

A recent meta-analysis included five case-control or cohort studies specifically for green tea and bladder cancer and no association was found between bladder cancer risk and green tea consumption (Wu et al 2013), although a meta-analysis in the same year suggested that Asian people drinking green tea may benefit and a protective effect on bladder cancer was found in this subgroup (Wang et al 2013). More research is indicated to confirm this finding and to discover why the benefit may be only for Asian populations, but the type of green tea may be a possible reason.

A hospital-based case-control study was undertaken in China, in which 250 patients diagnosed with clear cell renal cell carcinoma were compared with healthy controls. The research found green tea consumption of 500 mL or more a day was inversely associated with clear cell renal cell carcinoma risk (Wang et al 2012a).

Oesophageal cancer

Ten epidemiological studies (eight case-control and two cohort studies; n = 33,731) were included in a meta-analysis of green tea consumption and oesophageal cancer risk. There was no association with low or high green tea consumption and oesophageal cancer, except in a subgroup analysis, where the authors reported a protective effect of any level of green tea drinking and oesophageal cancer for women (high green tea consumption: RR/OR = 0.32, 95% CI: 0.10–0.54; medium consumption: RR/OR = 0.43, 95% CI: 0.21–0.66; low consumption: RR/OR = 0.45, 95% CI: 0.10–0.79) (Zheng et al 2012). Another systematic review and meta-analysis of green tea, black tea and coffee and oesophageal cancer risk included 13 green tea studies (one cohort and the 12 case-controls) and the authors reported a significant association for the highest green tea drinkers in the case-control studies (OR = 0.70; 95% CI: 0.51–0.96, $P < 0.001$) and for the Chinese studies (OR = 0.64; 95% CI: 0.44–0.95, $P < 0.001$) and a more pronounced inverse association for women (Zheng et al 2013a). It is recommended that further studies with control of dose and the temperature of the tea be undertaken.

Gastric cancer

There is conflicting research on the benefit of green tea in reducing gastric cancer risk according to a Cochrane review on green tea and cancer (Boehm et al 2009). However, there may be a trend towards significance for higher green tea consumption (five or more cups per day) and this is especially noted in women and in Chinese populations. A recent review of epidemiological evidence included 17 Japanese and Chinese studies (10 case-control and seven cohort studies). This review concluded that the evidence was insufficient to suggest that green tea reduces the risk of gastric cancer. They found seven studies with no association, eight with an inverse association and one study showing a positive association; however, they do suggest that *Helicobacter pylori* infection may be a confounding factor and that future research should include this subgroup (Hou et al 2013). A pooled analysis of six Japanese cohort studies (total of 219,080 individuals) reported no significant association of green tea drinking and reduction in gastric cancer risk for men; however, women drinking five or more cups a day had a significant reduction in risk of distal gastric cancer (with no significant effect seen on proximal gastric cancer) (Inoue et al 2009b). A later systematic review of epidemiological studies in Japan agreed with this finding, reporting a protective effect for women reducing gastric cancer risk. They included eight cohort studies and three case-control studies and, when analysing only the case-control studies, they found a weak association with gastric cancer reduction and green tea but not in the cohort studies (Sasazuki et al 2012). This difference in results reported from case-control and cohort studies was also found in an earlier meta-analysis (Myung et al 2009). One meta-analysis (seven cohort, 10 case-control and one population-based nested case-control study) reported a statistically significant 14% reduced risk of stomach cancer for people drinking five or more cups of green tea. The five Chinese studies showed a stronger stomach cancer risk reduction than the Japanese studies. The authors recommend further research confined to higher green tea drinkers to confirm the findings (Kang et al 2010). A note of caution from a population-based case-control study ($n = 200$) found that drinking tea at a very hot temperature might be associated with an increased risk of gastric cancer (Mao et al 2011).

Cancer treatment

Studies have been conducted with various doses of green tea and GTCs in different cancers, producing mixed results.

Overall, the current evidence does not support the use of green tea as a cancer treatment; however, there are some exceptions, which suggest an adjunctive role.

Epithelial ovarian cancer

Green tea increased the survival rate of patients with epithelial ovarian cancer in a cohort of 309 Chinese women (Zhang et al 2004). Most (77.9%) of the women in the treatment group were alive at the 3-year follow-up, as compared with 47.9% of the control group.

G

Cervical cancer

In an RCT, 90 patients with cervical lesions infected with human papillomavirus were given either a capsule containing 200 mg EGCG and/or an ointment containing 200 mg Polyphenon E, to be applied daily (Ahn et al 2003). There was a 69% response rate (35 out of 51 patients) for those on treatment when compared with a 10% response rate for controls ($P < 0.05$), with the ointment showing the best effects.

Colorectal cancer

A pilot study was undertaken with 136 patients with colorectal adenomas, which are considered to be a precursor to colorectal cancers. This randomised trial in Japan increased green tea intake from an average of six cups a day to the equivalent of 10 cups a day by supplementing with green tea extract tablets. This involved supplementing the treatment group with 1.5 g of green tea extract per day for 12 months while both placebo and treatment group continued their green tea drinking. At the end of the intervention metachronous adenomas were evident in 31% (20 of 65) of the control and 15% (9 of 60) of the green tea extract group (RR 0.49; 95% CI, 0.24–0.99; $P < 0.05$) and the size of the relapsed adenomas was smaller in the treated group, illustrating a potential chemopreventive role for green tea extract (Shimizu et al 2008).

Oral premalignant lesions

A phase II RCT with 39 patients with oral premalignant lesions gave the treatment group of patients 500, 750 or 1000 mg of green tea extract three times a day for 12 weeks. On biopsy the green tea extract group had improved histology, especially at the two higher doses, although this was not statistically significant. During the follow-up (median time of 27.5 months) 15 of the patients developed oral cancer and there was no difference between oral cancer-free survival between the placebo and green tea extract groups. It is thought that the green tea extract may act through stromal vascular endothelial growth factor and the research suggests that longer-term trials are needed (Tsao et al 2009).

Prostate cancer

Several studies have been conducted in men with established prostate cancer. GTCs may have a role in arresting disease development in prostate cancer according to a double-blind, placebo-controlled study (Bettuzzi et al 2008). Sixty volunteers with high-grade prostate intraepithelial neoplasis and therefore at high risk of prostate cancer were treated with GTCs (three capsules of 200 mg/day) or placebo over 12 months. Of the 30 men in the GTC group, only one tumour was diagnosed, as opposed to nine cases in the placebo group. The GTC group also scored higher on the quality-of-life scores and had reduced lower urinary tract symptoms and no side effects were detected (Bettuzzi et al 2006). An update for this trial was undertaken 2 years later to see if the prostate cancer was merely delayed rather than prevented in the green tea group. Half the original subjects (equal numbers from placebo and green tea cohorts) agreed to further investigations, which detected one more tumour in the GTC group and two more in the placebo group. These results suggest that GTC given for a year may offer long-term protection within this at-risk group and might be useful as first-line preventive therapy. More recently, a small open-label study of 26 men (aged 41–68 years) with a recent diagnosis of prostate cancer (stage I, II or III) were given 800 mg EGCG (Polyphenon E) daily in the time between biopsy and radical prostatectomy and serum levels of prostate-specific antigen, hepatocyte growth factor, insulin-like growth factor-1 and vascular endothelial growth factor all decreased significantly with the median dosing period of 34.5 days. The authors also noted that there were no adverse effects on the liver observed during the study (McLarty et al 2009). This same trend was found in a RCT of 50 diagnosed prostate cancer patients given Polyphenon E or placebo for 3–6 weeks prior to surgery. Although not significant, biomarkers did show some chemopreventive potential with decreased prostate-specific antigen and insulin-like growth factors. However, it was found that apoptosis and angiogenesis did not differ in either group and the bioavailability of the polyphenols in the prostate tissue was low (Nguyen et al 2012). The authors suggested that longer term and larger controlled trials would be useful to verify findings.

In contrast, a small study testing green tea (6 g/day) in patients with pre-existing androgen-independent prostate cancer found little effect on PSA levels (Jatoi et al 2003). Similar results were obtained in a small study of 19 patients with hormone-refractory prostate cancer given a lower dose of 250 mg capsules of green tea twice a day (Choan et al 2005). It is likely that both these studies did not use a green tea treatment with sufficient concentrations of catechins or a high enough dose.

Leukaemia

A clinical trial with 42 patients with Rai stage 0–II early stage of chronic lymphocytic leukaemia, who were asymptomatic and not eligible to begin chemotherapy, were given Polyphenon E (2000 mg twice daily) for up to 6 months and found declines in the absolute lymphocyte count and lymphadenopathy in the majority of patients (Shanafelt et al 2013). This is a possible novel use as a low-toxicity early intervention, but randomised trials are needed to affirm these findings.

Adjunct in breast cancer treatment

Ten radiotherapy patients with non-inflammatory breast cancer (locally advanced) in a small 8-week study were randomly assigned to radiotherapy plus EGCG (400 mg three times daily) or radiotherapy plus placebo. The green tea treatment group showed serum changes, including suppression of cell proliferation and invasion, a reduction in metalloproteinase-9 and metalloproteinase-2 expression and lower serum vascular endothelial growth factor. This additive apoptotic effect with the radiation treatment suggests that green tea polyphenols have potential as an adjunctive treatment in breast cancer (Zhang et al 2012a).

Reducing cancer drug side effects

An animal study has suggested a possible novel use of green tea to protect against nephrotoxicity caused by the use of cisplatin, a chemotherapy drug used to treat a variety of cancers (Khan et al 2009b).

Some recent research has experimented with nanochemoprevention with encapsulated EGCG which enhanced the bioavailability of the EGCG by 10-fold. In the future this nanoparticle-mediated delivery could be used to reduce toxicity side effects of chemotherapy drugs (Siddiqui et al 2009).

Cardiovascular protection

Epidemiological studies suggest that green tea consumption is associated with a reduced risk of cardiovascular disease (CVD) (Kuriyama 2008, Maeda et al 2003). Its antioxidant effects may explain some of the CVD benefits and a recent systematic review of 31 RCTs found 0.6–1.5 L/day of green tea increased antioxidant capacity and reduced lipid peroxidation (Ellinger et al 2011). A systematic review of literature reported that observational studies indicated protection against stroke, atherosclerosis and hypertension for green tea drinkers (Clement 2009) and a recent review included four systematic reviews (Hooper et al 2008, Kim et al 2011, Wang et al 2011, Zheng et al 2011b) and meta-analysis, suggesting that, although evidence is not robust for a reduction in coronary artery disease (CAD), some RCTs do indicate that green tea may be effective in reducing LDLs and total cholesterol (Johnson et al 2012). This is confirmed by a recent Cochrane review reporting on 11 RCTs (n = 821), with seven of these trials on green tea alone (five on green tea tablets or capsules and two with tea drinking). The authors concluded that total cholesterol, LDL-cholesterol and blood pressure were significantly reduced with green tea consumption. They recommend caution in interpreting these results, as there were only a small number of studies in this analysis (Hartley et al 2013).

A 2000 prospective cohort study of 8552 people in Japan found that those consuming more than 10 cups a day, compared with those consuming fewer than three cups, had a decreased relative risk of death from CVD (Nakachi et al 2000). The Ohsaki National Health Insurance Cohort Study was a population-based study in Japan, spanning 11 years (1995–2005) with 40,530 Japanese adults aged 40–79 years. At baseline, no participants had cancer or coronary heart disease. The study identified an inverse association between green tea consumption and mortality due to CVD (especially mortality due to stroke) as well as all other causes. A significant protective effect was shown at a dose of five cups or more daily for men and three or more cups daily for women. Overall, the protective effects were greatest for women compared to men (Kuriyama et al 2006b). The investigators suggested higher smoking levels in men may have reduced potential benefits in this group (Cheng 2007).

Some 76,979 subjects from another Japanese study (Japan Collaborative Cohort Study for Evaluation of Cancer Risk) were included in a prospective study assessing tea drinking and mortality from CVD. The individuals did not have coronary heart disease nor had they had a stroke at the onset of the study. There were 1362 deaths from strokes and 650 deaths from CVD over the 13.1-year follow-up. The analysis found that a moderate intake of green tea was associated with lower CVD mortality. For coronary heart disease this benefit was more for women, who drank six or more cups of green tea a day (a 38% lower risk of mortality) (Mineharu et al 2011). Similarly, analysis from the Japan Public Health Center-Based Study, with a slightly larger cohort of 82,369, found that higher green tea drinkers had an inverse association with strokes (especially intracerebral haemorrhage) and CVD in the general population. The participants completed self-administered food frequency questionnaires over a 13-year period (Kokubo et al 2013).

Elderly people in a Japanese population-based study of 14,001 were followed for 6 years and drinking seven or more cups a day exerted a reduced risk of cardiovascular mortality (Suzuki et al 2009). A meta-analysis that included data from nine epidemiological studies with 4378 stroke incidences found a 21% lower risk of stroke among green or black tea drinkers if they consumed three or more cups a day (Arab et al 2009). These benefits of green tea drinking were not confirmed in a Dutch population study using a validated food frequency questionnaire (n = 37,514) over 13 years, where they found no correlation with tea drinking and stroke. The difference in findings with other population studies may be because most of the tea was black and not green tea (de Koning Gans et al 2010). Well-designed RCTs would be helpful to establish a benefit in reducing risk of stroke. However, this same large Dutch cohort of healthy men and women did appear to benefit from a reduction in coronary heart disease mortality by drinking three to six cups of tea a day (some green tea but mainly black tea). Relatively few people died from either stroke or coronary heart disease during the study, making associations with tea drinking difficult to evaluate (de Koning Gans et al 2010). In a later meta-analysis (13 studies on black tea and five studies with green tea), green but not black tea showed a significant association with reducing risk for the highest green tea drinkers. Including an additional cup of green tea per day was associated with a 10% decrease in CAD risk. This inverse association between green tea and CAD was found in the case-control studies, which may not be strong evidence given problems with recall or selection bias in retrospective studies. Thus the authors suggest the protective role of green tea is tentative and large prospective cohort studies are needed (Wang et al 2011). It may be that the catechins in green tea provide protection in CAD, whereas black tea benefits are more associated with heart disease (Di Castelnuovo et al 2012).

Lipid lowering

An increasing body of research suggests that green tea given to patients with hypercholesterolaemia may lower total and LDL-cholesterol levels but there is less robust evidence that triglycerides or high-density lipoproteins (HDLs) are impacted.

A recent Cochrane review included evidence from seven RCTs on green tea with varied doses (five studies with 375–600 mg daily of green tea extract and two studies on green tea beverages). The review reported a statistically significant reduction in total cholesterol (MD –0.62 mmol/L, 95% CI –0.77 to –0.46) and LDL-cholesterol (MD –0.64 mmol/L, 95% CI –0.77 to –0.52) compared to placebo, with a trend towards a reduction in triglycerides (Hartley et al 2013). A meta-analysis including 20 trials found that total and LDL-cholesterol levels were lowered with green tea but no effect was found on HDL-cholesterol or triglycerides. Subgroup analysis suggested that people with normal cholesterol levels found no benefit and there appeared to be no significant effect with green tea capsules. The heterogeneity of the studies limits the meta-analysis. It appears that higher-dose catechins may be more effective and further studies on dose and duration of green tea drinking are needed (Kim et al 2011). Another meta-analysis in the same year included 14 RCTs (n = 1136) and confirmed that green tea reduced both total and LDL-cholesterol but exerted no effect on HDLs, although these researchers found both green tea drinking and extracts were beneficial (Zheng et al 2011b).

A significant reduction in LDL-cholesterol and triglycerides and marked increase in HDL-cholesterol was also found for green tea consumption (400 mg given three times daily) in a double-blind, placebo, RCT of 78 obese women conducted over 12 weeks (Hsu et al 2008). Similar results were obtained in an early cross-sectional study involving 1371 men aged over 40 years (Imai & Nakachi 1995). The study showed that increased green tea consumption was associated with decreased serum concentrations of total cholesterol and triglyceride and an increase in HDL, together with a decrease in LDL and very-low-density lipoprotein cholesterols. Fifty-six obese hypertensive patients entered a randomised, double-blind, placebo-controlled trial and green tea supplementation did increase HDL-cholesterol as well as lower total and LDL-cholesterol. The treated group were given a green tea extract capsule (379 mg) daily for 3 months (Bogdanski et al 2012). Other studies have found no significant HDL effect which may be limited to patient subgroups.

In contrast, the inclusion of 3 g/day (145 mg of EGCG in 500 mL water daily) of green tea to a cholesterol-lowering diet provided no further lipid-lowering effects according to a study of 100 hypercholesterolaemic patients (Bertipaglia de Santana et al 2008). While green tea increased antioxidant potential, there was no significant reduction in any cholesterol parameters. This result may be explained by the low dose compared to other studies.

Hypertension

Research is now beginning to find antihypertensive benefits for green tea and large, longer-term, well-designed studies are needed. A recent Cochrane review included three trials which measured blood pressure (Bogdanski et al 2012, Nantz et al 2009) and on analysis found a statistically significant reduction in both systolic (MD −3.18 mmHg, 95% CI −5.25 to −1.11) and diastolic blood pressure (MD −3.42, 95% CI −4.54 to −2.30) (Hartley et al 2013). Blood pressure was significantly reduced in an RCT of 56 obese, hypertensive patients taking one capsule a day of 379 mg of a green tea extract (with 208 mg of EGCG from Olimp Labs, Debica, Poland) for over 3 months. At the end of the trial both systolic and diastolic blood pressure had reduced significantly, tumour necrosis factor-α and C-reactive protein were significantly reduced, fasting glucose and insulin levels had lowered, along with a reduction in LDL and total cholesterol and an increase in HDL-cholesterol. This small study shows promise for a multifaceted benefit for obese patients with hypertension (Bogdanski et al 2012). Another small trial with 46 obese male patients found a reduction in diastolic blood pressure (by a modest 2.5 mmHg) but no other metabolic effects were observed. The intervention was a 400 mg capsule twice a day for 8 weeks (Teavigo with 97% pure EGCG) (Brown et al 2009). In a randomised, double-blind placebo study of 111 healthy volunteers a green tea extract (200 mg decaffeinated catechin green tea extract Cardio Guard) was given twice daily. There was a reduction in systolic (5 mmHg) and diastolic (4 mmHg) blood pressure after only 3 weeks and after 3 months systolic blood pressure remained significantly lower. Other cardiovascular markers, including total and LDL-cholesterol-lowering effects, were also noted and there was a 42% reduction in serum amyloid-α (a marker of chronic inflammation) (Nantz et al 2009).

Weight loss

Animal studies have found that green tea consumption reduces food intake, decreases leptin levels and body weight and increases thermogenesis.

Clinical studies investigating the effects of green tea on weight loss have produced mixed results; however green tea in some studies suggests moderate weight loss, reduction in waist circumference and improvement in metabolic parameters and may be helpful when combined with an exercise program. The wide disparity in green teas, green tea extracts and dosage protocols hampers the pooling of results, in meta-analyses, in a meaningful way.

A recent Cochrane review included RCTs of overweight adults with trials of at least 12 weeks. They included six studies outside Japan; a small, non-significant reduction in weight, waist circumference and body mass index (BMI) was found which was unlikely to be clinically relevant. The data from the eight Japanese studies could not be pooled and again some small non-significant improvements in weight loss were seen in some studies. There was no significant benefit on weight maintenance (Jurgens et al 2012). A meta-analysis including 11 studies suggests that green tea has a small beneficial effect on weight loss and weight maintenance (Hursel et al 2009). A systematic review and meta-analysis comparing GTC benefits with and without caffeine found, of the 15 studies included, that the GTCs alone did not show anthropometric benefit; however GTCs with caffeine showed modest benefit with reduced weight, BMI and waist circumference compared with caffeine alone (Phung et al 2010).

One open study found that a green tea extract AR25 (80% ethanolic dry extract standardised at 25% catechins) taken by moderately obese patients resulted in a 4.6% decrease in body weight and 4.5% decrease in waist circumference after 3 months' treatment (Chantre & Lairon 2002). Both groups lost the same amount of weight and displayed similar metabolic parameters at the end of the study period. An RCT study in Thailand was undertaken over 12 weeks with 60 obese individuals all given a similar diet of three meals a day with 65% carbohydrates, 15% protein and 20% fat. There was no significant difference in weight loss at week 4 but at weeks 8 and 12 weight reduction was significantly greater in the green tea group than the placebo group. The difference in weight loss between the groups was 2.70 kg at 4 weeks, 5.10 kg at 8 weeks and 3.3 kg at 12 weeks. Researchers suggested the effects were due to changes in resting energy expenditure and fat oxidation (Auvichayapat et al 2008). However, two other studies produced negative findings. One double-blind, placebo-controlled parallel trial, with 46 women attempting a weight-loss program over 87 days, showed no difference between the green tea group and the placebo group (Diepvens et al 2005). Another double-blind, placebo RCT, with 78 obese women, also showed no significant difference in body weight, BMI or waist circumference after taking a green tea extract capsule of 400 mg three times a day for 12 weeks (Hsu et al 2008). An RCT (n = 104) of Chinese participants with high levels of visceral fat found a significant reduction in abdominal visceral fat and body weight by drinking a catechin-enriched green tea (609.3 mg catechins and 68.7 mg caffeine) daily for 12 weeks (Zhang et al 2012b).

A randomised clinical trial using a highly bioavailable form of green tea (Monoselect Camellia containing GreenSelect Phytosome) was used in a study with 100 overweight participants who were all assigned low-calorie diets and half of them given the green tea extract. After 90 days the diet-only group lost 5 kg in weight while the diet plus green tea group lost 14 kg. Males in the study also experienced a significant reduction in waistline measurement by 14% compared to 7% in the diet-only group. Other metabolic parameters were improved in both groups, including LDL, HDL-cholesterol, triglycerides, growth hormone, insulin and cortisol. This particular green tea extract appears to potentiate weight loss in combination with a calorie-controlled diet (Di Pierro et al 2009). More research is needed to confirm the findings of this bioavailable form of green tea.

There is some emerging research on benefit for obese patients with metabolic syndrome due to the effect green tea has on weight loss, lowering of lipids, improving blood glucose regulation and cardiovascular health (Thielecke & Boschmann 2009). A randomised, controlled prospective trial with 35 participants with obesity and metabolic syndrome were assigned placebo, four cups of green tea (equivalent of 440 mg EGCG) or green tea extract (two capsules a day totalling 460 mg EGCG). After 8 weeks a significant reduction in body weight and BMI was reported in both the green tea groups. Biomarkers of oxidative stress and lipid peroxidation including LDL-cholesterol also had a modest reduction. In this subgroup green tea may have potential, and further research would be recommended to confirm the findings (Basu et al 2010).

A small intervention study of elderly patients with metabolic syndrome found that drinking three cups of green tea a day for 60 days significantly reduced weight, waist circumference and BMI compared to placebo. There were no changes in biochemical parameters (Vieira Senger et al 2012). In a recent RCT with 46 obese participants given green tea extract (379 mg a day) or placebo over 3 months, the supplemented group had a reduction in BMI, waist circumference, total and LDL-cholesterol, triglycerides and glucose. The green tea extract group also saw an increase in antioxidant levels and zinc, HDL-cholesterol and magnesium, although iron levels were lower than the placebo group. This study shows potential for multieffect benefits for obese patients taking green tea extract (Suliburska et al 2012).

Combination of green tea with exercise for weight loss

Some small trials have shown additional benefits when dietary changes and exercise have been included in the studies. A recent double-blind, placebo-controlled trial with 36 overweight or obese women included dietary changes and resistance training over a 4-week period. They reported significant increases in resting metabolic rate, lean body mass and strength and significant reduction in waist circumference, body fat and triglycerides when combining green tea with resistance training compared with placebo and resistance training only (Cardoso et al 2013). Another study (n = 107) of overweight or obese participants over 12 weeks randomly assigned a green tea drink (625 mg catechins and 39 mg caffeine) or control drink (39 mg caffeine) and all participants were asked to do 180 minutes of moderate-intensity exercise each week. The trend (non-significant) was towards a reduction in weight, subcutaneous abdominal fat and triglycerides in the catechin group (Maki et al 2009). Further research is needed to see if green tea enhances the weight loss benefits of an exercise training program.

Diabetes

Animal studies have identified that green tea polyphenols reduce serum glucose levels and improve kidney function in diabetes (Rhee et al 2002, Sabu et al 2002) and may be helpful in preventing diabetic nephropathy (Kang et al 2012). Evidence from human trials has been contradictory and it may be that green tea is beneficial for some subgroups. A recent meta-analysis of 17 trials (including seven high-quality trials with the remainder low-quality) reported significant lowering of fasting glucose concentrations (−0.09 mmol/L; 95% CI: −015 to −0.03 mmol/L; $P < 0.01$) compared with controls and with HbA_{1C} (−0.30%; 95% CI: −0.37, −0.22%; $P \leq 0.01$). There was no significant change in fasting insulin or homeostatic model assessment of insulin resistance (HOMA-IR) values. Interestingly, subgroup analysis found that green tea lowered fasting glucose in those at risk of metabolic syndrome but not in healthy subjects and a high dose of catechins was more effective. In further analysis the higher-quality trials also showed green tea significantly reduced fasting insulin (Liu et al 2013). Another meta-analysis in the same year included 22 RCTs with 1584 participants and found a significant decrease in fasting blood glucose with GTCs (with or without caffeine) (−1.48 mg/dL; 95% CI: −2.57, −0.40 mg/dL) over a 12-week time period, but not in the shorter treatment protocols under 12 weeks. No significant effect was found with fasting blood insulin, HbA_{1C} or insulin resistance (HOMA-IR), but this could be because only a small number of the trials actually reported on these parameters. The trials included in this meta-analysis were pooled studies with diabetic, obese, metabolic syndrome and healthy patients; therefore outcome for diabetic patients alone may differ. The authors report conflicting results on dose of green tea consumption for the glucose metabolism effect and suggest further research is needed on the dose-response relationship and also to understand more about postprandial glycaemic variables (Zheng et al 2013b). One double-blind RCT with 49 individuals with type 2 diabetes mellitus found no significant hypoglycaemic effects for green tea given at 375 mg or 750 mg/day (MacKenzie et al 2007). Another RCT of 66 diabetic patients found 500 mg/day of green tea polyphenols had no clear effect on blood glucose or insulin resistance markers (Fukino et al 2005). A more recent randomised, double-blind and placebo-controlled trial with 68 obese type 2 diabetics found no significant difference in diabetic markers over 16 weeks with a decaffeinated green tea extract (500 mg three times daily 30 minutes after meals). However, some within-group comparisons did find significant reduction in HbA_{1C}, waist circumference, HOMA-IR index and insulin levels and increase in the appetite-regulating hormone ghrelin (Hsu et al 2011). A cross-over RCT with 60 borderline diabetic patients reported a significant reduction in HbA_{1C} levels and a borderline significant reduction in diastolic blood pressure after 2 months of green tea extract powder (456 mg catechins) daily. No changes were noted for weight, BMI, systolic blood pressure, lipids or fasting serum glucose levels (Fukino et al 2008). The bioavailability of some green tea extracts may vary and in some studies serum EGCG was detected in only half the subjects after early-morning testing, which could explain why some researchers report significant changes to diabetic markers and others non-significant changes. It appears that taking the green tea extract for at least 12 weeks is more beneficial and in most studies some of the diabetic markers are positively impacted, even if modestly so.

An epidemiological study of 542 men and women, aged over 65 years, from the Mediterranean islands found that tea consumption (green and black) was associated with reduced levels of fasting glucose but this was only in the non-obese subjects (Polychronopoulos et al 2008). The same MEDIS study in the Mediterranean islands evaluated 300 elderly men and women and found that long-term tea drinking (green and black) was associated with a reduction of risk of type 2 diabetes (Panagiotakos et al 2009).

Dental caries and gingivitis

Green tea extract tablets, gels, mouthwash and chewable oral preparations have been investigated for effects on dental plaque formation and gingival health under RCT conditions, overall producing favourable results (Liu & Chi 2000). Recent research also suggests potential for preventing caries.

A double-blind study investigated the effects of GTCs and polyphenols on the gingiva when used in the form of chewable oral sweets (Krahwinkel & Willershausen 2000). Compared with placebo, the green tea product chewed eight times a day significantly decreased gingival inflammation and improved periodontal structures before the 21-day test period was complete.

Another study investigated Chinese green tea polyphenol tablets for effects on plaque formation in 150 volunteers (Liu & Chi 2000). The randomised, controlled crossover study showed that green tea polyphenol tablets used for 2 weeks were able to reduce the plaque index compared with placebo treatment. Thirty chronic periodontitis patients were included in an RCT, with the treated group using a thermo-reversible sustained-release green tea gel. At the end of the 4-week trial the green tea group had a significant reduction in oral pocket depth and gingival index, showing a benefit and reduction in inflammation in these periodontitis patients (Chava & Vedula 2013).

A recent pilot study in a dental clinic concluded that rinsing with a green tea solution strongly inhibited *Streptococcus mutans* growth in saliva and plaque and reduced the gingival bleeding index score. The authors suggested further research to find out if a green tea mouthwash can reduce the prevalence of dental caries (Awadalla et al 2011). Another single-blinded RCT gave 25 high school female students, with gingivitis, a green tea mouthwash twice a day. They reported improvements on all periodontal indices over the 5-week study, although these improvements were not statistically significant (Jenabian et al 2012). In an RCT with 60 children a green tea mouthwash was as effective as sodium fluoride in reducing oral *S. mutans* and lactobacillus indicating a potential use for reduction in caries (Tehrani et al 2011).

Green tea drinking, in a study with 940 Japanese men, has also been found to have a small inverse association with periodontal disease (Kushiyama et al 2009).

Genital warts

A number of recent trials have shown good effectivity for a topical treatment (Polyphenon E, Medigene EU) containing a fixed amount of GTCs in the treatment of genital warts. The product is marketed as Veregen in the United States. It is thought the mechanism of action is a combination of immune enhancement, cell apoptosis and inhibition of human papillomavirus (Stockfleth & Meyer 2012).

A systematic review and meta-analysis included three RCTs of Polyphenon E (Gross 2008, Stockfleth et al 2008, Tatti et al 2008) with a total of 660 men and 587 women. It reported a significantly higher chance of complete clearance with the green tea product and very low recurrence rates with both the 10% ointment cream and 15% ointment. There was good tolerability, although some side effects were noted of erythema and localised skin itching (Tzellos et al 2011). Healing of genital warts occurred in 54.9% of patients using Polyphenon E ointment compared with 35.4% of patients receiving placebo in three placebo-controlled clinical studies (n = 1400) (Gross 2008). Another trial with the same Polyphenon E topical treatment evaluated 503 patients, with external genital and perianal warts, who were randomised to be treated with a 15% or 10% ointment or placebo. Treatment was applied three times a day for up to 16 weeks. After follow-up, 12 weeks later, 53% of patients with the 15% strength ointment had complete clearance, 51% for the 10% ointment and 37% for the control vehicle. A greater number of women experienced total clearance of all warts (with the Polyphenon E treatment compared to men, 60% compared to 45%: Stockfleth et al 2008). Another double-blind, placebo-controlled RCT of 502 patients with genital and perianal warts used a topical treatment of sinecatechins (a defined green tea extract), which was found to be effective and well tolerated. The findings were significant at weeks 4 and 6 and at subsequent visits over the 16-week trial. Complete clearance of warts was obtained in 57% of patients compared with only 33% with the control group (Tatti et al 2008).

Infections

Influenza

A potential novel use of green tea has been studied preventing influenza infection. A randomised, double-blind, placebo-controlled trial found the green tea group had significantly lower incidence of flu, a lower incidence of viral antigen measured in the laboratory and a significantly longer time free from the influenza infection from the start of the green tea intervention. This 5-month RCT with 200 health workers during the flu season administered six capsules of green tea extract a day (total catechins 378 mg/day and theanine 210 mg/day) or placebo. Larger trials are needed but this study may demonstrate a potential use as a prophylactic agent for influenza (Matsumoto et al 2011).

An observational study of 2663 schoolchildren in Japan gained information from questionnaires during the flu season and found an inverse association between drinking 1–5 cups a day of green tea and influenza infection (Park et al 2011).

Pneumonia

The Ohsaki cohort study in Japan followed up 19,079 men and 21,493 women (aged 40–79 years) and found 406 reported deaths from pneumonia and, although no significant association was found for men drinking green tea, it was found that green tea consumption for women did reduce the risk of dying from pneumonia (Watanabe et al 2009).

Tuberculosis

A study of 200 newly diagnosed patients with acid-fast bacilli-positive pulmonary tuberculosis were randomly assigned to receive catechin (500 mcg) or placebo. Patients were undergoing conventional treatment and after 1 and 4 months the patients with the green tea extract had a reduction in oxidative stress (Agarwal et al 2010). With further studies there may be a role for green tea extract as an adjuvant therapy in tuberculosis patients.

G

Sunburn protection and skin ageing

More than 150 in vitro and in vivo studies have reported the benefits of green tea for the skin (Hsu 2005). Many mechanisms appear to be responsible: green tea protects against ultraviolet and psoralen + ultraviolet A-induced carcinogenesis and DNA damage and is a potent antioxidant, anti-inflammatory, anticarcinogenic and vulnerary (Hsu 2005). Research with human volunteers has found that topical application of green tea to skin half an hour before ultraviolet exposure protects against the development of sunburn and epidermal damage (Elmets et al 2001). The effect is dose-dependent and strongest for the EGCG and epicatechin gallate polyphenols.

A 2-year, double-blind randomised placebo-controlled trial of oral supplementation of green tea reported significant improvement at 6 months in solar damage and improvement at 12 months in erythema and telangiectasias, although these improvements were not sustained to the 2-year end of the trial. At the end of 2 years there was no significant improvement in photoageing of the skin. The trial included 56 women who were randomised to take 250 mg of green tea polyphenols twice a day or placebo. This was a low dose of green tea extract and further research may be useful to confirm findings (Janjua et al 2009).

Liver disease

A recent meta-analysis reported borderline significance showing green tea was preventive (for both men and women) in reducing the risk of developing primary liver cancer (Fon Sing et al 2011). A systematic review of 10 studies showed that increased green tea consumption is associated with a reduced risk of liver disease. The studies were published between the years 1995 and 2005, with numbers of subjects ranging from 52 to 29,090. Of the 10 studies, four were RCTs, two cohort, one case–control and three cross-sectional studies. Among them, eight studies were conducted in China, one in Japan and the other in the United States. Most of the studies used adjustments such as age, sex, smoking and drinking to control potential confounders and the study periods varied from less than 6 months to more than 6 years. Eight studies yielded statistically significant results, showing a protective role of green tea against liver disease, whereas two studies only showed a partial tendency. Also, four studies showed a positive association between green tea intake and attenuation of liver disease. When considering the protective effects of green tea against subgroups of liver diseases, it seems that they are more effective in fatty liver disease and liver disorders (Jin et al 2008); The protective effect of green tea drinking to reduce liver cancer risk appears to be stronger for high-risk patients with hepatitis B or C and also for long-term green tea drinkers. Despite these promising results, more rigorous double-blind studies are still required to confirm the results as the studies used in the review were heterogeneous and differed in the design, outcome, tea dosage and other aspects.

OTHER USES

Green tea has many other uses, based on results of animal or in vitro tests or on the known pharmacological activity of constituents such as tannin and caffeine. Some of these other uses are treatment of diarrhoea, Crohn's disease, dyspepsia and other digestive symptoms, promoting alertness and cognitive performance, reducing symptoms of headache and promoting diuresis.

Allergic rhinitis

A novel study suggests drinking tea may provide benefits for seasonal allergic rhinitis. The trial was an open-label, single-dose, randomised study of 38 subjects in Japan. Half the participants drank the benifuuki green tea (34 mg *O*-methylated catechin) daily for 1.5 months before the cedar pollen season while the other group commenced at the start of the pollen season. The symptoms of throat pain, nose blowing and disturbance in daily life were significantly lower in the group taking the tea for the longer period pre-pollen season. This same group of researchers had previously reported that benifuuki green tea containing *O*-methylated catechin had reduced perennial or seasonal rhinitis whereas the placebo green tea did not. It may be the *O*-methylated catechins are required for this effect and more studies are warranted (Maeda-Yamamoto et al 2009).

Ulcerative colitis

Animal studies have shown anti-inflammatory activity in colitis (Varilek et al 2001, Westphal et al 2008). A double-blinded pilot study of 20 patients with mild to moderate ulcerative colitis achieved a 53% remission rate compared with 0% for placebo after daily doses of Polyphenon E (400 mg or 800 mg of EGCG daily) for 56 days. The remission results were based on the ulcerative colitis disease activity index and the inflammatory bowel disease questionnaire and 10 of the 15 patients in the Polyphenon E group responded to treatment. The authors suggest Polyphenon E may offer a novel therapy for mild to moderate ulcerative colitis (Dryden et al 2013).

Dementia/cognitive impairment

Several in vivo studies have demonstrated memory improvement in older animals for green tea extract and improvements in spatial cognition learning ability after long-term administration of GTCs (Haque et al 2006, Kaur et al 2008). In healthy adults a small RCT with 27 participants found a significant improvement in cerebral blood flow with the lower dose of 135 mg of EGCG (and not with the higher dose of 270 mg). These doses were given on two separate days and no significant improvement was found with mood or cognitive performance (Wightman et al 2012). A community-based self-administered questionnaire of 1003 Japanese geriatric people found that greater ingestion of green tea was associated with lower cognitive impairment (Kuriyama et al 2006a). Green tea intake was significantly associated with better cognitive performance in a 2-year follow-up study of Japanese elderly (Hasegawa et al 2005).

Depression

Novel research in Japan with 537 men and women in a cross-sectional study, using a validated dietary questionnaire, found a 51% lower prevalence of depression in those drinking four or more cups of green tea a day compared to one cup (Pham et al 2013).

Beta-thalassaemia

In vitro research shows green tea (tannins) chelates iron, which could prove useful in patients with conditions such as beta-thalassaemia (Srichairatanakool et al 2006). Beta-thalassaemic mice (with iron overload due to transfusions) were fed green tea extract and a reduction in liver iron content resulted. This may prove to be a novel therapy to chelate liver iron overload in beta-thalassaemia patients (Saewong et al 2010).

Amyloid light-chain amyloidosis

This rare disease, causing amyloid deposits in different organs, can affect the heart. Green tea's cardiac benefits may be useful in this condition when there is cardiac involvement. In a small longitudinal observational study of 59 patients with amyloid light-chain amyloidosis with cardiac involvement it was found that green tea polyphenol EGCG produced a significant reduction in left ventricular wall thickness. A reduction of 2 mm of wall thickness occurred in 11 patients; heart functionality was also improved, as was left ventricular ejection fraction. The patients either drank 1.5–2 L of green tea daily or consumed green tea extracts of 600–800 mg EGCG over a 6-month time period (Mereles et al 2010). This novel study requires more research to confirm findings.

Renal failure

Green tea extract blocks the development of cardiac hypertrophy in experimental renal failure and reduces oxidative stress, according to the results of investigation with animal models (Priyadarshi et al 2003, Yokozawa et al 1996).

Urinary stones

Two in vivo and in vitro studies have shown that green tea's antioxidant action may inhibit kidney stone formation (Itoh et al 2005, Jeong et al 2006).

Osteoporosis

There are several in vitro and animal studies as well as emerging human epidemiological research showing promise for green tea in improving bone health. Its mechanism of action is thought to be enhancing osteoblast activity, reducing osteoclasts plus osteoprotection through anti-inflammatory and antioxidant action, leading to a reduction in bone loss (Shen et al 2009, 2011, Tokuda et al 2008). Clinical studies are needed to confirm these findings and to assess if green tea results in fracture reduction. In a study, 150 postmenopausal women with osteopenia were randomised to have green tea supplement (500 mg daily) and/or tai chi exercise over 6 months. Muscle strength and bone formation biomarkers were improved by both green tea and tai chi exercise (Shen et al 2012).

DOSAGE RANGE

The dose varies depending on the indication it is being used for. Some research suggests 8–10 cups of green tea/day are required for effects whereas others indicate only 3–5 cups of green tea/day are required. It is likely that the dose also depends on the quality of the green tea and the concentration of GTCs in the preparation When used as a green tea extract in capsule form in high doses for long periods, green tea may have the potential to have adverse effects (Schonthal 2011).

- For external genital and perianal warts: Polyphenon E 10–15% strength ointment applied three times daily.
- For reduced risk of cancers: five or more cups daily.
- For CVD protection: 3–10 cups daily.
- For treatment for periodontal disease: use of gel, chewable tablets or mouthwash twice daily for 2–4 weeks.

ADVERSE REACTIONS

Due to the caffeine content of the herb, CNS stimulation and diuresis are possible when consumed in large amounts. Teeth staining is also possible due to the tannin content of the herb.

One clinical study found an absence of any severe adverse effects when 15 green tea tablets were taken daily (2.25 g green tea extracts, 337.5 mg EGCG and 135 mg caffeine) for 6 months (Fujiki et al 1999). One trial with high-dose green tea (600 mg/day) reported adverse effects in 69% of the patients with a range of adverse effects, including insomnia, fatigue, nausea, vomiting, diarrhoea, abdominal pain and confusion (Jatoi et al 2003).

There are rare, idiosyncratic reports of altered liver function with the consumption of green tea. A review of green tea and hepatic reactions found 34 cases of hepatitis with a positive rechallenge in 29 cases. There was one reported death (where there were other confounding factors, such as drugs and alcohol) and a positive rechallenge in seven cases. The authors suggest a causal association between green tea and liver damage which could be related to particular conditions and concomitant medications may be part of the picture (Mazzanti et al 2009). Frequently the green tea products were not fully analysed and others contained a herbal combination, making it difficult to definitively establish a causal relationship between green tea extracts and hepatotoxicity (Schonthal 2011). The US pharmacopeia similarly reports 27 cases where green tea is a possible causality and seven cases as a probable causality of liver damage. They reported that liver issues may be worse if the extract is taken under fasting conditions or on an empty stomach. This committee concluded that, when dietary supplements are formulated and manufactured appropriately, there are no significant safety issues with green tea but there should be caution with use (Sarma et al 2008). Another case report of acute hepatitis occurred in 2009 after consuming a green tea supplement; other causes were excluded and there was a rapid recovery after cessation of the supplement. However other studies have demonstrated no hepatotoxic effects, such as the placebo-controlled parallel study with healthy men taking six capsules of green tea extract daily (714 mg/day green tea polyphenols) for 3 weeks, where no significant changes in biomarkers of liver function or cardiovascular risk markers were found (Frank et al 2009). This was only a small study of 17 and so had no statistical power. Other studies have shown green tea to be effective in reducing liver disease (Jin et al 2008) and liver cancer (Ui et al 2009) and one trial using 1.3 g daily of GTCs reported no abnormalities in liver function tests when used for the duration of around 34 days (McLarty et al 2009).

There is one case report of thrombotic thrombocytopenic purpura after a 38-year-old woman consumed a weight loss product containing green tea extract (200 mg) for 2 months. After being hospitalised for 20 days and treated, her neurological symptoms reduced and platelet count and haematocrit levels normalised. The green tea preparation has been classed as a 'possible' cause of this condition developing in this woman and, as there are no other reported cases, it has been suggested that this could be an idiosyncratic drug reaction. The authors suggest that doctors be aware of this rare condition developing after ingesting green tea (Liatsos et al 2010).

When used over a 16-week period for genital warts, erythema and localised skin itching may occur (Tzellos et al 2011).

SIGNIFICANT INTERACTIONS

Few controlled studies are available for green tea, so interactions are speculative and based on evidence of pharmacological activity or known actions of key constituents such as caffeine and tannins.

Anticoagulants

Antagonistic interaction — a case of excessive consumption (2.25–4.5 L of green tea/day) was reported to inhibit warfarin activity and decrease the international normalised ratio (Taylor & Wilt 1999). Whether this is an exceptional case or representative of an expected interaction remains to be determined.

Hypoglycaemic agents

Caffeine-containing beverages can increase blood sugar levels when used in sufficient quantity (200 mg of caffeine); however, hypoglycaemic activity has been reported for green tea, which could theoretically negate this effect (Ulbricht & Basch 2005) — the outcome of this combination is uncertain, therefore observe the patient.

Iron

Tannins found in herbs such as *Camellia sinensis* can bind to iron and reduce its absorption — separate doses by at least 2 hours. Protein and iron have also been found to interact with tea polyphenols and decrease their antioxidant effects in vitro (Alexandropoulou et al 2006). The clinical significance of this is as yet unknown.

CNS stimulants

Based on the caffeine content of the herb, high intakes of green tea can theoretically increase the CNS stimulation effects of drugs such as nicotine and beta-adrenergic agonists (e.g. salbutamol); however, the clinical significance of this is unknown — observe patient.

CNS depressants

Based on the caffeine content of the herb, high intakes of green tea can theoretically decrease the CNS-depressant effects of drugs such as benzodiazepines; however, the clinical significance of this is unknown — observe patient.

Antidepressants

Based on theoretical considerations, caution is advised when using highly concentrated supplements with monoamine oxidase inhibitors or dopamimetic drugs because catechins are metabolised by catechol-*O*-methyltransferase (Shord et al 2009).

Bortezomib (BZM) and other boronic acid-based proteasome inhibitors

EGCG was tested in vitro and in vivo to investigate whether combining it with the proteasome inhibitor BZM, commonly used in the treatment of multiple myeloma, would result in an increase in the drug's antitumour activity (Golden et al 2009). Green tea extract almost completely blocked the effects of BZM both in vitro and in vivo — avoid.

Diuretics

Based on the caffeine content of the herb, high intakes of green tea can theoretically increase the diuretic effects of drugs such as frusemide; however, the clinical significance of this is unknown — observe patient.

Drugs metabolised by cytochrome P450 system

The inhibitory effect of caffeine on CYP1A2 may cause other interactions, but this is speculative for green tea. In vitro and animal research has shown that green tea inhibits CYP3A4 metabolism and a probable inhibition of intestinal CYP3A4, but clinical relevance is unknown (Engdal & Nilsen 2009, Fukuda et al 2009). A small trial with 42 volunteers giving 800 mg of green tea a day suggested that drugs metabolised by the CYP enzymes were unlikely to be significantly affected (Chow et al 2006).

CONTRAINDICATIONS AND PRECAUTIONS

Excessive intake will increase the likelihood of adverse effects due to the caffeine content and therefore is not recommended for people with hypertension, cardiac arrhythmias, severe liver disease, anxiety or psychiatric disorders or insomnia. It is considered safe when consumed as a tea in moderate amounts but should not be consumed to excess and is generally better on a full rather than empty stomach. However, if taken too close to meals, the tannin content of green tea will inhibit iron absorption.

PREGNANCY USE

Usual dietary intakes appear safe; however, excessive use is not recommended due to the caffeine content of green tea. It may also be prudent to avoid or drink small quantities of green tea in pregnancy due to its potential to chelate iron and a recent study linking high green tea intake with lower levels of folate in pregnant women (Shiraishi et al 2010).

PATIENTS' FAQs

What will this herb do for me?

Green tea has strong antioxidant effects and some population studies suggest that regular consumption may reduce the risk of cancer and CVD. Early research has found it may be useful for sunburn protection, reducing dental plaque formation, colitis,

Practice points/Patient counselling

- Green tea is made from the same plant as black tea, but it contains greater amounts of polyphenols and generally less caffeine.
- Green tea has been found to have significant antioxidant activity and protects against sunburn when applied topically.
- It has antibacterial activity and is used in oral preparations to reduce plaque and improve gingival health.
- Several in vitro and animal studies have shown anticarcinogenic activity for a range of cancers and some epidemiological evidence further suggests cancer-protective effects may occur, especially for reducing the risk of breast, prostate, endometrial, ovarian, colerectal and pancreatic cancers and leukaemia; however, further research is required. Patients with a high risk of prostate or liver cancer (due to hepatitis B) may benefit from regular green tea drinking.
- Epidemiological evidence suggests green tea may reduce CVD, especially stroke risk. Some clinical trials have demonstrated a reduction in LDL-cholesterol and antihypertensive effect.
- Preliminary evidence from animal studies has shown that it increases thermogenesis, decreases appetite, reduces inflammation in colitis, reduces glucose levels in diabetes, may be useful in renal failure and has the potential to improve cognitive function in the elderly and be used in Alzheimer's and Parkinson's diseases. Early clinical trials have shown specific green teas (benifuuki tea) may be preventive for allergic rhinitis and green tea drinking may reduce depression.
- Some clinical studies show inconsistent, but possibly modest, benefits in diabetes treatment.
- It is not known whether the use will promote weight loss in humans as research results are inconsistent; however, it may assist with modest weight reduction, especially when combined with exercise.
- A proprietary ointment made from a fixed concentration of GTCs is effective in the treatment of genital warts.

diabetes, flu prevention, renal disease, improving memory and cognition and as an antiseptic. However, further research is required.

When will it start to work?

This will depend on the reason it is being used. Preventive health benefits are likely to take several years of regular daily tea consumption. Effects on oral health care appear to develop more quickly, within 2 weeks.

Are there any safety issues?

Research suggests that green tea is a safe substance when used in usual dietary doses, but excessive consumption may produce side effects, chiefly because of the caffeine content.

REFERENCES

Adachi N et al. (–)-Epigallocatechin gallate attenuates acute stress responses through GABAergic system in the brain. Eur J Pharmacol 531.1–3 (2006): 171–175.

Afaq F et al. Inhibition of ultraviolet B-mediated activation of nuclear factor kappaB in normal human epidermal keratinocytes by green tea constituent (–)-epigallocatechin-3-gallate. Oncogene 22.7 (2003): 1035–1044.

Agarwal, A., et al. 2010. Effect of green tea extract (catechins) in reducing oxidative stress seen in patients of pulmonary tuberculosis on DOTS Cat I regimen. Phytomedicine, 17, 23–7.

Ahmed, S. 2010. Green tea polyphenol epigallocatechin 3-gallate in arthritis: progress and promise. Arthritis Res Ther, 12, 208.

Ahn WS et al. Protective effects of green tea extracts (polyphenon E and EGCG) on human cervical lesions. Eur J Cancer Prev 12.5 (2003): 383–390.

Alexandropoulou I, et al. Effects of iron, ascorbate, meat and casein on the antioxidant capacity of green tea under conditions of in vitro digestion. Food Chem 94 (2006): 359–365.

Alexopoulos, N., et al. 2008. The acute effect of green tea consumption on endothelial function in healthy individuals. Eur J Cardiovasc Prev Rehabil, 15, 300–5.

Andrade, J. P. & Assuncao, M. 2012. Protective effects of chronic green tea consumption on age-related neurodegeneration. Curr Pharm Des, 18, 4–14.

Antonello M et al. Prevention of hypertension, cardiovascular damage and endothelial dysfunction with green tea extracts. Am J Hypertens 20.12 (2007): 1321–1328.

Arab, L., et al. 2009. Green and black tea consumption and risk of stroke: a meta-analysis. Stroke, 40, 1786–92.

Araghizadeh, A., et al. 2013. Inhibitory Activity of Green Tea (*Camellia sinensis*) Extract on Some Clinically Isolated Cariogenic and Periodontopathic Bacteria. Med Princ Pract 22: 368–372.

Arts, I. C. 2008. A review of the epidemiological evidence on tea, flavonoids, and lung cancer. J Nutr, 138, 1561S-1566S.

Assuncao, M., et al. 2010. Green tea averts age-dependent decline of hippocampal signaling systems related to antioxidant defenses and survival. Free Radic Biol Med, 48, 831–8.

Assuncao, M., et al. 2011. Chronic green tea consumption prevents age-related changes in rat hippocampal formation. Neurobiol Aging, 32, 707–17.

Astill C et al. Factors affecting the caffeine and polyphenol contents of black and green tea infusions. J Agric Food Chem 49.11 (2001): 5340–5347.

Auvichayapat P et al. Effectiveness of green tea on weight reduction in obese Thais: a randomized, controlled trial. Physiol Behav 93.3 (2008): 486–491.

Avramovich-Tirosh Y et al. Neurorescue activity, APP regulation and amyloid-beta peptide reduction by novel multi-functional brain permeable iron-chelating antioxidants, M-30 and green tea polyphenol, EGCG. Curr Alzheimer Res 4.4 (2007): 403–411.

Awadalla, H. I., et al. 2011. A pilot study of the role of green tea use on oral health. Int J Dent Hyg, 9, 110–6.

Babu PV, Liu D. Green tea catechins and cardiovascular health: an update. Curr Med Chem 15.18 (2008): 1840–1850.

Bandyopadhyay D et al. In vitro and in vivo antimicrobial action of tea: the commonest beverage of Asia. Biol Pharm Bull 28.11 (2005): 2125–2127.

Basu, A., et al. 2010. Green tea supplementation affects body weight, lipids, and lipid peroxidation in obese subjects with metabolic syndrome. J Am Coll Nutr, 29, 31–40.

Bertipaglia de Santana M et al. Association between soy and green tea (*Camellia sinensis*) diminishes hypercholesterolemia and increases total plasma antioxidant potential in dyslipidemic subjects. Nutrition 24.6 (2008): 562–568.

Bettuzzi S et al. Chemoprevention of human prostate cancer by oral administration of green tea catechins in volunteers with high-grade prostate intraepithelial neoplasia: a preliminary report from a one-year proof-of-principle study. Cancer Res 66.2 (2006): 1234–1240.

Bettuzzi S et al. Inhibition of human prostate cancer progression by administration of green tea catechins: a two years later follow-up update. Eur Urol Supplements 7.3 (2008): 279.

Bhardwaj, P. & Khanna, D. 2013. Green tea catechins: defensive role in cardiovascular disorders. Chin J Nat Med, 11, 345–53.

Biasibetti, R., et al. 2013. Green tea (–)epigallocatechin-3-gallate reverses oxidative stress and reduces acetylcholinesterase activity in a streptozotocin-induced model of dementia. Behav Brain Res, 236, 186–93.

Boehm, K., et al. 2009. Green tea (*Camellia sinensis*) for the prevention of cancer. Cochrane Database Syst Rev, CD005004.

Bogdanski, P., et al. 2012. Green tea extract reduces blood pressure, inflammatory biomarkers, and oxidative stress and improves parameters associated with insulin resistance in obese, hypertensive patients. Nutr Res, 32, 421–7.

Brown, A. L., et al. 2009. Effects of dietary supplementation with the green tea polyphenol epigallocatechin-3-gallate on insulin resistance and associated metabolic risk factors: randomized controlled trial. Br J Nutr, 101, 886–94.

Butler, L. M. & Wu, A. H. 2011. Green and black tea in relation to gynecologic cancers. Mol Nutr Food Res, 55, 931–40.

Cardoso, G. A., et al. 2013. The effects of green tea consumption and resistance training on body composition and resting metabolic rate in overweight or obese women. J Med Food, 16, 120–7.

Chandra, A. K. & De, N. 2013. Catechin induced modulation in the activities of thyroid hormone synthesizing enzymes leading to hypothyroidism. Mol Cell Biochem, 374, 37–48.

Chang CW, et al. Inhibitory effects of polyphenolic catechins from Chinese green tea on HIV reverse transcriptase activity. J Biomed Sci 1.3 (1994): 163–166.

Chang LK et al. Inhibition of Epstein–Barr virus lytic cycle by (–)-epigallocatechin gallate. Biochem Biophys Res Commun 301.4 (2003): 1062–1068.

Chantre P, Lairon D. Recent findings of green tea extract AR25 (Exolise) and its activity for the treatment of obesity. Phytomedicine 9.1 (2002): 3–8.

Chava, V. K. & Vedula, B. D. 2013. Thermo reversible green tea catechin gel for local application in chronic periodontitis- a 4 week clinical trial. J Periodontol 84: 1290.

Chen, H., et al. 2013. Epigallocatechin gallate and sulforaphane combination treatment induce apoptosis in paclitaxel-resistant ovarian cancer cells through hTERT and Bcl-2 down-regulation. Exp Cell Res, 319, 697–706.

Cheng TO. Why is green tea more cardioprotective in women than in men? Int J Cardiol 122.3 (2007): 244.

Choan E et al. A prospective clinical trial of green tea for hormone refractory prostate cancer: An evaluation of the complementary/alternative therapy approach. Urol Oncol 23.2 (2005): 108–113.

Chou CC, et al. Antimicrobial activity of tea as affected by the degree of fermentation and manufacturing season. Int J Food Microbiol 48.2 (1999): 125–130.

Chow HH et al. Effects of repeated green tea catechin administration on human cytochrome P450 activity. Cancer Epidemiol Biomarkers Prev 15.12 (2006): 2473–2476.

Clement, Y. 2009. Can green tea do that? A literature review of the clinical evidence. Prev Med, 49, 83–7.

Dai, Q., et al. 2010. Is green tea drinking associated with a later onset of breast cancer? Ann Epidemiol, 20, 74–81.

De Koning Gans, J. M., et al. 2010. Tea and coffee consumption and cardiovascular morbidity and mortality. Arterioscler Thromb Vasc Biol, 30, 1665–71.

De Oliveira, A., et al. 2013. Inhibition of herpes simplex virus type 1 with the modified green tea polyphenol palmitoyl-epigallocatechin gallate. Food Chem Toxicol, 52, 207–15.

Di Castelnuovo, A., et al. 2012. Consumption of cocoa, tea and coffee and risk of cardiovascular disease. Eur J Intern Med, 23, 15–25.

Diepvens K et al. Effect of green tea on resting energy expenditure and substrate oxidation during weight loss in overweight females. Br J Nutr 94.6 (2005): 1026–1034.

Di Pierro, F., et al. 2009. Greenselect Phytosome as an adjunct to a low-calorie diet for treatment of obesity: a clinical trial. Altern Med Rev, 14, 154–60.

Dragicevic, N., et al. 2011. Green Tea Epigallocatechin-3-Gallate (EGCG) and Other Flavonoids Reduce Alzheimer's Amyloid-Induced Mitochondrial Dysfunction. Journal of Alzheimer's Disease, 26, 507–521.

Dryden, G. W., et al. 2013. A pilot study to evaluate the safety and efficacy of an oral dose of (–)-epigallocatechin-3-gallate-rich polyphenon e in patients with mild to moderate ulcerative colitis. Inflamm Bowel Dis, 19, 1904–12.

Dulloo AG et al. Green tea and thermogenesis: interactions between catechin-polyphenols, caffeine and sympathetic activity. Int J Obes Relat Metab Disord 24.2 (2000): 252–258.

Ellinger, S., et al. 2011. Consumption of green tea or green tea products: is there an evidence for antioxidant effects from controlled interventional studies? Phytomedicine, 18, 903–15.

Elmets CA et al. Cutaneous photoprotection from ultraviolet injury by green tea polyphenols. J Am Acad Dermatol 44.3 (2001): 425–432.

Engdal, S. & Nilsen, O. G. 2009. In vitro inhibition of CYP3A4 by herbal remedies frequently used by cancer patients. Phytother Res, 23, 906–12.

Erba D et al. Effectiveness of moderate green tea consumption on antioxidative status and plasma lipid profile in humans. J Nutr Biochem 16.3 (2005): 144–149.

Fassina G et al. Polyphenolic antioxidant (–)-epigallocatechin-3-gallate from green tea as a candidate anti-HIV agent. AIDS 16.6 (2002): 939–941.

Ferrazzano, G. F., et al. 2011. Antimicrobial properties of green tea extract against cariogenic microflora: an in vivo study. J Med Food, 14, 907–11.

Fon Sing, M., et al. 2011. Epidemiological studies of the association between tea drinking and primary liver cancer: a meta-analysis. Eur J Cancer Prev, 20, 157–65.

Frank, J., et al. 2009. Daily consumption of an aqueous green tea extract supplement does not impair liver function or alter cardiovascular disease risk biomarkers in healthy men. J Nutr, 139, 58–62.

Fritz, H., et al. 2013. Green tea and lung cancer: a systematic review. Integr Cancer Ther, 12, 7–24.

Fuhrman, B. J., et al. 2013. Green tea intake is associated with urinary estrogen profiles in Japanese-American women. Nutr J 12: 25.

Fujiki H et al. Mechanistic findings of green tea as cancer preventive for humans. Proc Soc Exp Biol Med 220.4 (1999): 225–228.

Fukino Y et al. Randomized controlled trial for an effect of green tea consumption on insulin resistance and inflammation markers. J Nutr Sci Vitaminol (Tokyo) 51.5 (2005): 335–42.

Fukino, Y., et al. 2008. Randomized controlled trial for an effect of green tea-extract powder supplementation on glucose abnormalities. Eur J Clin Nutr, 62, 953–60.

Fukuda, I., et al. 2009. Suppression of cytochrome P450 1A1 expression induced by 2,3,7,8-tetrachlorodibenzo-p-dioxin in mouse hepatoma hepa-1c1c7 cells treated with serum of (–)-epigallocatechin-3-gallate- and green tea extract-administered rats. Biosci Biotechnol Biochem, 73, 1206–8.

Gao J et al. [Green tea consumption and the risk of endometrial cancer: a population-based case-control study in urban Shanghai]. Zhonghua Liu Xing Bing Xue Za Zhi 26.5 (2005): 323–327.

Gao, M., et al. 2013. Meta-analysis of Green Tea Drinking and the Prevalence of Gynecological Tumors in Women. Asia Pac J Public Health.

Garcia F et al. Apoptosis induction by green tea compounds in cervical cancer cells. Eur J Cancer Supplements 4.1 (2006): 58.

Gillespie, K., et al. 2008. Effects of oral consumption of the green tea polyphenol EGCG in a murine model for human Sjogren's syndrome, an autoimmune disease. Life Sci, 83, 581–8.

Golden EB et al. Green tea polyphenols block the anticancer effects of bortezomib and other boronic acid-based proteasome inhibitors. Blood 113.23 (2009): 5927–37.

Gordon, N. C. & Wareham, D. W. 2010. Antimicrobial activity of the green tea polyphenol (–)-epigallocatechin-3-gallate (EGCG) against clinical isolates of *Stenotrophomonas maltophilia*. Int J Antimicrob Agents, 36, 129–31.

Graham HN. Green tea composition, consumption, and polyphenol chemistry. Prev Med 21.3 (1992): 334–350.

Gross G. [Polyphenon E. A new topical therapy for condylomata acuminata.] Hautarzt 59.1 (2008): 31–35.

Guo Q et al. Studies on protective mechanisms of four components of green tea polyphenols against lipid peroxidation in synaptosomes. Biochim Biophys Acta 1304.3 (1996): 210–222.

Guo S et al. Protective effects of green tea polyphenols in the 6-OHDA rat model of Parkinson's disease through inhibition of ROS-NO pathway. Biol Psychiatry 62.12 (2007): 1353–1362.

Gupta S, et al. Molecular pathway for (–)-epigallocatechin-3-gallate-induced cell cycle arrest and apoptosis of human prostate carcinoma cells. Arch Biochem Biophys 410.1 (2003): 177–185.

Han, D. H., et al. 2009. Anti-proliferative and apoptosis induction activity of green tea polyphenols on human promyelocytic leukemia HL-60 cells. Anticancer Res, 29, 1417–21.

Han, K. C., et al. 2011. Genoprotective effects of green tea (*Camellia sinensis*) in human subjects: results of a controlled supplementation trial. Br J Nutr, 105, 171–9.

Haque AM et al. Long-term administration of green tea catechins improves spatial cognition learning ability in rats. J Nutr 136.4 (2006): 1043–1047.

Hartley, L., et al. 2013. Green and black tea for the primary prevention of cardiovascular disease. Cochrane Database Syst Rev, 6, CD009934.

Hasegawa T et al. Protective effect of Japanese green tea against cognitive impairment in the elderly, a two-years follow-up observation. Alzheimers Dement 1.1 (Suppl 1) (2005): S100.

Henning, S. M., et al. 2011. Chemopreventive effects of tea in prostate cancer: green tea versus black tea. Mol Nutr Food Res, 55, 905–20.

Herges, K., et al. 2011. Neuroprotective effect of combination therapy of glatiramer acetate and epigallocatechin-3-gallate in neuroinflammation. PLoS One, 6, e25456.

Hirasawa M et al. Improvement of periodontal status by green tea catechin using a local delivery system: a clinical pilot study. J Periodontal Res 37.6 (2002): 433–8.

Ho C -T et al. Tea & tea products: chemistry & health promoting properties. CRC Press, Boka Raton, (2009).

Honicke, A. S., et al. 2012. Combined administration of EGCG and IL-1 receptor antagonist efficiently downregulates IL-1-induced tumorigenic factors in U-2 OS human osteosarcoma cells. Int J Oncol, 41, 753–8.

Hooper L et al. Flavonoids, fl avonoid-rich foods, and cardiovascular risk: a meta-analysis of randomized controlled trials. Am J Clin Nutr 88.1 (2008): 38–50.
Hou R-R et al. Neuroprotective effects of (-)-epigallocatechin-3-gallate (EGCG) on paraquat-induced apoptosis in PC12 cells. Cell Biol Int 32.1 (2008): 22–30.
Hou, I. C., et al. 2013. Green tea and the risk of gastric cancer: Epidemiological evidence. World J Gastroenterol, 19, 3713–22.
Hsu S. Green tea and the skin. J Am Acad Dermatol 52.6 (2005): 1049–59.
Hsu C -H et al. Effect of green tea extract on obese women: a randomized, double-blind, placebo-controlled clinical trial. Clin Nutr 27.3 (2008) : 363–70.
Hsu, C. H., et al. 2011. Does supplementation with green tea extract improve insulin resistance in obese type 2 diabetics? A randomized, double-blind, and placebo-controlled clinical trial. Altern Med Rev, 16, 157–63.
Hursel, R., et al. 2009. The effects of green tea on weight loss and weight maintenance: a meta-analysis. Int J Obes (Lond), 33, 956–61.
Imai K, Nakachi K. Cross sectional study of effects of drinking green tea on cardiovascular and liver diseases. BMJ 310.6981 (1995): 693–6.
Imanishi N et al. Additional inhibitory effect of tea extract on the growth of infl uenza A and B viruses in MDCK cells. Microbiol Immunol 46.7 (2002): 491–4.
Inoue, M., et al. 2009a. Effect of coffee and green tea consumption on the risk of liver cancer: cohort analysis by hepatitis virus infection status. Cancer Epidemiol Biomarkers Prev, 18, 1746–53.
Inoue, M., et al. 2009b. Green tea consumption and gastric cancer in Japanese: a pooled analysis of six cohort studies. Gut, 58, 1323–32.
Isaacs C E et al. Epigallocatechin gallate inactivates clinical isolates of herpes simplex virus. Antimicrob Agents Chemother 52.3 (2008): 962–70.
Ishihara N et al. Improvement of intestinal microfl ora balance and prevention of digestive and respiratory organ diseases in calves by green tea extracts. Livest Prod Sci 68.2–3 (2001): 217–29.
Itoh Y et al. Preventive effects of green tea on renal stone formation and the role of oxidative stress in nephrolithiasis. J Urol 173.1 (2005): 271–5.
Itoh, T., et al. 2011. (–)-Epigallocatechin-3-gallate protects against neuronal cell death and improves cerebral function after traumatic brain injury in rats. Neuromolecular Med, 13, 300–9.
Janjua, R., et al. 2009. A two-year, double-blind, randomized placebo-controlled trial of oral green tea polyphenols on the long-term clinical and histologic appearance of photoaging skin. Dermatol Surg, 35, 1057–65.
Jatoi A et al. A phase II trial of green tea in the treatment of patients with androgen independent metastatic prostate carcinoma. Cancer 97.6 (2003): 1442–6.
Jenabian, N., et al. 2012. The effect of *Camellia sinensis* (green tea) mouthwash on plaque-induced gingivitis: a single-blinded randomized controlled clinical trial. Daru, 20, 39.
Jeong BC et al. Effects of green tea on urinary stone formation: an in vivo and in vitro study. J Endourol 20.5 (2006): 356–361.
Jeong H-S et al. Effects of (–)-epigallocatechin-3-gallate on the activity of substantia nigra dopaminergic neurons. Brain Res 1130 (2007): 114–1118.
Jian L et al. Protective effect of green tea against prostate cancer: a case-control study in southeast China. Int J Cancer 108.1 (2004): 130–135.
Jin X, et al. Green tea consumption and liver disease: a systematic review. Liver Int 28.7 (2008): 990–996.
Johnson, R., et al. 2012. Green tea and green tea catechin extracts: an overview of the clinical evidence. Maturitas, 73, 280–7.
Jurgens, T. M., et al. 2012. Green tea for weight loss and weight maintenance in overweight or obese adults. Cochrane Database Syst Rev, 12, CD008650.
Kang, H., et al. 2010. Green tea consumption and stomach cancer risk: a meta-analysis. Epidemiol Health, 32, e2010001.
Kang, M. Y., et al. 2012. Preventive effects of green tea (*Camellia sinensis* var. assamica) on diabetic nephropathy. Yonsei Med J, 53, 138–44.
Katiyar, S. K. 2011. Green tea prevents non-melanoma skin cancer by enhancing DNA repair. Arch Biochem Biophys, 508, 152–8.
Kaur T et al. Effects of green tea extract on learning, memory, behavior and acetylcholinesterase activity in young and old male rats. Brain Cogn 67.1 (2008): 25–30.
Kavanagh KT et al. Green tea extracts decrease carcinogen-induced mammary tumor burden in rats and rate of breast cancer cell proliferation in culture. J Cell Biochem 82.3 (2001): 387–398.
Kazi A et al. Potential molecular targets of tea polyphenols in human tumor cells: significance in cancer prevention. In Vivo 16.6 (2002): 397–403.
Khan, N. & Mukhtar, H. 2010. Cancer and metastasis: prevention and treatment by green tea. Cancer Metastasis Rev, 29, 435–45.
Khan, N., et al. 2009a. Review: green tea polyphenols in chemoprevention of prostate cancer: preclinical and clinical studies. Nutr Cancer, 61, 836–41.
Khan, S. A., et al. 2009b. Studies on the protective effect of green tea against cisplatin induced nephrotoxicity. Pharmacological Research, 60, 382–391.
Kim, A., et al. 2011. Green tea catechins decrease total and low-density lipoprotein cholesterol: a systematic review and meta-analysis. J Am Diet Assoc, 111, 1720–9.
Kinjo J et al. Activity-guided fractionation of green tea extract with antiproliferative activity against human stomach cancer cells. Biol Pharm Bull 25.9 (2002): 1238–1240.
Kokubo, Y., et al. 2013. The impact of green tea and coffee consumption on the reduced risk of stroke incidence in Japanese population: the Japan Public Health Center-Based Study Cohort. Stroke 44: 1369–1374.
Krahwinkel T, Willershausen B. The effect of sugar-free green tea chew candies on the degree of inflammation of the gingiva. Eur J Med Res 5.11 (2000): 463–467.
Kumamoto M et al. Effects of pH and metal ions on antioxidative activities of catechins. Biosci Biotechnol Biochem 65.1 (2001): 126–132.
Kuo YC et al. A population-based, case-control study of green tea consumption and leukemia risk in southwestern Taiwan. Cancer Causes Control 20.1 (2009): 57–765.
Kurahashi N et al. Green tea consumption and prostate cancer risk in Japanese men: a prospective study. Am J Epidemiol 167.1 (2008): 71–77.
Kuriyama, S. 2008. The relation between green tea consumption and cardiovascular disease as evidenced by epidemiological studies. J Nutr, 138, 1548S-1553S.
Kuriyama S et al. Green tea consumption and cognitive function: a cross-sectional study from the Tsurugaya Project 1. Am J Clin Nutr 83.2 (2006a): 355–361.
Kuriyama S et al. Green tea consumption and mortality due to cardiovascular disease, cancer, and all causes in Japan: the Ohsaki study. JAMA 296.10 (2006b): 1255–1265.
Kushiyama, M., et al. 2009. Relationship between intake of green tea and periodontal disease. J Periodontol, 80, 372–7.
Lee, A. H. & Pasalich, M. 2013. Chapter 64 — Protective Aspects of Tea and Prostate Cancer: Emerging Evidence. Tea in Health and Disease Prevention. Amsterdam: Academic Press.
Lee, J. H., et al. 2009. In vitro anti-adhesive activity of green tea extract against pathogen adhesion. Phytother Res, 23, 460–6.
Leenen R et al. A single dose of tea with or without milk increases plasma antioxidant activity in humans. Eur J Clin Nutr 54.1 (2000): 87–92.
Li Q et al. Oral administration of green tea epigallocatechin-3-gallate (EGCG) reduces amyloid beta deposition in transgenic mouse model of Alzheimer's disease. Exp Neurol 198.2 (2006): 576.
Li, Y., et al. 2011. Green tea consumption, inflammation and the risk of primary hepatocellular carcinoma in a Chinese population. Cancer Epidemiol, 35, 362–8.
Liatsos, G. D., et al. 2010. Possible green tea-induced thrombotic thrombocytopenic purpura. Am J Health Syst Pharm, 67, 531–4.
Lin YS et al. Factors affecting the levels of tea polyphenols and caffeine in tea leaves. J Agric Food Chem 51.7 (2003): 1864–1873.
Liu T, Chi Y. Experimental study on polyphenol anti-plaque effect in humans. Zhonghua Kou Qiang Yi Xue Za Zhi 35.5 (2000): 383–384.
Liu S et al. Theaflavin derivatives in black tea and catechin derivatives in green tea inhibit HIV-1 entry by targeting gp41. Biochim Biophys Acta 1723.1–3 (2005): 270–281.
Liu, K., et al. 2013. Effect of green tea on glucose control and insulin sensitivity: a meta-analysis of 17 randomized controlled trials. Am J Clin Nutr 98: 340–348.
MacKenzie T, et al. The effect of an extract of green and black tea on glucose control in adults with type 2 diabetes mellitus: double-blind randomized study. Metabolism 56.10 (2007): 1340–13444.
Maeda K et al. Green tea catechins inhibit the cultured smooth muscle cell invasion through the basement barrier. Atherosclerosis 166.1 (2003): 23–30.
Maeda-Yamamoto, M., et al. 2009. The efficacy of early treatment of seasonal allergic rhinitis with benifuuki green tea containing O-methylated catechin before pollen exposure: an open randomized study. Allergol Int, 58, 437–44.
Maki, K. C., et al. 2009. Green tea catechin consumption enhances exercise-induced abdominal fat loss in overweight and obese adults. J Nutr, 139, 264–70.
Mandel S et al. Green tea catechins as brain-permeable, natural iron chelators-antioxidants for the treatment of neurodegenerative disorders. Mol Nutr Food Res 50.2 (2006): 229–234.
Mandel S et al. Iron dysregulation in Alzheimer's disease: multimodal brain permeable iron chelating drugs, possessing neuroprotective-neurorescue and amyloid precursor protein-processing regulatory activities as therapeutic agents. Prog Neurobiol 82.6 (2007): 348–360.

Mantena SK, et al. Epigallocatechin-3-gallate inhibits photocarcinogenesis through inhibition of angiogenic factors and activation of CD8 + T cells in tumors. Photochem Photobiol 81.5 (2005): 1174–1179.

Mao, X. Q., et al. 2011. Green tea drinking habits and gastric cancer in southwest China. Asian Pac J Cancer Prev, 12, 2179–82.

Masterjohn, C. & Bruno, R. S. 2012. Therapeutic potential of green tea in nonalcoholic fatty liver disease. Nutr Rev, 70, 41–56.

Matsubara S et al. Suppression of *Helicobacter pylori*-induced gastritis by green tea extract in Mongolian gerbils. Biochem Biophys Res Commun 310.3 (2003): 715–7119.

Matsumoto, K., et al. 2011. Effects of green tea catechins and theanine on preventing influenza infection among healthcare workers: a randomized controlled trial. BMC Complement Altern Med, 11, 15.

Mazzanti, G., et al. 2009. Hepatotoxicity from green tea: a review of the literature and two unpublished cases. Eur J Clin Pharmacol, 65, 331–41.

McLarty, J., et al. 2009. Tea polyphenols decrease serum levels of prostate-specific antigen, hepatocyte growth factor, and vascular endothelial growth factor in prostate cancer patients and inhibit production of hepatocyte growth factor and vascular endothelial growth factor in vitro. Cancer Prev Res (Phila), 2, 673–82.

Mereles, D., et al. 2010. Effects of the main green tea polyphenol epigallocatechin-3-gallate on cardiac involvement in patients with AL amyloidosis. Clin Res Cardiol, 99, 483–90.

Meydani, S. N. 2011. Green tea and autoimmune disorders: Impact on pathogenesis and the underlying mechanisms. Clinical Biochemistry, 44, S19-S20.

Mineharu, Y., et al. 2011. Coffee, green tea, black tea and oolong tea consumption and risk of mortality from cardiovascular disease in Japanese men and women. J Epidemiol Community Health, 65, 230–40.

Mukoyama A et al. Inhibition of rotavirus and enterovirus infections by tea extracts. Jpn J Med Sci Biol 44.4 (1991): 181–186.

Myung, S. K., et al. 2009. Green tea consumption and risk of s tomach cancer: a meta-analysis of epidemiologic studies. Int J Cancer, 124, 670–7.

Nagle, C. M., et al. 2010. Tea consumption and risk of ovarian cancer. Cancer Causes Control, 21, 1485–91.

Nakachi K et al. Preventive effects of drinking green tea on cancer and cardiovascular disease: epidemiological evidence for multiple targeting prevention. Biofactors 13.1–4 (2000): 49–54.

Nakachi K, et al. Can teatime increase one's lifetime? Ageing Res Rev 2.1 (2003): 1–110.

Nance, C. L., et al. 2009. Preclinical development of the green tea catechin, epigallocatechin gallate, as an HIV-1 therapy. J Allergy Clin Immunol, 123, 459–65.

Nantz, M. P., et al. 2009. Standardized capsule of *Camellia sinensis* lowers cardiovascular risk factors in a randomized, double-blind, placebo-controlled study. Nutrition, 25, 147–54.

Nath, S., et al. 2012. Catechins protect neurons against mitochondrial toxins and HIV proteins via activation of the BDNF pathway. J Neurovirol, 18, 445–55.

Neves, D., et al. 2008. Does regular consumption of green tea influence expression of vascular endothelial growth factor and its receptor in aged rat erectile tissue? Possible implications for vasculogenic erectile dysfunction progression. Age (Dordr), 30, 217–28.

Nguyen, M. M., et al. 2012. Randomized, double-blind, placebo-controlled trial of polyphenon E in prostate cancer patients before prostatectomy: evaluation of potential chemopreventive activities. Cancer Prev Res (Phila), 5, 290–8.

Ogunleye, A. A., et al. 2010. Green tea consumption and breast cancer risk or recurrence: a meta-analysis. Breast Cancer Res Treat, 119, 477–84.

Osterburg, A., et al. 2009. Highly antibiotic-resistant *Acinetobacter baumannii* clinical isolates are killed by the green tea polyphenol (–)-epigallocatechin-3-gallate (EGCG). Clin Microbiol Infect, 15, 341–6.

Ostrowska J et al. Green and black tea in brain protection. Oxidative Stress and Neurodegenerative Disorders. Amsterdam, Elsevier Science B.V. (2007), pp 581–605.

Otake S et al. Anticaries effects of polyphenolic compounds from Japanese green tea. Caries Res 25.6 (1991): 438–443.

Pae, M. & Wu, D. 2013. Immunomodulating effects of epigallocatechin-3-gallate from green tea: mechanisms and applications. Food Funct 4: 1287–1303.

Panagiotakos, D. B., et al. 2009. Long-term tea intake is associated with reduced prevalence of (type 2) diabetes mellitus among elderly people from Mediterranean islands: MEDIS epidemiological study. Yonsei Med J, 50, 31–8.

Park, M., et al. 2011. Green tea consumption is inversely associated with the incidence of influenza infection among schoolchildren in a tea plantation area of Japan. J Nutr, 141, 1862–70.

Persson IA et al. Tea flavanols inhibit angiotensin-converting enzyme activity and increase nitric oxide production in human endothelial cells. J Pharm Pharmacol 58.8 (2006): 1139–1144.

Pham, N. M., et al. 2013. Green tea and coffee consumption is inversely associated with depressive symptoms in a Japanese working population. Public Health Nutr, 1–9.

Phung, O. J., et al. 2010. Effect of green tea catechins with or without caffeine on anthropometric measures: a systematic review and meta-analysis. Am J Clin Nutr, 91, 73–81.

Polychronopoulos E et al. Effects of black and green tea consumption on blood glucose levels in non-obese elderly men and women from Mediterranean Islands (MEDIS epidemiological study). Eur J Nutr 47.1 (2008): 10–116.

Priyadarshi S et al. Effect of green tea extract on cardiac hypertrophy following 5/6 nephrectomy in the rat. Kidney Int 63.5 (2003): 1785–1790.

Qanungo S et al. Epigallocatechin-3-gallate induces mitochondrial membrane depolarization and caspase-dependent apoptosis in pancreatic cancer cells. Carcinogenesis 26.5 (2005): 958–967.

Qin J et al. A component of green tea, (–)-epigallocatechin-3-gallate, promotes apoptosis in T24 human bladder cancer cells via modulation of the PI3K/Akt pathway and Bcl-2 family proteins. Biochem Biophys Res Commun 354.4 (2007): 852–857.

Rasheed A, Haider M. Antibacterial activity of *Camellia sinensis* extracts against dental caries. Arch Pharm Res 21.3 (1998): 348–352.

Rezai-Zadeh K et al. Green tea epigallocatechin-3-gallate (EGCG) reduces [beta]-amyloid mediated cognitive impairment and modulates tau pathology in Alzheimer transgenic mice. Brain Res 1214 (2008): 177–187.

Reznichenko L et al. Reduction of iron-regulated amyloid precursor protein and beta-amyloid peptide by (–)-epigallocatechin-3-gallate in cell cultures: implications for iron chelation in Alzheimer's disease. J Neurochem 97.2 (2006): 527–536.

Rhee SJ, et al. Effects of green tea catechin on prostaglandin synthesis of renal glomerular and renal dysfunction in streptozotocin-induced diabetic rats. Asia Pac J Clin Nutr 11.3 (2002): 232–236.

Rietveld A, Wiseman S. Antioxidant effects of tea: evidence from human clinical trials. J Nutr 133.10 (2003): 3285–92S.

Sabu MC, et al. Anti-diabetic activity of green tea polyphenols and their role in reducing oxidative stress in experimental diabetes. J Ethnopharmacol 83.1–2 (2002): 109–116.

Sachinidis A, Hescheler J. Are catechins natural tyrosine kinase inhibitors? Drug News Perspect 15.7 (2002): 432–438.

Saewong, T., et al. 2010. Effects of green tea on iron accumulation and oxidative stress in livers of iron-challenged thalassemic mice. Med Chem, 6, 57–64.

Sakanaka S et al. Inhibitory effects of green tea polyphenols on growth and cellular adherence of an oral bacterium, *Porphyromonas gingivalis*. Biosci Biotechnol Biochem 60.5 (1996): 745–749.

Sannella AR et al. Antimalarial properties of green tea. Biochemical and Biochem Biophys Res Commun 353.1 (2007): 177–181.

Sarma, D. N., et al. 2008. Safety of Green Tea Extracts : A Systematic Review by the US Pharmacopeia. Drug Safety, 31, 469–484.

Sasazuki, S., et al. 2012. Green tea consumption and gastric cancer risk: an evaluation based on a systematic review of epidemiologic evidence among the Japanese population. Jpn J Clin Oncol, 42, 335–46.

Sayama K et al. Effects of green tea on growth, food utilization and lipid metabolism in mice. In Vivo 14.4 (2000): 481–484.

Schonthal, A. H. 2011. Adverse effects of concentrated green tea extracts. Mol Nutr Food Res, 55, 874–85.

Sen, T. & Chatterjee, A. 2011. Epigallocatechin-3-gallate (EGCG) downregulates EGF-induced MMP-9 in breast cancer cells: involvement of integrin receptor alpha5beta1 in the process. Eur J Nutr, 50, 465–78.

Shanafelt, T. D., et al. 2013. Phase 2 trial of daily, oral Polyphenon E in patients with asymptomatic, Rai stage 0 to II chronic lymphocytic leukemia. Cancer, 119, 363–70.

Shen, C. L., et al. 2009. Green tea and bone metabolism. Nutr Res, 29, 437–56.

Shen, C. L., et al. 2011. Green tea and bone health: Evidence from laboratory studies. Pharmacol Res, 64, 155–61.

Shen, C. L., et al. 2012. Effect of green tea and Tai Chi on bone health in postmenopausal osteopenic women: a 6-month randomized placebo-controlled trial. Osteoporos Int, 23, 1541–52.

Shimizu M et al. EGCG inhibits activation of the insulin-like growth factor-1 receptor in human colon cancer cells. Biochem Biophys Res Commun 334.3 (2005): 947–953.

Shimizu, M., et al. 2008. Green tea extracts for the prevention of metachronous colorectal adenomas: a pilot study. Cancer Epidemiol Biomarkers Prev, 17, 3020–5.

Shiraishi, M., et al. 2010. Association between the serum folate levels and tea consumption during pregnancy. Biosci Trends, 4, 225–30.

Shord, S. S., et al. 2009. Drug-botanical interactions: a review of the laboratory, animal, and human data for 8 common botanicals. Integr Cancer Ther, 8, 208–27.

Siddiqui, I. A., et al. 2009. Introducing nanochemoprevention as a novel approach for cancer control: proof of principle with green tea polyphenol epigallocatechin-3-gallate. Cancer Res, 69, 1712–6.

Siddiqui, I. A., et al. 2011. Green tea polyphenol EGCG blunts androgen receptor function in prostate cancer. FASEB J, 25, 1198–207.
Silva, K. C., et al. 2013. Green tea is neuroprotective in diabetic retinopathy. Invest Ophthalmol Vis Sci, 54, 1325–36.
Song J-M, et al. Antiviral effect of catechins in green tea on influenza virus. Antiviral Res 68.2 (2005): 66–74.
Song L et al. P345 Effects of green tea on lipids blood pressure and vasorelaxation in rats with hypercholesterolaemia-induced hypertension. Int J Cardiol 125 (Suppl 1) (2008): S64.
Srichairatanakool S et al. Iron-chelating and free-radical scavenging activities of microwave-processed green tea in iron overload. Hemoglobin 30.2 (2006): 311–327.
Srinivasan P et al. Chemopreventive and therapeutic modulation of green tea polyphenols on drug metabolizing enzymes in 4-Nitroquinoline 1-oxide induced oral cancer. Chem Biol Interact 172.3 (2008): 224–234.
Srividhya, R., et al. 2012. Impact of epigallo catechin-3-gallate on acetylcholine-acetylcholine esterase cycle in aged rat brain. Neurochem Int, 60, 517–22.
Stockfleth, E. & Meyer, T. 2012. The use of sinecatechins (polyphenon E) ointment for treatment of external genital warts. Expert Opin Biol Ther, 12, 783–93.
Stockfleth E et al. Topical Polyphenon E in the treatment of external genital and perianal warts: a randomized controlled trial. Br J Dermatol 158.6 (2008): 1329–1338.
Stoicov, C., et al. 2009. Green tea inhibits *Helicobacter* growth in vivo and in vitro. Int J Antimicrob Agents, 33, 473–8.
Suganuma, M., et al. 2011. New cancer treatment strategy using combination of green tea catechins and anticancer drugs. Cancer Sci, 102, 317–23.
Suliburska, J., et al. 2012. Effects of green tea supplementation on elements, total antioxidants, lipids, and glucose values in the serum of obese patients. Biol Trace Elem Res, 149, 315–22.
Sun CL et al. Green tea, black tea and breast cancer risk: a meta-analysis of epidemiological studies. Carcinogenesis 27.7 (2006): 1310–13115.
Sung H et al. In vivo antioxidant effect of green tea. Eur J Clin Nutr 54.7 (2000): 527–529.
Suzuki, E., et al. 2009. Green Tea Consumption and Mortality among Japanese Elderly People: The Prospective Shizuoka Elderly Cohort. Ann Epidemiol, 19, 732–739.
Tang, X. D., et al. 2008. [Effects of green tea extract on expression of human papillomavirus type 16 oncoproteins-induced hypoxia-inducible factor-1alpha and vascular endothelial growth factor in human cervical carcinoma cells.] Zhonghua Yi Xue Za Zhi, 88, 2872–7.
Tang, N., et al. 2009a. Green tea, black tea consumption and risk of lung cancer: a meta-analysis. Lung Cancer, 65, 274–83.
Tang, N. P., et al. 2009b. Tea consumption and risk of endometrial cancer: a metaanalysis. Am J Obstet Gynecol, 201, 605 e1–8.
Tao P. The inhibitory effects of catechin derivatives on the activities of human immunodeficiency virus reverse transcriptase and DNA polymerases. Zhongguo Yi Xue Ke Xue Yuan Xue Bao 14.5 (1992): 334–338.
Tatti S et al. Sinecatechins, a defined green tea extract, in the treatment of external anogenital warts: a randomized controlled trial. Obstet Gynecol 111.6 (2008): 1371–1379.
Taylor JR, Wilt VM. Probable antagonism of warfarin by green tea. Ann Pharmacother 33.4 (1999): 426–428.
Tehrani, M. H., et al. 2011. Comparing *Streptococcus mutans* and *Lactobacillus* colony count changes following green tea mouth rinse or sodium fluoride mouth rinse use in children (Randomized double-blind controlled clinical trial). Dent Res J (Isfahan), 8, S58–63.
Thakur, V. S., et al. 2012. The chemopreventive and chemotherapeutic potentials of tea polyphenols. Curr Pharm Biotechnol, 13, 191–9.
Thielecke, F. & Boschmann, M. 2009. The potential role of green tea catechins in the prevention of the metabolic syndrome - a review. Phytochemistry, 70, 11–24.
Tokuda, H., et al. 2008. (–)-Epigallocatechin gallate inhibits basic fibroblast growth factor-stimulated interleukin-6 synthesis in osteoblasts. Horm Metab Res, 40, 674–8.
Trudel, D., et al. 2012. Green tea for ovarian cancer prevention and treatment: a systematic review of the in vitro, in vivo and epidemiological studies. Gynecol Oncol, 126, 491–8.
Tsao, A. S., et al. 2009. Phase II randomized, placebo-controlled trial of green tea extract in patients with high-risk oral premalignant lesions. Cancer Prev Res (Phila), 2, 931–41.
Tzellos, T. G., et al. 2011. Efficacy, safety and tolerability of green tea catechins in the treatment of external anogenital warts: a systematic review and meta-analysis. J Eur Acad Dermatol Venereol, 25, 345–53.
Ueno, T., et al. 2009. Epigallocatechin-3-gallate improves nonalcoholic steatohepatitis model mice expressing nuclear sterol regulatory element binding protein-1c in adipose tissue. Int J Mol Med, 24, 17–22.
Ui, A., et al. 2009. Green tea consumption and the risk of liver cancer in Japan: the Ohsaki Cohort study. Cancer Causes Control, 20, 1939–45.
Ulbricht CE, Basch EM. Natural standard herb and supplement reference. St Louis: Mosby, 2005.
Valcic S et al. Inhibitory effect of six green tea catechins and caffeine on the growth of four selected human tumor cell lines. Anticancer Drugs 7.4 (1996): 461–468.
Varilek GW et al. Green tea polyphenol extract attenuates inflammation in interleukin-2-deficient mice, a model of autoimmunity. J Nutr 131.7 (2001): 2034–2039.
Vieira Senger, A. E., et al. 2012. Effect of green tea (*Camellia sinensis*) consumption on the components of metabolic syndrome in elderly. J Nutr Health Aging, 16, 738–42.
Vignes M et al. Anxiolytic properties of green tea polyphenol (–)-epigallocatechin gallate (EGCG). Brain Res 1110.1 (2006): 102–115.
Wang YC, Bachrach U. The specific anti-cancer activity of green tea (–)-epigallocatechin-3-gallate (EGCG). Amino Acids 22.2 (2002): 131–143.
Wang, Z. M., et al. 2011. Black and green tea consumption and the risk of coronary artery disease: a meta-analysis. Am J Clin Nutr, 93, 506–15.
Wang, G., et al. 2012a. Risk factor for clear cell renal cell carcinoma in Chinese population: a case-control study. Cancer Epidemiol, 36, 177–82.
Wang, J., et al. 2012b. Green tea drinking and risk of pancreatic cancer: A large-scale, population-based case–control study in urban Shanghai. Cancer Epidemiol, 36, e354–e358.
Wang, X. J., et al. 2012c. Association between green tea and colorectal cancer risk: a meta-analysis of 13 case-control studies. Asian Pac J Cancer Prev, 13, 3123–7.
Wang, Y., et al. 2012d. Coffee and tea consumption and risk of lung cancer: a dose-response analysis of observational studies. Lung Cancer, 78, 169–70.
Wang, Z. H., et al. 2012e. Green tea and incidence of colorectal cancer: evidence from prospective cohort studies. Nutr Cancer, 64, 1143–52.
Wang, X., et al. 2013. A meta-analysis of tea consumption and the risk of bladder cancer. Urol Int, 90, 10–6.
Watanabe, I., et al. 2009. Green tea and death from pneumonia in Japan: the Ohsaki cohort study. Am J Clin Nutr, 90, 672–9.
Weber JM et al. Inhibition of adenovirus infection and adenain by green tea catechins. Antiviral Res 58.2 (2003): 167–173.
Westphal S et al. S1753 EGCG, a Major Component of Green Tea Catechins Attenuates Inflammatory Responses in Two Different Mouse Colitis Models. Gastroenterology 134 (4 Suppl 1) (2008): A–263.
Wightman, E. L., et al. 2012. Epigallocatechin gallate, cerebral blood flow parameters, cognitive performance and mood in healthy humans: a double-blind, placebo-controlled, crossover investigation. Hum Psychopharmacol, 27, 177–86.
Williamson MP et al. Epigallocatechin gallate, the main polyphenol in green tea, binds to the T-cell receptor, CD4: Potential for HIV-1 therapy. J Allergy Clin Immunol 118.6 (2006): 1369–1374.
Wu, S., et al. 2013. The association of tea consumption with bladder cancer risk: a meta-analysis. Asia Pac J Clin Nutr, 22, 128–37.
Yamauchi, R., et al. 2009. Identification of epigallocatechin-3-gallate in green tea polyphenols as a potent inducer of p53-dependent apoptosis in the human lung cancer cell line A549. Toxicol In Vitro, 23, 834–9.
Yokozawa T et al. Effectiveness of green tea tannin on rats with chronic renal failure. Biosci Biotechnol Biochem 60.6 (1996): 1000–1005.
Yoo HG et al. Induction of apoptosis by the green tea flavonol (–)-epigallocatechin-3-gallate in human endothelial ECV 304 cells. Anticancer Res 22.6A (2002): 3373–3378.
Yu J et al. Chemoprevention trial of green tea polyphenols in high-risk population of liver cancer in southern Guangxi, China. AACR Meeting Abstracts 2006 (1) (2006): 1148–a.
Yuan, J. M., et al. 2011. Tea and cancer prevention: epidemiological studies. Pharmacol Res, 64, 123–35.
Zhang H et al. Modification of lung cancer susceptibility by green tea extract as measured by the comet assay. Cancer Detect Prev 26.6 (2002): 411–4118.
Zhang M et al. Green tea consumption enhances survival of epithelial ovarian cancer. Int J Cancer 112.3 (2004): 465–469.
Zhang M et al. Green tea and the prevention of breast cancer: a case-control study in Southeast China. Carcinogenesis 28.5 (2007a): 1074–1078.
Zhang, M., et al. 2007b. Possible protective effect of green tea intake on risk of adult leukaemia. Br J Cancer, 98, 168–170.
Zhang, G., et al. 2012a. Anti-cancer activities of tea epigallocatechin-3-gallate in breast cancer patients under radiotherapy. Curr Mol Med, 12, 163–76.
Zhang, Y., et al. 2012b. Effects of catechin-enriched green tea beverage on visceral fat loss in adults with a high proportion of visceral fat: A double-blind, placebo-controlled, randomized trial. Journal of Functional Foods, 4, 315–322.
Zheng, J., et al. 2011a. Green tea and black tea consumption and prostate cancer risk: an exploratory meta-analysis of observational studies. Nutr Cancer, 63, 663–72.
Zheng, X. X., et al. 2011b. Green tea intake lowers fasting serum total and LDL cholesterol in adults: a meta-analysis of 14 randomized controlled trials. Am J Clin Nutr, 94, 601–10.

Zheng, P., et al. 2012. Green tea consumption and risk of esophageal cancer: a meta-analysis of epidemiologic studies. BMC Gastroenterol, 12, 165.

Zheng, J. S., et al. 2013a. Effects of green tea, black tea, and coffee consumption on the risk of esophageal cancer: a systematic review and meta-analysis of observational studies. Nutr Cancer, 65, 1–16.

Zheng, X. X., et al. 2013b. Effects of green tea catechins with or without caffeine on glycemic control in adults: a meta-analysis of randomized controlled trials. Am J Clin Nutr 97: 750–762.

Zou, C., et al. 2010. Green tea compound in chemoprevention of cervical cancer. Int J Gynecol Cancer, 20, 617–24.

Guarana

HISTORICAL NOTE Guarana has been used by the Amazonian Indians of South America for centuries to enhance energy levels, suppress appetite, increase libido and protect them from malaria. More recently, hot and cold guarana beverages have been adopted by the greater population as a tonic to enhance wellbeing, in much the same way coffee is consumed in Australia.

COMMON NAME

Guarana

OTHER NAMES

Brazilian cocoa, guarana gum, guarana paste, quarana, quarane, uabano, uaranzeiro, zoom

BOTANICAL NAME/FAMILY

Paullinia cupana (family Sapindaceae)

PLANT PART USED

Seeds

CHEMICAL COMPONENTS

Guarana seeds are a rich source of caffeine, containing 3–6% on a dry-weight basis (Saldana et al 2002). Other major compounds include theobromine, theophylline, tannins, resins, protein, fat and saponins (Duke 2003).

MAIN ACTIONS

A review of the scientific literature reveals that guarana itself has only recently been the subject of clinical studies. As such, studies pertaining to caffeine are sometimes used to explain the herb's action, an approach that presupposes the other constituents are either inactive or of such weak effect they need not be recognised. Although this approach is convenient and provides us with some understanding of the herb's pharmacological effects, the results of clinical studies suggest that guarana's effects on cognitive function are due to more than its caffeine content. It has also been suggested that the effects of guarana are longer lasting than caffeine, possibly due to the saponin and tannin content (Babu et al 2008).

Central nervous system (CNS) stimulant

Although guarana has not been clinically investigated for its effects on the CNS, there is a great deal of evidence to show that caffeine is an antagonist of the adenosine receptor, which produces a net increase in CNS activity because the inhibitory action of adenosine is blocked (Smith 2002). This results in the release of a variety of neurotransmitters (e.g. noradrenaline, acetylcholine, dopamine, and the gamma-aminobutyric acid/benzodiazepine system).

OTHER ACTIONS

Inhibits platelet aggregation

Guarana inhibits platelet aggregation both in vitro and in vivo (Bydlowski et al 1988, 1991). Decreased thromboxane synthesis may in part explain this activity.

Gastric effects

Guarana may increase gastric acid secretion and delay gastric emptying. This has been demonstrated in a clinical study using a herbal combination known as YGD, which contains yerba mate (leaves of *Ilex paraguayensis*), guarana (seeds of *Paullinia cupana*) and damiana (leaves of *Turnera diffusa* var. *aphrodisiaca*) (Andersen & Fogh 2001). Whether stand-alone treatment with guarana will produce similar effects is unknown.

Chemoprotective

Guarana has been shown to be chemoprotective in a mouse hepatocarcinogenesis model (Fukumasu et al 2005). The herb was found to reduce the cellular proliferation of preneoplastic cells. It has also been demonstrated that guarana is protective against chemically-induced DNA damage in mouse liver. This effect was attributed to the tannin content of the herb (Fukumasu et al 2006). A later mouse experiment observed a decrease in proliferation and an increase in apoptosis of melanoma lung metastases, resulting in a reduction in tumour size (Fukumasu et al 2008).

Antibacterial

In vitro data have demonstrated the antibacterial and antioxidant effects of the ethanolic extract of guarana, thought to be due to the phenolic compounds (Basile et al 2005). Guarana was shown to be effective against many pathogens of the digestive tract, including *Escherichia coli*, *Salmonella typhimurium* and *Staphylococcus aureus*. This adds weight to the traditional use of guarana for diarrhoea. More recently in vitro research has demonstrated antibacterial activity against *Streptococcus mutans*, which could have applications in preventing dental plaque (Yamaguti-Sasaki et al 2007). Antimicrobial activity was further confirmed in vitro when testing guarana seed extracts against food-borne fungi and bacteria. This may have applications in food preservation (Majhenic et al 2007).

Antioxidant

A strong antioxidant activity has been demonstrated in vitro for guarana seeds (Majhenic et al 2007). This has been attributed to several processes, including an inhibitory effect on lipid peroxidation (Portella 2013) and nitric oxide metabolism (Bittencourt et al 2013).

Cardiovascular disease prevention

A recent observational study reported a lower prevalence of hypertension, obesity and metabolic syndrome in elderly individuals who habitually consumed guarana, compared to those who never ingested the herb. The guarana group also presented with lower cholesterol (total and low-density lipoprotein) and advanced oxidative protein product levels (Portella 2013).

Other actions relating to caffeine content

Although these have not been tested for guarana directly, the caffeine content, which is well absorbed from the herb, may cause mild dilation of the blood vessels; an increase in blood pressure, renin and catecholamine release, urine output, metabolic rate, lipolysis, respiration and intestinal peristalsis; and inhibition of CYP1A2. Caffeine also possesses thermogenic properties (Astrup 2000).

CLINICAL USE

Mood enhancing

For several years anecdotal evidence has suggested that guarana produces similar effects to caffeine on subjective feelings of wellbeing, energy, motivation and self-confidence (Mumford et al 1994). Tests with animal models indicate guarana exerts a mild antidepressant effect, thereby providing some support for the observed mood-elevating effects (Campos et al 2005, Otobone et al 2007).

Mood elevation was further demonstrated in a recent double-blind, placebo-controlled, multidose clinical study involving 26 volunteers which tested a low caffeine-containing guarana extract (PC-102) (Haskell et al 2007). Four strengths were investigated (37.5 mg, 75 mg, 150 mg and 300 mg). Treatment at each dose level produced a significant effect on mood. As there were low levels of caffeine measured in the guarana extract, mood elevation cannot be explained by the caffeine content alone.

Enhanced cognitive function and alertness

A growing number of clinical studies have been conducted to investigate whether guarana affects cognitive function, producing mixed results thus far. Four double-blind studies report that guarana has significant effects on cognitive function and provides evidence that these effects are not just mediated by the herb's caffeine content (Haskell et al 2005, 2007, Kennedy et al 2004, 2008). In contrast, two earlier double-blind studies failed to identify significant effects for guarana on cognitive function (Galduroz & Carlini 1994, 1996). Whether this is due to differences in the chemical profile and caffeine content of the tested extracts appears likely, but remains to be confirmed. Some studies have tested guarana in combination with other herbs or nutritional agents.

One double-blind, placebo-controlled study assessed the effects of four different doses of guarana (37.5 mg, 75 mg, 150 mg and 300 mg) in 22 subjects (Haskell et al 2005). Cognitive performance and mood were assessed at baseline and again 1, 3 and 6 hours after each dose using the Cognitive Drug Research computerised assessment battery, serial subtraction tasks, a sentence verification task and visual analogue mood scales. All doses improved picture and word recognition, results on the Bond–Lader visual analogue scales and caffeine research visual analogue scales showing improvements in alertness and reduced ratings of headache. The two lower doses produced better results than the two higher doses, which were associated with impaired accuracy of choice reaction and one of the subtraction tests. Several observations suggest that these effects were not due to caffeine alone. Firstly, effects were still apparent 6 hours after administration and secondly, better results were obtained with a dose of 37.5 mg than 300 mg with a caffeine content of less than 5 mg in the lowest dose. The study was replicated 2 years later, with a double-blind, counterbalanced, placebo-controlled study (Haskell et al 2007). In this study, 26 participants were given the same four doses of a standardised guarana extract. All doses improved mood; however, cognitive improvements were greatest for the two lower doses, with the 75 mg dose most effective. As there was only 9 mg of caffeine in this dose it is unlikely that the effects can be attributed solely to the caffeine content.

Another double-blind, placebo-controlled study investigated the effects of a single dose of guarana (75 mg) on cognition, in combination with and in comparison to ginseng (*Panax ginseng* 200 mg) in 28 healthy volunteers (Kennedy et al 2004). Guarana was shown to produce comparable effects to ginseng in improved task performance, with all three treatments better than placebo. However, guarana was superior to ginseng in improving the speed of performed tasks. Once again, given the low caffeine content (9 mg) of the guarana extract used in this study, the effects are unlikely to be attributable to its caffeine content alone, particularly as the dose

G

was shown to be as effective as a 16-fold dose of pure caffeine. A later double-blind, randomised, placebo-controlled study of 129 adults tested a multivitamin and mineral supplement with added guarana (Berocca Boost with 222 mg guarana containing 40 mg caffeine) and found it supported the previous findings that guarana improves cognitive performance. A single dose of the supplement also reduced mental fatigue after sustained mental effort (Kennedy et al 2008).

Two other randomised, double-blind studies have investigated the effects of guarana on cognitive function (Galduroz & Carlini 1994, 1996). One study involving 45 healthy elderly volunteers found that guarana treatment was ineffective (Galduroz & Carlini 1996), which confirmed the findings of a previous study conducted with younger subjects. Guarana 500 mg (12.5 mg caffeine) was given twice daily (Galduroz & Carlini 1994). Studies in some animal models have produced positive results for both single-dose and long-term administration of guarana, observing a positive effect on memory acquisition and memory maintenance (Espinola et al 1997).

A more recent double-blind randomised controlled trial of 129 volunteers found that treatment with an acute dose of a guarana and multivitamin mineral supplement increased speed and accuracy on a cognitive demand battery test and reduced the subjective feeling of fatigue (Scholey 2008). The study used Berocca Boost which contains caffeine (40 mg) derived from guarana (222 mg). As a combination supplement was used in this trial, the effects cannot be attributed to guarana alone.

Chemotherapy-related fatigue

Guarana has also been assessed in breast cancer patients experiencing fatigue during chemotherapy treatment. The randomised study involving 32 patients found a daily dose of 50 mg guarana taken over 21 days produced a significant reduction in fatigue during this period when compared to placebo and was not associated with toxicity or adverse effects (de Oliveira Campos 2011). Brief Fatigue Inventory (BFI) significantly improved after treatment with an oral purified dry extract of *P. cupana* (PC-18; 37.5 mg twice daily) given one week after starting chemotherapy. The study of 40 people with solid tumours found BFI fatigue scores improved or stabilised in 36 out of the 40 patients (mean BFI score difference = 2.503; $P = .0002$) (del Giglio et al 2013). Interestingly, the benefits continued for several weeks after ceasing guarana treatment.

Ergogenic aid

Guarana is also used as an ergogenic aid by some athletes, most likely because caffeine and theophylline have been used in this way, to improve performance in training and competition (Graham 2001). No human studies testing guarana for effects on physical performance could be located. Referring to caffeine studies, it appears that ergogenic effects are observed under some conditions but not under others (Doherty et al 2002, Hunter et al 2002, Ryu et al 2001). Testing guarana in several animal models has also produced contradictory results. Significant increases in physical capacity have been observed with a dose of 0.3 mg/mL of a guarana suspension after 100 and 200 days' treatment. However, the same effect was not seen with a concentration of 3.0 mg/mL nor with a solution of caffeine 0.1 mg/mL (Espinola et al 1997).

Appetite suppressant and weight-loss aid

Weight-loss products often contain guarana, in the belief that it suppresses appetite and may have thermogenic and diuretic activities. An animal study designed to evaluate the effects of guarana and decaffeinated guarana found that only the caffeinated herb was effective for weight loss (Lima et al 2005).

To date, most clinical studies have investigated the effects of guarana in combination with other herbs.

IN COMBINATION

A double-blind randomised controlled trial testing a combination of yerba mate (leaves of *Ilex paraguayensis*), guarana (seeds of *Paullinia cupana*) and damiana (leaves of *Turnera diffusa* var. *aphrodisiaca*) found that the preparation significantly delayed gastric emptying, reduced the time to perceived gastric fullness and induced significant weight loss over 45 days in overweight patients (Andersen & Fogh 2001). The same herbal combination (Zotrim) was tested in an open study of 73 overweight health professionals over 6 weeks. Active treatment resulted in a significant reduction in self-reported weight and waist and hip measurements, and increased satiety after meals. Significant weight loss was reported by 22% of volunteers.

Another randomised double-blind placebo-controlled trial evaluated the effects of guarana in combination with ma huang (*Ephedra* spp.) and concluded that the formula was effective for weight loss in overweight men after 8 weeks of treatment (Boozer et al 2001). A more recent double-blind, placebo-controlled, randomised study tested a multicomponent herbal combination containing extracts from asparagus, green tea, black tea, guarana, mate, kidney beans, *Garcinia cambogia* and chromium yeast and found that over a 12-week period there was a significant change in the Body Composition Improvement Index and decreased body fat compared to placebo (Opala et al 2006). The formula was more effective for those participants who were undertaking an exercise program at the same time than for those who remained sedentary.

A short-lived increase in metabolic rate was observed in a small double-blind, placebo-controlled, crossover study of 16 healthy subjects (Roberts et al 2005). A product containing primarily black tea (*Camellia sinensis*) and guarana extract providing 36% caffeine (plus vitamin C and some other trace nutrients and herbs) increased metabolic rate after 1 hour with no significant difference at the 2-hour check.

Although encouraging, the effects of guarana as a stand-alone treatment need to be confirmed.

Clinical note — Popular energy drinks and caffeine content

Adolescents in particular are high consumers of energy drinks, with a reported 30–50% of teens and young adults consuming these drinks in the United States alone (Seifert et al 2011). In the most recent American Drug Abuse Warning Network report, the number of emergency room visits associated with energy drinks doubled from just over 10,000 in 2007 to just over 20,000 in 2011 (SAMHSA 2013). In Australia, there also appears to be an increasing trend of adverse events associated with energy drink consumption (Gunja & Brown 2012). These drinks often contain a mixture of caffeine, guarana, taurine and other herbs and vitamins. According to product labels and websites, the following drinks contain varying amounts of caffeine:

• Coca Cola	34 mg per 355 mL can
• Diet Coke	45.6 mg per 355 mL
• Diet Pepsi	36 mg per 355 mL
• Diet Pepsi Max	69 mg per 355 mL
• Red Bull	151 mg per 475 mL can
• Mother	80 mg per 250 mL
• V	78 mg per 250 mL
• Brewed coffee	60–120 mg per cup

A large intake of these drinks can produce adverse effects based on their caffeine content such as headache, agitation, insomnia, anxiety, tremor, restlessness, seizures, tachycardia and nausea and other gastrointestinal disturbances. Four independent cases associating high consumption of energy drinks with seizures have been reported (Iyadurai & Chung 2007), and in 2009 a caffeine-related death from energy drinks was reported (Berger & Alford 2009). A prudent suggestion is to avoid a high intake of these drinks. There has been one reported case of intractable ventricular fibrillation in a young woman with a pre-existing mitral valve prolapse. This occurred after consuming an energy drink with guarana and high caffeine content (Cannon et al 2001).

OTHER USES

Traditionally, guarana has been used as an aphrodisiac, a treatment for diarrhoea, a diuretic and as a beverage in some cultures.

DOSAGE RANGE

According to clinical trials

- Cognition, alertness and mood: doses between 37.5 and 75 mg are sufficient to provide effects for at least 6 hours. However, doses of up to 300 mg have been used with varying concentrations of naturally present caffeine.
- For other indications, guarana has not been significantly researched. Based on its caffeine content, it is advised that doses should not exceed that amount that will provide approximately 250 mg of caffeine daily. This is equivalent to 2.5–4 g guarana/day, depending on the caffeine content of the preparation.

Clinical note — Is caffeine safe in pregnancy?

There have been numerous studies investigating the effects of caffeine in pregnancy, with inconsistent results. A meta-analysis of 32 case-control or cohort design studies found that there was a small, statistically significant increase in the risk of spontaneous abortion and of low-birth-weight babies where the pregnant mother consumed more than 150 mg of caffeine per day (equivalent to about 1.5 cups of freshly brewed coffee) (Fernandes et al 1998). Confounders such as maternal age, smoking and alcohol use could not be excluded. More recent studies have produced varying results, with one cohort study in Denmark concluding that high levels of coffee consumption were associated with a higher risk of fetal death, especially after 20 weeks (Bech et al 2005). A population-based case-control study in Uruguay also showed a significantly increased risk of fetal death when more than 300 mg caffeine per day is consumed (Matijasevich et al 2006). An increased risk of repeated miscarriage with high caffeine intake was reported in a Swedish study (George et al 2006) and a more recent study found an increased miscarriage risk even allowing for pregnancy-related symptoms (Weng et al 2008). The risk of small-for-gestational-age (SGA), especially for boys, was nearly doubled for mothers with high rather than low caffeine intake in the third trimester (Vik et al 2003). A UK study of 2643 women found that women whose pregnancies resulted in late miscarriage and stillbirth consumed more than 145 mg/day caffeine through the first trimester (Greenwood et al 2010).

In contradiction to these findings, other studies showed caffeine consumption was unlikely to be a major risk factor for SGA or low-birth-weight babies (Infante-Rivard 2007), and a systematic review showed no association between moderate caffeine consumption and fetal growth (Pacheco et al 2007). Another large prospective study confirmed no clinical importance was demonstrated looking at fetal growth, except for women consuming 600 mg caffeine daily (Bracken et al 2003).

It therefore seems prudent that caffeine intake should be avoided or limited throughout pregnancy and that the caffeine content of guarana products should be checked before use.

Practice points/Patient counselling

- Guarana has mild CNS-stimulant properties and increases alertness, cognitive function and mood.
- Current evidence is inconclusive as to whether guarana also enhances physical stamina.
- It has been used in combination with other herbs as a weight-loss aid with some degree of success. However, it is unknown what role guarana played in achieving these results.
- In some sensitive individuals, guarana may produce CNS-stimulant-related side effects, such as elevated heart rate and blood pressure, tremor, restlessness and excitability.

TOXICITY

Animal tests have shown that high doses of 1000–2000 mg/kg (intraperitoneal and oral) do not induce significant alterations in parameters for toxicological screening, suggesting an absence of toxicity (Mattei et al 1998). This has also been demonstrated with longer-term use (Antonelli-Ushirobira 2010).

ADVERSE REACTIONS

Due to a lack of clinical studies testing guarana as a stand-alone treatment, it is difficult to determine what adverse reactions may exist.

Based on caffeine content, the following adverse effects may theoretically occur at high doses: agitation, tremor, anxiety, restlessness, headache, seizures, hypertension, tachycardia and premature ventricular contractions, diarrhoea, gastrointestinal cramping, nausea and vomiting and diuresis.

SIGNIFICANT INTERACTIONS

Controlled studies are not available, therefore interactions are theoretical and based on evidence of pharmacological activity with uncertain clinical significance.

CNS stimulants

Additive stimulant activity is theoretically possible, so use with caution.

CNS sedatives

Antagonistic effects are theoretically possible due to the herb's CNS stimulant activity. However, one in vivo study found no interaction with pentobarbitone. Observe patients taking this combination.

Diuretics

Additive diuretic effects are theoretically possible — use this combination with caution.

Anticoagulants

Increased bleeding is theoretically possible, as in vitro and in vivo research has identified antiplatelet activity for guarana. Use this combination with caution.

CONTRAINDICATIONS AND PRECAUTIONS

Contraindicated in moderate to severe hypertension and cardiac arrhythmias.

Use with caution in anxiety states, hypertension, diabetes, gastric ulcers and chronic headache. Adverse reactions may be dose dependent. Suspend use of concentrated extracts 1 week before major surgery.

Under the World Anti-Doping Code 2007 Prohibited List, caffeine is not classified as a prohibited stimulant, unless specified by particular sports. Therefore athletes are recommended to check with their own sports federation about the status of caffeine-containing substances.

PREGNANCY USE

The use of caffeine-containing preparations should be limited during pregnancy and breastfeeding as it has the ability to cross the placenta and can be found in breast milk. Caffeine clearance is also delayed in the second and third trimesters, with the half-life of caffeine increasing to 10.5 hours from 2.5–4.5 hours in a non-pregnant woman. It also appears that the fetus has a reduced capacity to metabolise caffeine.

Antiplatelet drugs

Additive effects are theoretically possible as in vitro and in vivo research has identified antiplatelet activity for guarana. Observe patients taking this combination.

Digoxin

Long-term use of high-dose supplements can result in reduced potassium levels, which lowers the threshold for drug toxicity. Avoid long-term use of high-dose guarana preparations.

Drugs metabolised by CYP1A2

The inhibitory effect of caffeine on CYP1A2 may cause other interactions, but this is highly speculative for guarana.

PATIENTS' FAQs

What will this herb do for me?
Guarana is a herbal stimulant that increases alertness, cognitive function and possibly mood.

How quickly does it start working?
Effects are expected 1–2 hours after ingestion, although this will vary depending on the individual and the current level of wakefulness.

Are there any safety issues to be aware of?
Used in small amounts, it is likely to have a degree of stimulant activity and decrease fatigue; however, as with all stimulants, excessive use or long-term use can be detrimental to health. Guarana should be

used with caution in people with hypertension, anxiety states, gastric ulcers, diabetes and some types of cardiovascular disease. It may also interact with a variety of medicines and therefore it is recommended to consult your healthcare professional if you are currently taking pharmaceutical medication.

REFERENCES

Andersen T, Fogh J. Weight loss and delayed gastric emptying following a South American herbal preparation in overweight patients. J Hum Nutr Diet 14.3 (2001): 243–250.

Antonelli-Ushirobira T. Acute and subchronic toxicological evaluation of the semipurified extract of seeds of guaraná (*Paullinia cupana*) in rodents. Food Chem Toxicol 48.7 (2010): 1817–1820

Astrup A. Thermogenic drugs as a strategy for treatment of obesity. Endocrine 13.2 (2000): 207–212.

Babu KM et al. Energy drinks: the new eye-opener for adolescents. Clin Pediatr Emerg Med 9.1 (2008): 35–42.

Basile A et al. Antibacterial and antioxidant activities of ethanol extract from *Paullinia cupana* Mart. J Ethnopharmacol 102.1 (2005): 32–36.

Bech BH et al. Coffee and fetal death: a cohort study with prospective data. Am J Epidemiol 162.10 (2005): 983–990.

Berger A & Alford K. Cardiac arrest in a young man following excess consumption of caffeinated "energy drinks". MJA 190 (2009): 41–43.

Bittencourt L et al. The protective effects of guaraná extract (*Paullinia cupana*) on fibroblast NIH-3T3 cells exposed to sodium nitroprusside. Food Chem Toxico 53 (2013): 119–125.

Boozer CN et al. An herbal supplement containing Ma Huang–guarana for weight loss: a randomized, double-blind trial. Int J Obes Relat Metab Disord 25.3 (2001): 316–324.

Bracken MB et al. Association of maternal caffeine consumption with decrements in fetal growth. Am J Epidemiol 157.5 (2003): 456–466.

Bydlowski SP, et al. A novel property of an aqueous guarana extract (*Paullinia cupana*): inhibition of platelet aggregation in vitro and in vivo. Braz J Med Biol Res 21.3 (1988): 535–538.

Bydlowski SP, et al. An aqueous extract of guarana (*Paullinia cupana*) decreases platelet thromboxane synthesis. Braz J Med Biol Res 24.4 (1991): 421–424.

Campos AR et al. Acute effects of guarana (*Paullinia cupana* Mart.) on mouse behaviour in forced swimming and open field tests. Phytother Res 19.5 (2005): 441–443.

Cannon ME et al. Caffeine-induced cardiac arrhythmia: an unrecognised danger of healthfood products. Med J Aust 174.10 (2001): 520–521.

de Oliveira Campos M. Guarana (*Paullinia cupana*) improves fatigue in breast cancer patients undergoing systemic chemotherapy. J Altern Complement Med 17.6 (2011): 505–512.

Doherty M et al. Caffeine is ergogenic after supplementation of oral creatine monohydrate. Med Sci Sports Exerc 34.11 (2002): 1785–1792.

Duke JA. Dr Duke's Phytochemical and Ethnobotanical Databases. US Department of Agriculture-Agricultural Research Service-National Germplasm Resources Laboratory. Beltsville Agricultural Research Center, Beltsville, Maryland. Online. Available: www.ars-grin.gov/duke March 2003.

Espinola EB et al. Pharmacological activity of guarana (*Paullinia cupana* Mart.) in laboratory animals. J Ethnopharmacol 55.3 (1997): 223–229.

Fernandes OM et al. Moderate to heavy caffeine consumption during pregnancy and relationship to spontaneous abortion and abnormal fetal growth: a meta-analysis. Reprod Toxicol 12.4 (1998): 435–44.

Fukumasu H et al. Chemopreventive effects of *Paullinia cupana* Mart var. sorbilis, the guarana, on mouse hepatocarcinogenesis. Cancer Lett 233.1 (2005): 158–164.

Fukumasu H et al. Protective effects of guarana (*Paullinia cupana* Mart. var. sorbilis) against DEN-induced DNA damage on mouse liver. Food Chem Toxicol 44.6 (2006): 862–867.

Fukumasu H et al. *Paullinia cupana* Mart var. sorbilis, guarana, reduces cell proliferation and increases apoptosis of B16/F10 melanoma lung metastases in mice. Braz J Med Biol Res 41.4 (2008): 305–310.

Galduroz JC, Carlini EA. Acute effects of the *Paullinia cupana*, guarana on the cognition of normal volunteers. Rev Paul Med 112.3 (1994): 607–611.

Galduroz JC, Carlini EA. The effects of long-term administration of guarana on the cognition of normal, elderly volunteers. Rev Paul Med 114.1 (1996): 1073–1078.

George L et al. Risks of repeated miscarriage. Paediatr Perinat Epidemiol 20.2 (2006): 119–26.

Graham TE. Caffeine and exercise: metabolism, endurance and performance. Sports Med 31.11 (2001): 785–807.

Greenwood D et al. Caffeine intake during pregnancy, late miscarriage and stillbirth. Eur J Epidemiol 25.4 (2010): 275–280.

Gunja N & Brown J. Energy drinks: health risks and toxicity. MJA 196 (2012): 46–49.

Haskell CF et al. A 10 dose ranging study of the cognitive and mood effects of guarana. Behav Pharmacol 16 (Suppl 1) (2005): S26.

Haskell CF et al. A double-blind, placebo-controlled, multi-dose evaluation of the acute behavioural effects of guarana in humans. J Psychopharmacol 21.1 (2007): 65–70.

Hunter AM et al. Caffeine ingestion does not alter performance during a 100-km cycling time-trial performance. Int J Sport Nutr Exerc Metab 12.4 (2002): 438–452.

Infante-Rivard C. Caffeine intake and small-for-gestational-age birth: modifying effects of xenobiotic-metabolising genes and smoking. Paediatr Perinat Epidemiol 21.4 (2007): 300–309.

Iyadurai SJ, Chung SS. New-onset seizures in adults: possible association with consumption of popular energy drinks. Epilepsy Behav 10.3 (2007): 504–508.

Kennedy DO et al. Improved cognitive performance in human volunteers following administration of guarana (*Paullinia cupana*) extract: comparison and interaction with *Panax ginseng*. Pharmacol Biochem Behav 79.3 (2004): 401–411.

Kennedy DO et al. Improved cognitive performance and mental fatigue following a multi-vitamin and mineral supplement with added guaraná (*Paullinia cupana*). Appetite 50.2–3 (2008): 506–513.

Lima WP et al. Lipid metabolism in trained rats: Effect of guarana (*Paullinia cupana* Mart.) supplementation. Clin Nutr 24 (2005): 1019–1028.

Majhenic L et al. Antioxidant and antimicrobial activity of guarana seed extracts. Food Chem 104(3) (2007): 1258–1268.

Matijasevich A et al. Maternal caffeine consumption and fetal death: a case-control study in Uruguay. Paediatr Perinat Epidemiol 20.2 (2006): 100–109.

Mattei R et al. Guarana (*Paullinia cupana*): toxic behavioral effects in laboratory animals and antioxidants activity in vitro. J Ethnopharmacol 60.2 (1998): 111–1116.

Mumford GK et al. Discriminative stimulus and subjective effects of theobromine and caffeine in humans. Psychopharmacology (Berl) 115.1–2 (1994): 1–8.

Opala T et al. Efficacy of 12 weeks supplementation of a botanical extract-based weight loss formula on body weight, body composition and blood chemistry in healthy, overweight subjects – a randomised double-blind placebo-controlled clinical trial. Eur J Med Res 11.8 (2006): 343–350.

Otobone FJ et al. Effect of lyophilized extracts from guarana seeds [*Paullinia cupana* var. sorbilis (Mart.) Ducke] on behavioral profiles in rats. Phytother Res 21.6 (2007): 531–535.

Pacheco AH et al. Caffeine consumption during pregnancy and prevalence of low birth weight and prematurity: a systematic review. Cad Saude Publica 23.12 (2007): 2807–2819.

Portella R. Guarana (*Paullinia cupana* Kunth) effects on LDL oxidation in elderly people: an in vitro and in vivo study. Lipids Health Dis 12.1 (2013): 12.

Roberts AT et al. The effect of an herbal supplement containing black tea and caffeine on metabolic parameters in humans. Altern Med Rev 10.4 (2005): 321–325.

Ryu S et al. Caffeine as a lipolytic food component increases endurance performance in rats and athletes. J Nutr Sci Vitaminol (Tokyo) 47.2 (2001): 139–46.

Saldana MD et al. Extraction of methylxanthines from guarana seeds, mate leaves, and cocoa beans using supercritical carbon dioxide and ethanol. J Agric Food Chem 50.17 (2002): 4820–4826.

SAMHSA – Centre for Behavioural Health Statistics and Quality. The Dawn Report: Update on Emergency Department Visits Involving Energy Drinks: A Continuing Public Health Concern. January 10, 2013. Rockville, MD, SAMHSA.

Scholey A. A multivitamin–mineral preparation with guaraná positively effects cognitive performance and reduces mental fatigue during sustained mental demand. Appetite 50 (2008): 565.

Seifert S et al. Health Effects of Energy Drinks on Children, Adolescents, and Young Adults. Pediatrics 127.3 (2011): 511–528.

Smith A. Effects of caffeine on human behavior. Food Chem Toxicol 40.9 (2002): 1243–1255.

Vik T et al. High caffeine consumption in the third trimester of pregnancy: gender-specific effects on fetal growth. Paediatr Perinat Epidemiol 17.4 (2003): 324–331.

Weng X et al. Maternal caffeine consumption during pregnancy and the risk of miscarriage: a prospective cohort study. Am J Obstet Gynecol 198.3 (2008): 279.e1–8.

Yamaguti-Sasaki E et al. Antioxidant capacity and in vitro prevention of dental plaque formation by extracts and condensed tannins of *Paullinia cupana*. Molecules 12.8 (2007): 1950–1963.

Gymnema sylvestre

HISTORICAL NOTE Gymnema is a traditional Ayurvedic medicine used in India for over 2000 years. It has been called the sugar destroyer because the leaf demonstrates the ability to suppress sweet taste recognition on the tongue. It has been used to treat diabetes, as well as to aid metabolic control when combined with other herbal medicines. The first biological investigations were reported in 1930 where blood glucose lowering activity was observed for the leaves in animals with pancreatic function, thereby confirming traditional use (Shanmugasundaram et al. 1990).

COMMON NAME

Gymnema

OTHER NAMES

Asclepias geminate, gurmar (sugar destroyer), gemnema melicida, gokhru, gulrmaro, gurmara, gurmarbooti, kar-e-khask, kharak, merasingi, meshasringi, masabedda, *Periploca sylvestris*, sirukurinjan

BOTANICAL NAME/FAMILY

Gymnema sylvestre (family Asclepiadaceae)

PLANT PART USED

Leaf

CHEMICAL COMPONENTS

Gymnema contains gymnemasaponins, gymnemasides, gymnemic acids and gypenosides (Duke 2003), oleanane-type triterpenic acid (Peng et al 2005), flavonol glycosides (Liu et al 2004) and phenolic compounds (Kang et al 2012), as well as a range of nutrients, including ascorbic acid, beta-carotene, chromium, iron, magnesium and potassium. The main active chemical components appear to be the gymnemic acids, gymnemasaponins and the polypeptide gurmarin.

MAIN ACTIONS

Sweet-taste suppression

It appears that gymnema possesses a number of taste-suppressive substances, some of which are effective in certain animal species and not others. For example, in rats and mice, the constituent gumarin inhibits the ability to taste sweetness (Harada & Kasahara 2000, Kurihara 1969, 1992) but not in humans (Sigoillot et al 2012). In contrast, gymnemic acid, a triterpenoid saponin, increases sweet taste suppression in humans and chimpanzees (Hellekant et al 1996, 1985) but not in rodents (Hellekant et al 1976).

Antidiabetic

Extensive preclinical research has been conducted with gymnema and several of its isolated constituents in numerous diabetic models. Gymnema's antidiabetic activity appears to be due to a combination of mechanisms, including reduction of intestinal absorption of glucose (Shimizu et al 2001), inhibition of active glucose transport in the small intestine (Yoshioka 1986), suppression of glucose-mediated release of gastric inhibitory peptide (Fushiki et al 1992), increased activity of the enzymes responsible for glucose uptake and use (Shanmugasundaram et al 1983), stimulation of insulin secretion (Persaud et al 1999, Sugihara et al 2000) and increasing the number of islets of Langerhans and number of pancreatic beta cells (Prakash et al 1986, Shanmugasundaram et al 1990). *Gymnema montanum* (a related species) has also been shown to have antidiabetic, antiperoxidative and antioxidant effects in diabetic rats (Ananthan et al 2003) and antioxidant activity evident in the liver, kidney (Ananthan et al 2004) and brain tissues (Ramkumar et al 2004).

Animal studies suggest that gymnema will reduce blood glucose levels in response to a glucose load in streptozotocin-induced mildly diabetic rats (Okabayashi et al 1990) and alloxan-induced diabetic rats (Shanmugasundaram et al 1983, Srivastava et al 1985), but will not affect blood glucose levels in normal or spontaneously hypertensive rats (Preuss et al 1998). Gymnema extract has been found to return blood sugar and insulin levels to normal in streptozotocin-induced diabetic rats after 20–60 days and to double the number of pancreatic islet and beta cells (Shanmugasundaram et al 1990), as well as maintain stable blood glucose levels in rats given beryllium nitrate (Prakash et al 1986). One experimental rat model using streptozotocin to induce type 1 diabetes found that a standardised extract of gymnema, containing 70% of gymnemic acids, produced a significant decrease in blood glucose levels progressing for each of the 3 weeks of the experiment (Jain et al 2006).

In contrast, there are two in vivo studies that have not demonstrated efficacy in diabetic models. One study using a dose of 120 mg/kg/day oral gymnema did not find improvements in insulin resistance in insulin-resistant, streptozotocin-induced diabetic rats (Tominaga et al 1995) and the other study, from Brazil using dried powdered leaves of gymnema, found no effect on blood glucose, body weight or food or water consumption in non-diabetic and alloxan-diabetic rats (Galletto et al

2004). The concentration of gymnemic acids used in these studies is unknown.

Gymnemic acids have demonstrated hypoglycaemic activity in dexamethasone-induced hyperglycaemic mice (Gholap & Kar 2005) and gymnema, together with other Ayurvedic herbs, has been shown to have hypoglycaemic activity in streptozotocin-induced diabetic mice (Mutalik et al 2005) and rats (Babu & Prince 2004). Gymnema has also been shown to protect the lens against sugar-induced cataract by multiple mechanisms (Moghaddam et al 2005) and protect against the adverse effects of lipid peroxidation on brain and retinal cholinesterases, suggesting a use in preventing the cholinergic neural and retinal complications of hyperglycaemia in diabetes (Ramkumar et al 2005). In diabetic rats, gymnema extract decreased the activity of glutathione peroxidase in the liver and glutamate pyruvate transaminase in serum to normal levels and decreased lipid peroxidation levels in serum (31.7%), the liver (9.9%) and the kidney (9.1%). Phenolic compounds were thought to be responsible for this activity (Kang et al 2012).

Used in combination

A combination of gymnema, *Acacia catechu* and *Pterocarpus marsupium* was found to significantly elevate serum insulin levels in an animal model (Wadood et al 2007). The effect was thought to be due to beta cell regeneration. A polyformula of 18 herbs (Diabegon), including gymnema, was administered to rats resulting in improvement in insulin resistance and dyslipidaemia (Yadav et al 2007). Another polyherbal formula (Diakyur) also demonstrated significant hypoglycaemic activity and antilipid peroxidative effect (Joshi et al 2007). While these studies demonstrate the success of these specific herbal formulas, it is unclear what role gymnema had in producing these results.

Lipid lowering and weight loss activity

Gymnema extract reduces fat digestibility and increases faecal excretion of cholesterol, neutral sterols and acid steroids, as well as reducing serum cholesterol and triglyceride levels, according to animal studies (Nakamura et al 1999, Shigematsu et al 2001). A saponin-rich aqueous leaf extract of *Gymnema sylvestre* was studied in obese rats fed a high-fat diet for 8 weeks. An oral dose of 100 mg/kg of body weight was administered once a day to the treatment group (Reddy et al 2012). It significantly decreased food consumption, body weight and visceral organ weight and improved lipid profiles (decreased triglycerides, total cholesterol, low-density lipoproteins, very low-density lipoproteins, atherogenic index and increased levels of high-density lipoproteins). Another study in obese rats induced by a high-fat diet displayed similar findings. Rats fed a high fat diet for 28 days were treated with a standardised ethanolic extract of gymnema (200 mg/kg). The treatment group demonstrated a significant decrease in BMI, weight gain, organ weights and food intake, serum lipids (decreased total cholesterol, triglycerides, LDL-cholesterol, VLDL-cholesterol, apolipoprotein-B, atherogenic index and increased HDL-cholesterol and apolipoprotein-A1) and haemodynamic parameters (systolic, diastolic, mean arterial BP and heart rate). Other findings included significantly decreased serum leptin, insulin, glucose and lactate dehydrogenase (LDH), as well as decreased oxidative stress and prevention of myocardial apoptosis by decreasing cardiac caspase-3 levels, cardiac DNA fragmentation and increasing the cardiac Na-K ATPase levels (Kumar et al 2012).

G

Antimicrobial, antibacterial, antiviral and larvicidal

The ethanolic extract of *Gymnema sylvestre* leaves demonstrated antimicrobial activity against *Bacillus pumilis*, *B. subtilis*, *Pseudomonas aeruginosa* and *Staphylococcus aureus*, but was found inactive against *Proteus vulgaris* and *Escherichia coli* (Satdive et al 2003). This finding was confirmed in a later in vitro study which found that gymnemic acid extract exerted strong antibacterial activity against *Bacillus subtilis*, *Staphylococcus aureus*, *Klebsiella pneumoniae*, *Pseudomonas aeruginosa* and *Salmonella typhi* (Poonkothai et al 2005). Unlike the study by Satdive et al (2003), this study did identify activity against *Escherichia coli*. Antiviral activity has also been reported (Porchezhian & Dobriyal 2003). A larvicidal effect has been demonstrated for a 5% concentration of aqueous extract of *Gymnema sylvestre* leaves against *Culex quinquefasciatus* larvae (Gopiesh 2007). The treatment was 100% effective.

OTHER ACTIONS

Gymnema contains a constituent with ATPase inhibitor activity, which has been shown to block the effect of ATPase from snake venom (Manjunatha & Veerabasappa 1982). A significant anti-inflammatory activity was discovered for an aqueous extract of gymnema leaves, which was comparable to that of the drug phenylbutazone in a carrageenan-induced paw oedema animal model (Malik 2008).

CLINICAL USE

Several different gymnema extracts have been tested in clinical studies. An ethanolic acid-precipitated extract from gymnema, known as GS4, has been used in several human trials and been patented as the product ProBeta. Most commercial preparations are standardised for gymnemic acids.

Sweet-taste suppression and weight loss

A controlled trial of normal volunteers found that an aqueous gymnema extract with concentrated gymnemic acid reduced sweetness perception by 50%, resulting in reduced caloric consumption 1.5 hours after the sweetness-numbing effect stopped (Brala & Hagen 1983.

IN COMBINATION

In a 6-week randomised, double-blind, placebo-controlled study, a multiherbal formula that included gymnema was found to significantly reduce body weight and fat loss in obese adults after 6 weeks (Woodgate & Conquer 2003); however, the role of gymnema in achieving these results is unknown. A double-blind, placebo-controlled, RCT compared (–)-hydroxycitric acid (HCA-SX) with HCA plus a combination of chromium and *Gymnema sylvestre* extract. In this study, a group of 29 volunteers, in the obese BMI range, were divided into three groups and given the supplements or placebo for 8 weeks and all subjects were provided with a 2000 kcal diet per day and a supervised 30-minute walk for 5 days each week. The study combined data from two previous double-blind, placebo-controlled RCTs and reported that both the HCA-SX group and, to a greater degree, the group with the added chromium and gymnema experienced weight loss, decreased appetite, improvement in blood lipids, higher serum leptin and serotonin levels plus an increase in fat oxidation (Preuss et al 2005).). This result supports the findings of several animal studies.

Type 1 and type 2 diabetes

Orally, gymnema leaf is used to treat both type 1 and type 2 diabetes and hyperglycaemia. There are several clinical trials that suggest that gymnema may be useful in reducing blood glucose levels in both type 1 and type 2 diabetes.

Early clinical research was conducted in the 1980s, starting in India. In 1981, Shanmugasundaram et al showed that oral administration of the dried leaves of *G. sylvestre* (GS4) decreased blood glucose and raised serum insulin levels, during an oral glucose tolerance test in alloxan diabetic rabbits and in healthy human volunteers. Administration of dried leaves for a period of 10 days lowered blood glucose and increased the glucose-triggered rise in serum insulin levels in a single case of maturity onset diabetes, suggesting possible repair or regeneration of the *beta* cells in the Islets of Langerhans (Shanmugasundaram et al 1981).

This was followed by a second clinical study of 27 patients with type 1 diabetes who were treated with an aqueous extract of gymnema leaves (GS4 200 mg taken after breakfast and again after dinner) in addition to insulin and compared to 37 controls receiving insulin alone. Active treatment was for a minimum of 6 months. Over time, the groups receiving gymnema started to develop hypoglycaemia and insulin doses were reduced by 10 units at a time, ending at a dose nearly half the initial dose. Treatment also significantly reduced HbA_{1C} level in the first 6–8 months of therapy ($P < 0.001$) and reductions were also observed for glycosylated plasma protein levels, cholesterol, triglycerides and serum amylase. It was suggested that gymnema treatment enhanced endogenous insulin, possibly by regeneration/revitalisation of the residual beta cells as higher levels of serum C-peptide were found (Shanmugasundaram et al 1990).

In one study, the ability of the GS4 extract (400 mg/day) to supplement the use of conventional oral hypoglycaemic agents (glibenclamide or tolbutamide) was studied in 22 patients with type 2 diabetes over 18–20 months. Treatment resulted in a significant reduction in fasting blood glucose (174 ± 7 vs 124 ± 5 mg/dL), HbA_{1C} (11.91 ± 0.3 vs 8.48 ± 0.13%) and glycosylated plasma protein levels (3.74 ± 0.07 vs 2.46 ± 0.05 microgram hexose/mg protein) and raised insulin levels, whereas no changes were observed in the control group. This allowed for a decrease in conventional drug dosage and in five cases, blood glucose homeostasis was maintained with GS4 alone, suggesting that beta-cell function may have been restored (Baskaran et al 1990).

Recently, a novel high molecular weight gymnema extract (Om Santal Adivasi (OSA) was tested for effects on plasma insulin in 11 patients with type 2 diabetes (Al-Romaiyan et al 2010). In 10 of 11 patients, oral treatment with OSA (1 g/day, 60 days) was associated with a reduction in fasting blood glucose levels with a mean reduction from 162 ± 23 to 119 ± 17 mg/dL ($P < 0.005$). Postprandial blood glucose levels also showed significant reductions in 10 patients, with a reduction from 291 ± 10 to 236 ± 30 mg/dL ($P < 0.02$) and there was a mean increase in serum insulin from 24 ± 9 to 32 ± 6 U/mL ($P < 0.001$), Improvements in glycaemic control were associated with increased levels of insulin and/or C-peptide in all patients from 298 ± 42 to 447 ± 48 pmol/L ($P < 0.05$).

IN COMBINATION

A small, double-blind, randomised, placebo-controlled trial of a multiherbal Ayurvedic formula containing gymnema showed significantly improved glucose control and reduced HbA_{1C} levels in patients with type 2 diabetes within the 3-month test period (Hsia et al 2004).

Clinical note — Herbs and diabetes

Diabetes has been recognised since ancient times, and as early as 700–200 BC two types of diabetes were recorded in India, one of which was diet related and the other was described as genetic. Diabetes has also been recognised in China for thousands of years, where it is attributed to yin deficiency and treated with an integrated approach that involves more than lowering blood glucose. At least 30 different herbal medicines are used in the management of diabetes and its complications, with several of these having outstanding beneficial potential.

Hypercholesterolaemia and hypertriglyceridaemia

Short-term animal studies have shown that gymnema extracts are able to reduce serum cholesterol and triglyceride levels in experimentally induced hyperlipidaemic rats (Bishayee & Chatterjee 1994) and in spontaneously hypertensive rats (Preuss et al 1998), as well as in humans with type 2 diabetes (Shanmugasundaram et al 1990). These results have not yet been established by long-term studies. A recent rat experiment demonstrated reduced hyperlipidaemia and weight loss without rebound effect after the treatment was withdrawn for 3 weeks (Luo et al 2007).

OTHER USES

Gymnema has been used as a snakebite cure because it inhibits venom ATPase (Manjunatha & Veerabasappa 1982), and has also been used as a leaf paste to treat toe mycosis.

An insecticide against mosquitos may be another use due to its larvicidal properties.

In Ayurvedic medicine, gymnema is used as an antimalarial, digestive stimulant, laxative and diuretic and as a treatment for cough, fever, urinary conditions and diabetes.

DOSAGE RANGE

The typical therapeutic dose of an extract, standardised to contain 24% gymnemic acids, is 400–600 mg/day. When used to regulate blood sugar, gymnema may best be administered in divided doses with meals.

Diabetes

- Liquid extract (1:1): 25–75 mL/week or 3.6–11.0 mL/day.
- 6–60 g/day of dried leaf infusion.

Sweet craving and reducing sweet perception

- Liquid extract (1:1): 1–2 mL dropped onto the tongue and rinsed off — repeat every 2–3 hours as required.

ADVERSE REACTIONS

No clinically significant side effects have been reported in clinical trials lasting up to 3 years. At higher doses, gastric irritation can occur because of the saponin content. In this event, the dose should be decreased, or administered after eating. Gymnema liquid extracts will affect sweet-taste suppression of all foods, not just sugars. If gymnema is not being used as a sweet taste suppressor, it may be administered after eating to avoid decreasing the palatability of food.

Hepatotoxicity

There are two case reports of hepatotoxicity resulting from the consumption of a weight-loss formula containing gymnema and other herbs, including *Garcinia cambogia*, willow bark, glucomannan, green tea and guarana. Whether gymnema was the main causative factor remains unclear. There has been one case report in the literature linking gymnema to hepatotoxicity. A 60-year-old type 2 diabetic female with a BMI of 33 presented with fatigue, weakness, jaundice, anorexia and weight loss. Seventeen days prior she had started taking a *Gymnema sylvestre* tea (dose unknown, consumed three times per day). Her symptoms appeared on the seventh day and she discontinued use on the tenth day. The patient had also been taking acetazolamide for the past 2 years. Investigations found elevated bilirubin and transaminases; a minimally enlarged liver with steatosis on abdominal ultrasound and steatosis and inflammation on biopsy. The patient was prescribed prednisone and a proton-pump inhibitor. After monthly monitoring, bilirubin and transaminases returned to normal after 6 months. The gymnema was not re-challenged and was not tested to rule out adulteration, contamination or substitution (Shiyovich et al 2010).

G

SIGNIFICANT INTERACTIONS

Controlled studies are not available; therefore, interactions are based on evidence of activity and are largely theoretical and speculative.

Hypoglycaemic agents and insulin

Gymnema may enhance the blood glucose-lowering effects of insulin and hypoglycaemic agents, and so should be used with caution. In practice, the interaction may be useful, as a reduction in the drug dose could theoretically be achieved under professional supervision.

Contraindications and precautions

Blood glucose levels should be monitored closely when used in conjunction with insulin and hypoglycaemic agents.

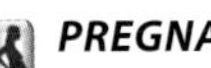

PREGNANCY USE

There is insufficient reliable information available about the safety of gymnema in pregnancy.

Practice points/Patient counselling

- Gymnema liquid extracts suppress the ability to taste sweet on the tongue.
- It may be useful as a weight-loss aid, according to preliminary research.
- Clinical studies have shown that gymnema may be useful to help control blood sugar levels in diabetes and also reduce lipid levels.
- When used with hypoglycaemic medications, blood sugar levels need to be monitored to prevent hypoglycaemia.
- Preliminary research suggests that it may also have a role in elevated cholesterol and triglyceride levels.

PATIENTS' FAQs

What will this herb do for me?

Gymnema has the ability to reduce the tongue's perception of sweetness. It may also improve blood glucose handling in diabetics, reduce lipid levels and possibly aid in weight loss.

When will it start to work?

Liquid extracts reduce the taste of sweetness rapidly, lasting for several hours, but effects on blood sugar regulation develop with long-term use.

Are there any safety issues?

Diabetic patients on medication should carefully monitor their blood sugar levels when taking this herb to avoid hypoglycemia.

REFERENCES

Al-Romaiyan A et al. A novel Gymnema sylvestre extract stimulates insulin secretion from human islets in vivo and in vitro. Phytother Res, 24.9 (2010): 1370–1376.

Ananthan R et al. Antidiabetic effect of Gymnema montanum leaves: effect on lipid peroxidation induced oxidative stress in experimental diabetes. Pharmacol Res 48.6 (2003): 551–556.

Ananthan R et al. Modulatory effects of Gymnema montanum leaf extract on alloxan-induced oxidative stress in Wistar rats. Nutrition 20.3 (2004): 280–285.

Babu PS, Prince PSM. Antihyperglycaemic and antioxidant effect of hyponidd, an ayurvedic herbomineral formulation in streptozotocin-induced diabetic rats. J Pharm Pharmacol 56.11 (2004): 1435–1442.

Baskaran K et al. Antidiabetic effect of leaf extract from Gymnema sylvestre in non-insulin-dependent diabetes mellitus patients. J Ethnopharmacol 30.3 (1990): 295–300.

Bishayee A, Chatterjee M. Hypolipidaemic and antiatherosclerotic effects of oral Gymnema sylvestre R. Br leaf extract in albino rats fed on a high fat diet. Phytother Res 8 (1994): 118–120.

Brala PM, Hagen RL. Effects of sweetness perception and calorie value of a preload on short term intake. Physiol Behav 30.1 (1983): 1–9.

Duke JA (ed). Dr Duke's Phytochemical and Ethnobotanical Databases. Beltsville, MD: US Department of Agriculture–Agricultural Research Service–National Germplasm Resources Laboratory, Beltsville Agricultural Research Center, 2003. www.ars-grin.gov/duke (accessed January 2008).

Fushiki T et al. An extract of Gymnema sylvestre leaves and purified gymnemic acid inhibits glucose-stimulated gastric inhibitory peptide secretion in rats. J Nutr 122.12 (1992): 2367–2373.

Galletto R et al. Absence of antidiabetic and hypolipidemic effect of Gymnema sylvestre in non-diabetic and alloxan-diabetic rats. Braz Arch Biol Technol 47.4 (2004): 545–551.

Gholap S, Kar A. Gymnemic acids from Gymnema sylvestre potentially regulates dexamethasone-induced hyperglycemia in mice. Pharm Biol 43.2 (2005): 192–195.

Gopiesh KV. Larvicidal effect of Hemidesmus indicus, Gymnema sylvestre, and Eclipta prostrate against Culex qinquifaciatus mosquito larvae. Afr J Biotechnol 6.3 (2007): 307–311.

Harada S, Kasahara Y. Inhibitory effect of gurmarin on palatal taste responses to amino acids in the rat. Am J Physiol Reg Integr Comp Physiol 278.6 (2000): R1513–R15117.

Hellekant G et al. On the effects of gymnemic acid in the hamster and rat. Acta Physiol Scand 98.2 (1976): 136–42.

Hellekant G et al. Effects of gymnemic acid on the chorda tympani proper nerve responses to sweet, sour, salty and bitter taste stimuli in the chimpanzee. Acta Physiol Scand 124.3 (1985): 399–408.

Hellekant G et al. Taste in chimpanzee: I. The summated response to sweeteners and the effect of gymnemic acid. Physiol Behav 60.2 (1996): 469–479.

Hsia SH et al. Effect of pancreas tonic (an Ayurvedic herbal supplement) in type 2 diabetes mellitus. Metab Clin Exp 53.9 (2004): 1166–1173.

Jain S et al. Efficacy of standardised herbal extracts in type 1 diabetes — an experimental study. Afr J Trad Comp Alt Med 3.4 (2006): 23–33.

Joshi C et al. Hypoglycemic and Antilipidperoxidative effects of a polyherbal formulation, Diakyur, in experimental animal models. J Health Sci 53.6 (2007): 734–739.

Kang MH et al. Hypoglycemic activity of Gymnema sylvestre extracts on oxidative stress and antioxidant status in diabetic rats. J Agric Food Chem 60.10 (2012): 2517–2524.

Kumar V et al. Evaluation of antiobesity and cardioprotective effect of Gymnema sylvestre extract in murine model. Indian J Pharmacol 44.5 (2012): 607–613.

Kurihara T. Antisweet activity of gymnemic acid A1 and its derivatives. Life Sci 8.9 (1969): 537–543.

Kurihara Y. Characteristics of antisweet substances, sweet proteins, and sweetness-inducing proteins. Crit Rev Food Sci Nutr 32.3 (1992): 231–252.

Liu X et al. Two new flavonol glycosides from Gymnema sylvestre and Euphorbia ebracteolata. Carbohydr Res 339.4 (2004): 891–895.

Luo H et al. Decreased bodyweight without rebound and regulated lipoprotein metabolism by gymnemate in genetic multifactor syndrome animal. Mol Cell Biochem 299.1–2 (2007): 93–98.

Malik J. Evaluation of anti-inflammatory activity of Gymnema sylvestre leaves extract in rats. Int J Green Pharm 2.2 (2008): 114–15.

Manjunatha Kini R, Veerabasappa Gowda T. Studies on snake venom enzymes. Part II: partial characterization of ATPases from Russell's viper (Vipera russelli) venom and their interaction with potassium gymnemate. Indian J Biochem Biophys 19.5 (1982): 342–346.

Moghaddam MS et al. Effect of Diabecon on sugar-induced lens opacity in organ culture: mechanism of action. J Ethnopharmacol 97.2 (2005): 397–403.

Mutalik S et al. Effect of Dianex, a herbal formulation on experimentally induced diabetes mellitus. Phytother Res 19.5 (2005): 409–415.

Nakamura Y et al. Fecal steroid excretion is increased in rats by oral administration of gymnemic acids contained in Gymnema sylvestre leaves. J Nutr 129.6 (1999): 1214–1222.

Okabayashi Y et al. Effect of Gymnema sylvestre. R.Br. on glucose homeostasis in rats. Diabetes Res Clin Pract 9.2 (1990): 143–148.

Peng S et al. A novel triterpenic acid from Gymnema sylvestre. Chin Chem Lett 16.2 (2005): 223–4.

Persaud SJ et al. Gymnema sylvestre stimulates insulin release in vitro by increased membrane permeability. J Endocrinol 163.2 (1999): 207–212.

Poonkothai M et al. Antibacterial activity of Gymnema sylvestre. J Ecotoxicol Environ Monit 15.1 (2005): 33–36.

Porchezhian E, Dobriyal RM. An overview on the advances of Gymnema sylvestre: chemistry, pharmacology and patents. Pharmazie 58.1 (2003): 5–12.

Prakash AO et al. Effect of feeding Gymnema sylvestre leaves on blood glucose in beryllium nitrate treated rats. J Ethnopharmacol 18.2 (1986): 143–146.

Preuss HG et al. Comparative effects of chromium, vanadium and Gymnema sylvestre on sugar-induced blood pressure elevations in SHR. J Am Coll Nutr 17.2 (1998): 116–123.

Preuss HG et al. Efficacy of a novel calcium/potassium salt of (-)-hydroxycitric acid in weight control. Int J Clin Pharmacol Res 25.3 (2005): 133–144.

Ramkumar KM et al. Modulatory effect of Gymnema montanum leaf extract on brain antioxidant status and lipid peroxidation in diabetic rats. J Med Food 7.3 (2004): 366–371.

Ramkumar KM et al. Modulation of impaired cholinesterase activity in experimental diabetes: effect of Gymnema montanum leaf extract. J Basic Clin Physiol Pharmacol 16.1 (2005): 17–35.

Reddy RM et al. The saponin-rich fraction of a Gymnema sylvestre R. Br. aqueous leaf extract reduces cafeteria and high-fat diet-induced obesity. Z Naturforsch C. 67.1–2 (2012): 39–46.

Satdive RK et al. Antimicrobial activity of Gymnema sylvestre leaf extract. Fitoterapia 74.7 (2003): 699–701.

Shanmugasundaram K.R et al. The insulinotropic activity of Gymnema sylvestre, R. Br. An Indian medical herb used in controlling diabetes mellitus. Pharmacol Res Commun 13.5 (1981): 475–486.

Shanmugasundaram KR et al. Enzyme changes and glucose utilisation in diabetic rabbits: the effect of Gymnema sylvestre R.Br. J Ethnopharmacol 7.2 (1983): 205–234.

Shanmugasundaram ER et al. Use of Gymnema sylvestre leaf extract in the control of blood glucose in insulin-dependent diabetes mellitus. J Ethnopharmacol 30.3 (1990): 281–294.

Shanmugasundaram KR et al. Possible regeneration of the islets of Langerhans in streptozotocin-diabetic rats given Gymnema sylvestre leaf extracts. J Ethnopharmacol 30.3 (1990): 265–279.

Shigematsu N et al. Effect of administration with the extract of Gymnema sylvestre R. Br leaves on lipid metabolism in rats. Biol Pharm Bull 24.6 (2001): 713–717.

Shimizu K et al. Structure-activity relationships of triterpenoid derivatives extracted from Gymnema inodorum leaves on glucose absorption. Jpn J Pharmacol 86.2 (2001): 223–229.

Shiyovich A et al. Toxic hepatitis induced by Gymnema sylvestre, a natural remedy for type 2 diabetes mellitus. Am J Med Sci 340.6 (2010): 514–517.

Sigoillot M et al. Sweet-taste suppressing compounds: current knowledge and perspectives of application. Appl Microbiol Biotechnol. 96.3 (2012): 619–630.

Srivastava Y et al. Hypoglycemic and life-prolonging properties of Gymnema sylvestre leaf extract in diabetic rats. Isr J Med Sci 21.6 (1985): 540–542.

Sugihara Y et al. Antihyperglycemic effects of gymnemic acid IV, a compound derived from Gymnema sylvestre leaves in streptozotocin-diabetic mice. J Asian Natural Prod Res 2.4 (2000): 321–327.

Tominaga M et al. Effects of seishin-renshi-in and Gymnema sylvestre on insulin resistance in streptozotocin-induced diabetic rats. Diabetes Res Clin Pract 29.1 (1995): 11–117.

Wadood N et al. Effect of a compound recipe (medicinal plants) on serum insulin levels of alloxan induced diabetic rabbits. J Ayub Med Coll Abbottabad 19.1 (2007): 32–38.
Woodgate DE, Conquer JA. Effects of a stimulant-free dietary supplement on body weight and fat loss in obese adults: a six-week exploratory study. Curr Ther Res 64.4 (2003): 248–262.
Yadav H et al. Preventive effect of diabegon, a polyherbal preparation, during progression of diabetes induced by high-fructose feeding in rats. J Pharmacol Sci 105.1 (2007): 12–21.Chapter
Yoshioka S. Inhibitory effects of gymnemic acid and an extract from the leaves of Zizyphus jujuba on glucose absorption in the rat small intestine. J Yonago Med Assoc 37 (1986): 142–154.

Hawthorn

HISTORICAL NOTE The name 'hawthorn' comes from 'hedgethorn', after its use as a living fence in much of Europe. Dioscorides and Paracelsus praised hawthorn for its heart-strengthening properties and it is also known in traditional Chinese medicine. It has since been shown to have many different positive effects on the heart and is a popular prescription medicine in Germany for heart failure (Rigelsky & Sweet 2002).

COMMON NAME

Hawthorn

OTHER NAMES

Aubepine, bianco spino, crataegi (azarolus, flos, folium, folium cum flore [flowering top], fructus [berry], nigra, pentagyna, sinaica boiss), English hawthorn, Chinese hawthorn, fructus oxyacanthae, fructus spinae albae, hagedorn, hedgethorn, maybush, maythorn, meidorn, oneseed hawthorn, shanzha, weissdorn, whitehorn

BOTANICAL NAME/FAMILY

Crataegus laevigata, C. cuneata, C. oxyacantha, C. monogyna, C. pinnatifida (family Rosaceae [Rose])

PLANT PARTS USED

Extracts of the leaf and flower are most commonly used, although the fruit (berries) may also be used.

CHEMICAL COMPONENTS

Leaves and flowers contain about 1% flavonoids, such as rutin, quercetin, vitexin, hyperoside, 1–3% oligomeric procyanidins, including catechin and epicatechin, triterpenes, sterols, polyphenols, coumarins, tannins (Blumenthal et al 2000). Although the therapeutic actions cannot be attributed to single compounds, the herb has been standardised to flavonoid content (hyperoside as marker) and procyanidins (epicatechin as marker). For example, RP WS 1442 is a hydroalcoholic extract of hawthorn prepared from leaves and blossoms and standardised to 18.75% oligomeric procyanidins. It has been found that bioequivalent extracts, as determined by noradrenaline-induced contraction of isolated guinea pig aorta rings, can be obtained using 40–70% ethanol or methanol as the extraction solvent, whereas aqueous extracts had markedly different constituents and pharmacological effects (Vierling et al 2003).

In vivo absorption studies found that oral administration of hawthorn phenolic extract resulted in detectable plasma levels of epicatechin whereas no hyperoside and isoquercetin were detected, indicating poor bioavailability of these compounds (Chang et al 2005). A year later the same authors, who used in vitro and in vivo experiments, showed that all three constituents have limited permeabilities and co-occurring extract components seem to have no significant effect on their intestinal absorption (Zuo et al 2006). Research with another important constituent, vitexin-2''-O-rhamnoside, showed that passive diffusion dominates its absorptive transport behaviour, and that the absorption and secretion are mediated by the efflux transport system P-glycoprotein (Xu et al 2008).

MAIN ACTIONS

Cardiovascular effects

The mechanisms of action for hawthorn have been extensively studied in vitro and in vivo. There is good research evidence to support cardiovascular actions that include increasing the force of myocardial contraction (positive inotropic action), increasing coronary blood flow, reducing myocardial oxygen demand, protecting against myocardial damage, improving heart rate variability and stroke volume, as well as hypotensive and antiarrhythmic effects (Garjani et al 2000, Mills & Bone 2000, Popping et al 1995).

Positive inotrope

Studies with animal models indicate that hawthorn exerts a positive inotropic effect similar to the beta-adrenergic agonist isoprenaline and the cardiac glycoside ouabain. The pharmacological mechanism appears to be comparable to the cAMP-independent positive inotropic action of cardiac glycosides which is mediated via inhibition of the sodium pump (Na^+/K^+-ATPase). Preclinical research shows it does not inhibit phosphodiesterases or a beta-sympathomimetic action (Koch & Malek 2011).

Antiarrhythmic effect and negative chronotropic effect

Crataegus extract blocks repolarising potassium currents in ventricular myocytes, an effect similar to the action of class III antiarrhythmic drugs, which might be the basis for its observed antiarrhythmic effects (Muller et al 1999). Hawthorn therefore differs from other inotropic agents, which reduce the refractory period and increase the risk of arrhythmias. In contrast, it increases the refractory period, which is thought to contribute to its arrhythmic effects (Joseph et al 1995). Additionally, hawthorn extract does not cause beta-adrenergic receptor blockade at concentrations which cause negative chronotropic effects (Long et al 2006). A study elucidated that the decreased chronotropic effect in rat cardiomyocytes may be mediated via muscarinic receptors (Salehi et al 2009).

Cardioprotective effect

In vitro and in vivo studies confirm that hawthorn extract has a significant cardioprotective effect against ischaemia and ischaemic reperfusion injury (Al Makdessi et al 1996, 1999, Jayachandran et al 2010, Jayalakshmi & Devaraj 2004, Min et al 2005, Swaminathan et al 2010, Veveris et al 2004). For example, pretreatment with alcohol-based hawthorn extract maintained mitochondrial status, and prevented mitochondrial lipid peroxidative damage and decrease in Kreb's cycle enzymes following induced myocardial infarction in rats (Jayalakshmi et al 2006).

Interestingly, hawthorn treatment modifies left ventricular remodelling and counteracts myocardial dysfunction in animal models of cardiac hypertrophy (Hwang et al 2008). In a rat study, hawthorn demonstrated marked suppression of aortic constriction and modest beneficial effects on cardiac remodelling and function in a long-term, pressure overload-induced model of heart failure (Hwang et al 2009).

Coronary blood flow

An increase in coronary blood flow for hawthorn extracts has repeatedly been demonstrated in multiple models.

When testing hawthorn extract WS 1442 for its effect on relaxation of rat aorta and human mammalian artery, it was shown to induce an endothelium-dependent, nitric oxide (NO)-mediated vasorelaxation (Anselm et al 2009, Brixius et al 2006, Rieckeheer et al 2011). The increase in coronary blood flow is dose-dependent (Siegel et al 1996). Moreover, long-term treatment with WS 1442 also reduced age-related endothelial dysfunction in rats by reducing the prostanoid-mediated contractile responses and decreasing cyclooxygenase-1 (COX-1) and COX-2 (Idris-Khodja et al 2012).

Much of hawthorn's cardiovascular activity is attributed to its flavonoid constituents (Nemecz 1999) and hawthorn extract is classified as a flavonoid drug in Germany. Studies using isolated guinea pig hearts suggest that the oligomeric procyanidins contribute to the vasodilating and positive inotropic effects of hawthorn (Schussler et al 1995), and ischaemia–reperfusion studies in rats suggest that these compounds are also responsible for cardioprotective effects (Chatterjee et al 1997).

It has been reported that hawthorn extracts prepared from dried leaves and those made from dried berries have similar chronotropic activities and that the extracts may contain multiple cardioactive components, because following various chromatographic steps, several fractions retained multiple cardiac activities (Long et al 2006).

Several procyanidins found in relatively high concentrations in hawthorn have shown angiotensin-converting enzyme (ACE) inhibition in vitro, in a reversible and non-competitive manner (Murray 1995, Uchida et al 1987).

Preventing restenosis

Hawthorn extract may prevent atherosclerosis and restenosis following angioplasty. Hawthorn extract WS 1442 (100 mcg/mL) taken from day 2 to day 13 after angioplasty reduced vascular smooth-muscle cell migration by 38% and proliferation by 44% and improved luminal volume compared to controls (Furst et al 2010).

No antiplatelet or antithrombotic activity

A small open, crossover trial testing *Crataegus laevigata* (2.4 g/day of Crataesor; equivalent to 50 mg of flavonoids and 134 mg of proanthocyanidins) found no inhibition of platelet aggregation or thromboxane A_2 synthesis compared to aspirin (100 mg/day) in 16 healthy volunteers after 15 days. Although *Crataegus laevigata* does not display antiplatelet effects as a stand-alone treatment, this has not been tested in patients with atherothrombotic vascular disease in conjunction with antiplatelet drugs (Dalli et al 2011b).

Antioxidant

Direct and indirect antioxidant activity plays a role in the herb's ability to exert cardioprotective effects. It can protect human low-density lipoprotein (LDL) from oxidation and maintain alpha-tocopherol (Periera et al 2000, Rajalakshmi et al 2000, Zhang et al 2001). The ethanolic hawthorn extract restores glutathione and the activity of endogenous antioxidant enzymes such as superoxide dismutase, catalase and glutathione peroxidase (Akila & Devaraj 2008, Ljubuncic et al 2005, Vijayan et al 2012).

Hawthorn's free radical-scavenging capacity is mainly related to its total phenolic proanthocyanidin and flavonoid content (Bahorun et al 1996, Kiselova et al 2006, Rakotoarison et al 1997). This is supported by a study that demonstrated that the capacity of hawthorn extracts to inhibit Cu^{2+}-induced LDL oxidation is linked to their content of total polyphenols, proanthocyanidins (global and oligomeric forms), as well as to their content of two individual phenolics: a flavonol, the dimeric procyanidin B_2, and a flavonol glycoside, hyperoside (Quettier-Deleu et al 2003). The highest antioxidant activity appears to be found in the flower buds, which are high in proanthocyanidin content, and the leaves, which are high in flavonoid content (Bahorun et al 1994), whereas the fresh and dried fruits possess less antioxidant activity.

When compared, epicatechin was found to be more efficient as an antioxidant than hyperoside or chlorogenic acid (Bernatoniene et al 2008, Sokól-Letowska et al 2007). Bernatoniene et al (2008) found that both aqueous and ethanolic hawthorn extracts have antioxidant activity, but that the effect displayed by the ethanolic extract was stronger. Moreover, the radical scavenging properties were higher for both extracts when a combination rather than individual constituents was compared (Bernatoniene et al 2008, Sokól-Letowska et al 2007).

Lipid lowering

Hawthorn extracts lower blood cholesterol levels in vivo, an effect mediated by several different mechanisms. Most recently, the effect was demonstrated in a study with diabetic volunteers.

One study identified that hawthorn extract given to rats while on an atherogenic diet (4% cholesterol, 1% cholic acid, 0.5% thiouracil) prevented the elevation of lipids in the serum and heart, and also significantly decreased lipid accumulation in the liver and aorta, thus reversing the rats' hyperlipidaemic conditions (Akila & Devaraj 2008). Similarly, rats fed dried fruit of *Crataegus pinnatifida* in conjunction with a high-cholesterol diet over 4 weeks displayed markedly suppressed total cholesterol and LDL and an increase in high-density lipoprotein (HDL) when compared to rats fed a high-cholesterol diet alone. In addition, rats in the treatment group demonstrated less hepatocyte enlargement, fatty deposits in the liver and improved antioxidant enzyme activities in liver and kidney (Kwok et al 2010).

The monomeric catechins and oligomeric procyanidins are thought to contribute to a hypocholesterolaemic effect. This may occur through a variety of mechanisms, including an upregulation of hepatic LDL receptors, increased degradation of cholesterol to bile acids and decreased cholesterol biosynthesis (Rajendran et al 1996), as well as inhibition of cholesterol absorption mediated by downregulation of intestinal acyl coenzyme A: cholesterol acyltransferase activity (Zhang et al 2002). Moreover, in mice hawthorn flavonoids increased lipoprotein lipase expression in muscular tissue and decreased it in adipose tissue (Fan et al 2006).

Antiviral

The *O*-glycosidic flavonoids and the oligomeric proanthocyanidins exhibited significant inhibitory activity against herpes simplex virus type 1 in vitro (Shahat et al 2002).

Antimicrobial

Hawthorn extracts showed moderate bactericidal activity, especially against Gram-positive bacteria *Micrococcus flavus*, *Bacillus subtilis* and *Lysteria monocytogenes*. Hawthorn was ineffective against *Candida albicans* (Tadic et al 2008).

Anti-inflammatory

Flavonoids from hawthorn have demonstrated anti-inflammatory and hepatoprotective activity in vitro and in vivo. In a model of carrageenan-induced rat paw oedema, orally administered hawthorn extract showed dose-dependent anti-inflammatory effects. Compared to an indomethacin dose producing 50% reduction of rat paw oedema, a dose of 200 mg/kg hawthorn extract produced 72.4% of anti-inflammatory activity (Tadic et al 2008). Hawthorn fruit has been shown to be protective in experimental models of inflammatory bowel disease in mice, with restoration of body weight and colon length, increased haemoglobin count, reduced signs of inflammation, such as infiltration by polymorphonuclear leukocytes and multiple erosive lesions, along with improved survival (Fujisawa et al 2005).

H

It is thought that anti-inflammatory effects are achieved by reducing the release of prostaglandin E_2 and NO in vitro, as well as decreasing the serum levels of the hepatic enzyme markers, reducing the incidence of liver lesions, such as neutrophil infiltration and necrosis, and decreasing the hepatic expression of inducible nitric oxide synthase (iNOS) and COX-2 in vivo (Kao et al 2005). A hydroalcoholic extract from the flower heads of *C. oxyacantha* has also been found to inhibit thromboxane A_2 biosynthesis in vitro (Nemecz 1999). An aqueous extract of *C. pinnatifida* inhibited NO and suppressed COX-2, tumour necrosis factor (TNF)-alpha, interleukin 6 (IL-6) and IL-1β expression in murine cell culture (Li & Wang 2011).

Chemopreventive effects have been postulated after the inhibition of skin tumour formation, a decrease in the incidence of tumour, inhibition of NF-kappaB and suppressed expression of COX-2 and iNOS were detected when using the polyphenol fraction of hot-water extracts from dried fruits of *C. pinnatifida* (Kao et al 2007).

A dry extract of leaves and flowers of *C. laevigata* inhibited *N*-formyl-Met-Leu-Phe (FMLP)-induced superoxide anion generation, elastase release and chemotactic migration in human neutrophils. It also reduced FMLP-induced leukotriene B_4 production and lipopolysaccharide-induced generation of TNF-alpha and IL-8 (Dalli et al 2008).

In a study using 62 male rats, no effect on IL-1ss, IL-6, IL-10 and leptin could be detected. However, there was a trend suggesting suppression of IL-2 plasma concentrations (Bleske et al 2007).

Radioprotective

A study using mouse bone marrow cells showed that a single intraperitoneal administration of hawthorn extract 1 hour prior to gamma radiation can significantly reduce the frequencies of micronucleated polychromatic erythrocytes and significantly increase the ratio of polychromatic erythrocyte/ polychromatic erythrocyte + normochromatic erythrocyte. Such a protective effect against genotoxicity appeared to be related to the antioxidant activity of the extract (Hosseinimehr et al 2007). The significant radioprotective potential of hawthorn was also detected in vitro using human peripheral blood lymphocytes. A reduced incidence of radiation-induced micronuclei, reduced levels of lipid peroxidation products and twofold enhanced apoptosis were observed. A stepwise slowdown of cell proliferation was seen as beneficial, thus enabling more time for repair (Leskovac et al 2007). Blood lymphocytes were extracted from human volunteers at different timeframes following ingestion of *C. microphylla*. Lymphocytes were exposed to gamma radiation, then assessed for binucleated cells. Hawthorn extract was most effective at reducing multinucleated cells 1 hour after ingestion (Hosseinimehr et al 2009).

Protection against ischaemic damage

Hawthorn flavonoids have also been shown to decrease the cytotoxicity of hypoxia to human umbilical vein endothelial cells in vitro (Lan et al 2005), as well as protect against delayed cell death caused by ischaemia-reperfusion brain injury in gerbils (Zhang et al 2004). These effects have been attributed to improving energy metabolism, scavenging oxygen free radicals and inhibiting production of free radicals in ischaemic myocardium (Min et al 2005, Zhang et al 2004). Hawthorn may also display neuroprotective effects. Rats pretreated with hawthorn extract displayed reduced brain damage and improved neurological behaviour after middle cerebral artery occlusion induced ischaemia-reperfusion injury (Elango et al 2009).

OTHER ACTIONS

The high procyanidin content in the herb provides a theoretical basis for other actions such as antiallergic and collagen-stabilising effects. Oligomeric procyanidins isolated from the leaves of *Crataegus pinnatifida* have demonstrated collagenase and gelatinase inhibitory activity (Moon et al 2010).

Moreover, a hawthorn extract has been shown to produce dose-dependent gastroprotective activity, with the efficacy comparable to ranitidine (Tadic et al 2008).

An aqueous extract of hawthorn leaves exhibited hypoglycaemic activity in streptozotocin-diabetic rats, but not in normal rats, without affecting basal plasma insulin concentrations (Jouad et al 2003). Hawthorn has also been found to have hepatoprotective effects in rats with myocardial infarction, with protection against alterations in tissue marker enzymes of experimentally-induced liver injury and a reversal of histological changes (Thirupurasundari et al 2005).

The dried fruit of *Crataegus monogyna* was investigated for effects on anxiety levels, motor coordination, spontaneous locomotor activity and nociceptive perception in mice. Findings suggested the treatment exhibited central nervous system-depressant activities, as well as central and peripheral analgesic effects. These were thought to be mediated by the endogenous opioid system (Can et al 2010). This correlates with the traditional use of hawthorn for nervous heart conditions and neurasthenia (Felter 1922).

CLINICAL USE

Congestive heart failure

There is considerable experimental and clinical evidence supporting the use of hawthorn as an effective treatment for congestive cardiac failure in patients with slight, mild limitation of activity who are comfortable at rest or with mild exertion (i.e. New York Heart Association [NYHA] class I-II). Systematic reviews and meta-analyses published since 2000 have consistently reported positive effects on a range of common symptoms and objective markers in mild congestive heart failure (CHF). Some studies have tested hawthorn extract as stand-alone therapy and others as an adjunct to standard treatment, mainly pharmaceutical diuretics. Some newer research also suggests that people with high-pressure-heart rate product increase and low maximal workload would be expected to benefit most.

The aqueous alcoholic extracts from the flowers and leaves of hawthorn that are most commonly used in trials are WS 1442 (Crataegutt forte, Schwabe Pharmaceuticals) which is standardised to 17.3–20.1% oligomeric procyanidins (4–6.6: 1 extracted in 45% ethanol) and LI 132 (70% methanol extract, MCM Klosterfrau Vertriebsgesellschaft).

A 2008 Cochrane systematic review of 14 randomised, placebo-controlled, double-blind clinical trials concluded that, in patients using hawthorn extract, symptoms such as shortness of breath and fatigue significantly improved, exercise tolerance significantly increased, the outcome measure of maximal workload significantly improved and the pressure-heart rate product (index for cardiac oxygen consumption) beneficially decreased. No data on relevant mortality and morbidity such as cardiac events were reported, except for one trial which reported deaths (three in active, one in control) without providing further details (Pittler et al 2008).

Since then, several new studies have been published which provide greater understanding of the benefits and limitations of treatment with hawthorn extracts. Eggeling et al (2011) conducted a combined analysis of 10 clinical trials (n = 687) with hawthorn extract (900 mg/day WS 1442) or placebo using pooled data from patients with early CHF (NYHA class I–III). The groups taking hawthorn showed significantly improved maximal workload compared to placebo ($P = 0.013$), with the benefits most significant in patients with the poorest baseline performance. Active treatment also significantly increased left ventricular ejection fraction (LVEF: +1.8) compared to placebo (+0.5) groups ($P < 0.001$). Pressure-heart rate product increase was more effective in the hawthorn group (−9.03 mmHg/

min) compared to placebo (+3.73 mmHg/min) ($P < 0.001$), with the treatment effect increasing with baseline severity. Overall, the majority of symptoms improved within the first 6 months, as measured with the von Zerssen scale, with significant improvements in physical symptoms of dyspnoea, weakness and fatigue, along with psychological symptoms such as worrying, irritability or restlessness. Researchers also confirmed the effects were similar for male and female patients (Eggeling et al 2011).

In contrast, Zick et al (2009) studied the effects of WS 1442 extract (450 mg twice daily) on 6-minute walking distance in a randomised, double-blind, placebo-controlled trial of 120 patients with NYHA class II or III CHF and an LVEF <40%. In the HERB CHF study, patients continued standard treatment (ACE inhibitor or angiotensin receptor antagonist, a beta-blocker and a diuretic) while also taking active treatment or placebo over 6 months. At the end of the test period, hawthorn treatment did not increase 6-minute walking distance compared to placebo. There were also no significant changes to secondary outcomes such as peak exercise oxygen consumption or anaerobic threshold by maximal cardiopulmonary testing, quality of life measures (measured with the Minnesota Living with Heart Failure Questionnaire scale) and no significant linear trend in the change in NYHA (Zick et al 2009).

A closer look at these reports and previous research suggests that the typical dose range used for hawthorn extracts in patients with CHF (NYHA class I–II) is between 160 and 900 mg daily, whereas the dose range tested and shown to work for patients with CHF NYHA class III is 900–1800 mg daily (Tauchert 2002). Since the effects on exercise capacity and clinical signs and symptoms are dose-dependent and nearly half the patients in the study by Zick et al (2009) had more severe CHF (NYHA class III), it is possible that a higher dosage was required to achieve positive results; however this remains to be confirmed. It is also possible that, since the HERB CHF study participants were also using contemporary pharmaceutical treatment (ACE inhibitor or angiotensin receptor antagonist, a beta-blocker and a diuretic for NYHA class II + spironolactone for NYHA III), few further benefits were possible.

Cardiac mortality and heart failure progression

Whether or not hawthorn, like phosphodiesterase inhibitors, has adverse effects on the prognosis of patients with chronic heart failure has been the subject of investigation recently.

Holubarsch et al (2008) conducted a large, international, multicentre, randomised, double-blind, placebo-controlled study involving 2681 patients with NYHA class II or III CHF and reduced LVEF (≤35%) despite being on standard treatment (Holubarsch et al 2008). Active treatment consisted of WS 1442 extract (900 mg daily) taken as add-on therapy, which did not alter the time to the first cardiac event but did significantly reduce cardiac mortality after 6 months ($P = 0.009$) and at 18 months ($P = 0.046$). For the subgroup of patients with LVEF ≥25%, sudden cardiac death was reduced by 39.7% ($P = 0.025$) in comparison to the placebo group. Treatment was well tolerated with effects similar to placebo.

Zick et al (2008) found that patients with CHF (NYHA classes II–III) and reduced LVEF (<40%) taking WS 1442 (900 mg/day) over 6 months had no difference in the clinical progression of heart failure compared to placebo ($P = 0.86$). Subgroup analysis of 68 participants with LVEF 35% found they were similar to the whole group, with no significant increase compared to placebo (Zick et al 2008). However, hawthorn treatment significantly increased the risk for progression of heart failure at baseline and in the more clinically compromised patients with LVEF ≤35% in this study. Communication with the authors identified that the test groups were not similar and further research is required to clarify these results.

Comparative studies

One study compared hawthorn extract LI 132 (Crataegutt novo 300 mg three times daily) to the ACE inhibitor captopril (12.5 mg three times daily) in 132 patients and found that the LI 132 extract improved exercise tolerance and decreased heart failure-related symptoms (Tauchert et al 1994).

Similarly, a prospective cohort study involving 952 patients with NYHA stage II heart failure compared the use of the WS 1442 extract of hawthorn either alone or in conjunction with conventional therapy to conventional medication. After 2 years, the hawthorn cohort was found to have similar or more pronounced improvements than the conventional medication group with reduced fatigue, stress dyspnoea and palpitations, along with marked reduction in the use of drugs such as ACE inhibitors, cardiac glycosides, diuretics and beta-blockers (Habs 2004).

Commission E supports the use of hawthorn leaf and flower to treat decreased cardiac output (NYHA class II) (Blumenthal et al 2000).

Arrhythmias, hypertension and atherosclerosis

In addition to treating congestive cardiac failure, hawthorn has traditionally been used to treat arrhythmias, hypertension and atherosclerosis (Petkov 1979). Blood pressure-lowering activity appears to take several weeks to establish and is not seen after acute dosing.

In one double-blind randomised controlled trial (RCT) of 92 subjects aged 40–60 years, a hydroalcoholic extract of Iranian hawthorn (*C. curvisepala* Lind) given three times daily was found to produce a significant decrease in both systolic and diastolic blood pressure after 3 months. Antihypertensive activity was also observed in one uncontrolled study that used hawthorn berry tincture (equivalent to 4.3 g/day of berry) (Mills & Bone 2000).

One study that focused primarily on mild hypertension compared the hypotensive effect of low-dose hawthorn extract (500 mg) and magnesium supplements, individually and in combination, to placebo. Walker et al (2002) found hawthorn treatment significantly reduced resting diastolic blood pressure at week 10 compared with the other groups. In addition, a trend towards a reduction in anxiety was also observed with hawthorn treatment, which is an interesting observation, as sedative effects have been observed in animal models.

A 2006 randomised, placebo-controlled, clinical trial ($n = 79$) focused for the first time on investigating possible hypotensive effects of hawthorn extract (1200 mg daily) in patients with type 2 diabetes while taking standard medication. Hypotensive drugs were used by 71% of the participants, with a mean intake of 4.4 hypoglycaemic and/or hypotensive drugs. The hawthorn group showed significantly greater reduction than the placebo group in mean diastolic blood pressure, but not in systolic blood pressure (Walker et al 2006).

Brachial artery flow-mediated dilation (FMD) and hypotensive activity were further investigated in an RCT crossover trial involving 21 volunteers with pre-hypertension or mildly elevated blood pressure (systolic 120–155 mmHg and diastolic 80–95 mmHg). Hawthorn extract (a 4:1 250 mg capsule standardised to 50 mg oligomeric procyanidins) was compared to placebo for effects on brachial artery FMD, an indirect measure of NO release and blood pressure. Each participant received four different dosage levels (placebo, hawthorn extract at 1000 mg, 1500 mg and 2500 mg) over 3½ days, with a 4-day washout period in between. The study found no evidence of a blood pressure-lowering effect or of a dose–response effect of hawthorn extract on FMD (Asher et al 2012). Limitations of this study include the extremely short treatment time.

Other studies have demonstrated hypotensive activity with treatment times between 10 and 16 weeks (Asgary et al 2004, Walker et al 2002, 2006) and the Commission E recommends a minimum treatment of 6 weeks.

IN COMBINATION FOR HYPOTENSION

Three double-blind RCTs have shown that a combination of natural D-camphor and an extract from fresh hawthorn berries was effective in treating orthostatic hypotension compared to placebo (Georg Belz & Loew 2003, Hempel et al 2005, Kroll et al 2005). Furthermore, when this combination of natural D-camphor and an extract from fresh hawthorn berries (marketed as Korodin) was given to hypotensive women in three randomised, double-blind, placebo-controlled, clinical trials, the treatment led to positive and differential effects on blood pressure and cognitive performance compared to placebo within 5 minutes (Schandry & Duschek 2008, Werner et al 2009).

Hyperlipidaemia

Hawthorn fruit extract has been reported to reduce serum lipid levels, as well as to reduce lipid deposits in the liver and aortas of rats (Shanthi et al 1994) and rabbits (Zhang et al 2002) fed a hyperlipidaemic diet. In combination with other traditionally used Chinese herbs, hawthorn has been shown to also reduce serum lipid levels in both animals (He 1990, La Cour et al 1995, Xu et al 2009) and humans (Chen et al 1995, Guan & Zhao 1995).

In a 2011 double-blind RCT of type 2 diabetic outpatients with chronic coronary heart disease, treatment with *Crataegus laevigata* (flower and leaf preparation, 400 mg three times a day, standardised to 5% of procyanidins and 2% flavonoids) over 6 months produced a significant reduction in total cholesterol ($P < 0.05$) and LDL ($P = 0.03$) compared to baseline, but no change in HDL-cholesterol or triglyceride levels. When compared to placebo, there was a trend to lower total cholesterol ($P = 0.11$) and LDL-cholesterol ($P = 0.054$). In addition, a statistically significant decrease in neutrophil elastase was observed (Dalli et al 2011a). Patients were also taking conventional treatment (including aspirin, statins, ACE inhibitors, beta-blockers or nitrates). No significant changes were observed for blood cell count, glucose, urea, creatinine, electrolytes, lipid peroxidation, C-reactive protein or malondialdehyde after 6 months.

Adjustment disorder

The results of a double-blind trial of 182 people suggest that hawthorn in combination with other herbs such as passionflower and valerian may be beneficial for people with adjustment disorder with anxious mood (Bourin et al 1996). Another double-blind trial of 264 people found that a combination containing *Crataegus oxyacantha* and *Eschscholzia californica* along with magnesium was effective in treating mild to moderate anxiety disorder (Hanus et al 2004).

OTHER USES

As it has a high flavonoid content, hawthorn is also used to strengthen connective tissue, decrease capillary fragility and prevent collagen destruction of joints and therefore may be beneficial in the treatment of certain connective tissue disorders (Mills & Bone 2000).

DOSAGE RANGE

- Infusion of dried herb: 0.2–2 g three times daily.
- Tincture of leaf (1:5): 3.5–17.5 mL/day.
- Fluid extract (1:2): 3–6 mL/day.
- Dry extract: 900–1200 mg/day.

According to clinical trials

LI 132 and WS 1442 are the most studied extracts.

- CHF (NYHA class I-II): 160–900 mg daily in divided doses.
- CHF (NYHA class III): 900–1800 mg daily in divided doses.
- Hyperlipidaemia: 1200 mg daily in divided doses.

TOXICITY

No target toxicity to 100-fold the human dose of the WS 1442 extract is defined (Schlegelmilch & Heywood 1994). This is in contrast to inotropic drugs, such as digoxin, which generally have a low therapeutic index. A preclinical toxicological assessment for a combination product consisting of hawthorn, passionflower and valerian demonstrated no toxicity, genotoxicity or mutagenicity in rats, mice and dogs at high doses over 180 days (Tabach et al 2009). No clinical, chemical, haematological, morphological or histological abnormalities could be identified in either dogs or rats following 26 weeks of oral treatment at doses of 30 mg, 90 mg or 300 mg/kg/day. There was no evidence of genotoxicity of any kind, including mutagenicity or clastogenicity. Postmarketing surveillance as well as animal and clinical studies has shown no safety signals for carcinogenicity (Koch & Malek 2011).

ADVERSE REACTIONS

A systematic review (24 clinical trials, n = 5577 patients) concluded that hawthorn extracts (mostly WS 1442, LI 132) were well tolerated at doses between 160 and 1800 mg daily for a duration of 3–24 weeks. Overall, 166 adverse events were reported, most of which were mild to moderate. Eight severe adverse effects had been reported with the LI 132 extract. The most frequent adverse effects were dizziness/vertigo (n = 15), gastrointestinal complaints (n = 24), headache (n = 9), migraine (n = 8) and palpitation (n = 11) (Daniele et al 2006). Similarly, a review of 14 clinical trials reported safe use of hawthorn with only infrequent, mild and transient adverse effects such as dizziness, cardiac and gastrointestinal complaints (Pittler et al 2008).

INTERACTIONS

WS 1442 (900 mg daily) was safe to use in patients (n > 2500) receiving optimal medication for heart failure (Holubarsch et al 2008). A systematic review (24 clinical trials) on the safety of hawthorn monopreparations found no reports of drug interactions (Daniele et al 2006).

Cardiac glycosides

Hawthorn may theoretically potentiate the effects of cardiac glycosides, as both in vitro and in vivo studies indicate that it has positive inotropic activity. Furthermore, the flavonoid components of hawthorn may also affect P-glycoprotein function and cause interactions with drugs that are P-glycoprotein substrates, such as digoxin. In practice, however, a randomised crossover trial with eight healthy volunteers evaluating digoxin 0.25 mg alone for 10 days and digoxin 0.25 mg with *Crataegus* special extract WS 1442 (hawthorn leaves with flowers) 450 mg twice daily for 21 days found no significant difference to any measured pharmacokinetic parameters, suggesting that hawthorn and digoxin in these doses may be co-administered safely (Tankanow et al 2003). Caution — use under professional supervision and monitor drug requirements.

Antiplatelet medication

A small open, crossover design trial investigated the antithrombotic effects of *Crataegus laevigata* compared to aspirin in 16 healthy volunteers. Patients were treated with either *C. laevigata* — a daily dose of 2.4 g of Crataesor (equivalent to 50 mg of flavonoids and 134 mg of proanthocyanidins), which is comparable to the standard dose of hawthorn used in most clinical trials for CHF (900 mg WS 1442 extract, equivalent to 70 mg of flavonoids and 153 mg of proanthocyanidins) — or aspirin (100 mg/day) for 15 days, with a washout period of 14 days between treatments. In contrast to aspirin, *C. laevigata* did not inhibit the synthesis of thromboxane A_2 or inhibit platelet aggregation. Although *C. laevigata* does not display antiplatelet effects as a stand-alone treatment, this has not been tested in patients with atherothrombotic vascular disease in conjunction with antiplatelet drugs. Monitor (Dalli et al 2011b).

H

Antihypertensive drugs

Theoretically, hawthorn may potentiate blood pressure-lowering effects, thereby requiring modified drug doses. However, hawthorn extract (1200 mg daily) was safe to use in patients with type 2 diabetes (n > 70) while taking their prescription drugs (mean intake of 4.4 hypoglycaemic and/or hypotensive drugs) (Walker et al 2006). In general, observe patients taking this combination and monitor drug requirements — interaction would be beneficial under professional supervision.

PREGNANCY USE

Hawthorn did not have an adverse effect on embryonic development in vitro and in vivo (Yao et al 2008). A combined extract of *Crataegus oxyacantha, Passiflora incarnata* and *Valeriana officinalis* in rats did not alter the oestrus cycle, did not affect fertility and did not induce teratogenesis in the offspring born from females treated during the entire pregnancy (Tabach et al 2009). Teratogenicity was not apparent in rats or rabbits following oral dosing with up to 1600 mg/kg WS 1442 (Koch & Malek 2011).

However, in vivo and in vitro evidence of uterine activity has been reported; therefore this herb should not be used in pregnancy until safety is established (Newell et al 1996).

PATIENTS' FAQs

What will this herb do for me?

Hawthorn appears to be useful in treating a variety of heart conditions, such as high blood pressure, hyperlipidaemia and mild heart failure.

Practice points/Patient counselling

- Hawthorn extract is an effective treatment for mild CHF and improves signs and symptoms of disease.
- Hawthorn has positive inotropic action, increases coronary blood flow, reduces myocardial oxygen demand, protects against myocardial damage and improves heart rate variability, as well as having hypotensive and antiarrhythmic effects.
- Although considered relatively effective, heart disease can be a very serious medical condition with a rapidly changing course and should not be treated without close medical supervision. In particular, chest pain and shortness of breath are extremely serious symptoms that require immediate medical attention.
- It may take 2–6 weeks' treatment to notice a benefit of treatment with hawthorn. For modest hypotensive effects at least 10 weeks are needed. Heart rate and blood pressure should be monitored.
- Hawthorn also exhibits antioxidant, anti-inflammatory, antiviral and lipid-lowering activity.
- Great care should be exercised if hawthorn is to be combined with other drugs that affect the heart.

When will it start to work?

Studies suggest it will start to have effects in 2–6 weeks. For modest hypotensive effects at least 10 weeks of treatment are needed.

Are there any safety issues?

Heart conditions are potentially serious, therefore professional supervision is required.

REFERENCES

Akila M, Devaraj H. Synergistic effect of tincture of *Crataegus* and *Mangifera indica* L. extract on hyperlipidemic and antioxidant status in atherogenic rats. Vascul Pharmacol 49 (2008): 173–7.

Al Makdessi S et al. Myocardial protection by pretreatment with *Crataegus oxyacantha*: an assessment by means of the release of lactate dehydrogenase by the ischemic and reperfused Langendorff heart. Arzneimittelforschung 46.1 (1996): 25–7.

Al Makdessi S et al. Protective effect of *Crataegus oxyacantha* against reperfusion arrhythmias after global no-flow ischemia in the rat heart. Basic Res Cardiol 94.2 (1999): 71–7.

Anselm E et al. *Crataegus* special extract WS 1442 causes endothelium-dependent relaxation via a redox-sensitive Src- and Akt-dependent activation of endothelial NO synthase but not via activation of estrogen receptors. J Cardiovasc Pharmacol 53.3 (2009): 253–60.

Asgary S et al. Antihypertensive effect of Iranian *Crataegus* curvisepala Lind.: a randomized, double-blind study. Drugs Exp Clin Res. 30.5–6(2004): 221–5.

Asher GN et al. Effect of hawthorn standardized extract on flow mediated dilation in prehypertensive and mildly hypertensive adults: a randomized, controlled cross-over trial. BMC Complementary and Alternative Medicine 12 (2012): 26.

Bahorun T et al. Antioxidant activities of *Crataegus monogyna* extracts. Planta Med 60.4 (1994): 323–8.

Bahorun T et al. Oxygen species scavenging activity of phenolic extracts from hawthorn fresh plant organs and pharmaceutical preparations. Arzneimittelforschung 46.11 (1996): 1086–9.

Bernatoniene J et al. Free radical-scavenging activities of *Crataegus monogyna* extracts. Medicina (Kaunas) 44.9 (2008): 706–12.

Bleske BE et al. Evaluation of hawthorn extract on immunomodulatory biomarkers in a pressure overload model of heart failure. Med Sci Monit 13.12 (2007): BR255–8.

Blumenthal M, et al. (eds). Herbal medicine: expanded Commission E monographs. Austin, TX: Integrative Medicine Communications, 2000.

Bourin M et al. A combination of plant extracts in the treatment of outpatients with adjustment disorder with anxious mood: controlled study versus placebo. Fundam Clin Pharmacol 11.2 (1996): 127–32.

Brixius K et al. *Crataegus* special extract WS 1442 induces an endothelium-dependent, NO-mediated vasorelaxation via eNOS-phosphorylation at serine 1177. Cardiovasc Drugs Ther 20.3 (2006): 177–84.

Can OD et al. Effects of hawthorn seed and pulp extracts on the central nervous system. Pharm Biol 48.8 (2010): 924–31.

Chang Q et al. Comparison of the pharmacokinetics of hawthorn phenolics in extract versus individual pure compound. J Clin Pharmacol 45.1 (2005): 106–12.

Chatterjee SS et al. In vitro and in vivo studies on the cardioprotective action of oligomeric procyanidins in a *Crataegus* extract of leaves and blooms. Arzneimittelforschung 47.7 (1997): 821–5.

Chen JD et al. Hawthorn (shan zha) drink and its lowering effect on blood lipid levels in humans and rats. World Rev Nutr Diet 77 (1995): 147–54.

Dalli E et al. Hawthorn extract inhibits human isolated neutrophil functions. Pharmacol Res 57.6 (2008): 445–50.

Dalli E et al. *Crataegus laevigata* decreases neutrophil elastase and has hypolipidemic effect: a randomized, double-blind, placebo-controlled trial. Phytomedicine 18.8–9 (2011a): 769–75.

Dalli E et al. Effects of hawthorn (*Crataegus laevigata*) on platelet aggregation in healthy volunteers. Thromb Res 128.4 (2011b): 398–400.

Daniele C et al. Adverse-event profile of *Crataegus* spp.: a systematic review. Drug Saf 29.6 (2006): 523–35.

Eggeling T et al. Baseline severity but not gender modulates quantified *Crataegus* extract effects in early heart failure — a pooled analysis of clinical trials. Phytomedicine 18.14 (2011): 1214–9.

Elango C, et al. Hawthorn extract reduces infarct volume and improves neurological score by reducing oxidative stress in ratbrain following middle cerebral artery occlusion. Int J Dev Neurosci 27.8 (2009): 799–803.

Fan C et al. Regulation of lipoprotein lipase expression by effect of hawthorn flavonoids on peroxisome proliferator response element pathway. J Pharmacol Sci 100.1 (2006): 51–8.

Felter HW 1922, The Eclectic Materia Medica, Pharmacology and Therapeutics. http://www.henriettesherbal.com/eclectic/felter/index.html

Fujisawa M et al. Protective effect of hawthorn fruit on murine experimental colitis. Am J Chin Med 33.2 (2005): 167–80.

Furst, R., et al. 2010. The *Crataegus* extract WS 1442 inhibits balloon catheter-induced intimal hyperplasia in the rat carotid artery by directly influencing PDGFR-beta. Atherosclerosis, 211, (2) 409–417.

Garjani A et al. Effects of extracts from flowering tops of *Crataegus meyeri* A. Pojark. on ischaemic arrhythmias in anaesthetized rats. Phytother Res 14.6 (2000): 428–31.

Georg Belz G, Loew D. Dose-response related efficacy in orthostatic hypotension of a fixed combination of D-camphor and an extract from fresh *Crataegus* berries and the contribution of the single components. Phytomedicine 10 (Suppl 4) (2003): 61–7.

Guan Y, Zhao S. Yishou jiangzhi (de-blood-lipid) tablets in the treatment of hyperlipidemia. J Trad Chin Med 15.3 (1995): 178–9.

Habs M. Prospective, comparative cohort studies and their contribution to the benefit assessments of therapeutic options: heart failure treatment with and without Hawthorn special extract WS 1442. Forsch Komplement Klass Naturheilk [Res Complement Nat Class Med] 11 (Suppl 1) (2004): 36–9.

Hanus M et al. Double-blind, randomised, placebo-controlled study to evaluate the efficacy and safety of a fixed combination containing two plant extracts (*Crataegus oxyacantha* and *Eschscholtzia californica*) and magnesium in mild-to-moderate anxiety disorders. Curr Med Res Opin 20.1 (2004): 63–71.

He G. Effect of the prevention and treatment of atherosclerosis of a mixture of hawthorn and motherworn. Zhong Xi Yi Jie He Za Zhi 10.6 (1990): 326–361.

Hempel B et al. Efficacy and safety of a herbal drug containing hawthorn berries and D-camphor in hypotension and orthostatic circulatory disorders/results of a retrospective epidemiologic cohort study. Arzneimittelforschung 55.8 (2005): 443–50.

Holubarsch CJ et al. The efficacy and safety of *Crataegus* extract WS(R) 1442 in patients with heart failure: The SPICE trial. Eur J Heart Fail 10.12 (2008): 1255–63.

Hosseinimehr SJ et al. Radioprotective effects of hawthorn fruit extract against gamma irradiation in mouse bone marrow cells. J Radiat Res (Tokyo) 48.1 (2007): 63–8.

Hosseinimehr SJ et al. Radioprotective effects of Hawthorn against genotoxicity induced by gamma irradiation in human blood lymphocytes. Radiat Environ Biophys 48.1 (2009): 95–8.

Hwang HS et al. Effects of hawthorn on cardiac remodeling and left ventricular dysfunction after 1 month of pressure overload-induced cardiac hypertrophy in rats. Cardiovasc Drugs Ther 22.1 (2008): 19–28.

Hwang HS et al. Effects of hawthorn on the progression of heart failure in a rat model of aortic constriction. Pharmacotherapy 29.6 (2009): 639–648.

Idris-Khodja N et al. *Crataegus* special extract WS(®)1442 prevents aging-related endothelial dysfunction. Phytomedicine 19.8–9 (2012): 699–706.

Jayachandran KS et al. *Crataegus oxycantha* extract attenuates apoptotic incidence in myocardial ischemia-reperfusion injury byregulating Akt and HIF-1 signaling pathways. J Cardiovasc Pharmacol 56.5 (2010):526–31.

Jayalakshmi R, Devaraj SN. Cardioprotective effect of tincture of *Crataegus* on isoproterenol-induced myocardial infarction in rats. J Pharm Pharmacol 56.7 (2004): 921–6.

Jayalakshmi R, et al. Pretreatment with alcoholic extract of *Crataegus oxycantha* (AEC) activates mitochondrial protection during isoproterenol-induced myocardial infarction in rats. Mol Cell Biochem 292.1–2 (2006): 59–67.

Joseph G, et al. Pharmacologic action profile of *Crataegus* extract in comparison to epinephrine, amirinone, milrinone and digoxin in the isolated perfused guinea pig heart. Arzneimittelforschung 45.12 (1995): 1261–5.

Jouad H et al. Hawthorn evokes a potent anti-hyperglycemic capacity in streptozotocin-induced diabetic rats. J Herb Pharmacother 3.2 (2003): 19–29.

Kao ES et al. Anti-inflammatory potential of flavonoid contents from dried fruit of *Crataegus pinnatifida* in vitro and in vivo. J Agric Food Chem 53.2 (2005): 430–6.

Kao ES et al. Effects of polyphenols derived from fruit of *Crataegus pinnatifida* on cell transformation, dermal edema and skin tumor formation by phorbol ester application. Food Chem Toxicol 45.10 (2007): 1795–804.

Kiselova Y et al. Correlation between the in vitro antioxidant activity and polyphenol content of aqueous extracts from Bulgarian herbs. Phytother Res 20.11 (2006): 961–5.

Koch, E. & Malek, F.A. 2011. Standardized extracts from hawthorn leaves and flowers in the treatment of cardiovascular disorders — preclinical and clinical studies. Planta Med, 77, (11) 1123–1128.

Kroll M et al. A randomized trial of Korodin® Herz-Kreislauf-Tropfen as add-on treatment in older patients with orthostatic hypotension. Phytomedicine 12.6–7 (2005): 395–402.

Kwok CY et al. Consumption of dried fruit of *Crataegus pinnatifida* (hawthorn) suppresses high-cholesterol diet-induced hypercholesterolemia in rats. J Funct Foods 2.3 (2010): 179–86

La Cour B, et al. Traditional Chinese medicine in treatment of hyperlipidaemia. J Ethnopharmacol 46.2 (1995): 125–9.

Lan W-J et al. Regulative effects of hawthorn leaves flavonoids on cytotoxicity, NO and Ca^{2+} in hypoxia-treated human umbilical vein endothelial cells. Hang Tian Yi Xue Yu Yi Xue Gong Cheng [Space Med Med Eng] 18.3 (2005): 157–60.

Leskovac A et al. Radioprotective properties of the phytochemically characterized extracts of *Crataegus monogyna*, *Cornus mas* and *Gentianella austriaca* on human lymphocytes in vitro. Planta Med 73.11 (2007): 1169–175.

Li C, Wang MH. Anti-inflammatory effect of the water fraction from hawthorn fruit on LPS-stimulated RAW 264.7 cells. Nutr Res Pract 5.2 (2011):101–6.

Ljubuncic P et al. Antioxidant activity of *Crataegus aronia* aqueous extract used in traditional Arab medicine in Israel. J Ethnopharmacol 101.1–3 (2005): 153–61.

Long SR et al. Effect of hawthorn (*Crataegus oxycantha*) crude extract and chromatographic fractions on multiple activities in a cultured cardiomyocyte assay. Phytomedicine 13.9–10 (2006): 643–650.

Mills S, Bone K. Principles and practice of phytotherapy. London: Churchill Livingstone, 2000.

Min Q et al. Protective effects of hawthorn leaves flavonoids on cardiac function in rats suffered from myocardial ischemia reperfusion injury. Chin Pharm J 40.7 (2005): 515–17.

Moon HI et al. Identification of potential and selective collagenase, gelatinase inhibitors from *Crataegus pinnatifida*. Bioorg Med Chem Lett 20.3 (2010): 991–3.

Muller A, et al. *Crataegus* extract blocks potassium currents in guinea pig ventricular cardiac myocytes. Planta Med 65.4 (1999): 335–9.

Murray M. The healing power of herbs. Rocklin, CA: Prima Health, 1995.

Nemecz G. Hawthorn. US Pharm 24.2 (1999). Online. Available: www.uspharmacist.com 1999.

Newell CA, et al. Herbal medicines: a guide for health care professionals. London, UK: The Pharmaceutical Press, 1996.

Periera DS et al. Antioxidants in medicinal plant extracts. A research study of the antioxidant capacity of *Crataegus*, *Hamamelis* and *Hydrastis*. Phytother Res 14.8 (2000): 612–16.

Petkov V. Plants and hypotensive, antiatheromatous and coronarodilatating action. Am J Chin Med 7.3 (1979): 197–236.

Pittler MH, et al. Hawthorn extract for treating chronic heart failure. Cochrane Database Syst Rev no. 1 (2008): CD005312.

Popping S et al. Effect of a hawthorn extract on contraction and energy turnover of isolated rat cardiomyocytes. Arzneimittelforschung 45.11 (1995): 1157–61.

Quettier-Deleu C et al. Hawthorn extracts inhibit LDL oxidation. Pharmazie 58.8 (2003): 577–81.

Rajalakshmi K, et al. Effect of eugenol and tincture of *Crataegus* (TCR) on in vitro oxidation of LDL + VLDL isolated from plasma of non-insulin dependent diabetic patients. Indian J Exp Biol 38.5 (2000): 509–11.

Rajendran S, et al. Effect of tincture of *Crataegus* on the LDL-receptor activity of hepatic plasma membrane of rats fed an atherogenic diet. Atherosclerosis 123.1–2 (1996): 235–41.

Rakotoarison DA et al. Antioxidant activities of polyphenolic extracts from flowers, in vitro callus and cell suspension cultures of *Crataegus monogyna*. Pharmazie 52.1 (1997): 60–4.

Rieckeheer E et al. Hawthorn special extract WS® 1442 increases red blood cell NO-formation without altering red blood cell deformability. Phytomedicine 15.19 (2011): 20–4.

Rigelsky JM, Sweet BV. Hawthorn: pharmacology and therapeutic uses. Am J Health Syst Pharm 59.5 (2002): 417–22.

Salehi S et al. Hawthorn (*Crataegus monogyna* Jacq.) extract exhibits atropine-sensitive activity in a cultured cardiomyocyte assay. Nat Med (Tokyo) 63.1 (2009): 1–8.

Schandry R, Duschek S. The effect of Camphor-*Crataegus* berry extract combination on blood pressure and mental functions in chronic hypotension — A randomized placebo controlled double blind design. Phytomedicine 15.11 (2008): 914–22.

Schlegelmilch R, Heywood R. Toxicity of *Crataegus* (hawthorn) extract (WS 1442). J Am Coll Toxicol 13.2 (1994): 103–11.

Schussler M, et al. Myocardial effects of flavonoids from *Crataegus* species. Arzneimittelforschung 45.8 (1995): 842–5.

Shahat AA et al. Antiviral and antioxidant activity of flavonoids and proanthocyanidins from *Crataegus sinaica*. Planta Med 68.6 (2002): 539–41.

Shanthi S et al. Hypolipidemic activity of tincture of *Crataegus* in rats. Indian J Biochem Biophys 31.2 (1994): 143–6.

Siegel G et al. Molecular physiological effector mechanisms of hawthorn extract in cardiac papillary muscle and coronary vascular smooth muscle. Phytother Res 10 (Suppl) (1996): S195–8.

Sokól-Letowska A, et al. Antioxidant activity of the phenolic compounds of hawthorn, pine and skullcap. Food Chemistry 103.3 (2007): 853–9.

Swaminathan JK et al. Cardioprotective properties of *Crataegus oxycantha* extract against ischemia-reperfusion injury. Phytomedicine 17.10 (2010):744–52.

Tabach R, et al. Preclinical toxicological assessment of a phytotherapeutic product — CPV (based on dry extracts of *Crataegus oxyacantha* L., *Passiflora incarnata* L., and *Valeriana officinalis* L.). Phytother Res 23.1 (2009): 33–40.

Tadic VM et al. Anti-inflammatory, gastroprotective, free-radical-scavenging, and antimicrobial activities of hawthorn berries ethanol extract. J Agric Food Chem 56.17 (2008): 7700–9.

Tankanow R et al. Interaction study between digoxin and a preparation of hawthorn (*Crataegus oxyacantha*). J Clin Pharmacol 43.6 (2003): 637–42.

Tauchert M. Efficacy and safety of *Crataegus* extract WS 1442 in comparison with placebo in patients with chronic stable New York Heart Association class-III heart failure. Am Heart J 143.5 (2002): 910–15.

Tauchert M, et al. High-dose *Crataegus* extract WS 1442 in the treatment of NYHA stage II heart failure. Herz 24.6 (1994): 465–74.

Thirupurasundari CJ et al. Liver architecture maintenance by tincture of *Crataegus* against isoproterenol-induced myocardially infarcted rats. J Med Food 8.3 (2005): 400–4.

Uchida S et al. Inhibitory effects of condensed tannins on angiotensin converting enzyme. Jpn J Pharmacol 43.2 (1987): 242–6.

Veveris M et al. *Crataegus* special extract WS(R) 1442 improves cardiac function and reduces infarct size in a rat model of prolonged coronary ischemia and reperfusion. Life Sci 74.15 (2004): 1945–55.

Vierling W et al. Investigation of the pharmaceutical and pharmacological equivalence of different Hawthorn extracts. Phytomedicine 10.1 (2003): 8–16.

Vijayan NA, et al. Anti-inflammatory and anti-apoptotic effects of *Crataegus oxyacantha* on isoproterenol-induced myocardialdamage. Mol Cell Biochem 367.1–2 (2012): 1–8.

Walker AF et al. Promising hypotensive effect of hawthorn extract: a randomized double-blind pilot study of mild, essential hypertension. Phytotherapy Res 16.1 (2002): 48–54.

Walker AF et al. Hypotensive effects of hawthorn for patients with diabetes taking prescription drugs: a randomised controlled trial. Br J Gen Pract 56.527 (2006): 437–43.
Werner NS, et al. D-camphor-*Crataegus* berry extract combination increases blood pressure and cognitive functioning in the elderly — a randomized, placebo controlled double blind study. Phytomedicine 16.12 (2009): 1077–82.
Xu YA et al. Assessment of intestinal absorption of vitexin-2''-o-rhamnoside in hawthorn leaves flavonoids in rat using in situ and in vitro absorption models. Drug Dev Ind Pharm 34.2 (2008): 164–70.
Xu H, et al. A study of the comparative effects of hawthorn fruit compound and simvastatin on lowering blood lipid levels. Am J Chin Med 37.5 (2009): 903–8.
Yao M, et al. A reproductive screening test of hawthorn. J Ethnopharmacol 118.1 (2008): 127–32.
Zhang Z et al. Characterization of antioxidants present in hawthorn fruits. J Nutr Biochem 12.3 (2001): 144–52.
Zhang Z et al. Hawthorn fruit is hypolipidemic in rabbits fed a high cholesterol diet. J Nutr 132.1 (2002): 5–10.
Zhang D-L et al. Oral administration of *Crataegus* flavonoids protects against ischemia/reperfusion brain damage in gerbils. J Neurochem 90.1 (2004): 211–219.
Zick SM, et al. The effect of *Crataegus* oxycantha Special Extract WS 1442 on clinical progression in patients with mild to moderate symptoms of heart failure. Eur J Heart Fail 10.6 (2008): 587–93.
Zick SM et al. Hawthorn Extract Randomized Blinded Chronic Heart Failure (HERB CHF) trial. Eur J Heart Fail 11.10 (2009): 990–9.
Zuo Z et al. Intestinal absorption of hawthorn flavonoids — in vitro, in situ and in vivo correlations. Life Sci 79.26 (2006): 2455–62.

Honey

HISTORICAL NOTE Honey has been used since ancient times as a healing agent for wounds and a treatment for gastric complaints. In ancient Greece, Hippocrates recommended honey and vinegar for pain and honey combinations for fever. Honey was included in about 500 remedies in ancient Egypt according to papyrus scrolls, from curing wounds to embalming the dead, and in ceremonies to promote fertility. Jars of honey have been found in ancient Egyptian temples, still edible after 3000 years. Early Ayurvedic, Chinese and Roman traditions also used honey in wound care and it is recommended in the Bible and the Koran as a medicinal agent (Lee et al 2011). Over the past few decades, scientific research has confirmed its role as a successful wound treatment.

CHEMICAL COMPONENTS

The composition of a particular honey greatly depends on the composition of the nectar it originated from, and therefore the plant species involved in its production.

Honey comprises a complex mix of glucose, fructose, sucrose, other carbohydrates, minerals, proteins, as well as other phytochemicals. It has a low pH and a significant osmolarity due to its low water content (Voidarou et al 2011).

The medicinal properties of honey have been attributed to various bioactive compounds including glucose oxidase, which generates hydrogen peroxide, flavonoid and phenolic compounds, methylglyoxal as well as methoxylated derivatives, with other active constituents still to be characterised (Fearnley et al 2011). The term 'unique manuka factor' (UMF) is used to describe the specific bioactive principles of manuka honey, derived from the tree genus *Leptospermum*, and is used as an indicator of relative potency of the specific honey (Fearnley et al 2011). A correlation between high concentrations of methylglyoxal and the notable antibacterial activity specific to manuka honey suggests that this may be a core active principle (Brudzynski et al 2011).

MAIN ACTIONS

Antibacterial

The type of plant species involved in honey production is significant, as some confer greater antibacterial properties than others. Currently, evidence suggests that honey produced from the tea trees *Leptospermum scoparium* (New Zealand manuka) and *Leptospermum polygalifolium* (Australian jelly bush), which are native to Australia and New Zealand, are the most clinically effective. However there is evidence to suggest that other honeys may also possess some antibacterial activity (Lusby et al 2005). Honey derived from the Malaysian tree *Koompassia excelsa* (Tualang tree), has shown particularly promising antibacterial activity (Tan et al 2009).

Research has demonstrated that honey has activity against a number of organisms, including *Escherichia coli*, *Pseudomonas aeruginosa*, *Staphylococcus aureus* (including methicillin-resistant strains), *Acinetobacter*, *Stenotrophomonas* and vancomycin-resistant *Enterococcus* (Lee et al 2011).

Several mechanisms of action account for the antibacterial effect of honey.

Hydrogen peroxide content

Honey contains a bee-derived enzyme, glucose oxidase, which, under certain conditions, can convert the glucose in honey to hydrogen peroxide. Researchers originally attributed much of the antibacterial activity of honey to this production of hydrogen peroxide. Factors such as dilution, the presence of a sodium from skin and body fluids and the pH of the body promote generation of hydrogen peroxide when honey is used in wound dressing. Clinically, however, it has been shown that the hydrogen peroxide is subsequently broken down by catalase, an enzyme present in wound fluids and in wound tissue cells, diminishing the amount available to support an antibacterial benefit. This suggests that although hydrogen peroxide may contribute towards the mechanism of action of honey, the main antibacterial activity may be due primarily to a non-peroxide-mediated mechanism (Brudzynski & Kim 2011, Packer et al 2012).

High osmolarity

Honey has a high sugar and low water content, with sugar concentration reaching up to 80% in some seasons. Its high sugar concentration is considered important because the honey draws fluid from the wound by osmosis, reducing the availability of water for bacteria. This results in inhibition of bacterial growth, while simultaneously creating a moist environment that promotes wound healing (Lusby et al 2002).

Low pH

Honey is an acidic substance (range 3.2–4.5) and therefore unfavourable to the growth of certain bacteria. *In vitro* testing shows that *Leptospermum* honey can inhibit the growth of several important bacterial pathogens, including *Escherichia coli*, *Salmonella typhimurium*, *Shigella sonnei*, *Listeria monocytogenes*, *Staphylococcus aureus*, *Bacillus cereus* and *Streptococcus mutans* (Steinberg et al 1996, Taormina et al 2001).

In a recent open-label, non-randomised prospective study, applying a manuka honey dressing to non-healing wounds was associated with a statistically significant decrease in wound pH and size. A reduction in pH of 0.1 was associated with an 8.1% reduction in wound size (Gethin et al 2008).

The antibacterial action of honey may be enhanced when combined with a synergistic compound. The antibacterial and antifungal activities of honey were increased by the addition of starch to the medium (Boukraa & Bouchegrane 2007, Boukraa & Amara 2008). When Royal Jelly was combined with four different samples of honey, the minimum inhibitory concentration (MIC) against *Staphylococcus aureus* was lowered by 50% (Boukraa et al 2008).

Honey has also been tested for efficacy against a range of drug-resistant bacteria, with positive results (Cooper et al 2002). Eighteen strains of methicillin-resistant *Staphylococcus aureus* and 27 strains of vancomycin-sensitive and -resistant enterococci, isolated from infected wounds and hospital surfaces, were sensitive to concentrations below 10% w/v of manuka honey and pasture honey. Artificial honey was also effective, but concentrations three times greater were required to produce similar results. In a study using a 10%–40% v/v medical-grade honey (Revamil®) applied to the skin of healthy volunteers colonised with antibiotic-susceptible and -resistant isolates of *Staphylococcus aureus*, *Staphylococcus epidermidis*, *Enterococcus faecium*, *Escherichia coli*, *Pseudomonas aeruginosa*, *Enterobacter cloacae* and *Klebsiella oxytoca*, bacterial levels were reduced 100-fold by day 2, and the number of positive skin cultures was reduced by 76% (Kwakman et al 2008).

Honey is effective (*in vitro*) against community-associated methicillin-resistant *Staphylococcus aureus* (CA-MRSA), which typically infects skin and soft tissues in healthy individuals. Culture counts of 10^6 colony-forming units were reduced to a non-detectable amount in 24 hours in the four honey samples tested, while levels in the control group (no honey) remained unchanged (Maeda et al 2008).

Phenolic compounds

The antioxidant activity of honey has been associated with the levels of phenolic compounds found in a range of floral honeys, with antioxidant activity varying between 43.0% and 95.7%. The responsible compounds suggested include p-coumaric acid, kaempferol, chrysin and apigenin (Baltrusaityte et al 2007).

The variation in the concentration of the phenolic compounds among different floral honeys is further confirmed through another study, which found that the concentration of millefiori honey is the highest in polyphenols, flavonoids and has a corresponding high antioxidant activity, when compared with *Acacia* honey (Blasa et al 2006). Manuka honey has been shown to contain significant levels of phenolic compounds and methoxylated derivatives such as methoxyphenyllactic acid, 2-methoxybenzoic acid and trimethoxybenzoic acid. It has been proposed that these phenolic compounds participate in scavenging of free radicals and in promoting wound healing.

Methylglyoxal

Recently, methylglyoxal, a bioactive compound found in high concentrations in manuka honey, has been identified as a significant contributing factor to the distinct antibacterial activity of manuka honey compared to other honeys. This compound confers a sustained non-peroxide antibacterial action to manuka honey, which is an advantage over the peroxide-derived action seen in other honeys, as it is not susceptible to catalase destruction from body fluids (Brudzynski & Kim 2011, Packer et al 2012).

Immunomodulation

An animal study has shown that both immunocompetent and immunodeficient mice had increased humoral immunity following administration with honey (Karmakar et al 2004). Tonks et al (2007) reported that manuka honey upregulates inflammatory cytokines: tumor necrosis factor-α, interleukin-1β, interleukin-6 and prostaglandin E_2 production, from monocytes, according to an *in vitro* study. The authors proposed that this immunomodulatory activity was mediated by a unique 5.8-kDa component found in manuka honey, via toll-like receptor 4 (TLR4) (Tonks et al 2007). Honey has been shown to reduce both acute and chronic inflammation, although the exact mechanism is not yet fully understood (Pieper 2009).

Antifungal

Honey has an antifungal action against three species of *Candida* in vitro (Irish et al 2006). Isolates of *C. albicans*, *C. glabrata* and *C. dubliniensis* were tested against four samples of honey: Jarrah honey with hydrogen peroxide activity, Medihoney Antibacterial Honey Barrier; a proprietary blend of

Leptospermum and hydrogen peroxide honeys, Comvita Wound Care; a pure *Leptospermum* honey; and an artificial honey. The natural honeys had a significantly greater antifungal effect compared to the artificial honey against *C. albicans* and *C. glabrata*, but only the Jarrah honey was effective against *C. dubliniesis*.

Deodorises wounds

Bacteria use the glucose found in honey in preference to amino acids, thereby producing lactic acid instead of malodorous products (Molan 2001).

Debriding

The topical application of honey to a wound may aid in wound debridement. Due to the osmolarity of honey, lymph fluid is pulled from wound tissue, debris is removed and slough and necrotic tissue is lifted off more easily. Hydrogen peroxide production may also contribute to honey's debridement properties (Pieper 2009). Honey does not adhere to the wound surface, allowing for easier and less painful wound dressing changes (Subrahmanyam 1998).

Enhances wound healing

Clinical evidence suggests that the application of honey hastens granulation and epithelialisation of necrotic tissue by various mechanisms. It appears to stimulate the growth of new blood capillaries and cytokine production, thereby stimulating tissue regeneration. The high viscosity of honey and its hygroscopic character allow it to form a physical barrier, creating a moist environment and a reduction in local oedema (Aysan et al 2002). Clinically, it appears that epithelialisation is accelerated between days 6 and 9 (Subrahmanyam 1998), and that honey is more beneficial than Edinburgh University solution of lime (EUSOL) as a wound-dressing agent (Okeniyi et al 2005). The upregulation of matrix metalloproteinase-9 and transforming growth factor-β in epidermal keratinocytes may also contribute to honey's wound-healing properties (Lee et al 2011).

Antioxidant

The phenolic compounds found in honey, namely the flavonoids, render it a good source of antioxidants (Al-Mamary et al 2002, Schramm et al 2003). The antioxidants in honey neutralise free radicals that arise through inflammatory processes (Molan 2001). In vitro tests have confirmed a significant link between absorbance and antioxidant power, with darker, more opaque honeys having stronger antioxidant power than lighter, clearer honeys (Taormina et al 2001). More specifically, manuka honey has been identified to be a specific scavenger of superoxide anions (Inoue et al 2005). A study examining different samples of honey for their ability to reduce reactive oxygen species (ROS) in vitro found significant variation in activity, with buckwheat honey most effective. This is possibly due to its high concentration of phenolic compounds, which have known antioxidant activity. Considering the fact that hydroxyl radicals and hypochlorite anions formed in the wound site impair wound healing, this honey should have superior wound-healing properties (van den Berg et al 2008). Regular daily consumption of honey (1.2 g/kg body weight) has been shown to increase serum levels of Vitamin C, beta-carotene, uric acid and glutathione reductase, according to the findings of a clinical study in 10 healthy individuals (Noori & Al-Waili 2004).

Bone metabolism

A study performed in ovariectomised rats showed that daily oral consumption of Tualang honey for two weeks promoted an increase in bone density, which was attributed to antioxidant effects and inhibition of proinflammatory cytokines (Zaid et al 2010). A subsequent study in experimental postmenopausal rats showed that daily oral administration of Tualang honey (0.2 mg/kg body weight) for 6 weeks resulted in a greater improvement in trabecular bone structure than calcium supplementation (1% in drinking water) (Zaid 2012). Based on these findings, it has been suggested that oral consumption of honey may confer protective effects against postmenopausal bone loss in women through antioxidant and anti-inflammatory action on osteoclast activity (Mohd Effendy et al 2012). There is, however, currently insufficient clinical evidence to recommend honey for this indication.

OTHER ACTIONS

An *in vitro* study showed that honey prevented binding of *Salmonella enteriditis* to intestinal epithelial cells (Alnaqdy et al 2005) at dilutions of up to 1:8.

Preliminary studies suggest that honey may have an impact on reducing the intoxicating effects of alcohol. Further, high quality research with more rigorous methodology is required to validate this effect (Onyesom 2004, 2005).

Honey may also have an antimutagenic activity against a common food carcinogen and mutagen, Trp-p-1 (Wang et al 2002).

CLINICAL USE

Honey is mainly used topically for wound healing, burns or dermatological conditions; however, it is now being used in mouthwashes, oral syrups and ocular preparations.

Wound healing

A recent Cochrane systematic review and meta-analysis of 25 trials was conducted to determine whether honey dressing increases the rate of healing in either acute wounds, such as lacerations and burns, or chronic wounds including skin ulcers and infected surgical wounds (Jull et al 2013). In summary, the review concluded that honey does not significantly increase healing in chronic leg ulcers and may delay healing of deep burns and ulcers caused by insect bites (cutaneous Leishmaniasis). It noted that there is currently insufficient evidence in other types of wounds to make clear recommendations (Jull et al 2013).

With respect to chronic venous leg ulcers, the Cochrane review (2013) reported that honey dressing does not significantly accelerate wound healing when used as an adjuvant to compression stockings, based on the evidence from two studies (Jull et al 2008, Gethin & Cowman 2008). The reviewers called for further research, given that a benefit may be possible, especially in population subgroups such as those with infected ulcers (Jull et al 2013).

Jull et al (2008) conducted an open-labelled, randomised controlled trial involving 368 patients with venous ulcers. This study found that honey dressings did not significantly decrease the time needed to heal compared to those treated with usual care (a range of dressings). After 12 weeks, 55.6% of ulcers healed in the honey-treated group and 49.7% in the usual care group. There were no significant differences found in the other parameters, including mean time to healing (63.5 days and 65.3 days in the honey and usual care groups, respectively), reduction in ulcer size, incidence of infections or quality of life between the groups (Jull et al 2008). There were also more adverse events reported in the honey-treated group, with 25% of participants reporting one or more episodes of discomfort.

The multi-centred open label randomised controlled study conducted by Gethin and Cowman (2009) recruited 108 participants with > 50% slough coverage on leg ulcers. Treatment consisted of either honey dressing plus compression, or hydrogel dressing plus compression for a period of 4 weeks, with a follow-up assessment at 12 weeks. After 4 weeks, there was a 67% mean reduction in slough area for the honey treated group compared to 52.9% in the hydrogel group ($P = 0.05$) and the median reduction in wound size was 34% compared to 13% respectively ($P = 0.001$). After 12 weeks, 44% of the ulcers had healed in the honey group versus 33% in the hydrogel group ($P = 0.04$). The authors concluded that manuka honey dressing resulted in a higher incidence of healing, with a lower incidence of infection (Gethin & Cowman 2009).

The Cochrane review (2013) also investigated the potential benefit of honey in abrasions, acute lacerations or minor surgical wounds. Three trials, with a combined total of 213 participants, were evaluated. The reviewers concluded that for these types of minor acute wounds, there is currently insufficient evidence to recommend honey dressing in preference to conventional therapy. It was suggested that further study was justified as a modest benefit in favour of honey dressing was considered possible (Jull et al 2013).

Data from some of the studies conducted with honey in wound management are presented below.

A case series of eight consecutive cases examined the efficacy of honey on non-healing lower limb ulcers. After 4 weeks of using a manuka honey dressing, ulcers decreased in size by a mean of 55% and were no longer malodorous. Patients whose ulcers had an arterial component reported the least benefit and also a stinging sensation following application (Gethin & Cowman 2005). One randomised study involving 40 patients with open or infected wounds compared honey to sugar dressings (Mphande et al 2007). In the honey group, 55% of patients had positive wound cultures at the start of treatment and 23% at one week, compared with 52% and 39% respectively in the sugar group. Additionally, the median rate of healing in the first 2 weeks of treatment was 3.8 cm^2/week for the honey group and 2.2 cm^2/week for the sugar group and after 3 weeks of treatment 86% of patients treated with honey had no pain during dressing changes, compared with 72% treated with sugar.

Emsen (2007) used medical honey for the fixation of the split-thickness skin grafts in 11 patients. Oedema and the amount of wound exudate were reduced, and no complications such as graft loss or infection were reported, either on the fifth day of grafting or at the end of the follow-up period (average 17 months).

Several studies have compared honey dressings to currently used treatments, finding it is as effective but not necessarily more effective.

A non-randomised, prospective, open study compared the effects of honey-impregnated gauze, paraffin gauze, hydrocolloid dressings and saline-soaked gauzes in 88 patients who underwent skin grafting (Misirlioglu et al 2003). Honey gauzes produced a faster epithelialisation and reduced the sensation of pain compared with paraffin and saline-soaked gauzes. This effect was the same as that observed for hydrocolloid dressings.

A RCT of 101 haemodialysis patients compared thrice-weekly application of Medihoney with mupirocin for the healing of catheter exit sites. This study found the honey to be safe, effective and more affordable than mupirocin for this group (Johnson et al 2005).

Burns

A recent Cochrane review (2013) concluded that honey dressing may reduce healing times in partial-thickness burns by an average of 4.68 days when compared to some conventional dressings such as polyurethane film dressing, impregnated gauze or saline soaks; however, the trials evaluated did not provide sufficient detail for findings to be considered conclusive (Jull et al 2013).

In the same review, efficacy of topical honey compared with that of silver sulfadiazine (SDD) was compared in six clinical trials. Although overall, evidence appears to be in favour of honey dressings, heterogeneity in trial design, burn assessment criteria, outcomes and follow-up periods make interpretation of the data challenging. It is still unclear whether honey either promotes healing, or is able to reduce healing times compared to SDD (Jull et al 2013).

The Cochrane review by Jull et al (2013) reports that current evidence indicates that for deeper or more extensive burns, surgical excision and skin grafting are a more suitable treatment approach than honey dressing. The recommendation is based on the findings of a small study (Subrahmanyam 1999) of 50 participants, where early excision and grafting resulted in significantly shorter hospital stays (weighted mean difference [WMD] 13.6 days, 95% CI 10.02 to 17.18 days) compared to use of honey wound dressings. In addition, 11 patients of the 25 assigned to treatment with honey dressing eventually required skin grafting. Three of the patients treated with honey dressing died of septicaemia, whereas none of the 25 patients in the excision group developed sepsis. At 3 months follow-up, 92% of the excision group had good to excellent functional and cosmetic results, compared to only 55% in the group treated with honey dressing (Subrahmanyam 1999).

Further research is required to determine the safety and efficacy of honey dressings in the management of burns, but current evidence suggests a possible role in minor burns, but that alternative treatments such as surgical excision and grafting are superior for deep or more extensive burns, unless the patient is unsuitable for surgery.

Coughs in children

A Cochrane review (2012) concluded that honey may be better than 'no treatment' and diphenydramine in relieving cough symptoms in children, but not better than dextromethorphan (Oduwole et al 2012).

In a randomised, partially double-blinded clinical trial involving 105 children, a single dose of buckwheat honey, given 30 minutes before bed, significantly reduced cough severity (47.3% versus 24.7%) and overall symptom score reduction (53.7% versus 33.4%) compared to no treatment (Warren & Cooper 2008). Similarly, Paul et al (2007) found that a single nighttime dose of buckwheat honey given to children with an upper respiratory tract infection resulted in greatest symptom improvement in nocturnal cough and sleeping difficulties compared to honey-flavoured dextromethorphan treatment or no treatment. A randomised controlled study involving 160 children demonstrated that a dose of 2.5 mL honey at bedtime was more effective than either dextromethorphan or diphenhydramine in alleviating night cough symptoms and sleep quality in children with upper respiratory infections (Shadkam et al 2010).

OTHER USES

Fournier's gangrene

The effects of topical honey has been investigated for the treatment of Fournier's gangrene (FG), a fulminating infection of the scrotum, perineum and abdominal wall in men. A study conducted in 30 male participants compared honey-soaked dressing to antiseptic EUSOL-soaked dressing (Subrahmanyam & Ugane 2004). Mean time to healing was reduced by 8 days in the honey-treated group (95% CI) compared to the EUSOL-treated group. Nine participants from each group required skin grafting and 1 patient from the honey-dressing group died, compared to 2 patients from the EUSOL dressing group. The authors concluded that honey dressings were beneficial in the treatment of Fournier's gangrene (Subrahmanyam & Ugane 2004). Validity of these findings have been questioned, however, since the comparator treatment, EUSOL dressings, has been shown to impair wound healing (Jull et al 2013). Further research is required to confirm a benefit before clear recommendations can be made.

Periodontal disease

In vitro tests show that honey can inhibit the growth of oral bacteria (Steinberg et al 1996). As a follow-up investigation, 10 volunteers were asked to swish 5 mL of honey around their mouths for 4 minutes and then swallow. At 10 minutes after honey use, oral bacterial counts were significantly decreased. A pilot study has also shown that manuka honey has potential in the treatment of gingivitis and periodontal disease (English et al 2004). Thirty subjects were given either a chewable 'honey leather' or a sugarless chewing gum to chew for 10 minutes after each meal for 3 weeks. The honey group had a statistically significant reduction in mean dental plaque scores and gingivitis (assessed by percentage of bleeding sites), with no significant changes in the control group (English et al 2004). Manuka honey has been shown to inhibit growth and adherence of *Streptococcus mutans*, an oral pathogen commonly associated with the formation of dental plaque (Badet et al 2011).

Eczema

Topically-applied honey is sometimes used to enhance skin healing and prevent infection in eczema. Although controlled trials are not available, the clinical evidence generally supporting efficacy in wound healing provides a theoretical basis for its use in this condition.

Anal fissures and haemorrhoids

A prospective pilot study examined the use of a topical preparation containing a mixture of honey, olive oil and beeswax in a ratio of 1:1:1 (v/v/v) on anal fissure or haemorrhoids. Treatment for up to 4 weeks significantly reduced the bleeding and itching in patients with haemorrhoids and pain, bleeding and itching in patients with anal fissures (Al-Waili et al 2006).

Colon cancer

Preliminary animal studies on experimentally-induced colon cancer show the potential for reduced disease development (Duleva & Bajkova 2005), but further study is necessary to validate this for clinical use.

Regulation of GI microflora

Honey may be of potential benefit in regulating gastrointestinal microflora. One in vitro study showed that honey promoted growth and activity of beneficial intestinal *bifidobacterium* spp (*B. longum*, *B. adolescentis*, *B. breve*, *B. bifidum* and *B. infantis*), while inhibiting the growth of the pathogenic bacteria *Clostridium perfringens* and *Eubacterium aerofaciens* (Shin & Ustunol 2005). Further in vitro, in vivo and human studies are needed to confirm this benefit.

Pain following tonsillectomy

In a prospective, randomised, placebo-controlled preliminary study involving 60 patients, 5 mL honey combined with paracetamol and antibiotics was found to be more effective in reducing postoperative pain following tonsillectomy than treatment with paracetamol and antibiotics only. The honey combination treatment group also demonstrated increased tonsillary fossa epithelialisation (Ozlugedik et al 2006).

Tear deficiency and meibomian gland disease

Topical application of honey (three times daily) was found to significantly reduce the total ocular bacterial colony-forming units (CFUs) of dry eye subjects caused by tear deficiency and/or meibomian gland disease. After 3 months, antibacterial effect was such that there was no significant difference in the CFUs of the patient groups and the non-dry eye (control) group (Albietz & Lenton 2006).

Radiation-induced oral mucositis

Several studies have examined the prophylactic effect of honey against oral mucositis in patients undergoing radiation therapy for the treatment for head and neck cancer. A meta-analysis of three trials (Biswal et al 2003, Khanal et al 2010, Rashad et al 2009) comprising a total of 120 patients reported that rinsing with honey before and after radiation therapy had an 80% protective effect against radiation-induced mucositis compared to the control group. These results, while favourable, should be interpreted cautiously due to a high risk of bias (Song 2012).

In another single-blind, randomised clinical trial of 40 patients, the honey treatment group swished 20 mL of honey around in their mouth and swallowed gradually 15 minutes before radiation therapy, and again 15 minutes and 6 hours after, while the control group rinsed with 20 mL of saline before and after radiation. The level of mucositis measured by the Oral Mucositis Assessing Scale (OMAS) was significantly lower in the honey-treated group compared to the control group (Motallebnejad et al 2008). More recently, a double-blind randomised study investigating the effect of manuka honey on radiation-induced mucositis in 131 patients with head and neck cancer reported no significant difference between the severity or duration of mucositis in the patients treated with manuka honey and the control group. The authors reported that poor compliance may have affected outcomes (Bardy et al 2012).

Radiotherapy and chemotherapy side effects

In a prospective, controlled, randomised study, 21 adult females who had radiotherapy to the breast or thoracic wall resulting in grade 3 skin toxicities greater than 15 mm in diameter were treated daily with either a honey or a paraffin gauze dressing. The honey-treated group reported less pain, itching or irritation as measured through daily visual analogue scale (VAS) (Moolenaar et al 2006).

Honey may help to reduce the extent of neutropenia experienced as a side effect of chemotherapy and thereby reduce the amount of colony-stimulating factors (CSFs) required. Thirty cancer patients who had undergone chemotherapy and developed grade 4 neutropenia requiring treatment with CSFs repeated this schedule of chemotherapy combined with 5 days of treatment with Life-Mel honey. The addition of the honey treatment resulted in improvement in all cell lines with fewer cases of neutropenia (40% of patients did not require treatment with CSFs), 64% of patients retaining haemoglobin levels above 11 g/dL and only 10% of patients developing thrombocytopenia. No side effects were reported with honey treatment (Zidan et al 2006).

DOSAGE RANGE

Topical use: Honey is usually applied topically (see 'Tips on how best to use honey in practice' below).

Oral use according to clinical studies:

- Coughs in children: 2.5–5 mL as a single dose up to 30 minutes before sleep.
- Mucositis: 20 mL, of honey as a rinse applied to oral mucosa then swallowed 15 minutes before radiation treatment, again 15 minutes after radiation treatment, then 6 hours later or at bedtime for up to 7 weeks.

TOXICITY

Not generally applicable when honey is used externally.

A rare type of food poisoning has been reported with oral ingestion of honey made from nectar of plants in the Rhodenendron genus, due to the presence of sodium channel blockers known as grayanotoxins. Described as 'mad honey', the dose-dependent toxic effects include mild symptoms such as hypersalivation, vomiting, dizziness and weakness, while severe intoxication can lead to potentially serious cardiac complications. No fatal cases have been reported (Koca & Koca 2007). Toxic hepatic pyrrolizidine alkaloids have also been identified in honey produced from nectar of flowers in the Rhododendron genus. These alkaloids are considered to be a health risk to humans as they are potentially mutagenic, teratogenic and carcinogenic. Pregnant women and young infants are considered most at risk (Edgar et al 2002).

CONTRAINDICATIONS AND PRECAUTIONS

Diabetics

Honey contains a large concentration of glucose. If applied to large open wounds, it may theoretically elevate blood sugar levels — monitor blood sugar levels. Caution is advised with oral ingestion of honey as it may alter plasma glucose levels. Use is potentially beneficial (Erejuwa et al 2012).

Children

Honey, honey flavouring and honey-containing supplements are not recommended for use in children under 12 months of age. Consumption of honey contaminated with spores from *Clostridium botulinum* may lead to infant botulism, which is potentially fatal if left untreated (Tanzi & Gabay 2002). However, older children and adults are not considered at risk.

PREGNANCY USE

Safety has not been scientifically established, but historical use suggests that it is generally safe. There are concerns over grayanotoxins found in some types of honey such as that produced from the flowering plants of the genus Rhododendron (Edgar et al 2002).

PATIENTS' FAQs

What will honey do for me?

If you apply a honey preparation that has tested positive for antibacterial activity, it may enhance wound healing, reduce pain and inflammation, and reduce the risk of wound infection.

Which honey should I use?

Honey produced from manuka trees has tested positive for antibacterial activity and is the most effective. Medicinal honey preparations are sterilised by gamma irradiation to destroy any contaminants, without loss of the antibacterial properties of the honey. Medicinal honey preparations are available as gels, pastes and impregnated wound dressings.

Will honey bought from the supermarket be effective if I applied it to a wound?

Not all honeys have the properties needed to heal wounds. In addition, commercial processed honeys undergo heat treatment before being sold as food in supermarkets, which destroys much of its potential antibacterial activity.

When will it start to work?

Studies have found that by the seventh day of use, most wounds show considerable improvement and healing.

Are there any safety issues?

Use of sterile laboratory-tested honey preparations is recommended.

Honey dressings are not recommended for use on deep burns where more aggressive strategies may be required to prevent complications, or on ulcers caused by insect bites.

Practice points/Patient counselling

- Topical application of honey has been used to enhance wound healing treatment of burns and infection control.
- Honey has a deodorising and debriding effect on wounds, accelerates epithelialisation and reduces inflammation and pain.
- Effects are generally seen within 7 days of use.
- Not all honeys have significant antibacterial properties; however, research has identified the New Zealand *Leptospermum* (manuka honey) and Australian jelly bush honey as having potent activity.
- The honey to be used as a topical wound-healing agent or dermatological treatment should ideally be sterile and tested for clinical activity.

Tips on how best to use honey in practice*

- Honey may be applied using manufactured sterile gauze dressings preimpregnated with honey (20–25 g of manuka honey on a 10 × 10 cm dressing).

For minor burns, these have been left in place for up to 25 days, but the wound should be inspected every 2 days. Use of honey dressings in deep burns is not recommended as current evidence suggests that treatment by surgical excision and skin grafting results in better outcomes.

Honey-medicated dressings have been used for longer periods of time (> 25 days) in wound management and skin ulcers.

The appropriateness of routine use of honey dressing in acute or chronic wounds is unclear based on insufficient evidence of a clear clinical benefit.

Where honey is applied directly:

- Ensure that there is an even coverage of the wound surface.
- Larger cavities may be filled by pouring in slightly warmed honey.
- Spreading honey on a dressing pad or gauze rather than on the wound directly will be more comfortable for the patient.
- The amount of honey needed depends on the amount of fluid leaking from the wound — if honey becomes diluted, it will be less effective; typically, 20 mL of honey is used on a 10 × 10 cm dressing.
- Cover with absorbent secondary dressings to prevent honey oozing out from the dressing. Change the dressings more frequently if the honey is being diluted — otherwise change every day or two.

*Adapted from www.worldwidewounds.com and www.manukahoney.co.uk.

ADVERSE REACTIONS

A mild transient stinging may occur when applied to open wounds. If this is too uncomfortable, honey can be washed away with warm water.

Allergic reactions have also been reported, but these are considered rare.

SIGNIFICANT INTERACTIONS

None known, but theoretically honey dressings used in combination with antibiotics may have an additive effect.

Oral intake may induce CYP3A4 enzyme activity, according to a small clinical study (Tushar et al 2007).

REFERENCES

Al-Mamary M et al. Antioxidant activities and total phenolics of different types of honey. Nutr Res 22.9 (2002): 1041–1047.

Al-Waili NS et al. The safety and efficacy of a mixture of honey, olive oil, and beeswax for the management of hemorrhoids and anal fissure: a pilot study. Scientific World Journal 6 (2006): 1998–2005.

Alanqdy A et al. Inhibition effect of honey on the adherence of Salmonella to intestinal epithelial cells in vitro. Int J Food Microbiol 103.3 (2005): 347–351.

Albietz JM, Lenton LM. Effect of antibacterial honey on the ocular flora in tear deficiency and meibomian gland disease. Cornea 25.9 (2006): 1012–1019.

Aysan E et al. The role of intra-peritoneal honey administration in preventing post-operative peritoneal adhesions. Eur J ObstetGynecolReprodBiol 104.2 (2002): 152.

Badet C, Quero F. The in vitro effects of manuka honeys on growth and adherence of oral bacteria. Anaerobe. 17 (2011): 19–22.

Baltrusaityte V, Venskutonis PR, Ceksteryte V. Radical scavenging activity of different floral origin honey and beebread phenolic extracts. Food Chem 101.2 (2007): 502–514.

Bardy J et al. A double-blind, placebo-controlled, randomised trial of active manuka honey and standard oral care for radiation-induced oral mucositis. Br J Oral & Maxillofac Surg 50 (2012): 221–226.

Biswal BM et al. Topical application of honey in the management of radiation mucositis: a preliminary study. Support Care cancer 11 (2003): 242–248.

Blasa M et al. Raw Millefiori is packed full of antioxidants. Food Chem 97.2 (2006): 217–222.

Boukraa L et al. Additive action of royal jelly and honey against Staphylococcus aureus. J Med Food 11.1 (2008): 190–192.

Boukraa L, Amara K. Synergistic effect of starch on the antibacterial activity of honey. J Med Food 11.1 (2008): 195–198.

Boukraa L, Bouchegrane S. Additive action of honey and starch against Candida albicans and Aspergillusniger. Rev IberoamMicol 24.4 (2007): 309–311.

Brudzynski K, Kim L. Storage-induced chemical changes in active components of honey de-regulate its antibacterial activity. Food Chemistry 126 (2011) 1155–1163.

Cooper RA et al. The sensitivity to honey of Gram-positive cocci of clinical significance isolated from wounds. J ApplMicrobiol 93.5 (2002): 857–863.

Duleva V, Bajkova D. Preventive action of honey on experimental colon tumorogenesis. Arch Balk Med Union 40.1 (2005): 49–51.

Edgar JA et al. Honey from plants containing alkaloids: a potential threat to health. J Agric Food Chem 50.10 (2002): 2719–2730.

Emsen IM. A different and safe method of split thickness skin graft fixation: medical honey application. Burns 33.6 (2007): 782–787.

English HK et al. The effects of manuka honey on plaque and gingivitis: a pilot study. J IntAcadPeriodontol 6.2 (2004): 63–67.

Erejuwa OO et al. Honey-a novel antidiabetic agent. Int J BiolSci 8.6 (2012): 913–934.

Fearnley L et al. Compositional analysis of manuka honeys by high-resolution mass spectrometry: Identification of a manuka-enriched archetypal molecule. Food Chemistry 132 (2011) 948–953.

Gethin G, Cowman S. Case series of use of Manuka honey in leg ulceration. Int Wound J 2.1 (2005): 10–15.

Gethin G, Cowman S. Manuka honey vs. hydrogel — a prospective, open label, multicentre, randomised controlled trial to compare desloughing efficacy and healing outcomes in venous ulcers. Journal of Clinical Nursing 18 (2009): 466–474.

Gethin GT et al. The impact of Manuka honey dressings on the surface pH of chronic wounds. Int Wound J 5.2 (2008): 185–194.

Inoue K et al. Identification of phenolic compound in manuka honey as specific superoxide anion radical scavenger using electron spin resonance (ESR) and liquid chromatography with coulometric array detection. J Sci Food Agric 85.5 (2005): 872–878.

Irish J et al. Honey has an antifungal effect against Candida species. Med Mycol 44.3 (2006): 289–291.

Johnson DW et al. Randomized, controlled trial of topical exit-site application of honey (Medihoney) verses mupirocin for the prevention of catheter-associated infections in hemodialysis patients. J Am SocNephrol 16.5 (2005): 1456–1462.

Jull A et al. Randomized clinical trial of honey-impregnated dressings for venous leg ulcers. Br J Surg 95.2 (2008): 175–182.

Jull AB et al. Honey as a topical treatment for wounds. Cochrane Database of Systematic Reviews (2013) Issue 2 CD005083. Doi:10.1002/14651858.

Karmakar S et al. Haematinic and immunomodulatory effects of honey on immunocompetent, immunodeficient and splenectomised experimental rodents. Phytomedica 5 (2004): 107–110.

Khanal B et al. Effect of topical honey on limitation of radiation-induced oral mucositis: an intervention study. Int J Oral MaxillofacSurg 39 (2010): 1181–1185.

Koca I, Koca AF. Poisoning by mad honey: a brief review. Food ChemToxicol 45.8 (2007): 1315–1318.

Kwakman PH et al. Medical-grade honey kills antibiotic-resistant bacteria in vitro and eradicates skin colonization. Clin Infect Dis 46.11 (2008): 1677–1682.

Lee DS et al. Honey and wound healing. Am J Clin Dermatol 12(3) (2011): 181–190.

Lusby PE et al. Honey: a potent agent for wound healing? Journal of Wound, Ostomy and Continence Nursing 29 (2002): 295–300.

Lusby PE et al. Bactericidal activity of different honeys against pathogenic bacteria. Arch Med Res 36.5 (2005): 464–467.

Maeda Y et al. Antibacterial activity of honey against community-associated methicillin-resistant Staphylococcus aureus (CA-MRSA). Complement TherClinPract 14.2 (2008): 77–82.

Misirlioglu A et al. Use of honey as an adjunct in the healing of split-thickness skin graft donor site. DermatolSurg 29.2 (2003): 168–172.

Mohd Effendy N et al. The effects of Tualang honey on bone metabolism of postmenopausal women. Evidence-Based Comp and Altern Med. (2012) doi.10.1155/2012/938574.

Molan PC. Potential of honey in the treatment of wounds and burns. Am J Clin Dermatol 2.1 (2001): 13–19.

Moolenaar M et al. The effect of honey compared to conventional treatment on healing of radiotherapy-induced skin toxicity in breast cancer patients. Acta Oncol 45.5 (2006): 623–624.

Motallebnejad M et al. The effect of topical application of pure honey on radiation-induced mucositis: a randomized clinical trial. J Contemp Dent Pract 9.3 (2008): 40–47.

Mphande AN et al. Effects of honey and sugar dressings on wound healing. J Wound Care 16.7 (2007): 317–3119.

Noori S, Al-Waili NS. Effects of daily consumption of honey solution on hematological indices and blood levels of minerals and enzymes in normal individuals. J Med Food 6 (2) (2004): 135–40.

Oduwole O et al. Honey for acute cough in children (review). Cochrane Library 2012, Issue 3.

Okeniyi JA et al. Comparison of healing of incised abscess wounds with honey and EUSOL dressing. J Altern Complement Med 11.3 (2005): 511–513.

Onyesom I. Effect of Nigerian citrus (Citrus sinensisOsbeck) honey on ethanol metabolism. S Afr Med J 94.12 (2004): 984–986.

Onyesom I. Honey-induced stimulation of blood ethanol elimination and its influence on serum triacylglycerols and blood pressure in man. Ann Nutr Metab 49.5 (2005): 319–324.

Ozlugedik S et al. Can postoperative pains following tonsillectomy be relieved by honey? A prospective, randomized, placebo controlled preliminary study. Int J Pediatr Otorhinolaryngol 70.11 (2006): 1929–1934.

Packer JM et al. Specific non-peroxide antibacterial effect of manuka honey on the Staphylococcus aureas proteome. Int J Antimicrob Agents 40 (2012):43–50

Paul IM et al. Effect of honey, dextromethorphan, and no treatment on nocturnal cough and sleep quality for coughing children and their parents. Arch Pediatr Adolesc Med 161.12 (2007): 1140–1146.

Pieper B. Honey-based dressings and wound care. J Wound Ostomy Continence Nurs. 36(1) (2009): 60–66.

Rashad UM et al. Honey as topical prophylaxis against radiochemotherapy-induced mucositis in head and neck cancer. J Laryngol Otol 123.2 (2009): 223–2228.

Schramm DD et al. Honey with high levels of antioxidants can provide protection to healthy human subjects. J Agric Food Chem 51.6 (2003): 1732–1735.

Shadkam MN, Mozaffari-Khosravi H, Mozayan MR. A comparison of the effect of honey, dextromethorphan, and diphenhyramine on nightly cough and sleep quality in children and their parents. J Altern Comp Med. 16.7 (2010): 787–793.
Shin H-S, Ustunol Z. Carbohydrate composition of honey with different floral sources and their influence on growth of selected intestinal bacteria: an in vitro comparison. Food Res Int 38.6 (2005): 721–8.
Song JJ et al. Systematic review and meta-analysis on the use of honey to protect from effects of radiation-induced oral mucositis. Adv Skin & Wound Care 25.1 (2012): 23–28.
Steinberg D, Kaine G, Gedalia I. Antibacterial effect of propolis and honey on oral bacteria. Am J Dent 9.6 (1996): 236–239.
Subrahmanyam M. Early tangential excision and skin grafting of moderate burns is superior to honey dressing: a prospective randomised trail. Burns 25.8 (1999): 729–31.
Subrahmanyam M, Ugane S. Honey dressing beneficial in treatment of Fournier's gangrene. Indian Journal of Surgery 66.2 (2004): 75–77.
Subrahmanyam M. A prospective randomised clinical and histological study of superficial burn wound healing with honey and silver sulfadiazine. Burns 24.2 (1998): 157–161.
Tan HT et al. The antibacterial properties of Malaysian tualang honey against wound and enteric microorganisms in comparison to manuka honey. BMC Compl and Altern Med 9.34 (2009).
Tanzi MG, Gabay MP. Association between honey consumption and infant botulism. Pharmacotherapy 22.11 (2002):1479–1483.
Taormina PJ et al. Inhibitory activity of honey against foodborne pathogens as influenced by the presence of hydrogen peroxide and level of antioxidant power. Int J Food Microbiol 69.3 (2001): 217–225.
Tonks AJ et al. A 5.8-kDa component of manuka honey stimulates immune cells via TLR4. J Leukocyte Biol. 82.5 (2007).
Tushar T et al. Effect of honey on CYP3A4, CYP2D6 and CYP2C19 enzyme activity in healthy human volunteers. Basic Clin Pharmacol Toxicol 100.4 (2007): 269–272.
van den Berg AJ et al. An in vitro examination of the antioxidant and anti-inflammatory properties of buckwheat honey. J Wound Care 17.4 (2008): 172–174, 176–178.
Voidarou C et al. Antibacterial activity of different honeys against pathogenic bacteria. Anaerobe. 17 (2011): 375–379.
Wang X-H, Andrae L, Engesteth NJ. Antimutagenic effect of various honeys and sugars against Trp-p-1. J Agric Food Chem 50.23 (2002): 6923–6928.
Warren MD, Cooper WO. Honey improves cough in children compared to no treatment. J Pediatr 152.5 (2008): 739–740.
Zaid SSM et al. Protective effects of Tualang honey on bone structure in experimental postmenopausal rats. Clinic 67.7 (2012): 779–784.
Zaid SSM et al. The effects of tualang honey on female reproductive organs, tibia bone and hormonal profile in ovariectomised rats-animal model for menopause. BMC Complementary and alternative Medicine. 10.82 (2010).
Zidan J et al. Prevention of chemotherapy-induced neutropenia by special honey intake. Med Oncol 23.4 (2006): 549–552.

Hops

HISTORICAL NOTE The cultivation of hops started from the middle of the ninth century, between AD 859 and 875, in Germany where it extended from north to south during the early and high Medieval period, as well as to other regions of central Europe. It was originally used as a beer additive and preservative in the European area and today, the beer-brewing industry accounts for 98% of the world's use of hops. Previously, the flower heads were also used to produce a fine brown dye and as a food flavouring agent in cereals, spices and sauces, whereas the fibrous stems were used in the manufacture of crude cloth and paper (Zanoli & Zavatti 2008). Although hops are most famous for producing the bitter flavour in beer, this plant has been used since ancient times in many different cultures (China, India and North America) as a sedative for insomnia, restlessness and nervousness, and also for digestive symptoms such as dyspepsia and lack of appetite. It is related botanically, though not pharmacologically, to cannabis. The climbing nature of the herb influenced its common name, as this is derived from the Anglo-Saxon *hoppan*, which means 'to climb'.

COMMON NAME

Hops

OTHER NAMES

Common hops, European hops, hop strobile, hopfen, houblon, humulus, lupulus, lupulin

BOTANICAL NAME/FAMILY

Humulus lupulus (family: Cannabaceae)

PLANT PART USED

Dried strobiles

CHEMICAL COMPONENTS

Resinous bitter principles (mostly alpha-bitter and beta-bitter acids comprising 5–20% of hop strobile weight) and their oxidative degradation products, polyphenolic condensed tannins, volatile oil, polysaccharides, mainly monoterpenes and sesquiterpenes, flavonoids (xanthohumol, isoxanthohumol, kaempferol, quercetin and rutin), phenolic acids and amino acids (Blumenthal et al 2000) and catechins (catechin gallate, epicatechin gallate). The main alpha acids are humulone (35–70% of total alpha-acids), cohumulone (20–65%) and adhumulone (10–15%); the corresponding beta-acids are lupulone (30–55% of total beta-acids), colupulone and adlupulone (Zanoli & Zavatti 2008). The volatile oil and bitter acids are the most significant components of hops, the latter providing its valuable quality in the brewing of beer. The prenylated flavonoids, particularly xanthohumol, have oestrogenic activity.

MAIN ACTIONS

Traditionally, hops are viewed as a bitter tonic with antispasmodic, relaxant and sedative actions.

Investigation into the mechanisms of action have focused on hops but also on several isolated constituents such as xanthohumol and 8-prenylnaringenin (Zanoli & Zavatti 2008).

Sedative and antidepressant

A long history of use within well-established systems of traditional medicine, together with scientific testing, have suggested that hops has significant sedative activity (Blumenthal et al 2000), probably through activation of melatonin receptors. Both the extract of hops and a fraction containing alpha-bitter acids demonstrates significant sedative properties in mice and antidepressant activity (Zanoli et al 2005). The hops beta-acids also exert antidepressant effects in vivo but have less sedative activity. A reduction in GABAergic activity was reported for the beta-acids in vivo (Zanoli et al 2007).

Research with a fixed herbal combination containing hops and valerian, known as Ze91019, demonstrated binding affinities at the melatonin ML_1 and serotonin 5-HT_6 receptor subtypes (Abourashed et al 2004).

Oestrogenic effects

In 1953, two German scientists followed up on a folk legend that women regularly began to menstruate 2 days after beginning to pick hops. Since then, there has been much research on the oestrogenic effects of hops. Hops showed significant competitive binding to alpha- and beta-oestrogen receptors and upregulation of progesterone receptors in vitro (Liu et al 2001). The oestrogenic activity is chiefly due to the constituent 8-prenylnaringenin (Milligan et al 1999, 2000), which is converted by intestinal microflora from isoxanthohumol (Possemiers et al 2005), and mimics the action of 17β-oestradiol, albeit with a 17-fold lesser potency in alpha-receptor sites (in the breast, liver, central nervous system and uterus), and a 20,000-fold lesser potency in the beta-receptor sites (mainly in the intestine, prostate, ovaries, testes and urogenital tract). The high oestrogenic activity of 8-prenylnaringenin has also been confirmed in different in vivo experiments and is considered one of the strongest phyto-oestrogens found in the plant kingdom (Zanoli & Zavatti 2008).

A small, double-blind randomised controlled trial (RCT) using standardised doses of 8-prenylnaringenin demonstrated systemic endocrine effects, including a decrease in luteinising hormone serum concentrations, in postmenopausal women. In vitro studies also show that hop extracts exert oestrogen-like activities on bone metabolism, although later in vivo studies on rats contradict this finding (Figard et al 2007).

Moderate beer consumption can provide enough 8-prenylnaringenin to ensure some biological activity in humans, with unknown consequences for health (Possemiers et al 2006).

Possible chemopreventive and anticancer effects

Hops exhibits potential anticancer activity by inhibiting cell proliferation and angiogenesis, by inducing apoptosis and by increasing the expression of cytochrome P450 detoxification enzymes (Van et al 2009).

Antiangiogenic activity is important because angiogenesis is necessary for solid tumour growth and dissemination. In addition to angiogenesis, it has become increasingly clear that inflammation is a key component in cancer insurgence that can promote tumour angiogenesis. The hops-derived chalcone, xanthohumol, prevents angiogenesis in vivo and induces detoxification enzymes, in particular quinone reductase, which may contribute to its chemoprotective effects (Dietz et al 2005).

Xanthohumol, a prenylated chalcone derived from hops, is a very promising, potential protective agent against genotoxicity of food-borne carcinogens and has been shown to inhibit the growth of the highly angiogenic Kaposi's sarcoma tumour cells in vivo. It also demonstrates antitumour activity on B-chronic lymphocytic leukaemia cells in vitro. The prenylflavonoids are able to modulate aromatase activity, thus decreasing oestrogen synthesis, and it is hypothesised that this may have relevance for the prevention and treatment of oestrogen-dependent disorders such as breast cancer. Xanthohumol also demonstrates growth-inhibitory and apoptosis-inducing activity in hormone-sensitive and hormone-refractory human prostate cancer cells lines at a concentration range of 20–40 microM (Deeb et al 2010). Additionally, xanthohumol from hops appears to induce apoptosis by increasing release of reactive oxygen species within the mitochondria of cancer cells, leading to a rapid breakdown of the mitochondrial membrane potential and release of cytochrome c (Strathmann et al 2010) This was demonstrated in three human cancer cell lines, whereby xanthohumol induced an immediate and transient increase in superoxide anion radical formation, followed by apoptosis.

Both hops and 8-prenylnaringenin have been found to significantly inhibit oestrogen-induced malignant transformation of MCF-10A cells, suggesting cancer chemopreventive activity (Hemachandra et al 2012). In addition, 8-prenylnaringenin was a potent inhibitor of oestrogen-induced expression of CYP450 1B1 and CYP450 1A1, further adding to a chemopreventive effect.

In vitro research shows that hop bitter acids exhibit a strong growth-inhibitory effect against human leukaemia HL-60 cells, with an estimated IC50 value of 8.67 mcg/mL, but were less effective against human histolytic lymphoma U937 cells (Chen & Lin 2004).

Antimicrobial

Hops extract and hops oil have activity against mainly Gram-positive bacteria (*Bacillus subtilis* and *Staphylococcus aureus*) and the fungus *Trichophyton mentagrophytes* var. *interdigitale*, but almost no activity against the Gram-negative bacterium *Escherichia coli* and the yeast *Candida albicans* (Langezaal et al 1992). Lupulone, in particular, has been found to have some action against Gram-positive bacteria and certain Gram-negative bacteria, but not against others, such as *E. coli*. A review of the antimicrobial properties concluded that hops was also effective against the parasite *Plasmodium falciparum* and a range of viruses, including herpes simplex virus types 1 and 2, cytomegalovirus and HIV (Gerhauser 2005). The mechanism of anti-HIV activity is not fully understood, but it is thought that the flavonoid, xanthohumol, may inhibit transcription (Wang et al 2004).

The activity of bitter acids from hops towards Gram-positive bacteria, including some species of *Micrococcus*, *Staphylococcus*, *Mycobacterium* and *Streptomycetes*, may involve primary membrane leakage, due to the interaction of the hydrophobic parts of the molecules with the bacterial cell wall. Antifungal activity has also been reported for the bitter acids against *Candida albicans*, *Trichophyton*, *Fusarium* and *Mucor* species (Mizobuchi & Sato 1985). The prenylchalcones XH and 6-PN were identified as the most potent agents against *Trychophyton* spp. and *Staphylococcus aureus*, but they were practically inactive against other human pathogenic fungi (*Candida albicans* and *Fusarium* spp.) (Mizobuchi & Sato 1984).

Cariogenic

Various components of hops have been studied for potential cariogenic activity and usefulness in dentistry. Cariogenic activity relies on a substance having an effect on dental plaque and the microorganisms involved, such as *Streptococcus mutans*. In vitro and in vivo research has shown inhibition of *S. mutans* and two clinical trials have confirmed cariogenic activity in humans (Shinada et al 2007, Yaegaki et al 2008).

OTHER ACTIONS

Cytochrome P450 induction and pregnane X receptor

Colupulone, a beta-bitter acid, was reported to induce the cytochrome P450 system and increase mRNA levels of cytochrome 2B and 3A in rats (Shipp et al 1994). The beta-bitter acid colupulone is also a direct activator of human pregnane X receptor (Teotico et al 2008). Another study found that the flavonoids from hops inhibit the cytochrome P450 system in vitro — in particular, cytochromes 1A1, 1B1 and 1A2, but not 2E1 or 3A4 (Henderson et al 2000). A review concluded that hops inhibits phase 1 detoxification and enhances phase 2 by inducing quinone reductase (Gerhauser et al 2002, Stevens & Page 2004). More recently, in vitro tests identified that hops extract at 5 mcg/mL with IC50 values of 0.8, 0.9, 3.3 and 9.4 mcg/mL inhibited CYP2C8 (93%), CYP2C9 (88%), CYP2C19 (70%) and CYP1A2 (27%) (Yuan et al 2013). The isoxanthohumol constituent was the most potent inhibitor of CYP2C8, whereas 8-prenylnaringenin was the most potent inhibitor of CYP1A2, CYP2C9 and CYP2C19. Clinical studies are not available to determine whether the effect on cytochromes is clinically relevant.

Anti-inflammatory

In clinical trials, hops has demonstrable anti-inflammatory action. A double-blind, randomised ex vivo study comparing hops extracts with ibuprofen demonstrated equivalence in cyclooxygenase (COX)-2 inhibitory action but with significant COX-1-sparing activity relative to ibuprofen, therefore, without the risk of gastrointestinal side effects found with other COX enzyme inhibitors, such as ibuprofen.

The same results were found in a study utilising a modified hops extract containing a defined mixture of rho iso-alpha-acids (RIAA) which significantly inhibited prostaglandin E_2 formation with >200-fold selectivity of COX-2 over COX-1 (Hall et al 2008). RIAA appears to inhibit inducible, but not constitutive, COX-2 and, overall, may have lower potential for gastrointestinal and cardiovascular toxicity observed with traditional pharmaceutical COX enzyme inhibitors. Gastric safety was confirmed in a 14-day human study, whereby oral RIAA (900 mg/day) produced no change to faecal calprotectin (a biomarker of gastric irritation) compared to naproxen (1000 mg/day), which increased faecal calprotectin 200%.

The chalcones from hops, including xanthohumol, significantly reduced nitric oxide by suppressing inducible nitric oxide synthase in mouse macrophage cells (Zhao et al 2003, 2005). Xanthohumol has also been reported to inhibit the production of prostaglandin E_2 Animal studies suggest that hops could be a useful agent for intervention strategies targeting inflammatory disorders and/or inflammatory pain in arthritis (Hougee et al 2006), but with low potential for gastrointestinal and cardiovascular toxicity. In fact, mouse studies indicate that hops extract may be useful for the prevention of gastric ulcer and inflammation, as it inhibits one of the important virulence factors responsible for *Helicobacter pylori*-induced gastritis and ulceration.

CLINICAL USE

In practice, the herb is prescribed in combination with other herbal medicines, such as valerian and passionflower. As is representative of clinical practice, most studies have investigated the effects of hops in combination with other herbs.

Restlessness and anxiety

Based on the herb's sedative activity, it is likely to have some effect in the treatment of restlessness and anxiety, but careful dosing would be required to avoid sedation. The relief of mild symptoms of mental stress is an indication that has been approved by Commission E and European Scientific Co-Operative on Phytotherapy (ESCOP) (Blumenthal 1998). It has also been approved as a treatment for excitability and restlessness.

Sleep disturbances and insomnia

Hops has been used as a bath additive for sleep disturbances. A double-blind RCT involving 40 patients found that taking three hops baths (4 g hops in a concentrated extract) on successive days significantly improved both objective and subjective sleep quality (Bone 1996).

Commission E and ESCOP support the use of hops for sleep disturbances, such as difficulty falling asleep and insomnia (Blumenthal et al 2000).

Studies on mice confirm that hops has a central sedating effect that can be attributed to the bitter acids and hop oil. Although there have been no human in vivo studies to support oral doses of hops as a stand-alone sedative agent, several studies have demonstrated that formulas combining hops with other sedative herbs are effective for insomnia.

IN COMBINATION

Numerous double-blind RCTs have investigated the effects of an oral preparation of hops and valerian in sleep disorders and currently, the evidence supports its use as a safe and effective treatment option for primary insomnia.

Four studies were included in a 2010 review (Salter & Brownie 2010), of which three were double-blind, placebo-controlled randomised studies and one was a single-blind randomised trial. Three of the four studies showed that the combination of valerian and hops was effective for some aspect of improving sleep. One study showed improved total sleep quantity, quality and deep sleep for valerian (480 mg) + hops (480 mg) over placebo, as calculated by electroencephalograph and subjective measures (Dimpfel & Suter 2008). Morin et al (2005) conducted a multicentre, randomised, placebo-controlled, parallel-group study in nine sleep disorder centres throughout the United States. The study, involving 184 adults with mild insomnia, used two tablets each night of standardised extracts of a valerian (187 mg native extracts; 5–8 : 1, methanol 45% m/m) and hops (41.9-mg native extracts; 7–10 : 1, methanol 45% m/m) taken for 28 days compared to placebo and two tablets of diphenhydramine (25 mg) for 14 days followed by placebo for 14 days. Modest improvements in subjective sleep parameters were obtained with the valerian-hops combination and people rated their insomnia as less severe with this treatment; quality of life (physical component) was significantly more improved in the valerian-hops group relative to the placebo group at the end of 28 days (Morin et al 2005). Koetter et al (2007) used a fixed combination of valerian (500 mg) and hops (120 mg) (Ze 91019) and found the herbal combination was significantly superior to placebo in reducing sleep latency (Koetter et al 2007). Finally, a study by Fussel et al (2000) testing the same valerian-hops preparation, Ze 91019, in 30 subjects with mild to moderate, non-organic insomnia found that treatment used at bedtime reduced sleep latency and nocturnal wakenings and improved sleep quality, as assessed by polysomnographic examination; however this study lacked a placebo group.

Comparisons with other treatments

One study observed equivalent efficacy and tolerability of a hops–valerian preparation comparable to benzodiazepine treatment, with withdrawal symptoms only reported for benzodiazepine use (Schmitz & Jackel 1998). Improvement in subjective perceptions of sleep quality was confirmed in another study, which also reported that a hops–valerian combination was well tolerated compared with flunitrazepam (Gerhard et al 1996).

More recently, a parallel-group, double-blind, RCT showed that treatment with NSF-3, a polyherbal sedative hypnotic (containing standardised extracts of valerian, passionflower and hops) was as effective as zolpidem (10 mg) in primary insomnia (Maroo et al 2013). Seventy-eight volunteers took part; they had primary insomnia with a perceived total sleep time of <6 hours per night and insomnia severity index >7. Treatment consisted of either NSF-3 (one tablet) or zolpidem (one 10 mg tablet) at bedtime for 2 weeks, There was significant improvement in total sleep time, sleep latency, number of nightly awakenings and insomnia severity index scores in both groups, with no statistically significant difference observed between them.

Menopause

Hop extract and especially 8-PN are promising candidates for the relief for menopausal symptoms based on demonstrated mechanisms of action and the available clinical evidence; however further research is still required before a definitive conclusion can be made (Keiler et al 2013).

A randomised, double-blind, placebo-controlled trial of a standardised extract of hops (100 mcg and 250 mcg 8-prenylnaringenin) demonstrated a significant reduction in menopausal discomfort, in particular hot flushes, after 12 weeks of treatment in 67 women (Heyerick et al 2005). Interestingly, no dose–response relationship could be made, as the lower standardised dose was shown to be more effective.

A 16-week double-blind placebo-controlled, crossover RCT was conducted with 36 menopausal women who were randomly allocated to either placebo or active treatment (hop extract) for a period of 8 weeks and then given the alternative treatment. After 8 weeks of active treatment following the placebo phase, a reduction in all outcome measures (Kupperman Index, the Menopause Rating Scale and a multifactorial visual analogue scale) was observed in comparison to placebo after active treatment, which resulted in an increase for all outcome measures (Erkkola et al 2010).

Single doses, from 50 to 750 mg, of 8-prenylnaringenin were orally given to healthy menopausal women in a randomised, double-blind, placebo-controlled study performed by Rad et al (2006). The decrease in luteinising hormone serum levels found after the highest dose demonstrated the ability of 8-prenylnaringenin to exert endocrine effects in menopausal women.

An open, non-controlled clinical trial in 100 postmenopausal women was performed over 12 weeks to investigate the effects of vaginal application of a gel (2.5 g/day for 1 week then two applications/

week for 11 weeks) containing phyto-oestrogens from hops extract, hyaluronic acid, liposomes and vitamin E, with the aim of testing its safety and efficacy in postmenopausal women with urogenital atrophy. The results showed a statistically significant reduction in vaginal dryness and other symptoms and signs associated with atrophic vaginitis (itching, burning, inflammation and rash) without any adverse effects (Morali et al 2006). The same group conducted a pilot study of 10 women with the same gel applied on the external genitals at a dose of 1–2 g/day for 30 days and confirmed acceptance of the treatment and a good safety profile, both locally and systemically (Morali et al 2006).

Indigestion

Due to the herb's bitter nature, it is used to stimulate digestion and in the treatment of common digestive complaints such as dyspepsia and indigestion. Animal studies on rats show that hops increases gastric juice volume.

Cariogenic — reducing dental plaque

Yaegaki et al (2008) demonstrated that hops polyphenols (HPP) significantly reduced the growth of *Streptococcus mutans* compared to controls ($P < 0.01$) and of lactic acid production ($P < 0.05$) and suppressed water-insoluble glucan formation in vitro (a major component of plaque) when used at all three test doses of 0.01%, 0.1%, and 0.5% ($P < 0.01$, $P < 0.001$ and $P < 0.001$, respectively). The same researchers conducted a single-blind RCT involving 28 healthy people and used either 20 mg or 7 mg HPP-containing tablets, representing high and low dosages, respectively, at a dose of one tablet seven times a day (before breakfast, after each meal, between meals and at bedtime) for 3 days. The study confirmed that high-strength treatment with HPP significantly reduced 3-day dental plaque regrowth ($P < 0.05$).

Positive results were also obtained in a double-blind, crossover clinical study utilising an HPP mouth rinse (0.1%) which significantly suppressed dental plaque regrowth in humans ($P < 0.001$) (Shinada et al 2007). Additionally, the number of mutans streptococci in the plaque samples after volunteers used the HPP mouth rinse was significantly lower than after they used the placebo ($P < 0.05$).

Allergy

A double-blind, placebo-controlled RCT showed that oral administration of a hop water extract during the allergy season significantly improved symptoms compared to placebo (Segawa et al 2007). The active treatment drink contained 100 mg of hop water extract, which was taken for 12 weeks. The effect had a slow onset, as a significant difference was observed in the symptom score and in the symptom medication score 10 weeks after the intervention in comparison with the placebo group. Improvements were observed in nasal swelling, nasal colour, amount of nasal discharge and characteristics of nasal discharge in the intervention group 12 weeks after the treatment. Additionally, no significant eosinophil infiltration into the nasal discharge was apparent in the intervention group throughout the study period, although it was observed in the placebo group.

Osteoarthritis

The anti-inflammatory activity of hops provides a rationale for its use in conditions characterised by inflammation such as osteoarthritis. At least two clinical studies have explored whether a preparation containing hops extracts with RIAA has any symptom-relieving benefits in osteoarthritis (Hall et al 2008, Minich et al 2007). In a 6-week open-label study of human subjects exhibiting knee osteoarthritis, a hops treatment containing RIAA (1000 mg/day) produced a 54% reduction in WOMAC global scores (Hall et al 2008). Additionally, results from a multicentre trial indicate that a herbal combination (NG440) containing RIAA from hops, rosemary and oleanolic acid reduced pain scores in patients with joint discomfort, as measured by visual analogue scale methodology (Minich et al 2007).

Double-blind studies utilising hops extract as a stand-alone treatment are warranted to explore the potential effects further.

OTHER USES

Traditionally, hops are also used to treat neuralgia, depression and pain and to wean patients off pharmaceutical sedative medicines. Topically it is used to treat leg ulcers and oedema.

Diabetes

Isohumulones, the bitter compounds in hops, have been shown to improve insulin resistance and hyperlipidaemia in several animal models and may prevent the progression of renal injury caused by hypertension via an antioxidative effect. Clinical studies are required to confirm significance.

Periodontitis

In vitro studies suggest that the hop-derived polyphenols are potent inhibitors of prostaglandin E_2 production by gingival epithelial cells stimulated with periodontal pathogen and may be useful for the prevention and treatment of periodontitis. The clinical significance of this finding is unknown and remains to be tested.

Deodorant

In vitro antibacterial activity of a hop extract against *Corynebacterium xerosis* and *Staphylococcus epidermidis* and the evaluation of the odour-reducing capacity of a hops/zinc ricinoleate-containing product by a sensory evaluation panel were employed to verify deodorant performance (Dumas et al 2009). The hops extract had good antibacterial activity against *C. xerosis* and *S. aureus*, In the clinical underarm odour reduction evaluation, the mean malodour score dropped from 6.28 (±0.70) to 1.80 (±0.71) 8 hours after application, with a noticeable effect lasting at both 12 and 24 hours after the application, with a score of 1.82 (±0.74) and 2.24 (±0.77), respectively.

Use in flavouring, preserving and colouring beer

The bitter acids of hops (*Humulus lupulus* L.) mainly consist of alpha-acids, beta-acids and their oxidation products that contribute the unique aroma of the beer beverage. The alpha-acids in particular are the crucial compounds for the quality of hops used in the brewing industry, contributing to foam stability as well as exerting antibacterial activity (Verzele & De Keukeleire 1991).

DOSAGE RANGE

- Infusion or decoction: 0.5 g in 150 mL water.
- Fluid extract (1 : 1) (g/mL): 0.5 mL/day; 0.5–1 mL three times daily.
- Tincture (1:5) (g/mL): 1–2.5 mL/day.
- Also used as a bath additive (4 g hops in a concentrated extract) and in pillows.

TOXICITY

Toxicological studies in animals stated that LD_{50} for orally administered hop extract in mice ranges from 500 to 3500 mg/kg (Hänsel et al 1993).

ADVERSE REACTIONS

Drowsiness is theoretically possible at excessive doses. Contact with the herb or oil has resulted in reports of systemic urticaria, allergic dermatitis, respiratory allergy and anaphylaxis (Pradalier et al 2002).

SIGNIFICANT INTERACTIONS

Interactions reported here are theoretical and yet to be tested clinically for significance.

Pharmaceutical sedatives

Additive effects are theoretically possible — observe the patient (this interaction may be beneficial).

Drugs metabolised chiefly with CYP2C8, CYP2C9 or CYP2C19

Altered drug effect — cytochrome (CYP) inhibition has been demonstrated in vitro. However, it is unknown whether these effects are clinically significant — observe the patient for signs of altered drug effectiveness.

Antioestrogenic drugs

Hops may alter the efficacy of these medicines; use with caution in patients taking antioestrogenic drugs. However the effect is theoretical and not anticipated to be significant — observe.

Practice points/Patient counselling

- Hops are often used as a mild sedative in combination with other herbs, such as valerian and passionflower.
- Several randomised trials have found that the combination of hops and valerian improves sleep quality, without next-day drowsiness; however, further investigation is required to determine the role of hops in achieving this effect.
- Although generally taken orally, it has also been successfully used as a bath additive and in aromatherapy pillows to induce sleep.
- It is traditionally used to treat anxiety, restlessness, pain, neuralgia and indigestion.
- It should not be used in patients with oestrogen-dependent tumours, and should be used with caution in pregnancy.

CONTRAINDICATIONS AND PRECAUTIONS

According to one source, hops should be used with caution in depression (Ernst 2001). Due to the herb's oestrogenic activity, disruption to the menstrual cycle is considered possible. While caution is advised in patients with oestrogen-dependent tumours, new research indicates chemopreventive activity against breast cancer cell lines.

PREGNANCY USE

Caution in pregnancy because of the possible hormonal effects.

PATIENTS' FAQs

What will this herb do for me?

Hops may be a useful treatment for anxiety and restlessness, and when combined with other sedative herbs, such as valerian or passionflower, improves sleep quality without inducing next-day hangover effects.

When will it start to work?

Several doses may be required; however, effects are generally seen within 2 weeks.

Are there any safety issues?

Constituents in the herb appear to have some oestrogenic activity; therefore, people with oestrogen-dependent tumours should avoid its use.

REFERENCES

Abourashed, E.A., et al. 2004. In vitro binding experiments with a Valerian, hops and their fixed combination extract (Ze91019) to selected central nervous system receptors. Phytomedicine, 11, (7–8) 633–638.

Blumenthal M (ed), The complete German commission E monographs: therapeutic guide to herbal medicines. Austin, TX: The American Botanical Council, 1998.

Blumenthal M, et al (eds). Herbal medicine: expanded commission E monographs. Austin, TX: Integrative Medicine Communications, 2000.

Bone K. Hops. Prof Monitor 16 (1996): 2.

Chen, W.J. & Lin, J.K. 2004. Mechanisms of cancer chemoprevention by hop bitter acids (beer aroma) through induction of apoptosis mediated by Fas and caspase cascades. J Agric.Food Chem., 52, (1) 55–64.

Deeb, D., et al. 2010. Growth inhibitory and apoptosis-inducing effects of xanthohumol, a prenylated chalone present in hops, in human prostate cancer cells. Anticancer Res., 30, (9) 3333–3339.

Dietz BM et al. Xanthohumol isolated from *Humulus lupulus* inhibits menadione-induced DNA damage through induction of quinone reductase. Chem Res Toxicol 18 (2005): 1296–305.

Dimpfel, W. & Suter, A. 2008. Sleep improving effects of a single dose administration of a valerian/hops fluid extract — a double blind, randomized, placebo-controlled sleep-EEG study in a parallel design using electrohypnograms. Eur J Med Res., 13, (5) 200–204.

Dumas, E.R., et al. 2009. Deodorant effects of a supercritical hops extract: antibacterial activity against *Corynebacterium xerosis* and *Staphylococcus epidermidis* and efficacy testing of a hops/zinc ricinoleate stick in humans through the sensory evaluation of axillary deodorancy. J Cosmet. Dermatol., 8, (3) 197–204.

Erkkola, R., et al. 2010. A randomized, double-blind, placebo-controlled, cross-over pilot study on the use of a standardized hop extract to alleviate menopausal discomforts. Phytomedicine, 17, (6) 389–396.

Ernst E (ed), The desktop guide to complementary and alternative medicine: an evidence-based approach. St Louis: Mosby, 2001.

Figard H et al. Effects of isometric strength training followed by no exercise and *Humulus lupulus* L-enriched diet on bone metabolism in old female rats. Metabolism 56.12 (2007): 1673–81.

Fussel A, et al. Effect of a fixed valerian-Hop extract combination (Ze 91019) on sleep polygraphy in patients with non-organic insomnia: a pilot study. Eur J Med Res 5 (2000): 385–390.

Gerhard U et al. Vigilance-decreasing effects of 2 plant-derived sedatives. Schweiz Rundsch Med Prax 85.15 (1996): 473–81.

Gerhauser C. Broad spectrum antiinfective potential of xanthohumol from hop (*Humulus lupulus* L.) in comparison with activities of other hop constituents and xanthohumol metabolites. Mol Nutr Food Res 49 (2005): 827–31.

Gerhauser C et al. Cancer chemopreventive activity of Xanthohumol, a natural product derived from hop. Mol Cancer Ther 1 (2002): 959–69.

Hall, A.J., et al. 2008. Safety, efficacy and anti-inflammatory activity of rho iso-alpha-acids from hops. Phytochemistry, 69, (7) 1534–1547.

Hänsel, R., et al 1993. Hagers Handbuch der Pharmazeutische Praxis, Hrsg. Springer Verlag, Berlin, pp. 447–458.

Hemachandra, L.P., et al. 2012. Hops (*Humulus lupulus*) inhibits oxidative estrogen metabolism and estrogen-induced malignant transformation in human mammary epithelial cells (MCF-10A). Cancer Prev. Res.(Phila), 5, (1) 73–81.

Henderson MC et al. In vitro inhibition of human P450 enzymes by prenylated flavonoids from hops, *Humulus lupulus*. Xenobiotica 30 (2000): 235–51.

Heyerick A et al. A first prospective randomized, double-blind, placebo-controlled study on the use of a standardized hop extract to alleviate menopausal discomforts. Maturitas 54.2 (2005): 164–75.

Hougee S et al. Selective inhibition of COX-2 by a standardized CO2 extract of *Humulus lupulus* in vitro and its activity in a mouse model of zymosan-induced arthritis. Planta Med 72.3 (2006): 228–33.

Keiler, A.M., et al 2013. Hop extracts and hop substances in treatment of menopausal complaints. Planta Med, 79, (7) 576–579.

Koetter, U., et al. 2007. A randomized, double blind, placebo-controlled, prospective clinical study to demonstrate clinical efficacy of a fixed valerian hops extract combination (Ze 91019) in patients suffering from non-organic sleep disorder. Phytother. Res., 21, (9) 847–851.

Langezaal CR, et al. Antimicrobial screening of essential oils and extracts of some *Humulus lupulus* L. cultivars. Pharm Week Sci 14.6 (1992): 353–6.

Liu J et al. Evaluation of estrogenic activity of plant extracts for the potential treatment of menopausal symptoms. J Agric Food Chem 49.5 (2001): 2472–9.

Maroo, N., et al. 2013. Efficacy and safety of a polyherbal sedative-hypnotic formulation NSF-3 in primary insomnia in comparison to zolpidem: a randomized controlled trial. Indian J Pharmacol, 45, (1) 34–39.

Milligan SR et al. Identification of a potent phytoestrogen in hops (*Humulus lupulus* L.) and beer. J Clin Endocrinol Metab 84.6 (1999): 2249–52.

Milligan SR et al. The endocrine activities of 8-prenylnaringenin and related hop (*Humulus lupulus* L.) flavonoids. J Clin Endocrinol Metab 85.12 (2000): 4912–15.

Minich, D.M., et al. 2007. Clinical safety and efficacy of NG440: a novel combination of rho iso-alpha acids from hops, rosemary, and oleanolic acid for inflammatory conditions. Can. J Physiol Pharmacol, 85, (9) 872–883.

Mizobuchi, S., Sato, Y., 1984. A new flavanone with antifungal activity isolated from hops. Agricultural and Biological Chemistry 48, 2771–2775.

Mizobuchi, S., Sato, Y., 1985. Antifungal activities of hop bitter resins and related compounds. Agricultural and Biological Chemistry 49, 399–403.

Morali, G., et al. 2006. Open, non-controlled clinical studies to assess the efficacy and safety of a medical device in form of gel topically and intravaginally used in postmenopausal women with genital atrophy. Arzneimittelforschung., 56, (3) 230–238.

Morin, C.M., et al. 2005. Valerian-hops combination and diphenhydramine for treating insomnia: a randomized placebo-controlled clinical trial. Sleep, 28, (11) 1465–1471.

Possemiers S et al. Activation of proestrogens from hops (*Humulus lupulus* L.) by intestinal microbiota; conversion of isoxanthohumol into 8-prenylnaringenin. J Agric Food Chem 53 (2005): 6281–8.

Possemiers S et al. The prenylflavonoid isoxanthohumol from hops (*Humulus lupulus* L.) is activated into the potent phytoestrogen 8-prenylnaringenin in vitro and in the human intestine. J Nutr 136.7 (2006): 1862–7.

Pradalier A, et al. Systemic urticaria induced by hops. Allerg Immunol (Paris) 34.9 (2002): 330–2.

Salter, S. & Brownie, S. 2010. Treating primary insomnia — the efficacy of valerian and hops. Aust.Fam.Physician, 39, (6) 433–437.

Schmitz M, Jackel M. Comparative study for assessing quality of life of patients with exogenous sleep disorders (temporary sleep onset and sleep interruption disorders) treated with a hops-valarian preparation and a benzodiazepine drug. Wien Med Wochenschr 148.13 (1998): 291–8.

Segawa, S., et al. 2007. Clinical effects of a hop water extract on Japanese cedar pollinosis during the pollen season: a double-blind, placebo-controlled trial. Biosci. Biotechnol. Biochem., 71, (8) 1955–1962.

Shinada, K., et al. 2007. Hop bract polyphenols reduced three-day dental plaque regrowth. J Dent.Res., 86, (9) 848–851.

Shipp EB, et al. The effect of colupulone (a HOPS beta-acid) on hepatic cytochrome P-450 enzymatic activity in the rat. Food Chem Toxicol 32.11 (1994): 1007–14.

Stevens JF, Page JE. Xanthohumol and related prenylflavonoids from hops and beer: to your good health! Phytochemistry 65 (2004): 1317–30.

Strathmann, J., et al. 2010. Xanthohumol-induced transient superoxide anion radical formation triggers cancer cells into apoptosis via a mitochondria-mediated mechanism. FASEB J, 24, (8) 2938–2950.

Teotico, D.G., et al. 2008. Structural basis of human pregnane X receptor activation by the hops constituent colupulone. Mol. Pharmacol, 74, (6) 1512–1520.

Van, C.M., et al. 2009. Hop (*Humulus lupulus*)-derived bitter acids as multipotent bioactive compounds. J Nat.Prod., 72, (6) 1220–1230.

Verzele, M., De Keukeleire, D., 1991. Chemistry and analysis of hop and beer bitter acids. Elsevier, Amsterdam.

Wang Q et al. Xanthohumol, a novel anti-HIV-1 agent purified from hops *Humulus lupulus*. Antiviral Res 64 (2004): 189–94.

Yaegaki, K., et al. 2008. Hop polyphenols suppress production of water-insoluble glucan by Streptococcus mutans and dental plaque growth in vivo. J Clin Dent., 19, (2) 74–78.

Yuan, Y., et al. 2013. Inhibition of human cytochrome P450 enzymes by hops (*Humulus lupulus*) and hop prenylphenols. Eur J Pharm.Sci., 53C, 55–61.

Zanoli, P. & Zavatti, M. 2008. Pharmacognostic and pharmacological profile of *Humulus lupulus* L. J Ethnopharmacol., 116, (3) 383–396.

Zanoli P et al. New insight in the neuropharmacological activity of *Humulus lupulus* L. J Ethnopharmacol 102.1 (2005): 102–6.

Zanoli, P., et al. 2007. Evidence that the beta-acids fraction of hops reduces central GABAergic neurotransmission. J Ethnopharmacol., 109, (1) 87–92.

Zhao F et al. Inhibitors of nitric oxide production from hops (*Humulus lupulus* L.). Biol Pharm Bull 26 (2003): 61–5.

Zhao F et al. Phenylflavonoids and phloroglucinol derivatives from hops (*Humulus lupulus*). J Nat Prod 68 (2005): 43–9.

Horse chestnut

HISTORICAL NOTE The horse chestnut tree is native to the countries of the Balkan Peninsula and is commonly found in ornamental gardens throughout Europe, growing up to 36 metres tall (Anonymous 2009). The seeds are not edible due to the presence of alkaloid saponins, but both the dried seeds and bark of the horse chestnut tree have been used medicinally since the 16th century. The seeds are also used for the children's game 'conkers' and were used to produce acetone during World War I and II. In modern times, a dry extract, referred to as horse chestnut seed extract (HCSE), is standardised to contain 16–21% triterpene glycosides (anhydrous aescin). HCSE has been extensively researched for its beneficial effects and is commonly used by general practitioners in Germany for the treatment of chronic venous insufficiency. Homeopathic preparations of both the leaf and the seed are also used for treating haemorrhoids, lower back pain and varicose veins, and the buds and flower are used to make the Bach flower remedies chestnut bud and white chestnut. The active component aescin is also used intravenously and topically in cosmetics (Bombardelli et al 1996, Herbalgram 2000, PDR Health 2006).

OTHER NAMES

Aescule, buckeye, chestnut, Castaño de Indias, graine de marronier d'inde, escine, eschilo, hestekastanje, hippocastani semen, marroneuropeen, marronnier, roßkastaniensamen, Spanish chestnut

BOTANICAL NAME/FAMILY

Aesculus hippocastanum (family [Sapindaceae] Hippocastanaceae).

It should be differentiated from *A. chinensis*, *A. turbinata*, *A. indica*, *A. californica* and *A. glabra*.

PLANT PARTS USED

Seed. Less commonly bark, flower and leaf.

CHEMICAL COMPONENTS

Horse chestnut seed contains 3–6% aescin (escin), a complex mixture of triterpene saponins (including the triterpeneoligoglycosides escins Ia, Ib, IIa, IIb and IIIa) (Yoshikawa et al 1996), the acylated polyhydroxyoleanenetriterpeneoligoglycosides aescins IIIb, IV, V and VI and isoaescins Ia, Ib and V (Yoshikawa et al 1998). Beta-aescin appears to be the active component of the triterpene saponins mixture and is the molecular form present in major available pharmaceutical products (Sirtori 2001). Horse chestnut also contains sapogenol shippocaesculin, barringtogenol-C (Konoshima & Lee 1986), flavonoids (flavonol oligosides of quercetin and kaempferol) (Dudek-Makuch & Matławska 2011, Hubner et al 1999), including 3-O-alpha-arabinofuranoside, 3-O-beta-glucopyranoside, 3-O-alpha-rhamnopyranoside, 3-O-alpha-rhamnopyranosyl (1 –> 6)-O-beta-glucopyranoside (Dudek-Makuch & Matławska 2011). Condensed tannins, quinines, sterols (including stigmasterol, alpha-spinasterol and beta-sitosterol) (Senatore et al 1989), sugars (including glucose, xylose and rhamnose) (Hubner et al 1999) and fatty acids (including linolenic, palmitic and stearic acids) (Herbalgram 2000). Horse chestnut bark and flowers also contain the sterols stigmasterol, alpha-spinasterol and beta-sitosterol (NMCD 2006).

Although the majority of trials in the scientific literature have focused on the benefits of the HCSE extract, some authors suggest that the flavonoids contained in horse chestnut may provide additional benefits (Mills & Bone 2000).

MAIN ACTIONS

HCSE and various key components such as aescin have been investigated for pharmacological activities.

Vasoprotective/normalises vascular permeability

Horse chestnut appears to prevent the activation of leucocytes and therefore inhibit the activity of lysosomal enzymes (hyaluronidase and elastase) involved in the degradation of proteoglycan (the main component of the extravascular matrix), thus reducing the breakdown of mucopolysaccharides in vascular walls (Pittler & Ernst 2004). Aescin is the major constituent thought to be responsible for the inhibitory effects on hyaluronidase. Interestingly, ruscogenins found in *Ruscus aculeatus* L. (butcher's broom), while ineffective on hyaluronidase activity, exhibit significant anti-elastase activity (Facino et al 1995), which may explain the practice by many herbalists of combining the two herbs. By reducing degradation, the synthesis of proteoglycans is able to occur, which reduces capillary hyperpermeability, preventing the leakage of fluid into intercellular spaces that results in oedema. The anti-exudative activity appears to be mediated by PGF_{2alpha} (Berti et al 1977). In animal studies the aescins Ia, Ib, IIa and IIb have been shown to reduce capillary hyperpermeability induced by histamine, ascetic acid, carrageenan and serotonin (Guillaume & Padioleau 1994, Matsuda et al 1997). In experimental rat aortic-ring models, aescin has been shown to increase endothelial cell permeability to calcium, which enhances the production of nitric oxide (NO) (due to the effect of endothelial NO synthase, a calcium-dependent enzyme), and results in enhanced endothelium-dependent relaxation. This is thought to contribute to aescin's beneficial effect in the treatment of venous insufficiency (Carrasco & Vidrio 2007). The mechanism of selective vascular permeabilisation can allow for a higher sensitivity to molecular ions, for example, calcium channels, resulting in increased venous and arterial tone in addition to enhanced venous contractile activity (Sirtori 2001).

Horse chestnut promotes the proliferation behaviour of human endothelial cells in vitro in a dose-dependent manner (Fallier-Becker et al 2002) and may therefore also play a role in maintaining as well as protecting vascular walls.

By improving vascular tone, HCSE may improve the flow of blood back to the heart, as demonstrated in animal studies in which it significantly increased, within normal arterial parameters, femoral venous pressure and flow, as well as thoracic lymphatic flow (Guillaume & Padioleau 1994).

Anti-oedema

Horse chestnut prevents the excessive exudation of fluid through the walls of the capillaries that result in oedema by inhibiting the degradation of vascular walls. In animal experiments, HCSE reduced oedema of both inflammatory and lymphatic origin (Guillaume & Padioleau 1994).

Anti-inflammatory

Under experimental conditions, aescin pretreatment reduced IL-6 release from vascular endothelium (Montopoli et al 2007). In animal studies the aescins Ia, Ib, IIa and IIb have been shown to reduce capillary hyperpermeability induced by histamine, ascetic acid, carrageenan and serotonin (Guillaume & Padioleau 1994, Matsuda et al 1997). A sterol extract of horse chestnut bark was shown to have anti-inflammatory effects comparable to phenylbutazone in an inflammatory animal study utilising carrageenan-induced paw oedema (Senatore et al 1989). Studies suggest that aescin can effectively alter the cellular phase of the inflammatory process, such as leucocyte activation (Sirtori 2001).

Antioxidant

Oxidative stress is increasingly recognised as a fundamental factor in inflammatory responses (Braga et al 2012). HCSE dose-dependently inhibits both enzymatic and non-enzymatic lipid peroxidation in vitro (Guillaume & Padioleau 1994).

Horse chestnut bark extract altered reactive oxygen/nitrogen species (ROS/RNS) production in a concentration-dependent manner with significant effects being observed for even very low concentrations, for example, 10 mcg/mL (Braga et al 2012).

The component aescin enhanced endogenous antioxidative capacity in mice with acute liver injury induced by endotoxin (established by injecting lipopolysaccharide (LPS)). Aescin also down-regulated levels of inflammation mediators (TNF-α, IL-1β and NO) and 11β-HSD2 expression in liver, up-regulated glucocorticoid receptor expression and it is suggested that aescin can alleviate the degree of necrosis and decrease serum ALT and AST activities (Jiang et al. 2011).

Chemopreventive, anti-angiogenic and anti-proliferative

Beta-aescin demonstrated in vitro potent inhibition of cell proliferation and induction of apoptosis in HL-60 acute myeloid leukaemia cells (Niu et al 2008b) and human chronic myeloid leukaemia K562 cells (Niu et al 2008a), in addition to inhibiting the growth of colon cancer cells in rats (Patlolla et al 2006). Beta-aescin sodium (40 micrograms/mL) also induced endothelial cell apoptosis and inhibited endothelial cell proliferation in a dose-dependent manner (10, 20, 40 micrograms/mL) (Wang et al 2008).

Anti-ageing

A number of studies by Fujimura and others (2006a, 2006b, 2007) have suggested that horse chestnut extract can generate contraction forces in fibroblasts through stress fibre formation followed by activation of Rho protein and Rho kinase (Fujimura et al 2006b), and thus act as a potent anti-ageing factor. In a controlled trial of 40 women using an eye gel (3% horse chestnut extract) applied around the eyes three times a day for 9 weeks a significant reduction in wrinkle scores around the corners of the eye and lower eyelids was observed after 6 weeks (Fujimura et al 2006a, 2007).

OTHER ACTIONS

Animal studies have demonstrated that isolated aescins Ia, Ib, IIa and IIb inhibit gastric emptying time and ethanol absorption, and exert a hypoglycaemic activity in the oral glucose tolerance test in rats (Matsuda et al 1999, Yoshikawa et al 1996). Aescin also appears to possess a weak diuretic activity (Mills & Bone 2000).

Blood-retinal barrier (BRB) breakdown is a hallmark of diabetic retinopathy. The aim of the study by Zhang et al. (2013) was to investigate whether aescin exhibited synergistic protective effects on BRB breakdown, when combined with glucocorticoids in a rat model of retinal ischaemia. Low concentrations of aescin and triamcinolone acetonide (TA) alone did not affect BRB permeability. However, when administered together, low-dose aescin and TA significantly reduced BRB permeability following ischaemia. Furthermore, low-dose aescin and TA alone did not affect the expression of occludin in the ischaemic retina; however, when administered together, they significantly increased occludin expression in the ganglion cell layer of the ischemic retina.

CLINICAL USE

The most commonly used preparation is a dry extract, referred to as horse chestnut seed extract (HCSE), which is standardised to contain 16–21% triterpene glycosides (anhydrous aescin). It is used internally and also in topical preparations. HCSE has been extensively researched, mainly in Europe, for its beneficial effects in conditions where improving circulation and blood vessel integrity would be beneficial. In particular, HCSE is chiefly used in chronic pathological conditions of the veins where there is increased activity of lysosomal enzymes resulting in damage to and hyperpermeability of vascular walls (Herbalgram 2000).

Chronic venous insufficiency

HCSE taken orally is an effective treatment for chronic venous insufficiency (CVI), reducing leg pain, fatigue and heaviness, volume and oedema and pruritic symptoms according to placebo controlled studies. Approximately 10–15% of men and 20–25% of women present signs and symptoms consistent with the diagnosis of CVI (Pittler & Ernst 2012). This supports its traditional use as a treatment of CVI and its associated symptoms, such as lower leg swelling. The ability of HCSE to inhibit the catalytic breakdown of capillary wall proteoglycans and reduce inflammation is thought in part to mediate this effect.

A Cochrane systematic review that assessed 17 RCTs utilising HCSE capsules (standardised to aescin) concluded that signs and symptoms of CVI improve with HCSE treatment as compared with placebo (Pittler & Ernst 2012). Of these trials, 10 were placebo-controlled. Leg pain was assessed in seven placebo-controlled trials with six of these trials (n = 543) reporting a significant reduction in leg pain for HCSE, another study reported a significant improvement compared with baseline and one study reported that HCSE may be as effective as treatment with compression stockings.

Meta-analysis of six trials (n = 502) suggested a reduction in leg volume compared with placebo, as did the studies in which the circumference at calf and ankle (n = 172) was assessed overall. Adverse events were usually mild and infrequent. From this analysis, patients given 100–150 mg aescin daily for 2–8 weeks led to a significant reduction in leg volume and the symptoms of pain, fatigue, sensation of tension and itching compared to placebo. Three of the studies using 100 mg aescin daily reported a statistically significant reduction of mean leg volume after 2 weeks of treatment compared with placebo ($P < 0.01$). In the eight placebo-controlled trials where pruritus was assessed, four trials (n = 407) showed a significant reduction compared with placebo ($P < 0.05$) and two trials showed a significant difference in favour of HCSE compared with baseline ($P < 0.05$), whereas one trial found no significant differences for a score including the symptom pruritus compared with compression. The results of this systematic review suggest that when compared with placebo and reference treatment, HCSE is an effective treatment option for CVI (Pittler & Ernst 2012).

An earlier meta-analysis of 13 RCTs (n = 1051) and three observational studies (n = 10,725) found that HCSE reduced leg volume by 46.4 mL (95% CI, 11.3–81.4 mL) and increased the likelihood of improvement in leg pain 4.1-fold (95% CI, 0.98–16.8), oedema 1.5-fold (95% CI, 1.2–1.9) and pruritus 1.7-fold (95% CI, 0.01–3.0). Observational studies reported significant improvements in pain, oedema and leg fatigue/heaviness (Siebert et al 2002).

A case observational study involving more than 800 general practitioners and more than 5000 patients with CVI taking HCSE reported that symptoms of pain, tiredness, tension and swelling in the leg, as well as pruritus and tendency to oedema, all improved markedly or disappeared completely, with the additional advantage of better compliance than compression therapy (Greeske & Pohlmann 1996). In an open study carried out to assess the safety and tolerability of horse chestnut, 91 subjects received a tablet (equivalent to 50 mg aescin) twice daily for 8 consecutive weeks. At the end of the study the majority of patients rated horse chestnut to be good or very good for Widmer stage I and II CVI (Dickson et al 2004).

A study was carried out to compare the efficacy (oedema reduction) and safety of compression stockings class II and HCSE (50 mg aescin, twice daily) in 240 patients with chronic venous insufficiency (Diehm et al 1996). The patients were treated over a period of 12 weeks in a randomised, partially blinded, placebo-controlled, parallel study design. Lower leg volume of the more severely affected limb decreased on average by 43.8 mL (n = 95) with HCSE and 46.7 mL (n = 99) with compression therapy, while it increased by 9.8 mL with placebo (n = 46) after 12 weeks therapy.

In patients suffering from CVI, oedema can give rise to trophic skin changes, inflammatory lesions and an increase in blood coagulability with the associated risk of thrombosis development. Therapy should therefore be aimed at providing protection against oedema at the earliest possible stage of venous disease (Widmer CVI stages I or II) to prevent complications (Pohlmann et al 2000). As HCSE therapy appears to provide more significant benefits in the earlier stages (less so with the advancement of the condition) (Ottillinger & Greeske 2001), it would appear prudent to initiate HCSE therapy early in order to prevent or delay the need for compression therapy, which is associated with discomfort and poor patient compliance. In the later stages, combined treatment with compression stockings and HCSE may provide added benefit (Blaschek 2004, Pittler & Ernst 2004).

Although the standard dose used in clinical trials appears to be equivalent to 50 mg aescin twice daily, one study observed that reducing the dose to 50 mg aescin once daily at 8 weeks appeared to maintain similar benefits to the twice-daily routine at the end of the 16-week observation period (Pohlmann et al 2000).

Venous leg ulceration

Chronic venous leg ulceration (VLU) is a common recurrent problem in the elderly population and may result in immobility, with 45% of patients being housebound (Baker & Stacey 1994). As a result, individuals with VLU frequently experience depression, anxiety, social isolation, sleeplessness and reduced working capacity (Leach 2004). CVI, which is characterised by an increase in capillary permeability, inflammatory reactions, decreased lymphatic reabsorption, oedema and malnutrition of tissues, is a precursor to VLU. As HCSE increases venous tone while reducing venous fragility and capillary permeability, and possesses anti-oedematous and anti-inflammatory properties, it has been speculated that by improving microcirculation, ulceration may be delayed or prevented (Blaschek 2004).

In a prospective triple-blind randomised placebo-controlled trial, 54 patients with venous leg ulcers received HCSE ($n = 27$) or placebo ($n = 27$) for 12 weeks. At weeks 4, 8 and 12 the difference between groups in the number of healed leg ulcers and change in wound surface area, depth, volume, pain and exudate was not statistically significant. There was, however, a significant effect on the percentage of wound slough over time ($P = 0.045$) and on the number of dressing changes at week 12 ($P = 0.009$) (Leach et al 2006a). As a result, after taking into account the cost of HCSE, dressing materials, travel, staff salaries and infrastructure for each patient, this study determined a cost benefit for the addition of HCSE to conventional therapy of AU$95 in organisational costs, and AU$10 in dressing materials per patient (Leach et al 2006b). Further large-scale trials are required to fully elucidate the potential use in practice.

Haemorrhoids

Horse chestnut is also used both internally and topically for the treatment of haemorrhoids. Although there are not many studies on the effectiveness of horse chestnut in the treatment of haemorrhoids, oral treatment with aescin has been shown to significantly improve signs and symptoms according to a placebo-controlled double-blind study of 72 volunteers with haemorrhoids. Symptom relief was experienced by 82% of subjects compared with 32% for placebo, and swelling improved in 87% compared with 38% for placebo (Sirtori 2001). Symptom improvement required at least 6 days of treatment to become established and the dose used was 40 mg aescin three times daily.

Bruising

In a double-blind, placebo-controlled, randomised crossover study, the influence of aescin on the capillary resistance was investigated in 12 males (aged 24–31) with healthy vessels. The dosage of HCSE was 500 mg three times per day (1500 mg daily). Using capillary-resistometry (petechiae test), under standardised conditions, the number and area of petechiae were significantly lower after 7 days. The study noted a carryover effect where it was found that HCSE may have had a more permanent impact on the reduction of petechiae. The authors of the study concluded that capillary resistance was significantly improved after horse chestnut administration.

Cosmetics

Horse chestnut extracts have anti-inflammatory and antioxidant activities, together with the ability to improve capillary fragility and reduce oedema, making it a good candidate for inclusion into topical cosmetic preparations. It also contains saponins (aescin) which have a gentle soapy feel (Wilkinson & Brown 1999).

A study involving 40 healthy women tested the use of an eye gel containing 3% horse chestnut extract, which was applied around the eyes three times a day for 9 weeks (Fujimura et al 2006). After 6 weeks, significant decreases in the wrinkle scores at the corners of the eye or in the lower eyelid skin were observed compared with controls, a result evaluated using visual scoring based on photo scales. After 9 weeks, similar results were obtained suggesting no further changes occurred.

OTHER USES

Traditionally the seeds are used to treat conditions affecting the veins, including haemorrhoids, phlebitis and varicose veins; bruising, diarrhoea, fever, enlarged prostate, eczema, menstrual pain, painful injuries, sprains, swelling and spinal problems. The leaf is used for soft tissue swelling from bone fracture and sprains, complaints after concussion, cough, arthritis and rheumatism, and the bark for malaria and dysentery, and topically for SLE and skin ulcers (NMCD 2006, PDR Health 2006).

There is some evidence to support its use for preventing postoperative oedema (Sirtori 2001) and the antioxidant, vascular toning and anti-inflammatory effects of *A. hippocastanum*, as well as the presence of flavonoids and other active constituents, may support some of the other traditional uses (Wilkinson & Brown 1999).

DOSAGE RANGE

- Chronic venous insufficiency: HCSE standardised to 50–100 mg aescin twice daily. The dose may be reduced to a maintenance dose of 50 mg aescin once daily after 8 weeks (Pohlmann et al 2000).
- Australian manufacturers recommend 2–5 mL/day of 1:2 liquid extract.
- 1–2 g dried seed daily (Mills & Bone 2005).

ADVERSE REACTIONS

According to clinical trials horse chestnut and oral HCSE appears to be well tolerated with only mild, infrequent reports of adverse reactions, including gastric irritation, skin irritation, dizziness, nausea, headache and pruritus. Postmarketing surveillance reports adverse effects of 0.7% (Micromedex 2003, NMCD 2006, PDR Health 2006, Pittler & Ernst 2004, Siebert et al 2002).

Practice points/Patient counselling

- Horse chestnut extract has been extensively researched for its beneficial effects and is commonly used by GPs in Germany for the treatment of chronic venous insufficiency. There is strong evidence to support its use for this indication.
- In practice, a dry extract is used (HCSE standardised to contain 16–21% triterpene glycosides (anhydrous aescin)).
- HCSE is also used for venous leg ulceration because it increases venous tone while reducing venous fragility and capillary permeability, and possesses anti-oedematous, antioxidant and anti-inflammatory properties.
- HCSE is also used in the treatment of haemorrhoids. Although it has not been investigated for this indication, aescin has been shown to significantly improve signs and symptoms under double-blind study conditions.
- HCSE is well tolerated with only mild, infrequent reports of adverse reactions, including gastric irritation, skin irritation, dizziness, nausea, headache and pruritus. Do not use on broken skin due to the irritant effect of the saponins.
- Horse chestnut can cause hypersensitivity reactions, which occur more commonly in people who are allergic to latex.

Horse chestnut contains a toxic glycoside aesculin (esculin), a hydroxycoumarin that may increase bleeding time because of its antithrombin activity and may be lethal when the raw seeds, bark, flower or leaves are used orally. Poisoning has been reported from children drinking tea made with twigs and leaves (NMCD 2006).

Symptoms of overdose include diarrhoea, vomiting, reddening of the face, severe thirst, muscle twitching, weakness, loss of coordination, visual disturbances, enlarged pupils, depression, paralysis, stupor and loss of consciousness (NMCD 2006, PDR Health 2006). Reports of poisoning with horse chestnut seeds are consequent to the presence of the toxic principle aesculoside, not to aescin (Sirtori 2001).

Horse chestnut can also cause hypersensitivity reactions, which occur more commonly in people who are allergic to latex (Diaz-Perales et al 1999).

Isolated cases of kidney and liver toxicity have occurred after intravenous and intramuscular administration (Micromedex 2003, Mills & Bone 2005, NMCD 2006).

Aescin has undergone toxicological studies in rodents. Toxic manifestations following IV administration of high doses were due to haemolysis. The LD_{50} following IV administration in rodents was equivalent to 28 times the maximum dose recommended for therapeutic use; the LD_{50} following oral dosing was over 100 mg/kg, equivalent to 59 times the recommended therapeutic range (Sirtori 2001).

SIGNIFICANT INTERACTIONS

In vitro studies have revealed that horse chestnut may inhibit CYP3A4-mediated metabolism and P-glycoprotein efflux transport activity (Hellum & Nilsen 2008). The clinical significance of these findings remains to be tested.

Antiplatelet/ anticoagulant medications

Properly prepared HCSE should not contain aesculin and should not carry the risk of antithrombin activity — observe. The clinical significance is unclear.

Hypoglycaemic agents

Due to possible hypoglycaemic activity, blood glucose levels should be monitored when horse chestnut or HCSE and hypoglycaemic agents are used concurrently (Yoshikawa et al 1996) — observe. The clinical significance is unclear.

CONTRAINDICATIONS AND PRECAUTIONS

As saponins may cause irritation to the gastric mucosa and skin, horse chestnut should be taken with food. It is suggested that it should be avoided by people with infectious or inflammatory conditions of the gastrointestinal tract, including coeliac disease and malabsorption disorders and should not be applied topically to broken or ulcerated skin.

Horse chestnut flower, raw seed, branch bark or leaf may be toxic and are not recommended (Tiffany et al 2002).

Avoid use in the presence of hepatic or renal impairment (Micromedex 2003, NMCD 2006, PDR Health 2006).

In toxicity studies in rats, aescin decreased white blood cells, increased the number of red blood cells and platelets and haemoglobin content and reduced prothrombin time and thrombin time (5, 10, 15 mg/kg) (Li et al 2006).

PREGNANCY USE

Safety in pregnancy and lactation has not been well established.

PATIENTS' FAQs

What will this herb do for me?

Horse chestnut standardised extract (HCSE) will relieve signs and symptoms of chronic venous insufficiency such as pain, pruritus and oedema. It may also be of benefit in alleviating signs and symptoms in people with haemorrhoids and has been used in venous leg ulceration.

When will it start to work?

Beneficial effects in chronic venous insufficiency have been reported within 3–6 weeks; however,

12 weeks may be required in some cases. Aescin provided symptom relief in haemorrhoids after 6 days of treatment.

Are there any safety issues?

HCSE is well tolerated with only mild, infrequent reports of adverse reactions including gastric irritation, skin irritation, dizziness, nausea, headache and pruritus. It can cause hypersensitivity reactions, which occur more commonly in people who are allergic to latex.

REFERENCES

Anonymous. Aesculus hippocastanum (Horse chestnut). Monograph. Altern Med Rev 14.3 (2009): 278–283.

Baker SR, Stacey MC. Epidemiology of chronic leg ulcers in Australia. Aust NZ J Surg 64.4 (1994): 258–261.

Berti F et al. The mode of action of aescin and the release of prostaglandins. Prostaglandins 14.2 (1977): 241–249.

Blaschek W. Aesculus hippocastanum: Horse chestnut seed extract in the treatment of chronic venous insufficiency. Z Phytother 25.1 (2004): 21–30.

Bombardelli E, Morazzoni P, Griffini A. Aesculus hippocastanum L. Fitoterapia 67.6 (1996): 483–511.

Braga PC et al. Characterisation of the antioxidant effects of Aesculus hippocastanum L. bark extract on the basis of radical scavenging activity, the chemiluminescence of human neutrophil bursts and lipoperoxidation assay. Eur Rev Med Pharmacol Sci 16.S3 (2012): 1–9.

Carrasco OF, Vidrio H. Endothelium protectant and contractile effects of the antivaricose principle escin in rat aorta. Vascul Pharmacol 47.1 (2007): 68–73.

Diaz-Perales A et al. Cross-reactions in the latex-fruit syndrome: A relevant role of chitinases but not of complex asparagine-linked glycans. J Allergy Clin Immunol 104.3 (1999): 681–687.

Dickson S et al. An open study to assess the safety and efficacy of Aesculus hippocastanum tablets (Aesculaforce 50 mg) in the treatment of chronic venous insufficiency. J Herb Pharmacother 4.2 (2004): 19–32.

Diehm C et al. Comparison of leg compression stocking and oral horse-chestnut seed extract therapy in patients with chronic venous insufficiency. Lancet 347.8997 (1996): 292–294.

Dudek-Makuch M, Matławska I. Flavonoids from the flowers of Aesculus hippocastanum. Acta Pol Pharm 68.3 (2011): 403–408.

Facino RM et al. Anti-elastase and anti-hyaluronidase activities of saponins and sapogenins from Hedera helix, Aesculus hippocastanum, and Ruscus aculeatus: factors contributing to their efficacy in the treatment of venous insufficiency. Arch Pharm (Weinheim) 328.10 (1995): 720–724.

Fallier-Becker P, Borner M, Weiser M. Proliferation modulating effect of Aesculus hippocastanum, Coenzyme Q10 and Heparsuis on endothelial cells. Biol Med 31.1 (2002): 10–14.

Fujimura T et al. A horse chestnut extract, which induces contraction forces in fibroblasts, is a potent anti-aging ingredient. J Cosmet Sci 57.5 (2006a): 369–376.

Fujimura T et al. Horse chestnut extract induces contraction force generation in fibroblasts through activation of rho/rho kinase. Biol Pharm Bull 29(6) (2006b): 1075–1081.

Fujimura T et al. A horse chestnut extract, which induces contraction forces in fibroblasts, is a potent anti-aging ingredient. Int J Cosmet Sci 29.2 (2007): 140.

Greeske K, Pohlmann BK. Horse chestnut seed extract: an effective therapy principle in general practice: Drug therapy of chronic venous insufficiency. Fortschr Med 114.15 (1996): 196–200.

Guillaume M, Padioleau F. Veinotonic effect, vascular protection, antiinflammatory and free radical scavenging properties of horse chestnut extract. Arzneimittelforschung 44.1 (1994): 25–35.

Hellum BH, Nilsen OG. In vitro inhibition of CYP3A4 metabolism and P-glycoprotein-mediated transport by trade herbal products. Basic Clin Pharmacol Toxicol 102.5 (2008): 466–475.

Herbalgram. Horse chestnut seed extract. In: Council AB, editor. Excerpt from: Blumenthal M, Goldberg A, Brinckmann J (eds). Herbal medicine: expanded Commission E monographs. Austin, TX: Integrative Medicine Communications, 2000.

Hubner G et al. Flavonol oligosaccharides from the seeds of Aesculus hippocastanum. Planta Med 65.7 (1999): 636–642.

Jiang N et al. Protective effect of aescin from the seeds of Aesculus hippocastanum on liver injury induced by endotoxin in mice. Phytomedicine 18.14 (2011):1276–1284.

Konoshima T, Lee KH. Antitumor agents, 82: Cytotoxic sapogenols from Aesculus hippocastanum. J Nat Prod 49.4 (1986): 650–656.

Leach MJ. The clinical feasibility of natural medicine, venotonic therapy and horsechestnut seed extract in the treatment of venous leg ulceration: a descriptive survey. Complement Ther Nursing Midwif 10.2 (2004): 97–109.

Leach MJ et al. Clinical efficacy of horsechestnut seed extract in the treatment of venous ulceration. J Wound Care 15.4 (2006a): 159–167.

Leach MJ et al. Using horsechestnut seed extract in the treatment of venous leg ulcers: a cost-benefit analysis. Ostomy Wound Manage 52.4 (2006b): 68–70, 72–4, 76–8.

Li C-m et al. Investigation of blood toxicity in association with aescin (the horse chestnut seed extract). Toxicology Letters 164 (Suppl 1) (2006): S90.

Matsuda H et al. Effects of escins Ia, Ib, IIa, and IIb from horse chestnut, the seeds of Aesculus hippocastanum L., on acute inflammation in animals. Biol Pharm Bull 20.10 (1997): 1092–1095.

Matsuda H et al. Effects of escins Ia, Ib, IIa, and IIb from horse chestnuts on gastric emptying in mice. Eur J Pharmacol 368.2–3 (1999): 237–243.

Micromedex. (Horse chestnut: Alternative Medicine Summary). Thomson, 2003.Online. Available: www.micromedex.com 10 January 2006.

Mills S, Bone K. Principles and practice of phytotherapy. London: Churchill Livingstone, 2000, pp 448–455.

Mills S, Bone K. The essential guide to herbal safety. St Louis: Elsevier, 2005.

Montopoli M et al. Aescin protection of human vascular endothelial cells exposed to cobalt chloride mimicked hypoxia and inflammatory stimuli. Planta Med 73.3 (2007): 285–288.

Natural Medicines Comprehensive Database (NMCD online). Horse chestnut: Monograph, 2006. Available: www.naturaldatabase.com 10 January 2006.

Niu YP, Li LD et al. Beta-aescin: a potent natural inhibitor of proliferation and inducer of apoptosis in human chronic myeloid leukemia K562 cells in vitro. Leuk Lymphoma 49.7 (2008a): 1384–1391.

Niu YP, Wu LM et al. Beta-escin, a natural triterpenoid saponin from Chinese horse chestnut seeds, depresses HL-60 human leukaemia cell proliferation and induces apoptosis. J Pharm Pharmacol 60.9 (2008b): 1213–1220.

Ottillinger B, Greeske K. Rational therapy of chronic venous insufficiency chances and limits of the therapeutic use of horse-chestnut seeds extract. BMC Cardiovasc Disord 1 (2001): 5.

Patlolla JM et al. Beta-escin inhibits colonic aberrant crypt foci formation in rats and regulates the cell cycle growth by inducing p21(waf1/cip1) in colon cancer cells. Mol Cancer Ther 5.6 (2006): 1459–1466.

PDR Health. Horse chestnut, 2006. Online. Available: www.pdrhealth 10 January 2006.

Pittler MH, Ernst E. Horse chestnut seed extract for chronic venous insufficiency. Cochrane Database Syst Rev. 4 (2012): CD003230.

Pittler M, Ernst E. Horse chestnut seed extract for chronic venous insufficiency. Cochrane Database Syst Rev 4 (2004): CD003230.

Pohlmann G, Bar H, Figulla H. Studies on dose dependency of the edema protective effect of extracts from horse chestnut in female patients suffering from chronic venous insufficiency. Vasomed 12.2 (2000): 69–75.

Senatore F et al. Steroidal constituents and anti-inflammatory activity of the horse chestnut (Aesculus hippocastanum L.) bark. Boll Soc Ital Biol Sper 65.2 (1989): 137–141.

Siebert U et al. Efficacy, routine effectiveness, and safety of horsechestnut seed extract in the treatment of chronic venous insufficiency: A meta-analysis of randomized controlled trials and large observational studies. Int Angiol 21.4 (2002): 305–315.

Sirtori CR. Aescin: pharmacology, pharmacokinetics and therapeutic profile. Pharmacol Res 44.3 (2001): 183–193.

Tiffany N et al. Horse chestnut: a multidisciplinary clinical review. J Herb Pharmacother 2.1 (2002): 71–85.

Wang XH et al. Effect of beta-escin sodium on endothelial cells proliferation, migration and apoptosis. Vascul Pharmacol 49.4–6 (2008): 158–165.

Wilkinson J, Brown A. Horse chestnut: Aesculus hippocastanum: Potential applications in cosmetic skin-care products. Int J Cosmet Sci 21.6 (1999): 437–447.

Yoshikawa M et al. Bioactive saponins and glycosides. III. Horse chestnut. (1): The structures, inhibitory effects on ethanol absorption, and hypoglycemic activity of escins Ia, Ib, IIa, IIb, and IIIa from the seeds of Aesculus hippocastanum L. Chem Pharm Bull (Tokyo) 44.8 (1996): 1454–1464.

Yoshikawa M et al. Bioactive saponins and glycosides. XII. Horse chestnut. (2): Structures of escins IIIb, IV, V, and VI and isoescins Ia, Ib, and V, acylatedpolyhydroxyoleanenetriterpeneoligoglycosides, from the seeds of horse chestnut tree (Aesculus hippocastanum L., Hippocastanaceae). Chem Pharm Bull (Tokyo) 46.11 (1998): 1764–1769.

Zhang F et al. Synergistic protective effects of escin and low-dose glucocorticoids on blood-retinal barrier breakdown in a rat model of retinal ischemia. Mol Med Rep 7.5 (2013): 1511–1515.

Horseradish

HISTORICAL NOTE Horseradish is a commonly used spice with a long history of use in traditional medicine. The leaves are used in cooking and as a salad green. Horseradish is one of the 'five bitter herbs' of the biblical Passover.

COMMON NAME

Horseradish

OTHER NAMES

Amoracia rusticanae radix, great mountain root, great raifort, mountain radish, pepperrot, red cole

BOTANICAL NAME/FAMILY

Armoracia rusticana, synonym *Armoracia lopathifolia*; *Cochlearia armoracia*, *Nasturtium armoracia*, *Roripa armoracia* (family Brassicaceae [Cruciferae])

PLANT PARTS USED

Fresh or dried roots and leaves

CHEMICAL COMPONENTS

Horseradish root contains volatile oils: glucosinolates (mustard oil glycosides); gluconasturtiin and sinigrin (S-glucosides); coumarins (aesculetin, scopoletin); phenolic acids, including caffeic acid derivatives and hydroxycinnamic acid derivatives, ascorbic acid; asparagin; resin; and peroxidase enzymes. Allyl isothiocyanate is the chief glucosinolate present in horseradish and responsible for most of its clinical activity. The concentration of allyl isothiocyanate in horseradish is dependent on the concentration of sulfate in the soil it is cultivated in (Alnsour et al 2013). Horseradish is one of the richest plant sources of peroxidase enzymes, in particular horseradish peroxidase, which are commonly used as oxidising agents in commercial chemical tests.

MAIN ACTIONS

Irritant

Horseradish is widely known for its pungent burning flavour. The pungency of horseradish is due to the release of allyl isothiocyanate and butyl thiocyanate upon crushing (Yu et al 2001). These mustard oil glycosides may irritate the mucous membranes upon contact or inhalation and may act as circulatory and digestive stimulants; however, the mechanism of action has not been fully elucidated (Blumenthal et al 2000, Jordt et al 2004). It has been found that topical application of allyl isothiocyanate to the skin activates sensory nerve endings producing pain, inflammation and hypersensitivity to thermal and mechanical stimuli due to depolarising the same sensory neurons that are activated by capsaicin and tetrahydrocannabinol (Jordt et al 2004).

Circulatory stimulant

The mustard oils released when horseradish is crushed may be responsible for this activity.

Digestive stimulant

Again, it is suspected that the mustard oils may be responsible as these act as irritants. Large doses may cause emesis (Pengelly 1996).

Antimicrobial activity

Allyl isothiocyanate has been well known to possess antimicrobial effects against *Escherichia coli* O157:H7, *Listeria monocytogenes*, *Salmonella typhimurium* and *Staphylococcus aureus* (Shin et al 2010).

Fungistatic and insecticidal activity

Horseradish extract, prepared from fresh plants in a solution of ethanol 80%, was found to have significant insecticidal activity against larvae of *Aedes albopictus* (Skuse) and when applied in a 10% ethanolic extract, a fungistatic activity against *Sclerotium rolfsii* Sacc., *Fusarium oxysporum* Schlecht. and *F. culmorum* (Wm. G. Sm) Sacc. (Tedeschi et al 2011).

Horseradish oil-derived compounds and several isothiocyanates are potential acaricides for the control of house dust mite populations as fumigants with contact action (Yun et al 2012).

OTHER ACTIONS

Isothiocyanates may inhibit thyroxine formation and be goitrogenic (Langer & Stole 1965), although this has not been demonstrated clinically.

The peroxidase enzymes assist in wound healing, whereas the sulfur-containing compounds may decrease the thickness of mucus by altering the structure of its mucopolysaccharide constituents (Mills & Bone 2000). Antispasmodic and antimicrobial effects have also been reported (Blumenthal et al 2000, Newell et al 1996). Horseradish has been found to lower plasma cholesterol and faecal bile acid excretion in mice fed with a cholesterol-enriched diet, possibly due to interference with exogenous cholesterol absorption (Balasinska et al 2005).

Horseradish has also been found to contain compounds that inhibit tumour cell growth and cyclooxygenase-1 enzymes (Weil et al 2005). In vivo trials testing a combination of herbs, including horseradish, has been found to protect against viral transmission of avian influenza (Oxford et al 2007).

Clinical note — Horseradish peroxidase: an important plant enzyme

Few plant enzymes are represented so widely in the scientific and patent literature as horseradish peroxidase. It is one of the most important enzymes obtained from a plant source and the subject of thousands of papers in the scientific literature. It is commercially produced from horseradish roots on a relatively large scale. This is due to its broad use, for example, as a component of clinical diagnostic kits and for immunoassays (Veitch 2004). Research is also being undertaken to understand how it may be used clinically.

CLINICAL USE

The therapeutic effectiveness of horseradish has not been significantly investigated.

Nasal congestion and sinusitis

Horseradish is widely used in combination with other ingredients such as garlic in herbal decongestant formulations. Anecdotal evidence suggests that a mild, transient decongestant effect occurs. It is reputed to eliminate excessive catarrh from the respiratory tract (Drew 2002, Tancred 2006), although clinical research is not available to confirm its efficacy.

OTHER USES

It has been used traditionally to treat both bronchial and urinary infections, joint and tissue inflammations, as well as treating gallbladder disorders, reducing oedema and as an abortifacient (Skidmore-Roth 2001).

An in vivo study in mice demonstrated that allyl isothiocyanate markedly inhibited the formation of gastric lesions (Matsuda et al 2007).

DOSAGE RANGE

- The typical dose of horseradish is 2–20 g/day of the root or equivalent preparations.
- Topical preparations with a maximum of 2% mustard oil content are commonly used (Blumenthal et al 2000).

ADVERSE REACTIONS

Despite the potential for severe irritation, horseradish is generally recognised as safe for human consumption in quantities used as food. Consuming large amounts of horseradish can cause gastrointestinal upset, vomiting and diarrhoea, and irritation of mucous membranes. Skin contact with fresh horseradish can cause irritation and blistering or allergic reactions. If used topically it should be diluted 50% with water and not applied for prolonged periods. Application to a small test area before wider application is recommended for people with sensitive skin.

Practice points/Patient counselling

- Horseradish has been used as a vegetable, condiment, diuretic and treatment for bronchial and urinary infections, joint and tissue inflammation and swelling.
- It is widely used together with other herbal ingredients, such as garlic, as a decongestant in the treatment of colds and sinusitis.
- No scientific investigation has been undertaken to support its use, although anecdotal evidence suggests that it may be useful.
- Horseradish is generally safe when the root is ingested in usual dietary amounts, although excessive intake may cause irritation to the stomach, respiratory tract and kidneys.

SIGNIFICANT INTERACTIONS

None known.

CONTRAINDICATIONS AND PRECAUTIONS

Internal use should be avoided in people with stomach and intestinal ulcers and kidney disorders, as well as in children under the age of 4 years (Blumenthal et al 2000).

Traditionally, horseradish is considered a warming herb that will exacerbate any 'hot' condition and is specifically indicated for 'cold' conditions.

PREGNANCY USE

The mustard oils released upon crushing are potentially toxic, therefore doses exceeding dietary intakes are contraindicated (Newell et al 1996).

PATIENTS' FAQs

What will this herb do for me?

Anecdotal evidence suggests that it may have decongestant effects and is a very popular treatment when combined with other herbs, such as garlic, to relieve the symptoms of colds and sinusitis.

When will it start to work?

It may relieve symptoms within the first few doses, but scientific tests are not available to confirm this.

Are there any safety issues?

Horseradish can be quite irritating for some people due to its bitter and pungent characteristics.

REFERENCES

Alnsour, M., et al. 2013. Sulfate determines the glucosinolate concentration of horseradish in vitro plants (*Armoracia rusticana* Gaertn., Mey. & Scherb.). J Sci. Food Agric., 93, (4) 918–923.

Balasinska B et al. Dietary horseradish reduces plasma cholesterol in mice. Nutr Res 25.10 (2005): 937–945.

Blumenthal M, et al (eds). Herbal medicine: expanded Commission E monographs. Austin, TX: Integrative Medicine Communications, 2000.

Drew A. Horseradish. Curr Ther 42.3 (2002).

Jordt S-E et al. Mustard oils and cannabinoids excite sensory nerve fibres through the TRP channel ANKTM1. Nature 427 (2004): 260–265.

Langer P, Stolc V. Goitrogenic activity of allylisothiocyanate: a widespread natural mustard oil. Endocrinology 76 (1965): 151–155.
Matsuda H et al. Effects of allyl isothiocyanate from horseradish on several experimental gastric lesions in rats. Eur J Pharmacol 561.1–3 (2007): 172–181.
Mills S, Bone K. Principles and practice of phytotherapy. London: Churchill Livingstone, 2000.
Newell CA, et al. Herbal medicines: a guide for health care professionals. London, UK: The Pharmaceutical Press, 1996.
Oxford JS et al. In vivo prophylactic activity of QR-435 against H3N2 influenza virus infection. Am J Ther 14.5 (2007): 462–468.
Pengelly A. The constituents of medicinal plants. Muswellbrook, NSW: Sunflower Herbals 1996.
Shin, I.S., et al. 2010. Effect of isothiocyanates from horseradish (*Armoracia rusticana*) on the quality and shelf life of tofu. Food Control, 21, (8) 1081–1086.
Skidmore-Roth L. Mosby's handbook of herbs and natural supplements. St Louis: Mosby, 2001.
Tancred J. Herbs for catarrh and congestion. JCM 5.5 (2006): 37–38, 40, 42.
Tedeschi, P., et al. 2011. Insecticidal activity and fungitoxicity of plant extracts and components of horseradish (*Armoracia rusticana*) and garlic (*Allium sativum*). J Environ. Sci. Health B, 46, (6) 486–490.
Veitch, N.C. 2004. Horseradish peroxidase: a modern view of a classic enzyme. Phytochemistry, 65, (3) 249–259.
Weil MJ, et al. Tumor cell proliferation and cyclooxygenase inhibitory constituents in horseradish (*Amoracia rusticana*) and Wasabi (*Wasabia japonica*). J Agric Food Chem 53.5 (2005): 1440–1444.
Yu EY et al. In situ observation of the generation of isothiocyanates from sinigrin in horseradish and wasabi. Biochim Biophys Acta 1527.3 (2001): 156–160.
Yun, Y.K., et al. 2012. Contact and fumigant toxicity of *Armoracia rusticana* essential oil, allyl isothiocyanate and related compounds to *Dermatophagoides farinae*. Pest. Manag. Sci., 68, (5) 788–794.

Iodine

BACKGROUND AND RELEVANT PHARMACOKINETICS

Iodine is an essential trace element required for proper functioning of the thyroid gland. It is mainly consumed as iodide salts obtained from sea salt, shellfish and seawater fish and vegetables, which are more bioavailable than the organic forms. The iodine content of soil is considered to be one of the most variable of all minerals, influenced by local geography and the type and quantity of fertiliser used in agriculture (Groff et al 2009). There is evidence of iodine-deficient soils in many regions of Australia. Dietary iodine content is also significantly influenced by agricultural iodine-containing compounds, used in irrigation products, fertiliser and livestock feeds (Zimmermann et al 2008).

Iodide is rapidly absorbed from the stomach to the small intestine and distributed via the blood to a range of tissues, most notably the thyroid, which traps iodide through an ATP-dependent iodide pump called the sodium iodide symporter. The thyroid contains 80% of the body's iodine pool, which is approximately 15 mg in adults. Also found in high concentrations in the salivary, gastric and mammary glands (exclusively during pregnancy and lactation in the latter), iodine's uptake is regulated by thyroid-stimulating hormone (TSH) (Groff et al 2009, Kohlmeier 2003).

Excess iodine is excreted via the kidneys when the needs of the thyroid have been met (Kohlmeier 2003), therefore urine concentrations are used as a means of assessing iodine status. Interestingly, there is no renal conservation mechanism for this mineral and the only evidence of iodine preservation comes from the scavenging and recycling of thyroid hormones by the selenium-dependent deiodinase DII (Kohlmeier 2003). Of the total amount excreted, 20% occurs via faeces and additional losses can occur through sweat, which, although a minor eliminatory pathway under normal circumstances, can be a significant contributor for people living in hot climates with low dietary consumption (Groff et al 2009).

FOOD SOURCES

Iodine can occur in foods as either an inorganic or organic salt, or as thyroxine in animal sources. Unlike many other essential nutrients, the organic form of iodine found in animal products has poor bioavailability, whereas the iodide salts found in the sea are almost completely absorbed (Jones 2002).

However, irrespective of whether it is animal or plant derived, food from the land has enormous variability in terms of iodine content, from 1 to 10 microgram/kg (Geissler & Powers 2005), due to iodine's high solubility and therefore susceptibility to leaching (Wahlqvist 2002).

Additionally, chemicals known as goitrogens are naturally found in some foods (e.g. brassica [cabbage] family), and these interfere with iodine utilisation and thyroid hormone production.

Best sources

Due to the high saltwater levels of bioavailable iodide, all sea-dwelling creatures, animal or plant, are considered as superior dietary sources.

- Seawater fish
- Shellfish
- Sea vegetables such as seaweeds
- Iodised salt (fortified form of table salt) — providing 20–40 microgram/g
- Recommended for use in Australia by the Foods Standard Australia New Zealand
- Commercially manufactured breads due to the iodate dough oxidisers
- Dairy milk (variable)

In Australia, milk no longer supplies a significant amount of iodine, whereas in the United Kingdom it is still an important dietary source because of the use of both supplemented feeds and iodine-based antiseptics in the dairy industry (Geissler & Powers 2005).

DEFICIENCY SIGNS AND SYMPTOMS

Primary deficiency

Iodine status is considered optimal in a population if the median urinary iodine concentration (MUIC) lies between 100 and 200 micrograms/L. An MUIC of between 50 and 100 micrograms/L is defined as a mild iodine deficiency; 29–49 micrograms/L as moderate deficiency and <20 micrograms/L as severe iodine deficiency. Intervention, such as fortification of salt, is recommended where a population MUIC is <100 micrograms/L. Urinary iodine concentration alone is not however considered an accurate measure of individual iodine status due to high intra-individual variability (Australian Population Health Development Principal Committee [APHDPC] 2007).

Inadequate intake of iodine leads to a decreased thyroid function which results in a collection of physical and mental disorders referred to as 'iodine deficiency disorders' (IDD). These disorders range from being mild to life-threatening (Groff et al 2009, Eastman 2012). A normal adult thyroid contains up to 20 mg of iodine, but this may drop as low as 20 micrograms in cases of chronic iodine deficiency (Zimmerman 2011).

In situations of moderate iodine deficiency, TSH induces thyroid hypertrophy in order to concentrate iodide, resulting in goitre. Most of these cases remain euthyroid, but in cases of severe iodine deficiency, myxoedema may result in adults and cretinism in infants, both of which are serious conditions.

Myxoedema is characterised by swelling of the hands, face, feet and peri-orbital tissues and can lead to coma and death if sufficiently severe and left untreated. Endemic cretinism is divided into two forms, neurological or myxoedematous, depending on the interplay of genetics and iodine deficiency. Usually, children with neurological cretinism are mentally deficient and often deaf–mute, but of normal height and strength and may have goitre. Myxoedematous cretinism is characterised by dwarfism, mental deficiency, dry skin, large tongue, umbilical hernia, muscular incoordination and puffy facial features. Concomitant selenium deficiency may be a contributing factor in myxoedematous cretinism. Early treatment with thyroid hormone supplementation can promote normal physical growth; however, intellectual disability may not be prevented and in very severe cases death may ensue.

Although severe iodine deficiency is rare in Australia and New Zealand, the Australian Population Health Development Principal Committee reports a high incidence of mild to moderate iodine deficiency in primary-school-aged children in Australia and New Zealand (APHDPC 2007). Many parts of the world have notoriously low iodine levels, which is attributed to factors such as depletion in soils, low intake of iodised salt and fish farming practices (Kotsirilos et al 2011). Countries where iodine deficiency is a primary concern include China, Latin America, Southeast Asia and the eastern Mediterranean (Wahlqvist 2002). A report conducted by the World Health Organization in 2007 found that while many countries had succeeded in reaching optimal iodine nutrition through enhanced monitoring and fortification programs over the past decade, worldwide, an estimated almost 2 billion people still have insufficient iodine intakes, including one-third of all school-going children (Zimmerman 2011). Iodine deficiency is considered the single most important cause of preventable mental retardation and brain damage worldwide (APHDPC 2007).

Fetal deficiency

The fetus depends solely on maternal thyroid hormones during the first trimester of pregnancy (Soldin et al 2002) and iodine deficiency uncorrected prior to mid-gestation results in irreversible brain damage (de Escobar et al 2007). To accommodate for this, increasing plasma volume, renal clearance and the increased thyroid hormone degradation secondary to hyperactivity of the uterine–placental deiodinases, healthy pregnant women exhibit a surge in T_4 production, partly under the stimulation of human chorionic gonadotrophin (HCG). From week 11 of gestation, fetal thyroid hormone synthesis usually begins, still dependent on maternal provision of iodine and at term a residual 20–40% of T_4 found in cord blood is of maternal origin (de Escobar et al 2008, Delange 2007, Glinoer 2007, Zimmermann 2008). These demands necessitate an approximately 100% increase (e.g. 250–300 microgram/day) (de Escobar et al 2008, Delange 2007) in maternal iodine intake from conception and throughout the pregnancy. Should such needs go unmet, the mother will adapt by preferentially producing T_3 to stave off both clinical and biochemical hypothyroidism. The fetus, however, yet to develop rapid adaptations to circulating iodine levels, will exhibit reductions of all thyroid hormones and develop hypothyroidism in spite of the mother's euthyroid state (de Escobar et al 2008).

Adequate iodine and healthy functioning of both the maternal and the fetal thyroid glands play a critical role in fetal neuropsycho-intellectual development, due to its role in neuronal migration and myelination, with brain damage risk secondary to a deficiency, peaking in the second trimester and the early neonatal period. Studies have also confirmed that 'mild but measurable' psychomotor deficits in early childhood can result from subclinical hypothyroidism and hypothyroxaemia caused by mild-to-moderate iodine deficiency in pregnancy (Glinoer 2007, Soldin et al 2002). Finally, severe iodine deficiency during pregnancy also increases risk of stillbirths, miscarriage, perinatal mortality and congenital abnormalities (Zimmermann 2008).

Because of the severe neurological consequences of untreated congenital hypothyroidism, neonatal screening programs have been established in some developed countries; however, early or pre-pregnancy detection of subclinical iodine deficiency would be most effective (Ares et al 2008).

Premature infant deficiency

Premature infants face a significantly elevated risk of iodine deficiency secondary to a collusion of factors: interruption of maternal supply (small amounts of breast milk provide substantially smaller quantities of iodine than placental transfer), immaturity of the hypothalamic pituitary thyroid axis and the deiodinase systems, maternal antibodies and postnatal exposure to drugs (e.g. dopamine, heparin, corticosteroids) (Ares et al 2008). Research suggests that 75% of premature neonates demonstrate a negative iodine balance at 5 days post-partum prior to intentional repletion.

Secondary deficiency

High consumption of goitrogens can induce a secondary deficiency state. Goitrogens are substances that inhibit iodine metabolism and include thiocyanates found in the cabbage family (e.g. cabbage, kale, cauliflower, broccoli, turnips and Brussels sprouts) and in linseed, cassava, millet, soybean and competing entities, such as other members of the halogen family (e.g. bromine, fluorine and lithium, as well as arsenic) (Groff et al 2009). Most researchers agree, however, that moderate intake of goitrogens in the diet is not an issue, except when accompanied by low iodine consumption (Groff et al 2009, Kohlmeier 2003). A very rare cause of secondary iodine deficiency and hypothyroidism is TSH deficiency.

Low selenium intake

Low dietary intake of selenium is a factor that exacerbates the effects of iodine deficiency. Selenium is found in the thyroid gland in high concentrations, and while iodine is required for thyroid hormone synthesis, selenium-dependent enzymes are required for the peripheral conversion of thyroxine (T_4) to its biologically active form triiodothyronine (T_3) (Higdon 2003), as well as the general recycling of iodine. Selenium deficiency results in decreased T_4 catabolism, which leads to increased production of peroxide and thyroid cell destruction, fibrosis and functional failure.

SIGNS AND SYMPTOMS

Overall, in addition to highly visible goitre, moderate-to-severe iodine deficiency produces subtle but widespread effects secondary to hypothyroidism, including reduced educability, apathy and impaired productivity, culminating ultimately in poor social and economic development (Zimmermann 2008).

Mild hypothyroidism

This refers to biochemical evidence of thyroid hormone deficiency in patients who have few or no apparent clinical features of hypothyroidism. Current literature does not adequately describe the health consequences of a mild iodine deficiency, although there is reasonable evidence of an association between a mild iodine deficiency and suboptimal neurological development in children such as a reduced IQ.

Congenital hypothyroidism

The majority of infants appear normal at birth and <10% are diagnosed with hypothyroidism based on the following clinical features:

- prolonged jaundice
- feeding problems
- hypotonia
- enlarged tongue
- delayed bone maturation
- umbilical hernia.

Importantly, permanent neurological damage results if treatment is delayed.

Adult hypothyroidism

According to Beers (2005), the clinical signs of hypothyroidism in adults are as follows:

- weakness, tiredness and sleepiness
- dry skin
- cold intolerance
- hair loss and diffuse alopecia
- poor memory and difficulty concentrating
- constipation
- reduced appetite and weight gain
- dyspnoea
- hoarse voice
- increased susceptibility to infectious diseases
- increased susceptibility to cardiovascular diseases
- paraesthesia
- puffy hands, feet and face and peripheral oedema
- impaired hearing
- menorrhagia (later amenorrhoea)
- carpal tunnel and other entrapment syndromes are common, as is impairment of muscle function with stiffness, cramps and pain
- reduced myocardial contractility and pulse rate, leading to a reduced stroke volume and bradycardia.

In adults, mild–moderate iodine deficiency also results in higher rates of more aggressive subtypes of thyroid cancer and an increased risk of (non) toxic goitre (Zimmermann 2008).

MAIN ACTIONS

Thyroid hormone production

Iodine is essential for the manufacture of T_4 and T_3, which are hormones that influence growth, maturation, thermogenesis, oxidation, myelination of the CNS and the metabolism of all tissues (Jones 2002). The thyroid hormones, especially T_3, exert their effects by binding to nuclear receptors on cell surfaces, which in turn trigger binding of the zinc fingers of the receptor protein to the DNA (Groff et al 2009).

OTHER ACTIONS

Due to the concentration of appreciable iodine levels in a range of other tissues, including salivary, gastric and lactating mammary glands, and the ovaries, questions remain about potential additional actions of iodine. One hypothesis postulates iodine as an indirect antioxidant, via its capacity to reduce elevated TSH, a trigger of increased peroxide levels in the body (Smyth 2003).

CLINICAL USE

Increased iodine intake can be achieved through dietary modification and supplementation with tablets. Dietary modification usually refers to increased intake of iodised salt, but may also refer to use of iodised water, iodised vegetable oil or seafood or the use of iodised salt in bread manufacture.

Treatment and prevention of deficiency

Iodine deficiency is accepted as the most common cause of brain damage worldwide, with IDD affecting 740 million people (Higdon 2003). Although it is well accepted that severe deficiency is responsible, evidence is now emerging that mild deficiency during pregnancy is also important and can have subtle effects on brain development, lowering intellectual functioning and inducing psychomotor deficits in early childhood (Glinoer 2007). Preliminary data are also emerging to suggest an association between iodine deficiency hypothyroidism of pregnancy and the incidence of attention-deficit/hyperactivity disorder (ADHD) in the offspring; however, this still requires confirmation in larger studies (Soldin et al 2002, Vermiglio et al 2004).

Pregnancy

Severe iodine deficiency is uncommon in Western countries, such as Australia and New Zealand, but several local surveys have identified that mild-to-moderate deficiency is more prevalent than once thought. The published studies on iodine status in pregnant Australians are limited to New South Wales, Victoria and Tasmania; however, the results are of concern as they consistently suggest that iodine intake is inadequate, with median urinary iodine concentrations (MUIC) ranging from 47–104 micrograms/L, well below the adequate range of 150–249 micrograms/L as defined by WHO for pregnant women (APHPDC 2007).

A research group at Monash Medical Centre in Melbourne screened 802 pregnant women and found that 48.4% of Caucasian women had urinary iodine concentration (UIC) below 50 microgram/L compared to 38.4% of Vietnamese women and 40.8% of Indian/Sri Lankan women (Hamrosi et al 2005). A study conducted at a Sydney hospital involving 81 women attending a 'high' risk clinic found moderate-to-severe iodine deficiency in 18.8% of subjects and mild iodine deficiency in another 29.6% (Gunton et al 1999), the former clearly too close to the WHO maximum acceptable level of 20%. This study also revealed that almost 5% of the sample had MUIC < 25 microgram/L.

Aside from fortification programs in populations affected by severe iodine deficiency, there have been several RCTs of iodine supplementation in mild-to-moderately deficient pregnant women (Zimmermann 2008). While treatment effects include reductions in maternal and newborn thyroid size and, in some, reduced maternal TSH, none of the studies have demonstrated a positive effect on T_4 and T_3 of mother or child, or measured longer term clinical outcomes. Future research needs to address these issues.

Infants

An investigation of infant TSH levels within 72 hours of birth at the Royal North Shore Hospital in Sydney suggests that endemic IDD may be emerging (McElduff et al 2002). Currently, the WHO recommends that less than 3% of newborns should have TSH levels greater than 5 mIU/L and of the 1773 infants enrolled in the study, 5–10% had a TSH reading > 5 mIU/L.

Children and adolescents

Evidence of iodine deficiency has also been demonstrated in Australian schoolchildren (Li et al 2006). Iodine status in schoolchildren is based on median UIC values and is categorised as normal (UIE ≥ 100 microgram/L), or as mild (UIE 50–99 microgram/L), moderate (UIE 20–49 microgram/L) or severe deficiency (UIE < 20 microgram/L). The UIC is considered in combination with the child's sex, year of school and presence of goitre.

A study of Melbourne schoolchildren aged 11–18 years found that 76% (439/577) had abnormal UIC values, with 27% (156/577) possessing values consistent with moderate-to-severe iodine deficiency (McDonnell et al 2003). The median UIC value in girls was lower than that in boys (64 microgram/L vs 82 microgram/L), and girls had significantly lower UIC values overall ($P < 0.002$). A study of 324 schoolchildren aged 5–13 years from the Central Coast of New South Wales produced similar results; there was a median UIC concentration of 82 microgram/L, with 14% of children having levels below 50 microgram/L (Guttikonda et al 2003).

These findings were confirmed in the Australian National Iodine Nutrition Study, which identified inadequate iodine intake in the Australian population and called for the urgent implementation of mandatory iodisation of all edible salt in Australia (Li et al 2006). The study consisted of a survey of 1709 schoolchildren aged 8–10 years in the five mainland Australian States and was conducted between July 2003 and December 2004. It found that, overall, children in mainland Australia are borderline iodine deficient, with a national median UIC of 104 microgram/L. On a state basis, children in Victoria and New South Wales are mildly iodine deficient, with median UIC levels of 89 microgram/L and 73.5 microgram/L, respectively; South Australian children are borderline iodine deficient, with a median UIC of 101 microgram/L, whereas both Queensland and Western Australian children are iodine sufficient, with median UIC levels of 136.5 microgram/L and 142.5 microgram/L, respectively. Researchers attributed the decline in iodine intake to changes within the dairy industry, with chlorine-containing sanitisers now replacing iodine-containing sanitisers and a decreased intake of iodised salt.

In 2001, an iodine supplementation program was initiated in Tasmania because it was identified as an area of endemic goitre by the Department of Health Services. The program involves the use of iodised salt in 80% of Tasmania's bread production and aims to reduce the incidence of iodine deficiency. Despite encouraging preliminary data (Doyle & Seal 2003), iodine levels are still inadequate according to the WHO standards. There have been conflicting opinions about the success of this program, with the largest study demonstrating evidence of ongoing iodine deficiency (Guttikonda et al 2002, Seal et al 2003).

Iodine deficiency in children and adolescents is associated with poorer school performance, reduced achievement motivation and a higher incidence of learning disabilities (Tiwari et al 1996, Zimmermann 2008). A meta-analysis of 18 studies from eight countries of people aged between 2 and 30 years showed that iodine deficiency alone reduced mean IQ scores by 13.5 points in children (Bleichrodt et al 1996). Iodine repletion studies in children have yielded improved somatic growth, partial reversal of cognitive impairment and normalisation of age of onset of puberty; however, the strength of the evidence is hampered by methodological issues (Markou et al 2008, Zimmermann et al 2006, Zimmermann 2008).

I

Clinical note — Why is iodine deficiency on the rise?

In spite of increased rates of household iodised salt use globally since 1990, iodine intakes in Australia are falling (Zimmermann 2008). The emergence or re-emergence of iodine deficiency, however, is not limited to Australia; median urinary iodine concentration had declined by more than 50% between 1971 and 1994 in the United States (Gunton et al 1999, Zimmerman 2008).

Several reasons have been proposed to explain the emergence of iodine deficiency in developed countries. Firstly, from the 1960s, milk had become an unplanned major dietary source of iodine due to residues left from sanitising agents used in the dairy industry. However, from the 1990s, the use of iodine-containing sanitisers were gradually replaced with chlorine-containing substitutes and better practice standards, resulting in significantly reduced iodine concentrations in milk. The significance of this change within the dairy industry was recently shown by Li et al (2006), who compared the iodine content of Australian milk products from 1975 and 2004. The researchers identified mean iodine concentrations of 593.5 microgram/L and 583 microgram/L from samples taken from Victoria and New South Wales (NSW), respectively in 1975 compared to a median concentration of 195 microgram/L in 2004 (250 mL providing 50–60 microgram iodine). Interestingly, the same researchers demonstrated that dairy products and water in northern and central Queensland contained higher iodine levels, which may explain the lower incidence of iodine deficiency in these areas (Li et al 2006). In spite of this, a survey of dietary habits of Tasmanian schoolchildren has revealed that consumption of dairy products is associated with improved iodine status (Hynes et al 2004), a case of some being better than none.

A second reason may relate to public health campaigns that have resulted in increased awareness of the potential adverse effects of salt and reduced its consumption, but failed to highlight the potential benefits of a moderate intake of iodised salt. The last decade has also seen the use of non-iodised rock salt in salt-grinders becoming more fashionable than the use of traditional iodised salt, although in recent years, iodised rock salt has become available. In addition, few food manufacturers use iodised salt in their products, further reducing exposure to iodine (Gunton et al 1999). The trend towards an increased consumption of processed foods has also impacted on iodine status, as only 0.5% of salt used in commercial manufacture is iodised.

Lastly, the mineral depletion of soils is another possible contributing factor, in particular, the depletion of selenium. Due to its role in iodine utilisation, a selenium deficiency would potentiate the effects of an iodine deficiency. Flooding, erosion and glaciation have also contributed to leaching of iodine from soil.

Other theoretical considerations include increased environmental exposure to halogens, such as fluorine and chlorine, and increased consumption of goitrogens, such as soy, in the diet.

Although identifying the key factors responsible for the increased incidence of iodine deficiency is important (Thomson 2004), many authors argue that implementation of national iodine monitoring and surveillance of the iodine content in foods are the most immediate concern (Li et al 2006, McDonnell et al 2003). Lessons learnt from Tasmania's iodine supplementation program, where statewide bread fortification failed to reduce the prevalence of iodine deficiency in children, indicate that greater efforts are required to create significant improvements in iodine status.

Adults

A study of non-pregnant adults in 1999 demonstrated iodine deficiency in 26.3% of 'healthy' subjects and 34.1% of diabetic subjects (Gunton et al 1999).

Non-toxic goitre thyroidectomy

One 12-month study involving 139 patients who had undergone thyroidectomy for non-toxic goitre identified that supplementing L-thyroxine therapy with iodised salt produced significant improvements in thyroid function compared with stand-alone L-thyroxine therapy (Carella et al 2002).

Antiseptic

Iodine solution has been used as a topical antiseptic in the treatment of superficial wounds for more than a century and is still widely used for this indication. It is a highly effective method of decontaminating intact skin and minor wounds and has a low toxicity profile. Povidone–iodine preparations have replaced older iodine solutions and are now the most commonly used form. Results from a systematic review of 27 randomised clinical trials on chronic and acute wound care demonstrated that iodine shows either equivalent or superior benefits to both non-antiseptic wound dressings (paraffin dressings, dextranomer or zinc paste) and other antiseptic agents (silver sulfadiazine cream or chlorhexidine dressings). The review also noted that use of topical iodine did not adversely affect thyroid function, cause significant allergic responses or reduce the speed of wound healing (Vermeulen et al 2010). Povidone–iodine has also been shown to be an effective disinfectant in ocular surgery as well as being an oral antibacterial agent.

Although the treatment is considered safe, a number of reports of iodine toxicity in newborns receiving ongoing treatment with topical iodine-based solutions suggest that it should be used with caution as an ongoing treatment in this group and TSH monitoring considered where appropriate.

Water purification

Iodine-releasing tablets and iodine tincture have been used for many years to decontaminate water and have been used by the United States Army since World War II. A weak aqueous solution of 3–5 ppm of elemental iodine can destroy a wide range of enteroviruses, amoebae and their cysts, bacteria and algae. Under temperate conditions of 25°C, the disinfection process takes 15 minutes, and longer in colder conditions. Adding to the versatility of iodine as a water decontamination agent is its ability to act over a wide range of pH and still be effective in the presence of ammonia and amino ions from nitrogenous wastes that may be also present in the water (Kahn & Visscher 1975). Heiner et al (2010) reported that a 10% povidone–iodine (PVI) solution at a concentration of at least 1:1000 in water is an effective bactericidal agent against *Escherichia coli* (*E. coli*), which is the most common cause of traveller's diarrhoea. Disinfection of the water occurred after 15 minutes of contact time with the iodine.

OTHER USES

Fibrocystic breast disease and cyclic mastalgia

A 1993 review that focused on three clinical studies suggested that iodine supplementation may improve objective and subjective outcomes, including pain and fibrosis, for women with fibrocystic breast disease and cyclic mastalgia (Ghent et al 1993). Together the trials involved 1000 women and used a variety of different forms, the most successful being molecular iodine at a dose of 0.08 mg/kg (approximately equivalent to 500 microgram/day in a 60 kg woman) (Ghent et al 1993).

Recently, a placebo-controlled trial conducted with 11 euthyroid women with cyclic mastalgia tested different doses of molecular iodine ranging from 1.5 to 6 mg/day and showed that after 3 months of treatment, 50% of patients consuming 3 or 6 mg/day experienced a significant decrease in pain (Kessler 2004). Although no dose-related adverse events were detected, further investigation is required to confirm both efficacy and safety.

Breast cancer

There is suggestive evidence of a preventive role for iodine in breast cancer. As far back as 1896, research suggested a link between iodine deficiency, thyroid disease and breast cancer (Gago-Dominguez & Castelao 2008, Smyth 2003, Stoddard et al 2008). Epidemiological data have demonstrated a correlation between increased incidence of breast cancer and a range of thyroid conditions, most notably hypothyroidism, with both conditions demonstrating peak incidence in postmenopausal women (Gago-Dominguez & Castelao 2008, Smyth 2003). A prospective study of peri- and postmenopausal women revealed that low free T_4 was an independent risk for the development of breast cancer (OR 2.3). Another study found that the premenopausal women treated for differentiated thyroid cancer with radioactive iodine were at an increased risk of developing breast cancer over the following 5–20 years (Gago-Dominguez & Castelao 2008). In addition, the observed low rates of breast cancer in Japanese women consuming a traditional diet are speculated to be partly due to a high dietary iodine intake, further suggesting a protective effect (Patrick 2008). Notably, this protection disappears when Japanese women consume a 'Western diet'.

It is noteworthy that both the thyroid and the breast share the capacity to concentrate iodide, which exerts both an oxidant effect, triggering and facilitating apoptosis, and antioxidant effect, protecting cells from peroxidative damage (Gago-Dominguez & Castelao 2008, Venturi 2001) and converting it to iodine. The thyroid retains this capacity throughout life, whereas the healthy breast can only concentrate iodide during pregnancy and lactation; states associated with a reduced risk of breast cancer. Curiously, approximately 80% of breast cancers also demonstrate iodide uptake (Stoddard et al 2008). It has been theorised that with iodine insufficiency during pregnancy and lactation, the protective effect of iodide may be compromised, concomitant with diminished oxidant and antioxidant activities. Researchers speculate that this scenario may be compounded by co-existing selenium deficiency (Turken et al 2003).

Besides the diminished antioxidant effect, studies with animal models show that iodine deficiency results in changes in the mammary gland that make it more sensitive to the effects of oestradiol (Stoddard et al 2008, Strum 1979). Iodine has been implicated in the synthesis of alpha-oestrogen receptors, down-regulation of several oestrogen-responsive genes and increased expression of the cytochrome P450 genes responsible for its phase I detoxification (Stoddard et al 2008). Together with other sources of evidence, it is clear that the potential protective effect of iodine against breast cancer is independent of its thyroid role (Stoddard et al 2008).

At present, the only interventional evidence comes from rat studies, demonstrating that administration of Lugol's iodine or iodine-rich Wakame seaweed suppressed the development of induced mammary tumours (Funahashi et al 2001) and in vitro evidence confirming that molecular iodine induces apoptosis in breast cancer cell lines (Shrivastava et al 2006). In light of ongoing evidence of a superior effect of molecular iodine rather than iodide in relation to breast pathology in both animals and humans, rigorous human studies using this form are required (Patrick 2008, Stoddard et al 2008).

Prevention of attention-deficit hyperactivity disorder

Emerging data from research conducted over the past 15 years suggest a possible link between low maternal iodine status and increased risk of ADHD in the offspring. According to a report published in 2004, 11 of 16 children born to women living in a moderately iodine-deficient region in Italy developed ADHD compared to no offspring from the 11 control mothers living in a marginally iodine-deficient region (Vermiglio et al 2004).

On the other hand, another group of researchers investigated whether T_4 levels at birth could represent a biomarker for later development of ADHD and found that all newborns in the sample had T_4 within the normal range and no correlation between values and risk could be demonstrated (Soldin et al 2002, Soldin et al 2003). This evidence invalidated TSH levels as a biomarker of risk, but does not disprove a link between iodine and ADHD, as earlier studies found that those newborns who later developed ADHD were all euthyroid at birth (Vermiglio et al 2004).

Although further investigation is required to clarify these observations, they have provided a new avenue for ADHD research.

DOSAGE RANGE

Australia and New Zealand recommended daily intake (RDI)

- Infants
  - 0–6 months: 90 microgram/day.
  - 7–12 months: 110 microgram/day.
- Children
  - 1–3 years: 90 microgram/day.
  - 4–8 years: 90 microgram/day.
  - 9–14 years: 120 microgram/day.
  - >14 years: 150 microgram/day.
- Adults: 150 microgram/day.
- Pregnancy: 220 microgram/day.
- Lactation: 270 microgram/day.
- Upper level of intake
  - 1–3 years: 200 microgram/day.
  - 4–8 years: 300 microgram/day.
  - 9–13 years: 600 microgram/day.
  - 14–18 years (including pregnancy, lactation): 900 microgram/day.
  - Adults >18 years (including pregnancy, lactation): 1100 microgram/day.

These are the revised Australian RDIs (2006), which are more closely aligned with the WHO recommendations than previously.

According to clinical studies

- ADHD prevention: adequate intake to prevent maternal deficiency (approximately 250 microgram/day)
- Topical antimicrobial: Various concentrations have been used depending on site, type and severity of the wound, with a range of 2–10% povidone-iodine being the most commonly used.
- Fibrocystic breast disease and cyclic mastalgia: 1.5–6 mg iodine/day for 6–18 months.
- Breast cancer prevention: dose is unknown; however, it is suggested that women meet RDI to prevent deficiency.
- Water disinfectant: Widely used practice suggests 3–10 drops iodine tincture per litre of water provides an antibacterial effect after 15 minutes.

TOXICITY

Chronic iodine toxicity results when iodide intake is approximately 2 mg daily or greater (Beers 2005). Overconsumption of iodine can cause gastrointestinal irritation, abdominal pain, nausea, vomiting and diarrhoea, cardiovascular symptoms and can induce both hypo- and hyperthyroidism, depending on the patient's preexisting susceptibility (Wahlqvist 2002, Zimmermann 2008). Excess iodine during pregnancy has also been associated with increased risk of postpartum thyroiditis (Guan et al 2005). Alternatively, there are many cases in which excesses have been tolerated without any overt consequences, particularly in individuals with healthy thyroid function (Geissler & Powers 2005, Groff et al 2009, Zimmermann 2008). Chronic ingestion of ≥500 microgram/day by children has resulted in increased thyroid size (Zimmermann 2008). Intake of very high doses can lead to a brassy taste in the mouth, increased salivation, gastric irritation and acneiform skin lesions.

SIGNIFICANT INTERACTIONS

Goitrogens

These are substances that interfere with iodine utilisation, uptake into the thyroid or thyroid hormone production. These include thiocyanates found in the cabbage family (e.g. cabbage, kale, cauliflower, broccoli, turnips and Brussels sprouts) and in linseed, cassava, millet and soybean — separate intake of iodine and goitrogens where possible. Smoking has also been shown to increase thiocyanate levels and reduce iodine content in the breastmilk of smoking mothers (Zimmermann et al 2008). Other chemical goitrogens include perchlorate and disulphides, the latter from coal processes and there is accumulating evidence of thyroid endocrine disruptors in the form of ingredients used in cosmetics, as pesticides or plasticisers. Major targets are the sodium–iodide symporter (NIS), the haemoprotein thyroperoxidase (TPO), the T_4 distributor protein transthyretin (TTR) and the deiodinases (Köhrle 2008).

Soy

The actions of this particular goitrogen are twofold: ingestion of soy appears to inhibit iodine absorption to some extent (particularly when presented in its thyroxine form in the gut) and also high levels of the isoflavones, genistein and daidzein, can inhibit T_3 and T_4 production — separate intake of iodine and goitrogens where possible. Particular attention should be paid to minimising soy consumption in individuals taking thyroid hormone supplementation, as it has been shown that soy consumption can increase dosage requirements.

Selenium

Selenium is intrinsic to the metabolism and activity of the thyroid hormones, facilitating the conversion of T_4 to T_3 and is also responsible for the only iodine recycling pathway of the body through the action of the deiodinases on excess or unnecessary thyroid hormones to release the iodine — beneficial interaction.

CONTRAINDICATIONS AND PRECAUTIONS

Thyroid conditions

Due to the complex and diverse causes of thyroid conditions, it is advised that iodine supplementation should be avoided unless under the supervision of a medical practitioner.

Practice points/Patient counselling

- Iodine is an essential trace element required for healthy functioning of the thyroid gland and for normal growth and development.
- It is mainly consumed as iodide salts from sea salt, shellfish, seawater fish and vegetables.
- Iodine is essential for the manufacture of thyroxine (T_4) and liothyronine (T_3), which are hormones that influence growth, maturation, thermogenesis, oxidation, myelination of the CNS and the metabolism of all tissues (Jones 2002).
- Iodine supplementation is commonly used to prevent and treat deficiency. There is also some evidence that it may reduce pain in fibrocystic breast disease and cyclic mastalgia and suggestive evidence of a protective role against breast cancer; however, rigorous research is required to confirm these observations.
- Current evidence points to widespread mild-to-moderate iodine deficiency in Australia, suggesting that dietary intake is inadequate and supplementation or fortification of foods with additional iodine may be required. Use of iodised salt is recommended.

PREGNANCY USE

Up until 2006, the Australian recommended daily intake of iodine was 150 micrograms for pregnant women and 170 micrograms for lactating women; however, reflecting new research, the Australian RDI levels for pregnancy and lactation have been revised and increased to 220 micrograms and 270 micrograms respectively. Care should be taken to avoid ingestion of excessive amounts during pregnancy due to suspected links with increased rates of postpartum thyroiditis and other disorders of thyroid function (Guan et al 2005).

PATIENTS' FAQs

What will this supplement do for me?

Adequate intake of iodine is critical for healthy thyroid function and normal growth and development. Ensuring adequate intake becomes critical during pregnancy and breastfeeding when the infant is solely dependent on the mother's intake for normal growth and brain development. Currently, there is some suggestive evidence that adequate iodine particularly during the female reproductive years may be protective against breast cancer and supplementation may relieve symptoms of breast pain in fibrocystic breast disease and cyclic mastalgia.

When will it start to work?

The time frames depend on the indication it is being used to treat and the level of deficiency. In the case of breast pain, studies suggest that 3 months of treatment are required to attain significant symptom relief.

Are there any safety issues?

People with preexisting thyroid conditions should only increase iodine intake under professional supervision. Doses in excess of the RDI should be avoided unless under the supervision of a medical practitioner.

REFERENCES

APHDPC. The prevalence and severity of iodine deficiency in Australia. Prepared for the Australian Population Health Development Principal Committee (APHDPC) (2007). Available online www.foodstandards.gov.au (accessed 24/01/2013)

Ares S, Quero J, de Escobar GM. Iodine balance, iatrogenic excess, and thyroid dysfunction in premature newborns. Semin Perinatol 32.6 (2008): 407–412.

Beers MH. Merck manual home edition. Whitehouse, NJ: Merck, 2005. www.merck.com (accessed 04-04-2006).

Bleichrodt N et al. The benefits of adequate iodine intake. Nutr Rev 54.4 (1996): S72–S78.

Carella C et al. Iodized salt improves the effectiveness of L-thyroxine therapy after surgery for nontoxic goitre: a prospective and randomized study. Clin Endocrinol (Oxf) 57.4 (2002): 507–513.

de Escobar GM et al. The changing role of national thyroid hormones in fetal brain development. Seminars in Perinatology 32.6 (2008): 407–412.

de Escobar GM, Obregon MJ, del Rey FE. Iodine deficiency and brain development in the first half of pregnancy. Public Health Nutr 10.12A (2007): 1554–1570.

Delange F. Iodine requirements during pregnancy, lactation and the neonatal period and indicators of optimal iodine nutrition. Public Health Nutr 10.12A (2007): 1581–1583.

Doyle Z, Seal J. The Tasmanian iodine monitoring program in schools. Asia Pacific J Clin Nutr 12 (Suppl) (2003): S14.

Eastman CJ. Screening for thyroid disease and iodine deficiency. Pathology 442. 2 (2012): 153–159.

Funahashi H et al. Seaweed prevents breast cancer? Jpn J Cancer Res 92.5 (2001): 483–487.

Gago-Dominguez M, Castelao JE. Role of lipid peroxidation and oxidative stress in the association between thyroid diseases and breast cancer. Crit Rev Oncol Hematol 68.2 (2008): 107–114.

Geissler C, Powers H (eds), Human nutrition, 11th edn. London: Elsevier, 2005.

Ghent WR et al. Iodine replacement in fibrocystic disease of the breast. Can J Surg 36.5 (1993): 453–460.

Glinoer D. The importancec of iodine nutrition during pregnancy. Public Health Nutr 10.12A (2007): 1542–1546.

Groff S et al. Advanced nutrition and human metabolism, 4th edn. Belmont, CA: Wadsworth Thomson Learning, 2009.

Guan H et al. High iodine intake is a risk factor of post-partum thyroiditis: result of a survey from Shenyang, China. J Endocrinol Invest 28.10 (2005): 876–881.

Gunton JE et al. Iodine deficiency in ambulatory participants at a Sydney teaching hospital: is Australia truly iodine replete? Med J Aust 171.9 (1999): 467–470.

Guttikonda K et al. Iodine deficiency in urban primary school children: a cross-sectional analysis. Med J Aust 179.7 (2003): 346–348.

Guttikonda K et al. Recurrent iodine deficiency in Tasmania, Australia: a salutary lesson in sustainable iodine prophylaxis and its monitoring. J Clin Endocrinol Metab 87.6 (2002): 2809–2815.

Hamrosi MA, Wallace EM, Riley MD. Iodine status in pregnant women living in Melbourne differs by ethnic group. Asia Pac J Clin Nutr 14.1 (2005): 27–31.

Heiner JD et al. 10% Povidine–iodine may be a practical field water disinfectant. Wilderness & Environmental Medicine 21 (2010): 332–336.

Higdon J. An evidence-based approach to vitamins and minerals. In: Iodine. New York: Thieme, 2003, pp 130–137.

Hynes KL et al. Persistent iodine deficiency in a cohort of Tasmanian school children: associations with socio-economic status, geographical location and dietary factors. Aust NZ J Public Health 28.5 (2004): 476–481.

Jones GP. Minerals. in: Wahlqvist M (ed). Food and nutrition, 2nd edn. Sydney: Allen & Unwin, 2002, pp 275–276.

Kahn FH, Visscher BR. Water disinfection in the wilderness: a simple, effective method of iodination. West J Med 122.5 (1975): 450–453.

Kessler JH. The effect of supraphysiologic levels of iodine on patients with cyclic mastalgia. Breast J 10.4 (2004): 328–336.

Kohlmeier M. Nutrient metabolism. London: Elsevier, 2003.

Köhrle J. Environment and endocrinology: the case of thyroidology. Ann Endocrinol (Paris) 69.2 (2008): 116–122.

Kotsirilos V et al. A guide to evidence-based integrative and complementary medicine. Chatsworth, NSW, Churchill Livingstone Elsevier (2011).

Li M et al. Are Australian children iodine deficient? Results of the Australian National Iodine Nutrition Study. Med J Aust 184.4 (2006): 165–169.

Markou K et al. Treating iodine deficiency: long-term effects of iodine repletion on growth and pubertal development in school-age children. Thyroid 18.4 (2008): 449–454.

McDonnell CM, Harris M, Zacharin MR. Iodine deficiency and goitre in schoolchildren in Melbourne, 2001. Med J Aust 178.4 (2003): 159–162.

McElduff A et al. Neonatal thyroid-stimulating hormone concentrations in northern Sydney: further indications of mild iodine deficiency? Med J Aust 176.7 (2002): 317–320.

Patrick L. Iodine: deficiency and therapeutic considerations. Altern Med Rev 13.2 (2008): 116–127.

Seal JA et al. Tasmania: doing its wee bit for iodine nutrition [Letter]. Med J Aust 179.8 (2003): 451–452.

Shrivastava A et al. Molecular iodine induces caspase-independent apoptosis in human breast carcinoma cells involving the mitochondria-mediated pathway. J Biol Chem 281.28 (2006): 19762–19771.

Smyth PP. The thyroid, iodine and breast cancer. Breast Cancer Res 5.5 (2003): 235–238 [Epub ahead of print].

Soldin OP et al. Lack of a relation between human neonatal thyroxine and pediatric neurobehavioral disorders. Thyroid 13.2 (2003): 193–198.

Soldin OP et al. Newborn thyroxine levels and childhood ADHD. Clin Biochem 35.2 (2002): 131–136.

Stoddard FR et al. Iodine alters gene expression in the MCF7 breast cancer cell line: evidence for an anti-estrogen effect of iodine. Int J Med Sci 5.4 (2008): 189–196.

Strum JM. Effect of iodide-deficiency on rat mammary gland. Virchows Arch B Cell Pathol Incl Mol Pathol 30.2 (1979): 209–220.

Thomson CD. Selenium and iodine intakes and status in New Zealand and Australia. Br J Nutr 91.5 (2004): 661–672.

Tiwari BD et al. Learning disabilities and poor motivation to achieve due to prolonged iodine deficiency. Am J Clin Nutr 63.5 (1996): 782–7816.

Turken O et al. Breast cancer in association with thyroid disorders. Breast Cancer Res 5.5 (2003): R110–R1113.

Venturi S. Is there a role for iodine in breast diseases? Breast 10.5 (2001): 379–382.

Vermeulen H et al. Benefit and harm of iodine in wound care: a systematic review. Journal of Hospital Infection 76 (2010): 191–199.

Vermiglio F et al. Attention deficit and hyperactivity disorders in the offspring of mothers exposed to mild-moderate iodine deficiency: a possible novel iodine deficiency disorder in developed countries. J Clin Endocrinol Metab 89.12 (2004): 6054–6060.

Wahlqvist M (ed). Food and nutrition, 2nd edn. Sydney: Allen & Unwin, 2002.

Zimmerman MB. The role of iodine in human growth and development. Seminars in Cell Development Biology 22 (2011): 645–652.

Zimmermann MB et al. Iodine supplementation improves cognition in iodine-deficient schoolchildren in Albania: a randomized, controlled, double-blind study. Am J Clin Nutr 83.1 (2006): 108–114.

Zimmermann MB, Jooste PL, Pandav CS. Iodine-deficiency disorders. Lancet 372.9645 (2008): 1251–1262.

Zimmermann MB. Iodine requirements and the risks and benefits of correcting iodine deficiency in populations. J Trace Elem Med Biol 22.2 (2008): 81–92.

Iron

BACKGROUND AND RELEVANT PHARMACOKINETICS

Iron is an essential mineral, vital to human health. The average human body contains 2–4 g of iron. Iron is found in the body in: haemoglobin (65%); myoglobin (10%); enzymes (1–5%); with the remaining approximately 20% of body iron being found in storage or in the blood (Gropper & Smith 2013).

Although the metal exists in several oxidation states in nature, only the ferrous (Fe^{2+}) and ferric (Fe^{3+}) forms are stable in the aqueous environment of the body (Gropper & Smith 2013).

Iron is found in the haem form, which comes from animal sources, and the non-haem form, derived from plants and dairy products.

The haem form of iron is more soluble than the non-haem form and is absorbed 2–3 times more readily. Absorption of haem iron occurs across the brush border of the small intestine, especially in the proximal region, and is facilitated by haem carrier protein 1 (hcp1). Non-haem iron is bound to other substances in food when ingested, and must first be enzymatically released by gastric secretions such as hydrochloric acid and pepsin before absorption can occur. Non-haem iron in the ferrous form (Fe^{2+}) is absorbed more readily than iron in the ferric (Fe^{3+}) form, and occurs primarily in the duodenum with the aid of divalent mineral transporter 1. Iron in the ferric form (Fe^{3+}) is susceptible to aggregation and precipitation in the alkaline environment of the small intestine which impairs absorption (Gropper & Smith 2013). Intestinal absorption of non-haem iron is influenced by a number of factors, as summarised below.

Solubility enhancers of non-haem iron

- Acids (including ascorbic acid) aid solubility of non-haem iron, thus improving absorption; the addition of 20 mg ascorbic acid has been shown to increase non-haem iron absorption by 39% (Hallberg et al 2003)
- Sugars (e.g. fructose and sorbitol) aid absorption
- Mucin
- Meat stimulates digestive secretions, and breakdown products such as cysteine-containing peptides aid absorption (Hurrell et al 1988). The addition of red meat increases non-haem iron absorption by 85% (Hallberg et al 2003). This appears to be dose-dependent, as a study found that the addition of 60 g Danish pork meat three times daily improved the absorption of non-haem iron from 5.3% to 7.9% (Bach-Kristensen et al 2005), although the addition of smaller amounts was not as effective (Baech et al 2003)
- The addition of fish to a high-phytate bean meal has also been shown to increase iron absorption (Navas-Carretero et al 2008)
- Alcohol improves iron uptake. The consumption of up to two alcoholic drinks per day is associated with reduced risk of iron deficiency and more than two can increase the risk of iron overload (Ioannou et al 2004).

Solubility inhibitors of non-haem iron

- Polyphenols, including tannin derivatives of gallic acid. A number of studies have shown that tea catechins can inhibit intestinal non-haem iron absorption (Ullmann et al 2005); however, polyphenols do not have chelating effects on cooked haem iron (Breet et al 2005). Overall, tea consumption has been reported to reduce non-haem iron absorption by 60% (Kaltwasser et al 1998) and coffee consumption by 40% when taken with or shortly after a meal (Gropper & Smith 2013).

Recent studies suggest that impaired absorption is unlikely to be significant in people with normal iron stores (Breet et al 2005, Ullmann et al 2005). The addition of milk to tea may reduce the chelating effects.

- Phytic acid or phytates (whole grains, legumes, maize) (Gropper & Smith 2013)
- Oxalic acid (spinach, chard, chocolate, berries, tea) (Gropper & Smith 2013)
- Phosvitin, a protein found in egg yolks (Gropper & Smith 2013)
- Calcium — a transient inhibitory effect has been observed which does not occur with long-term high-dose calcium intake (Lonnerdal 2010). This includes calcium found in dairy foods, and other forms such as calcium phosphate, calcium citrate, calcium carbonate and calcium chloride; when consumed in amounts of 300–600 mg, it significantly impairs iron absorption (ferrous sulfate and dietary iron) (Gropper & Smith 2013)
- Zinc competes with iron for absorption (Gropper & Smith 2013) — inorganic zinc supplements may reduce iron absorption by 66–80% (Crofton et al 1989), and supplements containing both iron and zinc may not be as efficacious as the same doses given in isolation (Fischer Walker et al 2005, Lind et al 2003). Nutrients consumed in a meal may not be as affected (Whittaker 1998)
- Manganese may reduce absorption by 22–40% (Rossander-Hulten et al 1991)
- Rapid intestinal transit time (Gropper & Smith 2013)
- Malabsorption syndromes (Gropper & Smith 2013)
- *Helicobacter pylori* infection (Ciacci et al 2004, Duque et al 2010)

- Gastrointestinal blood loss (Higgins & Rockey 2003)
- Insufficient digestive secretions (including achlorhydria), or raised gastric pH due to age-related decrease in gastric acid production
- Antacids, H_2 antagonists and proton pump inhibitor drugs due to raising pH within the gastrointestinal tract.

Systemic and local mechanisms have also been identified which regulate iron absorption and play a role in iron homeostasis. Hepcidin, a 25-amino-acid peptide, is the regulatory protein for systemic iron absorption from intestinal enterocytes as well as for the efflux of iron from macrophages. Factors that alter hepcidin levels, such as inflammation, infection and hypoxia, will in turn have an effect on iron levels, although exact mechanisms are yet to be fully elucidated. Local regulatory mechanisms involve an iron-responsive element/iron-regulatory protein system, which affects the regulation of proteins involved in iron metabolism. Disturbances in these local or systemic iron absorption regulatory mechanisms are implicated in both iron-loading and iron-deficiency disorders (Fuqua et al 2012).

> ***Clinical note — Factors affecting the absorption of iron***
> If the dietary intake of iron is adequate, it is often assumed that a patient's iron levels will be within the normal range. In practice, this is not always the case as absorption is significantly affected by a number of factors, thereby increasing or decreasing the amount of ingested dietary iron that reaches the systemic circulation.

CHEMICAL COMPONENTS

Ferrous sulfate is the most widely studied form and is generally considered the treatment of choice based on proven efficacy, cost and tolerability, especially when administered as oral sustained-release preparations (Santiago 2012). Other ferrous forms include ascorbate, carbonate, citrate, fumarate, gluconate, lactate, succinate and tartrate (non-haem iron). Iron from ferrous sulfate has a significantly greater bioavailability than ferrous glycine chelate or ferric ethylenediamine tetraacetic acid (EDTA) (Ferreira da Silva et al 2004). Other ferric forms include ammonium citrate, chloride, citrate, pyrophosphate and sulfate. Amino acid chelates, such as iron glycine, are also available. Dietary ferritin is as equally well absorbed as ferrous sulfate and therefore food sources are likely to be effective (Davila-Hicks et al 2004). Cooking in iron pots may also improve iron status (Geerligs et al 2003).

FOOD SOURCES

The average Western diet is estimated to contain 5–7 mg iron/1000 kcal.

Haem iron

About 50–60% of the iron in animal sources is in the haem form. Sources include liver, lean red meat, poultry, fish, oysters, clams, shellfish, kidney and heart.

Non-haem iron

This is found in plant and dairy products in the form of iron salts and makes up about 85% of the average intake. Sources include egg yolks, nuts, legumes, fruit, dried fruit, raisins, dark molasses, vegetables, including beetroot, grains and tofu. Dairy is a relatively poor source of iron.

A number of iron-fortified foods are also available and include wholegrain and enriched bread, pasta, cereal, soy sauce, Thai fish sauce, milk, orange juice and wines.

Considering that minerals such as calcium may reduce iron absorption, fortification of some foods may be relatively ineffectual unless absorption enhancers such as vitamin C are also included (Davidsson et al 1998).

DEFICIENCY SIGNS AND SYMPTOMS

Iron deficiency is the most common and widespread nutritional disorder in the world, affecting approximately 1.6 billion people according to World Health Organization reports (de Benoist et al 2008). Iron deficiency may occur with or without anaemia (Gillespie et al 1991); however an estimated 50% of all anaemias worldwide are attributed to a deficiency in iron (Stoltzfus 2003).

The term iron deficiency is used when there are no iron stores that can be mobilised and there are signs of a compromised supply of iron to tissues; however this has not yet led to a low haemoglobin level and thus a classification of 'anaemia' (Rattehalli et al 2013). A mild deficiency, without anaemia, will still result in symptoms such as mood changes, poor concentration, fatigue and reduced physical performance and may still warrant iron replenishment, especially in vulnerable patient groups (Rattehalli et al 2013).

Iron-deficiency anaemia results when an ongoing iron deficiency results in reduced erthyropoiesis and a drop in haemoglobin levels, which leads to a decrease in red blood cell count and mean corpuscle volume. The World Health Organization defines anaemia in terms of a haemoglobin concentration <13 g/dL for men and <12 g/dL for non-pregnant women. Iron-deficiency anaemia is associated with an increased risk of maternal and child mortality, especially in developing countries, and results in reduced work capacity and physical performance in adults, and in children leads to a reduced ability to learn and develop physically.

Signs and symptoms include:

- Fatigue and lethargy
- Decreased resistance to infection
- Cardiovascular and respiratory changes, which can progress to cardiac failure if left untreated
- Increased lead absorption, which in turn inhibits haem synthesis
- Decreased selenium and glutathione peroxidase levels

- Pale inside lower eyelid or mouth
- Pale-coloured nail bed
- Pale lines on stretched palm (palmar creases)
- Ridged, spoon-shaped, thin flat nails
- Brittle hair
- Impaired cognitive and motor function
- Adverse pregnancy outcomes and increased perinatal maternal mortality (NMCD 2005)
- Reduced thyroid function and ability to make thyroid hormones (Beard et al 1990)
- Difficulty maintaining body temperature in a cold environment.

Risk groups for iron deficiency

The four main population groups that are most at risk of developing iron deficiency are:

1. Young children (6 months–4 years), due to factors such as inadequate dietary intake, inadequate reserves to meet physiological requirements, rapid growth phases, low iron content in milk
2. Adolescents, due to pubertal growth spurts and increased need to match expansion in mass of red blood cells
3. Women during child-bearing years, due to menstrual blood loss
4. Pregnant women, due to increased fetal demands, expanding blood volume and blood loss associated with childbirth (Gropper & Smith 2013).

Primary deficiency

Primary deficiency is most common in vegetarians, the elderly, those with protein-calorie malnutrition, and during periods of increased iron requirement due to expanded blood volume in infancy, adolescence and pregnancy.

Secondary deficiency

Underlying causes of iron-deficiency anaemia include blood loss, inefficient absorption due to gastrointestinal disturbances and increased destruction of red blood cells.

- Blood loss (menstruation, menorrhagia, bleeding haemorrhoids, parasites, bleeding peptic ulcer, malignancy, *Helicobacter pylori* infection, gastrointestinal bleeding due to medication such as non-steroidal anti-inflammatory drugs)
- Inefficient absorption (chronic gastrointestinal disturbances, malabsorption syndromes, coeliac disease) (Annibale et al 2001)
- Increased destruction of red blood cells (malaria, high-intensity exercise).

Note: The majority of iron utilised in erythropoiesis is provided by recovered iron from old erythrocytes (Handelman & Levin 2008), thus a failure in this system will also impact on iron status.

MAIN ACTIONS

Iron plays a central role in many biochemical processes in the body.

> ***Clinical note — Testing for iron deficiency***
>
> In iron-deficiency anaemia, storage iron declines until the delivery of iron to bone marrow is insufficient for erythropoiesis to occur. In the early stages, blood tests will reveal low plasma ferritin, followed by decreased plasma iron and transferrin saturation, and ultimately low haemoglobin in red blood cells (Handelman & Levin 2008). As isolated haemoglobin has both low specificity and low sensitivity for determining iron status, the optimal diagnostic approach is to measure the serum ferritin as an index of iron stores and the serum transferrin receptor as an index of tissue iron deficiency (Cook 2005, Flesland et al 2004, Mei et al 2005). Iron deficiency is associated with a plasma ferritin concentration of <12 ng/mL. In the presence of infection or inflammation, however, plasma ferritin levels are a less reliable indicator of iron status. Inflammation or infection lead to a rise in plasma ferritin concentration and it may therefore still appear within normal range or high, even though iron levels are depleted (Gropper & Smith 2013).

Oxygen transport and storage

The key function of iron is to facilitate oxygen transport by haemoglobin, the oxygen-carrying pigment of erythrocytes. It is also involved in oxygen storage by myoglobin, an iron-containing protein that transports and stores oxygen within muscle and releases it to meet increased metabolic demands during muscle contraction.

Immunity

Iron is vital for the proliferation of all cells, including those of the immune system. In vitro and in vivo studies have indicated a link between iron deficiency and impaired T-lymphocyte proliferation. In anaemic children in Bolivia who received iron treatment for 3 months, the proportion of circulating immature T lymphocytes decreased from 18.3% to 9.2% (Sejas et al 2008).

Iron deficiency causes several defects in both humoral and cellular immunity (Bowlus 2003), including a reduction in peripheral T cells secondary to atrophy of the thymus and inhibition of thymocyte proliferation (Bowlus 2003) and a reduction in interleukin-2 (IL-2) production (Bergman et al 2004). Reduced IL-2 production may partly explain the increased susceptibility to infections and cancer in patients with iron-deficiency anaemia (Bergman et al 2004). Supplementation of ferrous sulfate (60 mg Fe) once daily for 8 weeks has been shown to reduce the incidence and duration of upper respiratory tract infections in children (De-Silva et al 2003).

However, there is also preliminary evidence that iron may be implicated in the pathogenesis of autoimmune disorders, including systemic lupus erythematosus, scleroderma, type 1 diabetes, Goodpasture's syndrome, multiple sclerosis and rheumatoid arthritis (Bowlus 2003). A review conducted by Recalcati et al (2012) highlights the importance of macrophages in autoimmune diseases, and the potential role that iron retention may play in promoting the proinflammatory, pathogenic activity of M1 macrophages, rather than allowing for modulation by the anti-inflammatory action of M2 macrophages. In this way, iron accumulation in macrophages may potentially exacerbate autoimmune disease (Recalcati et al 2012).

Protein and enzyme systems

Iron forms a part of several proteins and is a cofactor for many different enzymes. Processes in which iron plays a role include:

- Production of adenosine triphosphate and cellular respiration
- Amino acid metabolism (e.g. arginine, phenylalanine, tryptophan, tyrosine)
- Carbohydrate metabolism
- As a component of enzymes, including catalase, myeloperoxidase, thyroperoxidase and oxidoreductase, providing protection against free radical damage
- Synthesis of carnitine and niacin
- Synthesis of nitric oxide, which plays a role in blood pressure regulation, intestinal motility, macrophage function and inhibition of platelet aggregation
- Synthesis and function of hormones (e.g. thyroid hormone) and neurotransmitters (serotonin, dopamine and noradrenaline)
- Synthesis of procollagen and elastin.

CLINICAL USE

Iron supplementation is used to prevent deficiency in at-risk populations and also to rectify deficiency states. The best form of iron to use, administration form and dosage regimen are yet to be determined and likely to vary depending on the individual presentation. This review will mainly focus on oral supplementation as this is the most commonly used form. Oral ferrous iron supplements are a popular commercial form which is available in complexes as ferrous sulfate or ferrous fumarate, but may also be found in complexes with succinate, citrate, tartrate, lactate and gluconate. Amino acid-iron chelates such as iron glycine are also available. Administration in the chelate form has not been shown to provide better absorption than administration of iron as ferrous sulfate (Gropper & Smith 2013).

Iron deficiency and iron-deficiency anaemia

Ferrous sulfate is the most commonly used oral treatment for iron deficiency and iron-deficiency anaemia. Daily iron therapy has been shown to be the most effective treatment, but is associated with a higher incidence of adverse effects, such as nausea, constipation and dental discolouration, as well as poor compliance, and may not be feasible in all population groups (Fernandez-Gaxiola & De-Regil 2011). In practice, it is often prescribed in divided doses rather than a single, larger daily dose in an attempt to reduce the incidence and severity of these side effects.

Intermittent iron therapy is less effective than daily iron therapy in the prevention and treatment of iron-deficiency anaemia, but still a successful alternative strategy where daily supplementation is not possible, according to a recent Cochrane review of 21 trials involving 10,258 women in their menstrual years (Fernandez-Gaxiola & De-Regil 2011).

Previous evidence also suggested that weekly administration of iron was an effective strategy for the treatment and prevention of iron deficiency and iron-deficiency anaemia in most population groups, including pregnant women and children (Agarwal et al 2003, Mukhopadhyay et al 2004, Siddiqui et al 2004, Sungthong et al 2004, Yang et al 2004). Although this is associated with lower cost, fewer side effects and improved compliance (Haidar et al 2003), this notion has been challenged when twice-weekly doses of iron (ferrous dextran containing 60 mg elemental iron) for 12 months failed to improve haemoglobin or serum ferritin (iron stores) in children or adults (Olsen et al 2006). The results from some studies suggest that weekly doses may assist in maintenance but may not improve iron status (Wijaya-Erhardt et al 2007). To achieve a better result, it may be necessary to use higher weekly doses and also address concomitant nutritional deficiencies and other factors affecting iron absorption.

Children

According to a 2013 meta-analysis by Thompson et al, iron supplementation in children aged 2–5 years increases both haemoglobin and ferritin levels and may also lead to a small improvement in cognitive, but not physical, development in this age group (Thompson et al 2013). Benefits for growth appear most likely if iron is given together with a combination of micronutrients according to systematic reviews and meta-analyses (Allen et al 2009, Ramakrishnan et al 2004, 2009, Sachdev et al 2005).

Daily iron supplementation is more effective than intermittent supplementation in children under 12 years, according to a 2011 Cochrane systematic review (De-Regil et al 2011). Despite this, intermittent supplementation is still better than placebo and presents an effective solution should daily supplementation not be possible. It may also be associated with fewer side effects, according to a 2004 study of 60 children (age 5–10 years) with iron-deficiency anaemia given ferrous sulfate (200 mg) weekly for 2 months and compared to daily treatment with the same dose (Siddiqui et al 2004). Another study found that children receiving weekly doses of ferrous sulfate (300 mg) had similar improvements in haemoglobin, but a significantly higher increase in IQ, compared to those taking the same dose of iron 5 days per week (Sungthong et al 2004).

Preliminary data suggests that low iron status and low serum ferritin concentration should be investigated in children presenting with febrile seizures as these may be risk factors for the development of this condition (Zareifar et al 2012).

Elderly

The prevalence of iron-deficiency anaemia increases with age. This is mainly due to a combination of factors, including poor dietary intake together with decreased digestive function, use of medications affecting uptake and disease states associated with chronic inflammation, gastrointestinal bleeding and malabsorption, renal failure, portal hypertension, colorectal cancer and angiodysplasia (Andres et al 2008).

Elderly patients are particularly vulnerable to the dose-dependent adverse effects of iron supplementation, and should be given the lowest effective dose. A randomised controlled trial (RCT) of 90 hospitalised elderly patients demonstrated that 15 mg of liquid ferrous gluconate produced similar improvements in haemoglobin and ferritin over 60 days to 150 mg of ferrous calcium citrate tablets without the negative side effects (Rimon et al 2005). Iron supplementation appears to be effective and safe for the treatment of comorbid anaemia in elderly patients undergoing knee or hip surgery, according to recent meta-analysis (Yang et al 2011).

In all cases the lowest safe and effective dose at the lowest frequency of dosing should be used to correct iron deficiency with or without anaemia.

It is becoming clearer that long-term iron deficiency is also associated with an increased risk for cardiovascular disease and all-cause mortality in the elderly (Hsu et al 2013) and has implications in congestive heart failure (CHF). Anaemia is reported in over 50% of patients with CHF, and is associated with an increased risk of death compared to non-anaemic CHF patients (Avni et al 2012). Iron deficiency has also been highlighted as a potential problem in CHF patients, decreasing aerobic performance and exercise tolerance, and may be a predictor of disease severity and mortality (Klip et al 2012). A recent review reported that intravenous iron supplementation (1000–2000 mg total dose) may improve exercise capacity and quality of life and reduce the need for hospitalisation in CHF patients. Benefits were also reported in non-anaemic patients, suggesting that anaemia is not the only reason for improvement in symptoms of CHF with use of iron supplementation (Avni et al 2012).

Pregnancy

Women taking iron supplementation during pregnancy are at less risk of giving birth to babies of low birth weight (<2500 g) and more likely to have a baby with a higher mean birth weight than women not taking iron supplements, according to a recent Cochrane review of 43 trials (n = 27,400) (Pena-Rosas et al 2012). Prophylactic use of iron supplementation reduced the risk of iron deficiency at term by 57% and/or iron-deficiency anaemia by 70%. In the review, iron supplementation was also associated with a marginally higher risk of maternal adverse effects and raised haemoglobin levels, suggesting a need for updating recommendations on dosing and iron supplementation regimens. Improved birth weight with iron supplementation was also reported in a 2013 review of 48 RCTs (n = 17,793 women) and 44 cohort studies, involving almost 2 million women (Haider et al 2013). It was found to significantly decrease the risk of iron-deficiency anaemia in pregnancy and substantially improved birth weight in a linear dose–response manner.

Due to the possibility of uncontrolled lipid peroxidation, predictive of adverse effects for mother and fetus, iron supplementation should be prescribed on the basis of biological criteria, not on the assumption of anaemia alone (Lachili et al 2001) and the minimum dose possible should be used. Low-dose iron supplements (20 mg elemental iron) have demonstrated efficacy in treating anaemia in pregnancy with fewer gastrointestinal side effects (Zhou et al 2009).

According to trials, a supplement of 40 mg ferrous iron/day from 18 weeks' gestation appears adequate to prevent iron deficiency in 90% of women and iron-deficiency anaemia in at least 95% of women during pregnancy and postpartum (Milman et al 2004). A single weekly dose of 200 mg elemental iron, however, may be sufficient, as this has been shown to be comparable with 100 mg elemental iron daily on erythrocyte indices (Mukhopadhyay et al 2004). Other trials have found that low doses of sodium feredetate (33 mg and 66 mg of elemental iron given twice daily) produced comparable results to ferrous fumarate (100 mg elemental iron given twice daily), with no reports of adverse effects (Sarkate et al 2007).

Although iron supplementation is often used as stand-alone treatment in pregnant iron-deficient women, one RCT indicated that a combination of iron and folate therapy (80 mg iron protein succinylate, with 0.370 mg folinic acid daily) for 60 days produces a better therapeutic response than iron-only supplementation (Juarez-Vazquez et al 2002).

Postpartum anaemia

Postpartum anaemia is associated with breathlessness, tiredness, palpitations, maternal infections and impaired mood and cognition. A 2004 Cochrane review suggested that further high-quality trials were required before the benefits of iron supplementation or iron-rich diets in the treatment of postpartum anaemia could be established (Dodd et al 2004). Since then a randomised placebo-controlled study of iron sulfate (80 mg daily) for 12 weeks starting 24–48 hours after delivery demonstrated an improvement in haemoglobin levels and iron stores (Krafft et al 2005) and supplementation of ferrous sulfate (125 mg) with folate (10 mcg) and vitamin C (25 mg) demonstrated improvements in cognitive function, as well as depression and stress compared with folate and vitamin C alone (Beard et al 2005). However, further studies are still warranted.

Restless-leg syndrome

Low serum iron levels are frequently seen in patients with restless-leg syndrome. Whether this is a cause or consequence of the syndrome remains unclear. A Cochrane review of six RCTs (n = 192) concluded that currently there is insufficient evidence to determine whether iron supplementation would be of benefit in the treatment of restless-leg syndrome (Trotti et al 2012). The trials included patients with and without iron deficiency.

Unexplained fatigue without anaemia

Iron supplementation may be considered as a treatment in non-anaemic menstruating women with haemoglobin levels within normal range (>120 g/L) who complain of unexplained fatigue without identifiable secondary causes.

A recent multicentre RCT involving 198 women aged 18–53 years assessed the effect of oral iron therapy for 12 weeks in women with considerable fatigue without obvious clinical cause. Eligibility criteria included ferritin levels of <50 mcg/L and haemoglobin levels >12 g/dL (120 g/L). Iron supplementation (80 mg elemental iron/day as ferrous sulfate for 12 weeks) was shown to decrease fatigue by 47.7% in the treatment group compared to 28.8% in the placebo group (P = 0.02). No significant effects on anxiety or quality of life unrelated to fatigue were observed (Vaucher et al 2012). These findings support earlier research by Verdon and colleagues (2003), who conducted a double-blind, randomised placebo-controlled trial designed to determine the subjective response to iron therapy in non-anaemic women (haemoglobin > 117 g/L) with unexplained fatigue. This study found that supplementation with oral ferrous sulfate (80 mg/day elemental iron) for 4 weeks reduced the level of fatigue in the iron group by 29% compared with 13% in the placebo group. Subgroup analysis showed that only women with ferritin concentrations <50 mcg/L improved with oral supplementation. This was common in 85% of subjects and 51% of subjects had ferritin concentrations <20 mcg/L (Verdon et al 2003). It has been suggested that the current reference levels for women may need to be revised.

Improving athletic performance

Sports anaemia is a common finding among professional and non-professional athletes engaging in strenuous physical activity. Optimal iron balance is important to maintain athletic performance, yet elite athletes appear to be at greater risk of developing iron deficiency (Reinke et al 2012).

Possible mechanisms include: increased iron loss due to factors such as sweating, gastrointestinal bleeding and inflammation (McClung 2012). Proinflammatory cytokines such as IL-6 stimulate expression of hepcidin, a hormone that reduces absorption of iron in the enterocyte, while promoting the sequestering of iron in macrophages (McClung & Karl 2009). Some athletes may also consume carefully controlled diets which are low in meat and other sources of haem iron, yet high in grains and vegetable products that inhibit iron absorption (McClung 2012). Another possibility is dilutional pseudoanaemia, which is caused by plasma volume expansion greater than that of the red blood cell mass, but does not reflect actual blood loss and will generally normalise within 3–5 days of ceasing training; intravascular haemolysis due to mechanical trauma such as 'foot strike haemolysis', which can result in urinary loss of iron; or transient ischaemia resulting from vasoconstriction of the splanchnic and renal vessels, which can also result in blood loss from the gastrointestinal and urinary tracts (Merkel et al 2005).

In a placebo-controlled trial, iron supplementation (50 mg ferrous sulfate twice daily) for 6 weeks significantly improved iron status and maximal oxygen uptake (VO_{2max}) after 4 weeks' concurrent aerobic training in previously marginally deficient and untrained women (Brownlie et al 2002). In a later randomised double-blind placebo-controlled study of 41 untrained iron-deficient women without anaemia, ferrous sulfate (100 mg) for 6 weeks improved endurance capacity after aerobic training (Brownlie et al 2004). However, a review concluded that the current evidence does not justify the use of supplementation solely for the purpose of performance enhancement (Rodenberg & Gustafson 2007).

Due to the potential side effects of inappropriate iron supplementation and the possibility of masking more serious underlying complaints, athletes should only be supplemented if iron deficiency is established on the basis of biological criteria (Zoller & Vogel 2004). Short recuperation periods between intense athletic training may also allow for some recovery of iron storage; however, it may not be sufficient to fully normalise decreased iron levels and iron deficiency in athletes. Monitoring of iron status in elite athletes is recommended (Reinke et al 2012).

Anaemia of inflammation/chronic disease

In this form of anaemia storage iron is often abundant but not available for erythropoiesis. Thus, elevated markers of inflammation should be used for diagnosis. Treatment is difficult but often involves intravenous iron and erythropoietin (EPO) supplements (Handelman & Levin 2008). Emerging future therapies for anaemia associated with chronic inflammation and autoimmune disease may include iron chelation anticytokine administration, modulation of EPO receptors, use of erythropoietin-stimulating agents and agonists/antagonists to modulate the levels of the proteins hepcidin and ferroportin, which are involved with iron homeostasis (Recalcati et al 2012).

Cognitive function

Iron deficiency and iron-deficiency anaemia are associated with impaired cognitive function, which suggests that iron supplementation may have a potential role in improving cognitive function. Iron deficiency has been associated with delayed achievement of developmental motor milestones in a study of infants aged 9–10 months (Shafir et al 2008) and poor cognitive and motor development with behavioural problems (Otero et al 2004).

A systematic review and meta-analysis of 14 RCTs reported that iron supplementation results in a slight improvement (2.5 points) in IQ in anaemic participants ($P = 0.0002$), but not in non-anaemic ones (Falkingham et al 2010). Most of the studies included in the review were conducted on children or adolescents, but some studies in women were also included. Interestingly, iron supplementation may also improve attention and concentration in adolescents and women, irrespective of baseline iron status, although it was not found to have a significant effect on memory, psychomotor function or scholastic achievement (Falkingham et al 2010).

Modest improvements in mental development scores were found for iron supplementation according to a systematic review; however benefits were more prevalent in those who were initially anaemic or iron deficient (Sachdev et al 2005). Two-month supplementation of 15 mg iron (and multivitamin) was better than a multivitamin alone in preschoolers with iron-deficiency anaemia as it resulted in improvements to discrimination (specifically selective attention), accuracy and efficiency (Metallinos-Katsaras et al 2004). Another study found that iron deficiency was associated with compromised working memory in children between the ages of 8 and 10, with iron supplementation being able to restore attention and cognitive capabilities in this group (Otero et al 2008).

An increased incidence of iron deficiency and iron-deficiency anaemia has been reported in children with autistic spectrum disorders; this appears to be mainly due to low iron intake relating to feeding difficulties and food selectivity. These low iron levels may exacerbate the severity of psychomotor and behavioural problems in these children (Bilgic et al 2010).

In adults, iron deficiency in the absence of anaemia has been reported to impair cognitive function in a small study conducted on premenopausal women (Blanton et al 2011). Another study found that iron supplementation improved cognitive function and depression in postpartum anaemic women (Beard et al 2005).

Attention-deficit hyperactivity disorder (ADHD) in children

Whether iron supplementation has benefits in ADHD is difficult to determine at this stage due to a lack of RCTs; however, preliminary research suggests it may be of use in improving some aspects of ADHD. In particular, it appears that iron deficiency may contribute to behavioural problems, including ADHD (as well as restless-leg syndrome and Tourette's) due to an influence on the metabolism of dopamine and other catecholamines (Cortese et al 2008). As a result, children with ADHD and a positive family history of restless-leg syndrome appear to be at increased risk for severe ADHD symptoms (Konofal et al 2007). Iron supplementation (80 mg/day) for 12 weeks significantly improved ADHD symptoms in children with low serum ferritin levels but without anaemia. The mean Clinical Global Impression-Severity ($P < 0.01$) and ADHD Rating Scale ($P < 0.008$) were improved in a manner comparable to pharmaceutical stimulants (Konofal et al 2008).

Perioperative care

Iron is sometimes given before surgery to reduce postoperative decreases in haemoglobin (Andrews et al 1997). However, this use is contentious and numerous studies have failed to report benefits for preoperative autologous blood collection (Cid et al 2005) or for correcting anaemia associated with cardiac surgery (Madi-Jebara et al 2004) or orthopaedic surgery, such as hip or knee arthroplasty (Mundy et al 2005, Weatherall & Maling 2004). In a more recent randomised placebo-controlled trial in patients undergoing colorectal surgery, oral ferrous sulfate (200 mg TDS) for 2 weeks preoperatively resulted in increased mean haemoglobin and ferritin concentrations, and reduced the need for operative blood transfusion (mean 0 units transfused [range, 0–4 units] versus 2 units transfused [range, 0–11 units]; $P = 0.031$; 95% confidence interval 0.13–2.59) (Lidder et al 2007).

Gastric bypass patients

Iron deficiency may develop after gastric bypass due to red meat intolerance, diminished gastric acid secretion and exclusion of the duodenum from the gastrointestinal tract. Patients require lifelong follow-up of haematological and iron parameters since iron deficiency and anaemia may develop years after surgery and, once developed, may prove refractory to oral treatment, resulting in the need for parenteral iron, blood transfusions or surgical interventions (Love & Billett 2008).

Blood donors

Iron supplementation (150 mg ferrous sulfate three times daily) for 1 week following blood donation reduced the decline in haemoglobin concentration and maintained haematocrit, serum iron, serum ferritin and percentage saturation (Maghsudlu et al 2008). Normalisation of low haemoglobin, and thus blood donor retention, may be further enhanced by a standardised protocol offering iron supplementation and simple oral and written advice based on plasma ferritin measurements (Magnussen et al 2008).

OTHER USES

Breath-holding spells

According to one RCT in iron-deficient children, iron supplementation significantly reduced the incidence of breath-holding spells (Daoud et al 1997). No further research on this indication for iron supplements appears to have been conducted, according to a Cochrane review (Zehetner et al 2010).

Haemodialysis

Intravenous iron is frequently, but contentiously, prescribed for the aggressive management of anaemia associated with dialysis (Agarwal et al 2004, Gillespie & Wolf 2004, Ruiz-Jaramillo et al 2004). CYP3A4 activity is reduced in haemodialysis patients, which may be related to functional iron deficiency. However, with the exception of a subset of haemodialysis patients with low baseline CYP3A4 activity, intravenous iron does not appear to have a significant effect on hepatic CYP3A4 (Pai et al 2007). It has been suggested that strategies to improve vitamin C status and to decrease inflammation would lead to better utilisation of iron in these patients (Handelman 2007).

Hypothyroidism

Adjunct therapy in thyroid disorders

Iron supplementation as adjunct therapy to iodine supplementation results in greater improved thyroid function than giving iodine alone in populations that are deficient in both nutrients (Hess 2010). For patients with comorbid iron-deficiency anaemia and subclinical hypothyroidism, but raised thyroid-stimulating hormone levels, the addition of levothyroxine (50 mcg/day) to iron supplementation (ferrous sulfate 65 mg/day) resulted in better outcomes of both conditions than monotherapy with either iron or levothyroxine, according to one small study of 60 patients (Ravanbod et al 2013). The authors suggest that all patients with iron-deficiency anaemia of unknown aetiology should also be investigated for subclinical hypothyroidism.

DOSAGE RANGE

- Therapeutic dose: Generally 2–5 mg/kg/day; depending on the condition being treated. In many cases the equivalent of this dose may be given as a weekly dose rather than a daily dose. The duration of therapy may need to be individualised until iron stores are replenished.
- In cases of deficiency, initial effects on haemoglobin and erythrocyte concentrations take about 2 weeks but it may take 6–12 months to build iron stores (Gropper & Smith 2013).
- The Australian Iron Status Advisory Panel advocates dietary intervention as the first treatment option for mild iron deficiency (serum ferritin 10–15 mcg/L) (Patterson et al 2001). Trials have shown a significant increase in serum ferritin levels (26%) using dietary intervention alone (Heath et al 2001).

TABLE 1 AUSTRALIAN RECOMMENDED DAILY INTAKE (RDI) BY AGE AND SEX

Age	Australian RDI (mg/day)
Infants (0–6 months; breastfed)	0.2
Infants (7–12 months)	11
Children (1–8 years)	9–10
Girls (9–13 years)	8
Girls (14–18 years)	15
Boys (9–13 years)	8
Boys (14–18 years)	11
Men (>18 years)	8
Women (18 to menopause)	18
After menopause	8
Pregnancy	27
Lactation	9

In Table 1, the RDI of iron is expressed as a range to allow for differences in bioavailability of iron from different Australian foods.

Studies have shown that there can be a significant sex difference in haemoglobin and other indicators of iron status during infancy. Some of these may be genetically determined, whereas others seem to reflect an increased incidence of true iron deficiency in boys (Domellof et al 2002).

TOXICITY

Iron toxicity causes severe organ damage and eventually death. The most pronounced effects are haemorrhagic necrosis of the gastrointestinal tract, which manifests as vomiting, bloody diarrhoea and hepatotoxicity. Acute overdose or iron accumulation may progress to shock and/or impaired consciousness (Singhi & Baranwal 2003). Iron overdose in pregnant women has been associated with spontaneous abortion, preterm delivery and maternal death (Tran et al 2000). Excess iron accumulation is being investigated as a potential contributing factor for the development of diseases such as Parkinson's and Alzheimer's disease (Dwyer et al 2009, Rhodes & Ritz 2008, Sian-Hulsmann et al 2011). Some studies suggests that chronic iron overload may contribute to the development of type 2 diabetes and coronary heart disease; however, further research is required to confirm these associations (Mojiminiyi et al 2008).

Conditions that increase risk of toxicity include:

- Haemochromatosis (iron overload) — excess absorption and accumulation of iron in the body, which can cause organ and tissue damage (especially liver, heart and pancreas) and an increased risk for hepatic carcinoma. The most important

causes are a genetic disorder (hereditary haemochromatosis), which leads to abnormal iron absorption, or as a secondary consequence of a transfusion, or repeated transfusions.
- Haemosiderosis — iron overload without tissue damage.
- Iron-loading anaemias — thalassaemia and sideroblastic anaemia.

ADVERSE REACTIONS

Oral supplements may cause gastrointestinal disturbances such as nausea, diarrhoea, constipation, heartburn and upper gastric discomfort, and may cause stools to blacken.

Taking supplements with food appears to reduce the possibility of gastrointestinal side effects. Liquid iron preparations can discolour teeth — brush teeth after use.

Intermittent dosing on a weekly basis rather than a daily basis may also reduce side effects.

In the absence of appropriate storage or chelation, excess free iron can readily participate in the formation of toxic free radicals, inducing oxidative stress and apoptosis (Whitnall & Richardson 2006). Iron depletion leads to decreased availability of redox-active iron in vivo and appears to reduce atherosclerotic lesion size and increase plaque stability (Sullivan & Mascitelli 2007). Iron toxicity and subsequent organ damage can develop from long-term excessive intake.

There is preliminary evidence that iron may be implicated in the pathogenesis of autoimmune disorders (Bowlus 2003) and neurodegenerative diseases (Whitnall & Richardson 2006) and that moderately elevated iron stores may be associated with an overall increased risk for cancer, especially colorectal cancer (McCarty 2003). In younger people iron depletion is associated with a reduced risk of all-cause mortality (Sullivan & Mascitelli 2007), although numerous confounding factors cannot be ignored. While haem iron intake from red meat may present a risk for increased blood pressure, non-haem dietary intake may slightly reduce systolic blood pressure (Tzoulaki et al 2008). For the time being, supplementation without demonstrated biological need cannot be justified as the potential risks may outweigh any short-term benefits.

SIGNIFICANT INTERACTIONS

Iron interacts with a variety of foods, herbs and drugs through several different mechanisms. Most commonly, the formation of insoluble complexes occurs whereby both iron and drug absorption is hindered. Separation of doses by several hours will often reduce the severity of this type of interaction. Additionally, substances that alter gastric pH have the theoretical ability to reduce iron absorption. A summary of interactions is presented in Table 2 for easy reference.

TABLE 2 SUMMARY OF IRON INTERACTIONS

Drug/therapeutic substance	Mechanism	Possible outcome	Action required
Angiotensin-converting enzyme (ACE) inhibitors	Oral iron supplementation with ferrous sulfate 200 mg may suppress cough induced by ACE inhibitors through an effect on nitric oxide generation (Bhalla et al 2011, Lee et al 2001)	Reduced drug adverse effect	Beneficial interaction possible
Antacids and products containing aluminium, calcium or magnesium	Reduces iron absorption (O'Neil-Cutting & Crosby 1986)	Reduced effect of iron	Separate doses by at least 2 h
Ascorbic acid	Increases iron absorption	Increased effects of iron	Beneficial interaction is possible — caution in haemochromatosis
Cholestyramine and colestipol	In vitro investigations have shown that cholestyramine and colestipol both bind iron citrate (Leonard et al 1979)	Reduced drug and iron effect	Monitor for iron efficacy if cholestyramine is being used concurrently. Separate doses by 4 h. Increased iron intake may be required with long-term therapy
Cimetidine	Iron can bind cimetidine in the gastrointestinal tract and reduce its absorption (Campbell et al 1993)	Reduced drug and iron effect	Separate doses by at least 2 h
Dairy products and eggs	May reduce iron absorption	Reduced effect of iron	Monitor for iron efficacy

TABLE 2 SUMMARY OF IRON INTERACTIONS *(continued)*

Drug/therapeutic substance	Mechanism	Possible outcome	Action required
Erythropoietin	Pharmacodynamic interaction (Carnielli et al 1998). In patients with chemotherapy-related anaemia without iron deficiency, the addition of intravenous iron supplementation may improve the success of darbepoetin (92.5% versus 70% for darbepoetin alone; $P = 0.0033$) without increasing toxicity (Pedrazzoli et al 2008)	Additive pharmacological effect possible	Beneficial interaction is possible
H_2-receptor antagonists (antiulcer drugs)	Iron absorption is dependent upon gastric pH; therefore, medications that affect gastric pH may interfere with absorption of iron (Aymard et al 1988)	Reduced effect of iron	Monitor for iron efficacy if these drugs are being used concurrently
Haloperidol	May cause decreased blood levels of iron (Leenders et al 1994, Threlkeld 1999)	Reduced effect of iron	Monitor for iron efficacy if these drugs are being used concurrently. Increased iron intake may be required with long-term therapy
L-Dopa and carbidopa	May reduce bioavailability of carbidopa and L-dopa (van Woert et al 1977)	Reduced drug effect	Separate doses by 2 h
Omeprazole and other proton pump inhibitors	Reduced iron absorption due to changes in gastric pH	Reduced effect of iron	Monitor for iron efficacy if omeprazole is being used concurrently
Penicillamine	Reduced drug and iron absorption	Reduced drug and iron effect	Separate doses by at least 2 h. Sudden withdrawal of iron during penicillamine use has been associated with penicillamine toxicity and kidney damage (Harkness & Blake 1982) — caution
Quinolone antibiotics (e.g. norfloxacin)	Reduced drug absorption (Brouwers 1992)	Reduced drug effect	Take drug 2 h before or 4–6 h after iron dosing. Monitor patient for continued antibiotic efficacy
Sulfasalazine	May bind together, decreasing the absorption of both (Dukes & Duncan 1995)	Reduced drug and iron effect	Separate doses by at least 2 h
Tannins — herbs with significant tannin content (e.g. green tea, bilberry, raspberry leaf)	Tannin can bind to iron and reduce its absorption	Reduced effect of iron	Monitor for iron efficacy if these herbs are being used concurrently. Separate doses by 2 h
Tetracycline antibiotics (e.g. minocycline, doxycycline)	While early studies suggested reduced drug and iron absorption (Neuvonen 1976), more recent human data found no effect on erythrocyte iron uptake when in patients taking 100 mg iron orally and oral tetracycline (Potgieter et al 2007)	Reduced drug effect	Monitor for iron efficacy if tetracyclines are being used long-term. Separate doses by 4 h
L-Thyroxine	Decreased drug absorption possible. Iron supplements may decrease absorption of thyroid medication; however, iron deficiency may impair the body's ability to make thyroid hormones	Reduced drug effect	Thyroid function should be monitored and L-thyroxine dose may need alteration during treatment with iron. Separate doses by at least 2–4 h (Shakir et al 1997)
Vitamin A	Iron supplementation may cause a redistribution of retinol, inducing vitamin A deficiency in infants with marginal vitamin A status (Wieringa et al 2003)	Redistribution of retinol	Iron supplementation in infants should be accompanied by measures to improve vitamin A status

Practice points/Patient counselling

- Iron is an essential mineral that facilitates oxygen transport and storage in the body and is part of many enzyme systems.
- Haem iron, found in animal products, is absorbed two- to threefold better than non-haem forms found in vegetable sources. However, iron absorption is influenced by many factors, such as other foods ingested, medicines and gastric activity.
- Iron deficiency is the most common nutritional deficiency in the world and may occur with or without anaemia. Excessive blood loss during menstruation is the most common cause.
- Supplements are generally used to treat or prevent deficiency. Excess iron can be dangerous and can lead to organ damage and death.
- As inappropriate iron supplementation can inhibit growth in non-deficient children and adversely affect pregnancy outcomes, iron status should be tested before administration.
- Correction of iron deficiency with or without anaemia may be achieved with lower doses than those recommended in some trials. In many cases, once-weekly dosing of iron is as effective as daily dosing and improves compliance, while reducing side effects and cost.
- Oral liquid iron supplements should be diluted with water and drunk through a straw to prevent discolouration of teeth, especially if used long-term.

CONTRAINDICATIONS AND PRECAUTIONS

Iron poisoning can occur due to accidental ingestion of excess iron supplements. As such, iron supplements should be kept in childproof bottles and out of the reach of children.

Caution should be exercised when supplementing iron to infants or children with apparently normal growth when the iron status of the child is unknown. A double-blind placebo-controlled trial showed that, while iron therapy produced a significant improvement of mean monthly weight gain and linear growth in iron-deficient children, it significantly decreased the weight gain and linear growth of iron-replete children (Majumdar et al 2003). This study confirms the results of earlier studies (Dewey et al 2002).

Iron supplements should not be used in haemochromatosis, haemosiderosis or iron-loading anaemias (thalassaemia, sideroblastic anaemia).

Daily oral iron supplementation providing 50 mg elemental iron for 8 weeks did not result in increased oxidative damage in the plasma of college-aged women (Gropper et al 2003). However, more recently 100 mg doses of iron daily for 8 weeks were shown to increase lipid peroxidation. As iron status and duration of supplementation increased, so too did indicators of lipid peroxidation (King et al 2008). As the use of iron supplements may potentially result in oxidative damage, risk should always be assessed against benefit before prescribing iron supplements.

Elevated levels of serum ferritin have been implicated in the pathogenesis of vascular (and other) diseases, although this remains controversial (McCarty 2003, Zacharski et al 2004).

Haem-rich flesh foods may need to be limited in people with insulin resistance due to a possible link with increased cancer risk mediated by iron excess in such populations (McCarty 2003).

Iron supplementation should be prescribed on the basis of biological criteria, not on the assumption of anaemia alone, as unnecessary iron supplementation can result in adverse effects. The lowest safe and effective dose and frequency of dose should be recommended.

PREGNANCY USE

Oral iron preparations are considered safe in pregnancy; while adequate iron in pregnancy is important, unnecessary iron supplementation can result in uncontrolled lipid peroxidation (Lachili et al 2001), lowered serum levels of copper and zinc (Ziaei et al 2008), low birth weight and maternal hypertension disorder (Ziaei et al 2007). As a result, iron supplementation should be prescribed on the basis of biological criteria, and the woman's iron status should be assessed first, rather than basing it on the assumption of anaemia alone.

PATIENTS' FAQs

What will this supplement do for me?

Iron is necessary for health and wellbeing. It facilitates oxygen transport and storage in the body and is part of many enzyme systems. Iron deficiency is the most common nutrient deficiency in the world.

When will it start to work?

Iron deficiency responds to supplementation within 2 weeks; however, 6–12 months may be required to build up the body's iron stores.

Are there any safety issues?

Excess iron can be dangerous and ultimately can lead to severe organ damage and death.

REFERENCES

Agarwal KN et al. Anemia prophylaxis in adolescent school girls by weekly or daily iron-folate supplementation. Indian Pediatr 40.4 (2003): 296–301.

Agarwal R et al. Oxidative stress and renal injury with intravenous iron in patients with chronic kidney disease. Kidney Int 65.6 (2004): 2279–2289.

Allen LH, et al. Provision of multiple rather than two or few micronutrients more effectively improves growth and other outcomes in micronutrient-deficient children and adults. J Nutri 139.5 (2009): 1022–30

Andres E et al. Update of nutrient-deficiency anemia in the elderly. European Journal of Internal Medicine. 19 (2008): 488–493

Andrews CM, et al. Iron pre-load for major joint replacement. Transfus Med 7.4 (1997): 281–286.

Annibale B et al. Efficacy of gluten-free diet alone on recovery from iron deficiency anemia in adult celiac patients. Am J Gastroenterol 96.1 (2001): 132–137.

Avni T, et al. Iron supplementation for the treatment of chronic heart failure and iron deficiency: systematic review and meta-analysis. European Journal of Heart Failure 14 (2012):423–429

Aymard JP et al. Haematological adverse effects of histamine H2-receptor antagonists. Med Toxicol Adverse Drug Exp 3 (1988): 430–448.

Bach-Kristensen M et al. Pork meat increases iron absorption from a 5-day fully controlled diet when compared to a vegetarian diet with similar vitamin C and phytic acid content. Br J Nutr 94.1 (2005): 78–83.

Baech SB et al. Nonheme-iron absorption from a phytate-rich meal is increased by the addition of small amounts of pork meat. Am J Clin Nutr 77.1 (2003): 173–179.

Beard JL, et al. Impaired thermoregulation and thyroid function in iron-deficiency anaemia. Am J Clin Nutr 52 (1990): 813–8119.

Beard JL et al. Maternal iron deficiency anemia affects postpartum emotions and cognition. J Nutrition 135.2 (2005): 267–272.

Bergman M et al. In vitro cytokine production in patients with iron deficiency anemia. Clin Immunol 113.3 (2004): 340–344.

Bhalla P, et al. Attenuation of angiotensin converting enzyme inhibitor induced cough by iron supplementation: role of nitric oxide. J Renin Angiotensin Aldosterone Syst. 12.4 (2011):491–7

Bilgic A et al. Iron deficiency in preschool children with autistic spectrum disorders. Research in Autism Spectrum Disorders 4 (2010):639–644

Blanton CA, et al. Iron deficiency without anaemia impairs cognitive function in premenopausal women. Appetite 57 (2011): 553–569

Bowlus CL. The role of iron in T cell development and autoimmunity.Autoimmun Rev 2.2 (2003): 73–78.

Breet P et al. Actions of black tea and Rooibos on iron status of primary school children. Nutr Res 25.11 (2005): 983–994.

Brouwers J. Drug interactions with quinolone antibacterials. Drug Safety 7.4 (1992): 268–281.

Brownlie T et al. Marginal iron deficiency without anemia impairs aerobic adaptation among previously untrained women. Am J Clin Nutr 75.4 (2002): 734–742.

Brownlie T et al. Tissue iron deficiency without anemia impairs adaptation in endurance capacity after aerobic training in previously untrained women. Am J Clin Nutr 79.3 (2004): 437–443.

Campbell NR et al. Ferrous sulfate reduces cimetidine absorption. Dig Dis Sci 38.5 (1993): 950–954.

Carnielli VP, et al. Iron supplementation enhances responses to high doses of recombinant human erythropoietin in preterm infants.Arch Dis Child Fetal Neonatal Ed 79.1 (1998): F44–F48.

Ciacci C et al. *Helicobacter pylori* impairs iron absorption in infected individuals. Dig Liver Dis 36.7 (2004): 455–460.

Cid J et al. [Oral iron and folic acid supplements in a preoperative autologous blood collection program: a randomized study.] Med Clin (Barc) 124.18 (2005): 690–691.

Cook JD. Diagnosis and management of iron-deficiency anaemia. Best Pract Res Clin Haematol 18.2 (2005): 319–332.

Cortese S et al. Attention-deficit/hyperactivity disorder, Tourette's syndrome, and restless legs syndrome: the iron hypothesis. Med Hypotheses 70.6 (2008): 1128–1132.

Crofton R et al. Inorganic zinc and the absorption of ferrous iron. Am J Clin Nutr 50 (1989): 141–144.

Daoud AS et al. Effectiveness of iron therapy on breath-holding spells. J Pediatr 130.4 (1997): 547–550.

Davidsson L et al. Influence of ascorbic acid on iron absorption from an iron-fortified, chocolate-flavored milk drink in Jamaican children. Am J Clin Nutr May 67.5 (1998): 873–877.

Davila-Hicks P, et al. Iron in ferritin or in salts (ferrous sulfate) is equally bioavailable in nonanemic women. Am J Clin Nutr 80.4 (2004): 936–940.

de Benoist B, et al. (2008) Worldwide prevalence of anaemia 1993–2005. WHO global database on anaemia. Accessed March 2013. Available at URL: http://www.who.int/vmnis/publications/anaemia_prevalence/en/index.html

De-Regil LM et al. Intermittent iron supplementation for improving nutrition and development in children under 12 years of age. Cochrane Database of Syst Rev (2011) CD009085.

De-Silva A et al. Iron supplementation improves iron status and reduces morbidity in children with or without upper respiratory tract infections: a randomized controlled study in Colombo, Sri Lanka. Am J Clin Nutr 77.1 (2003): 234–241.

Dewey KG et al. Iron supplementation affects growth and morbidity of breast-fed infants: results of a randomized trial in Sweden and Honduras. J Nutr 132.11 (2002): 3249–3255.

Dodd J, et al. Treatment for women with postpartum iron deficiency anaemia. Cochrane Database Syst Rev 4 (2004): CD004222.

Domellof M et al. Sex differences in iron status during infancy. Pediatrics 110.3 (2002): 545–552.

Dukes DE Jr, Duncan BS. Applied Therapeutics: The clinical use of drugs, 6th edn. Philadelphia: Lippincott Williams & Wilkins, 1995, pp 24–7.

Duque X et al. Effect of eradication of *Helicobacter pylori* and iron supplementation on the iron status of children with iron deficiency. Archives of Medical Research 40 (2010): 38–45

Dwyer BE et al. Getting the iron out: phlebotomy for Alzheimer's disease?. Med Hypothesis 75.5 (2009): 504–9

Falkingham M et al. The effects of oral iron supplementation on cognition in older children and adults: a systematic review and meta-analysis. Nutrition Journal 9.4 (2010).

Fernandez-Gaxiola AC, De-Regil LM. Intermittent iron supplementation for reducing anaemia and its associated impairments in menstruating women. Cochrane Database of Syst Rev 12 (2011) CD009218

Ferreira da Silva L, et al. Serum iron analysis of adults receiving three different iron compounds. Nutr Res 24.8 (2004): 603–611.

Fischer Walker C et al. Interactive effects of iron and zinc on biochemical and functional outcomes in supplementation trials. Am J Clin Nutri 82 (2005):5–12

Flesland O et al. Transferring receptor in serum. A new tool in the diagnosis and prevention of iron deficiency in blood donors. Transf Aph Sci 31.1 (2004): 11–16.

Fuqua BK, et al. Intestinal iron absorption. Journal of Trace Elements in Medicine and Biology. 26 (2012):115–119

Geerligs PP et al. The effect on haemoglobin of the use of iron cooking pots in rural Malawian households in an area with high malaria prevalence: a randomized trial. Trop Med Int Health 8.4 (2003): 310–3115.

Gillespie RS, Wolf FM. Intravenous iron therapy in pediatric hemodialysis patients: a meta-analysis. Pediatr Nephrol 19.6 (2004): 662–666.

Gillespie S, et al (eds). Controlling iron deficiency. Geneva, Switzerland: United Nations Administrative Committee on Coordination/ Subcommittee on Nutrition. State-of-the-Art Series: Nutrition Policy, Discussion Paper No. 9, 1991.

Gropper SS, Smith JL, Advanced Nutrition and Human Metabolism, 6th edition. Belmont, CA: Wadsworth (2013): 481–500

Gropper SS, et al. Non-anemic iron deficiency, oral iron supplementation, and oxidative damage in college-aged females. J Nutr Biochem 14.7 (2003): 409–415.

Haidar J et al. Daily versus weekly iron supplementation and prevention of iron deficiency anaemia in lactating women. East Afr Med J 80.1 (2003): 11–116.

Haider BA et al. Anaemia, prenatal iron use, and risk of adverse pregnancy outcomes: systematic review and meta-analysis. BMJ. 346 (2013):f3443

Hallberg L et al. The role of meat to improve the critical iron balance during weaning. Pediatrics 111.4 Pt. 1 (2003): 864–870.

Handelman GJ. Newer strategies for anemia prevention in hemodialysis. Int J Artif Organs 30.11 (2007): 1014–10119.

Handelman GJ, Levin NW. Iron and anemia in human biology: a review of mechanisms. Heart Fail Rev 13.4 (2008): 393–404.

Harkness JAL, Blake DR. Penicillamine nephropathy and iron. Lancet 2 (1982): 1368–1369.

Heath AL et al. Can dietary treatment of non-anemic iron deficiency improve iron status? J Am Coll Nutr 20.5 (2001): 477–484.

Hess SY. The impact of common micronutrient deficiencies on iodine and thyroid metabolism: the evidence from human studies. Best Practice & Research Clinical Endocrinology & Metabolism. 24. 1 (2010):117–32

Higgins PDR, Rockey DC. Iron-deficiency anemia. Tech Gastrointest Endosc 5.3 (2003): 134–141.

Hsu HS et al. Iron deficiency with increased risk of cardiovascular disease an all-cause mortality in the elderly living in long-term care facilities. Nutrition (2013):29: 737–743.

Hurrell R et al. Iron absorption in humans: bovine serum albumin compared with beef muscle and egg white. Am J Clin Nutr 47 (1988): 102–107.

Ioannou GN et al. The effect of alcohol consumption on the prevalence of iron overload, iron deficiency, and iron deficiency anemia. Gastroenterology 126.5 (2004): 1293–1301.

Juarez-Vazquez J, et al. Iron plus folate is more effective than iron alone in the treatment of iron deficiency anaemia in pregnancy: a randomised, double blind clinical trial. Br J Obstet Gynaecol 109.9 (2002): 1009–1014.

Kaltwasser JP et al. Clinical trial on the effect of regular tea drinking on iron accumulation in genetic haemochromatosis. Gut 43.5 (1998): 699–704.

King SM et al. Daily supplementation with iron increases lipid peroxidation in young women with low iron stores. Exp Biol Med (Maywood) 233.6 (2008): 701–707.

Klip IT et al. Prevalence, predictors and prognosis of iron deficiency in patients with chronic heart failure: an international pooled analysis of 1,506 patients. Journal of American College of Cardiology. 59.13 (2012):E1045

Konofal E et al. Impact of restless legs syndrome and iron deficiency on attention-deficit/hyperactivity disorder in children. Sleep Med 8.7–8 (2007): 711–715.

Konofal E et al. Effects of iron supplementation on attention deficit hyperactivity disorder in children. Pediatr Neurol 38.1 (2008): 20–226.

Krafft A, et al. Effect of postpartum iron supplementation on red cell and iron parameters in non-anaemic iron-deficient women: a randomised placebo-controlled study. Br J Obstet Gynaecol 112.4 (2005): 445–450.

Lachili B et al. Increased lipid peroxidation in pregnant women after iron and vitamin C supplementation. Biol Trace Elem Res 83.2 (2001): 103–110.

Lee SC, et al. Iron supplementation inhibits cough associated with ACE Inhibitors. Hypertension 38 (2001): 166–170.

Leenders KL et al. Blood to brain iron uptake in one rhesus monkey using [Fe-52]-citrate and positron emission tomography (PET): influence of haloperidol. J Neural Transm 43 (Suppl) (1994): 123–132.

Leonard JP et al. In vitro binding of various biological substances by two hypocholesterolaemic resins: Cholestyramine and colestipol. Arzneim Forsch/Drug Res 29 (1979): 979–981.

Lidder PG et al. Pre-operative oral iron supplementation reduces blood transfusion in colorectal surgery — a prospective, randomised, controlled trial. Ann R Coll Surg Engl 89.4 (2007): 418–421.

Lind T et al. A community-based randomized controlled trial of iron and zinc supplementation in Indonesian infants: interactions between iron and zinc. Am J Clin Nutr 77.4 (2003): 883–890.

Lonnerdal B. Calcium and iron absorption-mechanisms and public relevance. International Journal for Vitamin & Nutrition Research 80 (2010):293–299

Love AL, Billett HH. Obesity, bariatric surgery, and iron deficiency: true, true, true and related. Am J Hematol 83.5 (2008): 403–409.

Madi-Jebara SN et al. Postoperative intravenous iron used alone or in combination with low-dose erythropoietin is not effective for correction of anemia after cardiac surgery. J Cardiothorac Vasc Anesth 18.1 (2004): 59–63.

Maghsudlu M et al. Short-term ferrous sulfate supplementation in female blood donors. Transfusion 48.6 (2008): 1192–1197.

Magnussen K, et al. The effect of a standardized protocol for iron supplementation to blood donors low in hemoglobin concentration. Transfusion 48.4 (2008): 749–754.

Majumdar I et al. The effect of iron therapy on the growth of iron-replete and iron-deplete children. J Trop Pediatr 49.2 (2003): 84–88.

McCarty MF. Hyperinsulinemia may boost both hematocrit and iron absorption by up-regulating activity of hypoxia-inducible factor-1[alpha]. Med Hypoth 61.5–6 (2003): 567–573.

McClung JP. Iron status and the female athlete. Journal of Trace Elements in Medicine and Biology. 26 (2012):124–126

McClung JP, Karl JP. Iron deficiency and obesity: the contribution of inflammation and diminished iron absorption. Nutri Rev 67 (2009):100–4

Mei Z et al. Hemoglobin and ferritin are currently the most efficient indicators of population response to iron interventions: an analysis of nine randomized controlled trials. J Nutr 135.8 (2005): 1974–1980.

Merkel D et al. Prevalence of iron deficiency and anemia among strenuously trained adolescents. J Adolesc Health 37.3 (2005): 220–223.

Metallinos-Katsaras E et al. Effect of iron supplementation on cognition in Greek preschoolers. Eur J Clin Nutr 58.11 (2004): 1532–1542.

Milman N et al. Iron prophylaxis during pregnancy: how much iron is needed? A randomized dose-response study of 20–80 mg ferrous iron daily in pregnant women. Acta Obstet Gynecol Scand 84.3 (2004): 238–247.

Mojiminiyi OA, et al. Body iron stores in relation to the metabolic syndrome, glycemic control and complications in female patients with type 2 diabetes. Nutrition, Metabolism & cardiovascular Diseases 18 (2008):559–566

Mukhopadhyay A et al. Erythrocyte indices in pregnancy: effect of intermittent iron supplementation. Natl Med J India 17.3 (2004): 135–137.

Mundy GM, et al. The effect of iron supplementation on the level of haemoglobin after lower limb arthroplasty. J Bone Joint Surg Br 87.2 (2005): 213–2117.

Navas-Carretero S et al. Oily fish increases iron bioavailability of a phytate rich meal in young iron deficient women. J Am CollNutr 27.1 (2008): 96–101.

Neuvonen PJ. Interactions with the absorption of tetracyclines. Drugs 11.1 (1976): 45–54.

NMCD (Natural Medicines Comprehensive Database) Iron. Available online: http://www.naturaldatabase.com 10 November 2005.

Olsen A et al. Failure of twice-weekly iron supplementation to increase blood haemoglobin and serum ferritin concentrations: results of a randomized controlled trial. Ann Trop Med Parasitol 100.3 (2006): 251–263.

O'Neil-Cutting MA, Crosby WH. The effect of antacids on the absorption of simultaneously ingested iron. JAMA 255 (1986): 1468–1470.

Otero GA et al. Iron supplementation brings up a lacking P300 in iron deficient children. Clin Neurophysiol 115.10 (2004): 2259–2266.

Otero GA et al. Working memory impairment and recovery in iron deficient children. Clinical Neurophysiology 119 (2008): 1739–1746

Pai AB et al. Effect of intravenous iron supplementation on hepatic cytochrome P450 3A4 activity in hemodialysis patients: a prospective, open-label study. Clin Ther 29.12 (2007): 2699–2705.

Patterson AJ et al. Dietary treatment of iron deficiency in women of childbearing age. Am J Clin Nutr 74.5 (2001): 650–656.

Pedrazzoli P et al. Randomized trial of intravenous iron supplementation in patients with chemotherapy-related anemia without iron deficiency treated with darbepoetin alpha. J Clin Oncol 26.10 (2008): 1619–1625.

Pena-Rosas JP et al. Daily oral iron supplementation during pregnancy. Cochrane Database Syst Rev (2012) doi:10/1002/14651858.CD004736. pub4

Potgieter MA et al. Effect of oral tetracycline on iron absorption from iron(III)-hydroxide polymaltose complex in patients with iron deficiency anemia /a single-centre randomized controlled isotope study. Arzneimittelforschung 57.6A (2007): 376–384.

Ramakrishnan U et al. Multimicronutrient interventions but not vitamin a or iron interventions alone improve child growth: results of 3 meta-analyses. J Nutr 134.10(2004): 2592–602

Ramakrishnan U, et al. Effects of micronutrients on growth of children under 5 y of age: meta-analyses of single and multiple nutrient interventions. Am J Clin Nutr 89.1 (2009): 191–203

Rattehalli D et al. Iron deficiency without anaemia: do not wait for the haemoglobin to drop? Health Policy and Technology 2 (2013):45–5

Ravanbod M et al. Treatment of iron-deficiency anaemia in patients with subclinical hypothyroidism. American Journal of Medicine 126 (2013): 420–424.

Recalcati S et al. Iron levels in polarized macrophages: regulation of immunity and autoimmunity. Autoimmun Rev 11.12 (2012): 883–889.

Reinke S et al. Absolute and functional iron deficiency in professional athletes during training and recovery. International Journal of cardiology 156 (2012):186–191

Rhodes SL, Ritz B. Genetics of iron regulation and the possible role of iron in Parkinson's disease. Neurobiology of Disease 32 (2008):183–195

Rimon E et al. Are we giving too much iron? Low-dose iron therapy is effective in octogenarians. Am J Med 118.10 (2005): 1142–1147.

Rodenberg RE, Gustafson S. Iron as an ergogenic aid: ironclad evidence? Curr Sports Med Rep 6.4 (2007): 258–264.

Rossander-Hulten L et al. Competitive inhibition of iron absorption by manganese and zinc. Am J Clin Nutr 54 (1991): 152–156.

Ruiz-Jaramillo M-L et al. Intermittent versus maintenance iron therapy in children on hemodialysis: a randomized study. Pediatr Nephrol 19.1 (2004): 77–81.

Sachdev H, et al. Effect of iron supplementation on mental and motor development in children: systematic review of randomised controlled trials. Public Health Nutr 8.2 (2005): 117–132.

Santiago P. Ferrous versus ferric oral iron formulations for the treatment of iron deficiency: A clinical overview. Scientific World Journal (2012) 2012: 846824.

Sarkate P et al. A randomised double-blind study comparing sodium feredetate with ferrous fumarate in anaemia in pregnancy. J Indian Med Assoc 105.5 (2007): 278, 280–281, 284.

Sejas E et al. Iron supplementation in previously anemic Bolivian children normalized hematologic parameters, but not immunologic parameters. J Trop Pediatr 54.3 (2008): 164–168.

Shafir T et al. Iron deficiency and infant motor development. Early Human Development 84 (2008):479–485

Shakir KM et al. Ferrous sulfate-induced increase in requirement for thyroxine in a patient with primary hypothyroidism. South Med J 90.6 (1997): 637–639.

Sian-Hulsmann J et al. The relevance of iron in the pathogenesis of Parkinson's disease. J Neurochem 118.6 (2011):939–57

Siddiqui IA, et al. Efficacy of daily vs. weekly supplementation of iron in schoolchildren with low iron status. J Trop Pediatr 50.5 (2004): 276–278.

Singhi S, Baranwal AK. Acute iron poisoning: clinical picture, intensive care needs and outcome. Indian Pediatr 40.12 (2003): 1177–82
Stoltzfus R. Iron deficiency: global prevalence and consequences. Food Nutr Bull 24.4 (2003):S99–103
Sullivan JL, Mascitelli L. [Current status of the iron hypothesis of cardiovascular diseases.] Recent Prog Med 98.7–8 (2007): 373–377.
Sungthong R et al. Once-weekly and 5-days a week iron supplementation differentially affect cognitive function but not school performance in Thai children. J Nutr 134.9 (2004): 2349–2354.
Thompson J, et al. Effects of daily iron supplementation in 2-to-5-year old children: systematic review and meta-analysis. Pediatrics 131.4 (2013):739–53
Threlkeld DS (ed.). Central nervous system drugs, antipsychotic agents. In: Facts and comparisons drug information. St Louis, MO: Wolter Kluwer Health, 1998, pp 266k–266m. Cited in: Lininger SW et al (eds). A–Z Guide to drug–herb–vitamin interactions. Roseville, CA: Healthnotes, 1999.
Tran T et al. Intentional iron overdose in pregnancy-management and outcome. J Emerg Med 18. 2 (2000): 225–8
Trotti LM, et al. Iron for restless leg syndrome (review). Cochrane Database Syst Rev 5 (2012): CD007834.
Tzoulaki I et al. Relation of iron and red meat intake to blood pressure: cross sectional epidemiological study. BMJ 337 (2008): a258.
Ullmann U et al. Epigallocatechingallate (EGCG) (TEAVIGO) does not impair nonhaem-iron absorption in man. Phytomedicine 12.6–7 (2005): 410–4115.
Van Woert MH et al. Long-term therapy of monoclonus and other neurological disorders with L-5-hydroxytryptophan and carbidopa. N Engl J Med 296 (1977): 70–75.
Vaucher P et al. Effect of iron supplementation on fatigue in anaemic menstruating women with low ferritin: a randomized controlled trial. CMAJ 184.11 (2012):1247–1254
Verdon F et al. Iron supplementation for unexplained fatigue in non-anaemic women: double blind randomised placebo controlled trial (Primary care). BMJ 326.7399 (2003): 1124.
Weatherall M, Maling TJ. Oral iron therapy for anaemia after orthopaedic surgery: randomized clinical trial. Aust NZ J Surg 74.12 (2004): 1049–1051.
Whitnall M, Richardson DR. Iron: a new target for pharmacological intervention in neurodegenerative diseases. Semin Pediatr Neurol 13.3 (2006): 186–197.
Whittaker P. Iron and zinc interactions in humans. Am J Clin Nutr 68 (1998): 442–6S.
Wieringa FT et al. Redistribution of vitamin A after iron supplementation in Indonesian infants. Am J Clin Nutr 77.3 (2003): 651–657.
Wijaya-Erhardt M et al. Effect of daily or weekly multiple-micronutrient and iron foodlike tablets on body iron stores of Indonesian infants aged 6–12 mo: a double-blind, randomized, placebo-controlled trial. Am J Clin Nutr 86.6 (2007): 1680–1686.
Yang Q, et al. Effect of daily or once weekly iron supplementation on growth and iron status of preschool children. Wei Sheng Yan Jiu 33.2 (2004): 205–207.
Yang Y et al. Efficacy and safety of iron supplementation for the elderly patients undergoing hip or knee surgery: A meta-analysis of randomized controlled trials. Journal of Surgical Research 171.2 (2011) e201-e207
Zacharski LR et al. Implementation of an iron reduction protocol in patients with peripheral vascular disease: VA cooperative study no. 410: The Iron (FE) and Atherosclerosis Study (FEAST). Am Heart J 148.3 (2004): 386–392.
Zareifar S et al. Association between iron status and febrile seizures in children. Seizure 21.8 (2012): 603–605.
Zehetner AA et al. Iron supplementation for breath-holding attacks in children. Cochrane Database Syst Rev 12.5 (2010): CD008132.
Zhou SJ et al. Should we lower the dose of iron when treating anaemia in pregnancy? A randomized dose-response trial. Eur J Clin Nutr (2009): 63: 183–190.
Ziaei S et al. A randomised placebo-controlled trial to determine the effect of iron supplementation on pregnancy outcome in pregnant women with haemoglobin> or = 13.2 g/dl. BJOG 114.6 (2007): 684–688.
Ziaei S et al. The effects of iron supplementation on serum copper and zinc levels in pregnant women with high-normal hemoglobin. Int J Gynaecol Obstet 100.2 (2008): 133–135.
Zoller H, Vogel W. Iron supplementation in athletes: first do no harm. Nutrition 20.7–8 (2004): 615–6119.

Kava

HISTORICAL NOTE For many centuries, Pacific Islanders have used the kava root to prepare a beverage used in welcoming ceremonies for important visitors. Drinking kava is not only done to induce pleasant mental states but also to reduce anxiety and promote socialising. It is believed that the first report about kava came to the West from Captain James Cook during his voyages through the Pacific region.

COMMON NAME

Kava, kava kava

OTHER NAMES

Kawa, awa, intoxicating pepper, rauschpfeffer, sakau, tonga, yagona

BOTANICAL NAME/FAMILY

Piper methysticum (family Piperaceae)

PLANT PARTS USED

Root and rhizome

CHEMICAL COMPONENTS

The most important constituents responsible for the pharmacological activity of kava rhizome are the fat-soluble kava lactones (kavapyrones), mainly methysticin, dihydromethisticin, kavain (kawain), dihydrokavain yangonin and desmethoxyangonin and flavonoids (flavokavains).

MAIN ACTIONS

Central nervous system (CNS) effects

The kava lactones reach a large number of targets that influence CNS activity and act centrally and peripherally. They interact with dopaminergic, serotonergic, GABAergic and glutamatergic neurotransmission, seem to inhibit monoamine oxidase B and exert multiple effects on ion channels, according to in vitro and in vivo research (Grunze et al 2001). Additionally, animal studies show that kava lactones are chiefly responsible for these effects that give rise to many of the herb's clinical actions (Cairney et al 2002).

Hypnotic

Although the exact mechanism of action is not yet understood, it has been observed that sleep promotion may be due to the preferential activity of D,L-kavain and kava extract on the limbic structures and, in particular, the amygdalar complex (Holm et al 1991) in the brain.

In an electroencephalogram brain-mapping study it was demonstrated that D,L-kavain could induce a dose-dependent increase in delta-, theta- and alpha-1 power, as well as a decrease in alpha-2 and beta power. These results indicate a sedative effect at the higher dose range (Frey 1991).

Anxiolytic effects

In vivo research showed that kava extract produces a statistically significant dose-dependent anxiolytic-like behavioural change in a rat model of anxiety (Garrett et al 2003). The effect is not mediated through the benzodiazepine-binding site on the GABA-A receptor complex, as flumazenil, a competitive benzodiazepine receptor antagonist, did not block this effect.

More recently, kava was shown to inhibit both noradrenaline uptake and sodium and potassium channels (Weeks 2009). Furthermore, kava appears to have a similar mechanism of action to the anxiolytic chlordiazepoxide, although it is less potent (Bruner & Anderson 2009). The yangonin constituent (a kavalactone) exhibits an affinity and selectivity for the human recombinant CB_1 receptor, indicating that the endocannabinoid system might contribute to kava's anxiolytic effects (Ligresti et al 2012).

Analgesic and local anaesthetic

Both the aqueous and lipid-soluble extracts of kava exhibit antinociceptive properties in experimental animal models (Jamieson & Duffield 1990). The effect is not mediated by an opiate pathway, as naloxone does not reduce the effects when administered in doses that reverse the effects of morphine. The lack of opioid activity was confirmed again in a rat model by Sullivan et al (2009), which also showed that the analgesic properties of kava were similar to morphine.

In vitro research has identified several compounds in kava that have the ability to inhibit cyclooxygenase-1 (COX-1) and, to a lesser extent, COX-2 enzyme activities (Wu et al 2002). A more recent study of various kava products (GNC, Sundown, Solaray) confirmed selective inhibition of COX-2 (Raman et al 2008).

The local anaesthetic effect of kava is well known for topical use and has been described as similar to procaine and cocaine (Mills & Bone 2000).

Antispasmodic activity

Antispasmodic activity for skeletal muscle has been observed in vitro and in vivo for both kava extract and kava lactones (Mills & Bone 2000). In vivo research suggests that kavain impairs vascular smooth-muscle contraction; this is likely to be through inhibition of calcium channels (Martin et al 2002).

OTHER ACTIONS

Anicancer/chemopreventive effects

Consumption of kava in the South Pacific Islands is inversely correlated with cancer incidence, even among smokers (Warmka et al 2012). Recently, it was found that men living in Fiji and drinking kava have low incidence of prostate cancer; however the incidence increased 5.1-fold when Fijian men migrated to Australia (Li et al 2012).

An early in vivo study (mice) showed that kava inhibited proliferation and enhanced apoptosis in lung tumours, as shown by a reduction in proliferating cell nuclear antigen, an increase in caspase-3 and cleavage of poly(ADP-ribose) polymerase. Kava treatment also inhibited the activation of nuclear factor kappaB (NF-κB), a potential upstream mechanism of kava chemoprevention (Johnson et al 2008). The same authors later confirmed, by analysing lung adenoma tissues derived from kava-treated mice, that kava significantly inhibited adenoma cell proliferation while it had no detectable effect on cell death, indicating that kava primarily suppressed lung tumorigenesis in A/J mice via inhibition of cell proliferation.

Investigation has begun in earnest to identify the key components in kava responsible for the anticancer/chemoprevention activities. A major class of compounds found in the beverage kava are the chalcones which have demonstrated anticancer properties in a variety of animal and cell culture models (Eskander et al 2012, Sakai et al 2012, Tang et al 2008, Warmka et al 2012, Zhao et al 2011). Chemoprevention activity has been identified for flavokawains A, B and C (Johnson et al 2011). Methysticin has also been identified as a potent and non-toxic NF-κB inhibitor, potentially responsible for kava's chemopreventive activity. Other kava constituents, including four kavalactones of similar structures to methysticin, demonstrate minimum activities in inhibiting NF-κB (Shaik et al 2009). A study in mice identified kava-derived compounds which mediate tumour necrosis factor-alpha suppression. For example, kavain was found to render mice immune to lethal doses of lipopolysaccharide (Pollastri et al 2009).

An in vivo study found that the consumption of kava or kava fractions reduces colon cancer risk in rats which were carcinogen-treated (Triolet et al 2012).

Due to the observation that kava-drinking Fijian men have a substantially increased rate of prostate cancer when migrating to Australia, Li et al (2012) investigated the effects of kava root extracts and its active components (kavalactones and flavokawains) on prostate cancer cell growth in an in vitro study. They found that the kava root extract and flavokawain B reduced tumour growth, AR expression in tumour tissues and levels of serum prostate-specific antigen in the patient-derived prostate cancer xenograft models (Li et al 2012). The same authors had demonstrated in an earlier study that flavokawain B induces apoptosis via upregulation of death receptor 5 and Bim expression in androgen receptor-negative, hormonal-refractory prostate cancer cell lines and reduced tumour growth (Tang et al 2010).

Antiparasite activity

Two phenolic compounds and three kava lactones possess an α-pyrone which inhibited *Trypanosoma brucei brucei* in vitro. In particular, β-phenethyl caffeate, farnesyl caffeate and dihydrokawain exhibited high or moderate selective and potent antitrypanosomal activity (Otoguro et al 2012).

Cytochromes and P-glycoprotein (P-gp)

There is no clinical evidence that kava affects substrates of CYP2C19, CYP3A4, CYP2D6 and P-gp, but further research is necessary to strengthen the evidence (Gurley et al 2005, 2008a, 2008b, Shi & Klotz 2012). It appears to mildly inhibit CYP2E1; however, whether this is sufficient to cause a major drug interaction has been questioned (Zadoyan & Fuhr 2012).

No significant effects were observed on digoxin pharmacokinetics when taken by healthy volunteers concomitantly with a standardised kava supplement (1227 mg daily) for 14 days (Gurley et al 2007).

CLINICAL USE

Kava extracts are popular in Europe and have been investigated in numerous clinical trials, primarily in European countries. As a result, many research papers have been published in languages other than English. In order to provide a more complete description of the evidence available, secondary sources have been used where necessary. The extract which has been most studied is kava extract WS 1490.

Anxiety

Several meta-analyses and systematic reviews have been published over the last two decades, evaluating the results of randomised trials investigating kava extract in anxiety. All have concluded that kava extract is an effective treatment for anxiety. The effect is not apparent after a single dose but requires treatment for at least 1 week to establish benefits. Importantly, no clinically significant changes to liver enzyme levels or hepatotoxic effects have been reported in clinical trials. As such, the expected benefits of treatment outweigh possible risks when aqueous extracts of the dried root and rhizome are used in recommended doses. Teschke et al (2011) recommend that safety may be further improved with the use of a noble kava cultivar such as Borogu, at least 5 years old at the time of harvest, and avoiding the use of poor-quality kava starting materials.

The first Cochrane systematic review published in 2000 assessed the results from seven double-blind, randomised, placebo-controlled trials and concluded that kava kava extract has significant anxiolytic activity and is superior to placebo for the symptomatic treatment of anxiety (Pittler & Ernst 2000). An update of this review was published in 2003 and analysed results from 12 clinical studies involving 700 subjects and once again concluded that kava treatment produces a significant reduction in anxiety when compared to placebo. The extract most commonly tested was WS 1490 at a dose of up to 300 mg daily.

According to the authors of the review, none of the trials reported any hepatotoxic events and seven trials measured liver enzyme levels as safety parameters and reported no clinically significant changes.

In 2005 a meta-analysis included data from six placebo-controlled, randomised trials with the kava extract WS 1490. The endpoints were the change in Hamilton Anxiety Scale (HAM-A) during treatment (continuous and binary). Kava significantly improved anxiety, with a mean improvement of 5.94 points on the HAM-A scale better than placebo. Interestingly, kava seemed to be more effective in females and in younger patients. The rigorous meta-analysis found no evidence of publication bias and no remarkable heterogeneity amongst the studies and concluded that trials had high methodological standards. Based on this impressive result, the authors concluded that kava remains as an effective alternative to benzodiazepines, selective serotonin reuptake inhibitors and other antidepressants in the treatment of non-psychotic anxiety disorders (Witte et al 2005).

In 2010, two more systematic reviews were published, both concluding that clinical evidence supports the use of kava extract for anxiety symptoms and disorders (Lakhan & Vieira 2010).

The Cochrane review analysed results of 12 double-blind, randomised trials using kava as a stand-alone treatment (n = 700). It concluded that, based on the current evidence, the effect size seems small; however treatment is relatively safe with short-term use (up to 24 weeks' use has been tested). Further research with larger participant numbers was called for to clarify the remaining uncertainties. A more recent comprehensive review of the literature which included research published in 2010 also concluded in favour of kava treatment for anxiety, with a significant result occurring for four out of six studies reviewed (Sarris et al 2011a).

Since then, another double-blind, placebo-controlled study has been published which involved 75 participants with generalised anxiety disorder (GAD), but no comorbid mood disorders, and utilised an aqueous extract of kava (120/240 mg of kavalactones per day depending on response) (Sarris et al 2013c). The 6-week study found a significant reduction in anxiety with active treatment compared to placebo with a moderate effect size (P = 0.046; Cohen d = 0.62). The effect was larger amongst people with moderate to severe GAD (P = 0.02; d = 0.82). The main side effects reported with kava treatment was headaches (P = 0.05), but no other significant differences were found between the groups for other adverse effects or liver function tests. Interestingly, they also found that specific GABA transporter polymorphisms appear to potentially modify the anxiolytic response to kava.

Anxiety with depression

In a placebo-controlled, double-blind crossover trial, 60 adult participants with 1 month or more of elevated GAD took five kava tablets per day (250 mg of kavalactones/day) for 3 weeks. This aqueous kava preparation produced significant anxiolytic and antidepressant activity compared to placebo and raised no safety concerns at the dose and duration studied. Importantly, a substantial effect size ($d = 2.24$) was identified with active treatment. As such, kava appeared equally effective in cases where anxiety was accompanied by depression (Sarris et al 2009b).

Increased female libido in GAD

Oral kava tablets made with an aqueous extract (delivering 120–240 mg kavalactones daily) significantly increased female libido compared to placebo ($P = 0.040$) on a subdomain of the Arizona Sexual Experience Scale (ASEX) in this randomised, placebo-controlled study ($n = 75$) in GAD. There was a highly significant correlation between ASEX reduction (improved sexual function and performance) and anxiety reduction in the whole sample, with no negative effects seen in males (Sarris et al 2013a).

Comparative studies

Comparative studies suggest the absence of significant differences between benzodiazepines and kavain or kava extract as treatments for anxiety when used in multiple doses. A 1993 double-blind, comparative study involving 174 subjects over 6 weeks demonstrated that 300 mg/day of a 70% kava lactone extract produced a similar improvement in anxiety level, as measured by HAM-A scores, to 15 mg oxazepam or 9 mg bromazepam taken daily (Woelk et al 1993). D,L-kavain produced equivalent anxiolytic effects to oxazepam in 38 outpatients with neurotic or psychosomatic disturbances, under double-blind study conditions (Lindenberg & Pitule-Schodel 1990).

It appears that a single dose of kava (180 mg kavalactones) is not as effective as oxazepam (30 mg) in moderately anxious volunteers (Sarris et al 2012). In this study, oxazepam significantly reduced anxiety whereas kava was ineffective.

An 8-week randomised, double-blind, multicentre clinical trial involving 129 outpatients with GAD showed that kava LI 150 (400 mg/day) was as effective as buspirone in the acute treatment of GAD, with about 75% of patients responding to treatment (Boerner et al 2003).

Benzodiazepine withdrawal

Kava may have a role in reducing anxiety and improving subjective wellbeing during benzodiazepine withdrawal, according to a 2001 randomised, double-blind, placebo-controlled study (Malsch & Kieser 2001). During the first 2 weeks of that study, kava dose was increased from 50 mg/day to 300 mg/day while benzodiazepine use was tapered off during the same period. Kava extract was superior to placebo in reducing anxiety as measured by the HAM-A scale and improved subjects' feelings of wellbeing according to a subjective wellbeing scale (Bf-S total scores).

Combination therapy

A combination of St John's wort (SJW) and kava was ineffective as a treatment for major depressive disorder with comorbid anxiety according to a randomised controlled trial ($n = 28$) conducted in 2009. After a placebo run-in of 2 weeks, the trial had a crossover design testing SJW and kava against placebo over two controlled phases, each of 4 weeks. SJW and kava gave a significantly greater reduction in self-reported depression on the Beck Depression Inventory over placebo in the first controlled phase. However, in the crossover phase, a replication of those effects in the delayed medication group did not occur. Nor were there significant effects on anxiety or quality of life. The authors postulated that a potential interaction with SJW, the presence of depression or an inadequate dose of kava could be explanations for the negative result (Sarris et al 2009a).

Menopausal and perimenopausal anxiety

A randomised, placebo-controlled study conducted with 40 menopausal women found that, using kava extract, together with hormone replacement therapy (HRT), led to significant reductions in anxiety, as measured by the HAM-A scale at both 3- and 6-month follow-up (De et al 2000). A 3-month, randomised, open study of 68 perimenopausal women showed that treatment with kava (100 mg/day) significantly reduced anxiety ($P < 0.001$) at 1 month and 3 months. This was significantly greater than that spontaneously occurring in controls ($P < 0.009$) (Cagnacci et al 2003).

Insomnia

The hypnotic activity of kava extract was confirmed in a randomised controlled trial in which a single dose of 300 mg kava extract was found to improve the quality of sleep significantly (Emser & Bartylla 1991, as reported by Ernst et al 2001). In vivo experiments with D,L-kavain have shown that it reduces active wakefulness and significantly prolongs sleep compared with placebo (Holm et al 1991).

OTHER USES

Traditionally, the herb has been used to treat urinary tract infections, asthma, conditions associated with pain, gonorrhoea and syphilis, and to assist with weight reduction, muscle relaxation and sleep. Topically, it has been used as a local anaesthetic and to treat pruritus.

DOSAGE RANGE

- Cut rhizome: 1.7–3.4 g/day.
- Dried rhizome: 1.5–3 g/day in divided doses or equivalent to 60–120 mg kavapyrones daily.
- Fluid extract (1:2): 3–8.5 mL/day in divided doses.

Ideally, ethanolic extracts should contain > 20 mg/mL kava lactones.

According to clinical studies:

- Anxiety: generally doses up to 300 mg daily of kava kava extract WS 1490 providing 105–210 mg kavalactones. A kava kava extract LI 150 (400 mg/day) and an aqueous kava extract (in solid-dose form) delivering 120/240 mg of kavalactones per day have successfully treated GAD.
- Anxiety with depression: an aqueous kava extract (in solid-dose form) delivering 250 mg of kavalactones per day.
- Insomnia — a single dose of 300 mg kava kava extract.
- Benzodiazepine withdrawal — 300 mg/day of kava kava extract.

ADVERSE REACTIONS

Two postmarketing surveillance studies involving more than 6000 patients found adverse effects in 2.3% and 1.5% of patients taking 120–240 mg standardised extract (Ernst 2002). The most common side effects appear to be gastrointestinal upset and headaches when used in recommended doses. Headaches were confirmed as a side effect with aqueous extract of kava (120/240 mg of kavalactones per day) taken over 6 weeks in a randomised controlled trial (Sarris et al 2013c). Clinical trials using therapeutic doses of kava extract have found no clinically significant changes to liver enzyme levels or hepatotoxic effects.

In contrast, the long-term use of high doses of water-based infusions of kava, such as sometimes seen amongst Pacific Islanders and those involved with kava abuse, are known to induce reversible, adverse outcomes such as kava dermopathy, raised gamma-glutamyltranspeptidase liver enzyme levels, nausea, loss of appetite or indigestion (Rychetnik & Madronio 2011). The reversible ichthyosiform eruption caused by heavy long-term use is known as kanikani in Fijian. This condition is characterised by yellow discolouration of the skin, hair and nails and reverses once kava intake ceases. A 2003 report found no evidence of brain dysfunction in heavy and long-term kava users (Cairney et al 2003).

Research with animal models has further explored the effects of long-term use. A 2011 study with a mouse model found that kava at all dosages and treatment regimens did not induce detectable adverse effects, particularly with respect to liver reactions. Specifically, kava treatment showed no effect on liver integrity indicator enzymes or liver weight, indicating that kava may be potentially safe for long-term use (Johnson et al 2011).

One case was reported which claimed that a patient presented with rhabdomyolysis related to the ingestion of a large amount of kava. The patient developed peak creatine phosphokinase levels in excess of 30,000 U/L, but had no significant renal damage. The amount of kava taken was not specified (Bodkin et al 2012).

Hepatotoxicity risk minimised

People in the Pacific Islands have used a kava rhizome preparation mixed with water as a ceremonial and social beverage for generations without reported hepatotoxicity. As a result, it was considered without serious side effects until 1998, when the first case reports of kava hepatotoxicity appeared. Causality of hepatotoxicity for kava, sometimes with concomitant use of other medicines, was evident after the use of predominantly ethanolic and acetonic kava extracts in Germany ($n = 7$), Switzerland ($n = 2$), United States ($n = 1$) and Australia ($n = 1$), as well as after aqueous extracts in New Caledonia ($n = 2$) (Teschke et al 2008a). Moreover, cases of tourists developing serious toxic liver disease after consumption of kava beverages in traditional Samoan kava ceremonies were reported (Christl et al 2009). For this reason, in 2002 the herb was withdrawn from various European countries (Sarris et al 2011b), and the US Food and Drug Administration issued a safety alert about kava and its potential to cause serious liver problems (Teschke 2010a).

To address the issue in Australia, in 2002 the Therapeutic Goods Administration restricted the amount of kavalactones present in each capsule or tablet to a maximum of 125 mg kava lactones and a maximum of 3 g of dried rhizome per tea bag. Additionally, commercial products must not provide more than a daily dose of 250 mg kava lactones. (Please note that the sale and supply are prohibited in Western Australia under a 1988 law, but exceptions apply for Pacific Islander people's traditional use.)

Various authors have evaluated the case reports; however, no clear mechanism for the hepatotoxic adverse effects has emerged. Similarly, research with animal models has not provided clear evidence of hepatotoxicity, further complicating the issue.

Stickel et al (2003) report that, in an analysis of 36 cases of hepatotoxicity, the pattern of injury was both hepatocellular and cholestasis, the majority of patients were women, the cumulative dose and latency were highly variable and liver transplant was necessary in eight of the cases (Stickel et al 2003). A 2007 report by the World Health Organization (WHO) entitled *Assessment of the Risk of Hepatotoxicity with Kava Products* evaluated data from 93 case reports (WHO 2007). Of these, eight were determined to have a close association between kava usage and liver dysfunction; 53 cases were classified as having a possible relationship, but they could not be fully assessed due to insufficient data or other potential causes of liver damage; five cases had a positive rechallenge. Most of the other case reports could not be evaluated due to lack of information. The WHO report concluded that there is 'significant concern' for a cause-and-effect relationship between kava products and hepatotoxity, especially for organic extracts. The report noted other risk factors such as heavy alcohol intake, pre-existing liver disease, genetic polymorphisms of cytochrome P450 enzymes, excessive dosage and comedication with other potentially hepatotoxic drugs and potentially interacting drugs. Similarly, Teschke et al analysed 26 suspected cases and concluded that kava taken as recommended is associated with rare hepatotoxicity, whereas overdose, prolonged treatment and comedication may carry an increased risk (Teschke et al 2008b, Teschke 2010). However, several papers outlined strengths and weaknesses of the current methods of causality evaluation (Teschke 2009, Teschke & Wolff 2011). The latest publications have accepted a causal relationship between the use of various kava extracts, including aqueous extracts, and liver injury, and have focused on an assessment of possible causes (Teschke et al 2009).

Various possible pathogenetic factors have been discussed, including metabolic interactions with exogenous compounds at the hepatic microsomal cytochrome P450 level; genetic enzyme deficiencies; toxic constituents and metabolites derived from the kava extract, including impurities and adulterations; cyclooxygenase inhibition; P-gp alterations; hepatic glutathione depletion; solvents and solubilisers of the extracts; and kava raw material of poor quality (Teschke 2010b). More recent reports have postulated that mould hepatotoxins present in kava raw material may be the cause of hepatotoxicity (Teschke et al 2012, 2013). This could be the case given that aflatoxins have been detected in kava samples (Rowe & Ramzan 2012, Trucksess & Scott 2008).

There are abundant data of in vitro cytotoxicity, including apoptosis by pipermethystine and flavokavain B added to the incubation media, yet evidence is lacking of in vivo hepatotoxicity in experimental animals under conditions similar to human kava use. Furthermore, in commercial Western kava extracts, pipermethystine was not detectable and flavokavain B was present as a natural compound in amounts much too low to cause experimental liver injury (Lechtenberg et al 2008, Teschke et al 2011).

A way forward?

Strict guidelines for kava standardisation have now been suggested by several researchers. They include: (1) use of a noble kava cultivar such as Borogu, at least 5 years old at time of harvest; (2) use of peeled and dried rhizomes and roots; (3) aqueous extraction; (4) dosage recommendation of ≤250 mg kavalactones per day (for medicinal use); (5) systematic rigorous future research; and (6) a Pan Pacific quality control system enforced by strict policing (Teschke et al 2011).

Lack of physical tolerance

A long-term, randomised, double-blind trial conducted over 25 weeks found that physical tolerance (effect diminishes over time) does not develop to kava extract (Volz & Kieser 1997).

No adverse effects on cognition

Evidence from a randomised, double-blind study conducted with 84 patients has shown that treatment with kavain (one of the active constituents of kava kava) produces continuous improvements in parameters such as memory function, vigilance, fluency of mental functions and reaction time. Interestingly, these effects were reported over a relatively short period of 3 weeks (Scholing & Clausen 1977). Another randomised, double-blind trial conducted with 52 patients over 28 days not only confirmed anxiolytic activity but also found that kavain promoted subjective vitality-related performance (Lehmann et al 1989). A more recent review of 10 clinical trials further concluded that available evidence suggests that kava has no replicated significant negative effects on cognition (LaPorte et al 2011).

SIGNIFICANT INTERACTIONS

Alcohol

Potentiation of CNS sedative effects has been reported in an animal study; however, one double-blind, placebo-controlled study found no additive effects on CNS depression or safety-related performance (Herberg 1993). Alternatively, a study of 10 subjects found that, when alcohol and kava were combined, kava potentiated both the perceived and the measured impairment compared to alcohol alone (Foo & Lemon 1997). Caution is advised when taking kava in therapeutic doses with moderate alcohol consumption. Avoidance of high doses of kava with alcohol is advised.

Barbiturates

Additive effects are theoretically possible. Use with caution and monitor drug dosage. However, interaction may be beneficial under professional supervision.

Benzodiazepines

Additive effects are theoretically possible. A potential pharmacodynamic interaction between alprazolam and kava has been reported (Izzo & Ernst 2009, Shi & Klotz 2012). Use with caution and monitor drug dosage. However, interaction may be beneficial under professional supervision. The combination has been used successfully to ease symptoms of benzodiazepine withdrawal.

Levodopa

A potential pharmacodynamic interaction between levodopa and kava was reported, leading to reduced efficacy of levodopa in four case reports (Izzo & Ernst 2009, Shi & Klotz 2012).

Paracetamol

Paracetamol overdose results in glutathione depletion and increased oxidative stress. A study with rat hepatocytes found that coadministration of kava with paracetamol caused further loss of cell viability by decreasing cellular adenosine triphosphate concentration and increasing reactive oxygen species formation (Yang & Salminen 2011). Avoid kava with high-dose paracetamol, as it may increase paracetamol-induced cell damage.

L-Dopa medication

Antagonistic effects are theoretically possible, thereby reducing the effectiveness of L-dopa. Avoid concurrent use unless under professional supervision until safety is confirmed.

Methadone and morphine

Additive effects with increased CNS depression are theoretically possible, so use with caution, although interactions may be beneficial under professional supervision.

Substrates for CYP2E1

Inhibition of CYP2E1 has been demonstrated in vivo — serum levels of CYP2E1 substrates may become elevated — use with caution.

Practice points/Patient counselling

- Kava kava is a scientifically proven treatment for the symptoms of anxiety and stress states. Its anxiety-reducing effects are similar to those of 15 mg oxazepam or 9 mg bromazepam when used for more than a week; yet physical tolerance and reduced vigilance have not been observed.
- It also reduces symptoms of anxiety related to menopause when used together with HRT, and reduces withdrawal symptoms associated with benzodiazepine discontinuation.
- It has anxiolytic, sedative, antispasmodic, analgesic and local anaesthetic activities.
- Although the herb is considered to have a low incidence of adverse effects, long-term use should be carefully supervised because of the possibility of developing adverse reactions.
- Kava should also be avoided in patients with heavy alcohol intake, pre-existing liver disease, genetic polymorphisms of cytochrome P450 enzymes, excessive dosage and comedication with other potentially hepatotoxic drugs and potentially interacting drugs.

CONTRAINDICATIONS AND PRECAUTIONS

Endogenous depression — according to Commission E (Blumenthal et al 2000).

Although clinical studies indicate no adverse effects on vigilance, the herb's CNS effects may slow some individuals' reaction times, thereby affecting ability to drive a car or operate heavy machinery. The decision as to whether people should avoid driving a car or operating heavy machinery when taking kava treatment should be considered on an individual basis.

Additionally, it should not be used by people with pre-existing liver disease and long-term continuous use should be avoided unless under medical supervision. It should be used with caution in the elderly and in those with Parkinson's disease.

PREGNANCY USE

Safety is unknown.

K

PATIENTS' FAQs

What will this herb do for me?

Kava is an effective herbal relaxant that reduces symptoms of anxiety and restlessness. It is also used to relieve anxiety in menopause, insomnia and symptoms of benzodiazepine withdrawal.

When will it start to work?

Anxiety-relieving effects are usually seen within the first few weeks of use.

Are there any safety issues?

Taking high doses long term has been associated with a number of side effects and should be avoided. Kava should also be avoided in patients with heavy alcohol intake, pre-existing liver disease, genetic polymorphisms of cytochrome P450 enzymes, excessive dosage and comedication with other potentially hepatotoxic drugs and potentially interacting drugs.

REFERENCES

Blumenthal M, et al. (eds). Herbal medicine: expanded Commission E monographs. Austin, TX: Integrative Medicine Communications, 2000.

Bodkin R, et al. Rhabdomyolysis associated with kava ingestion. Am J Emerg Med. 2012 May;30(4):635.

Boerner RJ et al. Kava-kava extract LI 150 is as effective as opipramol and buspirone in generalised anxiety disorder: an 8-week randomised, double-blind multi-centre clinical trial in 129 out-patients. Phytomedicine 10 (Suppl 4) (2003): 38–49.

Bruner NR, Anderson KG Discriminative-stimulus and time-course effects of kava-kava (*Piper methysticum*) in rats. Pharmacol Biochem Behav. 2009 Apr;92(2):297–303.

Cagnacci A et al. Kava-kava administration reduces anxiety in perimenopausal women. Maturitas 44.2 (2003): 103–109.

Cairney S, et al. The neurobehavioural effects of kava. Aust NZ J Psychiatry 36.5 (2002): 657–662.

Cairney S et al. Saccade and cognitive function in chronic kava users. Neuropsychopharmacology 28.2 (2003): 389–396.

Christl SU, et al. Toxic hepatitis after consumption of traditional kava preparation. J Travel Med. 2009 Jan-Feb;16(1):55–6.

De L et al. Assessment of the association of kava-kava extract and hormone replacement therapy in the treatment of postmenopause anxiety. Minerva Ginecol 52.6 (2000): 263–267.

Emser W, Bartylla K. Verbesserung der Schlafqualität: Zur Wirkung von Kava-extrakt WS1490 auf das Schlafmuster bei Gesunden. Tw

Neurologie Psychiatrie 5 (1991): 636–42, as cited by Ernst E et al. The Desktop Guide to Complementary and Alternative Medicine: An Evidence-based Approach. St Louis: Mosby, 2001.

Ernst E. The risk-benefit profile of commonly used herbal therapies: ginkgo, St. John's wort, ginseng, echinacea, saw palmetto, and kava. Ann Intern Med 136.1 (2002): 42–53.

Eskander RN, et al. Flavokawain B, a novel, naturally occurring chalcone, exhibits robust apoptotic effects and induces G2/M arrest of a uterine leiomyosarcoma cell line. J Obstet Gynaecol Res. 2012 Aug;38(8):1086–94.

Foo H, Lemon J. Acute effects of kava, alone or in combination with alcohol, on subjective measures of impairment and intoxication and on cognitive performance. Drug Alcohol Rev 16.2 (1997): 147–155.

Frey R. Demonstration of the central effects of D,L-kawain with EEG brain mapping. Fortschr Med 109.25 (1991): 505–508.

Garrett KM et al. Extracts of kava (*Piper methysticum*) induce acute anxiolytic-like behavioral changes in mice. Psychopharmacology (Berl) 170.1 (2003): 33–41.

Grunze H et al. Kava pyrones exert effects on neuronal transmission and transmembraneous cation currents similar to established mood stabilizers: a review. Prog Neuropsychopharmacol Biol Psychiatry 25.8 (2001): 1555–1570.

Gurley BJ et al. In vivo effects of goldenseal, kava kava, black cohosh, and valerian on human cytochrome P450 1A2, 2D6, 2E1, and 3A4/5 phenotypes. Clin Pharmacol Ther 77.5 (2005): 415–426.

Gurley BJ, et al. Effect of goldenseal (*Hydrastis canadensis*) and kava kava (*Piper methysticum*) supplementation on digoxin pharmacokinetics in humans. Drug Metab Dispos. 2007 Feb;35(2):240–5.

Gurley BJ et al. Clinical assessment of CYP2D6-mediated herb-drug interactions in humans: effects of milk thistle, black cohosh, goldenseal, kava kava, St. John's wort, and Echinacea. Mol Nutr Food Res 52.7 (2008a): 755–763.

Gurley BJ, et al. Supplementation with goldenseal (*Hydrastis canadensis*), but not kava kava (*Piper methysticum*), inhibits human CYP3A activity in vivo. Clin Pharmacol Ther. (2008b) Jan;83(1):61–9.

Herberg KW. Effect of kava-special extract WS 1490 combined with ethyl alcohol on safety-relevant performance parameters. Blutalkohol 30.2 (1993): 96–105.

Holm E et al. The action profile of D,L-kavain: cerebral sites and sleep-wakefulness-rhythm in animals. Arzneimittelforschung 41.7 (1991): 673–683.

Izzo AA, Ernst E. Interactions between herbal medicines and prescribed drugs: an updated systematic review. Drugs. 2009;69(13):1777–98

Jamieson DD, Duffield PH. The antinociceptive actions of kava components in mice. Clin Exp Pharmacol Physiol 17.7 (1990): 495–507.

Johnson TE, et al. Chemopreventive effect of kava on 4-(methylnitrosamino)-1-(3-pyridyl)-1-butanone plus benzo[a]pyrene-induced lung tumorigenesis in A/J mice. Cancer Prev Res (Phila). 2008 Nov;1(6):430–8.

Johnson TE, et al. Lung tumorigenesis suppressing effects of a commercial kava extract and its selected compounds in A/J mice. Am J Chin Med. 2011;39(4):727–42.

Lakhan SE, Vieira KF. Nutritional and herbal supplements for anxiety and anxiety-related disorders: systematic review. Nutr J. 2010 Oct 7;9:42

LaPorte E, et al. Neurocognitive effects of kava (*Piper methysticum*): a systematic review. Hum Psychopharmacol. 2011 Mar;26(2):102–11

Lechtenberg M, et al. Is the alkaloid pipermethystine connected with the claimed liver toxicity of Kava products? Pharmazie. 2008 Jan;63(1):71–4.

Lehmann E et al. The efficacy of Cavain in patients suffering from anxiety. Pharmacopsychiatry 22.6 (1989): 258–262.

Li X, et al. Kava components down-regulate expression of AR and AR splice variants and reduce growth in patient-derived prostate cancer xenografts in mice. PLoS One. 2012;7(2):e31213.

Ligresti A, et al. Kavalactones and the endocannabinoid system: the plant-derived yangonin is a novel CB_1 receptor ligand. Pharmacol Res. 2012 Aug;66(2):163–9.

Lindenberg D, Pitule-Schodel H. D,L-kavain in comparison with oxazepam in anxiety disorders. A double-blind study of clinical effectiveness. Fortschr Med 108.2 (1990): 49–54.

Malsch U, Kieser M. Efficacy of kava-kava in the treatment of non-psychotic anxiety, following pretreatment with benzodiazepines. Psychopharmacology (Berl) 157.3 (2001): 277–283.

Martin HB et al. Kavain attenuates vascular contractility through inhibition of calcium channels. Planta Med 68.9 (2002): 784–789.

Mills S, Bone K. Principles and practice of phytotherapy. London: Churchill Livingstone, 2000.

Otoguro K, et al. In vitro antitrypanosomal activity of some phenolic compounds from propolis and lactones from Fijian Kawa (*Piper methysticum*). J Nat Med. 2012 Jul;66(3):558–61.

Pittler MH, Ernst E. Kava extract versus placebo for treating anxiety. Cochrane Database Syst Rev 1 (2000): CD003383.

Pollastri MP et al. Identification and characterization of Kava-derived compounds mediating TNF-α suppressio. Chem Biol Drug Des 74.2 (2009): 121–128.

Raman P, et al. Lipid peroxidation and cyclooxygenase enzyme inhibitory activities of acidic aqueous extracts of some dietary supplements. Phytother Res. 2008 Feb;22(2):204–12.

Rowe A, Ramzan I. Are mould hepatotoxins responsible for kava hepatotoxicity? Phytother Res. 2012 Nov;26(11):1768–70.

Rychetnik L, Madronio CM. The health and social effects of drinking water-based infusions of kava: a review of the evidence. Drug Alcohol Rev. 2011 Jan;30(1):74–83

Sakai T, et al. Flavokawain B, a kava chalcone, induces apoptosis in synovial sarcoma cell lines. J Orthop Res. 2012 Jul;30(7):1045–50.

Sarris J, et al. St. John's wort and Kava in treating major depressive disorder with comorbid anxiety: a randomised double-blind placebo-controlled pilot trial. Hum Psychopharmacol. 2009 (a) Jan;24(1):41–8

Sarris J, et al. The Kava Anxiety Depression Spectrum Study (KADSS): a randomized, placebo-controlled crossover trial using an aqueous extract of *Piper methysticum*. Psychopharmacology (Berl). 2009 (b) Aug;205(3):399–407.

Sarris J, et al. Kava: a comprehensive review of efficacy, safety, and psychopharmacology. Aust N Z J Psychiatry. 2011 Jan;45(1):27–35.

Sarris J, et al. Re-introduction of kava (*Piper methysticum*) to the EU: is there a way forward? Planta Med 2011 (b) Jan; 77 (2): 107–10.

Sarris J, et al. The acute effects of kava and oxazepam on anxiety, mood, neurocognition; and genetic correlates: a randomized, placebo-controlled, double-blind study. Hum Psychopharmacol. 2012 May;27(3):262–9.

Sarris J, et al. Kava for the treatment of generalized anxiety disorder RCT: analysis of adverse reactions, liver function, addiction, and sexual effects. Phytother Res. 2013a; 27: 1723–1728.

Sarris J, et al. Does a medicinal dose of kava impair driving? A randomized, placebo-controlled, double-blind study. Traffic Inj Prev. 2013b;14(1):13–7.

Sarris, J., et al. 2013c. Kava in the treatment of generalized anxiety disorder: a double-blind, randomized, placebo-controlled study. J Clin. Psychopharmacol. 33: 643–648.

Scholing WE, Clausen HD. On the effect of D,L-kavain: experience with neuronika (author's transl). Med Klin 72.32–33 (1977): 1301–1306.

Shaik AA, et al. Identification of methysticin as a potent and non-toxic NF-kappaB inhibitor from kava, potentially responsible for kava's chemopreventive activity. Bioorg Med Chem Lett. 2009 Oct 1;19(19):5732–6.

Shi S, Klotz U. Drug interactions with herbal medicines. Clin Pharmacokinet. 2012 Feb 1;51(2):77–104

Stickel F, et al. Hepatitis induced by Kava (*Piper methysticum* rhizoma). J Hepatol. 2003 Jul;39(1):62–7.

Sullivan J, et al. A brief report of student research: mechanism of analgesic effect and efficacy and anesthesia interactions of kava in the male Sprague-Dawley rat. Dimens Crit Care Nurs. 2009 May-Jun;28(3):138–40.

Tang Y, et al. Effects of the kava chalcone flavokawain A differ in bladder cancer cells with wild-type versus mutant p53. Cancer Prev Res (Phila). 2008 Nov;1(6):439–51.

Tang Y, et al. Flavokawain B, a kava chalcone, induces apoptosis via up-regulation of death-receptor 5 and Bim expression in androgen receptor negative, hormonal refractory prostate cancer cell lines and reduces tumor growth. Int J Cancer. 2010 Oct 15;127(8):1758–68.

Teschke R Kava hepatotoxicity — a clinical review. Ann Hepatol. 2010a Jul-Sep;9(3):251–65.

Teschke R. Kava hepatotoxicity: pathogenetic aspects and prospective considerations. Liver Int. 2010b Oct;30(9):1270–9.

Teschke R, et al. Kava hepatotoxicity: a European view. N Z Med J. (2008a) Oct 3;121(1283):90–8

Teschke R, et al. Kava hepatotoxicity: a clinical survey and critical analysis of 26 suspected cases. Eur J Gastroenterol Hepatol 20.12 (2008b): 1182–1193.

Teschke R, et al. Kava hepatotoxicity: comparison of aqueous, ethanolic, acetonic kava extracts and kava-herbs mixtures. J Ethnopharmacol. 2009 Jun 25;123(3):378–84.

Teschke R, et al. Herbal hepatotoxicity by kava: update on pipermethystine, flavokavain B, and mould hepatotoxins as primarily assumed culprits. Dig Liver Dis. 2011 Sep;43(9):676–81

Teschke R, et al. Kava hepatotoxicity in traditional and modern use: the presumed Pacific kava paradox hypothesis revisited, Br J Clin Pharmacol. 2012 Feb;73(2):170–4.

Teschke R, et al. Contaminant hepatotoxins as culprits for kava hepatotoxicity — fact or fiction? Phytother Res. 2013 Mar;27(3):472–4.

Teschke R, Wolff A. Regulatory causality evaluation methods applied in kava hepatotoxicity: are they appropriate? Regul Toxicol Pharmacol 59.1(2011): 1–7.

Triolet J, et al. Reduction in colon cancer risk by consumption of kava or kava fractions in carcinogen-treated rats. Nutr Cancer. 2012 Aug;64(6):838–46

Trucksess MW, Scott PM. Mycotoxins in botanicals and dried fruits: a review. Food Addit Contam Part A Chem Anal Control Expo Risk Assess. 2008 Feb;25(2):181–92.

Volz HP, Kieser M. Kava-kava extract WS 1490 versus placebo in anxiety disorders: a randomised placebo-controlled 25-week outpatient trial. Pharmacopsychiatry 30.1 (1997): 1–5.

Warmka JK, et al. Inhibition of mitogen activated protein kinases increases the sensitivity of A549 lung cancer cells to the cytotoxicity induced by a kava chalcone analog. Biochem Biophys Res Commun. 2012 Aug 3;424(3):488–92.

Weeks BS. Formulations of dietary supplements and herbal extracts for relaxation and anxiolytic action: Relarian. Med Sci Monit. 2009 Nov; 15(11).RA256–62.

WHO. Assessment of the risk of hepatotoxicity with kava products. World Health Organization, May 2007. Available online: http://www.who.int/bookorders/anglais/detart1.jsp? sesslan=1&codlan=1&codcol=93&codcch=216 (accessed 26 February 09).

Witte S, et al. Meta-analysis of the efficacy of the acetonic kava-kava extract WS1490 in patients with non-psychotic anxiety disorders. Phytother Res 19.3 (2005): 183–188.

Woelk H et al. The treatment of patients with anxiety: a double-blind study – kava extract WS1490 vs benzodiazepine. Z. Allgemeinmed 69 (1993): 271–7; as cited in Nissen D (ed). Mosby's Drug Consult. St Louis: Mosby, 2003.

Wu D, et al. Novel compounds from *Piper methysticum* Forst (kava kava) roots and their effect on cyclooxygenase enzyme. J Agric Food Chem 50.4 (2002): 701–705.

Yang X, Salminen WF. Kava extract, an herbal alternative for anxiety relief, potentiates acetaminophen-induced cytotoxicity in rat hepatic cells. Phytomedicine. 2011 May 15;18(7):592–600.

Zadoyan G, Fuhr U. Phenotyping studies to assess the effects of phytopharmaceuticals on in vivo activity of main human cytochrome p450 enzymes. Planta Med. 2012 Sep;78(13):1428–57.

Zhao X, et al. Flavokawain B induces apoptosis of human oral adenoid cystic cancer ACC-2 cells via up-regulation of Bim and down-regulation of Bcl-2 expression. Can J Physiol Pharmacol. 2011 Nov 24.

L-Arginine

BACKGROUND AND RELEVANT PHARMACOKINETICS

L-Arginine is a basic, semiessential amino acid that was discovered in 1886 in lupin seedlings and then in 1895 in mammalian protein (Boger & Bode-Boger 2001). Arginine is a precursor to a variety of compounds, including nitric oxide (NO), creatine, urea, polyamines, proline, glutamate and agmatine (Morris 2009). For humans L-arginine is considered to be a semiessential amino acid or a conditionally essential amino acid, as requirements may increase during metabolic stress or when there is insufficient endogenous L-arginine for optimal growth or tissue repair; for birds and carnivores it is an essential amino acid. It is also the most abundant nitrogen carrier in animals and humans.

Ingested arginine is rapidly cleared from the plasma, and arginine metabolism occurs via a number of pathways, although not all pathways are well defined. Arginine is involved in two major metabolic pathways: the nitric oxide synthase (NOS) pathway and the arginase pathway.

In the NOS pathway, L-arginine is converted to NO and L-citrulline. Three isoforms of NOS (neuronal, inducible and endothelial) have been discovered, each with a different function. NO is a free radical that has vasodilatory and angiogenic characteristics. It regulates nutrient metabolism, plays a role in the circulatory and respiratory systems, especially endothelial function, and exerts numerous other effects in the body.

In the arginase pathway, conversion of L-arginine into L-ornithine and urea is catalysed by the activity of arginase, with the subsequent production of polyamines such as putrescine, spermidine and spermine. Polyamines are essential for cell proliferation and differentiation, tissue growth and development, and are involved in neurogenesis (Yi et al 2009). In mammals two isoforms of arginase play key roles in the regulation of most aspects of arginine metabolism. Arginases have been investigated for their effects in vascular disease, pulmonary disease, infectious disease, immune cell function and cancer (Morris 2009).

L-Arginine is an essential component in the urea cycle, which is the only pathway in mammals that allows elimination of continuously generated toxic ammonia. Arginine can be synthesised endogenously, mostly in the kidneys and to some degree in liver from the amino acids aspartate and citrulline by arginine synthase.

Arginine is incorporated in the synthesis of proteins, and L-arginine is also required for the production of creatine, which in its phosphorylated form plays an essential role in the energy metabolism of muscle, nerve and testis. Creatine degrades into creatinine, which is removed from the body by the kidneys. Homeostasis of plasma L-arginine is regulated by dietary arginine intake, arginine synthesis and metabolism and protein turnover.

Ingested arginine is rapidly absorbed and metabolised in the gastrointestinal tract. There is little urinary arginine excretion because it is mostly reabsorbed.

CHEMICAL COMPONENTS

2-amino-5-guanidino-pentanoic acid

FOOD SOURCES

Free arginine is found in dietary protein, commonly in meat, fish, poultry, milk and dairy products, and nuts and seeds (King et al 2008). Other dietary sources include barley, brown rice, buckwheat, chocolate, corn, oats, raisins and soy. It has been estimated that each gram of dietary protein provides 54 mg of L-arginine, and that 3–6 g of L-arginine is absorbed each day in adults who ingest a normal Western diet (Boger & Bode-Boger 2001, Visek 1986). Dietary lysine competes with arginine for uptake, so low-lysine diets are recommended for enhanced arginine absorption (Stargrove et al 2008).

DEFICIENCY SIGNS AND SYMPTOMS

Elevated arginase associated with arginine deficiency has been identified in an increasing number of diseases and conditions. Arginine deficiency syndromes may involve either T-cell dysfunction or endothelial dysfunction depending on the disease context. However the role of supplementation in ameliorating the effects of arginine deficiency requires further investigation (Morris 2012). A deficiency of arginine may affect growth and development, insulin production, lipid and protein metabolism or glucose tolerance. Arginine deficiency may be associated with poor wound healing, hair loss or breakage, liver disease, constipation or skin rash.

MAIN ACTIONS

Arginine is involved in numerous important and diverse biochemical pathways. L-Arginine and its metabolites produce a myriad of effects in the body, including pH regulation, depolarisation of endothelial cell membranes, macronutrient metabolism, cell-mediated immunity and antitumour activity, and it is an essential intermediate in the urea cycle (Wahlqvist 2002). L-Arginine also influences the release of hormones such as corticotrophin-releasing factor, insulin, glucagon, prolactin, aldosterone and somatostatin.

Growth hormone and immune function

Arginine triggers the release of growth hormone, which then increases the cytotoxic activity of macrophages, natural killer cells, cytotoxic T cells and neutrophils (Wahlqvist 2002).

Nitric oxide production

Although the arginine–NO pathway represents only a fraction of the total arginine metabolism, it has attracted considerable interest because of the many roles that NO plays in almost all organ systems. NO is a free radical molecule that is synthesised in all mammalian cells from L-arginine by NOS (Tapiero et al 2002). NO is recognised as an ubiquitous mediator, produced by many cell types, that has diverse and complex actions in multiple organ systems (Rawlingson 2003).

As a precursor of NO, L-arginine influences functions as varied as neurotransmission, vasodilation, inflammation, host defence, cytotoxicity, airway and vascular smooth-muscle relaxation, mucociliary clearance and airway mucus secretion and regulation of gene expression (Chionglo Sy et al 2006).

Cardiovascular disease

Arginine seems to exert its effects in the cardiovascular system mostly through the formation of NO, although it has NO-independent haemodynamic effects as well.

Through NO-dependent actions, arginine can increase smooth-muscle cell relaxation and endothelial cell proliferation, as well as promote angiogenesis and decrease platelet aggregation, leucocyte adhesion, superoxide production, endothelin-1 release and smooth-muscle proliferation (Chionglo Sy et al 2006). NO has also been known as endothelium-derived relaxing factor, which is responsible for maintaining vasomotor tone and systemic blood pressure. It also controls intravascular volume by enhancing renin secretion and natriuresis (Rawlingson 2003).

NO-independent actions include: increased plasmin generation or fibrinolysis; augmented release of insulin, growth hormone and glucagon; decreased blood viscosity and formation of fibrin; and decreased angiotensin-converting enzyme activity (Chionglo Sy et al 2006).

Antiobesity

In humans brown adipose tissue plays an important role in the oxidation of fatty acids and glucose. Dietary supplementation with L-arginine enhances brown adipose tissue growth, reduces white adipose tissue and improves metabolic profiles. As such it holds promise for preventing and treating obesity in humans (Wu et al 2012).

In a recent study of 20 obese women (aged ≥18 years and ≤40 years, body mass index ≥30 and ≤40 kg/m^2 and waist circumference ≥89 cm), 3 g of L-arginine was given three times a day for 12 weeks with lifestyle modification advice. At completion of study there was a significant reduction in waist circumference (mean ± SD: 115.6 ± 12.7 cm at baseline to 109.2 ± 11.7 cm at 12 weeks; P = 0.0004) and weight (mean ± SD: 98.6 ± 19.7 kg at baseline to 95.7 ± 18.6 kg at 12 weeks; P = 0.015) (Hurt et al 2014).

CLINICAL USE

Arginine can have one of two forms, the L-form and the D-form, as do most other amino acids. The majority of research literature focuses on oral L-arginine because it has a longer half-life and better long-term effects than systemic forms and would be the preferred route (Blum et al 1999). The role of arginine in NO production has formed the basis of its application in various disease states, such as cardiovascular disease, sexual dysfunction, peripheral arterial disease, asthma and interstitial cystitis.

Cardiovascular disease

In the management of cardiovascular disease, arginine supplementation is noted to improve endothelial function, particularly in hypercholesterolaemia and atherosclerosis (Boger & Bode-Boger 2001). Under- or overproduction of NO is considered to be a contributing factor to cardiovascular disease, or it may be a consequence of disease, leading to active investigations into the potential for the L-arginine–NO system as a therapeutic target for a variety of conditions such as hypertension, atherosclerosis and ischaemic stroke (Rawlingson 2003).

Numerous human studies have shown that arginine supplementation improves endothelial function. Some of the studies have been performed in people with poor flow-mediated dilation, smokers, people with diabetes or after cardiac surgery.

A meta-analysis of 12 studies (*n* = 492 subjects) investigating the effects of short-term supplementation of oral L-arginine on endothelial function reported that supplementation was effective in significantly improving vascular endothelial function only when the baseline flow-mediated dilation is low (<7%) (Bai et al 2009). In a small double-blind crossover trial 15 obese subjects with impaired glucose tolerance received a low-sugar and protein biscuit with or without 6.6 g of L-arginine in a 1600-kcal diet. Each study period lasted 2 weeks with a 2-week washout in between. During the active treatment phase recipients experienced enhanced endothelial function and improved glucose metabolism, insulin sensitivity and insulin secretion compared to the placebo phase (Monti et al 2013). In a short-term randomised, placebo-controlled, double-blind, crossover study investigating changes in smoking-induced endothelial function, oral supplementation of L-arginine (7 g/day) administered for 3 days in 10 healthy smokers (aged 24.3 ± 0.73 years) resulted in significantly improved arterial performance compared to placebo (Siasos et al 2008). A double-blind randomised parallel-order study investigating the effects of long-term oral L-arginine supplementation (6.4 g/day) on endothelial dysfunction and insulin sensitivity in 64 patients after an aortocoronary bypass who had stable coronary artery disease and without diabetes reported that L-arginine supplementation significantly improved endothelial function, insulin resistance and markers of inflammation after 6 months compared to placebo (Lucotti et al 2009). In a small study of young male patients (*n* = 10) with uncomplicated diabetes and control subjects (*n* = 20), L-arginine supplementation of 7 g/day for 1 week resulted in improved vascular function as determined by lower-limb blood flow. Resting lower-limb blood flow was lower in the patients (2.66 ± 0.3 vs 3.53 ± 0.35 mL/100 mL/min) and was restored to normal (2.66 ± 0.3 to 4.74 ± 0.86 mL/100 mL/min) by supplementation with arginine (Fayh et al 2013).

Numerous animal studies have investigated the effects of L-arginine supplementation on measures of atherosclerotic lesion formation and on several markers of endothelial health and function, such as macrophage function, platelet aggregation and adhesion and response to injury. L-Arginine supplementation appears to be of benefit regarding many parameters of vascular health: in particular, experimental models indicate slowed progression of the atherosclerotic disease process (Boger & Bode-Boger 2001, Preli et al 2002), although there is controversy as to whether pre-existing lesions are affected by L-arginine supplementation.

Human clinical trials have shown mixed results. A review of oral L-arginine supplementation identified 17 clinical studies that investigated its effects on vascular health (Preli et al 2002). The duration of supplementation varied from 3 days to 6 months, and doses varied from 6 g to 36 g daily, usually in divided doses. Studies were grouped into those investigating effects on small vessels, large vessels, coronary blood flow, adhesion molecule expression and monocyte adhesion, platelet aggregation and adhesion, limb ischaemia, exercise tolerance and myocardial infarction.

Of the 17 studies reviewed, 12 produced positive results and showed inhibition of platelet aggregation and adhesion, decreased monocyte adhesion resulting in decreased atherogenesis, improved endothelium-dependent vasodilation or greater painfree and total walking distance in intermittent claudication. In chronic heart failure patients, improvements in forearm blood flow, walking distance and subjective symptoms were reported. In hypercholesterolaemia, all four studies reviewed produced positive results, suggesting that this subgroup may be particularly responsive to therapy with oral L-arginine. The studies showing favourable effects involved subjects with or at risk of vascular disease, whereas two of the five studies showing no beneficial effect on vascular health were conducted with healthy volunteers who did not have endothelial dysfunction. Overall there are subgroups of patients who may gain vascular health benefits from supplementary arginine, particularly patients with less advanced disease (Boger 2008).

Hyperlipidaemia

Treatment with 9 g arginine daily for 6 months improved endothelial function and patient symptom scores in 26 adults with coronary artery disease (Lerman et al 1998). Similarly, in a study of 27 young hypercholesterolaemic adults, improved endothelial dilation was reported as a result of arginine supplementation (21 g/day) for 1 month (Clarkson et al 1996). Decreased serum total cholesterol levels were reported in a study of 45 healthy elderly adults who were treated with 30 g arginine aspartate/day (equivalent to 17 g arginine) for 2 weeks (Hurson et al 1995).

Hypertension

Both oral and intravenous administration of L-arginine may reduce blood pressure. A meta-analysis of 11 randomised, double-blind, placebo-controlled studies (*n* = 387 subjects) reported oral L-arginine supplementation (4–24 g/day) significantly lowers both systolic (by 5.39 mmHg; 95% confidence interval [CI] −8.54 to −2.25, $P = 0.001$) and diastolic (by 2.66 mmHg; 95% CI −3.77 to −1.54, $P < 0.001$) blood pressure compared to placebo (Dong et al 2011).

It is believed that supplementation with L-arginine stimulates NO biosynthesis, which leads to reduction of oxidative stress. In a randomised placebo-controlled study, 54 participants (24 women and 30 men) received either L-arginine (2 g tid or 4 g tid) or placebo for 28 days. In patients with mild arterial hypertension L-arginine significantly increased total antioxidant status and the plasma level of asymmetric dimethylarginine (Jabecka et al 2012).

Intravenous administration of L-arginine reduces blood pressure in both healthy subjects and patients with vascular disease. In a randomised, placebo-controlled, crossover study by West et al (2005), the benefit of oral arginine supplementation (12 g/day for 3 weeks) was investigated in 16 middle-aged men with hypercholesterolaemia. In contrast to the results of other studies, where arginine was administered intravenously, L-arginine supplementation did not affect lipids, glucose or inflammatory biomarkers; however, there was a reduction in homocysteine and blood pressure. Supplementation in normotensive people is not necessarily advantageous. In a randomised study of 19 healthy subjects, 6–12 g/day of L-arginine for 4 weeks resulted in a non-significant decrease in systolic and diastolic blood pressure (Ast et al 2011).

Pregnancy

A recent meta-analysis of five placebo-controlled studies that investigated the effects of L-arginine supplementation on blood pressure during pregnancy reported that diastolic blood pressure was reduced (mean decrease of 3.07 mmHg; $P = 0.004$) and there was an increase in gestational age at delivery (mean increase of 1.23 weeks; $P = 0.002$) with arginine supplementation, but there was no effect on systolic pressure ($P = 0.19$) (Zhu et al 2013).

Similarly, another recent systematic review and meta-analysis of seven randomised controlled trials with 916 patients administered different dosages (3–30 g) and administration routes (oral and intravenous) reported that L-arginine was effective in reducing pre-eclampsia or eclampsia incidence and prolonging pregnancy. Two of the studies reported adverse effects that included nausea, vomiting and headache in 1–10% of the subjects and one study reported diarrhoea during oral L-arginine treatment (Gui et al 2014).

Myocardial infarction

Some studies have reported that orally administered arginine improves cardiovascular function and reduces myocardial ischaemia in coronary artery disease, whereas others have noted increased mortality. A meta-analysis of two studies with 927 patients with acute myocardial infarction reported that oral supplementation of L-arginine had no significant effect on clinical outcomes in these patients with unstable coronary artery disease, although in an overall pooled estimate there was a reduction (7%) in mortality in the supplemented group compared with the control group (105/459, 22.9% vs 111/455, 24.4%; not significant) (Sun et al 2009).

In a randomised, controlled study by Schulman et al (2006) 153 patients with acute ST-segment elevation myocardial infarcts were given 9 g arginine (as arginine hydrochloride) a day or placebo for 6 months; however, this study was terminated while in progress, as a significant increase in death rate was noted (8.6% in the group given arginine versus zero in the placebo group; $P = 0.01$). The supplementary arginine was implicated by the authors, but this assumption was not verified.

In a large, multicentre, randomised, double-blind, placebo-controlled study, 792 patients with coronary artery disease were included within 24 h of the onset of acute myocardial infarction; the arginine group received 3 × 3 g L-arginine a day for 1 month. The results showed very little difference between the two groups with respect to various metabolic and clinical markers, although the arginine-supplemented group had favourable trends. However, positive results were seen in a subgroup of patients with hypercholesterolaemia (Bednarz et al 2005).

Angina

Not all studies report efficacy of arginine supplementation for the treatment of angina. A randomised, controlled study of 40 men with stable angina receiving 15 g arginine on a daily basis for 2 weeks did not show benefits for endothelium-dependent vasodilation, oxidative stress or exercise performance (Walker et al 2001). However, in a randomised controlled study, 10 patients with stable angina who were given 12 g arginine daily for 6 weeks demonstrated increased exercise tolerance benefits, decreased lactate accumulation and decreased heart rate (Doutreleau et al 2006).

Congestive heart failure

Studies report mixed findings regarding the benefits of supplemental arginine in congestive heart failure, although taking L-arginine orally, in combination with conventional treatment, seems to improve glomerular filtration rate, creatinine clearance and sodium and water elimination after saline loading.

A study of 21 patients with congestive heart failure who were given 9 g arginine daily for 7 days reported prolonged exercise capability (Bednarz et al 2004). However, in general, improvements in exercise tolerance, quality of life and peripheral vascular resistance are not consistently obtained. Oral arginine treatment did not have beneficial effects in endothelial function for 20 heart-failure patients who received 20 g/day for 4 weeks (Chin-Dusting et al 1996).

Peripheral arterial disease

Dietary supplementation of L-arginine has been reported to improve endothelium-dependent vasodilation, limb blood flow and walking distance in peripheral arterial disease. In one study (Oka et al 2005), 80 patients with peripheral arterial disease and intermittent claudication were randomly assigned oral doses of L-arginine in 3-g increments up to 9 g daily in three divided doses over a period of 12 weeks. No major differences were noted, although there was a trend for an improvement in walking speed in patients receiving L-arginine, and the group that was treated with 3 g L-arginine daily also demonstrated a moderate improvement in walking distance. On the other hand, in a randomised, controlled study of 133 patients with peripheral arterial occlusive disease who received L-arginine supplementation of 3 g daily for 6 months, no benefit was reported regarding vascular function and there was a significant decrease in the absolute walking distance (Wilson et al 2007).

Diabetes

Abnormal insulin modulation of L-arginine transport may contribute to vascular dysfunction in diabetes (Rajapakse et al 2013). Reduced arginine plasma levels have been noted in patients with diabetes mellitus, and reports indicate that endothelial function may be improved in such patients by supplementary arginine. Arginine may also counteract lipid peroxidation, thus reducing the long-term complications of diabetes. In a small study of 10 women with type 2 diabetes mellitus, improved endothelial function was noted after they were given 9 g arginine daily for 1 week (Regensteiner et al 2003).

In a recent long-term randomised, double-blind, parallel-group, placebo-controlled study of 144 subjects with impaired glucose tolerance and metabolic syndrome, arginine supplementation (6.4 g/day) for 18 months, including a follow-up at 12 months, did not reduce the incidence of diabetes, although the probability of normal glucose tolerance increased significantly because of improved insulin sensitivity and β-cell function (Monti et al 2012).

In a randomised placebo-controlled trial 60 patients with visceral obesity and 20 healthy lean control subjects received either 9 g of L-arginine or placebo for 3 months. Arginine treatment significantly decreased homeostasis model assessment-insulin resistance and insulin concentration in patients with visceral obesity, with no impact on tumour necrosis factor-alpha concentration (Bogdanski et al 2012).

However, in a small study of 38 patients with type 2 diabetes and atherosclerotic peripheral arterial disease of lower extremities and 12 healthy controls, L-arginine supplementation (3 × 2 g/day) for 2 months had no effect on fasting glucose and HbA_{1C}, but there was a significant increase in NO production and total antioxidant status (Jabłecka et al 2012).

Erectile dysfunction

Supplementary arginine has been investigated for its effect on erectile function, given the role of NO in the corpus cavernosum; the research in this area has mixed findings.

In a randomised double-blind, placebo-controlled, two-way crossover study, 26 patients were given 'on demand' 8 g L-arginine aspartate combined with 200 mg of adenosine monophosphate or placebo 1–2 h before sexual intercourse for the intermittent treatment of mild to moderate erectile dysfunction. In the active treatment phase participants experienced significant improvements in all International Index of Erectile Function domains, with the exception of the Sexual Desire and Orgasmic domains (Neuzillet et al 2013).

In a large prospective randomised, double-blind placebo-controlled study, a high dose of arginine (5 g/day) was administered for 6 weeks to 50 men with organic erectile dysfunction and significant improvement in sexual function was reported only in men with abnormal NO metabolism (Chen et al 1999). However, in a randomised, placebo-controlled, crossover oral study of 32 patients with mixed-type impotence who were treated with 3 × 500 mg L-arginine/day for 17 days, the results showed the supplement was no more effective than the placebo (Klotz et al 1999). Taking L-arginine orally in high doses, 5 g daily, seems to improve subjective assessment of sexual function in men with organic erectile dysfunction, but taking lower doses might not be effective. A combination of arginyl aspartate (equivalent to 1.7 g of L-arginine a day) with pycnogenol was administered to 40 men, aged 25–45 years, for 3 months; by the third month up to 92% of the men reported improved erectile function without any side effects (Stanislavov & Nikolova 2003).

Cancer

In a randomised prospective study, 37 ambulatory postsurgical patients (mean age 67.4 ± 13.1 years) with head and neck cancer and with recent weight loss (>5% during previous 3 months) received an oral supplement with omega-3 fatty acids and arginine (2 × 227 mL or 3 × 227 mL supplement containing either 8.4 or 12.6 g L-arginine and 1.2 or 1.8 g eicosapentaenoic acid and 0.8 or 1.2 g docosahexaenoic acid) for 12 weeks postdischarge from hospital. Both doses of the supplement were beneficial and resulted in improved levels of biomarkers, such as albumin, prealbumin and lymphocyte levels, and the higher-dose supplement also led to improved weight gain (de Luis et al 2013).

Chemotherapy adjunct

There are conflicting reports about the value of arginine supplementation during chemotherapy. As some studies have also used other supplementary constituents, it is difficult to attribute any benefits solely to arginine (Appleton 2002). Importantly, arginine has been implicated in promoting cancer growth, since polyamines can act as growth factors for cancers, and this might be of concern in long-term arginine treatment. Precautionary measures regarding L-arginine administration should be considered in cancer patients, although in recent years immunomodulating formulas containing supplementary arginine have been used safely (Aiko et al 2008, Marik & Zaloga 2008).

Necrotising enterocolitis

A small parallel-group double-blind randomised study of 83 very-low-birth-weight neonates (≤1500 g) and gestational age ≤34 weeks reported that enteral arginine supplementation (1.5 mmol/kg/day bid) between the third and 28th day of life (n = 40) compared to placebo (n = 43) resulted in significantly lower incidence of necrotising enterocolitis stage III (2.5% vs 18.6%, P = 0.030) (Polycarpou et al 2013).

Interstitial cystitis

The results of taking L-arginine for the management of interstitial cystitis are mixed. In a double-blind placebo-controlled crossover study (Cartledge et al 2000), 16 patients were randomised to receive L-arginine (2.4 g/day) or a placebo for 1 month. Although some patients reported improvement in their symptoms, the effects were only small and probably not clinically significant. A randomised, double-blind, placebo-controlled study with 53 patients who received 1500 mg L-arginine or a placebo orally for 3 months reported less pain and urgency in some of the patients (Korting et al 1999). A small study in which patients were treated with either 3 g or 10 g of supplementary arginine did not report any symptom improvements (Ehrén et al 1998). Overall, taking L-arginine orally may reduce symptoms, especially pain associated with interstitial cystitis, in only some patients.

Enhancing immune function

The results of the utility of supplemental arginine in immunonutrition are mixed. Numerous enteral formulas contain additional arginine for use in catabolic conditions and critical illness; most enteral feeds provide about 12–13 g per 1000 kcal.

A systematic review investigated the impact in critical illness of intramuscular formulas containing various supplementary nutrients such as arginine (ranging from 6.5 to 15 g arginine/L) and glutamine compared with a control diet. Analysis of 24 studies (3013 patients) found that intramuscular diets with supplementary arginine, with or without various supplementary nutrients, did not result in improved outcomes in intensive care, trauma and burn patients (Marik & Zaloga 2008).

Wound healing

A number of studies have reported that dietary L-arginine supplementation enhances wound healing and immunity. A randomised controlled study with 29 older adults receiving 15 g arginine daily for 4 weeks reported improved immune function (Moriguti et al 2005). Similarly, improved wound healing was reported in another randomised controlled study, in which 17 g arginine as arginine aspartate (30 g/day) was administered daily for 14 days to 30 healthy elderly people (Kirk et al 1993). Improved wound healing was noted in a randomised controlled trial of experimental surgical wounds in 36 healthy adults who were given 17–25 g oral arginine per day (Barbul et al 1990).

Renal failure

There are mixed reports about the benefit of supplemental L-arginine in the management of chronic renal failure. There was no improvement in renal function in a randomised, double-blind, placebo-controlled study of 24 patients who were given 200 mg/kg (14 g/70 kg) arginine daily for 6 months (De Nicola et al 1999). A study of 76 renal transplant patients who were given 9 g arginine a day and canola oil as a source of omega-3 fatty acids for 3 years noted reduced infections and transplant rejections (Alexander et al 2005).

Sports

A recent randomised, double-blind, placebo-controlled study investigating the acute effect of L-arginine supplementation (6 g) in 15 men during recovery from three sets of resistance exercise regarding biceps strength performance, indicators of NO production and muscle blood volume and oxygenation reported that supplementation significantly increased muscle blood volume but there was no difference between groups regarding the other measures (Alvares et al 2012). Similarly, in a randomised, double-blind crossover study investigating the effects of acute supplementation with L-arginine alpha-ketoglutarate (3000 mg) on muscular strength and endurance in eight resistance-trained and eight untrained men, it was reported that supplementation did not provide an ergogenic benefit regardless of the training status of the participants (Wax et al 2012).

In a further randomised, double-blind, placebo-controlled crossover study, 6 g arginine did not alter biomarkers of NO synthesis, oxygen cost of exercise or exercise tolerance in 15 healthy subjects (Vanhatalo et al 2013).

OTHER USES

HIV — general support

Supplementary arginine may have a beneficial role in the care of HIV infection and AIDS. A few studies have already been conducted investigating the effects of a combination of arginine with vitamins, minerals and glutamine; body weight was reported to increase, but other findings were mixed (Appleton 2002).

Asthma

Arginine supplementation may be beneficial to patients with asthma, although there are reports that such supplementation may also cause exacerbation of airway inflammation (Coman et al 2008). At present, it is unclear whether L-arginine supplementation results in any clinically significant benefit to patients with asthma.

Cystic fibrosis

In a small, double-blind, placebo-controlled crossover study of 10 patients with cystic fibrosis, arginine supplementation of 200 mg/kg administered for 6 weeks resulted in increased NO production (Grasemann et al 2005).

Dementia

Increased cognitive function and reduced lipid peroxidation were noted in 16 elderly patients with senile dementia who were administered arginine (1.6 g/day) (Ohtsuka & Nakaya 2000).

Subfertility

It has been well documented that arginine-deficient diets in adult men result in markedly decreased sperm counts. Infertile men given 500 mg arginine hydrochloride per day for 6–8 weeks were reported to have increased sperm counts, although such supplementation had no effect if the baseline sperm counts were less than 10 million/mL (Appleton 2002). Results of a single study note that supplementation of 16 g of arginine per day improved ovarian response and pregnancy rate in poor responders to in vitro fertilisation (Battaglia et al 1999).

DOSAGE RANGE

General guide

- Overall, L-arginine is well tolerated in doses <30 g administered orally, intravenously or via the intra-arterial route (Boger & Bode-Boger 2001). It is best taken in divided doses to improve overall absorption, reaching 1.5–6 g daily.
- In a risk assessment by Shao and Hancock (2008), the following recommendations have been made: no observed adverse effect level and lowest observed adverse effect level >42 g/day L-arginine; observed safe level 20 g/day. ULS 20 g/day.

According to clinical studies

- Angina pectoris: oral 12 g/day (uncertain efficacy).
- Coronary artery disease: 9 g/day.
- Erectile dysfunction: 5 g/day (in men with abnormal NO metabolism).
- Hyperlipidaemia: 30 g/day (uncertain efficacy).
- Wound healing: 17 g/day.

TOXICITY

Overall, arginine administration is considered safe for humans and animals (Wu & Meininger 2000). However, it must be noted that vasodilation and hypotension can result from the overproduction of NO due to excess administration of arginine.

ADVERSE REACTIONS

L-Arginine supplementation has been used safely and has been associated with only minor side effects in clinical studies lasting from a few days to months (Shao & Hathcock 2008). Orally, L-arginine can cause abdominal pain and bloating, diarrhoea and gout. Gastrointestinal disturbances have been reported as a result of arginine supplementation, although the studies have been of a mixed nature and involved a range of patients (Grimble 2007), whereas these effects have not been reported in controlled studies.

There has been only limited consideration of safety aspects of supplemental arginine, even though numerous animal studies have been conducted examining a wide range of diseases (Shao & Hathcock 2008). In humans only one study has used a high oral arginine dose of 42 g on a daily basis without any adverse effects being noted (Shao & Hathcock 2008). In patients with argininosuccinic aciduria, high doses (500 mg/kg body weight) of arginine may elevate liver enzymes (Nagamani et al 2012).

SIGNIFICANT INTERACTIONS

No controlled studies are available to determine the significance of the proposed interactions, so they remain speculative.

Antihypertensive medicines

Theoretically, additive hypotensive effects may occur — use with caution. Potential benefits under professional supervision.

Nitrates

Theoretically, additive vasodilation and hypotensive effects may occur — use with caution.

L-Lysine

A limited number of research studies report that high doses of arginine could be unfavourable, as arginine may compete with lysine uptake by tissues; caution is needed if considering the administration of both amino acids, since supplemental arginine has been reported to affect proliferation of the herpes simplex virus (Griffith et al 1981).

Sildenafil

Theoretically, additive vasodilation and hypotensive effects may occur — use with caution. Potential benefits under supervision.

CONTRAINDICATIONS AND PRECAUTIONS

Intravenous arginine needs to be administered with care, as overdose may result in adverse consequences such as severe hyponatraemia (Shao & Hathcock 2008), and high doses with high osmolality can cause local irritation and phlebitis (Boger & Bode-Boger 2001).

Other side effects that can occur as a result of administering arginine are metabolic acidosis associated with arrhythmias, and hyperkalaemia and increases in blood nitrogen urea in patients with liver disease and/or renal impairment (Boger & Bode-Boger 2001).

Hyperkalaemia and hypophosphataemia in patients with diabetes have also been reported (Boger & Bode-Boger 2001). Supplementary arginine may also be contraindicated in patients with systemic septic shock and hypotension due to NO production (Feihl et al 2001).

Caution is necessary in using high doses of 30 g/day in cancer patients, as even short-term use for 3 days may be linked to increased tumour growth.

PREGNANCY USE

At present there is insufficient reliable information available about the safety of L-arginine during pregnancy and for nursing mothers. Dietary intake levels are likely to be safe.

Practice points/Patient counselling

- L-Arginine is a conditionally essential amino acid for humans; requirements may be increased during metabolic stress or when there is insufficient endogenous L-arginine for optimal growth or tissue repair.
- Arginine deficiency can affect growth and development, insulin production, lipid and protein metabolism and glucose tolerance. Clinical symptoms include poor wound healing, hair loss or breakage, liver disease, constipation and skin rashes.
- The role of arginine in NO production forms the basis of its application in cardiovascular disease, peripheral arterial disease, sexual dysfunction, asthma and interstitial cystitis.
- Oral arginine supplementation shows promise in the treatment of angina, hyperlipidaemia, congestive heart failure, improving vascular health (reducing atherogenesis) and interstitial cystitis; however, results are not consistent.
- Oral arginine supplementation has shown benefits in erectile dysfunction and promoting wound healing.
- Arginine supplementation should be used with caution in people with cancer, kidney and/or liver impairment, schizophrenia, herpes simplex virus or a history of myocardial infarction.

PATIENTS' FAQs

What will this supplement do for me?

Arginine supplementation is used in cardiovascular disease, peripheral arterial disease, sexual dysfunction, wound healing and several other conditions. Its effects will depend on the dose used and indication for use.

When will it start to work?

This depends on the dose used and indication for use.

Are there any safety issues?

Arginine supplementation should be used with caution in people with cancer, kidney and/or liver impairment, schizophrenia, herpes simplex virus or a history of myocardial infarction. There are also several drug interactions that should be considered before use.

REFERENCES

Aiko S et al. Enteral immuno-enhanced diets with arginine are safe and beneficial for patients early after esophageal cancer surgery. Dis Esophagus 21.7 (2008): 619–627.

Alexander JW et al. The influence of immunomodulatory diets on transplant success and complications. Transplantation 79 (2005): 460–465.

Alvares TS et al. Acute l-arginine supplementation increases muscle blood volume but not strength performance. Appl Physiol Nutr Metab. 2012;37(1):115–26.

Appleton J. Arginine: clinical potential of a semi-essential amino acid. Alt Med Rev 7.6 (2002): 512–522.

Ast, J., et al. (2011). Supplementation with l-arginine does not influence arterial blood pressure in healthy people: A randomized, double blind, trial. Eur Rev Med Pharmacol Sci, 15(12), 1375–1384.

Bai Y et al. Increase in fasting vascular endothelial function after short-term oral L-arginine is effective when baseline flow-mediated dilation is low: a meta-analysis of randomized controlled trials. Am J Clin Nutr. 2009 Jan;89(1):77–84.

Barbul A et al. Arginine enhances wound healing and lymphocyte immune responses in humans. Surgery 108 (1990): 331–336.

Battaglia C et al. Adjuvant L-arginine treatment for the in vitro fertilization in poor responder patients. Hum Reprod 14 (1999): 1690–1697.

Bednarz B et al. L-arginine supplementation prolongs exercise capacity in congestive heart failure. Kardiol Pol 60 (2004): 348–353.

Bednarz B et al. Efficacy and safety of oral L-arginine in acute myocardial infarction. Results of the multicenter, randomized, double-blind, placebo controlled ARAMI pilot trial. Kardiol Pol 62 (2005): 421–427.

Blum A et al. Clinical and inflammatory effects of dietary-arginine in patients with intractable angina pectoris. Am J Cardiol 83 (1999): 1488–1490.

Bogdanski, P et al. (2012). Effect of 3-month l-arginine supplementation on insulin resistance and tumor necrosis factor activity in patients with visceral obesity. Eur Rev Med Pharmacol Sci, 16(6), 816–823.

Boger RH. L-Arginine therapy in cardiovascular pathologies: beneficial or dangerous? Curr Opin Clin Nutr Metab Care 11.1 (2008): 55–61.

Boger RH, Bode-Boger SM. The clinical pharmacology of L-arginine. Annu Rev Pharmacol Toxicol 41 (2001): 79–99.

Cartledge JJ, et al. A randomized double-blind placebo-controlled crossover trial of the efficacy of L-arginine in the treatment of interstitial cystitis. BJU Int 85 (2000): 421–426.

Chen J et al. Effect of oral administration of high-dose nitric oxide donor L-arginine in men with organic erectile dysfunction: results of a double-blind, randomized, placebo-controlled study. BJU Int 83.3 (1999): 269–273.

Chin-Dusting JP et al. Dietary supplementation with L-arginine fails to restore endothelial function in forearm resistance arteries of patients with severe heart failure. J Am Coll Cardiol 27 (1996): 1207–1213.

Chionglo Sy et al. Modern nutrition in health and disease. Philadelphia: Lippincott, Williams and Wilkins, 2006.

Clarkson P et al. Oral L-arginine improves endothelium-dependent dilation in hypercholesterolemic young adults. J Clin Invest 97.8 (1996): 1989–1994.

Coman D et al. New indications and controversies in arginine therapy. Clin Nutr 27 (2008): 489–496.

de Luis DA et al. A randomized clinical trial with two doses of a omega 3 fatty acids oral and arginine enhanced formula in clinical and biochemical parameters of head and neck cancer ambulatory patients. Eur Rev Med Pharmacol Sci. 2013;17(8):1090–4.

De Nicola L et al. Randomised, double-blind, placebo-controlled study of arginine supplementation in chronic renal failure. Kidney Int 56 (1999): 674–684.

Dong JY et al. Effect of oral L-arginine supplementation on blood pressure: a meta-analysis of randomized, double-blind, placebo-controlled trials. Am Heart J. 2011 Dec;162(6):959–65.

Doutreleau S et al. Chronic l-arginine supplementation enhances endurance exercise tolerance in heart failure patients. Int J Sports Med 27 (2006): 567–572.

Ehrén I et al. Effects of L-arginine treatment on symptoms and bladder nitric oxide levels in patients with interstitial cystitis. Urology 52.6 (1998): 1026–1029.

Fayh AP et al. Effects of L-arginine supplementation on blood flow, oxidative stress status and exercise responses in young adults with uncomplicated type I diabetes. Eur J Nutr. 2013;52(3):975–83.

Feihl F et al. Is nitric oxide overproduction the target of choice for the management of septic shock? Pharmacol Ther 91 (2001): 179–213.

Grasemann H et al. Oral l-arginine supplementation in cystic fibrosis patients: a placebo-controlled study. Eur Respir J 25 (2005): 62–68.

Griffith RS et al. Relation of arginine-lysine antagonism to herpes simplex growth in tissue culture. Chemother 27 (1981): 209–213.

Grimble GK. Adverse gastrointestinal effects of arginine and related amino acids. J Nutr 137 (2007): 1693S–1701S.

Gui S et al. Arginine supplementation for improving maternal and neonatal outcomes in hypertensive disorder of pregnancy: a systematic review. Journal of the Renin-Angiotensin-Aldosterone System 2014; 15(1): 88–96.

Hurson M et al. Metabolic effects of arginine in a healthy elderly population. JPEN J Parenter Enteral Nutr 19.3 (1995): 227–230.

Hurt RT et al. L-arginine for the treatment of centrally obese subjects: a pilot study. J Diet Suppl. 2014;11(1):40–52.

Jabecka, A. et al. (2012). Oral l-arginine supplementation in patients with mild arterial hypertension and its effect on plasma level of asymmetric dimethylarginine, l-citruline, l-arginine and antioxidant status. Eur Rev Med Pharmacol Sci, 16(12), 1665–1674.
Jabłecka A et al. The effect of oral L-arginine supplementation on fasting glucose, HbA1c, nitric oxide and total antioxidant status in diabetic patients with atherosclerotic peripheral arterial disease of lower extremities. Eur Rev Med Pharmacol Sci. 2012;16(3):342–50.
King D et al. Variation in L-arginine intake follow demographics and lifestyle factors that may impact cardiovascular disease risk. Nutr Res 28 (2008): 21–24.
Kirk SJ et al. Arginine stimulates wound healing and immune function in elderly human beings. Surg 114 (1993): 155–159.
Klotz T et al. Effectiveness of oral L-arginine in first-line treatment of erectile dysfunction in a controlled crossover study. Urol Int 63.4 (1999): 220–223.
Korting GE et al. A randomized double-blind trial of oral L-arginine for treatment of interstitial cystitis. J Urol 161 (1999): 558–565.
Lerman A et al. Long-term L-arginine supplementation improves small-vessel coronary endothelial function in humans. Circulation 97.21 (1998): 2123–2128.
Lucotti P et al. Oral L-arginine supplementation improves endothelial function and ameliorates insulin sensitivity and inflammation in cardiopathic nondiabetic patients after an aortocoronary bypass. Metabolism. 2009 Sep;58(9):1270–6.
Marik PE, Zaloga GP. Immunonutrition in critically ill patients: a systematic review and analysis of the literature. Intensive Care Med 34.11 (2008): 1980–1990.
Monti LD et al. Effect of a long-term oral l-arginine supplementation on glucose metabolism: a randomized, double-blind, placebo-controlled trial. Diabetes Obes Metab. 2012 Oct;14(10):893–900.
Monti, L.D et al. (2013). L-arginine enriched biscuits improve endothelial function and glucose metabolism: A pilot study in healthy subjects and a cross-over study in subjects with impaired glucose tolerance and metabolic syndrome. Metabolism, 62(2), 255–264.
Moriguti JC et al. Effects of arginine supplementation on the humoral and innate immune response of older people. Eur J Clin Nutr 59 (2005): 1362–1366.
Morris, S.M., Jr. (2009). Recent advances in arginine metabolism: Roles and regulation of the arginases. Br J Pharmacol, 157(6), 922–930.
Morris, S.M., Jr. (2012). Arginases and arginine deficiency syndromes. Curr Opin Clin Nutr Metab Care, 15(1), 64–70.
Nagamani, S.C et al. (2012). A randomized controlled trial to evaluate the effects of high-dose versus low-dose of arginine therapy on hepatic function tests in argininosuccinic aciduria. Mol Genet Metab, 107(3), 315–321.
Neuzillet, Y et al. (2013). A randomized, double-blind, crossover, placebo-controlled comparative clinical trial of arginine aspartate plus adenosine monophosphate for the intermittent treatment of male erectile dysfunction. Andrology, 1(2), 223–228.
Ohtsuka Y, Nakaya J. Effect of oral administration of L-arginine on senile dementia. Am J Med 108 (2000): 439.
Oka RK et al. A pilot study of L-arginine supplementation on functional capacity in peripheral arterial disease. Vasc Med 10.4 (2005): 265–274.
Polycarpou E et al. Enteral L-arginine supplementation for prevention of necrotizing enterocolitis in very low birth weight neonates: a double-blind randomized pilot study of efficacy and safety. JPEN J Parenter Enteral Nutr. 2013;37(5):617–22.
Preli RB, et al. Vascular effects of dietary L-arginine supplementation. Atherosclerosis 162 (2002): 1–115.
Rajapakse, N.W et al. (2013). Insulin-mediated activation of the l-arginine nitric oxide pathway in man, and its impairment in diabetes. PLoS One, 8(5), e61840.
Rawlingson A. Nitric oxide, inflammation and acute burn injury. Burns 29 (2003): 631–640.
Regensteiner JG et al. Oral L-arginine and vitamins E and C improve endothelial function in women with type 2 diabetes. Vasc Med 8 (2003): 169–175.
Schulman SP et al. L-Arginine therapy in acute myocardial infarction: the Vascular Interaction With Age in Myocardial Infarction (VINTAGE MI) randomized clinical trial. JAMA 295 (2006): 58–64.
Shao A, Hathcock JN. Risk assessment for the amino acids taurine, l-glutamine and l-arginine. Reg Tox Pharmol 50 (2008): 376–399.
Siasos G, et al. Short-term treatment with L-arginine prevents the smoking-induced impairment of endothelial function and vascular elastic properties in young individuals. Int J Cardiol. 2008 Jun 6;126(3):394–9.
Stanislavov R, Nikolova V. Treatment of erectile dysfunction with pycnogenol and L-arginine. J Sex Marital Ther 29.3 (2003): 207–213.
Stargrove M, et al. Herb, nutrient and drug interactions. St Louis: Mosby, Elsevier, 2008.
Sun T, et al. Oral L-arginine supplementation in acute myocardial infarction therapy: a meta-analysis of randomized controlled trials. Clin Cardiol. 2009 Nov;32(11):649–52.
Tapiero H et al. I. Arginine. Biomed Pharmacother 9.56 (2002): 439–445.
Vanhatalo, A., et al. (2013). No effect of acute l-arginine supplementation on o(2) cost or exercise tolerance. Eur J Appl Physiol, 113(7), 1805–1819.
Visek WJ. Arginine needs, physiological state and usual diets. A re-evaluation. J Nutr 116 (1986): 36–46.
Wahlqvist ML. Food & nutrition. Sydney: Allen & Unwin, 2002.
Walker HA et al. Endothelium-dependent vasodilation is independent of the plasma l-arginine/ADMA ratio in men with stable angina: lack of effect of oral l-arginine on endothelial function, oxidative stress and exercise performance. J Am Coll Cardiol 38 (2001): 499–505.
Wax B, et al. Acute L-arginine alpha ketoglutarate supplementation fails to improve muscular performance in resistance trained and untrained men. J Int Soc Sports Nutr. 2012 Apr 17;9(1):17.
West SG et al. Oral L-arginine improves hemodynamic responses to stress and reduces plasma homocysteine in hypercholesterolemic men. J Nutr 135 (2005): 212–217.
Wilson AM et al. L-arginine supplementation in peripheral arterial disease: no benefit and possible harm. Circulation 116 (2007): 188–195.
Wu G, Meininger CJ. Arginine nutrition and cardiovascular function. J Nutr 130 (2000): 2626–2629.
Yi J et al. L-arginine and Alzheimer's disease. Int J Clin Exp Pathol 3 (2009): 211–238.
Zhu Q, et al. Effect of L-arginine supplementation on blood pressure in pregnant women: a meta-analysis of placebo-controlled trials. Hypertens Pregnancy. 2013;32(1):32–41

Lavender

HISTORICAL NOTE Lavender, both the whole plant and its essential oils, has a long history of traditional use for a range of medical conditions. Lavender was used as an antiseptic in ancient Arabian, Greek and Roman medicines. Its generic name comes from the Latin *lavare*, to wash, and it was used as a bath additive as well as an antiseptic in the hospitals and sick rooms of ancient Persia, Greece and Rome (Blumenthal et al 2000), and as an antibacterial agent in World War I (Cavanagh & Wilkinson 2005). In the 17th century, Culpeper described lavender as having 'use for pains in the head following cold, cramps, convulsions, palsies and faintings' (Battaglia 1995). Lavender was also used traditionally to scent bed linen and to protect stored clothes from moths. This was such a well-accepted practice that the phrase 'laying up in lavender' was used metaphorically to mean 'putting away in storage' (Kirk-Smith 2003).

Lavender is now widely used in perfumes, potpourri, toiletries and cosmetics, to flavour food, as well as therapeutically. However, research produces a conflicting evidence base for lavender for a range of reasons, including the fact that the species of lavender is not always identified, that lavender is frequently adulterated and that little research has been conducted using species other than *Lavandula angustifolia*, which is also known as true lavender. *Lavandula angustifolia* is commonly adulterated with related species that vary in their chemical constituents. Spike lavender yields more oil, but is of lower quality than true lavender, and has a different chemical make-up. Lavandin is a hybrid of spike lavender and true lavender.

COMMON NAME

Lavender

OTHER NAMES

Common lavender, English lavender, French lavender, garden lavender, Spanish lavender, spike lavender, true lavender

BOTANICAL NAME/FAMILY

Lavandula angustifolia (synonyms: *L. officinalis*, *L. vera*, *L. spica*); *L. dentata*; *L. latifolia*; *L. pubescens*; *L. stoechas*, *L multifida* (family Labiatae)

PLANT PARTS USED

Flowers, leaves and stems

CHEMICAL COMPONENTS

Most lavender is extracted by steam distillation, but it can also be extracted using supercritical carbon dioxide extraction. Time and pressure affect the oil yield and antioxidant activity of lavender oil and both increase with pressure and time (Danh et al 2012).

Lavender flowers contain between 1% and 3% essential oil. The oil is a complex mixture of many different compounds, the amounts of which can vary between species. The most abundant compounds include linalyl acetate (30–55%), linalool (20–35%), cineole, camphor, coumarins and tannins (5–10%) (Schulz et al 1998), together with 1,8-cineole, thymol and carvacrol (Aburjai et al 2005) and borneol (Danh et al 2012). Perillyl alcohol and D-limonene have been shown to exert anticancer effects (see Clinical note). More recently, 39 constituents, accounting for 99% of total constituents, were extracted from *Lavandula multifida* (Rhaffari et al 2007). The main constituents were phenols such as thymol (32%), carvacrol (27.77%) and *p*-cymene (15.72%), and *γ*-terpinene (9.54%). Phenols are not commonly found in lavender. These constituents give the oil significant antibacterial activity similar to ampicillin and tetracycline in a dose-dependent manner (Rhaffari et al 2007).

MAIN ACTIONS

The pharmacological actions of various lavender extracts, essential oil and several of its constituents have been investigated. The true therapeutic benefit of the essential oil is difficult to ascertain as it is often combined with other oils or administered together with massage and other therapies such as acupressure, making interpretation of study results difficult.

Sedative/anxiolytic

The methanolic and aqueous extracts of *Lavandula officinalis* demonstrate potent sedative and hypnotic

> ***Clinical note — Perillyl alcohol and anticancer effects***
>
> Perillyl alcohol and D-limonene are monoterpenes found in lavender (also in cherries, mint and celery seeds) that have shown chemotherapeutic and chemoprotective effects in a wide variety of in vitro and animal models (Shi & Gould 2002) and are currently being examined in human clinical trials (Gould 1997, Kelloff et al 1999). Perillyl alcohol treatment has resulted in 70–99% inhibition of 'aberrant hyperproliferation', a late-occurring event preceding mammary tumorigenesis in vivo (Katdare et al 1997) and, together with limonene, perillyl alcohol has been shown to induce the complete regression of rat mammary carcinomas by what appears to be a cytostatic and differentiation process (Shi & Gould 1995). Perillyl alcohol has also been shown to inhibit human breast cancer cell growth in vitro and in vivo (Yuri et al 2004) and inhibit the expression and function of the androgen receptor in human prostate cancer cells (Chung et al 2006).
>
> A variety of mechanisms has been proposed to explain these effects. The compounds may act via interfering with Ras signal transduction pathways that regulate malignant cell proliferation (Hohl 1996) and have been found to promote apoptosis in pancreatic adenocarcinoma cells (Stayrook et al 1997) and liver tumours in vivo (Mills et al 1995). Perillyl alcohol, together with D-limonene, has been found to preferentially inhibit HMG-CoA reductase in tumour cells (Elson et al 1999), as well as inhibit ubiquinone synthesis and block the conversion of lathosterol to cholesterol, which may add to its antitumour activity (Ren & Gould 1994). Limonene is oxidised by the CYP2C9 and CYP2C19 enzymes in human liver microsomes (Miyazawa et al 2002a) and there are reported sex-related differences in the oxidative metabolism of limonene by liver microsomes in rats (Miyazawa et al 2002b).
>
> Although in vitro and animal studies have demonstrated the ability of perillyl alcohol to inhibit tumorigenesis in the mammary gland, liver and pancreas, the results are not yet conclusive and one animal study testing perillyl alcohol detected a weakly promoting effect early in nitrosamine-induced oesophageal tumorigenesis in rats (Liston et al 2003). In initial phase II clinical trials, perillyl alcohol administered orally, four times daily, at a dose of 1200 mg/m^2 had no clinical antitumour activity on advanced ovarian cancer (Bailey et al 2002), metastatic androgen-independent prostate cancer (Liu et al 2003) or metastatic colorectal cancer (Meadows et al 2002).

activities in vivo, thereby providing a pharmacological explanation for its therapeutic use in anxiety and insomnia (Alnamer et al 2012). Hritcu et al (2012) demonstrated that *L. angustifolia* ssp *angustifolia* and *L. hybrida* administered daily for 7 days significantly reduced anxiety, inhibited depression and improved spatial memory in male Wistar rats.

Lavender oil

The sedative properties of the essential oil and its main constituents (linalool and linalyl acetate) have a dose-dependent effect in mice and have been shown to reverse caffeine-induced hyperactivity in mice (Buchbauer et al 1991, Lim et al 2005), as well as reduce stress, as indicated by modulation of adrenocorticotrophic hormone (ACTH), catecholamine and gonadotrophin levels in experimental menopausal rats (Yamada et al 2005), and reduce cortisol responses in infant Japanese macaques (Kawakami et al 2002). Inhalation of lavender oil has also been shown to produce a dose-dependent anticonvulsant effect in both rats and mice (Yamada et al 1994).

In human trials, inhalation of lavender has been shown to induce relaxation and sedation (Schulz et al 1998) and to alter EEG responses (Diego et al 1998, Dimpfel et al 2004, Lee et al 1994, Sanders et al 2002, Yagyu 1994), enhance sleep and improve alertness on waking (Hirokawa et al 2012), as well as significantly decrease heart rate and increase high-frequency spectral components to produce calm and vigorous mood states in healthy volunteers (Kuroda et al 2005). Intermittent exposure to lavender over 30 minutes increased the proportion of beep and slow wave sleep in men and women (Goel et al 2005). In addition, Goel et al's subjects reported feeling more alert in the morning after inhaling lavender oil in the evening. Conversely, Sakamoto et al (2005) reported higher concentration levels in the afternoon in people receiving lavender at night compared to controls.

Transdermal absorption of linalool without inhalation produced a decrease in systolic blood pressure and a smaller decrease of skin temperature with no effects on subjective evaluation of wellbeing in healthy human subjects (Heuberger et al 2004), and another study found that lavender scent was associated with lower fatigue following an anxiety-provoking task (Burnett et al 2004). Lavender inhalation compared to sweet almond oil reduced autonomic arousal (e.g. heart and respiratory rates and blood pressure) and improved self-reported mood, supporting studies that reported on the relaxing effects of lavender (Sayorwan et al 2012).

Shaw et al (2011) also demonstrated anxiolytic effects in various parts of the hypothalamus and the central amygdala in rat brains, but the effect was not as significant as benzodiazepines. Shaw et al attributed the effects to linalool and linalyl acetate and recommended further study using single chemicals extracted from lavender. Similarly, Chioca et al (2011) demonstrated an anxiolytic effect of a combination of *L angustifolia* and *Citrus sinensis* administered via a vapouriser to Swiss mice without affecting locomotor activity and suggested the activity was not mediated through the GABA-A/benzodiazepine complex.

These positive studies are contrasted by studies with negative findings. Lavender aromatherapy did not significantly improve scores on the Hospital Anxiety and Depression Scale or the Somatic and Psychological Health Report (SPHERE) in a RCT of 313 patients undergoing radiotherapy (Graham et al 2003), and a study of 169 subjects, including both depressed and non-depressed subjects, showed that lavender increased fatigue, tension, confusion and total mood disturbance, and decreased vigour (Goel & Grasso 2004).

Lavender combined with sweet marjoram, patchouli and vetiver essential oils in a cream and applied as a massage five times per day for 4 weeks to 56 residents with moderate to severe dementia in an aged care facility demonstrated a significant but small improvement in Mini-Mental tests, increased alertness and less resistance, compared to the use of a massage cream without essential oils (Bowles et al 2002). The calming effects could be due to the large proportion of esters in *L. angustifolia* (26–56%) (Walsh et al 2011), but it is not clear which lavender species were used in the studies cited.

Antimicrobial

Various in vitro data suggest that lavender oil has antibacterial activity (Dadalioglu & Evrendilek 2004, Larrondo et al 1995), including against methicillin-resistant *Staphylococcus aureus* (MRSA) and vancomycin-resistant enterococcus (VRE) (Nelson 1997), antifungal activity (Inouye et al 2001), including against *Aspergillus nidulans* and *Trichophyton mega-trophytes* (Daferera et al 2000) and mitocidal activity (Perrucci et al 1996, Refaat et al 2002), with both lavender and linalool having fungistatic and fungicidal activities against *Candida albicans* strains at high concentrations and inhibiting germ tube formation and hyphal elongation at low concentrations, suggesting that it may be useful for reducing fungal progression and the spread of infection in host tissues (D'Auria et al 2005). Lavender has been shown to be active alone and to work synergistically with tea tree oil against the fungi responsible for tinea and onychomycosis (Cassella et al 2002). However, effective vapour concentrations have not yet been established for aromatherapy use.

The fungistatic properties of linalool have led to the suggestion that it could be used to complement environmental measures in preventing fungal contamination in storage areas of libraries (Rakotonirainy & Lavedrine 2005).

Carminative

Linalool, one of lavender's major components, demonstrated spasmolytic activity when tested on an in vitro preparation of guinea-pig ileum smooth muscle (Lis-Balchin & Hart 1999).

Antineoplastic effects

In vitro and animal studies suggest that perillyl alcohol and D-limonene (see Clinical note) may have useful chemotherapeutic and chemoprotective effects in a range of cancers, including cancers of the colon, liver, lung, breast, pancreas and prostate, as well as in melanoma (Micromedex 2003). These results have not yet been confirmed in human studies.

OTHER ACTIONS

When applied topically, lavender oil has rubefacient properties (Fisher & Painter 1996) and is thought to have analgesic, antihistaminic and anti-inflammatory activities. A small study comparing the effects of a bath containing lavender oil, synthetic lavender oil and distilled water in reducing perineal discomfort after childbirth found lower mean discomfort scores in the lavender group; however, the differences between groups were not significant (Cornwell & Dale 1995).

Traditionally, lavender oil is considered to have a balancing effect on the CNS, acting as an aromatic stimulant or calming agent.

Extracts of *L. multifida* have been found to have topical anti-inflammatory activity in mice, with some extracted compounds having activity comparable to that of indomethacin (Sosa et al 2005). At high concentrations (0.1%), lavender oil has also been found to suppress TNF-alpha-induced neutrophil adherence (Abe et al 2003). Lavender has also demonstrated powerful antioxidant activity (Gulcin et al 2004), as well as antimutagenic activity (Evandri et al 2005) and antiplatelet and antithrombotic properties demonstrated both in vitro and in vivo (Ballabeni et al 2004).

Insect bites

In vitro and animal studies suggest that lavender oil inhibits immediate-type allergic reactions by inhibition of mast cell degranulation (Kim & Cho 1999).

CLINICAL USE

Increasingly, clinical studies have been conducted with lavender oil in an oral dose form as well as externally applied essential oil and inhaled as an aromatherapy application. In particular, its potential therapeutic effect as an anxiolytic agent has gained much more attention than previously.

Anxiety

A number of controlled trials and observational studies suggest that inhalation of ambient lavender oil has a relaxing effect and is able to reduce anxiety and improve mood, concentration and sleep. It has been studied as a stand-alone treatment and in combination with other essential oils. Recent clinical research also shows that oral administration of lavender oil (Silexan) is an effective treatment for mild to moderate anxiety and is generally well tolerated. This product has been authorised for use in Germany for the treatment of states of restlessness during anxious mood (Uehleke et al 2012).

A 2012 systematic review of 15 randomised controlled trials (RCTs) (n = 1565) investigated various forms of lavender (inhaled as aromatherapy, essential oil combined with massage, oil added to bath and oral capsules) used with different cohorts (healthy, stress induced) and applied as acute treatment or as multiple doses/exposures. It concluded that limited specific effects of lavender inhalation and massage on anxiety measures are available and while reductions in anxiety measures were observed, methodological issues limit the extent to which firm conclusions can be drawn Alternately, the evidence available regarding the use of oral lavender oil is positive, supporting its use in anxiety (Perry et al 2012).

More specifically, RCTs using oral lavender oil capsules have reported beneficial effects in reducing mild to moderate anxiety (Bradley et al 2009, Kasper et al 2010, Uehleke et al 2012, Woelk & Schlafke 2010). All studies used a commercial product known as Silexan.

Woelk et al (2010) compared Silexan to lorazepam and found both groups significantly reduced anxiety as measured by the Hamilton Anxiety Rating Scale (HAM-A).While both treatments were well tolerated, there were marginally more side effects in the lavender group which were generally gastrointestinal disturbances. Kasper et al (2010) also tested the lavender oil capsules (Silexan) in this randomised double blind study, which used treatments for 10 weeks in volunteers with subsyndromal anxiety disorder (according to DMS-IV or ICD-10). Active treatment produced a significant reduction in anxiety levels (P < 0.01) compared to controls as measured by the HAM-A. Additionally, Bradley et al (2009) tested the same preparation (Silexan) in subjects with generalised anxiety disorder (GAD) over a 6-week treatment period and compared it to lorazepam. The mean of the HAM-A-total score decreased clearly and to a similar extent in both groups (by 11.3 ± 6.7 points (45%) in the silexan group and by 11.6 ± 6.6 points (46%) in the lorazepam group, from 25 ± 4 points at baseline in both groups. Both treatments were also comparable for a number of other outcomes such as SAS (Self-rating Anxiety Scale), PSWQ-PW (Penn State Worry Questionnaire), SF 36 Health Survey Questionnaire and Clinical Global Impressions of severity of disorder (CGI item 1, CGI item 2, CGI item 3), and the results of the sleep diary. It appeared to be most effective in cases of induced mild anxiety compared to more severe anxiety.

In 2012, Uehleke et al (2012) reported from an open label study that Silexan significantly increased mental wellbeing (SF-36) by 48.2% (P < 0.001), efficiency of sleep (P = 0.018) and mood (P = 0.03) and significantly reduced waking-up frequency (P = 0.002), waking-up duration (P < 0.001) and morning tiredness (P = 0.005). At baseline, patients suffered from restlessness (96%), depressed mood (98%), sleep disturbances (92%) or anxiety (72%). Of those, response rates were 62%, 57%, 51% and 62% respectively showing improvements during treatment (P < 0.001). The dose used was 80 mg/day Silexan over 6 weeks. The study involved 50 male and female patients with neurasthenia, post-traumatic stress disorder or somatisation disorder. For all patients, mean von Zerssen's Depression Scale score decreased by 32.7% and Symptom Checklist-90-Revised Global Severity Index by 36.4% as compared to baseline (P < 0.001).

Essential oil used externally

At least eight RCTs have investigated the effect of lavender oil inhalation with four trials reporting a significant decrease in anxiety for at least one outcome measure (Braden et al 2009, Kritsidima et al 2010, Kutlu et al 2008, Motomura et al 2001), whereas four other RCTs found no significant effect (Howard & Hughes 2008, Muzzarelli et al 2006, Sgoutas-Emch et al 2001, Toda & Morimoto 2008). A systematic review of these RCTs concluded that lavender oil inhalation and massage can reduce anxiety symptoms; however, the methodological shortcomings of the existing RCTs means a definitive conclusion cannot be made (Perry et al 2012).

More recently, a study conducted in an intensive care unit (ICU) involving 56 percutaneous coronary intervention (PCI) patients found that inhaling a combination of essential oils (lavender, roman chamomile and neroli with a 6:2:0.5 ratio) 10 times before PCI and another 10 times after PCI significantly lowered anxiety (P < 0.001) and improved sleep quality (P = 0.001) compared with conventional nursing interventions. The latter were not described (Cho et al 2013).

Veterinary use

Lavender oil has also been studied for veterinary applications. The ambient odour of lavender reduced travel-induced excitement in dogs, according to a study involving 32 dogs with a history of travel-induced excitement in owners' cars (Wells 2006). Dogs exposed to lavender spent significantly more time resting and sitting, and less time moving and vocalising during the experimental condition.

Lavender aromatherapy has also been found to produce increased resting and reduced movement and vocalisation in dogs housed in a rescue shelter (Graham et al 2005). Daily essential oil baths using *L. angustifolia* for 14 days led to lower stress and trait anxiety in both the experimental and the control groups, but a larger effect occurred in the lavender group (n = 37) (Morris 2008).

Insomnia

In Australia, lavender essential oil is the most popular aromatherapy oil, outselling the second most popular (orange) oil by more than seven times (Kheery (In Essence) pers. commun. 2002). It is often combined with bergamot and cedarwood oils for relieving anxiety and stress and combined with marjoram to induce sleep. A recent systematic review of four RCTs suggests lavender could be beneficial to promote sleep in people with insomnia compared to controls, but the differences in outcome measures, administration methods, other methodological inadequacies such as short duration of the studies and small sample size make it difficult to make definitive conclusions (Fismer & Pilkington 2012). It is most often used as part of an aromatherapy approach, applied topically or inhaled via ambient dispersion.

Since then, a study utilising a combination of essential oils (lavender, roman chamomile and neroli with a 6:2:0.5 ratio) with 56 ICU patients found that it significantly improved sleep quality (P = 0.001) compared with conventional nursing intervention (Cho et al 2013).

Commission E supports the use of oral lavender in mood disturbances such as restlessness and insomnia (Blumenthal et al 2000).

Depression and mood enhancement

According to a 4-week double-blind, RCT, oral lavender tincture (1:5 in 50% alcohol) taken as a dose of 60 drops/day was not as effective as imipramine for treating depression; however, a combination of lavender tincture and imipramine taken together was actually more effective than imipramine used alone and provided quicker improvement (Akhondzadeh et al 2003).

Another RCT of 80 non-depressed women tested the addition of lavender oil to a bath and found this procedure had a general mood-enhancing effect and produced a reduction in pessimism (Morris 2002). Similarly, improved mood and perceived anxiety were reported in a controlled trial of 122 ICU patients who received a massage with lavender oil (Dunn et al 1995).

Cardiovascular effects

Lavender aromatherapy reduced serum cortisol and improved coronary flow velocity reserve (CFVR) in healthy men, suggesting that lavender aromatherapy has relaxation effects and may have beneficial acute effects on coronary circulation (Shiina et al 2008). CFVR was measured with non-invasive transthoracic Doppler echocardiography (TTDE). CFVR was assessed at baseline and immediately after lavender aromatherapy (4 drops of essential oil diluted with 20 mL of hot water and inhaled for 30 minutes). Simultaneously, serum cortisol was measured.

Another study of healthy young women found that lavender aromatic treatment induced not only relaxation but also increased arousal level in these subjects as measured by continuous electrocardiographic (ECG) monitoring before and after (10, 20, 30 minutes) the lavender fragrance stimuli (Duan et al 2007). Increases in the parasympathetic tone were observed after the lavender fragrance stimulus, seen as increases in the heart function component and decreases in the low frequency (LF)/high frequency (HF). Additional measurement with positron emission tomography demonstrated the regional metabolic activation in the orbitofrontal, posterior cingulate gyrus, brainstem, thalamus and cerebellum, as well as the reductions in the pre/post-central gyrus and frontal eye field.

Hypertension — in combination

Seong et al (2013) demonstrated significant differences in systolic blood pressure between treatment and control groups in favour of the treatment group. The study involved 40 male soldiers with >140 mmHg of systolic or >90 mmHg diastolic blood pressure readings who were undergoing preliminary training and not taking antihypertensive medication. The active group used a combination of *L. angustifolia*, ylang ylang, marjoram and neroli for 2 weeks which was administered via inhalation using an aroma stone and aroma necklace. Hypertension was diagnosed using the American Society of Hypertension guidelines.

Dementia care

Managing difficult behaviours in aged care facilities is very challenging. A number of researchers have shown reductions in agitated behaviour using lavender in massage, baths, vaporisers and on bedclothes. These studies generally show positive effects; however, they are difficult to interpret because of the individual nature of behaviour and odour effects on individuals, as well as the methodological differences among the studies.

A placebo-controlled study found that lavender aromatherapy effectively reduced agitated behaviour in 15 patients with severe dementia (Holmes et al 2002), but it had no effect on reducing agitation in another controlled trial of seven severely demented patients (Snow et al 2004), nor was there an effect on reducing resistive behaviour in 13 people with dementia in a residential aged care facility (Gray & Clair 2002). Similarly, a crossover randomised trial of 70 Chinese older adults with dementia demonstrated that lavender inhalation for 3 weeks significantly decreased agitated behaviours (Lin et al 2007). As this patient population is particularly vulnerable to side effects of psychotropic medications, aromatherapy using lavender may offer an attractive alternative option.

In another controlled trial, a 2-week lavender aromatherapy hand massage program produced significant improvements in emotion and aggressive behaviour in elderly people with Alzheimer's type dementia (Lee 2005).

Reducing falls

Lavender administered in patches (n = 73) appears to reduce falls rates in residential aged care facilities compared to standard case (n = 72) when falls and falls incidence was monitored over 360 days (Sakamoto et al 2012). There were significantly fewer falls in the lavender group compared with controls. Likewise, the incident rate was lower: 1.04/person/year compared to 1.40/person per year. In addition, The Cohen-Mansfield Agency Inventory (CMAI) score was lower in the lavender group.

Improved concentration

In an RCT, exposure to lavender aromatherapy during breaks resulted in significantly higher concentration levels during the afternoon period when concentration was found to be lowest in a control group (Sakamoto et al 2005). Lavender oil aromatherapy has also been found to reduce mental stress and increase arousal rate (Motomura et al 2001), to elicit a subjective sense of 'happiness' (Vernet-Maury et al 1999) and to produce increased relaxation, less depressed mood and faster and more accurate mathematical computations (Field et al 2005). In an RCT, lavender aromatherapy tended to enhance calculating speed and calculating accuracy in female but not male subjects (Liu et al 2004); however, results from another study suggest that lavender reduced working memory and impaired reaction times for both memory and attention-based tasks compared with controls (Moss et al 2003).

IN COMBINATION

A controlled study of dementia patients found that a blend of lavender, sweet marjoram, patchouli and vetiver essential oils in a cream massaged five times/day for 4 weeks onto the bodies and limbs of 56 aged care facility residents with moderate-to-severe dementia produced a small but significant improvement in the Mini-Mental State Examination associated with increased mental alertness and awareness and resistance to nursing care procedures compared with massage with cream alone (Bowles et al 2002).

Migraine headache

Inhalation of lavender essential oil for 15 minutes significantly reduced the severity of migraine headache, based on a Visual Analogue Scale, compared with controls ($P < 0.0001$). The placebo-controlled study of 47 patients with a definite diagnosis of migraine headache showed that out of 129 headache attacks, 92 episodes responded entirely or partially to lavender compared to 32 out of 64 headaches responding to placebo. In other words, the percentage of responders was significantly higher in the lavender group than the placebo group ($P = 0.001$) (Sasannejad et al 2012).

Dyspepsia and bloating

Although there have been no clinical trials to investigate its use, lavender is commonly recommended for gastrointestinal disorders as a carminative and antiflatulent to soothe indigestion, colic, dyspepsia and bloating (Blumenthal et al 2000). Based on the antispasmodic actions of a key constituent, linalool, lavender may be useful in these conditions. No controlled clinical studies could be located to determine its effectiveness for these indications.

Alopecia — in combination

An RCT of scalp massage using thyme, rosemary, lavender and cedarwood essential oils in 86 patients with alopecia areata found a significant improvement in hair growth after 7 months (Hay et al 1998). Although the efficacy of lavender as a stand-alone treatment was not clarified with this trial, it is known that the herb has some antibacterial and antifungal activity that may play a role. In a single case study, topical application of lavender, together with other essential oils, was reported to assist in treating scalp eczema (De Valois 2004).

Perineal discomfort following childbirth

An RCT in 635 women following childbirth found that using lavender oil in bath water was safe and pleasant and that there was a tendency towards lower discomfort scores between the third and fifth day (Dale & Cornwell 1994). In that study, 6 drops of pure lavender oil was added to the bath. Vakilian et al (2011) demonstrated less perineal redness using lavender essential oil compared to povidone-iodine in 120 primiparous Pakastani women who had an episotomy. Lavender was administered in a sitz bath.

Likewise, Sheikhan et al (2012) demonstrated lavender 'essence' reduced perineal discomfort following episiotomy in 60 post partum primiparous women in a hospital setting in Iran. Lavender was administered in a sitz bath twice a day for 5 days. The women were randomly allocated to a treatment of control group and self-rated discomfort using a visual analogue scale. Nurses rated the appearance of the perineum for redness and discharge 4-hourly and 12-hourly for 5 days. However, it is not clear what lavender essence was, or even whether it was an essential oil.

Dysmenorrhoea and PMS

Ten minutes of aromatic inhalation with lavender significantly decreased depressive mood and feelings of dejection ($P = 0.045$) and confusion ($P = 0.049$) according to the Profile Of Moods (POMs) scale among women with mild to moderate subjective premenstrual symptoms. The randomised, crossover study of 17 women (20.6 ± 0.2 years) examined exposure to aromatic stimulation on two separate occasions (lavender and control) in the late-luteal phases. The beneficial effects lasted up to 35 minutes after exposure. Additionally, a 10-minute inhalation of the lavender scent significantly increased parasympathetic nervous system activity in comparison with water according to measures taken after 10–15 minutes and again after 20–25 minutes (Matsumoto et al 2013).

IN COMBINATION

Aromatherapy applied topically in the form of an abdominal massage using 2 drops of lavender (*Lavandula officinalis*), 1 drop of clary sage (*Salvia sclarea*) and 1 drop of rose (*Rosa centifolia*) in 5 cc of almond oil significantly decreased the severity of menstrual cramps, according to a randomised, placebo-controlled study (Han et al 2006). The study involved 67 female college students who rated their menstrual cramps to be greater than 6 on a 10-point visual analogue scale, who had no systemic or reproductive diseases and who did not use contraceptive drugs.

Acute external otitis — in combination

A randomised study of 70 subjects demonstrated that application of a combination herbal drop consisting of *Syzygum aromaticum*, *L angustifolia* and *Geranium robertainum* (Lamigex 1 drop) was as effective as Ciprofloxacin 0.3% drops after a week of treatment. Three drops were applied every 12 hours for a week ($n = 70$: 35 in each group). Tenderness, itching, erythema, oedema and discharge were all improved by the end of the treatment period ($P > 0.05$). Additionally, the rate of pain relief was the same with both treatments when evaluated on day 3 and day 7 ($P > 0.05$). Importantly, the number of positive cultures tested for micro-organisms were the same for both groups, indicating successful antibiotic effects (Panahi et al 2012).

Pain reduction

It has been suggested that the relaxing effects may be useful in the treatment of chronic pain (Buckle 1999), and this is supported by a study reporting that while lavender did not elicit a direct analgesic effect, it did alter affective appraisal of the pain experience with retrospective impression of pain intensity and pain unpleasantness from experimentally induced heat, pressure and ischaemic pain being reduced after treatment with lavender aromatherapy (Gedney & Glover 2004).

In an RCT, eight sessions of acupressure using lavender essential oil over 3 weeks was found to be effective in relieving pain, neck stiffness and stress in 32 adults with sub-acute non-specific neck pain (Yip & Tse 2006). Alternatively, one RCT involving 42 subjects found that the addition of lavender essential oil did not appear to increase the beneficial effects of massage for patients with advanced cancer (Soden et al 2004).

OTHER USES

Lavender has a long history of use as a sedative, an antidepressant, an antimicrobial agent, a carminative (smooth muscle relaxant), a topical analgesic agent for burns and insect bites (Cavanagh & Wilkinson 2002) and an insect repellent. Lavender has also been used to treat migraines and neuralgia, as an astringent to treat minor cuts and bruises, and is used externally for strained muscles, as well as acne, eczema and varicose ulcers (Fisher & Painter 1996). It is also used in a gargle for loss of voice.

DOSAGE RANGE

Probably no other herb is available in as many forms as lavender.

- Infusion (tea): 1.5 g dried flowers in 150 mL water, which is 1–2 teaspoons lavender flowers or

leaves in one cup of boiling water steeped for 5–10 minutes and strained before drinking.
- Internal: 1–4 drops (20–80 mg) on a sugar cube.
- Liquid extract (1:2): 2–4.5 mL/day.
- External use: mix 20 drops of oil with 20 mL of carrier oil such as almond oil. May be applied undiluted to insect bites or stings.
- As a bath additive: 20–100 g lavender flowers are commonly steeped in 2 L boiling water, strained, and then added to the bathwater. Alternatively 5–7 drops are added to the bath and stirred to mix the oil into the water.
- Aromatherapy: use 2–4 drops of lavender oil in a suitable oil diffuser or on a pillowcase to assist sleep.

Lavender oil is quickly absorbed by the skin and constituents linalool and linalyl acetate have been detected in the blood 5 minutes after administration. Blood levels peak after 19 minutes and are negligible by 90 minutes.

According to clinical studies

Anxiety, restlessness and depression: Silexan 80 mg/day

TOXICITY

McGuffin (1997) lists lavender as a Class I herb, a classification which represents herbs that can be 'safely consumed when used appropriately'. The acute oral toxicity dose (LD_{50}) in rats for lavender and linalool are 5 g/kg and 2.8 g/kg, respectively and the acute dermal toxicity in rabbits is 5 g/kg and 5.6 g/kg, respectively (Kiefer 2007). These doses would translate to approximately 350 g lavender oil or 1.5 cups. Although there are very few specific reports of toxicity, it is suggested that no more than 2 drops be taken internally.

ADVERSE EFFECTS

Topical use

The prevalence of dermatitis and skin allergies to essential oils, including lavender, increases with the duration of exposure, representing a cumulative risk: 1.1–13.9% over 13 years (Wu et al 2011). Dermatitis appears to be a cumulative occupational risk for aromatherapists applying essential oils in massage over long periods of time.

There is a potential for irritant or allergenic skin reactions with the topical use of lavender oil, as it has been found to be cytotoxic to human skin cells in vitro (endothelial cells and fibroblasts) at a concentration of 0.25% v/v, possibly due to membrane damage. The activity of linalool was found to reflect the cytotoxicity of the whole oil, whereas the cytotoxicity of linalyl acetate was found to be higher than that of the oil, suggesting suppression of its activity by an unknown factor in the oil (Prashar et al 2004). Three case reports have been published of gynaecomastia developing in boys aged four, seven and ten following regular topical use of lavender-containing products (soap, shampoo and lotions) (Henley et al 2007). Henley et al postulated that lavender has oestrogenic and antiandrogenic effects on several different cell lines. The implications for clinical practice and aromatherapy are unknown.

Skin sensitivity to lavender might develop with increased exposure and prolonged use (Sugiura et al 2000).

Oral use

Controlled studies with Silexan, a commercial lavender oil product manufactured for oral consumption, report that mild gastrointestinal symptoms are the most common side effect.

Practice points/Patient counselling

- The active part of lavender is the volatile oil, which has relaxing, sedative, antispasmodic and antiseptic activity.
- Lavender can be taken as a tincture or tea, or the oil can be applied topically, used in baths or inhaled from a diffuser.
- It is advised that topical preparations be tested on a small area of skin before widespread application.
- Lavender has traditionally been used for sleep disorders, anxiety and nervous stomach, as well as to treat minor cuts, burns, bruises and insect bites and is commonly found in cosmetics and toiletries.
- Ambient lavender induces a relaxation response in healthy people, the elderly with dementia, and agitation and also dogs with travel-induced excitement. It also may improve mood in women with mild to moderate PMS symptoms, enhance memory and concentration, reduce the severity of migraine headache.
- Abdominal massage with lavender oil (in combination with several others) has been shown to reduce menstrual cramps to a better degree than a non-aromatherapy oil.
- Recent studies with a commercial oral lavender preparation supports its use for insomnia.

SIGNIFICANT INTERACTIONS

Controlled studies are rarely available; however, the American Society for Pharmacology and Experimental Therapeutics (Doroshyenko et al 2013) found repeated doses of 160 mg/day of an oral lavender oil preparation Silexan did not significantly inhibit or induce the CYP 1A2, 2C9, 2C19, 2D6, or 3A4 liver enzymes in in vivo studies.

Pharmaceutical sedatives

Theoretically, lavender can potentiate the effects of sedatives, so observe patients taking this combination closely — beneficial interaction possible under professional supervision.

Antidepressants

Lavender tincture may have additive effects when used with these medicines — beneficial interaction possible.

PREGNANCY USE

No restrictions known for external use.

Safety of internal use has not been scientifically established.

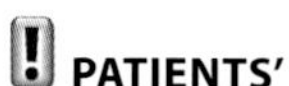

PATIENTS' FAQs

What will this herb do for me?

Lavender oil is often used together with other essential oils to assist relaxation, sleep disturbances, digestive problems and as first aid for minor skin conditions. Ambient lavender can improve mood in women with mild to moderate PMS, reduce the severity of migraine headache, induce a relaxation response in healthy people and older people with dementia and agitation, and also calms dogs during travel. Used as part of an aromatherapy massage, it also has antispasmodic activity. There is also research that a commercial lavender oil capsule has benefits in insomnia and when lavender is administered in patches, reduces falls rates in residential aged care.

When will it start to work?

As a relaxant, effects may be felt on the first day of use, but depends on the dose and dose form used.

Are there any safety issues?

Topical lavender oil is considered generally safe although skin irritation can occur whereas oral lavender (Silexan) has been associated with gastrointestinal discomfort in some people.

REFERENCES

Abe S et al. Suppression of tumor necrosis factor-alpha-induced neutrophil adherence responses by essential oils. Mediat Inflamm 12.6 (2003): 323–328.

Aburjai TM et al. Chemical composition of the essential oil from different aerial parts of lavender (Lavandula coronopofolia Poiert) (Lamiaceae) grown in Jordan. J Essent Oil Res 17.1 (2005): 49–51.

Akhondzadeh S et al. Comparison of Lavandula angustifolia Mill. tincture and imipramine in the treatment of mild to moderate depression: a double-blind, randomized trial. Prog Neuro-Psychopharmacol Biol Psychiatry 27.1 (2003): 123–127.

Alnamer R et al. Sedative and hypnotic activities of the methanolic and aqueous extracts of Lavandula officinalis from Morocco. Adv Pharmacol Sci (2012): 270824.

Bailey HH et al. A phase II trial of daily perillyl alcohol in patients with advanced ovarian cancer: Eastern Cooperative Oncology Group Study E2E96. Gynecol Oncol 85.3 (2002): 464–468.

Ballabeni V et al. Novel antiplatelet and antithrombotic activities of essential oil from Lavandula hybrida Reverchon grosso. Phytomedicine 11.7–8 (2004): 596–601.

Battaglia S. The complete guide to aromatherapy. Brisbane: The Perfect Potion, 1995.

Blumenthal M et al. (eds). Herbal medicine: expanded Commission E monographs. Austin, TX: Integrative Medicine Communications, 2000.

Bowles EJ et al. Effects of essential oils and touch on resistance to nursing care procedures and other dementia-related behaviours in a residential care facility. Int J Aromather 12.1 (2002): 22–29.

Braden R et al. The use of the essential oil lavandin to reduce preoperative anxiety in surgical patients. J Perianesth Nurs 24.6 (2009): 348–355.

Bradley BF et al. Effects of orally administered lavender essential oil on responses to anxiety-provoking film clips. Hum Psychopharmacol 24.4 (2009): 319–330.

Buchbauer G et al. Aromatherapy: evidence for sedative effects of the essential oil of lavender after inhalation. Z Naturforsch C 46.11–12 (1991): 1067–1072.

Buckle J. Use of aromatherapy as a complementary treatment for chronic pain. Altern Ther Health Med 5.5 (1999): 42–51.

Burnett KM et al. Scent and mood state following an anxiety-provoking task. Psychol Rep 95.2 (2004): 707–722.

Cassella SJ et al. Synergistic antifungal activity of tea tree (Melaleuca alternifolia) and lavender (Lavandula angustifolia) essential oils against dermatophyte infection. Int J Aromather 12.1 (2002): 2–15.

Cavanagh HM, Wilkinson JM. Biological activities of lavender essential oil. Phytother Res 16.4 (2002): 301–308.

Cavanagh H, Wilkinson J. Lavender essential oil: a review. Australian Infection Control 10.1 (2005): 35–37.

Chioca L et al. Anxiolytic-like effect of lavender and orange essential oil: participation of nitric oxide but not GABA-A benzodiazepine complex. European Pharmacology 21 (3) (2011): S538.

Cho MY et al. Effects of aromatherapy on the anxiety, vital signs, and sleep quality of percutaneous coronary intervention patients in intensive care units. Evid Based Complement Alternat Med (2013): 381381.

Chung B et al. Perillyl alcohol inhibits the expression and function of the androgen receptor in human prostate cancer cells. Cancer Lett 236.2 (2006): 222–228.

Cornwell S, Dale A. Lavender oil and perineal repair. Mod Midwife 5.3 (1995): 31–33.

D'Auria FD et al. Antifungal activity of Lavandula angustifolia essential oil against Candida albicans yeast and mycelial form. Med Mycol 43.5 (2005): 391–396.

Dadalioglu I, Evrendilek GA. Chemical compositions and antibacterial effects of essential oils of Turkish oregano (Origanum minutiflorum), bay laurel (Laurus nobilis), Spanish lavender (Lavandula stoechas L.), and fennel (Foeniculum vulgare) on common foodborne pathogens. J Agric Food Chem 52.26 (2004): 8255–8260.

Daferera DJ et al. GC-MS analysis of essential oils from some Greek aromatic plants and their fungitoxicity on Penicillin digitatum. J Agric Food Chem 48 (2000): 2576–2581.

Dale A, Cornwell S. The role of lavender oil in relieving perineal discomfort following childbirth: a blind randomized clinical trial. J Adv Nurs 19.1 (1994): 89–96.

Danh L et al. Antioxidant activity, yield and chemical composition of lavender essential oil extracted by supercritical CO2. J Supercritical Fluids 70 (2012) 27–34.

De Valois B. Using essential oils to treat scalp eczema. Int J Aromather 14.1 (2004): 45–47.

Diego MA et al. Aromatherapy positively affects mood, EEG patterns of alertness and math computations. Int J Neurosci 96.3–4 (1998): 217–224.

Dimpfel W et al. Effects of lozenge containing lavender oil, extracts from hops, lemon balm and oat on electrical brain activity of volunteers. Eur J Med Res 9.9 (2004): 423–431.

Doroshyenko O et al. Cocktail Interaction Study on the Effect of the Orally Administered Lavender Oil Preparation Silexan on Cytochrome P-450 Enzymes in Healthy Volunteers. Drug Metab Dispos. 2013

Duan X et al. Autonomic nervous function and localization of cerebral activity during lavender aromatic immersion. Technol Health Care 15.2 (2007): 69–78.

Dunn C et al. Sensing an improvement: an experimental study to evaluate the use of aromatherapy, massage and periods of rest in an intensive care unit. J Adv Nurs 21.1 (1995): 34–40.

Elson CE et al. Isoprenoid-mediated inhibition of mevalonate synthesis: Potential application to cancer. Proc Soc Exp Biol Med 221.4 (1999): 294–311.

Evandri MG et al. The antimutagenic activity of Lavandula angustifolia (lavender) essential oil in the bacterial reverse mutation assay. Food Chem Toxicol 43.9 (2005): 1381–1387.

Field T et al. Lavender fragrance cleansing gel effects on relaxation. Int J Neurosci 115.2 (2005): 207–222.

Fisher C, Painter G. Materia medica for the Southern Hemisphere. Auckland: Fisher-Painter Publishers, 1996.

Fismer K, Pilkington K. Lavender and sleep: a systematic review of the evidence. European Journal of Integrative Medicine 4 (2012) e436–477.

Gedney JJ et al. Sensory and affective pain discrimination after inhalation of essential oils. Psychosom Med 66.4 (2004): 599–606.

Goel N, Grasso DJ. Olfactory discrimination and transient mood change in young men and women: variation by season, mood state, and time of day. Chronobiol Int 21.4–5 (2004): 691–719.

Goel N et al. An olfactory stimulus modifies nighttime sleep in young men and women. Chronobiol Int 22.5 (2005): 889–904.

Gould MN. Cancer chemoprevention and therapy by monoterpenes. Environ Health Perspect 105 (Suppl 4) (1997): 977–979.

Graham P et al. Inhalation aromatherapy during radiotherapy: results of a placebo-controlled double-blind randomized trial. J Clin Oncol 21.12 (2003): 2372–2376.

Graham L et al. The influence of olfactory stimulation on the behaviour of dogs housed in a rescue shelter. Appl Anim Behav Sci 91.1–2 (2005): 143–153.
Gray SG, Clair AA. Influence of aromatherapy on medication administration to residential-care residents with dementia and behavioral challenges. Am J Alzheimers Dis Other Demen 17.3 (2002): 169–174.
Gulcin I et al. Comparison of antioxidant activity of clove (Eugenia caryophylata Thunb.) buds and lavender (Lavandula stoechas L.). Food Chem 87.3 (2004): 393–400.
Han SH et al. Effect of aromatherapy on symptoms of dysmenorrhea in college students: a randomized placebo-controlled clinical trial. J Altern Complement Med 12.6 (2006): 535–541.
Hay IC, Jamieson M, Ormerod AD. Randomized trial of aromatherapy. Successful treatment for alopecia areata [comment]. Arch Dermatol 134.11 (1998): 1349–1352.
Henley D et al. Prepubertal gynaecomastia linked to lavender and tee tree oils. N Engl J Med 356 (2007): 479–485.
Heuberger E, Redhammer S, Buchbauer G. Transdermal absorption of (-)-linalool induces autonomic deactivation but has no impact on ratings of well-being in humans. Neuropsychopharmacology 29.10 (2004): 1925–1932.
Hirokawa K et al. Effects of lavender aroma on sleep quality in healthy Japanese students. perceptual and motor skills 114.1 (2012): 111–122.
Hohl RJ. Monoterpenes as regulators of malignant cell proliferation. Adv Exp Med Biol 401 (1996): 137–146.
Holmes C et al. Lavender oil as a treatment for agitated behaviour in severe dementia: a placebo controlled study. Int J Geriatr Psychiatry 17.4 (2002): 305–308.
Howard S, Hughes BM. Expectancies, not aroma, explain impact of lavender aromatherapy on psychophysiological indices of relaxation in young healthy women. Br J Health Psychol 13 (Pt 4) (2008): 603–617.
Hritcu L et al. Effects of lavender oil inhalation on improving scopolamine-induced spatial memory impairment in laboratory rats. Phytomedicine 19 (2012) 529–534.
Inouye S et al. In-vitro and in-vivo anti-trichophyton activity of essential oils by vapour contact. Mycoses 44.3–4 (2001): 99–107.
Kasper S et al. Silexan, an orally administered Lavandula oil preparation, is effective in the treatment of 'subsyndromal' anxiety disorder: a randomized, double-blind, placebo controlled trial. Int Clin Psychopharmacol 25.5(2010): 277–287.
Katdare M et al. Prevention of mammary preneoplastic transformation by naturally-occurring tumor inhibitors. Cancer Lett 111.1–2 (1997): 141–147.
Kawakami K et al. The calming effect of stimuli presentation on infant Japanese Macaques (Macaca fuscata) under stress situation: a preliminary study. Primates 43.1 (2002): 73–85.
Kelloff GJ et al. Progress in cancer chemoprevention. Ann N Y Acad Sci 889 (1999): 1–113.
Kiefer D. Who needs benzos? Lavender and insomnia. Alternative Medicine Alert 10.7 (2007): 73–76.
Kim HM, Cho SH. Lavender oil inhibits immediate-type allergic reaction in mice and rats. J Pharm Pharmacol 51.2 (1999): 221–226.
Kirk-Smith M. The psychological effects of lavender II: scientific and clinical evidence. Int J Aromather 13.2–3 (2003): 82–89.
Kritsidima M et al. The effects of lavender scent on dental patient anxiety levels: a cluster randomised-controlled trial. Community Dent Oral Epidemiol 38.1 (2010): 83–87.
Kuroda K et al. Sedative effects of the jasmine tea odor and (R)-(-)-linalool, one of its major odor components, on autonomic nerve activity and mood states. Eur J Appl Physiol 95.2–3 (2005): 107–114.
Kutlu AK et al. Effects of aroma inhalation on examination anxiety. Teaching & Learning in Nursing 3.4 (2008): 125–130.
Larrondo JVA et al. Antimicrobial activity of essences from labiates. Microbios 82.332 (1995): 171–172.
Lee CF et al. Responses of electroencephalogram to different odors. Ann Physiol Anthropol 13.5 (1994): 281–291.
Lee SY. The effect of lavender aromatherapy on cognitive function, emotion, and aggressive behavior of elderly with dementia. Taehan Kanho Hakhoe Chi 35.2 (2005): 303–312.
Lim WC et al. Stimulative and sedative effects of essential oils upon inhalation in mice. Arch Pharm Res 28.7 (2005): 770–774.
Lin PW et al. Efficacy of aromatherapy (Lavandula angustifolia) as an intervention for agitated behaviours in Chinese older persons with dementia: a cross-over randomized trial. Int J Geriatr Psychiatry 22.5 (2007): 405–410.
Lis-Balchin M, Hart S. Studies on the mode of action of the essential oil of lavender (Lavandula angustifolia P. Miller). Phytother Res 13.6 (1999): 540–542.
Liston BW et al. Perillyl alcohol as a chemopreventive agent in N-nitrosomethylbenzylamine-induced rat esophageal tumorigenesis. Cancer Res 63.10 (2003): 2399–2403.
Liu G et al. Phase II trial of perillyl alcohol (NSC 641066) administered daily in patients with metastatic androgen independent prostate cancer. Invest New Drugs 21.3 (2003): 367–372.
Liu M et al. Influences of lavender fragrance and cut flower arrangements on cognitive performance. Int J Aromather 14.4 (2004): 169–174.
Matsumoto T et al. Does lavender aromatherapy alleviate premenstrual emotional symptoms?: a randomized crossover trial. Biopsychosoc Med 7.1 (2013): 12.
McGuffin M (ed). American Herbal Association's Botanical Safety Handbook. Boca Raton, FL: CRC Press, 1997.
Meadows SM et al. Phase II trial of perillyl alcohol in patients with metastatic colorectal cancer. Int J Gastrointest Cancer 32.2–3 (2002): 125–128.
Micromedex. Lavender. Thomson, 2003. Available online: www.micromedex.com.
Mills JJ et al. Induction of apoptosis in liver tumors by the monoterpene perillyl alcohol. Cancer Res 55.5 (1995): 979–983.
Miyazawa M et al. Metabolism of (+)- and (−)-limonenes to respective carveols and perillyl alcohols by CYP2C9 and CYP2C19 in human liver microsomes. Drug Metab Dispos 30.5 (2002a): 602–7.
Miyazawa M et al. Sex differences in the metabolism of (+)- and (−)-limonene enantiomers to carveol and perillyl alcohol derivatives by cytochrome P450 enzymes in rat liver microsomes. Chem Res Toxicol 15.1 (2002b): 15–20.
Morris N. The effects of lavender (Lavendula angustifolium) baths on psychological well-being: two exploratory randomised control trials. Complement Ther Med 10.4 (2002): 223–228.
Morris N. The effects of lavender (Lavandula angustifolia) essential oil baths on stress and anxiety. International Journal of Clinical Aromatherapy 5.1 (2008): 3–7.
Moss M et al. Aromas of rosemary and lavender essential oils differentially affect cognition and mood in healthy adults. Int J Neurosci 113.1 (2003): 15–38.
Motomura N et al. Reduction of mental stress with lavender odorant. Percept Mot Skills 93.3 (2001): 713–718.
Muzzarelli L et al. Aromatherapy and reducing preprocedural anxiety: A controlled prospective study. Gastroenterol Nurs 29.6 (2006): 466–471.
Nelson RR. In-vitro activities of five plant essential oils against methicillin-resistant Staphylococcus aureus and vancomycin-resistant Enterococcus faecium. J Antimicrob Chemother 40.2 (1997): 305–326.
Panahi Y et al. Investigation of the effectiveness of Syzygium aromaticum, Lavandula angustifolia and Geranium robertianum essential oils in the treatment of acute external otitis: A comparative trial with ciprofloxacin. J Microbiol Immunol Infect (2012): 1144–1150.
Perrucci S et al. The activity of volatile compounds from Lavandula angustifolia against psoroptes cuniculi. Phytother Res 10.1 (1996): 5–8.
Perry R et al. Is lavender an anxiolytic drug? A systematic review of randomised clinical traila. Phytomedicines 19 (2012) 825–835.
Prashar A et al. Cytotoxicity of lavender oil and its major components to human skin cells. Cell Prolif 37.3 (2004): 221–229.
Rakotonirainy MS, Lavedrine B. Screening for antifungal activity of essential oils and related compounds to control the biocontamination in libraries and archives storage areas. Int Biodeterior Biodegrad 55.2 (2005): 141–147.
Refaat AM et al. Acaricidal activity of sweet basil and French lavender essential oils against two species of mites of the family tetranychidae (Acari: Tetranychidae). Acta Phytopathol Entomol Hung 37.1–3 (2002): 287–298.
Ren Z, Gould MN. Inhibition of ubiquinone and cholesterol synthesis by the monoterpene perillyl alcohol. Cancer Lett 76.2–3 (1994): 185–190.
Rhaffari L et al. Chemical composition and antibacterial properties of the essential oil of Lavendula multifida L. International Journal of Essential Oil Therapeutics 1 (2007): 122–125.
Sakamoto R et al. Effectiveness of aroma on work efficiency: Lavender aroma during recesses prevents deterioration of work performance. Chem Senses 30.8 (2005): 683–691.
Sakamoto Y et al. Fall prevention using olfactory stimulation with lavender odor in elderly nursing home residents: a randomized controlled. J Am Geriatr Soc. 60.6 (2012):1005–1011.
Sanders C et al. EEG asymmetry responses to lavender and rosemary aromas in adults and infants. Int J Neurosci 112.11 (2002): 1305–1320.
Sasannejad P et al. Lavender essential oil in the treatment of migraine headache: a placebo-controlled clinical trial. Eur Neurol 67.5 (2012): 288–291.
Sayorwan W et al The effects of lavender oil inhalation on emotional states, autonomic nervous system, and brain electrical activity N. J Med Assoc Thai. 2 95 4 2012: 598–606.
Schulz V et al. Rational phytotherapy: a physician's guide to herbal medicine. Berlin: Springer, 1998.
Seong K et al. Two week aroma inhalation effects on blood pressure in young men with essential hypertension. European Journal of Integrative Medicine (2013)Doi.org/10.1016/eujm.2012.12.003

Sgoutas-Emch, S et al. Stress management: aromatherapy as an alternative. Scientific Review of Alternative Medicine 5.2 (2001): 90–95.
Shaw D et al. Chlordiazepoxide and lavender oil alter unconditioned anxiety-induced c-fos expression in rat brain. Behavioural Braon Research 224 (2011): 1–7.
Sheikhan F et al. Eposotomy pain relief: use of lavender oil essence in primiparous Iranian women. Complementary Therapies in Clinical Practice 18 (2012) 66–70.
Shi W, Gould MN. Induction of differentiation in neuro-2A cells by the monoterpene perillyl alcohol. Cancer Lett 95.1–2 (1995): 1–6.
Shi W, Gould MN. Induction of cytostasis in mammary carcinoma cells treated with the anticancer agent perillyl alcohol. Carcinogenesis 23.1 (2002): 131–142.
Shiina Y et al. Relaxation effects of lavender aromatherapy improve coronary flow velocity reserve in healthy men evaluated by transthoracic Doppler echocardiography. Int J Cardiol 129.2 (2008): 193–197.
Snow AL et al. A controlled trial of aromatherapy for agitation in nursing home patients with dementia. J Altern Complement Med 10.3 (2004): 431–437.
Soden K et al. A randomized controlled trial of aromatherapy massage in a hospice setting. Palliat Med 18.2 (2004): 87–92.
Sosa S et al. Extracts and constituents of Lavandula multifida with topical anti-inflammatory activity. Phytomedicine 12.4 (2005): 271–277.
Stayrook KR et al. Induction of the apoptosis-promoting protein Bak by perillyl alcohol in pancreatic ductal adenocarcinoma relative to untransformed ductal epithelial cells. Carcinogenesis 18.8 (1997): 1655–1658.
Sugiura M et al. Results of patch testing with lavender oil in Japan. Contact Dermatitis 43 (2000): 157–160.
Toda M, Morimoto K. Effect of lavender aroma on salivary endocrinological stress markers. Arch Oral Biol 53.10 (2008): 964–968.
Uehleke B et al. Phase II trial on the effects of Silexan in patients with neurasthenia, post-traumatic stress disorder or somatization disorder. Phytomedicine 19.8–9 (2012): 665–671.
Vakilian K et al. healing advantages of lavender essential oil during episiotomy recovery. Complementary Therapies in Clinical Practice 17 (2011): 50–53.
Vernet-Maury E et al. Basic emotions induced by odorants: a new approach based on autonomic pattern results. J Auton Nerv Syst 75.2–3 (1999): 176–183.
Walsh E et al. Integrating complementary and alternative medicine: use of essential oils in hypertension, Journal of Vascular Nursing (2011).
Wells DL. Aromatherapy for travel-induced excitement in dogs. J Am Vet Med Assoc 229.6 (2006): 964–967.
Woelk H, Schlafke S. A multi-center, double-blind, randomised study of the Lavender oil preparation Silexan in comparison to Lorazepam for generalized anxiety disorder. Phytomedicine 17.2 2010): 94–99.
Wu PA, James WD. Lavender. Dermatitis. 2011 Nov-Dec;22(6):344–7. doi: 10.2310/6620.2011.11040.
Yagyu T. Neurophysiological findings on the effects of fragrance: lavender and jasmine. Integr Psychiatry 10.2 (1994): 62–67.
Yamada K et al. Anticonvulsive effects of inhaling lavender oil vapour. Biol Pharm Bull 17.2 (1994): 359–360.
Yamada K et al. Effects of inhaling the vapor of Lavandula burnatii super-derived essential oil and linalool on plasma adrenocorticotropic hormone (ACTH), catecholamine and gonadotropin levels in experimental menopausal female rats. Biol Pharm Bull 28.2 (2005): 378–379.
Yip YB, Tse SH. An experimental study on the effectiveness of acupressure with aromatic lavender essential oil for sub-acute, non-specific neck pain in Hong Kong. Complement Ther Clin Pract 12.1 (2006): 18–26.
Yuri T et al. Perillyl alcohol inhibits human breast cancer cell growth in vitro and in vivo. Breast Cancer Res Treat 84.3 (2004): 251–260.

Lemon balm

HISTORICAL NOTE Lemon balm was used in ancient Greece and Rome as a topical treatment for wounds. In the Middle Ages it was used internally as a sedative and, by the 17th century, English herbalist Culpeper claimed it could improve mood and stimulate clear thinking (Myers 2007). Nowadays, it is still used to induce a sense of calm and help with anxiety, and it is also added to cosmetics, insect repellents, furniture polish and food.

COMMON NAME

Lemon balm

OTHER NAMES

Balm mint, bee balm, blue balm, common balm, cure-all, dropsy plant, garden balm, sweet balm

BOTANICAL NAME/FAMILY

Melissa officinalis (family Lamiaceae)

PLANT PART USED

Aerial parts

CHEMICAL COMPONENTS

Flavonoids, phenolic acids, tannins, triterpenes, essential oil and sesquiterpenes. Of note, the herb contains citronellal, caffeic acid, eugenol, rosmarinic acid, choline, ursolic acid and oleanolic acid (Wake et al 2000, Yoo et al 2011). Caftaric acid, *p*-cumaric acid, ferulic acid, luteolin and apigenin have also been identified (Hanganu et al 2008). Growing and harvesting methods have a major influence on the amount of volatile oil present in the leaves. It has been found that the oil content in the herb is highest in the top third and lowest in the bottom two-thirds (Mrlianova et al 2002).

> ***Clinical note***
> Long before the current biologically based theory of cholinergic abnormalities in Alzheimer's dementia emerged, Western European medicine systems traditionally used several herbs that are now known to exert cholinergic activity (such as sage and lemon balm) for their dementia-treating properties.

MAIN ACTIONS

Anxiolytic, sedative

Over the years, a number of studies involving rodents have suggested specific anxiolytic or sedative effects (Abuhamdah et al 2008, Ibarra et al 2010,

Kennedy et al 2002, Soulimani et al 1991, Taiwo et al 2012). A number of possible active components of the dried leaf and essential oil of the herb may be responsible for these effects, such as eugenol and citronellol, which bind to gamma-aminobutyric acid-A (GABA-A) receptors and increase the affinity of GABA to receptors (Aoshima & Hamamoto 1999).

A 2009 in vitro study found a methanol extract of lemon balm caused inhibition of rat brain GABA transaminase, the enzyme responsible for GABA degradation (Awad et al 2009). This effect was attributed to rosmarinic acid, a major constituent of lemon balm that has been shown to possess anti-anxiety properties in vivo (Pereira et al 2005).

Antidepressant activity

A rodent study investigated the antidepressant-like activity of an aqueous extract and the essential oil of lemon balm using a forced-swim test model. Both the aqueous extract and the essential oil demonstrated significant antidepressant effects. The antidepressant effect of the aqueous extract was similar to that of the reference drug imipramine. The aqueous extract also demonstrated a sedative effect not seen in the essential oil. The mechanism of the antidepressant effect of the aqueous extract and essential oil of lemon balm is unknown and requires further investigation (Emamghoreishi & Talebianpour 2009).

Antiviral

A lemon balm extract was found to have significant virucidal effects against herpes simplex virus-1 (HSV-1) within 3 and 6 hours of treatment in vitro and in animal tests (Dimitrova et al 1993). The volatile oils from *Melissa officinalis* have also been shown to inhibit the replication of HSV-2 in vitro (Allahverdiyer et al 2004).

A hydroalcoholic extract of lemon balm showed a significant virucidal effect against HSV-2 activity in vitro, and demonstrated a concentration-dependent inhibition of viral replication, with a maximum effect of 60% inhibition of viral replication achieved at 0.5 mg/mL (Mazzanti et al 2008).

An aqueous extract of lemon balm, as well as isolated phenolic compounds caffeic acid, *p*-coumaric acid and rosmarinic acid, exhibits strong antiviral activity against HSV-1 in vitro. Rosmarinic acid had the strongest effects; however the complete lemon balm extract demonstrated superior activity at lower doses than any of the isolated compounds, suggesting a synergistic effect (Astani et al 2012).

Two more studies have demonstrated the antiviral effects of lemon balm against HSV in plaque reduction assays. One study used an essential oil preparation, while the other used an aqueous extract (Nolkemper et al 2006, Schnitzler et al 2008). Both studies demonstrated > 90% inhibition of plaque formation for HSV-1 and HSV-2, and in one study an aciclovir-resistant strain of HSV-1 was reduced by 85% (Nolkemper et al 2006). Both studies also found that lemon balm affected HSV before adsorption, but had no effect on viral replication.

Lemon balm has demonstrated a virucidal effect against HIV-1 in T-cell lines and macrophages in vitro (Geuenich et al 2008). Inhibitory activity against HIV-1 reverse transcriptase has also been shown (Yamasaki et al 1998).

Antibacterial and antifungal

Lemon balm extract exhibited activity against bacteria, filamentous fungi and yeasts in vitro (Larrondo et al 1995). Lemon balm extracts have demonstrated moderate to strong antibacterial activity against *Sarcina lutea*, *Staphylococcus aureus* and *Bacillus cereus* in vitro (Canadanovic-Brunet et al 2008).

It is likely that the constituent eugenol is chiefly responsible, as it has well-established antibacterial activity against organisms such as *Escherichia coli* and *S. aureus* (Walsh et al 2003).

An in vitro study found that lemon balm essential oil exhibited a higher degree of antibacterial activity than lavender oil against Gram-positive strains, while both oil samples demonstrated a high activity against *Candida albicans*. Lemon balm oil displayed poor activity against Gram-negative bacteria. This study identified citral (a mixture of neral and geranial, 16.10%), citronellal (3.76%) and trans-caryophyllene (3.57%) as the chief antimicrobial constituents in lemon balm essential oil (Hancianu et al 2008).

An aqueous extract of lemon balm inhibited *Candida albicans* mycelial growth in vitro. However, green tea, cassia and lemon grass preparations demonstrated even greater antifungal activity against *C. albicans* (Taguchi et al 2010).

Cholinergic

Lemon balm appears to increase activity in the cholinergic system in the brain; this is necessary for memory and attention. Lemon balm exhibits central nervous system acetylcholine receptor activity, with both nicotinic and muscarinic-binding properties (Perry et al 1996, Wake et al 2000). In vitro data have demonstrated that lemon balm has a moderate affinity to the GABA-A benzodiazepine receptor site (Salah & Jager 2005). The essential oil has demonstrated reversible inhibition of GABA-induced currents in rat cortical neurons (Huang et al 2008) and inhibitory activities on both aetylcholinesterase and butyrylcholinesterase (Chaiyana & Okonogi 2012, Orhan et al 2008). Isolated compounds from lemon balm, including *cis*- and *trans*-rosmarinic acid, have shown a very high inhibitory activity against acetylcholinesterase in vitro (Dastmalchi et al 2009). These studies indicate that lemon balm may have a role to play in the treatment of Alzheimer's disease and epilepsy. However, a 2003 randomised, double-blind, placebo-controlled, crossover trial demonstrated that lemon balm did not inhibit cholinesterase. The trial demonstrated improved cognitive function and mood and concluded that for these reasons it was a valuable adjunct to Alzheimer's therapy (Kennedy et al 2003).

Anti-inflammatory, analgesic

The plant extract exerts analgesic activity at high doses in vivo (Soulimani et al 1991). A rodent study documented the dose-related analgesic effect of ethanolic extracts of lemon balm and rosmarinic acid produced via activation of cholinergic and inhibition of L-arginine-nitric oxide pathways (Guginski et al 2009).

Two constituents in lemon balm have documented anti-inflammatory activity, achieved through different mechanisms of action. Rosmarinic acid, a naturally occurring constituent found in *Melissa officinalis*, inhibits several complement-dependent inflammatory processes (Englberger et al 1988, Peake et al 1991). Eugenol, another important component, inhibits cyclooxygenase-1 (COX-1) and -2 activities in vitro (Huss et al 2002, Kelm et al 2000).

Presently, little clinical research has been conducted to determine whether topical application of lemon balm preparations have an anti-inflammatory effect.

To date, one randomised, placebo-controlled study of 40 healthy subjects investigated the anti-inflammatory activity of a topical lemon balm application for ultraviolet (UV)-induced erythema and found it was ineffective as used in the study. Test areas on the upper back were irradiated with 1.5-fold of the UV-B minimal erythema dose. A formulation of lemon balm was applied under occlusion to the irradiated areas and to a non-irradiated area on the contralateral side (Beikert et al 2013).

Antispasmodic

Both the whole volatile oil and its main component citral have demonstrated antispasmodic ability on isolated rat ileum (Sadraei et al 2003). Similarly, both the aqueous extract and rosmarinic acid component demonstrated vasorelaxant properties on isolated rat aorta (Ersoy et al 2008). An in vivo study has shown both an extract of lemon balm and the herbal formulation ColiMil (chamomile, fennel and lemon balm) may delay gastric emptying (Capasso et al 2007). The group treated with lemon balm exhibited 36% inhibition, chamomile 28% and fennel 9% as compared to 45% for the ColiMil group, suggesting a synergistic action.

Antioxidant

Lemon balm has shown antioxidant activity in several studies (Apak et al 2006, Canadanovic-Brunet et al 2008, Dastmalchi et al 2008, Ferreira et al 2006, Hohmann et al 1999, Koksal et al 2011, Lopez et al 2007, Marongiu et al 2004, Spiridon et al 2011). According to a 2003 study, concentrations of antioxidants within lemon balm are >75 mmol/100 g (Dragland et al 2003). Co-administration of an aqueous extract of lemon balm in manganese-treated mice resulted in a significant decrease in activity of the antioxidant enzymes superoxide dismutase and catalase in the hippocampus, striatum, cortex and cerebellum; and decreased oxidative stress marker levels in the hippocampus and striatum (Martins et al 2012). Lemon balm has demonstrated superior antioxidant activity compared to chamomile and lemongrass, and an aqueous extract of lemon balm has been found to have greater antioxidant potential than methanolic and ethanolic extracts (Pereira et al 2009).

Cardiovascular effects

Aqueous extracts of lemon balm have been shown to slow cardiac rate but not alter the force of contraction in isolated rat hearts (Gazola et al 2004). An aqueous extract of lemon balm was found to exhibit a vasodilatory effect on isolated rat aortic rings via the nitric oxide pathway (Ersoy et al 2008).

Hypolipidaemic

Lemon balm has been found to reduce blood cholesterol and lipid levels in rabbits fed a high-cholesterol diet (Karimi et al 2010). Interestingly, in a similar study using rats fed a high-fat and alcohol diet, the lemon balm extract also increased glutathione levels and reduced lipid peroxidation in the liver, demonstrating a hepatoprotective effect (Bolkent et al 2005).

The hypolipidaemic effects of lemon balm essential oil were investigated in vitro and in vivo using lipid-loaded HepG2 cells and human APOE2 transgenic mice, respectively. The HepG2 cells treated with lemon balm essential oil demonstrated increased bile acid synthesis, and decreased expression of HMG-CoA reductase and cellular triglyceride and cholesterol concentrations (Jun et al 2012).

The APOE2 transgenic mice treated with lemon balm essential oil for 2 weeks did not demonstrate a significant reduction in total cholesterol; however plasma triglyceride concentrations decreased by 36%, and the mouse livers showed increased expression of cholesterol metabolism genes. The authors suggest that longer-term treatment of APOE2 transgenic mice with lemon balm essential oil may have had hypocholesterolaemic effects (Jun et al 2012).

IN COMBINATION

In a 2008 study, mice fed a high-fat diet were supplemented with Ob-X, a herbal compound containing lemon balm, white mulberry and injin. At 12 weeks, mice supplemented with Ob-X had significantly decreased serum triglycerides and total cholesterol levels; significantly lower adipose tissue mass and body weight gain; and less hepatic lipid accumulation compared to mice fed a high-fat diet alone (Lee et al 2008). In two follow-up studies, Ob-X was found to inhibit angiogenesis and adipogenesis in vitro and in vivo (Hong et al 2011, Yoon & Kim 2011).

Dietary supplementation with 1% powdered clove flower combined with 0.2% lemon balm extract in broiler chickens had no influence on plasma low-density lipoproteins, serum cholesterol, total lipids, triglycerides or high-density lipoproteins. However, blood concentrations of vitamin E and sulfhydryl groups were found to increase (Petrovic et al 2012).

Promotes neurogenesis

Lemon balm enhances the neurogenic ability of cells of the hippocampal dentate gyrus in vivo: this is of relevance because this area is affected in several neurological disorders, including Alzheimer's disease. The study found administration of lemon balm extract resulted in increased GABA levels in the hippocampal dentate gyrus of mice, due to less GABA breakdown due to inhibition of GABA transaminase, the enzyme responsible for GABA degradation. Lemon balm was found to significantly increase cell proliferation and neuroblast differentiation in the mouse dentate gyrus. This is thought to be due to the increased GABA levels potentiating the survival of new cells, as GABA agonists have been found to increase maturation and survival of proliferating neuronal cells (Yoo et al 2011).

Hypoglycaemic

The hypoglycaemic potential of lemon balm essential oil was investigated in type 2 diabetic mice. Administration of 0.015 mg/day of lemon balm essential oil for 6 weeks resulted in significantly reduced blood glucose levels and triglyceride concentrations, improved glucose tolerance and significantly increased serum insulin levels. This action is mediated via activation of GCK, a key enzyme in the control of glucose homeostasis, and inhibition of G6Pase and PEPCK, two key enzymes in the gluconeogenesis pathway in the liver (Chung et al 2010).

Anticarcinogenic, antimutagenic

Ethanolic extracts of lemon balm have demonstrated both antigenotoxic and antimutagenic activity in mice (de Carvalho et al 2011). Antitumour activity has also been demonstrated (Chlabicz & Galasinski 1986, Dudai et al 2005, Galasinski 1996, Galasinski et al 1996, Saraydin et al 2012). Extracts of lemon balm were found to inhibit growth of cervix epithelial carcinoma cells and breast adenocarcinoma cells in vitro (Canadanovic-Brunet et al 2008).

Ethanolic and aqueous extracts of lemon balm demonstrated cytotoxic activity against human colon cancer cells in vitro. The ethanolic extract was found to reduce cell proliferation to values close to 40% and cell viability to 13% after 72 hours of treatment. Cytotoxic activity was largely attributed to rosmarinic acid (Encalada et al 2011).

Isolated extract of corchorifatty acid B (CFAB) from ethanolic preparations of lemon balm demonstrated antimelanogenic activity in both human melanocytes and mouse melanoma B16 cells. The inhibition of cellular pigmentation is likely to be induced by rapid degradation of tyrosinase, the rate-limiting enzyme for melanin production (Fujita et al 2011).

OTHER ACTIONS

Lemon balm inhibits the binding of thyroid-stimulating hormone to thyroid plasma membranes in vitro and the extrathyroidal enzymic T4-5'-deiodination to triiodothyronine (Auf'mkolk et al 1984a). Methanolic extracts of lemon balm exhibit moderate amoebicidal activity in vitro (Malatyali et al 2012).

Lemon balm extracts have demonstrated antiglycative activity in vitro. Ethanol extracts of lemon balm exhibited the highest inhibitory effects on the formation of advanced glycation end products, which induce cell and tissue damage and are known to promote diabetic complications, atherosclerosis, Alzheimer's disease and ageing (Miroliaei et al 2011).

CLINICAL USE

In clinical practice, lemon balm is often prescribed in combination with other herbal medicines. As a reflection of this, many clinical studies have investigated the effects of lemon balm as an ingredient of a herbal combination, making it difficult to determine the efficacy of this herb individually.

Anxiety

A small, double-blind, placebo-controlled, randomised, crossover trial involving 18 healthy volunteers investigated the effects of a whole extract of standardised *Melissa* extract (Pharmaton, Lugano, Switzerland) in two different doses (300 and 600 mg) and found a significant reduction in stress in the volunteers taking the larger dose; however alertness was also reduced at the higher dose (Kennedy et al 2004).

A prospective, open-label, 15-day pilot study evaluated the efficacy of a product called Cyracos, a standardised hydroalcoholic lemon balm extract containing >7% rosmarinic acid and >15% hydroxycinnamic acid derivatives, in 20 participants with mild to moderate anxiety disorders and sleep disturbances. Participants took 600 mg of active treatment per day in two divided doses. Anxiety levels were evaluated using the Free Rating Scale for Anxiety, and the Hamilton Rating Scale for Depression was used to assess insomnia. Cyracos reduced anxiety by 18%, anxiety-associated symptoms by 15% and insomnia by 42%. While significant improvements in associated symptoms of anxiety and insomnia were seen, these findings need to be replicated in a larger clinical trial that includes a placebo arm and double blinding (Cases et al 2011).

Commission E approves the use of lemon balm in the treatment of anxiety and restlessness (Blumenthal et al 2000).

IN COMBINATION

A combination of lemon balm and valerian (*Valeriana officinalis*) was examined for acute effects on anxiety in a double-blind, placebo-controlled, randomised, crossover experiment of 24 individuals (Kennedy et al 2006).

Three separate concentrations of the standardised product (600 mg, 1200 mg, 1800 mg) were given on separate days after a 7-day wash-out period. Any changes to mood and anxiety were assessed predose and at 1-, 3- and 6-h intervals. Interestingly, the lower dose (600 mg) was shown to decrease anxiety levels whereas the highest dose (1800 mg) increased anxiety. The exact effect of lemon balm in this preparation is hard to determine.

Cognitive function

Lemon balm has been used for centuries to improve cognitive function and encouraging results from a 2002 clinical study confirm that it can influence memory.

The randomised, double-blind crossover study involving 20 healthy young volunteers found that single doses of lemon balm (Pharmaton, Lugano Switzerland) were able to modulate both mood and cognitive performance in a dose- and time-dependent manner (Kennedy et al 2002). In this study, treatment with the lowest dose (300 mg) increased self-rated 'calmness' within 1 hour whereas the 600 mg and 900 mg doses produced significant effects on memory task performance, observable at both 2.5 hours and 4 hours after administration. The highest tested dose (900 mg) was found to significantly reduce alertness within 1 hour, suggesting a dose–response effect.

Alzheimer's disease

A randomised, double-blind, placebo-controlled trial demonstrated the efficacy and safety of *M. officinalis* in 42 patients aged 65–80 years with mild to moderate Alzheimer's disease: patients were given 60 drops/day for 4 months (Akhondzadeh et al 2003). The treatment consisted of a plant extract prepared as 1 : 1 in 45% alcohol and standardised to contain at least 500 mcg citral/mL. After week 4, the difference between placebo and active treatment was significant and became highly significant at the end point (week 16) ($P < 0.0001$) on the Alzheimer's disease assessment scale. By week 8, the difference was also significant on the clinical dementia rating scale and highly significant by week 16 ($P < 0.0001$).

Aromatherapy with lemon balm may not be as effective as oral use of the extract, according to a double-blind randomised controlled trial which compared lemon balm aromatherapy to donepezil or placebo aromatherapy in the treatment of agitation in people with Alzheimer's dementia. Participants were required to wear nose clips for the aromatherapy treatment to ensure that full blinding was maintained. The Pittsburgh Agitation Scale (PAS) and Neuropsychiatric Inventory (NPI) were completed at baseline, 4-week and 12-week follow-up. Of 114 participants, 94 completed the week 4 assessment and 81 completed the assessment at week 12. No significant differences were found between aromatherapy, donepezil and placebo either at week 4 or 12. However, the lack of significant differences between groups was due to an 18% improvement in the PAS and a 37% improvement in the NPI over 12 weeks in all three groups. The authors suggest that this may be attributed to potential non-specific benefits of touch and interaction in the treatment of agitation in people with Alzheimer's disease (Burns et al 2011).

In another study, lemon balm essential oil used as aromatherapy and applied twice daily to face and arms under double-blind placebo-controlled conditions was found to be a safe and effective treatment for clinically significant agitation in people with severe dementia (Ballard et al 2002). The trial, which involved 71 subjects, found that after 1 month's treatment, patients were less agitated, less socially withdrawn and spent more time in constructive activities than those in the placebo group. Quality-of-life ratings also improved.

Insomnia

In clinical practice, lemon balm is often prescribed in combination with other herbs such as valerian in the treatment of insomnia. As a reflection of this, a randomised, double-blind multicentre study investigated the effects of a commercial valerian and lemon balm herbal combination (Songha Night) in 98 healthy subjects (Cerny & Schmid 1999). Treatment was administered over a 30-day period and consisted of three tablets taken half an hour before bedtime, providing a total dose of 1–6 g valerian and 1–2 g lemon balm. Herbal treatment was found to significantly improve sleep quality and was well tolerated.

Another randomised, double-blind crossover study found that the same combination of valerian and lemon balm taken over 9 nights was as effective as triazolam in the treatment of insomnia (Dressing et al 1992). The dose used was equivalent to 1.4 g dried valerian and 0.9 g dried lemon balm.

As with all herbal combination studies, it is difficult to determine the contribution each individual herb made to the end result. As such, these studies are encouraging but the role of lemon balm as a stand-alone treatment for insomnia remains unclear.

Commission E approves the use of lemon balm in the treatment of insomnia (Blumenthal et al 2000).

Gastrointestinal conditions associated with spasm and nervousness

To date, lemon balm's activity in gastrointestinal conditions has only been studied in combination with other herbs.

A pilot study investigated the effects of Carmint, containing lemon balm, spearmint and coriander, in 32 patients with irritable bowel syndrome (Vejdani et al 2006). Patients were randomly assigned Carmint or placebo, plus loperamide or psyllium (based on their irritable bowel syndrome subtype) for 8 weeks. The severity and frequency of abdominal pain and bloating were significantly lower in the Carmint group as compared to placebo at the end of the 8 weeks. A larger follow-up trial is needed to confirm these results.

A 15-day open study involving 24 subjects with chronic non-specific colitis investigated whether a combination of lemon balm, St John's wort, dandelion, marigold and fennel could provide symptom relief (Chakurski et al 1981). Excellent results were obtained by the end of the study, with herbal treatment resulting in the disappearance of spontaneous and palpable pains along the large intestine in 95.83% of patients. A double-blind study using a herbal tea prepared from chamomile, lemon balm, vervain, licorice and fennel in infantile colic has also been conducted. A dose of 150 mL offered up to three times daily was found to eliminate symptoms of colic in 57% of infants, whereas placebo was helpful in only 26% after 7 days' treatment (Weizman et al 1993).

A randomised, double-blind, placebo-controlled trial was conducted to examine the effectiveness of ColiMil (lemon balm, chamomile and fennel) in 93 breastfed infants with colic (Savino et al 2005). The infants were randomised into two groups to receive either ColiMil or placebo, both twice a day at 5 p.m. and 8 p.m. before feeding (2 mL/kg/day) for 7 days. A reduction in crying time was observed in 85.4% subjects in the active treatment group as compared to 48.9% for placebo ($P < 0.005$). This is a significant result, especially considering the treatment period was only 7 days. No side effects were reported. Commission E supports the use of lemon balm for functional gastrointestinal conditions (Blumenthal et al 2000).

IN COMBINATION

A randomised, double-blind, placebo-controlled trial investigated the use of two herbal preparations in the treatment of somatoform disorders. A total of 182 patients with somatisation disorder and undifferentiated somatoform disorder were randomised into three treatment groups: (1) butterbur, valerian, passionflower and lemon balm; (2) valerian, passionflower and lemon balm; or (3) placebo, for a 2-week treatment period. Primary outcomes measured were anxiety (visual analogue scale) and depression (Beck's Depression Inventory). Clinical Global Impression was measured as a secondary outcome. Both herbal treatment groups showed significant improvement in anxiety and depression, yet the four-herb preparation was significantly superior to the three-herb preparation. There were no serious adverse events. While these results are promising, it is impossible to determine the individual efficacy of lemon balm in the treatment of somatoform disorders due to the herbal combinations used in each active treatment arm (Melzer et al 2009).

Herpes simplex type 1 — external use

The topical use of lemon balm preparations for HSV infection is very popular in Europe. Results from a randomised double-blind study in 66 subjects with a history of recurrent herpes labialis (>3 episodes/year) found that standardised lemon balm ointment (700 mg crude herb per gram) applied four times daily for 5 days significantly shortened healing time, prevented infection spread and produced rapid symptom relief (Koytchev et al 1999). Decreased symptoms and increased rate of healing were also observed in another double-blind study of lemon balm cream in 116 subjects (Woelbling & Leonhardt 1994).

Positive results were seen again in a 2008 double-blind randomised controlled trial of 60 patients with recurrent herpes simplex. In the study, volunteers applied either placebo or a lemon balm ointment five times daily for 5–10 minutes during herpes outbreaks until full recovery. The lemon balm ointment was found to significantly reduce healing time and the area of the lesion between day 1 and day 5 compared to placebo. No significant change was seen in the severity or duration of pain (Zolfaghari et al 2008).

Oxidative stress

A clinical trial involving 55 radiology staff found that a lemon balm infusion (1.5 g/100 mL) taken orally twice daily for 30 days resulted in significant increases in plasma levels of catalase, superoxide dismutase and glutathione peroxidase, and reductions in plasma DNA damage, myeloperoxidase and lipid peroxidation (Zeraatpishe et al 2011).

Another clinical trial evaluated the ability of lemon balm to reduce oxidative stress levels in 30 participants occupationally exposed to aluminium. Participants ingested an oral lemon balm infusion (1.5 g/100 mL) twice daily for 30 days. There was a significant increase in plasma levels of total antioxidant capacity and total thiol molecules, and a significant decrease in triglyceride, cholesterol and aspartate transaminase (AST). Lipid peroxidation levels did not differ before and after treatment (Fazli et al 2012).

OTHER USES

Animal studies have identified dose-dependent antiulcerogenic activity for lemon balm extract, which has been histologically confirmed. This activity is associated with a reduced acid output and an increased mucin secretion, an increase in prostaglandin E_2 release and a decrease in leukotrienes (Khayyal et al 2001).

A combination of lemon balm, cinnamon and nettle (1.5, 0.5 and 0.25 g/100 mL) was investigated in 35 patients with non-alcoholic fatty liver disease. An infusion of the combined herbs was consumed twice a day for 30 days. Plasma liver markers, including alanine transferase (ALT), AST and alkaline phosphatase (ALP), were measured before and after treatment. There was a significant decrease in ALT. AST and ALP also declined; however these decreases were not significant. While these results are encouraging, it is difficult to determine the degree to which lemon balm contributed to the outcome due to the use of a herbal combination (Malekirad et al 2012).

DOSAGE RANGE

- Fresh herb: 1.5–4.5 g two–three times daily.
- Infusion: 1.5–4.5 g in 150 mL water.
- Fluid extract (1 : 1) (g/mL): 6–12 mL/day.
- Ointment: 700 mg/g ointment applied four times daily for herpes simplex infection.

According to clinical studies

- Anxiety: Cyracos (a standardised hydroalcoholic lemon balm extract containing >7% rosmarinic acid and >15% hydroxycinnamic acid derivatives) 600 mg daily in divided doses; 600 mg daily of standardised *Melissa* extract (Pharmaton, Lugano, Switzerland)
- Alzheimer's dementia: 60 drops/day of *Melissa* extract (standardised to contain at least 500 mg citral/mL) taken internally.
- Herpes simplex infection: *Melissa* ointment applied five times daily.

TOXICITY

Not known.

ADVERSE REACTIONS

Lemon balm is well tolerated according to one double-blind, randomised crossover study (Kennedy et al 2002).

SIGNIFICANT INTERACTIONS

Controlled clinical studies are not available, so interactions are speculative and based on evidence of activity.

Barbiturates

Increased sedative effects: one animal study (Soulimani et al 1991) found that concomitant administration of lemon balm extract with pentobarbitone produced an increased sedative effect — observe patients taking this combination.

Cholinergic drugs

Additive effects are theoretically possible and may be beneficial — observe patients taking this combination.

CONTRAINDICATIONS AND PRECAUTIONS

Hypothyroidism — one in vitro study found that an extract of *M. officinalis* inhibited both the extrathyroidal enzymic T4-5'-deiodination to triiodothyronine and the T4-5'-deiodination (Auf'mkolk et al 1984b). At high doses (900 mg) oral *Melissa* extract was shown to reduce alertness, so caution is required if using this treatment together with alcohol, as it may potentiate sedative effects (Kennedy et al 2002).

PREGNANCY USE

Safety has not been scientifically established and is unknown.

Practice points/Patient counselling

- Lemon balm has been used traditionally to treat insomnia, irritability, restlessness, anxiety and dementia. It is also used to relieve gastrointestinal symptoms associated with spasms and nervousness.
- Used topically as a cold sore treatment, it significantly reduces symptoms, shortens the healing period and prevents infection spread. It may be suitable both as an active treatment and as a preventive agent in cases of chronic recurrent herpes simplex infections.
- Lemon balm may have some anti-inflammatory and antispasmodic activity.
- The essential oil is used in aromatherapy to relieve anxiety and promote calm and a sense of wellbeing.
- Clinical studies have demonstrated that, when taken internally, *Melissa* extract reduces stress and anxiety and can improve cognitive function.

PATIENTS' FAQs

What will this herb do for me?

Lemon balm has several different actions and is used for a number of different conditions. Taking the herb internally may help reduce anxiety and improve mood and mental concentration. When taken together with valerian, it can relieve insomnia. It may also relieve stomach spasms associated with nervousness, or in chronic, non-specific colitis when taken as part of a specific herbal combination. *Melissa* cream applied four to five times daily to herpes simplex infections can reduce symptoms, accelerate healing and reduce the chance of the infection spreading.

When will it start to work?

Approximately 1 month's treatment with the essential oil is required for calming effects on agitation in dementia to be seen. Taken internally with valerian, effects on sleep may be seen after 9 days' use. Improved memory occurred within 2.5 hours, according to one study; however, it is not known if and when effects are seen in dementia. *Melissa* cream has been shown to significantly reduce symptoms of herpes simplex within 2 days, when applied four times daily. Orally, 4-8 weeks of use with *Melissa* extract is required to see significant changes in Alzheimer's dementia, whereas improved cognitive function is seen after a single dose in healthy people.

Are there any safety issues?

One study using lemon balm in tablet form found that it was well tolerated. Drug interactions are theoretically possible and this herb should be used cautiously in people with hypothyroidism.

REFERENCES

Abuhamdah S et al. Pharmacological profile of an essential oil derived from *Melissa officinalis* with anti-agitation properties: focus on ligand-gated channels. J Pharm Pharmacol 60.3 (2008): 377–384.

L

Akhondzadeh S et al. *Melissa officinalis* extract in the treatment of patients with mild to moderate Alzheimer's disease: a double-blind, randomised, placebo controlled trial. J Neurol Neurosurg Psychiatry 74 (2003): 863–866.

Allahverdiyer A et al. Antioxidant activity of the volatile oils of *Melissa officinalis* L. against herpes simplex virus type-2. Phytomedicine 11 (2004): 657–661.

Aoshima H, Hamamoto K. Potentiation of GABAA receptors expressed in *Xenopus* oocytes by perfume and phytoncid. Biosci Biotechnol Biochem 63.4 (1999): 743–748.

Apak R et al. The cupric ion reducing antioxidant capacity and polyphenolic content of some herbal teas. Int J Food Sci Nutr 57.5–6 (2006): 292–304.

Astani A, et al. *Melissa officinalis* extract inhibits attachment of herpes simplex virus in vitro. Chemotherapy 58.1 (2012): 70–7.

Auf'mkolk M et al. Inhibition by certain plant extracts of the binding and adenylate cyclase stimulatory effect of bovine thyrotropin in human thyroid membranes. Endocrinology 115.2 (1984a): 527–534.

Auf'mkolk M et al. Antihormonal effects of plant extracts: iodothyronine deiodinase of rat liver is inhibited by extracts and secondary metabolites of plants. Horm Metab Res 16.4 (1984b): 188–192.

Awad R, et al. Bioassay-guided fractionation of lemon balm (*Melissa officinalis* L.) using an in vitro measure of GABA transaminase activity. Phytotherapy research 23.8 (2009): 1075–81.

Ballard CG et al. Aromatherapy as a safe and effective treatment for the management of agitation in severe dementia: the results of a double-blind, placebo-controlled trial with Melissa. J Clin Psychiatry 63.7 (2002): 553–558.

Beikert FC, et al. Antiinflammatory potential of seven plant extracts in the ultraviolet erythema test: A randomized, placebo-controlled study. Der Hautarzt; Zeitschrift Fur Dermatologie, Venerologie, Und Verwandte Gebiete 64.1 (2013): 40–6.

Blumenthal M, et al (eds). Herbal medicine: expanded Commission E monographs. Austin, TX: Integrative Medicine Communications, 2000.

Bolkent S et al. Protective role of *Melissa officinalis* L extract on liver of hyperlipidemic rats: A morphological and biochemical study. J Ethnopharmacol 99 (2005): 391–398.

Burns A et al. A double-blind placebo-controlled randomized trial of *Melissa officinalis* oil and donepezil for the treatment of agitation in Alzheimer's disease. Dementia And Geriatric Cognitive Disorders 31.2 (2011): 158–64.

Canadanovic-Brunet JG et al. Radical scavenging, antibacterial, and antiproliferative activities of *Melissa officinalis* L. extracts. J Med Food 11.1 (2008): 133–143.

Capasso R, et al. Effects of the herbal formulation ColiMil on upper gastrointestinal transit in mice in vivo. Phytother Res 21.10 (2007): 999–1101.

Cases J et al. Pilot trial of *Melissa officinalis* L. leaf extract in the treatment of volunteers suffering from mild-to-moderate anxiety disorders and sleep disturbances. Mediterranean journal of nutrition and metabolism 43 (2011): 211–8.

Cerny A, Schmid K. Tolerability and efficacy of valerian/lemon balm in healthy volunteers: a double-blind, placebo-controlled, multicentre study. Fitoterapia 70,3 (1999): 221–228.

Chaiyana W, Okonogi S. Inhibition of cholinesterase by essential oil from food plant. Phytomedicine: International Journal Of Phytotherapy And Phytopharmacology 19.8-9 (2012): 836–9.

Chakurski I et al. Treatment of chronic colitis with an herbal combination of *Taraxacum officinale, Hipericum perforatum, Melissa officinalis, Calendula officinalis* and Foeniculum vulgare. Vutr Boles 20.6 (1981): 51–54.b15.

Chlabicz J, Galasinski W. The components of *Melissa officinalis* L. that influence protein biosynthesis in-vitro. J Pharm Pharmacol 38.11 (1986): 791–794.

Chung M et al. Anti-diabetic effects of lemon balm (*Melissa officinalis*) essential oil on glucose- and lipid-regulating enzymes in type 2 diabetic mice. The British Journal of Nutrition 104.2 (2010): 180–8.

Dastmalchi K et al. Chemical composition and in vitro antioxidative activity of a lemon balm (*Melissa officinalis* L.) extract. LWT — Food Science and Technology 41.3 (2008): 391–400.

Dastmalchi K et al. Acetylcholinesterase inhibitory guided fractionation of *Melissa officinalis* L. Bioorganic & Medicinal Chemistry 17.2 (2009): 867–71.

de Carvalho NC et al. Evaluation of the genotoxic and antigenotoxic potential of *Melissa officinalis* in mice. Genetics And Molecular Biology 34.2 (2011) 290–7.

Dimitrova Z et al. Antiherpes effect of *Melissa officinalis* L. extracts. Acta Microbiol Bulg 29 (1993): 65–72.

Dragland S et al. Several culinary and medicinal herbs are important sources of dietary antioxidants. J Nutr 133.5 (2003): 1286–1290.

Dressing H et al. Insomnia: are valerian/balm combinations of equal value to benzodiazepine? Therapiewoche 42 (1992): 726–736.

Dudai N et al. Citral is a new inducer of caspase-3 in tumor cell lines. Planta Med 71.5 (2005): 484–488.

Emamghoreishi M, Talebianpour M. Antidepressant effect of *Melissa officinalis* in the forced swimming test. DARU Journal of Pharmaceutical Sciences 17.1 (2009): 42–7.

Encalada MA et al. Anti-proliferative effect of *Melissa officinalis* on human colon cancer cell line. Plant Foods For Human Nutrition 66.4 (2011): 328–34.

Englberger W et al. Rosmarinic acid: a new inhibitor of complement C3-convertase with anti-inflammatory activity. Int J Immunopharmacol 10.6 (1988): 729–737.

Ersoy S et al. Endothelium-dependent induction of vasorelaxation by *Melissa officinalis* L. ssp. *officinalis* in rat isolated thoracic aorta. Phytomedicine 15.12 (2008): 1087–92.

Fazli D et al. Effects of *Melissa officinalis* L. on oxidative status and biochemical parameters in occupationally exposed workers to aluminum: a before after clinical trial. International Journal of Pharmacology 8 (2012): 455–8.

Ferreira A et al. The in vitro screening for acetylcholinesterase inhibition and antioxidant activity of medicinal plants from Portugal. J Ethnopharmacol 108.1 (2006): 31–37.

Fujita H et al. Inhibitory effects of 16-hydroxy-9-oxo-10E,12E,14E-octadecatrienoic acid (Corchorifatty acid B) isolated from *Melissa officinalis* Linne on melanogenesis. Experimental Dermatology 20.5 (2011): 420–4.

Galasinski W. Eukaryotic polypeptide elongation system and its sensitivity to the inhibitory substances of plant origin. Proc Soc Exp Biol Med 212.1 (1996): 24–37.

Galasinski W et al. The substances of plant origin that inhibit protein biosynthesis. Acta Pol Pharm 53.5 (1996): 311–3118.

Gazola R, et al. *Lippa alba, Melissa officinalis, Cymbopogon citratus*: effects of the aqueous extracts on the isolated hearts of rats. Pharmacol Res 50 (2004): 477–480.

Geuenich S et al. Aqueous extracts from peppermint, sage and lemon balm leaves display potent anti-HIV-1 activity by increasing the virion density. Retrovirology 5 (2008): 27.

Guginski G et al. Mechanisms involved in the antinociception caused by ethanolic extract obtained from the leaves of *Melissa officinalis* (lemon balm) in mice. Pharmacology Biochemistry and Behavior 93.1 (2009): 10–16.

Hancianu M et al. Chemical composition and in vitro antimicrobial activity of essential oil of *Melissa officinalis* L. from Romania. Revista medico-chirurgicala a Societatii de Medici si Naturalisti din Iasi 112.3 (2008): 843–7.

Hanganu D et al. The study of some polyphenolic compounds from *Melissa officinalis* L. (Lamiaceae). Rev Med Chir Soc Med Nat Iasi 112.2 (2008): 525–9.

Hohmann J et al. Protective effects of the aerial parts of *Salvia officinalis, Melissa officinalis* and *Lavandula angustifolia* and their constituents against enzyme-dependent and enzyme-independent lipid peroxidation. Planta Med 65.6 (1999): 576–578.

Hong Y, et al. The anti-angiogenic herbal extracts Ob-X from *Morus alba, Melissa officinalis*, and *Artemisia capillaris* suppresses adipogenesis in 3T3-L1 adipocytes. Pharmaceutical Biology 49.8 (2011): 775–83.

Huang L et al. Pharmacological profile of essential oils derived from Lavandula angustifolia and *Melissa officinalis* with anti-agitation properties: focus on ligand-gated channels. Journal of Pharmacy and Pharmacology 60.11 (2008): 1515–22.

Huss U et al. Screening of ubiquitous plant constituents for COX-2 inhibition with a scintillation proximity based assay. J Nat Prod 65.11 (2002): 1517–1521.

Ibarra A et al. Effects of chronic administration of *Melissa officinalis* L. extract on anxiety-like reactivity and on circadian and exploratory activities in mice. Phytomedicine 17.6 (2010): 397–403.

Jun HJ et al. *Melissa officinalis* essential oil reduces plasma triglycerides in human apolipoprotein E2 transgenic mice by inhibiting sterol regulatory element-binding protein-1c-dependent fatty acid synthesis. The Journal Of Nutrition 142.3 (2012): 432–40.

Karimi I et al. Anti-hyperlipidaemic effects of an essential oil of *Melissa officinalis*. L in cholesterol-fed rabbits. J Appl Biologic Sci 4.1 (2010): 23–8.

Kelm MA et al. Antioxidant and cyclooxygenase inhibitory phenolic compounds from *Ocimum sanctum* Linn. Phytomedicine 7.1 (2000): 7–13.

Kennedy DO et al. Modulation of mood and cognitive performance following acute administration of *Melissa officinalis* (lemon balm). Pharmacol Biochem Behav 72.4 (2002): 953–964.

Kennedy DO et al. Modulation of mood and cognitive performance following acute administration of single doses of *Melissa officinalis* (Lemon balm) with human CNS nicotinic and muscarinic receptor-binding properties. Neuropsychopharmacology 28.10 (2003): 1871–1881.

Kennedy DO, et al. Attenuation of laboratory-induced stress in humans after acute administration of *Melissa officinalis* (lemon balm). Psychosom Med 66.4 (2004): 607–613.

Kennedy DO et al. Anxiolytic effects of a combination of *Melissa officinalis* and *Valeriana officinalis* during laboratory induced stress. Phytother Res 20.2 (2006): 96–102.
Khayyal MT et al. Antiulcerogenic effect of some gastrointestinally acting plant extracts and their combination. Arzneimittelforschung 51.7 (2001): 545–553.
Koksal E et al. Antioxidant activity of *Melissa officinalis* leaves. J. Med. Plant Res 5 (2011): 217–22.
Koytchev R, et al. Balm mint extract (Lo-701) for topical treatment of recurring herpes labialis. Phytomedicine 6.4 (1999): 225–230.
Larrondo JV, et al. Antimicrobial activity of essences from labiates. Microbios 82.332 (1995): 171–172.
Lee J et al. Regulation of obesity and lipid disorders by herbal extracts from *Morus alba*, *Melissa officinalis*, and *Artemisia capillaris* in high-fat diet-induced obese mice. Journal Of Ethnopharmacology 115.2 (2008): 263–70.
Lopez V et al. In vitro antioxidant and anti-rhizopus activities of Lamiaceae herbal extracts. Plant Foods Hum Nutr 62.4 (2007): 151–155.
Malatyali E et al. In vitro amoebicidal activities of *Satureja cuneifolia* and *Melissa officinalis* on *Acanthamoeba castellanii* cysts and trophozoites. Parasitology Research 110.6 (2012): 2175–80.
Malekirad AA et al. Effects of the mixture of *Melissa officinalis* L., *Cinnamomum zeylanicum* and *Urtica dioica* on hepatic enzymes activity in patients with nonalcoholic fatty liver disease. International Journal of Pharmacology 8.3 (2012): 204–8.
Marongiu B et al. Antioxidant activity of supercritical extract of *Melissa officinalis* subsp. *officinalis* and *Melissa officinalis* subsp. *inodora*. Phytotherapy Research 18.10 (2004): 789–92.
Martins EN et al. Protective effect of *Melissa officinalis* aqueous extract against Mn-induced oxidative stress in chronically exposed mice. Brain Research Bulletin 87.1 (2012): 74–9.
Mazzanti G et al. Inhibitory activity of *Melissa officinalis* L. extract on herpes simplex virus type 2 replication. Natural Product Research 22.16 (2008): 1433–40.
Melzer J et al. Fixed herbal drug combination with and without butterbur (Ze 185) for the treatment of patients with somatoform disorders: randomized, placebo-controlled pharmaco-clinical trial. Phytotherapy Research: PTR 23.9 (2009): 1303–08.
Miroliaei M et al. Inhibitory effects of lemon balm (*Melissa officinalis*, L.) extract on the formation of advanced glycation end products. Food Chemistry 129.2 (2011): 267–71.
Mrlianova M et al. The influence of the harvest cut height on the quality of the herbal drugs *Melissae folium* and *Melissae herba*. Planta Med 68.2 (2002): 178–180.
Michele Myers. Lemon Balm: An Herb Society of America Guide. Herb Society of America, Ohio, 2007: p. 8.
Nolkemper S et al. Antiviral effect of aqueous extracts from species of the Lamiaceae family against herpes simplex virus type 1 and type 2 in vitro. Planta Med 72.1 (2006): 1378–1382.
Orhan I et al. Activity of essential oils and individual components against acetyl- and butyrylcholinesterase. Journal Of Biosciences 63.7-8 (2008): 547–53.
Peake PW et al. The inhibitory effect of rosmarinic acid on complement involves the C5 convertase. Int J Immunopharmacol 13.7 (1991): 853–857.
Pereira P et al. Neurobehavioral and genotoxic aspects of rosmarinic acid. Pharmacol Res 52.3 (2005): 199–203.
Pereira RP et al. Antioxidant effects of different extracts from *Melissa officinalis*, *Matricaria recutita* and *Cymbopogon citratus*. Neurochemical Research 34.5 (2009): 973–83.
Perry N, et al. European herbs with cholinergic activities: Potential in dementia therapy. International journal of geriatric psychiatry 11.12 (1996): 1063–9.
Petrovic V et al. The effect of supplementation of clove and agrimony or clove and lemon balm on growth performance, antioxidant status and selected indices of lipid profile of broiler chickens. Journal Of Animal Physiology And Animal Nutrition 96.6 (2012): 970–7.
Sadraei H, et al. Relaxant effect of essential oil of *Melissa officinalis* and citral on rat ileum contractions. Fitoterapia 74 (2003): 445–452.
Salah S, Jager A. Screening of traditionally used Lebanese herbs for neurological activities. J Ethnopharmacol 97 (2005): 145–149.
Saraydin SU et al. Antitumoral effects of *Melissa officinalis* on breast cancer in vitro and in vivo. Asian Pacific Journal Of Cancer Prevention: APJCP 13.6 (2012): 2765–70.
Savino F et al. A randomized double-blind placebo-controlled trial of a standardized extract of *Matricariae recutita, Foeniculum vulgare* and *Melissa officinalis* (ColiMil) in the treatment of breastfed colicky infants. Phytother Res 19.4 (2005): 335–340.
Schnitzler P et al. *Melissa officinalis* oil affects infectivity of enveloped herpesviruses. Phytomedicine 15.9 (2008): 734–740.
Soulimani R et al. Neurotropic action of the hydroalcoholic extract of *Melissa officinalis* in the mouse. Planta Med 57.2 (1991): 105–109.
Spiridon I et al. Antioxidant capacity and total phenolic contents of oregano (*Origanum vulgare*), lavender (*Lavandula angustifolia*) and lemon balm (*Melissa officinalis*) from Romania. Natural Product Research 25.17 (2011): 1657–61.
Taguchi Y et al. Therapeutic effects on murine oral candidiasis by oral administration of cassia (*Cinnamomum cassia*) preparation. Japanese Journal Of Medical Mycology 51.1 (2010): 13–21.
Taiwo AE et al. Anxiolytic and antidepressant-like effects of *Melissa officinalis* (lemon balm) extract in rats: Influence of administration and gender. Indian Journal Of Pharmacology 44.2 (2012): 189–92.
Vejdani R et al. The efficacy of an herbal medicine, Carmint, on the relief of abdominal pain and bloating in patients with irritable bowel syndrome: a pilot study. Dig Dis Sci 51.8 (2006): 1501–1507.
Wake G et al. CNS acetylcholine receptor activity in European medicinal plants traditionally used to improve failing memory. J Ethnopharmacol 69.2 (2000): 105–114.
Walsh SE et al. Activity and mechanisms of action of selected biocidal agents on Gram-positive and -negative bacteria. J Appl Microbiol 94.2 (2003): 240–247.
Weizman Z et al. Efficacy of herbal tea preparation in infantile colic. J Pediatr 122.4 (1993): 650–652.
Woelbling RH, Leonhardt K. Local therapy of herpes simplex with dried extract from *Melissa officinalis*. Phytomedicine 1 (1994): 25–31.
Yamasaki K et al. Anti-HIV-1 activity of herbs in Labiatae. Biol Pharm Bull 21.8 (1998): 829–833.
Yoo DY et al. Effects of *Melissa officinalis* L. (lemon balm) extract on neurogenesis associated with serum corticosterone and GABA in the mouse dentate gyrus. Neurochemical Research 36.2 (2011): 250–7.
Yoon M, Kim MY. The anti-angiogenic herbal composition Ob-X from *Morus alba*, *Melissa officinalis*, and *Artemisia capillaris* regulates obesity in genetically obese ob/ob mice. Pharmaceutical Biology 49.6 (2011): 614–9.
Zeraatpishe A et al. Effects of *Melissa officinalis* L. on oxidative status and DNA damage in subjects exposed to long-term low-dose ionizing radiation. Toxicology And Industrial Health 27.3 (2011): 205–12.
Zolfaghari B et al. A randomized double-blind placebo controlled clinical trial of topical herbal drug against recurrent herpes simplex. Planta Medica 74.9 (2008): 215.

L

L-Glutamine

HISTORICAL NOTE Glutamine and glutamate were originally described in the mid 19th century and their functions began to be examined in the early 20th century. The role of glutamine in the immune system and gastrointestinal tract has been investigated since the 1980s.

BACKGROUND AND RELEVANT PHARMACOKINETICS

L-Glutamine is a conditionally essential amino acid found in all life forms and the most abundant amino acid in the human body. During conditions of metabolic stress characterised by catabolism and negative nitrogen balance, such as trauma (including surgical trauma), prolonged stress, glucocorticoid use, excessive exercise, starvation, infection, sepsis, cancer and severe burns, the body is unable to synthesise L-glutamine in sufficient quantities to meet biological needs and it becomes essential to have an exogenous intake (Miller 1999, PDRHealth 2006a).

L-Glutamine is absorbed from the lumen of the small intestine by active transport (Meng et al 2003) and is then transported to the liver via the portal circulation and enters the systemic circulation, where it is distributed to various tissues and transported into cells via an active process. Elimination occurs via glomerular filtration and it is almost completely reabsorbed by the renal tubules. Some metabolism of L-glutamine takes place in the enterocytes and hepatocytes and it is involved in various metabolic activities, including the synthesis of L-glutamate (catalysed by glutaminase), proteins, glutathione, pyrimidine and purine nucleotides and amino sugars. L-glutamate is converted to L-glutamine by glutamine synthase in the presence of ammonia, adenosine triphosphate (ATP) and magnesium or manganese.

L-Glutamine is synthesised endogenously from other amino acids, predominantly branched-chain amino acids and glutamate, and stored in skeletal muscles, where it comprises around 60% of the free amino acids and makes up 4–5% of muscle protein. In times of metabolic stress, glutamine is released into the circulation and transported to tissues in need (Kohlmeier 2003, Miller 1999, PDRHealth 2006a).

L-Glutamine is not very soluble or stable in solution, especially upon heating for sterilisation, and as a result, until recently, was not included in total parenteral nutrition (TPN). The more soluble and stable glutamine dipeptides are now commonly used as the delivery forms in TPN solutions and some nutritional supplements (Kohlmeier 2003, PDRHealth 2006b).

Common forms available

The terms L-glutamine and glutamine are often used interchangeably. L-glutamine is the amide form of L-glutamic acid and contains 15.7% nitrogen (Kohlmeier 2003). It is also known as 2-aminoglutaramic acid, levoglutamide, (S)-2,5-diamino-5-oxopentaenoic acid and glutamic acid 5-amide. Glutamic acid is a non-essential amino acid and glutamine is the aminated form of glutamic acid. Glutamic acid is found in many foods, such as grain cereals (barley, wheat, flax, sorghum, rye), nuts and seeds, dairy foods and meat. L-glutamic acid is commonly used as a supplement in sports nutrition. Salts and carboxylate anions of glutamic acid are known as glutamates (such as sodium glutamate, potassium glutamate). Glutamate is involved in cellular metabolism and it is an abundant neurotransmitter.

Two synthetic glutamine dipeptides that may be used in TPN are L-alanyl-L-glutamine and glycyl-L-glutamine. D-Glutamine, the stereoisomer of L-glutamine, has no known biological activity (Kohlmeier 2003, PDRHealth 2006b).

Since the late 1960s, L-glutamine has been manufactured for pharmaceutical use using a fermentation broth. The manufacture of high-quality, low-cost L-glutamine requires a strain of microorganism with good production efficiency and minimum byproducts. Impurities can then be removed from the broth using a nanofiltration membrane to obtain a fine crystalline powder (Kusumoto 2001, Li et al 2003).

FOOD SOURCES

Typical dietary intake of L-glutamine is 5–10 g/day (Miller 1999). Sources include animal and plant proteins, vegetable juices (especially cabbage), eggs, wheat, soybeans and fermented foods, such as miso and yoghurt (Kohlmeier 2003, PDRHealth 2006a).

DEFICIENCY SIGNS AND SYMPTOMS

Although traditionally considered a non-essential amino acid, L-glutamine is now considered 'conditionally essential' during periods of metabolic stress characterised by catabolism and negative nitrogen balance.

Critical illness, stress and injury can lead to a significant decrease in plasma levels of L-glutamine which, if severe, can increase the risk of mortality (Boelens et al 2001, Wischmeyer 2003).

Prolonged protein malnutrition may cause growth inhibition, muscle wasting and organ damage (Kohlmeier 2003). In the absence of sufficient plasma glutamine, the body will break down skeletal muscle stores, and gut integrity (gut mucosal barrier function) and immunity will be compromised. Because L-glutamine is utilised during exercise, a more recent phenomenon of deficiency has been explored and glutamine depletion has been linked with 'overtraining syndrome'.

MAIN ACTIONS

L-Glutamine has many important biological functions within the human body. It is an important fuel for the intestinal mucosal cells, hepatocytes and rapidly proliferating cells of the immune system, particularly lymphocytes and monocytes, assists in the regulation of acid balance, thus preventing acidosis, acts as a nitrogen shuttle protecting the body from high levels of ammonia, and is involved in the synthesis of amino acids (including L-glutamate), gamma-aminobutyric acid (GABA), glutathione (an important antioxidant), purine and pyramidine nucleotides, amino acid sugars in glycoproteins and glycans, and nicotinamide adenosine dinucleotide (NAD). It is also involved in protein synthesis and energy production (Boelens et al 2001, Kohlmeier 2003, Miller 1999, Niihara et al 2005, Patel et al 2001, PDRHealth 2006a).

Gastrointestinal protection/repair

According to in vitro and in vivo research, L-glutamine aids in the proliferation and repair of intestinal cells (Chun et al 1997, Rhoads et al 1997, Scheppach et al 1996) and is the preferred respiratory fuel for enterocytes (and also utilised by colonocytes) (Miller 1999). It is thus vital for maintaining the integrity of the intestinal lining and preventing the translocation of microbes and endotoxins into the body. In addition, L-glutamine helps to maintain secretory immunoglobulin A (IgA), which functions primarily by preventing the attachment of bacteria to mucosal cells (PDRHealth 2006a, Yu et al 1996).

According to evidence from animal studies, it may also assist in preventing atrophy following colostomy (Paulo 2002) and irradiation (Diestel et al 2005), and intestinal injury by inhibiting intestinal cytokine release (Akisu et al 2003). L-glutamine depletion induces apoptosis by triggering intercellular events that lead to cell death (Paquette et al 2005), resulting in altered epithelial barrier competence (increased intestinal permeability), bacterial translocation and increased mortality. Under experimental conditions, L-glutamine may assist in maintaining intestinal barrier function by increasing epithelial resistance to apoptotic injury, reducing oxidative damage, attenuating programmed cell death and promoting re-epithelialisation (Masuko 2002, Ropeleski et al 2005, Scheppach et al 1996) and may thus reduce bacterial and endotoxin translocation (Chun et al 1997).

Immunomodulation

L-Glutamine has demonstrated immunomodulatory activity in animal models of infection and trauma, as well as trauma in humans. L-Glutamine acts as the preferred respiratory fuel for lymphocytes, is essential for cell proliferation, and can enhance the function of stimulated immune cells.

Extracellular glutamine concentration affects lymphocyte, interleukin-2 and interferon-gamma proliferation, cytokine production, phagocytic and secretory macrophage activities and neutrophil bacterial killing (Miller 1999, Newsholme 2001, PDRHealth 2006a). In humans, L-glutamine may enhance both phagocytosis and reactive oxygen intermediate production by neutrophils (Furukawa et al 2000) and support the restoration of type-1T lymphocyte responsiveness following trauma (Boelens et al 2004). In a randomised trial, there was a reduced frequency of pneumonia, sepsis and bacteraemia in patients with multiple traumas who received glutamine-supplemented enteral nutrition (Houdijk et al 1998).

In addition, effects on the gastrointestinal tract may contribute significantly to immune defence by maintaining gut-associated lymphoid tissue and secretory IgA (preventing the attachment of bacteria to the gut mucosa) and maintaining gut integrity (thus preventing the translocation of microbes and their toxins, especially Gram-negative bacteria from the large intestine) (Miller 1999, Yu et al 1996).

Antioxidant

As a precursor to glutathione (together with cysteine and glycine), L-glutamine can assist in ameliorating the oxidation that occurs during metabolic stress. Glutathione protects epithelial cell membranes from damage, and its depletion can negatively affect gut barrier function and result in severe degeneration of colonic and jejunal epithelial cells (Iantomasi 1994, Ziegler et al 1999). In animal studies, it has also been shown to inhibit fatty acid oxidation, resulting in a reduction in body weight and alleviation of hyperglycaemia and hyperinsulinaemia in mice fed a high-fat diet (Opara et al 1996).

Anabolic/anticatabolic

As L-glutamine is stored primarily in skeletal muscles and becomes conditionally essential under conditions of metabolic stress, the anticatabolic/anabolic properties of supplemented L-glutamine are likely due to a sparing effect on skeletal muscle stores.

Following strenuous exercise, glutamine levels are depleted by approximately 20%, resulting in immunodepression (Castell 2003, Castell & Newsholme 1997, Rogero et al 2002). As a result supplemental L-glutamine may be of benefit in athletes to prevent the deleterious effects of glutamine depletion associated with 'overtraining syndrome'. Evidence supporting a direct ergogenic effect is currently lacking.

Cardioprotective

In vitro, L-glutamine has been shown to assist in the maintenance of myocardial glutamate, ATP and phosphocreatine, and in the prevention of lactate accumulation (Khogali et al 1998). In addition to its antioxidant properties and effects on hyperglycaemia and hyperinsulinaemia (Opara et al 1996), this may suggest a possible role as a cardioprotective agent.

A recent randomised, double-blind, placebo-controlled study by Lomivorotov et al (2013) reported no cardioprotective benefit of perioperative use of N_2-L-alanyl-L-glutamine (0.4 g/kg/day of 20% solution of N_2-L-alanyl-L-glutamine [Dipeptiven, Fresenius Kabi, Germany]) in 32 patients with type 2 diabetes who underwent cardiopulmonary bypass surgery compared to the control group of 32 patients who received 0.9% NaCl.

However glutamine supplementation was reported to be cardioprotective in the first 24 hours postoperatively, as assessed by dynamics of troponin I in a study of patients with ischaemic heart disease who underwent cardiopulmonary bypass surgery. The perioperative glutamine-supplemented group of 25 patients (0.4 g/kg glutamine [Dipeptiven, 20% solution] per day) was compared to 25 patients in the control group who were administered a placebo (0.9% NaCl) (Lomivorotov et al 2011) and the dynamics of troponin I were assessed at 30 minutes, and at 6, 24 and 48 hours after surgery.

In a small, randomised double-blind study, 14 patients who required cardiopulmonary bypass surgery were placed in two groups. One group of 7 patients received oral alanyl-glutamine (25 g twice daily) for 3 days prior to surgery and the other group served as a control and received maltodextrin. The glutamine-supplemented group was reported to have significantly reduced myocardial injury and clinical complications (Sufit et al 2012).

> ***Clinical note — Total parenteral nutrition***
> L-Glutamine is not very soluble or stable in solution, especially upon heating for sterilisation. As a result, until recently it was not included in TPN, resulting in compromised glutamine status in patients for whom reduced immune status and increased intestinal permeability could potentially increase the risk of morbid infection and mortality. The more soluble and stable synthetic glutamine dipeptides (L-alanyl-L-glutamine and glycyl-L-glutamine) have now been developed as delivery forms of L-glutamine for use in TPN. The dipeptide forms can also be used orally and have demonstrated a potential for greater bioavailability than glutamine alone (Macedo Rogero et al 2004).
>
> Numerous studies have now been conducted using glutamine dipeptides in TPN and have shown benefit in preventing deterioration of gut permeability and preserving mucosal structure (Hall et al 1996, Jiang et al 1999, PDRHealth 2006a, van der Hulst et al 1993). In addition, animal studies suggest that glutamine-enriched TPN may attenuate the suppression of CYP3A and CYP2C usually associated with TPN (Shaw et al 2002). The addition of glutamine to TPN in preterm infants also appears to hasten improvements in hepatic function (Wang et al 2013).
>
> In a meta-analysis of European and Asian randomised controlled trials (RCTs) in elective surgery patients, 13 studies (pooled $n = 355$) met inclusion criteria and demonstrated a significant reduction in infectious complication and length of hospital stay (weighted mean difference [WMD] of 3.86 days) (Jiang et al 2004). Conversely, a small study using glutamine (10 g) as part of home parenteral nutrition for 6 months did not reveal any significant effects compared to placebo for infective complications (36% vs 55%; $P = 0.67$), nutritional status, intestinal permeability or quality of life. It should be noted that plasma glutamine concentrations were also not affected in this study (Culkin et al 2008).

Neurotransmission

Disturbances of glutamine metabolism and/or transport may contribute to changes in glutamatergic or GABAergic transmission associated with different pathological conditions of the brain, such as epilepsy, hepatic encephalopathy and manganese encephalopathy. Glutamine appears to affect neurotransmission by interacting with the *N*-methyl-D-aspartate class of glutamine receptors (Albrecht et al 2010).

CLINICAL USE

Deficiency: prevention and treatment

During periods of increased need, L-glutamine is considered conditionally essential. Glutamine depletion can result in increased intestinal permeability, microbial translocation across the gut barrier, impaired wound healing, sepsis and multiple organ failure (Miller 1999). Experimental studies have proposed a number of benefits for patients with conditions that increase glutamine requirements. The suggested mechanisms include effects on proinflammatory cytokine expression, gut integrity, enhanced ability to mount a stress response and improved immune cell function, and studies have shown potential benefit with regard to mortality, length of hospital stay and infection.

To date, the results of studies using glutamine dipeptides in TPN have proven to be very promising in treating patients for whom enteral feeding is impossible. Benefits from studies of enteral glutamine supplementation have tended to be less pronounced, but preliminary trials have demonstrated benefits in some conditions, especially at high doses (e.g. 30 g/day enterally) (Wischmeyer 2003).

Critical care settings

A systematic review found trends to suggest that parenteral and enteral glutamine supplementation may reduce mortality, the development of infection and organ failure in critical illness; however, poor study design and possible publication bias limit what conclusions can be drawn from the current data (Avenell 2006).

A recent meta-analysis of 14 RCTs ($n = 587$) found that people given parenteral nutrition supplemented with glutamine dipeptide had a shorter length of hospital stay and a significant decrease in infectious complications (relative risk [RR] = 0.69; $P = 0.02$) compared to the group receiving standard parenteral nutrition (Wang et al 2010).

Similarly, in a recent meta-analysis by Bollhalder et al (2013) that included 40 RCTs, parenteral glutamine supplementation was associated with a significant reduction in infections (RR = 0.83) and a non-significant reduction in short-term mortality (RR = 0.89) and length of stay, although a significant reduction in mortality was not verified, in contrast to previous meta-analyses.

Likewise, a more recent meta-analysis by Chen et al (2014) that included 15 studies of 2862 critically ill patients in a number of settings, including surgical intensive care unit (ICU) subgroup and parenteral nutrition subgroup, reported that, compared to control groups, glutamine supplementation significantly reduced the incidence of hospital-acquired infections (RR 0.85; 95% confidence interval [CI] 0.74–0.97; $P = 0.02$). However, in 14 studies with 2777 patients, there was no benefit in overall mortality or length of hospital stay, although the mortality rate was significantly higher (RR 1.18; 95% CI

1.02–1.38; $P = 0.03$) in high glutamine dosage subgroup (above 0.5 g/kg/day).

Abdominal surgery and trauma

Parenteral supplementation of glutamine in critically ill patients has been shown to improve survival rate and minimise infectious complications, costs and length of hospital stay; however, the role of enteral glutamine supplementation remains controversial (Al Balushi et al 2013).

A meta-analysis of nine RCTs involving 373 patients was performed to assess the clinical and economical validity of glutamine dipeptide supplementation to parenteral nutrition in patients undergoing abdominal surgery. The review concluded that glutamine dipeptide has a positive effect in decreasing postoperative infectious morbidity (odds ratio [OR] = 0.24, $P = 0.04$), shortening the length of hospital stay (WMD = −3.55, 95% $P < 0.00001$) and improving postoperative cumulative nitrogen balance (WMD = 8.35, $P = 0.002$). No serious adverse effects were identified (Zheng 2006).

Enteral supplementation has not been shown to be as effective in abdominal trauma. In one trial, 120 patients with peritonitis or abdominal trauma were randomised to receive either enteral glutamine (45 g/day for 5 days) in addition to standard care ($n = 63$) or standard care alone ($n = 57$). No statistically significant benefits were noted in the treatment group for serum malondialdehyde or glutathione levels, infectious complications, survival rate or duration of hospital stay (Kumar et al 2007).

Trauma

Enteral glutamine has been shown to be protective to the gut in experimental models of shock and thus improve clinical outcomes. In a pilot study, enteral glutamine was administered during active shock resuscitation (0.5 g/kg/day during the first 24 hours) and continued for 10 days through the early postinjury period. The treatment was found to be safe and improved gastrointestinal tolerance (vomiting, nasogastric output, diarrhoea and distension). ICU and hospital length of stay were comparable (McQuiggan et al 2008). In a randomised trial using glutamine-enriched enteral nutrition in patients with multiple traumas, there was a reduction in the incidence of pneumonia, sepsis and bacteraemia (Houdijk et al 1998). Parenteral supplementation of alanyl-glutamine dipeptide may also result in better insulin sensitivity in multiple-trauma patients (Bakalar et al 2006).

Burns

Acute burn injury results in depletion of plasma and muscle glutamine, which contributes to muscle wasting, weight loss and infection. In critical illness, supplementation has been shown to minimise these effects and reduce the rate of mortality and length of stay (Windle 2006). In a double-blind controlled trial, 48 severely burned patients (total burn surface area 30–75%, full-thickness burn area 20–58%) were randomised into treatment ($n = 25$; 0.5 g/kg/day glutamine granules for 14 days with oral or tube feeding) or control group ($n = 23$; glycine placebo). The results indicated that significantly reduced plasma glutamine and damaged immunological function occurred and supplementation with glutamine granules increased plasma glutamine concentration and reduced the degree of immunosuppression. Glutamine improved immunological function (especially cellular immunity), wound healing and length of hospital stay (46.59 ± 12.98 days vs 55.68 ± 17.36 days, $P < 0.05$) (Peng et al 2006).

According to animal studies, oral glutamine supplementation may reduce bacterial and endotoxin translocation after burns by maintaining secretory IgA in the intestinal mucosa (Yu et al 1996). Systematic reviews and practice guidelines generally support glutamine supplementation in critical illness; however, in large or severe burns or inhalation injury there may be a prolonged critical illness phase (>4 weeks). Further research focusing on enteral and parenteral glutamine supplementation and long-term use is required (Windle 2006).

A recent meta-analysis of glutamine supplementation in critically ill patients with burns reported a reduction in mortality in hospital and complications due to Gram-negative bacteraemia (Lin et al 2013). The meta-analysis included four RCTs which involved 155 patients. The total burn surface area ($P = 0.34$) was similar in both glutamine and control groups at baseline; however, treatment with glutamine induced a significant decrease in the number of patients with Gram-negative bacteraemia (OR 0.27; $P = 0.04$) and hospital mortality (OR = 0.13; $P = 0.004$), and there was no statistical difference for the length of hospital stay.

Infants

Enteral and parenteral glutamine supplementation in preterm infants has been shown to have some beneficial effects on neonatal morbidity and mortality; however, these results are controversial (Korkmaz et al 2007).

In a short-term study of preterm infants (birth weight ≤ 1500 g) who received either enteral glutamine supplementation ($n = 36$; 300 mg/kg/day adjusted over time according to the current weight) or placebo ($n = 33$) between 8 and 120 days of life, the glutamine-supplemented group had significantly higher mean weight, length, head circumference, left upper mid-arm circumference and left mid-thigh circumference than the control group at the end of the fourth month. The effects appeared to occur in a time-dependent pattern (Korkmaz et al 2007). Another study reported that oral supplementation (0.25 mg/kg body weight) with glutamine did not improve growth or intestinal permeability (lactulose : mannitol ratio: 0.29 [95% CI 0.23–0.35] and 0.26 [95% CI: 0.21–0.32]) in malnourished Gambian infants (Williams et al 2007). It should be noted, however, that this dose is exceptionally low compared to other trials. The dose, route of

L

administration and length of supplementation require further elucidation in larger-scale trials before full assessment can be made.

Experimental data have suggested that, by stimulating the rate of recovery of the villi and lipid-synthesising enzymes, L-glutamine treatments could improve the efficacy of enteral feeding in infants recovering from bowel damage (Ahdieh et al 1998). However, a recent Cochrane review concluded insufficient data were available from RCTs to determine whether glutamine supplementation confers clinically significant benefits for infants with severe gastrointestinal disease (Wagner et al 2012).

Some authors have suggested that early glutamine supplementation may also provide longer-term benefits. Enteral glutamine supplementation (300 mg/kg/day) between 3 and 30 days of life has been shown to lower the incidence of atopic dermatitis (OR 0.13; 95% CI 0.02–0.97) but not the incidence of bronchial hyperreactivity and infectious diseases (upper respiratory, lower respiratory and gastrointestinal) during the first year of life (van den Berg et al 2007). Follow-up of 52 very preterm babies who received glutamine supplementation in their first month of life revealed that there was an increase in white matter, hippocampus and brainstem volumes at school age, and this was mediated by a decrease in serious neonatal infections (de Kieviet et al 2012).

Despite the many encouraging results, a recent Cochrane review of 11 RCTs (five trials of enteral glutamine supplementation and six trials of parenteral glutamine supplementation) that included 2771 preterm infants reported that glutamine supplementation did not have a significant effect on mortality or major neonatal morbidities, including the incidence of invasive infection and necrotising enterocolitis (Moe-Byrne et al 2012).

Strenuous exercise

Following strenuous exercise, glutamine levels are depleted approximately 20%, resulting in immunodepression (Castell 2003, Castell & Newsholme 1997, Rogero et al 2002). However the role of glutamine supplementation in preventing postexercise effects on immune function is controversial (Gleeson 2008). The type of training is important to note, as although previous reports suggest decreased glutamine concentrations in overtrained athletes, progressive endurance training may lead to steady increases in plasma glutamine levels (Kargotich et al 2007).

The provision of glutamine after exercise has been shown to improve immune status (Castell & Newsholme 1997). In a study of 200 elite runners and rowers given a glutamine or placebo drink immediately after and again 2 hours after strenuous exercise, 151 participants returned questionnaires reporting the incidence of infection over the subsequent 7 days. The percentage of athletes reporting no infections was considerably higher in the glutamine group (81%, $n = 72$) compared to the placebo group (49%, $n = 79$, $P < 0.001$) (Castell et al 1996).

During recovery from strenuous exercise, rates of lymphocyte apoptosis, hyperammonaemia and whole-body proteolysis may be affected by glutamine supplementation. In a small study of nine triathletes, glutamine supplementation (four tablets of 700 mg of hydrolysed whey protein enriched with 175 mg of glutamine dipeptide dissolved in 250 mL water) partially prevented lymphocyte apoptosis induced by exhaustive exercise, possibly by a protective effect on mitochondrial function (Cury-Boaventura et al 2008). Both intermittent and continuous-intensity exercises increase ammonia, urate, urea and creatinine in the blood stream. Chronic glutamine supplementation (100 mg/kg body weight) given immediately before exercise may partially protect against elevated ammonia but not urate, urea or creatinine (Bassini-Cameron et al 2008). The addition of glutamine (300 mg/kg body weight) to an oral carbohydrate (1 g/kg/h) and essential amino acid (9.25 g) solution had no effect on postexercise muscle glycogen resynthesis or muscle protein synthesis, but may suppress a rise in whole-body proteolysis during the later stages of recovery (Wilkinson et al 2006).

Conversely, a trial assessing the possible ergogenic effects of glutamine supplementation (300 mg/kg body weight) to improve high-intensity exercise performance in trained males was unable to determine a beneficial effect (Haub et al 1998). Currently, the use of glutamine to enhance exercise performance is speculative at best and the cost of the high doses indicated must be considered. Further large-scale research is required to elucidate any potentially beneficial effects.

Care should be taken in people with diabetes as a small study revealed an increase in postexercise overnight hypoglycaemia in adolescents with type 1 diabetes who received a glutamine drink (0.25 g/kg/dose) pre-exercise and at bedtime (Mauras et al 2010).

Gut repair

Preliminary research on enteral (as well as parenteral) glutamine supplementation suggested promise for the use of glutamine in gut repair by: (1) protecting the intestinal mucosa from damage and promoting repair, thus improving intestinal permeability and reducing subsequent microbial and endotoxin translocation, promoting glutathione and secretory IgA; and (2) improving gut immunity. However, while there is some evidence for the use of glutamine in TPN (Hall et al 1996), clinical evidence using oral supplementation is less convincing. As in vitro data suggest that the colonic mucosa receives its nutrients preferentially from the luminal (not vascular) side (Roediger 1986), it has been suggested that glutamine should be more effective when delivered by the enteral route (Kouznetsova et al 1999). This has yet to be determined in clinical trials.

L-Glutamine enemas, twice daily for 7 days, have been shown to reduce mucosal damage and inflammation in experimental models of colitis in rats

(Kaya et al 1999); however, preliminary trials in humans using parenteral glutamine (da Gama Torres et al 2008) and oral supplementation in malnourished preterm infants (Williams et al 2007) have not confirmed benefits for intestinal permeability.

Postoperative administration of TPN supplemented with a combination of glutamine and recombinant human growth hormone in patients following portal hypertension surgery prevented intestinal mucous membrane atrophy and preserved intestinal integrity, although the role of glutamine is unclear (Tang et al 2007). In a 1998 randomised, double-blind, placebo-controlled, 4-week trial of 24 HIV patients with abnormal intestinal permeability using 0, 4 or 8 g/day of glutamine, the authors reported a dose-dependent trend towards improved intestinal permeability and enhanced intestinal absorption with glutamine supplementation and recommended further studies to be carried out with higher doses (e.g. 20 g/day) over a longer study period (Noyer et al 1998). It is difficult to extrapolate the findings of this study to the wider community for the purpose of gut repair as there are factors involved in HIV/AIDS that may increase the biological demand for glutamine. Longer-term studies may provide more convincing results; however, it is possible that glutamine only stabilises gut barrier function under certain conditions and more research is required to elucidate these.

Crohn's disease

In a controlled trial, consecutive patients in remission from Crohn's disease with an abnormal intestinal permeability were randomised to receive oral glutamine or whey protein (0.5 g/kg ideal body weight/day). After 2 months intestinal permeability and morphology had improved significantly in both the glutamine and whey groups (Benjamin et al 2012). Previously a 4-week study on 18 children with active Crohn's disease fed a glutamine-enriched polymeric diet (Akobeng et al 2000) was unable to demonstrate benefits.

HIV

L-Glutamine has been shown to improve glutathione levels and significantly increase lean body mass in HIV patients (Patrick 2000); however, not all studies confirm this latter effect (Huffman & Walgren 2003). A recent study of 12 treated patients (six men and six women, 22–45 years old) and 20 healthy controls (10 men and 10 women, 20–59 years old) who were randomly assigned to 7-day dietary supplements containing *N*-acetylcysteine (1 g/day) or glutamine (20 g/day), with a 7-day washout period ingesting their usual diet, reported an increase in total glutathione by glutamine supplementation (Borges-Santos et al 2012). Improvements in intestinal absorption have also been reported in HIV patients receiving isonitrogenous doses of alanyl-glutamine (24 g/day for 10 days) (Leite et al 2013). Combined therapy with arginine and the leucine metabolite beta-hydroxy-beta-methylbutyrate has been shown to reverse lean tissue loss in HIV and cancer patients (Rathmacher et al 2004).

During initial HIV infection, the rapid turnover and proliferation of immune cells increase glutamine requirements and later the repeated episodes of infection, fever and diarrhoea may lead to further depletion. As a result, the doses used in the trial mentioned above (4 g and 8 g) may have been insufficient to meet the increased requirement in such patients (Noyer et al 1998).

Highly active antiretroviral therapy may be associated with diarrhoea and other gastrointestinal side effects. In a prospective, randomised, double-blind crossover study, HIV-infected patients with nelfinavir-associated diarrhoea (for >1 month) received L-glutamine (30 g/day) or placebo for 10 days. Glutamine supplementation resulted in a significant reduction in the severity of nelfinavir-associated diarrhoea (Huffman & Walgren 2003). A prospective 12-week trial of 35 HIV-positive men experiencing diarrhoea as a result of nelfinavir or lopinavir/ritonavir therapy was also conducted using probiotics and soluble fibre. When glutamine (30 g/day) was added to the regimen of non-responders at week 4, the response rate improved (Heiser et al 2004).

Cancer prevention

In addition to being the major fuel source for rapidly proliferating intestinal and immune cells, L-glutamine is the main fuel source for many rapidly growing tumours and, as a result, tumour growth is associated with a depletion in glutamine and glutathione stores and a depression of natural killer (NK) cell activity (Fahr et al 1994, Miller 1999). The increased intestinal permeability, immune suppression and oxidative damage that may result may further compromise the body's ability to deal with the tumour. While concerns exist, and are supported by in vitro evidence, that glutamine supplementation may feed the tumour, animal studies suggest that glutamine supplementation may assist in decreasing tumour growth by enhancing NK cell activity (Fahr et al 1994, Miller 1999). Animal studies have demonstrated that glutamine supplementation prevents the promotion of tumour cells in an implantable breast cancer model (Kaufmann et al 2003). The exact effects in different human tumour cell lines require further elucidation.

Gastrointestinal effects

A number of studies have reported that adding glutamine to chemotherapy appears to reduce the incidence and severity of oral mucositis, a frequent complication of mucotoxic cancer therapy, which causes significant oral pain, increased infection risk and impaired functioning (Peterson et al 2007). For instance, oral glutamine (30 g/day) appears to reduce the incidence of fluorouracil/leucovorin-induced mucositis/stomatitis (9% vs 38% in the control group; $P < 0.001$) (Choi et al 2007).

> ***Clinical note — Cancer therapy***
> Side effects of chemotherapy and radiation therapy can significantly affect the quality of life of patients undergoing treatment for cancer. A number of trials have demonstrated the benefits of glutamine supplementation for improving side effects such as oral pain and inflammation, increased gut permeability and reduced lymphocyte count.
>
> The provision of 15 g of oral glutamine three times daily appears to significantly reduce the incidence of severe radiation-induced diarrhoea (Kucuktulu et al 2013). Similarly, in a retrospective randomised experimental study of 46 patients with lung cancer who were treated with thoracic radiotherapy, the severity of acute radiotherapy-induced oesophagitis was significantly reduced ($P < 0.0001$) in those who were given 30 g prophylactic oral glutamine powder daily (Tutanc et al 2013).

Reduced oral pain and inflammation have also been observed in patients receiving radiation and chemotherapy during bone marrow transplantation taking oral glutamine (1 g four times daily) (Miller 1999). In a retrospective study involving 41 patients with stage III lung carcinoma treated with thoracic irradiation, prophylactic supplementation with powdered glutamine (10 g/8 h) was found to be associated with a 27% lower incidence of grade 2 or 3 acute radiation-induced oesophagitis (ARIE), a 6-day delay in ARIE (22 days vs 16 days) and weight gain during radiotherapy (Topkan et al 2009).

In another study, L-glutamine (4 g twice daily, swish and swallow) was given to 12 patients receiving doxorubicin, one receiving etoposide, and one receiving ifosfamide, etoposide and carboplatinum from day 1 of chemotherapy for 28 days or for 4 days past the resolution of any postchemotherapy mucositis. Oral supplementation with glutamine significantly decreased the severity of chemotherapy-induced stomatitis (Skubitz & Anderson 1996). In a small study, parenteral glutamine supplementation was shown to protect the gastrointestinal mucosa against fluorouracil/calcium-folinate chemotherapy-induced damage (Decker-Baumann et al 1999). Yoshida et al (1998, 2001) have also shown that 30 g/day L-glutamine for 28 days attenuates the increased gut permeability and reduced lymphocyte count observed in patients undergoing cisplatin and fluorouracil therapy for oesophageal cancer.

In a small phase I trial ($n = 15$), glutamine was co-administered in an attempt to escalate the dose of a chemoradiotherapy regimen (weekly paclitaxel and carboplatin with concurrent radiation therapy). The addition was deemed unsuccessful due to multiple severe toxicities, including haematological toxicities and oesophagitis (Jazieh et al 2007). The role of glutamine in reducing taxane-associated dysgeusia (taste alteration) appears limited (Strasser et al 2008).

In a double-blind, placebo-controlled, randomised trial, oral glutamine (18 g/day) or placebo was given to 70 chemotherapy-naive patients with colorectal cancer 5 days prior to their first cycle of fluorouracil (450 mg/m^2) in association with folinic acid (100 mg/m^2), which was administered intravenously for 5 days. Glutamine treatment was continued for 15 days and was shown to reduce the negative effects on intestinal absorption and permeability induced by the chemotherapy and to potentially reduce diarrhoea (Daniele et al 2001). L-Glutamine may also reverse the decrease in goblet cells induced by fluorouracil (Tanaka & Takeuchi 2002).

More recent studies have further investigated the utility of glutamine supplementation in different patient groups receiving various modes of nutrition support and a variety of glutamine dosages.

A randomised study of 70 patients (Chattopadhyay et al 2014) reported that oral glutamine (10 g in 1 L of water 2 hours before radiotherapy treatment for 5 days/week on treatment days only; $n = 35$) reduced the severity and duration of oral mucositis in head and neck cancer patients receiving primary or adjuvant radiation therapy compared to patients in the control group ($n = 35$) who did not receive the glutamine.

A recent systematic review of 131 studies that included 10,514 participants evaluated the effectiveness of a range of prophylactic agents, including glutamine supplementation for oral mucositis in patients with cancer receiving treatment, compared with other potentially active interventions, placebo or no treatment, and reported that there was some benefit with intravenous glutamine (Worthington et al 2011).

However a more recent systematic review investigating natural agents in the management of oral mucositis has made a recommendation against the use of intravenous glutamine in patients receiving high-dose chemotherapy prior to haematopoietic stem cell transplant (level II evidence) (Yarom et al 2013).

In particular an earlier study by Pytlík et al (2002) had reported that intravenous glutamine made mucositis worse and was significantly associated with more relapses ($P = 0.02$) and higher mortality ($P = 0.05$).

In contrast, Gibson et al (2013) reported in their systematic review that new research did not support earlier observations of toxicity associated with glutamine supplementation and therefore they were unable to make a clinical guideline regarding glutamine supplementation for gastrointestinal mucositis, whereas the previous guideline was not to use systemic glutamine.

In regard to use in children, the evidence is less clear. A recent systematic review by Qutob et al (2013) investigated the evidence for the use of agents regarding the prevention of oral mucositis in children and concluded that, due to conflicting results, certain agents such as oral or enteral glutamine should be avoided until their efficacy is confirmed by further research.

Chemotherapy-induced diarrhoea

Chemotherapy-induced diarrhoea is a significant adverse effect during treatment with chemotherapy. A recent meta-analysis of eight RCTs (five studies with glutamine administered intravenously and three studies where glutamine was taken orally) included 298 patients (147 patients who received glutamine supplementation [16–40 g/day] and 151 patients who received a placebo), and reported a statistically significant reduction in the duration of diarrhoea in the glutamine-supplemented group, although there was no significant difference in the severity of diarrhoea between the groups (Sun et al 2012).

In a small randomised double-blind, placebo-controlled pilot study of 33 patients with rectal cancer, 30 g of glutamine was given in three doses per day for 5 weeks during preoperative radiochemotherapy and the placebo was given as 30 g of maltodextrin. There was no difference between groups in the frequency and severity of diarrhoea during radiochemotherapy ($P = 0.5$ and $P = 0.39$ respectively) (Rotovnik Kozjek et al 2011).

Chemotherapy-induced peripheral neuropathy

Chemotherapy-induced peripheral neuropathy is a significant adverse effect associated with neurotoxic chemotherapy (especially taxanes, platinum compounds and vinca alkaloids). In a review, two studies were identified that suggested beneficial effects. In one study, oral glutamine was found to be effective in reducing peripheral neuropathy associated with high-dose paclitaxel, resulting in a reduction in numbness, dysaesthesias and motor weakness, as well as a smaller loss of vibratory sensation (Amara 2008). Another study found that the addition of oral glutamine (15 g twice daily for 7 consecutive days every 2 weeks, starting on the day of oxaliplatin infusion) resulted in a significant reduction in the incidence and severity of peripheral neuropathy, less interference with activities of daily living (16.7% versus 40.9%) and less need for oxaliplatin dose reduction due to adverse effects (7.1% vs 27.3%). The addition of glutamine did not affect response to chemotherapy or survival (Wang et al 2007).

Other benefits

In one report, L-glutamine (10 g three times daily), given 24 hours after receiving paclitaxel, appeared to prevent the development of myalgia and arthralgia associated with treatment (PDRHealth 2006a). In children with solid tumours receiving chemotherapy, oral glutamine supplementation (4 g/m^2/day) may improve nutritional and immunological parameters and reduce requirements for antibiotics (Okur et al 2006). Glutamine may also increase tumour methotrexate concentration and tumouricidal activity and reduce side effects and mortality rates (Miller 1999, PDRHealth 2006a).

OTHER USES

Growth and development

In a prospective randomised, double-blind, placebo-controlled 1-year study of 120 young Brazilian shantytown children aged from 2 months to 9 years who were given glutamine alone (16 g daily for 10 days at start of the study) or a combination of glutamine + zinc + vitamin, improved intestinal barrier function was seen, as measured by the percentage of lactulose urinary excretion and the lactulose : mannitol absorption ratio. Glutamine treatment significantly improved weight-for-height z-scores compared to the placebo-glycine control group (Lima et al 2014).

Radiation injury

In a recent double-blind study the beneficial effects of oral glutamine supplementation on radiation injury were investigated in women undergoing radiation therapy for breast cancer. In the 8-week study, 17 patients were randomised to receive either the supplementary glutamine (0.5 g/kg/day; $n = 9$) or a placebo (dextrose, 25 g/day; $n = 8$) three times daily during 6 weeks of radiation therapy. The patients were followed for 2 years for assessment of radiation injury using the Radiation Therapy Oncology Group scales. The study reported reduced acute radiation morbidity and pain in the glutamine-supplemented group (Rubio et al 2013).

Alcoholism

Preliminary studies suggested a potential for glutamine to reduce alcohol cravings; however, these effects have not yet been studied in controlled trials on humans (PDRHealth 2006a). More recently, in vitro research has suggested that glutamine supplementation may inhibit the deleterious effects of alcohol on the tight junctions of the gut mucosa and in turn reduce the increased risk for gastrointestinal cancers in alcoholics (Basuroy et al 2005, Seth et al 2004).

Acute pancreatitis

The enteral administration of L-glutamine (15 mg/kg/day) to rats with acute pancreatitis resulted in a reduction in necrosis and infectious complications by decreasing the bacterial translocation rate (Avsar et al 2001).

Sickle cell disease

Orally administered L-glutamine improves the NAD redox potential of sickle red blood cells. Investigations of blood samples taken from five adult patients with sickle cell anaemia who had been on L-glutamine (30 g/day) therapy for at least 4 weeks consistently resulted in improvement of sickle red blood cell adhesion to human umbilical vein endothelial cells compared to the control group. The authors conclude that these results suggest positive physiological effects for L-glutamine in sickle cell disease (Niihara et al 2005).

Other conditions

Glutamine is a popular supplement in naturopathic practice and sometimes used for conditions that may be associated with compromised intestinal permeability, such as food allergies, leaky gut syndrome and malabsorption syndromes, including diarrhoea. It may also be used for conditions such as dermatitis and general fatigue, based on the theory that compromised intestinal permeability provides the opportunity for undigested food particles (especially proteins) to enter the systemic circulation and gives rise to an unwanted immune response that manifests as a skin reaction or as lethargy.

DOSAGE RANGE

Naturally-occurring food proteins contain 4–8% of their amino acid residues as glutamine and so the daily consumption is usually less than 10 g/day (Hall et al 1996).

Supplemental L-glutamine is available for oral and enteral use (in capsules, tablets and powder form) and in a dipeptide form for parenteral use.

While solubility and stability are primarily factors for TPN solutions, several factors should also be considered when using oral supplements, as powder forms are often mixed into a solution to enable easy administration of higher doses: 1 g of L-glutamine dissolves in 20.8 mL of water at 30°C (PDRHealth 2006a) and is stable for up to 22 days if stored at 4°C (Hornsby-Lewis et al 1994). Ideally, powdered formulas should be consumed immediately after mixing.

- Gut repair: 7–21 g taken orally as a single dose or in divided doses.
- Cancer therapy: 2–4 g twice daily swished in the mouth and swallowed (up to 45 g has been used in trials and given orally in divided doses).
- Critical illness: 5 g/500 mL of enteral feeding solution.
- HIV: 30 g/day taken orally as a single dose or in divided doses.
- Infection: 12–30.5 g in an enteral feeding solution.
- Infants: 300 mg/kg/day added to breast milk or to preterm formula.

ADVERSE REACTIONS

Toxicity studies in rats fed up to 5% of their diet in L-glutamine showed no toxic events (Tsubuku et al 2004) and glutamine dose–response studies have demonstrated 'good tolerance without untoward clinical or biochemical effects' (Ziegler et al 1999). Based on the available published human clinical trial data, glutamine intakes up to 14 g/day appear to be safe in normal healthy adults. Higher levels have been tested without adverse effects and may be safe; however, the data for intakes above 14 g are not sufficient for a confident conclusion of long-term safety (Shao & Hathcock 2008).

Most adverse reactions are mild and uncommon; they include gastrointestinal complaints such as constipation and bloating (PDRHealth 2006a). No evidence of harm has been observed in the studies conducted to date (Wischmeyer 2003).

A report exists of mania in two hypomanic patients after self-medication with up to 4 g/day glutamine (Membane 1984). As glutamine is a precursor of GABA, this may provide a possible explanation.

Two cases of a transient increase in liver enzyme levels have also been reported (Hornsby-Lewis et al 1994).

SIGNIFICANT INTERACTIONS

Radiation and chemotherapy

Benefits have been observed for the use of L-glutamine during radiation and chemotherapy (see 'Clinical note — Cancer therapy', above).

Indomethacin/NSAIDs

Concomitant use of L-glutamine (7 g three times daily) and indomethacin may ameliorate the increased intestinal permeability caused by indomethacin. The inclusion of misoprostol may also have a synergistic effect with this combination (Hond et al 1999, PDRHealth 2006a, Tanaka & Takeuchi 2002) — beneficial interaction possible.

Human growth hormone

In patients with severe short-bowel syndrome, concomitant use of L-glutamine and human growth hormone may enhance nutrient absorption (PDRHealth 2006a).

CONTRAINDICATIONS AND PRECAUTIONS

It is contraindicated in patients with hypersensitivity to glutamine or hepatic disease or any condition where there is a risk of accumulation of nitrogenous wastes in the blood, thus increasing the risk of ammonia-induced encephalopathy and coma.

It should only be used in people with chronic renal failure under professional supervision.

PREGNANCY USE

Safety in pregnancy has not been established; however, doses in line with normal dietary intake (approximately 10 g/day) are unlikely to be cause for concern.

PATIENTS' FAQs

What will this supplement do for me?

L-Glutamine is an amino acid that is used by the immune systems and intestinal cells as a fuel source. People with critical illnesses, stress, burns, injury or having undergone surgery or undertaking strenuous physical exercise require an increased intake to restore glutamine levels to normal and avoid loss of muscle mass and compromised immune function. It also promotes gastrointestinal repair and may improve tolerance to some anticancer treatments.

When will it start to work?

This will depend on the indication for which it is being used.

Are there any safety issues?

Glutamine appears to be a safe supplement; however, it should not be used by people who are hypersensitive to this compound, those with liver disease or any condition where there is a risk of accumulation of nitrogenous wastes in the blood (e.g. Reye's syndrome).

It should be used only by people with chronic renal failure under professional supervision.

REFERENCES

Ahdieh N et al. L-glutamine and transforming growth factor-alpha enhance recovery of monoacylglycerol acyltransferase and diacylglycerol acyltransferase activity in porcine postischemic ileum. Pediatr Res 43.2 (X) (1998): 227–233.

Akisu M et al. The role of dietary supplementation with L-glutamine in inflammatory mediator release and intestinal injury in hypoxia/reoxygenation-induced experimental necrotizing enterocolitis. Ann Nutr Metab 47.6 (2003): 262–266.

Akobeng A et al. Double-blind randomized controlled trial of glutamine-enriched polymeric diet in the treatment of active Crohn's disease. J Pediatr Gastroenterol Nutr 30.1 (2000): 78–84.

Al Balushi, R.M., et al. (2013). The clinical role of glutamine supplementation in patients with multiple trauma: A narrative review. Anaesth Intensive Care, 41(1), 24–34.

Albrecht, J., et al. (2010). Roles of glutamine in neurotransmission. Neuron Glia Biol, 6(4), 263–276.

Amara S. Oral glutamine for the prevention of chemotherapy-induced peripheral neuropathy. Ann Pharmacother 42.10 (2008): 1481–1485.

Avenell A. Glutamine in critical care: current evidence from systematic reviews. Proc Nutr Soc 65.3 (2006): 236–241.

Avsar F et al. Effects of oral L-glutamine, insulin and laxative on bacterial translocation in acute pancreatitis. Turk J Med Sci 31.4 (2001): 297–301.

Bakalar B et al. Parenterally administered dipeptide alanyl-glutamine prevents worsening of insulin sensitivity in multiple-trauma patients. Crit Care Med 34.2 (2006): 381–386.

Bassini-Cameron A et al. Glutamine protects against increases in blood ammonia in football players in an exercise intensity-dependent way. Br J Sports Med 42.4 (2008): 260–266.

Basuroy S et al. Acetaldehyde disrupts tight junctions and adherens junctions in human colonic mucosa: protection by EGF and l-glutamine. Am J Physiol Gastrointest Liver Physiol 289.2 (2005): G367–G375.

Benjamin, J., et al. (2012). Glutamine and whey protein improve intestinal permeability and morphology in patients with Crohn's disease: A randomized controlled trial. Dig Dis Sci, 57(4), 1000–1012.

Boelens PG et al. Glutamine alimentation in catabolic state. J Nutr 131 (9 Suppl) (2001): 2569–77S; discussion 2590S.

Boelens PG et al. Glutamine-enriched enteral nutrition increases in vitro interferon-gamma production but does not influence the in vivo specific antibody response to KLH after severe trauma: A prospective, double blind, randomized clinical study. Clin Nutr 23.3 (2004): 391–400.

Bollhalder L, et al. A systematic literature review and meta-analysis of randomized clinical trials of parenteral glutamine supplementation. Clin Nutr.;32(2) (2013):213–23.

Borges-Santos MD, et al. Plasma glutathione of HIV+ patients responded positively and differently to dietary supplementation with cysteine or glutamine. Nutrition.28(7–8) (2012):753–6.

Castell L. Glutamine supplementation in vitro and in vivo, in exercise and in immunodepression. Sports Med 33.5 (2003): 323–345.

Castell LM, Newsholme EA. The effects of oral glutamine supplementation on athletes after prolonged, exhaustive exercise. Nutrition 13.7–8 (1997): 738–742.

Castell LM, et al. Does glutamine have a role in reducing infections in athletes?. Eur J Appl Physiol Occup Physiol 73.5 (1996): 488–490.

Chattopadhyay S, Saha A, Azam M, Mukherjee A, Sur PK. Role of oral glutamine in alleviation and prevention of radiation-induced oral mucositis: A prospective randomized study. South Asian J Cancer. 2014 Jan;3(1):8–12.

Chen QH, et al. The effect of glutamine therapy on outcomes in critically ill patients: a meta-analysis of randomized controlled trials. Crit Care. 2014 Jan 9;18(1):R8.

Choi K et al. The effect of oral glutamine on 5-fluorouracil/leucovorin-induced mucositis/stomatitis assessed by intestinal permeability test. Clin Nutr 26.1 (2007): 57–62.

Chun H et al. Effect of enteral glutamine on intestinal permeability and bacterial translocation after abdominal radiation injury in rats. J Gastroenterol 32 (1997): 189–195.

Culkin A et al. A double-blind, randomized, controlled crossover trial of glutamine supplementation in home parenteral nutrition. Eur J Clin Nutr 62.5 (2008): 575–583.

Cury-Boaventura MF et al. Effects of exercise on leukocyte death: prevention by hydrolyzed whey protein enriched with glutamine dipeptide. Eur J Appl Physiol 103.3 (2008): 289–294.

da Gama Torres HO et al. Efficacy of glutamine-supplemented parenteral nutrition on short-term survival following allo-SCT: a randomized study. Bone Marrow Transplant 41.12 (2008): 1021–1027.

Daniele B et al. Oral glutamine in the prevention of fluorouracil induced intestinal toxicity: a double blind, placebo controlled, randomised trial. Gut 48.1 (2001): 28–33.

Decker-Baumann C et al. Reduction of chemotherapy-induced side-effects by parenteral glutamine supplementation in patients with metastatic colorectal cancer. Eur J Cancer 35.2 (1999): 202–207.

de Kieviet, J.F., et al. (2012). Effects of glutamine on brain development in very preterm children at school age. Pediatrics, 130(5), e1121–1127.

Diestel CF et al. [Effect of oral supplement of L-glutamine in colonic wall of rats subjected to abdominal irradiation.] Acta Cir Bras 20 (Suppl 1) (2005): 94–100.

Fahr MJ, et al. Vars Research Award. Glutamine enhances immunoregulation of tumor growth. J Parenter Enteral Nutr 18.6 (1994): 471–476.

Furukawa S et al. Supplemental glutamine augments phagocytosis and reactive oxygen intermediate production by neutrophils and monocytes from postoperative patients in vitro. Nutrition 16.5 (2000): 323–329.

Gibson RJ, et al. Systematic review of agents for the management of gastrointestinal mucositis in cancer patients. Support Care Cancer. 2013 Jan;21(1):313–26.

Gleeson, M. (2008). Dosing and efficacy of glutamine supplementation in human exercise and sport training. J Nutr, 138(10), 2045S–2049S.

Hall J et al. Glutamine. Br J Surg 83 (1996): 305–312.

Haub MD et al. Acute l-glutamine ingestion does not improve maximal effort exercise. J Sports Med Phys Fitness 38.3 (1998): 240–244.

Heiser CR et al. Probiotics, soluble fiber, and l-Glutamine (GLN) reduce nelfinavir (NFV)- or lopinavir/ritonavir (LPV/r)-related diarrhea. J Int Assoc Physicians AIDS Care (Chic Ill) 3.4 (2004): 121–129.

Hond ED et al. Effect of glutamine on the intestinal permeability changes induced by indomethacin in humans. Aliment Pharmacol Ther 13.5 (1999): 679–685.

Hornsby-Lewis L et al. L-glutamine supplementation in home total parenteral nutrition patients: stability, safety and affects on intestinal absorption. J Parenter Enteral Nutr 18 (1994): 268–273.

Houdijk AP et al. Randomised trial of glutamine-enriched enteral nutrition on infectious morbidity in patients with multiple trauma. Lancet 352.9130 (1998): 772–776.

Huffman FG, Walgren ME. l-glutamine supplementation improves nelfinavir-associated diarrhea in HIV-infected individuals. HIV Clin Trials 4.5 (2003): 324–329.

Iantomasi T. Glutathione metabolism in Crohn's disease. Biochem Med Metab Biol 53 (1994): 87–91.

Jazieh AR et al. Phase I clinical trial of concurrent paclitaxel, carboplatin, and external beam chest irradiation with glutamine in patients with locally advanced non-small cell lung cancer. Cancer Invest 25.5 (2007): 294–298.

Jiang ZM et al. The impact of alanyl-glutamine on clinical safety, nitrogen balance, intestinal permeability, and clinical outcome in postoperative patients: a randomised, double blind, controlled study of 120 patients. J Parenter Enteral Nutr 23 (1999): S62–S66.

Jiang ZM et al. The impact of glutamine dipeptides on outcome of surgical patients: systematic review of randomized controlled trials from Europe and Asia. Clin Nutr Suppl 1.1 (2004): 17–23.

Kargotich S et al. Monitoring 6 weeks of progressive endurance training with plasma glutamine. Int J Sports Med 28.3 (2007): 211–216.

Kaufmann Y et al. Effect of glutamine on the initiation and promotion phases of DMBA-induced mammary tumor development. J Parenter Enteral Nutr 27.6 (2003): 411–4118.

Kaya E et al. L-glutamine enemas attenuate mucosal injury in experimental colitis. Dis Colon Rectum 42.9 (1999): 1209–1215.

Khogali SE et al. Effects of L-glutamine on post-ischaemic cardiac function: protection and rescue. J Mol Cell Cardiol 30.4 (1998): 819–827.

Kohlmeier M. Glutamine. In: Nutrient metabolism. St Louis: Elsevier, 2003, pp. 280–288.

Korkmaz A et al. Long-term enteral glutamine supplementation in very low birth weight infants: effects on growth parameters. Turk J Pediatr 49.1 (2007): 37–44.

Kouznetsova L et al. Glutamine reduces phorbol-12,13-dibutyrate-induced macromolecular hyperpermeability in HT-29Cl.19A intestinal cells. J Parenter Enteral Nutr 23.3 (1999): 136–139.

Kucuktulu, E., et al. (2013). The protective effects of glutamine on radiation-induced diarrhea. Support Care Cancer, 21(4), 1071–1075.

Kumar S et al. Effect of oral glutamine administration on oxidative stress, morbidity and mortality in critically ill surgical patients. Indian J Gastroenterol 26.2 (2007): 70–73.

Kusumoto I. Industrial production of L-glutamine. J Nutr 131 (9 Suppl) (2001): 2552–5S.

Li S et al. Separation of L-glutamine from fermentation broth by nanofiltration. J Membr Sci 222.1–2 (2003): 191–201.

Lima AA, et al. Effects of glutamine alone or in combination with zinc and vitamin A on growth, intestinal barrier function, stress and satiety-related hormones in Brazilian shantytown children. Clinics (Sao Paulo). 2014 Apr;69(4):225–33.

Lin JJ, et al. A meta-analysis of trials using the intention to treat principle for glutamine supplementation in critically ill patients with burn. Burns. 2013; 39: 565–570.

Lomivorotov VV et al Glutamine is cardioprotective in patients with ischemic heart disease following cardiopulmonary bypass. Heart Surg Forum. 2011 Dec;14(6):E384–8.

Lomivorotov VV, et al. Does glutamine promote benefits for patients with diabetes mellitus scheduled for cardiac surgery? Heart Lung Circ. 2013 May;22(5):360–5.

Macedo Rogero M et al. Plasma and tissue glutamine response to acute and chronic supplementation with L-glutamine and L-alanyl-L-glutamine in rats. Nutr Res 24.4 (2004): 261–270.

Masuko Y. Impact of stress response genes induced by L-glutamine on warm ischemia and reperfusion injury in the rat small intestine. Hokkaido Igaku Zasshi 77.2 (2002): 169–183.

Mauras, N., et al. (2010). Effects of glutamine on glycemic control during and after exercise in adolescents with type 1 diabetes: A pilot study. Diabetes Care, 33(9), 1951–1953.

McQuiggan M et al. Enteral glutamine during active shock resuscitation is safe and enhances tolerance of enteral feeding. J Parenter Enteral Nutr 32.1 (2008): 28–35.

Membane A. L-Glutamine and mania (letter). Am J Psychiatry 141 (1984): 1302–1303.

Meng Q et al. Regulation of intestinal glutamine absorption by transforming growth factor-beta. J Surg Res 114.2 (2003): 257–258.

Miller AL. Therapeutic considerations of L-glutamine: a review of the literature. Altern Med Rev 4.4 (1999): 239–247.

Moe-Byrne T, et al. Glutamine supplementation to prevent morbidity and mortality in preterm infants. Cochrane Database Syst Rev. 2012 Mar 14;3:CD001457.

Newsholme P. Why is L-glutamine metabolism important to cells of the immune system in health, postinjury, surgery or infection? J Nutr 131 (9 Suppl) (2001): 2515–222S: discussion 2523–4S.

Niihara Y et al. L-Glutamine therapy reduces endothelial adhesion of sickle red blood cells to human umbilical vein endothelial cells. BMC Blood Disord 5.4 (2005).

Noyer CM et al. A double-blind placebo-controlled pilot study of glutamine therapy for abnormal intestinal permeability in patients with AIDS. Am J Gastroenterol 93.6 (1998): 972–975.

Okur A et al. Effects of oral glutamine supplementation on children with solid tumors receiving chemotherapy. Pediatr Hematol Oncol 23.4 (2006): 277–285.

Opara EC et al. l-Glutamine supplementation of a high fat diet reduces body weight and attenuates hyperglycemia and hyperinsulinemia in C57BL/6J mice. J Nutr 126.1 (1996): 273–279.

Paquette JC, et al. Rapid induction of the intrinsic apoptotic pathway by L-glutamine starvation. J Cell Physiol 202.3 (2005): 912–921.

Patel AB et al. Glutamine is the major precursor for GABA synthesis in rat neocortex in vivo following acute GABA-transaminase inhibition. Brain Res 919.2 (2001): 207–220.

Patrick L. Nutrients and HIV. part three: N-acetylcysteine, alpha-lipoic acid, L-glutamine, and L-carnitine. Altern Med Rev 5.4 (2000): 290–305.

Paulo FL. Effects of oral supplement of L-glutamine on diverted colon wall. J Cell Mol Med 6.3 (2002): 377–382.

PDRHealth. L-Glutamine. PDRHealth [online]. Thomson Healthcare. www.pdrhealth (accessed 03–06), 2006a.

PDRHealth. Glutamine peptides. PDRHealth [online]. Thomson Healthcare. www.pdrhealth (accessed 03–06), 2006b.

Peng X et al. Glutamine granule-supplemented enteral nutrition maintains immunological function in severely burned patients. Burns 32.5 (2006): 589–593.

Peterson DE, et al. Randomized, placebo-controlled trial of Saforis for prevention and treatment of oral mucositis in breast cancer patients receiving anthracycline-based chemotherapy. Cancer 109.2 (2007): 322–331.

Pytlík R, et al (2002) Standardized parenteral alanyl-glutamine dipeptide supplementation is not beneficial in autologous transplant patients: a randomized, double-blind, placebo controlled study. Bone Marrow Transplant 30:953–961.

Qutob AF, et al. Prevention of oral mucositis in children receiving cancer therapy: a systematic review and evidence-based analysis. Oral Oncol.49(2) (2013):102–7.

Rathmacher JA et al. Supplementation with a combination of beta-hydroxy-beta-methylbutyrate (HMB), arginine, and glutamine is safe and could improve hematological parameters. J Parenter Enteral Nutr 28.2 (2004): 65–75.

Rhoads JM et al. L-glutamine stimulates intestinal cell proliferation and activates mitogen-activated protein kinases. Am J Physiol 272.5 (Pt 1) (1997): G943–G953.

Roediger WE. Metabolic basis of starvation diarrhoea: implications for treatment. Lancet 1.8489 (1986): 1082–1084.

Rogero M et al. Effect of L-glutamine and L-alanyl-L-glutamine supplementation on the response to delayed-type hypersensitivity test (DTH) in rats submitted to intense training. Rev Bras Cienc Farm 38.4 (2002): 487–497.

Ropeleski MJ et al. Anti-apoptotic effects of L-glutamine-mediated transcriptional modulation of the heat shock protein 72 during heat shock. Gastroenterology 129.1 (2005): 170–184.

Rotovnik Kozjek N, et al. Oral glutamine supplementation during preoperative radiochemotherapy in patients with rectal cancer: a randomised double blinded, placebo controlled pilot study. Clin Nutr.30(5) (2011):567–70.

Rubio I, et al. Oral glutamine reduces radiation morbidity in breast conservation surgery. JPEN J Parenter Enteral Nutr. 2013 Sep;37(5):623–30.

Scheppach W et al. Effect of L-glutamine and n-butyrate on the restitution of rat colonic mucosa after acid induced injury. Gut 38.6 (1996): 878–885.

Seth A et al. L-Glutamine ameliorates acetaldehyde-induced increase in paracellular permeability in Caco-2 cell monolayer. Am J Physiol Gastrointest Liver Physiol 287.3 (2004): G510–G517.

Shao A, Hathcock JN. Risk assessment for the amino acids taurine, L-glutamine and L-arginine. Regul Toxicol Pharmacol 50.3 (2008): 376–399.

Shaw AA et al. The influence of L-glutamine on the depression of hepatic cytochrome P450 activity in male rats caused by total parenteral nutrition. Drug Metab Dispos 30.2 (2002): 177–182.

Skubitz KM, Anderson PM. Oral glutamine to prevent chemotherapy induced stomatitis: A pilot study. J Lab Clin Med 127.2 (1996): 223–228.

Strasser F et al. Prevention of docetaxel- or paclitaxel-associated taste alterations in cancer patients with oral glutamine: a randomized, placebo-controlled, double-blind study. Oncologist 13.3 (2008): 337–346.

Sufit A, et al. Pharmacologically dosed oral glutamine reduces myocardial injury in patients undergoing cardiac surgery: a randomized pilot feasibility trial. JPEN J Parenter Enteral Nutr. 2012 Sep;36(5):556–61. 2012

Sun J, et al. Glutamine for chemotherapy induced diarrhea: a meta-analysis. Asia Pac J Clin Nutr. 21(3) (2012):380–5.

Tanaka A, Takeuchi K. Prophylactic effect of L-glutamine against intestinal derangement induced 5-fluorouracil or indomethacin in rats. Jpn Pharmacol Ther 30.6 (2002): 455–462.

Tang ZF et al. Glutamine and recombinant human growth hormone protect intestinal barrier function following portal hypertension surgery. World J Gastroenterol 13.15 (2007): 2223–2228.

Topkan E et al. Prevention of acute radiation-induced esophagitis with glutamine in non-small cell lung cancer patients treated with radiotherapy: evaluation of clinical and dosimetric parameters. Lung Cancer 2009, 63(3):393–399.

Tutanc, O.D., et al. (2013). The efficacy of oral glutamine in prevention of acute radiotherapy-induced esophagitis in patients with lung cancer. Contemp Oncol (Pozn), 17(6), 520–524.

Tsubuku S et al. Thirteen-week oral toxicity study of L-glutamine in rats. Int J Toxicol 23.2 (2004): 107–112.

van den Berg A et al. Glutamine-enriched enteral nutrition in very low-birth-weight infants: effect on the incidence of allergic and infectious diseases in the first year of life. Arch Pediatr Adolesc Med 161.11 (2007): 1095–1101.

van der Hulst RRWJ et al. Glutamine and the preservation of gut integrity. Lancet 341.8857 (1993): 1363–1365.

Wagner JV, et al. Glutamine supplementation for young infants with severe gastrointestinal disease. Cochrane Database Syst Rev. 2012 Jul 11;7:CD005947.

Wang WS et al. Oral glutamine is effective for preventing oxaliplatin-induced neuropathy in colorectal cancer patients. Oncologist 12.3 (2007): 312–319.

Wang Y, et al. The impact of glutamine dipeptide-supplemented parenteral nutrition on outcomes of surgical patients: a meta-analysis of randomized clinical trials. JPEN J Parenter Enteral Nutr. 34(5) (2010):521–9.
Wang, Y.,et al. (2013). Glutamine supplementation in preterm infants receiving parenteral nutrition leads to an early improvement in liver function. Asia Pac J Clin Nutr, 22(4), 530–536.
Wilkinson SB et al. Addition of glutamine to essential amino acids and carbohydrate does not enhance anabolism in young human males following exercise. Appl Physiol Nutr Metab 31.5 (2006): 518–529.
Williams EA, et al. A double-blind, placebo-controlled, glutamine-supplementation trial in growth-faltering Gambian infants. Am J Clin Nutr 86.2 (2007): 421–427.
Windle EM. Glutamine supplementation in critical illness: evidence, recommendations, and implications for clinical practice in burn care. J Burn Care Res 27.6 (2006): 764–772.
Wischmeyer PE. Clinical applications of L-glutamine: past, present, and future. Nutr Clin Pract 18.5 (2003): 377–385.
Worthington HV, et al. Interventions for preventing oral mucositis for patients with cancer receiving treatment. Cochrane Database Syst Rev. 2011 Apr 13;(4):CD000978.
Yarom N, et al. Systematic review of natural agents for the management of oral mucositis in cancer patients. study, 2013 Nov;21(11):3209–21.
Yoshida S et al. Effects of glutamine supplements and radiochemotherapy on systemic immune and gut barrier function in patients with advanced esophageal cancer. Ann Surg 227.4 (1998): 485–491.
Yoshida S et al. Glutamine supplementation in cancer patients. Nutrition 17.9 (2001): 766–768.
Yu B, et al. Enhancement of gut immune function by early enteral feeding enriched with L-glutamine in severe burned miniswine. Zhonghua Zheng Xing Shao Shang Wai Ke Za Zhi 12.2 (1996): 98–100.
Zheng YM. Glutamine dipeptide for parenteral nutrition in abdominal surgery: a meta-analysis of randomized controlled trials. World J Gastroenterol 12.46 (2006): 7537–7541.
Ziegler T et al. Interactions between nutrients and peptide growth factors in intestinal growth, repair and function. J Parenter Enteral Nutr 23 (1999): S174–S183.

Licorice

HISTORICAL NOTE Licorice root has been used in Europe since prehistoric times, and its medicinal use is well documented (Fiore et al 2005). References to licorice date back to approximately 2500 BC on Assyrian clay tablets and Egyptian papyri. It has been used as both a food and a medicine since ancient times. The genus name, meaning 'sweet root', is attributed to the 1st-century Greek physician Dioscorides. The herb is also popular in traditional Chinese and Ayurvedic medicines (Blumenthal et al 2000).

OTHER NAMES

Liquorice, licorice root, Chinese licorice, sweet root, gan cao, kanzo, kanzoh, radix glycyrrhizae, yashimadhu, yasti-madhu, alcacuz.

BOTANICAL NAME/FAMILY

Glycyrrhiza glabra L. (family Leguminosae)

There are around 30 species of *Glycyrrhiza* spp., so *G. glabra* should be differentiated from other medicinally used herbs such as: *G. uralensis* (synonyms: Chinese licorice, gan cao, licorice root, sweet root), *G. inflata* (synonyms: gan cao, zhigancao), *G. pallidiflora*, *G. glandulifera*, *G. pallida*, *G. typica* and *G. violacea*, although some studies do not always clearly state which form is used. In addition, there are three varieties of *G. glabra*: var. *violacea* (Persia, Turkey), var. *gladulifera* (Russia) and var. *typica* (Spain, Italy) (Asl & Hosseinzadeh 2008).

PLANT PARTS USED

Root and stolon

CHEMICAL COMPONENTS

Licorice contains several triterpenoid saponins (4–20%), the most studied of which is glycyrrhizin (GL, also known as glycyrrhizic acid or glycyrrhizinic acid), which is a mixture of potassium and calcium salts of glycyrrhetinic acid (GA). Other triterpenes include: liquiritic acid, glycyrretol, glabrolide and isoglabrolide (Asl & Hosseinzadeh 2008).

Other important constituents include: flavonoids (isoflavonoids, liquiritin, isoliquiritin, liquiritigenin, formononetin, glabridin, rhamnoliquiritin, neoliquiritin and the chalcones [isoliquiritigenin, licochalcone A and B]); sterols (beta-sitosterol, dihydrostigmasterol); polysaccharides (arabinogalactans); coumarins (liqcoumarin, glabrocoumarone A and B, herniarin,

> ***Clinical note — GL, GA and side effects***
>
> GL is mainly absorbed after presystemic hydrolysis to GA (18-beta-glycyrrhetinic acid [glycyrrhetic acid; the aglycone of GL]). On excretion via the bile it may be reconjugated to GA by commensal bowel flora and then reabsorbed (Gunnarsdottir & Johannesson 1997, Hattori et al 1983, Ploeger et al 2001). GL and GA are associated with the side effects encountered with high-dose or long-term licorice use, such as elevated blood pressure and fluid retention. In people with prolonged gastrointestinal transit time, GA can accumulate after repeated intake. As GA is 200- to 1000-fold more powerful in inhibiting 11-beta-hydroxysteroid dehydrogenase (11HSD) than GL, this may lead to more significant mineralocorticoid effects (Ploeger et al 2001). In order to minimise the risk of side effects, practitioners often use a deglycyrrhizinised form of licorice (DGL).
>
> While *G. glabra*, *G. uralensis* and *G. inflata* are often seen as similar remedies, there are some differences in the constituents, such as the phenolic contents (Mills & Bone 2000).

umbelliferone, glycerin, glycocoumarin, licofuranocoumarin, licopyranocoumarin and glabrocoumarin); phenols, fatty acids, glabrol; amines; glucose, sucrose; resin; and volatile oil. 5,8-Dihydroxy-flavone-7-*O*-beta-D-glucuronide, glychionide A, 5-hydroxy-8-methoxyl-flavone-7-*O*-beta-D-glucuronide, glychionide B, hispaglabridin A, hispaglabridin B, 4′-*O*-methylglabridin and 3′-hydroxy-4′-*O*-methylglabridin, glabroisoflavanone A and B and glabroisoflavanone B have also been isolated (Asl & Hosseinzadeh 2008, Blumenthal et al 2000).

Glycyrrhiza glabra should be differentiated from other species such as *G. inflata* and *G. uralensis*. While the constituent properties of *G. glabra* resemble that of *G. inflata*, they are not similar to *G. uralensis*. Furthermore, there are species-specific typical constituents including glabridin (*G. glabra*), licochalcone A (*G. inflata*) and glycycoumarin (*G. uralensis*) that may influence the pharmacological effects (Kondo et al 2007). Additionally, among different samples of *G. glabra* there may be significant differences in the content of active constituents and biological activity (Statti et al 2004). The lack of standardisation of herbs such as licorice provides a challenge for demonstrating reproducible efficacy in clinical settings.

MAIN ACTIONS

Mineralocorticoid effect

The GA constituent in licorice (and its metabolite 3-monoglucuronyl-glycyrrhetinic acid) inhibits the enzyme 11HSD (Kato et al 1995), which catalyses the conversion of cortisol into its inactive metabolite, cortisone. This results in delayed excretion and prolonged activity of cortisol. Additionally, GL and GA bind to mineralocorticoid and glucocorticoid receptors and may displace cortisol from its carrier molecule, transcortin (Nissen 2003).

Pseudohyperaldosteronism

As cortisol levels rise, they stimulate mineralocorticoid receptors in the distal renal tubule (Walker et al 1992). This creates pseudohyperaldosteronism, which has the same clinical features as primary aldosteronism, including sodium retention, fluid retention and oedema, hypertension, hypokalaemia and metabolic alkalosis (Armanini et al 1996, Heldal & Midtvedt 2002, Kato et al 1995, van Uum et al 1998, Walker & Edwards 1994).

A case report suggests that the symptoms occur despite low plasma levels of aldosterone (Nobata et al 2001). Decreased plasma renin activity (Bernardi et al 1994, Epstein et al 1977) and increased cortisol levels result in vasoconstriction of vascular smooth muscle (Dobbins & Saul 2000, Walker et al 1992), which may further exacerbate the hypertensive effects. This may be of particular significance in patients with prolonged intestinal transit time where GA levels can accumulate (Ploeger et al 2001).

Anti-inflammatory

The anti-inflammatory action of beta-glycyrrhetinic acid (β-GA), a major metabolite of GL, is largely mediated by cortisol, an endogenous hormone with anti-inflammatory action (Teelucksingh et al 1990). It inhibits glucocorticoid metabolism and therefore potentiates its effects.

Synergistic activity between GL and other constituents of licorice in suppressing the expression of inflammatory mediators nitric oxide and inducible nitric oxide synthase has also been identified (Uto et al 2012).

Attenuation of pro-inflammatory cytokine release by licorice or licorice constituents has been reported in a number of animal models (Chu et al 2013, Xie et al 2009). β-GA was shown to significantly suppress LPS-induced interleukin-12, as well as the expression of surface molecules CD80, CD86, major histocompatibility complex (MHC) class I and MHC class II molecules in dentritic cells in vitro (Kim ME et al 2013). The T-helper type 1 immune response was also reduced in response to β-GA.

Several studies have found that GA inhibits the activity of 11HSD and hepatic delta-4-5-beta-steroid reductase, preventing the conversion of cortisol to its inactive metabolite, cortisone (Kageyama et al 1997, MacKenzie et al 1990, Soma et al 1994, Whorwood et al 1993). As such, cortisol activity is prolonged and levels may rise, thereby increasing its anti-inflammatory effects. It may also inhibit classical complement pathway activation (Asl & Hosseinzadeh 2008). For these reasons, licorice has also been investigated for its ability to potentiate the effects of steroid medications (Teelucksingh et al 1990).

This mechanism alone does not fully account for the anti-inflammatory effects of licorice as oral doses of GL also appear to exert an effect in adrenalectomised rats (Gujral et al 2000). GL (10 mg/kg IP 5 min prior to carrageenan) exerts potent anti-inflammatory effects in mice by preventing the activation of nuclear factor (NF)-kappaB and STAT-3 (Menegazzi et al 2008). The DGL also exerts anti-inflammatory effects, and steroid-like activity has also been attributed to the liquiritin constituent (Bradley 1992).

Anti-allergic

The anti-allergic effects of licorice are mainly due to GL, β-GA and liquiritigenin, which can relieve IgE-induced allergic reactions, inhibit passive cutaneous anaphylactic reactions and scratching behaviour in mice (Shin et al 2007). A mouse model of asthma GL (5 mg/kg) markedly inhibited airway constriction and hyperreactivity, lung inflammation and infiltration of eosinophils in the peribronchial and perivascular areas. It decreased interleukin (IL)-4, IL-5 and ovalbumin-specific IgE levels (Ram et al 2006). This finding was supported by a more recent study, where GL (10 mg/kg) prevented chronic histopatholgical lung changes in a mouse model of asthma, including basement membrane thickness, and goblet and mass cell number (Hocaoglu et al 2011). These effects may prove beneficial for the treatment of allergic conditions such as asthma and dermatitis; however, further research is required.

Mucoprotective

Early investigation into the mucoprotective qualities of licorice led to the development of the anti-inflammatory and anti-ulcer medications, carbenoxolone (a hemisuccinate derivative of GA), and enoxolone (an analogue of carbenoxolone) used to treat gastric and oesophageal ulcer disease. Researchers have suggested that it may exert its mucoprotective effects by increasing mucosal blood flow as well as mucus production, and by interfering with gastric prostanoid synthesis (Guslandi 1985). Animal studies indicate that licorice preparations such as DGL improve the environment in the stomach by increasing mucus production, thereby allowing for proliferation of tissue and healing to occur. DGL increases mucus production by increasing the number of fundus glands and the number of mucus-secreting cells on each gland (van Marle et al 1981).

The increase in mucus production seen with carbenoxolone and licorice appears to occur in a number of epithelial tissues other than the digestive tract. It has been reported in the lungs and also bladder, according to in vivo studies (Mooreville & Fritz 1983), and in the trachea, accounting for its expectorant properties (Bradley 1992).

Anti-ulcer effects

Licorice demonstrates the ability to promote mucosal repair and reduce symptoms of active ulcer (Larkworthy & Holgate 1975).

The anti-ulcer effects of licorice are due to inhibition of 15-hydroxyprostaglandin dehydrogenase (which converts prostaglandin E_2 (PGE_2) and F_{2alpha} to their inactive forms) and delta-13-PG reductase. Licorice-derived compounds therefore increase the local concentration of PGs that promote mucus secretion and cell proliferation in the stomach, leading to healing of ulcers (Baker 1994).

Anti-inflammatory activity (as described above) further contributes to the herb's symptom-relieving action.

Antiviral

Both oral and injectable dose forms of licorice have been tested and found to have activity against a range of viruses. In human trials, GL and its derivatives reduce the liver sequelae associated with hepatitis B and C viruses; animal studies demonstrate a reduction in viral activity for herpes simplex virus, encephalitis and influenza A virus pneumonia; and in vitro studies reveal antiviral activity against HIV-1, severe acute respiratory syndrome (SARS) related coronavirus, respiratory syncytial virus, arboviruses, vaccinia virus, hand foot and mouth-related enterovirus and coxsackievirus, and vesicular stomatitis virus (Fiore et al 2008, Wang J et al 2013). The effects appear to be mediated by the constituents GL and GA (Jeong & Kim 2002). The proposed mechanisms for these antiviral effects include 'reduced transport to the membrane and sialylation of hepatitis B virus surface antigen, reduction of membrane fluidity leading to inhibition of fusion of the viral membrane of HIV-1 with the cell, induction of interferon gamma in T-cells, inhibition of phosphorylating enzymes in vesicular stomatitis virus infection and reduction of viral latency' (Fiore et al 2008). It should be noted that current studies focus largely on GL, which is converted in the gut to GA and may not produce the same results as those demonstrated for GL in vitro.

SARS-associated coronavirus

In vitro studies have shown GL to inhibit SARS-CV (clinical isolates FFM-1 and FFM-2) replication by inhibiting adsorption and penetration of the virus in the early steps of the replicative cycle. GL was most effective when given both during and after the adsorption period. High concentrations of GL (4000 mg/L) were found to completely block replication of the virus (Cinatl et al 2003). The ability of GL to reduce platelet accumulation in the lungs (Yu et al 2005) may also support this use and provide a possible therapeutic option for further investigation.

HIV

Preliminary evidence indicates that intravenous administration of GL may reduce replication of HIV. High-dose GL (1600 mg/day) was most effective in reducing HIV type 1 p24 antigen and increasing lymphocytes (Hattori et al 1989). In vitro, GL has the potential to inhibit viral replication in cultures of peripheral blood mononuclear cells from HIV-infected patients infected with a non-syncytium-inducing variant of HIV (Sasaki et al 2002–03).

Influenza

Animal studies have shown that GL offers protection against influenza virus in mice through stimulation of interferon-gamma production by T-cells (Utsunomiya et al 1997). While GL treatment has been shown to reduce the number of human lung cells infected with influenza A virus, this effect was limited to up to two viral replication cycles (Wolkerstorfer et al 2009). This study suggests that the antiviral activity of GL is via cell membrane interactions, reducing endocytotic activity and subsequent viral particle uptake.

Epstein–Barr virus

In vitro studies suggest that GL may interfere with an early step of the Epstein Barr Virus replication cycle (possibly penetration) (Lin JC 2003).

Herpes simplex virus 1

In Kaposi sarcoma-associated herpes virus (KSHV), GL reduced the synthesis of a viral latency protein and induced apoptosis of infected cells (Cohen 2005) terminating KSHV latent infection of B-lymphocytes (Bradbury 2005). Early in vitro studies found that GL inactivated herpes simplex virus irreversibly (Pompei et al 1979). Animal studies show that intraperitoneal administration of GL reduces HSV-1 viral replication and improves survival from herpetic encephalitis in mice (Sekizawa et al 2001). Whether GL may act against other latent herpes viruses or be suitable for clinical use against KSHV requires further elucidation (Bradbury 2005).

Antibacterial

A number of constituents in licorice, including phenolic compounds (glicophenone and glicoisoflavanone), licochalcone A and isoflavones, were found to have antibacterial effects on methicillin-resistant *Staphylococcus aureus* (MRSA) and methicillin-sensitive *Staphylococcus aureus* in vitro (Hatano et al 2000). GA has been shown to exhibit bactericidal activity against MRSA at concentration above 0.223 microM, and induced reduced expression of virulence genes saeR and hla at concentrations below this (Long et al 2013).

Glabridin has been identified as a potentially active agent against *Mycobacterium tuberculosis* (H(37) Ra and H(37)Rv strains), Gram-positive and Gram-negative bacteria (Gupta et al 2008). Additionally ether–water extracts of licorice have been found to have antibacterial activity against *E. coli*, *B. subtilis*, *E. aerogenes*, *K. pneumoniae* and *S. aureus* (Onkarappa et al 2005).

Antifungal

Licochalcone A and glabridin, but not GA, showed antifungal activity against *Candida albicans* in vitro (Messier & Grenier 2011). At high doses (100 mcg/mL), both licochalcone A and glabridin inhibited hyphal formation, with licochalcone A also inhibiting biofilm formation by 35–60% from 0.2 mcg/mL. It should be noted that glabridin and licochalcone A also induced toxicity in oral epithelial cells from 10 mcg/mL and 20 mcg/mL respectively.

Anti-parasitic

18βGA has been shown to possess anti-malarial properties both in vivo and in silico, *Plasmodium berghei*-infected mice showing 6.68 ± 2.19, 1.49 ± 1.04 and 0 ± 0% parasitaemia on day 8 following 62.5, 125 and 250 mg/kg doses respectively (control: 20.57 ± 3.13%) (Kalani et al 2013).

A preliminary study found that glabridin inhibited growth of *Plasmodium falciparum* in vitro, with the trophozoite stage of the erythrocytic cycle most sensitive to the compound (Cheema et al 2014). Due to an observed induction of apoptosis and increased markers of oxidative stress, it is thought these mechanisms underlie glabridin's anti-parasitic effect.

Expectorant

Expectorant effects may be attributed to the ability of licorice to stimulate tracheal mucus secretion, facilitating the elimination of mucus from the respiratory tract (Bradley 1992).

Antitussive

In animal studies licorice produces a persistent antitussive effect, which is mediated by liquiritin apioside in the earlier phase and liquiritin and liquiritigenin (a metabolite of liquiritin apioside) in the later phase (Kamei et al 2005). Isoliquiritigenin has also been shown to induce tracheal relaxation in guinea pig models (Liu et al 2008).

Antioxidant

In vitro research has identified seven antioxidant compounds from an acetone extract of licorice: four isoflavans (hispaglabridin A, hispaglabridin B, glabridin and 4′-*O*-methylglabridin), two chalcones (isoprenylchalcone derivative and isoliquiritigenin) and an isoflavone (formononetin) (Vaya et al 1997). Isoflavones from licorice were also shown to be effective in protecting mitochondrial function against oxidative stresses (Haraguchi et al 2000).

Flavanoids isolated from *Glycyrrhiza inflata* and *Glycyrrhiza uralensis* (namely licochalcone B, licochalcone A, echinatin, glycycoumarin, glyurallin B and 5-(1,1-dimethylallyl)-3,4,4′-trihydroxy-2-methoxychalcone) were tested in vitro for antioxidant activity (Fu et al 2013). Strong radical scavenging activity was shown by licochalcone B, echinatin and glycycoumarin, and potent inhibition of lipid peroxidation compared to control was shown in all compounds except echinatin.

Reduces lipid peroxidation

Macrophage-mediated oxidation of LDL cholesterol plays a major role in early atherogenesis. In animal models, glabridin accumulates in macrophages and inhibits macrophage-mediated oxidation of LDL by up to 80% (Aviram 2004). DGL (100 mg/day for 2 weeks) was found to reduce lipid peroxidation of LDL cholesterol after 1 week's use, according to a placebo-controlled trial (Fuhrman et al 1997).

Lipid-lowering

Dietary licorice flavonoid oil (2% in feed over 21 days) significantly decreased hepatic total cholesterol levels, as well as plasma VLDL and LDL cholesterol compared to control in rats fed a high-fat diet (Honda et al 2013). Through mRNA analysis, it was foud that this effect was likely to be mediated in part through significant up-regulation of the LDL receptor and LXRα, decreased HMG-CoA synthase and increased cholesterol metabolism via up-regulated CYP7A1.

Administration of licorice root powder (5 and 10 g in diet) to hypercholesterolaemic male albino rats for 4 weeks resulted in a 'significant reduction in plasma, hepatic total lipids, cholesterol, triglycerides and plasma low-density lipoprotein and VLDL cholesterol accompanied by significant increases in HDL cholesterol levels' (Visavadiya & Narasimhacharya 2006). These effects may have been due in part to increases in faecal cholesterol, neutral sterols and bile acid excretion and an increase in hepatic 3-hydroxy-3-methylglutaryl-coenzyme A (HMG-CoA) reductase activity and bile acid production. Additionally, decreased hepatic lipid peroxidation with a concomitant increase in superoxide dismutase (SOD) and catalase activities and total ascorbic acid content were noted. In normocholesterolaemic rats, the higher dose also led to a significant reduction in plasma lipid profiles and an increase in HDL cholesterol content (Visavadiya & Narasimhacharya 2006).

Anticancer effects

Licorice has demonstrated potent anti-angiogenic and antitumour activity in animal studies (Sheela et al 2006). Animal and in vitro studies have shown licorice components to be effective in reducing the occurrence and number of tumour cells in several cancer models (Shibata 1994, Wang & Mukhtar 1994, Wang & Nixon 2001, Wang K et al 2013, Wang et al 2014). The induction of apoptosis is frequently cited as a mechanism of cytotoxicity, although induction of caspase-dependent autophagy has also been implicated (Yo et al 2009). Licorice components have also been found to potentiate the effect of paclitaxel and vinblastine chemotherapy (Rafi et al 2000).

In vitro research reveals that chalcone and isoliquiritigenin significantly inhibit the proliferation of prostate cancer cell lines in a dose- and time-dependent manner and that beta-hydroxy-DHP inhibits breast and prostate tumour cells (Kanazawa et al 2003, Maggiolini et al 2002, Rafi et al 2002). Isoangustone A inhibited the growth of prostate cancer cells (5–20 microM) and xenograft tumour growth in mice (1–5 mg/kg), which was associated with G1 arrest, and inihibition of CDK2 and mTOR activity (Lee et al 2013).

In human epithelial carcinoma cell lines, 18βGA was found to potentiate trichostatin A-induced apoptosis and cell death, whereas GL had no effect on cell death or apoptotic activity (Lee et al 2010). Isoliquiritigenin has also been shown to significantly inhibit the proliferation of lung and colon cancer cells, restrain cell cycle progression and induce apoptosis (Chin et al 2007, Ii et al 2004, Takahashi et al 2004). Isoliquiritigenin reduced expression and secretion of vascular endothelial growth factor and inhibited migratory activity of metastatic breast cancer cells in vitro (Wang K et al 2013). Conversely, in a rat model of mammary tumorigenesis, isoliquiritigenin had no effect on the incidence of mammary tumours (Cuendet et al 2010).

Although the exact mechanism of action is still being determined, a 2001 review indicates that licorice and its derivatives may protect against carcinogen-induced DNA damage and that GA is an inhibitor of lipo-oxygenase and cyclo-oxygenase, inhibits protein kinase C and down-regulates the epidermal growth factor receptor (Wang & Nixon 2001).

Anti-diabetic

In an animal model of streptozotocin-induced diabetes, glabridin (10, 20 and 40 mg/kg) daily for 28 days significantly reduced fasting blood glucose levels and glucose tolerance compared to diabetic control mice. Glabridin treatment was also associated with significant increases in SOD activity and reduced MDA contents in the liver, kidneys and pancreas (Wu et al 2013).

Cognitive function

Glycyrrhiza glabra has shown promise as a memory-enhancing agent in both exteroceptive and interoceptive behavioural models of memory in mice. The effect is possibly due to facilitation of cholinergic transmission in the mouse brain (Dhingra et al 2004, Parle et al 2004).

In animal models, glabridin appears to reduce brain cholinesterase activity in mice (Cui et al 2008). Glabridin administration (25 mg/kg and 50 mg/kg) also improved memory and learning in control rats, and reversed induced memory and learning deficits in diabetic rats (Hasanein 2011). In rats, significant spatial memory retention enhancement has also been observed after 4 weeks of licorice administration (aqueous extract equivalent to 5 mg/mL of GL) in drinking water (Sharifzadeh et al 2008).

L

Neuroprotective

In a model of experimentally-induced ischaemic brain damage, oral GL (30 mg/kg) was shown to improve neurological scores and motor activity as well as attenuate ischaemia-induced learning and memory decifits compared to control ischaemic mice (Barakat et al 2014). GL has also been shown to reduce the development of inflammation and tissue injury associated with spinal cord trauma in mice, resulting in improved recovery of limb function (Genovese et al 2008). Neuroprotective effects in post-ischaemic rat brain following middle cerebral artery occlusion (MCAO) have also been found with GL, with improvements in motor function and neurological deficit, and reduced microglial activation (Kim et al 2012).

Several other constituents have also demonstrated possible neuroprotective effects. Glabridin (25 mg/kg by intraperitoneal injection) was able to modulate the cerebral injuries induced by MCAO in rats. The neuroprotective effect appeared to be at least in part associated with the modulation of multiple pathways associated with apoptosis (Yu et al 2008). In addition, pretreatment with isoliquiritigenin (5, 10 and 20 mg/kg, IG) significantly reduced cerebral infarct volume and oedema, and produced a significant reduction in neurological deficits due to MCAO-induced focal cerebral ischaemia-reperfusion injury in rats (Zhan & Yang 2006).

In vitro, isoliquiritigenin was shown to protect dopaminergic neurons from 6-hydroxydopamine-induced toxicity, which corresponded with suppression of reactive oxygen species, nitric oxide production and mediators of intrinsic apoptosis (Hwang et al 2012).

Antidepressant (serotonin reuptake inhibition)

Several flavonoid constituents in licorice (glabridin 60%, 4′-*O*-methylglabridin 53% and glabrene 47%) inhibit serotonin reuptake in a dose-dependent manner, according to in vitro research (Ofir et al 2003). However, animal models suggest that the effect may be on noradrenaline and dopamine. In rats, licorice extract (150 mg/kg) administered orally for 7 days exerted an antidepressant effect comparable to that of imipramine (15 mg/kg IP) and fluoxetine (20 mg/kg IP); the effect, however, appeared to be mediated by an increase of brain noradrenaline and dopamine, not serotonin. It is likely that licorice exerts a monoamine oxidase inhibiting effect (Dhingra & Sharma 2006).

Sedative

Licorice extract and glabrol have been shown to dose-dependently potentiate pentobarbitone-induced sleep in mice through positive allosteric modulation of $GABA_A$-benzodiazepine receptors (Cho et al 2012). In particular, the flavonoid glabrol was found to increase sleep duration and decrease sleep latency in a dose-dependent manner.

Hepatoprotective effects

RCTs have confirmed that GL and its derivatives reduce hepatocellular damage in chronic hepatitis B and C and reduce cirrhosis and hepatocellular carcinoma risk in hepatitis C (Fiore et al 2008). Animal studies demonstrate that licorice protects hepatocytes by inhibiting experimentally-induced lipid peroxidation (Rajesh & Latha 2004). Licorice water extract reduced enzymatic and histopathological changes associated with cadmium-induced hepatotoxicity in rats (Lee et al 2009). GL appears to alleviate carbon tetrachloride-induced liver injury by inducing haem oxygenase-1 and down-regulating pro-inflammatory mediators (tissue necrosis factor (TNF)-alpha, inducible nitric oxide synthase and cyclo-oxygenase-2 mRNA expression) (Lee et al 2007). Simiarly, glycyrrhetinic acid attenuated TNF-α-induced NF-κB activity, and reduced expression of iNOS and production of nitric oxide in rat primary hepatocytes (Chen et al 2014). In vitro studies have shown hepatoprotective effects of GL against aflatoxin B_1-induced cytotoxicity in human hepatoma cells (Chan et al 2003), and animal studies have shown GA exerts hepatoprotective effects against carbon tetrachloride-induced liver injury (Jeong et al 2002).

Several mechanisms appear to be responsible for the hepatoprotective effect. Glycyrrhizic acid enhances the detoxifying activity of the liver enzyme CYP1A1 and glutathione S-transferase and protects against oxidative stress, when induced by aflatoxin (Chan et al 2003). GA has also been found to prevent intracellular GSH depletion and inhibit mitochondrial membrane depolarisation in t-BHP-induced model of hepatocyte damage in vitro (Tripathi et al 2009).

Animal studies have found that GA inhibits expression of the liver enzyme CYP2E1. Once again, antioxidant mechanisms appear to be involved, as GA prevented glutathione depletion, an increase in ALT, AST activity, and hepatic lipid peroxidation in a dose-dependent manner when carbon tetrachloride exposure occurred (Jeong et al 2002). In addition, isoliquiritigenin may stimulate the proliferation of human hepatocytes according to in vitro studies (De Bartolo et al 2005).

Cardioprotective

An in vitro study has shown that both glycyrrhizin and glycyrrhetinic acid directly affect cardiac performance, although in opposing manners (Parisella et al 2012). Glycyrrhizin was found to induce significant positive inotropic and lusitropic effects, while glycyrrhetinic acid negatively affected both parameters. Both GL and GA increased heart rate.

Dehydroglyasperin C has been shown to have significant preventive effects against markers of cardiovascular disease in vitro, including reduction in platelet-derived growth factor-induced cell number, inhibition of cell migration, and inhibition of actin filament dissociation (Kim HJ et al 2013) and significantly decreased PDGF-induced cell number and DNA synthesis in a dose-dependent manner without any cytotoxicity.

In vivo, *Glycyrrhiza glabra* extract was found to significantly prevent the depletion of myocyte antioxidant enzymes, prevented glutathione depletion and inhibited lipid peroxidation within the rat heart following ischaemia-reperfusion injury (Ojha et al 2013). Significant restoration of mean arterial pressure, heart rate and left ventricular end diastolic pressure were also observed.

In mice treated with doxorubicin (20 mg/kg IP), *Glycyrrhiza uralensis* extract was found to protect against doxorubicin-induced cardiotoxicity, as indicated through improved tissue morphology, increased glutathione and glutathione peroxidase levels and reduced lactate dehydrogenase and creatine kinase (Zhang et al 2011). While this is promising, the authors did not acknowledge possible additive toxicity with respect to adverse cardiac effects associated with licorice, including hypertension and hypokalaemia-related events, or that doxorubicin is a CYP3A4 substrate, thus its metabolism may be affected by licorice intake.

Bone health

In vitro studies suggest the potential for glabridin to enhance osteoblast function (Choi 2005). As a result, glabridin has been proposed as a possible therapeutic aid in the prevention of osteoporosis and inflammatory bone diseases (Choi 2005), as well as cardiovascular diseases and bone disorders in postmenopausal women (Somjen et al 2004a, 2004b). Isoliquiritigenin was found to dose-dependently inhibit RANKL-induced osteoclast formation in vitro and prevent inflammatory bone loss in mice through attenuation of osteoclast activity (Zhu et al 2012). Similarly, formononetin has been shown to enhance bone mechanical properties and bone mineral content in vivo, suggesting it too may be of benefit in osteoporosis (Kaczmarczyk-Sedlak et al 2013).

Antiplatelet effect

Isoliquiritigenin purified from licorice has been shown to inhibit platelet aggregation in vitro and in vivo (Francischetti et al 1997, Kimura et al 1993, Tawata et al 1992). Whether the effect is clinically significant for licorice remains to be determined. Newer data indicate that GL is an effective thrombin inhibitor in vivo (Mendes–Silva et al 2003).

Anticoagulation effect

Several components of licorice have been identified in vitro as having anti-coagulant activity. Following a 90-day oral toxicity study in rats, licorice flavonoid oil was found to prolong prothrombin time (PT) and activated partial thromboplastin time (APTT) at high doses (from 400 mg/kg) through reduction of vitamin K-dependent coagulation factors (Nakagawa et al 2008). GL has been shown to act as a direct inhibitor of factor XA, both in vitro and in vivo (Jiang et al 2014).

Isolated compounds licoricone, isotrifoliol, glycyrrhiza-isoflavone B from *Glycyrrhiza uralensis* Fisher have also been found to have significant antithrombotic effects (Tao et al 2012).

OTHER ACTIONS

Sex hormones

Testosterone

Whether licorice consumption affects testosterone levels is still unknown, as conflicting results have been obtained from clinical studies. Armanini et al (1999, 2003a) have conducted a series of trials investigating the effects of licorice on testosterone levels in males with mixed results.

One study showed that licorice (7 g/day equivalent to 0.5 g GA) was able to reversibly reduce testosterone levels within 7 days, by inhibiting 17,20-lyase (involved in the conversion of 17-hydroxyprogesterone to androstenedione) and 17-beta-hydroxysteroid dehydrogenase (involved in the conversion of androstenedione to testosterone) (Armanini et al 1999). Another study twice attempted to replicate these results but was unable to detect an effect on testosterone levels in either study. The authors suggest that inappropriate use of statistical tests in the first study may explain the varying results (Josephs et al 2001).

Anti-androgenic effects of licorice root extract (150–300 mg/kg/day) were examined in male rats, with rats found to have a significantly reduced prostate weight, total testosterone and ventral prostate/stroma ratio after 7 days treatment (Zamansoltani et al 2009). There are limited studies that identify anti-androgenic effects of licorice outside of testosterone levels, therefore further studies are recommended to better elucidate these effects, and any clinical implications they may have.

More clinically promising are the results from a small trial of nine healthy women (22–26 years) in the luteal phase of their menstrual cycle. The women received 3.5 g licorice (containing 7.6% w/w of GL) daily for two cycles. Total serum testosterone decreased from 27.8 (± 8.2) to 19.0 (± 9.4) ng/dL in the first month and to 17 (± 6.4) ng/dL in the second month of therapy (Armanini et al 2004). Further larger scale trials are required to confirm these effects in women with conditions of elevated testosterone such as hirsutism and polycystic ovary syndrome (PCOS).

Oestrogen

The oestrogenic activity of different *Glycyrrhiza* species varies, with activity decreasing in the order *G. uralensis* > *G. inflata* > *G. glabra* (Hajirahimkhan et al 2013). Licorice contains isoflavones, including licochalcone A, which are also known as 'phyto-oestrogens' because they act as partial oestrogen agonists in the body (Setchell & Cassidy 1999). Additionally, in vitro studies suggest that stimulation of aromatase activity promotes oestradiol synthesis (Takeuchi et al 1991).

Liquiritigenin and isoliquiritigenin have displayed oestrogenic affinity to sex hormone-binding globulin and oestrogen receptors in vitro (Hillerns et al 2005) and glabridin and glabrene have both demonstrated oestrogen-like activities similar to 17β-oestradiol in animal studies (Somjen et al 2004a). In vitro, glabrene-rich fractions of licorice root extract only exhibited agonistic responses, preferentially towards oestrogen receptor-α however glabridin (6 microM) was found to reduce the oestrogenic response of 17β-oestradiol by approximately 80% (Simons et al 2011).

Anti-obesity

Glabridin has been shown to inhibit adipogenesis mouse fibroblast cells in vitro (Ahn et al 2013). This same study also found that a glabridin-rich supercritical fluid extract (SFE) of licorice (*Glycyrrhiza glabra* Linne) also showed a dose-dependent inhibitory effect on adipogenesis through inhibition of C/EBP-α and PPAR-α. When administered to rats fed a high-fat diet over 8 weeks, SFE significantly reduced weight gain, fat cell size and hypertrophy of white adipose tissue compared to untreated rats fed high-fat diets, suggesting a possible benefit of glabridin and glabridin-rich licorice extracts in reducing obesity.

Flavanoids isolated from *G. glabra* roots (isoliquiritigenin, 3,3′,4,4′-tetrahydroxy-2-methoxychalcone, licuroside, isoliquiritoside) showed strong inhibition of pancreatic lipase in vitro, with isoliquiritigenin shown to bind to amino acid residues within the enzyme active site (Birari et al

2011). Within the same study, rats fed a high-fat diet who received isoliquiritigenin and licuroside gained significantly less weight (23.2 ± 3.6 g and 28.2 ± 1.6 g respectively) compared to control high-fat diet rats (64.2 ± 0.5 g).

Immunomodulation

Although immunostimulating effects have been observed in experimental models (Lin et al 1996), elevated cortisol levels, which are also induced by licorice, may theoretically reduce this effect (Padgett & Glaser 2003).

Inhibition of aldolase reductase

In vitro studies show that licorice may suppress sorbitol accumulation in red blood cells by inhibiting aldolase reductase (Zhou & Zhang 1990). The isoliquiritigenin component appears to be responsible (Aida et al 1990a). This may have positive implications in diabetes.

Antispasmolytic

Isoliquiritigenin was found to exhibit concentration-dependent inhibition of spontaneous and pharmacologically-induced uterine contraction in the isolated rat uterus (Shi et al 2012). This relaxation was thought to be mediation through calcium channels, nitric oxide synthase and cyclooxygenase.

Protection against cisplatin-induced toxicities

In vivo, oral GA treatment (75 mg/kg and 150 mg/kg daily) for 7 days prior to cisplatin exposure (7 mg/kg IP) attenuated the induction of oxidative stress, including lipid peroxidation, hydrogen peroxide generation and glutathione depletion (Arjumand & Sultana 2011). Additionally, the restoration of normal kidney histology and dose-dependent reductions in DNS fragmentation and nephrotoxic markers, BUN, creatine and lactate dehydrogenase were observed, suggesting GA may play a role in protecting against cisplatin-induced nephrotoxicity and genotoxicity.

Cytochromes and P-glycoprotein

Several licorice components have been identified as possible cytochrome P450 modulators, including liquiritigenin, isoliquiritigenin, glycycoumarin, semilicoisoflavone B, licoisoflavone A, licoricone, glycyrol, licoflavonol and licoisoflavone B (Qiao et al 2014). Licorice inhibits CYP3A4 in vitro (Budzinski et al 2000), the glabridin constituent inhibits CYP2B6, 2C9 and 3A4 in vitro (Kent et al 2002), GA inhibits expression of CYP2E1 in animal studies (Jeong et al 2002) and GL enhances the detoxifying activity of CYP1A1 (Chan et al 2003).

CLINICAL USE

Peptic ulcer and dyspepsia

The anti-inflammatory, mucoprotective and anti-ulcer activities of licorice make it an attractive treatment for peptic ulcer. While these effects have been attributed to the GL and GA constituents, the DGL, which contains < 3% GL, has also been investigated and appears to produce the most promising results when used long term (Bardhan et al 1978, Larkworthy & Holgate 1975). DGL also promotes differentiation of undifferentiated cells to mucous cells and stimulates mucus production and secretion (van Marle et al 1981).

A placebo-controlled RCT ($n = 100$) determined that GutGard (root extract of *Glycyrrhiza glabra*) significantly decreased *Helicobacter pylori* load compared to placebo as assessed through ^{13}C-urea breath test and *H. pylori* stool antigen test (Puram et al 2013). Due to genetic differences in *H. pylori* strains, it is recommended that a similar trial be repeated at multiple centres and compared against gold standard treatment to help clarify any clinical benefit.

In an uncontrolled trial of 32 patients with chronic duodenal ulcer, 3800 mg/day of DGL (in five divided doses) produced signs of healing in all cases and total restoration of mucosa in a majority of subjects. Although treatment continued for 24 weeks, considerable improvement was seen in 56% of patients by week 12 and in 78% by week 16 (Larkworthy & Holgate 1975). A shorter 4-week trial of 96 patients with gastric ulcer failed to produce the same positive results (Bardhan et al 1978).

DGL plus antacid (Caved-S; two tablets chewed three times daily between meals) was as effective as cimetidine (200 mg three times daily plus 400 mg at night) after 6 weeks, according to one randomised single-blind trial of 100 volunteers with peptic ulcer. The two treatments continued to produce similar results after 12 weeks and recurrence rates after both medications were reduced were also similar (Morgan et al 1982).

Commission E approves the use of licorice for the treatment of gastric and duodenal ulcers (Blumenthal et al 2000).

Dermatitis

The anti-inflammatory effect induced by GA provides a theoretical basis for its use as a topical anti-inflammatory agent (much like hydrocortisone) in the treatment of dermatitis.

In practice, GA has been used to potentiate the effects of weak steroids (such as hydrocortisone) in order to increase pharmacological effects without the need for stronger corticosteroids (Teelucksingh et al 1990). It is assumed that increasing corticosteroid activity in this way will not attract an increase in adverse effects; however, no studies have yet confirmed this.

An early study comparing the effects of hydrocortisone- and GA-containing ointments in dermatitis found that hydrocortisone was usually superior in acute and infantile eczemas, whereas GA was superior for chronic and subacute conditions (Evans 1958).

It should be noted that GA is a many times more powerful inhibitor of 11HSD than GL and therefore should theoretically induce far stronger anti-inflammatory effects. GA is not present in licorice but is produced in the gastrointestinal tract from GL; therefore, it is uncertain whether topical preparations containing pure licorice are likely to produce significant anti-inflammatory effects.

Allergic conditions

The anti-allergic effects of licorice (Ram et al 2006, Shin et al 2007) provide a theoretical basis for the treatment of allergic conditions such as asthma and dermatitis; however, further research is required.

Viral infections

In human trials, GL and its derivatives reduce the liver sequelae associated with hepatitis B and C viruses; animal studies demonstrate a reduction in viral activity for herpes simplex virus, encephalitis and influenza A virus pneumonia; and in vitro studies reveal antiviral activity against HIV-1, SARS-related coronavirus, respiratory syncytial virus, arboviruses, vaccinia virus and vesicular stomatitis virus (Fiore et al 2008). However, until controlled studies are available, the clinical effectiveness of this treatment remains unknown.

Respiratory tract infections

Licorice increases mucus production within the respiratory tract and exerts an expectorant (Bradley 1992) and antitussive effect (Kamei et al 2005). When combined with its anti-inflammatory, antiviral and possible immune-enhancing effects, it is a popular treatment for upper and lower respiratory tract infections. In practice, it is often used to treat coughs (especially productive types) and bronchitis (Bradley 1992).

Commission E approves the use of licorice for catarrhs of the upper respiratory tract (Blumenthal et al 2000).

Chronic stress

Traditionally, licorice is viewed as an 'adrenal tonic', most likely due to its ability to slow cortisol breakdown. It may be of benefit in patients experiencing allostatic load due to chronic stress and who are therefore unable to mount a healthy stress response. This is also known as adrenocorticoid insufficiency. Controlled trials are not available to determine its effectiveness in this situation.

Whether this effect is desirable in patients without adrenocorticoid insufficiency and for whom increased cortisol levels may prove problematic is open to conjecture. Chronically high cortisol levels have been associated with desensitisation of the hypothalamic-pituitary-adrenal (HPA) axis, insulin resistance, depression and immunosuppression (Blackburn-Munroe 2001, Jessop 1999, Mitchell & Mitchell 2003). In the initial stages of stress, increased cortisol levels trigger negative feedback mechanisms to keep stress under control and, therefore, short-term use may be warranted but is unlikely to be beneficial unless some adrenocorticoid insufficiency exists.

(For more information see 'Clinical note — Allostasis' in the Siberian ginseng monograph.)

OTHER USES

Licorice has also been used traditionally as a sweetener and aromatic flavouring agent.

Although controlled trials are lacking, licorice is also used for a number of other conditions, largely based on evidence of pharmacological activity.

Chronic fatigue syndrome

The ability of licorice to slow cortisol catabolism may provide a theoretical basis for its use in cases of chronic fatigue syndrome (CFS) accompanied by low cortisol levels. A case report exists of a patient experiencing improved physical and mental stamina and recovery from CFS following use of licorice dissolved in milk (2.5 g/500 mL/day) (Baschetti 1995, 1996).

Polycystic ovary disease

The possibility that licorice may lower testosterone levels in women provides a theoretical basis for its use in PCOS (Armanini et al 2004). While trials using licorice as a stand-alone treatment are lacking, studies of licorice in combination with other herbal medicines such as peony have produced promising results, showing reductions in LH:FSH ratio, ovarian testosterone production and improvements in ovulation (Takahashi & Kitao 1994, Takahashi et al 1988).

Preventing diabetic complications

In diabetic patients with neuropathy, retinopathy or nephropathy, sorbitol:glucose ratios are significantly higher than in those without these complications and ratios increase as complications become more severe (Aida et al 1990b). As licorice and its component isoliquiritigenin have been shown to inhibit aldolase reductase and suppress sorbitol accumulation in red blood cells in vitro (Aida et al 1990b, Zhou & Zhang 1990), a theoretical basis exists for its use in the prevention of diabetic complications.

Menopause

Inhibition of serotonin reuptake and possible oestrogenic activity provide a theoretical basis for its use in pre- and postmenopausal women with mild to moderate depression (Ofir et al 2003, Takeuchi et al 1991).

Constituents in licorice may bind to oestrogen receptors, enhance osteoblast function and attenuate vascular injury and atherosclerosis (Choi 2005, Somjen et al 2004a, 2004b) suggesting a possible role in the prevention of bone disorders and cardiovascular diseases in postmenopausal women.

A pilot study found that administration of 330 mg licorice three times a day for 8 weeks reduced both severity and frequency of hot flushes in postmenopausal women (Nahidi et al 2012). Studies with appropriate power and more thorough end-point evaluations are recommended to better understand this preliminary finding.

Weight loss

The action of GA in blocking 11HSD type 1 at the level of fat cells may help to explain preliminary evidence suggesting an ability to reduce body fat mass and the thickness of thigh fat (Armanini et al 2003b, 2005). In vitro evidence suggests 18β-GA may also alter fat mass through direct effects on adipogenesis in maturing adipocytes and through lipolysis in mature adipocytes (Moon et al 2012).

An RCT of 84 participants found that in moderately overweight patients, 900 mg/day licorice flavonoid oil significantly decreased body weight, BMI, visceral fat area and LDL-cholesterol compared to placebo after 8 weeks (Tominaga et al 2009). Conversely, a small study investigating the effects of 300 mg/day licorice flavonoid oil supplementation over 8 weeks on body weight and body fat in both overweight/obese subjects (n = 22) and in athletic subjects (n = 23) found no significant effects on either parameter, suggesting the higher dose may be required for significant effects (Bell et al 2011). Further well-designed trials with appropriate power are recommended to clarify these findings.

Addison's disease

The ability of licorice to reduce cortisol breakdown provides a theoretical basis for its use in Addison's disease, either as a stand-alone treatment, when adrenocortical function is not severely impaired, or as an adjunct to cortisone therapy. While studies in the 1950s confirm this use (Borst et al 1953, Calvert 1954, Pelser et al 1953), recent studies are limited. In patients with Addison's disease (n = 17) on stable cortisone replacement therapy, a 3-day treatment of licorice significantly increased serum cortisol levels, with significant increase noticed within 3 hours of licorice ingestion (Methlie et al 2011). Based upon urinary cortisol excretion and the observed cortisol/cortisone ratio, this finding was attributed to licorice inihibiting 11β-HSD. A case report exists of an 11-year-old boy with hypoparathyroidism and Addison's disease developing hypermineralocorticoidism following excessive intake of licorice (300–400 g/day, equivalent to 600–800 mg GL) concurrently with hydrocortisone and 9-alpha-fluorocortisol. Pseudohyperaldosteronism persisted after treatment with 9-alpha-fluorocortisol was withdrawn and hydrocortisone was reduced; however, symptoms only diminished after the complete withdrawal of licorice. Similarly, it was also suggested that inhibition of 11HSD by licorice was responsible due to increased levels of free cortisol (Doeker & Andler 1999).

Hypercholesterolaemia

Preliminary studies in rats suggest a possible role for licorice root powder in the treatment of hypercholesterolaemia; however, clinical trials in humans need to be conducted to investigate this effect (Visavadiya & Narasimhacharya 2006).

Depression

Licorice extract (150 mg/kg) appears to exert a monoamine oxidase-inhibiting effect in rats, increasing brain noradrenaline and dopamine, and resulting in an antidepressant effect comparable to that of imipramine (15 mg/kg IP) and fluoxetine (20 mg/kg IP) (Dhingra & Sharma 2006). Whether the effects are clinically significant remains to be tested.

Hyperkalaemia

A 6-month prospective, double-blind, placebo-controlled crossover study (n = 10) found that patients supplemented with GA had increased cortisol/cortisone ratio in plasma, had lowered serum potassium relative to baseline and experienced less frequent episodes of severe hyperkalaemia (Farese et al 2009).

The use of GA or licorice may be of benefit in dialysis patients at risk of hyperkalaemia and associated sequelae (Ferrari 2009). It is recommended that the chronic toxicity of GA be further evaluated prior to any clinical implementation of this treatment.

DOSAGE RANGE

- Fluid extract (1 : 1): 2–4 mL three times daily or 15–40 mL/week (Australian manufacturer recommendations).
- Root: 5–15 g/day (equivalent to 200–600 mg of GL).
- Tea: pour 150 mL boiling water over one teaspoon (2–4 g) licorice root, simmer for 5 minutes and filter through a tea strainer after cooling.
- Chronic gastritis: one cup of licorice tea after each meal.

According to clinical studies

- Chronic duodenal ulcers: 3800 mg/day of DGL (in five divided doses) before meals and at bedtime.
- Ideally, licorice extracts should contain > 30 mg/mL GL.

ADVERSE REACTIONS

Many of the adverse effects attributed to licorice are due to GA at doses above 100–400 mg/day. For this reason, the DGL may be safer and more appropriate in cases where GL or GA is not required for efficacy.

Side effects may be more pronounced in people with essential hypertension who appear to be more sensitive to the inhibition of 11HSD by licorice than normotensive subjects (Sigurjonsdottir et al 2003).

- Hypercortisolism and pseudohyperaldosteronism — associated with sodium retention, potassium loss and suppression of the renin–angiotensin–aldosterone system and presenting as hypertension, fluid retention, breathlessness, hypernatraemia and hypokalaemia (Blachley & Knochel 1980, Dellow et al 1999, Kageyama et al 1997, Robles et al 2013, Ruiz-Granados et al 2012, Wash & Bernard 1975). A case of carpal tunnel syndrome following licorice-induced fluid retention has been reported (Tacconi et al 2009).

- Hypokalaemia — may present as hypotonia and flaccid paralysis, peripheral oedema, polyuria, proximal myopathy, lethargy, paraesthesiae, muscle cramps, headaches, tetany, breathlessness and/or hypertension (deKlerk et al 1997, Eriksson et al 1999). In practice, licorice is often mixed with the potassium-rich herb dandelion leaf, which also has mild diuretic effects.
- Hypokalaemic arrhythmia — rare cases of ventricular arrhythmia associated with licorice-induced hypokalaemia have been reported (Crean et al 2009, Kormann et al 2012, Yorgun et al 2010). One case of recurrent torsade de pointes associated with severe hypokalaemia has been described (Panduranga & Al-Rawahi 2013).
- Hypokalaemic paralysis — although rare, some cases have been reported as a result of chronic licorice use (Corsi et al 1983, Lin et al 2003, Shintani et al 1992, Templin et al 2009, van-den-Bosch et al 2005). A case report of a young female presenting with acute onset quadriparesis secondary to severe hypokalaemia has been attributed to a polyherbal preparation containing licorice (Mukherjee et al 2006).
- Rhabdomyolysis — a number of cases are reported in the scientific literature (Firenzuoli & Gori 2002, Shah et al 2012, Templin et al 2009, van-den-Bosch et al 2005) as a result of severe hypokalaemia.
- Thrombocytopenia — a case report of licorice-induced thrombocytopenia associated with hypokalaemia and oedema has been described. Following cessation of licorice, blood count returned to normal (Celik et al 2012).
- Dropped head syndrome — a case report exists of dropped head syndrome (isolated weakness of the extensor muscles of the neck) due to licorice-induced hypokalaemia (Yoshida & Takayama 2003).
- Hypertension encephalopathy — some cases associated with excessive licorice intake have been reported (Morgan et al 2011, van Beers et al 2011). This may occur even at low doses in susceptible patients with 11-beta-HSD deficiency (Russo et al 2000).
- Increased sodium retention — reduced 11-beta-HSD activity may play a role in increased sodium retention in preeclampsia, renal disease and liver cirrhosis. Reduced placental levels may explain the link between reduced birth weight and adult hypertension (the Barker hypothesis) (Quinkler & Stewart 2003).
- Juvenile hypertension — inhibition of 11HSD may also contribute to a rare form of juvenile hypertension (Chamberlain & Abolnik 1997, White et al 1997).
- Visual disturbance — ingestion of high doses of licorice (110–900 g) has been reported to elicit symptoms of visual disturbance in a case series of five patients. This may be attributed to the possible ability of licorice to 'stimulate retinal and occipital vasospasm and vasospasm of vessels supplying the optic nerve' (Dobbins & Saul 2000).
- Contact dermatitis — case reports of localised skin irritation with licorice-containing products have been reported, with patch testing confirming licorice as the causative irritant (Matsunaga et al 1995, Nishioka & Seguchi 1999, O'Connell et al 2008).

SIGNIFICANT INTERACTIONS

Controlled trials exist that have identified drug interactions. However, in most cases, the interactions are based on evidence of pharmacological activity, case reports or theoretical reasoning. The DGL form is considered safer and less likely to result in drug interactions.

Glabridin is a substrate of P-glycoprotein (P-gp/MDR1) (Cao et al 2007); therefore, potential drug–glabridin interactions need to be considered until more clinical data are available (Yu et al 2007).

Acetylsalicylic acid and other gastro-irritant anti-inflammatory drugs

Co-administration with licorice may reduce gastro-irritant effects induced by drug therapy — potentially beneficial interaction (Tawata et al 1992). Whether the effect is clinically significant for licorice remains to be determined — use high doses with caution.

Anticoagulants / antiplatelets

Licorice has been documented as having an anticoagulant effect, therefore high quantities should be avoid in patients taking any form of blood-thinning medication (Tsai et al 2013).

Antihypertensives

High-dose GL taken long term can lead to increased blood pressure, thereby reducing drug efficacy. Caution — monitor blood pressure when high-dose licorice preparations are taken for longer than 2 weeks.

Chemotherapy (paclitaxel and vinblastine)

A constituent of licorice has demonstrated significant potentiation of paclitaxel and vinblastine chemotherapy in vitro (Rafi et al 2000). Observe.

Cimetidine and other H_2 antagonists

Adjunctive licorice treatment may enhance ulcer-healing drug effects — potentially beneficial interaction.

Corticosteroids

Concurrent use of licorice preparations potentiates the effects of topical and oral corticosteroids (e.g. prednisolone). Caution should be advised to patients on acute and chronic corticosteroid therapy due to possible adverse additive effects (Liao et al 2010). Some practitioners employ licorice to minimise requirements for or aid in withdrawal from corticosteroid medications. Beneficial interaction is possible under professional supervision, but patients may require a reduction in corticosteroid dosage to avoid corticosteroid excess (Chen et al 1991, Homma et al 1994).

Cyclosporin

An in vivo study found that GA induced P-glycoprotein and CYP3A4, resulting in reduced oral bioavailability of cyclosporin (Hou et al 2012) — monitor cyclosporin levels closely.

Diclofenac sodium (NSAID)

In vitro studies have shown that the addition of GL enhanced the topical absorption of diclofenac sodium (Nokhodchi et al 2002), which may be a beneficial interaction.

Digoxin

Hypokalaemia increases sensitivity to cardiac glycoside drugs, therefore increased digoxin toxicity is possible when licorice is used in high doses for more than 2 weeks. A case report exists of congestive heart failure caused by digitalis toxicity in an elderly man taking a licorice-containing Chinese herbal laxative (Harada et al 2002). Avoid long-term use of high-dose licorice preparations and digoxin concurrently.

Diuretics (including loop, thiazide and potassium-depleting)

Case reports exist in which patients experience hypokalaemia and hypertension with concomitant use of licorice and diuretics (deKlerk et al 1997, Farese et al 1991, Folkerson et al 1996) due to increased potassium excretion. Avoid long-term use of licorice and diuretics concurrently unless under professional supervision — monitor potassium levels.

Methotrexate

An in vivo study has suggested that concurrent administration of methotrexate and either GL or licorice decoction can significantly increase MRT and AUC (Lin et al 2009). Until clarification of this interaction occurs, use combination with caution and monitor for signs of methotrexate toxicity.

Oral contraceptive pill

An increased risk of side effects such as hypokalaemia, fluid retention and elevated blood pressure due to increased mineralocorticoid effect exists. This has been demonstrated in case reports (Bernardi et al 1994, deKlerk et al 1997). Use this combination with caution when licorice is used in high dose or for more than 2 weeks and observe patients closely.

Potassium

Licorice may reduce the effect of potassium supplementation. A case report exists of a 69-year-old female developing hypokalaemia while taking potassium supplements and a mouth freshener containing licorice concurrently. The daily intake of GA was estimated at 6–10 mg/day (Kageyama et al 1997). In many cases potassium supplementation may be beneficial in reducing the hypokalaemic side effects of licorice.

Testosterone

Licorice may decrease testosterone levels, although clinical tests have produced conflicting results (Armanini et al 1999, 2003a, 2004, Sakamoto & Wakabayashi 1988, Takeuchi et al 1991) — observe and monitor patients for reduced testosterone effects.

Cytochrome P450 Substrates

In humans, GL has been shown to cause a moderate, clinically relevant, induction of CYP3A4 (Tu et al 2010). Other constituents have been found to affect various CYP P450 isoforms in vitro, including liquiritigenin, isoliquiritigenin, glycycoumarin, semilicoisoflavone B, licoisoflavone A, licoricone, glycyrol, licoflavonol and licoisoflavone B (Qiao et al 2014). Until studies in humans come to light, the clinical significance of this remains unclear (See chapter 8 on Interactions for more information.)

CONTRAINDICATIONS AND PRECAUTIONS

Licorice should be used with caution in people with hypertension (or a genetic predisposition to hypertension) or fluid retention, and is contraindicated in hypotonia, severe renal insufficiency, hypokalaemia, liver cirrhosis and cholestatic liver disease (Blumenthal et al 2000). The effects are likely to be dose-dependent and more likely in people with essential hypertension with a particular tendency to 11HSD inhibition by licorice (Sigurjonsdottir et al 2001, 2003). It is also contraindicated in people with a deficiency in 11HSD or with genetic mutation in the HSD11B2 gene (Harahap et al 2011, Russo et al 2000). A case report of severe hypokalaemia following low licorice intake was reported in a patient with anorexia nervosa, suggesting a possible increase in glycyrrhizin sensitivity in this population (Støving et al 2011).

Long-term use (>2 weeks) at therapeutic doses should be monitored closely due to the potential side effects. Additionally, a high-potassium low-sodium diet should be consumed during treatment (Bradley 1992, McGuffin et al 1997).

As licorice may questionably reduce testosterone levels in men, it should be used with caution in men with a history of impotence, infertility or decreased libido (Armanini et al 1999, Zava et al 1998).

Practice points/Patient counselling

- Licorice has been used as a food, flavouring agent and medicine since ancient times.
- It exhibits mineralocorticoid, anti-inflammatory, antioxidant, mucoprotective and ulcer-healing activity in humans. Antiviral, antibacterial, antitumour, expectorant and hepatoprotective effects have also been demonstrated in animal or test tube studies. Significant effects on oestrogen and testosterone levels remain to be established in controlled trials as evidence is inconsistent.
- Licorice is a popular treatment for respiratory tract infections, gastrointestinal ulcers and dyspepsia. It is also used to treat chronic stress and numerous other conditions, largely based on evidence of pharmacological activity.
- GA has been used topically as an anti-inflammatory agent and also together with cortisone preparations to increase effects.
- High-dose licorice (>100 mg GL) used for more than 2 weeks can induce hypokalaemia and pseudoaldosteronism in susceptible individuals. As such, it should be used with caution and under professional supervision. Additionally, it interacts with numerous medicines. The DGL form is considered safer.

PREGNANCY USE

Licorice is contraindicated in pregnancy. A Finnish trial found that high consumption of licorice during pregnancy increased the likelihood of early delivery, but did not significantly affect birth weight or maternal blood pressure (Strandberg et al 2001). A study by the same group found that compared with zero-low glycyrrhiza exposure, children who experience high prenatal exposure (500 mg/week and higher) had significantly reduced verbal and visuospatial ability, reduced narrative memory and had significantly increased tendencies towards externalising symptoms, inattention, rule-breaking and aggression problems (Räikkönen et al 2009). An association between children exposed to high GL due to maternal consumption during pregnancy and altered diurnal and stress-induced HPA-axis function at age 8 years has also been reported (Räikkönen et al 2010).

PATIENTS' FAQs

What will this herb do for me?

Licorice has many effects in the body, the most well-established ones being reducing inflammation, enhancing healing of peptic ulcers and treating infections such as bronchitis and cough.

When will it start to work?

Beneficial effects in peptic ulcer occur within 6–12 weeks, although DGL is usually used to avoid side effects. Symptoms of dyspepsia should respond within the first few doses. Effects in bronchitis will vary between individuals.

Are there any safety issues?

Used in high doses for more than 2 weeks, licorice can induce several side effects, such as raised blood pressure and fluid retention and may interact with a number of drugs. The DGL form is considered safer.

REFERENCES

Ahn J et al. Anti-obesity effects of glabridin-rich supercritical carbon dioxide extract of licorice in high-fat-fed obese mice. Food Chem Toxicol 51 (2013): 439–445.

Aida K et al. Isoliquiritigenin: a new aldose reductase inhibitor from glycyrrhizae radix. Planta Med 56.3 (1990a): 254–258.

Aida K et al. Clinical significance of erythrocyte sorbitol-blood glucose ratios in type II diabetes mellitus. Diabetes Care 13.5 (1990b): 461–467.

Arjumand W & Sultana S. Glycyrrhizic acid: A phytochemical with a protective role against cisplatin-induced genotoxicity and nephrotoxicity. Life Sciences 89.13–14 (2011): 422–429.

Armanini D et al. Further studies on the mechanism of the mineralocorticoid action of licorice in humans. J Endocrinol Invest 19.9 (1996): 624–629.

Armanini D et al. Licorice consumption and serum testosterone in healthy man. Exp Clin Endocrinol Diabetes 111.6 (2003a): 341–343.

Armanini D et al. Effect of licorice on the reduction of body fat mass in healthy subjects. J Endocrinol Invest 26.7 (2003b): 646–650.

Armanini D et al. Licorice reduces serum testosterone in healthy women. Steroids 69.11–12 (2004): 763–766.

Armanini D et al. Glycyrrhetinic acid, the active principle of licorice, can reduce the thickness of subcutaneous thigh fat through topical application. Steroids 70.8 (2005): 538–542.

Armanini D, Bonanni G, Palermo M. Reduction of serum testosterone in men by licorice. N Engl J Med 341.15 (1999): 1158.

Asl MN, Hosseinzadeh H. Review of pharmacological effects of *Glycyrrhiza* sp. and its bioactive compounds. Phytother Res 22.6 (2008): 709–724.

Aviram M. Flavonoids-rich nutrients with potent antioxidant activity prevent atherosclerosis development: the licorice example. Int Congr Ser 1262 (2004): 320–327.

Baker ME. Licorice and enzymes other than 11 beta-hydroxysteroid dehydrogenase: an evolutionary perspective. Steroids 59.2 (1994): 136–141.

Barakat W et al. Candesartan and glycyrrhizin ameliorate ischemic brain damage through downregulation of the TLR signaling cascade. Eur J Pharmacol 724 (2014): 43–50.

Bardhan KD et al. Clinical trial of deglycyrrhizinised licorice in gastric ulcer. Gut 19 (1978): 779–782.

Baschetti R. Chronic fatigue syndrome and licorice (letter). N Z Med J 108 (1995): 156–157.

Baschetti R. Chronic fatigue syndrome and neurally mediated hypotension (letter). JAMA 275 (1996): 359.

Bell ZW et al. A dual investigation of the effect of dietary supplementation with licorice flavonoid oil on anthropometric and biochemical markers of health and adiposity. Lipids Health Dis 10.29 (2011).

Bernardi M et al. Effects of prolonged ingestion of graded doses of licorice by healthy volunteers. Life Sci 55.11 (1994): 863–872.

Birari RB et al. Antiobesity and lipid lowering effects of Glycyrrhiza chalcones: Experimental and computational studies. Phytomedicine 18.8–9 (2011): 795–801.

Blachley JD, Knochel JP. Tobacco chewer's hypokalemia: licorice revisited. N Engl J Med 302.14 (1980): 784–785.

Blackburn-Munroe GRE. Chronic pain, chronic stress and depression: coincidence or consequence? J Neuroendocrinol 13 (2001): 1009–1023.

Blumenthal M et al (eds). Herbal medicine: expanded Commission E monographs. Austin, TX: Integrative Medicine Communications, 2000, p 237.

Borst JG et al. Synergistic action of liquorice and cortisone in Addisons and Simmonds' disease. Lancet 1.14 (1953): 657–663.

Bradbury J. Liquorice compound beats latent herpesvirus. Lancet Infect Dis 5.4 (2005): 201.

Bradley PR (ed). British herbal compendium, vol 1: A handbook of scientific information on widely used plant drugs. Bournemouth, Dorset, UK: British Herbal Medicine Association (1992).

Budzinski JW et al. An in vitro evaluation of human cytochrome P450 3A4 inhibition by selected commercial herbal extracts and tinctures. Phytomedicine 7 (2000): 273–282.

L

Calvert RJ. Liquorice extract in Addison's disease; successful, long-term therapy. Lancet 266.6816 (1954): 805–807.

Cao J et al. Role of P-glycoprotein in the intestinal absorption of glabridin, an active flavonoid from the root of Glycyrrhiza glabra. Drug Metab Dispos 35.4 (2007): 539–553.

Celik MM et al. Licorice induced hypokalemia, edema, and thrombocytopenia. Hum Exp Toxicol 31.12 (2012): 1295–1298.

Chamberlain J, Abolnik I. Pulmonary edema following a licorice binge (letter). West J Med 167.3 (1997): 184–185.

Chan HT et al. Inhibition of glycyrrhizic acid on aflatoxin B1-induced cytotoxicity in hepatoma cells. Toxicology 188.2–3 (2003): 211–2117.

Cheema HS et al. Glabridin induces oxidative stress mediated apoptosis like cell death of malaria parasite Plasmodium falciparum. Parasitol Int 63.2 (2014): 349–358.

Chen MF et al. Effect of oral administration of glycyrrhizin on the pharmacokinetics of prednisolone. Endocrinol Jpn 38.2 (1991): 167–174.

Chen HJ et al. Glycyrrhetinic Acid Suppressed NF-κB Activation in TNF-α-Induced Hepatocytes. J Agric Food Chem (2014) [ePub ahead of print].

Chin YW et al. Anti-oxidant constituents of the roots and stolons of licorice (Glycyrrhiza glabra). J Agric Food Chem 55.12 (2007): 4691–4697.

Cho S et al. Hypnotic effects and GABAergic mechanism of licorice (Glycyrrhiza glabra) ethanol extract and its major flavonoid constituent glabrol. Bioorg Med Chem 20.11 (2012): 3493–3501.

Choi E-M. The licorice root derived isoflavan glabridin increases the function of osteoblastic MC3T3-E1 cells. Biochem Pharmacol 70.3 (2005): 363–368.

Chu X et al. Attenuation of allergic airway inflammation in a murine model of asthma by Licochalcone A. Immunopharmaol Immunotoxicol 35.6 (2013): 653–661.

Cinatl J et al. Glycyrrhizin, an active component of licorice roots, and replication of SARS-associated coronavirus. (Research letters: possible treatment for severe acute respiratory syndrome.). Lancet 361 (2003): 2045–2046.

Cohen JI. Licking latency with licorice. J Clin Invest 115.3 (2005): 591–593.

Corsi FM et al. Acute hypokalemic myopathy due to chronic licorice ingestion: report of a case. Ital J Neurol Sci 4.4 (1983): 493–497.

Crean AM et al. Sweet tooth as the root cause of cardiac arrest. Can J Cardiol 25.10 (2009): e357–e358.

Cuendet M et al. Cancer chemopreventive activity and metabolism of isoliquiritigenin, a compound found in licorice. Cancer Prev Res (Phila) 3.2 (2010): 221–232.

Cui YM et al. Effect of glabridin from Glycyrrhiza glabra on learning and memory in mice. Planta Med 74.4 (2008): 377–380.

De Bartolo L et al. Effect of isoliquiritigenin on viability and differentiated functions of human hepatocytes maintained on PEEK-WC-polyurethane membranes. Biomaterials 26.33 (2005): 6625–6634.

deKlerk G et al. Hypokalemia and hypertension associated with use of liquorice flavoured chewing gum. BMJ 314.7082 (1997): 731–732.

Dellow EL et al. Pontefract cakes can be bad for you: refractory hypertension and liquorice excess. Nephrol Dial Transplant 14 (1999): 218–220.

Dhingra D et al. Memory enhancing activity of Glycyrrhiza glabra in mice. J Ethnopharmacol 91.2–3 (2004): 361–365.

Dhingra D, Sharma A. Antidepressant-like activity of Glycyrrhiza glabra L. in mouse models of immobility tests. Prog Neuropsychopharmacol Biol Psychiatry 30.3 (2006): 449–454.

Dobbins KRB, Saul RF. Transient visual loss after licorice ingestion. J Neuroophthalmol 20.1 (2000): 38–41.

Doeker BM, Andler W. Liquorice, growth retardation and Addison's disease. Horm Res 52.5 (1999): 253–255.

Epstein MT et al. Effect of eating licorice on the renin-angiotensin aldosterone axis in normal subjects. BMJ 1.6059 (1977): 488–490.

Eriksson JW et al. Life-threatening ventricular tachycardia due to liquorice-induced hypokalemia. J Intern Med 245.3 (1999): 307–310.

Evans FQ. The rational use of glycyrrhetinic acid in dermatology. Br J Clin Pract 12.4 (1958): 269–279.

Farese RV Jr et al. Licorice-induced hypermineralcorticoidism. N Engl J Med 325 (1991): 1223–1227.

Farese S et al. Glycyrrhetinic acid food supplementation lowers serum potassium concentration in chronic hemodialysis patients. Kidney Int 76.8 (2009): 877–884.

Ferrari P. Licorice: a sweet alternative to prevent hyperkalemia in dialysis patients? Kidney Int 76.8 (2009): 811–812.

Fiore C et al. A history of the therapeutic use of liquorice in Europe. J Ethnopharmacol 99.3 (2005): 317–324.

Fiore C et al. Antiviral effects of Glycyrrhiza species. Phytother Res 22.2 (2008): 141–148.

Firenzuoli F, Gori L. [Rhabdomyolysis due to licorice ingestion]. Recenti Prog Med 93.9 (2002): 482–483: (in Italian).

Folkerson L et al. Licorice. A basis for precautions one more time!. Ugeskr Laeger 158.51 (1996): 7420–7421.

Francischetti IM et al. Identification of glycyrrhizin as a thrombin inhibitor. Biochem Biophys Res Commun 235 (1997): 259–263.

Fu Y et al. Antioxidant and anti-inflammatory activities of six flavonoids separated from licorice. Food Chem 141.2 (2013): 1063–1071.

Fuhrman B et al. Licorice extract and its major polyphenol glabridin protect low-density lipoprotein against lipid peroxidation: in vitro and ex vivo studies in humans and in atherosclerotic apolipoprotein E-deficient mice. Am J Clin Nutr 66 (1997): 267–275.

Genovese TM et al. Glycyrrhizin reduces secondary inflammatory process after spinal cord compression injury in mice. Shock 31.4 (2008): 367–375.

Gujral ML et al. Ind J Med Sci 1961; 15: 624–9; as cited in: Mills S, Bone K. Principles and practice of phytotherapy. London: Churchill Livingstone (2000).

Gunnarsdottir S, Johannesson T. Glycyrrhetic acid in human blood after ingestion of glycyrrhizic acid in licorice. Pharmacol Toxicol 81 (1997): 300–302.

Gupta VK et al. Antimicrobial potential of Glycyrrhiza glabra roots. J Ethnopharmacol 116.2 (2008): 377–380.

Guslandi M. Ulcer-healing drugs and endogenous prostaglandins. Int J Clin Pharmacol Ther Toxicol 23 (1985): 398–402.

Hajirahimkhan A et al. Evaluation of estrogenic activity of licorice species in comparison with Hops used in botanicals for menopausal symptoms. PLoS One 8.7 (2013): e67947.

Harada T et al. Congestive heart failure caused by digitalis toxicity in an elderly man taking a licorice-containing Chinese herbal laxative. Cardiology 98.4 (2002): 218.

Harahap IS et al. Herbal Medicine Containing Licorice May Be Contraindicated for a Patient with an HSD11B2 Mutation. Evid Based Complement Alternat Med 2011 (2011): 646540.

Haraguchi H et al. Protection of mitochondrial functions against oxidative stresses by isoflavans from Glycyrrhiza glabra. J Pharm Pharmacol 52.2 (2000): 219–223.

Hasanein P. Glabridin as a major active isoflavan from Glycyrrhiza glabra (licorice) reverses learning and memory deficits in diabetic rats. Acta Physiol Hung 98.2 (2011): 221–230.

Hatano T et al. Phenolic constituents of licorice. VII: structures of glicophenone and glicoisoflavone, and effects of licorice phenolics on methicillin-resistant Staphylococcus aureus. Tokyo: Chem Pharm Bull 48.9 (2000): 1286–1292.

Hattori M et al. Metabolism of glycyrrhizin by human intestinal flora. Planta Med 48 (1983): 38–42.

Hattori T et al. Preliminary evidence for inhibitory effect of glycyrrhizin on HIV replication in patients with AIDS. Antiviral Res 11 (1989): 255–262.

Heldal K, Midtvedt K. [Licorice: not just candy]. Tidsskr Nor Laegeforen 122.8 (2002): 774–776 (in Norwegian).

Hillerns PI et al. Binding of phytoestrogens to rat uterine estrogen receptors and human sex hormone-binding globulins. Z Naturforsch (C) 60.7–8 (2005): 649–656.

Hocaoglu AB et al. Glycyrrhizin and long-term histopathologic changes in a murine model of asthma. Curr Ther Res 72.6 (2011): 250–261.

Homma M et al. A novel 11-beta-hydroxysteroid dehydrogenase inhibitor contained in Saiboku-To, a herbal remedy for steroid-dependent bronchial asthma. J Pharm Pharmacol 46.4 (1994): 305–309.

Honda K et al. Effect of licorice flavonoid oil on cholesterol metabolism in high fat diet rats. Biosci Biotechnol Biochem 77.6 (2013): 1326–1328.

Hou YC et al. Liquorice reduced cyclosporine bioavailability by activating P-glycoprotein and CYP 3A. Food Chem 135.4 (2012): 2307–2312.

Hwang CK et al. Isoliquiritigenin isolated from Glycyrrhiza uralensis protects neuronal cells against glutamate-induced mitochondrial dysfunction. Biosci Biotechnol Biochem 76.3 (2012): 536–543.

Ii T et al. Induction of cell cycle arrest and p21CIP1/WAF1 expression in human lung cancer cells by isoliquiritigenin. Cancer Lett 207.1 (2004): 27–35.

Jeong HG et al. Hepatoprotective effects of 18beta-glycyrrhetinic acid on carbon tetrachloride-induced liver injury: inhibition of cytochrome P450 2E1 expression. Pharmacol Res 46.3 (2002): 221–227.

Jeong HG, Kim JY. Induction of inducible nitric oxide synthase expression by 18b-glycyrrhetinic acid in macrophages. FEBS Lett 513 (2002): 208–212.

Jessop DS. Stimulatory and inhibitory regulators of the hypothalamo-pituitary-adrenocortical axis. Baillieres Clin Endocrinol Metab 13.4 (1999): 491–501.

Jiang L et al. Discovery of glycyrrhetinic acid as an orally active, direct inhibitor of blood coagulation factor xa. Thromb Res 133.3 (2014): 501–506.

Josephs RA et al. Licorice consumption and salivary testosterone concentrations. Lancet 358.9293 (2001): 1613–1614.

Kaczmarczyk-Sedlak I et al. Effect of formononetin on mechanical properties and chemical composition of bones in rats with ovariectomy-induced osteoporosis. Evid Based Complement Alternat Med (2013): 457052.

Kageyama K et al. A case of pseudoaldosteronism induced by a mouth refresher containing licorice. Endocr J 44.4 (1997): 631–632.

Kalani K et al. In silico and in vivo anti-malarial studies of 18β glycyrrhetinic acid from Glycyrrhiza glabra. PLoS One 8.9 (2013): e74761.

Kamei J et al. Pharmacokinetic and pharmacodynamic profiles of the antitussive principles of Glycyrrhizae radix (licorice), a main component of the Kampo preparation Bakumondo-to (Mai-men-dong-tang). Eur J Pharmacol 507.1–3 (2005): 163–168.

Kanazawa M et al. Isoliquiritigenin inhibits the growth of prostate cancer. Eur Urol 43.5 (2003): 580–586.

Kato H et al. 3-monoglucuronyl-glycyrrhetinic acid is a major metabolite that causes licorice-induced pseudoaldosteronism. J Clin Endocrinol Metab 80.6 (1995): 1929–1933.

Kent UM et al. The licorice root derived isoflavan glabridin inhibits the activities of human cytochrome P450S 3A4, 2B6, and 2C9. Drug Metab Dispos 30.6 (2002): 709–715.

Kim S-W et al. Glycyrrhizic acid affords robust neuroprotection in the postischemic brain via anti-inflammatory effect by inhibiting HMGB1 phosphorylation and secretion. Neurobiol Dis 46.1 (2012): 147–156.

Kim HJ et al. Dehydroglyasperin C, a component of liquorice, attenuates proliferation and migration induced by platelet-derived growth factor in human arterial smooth muscle cells. Br J Nutr 110.3 (2013): 391–400.

Kim ME et al. 18β-Glycyrrhetinic acid from licorice root impairs dendritic cells maturation and Th1 immune responses. Immunopharmacol Immunotoxicol 35.3 (2013): 329–335.

Kimura Y et al. Effects of flavonoids isolated from licorice roots (Glycyrrhiza inflata bat) on arachidonic acid metabolism and aggregation in human platelets. Phytother Res 7 (1993): 341–347.

Kondo KM et al. Constituent properties of licorices derived from Glycyrrhiza uralensis, G. glabra, or G. inflata identified by genetic information. Biol Pharm Bull 30.7 (2007): 1271–1277.

Kormann R et al. Dying for a cup of tea. BMJ Case Rep (2012).

Larkworthy W, Holgate PF. Deglycyrrizinised licorice in the treatment of chronic duodenal ulcer. Practitioner 215.1290 (1975): 787–792.

Lee CH et al. Protective mechanism of glycyrrhizin on acute liver injury induced by carbon tetrachloride in mice. Biol Pharm Bull 30.10 (2007): 1898–1904.

Lee JR et al. Hepatoprotective activity of licorice water extract against cadmium-induced toxicity in rats. Evid Based Complement Alternat Med 6.2 (2009): 195–201.

Lee CS et al. 18β-Glycyrrhetinic acid potentiates apoptotic effect of trichostatin A on human epithelial ovarian carcinoma cell lines. Eur J Pharmacol 649.1–3 (2010): 354–361.

Lee E et al. CDK2 and mTOR are direct molecular targets of isoangustone A in the suppression of human prostate cancer cell growth. Toxicol App Pharmacol 272.1 (2013): 12–20.

Liao HL et al. Concurrent use of corticosteroids with licorice-containing TCM preparations in Taiwan: a National Health Insurance Database study. J Altern Complement Med 16.5 (2010): 539–544.

Lin JC. Mechanism of action of glycyrrhizic acid in inhibition of Epstein-Barr virus replication in vitro. Antiviral Res 59.1 (2003): 41–47.

Lin IH et al. Chin Med J (Engl) 109.2 (1996): 138–42; as cited in: Mills S, Bone K. Principles and practice of phytotherapy. London: Churchill Livingstone, 2000.

Lin SP et al. Glycyrrhizin and licorice significantly affect the pharmacokinetics of methotrexate in rats. J Agric Food Chem 57.5 (2009): 1854–1859.

Lin SH et al. An unusual cause of hypokalemic paralysis: chronic licorice ingestion. Am J Med Sci 325.3 (2003): 153–156.

Liu B et al. Isoliquiritigenin, a flavonoid from licorice, relaxes guinea-pig tracheal smooth muscle in vitro and in vivo: role of cGMP/PKG pathway. Eur J Pharmacol 587.1–3 (2008): 257–266.

Long DR et al. 18β-Glycyrrhetinic acid inhibits methicillin-resistant Staphylococcus aureus survival and attenuates virulence gene expression. Antimicrob Agents Chemother 57.1 (2013): 241–247.

MacKenzie MA et al. The influence of glycyrrhetinic acid on plasma cortisol and cortisone in healthy young volunteers. J Clin Endocrinol Metab 70.6 (1990): 1637–1643.

Maggiolini M et al. Estrogenic and antiproliferative activities of isoliquiritigenin in MCF7 breast cancer cells. J Steroid Biochem Mol Biol 82.4–5 (2002): 315–322.

Matsunaga K et al. 2 cases with allergic contact dermatitis due to whitening agents. Aesthet Dermatol 5 (1995): 81–86.

McGuffin M et al (eds). American Herbal Products Association's botanical safety handbook. Boca Raton, FL: CRC Press, 1997; as cited in Micromedex. Thomson 2003. www.micromedex.com (accessed January 2009).

Mendes-Silva W et al. Antithrombotic effect of Glycyrrhizin, a plant-derived thrombin inhibitor. Thromb Res 112.1–2 (2003): 93–98.

Menegazzi M et al. Glycyrrhizin attenuates the development of carrageenan-induced lung injury in mice. Pharmacol Res 58.1 (2008): 22–31.

Messier C & Grenier D. Effect of licorice compounds licochalcone A, glabridin and glycyrrhizic acid on growth and virulence properties of Candida albicans. Mycoses 54.6 (2011): e801–e806.

Methlie P et al. Grapefruit juice and licorice increase cortisol availability in patients with Addison's disease. Eur J Endocrinol 165.5 (2011): 761–769.

Mills S, Bone K. Principles and practice of phytotherapy. London: Churchill Livingstone, 2000: 465–78.

Mitchell D, Mitchell P. Diabetes. J Comp Med 2.5 (2003): 14–19.

Moon M-H et al. 18β-Glycyrrhetinic acid inhibits adipogenic differentiation and stimulates lipolysis. Biochem Biophys Res Comm 420.4 (2012): 805–810.

Mooreville M et al. Enhancement of the bladder defense mechanism by an exogenous agent. J Urol 130.3 (1983): 607–609.

Morgan AG et al. Comparison between cimetidine and Caved-S in the treatment of gastric ulceration, and subsequent maintenance therapy. Gut 23 (1982): 545–551.

Morgan RD et al. Posterior reversible encephalopathy syndrome in a patient following binge liquorice ingestion. J Neurol 258.9 (2011): 1720–1722.

Mukherjee T et al. A young female with quadriparesis. J Assoc Physicians India 54 (2006): 400–402.

Nahidi F et al. Effects of licorice on relief and recurrence of menopausal hot flashes. Iran J Pharm Red 11.2 (2012): 541–548.

Nakagawa K et al. 90-Day repeated-dose toxicity study of licorice flavonoid oil (LFO) in rats. Food Chem Toxicol 46.7 (2008): 2349–2357.

Nishioka K, Seguchi K. Contact allergy due to oil-soluble liquorice extracts in cosmetic products. Contact Dermatitis 40.1 (1999): 56.

Nissen D (ed). Mosby's drug consult. St Louis, MO: Mosby, 2003.

Nobata S et al. [Licorice-induced pseudoaldosteronism in a patient with a non-functioning adrenal tumor]. Hinyokika Kiyo 47.9 (2001): 633–635 (in Japanese).

Nokhodchi A et al. The effect of glycyrrhizin on the release rate and skin penetration of diclofenac sodium from topical formulations. Farmaco 57.11 (2002): 883–888.

O'Connell RL et al. Liquorice extract in a cosmetic product causing contact allergy. Contact Dermatitis 59.1 (2008): 52.

Ofir R et al. Inhibition of serotonin re-uptake by licorice constituents. J Mol Neurosci 20.2 (2003): 135–140.

Ojha S et al. Glycyrrhiza glabra protects from myocardial ischemia–reperfusion injury by improving hemodynamic, biochemical, histopathological and ventricular function. Exp Toxicol Pathol 65.1–2 (2013): 219–227.

Onkarappa R et al. Efficacy of four medicinally important plant extracts (crude) against pathogenic bacteria. Asian J Microbiol Biotech Env Sci 7 (2005): 281–284.

Padgett DA, Glaser R. How stress influences the immune response. Trends Immunol 24.8 (2003): 444–448.

Panduranga P, Al-Rawahi N. Licorice-induced severe hypokalemia with recurrent torsade de pointes. Ann Noninvasive Electrocardiol 18.6 (2013): 593–596.

Parisella ML et al. Glycyrrhizin and glycyrrhetinic acid directly modulate rat cardiac performance. J Nutr Biochem 23.1 (2012): 69–75.

Parle M et al. Memory-strengthening activity of Glycyrrhiza glabra in exteroceptive and interoceptive behavioral models. J Med Food 7.4 (2004): 462–466.

Pelser HE et al. Comparative study of the use of glycyrrhizinic and glycyrrhetinic acids in Addison's disease. Metabolism 2.4 (1953): 322–334.

Ploeger B et al. The pharmacokinetics of glycyrrhizic acid evaluated by physiologically based pharmacokinetic modeling. Drug Metab Rev 33.2 (2001): 125–147.

Pompei R et al. Glycyrrhizic acid inhibits virus growth and inactivates virus particles. Nature 281.5733 (1979): 689–690.

Puram S et al. Effect of GutGard in the management of *Helicobacter pylori*: A randomized double blind placebo controlled study. Evid Based Complement Alternat Med 2013 (2013): 263805

Qiao X et al. Identification of key licorice constituents which interact with cytochrome P450: evaluation by LC/MS/MS cocktail assay and metabolic profiling. AAPS J 16.1 (2014): 101–113.

Quinkler M, Stewart PM. Hypertension and the cortisol-cortisone shuttle. J Clin Endocrinol Metab 88.6 (2003): 2384–2392.

Rafi MM et al. Modulation of Bcl-2 and cytotoxicity by licochalcone-A, a novel estrogenic flavonoid. Anticancer Res 20.4 (2000): 2653–2658.

Rafi MM et al. Novel polyphenol molecule isolated from licorice root (Glycrrhiza glabra) induces apoptosis, G2/M cell cycle arrest, and Bcl-2 phosphorylation in tumor cell lines. J Agric Food Chem 50.4 (2002): 677–684.

Räikkönen K et al. Maternal licorice consumption and detrimental cognitive and psychiatric outcomes in children. Am J Epidemiol 170.9 (2009): 1137–1146.

Räikkönen K et al. Maternal prenatal licorice consumption alters hypothalamic–pituitary–adrenocortical axis function in children. Psychoneuroendocrinology 35.10 (2010): 1587–1593.

Rajesh M, Latha M. Protective activity of Glycyrrhiza glabra Linn. on carbon tetrachloride-induced peroxidative damage. Indian J Pharmacol 36.5 (2004): 284–287.

Ram A et al. Glycyrrhizin alleviates experimental allergic asthma in mice. Int Immunopharmacol 6.9 (2006): 1468–1477.

Robles BJ et al. Lethal liquorice lollies (liquorice abuse causing pseudohyperaldosteronism). BMJ Case Reports (2013).

Ruiz-Granados ES et al. A salty cause of hypertension. BMJ (2012) pii.

Russo S et al. Low doses of licorice can induce hypertension encephalopathy. Am J Nephrol 20.2 (2000): 145–148.

Sakamoto K, Wakabayashi K. Inhibitory effect of glycyrrhetinic acid on testosterone production in rat gonads. Endocrinol Jpn 35 (1988): 333–342.

Sasaki H et al. Effect of glycyrrhizin, an active component of licorice roots, on HIV replication in cultures of peripheral blood mononuclear cells from HIV-seropositive patients. Pathobiology 70.4 (2002–2003): 229–236.

Sekizawa T et al. Glycyrrhizin increases survival of mice with herpes simplex encephalitis. Acta Virol 45.1 (2001): 51–54.

Setchell K, Cassidy A. Dietary isoflavones: Biological effects and relevance to human health. J Nutr 129 (1999): 758S–767S.

Shah M et al. Licorice-related rhabdomyolysis: a big price for a sweet tooth. Clin Nephrol 77.6 (2012): 491–495.

Sharifzadeh M et al. A time course analysis of systemic administration of aqueous licorice extract on spatial memory retention in rats. Planta Med 74.5 (2008): 485–490.

Sheela ML et al. Angiogenic and proliferative effects of the cytokine VEGF in Ehrlich ascites tumor cells is inhibited by Glycyrrhiza glabra. Int Immunopharmacol 6.3 (2006): 494–498.

Shi Y et al. Analgesic and uterine relaxant effects of isoliquiritigenin, a flavone from Glycyrrhiza glabra. Pytother Res 26.9 (2012): 1410–1417.

Shibata S. Antitumor-promoting and anti-inflammatory activities of licorice principles and their modified compounds, in food phytochemicals II: teas, spices, and herbs. Int J Pharmacog 32.1 (1994): 75–89.

Shin YW et al. In vitro and in vivo antiallergic effects of Glycyrrhiza glabra and its components. Planta Med 73.3 (2007): 257–261.

Shintani S et al. Glycyrrhizin (Licorice)-induced hypokalemic myopathy. Eur Neurol 32.1 (1992): 44–51.

Sigurjonsdottir HA et al. Licorice-induced rise in blood pressure: a linear dose-response relationship. J Hum Hypertens 15 (2001): 549–552.

Sigurjonsdottir HA et al. Subjects with essential hypertension are more sensitive to the inhibition of 11 beta-HSD by licorice. J Hum Hypertens 17.2 (2003): 125–131.

Simons R et al. Agonistic and antagonistic estrogens in licorice root (Glycyrrhiza glabra). Anal Bioanal Chem 401.1 (2011): 305–313.

Soma R et al. Effect of glycyrrhizin on cortisol metabolism in humans. Endocr Regul 28.1 (1994): 31–34.

Somjen D et al. Estrogenic activity of glabridin and glabrene from licorice roots on human osteoblasts and prepubertal rat skeletal tissues. J Steroid Biochem Mol Biol 91.4–5 (2004a): 241–246.

Somjen D et al. Estrogen-like activity of licorice root constituents: glabridin and glabrene, in vascular tissues in vitro and in vivo. J Steroid Biochem Mol Biol 91.3 (2004b): 147–155.

Statti GA et al. Variability in the content of active constituents and biological activity of Glycyrrhiza glabra. Fitoterapia 75.3–4 (2004): 371–374.

Støving RK et al. Is glycyrrhizin sensitivity increased in anorexia nervosa and should licorice be avoided? Case report and review of the literature. Nutrition 27.7–8 (2011): 855–858.

Strandberg TE et al. Birth outcome in relation to licorice consumption during pregnancy. Am J Epidemiol 153 (2001): 1085–1088.

Tacconi P et al. Carpal tunnel syndrome triggered by excessive licorice consumption. J Peripher Nerv Syst 14.1 (2009): 64–65.

Takahashi K et al. Effect of a traditional herbal medicine (Shakuyaku-Kanzo-To) on testosterone secretion in patients with polycystic ovary syndrome detected by ultrasound. Nippon Sanka Fujinka Gakkai Zasshi 40.6 (1988): 789–792.

Takahashi K, Kitao M. Effect of TJ-68 (Shakuyaku-Kanzo-To) on polycystic ovarian disease. Int J Fertil 39.2 (1994): 69–76.

Takahashi T et al. Isoliquiritigenin, a flavonoid from licorice, reduces prostaglandin E_2 and nitric oxide, causes apoptosis, and suppresses aberrant crypt foci development. Cancer Sci 95.5 (2004): 448–453.

Takeuchi T et al. Effect of paeoniflorin, glycyrrhizin and glycyrrhetic acid on ovarian androgen production. Am J Chin Med 19.1 (1991): 73–78.

Tao W-W et al. Antithrombotic phenolic compounds from Glycyrrhiza uralensis. Fitoterapia 83.2 (2012): 422–425.

Tawata M et al. Anti-platelet action of isoliquiritigenin, an aldose reductase inhibitor in licorice. Eur J Pharmacol 212.1 (1992): 87–92.

Teelucksingh S et al. Potentiation of hydrocortisone activity in skin by glycyrrhetinic acid. Lancet 335.8697 (1990): 1060–1063.

Templin C et al. Hypokalemic paralysis with rhabdomyolysis and arterial hypertension caused by liquorice ingestion. Clin Res Cardiol 98.2 (2009): 130–132.

Tominaga Y et al. Licorice flavonoid oil reduces total body fat and visceral fat in overweight subjects: A randomized, double-blind, placebo-controlled study. Obes Res Clin Pract 3.3 (2009): I-IV.

Tripathi M et al. Glycyrrhizic acid modulates t-BHP induced apoptosis in primary rat hepatocytes.Food Chem Tox 47.2 (2009): 339–347.

Tsai H-H et al. A Review of Potential Harmful Interactions between Anticoagulant/Antiplatelet Agents and Chinese Herbal Medicines. PLoS One 8.5 (2013): e64255.

Tu J-H et al. Effect of glycyrrhizin on the activity of CYP3A enzyme in humans. Eur J Clin Pharmacol 66.8 (2010): 805–810.

Uto T et al. Analysis of the synergistic effect of glycyrrhizin and other constituents in licorice extract on lipopolysaccharide-induced nitric oxide production using knock-out extract. Biochem Biophys Res Commun 417.1 (2012): 473–478.

Utsunomiya T et al. Glycyrrhizin, an active component of licorice roots, reduces morbidity and mortality of mice infected with lethal doses of influenza virus. Antimicrob Agents Chemother 41.3 (1997): 551–556.

van Beers EJ et al. Licorice consumption as a cause of posterior reversible encephalopathy syndrome: a case report. Crit Care 15.1 (2011): R64.

van Marle J et al. Deglycyrrhizinised licorice (DGL) and the renewal of rat stomach epithelium. Eur J Pharmacol 72.2–3 (1981): 219–225.

van-den-Bosch AE et al. Severe hypokalaemic paralysis and rhabdomyolysis due to ingestion of liquorice. Neth J Med 63.4 (2005): 146–148.

vanUum SHM et al. The role of 11-beta-hydroxysteroid dehydrogenase in the pathogenesis of hypertension. Cardiovasc Res 38 (1998): 16–24.

Vaya J et al. Antioxidant constituents from licorice roots: isolation, structure elucidation and antioxidative capacity toward LDL oxidation. Free Radic Biol Med 23 (1997): 302–313.

Visavadiya NP, Narasimhacharya AV. Hypocholesterolaemic and antioxidant effects of Glycyrrhiza glabra (Linn) in rats. Mol Nutr Food Res 50.11 (2006): 1080–1086.

Walker BR et al. Glucocorticoids and blood pressure: a role for the cortisol/cortisone shuttle in the control of vascular tone in man. Clin Sci 83.2 (1992): 171–178.

Walker BR, Edwards CRW. Licorice-induced hypertension and syndromes of apparent mineralcorticoid excess. Endocrinol Metab Clin North Am 23 (1994): 359–377.

Wang J et al. Glycyrrhizic acid as the antiviral component of Glycyrrhiza uralensis Fisch. against coxsackievirus A16 and enterovirus 71 of hand foot and mouth disease. J Ethnopharmacol 147.1 (2013): 114–121.

Wang K et al. Inhibitory effects of isoliquiritigenin on the migration and invasion of human breast cancer cells. Expert Opin Ther Targets 17.4 (2013): 337–349.

Wang D et al. 18beta-Glycyrrhetinic acid induces apoptosis in pituitary adenoma cells via ROS/MAPKs-mediated pathway. J Neurooncol 116.2 (2014): 221–230.

Wang ZY, Mukhtar H. Anticarcinogenesis of licorice and its major triterpenoid constituents. In: Huang MT et al (eds). Food Phytochemicals for Cancer Prevention II: teas, spices, and herbs. Washington: American Chemical Society, 1994, 329–334.

Wang ZY, Nixon DW. Licorice and cancer. Nutr Cancer 39.1 (2001): 1–11.

Wash LK, Bernard JD. Licorice-induced pseudoaldosteronism. Am J Hosp Pharm 32.1 (1975): 73–74.

White PC et al. 11 beta-hydroxysteroid dehydrogenase and the syndrome of apparent mineralocorticoid excess. Endocr Rev 18.1 (1997): 135–156.

Whorwood CB et al. Licorice inhibits 11 beta-hydroxysteroid dehydrogenase messenger ribonucleic acid levels and potentiates glucocorticoid hormone action. Endocrinology 132.6 (1993): 2287–2292.

Wolkerstorfer A et al. Glycyrrhizin inhibits influenza A virus uptake into the cell. Antiviral Res 83.2 (2009): 171–178.

Wu F et al. Hypoglycemic effects of glabridin, a polyphenolic flavonoid from licorice, in an animal model of diabetes mellitus. Mol Med Rep 7.4 (2013): 1278–1282.

Xie Y-C et al. Inhibitory effects of flavonoids extracted from licorice on lipopolysaccharide-induced acute pulmonary inflammation in mice.Int Immunopharmacol 9.2 (2009): 194–200.

Yo Y-T et al. Licorice and Licochalcone-A Induce Autophagy in LNCaP Prostate Cancer Cells by Suppression of Bcl-2 Expression and the mTOR Pathway. J Agric Food Chem 57.18 (2009): 8266–8273.

Yorgun H et al. Brugada syndrome with aborted sudden cardiac death related to liquorice-induced hypokalemia. Med Princ Pract 19.6 (2010): 485–489.

Yoshida S, Takayama Y. Licorice-induced hypokalemia as a treatable cause of dropped head syndrome. Clin Neurol Neurosurg 105.4 (2003): 286–287.

Yu Z et al. Critical roles of platelets in lipopolysaccharide-induced lethality: effects of glycyrrhizin and possible strategy for acute respiratory distress syndrome. Int Immunopharmacol 5.3 (2005): 571–580.

Yu XY et al. Role of P-glycoprotein in limiting the brain penetration of glabridin, an active isoflavan from the root of Glycyrrhiza glabra. Pharm Res 24.9 (2007): 1668–1690.
Yu XQ et al. In vitro and in vivo neuroprotective effect and mechanisms of glabridin, a major active isoflavan from Glycyrrhiza glabra (licorice). Life Sci 82.1–2 (2008): 68–78.
Zamansoltani F et al. Antiandrogenic activities of *Glycyrrhiza glabra* in male rats. Int J Androl 32.4 (2009): 417–422.
Zava DT, Dollbaum CM, Blen M. Estrogen and progestin bioactivity of foods, herbs, and spices. Proc Soc Exp Biol Med 217 (1998): 369–378.
Zhan C, Yang J. Protective effects of isoliquiritigenin in transient middle cerebral artery occlusion-induced focal cerebral ischemia in rats. Pharmacol Res 53.3 (2006): 303–309.
Zhang L et al. Cardioprotective effects of Glycyrrhiza uralensis extract against doxorubicin-induced toxicity. Int J Toxicol 30.2 (2011): 181–189.
Zhou Y, Zhang J. [Effects of baicalin and liquid extract of licorice on sorbitol level in red blood cells of diabetic rats]. Zhongguo Zhong Yao Za Zhi 15.7 (1990): 433–435, 448 (in Chinese).
Zhu L et al. Licorice isoliquiritigenin suppresses RANKL-induced osteoclastogenesis in vitro and prevents inflammatory bone loss in vivo. Int J Biochem Cell Biol 44.7 (2012): 1139–1152.

L-Lysine

BACKGROUND

L-Lysine is an amino acid which is absorbed from the small intestine and then transported to the liver via the portal circulation where it is involved in protein biosynthesis and is partly metabolised.

CHEMICAL COMPONENTS

L-Lysine is the biologically active stereoisomer of lysine.

MAIN ACTIONS

Essential amino acid

The human body cannot synthesise L-lysine so it must be taken through the diet. The richest sources of L-lysine are animal proteins such as meat and poultry. It is also found to lesser extents in eggs, beans and dairy products (Bratman & Kroll 2000).

Antiviral

L-Lysine has an inhibitory effect on the multiplication of herpes simplex virus (HSV) in cell cultures (Griffith et al 1981, Milman et al 1980). It appears to act as an antimetabolite and competes with arginine for inclusion into viral replicative processes (Griffith et al 1981). As such, lysine retards the viral growth-promoting action of arginine.

Calcium regulation

L-Lysine may be involved in the cellular absorption, regulation and use of calcium (Civitelli et al 1992). In vitro tests with human osteoblasts indicate that lysine has a positive effect on osteoblast proliferation, activation and differentiation (Torricelli et al 2003).

Inhibition of protein glycation and advanced glycation end products

L-Lysine inhibits protein glycation and the role of supplementary lysine has been investigated for the prevention of protein glycation and inhibition of the formation of advanced glycation end products. Under hyperglycaemic conditions, production of fibrin is increased by glycated fibrinogen and human studies report that lysine supplementation significantly reduces fibrinogen activity in diabetic patients ($P < 0.05$). As an inhibitor of glycation, lysine may therefore reduce fibrinogen's non-enzymatic glycation and rectify its structure and function (Mirmiranpour et al 2012).

OTHER ACTIONS

L-Lysine is required for biosynthesis of collagen, elastin and carnitine. Studies in animal models have reported that lysine deficiency can have a negative impact on carnitine synthesis which results in a reduction in carnitine levels and an increase in lipid levels. The addition of lysine in a lysine-deficient diet improves both triglyceride and carnitine levels (Khan & Bamji 1979). However in human studies supplementation of 1 g lysine daily for 12 weeks has failed to demonstrate benefits for lipid profiles (Hlais et al 2012).

L

CLINICAL USE

Herpes simplex — prevention and treatment

The most common use for oral lysine supplements in practice is to prevent and treat outbreaks of herpes simplex labialis. Most clinical research was conducted in the 1980s, generally producing positive results for reducing recurrences when used in high doses, long-term and possibly also reducing severity and improving healing time, but this is less consistent (Digiovanna & Blank 1984, Griffith et al 1978, 1987, McCune et al 1984, Milman et al 1978, 1980, Simon et al 1985, Thein & Hurt 1984, Walsh et al 1983, Wright 1994).

Preventing an outbreak

The majority of double-blind, placebo-controlled randomised controlled trials have shown oral L-lysine supplementation to be effective for decreasing the frequency of outbreaks.

One randomised, double-blind crossover study found that supplementation with 1000 mg/day of L-lysine together with a low arginine diet over 24 weeks decreased the recurrence rate of HSV attacks in non-immunocompromised subjects (McCune et al 1984). A group taking a lower dose of 500 mg daily experienced similar results to placebo. Another double-blind trial compared the effects of 1000 mg L-lysine three times daily for 6 months with placebo treatment in 52 subjects. Once again, oral L-lysine was found to decrease recurrence rates (Griffith et al 1987). An open study of 45 patients with recurring HSV infection found that L-lysine supplementation reduced recurrence when taken at concentrations between 312 and 1200 mg/day in single or multiple doses (Griffith et al 1978). Thein and Hurt (1984) conducted a 12-month, double-blind crossover trial involving 26 subjects with recurring herpes lesions and found that a dose of 1000 mg/day L-lysine in combination with dietary arginine restriction had protective effects against lesion formation. Furthermore, once supplementation ceased, an increase in lesion frequency occurred. This study went further than others, identifying that serum lysine levels need to exceed 165 nmol/mL in order for clinical effects to become significant.

An observational study of 1534 volunteers asking about the perceived effectiveness of lysine supplements to treat cold sores, canker sores or genital herpes over a 6-month trial period indicated positive results (Walsh et al 1983). Of those people with cold sores or fever blisters, 92% claimed lysine supplements were 'very effective' or 'an effective form' of treatment and 81% of those with genital herpes and who had tried other forms of treatment also claimed positive results.

A crossover study by Milman et al (1980) found that significantly more patients receiving treatment with L-lysine 500 mg twice daily for 12 weeks experienced a reduction in infection occurrence compared to placebo (27.7% versus 12.3%; $P < 0.05$). However, the total number of recurrences was 12.5% lower in the active treatment group compared to the placebo group, but not statistically significant.

In contrast, a small double-blind study of 21 participants found oral lysine hydrochloride therapy (400 mg three times a day) did not reduce the frequency, duration or severity of herpes simplex infections (Digiovanna & Blank 1984). A later study by Simon et al (1985) suggests that there is a dose response. In their study, 31 people with diagnosed herpes labialis or genitalis took two capsules twice a day for 3 months (1000 mg/day), then 18 patients took 750 mg/day for 3 more months (Simon et al 1985). The group taking the higher dose had fewer recurrences than predicted while taking 1000 mg/day (17 recurrences versus 42.6 predicted) but during the second 3-month period (750 mg/day or placebo) there was no significant difference between actual and predicted recurrences (17 recurrences versus 16.8 predicted in the treatment group and 16 recurrences versus 21.8 predicted in the placebo group).

Reducing severity and/or healing time

Griffith et al (1987) found that a higher dose of 1000 mg three times daily significantly reduced symptom severity and healing time. More specifically, healing time was reduced by a mean ± SD of 2.3 ± 0.7 days in the lysine group, versus 0.2 ± 0.6 day with placebo ($P < 0.1$). More patients in the lysine group than the placebo group reported their symptoms to be 'milder' (74% versus 28%; $P < 0.01$). The treatment group had been taking L-lysine long-term as a means of reducing outbreak frequency.

Previously, Griffith et al (1978) showed that L-lysine taken at doses between 312 mg/day and 1200 mg/day accelerated recovery time during an outbreak, whereas a double-blind, placebo-controlled study by Milman et al (1978) showed that the lower dose of L-lysine 1000 mg taken at the first sign of an outbreak was no better than placebo for reducing severity or enhancing healing rate. McCune et al (1984) also did not find that a daily dose of 1000 mg/day reduced healing time during an outbreak in non-immunocompromised volunteers.

The effect of lysine on herpes may depend on variables such as the overall dietary ratio of lysine to arginine and the additional dose of supplemental lysine. In practice, doses of >3000 mg/day are used as treatment during an acute episode, based on the positive findings of the Griffith study. This is combined with a diet low in arginine-rich foods, such as chocolate, peas, nuts and beer, and high in lysine-rich foods, such as baked beans and eggs.

A small pilot study examined the use of a topical preparation SuperLysine Plus+ cream containing lysine plus other nutrients (zinc oxide, vitamins A, D and E and lithium carbonate 3X) and botanicals (extracts of propolis, calendula, echinacea and goldenseal) in relieving the symptoms of herpes simplex. Patients with signs and symptoms of an active cold sore of less than 24 hours duration applied the ointment to the lesions 2-hourly during waking hours. Symptoms, including severity of tingling, burning and tenderness, showed significant improvement by day 3 except oozing, and 40% of patients had full resolution; 87% of patients had full resolution after day 6 (Singh et al 2005).

OTHER USES

Diabetes/hyperlipidaemia

Mirmiranpour et al (2012) investigated changes in fibrinogen activity in 50 subjects with type 2 diabetes mellitus (aged ≥40 years). The subjects were randomised to receive either 3 g of L-Lysine monohydrochloride or placebo daily for 3 months. Patients also received the antidiabetic drugs metformin and glibenclamide.The authors reported that fibrinogen activity in the diabetic patients was significantly reduced ($P < 0.05$) in the lysine-supplemented group compared to the placebo group, although there were no changes in the prothrombin time and partial thromboplastin time.

Body composition

A high-lysine diet (80 mg/kg/day) for 8 weeks in well and undernourished healthy males resulted in a small positive effect (~+7.5%) on muscle strength compared to those on low-lysine diets (Unni et al 2012). However most of the studies investigating lysine on body composition have used mixed formulations of amino acids.

Lysine has been reported to stimulate muscle protein anabolism; arginine stimulates whole-body protein synthesis and beta-hydroxy-beta-methylbutyrate has been shown to prevent excessive muscle proteolysis. A double-blind, randomised study (Flakoll et al 2004) investigated the effect of daily supplementation with lysine (1.5 g), arginine (5 g) and beta-hydroxy-beta-methylbutyrate (2 g) on strength, functionality, body composition and protein metabolism in 50 elderly women (mean age 76.7 years). The control group received an isocaloric isonitrogenous mixture (1.8 g of nitrogen) that contained non-essential amino acids (5.6 g of alanine, 0.9 g of glutamic acid, 3.1 g of glycine and 2.2 g of serine). The treatment group had increased measurements of functionality, lean tissue and protein synthesis ($P < 0.05$) after 12 weeks. Similarly, a subsequent double-blind randomised 1-year-long study (Baier et al 2009) investigated the effects of daily consumption of the same supplement in elderly men and women (76 ± 1.6 years) over 1 year. Compared to the control group ($n = 37$), there was a significant increase in protein turnover and fat-free mass ($P = 0.05$) in the treatment group ($n = 40$). Recently post hoc analysis of muscle strength based on the participants' vitamin D status was conducted because of the association of increased serum vitamin D levels with an increase in muscle function. The analysis revealed that vitamin D status did not affect fat-free mass, although muscle strength was increased significantly in the supplement group ($P < 0.01$) but only in those with adequate (≥30 ng 25OH-vitamin D_3/mL) vitamin D levels (Fuller et al 2011). The role that lysine plays in this combination is unclear.

Osteoporosis prevention

Two studies have investigated the effects of oral L-lysine supplementation on calcium use to determine whether L-lysine has a role in the prevention of osteoporosis. In these tests, oral L-lysine was shown to significantly increase intestinal absorption of calcium and decrease renal excretion in both healthy women and those with osteoporosis (Civitelli et al 1992).

Anxiety and mood disturbances

A systematic review of nutritional and herbal supplements for anxiety and anxiety-related disorder reported that there is evidence for the use of supplemental L-lysine in combination with L-arginine (Lakhan & Vieira 2010). According to a randomised, double-blind trial, fortification of lysine in a wheat-based (L-lysine-deficient) diet significantly reduced anxiety score in males, but not females with high baseline anxiety. It is suspected that L-lysine's action as a 5-HT_4 receptor antagonist and benzodiazepine receptor agonist is responsible for the observed effect (Smriga et al 2004). In a double-blind, randomised placebo-controlled study, Smriga et al (2007) evaluated the efficacy of combined lysine and arginine supplementation on reducing anxiety and stress response hormonal levels. Patients were given 1.32 g each of L-lysine and L-arginine twice daily for 1 week, estimated to be a 50% increase in total intake. Compared to placebo, long-term and stress-induced anxiety levels were reduced in both genders in the treatment group, and basal levels of salivary cortisol and chromogranin-A (a measure of sympathetic stress response) were significantly reduced in males (Smriga et al 2007). In contrast, a prospective study of 29,133 men (aged 50–69 years) found no association between L-lysine intake and depressed mood (Hakkarainen et al 2003).

It is believed that the brain's nitric oxide signalling system may be involved in the pathophysiology of schizophrenia. In a small, randomised single-blinded cross-over study, 10 patients with schizophrenia received L-lysine (6 g/day) or placebo in addition to their conventional antipsychotic medication for 4 weeks before being crossed over to the alternative phase of the study. During the lysine phase participants showed a significant decrease in positive symptoms, as assessed by the Positive and Negative Syndrome Scale. These encouraging results deserve further investigation in larger studies in future (Wass et al 2011).

Cancer treatment (in combination)

Preliminary research has been conducted into the possible protective or treatment effects of lysine in combination with other nutritional components.

A formulation of lysine combined with other compounds (proline, arginine, vitamin C and green tea extract) has been used in several in vitro and in vivo studies, suggesting it may be beneficial in cancer treatment by inhibiting the growth, invasion and metastasis of tumour cells via inhibiting metalloproteinases which trigger excellular matrix degradation (Roomi et al 2004, 2005a–e, 2006a–e, Roomi 2006). In contrast to this, however, an in vivo study conducted on mice found L-lysine and vitamin C Lysin C Drink, alone or in combination with epigallocatechin-gallate and amino acids Epican forte, was not effective as a prophylactic or treatment in reducing primary tumour growth (neuroblastoma model) or in preventing metastases (Lode et al 2008).

Lysinuric protein intolerance

Lysinuric protein intolerance is an autosomal recessive transport disorder of the cationic amino acids which leads to decreased intestinal absorption and excessive renal loss of lysine, arginine and ornithine. Usual treatment involves restriction of protein and citrulline supplementation, which corrects many side effects except those related to lysine deficiency. Long-term low-dose lysine supplementation improves plasma lysine concentration in patients and may help correct chronic lysine deficiency without causing side effects such as hyperammonaemia (Tanner et al 2007).

DOSAGE RANGE

Herpes simplex infections

- Prevention: 1000–3000 mg/day taken long-term (at least 6 months) together with a low-arginine diet.
- Acute treatment: minimum 3000 mg/day in divided doses taken between meals until lesions have healed.

Osteoporosis prevention

- 400–800 mg L-lysine taken together with calcium supplementation.

TOXICITY

Not known.

ADVERSE REACTIONS

Doses greater than 10–15 g/day may cause gastrointestinal discomfort with symptoms of nausea, vomiting and diarrhoea.

Practice points/Patient counselling

- L-Lysine is an essential amino acid found in foods such as animal proteins, eggs and milk.
- It has been shown to inhibit HSV multiplication in vitro.
- Supplemental L-lysine is popular as a prophylactic and treatment for HSV.
- Studies have yielded inconsistent results suggesting that there may be individual variation in responses. Due to its safety, a trial is worthwhile to determine individual response.
- Doses used as prophylaxis range from 1000 to 3000 mg/day, with treatment doses generally above 3000 mg/day.
- L-Lysine may also enhance intestinal absorption of calcium and reduces its renal excretion.

CONTRAINDICATIONS AND PRECAUTIONS

Contraindicated in people with the rare genetic disorder hyperlysinaemia/hyperlysinuria (Hendler & Rorvik 2001). High-dose lysine supplements should be used with caution in hypercalcaemic states, and by people with kidney or liver disease.

In children with pyridoxine-dependent epilepsy caused by antiquitin deficiency, a lysine-restricted diet as an adjunct to pyridoxine therapy appears to potentially decrease neurotoxic biomarkers and improve developmental outcomes (van Karnebeek et al 2012). As such lysine supplementation may not be suitable in such patients until more is known.

SIGNIFICANT INTERACTIONS

Calcium

Clinical tests have found L-lysine enhances intestinal absorption and decreases renal excretion of calcium (Civitelli et al 1992) — potentially beneficial interaction.

PREGNANCY USE

Safety is unknown for high-dose supplements; however, dietary intake levels are safe.

PATIENTS' FAQs

What will this supplement do for me?

L-Lysine supplements taken long-term appear to reduce the frequency of herpes simplex outbreaks and possibly reduce the severity and enhance healing. It may also improve the way the body absorbs and retains calcium.

When will it start to work?

Studies suggest that several months' treatment may be required, with a long-term approach recommended for prophylaxis against herpes simplex outbreaks.

Are there any safety issues?

L-Lysine appears to be a very safe supplement, although safety has not been established in pregnancy and lactation for high-dose supplements.

REFERENCES

Baier S, et al. Year-long changes in protein metabolism in elderly men and women supplemented with a nutrition cocktail of beta-hydroxy-beta-methylbutyrate (HMB), L-arginine, and L-lysine. JPEN J Parenter Enteral Nutr. 33(1) (2009):71–82.

Bratman S, Kroll D. Natural health bible. Rocklin, CA: Prima Health, 2000.

Civitelli R et al. Dietary L-lysine and calcium metabolism in humans. Nutrition 8.6 (1992): 400–405.

Digiovanna JJ, Blank H. Failure of lysine in frequently recurrent herpes simplex infection: Treatment and prophylaxis. Arch Dermatol 120.1 (1984): 48–51.

Flakoll P, et al. Effect of beta-hydroxy-beta-methylbutyrate, arginine, and lysine supplementation on strength, functionality, body composition, and protein metabolism in elderly women. Nutrition 20 (2004): 445–451.

Fuller JC Jr, et al. Vitamin D status affects strength gains in older adults supplemented with a combination of β-hydroxy-β-methylbutyrate, arginine, and lysine: a cohort study. JPEN J Parenter Enteral Nutr. 35(6) (2011):757–62.

Griffith RS, et al. A multicentered study of lysine therapy in herpes simplex infection. Dermatologica 156.5 (1978): 257–267.

Griffith RS, et al. Relation of arginine-lysine antagonism to herpes simplex growth in tissue culture. Chemotherapy 27.3 (1981): 209–213.

Griffith RS et al. Success of L-lysine therapy in frequently recurrent herpes simplex infection. Treatment and prophylaxis. Dermatologica 175.4 (1987): 183–190.

Hakkarainen R et al. Association of dietary amino acids with low mood. Depression Anxiety 18.2 (2003): 89–94.

Hendler SS, Rorvik D (eds). PDR for Nutritional Supplements. Montvale, NJ: Medical Economics Co., 2001.

Hlais S, et al. Effect of lysine, vitamin B(6), and carnitine supplementation on the lipid profile of male patients with hypertriglyceridemia: a 12-week, open-label, randomized, placebo-controlled trial. Clin Ther. 34(8) (2012):1674–82.

Khan L, Bamji MS. Tissue carnitine deficiency due to dietary lysine deficiency: triglyceride accumulation and concomitant impairment in fatty acid oxidation. J Nutr. 109 (1979):24–31.

Lakhan SE, Vieira KF. Nutritional and herbal supplements for anxiety and anxiety-related disorders: a systematic review. Nutrition Journal. 9 (2010): 42–55.

Lode HN et al. Nutrient mixture including vitamin C, L-lysine, L-proline, and epigallocatechin is ineffective against tumor growth and metastasis in a syngeneic neuroblastoma model. Pediatr Blood Cancer 50.2 (2008): 284–288.
McCune MA et al. Treatment of recurrent herpes simplex infections with L-lysine monohydrochloride. Cutis 34.4 (1984): 366–373.
Milman N, et al. Failure of lysine treatment in recurrent herpes simplex labialis. Lancet 2.8096 (1978): 942.
Milman N, et al. Lysine prophylaxis in recurrent herpes simplex labialis: a double-blind, controlled crossover study. Acta Derm Venereol 60.1 (1980): 85–87.
Mirmiranpour H, et al. Investigation of the mechanism(s) involved in decreasing increased fibrinogen activity in hyperglycemic conditions using L-lysine supplementation. Thromb Res. 130(3) (2012):e13–9.
Roomi MW. Antitumor effect of ascorbic acid, lysine, proline, arginine, and green tea extract on bladder cancer cell line T-24. Int J Urol 13.4 (2006): 415–19.
Roomi MW, et al. Anti-tumor effect of ascorbic acid, lysine, proline, arginine, and epigallocatechin gallate on prostate cancer cell lines PC-3, LNCaP, and DU145. Res Commun Mol Pathol Pharmacol 115–116 (2004): 251–264.
Roomi MW et al. Antitumor effect of a combination of lysine, proline, arginine, ascorbic acid, and green tea extract on pancreatic cancer cell line MIA PaCa-2. Int J Gastrointest Cancer 35.2 (2005a): 97–102.
Roomi MW et al. In vitro and in vivo antitumorigenic activity of a mixture of lysine, proline, ascorbic acid, and green tea extract on human breast cancer lines MDA-MB-231 and MCF-7. Med Oncol 22.2 (2005b): 129–38.
Roomi MW et al. In vivo antitumor effect of ascorbic acid, lysine, proline and green tea extract on human colon cancer cell HCT 116 xenografts in nude mice: evaluation of tumor growth and immunohistochemistry. Oncol Rep 13.3 (2005c): 421–5.
Roomi MW et al. In vivo antitumor effect of ascorbic acid, lysine, proline and green tea extract on human prostate cancer PC-3 xenografts in nude mice: evaluation of tumor growth and immunohistochemistry. In Vivo 19.1 (2005d): 179–83.
Roomi MW et al. Inhibitory effect of a mixture containing ascorbic acid, lysine, proline and green tea extract on critical parameters in angiogenesis. Oncol Rep 14.4 (2005e): 807–815.
Roomi MW et al. In vivo and in vitro antitumor effect of ascorbic acid, lysine, proline, arginine, and green tea extract on human fibrosarcoma cells HT-1080. Med Oncol 23.1 (2006a): 105–11.
Roomi MW et al. Inhibition of matrix metalloproteinase-2 secretion and invasion by human ovarian cancer cell line SK-OV-3 with lysine, proline, arginine, ascorbic acid and green tea extract. J Obstet Gynaecol Res 32.2 (2006b): 148–54.
Roomi MW et al. Inhibition of pulmonary metastasis of melanoma b16fo cells in C57BL/6 mice by a nutrient mixture consisting of ascorbic acid, lysine, proline, arginine, and green tea extract. Exp Lung Res 32.10 (2006c): 517–530.
Roomi MW et al. Suppression of human cervical cancer cell lines Hela and DoTc2 4510 by a mixture of lysine, proline, ascorbic acid, and green tea extract. Int J Gynecol Cancer 16 3 (2006d): 1241–47.
Roomi MW et al. In vivo and in vitro antitumor effect of ascorbic acid, lysine, proline and green tea extract on human melanoma cell line A2058. In Vivo 20.1 (2006e): 25–32.
Simon, C.A., et al. 1985. Failure of lysine in frequently recurrent herpes simplex infection. Arch.Dermatol., 121, (2) 167–168.
Singh BB et al. Safety and effectiveness of an L-lysine, zinc, and herbal-based product on the treatment of facial and circumoral herpes. Altern Med Rev 10.2 (2005): 123–127.
Smriga M et al. Lysine fortification reduces anxiety and lessens stress in family member in economically weak communities in Northwest Syria. Proc Natl Acad Sci USA 101.22 (2004): 8285–8288.
Smriga M et al. Oral treatment with L-lysine and L-arginine reduces anxiety and basal cortisol levels in healthy humans. Biomed Res 28.2 (2007): 85–90.
Tanner LM et al. Long-term oral lysine supplementation in lysinuric protein intolerance. Metabolism 56.2 (2007): 185–189.
Thein DJ, Hurt WC. Lysine as a prophylactic agent in the treatment of recurrent herpes simplex labialis. Oral Surg Oral Med Oral Pathol 58.6 (1984): 659–666.
Torricelli P et al. Human osteopenic bone-derived osteoblasts: essential amino acids treatment effects. Artif Cells Blood Substit Immobil Biotechnol 31.1 (2003): 35–46.
Unni, U.S., et al. (2012). The effect of a controlled 8-week metabolic ward based lysine supplementation on muscle function, insulin sensitivity and leucine kinetics in young men. Clin Nutr, 31(6), 903–910.
van Karnebeek, C.D., et al. (2012). Lysine restricted diet for pyridoxine-dependent epilepsy: First evidence and future trials. Mol Genet Metab, 107(3), 335–344.
Walsh DE, et al. Subjective response to lysine in the therapy of herpes simplex. J Antimicrob Chemother 12 (1983): 489–496.
Wass, C., et al. (2011). L-lysine as adjunctive treatment in patients with schizophrenia: A single-blinded, randomized, cross-over pilot study. BMC Med, 9, 40.
Wright EF. Clinical effectiveness of lysine in treating recurrent aphthous ulcers and herpes labialis. Gen Dent 42.1 (1994): 40–42.

Lutein and zeaxanthin

BACKGROUND AND RELEVANT PHARMACOKINETICS

Lutein and its isomer, zeaxanthin, are yellow-coloured, xanthophyll carotenoids that are not converted into vitamin A. The bioavailability of lutein and zeaxanthin from food sources is influenced by the food matrix and by the type and extent of food processing, but most notably by the presence of fat in the diet (Castenmiller et al 1999), with dietary fat intake being inversely related to serum levels (Nolan et al 2004). Cooking may increase their bioavailability by disrupting the cellular matrix and protein complexes, and supplemental sources may be significantly more bioavailable than food sources (Castenmiller et al 1999). It has also been observed that plasma responses to cholesterol and carotenoids are related (Clark et al 2006, Karppi et al 2010) and that the bioavailability of zeaxanthin from freeze-dried wolfberries is enhanced threefold when consumed in hot skimmed milk compared to hot water or warm milk (Benzie et al 2006). One clinical study found that plasma lutein was higher when lutein was consumed with a high-fat spread (207% increase) than with a low-fat spread (88% increase) (Roodenburg et al 2000). This was supported by a small in vitro study showing that dietary lutein is absorbed more efficiently with 24 g of avocado oil or 150 g of avocado fruit (Unlu et al 2005). For each 10% increase in dietary lutein and zeaxanthin, serum levels are seen to increase by 1% (Gruber et al 2004).

When ingested, lutein and zeaxanthin are transported from the intestine to the liver via chylomicrons. They are then transported via low-density lipoproteins (LDL) and high-density lipoproteins (HDL) to various parts of the body (Yeum & Russell 2002). Lutein and zeaxanthin are present in the eye, blood serum, skin, cervix, brain, breast and adipose tissue. In the eye, lutein is more prominent at the edges of the retina and in the rods (Bernstein et al 2001, Bone et al 1997). Lutein appears to undergo some metabolism in the retina to *meso*-zeaxanthin in most, but not all people. This accounts for lower retinal levels of lutein and higher relative levels of meso-zeaxanthin in the central macular and visa versa in the peripheral macular (Bone et al 1993). As such, meso-zeaxanthin and zeaxanthin are the predominant carotenoids in the foveal region, whereas lutein predominates in the parafoveal region (Bone et al 1988, Snodderly et al 1991). In particular, zeaxanthin is primarily concentrated in the centre of the retina and the cones, where it is present in concentrations nearly 1000-fold of those found in other tissues, thus giving the macula lutea or yellow spot of the retina its characteristic colour (Krinsky et al 2003). It is suggested, however, that during supplementation with xanthophylls, lutein is predominantly deposited in the fovea, while zeaxanthin deposition appears to cover a wider retinal area (Schalch et al 2007).

Lower serum concentrations of zeaxanthin have been associated with male gender, smoking, younger age, lower non-HDL cholesterol, greater ethanol consumption and higher body mass index (Brady et al 1996). Lutein and zeaxanthin, together with other carotenoids, have also been found to be lower in people with chronic cholestatic liver disease, which can be attributed to malabsorption of fat-soluble vitamins, as well as other mechanisms of hepatic release (Floreani et al 2000). In an epidemiological study involving 7059 participants, lower serum lutein and zeaxanthin levels were significantly associated with smoking, heavy drinking, being white, female, not physically active, having lower dietary lutein and zeaxanthin, a higher percentage of fat mass, a higher waist–hip ratio, lower serum cholesterol, a higher white blood cell count and high levels of C-reactive protein (Gruber et al 2004).

In a pharmacokinetic study involving 20 healthy volunteers, serum zeaxanthin levels were found to have an effective half-life for accumulation of 5 days and a terminal elimination half-life of around 12 days (Hartmann et al 2004). This was confirmed by another study that also found that lutein did not affect the concentrations of other carotenoids in healthy volunteers (Thurmann et al 2005). Similarly, high doses (50 mg) of beta-carotene over 5 years were not found to influence serum levels of lutein and zeaxanthin (Mayne et al 1998). It has been suggested that the associations between macula pigment density and serum lutein, serum zeaxanthin and adipose lutein concentrations are stronger in men (Broekmans et al 2002, Johnson et al 2000) and that the processes governing accumulation and/or stabilisation of zeaxanthin in fat tissue are different for males and females (Nolan et al 2004). This is supported by the finding that serum lutein and zeaxanthin concentrations vary with the menstrual cycle, with levels being higher in the late follicular than in the luteal phase (Forman et al 1998).

CHEMICAL COMPONENTS

Lutein and zeaxanthin are isomers and have identical chemical formulas, differing only in the location of a double bond in one of the hydroxyl groups. Lutein is known as beta, epsilon-carotene-3,3′-diol, whereas zeaxanthin is known as all-*trans* beta-carotene-3,3′-diol.

FOOD SOURCES

Foods differ in their relative amounts of lutein and zeaxanthin, with lutein generally being more abundant. Lutein is found in dark green leafy vegetables such as spinach and kale, as well as in sweetcorn and egg yolks, whereas zeaxanthin is found in sweetcorn, egg yolk, orange peppers (capsicums), persimmons, tangerines, mandarins and oranges. Goji berries are a very rich source of zeaxanthin.

Lutein, zeaxanthin and *meso*-zeaxanthin are primarily extracted from marigold flowers (*Tagetes erecta*) for use in supplements and are available in either free or esterified form. The esters typically contain two fatty acid groups that must be cleaved by pancreatic esterases and their absorption requires higher levels of dietary fat (Roodenburg et al 2000); however, addition of omega-long-chain polyunsaturated fatty acids to oral supplementation of lutein/zeaxanthin has not been found to change serum levels of lutein and zeaxanthin (Huang et al 2008).

DEFICIENCY SIGNS AND SYMPTOMS

Zeaxanthin and lutein can be considered conditionally essential nutrients because low serum levels or low dietary intakes are associated with low macular pigment density (Mares et al 2006) and increased risk of age-related macular degeneration (ARMD) (Semba & Dagnelie 2003).

Epidemiological studies have also found an association between low serum carotenoid levels, including lutein and zeaxanthin levels, with all-cause mortality (De Waart et al 2001), the risk of inflammatory polyarthritis (Pattison et al 2005), breast cancer (Tamimi et al 2005), prostate cancer (Jian et al 2005), colon cancer (Nkondjock & Ghadirian 2004), cervical cancer (Garcia-Closas et al 2005, Kim et al 2004), human papillomavirus persistence (Garcia-Closas et al 2005), type 2 diabetes and impaired glucose metabolism (Coyne et al 2005), chronic cholestatic liver diseases (Floreani et al 2000), Alzheimer's disease and vascular dementia (Polidori et al 2004) and low fruit and vegetable consumption (Al-Delaimy et al 2005).

Carotenoids have also emerged as an excellent tissue marker for a diet rich in fruit and vegetables, and measurement of plasma and tissue carotenoids is considered to have an important role in defining optimal diets (Al-Delaimy et al 2005, Brevik et al 2004, Handelman 2001).

MAIN ACTIONS

Antioxidant

Lutein and zeaxanthin are both powerful antioxidants, with activity having been demonstrated in a number of in vitro and in vivo tests (Higashi-Okai et al 2001, Iannone et al 1998, Muriach et al 2008, Naguib 2000). In vitro studies of human lens epithelial cells also indicate that their antioxidant activity may protect the lens from ultraviolet (UV) B radiation (Chitchumroonchokchai et al 2004). According to animal studies, lutein increases glutathione levels and reduces retinal apoptosis following ischaemic reperfusion (Dilsiz et al 2005). Lutein was also found to significantly protect against injury associated with oxidative stress in rat intestinal tissues following ischaemia-reperfusion (Sato et al 2011).

Lutein supplementation of 20 mg daily over 12 weeks was shown to significantly reduce C-reactive protein levels and lipid peroxidation, as well as increase total antioxidant capacity, in a randomised placebo-controlled trial of healthy volunteers (n = 117; Wang et al 2013). In contrast, a smaller study of 20 well-nourished adults aged 50–70 years found that supplementation of lutein (12 mg daily) for 112 days resulted in increased plasma antioxidant concentration but no significant changes in antioxidant activity or lipid peroxidation (Li et al 2010).

Blue light filter

The yellow colour of lutein and zeaxanthin is due to their ability to absorb blue light, which is believed to contribute to their protective function because blue light is at the high-energy, and therefore the most damaging, end of the visible spectrum (Krinsky et al 2003). Lutein and zeaxanthin thus serve as 'natural sunglasses' (Rehak et al 2008) that act as an optical filter for blue light, reducing chromatic aberration and preventing damage to the photoreceptor cell layer (Krinsky et al 2003). An in vivo study confirmed that lutein afforded protection against light-induced retinal damage in mice, which was associated with reduced markers of DNA damage in photoreceptor cells, and upregulation of the prosurvival gene 'eyes absent' (Sasaki et al 2012). The reduction of light-induced oxidative stress was thought to contribute to protection against DNA strand damage.

Macular pigment development

Lutein and zeaxanthin are entirely of dietary origin and are initially absent in newborns but gradually accumulate over time (Nussbaum et al 1981). It has been generally accepted that macular pigment density decreases with age; however, there are conflicting results. In one prospective, observational study involving 390 patients, macular pigment density was not found to change significantly with age, even when elderly subjects with cataracts and ARMD were considered (Ciulla & Hammond 2004). Other studies, however, have found that macular pigment does indeed decline with age in both normal eyes (Beatty et al 2001, Bernstein et al 2002) and those with ARMD (Bernstein et al 2002) and Stargardt macular dystrophy (Zhao et al 2003), but not in retinitis pigmentosa or choroideraemia (Zhao et al 2003).

Although lutein and zeaxanthin levels in the serum, diet and retina correlate, the nature of the relationships between lutein and zeaxanthin in foodstuffs, blood and the macula is confounded by many variables, including processes that influence digestion, absorption and transport and accumulation and stabilisation of the carotenoids in the tissues (Beatty et al 2004). It is suggested, however, that lutein and zeaxanthin are transported into an individual's retina in the same proportions found in his or her blood (Bone et al 1997). An in vitro study using retinal pigment epithelial cells found that both lutein and zeaxanthin modulate inflammatory responses to photo-oxidation, providing a possible mechanism for these compounds' effects in ARMD (Bain et al 2012).

Immunomodulation

Lutein modulates cellular and humoral-mediated immune responses, according to animal studies (Kim et al 2000a, 2000b). In particular, high levels of C-reactive protein and a high white blood cell count have been identified in individuals with low serum levels of lutein (Gruber et al 2004). In a case-controlled study, serum lutein and zeaxanthin, together with other carotenoids, were also found to be lower in children with acute-phase infections compared to healthy controls (Cser et al 2004).

Anti-inflammatory

Lutein supplementation (20 mg daily) in early atherosclerosis patients (n = 65) was found to significantly reduce serum cytokines interleukin-6 and monocyte chemotactic protein-1 after 3 months compared to placebo (Xu et al 2013). This also correlated with reduced serum LDL and triglyceride levels in patients receiving lutein, though this study may be insufficiently powered to draw meaningful conclusions. Further studies are recommended to clarify lutein's anti-inflammatory effects.

Photoprotection

According to animal studies, lutein reduces the risk of sunburn, as well as local UVB radiation-induced immune suppression and reactive oxygen species generation (Lee et al 2004), and directly protects against photoageing and photocarcinogenesis (Astner et al 2007). A protective effect on skin cancer, however, has not been observed in human cohort studies. One prospective cohort study involving 43,867 men and 85,944 women found no significant inverse association between intake of lutein and squamous cell carcinoma (Fung et al 2003), while an increased risk of squamous cell carcinoma was observed for people with multiple prior non-melanoma skin cancers and high serum levels of lutein and zeaxanthin (Dorgan et al 2004).

While a protective effect against skin cancer is uncertain, there is evidence to suggest that supplementation with lutein and zeaxanthin may improve general skin health and simultaneously help to minimise signs of premature ageing (Maci 2007). A double-blind, placebo-controlled study that examined surface lipids, hydration, photoprotective activity, skin elasticity and skin lipid peroxidation found that oral and/or topical administration of either lutein or zeaxanthin provided antioxidant protection, with the greatest protection being seen with combined administration of lutein and zeaxanthin (Palombo et al 2007). The clinical significance of these findings is uncertain.

CLINICAL USE

Lutein and zeaxanthin supplementation is most often used for preventing and/or treating various ocular conditions.

Age-related macular degeneration

ARMD is the leading cause of irreversible visual dysfunction in individuals over 65 years in Western society. People with ARMD are classified as having early-stage disease (early ARMD), in which visual function is affected, or late ARMD (generally characterised as either 'wet' neovascular ARMD or 'dry' atrophic ARMD, or both) in which central vision is severely compromised or lost (Bowes et al 2013). Atrophic ARMD accounts for 90% of all ARMD cases (Richer et al 2004).

The evidence that lifetime oxidative stress plays an important role in the development of ARMD is now compelling (Hogg & Chakravarthy 2004). ARMD is thought to be the result of free radical damage to photoreceptors within the macula, and therefore it is suspected that inefficient macular antioxidant systems play a role in disease development. After ageing, smoking is the next significant risk factor, most likely due to antioxidant depletion and increased oxidative stress. Smoking is also associated with lower levels of macular xanthophyll pigments such as lutein. Diets low in fruit and vegetables, excessive exposure to sunlight and blue light and use of photosensitising medicines are other factors known to increase the risk of developing ARMD (Richer et al 2004).

Epidemiological and autopsy studies have found an inverse relationship between lutein and zeaxanthin intake and macular pigment density (Bone et al 2001, Curran-Celentano et al 2001). The presence of unusually high levels of macular carotenoids in older donors who were regularly consuming high-dose lutein supplements further supports the hypothesis that long-term high intake of lutein can raise levels of macular pigment (Bhosale et al 2007). Similarly, clinical studies have also confirmed the association between macular pigmentation, dietary lutein intake and serum lutein levels (Burke et al 2005, Mares et al 2006, Yao et al 2013).

Lutein supplementation can also effectively increase plasma lutein and macular pigment density in most people with established ARMD (Bernstein et al 2002, Richer et al 2004, 2011, Wang et al 2007) and also in healthy controls (Koh et al 2004), demonstrating that both a diseased and a healthy macula can accumulate and stabilise lutein and/or zeaxanthin (Koh et al 2004). An increase in macular pigment density develops within 4 weeks of increasing lutein, according to clinical studies (Berendschot et al 2000, Hammond et al 1997). Interestingly, it was recently discovered that the variability in retinal macular pigment response to increased lutein intake is due to underlying genetic variants (Yonova-Doing et al 2013). Clinical research further indicates that people with lower starting lutein levels experience greater protective effects when increasing lutein consumption in regard to age-related maculopathy (which precedes ARMD) (Cho et al 2004). There is also evidence from the Lutein Antioxidant Supplementation Trial (LAST) II that people with established atrophic ARMD starting with the lowest macular pigment optical density (MPOD) experience the greatest increases in MPOD when taking lutein or lutein + antioxidant supplements over 12 months (Richer et al 2007). These combined results are helping to clarify who is most likely to experience benefits from increased lutein intake and the variability in clinical trial results to date.

At least 16 epidemiological studies have reported a link between lutein and zeaxanthin and ARMD risk, supporting the theory that higher intakes and/or plasma levels of these macular pigments may be protective (Elliott & Williams 2012). A 2012 systematic review and meta-analysis concluded that, while dietary intake of lutein and zeaxanthin was not significantly associated with reduced risk of early ARMD onset, it was associated with protection in late ARMD (relative risk 0.74; Ma et al 2012). Joachim et al (2014) reported that dietary lutein-zeaxanthin intake was associated with decreased likelihood of progression from reticular drusen to late ARMD (adjusted odds ratio 0.5; 95% confidence interval 0.3–1.0), as based on the most recent results from the Blue Mountains Eye Study (n = 3654), which involves 5-year, 10-year and 15-year follow-up examinations. Using data from the same study cohort together with data from the Rotterdam Study, Wang et al (2014) reported that people with a high ARMD genetic risk and the highest intake of lutein/zeaxanthin had a >20% reduced risk of early ARMD compared to people with a low genetic risk having a high intake of lutein/zeaxanthin.

For people with established ARMD, several important benefits have been reported with increased lutein intake, often when combined with other antioxidant nutrients. Improvements of up to 92% in visual acuity tests were observed when subjects with atrophic ARMD consumed a diet designed to contain approximately 150 g of spinach 4–7 times a week, according to an early pilot study (Richer 1999). A small pilot study by Falsini et al (2003) involving 30 patients with early ARMD and visual acuity of 6/9 or better experienced improved macular function with the use of daily lutein (15 mg) + vitamin E (20 mg) and nicotinamide (18 mg) for 180 days; this improvement was lost when supplementation was stopped (Falsini et al 2003).

Richer et al (2004) subsequently conducted a much larger study which found that lutein supplements (10 mg/day) improved some symptoms of atrophic ARMD after 12 months, such as contrast sensitivity, glare recovery and near vision acuity, while also increasing macular pigment density. The groups receiving lutein + antioxidants (including zinc) demonstrated even broader effects compared to lutein alone or placebo. LAST, conducted by Richer et al (2004), was a double-blind, randomised, placebo-controlled study involving 90 subjects. In addition to improving most measures of quality of vision, both the lutein (FloraGloB, Kemin Foods International, USA) and lutein plus antioxidant (OcuPower, Nutraceutical Sciences Institute (NSI), USA) groups achieved an increase of 36% and 43%, respectively, in macular pigment density, whereas the placebo group experienced a slight decrease (Richer et al 2004). In other studies, lutein supplementation has been shown to increase macular pigment optical density and contrast and glare sensitivity compared to placebo (Yao et al 2013), and was seen to improve visual performance at low illumination, yet this was not correlated with macular pigment density (Kvansakul et al 2006).

More recently, a double-blind, placebo-controlled trial reported that macular pigment optical density and best-corrected visual acuity were significantly improved in patients with non-exudative ARMD ($n = 172$) after taking a combination of lutein (10–20 mg) + zeaxanthin (1–2 mg) + omega-3 fatty acids (100–200 mg docosahexaenoic acid and 30–60 mg eicosapentaenoic acid) + antioxidants over 12 months (Dawczynski et al 2013). Two doses were used and both were as effective as each other but better than placebo, suggesting the lower dose saturated retinal levels and no further benefits could be achieved with a higher dose. A low dose of 6 mg daily of lutein is not effective according to a small double-blind, randomised controlled trial conducted over 60 weeks involving people with ARMD (Bartlett & Eperjesi 2007).

In regard to delaying the progression of ARMD, the AREDS2 study found that general antioxidant supplementation (original AREDS formula) was not enhanced by the addition of lutein (10 mg) and zeaxanthin (2 mg) (The AREDS2 Research Group 2013b). More recently, combinations of lutein and zeaxanthin combined with meso-xanthin have been tested in AMD. The Central Retinal Enrichment Supplementation Trials (CREST) are underway and will investigate the potential impact of macular pigment (MP) enrichment, following supplementation with a formulation containing 10 mg lutein (L), 2 mg zeaxanthin (Z) and 10 mg meso-zeaxanthin (MZ), on visual function in normal subjects and in subjects with early age-related macular degeneration (Akuffo et al 2014).

Cataracts

Lens density has been found to inversely correlate with macular lutein and zeaxanthin levels (Hammond et al 1997) and numerous observational studies have found that increased consumption of foods high in lutein and zeaxanthin is associated with a decreased risk for cataracts (Brown et al 1999, Delcourt et al 2006, Tavani et al 1996). In one study involving 77,466 female nurses from the Nurses' Health Study, those with the highest quintile for consumption of zeaxanthin and lutein were found to have a 22% reduction in the risk of cataract extraction (Chasan-Taber et al 1999). Similarly, a study of 1802 women aged 50–79 years found that women in the highest quintile category of diet or serum levels of lutein and zeaxanthin were 32% less likely to have nuclear cataract as compared with those in the lowest quintile category (Moeller et al 2008). A further epidemiological study of 3271 Melbourne residents found that, while cortical and posterior subcapsular cataracts were not significantly associated with lutein or zeaxanthin intake, high dietary lutein and zeaxanthin intake was inversely associated with the prevalence of nuclear cataract (Vu et al 2006). The link between lutein and cataracts is further supported by a small randomised, placebo-controlled trial of 17 patients with clinically diagnosed age-related cataracts that found that supplementation with lutein 15 mg three times weekly for up to 2 years resulted in improved visual performance (visual acuity and glare sensitivity) compared with placebo (Olmedilla et al 2003).

These results contrast with those from a cohort study of 478 women without previously diagnosed cataracts, which failed to detect a significant inverse relationship between lutein intake and lens opacities over a 13–15-year follow-up period (Jacques et al 2001). The AREDS2 randomised clinical trial also determined that daily supplementation with lutein (10 mg) and zeaxanthin (2 mg) had no statistically significant effects on rates of cataract surgery or vision loss in adults aged 50–85 years at risk for progression to advanced ARMD (The AREDS2 Research Group 2013a).

Retinitis pigmentosa

In a double-blind, randomised, placebo-controlled crossover trial, supplementation with lutein (10 mg/day) for 12 weeks followed by 30 mg/day for 12 weeks was found to improve visual field and possibly visual acuity in 34 patients with retinitis pigmentosa (Bahrami et al 2006). A further study found that daily supplementation with 40 mg of lutein over 9 weeks followed by 20 mg for a further 16 weeks significantly improved visual acuity in 16 subjects with retinitis pigmentosa, many of whom were also taking other supplements (Dagnelie et al 2000).

Clinical note

The macula (central retina) contains a yellow pigment comprising the dietary carotenoids lutein (L), zeaxanthin (Z), and meso-zeaxanthin, known as macular pigment (MP). The concentrations of MP's constituent carotenoids in retina and brain tissue correlate, and there is a biologically plausible rationale, supported by emerging evidence, that MP's constituent carotenoids are also important for cognitive function (Nolan et al 2014).

Retinopathy of prematurity

Supplementation of lutein and zeaxanthin in preterm infants did not prevent the occurrence of retinopathy of prematurity or outcome at hospital discharge compared to placebo in a randomised controlled trial of 114 infants of ≤32 weeks' gestation (Dani et al 2012).

Cancer prevention

High dietary intake of lutein has been associated with reduced risk of some cancers, most notably endometrial and ovarian cancer, but not all cancers, according to epidemiological evidence (Freudenheim et al 1996, Fung et al 2003, Gann et al 1999, Giovannucci et al 1995, Huang et al 2003, Ito et al 2003, Lu et al 2001, McCann et al 2000, Michaud et al 2000, Nomura et al 1997, Schuurman et al 2002, Terry et al 2002).

Lung cancer

Three large population studies of diet and lung cancer have revealed a non-significant association between high lutein intake and lower risk of lung cancer (Ito et al 2003, Michaud et al 2000, Ziegler et al 1996), and a significant trend was observed in another population-based case–control study (Le Marchand et al 1993). A nested case–control study also found that serum lutein and zeaxanthin were lower in those with lung cancer than in controls (Comstock et al 1997). These results are contrasted with those from a case–control study of 108 cases of lung cancer in a Chinese occupational cohort that found that higher serum carotenoid levels, including lutein and zeaxanthin, were significantly associated with increased lung cancer risk among alcohol drinkers, while having a possible protective association among non-drinkers (Ratnasinghe et al 2000).

Cervical cancer

A 2005 systematic review suggests that lutein/zeaxanthin is likely to have a protective effect for cervical neoplasia and possibly for human papillomavirus persistence (Garcia-Closas et al 2005).

Endometrial cancer

An epidemiological study involving 232 patients with endometrial cancer and 639 controls found that an intake of more than 7.3 mg/day of lutein was associated with a 70% reduced risk of endometrial cancer (McCann et al 2000).

Ovarian cancer

A case–control study found that weekly intake of lutein of more than 24 mg was associated with a 40% reduction in the risk for developing ovarian cancer compared with weekly consumption of less than 3.8 mcg (Bertone et al 2001).

Breast cancer

High lutein and zeaxanthin intake has been related to reduced risk of breast cancer (Dorgan et al 1998, Toniolo et al 2001). High lutein intake (>7 mg/day) was associated with a 53% reduction in the risk of developing breast cancer compared with low consumption (<3.7 mg/day) in a population-based case-control study of 608 premenopausal women over age 40 (Freudenheim et al 1996). Similar risk reductions were found in a nested case-control study of 540 New York women (Toniolo et al 2001) and another nested case–control study of 969 cases of breast cancer and matched controls from the Nurses' Health Study found that the risk of breast cancer was 25–35% less for women with the highest quintile compared with that for women with the lowest quintile of lutein/zeaxanthin and total carotenoid intake (Tamimi et al 2005). Although this association is encouraging, another study of 4697 women followed over 25 years found no significant relationships between lutein intake and breast cancer risk (Jarvinen et al 1997).

Gastric cancer

High serum lutein levels have been associated with a higher incidence of gastric carcinoma, according to a cohort study of 29,584 patients with oesophageal and stomach cancer (Abnet et al 2003); however, this association requires further investigation.

Bowel cancer

The relationship between lutein and zeaxanthin intake and colon cancer is uncertain. A case-control study involving 1993 cases of colon cancer and 2410 controls found that lutein intake, as measured by a food frequency score, was inversely associated with colon cancer and another case–control study of 223 subjects with histologically confirmed colon or rectal cancer identified a non-significant inverse association with lutein (Levi et al 2000). A cohort analysis of 5629 women, however, found no such association (Terry et al 2002). A case-controlled study found that women with high intakes of long-chain polyunsaturated fatty acids had an inverse association between lutein and zeaxanthin intake and the risk of colon cancer (Nkondjock & Ghadirian 2004). Further investigation is required to clarify these findings because animal studies suggest low doses of lutein inhibit aberrant crypt foci formation, whereas high doses may increase the risk by 9–59% (Raju et al 2005).

Prostate cancer

Overall, epidemiological evidence suggests that lutein and zeaxanthin intake has no influence over the risk of prostate cancer (Bosetti et al 2004, Gann et al 1999, Giovannucci et al 1995, Huang et al 2003, Lu et al 2001, Nomura et al 1997, Schuurman et al 2002). However, when lutein was included as part of a mixed carotenoid and tocopherol extract, the combination was effective in an in vitro study of prostate cancer cell lines (Lu et al 2005). A case-controlled study of 130 patients with adenocarcinoma of the prostate found that prostate cancer risk was seen to decline with increasing consumption of carotenoids, including lycopene, alpha-carotene, beta-carotene, beta-cryptoxanthin, lutein and zeaxanthin (Jian et al 2005).

Laryngeal cancer

A case–control study involving 537 subjects identified an inverse relationship between dietary lutein and zeaxanthin intake, together with the intake of other carotenoids, and the risk of laryngeal cancer (Bidoli et al 2003).

OTHER USES

Lutein and zeaxanthin may be used as part of a general antioxidant supplement, often taken in conjunction with other carotenoids in cases where there is known or suspected increased oxidative load.

Sleep duration

Reduced lutein and zeaxanthin intake may be associated with reduced sleep duration; however more studies are needed to confirm this preliminary finding (Grandner 2013).

Cognitive impairment

Dementia has been found to be associated with increased protein oxidative modification and the depletion of a large spectrum of antioxidant micronutrients, including lutein and zeaxanthin (Polidori et al 2004). In a clinical study of 25 subjects with mild cognitive impairment, 63 subjects with Alzheimer's disease and 56 healthy individuals found that serum lutein levels were lowest in the first two groups, particularly those with Alzheimer's disease (Rinaldi et al 2003), while a double-blind trial of 49 women aged 60–80 years found improved cognitive function after supplementation with a combination of docosahexaenoic acid and lutein (Johnson et al 2008).

A large, population-based study of adults aged over 50 years identified that low macular pigment density was associated with lower cognitive performance (Feeney et al 2013). This, however, was not an intervention-based study and therefore was not able to determine the effect of exogenous lutein supplementation in acutely improving cognitive parameters.

Atherosclerosis

The relationship between lutein and zeaxanthin status and atherosclerosis is being investigated but remains unclear. Plasma levels of lutein, beta-cryptoxanthin and zeaxanthin were correlated to carotid intima media thickness in a 3-year case-controlled study of 231 subjects (Iribarren et al 1997), as well as in an 18-month epidemiological study of 573 subjects, suggesting that these carotenoids may be protective against early atherosclerosis (Dwyer et al 2004). Lutein intake has also been found to be inversely associated with the risk of ischaemic stroke in an observational study involving 43,738 males (Ascherio et al 1999), as well as being inversely associated with the risk of subarachnoid haemorrhage in a cohort study of 26,593 male smokers (Hirvonen et al 2000). Serum levels of lutein and zeaxanthin, however, were not associated with atherosclerosis risk in a case–control study involving 108 cases of aortic atherosclerosis in an elderly population (Klipstein-Grobusch et al 2000).

The foregoing findings contrast with those from two case-controlled studies that found a positive correlation between lutein and zeaxanthin levels and cardiovascular risk. A nested, case-control study of 499 cases of cardiovascular disease with matched controls taken from the Physicians' Health Study found that concentrations of plasma lutein, zeaxanthin and retinol corresponded to a moderate increase in cardiovascular disease (Sesso et al 2005). Similarly, myocardial infarction risk was positively associated with lutein and zeaxanthin levels in adipose tissue and diet in a case-controlled study of 1456 cases of first acute myocardial infarction and matched controls (Kabagambe et al 2005). The clinical significance of these findings is unclear and requires further investigation.

DOSAGE RANGE

According to clinical studies

- Macular protection: lutein 6–20 mg/day; zeaxanthin 2–5 mg/day.
- The original AREDS formulation contained vitamin C, vitamin E, beta-carotene, zinc and copper.
- The successful AREDS2 formulation contained lutein and zeaxanthin instead of beta-carotene.
- Atrophic ARMD: improving visual quality — 10 mg lutein daily, ideally in combination with other antioxidants and possibly omega-3 essential fatty acids for better effects.
- Cataracts — improving visual performance: lutein 15 mg three times weekly.

L

TOXICITY

Dietary amounts and those used in clinical studies are considered safe.

ADVERSE REACTIONS

Lutein and zeaxanthin supplements are well tolerated.

SIGNIFICANT INTERACTIONS

Vitamin C

Lutein showed increased antioxidant efficacy with vitamin C in an animal study (Blakely et al 2003). Further to this, a small in vivo study showed that 2000 mg of vitamin C enhanced the absorption of lutein (Tanumihardjo et al 2005).

Vitamin E

Vitamin E showed increased antioxidant efficacy with lutein according to an animal study (Blakely et al 2003).

Phytosterols

High dietary intake of phytosterol esters (6.6 g/day) reduced plasma levels of lutein by 14% in a small clinical trial; however, this was reversed by increasing fruit and vegetable intake (Clifton et al 2004).

Orlistat

Theoretically, long-term use of orlistat leads to reduced plasma levels of lutein due to reduced gastric absorption (Australian Medicines Handbook) — increased dietary intake of lutein should be considered.

Olestra

Lutein and zeaxanthin levels have been found to decrease with long-term use of olestra (Tulley et al 2005) — increased dietary intake of lutein should be considered.

CONTRAINDICATIONS AND PRECAUTIONS

Lutein and zeaxanthin are contraindicated in people with a hypersensitivity to these carotenoids or their food sources.

PREGNANCY USE

Eating dietary amounts of foods rich in lutein and zeaxanthin is likely to be safe. Women at risk of premature rupture of the membranes are cautioned against very high intake because one study observed a fourfold greater risk of membrane rupture with high serum lutein levels (Mathews & Neil 2005).

Practice points/Patient counselling

- Lutein and zeaxanthin are antioxidant carotenoids found in spinach, corn, egg yolk, squash and greens. Goji berries are a particularly rich source of zeaxanthin.
- Lutein and zeaxanthin are essential for the development of macular pigment, which protects photoreceptor cells in the retina from free radical damage.
- Epidemiological studies have generally found an inverse relationship between lutein and zeaxanthin intake and macular degeneration; increased intakes will reduce the incidence of ARMD in some populations, but not all.
- People with established 'dry' macular degeneration may experience improved visual quality with lutein supplementation.
- Long-term use of lutein supplements may increase visual performance in people with pre-existing cataracts.
- High dietary intake of lutein has been associated with reduced risk of some cancers, most notably endometrial and ovarian cancer, but not all cancers, according to epidemiological evidence.
- Supplements containing lutein and zeaxanthin should be taken with food as dietary fat improves their absorption.

PATIENTS' FAQs

What will this supplement do for me?

Lutein and zeaxanthin are important for eye health. They improve visual quality in people with established 'dry' ARMD and may reduce the risk of progressing to ARMD in some at-risk people. There may also be some protection against developing certain cancers when consumed over time.

When will it start to work?

Increased intake of lutein can improve macular health within 4 weeks; however, clinical effects develop slowly and may not be detected for 6 months. In regard to improving visual performance in people with pre-existing cataracts, effects take even longer (≈2 years).

Are there any safety issues?

Lutein and zeaxanthin are generally considered safe.

REFERENCES

Abnet CC et al. Prospective study of serum retinol, beta-carotene, beta-cryptoxanthin, and lutein/zeaxanthin and esophageal and gastric cancers in China. Cancer Causes Control 14.7 (2003): 645–655.

Al-Delaimy WK et al. Plasma carotenoids as biomarkers of intake of fruits and vegetables: ecological-level correlations in the European Prospective Investigation into Cancer and Nutrition (EPIC). Eur J Clin Nutr 59.12 (2005): 1397–1408.

Akuffo KO et al. Central Retinal Enrichment Supplementation Trials (CREST): design and methodology of the CREST randomized controlled trials. Ophthalmic Epidemiol 21.2 (2014): 111-123.

Ascherio A et al. Relation of consumption of vitamin E, vitamin C, and carotenoids to risk for stroke among men in the United States. Ann Intern Med 130.12 (1999): 963–970.

Astner S et al. Dietary lutein/zeaxanthin partially reduces photoaging and photocarcinogenesis in chronically UVB-irradiated Skh-1 hairless mice. Skin Pharmacol Physiol 20.6 (2007): 283–291.

Australian Medicines Handbook. Royal Australian College of General Practitioners, the Pharmaceutical Society of Australia and the Australasian Society of Clinical and Experimental Pharmacologists and Toxicologists. www.amh.hcn.net.au (accessed 06-12-05).

Bahrami H, et al. Lutein supplementation in retinitis pigmentosa: PC-based vision assessment in a randomized double-masked placebo-controlled clinical trial [NCT00029289]. BMC Ophthalmol 6 (2006): 23.

Bain Q et al. Lutein and zeaxanthin supplementation reduces photooxidative damage and modulates the expression of inflammation-related genes in retinal pigment epithelial cells. Free Radic Biol Med 53.6 (2012): 1298–1307.

Bartlett HE, Eperjesi F. Effect of lutein and antioxidant dietary supplementation on contrast sensitivity in age-related macular disease: a randomized controlled trial. Eur J Clin Nutr 61.9 (2007): 1121–1127.

Beatty S et al. Macular pigment and risk for age-related macular degeneration in subjects from a Northern European population. Invest Ophthalmol Vis Sci 42.2 (2001): 439–446.

Beatty S et al. Macular pigment optical density and its relationship with serum and dietary levels of lutein and zeaxanthin. Arch Biochem Biophys 430.1 (2004): 70–76.

Benzie IF et al. Enhanced bioavailability of zeaxanthin in a milk-based formulation of wolfberry (Gou Qi Zi; *Fructus barbarum* L.). Br J Nutr 96.1 (2006): 154–160.

Berendschot TT et al. Influence of lutein supplementation on macular pigment, assessed with two objective techniques. Invest Ophthalmol Vis Sci 41.11 (2000): 3322–3326.

Bernstein PS et al. Identification and quantification of carotenoids and their metabolites in the tissues of the human eye. Exp Eye Res 72.3 (2001): 215–223.

Bernstein PS et al. Resonance Raman measurement of macular carotenoids in normal subjects and in age-related macular degeneration patients. Ophthalmology 109.10 (2002): 1780–1787.

Bertone ER et al. A population-based case-control study of carotenoid and vitamin A intake and ovarian cancer (United States). Cancer Causes Control 12.1 (2001): 83–90.

Bhosale P, et al. HPLC measurement of ocular carotenoid levels in human donor eyes in the lutein supplementation era. Investigative Ophthalmology and Visual Science 48.2 (2007): 543–54549.

Bidoli E et al. Micronutrients and laryngeal cancer risk in Italy and Switzerland: a case control study. Cancer Causes Control 14.5 (2003): 477–484.

Blakely S et al. Lutein interacts with ascorbic acid more frequently than with (alpha)-tocopherol to alter biomarkers of oxidative stress in female Zucker obese rats. J Nutr 133.9 (2003): 2838–2844.

Bone R et al. Distribution of lutein and zeaxanthin stereoisomers in the human retina. Exp Eye Res 64.2 (1997): 211–2118.

Bone R et al. Macular pigment in donor eyes with and without AMD: a case-control study. Invest Ophthalmol Vis Sci 42.1 (2001): 235–240.

Bosetti C et al. Retinol, carotenoids and the risk of prostate cancer: a case-control study from Italy. Int J Cancer 112.4 (2004): 689–692.

Bowes, R.C., et al. 2013. Dry age-related macular degeneration: mechanisms, therapeutic targets, and imaging. Invest Ophthalmol.Vis. Sci., 54, (14) ORSF68–ORSF80.

Brady WE et al. Human serum carotenoid concentrations are related to physiologic and lifestyle factors. J Nutr 126.1 (1996): 129–137.
Brevik A et al. Six carotenoids in plasma used to assess recommended intake of fruits and vegetables in a controlled feeding study. Eur J Clin Nutr 58.8 (2004): 1166–1173.
Broekmans WM et al. Macular pigment density in relation to serum and adipose tissue concentrations of lutein and serum concentrations of zeaxanthin. Am J Clin Nutr 76.3 (2002): 595–603.
Brown L et al. A prospective study of carotenoid intake and risk of cataract extraction in US men. Am J Clin Nutr 70.4 (1999): 517–524.
Burke JD, et al. Diet and serum carotenoid concentrations affect macular pigment optical density in adults 45 years and older. J Nutr 135.5 (2005): 1208–1215.
Castenmiller JJ et al. The food matrix of spinach is a limiting factor in determining the bioavailability of beta-carotene and to a lesser extent of lutein in humans. J Nutr 129.2 (1999): 349–355.
Chasan-Taber L et al. A prospective study of vitamin supplement intake and cataract extraction among U.S. women. Epidemiology 10.6 (1999): 679–684.
Chitchumroonchokchai C et al. Xanthophylls and [alpha]-tocopherol decrease UVB-induced lipid peroxidation and stress signaling in human lens epithelial cells. J Nutr 134.12 (2004): 3225–3232.
Cho E, et al. Prospective study of intake of fruits, vegetables, vitamins, and carotenoids and risk of age-related maculopathy. Arch Ophthalmol 2004;122:883–92.
Ciulla TA, Hammond BR Jr. Macular pigment density and aging, assessed in the normal elderly and those with cataracts and age-related macular degeneration. Am J Ophthalmol 138.4 (2004): 582–587.
Clark RM et al. Hypo- and hyperresponse to egg cholesterol predicts plasma lutein and beta-carotene concentrations in men and women. J Nutr 136.3 (2006): 601–607.
Clifton PM et al. High dietary intake of phytosterol esters decreases carotenoids and increases plasma plant sterol levels with no additional cholesterol lowering. J Lipid Res 45.8 (2004): 1493–1499.
Comstock GW et al. The risk of developing lung cancer associated with antioxidants in the blood: ascorbic acid, carotenoids, alpha-tocopherol, selenium, and total peroxyl radical absorbing capacity. Cancer Epidemiol Biomarkers Prev 6.11 (1997): 907–916.
Coyne T et al. Diabetes mellitus and serum carotenoids: findings of a population-based study in Queensland. Australia. Am J Clin Nutr 82.3 (2005): 685–693.
Cser MA et al. Serum carotenoid and retinol levels during childhood infections. Ann Nutr Metab 48.3 (2004): 156.
Curran-Celentano J et al. Relation between dietary intake, serum concentrations, and retinal concentrations of lutein and zeaxanthin in adults in a Midwest population. Am J Clin Nutr 74.6 (2001): 796–802.
Dagnelie G, et al. Lutein improves visual function in some patients with retinal degeneration: a pilot study via the Internet. Optometry 71 (2000): 147–164.
Dani C et al. Lutein and zeaxanthin supplementation in preterm infants to prevent retinopathy of prematurity: a randomized controlled study. J Matern Fetal Neonatal Med 25.5 (2012): 523–527
Dawczynski J et al. Long term effects of lutein, zeaxanthin and omega-3-LCPUFAs supplementation on optical density of macular pigment in AMD patients: the LUTEGA study. Graefes Arch Clin Exp Ophthalmol 251.12 (2013): 2711–2723
Delcourt C et al. Plasma lutein and zeaxanthin and other carotenoids as modifiable risk factors for age-related maculopathy and cataract: The POLA study. Investigative Ophthalmology and Visual Science 47.6 (2006): 2329–2335.
De Waart FG et al. Serum carotenoids, [alpha]-tocopherol and mortality risk in a prospective study among Dutch elderly. Int J Epidemiol 30.1 (2001): 136–143.
Dilsiz N et al. Protective effects of various antioxidants during ischemia-reperfusion in the rat retina. Graefe's Arch Clin Exp Ophthalmol (2005): 1–7.
Dorgan JF et al. Relationships of serum carotenoids, retinol, [alpha]-tocopherol, and selenium with breast cancer risk: results from a prospective study in Columbia, Missouri (United States). Cancer Causes Control 9.1 (1998): 89–97.
Dorgan JF et al. Serum carotenoids and (alpha)-tocopherol and risk of nonmelanoma skin cancer. Cancer Epidemiol Biomarkers Prev 13.8 (2004): 1276–1282.
Dwyer JH et al. Progression of carotid intima-media thickness and plasma antioxidants: the Los Angeles Atherosclerosis Study. Arterioscler Thromb Vasc Biol 24.2 (2004): 313–3119.
Elliott, J.G. & Williams, N.S. 2012. Nutrients in the battle against age-related eye diseases. Optometry., 83, (1) 47–55.
Falsini B et al. Influence of short-term antioxidant supplementation on macular function in age-related maculopathy: a pilot study including electrophysiologic assessment. Ophthalmology 110.1 (2003): 51–60.
Feeney J et al. Low macular pigment opticl density is associated with lower cognitive performance in a large, population-based sample of older adults. Neurobiol Aging 34.11 (2013): 2449–2456
Floreani A et al. Plasma antioxidant levels in chronic cholestatic liver diseases. Aliment Pharmacol Ther 14.3 (2000): 353–358.
Forman MR et al. Effect of menstrual cycle phase on the concentration of individual carotenoids in lipoproteins of premenopausal women: a controlled dietary study. Am J Clin Nutr 67.1 (1998): 81–87.
Freudenheim JL et al. Premenopausal breast cancer risk and intake of vegetables, fruits, and related nutrients. J Natl Cancer Inst 88.6 (1996): 340–348.
Fung TT et al. Vitamin and carotenoid intake and risk of squamous cell carcinoma of the skin. Int J Cancer 103.1 (2003): 110–1115.
Gann PH et al. Lower prostate cancer risk in men with elevated plasma lycopene levels: results of a prospective analysis. Cancer Res 59.6 (1999): 1225–1230.
Garcia-Closas R et al. The role of diet and nutrition in cervical carcinogenesis: a review of recent evidence. Int J Cancer 117.4 (2005): 629–637.
Giovannucci E et al. Intake of carotenoids and retinol in relation to risk of prostate cancer. J Natl Cancer Inst 87.23 (1995): 1767–1776.
Grandner MA. Dietary nutrients associated with short and long sleep duration. Data from a nationally representation sample. Appetite 64 (2013): 71–80
Gruber M et al. Correlates of serum lutein + zeaxanthin: findings from the Third National Health and Nutr Examination Survey. J Nutr 134.9 (2004): 2387–2394.
Hammond BR Jr et al. Dietary modification of human macular pigment density. Invest Ophthalmol Vis Sci 38.9 (1997): 1795–1801.
Handelman GJ. The evolving role of carotenoids in human biochemistry. Nutrition 17.10 (2001): 818–822.
Hartmann D et al. Plasma kinetics of zeaxanthin and 3′-dehydro-lutein after multiple oral doses of synthetic zeaxanthin. Am J Clin Nutr 79.3 (2004): 410–417.
Higashi-Okai K et al. Identification and antioxidant activity of several pigments from the residual green tea (*Camellia sinensis*) after hot water extraction. J Univ Occup Environ Health 23.4 (2001): 335–344.
Hirvonen T et al. Intake of flavonoids, carotenoids, vitamins C and E, and risk of stroke in male smokers. Stroke 31.10 (2000): 2301–2306.
Hogg R, Chakravarthy U. AMD and micronutrient antioxidants. Current Eye Res 29.6 (2004): 387–401.
Huang HY et al. Prospective study of antioxidant micronutrients in the blood and the risk of developing prostate cancer. Am J Epidemiol 157.4 (2003): 335–344.
Huang LL et al. Oral supplementation of lutein/zeaxanthin and omega-3 long chain polyunsaturated fatty acids in persons aged 60 years or older, with or without AMD. Invest Ophthalmol & Vis Sci 49.9 (2008): 3864–3869.
Iannone A et al. Antioxidant activity of carotenoids: an electron-spin resonance study on beta-carotene and lutein interaction with free radicals generated in a chemical system. J Biochem Mol Toxicol 12.5 (1998): 299–304.
Iribarren C et al. Association of serum vitamin levels, LDL susceptibility to oxidation, and autoantibodies against MDA-LDL with carotid atherosclerosis: a case-control study: the ARIC Study Investigators (Atherosclerosis Risk in Communities). Arterioscler Thromb Vasc Biol 17.6 (1997): 1171–1177.
Ito Y et al. Serum carotenoids and mortality from lung cancer: a case-control study nested in the Japan Collaborative Cohort (JACC) study. Cancer Sci 94.1 (2003): 57–63.
Jacques PF et al. Long-term nutrient intake and early age-related nuclear lens opacities. Arch Ophthalmol 119.7 (2001): 1009–1019.
Jarvinen R et al. Diet and breast cancer risk in a cohort of Finnish women. Cancer Lett 114.1–2 (1997): 251–253.
Jian L et al. Do dietary lycopene and other carotenoids protect against prostate cancer? Int J Cancer 113.6 (2005): 1010–10114.
Joachim, N., et al. 2014. Incidence and progression of reticular drusen in age-related macular degeneration: findings from an older Australian cohort. Ophthalmology 121: 917–925.
Johnson E et al. Relation among serum and tissue concentrations of lutein and zeaxanthin and macular pigment density. Am J Clin Nutr 71.6 (2000): 1555–1562.
Johnson EJ et al. Cognitive findings of an exploratory trial of docosahexaenoic acid and lutein supplementation in older women. Nutr Neurosci 11.2 (2008): 75–83.
Kabagambe EK et al. Some dietary and adipose tissue carotenoids are associated with the risk of nonfatal acute myocardial infarction in Costa Rica. J Nutr 135.7 (2005): 1763–1769.
Karppi J et al. Lycopene, lutein and β-carotene as determinants of LDL conjugated dienes in serum. Atherosclerosis 209.2 (2010): 565–572
Kim HW et al. Dietary lutein stimulates immune response in the canine. Vet Immunol Immunopathol 74.3–4 (2000a): 315–27.
Kim HW et al. Modulation of humoral and cell-mediated immune responses by dietary lutein in cats. Vet Immunol Immunopathol 73.3–4 (2000b): 331–41.
Kim YT et al. Relation between deranged antioxidant system and cervical neoplasia. Int J Gynecol Cancer 14.5 (2004): 889–895.
Klipstein-Grobusch K et al. Serum carotenoids and atherosclerosis: the Rotterdam Study. Atherosclerosis 148.1 (2000): 49–56.
Koh HH et al. Plasma and macular responses to lutein supplement in subjects with and without age-related maculopathy: a pilot study. Exp Eye Res 79.1 (2004): 21–27.

Krinsky NI, et al. Biologic mechanisms of the protective role of lutein and zeaxanthin in the eye. Annu Rev Nutr 23 (2003): 171–201.
Kvansakul J et al. Supplementation with the carotenoids lutein or zeaxanthin improves human visual performance. Ophthalmic and Physiological Optics 26.4 (2006): 362–371.
Lee EH et al. Dietary lutein reduces ultraviolet radiation-induced inflammation and immunosuppression. J Invest Dermatol 122.2 (2004): 510–5117.
Le Marchand L et al. Intake of specific carotenoids and lung cancer risk. Cancer Epidemiol Biomarkers Prev 2.3 (1993): 183–187.
Levi F et al. Selected micronutrients and colorectal cancer. a case-control study from the canton of Vaud. Switzerland. Eur J Cancer 36.16 (2000): 2115–21119.
Li L et al. Supplementation with lutein or lutein plus green tea extracts does not change oxidative stress in adequately nourished older adults. J Nutr Biochem 21.6 (2010): 544–549
Lu QY et al. Inverse associations between plasma lycopene and other carotenoids and prostate cancer. Cancer Epidemiol Biomarkers Prev 10.7 (2001): 749–756.
Lu QY et al. Inhibition of prostate cancer cell growth by an avocado extract: role of lipid-soluble bioactive substances. J Nutr Biochem 16.1 (2005): 23–30.
Ma L et al. Lutein and zeaxanthin intake and the risk of age-related macular degeneration: a systematic review and meta-analysis. Br J Nutr 107.3 (2012): 350–359
Maci S. Nutritional support against skin ageing: New scientific evidence for the role of lutein. Agro Food Industry Hi-Tech 18.5 (2007): 42–44.
Mares J et al. Predictors of optical density of lutein and zeaxanthin in retinas of older women in the Carotenoids in Age-Related Eye Disease Study, an ancillary study of the Women's Health Initiative. Am J Clin Nutr 84.5 (2006): 1107–1122.
Mathews F, Neil A. Antioxidants and preterm prelabour rupture of the membranes. Br J Obstet Gynaecol 112.5 (2005): 588–594.
Mayne ST et al. Effect of supplemental [beta]-carotene on plasma concentrations of carotenoids, retinol, and [alpha]-tocopherol in humans. Am J Clin Nutr 68.3 (1998): 642–647.
McCann SE et al. Diet in the epidemiology of endometrial cancer in western New York (United States). Cancer Causes Control 11.10 (2000): 965–974.
Michaud DS et al. Intake of specific carotenoids and risk of lung cancer in 2 prospective US cohorts. Am J Clin Nutr 72.4 (2000): 990–997.
Moeller SM et al. Associations between age-related nuclear cataract and lutein and zeaxanthin in the diet and serum in the carotenoids in the age-related eye disease study (CAREDS), an ancillary study of the Women's Health Initiative. Arch Ophthalmol 126.3 (2008): 354–364.
Muriach M et al. Lutein prevents the effect of high glucose levels on immune system cells in vivo and in vitro. J Physiol Biochem 64.2 (2008): 149–158.
Naguib YM. Antioxidant activities of astaxanthin and related carotenoids. J Agric Food Chem 48.4 (2000): 1150–1154.
Nkondjock A, Ghadirian P. Dietary carotenoids and risk of colon cancer: Case-control study. Int J Cancer 110.1 (2004): 110–1116.
Nolan JM et al. Macular pigment, visual function, and macular disease among subjects with Alzheimer's disease: An exploratory study. J Alzheimers Dis 2014. [Epub ahead of print]
Nolan J et al. Macular pigment and percentage of body fat. Invest Ophthalmol Vis Sci 45.11 (2004): 3940–3950.
Nomura AM et al. Serum micronutrients and prostate cancer in Japanese Americans in Hawaii. Cancer Epidemiol Biomarkers Prev 6.7 (1997): 487–491.
Nussbaum JJ, et al. Historic perspectives: Macular yellow pigment: the first 200 years. Retina 1.4 (1981): 296–310.
Olmedilla B et al. Lutein, but not alpha-tocopherol, supplementation improves visual function in patients with age-related cataracts: a 2-y double-blind, placebo-controlled pilot study. Nutr 19.1 (2003): 21–24.
Palombo P et al. Beneficial long-term effects of combined oral/topical antioxidant treatment with the carotenoids lutein and zeaxanthin on human skin: A double-blind, placebo-controlled study. Skin Pharmacol Physiol 20.4 (2007): 199–210.
Pattison DJ et al. Dietary beta-cryptoxanthin and inflammatory polyarthritis: results from a population-based prospective study. Am J Clin Nutr 82.2 (2005): 451–455.
Polidori MC et al. Plasma antioxidant status, immunoglobulin G oxidation and lipid peroxidation in demented patients: Relevance to Alzheimer disease and vascular dementia. Dementia Geriatr Cognitive Disord 18.3–4 (2004): 265–270.
Raju J et al. Low doses of beta-carotene and lutein inhibit AOM-induced rat colonic ACF formation but high doses augment ACF incidence. Int J Cancer 113.5 (2005): 798–802.
Ratnasinghe DM et al. Serum carotenoids are associated with increased lung cancer risk among alcohol drinkers, but not among non-drinkers in a cohort of tin miners. Alcohol Alcoholism 35.4 (2000): 355–360.
Rehak M, et al. Lutein and antioxidants in the prevention of age-related macular degeneration. Lutein und Antioxidantien zur Pravention der AMD 105.1 (2008): 37–45.
Richer S. ARMD-pilot (case series) environmental intervention data. J Am Optom Assoc 70 (1999): 24–36.
Richer S et al. Double-masked, placebo-controlled, randomized trial of lutein and antioxidant supplementation in the intervention of atrophic age-related macular degeneration: the Veterans LAST study (Lutein Antioxidant Supplementation Trial). Optometry 75 (2004): 216–230.
Richer, S., et al. 2007. LAST II: Differential temporal responses of macular pigment optical density in patients with atrophic age-related macular degeneration to dietary supplementation with xanthophylls. Optometry., 78, (5) 213–219.
Richer SP et al. Randomised, double-blind, placebo-controlled study of zeaxanthin and visual function in patients with atrophic age-related macular degeneration: The Zeaxanthin and Visual Function Study (ZVF) FDA IND #78, 973. J Am Optom Assoc 82.11 (2011): 667–680
Rinaldi P et al. Plasma antioxidants are similarly depleted in mild cognitive impairment and in Alzheimer's disease. Neurobiol Aging 24.7 (2003): 915–9119.
Roodenburg AJ et al. Amount of fat in the diet affects bioavailability of lutein esters but not of alpha-carotene, beta-carotene, and vitamin E in humans. Am J Clin Nutr 71.5 (2000): 1187–1193.
Sasaki M et al. Biological role of lutein in the light-induced retinal degeneration. J Nutr Biochem 23.5 (2012): 423–429
Sato Y et al. Protective effect of lutein after ischemia-reperfusion in the small intestine. Food Chem 127.3 (2011): 893–898
Schalch W et al. Xanthophyll accumulation in the human retina during supplementation with lutein or zeaxanthin — the LUXEA (LUtein Xanthophyll Eye Accumulation) study. Arch Biochem Biophys 458.2 (2007): 128–135.
Schuurman AG et al. A prospective cohort study on intake of retinol, vitamins C and E, and carotenoids and prostate cancer risk (Netherlands). Cancer Causes Control 13.6 (2002): 573–582.
Semba RD, Dagnelie G. Are lutein and zeaxanthin conditionally essential nutrients for eye health? Med Hypotheses 61.4 (2003): 465–472.
Sesso HD et al. Plasma lycopene, other carotenoids, and retinol and the risk of cardiovascular disease in men. Am J Clin Nutr 81.5 (2005): 990–997.
Tamimi RM et al. Plasma carotenoids, retinol, and tocopherols and risk of breast cancer. Am J Epidemiol 161.2 (2005): 153.
Tanumihardjo SA, et al. Lutein absorption is facilitated with cosupplementation of ascorbic acid in young adults. J Am Dietetic Assoc 105.1 (2005): 114–1118.
Tavani A, et al. Food and nutrient intake and risk of cataract. Ann Epidemiol 6 (1996): 41–46.
Terry P et al. Dietary carotenoid intake and colorectal cancer risk. Nutr Cancer 42.2 (2002): 167–172.
The AREDS2 Research Group. Lutein / zeaxanthin for the treatment of age-related cataract: AREDS2 randomised trial report no. 4. JAMA Ophthalmol 131.7 (2013a): 843–850.
The AREDS2 Research Group. Lutein + zeaxanthin and omega-3 fatty acids for age-related macular degeneration: the Age-Related Eye Disease Study 2 (AREDS2) randomized clinical trial. JAMA 309.19 (2013b): 2005–2015
Thurmann PA et al. Plasma kinetics of lutein, zeaxanthin, and 3-dehydro-lutein after multiple oral doses of a lutein supplement. Am J Clin Nutr 82.1 (2005): 88–97.
Toniolo P et al. Serum carotenoids and breast cancer. Am J Epidemiol 153.12 (2001): 1142–1147.
Tulley RT et al. Daily intake of multivitamins during long-term intake of olestra in men prevents declines in serum vitamins A and E but not carotenoids. J Nutr 135.6 (2005): 1456–1461.
Unlu NZ et al. Carotenoid absorption from salad and salsa by humans is enhanced by the addition of avocado or avocado oil. J Nutr 135.3 (2005): 431.
Vu HT et al. Lutein and zeaxanthin and the risk of cataract: the Melbourne Visual Impairment Project. Invest Ophthalmol Vis Sci 47.9 (2006): 3783–3786.
Wang W et al. Effect of dietary lutein and zeaxanthin on plasma carotenoids and their transport in lipoproteins in age-related macular degeneration. Am J Clin Nutr 85.3 (2007): 762–769.
Wang MX et al. Lutein supplementation reduces plasma lipid peroxidation and C-reactive protein in healthy nonsmokers. Atherosclerosis 227.2 (2013): 380–385
Wang, J.J., et al. 2014. Genetic susceptibility, dietary antioxidants, and long-term incidence of age-related macular degeneration in two populations. Ophthalmology 121: 667–675.
Xu XR et al. Effects of lutein supplement on serum inflammatory cytokines, ApoE and lipid profiles in early atherosclerosis population. J Atheroscler Thromb 20.2 (2013): 170–177
Yao Y et al. Lutein supplementation improves visual performance in Chinese drivers: 1 year randomised, double-blind, placebo-controlled study. Nutrition 29.7–8 (2013): 958–964.
Yeum KJ, Russell RM. Carotenoid bioavailability and bioconversion. Ann Rev Nutr 22 (2002): 483–504.
Yonova-Doing, E., et al. 2013. Candidate gene study of macular response to supplemental lutein and zeaxanthin. Exp.Eye Res., 115, 172–177
Zhao D-Y et al. Resonance Raman measurement of macular carotenoids in retinal, choroidal, and macular dystrophies. Arch Ophthalmol 121.7 (2003): 967–972.
Ziegler RG et al. Importance of alpha-carotene, beta-carotene, and other phytochemicals in the etiology of lung cancer. J Natl Cancer Inst 88.9 (1996): 612–6115.

Maca

HISTORICAL NOTE Maca is a biennial plant native to the central Peruvian Andean plateaus that resembles a radish. It has thousands of years of cultivation and traditional use as a medicinal food. Its growing conditions are harsh, at altitudes of over 3300 m, with extreme weather conditions. It is a herbaceous plant with its flat and small overground leaves, an adaption to the strong, cold winds of the mountains. The first written description about maca as a food was in 1553, and in 1653 its properties were recorded as fertility-enhancing and energy and mood-stimulating (Gonzales 2012). Other traditional uses include promoting mental clarity, regulating menstrual cycles and relieving menopausal symptoms (Cicero et al 2001). Legend has it that the Inca warriors used to eat maca to increase their energy for battle, but were prohibited from consuming it postconquest, as a measure to protect the women of the conquered city from the warriors' enhanced sexual impulses (Wang et al 2007).

OTHER NAMES

Ayuk willku, Ayak chicira, *Maca maca*, maka, maino, Peruvian maca, Peruvian ginseng, maca peruvien, ginseng andin.

BOTANICAL NAME/FAMILY

Lepidium meyenii; synonym: *Lepidium peruvianum* (family: Cruciferae/Brassicaceae)

There are many ecotypes of maca, characterised by their colour. Over 13 colours have been described, ranging from white, yellow, purple, red to black, and they possess different biological properties (Gonzales 2012). The yellow ecotype is the most common cultivar in the Peruvian Andes (Wang et al 2007).

PLANT PARTS USED

The hypocotyl-root axis is used (radish-like tuber). This is 10–14 cm long and 3–5 cm wide. When dried, it is reduced in size to 2–8 cm in diameter. Traditionally, the root is naturally dried and can be stored for many years. To prepare for use, it is boiled or extracted in alcohol prior to consumption (Gonzales 2012).

CHEMICAL COMPONENTS

Dried root contains 54.6–60% carbohydrates, 8.87–16% protein, 8.23–9.08% fibre and 1.09–2.2% lipids. The carbohydrate breakdown is 23.4% sucrose, 1.55% glucose, 4.56% oligosaccharides and 30.4% polysaccharides. Fatty acids include oleic, linolenic, palmic and oleic acids, and both saturated (40%) and unsaturated (52.7%) fatty acids are present. It is a rich source of amino acids, containing up to 19 different ones: leucine, arginine, phenylalanine, lysine, glycine, alainine, valine, isoleucine, glutamic acid, serine, aspartic acid and others in lesser proportions. Mineral content includes significant levels of iron, calcium, manganese, sodium, potassium, copper and zinc. Maca has an energy content of 663 kJ/100 g (Gonzales 2012, Wang et al 2007).

Maca also has some unique secondary metabolites, including specific polyunsaturated fatty acids, alkaloids, steroids, glucosinolates and isothiocyanates. Macaene and macamides are unique polyunsaturated fatty acids and their amides, often used as markers (Wang et al 2007, Wu et al 2013). Macaridine and other maca alkaloids are among the other unique constituents isolated and characterised (Muhammad et al 2002). Its sterol profile includes campesterol, beta-sisosterol, brassicasterol and stigmasterol. Maca root also contains nine different types of glucosinolates (Wang et al 2007). Most likely other compounds will be discovered in the future (Pino-Figueroa et al 2010).

Levels of macaene, macamides, sterols and glucosinolates, and their proportions, vary in different-coloured maca, which may explain the different biological properties of maca. The processing of the product affects the active secondary metabolites, particularly the glucosinolates. For example, sulforophane formation is increased at boiling point, and epithiospecifier protein activity is decreased (Gonzales 2012).

Macamides are chemically neutral lipids in a carbohydrate-rich plant, which means they should easily cross the intestinal wall and the brain–blood barrier (Wu et al 2013).

Another identified compound is (1R,3S)-1-methyl-1,2,3,4-tetrahydro-B-carboline-3-carboxylic acid (MTCA), which is a member of the tetrahydro-β-carbolines, and a potential monoamine oxidase enzyme inhibitor. MTCA can accumulate in mammalian tissues and in the presence of nitrates becomes a mutagenic precursor. When consumed as a multi-component within the whole maca plant extract, MTCA loses its adverse drug reaction and has beneficial effects (Gonzales-Castaneda & Gonzales 2008). This inhibition of MTCA mutagenicity may in part be due to the polyphenol content.

MAIN ACTIONS

Maca has many different active constituents, and thus its pharmacological activities are numerous. Antioxidant modulation appears to be a major action, contributing to its many demonstrated effects.

Schaeffer et al (2013) cite varying levels of evidence from animal and in vitro experiments for actions affecting the nervous system (antidepressant, energising, antistress, central nervous system stimulation, enhanced cognitive function), reproductive system (antierectile dysfunction, oestrogenic properties, female fertility, enhancement of progesterone levels and enhanced sexual function and spermatogenesis effects) and other systems (antioxidant, hepatoprotective activity, immunostimulant effects, joint disease effects, improved growth rates and prevention of postmenopausal osteoporosis). Wang et al (2007) summarised maca's actions as improving fertility, sexual performance and antiproliferative function, supporter of vitality and stress tolerance, improving growth rate (in rainbow trout) and reducing postmenopausal osteoporosis.

Antioxidant

Maca has the capacity to scavenge free radicals and protect cells against oxidative stress. In vitro tests indicate that maca's antioxidant action contributes to adenosine triphosphate production and may help to maintain a balance between oxidants and antioxidants (Sandoval et al 2002).

Tests with preclinical models using traditionally prepared aqueous extracts of maca demonstrated epithelial cell protection from ultraviolet A, B and C radiation (Gonzales-Castaneda & Gonzales 2008). The MTCA component found in maca has significant antioxidant activity, considered greater than vitamin E and most likely contributes to the protective effect against ultraviolet radiation (Gonzales-Castaneda & Gonzales 2008). Maca polyphenols are also thought to be responsible for the antioxidant effect.

Neuroprotection

Black maca exhibited a neuroprotective effect in an animal model of scopolamine-induced memory impairment. The activity was possibly due to the polyphenols, quercetin and anthocyanins (Rubio et al 2007). In vitro studies on crayfish neurons demonstrated potential neuroprotective properties in a dose-dependent manner. The same paper tested rats with a pentane extraction of maca, containing mostly liposoluble constituent alkaloids (macamides, macaenes and isothiocyanates) which indicated at low dose inhibitory, antioxidative or antiapoptotic mechanisms preventing the experimental ischaemic insult. High concentrations showed some deleterious effects (Pino-Figueroa et al 2010).

Antiproliferative actions

Like other cruciferous vegetables, maca may be antiproliferative due to its high concentration of glucosinolates, as these are known to have both antiproliferative and proapoptotic actions and polyphenols (Gonzales 2012). The polyphenols, alkaloids and sterols in maca may further contribute to its proposed anticancer properties (Wang et al 2007).

Reducing prostate size in benign prostatic hypertrophy

Both aqueous and hydroalcoholic extracts of red maca reduced prostate size but not yellow or black maca in a preclinical study. Interestingly, serum testosterone and oestradiol levels were not affected by any of the maca types assessed; however, red maca prevented an increase in prostate weight induced by testosterone treatment (Gonzales 2012). Previously, Gasco et al (2007b) suggested that red maca may inhibit dihydrotestosterone conversion by 5-alpha-reductase 2; however, this remains uncertain. A study investigating the mechanism further compared red maca to finasteride (a 5-alpha-reductase inhibitor), where it was shown to reduce prostate weight but not seminal vesicles, unlike finasteride, which reduced both. The study indicated a need for a direct measure of levels of reductase to clarify the mechanism of action (Gasco et al 2007b, Shrivastava & Gupta 2012).

Aphrodisiac and sexual and reproductive enhancement

Traditionally, maca has been used to enhance fertility in livestock living at high altitudes, and also as an aphrodisiac for both men and women (Wang et al 2007).

Different variants of maca appear to affect reproductive function differently. Black maca significantly enhanced spermatogenesis, measured in daily sperm production in vivo (Gonzales et al 2006). While studies in both men (Dording et al 2008, Gonzales et al 2003, Stone et al 2009) and mice (Cicero et al 2001, Gonzales et al 2006, Yucra et al 2008, Zheng et al 2000) suggest an aphrodisiac action, the mechanism involved has not been fully elucidated. In particular, the lipid extracts of macaene and macamide seem to increase sexual activity and correct erectile dysfunction in experimental animals (National Medicines Comprehensive Database 2012).

Spermatogenesis studies in rats observed the greatest effect with the ethyl acetate fraction from the hydroalcoholic extract of black maca (Yucra et al 2008). The effect may be mediated via an oxidant/antioxidant homeostatic mechanism, possibly in the epididymis (Yucra et al 2008). Wang et al (2007) further suggest that maca does not act on the hypothalamic-pituitary axis to regulate secretion, nor does it activate human androgen receptors or influence genes regulated by androgens.

Studies in female animal models show that rats fed high doses of maca (more than 15 g/kg) had increased luteinising hormone serum levels during the pro-oestrus and the luteinising hormone surge occurred in a dose-dependent manner (Uchiyama et al 2013). This high dose is consistent with traditional intakes of up to 100 g a day. Similarly, in vitro tests reveal that maca extract exhibits oestrogenic activity (Valentova et al 2006).

Adaptogenic action

Maca can reduce the effects of stress, including preventing increases in corticosterone and adrenal gland size, and exhibits an antitiredness effect (Wang et al 2007). The highly nutritious profile of maca is proposed as one reason for these effects; however it is likely that more specific mechanisms are at work. Lopez-Fando et al (2004) hypothesised that maca may lead to activation of the hypothalamic-pituitary-adrenal (HPA) axis to increase generalised resistance to various noxious and stressful stimuli, although no clear mechanism has been proven.

Lipid and glucose metabolism

Experimentation on hereditary hypertriglyceridaemic rats administered maca with a high-sucrose diet showed decreased levels of very-low-density lipoprotein, low-density lipoprotein and total cholesterol, an improvement in glucose metabolism, enhanced glutathione levels in blood and liver and increased superoxide dismutase activity in the liver (Vecera et al 2007).

Improving bone density

Maca increases bone density in overiectomised rats and works in a different manner to hormone replacement therapy (HRT). Maca did not significantly increase uterine weight or oestrogen levels in the studies reviewed (Wang et al 2007). The effect of maca was more obvious in cancellous bone-rich regions than in cortical bone-rich ones. The exact mechanisms regulating the endocrine are unclear; some investigators suggest that the effect is not due to the phyto-oestrogens or plant hormones, but to the maca alkaloids acting on the HPA axis (Zhang et al 2006).

CLINICAL USES

Improvement in sexual function

Maca is used within Peru as a sexual stimulant, energiser and nutritional food. Due to the lack of large randomised controlled trials testing the effects of maca for sexual function, it is difficult to draw firm conclusions about its effectiveness (Bella & Shamloul 2014); however the available evidence is promising and supported by animal and human research (Gonzales 2012, Shin et al 2010).

A 12-week, double-blind placebo-controlled, randomised, parallel trial involving 57 healthy males aged 21–56 years, testing doses of 1.5 and 3 g maca gelatinizada/day, concluded that maca improves sexual desire in men. The self-reported increase in desire was 40% and 42.2% over 8 and 12 weeks respectively (Gonzales et al 2002). Another double-blind clinical trial of 50 Caucasian men with mild erectile dysfunction, using 2400 mg dried maca over 12 weeks, concluded that there was a small but significant effect of maca supplementation on subjective perception of general and sexual wellbeing (Zenico et al 2009).

Sportsmen taking 2 g/day of maca root extract for 14 days increased their sexual desire, and reduced their cycling time for 40 km, compared to placebo in a randomised crossover design (Stone et al 2009). Evaluation of reproductive hormones found that maca did not alter serum concentrations of testosterone, oestradiol or 17-hydroxyprogesterone throughout the 12-week trial (Gonzales et al 2003).

Maca root may help alleviate selective serotonin reuptake inhibitor (SSRI)-induced sexual dysfunction. A small trial of 10 remitting depressed patients showed improvement in sexual dysfunction and libido when taking 3 g/day over 12 weeks. No improvement was noticed at doses of 1.5 g/day (Dording et al 2008).

Fertility

No randomised controlled trials are available to determine whether maca has any benefits in improving male or female fertility. Research with animal models is promising and suggests improvements in spermatogenesis in a number of models (Gasco et al 2007a, Gonzales 2012, Rubio et al 2006). Additionally, Peruvian researchers have shown that maca helps alleviate altitude-related compromises in sheep and guinea pig fertility through actions on both the female and the male reproductive systems (Sandoval et al 2002).

Menopausal symptom relief

Maca has been used to reduce menopausal symptoms as an alternative to HRT and also when women are reducing their HRT dose (Meissner et al 2006). Two randomised controlled trials provide support for the use of maca in alleviating several menopausal symptoms (Brooks et al 2008, Meissner et al 2006).

A large (n = 124) double-blind, randomised, placebo-corrected, outpatient, multicentre clinical study of early postmenopausal women taking maca (2 × 1000 mg/day with meals) resulted in significant reduction in menopausal symptoms over the 8-week trial (Meissner et al 2006). The symptoms most significantly improved were excessive night sweating, hot flushes, nervousness, excessive alertness, lack of energy, tiredness and, to a lesser degree, irritability and headaches. The second month of treatment magnified the positive effect, and the cessation of maca showed a 'residual effect' for 1 month. Maca treatment was found to stimulate production of oestradiol, suppress blood follicle-stimulating hormone and increase high-density lipoprotein cholesterol. The maca used in this study was pregelatinised organic maca, a combination of three main root ecotypes, 16% black, 48% yellow, 9% purple/red and 27% other colours, dried and processed at a Peruvian university.

A smaller double-blind, placebo-controlled, crossover randomised controlled trial of 14 postmenopausal women showed that treatment with 3.5 g/day powdered maca for 6 weeks significantly reduced psychological symptoms, including anxiety and depression, together with measures of sexual dysfunction, when compared to placebo. Interestingly, the women's blood samples showed no differences in the concentrations of oestradiol, follicle-stimulating hormone, luteinising hormone and sex hormone-binding globulin. Additionally, the maca extracts were tested in in vitro yeast assays, and showed no androgenic or oestrogenic activity (Brooks et al 2008).

OTHER USES

As a food, maca can be eaten baked, roasted, in soup or made into fermented drinks or coffee.

DOSAGE RANGE

Traditionally, prepared maca was consumed at levels of 50–100 g/day.

According to clinical trials

- Male libido enhancement: 2 g daily in three divided doses.
- SSRI-induced sexual dysfunction: 3 g/day.
- Menopausal symptom relief: 2–3.5 g daily for 8 weeks.

TOXICITY

Toxicity studies showed safety for use at 7.5 g/kg (on rats) and 15 g/kg (on mice), suggesting maca is safe in high doses (Meissner et al 2006).

ADVERSE REACTIONS

Peruvian highlanders state that fresh maca may have adverse effects on health (Valerio & Gonzales 2005); however this has not been scientifically validated (Gonzales 2012).

SIGNIFICANT INTERACTIONS

Theoretical interactions have been suggested to be plausible in people taking antidepressants, blood thinners and blood pressure medications (Health Canada 2013).

No reported drug interactions.

Practice points/Patient counselling

Maca is a traditional food and medicine from the Peruvian Andes used for thousands of years. Traditional uses include to enhance sexual behaviour in men and women, support fertility, enhance energy and reduce the adverse symptoms of menopause. It is rich in nutrients and contains many unique plant chemicals that have multiple benefits on health. There is still much scientific research needed to understand its actions and validate its effectiveness in humans. As with any natural medicine, the effect is gradual and subtle, so it may take 6–12 weeks of dosing before effect will be noted. Maca tastes slightly nutty when taken as a powder mixed in drinks. Other preparations are available (tablets and capsules). General dosage is 1.5–3 g/day for 6–12 weeks.

CONTRAINDICATIONS AND PRECAUTIONS

Allergy to cruciferous family.

Some plants in the *Brassica* genus have goitrogenic effect, due to a range of constituents such as thiocyanates and isothiocyanates. To date there are no studies on whether maca exerts a goitrogenic effect. Goitrogens may become inactive after cooking (Srilakshmi 2006). Epidemiological surveys of the Andean region revealed endemic goitre and cretinism; however a wide range of factors contributed to this (Fierro-Benítez et al 1969). Ensure maca is correctly prepared and not used as a food staple.

PREGNANCY USE

Insufficient information regarding use in pregnancy and lactation. Avoid use.

PATIENTS' FAQs

What will this do for me?
Maca may improve libido and sexual function and also reduce menopausal symptoms; however more clinical research is required to be certain.

When will it work?
Most studies show that maca works after 6–8 weeks of dosing at the correct levels.

Are there any safety issues?
Maca has been used for centuries as a food at high doses with no safety issues.

REFERENCES

Bella AJ, Shamloul R (2014) Traditional Plant Aphrodisiacs and Male Sexual Dysfunction, Phytotherapy Research 28: 831–835.

Brooks, N.A., et al. Beneficial effects of *Lepidium meyenii* (Maca) on psychological symptoms and measures of sexual dysfunction in postmenopausal women are not related to estrogen or androgen content. Menopause 2008 15(6); 1157–62.

Cicero AFG, et al. *Lepidium meyenii* Walp. Improves sexual behaviour in male rats independently from its action on spontaneous locomotor activity, Journal of Ethnopharmacology 75 (2001); 225–229.

Dording CM, et al.A double-blind, randomised, piolet dose-finding study of maca root (*L. meyenii*) for the management of SSRI-induced sexual dysfunction. CNS Neurosci Ther 14.3 (2008); 182–91.

Fierro-Benítez R, et al. Endemic Goiter and Endemic Cretinism in the Andean Region, N Engl J Med 1969; 280:296–302.

Gasco M, et al. (2007a) Effect of chronic treatment with three varieties of *Lepidium meyenii* (Maca) on reproductive parameters and DNA quantification in adult male rats. Andrologia 39, 151–158.

Gasco M, et al. Dose-response effect of Red Maca (*Lepidium meyenii*) on benign prostatic hyperplasia induced by testosterone enanthate, Phytomedicine 14 (2007b); 460–464.

Gonzales, G.F., Ethnobiology and Ethnopharmacology of *Lepidium meyenii* (Maca), a Plant from the Peruvian highlands. Evidence-based Complementary and Alternative Medicine, 2012 (2012), 10.1155/2012/193496.

Gonzales GF, et al. (2002) Effect of *Lepidium meyenii* (MACA) on sexual desire and its absent relationship with serum testosterone levels in adult healthy men, Andrologia 34; 367–373.

Gonzales, GF, et al. Effect of *Lepidium meyenii* (Maca), a root with aphrodisiac and fertility-enhancing properties, on serum reproductive hormone levels in adult healthy men, Journal of Endocrinology (2003) 176; 163–168.

Gonzales C, et al. (2006) Effect of short-term and long-term treatments with three ecotypes of *Lepidium meyenii* (Maca) on spermatogenesis in rats, Journal of Ethnopharmacology 103; 448–454.

Gonzales-Castaneda C, Gonzales GF Hypocotyls of *Lepidium meyenii* (Maca), a plant of the Peruvian highlands, prevents ultraviolet A-, B-,

and C-induced skin damage in rats. Photodermatol Photoimmunol Photomed 2008; 24.2:24–31.
Health Canada (2013) Maca Monograph, accessed 14 May 2014, http://webprod.hc-sc.gc.ca/nhpid-bdipsn/monoReq.do?id=1903&lang=eng
Lopez-Fando A, et al. (2004) *Lepidium peruvianum* chacon restores homeostasis impaired by restraint stress. Phytotherapy Research, 18, 471–474.
Meissner HO, et al. Hormone-Balancing Effect of Pre-Gelatinized Organic Maca (*Lepidium peruvianum* chacon): Physiological and Symptomatic responses of early-postmenopausal women to standardized doses of maca in double blind, ramdomized, placebo-controlled, multi-centre clinical study, International Journal of Biomedical Science, 2006; 360–374.
Muhammad I, et al. Constituents of *Lepidium meyenii* 'maca', Phytochemistry 59 (2002) 105–110.
National Medicines Comprehensive Database 2012, http://naturaldatabase.therapeuticresearch.com/
Pino-Figueroa A et al. (2010) Neuroprotective effects of *Lepidium meyenii* (Maca), Annals of the New York Academy of sciences, 1199;77–85.
Rubio, J, et al. *Lepidium meyenii* (Maca) reversed the lead acetate induced-damage on reproductive function in male rats, Food and Chemical Toxicology 44 (2006), 1114–1122.
Rubio J, et al. Aqueous and hydroalcoholic extracts of Black Maca (*Lepidium meyenii*) improve scopolamine-induced memory impairment in mice, Food and Chemical Toxicology 45 (2007) 1882–1890.
Sandoval M, et al. Antioxidant activity of the cruciferous vegetable Maca (*Lepidium meyenii*), Food Chemistry 79 (2002) 207–213.
Schaeffer T, et al. Maca (*Lepidium meyenii*). Natural Standard Professional Monograph, 2013 www.naturalstandard.com
Shin BC, et al. Maca (*L. meyenii*) for improving sexual function: a systematic review. BMC Complementary and Alternative Medicine, 2010, 10:44.
Shrivastava A, Gupta VB, Various treatment options for benign prostatic hyperplasia: A current update, J Midlife Health 2012, 3(1): 10–19.
Srilakshmi, B Nutritional Science, New Age International, 2006
Stone, M, et al. A pilot investigation in the effect of maca supplementation on physical activity and sexual desire in sportsmen, Journal of Ethnopharmacology (2009) 126, 574–576.
Uchiyama F, et al. *Lepidium meyenii* (Maca) enhances the serum levels of luteinising hormone in female rats, Journal of Ethnopharmacology (2013), http://dx.doi.org/10.1016/j.jep.2013.11.058.
Valentova, K., et al.. 2006. The in vitro biological activity of *Lepidium meyenii* extracts. Cell Biol.Toxicol., 22, (2) 91–99.
Valerio, LG & Gonzales, GF, Toxicological aspects of the South American Herbs cat's claw (*Uncaria tomentosa*) and maca (*Lepidium meyenii*): a critical synopsis, Toxicological Reviews, 2005, 24, 11–35.
Vecera R, et al. The influence of Maca (*Lepidium meyenii*) on antioxidant status, lipid and glucose metabolism in rat, Plant Foods Hum Nutr 2007; 62(2):59–63.
Wang Y, et al. Maca: An Andean crop with multi-pharmacological functions, Food Research International 2007, 40 (207), 783–792.
Wu H, et al. Macamides and their synthetic analogs: Evaluation of in vitro FAAH inhibition, Bioorganic & Medicinal Chemistry 21 (2013) 5188–5197.
Yucra S, et al. Effect of different fractions from hydroalcoholic extract of Black Maca (*Lepidium meyenii*) on testicular function in adult male rats, Fertillity and Sterility, Vol 89 Supp 3, 2008.
Zenico T, et al. Subjective effects of *Lepidium meyenii* (Maca) extract on well-being and sexual performance in patients wild mild erectile dysfunction: a randomised, double-blind clinical trial. Andrologia 2009; 41 (2): 95–99
Zhang Y, et al. (2006) Effect of ethanol extract of *Lepidium meyenii* Walp on osteoporosis in ovariectomized rat. Journal of ethnopharmacology 105 (2006) 274–279.
Zheng BL, et al. Effect of a lipidic extract from *Lepidium meyenii* on sexual behaviour in mice and rats, Urology (2000) 55 (4):598–602.

Magnesium

HISTORICAL NOTE 'Magnesium' comes from the name of the ancient Greek city Magnesia, where large deposits of magnesium were found. In the form of Epsom salts, magnesium has long been used therapeutically as a laxative although it is also used in many other ways, such as a foot soak to soften rough spots and absorb foot odour and as a bath additive to ease muscle aches and pains. Supplemental magnesium in recent years is commonly ingested to alleviate musculoskeletal pains and cramping.

BACKGROUND AND RELEVANT PHARMACOKINETICS

Magnesium is an essential mineral and critical cofactor for over 300 biochemical processes, such as adenosine triphosphate (ATP) manufacture, critical to phosphorylation reactions. It is also necessary for DNA, RNA protein synthesis, carbohydrate metabolism, bone formation and cellular signal transduction (Allen 2013, Hartwig 2001, Rude et al 2009). Magnesium may also serve as an immunomodulator regulating NF-κB activation and cytokine production. In this role it may limit systemic inflammation and corresponding general markers such as C-reactive protein (Chacko et al 2010, Song et al 2007). It is the fourth most abundant cation in the body, with 50–60% sequestered in the bone, the remainder distributed equally between muscle and non-muscular soft tissue. Only about 1% of total body magnesium is found in the extracellular fluid. Dietary intake, renal and intestinal function finely balance and maintain plasma magnesium concentrations.

Absorption of dietary magnesium starts within 1 hour of ingestion, and occurs along the entire length of the bowel, with salts of high solubility having the most complete absorption (e.g. magnesium citrate). Normal magnesium absorption occurs passively at a rate of approximately 90% through the paracellular pathway. Active transport may occur only where extremely low dietary magnesium magnesium intake is observed, i.e. it is thought that magnesium absorption may be enhanced in bowel disorders, which must be considered when suggesting magnesium supplementation for these conditions (Allen 2013, Swaminathan 2003, Topf & Murray 2003). Magnesium absorption requires selenium, parathyroid hormone (PTH) and vitamins B_6 and D and is hindered by phytate, fibre, alcohol, excess saturated fat and the presence of unabsorbed fatty acids, high phosphorus or calcium intake (Johnson 2001, Saris et al 2000). However, calcium is no longer perceived to be as antagonistic to magnesium uptake as previously thought, while research using test meals may show negative interaction — in contrast to long-term balance studies (Andon et al 1996, Fine et al 1991, Gropper et al 2009, Lewis et al 1989). Some authors suggest that such nutrient interactions only become significant in situations of low magnesium intake (Gropper et al 2009, Lewis et al 1989). Healthy people absorb 30–50% of ingested magnesium; increasing to 70% bioavailability in cases of low intake or deficiency (Allen 2013, Braunwald et al 2003). Other research suggests that fructo-oligosaccharides may improve magnesium absorption, particularly in adolescent girls (Ellen 2009).

Although currently it is undisputed that magnesium metabolism is regulated, the identity of such regulators remains largely obscured (Gropper et al 2009). While a number of hormones affect magnesium homeostasis they fail to explain every facet. What is understood to date is that magnesium homeostasis is regulated via a filtration–reabsorption process in the kidneys. Magnesium conservation is facilitated when magnesium is deficit, and excreted when surfeit (Quamme 2008). Reabsorption occurs in the ascending loop of Henle mediated by mechanisms involving paracellin-1, where sodium-assisted potential is generated to enhance transepithelial transport. Therefore medications that impact sodium resorption, such as loop diuretics, osmotic diuretics and changes in extracellular fluid volume expansion, may enhance the excretion of magnesium (Allen 2013).

While hormones central to calcium homeostasis, e.g. PTH, play a role in magnesium metabolism, this is a greatly diminished one compared to calcium (Shils & Rude 1996). Additional regulators include adrenergic signalling pathways, insulin, oestrogen and growth hormone (Rude & Shils 2006). Some researchers suggest that the real locus of control over magnesium homeostasis may be independent of hormones; instead there may be a combination of fractional absorption, renal excretion and transmembranous cation flux (Gropper et al 2009).

Once absorbed, magnesium travels to the liver, enters the systemic circulation and is transported around the body, to be ultimately excreted via the kidneys, with urine representing the major excretory pathway. Consequently, the kidney is pivotal in homeostatic control, rapidly adjusting to changing dietary intake (Rude & Shils 2006). Renal handling of magnesium is subject to additional negative influences. For example, increased calcium (≈ 2600 mg/day) (NHMRC 2005), sodium, protein, caffeine and alcohol consumption (Allen 2013, Gropper et al 2009, Rude 2010, Rude & Shils 2006), B_6 depletion (Turnlund et al 1992), glycosuria, stress (Allen 2013, Khan et al 1999, Rude & Shils 2006, Turnlund et al 1992, Walti et al 2003), elevated thyroid hormones (Wester 1987), protein intakes either above or below recommended levels (Wester 1987) and increases in net endogenous acid production (Rylander et al 2006) all impair the kidney's capacity to reabsorb magnesium. Additional minor losses occur through sweat and faeces (Gropper et al 2009, Rude & Shils 2006).

Magnesium assessment

In spite of intense ongoing research, there is still no simple, rapid and accurate laboratory test to determine total body magnesium status in humans (Arnaud 2008, Feillet-Coudray et al 2000). In particular, as with many of the minerals, there is an urgent need to identify a functional or biological marker of magnesium status, similar to the role of ferritin in iron assessment (Arnaud 2008). While serum testing is still frequently performed, it is only indicative of severe depletion, as evidenced by values <0.75 mmol/L and while some studies demonstrate a correlation between these values and the magnesium content of other tissues, many do not (Arnaud 2008). Some researchers suggest that serum values 0.75–0.85 mmol/L warrant further investigation with more sensitive tests.

Erythrocytes naturally contain large amounts of magnesium and experimental depletion is reflected by declining red blood cell (RBC) concentrations within weeks. A criticism of this method relates to repletion studies which found greater increases in serum magnesium following supplementation than reflected in the RBC; however, one could argue that the diminished response is a more accurate reflection of delayed intracellular recovery. Both animal and human studies have shown magnesium concentrations in white blood cells, e.g. lymphocytes, to be a particularly accurate indicator of magnesium content of both skeletal and cardiac tissues, which, given their functional significance, represents an attractive option. Actual muscle biopsies are believed to be an excellent indicator of body status; however, due to their invasive nature, they are rarely used (Arnaud 2008).

Increasingly, however, magnesium loading tests are probably the best assessment (Allen 2013, Arnaud 2008). The procedure involves either oral or intravenous (IV) loading with magnesium (e.g. 500–700 mg) followed by collection of 24-hour urine. Generally, excretion of <70% is considered indicative of magnesium deficiency. One of the significant disadvantages of this method is the lack of standardisation, e.g. form and dose of magnesium administered, which is critical for ensuring its sensitivity and reproducibility. Additionally, this test should only be used in individuals with healthy renal function generally and absorptive capacity specifically in oral loading. Exchangeable magnesium pool tests requiring magnesium stable isotopes is a novel approach to magnesium assessment; more studies and human trials are needed (Allen 2013).

FOOD SOURCES

Good dietary sources of magnesium include, in descending order, dark green leafy vegetables, legumes, wholegrain cereals, nuts, fruit, fish, most meat, whole full-fat milk, cheese, eggs, cocoa, soy flour, mineral water and hard water (Allen 2013).

In some communities, 'hard tap water' contains significant amounts of magnesium. Food processing and refining remove a substantial amount of naturally occurring magnesium from the food chain — up to 80% in refined grains (Insel et al 2013). High-fibre foods can limit the amount of magnesium absorbed from food but those containing fermentable carbohydrates (e.g. oligosaccharides, pectin) can improve magnesium absorption.

DEFICIENCY SIGNS AND SYMPTOMS

When reduced intakes or increased losses of magnesium, potassium or phosphorus occur (the three major intracellular elements), losses of the others generally follow. As such, many deficiency symptoms are also due to alterations in potassium and/or phosphorus status and manifest as neurological or neuromuscular symptoms.

Symptoms of deficiency include:

- anorexia and weight loss
- nausea and vomiting
- muscular weakness and spasms
- numbness, tingling, cramps
- spontaneous carpal–pedal spasm
- vertigo, ataxia, athetoid, choreiform movements
- lethargy
- difficulty remembering things
- apathy and melancholy
- confusion
- dysregulation of biorhythms (some sleep and mental health disorders, including insomnia)
- depression
- mental confusion, decreased attention span and poor concentration
- personality changes
- hyperirritability and excitability
- vertigo
- cardiac arrhythmia, tetany and ultimately convulsions can develop if deficiency is prolonged.

Although magnesium deficiency is a common clinical problem, serum levels are often overlooked or not measured in patients at risk for the disorder. About 10% of patients admitted to hospitals and up to 65% of patients in intensive care units may be magnesium-deficient (Braunwald et al 2003).

Low magnesium states are associated with several serious diseases such as congestive heart failure, ischaemic heart disease, atherogenesis, atherosclerosis, cardiac arrhythmias, hypertension, mitral valve prolapse, metabolic syndrome, diabetes mellitus, hyperlipidaemia, pre-eclampsia (PE) and eclampsia and osteoporosis, although the latter demonstrates conflicting evidence (Allen 2013, Fox et al 2001, Guerrero-Romero & Rodriguez-Moran 2002, Rude & Shils 2006). Epidemiological evidence suggests that a low dietary intake of magnesium is also associated with impaired lung function, bronchial hyperreactivity and wheezing, and risk of stroke (Ascherio et al 1998, Hill et al 1997). Magnesium deficiency may also play a role in the pathophysiology of Tourette's syndrome (Grimaldi 2002).

Primary deficiency

A primary deficiency is rare in healthy people as the kidneys are extremely efficient at maintaining magnesium homeostasis. Studies of experimental magnesium depletion demonstrate that it takes months of intentional magnesium deprivation to induce a deficiency and even then, its presentation is 'vague' and idiosyncratic (Shils & Rude 1996, Wester 1987).

Marginal deficiencies are far more common and very often undiagnosed. There is evidence that daily magnesium intake has declined substantially since the beginning of the last century, with dietary surveys showing the average intake in Western countries is often below the recommended dietary intake (RDI) (Ford & Mokdad 2003, Lukaski 2000, Rude & Shils 2006, Saris et al 2000). Those particularly susceptible to inadequate dietary intakes are institutionalised elderly and the elderly in general (McKeown et al 2008, Woods et al 2009).

Secondary deficiency

In contrast to the low rates of reported primary magnesium deficiency, secondary deficiency is far more common and seen in both the acutely and the chronically ill (Gropper et al 2009, Shils 1964). Most magnesium deficiencies occur due to a combination of insufficient dietary intake and/or intestinal malabsorption and increased magnesium depletion or excretion. There are many factors that predispose to deficiency and the most common are listed in Table 1.

Medicines increasing risk of deficiency

Many pharmaceutical drugs have the potential to cause hypomagnesaemia.

MAIN ACTIONS

Magnesium plays an essential role in a wide range of fundamental biological reactions in the body. It is involved in over 300 essential enzymatic reactions and is necessary for every major biological process. It is especially important for those enzymes that use nucleotides as cofactors or substrates and plays a role in many processes that are of central importance in the biochemistry of each cell, particularly in energy metabolism. It is also required for many other important biological functions, such as:

- nerve conduction
- regulation of vascular tone
- muscle activity
- amino acid and protein synthesis
- DNA synthesis and degradation
- immune function
- ATP production
- blood clotting
- natural calcium antagonist.

Interaction with other nutrients

Magnesium is extremely important for the metabolism of calcium, potassium, phosphorus, zinc, copper, iron, sodium, lead and cadmium and the

TABLE 1 RISK FACTORS FOR MAGNESIUM DEPLETION AND DEFICIENCY	
Dietary	Excessive intake of ethanol, salt, phosphoric acid (soft drinks), caffeine Sodium deficit (via drug administration) Protein-energy malnutrition. There is evidence that magnesium balance remains positive despite reduced recommended dietary intake as long as protein >30 g/day Chronic excessive magnesium intake
Endocrine disorders	Hyperaldosteronism Hyperparathyroidism with hypercalcaemia Hyperthyroidism Diabetes mellitus and glycosuria
Lifestyle	Profuse sweating Intense, prolonged stress Alcohol ingestion
Gastrointestinal disorders (gastrointestinal tract [GIT] absorptive surface pathology or reduced transit time or increased upper GIT loss)	Coeliac disease Infections Inflammatory bowel disease Malabsorption syndromes Biliary and intestinal fistula Pancreatitis Partial bowel obstruction Vomiting/diarrhoea
Elevated cortisol levels	Chronic stress Sleep deprivation Athletes and high-frequency exercise
Pharmaceutical drugs	Aminoglycoside antibiotics Amphotericin B Antivirals (ribavirin, foscavir) Carboplatin, cisplatin Cetuximab, panitumumab Corticosteroids Cyclosporin Digoxin Loop diuretics Oestrogens Osmotic diuretics Penicillamine Pentamidine Proton pump inhibitors Tacrolimus Tetracycline antibiotics
Renal	Metabolic disorders Renal failure Acidosis Nephrotoxic drugs (e.g. cisplatin, cyclosporin)
Other	Hyperthermia Hypercatabolic states such as burns Phosphate depletion Potassium depletion Pregnancy Lactation (prolonged (>12 months) or excessive lactation) Excessive menstruation Long-term parenteral nutrition combined with loss of body fluids (e.g. diarrhoea) Parasitic infection (e.g. pinworms)

Source: Allen (2013), Braunwald et al (2003), Johnson (2001), McDermott et al (1991), Sanders et al (1999), Shils et al (1999).

intracellular homeostasis and activation of thiamine (Johnson 2001). It acts as a calcium antagonist and positively interacts with nutrients such as potassium, phosphorus, vitamin B_6 and boron.

OTHER ACTIONS

In its macro form, oral inorganic magnesium salts have a laxative and antacid activity and are practically insoluble in water.

CLINICAL USE

In practice, magnesium is administered by various routes, such as intramuscular injection and intravenous infusion. This review will focus only on oral magnesium, as this is the form most commonly used by healthcare professionals and the general public, outside the hospital setting.

Deficiency: treatment and prevention

Magnesium supplementation is used to prevent and/or treat magnesium deficiency. This is achieved using either oral or parenteral administration forms. Ideally, forms of magnesium less likely to induce diarrhoea are recommended for long-term use. Table 1 lists the diet, lifestyle, comorbidities and pharmaceutical medications which can increase the risk of hypomagnesaemia. Sometimes, suboptimal magnesium states are associated with other electrolyte imbalances, such as calcium and potassium.

Healthy representation of total plasma magnesium levels are 0.86 mmol/L, between a reference value of 0.75–0.96 mmol/L. Low total plasma magnesium levels <0.7 mmol/L (1.8 mg/dL, 1.5 mEq/L) are indicative of magnesium deficiency, although symptoms occur when total plasma magnesium is <0.5 mmol/L (1.2 mg/dL, 1.0 mEq/L). It should be noted that total plasma magnesium may not be a good indicator of magnesium status, as low plasma levels may exist with low intracellular magnesium. Further investigation is needed to ascertain accurate measurement of magnesium status (Allen 2013, Braunwald et al 2003).

Constipation

In high doses magnesium exerts a laxative effect, which is used in practice for the short-term treatment of constipation and in order to get the bowel ready for surgical or diagnostic procedures. It is often used in the form of magnesium hydroxide (milk of magnesia) or magnesium sulfate (Epsom salts) (Guerrera et al 2009).

Dyspepsia

As magnesium hydroxide (milk of magnesia), oral magnesium is used to reduce symptoms of dyspepsia and gastric acidity and acts as an antacid by forming magnesium chloride in the stomach. Magnesium oxide is also used for its antacid properties, which are greater than magnesium carbonate and sodium bicarbonate (Coffin et al 2011, Reynolds et al 1982). Magnesium trisilicate is the form used when a prolonged antacid activity is required.

Clinical note — Magnesium citrate and orotate: superior supplements?

Magnesium supplements come in a variety of salts (e.g. citrate, oxide, gluconate, acetate, orotate); however their bioavailability varies. Current evidence, although not clearly demonstrating superiority of one preparation over another, supports the use in general of organic over inorganic forms (Coudray et al 2005, Firoz & Graber 2001, Lindberg et al 1990, Walker et al 2003). In particular, investigations of magnesium orotate (Lindberg et al 1990), citrate (Walker et al 2003) and gluconate (Coudray et al 2005) demonstrate high solubility and bioavailability. Magnesium orotate has attracted further attention regarding its potential synergism with magnesium in terms of repair of damaged myocardium (Classen 2004, Zeana 1999).

According to one randomised, double-blind, placebo-controlled study, magnesium amino chelate and magnesium citrate are better absorbed than magnesium oxide in healthy individuals (Walker et al 2003). Of the three, magnesium citrate led to the greatest increase in mean serum magnesium, a result evident after acute dosing (24 hours) and chronic dosing (60 days). Furthermore, although mean erythrocyte magnesium concentration showed no differences among groups, chronic magnesium citrate supplementation resulted in the greatest mean salivary magnesium concentration compared with all other treatments.

Cardiovascular disease (CVD)

Whether adequate magnesium intake has a protective effect against the development of CVD appears likely, based on the balance of evidence; however some studies remain inconclusive. This is largely based on epidemiological evidence which continues to strongly link magnesium deficiency to numerous CVD presentations, including congestive heart failure, ischaemic heart disease, cardiac arrhythmias, hypertension, mitral valve prolapse, stroke, non-occlusive myocardial infarction and hyperlipidaemia (Alon et al 2006, Flight & Clifton 2006, Fox et al 2001, Frishman et al 2005, Gropper et al 2009, Guerrero-Romero & Rodriguez-Moran 2002, Haenni et al 1998, Klevay & Milne 2002, Ma et al 1995, Rasmussen et al 1988, Rude & Shils 2006, Saris et al 2000, Song et al 2006, Xu et al 2012, Zhang et al 2012).

Xu et al (2012), in their meta-analysis of >210,000 people with cardiovascular history and CVD incidence and mortality, suggest that the evidence is weighted more towards protective factors in women than men. The Japan Collaborative Cohort study produced similar findings; however the authors state that this may be due to confounders such as a propensity of men to more risky lifestyle factors such as high-energy drinks, smoking and alcohol consumption (Zhang et al 2012).

A protective effect from hard water consumption, and in particular magnesium intake from this source, against CVD has been hypothesised for many years, culminating in a meta-analysis which determined a pooled odds ratio of 0.75 for cardiovascular mortality (Catling et al 2008).

Although the pathophysiology of each condition is multifactorial, the multiple biological effects of magnesium in the cardiovascular system suggest an important cardioprotective role. In the heart, magnesium acts as a calcium-channel blocker and promotes resting polarisation of the cell membrane, thereby reducing arrhythmias (Shattock et al 1987). It also helps to prevent serum coagulation (Frishman et al 2005). Low magnesium selectively impairs the release of nitric oxide from the coronary endothelium, resulting in vasoconstriction and possibly coronary embolism. Magnesium plays a role in blood lipid levels with detrimental changes, e.g. increased oxidation of low-density lipoproteins (LDLs), as well as generally increased oxidation, evident in hypomagnesaemia (Rude & Shils 2006). In experimental animals, dietary magnesium deficiency exacerbates atherosclerosis and vascular damage because it has a modulatory role in controlling lipid metabolism in the arterial wall.

Mitral valve prolapse

It has been suggested that hypomagnesaemia is common in patients with mitral valve prolapse and therefore supplementation to correct this deficiency could exert beneficial clinical effects (Kitlinski et al 2004). In 1997, one study of 141 subjects with symptomatic mitral valve prolapse confirmed this suspicion by identifying hypomagnesaemia in 60% of patients (Lichodziejewska et al 1997). A randomised, double-blind, crossover study followed those magnesium-deficient people and found that 5 weeks' magnesium supplementation significantly alleviated symptoms of weakness, chest pain, dyspnoea, palpitation and anxiety (Lichodziejewska et al 1997). The dose regimen used was three tablets of magnesium carbonate 600 mg (7 mmol elementary magnesium) daily for the first week followed by two tablets daily until the fifth week. New research in this area is sadly lacking; the most recent article was presented in a paediatric study of the prevalence of hypomagnesaemia in mitral valve prolapse syndrome. A small percentage of the patients had serum magnesium levels <1.5 mg/dL after therapy symptoms of chest pain decreased (Amoozagar et al 2012).

Symptoms of coronary artery disease (CAD)

In 2003, the results from a multicentre, double-blind randomised controlled trial (RCT) showed that 6 months' oral magnesium supplementation in patients with CAD resulted in a significant improvement in exercise tolerance, exercise-induced chest pain and quality of life compared to placebo (Shechter et al 2003). The study used oral magnesium citrate (15 mmol twice daily) as Magnosolv-Granulat (total magnesium 365 mg). Previously, randomised placebo-controlled studies have shown that oral magnesium supplementation in CAD patients is associated with significant improvement in brachial artery endothelial function and inhibits platelet-dependent thrombosis, providing several potential mechanisms by which magnesium could beneficially alter outcomes in these patients. Additionally, Shechter (2010) suggests magnesium supplementation has theoretical benefits in hospitalised and elderly patients as cardioprotective therapy in CAD (Shechter et al 1999, 2000, 2010).

Hypertension

Epidemiological evidence suggests an inverse relationship between blood pressure and serum magnesium, while large well-designed prospective studies report that magnesium-rich diets may lower blood pressure, particularly in older individuals (Sontia & Touryz 2007). Magnesium modulates vascular tone and reactivity both directly, e.g. calcium-channel blocker, and indirectly, e.g. prostacyclin, and alters vascular responsivity to vasoactive agonists. However, magnesium deficiency does not appear universal amongst hypertensive patients and several subgroups have been identified as characteristically demonstrating both pathologies. These include individuals of African descent, obese patients, patients with severe or malignant presentations and those also diagnosed with metabolic syndrome.

This may partly explain the mixed findings produced from magnesium supplementation studies, as well as additional heterogeneities in study designs, such as the salts used, dose administered, sample size and trial duration (Sontia & Touryz 2007). Modest but significant success (≈ −2 to −5 mmHg), however, has been achieved, particularly in those patients deficient at baseline, African American individuals and those patients with diuretic-associated hypertension (Rude & Shils 2006, Sontia & Touryz 2007, Witteman et al 1994). Patients who are considered metabolically obese normal-weight people (also deficient at baseline) demonstrate lowered mean systolic (−2.1 vs 3.9% mmHg, $P < 0.05$) and diastolic (−3.8 vs 7.5% mmHg, $P < 0.05$) benefit from IV magnesium supplementation (equivalent: 382 mg magnesium) when compared to controls (Rodriguez-Moran & Guerrero-Romero 2014).

Stroke protection

A prospective study of 43,738 men (Health Professional Follow-up Study) conducted over 8 years showed an inverse association between dietary magnesium intake and the risk of total stroke (Ascherio et al 1998). This association was stronger in hypertensive than normotensive men and was not materially altered by adjustments for blood pressure levels. This association was confirmed in a later study of male smokers (Larsson et al 2008). Following adjustment for age and other cardiovascular risks, high magnesium intake was associated with a statistically significant reduced risk of cerebral infarct, with a relative risk of 0.85 across men of all ages or 0.76 in those men aged <60 years, while the dietary intake of other minerals did not appear to convey any protection. It is also interesting to note that low concentrations of magnesium in the serum or cerebrospinal fluid in acute ischaemic stroke patients at admission or within 48 hours of onset of the stroke predict both greater neurological deficits, e.g. paresis, and higher 1-week mortality (Bayir et al 2009, Cojocaru et al 2007). In a meta-analysis of eight cohort studies — 8367 stroke cases amongst 304,551 people — a significant inverse association between high magnesium intake (range 228–471 mg magnesium day) and risk of stroke was found. More specifically, the people with the highest magnesium intake experienced an 11% reduction in the relative risk of stroke (Nie et al 2012). Findings were confirmed by the National Institutes of Health Stroke Scale, appearing as a dose–response relationship between magnesium serum levels and risk of death, in an epidemiological study in China (Feng et al 2012).

Dyslipidaemia

Oral magnesium supplementation (magnesium oxide 12 mmol/day) taken over 3 months effectively reduced plasma lipids compared with placebo in people with ischaemic heart disease (Rasmussen et al 1989). The double-blind study showed that magnesium produced a statistically significant 13% increase in molar ratio of apolipoprotein A1:apolipoprotein B, compared with a 2% increase in the placebo group. This was caused by a decrease in apolipoprotein B concentrations, which were reduced by 15% in the magnesium group as compared with a slight increase in the placebo group. Additionally, triglyceride levels decreased by 27% after magnesium treatment.

In a later study measuring serum lipids and insulin sensitivity (IS) in 48 patients with mild uncomplicated hypertension, oral magnesium (600 mg pidolate) was administered with concurrent lifestyle recommendations. In the control group there were no changes to oral glucose tolerance test-derived IS indices, nor serum lipids, whereas the active treatment group experienced increased IS indices and decreased triglycerides, LDL and total cholesterol, with elevated high-density lipoprotein (HDL) levels (Hadjistavri et al 2010).

A study of 50 healthy volunteers by Marken et al (1989) found no change in lipid profile in a double-blind, crossover RCT using magnesium oxide (400 mg twice daily) for 60 days. This may be due to the fact that participants had lipid levels within the normal range at baseline.

Arrhythmia prevention

In congestive heart failure

Although magnesium is usually administered intravenously when indicated in this condition, one controlled study using oral magnesium showed that it significantly reduced the incidence of arrhythmias in patients with stable congestive heart failure (Bashir et al 1993). The double-blind crossover study used magnesium chloride (3204 mg/day in divided doses). Its role in sudden cardiac death as a result of fatal ventricular arrhythmia was observed in a prospective women's cohort, where higher plasma magnesium from dietary intake was associated with lower risk of sudden cardiac death (Chiuve et al 2011).

Postoperative recovery from cardiac surgery

An interesting Australian study employed a range of preoperative treatments addressing mental, physical and metabolic components, including magnesium. The results of this RCT, using 1200 mg magnesium orotate, together with 300 mg CoQ10, 300 mg alpha-lipoic acid and 3 g omega-3 essential fatty acids administered daily 1 month prior to surgery, suggest an enhanced postoperative recovery and improved quality of life (Hadj et al 2006). IV administration of magnesium sulfate is also used to reduce the risk of atrial fibrillation postsurgery (Burgess et al 2006).

Postsurgical pain

Systemic magnesium has been used with some scepticism in the management of postoperative pain management. Magnesium was examined in both intraoperative and postoperative patient observations in a vast variety of surgical procedures. The perioperative meta-analysis of 20 RCTs suggests a use for magnesium to reduce opioid consumption and mitigate postoperative pain. In the cardiac patients (three studies) no adverse effects were noted (De Oliveira et al 2013).

Migraine headaches: prevention

People who suffer with recurrent migraines appear to have lower intracellular magnesium levels (demonstrated in both red and white blood cells) than those who do not experience migraines. (See Feverfew monograph for more information about migraine aetiology.) The low magnesium level is believed to result in cerebral artery spasm and increased release of substance P and other pain mediators (Woolhouse 2005).

Two randomised, double-blind studies using high-dose oral magnesium have found it to be useful in migraine sufferers, reducing frequency and/or number of days with migraine headache (Peikert et al 1996, Taubert 1994). One placebo-controlled study using a lower dose found no benefit in reducing the frequency of migraine headaches (Pfaffenrath et al 1996).

A dose of 24 mmol/L magnesium (600 mg trimagnesium dicitrate) taken daily over 12 weeks produced a 42% reduction in frequency of attack compared with 16% with placebo in one study of 81 patients, with a mean attack frequency of 3.6 migraine headaches each month (Peikert et al 1996).

Effects were observed after week 9 and treatment also significantly decreased the duration of each migraine. Significant decreases in migraine frequency were also observed in a crossover study that used the same dose and form of oral magnesium (Taubert 1994). In a recent study, 300 mg magnesium, in combination with other B vitamins and a standardised extract of feverfew magnesium, was stated as probably prophylactic for migraine treatment (Holland et al 2012). However research on the use of single magnesium supplementation in the reduction of migraine headaches is limited.

Clinical note — What is the link between magnesium and migraine?

Magnesium seems to play a significant role in the pathogenesis of migraine, with low brain levels and impaired magnesium metabolism reported in migraine sufferers (Thomas et al 2000). Magnesium has an effect on serotonin receptors, nitric oxide synthesis and release and a variety of other migraine-related receptors and neurotransmitters. It is also essential for mitochondrial function within the cell. The available evidence suggests that up to 50% of patients during an acute migraine attack have lowered levels of ionised magnesium (Mauskop & Altura 1998). Pilot studies of migraine patients have suggested that disordered energy metabolism or magnesium deficiencies may be responsible for hyperexcitability of neuronal tissue in migraine patients (Boska et al 2002). As such, factors that decrease neuronal excitability, such as magnesium, may alter the threshold for triggering attacks (Boska et al 2002). The efficacy of magnesium is stated as probably effective for migraine prevention (Holland et al 2012).

Menstrual migraine headache

Oral magnesium supplementation decreases pain, premenstrual symptoms and the number of days with migraine headache, according to two double-blind, placebo-controlled studies (Facchinetti et al 1991a, Peikert et al 1996). In the earlier study, treatment consisted of 360 mg/day of magnesium (pyrrolidone carboxylic acid) starting on day 15 of the menstrual cycle and continuing until the onset of menses. In the second study 600 mg of trimagnesium dicitrate was administered every morning. Both studies suggest a benefit in the reduction of symptoms (Mauskop & Varughese 2012).

Migraine prophylaxis in children

Oral magnesium oxide (9 mg/kg/day) given in three divided doses with food may decrease headache frequency and severity, according to a multicentre, randomised, double-blind, placebo-controlled trial (Wang et al 2003). The 16-week study involved children aged 3–17 years who reported a 4-week history of at least weekly moderate to severe headache with a throbbing or pulsatile quality, associated anorexia/nausea, vomiting, photophobia, sonophobia or relief with sleep, but no fever or evidence of infection. Of note, 27% of subjects (n = 42 magnesium oxide; n = 44 placebo) failed to complete the study, thereby hindering interpretation of the results. While promising, there has been little further investigation so the evidence to date can be described as limited, with further research required (Orr & Venkateswaran 2014).

Attention-deficit hyperactivity disorder (ADHD)

The role of magnesium status and supplementation in ADHD remains unclear.

Several studies have demonstrated a positive correlation between magnesium status and ADHD pathology. Reported prevalence of hypomagnesaemia varies between 50% and 95% (Kozielec & Starobrat-Hermelin 1997, Mousain-Bosc et al 2004). It has been hypothesised that a genetic mutation involving the TRPM6 gene, which is crucial for magnesium transport and homeostasis, may be implicated, therefore making deficiency possible irrespective of adequate dietary intake (Mousain-Bosc et al 2004). There have been three magnesium supplementation studies in combination with vitamin B_6 (6 mg/kg/day magnesium ± 0.6–0.8 mg/kg/day vitamin B_6), producing significant behavioural improvement (Mousain-Bosc et al 2004). Magnesium–B_6 treatment led to a rise in erythrocyte magnesium levels; when treatment ceased, behavioural symptoms reappeared within a few weeks, concurrent with lowered erythrocyte magnesium levels (Mousain-Bosc et al 2006).

More recently, a systematic review of magnesium monotherapy in ADHD by Ghanizadeh (2013) concluded there are no well-controlled trials available to support the efficacy of magnesium in ADHD, even though preliminary reports are promising. Part of the difficulties arise from the fact that some pharmaceutical stimulants affect magnesium plasma levels, baseline levels of children with ADHD in the studies are unknown and confounders such as B_6 deficiency (which negatively affects magnesium balance), dietary intake and kidney/liver function are not usually taken into account.

Autism spectrum disorders (ASD)

Research suggests that people with ASD generally demonstrate RBC magnesium depletion (Mousain-Bosc et al 2006, Priya 2011, Strambi et al 2006). In spite of two negative reviews published 10 years apart (Nye & Brice 2005, Pfeiffer et al 1995), enthusiasm regarding the use of magnesium as an adjunct to high-dose vitamin B_6 therapy (6 mg/kg/day with 0.6–0.8 mg/kg/day vitamin B_6) in ASD continues (Kidd 2002, Mousain-Bosc et al 2006). Whether magnesium ultimately proves to be a successful adjunctive treatment remains unclear as currently there are limited trials and poor methodological rigour (Ghanizadeh 2103, Kidd 2002, Nye & Brice 2005, Pfeiffer et al 1995).

It has been proposed by Yasuda and Tsutsui (2013) that the pathogenesis of autism may somehow relate to low zinc and magnesium levels coupled with high aluminium, cadmium, lead, mercury and arsenic. This complex interplay of nutritional factors needs further exploration to be confirmed.

Kidney stone prevention

Magnesium deficiency is one of many risk factors for the development of kidney stones (Anderson 2002, Seiner 2005). Others include nutritional deficiencies of water, calcium, potassium and vitamin B_6, excessive intakes of animal protein, fat, sugar, oxalates, colas, alcohol, caffeine, salt and vitamin D, lifestyle factors and a positive family history.

A prospective double-blind study of 64 patients who were randomly assigned to receive placebo or potassium–magnesium citrate (42 mEq potassium, 21 mEq magnesium and 63 mEq citrate) daily for up to 3 years showed that the combination supplement reduced the risk of developing recurrent calcium oxalate kidney stones by 85% (Ettinger et al 1997). In a recent epidemiological study (European Prospective Investigation into Cancer and Nutrition: EPIC), participants with higher levels of fresh fruit, wholegrain fibre and dietary magnesium (low range 282, higher range 481 mg/day) were found to have a lower risk of kidney stone formation (Turney et al 2014).

Premenstrual syndrome (PMS)

Three early double-blind studies using oral magnesium supplements in women with PMS produced positive results for decreasing symptoms such as fluid retention and mood swings (Facchinetti et al 1991b, Rosenstein et al 1994, Walker et al 1998). According to these, clinical effects develop slowly, starting during the second menstrual cycle. More recently, an open-label study of magnesium (250 mg) in PMS showed a 35% reduction in symptoms as assessed by investigators and 33.5% improvement as assessed by participants (Quaranta et al 2007). The study of 41 women with PMS used a modified-release magnesium tablet taken at intermittent times over three menstrual cycles, beginning 20 days after the start of their last menstrual period and continuing until the start of their next menstrual period.

Although it is not clear what mechanism of action is responsible, some, but not all, studies have identified decreased magnesium concentrations in both RBC and mononuclear blood cells of women with PMS (Khine et al 2006, Rosenstein et al 1994).

To date, the evidence overall remains promising for magnesium supplementation for some women with PMS; however further studies are required for a definitive conclusion to be made (Whelan et al 2009).

Dysmenorrhoea

A Cochrane review of seven RCTs investigating the effects of various treatments for dysmenorrhoea included three trials comparing magnesium with placebo. Overall, magnesium was found to be more effective than placebo for pain relief and resulted in less extra medication being required (Doty & Attaran 2009, Wilson & Murphy 2001). It appears that decreased serum magnesium is associated with dysmenorrhoea in young female adults; however evaluation of effective dosing is not available (Kibirian 2011, Yakubova 2012).

Osteoporosis prevention

Magnesium comprises about 1% of bone mineral and is involved in a number of activities supporting bone strength, preservation and remodelling. Epidemiological studies have linked increased magnesium consumption, as part of an alkaline diet, with improved bone mineral density (BMD) (Tucker et al 1999). Chronic magnesium deficiency compromises bone health by increasing the size and brittleness of the bone crystals, inducing hypocalcaemia and possibly increasing inflammatory cytokines (Rude & Shils 2006). Therefore, low magnesium states increase the risk of osteoporosis. Several studies have investigated the effects of supplemental magnesium on bone density, generally yielding positive effects in both men and women (Tucker 2009).

One long-term study has reported an increase in bone density for magnesium hydroxide supplementation in a group of menopausal women (Sojka & Weaver 1995). After the 2-year test period, fracture incidence was also reduced. Another 2-year study showed that magnesium supplementation in postmenopausal women with osteoporosis results in increased bone mass at the wrist after 1 year, with no further increase after 2 years of supplementation (Stendig-Lindberg et al 1993). The regimen used here was oral magnesium 750 mg/day for the first 6 months, followed by 250 mg/day thereafter. In the Women's Health Initiative Observational Study, observing risk factors for osteoporotic fractures and altered BMD, low magnesium intake was associated with lower-bone (whole body, including hip) mineral density, but this did not translate to increased risk of fracture. In women who consumed magnesium via food and supplementation, baseline hip BMD and whole-body BMD was 2–3% higher than controls (Orchard et al 2014).

Clinical note — Peak bone mass

The best opportunity to influence bone mass occurs early in life. It has been estimated that approximately 40% of peak bone mass is accumulated during adolescence, with peak bone mass in the hip achieved by age 16–18 years (Weaver 2000). The spinal vertebrae are still able to increase in mass until the third decade of life, when total peak bone mass reaches 99% by age 26.6 years (± 3.7 years). As such, ensuring an adequate intake of calcium and magnesium early in life is essential for attaining optimal bone mass.

Fibromyalgia

A study of 60 premenopasual women diagnosed with fibromyalgia according to the American College of Radiology criteria and 20 healthy women matched for age and weight found that oral magnesium citrate (300 mg/day) significantly reduced the number of tender points, tender point index and Beck depression scores by the end of the 8-week treatment period (Bagis et al 2013). Interestingly, the serum and erythrocyte magnesium levels were significantly lower in patients with fibromyalgia than in the controls and there was a negative correlation between the magnesium levels and fibromyalgia symptoms.

Asthma

There is some evidence that asthmatics have low intracellular (both red and white blood cells) magnesium (Dominguez et al 1998, Mircetic et al 2001, Sedighi et al 2006). This has relevance in asthma because healthy magnesium concentrations inhibit calcium entering smooth muscles such as those in the airways and therefore potentially reduce bronchospasm (Dominguez et al 1998, Gropper et al 2009). In addition, magnesium influences pulmonary vascular muscle contractility, mast cell granulation and neurohumoral mediator release (Mathew & Altura 1988).

Results of two randomised, double-blind studies suggest that oral supplements may also significantly alleviate asthma symptoms (Bede et al 2003, Hill et al 1997). Hill et al found that treatment improved symptoms, although it failed to change objective measures of air flow or airway reactivity, and Bede et al found a significant decrease in bronchodilator use after 8 weeks compared with placebo. This was a 12-week study using oral magnesium citrate in 89 children (4–16 years) with mild or moderate persistent bronchial asthma. The dose used was 200 mg daily for children aged 7 years and 290 mg for those older than 7 years. Adding to this, a randomised double-blind trial of magnesium glycine (300 mg/day) in 37 subjects aged 7–19 years over 2 months resulted in a statistically significant reduction in bronchial reactivity, skin responses to recognised antigens and salbutamol use in the treatment group compared to placebo (Gontijo-Amaral et al 2007). Kasaks (2013) suggests magnesium supplementation may be a useful adjunct to medical management to reduce airway hyperresponsiveness and improve perceived quality of life and asthma control.

Pregnancy

Six studies suggest magnesium intake in pregnant women is less than the recommended values and gene expression at week 37 of TRPM6 denotes higher urinary excretion of magnesium, indicating an increased demand in pregnant women (Rylander 2014).

Pregnancy-induced hypertension

A double-blind RCT of pregnant primagravida women given an oral supply of 300 mg magnesium citrate from pregnancy week 25 found that the average diastolic blood pressure at week 37 was significantly lower than in the placebo group ($P = 0.031$) and the number of women with an increase in diastolic blood pressure of ≥15 mmHg was also significantly lower than with placebo ($P = 0.011$) (Bullarbo et al 2013).

Pregnancy-induced leg cramps

A 2002 Cochrane review of five RCTs of treatments for leg cramps in pregnancy concluded that the best evidence is for magnesium lactate or citrate taken as 5 mmol in the morning and 10 mmol in the evening (Young & Jewell 2002). According to a more recent double-blind RCT involving 45 women, short-term use of magnesium supplementation (120 mg magnesium citrate and magnesium lactate 360 mg daily) over 2 weeks was insufficient to modify the intensity or frequency of leg cramps compared to placebo (Nygaard et al 2008). Possibly another dose or longer-term use would be more beneficial; however this remains to be tested.

Preterm birth and low birth weight

A 2001 Cochrane review of seven studies involving 2689 women concluded that, although not all trials were positive, oral magnesium taken before the 25th week of gestation was associated with a lower frequency of preterm birth, a lower frequency of low birth weight and fewer small-for-gestational-age infants. Additionally, fewer hospitalisations during pregnancy and fewer cases of antepartum haemorrhage were associated with magnesium use (Makrides & Crowther 2014).

Pre-eclampsia and eclampsia

Parenteral magnesium is used for preventing and managing PE and eclampsia. In particular, magnesium sulfate administered intravenously or intramuscularly is used.

An interesting longitudinal study revealed that, while serum magnesium levels decline in both healthy and pre-eclamptic pregnant women, such a decrease occurs earlier in those women who later develop PE (Sontia & Touryz 2007). Lower measures of erythrocyte, brain and muscle magnesium have recently been observed in PE women compared to those with normal pregnancies. In addition, there was a lower risk of hypertension in PE women with higher magnesium intake. More specifically, the study of 50 patients with PE and 50 controls demonstrated severe PE with erythrocyte magnesium levels 0.62 mmol/L, mild PE with erythrocyte magnesium of 0.67 mmol/L, and normal with 0.79 mmol/L (Rylander 2014).

Diabetes mellitus

A strong association between magnesium, diabetes and hypertension has been established (Ascherio et al 1998, Dasgupta et al 2012, Sontia & Touryz 2007). Deficiency aggravates insulin resistance and contributes to an increased risk of CVD in people with diabetes.

Type 1 diabetes mellitus (T1DM)

Hypomagnesaemia is present in 25–38% of all diabetic patients secondary to glycosuria and magnesium redistribution (Paolisso et al 1992). Such depletion may occur early in the pathology, with T1DM children demonstrating progressive deterioration of serum levels within 2 years of diagnosis in some (Tuvemo et al 1997), but not all, studies. Magnesium depletion in T1DM has also been linked to earlier atherosclerotic development (Atabek et al 2006, Djurhuus et al 1999), polyneuropathy (De Leeuw et al 2004), advanced retinopathy (de Valk et al 1999) and immunosuppression (Cojocaru et al 2006). Supplementation studies have produced mixed results (Eibl et al 1998); however, magnesium supplementation may reduce risks of secondary pathology.

Consistent with these findings, some researchers suggest T1DM patients receive a high dose in the first month of treatment to normalise RBC and serum magnesium and then remain on continuous lower-dose supplementation (e.g. 300 mg/day) in order to avoid a return to hypomagnesaemia (Eibl et al 1998). Lower serum magnesium levels are found in young patients with poor glycaemic control (0.79 ± 0.09 vs 0.82 ± 0.09 mmol/L, respectively; $P = 0.002$). In youths with T1DM, low magnesium levels provide inadequate glycaemic control ($HbA_{1C} > 7.5\%$). Higher levels of magnesium concentration present a decrease of 1.7% in HbA_{1C} (Galli-Tsinopoulou et al 2014).

Type 2 diabetes mellitus (T2DM)

Epidemiological studies have drawn a link between poor dietary and/or serum magnesium and an increased risk of T2DM (Chambers et al 2006, Dasgupta et al 2012, He et al 2006, van Dam et al 2006). In one large study those in the lowest tertile of magnesium and fibre intakes exhibited a three to four times greater risk (Bo et al 2006). Serum magnesium depletion is also evident in ≈ 25–38% patients. Hypomagnesaemia in diabetic patients appears to exacerbate impaired insulin resistance, elevated fasting blood glucose and HbA_{1C} concentrations (He et al 2006, Walti et al 2003). Oral magnesium (magnesium chloride 2.5 g/day for 4 months) adjunctive to hypoglycaemic medication has produced reductions of fasting glucose (–37.5%), HbA_{1C} (–30.4%), homeostasis model assessment-insulin resistance index (–9.5%) and insulin (Rodriguez-Moran & Guerrero-Romero 2003), while other studies demonstrate increased insulin levels with improved action (Paolisso et al 1992). In another study, a combination of magnesium (200 mg/day), zinc (30 mg/day) and vitamins (C 200 mg/day and E 150 mg/day) over 3 months significantly increased levels of HDL and apo-A1 24% and 8.8%, respectively (Farvid et al 2004).

Several RCTs and a meta-analysis of prospective cohort studies investigating oral magnesium supplementation have shown improvements in diabetic control (Dong et al 2011, Paolisso et al 1992, Rodriguez-Moran & Guerrero-Romero 2003). A double-blind trial that involved 63 patients with T2DM and reduced serum magnesium levels (treated with glibenclamide) demonstrated that the addition of oral magnesium over 16 weeks significantly improves IS and metabolic control (Rodriguez-Moran & Guerrero-Romero 2003). In a meta-analysis of prospective cohort studies involving 536,318 participants, a dose-responsive relative risk for type 2 diabetes for 100 mg/day increment in magnesium intake was 0.86 (95% confidence interval 0.82–0.89) (Dong et al 2011).

Chronic leg cramps

Two randomised, double-blind studies have investigated the use of oral magnesium supplements in people with leg cramps. Frusso et al (1999) conducted a crossover trial involving 45 individuals who had experienced at least six cramps during the previous month. Subjects were given 1 month of oral magnesium citrate (900 mg twice daily) followed by a matching placebo for 1 month, or vice versa. This treatment regimen failed to reduce the severity, duration or number of nocturnal leg cramps. In contrast, Roffe et al (2002) tested magnesium citrate equivalent to 300 mg magnesium in subjects suffering regular leg cramps and identified a trend towards fewer cramps with active treatment ($P = 0.07$). Significantly more subjects thought that the treatment had helped after magnesium than after placebo — 36 (78%) and 25 (54%) respectively. Interestingly, in both studies patients improved over time regardless of the treatment they received.

Although two additional studies in athletes found no correlation between cramping incidence and serum magnesium, the authors suggest that the cramping was caused by increased neuromuscular excitability (Schwellnus et al 2004, Sulzer et al 2005), which is a classic feature of magnesium deficiency (Rude & Shils 2006). As is the case with much magnesium research, more accurate and validated assessment methods may be required to elicit the true relationship between magnesium status and this presentation.

Cancer

Colorectal cancer (CRC)

A meta-analysis of prospective studies suggests that higher magnesium intake is inversely related to the risk of CRC. In dose–response analyses, summary relative risks for incremental magnesium intake of 50 mg/day in colorectal, colon and rectal cancer were 0.95, 0.93 and 0.93 respectively. In a case–control study on colorectal adenomas (three) and carcinomas (six prospective cohort studies) meta-analysis, for every 100-mg/day elevation in magnesium intake, there was an associated 13% lower risk of colorectal adenomas and 12% lower risk of CRC (Chen et al 2012, Wark et al 2012).

Lung cancer

There is limited evidence to suggest an association between risk of lung cancer and lower calcium and magnesium levels (Cheng et al 2012).

Prostate cancer

There is a possible relationship between low blood magnesium levels and high calcium-to-magnesium ratio and high-grade prostate cancer. More studies are needed (Dai et al 2011).

OTHER POSSIBLE USES

Oral magnesium supplements are used in a variety of different conditions, most notably those involving muscle spasm or tension, pain and/or psychological and physical symptoms of stress and hyperexcitability. This includes irritable bowel syndrome, restless legs syndrome, chronic fatigue syndrome, anxiety states, tension headaches and insomnia. Preliminary evidence suggests that it may be beneficial for women with detrusor muscle instability (incontinence) or sensory urgency.

DOSAGE RANGE

Australian RDI for adults

Men

- 19–30 years: 400 mg/day.
- >30 years: 420 mg/day.

Women

- 19–30 years: 310 mg/day.
- >30 years: 320 mg/day.

Pregnancy

- ≤18 years: 400 mg/day.
- >19–30 years: 350 mg/day.
- >31–50 years: 360 mg/day.

Lactation

- ≤18 years: 360 mg/day.
- >18–30 years: 310 mg/day.
- >31–50 years: 320 mg/day.

According to clinical studies

- ADHD: 6 mg/kg/day ± 0.6–0.8 mg/kg/day vitamin B_6.
- Arrhythmia prevention in congestive heart failure: magnesium chloride 3204 mg/day in divided doses.
- ASD: 6 mg/kg/day ± 0.6–0.8 mg/kg/day vitamin B_6.
- CAD symptoms: oral magnesium citrate (15 mmol twice daily as Magnosolv-Granulat, total magnesium 365 mg).
- Cancer risk reduction CRC: >100 mg/day.
- Dyslipidaemia: 600 mg/day magnesium pidolate.
- Fibromylagia: 300 mg/day.
- Hypertension: 360–600 mg/day.
- Kidney stone prevention: magnesium hydroxide 400–500 mg/day.
- Migraine: 600 mg trimagnesium dicitrate daily.
- Migraine prophylaxis in children: magnesium oxide (9 mg/kg/day).
- Mitral valve prolapse: three tablets magnesium carbonate 600 mg (7 mmol of elementary magnesium) daily for the first week followed by two tablets daily.
- Nocturnal leg cramps: magnesium citrate equivalent to 300 mg magnesium daily.
- Osteoporosis prevention: taken on an empty stomach, 250 mg three times daily for 6 months, followed by 250 mg/day for 18 months.
- Paediatric asthma: magnesium citrate 200–300 mg daily.
- PMS general symptoms: 260 mg/day.
- PMS fluid retention symptoms: 200 mg magnesium (as magnesium oxide) daily.
- PMS mood swings: magnesium pyrrolidone carboxylic acid (360 mg) taken three times daily, from day 15 of the menstrual cycle to the onset of menstrual flow.
- Postoperative recovery from cardiac surgery: 1200 mg magnesium orotate in combination with 300 mg CoQ10, 300 mg alpha-lipoic acid and 3 g omega-3 oils taken daily 1 month prior to surgery.
- Stroke prevention 228–471 mg/day.
- T1DM: initial high dose to normalise serum levels and then continuous 300 mg daily.
- T2DM: 2.5 g magnesium dichloride daily or 300 mg elemental magnesium in combination with 30 mg zinc, 250 mg vitamin C and 150 mg vitamin E daily.

ADVERSE REACTIONS

The most common adverse effects of oral supplements are diarrhoea (18.6%) and gastric irritation (4.7%) (Peikert et al 1996). It can be found as a primary ingredient in some laxatives (magnesium hydroxide) providing 500 mg of elemental magnesium (Guerrera et al 2009). Typically, doses of inorganic preparations supplying above 350 mg/day (elemental) may be associated with adverse effects. Dividing total daily supplemental amounts over two to three separate doses may help to reduce this risk and maximise bioavailability.

TOXICITY

The possibility of hypermagnesaemia is rare, and is seen mostly in the elderly, people with renal insufficiency, dialysis or with serious bowel disorders.

Mild hypermagnesaemia signs and symptoms are subtle, such as light-headedness, headache, nausea, flushing and warmth.

At levels between 6 and 12 mg/dL (5–10 mEq/L), electrocardiographic changes occur with prolonged reportedly similar changes to hyperkalaemia. Concentrations of 9–12 mg/dL may increase hypotension, loss of deep tendon reflex and somnolence. Levels >12 mg/dL (10 mEq/L) may initiate muscle paralysis, arrhythmias, hypoventilations, stupor, sinoatrial and atrioventricular block and ventricular arrhythmias. Levels exceeding 15.6 mg/dL (13 mEq/L) may result in coma, respiratory arrest and cardiac asystole (Jhang et al 2013).

SIGNIFICANT INTERACTIONS

The interactions included in this section are relevant for oral supplementation and do not refer to other administration routes, although there may be an overlap.

Alcohol

Alcohol consumption results in increased urinary losses of magnesium and therefore with higher chronic ingestion additional magnesium replacement may be necessary.

Aminoglycosides (e.g. gentamicin)

Drug may reduce absorption of magnesium — monitor for signs and symptoms of magnesium deficiency, as increased magnesium intake may be required with long-term therapy.

Calcium

Magnesium and calcium deficiencies usually coexist due to magnesium's key role in active PTH and vitamin D production (Gropper et al 2009, Rude & Shils 2006, Wester 1987). Conversely, if magnesium intakes are excessive, calcium levels decline due to inhibition of PTH release and increased renal excretion. There is additional redistribution with impaired calcium influx and release from intracellular stores. Magnesium can also bind calcium-binding sites and mimic its actions (Gropper et al 2009, Rude & Shils 2006).

Calcium-channel blockers

Magnesium may enhance the hypotensive effect of calcium-channel blockers: monitor patients and their drug requirements — possible beneficial interaction under supervision.

Fluoroquinolones

Magnesium may decrease absorption of fluoroquinolone antibiotics — separate doses by at least 2 hours before or 4 hours after oral magnesium.

Loop diuretics and thiazide diuretics

Increased magnesium intake may be required with long-term therapy because of increased urinary excretion — monitor magnesium efficacy and status with long-term drug use.

Potassium

Hypomagnesaemia results in hypokalaemia due to increased potassium efflux from cells and renal excretion (Gropper et al 2009, Rude & Shils 2006).

Potassium-sparing diuretics

May increase the effects of supplemental magnesium — observe patients taking this combination.

Tetracycline antibiotics

Tetracyclines form insoluble complexes with magnesium, thereby reducing absorption of both — separate doses by at least 2 hours.

Dasatinib

May increase magnesium blood levels — observe (Vest & Cho 2012).

Neuromuscular blockers

May potentiate effects of neuroblockers — observe (Amgen Inc 2012, Kim et al 2012).

L-thyroxine

Case studies suggest reduced effectiveness of levothyroxine with magnesium-containing antacids and laxatives (Pinard et al 2003) — observe.

CONTRAINDICATIONS AND PRECAUTIONS

- Magnesium supplementation should be done cautiously in people with compromised renal function and is contraindicated in renal failure and heart block (unless a pacemaker is present).
- Hypermagnesaemia can develop in patients with renal failure and receiving magnesium-containing antacids or laxatives and with accidental Epsom salt ingestion.
- Overuse of magnesium hydroxide or magnesium sulfate may cause deficiencies of other minerals or lead to toxicity.

PREGNANCY USE

Pregnant women and nursing mothers are advised to consume sufficient magnesium (see Australian RDI under Dosage range, above).

PATIENTS' FAQs

What will this supplement do for me?

Magnesium is essential for health and wellbeing. Although used to prevent or treat deficiency states, it is also used to alleviate many conditions, such as CVD and PMS, and prevent migraine and muscular spasms.

When will it start to work?

This will depend on the indication it is being used to treat.

Are there any safety issues?

In high doses, some magnesium supplements can cause diarrhoea. High-dose supplements should not be used by people with severe kidney disease or heart block.

Practice points/Patient counselling

- Magnesium is an essential mineral in human nutrition with a wide range of biological functions.
- Low magnesium states are associated with several serious diseases, such as congestive heart failure, ischaemic heart disease, cardiac arrhythmias, hypertension, mitral valve prolapse, metabolic syndrome, stroke, diabetes mellitus, hyperlipidaemia, pre-eclampsia and eclampsia.
- Although supplementation is traditionally used to correct or avoid deficiency states, research has also shown a role in the management of numerous disease states, e.g. asthma, CVD, PMS, dysmenorrhoea, migraine prevention, diabetes, kidney stone prevention, osteoporosis prevention, dyspepsia and constipation. Preliminary research also suggests a possible benefit in ADHD, autism, women with detrusor muscle instability (incontinence) and pregnancy-induced leg cramps.
- Oral magnesium supplements are also used in a variety of different conditions, most notably those involving muscle spasm or tension, pain and/or psychological and physical symptoms of stress and hyperexcitability.
- Numerous drug interactions exist, so care should be taken to ensure safe use.

REFERENCES

Allen LH Magnesium. Encyclopedia of Human Nutrition (3rd edn) 2013;131–135.

Alon I et al. Intracellular magnesium in elderly patients with heart failure: effects of diabetes and renal dysfunction. J Trace Elem Med Biol 20.4 (2006): 221–226.

Amgen Inc. Vectibix (panitumumab) prescribing information (revised 08/2012). Available at http://pi.amgen.com/united_states/vectibix/vectibix_pi.pdf. Accessed October 3, 2012.

Amoozagar H, et al. The prevalence of hypomagnesaemia in pediatric patients with mitral valve prolapse syndrome and the effect of Mg therapy, 2012. Int Cardiovasc Res J 6:3;92–5.

Anderson RA. A complementary approach to urolithiasis prevention. World J Urol 20.5 (2002): 294–301.

Andon M et al. Magnesium balance in adolescent females consuming a low- or high-calcium diet. AJCN 63 (1996): 950–953.

Arnaud MJ. Update on the assessment of magnesium status. Br J Nutr 99 (Suppl 3) (2008): S24–S36.

Ascherio A et al. Intake of potassium, magnesium, calcium, and fiber and risk of stroke among US men. Circulation 98.12 (1998): 1198–1204.

Atabek M et al. Serum magnesium concentrations in type 1 diabetic patients: relation to early atherosclerosis (abstract). Diabetes Res Clin Pract 72.1 (2006): 42–47.

Bagis, S., et al. 2013. Is magnesium citrate treatment effective on pain, clinical parameters and functional status in patients with fibromyalgia? Rheumatol.Int., 33, (1) 167–172.

Bashir Y et al. Effects of long-term oral magnesium chloride replacement in congestive heart failure secondary to coronary artery disease. Am J Cardiol 72.15 (1993): 1156–1162.

Bayir A et al. Serum and cerebrospinal fluid magnesium levels, Glasgow coma scores, and in-hospital mortality in patients with acute stroke. Biol Trace Elem Res (2009 Jan 23): Epub ahead of print.

Bede O et al. Urinary magnesium excretion in asthmatic children receiving magnesium supplementation: a randomized, placebo-controlled, double-blind study. Magnes Res 16.4 (2003): 262–270.

Bo S et al. Dietary magnesium and fiber intakes and inflammatory and metabolic indicators in middle-aged subjects from a population-based cohort. AJCN 84.5 (2006): 1062–1069.

Boska MD et al. Contrasts in cortical magnesium, phospholipid and energy metabolism between migraine syndromes. Neurology 58.8 (2002): 1227–1233.

Braunwald E et al. Harrison's principles of internal medicine. New York: McGraw Hill, 2003.

Bullarbo, M., et al. 2013. Magnesium supplementation to prevent high blood pressure in pregnancy: a randomised placebo control trial. Arch. Gynecol.Obstet., 288, (6) 1269–1274.

Burgess DC, et al. Interventions for prevention of post-operative atrial fibrillation and its complications after cardiac surgery: a meta-analysis. Eur Heart J 27.23 (2006): 2846–2857.

Catling LA et al. A systematic review of analytical observational studies investigating the association between cardiovascular disease and drinking water hardness. J Water Health 6.4 (2008): 433–42.

Chacko SA, et al. Relations of dietary magnesium intake to biomarkers of inflammation and endothelial dysfunction in an ethnically diverse cohort of postmenopausal women. Diabetes Care 2010;33(2):304–310.

Chambers E et al. Serum magnesium and type-2 diabetes in African Americans and Hispanics: a New York Cohort. J Am Coll Nutr 25.6 (2006): 509–513.

Chen, G. C., et al. Magnesium intake and risk of colorectal cancer: a meta-analysis of prospective studies. Eur J Clin Nutr. 2012. 66(11):1182–6.

Cheng, M. H., et al. Calcium and magnesium in drinking-water and risk of death from lung cancer in women. Magnesium Research. 25(3):112–119, 2012.

Chiuve, S. E., et al. Plasma and dietary magnesium and risk of sudden cardiac death in women. American Journal of Clinical Nutrition. 93(2):253–260, 2011.

Classen H. Magnesium orotate — experimental and clinical evidence. Rom J Intern Med 42.3 (2004): 491–501.

Coffin B, et al. Efficacy of a simethicone, activated charcoal and magnesium oxide combination (Carbosymag ®) in functional dyspepsia: Results of a general practice-based randomized trial. Clinics and Research in Hepatology and Gastroenterology 2011: 35;6–7;494–499.

Cojocaru M et al. The effect of magnesium deficit on serum immunoglobulin concentrations in type 1 diabetes mellitus. Rom J Intern Med 44.1 (2006): 61–67.

Cojocaru IM et al. Serum magnesium in patients with acute ischemic stroke. Rom J Intern Med 45.3 (2007): 269–273.

Coudray C et al. Study of magnesium bioavailability from the organic and inorganic Mg salts in Mg-depleted rats using a stable isotope approach. Magnes Res 18.4 (2005): 215–223.

Dai, Q., et al. Blood magnesium, and the interaction with calcium, on the risk of high-grade prostate cancer. PLoS One. 6(4):e18237, 2011.

Dasgupta A, et al. Hypomagnesemia in type 2 diabetes mellitus. Indian J Endocrin Metab. 2012; 16:6; 1000–1003.

Djurhuus MS et al. Effect of moderate improve- ment in metabolic control on magnesium and lipid concen- trations in patients with type 1 diabetes. Diabetes Care 22.4 (1999): 546–554.

De Leeuw I et al. Long term magnesium supplementation influences favourably the natural evolution of neuropathy in Mg-depleted type 1 diabetic patients (1DM). (abstract). Magnes Res 17.2 (2004): 109–114.

de Valk H et al. Plasma magnesium concentration and progression of retinopathy. Diabetes Care 22.5 (1999): 864–865.

Dominguez L et al. Bronchial reactivity and intracellular magnesium: a possible mechanism for the bronchodilating effects of magnesium in asthma (abstract). Clin Sci (Lond) 95.2 (1998): 137–142.

Dong Jy, et al. Magnesium intake and risk of type 2 diabetes:meta-analysis of prospective cohort studies. Diabetes Care 2011. 34:9;2116–22.

Doty E. & Attaran C. (2009). Managing primary dysmenorrhea. Journal of Pediatric and Adolescent Gynecology 19 (5): 341–344.

Eibl N, et al. Magnesium supplementation in type 2 diabetes (Letter). Diabetes Care 21 (1998): 2031–2032.

Ellen GHM. Short-chain fructo-oligosaccharides improve magnesium absorption in adolescent girls with a low calcium intake. Nutr Res 29.4 (2009): 229–237.

Ettinger B et al. Potassium-magnesium citrate is an effective prophylaxis against recurrent calcium oxalate nephrolithiasis. J Urol 158.6 (1997): 2069–2073.

Facchinetti F et al. Magnesium prophylaxis of menstrual migraine: effects on intracellular magnesium. Headache 31.5 (1991a): 298–301.

Facchinetti F et al. Oral magnesium successfully relieves premenstrual mood changes. Obstet Gynecol 78.2 (1991b): 177–81.

Farvid MS et al. The impact of vitamins and/or mineral supplementation on blood pressure in type 2 diabetes. J Am Coll Nutr 23.3 (2004): 272–9.

Feillet-Coudray C et al. Exchangeable magnesium pool masses reflect the magnesium status of rats. J Nutr 130.9 (2000): 2306–2311.

Feng, P., et al. Association between concentrations of serum magnesium and the short-term outcome of patients with acute ischemic stroke. Department of Epidemiology, School Of Public Health of medical College, China 2012. 33(11):1171–1175.

Fine K et al. Intestinal absorption of magnesium from food and supplements. J Clin Invest 88 (1991): 396–402.

Firoz M, Graber M. Bioavailability of US commercial magnesium preparations. Magnes Res 14.4 (2001): 257–262.

Flight I, Clifton P. Cereal grains and legumes in the prevention of coronary heart disease and stroke: a review of the literature. Eur J Clin Nutr 60.10 (2006): 1145–1159.

Ford E, Mokdad A. Dietary magnesium intake in a national sample of U.S. adults. J.Nutr 133 (2003): 2879–2882.

Fox C, et al. Magnesium: its proven and potential clinical significance. South Med J 94.12 (2001): 1195–1201.
Frishman WH, et al. Alternative and complementary medical approaches in the prevention and treatment of cardiovascular disease. Current Prob Cardiol 30.8 (2005): 383–459.
Frusso R et al. Magnesium for the treatment of nocturnal leg cramps: a crossover randomized trial. J Fam Pract 48.11 (1999): 868–871.
Galli-Tsinopoulou A et al., Association between magnesium concentration and HbA1c in children and adolescents with type 1 diabetes mellitus. Journal of Diabetes 2014 ;6;4; 369–377.
Ghanizadeh A. A systematic review of magnesium therapy for treating ADHD. Archives of Iranian Medicine 2013 16:7; 412–417.
Gontijo-Amaral C et al. Oral magnesium supplementation in asthmatic children: a double-blind randomized placebo-controlled trial. Eur J Clin Nutr 61.1 (2007): 54–60.
Grimaldi BL. The central role of magnesium deficiency in Tourette's syndrome: causal relationships between magnesium deficiency, altered biochemical pathways and symptoms relating to Tourette's syndrome and several reported comorbid conditions. Med Hypotheses 58.1 (2002): 47–60.
Gropper S, et al. Advanced nutrition and human metabolism, 5th edn. Belmont: Thomson Wadsworth, 2009.
Guerrera MP, et al. Therapeutic uses of magnesium. Am Fam Physician 2009;80:157–62.
Guerrero-Romero F, Rodriguez-Moran M. Low serum magnesium levels and metabolic syndrome. Acta Diabetol 39.4 (2002): 209–213.
Hadj A et al. Pre-operative preparation for cardiac surgey utilising a combination of metabolic, physical and mental therapy. Heart Lung Circ 15.3 (2006): 172–181.
Hadjistavri, L. S., et al. Beneficial effects of oral magnesium supplementation on insulin sensitivity and serum lipid profile. Med Sci Monit. 16(6):13–18, 2010.
Haenni A, et al. Atherogenic lipid fractions are related to ionized magnesium status. AJCN 67 (1998): 202–207.
Hartwig A. Role of magnesium in genomic stability. Mutat Res. 2001;475(1–2):113–121.
He K et al. Magnesium intake and incidence of metabolic syndrome among young adults. Circulation 113 (2006): 1675–1682.
Hill J et al. Investigation of the effect of short-term change in dietary magnesium intake in asthma. Eur Respir J 10.10 (1997): 2225–2229.
Holland S, et al. Evidence-based guideline update: NSAIDs and other complementary treatments for episodic migraine prevention in adults. Neurology 2012;78:1346–53.
Jhang WK, et al. Severe hypermagnesemia presenting with abnormal electrocardiographic findings similar to those of hyperkalemia in a child undergoing peritoneal dialysis. Korean J Pediatr. 2013:56;7:308–311.
Johnson S. The multifaceted and widespread pathology of magnesium deficiency. Med Hypotheses 56.2 (2001): 163–170.
Khan L et al. Serum and urinary magnesium in young diabetic subjects in Bangladesh. AJCN 69 (1999): 70–73.
Khine K et al. Magnesium (Mg) retention and mood effects after intravenous Mg infusion in premenstrual dysphoric disorder. Biol Psychiatry 59.4 (2006): 327–333.
Kidd P. Autism, an extreme challenge to integrative medicine. Part II: Medical management. Alt Med Rev 7.6 (2002): 472–499.
Kim MH, et al. A randomised controlled trial comparing rocuronium priming, magnesium pre-treatment and a combination of the two methods. Anaesthesia. 2012;67(7):748–754.
Kitlinski M et al. Is magnesium deficit in lymphocytes a part of the mitral valve prolapse syndrome? Magnes Res 17.1 (2004): 39–45.
Klevay L, Milne D. Low dietary magnesium increases supraventricular ectopy. AJCN 75 (2002): 550–554.
Kozielec T, Starobrat-Hermelin B. Assessment of magnesium levels in children with attention deficit hyperactivity disorder (ADHD). Magnes Res 10.2 (1997): 143–148.
Larsson SC et al. Magnesium, calcium, potassium, and sodium intakes and risk of stroke in male smokers. Arch Intern Med 168.5 (2008): 459–465.
Lewis N et al. Calcium supplements and milk: effects on acid-base balance and on retention of calcium magnesium, phosphorus. AJCN 49 (1989): 527–533.
Lichodziejewska B et al. Clinical symptoms of mitral valve prolapse are related to hypomagnesemia and attenuated by magnesium supplementation. Am J Cardiol 79.6 (1997): 768–772.
Lindberg J et al. Magnesium bioavailability from magnesium citrate and magnesium oxide. J Am Coll Nutr 9.1 (1990): 48–55.
Lukaski H. Magnesium, zinc, and chromium nutriture and physical activity. AJCN 72 (Suppl) (2000): 585S–593S.
Ma J et al. Associations of serum and dietary magnesium with cardiovascular disease, hypertension, diabetes, insulin, and carotid arterial wall thickness: the ARIC study. (Atherosclerosis Risk in Communities Study). J Clin Epidemiol 48.7 (1995): 927–940.
Makrides M., Crowther CA. Magnesium supplementation in pregnancy. Cochrane Database Syst Rev. 2014;4:CD000937.
Marken PA et al. Effects of magnesium oxide on the lipid profile of healthy volunteers. Atherosclerosis 77 (1989): 37–42.
Mathew R, Altura BM. Magnesium and the lungs. Magnesium 7.4 (1988): 173–187.
Mauskop A, Altura BM. Role of magnesium in the pathogenesis and treatment of migraines. Clin Neurosci 5.1 (1998): 24–27.
Mauskop A, Varughese J. Why all migraine patients should be treated with magnesium. Journal of Neural Transmission 2012; 119:5:575–9.
McDermott KC, et al. The diagnosis and management of hypomagnesemia: a unique treatment approach and case report. Oncol Nurs Forum 18.7 (1991): 1145–1152.
McKeown NM, et al. Dietary magnesium intake is related to metabolic syndrome in older Americans. Eur J Nutr. Jun 2008;47(4):210–216.
Mircetic R et al. Magnesium concentration in plasma, leukocytes and urine of children with intermittent asthma (abstract). Clin Chim Acta 312.1–2 (2001): 197–203.
Mousain-Bosc M et al. Magnesium VitB6 Intake reduces central nervous system hyperexcitability in children. J Am Coll Nutr 23.5 (2004): 545S–548S.
Mousain-Bosc M et al. Improvement of neurobehavioural disorders in children supplemented with magnesium-vitamin B6. II. Pervasive developmental disorder (abstract). Magnes Res 19.1 (2006a): 53–62.
Mousain-Bosc, M., et al. Improvement of neurobehavioral disorders in children supplemented with magnesium-vitamin B6. I. Attention deficit hyperactivity disorders. Magnesium Research. 19(1):46–52, 2006b.
NHMRC. Nutrient reference values for Australia and New Zealand including recommended dietary intakes: Australian Government Department of Health and Ageing, Canberra, 2005.
Nie ZL, et al. Magnesium intake and incidence of stroke: Meta analysis of cohort studies. Nutrition, Metabolism and Cardiovascular Diseases 2013. 23:3; 169–176.
Nye C, Brice A. Combined vitamin B6-magnesium treatment in autism spectrum disorder. Cochrane Database Syst Rev 19.4 (2005): CD003497.
Nygaard IH, et al. Does oral magnesium substitution relieve pregnancy-induced leg cramps? European Journal of Obstetrics & Gynecology and Reproductive Biology 2008:141;1;23–26.
Orchard TS et al. Magnesium intake, bone mineral density, and fractures: results from the Women's Health Initiative Observational Study. Am J Clin Nutr 2014: 99;4;926–933.
Orr SL, Venkateswaran S. Nutraceuticals in the prophylaxis of pediatric migraine: Evidence-based review and recommendations. 2014 Cephalalgia. abstract available online http://www.ncbi.nlm.nih.gov/pubmed/24443395?dopt=Abstract accessed 14 th June 2014.
Paolisso G et al. Daily magnesium supplements improve glucose handling in elderly subjects. Am J Clin Nutr 55.6 (1992): 1161–1167.
Peikert A, et al. Prophylaxis of migraine with oral magnesium: results from a prospective, multi-center, placebo-controlled and double-blind randomized study. Cephalalgia 16.4 (1996): 257–263.
Pfaffenrath V et al. Magnesium in the prophylaxis of migraine: a double-blind placebo-controlled study. Cephalalgia 16.6 (1996): 436–440.
Pfeiffer S et al. Efficacy of vitamin B6 and magnesium in the treatment of autism: a methodology review and summary of outcomes. J Autism Dev Disord 25.5 (1995): 481–493.
Pinard AM, et al. Magnesium potentiates neuromuscular blockade with cisatracurium during cardiac surgery. Can J Anaesth. Feb 2003;50(2):172–178.
Quamme GA. Recent developments in intestinal magnesium absorption. Curr Opin Gastroenterol. Mar 2008;24(2):230–235.
Quaranta S et al. Pilot study of the efficacy and safety of a modified-release magnesium 250 mg tablet (Sincromag) for the treatment of premenstrual syndrome. Clin Drug Investig 27.1 (2007): 51–58.
Rasmussen HS et al. Magnesium deficiency in patients with ischemic heart disease with and without acute myocardial infarction uncovered by an intravenous loading test. Arch Intern Med 148.2 (1988): 329–332.
Rasmussen HS et al. Influence of magnesium substitution therapy on blood lipid composition in patients with ischemic heart disease: a double-blind, placebo controlled study. Arch Intern Med 149.5 (1989): 1050–1053.
Reynolds JEF et al. Martindale extra pharmacopoeia, 28th edn. London: The Pharmaceutical Press, 1982.
Rodriguez-Moran M, Guerrero-Romero F. Oral magnesium supplementation improves insulin sensitivity and metabolic control in type 2 diabetic subjects: a randomized double-blind controlled trial. Diabetes Care 26.4 (2003): 1147–1152.
Rodriguez-Moran M, Guerrero-Romero F. Oral magnesium supplementation improves the metabolic profile of metabolically obese, normal weight individuals: A randomized double blind, placebo-controlled trial. Archives of Medical Research 2014. Online http://www.sciencedirect.com/science/article/pii/S0188440914000782 accessed 12th June 2014.
Roffe C et al. Randomised, cross-over, placebo controlled trial of magnesium citrate in the treatment of chronic persistent leg cramps. Med Sci Monit 8.5 (2002): CR326–CR330.
Rosenstein DL et al. Magnesium measures across the menstrual cycle in premenstrual syndrome. Biol Psychiatry 35.8 (1994): 557–561.

Rude RK. Magnesium. In: Coates PM et al. eds. Encyclopedia of dietary supplements, 2nd edn. New York, NY: Informa Healthcare; 2010:527–37.

Rude R, Shils M. Magnesium. In: Shils M (ed), Modern nutrition in health and disease, 10th edn. Baltimore: Lippincott, Williams & Wilkins, 2006, pp 223–47.

Rude RK, et al. Skeletal and hormonal effects of magnesium deficiency. J Am Coll Nutr 2009;28(2):131–141.

Rylander R, Magnesium in pregnancy blood pressure and pre-eclampsia — A review. Pregnancy Hypertension 4, (2), 2014, 146–149.

Rylander R et al. Acid-base status affects renal magnesium losses in healthy, elderly persons. J.Nutr 136.9 (2006): 2374–2377.

Sanders GT, et al Magnesium in disease: a review with special emphasis on the serum ionized magnesium. Clin Chem Lab Med 37.11–12 (1999): 1011–1033.

Saris NE et al. Magnesium: an update on physiological, clinical and analytical aspects. Clin Chim Acta 294.1–2 (2000): 1–26.

Schwellnus M et al. Serum electrolyte concentrations and hydration status are not associated with exercise associated muscle cramping (EAMC) in distance runners. Br J Sports Med 38.4 (2004): 488.

Sedighi M et al. Low magnesium concentration in erythrocytes of children with acute asthma (abstract). Iran J Allergy Asthma Immunol 5.4 (2006): 183–186.

Shattock MJ, et al. The ionic basis of the anti-ischemic and anti-arrhythmic properties of magnesium in the heart. J Am Coll Nutr 6.1 (1987): 27–33.

Shechter M, Magnesium and cardiovascular system. Magnesium Research 2010, 23:2;60–72.

Shechter M et al. Oral magnesium supplementation inhibits platelet-dependent thrombosis in patients with coronary artery disease. Am J Cardiol 84.2 (1999): 152–156.

Shechter M et al. Oral magnesium therapy improves endothelial function in patients with coronary artery disease. Circulation 102.19 (2000): 2353–2358.

Shechter M et al. Effects of oral magnesium therapy on exercise tolerance, exercise-induced chest pain, and quality of life in patients with coronary artery disease. Am J Cardiol 91.5 (2003): 517–521.

Shils M. Experimental human magnesium depletion. AJCN 15 (1964): 133–143.

Shils M, Rude R. Deliberations and evaluations of the approaches endpoints and paradigms for magnesium dietary recommendations. J Nutr 126 (1996): 2398S–2403S.

Shils ME et al. Magnesium. In: Modern nutrition in health and disease, 9th edn. Baltimore: Williams and Wilkins, 1999; Ch 9.

Sojka JE, Weaver CM. Magnesium supplementation and osteoporosis. Nutr Rev 53.3 (1995): 71–74.

Song Y et al. Dietary magnesium intake and risk of incident hypertension among middle-aged and older US women in a 10-year follow-up study. Am J Cardiol 98.12 (2006): 1616–1621.

Song Y, et al. Magnesium intake and plasma concentrations of markers of systemic inflammation and endothelial dysfunction in women. Am J Clin Nutr 2007;85(4):1068–1074.

Sontia B, Touryz RM. Role of magnesium in hypertension. Arch Biochem Biophys 458.1 (2007): 33–39.

Stendig-Lindberg G, et al. Trabecular bone density in a two year controlled trial of perioral magnesium in osteoporosis. Magnes Res 6.2 (1993): 155–163.

Strambi M et al. Magnesium profile in autism. Biol Trace Elem Res 109.2 (2006): 97–104.

Sulzer N, et al. Serum electrolytes in Ironman triathletes with exercise-associated muscle cramping (abstract). Med Sci Sports Exerc 37.7 (2005): 1081–1085.

Swaminathan R. Magnesium metabolism and its disorders. Clin Biochem Rev 2003;24(2):47–66.

Taubert K. Magnesium in migraine: results of a multicenter pilot study. Fortschr Med 112.24 (1994): 328–330.

Thomas J et al. Free and total magnesium in lymphocytes of migraine patients: effect of magnesium-rich mineral water intake. Clin Chim Acta 295.1–2 (2000): 63–75.

Topf JM, Murray PT. Hypomagnesemia and hypermagnesemia. Rev Endocr Metab Disord. May 2003;4(2):195–206.

Tucker KL. Osteoporosis prevention and nutrition. Curr Osteoporos Rep 2009; 7:111–7.

Tucker K et al. Potassium magnesium, and fruit and vegetable intakes are associated with greater bone mineral density in elderly men and women. AJCN 69 (1999): 727–736.

Turney BW et al. Diet and risk of kidney stones in the Oxford cohort of the European Prospective Investigation into Cancer and Nutrition (EPIC). Eur J Epidemiol 2014, 29: 363–369.

Turnlund J et al. Vitamin B-6 depletion followed by repletion with animal- or plant-source diets and calcium and magnesium metabolism in young women. AJCN 56 (1992): 905–910.

Tuvemo T et al. Serum magnesium and protein concentrations during the first five years of insulin-dependent diabetes in children. Acta Paediatr 418 (Suppl) (1997): 7–10.

van Dam R et al. Dietary calcium and magnesium, major food sources, and risk of type 2 diabetes in U.S. black women. Diabetes Care 29 (2006): 2238–2243.

Vest AR, Cho LS. Hypertension in pregnancy. Cardiol Clin 2012;30(3):407–423.

Walker AF et al. Magnesium supplementation alleviates premenstrual symptoms of fluid retention. J Womens Health 7.9 (1998): 1157–1165.

Walker AF et al. Mg citrate found more bioavailable than other Mg preparations in a randomised, double-blind study. Magnes Res 16.3 (2003): 183–191.

Walti M et al. Measurement of magnesium absorption and retention in type 2 diabetic patients with the use of stable isotopes. AJCN 78 (2003): 448–453.

Wang F et al. Oral magnesium oxide prophylaxis of frequent migrainous headache in children: a randomized, double-blind, placebo-controlled trial. Headache 43.6 (2003): 601–610.

Wark, P. A., et al. Magnesium intake and colorectal tumor risk: a case-control study and meta-analysis. American Journal of Clinical Nutrition. 96(3):622–631, 2012.

Weaver CM. Calcium and magnesium requirements of children and adolescents and peak bone mass. Nutrition 16.7–8 (2000): 514–5116.

Wester P. Magnesium. AJCN 45 (1987): 1305–1312.

Whelan AM, et al. Herbs, vitamins and minerals in the treatment of premenstrual syndrome: a systematic review. Canadian Journal of Clinical Pharmacology 2009; 16;3;e 407–429.

Wilson ML, Murphy PA. Herbal and dietary therapies for primary and secondary dysmenorrhoea. Cochrane Database Syst Rev 3 (2001): CD002124.

Witteman J et al. Reduction of blood pressure with oral magnesium supplementation in women with mild to moderate hypertension. AJCN 60 (1994): 129–135.

Woods JL, et al. Malnutrition on the menu: Nutritional status of institutionalized elderly Australians in low level care. 2009 JNHA: Geriatric Science 13:8 p 693.

Woolhouse M. Migraine and tension headache — a complementary and alternative approach. Aust Fam Physician 34.8 (2005): 647–651.

Xu T, et al. Magnesium intake and cardiovascular disease mortality: A meta-analysis of prospective cohort studies. International Journal of Cardiology, 2012. 167:6:3044–3047.

Yakubova O. Relationship of connective tissue dysplasia and hypomagnesemia in genesis of juvenile dysmenorrhea. European Medical, Health and Pharmaceutical Journal 2012;3;5–6.

Yasuda H, and Tsutsui T. Assessment of infantile mineral imbalances in austism spectrum disorders (ASDs). Int J Environ Res Public Health 2013:10: 6027–6043.

Young GL, Jewell D. Interventions for leg cramps in pregnancy. Cochrane Database Syst Rev 1 (2002): CD000121.

Zeana C. Magnesium orotate in myocardial and neuronal protection. Rom J Intern Med 37.1 (1999): 91–97.

Zhang W, et al. Associations of dietary magnesium intake with mortality from cardiovascular disease: The JACC study 2012. Atherosclerosis 221;2; 587–695.

Meadowsweet

HISTORICAL NOTE Meadowsweet is a medicinal herb indigenous to Europe that has been used traditionally as an anti-inflammatory agent. The health benefits of meadowsweet may be due to the polyphenol content, which is well known for its antioxidative and anti-inflammatory characteristics (Drummond et al 2013). Meadowsweet was one of the most sacred herbs used by ancient Celtic druid priests, hundreds of years ago (Blumenthal et al 2000). Modern-day aspirin owes its origins to the salicin content isolated from meadowsweet in the early 1800s. In fact, the name aspirin relates to this herb's former genus name 'Spiracea'.

COMMON NAME

Meadowsweet

OTHER NAMES

Bridewort, dolloff, dropwort, fleur d'ulmaire, gravel root, lady of the meadow, meadow-wort, queen of the meadow, spireaeflos.

BOTANICAL NAME/FAMILY

Filipendula ulmaria (family Rosaceae)

PLANT PART USED

Aerial parts

CHEMICAL COMPONENTS

Phenolic glycosides, essential oil, tannins, mucilage, flavonoids (up to 6% in fresh flowers) and ascorbic acid. Hydrolysable tannins (rugosins A, B, D, E) (Fecka 2009). The herb also contains various salicylate constituents, including methyl salicylate, salicin and salicylic acid. Fecka (2009) states that a dose of 3 g of meadowsweet flowers yielded an average of 394.9 mg of the polyphenols, of which 265.2 mg are ellagitannins and 107.9 mg are flavonoids.

MAIN ACTIONS

Antibacterial

Bacteriostatic activity has been reported in vitro against *Staphylococcus aureus*, *S. epidermidis*, *Escherichia coli*, *Proteus vulgaris* and *Pseudomonas aeruginosa* (Rauha et al 2000). The essential oil of *Filipendula vulgaris* has been found to inhibit the growth of *Aspergillus niger*, *Candida albicans*, *Escherichia coli*, *Klebsiella pneumoniae*, *Pseudomonas aeruginosa*, *Salmonella enteritidis* and *Staphylococcus aureus* (Radulović et al 2007). It seems the antimicrobial activity of *F. vulgaris* essential oil can be attributed to the synergistic interaction of the compounds within the oil rather than to the presence of a single inhibitory agent (Radulović et al 2007).

Anti-inflammatory

Meadowsweet has been shown to reduce complement activity and T-cell activation (Drummond et al 2013).

Gastroprotective effects

In vivo tests have identified protective effects against stomach ulcers induced by acetylsalicylic acid, but no protection was seen against ulcers produced under high-acid environments or due to stimulation by histamine (Barnaulov & Denisenko 1980). Based on these observations, it appears that the effect may involve a prostaglandin (PG)-mediated mechanism.

Hepatoprotective

An in vivo trial has demonstrated the hepatoprotective and antioxidant effects of meadowsweet (Shilova et al 2006). Meadowsweet extract (70% ethanol, 100 mg/kg) was shown to improve liver function in carbon tetrachloride (CCl_4)-induced hepatitis in rats. In many parameters, the extract was shown to be more effective than Carsil, a silymarin preparation well known for its hepatoprotective ability.

OTHER ACTIONS

In vitro tests have identified antioxidant and anticoagulant activities (Calliste et al 2001, Liapina & Koval'chuk 1993).

Whether meadowsweet exerts anti-inflammatory and analgesic effects because of its high salicylate content is unknown and remains to be tested. The ethyl acetate extract of the petal of meadowsweet was investigated on whether it inhibited histidine decarboxylase (HDC) (Nitta et al 2013). HDC catalyses the formation of histamine and by controlling HDC, histamine-mediated symptoms, such as allergies and stomach ulceration, may be reduced. Future research is suggested in a clinical setting.

CLINICAL USE

Meadowsweet has not been significantly investigated under clinical trial conditions, so evidence is largely derived from traditional, in vitro and animal studies.

Supportive therapy for colds

Commission E approval for this condition is based on historical use in well-established systems of medicine, in vitro tests and animal studies (Blumenthal et al 2000).

M

Acne

Researchers believe that meadowsweet may stimulate the skin's natural immune mechanisms, reducing bacterial colonies and therefore limiting the complications of acne (Lenaers et al 2007). Volunteers used a meadowsweet preparation twice a day for 28 days and found a reduction in acne spots by 10%, an improvement in the homogeneity of the skin grain by 21% and a reduction of inflammatory lesions by 20%. Bacterial infiltration of lesions was also reduced by 22%.

Gastrointestinal symptoms

Meadowsweet is often used to treat gastrointestinal conditions associated with hyperacidity, such as gastritis, acidic dyspepsia and peptic ulceration. In vivo testing has found a decoction made from flowers of meadowsweet reduced experimentally-induced ulcers caused by acetylsalicylic acid. Additionally, it promoted healing of chronic stomach ulcers induced by ethanol (Barnaulov & Denisenko 1980). Currently, there is no evidence available to confirm an antacid activity.

Conditions associated with mild-to-moderate pain

Based on its significant salicylate content, meadowsweet is also prescribed for conditions associated with mild-to-moderate pain. However, no clinical research is available to confirm efficacy.

OTHER USES

Meadowsweet has traditionally been used as a treatment for diarrhoea based on the herb's appreciable tannin content. It has also been used for conditions associated with mild-to-moderate pain (most likely due to the herb's significant salicylate content), fever and inflammation.

DOSAGE RANGE

As no clinical trials are available to determine effective doses, the following doses are a general guideline.

- Fresh flowers: 2.5–3.5 g/day.
- Fresh herb: 4–5 g/day.
- Infusion: steep 2–3 g in 150 mL boiled water for 10 minutes and drink as hot as tolerable.
- Fluid extract (1 : 1) (g/mL): 2–3 mL/day.

TOXICITY

Not known.

ADVERSE REACTIONS

Although salicylates are present, they appear to cause less gastrointestinal irritation than acetylsalicylic acid. In fact, a meadowsweet preparation protected against acetylsalicylic acid-induced stomach ulcers in vivo (Barnaulov & Denisenko 1980).

SIGNIFICANT INTERACTIONS

Controlled studies are not available; therefore, interactions are based on evidence of activity and are largely theoretical and speculative.

Aspirin and simple analgesics

Theoretically, meadowsweet may enhance anti-inflammatory and antiplatelet effects. Observe patients taking this combination — beneficial interaction possible.

Iron

Separate doses of iron and meadowsweet by 2 hours – this is due to the tannin content of meadowsweet potentially forming an insoluble complex with iron and reducing its absorption.

Warfarin

It is uncertain whether internal use of the herb will increase bleeding risk, so it is advised to observe patients taking warfarin concurrently. The herb has been shown to exert anticoagulant activity in vitro and in vivo, but human studies combining use with warfarin have not been conducted, so the clinical significance of this theoretical interaction remains unknown (Liapina & Koval'chuk 1993).

CONTRAINDICATIONS AND PRECAUTIONS

Meadowsweet should not be taken by people with salicylate sensitivity. Suspend use of concentrated extracts 1 week before major surgery to avoid increasing bleeding risk.

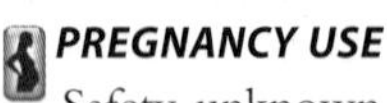

PREGNANCY USE

Safety unknown.

Practice points/Patient counselling

- Meadowsweet is traditionally used as a herbal antacid, analgesic and antipyretic, antidiarrhoeal and treatment for urinary tract infections.
- Commission E approves its use as supportive therapy for the common cold.
- It contains several different salicylates that are thought to be responsible for much of its clinical activity; however, this remains to be proven.
- Although it contains salicylates, the herb does not appear to cause significant gastrointestinal irritation and may, in fact, have anti-ulcer activity.
- People who are salicylate sensitive should not take this herbal medicine.
- In practice, it is often combined with herbs such as chamomile and marshmallow in the treatment of gastrointestinal complaints.

PATIENTS' FAQs

What will this herb do for me?

Traditionally, the herb has been used to treat gastrointestinal complaints such as dyspepsia and diarrhoea, urinary tract infections and joint aches and pains. It is also used as supportive therapy for the common cold.

When will it start to work?

Symptomatic relief should be experienced within the first few doses.

Are there any safety issues?

People who are salicylate-sensitive should not take meadowsweet. People taking anticoagulant medicines should use this herb with caution as increased bruising is theoretical possibility.

REFERENCES

Barnaulov OD, Denisenko PP. Anti-ulcer action of a decoction of the flowers of the dropwort, Filipendula ulmaria (L.) Maxim. Farmakol Toksikol 43.6 (1980): 700–705.

Blumenthal M, Goldberg A, Brinckmann J (eds). Herbal medicine: expanded commission E monographs. Austin, TX: Integrative Medicine Communications (2000).

Calliste CA et al. Free radical scavenging activities measured by electron spin resonance spectroscopy and B16 cell antiproliferative behaviors of seven plants. J Agric Food Chem 49.7 (2001): 3321–3327.

Drummond EM et al. Inhibition of Proinflammatory Biomarkers in THP1 Macrophages by Polyphenols Derived From Chamomile, Meadowsweet and Willow bark. Phytother Res 27.4 (2013): 588–594.

Fecka I. Qualitative and quantitative determination of hydrolysable tannins and other polyphenols in herbal products from meadowsweet and dog rose. Phytochem Anal. 20.3 (2009): 177–190.

Lenaers C et al. Presented at the 16(th) DGK Symposium, March 2–4, 2005, Leipzig, Germany — Received the Award for the Best Poster Presentation 1 Influencing the equilibrium of the cutaneous ecosystem to improve the properties of skin prone to acne. Int J Cosmet Sci 29.2 (2007): 143–144.

Liapina LA, Koval'chuk GA. A comparative study of the action on the hemostatic system of extracts from the flowers and seeds of the meadowsweet (Filipendula ulmaria (L.) Maxim.). Izv Akad Nauk Ser Biol 4 (1993): 625–628.

Nitta Y et al. Inhibitory activity of Filipendula ulmaria constituents on recombinant human histidine decarboxylase. Food Chem. 138.2–3 (2013): 1551–1556.

Radulović N et al. Antimicrobial synergism and antagonism of salicylaldehyde in Filipendula vulgaris essential oil. Fitoterapia 78.7–8 (2007): 565–570.

Rauha JP et al. Antimicrobial effects of Finnish plant extracts containing flavonoids and other phenolic compounds. Int J Food Microbiol 56.1 (2000): 3–12.

Shilova IV et al. Hepatoprotective and antioxidant activity of meadowsweet extract during experimental toxic hepatitis. Bull Exp Biol Med 142.2 (2006): 216–218.

Mullein

HISTORICAL NOTE Over the centuries mullein has been used in various ways. Taken internally, it has been used to treat respiratory conditions and tumours; applied topically, its use has been to relieve itch and dress wounds. It was also used to make candlewicks for casting out evil spirits. Due to its robust nature, mullein is now considered a serious weed pest of roadsides and industrial areas in countries such as the USA.

> ***Clinical note — Natural mucilages found in herbs***
> Mucilages are large, highly branched polymeric structures made from many different sugar and uronic acid units. They are hydrophilic and are capable of trapping water, causing them to swell in size and develop a gel-like consistency. The gels tend to have soothing properties and can be broken down by bowel flora when taken internally (Mills & Bone 2000). They are known to have beneficial effects on burns, wounds and ulcers when applied externally, and on gastric inflammation and irritation and diarrhoea when taken internally.

OTHER NAMES

Aaron's rod, Adam's flannel, blanket herb, bunny's ears, candlewick plant, flannel-leaf, great mullein, Jacob's staff, flannelflower, gidar tamaku, gordolobo, hare's beard, hedge taper, longwort, Our Lady's flannel, rag paper, shepherd's club, shepherd's staff, torch weed, velvet plant, wild ice leaf, woollen, woolly mullein.

BOTANICAL NAME/FAMILY

Verbascum densiflorum (syn *Verbascum thapsiforme*), *Verbascum phlomoides*, *Verbascum thapsus* (family Scrophulariaceae)

Note that although there are many species within the *Verbascum* genus utilised in various traditional medicinal systems (Akdemir et al 2011), this monograph focuses on the above three species as outlined in British Pharmacopoeia (2012).

PLANT PARTS USED

Flower — dried petals, leaves

CHEMICAL COMPONENTS

The constituents of the plant mullein include water-soluble mucilage, polysaccharides, flavonoids (including glycosides of quercetin, apigenin, luteolin, kaempferol and rutin), phenolic acids, iridoid glycosides (ajugol, harpagide and aucubin), phenylethanoid glycosides (including verbascoside), triterpene saponins (verbascosaponin) and sterols (Panchal et al 2010, Hussain et al 2009, Turker et al 2005, Georgiev et al 2011).

One of the most investigated constituents isolated from *Verbascum* spp. plants is verbascoside. Whether the pharmacological effects demonstrated for this single constituent can be extrapolated to explain those for mullein is uncertain, as the effects of any herb are due to a number of phyto-constituents and their interaction with each other and the body. As such, information about verbascoside is included here in order to provide a further insight into the herb, but it should be interpreted accordingly.

Verbascoside has also been isolated from other herbs such as *Verbena officinalis*, *Echinacea purpurea* roots, *Euphrasia pectinata*, *Phlomis longifolia*, *Pedicularis plicata*, *Duranta erecta*, *Marrubium alysson*, *Leonurus glaucescens* and *Ballota nigra* (Calis et al 1992a, 1992b, Deepak & Handa 2000, Ersoz et al 2000, 2001, Liao et al 1999, Seidel et al 2000, Sloley et al 2001, Takeda et al 1995).

MAIN ACTIONS

Mullein has not been significantly investigated under clinical trial conditions, so evidence is derived from traditional, in vitro and animal studies.

Demulcent and emollient

Traditionally, these actions were thought to occur primarily within the respiratory system, especially the lungs. However, topical preparations of mullein also exert an emollient action on the skin (Blumenthal et al 2000). This is most likely due to the herb's high mucilaginous content.

Antiviral

Mullein extract exhibits in vitro antiviral activity against fowl plague virus, several influenza A strains and influenza B strain, HSV and pseudorabies virus (Escobar et al 2012, McCutcheon et al 1995, Serkedjieva 2000, Slagowska et al 1987, Zanon et al 1999, Zgorniak-Nowosielska et al 1991). Antiviral activity has been demonstrated for both infusions and alcoholic extracts (Serkedjieva 2000).

Antibacterial

In vitro studies have demonstrated antibacterial activity for mullein extracts (aqueous, ethanol and methanol) against *Klebsiella pneumonia*, *Staphylococcus aureus*, *Staphylococcus epidermidis* and *Escherichia coli* (Turker & Camper 2002). Of the three extracts tested, the aqueous extract exhibited the strongest antibacterial action.

Anthelmintic

Crude methanolic extracts of *Verbascum thapsus* demonstrated in vitro anthelmintic activity against

Ascaridia galli (roundworm) and *Rallietina spiralis* (tapeworm) (Ali et al 2012).

Antitumour

Some plants, such as mullein, were used in folk medicine as sources of antitumour remedies. An in vitro study has identified inhibitors of protein biosynthesis in *Verbascum thapsiforme* flowers. Researchers found that a saponin glycoside and its aglycon, isolated from the flowers, directly inactivates ribosomes (Galasinski et al 1996). The constituent, verbascoside, has been shown to inhibit telomerase activity in human gastric carcinoma cells in test tube studies, resulting in inhibition of tumour growth (Zhang et al 2002). Cytotoxic effects for verbascoside have also been identified against rat hepatoma and sarcoma cells, and cytostatic activity on human epithelial carcinoma cells (Saracoglu et al 1995).

OTHER ACTIONS

The verbascoside constituent demonstrates antioxidant activity in vitro (Gao et al 1999). The saponins in mullein are thought to exert an expectorant activity; however, further investigation is required to confirm this.

CLINICAL USE

Mullein has not been subjected to significant clinical investigation; therefore, information is generally derived from traditional usage, phytochemical research or evidence of pharmacological activity. In practice, this herbal medicine is often combined with other herbs in order to strengthen clinical effects.

Chronic otitis media

To date, no controlled studies are available to determine the clinical effectiveness of mullein as a standalone treatment. However, two double-blind studies that tested a herbal combination ear-drop product (containing mullein) in children have produced positive results. The first study involved 103 children aged 6–18 years, and found that a naturopathic herbal ear drop, known commercially as Otikon (consisting of *Allium sativum*, *Verbascum thapsus*, *Calendula* flowers and *Hypericum perforatum* in olive oil), was as effective as local anaesthetic ear drops (containing ametocaine and phenazone in glycerin) in the management of ear pain associated with acute otitis media. Treatment lasted for 3 days and produced a statistically significant improvement (Sarrell et al 2001). The second was a randomised, double-blind study involving 171 children aged 5–18 years who had otalgia and clinical findings associated with middle-ear infection (Sarrell et al 2003). Children receiving herbal ear drops containing *Allium sativum*, *Verbascum thapsus*, *Calendula* flowers, *Hypericum perfoliatum*, lavender and vitamin E in olive oil achieved better pain relief than controls; however, the pain appeared to be self-limiting with significant improvements seen in all groups over 3 days. The dose used was 5 drops three times daily.

Productive and dry cough

Traditionally, mullein is combined with other demulcent or expectorant herbal medicines such as *Glycyrrhiza glabra*, *Tussilago farfara* and *Althaea officinalis* in the treatment of productive cough.

Commission E approves the use of mullein flowers for catarrhs of the respiratory tract (Blumenthal et al 2000). This is largely based on traditional use extending back to ancient times, and phytochemical investigation from in vitro and in vivo studies.

Topical use

Mullein is used topically for wounds, burns, bruises, haemorrhoids and pruritus, and to soften the skin. The high mucilage and tannin content of the herb provides a theoretical basis for its use in these situations as an antipruritic and astringent agent. The leaves are used topically to soften and protect the skin. To date, no controlled studies are available to determine its effectiveness.

OTHER USES

Mullein is included in herbal combination treatments for a variety of respiratory conditions such as bronchitis, asthma and tracheitis. Traditionally it is also used for diarrhoea, dysentery, haemorrhoids and laryngitis. In manufacturing, mullein is used as a flavouring component in alcoholic beverages.

DOSAGE RANGE

- Fluid extract (1 : 1): 1.5–2 mL twice daily.
- Tincture (1 : 5): 7.5–10 mL twice daily.
- Dried leaf: 12–24 g/day.
- Decoction: 1.5–2 g of herb in 250 mL of cold water, brought to the boil for 10 minutes, taken twice daily.

ADVERSE REACTIONS

A case of contact dermatitis has been reported (Romaguera et al 1985).

SIGNIFICANT INTERACTIONS

Controlled studies are not available.

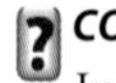

CONTRAINDICATIONS AND PRECAUTIONS

Insufficient reliable information is available.

PREGNANCY USE

Insufficient reliable information is available; however, Commission E states that no restrictions are known (Blumenthal et al 2000).

PATIENTS' FAQs

What will this herb do for me?

Mullein has been used since ancient times as a treatment for productive coughs and catarrhal states. In modern times, it is also used to treat chronic otitis media, and has antiviral action against influenza virus and HSV. Currently, more scientific investigation is required to confirm efficacy for these indications.

When will it start to work?

Mullein has not been subjected to significant clinical investigation so it is unclear.

Are there any safety issues ?

None are currently known.

Practice points/Patient counselling

- Mullein flowers have been used since ancient times as an expectorant and anticatarrhal agent in conditions of productive cough and respiratory infections.
- It is most commonly used in combination with other demulcent and expectorant herbal medicines in the treatment of productive and dry cough.
- In vitro studies have identified antiviral and antibacterial activity.
- Mullein has not been subjected to significant clinical investigation; therefore, information is generally derived from traditional usage or evidence of pharmacological activity. As such, Commission E approves its use for catarrhs of the respiratory tract.
- Used in the form of a herbal combination ear drop, significant anaesthetic activity has been demonstrated.

REFERENCES

Akdemir Z et al. Bioassay-guided isolation of anti-inflammatory, antinociceptive and wound healer glycosides from the flowers of Verbascum mucronatum Lam. J Ethnopharmacol 136 (2011): 436–443.

Ali N et al. Anthelmintic and relaxant activities of Verbascum Thapsus Mullein. BMC complementary and alternative medicine, 12 (2012): 29.

Blumenthal M et al. (eds). Herbal medicine: expanded Commission E monographs. Austin, TX: Integrative Medicine Communications, 2000.

British Pharmacopoeia, Mullein, vol IV (2012).

Calis I et al. Phenylpropanoid glycosides from Marrubium alysson. Phytochemistry 31.10 (1992a): 3624–3626.

Calis I et al. Two phenylpropanoid glycosides from Leonurus glaucescens. Phytochemistry 31.1 (1992b): 357–359.

Deepak M, SS Handa. Antiinflammatory activity and chemical composition of extracts of Verbena officinalis. Phytother Res 14.6 (2000): 463–465.

Ersoz T et al. An iridoid glucoside from Euphrasia pectinata. J Nat Prod 63.10 (2000): 1449–1450.

Ersoz T et al. Iridoid and phenylethanoid glycosides from Phlomis longifolia var. longifolia. Nat Prod Lett 15.5 (2001): 345–351.

Escobar MF et al. Antiviral effect and mode of action of methanolic extract of Verbascum thapsus L. on pseudorabies virus (strain RC/79). Natural Product Research, 26:17 (2012): 1621–1625.

Galasinski W et al. The substances of plant origin that inhibit protein biosynthesis. Acta Pol Pharm 53.5 (1996): 311–318.

Gao JJ et al. Radical scavenging activity of phenylpropanoid glycosides in Caryopteris incana. Biosci Biotechnol Biochem 63.6 (1999): 983–988.

Georgiev MI et al. Metabolic differentiations and classification of Verbascum species by NMR-based metabolomics. Phytochemistry, 72 (2011) 2045–2051.

Hussain H et al. Minor chemical constituents of Verbascum thapsus. Biochemical Systematics and Ecology, 37 (2009): 124–126.

Liao F et al. Retardation of skeletal muscle fatigue by the two phenylpropanoid glycosides: verbascoside and martynoside from Pedicularis plicata maxim. Phytother Res 13.7 (1999): 621–623.

McCutcheon AR et al. Antiviral screening of British Columbian medicinal plants. J Ethnopharmacol 49.2 (1995): 101–110.

Mills S, Bone K. Principles and practice of phytotherapy. London: Churchill Livingstone, 2000.

Panchal MA et al. 2010. Pharmacological properties of Verbascum thapsus — A review. International Journal of Pharmaceutical Sciences Review and Research, 5, 73–77.

Romaguera C et al. Occupational dermatitis from Gordolobo (Mullein). Contact Dermatitis 12.3 (1985): 176.

Saracoglu I et al. Studies on constituents with cytotoxic and cytostatic activity of two Turkish medicinal plants Phlomis armeniaca and Scutellaria salviifolia. Biol Pharm Bull 18.10 (1995): 1396–1400.

Sarrell EM et al. Naturopathic treatment for ear pain in children. Pediatrics 111.5 (Pt 1) (2003): e574–e579.

Sarrell EM et al. Efficacy of naturopathic extracts in the management of ear pain associated with acute otitis media. Arch Pediatr Adolesc Med 155.7 (2001): 796–799.

Seidel V et al. Phenylpropanoids from Ballota nigra L. inhibit in vitro LDL peroxidation. Phytother Res 14.2 (2000): 93–98.

Serkedjieva J. Combined antiinfluenza virus activity of Flos verbasci infusion and amantadine derivatives. Phytother Res 14.7 (2000): 571–574.

Slagowska A, Zgorniak-Nowosielska I, Grzybek J. Inhibition of herpes simplex virus replication by Flos verbasci infusion. Pol J Pharmacol Pharm 39.1 (1987): 55–61.

Sloley BD et al. Comparison of chemical components and antioxidants capacity of different Echinacea species. J Pharm Pharmacol 53.6 (2001): 849–857.

Takeda Y et al. Iridoid glucosides from the leaves and stems of Duranta erecta. Phytochemistry 39.4 (1995): 829–833.

Turker AU, Camper ND. Biological activity of common mullein, a medicinal plant. J Ethnopharmacol 82.2–3 (2002): 117–125.

Turker A U, Gurel E. 2005. Common Mullein (Verbascum thapsus L.): Recent advances in research. Phytotherapy Research, 19, 733–739.

Zanon SM et al. Search for antiviral activity of certain medicinal plants from Cordoba, Argentina. Rev Latinoam Microbiol 41.2 (1999): 59–62.

Zgorniak-Nowosielska I et al. Antiviral activity of Flos verbasci infusion against influenza and Herpes simplex viruses. Arch Immunol Ther Exp (Warsz) 39.1–2 (1991): 103–108.

Zhang F et al. In vitro modulation of telomerase activity, telomere length and cell cycle in MKN45 cells by verbascoside. Planta Med 68.2 (2002): 115–118.

Myrrh

HISTORICAL NOTE Myrrh is the resin that seeps out of the secretory tissue in the bark of the *Commiphora* plant and has been considered an important medicinal product throughout the Middle East, China and India since biblical times. Because of its antimicrobial activity, myrrh has historically been used, alone and in combination with other herbs, to treat infections and inflammations of the oral cavity, in purification rituals, to embalm bodies, dress infected wounds and as a treatment for leprosy. Myrrh was one botanical ingredient in ocular applications from the Pharaonic pharmacopoeia of Egypt (Murube 2013) and in combination with aniseed, fennel, thyme and parsley, sweet myrrh was in one of the earliest formulations for a theriac (ointment or potion to antidote poisonous bites from wild animals), detailed on a stone in the Temple of Asclepios on the Kos island (Karaberopoulos et al 2012).

COMMON NAME

Myrrh

OTHER NAMES

Abyssinian myrrh, bal, bol, common myrrh, heerabol, hirabol myrrh, gum myrrh tree, gummi myrrh, Somali myrrh, Yemen myrrh

BOTANICAL NAME/FAMILY

Genus: Commiphora
Species: There are over 150 species of Commiphora. The three species most used medicinally are:
Commiphora molmol (commonly farmed species)
Commiphora myrrha (native to Yemen, Somalia, Eritrea and Ethiopia)
Commiphora mukul guggul (native to India, used in Ayurveda)
Family: Burseraceae

PLANT PARTS USED

Essential oil (called oleoresin), gum resin, stem, leaves

CHEMICAL COMPONENTS

More than 300 molecules have been identified in this genus, including a diverse range of secondary metabolites, such as terpenoids, steroids, flavonoids, sugars and lignans (Shen et al 2012). Myrrh contains three main components: gum resin 30–60% (containing polysaccharides and proteins), alcohol-soluble resins 20–40% and volatile oils (2–10%) (composed of steroids, sterols and terpenes).

Sesquiterpenes have been identified as active constituents in the volatile oil. Resins are sticky, water-insoluble substances that are secreted where a plant is damaged by incision or natural causes. The viscous substance hardens shortly after secretion, but may be returned to a liquid state with heating. Resins tend to be soluble in alcohol. Each species has its unique constituent profile, which contribute to their specific therapeutic actions.

C. molmol oleo-gum resin contains volatile oils, resins and gum. Resins contain a wide range of constituents, including commiphoric acids and compesterol. The gum constituents include arabinose, galactose and xylose (Al-Harbi et al 1997). *C. molmol* is known for its anti-inflammatory, antipyretic and antihistamine effects (Al-Harbi et al 1997). *C. mol mol* and *C. myrrha* are known for their antiparasitic actions.

Four new sesquiterpenes have been isolated from the resin of *C. myrrha*, called myrrhterpenoids K-N(1-4) (Xu et al 2012). Triterpenoids have also been identified in *C. myrrha*.

Guggulipid is extracted from guggul, oleo-gum-resin exudate from *C. mukul*. It contains plant sterols (guggulsterones E and Z), thought to be its main pharmacologically active constituents (Ulbricht et al 2005). Diterpenoids, such as camphorene, and steroids have been identified in guggul (Shen et al 2012). This species is known for its actions as an anti-inflammatory and lipid-lowering agent and for its role in obesity management.

MAIN ACTIONS

Antiseptic

Antifungal and antibacterial activities have been observed in vitro against standard pathogenic strains of *Escherichia coli*, *Staphylococcus aureus*, *Pseudomonas aeruginosa* and *Candida albicans* (Dolara et al 2000). The oleo-gum-resin of *C. mukul* was shown to be comparable to kanamycin against both Gram-positive and Gram-negative bacteria in vitro (Saeed & Sabir 2004). Myrrh essential oil (species not identified in abstract) demonstrated some antifungal activity against *C. albicans* isolates in vitro (Carvalhinho et al 2012).

Antiparasitic

The use of *C. molmol* as an antiparasitic agent in Egypt resumed in the 1990s after numerous studies provided good evidence; however, the mode of action is still unclear (Abdul-Ghani et al 2009). The preparation called *Mirazid*, an oleo-resin containing 300 mg of purified *C. molmol*, has proven to be 100% effective against *Giardia lamblia* in rats, and had effect on hepatic coccidiosis induced by the parasite *Eimeria stiedae* in rabbits (Shen et al 2012). It was also considered to be effective against heterophyiasis with an animal study reporting a 100% reduction in worm load after 3 days (Fathy et al 2005).

Antiparasitic effects have been shown against *Schistosoma mansoni* in mouse livers in vitro (Hamed & Hetta 2005). Liver enzymes were significantly decreased after treatment with myrrh (*C. molmol*), while ova and worms' numbers were noticeably decreased. An in vivo study in the same year also produced promising results (Massoud et al 2005). Myrrh (500 mg/kg) was given for 5 days, 8 weeks postinfection. The animals were sacrificed after 12 weeks from the beginning of the experiment and myrrh was found to be comparable to cremophor EL, both producing approximate normal liver histology as compared to untreated animals. Another study compared the toxicity of myrrh to the commonly used antischistosoma drug Praziquantel. Praziquantel is well known for its toxicity and it would be a distinct advantage if another safer product could be found. The researchers reported that myrrh is a safe and promising alternative without hepatotoxic, genotoxic and carcinogenic consequences.

Lipid-lowering effects

Several mechanisms of action are responsible for this effect. The guggulsterones act as antagonists of the bile-acid receptor and of the farnesoid X receptor (FXR), which are involved in bile-acid regulation and cholesterol metabolism. Crude guggul contains ion-exchange resins that may remove bile from the intrahepatic circulation (Urizar et al 2002, Wu et al

2002). Additionally, two diterpenoids have been identified which act on pancreatic enzymes (PLA2) to control absorption of fat and cholesterol from the gastrointestinal tract (Shen et al 2012).

According to one review, 11 clinical studies have generally demonstrated that guggulipid from *C. mukul* significantly reduces triglyceride and total cholesterol levels; however, results from a recent double-blind randomised study were negative (Ulbricht et al 2005). Conflicting clinical results in the effects on total cholesterol, HDL, TG and LDL levels may be due to administration of different *C. mukul* materials (Shen et al 2012).

Anti-diabetic

A recent review (Shen et al 2012) detailed the evidence for the use of *C. mukul* for diabetes. The ethanolic resin extract of *C. mukul* exhibited anti-hyperglycaemic and antioxidant effects in diabetic rat models. Guggulsterones 21 and 22 were identified as protective for the pancreatic beta cell function and prevented any impairment of glucose-stimulated insulin secretion. In vivo studies showed 21 and 22 reduced plasma insulin and blood glucose levels, and increased the glycogen content in induced DM2 models with high fat diets. Additionally, the antidiabetic target G6Pase has been inferred by 21 and 22 (Shen et al 2012).

Anti-inflammatory

Myrrhanol A, a triterpene isolated from *C. mukul* gum resin, produces potent anti-inflammatory activity, as observed in an animal model of inflammation. In this study, anti-inflammatory activity was more marked than that of hydrocortisone (Kimura et al 2001). An animal model of rheumatoid arthritis (RA) confirmed significant anti-inflammatory effects with oral administration, also resulting in decreased joint swelling (Sharma & Sharma 1977). The essential oil of myrrh has also been shown to inhibit IL-6, probably due to down-regulating PGE_2 production, but not via nuclear factor kappaB inhibition in human gingival fibroblasts (Tipton et al 2006). Conversely, guggulsterone from *C. mukul* has demonstrated anti-inflammatory effects by decreasing nuclear factor kappaB and therefore tumour cell-induced osteoclastogenesis in vitro (Ichikawa & Aggarwal 2006).

Ethanolic and petroleum ether extracts of *C. myrrha* both demonstrated analgesic and anti-inflammatory activities in mice studies, providing some evidence to support the traditional use of myrrh for inflammatory pain (Su et al 2011). A water extraction of powdered resin of myrrh displayed anti-inflammatory and analgesic activities in mice models of inflammation. A combination of *C. myrrha* and *Boswellia carterii* (frankincense) demonstrated more potent anti-inflammatory and analgesic effect than the single herb. The suggested mechanism was the inhibition of inflammatory mediator overproduction, including nitrite and PGEs (Su et al 2012).

Anti-oxidant

Essentially oil of *C. myrrha* showed potent antioxidant activity, and exceeded that of α-tocopherol. The furano ring of *C. myrrha* constituents (namely furano sesquiterpenoids) reacted with singlet oxygen as the mechanism for the antioxidant activity. Three furano sesquiterpenoids showed significant radical scavenging activity (Shen et al 2012).

An emulsion of *C. molmol* displayed protective effects in rabbits poisoned with lead. The study showed that the rabbits given 50 mg/kg of *C. molmol* emulsion were protected from lead-induced hepatic oxidative damage and immunotoxicity, via reducing lipid peroxidation and enhancing antioxidant and immune defences (Ashry et al 2010).

Local anaesthetic

Several compounds found within myrrh exert local anaesthetic activity, chiefly by blocking the inward sodium current across membranes (Dolara et al 2000).

OTHER ACTIONS

Antispasmodic

One major component, T-cadinol, and several minor components possess smooth muscle-relaxing properties according to ex vivo tests (Andersson et al 1997, Claeson et al 1991).

Increases glucose tolerance

An extract of myrrh effectively increased glucose tolerance in both normal and diabetic rats (Al-Awadi & Gumaa 1987). Guggulipid (20 g/kg) improved glucose tolerance in another in vivo study (Cornick et al 2008). The purified ethyl ester of commipheric acid (150 mg/kg, twice daily) also lowered fasting blood glucose, insulin and triglycerides, leading researchers to propose that this constituent may be at least partly responsible for the antidiabetic effects; however, oral bioavailability is poor.

Local astringent and enhanced wound healing

Myrrh has astringent activity, promotes tissue granulation and enhances wound healing (Blumenthal 2000). In mice studies, myrrh (*C. molmol*) suspension promoted healing and repair of damaged (buccal) tissue over a 2-week period at low concentration (0.2% myrrh in sodium chloride solution). The mice had surgical incisions imposed on their buccal mucosa, which was irrigated every second day with the myrrh solution (Al-Mobeeriek 2011).

Chemoprotective

In vitro tests of myrrh-terpenoids K-N 1 and 4 from *C. myrrha*, on dopaminergic neuroblastoma cells, exhibited some neuroprotective effects without any cytotoxicity (Xu et al 2012). Another study showed guggulsterone from *C. mukul* was cardioprotective through its antioxidative activity against a potent anti-neoplastic drug (doxorubicin) in vitro (Wang et al 2012).

Antiproliferative/anticancer

A study of the protective effects of *C. molmol* against nitrosamine-induced hepatocarcinogenesis in rats showed that it did not prevent or delay the progression of hepatocarcinogenesis. Additionally, the study showed that, unlike earlier studies showing the contrary, *C. molmol* did not improve biochemical parameters nor the histological profile regarding antitumour efficacy, but actually negatively affected them (El-Shahat et al 2012).

CLINICAL USE

Topical treatment of oral or pharyngeal inflammation

Often used as a component of gargles, mouthwashes or paints for these indications, there are few controlled clinical trials or in vitro studies on the effects of myrrh on cells derived from the human oral cavity. A 2003 in vitro study investigating the effects of myrrh oil on a number of key cells implicated in gingivitis found that low concentrations of myrrh oil reduced gingival fibroblast production of proinflammatory cytokines and, therefore, the participation of these cells in gingival inflammation associated with gingivitis and periodontitis (Tipton et al 2003). This is thought to be, at least in part, due to inhibition of PGE_2. Taheri et al (2011) report that myrrh resin has potential use as a topical preparation in dentistry for small wound treatment, anodyne for the buccal cavity or for oropharyngeal infections, by soothing and astringing inflamed tissues of the oral cavity and throat (Taheri et al 2011). Commission E approved myrrh for these indications (Blumenthal 2000).

External treatment of minor inflammatory conditions and wounds

Myrrh is incorporated into salves and topical preparations for the treatment of bed sores, minor wounds and haemorrhoids. Although no clinical trials are available, the antimicrobial, anti-inflammatory, astringent and local anaesthetic activities of myrrh provide a theoretical basis for efficacy.

Osteoarthritis

A small, uncontrolled trial of *C. mukul* for patients with osteoarthritis ($n = 30$) demonstrated that treatment with 500 mg (3.5% guggulsterones) of the herb, three times daily for 2 months resulted in reduced joint inflammation, swelling and pain (Singh et al 2003). Although this suggests that the effects may be clinically significant, further investigation is required.

Hyperlipidaemia, hypercholesterolaemia, hypertriglyceridaemia

Various RCTs have investigated the effects of guggulipid on high-blood levels of lipids, cholesterol and triglycerides with inconsistent results. Overall, effects seem to be more likely in Indian populations than people eating Western diets; however, the reason for the discrepancy is unknown. A review of nonpharmacological treatments of cardiovascular diseases suggested that guggulipid (*C. mukul*) merits further clinical research; however, it was not recommended for the treatment of dyslipidaemia, due to the non-significant and often paradoxical results in Western populations according to double-blind trials and also due to concerns about bioavailability of concomitantly administered propanolol and diltiazem (Houston et al 2009).

Szapary et al (2003) conducted a double-blind, placebo-controlled, randomised trial with 103 subjects with LDL cholesterol levels of 3.37–5.19 mmol/L. A standardised dose of 1000 mg of guggulipid (containing 2.5% guggulsterones) was given to one treatment group, while a higher standardised dose of 2000 mg was given to the other, three times daily for 8 weeks. Results showed a decrease of LDL cholesterol in the placebo group of 5%, an increase of 4% in the 1000 mg group and an increase of 5% in the 2000 mg group. Overall, this constituted a 9% and a 10% increase in LDL cholesterol with guggulipid treatment. By comparison, several randomised clinical trials and in vivo tests using various extracts of guggul have reported significant lowering of total cholesterol, triglycerides and LDL cholesterol levels and increases in HDL cholesterol (Gopal et al 1986, Malhotra et al 1977, Nityanand et al 1989, Singh et al 1990). In two reports, the duration of the lipid-lowering effect continued for 6–20 weeks after discontinuation of therapy (Gopal et al 1986, Nityanand et al 1989). One clinical study showed that the lipid-lowering effects of a preparation of guggul fraction A (1.5 g/day) were similar to clofibrate (2 g/day) (Malhotra et al 1977). A larger study of 235 volunteers, conducted under double-blind randomised conditions, showed that patients with hypercholesterolaemia responded better to guggulipid (1.5 g/day) than to clofibrate (1.5 g/day). However, those with hypertriglyceridaemia responded better to clofibrate (Nityanand et al 1989). Many of these trials have been criticised for being small and methodologically flawed or poorly reported (Ulbricht et al 2005).

However, a more recent review stated a difference in opinion and concluded that the trials were of reasonable quality (Singh et al 2007). They found that over 80% of trials using guggul produced favorable results. A 2009 placebo-controlled RCT conducted in Norway ($n = 43$) using 2160 mg guggul (4 caps) daily over 12 weeks resulted in a significant reduction in total cholesterol and HDL-C, with no significant changes to LDL-C, triglycerides and total cholesterol/HDL-C ratios over placebo. Authors concluded that the clinical significance of reducing total cholesterol or HDL-C around 3–6% was questionable, especially because the ratio between them remained unchanged. Additionally, there were reported side effects from 10 of the guggul users, including GIT discomfort, thyroid problems and generalised skin rash (Nohr et al 2009).

Again, more large-scale clinical trials need to be done to assess the efficacy of guggulipid in hypercholesterolaemia.

OTHER USES

Traditional indications

Myrrh has been used in traditional medicine in China, Tibet, Ayurveda, the Middle East and Europe and consequently has numerous traditional indications. Myrrh has been used to treat infections, respiratory conditions, mouth ulcers, gingivitis, pharyngitis, respiratory catarrh, dysmenorrhoea, amenorrhoea, menopausal symptoms, wounds and haemorrhoids. It has also been used to treat arthritis and as an embalming agent.

Parasitic diseases

Schistosomiasis

Schistosomiasis is an important trematode infection affecting over 200 million people in the tropics and subtropics (Kumar & Clark 2002). After malaria, it is the next most important parasitic disease with chronic infection causing significant morbidity. Currently, the drug praziquantel is often recommended, but it does not affect the immature stage and may not abort an early infection. Additionally, a drug-resistant strain has developed (Beers & Berkow 2003). Due to these factors, there is great interest in discovering alternative treatments.

One clinical study involving 204 patients with schistosomiasis produced impressive results with a 3-day oral dose regimen producing a cure rate of 92% (Sheir et al 2001). Re-treatment of non-responders increased the overall cure rate to 98%. A field study produced similar results with 97.4% of subjects infected with the *Schistosoma haematobium* strain and 96.2% infected with the *S. mansoni* strain successfully clearing the parasite after ingesting 1200 mg of *Commiphora molmol* daily for 6 days (Abo-Madyan et al 2004a). However, two randomised trials, controlled with the drug praziquantel, have both shown little effectiveness of myrrh against the parasite (Barakat et al 2005, Botros et al 2005).

A 2009 review identified some discrepancies in the published clinical trials of myrrh's effect against *schistosomes*. One large open-label field trial (n = 1091) found that a 600-mg dose of commercial myrrh preparation (Mirazid) on an empty stomach 1 hour before breakfast for 6 consecutive days was effective against both types of schistosomiasis in Egypt, with cure rates of 97.4% and 96.2% for *S. haematobium* and *S. mansoni* respectively. Despite many initial studies showing great success of myrrh, subsequent multicentre investigations and RCTs comparing commercial myrrh with the conventional drug praziquantel have suggested myrrh cure rates were not as efficient against worms and their eggs as originally believed. However, these clinical trials involved dosing regimens of two administrations of a commercially-available myrrh product, over a 3-week period; significantly less than the earlier studies affirming its efficacy. A re-evaluation of myrrh as a schistosomicidal was recommended (Abdul-Ghani et al 2009).

Fascioliasis

Human fascioliasis occurs in Europe, Africa, China and South America and is an infection with *Fasciola hepatica*, which is acquired by eating contaminated watercress. The flukes mature in the bile ducts and cause biliary tract obstruction and liver damage (Beers & Berkow 2003).

A small study of seven infected patients found that treatment with myrrh over 6 consecutive days produced alleviation of all symptoms and signs, and a dramatic drop in egg count, with eggs no longer detected 3 weeks after treatment (Massoud et al 2001a). Furthermore, high-eosinophil counts elevated liver enzymes and *Fasciola* antibody titres returned to normal. A field study showed that myrrh (1200 mg daily for 6 days) cleared the parasite in 94.1% of infected people at the 3-month follow-up (Abo-Madyan et al 2004b). A 2009 review, drawing from promising results of myrrh in animal studies, clinical trials and field studies, concluded that myrrh is an excellent fasciolicidal drug free of side effects (Abdul-Ghani et al 2009).

Heterophycide

Heterophyes heterophyes is a common Egyptian parasite (fluke) which finds an intermediate host in snails and fish. A review detailed that, both clinically and experimentally, myrrh (in the commercial form of Mirazid made from *C. molmol*) was effective. The clinical study used a dose of 300 mg twice daily for 9 consecutive days after overnight fasting and had a 94% efficacy in the first instance (Abdul-Ghani et al 2009).

Dicrocoeliasis

Dicrocoelium dendriticum is a small liver fluke that infects animals and humans after ingestion of an infected second intermediate host (i.e. an ant) through raw vegetables or herbs or in drinking water. A number of both small and larger human studies, using 600 mg Mirazid/kg 1 hour before breakfast daily for 6 days, demonstrated efficacy in clearing the fluke in both stool analysis and clinical symptoms (Abdul-Ghani et al 2009).

> ***Historical note — Myrrh and mummification***
> Chemical treatments were an essential part of the mummification process in ancient Egypt. Several different plant products were used in the process, one of which was oil of myrrh. Interestingly, modern-day research has discovered that the oil has molluscicidal properties against several Egyptian snail species, suggesting that it may have been a wise choice for protecting mummified remains against destruction (Allam et al 2001).

Mosquitocidal

The oil and oleo-resin from the plant extract of *C. molmol* exhibit larvicidal activity against *Culex pipiens* larvae (Massoud et al 2001b).

Acne

Three months' treatment with guggulipid (equivalent to 25 mg guggulsterone) was found to be as effective as tetracycline in the treatment of nodulocystic acne in a randomised clinical study of 20 patients (Thappa & Dogra 1994).

Ulcerative colitis (UC) — in combination

Maintenance of UC remission was tested (n = 96) using a blend of 100 mg myrrh (species not specified), 70 mg chamomile extract and 50 mg coffee charcoal (3 × 4/day) over 12 months in a randomised, double-blind, double-dummy, multicentre, non-inferiority study, comparing it with mesalamine 500 mg (3 × 1/day). The herbal blend demonstrated efficacy and safety comparable to gold standard pharmaceutical treatment, and is an alternative option for maintenance therapy of UC (Langhorst et al 2011).

DOSAGE RANGE

Internal preparations — *Commiphora molmol*

- Fluid extract (1 : 1) (g/mL): 2 mL/day.
- Tincture (1 : 5): 0.5–2 mL three times daily.
- Commercial tablet Mirazid 300 mg twice daily.

Internal preparations — guggulipid

- Acne: a dose equivalent to 25 mg guggulsterone taken once to twice daily.
- Hyperlipidaemia — 500–1000 mg of standardised guggulipid administered two to three times daily.
- (Guggulipid preparations are often standardised to 2.5–5% of guggulsterones.)

External preparations

- Tincture (1 : 5) (g/mL) in 90% ethanol can be used in different concentrations to produce different therapeutic products.
- Mouthwash or gargle: 30–60 drops tincture in a glass of warm water.
- Paint: the undiluted tincture can be applied directly to gums or mucous membranes of the mouth two to three times a day.

TOXICITY

A dose of 10 mg/kg/day was given to subjects in one study with no serious adverse effects (Sheir et al 2001). *C. myrrha* and *C. molmol* are considered free from hepatotoxic, genotoxic and carcinogenic effects, even after long-term use. However, high doses (3.139 mg/kg) of the preparation Mirazid was acutely toxic (Abdul-Ghani et al 2009). Combining *C. molmol* with nitrosamine (diethylnitrosamine (DENA)) increased the rate of hepatocarcinogenesis in rats.

ADVERSE REACTIONS

Restlessness, mild abdominal discomfort and gastrointestinal symptoms, such as diarrhoea and nausea, have been reported, mainly with orally-administered extracts. Allergic dermatitis has also been reported for topical usage. Skin rash and possible thyroid problems were recorded in a small percentage of people in a trial using guggul internally (Nohr et al 2009). The standardised guggulsterone (guggulipid) preparations tend to be far better tolerated.

SIGNIFICANT INTERACTIONS

Interactions are theoretical and based on in vitro and in vivo data; therefore, clinical significance is unclear and remains to be confirmed.

Diabetic medication

In vivo studies suggest myrrh (*C. mukul*) may have hypoglycaemic effects and therefore would have additive effects with diabetic medications. Changes in serum glucose in patients taking these medications should therefore be monitored.

Lipid-lowering medication

Guggul may have cholesterol-lowering activity and therefore have additive effects with other lipid-lowering medications — observe patients taking this combination and monitor drug requirements. Beneficial interaction is possible.

Anticoagulant and antiplatelet medication

Guggul inhibited platelet aggregation in vitro and in a clinical study; therefore, concurrent use may theoretically increase the risk of bruising and bleeding (Bordia & Chuttani 1979) and interfere with anticoagulant medications, particularly in geriatric clients (Zarowitz 2010). It is uncertain what implications this observation has for *C. molmol* use. Observe patients taking these combinations.

Diltiazem

Reduced efficacy possible. A clinical study confirmed that guggulipid reduces bioavailability of this medicine (Dalvi et al 1994). It is uncertain what implications this observation has for *C. molmol* use. Observe patients taking this combination.

Propranolol

Reduced efficacy possible. A clinical study confirmed that guggulipid reduces bioavailability of this medicine (Dalvi et al 1994). It is uncertain what implications this observation has for *C. molmol* use. Observe patients taking this combination.

CONTRAINDICATIONS AND PRECAUTIONS

Do not use in cases of known allergy. Suspend use of guggul preparations 1 week before major surgery.

PREGNANCY USE

Safety is unknown.

Practice points/Patient counselling

- Myrrh has been used since ancient times in a variety of forms as an antiseptic, anti-inflammatory and analgesic medicine.
- It has been used as a topical preparation to reduce inflammation and enhance wound healing — in vivo evidence suggests that the anti-inflammatory activity of one of the main constituents is stronger than hydrocortisone and local anaesthetic activity is likely.
- Preliminary evidence suggests that it may be a useful treatment in gingivitis and periodontal disease.
- The preparation known as guggulipid, which comes from *Commiphora* species, may have lipid-lowering effects according to clinical studies; however, evidence is contradictory and further research is required to confirm this.
- Myrrh may interact with a number of medications when used orally.

PATIENTS' FAQs

What will this herb do for me?

Traditionally, the herb has been used as a mouthwash or topical paint to relieve symptoms of mouth ulcers, sore throats and gum disease. It has also been used as a topical application for inflamed skin conditions and wounds. Scientific research confirms antiseptic, anti-inflammatory and local anaesthetic effects and significant antiparasitic effects. The preparation known as guggulipid, which comes from *Commiphora* species, may lower total cholesterol levels.

When will it start to work?

A mouthwash or paint should provide rapid symptom relief.

Antiparasitic activity has been reported within 3 days' use in some parasitic infestations.

The lipid-lowering effects of guggulipid have been reported within 12 weeks.

Are there any safety issues?

The herb should not be taken during pregnancy until safety is confirmed. It may interact with some medications.

REFERENCES

Abdul-Ghani RA et al. Myrrh and trematodoses in Egypt: An overview of safety, efficacy and effectiveness profiles, Parasitology International 58 (2009): 210–214.

Abo-Madyan AA et al. Efficacy of Myrrh in the treatment of schistosomiasis (haematobium and mansoni) in Ezbet El-Bakly, Tamyia Center, El-Fayoum Governorate, Egypt. J Egypt Soc Parasit 34.2 (2004a): 423–46.

Abo-Madyan AA et al. Clinical trial of Mirazid in treatment of human fascioliasis, Ezbet El-Bakly (Tamyia Center) Al-Fayoum Governorate. J Egypt Soc Parasit 34.3 (2004b): 807–818.

Al-Awadi FM, Gumaa KA. Studies on the activity of individual plants of an antidiabetic plant mixture. Acta Diabetol Lat 24.1 (1987): 37–41.

Allam AF et al. Laboratory assessment of the molluscicidal activity of Commiphora molmol (Myrrh) on Biomphalaria alexandrina, Bulinus truncatus and Lymnaea cailliaudi. J Egypt Soc Parasitol 31.3 (2001): 683–690.

Al-Harbi, MM et al. Gastric antiulcer and cytoprotective effect of Commiphora molmol in rats. J Ethnopharmacol 55 (1997): 141–150.

Al-Mobeeriek A. Effects of myrrh on intra-oral mucosal wounds compared with tetracycline- and chlorhexidine-based mouthwashes, Clin Cosmet Investig Dent. 3 (2011): 53–58.

Andersson M et al. Minor components with smooth muscle relaxing properties from scented myrrh (Commiphora guidotti). Planta Med 63.3 (1997): 251–254.

Ashry KM et al. Oxidative stress and immunotoxic effects of lead and their amelioration with myrrh (Commiphora molmol) emulsion. Food Chem Toxicol 48 (2010): 236–241.

Barakat R et al. Efficacy of myrrh in the treatment of human schistosomiasis mansoni. Am J Trop Med Hyg 73.2 (2005): 365–367.

Beers MH, Berkow R (eds). The Merck manual of diagnosis and therapy, 17th edn; Rahway, NJ: Merck and C, 2003.

Bordia A, Chuttani SK. Effect of gum guggulu on fibrinolysis and platelet adhesiveness in coronary heart disease. Indian J Med Res 70 (1979): 992–996.

Blumenthal M (ed). Herbal medicine expanded commission E monographs. Austin, TX: Integrative Medicine Communications, 2000.

Botros S et al. Efficacy of mirazid in comparison with praziquantel in Egyptian Schistosoma mansoni-infected school children and households. Am J Trop Med Hyg 72.2 (2005): 119–123.

Carvalhinho S et al. Susceptibilities of Candida albicans mouth isolates to antifungal agents, essential oils and mouth rinses, Mycopathologia, 174.1 (2012): 69–76.

Claeson P et al. T-cadinol: a pharmacologically active constituent of scented myrrh: introductory pharmacological characterization and high field ^{1}H- and ^{13}C-NMR data. Planta Med 57.4 (1991): 352–356.

Cornick CL et al. Identification of a novel agonist of peroxisome proliferator-activated receptors alpha and gamma that may contribute to the anti-diabetic activity of guggulipid in Lep(ob)/Lep(ob) mice. J Nutr Biochem (2008) [epub ahead of print].

Dalvi SS et al. Effect of gugulipid on bioavailability of diltiazem and propranolol. J Assoc Physicians India 42.6 (1994): 454–455.

Dolara P et al. Local anaesthetic, antibacterial and antifungal properties of sesquiterpenes from myrrh. Planta Med 66.4 (2000): 356–358.

El-Shahat, M et al. Potential chemoprevention of diethylnitrosamine-induced hepatocarcinogenesis in rats: Myrrh (Commiphora molmol) vs turmeric (Curcuma longa), Acta Histochemica 114 (2012): 421–428.

Fathy FM et al. Effect of Mirazid (Commiphora molmol) on experimental heterophyidiasis. J Egypt Soc Parasitol 35.3 (2005): 1037–1050.

Gopal K et al. Clinical trial of ethyl acetate extract of gum gugulu (gugulipid) in primary hyperlipidemia. J Assoc Physicians India 34.4 (1986): 249–251.

Hamed MA, Hetta MH. Efficacy of Citrus reticulata and Mirazid in treatment of Schistosoma mansoni. Mem Inst Oswaldo Cruz 100.7 (2005): 771–778.

Houston MC et al. Nonpharmacologic Treatment of Dyslipidemia, Progress in Cardiovascular Diseases 52 (2009): 61–94.

Ichikawa H, Aggarwal BB. Guggulsterone inhibits osteoclastogenesis induced by receptor activator of nuclear factor-kappaB ligand and by tumor cells by suppressing nuclear factor-kappaB activation. Clin Cancer Res 12.2 (2006): 662–668.

Karaberopoulos D et al. The Art of medicine; The theriac in antiquity, The Lancet 379 (2012): 1942–1943.

Kimura I et al. New triterpenes, myrrhanol A and myrrhanone A, from guggul-gum resins, and their potent anti-inflammatory effect on adjuvant-induced air-pouch granuloma of mice. Bioorg Med Chem Lett 11.8 (2001): 985–989.

Kumar P, Clark M. Clinical medicine, 5th edn. WB Saunders, 2002.

Langhorst J et al. Randomized, Double-Blind, Double-Dummy, Multicenter Trial of a Herbal Preparation of Myrrh, Camomile and Coffee Coal Compared to Mesalamine in Maintaining Remission in Ulcerative Colitis, Gastroenterology 140.5 (2011): Sup1:pS-264.

Malhotra SC et al. Long term clinical studies on the hypolipidaemic effect of Commiphora mukul (Guggulu) and clofibrate. Indian J Med Res 65.3 (1977): 390–395.

Massoud A et al. Preliminary study of therapeutic efficacy of a new fasciolicidal drug derived from Commiphora molmol (myrrh). Am J Trop Med Hyg 65.2 (2001a): 96–99.

Massoud AM et al. Biochemical changes of Culex pipiens larvae treated with oil and oleo-resin extracts of Myrrh Commiphora molmol. J Egypt Soc Parasitol 31.2 (2001b): 517–529.

Massoud AM et al. Light microscopic study of the effect of new antischistomal drug (myrrh extract) on the liver of mice. J Egypt Soc Parasitol 35.3 (2005): 971–988.

Murube J. Ocular cosmetics in ancient times, the ocular surface 11.1 (2013): 2–7.

Nityanand S, Srivastava JS, Asthana OP. Clinical trials with gugulipid. A new hypolipidaemic agent. J Assoc Physicians India 37.5 (1989): 323–328.

Nohr LA et al. Resin from the mukul myrrh tree, guggul, can it be used for treating hypercholesterolemia? A randomized, controlled study, Complmentary Therapies in Medicine 17 (2009): 16–22.

Saeed MA, Sabir AW. Antibacterial activities of some constituents from oleo-gum-resin of Commiphora mukul. Fitoterapia 75.2 (2004): 204–208.

Sharma JN, Sharma JN. Comparison of the anti-inflammatory activity of Commiphora mukul (an indigenous drug) with those of phenylbutazone and ibuprofen in experimental arthritis induced by mycobacterial adjuvant. Arzneimittelforschung 27.7 (1977): 1455–1457.

Sheir Z et al. A safe, effective, herbal antischistosomal therapy derived from myrrh. Am J Trop Med Hyg 65.6 (2001): 700–704.

Shen T et al. The genus Commiphora: A review of its traditional uses, phytochemistry and pharmacology, J Ethnopharmacol 142 (2012): 319–330.

Singh BB et al. The effectiveness of Commiphora mukul for osteoarthritis of the knee: an outcomes study. Altern Ther Health Med 9.3 (2003): 74–79.

Singh BB et al. Ayurvedic and collateral herbal treatments for hyperlipidemia: a systematic review of randomized controlled trials and quasi-experimental designs. Altern Ther Health Med 13.4 (2007): 22–28.

Singh V et al. Stimulation of low density lipoprotein receptor activity in liver membrane of guggulsterone treated rats. Pharmacol Res 22.1 (1990): 37–44.

Su S et al. Anti-inflammatory and analgesic activity of different extracts of Commiphora myrrha, J Ethnopharmacol 134 (2011): 251–258.

Su S et al. Evaluation of the anti-inflammatory and analgesic properties of individual and combined extracts from Commiphora myrrha and Boswellia carterii, J Ethnopharmacol 139 (2012): 649–656.

Szapary PO et al. Guggulipid for the treatment of hypercholesterolemia: a randomized controlled trial. JAMA 290.6 (2003): 765–772.

Taheri JB et al. Herbs in dentistry. Int Dent J 61 (2011): 287–296.

Thappa DM, Dogra J. Nodulocystic acne: oral gugulipid versus tetracycline. J Dermatol 21.10 (1994): 729–731.

Tipton DA et al. In vitro cytotoxic and anti-inflammatory effects of myrrh oil on human gingival fibroblasts and epithelial cells. Toxicol In Vitro 17.3 (2003): 301–310.

Tipton DA et al. Effect of myrrh oil on IL-1beta stimulation of NF-kappaB activation and PGE2 production in human gingival fibroblasts and epithelial cells. Toxicol In Vitro 20.2 (2006): 248–255.

Ulbricht C et al. Guggul for hyperlipidemia: a review by the Natural Standard Research Collaboration. Complement Ther Pract 13 (2005): 279–290.

Urizar NL et al. A natural product that lowers cholesterol as an antagonist ligand for FXR. Science 296.5573 (2002): 1703–1706.

Wang, WC, et al. Protective effect of guggulsterone against cardiomyocyte injury induced by doxorubicin in vitro BMC Complementary and Alternative Medicine. 12 (2012): 138.

Wu J et al. The hypolipidemic natural product guggulsterone acts as an antagonist of the bile acid receptor. Mol Endocrinol 16.7 (2002): 1590–1597.

Xu J et al. Four new sesquiterpenes from Commiphora myrrha and their neuroprotective effects, Fitoterapia 83 (2012): 801–805.

Zarowitz BJ, Pharmacy Column Complementary and Alternative Medicine: Dietary Supplement Interactions with Medication, Geriatric Nursing 31 (2010): 206–211.

New Zealand green-lipped mussel

HISTORICAL NOTE The Mytilidae are a family of bivalve molluscs that first appeared approximately 400 million years ago (Scotti et al 2001). In New Zealand, they include the green-lipped mussel, which is also known as *Perna canaliculus* and has the Māori name kuku. Green-lipped mussel forms an important component of the traditional diet of coastal Māori people in New Zealand. Interest in the potential therapeutic use of green-lipped mussel as a natural anti-inflammatory began about four decades ago when it was observed that coastal Māoris had a lower incidence of arthritis than those living inland.

BACKGROUND AND RELEVANT PHARMACOKINETICS

There is insufficient reliable information available.

CHEMICAL COMPONENTS

Green-lipped mussel contains a number of constituents, of which the protein (61%) and lipid content (5%) are considered the most important for pharmacological activity. Virtually all of the protein content is comprised of pernin, a self-aggregating glycoprotein rich in histidine and aspartic acid, while the lipid content is comprised of polyunsaturated fatty acids including omega-3 EFAs, free fatty acids, furan fatty acid, sterols, sterol esters and triglycerides. Other constituents include carbohydrates (13%), glucosaminoglycans (12%), minerals (5%) and water (4%) (Scotti et al 2001, Wakimoto et al 2011).

The green-lipped mussel also contain toxins, including BTXB4, a B4 analogue of brevetoxin, yessotoxins, pectenotoxin and okadaic acid (Mackenzie et al 2002, Morohashi et al 1999). BTXB4 has been associated with neurotoxic shellfish poisoning and has been identified as the most significant toxin in green-lipped mussel (Morohashi et al 1999).

MAIN ACTIONS

Most investigation has been conducted with the commercial preparations: Seatone and Lyprinol.

Anti-Inflammatory

Significant anti-inflammatory activity has been observed with the New Zealand green-lipped mussel, which forms the basis of much of its clinical use (Halpern 2000, McPhee et al 2007, Miller & Ormrod 1980, Miller et al 1993). Multiple mechanisms of action have been demonstrated in preclinical tests and include inhibition of the 5-lipoxygenase pathway and synthesis of leukotriene B_4, as well as inhibition of PGE_2 production by activated macrophages and prostaglandin inhibitor actions (Miller & Wu 1984, Miller et al 1993), and potent inhibition of the cyclo-oxygenase COX-1 and COX-2 enzyme pathways (Lawson et al 2007, Mani & Lawson 2006, McPhee et al 2007), with some findings suggesting preferential blockade of COX-2 enzyme activity over COX-1 activity (Efthimiou & Kukar 2010).

Inhibition of IgG, TNF-α, IL-1, IL-2 and IL-6 by green-lipped mussel extract has been demonstrated in an in vitro study by Mani and Lawson

(2006) and in vivo research indicates that green-lipped mussel decreases anti-collagen antibody levels, inhibiting production of pro-inflammatory cytokines (TNF-α, IL-12p40) and reduces superoxide release (Lawson et al 2007).

The most important constituents responsible for these mechanisms of action are the various fatty acids found in green-lipped mussel.

The omega-3 fatty acids EPA and DHA have been isolated in green-lipped mussel (Murphy et al 2003), in addition to a unique series of other omega-3 polyunsaturated fatty acids (C18:4, C19:4, C20:4, C21:5) which may confer a more potent anti-inflammatory action than DHA and EPA, via competitive inhibition of arachidonic acid metabolism, reducing both leukotriene and prostaglandin synthesis (Treschow et al 2007). Furan fatty acids (F-acids), compounds found only in algae and in a limited number of marine animals, are thought to be other key therapeutic components of green-lipped mussel, which exhibits more potent anti-inflammatory activity than the omega-3 fatty acid, EPA (Wakimoto et al 2011). These unstable fatty acids also have potent free-radical-scavenging activity, especially reducing lipid peroxidation.

OTHER ACTIONS

In addition to anti-inflammatory and antioxidant activity, green-lipped mussel has demonstrated antihistamine activity and immunomodulatory properties, as well as endocrine actions and uterine effects (Ulbricht et al 2009). The protein, polysaccharide and lipid fractions are reportedly the bioactive components responsible for these actions (McPhee et al 2007).

CLINICAL USE

In clinical practice, green-lipped mussel is chiefly used for indications characterised by inflammation.

Osteoarthritis

The clinical evidence to support the use of green-lipped mussel (GLM) in osteoarthritis is promising and supported by mechanistic studies demonstrating an effect on inflammatory pathways.

In 2013, a non-blinded randomised clinical trial (RCT) was conducted with 38 subjects diagnosed with knee osteoarthritis (OA) (Coulson et al 2013). Each volunteer received either 3000 mg/day of a whole GLM extract or 3000 mg/day of glucosamine sulphate (GS) orally for 12 weeks. A significant improvement was seen with GLM treatment using the Western Ontario McMaster Universities Arthritis Index (WOMAC) and the Lequesne algofunctional indices ($P < 0.05$) after the test period.

Previously, an open study of 21 subjects with knee OA found that treatment with 3000 mg/day of green-lipped mussel extract for 8 weeks provided a significant improvement for the Lequesne and WOMAC ($P < 0.001$), thereby demonstrating improvements in knee joint pain, stiffness and mobility. The doses used by Coulson and colleagues exceeded those previously tested (maximum 1150 mg/day), which may have contributed to the positive findings.

A 2008 systematic review by Brien et al identified four RCTs where green-lipped mussel was used as an adjunct to standard therapy in mild to moderate osteoarthritis. In three studies, GLM was compared to placebo and in the fourth, a GLM lipid extract was compared to a stabilised powder extract. Results from the two studies considered to be of higher quality suggested that GLM may be superior to placebo for the treatment of mild to moderate OA (Brien et al 2008).

Rheumatoid arthritis (RA)

In contrast, evidence is less supportive of the use of GLM in RA as clinical studies with Seatone have produced inconsistent results. Whether the negative results are due to insufficient dosage or lack of any real effect remains to be tested further.

The first clinical trials testing Seatone in RA were conducted in the 1980s. Huskisson et al (1981) conducted a 4-week study of Seatone 300 mg three times a day as an adjunct to standard therapy in RA (n = 26). It failed to show a significant benefit compared to placebo (Huskisson et al 1981). Another RCT using Seatone in 35 patients with RA found no significant difference in chemical or clinical parameters compared with placebo, after 6 months' use (Larkin et al 1985). A more recent RCT of 28 patients using Seatone over 3 months, with a follow-up phase of another 3 months, reported that active treatment was effective in reducing symptoms of RA in 68% of the treatment group (Gibson & Gibson 1998). This study was subsequently criticised as the subjects served as their own controls in the second phase of the study, and because treatment group were further subdivided into responders and non-responders making interpretation of the results difficult (Cobb & Ernst 2006).

Asthma

To date, two studies have investigated GLM in asthma, producing promising results. A 2002 study of 46 patients with asthma compared Lyprinol (2 capsules twice daily) to placebo twice daily over 8 weeks under double-blind randomised test conditions (Emelyanov et al 2002). Active treatment resulted in a significant improvement on several parameters, such as daytime wheeze, reduced concentration of exhaled H_2O_2 (marker of airway inflammation) and an increase in morning peak expiratory flow (PEF), compared with placebo, but it did not improve night awakenings or reduce the use of beta-agonist bronchodilators or forced expiratory volume in 1-sec (FEV_1).The Lyprinol product contains GLM oil as 50 mg per capsule.

More recently in 2013, treatment with a GLM product (Lyprinol/Omega XL) was tested for effects on airway inflammation and the bronchoconstrictor response to eucapnic voluntary hyperpnoea (EVH) in asthmatics (Mickleborough et al 2013). The placebo controlled double-blind randomised crossover trial involved 23 asthmatic volunteers with clinically treated mild to moderate persistent asthma and a resting forced expiratory volume in 1-sec (FEV_1) of >65% predicted, and EIB as demonstrated by a greater than 10% drop in FEV_1 following a eucapnic voluntary hyperventilation (EVH) challenge. All subjects had a history of shortness of breath, chest tightness and intermittent wheezing following exercise, which was relieved by bronchodilator therapy and none were taking any maintenance medications (e.g. corticosteroids and leukotriene modifiers) at the time of the study.

Treatment consisted of 3 weeks of Lyprinol/Omega XL (8 capsules daily) or placebo followed by a 2-week washout period, before crossing over to the alternative arm. Additionally, all subjects were reviewed to ensure dietary intake was unchanged during the test period, in particular omega-3 EFA intake. Active treatment was found to significantly improve asthma symptom scores ($P < 0.05$), reduce bronchodilator use ($P < 0.05$) and reduce the maximum fall in post-EVH FEV_1 compared to usual and placebo ($P < 0.05$). It appears that effects are slow-acting as a reduction in bronchodilator use was only evident after 1 week of treatment.

OTHER USES

Veterinary use for osteoarthritis

New Zealand GLM shows promise as a treatment option for dogs, cats and horses with joint disease. In dogs, the most common form of joint disease is OA, which has been successfully treated by green-lipped mussel powder in one double-blind RCT (Bierer & Bui 2002). Active treatment was shown to significantly improve total arthritic score, and alleviate joint pain and swelling at the end of week six compared with controls. More specifically, 83% of dogs in the active treatment group experienced a 30% or greater reduction in total arthritic scores and of these, 18% showed a 70% or greater improvement. Only 7% of controls showed a 30% or greater improvement, with no dogs showing a 50% or greater improvement. The doses of GLM powder ranged from 450 mg to 1000 mg/day, depending on body weight. Another randomised double-blind study of 45 dogs with OA reported that the dogs treated with green-lipped mussel showed significant improvements according to veterinary pain and mobility scales compared to placebo. However, these benefits were not as great as those observed in the dogs treated with carprofen, a non-steroidal anti-inflammatory drug (Hielm-Bjorkman et al 2009). A further study was conducted including 81 dogs with a diagnosis of mild-moderate degenerative joint disease. Daily oral consumption of an extract of green lipped mussel appeared to reduce clinical signs of disease (Pollard et al 2006).

GLM extract has also been evaluated in cats diagnosed with degenerative joint disease. In one study of 45 cats, the animals in the treatment group were given a diet high in EPA/DHA, green-lipped mussel extract and supplemental glucosamine/chondroitin. Although improvements in mobility were reported, it is unclear how much of this benefit can be attributed to green-lipped mussel (Lascelles et al 2010).

Lyophilised products from green-lipped mussel (*Perna canaliculus* [LPPC]) are also used in horses to treat OA. A double-blind, multi-centre RCT evaluating horses with primary fetlock lameness found treatment with oral LPPC 25 mg/kg bwt/day for 56 days produced a significant reduction in severity of lameness ($P < 0.001$), improved response to the joint flexion test ($P < 0.001$) and reduced joint pain ($P = 0.014$) when compared with horses treated with placebo (Cayzer et al 2012).

Inflammatory bowel disease

Findings from a preliminary animal study suggest green-lipped mussel may be of potential benefit in inflammatory bowel disease (IBD). A study compared the anti-inflammatory effects of green-lipped mussel (Lyprinol containing <1 mg omega-3 fatty acids/day) to that of fish oils (given at a dose 55 mg omega-3 fatty acids/day) in mice with experimentally induced IBD. The mice treated with Lyprinol showed significantly less weight loss, disease activity index scores and colonic damage than those treated with omega-3 fatty acids ($P < 0.05$) after 13 days (Tenikoff et al 2005). Based on these results, the researchers proposed that GLM has a potential therapeutic benefit in IBD due to a mechanism or constituent unrelated to omega-3 fatty acids content (Tenikoff et al 2005). Human trials are now required to determine whether the effect is clinically significant.

Muscle damage and soreness in athletes — no effect

A double-blind RCT found GLM was ineffective in reducing delayed onset muscle soreness, inflammatory markers or muscle damage after exercise. Twenty well-trained male athletes from various sports disciplines were randomly assigned to either Lyprinol 200 mg/day or placebo, taken for 8 weeks prior to an intense exercise intervention (Pumpa et al 2011).

Cancer — no effect

Some research has been conducted with New Zealand GLM in the management of certain cancers as in vivo and in vitro studies suggest that inhibition of lipo-oxygenase pathways may arrest tumour growth in some cancers, especially prostate cancer and green-lipped mussel is a potent natural lipo-oxygenase inhibitor (Sukumaran et al 2010). An open-labelled clinical study involving 19 subjects found that GLM (Lyprinol) produced no clinical benefits in the management of advanced, treatment-refractory, prostate or breast cancer (Sukumaran et al 2010).

DOSAGE RANGE

Doses provided are based on the available clinical research. In addition, there is no well-known standardisation for green lipped mussel and efficacy may vary between manufacturers and between different batches (Ulbricht et al 2009).

- Asthma — Lyprinol/Omega XL taken as 8 capsules daily or Lyprinol taken as 4 capsules daily.
- Osteoarthritis — two studies showed significant symptomatic improvement at a dose of 3000 mg/day.

TOXICITY

GLM contain the toxin brevetoxin B4 (BTXB4), which has been associated with neurotoxic shellfish poisoning (Morohashi et al 1999). Regular ingestion of New Zealand green-lipped mussels does not appear to lead to heavy metal toxicity according to traditional dietary use by Māori people, nor according to a preliminary laboratory investigation (Whyte et al 2009). Insufficient reliable information is available to determine toxicity of supplemental green-lipped mussel.

ADVERSE REACTIONS

Gastrointestinal discomfort, nausea, gout and skin rashes have been reported (Ahern et al 1980, Brooks 1980). There have been three case reports in the literature suggesting that green-lipped mussel may be associated with rare incidences of liver dysfunction, however causality is difficult to ascertain (Abdulazim et al 2012). Raised liver enzymes were reported in two cancer patients participating in a small study (n = 17) on the safety and tolerability of green-lipped mussel as adjunct therapy. One of the two patients had significant metastatic liver involvement and this was reported as the most likely reason for raised liver enzymes. The other patient had normal liver function at baseline and no liver cancer involvement. The dose of green-lipped mussel at which liver abnormalities were reported was not specified, nor were any other medications taken by the patients described (Sukumaran et al 2010).

SIGNIFICANT INTERACTIONS

Insufficient reliable information exists regarding clinical interactions with green lipped mussel; however, in vivo studies suggest possible interactions with some medications.

Anti-inflammatory agents

Due to the anti-inflammatory activity of GLM, concomitant use with these medications can theoretically result in enhanced anti-inflammatory effects or a reduction in drug dosage — beneficial.

CONTRAINDICATIONS AND PRECAUTIONS

Contraindicated in people with allergies to shellfish. Rash, swelling of extremities and mouth, tingling, chest tightness and breathing difficulties have been reported (Ulbricht et al 2009). Lung dysfunction and a range of respiratory symptoms were reported in 32.3% of workers employed as New Zealand mussels openers, according to one study of 224 employees (Glass et al 1998). Whether the same effect is seen with manufactured GLM extracts taken orally remains to be seen.

Use with caution in people with hypertension, as the sodium content could theoretically raise blood pressure.

PREGNANCY USE

Insufficient reliable information is available to assess safety.

Practice points/Patient counselling

- New Zealand green-lipped mussel has been used to treat arthritis by the New Zealand Māoris for many years.
- Significant anti-inflammatory activity has been observed in both animals and humans.
- Several clinical trials have produced promising results for GLM in the symptomatic treatment of OA.
- Two clinical trials also suggest a possible role in asthma management.
- Significant symptom relief has been observed for GLM in dogs with osteoarthritis and cats and horses with joint disease.
- The most common side effects associated with GLM are gastrointestinal discomfort, nausea, gout and skin rashes.

PATIENTS' FAQs

What will this supplement do for me?
Some studies have shown that NZ green-lipped mussel exerts significant anti-inflammatory activity and is likely to relieve symptoms of OA when taken for several weeks, Two studies also suggest a possible role in the treatment of asthma.

When will it start to work?
Effects in osteoarthritis are likely to be seen within 8 weeks of use. Effects with a combination of GLM and omega-3 EFAS developed within 3 weeks in the management of mild-to-moderate asthma.

Are there any safety issues?
GLM should not be taken by people with allergies to shellfish and should be used with caution by people with high blood pressure due to the sodium content.

REFERENCES

Abdulazim A et al. Acute hepatitis induced by Lyprinol, the lipid extract of the green-lipped mussel (Pernacanaliculus), in a patient with polyarthrosis. Case Reports in Hepatology. Article 135146 (2012). doi:10.1155/2012/135146

Ahern MJ et al. Granulomatous hepatitis and Seatone. Med J Aust 2.3 (1980): 151–152.

Bierer TL, Bui LM. Improvement of arthritic signs in dogs fed green-lipped mussel (Pernacanaliculus). J Nutr 132.6 Suppl 2 (2002): 1634–1636S.

Brien S et al. Systematic review of the nutritional supplement Pernacanaliculus (green-lipped mussel) in the treatment of osteoarthritis. Q J Med 101 (2008):167–179. doi:10.1093/qjmed/hcm108.

Brooks PM. Side effects from Seatone. Med J Aust 2.3 (1980): 158.

Cayzer J et al. A randomised, double-blinded, placebo-controlled study on the efficacy of a unique extract of green-lipped mussel (Perna canaliculus) in horses with chronic fetlock lameness attributed to osteoarthritis. Equine Vet J 44.4 (2012) 393–398.

Cobb CS, Ernst E. Systematic review of a marine nutriceitical supplement in clinical trials for arthritis: the effectiveness of the New Zealndgree-lipped mussel Pernacanaliculus. Clinical Rheumatology 25 (2006): 275–284.

Coulson S et al. Green-lipped mussel extract (Perna canaliculus) and glucosamine sulphate in patients with knee osteoarthritis: therapeutic efficacy and effects on gastrointestinal microbiota profiles. Inflammopharmacology 21.1 (2013): 79–90.

Efthimiou P, Kukar M. Complementary and alternative medicine use in rheumatoid arthritis: prosed mechanism of action and efficacy of commonly used modalities. RheumatolInt 30.(2010): 571–586.

Emelyanov A et al. Treatment of asthma with lipid extract of New Zealand green-lipped mussel: a randomised clinical trial. EurRespir J 20.3 (2002): 596–600.

Gibson SLM, Gibson RG. The treatment of arthritis with a lipid extract of Perna canaliculis: a randomised trial. Comp Ther Med 6 (1998):122–126.

Glass WI et al. Work-related respiratory symptoms and lung function in New Zealand mussel openers. Am J Ind Med. 34.2 (1998):163–168.

Halpern GM. Anti-inflammatory effects of a stabilized lipid extract of Pernacanaliculus (Lyprinol). AllergImmunol (Paris) 32.7 (2000): 272–278.

Hielm-Bjorkman A et al. Evaluating complementary therapies for canine osteoarthritis Part 1: green-lipped mussel (Pernacanaliculus). eCam 6.3 (2009): 365–373.

Huskisson EC et al. Seatone is ineffective in rheumatoid arthritis. Br Med J (Clin Res Ed) 4.25 (1981): 1358–1359.

Larkin JG, Capell HA, Sturrock RD. Seatone in rheumatoid arthritis: a six-month placebo-controlled study. Ann Rheum Dis 44.3 (1985): 199–201.

Lascelles BDX et al. Evaluation of a therapeutic diet for feline degenerative joint disease. J Vet Intern Med 24 (2010): 487–495.

Lawson BR et al. Immunomodulation of murine collagen-induced arthritis by N,N-dimethylglycine and a preparation of Pernacanaliculus. BMC Complementary and Alternative Medicine 7.20 (2007).

Mackenzie L et al. Complex toxin profiles in phytoplankton and greenshell mussels (Pernacanaliculus) revealed by LC-MS/MS analysis. Toxicon. 40.9 (2002): 1321–1330.

Mani S, Lawson JW. In vitro modulation of inflammatory cytokine and IgG levels by extracts of Pernacanaliculus. BMC Complemen Alt Med 6.1 (2006).

McPhee S et al. Anti-cyclooxygenase effects of lipid extarcts from the New Zealand green-lipped mussel, Pernacanaliculus. Comparative Biochemistry and Physiology, part B 146 (2007): 346–356.

Mickleborough TD et al. Marine lipid fraction PCSO-524 (lyprnol/ omega XL) of the New Zealand green lipped mussel attenuates hyperpnea-induced bronchoconstriction in asthma. Respir Med, 107.8 (2013): 1152–1163.

Miller T, Wu H. In vivo evidence for prostaglandin inhibitory activity in New Zealand green-lipped mussel extract. NZ Med J 97.757 (1984): 355–357.

Miller TE et al. Anti-inflammatory activity of glycogen extracted from Pernacanaliculus (NZ green-lipped mussel). Agents Actions 38 (1993): C139–42.

Miller TE, Ormrod D. The anti-inflammatory activity of Pernacanaliculus (NZ green lipped mussel). NZ Med J 92.667 (1980): 187–193.

Morohashi A et al. Brevetoxin B4 isolated from greenshell mussels Pernacanaliculus, the major toxin involved in neurotoxic shellfish poisoning in New Zealand. Natural Toxins 7.2 (1999): 45–48.

Murphy KJ et al. Fatty acid and sterol composition of frozen and freeze-dried Mew Zealand green lipped mussel (Pernacanaliculus) from three sites in New Zealand. Asia Pac. J. Clin. Nutr. 12 (2003): 50–60.

Pollard B et al. Clinival efficacy and tolerance of an extract of green-lipped mussel (Pernacanaliculus) in dogs presumptively diagnosed with degenerative joint disease. New Zealand Veterinary Journal 54.3 (2006): 114–118.

Pumpa KL et al. The effects of Lyprinol® on delayed onset musclesoreness and muscle damage in well trainedathletes: A double-blind randomised controlled trial. Complemen Ther Med 19 (2011): 311–318.

Scotti PD et al. Pernin: a novel, self-aggregating haemolymph protein from the New Zealand green-lipped mussel, Pernacanaliculus (Bivalvia: Mytilidae). Comp Biochem Physiol B Biochem Mol Biol 128.4 (2001): 767–779.

Sukumaran S et al. A phase 1 study to determine the safety, tolerability and maximum tolerated dose of green-lipped mussel (Pernacanaliculus) lipid extract in patients with advanced prostate and breast cancer. Annals Oncol 21.5 (2010): 1089–1093.

Tenikoff D et al. Lyprinol (stabilized lipid extract of New Zealand green-lipped mussel): a potential preventative treatment modality for inflammatory bowel disease. J Gastroenterol 40.4 (2005): 361–365.

Treschow AP et al. Novel anti-inflammatory ω-3 PUFA's from the New Zealand green-lipped mussel, Pernacanaliculus. Comparative Biochemistry and Physiology, part B 147 (2007): 645–656.

Ulbricht C et al. An Evidence-based systematic review of green-lipped mussel (Pernacanaliculus) by the Natural Standard Research Collaboration. J Diet Supplements 6.1 (2009): 54–90.

Wakimoto T et al. Furan fatty acid as an anti-inflammatory component from the green-lipped mussel Pernacanaliculus. PNAS 108.42 (2011).

Whyte ALH et al. Human dietary exposure to heavy metals via the consumption of greenshell mussels (PernacanaliculusGmelin 1791) from the Bay of Islands, Northern New Zealand. Science of the Total Environment 407 (2009): 4348–4355.

Nigella

HISTORICAL NOTE Records suggest that black seed has been used medicinally for thousands of years, especially in the Middle East and Southeast Asia. Black seed (nigella) is referred to in the Old Testament in the Book of Isaiah, where Isaiah compares nigella to wheat (Isaiah 28:25, 27). It is also reported that the Islamic prophet Mohammed claimed that black seed (kalonji) was a remedy for all diseases except death. Black seed was used in Ancient Egypt, with extracts being found at various sites, including King Tutankhamun's tomb, and in Turkey, a Hittite flask of black seed dating back to 1650 BC was recovered by archaeologists. Black seed was also reportedly used by both Hippocrates (460–370 BC) and Dioscorides (40–90 AD) for a range of conditions.

LATIN BINOMIAL/CLASS

Nigella sativa (family Ranunculeae)

OTHER NAMES

Nigella, black cumin, black caraway, blessed seed or seed of blessing, fennel flower, nutmeg flower, roman coriander, habbatul baraka, habat-ul-sauda, kalonji, nigelle de Crête, nigelle cultivée, Roman-coriander, Schwarzkummel.

Plant part used

Seed

CHEMICAL COMPONENTS

Thymoquinone, a component of the essential oil found in *Nigella sativa* seeds, has been identified as the main active constituent (Edris 2009). Other important constituents include dithymoquinone (nigellone), thymohydroquinone, *p*-cymene, carvacrol, 4-terpineol, *t*-anethol, sesquiterpene longifolene, α-pinene, thymol, α-hederin, isoquinoline and pyrazol alkaloids (Ahmad et al 2013). In addition, trace amounts are found of other compounds, including monosaccharides (glucose, rhamnose, xylose, arabinose), unsaturated fatty acids (linoleic acid, linolenic acid, oleic acid), alpha-spinasterol, arabic acid, aspartic acid, beta-sitosterol, campesterol, carvone, cholesterol, D-limonene, dehydroascorbic acid, eicosadienoic acid, melanthigenin, melanthin, myristic acid, palmitic acid, stearic acid, stigmasterol, various amino acids, vitamins and minerals.

MAIN ACTIONS

Antiallergic

Antihistamine effects have been demonstrated in human and animal study (Isik et al 2010, Kalus et al 2003, Nikakhlagh et al 2011). Decreased synthesis of proinflammatory leukotrienes via an inhibitory action on the arachidonic pathway has been described (Kalus et al 2003). Immunomodulatory effects were described by Isik and colleagues, with administration of black seed leading to an increase in phagocytic and intracellular killing activities of polymorphonuclear leucocytes in patients receiving allergen-specific immunotherapy (Isik et al 2010).

Anticarcinogenic effects

Thymoquinone, the main active constituent of black seed, has been shown to possess a number of anticancer properties, mediated through a number of different mechanisms. In vitro and in vivo studies have identified antiproliferative actions, induction of apoptosis, cell cycle arrest, reactive oxygen species generation and antimetastasis/antiangiogenesis. Thymoquinone also appears to modulate various molecular targets, including p53, p73, PTEN, STAT3, PPAR-g and activation of caspases (Ahmad et al 2013, Randhawa & Alghamdi 2011, Woo et al 2012).

Thymoquinone has been shown to inhibit proliferation of a variety of tumour cells, including neuroblastoma (Paramasivam et al 2012), human pancreatic adenocarcinoma, neoplastic keratinocytes (Worthen et al 1998), breast adenocarcinoma, ovarian adenocarcinoma (Shoieb et al 2003), colorectal cancer (Gali-Muhtasib et al 2004), human osteosarcoma (Roepke et al 2007), fibrosarcoma, lung carcinoma (Kaseb et al 2007) and myeloblastic leukaemia (El-Mahdy et al 2005). Researchers demonstrated that thymoquinone inhibited tumour growth and induced apoptosis via generation of reactive oxygen species in primary effusion lymphoma cell lines (Hussain et al 2011). According to the findings of laboratory research conducted using multiple myeloma cells, thymoquinone inhibited phosphorylation of the STAT3 signalling pathway, both constitutive and interleukin-6 (IL-6)-induced. Downregulation of the expression of STAT3-regulated gene products (cyclin D1, Bcl-2, Bcl-xL, survivin, Mcl-1 and vascular endothelial growth factor) were also observed (Li et al 2010). Thymoquinone was shown to attenuate haematological changes and oxidative stress in animal models with colon cancer (Harzallah et al 2012).

Use of thymoquinone in combination with other cytotoxic drugs to enhance drug efficacy is a promising area of research. One laboratory study demonstrated that thymoquinone induced apoptosis in doxorubicin-resistant human breast cells, primarily via upregulation of the tumour suppressor gene PTEN (El-Shaimaa et al 2011). Thymoquinone was also shown to be protective against doxorubicin-induced cardiotoxicity, which the authors proposed was due primarily to antioxidant activity (Nagi & Mansour 2000).

An animal study investigating thymoquinone in combination with 5-fluorouracil (5-FU) in gastric cancer cells demonstrated a significantly more effective antitumour benefit when the two agents were combined, than either used alone. It was proposed that this was due to thymoquinone enhancing the activation of caspase-3 and caspase-9 in gastric cancer cells, which resulted in the chemosensitisation of gastric cancer cells to 5-FU treatment (Lei et al 2012).

Synergistic effects were observed when thymoquinone was used in combination with cisplatin in lung cancer cells and in animal models (Jafri et al 2010).

Researchers also reported that thymoquinone significantly potentiated the apoptotic effects of thalidomide and bortezomib in multiple myeloma cells (Li et al 2010).

Banerjee et al (2009) report that thymoquinone potentiated the effects of gemcitabine and oxaliplatin in pancreatic cancer cells, possibly due to downregulation of NF-kappaB, which resulted in chemosensitisation.

Encapsulation of thymoquinone into nanoparticles appears to enhance the antiproliferative, anti-inflammatory and chemosensitising effects of thymoquinone, according to findings of one study (Ravindran et al 2010). While thymoquinone appears to be the most promising anticarcinogenic constituent of black seed, other constituents such as α-hederin and derivatives of both of these compounds have also been identified as holding therapeutic potential (Randhawa & Alghamdi 2011).

Antidiabetic effects

Animal and preliminary human studies with black seed and the constituent thymoquinone have demonstrated improved glucose tolerance, antioxidant status, renal function, decreased blood glucose, serum insulin and glycated haemoglobin levels (Bamosa et al 2010, Fararh et al 2010, Kaleem et al 2006, Meddah et al 2009, Najimi et al 2006). The mechanism of action is yet to be elucidated, but decreased hepatic gluconeogenesis and inhibition of nitric oxide pathways have been proposed by researchers in this field (El-Mahmoudy et al 2005, Fararh et al 2005).

Antihypertensive effects

Antihypertensive effects have been demonstrated in an animal study, and appeared to be centrally mediated via direct and indirect mechanisms involving muscarinic and 5-hydroxytryptaminergic action (El-Tahir et al 1993). Mild antihypertensive effects were reported in one clinical study, which the authors proposed may be related to the antioxidant properties of black seed.

Antimicrobial actions

Antibacterial actions have been observed in vitro against *Staphylococcus aureus*, *Helicobacter pylori* and *Streptococcus* spp. Antiparasitic effects were identified in animal and human studies against *Schistosoma mansoni*, which may be due to antioxidant and immunomodulatory effects. In vitro study using methanolic extracts of *Nigella sativa* has shown antifungal activity against *Candida albicans*, and ether extracts showed activity against dermatophytes, supporting traditional folk use of black seed for fungal skin infections (Ahmad et al 2013).

Antioxidant

Antioxidant effects have been reported in several in vitro and animal studies, mainly attributed to the constituent thymoquinone (Ahmad et al 2013). Black seed oil extracted by cold pressing has been shown to possess significant antioxidant properties, and appears to yield higher levels of thymoquinone than black seed oil extracted via other techniques (Lutterodt et al 2010). One preliminary clinical study of 30 postmenopausal women reported that black seed 3 g/day for 12 weeks increased levels of superoxide dismutase and glutathione peroxidase enzymes (Mostafa & Moustafa 2012).

Hyperlipidaemic actions

Clinical studies have demonstrated that black seed reduces total cholesterol, low-density lipoprotein (LDL) cholesterol and triglyceride levels, and induces a slight increase in high-density lipoprotein (HDL) cholesterol (Kaatabi et al 2012, Najmi et al 2008). One animal study suggests that this may be due to inhibition of the HMG-CoA reductase enzyme and of LDL lipoprotein receptor upregulation (Al Naqeep et al 2009).

OTHER ACTIONS

Analgesic and neurological effects

Analgesic activity has been observed in experimental models and animal studies (Abdel-Fattah et al 2000, Al-Naggar et al 2003, Bashir & Qureshi 2010). Anxiolytic activity has been reported in animal study, with increased levels of gamma-aminobutyric acid, 5-hydroxytryptamine and trytophan having been recorded (Ahmad et al 2013).

Antiasthmatic effects

Tracheal relaxation has been observed in animal studies. The mechanism is unclear, but it has been proposed to be due to lipooxygenase inhibition of arachidonic acid metabolism and a non-selective histamine and serotonin blockade (Al-Majed et al 2001).

Anticoagulant effects

Inhibition of platelet aggregation and blood coagulation has been demonstrated in vitro and in vivo (Al-Jishi & Abuo Hozaifa 2003, Enomoto et al 2001).

Anti-inflammatory effects

Anti-inflammatory effects have been identified in vitro and in vivo. The main constituents involved are thymoquinone, carvacrol, dithymoquinone, thymohydroquinone and thymol. Observed anti-inflammatory effects according to various studies include inhibition of IL-1, IL-6, transcription factor, NF-κB, cyclooxygenase-1 and/or cyclooxygenase 2, nitric oxide release and leukotrienes (Ahmad et al 2013, El Gazzar et al 2007).

Bone metabolism

A recent experimental laboratory study reported that the constituent thymoquinone induced proliferation and mineralisation of MC3T3-E1 osteoblastic cells, which the authors proposed was mediated by an increased expression of bone morphogenetic protein-2 (BMP-2), associated with phosphorylation of the ERK signalling pathway (Wirries et al 2013). Acceleration of bone formation with use of thymoquinone has been shown in an animal study (Kara et al 2012).

Gastroprotective effects

Gastroprotective mechanisms have been observed in one animal study. Thymoquinone is reported to have inhibited proton pump activity and acid secretion, while increasing secretion of mucin and nitric oxide production (Mahmoud-Awny et al 2012).

Hepatoprotective

Based on animal studies, black seed appears to confer hepatoprotective effects against a number of agents, including aflatoxin B_1 (Sabzevari et al 2011), D-galactosamine, carbon tetrachloride (El-Dakhakhny et al 2000, Ibrahim et al 2008), lead (Farraq et al 2007), isoniazid (Hassan et al 2012) and sodium valproate (Raza et al 2006). Conversely, one in vitro study cautions that the constituent thymoquinone may be metabolised to a reactive species and increase oxidative stress, leading to DNA damage in hepatocytes (Khader et al 2009). One laboratory study demonstrated that thymoquinone attenuated liver fibrosis via Toll-like receptor 4 blockade and phosphatidylinositol 3-kinase, suggesting a potential role in hepatic fibrosis (Bai et al 2013). Further study is required to determine the clinical significance of black seed in hepatic disorders or as a hepatoprotective agent.

Heavy-metal toxicity

Animal studies have shown that thymoquinone, the active constituent of black seed, provides hepatoprotective effects against toxicity due to heavy metals such as cadmium and lead (Farraq et al 2007, Waseem et al 2012). Further research is required to confirm clinical significance.

Immunomodulatory effects

Immunomodulatory effects have been identified in vitro and in vivo. Observed effects according to different studies include enhanced splenocyte proliferation; enhanced natural killer cytotoxic activity, including action against YAC-1 tumour cells, preferential secretion of Th2 over Th1 cytokines, suppression of proinflammatory mediator secretion (IL-6, tumour necrosis factor-alpha and nitric oxide), induction of IL-8, possibly due to involvement of Toll-like receptor 4, increased white blood cell count and radioprotective effects (Ahmad et al 2013, El-Obeid et al 2006, Majdalawieh et al 2010).

CLINICAL USAGE

Most research regarding black seed has been done in vitro and with animal models and relatively few clinical trials are available. The clinical studies that are available suggest a potential therapeutic role in a range of conditions and warrant further investigation.

Asthma

Preliminary research with black seed aqueous extract suggests it may be beneficial as an adjunct therapy in asthmatic patients. A randomised double-blind study investigated the effect of black seed on asthma symptoms in 29 patients as adjunct therapy to their conventional asthma medication over a period of 3 months. The addition of black seed extract (15 mL/kg of 1 g% extract) resulted in a significant decrease in frequency of asthma symptoms, chest wheezing and lung function test values compared to baseline ($P < 0.05$), allowing for a reduction in usage of drug therapy in the treatment group (Boskabady et al 2007). A subsequent smaller study ($n = 15$) compared the bronchodilatory effects of black seed aqueous extract (50 mg/kg and 100 mg/kg) to theophylline 6 mg/kg) as adjunct therapy to inhaled corticosteroids in patients with diagnosed moderate to severe asthma. Analysis of lung function test results showed that onset of bronchodilatory action and duration of action were similar for both black seed and theophylline (30 min and 150 min respectively); however the magnitude of benefit was greater with theophylline. There was no significant difference in effect between the two doses of black seed used in the study (Boskabady et al 2010). These findings are suggestive of a beneficial effect for black seed as adjunctive asthma therapy; however further larger-scale research with more rigorous methodology is required before conclusions can be drawn. These preliminary human study data are supported by animal studies in which observations include tracheal-relaxant effects (Al-Majed et al 2001, Boskabady et al 2008) and inhibitory effects on inflammation, nitric oxide synthetase, tumour necrosis factor-alpha, immunoglobulin E levels and transforming growth factor-β_1 (El-Sayed et al 2011).

Allergies

Results from clinical studies suggest that oral use of black seed oil may be of benefit in the treatment of various allergic conditions. In a double-blind study of 66 patients, administration of black seed oil was shown to reduce symptoms of allergic rhinitis, including itching, nasal congestion, sneezing and runny nose, as determined by subjective questionnaires. The dose of black seed oil was not described in the research methodology (Nikakhlagh et al 2011). These findings support prior research in which black seed oil taken at doses ranging from 500 to 2000 mg three times a day (40–80 mg/kg/day) for up to 8 weeks provided subjective improvement of the symptoms of allergic rhinitis, atopic eczema and bronchial asthma (Kalus et al 2003). According to findings in another study, supplementation with black seed oil (2 g/day) increased the phagocytic and intracellular killing activities of polymorphonuclear leucocyte functions in patients with allergic rhinitis on allergen-specific immunotherapy (Isik et al 2010).

Diabetes mellitus

Clinical studies suggest a potential benefit of black seed as adjunct therapy in patients with type 2 diabetes mellitus within 6–12 weeks of oral use. In one study of 94 patients, black seed was administered as adjunct therapy in patients with diagnosed type 2 diabetes, given at doses of 1, 2 or 3 g/day. Optimal benefits were at the 2 g/day dose, with significant reductions reported in fasting blood glucose, 2 hours postprandial blood glucose and glycosylated haemoglobin levels. Improvements in β-cell function and insulin resistance were also reported after 12 weeks of treatment (Bamosa et al 2010). An open, non-randomised, non-blinded study was conducted by Najimi et al to investigate potential benefits of black seed as adjunct therapy in 60 patients with hyperlipidaemia and type 2 diabetes mellitus and insulin resistance syndrome (Najimi et al 2006). The control group received atorvastatin 10 mg/day and metformin 500 mg twice daily for 6 weeks. The treatment group received the same drug therapy, as well as black seed oil 2.5 mL twice daily. Significant reductions in fasting blood glucose were reported ($P < 0.05$), as well as reductions in total cholesterol and LDL cholesterol. In another open study, administration of black seed powder for 40 days to type 2 diabetic patients was reported to result in significant reductions in fasting blood glucose levels ($P < 0.001$), LDL cholesterol ($P = 0.001$) and triglyceride ($P < 0.001$) levels, and to increase insulin ($P < 0.001$) and HDL levels ($P = 0.011$). These benefits reversed after withdrawal of black seed powder. Further data regarding research methodology are not available (Bilal et al 2008). Improved glucose tolerance and a reduction in blood glucose levels have also been reported in animal studies (Fararh et al 2010, Kaleem et al 2006, Meddah et al 2009).

Epilepsy

Anticonvulsant properties have been observed in animal studies conducted with black seed and the constituent thymoquinone, suggesting a possible role in epilepsy (Hosseinzadeh et al 2005, Hosseinzadeh & Parvardeh 2004, Illhan et al 2005). To date, only one randomised study was located which has explored this in humans. The double-blind, randomised crossover study was conducted in 23 children with refractory epilepsy using an aqueous extract of black seed. This extract was given as a syrup, standardised to 0.5 mg/kg/12 h thymoquinone, and compared to a placebo syrup, as adjunct therapies to their regular anticonvulsant medication. One group of participants received thymoquinone for 4 weeks, while the other received placebo. After a 2-week washout period, the groups were crossed over and treatment continued for another 4 weeks. Seizure frequency was assessed during treatment periods for both groups. A 30% reduction in mean frequency of seizures was reported in both groups when treated with black seed extract ($P \leq 0.04$), supported by a 75% parental satisfaction, compared to 30% satisfaction in the placebo group ($P = 0.03$; Akhondian et al 2011). Further study is needed before conclusions can be drawn.

Hyperlipidaemia

A clinical study ($n = 94$) showed that ingestion of black seed 2 g/day for 12 weeks resulted in a significant reduction in total cholesterol, LDL cholesterol and triglyceride levels in type 2 diabetic patients. A slight increase in HDL cholesterol was also reported. Black seed was administered as 500 mg capsules containing ground black seed powder in this study (Kaatabi et al 2012). In another small-scale randomised double-blind study ($n = 73$), black seed (1 g/twice daily as encapsulated powder) was administered as adjunctive therapy to statin therapy in patients with hypercholesterolaemia over 6 weeks. Reductions in total cholesterol, LDL cholesterol and trigylceride levels were observed; however these effects were not clinically significant. No adverse renal or hepatic effects were reported and no significant reductions in either systolic or diastolic blood pressure were recorded (Qidwai et al 2009). Further study is needed before conclusions can be drawn.

Hypertension

Hypotensive benefits were reported in animal study (Zaoui et al 2000) which have been demonstrated in humans. A subsequent randomised double-blind placebo-controlled clinical study ($n = 108$) showed that administration of black seed extract (100 mg or 200 mg/day) for 8 weeks reduced both systolic and diastolic blood pressure slightly (2.8 mmHg and 1.1 mmHg respectively). However, in another study using a higher dose of 2 g/day for 6 weeks, no clinically significant reductions in blood pressure were observed (Qidwai et al 2009). Further study is needed to establish therapeutic doses and magnitude of benefit.

OTHER USES

Addiction

Preliminary evidence suggests that black seed may be of benefit in reducing the symptoms of withdrawal in opiate-dependent patients. A significant reduction ($P \leq 0.05$) in opioid withdrawal symptoms was reported in a randomised single-blind study of 35 known male addicts administered dried black seed 500 mg three times a day for up to 12 days. There were no physiological changes to pulse rate, blood pressure or weight during treatment (Sangi et al 2008). Findings of a study conducted with mice suggest that black seed oil may protect against tramadol-induced tolerance and dependence (Abdel-Zaher et al 2011). Further well-designed study is required before conclusions can be drawn.

Atopic dermatitis

In vitro study suggests that the constituent nigellone may inhibit histamine release; however results from one small clinical study found that an ointment made with 15% black seed oil did not reduce symptoms of atopic dermatitis compared to placebo (Stern et al 2002). There are also two case study reports where topical use of black seed oil caused allergic contact dermatitis (Ali & Blunden 2003). Further study is required, but a benefit seems unlikely.

Helicobacter pylori eradication

One small-scale randomised study of non-ulcer dyspepsia patients found that a combination of *Nigella sativa* 2 g/day with omeprazole 40 mg/day resulted in a 66.7% eradication of *H. pylori*, compared to a 82.6% eradication rate in the group treated with triple therapy (clarithromycin, amoxicillin, omeprazole) (Salem et al 2010).

DOSAGE RANGE

Doses provided are suggestive, based on limited clinical study. There are insufficient data available at this stage to make conclusive recommendations.

According to clinical studies:

- Allergies: black seed oil at doses of 40–80 mg/kg/day in divided dose has been used for up to 8 weeks.
- Asthma: 50–100 mg/kg/day has been used as adjunct therapy.
- Hyperlipidaemia: 1 g twice daily for 12 weeks has been used as adjunct therapy.
- Hypertension: 100–200 mg/day for 8 weeks led to a minor reduction in systolic and diastolic blood pressure.
- Refractory paediatric epilepsy: aqueous extract, given as a syrup at a dose of 0.02 mL/kg/12 h (equivalent to 0.5 mg/kg/12 h of thymoquinone), has been used as adjunct therapy for 4 weeks.
- Type 2 diabetes mellitus: 2 g/day for 3 months has been used as adjunct therapy.

ADVERSE REACTIONS

Insufficient reliable information exists about adverse reactions with black seed; however there are two case study reports of allergic contact dermatitis following topical use of black seed oil (Ali & Blunden 2003). One study suggests that doses exceeding 80 mg/kg/day may result in gastrointestinal adverse effects (Kalus et al 2003).

A review of the toxicological profile of black seed suggests a wide margin of safety at therapeutic doses, but cautions against potential changes in haemoglobin metabolism, platelet count and leucocyte levels (Zaoui et al 2002).

SIGNIFICANT INTERACTIONS

Analgesics

Theoretically, potentiation effects are possible when using black seed at high doses based on animal models (Abdel-Fattah et al 2000, Al-Ghamdi 2001) — interaction may be beneficial. Clinical significance unknown.

Anticoagulants

Theoretical interaction predicted based on antiplatelet, anticoagulant and conversely coagulant effects observed in vitro and in vivo (Al-Jishi & Abuo Hozaifa 2003, Asgary et al 2012, Awad & Binder 2005, Enomoto et al 2001). Clinical significance unknown — caution advised.

Anticonvulsants

A small clinical study shows that black seed had anticonvulsant effects in epileptic children refractory to their antiepileptic medication (Akhondian 2007). The constituent thymoquinone was reported to reduce sodium valproate-induced hepatotoxicity in one animal study (Raza et al 2006). Observe — however, interaction may be beneficial.

Antidiabetic agents

Preliminary clinical studies suggest that black seed reduces blood glucose levels and improves glucose tolerance in type 2 diabetes mellitus patients (Bamosa et al 2010), including those with diabetes as a comorbidity in dyslipidaemic patients (Kaatabi et al 2012, Najimi et al 2006). Caution — however, interaction may be beneficial.

Antihypertensives

A clinical study reported that black seed reduced blood pressure in patients with mild hypertension to a small extent (Dehkordi & Kamkhah 2008). Observe — however, interaction may be beneficial.

Antineoplastic agents

A theoretical and speculative interaction exists between black seed when used in combination with antineoplastic agents. Cytotoxic, apoptotic and necrotic effects have been observed in laboratory studies with the constituents thymoquinone and alpha-hederin (El-Mahdy et al 2005, Gali-Muhtasib et al 2004). The anticancer activity of thymoquinone has also been observed in animal studies (Ahmad et al 2013, Banerjee et al 2010, Randhawa & Alghamdi 2011, Woo et al 2012). Thymoquinone potentiated the antineoplastic effects of gemcitabine and oxaliplatin in one animal study (Banerjee et al 2009) and of ifosfamide in another animal study (Badary 1999). Theoretically, beneficial interactions exist, but further research is required to determine significance in humans.

N

Cisplatin

The constituent thymoquinone is theoretically protective against cisplatin-induced nephrotoxicity and deleterious drug effects on haemoglobin levels and leucocyte count, based on animal study findings (Badary et al 1997, Nair et al 1991). Synergistic effects were observed when thymoquinone was used in combination with cisplatin in lung cancer cells and in animal models (Jafri et al 2010). Observe — interaction theoretically beneficial. Clinical significance unknown.

Cytochrome P450-metabolising agents

Preliminary animal study data suggest that black seed may be protective against carbon tetrachloride-induced downregulation of cytochrome P450 enzymes CYP2B, CYP3A2, CYP2C11 and CYP1A2 (Ibrahim et al 2008). A potential interaction with drugs with cytochrome P450-metabolising activity is theoretical and speculative. Further research is required to determine clinical significance.

Doxorubicin

The constituent thymoquinone is theoretically protective against doxorubicin-induced cardiotoxicity and renal toxicity based on findings in animal studies (Al-Shabanah et al 1998, Badary et al 2000, Nagi & Mansour 2000). Observe — interaction theoretically beneficial. Clinical significance unknown.

Gentamicin

Black seed is theoretically protective against gentamicin-induced nephrotoxicity, based on findings in animal studies, but the clinical significance is unknown (Ali 2004, Sayed-Ahmed & Nagi 2007, Yaman & Balikci 2010). Observe — interaction theoretically beneficial.

Hepatotoxic agents

Based on animal studies, black seed appears to confer hepatoprotective effects against a number of agents. A theoretically beneficial interaction exists, but further research is required to determine significance in humans and with other hepatotoxic drugs.

Hypolipidaemic drugs

Black seed has been shown to modulate lipid levels according to clinical trials (Kaatabi et al 2012, Najmi et al 2008). Observe — however, interaction may be beneficial.

Immunomodulatory agents

Based on laboratory and animal studies, black seed displays immunomodulatory activity and may theoretically interact with either immunostimulant or immunosuppressant drugs (Abbas et al 2005, El-Obeid et al 2006, Gali-Muhtasib et al 2006, Islam et al 2004). Human studies are not available, therefore interactions are currently speculative and based on evidence of pharmacological activity. Clinical significance unknown.

Iron

Increased iron status possible with consumption of black seed, based on limited animal study (Jadayil et al 1999). Clinical significance is unknown, but theoretically beneficial in iron deficiency.

Non-steroidal anti-inflammatory drugs and cyclooxygenase-2 inhibitors

Based on laboratory and animal studies, black seed displays anti-inflammatory activity and may therefore theoretically interact with non-steroidal anti-inflammatory agents and cyclooxygenase-2 inhibitors (Al-Ghamdi 2001, El-Dakhakhny et al 2002, Houghton et al 1995, Mansour & Tornhamre 2004, Marsik et al 2005, Tekeoglu et al 2006). Human studies are not available, therefore interactions are currently speculative and based on evidence of pharmacological activity, but may theoretically be beneficial.

Methotrexate

Theoretically, the antioxidant properties of black seed may ameliorate the gastrointestinal adverse effects associated with methotrexate, according to preliminary animal studies (Labib et al 2009). Clinical studies

CONTRAINDICATIONS AND PRECAUTIONS

Avoid if known allergy or hypersensitivity to plants of the Ranunculaceae family. There are case study reports of allergic contact dermatitis following topical use of black seed oil (Ali & Blunden 2003). Black seed has been shown to alter levels of inflammatory mediators and various cytokines, although the clinical significance is still to be fully investigated (El-Obeid et al 2006, Gali-Muhtasib et al 2006). Caution is advised in patients with immune disorders, although dietary intake appears safe.

PREGNANCY USE

When taken in usual dietary amounts, black seed is likely to be safe; however the safety of larger doses has not been scientifically evaluated.

Animal studies suggest that the volatile oil of *Nigella sativa* seeds may suppress uterine contractions (Aqel & Shaheen 1996) and may also confer some contraceptive properties (Keshri et al 1995). There are insufficient data to extrapolate these data to humans; however it is suggested that large doses should be avoid in women trying to conceive.

Practice points/Patient counselling

- Black seed has been used for thousands of years to flavour food and for medicinal purposes, mostly in the Middle East and Southeast Asia.
- It has been referred to as a 'miracle herb' and has been used traditionally as a natural remedy for a range of conditions, including asthma, hypertension, diabetes, inflammation, cough, bronchitis, headache, eczema, fever, dizziness and influenza, as a carminative, a diuretic, a galactogogue, a vermifuge and for general wellbeing.
- A wide spectrum of pharmacological actions has been identified, including antiallergic, antidiabetic, antihypertensive, antimicrobial, antioxidant, lipid-lowering, antiepileptic, anti-inflammatory, immunomodulatory and anticancer properties.
- Currently. traditional folk use is supported by limited clinical evidence, but preliminary research suggests a potential role of black seed as adjunct therapy in asthma, allergy, type 2 diabetes mellitus, hyperlipidaemia and epilepsy.
- Appropriate therapeutic doses and potential for interactions and adverse effects are still to be confirmed.
- There is considerable interest in the potential of black seed as an innovative anticancer therapy and this is an area of current research.

are not yet available — however, beneficial interaction is possible.

Respiratory agents

Black seed has been shown to have antiasthmatic effects according to preliminary human study (Boskabady et al 2007, 2010). Observe — adjunctive use may be beneficial.

Warfarin

Theoretically, black seed may interact with warfarin, based on an in vitro study in which warfarin binding was displaced by the constituent thymoquinone (Lupido et al 2010). Caution — monitor concurrent use.

PATIENTS' FAQs

What will this herb do for me?
Black seed has a long history of traditional use as a folk medicine. It may be used in combination with drug therapies to support the treatment of a range of conditions, including allergy, asthma, diabetes and high cholesterol.

When will it start to work?
Benefits have been reported after 6 weeks of use, although further scientific evidence is required to confirm this and to determine suitable therapeutic doses.

Are there any safety issues?
Black seed is generally considered to be a very safe treatment based on historical use as a food and traditional medicine, although further research at therapeutic doses is required to confirm safety of black seed.

REFERENCES

Abbas AT et al. Effect of dexamethasone and *Nigella sativa* on peripheral blood eosinophil count, IgG1 and IgG2a, cytokine profiles and lung inflammation in murine model of allergic asthma. Egypt J Immunol. 12.1 (2005):95–102.

Abdel-Fattah AM, et al. Antinociceptive effects of *Nigella sativa* oil and its major component, thymoquinone, in mice. Eur J Pharmacol 14.400 (2000):89–97.

Abdel-Zaher AO et al. Protective effect of *Nigella sativa* oil against tramadol-induced tolerance and dependence in mice: role of nitric oxide and oxidative stress. Neurotoxicology 32.6 (2011):725–733.

Ahmad A et al. A review on therapeutic potential of *Nigella sativa*: A miracle herb. Asian Pac J Trop Biomed 3.5 (2013):337–352.

Akhondian J et al. The effect of thymoquinone on intractable pediatric seizures. Epilepsy Res. 93.1 (2011):39–43.

Akhondian J et al. The effect of Nigella sativa L. (black cumin seed) on intractable pediatric seizures. Med Sci Monit 13.12 (2007): CR555–559.

Ali BH. The effect of *Nigella sativa* oil on gentamicin nephrotoxicity in rats. Am J Chin Med 32.1. (2004): 49–55.

Ali BH, Blunden G. Pharmacological and toxicological properties of *Nigella sativa*. Phytother. Res. 17.4 (2003):299–305.

Al-Ghamdi MS. The anti-inflammatory, analgesic and antipyretic activity of *Nigella sativa*. J Ethnopharmacol 76.1 (2001):45–8.

Al-Jishi SA, Abuo Hozaifa B. Effect of *Nigella sativa* on blood hemostatic function in rats. J Ethnopharmacol. 85.1 (2003):7–14.

Al-Majed AA et al. Thymoquinone-induced relaxation of guinea-pig isolated trachea. Res Commun Mol Pathol Pharmacol 110. 5–6 (2001):333–45.

Al-Naggar TB et al. Neuropharmacological activity of *Nigella sativa* L. extracts. J Ethnopharmacol. 88.1 (2003):63–8.

Al Naqeep G, et al. Effects of thymoquinone rich fraction and thymoquinone on plasma lipoprotein levels and hepatic low density lipoprotein receptor and 3-hydroxy-3-methylglutaryl coenzyme A reductase gene expression. J Functional Foods 1 (2009): 298–303.

Al-Shabanah OA et al. Thymoquinone protects against doxorubicin-induced cardiotoxicity without compromising its antitumor activity. J Exp Clin Cancer Res 17.2 (1998): 193–8.

Aqel M, Shaheen R. Effects of volatile oil of *Nigella sativa* seeds on the uterine smooth muscle of rat and guinea pig. Journal of Ethnopharmacology. 52 (1996): 23–26.

Asgary S et al. Efficiency of black cumin seed on hematological factors in normal and hypercholesterolemic rabbits. ARYA Atheroscler 7.4 (2012):146–50.

Awad EM, Binder BR. In vitro induction of endothelial cell fibrinolytic alterations by *Nigella* seed. Phytomedicine 12.3 (2005):194–202.

Badary OA. Thymoquinone attenuates ifosfamide-induced Fanconi syndrome in rats and enhances its antitumor activity in mice. J Ethnopharmacol 67.2 (1999):135–42.

Badary OA et al. Thymoquinone ameliorates the nephrotoxicity induced by cisplatin in rodents and potentiates its antitumor activity. Can J Physiol Pharmacol 75.12 (1997): 1356–61.

Badary OA et al. The influence of thymoquinone on doxorubicin-induced hyperlipidemic nephropathy in rats. Toxicology 143.3 (2000): 219–26.

Bai T et al. Thymoquinone attenuates liver fibrosis via PI3K and TLR4 signalling pathways in activated hepatic stellate cells. International Immunopharmacology 15 (2013):275–281.

Bamosa AO et al. Effect of *Nigella sativa* seed on the glycemic control of patients with type 2 diabetes mellitus. Indian J Physiol Pharmacol 54.4 (2010):344–54.

Banerjee S et al. Antitumor activity of gemcitabine and oxaliplatin is augmented by thymoquinone in pancreatic cancer. Cancer Res. 69.13 (2009):5575–83.

Banerjee S et al. Review on molecular and therapeutic potential of thymoquinone in cancer. Nutr Cancer 62.7 (2010):938–46.

Bashir MU, Qureshi HJ. Analgesic effect of *Nigella sativa* seeds extract on experimentally induced pain in albino mice. J Coll Physicians Pak 20.7 (2010):464–7.

Bilal A, et al. Black seed (*Nigella sativa*) regulates glucose, insulin level and lipd profile in patients with Type 2 diabetes. Diabetes Research and Clinical Practice 79 (2008):S1–S127.

Boskabady MH et al. The possible prophylactic effect of *Nigella sativa* seed extract in asthmatic patients. Fundam Clin Pharmacol 21.5 (2007): 559–66.

Boskabady MH, et al. Relaxant effects of different fractions from *Nigella sativa* L. on guinea pig tracheal chains and its possible mechanism(s). Indian J Exp Biol 46.12 (2008):805–10.

Boskabady MH, et al. Antiasthmatic effect of *Nigella sativa* in airways of asthmatic patients. Phytomedicine. 17.10 (2010):707–13.

Dehkordi FR, Kamkhah AF. Antihypertensive effects of *Nigella sativa* seed extract in patients with mild hypertension. Fundam Clin. Pharmacol 22.4 (2008):447–52.

Edris AE. Anti-cancer properties of *Nigella* spp. essential oils and their major constituents, thymoquinone and β-elemene. Current Clinical Pharmacology (2009) 4: 43–46.

El-Dakhakhny M, et al. *Nigella sativa* L. oil protects against induced hepatoxicity and improves lipid profile in rats. Arzneimittelforschung 50.9 (2000): 832–6.

El-Dakhakny M et al. *Nigella sativa* oil, nigellone and derived thymoquinone inhibit synthesis of 5-lipoxygenase products in polymorphonuclear leukocytes from rats. J Ethnopharmacol 81.2 (2002): 161–4.

El Gazzar MA et al. Thymoquinone attenuates proinflammatory responses in lipopolysaccharide-activated mast cells by modulating NF-kappaB nuclear transactivation. Biochimica et Biophysica Acta 1770 (2007):556–564.

El-Mahdy MA et al. Thymoquinone induces apoptosis through activation of caspase-8 and mitochondrial events in p53-null myeloblastic leukemia HL-60 cells. Int J Cancer 117.3 (2005): 409–17.

El-Mahmoudy A et al. Successful abrogation by thymoquinone against induction of diabetes mellitus with streptozotocin via nitric oxide inhibitory mechanism. Int Immunopharmacol 5.1 (2005): 195–207.

El-Obeid A et al. Herbal melanin modulates tumor necrosis factor alpha (TNF-alpha), interleukin 6 (IL-6) and vascular endothelial growth factor (VEGF) production. Phytomedicine 13. 5 (2006): 324–33.

El-Sayed M et al. Comparative evaluation of anti-inflammatory properties of thymoquinone and curcumin using an asthmatic murine model. International Immunopharmacology. 11 (2011):2232–2236.

El-Shaimaa AA et al. Thymoquinone up-regulates PTEN expression and induces apoptosis in doxorubicin-resistant human breast cancer cells. Mutation Research 706 (2011): 28–35.

El-Tahir KEH, et al. The cardiovascular actions of the volatile oil of the black seed (*Nigella sativa*) in rats: elucidation of the mechanism of action. Gen Pharmac 24: 5 (1993): 1123–1131.

Enomoto S et al. Hematological studies on black cumin oil from the seeds of *Nigella sativa* L. Biol Pharm Bull 4.3 (2001):307–10.

Fararh KM et al. Thymoquinone reduces hepatic glucose production in diabetic hamsters. Res Vet Sci 79.3 (2005):219–23.

Fararh KM, et al. Thymoquinone enhances the activities of enzymes related to energy metabolism in peripheral leucocytes of diabetic rats. Res Vet Sci. 88.3 (2010):400–4.

Farraq AR et al. Protective effect of *Nigella sativa* seeds against lead-induced hepatorenal damage in male rats. Pak J Biol Sci 1.10 (2007):2809–16.

Gali-Muhtasib H et al. Thymoquinone extracted from black seed triggers apoptotic cell death in human colorectal cancer cells via a p53-dependent mechanism. Int J Oncol 25.4 (2004): 857–66.

Gali-Muhtasib H, et al. Thymoquinone: a promising anti-cancer drug from natural sources. Int J. Biochem Cell Biol. 38.8 (2006):1249–53.

Harzallah HJ et al. Thymoquinone, the *Nigella sativa* bioactive compound, prevents circulatory oxidative stress caused by 1,2-dimethylhydrazine in erythrocyte during colon postinitiation carcinogenesis. Oxidative Medicine and Cellular Longevity (2012); 2012: 854065.

Hassan AS, et al. A study of the effect of *Nigella sativa* (black seeds) in isoniazid (INH)-induced hepatotoxicity in rabbits. Indian J Pharmacol 44.6 (2012):678–82.

Hosseinzadeh H, Parvardeh S. Anticonvulsant effects of thymoquinone, the major constituent of *Nigella sativa* seeds, in mice. Phytomedicine 11.1 (2004): 56–64.

Hosseinzadeh H et al. Intracerebroventricular administration of thymoquinone, the major constituent of *Nigella sativa* seeds, suppresses epileptic seizures in rats. Med Sci Monit 11.4 (2005):BR106–10.

Houghton PJ et al. Fixed oil of *Nigella sativa* and derived thymoquinone inhibit eicosanoid generation in leukocytes and membrane lipid peroxidation. Planta Med 61.1 (1995):33–6.

Hussain AR et al. Thymoquinone suppresses growth and induces apoptosis via generation of reactive oxygen species in primary effusion lymphoma. Free Radical Biology & Medicine 50 (2011):978–987.

Ibrahim ZS et al. Protection by *Nigella sativa* against carbon-tetrachloride-induced downregulation of hepatic cytochrome P450 isoenzymes in rats. Jpn J Vet Res 56.3 (2008):119–28.

Illhan A et al. Antiepileptogenic and antioxidant effects of *Nigella sativa* oil against pentylenetetrazol-induced kindling in mice. Neuropharmacology 49.4 (2005): 456–64.

Isik H et al. Potential adjuvant effects of *Nigella sativa* seeds to improve specific immunotherapy in allergic rhinitis patients. Med Princ Pract 19 (2010):206–211.

Islam SN et al. Immunosuppressive and cytotoxic properties of *Nigella sativa*. Phytother Res 18.5 (2004):395–8.

Jadayil SA, et al. Bioavailability of iron from four different local food plants in Jordan. Plant foods Hum Nutr 54.4 (1999):285–94.

Jafri SH et al. Thymoquinone and cisplatin as a therapeutic combination in lung cancer: in vitro and in vivo. Journal of Experimental and Clinical Cancer Research 29.1(2010):87.

Kaatabi H et al. Favourable impact of *Nigella sativa* seeds on lipid profile in type 2 diabetic patients. J Family Community Med. 19.3 (2012):155–161.

Kaleem M et al. Biochemical effects of *Nigella sativa* L seeds in diabetic rats. Indian J Exp Biol. 44.9 (2006):745–8.

Kalus U et al. Effect of *Nigella sativa* (black seed) on subjective feeling in patients with allergic diseases. Phytother Res 17.10 (2003): 1209–14.

Kara MI et al. Thymoquinone accelerates new bone formation in the rapid maxillary expansion procedure. Archives of Oral Biology 57 (2012):357–363.

Kaseb AO et al. Androgen receptor and E2F-1 targeted thymoquinone therapy for hormone-refractory prostate cancer. Cancer Res 67 (2007): 7782–7788.

Keshri G et al. Post-coital contraceptive efficacy of the seeds of *Nigella sativa* in rats. Indian J Physiol Pharmacol. 39.1 (1995): 59–62.

Khader M, et al. In vitro toxicological properties of thymoquinone. Food and Chemical Toxicology. 47 (2009): 129–133.

Labib R, et al. *Nigella sativa* oil ameliorates methotrexate intestinal toxicity through antioxidant activity. European Journal of Cancer Supplements. 7. 2 (2009):106.

Lei X et al. Thymoquinone inhibits growth and augments 5-fluorouracil-induced apoptosis in gastric cancer cells both in vitro and in vivo. Biochemical and Biophysical Research Communications 417 (2012):864–868.

Li F, et al. Thymoquinone inhibits proliferation, induces apoptosis and chemosensitizes human multiple myeloma cells through suppression of signal transducer and activator of transcription 3 activation pathway. Br J Pharmacol 161 (2010):541–554.

Lupido G et al. Thymoquinone, a potential therapeutic agent of *Nigella sativa,* binds to site I of human serum albumin. Phytomedicine 17.10 (2010): 714–720.

Lutterodt H et al. Fatty acid profile, thymoquinone content, oxidative stability, and antioxidant properties of cold-pressed black cumin seed oils. LWT-Food Science and Technology 43 (2010):1409–1413.

Mahmoud-Awny M, et al. Thymoquinone: Novel gastroprotective mechanisms. European Journal of Pharmacology 697 (2012):126–131.

Majdalawieh AF, et al. *Nigella sativa* modulates plenocyte proliferation, Th1/Th2 cytokine profile, macrophage function and NK anti-tumor activity. Journal of Ethnopharmacology 131 (2010):268–275.

Mansour M, Tornhamre S. Inhibition of 5-lipoxygenase and leukotriene C4 synthase in human blood cells by thymoquinone. J Enzyme Inhib Med Chem 19.5 (2004): 431–436.

Marsik P et al. In vitro inhibitory effects of thymol and quinones of *Nigella sativa* seeds on cyclooxygenase-1- and -2-catalyzed prostaglandin E2 biosyntheses. Planta Med 71.8 (2005):739–42.

Meddah B et al. *Nigella sativa* inhibits intestinal glucose absorption and improves glucose tolerance in rats. J Ethnopharmacol. 121.3 (2009):419–24.

Mostafa R, Moustafa Y. Oxidants and antioxidants balance modulation by *Nigella sativa* seeds consumption in healthy postmenopausal women. Maturitas 71, Supplement 1 (2012):S1–S82.

Nagi MN, Mansour MA. Protective effect of thymoquinone against doxorubicin-induced cardiotoxicity in rats: a possible mechanism of protection. Pharmacological research 41. 3 (March 2000): 283–289.

Nair SC et al. Modulatory effects of Crocus sativus and *Nigella sativa* extracts on cisplatin-induced toxicity in mice. J Ethnopharmacolo 31.1 (1991): 75–83.

Najmi A et al. Effect of *Nigella sativa* oil on various clinical and biochemical parameters of insulin resistance syndrome. Int J Diabetes Dev Ctries 28.1 (2008):11–4.

Nikakhlagh S et al. Herbal treatment of allergic rhinitis: the use of *Nigella sativa*. American Journal of Otolaryngology-Head and Neck Medicine Surgery 32 (2011):402–407.

Paramasivam A et al. Induction of apoptosis in mouse neuroblastoma (Neuro-2a) cells by thymoquinone. Biomedicine & Preventative Nutrition 2 (2012):223–227.

Qidwai W et al. Effectiveness, safety, and tolerability of powdered *Nigella sativa* (kalonji) seed in capsules on serum lipid levels, blood sugar, blood pressure, and body weight in adults: results of a randomized, double-blind controlled trial. The Journal of Alternative and Complementary Medicine. 15.6 (2009):639–644.

Randhawa MA, Alghamdi MS. Anticancer activity of *Nigella sativa* (black seed) — a review. The American Journal of Chinese Medicine 39.6 (2011):1075–1091.

Ravindran J et al. Thymoquinone poly (lactide-co-glycolide) nanoparticles exhibit enhanced anti-proliferative, anti-inflammatory, and chemosensitization potential. Biochemical Pharmacology 79 (2010):1640–1647.

Raza M et al. Beneficial interaction of thymoquinone and sodium valproate in experimental models of epilepsy: reduction in hepatotoxicity of valproate. Scientia Pharmaceutica (Austria) 17 (2006):159–173.

Roepke M et al. Lack of p53 augments thymoquinone-induced apoptosis and caspase activation in human osteosarcoma cells. Cancer Biol Ther 6(2007):160–169.

Sabzevari O et al. Protective effect of thymoquinone against liver toxicity induced by aflatoxin B1 in mice. Toxicology Letters. 205d (2011):S180–S300.

Salem EM et al. Comparative Study of *Nigella sativa* and triple therapy in eradication of *Helicobacter pylori* in patients with non-ulcer dyspepsia. Saudi Journal of Gastroenterology 16. 3 (2010):207–14.

Sangi S et al. A new and novel treatment of opioid dependence: *Nigella sativa* 500 mg. J Ayub Med Coll Abbotabad 20.2 (2008):118–24.

Sayed-Ahmed MM and Nagi MN. Thymoquinone supplementation prevents the development of gentamicin-induced acute renal toxicity in rats. Clin Exp Pharmacol Physiol 34 (2007):399–405.

Shoieb AM et al. In vitro inhibition of growth and induction of apoptosis in cancer cell lines by thymoquinone. Int J Oncol 22 (2003): 107–113.

Stern T et al. Black seed oil ointment - a new approach for the treatment of atopic dermatitis? Akttuelle Dermatologie 28. 3 (2002):74–79.

Tekeoglu I, et al. Effects of thymoquinone (volatile oil of black cumin) on rheumatoid arthritis in rat models. Phytother Res 20.10 (2006):869–71.

Waseem M et al. Heavy metal toxicity: mitagatory role of thymoquinone. Int J Devl Neuroscience 20 (2012):640–671.

Wirries A et al. Thymoquinone accelerates osteoblast differentiation and activates bone morphogenetic protein-2 and ERK pathway. International Immunopharmacology 15 (2013):381–386.

Woo CC et al. Thymoquinone: Potential cure for inflammatory disorders and cancer. Biochemical Pharmacology 83 (2012): 443–451.

Worthen DR et al. The *in vitro* anti-tumor activity of some crude and purified components of blackseed, *Nigella sativa* L. Anticancer Res 18.3A (1998): 1527–1532.

Yaman I, Balikci E. Protective effects of *Nigella sativa* against gentamicin-induced nephrotoxicity in rats. Exp Toxicol Pathol 62.2 (2010): 183–90.

Zaoui A et al. Diuretic and hypotensive effects of *Nigella sativa* in the spontaneously hypertensive rat. Therapie 55.3 (2000): 379–82.

Zaoui A et al. Acute and chronic toxicity of *Nigella sativa* fixed oil. Phytomedicine 9 (2002):69–74.

Noni

HISTORICAL NOTE Noni has been used throughout Southeast Asia and Polynesia for more than 2000 years as a food source, a medicine and a dye. Noni fruit was traditionally used by Polynesians to combat fatigue (Ma et al 2007) and legends tell of Polynesian heroes and heroines that used noni to survive from famine (Wang et al 2002). Based on existing Bishop Museum records, it has been stated that the juice of the ripe fruit boiled is used as a remedy for diabetes, and fermented, as a tonic for cardiac complications and high blood pressure (Brown 2012).

COMMON NAME

Noni

OTHER NAMES

Ba Ji Tian, cheese fruit, Indian mulberry, mengkudu, nhau, nono, nonu.

BOTANICAL NAME/FAMILY

Morinda citrifolia (family Rubiaceae)

PLANT PARTS USED

Roots, stems, bark, leaves, flowers, fruit and juice.

CHEMICAL COMPONENTS

Noni contains terpenoids, alkaloids, anthraquinones (e.g. damnacanthal, morindone and rubiadin), the coumarin scopoletin, beta sitosterol, carotene, vitamin A, flavone glycosides, linoleic acid, the orange-red pigment alizarin, L-asperuloside, caproic acid, caprylic acid, ursolic acid, octanoic acid, potassium, vitamin C, rutin (Hiramatsu et al 1993, Wang et al 2002), as well as a natural precursor for xeronine named proxeronine (Heinicke 1985, 2001). In vitro studies suggest that the antioxidant activity is due to several compounds such as coumarin derivatives (Ikeda et al 2009) and phenolic compounds (Liu et al 2007) that may contribute individually or synergistically.

Scopoletin has been suggested as a bioactive marker and a candidate for product standardisation and pharmacokinetic studies (Issell et al 2008).

MAIN ACTIONS

Noni is purported to have many different effects including analgesic, anti-inflammatory, antioxidant, anticancer, antimicrobial, immune enhancement and antihypertensive activity.

Analgesic and anti-inflammatory

Noni root extract has exhibited opioid-like properties, with dose-dependent analgesic properties in mice that were reversible by naloxone, together with sedative effects at higher doses (Younos et al 1990). Analgesic activity has also been reported in controlled trials using rats and mice (Wang et al 2002). The analgesic effect of noni is also due to its ability to inhibit cyclooxygenase and may be as potent as some NSAIDs (McKoy et al 2002).

Antioxidant

Fruit, leaf and root extracts have all been shown to exhibit antioxidant activity (Kamiya et al 2004, Zin et al 2006) and NO scavenging activity in vitro (Jagetia & Baliga 2004), with some extracts showing comparable antioxidant activity to tocopherol (Zin et al 2002, 2006), grape seed powder and pycnogenol (Wang et al 2002). The neolignan, americanin A, has shown to be a particularly potent antioxidant in vitro (Su et al 2005).

A 1-month double-blind, randomised, placebo-controlled trial involving 68 smokers found that 50 mL of noni juice twice daily significantly reduced plasma superoxide radicals and lipid peroxides (Wang et al 2002). Noni juice has also been shown to reduce oxidative stress and liver damage in carbon tetrachloride-treated rats (Wang et al 2002, 2008a, 2008b), as well as inhibit the in vitro enzymatic activity of cyclooxygenase-1 (COX-1) (Li et al 2003) and cyclooxygenase-2 (COX-2) (Wang et al 2002). The clinical significance of these findings is yet to be determined.

Gastroprotective

One in vivo study which evaluated the effect of an aqueous extract of dried noni fruit as well as its biomarker (scopoletin) demonstrated that noni may be beneficial as a potential preventive and therapeutic agent for gastro-oesophageal inflammation, mainly through its ability to enhance the mucosal defensive mechanisms via suppression of serotonin, free radicals and cytokine-mediated inflammation. Moreover, the efficacy was comparable to that of a standard potent anti-secretory proton pump inhibitor (lansoprazole) (Mahattanadul et al 2011). Further research is required to establish efficacy in humans with GORD.

Antitumour/anticancer

A review by Brown et al (2012) investigated 19 (both in vitro and in vivo) studies related to cancer. Of these studies, noni was tested in various forms (extract, powder and precipitate). Only nine studies were conducted on noni extract and the results suggest a bioactive component in noni juice extract (not leaves, roots or other plant parts) may be effective against cancer up to 30% of the time in laboratory rodents. However, the noni precipitate or

N

extract was injected into these animals, so the results may not be clinically relevant.

Several in vitro studies found anti-proliferative compounds in the leaves and roots of noni. Furthermore, the polysaccharide ethanol precipitate of noni has been shown to stimulate the immune system through macrophages, which were reported to release cytokines, nitric oxide (NO), interleukin-1 and interleukin 12 (IL-1, IL-12) and tumour necrosis factor (TNF) (Furusawa et al 2003, Hirazumi et al 1994). More recent in vitro data suggests that noni juice can enhance treatment responses in women with existing HER2/neu breast cancer as it significantly reduces tumour weight and volume, and has the ability to inhibit the growth of this aggressive form of cancer at an equivalent human dose of between 45 and 80 mL/day (Clafshenkel et al 2012).

In another study, cisplatin, an antitumour agent, showed only a slightly higher cell-killing activity against human cervical carcinoma HeLa and SiHa cells when compared to noni juice in vitro (Gupta et al 2013). The combination of noni juice and cisplatin showed additive effects through the upregulation of pro-apoptotic members and down-regulation of the anti-apoptotic members suggesting noni may be a potential adjuvant agent for chemotherapy.

Older research reveals that an alcoholic precipitate of noni juice significantly prolonged the life of mice with implanted tumours (Furusawa et al 2003, Hirazumi et al 1994). It is suggested that this antitumour activity is due to immunostimulatory activity because the noni precipitate was not directly cytotoxic to tumour cells, but did activate immune cells in vitro with its activity reduced by immunosuppressant drugs (Furusawa et al 2003, Hirazumi et al 1996). Noni juice has also been observed to increase the wet weight of thymus tissue in animals (Wang et al 2002) and to protect against 7,12-dimethylbenz(*a*)anthracene (DMBA)-induced DNA adduct formation in rats (Wang & Su 2001).

Noni improved survival times in cancer-implanted mice when combined with suboptimal doses of standard chemotherapeutic agents (Hirazumi & Furusawa 1999) and this is supported by in vitro studies demonstrating synergistic effects with chemotherapeutic agents (Furusawa et al 2003, Wang et al 2002).

In vitro studies have also found that noni fruit has antiproliferative activity against SKBR3 human breast adenocarcinoma cells (Moongkarndi et al 2004), and that glycosides extracted from noni inhibit cell transformation (Liu et al 2001) and ultraviolet-B (UVB)-induced activator protein-1 activity (Sang et al 2001, 2003). The anthraquinone, damnacanthal, is reported to stimulate UV-induced apoptosis in vitro (Hiwasa et al 1999).

Antimicrobial

Constituents of noni show activity against *Escherichia coli* in vitro (Duncan et al 1998) and *Mycobacterium tuberculosis* (National Library of Medicine 2001), as well as the parasite *Ascaris lumbricoides* (Raj 1975); however, the clinical significance of this is undetermined. In vitro testing found that noni juice was as effective as sodium hypochlorite in reducing the smear layer when used as an endodontic irrigant (Murray et al 2008).

Hepatoprotective

In vivo evidence (Lin et al 2013) suggests that noni juice significantly ameliorates ($P < 0.05$) the increased liver size and visceral fat levels in hamsters fed a high-fat diet compared to hamsters fed a normal-fat diet over a 6-week period. The hamsters were put into five groups (including the control group), and the high-fat diet hamsters received distilled water, and 3, 6 and 9 mL of noni juice/kg of body weight, respectively. Supplementation with noni juice decreased serum and liver lipid levels, and also lipid deposits in hepatohistological examination, and diminished overall liver damage induced by a high-fat diet.

Anti-psychotic

Studies have demonstrated that a methanolic extract of noni fruit, which was orally administered to mice (at doses of 1, 3, 5, 10 g/kg) significantly decreased methamphetamine and apomorphine-induced behaviour (licking, biting, gnawing and sniffing) and climbing time in mice in a dose-dependent manner (Pandy et al 2012). Conversely, when noni juice was made freely available in drinking water at a volume concentration of 50% and 100%, there were significant reductions in apomorphine-induced climbing behaviour and time. This data demonstrates the anti-dopaminergic effect of noni juice in mice, and supports anecdotal evidence which suggests that noni is effective in the treatment of CNS disorders. Further studies are required to identify the actions responsible for the observed antipsychotic activity of noni.

Ergogenic

Animal studies in aged mice have shown that noni juice improved endurance, balance and flexibility (Ma et al 2007).

Antihypertensive

The antihypertensive effects of the root extract of noni were first investigated in the 1950s (Ho 1955) and a hot-water extract of noni root is reported to have lowered the blood pressure of an anaesthetised dog (Youngken 1958). Antispasmodic and vasodilator activities of noni root extract are believed to be mediated through a blockade of voltage-dependent calcium channels (Gilani et al 2010). However, the root is not a component of commercial preparations, and this study used a vacuum-dried 70% aqueous-ethanolic extract.

Antidiabetic

In experimental diabetic models, noni extract displayed antihyperglycaemic as well as antioxidant effects (Kamiya et al 2008, Mahadeva Rao & Subramanian 2008). When fermented as a soybean paste, noni has shown benefit in murine models as a functional food for the management of type 2 diabetes (Lee et al 2012). Over a 90-day period the fermented noni paste reduced blood glucose levels to 211.60–252.20 mg/dL (11.8 mmol/ L–14.0 mmol /L) after 90 days, while those in the control group were in excess of 400 mg/dL (22.2 mmol/L) after 20 days. In addition, supplementation with the fermented noni paste reduced glycosylated haemoglobin (HbA_{1C}) levels, enhanced insulin sensitivity and significantly decreased serum triglycerides and low-density lipoprotein (LDL) cholesterol (Lee et al 2012).

Cardioprotective

In vitro evidence suggests that noni juice exerts a cardio-protective effect in hamsters consuming a high-fat/cholesterol diet (Lin et al 2012). In this study, noni juice supplementation decreased serum triacylglycerol, cholesterol, atherogenic index, malondialdehyde levels and hepatic lipids, while glutathione and faecal lipids were increased ($P < 0.05$).

OTHER ACTIONS

Noni has been shown to inhibit gastric emptying in male rats via a mechanism involving stimulation of cholecystokinin (CCK) secretion and CCK1 receptor activation (Pu et al 2004) and in vitro studies demonstrate inhibition of lipoprotein lipase suggesting potential use in weight management (Pak-Dek et al 2008).

CLINICAL USE

In recent years noni juice has been touted as a 'super juice' that enhances wellbeing. Noni has been reported to be of benefit for people with arthritis, diabetes, hypertension, muscle aches and pains, menstrual difficulties, headache, heart disease, atherosclerosis, AIDS, cancers, gastric ulcers, poor digestion, depression, senility and drug addiction (Wang et al 2002). Since noni has not been significantly investigated in human studies, uncertainty remains about its potential benefits in these conditions and diseases. At this stage, evidence for its use is mostly derived from traditional, in vitro and animal studies and a handful of trials of varying quality.

Osteoarthritis

Based on its demonstrated anti-inflammatory and analgesic properties, a benefit in osteoarthritis seems possible. Wang et al (2011) have investigated this further in an open label pilot study of 82 patients with diagnosed knee or hip osteoarthritis (OA), which revealed that Tahitian Noni Juice (TNJ, produced by Morinda Holding Inc.) improved both quality of life and symptoms as measured by two validated scales, SF-36 and the Arthritis Impact Measurement Scales (AIMS 2).

The 21 male and 61 female participants (aged 40–75 years) received 88 mL of TNJ per day for 90 days, and were not taking any other prescription medication for arthritis. The results indicated that there were statistically significant improvements in OA patient satisfaction with mobility, walking and bending, hand and finger functions, arm function, self-care, household tasks, social activity, arthritis pain, work, level of tension and mood (Wang et al 2011). Since the study lacked a placebo arm, it can only be described as suggestive of a benefit. Double-blind, placebo-controlled studies are now warranted.

Primary dysmenorrhoea

A prospective, randomised, double-blind placebo-controlled trial of 100 university students (aged 18 years or older) found that 3 months treatment with noni capsules (400 mg twice daily; Vitamin World, USA) provided no benefits for primary dysmenorrhoea (Fletcher et al 2013). Interestingly, the placebo group had a greater decrease in mean pain scores than the noni group after 3 months and there were no significant differences in the mean bleeding score. The fact that the subjects using noni had a better decrease in their ESR (an acute phase reactant) suggests that it does have some anti-inflammatory effects; however, this was not manifested in clinically improved pain or bleeding scores during the time of the study. The authors suggested that poor treatment compliance may have been a limitation of the study. Whether a higher dose or longer treatment term may have produced different results remains to be tested.

N

Smoking-induced dyslipidaemia

Noni juice has been shown to mitigate cigarette smoke-induced dyslipidaemia (Wang et al 2012). A randomised, double-blind, placebo-controlled clinical trial investigated the antioxidant activity of noni juice in 100 heavy smokers who smoked more than 20 cigarettes per day. The study, which used a blend of grape and blueberry juices as placebo, found that noni juice (29.5–188 mL/day for 30 days) significantly reduced cholesterol levels, triglycerides and high-sensitivity C reactive protein. It is theorised that noni juice inhibits cigarette smoke-induced oxidative stress by increasing the activity of glutathione-utilising enzymes (Wang et al 2012).

Hearing and mental health

A small placebo-controlled pilot study involving nine hearing-impaired osteopenic or osteoporotic women found that ingestion of approximately 50 mL of noni juice over 3 months resulted in improved mental health and a mild protective effect on hearing. Further studies are required to determine the clinical significance of these findings (Langford et al 2004).

Practice points/Patient counselling

- Noni has been traditionally used as food and medicine for a wide range of medical conditions.
- Noni has not been significantly investigated in clinical studies, so its use is based on traditional evidence and laboratory and animal studies demonstrating various actions.
- Although it is likely to be safe, it is prudent to avoid using noni in amounts greater than those ingested as a food during pregnancy and to monitor clotting profiles if noni is used with anticoagulant medications.

OTHER USES

Noni fruit may be used as a food source.

DOSAGE RANGE

There is little human research upon which to make accurate dosage recommendations, however, successful studies have used in the vicinity of 30–190 mL/day (Wang et al 2012).

Noni juice can also be used to create freeze-dried pills, concentrated extracts, powders, tinctures and even fruit leather similar to dried fruit strips (Brown 2012).

TOXICITY

Human clinical trials have shown the maximum tolerated dose of noni was 12 g (tablet form) with no dose-limiting toxicity found in seven of eight patients who ingested 14 g (Issell et al 2009). No toxic effects have been found in rats (Mancebo et al 2002), even when given doses up to 80 mL/kg (Wang et al 2002).

Idiosyncratic adverse events have been reported for noni juice; however, these appear to be rare.

Several cases of hepatotoxicity related to noni juice consumption have been reported, with one case requiring urgent liver transplantation (Millonig et al 2005, Stadlbauer et al 2005, Yu et al 2011), and others spontaneously recovering after ceasing noni consumption (Millonig et al 2005, Stadlbauer et al 2005). More recently, a case was reported of a 38-year-old woman who developed acute liver injury and jaundice associated with noni juice (cumulative amount approximately 400 mL) in a patient on long-term (9 months) anticonvulsant therapy (Mrzljak et al 2013). It is unknown whether this toxic effect is a result of the synergistic effect of both the medication prescribed and noni juice consumption. Such case reports are in contrast to studies that indicate that the no-observed-adverse-effect level (NOAEL) for freeze-dried noni fruit puree is greater than 6.86 g/kg body weight, equivalent to approximately 90 mL of noni fruit juice/kg (West et al 2009).

More safety data is required before clinical conclusions can be made.

ADVERSE REACTIONS

Noni appears to be well tolerated. A safety study conducted on 96 healthy volunteers who consumed up to 750 mL Tahitian Noni Juice per day revealed no adverse effects (West et al 2009). Similarly no adverse events were reported in a clinical trial using 29.5 to 188 mL daily for 30 days (Wang et al 2012). Allergenicity studies using guinea pigs report no allergic responses (Wang et al 2002).

SIGNIFICANT INTERACTIONS

There is one case report of noni juice consumption causing resistance to warfarin (Carr et al 2004). Further investigation is required to determine the certainty of this causal association.

CONTRAINDICATIONS AND PRECAUTIONS

Noni juice is high in potassium and use needs to be monitored in patients with kidney, liver or heart problems (Brown 2012).

PREGNANCY USE

Likely to be safe when consumed in dietary amounts; however, safety is not known when used in larger quantities. In vivo studies suggest the possibility of reproductive toxicity in rats (Muller et al 2009) while prenatal toxicity in developing rat embryos or fetuses revealed no evidence of toxicity (West et al 2008).

PATIENTS' FAQs

What will this herb do for me?

Noni has not been significantly investigated under clinical trial conditions, so its use is largely based on traditional evidence and laboratory and animal studies. Preliminary research suggests it may be useful in osteoarthritis and reducing cholesterol levels in heavy smokers, but benefits remain unclear and further clinical studies are required to confirm effects.

When will it start to work?

There is little published evidence to indicate its speed of action, which will depend on the clinical use.

Are there are any safety issues?

Noni is generally considered safe and can be consumed as a food; however, the safety of large intakes is unknown. The available human studies show it is well tolerated.

REFERENCES

Brown AC. Anticancer activity of Morinda citrifolia (Noni) fruit: a review. Phytother Res. 26.10 (2012): 1427–1440.

Carr ME et al. Coumadin resistance and the vitamin supplement Noni. Am J Hematol 77.1 (2004): 103.

Clafshenkel WP et al. *Morinda citrifolia* (Noni) juice augments mammary gland differentiation and reduces mammary tumor growth in mice expressing the Unactivated c-erbB2 Transgene. Evid Based Complement Alternat Med. (2012):487423.

Duncan SH et al. Inhibitory activity of gut bacteria against Escherichia coli O157 mediated by dietary plant metabolites. FEMS Microbiol Lett 164.2 (1998): 283–288.

Fletcher HM et al. Morinda citrifolia (Noni) as an Anti-Inflammatory Treatment in Women with Primary Dysmenorrhoea: A Randomised Double-Blind Placebo-Controlled Trial. Obstet Gynecol Int. (2013): 195454. doi: 10.1155/2013/195454

Furusawa E et al. Antitumour potential of a polysaccharide-rich substance from the fruit juice of Morinda citrifolia (Noni) on sarcoma 180 ascites tumour in mice. Phytother Res 17.10 (2003): 1158–1164.

Gilani AH et al. Antispasmodic and vasodilator activities of Morinda citrifolia root extract are mediated through blockade of voltage dependent calcium channels. BMC Complement Altern Med. Jan 13 (2010): 10:2.

Gupta RK et al. Induction of mitochondrial-mediated apoptosis by Morinda citrifolia (Noni) in human cervical cancer cells. Asian Pac J Cancer Prev. 14.1 (2013): 237–242.

Heinicke R. The pharmacologically active ingredient of Noni. Bull Ntl Trop Bot Gardens; as cited in Wang MY et al (2002). Morinda citrifolia (Noni): a literature review and recent advances in Noni Res. Acta Pharmacol Sin 23.12 (1985): 1127–1141.

Heinicke R. The xeronine system: a nex cellular mechanism that explains the health promoting action of NONI and Bromelain. USA: Direct Source Publishing [online], 2001.

Hiramatsu T et al. Induction of normal phenotypes in ras-transformed cells by damnacanthal from Morinda citrifolia. Cancer Lett 73.2–3 (1993): 161–166.

Hirazumi A, Furusawa E. An immunomodulatory polysaccharide-rich substance from the fruit juice of Morinda citrifolia (noni) with antitumour activity. Phytother Res 13.5 (1999): 380–387.

Hirazumi A et al. Anticancer activity of Morinda citrifolia (noni) on intraperitoneally implanted Lewis lung carcinoma in syngeneic mice. Proc West Pharmacol Soc 37 (1994): 145–146.

Hirazumi A et al. Immunomodulation contributes to the anticancer activity of morinda citrifolia (noni) fruit juice. Proc West Pharmacol Soc 39 (1996): 7–9.

Hiwasa T et al. Stimulation of ultraviolet-induced apoptosis of human fibroblast UVr-1 cells by tyrosine kinase inhibitors. FEBS Lett 444.2–3 (1999): 173–176.

Ho DV. Treatment and prevention of hypertension and its cerebral complications by total root extracts of Morinda citrifolia. Presse Med 63.72 (1955): 1478.

Ikeda R et al. Quantification of coumarin derivatives in Noni (Morinda citrifolia) and their contribution of quenching effect on reactive oxygen species. Food Chem 113.4 (2009): 1169–1172.

Issell BF et al. Pharmacokinetic study of noni fruit extract. J Diet Suppl 5.4 (2008): 373–382.

Issell BF et al. Using quality of life measures in a Phase I clinical trial of noni in patients with advanced cancer to select a Phase II dose. J Diet Suppl. 6.4 (2009): 347–359.

Jagetia GC, Baliga MS. The evaluation of nitric oxide scavenging activity of certain Indian medicinal plants in vitro: a preliminary study. J Med Food 7.3 (2004): 343–348.

Kamiya K et al. Chemical constituents of Morinda citrifolia fruits inhibit copper-induced low-density lipoprotein oxidation. J Agric Food Chem 52.19 (2004): 5843–5848.

Kamiya K et al. Chemical constituents of Morinda citrifolia roots exhibit hypoglycemic effects in streptozotocin-induced diabetic mice. Biol Pharm Bull 31.5 (2008): 935–938.

Langford J et al. Effects of Morinda citrifolia on quality of life and auditory function in postmenopausal women. J Altern Complement Med 10.5 (2004): 737–739.

Lee SY et al. Antidiabetic Effect of Morinda citrifolia (Noni) Fermented by Cheonggukjang in KK-A(y) Diabetic Mice. Evid Based Complement Alternat Med. (2012): 163280.

Li RW et al. A cross-cultural study: anti-inflammatory activity of Australian and Chinese plants. J Ethnopharmacol 85.1 (2003): 25–32.

Lin YL et al. Hypolipidemic and antioxidative effects of noni (Morinda citrifolia L.) juice on high-fat/cholesterol-dietary hamsters. Plant Foods Hum Nutr. 67.3 (2012):294–302.

Lin YL et al. Beneficial effects of noni (Morinda citrifolia L.) juice on livers of high-fat dietary hamsters. Food Chem. 140.1–2 (2013): 31–8

Liu G et al. Two novel glycosides from the fruits of Morinda Citrifolia (noni) inhibit AP-1 transactivation and cell transformation in the mouse epidermal JB6 cell line. Cancer Res 61.15 (2001): 5749–5756.

Liu CH et al. Extraction and characterization of antioxidant compositions from fermented fruit juice of Morinda citrifolia (Noni). Agric Sci China 6.12 (2007): 1494–1501.

Ma DL et al. Evaluation of the ergogenic potential of noni juice. Phytother Res 21.11 (2007): 1100–1101.

Mahadeva Rao US, Subramanian S. Biochemical evaluation of antihyperglycemic and antioxidative effects of Morinda citrifolia fruit extract studied in streptozotocin-induced diabetic rats. Med Chem Res 18.6 (2008): 1–14.

Mahattanadul S et al. Effects of Morinda citrifolia aqueous fruit extract and its biomarker scopoletin on reflux esophagitis and gastric ulcer in rats. J Ethnopharmacol. 134.2 (2011): 243–250.

Mancebo A et al. Repeated dose oral toxicity assay (28 days) of the aqueous extract of Morinda citrifolia in Sprague Dawley rats. Rev Toxicol 19.2 (2002): 73–78.

McKoy ML et al. Preliminary investigation of the anti-inflammatory properties of an aqueous extract from Morinda citrifolia (noni). Proc. West Pharmacol.Soc. 45 (2002): 76–78.

Millonig G et al. Herbal hepatotoxicity: acute hepatitis caused by a Noni preparation (Morinda citrifolia). Eur J Gastroenterol Hepatol 17.4 (2005): 445–447.

Moongkarndi P et al. Antiproliferative activity of Thai medicinal plant extracts on human breast adenocarcinoma cell line. Fitoterapia 75.3–4 (2004): 375–377.

Muller JC et al. Morinda citrifolia Linn (Noni): in vivo and in vitro reproductive toxicology. J Ethnopharmacol 121.2 (2009): 229–233.

Murray PE et al. Evaluation of Morinda citrifolia as an endodontic irrigant. J Endod 34.1 (2008): 66–70.

Mrzljak A et al. Drug-Induced Liver Injury Associated with Noni (Morinda citrifolia) Juice and Phenobarbital. Case Rep Gastroenterol. 7.1 (2013): 19–24.

National Library of Medicine. Noni plant may help TB. AIDS Patient Care STDs 15.3 (2001): 175.

Pak-Dek MS et al. Inhibitory effect of Morinda citrifolia L. on lipoprotein lipase activity. J Food Sci 73.8 (2008): C595–C598.

Pandy V et al. Antipsychotic-like activity of noni (Morinda citrifolia Linn.) in mice. BMC Complement Altern Med. 12 (2012): 186.

Pu HF et al. Effects of juice from Morinda citrifolia (Noni) on gastric emptying in male rats. Chin J Physiol 47.4 (2004): 169–174.

Raj RK. Screening of indigenous plants for anthelmintic action against human Ascaris lumbricoides: part II. Indian J Physiol Pharmacol 19.1 (1975): 47–49.

Sang S et al. Citrifolinin A, a new unusual iridoid with inhibition of activator protein-1 (AP-1) from the leaves of noni (Morinda citrifolia L.). Tetrahedron Lett 42.10 (2001): 1823–1825.

Sang S et al. New unusual iridoids from the leaves of noni (Morinda citrifolia L.) show inhibitory effect on ultraviolet B-induced transcriptional activator protein-1 (AP-1) activity. Bioorg Med Chem 11.12 (2003): 2499–2502.

Stadlbauer V et al. Hepatotoxicity of NONI juice: report of two cases. World J Gastroenterol 11.30 (2005): 4758–4760.

Su BN et al. Chemical constituents of the fruits of Morinda citrifolia (Noni) and their antioxidant activity. J Nat Prod 68.4 (2005): 592–595.

Wang MY, Su C. Cancer preventive effect of Morinda citrifolia (Noni). Ann N Y Acad Sci 952 (2001): 161–168.

Wang MY et al. Morinda citrifolia (Noni): a literature review and recent advances in Noni Res. Acta Pharmacol Sin 23.12 (2002): 1127–1141.

Wang MY et al. Hepatic protection by noni fruit juice against CCl4-induced chronic liver damage in female SD rats. Plant Foods Hum Nutr 63.3 (2008a): 141–145.

Wang MY et al. Liver protective effects of Morinda citrifolia (Noni). Plant Foods Hum Nutr 63.2 (2008b): 59–63.

Wang MY et al. Morinda citrifolia L. (noni) improves the Quality of Life in adults with Osteoarthritis. Functional Foods in Health and Disease. 1.2 (2011):75–90.

Wang MY et al. Noni juice improves serum lipid profiles and other risk markers in cigarette smokers. Scientific World Journal. (2012): 594657.

West BJ et al. Prenatal toxicity test of Morinda citrifolia (noni) fruit. J Toxicol Sci 33.5 (2008): 647–649.

West BJ et al. Hepatotoxicity and subchronic toxicity tests of Morinda citrifolia (noni) fruit. J Toxicol Sci. 34.5 (2009): 581–585.

West BJ et al. A double-blind clinical safety study of noni fruit juice. Pac Health Dialog. 15.2 (2009): 21–32.

Yu EL et al. Acute hepatotoxicity after ingestion of Morinda citrifolia (Noni Berry) juice in a 14-year-old boy. J Pediatr Gastroenterol Nutr. 52.2 (2011): 222–224.

Youngken HW Sr. A study of the root of Morinda citrifolia Linne. I. J Am Pharm Assoc Am Pharm Assoc (Baltim) 47.3 (1958): 162–165.

Younos C et al. Analgesic and behavioural effects of Morinda citrifolia. Planta Med 56.5 (1990): 430–434.

Zin ZM et al. Antioxidative activity of extracts from Mengkudu (Morinda citrifolia L.) root, fruit and leaf. Food Chem 78.2 (2002): 227–231.

Zin ZM et al. Antioxidative activities of chromatographic fractions obtained from root, fruit and leaf of Mengkudu (Morinda citrifolia L.). Food Chem 94.2 (2006): 169–178.

Oats

HISTORICAL NOTE Culpeper (1652) recommended that 'a poultice made of meal of oats and some oil of bay helpeth the itch and the leprosy'. By the end of the 18th century oats was the main grain used by all levels of the population in Scotland. Students would arrive at university after the summer with a bag of oatmeal to live on during the term. The older Scottish universities still call the autumn midterm break 'Meal Monday' because traditionally at that time the students would return home to replenish their supplies. In recent years oats has gained a reputation as a superfood due to its high nutritional content and cardiovascular benefits. It is a good source of B-complex vitamins, protein, fat and minerals as well as the heart-healthy soluble fibre known as beta-glucan, which appears to improve blood glucose and cholesterol levels (Sadiq Butt et al 2008).

OTHER NAMES

Groats, green oats, green tops, haver, oat herb, oatmeal

BOTANICAL NAME/FAMILY

Avena sativa (family Poaceae [Graminaceae])

PLANT PARTS USED

The whole flowering plant, including the oat straw and the seed (also used for porridge). Oat bran is also used in some clinical trials.

CHEMICAL COMPONENTS

Beta-glucan (soluble fibre), triterpenoid saponins (including avenacosides A and B), phenolic compounds (avenanthramides A, B, C), alkaloids (including indole alkaloid, gramine, trigonelline, avenine), sterol (avenasterol), flavonoids, starch, phytates, protein (avenalin, a water-soluble globulin; avenin, a prolamine protein) (Mahmood et al 2013) (including gluten) and coumarins.

Nutrients such as silicic acid, calcium, potassium, phosphorus, iron (39 mg/kg), manganese (8.5 mg/kg), zinc (19.2 mg/kg) (Witchl & Bisset 1991), vitamins A, B-complex, C, E and K and amino acids.

MAIN ACTIONS

The actions of oats, oatbran and key constituents such as beta-glucan have been investigated in various models.

Lipid lowering

Beta-glucans increase bile acid synthesis and thus decrease serum cholesterol (Andersson et al 2002). The fibre binds to cholesterol, preventing initial absorption and enterohepatic recirculation of cholesterol, and the two are excreted together. A recent animal study examining the lipid-lowering properties of oats reported that increased bile acid production occurs by upregulating cholesterol -7 α-hydroxylase and sterol-12 α-hydroxylase (Andersson et al 2012). This study also noted that intestinal microbial flora may alter bile acid or cholesterol metabolism (Andersson et al 2012).

Clinical trials have shown that oat bran contains soluble fibres, such as beta-glucan (e.g. 75 g extruded oat bran, equivalent to 11 g beta-glucan), which nearly double the serum alpha-HC (7 alpha-hydroxy-4-cholesten-3-one) concentration within 8 hours, indicating increased bile acid synthesis and thus decreased serum cholesterol (Andersson et al 2002). Recent human studies using 75 g extruded oat bran breakfast cereal daily (containing 11.6 g native beta-glucans) have confirmed similar effects. Administration of oat bran significantly increased median excretion of bile acids by 144%, decreased cholesterol absorption by 19%, increased the sum of bile acid and cholesterol excretion by 40% and increased alpha-HC concentration (reflecting bile acid synthesis) by 57% within 24 hours of consumption (Ellegard & Andersson 2007).

Beta-glucan added to a fruit drink appears to significantly reduce both total and low-density lipoprotein (LDL) cholesterol in human subjects without affecting fat-soluble antioxidant levels (Naumann et al 2006). Triglyceride levels may also be reduced. In a randomised crossover study, 27 healthy men added oat (providing 5.7 g/day beta-glucan) or wheat (control) cereal products to their usual diet for 2 weeks. Peak triglyceride concentration was significantly lower in the oats group compared to controls (Maki et al 2007a).

Antiatherogenic effects

In vitro studies suggest that the polyphenolic antioxidants known as avenanthramides, present in oats, may exert anti-inflammatory and antiatherogenic effects (Andersson & Hellstrand 2012, Liu et al 2004). Avenanthramides have been shown to decrease the expression of endothelial proinflammatory cytokines. This is in part due to inhibition of nuclear factor-kappaB activation via inhibiting phosphorylation of IkappaB kinase and IkappaB, and suppressing proteasome activity (Guo et al 2008). Additionally, avenanthramide C inhibits the serum-induced proliferation of vascular smooth-muscle cells and increases nitric oxide production (Nie et al 2006a, 2006b). As chronic inflammation and proliferation of vascular smooth-muscle cells are involved in the initiation and development of atherosclerosis, these mechanisms may reduce atherogenesis.

Antihypertensive effects

Reviews report that supplementation of oat β-glucan daily reduces systolic and diastolic blood pressure as well as the need for antihypertensive medication (Daou & Zhang 2012). Oats are known to contain angiotensin-converting enzyme-inhibiting dipeptides and tripeptides (Pihlanto & Mäkinen 2013). While a reduction in blood pressure has been observed in clinical trials, the mechanism of action has not been fully elucidated (Keenan et al 2002, Pins et al 2002, Saltzman et al 2001).

Blood glucose control

Oats have been shown in clinical trials to reduce the postprandial glycaemic response (Brummer et al 2012, Jenkins et al 2002, Pins et al 2002, Tapola et al 2005). This is most likely to be due to the ability of beta-glucans to slow stomach emptying and increase the viscosity of food in the small intestine, resulting in delayed glucose absorption (Rakel 2003, Regand et al 2011). The fat content of rolled oats does not appear to be responsible for either the glycaemic or the insulinaemic response (Tuomasjukka et al 2007).

While some studies have suggested that a minimum of 4 g of beta-glucans is required to produce a significant decrease in glucose and insulin responses in healthy people (Granfeldt et al 2008), other studies suggest this dose may not exert a significant response (Biorklund et al 2008). The effect is likely to be dependent not only on the amount of beta-glucan but on the amount of extractable beta-glucan in oat products (Makelainen et al 2007). In humans this extraction is dependent upon the solubility of beta-glucans, and a recent study noted that beta-glucans of higher molecular weight were more soluble than beta-glucans of lower molecular weight (Kwong et al 2013, Regand et al 2011). This may explain inconsistent results in clinical studies using different formulations of oats (Tosh et al 2008).

Antioxidant

In human trials, avenanthramides (A–C) in oats have been found to be bioavailable and increase antioxidant capacity in healthy older adults. A randomised controlled trial (RCT) of healthy adults who received daily supplementation of 3.12 mg oat-extracted avenanthramides for 1 month reported potent antioxidant activity. The intervention resulted in an increase in serum superoxide dismutase of 8.4% ($P < 0.05$); a reduction in glutathione hormone of 17.9% ($P < 0.05$); and a decrease in malondialdehyde of 28.1% (Liu et al 2011). After consumption of an avenanthramide-enriched mixture extracted from oats, plasma-reduced glutathione was elevated by 21% at 15 minutes ($P \leq 0.005$) and by 14% at 10 hours ($P \leq 0.05$) in another study (Chen et al 2007). In a further study whole oat grains (seven different varieties) showed superior antioxidant activity compared to other whole grains but the antioxidant capacity did not correlate with avenanthramide content, suggesting that other compounds in oats may potentially contribute to synergistic or matrix effects (Chu et al 2013).

Antipruritic/anti-inflammatory effects

External application of oat preparations has been shown to relieve itch (Matheson et al 2001). These effects are most likely to be due to the potent anti-inflammatory effects of the avenanthramide constituents (Sur et al 2008). Experimental studies demonstrate that avenanthramides can inhibit the activity of nuclear factor-kappaB and the release of proinflammatory cytokines and histamine (Cerio et al 2010). Topical application of 1–3 ppm avenanthramides has been shown to alleviate inflammation in experimental models of contact hypersensitivity, neurogenic inflammation and itch (Sur et al 2008). The high concentration of starch and beta-glucan in colloidal oatmeal (produced by finely grinding the oats and boiling to extract the colloidal material) is responsible for the protective and water-holding functions of oats (Kurtz & Wallo 2007).

Anticarcinogenic

The consumption of oats and oat bran has been shown to reduce the risk of colon cancer, not only because of their high fibre content, but also because in vitro studies suggest that avenathramides attenuate the proliferation of colon cancer cells (Guo et al 2010). The beta-glucans in oats have demonstrated anticytotoxic, antimutagenic and antitumorogenic activity (Mantovani et al 2008). An in vitro study using an inflammation-related cancer model in mice demonstrated that whole oats reduced aberrant crypt foci and colon tumours, indicating a protective effect of oats against colon cancer and the potential to act as a chemoprotective agent (Wang et al 2011). However, further investigation is needed to confirm these effects.

O

OTHER ACTIONS

Due to its vitamin, mineral and amino acid content, oats are a nutritious food. Internally, oats also act as a bulk-forming laxative. Wholegrain oat-based breakfast cereals may also act as prebiotics, increasing the proliferation of the *Bifidobacterium* genus (Connolly et al 2012).

CLINICAL USE

Oats are sometimes used in clinical practice in tincture form, often as part of an overall management program, combined with other herbal medicines. It is also used in topical preparations and, most recently, the beta-glucan component in oats has received a lot of attention, whereby dietary oats are used as a means of increasing beta-glucan uptake and conferring health benefits.

Hyperlipidaemia

In 1997 the US Food and Drug Administration approved a health claim for β-glucan soluble fibre from oats for reducing plasma cholesterol levels and risk of heart disease, and this was followed by similar approvals in 2004 from the UK Joint Health Claims Initiative. Recent reviews have confirmed that intake of oat β-glucan at daily doses of at least 3 g may reduce plasma total and LDL cholesterol levels by 5–10% in normocholesterolaemic or hypercholesterolaemic people (Othman et al 2011, Tiwari & Cummins 2011).

A Cochrane review estimating the effect of wholegrain foods on risk factors for coronary heart disease summarised the results of eight RCTs, which had used an oatmeal-based intervention in individuals with raised cholesterol levels (Kelly et al 2007). The duration of the studies varied between 4 and 12 weeks. The review found evidence that oatmeal-based foods lower total cholesterol and LDL-cholesterol. Combined results from the eight studies showed a weighted mean difference of –0.19 mmol/L (95% confidence interval [CI] –0.30 to –0.08, P = 0.0005) in the reduction of total cholesterol. The combined result for reduction in LDL showed a weighted mean difference of –0.18 mmol/L (95% CI –0.28 to –0.09, $P < 0.0001$).

Several clinical trials have shown a marked reduction in total and/or LDL cholesterol using oat-based beta-glucan-containing products (Karmally et al 2005, Queenan et al 2007, Saltzman et al 2001).

In a double-blind, randomised crossover study in 24 young adults (age 25.2 ± 2.7 years; body mass index [BMI] 24.9 ± 2.9 kg/m^2), the addition of oat bran (6 g soluble fibre/day) to a low-fibre diet for 2 weeks lowered total cholesterol by 14% compared with 4% during the control period ($P < 0.001$) (Kristensen & Bugel 2011). There were also decreases in non-high-density lipoprotein (HDL) cholesterol (16% vs 3%; $P < 0.01$), total triacylglycerol (21% vs 10%, $P < 0.05$), very-low-density lipoprotein triacylglycerol (33% vs 9%, $P < 0.01$), plasminogen activator inhibitor-1 (30 vs 2.3%, $P < 0.01$) and factor VII (15 vs 7.6%, $P < 0.001$). Faecal volume and dry matter were greater when consuming the oat bran diet ($P < 0.001$), and energy excretion was increased by 37% ($P < 0.001$); although changes in body weight were not significantly different.

In a randomised, controlled, parallel-arm study of 166 Asian adults with mild to moderate hypercholesterolaemia, participants received 100 g of instant oat cereal or 100 g of wheat flour-based noodles daily for 6 weeks. Total, LDL-cholesterol and waist circumference decreased significantly and dietary fibre intake increased significantly in the oat group compared to the control group at the end of the 6-week intervention. Conversely, HDL-cholesterol decreased significantly in the control group compared to the oat group (Zhang et al 2012). Oat bran has been shown to reduce LDL-cholesterol by 16% in 140 hypercholesterolaemic subjects consuming 56 g oat bran/day for 12 weeks (Davidson et al 1991). In overweight men consuming an oat-based cereal (14 g dietary fibre) for 12 weeks, LDL-cholesterol was most significantly affected, with a reduction in concentrations of small, dense LDL-cholesterol and LDL particle number. No adverse changes occurred in blood triacylglycerol or HDL-cholesterol concentration (Davy et al 2002). In another clinical trial, a group consuming wholegrain oat-based cereals experienced a 24.2 mg/dL reduction in total cholesterol levels and a 16.2 mg/dL decrease in LDL-cholesterol levels (Pins et al 2002).

In a controlled trial 75 hypercholesterolaemic subjects were randomised to receive 6 g/day of concentrated oat beta-glucan or placebo (dextrose) for 6 weeks. Oat beta-glucan significantly reduced total cholesterol (–0.3 ± 0.1 mmol/L) and LDL-cholesterol (–0.3 ± 0.1 mmol/L), but only the reduction in LDL-cholesterol was significantly greater than in the control group. In an intestinal fermentation model the concentrated oat beta-glucan also produced higher concentrations of the short-chain fatty acid known as butyrate than guar gum and inulin, suggesting it may have benefits for colonic health (Queenan et al 2007).

A clinical trial of 38 normotensive males (mean age 59.8 years) with mild to moderate hypercholesterolaemia and a mean BMI of 28.3 kg/m^2 was conducted over 8 weeks. The study investigated the effects of adding high levels of monounsaturated fatty acids plus bread formulated with 6 g of beta-glucan to the American Heart Association Step II diet plus 60 min walking per day. While results were impressive, it is unclear what part the beta-glucan played in isolation (Reyna-Villasmil et al 2007).

The lipid-lowering effects of a hypocaloric diet containing oats have been shown in a clinical trial to result in significantly greater decreases in total and LDL-cholesterol than a hypocaloric diet alone (Saltzman et al 2001). In addition, an RCT of moderately hypercholesterolaemic men consuming oat milk, deprived of insoluble fibre but still containing 0.5 g/100 g beta-glucan (750 mL/day) for 5 weeks, also showed a 6% reduction in total and LDL-cholesterol (Onning et al 1999). Effects on serum lipid levels in people without hypercholesterolaemia are not well supported in clinical trials (Chen et al 2006). (See Clinical note: Major lipids affecting cardiovascular disease risk, in monograph on vitamin B_3.)

Hypertension

Daily consumption of three portions of wholegrains, including oats, has been shown to significantly reduce systolic blood pressure (SBP) and pulse pressure (Tighe et al 2010). Results of RCTs suggest that consumption of oat-based cereals may reduce SBP and reduce or eliminate requirements for antihypertensive medications in some people (Pins et al 2002, Saltzman et al 2001).

The inclusion of wholegrain oat-based cereals was found in an RCT to decrease blood pressure in hypertensive patients and reduce requirements for antihypertensive medications. 'Seventy-three percent of participants in the oats group versus 42% in the control group were able to stop or reduce their medication by half. Treatment group participants whose medication was not reduced had substantial decreases in blood pressure' (Pins et al 2002). In another RCT, overweight subjects consuming a hypocaloric diet containing oats (45 g/4.2 MJ dietary energy/day) for 6 weeks experienced a reduction in SBP that was more significant than a hypocaloric diet alone (oats −6 ± 7 mmHg, control −1 ± 10 mmHg, $P = 0.026$). Lipid-lowering effects were also noted (Saltzman et al 2001). In another double-blind, multicentre clinical trial, 97 hypertensive patients were randomly assigned to receive a control diet or one containing oat beta-glucan for 12 weeks. Subgroup analysis revealed that only obese patients with a BMI > 31.5 kg/m^2 experienced a significant decrease in blood pressure (SBP −8.3 mmHg, diastolic blood pressure −3.9 mmHg) compared to controls (Maki et al 2007b). Overall, results appear to suggest greater benefits for overweight or obese individuals.

Blood sugar regulation

The ability of oats to delay glucose absorption, and therefore reduce the postprandial glycaemic response, provides a theoretical basis for their use as part of an overall treatment protocol in diabetes and hypoglycaemic conditions.

In a crossover RCT, 35 patients with type 2 diabetes and dyslipidaemia received a breakfast consisting of 250 g of oat bread (50% oat flour, 50% white flour) or barley bread (50% barley flour, 50% white flour) daily for 3 weeks (with a washout period of 3 weeks). Both oat and barley bread reduced fasting blood sugar (FBS) ($P < 0.0001$) and improved HDL-cholesterol ($P < 0.01$). However, the beneficial effect of oat bread on reducing serum FBS (mean difference 6.2 ± 9.2 mg/dL) and improving HDL-C (mean difference 1.34 ± 0.2 mg/dL) was greater than for barley bread (mean difference in FBS, 32 ± 2.7 mg/dL; HDL-C, 9.2 ± 1.8 mg/dL). Neither of the interventions demonstrated significant differences for LDL-C, insulin sensitivity or triglycerides (Hajifaraji et al 2012). Animal studies have also reported that the effects of oat bran are superior to barley bran (El Rabey et al 2013). An RCT of 12 patients with type 2 diabetes demonstrated that 30 g oat bran flour, high in beta-glucan, had a low glycaemic response and decreased the postprandial glycaemic response of an oral glucose load in a series of 2-hour meal glucose tolerance tests (Tapola et al 2005).

Another trial showed a 15.03 mg/dL drop in plasma glucose levels versus controls when consuming wholegrain oat-based cereals (Pins et al 2002). Processing methods may affect the benefits of oats, with a small study demonstrating that processing oat beta-glucan through enzymatic, rather than aqueous, methods preserves the viscosity and improves post-prandial glycaemic control (Panahi et al 2007). In a 50 g portion of carbohydrate, each gram of beta-glucan reduces the glycaemic index by 4 units, making it a useful adjunct to reduce the postprandial glycaemic response without affecting palatability (Jenkins et al 2002).

In an uncontrolled pilot study, 14 hospitalised patients with metabolic syndrome were given a diabetes-adapted hypocaloric diet (1500 kcal/day; 50–55% carbohydrate, 15–20% protein, 30% fat) for 5 days with or without a 2-day period (third and fourth day), where the diet included 15 carbohydrate units of oatmeal (1200 kcal/day; 63% carbohydrate, 12% protein, 6% fat and 16.2 g fibre). The oatmeal intervention reduced insulin requirements by 42.5% and the effect persisted after a 4-week outpatient period (Lammert et al 2008). The differences in calorie intake and nutritional breakdown make it difficult to attribute the observed effects to oatmeal alone and more controlled studies are warranted.

Recent studies suggest that porridge made from pinhead oats compared to rolled oats may have better effects on glycaemic control and sense of fullness (Gonzalez & Stevenson 2012). In addition different food formats that deliver similar amounts of soluble β-glucan may have similar effects. For instance, 1.5 g/day β-glucan from ready-to-eat oat flakes was reported to be as effective in lowering cholesterol as 3.0 g/day from oats porridge in a 6-week RCT of 87 mildly hypercholesterolaemic adults (≥5 mmol/L and <7.5 mmol/L) (Charlton et al 2012).

Obesity

In a recent RCT of 34 adult participants with a BMI ≥ 27, beta-glucan-containing oat cereal was compared to placebo daily for 12 weeks. Consumption of the oat cereal reduced body weight, BMI, body fat and the waist-to-hip ratio. Liver function tests revealed a reduction in aspartate transaminase, and especially alanine transaminase, with oat consumption. Oats were well tolerated and the authors concluded that consumption of oats reduced obesity and abdominal fat and improved lipid profiles and liver function (Chang et al 2013). Further research is required to confirm and elucidate these effects.

Pruritus

Topical oatmeal has been used traditionally to relieve the itch and irritation associated with various dry, itchy skin conditions. Colloidal oatmeal lotion, Aveeno (Johnson & Johnson, Maidenhead, Berkshire, UK) has been shown to be an effective treatment for pruritus (Talsania et al 2008). These effects may be explained by the avenanthramides, potent anti-inflammatory agents that appear to mediate the anti-irritant effects of oats (Sur et al 2008). In addition, the beta-glucan and starch in colloidal oatmeal are thought to possess water-holding effects (Kurtz & Wallo 2007).

A clinical trial assessing the itch experienced by burns patients found that the group using a product with 5% colloidal oatmeal reported significantly less itch and requested significantly less antihistamine treatment than the control group (Matheson et al 2001).

Commission E approves topical use in baths for inflammatory and seborrhoeic skin disease, especially with itch (Blumenthal et al 2000).

Atopic dermatitis

Daily use of moisturisers and/or cleansers containing colloidal oatmeal appears to improve many clinical outcomes of atopic dermatitis, including the size and severity of the affected area, itch and dryness (Fowler et al 2012). In a controlled trial, an emollient treatment (containing oat extract) for 6 weeks significantly reduced high-potency topical corticosteroid consumption (−42%; $P < 0.05$) in infants with atopic dermatitis. Significant effects were not demonstrated for moderate-potency corticosteroids (Grimalt et al 2007). However, it should be noted that percutaneous sensitisation to oats used in emollients and moisturisers has been reported and one study found that 32% of children with atopic dermatitis using oat-based creams had an oat-positive atopy patch test vs 0% of non-users (Boussault et al 2007). Given the hyperpermeability of infant skin, topical products containing potentially allergenic food proteins should be used cautiously (Codreanu et al 2006).

OTHER USES

Traditionally, oats are considered a nervous system nutritive and therefore used during times of convalescence. More specifically, the straw is prescribed for nervous debility and exhaustion, whereas the seed is considered more stimulating and said to gently improve energy and support an overly stressed nervous system (Chevallier 1996). An animal study on rats showed that beta-glucan enhanced endurance and significantly improved recovery from fatigue (Xu et al 2013).

Preliminary trials have suggested an improvement in sexual interest and performance in people taking oats in combination with nettles. The effects were more consistent in males than females. Further trials are required to confirm the benefits of oats in isolation (Haroian et al 1987).

Interestingly, oats are also used as supportive therapy during nicotine (Beglinger et al 1977, Schmidt & Geckeler 1976) and morphine withdrawal; however, reliable clinical evidence is currently limited and does not fully support these recommendations.

Due to its high soluble fibre content, oats are also used as an aid to weight loss. Taken before meals, they increase satiety and therefore enable smaller food portions to satisfy hunger.

DOSAGE RANGE

- 1–4 g three times daily of oatmeal or straw (Mills 1991).
- Australian manufacturers recommend 20–40 mL/week 1:2 tincture.
- Topically for itch: 5% colloidal oatmeal in a suitable carrier (Matheson et al 2001) or 100 g cut herb in a bath (Blumenthal et al 2000).
- The inclusion of wholegrain oat-based cereals or oat bran may be a useful adjunct to the treatment of hyperlipidaemia and hypertension and to delay glucose absorption — 75 g dried oatmeal (equivalent to ≈ 3 g soluble fibre daily) (Rakel 2003). Some research indicates 6 g/day of concentrated oat beta-glucan is required for lipid-lowering effects.

ADVERSE REACTIONS

Excessive oral intake of fibre from oats or oat bran may cause flatulence and anal irritation.

SIGNIFICANT INTERACTIONS

Controlled studies are largely unavailable; therefore, interactions are based on evidence of activity and are largely theoretical and speculative.

Antihypertensives

Additive effects are theoretically possible (Pins et al 2002); beneficial interaction is possible — observe.

Lipid-lowering medications

Additive effects are theoretically possible — beneficial interaction is possible.

Insulin and diabetic medications

In an uncontrolled pilot study, an oatmeal intervention reduced insulin requirements by 42.5% in hospitalised patients with metabolic syndrome; the effect persisted after a 4-week outpatient period (Lammert et al 2008). Insulin requirements should be monitored in patients taking oat beta-glucans as a change to medication dose could be required. Beneficial interaction possible under supervision.

CONTRAINDICATIONS AND PRECAUTIONS

Given the hyperpermeability of infant skin, topical products containing potentially allergenic oat proteins should be used cautiously (Codreanu et al 2006). Dietary oats should not be used in cases of intestinal obstruction (Skidmore-Roth 2001).

Clinical note — Do oats interfere with nutrient absorption?

Although the high phytate content of oats would indicate a potential for reduced absorption of trace elements such as zinc, calcium and iron, one clinical trial investigating the effects of oat bran on zinc absorption found no evidence of reduced absorption (Sandstrom et al 2000).

Coeliac disease and oats consumption

In the past oats were generally contraindicated in people with coeliac disease due to their gluten content. Recent studies however have demonstrated that oats appear to be well tolerated by the majority of adults (Cooper et al 2013, Guttormsen et al 2008, Kemppainen et al 2007, Lundin et al 2003, Pulido et al 2009) and children (Benkebil & Nydegger 2007, Hogberg et al 2004, Holm et al 2006) with coeliac disease. For instance, a recent study of 46 patients with coeliac disease who consumed oats for 1 year reaffirmed the lack of oats immunogenicity and toxicity (Cooper et al 2013).

However, some patients display a specific small intestinal T-cell response to oat peptides that cannot be explained by contamination with other cereals (Ellis & Ciclitira 2008) and may experience intestinal discomfort, diarrhoea, bloating and subtotal villous atrophy (Lundin et al 2003, Peraaho et al 2004, Storsrud et al 2003).

Food-processing techniques such as kilning do not appear to either increase or decrease the antigenic potential (Kemppainen et al 2008); however some species such as the Italian variety, Astra, and the Australian variety, Mortlock, may be more reactive (Silano et al 2007).

Two recent reviews of the literature concluded that oats are well tolerated by most patients with coeliac disease (Garsed & Scott 2007, Haboubi et al 2006) but recommended the avoidance of oat products that may have been contaminated by wheat (Garsed & Scott 2007) and regular follow-up, including small-bowel biopsy (Haboubi et al 2006). The Canadian Coeliac Association recommends consumption of uncontaminated oats up to 70 g (½–¾ cup)/day for adults and up to 25 g (¼ cup)/day for children (Rashid et al 2007).

PREGNANCY USE

Oral use is considered to be safe in pregnancy and lactation.

Practice points/Patient counselling

- Oats are a rich source of nutrients, such as calcium, potassium, phosphorus, iron, manganese and zinc, vitamins A, B-complex, C, E and K and amino acids. Dietary oats also contain a significant amount of soluble fibre.
- Regular intake of wholegrain oat-based beta-glucan-containing cereals may have positive effects on cardiovascular disease risk factors such as hypertension, hyperlipidaemia and glucose regulation.
- Topical use of the cut herb in the bath or 5% colloidal oatmeal in a suitable carrier is used to relieve itch.
- Traditionally, oats are viewed as a nervous system nutritive and therefore used during times of convalescence.
- Patients with coeliac disease should be able to tolerate moderate amounts of oats in the diet.

PATIENTS' FAQs

What will this herb do for me?

Oats are a concentrated nutrient source and also contain soluble fibre. They not only provide a range of vitamins and minerals, but can reduce blood pressure and cholesterol and improve blood sugar regulation.

When will it start to work?

Scientific studies have shown that oatbran and oat-based cereals containing beta-glucan may reduce cholesterol levels and blood pressure within 5–6 weeks.

Are there any safety issues?

Dietary oats should be avoided in cases of intestinal obstruction.

REFERENCES

Andersson, KE, & Hellstrand, P. (2012). Dietary oats and modulation of atherogenic pathways. Molecular nutrition & food research, 56(7), 1003–1013.

Andersson M, et al. Oat bran stimulates bile acid synthesis within 8 h as measured by 7alpha-hydroxy-4-cholesten-3-one. Am J Clin Nutr 76.5 (2002): 1111–11116.

Andersson, KE, et al (2012). Diverse effects of oats on cholesterol metabolism in C57BL/6 mice correlate with expression of hepatic bile acid-producing enzymes. European journal of nutrition, 1–15.

Beglinger C, et al. Modification of smoking behavior using long-distance methods. Soz Praventivmed 22.4 (1977): 182–183 [in German].

Benkebil F, Nydegger A. [Coeliac disease in children — an update.] Rev Med Suisse 3.100 (2007): 515–5119.

Biorklund M et al. Serum lipids and postprandial glucose and insulin levels in hyperlipidemic subjects after consumption of an oat beta-glucan-containing ready meal. Ann Nutr Metab 52.2 (2008): 83–90.

Blumenthal M, et al (eds). Herbal medicine: expanded Commission E monographs. Austin, TX: Integrative Medicine Communications, 2000.

Boussault P et al. Oat sensitization in children with atopic dermatitis: prevalence, risks and associated factors. Allergy 62.11 (2007): 1251–1256.

Brummer, Y et al. (2012). Glycemic response to extruded oat bran cereals processed to vary in molecular weight. Cereal Chemistry, 89(5), 255–261.

Cerio R, et al. (2010). Mechanism of action and clinical benefits of colloidal oatmeal for dermatologic practice. J Drugs Dermatol, 9(9), 1116–1120.

Chang HC, et al. Oat prevents obesity and abdominal fat distribution, and improves liver function in humans. Plant foods for human nutrition (Dordrecht, Netherlands) 2013;68(1):18–23.

Charlton KE, et al. Effect of 6 weeks' consumption of beta-glucan-rich oat products on cholesterol levels in mildly hypercholesterolaemic overweight adults. Br J Nutr 2012;107(7):1037–47.

Chen J et al. A randomized controlled trial of dietary fiber intake on serum lipids. Eur J Clin Nutr 60.1 (2006): 62–68.

Chen CY et al. Avenanthramides are bioavailable and have antioxidant activity in humans after acute consumption of an enriched mixture from oats. J Nutr 137.6 (2007): 1375–1382.

Chevallier A. The encyclopedia of medicinal plants. London: Dorling Kindersley, 1996.

Chu, Y-F et al. (2013). In vitro antioxidant capacity and anti-inflammatory activity of seven common oats. Food Chemistry 139: 426–431.

Codreanu F et al. Risk of allergy to food proteins in topical medicinal agents and cosmetics. Eur Ann Allergy Clin Immunol 38.4 (2006): 126–130.

Connolly ML, et al. Wholegrain oat-based cereals have prebiotic potential and low glycaemic index. Br J Nutr 2012;108(12):2198–206.

Cooper SE, et al. Immunological indicators of coeliac disease activity are not altered by long-term oats challenge. Clinical and experimental immunology 2013;171(3):313–8.

Culpeper N. The English physician, 1652.

Daou, C & Zhang, H. (2012). Oat beta-glucan: its role in health promotion and prevention of diseases. Comprehensive Reviews in Food Science and Food Safety, 11(4), 355–365.

Davidson MH et al. The hypocholesterolaemic effects of beta-glucan in oatmeal and oat bran: A dose-controlled study. JAMA 265 (1991): 1833–1839.

Davy BM et al. High-fiber oat cereal compared with wheat cereal consumption favorably alters LDL-cholesterol subclass and particle numbers in middle-aged and older men. Am J Clin Nutr 76.2 (2002): 351–358.

Ellegard L, Andersson H. Oat bran rapidly increases bile acid excretion and bile acid synthesis: an ileostomy study. Eur J Clin Nutr 61.8 (2007): 938–945.

Ellis HJ, Ciclitira PJ. Should coeliac sufferers be allowed their oats? Eur J Gastroenterol Hepatol 20.6 (2008): 492–493.

El Rabey HA, et al. Efficiency of barley bran and oat bran in ameliorating blood lipid profile and the adverse histological changes in hypercholesterolemic male rats. BioMed research international 2013;2013:263594.

Fowler JF, et al Colloidal oatmeal formulations as adjunct treatments in atopic dermatitis. J Drugs Dermatol 2012;11(7):804–7.

Garsed K, Scott BB. Can oats be taken in a gluten-free diet? A systematic review. Scand J Gastroenterol 42.2 (2007): 171–178.

Gonzalez JT, Stevenson EJ. Postprandial glycemia and appetite sensations in response to porridge made with rolled and pinhead oats. J Am Coll Nutr 2012;31(2):111–6.

Granfeldt Y et al. Muesli with 4 g oat beta-glucans lowers glucose and insulin responses after a bread meal in healthy subjects. Eur J Clin Nutr 62.5 (2008): 600–607.

Grimalt R et al. The steroid-sparing effect of an emollient therapy in infants with atopic dermatitis: a randomized controlled study. Dermatology 214.1 (2007): 61–67.

Guo W et al. Avenanthramides, polyphenols from oats, inhibit IL-1beta-induced NF-kappaB activation in endothelial cells. Free Radic Biol Med 44.3 (2008): 415–429.

Guo, W., et al. (2010). Avenanthramides inhibit proliferation of human colon cancer cell lines in vitro. Nutr Cancer, 62(8), 1007–1016.

Guttormsen V et al. No induction of anti-avenin IgA by oats in adult, diet-treated coeliac disease. Scand J Gastroenterol 43.2 (2008): 161–165.

Haboubi NY et al. Coeliac disease and oats: a systematic review. Postgrad Med J 82.972 (2006): 672–678.

Hajifaraji, M, et al. (2012). Comparison study between the effect of oat and barley breads on serum glucose and lipid profiles in dyslipidemic and type 2 diabetic subjects: a short-term trial. Mediterranean Journal of Nutrition and Metabolism, 5(3), 247–252.

Haroian L et al. Institute for Advanced Study of Human Sexuality research report: The exsativa project (Swiss formula A111). Specific Press, 1987.

Hogberg L et al. Oats to children with newly diagnosed coeliac disease: a randomised double blind study. Gut 53.5 (2004): 649–654.

Holm K et al. Oats in the treatment of childhood coeliac disease: a 2-year controlled trial and a long-term clinical follow-up study. Aliment Pharmacol Ther 23.10 (2006): 1463–1472.

Jenkins AL et al. Depression of the glycemic index by high levels of beta-glucan fiber in two functional foods tested in type 2 diabetes. Eur J Clin Nutr 56.7 (2002): 622–628.

Karmally W et al. Cholesterol-lowering benefits of oat-containing cereal in Hispanic Americans. J Am Diet Assoc 105.6 (2005): 967–970.

Keenan, J. M., et al. (2002). "Oat ingestion reduces systolic and diastolic blood pressure in patients with mild or borderline hypertension: a pilot trial." J Fam Pract 51(4): 369.

Kelly SA et al. Wholegrain cereals for coronary heart disease. Cochrane Database Syst Rev (2) (2007): CD005051.

Kemppainen T et al. No observed local immunological response at cell level after five years of oats in adult coeliac disease. Scand J Gastroenterol 42.1 (2007): 54–59.

Kemppainen TA et al. Unkilned and large amounts of oats in the coeliac disease diet: a randomized, controlled study. Scand J Gastroenterol 43.9 (2008): 1094–1101.

Kristensen M, Bugel S. A diet rich in oat bran improves blood lipids and hemostatic factors, and reduces apparent energy digestibility in young healthy volunteers. Eur J Clin Nutr 2011;65(9):1053–8.

Kurtz ES, Wallo W. Colloidal oatmeal: history, chemistry and clinical properties. J Drugs Dermatol 6.2 (2007): 167–170.

Kwong, MGY et al. (2013). Attenuation of glycemic responses by oat β-glucan solutions and viscoelastic gels is dependent on molecular weight distribution. Food & function 4: 401–408.

Lammert A et al. Clinical benefit of a short term dietary oatmeal intervention in patients with type 2 diabetes and severe insulin resistance: a pilot study. Exp Clin Endocrinol Diabetes 116.2 (2008): 132–134.

Liu L et al. The antiatherogenic potential of oat phenolic compounds. Atherosclerosis 175.1 (2004): 39–49.

Liu, S, et al. (2011). Antioxidant effects of oats avenanthramides on human serum. Agricultural Sciences in China, 10(8), 1301–1305.

Lundin KE et al. Oats induced villous atrophy in coeliac disease. Gut 52.11 (2003): 1649–1652.

Mahmood, K, et al. (2013). Nutrient-Rich Botanicals in Skin Health: Focus on *Avena sativa*. Bioactive Dietary Factors and Plant Extracts in Dermatology, 153–168.

Makelainen H et al. The effect of beta-glucan on the glycemic and insulin index. Eur J Clin Nutr 61.6 (2007): 779–785.

Maki KC, et al. Effects of high-fiber oat and wheat cereals on postprandial glucose and lipid responses in healthy men. Int J Vitam Nutr Res 77.5 (2007a): 347–356.

Maki KC, et al. Effects of consuming foods containing oat beta-glucan on blood pressure, carbohydrate metabolism and biomarkers of oxidative stress in men and women with elevated blood pressure. Eur J Clin Nutr 61.6 (2007b): 786–795.

Mantovani MS et al. beta-Glucans in promoting health: prevention against mutation and cancer. Mutat Res 658.3 (2008): 154–161.

Matheson JD, et al. The reduction of itch during burn wound healing. J Burn Care Rehabil 22.1 (2001): 76–81.

Mills S. The essential book of herbal medicine. Harmondsworth, Middlesex: Penguin, 1991.

Naumann E et al. Beta-glucan incorporated into a fruit drink effectively lowers serum LDL-cholesterol concentrations. Am J Clin Nutr 83.3 (2006): 601–605.

Nie L et al. Mechanism by which avenanthramide-c, a polyphenol of oats, blocks cell cycle progression in vascular smooth muscle cells. Free Radic Biol Med 41.5 (2006a): 702–8.

Nie L et al. Avenanthramide, a polyphenol from oats, inhibits vascular smooth muscle cell proliferation and enhances nitric oxide production. Atherosclerosis 186.2 (2006b): 260–6.

Onning G et al. Consumption of oat milk for 5 weeks lowers serum cholesterol and LDL cholesterol in free-living with moderate hypercholesterolemia. Ann Nutr Metab 43.5 (1999): 301–309.

Othman RA, et al. Cholesterol-lowering effects of oat beta-glucan. Nutrition reviews 2011;69(6):299–309.

Panahi S et al. Beta-glucan from two sources of oat concentrates affect postprandial glycemia in relation to the level of viscosity. J Am Coll Nutr 26.6 (2007): 639–644.

Peraaho M et al. Effect of an oats-containing gluten-free diet on symptoms and quality of life in coeliac disease: A randomized study. Scand J Gastroenterol 39.1 (2004): 27–31.

Pihlanto, A, & Mäkinen, S. (2013). Antihypertensive Properties of Plant Protein Derived Peptides. Available online at: http://www.intechopen.com/books/bioactive-food-peptides-in-health-and-disease/antihypertensive-properties-of-plant-protein-derived-peptides

Pins JJ et al. Do whole-grain oat cereals reduce the need for antihypertensive medications and improve blood pressure control? J Fam Pract 51.4 (2002): 353–3559.

Pulido, OM et al. (2009). Chapter 6 Introduction of oats in the diet of individuals with celiac disease: a systematic review. In S.L Taylor (Ed.), Advances in Food and Nutrition Research (Vol. 57, pp. 235–285): Academic Press.

Queenan KM et al. Concentrated oat beta-glucan, a fermentable fiber, lowers serum cholesterol in hypercholesterolemic adults in a randomized controlled trial. Nutr J 6 (2007): 6.

Rakel D. Integrative medicine. Philadelphia: Saunders, 2003.

Rashid M et al. Consumption of pure oats by individuals with celiac disease: a position statement by the Canadian Celiac Association. Can J Gastroenterol 21.10 (2007): 649–651.

Regand, A et al (2011). The molecular weight, solubility and viscosity of oat beta-glucan affect human glycemic response by modifying starch digestibility. Food Chemistry, 129(2), 297–304.

Reyna-Villasmil N et al. Oat-derived beta-glucan significantly improves HDLC and diminishes LDLC and non-HDL cholesterol in overweight individuals with mild hypercholesterolemia. Am J Ther 14.2 (2007): 203–212.

Sadiq Butt M et al. Oat: unique among the cereals. Eur J Nutr 47.2 (2008): 68–79.

Saltzman E et al. An oat-containing hypocaloric diet reduces systolic blood pressure and improves lipid profile beyond effects of weight loss in men and women. J Nutr 131.5 (2001): 1465–1470.

Sandstrom B et al. A high oat-bran intake does not impair zinc absorption in humans when added to a low-fiber animal protein-based diet. J Nutr 130.3 (2000): 594–599.

Schmidt K, Geckeler K. Pharmacotherapy with avena sativa: a double blind study. Int J Clin Pharmacol Biopharm 14.3 (1976): 214–2116.

Silano M et al. In vitro tests indicate that certain varieties of oats may be harmful to patients with coeliac disease. J Gastroenterol Hepatol 22.4 (2007): 528–531.

Skidmore-Roth L. Mosby's handbook of herbs and natural supplements. St Louis: Mosby, 2001.

Storsrud S et al. Adult coeliac patients do tolerate large amounts of oats. Eur J Clin Nutr 57.1 (2003): 163–169.

Sur R et al. Avenanthramides, polyphenols from oats, exhibit anti-inflammatory and anti-itch activity. Arch Dermatol Res 300.10 (2008): 569–574.

Talsania N et al. Colloidal oatmeal lotion is an effective treatment for pruritus caused by erlotinib. Clin Exp Dermatol 33.1 (2008): 108.

Tapola N et al. Glycemic responses of oat bran products in type 2 diabetic patients. Nutr Metab Cardiovasc Dis 15.4 (2005): 255–261.

Tighe, P., et al (2010). Effect of increased consumption of whole-grain foods on blood pressure and other cardiovascular risk markers in healthy middle-aged persons: a randomized controlled trial. Am J Clin Nutr, 92(4), 733–740.

Tiwari, U., & Cummins, E. (2011). Meta-analysis of the effect of beta-glucan intake on blood cholesterol and glucose levels. Nutrition, 27(10), 1008–1016.

Tosh, SM et al. (2008). Glycemic response to oat bran muffins treated to vary molecular weight of β-glucan. Cereal Chemistry, 85(2), 211–217.

Tuomasjukka S et al. The glycaemic response to rolled oat is not influenced by the fat content. Br J Nutr 97.4 (2007): 744–748.

Wang, H-C et al. (2011). Inhibitory effect of whole oat on aberrant crypt foci formation and colon tumor growth in ICR and BALB/c mice. Journal of Cereal Science, 53(1), 73–77.

Witchl M, Bisset NG (eds). Herbal drugs and phytopharmaceuticals, Stuttgart: Medpharm Scientific Publishers, 1991.

Xu, C et al. (2013). Effects of oat β-glucan on endurance exercise and its anti-fatigue properties in trained rats. Carbohydrate Polymers, 92(2), 1159–1165.

Zhang J, et al. Randomized controlled trial of oatmeal consumption versus noodle consumption on blood lipids of urban Chinese adults with hypercholesterolemia. Nutr J 2012;11:54.

Passionflower

HISTORICAL NOTE Legend has it that this herb received its name because the corona resembles the crown of thorns worn by Christ during the crucifixion. A popular sedative medicine in the early 20th century, it was listed in the US National Formulary until 1936.

COMMON NAME

Passionflower

OTHER NAMES

Apricot vine, granadilla, Jamaican honeysuckle, Maypop passion flower, maracuja, passion vine, water lemon

BOTANICAL NAME/FAMILY

Passiflora incarnata (family Passifloraceae)

PLANT PARTS USED

Aerial parts, particularly leaves

CHEMICAL COMPONENTS

Flavonoids and related compounds (including apigenin, quercetin, kaempferol and chrysin), maltol, coumarin derivatives, indole alkaloids (mainly harman, harmaline, harmine), phytosterols (stigmasterol), sugars and small amounts of essential oil.

Note: Some research trials use other species of *Passiflora*, notably *P. edulis*, *P. alata* or *P. caerulea*. Each species contains similar, but not equivalent, constituents and may have different pharmacological properties and effects.

Harmine

Research has been conducted with several key constituents found in passionflower, in particular harmine and harman. Harmine is a β-carboline alkaloid, a compound class known to be strong inhibitors of monoamine oxidase which metabolises catecholamine neurotransmitters. Harmine exhibits various pharmacological effects both in vitro and in vivo, such as improvement of insulin sensitivity, a vasorelaxant effect and an antidepressant effect. In vitro and ex vivo models also show that harmine inhibits osteoclast differentiation and suppresses bone loss. In vivo studies on mice have demonstrated that harmine was able to prevent bone loss in osteoporosis models (Yonezawa et al 2011).

Harman

Numerous in vitro and in vivo trials have been conducted on the constituent known as harman suggesting mild monoamine oxidase A inhibitory activity (Adell et al 1996), inhibition of HIV replication (Ishida et al 2001), vasorelaxant activity (Shi et al 2000) and effects on gamma-aminobutyric acid (GABA) release (Dolzhenko & Komissarov 1984).

However, harman is not considered to be one of the main active constituents in the herb and is not present in biologically active concentrations in the dosage range used for passionflower. As such, results obtained using isolated harman in vitro and in vivo cannot necessarily be extrapolated to the use of passionflower in humans.

Harman has also been identified in beer, and to a lesser extent in wine, both of which contain levels far in excess of those found in passionflower at therapeutic doses.

MAIN ACTIONS

Anxiolytic and sedative activity

Several in vivo studies have demonstrated the anxiolytic effects of *Passiflora* extract (Della Loggia et al 1981, Dhawan et al 2001, Soulimani et al 1997). Behavioural tests in mice have also demonstrated that high doses have a sedative effect (Soulimani et al 1997).

The mechanism of action has been unclear until recently, as some research suggested stimulation of GABA release or an interaction with GABA receptors, and other research observed no interaction with GABA benzodiazepine receptors (Zanoli et al

2000). This may be due to different *Passiflora* species being used in research, as well as different routes of administration.

In 1999, an in vitro study showed inhibition of GABA-A binding with *Passiflora* extract (Simmen et al 1999). A more recent study has determined that, indeed, the anxiolytic effects of *P. incarnata* are mediated via the GABAergic system (Grundman et al 2008). This was confirmed yet again in 2011, whereby numerous pharmacological effects of *Passiflora incarnata* were shown to be mediated via modulation of the GABA system including affinity to GABA-A and GABA-B receptors, and effects on GABA uptake in vitro (Appel et al 2011).

Anticonvulsant

A hydroalcoholic extract of *Passiflora* (Pasipay 0.4 mg/kg) has demonstrated anticonvulsant activity in vivo (Nassiri-Asl et al 2007). The extract was shown to delay onset and decrease the duration of seizures compared to placebo. It appeared to work through GABAergic and opioid pathways; however more research is needed to confirm the mechanism.

OTHER ACTIONS

Recent in vitro and rat studies demonstrated that *Passiflora* enhances the potency of St John's wort's antidepressant action (Fiebich et al 2011).

Antiepileptic

Passiflora significantly reduced the severity of seizures in vivo, and ameliorated postictal (the period immediately after a seizure) depression, possibly due to its ability to retain serotonin and noradrenaline levels of the brain. This is worthy of further consideration as the standard anticonvulsive therapies such as diazepam tend to worsen postictal depression (Singh et al 2012).

Aphrodisiac

Tests in mice have identified significant aphrodisiac properties associated with high doses of *Passiflora* extract (Dhawan et al 2003a). A benzoflavone moiety may be chiefly responsible, as tests with this isolated compound were found to increase libido and fertility of male rats after 30 days' treatment (Dhawan et al 2002a).

Antitussive and antiasthmatic activity

P. incarnata was as effective as codeine phosphate in suppressing a sulfur dioxide-induced cough in mice (Dhawan & Sharma 2002). Passionflower (100 mg/kg) was also able to prevent dyspnoea-related convulsions in guinea pigs with acetylcholine-induced bronchospasm (Dhawan et al 2003b).

Antidiabetic

In the Ayurvedic system, the leaves of *P. incarnata* are used for their antidiabetic properties. Recent tests using mice confirm hypoglycaemic and hypolipidaemic effects, with improvement in glucose tolerance and lipid profile as well as regeneration of pancreatic islets of Langerhans (Gupta et al 2012).

Nicotine withdrawal

Promising new in vivo research suggests that passionflower extract has the potential to ameliorate the signs of nicotine sensitisation (Breivogel & Jamerson 2012). This builds on previous research which identified a benzoflavone moiety in *Passiflora* which, when given acutely to test animals as a single 20 mg/kg dose, prevented some of the nicotine withdrawal effects (Dhawan et al 2002c).

CLINICAL USE

Preclinical research and traditional evidence suggest *Passiflora* can play a role in the symptomatic relief of anxiety. The clinical evidence currently available supports this and shows benefits for anxiety and possibly insomnia and opiate withdrawal. However, evidence comes from only a handful of randomised controlled trials, so ideally, larger controlled trials are required to further clarify its role in practice.

Anxiety and nervous restlessness

Passiflora extract is a popular herb for nervousness and anxiety and is most often prescribed in combination with other herbs such as valerian and St John's wort.

At least three clinical trials have confirmed the efficacy of passionflower treatment for symptoms of anxiety. Two trials found that treatment with passiflora before surgery relieved anxiety and one trial investigated its use in generalised anxiety disorder (GAD), finding positive results (Lakhan & Vieira 2010).

Treatment with passionflower extract (45 drops/day) was compared to oxazepam (30 mg/day) in a double-blind study involving 36 volunteers with GAD and found both treatments were equally effective anxiolytics in this population. Both treatments were used for 4 weeks. Passionflower treatment had a slower onset of action compared to oxazepam; however, the herbal group also reported less job impairment (Akhondzadeh et al 2001a).

Commission E approved passionflower for this indication (Blumenthal et al 2000).

Presurgery use

Two studies have investigated the use of passiflora to relieve anxiety before surgery. In the first study, 60 patients were randomised to two groups and given passionflower (500 mg; Passipy Iran Darouk) or placebo 90 minutes before surgery (Movafegh et al 2008). Anxiety scores were significantly lower in the active treatment group compared to the placebo group, while other parameters such as psychological and physiological recovery were the same for both groups.

Anxiolytic activity was confirmed in a more recent randomised, double-blind, placebo-controlled study involving 60 patients about to undergo spinal anaesthesia. Thirty minutes before the procedure, patients were randomly assigned to receive either oral *Passiflora incarnata* extract or placebo. The passiflora extract was found to reduce the increase in anxiety before spinal anaesthesia without changing psychomotor function test results, sedation level or haemodynamics (Aslanargun et al 2012).

IN COMBINATION

A formulated extract containing passionflower, St John's wort and valerian was tested on 16 healthy adults in a randomised, placebo-controlled crossover study. Electroencephalogram (EEG) recordings were performed 0.5, 1.5, 3 and 4 hours after administration of the preparation and analysis revealed a difference to placebo 3 and 4 hours after intake. Analysis of the neurophysiological changes following the intake of the preparation showed a similarity of brain frequency changes on the EEG to those of calming and antidepressive drugs without impairment of cognition (Dimpfel et al 2011).

Previously, an anxiolytic effect was observed in a randomised, placebo-controlled study of 182 people diagnosed with adjustment disorder and anxious mood who were treated with a combination of *Crataegus oxyacantha, Ballota foetida, Valeriana officinalis, Cola nitida* and *Paullinia cupana* in a commercial product known as Euphytose, taken as two tablets three times daily for 28 days (Bourin et al 1997).

Opiate withdrawal

A randomised double-blind study involving 65 subjects with opiate addiction compared the effects of clonidine and placebo with clonidine and passiflora extract over a 14-day period. The fixed daily dose was 60 drops of passiflora extract and a maximum daily dose of 0.8 mg of clonidine administered in three divided doses.

The combination treatment of clonidine and passiflora extract was significantly better at alleviating the psychological symptoms associated with withdrawal; however, no differences in physical symptoms were seen between the groups (Akhondzadeh et al 2001b).

Insomnia

Currently, in vivo evidence supports the sedative activity of passiflora when used in high doses. There has been only one small randomised controlled trial ($n = 41$) that compared 2 g of passionflower tea to placebo before sleep and demonstrated an improvement for subjective sleep quality but no other significant findings on other sleep outcomes (Ngan & Conduit 2011). Preclinical research suggests it should have potential for this indication.

IN COMBINATION

A herbal combination consisting of standardised extracts of *Valeriana officinalis* (300 mg; standardised to 0.8% total valerinic acid), *Passiflora incarnata* (80 mg; standardised to 4% isovitexin) and *Humulus lupulus* (30 mg; standardised to 0.35% rutin) may be a suitable alternative to zolpidem as a treatment for primary insomnia, according to a recent randomised, double-blind study (Maroo et al 2013). The study of 91 people with primary insomnia identified that the herbal combination was as effective as zolpidem in significantly improving total sleep time, sleep latency, number of nightly awakenings and insomnia severity index scores. Interestingly, the Epworth sleepiness scores did not change significantly over the study period for either group.

In regard to safety, 12 people in the herbal group and 16 treated with zolpidem reported side effects, with drowsiness the most common. Most were mild and not serious.

OTHER USES

Traditional uses

Traditionally, passionflower has been used to treat neuralgia, generalised seizures, hysteria and insomnia. It has also been used to treat diarrhoea, dysentery and dysmenorrhoea by acting on the nervous system.

DOSAGE RANGE

- Dried herb: 2 g three to four times daily.
- Infusion of dried herb: 0.25–2 g three to four times daily.
- Fluid extract (1 : 1) (g/mL): 2 mL three to four times daily in 150 mL of water.
- Tincture (1 : 5) (g/mL): 10 mL three to four times daily.

TOXICITY

Not known.

ADVERSE REACTIONS

Drowsiness is the most common side effect according to the available clinical research.

One human study found that *Passiflora* extract has a significantly lower incidence of impairment of job performance compared with oxazepam (Akhondzadeh et al 2001b). One case reports a 34-year-old woman who developed severe nausea, vomiting, drowsiness and episodes of non-sustained ventricular tachycardia following administration of passionflower at therapeutic doses (Fisher et al 2000).

SIGNIFICANT INTERACTIONS

Controlled studies are not available; therefore, interactions are based on evidence of pharmacological activity and are theoretical.

Benzodiazepines

Additive effects are theoretically possible at high doses. There has been one case report of a patient taking passiflora and valerian while also taking lorazepam and developing shaking hands, dizziness, throbbing and muscular fatigue (Carrasco et al 2009). It is not known if the treatment was tested for authenticity or contamination, so causality is difficult to ascertain.

Use with caution and monitor drug dosage — possible beneficial interaction under medical supervision.

Note: *Passiflora* may be a useful support during benzodiazepine withdrawal.

Barbiturates

Additive central nervous system sedation is theoretically possible. Use with caution and monitor drug dosage — possible beneficial interaction under medical supervision.

Practice points/Patient counselling

- Both human and animal studies confirm passionflower has significant anxiolytic activity and reduces the symptoms of anxiety.
- When used 30 minutes before surgery, it appears to reduce nervousness.
- One randomised study found that it has significantly less negative effects on performance than 30 mg oxazepam, yet is as effective for GAD.
- Maximal effects may require several days of regular intake.
- It is not known whether physical tolerance develops.
- One study has shown it improves psychological symptoms during opiate withdrawal when used together with clonidine.
- In practice, it is often prescribed with other herbs for stronger effects in anxiety and insomnia.

CONTRAINDICATIONS AND PRECAUTIONS

Whether concomitant use of high doses of passiflora adversely affects people's ability to drive a car or operate heavy machinery should be evaluated on an individual case-by-case basis.

PREGNANCY USE

Passionflower has demonstrated the ability to increase uterine contractions in an isolated rat uterus model when compared to control tissue (Sadraei et al 2003). Whether this has any adverse effects in pregnancy remains unknown. Caution is advised until safety is better established.

PATIENTS' FAQs

What will this herb do for me?

Passionflower has anxiolytic effects that help reduce symptoms of anxiety. It might also be useful for insomnia, especially when used as part of a herbal combination. There is some research suggesting it may help ease the symptoms of opiate withdrawal.

When will it start to work?

When being used for anxiety, it may take 3–4 weeks before significant effects are seen.

Are there any safety issues?

Overall, passionflower does not appear to impair job performance but some people have reported drowsiness. However, it may theoretically interact with other sedative medicines when used in high doses. Other interactions are theoretically possible, so use should be monitored by a healthcare professional.

REFERENCES

Adell A, et al. Action of harman (1-methyl-beta-carboline) on the brain: body temperature and in vivo efflux of 5-HT from hippocampus of the rat. Neuropharmacology 35.8 (1996): 1101–1107.

Akhondzadeh S et al. Passionflower in the treatment of opiates withdrawal: a double-blind randomized controlled trial. J Clin Pharm Ther 26.5 (2001a): 369–73.

Akhondzadeh S et al. Passionflower in the treatment of generalized anxiety: a pilot double-blind randomized controlled trial with oxazepam. J Clin Pharm Ther 26.5 (2001b): 363–7.

Appel, K., et al. 2011. Modulation of the gamma-aminobutyric acid (GABA) system by *Passiflora incarnata* L. Phytother.Res., 25, (6) 838–843.

Aslanargun, P., et al. (2012). *Passiflora incarnata* Linneaus as an anxiolytic before spinal anesthesia. J Anesth., 26(1), 39–44.

Blumenthal M, et al (eds). Herbal medicine: expanded Commission E monographs. Austin, TX: Integrative Medicine Communications, 2000.

Bourin, M., et al. 1997. A combination of plant extracts in the treatment of outpatients with adjustment disorder with anxious mood: controlled study versus placebo. Fundam.Clin. Pharmacol., 11, (2) 127–132.

Breivogel, C., & Jamerson, B. (2012). Passion flower extract antagonizes the expression of nicotine locomotor sensitization in rats. Pharm Biol., 50(10), 1310–1316.

Carrasco, M. C., et al. (2009). Interactions of *Valeriana officinalis* L. and *Passiflora incarnata* L. in a patient treated with lorazepam. Phytother. Res., 23, 1795–1796.

Della Loggia R, et al. Evaluation of the activity on the mouse CNS of several plant extracts and a combination of them. Riv Neurol 51.5 (1981): 297–310.

Dhawan K, Sharma A. Antitussive activity of the methanol extract of *Passiflora incarnata* leaves. Fitoterapia 73.5 (2002): 397–399.

Dhawan K, et al. Anxiolytic activity of aerial and underground parts of *Passiflora incarnata*. Fitoterapia 72.8 (2001): 922–926.

Dhawan K, et al. Beneficial effects of chrysin and benzoflavone on virility in 2-year-old male rats. J Med Food 5.1 (2002a): 43–8.

Dhawan K, et al. Suppression of alcohol-cessation-oriented hyper-anxiety by the benzoflavone moiety of *Passiflora incarnata* Linneaus in mice. J Ethnopharmacol 81.2 (2002c): 239–44.

Dhawan K, et al. Aphrodisiac activity of methanol extract of leaves of *Passiflora incarnata* Linn. in mice. Phytother Res 17.4 (2003a): 401–3.

Dhawan K, et al. Antiasthmatic activity of the methanol extract of leaves of Passiflora incarnata. Phytother Res 17.7 (2003b): 821–2.

Dimpfel, W., et al. (2011). Early effect of NEURAPAS® balance on current source density (CSD) of human EEG. Links Export Central Citation BMC psychiatry, 11, 123.

Dolzhenko AT, Komissarov IV. GABA-ergic effects of harman independent of its influence on benzodiazepine receptors. Bull Eksp Biol Med 98.10 (1984): 446–448.

Fiebich, B., et al. (2011). Pharmacological studies in an herbal drug combination of St. John's Wort (*Hypericum perforatum*) and passion flower (*Passiflora incarnata*): In vitro and in vivo evidence of synergy between *Hypericum* and *Passiflora* in antidepressant pharmacological models. Fitoterapia, 82(3), 474–480.

Fisher AA, et al. Toxicity of *Passiflora incarnata* L. J Toxicol Clin Toxicol 38.1 (2000): 63–66.

Grundman, O., et al. (2008). Anxiolytic activity of a phytochemically characterized *Passiflora incarnata* extract is mediated via the GABAergic system. Planta medica, 74(15).

Gupta, K., et al. (2012). Antidiabetic activity of *Passiflora incarnata* Linn. in streptozotocin-induced diabetes in mice. Journal of Ethnopharmacology, 139, 801–806.

Ishida J et al. Anti-AIDS agents. 46: Anti-HIV activity of harman, an anti-HIV principle from *Symplocos setchuensis*, and its derivatives. Nat Prod 64.7 (2001): 958–960.

Lakhan, S.E. & Vieira, K.F. 2010. Nutritional and herbal supplements for anxiety and anxiety-related disorders: systematic review. Nutr.J, 9, 42.

Maroo, N., et al. 2013. Efficacy and safety of a polyherbal sedative-hypnotic formulation NSF-3 in primary insomnia in comparison to zolpidem: a randomized controlled trial. Indian J Pharmacol., 45, (1) 34–39.

Movafegh A et al. Preoperative oral *Passiflora incarnata* reduces anxiety in ambulatory surgery patients: a double-blind, placebo-controlled study. Anesth Analg 106.6 (2008): 1728–1732.

Nassiri-Asl M, et al. Anticonvulsant effects of aerial parts of *Passiflora incarnata* extract in mice: involvement of benzodiazepine and opioid receptors. BMC Complement Altern Med 7 (2007): 26.

Ngan, A., & Conduit, R. (2011). A double-blind placebo-controlled investigation of the effects of *Passiflora incarnata* (passionflower) herbal tea on subjective sleep quality. Phtyotherapy Research. 25: 1153–1159.

Sadraei H, et al. Extract of *Zataria multiflora* and *Carum carvi* essential oils and hydroalcoholic extracts of *Passiflora incarnata, Berberis intejerrimat* and *Crocus sativus* on rat isolated uterus contractions. Int J Aromather 13.2–3 (2003): 121–127.

Shi CC et al. Vasorelaxant effect of harman. Eur J Pharmacol 390.3 (2000): 319–325.

Simmen U et al. Extracts and constituents of *Hypericum perforatum* inhibit the binding of various ligands to recombinant receptors expressed with the Semliki Forest virus system. J Recept Signal Transduct Res 19.1–4 (1999): 59–74.

Singh, B., et al. (2012). Dual protective effect of *Passiflora incarnata* in epilepsy and associated post-ictal depression. Journal of Ethnopharmacology, 139(1), 273–279.

Soulimani R et al. Behavioural effects of *Passiflora incarnata* L. and its indole alkaloid and flavonoid derivatives and maltol in the mouse. J Ethnopharmacol 57.1 (1997): 11–20.

Yonezawa, T., et al. (2011). Harmine, a β-carboline alkaloid, inhibits osteoclast differentiation and bone resorption in vitro and in vivo. European Journal of Pharmacology, 650, 511–518.

Zanoli P, Avallone R, Baraldi M. Behavioral characterisation of the flavonoids apigenin and chrysin. Fitoterapia 71 (Suppl 1) (2000): S117–S123.

Pelargonium

HISTORICAL NOTE *Pelargonium sidoides* DC. (Geraniaceae) is an important traditional medicine in South Africa where it has been used to treat diarrhoea, dysentery, coughs and colds, tuberculosis and gastrointestinal conditions. This and other South African traditional medicines were often referred to by their original Khoi-Khoi name *rabas*, and were amongst the first to be recorded by early explorers such as van der Stel (1685) and Thunberg (1773). The most detailed account of the value and uses of *P. sidoides* is that of Smith (1895), who listed *P. reniforme/P. sidoides* as the first of five species used in the treatment of dysentery (Brendler & van Wyk 2008). The herb was introduced to Europe by the Englishman Charles Henry Stevens and is now a popular, commercially produced herbal medicine, listed in the European Pharmacopoeia (Brendler & van Wyk 2008).

***Clinical note — Is it* P. sidoides *or* P. reniforme?**

P. sidoides is predominantly found over large parts of the interior of southern Africa, but also occurs in coastal mountain ranges. The product may be adulterated with the very similar-looking *P. reniforme* and the two species often grow side by side. The phytochemical composition of the roots of *P. sidoides* is similar to *P. reniforme*, reflecting the close botanical relationship between the two species (Brendler & van Wyk 2008, Kolodziej 2007). Morphological distinction of the dried product is extremely difficult and chemical analysis is the only reliable method of telling them apart.

COMMON NAME

South African geranium

OTHER NAMES

Geranium, EPs 7630, Geranien, geranium root, Ikhubalo, Icwayiba, i-Yeza lezikali, Kaloba, Kalwerbossie, Pelargonien, pelargonium root, Rabas, Rabassam, silverleaf geranium, Umckaloabo, Uvendle

BOTANICAL NAME/FAMILY

Pelargonium sidoides (family: Geraniaceae)

PLANT PARTS USED

Root

CHEMICAL COMPONENTS

Oligomeric and polymeric proanthocyanidins are present in significant amounts: the putative precursors afzelechin, catechin and gallocatechin have been isolated; and highly oxygenated coumarins. Gallic acid is consistently found in high concentrations in the plant material and the minerals calcium and silica (Kolodziej 2007, Kolodziej et al 2003).

Coumarins and phenolic compounds, including simple phenolic acids and proanthocyanidins, are the principal compounds found in the special extract, EPs 7630 (Kolodziej 2007). Gallic acid occurs in low amounts in EPs 7630 (Kolodziej 2007).

MAIN ACTIONS

Antibacterial activity

Different in vitro evaluations of the herbal preparation from the roots of *P. sidoides* and its isolated constituents demonstrated pharmacological activities, including moderate, direct antibacterial effects against a panel of pathogenic bacteria that are responsible for numerous respiratory tract infections (RTIs), several multiresistant strains of *Staphylococcus aureus*, also *Streptococcus pneumoniae*, *Haemophilus influenzae*, *Moraxella catarrhalis* and *Mycobacterium tuberculosis* (Kolodziej et al 2003, Lizogub et al 2007, Mativandlela et al 2006).

Antiadhesion properties

Antiadhesive properties of pelargonium have been demonstrated for several bacteria, including *Helicobacter pylori,* and is thought to be one of the mechanisms responsible for its antimicrobial activity (Beil & Kilian 2007, Wittschier et al 2007).

Immune enhancement

The root extract also exhibits notable immune modulatory capabilities. The immune modulatory activities are mediated mainly by the release of tumour necrosis factor-alpha and nitric oxides, the stimulation of interferon-beta, the increase of natural killer cell activity and interferon-like activity (Kolodziej et al 2003, Lizogub et al 2007). Improved phagocytosis has also been demonstrated in vitro.

Antiviral activity

Direct antiviral activity against herpesvirus 1 and 2 has been demonstrated (Schnitzler et al 2008). *P. sidoides* extract affects the virus before penetration into the host cell and reveals a different mode of action when compared to aciclovir; it might be suitable for topical therapeutic use as antiviral drug in both labial and genital herpes infection. Through induction of the interferon system and upregulation of cytokines, important in protecting host cells from viral infection, the herb can be expected to exhibit antiviral activity in vivo (Engler et al 2009).

OTHER ACTIONS

A variety of mechanisms account for its symptom-relieving effects in RTIs.

The liquid extract acts as an expectorant and reduces sputum production, allowing the body to expel mucus, thereby making conditions less suitable for the multiplication of the bacteria and viruses. It has also been shown to increase cilia beat frequency in nasal epithelia.

> ***Clinical note — The difficult and winding road to successful commercialisation***
>
> It is believed that the medicinal properties of *Pelargonium sidoides* were first recognised and applied by traditional tribal healers in South Africa many centuries ago. It first came to the attention of Europeans in the early 1900s, as a result of a serendipitous meeting between an Englishman, Charles Henry Stevens, and a traditional Zulu healer. In 1897, Stevens was sent to South Africa by his doctor to recover from pulmonary tuberculosis. While there, he was treated by a traditional Zulu healer with a root concoction that successfully cured his condition (Bladt & Wagner 2007). Seeing the need for such a medicine back home and no doubt the commercial opportunity, Stevens called the tuberculosis treatment 'Umckaloabo', which he commercially manufactured once back in England. The treatment also became known as the 'Stevens' cure' and caused controversy amongst the medical establishment, which sought to discredit him by labelling Stevens a 'quack'. After his death in 1942, Stevens' son sold the business to a drug manufacturer in Germany. The exact herbal ingredient in the remedy and its source were kept secret and shrouded in mystery until well into the 1970s, when the plant ingredient was finally identified as *P. sidoides* by S. Bladt, while undertaking research for her thesis in Germany (Bladt & Wagner 2007). After the conduct of scientific and clinical trials, the herb was once again commercially manufactured in Europe with great success, with an annual turnover in Germany of 80 million Deutschmark in 2006 (Brendler & van Wyk 2008).

CLINICAL USE

Most research has been conducted with a standardised liquid herbal extract of the roots of *P. sidoides* (1:8–10), extraction solvent: ethanol 11% (wt/wt) produced by Willmar Schwabe Pharmaceuticals, Karlsruhe, Germany, also known as EPs 7630 (Umckaloabo, marketed by Spitzner Arzneimittel, Ettlingen, Germany). It has been approved for use in over 30 countries, including Australia.

Respiratory tract infections — bronchitis, common cold, sinusitis

In the light of inappropriate antibiotic use and increasing drug resistance rates worldwide, the need for an alternative, effective remedy for respiratory tract conditions is crucial. *P. sidoides* has been investigated as one such medicine and represents a promising treatment for the management of RTIs. It has achieved widespread popularity in Germany over the last 50 years, where it is approved for the treatment of acute bronchitis, acute tonsillopharyngitis and acute sinusitis. The standardised, liquid extract is now a registered medicine on the Australian Register of Therapeutic Goods and has been given an AUST R number, signifying claims have been evaluated by the Therapeutic Goods Administration for which there is good supportive scientific evidence.

Overall, the available evidence indicates that pelargonium is likely to be beneficial in the treatment of acute, mild to moderate bronchitis, acute rhinosinusitis and the common cold in adults. Paediatric trials suggest a potential benefit in acute bronchitis and in alleviating several common RTI symptoms, in particular, nasal congestion.

The scientific investigation of *P. sidoides* in the treatment of various RTIs really began in earnest in the 1990s (Brendler & van Wyk 2008). The earliest trials were mainly observational studies, whereas more recent studies tend to be placebo-controlled randomised trials and focus on acute bronchitis, although observational studies are still performed. The results of the individual research reports are compelling, particularly as there are no good treatment options for viral RTIs and bacterial RTIs are becoming increasingly difficult to treat.

One of the largest adult studies published to date was a randomised, double-blind, placebo-controlled, multicentre study of 406 adults with acute bronchitis published in 2010 (Matthys et al 2010). Patients were randomly assigned to one of four parallel treatment groups to receive different doses of EPs 7630 tablets (10 mg EPs 7630 tablets three times a day (30 mg group), 20 mg EPs 7630 tablets three times a day (60 mg group), 30 mg EPs 7630 tablets three times a day (90 mg group)) or placebo three times a day for a treatment period of 7 days. Bronchitis-specific symptoms were measured from baseline to day 7 and the groups were compared. Overall, the participants receiving EPs 7630 tablets had a statistically significant improvement in symptoms compared to the placebo group. The best results were obtained for the two higher-dosage regimens. When the incidence of side effects was considered, the optimal dose was 20 mg tablets of EPs 7630 taken three times daily.

Two new paediatric studies have been published since 2009, both in 2012. They continue to build the supportive evidence base for *Pelargonium sidoides* as a medicine for the treatment of common symptoms associated with RTIs, in particular, nasal congestion.

A randomised, placebo-controlled study by Patiroglu et al (2012) involved 28 children aged between 1 and 5 years with transient hypogammaglobulinaemia of infancy, one of the more common immune deficiencies of childhood. In this study, 14 participants were treated with *Pelargonium sidoides* for 1 week (10 drops three times a day), while 14 were given placebo during an episode of upper RTI. Active treatment with *P. sidoides* resulted in significantly improved appetite by day 5, a good representative factor in terms of indicating the general state of health of children. A highly relevant improvement was observed for nasal congestion in the *P. sidoides* extract group, compared to no improvement in the placebo group. On day 7, 71.4% of children taking active treatment had no nasal congestion compared with 21.5% in the placebo group. In contrast, no improvements were detected between the *P. sidoides* extract group and the placebo group for daily and nocturnal cough, fever or pain.

The prevention of an asthma attack during an upper RTI by 5 days of pelargonium treatment was tested in a randomised study of 61 children (Tahan et al 2012). This is based on the fact that viral infections have been implicated in most (>80%) asthma exacerbations in children. When the active treatment and placebo groups were compared, those receiving liquid *P. sidoides* had a significant decrease in cough frequency and nasal congestion and a statistically significant reduced frequency of developing an asthma attack. No significant changes were reported for fever or muscle aches and pains. The dosage schedule used was: for 1–5 years, 10 drops three times a day; for 6–12 years, 20 drops three times a day; for 12 years and above, 30 drops three times a day.

Previously, in 2008 a Cochrane systematic review was published in which authors evaluated data from eight randomised control trials (RCTs) and concluded that *P. sidoides* may be effective in alleviating symptoms of acute bronchitis, rhinosinusitis and the common cold in adults, but the findings were not yet definitive (Timmer et al 2008). The authors identified two RCTs that showed *P. sidoides* was effective in relieving all symptoms, and in particular cough and sputum production in adults with acute bronchitis, although a third study showed that the preparation was only effective for treating sputum reduction. Similarly, *P. sidoides* was effective in resolving symptoms of acute bronchitis in two out of three paediatric studies. One RCT of 104 adults was included in the review, showing significant treatment effects in acute rhinosinusitis for the resolution of all symptoms as well as the key symptoms of nasal discharge and headache resolution.

The results obtained by studies using tablet preparations included in this review were different from those using the liquid preparation. Based on this, the authors stated that the liquid preparation (alcoholic solution) may be associated with improvement in some symptoms of acute bronchitis in both children and adults — in particular sputum production and cough — but tablet preparations produced fewer or no potential beneficial effects in both children and adults. The cause of this difference is unknown and may be due to chance or differences in constituent bioavailability or in the product's phytochemical constituents. Another caution expressed by the review authors was of the use of non-validated symptom scales as a primary end point and the subjective nature of the results.

The same year, a review was published in *Phytomedicine* that analysed six RCTs, of which four were suitable for statistical pooling (Agbabiaka et al 2008). One study compared EPs 7630 against conventional non-antibiotic treatment (acetylcysteine); the other five studies tested EPs 7630 against placebo. All RCTs reported findings suggesting the effectiveness of EPs 7630 in treating acute bronchitis. When a meta-analysis of the four placebo-controlled RCTs was conducted, the results confirmed that EPs 7630 significantly reduced bronchitis symptom scores in patients with acute bronchitis by day 7.

P

Common cold

A multicentre, randomised, double-blind trial by Lizogub et al (2007) involved 107 participants with cold symptoms present for between 24 and 48 hours. It demonstrated that treatment with liquid extract of *P. sidoides* significantly hastened recovery from the common cold, and markedly improved individual symptoms, most notably nasal congestion and drainage, sneezing, sore throat, hoarseness and headache. The group receiving active treatment also experienced significantly higher remission and improvement in rates of other cold-related symptoms compared to placebo, such as limb pain (95.5% vs 74%), general weakness (79% vs 35%), exhaustion

(85% vs 43%) and fatigue (89% vs 60.5%) (Lizogub et al 2007). The study compared 30 drops (1.5 mL) of liquid herbal pelargonium three times daily to placebo for a maximum of 10 days. After 10 days, substantially more people receiving the herbal treatment were considered clinically cured than the placebo group (78.8% vs 31.4%; $P < 0.0001$). All (100%) of patients receiving pelargonium judged tolerability of treatment as good or very good.

Immune modulation in athletes

Exhaustive physical exercise is associated with increased frequency of upper RTIs, probably due to a compromised immune response. A double-blind, placebo-controlled study involving male marathon runners found that treatment with *P. sidoides* extract modulated the production of secretory immunoglobulin A in saliva, both interleukin-15 (IL-15) and IL-6 in serum, and IL-15 in the nasal mucosa after an intense running session. Secretory immunoglobulin A levels were increased, while levels of IL-15 and IL-6 were decreased, thereby indicating a strong modulating influence on the immune response (Luna et al 2011). The treatment schedule consisted of umckaloabo or placebo (3 × 30 drops/day) for 28 consecutive days before training and testing.

OTHER USES

The traditional uses of tuberous *Pelargonium* species mainly involve ailments of the gastrointestinal tract (diarrhoea and dysentery) and respiratory tract, although Smith (1895) made a case for it being used as a general tonic.

It is also used as a gripe water for infants ('upset stomach', 'air in the intestine'). The crushed root is mixed with water and a teaspoonful of the red infusion is taken orally (Brendler & van Wyk 2008).

The aerial parts have also been used traditionally as a wound-healing agent. This may be due to their high tannin content that would contribute to its astringent effect (Kolodziej 2007).

DOSAGE RANGE

Dried herb: 0.4 g/day

According to clinical studies

Treatment of acute bronchitis

General dosage: Adults and children over 12 years: 30 drops (1.5 mL) of liquid extract herbal pelargonium three times daily before meals for up to 10 days.

Adults — for acute bronchitis symptoms: 20 mg tablets of EPs 7630 taken three times daily.

Children aged 6–12 years: 20 drops (1.0 mL) three times per day.

Children aged 2–5 years: 10 drops three times a day.

Treatment for the common cold

Adults: 30 drops (1.5 mL) of liquid herbal pelargonium three times daily.

Acute sinusitis treatment

Adults: 60 drops three times a day.

Reducing the frequency of an asthma attack during respiratory tract infection in children with mild asthma

1–5 years: 10 drops three times a day.

6–12 years: 20 drops three times a day.

Over 12 years of age: 30 drops three times a day.

Practice points/Patient counselling

- *P. sidoides* is a traditional herbal medicine originating from South Africa and now extremely popular in Europe, particularly Germany, and available in Australia.
- The herb demonstrates antibacterial and antiviral activity and enhances non-specific immune function; it also has activity against herpesvirus 1 and 2.
- Observational and randomised studies indicate *Pelargonium sidoides* liquid extract EPs 7630 may provide benefits in the treatment in acute, mild to moderate bronchitis, acute rhinosinusitis and possibly the common cold in adults, acute bronchitis in children and in alleviating several common RTI symptoms, in particular, nasal congestion.
- It appears to hasten recovery from the common cold, reduce symptoms and improve associated fatigue and weakness and may have a role in the acute treatment of other, uncomplicated respiratory infections.
- It is generally well tolerated; however, gastrointestinal side effects and allergic skin reactions have been reported with use.

TOXICITY

Not known.

ADVERSE REACTIONS

Evidence from clinical trials and postmarket surveillance studies indicates few serious adverse events, all found to be unrelated to the medicine, and only mild side effects, which tended to be limited to gastrointestinal symptoms such as nausea, vomiting, diarrhoea or heartburn, and rashes. Allergic skin reactions with pruritus and urticaria have been reported in trials.

SIGNIFICANT INTERACTIONS

Controlled clinical studies are not available; therefore, interactions are based on evidence of activity and are largely theoretical and speculative.

Immunosuppressant drugs

Theoretically, use of this herb may reduce the effectiveness of immunosuppressant medication — avoid until safety can be established.

CONTRAINDICATIONS AND PRECAUTIONS

People with an allergy to the geranium family of plants should avoid this herb.

PREGNANCY USE

It appears safe in pregnancy based on studies using animal models of reproduction and development whereby no effects on fertility or development were detected at up to 2700 mg/kg body weight/day EPs 7630.

PATIENTS' FAQs

What will this herb do for me?
Pelargonium sidoides has antibacterial and antiviral actions and will enhance immune function. It may provide benefits in the treatment in acute, mild to moderate bronchitis, acute rhinosinusitis and possibly the common cold in adults, acute bronchitis in children and in alleviating several common RTI symptoms, in particular, nasal congestion.

When will it start to work?
It should be started at the first sign of infection and a course of treatment is 6–10 days. When used as acute treatment for the common cold, symptom relief may be noticeable within 3 days and significant after 5 days. Symptom relief may take longer to fully establish in cases of acute bronchitis and rhinosinusitis.

Are there any safety issues?
It is generally well tolerated; however; gastrointestinal side effects and allergic skin reactions have been reported with use.

REFERENCES

Agbabiaka TB, et al. *Pelargonium sidoides* for acute bronchitis: a systematic review and meta-analysis. Phytomedicine 15.5 (2008): 378–385.

Beil, W. & Kilian, P. 2007. EPs 7630, an extract from *Pelargonium sidoides* roots inhibits adherence of *Helicobacter pylori* to gastric epithelial cells. Phytomedicine, 14 (Suppl 6), 5–8.

Bladt S, Wagner H. From the Zulu medicine to the European phytomedicine Umckaloabo. Phytomedicine 14 (Suppl 6) (2007): 2–4.

Brendler T, van Wyk BE. A historical, scientific and commercial perspective on the medicinal use of *Pelargonium sidoides* (Geraniaceae). J Ethnopharmacol 119.3 (2008): 420–433.

Engler RJM et al. Complementary and alternative medicine for the allergist-immunologist: where do I start? J Allergy Clin Immunol 123.2 (2009): 309–316.

Kolodziej H et al. Pharmacological profile of extracts of *Pelargonium sidoides* and their constituents. Phytomedicine 10 Suppl 4 (2003): 18–24.

Kolodziej H. Fascinating metabolic pools of *Pelargonium sidoides* and *Pelargonium reniforme*, traditional and phytomedicinal sources of the herbal medicine Umckaloabo. Phytomedicine 14.Suppl 6 (2007): 9–17.

Lizogub VG, et al. Efficacy of a *Pelargonium sidoides* preparation in patients with the common cold: a randomized, double blind, placebo-controlled clinical trial. NY: Explore 3.6 (2007): 573–84.

Luna, L.A., Jr., et al. 2011. Immune responses induced by *Pelargonium sidoides* extract in serum and nasal mucosa of athletes after exhaustive exercise: modulation of secretory IgA, IL-6 and IL-15. Phytomedicine, 18, (4) 303–308.

Mativandlela SPN, et al. Antibacterial, antifungal and antitubercular activity of (the roots of) *Pelargonium reniforme* (CURT) and *Pelargonium sidoides* (DC) (Geraniaceae) root extracts. S Afr J Bot 72.2 (2006): 232–237.

Matthys H, et al. [*Pelargonium sidoides* in acute bronchitis — Health related quality of life and patient-reported outcome in adults receiving EPs 7630 treatment.] Wien Med Wochenschr 2010;160(21–22):564–570.

Patiroglu T, et al. The efficacy of *Pelargonium sidoides* in the treatment of upper respiratory tract infections in children with transient hypogammaglobulinemia of infancy. Phytomedicine 2012;19(11):958–961.

Schnitzler P et al. Efficacy of an aqueous *Pelargonium sidoides* extract against herpesvirus. Phytomedicine 15.12 (2008): 1108–1116.

Tahan F, Yaman M. Can the *Pelargonium sidoides* root extract EPs((R)) 7630 prevent asthma attacks during viral infections of the upper respiratory tract in children? Phytomedicine 2012; 20: 148–150.

Timmer A et al. *Pelargonium sidoides* extract for acute respiratory tract infections. Cochrane Database Syst Rev 3 (2008): CD006323.

Wittschier, N., et al. 2007. An extract of *Pelargonium sidoides* (EPs 7630) inhibits in situ adhesion of *Helicobacter pylori* to human stomach. Phytomedicine, 14, (4) 285–288.

P

Peppermint

HISTORICAL NOTE The written record of mint dates back to an ancient Greek myth in which the Greek god Pluto was said to have affections for a beautiful nymph named Minthe. His jealous wife Persephone cast a spell on the nymph, transforming her into a plant. When Pluto could not reverse the spell, he gave her a sweet scent that would emanate throughout the garden (Murray & Pizzorno 1999). Peppermint has been used medicinally for generations as a digestive aid and carminative. More recently, enteric-coated peppermint oil capsules have been widely prescribed for the relief of irritable bowel syndrome (IBS).

BOTANICAL NAME/FAMILY

Mentha × piperita (family [Labiatae] Lamiaceae)

PLANT PARTS USED

Leaf or stem — essential oil is distilled from the aerial parts.

CHEMICAL COMPONENTS

Peppermint leaves contain about 2.5% essential oil, 19% total polyphenolic compounds, 12% total flavonoid compounds (eriocitrin, luteolin-7-O-rutinoside and hesperidoside) and 7% total hydroxycinnamic compounds (including rosmarinic acid) (Duband et al 1992). The biochemistry, organisation and regulation of essential oil metabolism in the epidermal oil glands of peppermint have been defined, and research is underway to create 'super' transgenic peppermint plants with improved oil composition and yield (Wildung & Croteau 2005).

Essential oil

Over 100 constituents have been identified in peppermint oil. The principal constituents are terpenes; menthol (35–55%), menthones (10–35%), isomenthone, menthyl acetate, menthofuran and cineole. To comply with the European Pharmacopoeia, the oil must not contain more than 4% pulegone and not more than 1% carvone.

MAIN ACTIONS

The actions of the leaf as an infusion (tea) or liquid extract are largely dependent on the essential oil content. Other compounds, such as the flavonoids, also contribute to the overall activity, especially the antioxidant activity. Peppermint oil is relatively rapidly absorbed after oral administration and eliminated mainly via bile (Grigoleit & Grigoleit 2005a).

Antispasmodic

Peppermint essential oil, ethanol extracts and flavonoids isolated from the leaf have all shown antispasmodic effects in vitro (ESCOP 1997). The antispasmodic effect of various peppermint preparations has been confirmed in human clinical trials. An antispasmodic effect on gastric smooth muscle was demonstrated for peppermint oil when used topically (intraluminal) or ingested orally in doses of 0.1–0.24 mL (Grigoleit & Grigoleit 2005). According to a double-blind RCT, oral administration of 182 mg peppermint oil significantly reduced intragastric pressure, proximal phasic contractility and appetite, but had no effect on gastric sensitivity, tone and nutrient tolerance (Papathanasopoulos et al 2013). In healthy volunteers, intragastric administration of a dose equivalent to 180 mg peppermint oil reduced intraoesophageal pressure within 1–7 minutes of infusion (Kingham 1995). Investigation with a peppermint leaf extract found it reduced the frequency of slow wave motion in the small intestine but not the amplitude (Sibaev et al 2006).

Gastric smooth muscle relaxation was also seen for a combination product, Enteroplant, an enteric-coated capsule containing 90 mg peppermint and 50 mg caraway oil (Micklefield et al 2003).

The antispasmodic activity is believed to be mediated via activation of sensory neurons of transient receptor potential (TRP) channels, in particular melstatin8 (TRPM8) (Farco & Grundmann 2013). The active constituent menthol induces Ca^{2+} ion influx through the TRPM8 channels expressed in sensory neurons, the dorsal root ganglia, vagal afferent neurons, the gastric fundus, colon and small intestine (Papathanasopoulos et al 2013). Although menthol has been shown to induce Ca^{2+} release from intracellular stores in several TRPM8-expressing cell types, a TRPM8-independent pathway of Ca^{2+} release, originating from the endoplasmic reticulum and the Golgi compartments, has also been postulated (Kim et al 2009, Mahieu et al 2007).

Carminative

Peppermint has a carminative activity, which refers to its ability to relax the gastrointestinal sphincters. Carminatives are thought to alleviate symptoms of bloating and gas by facilitating eructation and passage of flatus and by inducing relaxation of the lower oesophageal sphincter (LES) (Massey 2001). An early study demonstrated that peppermint oil canalised into the gall bladder and duodenal areas was able to counteract morphine hydrochloride-induced constriction of the sphincter of Oddi (Giachetti et al 1988). In patients with diffuse oesophageal spasm, peppermint oil orally (10 drops in water) did not affect lower oesophageal sphincter contractile pressure but completely eliminated simultaneous oesophageal contractions in all patients (Pimentel et al 2001).

Choleretic

Choleretic activity has been demonstrated for peppermint tea, flavonoids and the essential oil (ESCOP 1997). Hydrophilic compounds may contribute to the gastrointestinal effects, with aqueous extracts from peppermint leaves having antiulcerogenic and choleretic effects (Grigoleit & Grigoleit 2005c, Van Rensen 2004). Peppermint oil has a relaxing effect on the gall bladder and small intestine, inhibiting gall bladder emptying and prolonging orocaecal transit time in a manner comparable to *N*-butylscopolamine (Goerg & Spilker 2003). Peppermint oil strongly promotes bile acid secretion and decreases cholesterol levels in bile. The oil has been shown to up-regulate bile acid synthesis-related genes CYP7A1, and FXR mRNA levels, suggesting that the molecular mechanisms are related to gene expression involved in bile acid synthesis (Zong et al 2011).

Antimicrobial

Peppermint oil and its main constituent menthol have significant antibacterial, antifungal and antiplasmid activity and are able to potentiate the effect of some antibiotics (Schelz et al 2006).

Antibacterial

Peppermint oil has significant antibacterial activity (Mimica-Dukic et al 2003), as has the juice of peppermint leaves (Rakover et al 2008, Saeed & Tariq 2005). Peppermint oil has been shown to inhibit *Helicobacter pylori*, *Staphylococcus aureus* (Betoni et al 2006, Imai et al 2001, Mohsenzadeh 2007, Yadegarinia et al 2006), *Escherichia coli* (Mohsenzadeh 2007, Pattnaik et al 1995, Yadegarinia et al 2006), *Salmonella enteritidis*, *Listeria monocytogenes* and multiresistant strains of *Shigella sonnei* and *Micrococcus flavus* (Mimica-Dukic et al 2003). Peppermint oil has further been shown to have a significant antimycobacterial activity in vitro, and inhalation of peppermint oil has been used successfully as a supplement to combined multidrug therapy for pulmonary tuberculosis (Shkurupii et al 2002). In a recent study, peppermint oil showed stronger antimicrobial and antibiofilm properties than chlorhexidine against *Streptococcus mutans* and *Streptococcus pyogenes* (Rasooli et al 2008).

Peppermint oil has been tested in conjunction with various antibiotics to determine whether antimicrobial effects are enhanced.. The notion that concurrent use may be beneficial began with the observation that peppermint extract produced a synergistic antibacterial effect against *Staphylococcus aureus* when used in conjunction with a variety of antimicrobial drugs (Betoni et al 2006). More recently, peppermint oil was tested with piperacillin and meropenem, which resulted in a substantial increase in the susceptibility of *Escherichia coli* to antibiotic therapy. There was also a considerable reduction in the minimum inhibitory concentrations (MIC) of the antibiotics (Yap et al 2013).

Fungistatic, fungicidal

Peppermint is also fungistatic and fungicidal (Pattnaik et al 1996, Positive Health News 1998) with its activity against *Trichophyton tonsurans*, *Candida albicans* being considerably greater than the commercial fungicide bifonazole (Mimica-Dukic et al 2003, Sokovic et al 2009, Yadegarinia et al 2006). Fungicidal activity similar to lavender and clove oil was reported for peppermint oil against *Trichophyton mentagrophytes* when used in combination with salt and heat (Inouye et al 2007). Peppermint oil showed high antifungal activity against *Candida albicans* (Yigit et al 2008), with one study reporting a 74% *Candida albicans* (strain CA I) biofilm reduction due to the effects of peppermint oil (Agarwal et al 2008). Moderate antifungal activity was observed for peppermint oil against *Rhizopus stolonifer, Botrytis cinerea, Aspergillus niger, Aspergillus candidus, Penicillium* spp and *Fusarium culmorum* (Behnam et al 2006, Magro et al 2006). Moreover, peppermint oil at various concentrations has been shown to inhibit aflatoxin B production by 85–90% when evaluated for activity against *Aspergillus parasiticus* and *Aspergillus flavus* (Bluma et al 2008).

Antiviral

Peppermint oil also has virucidal activity against herpes simplex virus (HSV)-1 and -2, including activity against an aciclovir-resistant strain of HSV-1 (ACV_{res}) with a 50% inhibitory concentration determined at 0.002 and 0.0008% for HSV-1 and HSV-2, respectively. The oil was also found to affect the virus before, but not after, penetration into the host cell indicating it acts on free HSV (Schuhmacher et al 2003). This suggests the potential for topical use against recurrent herpes infections (Nolkemper et al 2006). Aqueous extract (Geuenich et al 2008, Nolkemper et al 2006) and 80% ethanolic extract of peppermint (Reichling et al 2008) at maximum non-cytotoxic concentrations reduced plaque formation of HSV-1, HSV-2 and ACV_{res} significantly following exposure of free virions as well as host cells to the extracts prior to infection.

Insecticidal

Peppermint oil shows moderate repellent activity against *Culex pipiens* (Erler et al 2006), and menthol and its derivatives show mosquitocidal activity against *Culex quinquefasciatus, Aedes aegypti* and *Anopheles tessellatus* (Samarasekera et al 2008). This preliminary research shows promise for the development of insecticidal and repellant agents. Peppermint oil was shown to only exert some repellence against head lice (*Pediculus humanus* var. *capitis*), which was due to the slippery nature of the oil rather than specific repellent activity (Canyon & Speare 2007). However, a combination product of 5% eucalyptus and 5% peppermint oil in 50% ethanol showed effectiveness against the head lice (Gonzalez Audino et al 2007).

Antiparasitic

Aqueous extracts of peppermint showed activity against gastrointestinal nematodes in goats and pigs (De Almeida et al 2007, Lans et al 2007). In vitro, dichlormethane extracts, but not water extracts, of peppermint showed antigiardial activity by causing alterations on the plasma membrane surface of the parasite and inhibiting its adhesion (Vidal et al 2007). The antigiardial action is comparatively weaker than other essential oils of plants with high levels of phenolic compounds (Machado et al 2010). Research on the anthelmintic action of peppermint remains limited to in vitro testing and suitable doses appear to have no affect when administered in vivo (Carvalho et al 2012).

Antioxidant

P

The polyphenolic compounds in peppermint, such as luteolin-7-O-rutinoside, eriocitrin and rosmarinic acid, have been shown to have antioxidant and free radical scavenging activity (Sroka et al 2005). Peppermint oil and its constituents menthone and isomenthone exert antioxidant activity (Mimica-Dukic et al 2003). Interestingly, peppermint and lemon balm exerted the strongest antioxidant and radical scavenging effects when examining all individual herbs from a herbal combination preparation (STW 5 — Iberogast: 9 plant extracts from *Mentha piperita, Iberis amara, Chelidonii herba, Cardui mariae fructus, Melissae folium, Carvi fructus, Liquiritiae radix, Angelicae radix, Matricariae flos*) (Germann et al 2006, Schempp et al 2006).

Stimulant

Intraperitoneal and intravenous injections of peppermint oil and its constituents, 1,8-cineol, menthone, isomenthone, menthol, pulegone, menthyl acetate and caryophyllene, dramatically increased ambulatory activity in mice, which may explain the traditional use of peppermint for mental fatigue (Umezu & Morita 2003, Umezu et al 2001). A recent study suggests that this effect exerted by menthone is mediated via dopamine (Umezu 2009). Inhalation of peppermint oil has also been shown to have a stimulant effect on mice in a forced swimming test (Lim et al 2005).

Coolant

The active constituent menthol is considered responsible for the cooling sensation brought about by peppermint, and is achieved via the same mechanism responsible for its antispasmodic action. Activation of sensory neurons TRPM8 and transient receptor potential subfamily A, member 1 (TRPA1) rapidly increases intracellular calcium and mobilises calcium flux through the channels to induce cold response signals at the application site (Farco & Grundmann 2013). In the peripheral nerves, this effect may be responsible for the characteristic cooling sensation experienced on oral ingestion of mint. Interestingly, menthol's cold sensitivity response mechanism has been shown to inhibit mucosal recognition of nicotine and cigarette toxins common in mentholated cigarette brands. Menthol has been investigated for its action on airway epithelium and was found to regulate cAMP-activated anion transporters on the apical and basolateral membranes, independent of the transient receptor potential (TRP) channels. This action directly relates to the airway lumen forming low viscosity mucus and contributing to overall mucociliary clearance (Morise et al 2010). A second proposed mechanism of action is the antioxidant action of peppermint oil.

IN COMBINATION

A combination of essential oils (soy oil — 69.18%; coconut oil — 20.00%; orange oil — 4.90%; aloe vera oil — 4.90%; peppermint oil — 0.75%; vitamin E — 0.27%) was shown to effectively reduce inflammation associated with oxidant stress-related challenge to the nasal mucosa (Gao et al 2011), however the role of peppermint alone is unclear. A double-blind randomised controlled trial (RCT) investigated a spray containing aromatic essential oils of five plants (*Eucalyptus citriodora, Eucalyptus globulus, Mentha piperita, Origanum syriacum,* and *Rosmarinus officinalis*) applied five times a day for 3 days and compared with a placebo spray. The treatment group reported a significantly greater improvement in symptom severity compared to participants in the placebo group ($P = 0.019$) after 20 minutes; however, there was no difference in symptom severity between the two groups after 3 days of treatment (Ben-Arye et al 2011).

Analgesic

Peppermint and caraway oil have been shown to synergistically modulate post-inflammatory visceral hyperalgesia in a rat model (Adam et al 2006). A significant analgesic effect, with a reduction in sensitivity to headache, was observed in a double-blind, placebo-controlled, randomised, 7-day crossover study that used a combination of peppermint oil and ethanol applied externally in 32 healthy males undergoing artificial pain stimulation (Gobel et al 1994). Research reports menthol engages in synergistic excitation of GABA receptors and sodium ion channels resulting in analgesia (Farco & Grundmann 2013).

OTHER ACTIONS

A spray-dried peppermint infusion has been found to be mildly diuretic and produce weak sedative action in several tests when administered orally to mice (Della et al 1990). Peppermint tea has been found to significantly increase follicle stimulating hormone (FSH) and luteinising hormone (LH) levels and reduce total testosterone levels in rats (Akdogan et al 2004). Concomitant topical exposure to low concentrations of peppermint oil reduced the percutaneous penetration of benzoic acid; however, with increased peppermint oil doses, penetration of benzoic acid increased (Nielsen 2006). Peppermint extract was shown to reduce the side effects of arsenic-induced hepatopathy (Sharma et al 2007). In a more recent study, peppermint oil displayed acetylcholinesterase and butyrylcholinesterase inhibitory activities, which was more than the activity exerted by individual components of the oil (Orhan et al 2008).

Mentha piperita protects against radiation-induced lethality, lipid peroxidation and DNA damage (Jagetia 2007) through its antioxidant and free radical scavenging activities (Samarth et al 2006b). The same authors suggest that these activities are also responsible for a significant reduction in the number of lung tumours observed in mice following oral administration of peppermint extract (Samarth et al 2006a). It has also been reported that peppermint protected against radiation-induced haematopoietic damage in bone marrow of mice by increasing erythropoietin.

CLINICAL USE

In practice, peppermint and its derivatives are used in many forms and administered by various routes. This review will focus only on those methods that are commonly used by the public and preparations that are available over the counter (OTC), such as oral dose forms, topical applications and inhalations. In many cases, peppermint is used as part of a multiherbal combination, which is reflected in some of the studies presented here.

Irritable Bowel Syndrome (IBS)

Since the late 1970s, clinical studies have been conducted to determine the role of various peppermint preparations in the treatment of IBS (Dew et al 1984, Rees et al 1979). Generally, the oil was used in the early studies with more recent research utilising other forms such as pH-triggered, enteric-coated peppermint oil capsules that prevent dissolution of the capsules until they have reached the small intestine, and release into the colon over 10–12 hours (Grigoleit & Grigoleit 2005c). Enteric coating also has the advantage of allowing administration of a higher dose than would otherwise be possible to tolerate and, importantly, avoids the risk of excessively relaxing the lower oesophageal sphincter and causing reflux.

Multiple systematic reviews and meta-analyses have been published since 1998, concluding that peppermint oil is a worthwhile symptomatic treatment in IBS (Pittler & Ernst 1998, Grigoleit & Grigoleit 2005a, Khanna et al 2014, Ruepert et al 2011). One systematic review of 16 clinical trials investigating peppermint oil in IBS showed statistically significant effects in favour of peppermint oil, with an average response for 'overall success' being 58% for peppermint oil and 29% for placebo. Three studies that compared peppermint oil to smooth muscle relaxants showed no difference between these treatments (Grigoleit & Grigoleit 2005a).

In 2013, a more recent meta-analysis of nine RCTs (n = 726 patients) concluded that peppermint oil was significantly superior to placebo for global improvement of IBS symptoms (five studies, 392 patients, relative risk 2.23) and improvement in abdominal pain (five studies, 357 patients, RR 2.14) using a minimum treatment time-frame of 2 weeks (Khanna et al 2014). When side effect incidence was compared, the group receiving active treatment was more likely to experience mild transient adverse events, most commonly heartburn; however, the treatment is considered safe and effective for the short-term treatment of IBS.

Clinical note — Pathophysiology of IBS

The pathophysiology of IBS is poorly understood, but it is believed to occur when the intestinal muscles are contracting faster or more slowly than normal. Colonic contractions cause abdominal pain, cramping, wind and diarrhoea or constipation. It has been proposed that IBS may result from dysregulation of gastrointestinal motor and enhanced sensory functions, as modulated by the central nervous system (CNS). However, clinical and laboratory investigations have failed to uncover any histological, microbiological or biochemical abnormalities in patients with IBS. Patients with IBS demonstrate increased motility and abnormal contractions of the intestinal muscles when faced with an emotionally or physically stressful situation (Greenberg et al 2002). It is likely that IBS is also associated with dietary habits, poor upper digestion and intestinal dysbiosis (bacterial overgrowth of the bowels).

Common symptoms of IBS are (Greenberg et al 2002) as follows:

- cramping pain in the lower abdomen
- bloating and excess gas (wind)
- changes in bowel habits
- diarrhoea or constipation, either one dominant or both alternating
- immediate need for a bowel movement on awakening or during or after meals
- relief of pain after bowel movements
- feeling of incomplete emptying after bowel movements
- mucus in the stool.

IN COMBINATION

An early placebo-controlled trial of 223 patients with nonulcer dyspepsia and IBS tested a caraway (*Carum carvi*) and peppermint oil combination which was found to significantly reduce pain compared to placebo (P < 0.001) (Freise & Kohler 1999). The herbal combination commercially available as Iberogast contains peppermint leaf in addition to other herbs and has also been tested in IBS.

A 2013 systematic review of RCTs concluded that Iberogast produces symptomatic relief in IBS and is well tolerated (Ottillinger et al 2013). Since peppermint is only one component of this multi-component herbal product, it is uncertain what contribution this herb made to achieving the beneficial outcomes.

Dyspepsia

A two-way crossover study with 10 healthy male volunteers showed that peppermint oil enhances gastric emptying during the early phase, suggesting the potential use of peppermint oil in functional gastrointestinal disorders (Inamori et al 2007).

IN COMBINATION

Peppermint is often combined with other herbal ingredients, such as caraway (*Carum carvi*) in the treatment of dyspepsia. As a reflection of practice, nearly all studies have tested a herbal combination containing peppermint oil or leaf as one of the ingredients and there is little research available that has used peppermint as a standalone treatment.

A popular herbal combination preparation (STW 5 — Iberogast) that includes peppermint leaf extract and eight other plant extracts (*Iberis amara, Chelidonii herba, Cardui mariae fructus, Melissae folium, Carvi fructus, Liquiritiae radix, Angelicae radix* and *Matricariae flos*) has been demonstrated to significantly relieve dyspepsia in a number of RCTs, including a meta-analysis of three trials (Melzer et al 2004), with a fourth RCT showing similar effects to cisapride (Rosch et al 2002). In a newer study, it was shown that STW 5 lowered gastric acidity as effectively as commercial antacid preparations (i.e. Rennie, Talcid and Maaloxan), prevented secondary hyperacidity more effectively and additionally inhibited serum gastrin levels in rats (Khayyal et al 2006). A more recent 2013 systematic review of RCTs further concluded that Iberogast produces symptomatic relief in functional dyspepsia and is well tolerated with a side effect incidence of 0.04% when considering worldwide spontaneous reporting schemes (Ottillinger et al 2013). Since peppermint is only one component of this multicomponent herbal product, it is uncertain what contribution this herb made towards achieving the beneficial outcomes.

The combination of peppermint and caraway has also been the subject of numerous trials. Previously, in a systematic review of herbal medicines for functional dyspepsia, Coon and Ernst (2002) identified four RCTs of a fixed combination of peppermint and caraway oils; five which tested the herbal combination known as Iberogast; one trial of a combination of extracts of peppermint leaves, caraway fruit, fennel fruit and wormwood herbs; and one trial of a combination of peppermint oil and ginger extract. Various clinical benefits were found for all treatments.

The commercial peppermint and caraway combination products tested were found to produce significant symptomatic relief. These were Enteroplant products delivering 180 mg/day peppermint oil and 100 mg/day caraway oil; 270 mg/day peppermint oil and 150 mg/day caraway oil; or an enteric soluble formulation providing 108 mg/day peppermint oil and 60 mg/day caraway oil (Dr Willmar Schwabe, Karlsruhe, Germany).

One of the studies included in the review was by May et al (2000), which involved 96 outpatients and used Enteroplant (180 mg/day peppermint oil and 100 mg/day caraway oil; (Dr Willmar Schwabe GmbH, Karlsruhe, Germany), which significantly improved symptoms of functional dyspepsia. After 4 weeks the average intensity of pain was reduced by 40% versus baseline in the active group and by 22% in the placebo group. The peppermint combination also reduced pressure, heaviness and fullness (May et al 2000). A subgroup analysis from this study revealed that *Helicobacter pylori*-positive patients had a substantially better treatment response (May et al 2003). In a further double-blind, placebo-controlled trial, the same oil combination was found to significantly improve disease-specific quality of life (QOL), as measured by the validated Nepean Dyspepsia Index compared to placebo (Holtmann et al 2003).

The peppermint oil and caraway oil product (Enteroplant; 180/100 mg) has been compared to cisapride (30 mg/day) in a double blind RCT involving 120 people with functional dyspepsia and moderate pain and one other gastric symptom over the last 14 days. In the 4-week study, the peppermint and caraway oil combination (Enteroplant, 2 capsules daily) was shown to be as effective as cisapride in reducing both the magnitude and the frequency of epigastric pain and dyspeptic discomfort. Doctors rated the two treatments comparable in regard to other dyspeptic symptoms, in addition to intestinal and extraintestinal autonomic symptoms. Corresponding results were also found in *H. pylori*-positive patients and patients who initially presented with intense epigastric pain in the two treatment groups. Both medications were well tolerated (Madisch et al 1999).

Infantile colic

Peppermint (1 drop/kg body weight) was compared with simethicone in a double-blind crossover study of 30 infants experiencing infantile colic for a period of 14 days. At the end of the treatment period, the number of daily episodes of colic fell and the crying duration decreased in both groups. All mothers reported a decrease in frequency and duration of episodes of infantile colic, and both treatments seemed to be as effective as each other. The extract of peppermint was not specified in this report. These preliminary findings justify further clinical trials using peppermint for the treatment of infantile colic (Alves et al 2012).

Diffuse oesophageal spasm

Diffuse oesophageal spasm (DES) is a relatively rare motor disorder. Associated manometric abnormalities may include hypertensive and repetitive contractions. The lower oesophageal sphincter (LES) may also be hypertensive. Although LES relaxation with deglutition is generally normal, disturbances in LES function are often seen. These abnormalities are, however, not required for the diagnosis (Massey 2001). In a study of eight DES patients with chest pain or dysphagia, peppermint oil had no effect on LES pressures or contractile pressures and durations in the oesophagus, yet completely eliminated simultaneous oesophageal contractions in all patients ($P < 0.01$). The number of multiphasic, spontaneous and missed contractions also improved. Two of the eight patients had their chest pain resolved after taking the peppermint oil (Pimentel et al 2001).

Aid for endoscopic procedures

Results from double-blind RCTs suggest that the antispasmodic properties of peppermint oil can be utilised intraluminally during upper endoscopy with superior efficacy and fewer side-effects than hyoscine-N-butylbromide (Buscopan) administered by intramuscular injection (Hiki et al 2003a, 2003b). The use of peppermint oil solution was used to successfully extend an endoscope past an area of severe antral stenosis in a case that was unresponsive to Buscopan. In a study of 383 patients receiving double-contrast barium enemas, which compared peppermint oil in the barium, peppermint in the enema tube, Buscopan and no treatment, found that peppermint oil in the barium or the enema tube could be safely and effectively used instead of Buscopan and that the oil had a stronger antispasmodic effect in the caecum and the ascending colon than a Buscopan injection (Asao et al 2003). Similarly, orally-administered peppermint oil was an effective and safe antispasmodic agent for double-contrast barium meal examination in a controlled study with 420 participants (Mizuno et al 2006). In another study ($n = 40$) peppermint oil (20 mL, 1.6%) was effective and safe in inhibiting duodenal motility during endoscopic retrograde cholangiopancreatography, but additional administration was recommended for future procedures. The effect was identical to that of glucagon (Yamamoto et al 2006). A non-randomised prospective study compared the anti-spasmodic scores between non-elderly patients (younger than 70) and elderly patients (70 years old or older) treated with buscopan, peppermint oil or glucagon, while undergoing an oesophagogastroduodenoscopy procedure. A total of 8269 procedures were performed and analysis revealed peppermint oil in the elderly was as effective as Buscopan and more effective than glucagon in providing antispasmodic relief (Imagawa et al 2012).

Headache/migraine

Topical application of a solution of 10% peppermint oil in ethanol has been shown in a randomised, placebo-controlled, double-blind, crossover study to efficiently alleviate tension-type headache. The study analysed 164 headache attacks in 41 patients of both sexes ranging from 18 to 65 years of age, suffering from tension-type headache. The peppermint oil was spread largely across forehead and temples and repeated after 15 and 30 minutes. Using a headache diary, the headache parameters were assessed after 15, 30, 45 and 60 minutes. Compared with the application of a placebo, the peppermint oil significantly reduced the intensity of the headache after 15 minutes ($P < 0.01$). The analgesic effect of the peppermint oil was comparable to 1000 mg paracetamol (acetaminophen). Simultaneous ingestion of 1000 mg of paracetamol and application of 10% peppermint oil in ethanol solution led to a slight additive effect (Gobel et al 1996).

One of the main active constituents in peppermint is menthol, which has been investigated as a stand-alone, topical treatment in migraine headache. A randomised, triple-blind, placebo-controlled, crossover study found cutaneous application of menthol 10% as a treatment for migraine without aura produced an acute and significant effect on pain. Thirty-five patients were involved and a total of 118 migraine attacks were reported. The menthol solution was statistically superior to the placebo on 2-hour pain-free ($P = 0.001$), 2-hour pain relief ($P = 0.000$), sustained pain-free and sustained pain relief end-points ($P = 0.008$). The menthol solution was also more efficacious in alleviating nausea and/or vomiting and phonophobia and/or photophobia ($P = 0.02$). No significant difference was observed between the adverse effects of the drug and the placebo groups ($P = 0.13$). The authors report that menthol may inhibit the transmission of nociceptive impulses from the pain-producing cranial vessels, via branches of the trigeminal nerve, to higher brain centres (Borhani Haghighi et al 2010).

Nausea

A review of scientific evidence of essential oils for the alleviation of nausea and vomiting found that the inhaled vapour of peppermint or ginger essential oils not only reduced the incidence and severity of nausea and vomiting but also decreased antiemetic requirements. However, the authors did acknowledge methodological flaws in the existing research articles and determined the results were not yet fully substantiated (Lua & Zakaria 2012). Furthermore, a Cochrane review of aromatherapy for the treatment of postoperative nausea and vomiting found no reliable evidence for the use of peppermint oil (Hines et al 2012).

Postoperative nausea

Inhalation of peppermint oil vapours has been shown in a study to reduce postoperative nausea in gynaecological patients in a placebo-controlled trial in which patients were able to inhale peppermint oil as frequently as desired (Tate 1997). A more recent study examined peppermint spirits (ethyl alcohol 82%, peppermint oil, purified water, peppermint leaf extract) for the treatment of nausea following postoperative C-section. The women who inhaled peppermint had significantly lower nausea levels compared with controls after 2 and 5 minutes, indicating a quick-acting effect (Lane et al 2012).

In another placebo-controlled trial, a reduction in postoperative nausea was seen equally with inhalation of isopropyl alcohol, peppermint oil or saline, with the authors attributing the effect to the controlled breathing used during inhalation (Anderson & Gross 2004).

A hot peppermint oil compress is used in China to prevent abdominal distension in postoperative gynaecological patients (Feng 1997).

Nausea in cancer treatment

Inhalation of peppermint significantly reduced the intensity and number of emetic events in the first 24 hours following chemotherapy treatment in cancer patients when compared with a control group (Tayarani-Najaran et al 2013).

Nausea in pregnancy

In a double-blind RCT, peppermint essential oil was shown to have no significant effects on nausea and vomiting during pregnancy when compared to saline (Pasha et al 2012).

Respiratory tract infections

Peppermint and menthol have an established tradition in the treatment of respiratory infections. Chest rubs containing menthol are frequently used to treat coughs and bronchitis. Inhalation of various antiseptic and anti-inflammatory essential oils is often used in the treatment of respiratory infections, including bronchitis (Shubina et al 1990). In a recent study conducted with 18 healthy volunteers, it was shown that menthol inhalation did not affect nasal mucosal temperature and nasal airflow but supported the fact that menthol leads to direct stimulation of cold receptors modulating the cool sensation, thus inducing a feeling of clear and open nasal passages (Lindemann et al 2008).

Peppermint oil has been found to have a pronounced antimycobacterial effect in vitro, and long-term use of peppermint oil in a humidifier has been used in Ukraine as an adjunctive treatment to multidrug therapy for pulmonary tuberculosis (Shkurupii et al 2002). A more recent study shows that inhaling peppermint oil by patients with infiltrative pulmonary tuberculosis in the penitentiary system was most effective in the phase of resorption of infiltrates and/or closure of decay cavities (Shkurupii et al 2006).

Exercise performance

Peppermint oil was investigated for its ability to enhance sports performance in 12 healthy male students. The students consumed a 500-mL bottle of mineral water, containing 0.05 mL peppermint essential oil for 10 days, after which there were significant changes to forced vital capacity (FVC), peak expiratory flow rate (PEF) and peak inspiratory flow (PIF). Exercise performance evaluated by time to exhaustion, work and power also significantly increased. In addition, the results of respiratory gas analysis exhibited significant differences in VO_2 and VCO_2. Authors referred to a number of possible explanations for peppermint's action on exercise performance including: a stimulating effect on the CNS including cognitive performance, perceived physical workload and analgesic effects. They also suggested peppermint may improve muscular energy metabolism, lower heart rate and systolic BP and reduce arterial smooth muscle tonicity (Meamarbashi & Rajabi 2013). While these results are interesting, the absence of a placebo group make it difficult to interpret.

Enhance cognitive performance

Peppermint odour has also been shown to reduce daytime sleepiness (Norrish & Dwyer 2005) and fatigue and to improve mood (Goel & Lao 2006), as well as significantly improve performance in difficult tactile tasks (Ho & Spence 2005) and promote a general arousal of attention with improved typing speed and accuracy (Barker et al 2003). Similarly, in a recent study with healthy volunteers (n = 144), peppermint oil inhalation enhanced memory and alertness when measured by the Cognitive Drug Research computerised assessment battery (Moss et al 2008).

IN COMBINATION

A combination of peppermint oil, eucalyptus oil and ethanol was shown in a crossover double-blind study to increase cognitive performance and promote relaxation in 32 healthy subjects (Gobel et al 1994). A randomised, double-blind pilot trial determined the effectiveness of a combination of essential oils (peppermint, basil and helichrysum) on mental exhaustion, or moderate burnout (ME/MB) using a personal inhaler. While both groups had a reduction in perception of ME/MB, the aromatherapy group had a much greater reduction compared to placebo (Varney & Buckle 2013).

Traditional uses

Traditionally, peppermint was believed to increase libido and used to stop hiccups, relieve pain in childbirth, reduce bleeding and treat menorrhagia (Fisher & Painter 1996). It was also used externally to repress lactation, to treat dermatological conditions, as a mouthwash for painful gums and mouth and applied to the temples to relieve headaches.

OTHER USES

Peppermint or pure menthol is commonly used in heat rub ointments for arthritis, fibromyositis, tendonitis and other musculoskeletal conditions. Commission E approved peppermint oil externally for neuralgia and myalgia (Blumenthal et al 2000). A case report describes the treatment of postherpetic neuralgia with the direct application of undiluted peppermint oil containing 10% menthol to the affected area. The pain relief persisted for 4–6 hours after application of the oil. At a 2-month follow-up, the patient had only minor side effects and continued to use the medication (Davies et al 2002). An aromatherapy acupressure intervention using peppermint oil displayed positive effects on hemiplegic shoulder pain, compared to acupressure alone, in patients with stroke (Shin & Lee 2007).

An oral spray or gargle containing a range of essential oils including peppermint oil is reported to reduce snoring in one double-blind study (Prichard 2004). A mixture of tea tree, peppermint and lemon oil seemed effective in reducing malodour and volatile sulphur compounds in intensive care unit patients (Hur et al 2007).

Two studies conducted with breastfeeding women found that topical application of peppermint water and peppermint gel prevented nipple cracks and associated pain more effectively than lanolin and placebo (Melli et al 2007a, 2007b).

A small study (n = 44) conducted with patients undergoing breast cancer treatment showed that 18 of them (41%) chose peppermint and neroli hydrolat spray over plain water spray to manage their hot flushes (Dyer et al 2008).

Antimicrobial and antibiofilm properties of peppermint oil against *Streptococcus mutans* and *Streptococcus pyogenes* were evident, when an in vivo study with healthy volunteers showed that brushing teeth with peppermint oil-blended toothpastes was more effective than using a chlorhexidine mouthwash (Shayegh et al 2008).

DOSAGE RANGE

Leaf

- Infusion: 3–6 g three times daily (Blumenthal et al 2000).
- Liquid extract (1:2): 1.5–4.5 mL/day.

These dosages are for adults; adjust according to size for children.

Essential oil

- Digestive disorders: 0.2–0.4 mL three times daily in dilute preparations or in suspension (ESCOP 1997). Often used in combination with caraway and other herbs.
- IBS: Most studies report doses of approx. 0.2–0.5 mL two to four times daily in enteric-coated capsules or tablets (Ruepert et al 2011).
- Inhalation: 3–4 drops added to hot water.
- Lozenge: 2–10 mg.
- External use (for analgesic, anaesthetic or antipruritic activity): 0.1–1.0% m/m (ESCOP 1997).
- External use (counterirritant): 1.25–16% m/m (ESCOP 1997).

ADVERSE REACTIONS

A single dose of 4000 mg/kg of a spray-dried infusion did not produce any macroscopic signs of toxicity in mice (Della et al 1990). Peppermint oil taken orally has been shown to be well tolerated at the commonly recommended dosage but may cause significant adverse effects at higher doses (Kligler & Chaudhary 2007).

Short-term and subchronic oral studies reported brain lesions in rats that were given very large doses of peppermint oil containing pulegone, pulegone alone or large amounts (>200 mg/kg/day) of menthone. Pulegone is also a recognised hepatotoxin, and large doses of peppermint oil have been shown to be hepatotoxic in cultured human hepatoma cells (Vo et al 2003). Peppermint oil was negative in an Ames test and a mouse lymphoma mutagenesis assay, but gave equivocal results in a Chinese hamster fibroblast cell chromosome aberration assay. There is a case report of acute lung injury following intravenous injection of peppermint oil (Behrends et al 2005).

Although sensitisation to peppermint oil and/or its constituents has been reported, a solution containing 8% peppermint oil was shown not to be a sensitiser (Nair 2001). Cases of allergic contact dermatitis to peppermint and menthol have been reported following intraoral application (Morton et al 1995, Tamir et al 2005), with one case reporting vulval allergic contact dermatitis following long-term (6 years) high oral consumption of peppermint tea (Vermaat et al 2008). Moreover, the application of a transcutaneous patch (Foti et al 2003) or foot spray (Kalavala et al 2007) caused allergic contact dermatitis. However, the incidence of allergic contact dermatitis due to peppermint and its components is low considering its widespread use and seems to be more common in patients with a history of allergic reactions (Kalavala et al 2007, Vermaat et al 2008). As long as the pulegone content is kept to a minimum, peppermint oil and peppermint extract are considered to have a very good safety profile.

SIGNIFICANT INTERACTIONS

Controlled studies are not available; therefore, interactions are based on evidence of activity and are largely theoretical and speculative.

Felodipine

Peppermint oil has been shown to increase the oral bioavailability of felodipine in animal studies (Dresser et al 2002b) — use this combination with caution.

Simvastatin

Peppermint oil has been shown to increase the oral bioavailability of simvastatin in animal studies (Dresser et al 2002b). Observe the patient and monitor drug requirements — possible beneficial interaction.

Cyclosporin

Peppermint oil has been shown to increase the oral bioavailability of cyclosporin in animal studies (Dresser et al 2002b) — avoid concurrent use, unless under medical supervision.

Drugs metabolised by CYP3A4 liver enzyme

Peppermint may increase the oral bioavailability of certain drugs by inhibition of CYP3A4-mediated drug metabolism, which has been demonstrated in vitro but not in test animals (Dresser et al 2002a, Maliakal & Wanwimolruk 2001). Although these studies seem to suggest that peppermint may modulate drug-metabolising enzymes, the clinical significance of this is unknown and requires further investigation. Observe.

Practice points/Patient counselling

- Peppermint oil and/or peppermint leaf extracts can be used for IBS, dyspepsia, flatulence, intestinal colic and biliary disorders as it exerts an antispasmodic and carminative effect.
- Although enteric-coated peppermint oil capsules may prevent side effects such as reflux and allow higher doses to be used, traditional extracts of peppermint, including hydroethanolic extracts and infusions, may also be effective.
- Peppermint leaf extract combines well with chamomile, caraway, licorice, lemon balm, angelica, St Mary's thistle and the bitter candytuft (*Iberis amara*) in the treatment of functional dyspepsia (Madisch et al 2001).
- Peppermint oil can be used as an inhalation or chest rub for coughs, sinusitis and bronchitis. Commission E approved peppermint oil for internal use in the treatment of respiratory tract inflammation (Blumenthal et al 2000), and hot peppermint leaf infusion is used as a diaphoretic tea in the treatment of colds and influenza.
- Peppermint oil can be inhaled to reduce nausea and may enhance cognitive performance and tactile tasks.
- Ten per cent peppermint oil in ethanol solution can be applied externally for tension headaches and over affected areas for postherpetic neuralgia.

CONTRAINDICATIONS AND PRECAUTIONS

Hypersensitivity to peppermint oil (Morton et al 1995).

Non-enteric-coated peppermint may be best avoided in patients with gastro-oesophageal reflux symptoms (McKay & Blumberg 2006). Avoid chewing enteric-coated capsules as it may cause heartburn (Liu et al 1997). Avoid the use of peppermint oil on the face of infants and small children. Capsules containing peppermint oil are contraindicated in biliary duct occlusion, gall bladder inflammation and severe liver damage (Blumenthal et al 2000). Similarly, caution has been urged in patients with hiatal hernia and kidney stones (McKay & Blumberg 2006).

PREGNANCY USE

Safe dosages in pregnant women have not been determined; however, external use and inhalation is likely to be safe.

PATIENTS' FAQs

What will this herb do for me?

Peppermint is a safe herb for gastrointestinal disorders, including dyspepsia and IBS. It is also safe for children, particularly as a herbal tea.

When will it start to work?

Peppermint will generally have an immediate effect, with the condition continuing to improve with long-term use.

Are there any safety issues?

Concentrated peppermint oil preparations may theoretically interact with a number of different medications. It is unlikely that any interaction will occur with peppermint tea or simple liquid extracts. Avoid the use of peppermint oil on the face of infants and small children. Allergic reactions may occur in hypersensitive individuals.

REFERENCES

Adam B et al. A combination of peppermint oil and caraway oil attenuates the post-inflammatory visceral hyperalgesia in a rat model. Scand J Gastroenterol 41.2 (2006): 155–160.

Agarwal V et al. Prevention of Candida albicans biofilm by plant oils. Mycopathologia 165.1 (2008): 13–19.

Akdogan M et al. Effects of peppermint teas on plasma testosterone, follicle-stimulating hormone, and luteinizing hormone levels and testicular tissue in rats. Urology 64.2 (2004): 394–398.

Alves JG et al. Effectiveness of Mentha piperita in the Treatment of Infantile Colic: A Crossover Study. Evid Based Complement Alternat Med (2012): 981352.

Anderson LA, Gross JB. Aromatherapy with peppermint, isopropyl alcohol, or placebo is equally effective in relieving postoperative nausea. J Perianesth Nurs 19.1 (2004): 29–35.

Asao T et al. Spasmolytic effect of peppermint oil in barium during double-contrast barium enema compared with Buscopan. Clin Radiol 58.4 (2003): 301–305.

Barker S et al. Improved performance on clerical tasks associated with administration of peppermint odor. Percept Mot Skills 97.3 (2003): 1007–1010.

Behnam S et al. Composition and antifungal activity of essential oils of Mentha piperita and Lavendula angustifolia on post-harvest phytopathogens. Commun Agric Appl Biol Sci 71.3 Pt B (2006): 1321–1326.

Behrends M et al. Acute lung injury after peppermint oil injection. Anesth Analg 101.4 (2005): 1160–1162.

Ben-Arye E et al. Treatment of upper respiratory tract infections in primary care: a randomized study using aromatic herbs. Evid Based Complement Alternat Med (2011): 690346.

Betoni JE et al. Synergism between plant extract and antimicrobial drugs used on Staphylococcus aureus diseases. Mem Inst Oswaldo Cruz 101.4 (2006): 387–390.

Bluma R et al. Control of Aspergillus section Flavi growth and aflatoxin accumulation by plant essential oils. J Appl Microbiol 105.1 (2008): 203–214.

Blumenthal M et al. (eds). Herbal medicine: expanded Commission E monographs. Austin, TX: Integrative Medicine Communications, 2000.

Borhani Haghighi A et al. Cutaneous application of menthol 10% solution as an abortive treatment of migraine without aura: a randomised, double-blind, placebo-controlled, crossed-over study. Int J Clin Pract, 64 (2010): 451–456.

Canyon DV, Speare R. A comparison of botanical and synthetic substances commonly used to prevent head lice (Pediculus humanus var. capitis) infestation. Int J Dermatol 46.4 (2007): 422–426.

Carvalho CO et al. The anthelmintic effect of plant extracts on Haemonchus contortus and Strongyloides venezuelensis. Vet Parasitol, 183 (2012): 260–268.

Coon JT, Ernst E. Systematic review: herbal medicinal products for non-ulcer dyspepsia. Aliment Pharmacol Ther 16.10 (2002): 1689–1699.

Davies SJ et al. A novel treatment of postherpetic neuralgia using peppermint oil. Clin J Pain 18.3 (2002): 200–202.

De Almeida MA et al. [Effects of aqueous extracts of Mentha piperita L. and Chenopodium ambrosioides L. leaves in infective larvae cultures of gastrointestinal nematodes of goats]. Rev Bras Parasitol Vet 16.1 (2007): 57–59.

Della LR et al. Evaluation of some pharmacologica activities of a peppermint extract. Fitoterapia 61.3 (1990): 215–221.

Dew MJ et al. Peppermint oil for the irritable bowel syndrome: a multicentre trial. Br J Clin Pract 38.11–12 (1984): 394, 398.

Dresser GK et al. Evaluation of peppermint oil and ascorbyl palmitate as inhibitors of cytochrome P4503A4 activity in vitro and in vivo. Clin Pharmacol Ther 72.3 (2002a): 247–255.

Dresser GK et al. Peppermint oil increases the oral bioavailability of felodipine and simvastatin. Clin Pharmacol Ther 71.2 (2002b): P67.

Duband F et al. Aromatic and polyphenolic composition of infused peppermint. Mentha × piperita L. Ann Pharm Fr 50.3 (1992): 146–155.

Dyer J et al. A study to look at the effects of a hydrolat spray on hot flushes in women being treated for breast cancer. Complement Ther Clin Pract 14.4 (2008): 273–279.

Erler F et al. Repellent activity of five essential oils against Culex pipiens. Fitoterapia 77.7–8 (2006): 491–494.

ESCOP. Menthae Piperitae folium: peppermint leaf. European Scientific Co-operative On Phytomedicine (ESCOP), 2nd edn. Stuttgart: Thieme, 1997.

Farco JA, Grunmann, O. 2013. Menthol–pharmacology of an important naturally medicinal 'cool'. Mini Rev Med Chem, 13, 124–131.

Feng XZ. Effect of peppermint oil hot compresses in preventing abdominal distension in postoperative gynecological patients. Zhonghua Hu Li Za Zhi 32.10 (1997): 577–578.

Fisher C, Painter G. Materia Medica for the Southern Hemisphere. Auckland: Fisher-Painter Publishers, 1996.

Foti C et al. Contact dermatitis from peppermint and menthol in a local action transcutaneous patch. Contact Dermatitis 49.6 (2003): 312–313.

Freise J, Kohler S. Peppermint oil-caraway oil fixed combination in non-ulcer dyspepsia: comparison of the effects of enteric preparations. Pharmazie 54.3 (1999): 210–215.

Gao M et al. Antioxidant components of naturally-occurring oils exhibit marked anti-inflammatory activity in epithelial cells of the human upper respiratory system. Respir Res, 12 (2011): 92.

Germann I et al. Antioxidative properties of the gastrointestinal phytopharmaceutical remedy STW 5 (Iberogast). Phytomedicine 13 Suppl 5 (2006): 45–50.

Geuenich S et al. Aqueous extracts from peppermint, sage and lemon balm leaves display potent anti-HIV-1 activity by increasing the virion density. Retrovirology 5 (2008): 27.

Giachetti D et al. Pharmacological activity of essential oils on Oddi's sphincter. Planta Med 54.5 (1988): 389–392.

Gobel H et al. Effect of peppermint and eucalyptus oil preparations on neurophysiological and experimental algesimetric headache parameters. Cephalalgia 14.3 (1994): 228–234.

Gobel H et al. Effectiveness of Oleum menthae piperitae and paracetamol in therapy of headache of the tension type. Nervenarzt 67.8 (1996): 672–681.

Goel N, Lao RP. Sleep changes vary by odor perception in young adults. Biol Psychol 71.3 (2006): 341–349.

Goerg KJ, Spilker T. Effect of peppermint oil and caraway oil on gastrointestinal motility in healthy volunteers: a pharmacodynamic study using simultaneous determination of gastric and gall-bladder emptying and orocaecal transit time. Aliment Pharmacol Ther 17.3 (2003): 445–451.

Gonzalez Audino P et al. Effectiveness of lotions based on essential oils from aromatic plants against permethrin resistant Pediculus humanus capitis. Arch Dermatol Res 299.8 (2007): 389–392.

Greenberg MM et al. A contemporary review of irritable bowel syndrome. Physician Assist 26.8 (2002): 26–33.

Grigoleit HG, Grigoleit P. Gastrointestinal clinical pharmacology of peppermint oil. Phytomedicine 12.8 (2005a): 607–611.

Grigoleit HG, Grigoleit P. Peppermint oil in irritable bowel syndrome. Phytomedicine 12.8 (2005b): 601–606.

Grigoleit HG, Grigoleit P. Pharmacology and preclinical pharmacokinetics of peppermint oil. Phytomedicine 12.8 (2005c): 612–616.

Hiki N et al. Peppermint oil reduces gastric spasm during upper endoscopy: a randomized, double-blind, double-dummy controlled trial. Gastrointest Endosc 57.4 (2003a): 475–482.

Hiki N et al. Case of gastric outlet stenosis with features of pyloric stenosis diagnosed by using peppermint oil solution as a new antispasmodic. Dig Endosc 15.3 (2003b): 224–227.

Hines S et al. Aromatherapy for treatment of postoperative nausea and vomiting. Cochrane Database Syst Rev, 4 (2012): CD007598.

Ho C, Spence C. Olfactory facilitation of dual-task performance. Neurosci Lett 389.1 (2005): 35–40.

Holtmann G et al. Effects of a fixed combination of peppermint oil and caraway oil on symptoms and quality of life in patients suffering from functional dyspepsia. Phytomedicine 10 (Suppl 4) (2003): 56–57.

Hur MH et al. Reduction of mouth malodour and volatile sulphur compounds in intensive care patients using an essential oil mouthwash. Phytother Res 21.7 (2007): 641–643.

Imagawa, A et al. Peppermint oil solution is useful as an antispasmodic drug for esophagogastroduodenoscopy, especially for elderly patients. Dig Dis Sci, 57 (2012): 2379–2384.

Imai H et al. Inhibition by the essential oils of peppermint and spearmint of the growth of pathogenic bacteria. Microbios 106 (Suppl 1) (2001): 31–39.

Inamori M et al. Early effects of peppermint oil on gastric emptying: a crossover study using a continuous real-time 13C breath test (BreathID system). J Gastroenterol 42.7 (2007): 539–542.

Inouye S et al. Combined effect of heat, essential oils and salt on fungicidal activity against Trichophyton mentagrophytes in a foot bath. Nippon Ishinkin Gakkai Zasshi 48.1 (2007): 27–36.

Jagetia C. Radioprotective potential of plants and herbs against the effects of ionizing radiation. J Clin Biochem Nutr 40.2 (2007): 74–81.

Kalavala M et al. Allergic contact dermatitis to peppermint foot spray. Contact Dermatitis 57.1 (2007): 57–58.

Khanna, R et al. Peppermint Oil for the Treatment of Irritable Bowel Syndrome: A Systematic Review and Meta-analysis. J Clin. Gastroenterol. 48.6 (2014): 505–512.

Khayyal MT et al. Mechanisms involved in the gastro-protective effect of STW 5 (Iberogast) and its components against ulcers and rebound acidity. Phytomedicine 13 Suppl 5 (2006): 56–66.

Kim SH et al. Menthol regulates TRPM8-independent processes in PC-3 prostate cancer cells. Biochim Biophys Acta 1792.1 (2009): 33–38.

Kingham JG. Peppermint oil and colon spasm. Lancet 346.8981 (1995): 986.

Kligler B, Chaudhary S. Peppermint oil. Am Fam Physician 75.7 (2007): 1027–1030.

Lane B et al. Examination of the effectiveness of peppermint aromatherapy on nausea in women post C-section. J Holist Nurs, 30 (2012): 90–104.

Lans C et al. Ethnoveterinary medicines used to treat endoparasites and stomach problems in pigs and pets in British Columbia. Canada. Vet Parasitol 148.3–4 (2007): 325–340.

Lim WC et al. Stimulative and sedative effects of essential oils upon inhalation in mice. Arch Pharmacol Res 28.7 (2005): 770–774.

Lindemann J et al. Impact of menthol inhalation on nasal mucosal temperature and nasal patency. Am J Rhinol 22.4 (2008): 402–405.

Liu JH et al. Enteric-coated peppermint-oil capsules in the treatment of irritable bowel syndrome: a prospective, randomized trial. J Gastroenterol 32.6 (1997): 765–768.

Lua PL, Zakaria NS. A brief review of current scientific evidence involving aromatherapy use for nausea and vomiting. J Altern Complement Med, 18 (2012): 534–540.

Machado, M et al. C. Effects of essential oils on the growth of Giardia lamblia trophozoites. Nat Prod Commun, 5 (2010): 137–141.

Madisch A et al. Treatment of functional dyspepsia with a fixed peppermint oil and caraway oil combination preparation as compared to cisapride: a multicenter, reference-controlled double-blind equivalence study. Arzneimittelforschung 49.11 (1999): 925–932.

Madisch A et al. A plant extract and its modified preparation in functional dyspepsia. Results of a double-blind placebo controlled comparative study. Z Gastroenterol 39.7 (2001): 511–517.

Magro A et al. Efficacy of plant extracts against stored-products fungi. Rev Iberoam Micol 23.3 (2006): 176–178.

Mahieu F et al. TRPM8-independent menthol-induced Ca2+ release from endoplasmic reticulum and Golgi. J Biol Chem 282.5 (2007): 3325–3336.

Maliakal PP, Wanwimolruk S. Effect of herbal teas on hepatic drug metabolizing enzymes in rats. J Pharm Pharmacol 53.10 (2001): 1323–1329.

Massey BT. Diffuse esophageal spasm: a case for carminatives? J Clin Gastroenterol 33.1 (2001): 8–10.

May BL et al. Efficacy and tolerability of a fixed combination of peppermint oil and caraway oil in patients suffering from functional dyspepsia. Aliment Pharmacol Ther 14.12 (2000): 1671–1677.

May B et al. Peppermint oil and caraway oil in functional dyspepsia: efficacy unaffected by H. pylori. Aliment Pharmacol Ther 17.7 (2003): 975–976.

McKay DL, Blumberg JB. A review of the bioactivity and potential health benefits of peppermint tea (Mentha piperita L.). Phytother Res 20.8 (2006): 619–633.

Meamarbashi A, Rajabi A. The effects of peppermint on exercise performance. J Int Soc Sports Nutr 10 (2013): 15.

Melli MS et al. A randomized trial of peppermint gel, lanolin ointment, and placebo gel to prevent nipple crack in primiparous breastfeeding women. Med Sci Monit 13.9 (2007a): CR406–11.

Melli MS et al. Effect of peppermint water on prevention of nipple cracks in lactating primiparous women: a randomized controlled trial. Int Breastfeed J 2 (2007b): 7.

Melzer J et al. Meta-analysis: phytotherapy of functional dyspepsia with the herbal drug preparation STW 5 Iberogast. Aliment Pharmacol Ther 20.11–12 (2004): 1279–1287.

Micklefield G et al. Effects of intraduodenal application of peppermint oil (WS® 1340) and caraway oil (WS® 1520) on gastroduodenal motility in healthy volunteers. Phytother Res 17.2 (2003): 135–140.

Mimica-Dukic N et al. Antimicrobial and antioxidant activities of three Mentha species essential oils. Planta Med 69.5 (2003): 413–419.

Mizuno S et al. Oral peppermint oil is a useful antispasmodic for double-contrast barium meal examination. J Gastroenterol Hepatol 21.8 (2006): 1297–1301.

Mohsenzadeh M. Evaluation of antibacterial activity of selected Iranian essential oils against Staphylococcus aureus and Escherichia coli in nutrient broth medium. Pak J Biol Sci 10.20 (2007): 3693–3697.

Morise, M et al. Heterologous regulation of anion transporters by menthol in human airway epithelial cells. Eur J Pharmacol, 635 (2010): 204–211.

Morton CA et al. Contact sensitivity to menthol and peppermint in patients with intra-oral symptoms. Contact Dermatitis 32.5 (1995): 281–284.

Moss M et al. Modulation of cognitive performance and mood by aromas of peppermint and ylang-ylang. Int J Neurosci 118.1 (2008): 59–77.

Murray MT, Pizzorno JE. Mentha piperita peppermint. In: Textbook of natural medicine. Philadelphia: Churchill Livingstone, 1999, pp 827–829.

Nair B. Final report on the safety assessment of Mentha piperita (peppermint) oil, Mentha piperita (Peppermint) leaf extract, Mentha piperita (peppermint) leaf, and Mentha piperita (peppermint) leaf water. Int J Toxicol 20 (Suppl 3) (2001): 61–73.

Nielsen JB. Natural oils affect the human skin integrity and the percutaneous penetration of benzoic acid dose-dependently. Basic Clin Pharmacol Toxicol 98.6 (2006): 575–581.

Nolkemper S et al. Antiviral effect of aqueous extracts from species of the Lamiaceae family against Herpes simplex virus type 1 and type 2 in vitro. Planta Med 72.15 (2006): 1378–1382.

Norrish MIK, Dwyer KL. Preliminary investigation of the effect of peppermint oil on an objective measure of daytime sleepiness. Int J Psychophysiol 55.3 (2005): 291–298.

Orhan I et al. Activity of essential oils and individual components against acetyl- and butyrylcholinesterase. Z Naturforsch C 63.7–8 (2008): 547–553.

Ottillinger B et al. STW 5 (Iberogast(R)) — a safe and effective standard in the treatment of functional gastrointestinal disorders. Wien.Med Wochenschr 163 (3–4) (2013): 65–72.

Papathanasopoulos A. et al. Effect of acute peppermint oil administration on gastric sensorimotor function and nutrient tolerance in health. Neurogastroenterol Motil, 25 (2013): e263–271.

Pasha H et al. Study of the effect of mint oil on nausea and vomiting during pregnancy. Iran Red Crescent Med J, 14 (2012): 727–730.

Pattnaik S et al. Effect of essential oils on the viability and morphology of Escherichia coli (SP-11). Microbios 84.340 (1995): 195–199.

Pattnaik S et al. Antibacterial and antifungal activity of ten essential oils in vitro. Microbios 86.349 (1996): 237–246.

Pimentel M et al. Peppermint oil improves the manometric findings in diffuse esophageal spasm. J Clin Gastroenterol 33.1 (2001): 27–31.

Pittler MH, Ernst E. Peppermint oil for irritable bowel syndrome: a critical review and metaanalysis. Am J Gastroenterol 93.7 (1998): 1131–1135.

Positive Health News. Essential oils of peppermint, orange or lemongrass kill most strains of fungal and bacterial infections. Posit Health News 17 (1998): 26–27.

Prichard AJN. The use of essential oils to treat snoring. Phytother Res 18.9 (2004): 696–699.

Rakover Y et al. [The treatment of respiratory ailments with essential oils of some aromatic medicinal plants]. Harefuah 147.10 (2008): 783–788, 838.

Rasooli I et al. Phytotherapeutic prevention of dental biofilm formation. Phytother Res 22.9 (2008): 1162–1167.

Rees WD et al. Treating irritable bowel syndrome with peppermint oil. Br Med J 2.6194 (1979): 835–836.

Reichling J et al. Impact of ethanolic lamiaceae extracts on herpesvirus infectivity in cell culture. Forsch Komplementmed 15.6 (2008): 313–320.

Rosch W et al. A randomised clinical trial comparing the efficacy of a herbal preparation STW 5 with the prokinetic drug cisapride in patients with dysmotility type of functional dyspepsia. Z Gastroenterol 40 (2002): 401–408.

Ruepert, L et al. Bulking agents, antispasmodics and antidepressants for the treatment of irritable bowel syndrome. Cochrane Database Syst Rev (2011): CD003460.

Saeed S, Tariq P. Antibacterial activities of Mentha piperita, Pisum sativum and Momordica charantia. Pakistan J Botany 37.4 (2005): 997–1001.
Samarasekera R et al. Insecticidal activity of menthol derivatives against mosquitoes. Pest Manag Sci 64.3 (2008): 290–295.
Samarth RM et al. Modulatory effects of Mentha piperita on lung tumor incidence, genotoxicity, and oxidative stress in benzo[a]pyrene-treated Swiss albino mice. Environ Mol Mutagen 47.3 (2006a): 192–198.
Samarth RM et al. Radioprotective influence of Mentha piperita (Linn) against gamma irradiation in mice: antioxidant and radical scavenging activity. Int J Radiat Biol 82.5 (2006b): 331–337.
Schelz Z, Molnar J, Hohmann J. Antimicrobial and antiplasmid activities of essential oils. Fitoterapia 77.4 (2006): 279–285.
Schempp H et al. Radical scavenging and anti-inflammatory properties of STW 5 (Iberogast) and its components. Phytomedicine 13 Suppl 5 (2006): 36–44.
Schuhmacher A et al. Virucidal effect of peppermint oil on the enveloped viruses herpes simplex virus type 1 and type 2 in vitro. Phytomedicine 10.6–7 (2003): 504–510.
Sharma A et al. Protective effect of Mentha piperita against arsenic-induced toxicity in liver of Swiss albino mice. Basic Clin Pharmacol Toxicol 100.4 (2007): 249–257.
Shayegh S et al. Phytotherapeutic inhibition of supragingival dental plaque. Nat Prod Res 22.5 (2008): 428–439.
Shin BC, Lee MS. Effects of aromatherapy acupressure on hemiplegic shoulder pain and motor power in stroke patients: a pilot study. J Altern Complement Med 13.2 (2007): 247–251.
Shkurupii VA et al. [Efficiency of the use of peppermint (Mentha piperita L.) essential oil inhalations in the combined multi-drug therapy for pulmonary tuberculosis]. Probl Tuberk 4 (2002): 36–39.
Shkurupii VA et al. [Use of essential oil of peppermint (Mentha piperita) in the complex treatment of patients with infiltrative pulmonary tuberculosis]. Probl Tuberk Bolezn Legk 9 (2006): 43–45.
Shubina LP et al. [Inhalations of essential oils in the combined treatment of patients with chronic bronchitis] Vrach Delo 5 (1990): 66–67.
Sibaev A et al. STW 5 (Iberogast) and its individual herbal components modulate intestinal electrophysiology of mice. Phytomedicine 13 Suppl 5 (2006): 80–89.
Sokovic MD et al. Chemical composition of essential oils of Thymus and Mentha species and their antifungal activities. Molecules 14.1 (2009): 238–249.
Sroka Z et al. Antiradical and anti-H_2O_2 properties of polyphenolic compounds from an aqueous peppermint extract. Z Naturforsch C 60.11–12 (2005): 826–832.
Tamir S et al. Peppermint oil chemical burn. Otolaryngol Head Neck Surg 133.5 (2005): 801–802.
Tate S. Peppermint oil: a treatment for postoperative nausea. J Adv Nurs 26.3 (1997): 543–549.
Tayarani-Najaran, Z et al. Antiemetic activity of volatile oil from Mentha spicata and Mentha x piperita in chemotherapy-induced nausea and vomiting. Ecancermedicalscience, 7 (2013): 290.
Umezu T et al. Ambulation-promoting effect of peppermint oil and identification of its active constituents. Pharmacol Biochem Behav 69.3–4 (2001): 383–390.
Umezu T, Morita M. Evidence for the involvement of dopamine in ambulation promoted by menthol in mice. J Pharmacol Sci 91.2 (2003): 125–135.
Umezu T. Evidence for dopamine involvement in ambulation promoted by menthone in mice. Pharmacol Biochem Behav 91.3 (2009): 315–320.
Van Rensen I. Mentha × piperita: peppermint in indigestion. Z Phytother 25.3 (2004): 118–127.
Varney E, Buckle J. Effect of inhaled essential oils on mental exhaustion and moderate burnout: a small pilot study. J Altern Complement Med, 19 (2013): 69–71.
Vermaat H et al. Vulval allergic contact dermatitis due to peppermint oil in herbal tea. Contact Dermatitis 58.6 (2008): 364–365.
Vidal F et al. Giardia lamblia: the effects of extracts and fractions from Mentha x piperita Lin. (Lamiaceae) on trophozoites. Exp Parasitol 115.1 (2007): 25–31.
Vo LT et al. Investigation of the effects of peppermint oil and valerian on rat liver and cultured human liver cells. Clin Exp Pharmacol Physiol 30.10 (2003): 799–804.
Wildung MR, Croteau RB. Genetic engineering of peppermint for improved essential oil composition and yield. Transgenic Res 14.4 (2005): 365–372.
Yadegarinia D et al. Biochemical activities of Iranian Mentha piperita L. and Myrtus communis L. essential oils. Phytochemistry 67.12 (2006): 1249–1255.
Yamamoto N et al. Efficacy of peppermint oil as an antispasmodic during endoscopic retrograde cholangiopancreatography. J Gastroenterol Hepatol 21.9 (2006): 1394–1398.
Yap PS et al. 2013. Combination of essential oils and antibiotics reduce antibiotic resistance in plasmid-conferred multidrug resistant bacteria. Phytomedicine, 20, 710–713.
Yigit D et al. An investigation on the anticandidal activity of some traditional medicinal plants in Turkey. Mycoses 522 (2008): 135–140.
Zong, L et al. Preliminary experimental research on the mechanism of liver bile secretion stimulated by peppermint oil. J Dig Dis, 12 (2011): 295–301.

Perilla

HISTORICAL NOTE Perilla is an annual plant native to Eastern Asia. It was introduced to Japan from China and is now cultivated extensively in Japan, India and Korea. The seed is mainly used for its high oil content (*Perilla frutescens* var. *frutescens*), and the leaves of *Perilla frutescens* var. *crispa* are used as a vegetable and food colouring in gourmet cooking. The salty umeboshi plum is coloured by the addition of special red perilla leaves. The leaves of var. *crispa* are also used medicinally. In China, perilla has been used to reduce the risk of food poisoning by cooking seafood with the leaf (Bensky & Gamble 1986). In recent times, certain compounds (monoterpenes) isolated from the oil are being investigated as an anticancer treatment, and the defatted seed extract is used in the treatment of allergies.

COMMON NAME

Perilla

OTHER NAMES

Different names are used for the different varieties of perilla. *Perilla frutescens* var *frutescens*: Chinese: Ren; Korean: Deulggae; Japanese: Egoma. *P. frutescens* var. *crispa* — Chinese: Zisu; Korean: Cha-Jo-Ki; Japanese: Shiso. In English, wild sesame refers to var. *frutescens*, while beefsteak plant refers to var. *crispa*.

BOTANICAL NAME/FAMILY

Perilla frutescens (L.) Britt.

There are several botanical variants: *P. frutescens* var. *frutescens and P. frutescens* var. *japonica* are used interchangeably; the use is for the seed and oil crop, as well as a traditional vegetable and is the most important crop in Korea; *P. crispa* represents another variety, and the leaf is used for nutritional and medicinal purposes. (family Lamiaceae [mint family]).

PLANT PARTS USED

Leaf, stem and the fruit (seed) are used.

Some genotypes of perilla are not suitable for consumption as they contain a toxic perilla ketone.

CHEMICAL COMPONENTS

A study of the five most common genotypes of var. *frutescens* and var. *crispa* found that the phenolic content and corresponding antioxidant capacity of perilla is relatively high compared to other vegetables. In particular, they contain high concentrations of carotenoids, especially lutein and β-carotene, with concentrations up to five-fold higher than in other carotenoid rich vegetables.

A study of eight cultivars of the two *Perilla frutescens* varieties showed variations in major phenolic acids and flavones were quite marked between green and red cultivars (Meng et al 2009). No obvious relationships between genotypes and geographical origin of *P. frutescens* were noted by the authors.

As different parts of the plant are used, the rest of this section will deal with each part individually.

Raw oil

Perilla seed contains 25–51% lipids. The raw perilla oil has been used as a drying oil in paints, varnishes, linoleum, printing ink and lacquers and for protective waterproof coatings on cloth. It has also been used for cooking and as a fuel.

Refined oil

The purified oil is rich in fatty acids including palmitic acid, linoleic acid, alpha-linolenic acid, stearic acid, eicosanoic acid and arachidic acid. The omega-3 essential fatty acid, alpha-linolenic acid, comprises over 60% of the oil (Tan et al 1998).

Defatted perilla seed extract

Defatted perilla seed extract is a concentrated ethanolic extract rich in polyphenolic compounds including rosmarinic acid and rosmarinic acid methyl ester and the flavones apigenin, luteolin and chrysoeriol. Normally, flavonoids exist as glycosides in plants; however, in perilla seed extract, they occur as aglycones (free flavonoids), which have more potent activity. The defatted extract is free of perillyl ketone, perillyl aldehyde and perillyl alcohol (Oryza Co 2003). Individual and total phenolic content in the seed varies significantly between *Perilla frutescens* cultivars and therefore affects antioxidant activity (Lee et al 2013).

Leaf

The leaf contains flavones, including apigenin and luteolin; flavone glycosides, anthocyanins, phenolic compounds, including rosmarinic acid, and aldehydes including perillyl aldehyde (Makino et al 2003a).

Essential oil

The volatile oil is distilled from the dried foliage of perilla. It contains perillyl aldehyde, elsholtzia ketone, perillyl ketone, citral and perillene, in addition to more than 70 other compounds (Ito et al 1999). Notably, rosmarinic acid is one of the major polyphenolic ingredients of perilla leaf. Perillyl aldehyde is used as a sweetener and flavouring agent. One of the aldehyde isomers is 2000-fold sweeter than sugar and four–eight-fold sweeter than saccharin. Perillyl alcohol, prepared from perillyl aldehyde, is used in fragrances (Misra & Husain 1987). There are different chemotypes of perilla; one genotype lacks perillyl aldehyde but has perillyl ketone (Brenner 1993).

MAIN ACTIONS

The herb has several different actions demonstrated in vitro and in vivo, and the part of the plant used will determine which is exhibited. As such, this review specifies which part of the herb is responsible for the activity listed. Additionally, much research has been conducted with the rosmarinic acid and luteolin components isolated from perilla.

Anti-inflammatory action

Both the refined oil and seed extract demonstrate anti-inflammatory activity in vitro and in vivo.

Refined oil

The pharmacological effects of the refined oil are associated with its high level of alpha-linolenic acid, which is metabolised in the body to eicosapentaenoic acid (EPA) and docosahexaenoic acid. EPA is a precursor of the series 3 prostaglandins, the series 5 leukotrienes and the series 3 thromboxanes, which have anti-inflammatory and anti-atherogenic properties. The effects have been shown clinically, as perilla seed oil significantly suppressed the generation of leukotrienes in patients with asthma in an observational study comparing two groups of patients with asthma, one of whom received perilla oil for 4 weeks. Ventilatory parameters, such as peak expiratory flow (PEF), forced vital capacity (FVC) and forced expiratory volume (FEV_1), increased significantly after 4 weeks' dietary supplementation in the treated group (Okamoto et al 2000). In vivo dietary perilla oil has been shown to alleviate inflammation in mice by decreasing the secretion of pro-inflammatory cytokines (Chang et al 2008).

Seed extract

Perilla seed extract, as well as its constituents luteolin, rosmarinic acid and chrysoeriol, has been shown to inhibit 5-lipoxygenase in vitro and therefore leukotriene synthesis. Leukotrienes are associated with both allergic and inflammatory disorders, including hay fever, asthma and inflammatory bowel disorders.

Anti-allergic activity

In both in vitro and animal models of allergy, perilla preparations have demonstrated anti-allergic effects. Luteolin and rosmarinic and caffeic acids are chiefly responsible for this activity.

Seed extract

The defatted seed extract has been shown to inhibit chemically induced type IV allergy and inflammation in vivo, with the luteolin constituent exhibiting the most potent activity.

Perilla seed extract has also been shown to inhibit histamine release from mast cells in a dose-dependent manner. The effect is more potent than for isolated flavonoids including catechin, quercetin and caffeic acid. Additionally, in a case report of perilla seed extract, 150 mg/day for 2 weeks selectively inhibited the production of serum IgE in two human subjects suffering allergic symptoms including sneezing, nasal obstruction and itchy eyes (Oryza Co 2003).

Leaf

Perilla leaf extract is thought to down-regulate Th2-type cytokine production and prevent the Th1/Th2 balance from shifting towards Th2-type immune responses. A study on the effects of perilla leaf extract on cytokine production in allergic reaction in mice found that it suppressed IgE and IgG antibodies as well as IL-4, IL-5 and IL-10 (Ishihara et al 1999).

An aqueous extract of perilla leaf was shown in vitro and in vivo to inhibit local and systemic reactions in a mast cell-mediated immediate-type allergic reaction. Plasma histamine levels and cyclic adenosine monophosphate (AMP) were reduced in a dose-dependent manner. Perilla also inhibited IgE-induced tumour necrosis factor (TNF)-alpha production (Shin et al 2000). Oral administration of a hot water extract of perilla leaf was also shown to inhibit histamine release from mast cells and reduce scratching in an animal model of dermatitis (Wakame et al 2000).

Oral administration of a perilla leaf extract inhibited the inflammatory response in an induced allergic reaction in animals. Luteolin, rosmarinic and caffeic acids were isolated and identified as active constituents. Luteolin has been shown in vivo to inhibit TNF-alpha and arachidonic acid and reduce oedema (Ueda et al 2002). In another inflammatory model, perilla dose-dependently reduced the allergic response in mice by over 40%. Rosmarinic acid was identified as the main active constituent (Makino et al 2001) and has been shown to decrease the inflammatory response and increase superoxide radical scavenging in vivo (Osakabe et al 2004a). An extract of perilla leaf with high levels of rosmarinic acid decreased cytokine activity in asthma-induced rats (Sanbongi et al 2004). A perilla leaf decoction was found to suppress IgA nephropathy in genetically predisposed rats, possibly through modulation of the intestinal mucosal immune system. Perilla suppressed proteinuria, proliferation of glomerular cells, serum levels of IgA, glomerular IgA and IgG depositions in the mice. Rosmarinic acid seems to produce this effect synergistically with other constituents (Makino et al 2003b).

Antioxidant activity

A methanolic extract of roasted defatted perilla seed has been shown to exert strong antioxidant activity, and upon fractionation, luteolin was identified as one of the active antioxidant constituents (Jung et al 2001). Rosmarinic acid inhibits NO and nitric oxide synthase (iNOS) in vitro (Qiao et al 2005, Renzulli et al 2004). Aqueous extract of perilla significantly inhibits free radical production by neutrophil leucocytes (Zekonis et al 2008). In vitro, isolated luteolin from *P. frutescens* showed non-competitive inhibition of aldose reductase (involved in diabetic complications and α-glucosidase) (Ha et al 2012).

A small study of eight healthy non-smoking females showed that a water extract of a red cultivar of *P. frutescens* var. *crispa* standardised at 1000 mg of polyphenols prolonged LDL peroxidation lag time by 5 minutes at 4 hours post-ingestion indicating a clinical effect (Saita et al 2012). In vitro, the comparative study of red and green perilla showed the red cultivar had a higher polyphenol content and increased antioxidant activity in endothelial cells (Saita et al 2012).

Neuroprotective

Oral ingestion of perilla seed oil caused brain cells to be significantly less sensitive to reactive oxygen species, reactive nitrogen species and mitochondrial dysfunction according to an animal model. Furthermore, an increase in oleic and linoleic acid brain content was observed, as well as increased in-situ biosynthesis of arachadonic acid (AA) and DHA (Eckert et al 2010). Despite these changes in fatty acid content, synapse membrane fluidity was unchanged.

Immunostimulant

Perilla leaf extract stimulates phagocytosis in vitro and in vivo (Simoniene et al 2005). An increase in neutrophil phagocytosis was noted after 7 days, but was strongest after 4 weeks of treatment. A polysaccharide extract from perilla leaf has also demonstrated phagocytic ability both in vitro and in vivo (Kwon et al 2002).

Antimicrobial activity

Perilla may help prevent dental caries and periodontal disease. Perilla seed extract has been shown to have antimicrobial activity against oral cariogenic streptococci and periodontopathic *Porphyromonas gingivalis*. The luteolin constituent showed the strongest antimicrobial effect among the phenolic compounds tested (Yamamoto & Ogawa 2002).

Hepatoprotective effects

Perilla extract and its constituent rosmarinic acid showed hepatoprotective activity against lipopolysaccharide-induced liver damage in mice, possibly due to an antioxidant mechanism (Osakabe et al 2002).

Lipid lowering activity

Perilla and perilla flavonoids demonstrate lipid lowering activity in vivo. Perilla oil lowers cholesterol by suppressing hepatic beta-hydroxy-beta-methylglutaryl-CoA (HMG-CoA) reductase activity (Du et al 2003). Perilla oil also lowers plasma triacylglycerol by suppressing fatty acid synthase (Kim et al 2004) and stimulating acyl-CoA oxidase (Kim & Choi 2005) in the liver. Perilla oil mixed with borage and evening primrose oil has been shown to reduce cholesterol in older rats (Fukushima et al 2001). Similarly, a dose of 200 mg/kg of perilla flavonoids given to test animals over 30 days and fed a high fat diet for 4 weeks was shown to normalise lipid levels (Feng et al 2011).

Anticancer effects

Several constituents found in perilla have demonstrated anticancer effects in vitro and in experimental cancer models. This has prompted phase I and phase II clinical testing with one key active constituent, perillyl alcohol.

Conjugated alpha-linolenic acid from perilla oil has been shown to reduce the rate of carcinogenesis in a chemically-induced rat mammary cancer model (Futakuchi et al 2002). The fibrinolytic and antioxidative activities of rosmarinic acid suppress the proliferation of mesangial cells in vivo (Makino et al 2002, Osakabe et al 2004b). Animal studies have demonstrated the ability of perillyl alcohol to inhibit tumorigenesis in the mammary gland (Yuri et al 2004) and skin (Lluria-Prevatt et al 2002). The precise mechanism of action is unclear, but it is thought that compounds other than the rosmarinic acid stimulate apoptosis (Lin et al 2007). Perillyl alcohol has been shown to inhibit part of the signal transduction cascade involved in uncontrolled cell proliferation, upregulate the mannose-6-phosphate receptor and induce apoptosis (Liston et al 2003, Xu et al 2004). Perillyl alcohol has also demonstrated an ability to decrease the release of vascular endothelial growth factor from cancer cells and encourage the expression of angiopoietin-2 by endothelial cells (Loutrari et al 2004). This indicates that perilla may play a role in decreasing the vascularisation of tumours and inducing regression. The effects of perillyl alcohol and its metabolite perillic acid on the proliferation of non-small cell lung cancer cells were investigated in vivo. Both elicited dose-dependent cytotoxicity, induced cell cycle arrest and apoptosis in a dose-dependent manner (Yeruva et al 2007).

Perillyl alcohol increases the sensitivity of cancer cells in vitro to radiation treatment of prostate cancer (Rajesh & Howard 2003), glioma (Rajesh et al 2003) and certain neck and head cancers (Samaila et al 2004).

Antidepressant activity

Several different constituents within perilla leaf have demonstrated effects on behaviour in vivo, most notably antidepressant effects. Perilla demonstrated an antidepressant-like property in animal models of depression, possibly through cell proliferation in the hippocampus (Ito et al 2008b). Rosmarinic acid and caffeic acid have demonstrated antidepressant activity in a forced swimming test in mice. The activity is thought to be via some mechanism other than the inhibition of monoamine transporters and monoamine oxidase (Takeda et al 2002a). Apigenin from perilla significantly reduced immobility in a forced swimming test in mice, an effect mediated by dopaminergic mechanisms (Nakazawa et al 2003). Inhalation of L-perillaldehyde, a major component in the essential oil, shows antidepressant-like activity in mice through the olfactory nervous function (Ito et al 2008a).

Rosmarinic acid and caffeic acid have been shown to decrease the duration of the defensive freezing behaviour caused by fear and stress in animals (Takeda et al 2002b).

OTHER ACTIONS

Perilla oil has been shown to reduce the excessive growth of visceral adipose tissue in rats by downregulating adipocyte differentiation in animals (Okuno et al 1997). This has direct relevance to obesity, as a high-fat diet not only accelerates the filling process of preexisting preadipocytes but also stimulates the proliferation of adipose precursor cells. Adipocyte differentiation, from adipoblasts to adipocytes, is a key factor underlying obesity.

P

A glycoprotein isolated from perilla oil has been shown to inhibit an early stage of HIV-1 replication without blocking viral adsorption in vitro (Kawahata et al 2002, Yamasaki et al 1998).

Perilla aldehyde has demonstrated vasodilatory activity in isolated rat aorta and appears to work by blocking Ca^{2+} channels (Takagi et al 2005). The clinical significance of this is currently unknown.

CLINICAL USE

The form most commonly used at the moment is the extract of defatted perilla seed; however, this review will also include information regarding other forms.

Cancer

The main form tested is the perillyl alcohol in various vehicles such as topical creams and intranasal delivery.

Perillyl alcohol (POH)

Phase I clinical trials have shown a favourable toxicity profile, and preliminary data have suggested some chemotherapeutic efficacy in cancer, but no definitive conclusions can be made just yet as to the potential use of POH as there are few clinical trials and results to date have been dissappointing.

In vitro studies suggest that POH inhibits the expression and function of androgen receptors in human prostate cancer cell line, suggesting that POH could be useful for intervention of prostate cancer (Chung et al 2006). Another in vitro study of a combination of POH with a virally delivered therapeutic cytokine shows promise for both preventing and treating human pancreatic cancer without toxic effects (Lebedeva et al 2008). In a small pilot study of eight patients with adenocarcinomas of the exocrine pancreas treated perioperatively with POH 1200 mg/m^2 four times daily, there was a non-statistical increase in survival time and greater local apoptosis; however, tumour size and CA 19.9, a commonly used pancreatic cancer marker, remained unchanged (Matos et al 2008).

Similarly, POH (1200 mg/m^2 four times daily) failed to extend the time-to-progression in three phase II studies in patients with advanced ovarian carcinoma (Bailey et al 2002), refractory metastatic breast cancer (Bailey et al 2008), prostate cancer (Liu et al 2003) and colorectal cancer. All trials were very small and had to contend with high dropout rates due to intolerability of the medicine. Despite encouraging preclinical results, perilla does not appear to be an effective treatment for advanced cancer based on the small amount of clinical investigation conducted thus far.

Topical POH inhibits ultraviolet B-induced skin carcinogenesis in vivo so has been tested clinically for activity. A 1-month, double-blind, phase 1 trial of topically administered perillyl alcohol cream was tested in 25 human subjects. They were monitored for toxicity and underwent histopathological evaluation. The topical cream was well tolerated and no serious cutaneous toxicities, systemic toxicities or histopathological abnormalities were observed. However, there was no significant difference between lesions appearing on the treated forearm versus the placebo-treated forearm (Stratton et al 2008). In a phase IIa trial comparing placebo against a low dose POH (0.3%) cream and a high dose POH (0.76%) topical cream for chemoprevention on participants with sun damaged skin, there was a borderline statistical significance in histopathological score in the groups using 0.3% cream but no change with use of 0.76% cream, although a decrease in nuclear abnormalities was demonstrated in karyotyping analysis (Stratton et al 2010).

The 6-month treatment of recurrent malignant glioma in a phase I/II study of 37 patients with intranasal POH spray demonstrated antitumour activity and decrease in peritumoral brain oedema. While no toxicity was noted, nausea, early satiety, eructation and fatigue side effects interfered with compliance (Da Fonseca et al 2008). Further research is required to further investigate the effects of intranasal POH in this cohort.

Allergy

Based on traditional use, in vitro and in vivo studies and human trials, perilla leaf and defatted seed extracts are used for allergic respiratory disorders including hay fever, asthma and sinusitis. The refined oil may also help allergic and inflammatory respiratory conditions by regulating the arachidonic acid metabolism pathways and suppressing leukotriene generation.

A double-blind, randomised, placebo-controlled clinical trial showed a significant reduction in symptoms such as watery eyes, itchy eyes and itchy nose in 29 patients with seasonal allergic rhinoconjunctivitis, taking 50 or 200 mg of rosmarinic acid-enriched perilla for 21 days (Takano et al 2004). Responder rates were 55.6 and 70%, respectively. A drastic reduction in the number of neutrophils and eosinophils in nasal fluid was also demonstrated.

In an open clinical trial, 20 human subjects suffering allergic symptoms, including sneezing, nasal obstruction and itchy eyes and skin, were treated with 100–150 mg perilla seed extract daily (higher dose for persons over 60 kg) for 2 weeks. The subjects themselves evaluated changes in the severity of symptoms. Significant improvement was noted in 80% of the subjects for nasal obstructive symptoms, 40% reported a significant improvement in sneezing and half reported a significant reduction of itchy eyes (Oryza Co 2003).

A systematic review of double-blind randomised trials evaluating various herbal medicines in patients with allergic rhinitis concluded that perilla (part used not specified) showed promising results (Guo et al 2007).

Perilla leaf extract cream and dermatitis

Open studies of more than 100 children with atopic dermatitis found that perilla leaf extract cream improved symptoms in 80% of cases after 3 months' treatment (Yu et al 1997). Another open study with 20 allergic patients, using perilla leaf cream topically and perilla leaf extract orally, showed a general improvement in 90% of the patients after 2 months, with 30% reporting significant improvements (Yu et al 1997).

Dental caries and periodontal disease

Perilla seed extract inhibits the growth of cariogenic and inflammatory microorganisms including oral streptococci and *Porphyromonas gingivalis* (Yamamoto & Ogawa 2002). Perilla seed extract also reduces inflammation through inhibition of leucocyte production and radical scavenging activity. As such, application of the extract in the oral cavity is used to reduce dental caries and pericoronitis.

OTHER USES

Refined perilla oil is a good source of omega-3 series alpha-linolenic acid.

Clinical note — Perilla and traditional medicine systems

Perilla is an important ingredient of several traditional Chinese medicine (TCM) formulas. Perilla leaf is a key ingredient in Saiboku-to, a traditional Chinese formulation used in the treatment of type 1 hypersensitivity disorders, including asthma (Nishiyori et al 1985). Saiboku-to contains *Bupleurum falcatum*, *Pinellia ternata*, *Poria cocos*, *Scutellaria baicalensis*, *Magnolia officinalis*, *Zizyphus spinosa*, *Panax ginseng*, *Glycyrrhiza uralensis*, *Zingiber officinale* and perilla. Another TCM formula containing perilla, Sam So Eum, is used to treat asthma and has been shown in an animal model to decrease airway hyperresponsiveness by restoring the immunomodulating cytokines. The anti-inflammatory effects of this formula are similar in effectiveness to prednisolone (Cho et al 2008). Perilla is also a component of the Banxia Houpu Decoction used for depression. It contains *Pinellia ternata*, *Poria cocos*, *Magnolia officinalis*, *Perilla frutescens and Zingiber officinale* (Luo et al 2000). Perilla leaf has been prescribed as one of the component herbs in certain Kampo (Japanese herbal) medicines that are used clinically for the improvement of depressive mood. These formulae demonstrate antidepressant-like effect in mice models through suppressing the hyperactivity of the hypothalamic-pituitary-adrenal (HPA) axis (Ito et al 2006).

DOSAGE RANGE

- Perilla leaf: extract equivalent to 4–9 g/day (Bensky & Gamble 1986).
- Refined perilla oil: 1000 mg capsules taken three to six times daily.
- Perilla seed extract (containing a minimum of 3.0% polyphenols): 100–150 mg/day (Oryza Co 2003).
- External use (dental caries and periodontal disease): 80–160 mg defatted perilla seed daily delivered directly into the oral cavity in the form of toothpaste, chewing gum or mouth rinse.

ADVERSE REACTIONS

Defatted perilla seed extract has very low toxicity. After administering 2000 mg/kg to mice for 2 weeks, no toxic effects were observed (LD_{50} for mice is therefore more than 2000 mg/kg). Dosage of 7.0 g/kg for 2 weeks did not produce any toxic effects in humans.

In Japan, 20–50% of long-term workers in the perilla industry develop dermatitis on their hands due to contact with perillyl aldehyde (Brenner 1993).

A 13-week subchronic oral toxicity study of perilla leaf extracts in drinking water did not show any acute toxicity. There were no treatment-related changes in body weight gain or in haematological or blood biochemistry values. Nor were there any treatment-related histopathological changes observed in the highest dose group (Yun et al 1999).

Phase I and II clinical trials of perillyl alcohol for certain cancers have shown that gastrointestinal side effects and fatigue are the most common adverse reactions (Azzoli et al 2003, Bailey et al 2002, 2004, Liu et al 2003, Meadows et al 2002). Gastrointestinal effects are usually mild and include nausea, vomiting, bloating and belching. Doses were usually between 1200 and 1600 mg/m^2 four times daily.

The refined perilla oil is clear golden yellow. It is fully refined (neutralised, bleached and deodorised) and should be free of perillyl ketone, which is a potent lung toxin that causes increased microvascular permeability and pulmonary oedema in grazing animals (Waters et al 1993).

There has been a report of lipoid pneumonia in a 57-year-old man who had a history of ingesting green perilla oil, and there was also residual neurological deficit of cerebral infarction with right hemiparesis (Kwang et al 1999).

Anaphylactic reactions to *Perilla frutescens* seeds were reported in 2006 (Jeong et al) in two atopic subjects with high serum-specific IgE response.

A separate report of a 21-year-old atopic man who presented with bronchospasms and periorbital urticaria after ingestion of Shiso leaves (botanical name and chemotype not supplied) concluded the reaction was mediated by direct histamine release from basophils; there was no detection of serum IgE antibodies (Shin et al 2009). None of these reports gave specific information about the variety, cultivar or PK content taken.

P

SIGNIFICANT INTERACTIONS

Controlled studies are not available, so interactions are based on evidence of activity and are largely theoretical and speculative.

Antihistamine agents

Theoretical additive effect is possible. Patients taking perilla concurrently with antihistaminic should be observed and drug doses modified if required.

CONTRAINDICATIONS AND PRECAUTIONS

None reported for perilla seed extract or refined oil; however, perilla leaf extract is contraindicated in diarrhoea (Bensky & Gamble 1986).

PREGNANCY USE

Insufficient information is available to determine the safety of perilla during pregnancy.

Practice points/Patient counselling

- Perilla exhibits anti-inflammatory, anti-allergic, antioxidant and anticariogenic activity. Preliminary evidence also suggests hepatoprotective and behavioural effects.
- Perilla leaf and defatted seed extracts are specifically used for allergic respiratory disorders including hay fever, asthma and sinusitis.
- Perilla leaf and defatted seed extract may down-regulate Th2-type cytokine production and prevent the Th1/Th2 balance from shifting towards Th2-type immune responses that may be associated with a range of allergic reactions and autoimmune disorders.
- Refined perilla oil is a good source of omega-3 series alpha-linolenic acid, and extracts should be free of perillyl ketones and aldehydes.

PATIENTS' FAQs

What can this herb do for me?

Perilla leaf and defatted seed extracts are used in the treatment of allergic respiratory conditions, such as hay fever, asthma and sinusitis. Preliminary evidence suggests that it may be beneficial; however, more rigorous studies are still required to confirm effectiveness.

When will it start to work?

Relief of allergic symptoms should be noticed within the first week, although it may take a couple of weeks to show a significant effect. For hayfever, it would be beneficial to start taking perilla at least 1 month before the onset of the hayfever season.

Are there any safety issues?

Perilla is generally well tolerated and nontoxic. It can be used long term if indicated.

REFERENCES

Azzoli CG et al. A phase I trial of perillyl alcohol in patients with advanced solid tumors. Cancer Chemother Pharmacol 51.6 (2003): 493–498.

Bailey HH et al. Phase II trial of daily perillyl alcohol in patients with advanced ovarian cancer: Eastern Cooperative Oncology Group Study E2E96. Gynecol Oncol 85 (2002): 464–468.

Bailey HH et al. A phase I trial of perillyl alcohol administered four times daily for 14 days out of 28 days. Cancer Chemother Pharmacol 54.4 (2004): 368–376.

Bailey HH et al. Phase II trial of daily oral perillyl alcohol (NSC 641066) in treatment-refractory metastatic breast cancer. Cancer Chemother. Pharmacol 62.1 (2008): 149–157.

Bensky D, Gamble A. Chinese herbal medicine: Materia Medica. Seattle: Eastland Press, 1986, pp 294–295.

Brenner DM. New crops. New York: Wiley, 1993, pp. 322–328.

Chang HH et al. Dietary perilla oil inhibits proinflammatory cytokine production in the bronchoalveolar lavage fluid of ovalbumin-challenged mice. Lipids 43.6 (2008): 499–506.

Cho SJ et al. Sam So Eum, a herb extract, as the remedy for allergen-induced asthma in mice. Pulm Pharmacol Ther 21.3 (2008): 578–583.

Chung BH et al. Perillyl alcohol inhibits the expression and function of the androgen receptor in human prostate cancer cells. Cancer Lett 236.2 (2006): 222–228.

Da Fonseca et al. Preliminary results from a phase I/II study of perillyl alcohol intranasal administration in adults with recurrent malignant gliomas. Surgical Neurology 70.3 (2008): 259–266.

Du C et al. Cholesterol synthesis in mice is suppressed but lipofuscin formation is not affected by long-term feeding of n-3 fatty acid-enriched oils compared with lard and n-6 fatty acid-enriched oils. Biol Pharm Bull 26.6 (2003): 766–770.

Eckert GP et al. Plant derived omega-3 fatty acids protect mitochondrial function in the brain. Pharmacological Research 61.3 (2010): 234–241.

Feng LJ et al. Hypolipidemic and antioxidant effects of total flavonoids of Perilla Frutescens leaves in hyperlipidemia rats induced by high-fat diet. Food research international 44 (2011): 404–409.

Fukushima M, Ohhashi T, Ohno S et al. Effects of diets enriched in n-6 or n-3 fatty acids on cholesterol metabolism in older rats chronically fed a cholesterol-enriched diet. Lipids 36.3 (2001): 261–266.

Futakuchi M et al. Inhibition of conjugated fatty acids derived from safflower or perilla oil of induction and development of mammary tumors in rats induced by 2-amino-1-methyl-6-phenylimidazo [4,5-b] pyridine (PhIP). Cancer Lett 178.2 (2002): 131–139.

Guo R et al. Herbal medicines for the treatment of allergic rhinitis: a systematic review. Ann Allergy Asthma Immunol 99.6 (2007): 483–495.

Ha TJ et al. Isolation and identitification of phenolic compounds from the seeds of Perilla frutescens (L.) and their inhibitory activities against α-glucosidase and aldose reductase. 135.3 (2012): 1397–1403.

Ishihara T et al. Inhibition of antigen-specific T helper type 2 responses by Perilla frutescens extract. Jpn J Allergol 48.4 (1999): 443–450 [in Japanese].

Ito M et al. Chemical composition of the essential oil of Perilla frutescens. Nat Med 53.1 (1999): 32–36.

Ito N et al. Antidepressant-like activity of a Kampo (Japanese herbal) medicine, Koso-san (Xiang-Su-San), and its mode of action via the hypothalamic-pituitary-adrenal axis. Phytomedicine 13.9–10 (2006): 658–667.

Ito N et al. Antidepressant-like effect of l-perillaldehyde in stress-induced depression-like model mice through regulation of the olfactory nervous system. Evid Based Complement Alternat Med (2008a) [Epub ahead of print].

Ito N et al. Rosmarinic acid from Perillae Herba produces an antidepressant-like effect in mice through cell proliferation in the hippocampus. Biol Pharm Bull 31.7 (2008b): 1376–1380.

Jeong YY et al. Two cases of anaphylaxis caused by perilla seed. J Allergy Clin Immunol, 117 (2006): 1505–1506.

Jung MJ et al. Antioxidant activity of roasted defatted perilla seed. Nat Prod Sci 7.3 (2001): 72–75.

Kawahata T et al. A novel substance purified from Perilla frutescens Britton inhibits an early stage of HIV-1 replication without blocking viral adsorption. Antivir Chem Chemother 13.5 (2002): 283–288.

Kim HK, Choi H. Stimulation of acyl-CoA oxidase by alpha-linolenic acid-rich perilla oil lowers plasma triacylglycerol level in rats. Life Sci 77.12 (2005): 1293–1306.

Kim HK et al. Suppression of hepatic fatty acid synthase by feeding alpha-linolenic acid rich perilla oil lowers plasma triacylglycerol level in rats. J Nutr Biochem 15.8 (2004): 485–492.

Kwang JJ et al. A case of lipoid pneumonia after ingestion of green perilla oil. Tuberculosis Resp Dis 47.1 (1999): 123–126 [in Korean].

Kwon KH et al. In vitro and in vivo effects of macrophage-stimulatory polysaccharide from leaves of Perilla frutescens var. crispa. Biol Pharm Bull 25.3 (2002): 367–371.

Lebedeva IV et al. Chemoprevention by perillyl alcohol coupled with viral gene therapy reduces pancreatic cancer pathogenesis. Mol Cancer Ther 7.7 (2008): 2042–2050.

Lee JH et al. Identification, characterization, and quantification of phenolic compounds in the antioxidant activity-containing fraction from the seeds of Korean perilla (Perilla frutescens) cultivars. Food chem. 136.2 (2013): 843–852.

Lin CS et al. Growth inhibitory and apoptosis inducing effect of Perilla frutescens extract on human hepatoma HepG2 cells. J Ethnopharmacol 112.3 (2007): 557–567.

Liston BW et al. Perillyl alcohol as a chemopreventive agent in N-nitrosomethylbenzylamine-induced rat esophageal tumorigenesis. Cancer Res 63 (2003): 2399–2403.

Liu G et al. Phase II trial of perillyl alcohol (NSC 641066) administered daily in patients with metastatic androgen independent prostate cancer. Invest New Drugs 21.3 (2003): 367–372.

Lluria-Prevatt M et al. Effects of perillyl alcohol on melanoma in the TPras mouse model. Cancer Epidemiol Biomarkers Prev 11.6 (2002): 573–579.

Loutrari H et al. Perillyl alcohol is an angiogenesis inhibitor. J Pharmacol Exp Ther 311.2 (2004): 568–575.

Luo L et al. Antidepressant effects of Banxia Houpu decoction, a traditional Chinese medicinal empirical formula. J Ethnopharmacol 73.1–2 (2000): 277–281.

Makino T et al. Effect of oral treatment of Perilla frutescens and its constituents on type-I allergy in mice. Biol Pharm Bull 24.10 (2001): 1206–1209.

Makino T et al. Suppressive effects of rosmarinic acid on mesangioproliferative glomerulonephritis in rats. Nephron 92.4 (2002): 898–904.

Makino T et al. Anti-allergic effect of Perilla frutescens and its active constituents. Phytother Res 17 (2003a): 240–3.

Makino T et al. Suppressive effects of Perilla frutescens on IgA nephropathy in HIGA mice. Nephrol Dial Transplant 18.3 (2003b): 484–90.
Matos JM et al. A pilot study of perillyl alcohol in pancreatic cancer. Journal of Surgical Research 147 (2008): 194–199.
Meadows SM et al. Phase II trial of perillyl alcohol in patients with metastatic colorectal cancer. Int J Gastrointest Cancer 32.2–3 (2002): 125–128.
Meng L et al. Polyphenol extracton from eight Perilla frutescens cultivars. Compte rendus chimie, 12.5 (2009): 602–611.
Misra LN, Husain A. The essential oil of Perilla ocimoides: a rich source of rosefuran. Planta Med 53.4 (1987): 379–380.
Nakazawa T et al. Antidepressant-like effects of apigenin and 2,4,5-trimethoxycinnamic acid from Perilla frutescens in the forced swimming test. Biol Pharm Bull 26 (2003): 474–480.
Nishiyori T et al. Effect of Saiboku-to, a blended Chinese traditional medicine, on type I hypersensitivity reactions, particularly on experimentally-caused asthma. Nippon Yakurigaku Zasshi 85.1 (1985): 7–16.
Okamoto M et al. Effects of perilla seed oil supplementation on leukotriene generation by leucocytes in patients with asthma associated with lipometabolism. Int Arch Allergy Immunol 122.2 (2000): 137–142.
Okuno M et al. Perilla oil prevents the excessive growth of visceral adipose tissue in rats by down-regulating adipocyte differentiation. J Nutr 127 (1997): 1752–1757.
Oryza Co. Perilla seed extract: product monograph. Version 5.0 TS edn. Japan: Oryza Oil & Fat Chemical Co, 2003.
Osakabe N et al. Rosmarinic acid, a major polyphenolic component of Perilla frutescens, reduces lipopolysaccharide (LPS)-induced liver injury in D-galactosamine (D-GalN)-sensitized mice. Free Radical Biol Med 33.6 (2002): 798–806.
Osakabe N et al. Anti-inflammatory and anti-allergic effect of rosmarinic acid (RA); inhibition of seasonal allergic rhinoconjunctivitis (SAR) and its mechanism. Biofactors 21.1–4 (2004a): 127–31.
Osakabe N et al. Rosmarinic acid inhibits epidermal inflammatory responses: anticarcinogenic effect of Perilla frutescens extract in the murine two-stage skin model. Carcinogenesis 25.4 (2004b): 549–57.
Qiao S et al. Rosmarinic acid inhibits the formation of reactive oxygen and nitrogen species in RAW264.7 macrophages. Free Radic Res 39.9 (2005): 995–1003.
Rajesh D, Howard SP. Perillyl alcohol mediated radiosensitization via augmentation of the Fas pathway in prostate cancer cells. Prostate 57.1 (2003): 14–23.
Rajesh D, Stenzel RA, Howard SP. Perillyl alcohol as a radio-chemosensitizer in malignant glioma. J Biol Chem 278.38 (2003): 35968–35978.
Renzulli C et al. Effects of rosmarinic acid against aflatoxin B1 and ochratoxin-A-induced cell damage in a human hepatoma cell line (Hep G2). J Appl Toxicol 24.4 (2004): 289–296.
Saita E et al. Antioxidant activities of Perilla frutescens against low-density lipoprotein oxidation in vitro and in human subjects. J Oleo Sci. 61.3 (2012): 11320.
Samaila D et al. Monoterpenes enhanced the sensitivity of head and neck cancer cells to radiation treatment in vitro. Anticancer Res 24 (2004): 3089–3095: 5A.
Sanbongi C et al. Rosmarinic acid in perilla extract inhibits allergic inflammation induced by mite allergen, in a mouse model. Clin Exp Allergy 34.6 (2004): 971–977.
Shin TY et al. Inhibitory effect of mast cell-mediated immediate-type allergic reactions in rats by Perilla frutescens. Immunopharmacol Immunotoxicol 22.3 (2000): 489–500.
Shin YS et al. A case of bronchospasm and urticaria casued Shiso ingestion. Annals of Allergy, Asthma & Immunology, 102.2 (2009): 16.
Simoniene G et al. [The influence of common perilla (Perilla frutescens (L.) Britton) on non-specific cell-mediated immunity phagocytosis activity]. Kaunas: Medicina 41.12 (2005): 1042–7.
Stratton SP et al. Phase 1 study of topical perillyl alcohol cream for chemoprevention of skin cancer. Nutr Cancer 60.3 (2008): 325–330.
Stratton SP et al. A Phase 2a Study of topical Perillyl Alcohol Cream for chemoprevention of skin cancer. Cancer Prev Res 3 (2010): 160–169.
Takagi S et al. Vasodilative effect of perillaldehyde on isolated rat aorta. Phytomedicine 12.5 (2005): 333–337.
Takano H et al. Extract of Perilla frutescens enriched for rosmarinic acid, a polyphenolic phytochemical, inhibits seasonal allergic rhinoconjunctivitis in humans. Exp Biol Med (Maywood) 229.3 (2004): 247–254.
Takeda H et al. Rosmarinic acid and caffeic acid produce antidepressive-like effect in the forced swimming test in mice. Eur J Pharmacol 449.3 (2002a): 261–267.
Takeda H et al. Rosmarinic acid and caffeic acid reduce the defensive freezing behavior of mice exposed to conditioned fear stress. Psychopharmacology (Berl) 164.2 (2002b): 233–235.
Tan YF, Lai BS, Yan XL. Analysis of fatty acids in Perilla frutescens seed oil. Chin Pharm J 33.7 (1998): 400–402 [in Chinese].
Ueda H et al. Luteolin as an anti-inflammatory and anti-allergic constituent of Perilla frutescens. Biol Pharm Bull 25 (2002): 1197–1202.
Wakame K et al. Effects of perilla extracts on compound 48/80-induced scratching behavior in mice and histamine release from peritoneal cells. Dokkyo J Med Sci 27.2 (2000): 373–378.
Waters CM et al. Perilla ketone increases endothelial cell monolayer permeability in vitro. J Appl Physiol 74.5 (1993): 2493–2501.
Xu M et al. Perillyl alcohol-mediated inhibition of lung cancer cell line proliferation: potential mechanisms for its chemotherapeutic effects. Toxicol Appl Pharmacol 195.2 (2004): 232–246.
Yamamoto H, Ogawa T. Antimicrobial activity of perilla seed polyphenols against oral pathogenic bacteria. Biosci Biotechnol Biochem 66 (2002): 921–924.
Yamasaki K et al. Anti-HIV-1 activity of herbs in Labiatae. Biol Pharm Bull 21.8 (1998): 829–833.
Yeruva L et al. Perillyl alcohol and perillic acid induced cell cycle arrest and apoptosis in non small cell lung cancer cells. Cancer Lett 257.2 (2007): 216–226.
Yu H-C et al. Perilla—the genus Perilla. Medicinal and aromatic plants. Industrial profiles. Amsterdam: Hardwood Academic, 1997.
Yun L et al. A 13-week subchronic oral toxicity study of Perilla extracts in F344 rats. Kokuritsu Iyakuhin Shokuhin Eisei Kenkyusho Hokoku 117 (1999): 104–107 [in Japanese].
Yuri T et al. Perillyl alcohol inhibits human breast cancer cell growth in vitro and in vivo. Breast Cancer Res Treat 84.3 (2004): 251–260.
Zekonis G et al. Effect of Perilla frutescens aqueous extract on free radical production by human neutrophil leukocytes. Kaunas: Medicina 44.9 (2008): 699–705.

Policosanol

BACKGROUND AND RELEVANT PHARMACOKINETICS

Policosanol is isolated from the waxes of plants such as sugar cane. The main component, octacosanol, has variable absorption from the small intestine and is chiefly metabolised by the liver and excreted in the faeces.

CHEMICAL COMPONENTS

Policosanol is a mixture of long-chain primary aliphatic alcohols (Arruzazabala et al 1993a). The alcohols have a chain length ranging from 24 to 34 carbons and the major components of the mixture are octacosanol (60–70%, w/w), triacosanol (10–15%, w/w) and hexacosanol (4–10%, w/w) (Francini-Pesenti et al 2008). Octacosanol is regarded as the main active constituent.

MAIN ACTIONS

Lipid lowering — questionable

Cuban sugar cane policosanol (CSP), derived from the waxy coating of stems and leaves of sugar cane and other plant materials, has been shown to exert significant lipid-lowering effects in animals and humans in numerous studies conducted by a single laboratory and using a CSP product manufactured by Dalmer Laboratories (Havana, Cuba). Tests investigating CSP with experimental models, including rats, rabbits, dogs and monkeys, have demonstrated reductions in circulating total cholesterol levels consistently greater than 13% (Kassis et al 2007). Early human studies using CSP showed significant reductions in total cholesterol and low-density lipoprotein (LDL)-cholesterol; however, these findings are being questioned because there has been a plethora of negative clinical and experimental studies published since 2006 which have been unable to detect lipid-lowering activity for CSP and other policosanol preparations.

Reduces oxidation of LDL-cholesterol

This has been demonstrated in vitro at an equivalent dose of 5 and 10 mg/day (Menendez et al 2000).

Reduces platelet aggregation

This has been confirmed in animal models and randomised double-blind studies, with effects starting at 10 mg/day (Arruzazabala et al 1993b, 2002, Castano et al 1999a). One clinical study found that a dose of 20 mg/day policosanol produces the same inhibitory effects on platelet aggregation as 100 mg aspirin daily (Arruzazabala et al 1997). A higher dose of 40 mg policosanol does not appear to produce any further antiplatelet effects according to another double-blind study (Arruzazabala et al 2002). Thromboxane, but not prostacyclin, generation induced by collagen is also inhibited by policosanol in clinical studies (Carbajal et al 1998a).

OTHER ACTIONS

Endothelial protection

Oral administration of policosanol to spontaneously hypertensive rats resulted in a significant reduction in circulating endothelial cells compared with controls. Moreover, comparison between groups revealed a lower frequency of aortic lesions in policosanol-treated animals than in untreated animals (Noa et al 1997).

Antihypertensive effects at very high doses

Tests in animal models have identified enhancement of propranolol-induced hypotensive effects with pretreatment at 200 mg/kg policosanol (Molina et al 1999), which is an extremely high dose and clinically irrelevant in humans.

Reduces atherosclerotic lesion development

According to one animal study, most policosanol-treated animals did not develop atherosclerotic lesions compared with an untreated group, and the thickness of fatty streaks that did develop with treatment had fewer foam cell layers than in controls (Arruzazabala et al 2000).

CLINICAL USE

Policosanol is most often used in the management of hyperlipidaemia and was sold as a lipid-lowering agent in over 40 countries worldwide.

Hyperlipidaemia

Policosanol has been the focus of multiple clinical trials in an attempt to clarify its role as a potential treatment in hyperlipidaemia. Initial results published prior to 2006 and conducted with CSP, manufactured by Dalmer Laboratories (Havana, Cuba), supported its use and indicated significant lipid-lowering activity. However, studies conducted by other research groups outside Cuba have not been able to reproduce the results obtained in the original studies, casting doubt on the product's lipid-lowering activity. Since 2007 several new double-blind studies have been published with policosanol producing negative results again, thereby confirming that policosanol is not an effective treatment for hyperlipidaemia.

Prior to 2006

Numerous randomised, double-blind clinical trials conducted prior to 2006 demonstrated significant cholesterol-lowering effects of oral policosanol (Castano et al 2001b, Mas et al 1999, Menendez et al 2000, Pons et al 1994, Torres et al 1995). Several previous studies conducted with postmenopausal women confirmed benefits in this population (Castano et al 2000, Mas et al 1999, Menendez et al 2000, Mirkin et al 2001, Pons et al 1994, Torres et al 1995). Overall, these early results showed that a daily dose of 5 mg policosanol may: reduce LDL-cholesterol by 11–18%, reduce total cholesterol by 8–15% and increase high-density lipoprotein (HDL) by 8–15%, whereas a higher dose of 20 mg policosanol daily can: reduce LDL-cholesterol by 31%, reduce total cholesterol by 23% and increase HDL by 27%. These studies used the same specific policosanol product.

Since 2006 the body of evidence has shifted significantly

In 2006 five negative clinical studies were published which were conducted by different research teams around the world, using either Cuban or non-Cuban policosanol products.

In Germany, Berthold et al (2006) conducted a 12-week randomised study of 143 Caucasian subjects with hypercholesterolaemia or combined hyperlipidaemia. The multicentre study used CSP at doses of 10, 20, 40 and 80 mg/day. In contrast to previous studies, policosanol failed to significantly reduce LDL-cholesterol, total cholesterol, HDL-cholesterol, triglycerides and other lipid parameters at all test doses. In a US double-blind, placebo-controlled trial of 40 healthy adults with mild hypercholesterolaemia, conducted by Dulin et al (2006), subjects were assigned to receive oral policosanol 20 mg or placebo once daily for 8 weeks. No significant changes were seen for LDL-cholesterol, total cholesterol, HDL-cholesterol, triacylglycerol, C-reactive protein and nuclear magnetic resonance spectroscopy-determined profiles. Also in the United States, Cubeddu et al (2006) divided subjects with LDL-cholesterol levels from 140 to 189 mg/dL into four groups and compared policosanol 20 mg to atorvastatin 10 mg, combination therapy or placebo for 12 weeks (Cubeddu et al 2006). In total, 99 patients took part and groups were well matched at baseline. Yet again, policosanol failed to have a significant effect on any lipid parameter and produced no additional lipid-lowering effects when added to atorvastatin. In Canada, Kassis and Jones (2006) compared policosanol 10 mg/day to placebo in 21 people over a period of 28 days. The double-blind, crossover study also failed to find significant changes to plasma lipid levels for total, LDL-cholesterol, HDL-cholesterol and triacylglycerol concentrations with policosanol treatment. In South Africa, Greyling et al (2006) conducted a double-blind study involving 19 hypercholesterolaemic and familial hypercholesterolaemic subjects who received either policosanol 20 mg/day or placebo for 12 weeks. After a 4-week wash-out period, the interventions were crossed over and treatment recommenced. No significant differences in total cholesterol and LDL-cholesterol from baseline to end or between policosanol and placebo were seen in the hypercholesterolaemic or familial hypercholesterolaemic groups.

Since 2006, the negative evidence has continued to accumulate as studies using animal models and clinical trials consistently fail to find significant lipid-lowering activity for either CSP or its other forms (Backes et al 2011, Francini-Pesenti et al 2008, Kassis 2008, Kassis & Jones 2008, Kassis et al 2007, Marinangeli et al 2007, Martino et al 2013, Swanson et al 2011).

In 2011, two more negative clinical trials were published. Backes et al (2011) used a modified policosanol (MP) product in an attempt to improve the absorption of policosanol and determine if this new form would produce better results. MP was administered as stand-alone treatment (20 mg/daily) or together with statins and compared to a placebo group over an 8-week test period. In both groups receiving MP there were no significant changes to major lipoproteins.

Swanson et al (2011) found that a dose of 20 mg daily of standard policosanol failed to normalise any of the dyslipidaemic parameters measured (LDL-cholesterol, HDL-cholesterol, triglycerides) in their randomised, double-blind, crossover study. The study involved 54 people with HIV who received either 20 mg of policosanol or placebo for 12 weeks, followed by a 4-week washout period and 12 more weeks of the alternative treatment (Swanson et al 2011). No adverse effects were reported.

Clinical note — Policosanol controversy

It is now certain that policosanol does not have significant lipid-lowering activity as the more recent clinical trials have failed to confirm earlier positive results. Several theories may explain the discrepancy, such as differences in the purity and composition of different policosanol products, insufficient test timeframes, differences between test subjects and, of course, researcher bias or contamination of product.

Researchers external to the original Cuban research groups began testing these different theories to uncover the answer. Theories proposing differences in octacosanol content have been discounted as the various policosanol products tested externally have contained similar concentrations to the original Cuban blend. Another suggestion is that products may have differed in minor alcohol content, explaining the disparate results. To test this theory, Cuban policosanol has been directly compared to other policosanol products in various animal models. Using a hamster model, Kassis et al (2007) compared Dalmer Cuban policosanol to an alternative Degussa policosanol mixture and found that neither treatment had a significant effect on lipids. A second research team, headed by Marinangeli, also compared Cuban policosanol to another product with a similar amount of octacosanol and found no differences between them for tissue, plasma and faecal policosanol levels in an animal model (Marinangeli et al 2007). In regard to timeframes, Cuban clinical studies indicate that lipid-lowering activity can be observed by 4 weeks of treatment and reaches a maximal effect between 6 and 8 weeks. Studies conducted by Berthold et al (2006), Greyling et al (2006) and Cubeddu et al (2006) lasted 12 weeks and still found no significant activity, so this theory can also be discounted.

More recently, a modified form of policosanol with improved absorption was tested by Backes et al (2011), but no significant lipid-lowering activity was observed. Finally, genetic differences between test subjects and differences in dietary habits could account for the varied responses between test subjects; however this appears unlikely.

Wheatgerm-derived policosanol

No beneficial effects on blood lipid profiles were observed in a double-blind, randomised study of 58 subjects with normal to mildly elevated plasma cholesterol who were given 20 mg wheatgerm policosanol in a short, 4-week study (Lin et al 2004).

Intermittent claudication

Policosanol treatment for intermittent claudication has produced encouraging results in several randomised studies (Castano et al 1999b, 2001a, 2003a).

Policosanol 10 mg/day taken for 6 months significantly increased initial claudication walking distance by approximately 70 metres and absolute claudication by approximately 140 metres in one double-blind study, whereas placebo produced no changes (Castano et al 1999b). A single-blind study using 20 mg policosanol daily showed significant improvements after 6 months' treatment, which further increased after 12 months (Castano et al 2001b). In both studies patients in the policosanol group reported improvements in lower-limb symptoms that were greater than those in the placebo group.

More recently, policosanol (10 mg twice daily) was shown to be as effective as ticlopidine (250 mg twice daily) for improving walking distances of claudicant patients (Castano et al 2004b). In the 20-week double-blind, randomised study of 28 subjects, policosanol significantly increased mean values of initial and absolute claudication distances from 162.1 to 273.2 metres and from 255.8 to 401.0 metres, respectively, which was not significantly different to ticlopidine. Both treatments were well tolerated.

In 2008, a randomised, double-blind study comparing policosanol (10 mg/day) to aspirin (100 mg/day) was published showing that policosanol modestly but significantly increased the initial and absolute claudication walking distances whereas no change occurred with aspirin (Illnait et al 2008). The study involved 39 volunteers and treatment lasted for 10 weeks.

Until these results can be confirmed by other research groups, these results remain uncertain.

Practice points/Patient counselling

- Policosanol can no longer be considered an efficacious lipid-lowering treatment because of a spate of negative studies showing no significant effect.
- It is a potentially useful treatment in claudication; however, more research is required to confirm its effects.
- Policosanol may have platelet aggregation inhibitor activity.
- Safety studies indicate that it is well tolerated and has a wide safety margin.

OTHER USES

Pre-existing coronary heart disease

A randomised double-blind study of 45 subjects with documented coronary heart disease found that a dose of 10 mg policosanol daily increased maximum oxygen uptake and exercise electrocardiograph responses. The effects were further enhanced by co-administration of 125 mg aspirin (Stusser et al 1998).

Cerebrovascular disease

In two different experimental models, policosanol had anti-ischaemic activity when administered after induction of cerebral ischaemia, suggesting a possible therapeutic effect in cerebrovascular disease (Molina et al 1999).

DOSAGE RANGE

The doses tested in clinical trials range from 5 to 20 mg/day.

More specific doses

- Hypercholesterolaemia: 5–20 mg/day has been tested (recent evidence now indicates it is ineffective).
- Intermittent claudication: 10–20 mg/day — 3 months' continual use may be required before effects are observed (uncertain efficacy).

TOXICITY

Studies using several animal models have confirmed no carcinogenic effects and no signs of toxicity at doses as high as 500 mg/kg (Aleman et al 1994a, 1994b). This dose is hundreds of times greater than the maximal recommended therapeutic dose (20 mg/day), thereby indicating an excellent safety profile (Mesa et al 1994).

ADVERSE REACTIONS

A pharmacovigilance study of 2252 subjects aged 60 or more years with coronary, cerebrovascular and peripheral artery disease and treated with policosanol (5, 10 or 20 mg/day) at seven major medical centres found that long-term tolerability of policosanol in elderly patients at high vascular risk was very good (Fernandez et al 2004).

SIGNIFICANT INTERACTIONS

Aspirin

Increased antiplatelet effects may develop — patients taking aspirin and policosanol concurrently should be observed for increased bleeding or bruising.

Warfarin

Current evidence suggests that there is no interaction between policosanol and warfarin. One clinical study confirmed that the addition of policosanol to warfarin therapy does not enhance the prolongation of the bleeding time induced by warfarin alone (Carbajal et al 1998b). Caution with doses > 10 mg/day.

CONTRAINDICATIONS AND PRECAUTIONS

Suspend use of high doses 1 week before major surgery.

PREGNANCY USE

Safety has been investigated in animal tests with no evidence of teratogenicity or any other embryonal toxicity (Rodriguez & Garcia 1994, 1998, Rodriguez et al 1997).

PATIENTS' FAQs

What can this supplement do for me?

It now appears unlikely that policosanol can significantly lower cholesterol levels. Early studies suggested this effect was as strong as conventional cholesterol-lowering medications; however, more recent studies have found no effect. It may also be useful in intermittent claudication but confirmation is required by other researchers before this is certain.

When will it start to work?

Early studies suggest that maximal lipid-lowering effects are seen after 6–8 weeks of continuous use; however, new evidence casts doubt over its efficacy.

Are there any safety issues?

Policosanol has a wide safety margin and is well tolerated.

REFERENCES

Aleman CL et al. Carcinogenicity of policosanol in Sprague Dawley rats: a 24 month study. Teratog Carcinog Mutagen 14.5 (1994a): 239–249.

Aleman CL et al. A 12-month study of policosanol oral toxicity in Sprague Dawley rats. Toxicol Lett 70.1 (1994b): 77–87.

Arruzazabala ML et al. Effect of policosanol on cerebral ischemia in Mongolian gerbils: role of prostacyclin and thromboxane A2. Prostaglandins Leukot Essent Fatty Acids 49.3 (1993a): 695–697.

Arruzazabala ML et al. Effects of policosanol on platelet aggregation in rats. Thromb Res 69.3 (1993b): 321–327.

Arruzazabala ML et al. Comparative study of policosanol, aspirin and the combination therapy policosanol-aspirin on platelet aggregation in healthy volunteers. Pharmacol Res 36.4 (1997): 293–297.

Arruzazabala ML et al. Protective effect of policosanol on atherosclerotic lesions in rabbits with exogenous hypercholesterolemia. Braz J Med Biol Res 33.7 (2000): 835–840.

Arruzazabala ML et al. Antiplatelet effects of policosanol (20 and 40 mg/day) in healthy volunteers and dyslipidaemic patients. Clin Exp Pharmacol Physiol 29.10 (2002): 891–897.

Backes, J.M., et al. 2011. Modified-policosanol does not reduce plasma lipoproteins in hyperlipidemic patients when used alone or in combination with statin therapy. Lipids, 46, (10) 923–929.

Berthold HK et al. Effect of policosanol on lipid levels among patients with hypercholesterolemia or combined hyperlipidemia: a randomized controlled trial. JAMA 295.19 (2006): 2262–2269.

Carbajal D et al. Effect of policosanol on platelet aggregation and serum levels of arachidonic acid metabolites in healthy volunteers. Prostaglandins Leukot Essent Fatty Acids 58.1 (1998a): 61–64.

Carbajal D et al. Interaction policosanol-warfarin on bleeding time and thrombosis in rats. Pharmacol Res 38.2 (1998b): 89–91.

Castano G et al. Effects of policosanol and pravastatin on lipid profile, platelet aggregation and endothelemia in older hypercholesterolemic patients. Int J Clin Pharmacol Res 19.4 (1999a): 105–116.

Castano G et al. A double-blind, placebo-controlled study of the effects of policosanol in patients with intermittent claudication. Angiology 50.2 (1999b): 123–130.

Castano G et al. Effects of policosanol on postmenopausal women with type II hypercholesterolemia. Gynecol Endocrinol 14.3 (2000): 187–195.

Castano G et al. Effects of policosanol in older patients with type II hypercholesterolemia and high coronary risk. J Gerontol A Biol Sci Med Sci 56.3 (2001a): M186–M192.

Castano G et al. A long-term study of policosanol in the treatment of intermittent claudication. Angiology 52.2 (2001b): 115–125.

Cubeddu LX et al. Comparative lipid-lowering effects of policosanol and atorvastatin: a randomized, parallel, double-blind, placebo-controlled trial. Am Heart J 152.5 (2006): 982–985.

Dulin MF, et al. Policosanol is ineffective in the treatment of hypercholesterolemia: a randomized controlled trial. Am J Clin Nutr 84.6 (2006): 1543–1548.

Fernandez S et al. A pharmacological surveillance study of the tolerability of policosanol in the elderly population. Am J Geriatr Pharmacother 2.4 (2004): 219–229.

Francini-Pesenti F et al. Sugar cane policosanol failed to lower plasma cholesterol in primitive, diet-resistant hypercholesterolaemia: A double blind, controlled study. Complementary Therapies in Medicine. 2008; 16: 61–65.

Greyling A et al. Effects of a policosanol supplement on serum lipid concentrations in hypercholesterolaemic and heterozygous familial hypercholesterolaemic subjects. Br J Nutr 95.5 (2006): 968–975.

Illnait J et al. Effects of policosanol (10 mg/d) versus aspirin (100 mg/d) in patients with intermittent claudication: a 10-week, randomized, comparative study. Angiology 59.3 (2008): 269–277.

Kassis AN. Evaluation of cholesterol-lowering and antioxidant properties of sugar cane policosanols in hamsters and humans. Appl Physiol Nutr Metab 33.3 (2008): 540–541.

Kassis AN, Jones PJ. Lack of cholesterol-lowering efficacy of Cuban sugar cane policosanols in hypercholesterolemic persons. Am J Clin Nutr 84.5 (2006): 1003–1008.

Kassis AN, Jones PJ. Changes in cholesterol kinetics following sugar cane policosanol supplementation: a randomized control trial. Lipids Health Dis 7 (2008): 17.

Kassis AN et al. Lack of effect of sugar cane policosanol on plasma cholesterol in golden syrian hamsters. Atherosclerosis 194.1 (2007): 153–158.

Lin Y et al. Wheat germ policosanol failed to lower plasma cholesterol in subjects with normal to mildly elevated cholesterol concentrations. Metabolism 53.10 (2004): 1309–1314.

Marinangeli CP et al. Comparison of composition and absorption of sugarcane policosanols. Br J Nutr 97.2 (2007): 381–388.

Martino, F., et al. Low dose chromium-polynicotinate or policosanol is effective in hypercholesterolemic children only in combination with glucomannan. Atherosclerosis (2013) 228: 198–202

Mas R et al. Effects of policosanol in patients with type II hypercholesterolemia and additional coronary risk factors. Clin Pharmacol Ther 65.4 (1999): 439–447.

Menendez R et al. Effects of policosanol treatment on the susceptibility of low density lipoprotein (LDL) isolated from healthy volunteers to oxidative modification in vitro. Br J Clin Pharmacol 50.3 (2000): 255–262.

Mesa AR et al. Toxicity of policosanol in beagle dogs: one-year study. Toxicol Lett 73.2 (1994): 81–90.

Mirkin A et al. Efficacy and tolerability of policosanol in hypercholesterolemic postmenopausal women. Int J Clin Pharmacol Res 21.1 (2001): 31–41.

Molina V et al. Effect of policosanol on cerebral ischemia in Mongolian gerbils. Braz J Med Biol Res 32.10 (1999): 1269–1276.

Noa M, et al. Effect of policosanol on circulating endothelial cells in experimental models in Sprague-Dawley rats and in rabbits. J Pharm Pharmacol 49.10 (1997): 999–1002.

Pons P et al. Effects of successive dose increases of policosanol on the lipid profile of patients with type II hypercholesterolaemia and tolerability to treatment. Int J Clin Pharmacol Res 14.1 (1994): 27–33.

Rodriguez MD, Garcia H. Teratogenic and reproductive studies of policosanol in the rat and rabbit. Teratog Carcinog Mutagen 14.3 (1994): 107–113.

Rodriguez MD, Garcia H. Evaluation of peri- and post-natal toxicity of policosanol in rats. Teratog Carcinog Mutagen 18.1 (1998): 1–7.

Rodriguez MD, et al. Multigeneration reproduction study of policosanol in rats. Toxicol Lett 90.2–3 (1997): 97–106.

Stusser R et al. Long-term therapy with policosanol improves treadmill exercise-ECG testing performance of coronary heart disease patients. Int J Clin Pharmacol Ther 36.9 (1998): 469–473.

Swanson, B., et al. 2011. Policosanol for managing human immunodeficiency virus-related dyslipidemia in a medically underserved population: a randomized, controlled clinical trial. Altern. Ther. Health Med, 17, (2) 30–35.

Torres O et al. Treatment of hypercholesterolemia in NIDDM with policosanol. Diabetes Care 18.3 (1995): 393–397.

Prebiotics

HISTORICAL NOTE Gibson & Roberfroid (1995) introduced the concept of prebiotic as 'a non-digestible food ingredient that beneficially affects the host by selectively stimulating the growth and/or activity of one or a limited number of bacteria in the colon and thus improves health'. This concept has been further developed to define prebiotics as 'selectively fermented ingredients that allow specific changes, both in the composition and/or activity of the gastrointestinal microflora that confer benefits upon host wellbeing and health' (Roberfroid 2007b).

BACKGROUND AND RELEVANT PHARMACOKINETICS

Numerous components appear to have prebiotic characteristics, but some will not be classified as prebiotics because they may not meet all the criteria, i.e. not metabolised (hydrolysed or absorbed) in the upper gastrointestinal tract (GIT), demonstrate selective fermentation by one or a limited number of potentially beneficial intestinal bacteria and change the colonic microflora to a healthier composition (Gibson & Roberfroid 1995, Roberfroid 2007b). To date, the most well-researched prebiotics are inulin, lactulose, fructooligosaccharides (FOS) and galactooligosaccharides (GOS) (Roberfroid 2007a).

One of the key characteristics of prebiotics is to stimulate the selective growth of intestinal microorganisms and, in particular, the growth of lactobacilli and bifidobacteria.

Studies have demonstrated that the intestinal microflora of breastfed infants is characterised by high levels of bifidobacteria and lactic acid bacteria because oligosaccharides occur naturally in breastmilk. Formula-fed infants were found to have more *Bacteroides*, clostridia and Enterobacteriaceae and lower levels of the beneficial microorganisms (Coppa et al 2006).

Bifidobacteria are well-known defences against pathogenic bacteria and are significant for promoting gut health (Brunser et al 2006, Cummings & Macfarlane 2002, Gibson 1998, Gibson & Roberfroid 1995). In addition to stabilising the gut microflora, prebiotics may have a role in allergy: reports indicate that infants with allergy had lower levels of lactobacilli and bifidobacteria (Bjorksten et al 2001) and feeding prebiotics was able to rectify this. Increasingly, prebiotics have been added to infant milk formulas in order to simulate the composition of human breastmilk prebiotic oligosaccharides.

In recent years, there has been a focus on using multiple prebiotics together rather than a single component; combinations of long-chain FOS and short-chain GOS have been utilised mainly because different gastrointestinal microorganisms may require different substrates for optimal growth.

In both adults and the young, prebiotics are reported to have other health-promoting properties and they may have a role in the management of a number of diseases and conditions. Altered gastrointestinal microflora and abnormal colonic fermentation are also noted in some conditions, such as inflammatory bowel disease (IBD) and irritable bowel syndrome (IBS) (King et al 1998); treatment with prebiotics or synbiotics may normalise the altered microflora.

Prebiotics as indigestible components are known to have laxative properties and are used as bulking agents for gastrointestinal health. The end products of the prebiotic fermentation in the colon are short-chain fatty acids (SCFAs), while have direct effects on the intestinal cells and stimulate intestinal peristalsis (Gibson 1998, 1999, Gibson & Roberfroid 1995, Gibson et al 1995).

Both lactobacilli and bifidobacteria species in the colon have important roles in immune stimulation and prevention of infection and diarrhoea (Gorbach et al 1987, Macfarlane et al 2006, Saavedra et al 1994). Some bifidobacteria and lactobacilli strains may have antimutagenic and antitumour properties; prebiotics such as inulin appear to inhibit colonic cancer cell growth (Pool-Zobel & Sauer 2007).

Prebiotics also demonstrate anti-inflammatory activity in the GIT, with lactulose, inulin and FOS all demonstrating GIT anti-inflammatory activity in animal models and/or human research (Cherbut et al 2003, Koleva et al 2012, Lara-Villoslada et al 2006, Looijer–Van Langen & Dieleman 2009, Yasuda et al 2012).

CHEMICAL COMPONENTS

Prebiotics are principally oligosaccharides or disaccharides, of which there are various types: oligofructose, inulins, isomaltooligosaccharides, lactosucrose, GOS, lactulose, pyrodextrins and xylooligosaccharides. Potential prebiotics, their food sources and their targeted microorganisms are highlighted in Table 1.

Inulins are multiple fructose units and inulin degradation results in oligofructose. GOS occur naturally in breastmilk. Fructans are linear or branched fructose polymers and the GOS are synthesised from lactose by the action of beta-galactosidase. FOS are the inulin-type fructans that can be readily obtained from plant sources. Both GOS and FOS are widely used in the food industry (Yang & Silva 1995).

TABLE 1 PREBIOTIC SUBSTANCES AND THE ORGANISMS WHOSE GROWTH THEY PROMOTE (HUDSON & MARSH 1995, TERAMOTO ET AL 1996, TEURI & KORPELA 1998, VAN LOO ET AL 1995, 1998)

Prebiotic compound	Food sources	Targeted microorganisms
β-glucooligomers	Oats	*Lactobacillus* spp.
Fructooligosaccharides and inulin	Jerusalem artichokes, garlic, onions, chicory roots, asparagus, wheat	*Bifidobacterium* spp.
Galactooligosaccharides	Cow's milk, yoghurt, human milk	*Bifidobacterium* spp.
Galactosyl lactose	Human milk	*Bifidobacterium* spp.
Lactitol	None known	*Lactobacillus* spp.; *Bifidobacterium* spp.
Lactosucrose	None	*Bifidobacterium* spp.
Lactulose	UHT milk	*Lactobacillus* spp.; *Bifidobacterium* spp.
Polydextrose	None known	*Lactobacillus* spp.; *Bifidobacterium* spp.
Raffinose	Legumes, beets	*Lactobacillus* spp.; *Bifidobacterium* spp.
Xylooligosaccharides	Oats	*Bifidobacterium* spp.

Clinical note — The hygiene hypothesis

The intestinal microflora is crucial for the development of the immune system (Ouwehand et al 2002) and the 'hygiene theory' suggests that exposure to microorganisms is required for this. The consumption of foods containing microorganisms for health-promoting properties has a long history. Probiotics are microorganisms that can 'beneficially affect the host physiology by modulating mucosal and systemic immunity, as well as improving nutritional and microbial balance of the intestinal tract' (Gibson & Roberfroid 1995, Salminen et al 1998).

Clinical note — Synbiotics

Synbiotics are products that contain both probiotic and prebiotic agents (Schrezenmeir & de Vrese 2001). The combination is supposed to enhance the survival of the probiotic bacteria through the upper GIT, improve implantation of the probiotic in the colon and have a stimulating effect on the growth and/or activities of both the exogenously-provided probiotic strain(s) and the endogenous inhabitants of the bowel (Casiraghi et al 2007). In recent years, there has been a trend to increasingly use synbiotics for a synergistic health-promoting effect, but this also makes it difficult to evaluate the individual effects of each component.

FOOD SOURCES

Low levels of prebiotic compounds can be found in artichokes, asparagus, bananas, chicory root, garlic, leek, onions and wheat. Inulin and oligofructose occur naturally in these foods. Commercially produced prebiotics are extracted from chicory roots or Jerusalem artichokes or synthesised from sucrose and are used widely in the food industry. Dietary intake of prebiotics is variable, with the intake for Americans being in the range 1–4 g/day and on average a higher intake among Europeans, who consume 3–10 g/day (Delzenne 2003).

DEFICIENCY SIGNS AND SYMPTOMS

Clear deficiency signs are difficult to establish because the symptoms may vary enormously. Local signs and symptoms of disruption of the intestinal microflora leading to an imbalance (intestinal dysbiosis) include bloating, flatulence, abdominal pain, diarrhoea and/or constipation and fungal overgrowth (such as *Candida*). An imbalance in the gastrointestinal microflora can be caused by the use of antibiotics, GIT infections, stress and dietary factors (Hawrelak & Myers 2004). Administration of prebiotics, probiotics or synbiotics is used as a means of restoring this microflora imbalance.

MAIN ACTIONS

The health benefits claimed for prebiotics mainly stem from their ability to increase numbers of beneficial organisms in the colon, modulate the immune response, reduce numbers of potentially pathogenic microorganisms (PPMs) in the GIT and stimulate SCFA production.

Stimulation of beneficial bacteria and prevention of GIT infections

Many animal and human studies have demonstrated that prebiotics modulate the gut microflora by increasing bifidobacteria and lactobacilli levels (Bouhnik et al 1997, Gibson & Wang 1994, Langlands et al 2004).

Prebiotics are fermented by the microflora in the proximal colon, resulting in the production of SCFAs (acetic, propionic and butyrate acids) and gas (CO_2 and H_2). Consequently, the lower intraluminal pH inhibits the growth of PPMs while simultaneously creating an atmosphere more conducive to the growth of lactobacilli and bifidobacteria (Walker et al 2005). As a result of prebiotics stimulating the growth of beneficial bacteria, these microorganisms secrete antimicrobial compounds and can inhibit colonisation of the pathogenic bacteria and prevent their adherence to the intestinal epithelium (Shoaf-Sweeney & Hutkins 2009). Adherence can also be limited as a result of the oligosaccharide's terminal sugars interfering with the receptors on the pathogenic bacteria (Hopkins & Macfarlane 2003, Zopf & Roth 1996): reduced adherence of enteropathogenic *Escherichia coli* in HeP and Caco-2 cells has been noted with GOS, for example (Shoaf et al 2006). GOS have also been shown to inhibit binding of *Vibrio cholerae* toxin to its receptor in the human GIT (Sinclair et al 2009) and reduce colonisation and pathology associated with *Salmonella typhimurium* infection in a murine model (Searle et al 2009).

Immunomodulation and enhanced mucin production

The mechanisms whereby prebiotics have immunomodulatory effects (modulate cytokine and antibody production) are largely unknown and the proposed mechanisms include beneficial changes in the intestinal microflora and increased production of both mucin and SCFAs. There may also be changes in the gut-associated lymphoid tissues (GALT) as a result of prebiotic fermentation in the colon (Forchielli & Walker 2005). The SCFAs are beneficial to the host as an energy source and enhance mucosal integrity with increased production of mucin, binding to receptors on immune cells within GALT and limiting translocation. Mucin may limit bacterial translocation and acts as a barrier against luminal contents by protectively covering the intestinal epithelial cells. There is little information about the effects of prebiotics on mucin production, but both animal and human research has noted increased mucin production associated with inulin and FOS supplementation (Fontaine et al 1996, Ten Bruggencate et al 2006). This increase appears to be mediated via increases in mucin 3 gene expression, as well as increases in colon crypt depth with more mucin-secreting goblet cells per crypt (Paturi et al 2012).

Both prebiotics and probiotics are reported to have beneficial effects in reducing the effects of colitis by altering the gastrointestinal microflora due to stimulating growth of the protective bacteria and reducing colonisation with potentially hazardous bacteria (Sartor 2004). Prebiotics (mainly inulin and FOS) may also ameliorate inflammation as a result of reducing the activity of proinflammatory transcription factors (e.g. NF-κB), and by the increased production of SCFAs (Cavin et al 2005, Holma et al 2002, Kinoshita et al 2002, Millard et al 2002). Animal studies show conflicting findings, with the majority reporting a reduction in inflammation with prebiotic supplementation (Cherbut et al 2003) and others reporting that there is no protection from FOS or GOS in rat models of colitis (Looijer-Van Langen & Dieleman 2009). In recent years, some human studies have been undertaken and mixed results are reported. Butyrate is a major source of energy for colonocytes, and in vitro studies indicate that butyrate has anti-inflammatory effects (Saemann et al 2000, Segain et al 2000); butyrate and acetate also enhance mucin secretion.

Cancer prevention

Various in vitro and animal studies have been conducted to investigate the role of prebiotics and synbiotics for their anticancer effects, but there are only a limited number of studies in humans (Pool-Zobel & Sauer 2007). Animal studies have shown that prebiotic treatment is beneficial in reducing precancerous aberrant crypt foci and the effects may be more pronounced with synbiotics. Rowland et al (1998) reported that the effect is enhanced with synbiotics such as inulin plus *Bifidobacterium longum* in their study of azoxymethane-induced aberrant crypt foci in rats. Oligofructose-enriched inulin plus *Lactobacillus rhamnosus* and *B. lactis* treatment prevented azoxymethane-induced suppression of natural killer (NK) cell activity in Peyer's patches (Roller et al 2004) and, similarly, a study (Le Leu et al 2005) demonstrated increased apoptotic response with resistant starch plus *B. lactis* treatment.

OTHER ACTIONS

Mineral metabolism

Animal studies have indicated that prebiotics such as inulin and oligofructose can affect calcium bioavailability and increase calcium absorption. A number of mechanisms have been proposed for this action, including the increased production of SCFAs, which increase the solubility of minerals and also facilitate the colonic absorption of calcium and magnesium (Demigne et al 2008).

Improved bioavailability of phyto-oestrogens

An interesting animal (rat) study has found that concurrent consumption of FOS and the soy isoflavones, genistein and daidzein, significantly improved the bioavailability of these compounds. The relative absorption of genistein was ~20% higher in FOS-fed rats than in controls. In addition, the presence of both phyto-oestrogens in serum was maintained for longer in FOS-fed rats than in controls, suggesting that FOS enhanced colonic absorption of these compounds (Uehara et al 2001).

This result may be especially relevant to women postantibiotic therapy, where the metabolism and subsequent absorption of phyto-oestrogens appear to be impaired (Kilkkinen et al 2002). Bifidobacteria have been shown to possess β-glucosidase activity, and FOS administration has resulted in enhanced β-glucosidase activity in animal models (Rowland et al 1998) as well as improved phyto-oestrogen bioavailability (Ohta et al 2002). FOS consumption not only aids in the re-establishment of a healthy GIT microflora, but its consumption also increases colonic β-glucosidase activity, resulting in enhanced deglycosylation and thus increased colonic concentrations of the medicinally active aglycones.

The synergistic effect of FOS supplementation with soy isoflavones on bone health has been observed in an osteopenic rat model, where coadministration of the two agents was found to exert the strongest effect in inhibiting bone loss in rats. This was due, at least in part, to FOS-induced increases in calcium absorption and equol production (Kimira et al 2012). Another study utilising an ovariectomised rat model of osteoporosis also found a strong synergistic effect between soy isoflavones and FOS supplementation in preventing bone loss (Hooshmand et al 2010).

CLINICAL USE

Irritable bowel syndrome

A multicentre, double-blind randomised controlled trial (RCT) by Olesen and Gudmand-Hoyer (2000) did not find benefits for the use of FOS in the treatment of IBS, similar to the findings of Hunter et al (1999), who utilised oligofructose in their double crossover study investigating IBS.

Conversely, in a randomised, single-blind, placebo-controlled, crossover trial, supplementation of 3.5 g/day of GOS to subjects with IBS significantly improved stool consistency, flatulence scores, bloating scores and overall IBS symptom scores compared to placebo (all $P < 0.05$) over a 4-week treatment period. Supplementation of 7 g/day resulted in significant improvements in overall IBS symptom scores and a reduction in anxiety levels compared to placebo (both $P < 0.05$). However, there was also a significant increase in bloating scores relative to baseline when subjects were taking the higher dosage ($P < 0.05$) (Silk et al 2009).

Inflammatory bowel disease

In a study of patients with active IBD, 14 patients presenting with ulcerative colitis (UC) and 17 patients presenting with Crohn's disease (CD) received either standard medication treatment or the medications with an additional 10 g/day lactulose dose for 4 months. At the end of the study there were no differences in the clinical or endoscopic score, although the UC group receiving the lactulose treatment reported an improved quality of life compared to the control group ($P = 0.04$) (Hafer et al 2007).

Crohn's disease

At present, the role of prebiotics in the management of CD remains unknown due to a limited number of studies.

A small open-label study of 10 patients with active ileocolonic CD who were treated with FOS (15 g/day for 3 weeks) reported a significant reduction in disease activity scores (30% reduction; $P < 0.01$) and inflammation, with an increase in interleukin-10 (IL-10)-positive dendritic cells and Toll-like receptor 2 and Toll-like receptor 4 expression. It is noteworthy that patients entering remission had increased mucosal-associated bifidobacteria (Lindsay et al 2006).

This positive, but small, open-label trial was followed up with a double-blind, placebo-controlled RCT. One hundred and three subjects with active CD were supplemented with 15 g/day FOS or placebo for 4 weeks in conjunction with standard medications. While there was an increased percentage of IL-10-positive dendritic cells ($P = 0.035$), there was no significant difference in response rate or rate of remission. Surprisingly, there were no changes in faecal bifidobacterial concentrations in the FOS-treated group. It is also worth noting that 19% of the FOS-treated group withdrew from the trial due to adverse gastrointestinal effects (flatulence, borborygmi and abdominal pain) (Benjamin et al 2011).

In a small, randomised, open-label trial, Hafer et al (2007) investigated the efficacy of lactulose therapy (10 g/day for 4 months) compared to standard care in patients with CD ($n = 17$). No significant improvements in clinical activity index, endoscopic score or immunohistochemical parameters were observed in CD patients receiving lactulose, in comparison to controls (Hafer et al 2007).

P

A RCT of 30 patients with CD postoperative ileocaecal resection, who were treated with Synbiotic 2000, a combination of four prebiotic components plus a probiotic mixture of four lactic acid strains (*Pediococcus pentosaceus*, *Lactobacillus raffinolactis*, *Lactobacillus paracasei* subsp. *paracasei* F19, *Lactobacillus plantarum*, 2.5 g beta-glucans, 2.5 g inulin, 2.5 g pectin, 2.5 g resistant starch), did not show prevention of relapse 24 months later (Chermesh et al 2007). In another study (duration: 13.0 ± 4.5 months) (Fujimori et al 2007), 10 non-hospitalised patients with active CD were treated with high-dose synbiotic therapy consisting of bifidobacterium and lactobacillus (75 billion colony-forming units (CFU)/day) plus psyllium (9.9 g/day); only three patients did not experience any benefit.

These differing results may be due to the variation in fibres used in the trials, as well as differences in the probiotic strains utilised.

Ulcerative colitis

The results from a number of animal studies have indicated that prebiotics may be of therapeutic value in UC and preliminary human studies appear to show similar results. A small randomised, double-blind, placebo-controlled trial evaluated 19 patients with active UC (mild/moderate). Subjects received prebiotic treatment (12 g/day of oligofructose-enriched inulin, ratio 1 : 1) or placebo plus 3 g/day of mesalazine for 2 weeks. Subjects in the prebiotic group experienced significantly fewer dyspeptic symptoms and a reduction of intestinal inflammation, as determined by faecal calprotectin levels, which decreased after 1 week of treatment (from 4377 to 1033; $P < 0.05$). However, there was no change in prostaglandin E_2 secretion and IL-8 production (Casellas et al 2007).

The effectiveness of lactulose therapy in UC was evaluated in a small, randomised, open-label trial. Seven subjects consumed 10 g/day of lactulose in conjunction with their standard medications for 4 months, while another seven received standard care only. There was a significant improvement seen in the clinical activity index in the lactulose-treated group (54% reduction; $P = 0.047$ compared to baseline). The decrease in the clinical activity index was not significant when compared to controls, however ($P = 0.09$). Four patients in the lactulose group achieved remission versus none in the control group. Quality-of-life scores significantly improved in the lactulose group compared to controls ($P = 0.037$) and there was also a trend for a reduction in steroid dose ($P = 0.063$) in this group (Hafer et al 2007).

In a double-blind RCT of 18 patients with active UC, synbiotic treatment with 12 g oligofructose-enriched inulin (1 : 1) plus *Bifidobacterium longum* for 4 weeks resulted in reduced colonic inflammation, decreased human beta-defensin mRNA, tumour necrosis factor-alpha and IL-1alpha, and improved sigmoidoscopy scores, although there was no difference in clinical measures (Furrie et al 2005).

In another RCT, the efficacy of synbiotic therapy was compared to either prebiotics or probiotics and involved 120 outpatients with UC in remission (Fujimori et al 2009). Each group of patients enrolled in the study were treated with either one capsule per day consisting of *B. longum* 2×10^9 CFU (probiotic group) or 2×4 g doses of psyllium (prebiotic group) or both the probiotic plus prebiotic (synbiotic group) for 4 weeks. At the end of the study, C-reactive protein decreased significantly ($P = 0.04$) and the quality-of-life scores in the Inflammatory Bowel Disease Questionnaires were also significantly improved for the synbiotic treated group; the score for bowel function was significant in the prebiotic group ($P = 0.04$).

Pouchitis

There are only a limited number of studies that have investigated the role of prebiotics or synbotics in pouchitis.

A small open-label study of 10 patients with pouchitis (antibiotic-refractory or antibiotic-dependent) treated with a synbiotic mixture of FOS plus *Lactobacillus rhamnosus* GG reported complete remission as determined by clinical and endoscopic criteria (Friedman & George 2000). In a crossover study of 20 patients with ileal pouch–anal anastomosis, daily treatment with 24 g of inulin or placebo for 3 weeks did not change the clinical activity scores, although there was a reduction in inflammation ($P = 0.01$) and increased faecal butyrate concentrations. Lactobacilli and bifidobacteria levels were not affected, although a significant reduction in faecal levels of *Bacteroides fragilis* was reported (Welters et al 2002).

Constipation

The use of lactulose has a long history and it has been used successfully as an osmotic laxative to treat constipation (de Schryver et al 2005, Petticrew et al 1997). Likewise, FOS and GOS also have laxative effects: Gibson et al (1995) demonstrated that feeding 15 g of FOS or 15 g inulin per day could significantly increase stool output. Utilising 9 g GOS/day, one study found an increase in defecation frequency (from 5.9 to 7.1 movements/week) in elderly subjects over a 2-week treatment period. There was also a trend for easier defecation ($P = 0.07$) during the GOS phase of the trial (Teuri & Korpela 1998).

Two RCTs evaluated the laxative effects of GOS in healthy adult subjects with a tendency to constipation. At a daily dose of 5 and 10 g there were significant improvements in defecation frequency — from 0.92 to 1.07 movements daily ($P < 0.05$) and from 0.85 to 0.97 times per day ($P < 0.05$), respectively (Niittyen et al 2007).

Diarrhoea

Various prebiotic components have been utilised in clinical trials to evaluate their efficacy in diarrhoea of different origins.

Traveller's diarrhoea

A double-blind RCT of 244 people travelling to medium–high-risk destinations and at risk of traveller's diarrhoea reported that those subjects who were treated with FOS (10 g) experienced increased wellbeing and less severe diarrhoea, although there was no significant difference in the incidence of diarrhoea (Cummings et al 2001).

A more recent double-blind RCT evaluated the potential of GOS administration to prevent traveller's diarrhoea. Subjects ingested 2.6 g GOS once daily starting 7 days before reaching their holiday destination and continued taking it daily throughout their holiday. Compared to the placebo group, subjects in the GOS group experienced a 40% decrease in the incidence ($P < 0.05$) and a 48% reduction in duration of traveller's diarrhoea ($P < 0.05$). Additionally, they suffered less abdominal pain ($P < 0.05$) and experienced improved quality of life ($P < 0.05$) (Drakoularakou et al 2009).

Clostridium difficile-associated diarrhoea (CDAD)

In a double-blind RCT, 142 patients with CDAD in hospital were randomised to receive oligofructose or placebo as well as the standard antibiotic treatment for 30 days and followed up 30 days later. It was found that the prebiotic-treated patients had increased bifidobacteria levels and reduction in the rate of relapse and experienced significantly less diarrhoea compared to placebo (8% vs 34%, $P <$ 0.001) (Lewis et al 2005a).

In another double-blind RCT of 435 hospitalised patients who were receiving antibiotics, treatment with oligofructose for 7 days was compared to placebo. After a 7-day follow-up period, there was a significant increase in bifidobacteria concentrations in the prebiotic group, although there was no difference in the incidence of *Clostridium difficile* (Lewis et al 2005b).

Allergic disease and food hypersensitivity

Clinical trials confirm that prebiotic-enhanced infant formula ingested during the first 6 months of life reduces the risk of atopic disease. The effect is not limited to the 6-month treatment period but seems to provide longer-term protection.

In a double-blind RCT, Moro et al (2006) evaluated the effects of a prebiotic-enhanced infant formula (FOS and GOS combination) on the incidence of atopic dermatitis during the first 6 months of life in formula-fed infants at high risk of atopy development. Atopic dermatitis developed in 23% of infants in the control group compared to 10% in the prebiotic group ($P = 0.014$) over the 6-month intervention period. Subjects in the prebiotic group were also found to have significantly reduced plasma levels of total IgE ($P = 0.007$), IgG_2 ($P = 0.029$) and IgG_3 ($P = 0.0343$), as well as cow's milk protein-specific IgG_1 ($P = 0.015$), suggesting that FOS and GOS supplementation induces an antiallergic antibody profile (Nauta et al 2008).

These same infants were followed up over the next 18 months. Those infants who received the prebiotic-enhanced formula for the first 6 months of life were at reduced risk of developing atopic disease over the follow-up period. Infants in the control group experienced a significantly higher rate of atopic disease, such as atopic dermatitis (27.9% vs 13.6%), recurrent wheezing (20.6% vs 7.6%) and allergic urticaria (10.3% vs 1.5%) compared to infants in the prebiotic group (all $P < 0.05$) (Arslanoglu et al 2010).

A Cochrane systematic review (Osborn & Sinn 2013) investigated the effectiveness of prebiotics for the prevention of allergic disease or food hypersensitivity in infants. Four studies including 1428 infants were eligible for inclusion. Meta-analysis of two studies (226 infants) found no significant difference in rates of infant asthma, although significant heterogeneity was observed between the two studies. Meta-analysis of four studies found a significant reduction in eczema incidence in the prebiotic-treated groups (1218 infants, typical risk ratio 0.68; $P = 0.03$), with no statistically significant heterogeneity found between studies.

Improved immune response

Prebiotics, like FOS, have long been suggested to have immune-enhancing effects (Bornet & Brouns 2002, Watz et al 2005). It is, however, only recently that human trials with hard end points have been completed, in both children and adults.

Use in children

Various studies have evaluated whether long-term prebiotic use reduces the incidence of various infections and reduces the use of antibiotic medication, overall producing positive results.

One of the first of these trials investigated the effects of a prebiotic mixture (containing a combination of FOS and GOS) in protecting against infection during the first 6 months of life in formula-fed infants. In this randomised, double-blind, placebo-controlled trial, infants allocated to the prebiotic group experienced significantly fewer episodes of all types of infections combined ($P = 0.01$) compared to those in the placebo group. There was also a trend for fewer episodes of upper respiratory tract infection ($P = 0.07$) and fewer infections requiring antibiotic treatment ($P = 0.10$) in the prebiotic group. Additionally, the cumulative incidence of recurring infection and recurring respiratory tract infection was 3.9% and 2.9% in the prebiotic group versus 13.5% and 9.6% in the placebo group, respectively ($P < 0.05$) (Arslanoglu et al 2008).

This same infant cohort was followed up over the next 1.5 years. Those infants who received the prebiotic-enhanced formula for the first 6 months of life experienced significantly fewer episodes of medically-diagnosed respiratory tract infections ($P <$ 0.01), fever episodes ($P < 0.00001$) and fewer antibiotic prescriptions ($P < 0.05$) compared to those in the placebo group (Arslanoglu et al 2010).

In an open-label, placebo-controlled, randomised study, Bruzzese et al (2009) also investigated the efficacy of a prebiotic-enhanced infant formula (a combination of GOS and FOS) on infection incidence in infants. The prebiotic-enhanced formula or a standard infant formula was consumed over the initial 12 months of life. During this period, the incidence of gastroenteritis was 59% lower in the prebiotic group ($P = 0.015$). Additionally, the number of children suffering from recurrent upper respiratory tract infections tended to be lower in the prebiotic group (28% vs 45%; $P = 0.06$) and the number of children prescribed multiple antibiotic courses per year was also lower (40% vs 66%; $P =$ 0.004).

A shorter double-blind RCT was conducted involving children (aged 7–19 months) attending day-care centres. The authors found that 21 days of treatment with FOS significantly reduced the number of infectious diseases requiring antibiotic treatment ($P < 0.001$), episodes of diarrhoea and vomiting ($P < 0.001$) and episodes of fever ($P <$ 0.05) compared to controls (Waligora-Dupriet et al

2007). In another RCT investigating the effects of FOS in toddlers (4–24-month-olds) attending day care, FOS administration was found to significantly reduce antibiotic use (32% reduction; $P = 0.001$) and day-care absenteeism (61% decrease; $P = 0.025$) compared to those in the control group. There was also a 34% reduction in episodes of fever in combination with any cold symptoms ($P = 0.001$) and a 61% decrease in episodes of fever in association with diarrhoea ($P < 0.05$) in the FOS-supplemented group (Saavedra & Tschernia 2002).

Use in adults

Treatment with GOS for 8 weeks around exam time had multiple beneficial effects according to a double-blind RCT involving 427 academically stressed undergraduate students. Students received placebo, 2.5 or 5.0 g GOS daily for 8 weeks. Active treatment resulted in a significant reduction in stress-induced gastrointestinal symptoms such as diarrhoea ($P = 0.0298$) and constipation ($P = 0.0003$). Additionally, the lower dose of GOS was associated with lower cold and flu symptom intensity. The higher dose was found to reduce the probability of having a sick day by 40% in normal-weight individuals ($P = 0.0002$). However, this protective effect was not observed in overweight or obese patients. The authors theorised that the lack of efficacy in overweight patients was due to differences in the baseline microbiota (e.g. fewer bifidobacteria) (Hughes et al 2011).

In another randomised, double-blind, placebo-controlled, crossover trial, the impact of GOS supplementation (2.75 g/day) on immune parameters in healthy elderly subjects was assessed. Forty-four subjects took part in this 24-week trial (2 × 10-week treatment periods with a 4-week washout in between). Ten weeks of GOS supplementation was found to not only significantly increase faecal populations of bifidobacteria and decrease the quantity of less beneficial bacteria (*E. coli*, *Bacteroides* spp., *Clostridium* spp. and *Desulfovibrio* spp.) compared to the control period, but also significantly increase NK cell activity, phagocytic activity of leucocytes and the production of the anti-inflammatory cytokine IL-10. GOS supplementation also resulted in a significant reduction in the production of proinflammatory cytokines (IL-6, IL-1beta and tumour necrosis factor-alpha) (Vulevic et al 2008).

Prebiotic supplementation has also been tested in an HIV-positive population, showing benefits. In a double-blind RCT, 57 highly active antiretroviral therapy (HAART)-naive HIV-1-infected adults received either a unique prebiotic mixture (GOS, long-chain FOS and pectin hydrolysate-derived acidic oligosaccharides) or placebo for 12 weeks. Subjects in the prebiotic group demonstrated significant improvements in the gut microbiota composition, a reduction of soluble CD14 and $CD4^+$ T-cell activation and increased NK cell activity compared to controls (Gori et al 2011).

Cancer of the colon

Administration of lactulose or oligofructose-enriched inulin to healthy volunteers resulted in a significant decrease in colonic beta-glucuronidase activity, which is considered protective against colon cancer development (De Preter et al 2008). A randomised, double-blind, placebo-controlled study investigated the effects of a synbiotic mixture on immune modulation in patients with colon cancer ($n = 34$) post 'curative resection' and polypectomised patients ($n = 40$). The synbiotic-treated group received encapsulated *Lactobacillus rhamnosus* GG 1×10^{10} CFU + *Bifidobacterium lactis* Bb12 1×10^{10} CFU plus 10 g of inulin enriched with oligofructose on a daily basis for 12 weeks. Overall, both groups receiving the synbiotic treatment demonstrated minor effects on some of the immune markers (Roller et al 2007). Likewise, in another randomised, double-blind, placebo-controlled study of 80 patients (37 colon cancer and 43 polypectomised) by this group, a number of colorectal cancer biomarkers were positively affected by 12 weeks' synbiotic treatment (Rafter et al 2007).

A randomised clinical trial conducted by Roncucci et al (1993) demonstrated the ability of lactulose to prevent the growth of resected colorectal polyps. Lactulose administration (20 g/day) reduced the recurrence rates of colonic polyps by 66% ($P < 0.02$) as compared to controls.

Prevention of urinary tract infections

Two human studies have demonstrated the efficacy of lactulose therapy in the prevention of urinary tract infections. McCutcheon and Fulton (1989) conducted a retrospective study using 45 elderly, long-term hospital patients as subjects. The study found that daily lactulose therapy for 6 months (30 mL lactulose syrup/day) resulted in a significant reduction in urinary tract infections compared to controls ($P < 0.025$). Sixteen of the 17 lactulose-treated patients (94%) remained infection-free over the 6 months, compared to 16 of the 28 control patients (57%) ($P < 0.005$). In addition, there was a significant reduction in the number of antibiotic prescriptions ($P < 0.05$) and in the number of patients receiving antibiotics ($P < 0.005$) in the lactulose group.

In the second study, Mack et al (cited in Conn 1997) enrolled 75 elderly, hospitalised patients in a randomised, placebo-controlled trial. Thirty-eight patients received the placebo and 58 received lactulose therapy. Twelve per cent of the lactulose group developed urinary tract infections during the period of follow-up, compared to 32% in the control group ($P < 0.01$).

Bone health

Calcium absorption was significantly increased ($P = 0.04$) in women ingesting a yoghurt drink (2 × 200 mL/day) rich in GOS (20 g/day) according to a double-blind, crossover RCT. The study used a

9-day intervention period and involved 12 menopausal women (van den Heuvel et al 2000).

Griffin et al (2002) conducted a larger, randomised, crossover study of 59 young girls to investigate the effect of either inulin or inulin plus oligofructose (8 g/day) taken for 3 weeks in addition to 1500 mg/day calcium (two glasses of calcium-fortified orange juice); at the end of the study, the inulin plus oligofructose-treated group was reported to have significantly higher calcium absorption. Research by Abrams et al (2005) has supported these findings.

Promotion of satiety

FOS supplementation affects satiety and hunger, according to a single-blind, crossover, placebo-controlled trial (Cani et al 2006). Subjects who ingested 8 g of FOS twice daily (with breakfast and dinner) experienced a significant increase in satiety at both meals (both $P = 0.04$), but not at lunch. At dinner, FOS supplementation was also found to reduce hunger ($P = 0.04$) and prospective food consumption ($P = 0.05$). Energy intake at breakfast ($P = 0.01$) and lunch ($P = 0.03$) was also found to be significantly reduced after FOS supplementation, resulting in a 5% decrease in total energy intake per day.

A later double-blind RCT investigated the effects of a higher dose (21 g/day) of FOS over a 12-week period and found that active treatment resulted in a mean reduction of 1.03 kg bodyweight compared to a 0.45 kg increase in weight in the placebo group ($P = 0.01$). FOS consumption was also associated with a lower area under the curve (AUC) for ghrelin ($P = 0.004$) and a higher AUC for peptide YY ($P = 0.03$), suggesting an upregulation of satiety hormone secretion. These changes coincided with a reduction in self-reported caloric intake ($P < 0.05$). Serum glucose concentrations and insulin levels also significantly improved in the FOS group compared to baseline measures (both $P < 0.05$) (Parnell & Reimer 2009).

Metabolic syndrome

Treatment with GOS (2.75 g/day) for 12 weeks resulted in significant decreases in levels of plasma C-reactive protein ($P < 0.0012$), insulin ($P < 0.005$), total cholesterol ($P < 0.001$) and triglycerides ($P < 0.0005$) compared to placebo in a double-blind, crossover RCT involving 45 overweight adults with three or more risk factors associated with metabolic syndrome. The decreases in total cholesterol and triglycerides, while statistically significant, was not of a magnitude considered clinically significant (Vulevic et al 2013).

OTHER USES

Liver disease — hepatic encephalopathy

Lactulose has been used routinely as part of the treatment for hepatic encephalopathy, although the exact mechanism of its action is still undetermined. Lactulose treatment results in normalising of the intestinal microflora, lowering faecal pH, decreasing colonic ammonia production and increasing nitrogen excretion (Ballongue et al 1997, Elkington et al 1969). A meta-analysis of prebiotics in the treatment of minimal hepatic encephalopathy found lactulose treatment (five studies) to be associated with significant improvement in the condition (Shukla et al 2011). Lactulose therapy has also recently found in RCTs to effectively prevent the development of hepatic encephalopathy in patients with liver cirrhosis (Sharma et al 2012, Wen et al 2013).

Pancreatitis

Some studies have found that synbiotic supplementation was more beneficial than prebiotics alone for improved systemic inflammatory response in patients with acute pancreatitis (Olah et al 2005).

DOSAGE RANGE

Lactulose, FOS and GOS have all demonstrated dose-dependent responses in terms of altering the GIT microbiota, with larger doses inducing greater beneficial changes in the ecosystem. However, prebiotics are known to induce gastrointestinal side effects, such as abdominal pain, bloating, borborygmi and excessive flatulence when used in high doses; these symptoms tend to diminish over time or with dose reduction. Hence, the initial dose should be small and increased gradually dependent on gastrointestinal tolerance. Therapeutic dosage ranges are as follows: GOS: 2.5–20 g/day; FOS: 4–40 g/day; lactulose: 3–40 g/day.

TOXICITY

Overall, prebiotics have a good profile but their consumption can result in some adverse gastrointestinal side effects. (See Adverse reactions, below.)

P

ADVERSE REACTIONS

There are many reports of transient gastrointestinal side effects of prebiotic treatment; symptoms such as abdominal pain, bloating, diarrhoea and increased flatulence are commonly reported. The severity of the symptoms is dose-dependent.

A potentially more troubling aspect of prebiotic prescription is their possible enhancement of bacterial translocation, although the research results have been mixed, with some research finding a protective effect and other research finding the opposite, and others no effect. Studies in rats have shown that both inulin and FOS supplementation not only increased intestinal lactobacilli and bifidobacteria colonisation, but also enhanced translocation of *Salmonella enterica* serovar *enteritidis* and the caecal contents also contained *Salmonella*, although concurrent calcium intake was noted to resolve this problem (Bovee-Oudenhoven et al 2003, Ten Bruggencate et al 2004). On the other hand, reduced bacterial translocation to the liver has been reported in rats with dextran sulfate sodium-induced colitis when fed FOS (Osman et al 2006) and feeding mice a combination of FOS and inulin was found to protect against *Klebsiella pneumoniae* translocation (Silva et al 2009). In piglets, the addition of GOS or polydextrose to their diet had no impact on rates of bacterial translocation (Monaco et al 2011). In a human study of 72 elective surgery patients, synbiotic feeding (FOS in combination with four strains of probiotic bacteria) did not result in increased bacterial translocation (Anderson et al 2004).

A published case study has described an instance of anaphylaxis attributed to inulin found in vegetables and processed foods. This was later confirmed with skinprick testing and blinded food provocation testing (Gay-Crosier et al 2000). This allergy appears to be extremely rare considering the widespread consumption of FOS-containing foods. There is also one report describing an allergic reaction to lactulose ingestion in a child with severe milk allergy, presumably due to contamination of trace amounts of cow's milk protein in the preparation used (Maiello et al 2011).

SIGNIFICANT INTERACTIONS

Controlled studies are not available and at present there are no known drug interactions with prebiotics.

CONTRAINDICATIONS AND PRECAUTIONS

Prebiotics/synbiotics are contraindicated in those people who are hypersensitive to any component of the prebiotics/synbiotics-containing product. People with IBS who may have increased gas production should avoid high intakes of prebiotics (Serra et al 2001); low doses of GOS have, however, been found to decrease gas-related symptoms in IBS patients (Silk et al 2009). People with lactose intolerance should use lactulose with caution, as its use may cause more gastrointestinal adverse events than in lactose digesters (Teuri et al 1999). On the other hand, long-term ingestion of lactulose in lactose maldigesters has been found to increase their tolerance to lactose (Szilagyi et al 2001). Patients with fructose intolerance may also be more sensitive to the gastrointestinal adverse effects of FOS (Shepherd et al 2008).

One research group has found FOS intake to promote bacterial translocation and increase mucosal irritation in an animal model of *Salmonella* infection (Bovee-Oudenhoven et al 2003, Ten Bruggencate et al 2005). Hence, FOS supplementation may be contraindicated in patients with *Salmonella* enteritis.

PREGNANCY USE

Prebiotics found in the food chain (FOS, inulin and GOS) are considered safe to consume in pregnancy. Lactulose in laxative doses (10–20+ g in a single dose) carries a category B classification (Prather 2004).

Practice points/Patient counselling

- Prebiotics can be obtained from foods such as artichoke, Jerusalem artichokes, asparagus, bananas, chicory root, garlic, leek, onions and wheat, although not necessarily in clinically relevant amounts.
- Prebiotics may be combined with probiotics to produce synbiotics that will enable the two components to work together in synergy.
- Although prebiotics may improve the long-term bowel flora, prebiotic supplementation has many other benefits not associated with improvement in the ecosystem of the GIT.
- There is some evidence that prebiotics support both the development and the maintenance of a healthy immune system.
- Prebiotics have been used in the management of diarrhoea, constipation, other gastrointestinal disorders, bone health, allergic disease and food sensitivity.
- Continuous intake of prebiotics is required in order to maintain their health benefits.
- Some individuals may experience greater gastrointestinal discomfort with use, although some symptoms may subside over time and dose reduction can improve tolerance.

PATIENTS' FAQs

What will this supplement do for me?

Studies have shown that prebiotics are beneficial in the treatment of digestive disorders such as diarrhoea, constipation and some IBDs, such as ulcerative colitis, and also other conditions, such as IBS, food allergies and eczema. There is some evidence that prebiotics may be useful for bone health.

When will it start to work?

Usually prebiotics can exert beneficial effects for digestive disorders such as constipation and diarrhoea within 1–2 weeks, although continuous use for several weeks/months may produce long-term benefits and be necessary in the treatment of other disorders.

Are there any safety issues?

Generally, prebiotics have a good safety profile; however, high-dose supplementation can cause a number of gastrointestinal adverse effects, such as bloating, distension and increased flatulence. These effects are most often noted at the beginning of prebiotic therapy and are generally dose-related. Hence, in some patients it is advisable to commence prebiotic supplementation at a low dose and slowly increase to achieve the optimal dose over several weeks.

REFERENCES

Abrams SA et al. A combination of prebiotic short- and long-chain inulin-type fructans enhances calcium absorption and bone mineralization in young adolescents. Am J Clin Nutr 82.2 (2005): 471–476.

Anderson AD et al. Randomised clinical trial of synbiotic therapy in elective surgical patients. Gut 53 (2004): 241–245.

Arslanoglu S et al. Early dietary intervention with a mixture of prebiotic oligosaccharides reduces the incidence of allergic manifestations and infections during the first two years of life. J Nutr 138 (2008): 1091–1095.

Arslanoglu, S., et al. 2010. Early dietary intervention with a mixture of prebiotic oligosaccharides reduces the incidence of allergic manifestations and infections during the first two years of life. J Nutr, 138, 1091–1095.

Ballongue et al. Effects of lactulose and lactitol on colonic microflora and enzymatic activity. Scand J Gastroenterol 32.222 (1997): 41–44.

Benjamin, J. L., et al. 2011. Randomised, double-blind, placebo-controlled trial of fructo-oligosaccharides in active Crohn's disease. Gut, 60, 923–929.

Bjorksten B et al. Allergy development and the intestinal microflora during the first year of life. J Allergy Clin Immunol 108 (2001): 516–520.

Bornet, F. R. & Brouns, F. 2002. Immune-stimulating and gut health-promoting properties of short-chain fructo-oligosaccharides. Nutrition Reviews, 60, 326–334.

Bouhnik Y et al. Administration of transgalacto-oligosaccharides increases fecal bifidobacteria and modifies colonic fermentation metabolism in healthy humans. J Nutr 127 (1997): 444–448.

Bovee-Oudenhoven IM et al. Dietary fructo-oligosaccharides and lactulose inhibit intestinal colonisation but stimulate translocation of salmonella in rats. Gut 52 (2003): 1572–1578.

Brunser O et al. Effects of probiotic or prebiotic supplemented milk formulas on fecal microbiota composition of infants. Asia Pac J Clin Nutr 15 (2006): 368–376.

Bruzzese, E., et al. 2009. A formula containing galacto- and fructo-oligosaccharides prevents intestinal and extra-intestinal infections: An observational study. Clin Nutr, 28, 156–161.

Cani, P. D., et al. 2006. Oligofructose promotes satiety in healthy human: a pilot study. European Journal of Clinical Nutrition, 60, 567–572.

Casellas F et al. Oral oligofructose-enriched inulin supplementation in acute ulcerative colitis is well tolerated and associated with lowered faecal calprotectin. Aliment Pharmacol Ther 25 (2007): 1061–1067.

Casiraghi, M. C., et al. 2007. Effects of a synbiotic milk product on human intestinal ecosystem. Journal of Applied Microbiology, 103, 499–506.

Cavin C et al. Inhibition of the expression and activity of cyclooxygenase-2 by chicory extract. Biochem Biophys Res Commun 327 (2005): 742–749.

Cherbut C, et al. The prebiotic characteristics of fructooligosaccharides are necessary for reduction of TNBS-induced colitis in rats. J Nutr 133 (2003): 21–27.

Chermesh I et al. Failure of synbiotic 2000 to prevent postoperative recurrence of Crohn's disease. Dig Dis Sci 52 (2007): 385–389.

Coppa GV et al. Prebiotics in human milk: a review. Dig Liver Dis 38 (Suppl 2) (2006): S291–S294.

Cummings JH, Macfarlane GT. Gastrointestinal effects of prebiotics. Br J Nutr 87 (Suppl 2) (2002): S145–S151.

Cummings JH, et al. A study of fructo-oligosaccharides in the prevention of traveller's diarrhoea. Aliment Pharmacol Ther 15 (2001): 1139–1145.

Delzenne NM. Oligosaccharides: state of the art. Proc Nutr Soc 62 (2003): 177–182.

Demigne C et al. Comparison of native or reformulated chicory fructans, or non-purified chicory, on rat cecal fermentation and mineral metabolism. Eur J Nutr 47 (2008): 366–374.

de Preter, V., et al 2008. Effect of dietary intervention with different pre- and probiotics on intestinal bacterial enzyme activities. Eur J Clin Nutr, 62, 225–31.

de Schryver AM et al. Effects of regular physical activity on defecation pattern in middle-aged patients complaining of chronic constipation. Scand J Gastroenterol 40 (2005): 422–429.

Drakoularakou, A., et al. 2009. A double-blind, placebo-controlled, randomized human study assessing the capacity of a novelgalacto-oligosaccharide mixture in reducing travellers' diarrhoea. European Journal of Clinical Nutrition, 64, 146–152.

Elkington SG, et al. Lactulose in the treatment of chronic portal-systemic encephalopathy. N Engl J Med 281 (1969): 408–411.

Fontaine N et al. Intestinal mucin distribution in the germ-free rat and in the heteroxenic rat harbouring a human bacterial flora: effect of inulin in the diet. Br J Nutr 75.6 (1996): 881–892.

Forchielli ML, Walker WA. The role of gut-associated lymphoid tissues and mucosal defence. Br J Nutr 93 (Suppl 1) (2005): S41–S48.

Friedman G, George J. Treatment of refractory 'pouchitis' with prebiotic and probiotic therapy. Gastroenterology 118 (2000) G4167.

Fujimori S et al. High dose probiotic and prebiotic cotherapy for remission induction of active Crohn's disease. J Gastroenterol Hepatol 22.8 (2007): 1199–1204.

Fujimori S et al. A randomised controlled trial on the efficacy of synbiotic versus probiotic or prebiotic treatment to improve the quality of life in patients with ulcerative colitis. Nutrition 25.5 (2009): 520–5.

Furrie E et al. Synbiotic therapy (*Bifidobacterium longum*/Synergy 1) initiates resolution of inflammation in patients with active ulcerative colitis: a randomised controlled pilot trial. Gut 54 (2005): 242–249.

Gay-Crosier, F., et al. 2000. Anaphylaxis from inulin in vegetables and processed food [Letter]. New England Journal of Medicine, 342, 1372.

Gibson GR. Dietary modulation of the human gut microflora using prebiotics. Br J Nutr 80 (1998): S209–S212.

Gibson GR. Dietary modulation of the human gut microflora using the prebiotics oligofructose and inulin. J Nutr 129 (1999): 1438S–41S.

Gibson GR, Roberfroid MB. Dietary modulation of the human colonic microbiota: introducing the concept of prebiotics. J Nutr 125 (1995): 1401–1412.

Gibson GR, Wang X. Regulatory effects of bifidobacteria on the growth of other colonic bacteria. J Appl Bacteriol 77 (1994): 412–420.

Gibson GR et al. Selective stimulation of bifidobacteria in the human colon by oligofructose and inulin. Gastroenterology 108 (1995): 975–982.

Gorbach SL, Chang TW, Goldin B. Successful treatment of relapsing *Clostridium difficile* colitis with Lactobacillus GG. Lancet 262.8574 (1987): 1519.

Gori, A., et al. 2011. Specific prebiotics modulate gut microbiota and immune activation in HAART-naive HIV-infected adults: results of the "COPA" pilot randomized trial. Mucosal Immunol, 4, 554–63.

Griffin IJ, et al. Non-digestible oligosaccharides and calcium absorption in girls with adequate calcium intakes. Br J Nutr 87 (Suppl 2) (2002): S187–S191.

Hafer A et al. Effect of oral lactulose on clinical and immunohistochemical parameters in patients with inflammatory bowel disease: a pilot study. BMC Gastroenterol 7 (2007): 36.

Hawrelak, J. A. & Myers, S. P. 2004. Intestinal dysbiosis: A review of the literature. Alternative Medicine Review, 9, 180–197.

Holma R et al. Galacto-oligosaccharides stimulate the growth of bifidobacteria but fail to attenuate inflammation in experimental colitis in rats. Scand J Gastroenterol 37 (2002): 1042–1047.

Hooshmand, S., et al. 2010. Combination of genistin and fructooligosaccharides prevents bone loss in ovarian hormone deficiency. J Med Food, 13, 320–5.

Hopkins MJ, Macfarlane GT. Nondigestible oligosaccharides enhance bacterial colonisation resistance against *Clostridium difficile* in vitro. Appl Environ Microbiol 69 (2003): 1920–1927.

Hudson, M. J. & Marsh, P. D. 1995. Carbohydrate metabolism in the colon. In: Gibson, G. R. & Macfarlane, G. T. (eds.) Human Colonic Bacteria: Role in Nutrition, Physiology, and Pathology. Boca Raton: CRC Press.

Hughes, C., et al. 2011. Galactooligosaccharide supplementation reduces stress-induced gastrointestinal dysfunction and days of cold or flu: a randomized, double-blind, controlled trial in healthy university students. Am J Clin Nutr, 93, 1305–11.

Hunter JO, et al. Controlled trial of oligofructose in the management of irritable bowel syndrome. J Nutr 129 (7 Suppl) (1999): 1451S–3S.

Kilkkinen, A., et al. 2002. Use of oral antimicrobials decreases serum enterolactone concentration. American Journal of Epidemiology, 155, 472–477.

Kimira, Y., et al. 2012. Synergistic effect of isoflavone glycosides and fructooligosaccharides on postgastrectomy osteopenia in rats. J Clin Biochem Nutr, 51, 156–60.

King TS, et al. Abnormal colonic fermentation in irritable bowel syndrome. Lancet 352 (1998): 1187–1189.

Kinoshita M, et al. Butyrate reduces colonic paracellular permeability by enhancing PPARgamma activation. Biochem Biophys Res Commun 293 (2002): 827–831.

Koleva, P. T., et al. 2012. Inulin and fructo-oligosaccharides have divergent effects on colitis and commensal microbiota in HLA-B27 transgenic rats. Br J Nutr, 108, 1633–43.

Langlands SJ et al. Prebiotic carbohydrates modify the mucosa associated microflora of the human large bowel. Gut 53 (2004): 1610–1616.

Lara-Villoslada, F., et al. 2006. Short-chain fructooligosaccharides, in spite of being fermented in the upper part of the large intestine, have anti-inflammatory activity in the TNBS model of colitis. Eur J Nutr, 45, 418–25.

Le Leu RK et al. A synbiotic combination of resistant starch and *Bifidobacterium lactis* facilitates apoptotic deletion of carcinogen-damaged cells in rat colon. J Nutr 135 (2005): 996–1001.

Lewis S, et al. Effect of the prebiotic oligofructose on relapse of *Clostridium difficile*-associated diarrhoea: a randomised controlled study. Clin Gastroenterol Hepatol 3 (2005a): 442–8.

Lewis S et al. Failure of dietary oligofructose to prevent antibiotic-associated diarrhoea. Aliment Pharmacol Ther 21 (2005b): 469 77.

Lindsay JO et al. Clinical, microbiological, and immunological effects of fructo-oligosaccharide in patients with Crohn's disease. Gut 55 (2006): 348–355.

Looijer–Van Langen, M. A. C. & Dieleman, L. A. 2009. Prebiotics in chronic intestinal inflammation. Inflammatory Bowel Diseases, 15, 454–462.

P

Macfarlane S, et al. Review article: prebiotics in the gastrointestinal tract. Aliment Pharmacol Ther 24.5 (2006): 701–714.
Maiello, N., et al. 2011. Severe allergic reaction to lactulose in a child with milk allergy. Annals of Allergy, Asthma & Immunology, 107, 85.
McCutcheon, J. & Fulton, J. D. 1989. Lowered prevalence of infection with lactulose therapy in patients in long-term hospital care. Journal of Hospital Infection, 13, 81–86.
Millard AL et al. Butyrate affects differentiation, maturation and function of human monocyte-derived dendritic cells and macrophages. Clin Exp Immunol 130 (2002): 245–255.
Monaco, M. H., et al. 2011. Addition of polydextrose and galactooligosaccharide to formula does not affect bacterial translocation in the neonatal piglet. J Pediatr Gastroenterol Nutr, 52, 210–6.
Moro G et al. A mixture of prebiotic oligosaccharides reduces the incidence of atopic dermatitis during the first six months of age. Arch Dis Child 91 (2006): 814–819.
Nauta, A. J., et al. 2008. A specific mixture of short-chain galacto-oligosaccharides and long-chain fructo-oligosaccharides induced an anti-allergic Ig profile in infants at risk for allergy. Proceedings of the Nutrition Society, 67, E82.
Niittyen, L., et al. 2007. Galacto-oligosaccharides and bowel function. Scandinavian Journal of Food and Nutrition, 51, 62–66.
Ohta, A., et al. 2002. A combination of dietary fructooligosaccharides and isoflavone conjugates increases femoral bone mineral density and equol production in ovariectomized mice. Journal of Nutrition, 132, 2048–2054.
Olah A et al. Combination of early nasojejunal feeding with modern synbiotic therapy in the treatment of severe acute pancreatitis (prospective, randomised, double-blind study). Magy Seb 58 (2005): 173–178.
Olesen M, Gudmand-Hoyer E. Efficacy, safety, and tolerability of fructooligosaccharides in the treatment of irritable bowel syndrome. Am J Clin Nutr 72.6 (2000): 1570–1575.
Osborn DA, Sinn JK. Prebiotics in infants for prevention of allergic disease and food sensitivity. Cochrane Database Syst Rev Oct 17.4 (2013): CD006474.
Osman N et al. Bifidobacterium infantis strains with and without a combination of oligofructose and inulin (OFI) attenuate inflammation in DSS-induced colitis in rats. BMC Gastroenterol 6 (2006): 31.
Ouwehand A, et al. The role of the intestinal microflora for the development of the immune system in early childhood. Eur J Nutr 41 (Suppl 1) (2002): 132–137.
Parnell, J. A. & Reimer, R. A. 2009. Weight loss during oligofructose supplementation is associated with decreased ghrelin and increased peptide YY in overweight and obese adults. Am J Clin Nutr, 89, 1751–1759.
Paturi, G., et al. 2012. Effects of early dietary intervention with a fermentable fibre on colonic microbiota activity and mucin gene expression in newly weaned rats. Journal of Functional Foods, 4, 520–530.
Petticrew M, et al. Systematic review of the effectiveness of laxatives in the elderly. Health Technol Assess 1 (1997): 1–52.
Pool-Zobel BL, Sauer J. Overview of experimental data on reduction of colorectal cancer risk by inulin-type fructans. J Nutr 137 (2007): 2580S–4S.
Prather, C. 2004. Pregnancy-related constipation. Current Gastroenterology Reports, 6, 402–404.
Rafter J et al. Dietary synbiotics reduce cancer risk factors in polypectomized and colon cancer patients. Am J Clin Nutr 85.2 (2007): 488–496.
Roberfroid MB. Inulin-type fructans: functional food ingredients. J Nutr 137.11 (2007a): 2493S–502S.
Roberfroid, M. 2007b. Prebiotics: the concept revisited. J Nutr, 137, 830S-7S.
Roller M et al. Intestinal immunity of rats with colon cancer is modulated by oligofructose-enriched inulin combined with *Lactobacillus rhamnosus* and *Bifidobacterium lactis*. Br J Nutr 92 (2004): 931.
Roller M et al. Consumption of prebiotic inulin enriched with oligofructose in combination with the probiotics *Lactobacillus rhamnosus* and *Bifidobacterium lactis* has minor effects on selected immune parameters in polypectomised and colon cancer patients. Br J Nutr 97.4 (2007): 676–684.
Roncucci, L., et al. 1993. Antioxidant vitamins or lactulose for the prevention of the recurrence of colorectal polyps. Diseases of the Colon and Rectum, 67, 227–234.
Rowland IR et al. Effect of *Bifidobacterium longum* and inulin on gut bacterial metabolism and carcinogen-induced aberrant crypt foci in rats. Carcinogenesis 19 (1998): 281–285.
Saavedra, J. M. & Tschernia, A. 2002. Human studies with probiotics and prebiotics: clinical implications. Br J Nutr, 87 (suppl 2), S241–S246.
Saavedra JM et al. Feeding of *Bifidobacterium bifidum* and *Streptococcus thermophilus* to infants in hospital for prevention of diarrhea and shedding of rotavirus. Lancet 344 (1994): 1046–1049.
Saemann MD et al. Anti-inflammatory effects of sodium butyrate on human monocytes: potent inhibition of IL-12 and up-regulation of IL-10 production. FASEB J 14 (2000): 2380–2382.
Salminen S et al. Demonstration of safety of probiotics: a review. Int J Food Microbiol 44.1–2 (1998): 93–106.
Sartor RB. Therapeutic manipulation of the enteric microflora in inflammatory bowel diseases: antibiotics, probiotics, and prebiotics. Gastroenterology 126 (2004): 1620–1633.
Schrezenmeir, J. & de Vrese, M. 2001. Probiotics, prebiotics, and synbiotics-approaching a definition. American Journal of Clinical Nutrition, 73, 361–364.
Searle, L. E., et al. 2009. A mixture containing galactooligosaccharide, produced by the enzymic activity of *Bifidobacterium bifidum*, reduces *Salmonella enterica* serovar *Typhimurium* infection in mice. Journal of Medical Microbiology, 58, 37–48.
Segain JP et al. Butyrate inhibits inflammatory responses through NFkappaB inhibition: implications for Crohn's disease. Gut 47 (2000): 397–403.
Serra J, et al. Impaired transit and tolerance of intestinal gas in the irritable bowel syndrome. Gut 48 (2001): 14–19.
Sharma, P., et al. 2012. Primary prophylaxis of overt hepatic encephalopathy in patients with cirrhosis: an open labeled randomized controlled trial of lactulose versus no lactulose. J Gastroenterol Hepatol, 27, 1329–35.
Shepherd, S. J., et al. 2008. Dietary Triggers of Abdominal Symptoms in Patients With Irritable Bowel Syndrome: Randomized Placebo-Controlled Evidence. Clinical Gastroenterology and Hepatology, 6, 765–771.
Shoaf K et al. Prebiotic galactooligosaccharides reduce adherence of enteropathogenic *Escherichia coli* to tissue culture cells. Infect Immun 74 (2006): 6920–6928.
Shoaf-Sweeney KD, Hutkins RW. Adherence, anti-adherence, and oligosaccharides preventing pathogens from sticking to the host. Adv Food Nutr Res 55 (2009): 101–161.
Shukla, S., et al. 2011. Meta-analysis: the effects of gut flora modulation using prebiotics, probiotics and synbiotics on minimal hepatic encephalopathy. Aliment Pharmacol Ther, 33, 662–71.
Silk, D. B., et al. 2009. Clinical trial: the effects of a trans-galactooligosaccharide prebiotic on faecal microbiota and symptoms in irritable bowel syndrome. Alimentary Pharmacology & Therapeutics, 29, 508–518.
Silva, D. F. D., et al. 2009. Translocation of *Klebsiella* sp. in mice fed an enteral diet containing prebiotics. Revista de Nutrição, 22, 229–235.
Sinclair, H. R., et al. 2009. Galactooligosaccharides (GOS) inhibit *Vibrio cholerae* toxin binding to its GM1 receptor. J Agric Food Chem, 57, 3113–3119.
Szilagyi, A., et al. 2001. Improved parameters of lactose maldigestion using lactulose. Dig Dis Sci, 46, 1509–19.
Ten Bruggencate SJ et al. Dietary fructo-oligosaccharides and inulin decrease resistance of rats to salmonella: protective role of calcium. Gut 53 (2004): 530–535.
Ten Bruggencate, S. J. M., et al. 2005. Dietary Fructooligosaccharides Increase Intestinal Permeability in Rats. The Journal of Nutrition, 135, 837–842.
Ten Bruggencate, S. J. M., et al. 2006. Dietary Fructooligosaccharides Affect Intestinal Barrier Function in Healthy Men. The Journal of Nutrition, 136, 70–74.
Teramoto, F., et al. 1996. Effect of 4- B -D-galactosylsucrose (lactosucrose) on fecal microflora in patients with chronic inflammatory bowel disease. Journal of Gastroenterology, 31, 33–39.
Teuri, U. & Korpela, R. 1998. Galacto-oligosaccharides relieve constipation in elderly people. Annals of Nutrition and Metabolism, 42, 319–327.
Teuri, U., et al. 1999. Fructooligosaccharides and lactulose cause more symptoms in lactose maldigesters and subjects with pseudohypolactasia than in control lactose digesters. The American Journal of Clinical Nutrition, 69, 973–979.
Uehara, M., et al. 2001. Dietary fructooligosaccharides modify intestinal bioavailability of a single dose of genistein and daidzein and affect their urinary excretion and kinetics in blood of rats. Journal of Nutrition, 131, 787–795.
Van den Heuvel EG, et al. Transgalactooligosaccharides stimulate calcium absorption in postmenopausal women. J Nutr 130.12 (2000): 2938–2942.
Van Loo, J., et al. 1995. On the presence of inulin and oligofructose as natural ingredients in the Western diet. Critical Reviews in Food Science and Nutrition, 35, 525–552.
Van Loo, J., et al. 1998. Functional food properties of non-digestible oligosaccharides: a consensus report from the ENDO project (DGXII AIRII-CT94-1095). British Journal of Nutrition, 81, 121–132.
Vulevic, J., et al. 2008. Modulation of the fecal microflora profile and immune function by a novel trans-galactooligosaccharide mixture (B-GOS) in healthy elderly volunteers. Am J Clin Nutr, 88, 1438–46.

Vulevic, J., et al. 2013. A Mixture of trans-Galactooligosaccharides Reduces Markers of Metabolic Syndrome and Modulates the Fecal Microbiota and Immune Function of Overweight Adults. J Nutr, 143, 324–31.
Waligora-Dupriet, A. J., et al. 2007. Effect of oligofructose supplementation on gut microflora and well-being in young children attending a day care centre. Int J Food Microbiol, 113, 108–113.
Walker AW et al. pH and peptide supply can radically alter bacterial populations and short-chain fatty acid ratios within microbial communities from the human colon. Appl Environ Microbiol 71 (2005): 3692–3700.
Watz, B., et al. 2005. Inulin, oligofructose and immunomodulation. Br J Nutr, 93, S49–S55.
Welters CF et al. Effect of dietary inulin supplementation on inflammation of pouch mucosa in patients with an ileal pouch-anal anastomosis. Dis Colon Rectum 45 (2002): 621–627.
Wen, J., et al. 2013. Lactulose is highly potential in prophylaxis of hepatic encephalopathy in patients with cirrhosis and upper gastrointestinal bleeding: results of a controlled randomized trial. Digestion, 87, 132–8.
Yang ST, Silva EM. Novel products and new technologies for use of a familiar carbohydrate, milk lactose. J Dairy Sci 78 (1995): 2541–2562.
Yasuda, A., et al. 2012. Dietary supplementation with fructooligosaccharides attenuates allergic peritonitis in mice. Biochemical and Biophysical Research Communications, 422, 546–550.
Zopf D, Roth S. Oligosaccharide anti-infective agents. Lancet 347 (1996): 1017–1021.

Probiotics

HISTORICAL NOTE There is a long history of consuming fermented foods and beverages containing microorganisms to improve health. The term 'probiotic' is derived from Greek and means 'for life'. As far back as 1907, Metchnikoff, the Nobel laureate, popularised the idea that fermented milk products could beneficially alter the microflora of the gastrointestinal tract (GIT). He believed that many diseases, and even ageing itself, were caused by putrefaction of protein in the bowel by intestinal bacteria. Lactic acid-producing bacteria were thought to be able to inhibit the growth of putrefactive bacteria in the intestines and, thus, yoghurt consumption was recommended to correct this 'autointoxication' and improve the composition of the microflora (Metchnikoff 1907). The term 'probiotics' was first coined in 1965 and has since been applied to those live microorganisms that are able to promote health when consumed in sufficient quantities (FAO/WHO 2001). This definition includes fermented foods, as well as specific supplements containing freeze-dried bacteria. Although it has taken more than a century for scientists to investigate their health benefits, there are now several thousand studies published on probiotics, the majority published since 2000.

BACKGROUND AND RELEVANT PHARMACOKINETICS

Prior to birth, the GIT of the neonate is generally considered completely sterile, although new research findings suggest that there may be some degree of transfer from the mother's microbiota in utero. During delivery, the newborn is inoculated with microorganisms from the birth canal (ideally) and the mother's faecal flora, as well as from organisms in the environment (Matamoros et al 2013). Subsequently, growth of normal gut flora is influenced by factors such as composition of the maternal GIT microbiota, diet (breast milk vs formula), degree of hygiene, use of antibiotics or other medication, the environment and possibly genetic aspects. These microorganisms confer many health benefits by preventing the colonisation of the GIT with pathogenic microorganisms and by carrying out a number of biochemical functions, such as deconjugation and dehydroxylation of bile acids, the conversion of bilirubin to urobilinogen, generation of short-chain fatty acids (SCFA) and the metabolism of cholesterol to coprostanol (Bengmark 1998, Hill 1997). Additionally the microbiota modulates immune function, enhances GIT motility and gut barrier function, induces mucin production, improves digestion and nutrient absorption, metabolises xenobiotics (e.g. phyto-oestrogens), and produces vitamins K, B_1, B_2, B_6 and B_{12} (Fotiadis et al 2008, Hawrelak & Myers 2004, Isolauri 2012).

The gastrointestinal microbiota is reasonably resilient to change and remains fairly constant in adults, although research has shown that components such as pre- and probiotics can beneficially modulate the gut microflora, while antibiotics, chemotherapy, stress and a Western diet can negatively impact the ecosystem (Hawrelak & Myers 2004). It has been estimated that the intestines are host to 10^{14} microbes representing over 1000 different species (Rajilic-Stojanovic et al 2007), which includes yeasts, mostly *Candida albicans* (<0.1% of the microbiota) (Vandenplas et al 2007).

Probiotics can be obtained from the consumption of fermented foods as well as supplements. It is important to note, however, that probiotic organisms require certain characteristics to enable them to exert maximum therapeutic effects. These qualities are summarised in Table 1.

Out of these characteristics, there are some that are considered most important for a probiotic to have therapeutic effects. These are: (1) gastric acid and bile salt stability; (2) an ability to adhere to the intestinal mucosa; and (3) an ability to colonise the intestinal tract (Dunne et al 2001). Some commercially available probiotic supplements and yoghurts contain strains that do not exhibit these vital characteristics. If a probiotic strain does not exhibit these

TABLE 1 THE DESIRABLE CHARACTERISTICS OF EFFECTIVE PROBIOTIC STRAINS

Characteristics	Functional benefit
Gastric acid and bile salt stability	Survival through stomach and small intestine
Adherence to intestinal mucosa	Believed to be essential for immune cell modulation and competitive inhibition of pathogens
Colonisation of intestinal tract	Multiplication in the intestines suggests that daily ingestion may not be needed; immune cell modulation
Human origin	Human origin should translate to the ability to survive conditions in the human gastrointestinal tract, as well as the possibility of species-specific health effects
Safety in food and documented clinical safety	Adverse effects absent or minimal; accurate identification (genus, species, strain)
Production of antimicrobial compounds	Normalisation of gastrointestinal tract flora; suppressed growth of pathogens
Antagonism against pathogenic organisms	Prevention of adhesion and toxin production by pathogens
Clinically documented and validated health effects	Clinicians can be confident of therapeutic effects; dose-response data for minimum effective dosage in different formulations are known
Increased shelf-life and stability during processing	All of the above properties should be maintained during storage and processing

Adapted from Mattila-Sandholm & Salminen (1998).

characteristics, then it will be less effective than strains that do.

Recently, the concept that probiotics should be viable/live has been re-evaluated. Studies have shown that bacterial DNA sequences may have similar effects as the live bacteria in some situations, and therefore colonisation of the intestinal tract may not be a prerequisite for the action of probiotics (Jijon et al 2004, Rachmilewitz et al 2002). In addition, the mucosal immune system may not require direct contact with probiotics for beneficial effects as other routes of administration (such as the parenteral route) are also effective (Rachmilewitz et al 2004, Sheil et al 2004). However, there are significant species and strain differences between the probiotic microorganisms, and therefore, they do not all share the same characteristics.

At present, there are numerous uses of probiotics, and reports of their beneficial effects cover a wide range of diseases and conditions.

> ***Clinical note — Prebiotics and synbiotics***
> Prebiotics are components that modify the environment of the GIT to selectively favour proliferation of the beneficial intestinal microflora, lactobacilli and bifidobacteria (Gibson & Roberfroid 1995). Prebiotics include oligofructose (fructooligosaccharides), inulin, lactulose and galactooligosaccharides. (See Prebiotics monograph.) Synbiotics contain both pre- and probiotics.

CHEMICAL COMPONENTS

There are many different microorganisms currently used as probiotics in supplement and functional food form. Table 2 provides examples of commonly used probiotic species.

Common probiotic microorganisms

To better understand how bacteria are named and classified, the following discussion may be helpful. Genus is the first name of a bacterium (e.g. *Lactobacillus*). It is somewhat general and refers to a grouping of organisms based on similarity of qualities, such as physical characteristics, metabolic needs and metabolic end products. Species is a bacterium's second name (e.g. *acidophilus*). It is a much more narrow classification based on shared common characteristics that distinguish them from other species. Strain is an even more specific classification that divides members of the same species into subgroups based on several properties that a bacterial strain has that are distinct from other members of that species (e.g. strain LA5) (McKane & Kandel 1986).

FOOD SOURCES

Traditional fermented foods, such as sauerkraut (Dedicatoria et al 1981), kim chi (Cheigh et al 1994), ogi (Oyewole 1997) and kefir (Garrote et al 2001), are rich sources of probiotic organisms. The most commonly consumed probiotic food in Australia and New Zealand is yoghurt. As research has suggested that the main yoghurt-producing bacteria (*Lactobacillus delbrueckii* ssp. *bulgaricus* and *Streptococcus thermophilus*) have limited therapeutic potential,

TABLE 2 SOME ORGANISMS THAT ARE CURRENTLY USED AS PROBIOTICS (LISTED BY GENUS AND SPECIES) (GOLDIN 1998, MACFARLANE & CUMMINGS 1999, MATTILA-SANDHOLM & SALMINEN 1998)

Lactobacillus spp.	*Bifidobacterium* spp.	*Bacillus* spp.	*Streptococcus* spp.	*Enterococcus* spp.	*Saccharomyces* spp.
acidophilus	*breve*	*coagulans*	*thermophilus*	*faecium*	*cerevisiae*
plantarum	*infantis*				
rhamnosus	*longum*				
paracasei	*bifidum*				
fermentum	*thermophilum*				
reuteri	*adolescentis*				
johnsonii	*animalis*				
brevis	*lactis*				
casei					
lactis					
delbrueckii					
gasseri					

Strain selectivity of action

Within each species of bacteria there is a multitude of strains. Some probiotic strains are resilient and strong, with a demonstrated capacity to survive passage through the upper GIT and inhibit pathogenic bacteria, whereas others are weak and cannot even survive transit through the stomach. It is vital to note that, just because one strain of bacteria in a given species has a proven action or characteristic, it does not always mean that another strain will too, even if they are closely related. Strains of bacteria within the same species can have significantly different actions, properties and characteristics, as these are all essentially strain-specific qualities (Guarner et al 2011, Marteau 2011). For example, *Lactobacillus plantarum* strain 299v has been shown to effectively reduce irritable bowel syndrome (IBS) symptoms (Ducrotte et al 2012), whereas administration of *L. plantarum* strain MF1298 may actually worsens IBS symptoms (Ligaarden et al 2010). Thus, to achieve the desired therapeutic result, it is imperative to prescribe the precise probiotic strains that have demonstrated therapeutic and clinical efficacy in the condition in question. Additionally, strains that work in one condition will not necessarily be as effective in other conditions. For example, *Lactobacillus rhamnosus* GG (LGG) appears to be effective in the prevention of antibiotic-associated side effects (Arvola et al 1999) but not of any demonstrable benefit in urinary tract infections (Kontiokari et al 2001). When reviewing the Clinical Use section below, it is important to take note of the strains that were used in the summarised trials, not just the species.

human GIT-derived probiotic strains are now commonly added to yoghurt in an attempt to increase its therapeutic potential (e.g. strains of *Lactobacillus acidophilus* and *Bifidobacterium* spp.) (Molin 2001).

DEFICIENCY SIGNS AND SYMPTOMS

Clear deficiency signs are difficult to establish because the symptoms may vary enormously. Local signs and symptoms of disruption of the intestinal microflora leading to an imbalance (intestinal dysbiosis) include bloating, flatulence, abdominal pain, diarrhoea and/or constipation and fungal overgrowth (such as *Candida*). An imbalance in the gastrointestinal microflora can be caused by the use of antibiotics, GIT infections, stress and dietary factors (Hawrelak & Myers 2004). Administration of probiotics is often used as a means of restoring this microflora imbalance (Bengmark 1998, Hedin et al 2007, Hoveyda et al 2009, Kajander et al 2008, McFarland 2006, 2007, McFarland & Dublin 2008).

MAIN ACTIONS

The exact mechanisms by which probiotics accomplish their myriad of beneficial actions have become clearer over the past decade and we now know of several mechanisms that explain many of their favourable effects.

Immune modulation

A growing body of evidence indicates that some probiotic strains are capable of modulating the immune system at both the systemic and the mucosal level, affecting many cell types (e.g. epithelial cells, dendritic cells, natural killer cells). This immune response may take the form of increased secretion of immunoglobulin A (IgA) via interaction with mesenteric lymph nodes (Link-Amster et al 1994,

Walker 2008), elevated numbers of natural killer cells or enhanced phagocytic activity of macrophages (Schiffrin et al 1997). Recent research has demonstrated that dendritic cells in the lamina propria can extend their appendices between epithelial cells, and, via Toll-like receptors on their surface, sample probiotic-bacterial molecular patterns. This interaction leads to the maturation of the dendritic cells and to the release of cytokines, which orchestrate the conversion of naive T-helper cells (Th0) into a mature, balanced response of T-helper cells (Th1, Th2 and Th3/Tr1) (Walker 2008).

Anti-inflammatory activity

Probiotic strains have been shown to have anti-inflammatory effects via a number of different mechanisms. They can secrete metabolites with anti-inflammatory properties (anti-tumour necrosis factor-α [TNF-α] effects) (Ménard et al 2004), they can interact with Toll-like receptors (Rachmilewitz et al 2004), downregulate the transcription of a number of genes encoding proinflammatory effectors (Tien et al 2006) and upregulate the production of anti-inflammatory cytokines (Imaoka et al 2008).

GIT transit time modification

Some probiotic strains can modify GIT transit. Two strains of bifidobacteria have been found to significantly speed colonic transit time (Meance et al 2001, Waller et al 2011), while a strain of propionibacteria has been shown to slow descending colon transit (Bougle et al 1999). The mechanisms by which probiotics alter GIT transit time have not yet been fully elucidated; however, it is postulated that a bacterial metabolite may impact sigmoid tone and alter colonic motility (Marteau et al 2002).

Induction of oral tolerance

The GIT microflora has been shown to play a crucial role in generating an adequate population of Th2 cells that are capable of oral tolerance induction (Sudo et al 1997). In the presence of intestinal dysbiosis, some probiotic strains can also help induce oral tolerance and help protect against the development of food allergies (Prioult et al 2003).

Decrease visceral hypersensitivity

Animal research has suggested that some probiotic strains are capable of decreasing visceral hypersensitivity, believed to be one of the main contributing factors in IBS and other functional gastrointestinal disorders (Ait-Belgnaoui et al 2006, Johnson et al 2011, McKernan et al 2010). The exact mechanisms are unknown, but another lactobacilli strain has been shown to decrease visceral hypersensitivity by inducing cannabinoid and opioid receptor expression in the colonic epithelium (Rousseaux et al 2007).

Competition for gastrointestinal adhesion sites

Many pathogenic organisms must associate with the GIT epithelium in order to colonise effectively. However some strains of bifidobacteria and lactobacilli can adhere to the epithelium and act as 'colonisation barriers' by preventing pathogens from adhering to the mucosa (Fuller & Gibson 1997). This effect has been demonstrated with LGG and *L. plantarum* 299v. Both of these organisms have shown the ability to inhibit attachment of *Escherichia coli* to human colon cells (Mack et al 1999).

Antagonism against potentially pathogenic microorganisms and viruses

One of the mechanisms by which probiotics exert their beneficial effects is via inducing changes to the GIT microflora; specifically by inhibiting the growth of potentially pathogenic organisms. Some probiotic strains are capable of producing inhibitory substances such as bacteriocins, lactic acid and toxic oxygen metabolites. Of the toxic oxygen metabolites, hydrogen peroxide is of major importance as it exerts a bactericidal effect on many pathogens (Kaur et al 2002). The ability to produce bacteriocins, hydrogen peroxide and other antimicrobial compounds is strain-dependent. Probiotics have demonstrated in vitro inhibitory activity against a range of potentially pathogenic microorganisms, such as *Helicobacter pylori, Clostridium difficile, Escherichia coli, Candida albicans, Salmonella enterica, Shigella sonnei* and *Vibrio cholerae* (Hasslof et al 2010, Naaber et al 2004, Sgouras et al 2004, Spinler et al 2008). Some probiotic strains (LGG and *Bifidobacterium lactis* Bb12) can also bind to viruses, such as rotaviruses, helping to prevent mucosa-associated viral infections (Salminen et al 2010). Several probiotic strains have also demonstrated the ability to bind or remove toxins, such as aflatoxins and cyanotoxins (Salminen et al 2010), as well as inhibit the effects of bacterial toxins, such as *Clostridium difficile* toxins A and B (Castagliuolo et al 1999). Specific strains have also been found to reduce the expression of virulence factors via inhibition of pathogen gene encoding (Corr et al 2009).

Selective gastrointestinal antimicrobial activity

Ingestion of selected probiotic strains has been found to significantly increase gastrointestinal populations of beneficial bacteria (i.e. lactobacilli or bifidobacteria), while simultaneously decreasing populations of less health-promoting genera (Ahmed et al 2007, Benno et al 1996, Mohan et al 2006).

Production of beneficial compounds

The production of SCFAs as metabolic byproducts is a characteristic which almost all probiotic strains share. These SCFAs help create a healthier colonic milieu by decreasing the luminal pH and some (e.g. butyrate) are used as energy sources by colonocytes (D'Argenio & Mazzacca 1999, Ng et al 2009). Other probiotic strains can help restore normal small intestinal architecture and upregulate intestinal brush border enzyme expression via the luminal release of polyamines (Buts et al 1986, 1994, Guillot et al 1995). These strains will have clinical utility in situations of small intestinal damage and decreased brush border enzyme activity, such as coeliac disease, Crohn's disease, or after small intestinal infections.

Strengthen the intestinal barrier

A number of probiotic strains have been found to increase mucin production in the gut via increases in mucin gene expression, which provides a protective coating between the lumen and intestinal epithelial cells (Caballero-Franco et al 2007, Mack et al 2003). Probiotics are also capable of directly strengthening the intestinal barrier. A strain of *Lactobacillus plantarum* (WCSF1) has been found to decrease paracellular intestinal permeability by increasing the relocation of occludin and zonulin into the tight junction between duodenal epithelial cells (Ahrne & Hagslatt 2011). Other strains appear to enhance barrier function via the preservation of enterocyte cytoskeleton architecture and enhancement of tight junctional protein structures (Ng et al 2009). Such strains should prove useful in the treatment and prevention of intestinal permeability.

Chemopreventive effects

Select probiotics may have anticancer properties. Different strains of *Lactobacillus acidophilus* and bifidobacteria have been studied to investigate their antimutagenic activity against chemical mutagens (Lankaputhra & Shah 1998).

Antimutagenic activity against chemical mutagens and promutagens has been demonstrated for different strains of *Lactobacillus acidophilus*, bifidobacteria and the organic acids usually produced by these probiotics, with live cells producing the most positive results (Lankaputhra & Shah 1998). Some probiotics also reduce faecal enzymes implicated in cancer initiation, while others produce butyric acid, which affects the turnover of colonocytes and neutralises the activity of dietary carcinogens, such as nitrosamines. Additionally, enhancing host immunity and qualitative and quantitative changes to the intestinal microflora and physicochemical conditions are important contributing factors (Hirayama & Rafter 1999).

OTHER ACTIONS

Several clinical studies have investigated lipid-lowering activity of probiotics (see section on Clinical Use, below).

CLINICAL USE

Restoring GIT microflora after antibiotic use

Antibiotic use frequently results in significant perturbations in the GIT microflora and gastrointestinal adverse events, such as diarrhoea (Rafii et al 2008). It was once believed that taking probiotics concurrently with antibiotics would be a waste of time and money as the antibiotic would be likely to destroy all the administered probiotic bacteria. However, research conducted over the past 20 years clearly shows that concurrent administration of specific probiotic strains alongside antibiotics is effective and significantly decreases the incidence of antibiotic-related side effects. Table 3 highlights the research examining the impact of probiotics on antibiotic-related gastrointestinal adverse events, primarily antibiotic-associated diarrhoea. As can be seen, the probiotic strains with the highest level of substantiating evidence are *L. rhamnosus* GG and *Saccharomyces cerevisiae* var. *boulardii* Biocodex, but a number of other strains have also demonstrated efficacy.

> ***How to choose an effective probiotic supplement***
>
> Firstly, one needs to know not only the genera and species details of the organisms contained in the supplement, but also the strain details. Ideally, this should be detailed on the label, but if this is not clear, contact the manufacturer for further information. Secondly, the strains contained in the supplement will ideally display the desirable characteristics highlighted in Table 1. Thirdly, the right strain(s) with the desired action should be chosen for the clinical scenario at hand. Fourthly, there should be adequate amounts of viable organisms contained in the supplement at the time of consumption — for most strains this is currently considered to be $\geq 10^9$ colony-forming units of each organism per dose, but will vary depending on indication (see Dosage Range section below for more details).

Abdominal pain (functional)

A meta-analysis of trials evaluating LGG in the treatment of functional abdominal pain in children found LGG effective. LGG supplementation was associated with a significantly higher rate of treatment responders (defined as no pain or a decrease in pain intensity) in the overall population of children with abdominal pain-related functional gastrointestinal disorders (three trials: $n = 290$; relative risk [RR] 1.31, 95% confidence interval [CI] 1.08–1.59) and in the IBS subgroup (three randomised controlled trials; $n = 167$; RR 1.70, 95% CI 1.27–2.27, number needed to treat 4, 95% CI 3–8). There was also a significant decrease in the perception of pain intensity in children with functional abdominal pain (Horvath et al 2011).

Atopic eczema

The intestinal microflora plays a major protective role against the development of allergy because it reduces antigen transport through the intestinal mucosa and helps induce oral tolerance (Tanaka & Ishikawa 2004). Consequently, probiotics may have a protective role in the prevention and/or management of atopic dermatitis and eczema because of their proposed actions (Rosenfeldt et al 2004).

A number of clinical trials have investigated probiotic therapy to prevent atopic eczema development, and some have evaluated the efficacy of probiotic therapy in the treatment of atopic eczema.

TABLE 3 IMPACT OF PROBIOTICS ON ANTIBIOTIC-RELATED GASTROINTESTINAL ADVERSE EVENTS (comments in italics)

Trial methodology	Strain(s) utilised	Results and comments
Meta-analysis 16 studies *n* = 3432 paediatric subjects	Various	In the per protocol analysis, the incidence of antibiotic-associated diarrhoea (AAD) in the probiotic group was 9% compared to 18% in the control group (2874 participants; relative risk [RR] 0.52; 95% confidence interval [CI] 0.38–0.72). An extreme-plausible intention to treat (ITT) analysis, where 60% of the drop-outs in the probiotic group was assumed to have AAD compared to only 20% of drop-outs in the control group, revealed no significant benefit to probiotic therapy (RR 0.81; 95% CI 0.63–1.04) (Johnston et al 2011). *The considerable bias against probiotic therapy built into the ITT analysis made the chance of a positive outcome very remote. Additionally, meta-analyses that combine the results of studies utilising different probiotic strains (such as this one) are actively discouraged as they are fundamentally flawed and fail to provide clinically relevant conclusions. Each strain is a unique therapeutic agent and should be evaluated as such. Meta-analyses such as this can only provide proof of concept data*
Meta-analysis 63 studies *n* = 11,811 subjects of all ages	Various	Probiotic administration was associated with a significant reduction in risk of AAD (RR = 0.58; 95% CI 0.50–0.68; $P < 0.001$) (Hempel et al 2012). *The same criticism of combining results on different probiotic strains is valid for this meta-analysis as well*
Meta-analysis two studies *n* = 307 paediatric subjects	*Lactobacillus rhamnosus* GG	70% reduced risk of developing AAD in children (95% CI 0.15–0.6; $P = 0.00003$) (Szajewska et al 2010). *This meta-anlaysis combines the data on a single probiotic strain, providing valuable clinically relevant information, demonstrating that this strain is effective in the prevention of AAD in paediatric populations being administered antibiotics*
Meta-analysis five studies *n* = 1076 subjects of all ages	*Saccharomyces cerevisiae* var. *boulardii* Biocodex	Supplementation reduced the risk of AAD from 17.2% in controls to 6.7% (RR = 0.43; 95% CI 0.23–0.78) (Szajewska & Mrukowicz 2005)
R, DB, PC *n* = 162 adult subjects receiving antibiotic treatment for *Helicobacter pylori* infection	*Lactobacillus acidophilus* strains CUL-60 and CUL-21, *Bifidobacterium lactis* CUL-34 and *Bifidobacterium bifidum* CUL-20 (Lab4)	Coadministration of the probiotic combination with antibiotics prevented the increase in faecal *Candida albicans* populations immediately following antibiotic therapy ($P = 0.049$) (Plummer et al 2005)
R, DB, PC *n* = 239	*Lactobacillus plantarum* 299v	31% reduced risk of developing loose or watery stools (95% CI 0.52–0.92; $P = 0.012$); 49% reduced risk of experiencing nausea (95% CI 0.30–0.85; $P = 0.0097$) (Lonnermark et al 2010)
R, DB, PC *n* = 40 paediatric subjects	*Lactobacillus reuteri* MM53	Reduced incidence of a number of gastrointestinal symptoms relative to placebo in triple therapy-treated children — epigastric pain (15% vs 45%; $P < 0.04$), abdominal distension (0% vs 25%; $P < 0.04$), disorders of defecation (15% vs 45%; $P < 0.04$) and halitosis (5% vs 35%; $P < 0.04$) (Lionetti et al 2006)
R, DB, PC *n* = 87 subjects	*Lactobacillus rhamnosus* GG, *Lactobacillus acidophilus* LA5 and *Bifidobacterium lactis* Bb12	79% reduced risk of developing AAD ($P = 0.035$) (Wenus et al 2008)

R, randomised; DB, double-blind; PC, placebo-controlled.

TABLE 4 ROLE OF *LACTOBACILLUS RHAMNOSUS* GG (LGG) IN THE PREVENTION OF ATOPIC ECZEMA

Trial design	Intervention details	Results
R, DB, PC n = 159 pregnant women with an atopic family history	1 × 10^{10} CFU/day LGG for 2–4 weeks before expected delivery. After delivery, breastfeeding mothers could take the capsules; otherwise infants received the agent directly for the following 6 months	There was a 49% reduced risk of eczema development at 2 years of age (P = 0.008), 43% reduced risk of eczema at 4 years of age (P < 0.05) and a 36% reduced risk at 7 years of age (Kalliomaki et al 2001, 2003, 2007)
R, DB, PC n = 105 pregnant women with an atopic family history	1 × 10^{10} CFU/day LGG for 4–6 weeks before expected delivery. After delivery, exclusively breastfeeding mothers took the LGG directly for the initial 3 months and it was administered directly to the infant for the following 3 months. Formula-fed infants received LGG directly for 6 months	The risk of atopic dermatitis in children on LGG was not decreased relative to placebo (relative risk [RR] = 0.96; confidence interval [CI] 0.38–2.33) (Kopp et al 2008)
R, DB, PC n = 250 pregnant women with an atopic family history	LGG 1.8 × 10^{10} CFU/day from 36 weeks' gestation until delivery only	Prenatal LGG treatment was not associated with reduced risk of eczema (34% probiotic, 39% placebo; RR 0.88; 95% CI 0.63–1.22) or immunoglobulin E-associated eczema (18% probiotic, 19% placebo; RR 0.94; 95% CI 0.53–1.68) (Boyle et al 2011)

R, randomised; DB, double-blind; PC, placebo-controlled; CFU, colony-forming unit.

Prevention of atopic eczema

The initial research detailing the efficacy of probiotics in the prevention of atopic eczema utilised the probiotic strain LGG (Kalliomaki et al 2001). Other studies assessing this same strain have since been published, with conflicting results (Boyle et al 2011, Kopp et al 2008). Table 4 provides details on these trials. As can be seen, the studies by Kalliomaki et al and Kopp et al had similar protocols, but contrasting results. The small differences in protocol are unlikely to explain the differences. The trial by Boyle et al only gave LGG to the mother from week 36 until delivery. Lack of apparent efficacy in this study might suggest that LGG needs to be given to the infant (either directly or via breast milk) for efficacy to be seen. More research is needed, however, to clearly define the role of LGG in the prevention of atopic eczema development.

A number of other probiotic strains have been evaluated for their effectiveness in the prevention of atopic eczema, with conflicting results. Pelucchi et al (2012) performed a meta-analysis of randomised controlled trials to investigate whether probiotic use during pregnancy and early life decreases the incidence of atopic eczema and IgE-associated atopic eczema in infants and young children. Eighteen publications based on 14 studies were included in the analysis. Meta-analysis demonstrated that probiotic use decreased the incidence of atopic dermatitis (RR = 0.79; 95% CI 0.71–0.88). The corresponding RR of IgE-associated atopic dermatitis was 0.80 (95% CI 0.66–0.96) (Pelucchi et al 2012). While the evidence on the whole supports the use of probiotics to decrease the incidence of atopic dermatitis in infancy and early childhood, some strains were not effective.

In a randomised, double-blind, placebo-controlled trial, Taylor et al (2007) administered *Lactobacillus acidophilus* strain LAVRI-A1 (3 × 10^9 colony-forming units [CFU]/day) to infants at high risk of allergic disease for the first 6 months of life. At both 6 and 12 months, the incidence of atopic dermatitis was similar in both the probiotic and the placebo group. The proportion of children with a positive skin prick test and atopic eczema was significantly higher in the probiotic group (P = 0.045) at 12 months, as was the rate of allergen sensitisation (P = 0.030). Hence, this strain was not effective in decreasing the incidence of atopic dermatitis development and may have actually increased allergen sensitisation, despite promising preliminary in vitro results (Taylor et al 2007).

Abrahamsson et al (2007) conducted a double-blind, randomised, placebo-controlled trial investigating the role of *Lactobacillus reuteri* strain ProGaia (MM53) in the prevention of atopic dermatitis development (n = 232). The mothers received *L. reuteri* ProGaia (1 × 10^8 CFU) daily from gestational week 36 until delivery. Their babies then continued with the same product from birth until 12 months of age. The incidence of eczema was found to be similar in both groups at 2 years of age. However, infants in the probiotic group did have less IgE-associated eczema (8 vs 20%; P = 0.02) and, in infants with allergic mothers, less skin prick test reactivity (14 vs 31%; P = 0.02) (Abrahamsson et al 2007).

Wickens et al (2008) performed a randomised, double-blind, placebo-controlled trial to assess the impact of two different probiotic strains on the development of atopic eczema. Pregnant women with an atopic family history were randomised to take *Lactobacillus rhamnosus* HN001, *Bifidobacterium animalis* subsp. *lactis* strain HN019 or placebo daily from 35 weeks' gestation until 6 months if breastfeeding, and their infants were randomised to receive the same treatment from birth to 2 years (n = 474). Infants in the *L. rhamnosus* HN001 group had a 49% reduced risk of eczema development at 2 years of age (95% CI 0.30–0.85; P = 0.01). On the other hand, there was no reduced risk of eczema development in infants receiving *Bifidobacterium animalis* subsp. *lactis* strain HN019 (Wickens et al 2008).

In another randomised, placebo-controlled, double-blind trial, the efficacy of *Lactobacillus paracasei* F-19 was evaluated. In this trial, the probiotic was administered to the infant (n = 179) directly at the time of weaning (mixed into food). Infants consumed the probiotic agent (1×10^8 CFU/day) from 4 to 13 months of age. Probiotic supplementation resulted in a significantly reduced cumulative incidence of eczema at 13 months of age (11 vs 22%; $P < 0.05$) and an improved Th1/Th2 ratio (West et al 2009).

In a further double-blind trial, women (n = 415) were randomised to receive either placebo or a probiotic milk (containing LGG, *Lactobacillus acidophilus* La5 and *Bifidobacterium lactis* Bb12) from 36 weeks' gestation to 3 months postnatally during breastfeeding. At 2 years old, the odds ratio (OR) for the cumulative incidence of atopic eczema was 0.51 in the probiotic group compared with the placebo (95% CI 0.30–0.87; P = 0.013). There were no significant effects on rates of asthma or atopic sensitisation (Dotterud et al 2010).

Treatment of atopic eczema

To determine whether probiotics are efficacious in treating atopic eczema, Michail et al (2008) performed a meta-analysis of randomised controlled trials. Eleven studies were located and data from 10 trials were available to pool and analyse (n = 678). There was an overall statistically significant difference favouring probiotics compared with placebo in reducing the Scoring of Atopic Dermatitis Severity Index score (mean change from baseline, −3.01; 95% CI −5.36 to −0.66; P = 0.01). Children with moderately severe disease appeared more likely to benefit. There was also a trend for greater improvement in IgE-sensitised patients (P = 0.07) (Michail et al 2008).

A randomised, double-blind study of 56 young children (aged 6–18 months) with moderate or severe atopic eczema found that treatment with *L. fermentum* VRI-003 PCC (1×10^9 twice daily) produced a significant reduction in the Severity Scoring of Atopic Dermatitis (SCORAD) index (Weston et al 2005). At week 16, 92% of children receiving probiotics had a SCORAD index that was significantly better than baseline compared with the placebo group (n = 17, 63%; P = 0.01). Another randomised double-blind study has found that supplementation of infant formula with viable, but not heat-inactivated, LGG may have benefits for the management of atopic eczema and cow's milk allergy, particularly in terms of acceleration of improvement (Kirjavainen et al 2003).

According to two other placebo-controlled studies, it appears that people with greater allergic responses may be better suited to treatment and experience superior effects. Rosenfeldt et al (2003) found that treatment with two *Lactobacillus* strains (lyophilised *L. rhamnosus* 19070-2 and *L. reuteri* DSM 122460) given in combination for 6 weeks to children aged 1–13 years with atopic dermatitis resulted in 56% experiencing improvement. Interestingly, the total SCORAD score did not change significantly. Allergic patients with a positive skin prick test response and increased IgE levels experienced a more pronounced response to treatment.

Similarly, a randomised, controlled trial by Sistek et al (2006) found that a combination of two probiotic strains (*Lactobacillus rhamnosus* HN001 and *Bifidobacterium lactis* HN019) given to children with established atopic eczema effectively reduced the SCORAD index among the food-sensitised children, but not in other children. Children in this study received 2×10^{10} CFU/g of probiotics or placebo daily as a powder mixed with food or water.

Gastrointestinal infections

Probiotics have a role in the management of various gastrointestinal infections, such as bacterial and viral-induced diarrhoea, *Helicobacter pylori*, traveller's diarrhoea (TD), recurrent *Clostridium difficile*-associated disease (CDAD) and pancreatitis.

Diarrhoea

Various probiotic strains have been subjected to clinical trials to evaluate their efficacy in diarrhoea of different origins.

Viral gastroenteritis — prevention

In a randomised, double-blind, placebo-controlled trial, infants admitted to a chronic medical hospital (average duration of stay 80 days) ingested formula that was supplemented with either placebo or a combination probiotic. The probiotic contained *Bifidobacterium lactis* Bb12 (1.9×10^8 CFU/g powdered formula) and the TH-4 strain of *Streptococcus thermophilus* (0.14×10^8 CFU/g powdered formula). Probiotic supplementation was found to significantly reduce diarrhoea incidence (7 vs 31%; P = 0.035) and rotavirus shedding (10 vs 39%; P = 0.025) (Saavedra et al 1994).

Another randomised, controlled trial found that the administration of LGG to hospitalised children reduced the risk of rotavirus gastroenteritis by 87% (P = 0.02) (Szajewska et al 2001).

Treatment

A meta-analysis of eight randomised controlled trials (n = 988) by Szajewska et al (2007) found that supplementation of LGG significantly reduced duration of rotavirus diarrhoea by 2.1 days in children ($P = 0.006$) and the risk of diarrhoea lasting >7 days was reduced by 75% ($P = 0.01$). The authors did caution, however, that the heterogeneity and methodological considerations of the studies limited the strength of the conclusions (Szajewska et al 2007).

In order to determine the dose-dependent effect of LGG on faecal rotavirus shedding, Fang et al (2009) conducted an open-label randomised study where 23 children with rotavirus gastroenteritis were treated for 3 days with a daily dose of LGG: 0 CFU/day (control group, $n = 6$); 2×10^8 CFU/day (low-dose group, $n = 9$); or 6×10^8 CFU/day (high-dose group, $n = 8$). The high-dose LGG group was the only group who experienced a significant reduction of rotavirus levels in stool samples (86% after 3 days).

A randomised, placebo-controlled trial comparing the efficacy of two different doses of *Lactobacillus reuteri* MM53 (1×10^{10} CFU/day or 1×10^7 CFU/day) with placebo in children with rotavirus-associated diarrhoea ($n = 66$) found that probiotic treatment reduced the duration of viral gastroenteritis-induced diarrhoea from 2.5 days in the placebo group to 1.9 days in the low-dose group and 1.5 days in the high-dose group ($P = 0.01$). By the second day of treatment watery diarrhoea persisted in 80% of the placebo, 70% of the low-dose group and 48% of the large-dose group ($P = 0.04$, large dosage vs. placebo) (Shornikova et al 1997).

Another double-blind, randomised, placebo-controlled study evaluated the efficacy of the multistrain probiotic preparation (VSL#3) in the treatment of rotavirus diarrhoea in children. Two hundred and thirty children were enrolled in the trial. By day 2, a lower mean stool frequency and improved stool consistency were noted in the VSL#3 group (both $P \leq 0.05$). On day 4 of treatment, 89% of VSL#3-treated children were recovered vs 40% of controls ($P < 0.001$) (Dubey et al 2008).

Bacterial gastroenteritis — traveller's diarrhoea

TD is the most common health problem in those visiting developing countries, affecting between 20% and 50% of tourists. Although it is usually short-lived and self-limiting, TD represents a considerable socioeconomic burden for both the traveller and the host country. The most common enteropathogen is *Escherichia coli*, but a number of other microorganisms are also implicated (Ardley & Wright 2010). Recent research has highlighted the causative role of TD in the development of postinfectious IBS (Stermer et al 2006). Thus agents capable of preventing the development of TD are much needed.

Clinical trials with probiotics have thus far produced mixed results. In an attempt to clarify the role of probiotics in the prevention of TD, McFarland (2007) conducted a systematic review and meta-analysis on the area. Combining the data from 12 randomised, controlled trials indicated that probiotics significantly prevent the development of TD, with a pooled RR of 0.85 (95% CI 0.79–0.91; $P < 0.001$). While the data for probiotics as a whole were positive, a number of preparations were found to be ineffective: *Lactobacillus fermentum* VRI-003 (Katelaris & Salam 1995), Lactinex (unspecified strains of *Lactobacillus acidophilus* and *Lactobacillus helveticus* in combination) (de Dios Pozo-Olano et al 1978) and an unspecified strain of *Lactobacillus acidophilus* (Antibiophilus-Kapsein) (Kollaritsch et al 1989). Only strains with proven efficacy in TD should be utilised clinically (see below).

In a randomised, double-blind, placebo-controlled trial by Black et al (1989), the combination of *Lactobacillus acidophilus* La5 and *Bifidobacterium lactis* Bb12 was evaluated for the prevention of TD. Ninety-five Danish travellers touring Egypt took part in the trial and consumed either placebo or a probiotic preparation containing 1.8×10^{10} CFU/day of a combination of *Lactobacillus acidophilus* La5, *Bifidobacterium lactis* Bb12, *Lactobacillus delbrueckii* ssp. *bulgaricus* and *Streptococcus thermophilus* starting 2 days prior to travel. The first two strains constituted 90% of the mixture. The number of tourists developing diarrhoea was significantly reduced in the probiotic group — from 71% in controls to 43% ($P = 0.019$). This equated to a protection rate of 39.4% (Black et al 1989).

A large, randomised, placebo-controlled, double-blind study of the efficacy of LGG in preventing TD involved 820 people on holiday to Turkey to two destinations. The group was randomly assigned either LGG (2×10^9 CFU/day) or placebo in identical sachets. On the return flight, each participant completed a questionnaire indicating the incidence of diarrhoea and related symptoms during the trip. Of the original group, 756 (92%) subjects completed the study. The overall incidence of diarrhoea was 43.8% (331 cases), and the total incidence of diarrhoea in the LGG group was 41.0% compared with 46.5% in the placebo group, indicating an overall protection of 11.8%. Protection rates varied between two different destinations, with the maximum protection rate reported as 39.5% and no side effects reported (Oksanen et al 1990).

In another randomised, placebo-controlled trial investigating the efficacy of LGG (2×10^9 CFU/day) in the prophylaxis of TD, 245 subjects travelling from Finland to developing nations were enrolled. The risk of TD development for subjects taking LGG was reduced by 47% compared to the placebo-treated controls ($P = 0.05$) (Hilton et al 1997).

Utilising a randomised, placebo-controlled, double-blind trial design, Kollaritsch et al (1989) investigated the efficacy of two different doses of *Saccharomyces cerevisiae* var. *boulardii* strain Biocodex (250 mg/day and 500 mg/day) in the prevention of

TD. Four hundred and six Austrian subjects travelling to tropical locales were enrolled. The rate of TD in the placebo group was 42.6%, versus 33.6% in the low-dose group and 31.8% in the high-dose group. This equates to a 21% reduction in incidence in the 250 mg/day group ($P < 0.007$) and 25% reduction with 500 mg/day ($P < 0.002$) compared to placebo (Kollaritsch et al 1989).

In another placebo-controlled double-blind study, two doses (250 and 1000 mg) of *Saccharomyces cerevisiae* var. *boulardii* strain Biocodex were administered prophylactically to 3000 Austrian travellers. A significant reduction in the incidence of diarrhoea was observed, with success depending directly on the rigorous use of the preparation. A tendency was noted for *S. cerevisiae* var. *boulardii* Biocodex to have a regional effect, which was particularly marked in North Africa and in Turkey. The effect was also dose-dependent, with participants taking the higher dose of probiotics experiencing the lowest incidence of TD (29%); little difference was observed between low-dose supplementation (34%) and placebo (39%). Treatment was considered very safe (Kollaritsch et al 1993).

Clostridium difficile-associated diarrhoea

Clostridium difficile is a common cause of diarrhoea associated with treatment with antimicrobial and/or antibiotic medication and can potentially progress to colitis, pseudomembranous colitis, toxic megacolon and death. In spite of antimicrobial therapy, recurrence is common, and increasingly, probiotic supplementation has been investigated as a potential treatment for CDAD.

A meta-analysis by McFarland (2006) assessed six blinded randomised controlled trials (n = 354 patients) that used a mixture of probiotics in the management of CDAD. The results showed that only *S. cerevisiae* var. *boulardii* supplementation resulted in a significant reduction in recurrence. These findings are in contrast to an earlier meta-analysis by Dendukuri et al (2005), where a role for probiotic use in CDAD was not supported in all the studies; the authors of this meta-analysis reported methodological flaws in some of the studies, although some benefit of probiotic therapy was seen in patient subgroups, particularly those characterised by severe CDAD and high use of vancomycin. Individual strains that have demonstrated efficacy in randomised, controlled trials for the prevention or treatment of CDAD include *S. cerevisiae* var. *boulardii* Biocodex (McFarland et al 1994, Surawicz et al 2000) and *Lactobacillus plantarum* 299v (Klarin et al 2008).

Vancomycin-resistant enterococci

Over the past 15–20 years, there has been a rapid increase in the prevalence of vancomycin-resistant enterococci (VRE). This has been associated with the widespread use of broad-spectrum antibiotics. VRE can be involved in the pathogenesis of persistent, hospital-acquired infections that often have poor outcomes. Additionally, they have the capacity to transfer their antibiotic resistance factors to other organisms. Non-antibiotic control measures of VRE are much needed. This randomised, double-blind, placebo-controlled trial was performed to assess the efficacy of LGG in the eradication of VRE. Twenty-seven VRE-positive hospital inpatients were randomly allocated to consume either a yoghurt containing LGG (100 g daily for 4 weeks) or an equivalent amount of pasteurised yoghurt. All subjects who received LGG yoghurt were cleared of VRE, compared to only 8% of controls ($P < 0.001$) (Manley et al 2007).

Pancreatitis

Probiotic therapy has been investigated in pancreatitis because of the increased risk of bacterial infections. Some animal studies have shown that the use of *L. plantarum* 299v (Mangiante et al 2001) and *S. cerevisiae* var. *boulardii* (Akyol et al 2003) reduced bacterial translocation. Human studies have investigated the use of single probiotic agents such as live *L. plantarum* 299v given to 22 patients compared with an inactivated form given to 23 patients; the probiotic-supplemented group had reduced rates of infection and abscess formation (Olah et al 2002).

However, these findings are in contrast to those of Besselink et al (2008), who used a novel preparation consisting of six different strains from six different species of lactic acid bacteria — *Lactobacillus acidophilus, L. casei, L. salivarius, Lactococcus lactis, Bifidobacterium bifidum* and *B. lactis* — in patients with severe acute pancreatitis. Use of this probiotic preparation was associated with significantly increased risk of bowel ischaemia (see section on Adverse Reactions, below). Thus not all probiotic preparations have a role for use as an adjunct treatment in pancreatitis.

Chemotherapy-induced diarrhoea

In an open-label trial, subjects (n = 150) undergoing 5-fluorouracil-based chemotherapy for colorectal cancer were randomly assigned to receive supplementation with LGG ($1–2 \times 10^{10}$ CFU/day). LGG supplementation was associated with a 41% reduced frequency of severe diarrhoea ($P = 0.027$), an 83% reduction in abdominal discomfort scores ($P = 0.025$) and 55% decreased frequency in bowel toxicity-induced dose reductions ($P = 0.0008$) compared to untreated controls (Osterlund et al 2007).

AIDS-related diarrhoea

In a small double-blind, placebo-controlled study, 24 women with AIDS/HIV, aged 18–44 years, who were not being treated with antiretrovirals and had moderate diarrhoea, were given either a yoghurt fermented with *Lactobacillus delbrueckii* ssp. *bulgaricus* and *Streptococcus thermophilus* (the typical yoghurt-making bacteria), supplemented with the probiotic strains *Lactobacillus rhamnosus* GR-1 and *L. reuteri* RC-14 or an unsupplemented yoghurt for 15 days. Women receiving the supplemented probiotic yoghurt experienced less diarrhoea, flatulence and nausea compared to those receiving the unsupplemented yoghurt. All probiotic-treated subjects were free of diarrhoea after 15 days' treatment vs 9% of controls. Additionally, there was an increase in CD4 counts observed in probiotic-treated subjects compared to a decrease in controls ($P < 0.02$) (Anukam et al 2008).

In an open-label trial, 17 HIV-positive patients with chronic diarrhoea were given *Saccharomyces cerevisiae* var. *boulardii* Biocodex strain (3 g/day) for 15 days. The mean number of stools per day decreased from 9.0 on enrolment to 2.1 on day 15. Patients gained a mean of 3.6 kg during the trial (McFarland & Bernasconi 1993, Saint-Marc et al 1991).

Trois et al (2008) investigated the effect of probiotics on the immune response in a randomised, double-blind, controlled trial of two groups of children (2–12 years) infected with HIV. The study of 77 children administered either a formula containing unspecified strains of *Bifidobacterium bifidum* and *Streptococcus thermophilus* — 2.5×10^{10} CFU/day (NAN2 probiotico Nestlé) — or a standard formula on a daily basis for 2 months. At the end of the study, there was an increase in CD4 cell count in the probiotic group (+118 cells/mm vs −42 cells/mm in controls; $P = 0.049$), suggesting that this probiotic combination has immunostimulatory properties.

Constipation

Constipation affects a significant proportion of the population. Probiotics have long been touted as useful for the treatment of constipation and recent randomised controlled trials have demonstrated efficacy for some probiotic strains.

In a randomised, controlled trial, Yang et al (2008) evaluated the effect of consuming a fermented milk containing *Bifidobacterium animalis* DN-173010 (1.25×10^{10} CFU/day) on stool parameters in constipated women ($n = 135$). Compared to controls, stool frequency was significantly increased in the bifidobacteria group after 1 week (3.5 movements/week vs 2.5; $P < 0.01$) and after 2 weeks' consumption (4.17 vs 2.6; $P < 0.01$). Defecation condition and stool consistency also significantly improved after 1 and 2 weeks (all $P < 0.01$) of bifidobacteria consumption (Yang et al 2008).

Another randomised, double-blind, placebo-controlled trial compared the efficacy of placebo to a probiotic drink containing *Lactobacillus casei* Shirota (6.5×10^9 CFU/day) in constipated subjects ($n = 70$). After a 4-week treatment period, there was a significant decrease in the occurrence of moderate and severe constipation ($P < 0.001$) and in occurrence of hard stools ($P < 0.001$) in the probiotic group. There was also an increase in defecation frequency ($P = 0.004$) and improvement in stool consistency ($P < 0.001$). General wellbeing was also significantly improved in the probiotic group ($P = 0.008$) (Koebnick et al 2003).

Immune enhancement/infection prevention

The potential role of probiotics in the enhancement of immune function has been under investigation over the past few decades. The process started with in vitro and animal research, followed by studies evaluating the effects of probiotic administration on immune cell function in human subjects. More recently, well-conducted human trials with hard outcomes have been published.

In a systematic review, Vouloumanou et al (2009) assessed the data from randomised controlled trials (14 trials) that had investigated the role of probiotics for the prevention and treatment of respiratory tract infections (RTIs). Ten of the 14 trials did not find that the probiotic agents trialled reduced the incidence of RTIs compared to placebo; the remaining four trials found the incidence of RTIs to be significantly lower in probiotic-treated patients. A significant reduction in the severity of RTI symptoms associated with probiotic treatment was found in five of six randomised controlled trials that provided relevant data. In the remaining randomised controlled trial, no difference was noted. Three randomised controlled trials reported a significant decrease in duration of RTI symptoms associated with probiotic therapy, whereas nine did not (Vouloumanou et al 2009). The data suggest that some, but not all, probiotic preparations have the capacity to enhance immune function and decrease risk and duration of RTIs.

A number of probiotic strains have demonstrated the capacity to reduce the incidence of infections and/or shorten their duration. The results of these trials are detailed in Table 5.

Infantile colic

In a randomised, open-label trial, colicky breastfed infants ($n = 90$; aged 21–90 days) were supplemented with either simethicone (active control) or *Lactobacillus reuteri* MM53 (1×10^8 CFU/day) for 4 weeks. Significant reductions in daily crying time were noted by day 7 in the MM53 group compared to the simethicone group ($P = 0.005$). This improvement continued until day 28, when median crying time was reduced to 51 min/day in the MM53 group vs 145 min/day in controls ($P < 0.001$) On day 28, 95% of patients were responders in the probiotic group versus 7% in the simethicone group (Savino et al 2007).

Irritable bowel syndrome

Although the aetiology of IBS is still unknown, there is growing evidence that there is a persistent, mild inflammatory state with changes in mucosal function or structure and an associated imbalance of intestinal flora (Camilleri 2006). Dysbiosis has long been theorised to play a role in the pathophysiology of IBS and the first trial conducted investigating the efficacy of probiotics in IBS was published in 1955 (Rafsky & Rafsky 1955). Many trials have been conducted since this time.

TABLE 5 PROBIOTICS IN THE PREVENTION OF INFECTIONS

Trial methodology	Strain(s) utilised	Results
R, DB, PC *n* = 201 infants 4–10 months old	*Bifidobacterium lactis* Bb12	Over a 3-month period, there was a reduction in fever episodes by 34% ($P < 0.001$), diarrhoea episodes by 58% ($P < 0.001$) and duration of diarrhoea episodes by 37% ($P < 0.001$) (Weizman et al 2005)
R, DB, PC *n* = 326 children 3–5 years of age	*Lactobacillus acidophilus* NCFM	Over a 6-month period, fever incidence was reduced by 53% ($P = 0.0085$) and coughing incidence by 41% ($P = 0.027$); use of antibiotics reduced by 68% ($P = 0.0002$); 32% reduction in days absent from child care ($P = 0.002$) (Leyer et al 2009)
R, DB, PC *n* = 326 children 3–5 years of age	*Lactobacillus acidophilus* NCFM and *Bifidobacterium lactis* Bi07	Over a 6-month period, fever incidence was reduced by 73% ($P = 0.0009$), coughing incidence by 62% ($P = 0.005$) and rhinorrhoea incidence by 59% ($P = 0.03$); use of antibiotics reduced by 84% ($P < 0.0001$); 28% reduction in days absent from child care ($P < 0.001$) (Leyer et al 2009)
R, DB, PC *n* = 215 infants aged 6–12 months	*Lactobacillus fermentum* CECT5716	Over a 6-month period, there was a 46% reduced incidence of gastrointestinal infections ($P = 0.032$), a 26% reduction in respiratory tract infections ($P = 0.022$) and a 30% reduction in the total number of infections ($P = 0.003$); the incidence of recurrent respiratory tract infections was reduced by 72% (Maldonado et al 2012)
R, DB, PC, CO *n* = 20 elite, male distance runners	*Lactobacillus fermentum* VRI-003	Over a 4-month winter period, distance runners taking the probiotic reported less than half the number of days of respiratory symptoms (30 vs 72; $P = 0.00006$) compared with placebo; illness severity was also decreased ($P = 0.06$) (Cox et al 2010).
R, DB, PC *n* = 201 infants 4–10 months old	*Lactobacillus reuteri* MM53	Over a 3-month period, fever episodes were reduced by 73% ($P < 0.001$), diarrhoea episodes by 94% ($P < 0.001$), duration of diarrhoea by 75% ($P < 0.001$) and child care absences by 67% ($P = 0.015$) in infants (Weizman et al 2005)
R, DB, PC *n* = 262 healthy adults	*Lactobacillus reuteri* MM53	Over the 80-day trial period, there was a 58% reduction in number of subjects reporting sick days in the MM53 group compared to placebo ($P < 0.01$); amongst shift workers, 33% of those in the placebo group reported sick over the study period vs none in the MM53 group ($P < 0.005$) (Tubelius et al 2005)
R, DB, PC *n* = 571 children aged 1–6 years	*Lactobacillus rhamnosus* GG (LGG)	Over the 7-month winter period, there were 16% fewer days absent from day care in children in the LGG group ($P = 0.03$) and a 19% reduction in antibiotic use for respiratory tract infections ($P = 0.03$) (Hatakka et al 2001)
R, DB, PC *n* = 281 day-care-aged children	*Lactobacillus rhamnosus* GG	Over the 3-month intervention period, there was a 34% reduced risk of upper respiratory tract infections in toddlers in the LGG group, a 43% reduced risk of respiratory tract infections lasting longer than 3 days and significantly fewer number of days with respiratory tract symptoms (all $P < 0.001$). There was a trend for reduced number of days with gastrointestinal symptoms ($P = 0.06$) (Hojsak et al 2009)
R, DB, PC *n* = 81 infants < 2 months old	*Lactobacillus rhamnosus* GG and *Bifidobacterium lactis* Bb12	Over the 10-month period, there was a 56% reduced risk of otitis media in infants ($P = 0.014$), a 48% reduced risk of antibiotic prescription ($P = 0.015$) and a 49% reduced risk of recurrent respiratory tract infection ($P = 0.022$) (Rautava et al 2009)

R, randomised; DB, double-blind; PC, placebo-controlled; CO, crossover.

Moayyedi et al (2010) performed a systematic review and meta-analysis of randomised controlled trials that investigated the efficacy of probiotics in the treatment of IBS. Nineteen randomised controlled trials were included ($n = 1650$) in the review. Combining the data found probiotics to be significantly better than placebo in relieving IBS symptoms (relative risk of IBS not improving = 0.71; 95% CI 0.57–0.88) with a number needed to treat of four (95% CI 3–12.5). The authors concluded that probiotics appear to be efficacious in the treatment of IBS, but the magnitude of benefit and the most effective strains are uncertain (Moayyedi et al 2010).

A 2008 meta-analysis concluded that the use of probiotics can result in improved symptom relief in patients with IBS (McFarland & Dublin 2008). Twenty randomised controlled clinical trials (n = 1404) were reviewed, and either single or multiple probiotics were used for varying time periods ranging from 2 to 24 weeks (median = 4 weeks). Probiotic use was associated with improvement in global IBS symptoms compared to placebo (pooled relative risk [RRpooled] 0.77, 95% CI 0.62–0.94). Probiotic use was also associated with less abdominal pain compared to placebo (RRpooled 0.78 [0.69–0.88], 95% CI 0.45–0.81). There were insufficient data, however, to draw conclusions about the most effective probiotic strains or the assessment of individual IBS symptoms.

Similarly, a systematic review and meta-analysis by Hoveyda et al (2009) reported that probiotic therapy for several weeks may result in modest improvement in the overall symptoms of IBS. A total of 14 randomised placebo-controlled trials of varying length (from 4 weeks to 6 months; although the majority lasted 8 weeks or less) were included in the analyses. The probiotic therapy varied in the strains utilised as well as the dose and strength; in addition, some studies used a single agent and others used combinations of multiple strains. It is important to note, however, that not all clinical studies have produced positive results. A large randomised, parallel-group, double-blind study by Drouault-Holowacz et al (2008) investigated the effects of four strains of lactic acid (LA) bacteria (1×10^{10} CFU *Bifidobacterium longum* LA 101 [29%], *Lactobacillus acidophilus* LA 102 [29%], *Lactococcus lactis* LA 103 [29%] and *Streptococcus thermophilus* LA 104 [13%]) on symptoms of IBS in 100 patients over a 4-week period. The probiotic combination was not significantly superior to the placebo in relieving symptoms of IBS, although symptomatic improvement was noted in some patient subgroups. Studies utilising LGG (in isolation) (O'Sullivan & O'Morain 2000), *Lactobacillus salivarius* UCC4331 (O'Mahony et al 2005a, 2005b) and *Lactobacillus acidophilus* NCFM (Newcomer et al 1983) also failed to demonstrate positive results. Probiotic preparations that have shown efficacy in the treatment of IBS are detailed in Table 6.

Inflammatory bowel disease

Probiotics are also being used as adjunctive therapy for Crohn's disease and ulcerative colitis (Goh & O'Morain 2003, Guslandi 2003a, 2003b, Kanauchi et al 2003, Karthik 2003, Marteau et al 2003, Rutgeerts 2003). Overall, present research indicates a limited role for probiotics in Crohn's disease; the results for ulcerative colitis are more promising, and there does seem to be a beneficial effect in pouchitis.

Crohn's disease

Only a limited number of studies have indicated a role for probiotics in the remission of Crohn's disease. In an open-label study, Guslandi et al (2000) compared *Saccharomyces cerevisiae* var. *boulardii* Biocodex plus mesalazine with mesalazine alone and found that adjunctive probiotic treatment resulted in fewer relapses (6% vs 38%; $P = 0.04$).

Supplementation with VSL#3 has also been evaluated. VSL#3 contains a high concentration of eight strains of lactic acid bacteria — *Bifidobacterium breve*, *B. longum*, *B. infantis*, *Lactobacillus acidophilus*, *L. plantarum*, *L. casei*, *L. bulgaricus* and *Streptococcus thermophilus*. A study of 40 patients randomised to 3 months of rifaximin followed by 9 months of VSL#3 or to 12 months of mesalazine also reported relapse prevention with probiotic therapy (Campieri et al 2000).

Other studies, including randomised, double-blind placebo-controlled trials, have suggested that LGG and *Lactobacillus johnsonii* La1 have no role to play in maintaining Crohn's disease in remission (Hedin et al 2007). Similarly, studies that have administered probiotics for the treatment of active Crohn's disease have also provided mixed results, mainly because of concurrent use of medications during the intervention period (e.g. prednisolone use or metronidazole) (Gupta et al 2000).

A Cochrane systematic review by Rolfe et al (2006) did not advocate a role for probiotics in Crohn's disease based on the available evidence, suggesting that, because all studies enrolled small numbers of patients, they may have lacked statistical power to show differences should they exist. Seven randomised controlled trials were identified that had utilised a variety of probiotics, such as LGG, *Escherichia coli* Nissle 1917 and *Saccharomyces cerevisiae* var. *boulardii*; most of the studies had a relatively small number of participants with different treatment protocols, probiotic strains and outcome measures, making it difficult for comparisons to be made.

Similar conclusions were reached in a recent systematic review of probiotics in Crohn's disease, where the authors stated there was no evidence from randomised controlled trials to support the use of probiotic therapy in Crohn's disease (Jonkers et al 2012).

Given the promising preliminary research on *Saccharomyces cerevisiae* var. *boulardii* Biocodex in Crohn's disease, the strain was evaluated using a more rigorous randomised, double-blind, placebo-controlled trial design. One hundred and sixty-five subjects with Crohn's disease that was currently in remission after treatment with steroids or salicylates were randomly allocated to receive either placebo or probiotic (1 g/day) for 12 months. Over the 12 months, the relapse rates were 47.5% in the probiotic group and 53.2% in the placebo group (a non-significant difference). The median time to relapse did not differ significantly between patients given probiotics (40.7 weeks) vs placebo (39.0 weeks). There were also no significant differences between groups in mean Crohn's disease activity index scores or erythrocyte sedimentation rates or in median levels of C-reactive protein. A post hoc analysis did reveal, however, that non-smokers given *S. cerevisiae* var. *boulardii* Biocodex were less likely to experience a relapse of Crohn's disease than non-smokers given placebo (OR 0.22, 95% CI 0.07–0.70; $P = 0.01$) (Bourreille et al 2013). The latter result requires confirmation in future research to ensure it was not

TABLE 6 PROBIOTICS IN THE TREATMENT OF IRRITABLE BOWEL SYNDROME (IBS)

Trial methodology	Strain(s) utilised	Results
R, DB, PC *n* = 34 female subjects with C-IBS	*Bifidobacterium animalis* strain DN-173010	After a 4-week treatment period, there was a significant reduction in abdominal distension (*P* = 0.02), an acceleration of gut transit time (*P* = 0.049) and a reduction in overall IBS symptom severity (*P* = 0.032). There were also reductions in abdominal pain/discomfort (*P* = 0.044), bloating (*P* = 0.059) and flatulence scores (*P* = 0.092) (Agrawal et al 2009)
R, DB, PC *n* = 362 female subjects with IBS	*Bifidobacterium infantis* 35624	After a 4-week treatment phase, there were significant reductions in abdominal pain/discomfort (*P* = 0.023), bloating/distension (*P* = 0.046), feeling of incomplete evacuation (*P* < 0.04), sense of straining at stool (*P* < 0.02), passage of gas (*P* < 0.04) and composite IBS symptom scores (*P* = 0.013) compared to controls. There was also a significant improvement in bowel habit satisfaction (*P* < 0.02) (Whorwell et al 2006)
R, DB, PC *n* = 52 subjects with IBS	*Lactobacillus acidophilus* strains CUL-60 and CUL-21, *Bifidobacterium lactis* CUL-34, and *Bifidobacterium bifidum* CUL-20 (Lab4)	After an 8-week treatment period, there were significant reductions in composite IBS symptom scores (*P* = 0.0217) and improvements in quality-of-life scores (*P* = 0.0068) compared to controls (Williams et al 2008)
R, DB, PC *n* = 48 subjects with IBS and bloating	VSL#3	After either a 4- or an 8-week treatment phase, there was a significant reduction in flatulence scores (*P* = 0.011). There were no significant changes in other IBS symptoms or bowel function, although colonic transit time was retarded in the VSL#3 group (Kim et al 2005)
R, DB, PC *n* = 214 subjects with IBS	*Lactobacillus plantarum* 299V	After a 4-week treatment phase, the frequency and severity of abdominal pain, bloating and feeling of incomplete evacuation scores were significantly reduced in the 299V group compared to controls (all *P* < 0.05). Stool frequency was significantly reduced in the 299V group (*P* < 0.05), and 78% of subjects in the 299V group scored the symptomatic effect as excellent or good vs 8% of controls (*P* < 0.01) (Ducrotte et al 2012)

R, randomised; DB, double-blind; PC, placebo-controlled; CO, crossover; C-IBS, constipation-predominant irritable bowel syndrome.

a random finding, but in the meantime a trial of this probiotic strain would be warranted in non-smoking Crohn's disease patients.

Ulcerative colitis

A Cochrane review conducted in 2011 found four randomised controlled trials (*n* = 587) that evaluated probiotics for the maintenance of remission in ulcerative colitis. Combining the data from the three trials comparing probiotics to mesalazine found no significant difference in recurrence rates between the two treatments: 40.1% of subjects in the probiotics group and 34.1% in the mesalazine group relapsed over the treatment period. The final trial included a small placebo controlled trial (*n* = 32), and found no statistically significant difference in efficacy — 75% of probiotic patients relapsed at 1 year compared to 92% of placebo patients. The authors concluded that there is currently insufficient evidence to draw conclusions about the efficacy of probiotics for maintenance of remission in ulcerative colitis (Naidoo et al 2011).

A recent meta-analysis of randomised, controlled trials assessed the impact of probiotics on remission induction and maintenance in ulcerative colitis. Thirteen randomised controlled trials were included in the analysis. Seven reports evaluated remission rates (*n* = 399). When combined, the adjunct use of probiotics alongside standard care did not significantly alter remission rates. There was, however, marked heterogeneity in the results. Eight reports assessed the recurrence rate (*n* = 709). Compared to the placebo group, the use of probiotics was found to significantly reduce the ulcerative colitis recurrence rate (recurrence rate: 0.69, 95% CI 0.47–1.01; *P* = 0.05). Heterogeneity was again observed. The results suggest that using probiotics provides no additional benefit in inducing remission of ulcerative colitis, but probiotics auxiliary therapy is much better than non-probiotics therapy for maintenance of remission (Sang et al 2010). The significant heterogeneity observed in this study, which should have precluded the conduction of a meta-analysis, was most likely caused by the all-too-common error

TABLE 7 PROBIOTICS IN THE TREATMENT OF ULCERATIVE COLITIS (UC) — INDUCTION OF REMISSION

Trial methodology	Strain(s) utilised	Results
R, DB, C *n* = 116 patients with active UC	*Escherichia coli* Nissle 1917	Over a 12-month treatment period, *Escherichia coli* Nissle 1917 supplementation, in conjunction with standard inflammatory bowel disease therapy (corticosteroids), was equivalent to mesalazine in terms of remission rate ($P = 0.05$) and time to remission ($P = 0.009$). The duration of remission was also equivalent ($P = 0.017$) (Rembacken et al 1999)
R, DB, PC *n* = 90 patients with moderately active distal UC	*Escherichia coli* Nissle 1917	Intrarectal administration (via enema) of three different doses of *E. coli* Nissle 1917 (40, 20, or 10 mL) daily for 2 weeks did not significantly impact rates of remission in intention to treat analysis. There were a large number of protocol violations, however, and a per protocol analysis demonstrated a significant dose-dependent effect ($P = 0.0446$). Remission rates in the 40 mL group were 53%, 44% in the 20 mL group and 27% in the 10 mL group, compared to 18% in the placebo group (Matthes et al 2010)
R, DB, PC *n* = 147 subjects with mild to moderate active UC	VSL#3	At 6 weeks, 33% of VSL#3-treated subjects achieved >50% in the UC disease activity index versus 10% of controls ($P = 0.001$). At week 12, 43% of subjects in the VSL#3 group were in remission vs 16% of controls ($P < 0.001$) (Sood et al 2009)
R, DB, PC *n* = 29 children with active UC	VSL#3	In conjunction with standard UC therapy (steroids and mesalamine), remission was achieved in 93% of VSL#3-treated children vs 36% of controls ($P < 0.001$). Twenty-one per cent of VSL#3-treated subjects relapsed within 1 year versus 73% of controls ($P = 0.014$) (Miele et al 2009)
R, DB, PC *n* = 144 subjects with mild to moderate relapsing UC	VSL#3	In conjunction with standard UC therapy (stable doses of 5-aminosalicylic acid and/or immunosuppressants), the number of subjects experiencing a decrease in UC disease activity index scores of 50% or more was higher in the VSL#3 group than in the placebo group ($P = 0.031$). Rectal bleeding also improved significantly more in the VSL#3 group than controls ($P = 0.036$). Rates of remission were higher in the VSL#3 group, but not significantly so (43.6% vs 31.5%; $P = 0.132$) (Miele et al 2009)

R, randomised; DB, double-blind; PC, placebo-controlled.

of combining research conducted on different probiotic strains or variations in study designs. Each strain must be viewed as a separate therapeutic agent.

Probiotic preparations that have shown efficacy in the treatment of ulcerative colitis are detailed in Tables 7 and 8.

Pouchitis

Probiotics have also been used in patients with relapsing or chronic pouchitis (Kailasapathy & Chin 2000). While studies have produced inconsistent results, overall there appears to be some evidence to support the therapeutic use of probiotics in postoperative pouchitis (Penner et al 2005) and the general view is that VSL#3 treatment can be effective in controlling this condition.

Studies by Gionchetti et al (2000, 2003) assessed the use of VSL#3 in both primary prevention of pouchitis and maintenance therapy for chronic relapsing pouchitis, demonstrating some success. In their randomised, controlled, double-blind study, 40 patients with relapsing pouchitis in remission received a 6 g daily dose of VSL#3 or a placebo for 9 months. Probiotic treatment resulted in a significantly reduced incidence of pouchitis (Gionchetti et al 2000), but when VSL#3 treatment was ceased, all patients relapsed 3 months later. In a subsequent randomised controlled study to investigate VSL#3 treatment for primary prophylaxis of pouchitis in 40 patients, Gionchetti et al (2003) reported that treatment with VSL#3 resulted in fewer relapses.

In another randomised, double-blind, controlled trial, Mimura et al (2004) also utilised VSL#3 in 36 patients with more severe recurrent pouchitis over a 1-year follow-up period and reported good results regarding maintenance of remission and improved quality of life in the patients.

A combination of probiotics also has been reported to result in beneficial effects; lactobacilli and bifidobacteria in fermented milk were administered to patients who had pouchitis after ulcerative colitis surgery, resulting in some resolution of disease activity (Laake et al 2005).

In contrast, in an uncontrolled study of 31 patients who were treated with antibiotics and were in remission, Shen et al (2005) found little benefit with VSL#3 administered for 8 months.

TABLE 8 PROBIOTICS IN THE TREATMENT OF ULCERATIVE COLITIS (UC) — MAINTENANCE OF REMISSION

Trial methodology	Strain(s) utilised	Results
R, DB, C *n* = 327 UC patients in remission	*Escherichia coli* Nissle 1917	Over the 12-month trial period, *E. coli* Nissle 1917 treatment was found to be equally effective as mesalazine in preventing relapse (36.4% relapse vs 33.9%; *P* = 0.003) (Kruis et al 2004)
R, DB, C *n* = 120 UC patients in remission	*Escherichia coli* Nissle 1917	Over a 12-week period, relapse rates were 11.3% under mesalazine and 16.0% under *E. coli* Nissle 1917 (not significantly different). The mean relapse-free time was 103 ± 4 days for mesalazine and 106 ± 5 days for *E. coli* Nissle 1917 (not significantly different) (Kruis et al 1997)
R, OL *n* = 187 UC patients in remission	*Lactobacillus rhamnosus* GG	Subjects were randomised to receive either *Lactobacillus rhamnosus* GG (LGG) alone or in combination with mesalazine, or mesalazine alone. Over the 12-month trial period, there was no difference in relapse rates between the three groups. LGG supplementation was equally effective as mesalazine in maintaining clinical remission, but significantly more effective than mesalazine in prolonging the relapse-free time (*P* < 0.05) (Zocco et al 2006)
OL *n* = 34 UC patients in remission aged 11–18 years	*Escherichia coli* Nissle 1917	Over the 12-month treatment period, the relapse rate was 25% in probiotic-treated subjects vs 30% in the mesalazine group (Henker et al 2008)
OL *n* = 20 UC patients in remission	VSL#3	After 12 months, 15 of the 20 participants remained in remission, which compares favourably to rates of remission observed during long-term mesalazine therapy (Venturi et al 1999)

R, randomised; DB, double-blind; C, controlled; OL, open-label.

An open-label trial evaluated the efficacy of LGG in preventing pouchitis. Subjects with ulcerative colitis who had undergone an ileal pouch-anal anastomosis (*n* = 117) took part in the trial. LGG supplementation (1–2 × 10^{10} CFU/day) significantly delayed first onset of pouchitis compared to no-treatment controls (cumulative risk at 3 years: 7 vs 29%; *P* = 0.011) (Gosselink et al 2005).

Probiotics and diverticular disease

It has been suggested that altered bacterial flora is one of the causes of diverticular inflammation (White 2006). Consequently, some investigators have evaluated the role of probiotics in diverticular disease. In an open-label study, 15 patients with diverticular disease were treated with an antimicrobial and charcoal for the first symptomatic episode after enrolment and the second episode was treated with the same therapy, followed by *Escherichia coli* Nissle 1917 for 6 weeks. This second treatment resulted in a longer symptom-free duration of a mean of 14 months compared to a mean of 2.4 months in the control group (Fric & Zavoral 2003).

Various studies have attempted to restore the altered microflora using probiotics, but most of these studies have been limited in their design and methods (Sheth & Floch 2009). However, results from these studies appear to be mostly positive, and randomised placebo-controlled studies are needed in order to make recommendations.

Alcohol-induced liver disease

In a prospective, randomised, clinical study, 66 men with advanced alcohol-induced liver disease received either *Bifidobacterium bifidum* (unspecified strain) and *Lactobacillus plantarum* 8PA3 or standard therapy (no probiotics) for 5 days. At the end of the study, patients who had received the probiotic therapy had significantly increased numbers of both bifidobacteria (7.9 vs 6.81 log 10^9 CFU/g) and lactobacilli (4.2 vs 3.2 log 10^9 CFU/g) compared to the standard therapy group; likewise, the former group had a significant improvement in hepatic enzyme levels (Kirpich et al 2008).

Non-alcoholic fatty liver disease (NAFLD)

NAFLD comprises a spectrum of diseases ranging from simple steatosis to non-alcoholic steatohepatitis, fibrosis and cirrhosis. Probiotics have been proposed as a treatment option because of their modulating effect on the gut flora that could influence the gut-liver axis and there are now considerable data from animal models in support of this idea. A Cochrane systematic review conducted in 2007 found no human randomised controlled trials that evaluated probiotics in the treatment of NAFLD. The authors concluded that the lack of randomised controlled trials makes it impossible to support or refute the use of probiotics in NAFLD (Lirussi et al 2007).

In a randomised, double-blind, placebo-controlled trial, supplementation of obese children (*n* = 20; mean age 10.7 years) with persisting hypertransaminasaemia and ultrasonographic changes suggestive of NAFLD with LGG (1.2×10^{10} CFU/day) for 8 weeks resulted in a decrease in alanine aminotransferase concentration ($P = 0.03$) and in antipeptidoglycan-polysaccharide antibody levels ($P = 0.03$). Alanine aminotransferase levels normalised in 80% of LGG-treated subjects (Vajro et al 2011).

Hepatic encephalopathy

To date, there are only a few reports about the role of probiotics in hepatic encephalopathy; in addition to the conventional management with antibiotics and lactulose, probiotics may confer favourable changes in intestinal microflora in patients with hepatic encephalopathy.

A recent randomised, controlled, single tertiary centre study with open allocation by Bajaj et al (2008) investigated the effects of a probiotic yoghurt on minimal hepatic encephalopathy (MHE), a pre-clinical stage prior to full-blown hepatic encephalopathy. The probiotics *Streptococcus thermophilus*, *L. bulgaricus*, *L. acidophilus*, bifidobacteria and *L. casei* (unspecified strains) were administered in the form of a commercial yoghurt to a group of non-alcoholic MHE cirrhotic patients for 60 days; the study demonstrated a significant rate of MHE reversal (71% vs 0% in controls; $P = 0.003$).

Colon cancer

A number of factors may be involved in colon cancer risk, and it has been suggested that the colonic microbiota may be involved in the aetiology of colorectal cancer. A lower incidence of colon cancer has been associated with the consumption of lactobacilli or bifidobacteria. The exact mechanisms have not been fully elucidated (Fotiadis et al 2008), but may have to do with probiotic-induced reductions in colonic expression of β-glucuronidase, nitroreductase and azoreductase (Marotta et al 2003).

A randomised, controlled trial evaluated the efficacy of *Lactobacillus casei* Shirota in the prevention of colorectal cancer in patients ($n = 398$) who had had at least two colorectal tumours removed. Daily consumption of the probiotic over a 4-year period resulted in a significant reduction in the occurrence of colorectal tumours with moderate or severe atypia compared to the dietary instruction only group ($P < 0.05$) (Ishikawa et al 2005).

High cholesterol

Some probiotics may have cholesterol-lowering effects due to several mechanisms, including enzymatic deconjugation of bile acids and metabolic

Clinical note — The hygiene hypothesis

The intestinal tract is the largest immune organ of the body. It produces more antibodies than any other part of the body and contains 80% of all antibody-producing cells. The intestinal mucosa functions as a barrier against infections, but it also provides communication between the different mucosal surfaces of the body (Ouwehand et al 2002).

At birth, the GIT is sterile. Normal gut flora develops gradually over time and is influenced by factors such as composition of the maternal gut microbiota, diet, degree of hygiene, use of antibiotics or other medications, the environment and possibly genetic aspects. Studies in germ-free mice have shown that, without these bacteria, the systemic immune system will not function normally (Vanderhoof & Young 2002).

In the absence of microbes, a mammal develops fewer Peyer's patches (part of the gut-associated lymphoid tissue) and less than 10% of the number of IgA-producing B cells compared with normal. However, on exposure to a normal microflora, previously germ-free animals develop their immune system very much like other animals. This indicates that the intestinal microflora is instrumental in the proper development of the immune system (Ouwehand et al 2002) and has led to the emergence of the 'hygiene theory of immune disorders'.

More specifically, the hygiene hypothesis suggests that improved hygienic conditions and vaccinations, which reduce early-life exposure to microbes, are associated with a heightened risk of allergic disease and other immune disorders. This is because reduced exposure may result in reduced stimulation of the immune system. As a result, lymphocytes that would normally differentiate to become Th1-type differentiate to Th2-type cells and produce inflammatory cytokines in the allergic response in much greater quantities. As such, very early stimulation of the immune system is important in dampening the Th2 dominance and reducing the development of IgE-mediated food reactions as well as other allergic reactions. In a closely observed cohort of 329 Finnish children, it was shown that the earlier an acute respiratory infection occurred, the greater the protective effect was against atopic eczema (Vanderhoof & Young 2003).

The obvious solution for increasing microbial exposure without increasing the health risk is the use of prebiotics and probiotics. Supplementation with probiotics has been shown to both reduce the risk and treat the symptoms of childhood eczema (see Atopic Eczema, above).

Modulating the intestinal microflora with probiotics and prebiotics may be an effective and safe therapy for the natural development of a balanced immune defence in infants and children. In adults and the elderly, prebiotics and probiotics may be used to improve the general functioning of the immune system.

utilisation of cholesterol (Brashears et al 1998, Liong & Shah 2005).

According to a meta-analysis of six studies of a probiotic dairy product containing *Enterococcus faecium*, treatment with the fermented yoghurt product produced a 4% decrease in total cholesterol and a 5% decrease in low-density lipoprotein cholesterol (Agerholm-Larsen et al 2000).

Since then, mixed findings have been reported regarding the use of encapsulated probiotics; a hypocholesterolaemic effect was not observed in some studies (Greany et al 2008, Hatakka et al 2008, Larsen et al 2006, Lewis & Burmeister 2005, Simons et al 2006), but Hlivak et al (2005) provided a daily dose of 10^9 CFU of probiotic bacteria and noted a hypocholesterolaemic effect. It is possible that lipid-lowering activity induced by probiotics is dependent on whether patients have high cholesterol levels (>6.0 mmol/L) (Agerback et al 1995, Bertolami et al 1999, Hlivak et al 2005, Xiao et al 2003) or lower to normal cholesterol levels (<5.4 mmol/L) (de Roos et al 1999, Greany et al 2004), although further randomised trials are required to confirm this observation. It is also possible that some probiotic strains have the capacity to lower serum cholesterol levels while others do not.

Most recently, two randomised, placebo-controlled studies failed to detect a significant lipid-lowering activity for different strains of probiotics. Greany et al (2008) conducted a randomised, single-blinded, placebo-controlled, parallel-arm study of 33 normocholesterolaemic women and 22 men aged 18–36 years. Subjects in the intervention group were treated for 3 months with probiotic capsules (three capsules daily) containing a total of 10^9 CFU *Lactobacillus acidophilus* strain DDS-1 and *Bifidobacterium longum* strain UABL-14 and 10–15 mg fructooligosaccharide. These probiotic strains had no effect on plasma lipid concentrations (Greany et al 2008).

Likewise, Hatakka et al (2008) conducted a double-blind, randomised, placebo-controlled, two-period crossover study to investigate the effects of taking on a daily basis two probiotic capsules containing viable *Lactobacillus rhamnosus* LC705 and *Propionibacterium freudenreichii* ssp. *shermanii* JS (2×10^{10} CFU of each strain) on serum cholesterol and triglyceride levels: the study of 38 mildly or moderately hypercholesterolaemic men aged 24–55 years found that probiotic treatment over 4 weeks did not have any effect on serum lipids.

Mastitis

Mastitis is an inflammatory condition of the breast that may, or may not, be associated with infection. It is a common reason for premature cessation of breastfeeding (Academy of Breastfeeding Medicine 2008). Recent research has found some probiotic strains to be of benefit in the treatment of mastitis and the prophylaxis of recurrent mastitis.

In a randomised, double-blind, placebo-controlled trial, 352 women with lactational mastitis were allocated into one of three groups: antibiotics, *Lactobacillus fermentum* CECT5716 or *L. salivarius* CECT (both at 1.0×10^9 CFU/day). After 3 weeks' treatment, both probiotic strains were found to be superior to antibiotics in decreasing levels of pathogenic bacteria in breast milk, increasing lactobacilli counts in breast milk and decreasing breast pain scores (all $P < 0.001$). They also significantly reduced the rate of recurrence compared to antibiotics: 10.5% in the *L. fermentum* CECT5716 group and 7.1% in the *L. salivarius* CECT5713 group versus 30.7% in the antibiotic group (both $P < 0.001$) (Arroyo et al 2010).

In another randomised, placebo-controlled trial, women ($n = 20$) with antibiotic-resistant mastitis were allocated to receive either placebo or a probiotic preparation (*Lactobacillus salivarius* CECT5713 and *L. gasseri* CECT5714; 2.0×10^{10} CFU/day) for 14 days. All mastitis signs were eliminated by day 14 in the probiotic group, whereas mastitis persisted in all women in the control group. There was also an ~100-fold decrease in milk staphylococcal counts in probiotic group (Jimenez et al 2008).

Postpartum obesity

Another novel area of research is using probiotics to prevent postpartum obesity. Ilmonen et al investigated the use of a probiotic combination product (containing LGG and *Bifidobacterium lactis* Bb12) in the prophylaxis of postpartum obesity. In the first trimester of pregnancy, 256 women were randomly assigned to receive no dietary counselling or nutritional counselling (low-fat and high-fibre diet) plus probiotics (LGG and Bb12; 2.0×10^{10} CFU/day) or counselling plus placebo. Interventions lasted until the end of exclusive breastfeeding for up to 6 months. At 6 months postpartum, the risk of central adiposity (defined as waist circumference 80 cm or more) was lowered in women in the diet/probiotics group compared with the control/placebo group (OR 0.30, 95% CI 0.11–0.85; $P = 0.023$ adjusted for baseline body mass index), while the diet/placebo group did not differ from the controls (OR 1.00, 95% CI 0.38–2.68; $P = 0.994$). The number needed to treat with diet/probiotics to prevent one woman from developing a waist circumference of 80 cm or more was four (Ilmonen et al 2011). At 12 months postpartum, central obesity occurred in 25% of diet/probiotic subjects versus 43% in the diet/placebo group. The proportion of body fat was also 3.5% lower in the diet/probiotic group ($P = 0.018$) (Laitinen et al 2009).

Urogenital infections

Probiotics are widely used in the treatment and prevention of urogenital infections. They can be administered both orally and locally, with several trials supporting their use. There are additional criteria needed for probiotic strains to be efficacious in urogenital applications. Strains must demonstrate the capacity to adhere to uroepithelial and vaginal cells, colonise the vagina, inhibit urogenital pathogen growth and/or attachment and ideally should produce hydrogen peroxide. Strains that will be administered orally must have sufficient tolerance to gastric acid and bile salts and the capacity to colonise the vagina after oral intake (Reid & Bruce 2001). Probiotic strains that do not exhibit these characteristics are unlikely to be therapeutic for urogenital applications.

The mechanisms by which some *Lactobacillus* strains reduce bacterial vaginosis, vaginal candidiasis and urinary tract infectionss appear to involve a combination of antiadhesion factors, byproducts such as hydrogen peroxide, bacteriocins and lactic acid, and destruction of urogenital pathogen biofilms, as well as immune modulation or modification of vaginal epithelial cell cytokine production (Kohler et al 2012, Korshunov et al 1999, McMillan et al 2011, Wagner & Johnson 2012).

Bacterial vaginosis

Bacterial vaginosis is the most prevalent vaginal infection worldwide and is characterised by an altered vaginal ecosystem — specifically depletion of the indigenous lactobacilli. Administration of exogenous lactobacilli strains has thus been an area of research interest (Martinez et al 2009a).

A Cochrane systematic review conducted in 2009 included four randomised controlled trials that examined probiotic agents in the treatment of bacterial vaginosis. Analysis suggested that probiotics were effective in enhancing microbiological cure rates, with the oral metronidazole/probiotic (*Lactobacillus rhamnosus* GR-1 and *L. reuteri* RC-14) regimen (OR 0.09; 95% CI 0.03–0.26) and the probiotic (unspecified strain of *Lactobacillus acidophilus*)/oestriol preparation (OR 0.02; 95% CI 0.00–0.47) showing effectiveness. The authors cautioned, however, that larger well-designed trials were needed before any firm conclusions could be made (Senok et al 2009). Research on specific strains that have demonstrated efficacy is highlighted below.

A randomised, controlled, open-label trial evaluated the efficacy of a probiotic combination (*Lactobacillus rhamnosus* GR-1 and *L. reuteri* RC-14; 2 × 10^9 CFU/day) in women with bacterial vaginosis. Women received either metronidazole gel or the probiotic preparation. Both preparations were applied intravaginally for 5 days. Application of probiotics resulted in a 90% cure rate by day 30. Follow-up at day 6, 15 and 30 showed cure of bacterial vaginosis in significantly more probiotic-treated subjects (16, 17 and 18/20, respectively) compared to metronidazole gel treatment (9, 9 and 11/20, respectively; $P = 0.016$ at day 6, $P = 0.002$ at day 15 and $P = 0.056$ at day 30) (Anukam et al 2006).

In a randomised, double-blind, placebo-controlled trial, 64 women diagnosed with bacterial vaginosis were randomly assigned to receive a single dose of tinidazole supplemented with either two placebo capsules or two capsules containing *Lactobacillus rhamnosus* GR-1 and *L. reuteri* RC-14 (2 × 10^9 CFU/day) taken orally every morning for the following 4 weeks. At the end of the trial, subjects in the probiotic group had a higher rate of bacterial vaginosis cure (88% vs 50%; $P = 0.001$). Vaginal flora normalised in 75% of probiotic-treated subjects compared to only 34% of controls ($P = 0.011$) (Martinez et al 2009a).

A more recent randomised, double-blind, placebo-controlled trial evaluated the efficacy of probiotics in isolation on bacterial vaginosis. Women diagnosed with bacterial vaginosis ($n = 544$) were randomly assigned to receive either oral placebo or probiotic therapy (*Lactobacillus rhamnosus* GR-1 and *L. reuteri* RC-14; ~1 × 10^9 CFU/day) for 6 weeks. Restitution of a balanced vaginal ecosystem was reported in 27% of subjects in the placebo group compared to 62% in the probiotic group ($P < 0.001$). After an additional 6 weeks of follow-up, a normal vaginal ecosystem was still present in more than half (51%) of subjects in the probiotic group, but only in around one-fifth (21%) of subjects who were taking placebo ($P < 0.001$) (Vujic et al 2013).

A randomised, double-blind, placebo-controlled trial investigating the potential role of probiotics in the prevention and cure of bacterial vaginosis in women with HIV ($n = 65$) found 6 months' daily treatment with a probiotic preparation (*Lactobacillus rhamnosus* GR-1 and *Lactobacillus reuteri* RC-14; 2 × 10^9 CFU/day) to be ineffective in enhancing bacterial vaginosis cure rates in this population. Nor was there a difference in recurrence rates of bacterial vaginosis between the probiotics and the placebo groups. There was, however, a trend for a higher prevalence of normal vaginal flora in the probiotic group (53% normalised vs 25%; $P = 0.08$) (Hummelen et al 2010).

The strains to use in the prevention and treatment of bacterial vaginosis appear to be *Lactobacillus rhamnosus* GR-1 and *L. reuteri* RC-14.

P

Urinary tract infections

Grin et al (2013) performed this systematic review and meta-analysis to review the data on the potential effectiveness of lactobacilli in the prevention of recurrent urinary tract infections in women. Five randomised, controlled trials were included in the analysis. Combining the data from all the trials (294 patients) found no preventive effect of lactobacilli supplementation (RR = 0.85, 95% CI 0.58–1.25; $P = 0.41$). However, a sensitivity analysis was performed, excluding studies using ineffective strains and studies testing for safety only. Data from 127 patients in two trials were included. A statistically significant decrease in recurrent urinary tract infections was found in patients given lactobacilli, denoted by the pooled risk ratio of 0.51 (95% CI 0.26–0.99; $P = 0.05$) (Grin et al 2013).

A significant reduction in urinary tract infection recurrence rate was reported in a randomised, double-blind study involving 55 premenopausal women (Reid 2001). The study investigated the effectiveness of treatment for 1 year with a weekly suppository containing either 0.5 g *L. rhamnosus* GR-1 and *L. fermentum* B-54 or a *Lactobacillus* growth factor (skim milk). Treatment resulted in the urinary tract infection rate decreasing by 73% and 79%, respectively, with no adverse effects reported.

A recent, randomised, double-blind, non-inferiority trial compared the efficacy of 12 months of prophylaxis with antibiotics (trimethoprim-sulfamethoxazole; 480 mg/day) or oral probiotics (2 × 10^9 CFU/day of *Lactobacillus rhamnosus* GR-1 and *L. reuteri* RC-14) in the prevention of urinary tract infections in postmenopausal women with recurrent cystitis (*n* = 252). The number of symptomatic urinary tract infections over the 12-month treatment period was 2.9 in the antibiotic group and 3.3 in the lactobacilli group — a between-treatment difference of 0.4 episodes (95% CI −0.4 to 1.5) or 13.8%. In the year preceding the trial, the subjects experienced a mean of 6.9 urinary tract infections. The percentage of patients with at least one urinary tract infection at 12 months was 69.3% in the trimethoprim-sulfamethoxazole group and 79.1% in the lactobacilli group. The median times to first recurrence were 6 and 3 months, respectively. After 12 months of trimethoprim-sulfamethoxazole prophylaxis, all urinary *E. coli* isolates of asymptomatic women were resistant to trimethoprim-sulfamethoxazole and trimethoprim. Probiotic use, however, was not associated with increased antibiotic resistance. The authors stated that this lactobacilli combination may be an acceptable alternative for the prevention of urinary tract infections, especially in women who dislike taking antibiotics (Beerepoot et al 2012). While probiotic therapy appeared slightly less effective than antibiotic prophylaxis in postmenopausal women with recurrent urinary tract infections, their use does not damage the GIT ecosystem, nor create antibiotic-resistant organisms, and for these reasons, some have argued that this probiotic combination has a role to play in the prevention of recurrent urinary tract infections (Trautner & Gupta 2012).

The probiotic combination of *Lactobacillus rhamnosus* GR-1 and *L. reuteri* RC-14 appears to have the greatest evidence supporting its use in the prevention of urinary tract infections.

Vaginal candidiasis

Lactobacilli can impair the growth of *Candida albicans* via the production of lactic acid, which creates a low-pH environment, resulting in suppressed fungal growth. Cocultures of specific lactobacilli strains with *C. albicans* revealed that *C. albicans* cells lost metabolic activity and eventually died. Transcriptome analyses showed increased expression of stress-related genes and lower expression of genes involved in antifungal resistance (Kohler et al 2012).

A systematic review examining the role of lactobacilli probiotics in the treatment and prevention of vulvovaginal candidiasis (and other urogenital infections) was conducted by Abad and Safdar in 2009. Only four studies were found that evaluated lactobacilli supplementation in vulvovaginal candidiasis — two assessed preventive effects and two treatment effects. Only one prospective crossover trial found a significant benefit of probiotic therapy for the prevention of vulvovaginal candidiasis (RR 0.39; 95% CI 0.17–0.70). The authors concluded that there were insufficient data to make definitive conclusions at this point in time (Abad & Safdar 2009).

Some probiotic preparations have been shown to be ineffective in the treatment of vulvovaginal candidiasis — Lactobac (unspecified strains of *Lactobacillus rhamnosus* and *Bifidobacterium longum*) and Femilac (unspecified strains of *L. rhamnosus*, *L. delbrueckii* ssp. *bulgaricus*, *L. acidophilus* and *Streptococcus thermophilus*) (Pirotta et al 2004). Probiotic preparations that have shown efficacy in the treatment of vulvovaginal candidiasis are detailed in Table 9, although it should be highlighted that most of these trials were small in size.

OTHER USES

Probiotics may have many potentially important clinical applications, and current areas of active research include mostly animal studies investigating a range of diseases, including control or prevention of cancer (Fotiadis et al 2008) and prevention or treatment of graft-versus-host disease in transplant recipients (Gerbitz et al 2004).

DOSAGE RANGE

Probiotic doses are usually standardised in terms of the amount of living bacteria per unit of volume. Each living bacterium is referred to as a colony-forming unit or CFU.

The minimum concentration of probiotic bacteria needed to achieve therapeutic effects appears to be somewhat strain-dependent, in that, for some strains (e.g. *L. reuteri* MM53), 10^7 bacteria is a sufficient quantity to produce beneficial effects (Shornikova et al 1997), while for other strains, 10^9 viable bacteria is needed (e.g. *L. rhamnosus* GG) (Saxelin 1996). This situation, unfortunately, makes it hard to give firm dosage recommendations, as the minimum effective dosage appears to differ by strain. Thus it is best practice to ensure that supplements contain bacteria in concentrations $>10^9$ bacteria/dose, unless research has demonstrated that the specific strain contained in the supplement is effective in smaller amounts.

If a product contains multiple strains, then each strain should be present at levels of $\geq 10^9$ to ensure effectiveness. The viable bacteria are typically mixed in a suitable matrix, which may contain maltodextrin, cellulose, and small amounts of prebiotics, such as fructooligosaccharides and inulin.

Supplements are best taken with meals to enhance bacterial survival.

A serving of yoghurt containing fewer than 10^8 viable bacteria is unlikely to have any therapeutic activity beyond acting as a nutritional source.

TABLE 9 PROBIOTICS IN THE TREATMENT OF VULVOVAGINAL CANDIDIASIS (VC)

Trial methodology	Strain(s) utilised	Results
R, DB, PC $n = 27$ women with a history of recurrent VC	*Lactobacillus acidophilus* NAS as a vaginal suppository in isolation or with *L. acidophilus* NAS strain; *Bifidobacterium bifidum* Malyoth strain, and *Lactobacillus bulgaricus* LB-51 strain taken orally	In women who used the *L. acidophilus* NAS vaginal suppository, the incidence of recurrent VC was significantly reduced compared to controls ($P = 0.005$). Subjects who took both the suppository and the oral probiotic supplement also had a significant reduction in the number of infections compared to controls ($P = 0.011$). There was, however, no extra benefit seen from taking the oral probiotic preparation (Metts et al 2003)
R, DB, PC $n = 55$ women with VC	*Lactobacillus rhamnosus* GR-1 and *Lactobacillus reuteri* RC-14	After a single dose of fluconazole and 4 weeks' oral treatment with either probiotic or placebo, subjects in the probiotic group had reduced *Candida* colonisation (10% vs 39%; $P = 0.014$) and decreased vaginal discharge (10% vs 35%; $P = 0.03$) (Martinez et al 2009b)
R, PC, CO $n = 33$ women with a history of recurrent VC	*Lactobacillus acidophilus* LA5	The mean number of infections per 6 months decreased while in the probiotic phase compared to control phase of trial (0.38 vs 2.54; $P = 0.001$). The incidence of *Candida* colonisation also decreased during probiotic treatment (0.84 vs 3.23 per 6 months; $P = 0.001$) (Hilton et al 1992)
OL $n = 28$ women with a history of recurrent VC	*Lactobacillus rhamnosus* GG (LGG)	Twice-daily intravaginal application of LGG resulted in decreased symptoms of vulvovaginal candidiasis, as well as less erythema and discharge; 4/5 women who were positive for *Candida* at baseline had negative cultures at the end of 7 days (Hilton et al 1995)

R, randomised; DB, double-blind; PC, placebo-controlled; CO, crossover; OL, open-label.

Practice points/Patient counselling

- Some probiotics may improve the long-term bowel flora; however, the benefits of probiotics extends well beyond this role.
- Studies have shown that probiotics are beneficial in the treatment of digestive disorders such as diarrhoea and some inflammatory bowel diseases and also other conditions, such as urogenital infections, antibiotic-induced and TD, IBS, ulcerative colitis, food allergies, eczema and the prevention and treatment of paediatric atopic dermatitis.
- It is vital to note that, just because one strain of bacteria in a given species has a proven action or characteristic, it does not mean that another strain will too, even if they are closely related. Strains within the same species can have significantly different actions, properties and characteristics, as these are all essentially strain-specific qualities.
- Probiotics can be administered orally or intravaginally. They can also be taken as yoghurt or other cultured dairy products. It should be noted that only products containing actual probiotic strains will be beneficial. The so-called starter cultures (strains of *Lactobacillus delbrueckii* ssp. *bulgaricus* and *Streptococcus thermophilus*) have limited beneficial effects.
- For traveller's diarrhoea prevention, , it is recommended that the probiotic dose be started some days before travelling to ensure that the beneficial bacteria have colonised the gut; the dosage may vary depending on the probiotic strain.

ADVERSE REACTIONS

Probiotics are generally regarded as safe. However, probiotic therapy should be used with caution in the immunocompromised, as they may be at increased risk of adverse reactions. Infections, sepsis and meningitis have been reported in adult cases when administered lactobacilli (Land et al 2005, Mackay et al 1999, Rautio et al 1999). Cases of young children and infants have also been reported (Borriello et al 2003). Opportunistic pathogenicity is, however, considered low (Shanahan 2012).

There have been a number of cases of fungaemia reported in the literature from the oral administration of *Saccharomyces cerevisiae* var. *boulardii* (aka *S. boulardii*). These have occurred almost exclusively in immunocompromised or critically ill individuals, in particular those with intravascular catheters. Thus administration of strains of *S. cerevisiae* var.

boulardii may best be limited to immunocompetent individuals — i.e. those with well-functioning immune systems (Enache-Angoulvant & Hennequin 2005, Lherm et al 2002, Riquelme et al 2003). Additionally, in hospitalised patients with a central venous catheter, supplementation with a strain of *S. cerevisiae* var. *boulardii* should be avoided to prevent inadvertent catheter contamination (Venugopalan et al 2010).

There is also concern in critically ill patients because impaired intestinal barrier function could result in infection as a result of bacterial translocation (Land et al 2005, Munoz et al 2005). Recently, there has been one report citing increased mortality in patients with severe acute pancreatitis who were administered a novel multispecies probiotic (Besselink et al 2008).

SIGNIFICANT INTERACTIONS

Antibiotics

Concomitant administration of some strains of probiotics reduces gastrointestinal and genitourinary side effects according to clinical studies — combination can be safely used together and a beneficial interaction is likely.

CONTRAINDICATIONS AND PRECAUTIONS

Specific strains of probiotics are appropriate for different disorders. Probiotics are contraindicated in those people who are hypersensitive to any component of the probiotics-containing product. Strains of *Saccharomyces cerevisiae* var. *boulardii* may best be avoided in immunocompromised individuals

PREGNANCY USE

Likely to be safe in pregnancy; however, it is best practice to utilise strains that have demonstrated excellent safety profiles in clinical trials conducted on pregnant women.

PATIENTS' FAQs

What can probiotics do for me?

Studies have shown that probiotics are beneficial in the treatment of digestive disorders such as diarrhoea and some inflammatory bowel diseases and also other conditions not directly connected with the digestive tract, such as vaginal thrush and recurrent cystitis, antibiotic-induced and TD, IBS, food allergies and eczema.

When will they start to work?

Usually, probiotics can exert beneficial effects in digestive disorders within days, although continuous use for several weeks/months may produce long-term benefits and be necessary in the treatment of other disorders.

Are there any safety issues?

Generally, probiotics have a good safety profile; however, supplements should be used under supervision in the immunocompromised.

REFERENCES

Abad, C. L. & Safdar, N. 2009. The role of lactobacillus probiotics in the treatment or prevention of urogenital infections — a systematic review. J Chemother, 21, 243–52.

Abrahamsson, T. R., et al. 2007. Probiotics in prevention of IgE-associated eczema: a double-blind, randomized, placebo-controlled trial. J Allergy Clin Immunol, 119, 1174–1180.

Academy of Breastfeeding Medicine 2008. ABM clinical protocol #4: mastitis. Revision, May 2008. Breastfeed Med, 3, 177–80.

Agerback M, et al. Hypocholesterolemic effect of a new fermented milk product in healthy middle-aged men. Eur J Clin Nutr 49 (1995): 346–352.

Agerholm-Larsen L et al. The effect of a probiotic milk product on plasma cholesterol: A meta-analysis of short-term intervention studies. Eur J Clin Nutr 54.11 (2000): 856–860.

Agrawal, A., et al. 2009. Clinical trial: the effects of a fermented milk product containing *Bifidobacterium lactis* DN-173010 on abdominal distension and gastrointestinal transit in irritable bowel syndrome with constipation. Aliment Pharmacol Ther, 29, 104–14.

Ahmed, M., et al. 2007. Impact of consumption of different levels of *Bifidobacterium lactis* HN019 on the intestinal microflora of elderly human subjects. Journal of Nutrition, Health & Aging, 11, 26–31.

Ahrne, S. & Hagslatt, M. L. 2011. Effect of lactobacilli on paracellular permeability in the gut. Nutrients, 3, 104–17.

Ait-Belgnaoui, A., et al. 2006. *Lactobacillus farciminis* treatment suppresses stress induced visceral hypersensitivity: a possible action through interaction with epithelial cell cytoskeleton contraction. Gut, 55, 1090–4.

Akyol S et al. The effect of antibiotic and probiotic combination therapy on secondary pancreatic infections and oxidative stress parameters in experimental acute necrotizing pancreatitis. Pancreas 26.4 (2003): 363–367.

Anukam, K. C., et al. 2006. Clinical study comparing probiotic *Lactobacillus* GR-1 and RC-14 with metronidazole vaginal gel to treat symptomatic bacterial vaginosis. Microbes & Infection, 8, 2772–2776.

Anukam KC et al. Yogurt containing probiotic *Lactobacillus rhamnosus* GR-1 and *L. reuteri* RC-14 helps resolve moderate diarrhoea and increases CD4 count in HIV/AIDS patients. J Clin Gastroenterol 42.3 (2008): 239–243.

Ardley, C. & Wright, S. 2010. Travellers' diarrhoea. Medicine, 38, 26–29.

Arroyo, R., et al. 2010. Treatment of infectious mastitis during lactation: antibiotics versus oral administration of Lactobacilli isolated from breast milk. Clin Infect Dis, 50, 1551–8.

Arvola, T., et al. 1999. Prophylactic *Lactobacillus* GG reduces antibiotic-associated diarrhea in children with respiratory infections: a randomized study. Pediatrics, 104, 1–4.

Bajaj JS et al. Probiotic yogurt for the treatment of minimal hepatic encephalopathy. Am J Gastroenterol 103.7 (2008): 1707–1715.

Beerepoot, M. A., et al. 2012. Lactobacilli vs antibiotics to prevent urinary tract infections: a randomized, double-blind, noninferiority trial in postmenopausal women. Arch Intern Med, 172, 704–12.

Bengmark S. Ecological control of the gastrointestinal tract: the role of probiotic flora. Gut 42 (1998): 2–7.

Benno, Y., et al. 1996. Effects of *Lactobacillus* GG yoghurt on human intestinal microecology in Japanese subjects. Nutrition Today, 31, 9S–12S.

Bertolami MC, et al. Evaluation of the effects of a new fermented milk product (Gaio) on primary hypercholesterolemia. Eur J Clin Nutr 53 (1999): 97–101.

Besselink MG et al. Probiotic prophylaxis in predicted severe acute pancreatitis: a randomized, double-blind, placebo-controlled trial. Lancet 371 (2008): 651–659.

Black, F., et al. 1989. Prophylactic efficacy of Lactobacilli on travellers' diarrhea. Travel Med, 7, 333–335.

Borriello SP et al. Safety of probiotics that contain Lactobacilli or Bifidobacteria. Clin Infect Dis 36 (2003): 775–780.

Bougle, D., et al. 1999. Effect of propionibacteria supplementation on fecal bifidobacteria and segmental colonic transit time in healthy human subjects. Scand J Gastroenterol, 34, 144–8.

Bourreille, A., et al. 2013. *Saccharomyces boulardii* does not prevent relapse of Crohn's disease. Clinical Gastroenterology and Hepatology 11.8 982–987.

Boyle, R. J., et al. 2011. Lactobacillus GG treatment during pregnancy for the prevention of eczema: a randomized controlled trial. Allergy, 66, 509–516.

Brashears MM, et al. Bile salt deconjugation and cholesterol removal from media by *Lactobacillus casei*. J Dairy Sci 81 (1998): 2103–2110.

Buts, J. P., et al. 1986. Response of human and rat small intestinal mucosa to oral administration of *Saccharomyces boulardii*. Pediatr Res, 20, 192–6.

Buts, J. P., et al. 1994. *Saccharomyces boulardii* enhances rat intestinal enzyme expression by endoluminal release of polyamines. Pediatric Research, 36, 522–527.

Caballero-Franco, C., et al. 2007. The VSL#3 probiotic formula induces mucin gene expression and secretion in colonic epithelial cells. American Journal of Physiology — Gastrointestinal and Liver Physiology, 292, G315–G322.

Camilleri M. Probiotics and irritable bowel syndrome: rationale, putative mechanisms, and evidence of clinical efficacy. J Clin Gastroenterol 40.3 (2006): 264–269.

Campieri M et al. Combination of antibiotic and probiotic treatment is efficacious in prophylaxis of post-operative recurrence of Crohn's disease: A randomized controlled study vs mesalamine. Gastroenterology 118 (2000): G4179.

Castagliuolo, I., et al. 1999. *Saccharomyces boulardii* protease inhibits the effects of *Clostridium difficile* toxins A and B in human colonic mucosa. Infect Immun, 67, 302–7.

Cheigh, H. S., et al. 1994. Biochemical, microbiological, and nutritional aspects of kimchi (Korean fermented vegetable products). Critical Reviews in Food Science and Nutrition, 34, 175–203.

Corr, S. C., et al. 2009. Understanding the mechanisms by which probiotics inhibit gastrointestinal pathogens. Adv Food Nutr Res, 56, 1–15.

Cox, A. J., et al. Oral administration of the probiotic *Lactobacillus fermentum* VRI-003 and mucosal immunity in endurance athletes. Br J Sports Med, 14 (2010): 222–226.

D'Argenio, G. & Mazzacca, G. 1999. Short-chain fatty acid in the human colon. *In:* Zappia, V., et al. (eds.) Advances in Nutrition and Cancer, vol. 2. Springer US.

Dedicatoria RF, et al. The fermentation inoculation with lactic acid bacteria to increase the nutritive value of sauerkraut. Kalikasan 10 (1981): 214–2119.

De Dios Pozo-Olano, J., et al. 1978. Effect of a lactobacilli preparation on traveler's diarrhea. A randomized, double blind clinical trial. Gastroenterology, 74, 829–30.

Dendukuri N et al. Probiotic therapy for the prevention and treatment of *Clostridium difficile*-associated diarrhoea: a systematic review. CMAJ 173.2 (2005): 167–170.

de Roos NM, et al. Yoghurt enriched with *Lactobacillus acidophilus* does not lower blood lipids in healthy men and women with normal to borderline high serum cholesterol levels. Eur J Clin Nutr 53 (1999): 277–280.

Dotterud, C. K., et al. 2010. Probiotics in pregnant women to prevent allergic disease: a randomized, double-blind trial. Br J Dermatol, 163, 616–23.

Drouault-Holowacz S et al. A double blind randomized controlled trial of a probiotic combination in 100 patients with irritable bowel syndrome. Gastroenterol Clin Biol 32.2 (2008): 147–152.

Dubey, A. P., et al. 2008. Use of VSL#3 in the treatment of rotavirus diarrhea in children. J Clin Gastroenterol, 42, S126–S129.

Ducrotte, P., et al. 2012. Clinical trial: *Lactobacillus plantarum* 299v (DSM 9843) improves symptoms of irritable bowel syndrome. World J Gastroenterol, 18, 4012–8.

Enache-Angoulvant A, Hennequin C. Invasive *Saccharomyces* infection: a comprehensive review. Clin Infect Dis 41.11 (2005): 1559–1568.

Fang SB et al. Dose-dependent effect of *Lactobacillus* GG on quantitative reduction of faecal rotavirus shedding in children. J Trop Pediatr 55.5 (2009): 297–301.

FAO/WHO (Food and Agriculture Organization and World Health Organization). Expert consultation on evaluation of health and nutritional properties of probiotics in food including powder milk with live lactic acid bacteria. WHO: Geneva, 2001. Available online from www.who.int/foodsafety/publications/fs_management/en/probiotics.pdf (accessed September 2009).

Fotiadis CI et al. Role of probiotics, prebiotics and synbiotics in chemoprevention for colorectal cancer. World J Gastroenterol 14.42 (2008): 6453–6457.

Fric P, Zavoral M. The effect of non-pathogenic *Escherichia coli* in symptomatic uncomplicated diverticular disease of the colon. Eur J Gastroenterol Hepatol 15 (2003): 313–3115.

Fuller, R. & Gibson, G. R. 1997. Modification of the intestinal microflora using probiotics and prebiotics. Scandinavian Journal of Gastroenterology, 32(suppl 222), 28–31.

Garrote GL, et al. Chemical and microbiological characterisation of kefir grains. J Dairy Res 68 (2001): 639–652.

Gerbitz A, et al. Probiotic effects on experimental graft-versus-host disease: let them eat yogurt. Blood 103 (2004): 4365–4367.

Gibson GR, Roberfroid MB. Dietary modulation of the human colonic microbiota: introducing the concept of prebiotics. J Nutr 125.6 (1995): 1401–1412.

Gionchetti P, et al. Oral bacteriotherapy as maintenance treatment in patients with chronic pouchitis: a double-blind, placebo-controlled trial. Gastroenterology 119.2 (2000): 305–309.

Gionchetti P, et al. Prophylaxis of pouchitis onset with probiotic therapy: a double-blind, placebo-controlled trial. Gastroenterology 124.5 (2003): 1202–1209.

Goh J, O'Morain CA. Review article: nutrition and adult inflammatory bowel disease. Aliment Pharmacol Ther 17.3 (2003): 307–320.

Goldin, B. R. 1998. Health benefits of probiotics. British Journal of Nutrition, 80(suppl 2), S203–S207.

Gosselink, M. P., et al. 2005. Delay of the first onset of pouchitis by oral intake of the probiotic strain *Lactobacillus rhamnosus* GG. Diseases of the Colon & Rectum, 47, 876–884.

Greany KA et al. Probiotic consumption does not enhance the cholesterol-lowering effect of soy in postmenopausal women. J Nutr 134 (2004): 3277–3283.

Greany KA et al. Probiotic capsules do not lower plasma lipids in young women and men. Eur J Clin Nutr 62.2 (2008): 232–237.

Grin, P. M., et al. 2013. Lactobacillus for preventing recurrent urinary tract infections in women: meta-analysis. Can J Urol, 20, 6607–14.

Guarner, F., et al. 2011. Probiotics and prebiotics. World Gastroenterology Organisation Global Guideline 46.6 (2012); 468–481.

Guillot, C. C., et al. 1995. Effects of *Saccharomyces boulardii* in children with chronic diarrnea, especially cases due to giardiasis. Rev Mex de Puercultura y Pediatria, 2, 1–5.

Gupta P et al. Is lactobacillus GG helpful in children with Crohn's disease? Results of a preliminary, open-label study. J Pediatr Gastroenterol Nutr 31 (2000): 453–457.

Guslandi M. Of germs in inflammatory bowel disease and of how to fight them. J Gastroenterol Hepatol 18.1 (2003a): 115–16.

Guslandi M. Probiotics for chronic intestinal disorders. Am J Gastroenterol 98.3 (2003b): 520–1.

Guslandi M et al. *Saccharomyces boulardii* in maintenance treatment of Crohn's disease. Dig Dis Sci 45 (2000): 1462–1464.

Hasslof, P., et al. 2010. Growth inhibition of oral mutans streptococci and candida by commercial probiotic lactobacilli — an in vitro study. BMC Oral Health, 10, 18.

Hatakka, K., et al. 2001. Effect of long-term consumption of probiotic milk on infections in children attending day care centres: double-blind, randomised trial. British Medical Journal, 322, 1327.

Hatakka K et al. *Lactobacillus rhamnosus* LC705 together with *Propionibacterium freudenreichii* ssp *shermanii* JS administered in capsules is ineffective in lowering serum lipids. J Am Coll Nutr 27.4 (2008): 441–447.

Hawrelak, J. A. & Myers, S. P. 2004. Intestinal dysbiosis: A review of the literature. Alternative Medicine Review, 9, 180–197.

Hedin C, et al. Evidence for the use of probiotics and prebiotics in inflammatory bowel disease: a review of clinical trials. Proc Nutr Soc 66.3 (2007): 307–315.

Hempel, S., et al. 2012. Probiotics for the prevention and treatment of antibiotic-associated diarrhea: a systematic review and meta-analysis. JAMA, 307, 1959–69.

Henker, J., et al. 2008. Probiotic *Escherichia coli* Nissle 1917 (EcN) for successful remission maintenance of ulcerative colitis in children and adolescents: an open-label pilot study. Z Gastroenterol, 46, 874–875.

Hill MJ. Intestinal flora and endogenous vitamin synthesis. Eur J Cancer Prev 6 (1997): S43–S45.

Hilton E et al. Ingestion of yogurt containing *Lactobacillus acidophilus* as prophylaxis for candidal vaginitis. Ann Intern Med 116.5 (1992): 353–357.

Hilton, E., et al. 1995. Lactobacillus GG vaginal suppositories and vaginitis. Journal of Clinical Microbiology, 33, 1433.

Hilton, E., et al. 1997. Efficacy of Lactobacillus GG as a diarrheal preventive in travelers. Journal of Travel Medicine, 4, 41–43.

Hirayama K, Rafter J. The role of lactic acid bacteria in colon cancer prevention: mechanistic considerations. Antonie Van Leeuwenhoek 76.1–4 (1999): 391–394.

Hlivak P et al. One-year application of probiotic strain *Enterococcus faecium* M-74 decreases serum cholesterol levels. Bratisl Lek Listy 106 (2005): 67–72.

Hojsak, I., et al. 2009. Lactobacillus GG in the prevention of gastrointestinal and respiratory tract infections in children who attend day care centers: A randomized, double-blind, placebo-controlled trial. Clin Nutr, 125.5 (2010); 171–177.

Horvath, A., et al. 2011. Meta-analysis: *Lactobacillus rhamnosus* GG for abdominal pain-related functional gastrointestinal disorders in childhood. Aliment Pharmacol Ther, 33, 1302–10.

Hoveyda N et al. A systematic review and meta-analysis: probiotics in the treatment of irritable bowel syndrome. BMC Gastroenterol Feb 16.9 (2009): 15.

Hummelen, R., et al. 2010. *Lactobacillus rhamnosus* GR-1 and L. reuteri RC-14 to prevent or cure bacterial vaginosis among women with HIV. International Journal of Gynecology & Obstetrics, 111, 245–248.

Ilmonen, J., et al. 2011. Impact of dietary counselling and probiotic intervention on maternal anthropometric measurements during and after pregnancy: A randomized placebo-controlled trial. Clinical Nutrition, 30, 156–164.

Imaoka, A., et al. 2008. Anti-inflammatory activity of probiotic *Bifidobacterium*: enhancement of IL-10 production in peripheral blood

P

mononuclear cells from ulcerative colitis patients and inhibition of IL-8 secretion in HT-29 cells. World J Gastroenterol, 14, 2511–6.

Ishikawa, H., et al. 2005. Randomized trial of dietary fiber and *Lactobacillus casei* administration for prevention of colorectal tumors. International Journal of Cancer, 116, 762–767.

Isolauri, E. 2012. Development of healthy gut microbiota early in life. Journal of Paediatrics and Child Health, 48, 1–6.

Jijon H et al. DNA from probiotic bacteria modulates murine and human epithelial and immune function. Gastroenterology 126 (2004): 1358–1373.

Jimenez, E., et al. 2008. Oral administration of *Lactobacillus* strains isolated from breast milk as an alternative for the treatment of infectious mastitis during lactation. Appl Environ Microbiol, 74, 4650–4655.

Johnson, A. C., et al. 2011. Effects of *Bifidobacterium infantis* 35624 on post-inflammatory visceral hypersensitivity in the rat. Dig Dis Sci, 56, 3179–86.

Johnston, B. C., et al. 2011. Probiotics for the prevention of pediatric antibiotic-associated diarrhea. Cochrane Database Syst Rev, CD004827.

Jonkers, D., et al. 2012. Probiotics in the management of inflammatory bowel disease: a systematic review of intervention studies in adult patients. Drugs, 72, 803–23.

Kailasapathy K, Chin J. Survival and therapeutic potential of probiotic organisms with reference to *Lactobacillus acidophilus* and *Bifidobacterium* spp. Immunol Cell Biol 78.1 (2000): 80–88.

Kajander K et al. Clinical trial: multispecies probiotic supplementation alleviates the symptoms of irritable bowel syndrome and stabilizes intestinal microbiota. Aliment Pharmacol Ther 27.1 (2008): 48–57.

Kalliomaki, M., et al. 2001. Probiotics in primary prevention of atopic disease: a randomised, placebo-controlled trial. Lancet, 357, 1076–1079.

Kalliomaki M et al. Probiotics and prevention of atopic disease: 4-year follow-up of a randomised placebo-controlled trial. Lancet 361.9372 (2003): 1869–1871.

Kalliomaki, M., et al. 2007. Probiotics during the first 7 years of life: A cumulative risk reduction of eczema in a randomized, placebo-controlled trial. J Allergy Clin Immunol, 119, 1019–1021.

Kanauchi O et al. Modification of intestinal flora in the treatment of inflammatory bowel disease. Curr Pharm Des 9.4 (2003): 333–346.

Karthik SV. Probiotics in inflammatory bowel disease. J R Soc Med 96.7 (2003): 370.

Katelaris, P. H. & Salam, I. 1995. Lactobacilli to prevent traveler's diarrhea. New England Journal of Medicine, 333, 1360–1361.

Kaur IP, et al. Probiotics: potential pharmaceutical applications. Eur J Pharm Sci 15.1 (2002): 1–9.

Kim, H. J., et al. 2005. A randomized controlled trial of a probiotic combination VSL#3 and placebo in irritable bowel syndrome with bloating. Neurogastroenterolgy and Motility, 17, 1–10.

Kirjavainen PV, et al. Probiotic bacteria in the management of atopic disease: underscoring the importance of viability. J Pediatr Gastroenterol Nutr 36.2 (2003): 223–227.

Kirpich IA et al. Probiotics restore bowel flora and improve liver enzymes in human alcohol-induced liver injury: a pilot study. Alcohol 42.8 (2008): 675–682.

Klarin, B., et al. 2008. *Lactobacillus plantarum* 299v reduces colonisation of *Clostridium difficile* in critically ill patients treated with antibiotics. Acta Anaesthesiol Scand, 52, 1096–1102.

Koebnick, C., et al. 2003. Probiotic beverage containing *Lactobacillus casei* Shirota improves gastrointestinal symptoms in patients with chronic constipation. Canadian Journal of Gastroenterology, 17, 655–659.

Kohler, G. A., et al. 2012. Probiotic interference of *Lactobacillus rhamnosus* GR-1 and *Lactobacillus reuteri* RC-14 with the opportunistic fungal pathogen *Candida albicans*. Infect Dis Obstet Gynecol, 2012, 636474.

Kollaritsch, H., et al. 1989. Prevention of traveller's diarrhea: comparison of different nonantibiotic preparations. Travel Med Int, 9–17.

Kollaritsch H et al. [Prevention of traveler's diarrhea with *Saccharomyces boulardii*: Results of a placebo controlled double-blind study.] Fortschr Med 111.9 (1993): 152–156.

Kontiokari, T., et al. 2001. Randomised trial of cranberry-lingonberry juice and *Lactobacillus* GG drink for the prevention of urinary tract infections in women. British Medical Journal, 322, 1571.

Kopp, M. V., et al. 2008. Randomized, double-blind, placebo-controlled trial of probiotics for primary prevention: no clinical effects of Lactobacillus GG supplementation. Pediatrics, 121, e850–e856.

Korshunov VM et al. The vaginal *Bifidobacterium* flora in women of reproductive age. Zh Mikrobiol Epidemiol Immunobiol 4 (1999): 74–78.

Kruis, W., et al. 1997. Double-blind comparison of an oral *Escherichia coli* preparation and mesalazine in maintaining remission of ulcerative colitis. Aliment Pharmacol Ther, 11, 853–8.

Kruis, W., et al. 2004. Maintaining remission of ulcerative colitis with the probiotic *Escherichia coli* Nissle 1917 is as effective as with standard mesalazine. Gut, 53, 1617–1623.

Laake KO et al. Outcome of four weeks' intervention with probiotics on symptoms and endoscopic appearance after surgical reconstruction with a J-configurated ileal-pouch-anal-anastomosis in ulcerative colitis. Scandinavian J Gastroenterol 40 (2005): 43–51.

Laitinen, K., et al. 2009. Dietary counselling and probiotic intervention initiated in early pregnancy modifies maternal adiposity over 12 months postpartum. Obesity Facts, 2 (suppl 2), 4.

Land MH et al. Lactobacillus sepsis associated with probiotic therapy. Pediatrics 115 (2005): 178–181.

Lankaputhra WE, Shah NP. Antimutagenic properties of probiotic bacteria and of organic acids. Mutat Res 397.2 (1998): 169–182.

Larsen CN et al. Dose-response study of probiotic bacteria *Bifidobacterium animalis* subsp *lactis* BB-12 and *Lactobacillus paracasei* subsp *paracasei* CRL-341 in healthy young adults. Eur J Clin Nutr 60 (2006): 1284–1293.

Lewis SJ, Burmeister S. A double-blind placebo-controlled study of the effects of *Lactobacillus acidophilus* on plasma lipids. Eur J Clin Nutr 59 (2005): 776–780.

Leyer, G. J., et al. 2009. Probiotic effects on cold and influenza-like symptom incidence and duration in children. Pediatrics, 124, e172–e179.

Lherm, T., et al. 2002. Seven cases of fungemia with *Saccharomyces boulardii* in critically ill patients. Intensive Care Medicine, 28, 797–801.

Ligaarden SC et al. A candidate probiotic with unfavourable effects in subjects with irritable bowel syndrome: a randomised controlled trial. BMC Gastroenterology 2010, 10:16

Link-Amster, H., et al. 1994. Modulation of a specific humoral immune response and changes in intestinal flora mediated through fermented milk intake. FEMS Immunology and Medical Microbiology, 10, 55–64.

Lionetti, E., et al. 2006. *Lactobacillus reuteri* therapy to reduce side-effects during anti-*Helicobacter pylori* treatment in children: a randomized placebo controlled trial. Aliment Pharmacol Ther, 24, 1461–1468.

Liong MT, Shah NP. Acid and bile tolerance and cholesterol removal ability of lactobacilli strains. J Dairy Sci 88 (2005): 55–66.

Lirussi, F., et al. 2007. Probiotics for non-alcoholic fatty liver disease and/or steatohepatitis. Cochrane Database Syst Rev, CD005165.

Lonnermark, E., et al. 2010. Intake of *Lactobacillus plantarum* reduces certain gastrointestinal symptoms during treatment with antibiotics. J Clin Gastroenterol, 44, 106–112.

Macfarlane, G. T. & Cummings, J. H. 1999. Probiotics and prebiotics: can regulating the activities of the intestinal bacteria benefit health. British Medical Journal, 318, 999–1003.

Mack, D. R., et al. 1999. Probiotics inhibit enteropathogenic E. coli adherence in vitro by inducing intestinal mucin gene expression. American Journal of Physiology, 276, G941–G950.

Mack, D. R., et al. 2003. Extracellular MUC3 mucin secretion follows adherence of *Lactobacillus* strains to intestinal epithelial cells in vitro. Gut, 52, 827–833.

Mackay AD et al. Lactobacillus endocarditis caused by a probiotics organism. Clin Microbiol Infect 5 (1999): 290–292.

Maldonado, J., et al. 2012. Human milk probiotic *Lactobacillus fermentum* CECT5716 reduces the incidence of gastrointestinal and upper respiratory tract infections in infants. J Pediatr Gastroenterol Nutr, 54, 55–61.

Mangiante G et al. *Lactobacillus plantarum* reduces infection of pancreatic necrosis in experimental acute pancreatitis. Dig Surg 18 (2001): 47–50.

Manley, K. J., et al. 2007. Probiotic treatment of vancomycin-resistant enterococci: a randomised controlled trial. MJA, 186, 454–457.

Marotta, F., et al. 2003. Chemopreventive effect of a probiotic preparation on the development of preneoplastic and neoplastic colonic lesions: an experimental study. Hepatogastroenterology, 50, 1914–8.

Marteau, P. 2011. Evidence of probiotic strain specificity makes extrapolation of results impossible from a strain to another, even from the same species. Annals of Gastroenterology & Hepatology, 2, 34–36.

Marteau, P., et al. 2002. *Bifidobacterium animalis* strain DN-173010 shortens the colonic transit time in healthy women: a double-blind, randomized, controlled study. Alimentary Pharmacology & Therapeutics, 16, 587–593.

Marteau P, et al. Manipulation of the bacterial flora in inflammatory bowel disease. Best Pract Res Clin Gastroenterol 17.1 (2003): 47–61.

Martinez, R. C., et al. 2009a. Improved cure of bacterial vaginosis with single dose of tinidazole (2 g), *Lactobacillus rhamnosus* GR-1, and *Lactobacillus reuteri* RC-14: a randomized, double-blind, placebo-controlled trial. Can J Microbiol, 55, 133–138.

Martinez, R. C., et al. 2009b. Improved treatment of vulvovaginal candidiasis with fluconazole plus probiotic *Lactobacillus rhamnosus* GR-1 and *Lactobacillus reuteri* RC-14. Lett Appl Microbiol, 48, 269–274.

Matamoros, S., et al. 2013. Development of intestinal microbiota in infants and its impact on health. Trends in Microbiology, 21, 167–173.

Matthes, H., et al. 2010. Clinical trial: probiotic treatment of acute distal ulcerative colitis with rectally administered *Escherichia coli* Nissle 1917 (EcN). BMC Complement Altern Med, 10, 13.

Mattila-Sandholm, T. & Salminen, S. 1998. Up-to-date on probiotics in Europe. Gastroenterology International, 11(suppl), 8–16.

McFarland LV. Meta-analysis of probiotics for the prevention of antibiotic associated diarrhoea and the treatment of *Clostridium difficile* disease. Am J Gastroenterol 101 (2006): 812–822.

McFarland LV. Meta-analysis of probiotics for the prevention of traveller's diarrhoea. Travel Med Infect Dis 5.2 (2007): 97–105.
McFarland, L. V. & Bernasconi, P. 1993. *Saccharomyces boulardii*'. A review of an innovative biotherapeutic agent. Microbial Ecology in Health and Disease, 6, 157–171.
McFarland LV, Dublin S. Meta-analysis of probiotics for the treatment of irritable bowel syndrome. World J Gastroenterol 14 (2008): 2650–2661.
McFarland, L. V., et al. 1994. A randomized placebo-controlled trial of *Saccharomyces boulardii* in combination with standard antibiotics for *Clostridium difficile* disease. JAMA: The Journal of the American Medical Association, 271, 1913–1918.
McKane, L. & Kandel, J. 1986. Microbiology: Essentials and Applications, New York, McGraw-Hill.
McKernan, D. P., et al. 2010. The probiotic *Bifidobacterium infantis* 35624 displays visceral antinociceptive effects in the rat. Neurogastroenterol Motil, 22, 1029–35, e268.
McMillan, A., et al. 2011. Disruption of urogenital biofilms by lactobacilli. Colloids and Surfaces B: Biointerfaces, 86, 58–64.
Meance, C. C., et al. 2001 A fermented milk with a Bifidobacterium probiotic strain DN-173010 shortened oro-fecal gut transit time in elderly. Microbial Ecology in Health and Disease, 13, 217–222.
Ménard, S., et al. 2004. Lactic acid bacteria secrete metabolites retaining anti-inflammatory properties after intestinal transport. Gut, 53, 821–828.
Metchnikoff, E. 1907. The Prolongation of Life: Optimistic Studies, London, William Heinemann.
Metts, J., et al. 2003. *Lactobacillus acidophilus*, strain NAS (H2O2 positive), in reduction of recurrent candidal vulvovaginitis. Journal of Applied Research, 3, 340–348.
Michail, S. K., et al. 2008. Efficacy of probiotics in the treatment of pediatric atopic dermatitis: a meta-analysis of randomized controlled trials. Annals of Allergy, Asthma & Immunology, 101, 508–516.
Miele, E., et al. 2009. Effect of a probiotic preparation (VSL#3) on induction and maintenance of remission in children with ulcerative colitis. Am J Gastroenterol, 104, 437–443.
Mimura T et al. Once daily high dose probiotic therapy (VSL#3) for maintaining remission in recurrent or refractory pouchitis. Gut 53.1 (2004): 108–114.
Moayyedi, P., et al. 2010. The efficacy of probiotics in the treatment of irritable bowel syndrome: a systematic review. Gut, 59, 325–32.
Mohan, R., et al. 2006. Effects of *Bifidobacterium lactis* Bb12 supplementation on intestinal microbiota of preterm infants: a double-blind, placebo-controlled, randomized study. J Clin Microbiol, 44, 4025–4031.
Munoz P et al. *Saccharomyces cerevisiae* fungemia: an emerging infectious disease. Clin Infect Dis 40 (2005): 1625–1634.
Naaber, P., et al. 2004. Inhibition of *Clostridium difficile* strains by intestinal *Lactobacillus* species. Journal of Medical Microbiology, 53, 551–554.
Naidoo, K., et al. 2011. Probiotics for maintenance of remission in ulcerative colitis. Cochrane Database Syst Rev, CD007443.
Newcomer, A. D., et al. 1983. Response of patients with irritable bowel syndrome and lactase deficiency using unfermented acidophilus milk. American Journal of Clinical Nutrition, 38, 257–263.
Ng, S. C., et al. 2009. Mechanisms of action of probiotics: Recent advances. Inflammatory Bowel Diseases, 15, 300–310.
Oksanen PJ et al. Prevention of travellers' diarrhoea by *Lactobacillus* GG. Ann Med 22.1 (1990): 53–56.
Olah A et al. Randomized clinical trial of specific lactobacillus and fibre supplement to early enteral nutrition in patients with acute pancreatitis. Br J Surg 89.9 (2002): 1103–1107.
O'Mahony L et al. A randomized, placebo-controlled, double-blind comparison of the probiotic bacteria lactobacillus and bifidobacterium in irritable bowel syndrome (IBS): symptom responses and relationship to cytokine profiles. Gastroenterology 128 (2005a): 541–551.
O'Mahony, L., et al. 2005b. Lactobacillus and *Bifidobacterium* in irritable bowel syndrome: symptom responses and relationship to cytokine profiles. Gastroenterology, 128, 541–551.
Osterlund, P., et al. 2007. Lactobacillus supplementation for diarrhoea related to chemotherapy of colorectal cancer: a randomised study. Br J Cancer, 97, 1028–1034.
O'Sullivan, M. A. & O'Morain, C. A. 2000. Bacterial supplementation in the irritable bowel syndrome: a randomised double-blind placebo-controlled crossover study. Digestive and Liver Disease, 32, 294–301.
Ouwehand A, et al. The role of the intestinal microflora for the development of the immune system in early childhood. Eur J Nutr 41.Suppl 1 (2002): 132–137.
Oyewole, O. B. 1997. Lactic fermented foods in Africa and their benefits. Food Control, 8, 289–297.
Pelucchi, C., et al. 2012. Probiotics supplementation during pregnancy or infancy for the prevention of atopic dermatitis: a meta-analysis. Epidemiology, 23, 402–14.
Penner R, et al. Probiotics and nutraceuticals: non-medicinal treatments of gastrointestinal diseases. Curr Opin Pharmacol 5.6 (2005): 596–603.
Pirotta, M., et al. 2004. Effect of lactobacillus in preventing post-antibiotic vulvovaginal candidiasis: a randomised controlled trial. BMJ, 329, 548.
Plummer, S. F., et al. 2005. Effects of probiotics on the composition of the intestinal microbiota following antibiotic therapy. Int J Antimicrob Agents, 26, 69–74.
Prioult, G., et al. 2003. Effect of probiotic bacteria on induction and maintenance of oral tolerance to β-lactoglobulin in gnotobiotic mice. Clinical and Diagnostic Laboratory Immunology, 10, 787–792.
Rachmilewitz D et al. Immunostimulatory DNA ameliorates experimental and spontaneous murine colitis. Gastroenterology 122 (2002): 1428–1441.
Rachmilewitz D et al. Toll-like receptor 9 signaling mediates the anti-inflammatory effects of probiotics in murine experimental colitis. Gastroenterology 126 (2004): 520–528.
Rafii, F., et al. 2008. Effects of treatment with antimicrobial agents on the human colonic microflora. Ther Clin Risk Manag, 4, 1343–58.
Rafsky, H. A. & Rafsky, J. C. 1955. Clinical and bacteriological studies of a new *Lactobacillus acidophilus* concentrate in functional gastrointestinal disturbances. American Journal of Gastroenterology, 24, 87–92.
Rajilic-Stojanovic, M., et al. 2007. Diversity of the human gastrointestinal tract microbiota revisited. Environ Microbiol, 9, 2125–36.
Rautava, S., et al. 2009. Specific probiotics in reducing the risk of acute infections in infancy — a randomised, double-blind, placebo-controlled study. Br J Nutr, 101, 1722–1726.
Rautio M et al. Liver abcess due to a *Lactobacillus rhamnosus* strain indistinguishable from a *L. rhamnosus* strain GG. Clin Infect Dis 28 (1999): 1159–1160.
Reid G. Probiotic agents to protect the urogenital tract against infection. Am J Clin Nutr 73 (Suppl) (2001): 437S–443S.
Reid, G. & Bruce, A. W. 2001. Selection of *Lactobacillus* strains for urogenital applications. Journal of Infectious Diseases, 183 (suppl 1), S77–S80.
Rembacken, B. J., et al. 1999. Non-pathogenic *Escherichia coli* versus mesalazine for the treatment of ulcerative colitis: a randomized trial. Lancet, 354, 635–639.
Riquelme, A. J., et al. 2003. *Saccharomyces cerevisiae* fungemia after *Saccharomyces boulardii* treatment in immunocompromised patients. Journal of Clinical Gastroenterology, 36, 41–43.
Rolfe VE et al. Probiotics for maintenance of remission in Crohn's disease. Cochrane Database Syst Rev 4 (2006): CD004826.
Rosenfeldt V et al. Effect of probiotic *Lactobacillus* strains in children with atopic dermatitis. J Allergy Clin Immunol 111.2 (2003): 389–395.
Rosenfeldt V et al. Effect of probiotics on gastrointestinal symptoms and small intestinal permeability in children with atopic dermatitis. J Pediatr 145.5 (2004): 612–6116.
Rousseaux C, et al. *Lactobacillus acidophilus* modulates intestinal pain and induces opioid and cannabinoid receptors. Nat Med 13 (2007): 35–37.
Rutgeerts P. Modern therapy for inflammatory bowel disease. Scand J Gastroenterol Suppl 237 (2003): 30–33.
Saavedra, J. M., et al. 1994. Feeding of *Bifidobacterium bifidum* and *Streptococcus thermophilus* to infants in hospital for prevention of diarrhoea and shedding of rotavirus. Lancet, 344, 1046–1049.
Saint-Marc T, et al. Efficacy of *Saccharomyces boulardii* in the treatment of diarrhoea in AIDS. Ann Med Interne (Paris) 142 (1991): 64–5.
Salminen, S., et al. 2010. Interaction of probiotics and pathogens — benefits to human health? Current Opinion in Biotechnology, 21, 157–167.
Sang, L. X., et al. 2010. Remission induction and maintenance effect of probiotics on ulcerative colitis: a meta-analysis. World J Gastroenterol, 16, 1908–15.
Savino, F., et al. 2007. *Lactobacillus reuteri* (American type culture collection strain 55730) versus simethicone in the treatment of infantile colic: A prospective randomized study. Pediatrics, 119, e124–e130.
Schiffrin, E. J., et al. 1997. Immune modulation of blood leukocytes in humans by lactic acid bacteria: criteria for strain selection. American Journal of Clinical Nutrition, 66, 515S–520S.
Senok, A. C., et al. 2009. Probiotics for the treatment of bacterial vaginosis. Cochrane Database Syst Rev, CD006289.
Sgouras, D., et al. 2004. In vitro and in vivo inhibition of *Helicobacter pylori* by *Lactobacillus casei* strain Shirota. Applied and Environmental Microbiology, 70, 518–526.
Shanahan, F. 2012. A commentary on the safety of probiotics. Gastroenterology Clinics of North America, 41, 869–876.
Sheil B et al. Is the mucosal route of administration essential for probiotic function? Subcutaneous administration is associated with attenuation of murine colitis and arthritis. Gut 53 (2004): 694–700.
Shen B et al. Maintenance therapy with a probiotic in antibiotic-dependent pouchitis: experience in clinical practice. Aliment Pharmacol Ther 22.8 (2005): 721–728.
Sheth A, Floch M. Probiotics and diverticular disease. Nutr Clin Pract 24.1 (2009): 41–44.
Shornikova, A. V., et al. 1997. Bacteriotherapy with *Lactobacillus reuteri* in rotavirus gastroenteritis. Pediatr Infect Dis, 16, 1103–1107.

Simons LA, et al. Effect of *Lactobacillus fermentum* on serum lipids in subjects with elevated serum cholesterol. Nutr Metab Cardiovasc Dis 16 (2006): 531–535.
Sistek D et al. Is the effect of probiotics on atopic dermatitis confined to food sensitized children? Clin Exp Allergy 36.5 (2006): 629–633.
Sood, A., et al. 2009. The probiotic preparation, VSL#3 induces remission in patients with mild-to-moderately active ulcerative colitis. Clin Gastroenterol Hepatol, 7, 1202–1209.
Spinler, J. K., et al. 2008. Human-derived probiotic *Lactobacillus reuteri* demonstrate antimicrobial activities targeting diverse enteric bacterial pathogens. Anaerobe, 14, 166–171.
Stermer, E., et al. 2006. Is traveler's diarrhea a significant risk factor for the development of irritable bowel syndrome? A prospective study. Clin Infect Dis, 43, 898–901.
Sudo, N., et al. 1997. The requirement of intestinal bacterial flora for the development of an IgE production system fully susceptible to oral tolerance induction. The Journal of Immunology, 159, 1739–45.
Surawicz, C. M., et al. 2000. The search for a better treatment for recurrent *Clostridium difficile* disease: use of high-dose vancomycin combined with *Saccharomyces boulardii*. Clinical and Infectious Disease, 31, 1012–1017.
Szajewska, H. & Mrukowicz, J. 2005. Meta-analysis: non-pathogenic yeast *Saccharomyces boulardii* in the prevention of antibiotic-associated diarrhoea. Aliment Pharmacol Ther, 22, 365–72.
Szajewska, H., et al. 2001. Efficacy of *Lactobacillus* GG in prevention of nosocomial diarrhea in infants. J Pediatr, 138, 361–365.
Szajewska H et al. Meta-analysis: *Lactobacillus* GG for treating acute diarrhoea in children. J Aliment Pharmacol Ther 25.8 (2007): 871–881.
Szajewska, H., et al. 2010. Probiotics in the prevention of antibiotic-associated diarrhea in children: a meta-analysis of randomized controlled trials. J Pediatr, 149, 367–372.
Tanaka, K. & Ishikawa, H. 2004. Role of intestinal bacterial flora in oral tolerance induction. Histol Histopathol, 19, 907–14.
Taylor Al, et al. Probiotic supplementation for the first 6 months of life fails to reduce the risk of atopic dermatitis and increases the risk of allergen sensitization in high-risk children: A randomised controlled trial. J Allergy Clin Immunol 119 (2007): 184–191.
Tien, M.-T., et al. 2006. Anti-inflammatory effect of *Lactobacillus casei* on Shigella-infected human intestinal epithelial cells. The Journal of Immunology, 176, 1228–1237.
Trautner, B. W. & Gupta, K. 2012. The advantages of second best: comment on "Lactobacilli vs antibiotics to prevent urinary tract infections". Arch Intern Med, 172, 712–4.
Trois L, et al. Use of probiotics in HIV-infected children: a randomized double-blind controlled study. J Trop Pediatr 54.1 (2008): 19–24.
Tubelius, P., et al. 2005. Increasing work-place healthiness with the probiotic *Lactobacillus reuteri* : A randomised, double-blind placebo-controlled study. Environmental Health: A Global Access Science Source, 4, 25.
Vajro, P., et al. 2011. Effects of *Lactobacillus rhamnosus* strain GG in pediatric obesity-related liver disease. J Pediatr Gastroenterol Nutr, 52, 740–3.
Vandenplas Y et al. Probiotics in infectious diarrhoea in children: are they indicated? Eur J Pediatr 166.12 (2007): 1211–1218.
Vanderhoof JA, Young RJ. Probiotics in pediatrics. Pediatrics 109.5 (2002): 956–958.
Vanderhoof JA, Young RJ. Role of probiotics in the management of patients with food allergy. Ann Allergy Asthma Immunol 90.(6 Suppl 3) (2003): 99–103.
Venturi, A., et al. 1999. Impact on the composition of the faecal flora by a new probiotic preparation: preliminary data on maintenance treatment of patients with ulcerative colitis. Alimentary Pharmacology and Therapeutics, 13, 1103–1108.
Venugopalan, V., et al. 2010. Regulatory oversight and safety of probiotic use. Emerg Infect Dis, 16, 1661–5.
Vouloumanou, E. K., et al. 2009. Probiotics for the prevention of respiratory tract infections: a systematic review. International Journal of Antimicrobial Agents, 34, 197.e1–197.e10.
Vujic, G., et al. 2013. Efficacy of orally applied probiotic capsules for bacterial vaginosis and other vaginal infections: a double-blind, randomized, placebo-controlled study. Eur J Obstet Gynecol Reprod Biol, 168, 75–9.
Wagner, R. D. & Johnson, S. J. 2012. Probiotic lactobacillus and estrogen effects on vaginal epithelial gene expression responses to *Candida albicans*. J Biomed Sci, 19, 58.
Walker, W. A. 2008. Mechanisms of action of probiotics. Clinical Infectious Diseases, 46, S87–S91.
Waller, P. A., et al. 2011. Dose-response effect of *Bifidobacterium lactis* HN019 on whole gut transit time and functional gastrointestinal symptoms in adults. Scand J Gastroenterol, 46, 1057–64.
Weizman, Z., et al. 2005. Effect of a probiotic infant formula on infections in child care centers: comparison of two probiotic agents. Pediatrics, 115, 5–9.
Wenus, C., et al. 2008. Prevention of antibiotic-associated diarrhoea by a fermented probiotic milk drink. Eur J Clin Nutr, 62, 299–301.
West, C. E., et al. 2009. Probiotics during weaning reduce the incidence of eczema. Pediatr Allergy Immunol, 20, 430–437.
Weston S et al. Effects of probiotics on atopic dermatitis: a randomised controlled trial. Arch Dis Child 90.9 (2005): 892–897.
White JA. Probiotics and their use in diverticulitis. J Clin Gastroenterol 40 suppl 3 (2006): S160–S162.
Whorwell PJ et al. Efficacy of an encapsulated probiotic *Bifidobacterium infantis* 35624 in women with irritable bowel syndrome. Am J Gastroenterol 101 (2006): 326–333.
Wickens, K., et al. 2008. A differential effect of 2 probiotics in the prevention of eczema and atopy: A double-blind, randomized, placebo-controlled trial. J Allergy Clin Immunol, 122, 788–794.
Williams, E. A., et al. 2008. Clinical trial: a multistrain probiotic preparation significantly reduces symptoms of irritable bowel syndrome in a double-blind placebo-controlled study. Aliment Pharmacol Ther, 29, 97–103.
Xiao JZ et al. Effects of milk products fermented by *Bifidobacterium longum* on blood lipids in rats and healthy adult male volunteers. J Dairy Sci 86.7 (2003): 2452–2461.
Yang, Y. X., et al. 2008. Effect of a fermented milk containing *Bifidobacterium lactis* DN-173010 on Chinese constipated women. World J Gastroenterol, 14, 6237–43.
Zocco, M. A., et al. 2006. Efficacy of *Lactobacillus* GG in maintaining remission of ulcerative colitis. Aliment Pharmacol Ther, 23, 1567–1574.

Psyllium

HISTORICAL NOTE Psyllium has a long history of use in both conventional and traditional medical systems and has been listed in various pharmacopoeias around the world.

OTHER NAMES

Psyllium seed, Blonde *Plantaginis ovatae* semen — ripe seeds of *Plantago ovata* (*P. isphagula*).

Plantago ovata semen refers to the unprocessed seed.

White or *blond* psyllium, also known as Indian plantago.

Psyllium seed husk, Blonde *Plantaginis ovatae testa* — referring to the epidermis layers of *Plantago ovata* (*P. isphagula*)

Psyllium seed, Black *Psyllii semen* — referring to the dried ripe seed of *Plantago psyllium* (*P. afra*, *P. arenaria* and *P. indica*)

Black, French or Spanish psyllium comes from *P. psyllium* (syn. *P. afra*) and *P. arenaria* (*P. indica*).

BOTANICAL NAME/FAMILY

Plantago ovata, *P. psyllium*, *P. arenaria* (family Plantago)

PLANT PART USED

Seed coat and seed

CHEMICAL COMPONENTS

Plantago ovata seed husk generally consists of 67–71% fibre; constituents includes 10–30% mucilage (arabinoxylans), iridoid glycosides (≈ aucubin), trace monoterpene alkaloids, sugars, protein, sterols, triterpenes, fatty acids and tannins. Phytosterol and beta-sitosterol (Nakamura et al 2005). The seeds contain a 20:80 ratio of soluble to insoluble fibre, and the husks a 70:30 ratio (Lopez et al 2009).

MAIN ACTIONS

Bulking agent

Psyllium husk is commonly used throughout the world as a bulking agent in the treatment of both constipation and diarrhoea. A component of psyllium husk is incompletely fermented, forming a mucilaginous gel which provides lubrication, increases moisture content and facilitates propulsion of the colon contents (Marlett et al 2000).

Psyllium promotes stools that are more frequent and softened, and reduces pain on defecation. Psyllium has been shown to be more beneficial in maintaining regularity than bran (Singh 2007).

Promotes satiety

A placebo-controlled study of a *P. ovata* preparation administered in water found a significant difference in satiety 1 hour after consumption (Turnbull & Thomas 1995). Increased satiety was apparent up to 6 hours after consumption. A recent animal study showed that among its proposed range of action psyllium had the potential to attenuate weight gain (Wang et al 2007).

Lipid lowering

Psyllium husk effectively reduces lipid levels by altering cholesterol metabolism, increasing hepatic cholesterol catabolism and increasing faecal bile acid excretion (Romero et al 2002). *Psyllium* sequesters bile salts during passage through the intestinal lumen as well as physically disrupts the intraluminal formation of micelles, thereby reducing the absorption of cholesterol and reabsorption of bile salts. As a result, bound bile acids are moved to the terminal ileum and colon, thereby interrupting the enterohepatic circulation so that more cholesterol is converted into newly produced bile acids (Rodriguez-Moran et al 1998). It is postulated that this increased hepatic conversion of cholesterol into bile acids results in increased LDL uptake by the liver, leading to decreased levels of serum LDL cholesterol and total cholesterol (Theuwissen & Mensink 2008). Reduced cholesterol biosynthesis results in an upregulation of LDL receptors and enhanced uptake of LDL cholesterol (Shrestha et al 2007). Both the unfermented and viscous components of psyllium are considered responsible for the observed lipid-lowering effects (Marlett & Fischer 2003, Dikeman & Fahey 2006).

Slows glucose absorption

Animal and human models have demonstrated that psyllium modulates the glycaemic response through various mechanisms. Psyllium supplementation delays gastric emptying, small bowel motility and reduces intestinal mixing, thereby slowing and reducing glucose absorption across the intestinal lumen of the small intestine (Dikeman & Fahey 2006). Psyllium has induced an upregulation of GLUT-4 receptors in skeletal muscle cell membranes in vitro (Song et al 2000), and has been shown to improve glycaemic response by modulating postprandial glucose concentrations and insulin requirements (Anderson et al 1999, Frati-Munari et al 1989, Sierra et al 2001). Wang et al demonstrated in vivo that psyllium enhances insulin sensitivity, reduces weight gain and modulates GLP-1 secretion (Wang et al 2007).

Metabolic syndrome

Psyllium husk administration may beneficially alter many of the abnormalities observed in metabolic syndrome through the actions detailed above, but recent animal research also suggests a capacity to upregulate hepatic AMP-activated protein kinase phophorylation, reduce secretion of tumour-necrosis factor-alpha (TNF-α), increase production of adiponectin, and enhance expression of its receptors in visceral adipose tissue (Galisteo et al 2010).

Colonic anti-inflammatory effects

In a rat model of ulcerative colitis, administration of psyllium seeds resulted in increased concentrations of short-chain fatty acids (particularly butyrate) in the colonic lumen, ameliorated the development of colonic inflammation, and decreased colonocyte production of pro-inflammatory mediators leukotriene B_4 and tumour-necrosis factor-alpha (Rodriguez-Cabezas et al 2003).

P

Promotes apoptosis of colorectal cancer cells

The fermentation products of psyllium husks (representative of what occurs in the colon after ingestion) were found to induce apoptosis in primary colorectal tumour cells and metastatic cell lines (Caco-2, HCT116, LoVo, HT-29 and SW480). Apoptosis was caspase-dependent and both intrinsic and extrinsic pathways were involved (Sohn et al 2012).

CLINICAL USE

Psyllium is used mainly for its mucilage content, which comes from the seed coat (husk).

Bulking agent

Psyllium is commonly used as a bulking agent to treat constipation or diarrhoea and to regulate stool consistency in people with a colostomy or ileostomy. As a bowel regulator, psyllium husk absorbs water in the colon to increase faecal bulk, which stimulates peristaltic activity. Alternatively, psyllium can be used to promote normal stool formation in people with diarrhoea by decreasing the frequency of fluid stools. Commission E approves the use of black psyllium seed and blond psyllium seed for chronic constipation and when a soft stool is desirable, such as in patients with haemorrhoids, anal fissures or postrectal surgery (Blumenthal et al 2000).

The symptoms associated with constipation-induced haemorrhoids may also be reduced through administration of psyllium. A reduction of pain and length of hospital stay following open haemorrhoidectomy were achieved through supplementation of laxomucil (3.26 g psyllium) (Kecmanovic et al 2004). A subsequent study further identified a reduction of postsurgical tenesmus rate (Kecmanovic et al 2006).

Weight loss aid

Psyllium is used to increase the subjective feeling of satiety before and between meals in an attempt to reduce total caloric intake. One study comparing *Plantago ovata* preparation (20 g granules with 200 mL water) to water or a placebo preparation found a significant difference in fullness 1 hour after consumption (Turnbull & Thomas 1995). Other studies have confirmed a suppressant effect on hunger and increased satiety that remains apparent up to 6 hours after consumption. Psyllium also significantly delays gastric emptying from the third hour after a meal (Bergmann et al 1992, Delargy et al 1997).

Metabolic syndrome

Psyllium husks also appear able to beneficially alter a number of metabolic syndrome abnormalities. In a randomized, double-blind, placebo-controlled trial, Sola et al administered psyllium husks (14 g/day) or placebo to hypercholesterolaemic patients (n = 254) for 8 weeks. Relative to placebo, administration of psyllium husks reduced plasma LDL cholesterol by 6% ($P < 0.0002$), total cholesterol by 6% ($P < 0.0001$), triglycerides by 22% ($P = 0.0004$), apolipoprotein B-100 by 7% ($P < 0.0001$), oxidised LDL by 7% ($P = 0.0003$), insulin by 4.7 pmol/L ($P = 0.02$) and systolic blood pressure by 4.0 mmHg (95% CI 1.2–6.7; $P < 0.05$) (Sola et al 2010).

Hyperlipidaemia

Psyllium is also used as a cholesterol-lowering agent, usually as an adjunct to a low-fat diet (Reid et al 2002). Soluble fibres, such as psyllium husk, increase the cholesterol-lowering effect of a low-fat diet in people with elevated cholesterol (Anderson et al 2000). A meta-analysis of 21 controlled clinical trials (n = 1697) testing psyllium dosages ranging between 3.0 and 20.4 g daily confirmed that psyllium produced a time- and dose-dependent serum cholesterol-lowering effect in patients with mild-to-moderate hypercholesterolaemia (Wei et al 2009). Reductions in serum cholesterol occurred more quickly than changes in LDL cholesterol with psyllium supplementation.

Similar results were obtained in two previously published meta-analyses. Davidson et al (1996) evaluated data from eight studies and found that psyllium (10.2 g/day) lowered serum total cholesterol by 4%, LDL cholesterol by 7% and the ratio of apolipoprotein (apo) B to apo A–I by 6% relative to placebo. This was achieved together with a low-fat diet over 8 weeks. It has also been used with some success in the paediatric population and is easy to incorporate into various foods (Davidson et al 1996). Olson et al (1997), using the data from 404 subjects with mild-to-moderate hypercholesterolaemia, concomitantly consuming a high-fat diet supplemented with psyllium in the form of cereal, found psyllium to be beneficial in lowering both LDL and total cholesterols; however, HDL concentrations were unaffected (Olson et al 1997).

Studies with statin drugs

A 12-week blinded, placebo-controlled study comprising 68 patients demonstrated that supplementation of dietary psyllium 15 g (Metamucil) daily in patients taking 10 mg of simvastatin was as effective in lowering cholesterol as 20 mg of simvastatin alone (Moreyra et al 2005). However, a 4-week open-label, randomised, parallel study of 36 subjects demonstrated that 10 g of psyllium daily added to 20 mg of lovastatin provided an additive effect in cholesterol-lowering than lovastatin alone, although the difference was not statistically significant (Agrawal et al 2007). The duration of the supplementation may offer some insight into conflicting outcomes. In a 12-week study involving 100 subjects with hyperlipidaemia randomised to receive either a combination of isapgol powder (Naturolax) 5.6 g twice daily and atorvastatin 10 mg once daily or atorvastatin 10 mg daily alone, significant reduction in LDL cholesterol was achieved at the end of week 8; there was, however, no difference between treatment groups. However, at the end of week 12, the combination of isapgol and atorvastatin produced significantly greater reduction in LDL when compared to atorvastatin alone (Jayaram et al 2007).

Colorectal cancer

A 2002 case-control study (n = 424) found the consumption of psyllium husks to be inversely proportional to the risk of colorectal cancer (OR = 0.17, 95% CI 0.03–0.81; $P = 0.01$). The effect was even stronger in constipated individuals (OR = 0.08, 95% CI 0.01–0.38; $P = 0.001$) (Juarranz et al 2002). This was followed by another epidemiological study in 2009 correlating the rate of mortality from colorectal cancer in a number of Spanish provinces to the consumption of psyllium husks in these same areas. The highest quintile intake of psyllium husks was found to be inversely correlated with mortality from colorectal cancer (RR = 0.746, 95% CI 0.416–0.908; $P = 0.042$) (Lopez et al 2009).

Diabetes

Fibre products, such as psyllium, have been used as an aid to metabolic control in patients with diabetes (Pittler & Ernst 2004, Sierra et al 2002). Epidemiological and clinical data suggest a role for both soluble and insoluble fibre products in the management of hyperglycaemia. It appears that soluble fibre has a dose-dependent effect on serum glucose levels and the insulin response to a meal, improves glycaemic control in type 2 diabetes and can reduce the amount of medication required (Pastors et al 1991).

The adjunct use of 5.1 g psyllium twice daily for 8 weeks with a traditional diet for 34 men with type 2 diabetes and mild-to-moderate hypercholesterolaemia was well tolerated and shown to improve glycaemic and lipid levels as compared to placebo (Anderson et al 1999). One clinical study using 14 g/day of psyllium (Plantaben, ALTANA Pharma, Mexico) showed a significant 12.2% reduction in glucose absorption, as well as a significant reduction in total cholesterol and LDL cholesterol, and also uric acid (Sierra et al 2002). Another study identified that a higher dose (20 g/day in divided doses) may produce better results, and it significantly lowers both basal and postprandial hyperglycaemia (Frati-Munari et al 1989). In an 8-week double-blind, placebo-controlled study of 49 subjects, psyllium (5.1 g twice daily) was evaluated as an adjunct to the use of diet and pharmaceutical hypoglycaemic therapy in patients with type 2 diabetes. Fasting blood glucose and glycosylated haemoglobin were significantly reduced following psyllium administration and improved gastric tolerance to metformin was identified in the psyllium group. The authors concluded psyllium to be safe, well tolerated and improved glycaemic control in patients with type 2 diabetes (Ziai et al 2005). Psyllium significantly improved the breakfast postprandial glycaemic, insulinaemic and free fatty acid response in 45 patients with type 2 diabetes mellitus participating in a randomised, crossover intervention trial of a low-glycaemic-load breakfast meal containing soluble psyllium fibre 6.6 g for 3 weeks duration (Clark et al 2006).

Irritable bowel syndrome (IBS)

In a systematic review examining the effects of fibre supplementation in IBS, Bijkerk et al identified 17 randomised, controlled trials including a total of 1363 IBS patients. Nine studies investigated soluble fibre supplementation (eight of these studies utilised psyllium husks) and eight insoluble fibres. A meta-analysis was performed looking at the effects of fibre (as a whole), and soluble fibre and insoluble fibre specifically on global IBS symptoms, abdominal pain and constipation. Fibre (as a whole) was found to significantly improve global IBS symptoms (RR = 1.33, 95% CI 1.19–1.50) and IBS-related constipation (RR = 1.56, 95% CI 1.21–2.02). However, fibre supplementation was found to significantly worsen abdominal pain (RR = 0.78, 95% CI 0.64–0.95). When soluble fibre was examined in isolation, it was found to induce a greater reduction in global IBS symptoms (RR = 1.55, 95% CI 1.35–1.78) and to improve constipation in constipation-predominant IBS subjects (RR = 1.60, 95% CI 1.06–2.42). Conversely, insoluble fibre supplementation was found to have no significant impact upon global IBS symptoms, although it did improve constipation (RR = 1.54, 95% CI 1.10–2.14) (Bijkerk et al 2004).

The superiority of soluble fibre over insoluble was further confirmed in a 12-week randomised, double-blind, placebo-controlled trial (n = 275) comparing psyllium husks (10 g/day), wheat bran (10 g/day) and placebo in IBS patients. The proportion of subjects describing their IBS symptoms as 'adequately relieved' was significantly greater in the psyllium group than the bran or placebo groups in the first 2 months of treatment, but not the third. At the end of the 12-week treatment period, total IBS symptom severity was significantly reduced only in the psyllium group. However, abdominal pain scores and quality of life scores were not (Bijkerk et al 2009).

Black and blond psyllium seed is approved for use by Commission E in IBS and recommended when a soft stool is desired (Blumenthal et al 2000).

Ulcerative Colitis

A limited number of studies have examined the role of psyllium in the treatment of ulcerative colitis (UC).

A randomised, open-label trial in 1999 (n = 105) compared the efficacy of psyllium seeds (10 g bid) to mesalamine and the combination of mesalamine and psyllium seeds over a 12-month period. Over the trial period, there was no significant difference in remission rates between the three groups — 60% of subjects in the psyllium seed group remained in remission, versus 65% in the mesalamine group and 70% in the combination group. Faecal butyrate concentrations increased significantly in the psyllium seed treated groups (P = 0.018) (Fernandez-Banares et al 1999).

A randomised controlled trial of 120 patients with ulcerative colitis demonstrated that patients receiving treatment with a synbiotic therapy of *Bifidobacterium longum* (2×10^9 colony-forming units per day; unspecified strain) and psyllium (8 g daily) reported greater 'quality-of-life' changes than those treated with the probiotic strain or psyllium alone, as well as significant decreases in C-reactive protein levels (Fujimori et al 2009).

Hypertension

Participants in a randomised controlled trial of 41 hypertensive patients increased their intake of dietary protein and psyllium (additional 12 g/day) for 8 weeks. A net reduction in 24-hour systolic blood pressure of 5.9 mmHg was demonstrated (Burke et al 2001). In a 6-month, randomised, open-label clinical trial involving 141 hypertensive and overweight patients, treatment with psyllium powder as compared to guar gum appeared to significantly reduce systolic and diastolic blood pressures (Cicero et al 2007).

OTHER USES

In the confectionery industry psyllium is used as a thickening agent in ice cream and frozen desserts.

DOSAGE RANGE

General recommendations

- Blond psyllium seed: 12–40 g of whole seeds or equivalent taken in divided doses daily.
- Black psyllium seed: 10–30 g of whole or ground seeds or equivalent taken in divided doses daily.
- Seeds should be presoaked in 100–150 mL of warm water for several hours before ingestion. Each dose should be followed by another full glass of water.
- Powdered blond psyllium seed husk: 4–5 g taken up to four times daily. Stir desired dose into 150 mL of water and drink immediately. Follow each dose with ½–1 glass of water.

According to clinical studies

- Weight loss: *Plantago ovata* preparation (20 g granules with 200 mL water).
- Constipation: 7–11 g daily in divided doses with water.
- Hyperlipidaemia: 7–20 g daily in divided doses with water.
- Hyperglycaemia: 10–15 g daily in divided doses with water.
- Diabetes: 14–20 g daily in divided doses.
- Metabolic syndrome: 14 g daily in divided doses with water.
- Diarrhoea: 7–30 g in divided doses for 7 days with water.
- Haemorrhoids: 7 g daily for 6 weeks with water.
- Children 6–12 years: 3–8 g in divided doses.

SIGNIFICANT INTERACTIONS

Calcium

Animal studies suggest that soluble fibre from sources of purified psyllium negatively impact calcium balance by decreasing the bioavailability of calcium from the diet (Luccia & Kunkel 2002) — psyllium and other soluble fibre supplements should be taken at least 1 hour before or after calcium.

Lithium

Soluble fibre may decrease the bioavailability of lithium (EMEA 2003) — take psyllium at least 1 hour before or after lithium.

Levodopa

Animal research suggests that concomitant administration of psyllium husks with levodopa results in an improvement in the levodopa kinetic profile with higher final concentrations and a longer plasma half-life (Diez et al 2008).

Coumarin derivatives

Soluble fibre may decrease the bioavailability of coumarin derivatives (EMEA 2003) — take psyllium at least 1 hour before or after coumarin derivatives.

Vitamin B_{12}

Soluble fibre may decrease the bioavailability of vitamin B_{12} (EMEA 2003) — take psyllium at least 1 hour before or after vitamin B_{12}.

Cardiac glycosides

Soluble fibre may decrease the bioavailability of cardiac glycosides (EMEA 2003) — take psyllium at least 1 hour before or after cardiac glycosides.

Hypoglycaemic agents

Additive hypoglycaemic effects are theoretically possible — drug dose may need modification and the outcome can be favourable under professional supervision.

Anticonvulsant medication

Absorption concomitantly administered with psyllium may be delayed (EMEA 2007) — product taken 1 hour to half an hour before or after the medicinal product.

Thyroid hormones

Medication dose may need to be adjusted — seek medical supervision (EMEA 2007).

Lipid lowering agents

Concurrent use of psyllium with lipid-lowering drugs may lead to a reduction in drug dose and further lipid-lowering effects — beneficial interaction.

Other vitamins and minerals

Given the known capacity of psyllium husks to decrease the absorption of calcium, it would be prudent to avoid coadministration of psyllium husks with any vitamin or mineral supplement. Ensure administration is at least 1 hour before or after nutritional supplementation.

ADVERSE REACTIONS

Allergy is possible, although rare and is characterised by tightness in the chest, wheezing and urticaria. According to a study of healthcare workers, daily exposure to laxatives containing *Plantago ovata* causes sensitisation to *Plantago ovata* seed in approximately 14% of people (Bernedo et al 2008). Psyllium should not be consumed dry, as it may cause oesophageal obstruction. In practice, it is not unusual for people to experience flatulence, bloating and mild abdominal discomfort when they start to use psyllium; however, these symptoms can reduce with long-term use. It is also worth noting that patients can experience a worsening in their constipation if they consume psyllium husks without a concomitant increase in water intake.

A rare adverse effect noted in the literature is intestinal obstruction. A handful of cases of intestinal obstruction have been reported in the medical literature over the past 80 years secondary to the ingestion of psyllium, typically in individuals with a very low fluid intake (Fisher 1938, Souter 1965). Hence, all individuals should be strongly advised to significantly increase their fluid intake upon commencement of psyllium therapy.

CONTRAINDICATIONS AND PRECAUTIONS

Although psyllium is considered a safe substance, it should not be used by people with partial or complete bowel obstruction, colonic impaction or stenosis of the gastrointestinal tract.

According to Commission E, blond psyllium seed is contraindicated if there is difficulty regulating diabetes mellitus.

PREGNANCY USE

May be used during pregnancy and lactation.

Practice points/Patient counselling

- Psyllium seed husk contains a water-soluble fibre that forms a mucilaginous gel on contact with aqueous fluids and is degraded by human intestinal flora.
- It is most commonly used to treat constipation or diarrhoea and to regulate stool consistency.
- It is also used to promote satiety and weight loss, and as an aid to metabolic control in diabetes and metabolic syndrome, as well as hyperlipidaemia when combined with a low-fat diet.
- The seeds and husks should be presoaked in warm water before ingestion. Each dose should be followed by at least a full glass of water and patients should be instructed to ensure their water intake is adequate while taking psyllium husks. Ingesting it dry may cause oesophageal obstruction.
- Although generally safe, it should not be used by people with partial or complete bowel obstruction, colonic impaction or stenosis of the gastrointestinal tract.

PATIENTS' FAQs

What will this herb do for me?

Psyllium is a bulking agent that can regulate stool consistency, increase satiety, improve metabolic control in diabetes and reduce cholesterol when combined with a low-fat diet.

When will it start to work?

As a bulking agent, it will start to have an effect within several hours. It will improve satiety within 30–60 minutes and has a mild cholesterol-lowering effect after 8 weeks of use.

Are there any safety issues?

Although generally safe, it should not be ingested dry or used by people with partial or complete bowel obstruction, colonic impaction or stenosis of the gastrointestinal tract.

REFERENCES

Agrawal AR et al. Effect of combining viscous fibre with lovastatin on serum lipids in normal human subjects. Int J Clin Pract 61.11 (2007): 1812–1818.

Anderson JW et al. Effects of psyllium on glucose and serum lipid responses in men with type 2 diabetes and hypercholesterolemia. Am J Clin Nutr 70.4 (1999): 466–473.

Anderson JW et al. Cholesterol-lowering effects of psyllium intake adjunctive to diet therapy in men and women with hypercholesterolemia: meta-analysis of 8 controlled trials. Am J Clin Nutr 71 (2000): 472–479.

Bergmann JF et al. Correlation between echographic gastric emptying and appetite: influence of psyllium. Gut 33 (1992): 1042–1043.

Bernedo N et al. Allergy to laxative compound (Plantago ovata seed) among health care professionals. J Investig Allergol Clin Immunol 18.3 (2008): 181–189.

Bijkerk CJ et al. Systematic review: the role of different types of fibre in the treatment of irritable bowel syndrome. Aliment Pharmacol Ther, 19 (2004): 245–251.

Bijkerk CJ et al. Soluble or insoluble fibre in irritable bowel syndrome in primary care? Randomised placebo controlled trial. BMJ 339 (2009): B3154.

Blumenthal M et al. (eds). Herbal medicine: expanded commission E monographs. Austin, TX: Integrative Medicine Communications, 2000.

Burke V et al. Dietary protein and soluble fiber reduce ambulatory blood pressure in treated hypertensives. Hypertension 38.4 (2001): 821–826.

Cicero AF et al. Different effect of psyllium and guar dietary supplementation on blood pressure control in hypertensive overweight patients: a six-month, randomized clinical trial. Clin Exp Hypertens 29.6 (2007): 383–394.

Clark CA et al. Effects of breakfast meal composition on second meal metabolic responses in adults with Type 2 diabetes mellitus. Eur J Clin Nutr 60.9 (2006): 1122–1129.

Davidson MH et al. A psyllium-enriched cereal for the treatment of hypercholesterolemia in children: a controlled, double-blind, crossover study. Am J Clin Nutr 63 (1996): 96–102.

Delargy HJ et al. Effects of amount and type of dietary fibre (soluble and insoluble) on short-term control of appetite. Int J Food Sci Nutr 48 (1997): 67–77.

Diez MJ et al. The hydrosoluble fiber plantago ovata husk improves levodopa (with carbidopa) bioavailability after repeated administration. J Neurol Sci, 271 (2008): 15–20.

Dikeman CL, Fahey GC. Viscosity as related to dietary fiber: a review. Crit Rev Food Sci Nutr 46.8 (2006): 649–663.

EMEA (European agency for the evaluation of medicinal products). London UK: EMEA, 1995–2009. www.emea.eu.int (accessed February 2009).

Fernandez-Banares F et al. Randomized clinical trial of Plantago ovata seeds (dietary fiber) as compared with mesalamine in maintaining remission in ulcerative colitis. Spanish Group for the Study of Crohn's Disease and Ulcerative Colitis (GETECCU). Am J Gastroenterol 94.2 (1999): 427–433.

Fernandez-Banares F et al. Randomized clinical trial of plantago ovata seeds (dietary fiber) as compared with mesalamine in maintaining remission in Ulcerative Colitis. Am J Gastroenterol, 94 (1999): 427–433.

Fisher RE. Psyllium seeds: intestinal obstruction. Cal West Med 48 (1938) 190.

Frati-Munari AC et al. [Effect of different doses of Plantago psyllium mucilage on the glucose tolerance test]. Arch Invest Med (Mex) 20.2 (1989): 147–152.

Fujimori S et al. A randomised controlled trial on the efficacy of synbiotic versus probiotic or prebiotic treatment to improve the quality of life in patients with ulcerative colitis. Nutrition 25.5 (2009): 520–525.

Galisteo M et al. Plantago ovata husks-supplemented diet ameliorates metabolic alterations in obese zucker rats through activation of amp-activated protein kinase. Comparative study with other dietary fibers. Clin Nutr 29 (2010): 261–267.

Jayaram S et al. Randomised study to compare the efficacy and safety of isapgol plus atorvastatin versus atorvastatin alone in subjects with hypercholesterolaemia. J Indian Med Assoc 105.3 (2007): 142–145, 150.
Juarranz M et al. Physical exercise, use of plantago ovata and aspirin, and reduced risk of colon cancer. Eur J Cancer Prev 11 (2002): 465–472.
Kecmanovic D et al. [Plantago ovata (Laxomucil) after hemorrhoidectomy]. Acta Chir Iugosl 51.3 (2004): 121–123.
Kecmanovic DM et al. Bulk agent Plantago ovata after Milligan-Morgan hemorrhoidectomy with Ligasure. Phytother Res 20.8 (2006): 655–658.
Lopez JC et al. Plantago ovata consumption and colorectal mortality in Spain, 1995–2000. J Epidemiol 19 (2009): 206–211.
Luccia BHD, Kunkel ME. Psyllium reduces relative calcium bioavailability and induces negative changes in bone composition in weanling Wistar rats. Nutr Res 22 (2002): 1027–1040.
Marlett JA et al. An unfermented gel component of psyllium seed husk promotes laxation as a lubricant in humans. Am J Clin Nutr 72.3 (2000): 784–789.
Marlett JA, Fischer MH. The active fraction of psyllium seed husk. Proc Nutr Soc 62.1 (2003): 207–209.
Moreyra AE et al. Effect of combining psyllium fiber with simvastatin in lowering cholesterol. Arch Intern Med 165.10 (2005): 1161–1166.
Nakamura Y et al. Beta-sitosterol from psyllium seed husk (Plantago ovata Forsk) restores gap junctional intercellular communication in Ha-ras transfected rat liver cells. Nutr Cancer 51.2 (2005): 218–225.
Olson BH et al. Psyllium-enriched cereals lower blood total cholesterol and LDL cholesterol, but not HDL cholesterol, in hypercholesterolemic adults: results of a meta-analysis. J Nutr 127.10 (1997): 1973–1980.
Pastors JG et al. Psyllium fiber reduces rise in postprandial glucose and insulin concentrations in patients with non-insulin-dependent diabetes. Am J Clin Nutr 53 (1991): 1431–1435.
Pittler MH, Ernst E. Dietary supplements for body-weight reduction: a systematic review. Am J Clin Nutr 79 (2004): 529–536.
Reid R et al. Dietary counselling for dyslipidemia in primary care: results of a randomized trial. Can J Diet Pract Res 63 (2002): 169–175.
Rodriguez-Cabezas ME et al. Intestinal anti-inflammatory activity of dietary fiber (plantago ovata seeds) in HLA-B27 transgenic rats. Clin Nutr 22 (2003): 463–471.
Rodriguez-Moran M et al. Lipid- and glucose-lowering efficacy of plantago psyllium in type II diabetes. J Diabetes Complications 12 (1998): 273–278.
Romero AL et al. The seeds from Plantago ovata lower plasma lipids by altering hepatic and bile acid metabolism in guinea pigs. J Nutr 132.6 (2002): 1194–1198.
Shrestha S et al. A combination of psyllium and plant sterols alters lipoprotein metabolism in hypercholesterolemic subjects by modifying the intravascular processing of lipoproteins and increasing LDL uptake. J Nutr 137.5 (2007): 1165–1170.
Sierra M et al. Effects of ispaghula husk and guar gum on postprandial glucose and insulin concentrations in healthy subjects. Eur J Clin Nutr 55.4 (2001): 235–243.
Sierra M et al. Therapeutic effects of psyllium in type 2 diabetic patients. Eur J Clin Nutr 56.9 (2002): 830–842.
Singh B. Psyllium as therapeutic and drug delivery agent. Int J Pharm 334.1–2 (2007): 1–14.
Sohn VR et al. Stool-fermented plantago ovata husk induces apoptosis in colorectal cancer cells independently of molecular phenotype. Br J Nutr 107 (2012): 1591–1602.
Sola R et al. Soluble fibre (plantago ovata husk) reduces plasma low-density lipoprotein (ldl) cholesterol, triglycerides, insulin, oxidised ldl and systolic blood pressure in hypercholesterolaemic patients: a randomised trial. Atherosclerosis 211 (2010): 630–637.
Song Y et al. Soluble dietary fibre improves insulin sensitivity by increasing muscle GLUT-4 content in stroke-prone spontaneously hypertensive rats. Clin Exp Pharmacol Physiol 27.1–2 (2000): 41–45.
Souter WA Bolus obstruction of gut after use of hydrophilic colloid laxatives. Br Med J 1 (1965): 166–168.
Theuwissen E, Mensink RP. Water-soluble dietary fibers and cardiovascular disease. Physiol Behav 94.2 (2008): 285–292.
Turnbull WH, Thomas HG. The effect of a Plantago ovata seed containing preparation on appetite variables, nutrient and energy intake. Int J Obes Relat Metab Disord 19 (1995): 338–342.
Wang ZQ et al. Effects of dietary fibers on weight gain, carbohydrate metabolism, and gastric ghrelin gene expression in mice fed a high-fat diet. Metabolism 56.12 (2007): 1635–1642.
Wei ZH et al. Time- and dose-dependent effect of psyllium on serum lipids in mild-to-moderate hypercholesterolemia: a meta-analysis of controlled clinical trials. Eur J Clin Nutr 63 (2009): 82.
Ziai SA et al. Psyllium decreased serum glucose and glycosylated hemoglobin significantly in diabetic outpatients. J Ethnopharmacol 102.2 (2005): 202–207.

Pygeum

HISTORICAL NOTE *Pygeum africanum* is a large, evergreen tree native to Africa. Its bark has been used medicinally for thousands of years by traditional African healers to treat bladder disorders, kidney disease, prostate disorders and malaria, as well as male baldness, and to enhance sexual functioning. Since the late 1960s, the extract has been used in clinical practice in Europe; however, because of overharvesting, the plant is now considered an endangered species and efforts are under way to protect it.

Clinical note — Popular to the point of extinction?

For the past 35 years, pygeum has been used in Europe for the treatment of benign prostatic hyperplasia (BPH) and other disorders. The bark is entirely wild-collected, mainly from Cameroon, Madagascar, Equatorial Guinea and Kenya, and exported principally to Europe for production into commercial medicinal extracts (Stewart 2003). Since 1995, it has been considered an endangered species, so attempts at cultivation are under way to protect the plant from extinction. Prior to 1966, when it was discovered to have significant medicinal effects, *P. africana* was a relatively common, but never abundant, species. The reasons for its demise include economic, social and ecological factors. Currently, wildcrafting is no longer commercially viable in Cameroon, and harvest has ceased in both Uganda and Kenya.

COMMON NAME

Pygeum

OTHER NAMES

African plum tree, African prune tree, *Pygeum africanum*, alumty, iluo, kirah, Natal tree, Pignil, Pronitol, Tanaden

BOTANICAL NAME/FAMILY

Prunus africana (Hook. f.) KalRm (family Rosaceae)

PLANT PART USED

Bark

CHEMICAL COMPONENTS

Phytosterols (beta-sitosterol, beta-sitostenone), pentacyclic triterpenes (oleanolic and ursolic acids) and ferulic esters (*n*-docosanol and *n*-tetracosanol) (Stewart 2003), atraric acid (AA) and *N*-butylbenzene sulfonamide (NBBS) (Daniela & Baniahmad 2011, Papaioannou et al 2010).

MAIN ACTIONS

Pygeum has demonstrated several different pharmacological effects according to in vitro and in vivo data. The majority of initial studies conducted on *P. africanum* were investigating its role in the symptomatic relief of BPH. More recent research is seeking to elucidate pygeum's pharmacological capacity in the modulation and restoration of bladder function, androgen receptor modification and attenuating prostatic cancer cell line replication.

Hormonal effects

In vivo studies have shown that orally administered pygeum extract has a significant effect on dihydrotestosterone (DHT)-induced prostatic enlargement (Choo et al 2000, Yoshimura et al 2003). Pretreatment with pygeum extract counteracted the effect of DHT-induced prostate enlargement (Choo et al 2000), and the more recent study found that oral administration of pygeum extract suppressed the effects of DHT on micturition (Yoshimura et al 2003) and effectively suppressed prostatic growth when coadministered with DHT; however, it did not reverse established prostatic growth when administered after DHT. A comparative study found that pygeum exerted only a weak inhibition of 5-alpha reductase compared to that of finasteride (Rhodes et al 1993). Phyto-oestrogens isolated in pygeum can exert a dose-dependent oestrogenic or antioestrogenic effect, according to other in vivo tests (Mathe et al 1995), and may also contribute to its effects in the prostate.

Antiandrogenic

Recent in vitro investigations have confirmed the antiandrogenic activity of pygeum. When compared to *Serenoa repens* and *Cucurbita pepo*, pygeum exhibited the highest androgen antagonistic activity (Schleich et al 2006). AA and NBBS, isolated from pygeum, has been shown to selectively competitively inhibit transactivation-mediated ligand-activated human androgen receptor, inhibiting the expression of endogenous prostate-specific antigen. Its effects have proved more potent than currently used clinical antiandrogens such as flutamide and do not display the molecular mechanisms of current antiandrogens associated with resistance. Therefore not only might AA and NBBS be useful novel antiandrogens, but they may also increase the effectiveness of current treatments (Daniela & Baniahmad 2011, Papaioannou et al 2010, Quiles et al 2010).

Anti-inflammatory

Phytosterols (beta-sitosterol, beta-sitostenone) reportedly inhibit the production of prostaglandins in the prostate, which suppresses the inflammatory symptoms associated with BPH and chronic prostatitis. The pentacyclic triterpenes (oleanolic and ursolic acids) are believed to inhibit the activity of glucosyltransferase, an enzyme involved in the inflammation process (Stewart 2003).

Studies with pygeum extract confirm that it decreases production of leukotrienes and other 5-lipoxygenase metabolites (Cristoni et al 2000).

Bladder effects

Pygeum protects the bladder from contractile dysfunction induced by ischaemia and reperfusion according to in vivo animal studies (Chen et al 1999). Pretreatment with pygeum prior to induced partial outlet obstruction in animal models prevents the development of contractile dysfunction, possibly by protecting the bladder from ischaemic injury (Levin et al 2005). Administration of pygeum was found to reverse already ischaemic compromised bladder function in a dose-dependent manner (Levin et al 2002).

Inhibition of fibroblast proliferation and apoptosis

Pygeum is a potent inhibitor of prostatic growth factor-mediated fibroblast proliferation, as demonstrated in animal models (Szolnoki et al 2001, Yablonsky et al 1997). A dose-dependent inhibition of fibroblastic growth was exerted in human stromal cells treated with pygeum extract (Boulbes et al 2006).

Further study comparing cell lines harvested from prostatic tissue with or without BPH and treated with pygeum extract demonstrated apoptosis via alpha-smooth-muscle actin, found in greater amounts in those with BPH. Transforming growth factor-beta$_1$ and fibroblast growth factor 2 were both downregulated. Smooth-muscle tissue was unaffected (Quiles et al 2010).

P

Chemopreventive

Recent investigations have focused primarily upon *P. africanum* regulation of cancer cell growth in vitro and in vivo. Treatment with pygeum extract exhibited a significant and dose-dependent inhibition of human prostate cancer cell lines and BPH-derived epithelial cells. Pygeum also exerted a potent antimitogenic action in this study (Santa Maria Margalef et al 2003). Pygeum-treated mice displayed a significant reduction in prostate cancer incidence (35%) in comparison to the casein-fed mice (62.5%) (Shenouda et al 2007).

OTHER ACTIONS

Ferulic esters (*n*-docosanol and *n*-tetracosanol) reportedly lower blood levels of cholesterol, from which testosterone is produced (Stewart 2003).

New metabolomics studies may soon shed further light on the action of pygeum on the prostate. Cornu et al (2012) compared the urine of 15 newly diagnosed men with BPH pre- and posttreatment with pygeum. The result was the identification of three novel compounds that were increased and one that was reduced in the urine samples treated with pygeum only.

CLINICAL USE

The most commonly investigated form of *P. africanum* is Tanenan (DEBAT Pharmaceuticals, France), which is a lipophilic extract standardised to contain 13% total plant sterols. One capsule of Tadenan contains 50 mg of standardised extract.

Benign prostatic hyperplasia

Clinical trials since the late 1970s have been encouraging, most reporting improvement in BPH symptoms.

A Cochrane systematic review analysed the results of 18 clinical trials that involved a total of 1562 participants (Wilt et al 2002). Seventeen studies were double-blinded, and the mean treatment duration was 61 ± 21 days (range 30–122 days). Most studies used a standardised extract of *P. africanum* in doses ranging from 75 to 200 mg/day.

The overall summary effect size indicated a large and statistically significant improvement with *P. africanum*. More specifically, active treatment increased peak urine flow by 23% and reduced residual urine volume by 24%, and doctors were twice as likely to report that their patients were experiencing an overall improvement in symptoms when pygeum was being used. The authors report that these findings are similar to other widely used treatment options and that treatment was well tolerated.

An observational study (TRIUMPH trial) in six European countries including 2559 newly-presented BPH patients compared treatment with either *P. africanum*, *Serenoa repens*, finasteride or alpha-blocker drugs (tamsulosin etc.) to untreated men (watchful waiters). Follow-up was at 1 year, with significant improvement (IPSS change >4) seen in all categories for the treatments: *P. africanum* 43.3%, *S. repens* 42.7%, finasteride 57% and alpha-blockers 68%, when compared to watchful waiters (Hutchison et al 2007).

IN COMBINATION

In 2013, a randomised, double-blind placebo-controlled trial was published which investigated the effects of a combination supplement ProstateEZE Max — *Cucurbita pepo* seed oil (160 mg), *Epilobium parviflorum* extract (equivalent to 500 mg dry herb), lycopene (2.1 mg), *Prunus africana* (equivalent to 15 g dry stem, standardised to β-sitosterol) and *S. repens* (equivalent to 660 mg dry leaf) on 57 patients with newly medically diagnosed BPH. At the end of 3 months, active treatment resulted in a symptom reduction in the median score (IPSS) of 36% compared to placebo 8% ($P < 0.05$). Daytime frequency of urination was reduced by 15.5% compared to no significant reduction in placebo group ($P < 0.03$) and nighttime frequency was reduced by 39.3% compared to placebo 7% ($P < 0.004$) (Coulsen et al 2013).

OTHER USES

Fertility disorders

Pygeum extract was used experimentally in the treatment of 22 men with reduced fertility and diminished prostatic secretion and proved to have a beneficial effect (Lucchetta et al 1984). Treatment was administered every day over 2 months and was most effective in men who did not have prostatitis.

DOSAGE RANGE

According to clinical studies:

- BPH: 50–100 mg of extract twice daily standardised to 12–13% total sterols.

ADVERSE REACTIONS

Pygeum is well tolerated, with side effects similar to placebo (Wilt et al 2002). Mild gastrointestinal discomfort has been reported.

SIGNIFICANT INTERACTIONS

None known.

CONTRAINDICATIONS AND PRECAUTIONS

People with known allergies should avoid use.

PREGNANCY USE

Safety not scientifically established; however, it is not used for any indication that would cause a pregnant woman to use it.

Practice points/Patient counselling

- Pygeum is a popular treatment in Europe for BPH.
- A systematic review of 18 clinical studies found that it has significant effects in BPH, such as increasing peak urine, reducing residual urine volume and producing an overall improvement in symptoms.
- Several different mechanisms of action have been identified using animal models, which would explain its effectiveness in BPH.
- According to clinical studies, the dose used is 50–100 mg of standardised extract twice daily for BPH and the treatment is well tolerated.
- Overharvesting has meant the tree is now considered endangered and efforts are being made to protect it from extinction.

PATIENTS' FAQs

What will this herb do for me?

Standardised pygeum extract is an effective treatment in benign prostate enlargement or inflammation and improves several symptoms.

When will it start to work?

Some men will notice an improvement in symptoms after 4 weeks; however, others will require a long-term treatment.

Are there any safety issues?

It is a well-tolerated treatment but should not be used by people with a known allergy to the plant. If symptoms worsen, seek professional advice.

REFERENCES

Boulbes D et al. *Pygeum africanum* extract inhibits proliferation of human cultured prostatic fibroblasts and myofibroblasts. BJU Int 98.5 (2006). 1106–1113.

Chen MW et al. Effects of unilateral ischemia on the contractile response of the bladder: protective effect of Tadenan (*Pygeum africanum* extract). Mol Urol 3.1 (1999): 5–10.

Choo MS, et al. Functional evaluation of Tadenan on micturition and experimental prostate growth induced with exogenous dihydrotestosterone. Urology 55 (2000): 292–298.

Cornu JN, et al. Metabolomics profiles of prostatic secretions from patients treated by *Pygeum africanum* for low urinary tract symptoms related to benign prostatic hyperplasia. Eur Urol Suppl 11.1 (2012): e10.

Coulsen S et al. A phase II randomised double-blind placebo controlled clinical trial investigating the efficacy and safety of ProstateEZE Max: A herbal medicine preparation for the management of symptoms of benign prstatic hypertrophy. Complement Ther Med 21.3 (2013): 172–179.

Cristoni A, et al. Botanical derivatives for the prostate. Fitoterapia 71 (Suppl 1) (2000): S21–S28.

Daniela R., A. Baniahmad, The natural compounds atraric acid and N-butylbenzene-sulfonamide as antagonists of the human androgen receptor and inhibitors of prostate cancer cell growth. Mol. Cell. Endocrinol, 332.1–2 (2011): 1–8

Hutchison, A., et al. The efficacy of drugs for the treatment of LUTS/BPH, A study in 6 European countries. Eur Urol 51 (2007): 207–216

Levin RM et al. Effect of oral Tadenan treatment on rabbit bladder structure and function after partial outlet obstruction. J Urol 167.5 (2002): 2253–2259.

Levin RM et al. Low-dose tadenan protects the rabbit bladder from bilateral ischemia/reperfusion-induced contractile dysfunction. Phytomedicine 12 (2005): 17–24.

Lucchetta G et al. Reactivation of the secretion from the prostatic gland in cases of reduced fertility. Biological study of seminal fluid modifications. Urol Int 39 (1984): 222–224.

Mathe GS et al. The so-called phyto-estrogenic action of *Pygeum africanum* extract. Biomed Pharmacother 49.7–8 (1995): 339–340.

Papaioannou, M., et al. NBBS isolated from *Pygeum africanum* bark exhibits androgen antagonistic activity, inhibits AR nuclear translocation and prostate cancer cell growth. Invest. New Drugs, 28.6 (2010): 729–743.

Quiles, M.T., et al. Antiproliferative and apoptotic effects of the herbal agent *Pygeum africanum* on cultured prostate stromal cells from patients with benign prostatic hyperplasia (BPH). Prostate 70:10 (2010): 1044–1053

Rhodes L et al. Comparison of finasteride (Proscar), a 5 alpha reductase inhibitor, and various commercial plant extracts in in vitro and in vivo 5 alpha reductase inhibition. Prostate 22.1 (1993): 43–51.

Santa Maria Margalef A et al. [Antimitogenic effect of *Pygeum africanum* extracts on human prostatic cancer cell lines and explants from benign prostatic hyperplasia.] Arch Esp Urol 56.4 (2003): 369–378.

Schleich S et al. Extracts from *Pygeum africanum* and other ethnobotanical species with antiandrogenic activity. Planta Med 72.9 (2006): 807–13.

Shenouda NS et al. Phytosterol *Pygeum africanum* regulates prostate cancer in vitro and in vivo. Endocrine 31.1 (2007): 72–81.

Stewart KM. The African cherry (*Prunus africana*): can lessons be learned from an over-exploited medicinal tree? J Ethnopharmacol 89 (2003): 3–13.

Szolnoki E et al. The effect of *Pygeum africanum* on fibroblast growth factor (FGF) and transforming growth factor beta (TGF beta 1/LAP) expression in animal model. Acta Microbiol Immunol Hung 48.1 (2001): 1–9.

Wilt T et al. *Pygeum africanum* for benign prostatic hyperplasia. Cochrane Database Syst Rev (2002): CD001044.

Yablonsky F et al. Antiproliferative effect of *Pygeum africanum* extract on rat prostatic fibroblasts. J Urol 157.6 (1997): 2381–2387.

Yoshimura Y et al. Effect of *Pygeum africanum* tadenan on micturition and prostate growth of the rat secondary to coadministered treatment and post-treatment with dihydrotestosterone. Urology 61 (2003): 474–478.

Quercetin

BACKGROUND AND RELEVANT PHARMACOKINETICS

Quercetin is a flavanol belonging to a group of polyphenolic substances known as flavonoids or bioflavonoids, the first of which were identified in 1936 by Albert Szent-Györgyi, who was awarded the Nobel Prize for his discovery of vitamin C (Challem 1998).

Quercetin is regarded generally to exhibit poor solubility and instability, making it the target of research involving the use of several modified forms, e.g. liposomes, nanoparticles or micelles, which appear to provide higher solubility and bioavailability (Cai et al 2013).

Studies on the absorption, bioavailability and metabolism of quercetin after oral intake in humans to date therefore have produced contradictory results (Graefe et al 1999). It is thought that quercetin is extensively metabolised in the gut and liver after absorption, and occurs in the blood stream mainly as conjugated metabolites (Meng et al 2013). In human trials, supplementation increased plasma quercetin concentrations in a dose-dependent manner — 178% (50 mg), 359% (100 mg) and 570% (150 mg) — and maximum plasma concentrations were reached 6 hours after intake of a 150 mg dose. There was also a significant interindividual variability in plasma quercetin concentrations (36–57%) (Egert et al 2008, Jin et al 2010). The main determinant of absorption of quercetin conjugates is the nature of the sugar moiety. Glucose-bound glycosides (quercetin glucosides) are effectively absorbed from the small intestine because the cells possess glucoside-hydrolysing activity and their glucose transport system is capable of participating in glucoside absorption, whereas quercetin glycosides are subject to deglycosidation by enterobacteria before absorption in the large intestine (Murota & Terao 2003).

After absorption, quercetin is transported to the liver via the portal circulation, where it undergoes significant first-pass metabolism. Peak plasma levels of quercetin occur from 0.7 to 9 hours following ingestion, and the elimination half-life of quercetin is approximately 23–28 hours (Hollman et al 1997, PDRHealth 2005). Due to its long half-life, repeated consumption of quercetin-containing foods should cause accumulation of quercetin in the body. Excretion is likely to be via the biliary system (Erlund 2004).

> ***Clinical note — Improving quercetin bioavailability***
> Human studies have also been undertaken to find combinations which improve quercetin bioavailability, with quercetin from quercetin-enriched cereal bars significantly more bioavailable than from quercetin powder-filled hard capsules (Egert et al 2012), and a threefold increase in bioavailability when ingested via onions compared to apples (Hollman et al 1997) and twofold increase with black tea (deVries et al 1998). Ingestion of quercetin with onion powder results in faster absorption and higher plasma levels compared to apple peel powder (Lee & Mitchell 2012). Other factors that may improve bioavailability include gender (especially females taking oral contraceptives), gastrointestinal flora (Duda-Chodak 2012, Erlund 2004) and concurrent intake of dietary fat (Guo et al 2013) or bromelain and papain (Shoskes et al 1999).

CHEMICAL COMPONENTS

Quercetin, also known as meletin and sophretin, is known chemically as 2-(3,4-dihydroxyphenyl)-3,5,7-trihydroxy-^{4}H-1-benzopyran-4-one and 3,3′,4′5,7-penthydroxyflavone. It is typically found in plants as a glycone or carbohydrate conjugate but does not in itself possess a carbohydrate moiety in its structure. Quercetin glycone conjugates include rutin (quercetin-3-rutinoside) and quercitrin (thujin, quercetin-3-L-rhamnoside or 3-rhamnosylquercetin) (Erlund et al 2000, PDRHealth 2005).

FOOD SOURCES

Food sources include apples, berries (blackcurrants, lingonberries and bilberries), beans, black tea, broccoli, grapes, green tea, onions and red wine (Duda-Chodak 2012, Somerset & Johannot 2008).

Herbal medicines such as St John's wort, *Ginkgo biloba*, *Vaccinium macrocarpon* (cranberry) and *Oenothera biennis* (evening primrose) also contain quercetin and this may help to explain part of their therapeutic benefits.

MAIN ACTIONS

Antioxidant/pro-oxidant

Quercetin is a phenolic antioxidant shown to inhibit lipid peroxidation, protecting the lens of the eye (Cornish et al 2002) and renal tubular epithelial cells from oxidant-induced injury (Pietruck et al 2003). The antioxidant activity may be the result of free radical scavenging, metal chelation, enzyme inhibition or the induction of protective enzymes (Erlund 2004). When compared to curcumin, quercetin exhibits higher reduction potential at three different pH settings, with a total antioxidant capacity 3.5-fold higher than curcumin (Zhang et al 2011).

While some studies demonstrate that quercetin treatment at low concentrations or for short periods may exert an antioxidant effect, other trials suggest that higher concentrations (>0.5% in rats fed a 1.0% Met-supplemented diet) or treatment which lasts longer than 6 weeks may produce a pro-oxidant effect (Ferraresi et al 2005, Meng et al 2013, Robaszkiewicz et al 2007). These effects may be due to induction of oxidative stress due to formation of reactive oxygen species in the extracellular medium (Robaszkiewicz et al 2007) or increasing oxidant activity due to a reduction in glutathione (GSH) levels (Ferraresi et al 2005). The paradox is that, in the process of offering protection, quercetin depletes GSH levels and is converted into potentially toxic products (thiol-reactive quercetin metabolites) (Boots et al 2007). In the absence of GSH, potentially harmful oxidation products such as orthoquinone may be produced when quercetin exerts its antioxidant activity. Therefore, adequate GSH levels should be maintained when quercetin is supplemented (Boots et al 2003).

In human trials, while daily supplementation of quercetin (50, 100 and 150 mg/day) for 2 weeks dose-dependently increased plasma quercetin concentrations, it did not appear to affect antioxidant status, oxidised low-density lipoprotein (LDL), inflammation or metabolism (Egert et al 2008). Research also suggests that the effects of antioxidant supplementation reducing oxidative stress can only be expected in people with enhanced oxidative stress or inflammation (Boots et al 2011), potentially explaining the negative outcome of many clinical studies (Egert et al 2008, Shanely et al 2010), where antioxidants were supplied to healthy subjects.

Anti-inflammatory

In animal and in vitro studies, quercetin inhibits inflammation by modulating neutrophil function, prostanoid synthesis, cytokine production and inducible nitric oxide synthase (iNOS) expression via the inhibition of the neutrophil factor (NF)-kappa-B pathway (Busse et al 1984, Comalada et al 2005, Morikawa et al 2003). In vitro studies on human adipocytes and grape powder extract, containing both quercetin and *trans*-resveratrol (trans-RSV), have demonstrated that quercetin is equally as or more effective than trans-RSV in attenuating tumour necrosis factor-alpha (TNF-α)-mediated inflammation and insulin resistance (Chuang et al 2010).

While quercetin supplementation has been shown to decrease circulating markers of inflammation in mice (Stewart et al 2008), these effects have not been consistently replicated in humans (Egert et al 2008, McAnulty et al 2008, Pfeuffer et al 2013). Further clinical trials are required to clarify these findings.

Antiviral

Quercetin causes a dose-dependent reduction in the infectivity and intracellular replication of herpes simplex virus-1, poliovirus type 1, parainfluenza virus type 3 and respiratory syncytial virus in vitro

(Kaul et al 1985); however, pretreatment with quercetin does not appear to provide any additional benefit. In vitro and in vivo evidence also suggests that quercetin has the ability to block the replication of rhinovirus, responsible for producing the common cold (Ganesan et al 2012). Animal studies have also suggested that the antioxidant effects of quercetin may protect the lungs from the deleterious effects of oxygen-derived free radicals released during influenza infection (Kumar et al 2005).

Immunomodulation

Results from animal and in vitro studies have produced contradictory findings, suggesting both an induction and an inhibition of Th1 cytokines (Muthian & Bright 2004, Nair et al 2002).

According to in vitro research, quercetin induces Th1-derived cytokines (promoting cellular immunity) and inhibits Th2-derived cytokines, which exert negative effects on cellular immunity (Nair et al 2002). An excess of Th2 cytokines has also been implicated in allergic tendencies, and this provides a theoretical basis for the use of quercetin as an antiallergic substance. Conversely, animal studies have demonstrated that quercetin is able to inhibit Th1 differentiation and signalling of interleukin (IL)-12 (Muthian & Bright 2004) and appears to exert an effect on Th1-mediated immune responses through suppression of both interferon-gamma and IL-2 cytokine production (Yu et al 2008). As a result, a possibility exists that quercetin actually exerts an immunomodulatory effect on these cells.

Antiallergy

Quercetin is structurally similar to the antiallergic drug disodium cromoglycate (available as Intal or Cromese in Australia) and has been proposed as a useful treatment for mast cell-derived allergic inflammatory diseases, including contact dermatitis and photosensitivity, especially in formulations that have enhanced oral absorption (Min et al 2007, Weng et al 2012). Antiasthmatic activity similar to cromolyn sodium and dexamethasone has been demonstrated in guinea pigs (Moon et al 2008) and a greater effect on inhibiting IL-8 and TNF release from LAD2 mast cells stimulated by substance P for quercetin than cromolyn in vitro (Weng et al 2012).

In vitro and animal studies demonstrate that quercetin stabilises mast cells, neutrophils and basophils inhibiting antigen as well as mitogen-induced histamine release (Blackburn et al 1987, Busse et al 1984, Middleton & Drzewiecki 1982, Middleton et al 1981, Ogasawara et al 1996, Pearce et al 1984). Inhibition of inflammatory enzymes, prostaglandins and leukotrienes and modulation of Th2 excess may further contribute to the antiallergic effects. Pretreatment with quercetin does not appear to produce any additional benefits.

Antihypertensive

Chronic treatment with quercetin lowers blood pressure and restores endothelial dysfunction in animal models of hypertension (Garcia-Saura et al 2005, Sanchez et al 2006). This effect may be in part due to modulation of renal function, including increased urinary and sodium output (Mackraj et al 2008). Several small clinical trials have confirmed a moderate blood pressure-lowering activity (Edwards et al 2007, Egert et al 2009).

Cardioprotective

During inflammation, circulating conjugates of quercetin pass through the endothelium to reach vascular smooth-muscle cells, where they exert their biological effects and are then deconjugated (Mochizuki et al 2004). The cardioprotective effects of quercetin may be related to its vasorelaxant (Ke Chen & Pace-Asciak 1996, Roghani et al 2004), anti-inflammatory and antioxidant properties and inhibition of vascular smooth-muscle cell proliferation and migration (Alcocer et al 2002, Moon et al 2003), as demonstrated in animal and in vitro models.

Animal experiments indicate that doses of quercetin equivalent to one to two glasses of red wine (approximately 2 mg) exert a cardioprotective effect following ischaemia-reperfusion by improving the function of mitochondria, which plays a critical role in myocardial recovery (Brookes et al 2002), and may also prevent the development of atherosclerosis through several indirect mechanisms (Auger et al 2005).

In humans, quercetin inhibits platelet aggregation and signalling and thrombus formation at a dose of 150 or 300 mg quercetin-4′-*O*-beta-D-glucoside (Hubbard et al 2004). One small crossover randomised controlled trial (RCT) involving 12 healthy men testing the acute effects of oral administration of 200 mg quercetin, (−)-epicatechin or epigallocatechin gallate on nitric oxide, endothelin-1 and oxidative stress found that quercetin augmented nitric oxide status and reduced endothelin-1 concentrations, thereby having the potential to improve endothelial function (Loke et al 2008).

Q

Antiatherogenic

Adhesion of circulating monocytes to vascular endothelial cells is a critical step in both inflammation and atherosclerosis. Experimental studies have indicated that both quercetin and its metabolites can inhibit the expression of key molecules involved in monocyte recruitment during the early stages of atherosclerosis (Tribolo et al 2008), suggesting a theoretical basis for the use of quercetin in preventing this condition. Further human trials are required to examine this effect.

Neuroprotective

Quercetin protects neuronal cells from oxidative stress-induced neurotoxicity (Heo & Lee 2004) and inflammatory-related neuronal injury (Chen et al 2005). In vitro studies have found that quercetin protects against elevated reactive oxygen species induced by $H_2O_2^-$ and changes in plasma membrane integrity and nuclear morphology as a result of increased oxidative stress (Jazvinšćak Jembrek et al 2012). At lower doses (5 and 10 microM), it has been proposed as a treatment worthy of further investigation for Alzheimer's disease and other oxidative stress-related neurodegenerative diseases; however, at higher doses (20 and 40 microM) it may be neurotoxic (Ansari et al 2008). A key consideration remains the bioavailability of oral quercetin. A comprehensive review of the neuroprotective effects of quercetin concluded that, although quercetin and quercetin-containing plants exhibit potential as therapeutic modalities in neuropathology, the data collectively highlight the need to elucidate issues such as low bioavailability in plasma and in the brain (Dajas 2012). Whether quercetin needs to actually cross the blood–brain barrier to a large extent to exert benefits remains to be seen, as accumulating research suggests that peripheral reductions in inflammation can have potent reciprocal effects in the central nervous system (Kang et al 2011).

Mood and cognitive enhancement

Anxiolytic effects have been demonstrated in stress-affected mice (Kumar & Goyal 2008) and both anxiolytic and cognitive-enhancing effects have been shown in rats following both oral and intranasal-administered quercetin treatment (Priprem et al 2008).

Gastroprotective

Quercetin treatment (100 mg/kg/day by intragastric gavage) inhibits hyperproliferation of gastric mucosal cells in rats treated with chronic oral ethanol (Liu et al 2008). It has been suggested that the gastroprotective effect of quercetin in animal models may be due to its antiperoxidative, antioxidant and antihistamine effects, resulting in a significant reduction in the number of mast cells and size of gastric erosions (Kahraman et al 2003). More recent studies demonstrate the inhibition of gastric tumour promotion by inducing cell cycle arrest and promoting apoptotic cell death, while exposure of gastric cancer cells AGS and MKN28 to quercetin results in pronounced proapoptotic effects through mitochondrial pathway activation (Wang et al 2011).

Hepatoprotective

In vitro and animal studies have demonstrated the hepatoprotective effects of quercetin. It protects the liver from oxidative damage and may reduce biliary obstruction (Alia et al 2006, Peres et al 2000). In experimental models, quercetin protects human hepatocytes from ethanol-induced oxidative stress (Yao et al 2007) and reduces liver fibrosis in rats by enhancing antioxidant enzyme activity (Amalia et al 2007). Pretreatment of rats with quercetin (10 mg/kg) reduced the mortality rate for paracetamol (1 g/kg) from 100% to 30% and prevented liver damage at sublethal doses (640 mg/kg) (Janbaz et al 2004).

Chemoprotective

In the 1970s, quercetin was considered to be carcinogenic after demonstrating mutagenicity in the Ames test; however, subsequent long-term studies have refuted this and demonstrated an anticarcinogenic effect in laboratory animals (Erlund 2004). Epidemiological and experimental studies have demonstrated potential benefits for melanoma (Thangasamy et al 2007), colon, lung (Murakami et al 2008), breast (Lin et al 2008), gastric (Ekström et al 2011), prostate (Wang et al 2012) and liver cancer (Mu et al 2007).

In vitro and preliminary animal and human data indicate that quercetin inhibits tumour growth and induces apoptosis. The anticarcinogenic effects may be due to its antioxidant properties, protection against DNA damage, inhibition of angiogenesis, effects on gene expression, effects on cell cycle regulation, phyto-oestrogen-like activity, interaction with type II oestrogen-binding sites and tyrosine kinase inhibition (Duraj et al 2005, Erlund 2004, Igura et al 2001, Lamson & Brignall 2000, Lee et al 2003, 2006, Tan et al 2003, van der Woude et al 2005, Wilms et al 2005, Zhang et al 2008). Quercetin is also believed to block the activation of procarcinogens by modulating the expression of cytochrome P450 (Scalbert et al 2005). Moreover, a natural inhibitor of catechol-*O*-methyl transferase, quercetin has been shown to inhibit epigallocatechin gallate (EGCG) methylation, leading to enhanced antiproliferative activity of EGCG in prostate cancer cells. Quercetin and EGCG synergistically inhibit cell proliferation, cause cell cycle arrest and induce apoptosis in prostate cancer-3 cells (Wang et al 2012).

Quercetin may also protect against nicotine-induced cellular and DNA damage in rats (Muthukumaran et al 2008a, 2008b) and radioprotective effects have also been reported (Devipriya et al 2008). In vivo and in vitro evidence also suggests that quercetin increases tumour radiosensitivity and inhibits ataxia telangiectasia-mutated activation in the DNA damage response pathways, thus enhancing the effectiveness of radiotherapy (Lin et al 2012).

Antidiabetic effects

Oral administration of quercetin (10 mg/kg body weight) to diabetic rats restores vascular function, and this is thought to be due to enhancement in the bioavailability of endothelium-derived nitric oxide as well as a reduction in blood glucose levels and oxidative stress (Machha et al 2007). Diabetic rats receiving quercetin (15 mg/kg/day) for 4 weeks also experienced a decrease in blood glucose and an increase in plasma insulin, calcium and magnesium (Kanter et al 2007). A similar trial investigated the hypoglycaemic, hypolipidaemic and antioxidant effects of dietary quercetin in an animal model of type 2 diabetes over a 4-week period (Jeong et al 2012). A reduction of plasma glucose levels, triglycerides and total cholesterol, as well as an increase in high-density lipoprotein (HDL) cholesterol, were observed in the low (0.04% of diet) and high (0.08% of diet) quercetin groups when compared to the control group.

Preventing bone loss

Quercetin is claimed to play an important role in preventing bone loss by affecting osteoclastogenesis and regulating many systemic and local factors, including hormones and cytokines (Son et al 2006), providing a theoretical basis for its use in the prevention of postmenopausal bone loss. In vitro studies reveal that bone resorption is mediated by oestrogen receptor proteins via inhibition of nuclear factor kappa beta (RANK) protein and/or the activation of caspases (Rassi et al 2005, Wattel et al 2003). However, in vitro studies also suggest that quercetin inhibits the metabolism of not only osteoclasts (bone resorption cells) but also osteoblasts (bone-forming cells) in a dose-dependent manner, and therefore further research is required to elucidate whether quercetin increases or decreases bone mass (Notoya et al 2004).

Sperm quality

An injected form of high-dose quercetin (270 mg/kg body weight/day over 14 days) resulted in improved sperm motility, viability and concentration and increased the weight of the testes, epididymis and ductus deferens in a rat model (Taepongsorat et al 2008). Oral administration of quercetin and onions to mice has also been shown to reduce the male reproductive toxicity (sperm abnormalities) induced by diesel exhaust particles (Izawa et al 2008). Although quercetin has the ability to attenuate the negative effects of heavy metals and maintain membrane integrity, one review (Ranawat et al 2013) concluded that overall there are conflicting biological effects of quercetin, and thus more research is required.

OTHER ACTIONS

Quercetin has been shown to reduce oxalate-induced urinary crystal formation and increase catalase and superoxide dismutase activities in rats (Park et al 2005).

CLINICAL USE

Quercetin is mainly consumed as part of the food chain as it is present in many fruits and vegetables. It is also an ingredient in some nutritional supplements.

Allergies

Quercetin is used in the treatment of acute and chronic allergic symptoms, such as hayfever and chronic rhinitis. The anti-inflammatory activity of quercetin and its ability to block allergic mediators provide a rationale for its use in these indications. Quercetin stabilises mast cells, neutrophils and basophils and inhibits histamine release (Blackburn et al 1987, Busse et al 1984, Middleton & Drzewiecki 1982, Middleton et al 1981, Ogasawara et al 1996, Pearce et al 1984). It acts as an inhibitor of mast cell secretion; reduces the release of tryptase, monocyte chemotactic protein-1 and IL-6 and downregulates histidine decarboxylase mRNA from several mast cell lines (Shaik et al 2006).

In a study of 123 patients sensitised to house dust mite and displaying nasal symptoms of mild to severe perennial allergic rhinitis, nasal scrapings were taken and histamine release measured as a percentage of the total content in the specimen (Otsuka et al 1995). Antigen exposure resulted in an increase in mast cells of the epithelial layer of the nasal mucosa, resulting in nasal hypersensitivity. Quercetin inhibited histamine release by 46–96% in a dose-dependent manner.

Further human trials are required to further explore the potential for quercetin to act as an antihistaminic agent in various allergic conditions.

Upper respiratory tract infections (URTIs)

A clinical trial of 40 trained male cyclists receiving 1000 mg/day of quercetin or placebo for 2 weeks found that active treatment resulted in a significantly reduced incidence of URTIs during a 2-week postexercise period (quercetin = 1/20 vs placebo = 9/20; $P = 0.004$), despite there being no significant differences in immune markers such as natural killer cells, phytohaemagglutinin-stimulated lymphocyte proliferation and salivary IgA output (Nieman et al 2007).

More recently, a double-blind RCT investigated the effect of two different doses of quercetin (500 mg/day and 1000 mg/day) on the incidence and severity of URTIs in a large community group ($n = 1002$) of adults (aged 18–85 years). Overall, quercetin supplementation over the 12-week study period had no significant influence on URTI rates or symptomatology when compared to placebo. However, a reduction in number of URTI-related sick days and severity was observed in a subgroup of middle-aged and older subjects ingesting 1000 mg quercetin/day who rated themselves as physically fit (Heinz et al 2010).

Asthma

Quercetin has also been used as an adjunct in the management of asthma, often in combination with vitamin C because of its antiallergic activity and ability to inhibit leukotriene synthesis (Formica & Regelson 1995). While preclinical studies have demonstrated antihistamine, antioxidant and anti-inflammatory activity, there has been a paucity of clinical trials investigating the potential of quercetin in the management of asthma.

Preventing diabetic complications

As quercetin has been shown to inhibit aldose reductase, the first enzyme in the polyol pathway, a theoretical basis exists for its use in the prevention of long-term diabetic complications such as cataracts, nephropathy, retinopathy and neuropathy

(Chaudhry et al 1983). Quercetin may also provide beneficial effects in people with diabetes by decreasing oxidative stress and preserving pancreatic beta-cell integrity (Coskun et al 2005). In vivo evidence also reveals that quercetin attenuates the damage caused by diabetes by promoting a neuroprotective effect and reducing enteric glial loss in the duodenum (Lopes et al 2012).

Preliminary evidence suggests a possible antinociceptive activity of quercetin, probably through modulation of opioidergic mechanism, suggesting a potential for the treatment of diabetic neuropathic pain (Anjaneyulu & Chopra 2003). Topical application of quercetin, in combination with ascorbyl palmitate and vitamin D_3, has been tested in a randomised, placebo-controlled, double-blind trial of 34 men and women (age 21–71 years) with diabetic neuropathy. The QR-333 preparation or placebo was applied three times daily for 4 weeks to each foot experiencing symptoms. QR-333 was well tolerated and reduced the severity of numbness, jolting pain and irritation from baseline values and improved quality-of-life scores (Valensi et al 2005).

The diabetic status of rats fed high-dose quercetin (1 g/kg) was found to be ameliorated by approximately 25%; however, the amounts used were considerably higher than those commonly used in humans (Shetty et al 2004) and these results cannot be applied to oral doses in humans. Further research is required to confirm any potential benefits.

Cataracts

In addition to the potential reduction in diabetic cataract formation afforded by the inhibition of aldose reductase (Chaudhry et al 1983, Ramana et al 2007), quercetin may reduce oxidative stress associated with the initiation of maturity-onset cataracts.

Cataracts may result from oxidative damage to the lens, which causes a disruption of the redox system, membrane damage, proteolysis, protein aggregation and a loss of lens transparency. Quercetin has been shown to inhibit oxidative damage to the lens and maintain lens transparency in vitro (Cornish et al 2002, Sanderson et al 1999). In rats with galactosaemic cataracts, quercetin improves lens transparency by maintaining the characteristic osmotic ion (calcium, sodium and potassium) equilibrium and protein levels of the lens (Ramana et al 2007). Further trials are warranted to confirm the effects of oral doses in humans.

Preventing cardiovascular disease

The cardioprotective properties of quercetin, as demonstrated in human, animal and in vitro studies, provide a basis for investigating quercetin in the prevention of cardiovascular disease; however, current evidence is unclear as to whether benefits are clinically relevant.

A double-blind, placebo-controlled study investigating the effects of a quercetin-containing supplement on plasma quercetin status, risk factors for heart disease and serum/platelet fatty acid levels was conducted on 27 healthy men and women with cholesterol levels of 4.0–7.2 mmol/L (Conquer et al 1998). The subjects consumed a quercetin-containing supplement (1 g quercetin/day) or rice flour placebo for 28 days. Quercetin intakes were approximately 50-fold greater than dietary intakes previously associated with lower coronary heart disease mortality in epidemiological studies. Plasma quercetin concentrations were approximately 23-fold greater in subjects consuming the quercetin capsules than in the placebo group. No effect was observed on the levels of omega-3 or omega-6 polyunsaturated fatty acids in serum or platelet phospholipids, nor did quercetin supplementation alter serum total, LDL or HDL cholesterol or triglyceride levels or other cardiovascular disease or thrombogenic risk factors, such as platelet thromboxane B_2 production, blood pressure or resting heart rate. This is in contrast to the findings of other trials (Hubbard et al 2004, Pfeuffer et al 2013), which demonstrated inhibition of platelet aggregation and signalling and thrombus formation at a dose of 150 or 300 mg quercetin-4′-*O*-beta-D-glucoside (Hubbard et al 2004); as well as decreased postprandial triacylglycerol concentrations.

IN COMBINATION

Another clinical trial which involved a large group of community-dwelling adults (n = 1000) who were randomised into one of three groups, and given placebo or a combination of quercetin (500 mg), vitamin C (125 mg) and niacin supplements (5 mg) or the same combination at double the dosage over a 12-week period also yielded non-significant results. A difference in serum total cholesterol was measured between Q-500 and placebo groups, and there was a small decrease in HDL cholesterol levels in the Q-1000 group. Change in inflammatory measures did not differ between groups, except for a slight decrease in IL-6 for the Q-1000 group (Knab et al 2011).

Metabolic syndrome

One double-blind, randomised trial involving 200 healthy persons with dyslipidaemia evaluated the effects of regular consumption of quercetin (over 2 months) on blood lipids. Upon completion of therapy, the test group demonstrated a decrease in cholesterol, triglyceride and LDL values, with a parallel increase in HDL (Talirevic & Jelena 2012). Although quercetin was used in supplemental form, no doses are mentioned in this study.

Hypertension

In a small randomised, double-blind, placebo-controlled, crossover study, 730 mg quercetin/day for 4 weeks resulted in reductions in mean systolic (−7 ± 2 mmHg), diastolic (−5 ± 2 mmHg) and arterial blood pressures (−5 ± 2 mmHg) ($P < 0.01$) in patients with stage 1 hypertension. Significant effects were not demonstrated in prehypertensive subjects, and indices of oxidative stress were not affected by quercetin (Edwards et al 2007). A more recent clinical trial revealed that quercetin supplementation (150 mg/day over 6 weeks) reduced systolic blood pressure by an average of 2.6 mmHg ($P < 0.01$) (Egert et al 2009). The same double-blind, crossover RCT showed that quercetin supplementation reduced plasma oxidised LDL concentrations in overweight subjects with a high-cardiovascular disease risk phenotype. At this dose, no adverse effects were seen.

Performance enhancing

Some evidence suggests that quercetin supplementation increases performance in humans (Dumke et al 2009); however, not all studies are positive, A meta-analysis which reviewed 11 studies involving 254 human subjects of differing fitness levels found that quercetin (median treatment duration of 14 days; median dosage of 1083 mg/day) provides a significant benefit in human endurance exercise capacity, but the effect is small, with greater effects observed in subjects with a lower fitness level (Kressler et al 2011).The proposed mechanisms for ergogenic effects of quercetin are the antagonism of adenosine receptors, and improved mitochondrial biogenesis (through peroxisome proliferator-activated receptor gamma coactivator 1-alpha), which in turn would increase oxidative capacity and subsequently endurance performance (Kressler et al 2011).

Interestingly, previously a placebo-controlled trial of 40 athletes found that 6 weeks of treatment with quercetin (1000 mg/day) did not protect against exercise-induced oxidative stress and inflammation (McAnulty et al 2008). Additionally, a recent small crossover study of soldiers found that oral quercetin (1000 mg/day) taken for 8.5 days had no effects on aerobically-demanding soldier performance compared to placebo (Casuso et al 2013, Sharp et al 2012).

Recent research using an animal model found that quercetin supplementation during exercise provided a disadvantage to exercise-induced muscle adaptations (Casuso et al 2013), a finding which should be investigated in humans to better understand the benefit: risk considerations in athletes.

Chronic prostatitis

Thirty men with category IIIa or IIIb chronic pelvic pain syndrome received either placebo or quercetin 500 mg twice daily for 1 month. Sixty-seven per cent of the treated subjects had at least a 25% improvement in symptoms compared to 20% of the placebo group. In a follow-up, unblinded, open-label study, 17 additional men received the same dose of quercetin (combined with bromelain and papain to enhance absorption) for 1 month. The combination increased the response rate from 67% to 82% (Shoskes et al 1999). The anti-inflammatory, antioxidant and immunomodulating activities of quercetin may help to explain these results.

Cancer

Early concerns that quercetin may be carcinogenic have not been supported by recent research. Quercetin is primarily found in fruit and vegetables, which have been shown to decrease the risk of certain human cancers when consumed regularly (Ekström et al 2011, Morrow et al 2001), thereby casting doubt on this proposition. In fact, the anti-carcinogenic effects of quercetin seen in laboratory animals suggest a possible preventive role (Erlund 2004), and in vitro and epidemiological studies have suggested potential benefits in the prevention of colon (Kim et al 2005, Park et al 2005), lung (Schwarz et al 2005), prostate (Yuan et al 2004) and breast cancer (Otake et al 2000).

Sarcoidosis

Oral quercetin supplementation (4 × 500 mg over 24 hours) increased total plasma antioxidant capacity, and reduced markers of oxidative stress and inflammation according to a double-blind, placebo-controlled study of non-smoking, untreated sarcoidosis patients, matched for age and gender ($n = 18$). The effects of quercetin supplementation appeared to be more pronounced when the levels of the oxidative stress and inflammation markers were higher at baseline (Boots et al 2011).

Aphthous ulcers

One clinical trial involving 40 male patients found that daily (2–3 times) topical application of a quercetin-based cream may be useful in accelerating the healing process of minor aphthous ulcers (Hamdy & Ibrahem 2010).

OTHER USES

Although the potential benefits of quercetin in allergic conditions have yet to be confirmed by large human trials, quercetin is often used to treat conditions such as hayfever and other respiratory allergies and histamine-related conditions based on demonstrated pharmacological properties. In practice, quercetin is also commonly used to stabilise the integrity of blood vessel walls and address conditions resulting from capillary fragility, and used in conjunction with vitamin C for the treatment of viral infections. It is sometimes considered as a means of reducing the toxic effects of exposure to heavy metals. In vivo research suggests that quercetin consumption may attenuate the toxicity of environmental cadmium by decreasing lipid peroxidation and restoring the activities of antioxidant enzymes such as glutathione peroxidase and superoxide dismutase (Bu et al 2011).

DOSAGE RANGE

General dose range

- 200–1500 mg daily taken in divided doses (PDRHealth 2005, Spoerke & Rouse 2004).

Specific doses

- Chronic prostatitis: 500 mg (combined with bromelain and papain to enhance absorption) twice daily (Shoskes et al 1999).
- Acute allergies: 2 g every 2 hours for 2 days (often used with vitamin C) in practice.
- Chronic allergies: 2 g daily used in practice.
- Asthma: as an adjunct to standard treatment 2 g daily used in practice.
- Sarcoidosis: 2000 mg/day oral quercetin.
- Cardiovascular disease prevention: 3 × 200 mL of black tea per day, or two medium-sized apples per day.
- Hypertension: 150 mg/day for 6 weeks.
- Aphthous ulcers: topical quercetin cream, three times a day.

ADVERSE REACTIONS

Quercetin is generally well tolerated and appears to be associated with little toxicity when administered orally or intravenously (Lamson & Brignall 2000). Adverse effects are rare and include nausea, dyspnoea, headache and mild tingling of the extremities (PDRHealth 2005, Spoerke & Rouse 2004).

SIGNIFICANT INTERACTIONS

Possible modulation of P-glycoprotein (Choi & Li 2005, Hsiu et al 2002, Limtrakul et al 2005) and inhibition of CYP1A1 (Schwarz et al 2005) and CYP1A2 (Chang et al 2006) activity should be considered when prescribing. According to a recent crossover RCT, 500 mg of oral quercetin significantly induces CYP3A4; therefore healthcare providers should carefully monitor the concurrent use of all drugs chiefly metabolised by CYP3A4 to avoid drug interactions (Duan et al 2012).

Note: Phase II metabolites of quercetin appear to inhibit human multidrug resistance-associated protein 1 (MRP1) and 2 (MRP2), which may prove beneficial in MRP-mediated multidrug resistance (van Zanden et al 2007). For instance, the combined effect of quercetin with hyperthermia in human myelogenous leukaemia cells may assist in the reversal of multidrug resistance (Shen et al 2008).

Iron

Quercetin is a powerful iron chelator so should not be ingested at the same time as iron supplements or iron-rich foods to avoid reducing absorption (Vanhees et al 2011). Separate dose by 2 hours.

Adriamycin

Quercetin has demonstrated to have a protective effect against Adriamycin-induced cardiotoxicity in mice. The effect is likely to be related to enhanced myocardial superoxide dismutase activity, decreased iNOS activity and inhibition of myocardial apoptosis (Pei et al 2007).

Cisplatin

Quercetin pretreatment may sensitise human cervix carcinoma cells to cisplatin-induced apoptosis (Jakubowicz-Gil et al 2005). Beneficial interaction is theoretically possible under professional supervision, but clinical significance is unknown.

Cyclosporin

Animal studies demonstrate that coadministration of quercetin significantly decreases the oral bioavailability of cyclosporin (Hsiu et al 2002) — avoid concurrent use.

Digoxin

An increase in drug bioavailability is theoretically possible and has been observed in an in vivo study. Although human studies at lower doses are not available, the narrow therapeutic range of digoxin and the serious nature of the interaction should not be underestimated. Avoid concurrent use.

Diltiazem

Pretreatment of rabbits with quercetin resulted in an increased bioavailability of the calcium channel blocker diltiazem, which may be the result of inhibition of P-glycoprotein and CYP 3A4 (Choi & Li 2005). Caution — use under professional supervision; doses may need to be adjusted accordingly.

Doxorubicin

A positive interaction has been observed. When combined with doxorubicin, quercetin potentiated antitumour effects, specifically in the highly invasive breast cancer. Moreover, in non-tumour cells, quercetin reduced doxorubicin cytotoxic side effects (Staedler et al 2011). Therefore, it theoretically may have benefits in reducing doxorubicin-mediated toxicity (Vaclavikova et al 2008); however, further investigation is required to confirm.

Haloperidol

Tardive dyskinesia (rhythmical involuntary movements of the tongue, face, mouth or jaw, e.g. protrusion of tongue, puffing of cheeks, puckering of mouth and chewing movements) may result from long-term therapy with the traditional antipsychotic medication haloperidol and may be irreversible in some individuals. Oxidative stress and the products of lipid peroxidation have been implicated in the pathophysiology of tardive dyskinesia, and coadministration of quercetin (25–100 mg/kg) has been shown to dose-dependently reduce haloperidol-induced vacuous chewing movements and tongue protrusions in animal models (Naidu et al 2003). Beneficial interaction is theoretically possible under professional supervision.

Paclitaxel

Pretreatment with quercetin may increase the bioavailability of paclitaxel according to animal studies (Choi et al 2004). Caution — use under professional supervision; doses may need to be adjusted accordingly.

Paracetamol

According to animal data, pretreatment with quercetin may reduce the risk of mortality from paracetamol overdose (Janbaz et al 2004). However, effects in humans have not been studied —beneficial interaction theoretically possible.

Pioglitazone

Quercetin may increase the bioavailability of pioglitazone (Actos) (Umathe et al 2008). Due to the potential for toxicity, careful monitoring of hepatic and cardiac function is required — caution.

Quinolone antibiotics

In vitro, quercetin binds to the DNA gyrase site in bacteria and therefore may theoretically compete with quinolone antibiotics that also bind to this site (PDRHealth 2005) — caution.

Saquinavir

Despite the inhibition of P-glycoprotein by quercetin, coadministration does not appear to alter plasma saquinavir concentrations. However, as there appears to be a substantial inter- and intrasubject variability in saquinavir intracellular concentrations, caution should be exerted until more is known (DiCenzo et al 2006).

Stibanate

Concurrent use of quercetin with the antileishmanial drug stibanate appears to improve the efficacy of the drug and reduce anaemia and parasitaemia associated with the condition (Sen et al 2005) — beneficial interaction theoretically possible.

CONTRAINDICATIONS AND PRECAUTIONS

Hypersensitivity to quercetin.

According to experimental studies, quercetin may possess some antithyroid properties, inhibiting thyroid cell growth in association with inhibition of insulin-modulated phosphatidylinositol 3-kinase-Akt kinase activity. While these findings are preliminary, quercetin should be used with caution in thyroid disease and therapy until more is understood about these effects in humans (Giuliani et al 2008).

PREGNANCY USE

Quercetin is widely available in the food chain and considered safe when consumed in dietary amounts (4–68 mg per day). The safety of higher oral doses is unclear, as some in vivo research indicates that quercetin crosses the placenta and accumulates in the fetus, and a relatively high intake of quercetin (302 mg/kg feed, which is comparable to supplemental intake of between 200 and 1800 mg/day) may have detrimental effects later in life (Vanhees et al 2011). However doses greater than this (333 mg/kg feed) did not exhibit teratogenic effects in other in vivo trials (Prater et al 2008).

Practice points/Patient counselling

- Quercetin is a flavanol belonging to a group of polyphenolic substances known as flavonoids or bioflavonoids and is found in many fruits and vegetables and some herbal medicines.
- According to experimental studies, it has antioxidant, anti-inflammatory, antiviral, mast cell stabilisation and inhibition, neuroprotective, gastroprotective, hepatoprotective and possibly cardioprotective actions.
- In practice, it is used for respiratory allergies such as hayfever, as an adjunct in asthma management, preventing diabetic complications such as cataracts and symptom relief in prostatitis; however, large controlled studies are not available to determine its effectiveness.
- Numerous drug interactions are possible, mainly due to CYP3A4 induction.
- Quercetin is generally well tolerated, although adverse effects may include nausea, dyspnoea, headache and mild tingling of the extremities.
- The daily intake of quercetin from food sources ranges from 5 to 40 mg but can reach up to 500 mg/day when consumption of fruits and vegetables is high, especially when the peel of the fruit is consumed (Harwood et al 2007).

PATIENTS' FAQs

What will this supplement do for me?

Quercetin has several pharmacological effects, may provide some symptom relief in allergic conditions and prostatitis and may be beneficial in the prevention of many chronic diseases, such as diabetes, osteoarthritis, neurodegeneration, cancer (as an adjunct) and cardiovascular disease; however, further research is required to clarify its effectiveness.

When will it start to work?

This will depend on the indication it is being used to treat.

Are there any safety issues?

Although it is generally well tolerated, numerous drug interactions are possible, so seek professional advice if taking other medication.

Q

REFERENCES

Alcocer F et al. Quercetin inhibits human vascular smooth muscle cell proliferation and migration. Surgery 131.2 (2002): 198–204.

Alia M et al. Quercetin protects human hepatoma HepG2 against oxidative stress induced by tert-butyl hydroperoxide. Toxicol Applied Pharmacol 212.2 (2006): 110–1118.

Amalia PM et al. Quercetin prevents oxidative stress in cirrhotic rats. Dig Dis Sci 52.10 (2007): 2616–2621.

Anjaneyulu M, Chopra K. Quercetin, a bioflavonoid, attenuates thermal hyperalgesia in a mouse model of diabetic neuropathic pain. Prog Neuropsychopharmacol Biol Psychiatry 27.6 (2003): 100–105.

Ansari MA et al. Protective effect of quercetin in primary neurons against Abeta(1–42): relevance to Alzheimer's disease. J Nutr Biochem 20.4 (2008): 269–275.

Auger C et al. Dietary wine phenolics catechin, quercetin, and resveratrol efficiently protect hypercholesterolemic hamsters against aortic fatty streak accumulation. J Agric Food Chem 53.6 (2005): 2015–2021.

Blackburn W, et al. The bioflavonoid quercetin inhibits neutrophil degranulation, superoxide production, and the phosphorylation of specific neutrophil proteins. Biochem Biophys Res Commun 144.3 (1987): 1229–1236.

Boots AW et al. Oxidized quercetin reacts with thiols rather than with ascorbate: implication for quercetin supplementation. Biochem Biophys Res Commun 308.3 (2003): 560–565.

Boots AW et al. The quercetin paradox. Toxicol Appl Pharmacol 222.1 (2007): 89–96.

Boots AW et al. Quercetin reduces markers of oxidative stress and inflammation in sarcoidosis. Clin Nutr. 30.4 (2011):506–12.

Brookes PS et al. Mitochondrial function in response to cardiac ischemia-reperfusion after oral treatment with quercetin. Free Radic Biol Med 32.11 (2002): 1220–1228.

Bu T et al. Protective effect of quercetin on cadmium-induced oxidative toxicity on germ cells in male mice. Anat Rec (Hoboken) 294 (2011): 520–526.

Busse W, et al. Flavonoid modulation of human neutrophil function. J Allergy Clin Immunol 73.6 (1984): 801–809.

Cai X et al. Bioavailability of quercetin: problems and promises. Curr Med Chem. 2013 20: 2572–2582.

Casuso, R.A., et al. 2013. Oral quercetin supplementation hampers skeletal muscle adaptations in response to exercise training. Scand. J Med Sci. Sports doi. 10.1111/sms.12136 (epub ahead of print).

Challem J. The power of flavonoids: antioxidant nutrients in fruits, vegetables, and herbs. The Nutrition Reporter (1998).

Chang TK, et al. Effect of *Ginkgo biloba* extract on procarcinogen-bioactivating human CYP1 enzymes: Identification of isorhamnetin, kaempferol, and quercetin as potent inhibitors of CYP1B1. Toxicol Appl Pharmacol (2006)213: 18–26.

Chen JC et al. Inhibition of iNOS gene expression by quercetin is mediated by the inhibition of I(kappa)B kinase, nuclear factor-kappa B and STAT1, and depends on heme oxygenase-1 induction in mouse BV-2 microglia. Eur J Pharmacol 521.1–3 (2005): 9–20.

Choi JS, Li X. Enhanced diltiazem bioavailability after oral administration of diltiazem with quercetin to rabbits. Int J Pharm 297.1–2 (2005): 1–8.

Choi JS, et al. Enhanced paclitaxel bioavailability after oral administration of paclitaxel or prodrug to rats pretreated with quercetin. Eur J Pharm Biopharm 57.2 (2004): 313–3118.

Chuang CC et al. Quercetin is equally or more effective than resveratrol in attenuating tumor necrosis factor-{alpha}-mediated inflammation and insulin resistance in primary human adipocytes. Am. J. Clin. Nutr. 92.6 (2010): 1511–21

Comalada M et al. In vivo quercitrin anti-inflammatory effect involves release of quercetin, which inhibits inflammation through down-regulation of the NF-kappaB pathway. Eur J Immunol 35.2 (2005): 584–592.

Conquer JA et al. Supplementation with quercetin markedly increases plasma quercetin concentration without effect on selected risk factors for heart disease in healthy subjects. J Nutr 128.3 (1998): 593–597.

Cornish KM, et al. Quercetin metabolism in the lens: role in inhibition of hydrogen peroxide induced cataract. Free Radic Biol Med 33.1 (2002): 63–70.

Coskun O et al. Quercetin, a flavonoid antioxidant, prevents and protects streptozotocin-induced oxidative stress and (beta)-cell damage in rat pancreas. Pharmacol Res 51.2 (2005): 117–123.

Dajas F. Life or death: neuroprotective and anticancer effects of quercetin. J Ethnopharmacol. 143. 2 (2012):383–96.

Devipriya N et al. Quercetin ameliorates gamma radiation-induced DNA damage and biochemical changes in human peripheral blood lymphocytes. Mutat Res 654.1 (2008): 1–7.

deVries J et al. Plasma concentrations and urinary excretion of the antioxidant flavonols quercetin and kaempferol as biomarkers for dietary intake. Am J Clin Nutr 68.1 (1998): 60–65.

DiCenzo R et al. Effect of quercetin on the plasma and intracellular concentrations of saquinavir in healthy adults. Pharmacotherapy 26.9 (2006): 1255–1261.

Duan KM et al. Effect of quercetin on CYP3A activity in Chinese healthy participants. J Clin Pharmacol.52.6 (2012); 940–6

Duda-Chodak A. The inhibitory effect of polyphenols on human gut microbiota. J Physiol Pharmacol. 63.5 (2012):497–503.

Dumke CL et al. Quercetin's effect on cycling efficiency and substrate utilization. Appl Physiol Nutr Metab. 34.6 (2009): 993–1000

Duraj J et al. Flavonoid quercetin, but not apigenin or luteolin, induced apoptosis in human myeloid leukemia cells and their resistant variants. Neoplasma 52.4 (2005): 273–279.

Edwards RL et al. Quercetin reduces blood pressure in hypertensive subjects. J Nutr 137.11 (2007): 2405–2411.

Egert S et al. Daily quercetin supplementation dose-dependently increases plasma quercetin concentrations in healthy humans. J Nutr 138.9 (2008): 1615–1621.

Egert S et al. Quercetin reduces systolic blood pressure and plasma oxidised low-density lipoprotein concentrations in overweight subjects with a high-cardiovascular disease risk phenotype: a double-blinded, placebo-controlled cross-over study. Br J Nutr. 102.7 (2009): 1065–74

Egert S et al. Enriched cereal bars are more effective in increasing plasma quercetin compared with quercetin from powder-filled hard capsules.Br J Nutr. 107.4 (2012):539–46.

Erlund I. Review of the flavonoids quercetin, hesperetin, and naringenin. Dietary sources, bioactivities, bioavailability, and epidemiology. Nutr Res 24.10 (2004): 851–874.

Erlund I et al. Pharmacokinetics of quercetin from quercetin aglycone and rutin in healthy volunteers. Eur J Clin Pharmacol 56.8 (2000): 545–553.

Ferraresi R et al. Essential requirement of reduced glutathione (GSH) for the anti-oxidant effect of the flavonoid quercetin. Free Radic Res 39.11 (2005): 1249–1258.

Formica JV, Regelson W. Review of the biology of quercetin and related bioflavonoids. Food Chem Toxicol 33 (1995): 1061–1080.

Ganesan S et al. Quercetin inhibits rhinovirus replication in vitro and in vivo. Antiviral Res. 94.3(2012):258–71.

Garcia-Saura MF et al. Effects of chronic quercetin treatment in experimental renovascular hypertension. Mol Cell Biochem 270.1–2 (2005): 147–155.

Giuliani C et al. The flavonoid quercetin regulates growth and gene expression in rat FRTL-5 thyroid cells. Endocrinology 149.1 (2008): 84–92.

Graefe EU, et al. Pharmacokinetics and bioavailability of the flavonol quercetin in humans. Int J Clin Pharmacol Ther 37.5 (1999): 219–233.

Guo et al. Dietary fat increases quercetin bioavailability in overweight adults. Mol Nutr Food Res. 57.5 (2013):896–905.

Hamdy AA, Ibrahem AA. Management of aphthous ulceration with topical quercetin: a randomized clinical trial. J Contemp Dent Pract. 11.4 (2010): E009–16

Harwood M et al. A critical review of the data related to the safety ofquercetin and lack of evidence of in vivo toxicity, including lack of genotoxic/carcinogenic properties. Food Chem Toxicol (2007): 45: 2179–2205.

Heinz SA et al. Quercetin supplementation and upper respiratory tract infection: A randomized community clinical trial. Pharmacol Res. 62.3 (2010): 237–42.

Heo HJ, Lee CY. Protective effects of quercetin and vitamin C against oxidative stress-induced neurodegeneration. J Agric Food Chem 52.25 (2004): 7514–75117.

Hollman PCH et al. Bioavailability of the dietary antioxidant flavonol quercetin in man. Cancer Lett 114.1–2 (1997): 139–140.

Hsiu SL et al. Quercetin significantly decreased cyclosporin oral bioavailability in pigs and rats. Life Sci 72.3 (2002): 227–235.

Hubbard GP et al. Ingestion of quercetin inhibits platelet aggregation and essential components of the collagen-stimulated platelet activation pathway in humans. J Thromb Haemost 2.12 (2004): 2138–2145.

Igura K et al. Resveratrol and quercetin inhibit angiogenesis in vitro. Cancer Lett 171.1 (2001): 11–116.

Izawa H et al. Alleviative effects of quercetin and onion on male reproductive toxicity induced by diesel exhaust particles. Biosci Biotechnol Biochem 72.5 (2008): 1235–1241.

Jakubowicz-Gil J et al. The effect of quercetin on pro-apoptotic activity of cisplatin in HeLa cells. Biochem Pharmacol 69.9 (2005): 1343–1350.

Janbaz KH, et al. Studies on the protective effects of caffeic acid and quercetin on chemical-induced hepatotoxicity in rodents. Phytomedicine 11.5 (2004): 424–430.

Jazvinšćak Jembrek M et al. Neuroprotective effect of quercetin against hydrogen peroxide-induced oxidative injury in P19 neurons. J Mol Neurosci. 47.2 (2012):286–99.

Jeong SM et al. Quercetin ameliorates hyperglycemia and dyslipidemia and improves antioxidant status in type 2 diabetic db/db mice.Nutr Res Pract. 6.3 (2012):201–7.

Jin F et al. The variable plasma quercetin response to 12-week quercetin supplementation in humans. Eur J Clin Nutr. 64.7 (2010): 692–7

Kahraman A et al. The antioxidative and antihistaminic properties of quercetin in ethanol-induced gastric lesions. Toxicology 183.1–3 (2003): 133–142.

Kang, A., et al. 2011. Peripheral anti-inflammatory effects explain the ginsenosides paradox between poor brain distribution and anti-depression efficacy. J Neuroinflammation., 8, 100.

Kanter M et al. The effects of quercetin on bone minerals, biomechanical behavior, and structure in streptozotocin-induced diabetic rats. Cell Biochem Funct 25.6 (2007): 747–752.

Kaul T, et al. Antiviral effect of flavonoids on human viruses. J Med Virol 15.1 (1985): 71–79.

Ke Chen C, Pace-Asciak CR. Vasorelaxing activity of resveratrol and quercetin in isolated rat aorta. Gen Pharmacol Vasc Syst 27.2 (1996): 363–366.

Kim WK et al. Quercetin decreases the expression of ErbB2 and ErbB3 proteins in HT-29 human colon cancer cells. J Nutr Biochem 16.3 (2005): 155–162.

Knab AM et al. Influence of quercetin supplementation on disease risk factors in community-dwelling adults. J Am Diet Assoc. 111.2 (2011):542–9.

Kressler J et al. Quercetin and endurance exercise capacity: a systematic review and meta-analysis. Med Sci Sports Exerc. 43.12 (2011): 2396–404

Kumar A, Goyal R. Quercetin protects against acute immobilization stress-induced behaviors and biochemical alterations in mice. J Med Food 11.3 (2008): 469–473.

Kumar P et al. Effect of quercetin supplementation on lung antioxidants after experimental influenza virus infection. Exp Lung Res 31.5 (2005): 449–459.

Lamson DW, Brignall MS. Antioxidants and cancer. Part 3: quercetin. Altern Med Rev 5.3 (2000): 196–208.

Lee J, Mitchell AE. Pharmacokinetics of quercetin absorption from apples and onions in healthy humans. J. Agric. Food Chem. 60.15 (2012): 3874–81

Lee JC et al. The antioxidant, rather than prooxidant, activities of quercetin on normal cells: quercetin protects mouse thymocytes from glucose oxidase-mediated apoptosis. Exp Cell Res 291.2 (2003): 386–397.

Lee TJ et al. Quercetin arrests G2/M phase and induces caspase-dependent cell death in U937 cells. Cancer Lett 2006: 240: 234–242.

Limtrakul P, et al. Inhibition of P-glycoprotein function and expression by kaempferol and quercetin. J Chemother 17.1 (2005): 86–95.

Lin CW et al. Quercetin inhibition of tumor invasion via suppressing PKC delta/ERK/AP-1-dependent matrix metalloproteinase-9 activation in breast carcinoma cells. Carcinogenesis 29.9 (2008): 1807–1815.

Lin C et al. Combination of quercetin with radiotherapy enhances tumor radiosensitivity in vitro and in vivo. Radiother Oncol. 104.3 (2012): 395–400.

Liu JL et al. Effects of quercetin on hyper-proliferation of gastric mucosal cells in rats treated with chronic oral ethanol through the reactive oxygen species-nitric oxide pathway. World J Gastroenterol 14.20 (2008): 3242–3248.

Loke WM et al. Pure dietary flavonoids quercetin and (−)-epicatechin augment nitric oxide products and reduce endothelin-1 acutely in healthy men. Am. J. Clin. Nutr.88.4 (2008): 1018–25

Lopes CR et al. Neuroprotective effect of quercetin on the duodenum enteric nervous system of streptozotocin-induced diabetic rats. Dig. Dis. Sci. 57.12 (2012): 3106–15

Machha A et al. Quercetin, a flavonoid antioxidant, modulates endothelium-derived nitric oxide bioavailability in diabetic rat aortas. Nitric Oxide 16.4 (2007): 442–447.

Mackraj I, et al. The antihypertensive effects of quercetin in a salt-sensitive model of hypertension. J Cardiovasc Pharmacol 51.3 (2008): 239–245.

McAnulty SR et al. Chronic quercetin ingestion and exercise-induced oxidative damage and inflammation. Appl Physiol Nutr Metab 33.2 (2008): 254–262.

Meng B et al. Quercetin reduces serum homocysteine level in rats fed a methionine-enriched diet. Nutrition. 29.4 (2013):661–6.

Middleton E, Drzewiecki G. Effects of flavonoids and transitional metal cations on antigen-induced histamine release from human basophils. Biochem Pharmacol 31.7 (1982): 1449–1453.

Middleton C, et al. Quercetin: an inhibitor of antigen-induced human basophil histamine release. J Immunol 127 (1981): 546–550.

Min YD et al. Quercetin inhibits expression of inflammatory cytokines through attenuation of NF-kappaB and p38 MAPK in HMC-1 human mast cell line. Inflamm Res 56.5 (2007): 210–215.

Mochizuki M et al. Effect of quercetin conjugates on vascular permeability and expression of adhesion molecules. Biofactors 22.1–4 (2004): 201–204.

Moon SK et al. Quercetin exerts multiple inhibitory effects on vascular smooth muscle cells: role of ERK1/2, cell-cycle regulation, and matrix metalloproteinase-9. Biochem Biophys Res Commun 301.4 (2003): 1069–1078.

Moon H et al. Quercetin inhalation inhibits the asthmatic responses by exposure to aerosolized-ovalbumin in conscious guinea-pigs. Arch Pharm Res 31.6 (2008): 771–778.

Morikawa K et al. Inhibitory effect of quercetin on carrageenan-induced inflammation in rats. Life Sci 74.6 (2003): 709–721.

Morrow DM et al. Dietary supplementation with the anti-tumour promoter quercetin: its effects on matrix metalloproteinase gene regulation. Mutat Res 480–1 (2001): 269–276.

Mu C et al. Quercetin induces cell cycle G1 arrest through elevating Cdk inhibitors p21 and p27 in human hepatoma cell line (HepG2). Methods Find Exp Clin Pharmacol 29.3 (2007): 179–183.

Murakami A, et al. Multitargeted cancer prevention by quercetin. Cancer Lett 269.2 (2008): 315–325.

Murota K, Terao J. Antioxidative flavonoid quercetin: implication of its intestinal absorption and metabolism. Arch Biochem Biophys 417.1 (2003): 12–117.

Muthian G, Bright JJ. Quercetin, a flavonoid phytoestrogen, ameliorates experimental allergic encephalomyelitis by blocking IL-12 signaling through JAK-STAT pathway in T lymphocyte. J Clin Immunol 24.5 (2004): 542–552.

Muthukumaran S et al. Protective effect of quercetin on nicotine-induced prooxidant and antioxidant imbalance and DNA damage in Wistar rats. Toxicology 243.1–2 (2008a): 207–215.

Muthukumaran S, et al. Effect of quercetin on nicotine-induced biochemical changes and DNA damage in rat peripheral blood lymphocytes. Redox Rep 13.5 (2008b): 217–224.

Naidu PS, et al. Quercetin, a bioflavonoid, attenuates haloperidol-induced orofacial dyskinesia. Neuropharmacology 44.8 (2003): 1100–1106.

Nair MPN et al. The flavonoid, quercetin, differentially regulates Th-1 (IFN(gamma)) and Th-2 (IL4) cytokine gene expression by normal peripheral blood mononuclear cells. Biochim Biophys Acta Mol Cell Res 1593.1 (2002): 29–36.

Nieman DC et al. Quercetin reduces illness but not immune perturbations after intensive exercise. Med Sci Sports Exerc 39.9 (2007): 1561–1569.

Notoya M et al. Quercetin, a flavonoid, inhibits the proliferation, differentiation, and mineralization of osteoblasts in vitro. Eur J Pharmacol 485.1–3 (2004): 89–96.

Ogasawara H et al. The role of hydrogen peroxide in basophil histamine release and the effect of selected flavonoids. J Allergy Clin Immunol 78 (1996): 321–328.

Otake Y et al. Quercetin and resveratrol potently reduce estrogen sulfotransferase activity in normal human mammary epithelial cells. J Steroid Biochem Mol Biol 73.5 (2000): 265–270.

Otsuka H et al. Histochemical and functional characteristics of metachromatic cells in the nasal epithelium in allergic rhinitis: studies of nasal scrapings and their dispersed cells. J Allergy Clin Immunol 96.4 (1995): 528–536.

Park CH et al. Quercetin, a potent inhibitor against (beta)-catenin/Tcf signaling in SW480 colon cancer cells. Biochem Biophys Res Commun 328.1 (2005): 227–234.

PDRHealth [online]. Thomson Healthcare, 2005. http://www.pdrhealth.com (accessed 04-02-06).

Pearce FL, et al. Mucosal mast cells: effect of quercetin and other flavonoids on antigen-induced histamine secretion from rat intestinal mast cells. J Allergy Clin Immunol 73.6 (1984): 819–823.

Peres W et al. The flavonoid quercetin ameliorates liver damage in rats with biliary obstruction. J Hepatol 33.5 (2000): 742–750.

Pfeuffer M et al. Effect of quercetin on traits of the metabolic syndrome, endothelial function and inflammation in men with different APOE isoforms.Nutr Metab Cardiovasc Dis. 23.5 (2013):403–9.

Pietruck F et al. Effect of quercetin on hypoxic injury in freshly isolated rat proximal tubules. J Lab Clin Med 142.2 (2003): 106–112.

Prater, MR et al. Placental oxidative stress alters expression of murine osteogenic genes and impairs fetal skeletal formation. Placenta 29 (2008): 802–808.

Priprem A et al. Anxiety and cognitive effects of quercetin liposomes in rats. Nanomedicine 4.1 (2008): 70–78.

Ramana BV et al. Defensive role of quercetin against imbalances of calcium, sodium, and potassium in galactosemic cataract. Biol Trace Elem Res 119.1 (2007): 35–41.

Ranawat P, et al. A new perspective on the quercetin paradox in male reproductive dysfunction. Phytother Res. 27.6 (2013):802–10.

Rassi CM et al. Modulation of osteoclastogenesis in porcine bone marrow cultures by quercetin and rutin. Cell Tissue Res 319.3 (2005): 383–393.

Robaszkiewicz A, et al. Antioxidative and prooxidative effects of quercetin on A549 cells. Cell Biol Int 31.10 (2007): 1245–1250.

Roghani M et al. Mechanisms underlying quercetin-induced vasorelaxation in aorta of subchronic diabetic rats: an in vitro study. Vasc Pharmacol 42.1 (2004): 31–35.

Sanchez M et al. Quercetin downregulates NADPH oxidase, increases eNOS activity and prevents endothelial dysfunction in spontaneously hypertensive rats. J Hypertens 24.1 (2006): 75–84.

Sanderson J, et al. Quercetin inhibits hydrogen peroxide-induced oxidation of the rat lens. Free Radic Biol Med 26.5–6 (1999): 639–645.

Scalbert A et al. Dietary polyphenols and the prevention of diseases. Crit Rev Food Sci Nutr. 45.4 (2005): 287–306.

Schwarz D, et al. CYP1A1 genotype-selective inhibition of benzo(a) pyrene activation by quercetin. Eur J Cancer 41.1 (2005): 151–158.

Sen G et al. Therapeutic use of quercetin in the control of infection and anemia associated with visceral leishmaniasis. Free Radic Biol Med 38.9 (2005): 1257–1264.

Shaik YB et al. Role of quercetin (a natural herbal compound) in allergy and inflammation. J Biol Regul Homeost Agents 20.3–4 (2006): 47–52.

Shanely RA et al. Quercetin supplementation does not alter antioxidant status in humans. Free Radic Res. 44 (2010): 224–31.

Sharp, M.A., et al. 2012. Effects of short-term quercetin supplementation on soldier performance. J Strength. Cond. Res., 26 Suppl 2, S53–S60.

Shen J et al. The synergistic reversal effect of multidrug resistance by quercetin and hyperthermia in doxorubicin-resistant human myelogenous leukemia cells. Int J Hyperthermia 24.2 (2008): 151–159.
Shetty AK et al. Antidiabetic influence of quercetin in streptozotocin-induced diabetic rats. Nutr Res 24.5 (2004): 373–381.
Shoskes DA et al. Quercetin in men with category III chronic prostatitis: a preliminary prospective, double-blind, placebo-controlled trial. Urology 54.6 (1999): 960–963.
Somerset SM, Johannot L. Dietary flavonoid sources in Australian adults. Nutr Cancer 60.4 (2008): 442–449.
Son YO et al. Quercetin, a bioflavonoid, accelerates TNF-(alpha)-induced growth inhibition and apoptosis in MC3T3-E1 osteoblastic cells. Eur J Pharmacol 529.1–3 (2006): 24–32.
Spoerke D, Rouse J. Quercetin: alternative medicine summary. Micromedex, 2004.www.micromedex.com (accessed 04-02-06).
Staedler D et al. Drug combinations with quercetin: doxorubicin plus quercetin in human breast cancer cells. Cancer Chemother Pharmacol. 68. 5 (2011):1161–72.
Stewart LK et al. Quercetin transiently increases energy expenditure but persistently decreases circulating markers of inflammation in C57BL/6J mice fed a high-fat diet. Metabolism 57.7 (Suppl 1) (2008): S39–S46.
Taepongsorat L et al. Stimulating effects of quercetin on sperm quality and reproductive organs in adult male rats. Asian J Androl 10.2 (2008): 249–258.
Talirevic E, Jelena S. Quercetin in the treatment of dyslipidemia. Med Arh 66.2 (2012): 87–88.
Tan W-F et al. Quercetin, a dietary-derived flavonoid, possesses antiangiogenic potential. Eur J Pharmacol 459.2–3 (2003): 255–262.
Thangasamy T et al. Quercetin selectively inhibits bioreduction and enhances apoptosis in melanoma cells that overexpress tyrosinase. Nutr Cancer 59.2 (2007): 258–268.
Tribolo S et al. Comparative effects of quercetin and its predominant human metabolites on adhesion molecule expression in activated human vascular endothelial cells. Atherosclerosis 197.1 (2008): 50–56.
Umathe SN et al. Quercetin pretreatment increases the bioavailability of pioglitazone in rats: involvement of CYP3A inhibition. Biochem Pharmacol 75.8 (2008): 1670–1676.
Vaclavikova R et al. The effect of flavonoid derivatives on doxorubicin transport and metabolism. Bioorg Med Chem 16.4 (2008): 2034–2042.
Valensi P et al. A multicenter, double-blind, safety study of QR-333 for the treatment of symptomatic diabetic peripheral neuropathy: a preliminary report. J Diabetes Complications 19.5 (2005): 247–253.
van der Woude H et al. The stimulation of cell proliferation by quercetin is mediated by the estrogen receptor. Mol Nutr Food Res 49.8 (2005): 763–771.
Vanhees et al. Maternal quercetin intake during pregnancy results in an adapted iron homeostasis at adulthood. Toxicology. 290.2–3 (2011):350–8.
van Zanden JJ et al. The effect of quercetin phase II metabolism on its MRP1 and MRP2 inhibiting potential. Biochem Pharmacol 74.2 (2007): 345–351.
Wang K et al. Quercetin induces protective autophagy in gastric cancer cells: involvement of Akt-mTOR- and hypoxia-induced factor 1α-mediated signaling. Autophagy. 7.9 (2011): 966–78
Wang P, et al. Quercetin increased the antiproliferative activity of green tea polyphenol (-)-epigallocatechin gallate in prostatecancer cells. Nutr Cancer. 64.4 (2012):580–7.
Wattel A et al. Potent inhibitory effect of naturally occurring flavonoids quercetin and kaempferol on in vitro osteoclastic bone resorption. Biochem Pharmacol 65.1 (2003): 35–42.
Weng Z et al. Quercetin is more effective than cromolyn in blocking human mast cell cytokine release and inhibits contact dermatitis and photosensitivity in humans. PLoS ONE.7.3 (2012); e33805
Wilms LC et al. Protection by quercetin and quercetin-rich fruit juice against induction of oxidative DNA damage and formation of BPDE-DNA adducts in human lymphocytes. Mutat Res 582.1–2 (2005): 155–162.
Yao P et al. Quercetin protects human hepatocytes from ethanol-derived oxidative stress by inducing heme oxygenase-1 via the MAPK/Nrf2 pathways. J Hepatol 47.2 (2007): 253–261.
Yu ES et al. Regulatory mechanisms of IL-2 and IFNgamma suppression by quercetin in T helper cells. Biochem Pharmacol 76.1 (2008): 70–78.
Yuan H, et al. Overexpression of c-Jun induced by quercetin and resverol inhibits the expression and function of the androgen receptor in human prostate cancer cells. Cancer Lett 213.2 (2004): 155–163.
Zhang F, et al. Effect of quercetin on proliferation and apoptosis of human nasopharyngeal carcinoma HEN1 cells. J Huazhong Univ Sci Technolog Med Sci 28.3 (2008): 369–372.
Zhang M et al. Antioxidant properties of quercetin.Adv Exp Med Biol. 701 (2011):283–9.

Raspberry leaf

HISTORICAL NOTE Although the fruits of the raspberry are used as a luxury food source and in dietary drinks, midwives have used raspberry leaves since ancient times to prepare the uterus for childbirth. Raspberry has also been used as an antidiarrhoeal agent and an astringent to treat inflammations of the mucous membranes of the mouth and throat.

COMMON NAME

Red raspberry

OTHER NAMES

Framboise, *Rubi idaei folium*, rubus

BOTANICAL NAME/FAMILY

Rubus idaeus (synonym: *Rubus strigosus*) (family Rosaceae [roses])

PLANT PART USED

Leaf

CHEMICAL COMPONENTS

Raspberry leaves have a tannin content of between 13% and 15%, as well as phenolic compounds like the flavonoids rutin and quercetin, volatile oils, organic acids and vitamin C.

MAIN ACTIONS

Raspberry leaf contains a number of active constituents and their therapeutic actions have been reviewed (Patel et al 2004). Currently, evidence of activity comes from in vitro and in vivo studies.

Uterine effects

Raspberry leaf has demonstrated a variable effect on uterine muscle tone, as it contains a smooth-muscle stimulant, an anticholinesterase and an antispasmodic. The results of animal studies indicate that raspberry can either reduce or initiate uterine contractions (Bamford et al 1970). It appears to inhibit uterine contractions in samples from pregnant test animals, but has no effect in non-pregnant ones. Samples from human pregnant uteri respond with contraction effects; however, no effect was seen on non-pregnant uteri samples. Overall, it appeared that raspberry leaf extract promoted more regular contractions that generally became less frequent (Newell et al 1996). A more recent preliminary study produced similar results with fractions of raspberry leaf extract, both stimulating and relaxing uterine muscle in pregnant rats (Briggs & Briggs 1997). There is evidence of at least two components of raspberry leaf extract that exhibit relaxant activity in an in vitro guinea pig ileum preparation (Rojas-Vera et al 2002). Results imply a regulatory action on contractions.

Antidiarrhoeal

In addition to the high tannin content of the leaves which may exert an antidiarrhoeal action, raspberry cordial and juice, made from the fruits, were found to significantly reduce the growth of several species of gut bacteria, including *Salmonella*, *Shigella* and *Escherichia coli*. However, no antimicrobial activity was detected in the leaf extract or tea (Ryan et al 2001).

Anti-inflammatory

Raspberry leaf exhibits anti-inflammatory activity because of its high tannin content, which has been found to inhibit cyclooxygenase (Duke 2003). When applied topically to mucous membranes, tannins have a local anti-inflammatory effect, produce capillary vasoconstriction and decrease vascular permeability (Halvorsen et al 2001).

Astringent

The high tannin content of the leaf is responsible for the astringent activity.

Antioxidant

The polyphenols in raspberry leaf demonstrate cytotoxic effects through antioxidant action in in vitro studies (Durgo et al 2012).

OTHER ACTIONS

The phenolic content of raspberry leaves may provide antioxidant protection against oxidative stress that can induce neuronal damage. Raspberry ketone, which is an aromatic compound with similar structure to capsaicin and synephrine, has been shown in vivo to prevent and improve obesity and fatty liver though increasing noradrenaline-induced lipolysis in white adipocytes (Morimoto et al 2005).

CLINICAL USE

The therapeutic effects of raspberry have not been significantly investigated under clinical trial conditions, so most evidence is derived from traditional, in vitro and animal studies.

Uterine tonic

Raspberry leaf is commonly used as a 'partus preparator' to prepare the uterus for delivery and to facilitate labour, as well as for treating morning sickness, dysmenorrhoea, leucorrhoea and menorrhagia (McFarlin et al 1999). A study of 588 pregnant women of 36–38 weeks' gestation who were attending a public tertiary maternity hospital in Melbourne, Australia were surveyed to measure the prevalence of herbal medicine use in pregnancy. Thirty-six per cent of women took at least one herbal supplement during the current pregnancy, their most common supplement being raspberry leaf (14%).

In vitro studies using pregnant rat and human uteri preparations suggest that raspberry may increase the regularity and decrease the frequency of uterine contractions (Bamford et al 1970), although a recent trial suggests that this varies depending on the herbal preparation used and pregnancy status (Jing et al 2010). In a double-blind trial of 192 low-risk nulliparous women, raspberry leaf (2 × 1.2 g/day), consumed from 32 weeks' gestation until labour, was associated with a lower rate of interventions with no adverse effects for mother or baby (Simpson et al 2001). Raspberry leaf did not shorten the first stage of labour; however, it did significantly reduce the second stage. A retrospective, observational study of 108 mothers also found that treatment with raspberry leaf was associated with a lower rate of medical intervention (Parsons et al 1999). This study further suggested that treatment may shorten labour, and reduce the incidence of pre- and post-term labour. Some pregnant women commenced use of raspberry leaf from 8 weeks' gestation; however, most chose to start it between 30 and 34 weeks' gestation.

A more recent finding from a survey of 600 Norwegian women after delivery in a regional hospital found 5.7% had taken raspberry leaf during their pregnancy. A significant association was found between the use of raspberry leaf and caesarean delivery (23.5% vs 9.1% among women with no use of herbal medicines). The authors conclude that this finding should be explored further where information about the reason for caesarean section and the amount, timing and duration of raspberry leaf intake are included (Nordeng et al 2011).

Topical inflammatory conditions

The high tannin content of raspberry supports its traditional use as a topical treatment for inflammation of the mouth, throat, eye and skin, as well as to treat cuts and wounds.

Diarrhoea

Once again, the high tannin content of raspberry supports its traditional use as an antidiarrhoeal agent.

Dyspeptic complaints

Traditionally understood to act as a choleretic, raspberry leaf is used to improve digestion and detoxifying processes, but controlled studies are not available to determine its effectiveness.

OTHER USES

Raspberry leaf is commonly recommended for nausea and vomiting in pregnancy, but this advice is based more on anecdotal evidence than rigorous scientific evidence, highlighting a need for more research in this area.

Cold infusions of raspberry leaf have been used to treat diarrhoea, loose bowels and stomach complaints in children. Raspberry leaf has traditionally been incorporated into mouthwashes to treat inflammation of the mouth and throat, used as a diaphoretic for fever, as a choleretic to improve digestion and detoxification, and as a food and flavouring agent.

In a small, uncontrolled, prospective pilot study of eight women, raspberry leaf in combination with 11 other botanical extracts was found to relieve menopausal symptoms (Smolinski et al 2005).

Practice points/Patient counselling

- Raspberry leaves have been traditionally used to prepare the uterus for childbirth, with some modern research suggesting that they may be useful.
- When used in this way, raspberry leaf is often combined with other herbs and used during the last 6–8 weeks of pregnancy under close supervision.
- Raspberry leaves are high in tannins, which may make them useful as a mouthwash and to treat diarrhoea, although this has not been confirmed in clinical trials.
- As tannins may reduce the absorption of other substances, it is recommended to take raspberry leaf preparations separately from other medications. Raspberry leaf preparations can be considered safe and non-toxic.

DOSAGE RANGE

Internal use

- Infusion of dried leaf: 4–8 g taken up to three times daily.
- Liquid extract: (1 : 1): 4–8 mL three times daily.

External use

- Topically, the tea can be used as a mouth or eye wash, or to clean wounds.

TOXICITY

There is no evidence that raspberry leaf tea is toxic.

ADVERSE REACTIONS

Owing to the tannin content of the herb, it may cause gastrointestinal discomfort.

SIGNIFICANT INTERACTIONS

Iron, calcium, magnesium

Due to its high tannin content, raspberry leaf may decrease absorption of iron, calcium and magnesium, as well as some drugs. As such, it is advised to separate the administration of these substances by at least 2 hours.

CONTRAINDICATIONS AND PRECAUTIONS

The high tannin concentration within the herb means it should be avoided in constipation and used cautiously in active peptic ulcer and gastrointestinal conditions associated with inflammation.

PREGNANCY USE

A systematic review of raspberry leaf and safety or efficacy during pregnancy, pharmacology and in vitro tests explaining mode of action or constituents looked at 12 original publications, some of which were 50 years old or older. Six of the studies were in vitro or animal experiments, five were clinical trials or other human studies and one proposed possible pharmacological actions. All the studies were small and only the latest animal study (Johnson et al 2009) indicated any potential for increased risk (Holst et al 2009). There is no evidence of harmful effects on the fetus, despite consumption by a large number of women. Clinical studies suggest that it is safe to use after the first trimester, although it is prudent to ensure close professional supervision.

PATIENTS' FAQs

What will this herb do for me?
Raspberry leaf preparations have been used since ancient times to prepare the uterus for birth in an attempt to facilitate a complication-free labour. It is also used to treat diarrhoea and dyspeptic complaints, and incorporated into a mouthwash to reduce inflammation of the mouth and throat.

When will it start to work?
Currently, there is insufficient research to answer this question. However, it is used in increasing doses during the last few weeks of pregnancy. Symptomatic relief of diarrhoea and inflammation of the oral cavity is likely to occur within the first few doses.

Are there any safety issues?
Considering that raspberry leaf has uterine activity, it is recommended that pregnant women wanting to use it do so under the careful supervision of an experienced healthcare professional.

REFERENCES

Bamford DS, et al. Raspberry leaf tea: a new aspect to an old problem. Br J Pharmacol 40.1 (1970): 161–162.

Briggs CJ, Briggs K. Raspberry. Can Pharm J 130.3 (1997): 41–43.

Duke JA. Dr Duke's phytochemical and ethnobotanical databases. Beltsville, MD: US Department of Agriculture–Agricultural Research Service–National Germplasm Resources Laboratory, Beltsville Agricultural Research Center, 2003. Available online: www.ars-grin.gov/duke.

Durgo, K., et al. (2012). The Bioactive Potential of Red Raspberry (*Rubus idaeus* L.) Leaves in Exhibiting Cytotoxic and Cytoprotective Activity on Human Laryngeal Carcinoma and Colon Adenocarcinoma. Journal of Medicinal Food, 15(3), 258–268.

Halvorsen BL et al. A systematic screening of total antioxidants in dietary plants. J Nutr 142.3 (2001): 461–471.

Holst, L., et al. (2009). Raspberry leaf — Should it be recommended to pregnant women? Complementary Therapies in Clinical Practice, 15(4), 204–208.

Jing, Z., et al. (2010). The effects of commercial preparations of red raspberry leaf on the contractility of the rat's uterus in vitro. Reproductive Sciences, 17(5), 494–501.

Johnson, J., et al. (2009). Effect of maternal raspberry leaf consumption in rats on pregnancy outcome and the fertility of the female offspring. Reprod Sci, 16(6), 605–609.

McFarlin BL et al. A national survey of herbal preparation use by nurse-midwives for labor stimulation: review of the literature and recommendations for practice. J Nurse Midwifery 44.3 (1999): 205–216.

Morimoto C et al. Anti-obese action of raspberry ketone. Life Sci 77.2 (2005): 194–204.

Newell CA, et al. Herbal medicines: a guide for health care professionals. London, UK: The Pharmaceutical Press, 1996.

Nordeng, H., et al. (2011). Use of herbal drugs during pregnancy among 600 Norwegian women in relation to concurrent use of conventional drugs and pregnancy outcome. Complementary Therapies in Clinical Practice, 17(3), 147–151.

Parsons M, et al. Raspberry leaf and its effect on labour: safety and efficacy. Aust Coll Midwives Inc J 12.3 (1999): 20–25.

Patel AV, et al. Therapeutic constituents and actions of *Rubus* species. Curr Med Chem 11.11 (2004): 1501–1512.

Rojas-Vera J, et al. Relaxant activity of raspberry (*Rubus idaeus*) leaf extract in guinea-pig ileum in vitro. Phytother Res 16.7 (2002): 665–668.

Ryan T, et al. Antibacterial activity of raspberry cordial in vitro. Res Vet Sci 71.3 (2001): 155–159.

Simpson M et al. Raspberry leaf in pregnancy: its safety and efficacy in labor. J Midwifery Womens Health 46.2 (2001): 51–59.

Smolinski D et al. A pilot study to examine a combination botanical for the treatment of menopausal symptoms. J Altern Complement Med 11.3 (2005): 483–489.

Red clover

HISTORICAL NOTE Red clover has been used for a long time as an animal fodder as well as a human medicine. Traditionally, it is considered as an alternative remedy with blood-cleansing properties useful in the treatment of skin diseases such as psoriasis, eczema and rashes. A strong infusion was used to ease whooping cough and other spasmodic coughs due to measles, bronchitis and laryngitis. It was recommended for 'ulcers of every kind, and deep, ragged-edged, and otherwise badly conditioned burns. It possesses a peculiar soothing property, proves an efficient detergent, and promotes a healthful granulation'. Combined with other herbs, red clover was recommended for syphilis, scrofula, chronic rheumatism, glandular and various skin afflictions (Felter & Lloyd 1983). Interestingly, red clover was not traditionally used for the treatment of menopausal symptoms.

OTHER NAMES

Cow clover, meadow clover, purple clover, trefoil

BOTANICAL NAME/FAMILY

Trifolium pratense L. (family Fabaceae)

PLANT PARTS USED

Flower head or leaf

CHEMICAL COMPONENTS

Flower head

Flavanoids, including formononetin; flavonols, including isorhamnetin and quercetin glucosides; phenolic acids, including salicylic and *p*-coumaric acids; volatile oils and other constituents, including sitosterol, starch, fatty acids (British Herbal Medicine Association Scientific Committee 1983).

Leaf

Isoflavones, including biochanin A, daidzein, formononetin and genistein; caffeic acid derivatives; and coumestrol (trace) (Clifton-Bligh et al 2001, He et al 1996).

In the plant, the isoflavones are attached to a sugar molecule, usually glucose. The chemical term for any compound attached to a sugar is glycoside. The free isoflavone form is known as an aglycone. The active aglycone is liberated in the gut. Isoflavones are readily absorbed from the gut; they circulate freely in the blood and are excreted in the urine; 50% of ingested isoflavones are eliminated within 12 hours (Joannou et al 1995).

The aglycone forms of the four main oestrogenic isoflavones are genistein, daidzein, biochanin and formononetin.

Bioavailability

The isoflavone content of the marketed red clover products is highly variable and this has been shown to significantly affect the metabolism of red clover isoflavones by altering their absorption and excretion rates (S Wang et al 2008). New research testing the bioavailability of three isoflavones from a commercial red clover dietary supplement (MenoStabil) found a relatively high bioavailability of irilone, compared to the main isoflavone metabolites expected in plasma, daidzein and genistein, even after a single dose (Maul & Kulling 2010).

MAIN ACTIONS

Oestrogenic activity

The pharmacological investigation of red clover has mainly centred around the activity of the isoflavone constituents, especially their oestrogenic activity (Miksicek 1994). Red clover products contain primarily formononetin and biochanin A. The isoflavones have varying levels of subtle oestrogenic activity, with biochanin A having the strongest effect. Red clover isoflavones have been shown to have an affinity for oestrogen alpha- and beta-receptors and may act as both agonists and antagonists, depending on the level of endogenous oestrogens (Nelson et al 2006, Yatkin & Diaglioglu 2011, Zava et al 1998). The isoflavones in red clover (and soy extracts) act as selective oestrogen receptor modulators as well as selective oestrogen enzyme modulators. The higher affinity of isoflavones to oestrogen beta-receptors compared to oestrogen alpha-receptors has been used to explain why red clover extracts treat menopausal disorders, reduce risk of breast cancer and have protective effects on osteoporosis and the cardiovascular system (Beck et al 2005). Animal studies show that red clover extract, standardised to contain 15% isoflavones, produced a dose-dependent increase in uterine weight and differentiated vaginal cells, but did not stimulate cell proliferation in mammary glands in an ovariectomised rat model. The extract did not produce any antioestrogenic or additive oestrogenic effects when combined with 17-beta-oestradiol (Burdette et al 2002). Another animal study showed that formononetin had antioxidant and oestrogenic effects and, further, the oestrogenic effect was not dosage-related (Mu et al 2009). Supplementing isoflavones, either daidzein (at 100 mg/kg) or red clover extract (at 6.68 mg/kg), in menopausal rabbits also showed significant improvements in bone density, tissue integrity and vaginal blood flow, with minimal effect on uterine weight (Adaikan et al 2009). Animal studies have also demonstrated that red clover stimulates oestrogen receptors in the endometrium without increasing cell proliferation (Alves et al 2008).

Antioxidant activity

The isoflavones in red clover display antioxidant activity at concentrations well within the range found in the plasma of subjects consuming soy products, even though they undergo extensive metabolism in the intestine and the liver (Rufer & Kulling 2006).

Opioid activity

A new understanding of a potential mechanism of action for red clover has been identified which involves interaction with opiate receptors. Red clover extract has high binding affinity for the mu-opiate receptor and also affinity at the delta-opiate receptor. Given the essential role of the opioid system in regulating temperature, mood and hormonal levels, this newly identified activity provides further rationale for its investigation as a treatment for relieving menopausal symptoms (Nissan et al 2007).

> ***Clinical note — Phyto-oestrogens and isoflavones***
> Phyto-oestrogens are plant-based compounds that are structurally similar to oestradiol. The term phyto-oestrogen encompasses isoflavone compounds, such as genistein and daidzein, found predominantly in soy and red clover, and the lignans, such as matairesinol and secoisolariciresinol, found in many fruits, cereals and in linseed. Phyto-oestrogens have been investigated for their potential to reduce the risk of hormone-dependent diseases such as breast and prostate cancers and osteoporosis. The metabolism of isoflavones and lignans is complex and involves gut microbial processes. Isoflavones are present predominantly as glucosides; however, their bioavailability requires initial hydrolysis of the sugar moiety by intestinal beta-glucosidases. After absorption, phyto-oestrogens are reconjugated predominantly to glucuronic acid and, to a lesser degree, to sulfuric acid. There is further metabolism of isoflavones (to equol and *O*-desmethylangolensin) and lignans (to enterodiol and enterolactone) by gut bacteria. In humans, even those on controlled diets, there is large inter-individual variation in the metabolism of isoflavones and lignans, particularly in the production of the gut bacterial metabolite equol (from daidzein). Dietary factors and gut microflora directly influence the absorption and metabolism of phyto-oestrogens and are likely to influence the clinical benefits of supplementation with phyto-oestrogens (Rowland et al 2003).

Reducing cancer risk

As red clover has various antiangiogenic active compounds with different modes of action, it may be useful as a chemoprotective agent against carcinogenesis; however, the evidence is still not definitive (Adlercreutz et al 1995, Clarke et al 1996, Ingram et al 1997, Pagliaaci et al 1994). Biochanin A isolated from red clover has been shown to be antimutagenic, as well as protective against chemically induced DNA damage in vitro (Chan et al 2003, Kole et al 2011) and inhibitory on melanogenesis in vitro and in vivo (Lin et al 2011). Genistein has been shown to inhibit cell proliferation and in vitro angiogenesis (Fotsis et al 1995) and the antiangiogenic effect of genistein and daidzein has been confirmed in an in vivo study using hen's eggs (Krenn & Paper 2009). Formononetin has been found in breast cancer cell models, both in vitro and in vivo, to cause cell cycle arrest by inactivating some insulin-like growth factor pathways and decreasing protein expression, indicating its potential use in the prevention of breast cancer carcinogenesis (Chen et al 2011).

An animal study has found that red clover isoflavones significantly increase oestrogen beta-receptor and E-cadherin expression, but decrease transforming growth factor beta-1. These proteins are markers of oestrogen-induced proliferation, preservation of cell phenotype and reduction of the potential for neoplastic and metastatic transformation. These results suggest that red clover isoflavones may be useful in the treatment of prostatic hyperplasia and reduce the risk of neoplastic transformation (Slater et al 2002). A study has reported that red clover-derived isoflavones significantly reduced non-malignant prostatic growth in mice by acting as antiandrogenic agents rather than weak oestrogenic substances (Jarred et al 2003). The metabolites of the red clover isoflavone, biochanin, are thought to contribute to its chemopreventive effects.

Biochanin A, daidzein and genistein have demonstrated antiproliferative activity in vitro (Hempstock et al 1998). In an in vitro study, red clover isoflavones were tested for their potential in transactivating aryl hydrocarbon receptor (AhR), which is known to affect the cell cycle and drive cells to apoptosis. Selective AhR modulators have previously been implicated in cancer therapy and prevention, particularly for hormone-dependent cancers. It was found that the isoflavones biochanin A and formononetin were potent AhR agonists in vitro — 10 times more potent compared to the indole compounds (Medjakovic & Jungbauer 2008). Red clover isoflavones (50 mg total isoflavones), however, were found not to be antiproliferative in a double-blind, randomised study of 30 perimenopausal women (Hale et al 2001).

CLINICAL USE

Considerable research has been carried out on the constituents of red clover; however, very few investigations have concentrated specifically on the flower heads and the traditional uses.

Relief of menopausal symptoms

Numerous clinical studies have been conducted using red clover extracts or isoflavones, which are found in red clover in varying concentrations. Many isoflavone studies do not report whether these constituents were derived from red clover or other sources, making interpretation of the data difficult. Additionally, inferences about red clover based on soy isoflavone studies may not be valid because the two substances differ in their balance of individual isoflavones.

Red clover extract studies

The general consensus from systematic reviews and meta-analyses is that there is a lack of evidence to support the use of monopreparations containing *Trifolium pratense* isoflavones as a means of significantly reducing hot-flush frequency, severity or other menopausal symptoms (Booth et al 2006, Cheema et al 2007, Coon et al 2007, Low Dog 2005, Nelson et al 2006). A Cochrane review also supported this conclusion (Lethaby et al 2007).

The most recent meta-analysis evaluated data from five randomised clinical trials of monopreparations containing *T. pratense* isoflavones (40–82 mg daily) and concluded that active treatment resulted in a marginally significant effect, reducing frequency of hot flushes in menopausal women, although the size of this effect may not be considered clinically relevant (Coon et al 2007). In 2007, Lethaby et al also reported in their systematic review that, of the five trials with data suitable for pooling that assessed daily frequency of hot flushes, there was no significant difference overall in the frequency of hot flushes between Promensil (a red clover extract) and placebo. Furthermore, a systematic review by Low Dog (2005) stated that the largest study showed minimal to no effect in reducing menopausal symptoms.

Three recent placebo-controlled studies again demonstrated that red clover had no significant effect in reducing menopausal symptoms. In each of these studies improvements in vasomotor symptoms were observed from baseline in both red clover and placebo groups; however, there were no significant differences between groups. In a randomised, triple-blind, placebo-controlled clinical trial, 55 menopausal women were randomly allocated to receive either placebo or 45 mg of red clover isoflavones for 8 weeks. Before the treatment and at the end of the study, a menopause-specific quality of life questionnaire was completed in both groups; however, the differences between two groups were not significant for total quality of life, nor for its domains (Ehsanpour et al 2012). A prospective, randomised, double-blind, placebo-controlled study in which 120 postmenopausal women received either 40 mg red clover or placebo over a 12-month trial period did not show significant improvement in menopausal symptoms or sexual satisfaction in women in the red clover group compared with placebo (del Giorno et al 2010).

A four-arm, randomised, double-blind clinical trial of standardised black cohosh, red clover, placebo and oestrogen/progesterone found that neither black cohosh nor red clover reduced the number of vasomotor symptoms compared with placebo, but that both herbal extracts were safe during daily administration for 12 months (Geller et al 2009). In a discussion paper about this study it was suggested that particular aspects of methodology may have led to these negative results, such as a large proportion of non-Caucasian participants (perhaps women with genomic differences from those women historically included in menopausal studies), long trial period and rigorous authentication of the herbal preparations could have led to marked differences in clinical outcomes from earlier trials. The authors of this discussion paper conclude that, because of these factors, further studies could be of value to determine if there are specific populations that may find such interventions of clinical value. They suggest, for example, that studies with different primary and secondary clinical outcomes, or studies determining if earlier trials used herbal products that may have contained different active compounds, may result in clinical outcomes different from those reported (Shulman et al 2011).

In a study to test whether phyto-oestrogens had any impact on cognition in menopausal women, 66 women with 35 or more weekly hot flushes were enrolled in a randomised, double-blind, placebo-controlled study and received red clover (120 mg) or black cohosh (128 mg) or 0.625 mg conjugated equine oestrogens plus 2.5 mg medroxyprogesterone acetate or placebo. Participants completed measures of verbal memory (primary outcome) and other cognitive measures (secondary outcomes) before and during 12 months of treatment. Neither of the herbal treatments was found to have an impact on any cognitive measures (Maki et al 2009).

Isoflavone studies

Several reviews have evaluated the clinical evidence relating to isoflavone treatment in the relief of menopausal hot flushes, finding conflicting and ambiguous results. Some of this confusion may arise from the fact that a variety of isoflavone sources have been tested, often without discriminating between the identities of individual isoflavones or the different concentrations contained in the tested intervention product. As such, volunteers may be receiving greatly different doses or ranges of specific isoflavones from the different test products, but researchers have not taken this into account when evaluating and comparing results.

A review by Williamson-Hughes et al (2006) highlights this issue and the importance of clearly defining the chemical composition of isoflavone treatments in research reports. The authors evaluated results from 11 studies that tested similar total isoflavone doses. Five of the 11 studies (n = 177) reported a statistically significant decrease in hot-flush symptoms. Later evaluation revealed that the test products used in these studies provided more than 15 mg genistein (calculated as aglycone equivalents) per treatment. Of the remaining six studies (n = 201), five failed to find a significant decrease in hot-flush symptoms. Participants in these studies received less than 15 mg genistein per treatment. Thus, the reduction in hot flushes was related to genistein content and not total isoflavone content of the treatments.

To demonstrate this point, a 12-month, prospective, randomised, double-blind, placebo-controlled study showed that the phyto-oestrogen genistein (54 mg/day) from red clover reduced the number and severity of hot flushes in postmenopausal women, with no adverse effect on the endometrium (D'Anna et al 2007). Similarly, another prospective randomised, double-blind, placebo-controlled trial (n = 109) demonstrated that 40 mg mixed aglyconic isoflavones from red clover produced superior results over placebo in the treatment of vasomotor and menopausal symptoms, with a concomitant decrease in depression and anxiety symptoms (Lipovac et al 2012).

Red clover-derived isoflavones have been shown to be effective in reducing depressive and anxiety symptoms among postmenopausal women. A randomised placebo control study evaluated the effect of isoflavones derived from red clover extracts (MF11RCE) on anxiety and depressive symptoms in 109 postmenopausal women. Participants were given 80 mg red clover isoflavones or placebo for a 90-day period; then, after a washout period of 7 days, medication was crossed over and taken for 90 days more. Anxiety and depressive symptoms were measured at baseline, 90 and 187 days with the Hospital Anxiety and Depression Scale and Zung's Self-rating Depression Scale. After adjustment for the placebo response the red clover isoflavone extract was shown to cause a significant decrease on both scales by an average 21.7% in comparison to baseline (Lipovac et al 2010).

IN COMBINATION

A nutritional supplement containing isoflavones from kudzu and red clover, along with other targeted nutrients, produced a 46% decrease in hot-flush frequency, and quality of life, as assessed by the standardised Greene Questionnaire, showed similar improvement in a small pilot study of 25 menopausal women suffering from severe hot flushes and night sweats (Lukaczer et al 2005). A modest improvement in the ratio of total cholesterol to high-density lipoprotein (HDL) cholesterol was also observed and a statistical improvement in a proposed marker of breast cancer risk (the ratio of 2-hydroxyestrone to 16 alpha-hydroxyestrone) was also demonstrated. While promising, the role of red clover in achieving these results remains unknown.

Other potential benefits in menopause

A randomised controlled trial using a standardised extract of red clover found that red clover exerts a moderate effect on testosterone levels in postmenopausal women, while oestradiol levels remained unchanged (Imhof et al 2006). The significance of this finding for clinical practice remains unknown.

There is some evidence from animal studies that oestrogen deprivation reduces the pain threshold and administration of phyto-oestrogens may reverse this. A methanol extract of isoflavones from red clover was administered orally (500 mg/kg of body weight) to ovariectomised and normal (controls) rats for 90 and 180 days. The pain threshold levels in ovariectomised rats treated with isoflavones extract were found to be similar to those of the control animals (Vishali et al 2011).

Cardiovascular effects

Lipid lowering

The isoflavones in red clover regulate genes involved in lipid metabolism and antioxidation (Pakalapati et al 2009). Red clover isoflavones have anti-inflammatory effects and activate peroxisome proliferator-activated receptor-alpha, which leads to an improved blood lipid profile (Mueller et al 2010).

A 2006 systematic review of randomised controlled trials, which included peri- and postmenopausal women, concluded that red clover extracts reduce levels of triglycerides and increase HDL cholesterol (Geller & Studee 2006). A randomised, placebo-controlled, crossover study of 60 postmenopausal women found that red clover isoflavones (80 mg/day) significantly decreased total cholesterol, low-density lipoprotein (LDL) cholesterol and lipoprotein A levels in women with body mass index (BMI) > 25 kg/m^2, but not women with lower BMI (Chedraui et al 2008).

In a prospective open randomised controlled clinical trial, 40 healthy postmenopausal women were given one capsule daily of either placebo or 40 mg of red clover-derived isoflavones (containing 23 mg biokain A, 1 mg diadzein, 15 mg formononetin and 1 mg genistein). All participants had total blood cholesterol, LDL and HDL cholesterol and triglycerides tested at baseline and at 4-month intervals over the following 12 months. Total serum cholesterol, LDL cholesterol and triglyceride levels significantly decreased and HDL cholesterol levels significantly increased in the group receiving phyto-oestrogens (Terzic et al 2009).

Despite these positive results, a 2013 Cochrane review found no evidence of cholesterol-lowering effects of isoflavones (red clover- or soy-derived) in people with hypercholesterolaemia. Five randomised trials (n = 208) with interventions ranging from 3 to 6 months were analysed. There was a slight significant effect of isoflavones on triglycerides compared with placebo, but no statistically significant effects on total cholesterol, LDLs or HDLs. None of the trials found serious adverse events. The authors suggest their results be interpreted cautiously due to the low number of participants in the trials (Qin et al 2013).

Blood pressure

Clinical studies have not consistently shown red clover isoflavones to significantly reduce blood pressure (Atkinson et al 2004b, Teede et al 2003); however, there is evidence that red clover isoflavones reduce arterial stiffness and total vascular resistance (Fugh-Berman & Kronenberg 2001, Nestel et al 1999, Teede et al 2003). A reduction in blood pressure and improved endothelial function were reported for red clover isoflavones (approximately 50 mg/day) in a small randomised, double-blind, crossover trial (n = 16) involving postmenopausal women with type 2 diabetes (Howes et al 2003).

Given the lack of serious safety concerns, red clover supplementation might be beneficial for postmenopausal women to reduce cardiovascular risk.

Antiatherogenic

In vitro studies on cultured human endothelial cells have shown that phyto-oestrogens contained in red clover extracts act as anti-inflammatory and antiatherogenic agents by reducing the expression of the leucocyte adhesion molecules (Simoncini et al 2008).

Reducing cancer risk

Much of the research in this area has focused on isoflavones generally derived from soy products rather than red clover sources. As such, it is uncertain whether the results from these studies can be extrapolated to red clover extracts. For more information about the association between soy isoflavones and cancer risk, refer to the soy monograph.

Prostate cancer

In vitro models have confirmed that transforming growth factor 1 (TGF-1) increases dehydroepiandrosterone metabolism to androgens and prostate-specific antigen (PSA) in prostate tissue. Red clover isoflavones inhibit TGF-induced androgenicity and are therefore protective of prostate tissue (Liu et al 2011). Investigation of the mechanism involved in the apoptosis effect of formononetin on human prostate cancer cells found it inactivated the extracellular signal-regulated kinase1/2 (ERK1/2) mitogen-activated protein kinase (MAPK) signalling pathway in a dose-dependent manner (Ye et al 2012). These studies suggest that further research on the use of red clover isoflavones in the prevention and treatment of prostate cancer is warranted.

A non-randomised, non-blinded trial of 38 men with clinically significant prostate cancer found that 160 mg/day red clover-derived dietary isoflavones, containing a mixture of genistein, daidzein, formononetin and biochanin A, significantly increased apoptosis compared with matched controls (P = 0.0018). There were no significant differences between pre- and posttreatment serum levels of PSA, testosterone or biochemical factors or Gleason score in the treated patients ($P > 0.05$). The study was performed in men undergoing radical prostatectomy; however, it indicates that the isoflavones may halt the progression of prostate cancer by inducing apoptosis in low-to-moderate-grade tumours (Gleason grade 1–3) (Jarred et al 2002).

Breast cancer

An antioestrogenic effect on breast tissue is particularly important in women at high risk, or with a history, of breast cancer. A 2010 systematic review and meta-analysis assessing the effects of isoflavone-rich foods or supplements on mammographic density, a biomarker of breast cancer risk, looked at eight randomised controlled trials (n = 1287 women) comparing isoflavones with placebo for between 6 months and 3 years. The meta-analysis suggested no overall effect of dietary isoflavones on breast density in all women combined or postmenopausal women; however, there was a modest increase in mammographic density in premenopausal women. The authors concluded that isoflavone intake does not alter breast density in postmenopausal women, but may cause a small increase in breast density in premenopausal women and that larger, long-term trials are required to determine if these small effects are clinically relevant (Hooper et al 2010).

Overexposure of oestrogen is a major contributing factor in the development of breast cancer, and cytochrome P450 (CYP) 19 enzyme, or aromatase, catalyses the reaction converting androgen to oestrogen. Biochanin A, isolated from red clover, has been shown to inhibit CYP19 activity and gene expression (Y Wang et al 2008). In vitro studies have shown that genistein slightly increases breast cancer cell migration and invasion, but in the presence of oestradiol its effect is antioestrogenic (Mannella et al 2012). In another in vitro study, isoflavones were added to 11 human cancer cell lines and one human fibroblast cell line, and their effects on cell proliferation, apoptosis induction and cell cycle were measured. It was found that high isoflavone concentrations did not promote the growth of these human cancer cells in vitro. Furthermore, oestrogen receptor-positive MCF-7 breast cancer cells grown under pre- and postmenopausal conditions showed decreased rather than increased cell proliferation (Reiter et al 2011). Another in vitro study found that formononetin inhibits the proliferation of oestrogen receptor-positive, but not oestrogen receptor-negative, breast cancer cells (Chen & Sun 2012).

A large prospective study (the HEAL study: n = 1183) conducted surveys of women with breast cancer within 12 months of diagnosis and again at 30 and 40 months after diagnosis, in particular seeking information about quality of life and levels of fatigue. At 30 months after diagnosis, 39.5% of women were using phyto-oestrogenic supplements, but only 38 women were taking supplements of red clover. In this small sample only three symptoms — weight gain, night sweats, and difficulty concentrating — were less common than in women not consuming any phyto-oestrogens (Ma et al 2011).

A 2006 systematic review of complementary and alternative therapeutic approaches, including the use of red clover, in patients with early breast cancer drew the conclusion that available data on complementary and alternative medicine modalities in the treatment of early-stage breast cancer did not support their application (Gerber et al 2006). However more recent in vitro research on isoflavones from red clover suggests that further investigation for their use in treating oestrogen receptor-positive breast cancer may be warranted.

Benign prostatic hypertrophy

Isoflavone-containing food and supplements are widely used in patients with benign prostatic hypertrophy (BPH). An in vivo study using mice showed that red clover-derived isoflavones have a significant effect on prostatic growth, and are capable of reducing the tendency to enlarged non-malignant prostate, by acting as antiandrogenic agents rather than weak oestrogenic substances (Jarred et al 2003). An ex vivo study investigating the effect on contractility of rat prostatic smooth muscle concluded that, as well as having antiproliferative effects, red clover isoflavones cause inhibition of prostatic smooth-muscle contractions; however, such high concentrations were required that this may be of limited clinical use (Brandli et al 2010).

A case series (n = 29) presented at the Endocrine Society's 82nd Annual Meeting in 2000 suggested that 3 months of treatment with one or two tablets of Trinovin (standardised to 40 mg red clover isoflavones per tablet) significantly decreased nocturia frequency, the International Prostate Symptom Score, increased urinary flow rates and quality-of-life score. PSA values and prostate size did not alter from baseline (Ulbricht & Basch 2005). A small clinical trial involving 20 men aged over 65 years with elevated PSA levels and negative prostate biopsy findings showed that oral administration of a red clover isoflavone extract (60 mg/day) significantly decreased total PSA levels by >30%. During the 1-year treatment period, active treatment was well tolerated and caused no side effects, and significantly increased liver transaminases (an indication of improved liver function) were observed (Engelhardt & Riedl 2008).

Osteoporosis prevention

Pharmaceutical hormone replacement therapy (HRT) is sometimes used to prevent loss of bone following menopause; however, a growing number of users are concerned about the increased risk of breast cancer associated with long-term HRT. As such, phyto-oestrogens have been used as an alternative to prevent osteoporosis. Most research has focused on soy isoflavones, although there is some evidence that red clover-derived isoflavones may also be of benefit.

Animal studies have demonstrated that red clover isoflavones are effective in reducing bone loss, probably by reducing bone turnover via inhibition of bone resorption (Kawakita et al 2009, Occhiuto et al 2007). However, human studies show variable results. In a trial by Atkinson et al (2004a), loss of lumbar spine bone mineral content and bone mineral density was significantly reduced in women taking red clover-derived isoflavones (43.5 mg/day) compared to placebo in a double-blind, placebo-controlled, randomised trial in 205 women over 12 months. Bone formation markers were also significantly increased; however, no improvement in hip bone mineral content or bone mineral density was noted. A double-blind study of 46 postmenopausal women investigated the effects of a red clover isoflavone preparation (Rimostil) containing genistein, daidzein, formononetin and biochanin A after a single-blind placebo phase and followed by a single-blind washout phase. Patients were randomly assigned to receive 28.5 mg, 57 mg or 85.5 mg phyto-oestrogens daily for a 6-month period. After the test period, the bone mineral density of the proximal radius and ulna rose significantly — by 4.1% with a dose of 57 mg/day and by 3.0% with a dose of 85.5 mg/day isoflavones. The response with 28.5 mg/day isoflavones was not significant (Clifton-Bligh et al 2001).

No significant difference in bone turnover markers was apparent after 12 weeks of treatment with Promensil and Rimostil in a double-blind, placebo-controlled, randomised clinical trial in 252 menopausal women aged between 45 and 60 years (Schult et al 2004).

OTHER USES

Several human and animal studies have attributed hypolipidaemic, hypoglycaemic or antiatherosclerotic effects to red clover extract or isoflavones. A recent in vivo study, however, showed that red clover extract, biochanin A and formononetin had no hypoglycaemic effect in diabetic mice (Qiu et al 2012). A recent small randomised controlled trial ($n = 43$) compared the effects of transdermal oestrogen with Promensil (40 mg or 80 mg/day) on plasma glucose, insulin sensitivity, plasma testosterone, oestradiol and sex hormone-binding globulin (SHBG) over a 12-week period. In contrast to prior studies on red clover-based phyto-oestrogens, this study found that red clover was associated with a significant decrease in insulin sensitivity, but had no effect on SHBG, oestradiol or testosterone levels in healthy non-diabetic postmenopausal women (Lee et al 2012).

In vitro research suggests that red clover isoflavones have a protective effect on dopaminergic neurons through inhibition of the generation of proinflammatory factors (Chen et al 2008) and exert a neuroprotective effect in human cortical neurons, possibly due to antioxidant and oestrogenic actions (Occhiuto et al 2008, 2009).

An animal study to investigate the effects of red clover isoflavones on skin ageing, the histology of the skin, skin thickness and the amount of total collagen, with a red clover extract standardised to contain 11% isoflavones, concluded that red clover isoflavones are effective in reducing skin ageing induced by oestrogen deprivation (Circosta et al 2006). A combination of red clover isoflavones from various *Trifolium* species, including *T. pratense*, demonstrated wound-healing properties in animal models (Renda et al 2013).

TRADITIONAL USES

Red clover flower heads are traditionally used for indications not related to the potential hormonal activity of the herb. The alterative or blood-cleansing action is used in skin eruptions and as part of treatment for cancer. A poultice of red clover flowers can be used to soothe local inflammations such as acne, burns or ulcers.

The British Herbal Pharmacopoeia lists red clover as a dermatological agent, mild antispasmodic and expectorant (British Herbal Medicine Association Scientific Committee 1983). The specific indications are for eczema and psoriasis. Red clover is said to combine well with yellow dock for the treatment of chronic skin disease.

DOSAGE RANGE

- 4 g as infusion or extract.
- Liquid extract (1 : 1) in 25% alcohol: 1.5–3.0 mL/day.
- Concentrated isoflavone extract containing 40–80 mg total isoflavones is recommended, based on the daily intake of phyto-oestrogens in a traditional Japanese diet.

Note: The isoflavone content of the marketed red clover products is highly variable and this alone may significantly affect absorption rates.

According to clinical reports

- Menopausal symptoms: 40–82 mg daily of red clover-derived isoflavones.
- Lipid lowering: 40–86 mg daily of red clover-derived isoflavones.
- Osteoporosis prevention: 44–86 mg daily of red clover-derived isoflavones.
- BPH symptom relief: 40–80 mg daily of red clover-derived isoflavones.

Practice points/Patient counselling

- Red clover flower heads are traditionally considered a dermatological agent, mild antispasmodic and expectorant and specifically used for eczema and psoriasis. In practice, red clover is often combined with yellow dock for the treatment of chronic skin disease.
- In recent years, red clover isoflavones have been studied and shown to have an affinity for oestrogen alpha- and beta-receptors and may act as both agonists and antagonists, depending on the level of endogenous oestrogens.
- Evidence that red clover-derived isoflavones reduce hot-flush frequency in menopause is unconvincing.
- Preliminary evidence suggests a possible preventive role in osteoporosis; however, further research is required.
- Concentrated isoflavone extracts from red clover are used in cardiovascular disease as there is weak evidence that it may reduce arterial stiffness, increase HDL cholesterol and decrease triglycerides.
- Evidence from animal studies and case series suggests a potential role in BPH, but further research is required.
- There is weak evidence that red clover isoflavone extracts may reduce the risk of hormone-sensitive cancers and that they may be beneficial in the treatment of prostate cancer.

ADVERSE REACTIONS

The oestrogenic potency of the isoflavones has been well documented. Overgrazing cattle or sheep on red clover can be detrimental to their fertility. In 'clover disease', ewes are made permanently infertile by clover consumption. In animals with clover disease, the uterine response to oestrogen is reduced, as is the surge in luteinising hormone. Clover disease has not been observed with normal therapeutic doses in humans. None of the trials has reported adverse effects. An isoflavone preparation from soy bean, and red clover extracts containing genistein, daidzein, biochanin A and formononetin, did not modify the endometrial architecture in 25 postmenopausal women taking the preparation for 1 year (Aguilar et al 2002).

SIGNIFICANT INTERACTIONS

Controlled studies are not available; therefore, interactions are based on evidence of activity and are largely theoretical and speculative.

Anticoagulant agents

The byproduct, dicoumarol (produced by microorganisms in poorly dried sweet clover), has established anticoagulant effects. Therefore, only red clover extracts made from poorly dried raw materials may pose an interaction risk. Observe patients taking red clover and anticoagulants concurrently.

Oestrogens

Theoretically, if taken in large quantities, phyto-oestrogens may compete with synthetic oestrogens for receptor binding, but the clinical significance of this remains unknown. One review concluded that up to 2 mg of red clover-derived isoflavones per kg should be considered a safe dose for most patient groups (Barnes 2003).

CONTRAINDICATIONS AND PRECAUTIONS

There are no known contraindications for the flower head extracts. Concentrated isoflavone extracts should only be used by people with oestrogen-sensitive cancers under professional supervision because of the possible proliferative effects. Additionally, people with conditions that may be aggravated by increased oestrogen levels, such as endometriosis or uterine fibroids, should use this herb under professional supervision only. Importantly, no randomised controlled trials have addressed the long-term safety of phyto-oestrogens in patients after a diagnosis of breast cancer (Boekhout et al 2006).

Red clover isoflavones are well tolerated in healthy women, according to a 3-year study of 400 women. Supplements containing red clover isoflavones did not adversely affect breast density, skeletal strength or cardiovascular status. In postmenopausal women, endometrial status was not adversely affected. The adverse event profile was similar between red clover isoflavones and placebo and endocrine status did not differ (Powles et al 2008).

There are some concerns whether isoflavones exert oestrogen-like effects in men by lowering bioavailable testosterone. A recent meta-analysis evaluated the effects of soy protein or isoflavones from red clover on testosterone, SHBG, free testosterone and free androgen index in men. Fifteen placebo-controlled trials and 32 reports were assessed and no significant effects were detected (Hamilton-Reeves et al 2010).

PREGNANCY USE

Scientific evidence for the use of red clover during pregnancy has not been established, so safety is unknown.

PATIENTS' FAQs

What will this herb do for me?
Red clover is traditionally used for skin disorders. In recent years, concentrated red clover isoflavone extracts have been promoted for use in the treatment of menopausal symptoms, although clinical studies are inconsistent and generally unsupportive.

When will it start to work?
Red clover tea or extract for skin diseases requires long-term use. Improvement may occur within several weeks, with the condition continuing to improve with long-term use. Improvement in menopausal symptoms from the use of concentrated isoflavone extracts may take 2–3 months, although results are inconsistent.

Are there any safety issues?
Short- or long-term use of red clover tea or flower head extract is not thought to be associated with any adverse reactions and its use is considered safe. Concentrated red clover isoflavone extracts may have subtle oestrogenic activity and little is known about drug interactions or long-term use. As a result, they should not be used by people with oestrogen-sensitive tumours or conditions that may be aggravated by increased oestrogen levels, such as endometriosis, unless under professional supervision. People with breast cancer should only use red clover extracts under professional supervision.

REFERENCES

Adaikan PG, et al. Efficacy of red clover isoflavones in the menopausal rabbit model. Fertil Steril (2009): 92: 2008–2013.

Adlercreutz H et al. Soybean phytoestrogen intake and cancer risk. J Nutr 125 (Suppl 3) (1995): 757–770.

Aguilar JG et al. Histeroscopic prospective study of the action of isoflavones on the endometrium. Acta Ginecologica 59.7 (2002): 217–220.

Alves, D., et al. (2008). Effects of *Trifolium pratense* and *Cimicifuga racemosa*on the endometrium of wistar rats. Maturitas, 61(3), 364–370.

Atkinson C et al. Red-clover-derived isoflavones and mammographic breast density: a double-blind, randomized, placebo-controlled trial [ISRCTN42940165]. Breast Cancer Res 6.3 (2004a): R170–9.

Atkinson C et al. Modest protective effects of isoflavones from a red clover-derived dietary supplement on cardiovascular disease risk factors in perimenopausal women, and evidence of an interaction with

ApoE genotype in 49-65-year-old women. J Nutr 134.7 (2004b): 1759–64.

Barnes S. Phyto-oestrogens and osteoporosis: what is a safe dose? Br J Nutr 89 (Suppl 1) (2003): S101–S108.

Beck V, et al. Phytoestrogens derived from red clover: an alternative to estrogen replacement therapy? J Steroid Biochem Mol Biol 94.5 (2005): 499–518.

Boekhout AH, et al. Symptoms and treatment in cancer therapy-induced early menopause. Oncologist 11.6 (2006): 641–654.

Booth NL et al. Clinical studies of red clover (*Trifolium pratense*) dietary supplements in menopause: a literature review. Menopause 13.2 (2006): 251–264.

Brandli, A., et al. (2010). Isoflavones isolated from red clover (*Trifolium pratense*) inhibit smooth muscle contraction of the isolated rat prostate gland. Phytomedicine, 17(11), 895–901.

British Herbal Medicine Association Scientific Committee. British herbal pharmacopoeia. Lane House. Cowling, UK: BHMA, 1983.

Burdette JE et al. *Trifolium pratense* (red clover) exhibits estrogenic effects in vivo in ovariectomized Sprague-Dawley rats. J Nutr 132.1 (2002): 27–30.

Chan HY, et al. The red clover (*Trifolium pratense*) isoflavone biochanin A modulates the biotransformation pathways of 7,12-dimethylbenz[a] anthracene. Br J Nutr 90.1 (2003): 87–92.

Chedraui P et al. Effect of *Trifolium pratense*-derived isoflavones on the lipid profile of postmenopausal women with increased body mass index. Gynecol Endocrinol 24.11 (2008): 620–624.

Cheema D, et al. Non-hormonal therapy of post-menopausal vasomotor symptoms: a structured evidence-based review. Arch Gynecol Obstet 276.5 (2007): 463–469.

Chen, J., & Sun, L. (2012). Formononetin-induced apoptosis by activation of Ras/p38 mitogen-activated protein kinase in estrogen receptor-positive human breast cancer cells. Hormone & Metabolic Research, 44(13), 943–948.

Chen, H.-Q., et al. (2008). Protective effect of isoflavones from *Trifolium pratense* on dopaminergic neurons. Neuroscience Research, 62(2), 123–130.

Chen, J., et al. (2011). Formononetin induces cell cycle arrest of human breast cancer cells via IGF1/PI3K/Akt pathways in vitro and in vivo. Horm Metab Res 43(10), 681–686.

Circosta C et al. Effects of isoflavones from red clover (*Trifolium pratense*) on skin changes induced by ovariectomy in rats. Phytother Res 20.12 (2006): 1096–1099.

Clarke R et al. Estrogens, phytoestrogens and breast cancer. Adv Exp Med Biol 401 (1996): 63–85.

Clifton-Bligh PB et al. The effect of isoflavones extracted from red clover (Rimostil) on lipid and bone metabolism. Menopause 8.4 (2001): 259–265.

Coon JT, et al. *Trifolium pratense* isoflavones in the treatment of menopausal hot flushes: a systematic review and meta-analysis. Phytomedicine 14.2–3 (2007): 153–159.

D'Anna RCM et al. Effects of the phytoestrogen genistein on hot flushes, endometrium, and vaginal epithelium in postmenopausal women: a 1-year randomized, double-blind, placebo-controlled study. Menopause 14.4 (2007): 648–655.

del Giorno, C., et al. (2010). Effects of *Trifolium pratense* on the climacteric and sexual symptoms in postmenopause women. Rev Assoc Med Bras, 56(5), 558–562.

Ehsanpour, S., et al. (2012). The effects of red clover on quality of life in post-menopausal women. Iran J Nurs Midwifery Res., 17(1), 34–40.

Engelhardt PF, Riedl CR. Effects of one-year treatment with isoflavone extract from red clover on prostate, liver function, sexual function, and quality of life in men with elevated PSA levels and negative prostate biopsy findings. Urology 71.2 (2008): 185–190; discussion 190.

Felter HW, Lloyd JU. King's American dispensatory, 18th edn. Portland: Eclectic Medical Publications, 1983.

Fotsis T, et al. Genistein, a dietary ingested isoflavonoid, inhibits cell proliferation and in vitro angiogenesis. J Nutr 125 (1995): 790–797.

Fugh-Berman A, Kronenberg F. Red clover (*Trifolium pratense*) for menopausal women: current state of knowledge. Menopause 8.5 (2001): 333–337.

Geller SE, Studee L. Soy and red clover for mid-life and aging. Climacteric 9.4 (2006): 245–263.

Geller, S., et al. (2009). Safety and efficacy of black cohosh and red clover for the management of vasomotor symptoms: a randomized controlled trial. Menopause, 16(6), 1156–1166.

Gerber B et al. Complementary and alternative therapeutic approaches in patients with early breast cancer: a systematic review. Breast Cancer Res Treat 95.3 (2006): 199–209.

Hale GE et al. A double-blind randomized study on the effects of red clover isoflavones on the endometrium. Menopause 8.5 (2001): 338–346.

Hamilton-Reeves, J., et al. (2010). Clinical studies show no effects of soy protein or isoflavones on reproductive hormones in men: results of a meta-analysis. Fertility & Sterility, 94(3), 997–1007.

He X, et al. Analysis of flavonoids from red clover by liquid chromatography-electrospray mass spectrometry. J Chromatogr A 755.1 (1996): 127–132.

Hempstock JP, et al. Growth inhibition of prostate cell lines in vitro by phyto-oestrogens. Br J Urol 82.4 (1998): 560–563.

Hooper, L., et al. (2010). Effects of isoflavones on breast density in pre- and post-menopausal women: a systematic review and meta-analysis of randomized controlled trials. Human Reproduction Update, 16(6), 745–760.

Howes JB et al. Effects of dietary supplementation with isoflavones from red clover on ambulatory blood pressure and endothelial function in postmenopausal type 2 diabetes. Diabetes Obes Metab 5.5 (2003): 325–332.

Imhof M et al. Effects of a red clover extract (MF11RCE) on endometrium and sex hormones in postmenopausal women. Maturitas 55.1 (2006): 76–81.

Ingram D et al. Case control study of phyto-oestrogens and breast cancer. Lancet 350.9083 (1997): 990–994.

Jarred RA et al. Induction of apoptosis in low to moderate-grade human prostate carcinoma by red clover-derived dietary isoflavones. Cancer Epidemiol Biomarkers Prev 11.12 (2002): 1689–1696.

Jarred RA et al. Anti-androgenic action by red clover-derived dietary isoflavones reduces non-malignant prostate enlargement in aromatase knockout (ArKo) mice. Prostate 56.1 (2003): 54–64.

Joannou GE et al. A urinary profile study of dietary phytoestrogens: the identification and mode of metabolism of new isoflavonoids. J Steroid Biochem Mol Biol 54.3–4 (1995): 167–184.

Kawakita, S., et al. (2009). Effect of an isoflavones-containing red clover preparation and alkaline supplementation on bone metabolism in ovariectomized rats. Clinical Interventions In Aging, 4, 91–100.

Kole, L., et al. (2011). Biochanin-A, an isoflavon, showed anti-proliferative and anti-inflammatory activities through the inhibition of iNOS expression, p38-MAPK and ATF-2 phosphorylation and blocking NFκB nuclear translocation. European Journal of Pharmacology, 653(1–3), 8–15.

Krenn, L., & Paper, D. (2009). Inhibition of angiogenesis and inflammation by an extract of red clover (*Trifolium pratense* L.). Phytomedicine, 16, 1083–1088.

Lee, C., et al. (2012). Effect of oral phytoestrogen on androgenicity and insulin sensitivity in postmenopausal women. Diabetes, Obesity and Metabolism, 14, 315–319.

Lethaby AE et al. Phytoestrogens for vasomotor menopausal symptoms. Cochrane Database Syst Rev 4 (2007): CD001395.

Lin, V., et al. (2011). In vitro and in vivo melanogenesis inhibition by biochanin A from *Trifolium pratense*. Bioscience, Biotechnology & Biochemistry, 75(5), 914–918.

Lipovac, M., et al. (2010). Improvement of postmenopausal depressive and anxiety symptoms after treatment with isoflavones derived from red clover extracts. Maturitas, 65(3), 258–261.

Lipovac, M., et al. (2012). The effect of red clover isoflavone supplementation over vasomotor and menopausal symptoms in postmenopausal women. Gynecological Endocrinol, 28(3), 203–207.

Liu, X., et al. (2011). Transforming growth factor 1 increase of hydroxysteroid dehydrogenase proteins is partly suppressed by red clover isoflavones in human primary prostate cancer-derived stromal cells. Carcinogenesis, 32(11), 1648–1654.

Low Dog T. Menopause: a review of botanical dietary supplements. Am J Med 118 (Suppl 12B) (2005): 98–108.

Lukaczer D et al. Clinical effects of a proprietary combination isoflavone nutritional supplement in menopausal women: a pilot trial. Altern Ther Health Med 11.5 (2005): 60–65.

Ma, H., et al. (2011). Estrogenic botanical supplements, health-related quality of life, fatigue, and hormone-related symptoms in breast cancer survivors: a HEAL study report. BMC Complementary and Alternative Medicine, 11, 109.

Maki, P., et al. (2009). Effects of botanicals and combined hormone therapy on cognition in postmenopausal women. Menopause, 16(6), 1167–1177.

Mannella, P., et al. (2012). Effects of red clover extracts on breast cancer cell migration and invasion. Gynecological Endocrinology, 28(1), 29–33.

Maul, R., & Kulling, S. (2010). Absorption of red clover isoflavones in human subjects: results from a pilot study. British Journal of Nutrition, 103(11), 1569–1572.

Medjakovic S, Jungbauer A. Red clover isoflavones biochanin A and formononetin are potent ligands of the human aryl hydrocarbon receptor. J Steroid Biochem Mol Biol 108.1–2 (2008): 171–177.

Miksicek RJ. Interaction of naturally occurring nonsteroidal estrogens with expressed recombinant human estrogen receptor. J Steroid Biochem Mol Biol 49.2–3 (1994): 153–160.

Mu, H., et al. (2009). Research on antioxidant effects and estrogenic effect of formononetin from *Trifolium pratense* (red clover). Phytomedicine, 16(4), 314–319.

R

Mueller, M., et al. (2010). Red clover extract: a source for substances that activate peroxisome proliferator-activated receptor alpha and ameliorate the cytokine secretion profile of lipopolysaccharide-stimulated macrophages. Menopause, 17(2), 379–387.
Nelson HD et al. Nonhormonal therapies for menopausal hot flashes: systematic review and meta-analysis. JAMA 295.17 (2006): 2057–2071.
Nestel PJ et al. Isoflavones from red clover improve systemic arterial compliance but not plasma lipids in menopausal women. J Clin Endocrinol Metab 84.3 (1999): 895–898.
Nissan HP et al. A red clover (*Trifolium pratense*) phase II clinical extract possesses opiate activity. J Ethnopharmacol 112.1 (2007): 207–210.
Occhiuto F et al. Effects of phytoestrogenic isoflavones from red clover (*Trifolium pratense* L.) on experimental osteoporosis. Phytother Res 21.2 (2007): 130–134.
Occhiuto F et al. The phytoestrogenic isoflavones from *Trifolium pratense* L. (Red clover) protects human cortical neurons from glutamate toxicity. Phytomedicine 15.9 (2008): 676–682.
Occhiuto F et al. The isoflavones mixture from *Trifolium pratense* L. protects HCN 1-A neurons from oxidative stress. Phytother Res 23.2 (2009): 192–196.
Pagliaaci MC, et al. Growth inhibitory effects of the natural phyto-oestrogen genistein in MCF-7 human breast cancer cells. Eur J Cancer 30A.11 (1994): 1675–1682.
Pakalapati, G., et al. (2009). Influence of red clover (*Trifolium pratense*) isoflavones on gene and protein expression profiles in liver of ovariectomized rats. Phytomedicine, 16, 845–855.
Powles TJ et al. Red clover isoflavones are safe and well tolerated in women with a family history of breast cancer. Menopause Int 14.1 (2008): 6–12.
Qin, Y., et al. (2013). Isoflavones for hypercholesterolaemia in adults. Cochrane Metabolic and Endocrine Disorders Group. Cochrane Library doi: 10.1002/14651858.CD009518.pub2.
Qiu, L., et al. (2012). Red clover extract ameliorates dyslipidemia in streptozotocin-induced diabetic C57BL/6 mice by activating hepatic PPAR. Phytotherapy Research, 26(6), 860–864.
Reiter, E., et al. (2011). Red clover and soy isoflavones — an in vitro safety assessment. Gynecological Endocrinology, 27(12), 1037–1042.
Renda, G., et al. (2013). Comparative assessment of dermal wound healing potentials of various Trifolium L. extracts and determination of their isoflavone contents as potential active ingredients. J Ethnopharmacol 148: 423–432.
Rowland I et al. Bioavailability of phyto-oestrogens. Br J Nutr 89 (Suppl 1) (2003): S45–S58.
Rufer CE, Kulling SE. Antioxidant activity of isoflavones and their major metabolites using different in vitro assays. J Agric Food Chem 54.8 (2006): 2926–2931.
Schult TM et al. Effect of isoflavones on lipids and bone turnover markers in menopausal women. Maturitas 48.3 (2004): 209–218.
Shulman, L., et al. (2011). Discussion of a well-designed clinical trial which did not demonstrate effectiveness: UIC center for botanical dietary supplements research study of black cohosh and red clover. Fitoterapia, 82(1), 88–91.
Simoncini, T., et al. (2008). Effects of phytoestrogens derived from red clover on atherogenic adhesion molecules in human endothelial cells. Menopause, 15(3), 542–550.
Slater M, et al. In the prostatic epithelium, dietary isoflavones from red clover significantly increase estrogen receptor beta and E-cadherin expression but decrease transforming growth factor beta1. Prostate Cancer Prostatic Dis 5.1 (2002): 16–21.
Teede HJ et al. Isoflavones reduce arterial stiffness: a placebo-controlled study in men and postmenopausal women. Arterioscler Thromb Vasc Biol 23.6 (2003): 1066–1071.
Terzic, M., et al. (2009). Influence of red clover-derived isoflavones on serum lipid profile in postmenopausal women. Journal of Obstetrics & Gynaecology Research, 35(6), 1091–1095.
Ulbricht CE, Basch EM. Natural standard herb and supplement reference. St Louis: Mosby, 2005.
Vishali, N., et al. (2011). Red clover *Trifolium pratense* (Linn.) isoflavones extract on the pain threshold of normal and ovariectomized rats — a long-term study. Phytotherapy Research, 25(1), 53–58.
Wang, S., et al. (2008). Variable isoflavone content of red clover products affects intestinal disposition of biochanin A, formononetin, genistein, and daidzein. Journal of Alternative & Complementary Medicine, 14(3), 287–297.
Wang, Y., et al. (2008). The red clover (*Trifolium pratense*) isoflavone biochanin A inhibits aromatase activity and expression. British Journal of Nutrition, 99(2), 303–310.
Williamson-Hughes PSF et al. Isoflavone supplements containing predominantly genistein reduce hot flash symptoms: a critical review of published studies. Menopause 13.5 (2006): 831–839.
Yatkin, E., & Diaglioglu, C. (2011). Evaluation of the estrogenic effects of dietary perinatal *Trifolium pratense*. Journal of Veterinary Science, 12(2), 121–126.
Ye, Y., et al. (2012). Formononetin-induced apoptosis of human prostate cancer cells through ERK1/2 mitogen-activated protein kinase inactivation. Hormone & Metabolic Research, 44(4), 263–267.
Zava DT, et al. Estrogen and progestin bioactivity of foods, herbs, and spices. Proc Soc Exp Biol Med 217.3 (1998): 369–378.

Red yeast rice

HISTORICAL NOTE Red yeast rice (RYR), also known as red Koji or 'Hongqu', is a dietary staple in many Asian countries, including China and Japan, and has been used as a food, medicine and seasoning for more than a thousand years. Li Shizhen, the great pharmacologist of the Ming Dynasty (1368–1644), reported that 'Hongqu' promotes 'digestion and blood circulation, and can strengthen the spleen and dry the stomach' (Ma et al 2000). RYR, which is produced by fermenting steamed, non-glutinous rice with *Monascus* species of food fungus, is widely used in making pickled tofu, for brewing rice wine and as a preservative for meat and fish, thereby giving many dishes such as Peking duck their characteristic red colour. In recent years, several commercial versions of RYR have been made available and it has been included by the Chinese Ministry of Health into food additive standards to increase the colour and delicacy of meat, fish and soybean products.

In 1979, Professor Akira Endo, working in Japan on fungicides, found that *Monascus purpureus* on rice contained a compound that he called 'monacolin K', which was identified as a new hypocholesterolaemic agent that specifically inhibits HMG-CoA reductase (Endo 1980). It is now known as lovastatin. This discovery led to the development of a new class of lipid-lowering drugs, called statins.

Due to concerns about the quality and safety of RYR, it is no longer a listable ingredient for use in over-the-counter products in Australia (www.tga.gov.au/archive/committees-cmec-resolutions-34.htm).

COMMON NAME

Red yeast rice (RYR)

OTHER NAMES

Chinese red yeast rice, red Koji, Hongqu, Hon-Chi, Beni-koji. Zhi Tai is the dried, powdered form, while Xuezhikang is a standardised ethanolic extract.

BOTANICAL NAME/FAMILY

RYR is produced by fermenting cooked rice with various *Monascus* species, most commonly *M. pilous* and *M. purpureus*.

CHEMICAL COMPONENTS

RYR is a food and medicine with a range of potentially active and synergistic constituents whose amounts vary widely depending on preparation.

While it is assumed that the main active constituents are the monacolins, particularly monacolin K or lovastatin, there are a number of other potentially active constituents, including 13 kinds of natural statins, anti-inflammatory pigments ankaflavin and monascin; amino acids, gamma-aminobutyric acid, unsaturated fatty acids, plant sterols, isoflavones and isoflavone glycosides, tannins, alkaloids and other phytochemicals and trace elements that may act synergistically to produce clinical effects (Feng et al 2012, Lee & Pan 2012).

Quality concerns

The monacolin content of traditionally produced RYR has been found to vary widely (Huang et al 2006, Li et al 2004). This may be due to variations in *Monascus* species or growing and storage conditions, as monacolin levels are influenced by exposure to light and heat (Li et al 2005). RYR, as both a food and supplement, may also contain a toxic fermentation by-product, citrinin, a mycotoxin. Citrinin is a hepatonephrotoxin, which causes functional and structural damage through alterations in liver and kidney metabolism (Nigovic et al 2013). Levels of citrinin vary based on preparation method (Childress et al 2013).

A 2010 study tested 12 commercially available 600 mg RYR products, with the amount of monacolins ranging from 0.31 to 11.15 mg per capsule (Gordon et al 2010); many failed to contain the anticipated or effective quantities. The study also found four of the 12 products had levels of citrinin many times higher than allowed in Japan and Europe (Gordon et al 2010).

Interestingly, other constituents of RYR have been identified which may be protective against the cytotoxicity of citrinin, such as deferricoprogen, which has strong antiapoptotic properties in human embryonic kidney cells (Hsu et al 2012b). Improved production (Suh et al 2007) and testing methods are being developed which should help standardise the monacolin content and minimise the citrinin content in RYR products in the future (Lee et al 2006, Nigovic et al 2013, Wu et al 2011) and allay quality and safety concerns.

MAIN ACTIONS

RYR has many different actions with potential benefits on human health. As a consequence, Feng et al (2012) suggest that Xuezhikang (a RYR product standardised to 2.5–3.2 mg of monacolin K/capsule) should be considered a natural 'polypill' as it seems to assist in so many areas — in cardiovascular disease, such as improving lipid profile management and inhibiting atherosclerosis, liver protection, anticancer, antidiabetic, neural and kidney protection (Feng et al 2012).

Cholesterol lowering

RYR has significant lipid-lowering activity which is due to multiple mechanisms. One of the most studied is its inhibition of HMG-CoA reductase, which is the rate-limiting enzyme in cholesterol biosynthesis. Inhibition of the enzyme causes a decrease in endogenous cholesterol production, which leads to upregulation of low-density lipoprotein (LDL) receptors, increasing the rate of removal of LDL from plasma. RYR contains natural statin components that inhibit HMG-CoA reductase in a dose-dependent manner and hence reduce cholesterol synthesis in human hepatic cells (Feng et al 2012, Man et al 2002).

RYR has also been found to reduce serum total cholesterol and triglycerides in rabbits and quails with experimental hyperlipidaemia and suppress atherosclerosis induced by atherogenic diets (Li et al 1997, Wei et al 2003). Investigation with an animal model suggests the antiatherogenic effects are superior to the isolated chemical, lovastatin (Wei et al 2003).

As well as reducing cholesterol, RYR may have positive effects on endothelial function by reducing homocysteine-stimulated endothelial adhesiveness, as well as downregulating intracellular reactive oxygen species formation (Lin et al 2008). RYR extract (Xuezhikang) significantly enhanced the proliferation and adhesion capacity of endothelial progenitor cells derived from the peripheral blood of patients with stable coronary artery disease, to the same extent as atorvastatin (Kong et al 2008).

Anti-inflammatory

Studies suggest that, in addition to lowering cholesterol, the statin drugs may have potent vascular anti-inflammatory actions that produce reductions in vascular plaque adherence and migration to sites of inflammation in atherosclerosis. This has led to the suggestion that low-dose statins may be used for long-term treatment of cardiovascular disease in susceptible individuals (Liao 2004).

In a randomised controlled trial (RCT) involving 36 patients with cardiovascular disease, 1200 mg/day of an RYR extract (Xuezhikang) was found to significantly reduce C-reactive protein (CRP) and other inflammatory markers and prolong exercise tolerance and time, in addition to significantly reducing total cholesterol, LDL cholesterol and triglycerides (Li et al 2007). Other studies support

Xuezhikang's CRP-lowering actions (Kao et al 2006, Li et al 2007), as well as the attenuation of additional inflammatory mediators such as tumour necrosis factor-α (TNF-α), interleukin-6 (IL-6) and fibrinogen (Feng et al 2012).

Treatment with Xuezhikang improves preprandial and postprandial endothelial function after 6 weeks of use in patients with coronary heart disease (CHD) (Liu et al 2003, Zhao et al 2004). These findings have led to the suggestion that the inclusion of RYR in Asian diets may contribute to the median CRP level of Asians being only one-tenth that of Westerners (Kao et al 2006).

Hsu et al (2012b) suggest that monascin is one of the key components responsible for the anti-inflammatory mechanism.

Anticancer

In vitro studies indicate that RYR and some of its individual constituents exert anticancer activity. The effect is not simply attributed to the lovastatin content but also to other monacolins, pigments or the combined matrix effects of multiple constituents which may affect intracellular signalling pathways differently from lovastatin (Hong et al 2008a, 2008b) This suggestion is supported by an in vitro study using prostate cancer cells, which found that RYR had a more potent inhibitory action on cell growth compared to isolated lovastatin (Hong et al 2008b).

Hsu et al (2012a) proposed that monascus-fermented metabolites may be developed into a topical application to prevent or cure oral carcinogenesis. This is a novel therapeutic approach focusing on tumour growth attenuation to improve patient survival and quality of life. Their results suggest that functional secondary metabolites of monascus, including monacolin K, citrinin, ankaflavin and monascin, have shown anti-inflammatory, antioxidative and antitumour activities (Hsu & Pan 2012). Additionally, a new derivative, monapurpyridine A, which has been isolated from RYR, shows moderate cytotoxicity against breast cancer cells (MCF-7) in vitro (Hsu et al 2012a).

Osteogenesis

Just as statins demonstrate an ability to stimulate bone formation, similarly, RYR preparations have also been shown to produce strong bone anabolic effects, both in vitro and in vivo (Gutierrez et al 2006, Wong & Rabie 2008). As a result, RYR may provide a dietary intervention to stimulate bone formation and prevent osteoporosis (Mundy 2006). In vitro studies suggest that RYR extract may increase osteogenic effect by stimulating cell proliferation and alkaline phosphatase activity in osteoblastic cells (Cho et al 2010).

Antidiabetic

In vivo research with RYR and its ankaflavin component demonstrate several different mechanisms of action with potential benefits in diabetes.

Oral administration of RYR (Hon-Chi) decreased plasma glucose in a dose-dependent manner and delayed the development of insulin resistance in rats fed a fructose-rich diet. Oral administration of Hon-Chi (150 mg/kg) three times daily improved insulin sensitivity in streptozotocin-induced diabetic rats (Su et al 2007).

RYR attenuated the elevation of plasma glucose induced by an intravenous glucose challenge test in normal rats and reversed hyperphagia in streptozotocin-diabetic rats (Chang et al 2006). Further rat studies suggest that the plasma glucose-lowering action of RYR is due to release of acetylcholine and subsequent stimulation of muscarinic M_3 receptors in pancreatic cells that affect insulin release (Chen & Liu 2006), as well as decreasing hepatic gluconeogenesis to lower plasma glucose in diabetic rats lacking insulin (Chang et al 2006). The ankaflavin component attenuated insulin resistance in high-fat diet-induced mice by increased glucose uptake by adipocytes through peroxisome proliferator-activated receptor-gamma activation of insulin receptors and p-Akt (Hsu et al 2013).

Hepatoprotective

Used in combination with conventional therapies, Xuezhikang can positively affect patients with fatty liver, relieving clinical syndromes and improving liver function (Feng et al 2012), as it can reverse aminotransferase abnormalities and inhibit hepatic expression of TNF-α. The high levels of selenium and flavonoids in Xuezhikang may also be important due to their antioxidant actions (Feng et al 2012). RYR was also effective against obesity-related inflammation, insulin resistance and non-alcoholic fatty liver disease in mice (Fujimoto et al 2012).

CLINICAL USE

RYR and its various preparations are gaining a reputation as a natural polypill due to its wide range of biologically active constituents with multiple mechanisms of action, such as lipid lowering, anti-inflammatory, antioxidant, atherosclerotic prevention and effects on blood glucose regulation and endothelial activity. Recent research in China indicates significant decreases in cardiovascular events and mortality amongst people with established cardiovascular disease, lending weight to this description.

Hyperlipidaemia, reducing coronary events and mortality

RYR preparations induce a significant reduction in serum total cholesterol levels, triglyceride levels and LDL cholesterol levels and an increase in high-density lipoprotein (HDL) cholesterol levels compared to placebo, according to a meta-analysis of 93 RCTs involving 9625 participants. The three RYR preparations tested were Cholestin, Xuezhikang and Zhibituo. These studies found that the lipid modification effects of RYR were comparable to standard statin medications and RYR treatment is generally safe and well tolerated. When compared with non-statin lipid-lowering agents, RYR preparations are superior to nicotinate and fish oils, but equal to or less effective than fenofibrate and gemfibrozil (Liu et al 2006). Three more recent placebo-controlled studies with RYR have shown a significant reduction in total cholesterol by up to 23.7% as well as a significant reduction in LDL cholesterol (Yang & Mousa 2012).

The large China Coronary Secondary Prevention Study (CCSP), a multicentre, placebo-controlled trial involving 4870 Chinese patients with a history of myocardial infarction (MI), found that 4.5 years of supplementation with Xuezhikang 600 mg twice daily (standardised to 2.5–3.2 mg of monacolin K/capsule) significantly reduced total cholesterol (11.3%) and LDL cholesterol (21.2%), respectively, compared with only 2.3% and 2.3% in the placebo group ($P < 0.0001$). Triglyceride levels fell 12.1% with active treatment compared with 3.1% for placebo ($P = 0.0031$) and there was a significant increase in HDL cholesterol by 4.0% compared with baseline ($P = 0.0043$) (Lu et al 2008). A daily dose of Xuezhikang 1200 mg naturally contains 10–13 mg of lovastatin, together with other bioactive natural compounds displaying different mechanisms of action.

All-cause mortality and CHD mortality

A systematic review of 22 RCTs of Xuezhikang in patients with CHD, complicated by dyslipidaemia, concluded that there were significant benefits with regard to all-cause mortality, CHD mortality, MI and revascularisation as compared with placebo. Placebo was based on conventional treatment for CHD. Active treatment with RYR lowered total cholesterol, triglyceride and LDL cholesterol compared with placebo or inositol nicotinate. It raised HDL cholesterol compared to placebo or no intervention and was found to be safe (Shang et al 2012).

Supplementation with Xuezhikang 600 mg twice daily (standardised to 2.5–3.2 mg of monacolin K/capsule) over 4.5 years significantly decreased the recurrence of coronary events and the occurrence of new cardiovascular events and deaths in the CCSP study, involving 4870 Chinese patients with a history of MI (Lu et al 2008). Besides a significant lipid-lowering effect on total cholesterol, triglyceride and LDL cholesterol, this study found a relative risk reduction of 45% and an absolute risk reduction of 4.7% for coronary events, along with a 33% reduction in total mortality in those taking the RYR extract. Interestingly, a marked 45% reduction of cancer-related deaths was also observed in the treatment group (Lu et al 2008). The participants in this study had experienced an acute MI between 28 days and 5 years before entering the study and were aged between 18 and 75 years. Patients maintained a stable diet and lifestyle during the test period and all medical treatments for hypertension or CHD or complications of CHD were continued throughout the study and only lipid-lowering medication was prohibited.

A subgroup analysis of the 1530 elderly (>65 years) hypertensive patients in the CCSP study found that treatment with Xuezhikang significantly decreased the risk of a coronary event by 38.2% ($P = 0.0009$), risk of non-fatal MI by 53.4% ($P = 0.0042$) and risk of death due to CHD by 29.2% ($P = 0.0503$) compared with placebo (Li et al 2009). Furthermore, the risk for all-cause death was 36.3% lower in the active treatment group compared to placebo ($P = 0.0030$). Beyond the effects on CVD, the total events from cancer were 49.2% less with RYR treatment compared to controls ($P = 0.0395$). Interestingly, when these results are compared to studies utilising statin therapy in a Western population, treatment with Xuezhikang produced a greater reduction in mortality from all-cause and coronary events. This RCT compared placebo ($n = 758$) to active treatment ($n = 772$) and found no significant changes to blood pressure with treatment, indicating that other mechanisms were at work. At baseline, the two groups were well matched for age, body mass index, blood lipids, fasting blood glucose and blood pressure, prevalence of smoking or diabetes and use of antihypertensive medications and aspirin. The incidence of adverse effects was comparable between the groups.

Another subgroup analysis of the 591 diabetic patients in the CCSP study found even more dramatic results with a 50.8% reduction for CHD events ($P < 0.001$) and 63.8% reduction in risk of non-fatal MI ($P < 0.05$) (Zhao et al 2007). Additionally, the risk of CHD death reduced by 44.1% ($P < 0.05$) for patients taking RYR compared to the placebo group. The beneficial effect on reducing mortality was observed after the first year of treatment and overall, the risk for all-cause mortality was 44.1% lower in the active treatment group compared to placebo ($P < 0.01$). Once again, the incidence of side effects was comparable between the groups.

R

OTHER USES

It has been suggested that, in addition to reducing cholesterol, it is possible that monacolins could prevent stroke and reduce the development of peripheral vascular disease. This class of molecules has antithrombotic and anti-inflammatory effects, which may offer protection against atherosclerotic plaque growth as well as being used for the treatment of hypertension, osteoporotic fractures, ventricular arrhythmia and immune response (Manzoni & Rollini 2002).

DOSAGE RANGE

RYR is a dietary staple in many Asian countries, with typical consumption ranging from 14 to 55 g/person/day. The average dose of RYR products is 2.4 g/day depending on the product used.

Supplemental forms

Xuezhikang 300 mg capsules, also known as lipascor, is standardised to 2.5–3.2 mg of monacolin K/capsule. Doses range from 600 to 2400 mg per day (Lu et al 2008, Shang et al 2012).

ADVERSE REACTIONS

The American College of Cardiology Task Force on integrating complementary medicine into cardiovascular medicine suggested that RYR should be 'treated as an HMG-CoA reductase inhibitor, with all the possible side effects, drug interactions, and precautions associated with this class of drugs' (Vogel et al 2005). While this approach simplifies the issue, consideration should be made for the fact that RYR contains multiple active components and is not just a natural source of low-dose statin-like compounds. RCTs indicate that it is well tolerated and not associated with serious adverse effects.

A meta-analysis of 77 controlled trials reported that there were no serious adverse events and non-serious adverse effects were limited to dizziness, low appetite, nausea, stomach ache, abdominal distension and diarrhoea, with a small proportion of participants having increased serum blood urea nitrogen and alanine aminotransferase levels (Liu et al 2006). More recently, an RCT of elderly (>65 years) Chinese patients with previous MI and hypertension found that the most common side effects were gastrointestinal discomfort, allergic reactions, myalgias, oedema, psychoneurological symptoms and erectile dysfunction, although the incidence of side effects was comparable to placebo (Li et al 2009). Another RCT of diabetic Chinese patients with previous MI confirmed that the incidence of side effects was similar to placebo. When side effects were reported, they were limited to gastrointestinal disorders, oedema and a case of mental-neurological symptoms (Zhao et al 2007).

A number of cases of statin-like muscle damage have been reported in patients taking RYR (Smith & Olive 2003, Vercelli et al 2006), and animal studies have demonstrated a dose-dependent reduction in coenzyme Q10 (CoQ10) levels with high levels of RYR (Yang et al 2005). Also, in a randomised, double-blind placebo-controlled trial of 62 patients with known statin-associated myalgias, RYR (3600 mg/day, 13 mg monacolins, 6 mg monacolin K for 24 weeks) was better tolerated than statins (Becker et al 2009).

SIGNIFICANT INTERACTIONS

Statin drugs

RYR products contain low doses of natural statins and, as such, a pharmacodynamic interaction is possible with other statin medications with increased lipid-lowering effects — observe.

Cyclosporin and P450 inhibitors

Monacolins are metabolised by the cytochrome P450 system and therefore cyclosporin and other P450 inhibitors have the potential to increase the risk of rhabdomyolysis (Prasad et al 2002). This is a theoretical concern only — clinical significance unclear.

Coenzyme Q10

Similar to statin medications, RYR may reduce endogenous production of CoQ10 — a 3-month trial of CoQ10 supplementation may be worth considering with long-term use of RYR in people complaining of fatigue.

CONTRAINDICATIONS AND PRECAUTIONS

Patients with statin-induced muscle damage should be cautioned if using RYR (Becker et al 2009, Vercelli et al 2006).

PREGNANCY USE

Avoid use during pregnancy. The major ingredient in RYR is monacolin K, which is also known as mevinolin or lovastatin and has statin-like activity. Statins are potential teratogens based on theoretical considerations and, in small case studies, central nervous system and limb defects have been reported in newborns exposed to statins in utero (Childress et al 2013, http://www.drugs.com/npp/red-yeast.html).

Practice points/Patient counselling

- RYR is a complex whole-food substance that has a long traditional use as a food and medicine and is still a common feature of Asian diets.
- RYR has been found to naturally contain monacolins (statins) together with a variety of other bioactive constituents. It has demonstrated beneficial effects on blood lipids, atherosclerosis, blood glucose regulation and endothelial function, free radical scavenging and bone mineral density.
- Meta-analyses confirm that RYR preparations (Cholestin, Xuezhikang and Zhibituo) significantly reduce total and LDL cholesterol and triglycerides and increase HDL cholesterol.
- Significant reductions in coronary events, total mortality and cancer-related deaths have been observed in a large, randomised, placebo-controlled study of elderly Chinese patients with a previous MI, using Xuezhikang long-term.
- There are quality concerns regarding RYR products, with variable amounts of both the active monacolins and potential toxic byproducts and therefore standardisation and quality control of RYR supplements are imperative.
- RYR products should be stored away from heat and light and not used in pregnancy.

PATIENTS' FAQs

What will this supplement do for me?

RYR will effectively lower total cholesterol levels and reduce the risk of atherosclerosis. It may also have beneficial effects for people with diabetes, osteoporosis, inflammatory disease and cancer.

When will it start to work?

Lipid-lowering effects will take 6–8 weeks to become fully established.

Are there any safety issues?

RYR may have rare adverse effects similar to the statin medications, such as unexplained muscle pain and weakness and, depending on the preparation of the supplement and ultimate quality, can lead to kidney damage. In general, it is well tolerated.

REFERENCES

Becker, D. J., et al. 2009. Red yeast rice for dyslipidemia in statin-intolerant patients: a randomized trial. Ann Intern Med, 150, 830–9, W147–9.

Chang JC et al. Plasma glucose-lowering action of Hon-Chi in streptozotocin-induced diabetic rats. Horm Metab Res 38.2 (2006): 76–81.

Chen CC, Liu IM. Release of acetylcholine by Hon-Chi to raise insulin secretion in Wistar rats. Neurosci Lett 404.1–2 (2006): 117–21.

Childress, L., et al. 2013. Review of red yeast rice content and current Food and Drug Administration oversight. J Clin Lipidol, 7, 117–22.

Cho, Y. E., et al. 2010. Red yeast rice stimulates osteoblast proliferation and increases alkaline phosphatase activity in MC3T3-E1 cells. Nutr Res, 30, 501–10.

Endo A. Monacolin K, a new hypocholesterolemic agent that specifically inhibits 3-hydroxy-3-methylglutaryl coenzyme A reductase. J Antibiot (Tokyo) 33.3 (1980): 334–6.

Feng, Y., et al. 2012. Natural polypill Xuezhikang: its clinical benefit and potential multicomponent synergistic mechanisms of action in cardiovascular disease and other chronic conditions. J Altern Complement Med, 18, 318–28.

Fujimoto, M., et al. 2012. Study of the effects of monacolin k and other constituents of red yeast rice on obesity, insulin-resistance, hyperlipidemia, and nonalcoholic steatohepatitis using a mouse model of metabolic syndrome. Evid Based Complement Alternat Med, 2012, 892697.

Gordon, R. Y., et al. 2010. Marked variability of monacolin levels in commercial red yeast rice products: buyer beware! Archives of internal medicine, 170, 1722–7.

Gutierrez GE et al. Red yeast rice stimulates bone formation in rats. Nutr Res 26.3 (2006): 124–9.

Hong MY et al. Anticancer effects of Chinese red yeast rice versus monacolin K alone on colon cancer cells. J Nutr Biochem 19.7 (2008a): 448–58.

Hong MY et al. Chinese red yeast rice versus lovastatin effects on prostate cancer cells with and without androgen receptor overexpression. J Med Food 11.4 (2008b): 657–66.

Hsu, W. H. & Pan, T. M. 2012. *Monascus purpureus*-fermented products and oral cancer: a review. Appl Microbiol Biotechnol, 93, 1831–42.

Hsu, L. C., et al. 2012a. Induction of apoptosis in human breast adenocarcinoma cells MCF-7 by monapurpyridine A, a new azaphilone derivative from *Monascus purpureus* NTU 568. Molecules, 17, 664–73.

Hsu, L. C., et al. 2012b. Protective effect of deferricoprogen isolated from *Monascus purpureus* NTU 568 on citrinin-induced apoptosis in HEK-293 cells. J Agric Food Chem, 60, 7880–5.

Hsu, W. H., et al. 2013. Ankaflavin regulates adipocyte function and attenuates hyperglycemia caused by high-fat diet via PPAR-γ activation. J Functional Foods, 5, 124–132.

Huang HN et al. The quantification of monacolin K in some red yeast rice from Fujian province and the comparison of the other product. Tokyo: Chem Pharm Bull 54.5 (2006): 687–9.

Kao PC, et al. Review: serum C-reactive protein as a marker for wellness assessment. Ann Clin Lab Sci 36.2 (2006): 163–9.

Kong XQ et al. Effects of xuezhikang on proliferation and adhesion capacity of cultured endothelial progenitor cells: an in vitro study. Curr Ther Res Clin Exp 69.3 (2008): 252–9.

Lee, B. H. & Pan, T. M. 2012. Benefit of *Monascus*-fermented products for hypertension prevention: a review. Appl Microbiol Biotechnol, 94, 1151–61.

Lee, C. L., et al. 2006. Synchronous analysis method for detection of citrinin and the lactone and acid forms of monacolin K in red mold rice. Journal of AOAC International, 89, 669–77.

Li C et al. *Monascus purpureus*-fermented rice (red yeast rice): a natural food product that lowers blood cholesterol in animal models of hypercholesterolemia. Nutr Res 18.1 (1997): 71–81.

Li YG et al. Identification and chemical profiling of monacolins in red yeast rice using high-performance liquid chromatography with photodiode array detector and mass spectrometry. J Pharm Biomed Anal 35.5 (2004): 1101–12.

Li YG, et al. A validated stability-indicating HPLC with photodiode array detector (PDA) method for the stress tests of *Monascus purpureus*-fermented rice, red yeast rice. J Pharm Biomed Anal 39.1–2 (2005): 82–90.

Li JJ et al. Xuezhikang, an extract of cholestin, decreases plasma inflammatory markers and endothelin-1, improve exercise-induced ischemia and subjective feelings in patients with cardiac syndrome X. Int J Cardiol 122.1 (2007): 82–4.

Li, J.J., et al. 2009. Beneficial impact of Xuezhikang on cardiovascular events and mortality in elderly hypertensive patients with previous myocardial infarction from the China Coronary Secondary Prevention Study (CCSPS). J Clin. Pharmacol., 49, (8) 947–956.

Liao JK. Statins: potent vascular anti-inflammatory agents. Int J Clin Pract Suppl 58 (Suppl 143) (2004): 41–8.

Lin CP et al. Cholestin (*Monascus purpureus* rice) inhibits homocysteine-induced reactive oxygen species generation, nuclear factor-κB activation, and vascular cell adhesion molecule-1 expression in human aortic endothelial cells. J Biomed Sci 15.2 (2008): 183–96.

Liu L et al. Xuezhikang decreases serum lipoprotein(a) and C-reactive protein concentrations in patients with coronary heart disease. Clin Chem 49.8 (2003): 1347–52.

Liu J et al. Chinese red yeast rice (*Monascus purpureus*) for primary hyperlipidemia: a meta-analysis of randomized controlled trials. Chin Med 1 (2006): 4.

Lu Z et al. Effect of xuezhikang, an extract from red yeast Chinese rice, on coronary events in a Chinese population with previous myocardial infarction. Am J Cardiol 101.12 (2008): 1689–93.

Ma J et al. Constituents of red yeast rice, a traditional Chinese food and medicine. J Agric Food Chem 48.11 (2000): 5220–5.

Man RY et al. Cholestin inhibits cholesterol synthesis and secretion in hepatic cells (HepG2). Mol Cell Biochem 233.1–2 (2002): 153–8.

Manzoni M, Rollini M. Biosynthesis and biotechnological production of statins by filamentous fungi and the application of these to cholesterol-lowering drugs. Appl Microbiol Biotechnol 58 (2002): 555–64.

Mundy GR. Nutritional modulators of bone remodeling during aging. Am J Clin Nutr 83.2 (2006): 427S–30S.

Nigovic, B., et al. 2013. Simultaneous determination of lovastatin and citrinin in red yeast rice supplements by micellar electrokinetic capillary chromatography. Food chemistry, 138, 531–8.

Prasad GV et al. Rhabdomyolysis due to red yeast rice (*Monascus purpureus*) in a renal transplant recipient. Transplantation 74.8 (2002): 1200–1.

Shang, Q., et al. 2012. A systematic review of xuezhikang, an extract from red yeast rice, for coronary heart disease complicated by dyslipidemia. Evid Based Complement Alternat Med, 2012, 636547.

Smith DJ, Olive KE. Chinese red rice-induced myopathy. South Med J 96.12 (2003): 1265–7.

Su CF, et al. Improvement of insulin resistance by Hon-Chi in fructose-rich chow-fed rats. Food Chem 104.1 (2007): 45–52.

Suh, S. H., et al. 2007. Optimization of production of monacolin K from gamma-irradiated *Monascus* mutant by use of response surface methodology. Journal of medicinal food, 10, 408–15.

Vercelli L et al. Chinese red rice depletes muscle coenzyme Q10 and maintains muscle damage after discontinuation of statin treatment. J Am Geriatr Soc 54.4 (2006): 718–20.

Vogel JH et al. Integrating complementary medicine into cardiovascular medicine: a report of the American College of Cardiology Foundation Task Force on clinical expert consensus documents (Writing Committee to develop an expert consensus document on complementary and integrative medicine). J Am Coll Cardiol 46.1 (2005): 184–221.

Wei W et al. Hypolipidemic and anti-atherogenic effects of long-term cholestin (*Monascus purpureus*-fermented rice, red yeast rice) in cholesterol fed rabbits. J Nutr Biochem 14.6 (2003): 314–18.

Wong RWK, Rabie B. Chinese red yeast rice (*Monascus purpureus*-fermented rice) promotes bone formation. Chin Med 3 (2008): 16.

Wu, C. L., et al. 2011. Synchronous high-performance liquid chromatography with a photodiode array detector and mass spectrometry for the determination of citrinin, monascin, ankaflavin, and the lactone and acid forms of monacolin K in red mold rice. Journal of AOAC International, 94, 179–90.

Yang, C. W. & Mousa, S. A. 2012. The effect of red yeast rice (*Monascus purpureus*) in dyslipidemia and other disorders. Complement Ther Med, 20, 466–74.

Yang HT et al. Acute administration of red yeast rice (*Monascus purpureus*) depletes tissue coenzyme Q10 levels in ICR mice. Br J Nutr 93.1 (2005): 131–5.
Zhao SP et al. Xuezhikang, an extract of cholestin, protects endothelial function through antiinflammatory and lipid-lowering mechanisms in patients with coronary heart disease. Circulation 110.8 (2004): 915–20.
Zhao SP et al. Xuezhikang, an extract of cholestin, reduces cardiovascular events in type 2 diabetes patients with coronary heart disease: subgroup analysis of patients with type 2 diabetes from China Coronary Secondary Prevention Study (CCSPS). J Cardiovasc Pharmacol 2 (2007): 81–4.

Rhodiola

HISTORICAL NOTE Rhodiola is a popular herb in the traditional medicine of Eastern Europe, Asia and Scandinavia where it has been used to stimulate the nervous system, enhance physical and mental performance and improve resistance to high-altitude sickness (van Diermen et al 2009). It grows in high-altitude Arctic regions of Europe and Asia (Goel et al 2006) and is reported to have been used by the Vikings to enhance physical strength and endurance (Darbinyan et al 2007). It is also mentioned by Dioscorides as early as the 1st century AD. Rhodiola has been categorised as an 'adaptogen' in traditional systems due to its ability to increase resistance to a variety of chemical, biological and physical stressors, and is noted for its antidepressant, anticancer and cardioprotective properties (Kelly 2001). It has a reputation for improving depression, enhancing work performance, eliminating fatigue and treating symptoms of debility following intense physical and psychological stress (Perfumi & Mattioli 2007).

OTHER NAMES

Arctic root, golden root, Hongjingtian, king's crown, Lignum rhodium, rose root, rosenroot, orpin rose, Russian rhodiola, Siberian golden root

BOTANICAL NAME/FAMILY

Rhodiola rosea (family Crassulaceae)

A number of rhodiola species can be identified in the scientific literature and may possess varying pharmacological activities, chemical constituents and efficacy in clinical application (Kucinskaite et al 2007, Li & Zhang 2008). These include: the Indian herb *Rhodiola imbricata* (Goel et al 2006) and the Tibetan herb *Rhodiola sacra* (Shih et al 2008), *Rhodiola quadrifida* (Skopnska-Rozewska et al 2008), *Rhodiola sachalinensis* (Wu et al 2008), *Rhodiola crenulata* (Song et al 2008) and *Rhodiola dumulosa* (Liu et al 2008).

The characteristic feature of *R. rosea* is the presence of cynnamic alcohol glucosides and relatively high content of phenylpropanoids rosavin, whereas salidroside is common to most other *Rhodiola* species. In particular, *R. rosea* extracts contain a substantial concentration of proanthocyandins, including (-)-epigallocatechin and its 3-O-gallate esters (Yousef et al 2006).

PLANT PART USED

Root

CHEMICAL COMPONENTS

Salidroside (aka rhodiolosides A-F, monoterpene glycosides), and their aglycones; rhodiolol A, rosiridol and sachalinol A (Ali et al 2008, Li HB et al 2008, Li W et al 2008, Ma et al 2006, Yu et al 2008); rosavins (rasavin, rosin, rosarin; phenylpropanoids) (Kucinskaite et al 2007); gossypetin-7-O-L-rhamnopyranoside, rhodioflavonoside, gallic acid, trans-p-hydroxycinnamic acid and p-tyrosol (Ming et al 2005); cinnamic alcohol, cinnamaldehyde and cinnamic acid (Panossian et al 2008); hydroquinone (Wang et al 2007).

Most commercial preparations are standardised to specific levels of marker compounds rosavin, salidroside or both. The balance of rosavins to salidrosides is usually 3:1.

MAIN ACTIONS

Adaptogenic (modulates stress response)

Prolonged exposure to stressful life events and depression may contribute to significant behavioural, endocrinological and neurobiological changes in both humans and animals. Animal studies have suggested that chronic administration of rhodiola extract (standardised to 3% rosavin and 1% salidroside; 10, 15 and 20 mg/kg by gavage) results in potent inhibition of the behavioural and physiological changes induced by chronic exposure to mild stressors in a manner comparable to those of fluoxetine (oral 10 mg/kg) (Mattioli et al 2009). Other studies suggest an ability to selectively attenuate stress-induced anorexia (Mattioli & Perfumi 2007). In experimental studies, extracts of rhodiola appear to increase stress resistance and contribute to a longer lifespan. The extract induces translocation of the DAF-16 transcription factor from the cytoplasm into the nucleus, suggesting a reprogramming of transcriptional activities favouring the synthesis of proteins involved in stress resistance and longevity (Wiegant et al 2009).

Single-dose studies of rhodiola extract (standardised to 3% rosavin and 1% salidroside; 10, 15 and 20 mg/kg) have demonstrated antidepressant, adaptogenic, anxiolytic and stimulating effects in mice (Perfumi & Mattioli 2007). In addition, rhodiola has been reported to prevent catecholamine release and subsequent cyclic AMP elevation in the myocardium, and the depletion of adrenal catecholamines induced by acute stress in vivo (Maslova et al 1994). According to Panossian and Wagner (2005), the beneficial effects of multidose administration of adaptogens, such as rhodiola, are mainly associated with the hypothalamic–pituitary–adrenal (HPA) axis, while single-dose applications are more useful in situations that require a rapid response to tension or to a stressful situation via the sympatho-adrenal system (SAS). Rhodiola exerts a stimulating effect within 30 minutes of administration that continues for approximately 4–6 hours. This activity appears to be due to salidroside and rosavin (Panossian & Wagner 2005).

Improved physical performance

While earlier animal studies seemed promising (Abidov et al 2003, Azizov & Seifulla 1998), rhodiola has produced mixed results when attempting to demonstrate an ergogenic effect during exercise in humans (Walker & Robergs 2006). Rhodiola is purported to enhance physical performance, possibly by improving adenosine triphosphate (ATP) turnover; however, several small-scale human trials have produced inconsistent results.

Improved mental performance

It has been suggested that rhodiola extract promotes the release of monoamine neurotransmitters in the ascending pathways of the brainstem, thus activating the cerebral cortex and limbic system. As a result, cognitive function, attention, memory and learning may be enhanced (Panossian & Wagner 2005). Animal experiments have demonstrated improvements in learning and retention after 24 hours following a single dose (0.10 mL/rat) and long-term memory after 10 days treatment at the same dose. Higher (1.0 mL) and lower (0.02 mL) doses did not appear to be effective (Petkov et al 1986).

Anticholinesterase

Spectral methods (NMR, UV and MS) have identified a strong anticholinesterase activity for hydroquinone, a component of rhodiola (Wang et al 2007).

Antidepressant

Rhodiola is one of the more promising herbal medicines for the treatment of monopolar depression (Kelly 2001, Kucinskaite et al 2004, Sarris 2007). It appears to influence the levels and activity of monoamine neurotransmitters such as serotonin, noradrenalin and dopamine (Stancheva & Mosharrof 1987).

Extracts of rhodiola exhibit potent anti-depressant activity by inhibiting monoamine oxidase (MAO)-A in vitro which may partly explain its effects (van Diermen et al 2009). It increases serotonin levels and significantly increases serotonin receptor 1A according to research with a nicotine withdrawal model (Mannucci et al 2012). It is suspected that rhodiola also facilitates neurotransmitter transport within the brain (Stancheva & Mosharrof 1987). Other studies indicate that antidepressant effects are likely to be due to salidroside on stress-activated protein kinases (SAPK), which play a key role in HPA axis overactivity by inhibiting the sensitivity of glucocorticoid receptors to cortisol (Darbinyan et al 2007).

Immunomodulation

While studies using rhodiola alone for immune modulation could not be located, several polyherbal preparations containing rhodiola have been tested producing good results. In a placebo-controlled trial, a combined preparation known as Admax (Nulab Inc), containing *Rhodiola rosea* in combination with *Eleutherococcus senticosus*, *Schisandra chinensis* and *Leuzea carthamoides* (270 mg/day) was given to 28 patients with stage III–IV epithelial ovarian cancer receiving a one-off dose of cisplatin (75 mg/m^2) and cyclophosphamide (600 mg/m^2). Subjects received treatment or placebo for 4 weeks. In patients who took Admax, the mean numbers of four T-cell subclasses (CD3, CD4, CD5 and CD8) and the mean amounts of IgG and IgM were increased, suggesting attenuation of the suppressed immunity experienced by ovarian cancer patients undertaking chemotherapy (Kormosh et al 2006). Additionally, a double-blind, placebo-controlled, randomised trial of Chisan (a standardised combination of *Rhodiola rosea*, *Schisandra chinensis* and *Eleutherococcus senticosus*) was carried out on 60 patients receiving cephazoline, bromhexine and theophylline for acute non-specific pneumonia. The addition of Chisan twice daily for 10–15 days in the treatment group resulted in a 2-day reduction in the mean time required to bring about recovery from the acute phase and improved quality-of-life (QOL) scores during convalescence (Narimanian et al 2005).

Antibacterial

The methanolic extract of rhodiola root has been shown to inhibit the activity of *Staphylococcus aureus* in Microbial Sensitivity Tests. The active compounds were identified as gossypetin-7-O-L-rhamnopyranoside and rhodioflavonoside at concentrations of 50 microgram/mL and 100 microgram/mL, respectively (Ming et al 2005).

Cardioprotective

Rhodiola extract has been shown to exert cardioprotective effects in vivo. More specifically, rhodiola extract demonstrates protection against reperfusion injury after ischaemia, antiarrhythmic activity and increases serum levels of beta-endorphin and leu-enkephalin in myocardial tissue. The effects appear to be dependent on the occupancy of opioid receptors by endogenous opioid peptides (Maslov & Lishmanov 2007).

Salidroside isolated from rhodiola provided a protective effect on epirubicin-induced early left ventricular regional systolic dysfunction in patients with breast cancer according to a randomised placebo-controlled study (Zhang et al 2012). Participants received salidroside (600 mg/day) or placebo starting 1 week before chemotherapy and were investigated by means of echocardiography and strain rate (SR) imaging. Additionally, a significant increase in plasma concentrations of reactive oxygen species was found in the placebo group, but levels remained unchanged with salidroside, indicating an antioxidant mechanism.

Combination preparations, such as tonizid (containing *Rhodiola rosea* in combination with *Aralia mandshurica*, *Panax ginseng* and *Eleutherococcus senticosus*), have also demonstrated cardioprotective and antifibrillatory properties during acute cardiac ischaemia/reperfusion and postinfarction cardiac fibrosis (Arbuzov et al 2006, Lishmanov et al 2008).

Improved cardiac function

Oral administration of a *Rhodiola rosea* ethanolic extract (75 mg/kg) for 21 days increased the cardiac output of streptozocin-induced diabetic rats showing heart failure without modifying the diabetic parameters (Cheng et al 2012). Mean arterial pressures in STZ-diabetic rats were significantly increased after treatment with rhodiola. The effect was abolished after administration of an antagonist of PPARδ. Previously, oral administration of *R. rosea* extract (3.5 mg/kg) was shown to improve heart contractility and coronary flow parameters, thought to be due to an increase in the level of endogenous opioid peptides (Lishmanov et al 1997). The anti-arrhythmic effect of rhodiola extract is a result of activation of both central and peripheral opioid receptors (Maimeskulova & Maslov 2000) and stimulation of kappa-opioid receptor (Maimeskulova et al 1997).

OTHER ACTIONS

Antioxidant

Rhodiola extract reduces oxidative stress in vitro (Battistelli et al 2005) and increases endogenous antioxidant production in vivo. Rhodiola was able to significantly protect human erythrocytes from glutathione (GSH) depletion, glyceraldehyde-3-phosphate dehydrogenase (GAPDH) inactivation and haemolysis induced by the oxidant hypochlorous acid (HOCl), in a dose-dependent manner (De Sanctis et al 2004). In animal studies, rhodiola extract (200 mg/kg/day for 12 weeks) increased the levels of reduced glutathione and the activity of glutathione reductase, glutathione S-transferase, glutathione peroxidase, catalase and superoxide dismutase in the liver (Kim et al 2006). In human trials, a trend towards decreased lipid peroxidation has been observed following 7-day treatment with *Rhodiola rosea* (Wing et al 2003). Additionally, a placebo-controlled study utilising salidroside isolated from rhodiola acted via an antioxidant mechanism to provide a cardioprotective effect on epirubicin-induced early left ventricular regional systolic dysfunction (Zhang et al 2012).

Antidiabetic

Rhodiola extract (200 mg/kg/day for 12 weeks) significantly decreases blood glucose and lipid peroxidation in vivo. It also increases levels of reduced glutathione and the activity of glutathione reductase, glutathione S-transferase, glutathione peroxidase, catalase and superoxide dismutase in the liver (Kim et al 2006). Further in vivo studies have revealed that water-soluble rhodiola extract inhibits alpha-glucosidase and pancreatic alpha-amylase (Apostolidis et al 2006). Ethanolic extracts also inhibit alpha-amylase, alpha-glucosidase and also angiotensin-converting enzyme (ACE) (Kwon et al 2006). The effect appears to be dependent on the phenolic content and profile (Apostolidis et al 2006, Kwon et al 2006). In experimental studies, salidroside, one of the major active components of rhodiola, has a dose-dependent effect on glucose transport activation and insulin sensitivity via AMP-activated protein kinase (AMPK) activation (Li HB et al 2008) and may inhibit lipid peroxidation (Zhang & Liu 2005).

Anti-inflammatory

Salidroside demonstrates significant anti-inflammatory activity (Li et al 2013).

Neuroprotective

Salidroside, an isolated component of rhodiola, has demonstrated a dose-dependent neuroprotective effect in animal models (Bocharov et al 2008). Salidroside has protective effects against oxidative stress-induced cell apoptosis (Zhang et al 2007), inhibits intracellular reactive oxygen species (ROS) production and restores mitochondrial membrane potential (Yu et al 2008) and decreases intracellular free calcium concentration (Zhang et al 2004). As a result, salidroside may warrant further investigation for preventing and treating cerebral ischaemic and neurodegenerative diseases (Yu et al 2008).

Cytoprotective

Salidroside, extracted from *R. rosea*, may protect PC12 cells against glutamate excitotoxic damage through suppressing the excessive entry of calcium and the release of the calcium stores (Cao et al 2006).

Hepatoprotective

Hepatoprotective effects have been demonstrated in rats with experimental toxic hepatitis: normalising the activity of aspartate aminotransferase (AST) and alkaline phosphatase (ALP); reducing the activity of alanine aminotransferase (ALT) and glutathione-S-transferase; and normalising the content of medium-molecular-weight peptides, urea and bilirubin in plasma (Iaremii & Grigor'eva 2002). Rhodiola extract has also been shown to reduce the liver dysfunction associated with adriamycin (an anthracycline antibiotic) in mice without affecting the drug's antitumour activity (Udintsev et al 1992).

Anticancer effects (antimutagenic, cytostatic, antiproliferative, antimetastatic)

Rhodiola extract demonstrates anticancer activity according to test tube and animal studies, which is due to a combination of mechanisms. The main constituent attracting attention for its anticancer activity is salidroside, which has been studied in a variety of models. However, it is not the only active constituent with anticancer activity; for example, gossypetin-7-O-L-rhamnopyranoside and rhodioflavonoside have cytotoxic activity against prostate cancer cell lines (Ming et al 2005a).

R. rosea extracts reduce experimentally-induced mutations, most likely due to increased efficiency of intracellular DNA repair mechanisms (Salikhova et al 1997). The cytostatic and antiproliferative effects of rhodiola extract have been demonstrated in experimental models. Rhodiola has been shown to inhibit the division of HL-60 cells leading to induction of apoptosis and necrosis, and to a marked reduction in their survival. After treatment with the extract, no chromosome aberrations or micronuclei were observed (Majewska et al 2006). Antiproliferative and antimetastatic effects have been noted in animal models of Pliss lymphosarcoma (Udintsev & Shakhov 1991b).

In a small human trial, oral administration of rhodiola extract to 12 patients with superficial bladder carcinoma (T1G1-2) resulted in improvements in urothelial tissue integration, parameters of leucocyte integrins and T-cell immunity. A non-significant reduction in the average frequency of relapse was also noted (Bocharova et al 1995).

Salidroside

Salidroside inhibits the growth of various human cancer cell lines in concentration- and time-dependent manners, and the sensitivity to salidroside is different for different cancer cell lines (Hu et al 2010a).

Hu et al (2010a) report that salidroside causes G1-phase or G2-phase arrest in different cancer cell lines, a decrease of CDK4, cyclin D1, cyclin B1 and Cdc2, and upregulation of the levels of p27(Kip1) and p21(Cip1). Taken together, salidroside appears to inhibit the growth of cancer cells by modulating CDK4-cyclin D1 pathway for G1-phase arrest and/ or modulating the Cdc2-cyclin B1 pathway for G2-phase arrest.

The salidroside constituent from *Rhodiola rosea* has cytotoxic effects on human breast cancer MDA-MB-231 cells (oestrogen receptor negative) and human breast cancer MCF-7 cells (oestrogen receptor positive) by inducing cell-cycle arrest and apoptosis (Hu et al 2010b).

A study by Liu et al (2012) showed that both *R. rosea* extracts and salidroside could decrease the growth of bladder cancer cell lines with minimal effect on non-malignant bladder epithelial cells TEU-2 via inhibition of the mTOR pathway and induction of autophagy (Liu et al 2012).

Effect on cytochromes and p-glycoprotein

In vitro tests reveal that *R. rosea* extract inhibits CYP 3A4 and p-glycoprotein (Hellum et al 2010). These effects have not been investigated in clinical studies so the significance of the findings are unknown.

An in vivo study showed that *R. rosea* extract did not affect the metabolism of warfarin or theophylline, therefore it is unlikely to significantly affect CYP 1A2 or CYP 2C9 (Panossian et al 2009). Recently, an in vivo test showed that *R. rosea* significantly alters the pharmacokinetic properties of losartan after concurrent oral administration to rabbits, increasing the maximum plasma concentration (C_{max}), the area under the curve (AUC) and the apparent total body clearance (CL/F) (Spanakis et al 2013). Losartan is metabolised by CYP2C9 and 3A4. Based on negative results for activity on CYP2C9, it is likely that the interaction is mainly due to inhibition of CYP3A4. Clinical tests are now warranted to further investigate this drug interaction.

CLINICAL USE

Both *Rhodiola rosea* liquid extract and solid dose forms have been investigated in clinical studies. Some recent clinical research has been conducted with the *R. rosea* rhizome product known as SHR-5 which is standardised to provide a minimum 3% rosavins and 0.8% salidroside, because the naturally occurring ratio of these compounds in *R. rosea* root is approximately 3:1.

Unfortunately, conclusions about the body of evidence are difficult to make as studies use a wide range of doses, so are not easy to compare. As with all pharmacologically active treatments, a dose-response is likely to occur. Results from several studies investigating mental and physical performance effects suggest the dose response is not linear but instead a bell-shaped curve whereby very low and high doses are less effective than moderate doses. Further investigation is required to confirm the clinical effects and discover the optimal dosage range for use in various indications.

The variation in chemical makeup for the test extracts may be another factor contributing to the inconsistent findings observed. The stimulating and adaptogenic properties of *R. rosea* are attributed specifically to p-tyrosol, salidroside, rosavins, and additional phenolic compounds, while the high content in organic acids and flavonoids contributes to the strong antioxidant properties of the plant (Ming et al 2005b).

Adaptogen

Rhodiola rosea was first investigated in human studies in the 1960s as a possible adaptogenic agent. Based on positive results in these early studies, it was recommended as a stimulant for fatigue in 1969 by the Pharmacological Committee of the Ministry of Health of the USSR and it remains a very popular adaptogen in Russia today (Panossian et al 2010). It is also very popular in Sweden where it is a recognised herbal medicinal product by authorities. *Rhodiola rosea* is used by healthy people during periods of high mental stress or physical exertion. The adaptogenic activity of *R. rosea* has been demonstrated in numerous preclinical trials and attributed primarily due to its ability to influence levels and activity of biogenic monoamines such as serotonin, dopamine and noradrenaline in the central nervous system (Kelly 2001).

The European Food Safety Authority (EFSA) allows rhodiola treatment to carry the functional claim 'contributes to optimal mental and cognitive activity'.

The human clinical trials conducted to date tend to focus on mental stress and fatigue, response to physical stress, physical fatigue or ergogenic activity.

Mental stress and fatigue

In the 1960s, two non-randomised, placebo-controlled studies were conducted which demonstrated that a single dose of rhodiola liquid extract or salidroside (2.5 mg) improved mental performance for at least 4 hours and reduced the number of errors in Anfimov's correction test (Panossian et al 2010). In the study by Zatova, doses of 5–10 drops were found to be the most effective, reducing the number of errors by an average of 46%. At a dose of 5 drops, the rhodiola extract led to a reduction in the number of errors in 88% of the subjects tested, but to an increase in the remaining 12%. This was in comparison to placebo, which produced a reduction in the number of errors in 35% of the subjects, an increase in 58% and no change in the remaining 7% (Panossian & Wagner 2005).

A 28-day course of SHR-5 extract (576 mg/day) demonstrated a significant improvement in fatigue scores (Pines burnout scale) and a significant improvement in mental performance, particularly the ability to concentrate according to a randomised, double-blind study of 60 people aged between 20 and 55 years with fatigue syndrome (Olsson et al 2008). Treatment also decreased cortisol response to awakening stress.

A randomised, double-blind, placebo-controlled study involving 161 cadets aged 19–21 years found that single doses of SHR-5 extract produced a highly significant antifatigue effect using the antifatigue index (AFI). Both the standard (9 mg/day salidroside) and high dose (13.5 mg/day salidroside) treatment regimens were significantly superior to placebo, but were as effective as each other (Shevtsov et al 2003).

The same extract (SHR-5) was also used in a double-blind, randomised, placebo-controlled trial of 40 foreign students during a stressful examination period. A repeated low-dose regimen (100 mg/day) was administered for 20 days resulting in significant improvements in hand-eye co-ordination ($P < 0.01$), self-reported mental fatigue ($P < 0.01$) and general wellbeing. There were no significant differences for speed or accuracy of mental performance between the groups or physical performance (Spasov et al 2000).

A randomised, double blind, crossover study of 56 young, healthy doctors tested a dose of 170 mg of SHR-5 extract. Placebo or active treatment was taken for 2 weeks with a 2-week washout period between crossing over to the alternative treatment (Darbinyan et al 2000). Authors reported that two weeks of active treatment in the first period improved performance by approximately 20% ($P < 0.01$). It was effective at relieving mental fatigue symptoms and improving concentration and speed of audio–visual perception. When active treatment was taken by the alternative group in the second 2-week treatment term, no significant changes were found. It is possible that after 6 weeks of night duty, the test dose used was insufficient to have a significant effect, whereas it was sufficient after only 2 weeks of night duty. While these results are promising, the study did not use a validated fatigue scale.

IN COMBINATION

During a 12-week study, the efficacy and safety of rhodiola extract given in combination with vitamins and minerals (Vigodana) was tested in 120 adults (83 women and 37 men aged 50–89 years) with physical and cognitive deficiencies (Fintelmann & Gruenwald 2007). Two different dosage regimens were chosen: 2 capsules orally in the morning after breakfast, or 1 capsule after breakfast and 1 after lunch. A significant improvement in physical and cognitive performance was observed in both groups ($P < 0.001$), but it was more pronounced in the group taking both capsules after breakfast. No adverse events occurred during the course of the study (Fintelmann & Gruenwald 2007). While the results of this study are promising, this was not a placebo-controlled clinical trial of stand-alone rhodiola treatment.

Results of four double-blind studies with rhodiola extract (SHR-5) are promising but not decisive, as some studies indicate significant antifatigue effects, whereas others are inconclusive or show no changes in aspects of mental performance.

Physical fatigue and enhanced physical performance

Randomised clinical trials involving both trained and untrained people have been published with wide ranging test doses.

A double-blind, placebo-controlled study demonstrated beneficial effects with acute but not with chronic dosing of rhodiola. A single dose of rhodiola extract (200 mg standardised to 3% rosavin and 1% salidroside) significantly increased time to exhaustion (16.8 ± 0.7 min to 17.2 ± 0.8 min; $P <$

0.05), VO_{2peak} and VCO_{2peak} compared to placebo, and also tended to increase pulmonary ventilation ($P = 0.07$) (124.8 ± 7.7 L/min versus 115.9 ± 7.7 L/min). Prior administration of the same dose daily for 4 weeks did not alter any of the variables measured (De Bock et al 2004).

Treatment with a higher dose (340 mg/day) of *Rhodiola rosea* extract containing 30 mg active RR (including rosavin) for 30 days before and 6 days after exhausting physical exercise significantly reduced C-reactive protein levels when tested 5 hours and 5 days after exercise when compared to controls (Abidov et al 2004). The double-blind study of 36 untrained people also found blood CK levels decreased after 5 days only in the active treatment group and not in controls. These results suggest active treatment reduced inflammation and protected muscle tissue from damage during exercise.

A significant decrease in reported level of fatigue and tiredness was demonstrated after 1 week of treatment with SHR-5 (280 mg/day) according to another double blind, placebo-controlled study (Schutgens et al 2009).

In contrast, two studies found no significant effect on various aspects of physical performance; however, one study used a very high dose (1500 mg/day) and the other a very low dose (100 mg/day), making conclusions difficult to draw (Walker et al 2007, Spasov et al 2000).

Walker et al (2007) conducted a placebo-controlled trial of 12 resistance-trained men, aged 19–39 years that completed an incremental forearm wrist flexion exercise to fatigue, after ingesting very high dose rhodiola (1500 mg/day) or placebo for 4 days (Walker et al 2007). At this dose there were no significant differences between groups for time to exhaustion or recovery. Negative results were also obtained by Spasov et al (2000) in another double-blind, randomised, placebo-controlled trial. This study involved 40 foreign students during a stressful examination period and found that treatment with low dose SHR-5 extract (100 mg/day) for 20 days did not produce any significant changes in physical performance as measured by work capacity using a stationary bicycle and pulse rate immediately after the ergometric test. It did, however, produce a significant improvement in hand–eye coordination ($P < 0.01$) (Spasov et al 2000).

IN COMBINATION

Two double-blind RCTs using a formula containing *R. rosea* and *Cordyceps sinensis* failed to observe any significant changes to various aspects of physical performance.

Earnest et al (2004) found that competitive amateur cyclists given 14 days of treatment with a commercial herbal product, taken as 6 capsules daily for 4 days then 3 capsules daily for 11 days (3 capsules = *Rhodiola rosea* 300 mg; *Cordyceps sinensis* 1000 mg and assorted nutrients), produced no significant change for oxygen consumption (VO_2), time to exhaustion, peak power output or peak heart rate compared to placebo (Earnest et al 2004). Similarly, a double-blind, RCT of the same combination of herbs (*Rhodiola rosea* 300 mg and *Cordyceps sinensis* 1000 mg per 3 capsules) failed to demonstrate significant effects on muscle tissue oxygen saturation, VO_{2max}, ventilatory threshold or time to exhaustion (Colson et al 2005). The dose used was 6 capsules daily for 6 days and 3 capsules daily for 7 days.

Depression

Several studies with experimental models have shown that rhodiola exhibits significant antidepressant activity and in vitro tests provide plausible mechanisms of action (Panossian & Wagner 2005, Perfumi & Mattioli 2007). In one study, rhodiola exhibited a stronger antidepressant effect than either imipramine (30 mg/kg) or *Hypericum perforatum* (20 mg/kg). Rhodioloside and tyrosol were identified as active principles (Panossian et al 2008). Despite this encouraging preliminary evidence, clinical investigation has only just begun and produced inconsistent results.

In a double-blind RCT conducted over 6 weeks, 89 participants aged 18–70 years were selected according to Diagnostic and Statistical Manual of Mental Disorders (DSM)-IV diagnostic criteria for mild-to-moderate depression (Darbinyan et al 2007). The severity of the depression was determined by scores gained in the Beck Depression Inventory (BDI) and Hamilton Rating Scale for Depression (HAM-D) questionnaires. Patients with initial HAM-D scores between 21 and 31 were randomised to receive either *Rhodiola rosea* extract SHR-5 (340 mg/day) or SHR-5 (680 mg/day) or placebo. At the end of the 6-week trial, participants in both treatment groups experienced significant improvements ($P < 0.0001$) in overall depression, insomnia, emotional instability and somatisation compared to the placebo group. The high-dose group also experienced improvements in self-esteem. There was a dose-dependent effect for the BDI but not for the HAM-D and no serious side effects were reported in any of the groups (Darbinyan et al 2007).

In contrast, a 28-day course of SHR-5 extract (576 mg/day) demonstrated no significant effect on the Montgomery-Asberg Depression Rating Scale (MADRS) in a randomised, double-blind study of 60 people aged between 20 and 55 years with fatigue syndrome (Olsson et al 2008). Whether this means a longer treatment period is required to see effects (as per Darbinyan et al) or that the treatment is ineffective requires further investigation.

Generalised anxiety disorder (GAD)

In a small pilot study, 10 participants aged 34–55 years were selected according to DSM-IV diagnostic criteria for generalised anxiety disorder (GAD). Participants received rhodiola extract (340 mg/day) for 10 weeks after which time there was a significant decrease in mean Hamilton Anxiety Rating Scale (HAM-A) scores. Only mild-to-moderate adverse effects were noted, most commonly dizziness and dry mouth, and no drug interaction was observed in the three patients taking benzodiazepines (Bystritsky et al 2008). Larger well-designed trials should be conducted to confirm these effects.

OTHER USES

Reward deficiency syndrome (RDS)

Reward deficiency syndrome (RDS), associated with low dopamine 2 (D_2) receptors, may increase craving behaviour, causing the individual to seek out substances that increase the release of dopamine. Researchers in this area have suggested that the addition of rhodiola, a known catechol-O-methyltransferase (COMT) inhibitor, may be a useful adjunct to the treatment of this condition. It is thought that during recovery or rehabilitation from alcohol or other psychoactive drugs (dopamine releasers), decreasing COMT activity should result in 'enhanced synaptic dopamine, thereby proliferating D_2 receptors while reducing stress, increasing wellbeing, reducing craving behaviour and preventing relapse' (Blum et al 2007).

Opioid addiction

Results from two studies with experimental mouse models indicate that *Rhodiola rosea* L. extract significantly and dose-dependently attenuates both the development and the expression of morphine dependence after chronic or acute administration and reduced opioid craving and vulnerability to relapse (Mattioli & Perfumi 2011a, Mattioli et al 2012). Based on these preliminary results, *R. rosea* extract has potential as a treatment for opioid addiction and should be investigated further.

Nicotine withdrawal

In an experimental model of nicotine dependence, *Rhodiola rosea* extract abolished both affective and somatic signs induced by nicotine withdrawal in a dose-dependent fashion, during both nicotine exposure and nicotine cessation (Mattioli & Perfumi 2011b). Positive results were also obtained in another study which found *R. rosea* or isolated salidroside significantly reduced the rewarding properties of nicotine at all doses tested and prevented relapse to nicotine through both priming and stress-induced influences (Titomanlio et al 2013). Currently, no human studies have been published to determine whether the effects are clinically significant.

Cardiovascular disease prevention

In animal studies, rhodiola extract has demonstrated cardioprotective, antiarrhythmic and antioxidant effects (Lishmanov et al 1997, Maimeskulova & Maslov 2000, Maslov & Lishmanov 2007, Wing et al 2003). Whether these effects are clinically relevant in human populations at risk of cardiovascular disease remains to be tested.

Diabetes

In animal studies, rhodiola extract (200 mg/kg/day for 12 weeks) significantly decreased blood glucose and lipid peroxidation. It also increased the levels of reduced glutathione and the activities of glutathione reductase, glutathione S-transferase, glutathione peroxidase, catalase and superoxide dismutase in the liver. As increased oxidative stress has been shown to play an important role in the pathogenesis and long-term complications of diabetes mellitus, rhodiola shows potential as a useful treatment in diabetes with multiple mechanisms of relevance (Kim et al 2006).

Practice points/Patient counselling

- Rhodiola may have beneficial effects on physical and mental performance and fatigue; preclinical trials are supportive; however, results from clinical trials have been inconsistent. This may relate to incorrect dosage and/or variations in herbal test substances.
- Rhodiola has antidepressant activity according to preclinical studies and improves mood, reduces irritability, insomnia and emotional instability according to a placebo-controlled study of people with depression. However, it had no antidepressant effect in a study of people with fatigue syndrome.
- It may also be a useful treatment in generalised anxiety disorder, according to a small clinical study.
- Rhodiola is safe and well tolerated, but it has the potential to interact with some medications.
- Preliminary research also shows it has potential in opioid dependency, nicotine withdrawal, diabetes, cardioprotection, improves heart function in heart failure and kills various cancer cells.

DOSAGE RANGE

- Fluid extract (1:2): 20–40 mL/wk (Australian manufacturer recommendations).
- In clinical trials, extracts are often standardised to 3% rosavin and 1% salidroside (Perfumi & Mattioli 2007).

Doses used in clinical trials

Mental fatigue: 100–576 mg/day
Physical fatigue and performance: 200 mg/day–1500 mg/day

- Positive results on various aspects of mental performance have been seen for the dose range 100–576 mg daily.
- For physical fatigue and performance, the most effective dose range appears to be 200 mg–340 mg daily with no significant results seen for doses of 600 mg or higher.

- Depression and anxiety: rhodiola extract 340 mg/day (equiv 1500 mg dried root) (Bystritsky et al 2008, Darbinyan et al 2007).

Note: One study suggested improved results from taking rhodiola after breakfast rather than in divided doses after breakfast and lunch (Fintelmann & Gruenwald 2007). This may be due to diurnal variations in HPA and adrenal function.

ADVERSE REACTIONS

Serious adverse events have not been reported to this herbal medicine and side effects tend to be uncommon and mild and can include allergy, insomnia, irritability, fatigue and unpleasaent sensations at high doses. An increase in irritability and insomnia has been reported within several days in some individuals taking high doses (1500 mg–2000 mg, standardised to 2% rosavin) (Iovieno et al 2011).

A review of 11 clinical studies involving 446 volunteers identified only 2 adverse events among those taking active rhodiola treatment — one was mild headache and another severe headache when taking a dose of 200 mg daily for 4 weeks. Similarly, headaches were reported in the placebo groups, so it is not considered serious (Ishaque et al 2012).

SIGNIFICANT INTERACTIONS

As controlled human studies are not available, interactions are currently speculative and based on evidence of pharmacological activity, test tube and animal studies.

Adriamycin

Rhodiola extract has been shown to reduce the liver dysfunction (suggested by a sharp increase in blood transaminase levels) associated with Adriamycin in vivo without affecting the drug's antitumour effects (Udintsev et al 1992). Theoretically, a beneficial interaction is possible under clinical supervision.

Cyclophosphamide

Rhodiola rosea root extract synergises the antitumour activity of cyclophosphamide and decreases its hepatotoxicity in an experimental rodent model (Udintsev & Schakhov 1991a).

Whether the effects are clinically relevant remains to be tested.

Antidepressants

In vitro tests suggest an inhibition of MAO-A by rhodiola extracts (van Diermen et al 2009), a theoretical interaction exists with MAOI antidepressants. The clinical significance of this and whether other antidepressants may be affected is as yet unclear. Observe.

P-glycoprotein substrates

In vitro tests reveal that *R. rosea* extract inhibits P-gp — clinical significance is unknown (Hellum et al 2010).

Cytochrome 3A4 substrates

In vitro tests reveal that *R. rosea* extract inhibits CYP 3A4; this has also been suggested in vivo — clinical significance is unknown (Hellum et al 2010).

Until further tests have been conducted, caution is advised when concurrently using medicines chiefly metabolised by CYP3A4 as the interaction could result in raised drug serum levels.

Losartan

R. rosea significantly alters the pharmacokinetic properties of losartan after concurrent oral administration to rabbits (Spanakis et al 2013). The results indicate that rhodiola is likely to inhibit CYP3A4, resulting in increased drug serum levels. Avoid — until further research is available to determine the seriousness of the interaction.

CONTRAINDICATIONS AND PRECAUTIONS

While the administration of rhodiola may be beneficial in monopolar depression, use is not recommended for bipolar states.

Theoretically, the possibility of the herb exerting MAO-inhibiting effects may require consumers to adhere to dietary restriction of tyramine-rich foods (e.g. some cheeses, pickled foods, chocolates, meats, beer, wine etc), as the interaction of tyramine with MAOIs can result in a significant elevation in blood pressure.

PREGNANCY USE

Safety in pregnancy and lactation has not been established.

PATIENTS' FAQs

What will this herb do for me?

Rhodiola may be of assistance in the treatment of stress-related conditions, in particular depression, mental and/or physical and fatigue and also generalised anxiety disorder. It may also be of benefit in depression.

When will it start to work?

Rhodiola exerts a stimulating effect within 30 minutes of administration that continues for approximately 4–6 hours.

In mild-to-moderate depression, the benefits of *Rhodiola rosea* extract SHR-5 (340 mg/day) or SHR-5 (680 mg/day) were noted at the end of a 6-week trial.

Are there any safety issues?

It is generally considered very safe and well tolerated with side effects being rare and mild. People taking MAOI antidepressants or drugs chiefly metabolised by cytochrome 3A4 should be closely monitored until more is known about the mechanism of action of this herb and its drug interactions. Safety in pregnancy and lactation has not been established.

REFERENCES

Abidov M et al. Extract of rhodiola rosea radix reduces the level of C-reactive protein and creatinine kinase in the blood. Bull Exp Biol Med 138.1 (2004): 63–64.

Abidov M et al. Effect of extracts from rhodiola rosea and rhodiola crenulata (Crassulaceae) roots on ATP content in mitochondria of skeletal muscles. Bull Exp Biol Med 136.6 (2003): 585–587.

Ali Z et al. Phenylalkanoids and monoterpene analogues from the roots of rhodiola rosea. Planta Med 74.2 (2008): 178–181.

Apostolidis E et al. Potential of cranberry-based herbal synergies for diabetes and hypertension management. Asia Pac J Clin Nutr 15.3 (2006): 433–441.

Arbuzov AG et al. Antihypoxic, cardioprotective, and antifibrillation effects of a combined adaptogenic plant preparation. Bull Exp Biol Med 142.2 (2006): 212–215.

Azizov AP, Seifulla RD. [The effect of elton, leveton, fitoton and adapton on the work capacity of experimental animals]. Eksp Klin Farmakol 61.3 (1998): 61–63.

Battistelli M et al. rhodiola rosea as antioxidant in red blood cells: ultrastructural and hemolytic behaviour. Eur J Histochem 49.3 (2005): 243–254.

Blum K et al. Manipulation of catechol-O-methyl-transferase (COMT) activity to influence the attenuation of substance seeking behavior, a subtype of Reward Deficiency Syndrome (RDS), is dependent upon gene polymorphisms: a hypothesis. Med Hypotheses 69.5 (2007): 1054–1060.

Bocharov EV et al. [Neuroprotective features of phytoadaptogens]. Vestn Ross Akad Med Nauk 4 (2008): 47–50.

Bocharova OA et al. [The effect of a rhodiola rosea extract on the incidence of recurrences of a superficial bladder cancer (experimental clinical research)]. Urol Nefrol (Mosk) 2 (1995): 46–47.

Bystritsky A et al. A pilot study of rhodiola rosea (Rhodax) for generalized anxiety disorder (GAD). J Altern Complement Med 14.2 (2008): 175–180.

Cao LL et al. The effect of salidroside on cell damage induced by glutamate and intracellular free calcium in PC12 cells. J Asian Nat Prod Res 8.1–2 (2006): 159–165.

Cheng YZ et al. Increase of myocardial performance by Rhodiola–ethanol extract in diabetic rats. J Ethnopharmacol 144.2 (2012): 234–239.

Colson SN et al. Cordyceps sinensis- and rhodiola rosea-based supplementation in male cyclists and its effect on muscle tissue oxygen saturation. J Strength Cond Res 19.2 (2005): 358–363.

Darbinyan V et al. Clinical trial of rhodiola rosea L. extract SHR-5 in the treatment of mild to moderate depression. Nord J Psychiatry 61.5 (2007): 343–348.

Darbinyan V et al. Rhodiola rosea in stress induced fatigue — a double blind cross-over study of a standardized extract SHR-5 with a repeated low-dose regimen on the mental performance of healthy physicians during night duty. Phytomedicine 7.5 (2000): 365–371.

De Bock K et al. Acute rhodiola rosea intake can improve endurance exercise performance. Int J Sport Nutr Exerc Metab 14.3 (2004): 298–307.

De Sanctis R et al. In vitro protective effect of rhodiola rosea extract against hypochlorous acid-induced oxidative damage in human erythrocytes. Biofactors 20.3 (2004): 147–159.

Earnest CP et al. Effects of a commercial herbal-based formula on exercise performance in cyclists. Med Sci Sports Exerc., 36.3 (2004): 504–509.

Fintelmann V, Gruenwald J. Efficacy and tolerability of a rhodiola rosea extract in adults with physical and cognitive deficiencies. Adv Ther 24.4 (2007): 929–939.

Goel HC et al. Radioprotection by rhodiola imbricata in mice against whole-body lethal irradiation. J Med Food 9.2 (2006): 154–160.

Hellum BH et al. Potent in vitro inhibition of CYP3A4 and P-glycoprotein by Rhodiola rosea. Planta Med, 76.4 (2010): 331–338.

Hu, X et al. A preliminary study: the anti-proliferation effect of salidroside on different human cancer cell lines. Cell Biol Toxicol., 26.6 (2010a): 499–507.

Hu, X et al. Salidroside induces cell-cycle arrest and apoptosis in human breast cancer cells. Biochem Biophys Res Commun, 398.1 (2010b): 62–67.

Iaremii IN, Grigor'eva NF. [Hepatoprotective properties of liquid extract of rhodiola rosea]. Eksp Klin Farmakol 65.6 (2002): 57–59.

Iovieno N et al. Second-tier natural antidepressants: review and critique. J Affect Disord 130.3 (2011): 343–357.

Ishaque S et al. Rhodiola rosea for physical and mental fatigue: a systematic review. BMC Complement Altern Med 12 (2012): 70.

Kelly GS. Rhodiola rosea: a possible plant adaptogen. Altern Med Rev 6.3 (2001): 293–302.

Kim SH et al. Antioxidative effects of Cinnamomi cassiae and rhodiola rosea extracts in liver of diabetic mice. Biofactors 26.3 (2006): 209–219.

Kormosh N et al. Effect of a combination of extract from several plants on cell-mediated and humoral immunity of patients with advanced ovarian cancer. Phytother Res 20.5 (2006): 424–425.

Kucinskaite A et al. Evaluation of biologically active compounds in roots and rhizomes of rhodiola rosea L. cultivated in Lithuania. Kaunas: Medicina (Kaunas) 43.6 (2007):487–94.

Kucinskaite A et al. [Experimental analysis of therapeutic properties of rhodiola rosea L. and its possible application in medicine]. Medicina (Kaunas) 40.7 (2004): 614–6119.

Kwon YI et al. Evaluation of rhodiola crenulata and rhodiola rosea for management of type II diabetes and hypertension. Asia Pac J Clin Nutr 15.3 (2006): 425–432.

Li D et al. Salidroside attenuates inflammatory responses by suppressing nuclear factor-kappaB and mitogen activated protein kinases activation in lipopolysaccharide-induced mastitis in mice. Inflamm Res 62.1 (2013): 9–15.

Li HB et al. Salidroside stimulated glucose uptake in skeletal muscle cells by activating AMP-activated protein kinase. Eur J Pharmacol 588.2–3 (2008): 165–169.

Li T, Zhang H. Application of microscopy in authentication of traditional Tibetan medicinal plants of five rhodiola (Crassulaceae) alpine species by comparative anatomy and micromorphology. Microsc Res Tech 71.6 (2008): 448–458.

Li W et al. Revised absolute stereochemistry of rhodiolosides A-D, rhodiolol A and sachalinol A from rhodiola rosea. Chem Pharm Bull (Tokyo) 56.7 (2008): 1047–1048.

Lishmanov IUB et al. [Cardioprotective, inotropic, and anti-arrhythmia properties of a complex adaptogen. Tonizid®]. Eksp Klin Farmakol 71.3 (2008): 15–22.

Lishmanov IUB et al. [Contribution of the opioid system to realization of inotropic effects of rhodiola rosea extracts in ischemic and reperfusion heart damage in vitro]. Eksp Klin Farmakol 60.3 (1997): 34–36.

Liu Q et al. [Phenolic components from rhodiola dumulosa]. Zhongguo Zhong Yao Za Zhi 33.4 (2008): 411–413.

Liu Z et al. Rhodiola rosea extracts and salidroside decrease the growth of bladder cancer cell lines via inhibition of the mTOR pathway and induction of autophagy. Mol Carcinog 51.3 (2012): 257–267.

Ma G et al. Rhodiolosides A-E, monoterpene glycosides from rhodiola rosea. Chem Pharm Bull (Tokyo) 54.8 (2006): 1229–1233.

Maimeskulova LA et al. [The participation of the mu-, delta- and kappa-opioid receptors in the realization of the anti-arrhythmia effect of rhodiola rosea]. Eksp Klin Farmakol 60.1 (1997): 38–39.

Maimeskulova LA, Maslov LN. [Anti-arrhythmic effect of phytoadaptogens]. Eksp Klin Farmakol 63.4 (2000): 29–31.

Majewska A et al. Antiproliferative and antimitotic effect, S phase accumulation and induction of apoptosis and necrosis after treatment of extract from rhodiola rosea rhizomes on HL-60 cells. J Ethnopharmacol 103.1 (2006): 43–52.

Mannucci C et al. G. Serotonin involvement in Rhodiola rosea attenuation of nicotine withdrawal signs in rats. Phytomedicine 19.12 (2012): 1117–1124.

Maslov LN. Lishmanov IUB. [Cardioprotective and antiarrhythmic properties of rhodiolae roseae preparations]. Eksp Klin Farmakol 70.5 (2007): 59–67.

Maslova LV et al. [The cardioprotective and antiadrenergic activity of an extract of rhodiola rosea in stress]. Eksp Klin Farmakol 57.6 (1994): 61–63.

Mattioli L, Perfumi M. Effects of a Rhodiola rosea L. extract on acquisition and expression of morphine tolerance and dependence in mice. J Psychopharmacol 25.3 (2011a): 411–420.

Mattioli L, Perfumi M. Evaluation of Rhodiola rosea L. extract on affective and physical signs of nicotine withdrawal in mice. J Psychopharmacol 25.3 (2011b): 402–410.

Mattioli L, Perfumi M. Rhodiola rosea L. extract reduces stress- and CRF-induced anorexia in rats. J Psychopharmacol 21.7 (2007): 742–750.

Mattioli L et al. Effects of a Rhodiola rosea L. extract on the acquisition, expression, extinction, and reinstatement of morphine-induced conditioned place preference in mice. Psychopharmacology (Berl) 221.2 (2012): 183–193.

Mattioli L et al. Effects of rhodiola rosea L. extract on behavioural and physiological alterations induced by chronic mild stress in female rats. J Psychopharmacol 23.2 (2009): 130–142.

Ming DS et al. Bioactive compounds from rhodiola rosea (Crassulaceae). Phytother Res 19.9 (2005): 740–743.

Narimanian M et al. Impact of Chisan (ADAPT-232) on the quality-of-life and its efficacy as an adjuvant in the treatment of acute non-specific pneumonia. Phytomedicine 12.10 (2005): 723–729.

Olsson EM et al. A randomised, double-blind, placebo-controlled, parallel-group study of the standardised extract SHR-5 of the roots of rhodiola rosea in the treatment of subjects with stress-related fatigue. Planta Med (2008) [Epub].

Panossian A, Wagner H. Stimulating effect of adaptogens: an overview with particular reference to their efficacy following single dose administration. Phytother Res 19.10 (2005): 819–838.

Panossian, A et al. Rosenroot (Rhodiola rosea): traditional use, chemical composition, pharmacology and clinical efficacy. Phytomedicine 17.7 (2010): 481–493.

Panossian A et al. Pharmacokinetic and pharmacodynamic study of interaction of Rhodiola rosea SHR-5 extract with warfarin and theophylline in rats. Phytother Res 23.3 (2009): 351–357.

Panossian A et al. Comparative study of rhodiola preparations on behavioral despair of rats. Phytomedicine 15.1–2 (2008): 84–91.

Perfumi M, Mattioli L. Adaptogenic and central nervous system effects of single doses of 3% rosavin and 1% salidroside rhodiola rosea L. extract in mice. Phytother Res 21.1 (2007): 37–43.

Petkov VD et al. Effects of alcohol aqueous extract from rhodiola rosea L. roots on learning and memory. Acta Physiol Pharmacol Bulg 12.1 (1986): 3–16.

Salikhova RA et al. [Effect of rhodiola rosea on the yield of mutation alterations and DNA repair in bone marrow cells]. Patol Fiziol Eksp Ter 4 (1997): 22–24.

Sarris J. Herbal medicines in the treatment of psychiatric disorders: a systematic review. Phytother Res 21.8 (2007): 703–716.

Schutgens FW et al. 2009. The influence of adaptogens on ultraweak biophoton emission: a pilot-experiment. Phytother Res, 23, (8) 1103–1108 available from: PM:19170145

Shevtsov VA et al. A randomized trial of two different doses of a SHR-5 rhodiola rosea extract versus placebo and control of capacity for mental work. Phytomedicine 10.2–3 (2003): 95–105.

Shih CD et al. Autonomic nervous system mediates the cardiovascular effects of rhodiola sacra radix in rats. J Ethnopharmacol 112.2 (2008): 284–290.

Skopnska-Rozewska E et al. The effect of rhodiola quadrifida extracts on cellular immunity in mice and rats. Pol J Vet Sci 11.2 (2008): 105–111.

Song XW et al. [Purification and composition analysis of polysaccharide RCPS from rhodiola crenulata]. Guang Pu Xue Yu Guang Pu Fen Xi 28.3 (2008): 642–644.

Spanakis M et al. 2013. Pharmacokinetic Interaction between Losartan and Rhodiola rosea in Rabbits. Pharmacology, 91, (1–2) 112–116 available from: PM:23327826

Spasov AA et al. A double-blind, placebo-controlled pilot study of the stimulating and adaptogenic effect of rhodiola rosea SHR-5 extract on the fatigue of students caused by stress during an examination period with a repeated low-dose regimen. Phytomedicine 7.2 (2000): 85–89.

Stancheva S, Mosharrof A. Effect of the extract of rhodiola rosea L. on the content of the brain biogenic monamines. Med Physiol 40 (1987): 85–87.

Titomanlio F et al. 2013. Rhodiola rosea L. extract and its active compound salidroside antagonized both induction and reinstatement of nicotine place preference in mice. *Psychopharmacology (Berl)* available from: PM:24264566

Udintsev SN, Schakhov VP. Decrease of cyclophosphamide haematotoxicity by rhodiola rosea root extract in mice with Ehrlich and Lewis transplantable tumors. Eur J Cancer 27.9 (1991a): 1182.

Udintsev SN, Schakhov VP. The role of humoral factors of regenerating liver in the development of experimental tumors and the effect of rhodiola rosea extract on this process. Neoplasma 38.3 (1991b): 323–31.

Udintsev SN et al. [The enhancement of the efficacy of adriamycin by using hepatoprotectors of plant origin in metastases of Ehrlich's adenocarcinoma to the liver in mice]. Vopr Onkol 38.10 (1992): 1217–1222.

van Diermen D et al. Monoamine oxidase inhibition by rhodiola rosea L. roots. J Ethnopharmacol 122.2 (2009): 397–401.

Walker TB, Robergs RA. Does rhodiola rosea possess ergogenic properties? Int J Sport Nutr Exerc Metab 16.3 (2006): 305–315.

Walker TB et al. Failure of rhodiola rosea to alter skeletal muscle phosphate kinetics in trained men. Metabolism 56.8 (2007): 1111–1117.

Wang H et al. Acetylcholinesterase inhibitory-active components of rhodiola rosea L. Food Chem 105.1 (2007): 24–27.

Wiegant FA et al. Plant adaptogens increase lifespan and stress resistance in C. elegans. Biogerontology 10.1 (2009): 27–42.

Wing SL et al. Lack of effect of rhodiola or oxygenated water supplementation on hypoxemia and oxidative stress. Wilderness Environ Med 14.1 (2003): 9–16.

Wu YL et al. Protective effects of salidroside against acetaminophen-induced toxicity in mice. Biol Pharm Bull 31.8 (2008): 1523–1529.

Yousef GG et al. Comparative phytochemical characterization of three Rhodiola species. Phytochemistry 67.21 (2006): 2380–2391.

Yu S et al. Neuroprotective effects of salidroside in the PC12 cell model exposed to hypoglycemia and serum limitation. Cell Mol Neurobiol 28.8 (2008): 1067–1078.

Zhang H et al. Protective effects of salidroside on epirubicin-induced early left ventricular regional systolic dysfunction in patients with breast cancer. Drugs RD 12.2 (2012): 101–106 available from: PM:22770377

Zhang L et al. Protective effects of salidroside on hydrogen peroxide-induced apoptosis in SH-SY5Y human neuroblastoma cells. Eur J Pharmacol 564.1–3 (2007): 18–25.

Zhang WS et al. [Protective effects of salidroside on injury induced by hypoxia/hypoglycemia in cultured neurons]. Zhongguo Zhong Yao Za Zhi 29.5 (2004): 459–462.

Zhang Y, Liu Y. [Study on effects of salidroside on lipid peroxidation on oxidative stress in rat hepatic stellate cells]. Zhong Yao Cai 28.9 (2005): 794–796.

Rosehip

HISTORICAL NOTE Rosehips are fruits of the dog rose or wild briar rose that appear as orange-red oval berries and have been used traditionally to treat a range of conditions, including diarrhoea, bladder infections and diabetes. In foods and manufacturing, rosehips are used for tea, jam, jellies and soup, and as a natural source of vitamin C. Rosehips are one of the richest plant sources of vitamin C and rosehip syrup was used in Britain during World War II to help prevent scurvy when citrus supplies were limited. Rosehips are also fed to pet animals such as horses, chinchillas and guinea pigs to enhance their health.

COMMON NAME

Dog rose or wild briar rose

BOTANICAL NAME/FAMILY

Rosa canina / Rosaceae

PLANT PARTS USED

Berries/fruit of the rose plant

CHEMICAL COMPONENTS

Rosehip is a rich source of vitamins C, A, B_3, D and E, along with folate, flavonoids, carotenoids (including beta-carotene and lycopene and lutein), beta-sitosterol, fructose, malic acid, tannins, magnesium, zinc, copper and numerous other phytochemicals, including recently characterised galactolipids (Böhm et al 2003, Christensen 2009, Machmudah et al 2008, Rein et al 2004). These nutrients can be depleted or destroyed during processing and drying and the content of phytochemicals has been shown to be sensitive to maturity of the fruits as well as drying time, drying air temperature and moisture content (Erenturk et al 2005, Pirone et al 2007, Strålsjö et al 2003, Türkben et al 2010).

MAIN ACTIONS

Antioxidant

Rosehip is rich in polyphenolic compounds such as proanthocyanidins and flavonoids such as quercetin and catechin (Türkben et al 2010). The antioxidant activity of rosehip is attributed to its high phenolic and flavonoid content (Wenzig et al 2008) and when rosehip extract containing these phenolics is deprived of vitamin C it still shows considerable antioxidant activity (Daels-Rakotoarison et al 2002). This activity includes protective effects against oxidative stress, enhanced activity of antioxidant enzymes such as superoxide dismutase and catalase and protective effects on gap junction intercellular communication (Yoo et al 2008).

Anti-inflammatory

Rosehip has been found to have anti-inflammatory and antinociceptive activities in several in vivo experimental models (Deliorman Orhan et al 2007). The anti-inflammatory power of rosehip is reported to be similar to that of indomethacin, although its mode of action is different (Lattanzio et al 2011). The lipophilic constituents have particularly high anti-inflammatory activity, including actions on arachidonic acid metabolism and inhibition of both cyclooxygenase (COX)-1 and COX-2 (Wenzig et al 2008). A recent series of studies involving horses, dogs and double-blind, placebo-controlled, randomised controlled trials in humans found that rosehip seeds make an important contribution to rosehip's anti-inflammatory properties (Marstrand et al 2013).

Much of the anti-inflammatory action of rosehip has been attributed to high quantities of galactolipids, a class of compounds widely found in the plant kingdom as an important part of cell membranes and recently shown to possess antitumour-promoting and anti-inflammatory activity in both in vitro and in vivo studies (Christensen 2009). Rosehip and its constituent galactolipids have been found to inhibit the production of inflammatory mediators and confer chondroprotective effects in vitro (Schwager et al 2011). A particular galactolipid named GOPO has been shown to be the active principle responsible for the observed in vitro inhibition of chemotaxis and chemiluminescence of human peripheral blood leucocytes without any toxicity to the cells (Kharazmi 2008, Kharazmi & Winther 1999, Larsen et al 2003, Winther et al 1999). GOPO is suggested to play an important role in reducing inflammation, serum C-reactive protein and creatinine levels (Kharazmi & Winther 1999, Rossnagel & Willich 2001) and improving pain and joint movement in osteoarthritis patients (Rein et al 2004, Warholm et al 2003).

Unlike conventional non-steroidal anti-inflammatory drugs (NSAIDs), rosehip does not cause gastric ulceration, inhibit platelets or influence the coagulation cascade or fibrinolysis (Winther 2000). It has therefore been suggested that the anti-inflammatory properties of rosehip allow it to replace or supplement conventional anti-inflammatory drugs in patients who may be at increased risk from the gastrointestinal or cardiovascular side effects of NSAIDs (Cohen 2012, Kharazmi 2008).

OTHER ACTIONS

Antidiabetic

Antidiabetic, lipid-lowering and antiobesogenic activity

Rosehip's traditional use as a treatment for diabetes is supported by reports of hypoglycaemic effects in diabetic rats (Orhan et al 2009), as well as reduction of blood glucose levels after glucose loading in mice, without affecting food intake, weight gain or accumulation of visceral fat (Ninomiya et al 2007). While rosehip has been found to produce modest cholesterol-lowering effects in humans (Rein et al 2004), further confirmation is required in large human clinical trials (Chrubasik et al 2008b).

CLINICAL USES

Standardised patented rosehip powder is the only preparation that has been studied in clinical trials, although some laboratory studies have used other extracts. The standardised extract has been available for more than a decade in Scandinavia as a herbal remedy (Winther 2008) and is sold under the trade names LitoZin and LitoMove in Europe and i-flex throughout the rest of the world, and is available in Australia and New Zealand under the name Rose-Hip Vital. Since the patenting of standardised rosehip power, there have been a number of clinical trials exploring the efficacy of this preparation in conditions such as osteoarthritis, rheumatoid arthritis and inflammatory bowel disease, with all studies being supported by the manufacturer Hyben Vital.

Osteoarthritis

Clinical research into rosehip includes open-label and randomised controlled trials with durations of 6 months or less (Christensen et al 2013, Rein et al 2004, Warholm et al 2003, Winther & Thamsborg 2005), along with a number of corresponding systematic reviews and meta-analyses (Cohen 2012). These studies have consistently found rosehip to be extremely safe, with occasional mild allergic reactions or gastrointestinal complaints but no serious adverse effects (Chrubasik et al 2009) and rosehip is included in the Arthritis Australia Complementary Therapies Information Sheet as a therapy with moderate evidence of osteoarthritis (Arthritis Australia 2011). Reviews of controlled trials suggest that rosehip has a moderate effect in patients with osteoarthritis (Chrubasik et al 2006, Rossnagel et al 2007). Similarly, a meta-analysis of three randomised controlled trials involving 287 osteoarthritis patients reported that treatment for 3 months with patented rosehip powder consistently reduced pain scores and that patients allocated to rosehip powder were twice as likely to respond to rosehip (as indicated by a reduction in Western Ontario and McMaster Universities Arthritis Index [WOMAC] pain) compared to placebo (effect size of 0.37, 95% confidence interval 0.13–0.60) (Christensen et al 2008). A more recent meta-analysis indirectly compared the pain-reducing effect of glucosamine hydrochloride and standardised rosehip powder for osteoarthritis. This analysis, which was based on three studies on glucosamine hydrochloride involving a total of 933 patients and the three rosehip studies described above involving 287 patients, concluded that rosehip is more efficacious than glucosamine hydrochloride in reducing pain in osteoarthritis patients (Christensen 2009). These results are supported by a more recent 8-week randomised controlled trial involving 46 patients that found that 4500 mg/day of rosehip showed better efficacy than 1500 mg/day of glucosamine sulfate in terms of total WOMAC score reduction, and functional disability reduction at the end of the eighth week, with less evidence and severity of adverse reactions (Christensen et al 2013).

Rheumatoid arthritis

A 6-month, double-blind, placebo-controlled trial involving 89 patients with rheumatoid arthritis found that, compared to placebo, 5 g/day of standardised rosehip powder significantly improved scores on the Health Assessment Questionnaire Disability Index (HAQ-DI) along with various other patient- and doctor-reported scales, as well as significantly reducing erythrocyte sedimentation rate levels (Willich et al 2010). While these results appear promising, they are modest and larger studies with greater statistical power are needed to confirm these results.

A more recent and much smaller open, case-control study of 20 female patients with rheumatoid arthritis and 10 female controls found no significant effects on clinical symptoms, level of C-reactive protein or laboratory measures of antioxidant enzyme activity after 4 weeks' treatment with 10.5 g/day of rosehip powder (Kirkeskov et al 2011). The lack of significant improvements in this study may be due to a lack of effect or a slow onset of action, modest effect size, small sample size and lack of statistical power (Cohen 2012).

Back pain

A 1-year surveillance of 152 patients found that rosehip provided significant pain relief for patients with acute exacerbations of chronic back pain (Chrubasik et al 2008b).

DOSAGE

Dosage depends on the formulation and the indication. A commencement dose of around 5 g/day for 3–4 weeks followed by a maintenance dose of 2.5 g/day is recommended for treating osteoarthritis or chronic inflammation with the standardised extract. Rosehip should be taken with meals to enhance the absorption of its lipid elements.

TOXICITY

Modern clinical studies and widespread traditional use have not raised any significant safety concerns.

ADVERSE REACTIONS

Rosehip is considered safe and there are no documented interactions of major significance.

SIGNIFICANT INTERACTIONS

There are no documented interactions of significance, although some mild gastrointestinal side effects are reported.

PREGNANCY USE

There is little published on the use of rosehip in pregnancy. Rosehip tea has been traditionally recommended during pregnancy and there are no reports of ill effects.

Practice points/Patient counselling

- Rosehip is traditionally taken as a high-vitamin-C tea. A standardised rosehip extract has recently been shown to be an effective anti-inflammatory agent against osteoarthritis and rheumatoid arthritis.

PATIENTS' FAQs

What will this herb do for me?

Rosehip can serve as a source of vitamin C and an anti-inflammatory agent that may help to relieve the pain and disability of osteoarthritis and rheumatoid arthritis and the use of rosehip may reduce the need for anti-inflammatory drugs.

When will it start to work?

Rosehip may take 2–4 weeks to provide effective arthritis relief.

Are there any safety issues?

The growing evidence base for rosehip suggests that this traditional herbal remedy has a high safety profile.

REFERENCES

Arthritis Australia. (2011). "Arthritis Information Sheet: Complementary Therapies", from http://www.arthritisaustralia.com.au/images/stories/documents/info_sheets/2011/2011_updates/Complementary_therapies/Complementary_Therapies.pdf.

Böhm, V., et al. (2003). "Rosehip — A "new" source of lycopene?" Molecular Aspects of Medicine 24(6): 385–389.

Christensen, L. P. (2009). "Galactolipids as potential health promoting compounds in vegetable foods." Recent patents on food, nutrition & agriculture 1(1): 50–58.

Christensen, R., et al. (2008). "Does the hip powder of *Rosa canina* (rosehip) reduce pain in osteoarthritis patients? a meta-analysis of randomized controlled trials." Osteoarthritis and Cartilage 16(9): 965–972.
Christensen, R., et al. (2013). "Comparing different preparations and doses of rosehip powder in patients with osteoarthritis of the knee: an exploratory randomized active-controlled trial." Osteoarthritis and Cartilage 21, Supplement(0): S24.
Chrubasik, C., et al. (2006). "The evidence for clinical efficacy of rose hip and seed: A systematic review." Phytotherapy Research 20(1): 1–3.
Chrubasik, C., et al. (2008b). "A one-year survey on the use of a powder from *Rosa canina lito* in acute exacerbations of chronic pain." Phytotherapy Research 22(9): 1141–1148.
Chrubasik, S., et al. (2009). "The anti-inflammatory efficacy of powdered rose hip — A review." Zur antientzündlichen wirksamkeit von pulver aus der hagebutte 30(5): 227–231.
Cohen (2012). "Rosehip — an evidence based herbal medicine for inflammation and arthritis." Australian Family Physician 41(7): 495–498.
Daels-Rakotoarison, D. A., et al. (2002). "Effects of *Rosa canina* fruit extract on neutrophil respiratory burst." Phytotherapy Research 16(2): 157–161.
Deliorman Orhan, D., et al. (2007). "In vivo anti-inflammatory and antinociceptive activity of the crude extract and fractions from *Rosa canina* L. fruits." Journal of Ethnopharmacology 112(2): 394–400.
Erenturk, S., et al. (2005). "The effects of cutting and drying medium on the vitamin C content of rosehip during drying." Journal of Food Engineering 68(4): 513–518.
Kharazmi, A. (2008). "Laboratory and preclinical studies on the anti-inflammatory and anti-oxidant properties of rosehip powder — Identification and characterization of the active component GOPO®." Osteoarthritis and Cartilage 16(SUPPL. 1): S5–S7.
Kharazmi, A. and K. Winther (1999). "Rose hip inhibits chemotaxis and chemiluminescence of human peripheral blood neutrophils in vitro and reduces certain inflammatory parameters in vivo." Inflammopharmacology 7(4): 377–386.
Kirkeskov, B., et al. (2011). "The effects of rose hip (*Rosa canina*) on plasma antioxidative activity and C-reactive protein in patients with rheumatoid arthritis and normal controls: A prospective cohort study." Phytomedicine 18: 953–958.
Larsen, E., et al. (2003). "An antiinflammatory galactolipid from rose hip (*Rosa canina*) that inhibits chemotaxis of human peripheral blood neutrophils in vitro." Journal of Natural Products 66(7): 994–995.
Lattanzio, F., et al. (2011). "In vivo anti-inflammatory effect of *Rosa canina* L. extract." Journal of Ethnopharmacology 137(1): 880–885.
Machmudah, S., et al. (2008). "Process optimization and extraction rate analysis of carotenoids extraction from rosehip fruit using supercritical CO2." Journal of Supercritical Fluids 44(3): 308–314.
Marstrand, C., et al. (2013). "The anti-inflammatory capacity of Rose-hip is strongly dependent on the seeds — a comparison of animal and human studies." Osteoarthritis and Cartilage 21, Supplement(0): S216–S217.
Ninomiya, K., et al. (2007). "Potent anti-obese principle from *Rosa canina*: Structural requirements and mode of action of trans-tiliroside." Bioorganic and Medicinal Chemistry Letters 17(11): 3059–3064.
Orhan, N., et al. (2009). "Antidiabetic effect and antioxidant potential of *Rosa canina* fruits." Pharmacognosy Magazine 5(20): 309–315.
Pirone, B. N., et al. (2007). "Chemical characterization and evolution of ascorbic acid concentration during dehydration of rosehip (*Rosa eglanteria*) fruits." American Journal of Food Technology 2(5): 377–387.
Rein, E., et al. (2004). "A herbal remedy, Hyben Vital (stand. powder of a subspecies of *Rosa canina* fruits), reduces pain and improves general wellbeing in patients with osteoarthritis — A double-blind, placebo-controlled, randomised trial." Phytomedicine 11(5): 383–391.
Rossnagel, K. and S. N. Willich (2001). "Importance of complementary medicine exemplified by the use of rose hip." Bedeutung der komplementärmedizin am beispiel der hagebutte 63(6): 412–416.
Rossnagel, K., et al. (2007). "The clinical effectiveness of rosehip powder in patients with osteoarthritis. A systematic review." Klinische wirksamkeit von hagebuttenpulver bei patienten mit arthrose. Eine systematische übersicht 149(27-28 SUPPL.): 51–56.
Schwager, J., et al. (2011). "Rose hip and its constituent galactolipids confer cartilage protection by modulating cytokine, and chemokine expression." BMC Complementary and Alternative Medicine 11(105).
Strålsjö, L., et al. (2003). "Total folate content and retention in rosehips (*Rosa* ssp.) after drying." Journal of Agricultural and Food Chemistry 51(15): 4291–4295.
Türkben, C., et al. (2010). "Effects of different maturity periods and processes on nutritional components of rose hip (*Rosa canina* L.)." Journal of Food, Agriculture and Environment 8(1): 26–30.
Warholm, O.,et al. (2003). "The effects of a standardized herbal remedy made from a subtype of *Rosa canina* in patients with osteoarthritis: A double-blind, randomized, placebo-controlled clinical trial." Current Therapeutic Research — Clinical and Experimental 64(1): 21–31.
Wenzig, E. M., et al. (2008). "Phytochemical composition and in vitro pharmacological activity of two rose hip (*Rosa canina* L.) preparations." Phytomedicine. 15(10): 826–835.
Willich, S. N.,et al. (2010). "Patients with rheumatoid arthritis may benefit from a standardised powder of *Rosa canina* (rose hip)." Focus on Alternative and Complementary Therapies 15(2): 114–115.
Winther, K. (2000). Rose-hip in the form of HybenVital, has no impact on coagulation, platelet function and fibrinoloysis. Third International Exhibition and Conference on Nutraceuticals and Food for Vitality. Palexpo Exhibition and Conference Centre, Geneva, Switzerland.
Winther, K. (2008). "A standardized powder made from rosehips (*Rosa canina* L.) improves function and reduces pain and the consumption of rescue medication in osteoarthritis." Osteoarthritis and Cartilage 16(SUPPL. 1): S8–S9.
Winther, K. A., K., Thamsborg, G. (2005). "A powder made from seeds and shells of a rose-hip subspecies (*Rosa canina*) reduces symptoms of knee and hip osteoarthritis: a randomized, double-blind, placebo-controlled clinical trial." Scand J Rheumatol. 34(4): 302–308.
Winther, K., et al. (1999). "The anti-inflammatory properties of rose-hip." Inflammopharmacology 7(1): 63–68.
Yoo, K. M., et al. (2008). "Relative antioxidant and cytoprotective activities of common herbs." Food Chemistry 106(3): 929–936.

Rosemary

HISTORICAL NOTE Rosemary is an evergreen perennial shrub that is native to Europe (Dias et al 2000) and is grown in many parts of the world (Bakirel et al 2008). Since ancient times, rosemary has been used as a tonic and stimulant. The ancient Greeks used rosemary for stimulating the brain and strengthening memory function (Pengelly et al 2012). Furthermore, scholars wore garlands of rosemary during examinations in order to improve their memory and concentration (Blumenthal et al 2000). Nicolaus Copernicus (1473–1543) was noted to use rosemary, as well as nettle, clivers and pumpkin, for renal ailments (Popowska-Drojecka et al 2011). Rosemary was used in traditional Turkish folk medicine for the treatment of hyperglycaemia (Bakirel et al 2008). Folk medicine described the healing properties of rosemary as well as its use as a microbicide and for the treatment of gastrointestinal disturbances (Dias et al 2000). Some cemeteries have planted rosemary bushes, possibly as a sign to always remember those who have been buried there. It is widely used as a food spice and as an antioxidant to preserve foods.

COMMON NAME

Rosemary

OTHER NAMES

Compass plant, compass weed, garden rosemary, old man, polar plant, *Rosmarini folium*

BOTANICAL NAME/FAMILY

Rosmarinus officinalis (family Labiatae or Lamiaceae)

PLANT PART USED

Fresh or dried leaf

CHEMICAL COMPONENTS

Chemical components include phenolic acids and diterpenoid bitter substances, including rosmarinic acid (Nolkemper et al 2006, Tu et al 2013), carnosic acid and carnosol (Aruoma et al 1992, Bicchi et al 2000, Romo Vaquero et al 2013, Wei & Ho 2006), luteolin 3-glucuronide (Nolkemper et al 2006), triterpenoid acids, flavonoids, tannins and volatile oils (0.5–2.5%) that consist of 1,8-cineole (Kabouche et al 2005, Wang et al 2012), 2-ethyl-4,5-dimethylphenol gamma-terpinene (Kabouche et al 2005), pinene (Blumenthal et al 2000, Wang et al 2012), terpineol, camphor, camphene, borneol and bornyl acetate (Blumenthal et al 2000). Rosemary has also been found to contain high amounts of salicylates (Swain et al 1985).

MAIN ACTIONS

Preclinical research has been conducted with rosemary essential oil, leaves and other preparations. There has also been research with individual constituents such as rosmarinic acid, carnosol and carnosic acid.

Antioxidant

Rosemary has strong antioxidant activity and is widely used to preserve food and cosmetics (Etter 2004). The antioxidant activity of rosemary is due to a variety of compounds, most notably the phenolic abietane diterpenes and phenolic acids such as rosmarinic acid. These antioxidant effects may contribute to membrane stabilisation and the reduction of free radical production, which may assist with the electron donor ability of the rosemary diterpenes in protecting membranes against oxidative damage (Pérez-Fons et al 2010). Rosemary leaf extract has been shown to enhance superoxide dismutase activity (Kim et al 1995) and to have an effect stronger than vitamin E in scavenging oxygen radicals (Zhao et al 1989). The antioxidant activity of rosemary extract was measured by Trolox equivalent antioxidant capacity (TEAC) (Cheung & Tai 2007). The test is based on the reduction of the 2,2'-azino-*bis*(3-ethylbenzothiazoline-6-sulphonic acid) (ABTS) radical cation by antioxidants. Cell-free ABTS OH radical scavenging assay showed that 1/10 and 1/5 dilutions of the rosemary extract had substantial antioxidant activity. In the cell culture studies, rosemary extract at 1/2000 and 1/1000 concentrations significantly inhibited nitric oxide (NO) production by the lipopolysaccharide-activated RAW 264.7 cells in a dose-dependent manner. NO in the culture supernatant was also significantly reduced in the LPS-activated cells.

It is suggested that carnosol and carnosic acid account for over 90% of its antioxidant properties (Aruoma et al 1992, 1996). Carnosic acid has been shown to have a photoprotective action on human dermal fibroblasts exposed to ultraviolet A light in vitro (Offord et al 2002) and rosemary extract inhibits oxidative alterations to skin surface lipids, both in vitro and in vivo (Calabrese et al 2000), as well as enhancing cell-mediated immunity in rats under oxidative stress (Babu et al 1999). Rosmarinic acid has also been investigated for its antioxidant activities and plays an important role in the antioxidant capacities of the extracts containing very similar diterpene concentrations (Jordán et al 2012). In this study, extracts with a lower rosmarinic acid concentration (50:50) exhibited a poorer antioxidant capacity and antioxidant activity was further improved by the presence of carnosol as the major diterpene content.

Antioxidant activity has also been investigated in a model of macular degeneration (Organisciak et al 2013). Sprague-Dawley rats were administered with intraperitoneal rosemary test solution 1 hour before the start of light exposure tests. Rosemary powder extract (34 mg/kg) alone and when combined with zinc (1.3 mg/kg) effectively decreased the extent of retinal light damage. Rosemary (17 mg/kg) plus zinc (1.3 mg/kg) treatment reduced the expression of oxidative stress protein markers and enhanced visual cell survival, as shown by improved photoreceptor cell morphology and by decreased retinal DNA degradation.

Antibacterial

Both rosemary essential oil and rosemary extract exhibit antibacterial properties against a range of organisms, with both preparations being more effective against Gram-positive bacteria.

Rosemary extract demonstrates in vitro antibacterial activity against a variety of bacteria (Del Campo et al 2000, Erdogrul 2002, Ouattara et al 1997), including *Helicobacter pylori* (Mahady et al 2005), *Staphylococcus aureus* (Oluwatuyi et al 2004), *Klebsiella pneumoniae* and *Pseudomonas aeruginosa* (Kabouche et al 2005). The in vitro inhibitory activity of the rosemary methanolic extracts was found to be more effective against the Gram-positive than the Gram-negative food-borne pathogens assayed. A higher concentration of carnosol in relation to carnosic acid was found to improve the degree of the antibacterial activities of the rosemary extracts against *Listeria monocytogenes* and *Staphylococcus aureus* strains (Jordán et al 2012).

Rosemary essential oil and three of its main constituents, 1,8-cineole (27.23%), α-pinene (19.43%) and β-pinene (6.71%), were evaluated for their in vitro antibacterial activities (Wang et al 2012). Five microorganisms consisting of three Gram-positive bacteria (*Bacillus subtilis, Staphylococcus aureus, S. epidermidis*) and two Gram-negative bacteria (*Escherichia coli* and *Pseudomonas aeruginosa*) were tested. Gram-positive bacteria were more sensitive than Gram-negative bacteria to rosemary essential oil, α-pinene and β-pinene. Rosemary essential oil showed greater activity than its components.

Antiulcerogenic activity

Rosemary has potential antiulcer activity. Rosemary extract demonstrated in vitro antibacterial activity against *Helicobacter pylori* (Mahady et al 2005). Dias and colleagues (2000) investigated the antiulcerogenic activity of the crude hydroalcoholic extract (CHE) of rosemary in an experimental rat model. The extract was made from the dried aerial parts of rosemary that were processed to produce a CHE. In the ethanol-induced ulcer model, doses of 100 and 200 mg/kg CHE demonstrated no antiulcerogenic activity, whereas doses of 500 and 1000 mg/kg CHE inhibited the ulcerative lesion index in 70% and 74.6%, respectively. In the indomethacin-induced ulcer model, CHE (1000 mg/kg) inhibited the ulcerative lesion index by 44%. The antiulcerogenic activity of the CHE was also maintained in the ethanol-induced ulcer model, with previous administration of indomethacin, inhibiting the ulcerative lesion index by 70%. The results of this study suggest that the CHE of rosemary has active substances that increase the mucosal non-protein sulfhydryl group content (Dias et al 2000).

Antifungal activity

Topical application of rosemary essential oil preparations exerts antifungal activity (Ouraini et al 2005, Steinmetz et al 1988, Suleimanova et al 1995) and inhibits the growth and aflatoxin production of *Aspergillus* spp. at concentrations between 0.2% and 1% (Tantaoui-Elaraki & Beraoud 1994).

Antiviral

The carnosol constituent found in rosemary demonstrates anti-HIV activity (Aruoma et al 1996) and carnosic acid also demonstrates an inhibitory effect on HIV-1 protease in cell-free assays (Paris et al 1993). Rosemary extract has some antiviral activity against herpes simplex virus (HSV) (Vijayan et al 2004).

Herpes simplex virus

Rosemary and other herbs of the Lamiaceae family were examined for their antiviral activity against HSV. The in vitro testing was on plaque formation of HSV-1 and HSV-2 and an aciclovir-resistant strain of HSV-1. When rosemary extract was added during the adsorption period of viruses to host cells, the number of plaque-forming units was reduced by 36% for HSV-1 and 77% for HSV-2. Pretreatment of host cells with rosemary extracts prior to infection led to a 24% reduction for HSV-1. Pretreatment of HSV-1 and HSV-2 with rosemary extract prior to infection caused a significant decline in the amount of plaque. The results of this study indicate that rosemary extract affected HSV before adsorption but had no effect on intracellular virus replication. Rosemary extract exerted its antiviral effect on free HSV and this offers a potential use for topical therapeutic application against recurrent herpes infections (Nolkemper et al 2006).

Anti-inflammatory

Several different rosemary preparations have demonstrated anti-inflammatory activity using various models.

In vitro studies have found that rosemary extracts inhibited inflammatory-induced peroxynitrite radical and nitrite production (Chan et al 1995, Choi et al 2002) and that carnosol suppresses NO production (Lo et al 2002). Rosmarinic acid has been found to increase the production of prostaglandin E_2, reduce the production of leukotriene B_4 in human polymorphonuclear leucocytes and inhibit the complement system (al-Sereiti et al 1999). The anti-inflammatory and analgesic activity of rosemary essential oil has been confirmed in vivo using several different animal models (Lucarini et al 2013, Takaki et al 2008).

In cell culture studies, rosemary extract at a 1/500 dilution significantly reduced interleukin-1beta (IL-1β) ($P < 0.01$) and cyclooxygenase-2 ($P < 0.05$) mRNA expression and non-significantly reduced tumour necrosis factor-alpha (TNF-α) and inducible NO synthase mRNA expression in lipopolysaccharide-activated cells. Treatment with 1/1000 dilution of rosemary extract had no effect (Cheung & Tai 2007).

Acne

Propionibacterium acnes is a key pathogen involved in the progression of acne inflammation. Tsai et al (2013) investigated the inhibitory effect of rosemary extract on *P. acnes*-induced inflammation (TNF-α, IL-8, and IL-1β) in vitro and in vivo. Treatment with ethanolic rosemary extract significantly suppressed *P. acnes*-induced IL-8, IL-1β and TNF-α production. In addition, ethanolic rosemary extract suppressed the gene expression of IL-8, IL-1β and TNF-α in *P. acnes*-stimulated THP-1 cells. When individual constituents of rosemary were measured, rosmarinic acid significantly reduced the IL-8 production, but had no effect on the IL-1β level. Carnosol and carnosic acid significantly inhibited IL-1β levels at the concentration of 2.5 microM, but significantly increased IL-8 secretion at higher concentrations (10 microM). A mouse model was used to examine the in vivo anti-inflammatory effect of rosemary. Co-injection of ethanolic rosemary extract (1 mg/10 microL) attenuated the granulomatous response to *P. acnes* as compared to co-injection with an equal amount of vehicle, indicating a positive result.

Antispasmodic

Rosemary is widely acknowledged to be a carminative and is used internally as an antispasmodic for mild cramp-like gastrointestinal and biliary upsets, as well as for tension headache, renal colic and dysmenorrhoea (Blumenthal et al 2000). It is also used to relax bronchial smooth muscle in the treatment of asthma (al-Sereiti et al 1999). Antispasmodic activity has been confirmed in a study with isolated guinea pig ileum which tested the effects of different concentrations of an aqueous ethanolic extract of rosemary (Ventura-Martinez et al 2011). A significant dose-dependent activity was observed, which was mediated via calcium channels and muscarinic receptors but not nicotinic receptors, prostaglandins or NO.

Hepatoprotective

The hepatoprotective properties of rosemary extract are attributed to its antioxidant properties and improving detoxification systems dependent on glutathione S-transferase (Sotelo-Felix et al 2002). Rosemary extract has been shown to reduce thioacetamide-induced cirrhosis (Galisteo et al 2000) and azathioprine-induced toxicity in rats (Amin & Hamza 2005), as well as partially prevent carbon tetrachloride-induced liver damage in both rats (Sotelo-Felix et al 2002) and mice (Fahim et al 1999, Sotelo-Felix et al 2002). A water extract of rosemary (200 mg/kg body weight) was investigated for hepatoprotective properties in streptozotocin-induced diabetic rats for 21 days (Ramadan et al 2013). The fresh leaves of rosemary (5 g) were soaked in 50 mL of boiled water with 1 hour of stirring at room temperature. The supernatant was decanted and the residue was macerated for two more days with distilled water. The pooled supernatants were combined and filtered. The treatment group starting with elevated liver function enzymes (aspartate aminotransferase, alanine transaminase and alkaline phosphatase) experienced significantly restored levels, returning to near normal.

There was also a significant increase in total protein and albumin compared to the diabetic rats. The authors note that the hepatoprotective effects of rosemary could be due to the presence of the phenolic and flavonoid compounds and their antioxidant effects. Another thing to note in this study was that serum insulin and C-peptide levels decreased in diabetic animals, whereas rosemary water extract treatment brought about a marked increase in their serum levels in streptozotocin-induced diabetic rats. The water extract also lowered the glucose content to near normal.

Hypoglycaemic effects and activity in insulin resistance

Rosemary leaf extract significantly reduces blood glucose levels in vivo, according to a dose-response study utilising both normoglycaemic and alloxan-induced diabetic test animals (Bakirel et al 2008). Significant glucose-lowering effects were seen when using doses of 100 and 200 mg/kg in normoglycaemic rabbits whereas no significant effect was seen at the lower dose of 50 mg/kg. Two hours after treatment, the 100 mg/kg test dose reduced blood glucose levels by 14.5%, which was short-lived, whereas the higher dose of 200 mg/kg reduced the level by 20.4%, and this remained significant after 6 hours. None of these doses affected insulin levels in the normoglycaemic rabbits.

When the three different rosemary extract doses were tested in hyperglycaemic rabbits, the 50 mg/kg and 100 mg/kg treatments showed a significant effect, with blood glucose levels dropping by 12.4% and 19.9% respectively compared to placebo at 6 hours after glucose administration. At 200 mg/kg a comparatively more potent reduction was observed with the blood glucose levels 30.8% and 35.6%, respectively from that of control after 2 and 6 hours of glucose administration. Of note, the highest treatment dose produced an effect similar in magnitude to glibenclamide at 6 hours post glucose loading.

Further acute dose testing conducted with alloxan-diabetic animals showed significant effects for 200 mg/kg after 6 hours producing a blood glucose decrease of 28.3%, which was similar to glibenclamide, together with a significant increase in insulin levels. The maximal percentages of increase in insulin levels that occurred after 6 hours with rosemary extract or glibenclamide administration were 60.3% and 75.8% in diabetic rabbits, respectively.

A subacute study was then conducted which found the highest dose (200 mg/kg) produced the greatest reduction in blood glucose on the 8th day of treatment (29.5% drop), and this was greater than glibenclamide (18.2%). Interestingly, daily administration of the extract at 200 mg/kg dose to alloxan-diabetic rabbits induced a significant increase in the insulin level on the 5th day when compared with diabetic control rabbits. The magnitude of the increase of insulin after administration of the extract of 200 mg/kg (77.8%) was much closer to that of glibenclamide (75.6%). The doses of 100 mg/kg and 200 mg/kg showed a marked increase on insulin level in alloxan-diabetic rabbits (60.5% and 78.7%, respectively) on day 8. In addition, a significant elevation in serum superoxide dismutase was observed on the 5th day in alloxan-diabetic rabbits given glibenclamide and rosemary (200 mg/kg), which showed 22.1% and 24.4% increase, respectively. A more pronounced activity (25%) was recorded at the later stage for rosemary (200 mg/kg). Inhibition of lipid peroxidation was also observed.

In vivo research conducted by Ibarra et al (2011) showed that rosemary extract (standardised to 20% carnosic acid; 500 mg/kg body weight per day) given to test animals on a high-fat diet resulted in 72% ($P < 0.01$) less increase in plasma glucose levels and a rise in total cholesterol and a significant 12-fold increase ($P < 0.01$) in total faecal content compared with mice on a high-fat diet and not receiving rosemary extract. These results suggest that the reduction of weight gain induced by rosemary extract was mediated, at least partially, through a limitation of lipid absorption. More research is

R

required to understand this mechanism of action and its possible applications. Rosmarinic acid shows potential in reducing cardiovascular risk-associated insulin resistance and metabolic syndrome. Rosmarinic acid supplementation (oral dosage of 10 mg/kg/day) to fructose-fed rats significantly improved insulin sensitivity, reduced lipid levels and oxidative damage, and the expression of p22phox subunit of nicotinamide adenine dinucleotide phosphate reduced oxidase and prevented cardiac hypertrophy. Blood pressure was also lowered by rosmarinic acid through a decrease in endothelin-1 and angiotensin-converting enzyme activity and increase in NO levels (Karthik et al 2011).

Harach et al (2010) investigated the effects of rosemary leaf extract (20 or 200 mg/kg body weight) on the prevention of weight gain and associated metabolic disorders in mice fed a high-fat diet. The final weight gain of the mice treated with 200 mg/kg body weight of rosemary extract was significantly reduced by 64% when compared with the control group. The reduction of weight gain was associated with a significant reduction of body fat mass gain (–57%). Treatment with 200 mg/kg body weight of rosemary extract also increased lipid excretion in the faeces.

Carnosic acid and derived diterpenes abundant in rosemary extracts have been found to exert anti-obesity effects (Romo Vaquero et al 2013), with carnosic acid inhibiting adipogenesis in vivo (Wang et al 2011). Carnosic acid added to test animal chow significantly inhibited the gain of body weight after 3 weeks ($P < 0.01$). A magnetic resonance imaging (MRI) analysis revealed the areas of the abdomen ($P < 0.01$), abdominal cavity ($P < 0.05$) and visceral fat regions ($P < 0.05$) in mice fed the carnosic acid diet to be significantly smaller than those in the control mice. A significant reduction of the levels of serum triglycerides, cholesterol and alanine aminotransferase in mice of the carnosic acid group was also observed in comparison to controls. Active treatment also led to a significant decrease in the weight of liver mass in comparison to the controls (Wang et al 2011).

Neuroprotective effects

Carnosic acid and carnosol, which are major components of rosemary, have been found to markedly enhance synthesis of nerve growth factor in vitro (Kosaka & Yokoi 2003). Carnosic acid exhibits neuroprotective effects in vitro via its antioxidant activity and induction of antioxidant enzyme expression by means of activation of nuclear factor erythroid 2-related factor 2 transcription pathway. This neuroprotective effect is considered to be beneficial in the prevention of chronic neurodegenerative diseases (Kayashima & Matsubara 2012). For the development of carnosic acid as a protective agent against neurodegenerative diseases, penetration into the brain is an essential requirement. To examine this aspect, Satoh and colleagues (2008) administered carnosic acid orally to mice (3 mg per 25 g mouse) and measured the level of carnosic acid (catechol form) in serum and brain parenchyma by high-performance liquid chromatography. Within 1 hour, carnosic acid reached significant levels in the brain, suggesting that carnosic acid was able to penetrate the blood–brain barrier. In another section of the study, mice were allowed free access to food containing 0.03% carnosic acid for a week. Their brains were then removed and measured for reduced glutathione (GSH) and glutathione disulfide (GSSG) levels. Carnosic acid increased both total GSH + GSSG and the ratio of GSH/GSSG. More research is required on this potential pathway in neuroprotection.

A study investigated the protective mechanism of carnosic acid on ischaemia-reperfusion and hypoxia-induced neuronal cell injury. The results showed that carnosic acid reduced 52% of the infarct volume from brains under ischaemia-reperfusion in vivo and protected the PC12 cells from hypoxic injury in vitro. Carnosic acid at a concentration of 1.0 microM enhanced cell viability, scavenged reactive oxygen species, increased superoxide dismutase activity, prevented lactic dehydrogenase release and attenuated Ca^{2+} release, lipid peroxidation and prostaglandin E_2 production in hypoxic PC12 cells (Hou et al 2012).

Chemoprotection and antimutagenic effects

Evidence from animal and cell culture studies demonstrates the anticancer potential of rosemary extract, carnosol, carnosic acid, ursolic acid and rosmarinic acid against several types of cancers (Ngo et al 2011). The effects appear to be dose-related and not tissue- or species-specific. For example, rosemary has been shown to suppress the development of tumours in several organs, including the colon, breast, liver and stomach, as well as melanoma and leukaemia cells, and is most likely to be due to the modulation of different molecular target.

In vivo studies suggest that rosemary extract may reduce the effects of carcinogenic or toxic agents on many cell lines, including rat mammary gland (Amagase et al 1996, Singletary et al 1996), mouse liver and stomach (Singletary & Rokusek 1997), bone marrow (Fahim et al 1999) and skin (Huang et al 1994).

An in vitro study on human bronchial cells found that rosemary extract and its constituents, carnosol and carnosic acid, may have chemoprotective activity by decreasing carcinogen activation via inhibition of the enzyme cytochrome P450 (CYP1A1) and increasing carcinogen detoxification by induction of phase II enzymes (Offord et al 1995). Carnosol has been found to also restrict the invasive ability of mouse melanoma cells in vitro by reducing matrix metallopeptidase-9 expression and activity (Huang et al 2005).

Cigarette smoking is causally associated with a large number of human cancers and rosemary may reduce the risk of cigarette-induced lung cancer (Alexandrov et al 2006). Benzo(a)pyrene (BP) is a highly carcinogenic polycyclic aromatic hydrocarbon present in emission exhausts, charbroiled food, and in small quantities of cigarette smoke. It is metabolically activated into BP-7,8-diol-9,10-epoxide (BPDE), which reacts with DNA predominantly at the N^2 position of guanine to produce primarily N^2-guanine lesions. More research is suggested in this novel use of rosemary. The BPDE-dG adduct is exclusively concentrated in bronchial cells and has been implicated in the initiation of human lung cancer. The modified cigarette filter containing rosemary extract decreased BPDE-dG adduct level by >70% due to the cigarette smoke oxygen-generated radicals in MCF-7 cells. A 30% decrease in the hydroxyl radical was also observed.

Cheung and Tai (2007) investigated the antiproliferative properties of rosemary on several human cancer cell lines. Rosemary extract induced differential antiproliferative activity on the breast and leukaemia cell lines tested, with HL60 being the most susceptible, and MCF7 the most resistant. IC50 was estimated at 1/700, 1/500, 1/400 and 1/150 for the HL60, MDA-MB-468, K562 and MCF7 cells, respectively. In addition, a 1/1000 dilution of rosemary extract induced 9.5 ± 2.2% of HL60 cell differentiation along granulocyte lineage with $P < 0.01$ compared to the untreated control at 2.8 ± 0.8%.

Increases oestrogen metabolism

Feeding female mice a 2% rosemary diet enhanced the liver microsomal metabolism of endogenous oestrogens (Zhu et al 1998), thereby reducing oestrogen levels.

Antiobesity

Carnosic acid and derived diterpenes abundant in rosemary extracts have been found to exert anti-obesity effects (Romo Vaquero et al 2013), with carnosic acid inhibiting adipogenesis in vivo (Wang et al 2011).

Ob/ob mice were fed a chow diet supplemented with or without carnosic acid for 5 weeks. Carnosic acid significantly inhibited the gain of body weight after 3 weeks of treatment ($P < 0.01$). An MRI analysis revealed the areas of the abdomen ($P < 0.01$), abdominal cavity ($P < 0.05$) and visceral fat regions ($P < 0.05$) in mice fed the carnosic acid diet to be significantly smaller than those in the control mice. A significant reduction of the levels of serum triglycerides, cholesterol and alanine aminotransferase in mice of the carnosic acid group was observed in comparison to the mice of the non-carnosic acid group. In addition, the mice of the carnosic acid group showed a significant improvement in the non-fasting glucose levels and glucose tolerance 30 and 120 minutes after glucose loading. Mice of the carnosic acid group had a significant decrease in the weight of liver mass in comparison to the controls (Wang et al 2011). Ibarra et al (2011) investigated the effect of rosemary extract (standardised to 20% carnosic acid) in mice. Mice were given a low-fat diet, a high-fat diet or a high-fat diet supplemented with 500 mg rosemary extract/kg body weight per day. Mice in the high-fat diet plus rosemary group experienced 72% ($P < 0.01$) less increase in plasma glucose levels and 68% ($P < 0.001$) less rise in total cholesterol and a significant 12-fold increase ($P < 0.01$) in total faecal content compared with high-fat-diet mice. In vitro studies found rosemary extract (100 mcg/mL) inhibited pancreatic lipase activity and extracts at 30 and 100 mcg/mL activated peroxisome proliferator-activated receptor-γ. Harach et al (2010) investigated the effects of rosemary leaf extract (20 or 200 mg/kg body weight) on the prevention of weight gain and associated metabolic disorders in mice fed a high-fat diet. The final weight gain of the mice treated with 200 mg/kg body weight of rosemary extract was significantly reduced by 64% when compared with the control group. The reduction of weight gain was associated with a significant reduction of body fat mass gain (−57%). Treatment with 200 mg/kg body weight of rosemary extract also increased lipid excretion in the faeces. Rosemary extract was able to inhibit pancreatic lipase activity in vitro. The results of this study suggest that the reduction of weight gain induced by rosemary extract was mediated, at least partially, through a limitation of lipid absorption. More research is required on this action.

OTHER ACTIONS

Rosemary demonstrates significant antithrombotic activity in vitro and in vivo, possibly through a direct inhibitory effect on platelets (Yamamoto et al 2005).

Rosemary essential oil and its constituent monoterpenes, such as borneol, inhibit bone resorption in the rat (Muhlbauer et al 2003). Aqueous and ethanol extracts of rosemary have been found to produce significant antinociceptive activity and diminish morphine withdrawal syndrome in rats (Hosseinzadeh & Nourbakhsh 2003).

When used topically, rosemary essential oil is said to stimulate the skin and increase blood circulation (Blumenthal et al 2000).

Powdered rosemary leaves are said to be effective as a natural flea and tick repellent and rosemary essential oil has been found to be ovicidal and repellent towards mosquito (Prajapati et al 2005).

CLINICAL USE

Increased mental concentration

Several clinical trials of different designs have been conducted demonstrating that inhalation of rosemary oil affects various aspects of brain function generally, leading to improved memory and increased alertness with greater relaxation. Less research has been conducted with orally ingested rosemary extract.

In 2002, a small case series of 10 subjects found that rosemary essential oil had positive effects on mood concentration and memory (Svoboda et al

Clinical note — Carnosol investigation in cancer

The constituent carnosol found in rosemary has been the subject of extensive preclinical research as a potential treatment in various cancers, including prostate, breast, skin, leukaemia and colon cancer, with promising results (Johnson 2011). Multiple mechanisms of action have been discovered for carnosol which are associated with inflammation and cancer, such as antiangiogenic activity (Kayashima & Matsubara 2012) and effects on NF-κB, apoptotic-related proteins, phosphatidylinositol-3-kinase/Akt, androgen and oestrogen receptors, as well as molecular targets (Johnson 2011). When administered to test animals, it displays selective toxicity against tumour cells and is well tolerated.

2002). A 2003 randomised controlled trial of 140 subjects found that a 5-minute inhalation of rosemary essential oil placed on diffuser pads in an aroma stream produced a significant enhancement of performance for overall quality of memory and secondary memory factors, but also produced an impairment of speed of memory compared with controls (Moss et al 2003). Further support comes from an observational study in 40 adults where a 3-minute exposure to rosemary essential oil was seen to decrease frontal alpha and beta power, suggesting increased alertness. Subjects felt more relaxed and alert, had lower anxiety scores and were faster, but not more accurate, at completing mathematical computations (Diego et al 1998). Sayorwan et al (2013) examined the effects of rosemary oil inhalation on the nervous system in 10 males and 10 females (age range 18–28 years). Brain electrical activity and autonomic nervous system parameters (blood pressure, heart rate, respiratory rate and skin temperature) were recorded as the indicators of the arousal level of the nervous system. After rosemary oil exposure, heart rate, blood pressure and respiratory rate had significantly increased ($P < 0.010$). In contrast, skin temperature had decreased significantly. During the sessions of rosemary inhalation, the power of the alpha1 waves in the left and right anterior and right posterior regions was significantly decreased ($P < 0.05$). The power changes in the alpha2 waves were also significantly decreased during rosemary inhalation, and was shown in all areas of the brain ($P < 0.05$). In contrast, the power of the beta waves in the left and the right anterior brain regions was significantly increased. The participants felt fresher and became more active and less drowsy after exposure to the rosemary oil ($P < 0.05$). A small case series of 10 subjects also found that rosemary essential oil had positive effects on mood concentration and memory (Svoboda et al 2002). Moss et al (2003) demonstrated significantly enhanced overall memory quality but impaired memory speed using rosemary essential oil placed on diffuser pads in an aroma stream placed in test cubicles and switched on for 5 minutes prior to testing (n = 140, divided into three groups: lavender, rosemary and control).

Orally ingested rosemary extract

A double-blind crossover randomised controlled trial of 27 older adults (mean age 75 years) identified a biphasic dose-dependent effect in measures of speed of memory for acute oral rosemary treatment, with the lowest dose (750 mg) producing a statistically significant beneficial effect compared with placebo ($P = 0.01$), whereas the highest dose (6000 mg) had a significant impairing effect ($P < 0.01$). In regard to alertness, once again the lower dose of 750 mg produced a significant improvement ($P = 0.01$) compared with placebo, whereas an opposite effect was found at 6000 mg, which was worse than placebo ($P = 0.02$) (Pengelly et al 2012). This lower dose is more similar to levels found in culinary consumption. Less consistent were deleterious effects on other measures of cognitive performance. Further research using multiple doses of low concentrations may yield different effects and is worthy of greater exploration.

Alopecia — in combination

The traditional use of rosemary to stimulate hair growth is supported by a 7-month, randomised, double-blind study of 86 patients that found that rubbing oils (thyme, rosemary, lavender and cedarwood) into the scalp helped with alopecia for 44% of patients versus 15% of controls (Hay et al 1998).

While the role of rosemary as a stand-alone treatment in achieving these results is unclear, results from in vivo research indicate that topical rosemary leaf extract can improve hair regrowth, most likely by inhibition of dihydrotestosterone binding to androgen receptors (Murata et al 2013).

Chemoprotective and adjunct in cancer therapy

Rosemary was used topically to treat cancer in ancient Greece and South America. Although controlled trials are yet to be conducted, it has been suggested that rosemary may delay and inhibit tumour formation in women with breast cancer (Abascal & Yarnell 2001) and that it has potential as a preventive agent or as an adjunct in cancer therapy. An in vitro study in human breast cancer cells found that rosemary extract increased the intracellular accumulation of commonly-used chemotherapeutic agents, including doxorubicin and vinblastine via inhibition of P-glycoprotein, thereby overcoming multidrug resistance in tumour cells (Plouzek et al 1999). Clinical studies are required to determine whether the effect is significant.

Potential use in drug withdrawal

Solhi and colleagues (2013) investigated the efficacy of oral rosemary leaves in capsules as an adjunct therapy for alleviation of withdrawal syndrome in opium abuse (n = 81). People either received rosemary treatment or acted as controls and all were treated with methadone. The treatment regimen was 20 mg/day in the first week, then 15 mg/day in the second week, followed by 10 mg/day in the third week and 5 mg/day in the fourth week. The rosemary capsules were filled with 300 mg of dried powdered leaves and administrated to the patients in the case group as 16 capsules/day for the first 3 days, 12 capsules/day for the following 4 days, and then 8 capsules for the next week in divided doses. Subjects in the active treatment group had significantly better duration of sleep on the third and seventh days compared to the control group ($P < 0.001$ and $P < 0.002$, respectively) and experienced less severe withdrawal symptoms compared to those in the control group, particularly bone pain, perspiration and insomnia. The differences were statistically significant for the third and seventh days ($P < 0.05$).

OTHER USES

When applied topically, rosemary oil may stimulate the blood supply and act as supportive therapy for rheumatic conditions and circulatory problems (Blumenthal et al 2000). Topically, rosemary has also been used for wound healing, as an insect repellent and to treat toothache and eczema. Rosemary extract cream preparations have been shown to protect against sodium lauryl sulfate-induced irritant contact dermatitis (Fuchs et al 2005).

In a small, uncontrolled, prospective pilot study of eight women, rosemary in combination with 11 other botanical extracts was found to relieve menopausal symptoms (Smolinski et al 2005).

Acne

Rosemary shows potential in the treatment of acne. In vitro and mouse model studies showed that rosemary significantly suppressed *Propionibacterium acnes*-induced IL-8, IL-1β and TNF-α production and granulomatous response to *P. acnes*, respectively (Tsai et al 2013). Further research is warranted to determine its potential role in clinical practice for acne management.

Herpes simplex virus

In an in vitro study, rosemary extract exerted an antiviral effect on free HSV. This effect offers a potential use for topical therapeutic application of rosemary against recurrent herpes infections (Nolkemper et al 2006).

Cardiovascular disease

Rosmarinic acid shows potential in reducing cardiovascular disease risk, insulin resistance and metabolic syndrome as significantly improved insulin sensitivity, reduced lipid levels and oxidative damage have been exhibited in a preclinical model. Blood pressure was also lowered by rosmarinic acid through a decrease in endothelin-1 and angiotensin-converting enzyme activity and increase in NO levels (Karthik et al 2011). Additionally, rosmarinic acid (25 micromol/L) and carnosic acid (25 micromol/L) inhibited low-density lipoprotein (LDL) oxidation by 40.8% and 22.6%, respectively (Fuhrman et al 2000). Synergistic antioxidative effects with rosmarinic acid or carnosic acid (58.4% and 38.0%, respectively) were found against LDL oxidation when lycopene was added to LDL.

Age-related macular degeneration

Age-related macular degeneration is a multifactorial disease with an increased risk of vision loss associated with oxidation and inflammation (Organisciak et al 2013). Rosemary extract may have benefits in delaying or slowing the progression of macular degeneration according to results from research conducted with animal models that tested rosemary extract administered as an intraperitoneal injection before light exposure, which showed protection against macular changes by enhancing visual cell survival.

DOSAGE RANGE

- Infusion of dried leaf: 2–4 g three times daily.
- Fluid extract (45%): 1–4 mL three times daily.
- Topical preparations containing 6–10% essential oil can be applied directly to skin. Often a carrier oil, such as almond oil, is used as a vehicle for the essential oil.
- Bath additive: 10 drops essential oil added to bath.

ADVERSE REACTIONS

Rosemary is generally recognised as safe for human consumption in quantities used as food. Consuming large amounts of rosemary may cause stomach and intestinal irritation, as well as seizures, owing to the high content of highly reactive monoterpene ketones, such as camphor (Burkhard et al 1999). Topically, rosemary is not considered to be highly allergenic; however, allergic contact dermatitis from rosemary has been reported (Fernandez et al 1997, Hjorther et al 1997, Inui & Katayama 2005), as has asthma from repeated occupational exposure (Lemiere et al 1996). Rosemary essential oil should be diluted before topical application to minimise irritation.

R

SIGNIFICANT INTERACTIONS

Controlled studies are not available; therefore, interactions are based on evidence of activity and are largely theoretical and speculative.

Iron

Rosemary extracts are widely used as an antioxidant to preserve foods; however, the phenolic-rich extracts may reduce the uptake of dietary iron (Samman et al 2001). Separate doses by 2 hours.

Anticoagulants

Increased bruising and bleeding theoretically possible — use caution.

Drugs dependent on P-glycoprotein transport

Theoretically, increased drug uptake can occur with those drugs dependent on P-glycoprotein transport.

The clinical significance of this finding remains to be tested, although it has been suggested that this activity may be used to enhance the effects of chemotherapeutic agents (Plouzek et al 1999).

CONTRAINDICATIONS AND PRECAUTIONS

None known.

PREGNANCY USE

Rosemary has been shown to have an anti-implantation effect in rats, without interfering with normal fetal development postimplantation (Lemonica et al 1996). It is not recommended in pregnancy in doses higher than the usual dietary intake levels until safety is established or only under professional supervision.

Practice points/Patient counselling

- Rosemary is widely used as a food seasoning and preservative.
- Rosemary extract exhibits antioxidant, antibacterial, anti-inflammatory, hepatoprotective, neuroprotective and chemoprotective activities in various in vitro and experimental models.
- Rosemary oil is widely used to assist in concentration and memory and to stimulate blood flow. There is some research that low doses of powdered rosemary leaf taken orally can improve memory speed in older adults.
- Traditionally, it has been used to as an antispasmodic agent to relieve stomach, gallbladder and menstrual cramps. Preclinical research confirms rosemary has significant antispasmodic activity.
- Rosemary is generally safe when the leaves are consumed in dietary amounts, although excessive intake may cause stomach irritation and seizures in susceptible people.

REFERENCES

Alexandrov K et al. DNA damage by benzo(a)pyrene in human cells is increased by cigarette smoke and decreased by a filter containing rosemary extract, which lowers free radicals. Cancer Res 66.24 (2006): 11938–45.

al-Sereiti MR, et al. Pharmacology of rosemary (*Rosmarinus officinalis* Linn.) and its therapeutic potentials. Indian J Exp Biol 37.2 (1999): 124–30.

Amagase H et al. Dietary rosemary suppresses 7,12-dimethylbenz(a) anthracene binding to rat mammary cell DNA. J Nutr 126.5 (1996): 1475–80.

Amin A, Hamza AA. Hepatoprotective effects of *Hibiscus, Rosmarinus* and *Salvia* on azathioprine-induced toxicity in rats. Life Sci 77.3 (2005): 266–78.

Aruoma OI et al. Antioxidant and pro-oxidant properties of active rosemary constituents: carnosol and carnosic acid. Xenobiotica 22.2 (1992): 257–68.

Aruoma OI et al. An evaluation of the antioxidant and antiviral action of extracts of rosemary and Provencal herbs. Food ChemToxicol 34.5 (1996): 449–56.

Babu US, et al. Effect of dietary rosemary extract on cell-mediated immunity of young rats. Plant Foods Hum Nutr 53.2 (1999): 169–74.

Bakirel T et al. In vivo assessment of antidiabetic and antioxidant activities of rosemary (*Rosmarinus officinalis*) in alloxan-diabetic rabbits. J Ethnopharmacol 116.1 (2008): 64–73.

Bicchi C et al. Determination of phenolic diterpene antioxidants in Rosemary (*Rosmarinus officinalis* L.) with different methods of extraction and analysis. Phytochem Anal 11.4 (2000): 236–42.

Blumenthal M et al. (eds) Herbal medicine: expanded Commission E monographs. Austin, TX: American Botanical Council, 2000.

Burkhard PR et al. Plant-induced seizures: reappearance of an old problem. J Neurol 246.8 (1999): 667–70.

Calabrese V et al. Biochemical studies of a natural antioxidant isolated from rosemary and its application in cosmetic dermatology. Int J Tissue React 22.1 (2000): 5–13.

Chan M-Y, et al. Effects of three dietary phytochemicals from tea, rosemary and turmeric on inflammation-induced nitrite production. Cancer Lett 96.1 (1995): 23–9.

Cheung S and Tai J. Anti-proliferative and antioxidant properties of rosemary *Rosmarinus officinalis*. Oncol Rep 17.6 (2007): 1525–31.

Choi HR et al. Peroxynitrite scavenging activity of herb extracts. Phytother Res 16.4 (2002): 364–7.

Del Campo J, et al. Antimicrobial effect of rosemary extracts. J Food Protect 63.10 (2000): 1359–68.

Dias PC et al. Antiulcerogenic activity of crude hydroalcoholic extract of *Rosmarinus officinalis* L. J Ethnopharmacol. 69.1 (2000): 57–62.

Diego MA et al. Aromatherapy positively affects mood, EEG patterns of alertness and math computations. Int J Neurosci 96.3–4 (1998): 217–24.

Erdogrul OT. Antibacterial activities of some plant extracts used in folk medicine. Pharm Biol 40.4 (2002): 269–73.

Etter SC. *Rosmarinus officinalis* as an antioxidant. J Herbs Spices Med Plants 11.1–2 (2004): 121–59.

Fahim FA et al. Allied studies on the effect of *Rosmarinus officinalis* L. on experimental hepatotoxicity and mutagenesis. Int J Food SciNutr 50.6 (1999): 413–27.

Fernandez L et al. Allergic contact dermatitis from rosemary (*Rosmarinus officinalis* L.). Contact Dermatitis 37.5 (1997): 248–9.

Fuchs SM et al. Protective effects of different marigold (*Calendula officinalis* L.) and rosemary cream preparations against sodium-lauryl-sulfate-induced irritant contact dermatitis. Skin Pharmacol Physiol 18.4 (2005): 195–200.

Fuhrman B et al. Lycopene synergistically inhibits LDL oxidation in combination with vitamin E, glabridin, rosmarinic acid, carnosic acid, or garlic. Antioxid Redox Signal 2.3 (2000): 491–506.

Galisteo M et al. Antihepatotoxic activity of *Rosmarinus tomentosus* in a model of acute hepatic damage induced by thioacetamide. Phytother Res 14.7 (2000): 522–6.

Harach T et al. Rosemary (*Rosmarinus officinalis* L.) leaf extract limits weight gain and liver steatosis in mice fed a high-fat diet. Planta Med 76.6 (2010): 566–71.

Hay IC, et al. Randomized trial of aromatherapy: successful treatment for alopecia areata [comment]. Arch Dermatol 134.11 (1998): 1349–52.

Hjorther AB et al. Occupational allergic contact dermatitis from carnosol, a naturally-occurring compound present in rosemary. Contact Dermatitis 37.3 (1997): 99–100.

Hosseinzadeh H, Nourbakhsh M. Effect of *Rosmarinus officinalis* L. aerial parts extract on morphine withdrawal syndrome in mice. Phytother Res 17.8 (2003): 938–41.

Hou CW et al. Neuroprotective effects of carnosic acid on neuronal cells under ischemic and hypoxic stress. Nutr Neurosci. 2012 Jun 7 (epub ahead of print).

Huang MT et al. Inhibition of skin tumorigenesis by rosemary and its constituents carnosol and ursolic acid. Cancer Res 54.3 (1994): 701–8.

Huang S-C et al. Carnosol inhibits the invasion of B16/F10 mouse melanoma cells by suppressing metalloproteinase-9 through down-regulating nuclear factor-kappa B and c-Jun. Biochem Pharmacol 69.2 (2005): 221–32.

Ibarra A et al. Carnosic acid-rich rosemary (*Rosmarinus officinalis* L.) leaf extract limits weight gain and improves cholesterol levels and glycaemia in mice on a high-fat diet. Br J Nutr 106.8 (2011): 1182–9.

Inui S, Katayama I. Allergic contact dermatitis induced by rosemary leaf extract in a cleansing gel. J Dermatol 32.8 (2005): 667–9.

Johnson JJ. Carnosol: a promising anti-cancer and anti-inflammatory agent. Cancer Lett., 305.1 (2011): 1–7.

Jordán MJ et al. Relevance of carnosic acid, carnosol, and rosmarinic acid concentrations in the in vitro antioxidant and antimicrobial activities of *Rosmarinus officinalis* (L.) methanolic extracts. J Agric Food Chem 60.38 (2012): 9603–8.

Kabouche Z et al. Comparative antibacterial activity of five Lamiaceae essential oils from Algeria. Intl J of Aroma 15.3 (2005): 129–33.

Karthik D et al. Administration of rosmarinic acid reduces cardiopathology and blood pressure through inhibition of p22phox NADPH oxidase in fructose-fed hypertensive rats. J Cardiovasc Pharmacol 58.8 (2011): 514–21.

Kayashima T, Matsubara K. Antiangiogenic effect of carnosic acid and carnosol, neuroprotective compounds in rosemary leaves. Biosci Biotechnol Biochem 76.1 (2012):115–9.

Kim SJ et al. Measurement of superoxide dismutase-like activity of natural antioxidants. Biosci Biotech Biochem 59.5 (1995): 822–6.

Kosaka K, Yokoi T. Carnosic acid, a component of rosemary (*Rosmarinus officinalis* L.), promotes synthesis of nerve growth factor in T98g human glioblastoma cells. Biol Pharm Bull 26.11 (2003): 1620–2.

Lemiere C et al. Occupational asthma caused by aromatic herbs. Allergy 51.9 (1996): 647–9.

Lemonica IP, et al. Study of the embryotoxic effects of an extract of rosemary (*Rosmarinus officinalis* L.). Braz J Med Biol Res 29.2 (1996): 223–7.

Lo AH et al. Carnosol, an antioxidant in rosemary, suppresses inducible nitric oxide synthase through down-regulating nuclear factor-kappa B in mouse macrophages. Carcinogenesis 23.6 (2002): 983–91.

Lucarini R et al. In vivo analgesic and anti-inflammatory activities of *Rosmarinus officinalis* aqueous extracts, rosmarinic acid and its acetyl ester derivative. Pharm Biol. 2013 Jun 5. [Epub ahead of print].

Mahady GB et al. In vitro susceptibility of *Helicobacter pylori* to botanical extracts used traditionally for the treatment of gastrointestinal disorders. Phytother Res 19.11 (2005): 988–91.

Moss M et al. Aromas of rosemary and lavender essential oils differentially affect cognition and mood in healthy adults. Int J Neurosci 113.1 (2003): 15–38.

Muhlbauer RC et al. Common herbs, essential oils, and monoterpenes potently modulate bone metabolism. Bone 32.4 (2003): 372–80.

Murata K et al. Promotion of hair growth by *Rosmarinus officinalis* leaf extract. Phytother. Res 27.2 (2013): 212–217.

Ngo SN et al. Rosemary and cancer prevention: preclinical perspectives. Crit Rev. Food Sci. Nutr 51.10 (2011): 946–954.

Nolkemper S et al. Antiviral effect of aqueous extracts from species of the Lamiaceae family against herpes simplex virus type 1 and type 2 in vitro. Planta Med. 72.15 (2006): 1378–82.

Offord EA et al. Rosemary components inhibit benzo[a]pyrene-induced genotoxicity in human bronchial cells. Carcinogenesis 16.9 (1995): 2057–62.

Offord EA et al. Photoprotective potential of lycopene, beta-carotene, vitamin E, vitamin C and carnosic acid in UVA-irradiated human skin fibroblasts. Free Radic Biol Med 32.12 (2002): 1293–303.

Oluwatuyi M, et al. Antibacterial and resistance modifying activity of *Rosmarinus officinalis*. Phytochemistry 65.24 (2004): 3249–54.

Organisciak DT et al. Prevention of retinal light damage by zinc oxide combined with rosemary extract. Mol Vis 19 (2013): 1433–45.

Ouattara B et al. Antibacterial activity of selected fatty acids and essential oils against six meat spoilage organisms. Int J Food Microbiol 37.2–3 (1997): 155–62.

Ouraini D et al. Therapeutic approach to dermatophytoses by essential oils of some Moroccan aromatic plants. Phytotherapie 3.1 (2005): 3–12.

Paris A et al. Inhibitory effect of carnosic acid on HIV-1 protease in cell-free assays [corrected] [erratum appears in J Nat Prod 57.4 (1994): 552]. J Nat Prod 56.8 (1993): 1426–30.

Pengelly A et al. Short-term study on the effects of rosemary on cognitive function in an elderly population. J Med Food 15.1 (2012): 10–17.

Pérez-Fons L et al. Relationship between the antioxidant capacity and effect of rosemary (*Rosmarinus officinalis* L.) polyphenols on membrane phospholipid order. J Agric Food Chem 58.1 (2010):161–71.

Plouzek CA et al. Inhibition of P-glycoprotein activity and reversal of multidrug resistance in vitro by rosemary extract. Eur J Cancer 35.10 (1999): 1541–5.

Popowska-Drojecka J et al. Was the famous astronomer Copernicus also a nephrologist? J Nephrol 24.S17 (2011):S33–6.

Prajapati V et al. Insecticidal, repellent and oviposition-deterrent activity of selected essential oils against *Anopheles stephensi, Aedes aegypti* and *Culex quinquefasciatus*. Bioresource Technol 96.16 (2005): 1749–57.

Ramadan KS et al. Hypoglycemic and hepatoprotective activity of *Rosmarinus officinalis* extract in diabetic rats. J Physiol Biochem. 69.4 (2013): 779–83.

Romo Vaquero M et al. Bioavailability of the major bioactive diterpenoids in a rosemary extract: Metabolic profile in the intestine, liver, plasma, and brain of Zucker rats. Mol Nutr Food Res. 2013 57: 1834–1846.

Samman S et al. Green tea or rosemary extract added to foods reduces nonheme-iron absorption. Am J ClinNutr 73.3 (2001): 607–12.

Satoh T et al. Carnosic acid, a catechol-type electrophilic compound, protects neurons both in vitro and in vivo through activation of the Keap1/Nrf2 pathway via S-alkylation of targeted cysteines on Keap. J Neurochem 104.4 (2008): 1116–1131.

Sayorwan W et al. Effects of inhaled rosemary oil on subjective feelings and activities of the nervous system. Sci Pharm 81.2 (2013): 531–42.

Singletary KW, Rokusek JT. Tissue-specific enhancement of xenobiotic detoxification enzymes in mice by dietary rosemary extract. Plant Foods Hum Nutr 50.1 (1997): 47–53.

Singletary K et al. Inhibition by rosemary and carnosol of 7,12-dimethylbenz[a]anthracene (DMBA)-induced rat mammary tumorigenesis and in vivo DMBA-DNA adduct formation. Cancer Lett 104.1 (1996): 43–8.

Smolinski D et al. A pilot study to examine a combination botanical for the treatment of menopausal symptoms. J Alt Complement Med 11.3 (2005): 483–9.

Solhi H et al. Beneficial effects of *Rosmarinus officinalis* for treatment of opium withdrawal syndrome during addiction treatment programs: a clinical trial. Addict Health. 5.3–4 (2013): 90–4.

Sotelo-Felix JI et al. Evaluation of the effectiveness of *Rosmarinus officinalis* (Lamiaceae) in the alleviation of carbon tetrachloride-induced acute hepatotoxicity in the rat. J Ethnopharmacol 81.2 (2002): 145–54.

Steinmetz MD et al. Transmission and scanning electronmicroscopy study of the action of sage and rosemary essential oils and eucalyptol on *Candida albicans*. Mycoses 31.1 (1988): 40–51.

Suleimanova AB et al. Experimental assessment of fungicidal activity of 3% ointment with wild rosemary ether oil in external therapy of T. rubrum-induced mycosis of the soles. Vestn Dermatol Venerol 71.1 (1995): 17–18 (in Russian).

Svoboda KP et al. Case study: The effects of selected essential oils on mood, concentration and sleep in a group of 10 students monitored for 5 weeks. Int J Aromather 12.3 (2002): 157–61.

Swain AR et al. Salicylates in foods. J Am Diet Assoc 85.8 (1985): 950–60.

Takaki I et al. Anti-inflammatory and antinociceptive effects of *Rosmarinus officinalis* L. essential oil in experimental animal models. J Med Food 11.4 (2008): 741–746.

Tantaoui-Elaraki A, Beraoud L. Inhibition of growth and aflatoxin production in *Aspergillus parasiticus* by essential oils of selected plant materials. J Environ Pathol Toxicol Oncol 13.1 (1994): 67–72.

Tsai TH et al. *Rosmarinus officinalis* extract suppresses *Propionibacterium acnes*-induced inflammatory responses. J Med Food 16.4 (2013): 324–33.

Tu Z et al. Rosemary (*Rosmarinus officinalis* L.) extract regulates glucose and lipid metabolism by activating AMPK and PPAR pathways in HepG2 cells. J Agric Food Chem. 61.11 (2013): 2803–10.

Ventura-Martinez R et al. Spasmolytic activity of *Rosmarinus officinalis* L. involves calcium channels in the guinea pig ileum. J Ethnopharmacol 137.3 (2011): 1528–1532.

Vijayan P et al. Antiviral activity of medicinal plants of Nilgiris. Indian J Med Res 120.1 (2004): 24–9.

Wang T et al. Carnosic acid prevents obesity and hepatic steatosis in ob/ob mice. Hepatol Res 41.1 (2011): 87–92.

Wang W et al. Antibacterial activity and anticancer activity of *Rosmarinus officinalis* L. essential oil compared to that of its main components. Molecules 17.3 (2012): 2704–13.

Wei G-J, Ho C-T. A stable quinone identified in the reaction of carnosol, a major antioxidant in rosemary, with 2,2-diphenyl-1-picrylhydrazyl radical. Food Chem 96.3 (2006): 471–6.

Yamamoto J et al. Testing various herbs for antithrombotic effect. Nutrition 21.5 (2005): 580–7.

Zhao BL et al. Scavenging effect of extracts of green tea and natural antioxidants on active oxygen radicals. Cell Biophys 14.2 (1989): 175–85.

Zhu BT et al. Dietary administration of an extract from rosemary leaves enhances the liver microsomal metabolism of endogenous estrogens and decreases their uterotropic action in CD-1 mice. Carcinogenesis 19.10 (1998): 1821–7.

S-Adenosyl-L-methionine (SAMe)

HISTORICAL NOTE SAMe was first discovered in Italy in 1952. About 20 years later, a stable salt was commercially manufactured and produced for injectable use. At first, it was investigated as a treatment for schizophrenia, for which it proved inappropriate; however, successful trials in depressed patients began in the 1970s and it was inadvertently found to improve symptoms of arthritis. Since then, numerous studies have been undertaken to examine the role of SAMe in treating depression, osteoarthritis and liver pathology. To date, more than 75 clinical trials have been conducted using SAMe as a therapeutic agent, involving over 23,000 people.

BACKGROUND AND RELEVANT PHARMACOKINETICS

SAMe is a naturally occurring molecule synthesised in the cytosol of every cell, with the liver being the major site of biosynthesis and degradation. SAMe is derived from two acids: methionine (an amino acid) and adenosine triphosphate (ATP: a nucleic acid). Up to half the daily methionine is converted to SAMe in the liver, where it is metabolised to *S*-adenosylhomocysteine (SAH) and then homocysteine. Being a central part of the one-carbon metabolism cycle, SAMe is intrinsically linked with the other methyl donors such as betaine (choline), folate and B_{12}. SAMe also plays a role in the synthesis of choline, which plays a critical role in cell membrane structural integrity, cholinergic neurotransmission, cell signalling and lipid metabolism (Imbard et al 2013). SAMe is the second most used cofactor in the cells after ATP, and is used by over 100 methyl transferases that act on DNA, RNA, proteins and for the synthesis of polyamides that stabilise DNA (Smith et al 2010).

SAMe naturally exists as diastereoisomers and it is presently unclear whether both the R and the S forms are biologically active in humans. Evidence from a rat model suggests that they are equipotent (Dunne et al 1998). Oral doses achieve peak plasma concentrations within 3–5 hours after ingestion of an enteric-coated tablet (400–1000 mg). Enteric coating of SAMe supplements is essential to ensure product stability and potency. Oral SAMe has low systemic bioavailability due to first-pass effects and rapid metabolism. In vitro research by Wagner et al (2009) found that SAMe absorption and the subsequent anti-inflammatory effects are enhanced by encapsulating SAMe in liposomes derived from cholesterol. The half-life is reported to be 100 minutes, and excretion occurs via both urine and faeces (Najm et al 2004).

MAIN ACTIONS

SAMe is involved in myriad biochemical processes and metabolic pathways, chiefly as a methyl donor, where it is important for transmethylation reactions, including the synthesis of creatine, acetylcholine, carnitine, melatonin, glutathione (GSH), phospholipids, proteins, adrenaline, amino acids L-cysteine and taurine and many small molecules, such as neurotransmitters, and for RNA and DNA methylation (Stabler et al 2009). SAMe is closely linked with the metabolism of folate, vitamin B_{12} and all sulfur-containing compounds.

This review only discusses those actions that have been confirmed clinically.

Antidepressant activity

SAMe supplementation produces a clinically significant antidepressant activity that has been demonstrated in numerous randomised controlled trials (RCTs).

The mode of antidepressant action is likely to involve several mechanisms. As a methyl donor, SAMe plays a role in the metabolism and synthesis of various central nervous system neurotransmitters that play an integral part in synaptic transmission and behaviour, such as noradrenaline, dopamine and serotonin (Bottiglieri 1996, 2013, Stanger et al 2009). SAMe improves tetrahydrobiopterin function, a cofactor required for the synthesis of monoamines (Felger & Lotrich 2013). Administration of oral SAMe (800 mg daily) for 2 weeks significantly increased concentrations of 5-hydroxyindoleacetic acid in cerebrospinal fluid, a marker for increased serotonin in the brain (Bottiglieri 2013). Supplementation with SAMe in depressed patients raises serotonin, dopamine and phosphatidylserine and improves neurotransmitter binding to receptor sites, resulting in increased activity (Pizzorno & Murray 2006). Evidence suggests that the dopaminergic activity is most prominent. One human study confirmed that 7 days of supplemental SAMe (400 mg/day) decreased the exaggerated plasma noradrenaline levels found in depressed patients (Sherer et al 1986).

SAMe is also involved in the formation of phosphatidylcholine, a major component of cell membranes and neurotransmission (Carney et al 1987). A recent review suggested that one mode of action in depression may be via the methylation of plasma phospholipids, altering the fluidity of the neuronal membrane and thereby modifying the response to monoamine neurotransmitters that traverse the membrane (Papakostas et al 2012). The results of studies on genetic, epigenetic and environmental components of neuropsychiatric conditions such as depression, schizophrenia, bipolar disorder and autism point to the importance of the folate-methionine transsulfuration hub as a novel target pathway for treatment development (Ozbek et al 2008).

Additionally, SAMe displays antioxidant, anti-inflammatory and neuroprotective activities which may all contribute to the antidepressant effect.

Anti-inflammatory

A substantial body of evidence has identified clinically significant anti-inflammatory activity for SAMe, with comparative trials showing it to be as effective as standard non-steroidal anti-inflammatory drugs (NSAIDs).

Although the mechanism of action remains unclear, it does not appear to be mediated by prostaglandins. SAMe stimulates the synthesis of proteoglycans by articular chondrocytes and exerts a chondroprotective effect, according to in vitro research and tests with experimental animals (Barcelo et al 1987, Clayton 2007, Harmand et al 1987). In vitro studies using cultured rabbit synovial cells has found that SAMe reduces tumour necrosis factor-alpha and fibronectin RNA expression (Gutierrez et al 1997). Clinical responses suggest a concomitant analgesic property. The mechanism for this was previously unknown; however Tsao et al (2012) noted that serotonin-induced pain hypersensitivity in mice is reduced by either SAMe pretreatment or by the combined administration of SAMe with selective antagonists for β_2- and β_3-adrenergic receptors, which have previously been shown to mediate pain signalling. This result highlights a potential analgesic mechanism.

Hepatoprotective and restorative effects

SAMe indirectly reduces oxidative stress in the liver by serving as a precursor for GSH. GSH is particularly important for reducing the toxic effects of free radical molecules generated by various substances, including alcohol and paracetamol. The use of SAMe to prevent and reverse liver toxicity induced by paracetamol, cytokine, ethanol, carbon tetrachloride and ischaemia-reperfusion has been explored in animal models (Cederbaum 2010, Song et al 2004, Wallace et al 2002). An animal study confirmed that paracetamol reduces SAMe levels in liver tissue nuclei and mitochondria, and coadministration of SAMe prevented damage associated with paracetamol toxicity (Brown et al 2010). SAMe also acts as the main methylating agent in the liver. Research with people with alcoholic and non-alcoholic liver diseases confirms that SAMe supplementation significantly increases hepatic GSH levels (Vendemiale et al 1989). Additionally, in vitro and in vivo research has identified antifibrotic activity and enhanced production of interleukin-6, a key anti-inflammatory cytokine in the liver that assists regeneration and downregulation of tumour necrosis factor (Arteel et al 2003, Casini et al 1989, Song et al 2004). Furthermore, SAMe was found to minimise hepatic fibrogenesis by modulating nuclear factor-kappaB (NF-κB) signalling and inhibiting collagen processing (Thompson et al 2011).

Animal studies have shown that the availability of *S*-adenosylmethionine plays a critical role in the progression of liver regeneration via enhancement of GSH and polyamine synthesis (necessary for cell proliferation and differentiation), indicating that regulating hepatic transsulfuration reactions may be capable of modifying the recovery process after liver injury (Jung et al 2013).

Anticancer activity

Research using animal models demonstrates that SAMe is a natural growth regulator in hepatocytes and is antiapoptotic in healthy liver cells, but pro-apoptotic in hepatic carcinoma cells (Anstee & Day 2012, Lu & Mato 2005). SAMe has been shown to inhibit angiogenesis and endothelial cell proliferation in vitro and in vivo (Sahin et al 2011).

The folate-methionine transsulfuration hub has been found to be altered in cancer (Smith et al 2010). Aberrant DNA hypomethylation in the promoter regions of gene, which leads to inactivation of tumour suppressor and other cancer-related genes in cancer cells, has been shown to be one of the most well-defined epigenetic hallmarks in gastric cancer (Qu et al 2013) and epithelial ovarian cancer (Guerrero et al 2012). SAMe has been shown to ameliorate this hypomethylation in vitro and has also been shown to block mitogenic signalling in colon cancer cells in vitro (Chen et al 2007).

OTHER ACTIONS

Prolactin and thyroid-stimulating hormone (TSH) effects

A double-blind, placebo-controlled study involving 20 subjects with depression identified a significant reduction in prolactin concentrations following 14 days of SAMe treatment (Thomas et al 1987). The results of a study conducted in 1990, however, suggest that the effects on these hormones may be gender-specific, with women demonstrating an augmenting response of TSH and no effect on prolactin levels, whereas release of both TSH and prolactin was inhibited in male subjects (Fava et al 1990). If SAMe does exert dopaminergic effects, as presently suspected, then it should also be taken into consideration that dopamine naturally inhibits both TSH and prolactin secretion in humans.

Antioxidant

Previous in vitro experimental research suggested that SAMe acts as a direct antioxidant mainly by binding iron molecules in an inert form, thereby blocking iron-dependent interaction with molecular oxygen to generate reactive oxygen species (ROS), rather than by free radical scavenging (Caro & Cederbaum 2004). Recent in vitro research has shown that coadministration of SAMe and *Saccharomyces boulardii* (a probiotic yeast routinely used to prevent and treat gastrointestinal disorders) enhances the viability of *S. boulardii* in acidic environments, which may improve gastric survival in transit (possibly by preventing apoptosis via reduction of ROS) and the yeast's clinical efficacy (Cascio et al 2013).

CLINICAL USE

Although SAMe is administered as an oral supplement in Australia, it is also used in injectable dose forms in Europe. This is most likely to be because oral SAMe has poor bioavailability and is subject to significant first-pass effects. Manufacturers have been investigating different preparations to increase oral bioavailability, such as SAMe encapsulated in liposomes derived from cholesterol, which has demonstrated increased activity (Wagner et al 2009). This discussion will mainly focus on oral use.

Depression

Both oral and parenteral SAMe are effective treatments for major mood disorders according to a review of 45 RCTs involving depressed adults in Europe and the United States (Papakostas et al 2012). Papakostas et al (2012) and other authors' reviews have concluded that SAMe, at a dose of between 1200 and 1600 mg/day, is superior to placebo and as effective as standard tricyclic antidepressants (imipramine). It is also better tolerated in the treatment of depressive disorders, without any documented increased risk of suicide (Bressa 1994, Delle Chiaie et al 2002, De Vanna & Rigamonti 1992, Dhingra & Parle 2012, Qureshi et al 2013). There has been less research conducted with SAMe in combination with standard antidepressants, but what is available has been encouraging for partial responders to selective serotonin reuptake inhibitors (SSRIs) and serotonin noradrenaline reuptake inhibitors. Studies comparing SAMe to SSRIs found that SAMe has a faster onset of action (10 days) compared to SSRIs (21 days) and relatively few side effects, giving it an advantage (Mischoulon & Fava 2002).

SAMe alone or combined with other supplements has also been shown to alleviate depression associated with musculoskeletal disease, liver disease, Parkinson's disease and HIV/AIDS (Qureshi et al 2013).

Treatment-resistant depression

A number of early open-label studies found benefit of adjunctive treatment with SAMe in treatment-resistant depression, with remission rates ranging from 22% to 43% after treatment-resistant depression patients were augmented with SAMe (Alpert et al 2004, Rosenbaum et al 1990). A trial implementing 800–1600 mg/day SAMe as an adjunctive agent in 30 treatment-resistant patients over 6 weeks revealed a staggering 50% response rate, with 43% of the sample experiencing remission of symptoms (Alpert et al 2004).

More recently, a double-blind RCT of 73 patients with treatment-resistant major depressive disorder showed that coadministration of SAMe (800 mg twice daily) with SSRI treatment produced significantly higher response and remission rates compared to the addition of placebo, using the Hamilton Depression Rating and Clinical Global Impression scales. Furthermore, no serious adverse effects occurred during the trial (Papakostas et al 2010). A secondary analysis of this clinical trial by the same group also confirmed that the coadministration of SAMe improved the memory-related cognitive symptoms of major depressive disorder (Levkovitz et al 2012). Positive results such as these warrant further clinical investigation of SAMe in an adjunctive role in refractory depression, a view that was shared in recent reviews of treatment-resistant depression (Kupfer et al 2012, Shelton et al 2010).

Osteoarthritis

Treatment with SAMe (1200 mg/day) is effective in the management of osteoarthritis and equally as effective as standard treatments, including celecoxib, piroxicam, indomethacin, ibuprofen and naproxen, according to a 2011 meta-analysis of six RCTs (sample sizes 36–493 participants) (De Silva et al 2011). In all trials, SAMe was found to be equally as effective as the NSAID and more effective than placebo for pain and function. Drop-out rates were highest in the NSAID groups and lowest in the SAMe groups. Similar results were reported in a previous meta-analysis of 11 RCTs involving almost 1500 patients; it also concluded that SAMe was more effective than placebo and as effective as NSAIDs in reducing pain and improving functional limitation in patients with osteoarthritis of the knee. In addition, SAMe-treated patients were 58% less likely to experience adverse effects than those treated with NSAIDs (Soeken et al 2002). A 2009 Cochrane systematic review of the use of SAMe in osteoarthritis of the knee or hip ($n = 656$) was more conservative and acknowledged that the action of SAMe on both pain and function might be clinically significant; however larger trials are required for evidence to be definitive (Rutjes et al 2009).

The longest placebo-controlled study to date was conducted over 2 years and found that a loading dose of oral SAMe 600 mg/day taken over the first 2 weeks, followed by a maintenance dose of 400 mg, produced an improvement in symptoms within the first month and no serious adverse effects (Konig 1987).

Comparative studies

SAMe (1200 mg/day) was just as effective in reducing pain intensity as nabumetone (1000 mg/day) over a period of 8 weeks in a 2009 study of 134 Korean patients (Kim et al 2009). Other comparative studies in humans have found that oral SAMe (1200 mg) produces similar symptom-relieving effects as piroxicam (20 mg), ibuprofen (1200 mg), indomethacin (150 mg) or naproxen (750 mg) and celecoxib (200 mg/day) (Caruso & Pietrogrande 1987, Clayton 2007, Glorioso et al 1985, Maccagno et al 1987, Muller-Fassbender 1987, Vetter 1987).

In regard to celecoxib (200 mg/day), SAMe is as effective for symptom relief but has a slower onset of action according to a 16-week double-blind, crossover RCT of 61 individuals with osteoarthritis of the knee (Najm et al 2004). In this study, one month of treatment was required for full benefits to be observed.

Fibromyalgia

Four double-blind trials have investigated the effects of SAMe in fibromyalgia, with all reporting positive findings (Jacobsen et al 1991, Tavoni et al 1987, 1998, Volkmann et al 1997), such as reduced number of trigger points and areas of pain, improved mood and reduced fatigue (Sarac & Gur 2006). Two studies used injectable SAMe (200 mg daily).

The largest study involved 44 patients with primary fibromyalgia and found that, during week 5, the group receiving SAMe (800 mg/day) experienced improvements in clinical disease activity, pain, fatigue, morning stiffness and one measurement of mood. Although encouraging, not all parameters were improved beyond placebo, such as tender point score and isokinetic muscle strength (Jacobsen et al 1991).

These results should not be surprising, given that one-third of all fibromyalgia patients are reported to suffer from depression and a meta-analysis of the effectiveness of antidepressants (including SAMe) in fibromyalgia deemed them a successful treatment strategy (O'Malley et al 2000). It concluded that tricyclic antidepressants, SSRIs and SAMe all improved sleep, fatigue, pain and wellbeing, but not necessarily trigger points.

Schizophrenia

SAMe has been studied in the treatment of schizophrenia, largely based on biochemical considerations suggesting a possible benefit.

Meta-analyses have implicated polymorphisms in 5,10-methylenetetrahydrofolate reductase (MTHFR), encoding a critical enzyme in folate and homocysteine metabolism, in both schizophrenia and bipolar disorder (van Winkel et al 2010). These polymorphisms are functional and result in diminished enzyme activity, leading to lower folate and higher homocysteine levels, and both have been implicated in schizophrenia risk in two separate meta-analyses (Allen et al 2008, Shi et al 2008).

To date, only one small double-blind RCT has been conducted showing that SAMe (800 mg/day) taken for 8 weeks improved quality of life and reduced aggressive behaviour compared to placebo. The study included 18 people with long-term schizophrenia and also found female patients showed improvement of depressive symptoms and clinical improvement, but this did not correlate with serum SAMe levels. Additionally, two patients in the active group exhibited some exacerbation of irritability; however causality is difficult to determine (Strous et al 2009).

Parkinson's disease

High-dose SAMe (800–3600 mg/day) treatment was investigated in a pilot study involving 11 depressed patients with Parkinson's disease, all of whom had been previously treated with other antidepressant agents and had no significant benefit or intolerable side effects. After 10 weeks, 10 patients had at least a 50% improvement on the Hamilton Depression Scale, with only one patient showing no improvement. The mean score before treatment was 27.09 and was 9.55 after SAMe treatment (Di Rocco et al 2000).

Numerous studies have demonstrated that treatment with L-dopa in patients with Parkinson's disease induces high levels of homocysteine and depletes SAMe (Chao et al 2012, De Bonis et al 2010). When supplemented with SAMe, folate, vitamin B_{12} and vitamin B_6 homocysteine levels decrease in people with Parkinson's disease taking L-dopa (Lamberti et al 2005).

Further clinical trials in patients with Parkinson's are currently underway (Meissner et al 2011).

Liver cirrhosis

SAMe deficiency has been studied as a possible pathogenetic factor in several liver diseases, and its administration evaluated in the prevention and treatment of a variety of liver injuries, such as chronic hepatitis, pregnancy-induced liver injury, alcoholic hepatitis and paracetamol-induced liver damage (Vincenzi et al 2012). Depressed hepatic SAMe, especially together with a reduced SAM : SAH ratio, results in impaired transmethylation, producing increased fat deposition, apoptosis and accumulation of damaged proteins — all characteristic features of liver injury (Cave et al 2007, Kharbanda 2007). Primate studies have found that decreased hepatic SAMe concentrations and associated liver lesions, including mitochondrial injury, can be corrected with SAMe supplementation (Lieber et al 1990), with reduced markers of lipid peroxidation, histological evidence of liver injury and maintained mitochondrial GSH (Cave et al 2007).

Alcoholic liver disease

In alcoholic patients with advanced liver cirrhosis, hepatic SAMe concentration is greatly decreased through alcohol exposure, increasing the risk of nucleotide imbalance, apoptosis and carcinogenesis (Cave et al 2007, Gao & Bataller 2011, Halsted 2013, Kharbanda 2007, Lieber 2002). While transient SAMe depletion is necessary for the liver to regenerate, chronic hepatic SAMe depletion may lead to malignant transformation as SAMe is a substrate for all DNA and histone methyltransferases, including those involved in activation of liver injury/repair genes (Halsted 2013, Lu & Mato 2005, 2008). A 2010 double-blind RCT of 13 participants with alcoholic liver disease asked to abstain from alcohol showed that both placebo and SAMe (1200 mg/day) for 24 weeks improved serum aspartate aminotransferase (AST), alanine aminotransferase (ALT) and bilirubin levels (due to abstinence from alcohol), but no significant improvements in steatosis, fibrosis or inflammation were noted in the SAMe group. These results may be due to the small sample size and likely underpowering of the study, relatively short treatment timeframe or high dropout rate (30%) due to resumption of alcoholism during the study (Medici et al 2011).

A small follow-up expansion of this study found similar non-significant results; however this study was severely limited due to all 12 participants suffering severe fibrosis and/or metaplasia, with very few functioning hepatocytes at baseline (Le et al 2013). Two previous European clinical studies suggested that a longer treatment period with oral 1200 mg SAMe may be effective in alcoholic liver disease, and in a 6-month Italian RCT of 17 patients with initially low hepatic GSH levels, oral SAMe (1200 mg/day) normalised levels (Vendemiale et al 1989). In a subsequent 2-year European multicentre trial of 123 patients with alcoholic liver disease, total mortality or liver transplant incidence was reduced from 30% in the placebo group to 16% in the SAMe group, but this was only noted after excluding the most severely ill patients from the analysis (Mato et al 1999).

A 2006 Cochrane review (updated in 2009) of SAMe in alcoholic liver disease analysed results from nine RCTs that included a heterogeneous sample of 434 patients (Rambaldi & Gluud 2006). The methodological quality was considered low; however, eight of the trials were placebo-controlled. As a result, the analysis was based mainly on one trial that found no significant effects of SAMe on all-cause mortality, liver-related mortality, liver transplantation or complications. The authors concluded that, based on such limited evidence, more long-term, high-quality randomised trials of SAMe for these patients are required before SAMe may be recommended for clinical practice. More recent reviews note that improved survival and reduction in liver transplants in patients receiving SAMe are important positive outcomes (Halsted 2013, Vazquez-Elizondo & Bosques-Padilla 2012).

Non-alcoholic fatty liver disease (NAFLD) or non-alcoholic steatohepatitis (NASH)

Human studies have demonstrated that patients with liver disease have an impaired ability to convert methionine to SAMe and decreased plasma and hepatic GSH levels (Cave et al 2007). SAMe has been shown to improve GSH in patients with liver disease after 6 months of oral therapy. Of particular interest is recent evidence from animal studies which suggest that SAMe depletion in the early stages of NASH may be a key point of disease progression into NAFLD (Lu & Mato 2008, Wortham et al 2008). Clinical trials have demonstrated benefit from SAMe therapy in various forms of liver disease, including alcoholic cirrhosis, intrahepatic cholestasis of pregnancy and chemotherapy-induced NASH (Vincenzi et al 2012). SAMe supplementation has also demonstrated attenuation of inflammation and liver injury in a nutritional deficiency model of steatohepatitis and clinical trials were carried out in NASH patients (Cave et al 2007). In lieu of more solid evidence to support SAMe as a therapeutic agent in NASH and NAFLD, the preferred current treatment is betaine, which by virtue corrects methylation by serving as a methyl donor and reduces SAMe depletion (Kharbanda 2007, Kwon 2009, Singal et al 2011).

Prevention of drug-induced liver toxicity

Paracetamol is the leading cause of drug-induced liver failure, hepatotoxicity, and is known to be one of the most frequent side effects associated with different chemotherapy regimens. A recent clinical trial of 78 patients noted that administration of 800 mg/day SAMe as adjunctive therapy was effective in reducing chemotherapy-induced liver toxicity from oxaliplatin plus bevacizumab in patients with metastatic colorectal cancer. AST, ALT, lactate dehydrogenase and total bilirubin were significantly reduced in the SAMe group compared to placebo, and SAMe supplementation significantly reduced chemotherapy course delay and dosage reductions due to liver toxicity (Vincenzi et al 2012). This study confirmed earlier research by the same group that determined SAMe supplementation reduces chemotherapy-induced liver toxicity; similarly, in that trial, SAMe supplementation was found to be associated with a significant lowering of AST and ALT values in 70% of the treated patients and also reduced chemotherapy delays or dose reductions due to transaminase elevation (Santini et al 2003).

OTHER USES

SAMe is used to reduce pain in migraine headache because analgesic activity was reported at a dose of 400–800 mg/day in a group of migraine sufferers (Gatto et al 1986). A case report of 5 paediatric cases of Lesch–Nyhan disease (a rare X-linked recessive neurogenetic disorder) showed significant improvement in self-injury and aggressive behaviour as well as a milder reduction of dystonia when SAMe was administered at a dose of 21–33 mg/kg/day (Chen et al 2013). It is also used in AIDS-related myelopathy and coronary artery disease, as these conditions have been associated with depleted SAMe levels. Supplementation has also been prescribed in cases of general fatigue, poor digestion and allergies.

Alzheimer's dementia (AD)

AD has a multifactorial aetiology that includes nutritional, genetic and environmental risk factors, none of which in isolation is sufficient to account for all cases of AD (Shea & Chan 2008). There is a growing body of evidence indicating that some SAMe-mediated reactions are compromised in AD and age-related neurodegeneration: SAMe is diminished and its metabolites SAH and homocysteine are increased, the accumulation of which also impairs SAMe reactions (Kennedy et al 2004). In patients with AD, decreased SAMe concentrations have been observed in cerebrospinal fluid along with increased concentrations of SAH in brain tissue

(Bottiglieri 2013). Inhibited methylation reactions and hypomethylation of proteins that regulate levels of brain tissue phosphorylated-tau have also been noted in addition to hypomethylation of genes that affect the expression of β-amyloid protein (Bottiglieri 2013).

Interestingly, SAMe supplementation reduced amyloid production, increased spatial memory and reduced plaque spread in a 2012 in vivo study, suggesting a possible role in AD (Fuso et al 2012).

To date, no clinical trials have been published to investigate whether supplemental SAMe has benefits in AD, although the theoretical considerations make a good case for further investigation to be undertaken (Panza et al 2009).

Cholestasis of pregnancy

Cholestasis of pregnancy is characterised by elevated bilirubin and pruritus, and is associated with a high risk of a number of adverse perinatal outcomes, including preterm birth, meconium passage, fetal distress and fetal death (Anstee & Day 2012). A clinical trial of 78 pregnant volunteers with cholestasis showed that treatment with either SAMe or ursodeoxycholic acid (UDCA) effectively reduced pruritus; however the UDCA group showed greater improvement in bile acid secretion (Roncaglia et al 2004). However, a subsequent Cochrane review concluded that there was insufficient evidence to recommend either SAMe or UDCA for the treatment of cholestasis of pregnancy (Burrows et al 2010).

Hepatitis C management

An open-label pilot study of 29 patients with chronic hepatitis C who failed previous therapy with interferon-α and ribavirin were coadministered SAMe and betaine for 6–12 months, resulting in significant improvement of early virological response rates without significant additional adverse effects (Filipowicz et al 2010). SAMe was also found to improve early viral responses and interferon-stimulated gene induction in hepatitis C non-responders (Feld et al 2011). Larger trials are needed to confirm this combination as an effective adjunct treatment.

Cancer

There is a paucity of clinical trials exploring the role of SAMe supplementation in cancer; however, preclinical research and biochemical considerations provide a basis for its future investigation.

Hepatic cancer

Due to its role in the regulation of growth and apoptosis of hepatocytes, SAMe is being investigated as a possible preventive or treatment agent in hepatocellular carcinoma (Lu & Mato 2005, 2008), and has been administered in postradiofrequency ablation formulas to enhance recovery of hepatic tissue at an intravenous dose of 1000 mg for 2–3 days in conjunction with *Silybum marianum* (Feng et al 2012).

Colorectal cancer

There is considerable evidence that aberrant DNA methylation plays an integral role in oncogenesis, and genomic DNA hypomethylation has been reported in colorectal tumour tissue (Nagaraju & El-Rayes 2013). However few studies examine changes in intermediate methylation compounds: one study determined that folate concentration is diminished and SAMe and SAH is increased in neoplastic colonic mucosa when compared to healthy colon tissue (Alonzo-Aperte et al 2008). More studies are needed to confirm whether genomic DNA methylation measurements are functional biomarkers in colorectal cancer.

Breast and cervical cancer

A number of studies have explored the association between MTHFR C677T polymorphism and susceptibility to cervical and breast cancer and cervical intraepithelial neoplasia (Alshatwi 2010, Luo et al 2012). A recent meta-analysis confirmed that SAMe is known as an important DNA methylator, which may have a role in the prevention of pro-oncogene expression in cervical cancer; however, results remained controversial and further studies are needed (Luo et al 2012).

DOSAGE RANGE

Because SAMe is rapidly oxidised when exposed to air, the quality of the tablets is important in preserving potency. SAMe is better absorbed when taken at least 20 minutes before breakfast and 20 minutes before lunch. As an activating antidepressant, it can disturb sleep if taken after 4 pm (Bottiglieri 2013).

Based on clinical studies

- Depression: 1200–3200 mg/day in divided doses have been used in practice. Sometimes it is started as 200 mg twice daily, increased on day 2 to 400 mg twice daily and then increased again to 400 mg three times daily on day 10, until reaching a therapeutic dose of 400 mg four times daily by day 20.
- Osteoarthritis: 1200 mg/day in divided doses, taken as above, with a reduced dose of 400 mg/day used as a maintenance dose once a response occurs.
- Fibromyalgia: 600–800 mg/day in divided doses.
- Liver disease: 400–1200 mg/day in divided doses, although larger doses have been used.
- Parkinson's disease: 800–3600 mg/day in divided doses.
- Migraine: 400–800 mg/day in divided doses.
- Reducing aggression in schizophrenia: 800 mg/day (only under supervision).

ADVERSE REACTIONS

Orally, SAMe is generally well tolerated. Mild gastrointestinal discomfort (nausea) is the most common side effect reported in clinical studies, although anxiety, headache, urinary frequency, dizziness, nervousness, sweating and pruritus have also been reported (Ravindran & da Silva 2013). It has been reported that side effects are more likely with higher doses and may be minimised by consuming SAMe before food.

SIGNIFICANT INTERACTIONS

Controlled studies are not available; therefore, interactions are based on evidence of activity and are largely theoretical and speculative.

Tricyclic antidepressants and other serotonergic agents

Coadministration of SAMe with SSRIs has shown benefits in partial responders and may be a useful combination under professional supervision.

Hepatotoxic drugs

SAMe may reduce hepatic injury caused by agents such as paracetamol, alcohol and oestrogens — potentially beneficial interaction.

L-Dopa

SAMe methylates levodopa, which could theoretically reduce the effectiveness of levodopa given for Parkinson's disease; however, the effect has not been observed clinically — observe patients.

Thyroxine

Caution and monitoring may be warranted.

Betaine

In studies supplementing mice with betaine, significant increases in SAMe were observed with a threefold elevation of the activity of methionine adenosyltransferase — observe.

CONTRAINDICATIONS AND PRECAUTIONS

Previous case reports of agitation and mania in bipolar patients caution that SAMe should be avoided in people with bipolar disorder during the depressive phase (Andreescu et al 2008, Bogarapu et al 2008) and used with caution by people with schizophrenia or schizoaffective disorder (Guidotti et al 2007). However, separate research of coadministration of SAMe with SSRIs or venlafaxine reported no unmasking of hypomanic or manic symptoms (Alpert et al 2004, Papakostas et al 2010). Use under professional supervision to promote patient safety.

PREGNANCY USE

SAMe has been used intravenously in the last trimester of pregnancy with no adverse effects to mother or fetus. However, safety has not yet been conclusively established for either injectable or oral dose forms and possible effects on prolactin levels need to be considered.

PATIENTS' FAQs

What will this supplement do for me?

SAMe has anti-inflammatory, analgesic, antidepressant and protective effects on the liver. It effectively reduces pain and inflammation in osteoarthritis and elevates mood in depression. In fibromyalgia, SAMe reduces pain, fatigue and morning stiffness and may also reduce pain in migraine headache.

When will it start to work?

Beneficial effects are usually seen within 4–5 weeks for osteoarthritis, whereas antidepressant effects are experienced within 1 week. Benefits in fibromyalgia can take up to 6 weeks to establish.

Are there any safety issues?

SAMe should only be used under professional supervision by people with bipolar disorder, schizophrenia or schizoaffective disorder, Parkinson's disease or taking antidepressant medicines. Monitoring of homocysteine levels may be required with long-term supplementation.

Practice points/Patient counselling

- SAMe is involved in myriad biochemical reactions within the body. It is found within every cell and is a precursor for the synthesis of the antioxidant GSH and an important methyl donor.
- Clinically, it has significant anti-inflammatory, analgesic and antidepressant effects and is an effective treatment in depression and osteoarthritis.
- A 2011 meta-analysis concluded that SAMe is as effective as commonly used NSAIDs in reducing pain and improving functional limitation in patients with osteoarthritis without the adverse effects associated with NSAIDs. A recent study has found that it is as effective as celecoxib for providing symptom relief; however, SAMe has a slower onset of action.
- Clinical trials have also shown it to be a safe and effective treatment for depression — comparable with tricyclic antidepressant drugs, yet with a faster onset of action. SAMe also provides additional benefits when coadministered with SSRIs in treatment-resistant depression.
- It may also have benefits for patients with alcoholic liver disease and hepatitis C and for the prevention of drug-induced liver toxicity.
- SAMe may also be useful in fibromyalgia, and possibly migraine headache. Other uses include treatment of general fatigue, elevated homocysteine levels, allergies and poor digestion.

REFERENCES

Allen, NC et al. Systematic meta-analyses and field synopsis of genetic association studies in schizophrenia: the SzGene database. Nat. Genet. 40.7 (2008): 827–834.

Alonzo-Aperte E et al. Folate status and *S*-adenosylmethionine/*S*-adenosylhomocysteine ratio in colorectal adenocarcinoma in humans. Eur J Clin Nutr 62 (2008):295–298.

Alpert JE et al. *S*-adenosyl-L-methionine (SAMe) as an adjunct for resistant major depressive disorder: an open trial following partial or nonresponse to selective serotonin reuptake inhibitors or venlafaxine. J Clin Psychopharmacol 24.6 (2004): 661–664.

Alshatwi AA. Breast cancer risk, dietary intake, and methylenetetrahydrofolate reductase (MTHFR) single nucleotide polymorphisms. Food and Chem Toxicology 48 (2010):1881–1885.

Andreescu C, et al. Complementary and alternative medicine in the treatment of bipolar disorder — a review of the evidence. J Affect Disord 110.1–2 (2008): 16–26.

Anstee QM & Day CP. *S*-adenosylmethionine (SAMe) therapy in liver disease: A review of current evidence and clinical utility. J Hepatol 57 (2012): 1097–1109.

Arteel G et al. Advances in alcoholic liver disease. Best Pract Res Clin Gastroenterol 17 (2003): 625–647.

Barcelo HA et al. Effect of *S*-adenosylmethionine on experimental osteoarthritis in rabbits. Am J Med 83.5A (1987): 55–59.

Bogarapu S et al. Complementary medicines in pediatric bipolar disorder. Minerva Pediatr 60.1 (2008): 103–114.

Bottiglieri T. Folate, vitamin B_{12}, and neuropsychiatric disorders. Nutr Rev 54.12 (1996): 382–390.

Bottiglieri T. Folate, vitamin B_{12}, and *S*-adenosylmethionine. Psychiatric Clinics of North America (2013): 1–13.

Bressa GM. *S*-adenosyl-L-methionine (SAMe) as antidepressant: meta-analysis of clinical studies. Acta Neurol Scand Suppl 154 (1994): 7–14.

Brown JM et al. Temporal study of acetaminophen (APAP) and *S*-adenosyl-L-methionine (SAMe) effects on subcellular hepatic SAMe levels and methionine adenosyltransferase (MAT) expression and activity. Toxicol Appl Pharmacol. 247.1 (2010): 1–9.

Burrows RF et al. Interventions for treating cholestasis in pregnancy. Cochrane Database Sys Rev (2010).

Carney MW, et al. *S*-adenosylmethionine and affective disorder. Am J Med 83.5A (1987): 104–106.

Caro AA, Cederbaum AI. Antioxidant properties of *S*-adenosyl-methionine in Fe^{2+}-initiated oxidations. Free Radical Biol Med 36.10 (2004): 1303–1316.

Caruso I, Pietrogrande V. Italian double-blind multicenter study comparing *S*-adenosylmethionine, naproxen, and placebo in the treatment of degenerative joint disease. Am J Med 83.5A (1987): 66–71.

Cascio V et al. *S*-Adenosyl-L-Methionine protects the probiotic yeast, *Saccharomyces boulardii*, from acid-induced cell death. BMC Microbiology 13.35 (2013).

Casini A et al. *S*-adenosylmethionine inhibits collagen synthesis by human fibroblasts in vitro. Methods Find Exp Clin Pharmacol 11.5 (1989): 331–334.

Cave M et al. Nonalcoholic fatty liver disease: predisposing factors and the role of nutrition. J Nutr Biochem 18.3 (2007): 184–195.

Cederbaum AI. Hepatoprotective effects of *S*-adenosyl-L-methionine against alcohol- and cytochrome P450 2E1-induced liver injury. World J Gastroenterol 16.11(2010): 1366–1376.

Chao J et al Nutraceuticals and their preventive or potential therapeutic value in Parkinson's disease. Nutrition Reviews 70.7(2012):373–386.

Chen H et al Role of methionine adenosyltransferase 2A and *S*-adenosylmethionine in mitogen-induced growth of human colon cancer cells. Gastroenterology 133 (2007):207–218.

Chen BC et al. Treatment of Lesch–Nyhan disease with *S*-adenosylmethionine: Experience with five young Malaysians, including a girl. Brain & Development (2013) DOI: 10.1016/j.braindev.2013.08.013.

Clayton JJ. Nutraceuticals in the management of osteoarthritis. Orthopedics 30.8 (2007): 624–629.

Delle Chiaie R et al. Efficacy and tolerability of oral and intramuscular *S*-adenosyl-L-methionine 1,4-butanedisulfonate (SAMe) in the treatment of major depression: comparison with imipramine in 2 multicenter studies. Am J Cli Nutr. 76.5(2002): 1172S–1176S.

De Bonis ML et al. Impaired transmethylation potential in Parkinson's disease patients treated with L-dopa. Neuroscience Letters 468 (2010): 287–291.

De Silva V et al Evidence for the efficacy of complementary and alternative medicines in the management of osteoarthritis: a systematic review. Rheumatology 50 (2011):911–920.

De Vanna M, Rigamonti R. Oral *S*-adenosyl-L-methionine in depression. Curr Ther Res 52.3 (1992): 478–85.

Dhingra S, Parle M. Herbal remedies and nutritional supplements in the treatment of depression: a review. Bull Clinc Psychopharm 22.3 (2012): 286–92.

Di Rocco A et al. *S*-adenosyl-methionine improves depression in patients with Parkinson's disease in an open-label clinical trial. Mov Disord 15.6 (2000): 1225–1229.

Dunne JB et al. Evidence that *S*-adenosyl-L-methionine diastereoisomers may reduce ischaemia-reperfusion injury by interacting with purinoceptors in isolated rat liver. Br J Pharmacol 125 (1998): 225–233.

Fava M et al. Neuroendocrine effects of *S*-adenosyl-L-methionine: a novel putative antidepressant. J Psychiatr Res 24.2 (1990): 177–184.

Feld JJ, et al. *S*-adenosyl methionine improves early viral responses and interferon stimulated gene induction in hepatitis C nonresponders. Gastroenterology 140 (2011): 830–9.

Felger JC & Lotrich FE. Inflammatory cytokines in depression: neurobiological mechanisms and therapeutic implications. Neuroscience 246 (2013): 199–229.

Feng K et al A randomized controlled trial of radiofrequency ablation and surgical resection in the treatment of small hepatocellular carcinoma. J Hepatology 57 (2012): 794–802.

Filipowicz M et al. *S*-adenosyl-methionine and betaine improve early virological response in chronic hepatitis C patients with previous nonresponse. PLoS One 5.11 (2010): e15492.

Fuso A et al. *S*-adenosylmethionine reduces the progress of the Alzheimer-like features induced by B-vitamin deficiency in mice, Neurobiology of Aging 33 (2012):1482.e1–1482.e16.

Gao B, Bataller R. Alcoholic liver disease: pathogenesis and new therapeutic targets. Gastroenterology 141.5 (2011):1572–1585.

Gatto G et al. Analgesizing effect of a methyl donor (*S*-adenosylmethionine) in migraine: an open clinical trial. Int J Clin Pharmacol Res 6.1 (1986): 15–117.

Glorioso S et al. Double-blind multicentre study of the activity of *S*-adenosylmethionine in hip and knee osteoarthritis. Int J Clin Pharmacol Res 5.1 (1985): 39–49.

Guerrero K et al. A novel genome-based approach correlates TMPRSS3 overexpression in ovarian cancer with DNA hypomethylation. Gynecologic Oncology 125 (2012): 720–726.

Guidotti A et al. *S*-adenosyl methionine and DNA methyltransferase-1 mRNA overexpression in psychosis. Neuroreport 18.1 (2007): 57–60.

Gutierrez S et al. SAMe restores the changes in the proliferation and in the synthesis of fibronectin and proteoglycans induced by tumour necrosis factor alpha on cultured rabbit synovial cells. Br J Rheumatol 36 (1997): 27–31.

Halsted CH. B-vitamin dependent methionine metabolism and alcoholic liver disease. Clin Chem Lab Med 51.3(2013): 457–465.

Harmand MF et al. Effects of *S*-adenosylmethionine on human articular chondrocyte differentiation. An in vitro study. Am J Med 83.5A (1987): 48–54.

Imbard A et al. Plasma choline and betaine correlate with serum folate, plasma *S*-adenosyl-methionine and *S*-adenosyl-homocysteine in healthy volunteers. Clin Chem Lab Med 51.3 (2013): 683–692.

Jacobsen S, et al. Oral *S*-adenosylmethionine in primary fibromyalgia. Double-blind clinical evaluation. Scand J Rheumatol 20.4 (1991): 294–302.

Jung YS et al. Significance of alterations in the metabolomics of sulfur-containing amino acids during liver regeneration. Biochimie 95 (2013): 1605–1610.

Kennedy BP et al. Elevated *S*-adenosylhomocysteine in Alzheimer brain: influence on methyltransferases and cognitive function, J Neural Transm 111 (2004): 547–567.

Kharbanda KK. Role of transmethylation reactions in alcoholic liver disease. World J Gastroenterol 13.37 (2007): 4947–4954.

Kim J et al. Comparative clinical trial of *S*-adenosylmethionine versus nabumetone for the treatment of knee osteoarthritis: An 8-week, multicenter, randomized, double-blind, double-dummy, phase IV study in Korean patients. Clinical Therapeutics 31.12 (2009):2860–2872.

Konig BA. Long-term (two years) clinical trial with *S*-adenosylmethionine for the treatment of osteoarthritis. Am J Med 83.5A (1987): 89–94.

Kupfer D et al Major depressive disorder: new clinical, neurobiological, and treatment perspectives. Lancet 379 (2012): 1045–55.

Kwon DY. Impaired sulfur-amino acid metabolism and oxidative stress in nonalcoholic fatty liver are alleviated by betaine supplementation in rats. J Nutr (2009) 139(1):63–68.

Lamberti P et al. Hyperhomocysteinemia in L-dopa treated Parkinson's disease patients: effect of cobalamin and folate administration. Eur J Neurol. 12 (2005):365–368.

Le MD et al. Alcoholic liver disease patients treated with *S*-adenosyl-L-methionine: An in-depth look at liver morphologic data comparing pre and post treatment liver biopsies. Experimental and Molecular Pathology 95 (2013): 187–191.

Levkovitz Y et al Effects of *S*-adenosylmethionine augmentation of serotonin-reuptake inhibitor antidepressants on cognitive symptoms of major depressive disorder. Eur Psych 27 (2012): 518–521.

Lieber CS. *S*-Adenosyl-L-methionine and alcoholic liver disease in animal models: implications for early intervention in human beings. Alcohol 27.3 (2002): 173–177.

Lieber CS et al. *S*-adenosyl-L-methionine attenuates alcohol-induced liver injury in the baboon. Hepatology 11.2 (1990): 165–172.

Lu SC, Mato JM. Role of methionine adenosyltransferase and *S*-adenosylmethionine in alcohol-associated liver cancer. Alcohol 35.3 (2005): 227–234.

Lu SC, Mato JM. *S*-Adenosylmethionine in cell growth, apoptosis and liver cancer. J Gastroenterol Hepatol 23 (Suppl 1) (2008): S73–S77.

Luo YL et al Methylenetetrahydrofolate reductase C677T polymorphism and susceptibility to cervical cancer and cervical intraepithelial neoplasia: a meta-analysis. PLos One 7.9 (2012): e46272.

Maccagno A et al. Double-blind controlled clinical trial of oral *S*-adenosylmethionine versus piroxicam in knee osteoarthritis. Am J Med 83.5A (1987): 72–77.

Mato JM et al. *S*-adenosylmethionine in alcoholic liver cirrhosis: a randomized, placebo controlled, double-blinded, multicenter clinical trial. J Hepatol 30 (1999):1081–1089.

Medici V et al *S*-adenosyl-L-methionine treatment for alcoholic liver disease: A double-blinded, randomized, placebo-controlled trial. Alcohol Clin Exp Res 35.11 (2011): 1960–1965.

Meissner WG et al. Priorities in Parkinson's disease research. Nature Rev Drug Disc 10 (2011): 377–393.

Mischoulon D, Fava M. Role of *S*-adenosyl-L-methionine in the treatment of depression: a review of the evidence. Am J Clin Nutr 76.5 (2002): 1158S–61S.

Muller-Fassbender H. Double-blind clinical trial of *S*-adenosylmethionine versus ibuprofen in the treatment of osteoarthritis. Am J Med 83.5A (1987): 81–83.

Nagaraju GP, El-Rayes B. SPARC and DNA methylation: Possible diagnostic and therapeutic implications in gastrointestinal cancers. Cancer Letters 328 (2013):10–17.

Najm WI et al. *S*-adenosyl methionine (SAMe) versus celecoxib for the treatment of osteoarthritis symptoms: a double-blind cross-over trial. BMC Musculoskelet Disord 5 (2004): 6.

O'Malley PG et al. Treatment of fibromyalgia with antidepressants: a meta-analysis. J Gen Intern Med 15.9 (2000): 659–666.

Ozbek Z et al Effect of the methylenetetrahydrofolate reductase gene polymorphisms on homocysteine, folate and vitamin B_{12} in patients with bipolar disorder and relatives. Progress in Neuro-Psychopharmacology & Biological Psychiatry 32 (2008):1331–1337.

Panza F et al. Possible role of *S*-adenosylmethionine, *S*-adenosylhomocysteine, and polyunsaturated fatty acids in predementia syndromes and Alzheimer's disease. J Alz Dis 16 (2009): 467–470.

Papakostas GI et al. *S*-adenosyl methionine (SAMe) augmentation of serotonin reuptake inhibitors for antidepressant nonresponders with major depressive disorder: A double-blind, randomized clinical trial. Am J Psychiatry 167.8 (2010):942–948.

Papakostas GI et al. Folates and *S*-adenosylmethionine for major depressive disorder. Can J Psychiatry 57.7 (2012):406–413.

Pizzorno J, Murray M. Textbook of natural medicine, 3rd edn. St Louis: Elsevier, 2006.

Qu Y et al. Gene methylation in gastric cancer. Clinica Chimica Acta 424 (2013): 53–65.

Qureshi NA, Al-Bedah AM. Mood disorders and complementary and alternative medicine: a literature review. Neuropsych Dis Treat 9 (2013): 639–658.

Rambaldi A, Gluud C. *S*-adenosyl-L-methionine for alcoholic liver diseases. Cochrane Database Syst Rev 2 (2006): CD002235.pub2.

Ravindran AV, da Silva TL. Complementary and alternative therapies as add-on to pharmacotherapy for mood and anxiety disorders: A systematic review. J Affective Disorders 150 (2013): 707–719.

Roncaglia N et al. A randomized controlled trial of ursodeoxycholic acid and *S*-adenosyl-L-methionine in the treatment of gestational cholestasis. Br J Obstet Gynaecol 2 (2004): 17–21.

Rosenbaum JF et al. The antidepressant potential of oral *S*-adenosyl-L-methionine. Acta Psychiatr Scand 81.5 (1990): 432–6.

Rutjes AWS et al. *S*-adenosylmethionine for osteoarthritis of the knee or hip. CochraneDatabase of Systematic Reviews 4 (2009): CD007321.

Sahin M et al. Inhibition of angiogenesis by *S*-adenosylmethionine. Biochem Biophys Res Com 408 (2011): 145–148.

Santini D et al *S*-adenosylmethionine (AdoMet) supplementation for treatment chemotherapy-induced liver injury. Anticancer Res 23.6D (2003):5173–5179.

Sarac AJ, Gur A. Complementary and alternative medical therapies in fibromyalgia. Curr Pharm Des 12.1 (2006): 47–57.

Shea TB, Chan A. *S*-adenosyl methionine: a natural therapeutic agent effective against multiple hallmarks and risk factors associated with Alzheimer's disease. J Alz Dis 13 (2008): 67–70.

Sherer MA et al. Effects of *S*-adenosyl-methionine on plasma norepinephrine, blood pressure, and heart rate in healthy volunteers. Psychiatry Res 17.2 (1986): 111–1118.

Shelton RC et al Therapeutic options for treatment-resistant depression. CNS Drugs 24.2(2010): 131–161.

Shi J et al. Genetic associations with schizophrenia: meta-analyses of 12 candidate genes. Schizophr. Res. 104.1–3 (2008): 96–107.

Singal AK et al Antioxidants as therapeutic agents for liver disease. Liver Intl (2011):1432–48.

Smith CL et al Genomic and epigenomic instability, fragile sites, schizophrenia and autism. Current Genomics, 11 (2010): 447–469.

Soeken KL et al. Safety and efficacy of *S*-adenosylmethionine (SAMe) for osteoarthritis. J Fam Pract 51.5 (2002): 425–430.

Song Z et al. Modulation of endotoxin stimulated Interleukin 6 production in monocytes and Kupffer cells by *S*-adenosylmethionine (SAMe). Cytokine 28.6 (2004): 214–223.

Stabler SP et al. α-Lipoic acid induces elevated *S*-adenosylhomocysteine and depletes *S*-adenosylmethionine. Free Radical Biology & Medicine 47 (2009): 1147–1153.

Stanger O et al. Homocysteine, folate and B_{12} in neuropsychiatric diseases: review and treatment recommendations. Expert Rev. Neurother 9.9 (2009): 1393–1412.

Strous RD et al. Improvement of aggressive behavior and quality of life impairment following *S*-adenosyl-methionine (SAM-e) augmentation in schizophrenia. European Neuropsychopharmacology 19 (2009): 14–22.

Tavoni A et al. Evaluation of *S*-adenosylmethionine in primary fibromyalgia: a double-blind crossover study. Am J Med 83.5A (1987): 107–110.

Tavoni A, et al. Evaluation of *S*-adenosylmethionine in secondary fibromyalgia: a double-blind study. Clin Exp Rheumatol 16.1 (1998): 106–107.

Thomas CS et al. The influence of *S*-adenosylmethionine (SAM) on prolactin in depressed patients. Int Clin Psychopharmacol 2.2 (1987): 97–102.

Thompson KJ et al *S*-adenosyl-L-methionine inhibits collagen secretion in hepatic stellate cells via increased ubiquitination. Liver International (2011): 893–903.

Tsao D et al Serotonin-induced hypersensitivity via inhibition of catechol *o*-methyltransferase activity. Molecular Pain 8.25 (2012).

van Winkel R et al. MTHFR and risk of metabolic syndrome in patients with schizophrenia. Schizophrenia Research 121 (2010): 193–198.

Vazquez-Elizondo G, Bosques-Padilla FJ. Concise review: alcoholic hepatitis. Ann Gastro Hep 3.1(2012): 121–130.

Vendemiale G et al. Effects of oral *S*-adenosyl-L-methionine on hepatic glutathione in patients with liver disease. Scand J Gastroenterol 24.4 (1989): 407–415.

Vetter G. Double-blind comparative clinical trial with *S*-adenosylmethionine and indomethacin in the treatment of osteoarthritis. Am J Med 83.5A (1987): 78–80.

Vincenzi B et al The role of *S*-adenosylmethionine in preventing oxaliplatin-induced liver toxicity: a retrospective analysis in metastatic colorectal cancer patients treated with bevacizumab plus oxaliplatin-based regimen. Support Care Cancer 20 (2012):135–139.

Volkmann H et al. Double-blind, placebo-controlled cross-over study of intravenous *S*-adenosyl-L-methionine in patients with fibromyalgia. Scand J Rheumatol 26.3 (1997): 206–211.

Wagner EJ et al Liposome dependent delivery of *S*-adenosyl methionine to cells by liposomes: a potential treatment for liver disease. J Pharm Sc 98.2 (2009) 573–82.

Wallace KP et al. *S*-adenosyl-L-methionine (SAMe)for the treatment of acetaminophen toxicity in a dog. J Am Anim Hosp Assoc 38 (2002):246–254.

Wortham M et al. The transition from fatty liver to NASH associates with SAMe depletion in db/db mice fed a methionine choline-deficient diet. Dig Dis Sci 53.10 (2008): 2761–2774.

Saffron

HISTORICAL NOTE Saffron's name is derived from the Arab word for yellow, reflecting the high concentration of carotenoids present in the saffron flowers' stigmas, which contribute most to the colour profile of this spice (Melnyk et al 2010). Saffron has long been revered as both spice and medicine by many cultures including ancient Greece, the Middle East, China and Europe. Frescos uncovered in Greece clearly depict the use of saffron stigma as a medicine over 3600 years ago (Dwyer et al 2011). The famous Persian academic and physician Avicenna listed the traditional uses of saffron and its pharmacological activities in Book II, Canon of Medicine (al-Qanun fi al-tib) and described it as an antidepressant, hypnotic, anti-inflammatory, hepatoprotective, bronchodilatory and aphrodisiac and others. It is interesting to note that many of these effects have been tested in modern times and confirmed in vivo (Hosseinzadeh & Nassiri-Asl 2013). The mood elevating activity of saffron were also reported in a traditional Chinese medicine (TCM) text from the Mongol dynasty and in the mid-1800s by an English herbalist, Christopher Catton (Dwyer et al 2011). Today, saffron is cultivated in many countries such as Iran, Europe, Turkey, Central Asia, India, China, Algeria, Australia and New Zealand, and is considered the most expensive spice in the world.

LATIN BINOMIAL/CLASS

Crocus sativus — Iridaceae family

OTHER NAMES

Azafrán, azafron, crocus cultivé, Indian saffron, kashmira, kesar, kumkuma, safran cultivé, safran Espagnol, safran des Indes, safran véritable, Spanish saffron, true saffron, zafran.

PLANT PART USED

Dried stigma and petal.

It is estimated that it takes approximately 75,000 crocus blossoms or 225,000 stigmas to produce just one pound (454 g) of saffron. The stigmas must be hand-picked from the delicate blossoms upon opening to preserve the desirable volatile components before they evaporate in the heat of the day (Melnyk et al 2010).

CHEMICAL COMPONENTS

There are over 150 volatile and non-volatile compounds in saffron; however, not all have been identified. The most important constituents of stigmas of *C. sativus* are carotenoids (e.g. crocetin, crocins, a-carotene, lycopene, zeaxanthin), monoterpene aldehydes (e.g. picrocrocin and safranal), monoterpenoids (e.g. crocusatines), isophorones and flavonoids. The water-soluble crocins are the primary colouring pigment in saffron and make up ~10%. Picrocrocin is the precursor to safranal and provides the bitter taste, whereas safranal provides the aroma (Hosseinzadeh & Nassiri-Asl 2013). The crocin concentration varies depending on growing geographical location and processing methods. For example, Greek saffron has the highest concentration of crocins followed by India and New Zealand (Alavizadeh & Hosseinzadeh 2014).

MAIN ACTIONS

Many in vivo studies have been conducted for saffron, crocin and safranal and revealed numerous pharmacological effects.

Antidepressant

This has been demonstrated in numerous double-blind RCTs and confirmed in a recent meta-analysis (Hausenblas et al 2013). Both the saffron stigma and petal display antidepressant activity.

The antidepressant-like action appears to be due to increasing cAMP response element-binding protein (CREB), BDNF and VGF levels in hippocampus (Vahdati et al 2014). Crocin physically binds to a wide range of cellular proteins such as structural proteins, membrane transporters, and enzymes involved in ATP and redox homeostasis and signal transduction (Hosseinzadeh et al 2014). In vivo research has also identified that safranal and crocin induce uptake inhibition of dopamine, noradrenaline and serotonin (Hosseinzadeh et al 2004).

S

Improved learning, memory and neuroprotection

Multiple preclinical studies using different animal models consistently demonstrate that saffron and crocin improves various aspects of learning and memory. Saffron extract demonstrates moderate acetyl choline esterase inhibition with crocetin and dimethylcrocetin binding simultaneously to the catalytic and peripheral anionic sites and safranal interacting with only the binding site of the AChE (Geromichalos et al 2012).

Neuroprotection has also been demonstrated in vivo using different models chiefly via an antioxidant mechanism. In addition, the crocin constituent specifically inhibits neuronal cell death induced by both internal and external apoptotic stimuli. It modulates the expression of Bcl-2 family proteins which leads to a marked reduction in TNF-alpha-induced release of cytochrome c from the mitochondria. Crocin also blocks the cytochrome c-induced activation of caspase-3 (Soeda et al 2001).

One study showed that crocetin (8 mg/kg) protected cerebrocortical and hippocampus neurons against ischaemia resulting in improved spatial learning memory in rats after chronic cerebral hypoperfusion (Tashakori-Sabzevar et al 2013). Similarly, crocin (25 mg/kg) and saffron extract (250 mg/kg) given IP significantly improved spatial cognitive abilities following chronic cerebral hypoperfusion in another rat study, most likely due to an antioxidant mechanism (Hosseinzadeh et al 2012).

Crocin also prevented hippocampal neuron number loss in diabetic rats and improved learning and memory impairments (Tamaddonfard et al 2013). In addition, the long-term IP injection of crocin at doses of 15 and 30 mg/kg improved blood TCA, MDA, glucose, and insulin changes induced by streptozotocin. In vivo research also indicates that pretreatment with saffron saved many dopaminergic cells of the substantia nigra pars compacta (SNc) and retina in a mouse model of Parkinson's disease (Purushothuman et al 2013).

Oral crocin (100 mg/kg) administered for 21 consecutive days to streptozotocin-lesioned rats improved cognitive performance and resulted in a significant reduction in MDA levels and elevation in total thiol content and GPx activity indicating antioxidant activity (Naghizadeh et al 2013). A lower dose of crocin (30 mg/kg) given IP was also found to effectively ameliorate the cognitive deficits caused by streptozotocin-lesioned rats in another study (Khalili & Hamzeh 2010).

The memory impairing effects of chronic stress were attenuated by treatment with saffron and crocin according to another animal study (Ghadrdoost et al 2011). Those test animals that received saffron extract or crocin had significantly higher levels of lipid peroxidation products, significantly higher activities of antioxidant enzymes including glutathione peroxidase, glutathione reductase and superoxide dismutase and significantly lower total antioxidant reactivity capacity. Interestingly, crocin significantly decreased plasma levels of corticosterone compared to controls receiving vehicle.

Ethanol-induced learning impairment was improved with saffron extract in a study with test mice. It also prevented ethanol-induced inhibition of hippocampal long-term potentiation, a form of activity-dependent synaptic plasticity that may underlie learning and memory (Abe & Saito 2000).

Treatment with crocin (15 and 30 mg/kg) counteracted delay-dependent recognition memory deficits in normal rats, suggesting that these carotenoids modulate storage and/or retrieval of information. In further testing, crocins in high strength (30 mg/kg), and to a lesser extent a lower dose (15 mg/kg) attenuated scopolamine (0.2 mg/kg)-induced performance deficits in a different memory model (Pitsikas et al 2007).

Anticancer

Anticancer activity for saffron and its constituents has been demonstrated in various in vitro and in vivo studies (Rastgoo et al 2013). For example, crocin exhibits mild cytotoxic effects on a leukemia cell line which might be mediated through the increase of DNA fragmentation (Rezaee et al 2013). Saffron has also been shown to exert a significant chemopreventive effect against liver cancer through inhibition of cell proliferation and induction of apoptosis in vivo. The effect appears to be mediated by modulating oxidative damage and suppressing the inflammatory response (Amin et al 2011).

OTHER ACTIONS

Diazinon (DZN) is one of the most widely used insecticides in agricultural pest control and has been shown to induce hepatotoxicity and cardiotoxicity with subchronic exposure. Saffron has been shown to attenuate these toxic effects in vivo (Lari et al 2013, Razavi et al 2013).

Hypotensive activity has been reported for the aqueous extract of saffron stigma in vivo, which appear to be attributable, in part, to the actions of two major constituents, crocin and safranal (Imenshahidi et al 2010). It seems that safranal is more important than crocin for producing this effect.

Aqueous and ethanolic extracts of stigma and its constituents interact with the opioid system and reduced morphine withdrawal syndrome in an animal model (Hosseinzadeh & Jahanian 2010).

Anxiolytic and hypnotic activity has also been demonstrated for saffron aqueous extract and safranal in vivo (Hosseinzadeh & Noraei 2009).

Aphrodisiac activity was observed in a study of male rates for an aqueous saffron extract and crocin but not for safranal (Hosseinzadeh et al 2008).

Anti-tussive and anticonvulsant activities have also been demonstrated in vivo for saffron or its derivatives (Hosseinzadeh & Ghenaati 2006, Hosseinzadeh & Talebzadeh 2005).

Saffron showed some effects on blood coagulation and platelet aggregation in vitro and in vivo studies; however, a placebo controlled study of 60 healthy volunteers found that treatment with saffron tablets for 1 week at either 200 mg/day or 400 mg/day did not induce any significant changes to either coagulant or anticoagulant systems (Ayatollahi et al 2013).

CLINICAL USAGE

Saffron has gained popularity in the treatment of mental health disorders, particularly depression. It is also used for impaired memory in dementia and shows promise in PMS and early age-related macular degeneration.

Depression

Saffron has been used since antiquity for depression in several different cultures. Numerous controlled studies have been conducted with saffron, either stigma or petal, preparations and consistently report positive results showing superiority over placebo and effectiveness similar to standard antidepressant medications. The most studied preparations are by Novin Zaferan Co and IMIPRAN, Iran. Of note, studies tend to be small, last no longer than 6 weeks and most research has been conducted in one country, Iran. Ideally, the impressive results reported thus far should be confirmed in other countries involving a larger number of subjects.

A 2013 meta-analysis of five randomised controlled trials (RCTs) (n = 2 placebo controlled trials, n = 3 antidepressant controlled trials) found a large effect size for saffron supplementation compared to placebo for treating depressive symptoms in adults with major depressive disorder (MDD) ($P < 0.001$) (Hausenblas et al 2013). There was no significant difference between saffron and antidepressant treatment, indicating that both treatments were similarly effective in reducing depression symptoms. Importantly, the quality of the trials was considered high, using the Jadad score. Three studies investigated *Crocus sativus* (saffron) stigma, two investigated saffron petal, and one compared saffron stigma to petal.

A 6-week double-blind, placebo-controlled RCT of 40 outpatients with major depression (diagnosed as per structured clinical interview for DSM IV) found that treatment with saffron petal (30 mg/day) was significantly superior to placebo for improving patients' mood according to the Hamilton Depression Rating Scale (HAM-D) ($P < 0.001$) (Moshiri et al 2006). Significant superiority over placebo was observed by week 2 of treatment which continued at week 6. At the end of the study, HAM-D scores were reduced by 60% with saffron compared to 22% reduction with placebo ($P < 0.001$).

Previously, stigmas of saffron (30 mg/day) were found to be superior to placebo for producing a significantly better outcome using the HAM-D in a 6-week, double-blind RCT involving 40 outpatients with mild to moderate depression ($P < 0.001$) (Akhondzadeh et al 2005). Mean HAM-D scores reduced by 54% with saffron compared to 23% for placebo by week 6.

Compared to standard treatments

The efficacy and safety of saffron (30 mg/day; SaffroMoods, IMPIRAN) was compared to fluoxetine (40 mg/day) over 6 weeks in people with mild to moderate depression (n = 40) using a double-blind, RCT design (Shahmansouri et al 2014). Using the HAM-D at weeks 3 and 6, no significant difference was detected between two groups ($P = 0.62$), and remission and response rates were not significantly different either ($P = 1.00$ and $P = 0.67$ respectively). In regards to safety, there was no significant difference between two groups in the frequency of adverse events.

Previously, an 8-week pilot double-blind randomised trial of 40 adult outpatients who met the DSM-IV criteria for major depression found that saffron petal treatment (15 mg twice daily) was as effective as fluoxetine (10 mg twice daily) after 8 weeks ($P = 0.84$) (Akhondzadeh et al 2007). In addition, in both treatments, the remission rate was 25% and no significant differences were observed for side effects. Patients had a baseline HAM-D score of at least 18 in this study.

Saffron (30 mg/day) was found to be as effective as fluoxetine (20 mg/day) in another double-blind RCT of 40 outpatients with mild-to-moderate depression ($P = 0.71$) (Noorbala et al 2005). The 6-week study further confirmed no difference in side effects between the two groups.

Comparisons with imipramine have also been done in RCTs, finding that saffron is as effective a treatment (Akhondzadeh et al 2004). One double-blind RCT involving 30 patients with mild to moderate depression showed that saffron (30 mg/day) produced similar results to imipramine (100 mg/day) ($P = 0.09$). Both treatments reduced HAM-D scores to a similar extent compared to baseline, 55% reduction with saffron and 58% with imipramine (both $P < 0.0001$). As expected, the imipramine group experienced anticholinergic side effects such as dry mouth and sedation to a greater extent than with saffron treatment.

Reducing sexual dysfunction side effects of antidepressants

Saffron (30 mg/day) was used over 4 weeks in a double-blind RCT of 34 women stabilised on fluoxetine (40 mg/day) for at least 6 weeks and experiencing a subjective feeling of sexual dysfunction (Kashani et al 2013). By the end of 4 weeks, patients receiving saffron reported significant improvements using the Female Sexual Function Index (FSFI) ($P < 0.001$), arousal ($P = 0.028$), lubrication ($P = 0.035$) and pain ($P = 0.016$), but no changes in the domains for desire, satisfaction or orgasm compared to placebo.

Alzheimer's dementia (AD)

S

Two clinical trials have been conducted in people with Alzheimer's dementia, producing encouraging results (Akhondzadeh et al 2010a, 2010b).

One double-blind RCT involving people with mild to moderate AD compared oral saffron (15 mg twice per day) to placebo over 16 weeks. Active treatment with saffron produced a significantly better outcome on cognitive function than placebo and no significant differences in the two groups in terms of observed adverse events (Akhondzadeh et al 2010a).

Compared to standard treatments

Previously, a longer 22-week double-blind RCT involving 54 volunteers aged 55 years or older with mild to moderate AD found that saffron (30 mg/day) was as effective from a clinical and cognitive perspective as donepezil (5 mg twice daily). Saffron was the better tolerated treatment as donepezil was associated with significantly more episodes of vomiting (Akhondzadeh et al 2010b).

Premenstrual syndrome (PMS)

Positive results were obtained in a double-blind RCT using saffron stigma (30 mg/day) in women with PMS symptoms starting at least 6 months previously (Agha-Hosseini et al 2008). The treatment was compared to placebo over two menstrual cycles and found to reduce symptoms as measured by the Total Premenstrual Daily Symptoms and HAM-D.

Age-related macular degeneration (ARMD)

Due to the high concentration of carotenoids in saffron and its traditional history of use in improving vision, saffron has been investigated in ARMD with encouraging results.

A crossover RCT of 25 people with early ARMD found that supplementation with saffron (20 mg/day) over 3 months significantly improved retinal flicker sensitivity compared to placebo (Falsini et al 2010). Similar results were obtained in a recent pilot study of 33 people with early ARMD which also showed that oral saffron (20 mg/day) taken for 3 months significantly improved flicker sensitivity estimate compared to baseline ($P < 0.01$), a change which remained stable throughout the follow-up period of 8 months (Marangoni et al 2013). Piccardi et al (2012) followed the cohort from the previous study by Falsini et al (2010) and found that saffron (20 mg/day) taken over an average treatment period of 14 months maintained the improvements in flicker sensitivity seen at 3 months, suggesting long-term efficacy (Piccardi et al 2012).

Immunomodulation

A dose of 100 mg/day of saffron increased IgG levels and decreased IgM compared to baseline and placebo after 3 weeks ($P < 0.01$) in a double-blind RCT involving healthy male volunteers. The treatment also decreased the percentage of basophils compared with baseline, but increased the percentage of monocytes compared with placebo ($P < 0.05$).

The effects were short-lived as all parameters returned to baseline levels after 6 weeks (Kianbakht & Ghazavi 2011).

Other uses

Saffron is used as a culinary spice to colour food yellow and add flavour and also as a dye for clothing and to provide fragrance in perfumes. It is traditionally used as a medicine to improve digestion, elevate mood, as an aphrodisiac, relaxant and hypnotic, anti-inflammatory, hepatoprotective agent and bronchodilator (Hosseinzadeh & Nassiri-Asl 2013). It has also been used traditionally to relieve pain (e.g. toothache and teething infants), to treat both bacterial and fungal infections, for reproductive complaints ranging from amenorrhoea and impotency to pregnancy termination and contraception and used topically in skin conditions (e.g. psoriasis, eczema and wounds).

Topically, saffron is currently used as an ingredient in some cosmetic preparations in countries such as Japan and has demonstrated a sunscreen activity in vitro (Hosseinzadeh & Nassiri-Asl 2013).

DOSAGE RANGE

According to clinical studies

- Mild to moderate depression: saffron petal treatment (15 mg twice daily) or saffron stigma (30 mg/day) with effects starting within 2 weeks.
- Female sexual dysfunction due to fluoxetine: saffron 30 mg/day for at least 4 weeks.
- Alzheimer's dementia: saffron (15 mg twice daily) long-term.
- PMS: saffron (15 mg twice daily) with effects starting after 2 menstrual cycles.
- Early age-related macular degeneration: saffron 20 mg/day long-term.

ADVERSE REACTIONS

In RCTs for depression, saffron (30 mg/day) is as well tolerated as fluoxetine (20–40 mg/day) and better tolerated than imipramine (100 mg/day). Crocin tablets (20 mg/day) taken for 1 month did not induce any major adverse events or change haematological, biochemical, hormonal or urinary parameters when compared to placebo in healthy adult volunteers (Mohamadpour et al 2013). Less serious side effects reported include nausea and vomiting, diarrhoea and dizziness with high doses.

Toxicity

Saffron has a high LD_{50} = 20 g/kg, which explains why it is considered safe for human consumption (Bisset & Wichtl 1994).

Significant interactions

No clinical investigation has been undertaken into the potential for drug interactions with saffron.

Antidepressants

Due to the fact that saffron exhibits significant antidepressant activity, concomitant use should be carefully supervised. It is theoretically possible that pharmaceutical antidepressant dosage requirements will decrease with the addition of saffron in therapeutic doses.

CONTRAINDICATIONS AND PRECAUTIONS

Saffron should be used under professional supervision in the treatment of any mental health condition to promote safety. It should not be used by people with an allergy to saffron or its components.

PREGNANCY USE

Saffron has been used as a spice and food colouring agent for centuries and is likely to be safe when consumed in the usual dietary doses. Whether high dose saffron is safe in pregnancy remains to be confirmed.

An animal study utilising crocin and safranal found these substances reduced length and weight of fetuses, growth retardation and induced mainly skeletal malformations when administered to pregnant mice (Moallem et al 2013). The safety implications for saffron use during pregnancy should be investigated further.

Practice points/Patient counselling

- Saffron is an expensive and distinctive spice that has also been used as a medicine since ancient times by several different cultures.
- Double-blind studies show that saffron is effective in mild to moderate depression and as effective as fluoxetine, with benefits starting within 1–2 weeks. It may also improve some aspects of sexual dysfunction experienced by women taking fluoxetine.
- Saffron may also improve symptoms in PMS when used for at least two menstrual cycles and improve some aspects of age-related macular degeneration when used long-term.
- Preclinical studies and two human trials also indicate possible cognitive benefits in Alzheimer's dementia.
- Safety in pregnancy has not been confirmed for high-dose saffron treatment.

PATIENTS' FAQs

What will this herb do for me?

Saffron is an effective treatment for mild to moderate depression and possibly premenstrual syndrome and for improving cognition in Alzheimer's dementia.

When will it start to work?

Benefits in mild to moderate depression appear within 1–2 weeks of use, whereas benefits in PMS or dementia take several months of continued use.

Are there any safety issues?

Saffron is well tolerated. High doses are not recommended in pregnancy until safety can be confirmed.

REFERENCES

Abe K. & Saito H. Effects of saffron extract and its constituent crocin on learning behaviour and long-term potentiation. Phytother Res 14.3 (2000):149–152.

Agha-Hosseini M et al. Crocus sativus L. (saffron) in the treatment of premenstrual syndrome: a double-blind, randomised and placebo-controlled trial. BJOG 115.4 (2008): 515–519.

Akhondzadeh S et al. Comparison of Crocus sativus L. and imipramine in the treatment of mild to moderate depression: a pilot double-blind randomized trial [ISRCTN45683816]. BMC Complement Altern Med 4 (2004): 12.

Akhondzadeh S et al. Crocus sativus L. in the treatment of mild to moderate depression: a double-blind, randomized and placebo-controlled trial. Phytother Res 19.2 (2005): 148–151.

Akhondzadeh BA et al. Comparison of petal of Crocus sativus L. and fluoxetine in the treatment of depressed outpatients: a pilot double-blind randomized trial. Prog Neuropsychopharmacol Biol Psychiatry 31.2 (2007): 439–442.

Akhondzadeh S et al. Saffron in the treatment of patients with mild to moderate Alzheimer's disease: a 16-week, randomized and placebo-controlled trial. J Clin Pharm Ther 35. 5 (2010a): 581–588.

Akhondzadeh S et al. A 22-week, multicenter, randomized, double-blind controlled trial of Crocus sativus in the treatment of mild-to-moderate Alzheimer's disease. Psychopharmacology (Berl) 207.4 (2010b): 637–643.

Alavizadeh SH, Hosseinzadeh H. Bioactivity assessment and toxicity of crocin: A comprehensive review. Food Chem Toxicol 64 (2014): 65–80.

Amin, A et al. Saffron: a potential candidate for a novel anticancer drug against hepatocellular carcinoma. Hepatology 54.3 (2011): 857–867.

Ayatollahi, H et al. Effect of Crocus sativus L. (Saffron) on Coagulation and Anticoagulation Systems in Healthy Volunteers. Phytother Res. (2013).

Bisset N.G. Wichtl M. Herbal drugs and phytopharmaceuticals (3rd ed.) Medpharm GmbH Scientific Publishers, Stuttgart (1994).

Dwyer AV et al. Herbal medicines, other than St. John's Wort, in the treatment of depression: a systematic review. Altern Med Rev 16.1 (2011): 40–49.

Falsini B et al. Influence of saffron supplementation on retinal flicker sensitivity in early age-related macular degeneration. Invest Ophthalmol Vis Sci 51.12 (2010): 6118–6124.

Geromichalos G.D et al. Saffron as a source of novel acetylcholinesterase inhibitors: molecular docking and in vitro enzymatic studies. J Agric Food Chem 60.24 (2012): 6131–6138.

Ghadrdoost B et al. Protective effects of saffron extract and its active constituent crocin against oxidative stress and spatial learning and memory deficits induced by chronic stress in rats. Eur J Pharmacol 667.1–3 (2011): 222–229.

Hausenblas HA et al. Saffron (Crocus sativus L.) and major depressive disorder: a meta-analysis of randomized clinical trials. J Integr Med 11.6 (2013): 377–383.

Hosseinzadeh H et al. Antidepressant effects of crocus sativus stigma extracts and its constituents, crocin and safranal, in mice. J Med Plants 3 (2004): 48–58.

Hosseinzadeh H, Talebzadeh F. Anticonvulsant evaluation of safranal and crocin from Crocus sativus in mice. Fitoterapia, 76.7–8 (2005): 722–724.

Hosseinzadeh H, Ghenaati J. Evaluation of the antitussive effect of stigma and petals of saffron (Crocus sativus) and its components, safranal and crocin in guinea pigs. Fitoterapia 77.6 (2006): 446–448.

Hosseinzadeh H et al. The effect of saffron, Crocus sativus stigma, extract and its constituents, safranal and crocin on sexual behaviors in normal male rats. Phytomedicine, 15, (6–7) (2008): 491–495.

Hosseinzadeh H, Noraei NB. Anxiolytic and hypnotic effect of Crocus sativus aqueous extract and its constituents, crocin and safranal, in mice. Phytother Res 23.6 (2009): 768–774.

Hosseinzadeh H, Jahanian Z. Effect of Crocus sativus L. (saffron) stigma and its constituents, crocin and safranal, on morphine withdrawal syndrome in mice. Phytother Res 24.5 (2010): 726–730.

Hosseinzadeh H et al. Effects of saffron (Crocus sativus L.) and its active constituent, crocin, on recognition and spatial memory after chronic cerebral hypoperfusion in rats. Phytother Res 26.3 (2012): 381–386.

Hosseinzadeh H, Nassiri-Asl M. Avicenna's (Ibn Sina) the Canon of Medicine and saffron (Crocus sativus): a review. Phytother Res 27.4 (2013a): 475–483.

Hosseinzadeh H, Nassiri-Asl M. Avicenna's (Ibn Sina) the Canon of Medicine and saffron (Crocus sativus): a review. Phytother Res 27.4 (2013b): 475–483.

Hosseinzadeh H et al. Proteomic screening of molecular targets of crocin. Daru 22.1 (2014): 5.

Imenshahidi M et al. Hypotensive effect of aqueous saffron extract (Crocus sativus L.) and its constituents, safranal and crocin, in normotensive and hypertensive rats. Phytother. Res., 24, (7) (2010): 990–994.

Kashani L et al. Saffron for treatment of fluoxetine-induced sexual dysfunction in women: randomized double-blind placebo-controlled study. Hum.Psychopharmacol 28.1 (2013): 54–60.

Khalili M, Hamzeh F. Effects of active constituents of Crocus sativus L., crocin on streptozocin-induced model of sporadic Alzheimer's disease in male rats. Iran Biomed J 14.1–2 (2010): 59–65.

Kianbakht S, Ghazavi A. Immunomodulatory effects of saffron: a randomized double-blind placebo-controlled clinical trial. Phytother. Res., 25.12 (2011): 1801–1805.

Lari P et al. 2013. Evaluation of diazinon-induced hepatotoxicity and protective effects of crocin. Toxicol.Ind.Health.

S

Marangoni D et al. Functional effect of Saffron supplementation and risk genotypes in early age-related macular degeneration: a preliminary report. J Transl Med 11 (2013): 228.
Melnyk J et al. Chemical and biological properties of the world's most expensive spice: Saffron; Food Research International 43. 8 (2010): 1981–1989.
Moallem SA et al. Evaluation of teratogenic effects of crocin and safranal, active ingredients of saffron, in mice. Toxicol Ind Health (2013).
Mohamadpour AH et al. Safety Evaluation of Crocin (a constituent of saffron) Tablets in Healthy Volunteers. Iran J Basic Med Sci 16.1 (2013): 39–46.
Moshiri E et al. Crocus sativus L. (petal) in the treatment of mild-to-moderate depression: a double-blind, randomized and placebo-controlled trial. Phytomedicine 13.9–10 (2006): 607–611.
Naghizadeh B et al. Protective effects of oral crocin against intracerebroventricular streptozotocin-induced spatial memory deficit and oxidative stress in rats. Phytomedicine 20.6 (2013): 537–542.
Noorbala AA et al. Hydro-alcoholic extract of Crocus sativus L. versus fluoxetine in the treatment of mild to moderate depression: a double-blind, randomized pilot trial. J Ethnopharmacol 97.2 (2005): 281–284.
Piccardi M et al. A longitudinal follow-up study of saffron supplementation in early age-related macular degeneration: sustained benefits to central retinal function. Evid.Based.Complement Alternat. Med (2012): 429124.
Pitsikas, N et al. Effects of the active constituents of Crocus sativus L., crocins on recognition and spatial rats' memory. Behav Brain Res 183.2 (2007): 141–146.
Purushothuman S et al. Saffron pre-treatment offers neuroprotection to Nigral and retinal dopaminergic cells of MPTP-Treated mice. J Parkinsons Dis. 3.1 (2013): 77–83.
Rastgoo M et al.. Antitumor activity of PEGylated nanoliposomes containing crocin in mice bearing C26 colon carcinoma. Planta Med 79.6 (2013): 447–451.
Razavi BM et al. Protective effect of crocin on diazinon induced cardiotoxicity in rats in subchronic exposure. Chem Biol Interact 203.3 (2013): 547–555.
Rezaee R et al. Cytotoxic effects of crocin on MOLT-4 human leukemia cells. J Complement Integr Med, 10 (2013).
Shahmansouri N et al. A randomized, double-blind, clinical trial comparing the efficacy and safety of Crocus sativus L. with fluoxetine for improving mild to moderate depression in post percutaneous coronary intervention patients. J Affect Disord 155 (2014): 216–222.
Soeda S et al. Crocin suppresses tumor necrosis factor-alpha-induced cell death of neuronally differentiated PC-12 cells. Life Sci 69.24 (2001): 2887–2898.
Tamaddonfard E et al. Crocin improved learning and memory impairments in streptozotocin-induced diabetic rats. Iran J Basic Med Sci 16.1 (2013): 91–100.
Tashakori-Sabzevar F et al. Crocetin attenuates spatial learning dysfunction and hippocampal injury in a model of vascular dementia. Curr Neurovasc Res 10.4 (2013): 325–334.
Vahdati, H.F et al. Antidepressant effects of crocin and its effects on transcript and protein levels of CREB, BDNF and VGF in rat hippocampus. Daru 22.1 (2014): 16.

Sage

HISTORICAL NOTE The Salvia genus is one of the largest groups of the Lamiaceae family with over 700 species spread throughout the world (Nickavar et al 2005). Sage has been used since ancient times as an antiseptic, astringent, tonic, carminative, antispasmodic, anti-inflammatory and to reduce sweating in various traditional medicine systems. The name 'Salvia' derives from the Latin salvere (to be saved) (Blumenthal et al 2000). Sage oil is used as a culinary spice and as a fragrance in soaps and perfumes. The fragrance is said to suppress the odour of fish.

OTHER NAMES

Broad-leafed sage, common sage, dalmatian sage, garden sage, meadow sage, Spanish sage, true sage

BOTANICAL NAME/FAMILY

Salvia officinalis, Salvia lavandulaefolia, Salvia hypoleuca Benth (family Labiatae or Lamiaceae).

PLANT PART USED

Leaf

CHEMICAL COMPONENTS

The exact chemical constituents depend on geographical and climatic conditions, as well as harvesting conditions, distillation method and the part of the plant used (Nickavar et al 2005). The leaves contain up to 2.5% essential oil, which contains thujone, cineol and camphor, as well as humulene, pinene, camphene, limonene, carnosol and rosmarinic acid. In addition, the leaves contain catechin-type tannins, diterpene bitter principles, triterpenes, steroids, flavones, and flavonoid glycosides, together with polysaccharides. Sage is a rich source of beta-carotene, vitamins C and B-complex (Fisher & Painter 1996). The flowering parts of *S. hypoleuca* contain bicyclogermacrene, (E)-beta-caryophyllene, viridiflorol, spathulenol, beta-pinene and delta-pinene. Pharmacopoeial grade sage leaf must contain not less than 1.5% thujone-rich volatile oil (Blumenthal et al 2000).

MAIN ACTIONS

Antimicrobial

Sage is reported to have antimicrobial activity attributed to the thujone, thymol and eugenol contents of the volatile oil (Shapiro et al 1994), as well as its rosmarinic acid content (Petersen & Simmonds 2003). The phenolic acids, salvins and monomethyl ethers have also been attributed with antimicrobial activity. Overall, activity has been reported in vitro against *Escherichia coli*, *Salmonella* spp, *Shigella sonnei*, *Klebsiella ozanae*, *Bacillus subtilis* and various fungi, including *Candida albicans* (Newell et al 1996). Phenolic extracts have also shown antibacterial activity against *Enterococcus* (Feres et al 2005). There is some disagreement over whether sage is an effective bacteriostatic agent against *Staphylococcus aureus*. Sage had some in vitro antimicrobial effects on saliva samples from periodontally healthy and diseased subjects, although it had less activity than clove or propolis (Feres et al 2005). Sage essential oil has been shown to have effective inhibitory activity against microorganisms, such as *Klebsiella* spp, *Enterobacter* spp, *E. coli*, *Proteus mirabilis* and *Morganella morganii*, isolated from urinary tract infection (Santos Pereira et al 2004). There are also reports that sage may also be fungistatic and virustatic (Eidi et al 2005).

In vitro studies investigating the effect of digestive secretions on oral doses of sage concluded that any antimicrobial effects will probably be deactivated in the gastrointestinal tract after oral ingestion and thus *S. officinalis* is unlikely to demonstrate a systemic antibiotic action (Vermaak et al 2009).

Sage extracts are used as sources of antioxidant and antimicrobial protection against food decay in the food industry.

Antioxidant

Sage extracts have been shown to have strong antioxidant activity (Matsingou et al 2003, Pizzale et al 2002), with labiatic acid and carnosic acid reported to be the active compounds (Perry et al 2003). According to in vivo studies with animal models, ingestion of sage infusion improves the liver's antioxidant status (Lima et al 2005) and protects against azathioprine-induced toxicity (Amin & Hamza 2005). However, sage essential oil did not show protective effects against toxicity from an oxidative compound in isolated rat hepatocytes (Lima et al 2004).

Astringent

The high tannin content of sage supports its reported astringent activity.

Antispasmodic

Sage oil has antispasmodic effects in laboratory animals (Newell et al 1996) and this is likely to be due to the irritating effects of the volatile oil. There is some evidence that sage oil may also exert a centrally mediated antisecretory action.

Anxiolytic

Rosmarinic acid, which is a component of sage essential oil, produces an anxiolytic-like effect without exerting locomotor alterations or DNA damage in the brain tissue of rats (Pereira et al 2005). According to in vitro tests, compounds in the methanolic extract have an affinity for human brain benzodiazepine receptors (Kavvadias et al 2003).

Anticholinesterase

In vitro and in vivo studies suggest that sage essential oil and some individual monoterpenoid constituents inhibit acetylcholinesterase activity (Perry et al 2003). An extract of the sage leaf exhibited dose-dependent, in vitro inhibition of acetylcholinesterase (Kennedy & Scholey 2006).

Antidiabetic and lipid lowering effects

Sage ethanolic extract exhibits a number of mechanisms of relevance in diabetes according to animal studies. It significantly decreased serum glucose in diabetic rats without affecting insulin release (Eidi et al 2005). Oral administration of 0.2 and 0.4 g/kg body wt. of sage extract for 14 days exhibited a significant reduction in serum glucose, triglycerides, total cholesterol, urea, uric acid, creatinine, AST, ALT and increased plasma insulin in streptozotocin-induced diabetic rats but not in normal rats. Glibenclamide was used as reference and showed similar antidiabetic effect (Eidi & Eidi 2009).

It has been suggested that extracts of sage containing carnosic acid may act as a new class of lipid absorption inhibitor. A methanolic extract of sage has also shown significant inhibitory effect on serum triglyceride elevation in olive oil-loaded mice, and inhibitory activity against pancreatic lipase, mainly because of the carnosic acid content. Carnosic acid was also found to reduce the weight gain and accumulation of epididymal fat in high-fat diet-fed mice after 14 days (Ninomiya et al 2004).

OTHER ACTIONS

The water-soluble polysaccharide complex from sage has demonstrated immunomodulatory activity (Capek & Hribalova 2004) and the terpenoid fractions have shown antimutagenic properties in vivo (Vujosevic & Blagojevic 2004). In vitro and in vivo studies indicate that sage essential oil and some individual monoterpenoid constituents demonstrate antioxidant, anti-inflammatory and oestrogenic effects (Perry et al 2003).

Sage has demonstrated significant anti-inflammatory and antinociceptive effects in animal models (Rodrigues et al 2012).

CLINICAL USE

Although sage has not been the subject of many clinical studies, many of its constituents demonstrate significant pharmacological effects, providing a theoretical basis for some of its uses.

Reduces secretions

Sage has been traditionally used to treat excessive perspiration and salivation, dysmenorrhoea, diarrhoea, galactorrhoea and sweats associated with menopause and to cease lactation (Fisher & Painter 1996). An open study of 80 patients confirmed that it can reduce perspiration (Blumenthal et al 2000). The high tannin content of the herb provides a theoretical basis for its use.

Dyspepsia and lack of appetite

The reported antispasmodic action and bitter constituents of sage support its use in treating loss of appetite, gastritis, flatulence, bloating and dyspepsia. These uses await support from clinical research.

Inflammation of mucous membranes

Topically, sage is used as a gargle for laryngitis, pharyngitis, stomatitis, gingivitis, glossitis, minor oral injuries and inflammation of the nasal mucosa (Blumenthal et al 2000). These uses can be based on the pharmacological activity of its chemical components. In an open-label, single-blind randomised controlled trial (RCT) of 420 patients, the non-steroidal anti-inflammatory drug benzydamine hydrochloride was found to be more effective than sage in relieving postoperative pain when used as a mouthwash after tonsillectomy in children and adults (Lalicevic & Djordjevic 2004).

Sage has been found to have less antitussive effects than codeine, but a significantly higher or similar effect to dropropizine (Nosalova et al 2005). A small double-blind study suggested that use of an essential oil spray or gargle formulation that includes sage may help relieve snoring (Prichard 2004).

Pharyngitis

There have been two randomised trials of throat spray containing sage extract for the treatment of acute sore throat, both demonstrating efficacy. One was a multicentre, randomised, double-blind, double-dummy controlled trial (n = 154) in which patients presenting to general practice with acute sore throat >72 hours were given either an echinacea/sage spray or a chlorhexidine/lignocaine spray. Both sprays were well tolerated and found to have similar efficacy in reducing sore throat symptoms during the first 3 days, with the echinacea/sage group experiencing greater response rates after 3 days (Schapowal et al 2009). The other, a randomised, double-blind, parallel group study, compared the efficacy and tolerability of a spray containing sage against placebo in the treatment of patients with acute viral pharyngitis (Hubbert et al 2006). A total of 286 patients were randomised to receive placebo or treatment for 3 days, including one baseline visit and one final visit. The 15% spray containing 140 microlitre sage extract per dose was statistically significantly superior to placebo in reducing the throat pain intensity score. Symptomatic relief occurred within the first 2 hours after first administration and only minor side effects were seen, such as dry pharynx or burning of mild intensity.

Memory enhancement

Since ancient times, sage has been used to enhance memory and treat dementia. More recently, cholinergic activities have been demonstrated in vitro and in vivo, suggesting that it may be useful in treating Alzheimer's disease (Orhan et al 2013, Perry et al 2001). A randomised placebo-controlled study undertaken at three centres assessed the effects of sage extract (60 drops/day) in 42 subjects with mild-to-moderate Alzheimer's disease (Akhondzadeh et al 2003). Initially, subjects had a score of 12 or less on the cognitive subscale of Alzheimer's Disease Assessment Scale (ADAS-cog) and two or less on the Clinical Dementia Rating (CDR). At 4 months, sage extract produced a significantly better outcome on cognitive functions than placebo in both test scales and was well tolerated.

In 2003, two placebo-controlled, double-blind, crossover studies involving 44 healthy young adults investigated the effects of different strengths of standardised essential oil of *S. lavandulaefolia* on memory (Tildesley et al 2003). Both studies found that a 50-microlitre dose of Salvia essential oil significantly improved immediate word recall and was able to modulate cognition. In another placebo-controlled, double-blind, crossover study involving 24 subjects, Spanish sage (*S. lavandulaefolia*) essential oil was found to enhance cognitive performance and mood in healthy young adults (Tildesley et al 2005).

In 2006, results of a double-blind, placebo-controlled, crossover study were published involving 30 healthy participants who received a series of different treatments on each visit to the research laboratory (placebo, 300, 600 mg dried sage leaf) (Kennedy & Scholey 2006). The results confirm previous observations of the cholinesterase inhibiting properties of *S. officinalis*, and improved mood and cognitive performance following the administration of single doses to healthy young participants.

Hypercholesterolemia

Promising new research suggests that sage may be useful in lowering total cholesterol and triglyerides in hyperlipidaemic patients. A randomised double-blind placebo-controlled clinical trial (n = 67) using 500 mg of sage leaf extract (three times daily) standardised to 2.16% quercetin content significantly reduced total cholesterol ($P < 0.001$), triglyceride ($P = 0.001$), LDL ($P = 0.004$) and VLDL ($P = 0.001$), and increased the blood HDL levels ($P < 0.001$) significantly compared with the placebo control after 2 months of treatment. No toxic effects were observed on hepatic and renal functions and no adverse effects were reported by the patients (Kianbakht et al 2011).

Reducing hot flushes

Sage is commonly used by modern herbalists in prescriptions for menopause in order to treat hot flushes, night sweats, and for its oestrogenic effect. As yet, there is no clinical evidence available to confirm effectiveness for these indications (Blumenthal et al 2000).

A pilot study evaluating efficacy and safety of sage (150 mg three times daily) in controlling hot flushes in prostate cancer patients treated with androgen deprivation therapy (n = 10) found that hot flushes reduced significantly in the first 3 weeks of treatment, with the effect maintained for the rest of the 8-week trial. There was a non-significant decrease in LH and FSH levels and no significant effect on testosterone, free testosterone, SHBG, blood pressure, haemoglobin concentration or on cholesterol levels and no side effects were observed.

Despite this, there was no improvement on quality of life measures (Vandecasteele et al 2012).

OTHER USES

As an inhalant, sage is used for asthma. In foods, it is used as a culinary spice. In manufacturing, sage is used as a fragrance component in soaps and cosmetics. Topically, sage is used to treat herpes labialis, laryngitis, pharyngitis, stomatitis, gingivitis, glossitis, minor oral injuries and inflammation of the nasal mucosa. Sage oil exhibited anticandidal activity against *C. albicans* (Sookto et al 2013).

Cancer prevention

Promising in vitro research suggests that various constituents of sage may have a role in cancer prevention. The carnosic acid component has demonstrated cytotoxic activity, probably mediated by nitric oxide-induced apoptosis (Kontogianni et al 2013). Carnosic acid also efficiently suppresses the formation of PGE_2 which may contribute to its anti-inflammatory and anticarcinogenic properties (Bauer et al 2012). The linalyl acetate component demonstrated anticancer activities in another in vitro study, partly mediated through the suppression of NF-kappaB activation, suggestive that this could be utilised in combination with chemotherapeutic agents to induce apoptosis (Deeb et al 2011). Sage water extracts have demonstrated inhibitory effects on proliferation and induced apoptosis in human colorectal carcinoma cell lines (Xavier et al 2009) and sage tea was also found to be protective against oxidative DNA damage in HCT15 colon cells (Ramos et al 2012).

A case-control study in patients diagnosed with lung cancer evaluated the relationship between components of the Mediterranean diet and lung cancer. A decreased overall risk of developing lung cancer was associated with intake of some culinary herbs, particularly sage, presumed to be due to its polyphenol content, such as carnosol and carnosic acid (Johnson 2011).

DOSAGE RANGE

Internal use

- Infusion of dried herb: 1–4 g three times daily.
- Tincture (1 : 1): 1–4 mL three times daily.
- Essential oil: 2–3 drops in 100 mL water several times daily.
- Gargle or rinse (use warm infusion): 2.5 g cut leaf in 100 mL water; or 2–3 drops essential oil in 100 mL water; or use 5 mL fluid extract diluted in a glass of water, several times daily.

TOXICITY

Sage is likely to be safe when taken in amounts typically found in foods. Essential oil of sage may be toxic in large doses and any case reports of toxicity are usually due to ingestion of sage oil rather than sage extract. In large amounts, the camphor and thujone content of sage oil have been shown to have convulsant properties in rats (Millet et al 1981). When taken internally in large amounts, sage may cause restlessness and seizures in humans (Blumenthal et al 2000, Newell et al 1996) and there have been two case reports of epileptic seizures in young children caused by accidental ingestion of sage oil (Lachenmeier & Walch 2012). Sage tea has also been reported to cause cheilitis and stomatitis, dry mouth and local irritation.

A risk assessment of thujone in foods and medicines such as sage suggests that 0.11 mg/kg body weight/day is an acceptable daily intake (ADI), an amount unlikely to be consumed in normal dietary intake. Between 2 and 20 cups of sage tea would be required to reach this ADI (Lachenmeier & Uebelacker 2010).

ADVERSE REACTIONS

One double-blind, randomised trial found that sage was well tolerated and produced fewer side effects than placebo (Akhondzadeh et al 2003). There have been two case reports of contact dermatitis from sage products (Mayer et al 2011).

CONTRAINDICATIONS AND PRECAUTIONS

Sage oil can irritate the skin when used topically. Internal use of the essential oil should be closely monitored.

PREGNANCY USE

Traditionally, sage is reported to have abortifacient properties. Its use in pregnancy is therefore not recommended (Mills & Bone 2000, Newell et al 1996).

Practice points/Patient counselling

- Sage is a widely used, popular spice and sage oil is used in a variety of culinary applications. It has antioxidant, antibacterial and some antifungal activities.
- Sage has a long history of use in traditional medicine as an antispasmodic and carminative, to relieve excess sweating and as a gargle for inflammations of the mouth.
- It is also commonly prescribed in combination with other herbs to relieve menopausal symptoms such as night sweats with some preliminary research showing a reduction in hot flushes.
- Clinical research suggests it may be useful in mild-to-moderate Alzheimer's disease. Other studies report that it improves memory in healthy subjects.
- Standardised sage extract significantly reduces cholesterol levels according to a human study suggesting a possible benefit for people with elevated blood lipids.

SIGNIFICANT INTERACTIONS

Iron, calcium, magnesium.

Due to the tannin content, sage may reduce the absorption of these minerals — separate doses by 2–3 hours.

PATIENTS' FAQs

What will this herb do for me?

Sage is used to reduce symptoms of menopause such as night sweats; however, scientific testing has not been conducted to confirm whether it is effective. Recent research demonstrates effectiveness of sage spray for sore throat, a reduction in total cholesterol levels for people with elevated blood lipids and that it may improve memory in Alzheimer's disease and in healthy subjects.

When will it start to work?

The study in Alzheimer's disease found effects established within 4 months' use. In the case of menopause, a time frame is unknown.

Are there any safety issues?

When used in appropriate doses, it appears to be a safe herbal medicine; however, it should not be used in pregnancy.

REFERENCES

Akhondzadeh S et al. Salvia officinalis extract in the treatment of patients with mild to moderate Alzheimer's disease: a double blind, randomized and placebo-controlled trial. J Clin Pharm Ther 28.1 (2003): 53–59.

Amin A, Hamza AA. Hepatoprotective effects of Hibiscus, Rosmarinus and Salvia on azathioprine-induced toxicity in rats. Life Sci 77.3 (2005): 266–278.

Bauer J et al. Carnosol and carnosic acids from Salvia officinalis inhibit microsomal prostaglandin E2 synthase-1. J Pharmacol Experim Therapeut 342.1 (2012): 169–176.

Blumenthal M et al (eds). Herbal medicine: expanded Commission E monographs. Austin, TX: Integrative Medicine Communications, 2000.

Capek P, Hribalova V. Water-soluble polysaccharides from Salvia officinalis L. possessing immunomodulatory activity. Phytochemistry 65.13 (2004): 1983–1992.

Deeb S et al. Sage components enhance cell death through nuclear factor kappa-B signaling. Frontiers in Bioscience 3 (2011): 410–420.

Eidi A, Eidi M. Antidiabetic effects of sage (Salvia officinalis L.) leaves in normal and streptozotocin-induced diabetic rats. Diabetes & Metabolic Syndrome: Clinical Research & Reviews 3.1 (2009): 40–44.

Eidi M et al. Effect of Salvia officinalis L. leaves on serum glucose and insulin in healthy and streptozotocin-induced diabetic rats. J Ethnopharmacol 100.3 (2005): 310–313.

Feres ML et al. In vitro antimicrobial activity of plant extracts and propolis in saliva samples of healthy and periodontally-involved subjects. J Int Acad Periodontol 7.3 (2005): 90–96.

Fisher C, Painter G. Materia medica for the southern hemisphere. Auckland: Fisher-Painter Publishers, 1996.

Hubbert M et al. Efficacy and tolerability of a spray with Salvia officinalis in the treatment of acute pharyngitis — a randomised, double-blind, placebo-controlled study with adaptive design and interim analysis. Eur J Med Res 11.1 (2006): 20–26.

Johnson JJ Carnosol: A promising anti-cancer and anti-inflammatory agent. Cancer Letters, 305.1 (2011): 1–7.

Kavvadias D et al. Constituents of sage (Salvia officinalis) with in vitro affinity to human brain benzodiazepine receptor. Planta Med 69.2 (2003): 113–117.

Kennedy DO, Scholey AB. The psychopharmacology of European herbs with cognition enhancing properties. Curr Pharm Des 12.35 (2006): 4613–4623.

Kianbakht S et al.. Antihyperlipidemic Effects of Salvia officinalis L. Leaf Extract in Patients with Hyperlipidemia: A Randomized Double-Blind Placebo-Controlled Clinical Trial. Phytother Res 25.12 (2011) 1849–1853.

Kontogianni V et al. Phytochemical profile of Rosmarinus officinalis and Salvia officinalis extracts and correlation to their antioxidant and anti-proliferative activity. Food Chem 136.1 (2013): 120–129.

Lachenmeier DW, Uebelacker M. Risk assessment of thujone in foods and medicines containing sage and wormwood — Evidence for a need of regulatory changes? Regulat Toxicol Pharmacol, 58.3 (2010): 437–443.

Lachenmeier D, Walch S. Epileptic seizures caused by accidental ingestion of sage (Salvia officinalis) oil in children: a rare, exceptional case or a threat to public health? Ped Neurol, 46 (2012): 201.

Lalicevic S, Djordjevic I. Comparison of benzydamine hydrochloride and Salvia officinalis as an adjuvant local treatment to systemic nonsteroidal anti-inflammatory drug in controlling pain after tonsillectomy, adenoidectomy, or both: an open-label, single-blind, randomized clinical trial. Curr Ther Res 65.4 (2004): 360–372.

Lima CF et al. Evaluation of toxic/protective effects of the essential oil of Salvia officinalis on freshly isolated rat hepatocytes. Toxicol In Vitro 18.4 (2004): 457–465.

Lima CF et al. The drinking of a Salvia officinalis infusion improves liver antioxidant status in mice and rats. J Ethnopharmacol 97.2 (2005): 383–389.

Matsingou TC et al. Antioxidant activity of organic extracts from aqueous infusions of sage. J Agric Food Chem 51.23 (2003): 6696–6701.

Mayer E et al. Allergic contact dermatitis caused by Salvia officinalis extract. Contact Dermatitis 64.4 (2011): 237–238.

Millet Y et al. Toxicity of some essential plant oils: clinical and experimental study. Clin Toxicol 18.12 (1981): 1485–1498.

Mills S, Bone K. Principles and practice of phytotherapy. London: Churchill Livingstone, 2000.

Newell CA et al. Herbal medicines: a guide for health care professionals. London, UK: The Pharmaceutical Press, 1996.

Nickavar B et al. Volatile composition of the essential oil of Salvia hypoleuca Benth. Int J Aromather 15.1 (2005): 51–53.

Ninomiya K et al. Carnosic acid, a new class of lipid absorption inhibitor from sage. Bioorg Med Chem Lett 14.8 (2004): 1943–1946.

Nosalova G et al. Efficacy of herbal substances according to cough reflex. Minerva Biotechnol 17.3 (2005): 141–152.

Orhan I. E et al. Assessment of anticholinesterase and antioxidant properties of selected sage (Salvia) species with their total phenol and flavonoid contents. Industrial Crops and Products, 41.0 (2013): 21–30.

Pereira P et al. Neurobehavioral and genotoxic aspects of rosmarinic acid. Pharmacol Res 52.3 (2005): 199–203.

Perry N et al. In-vitro activity of S. lavandulaefolia (Spanish sage) relevant to treatment of Alzheimer's disease. J Pharm Pharmacol 53.10 (2001): 1347–1356.

Perry N et al. Salvia for dementia therapy: review of pharmacological activity and pilot tolerability clinical trial. Pharmacol Biochem Behav 75.3 (2003): 651–659.

Petersen M, Simmonds MSJ. Rosmarinic acid. Phytochemistry 62.2 (2003): 121–125.

Pizzale L et al. Antioxidant activity of sage (Salvia officinalis and S. fruticosa) and oregano (Origanum onites and O. indercedens) extracts related to their phenolic compound content. J Sci Food Agric 82.14 (2002): 1645–1651.

Prichard AJN. Use of essential oils to treat snoring. Phytother Res 18.9 (2004): 696–699.

Ramos A et al. Protection by Salvia extracts against oxidative and alkylation damage to DNA in human HCT15 and CO115 cells. Journal of Toxicology & Environmental Health, Part A. 75 (13–15) (2012): 765–775.

Rodrigues MRA et al. Antinociceptive and anti-inflammatory potential of extract and isolated compounds from the leaves of Salvia officinalis in mice. Journal of Ethnopharmacology, 139.2 (2012): 519–526.

Santos Pereira R et al. Antibacterial activity of essential oils on microorganisms isolated from urinary tract infection. Rev Saude Pub 38.2 (2004): 326–328.

Schapowal A et al. Echinacea/sage or chlorhexidine/lidocaine for treating acute sore throats: a randomized double-blind trial. Euro J Med Res 14.9 (2009): 406–412.

Shapiro S et al. The antimicrobial activity of essential oils and essential oil components towards oral bacteria. Oral Microbiol Immunol 9.4 (1994): 202–328.

Sookto T et al. In vitro effects of Salvia officinalis L. essential oil on Candida albicans. Asian Pacific J Tropical Biomed, 3.5 (2013): 376–380.

Tildesley NT et al. Salvia lavandulaefolia (Spanish Sage) enhances memory in healthy young volunteers. Pharmacol Biochem Behav 75.3 (2003): 669–674.

Tildesley NT et al. Positive modulation of mood and cognitive performance following administration of acute doses of Salvia lavandulaefolia essential oil to healthy young volunteers. Physiol Behav 83.5 (2005): 699–709.

Vandecasteele K et al. Evaluation of the Efficacy and Safety of Salvia officinalis in Controlling Hot Flashes in Prostate Cancer Patients Treated with Androgen Deprivation. Phytotherapy Research, 26.2 (2012): 208–213.

Vermaak I et al. Effect of simulated gastrointestinal conditions and epithelial transport on extracts of green tea and sage. Phytochem Letters 2.4 (2009): 166–170.

Vujosevic M, Blagojevic J. Antimutagenic effects of extracts from sage (Salvia officinalis) in mammalian system in vivo. Acta Vet Hung 52.4 (2004): 439–443.

Xavier C et al. Salvia fructicosa, Salvia officinalis and rosmarinic acid induce apoptosis and inhibit proliferation of human colorectal cell lines: the role in MAPK/ERK pathway. Nutrition & Cancer 61.4 (2009): 564–571.

Saw palmetto

HISTORICAL NOTE Saw palmetto was used traditionally as a treatment for urogenital irritations, impotence and male infertility, among other conditions, and was described by the American Eclectic physicians as the 'old man's friend'. Between 1906 and 1917 saw palmetto was listed in the US Pharmacopoeia and between 1926 and 1950 it was in the National Formulary as a treatment for urogenital ailments; however, it fell out of favour for several decades as pharmaceutical medicines came to the forefront of mainstream medicine. Not so in Europe where, in the 1960s, French researchers began to chemically analyse the saw palmetto berry, and a breakthrough lipophilic preparation was eventually developed and subjected to countless clinical trials.

COMMON NAME

Serenoa or saw palmetto

OTHER NAMES

American dwarf palm tree, cabbage palm, dwarf palmetto, fan palm, sabal fructus, sabal, serenoa

BOTANICAL NAME/FAMILY

Sabal serrulata, Serenoa repens (family Arecaceae or Palmaceae)

PLANT PART USED

Dried ripe fruit

CHEMICAL COMPONENTS

An ethanol extract of the berry contains free fatty acids rich in shorter-chain-length fatty acids, such as capric, caprylic, lauric and myristic acids (Nemecz 2003). Palmitic, stearic, oleic, linoleic and linolenic acids are also present in the extract. There are also lesser amounts of phytosterols (such as beta-sitosterol, stigmasterol, ampesterol and cycloartenol), aliphatic alcohols and polyprenic compounds. The lipophilic extract is used medicinally.

MAIN ACTIONS

The mechanism of action is not fully elucidated; however, it appears that several mechanisms are at work.

Inhibition of 5-alpha reductase

In different cell systems, the lipid-sterolic extract acts as a non-competitive inhibitor of both type 1 and type 2 5-alpha reductase activity, thereby preventing the conversion of testosterone to dihydrotestosterone (Bayne et al 2000, Raynaud et al 2002, Sultan et al 1984). However, it is currently unclear whether the effect is apparent in humans, as contradictory evidence exists. Raynaud et al (2002) explained that the discrepancies found by different authors were due to different experimental conditions and selectivity for fatty acids, as only specific aliphatic unsaturated fatty acids have been shown to inhibit 5-alpha reductase activity.

One study that analysed and compared benign prostatic hyperplasia (BPH) samples taken from both untreated and treated subjects (320 mg saw palmetto extract taken for 3 months) found that local levels of testosterone were raised, whereas dihydrotestosterone levels were reduced, suggestive of local 5-alpha reductase inhibition (Di Silverio et al 1998). An earlier short-term study found that a dose of 160 mg of a liposterolic extract (Permixon) produced no changes to serum dihydrotestosterone levels, whereas finasteride 5 mg induced a significant reduction (Strauch et al 1994). Since prostate levels were untested in this study, it is not known whether a local effect occurred, even though serum levels remained unchanged.

Unlike other 5-alpha reductase inhibitors, there is no interference with the cell's capacity to secrete prostate-specific antigens (PSAs) because it does not affect the transcription of the gene for PSA, as demonstrated both in vitro and in vivo (Maccagnano et al 2006). Although having an obvious clinical advantage with regard to PSA screening for prostate cancer, this also suggests that 5-alpha reductase inhibition is not a major mechanism of action.

Inhibits binding of dihydrotestosterone and testosterone to androgen receptors

Saw palmetto reduces receptor binding of dihydrotestosterone and testosterone by an average of 41%, as tested in 11 different tissue specimens from BPH patients (el Sheikh et al 1988). In 2003, results from two animal studies showed that saw palmetto (whole berry and extract) influenced prostatic hyperplasia via effects on androgen metabolism (Talpur et al 2003).

Inhibits prolactin

In vivo research has identified an inhibitory effect not only on androgens, but also on the trophic effect of prolactin in the rat prostate (Van

Coppenolle et al 2000). The inhibitory effect on prolactin activity appears to be due to inhibition of several steps in prolactin receptor signal transduction, according to one animal model (Vacher et al 1995).

Anti-inflammatory

Saw palmetto is a dual inhibitor of the cyclooxygenase (COX) and 5-lipoxygenase pathways, according to in vitro research (Breu et al 1992, Paubert-Braquet et al 1997). Decreased expression of COX-2 has also been identified, providing a further explanation for the observed anti-inflammatory activity (Goldmann et al 2001).

Antispasmodic

Both the lipid and the saponifiable fractions have demonstrated antispasmodic activity in several in vitro studies (WHO 2003).

Cytochromes

Saw palmetto failed to have a significant effect on CYP3A4 or CYP2D6 when tested in healthy individuals (Markowitz et al 2003).

Antiproliferative effects

In recent years, there has been interest in determining whether saw palmetto may have a role in prostate cancer, as an inhibitory activity has been observed in several test tube studies for prostatic cancer cell lines (Goldmann et al 2001, Ishii et al 2001, Scholtysek et al 2009).

In 2009, results of an in vitro study were published which tested a saw palmetto ethanolic berry extract (SPBE) and compared its activity on prostatic cancer cells (DU-145) to individual fatty sterol components β-sitosterol, stigmasterol and cholesterol. Most significant findings included an increased expression of nuclear protein p53, and a reduced expression of p27 and p21, with resulting inhibition of tumour cell growth greatest in SPBE, followed by β-sitosterol and β-stigmasterol respectively. It was also observed that p53 had a mechanical effect of binding to F-actin, increasing adhesive properties of cells, reducing the likelihood of cellular migratory effects. This may in the future have an impact on the knowledge and treatment of tumour invasion (Scholtysek et al 2009).

OTHER ACTIONS

Although alpha-1 adrenoreceptor activity has been reported in vitro, a clinical study found no evidence of this activity (Goepel et al 1999, 2001). Saw palmetto does not affect platelet function in vivo (Beckert et al 2007).

Traditionally, saw palmetto is believed to act as a mild diuretic, urinary antiseptic and expectorant.

CLINICAL USE

The most studied saw palmetto preparation is a commercial product known as Permixon (Pierre Fabre Médicament, France), which is a liposterolic extract consisting of 80% free (e.g. 94 g/100 g extract) and 7% esterified fatty acids, as well as small amounts of sterols (beta-sitosterol, campesterol, stigmasterol, cycloartenol), and a minimum percentage of polyprenic compounds, arabinose, glucose, galactose, uronic acid and flavonoids. More recently, some other saw palmetto extracts have also been studied; however, there is concern that variations in chemical constituents may be a key factor behind the inconsistent results sometimes seen. In particular, in the United States, common saw palmetto products include ethanol and CO_2 extracts, whereas in Germany, fruit extracts obtained with 90% ethanol are very popular, and contain a hexane extract. A study comparing saw palmetto extracts produced using 90% ethanol versus under an optimised CO_2 condition found that levels of free fatty acids differed and the ethanolic extract contained a large amount of ethyl esters that were not present in the CO_2-produced extract (Bombardelli & Morazzoni 1997).

Benign prostatic hypertrophy

Saw palmetto extracts are extremely popular in Europe where herbal preparations represent approximately one-third of total sales of all therapeutic agents sold for the treatment of BPH (Levin & Das 2000). In Germany, for instance, more than 30 different preparations containing saw palmetto are on the market. By far the most intensively studied product of this group is an *n*-hexane-liposterol-extract (Permixon), which is very popular in France and Italy. It is a complex mixture of free fatty acids and their esters, phytosterols, aliphatic alcohols and various polyprenic compounds (Madersbacher et al 2007).

Many clinical studies demonstrate mild to moderate improvements in several common urinary symptoms associated with BPH and with fewer side effects than alpha-blocker and 5-reductase inhibitor drugs. Some more recent study results are less consistent than previously, which is suspected to be mainly due to differences in chemical composition of test products. This is apparent when reviewing the Cochrane systematic reviews and other literature published in the last decade. In particular, differences in test dosages, treatment time frames, severity of disease and, importantly, herbal extract are likely to be contributing factors making the interpretation of results difficult. The possibility of inadequate blinding in some previous studies is yet another factor.

A 2002 Cochrane review assessing the results from 21 randomised controlled trials (RCTs) involving 3139 men concluded that saw palmetto improves urinary scores, symptoms and urinary flow measures compared with placebo, with effects on symptom scores and peak urine flow similar to the pharmaceutical drug finasteride (Wilt et al 2002). Additionally, its use is associated with fewer adverse effects compared with finasteride and, typically, symptomatic relief is reported more quickly.

In 2004, an updated meta-analysis of 14 RCTs and three open-label studies was published (Boyle et al 2004). The analysis used data from 4280 patients derived from clinical studies that had used Permixon. Three randomised trials had a study period of 6 months or longer. Peak urinary flow rate and nocturia were the two common endpoints. Active treatment was associated with a mean reduction in the International Prostate Symptom Score (IPSS) of 4.78, and a significant improvement in peak flow rate and reduction in nocturia were also reported.

In contrast to previous systematic reviews, a 2012 Cochrane review of 32 RCTs (27 double-blinded) concluded that saw palmetto was no better than placebo in the control of urinary symptoms, peak urine flow and nocturia (Wilt et al 2012). The review analysed results obtained from 5666 men. The negative CAMUS study had a substantial influence on the results. It involved 369 men and compared standardised saw palmetto extract (Prosta-Urgenin Uro) at three different daily doses (320 mg, 640 mg and 960 mg) over 72 weeks. In the CAMUS study, herbal treatment had no significant effect on the American Urological Association Symptom Index (AUASI) or secondary outcomes, including nocturia, peak urine flow and prostate size as compared to placebo (Barry et al 2011). Similarly, an earlier double-blind study of 1 year of continuous treatment with saw palmetto extract (160 mg twice daily containing 92.1% total fatty acids) failed to produce significant differences compared with placebo measured by AUASI, maximal urinary flow rate, prostate size, residual volume after voiding, quality of life or serum PSA levels in subjects with moderate to severe BPH (Bent et al 2006).

IN COMBINATION

In 2013, positive results were demonstrated for a combination product in a randomised, double-blind placebo-controlled trial of 57 men between the ages of 40 and 80 years with medically-diagnosed BPH (Coulsen et al 2013). The product tested was ProstateEze Max, a herbal formulation containing *Cucurbita pepo* seed oil (160 mg), *Epilobium parviflorum* extract (equivalent to 500 mg dry herb), lycopene (2.1 mg), *Prunus africana* (equivalent to 15 g dry stem, standardised to β-sitosterol) and *Serenoa repens* (equivalent to 660 mg dry leaf). At the end of the 12-week trial period the active treatment group had 35% symptom reduction in the median score (IPSS) of 36% compared to placebo (8%: $P < 0.05$). Daytime frequency of urination was reduced by 15.5% compared to no significant reduction in placebo group ($P < 0.03$) and night frequency was reduced by 39% compared to placebo 7% ($P < 0.004$).

Comparisons with alpha-adrenoreceptor antagonists

Although several comparative trials have been undertaken with finasteride, only a few have compared it with alpha-adrenoreceptor antagonist drugs, which are also commonly used in BPH (Adriazola et al 1992, Debruyne et al 2002).

A large, randomised, double-blind study involving 811 men with symptomatic BPH, who were recruited from 11 European countries, showed that Permixon 320 mg/day produced similar results to tamsulosin 0.4 mg/day (Omnic) (Debruyne et al 2002). More specifically, both treatments reduced the IPSS by an average of 4.4 in 80% of subjects. Those patients with the most severe disease experienced the greatest improvement in IPSS total score, with mean changes greater in the Permixon group than in the tamsulosin group (–8.0 and –6.8, respectively). With regard to safety, both treatments were considered well tolerated; however, ejaculation disorders were significantly more frequent with tamsulosin (4.2%) than with Permixon (0.6%). Although these results are promising, this study has been criticised for not including a placebo group as a comparator.

> ***Clinical note — BPH***
>
> BPH occurs in more than 50% of men over the age of 50 years. It is a slow, progressive enlargement of the fibromuscular and epithelial structures of the prostate gland, which can lead to obstruction of the ureter and urine retention. Symptoms such as frequent and/or painful urination, painful perineal stress and a decrease in urine volume and flow can develop. The condition has four stages, with stage 1 considered mild, stages 2 and 3 more severe and often requiring pharmacological treatment, and stage 4 severe and necessitating surgery.

In a short 3-week study, Grasso et al (1995) compared the effects of alfuzosin (7.5 mg/day) with saw palmetto (320 mg/day) in 63 BPH subjects under double-blind test conditions. Both treatments were found to be equally effective with regard to improving irritative score and with maximum and mean urine flow; however, alfuzosin was shown to more rapidly reduce symptoms of obstruction. Considering most studies have shown that 4–8 weeks' treatment with the herb is required to produce maximal effects, the effect seen at 3 weeks is encouraging.

An earlier study compared the effects of prazosin with saw palmetto in 45 patients with BPH over a 12-week period (Adriazola et al 1992). This study found that, although both treatments reduced symptoms, prazosin was slightly more effective.

In the TRIUMPH study, an observational study across six European countries involving 2351 men with newly diagnosed lower urinary tract symptoms suggestive of BPH, significant improvements were seen in 43% of patients taking *Serenoa repens*, 68% of people taking alpha blockers (tamsulosin), and 58% taking 5-alpha reductase (Hutchison et al 2007).

Changes to prostate size

It is still open to speculation as to whether saw palmetto affects prostate size, because studies have produced contradictory results (Aliaev et al 2002, Barry et al 2011, Bent et al 2006, Pytel et al 2002).

One open study of 155 men tested the effectiveness and tolerability of Permixon (160 mg twice daily) over 2 years (Pytel et al 2002) and not only detected a significant improvement in the IPSS and quality of life marker, but also a decrease in prostate size and significant improvement in sexual function after the first year of treatment.

A longer 5-year study using Permixon in 26 subjects with BPH showed that a total daily dose of 320 mg twice daily also significantly reduced disease symptoms and improved quality of life, while reducing prostate size by an average of 30% (Aliaev et al 2002). In 2003, results from animal models showed that saw palmetto (whole berry and extract) significantly diminished prostatic hyperplasia (Talpur et al 2003). In contrast, two previous studies from 2006 and 2011 failed to detect a significant effect on prostate size (Barry et al 2011, Bent et al 2006).

Androgenetic alopecia

The idea of using saw palmetto for androgenetic alopecia arose from the observation that finasteride appears to have some effect on this condition. One double-blind study has investigated the effects of saw palmetto as a potential therapeutic option, finding a highly positive response in 60% of subjects (Prager et al 2002). A second double-blind study of 48 men and women with androgenetic alopecia noted that mean hair density increased by 17% after 10 weeks of treatment with a topical lotion containing saw palmetto and by 27% after 50 weeks of treatment compared to baseline (Morganti et al, as reported in Linde et al 2006, Ulbricht & Basch 2006).

Chronic prostatitis and pelvic pain

Evidence to support the herb's use in prostatitis is scarce. However, in April 2003, positive findings from a preliminary study using Permixon to treat symptoms of chronic prostatitis and chronic pelvic pain syndrome (CP/CPPS) were presented at the annual meeting of the American Urological Association (AUA 2003). The RCT involving 61 patients with category IIIB CP/CPPS found that 75% receiving active treatment experienced at least mild improvement in symptoms, compared with 20% of the control group. Furthermore, 55% of patients receiving Permixon reported moderate or marked improvement, compared with 16% of the control group. In contrast, results from a 2004 prospective, randomised, open-label study failed to find benefits for saw palmetto (325 mg daily) in men diagnosed with category III CP/CPPS (Kaplan et al 2004). After 1 year, the mean total National Institutes of Health Chronic Prostatitis Symptom Index score decreased from 24.7 to 24.6 ($P = 0.41$) and no benefits were seen for quality of life or pain with saw palmetto treatment.

IN COMBINATION

More promising is a 2009 trial of 143 patients with chronic bacterial prostatitis which had two treatment arms, group A receiving the antibiotic prulifloxacin 600 mg, while group B were given the antibiotic plus saw palmetto 160 mg, nettle 120 mg, curcumin 200 mg and quercetin 100 mg extracts for 14 days. After 1 month 87% of group B had no further symptoms compared to 27% of group A (Cai et al 2009).

> ***Practice points/Patient counselling***
>
> - Many clinical studies demonstrate mild to moderate improvements in several common urinary symptoms associated with BPH, but the effect is most consistent for European preparations. Due to its good safety profile, a trial of treatment is still worthwhile for patients with mild to moderate BPH who have been advised to watch and wait with regard to conventional treatment.
> - Typically, if symptom reduction is experienced, this develops within 1–2 months' treatment. It is well tolerated and associated with fewer side effects than finasteride and tamsulosin.
> - The herb does not affect PSA levels; therefore PSA test results will be unaffected.
> - If symptoms worsen, blood is detected in the urine or acute urinary retention occurs, patients should be advised to seek professional advice.
> - If the patient is receiving radiotherapy for prostate cancer, saw palmetto supplementation should be ceased.

OTHER USES

Traditionally, saw palmetto has been used to treat a variety of urogenital conditions, such as impotence, male infertility and also as an aphrodisiac. It has also been used in female hirsutism, although its effectiveness in this condition is unknown.

DOSAGE RANGE

- Liposterolic extract: 320–960 mg/day in divided doses has been proved safe in a clinical trial (Barry et al 2011).
- Dried berry: 2–4 g.
- Liquid extract (1 : 2): 2–4.5 mL/day.

According to clinical studies

- 160 mg twice daily of liposterolic extract taken long term.

ADVERSE REACTIONS

The herb is generally well tolerated, with only non-specific symptoms reported, such as gastrointestinal upset, constipation, nausea, abdominal pain and diarrhoea. These minor complaints are generally resolved by taking the herb in association with meals (Agbabiaka et al 2009, Maccagnano et al 2006).

The 1-year STEP study provided a detailed assessment of the potential toxicity of saw palmetto, including both symptomatic adverse effects as well as asymptomatic laboratory abnormalities (Avins & Bent 2006). It found no evidence that consumption of saw palmetto extract (160 mg twice daily) over a period of 1 year was associated with any clinically important adverse effects. Relatively few participants suffered serious adverse events, and these were more common in the placebo-allocated participants. Additionally, no statistically significant differences were observed between the saw palmetto and placebo groups in the measured domains of sexual functioning, with the exception of the perception-of-sexual-problems domain, which showed a small but significantly greater improvement in the placebo group.

A 74-week trial which used doses up to 960 mg of a standardised extract daily produced no evidence of toxicity (Avins et al 2012).

SIGNIFICANT INTERACTIONS

No controlled studies are available and theoretical interactions are difficult to predict, due to the poorly understood nature of the herb's mechanism of action.

Finasteride (and other 5-alpha reductase inhibitor agents)

Additive effect theoretically possible — potential beneficial effect, although the clinical significance is unknown.

Androgenic drugs

Theoretically, saw palmetto may reduce the effectiveness of therapeutic androgens such as testosterone — observe patient for lack of drug effect.

CONTRAINDICATIONS AND PRECAUTIONS

If symptoms of BPH worsen, blood is detected in the urine or acute urinary retention occurs, professional reassessment is required.

Avoid saw palmetto products if undergoing radiotherapy for prostate cancer as preliminary in vitro studies suggest they may radiosensitise normal prostatic cells by inhibiting normal DNA repair (Hasan et al 2009).

PREGNANCY USE

Use of saw palmetto during pregnancy is contraindicated due to the herb's hormonal effects. In clinical practice, it is not used in pregnancy.

PATIENTS' FAQs

What will this herb do for me?

Saw palmetto has been extensively investigated as a treatment to relieve symptoms in BPH (enlarged prostate). Overall, it is more effective than placebo and most consistent results have been obtained for European preparations. There is some research suggesting that it may be useful in some forms of hair loss and prostatitis.

When will it start to work?

Symptom relief for enlarged prostate, if achieved, is generally experienced within 4–8 weeks.

Are there any safety issues?

Saw palmetto is well tolerated; however, occasionally mild gastrointestinal disturbances, headaches and rhinitis have been reported.

REFERENCES

Adriazola SM et al. Symptomatic treatment of benign hypertrophy of the prostate. Comparative study of prazosin and *Serenoa repens*. Arch Esp Urol 45.3 (1992): 211–2113.

Agbabiaka TB, et al. *Serenoa repens* (Saw palmetto): a systematic review of adverse events. Drug Saf. 32.8 (2009): 637–647.

Aliaev IG et al. Five-year experience in treating patients with prostatic hyperplasia patients with permixone (*Serenoa repens* Pierre Fabre Medicament). Urologiia 1 (2002): 23–25.

AUA (American Urological Association). Abstract 103937. In: Proceedings of American Urological Association 98th Annual Meeting, 26 April, 2003.

Avins AL, Bent S. Saw palmetto and lower urinary tract symptoms: what is the latest evidence? Curr Urol Rep 7.4 (2006): 260–265.

Avins AL et al. Safety and toxicity of saw palmetto in the CAMUS Trial. J Urol. 2012. http://dx.doi.org/10.1016/j.juro.2012.10.002, (accessed 20.02.13).

Barry M et al. The effect of increasing doses of a saw palmetto fruit extract on lower urinary tract symptoms attributed to benign prostatic hyperplasia: a randomized trial. JAMA 306.12 (2011): 1344–1351.

Bayne CW et al. The selectivity and specificity of the actions of the lipido-sterolic extract of *Serenoa repens* (Permixon) on the prostate. J Urol 164.3 (2000): 876–881.

Beckert BW et al. The effect of herbal medicines on platelet function: an in vivo experiment and review of the literature. Plast Reconstr Surg 120.7 (2007): 2044–2050.

Bent S et al. Saw palmetto for benign prostatic hyperplasia. N Engl J Med 354.6 (2006): 557–566.

Bombardelli E et al. Serenoa repens (Bartram). Small Fitoterapia 69.2 (1997): 99–113.

Boyle P et al. Updated meta-analysis of clinical trials of *Serenoa repens* extract in the treatment of symptomatic benign prostatic hyperplasia. BJU Int 93.6 (2004): 751–756.

Breu W et al. Anti-inflammatory activity of sabal fruit extracts prepared with supercritical carbon dioxide: in vitro antagonists of cyclooxygenase and 5-lipoxygenase metabolism. Arzneimittelforschung 42.4 (1992): 547–551.

Cai T et al. *Serenoa repens* associated with *Urtica dioica* (prostaMEVA®) and curcumin and Quercetin (FlogMEVA®) extract are able to improve patients results from a prospective randomised study. Int. J. Antimicrob. Agents 33.6 (2009): 549–553.

Coulsen S et al. A phase II randomised double –blind placebo controlled clinical trial investigating the efficacy and safety of ProstateEZE Max: A herbal medicine preparation for the management of symptoms of benign prostatic hypertrophy. Complement Ther Med (2013) 0965–2299.

Debruyne F et al. Comparison of a phytotherapeutic agent (Permixon) with an alpha-blocker (Tamsulosin) in the treatment of benign prostatic hyperplasia: a 1-year randomized international study. Eur Urol 41.5 (2002): 497–506.

Di Silverio F et al. Effects of long-term treatment with *Serenoa repens* (Permixon) on the concentrations and regional distribution of androgens and epidermal growth factor in benign prostatic hyperplasia. Prostate 37.2 (1998): 77–83.

el Sheikh MM, et al. The effect of Permixon on androgen receptors. Acta Obstet Gynecol Scand 67.5 (1988): 397–399.

Goepel M et al. Saw palmetto extracts potently and noncompetitively inhibit human alpha1-adrenoceptors in vitro. Prostate 38.3 (1999): 208–215.

Goepel M et al. Do saw palmetto extracts block human alpha1-adrenoceptor subtypes in vivo? Prostate 46.3 (2001): 226–232.

Goldmann WH et al. Saw palmetto berry extract inhibits cell growth and COX-2 expression in prostatic cancer cells. Cell Biol Int 25.11 (2001): 1117–1124.

Grasso M et al. Comparative effects of alfuzosin versus *Serenoa repens* in the treatment of symptomatic benign prostatic hyperplasia. Arch Esp Urol 48.1 (1995): 97–103.

Hutchison A et al. The efficacy of drugs for the treatment of LUTS/BPH, a study in 6 European countries. Eur Urol 51.1 (2007): 207–216.

Ishii K et al. Extract from *Serenoa repens* suppresses the invasion activity of human urological cancer cells by inhibiting urokinase-type plasminogen activator. Biol Pharm Bull 24.2 (2001): 188–190.

Kaplan SA, et al. A prospective, 1-year trial using saw palmetto versus finasteride in the treatment of category III prostatitis/chronic pelvic pain syndrome. J Urol 171.1 (2004): 284–288.

S

Levin RM, Das AK. A scientific basis for the therapeutic effects of *Pygeum africanum* and *Serenoa repens*. Urol Res 28.3 (2000): 201–209.
Linde K et al. Echinacea for preventing and treating the common cold. Cochrane Database Syst Rev 1 (2006): CD000530.
Maccagnano C et al. A critical analysis of Permixon (TM) in the treatment of lower urinary tract symptoms due to benign prostatic enlargement. Eur Urol Suppl 5.4 (2006): 430–440.
Madersbacher S et al. Medical management of BPH: role of plant extracts. EAU-EBU Update Series 5.5 (2007):1972–2205.
Markowitz JS et al. Multiple doses of saw palmetto (*Serenoa repens*) did not alter cytochrome P450 2D6 and 3A4 activity in normal volunteers. Clin Pharmacol Ther 74.6 (2003): 536–542.
Nemecz G. Saw palmetto. US Pharmacist (2003). Available online: www.uspharmacist.com (accessed 10-12-08).
Paubert-Braquet M et al. Effect of the lipidic lipidosterolic extract of *Serenoa repens* (Permixon) on the ionophore A23187- stimulated production of leukotriene B4 from human polymorphonuclear neutrophils. Prostaglandins Leukot Essent Fatty Acids 57.3 (1997): 299–304.
Prager N et al. A randomized, double-blind, placebo-controlled trial to determine the effectiveness of botanically derived inhibitors of 5-alpha-reductase in the treatment of androgenetic alopecia. J Altern Complement Med 8.2 (2002): 143–152.
Pytel YA et al. Long-term clinical and biologic effects of the lipidosterolic extract of *Serenoa repens* in patients with symptomatic benign prostatic hyperplasia. Adv Ther 19.6 (2002): 297–306.
Raynaud JP, et al. Inhibition of type 1 and type 2 5alpha-reductase activity by free fatty acids, active ingredients of Permixon. J Steroid Biochem Mol Biol 82.2–3 (2002): 233–239.
Scholtysek C et al. Characterizing components of the Saw Palmetto Berry Extract (SPBE) on prostate cancer cell growth and traction. Biochem Biophys ResCommun 379.3 (2009): 795–798.
Strauch G et al. Comparison of finasteride (Proscar) and *Serenoa repens* (Permixon) in the inhibition of 5-alpha reductase in healthy male volunteers. Eur Urol 26.3 (1994): 247–252.
Sultan C et al. Inhibition of androgen metabolism and binding by a liposterolic extract of *Serenoa repens* B in human foreskin fibroblasts. J Steroid Biochem 20.1 (1984): 515–5119.
Talpur N et al. Comparison of Saw Palmetto (extract and whole berry) and Cernitin on prostate growth in rats. Mol Cell Biochem 250.1–2 (2003): 21–26.
Ulbricht C, Basch E. Natural standards herb and supplement reference. St Louis: Mosby, 2006.
Vacher P et al. The lipidosterolic extract from *Serenoa repens* interferes with prolactin receptor signal transduction. J Biomed Sci 2.4 (1995): 357–365.
Van Coppenolle F et al. Pharmacological effects of the lipidosterolic extract of *Serenoa repens* (Permixon) on rat prostate hyperplasia induced by hyperprolactinemia: comparison with finasteride. Prostate 43.1 (2000): 49–58.
WHO. Monographs on selected medicinal plants. Geneva: World Health Organization, January 2003 update.
Wilt T et al. *Serenoa repens* for benign prostatic hyperplasia. Cochrane Database Syst Rev 3 (2002): CD001423.
Wilt T et al. *Serenoa repens* for benighn prostatic hyperplasia. Cochrane Database of Syst Rev 12 (2012) CD001423.

Schisandra

HISTORICAL NOTE Schisandra has an extensive history of use in traditional Chinese medicine (TCM). It has sour and warm qualities and is used to treat spleen and kidney 'deficiency', to restore Qi and also as a treatment for chronic cough, wheezing, diabetes, insomnia and palpitations.

OTHER NAMES

Chinese magnolia vine, gomishi, sheng-mai-san, wuweizi

BOTANICAL NAME/FAMILY

Schisandra chinensis (family Schisandraceae)

PLANT PART USED

Fruit

CHEMICAL COMPONENTS

Dibenzocyclooctene lignans (schisandrins A–C, deoxyshisandrin, γ-schisandrin, schizandrols, schisantherins, pregomisin, gomisins A–C, E–G, J, K and N), triterpenoids (schinchinenins A–H, schinchinenlactones A–C, henrischinins A–C, schicagenins A–C), essential oil, malic, tartaric, nigranoic and citric acids, resins, pectin, vitamins A, C and E, niacin, beta-carotene, sterols, tannins and several minerals (MG Kim et al 2010, Shi et al 2011, Song et al 2013, Waiwut et al 2011, Wei et al 2013).

MAIN ACTIONS

Studies have been conducted with schisandra and a number of its constituents in isolation, such as schisandrin B and gomisin A. Currently, most evidence is derived from in vitro and animal studies, as it has not been significantly investigated in clinical studies. Many studies have also been conducted on schisandra in combination with other herbs. It is difficult to determine the individual efficacy of schisandra in these cases, and further studies of schisandra in isolation are required.

Antioxidant

In vitro and in vivo tests have identified antioxidant activity (Y Chen et al 2008, Chiu et al 2011, Kim et al 2009, S Ko et al 2008, Leong et al 2012, Liu et al 2009, Meng et al 2008, Ohsugi et al 1999, Smejkal et al 2010, Steele et al 2013, M Wang et al 2008, Yan et al 2009). Seven lignans isolated from schisandra have demonstrated stronger antioxidant activity than vitamin E at the same concentrations, with schisanhenol exhibiting the strongest effects (Lu & Liu 1992). The essential oil from *Schisandra* berries has also demonstrated antioxidant activity (X Chen et al 2012, Liu et al 2012a, Ma et al 2012).

Protective effects against ethanol-induced oxidative stress have been demonstrated by schisandra extract in vitro (Chen et al 2010) and schisandrin B in vivo (Lam et al 2010). While an in vitro study found that schisandra did not protect against oxidative stress-induced lymphocyte DNA damage (Szeto et al 2011), the herb has demonstrated a protective effect against heat stress (KJ Kim et al 2012) and silica-induced lung damage (Li et al 2009) in rats via antioxidant mechanisms. It appears that several constituents also have indirect antioxidant activity and can increase hepatic and myocardial glutathione levels (Yim & Ko 1999).

An extract of schisandra and the isolated constituent schisandrin B have both demonstrated the ability to significantly decrease alanine aminotransferase and increase glutathione levels in CCL4-damaged liver in vivo (Chiu et al 2002). Schisandrins B and C protected rats against solar irradiation-induced oxidative damage to epithelial tissue (Lam et al 2011). Schisandrin B also demonstrated genoprotective activity in mice with cisplatin-induced oxidative stress (Giridharan et al 2012), and long-term supplementation with schisandrin B enhanced mitochondrial antioxidant capacity and functionality in ageing mice, suggesting schisandrin B may have potential as an antiageing therapy (KM Ko et al 2008).

Deoxyschisandrin protected human intestinal epithelial cells against oxidative stress-induced apoptosis (Gu et al 2010). Schisandra polysaccharides have demonstrated analgesic activity in vivo, which may be due to its antioxidant capacity (Ye et al 2013).

Hepatoprotective activity

Decreases hepatotoxic damage

In vitro and in vivo studies have identified hepatoprotective effects with schisandra against carbon tetrachloride toxicity (Cai et al 2010, Chang et al 2009, Cheng et al 2013, Chiu et al 2007, Ip et al 1995, Mak & Ko 1997, Y Xie et al 2010, Yan et al 2009, Zhu et al 1999, 2000) and mercuric chloride toxicity (Stacchiotti et al 2009). Research with schisandrin B suggests that it is the main constituent responsible for these beneficial effects (Chiu et al 2007, Ip et al 1995, Mak et al 1996, Pan et al 2002). Further investigation reveals that schisandrin B increases the efficiency of the hepatic glutathione antioxidant system, thereby inhibiting carbon tetrachloride-induced lipid peroxidation; however, additional mechanisms appear likely (Ip et al 1995). More recently, the whole extract of schisandra fruit was shown to induce glutathione S-transferases in vitro (EH Choi et al 2008). Several lignans have been found to induce expression of phase II detoxification enzymes in vitro, a factor believed to be important in the prevention of liver cancer (SB Lee et al 2009).

Protection against paracetamol-induced liver damage has been demonstrated in two animal models using gomisin A (Kim et al 2008, Yamada et al 1993). In one study, gomisin A inhibited not only the elevation of serum aminotransferase activity and hepatic lipoperoxide content, but also the appearance of histological changes such as degeneration and necrosis of hepatocytes (Yamada et al 1993). In 2003, protection against paracetamol-induced liver damage and D-galactosamine-induced liver damage was confirmed for a fractionated extract of *S. chinensis* in an experimental model (Nakagiri et al 2003).

The hepatoprotective effects of gomisin N and γ-schizandrin have been analysed in interleukin-1β (IL-1β)-treated rat hepatocytes. Gomisin N and γ-schizandrin suppressed genetic expression of nitric oxide synthase (NOS), and decreased the transcription of IL1β and inflammatory chemokines (Takimoto et al 2013).

Gomisin A protected against D-galactosamine-induced hepatotoxicity in vivo (Kim et al 2008). The latter also protected against carbon tetrachloride-induced liver fibrosis in rats (HY Kim et al 2011).

Schisandrin B decreased hepatic total cholesterol and triglyceride levels in hypercholesterolaemic mice (Pan et al 2008) and protected mouse hepatocytes against hypoxia/reoxygenation-induced apoptosis (Chiu et al 2009).

An extract of schisandra lignans protected against restraint-induced liver damage in mice. The hepatoprotective effect was potentially mediated via antioxidant mechanisms (Pu et al 2012).

IN COMBINATION

Shengmai San (comprised of *S. chinensis*, *Panax ginseng*, and *Ophiopogon japonicus*) reduced hepatic lipids and lipid peroxidation in rats fed a high-cholesterol diet (Yao et al 2008). Another herbal combination preparation (*S. chinensis*, *Vitis vinifera* and *Taraxacum officinale*) protected against D-galactosamine-induced hepatotoxicity in vivo (JW Kang et al 2012).

Liver regeneration

Two animal studies have demonstrated that oral administration of gomisin A, a lignan isolated from *S. chinensis*, accelerates liver regeneration after partial hepatectomy and hastens recovery of liver function (Kubo et al 1992, Takeda et al 1987). The mechanism for these effects is not fully elucidated; however, gomisin A increases ornithine decarboxylase activity, which is important during the early stages of regeneration and suppresses fibrosis proliferation.

Anti-inflammatory

Schisandrin inhibits nitric oxide (NO) production, prostaglandin E_2 release, cyclooxygenase-2, inducible iNOS and nuclear factor-kappaB (NF-κB) in vitro (Guo et al 2008). In vitro and in vivo studies have identified anti-inflammatory activity for gomisin A, gomisin J, wuweizi C (Yasukawa et al 1992), schisandrin B (Checker et al 2012), schisandrin C, gomisin N (Oh et al 2010), α-iso-cubebene (Choi et al 2009), α-iso-cubebenol (YJ Lee et al 2010) and schisandrin derivatives (Blunder et al 2010). Several lignans from schisandra, including gomisin N and schisandrol A, have shown potent inhibition of nuclear factor of activated T cells (NFAT) in vitro (Lee et al 2003). Excessive activation of NFAT has a significant role to play in autoimmune disease, but further study is needed to assess schisandra's usefulness in immunopathological disease states.

Aqueous extracts of schisandra inhibited lipopolysaccharide-induced lung inflammation in mice (Bae et al 2012), and demonstrated potent effects in a mast cell line (Kang et al 2006). The extracts were found to inhibit tumour necrosis factor alpha (TNF-α), IL-6, IL-1 and granulocyte-macrophage colony-stimulating factor production (Park et al 2011). These effects may be due to schisandra inhibiting the degradation of IkappaB and therefore the translocation and activation of NF-κB. This may indicate a potential role for schisandra in the treatment of allergy. Similarly, another study found that schisandrin decreased scratching behaviour by inhibiting the IgE-antigen complex in vivo (Lee et al 2007).

IN COMBINATION

A herbal combination containing schisandra (Jianpi Huoxue) was found to inhibit the liver cytokine secretion pathway in rats (Peng et al 2008).

Immunomodulatory

Animal studies have found schisandra to possess immune-modulating activity (D Ma et al 2009). In mice, α-iso-cubebenol isolated from schisandra protected against induced sepsis by increasing the bactericidal activity of phagocytes, attenuating inflammatory cytokine production and inhibiting leucocyte apoptosis (SK Lee et al 2012). An in vitro follow-up study suggested the immunomodulatory activity of α-iso-cubebenol was due to stimulated neutrophil activity, including calcium increase, degranulation and chemotactic migration via interaction with chemokine receptor CXCR2 (Jung et al 2013). Alpha-iso-cubebene has demonstrated similar activity in vitro (Y Lee et al 2009).

Administration of schisandra polysaccharides to cyclophosphamide-induced immunosuppressed mice resulted in improved parameters of immune function, including increased phagocytic activity of peritoneal macrophages, increased serum haemolysin (Yang et al 2008), increased organ weight of the thymus and spleen and increased splenocyte proliferation (Y Chen et al 2012).

Antidiabetic

Schisandra exhibits multiple mechanisms of relevance in diabetes.

In vitro studies indicate that schisandra possesses antidiabetic activity (Gao et al 2009, Lau et al 2008, S Park et al 2009). Various lignans have been found to improve basal glucose uptake of hepatic cells (HepG2) in vitro. In particular, gomisin N demonstrated a greater effect than rosiglitazone, which has been used as an antidiabetic drug (J Zhang et al 2010).

Moreover, in vivo studies show that schisandra extracts reduce blood glucose levels, improve lipid metabolism, increase liver glycogen content and attenuate diabetes-induced weight loss and polydipsia in alloxan-induced diabetic mice (Gao et al 2009, Xv et al 2008, Zhao et al 2013a). Aqueous extracts of schisandra reduced postprandial blood glucose levels in rats via inhibition of α-glucosidase and α-amylase, enzymes responsible for absorption of monosaccharides in the small intestine (Jo et al 2011).

A fraction containing schizandrin, gomisin A and angeloylgomisin H increased glucose disposal rates and enhanced hepatic insulin sensitivity in type 2 diabetic rats (Kwon et al 2011).

IN COMBINATION

A TCM formula containing *S. chinensis, Coptis chinensis, Psidium guajava* and *Morus alba* significantly decreased non-fasting blood glucose in insulin-resistant mice (Wang & Chiang 2012).

Antiobesity

Treatment with schisandra resulted in decreased weight gain and adiposity in obese rats fed a high-fat diet. In vitro results suggest this effect may be mediated by inhibition of adipogenesis and adipocyte differentiation (HJ Park et al 2012).

IN COMBINATION

Gyeongshingangjeehwan (GGEx), a product containing *S. chinensis, Liriope platyphylla, Platycodon grandiflorum* and *Ephedra sinica*, promoted weight loss in one study of obese rats (Shin et al 2010) and decreased food intake, weight and abdominal fat gain, circulating triglycerides and hepatic lipid accumulation in another (Jeong et al 2008).

Antiallergic

Schisandra has demonstrated various antiallergic effects, including inhibition of eosinophil recruitment to lung epithelial cells in vitro (Oh et al 2009) and reduced severity of atopic dermatitis in vivo (Kang & Shin 2012). An aqueous extract of schisandra inhibited β-hexosaminidase release and expression of IL-4, IL-13 and TNF-α mRNA and protein in immunoglobulin E-antigen complex-stimulated rat basophilic leukaemia cells (mucosal mast cell-type cells) (Chung et al 2012). It appears that schisandra ameliorates the production of reactive oxygen species that drives allergic inflammation.

In in vitro studies, gomisin N inhibited the production of prostaglandin D_2, leukotriene C_4, β-hexosaminidase, IL-6 and cyclooxygenase-2 in bone marrow-derived mast cells (Chae et al 2011) and schizandrin has been found to inhibit the production of thymic stromal lymphopoietin (TSLP) in human mast cell lines. TSLP plays a key role in allergic diseases such as asthma and atopic dermatitis (Moon et al 2012). In vivo, schizandrin demonstrated significant antiasthmatic activity via inhibition of airway eosinophil accumulation, reduction of IL-4, IL-5, interferon-γ and TNF-α levels in bronchoalveolar lavage fluid, reduced oxidative stress, and inhibition of goblet cell hyperplasia and inflammatory cell infiltration in lung tissue (MY Lee et al 2010).

IN COMBINATION

Antiasthmatic activity was demonstrated by Xiao Qing Long Tang, a preparation of eight herbs, including *S. chinensis* (Wang et al 2012).

Nephroprotective

Schisandra significantly decreased the urine albumin excretion rate and urinary albumin/creatinine ratio, attenuated glomerulosclerosis and protected against podocyte loss in a mouse model of diabetic nephropathy (Zhang et al 2012).

In vitro pretreatment with schisandrin B protected against cyclosporin A-induced nephrotoxicity in mice and human proximal tubular epithelial cell line via antioxidant effects (Zhu et al 2012), and in vivo schisandrin B was also found to protect against mercuric chloride-induced (Stacchiotti et al 2011) and gentamicin-induced (Chiu et al 2008a) nephrotoxicity in rats.

Schizandrin significantly attenuated high-glucose-induced murine mesangial cell (MMC) damage by reducing the proliferation and protein synthesis of MMCs, reducing production of reactive oxygen species and inhibiting the activity of NADPH oxidase. These results suggest that it may be useful in the treatment of diabetic nephropathy (Jeong et al 2012).

Cardiovascular effects

Schisandrin B demonstrated protective effects against ischaemia–reperfusion-induced myocardial damage in animal models (Chiu et al 2008b, Yim & Ko 1999). The myocardial protection was associated with an enhancement in myocardial glutathione antioxidant status. Schisandrin B has also been found to inhibit signalling of transforming growth factor-β_1 (TGF-β_1) in vascular smooth-muscle cells (EJ Park et al 2012). TGF-β_1 is implicated in the pathogenesis of a number of vascular disease processes, including hypertension, atherosclerosis and restenosis. Schisandrin B stereoisomers protected rat cardiomyocytes against hypoxia/reoxygenation-induced apoptosis.

The whole extract, deoxyschizandrin, schisantherin A and gomisin A, has demonstrated vasorelaxant properties in isolated rat thoracic aorta, suggesting cardioprotective effects (JY Park et al 2007, J Park et al 2009a, Rhyu et al 2006, Seok et al 2011, X Yang et al 2011). An aqueous schisandra extract restored endothelial function in rats that underwent balloon-induced carotid artery injury. Similar to oestradiol therapy, it also reduced serum cholesterol levels and exhibited hypotensive effects in ovariectomised rats (EY Kim et al 2011).

Gomisin J (J Park et al 2012a) and gomisin A (J Park et al 2009b) have demonstrated vasorelaxant effects in vitro via increased activation of calcium-dependent endothelial NOS and subsequent production of endothelial NO. Administration of gomisin A to hypertensive mice ameliorated the increase in blood pressure and reactive oxygen species production, and decrease in aortic vascular NO and phosphorylated endothelial NOS induced by treatment with angiotensin II (J Park et al 2012b).

IN COMBINATION

A Cochrane review of nine randomised controlled trials assessed the use of Shengmai (a TCM combination of *Panax ginseng*, *Ophiopogon japonicus* and *S. chinensis*) in patients with heart failure. While issues of poor study design, small sample size and heterogeneity of particular outcomes were cited, there was some evidence to show that Shengmai may improve heart function in patients with heart failure (Chen et al 2012).

Antitumour

Extracts of schisandra and several isolated constituents have demonstrated anticancer activity against various cancer lines, including leukaemia, breast, liver, gastric, colon and lung in vitro (Gnabre et al 2010, Hwang et al 2011, Jie et al 2009, JH Kim et al 2010, JE Kim et al 2012, SJ Kim et al 2010, Lin et al 2008, 2011, Min et al 2008, Nishida et al 2009, C Park et al 2009, Waiwut et al 2012, Yim et al 2009, Yuezhen 2010, Zhao et al 2013b). Several schisandra lignans have been found to inhibit fatty acid synthase, a potential oncogenic enzyme (Na et al 2010). Gomisins J and N inhibited Wnt/β-catenin signalling in human colon carcinoma cells. The Wnt/β-catenin signalling pathway is involved in regulating cell growth and apoptosis, and has been implicated in the aetiology and progression of various forms of cancer (K Kang et al 2012).

Gomisin N was found to enhance apoptosis induced by TNF-α (Waiwut et al 2011) and TNF-related apoptosis-inducing ligand (TRAIL) (Inoue et al 2012) in vitro. A schisandra polysaccharide, WSLSCP, significantly inhibited the proliferation of lymphoma cells, increased secretion level of serum TNF-α, and improved survival rate of lymphoma-bearing mice. WSLSCP was also found to enhance phagocytic activity and NO and TNF-α secretion of macrophages in vitro (C Xu et al 2012). Another isolated schisandra polysaccharide (SCPP11) exhibited indirect cytotoxic activity against tumour cells in vitro, and significantly inhibited the growth of hepatic tumour cells (HepS) in vivo. SCPP11 also increased thymus indexes, serum IL-2 and TNF-α levels in vivo, and significantly enhanced NO production and phagocytosis in mouse macrophage-like cell lines in vitro (Zhao et al 2013b). These results suggest that schisandra's immunomodulatory activity may contribute to its antitumour effects.

Other constituents of the herb, such as deoxyschizandrin and γ-schizandrin, restored the cytotoxic action of the chemotherapy drug doxorubicin in multidrug-resistant human lung carcinoma cell lines. They also enhanced cellular accumulation of doxorubicin, and induced cell cycle arrest when combined with subtoxic doses of doxorubicin (Slaninova et al 2009).

Schisandra has been found to inhibit the proliferation of cancer cells in rodents with induced hepatocellular carcinoma (He et al 2010, Loo et al 2007). An extract of schisandra lignans inhibited hepatic metastases of mastocytoma tumour cells in mice (Tang et al 2011).

An isolated compound from schisandra (1-O-MFF) inhibited melanogenic processes in mouse melanoma cells (Oh et al 2010), and gomisin A has been found to inhibit skin cancer formation in mice (Yasukawa et al 2009).

IN COMBINATION

Shu Gan Liang Xue decoction, a TCM product that contains schisandra and is often used in menopause, inhibited the growth of human mammary epithelial carcinoma cell line, but did not display any oestrogenic activity (Zhang & Li 2009).

Neuroprotective

In vitro data suggest that certain lignans from schisandra (Kim et al 2004) are protective against L-glutamate-induced neurotoxicity in rat cortical cells. Schisandrin C has been shown to decrease the membrane action potential in glioma and neuronal cells lines (Y Choi et al 2008). Schisandrin has demonstrated neurogenic activity in rat hippocampal neurons (SH Yang et al 2011). and demonstrated the ability to reverse hyoscine-induced memory impairment in vivo by enhancing cholinergic function (Egashira et al 2008). Extracts of schisandra ameliorated the depressed hippocampal acetylcholinesterase activity and behavioural learning impairments seen in ovariectomised mice (X Xie et al 2010).

Schizandrin (N Zhang et al 2010) and schisandrin B (Zeng et al 2012) have been found to inhibit lipopolysaccharide-induced microglia activation and significantly ameliorate neuronal cell death in vitro and in vivo via inhibition of the microglial-mediated neurotoxic inflammatory response. Microglia activation is implicated in the pathophysiology of Alzheimer's and Parkinson's disease.

Extracts of schisandra (M Miao et al 2009, Y Miao et al 2009) and schisandrin B (N Chen et al 2008) have been shown to improve the outcome in cerebral ischaemia/reperfusion models in vivo. Schisandrin B protected against damage by enhancing the cerebral antioxidant status. Schisandrin B also exhibited significant neuroprotective effects in a rat model of transient focal cerebral ischaemia. Schisandrin B demonstrated inhibition of TNF-α and IL-1β, and decreased expression of matrix metalloproteinases-2 and -9, all of which are involved in microglial activation after ischaemic events (TH Lee et al 2012).

Schisandrin B appears to improve cognition and hepatic functions in mice treated with tacrine, the common Alzheimer's dementia medication (Pan et al 2002). Pretreatment with schisandrin B prevented scopolamine-induced oxidative stress and impairment of learning and memory in vivo. Schisandrin B was found to ameliorate the scopolamine-induced increase in acetylcholinesterase activity, and maintain normal acetylcholine levels (Giridharan et al 2011). Similarly, schisandrin was found to prevent dexamethasone-induced cognitive deficits in vitro and in vivo (X Xu et al 2012).

Schisandrins B and C reversed beta-amyloid (Aβ) and homocysteine-induced neurotoxicity in vitro (Song et al 2011). Both deoxyschisandrin (Hu et al 2012) and ESP-806, a lignan-rich extract of schisandra (Jeong et al 2013), significantly ameliorated Aβ-induced memory impairment in mice. Deoxyschisandrin acted via antioxidative mechanisms, while ESP-806 attenuated the elevation of β-secretase activity, significantly inhibited hippocampal acetylcholinesterase activity and increased levels of reduced glutathione in the cortex and hippocampus. Deoxyschisandrin has also been found to inhibit the spontaneous and synchronous oscillations of intracellular Ca^{2+} in hippocampal neurons by depressing influx of extracellular calcium, and inhibiting spontaneous neurotransmitter release, suggesting deoxyschisandrin may be of benefit in regulating the excitability of neural networks (Fu et al 2008).

IN COMBINATION

A combined extract of *Schisandra chinensis, Angelica gigas* and *Saururus chinensis* is protective against L-glutamate-induced neurotoxicity in rat cortical cells (CJ Ma et al 2009). AdMax (Nulab, Florida), a product containing *Schisandra chinensis, Leuzea carthamoides, Rhodiola rosea* and *Eleutherococcus senticosus*, has been found to enhance expression of PANK2, which encodes the mitochondrial enzyme pantothenate kinase 2. Impaired PANK2 gene activity leads to pantothenate kinase-associated neurodegeneration (Antoshechkin et al 2008).

Gastrointestinal actions

Schisandra has demonstrated gastrointestinal antispasmodic activity in isolated rat colon (J Yang et al 2011a). Schisandra was also found to reverse visceral hypersensitivity in an irritable bowel syndrome rat model. The observed normalisation of elevated serotonin (5-HT) levels and a decline in the mRNA level of 5-HT receptors in the distal colon suggest the effect may be mediated via the colonic 5-HT pathway (Yang et al 2012). Extracts of schisandra inhibited acetylcholine- and 5-HT-induced contractions of guinea pig ileum, potentially via inhibition of both calcium ion influx and intracellular calcium ion mobilisation (J Yang et al 2011b).

Antibacterial

Schisandra has demonstrated bactericidal activity against *Staphylococcus epidermidis, S. aureus, Bacillus subtilis, Escherichia coli, Pseudomonas aeruginosa, Proteus vulgaris* (X Chen et al 2011, Wang 2008), *Bacillus anthracis, Shigella* (Wen-qiang 2009) and *Salmonella gallinarum* (Choi & Chang 2009).

OTHER ACTIONS

Lipid lowering

Schisandra may also help to reduce cholesterol, as it has been found to decrease triglycerides and low-density lipoprotein, and increase high-density lipoprotein cholesterol in vivo (Junshu & Anshan 2008). Schisandrin B (50–200 mg/kg) was coadministered with either a high-lipid diet or a cholesterol/bile salts mixture in vivo (Pan et al 2008). Hepatic total cholesterol and triglyceride levels were reduced by up to 50% and 52%, respectively, as compared to control animals. Similar results were found using an ethanol extract of schisandra (Pan 2011).

Improved erectile function

Corporeal smooth-muscle (CSM) relaxation is required for penile erection. Several schisandra lignans were found to induce CSM relaxation via inhibition of calcium ion influx (Han et al 2012). Schisandrol A, schisandrol B and an ethanol extract of schisandra were found to potentiate sildenafil citrate-induced relaxation of rabbit penile corpus cavernosum. Clinical studies are required to determine whether schisandra has a therapeutic role in patients with a poor response to sildenafil alone (HK Kim et al 2011).

IN COMBINATION

A combination of *Schisandra chinensis, Lycium chinense, Cornus officinalis, Rubus coreanus* and *Cuscuta chinensis* improved intracavernous pressure of corpus cavernosum in spontaneous hypertensive rats (Sohn et al 2008).

Anxiolytic and sedative

Schisandra has demonstrated sedative and hypnotic activity in mice, reducing sleep latency and prolonging sleep time (W Wang et al 2008a). Schisandra was found to decrease behavioural signs of anxiety in stressed mice, and ameliorated elevations in cerebral cortex noradrenaline, dopamine and 5-HT and plasma corticosterone levels (W Chen et al 2011). It is possible the anxiolytic effect is mediated by modulation of the hypothalamic-pituitary-adrenal axis activity.

Inhibits leukotriene formation

Various schisandra lignans decrease leukotriene production via inhibition of 5-lipoxygenase activity in vitro (Lim et al 2009). Gomisin A has been found to inhibit the biosynthesis of leukotrienes by preventing the release of arachidonic acid in vitro (Ohkura et al 1990).

Platelet-activating factor antagonist

Several lignans inhibit platelet-activating factor in vitro (Lee et al 1999). Pregomisin and gomisin N have demonstrated more potent inhibition of platelet-activating factor than aspirin (MG Kim et al 2010).

Enhanced exercise endurance

Schisandra (Cao et al 2009, W Wang et al 2008b) and ADAPT-232 (a standardised combination of *S. chinensis, Rhodiola rosea* and *Eleutherococcus senticosus*) (Panossian et al 2009) have been found to increase exercise endurance in mice.

Bone mineralisation

Lignans isolated from the fruit and seeds of schisandra may be able to protect against bone loss. An in vitro study using UMR 106 cells demonstrated that the lignans (extracted in 95% ethanol) stimulated the proliferation and activity of alkaline phosphatase in osteoblasts (Caichompoo et al 2009).

Cytochromes and P-glycoprotein

Schisandra extract and different isolated compounds have been tested for the effects of various cytochromes and P-glycoprotein in in vitro and animal model studies.

Cytochrome 3A4

In vitro evidence indicates that schisandrol A and gomisin A are inhibitors of CYP 3A4 (Wan et al 2010). Conflicting in vivo evidence has found schisandra to have both inhibitory and inducing effects on CYP 3A4 activity (Q Chen et al 2010, Iwata et al 2004, Li et al 2013, Su et al 2013, Wang et al 2011). In addition, schisandra has been found to increase the activation of the pregnane X receptor (PXR) signalling pathway. PXR is a transcription factor that, when activated, binds to the promoter region of CYP3A4 gene, resulting in increased CYP3A4 transcription (Yu et al 2011). The discrepancy between results from animal studies appears to be dependent on the duration of administration. Short-term treatment with schisandra (single dose) had an inhibitory effect on CYP 3A4, while longer-term treatment (6–14 consecutive days) resulted in induction of CYP 3A4 (Lai et al 2009, Yao et al 2011). Clinical studies are not available to clarify the effect of *S. chinensis* on CYP 3A4 in humans. One case study found that administration of deoxyschisandrin (22.5 mg after meals for 3 days) resulted in an increase of blood tacrolimus (a P-glycoprotein and CYP 3A4 substrate) concentration from 2.3 ng/mL to 17.7 ng/mL (Jiang et al 2010a). It was not clear whether the increased tacrolimus concentration was due to inhibition of P-glycoprotein, CYP 3A4, or a combination. Small-scale human studies have found that oral administration of *Schisandra sphenanthera* for 7–14 days resulted in increased area under the curve for tacrolimus (Jiang et al 2010b, Xin et al 2007) and midazolam (Xin et al 2009). Considering the two species share many of the same constituents (including deoxyschisandrin and schisandrin B), it is possible that *S. chinensis* may have the same effect.

It has been suggested that discrepancies between human and animal studies are due to lower mg/kg doses of schisandra in humans than animals, and the fact that gomisin C concentrations necessary for PXR activation in humans are twice those required for murine species (Gurley et al 2012). A 2012 review suggests that, based upon the human studies of *Schisandra sphenanthera*, *S. chinensis* is likely to have an inhibitory effect on CYP 3A4 in humans, and the potential for herb–drug interactions between schisandra extracts and drugs that are CYP 3A4 substrates is high (Gurley et al 2012).

P-glycoprotein

Various lignans from schisandra, including schisandrol A, gomisin A, schisandrin A and B and schisandrin B have demonstrated an inhibitory effect on P-glycoprotein in vitro (Fong et al 2007, Pan et al 2006, Qiangrong et al 2005, Wan et al 2006, Yoo et al 2007). Pretreatment with schisandrol B significantly increased the oral bioavailability of paclitaxel (a drug with notoriously poor oral bioavailability) in rodents, potentially via enhanced intestinal absorption due to inhibition of P-glycoprotein (Jin et al 2010). In vitro studies indicate that inhibition of P-glycoprotein by schisandra lignans can reverse multidrug resistance in cancer cells (Huang et al 2008); however clinical studies are required to confirm this.

In a small clinical trial ($n = 12$), pretreatment with schisandra extract (300 mg twice daily for 14 days) followed by a single dose of talinolol (100 mg) resulted in increased area under the curve and C_{max} of talinolol by 47% and 51% respectively, suggesting P-glycoprotein activity was inhibited (Fan et al 2009).

CLINICAL USE

While schisandra has not been extensively tested in clinical trials, it has been tested in numerous animal models and displays multiple mechanisms of action, thereby providing biological plausibility for some of its uses. It is often prescribed in combination with other herbal medicines, a factor which accounts for its investigation as part of multi-component treatments in some studies.

Liver damage, hepatoprotection

Traditionally, schisandra has been used to treat a variety of liver disorders. Hepatoprotective effects have been observed in test tube and animal studies; however, the clinical significance of these findings in humans remains unknown. Several encouraging clinical reports using an analogue of schisandrin C are available; however, it is not known whether these effects will be seen with *S. chinensis* (Akbar et al 1998). A pilot clinical study in 10 healthy subjects has evaluated the effects of schisandra and sesamin (a constituent of sesame oil) on blood fluidity due to the link between blood viscosity and liver dysfunction (Tsi & Tan 2008). The mixture was given for 1 week and blood fluidity was tested over 2 weeks, including 1 week postintervention. Blood passage time was reduced by 9.0% and 9.7% at 1 and 2 weeks, respectively, showing that the effect could be sustained for at least 1 week after cessation of treatment. The exact effects of schisandra in this formula are unknown.

Adaptogen

In TCM, schisandra is viewed as an adaptogen and prescribed with other herbs to increase resistance to physical and emotional stressors and to improve allostasis (see monographs on Korean ginseng and Siberian ginseng for further information about adaptogenic activity and allostasis).

IN COMBINATION

A randomised, double-blind, placebo-controlled pilot study assessed the effect of a single dose (270 mg) of ADAPT-232 (a standardised combination of *S. chinensis, Rhodiola rosea* and *Eleutherococcus senticosus*) on cognitive function in 40 healthy females aged 20–68 years. At 2 hours posttreatment, the treatment group demonstrated improvements in attention and increased speed and accuracy when performing stressful cognitive tasks compared to controls (Aslanyan et al 2010).

In a randomised, double-blind, placebo-controlled study, 30 subjects were assigned to three groups of 10: placebo group, *Rhodiola rosea* group (providing 144 mg SHR-5 extract twice daily) and ADAPT-232 group (140 mg of standardised combination twice daily) for 7 days. Experienced levels of fatigue significantly decreased in the *R. rosea* group but not in the ADAPT-232 group compared to placebo (Schutgens et al 2009).

Infection

Schisandra is also used in combination with other herbal medicines to treat infection. One double-blind, randomised, placebo-controlled pilot study found that a commercial product known as ImmunoGuard significantly reduced the duration, frequency and severity of attacks in patients with familial Mediterranean fever (Amaryan et al 2003). The dose regimen used was four tablets taken three times daily for 1 month. The ImmunoGuard product contains a fixed combination of *Andrographis paniculata* Nees., *Eleutherococcus senticosus* Maxim., *Schisandra chinensis* Bail. and *Glycyrrhiza glabra* L. special extracts, which are standardised for the content of andrographolide (4 mg/tablet), eleutheroside E, schisandrins and glycyrrhizin, respectively. Although these results are encouraging, it is not known to what extent schisandra contributed to the outcome.

A double-blind, placebo-controlled, randomised pilot study investigated the effects of another preparation known as Chisan (containing schisandra 51.0%, rhodiola 27.6% and Siberian ginseng 24.4%) on recovery time and quality-of-life scores in patients with acute non-specific pneumonia (Narimanian et al 2005). Sixty participants were randomised to receive the standard treatment of cephazoline, bromhexine and theophylline or the standard treatment plus the herbal mixture (20 mL twice a day standardised to contain schisandrin 0.177 mg/mL and gamma-schisandrin 0.105 mg/mL) for 10–15 days. Participants in the active group reported significant improvements in recovery time and quality-of-life scores. The requirement for antibiotics was on average 2 days shorter for those participants taking Chisan. All of these herbs have been celebrated for their adaptogenic effects and this may, at least in part, be responsible for the results. The individual effects of schisandra in this formula, however, are unknown.

OTHER USES

Traditionally, schisandra has been used to treat chronic cough and dyspnoea, diarrhoea, night sweats, irritability, palpitations and insomnia. Based on the herb's inhibitory effects on leukotriene biosynthesis and platelet-activating factor activity and anti-inflammatory effects, it is also used for asthmatic symptoms.

DOSAGE RANGE

As clinical research is lacking, the following dosages come from Australian manufacturers' recommendations.

- Dried fruit: 1.5–6 g/day.
- Liquid extract (1 : 2): 3.5–8.5 mL/day or 25–60 mL/week.

TOXICITY

Insufficient reliable information is available.

ADVERSE REACTIONS

Mild gastrointestinal discomfort

SIGNIFICANT INTERACTIONS

CYP3A4 substrates

Increased serum levels of drugs chiefly metabolised by CYP 3A4 are possible, based on current evidence. Practitioners are advised to carefully monitor patients who are already taking drugs that are CYP3A4 substrates to avoid inducing drug side effects caused by increased serum levels.

Schisandra should not be prescribed together with CYP3A4 substrates that have a narrow therapeutic index in order to avoid inducing drug toxicity.

P-glycoprotein substrates

Based on current evidence, it appears that P-glycoprotein inhibition is possible. As a result, serum levels of P-glycoprotein substrates could be increased. Practitioners are advised to carefully monitor patients who are already taking drugs that are P-glycoprotein substrates to avoid inducing drug side effects caused by increased serum levels.

Schisandra should not be prescribed together with P-glycoprotein substrates that have a narrow therapeutic index in order to avoid inducing drug toxicity.

Drugs metabolised by UGT1A3

Deoxyschizandrin and schisantherin A have demonstrated an inhibitory effect on UDP-glucuronosyltransferase 1A3 (UGT1A3) in vitro. This suggests a potential for herb–drug interactions between schisandra and drugs that mainly undergo UGT1A3-mediated metabolism; however the effect has not been confirmed clinically (Liu et al 2012b).

 ***CONTRAINDICATIONS AND PRECAUTIONS***

Insufficient reliable information is available.

 ***PREGNANCY USE***

Insufficient information is available to establish safety.

Practice points/Patient counselling

- *S. chinensis* is popular in TCM and is used to increase resistance to physical and emotional stressors and is regarded as an adaptogen.
- Traditionally, schisandra has been used to treat chronic cough and dyspnoea, diarrhoea, night sweats, irritability, palpitations and insomnia.
- It is commonly used as a liver tonic, and preliminary evidence has identified significant hepatoprotective effects.
- Schisandra exerts direct antioxidant activity and increases hepatic and myocardial glutathione levels, thereby increasing antioxidant systems within the heart and liver.
- Overall, little clinical evidence is available; therefore, much information is still speculative and based on in vitro and animal research and traditional use.

PATIENTS' FAQs

What will this herb do for me?

Schisandra is often prescribed to increase physical and emotional resilience and as a liver tonic. It has antioxidant activity, and early research suggests that it may have significant protective benefits for the liver.

When will it start to work?

This is uncertain due to insufficient research being available.

Are there any safety issues?

This is uncertain due to insufficient research being available.

REFERENCES

Akbar N et al. Effectiveness of the analogue of natural Schisandrin C (HpPro) in treatment of liver diseases: an experience in Indonesian patients. Chin Med J (Engl) 111.3 (1998): 248–251.

Amaryan G et al. Double-blind, placebo-controlled, randomized, pilot clinical trial of ImmunoGuard: a standardized fixed combination of *Andrographis paniculata* Nees, with *Eleutherococcus senticosus* Maxim, *Schizandra chinensis* Bail. and *Glycyrrhiza glabra* L. extracts in patients with familial Mediterranean fever. Phytomedicine 10.4 (2003): 271–285.

S

Antoshechkin A et al. Influence of the plant extract complex "AdMax" on global gene expression levels in cultured human fibroblasts. Journal of Dietary Supplements 5.3 (2008): 293–304.

Aslanyan G et al. Double-blind, placebo-controlled, randomised study of single dose effects of ADAPT-232 on cognitive functions. Phytomedicine 17.7 (2010): 494–9.

Bae H et al. Effects of *Schisandra chinensis* Baillon (Schizandraceae) on lipopolysaccharide induced lung inflammation in mice. Journal of Ethnopharmacology 142.1 (2012): 41–7.

Blunder M et al. Derivatives of schisandrin with increased inhibitory potential on prostaglandin E2 and leukotriene B4 formation in vitro. Bioorganic & Medicinal Chemistry 18.7 (2010): 2809–15.

Cai S et al. Protective effect of schisandrins extract on liver ultrastructure in rats with CCl_4 poisoning. Carcinogenesis, Teratogenesis & Mutagenesis 1.13 (2010).

Caichompoo W et al. Optimization of extraction and purification of active fractions from *Schisandra chinensis* (Turcz.) and its osteoblastic proliferation stimulating activity. Phytother Res 23.2 (2009): 289–292.

Cao S et al. Evaluation of anti-athletic fatigue activity of *Schizandra chinensis* aqueous extracts in mice. African Journal of Pharmacy and Pharmacology 3.11 (2009): 593–7.

Chae HS et al. Gomisin N has anti-allergic effect and inhibits inflammatory cytokine expression in mouse bone marrow-derived mast cells. Immunopharmacology and immunotoxicology 33.4 (2011): 709–13.

Chang C et al. Effect of schisandrin B and sesamin mixture on CCl4-induced hepatic oxidative stress in rats. Phytotherapy Research 23.2 (2009): 251–6.

Checker R et al. Schisandrin B exhibits anti-inflammatory activity through modulation of the redox-sensitive transcription factors Nrf2 and NF-ŒʃB. Free Radical Biology and Medicine 53.7 (2012): 1421–30.

Chen N, et al. Schisandrin B enhances cerebral mitochondrial antioxidant status and structural integrity, and protects against cerebral ischemia/reperfusion injury in rats. Biol Pharm Bull 31.7 (2008): 1387–1391.

Chen Y et al. Effects of Chinese herb medicine on performance, immune function and anti-oxidant capacity of broiler. Acta Ecologiae Animalis Domastici 4.16 (2008).

Chen ML et al. Biochemical mechanism of Wu-Zi-Yan-Zong-Wan, a traditional Chinese herbal formula, against alcohol-induced oxidative damage in CYP2E1 cDNA-transfected HepG2 (E47) cells. Journal Of Ethnopharmacology 128.1 (2010): 116–122.

Chen Q et al. Dual effects of extract of *Schisandra chinensis* Baill on rat hepatic CYP3A. Acta Pharmaceutica Sinica 45.9 (2010): 1194–8.

Chen W et al. Pharmacological studies on the anxiolytic effect of standardized schisandra lignans extract on restraint-stressed mice. Phytomedicine 18.13 (2011): 1144–7.

Chen X et al. Composition and biological activities of the essential oil from *Schisandra chinensis* obtained by solvent-free microwave extraction. LWT - Food Science and Technology 44.10 (2011): 2047–52.

Chen X et al. Chemical composition and antioxidant activity of the essential oil of *Schisandra chinensis* fruits. Natural Product Research 26.9 (2012): 842–9.

Chen Y et al. An immunostimulatory polysaccharide (SCP-IIa) from the fruit of *Schisandra chinensis* (Turcz.) Baill. International Journal of Biological Macromolecules. 50.3 (2012): 844–8.

Cheng N et al. Antioxidant and hepatoprotective effects of *Schisandra chinensis* pollen extract on CCl4-induced acute liver damage in mice. Food and Chemical Toxicology 55.0 (2013): 234–40.

Chiu PY et al. In vivo antioxidant action of a lignan-enriched extract of Schisandra fruit and an anthraquinone-containing extract of Polygonum root in comparison with schisandrin B and emodin. Planta Med 68.11 (2002): 951–956.

Chiu PY et al. Schisandrin B decreases the sensitivity of mitochondria to calcium ion-induced permeability transition and protects against carbon tetrachloride toxicity in mouse livers. Biol Pharm Bull 30.6 (2007): 1108–1112.

Chiu P et al. Schisandrin B enhances renal mitochondrial antioxidant status, functional and structural integrity, and protects against gentamicin-induced nephrotoxicity in rats. Biological & Pharmaceutical Bulletin 31.4 (2008a): 602–5.

Chiu P et al. Schisandrin B stereoisomers protect against hypoxia/reoxygenation-induced apoptosis and inhibit associated changes in Ca^{2+}-induced mitochondrial permeability transition and mitochondrial membrane potential in H9c2 cardiomyocytes. Life Sciences 82.21 (2008b): 1092–1101.

Chiu P et al. Schisandrin B stereoisomers protect against hypoxia/reoxygenation-induced apoptosis and associated changes in the Ca^{2+}-induced mitochondrial permeability transition and mitochondrial membrane potential in AML12 hepatocytes. Phytotherapy Research 23.11(2009): 1592–602.

Chiu P et al. Schisandrin B elicits a glutathione antioxidant response and protects against apoptosis via the redox-sensitive ERK/Nrf2 pathway in H9c2 cells. Molecular And Cellular Biochemistry 350.1–2 (2011): 237–50.

Choi I & Chang H. Antimicrobial activity of medicinal herbs against *Salmonella gallinarum* and Staphylococcus epidermidis. Korean Journal of Poultry Science 36.3 (2009): 231–8.

Choi EH et al. *Schisandra fructus* extract ameliorates doxorubicin-induced cytotoxicity in cardiomyocytes: altered gene expression for detoxification enzymes. Genes Nutr 2.4 (2008): 337–345.

Choi Y et al. Wuweizisu C from *Schisandra chinensis* decreases membrane potential in C6 glioma cells. Acta Pharmacologica Sinica 29.9 (2008): 1006–12.

Choi Y et al. Inhibition of endothelial cell adhesion by the new anti-inflammatory agent alpha-iso-cubebene. Vascular Pharmacology 51.4 (2009): 215–24.

Chung MJ et al. Suppressive effects of *Schizandra chinensis* Baillon water extract on allergy-related cytokine generation and degranulation in IgE-antigen complex-stimulated RBL-2H3 cells. Nutrition Research And Practice 6.2 (2012): 97–105.

Egashira N et al. Schizandrin reverses memory impairment in rats. Phytother Res 22.1 (2008): 49–52.

Fan L et al. Effect of *Schisandra chinensis* extract and Ginkgo biloba extract on the pharmacokinetics of talinolol in healthy volunteers. Xenobiotica; The Fate Of Foreign Compounds In Biological Systems 39.3 (2009): 249–54.

Fong WF et al. Schisandrol A from *Schisandra chinensis* reverses P-glycoprotein-mediated multidrug resistance by affecting Pgp-substrate complexes. Planta Med 73.3 (2007): 212–220.

Fu M et al. Deoxyschisandrin modulates synchronized Ca^{2+} oscillations and spontaneous synaptic transmission of cultured hippocampal neurons. Acta Pharmacologica Sinica 29.8 (2008): 891–8.

Gao X et al. Isolation, characterization and hypoglycemic activity of an acid polysaccharide isolated from *Schisandra chinensis* (Turcz.) Baill. Letters in Organic Chemistry 6.5 (2009): 428–33.

Giridharan VV et al. Prevention of scopolamine-induced memory deficits by schisandrin B, an antioxidant lignan from *Schisandra chinensis* in mice. Free Radical Research 45.8 (2011): 950–8.

Giridharan VV et al. Schisandrin B, attenuates cisplatin-induced oxidative stress, genotoxicity and neurotoxicity through modulating NF-κB pathway in mice. Free Radical Research 46.1 (2012): 50–60.

Gnabre J et al. Isolation of lignans from *Schisandra chinensis* with anti-proliferative activity in human colorectal carcinoma: Structure-activity relationships. Journal Of Chromatography. B, Analytical Technologies In The Biomedical And Life Sciences 878.28 (2010): 2693–700.

Gu BH et al. Deoxyschisandrin inhibits H2O2-induced apoptotic cell death in intestinal epithelial cells through nuclear factor-kappaB. International Journal Of Molecular Medicine 26.3 (2010): 401–6.

Guo LY et al. Anti-inflammatory effects of schisandrin isolated from the fruit of *Schisandra chinensis* Baill. Eur J Pharmacol 591.1–3 (2008): 293–299.

Gurley B, et al. Pharmacokinetic herb-drug interactions (part 2): drug interactions involving popular botanical dietary supplements and their clinical relevance. Planta Medica 78.13 (2012): 1490–514.

Han DH et al. Effects of *Schisandra chinensis* extract on the contractility of corpus cavernosal smooth muscle (CSM) and Ca^{2+} homeostasis in CSM cells. BJU International 109.9 (2012): 1404–13.

He Y, et al. The inhibit effect of *Fructus schizandrae* polysaccharide on the growth of tumor in mice with hepatocellular carcinoma and the primarily exploring on immunological mechanism. Information on Traditional Chinese Medicine 2.12. (2010).

Hu D et al. Deoxyschizandrin isolated from the fruits of *Schisandra chinensis* ameliorates AB1-42-induced memory impairment in mice. Planta Medica 78.12 (2012): 1332–6.

Huang M et al. Reversal of P-glycoprotein-mediated multidrug resistance of cancer cells by five schizandrins isolated from the Chinese herb *Fructus schizandrae*. Cancer chemotherapy and pharmacology 62.6 (2008): 1015–26.

Hwang D et al. A compound isolated from *Schisandra chinensis* induces apoptosis. Bioorganic & Medicinal Chemistry Letters 21.20 (2011): 6054–7.

Inoue H et al. Gomisin N enhances TRAIL-induced apoptosis via reactive oxygen species-mediated up-regulation of death receptors 4 and 5. International Journal Of Oncology 40.4 (2012): 1058–65.

Ip SP et al. Effect of schisandrin B on hepatic glutathione antioxidant system in mice: protection against carbon tetrachloride toxicity. Planta Med 61.5 (1995): 398–401.

Iwata H et al. Identification and characterization of potent CYP3A4 inhibitors in Schisandra fruit extract. Drug Metab Dispos 32.12 (2004): 1351–1358.

Jeong S et al. The Korean traditional medicine Gyeongshingangjeehwan inhibits obesity through the regulation of leptin and PPARα action in OLETF rats. Journal Of Ethnopharmacology 119.2 (2008): 245–51.

Jeong SI et al. Schizandrin prevents damage of murine mesangial cells via blocking NADPH oxidase-induced ROS signaling in high glucose. Food and Chemical Toxicology 50.3–4 (2012): 1045–53.

Jeong EJ et al. The effects of lignan-riched extract of *Schisandra chinensis* on amyloid-B-induced cognitive impairment and neurotoxicity in the cortex and hippocampus of mouse. Journal Of Ethnopharmacology 146.1 (2013): 347–54.

Jiang W, et al. The effect of deoxyschisandrin on blood tacrolimus levels: a case report. Immunopharmacology and immunotoxicology 32.1 (2010a): 177–8.

Jiang W et al. Effect of *Schisandra sphenanthera* extract on the concentration of tacrolimus in the blood of liver transplant patients. International Journal Of Clinical Pharmacology And Therapeutics 48.3 (2010b): 224.

Jie Y et al. Experimental study on isolation and purification of total lignans from *Schisandra chinensis* and the antitumor activity in vitro. China Pharmacist 12.18 (2009).

Jin J et al. Enhancement of oral bioavailability of paclitaxel after oral administration of Schisandrol B in rats. Biopharmaceutics & Drug Disposition 31.4 (2010): 264–8.

Jo SH et al. In vitro and in vivo anti-hyperglycemic effects of omija (*Schizandra chinensis*) fruit. International Journal of Molecular Sciences 12.2 (2011): 1359–70.

Jung YS et al. Role of CXCR2 on the immune modulating activity of Œ±-iso-cubebenol a natural compound isolated from the *Schisandra chinensis* fruit. Biochemical And Biophysical Research Communications 431.3 (2013): 433–6.

Junshu Y & Anshan S. Effect of *Schisandra chinensis* extract on blood biochemical index in broilers. Feed Industry 18.6 (2008).

Kang YH & Shin HM. Inhibitory effects of *Schizandra chinensis* extract on atopic dermatitis in NC/Nga mice. Immunopharmacology and immunotoxicology 34.2 (2012): 292–8.

Kang OH et al. Effects of the *Schisandra fructus* water extract on cytokine release from a human mast cell line. J Med Food 9.4 (2006): 480–486.

Kang JW et al. Protective effects of HV-P411 complex against D-galactosamine-induced hepatotoxicity in rats. The American Journal Of Chinese Medicine 40.3 (2012): 467–80.

Kang K et al. Dibenzocyclooctadiene lignans, gomisins J and N inhibit the Wnt/B-catenin signaling pathway in HCT116 cells. Biochemical And Biophysical Research Communications 428.2 (2012): 285–91.

Kim SR et al. Dibenzocyclooctadiene lignans from *Schisandra chinensis* protect primary cultures of rat cortical cells from glutamate-induced toxicity. J Neurosci Res 76.3 (2004): 397–405.

Kim S et al. Anti-apoptotic and hepatoprotective effects of gomisin A on fulminant hepatic failure induced by D-galactosamine and lipopolysaccharide in mice. Journal of pharmacological sciences 106.2 (2008): 225–33.

Kim SH, et al. Structural identification and antioxidant properties of major anthocyanin extracted from Omija (*Schizandra chinensis*) fruit. Journal of Food Science 74.2 (2009): C134–C140.

Kim JH et al. Apoptosis induction of human leukemia U937 cells by gomisin N, a dibenzocyclooctadiene lignan, isolated from *Schizandra chinensis* Baill. Food and Chemical Toxicology 48.3 (2010): 807–13.

Kim MG, et al. Anti-platelet aggregation activity of lignans isolated from *Schisandra chinensis* fruits. Journal of the Korean Society for Applied Biological Chemistry 53.6 (2010): 740–5.

Kim, SJ et al. Growth inhibition and cell cycle arrest in the G0/G1 by schizandrin, a dibenzocyclooctadiene lignan isolated from *Schisandra chinensis*, on T47D human breast cancer cells. Phytotherapy Research 24.2 (2010): 193–7.

Kim EY, et al. Cardioprotective effects of aqueous *Schizandra chinensis* fruit extract on ovariectomized and balloon-induced carotid artery injury rat models: Effects on serum lipid profiles and blood pressure. Journal Of Ethnopharmacology 134.3 (2011): 668–75.

Kim HK et al. The role of the lignan constituents in the effect of *Schisandra chinensis* fruit extract on penile erection. Phytotherapy Research 25.12 (2011): 1776–82.

Kim HY et al. Protective effect of HV-P411, an herbal mixture, on carbon tetrachloride-induced liver fibrosis. Food Chemistry 124.1 (2011): 248–53.

Kim JE et al. The a-iso-cubebenol compound isolated from *Schisandra chinensis* induces p53-independent pathway-mediated apoptosis in hepatocellular carcinoma cells. Oncology Reports 28.3 (2012): 1103–9.

Kim KJ et al. *Schisandra chinensis* prevents hepatic lipid peroxidation and oxidative stress in rats subjected to heat environmental stress. Phytotherapy Research 26.11 (2012): 1674–80.

Ko KM et al. Long-term schisandrin B treatment mitigates age-related impairments in mitochondrial antioxidant status and functional ability in various tissues, and improves the survival of aging C57BL/6J mice. Biofactors 34.4 (2008): 331–42.

Ko S et al. Comparison of anti-oxidant activities of seventy herbs that have been used in Korean traditional medicine. Nutrition Research And Practice 2.3 (2008): 143–51.

Kubo S et al. Effect of Gomisin A (TJN-101) on liver regeneration. Planta Med 58.6 (1992): 489–492.

Kwon DY et al. The lignan-rich fractions of Fructus Schisandrae improve insulin sensitivity via the PPAR-a pathways in in vitro and in vivo studies. Journal Of Ethnopharmacology 135.2 (2011): 455–62.

Lai L et al. Effects of short-term and long-term pretreatment of schisandra lignans on regulating hepatic and intestinal CYP3A in rats. Drug Metabolism and Disposition 37.12 (2009): 2399–407.

Lam PY et al. Schisandrin B co-treatment ameliorates the impairment on mitochondrial antioxidant status in various tissues of long-term ethanol treated rats. Fitoterapia 81.8 (2010): 1239–45.

Lam PY et al. Schisandrin B protects against solar irradiation-induced oxidative stress in rat skin tissue. Fitoterapia 82.3 (2011): 393–400.

Lau C et al. In vitro antidiabetic activities of five medicinal herbs used in Chinese medicinal formulae. Phytotherapy Research 22.10 (2008): 1383–8.

Lee IS et al. Structure-activity relationships of lignans from *Schisandra chinensis* as platelet activating factor antagonists. Biol Pharm Bull 22.3 (1999): 265–267.

Lee IS et al. Lignans with inhibitory activity against NFAT transcription from *Schisandra chinensis*. Planta Med 69.1 (2003): 63–64.

Lee B et al. Inhibitory effect of schizandrin on passive cutaneous anaphylaxis reaction and scratching behaviors in mice. Biol Pharm Bull 30.6 (2007): 1153–1156.

Lee SB et al. Induction of the phase II detoxification enzyme NQO1 in hepatocarcinoma cells by lignans from the fruit of *Schisandra chinensis* through nuclear accumulation of Nrf2. Planta Medica 75.12 (2009): 1314–8.

Lee Y et al. Identification of a novel compound that stimulates intracellular calcium increase and CXCL8 production in human neutrophils from *Schisandra chinensis*. Biochemical And Biophysical Research Communications 379.4 (2009): 928–32.

Lee MY et al. Anti-asthmatic effect of schizandrin on OVA-induced airway inflammation in a murine asthma model. International Immunopharmacology 10.1 (2010): 1374–9.

Lee YJ et al. Identification of a novel compound that inhibits iNOS and COX-2 expression in LPS-stimulated macrophages from *Schisandra chinensis*. Biochemical And Biophysical Research Communications 391.4 (2010): 1687–92.

Lee SK et al. a-Iso-cubebene, a natural compound isolated from *Schisandra chinensis* fruit, has therapeutic benefit against polymicrobial sepsis. Biochemical And Biophysical Research Communications 426.2 (2012): 226–31.

Lee TH, et al. Neuroprotective effects of Schisandrin B against transient focal cerebral ischemia in Sprague-Dawley rats. Food and Chemical Toxicology 50.12 (2012): 4239–45.

Leong PK et al. Cytochrome P450-catalysed reactive oxygen species production mediates the (-) schisandrin B-induced glutathione and heat shock responses in AML12 hepatocytes. Cell Biology International 36.3 (2012): 321–6.

Li SF et al. Protection of schisandrin B against silica-induced lung injury in rats. Chinese Journal of Comparative Medicine 5.7 (2009).

Li WL et al. In vivo effect of Schisandrin B on cytochrome P450 enzyme activity. Phytomedicine 20.8–9 (2013); 760–765.

Lim H et al. 5-Lipoxygenase-inhibitory constituents from *Schizandra fructus* and *Magnolia flos*. Phytotherapy Research 23.10 (2009): 1489–92.

Lin S, et al. Molecular mechanism of apoptosis induced by schizandrae-derived lignans in human leukemia HL-60 cells. Food Chem Toxicol 46.2 (2008): 590–597.

Lin RD et al. The immuno-regulatory effects of *Schisandra chinensis* and its constituents on human monocytic leukemia cells. Molecules 16.6 (2011): 4836–49.

Liu C, et al. Non-thermal extraction of effective ingredients from *Schisandra chinensis* Baill and the antioxidant activity of its extract. Natural Product Research 23.15 (2009): 1390–401.

Liu C et al. Chemical composition and antioxidant activity of essential oil from berries of *Schisandra chinensis* (Turcz.) Baill. Natural Product Research 26.23 (2012a): 2199–203.

Liu C et al. Strong inhibition of deoxyschizandrin and schisantherin A toward UDP-glucuronosyltransferase (UGT) 1A3 indicating UGT inhibition-based herb-drug interaction. Fitoterapia 83.8 (2012b): 1415–9.

Loo WT, et al. *Fructus schisandrae* (Wuweizi)-containing compound inhibits secretion of HBsAg and HBeAg in hepatocellular carcinoma cell line. Biomed Pharmacother 61.9 (2007): 606–610.

Lu H, Liu GT. Anti-oxidant activity of dibenzocyclooctene lignans isolated from Schisandraceae. Planta Med 58.4 (1992): 311–3113.

Ma CJ et al. ESP-102, a combined extract of *Angelica gigas, Saururus chinensis* and *Schizandra chinensis*, protects against glutamate-induced toxicity in primary cultures of rat cortical cells. Phytotherapy Research 23.11 (2009): 1587–91.

Ma D et al. Influence of an aqueous extract of *Ligustrum lucidum* and an ethanol extract of *Schisandra chinensis* on parameters of antioxidative metabolism and spleen lymphocyte proliferation of broilers. Archives Of Animal Nutrition 63.1 (2009): 66–74.

Ma C et al. Optimization of conditions of solvent-free microwave extraction and study on antioxidant capacity of essential oil from *Schisandra chinensis* (Turcz.) Baill. Food Chemistry 134.4 (2012): 2532–39.

Mak DH, Ko KM. Alterations in susceptibility to carbon tetrachloride toxicity and hepatic antioxidant/detoxification system in streptozotocin-induced short-term diabetic rats: effects of insulin and Schisandrin B treatment. Mol Cell Biochem 175.1–2 (1997): 225–232.

Mak DH et al. Effects of Schisandrin B and alpha-tocopherol on lipid peroxidation, in vitro and in vivo. Mol Cell Biochem 165.2 (1996): 161–165.

Meng X, et al. Study on extraction, purification and scavenging free radical of polysaccharide SCP-B II from *Schisandra chinensis*. Food Science 1.15 (2008).

Miao M, et al. Effect of *Schisandra chinensis* Baill distilled by ethanol on the ability of learning and memory in memory impairment mice model induced by repeated cerebral ischemia-reperfusion. Chinese Journal of Modern Applied Pharmacy 5.4 (2009).

Miao Y et al. Effect of *Schisandra chinensis* Baill distilled by ethanol on energy metabolism in brain of repeated cerebral ischemia-reperfusion model mice. China Journal of Traditional Chinese Medicine and Pharmacy 9.37 (2009).

Min HY et al. Antiproliferative effects of dibenzocyclooctadiene lignans isolated from *Schisandra chinensis* in human cancer cells. Bioorg Med Chem Lett 18.2 (2008): 523–526.

Moon PD, et al. Effects of schizandrin on the expression of thymic stromal lymphopoietin in human mast cell line HMC-1. Life Sciences 91.11–12 (2012): 384–8.

Na M et al. Fatty acid synthase inhibitory activity of dibenzocyclooctadiene lignans isolated from *Schisandra chinensis*. Phytotherapy Research 24.2 (2010): S225–S8.

Nakagiri R, et al. Small scale rat hepatocyte primary culture with applications for screening hepatoprotective substances. Biosci Biotechnol Biochem 67.8 (2003): 1629–1635.

Narimanian M et al. Impact of Chisan (ADAPT-232) on the quality-of-life and its efficacy as an adjuvant in the treatment of acute non-specific pneumonia. Phytomedicine 12.10 (2005): 723–729.

Nishida H et al. Inhibition of ATR protein kinase activity by schisandrin B in DNA damage response. Nucleic acids research 37.17 (2009): 5678–89.

Oh B et al. Inhibitory effects of Schizandrae Fructus on eotaxin secretion in A549 human epithelial cells and eosinophil migration. Phytomedicine 16.9 (2009): 814–22.

Oh SY et al. Anti-inflammatory effects of gomisin N, gomisin J, and schisandrin C isolated from the fruit of *Schisandra chinensis*. Bioscience, Biotechnology and Biochemistry 74.2 (2010): 285–291.

Ohkura Y et al. Effect of gomisin A (TJN-101) on the arachidonic acid cascade in macrophages. Jpn J Pharmacol 52.2 (1990): 331–336.

Ohsugi M et al. Active-oxygen scavenging activity of traditional nourishing-tonic herbal medicines and active constituents of *Rhodiola sacra*. J Ethnopharmacol 67.1 (1999): 111–1119.

Pan S. Ethanol extract of Fructus Schisandrae decreases hepatic triglyceride level in mice fed with a high fat/cholesterol diet, with attention to acute toxicity. Evidence-Based Complementary and Alternative Medicine (2011); 2011: 729412.

Pan SY et al. Schisandrin B protects against tacrine- and bis(7)-tacrine-induced hepatotoxicity and enhances cognitive function in mice. Planta Med 68.3 (2002): 217–220.

Pan Q et al. Dibenzocyclooctadiene lignans: a class of novel inhibitors of P-glycoprotein. Cancer Chemother Pharmacol 58.1 (2006): 99–106.

Pan SY et al. Schisandrin B from *Schisandra chinensis* reduces hepatic lipid contents in hypercholesterolaemic mice. J Pharm Pharmacol 60.3 (2008): 399–403.

Panossian A et al. Adaptogens exert a stress-protective effect by modulation of expression of molecular chaperones. Phytomedicine 16.6–7 (2009): 617–22.

Park JY et al. Gomisin A from *Schisandra chinensis* induces endothelium-dependent and direct relaxation in rat thoracic aorta. Planta Med 73.15 (2007): 1537–1542.

Park C et al. Induction of G1 arrest and apoptosis by schisandrin C isolated from *Schizandra chinensis* Baill in human leukemia U937 cells. International Journal Of Molecular Medicine 24.4 (2009): 495–502.

Park J et al. The mechanism of vasorelaxation induced by *Schisandra chinensis* extract in rat thoracic aorta. Journal Of Ethnopharmacology 121.1 (2009a): 69–73.

Park J et al. Gomisin A induces Ca^{2+}-dependent activation of eNOS in human coronary artery endothelial cells. Journal Of Ethnopharmacology 125.2 (2009b): 291–6.

Park S et al. Huang-Lian-Jie-Du-Tang supplemented with *Schisandra chinensis* Baill. and *Polygonatum odoratum* Druce improved glucose tolerance by potentiating insulinotropic actions in islets in 90% pancreatectomized diabetic rats. Bioscience, Biotechnology, And Biochemistry 73.11 (2009): 2384–92.

Park SY et al. *Schisandra chinensis* a-iso-cubebenol induces heme oxygenase-1 expression through PI3K/Akt and Nrf2 signaling and has anti-inflammatory activity in *Porphyromonas gingivalis* lipopolysaccharide-stimulated macrophages. International Immunopharmacology 11.11 (2011): 1907–15.

Park EJ et al. Schisandrin B suppresses TGF-α signaling by inhibiting Smad2/3 and MAPK pathways. Biochemical Pharmacology 83.3 (2012): 378–84.

Park HJ et al. Anti-obesity effect of *Schisandra chinensis* in 3T3-L1 cells and high fat diet-induced obese rats. Food Chemistry 134.1 (2012): 227–34.

Park J et al. Gomisin J from *Schisandra chinensis* induces vascular relaxation via activation of endothelial nitric oxide synthase. Vascular Pharmacology 57.2–4 (2012a): 124–30.

Park J et al. Antihypertensive effect of gomisin A from *Schisandra chinensis* on angiotensin II-induced hypertension via preservation of nitric oxide bioavailability. Hypertension Research 35.9 (2012b): 928–34.

Peng JH et al. Effect of Jianpi Houxue decoction on inflammatory cytokine secretion pathway in rat liver with lipopolysaccharide challenge. World journal of gastroenterology 14.12 (2008): 1851.

Pu HJ et al. Correlation between antistress and hepatoprotective effects of schisandra lignans was related with its antioxidative actions in liver cells. Evidence-Based Complementary and Alternative Medicine (2012); 2012: 161062.

Qiangrong P et al. Schisandrin B: a novel inhibitor of P-glycoprotein. Biochem Biophys Res Commun 335.2 (2005): 406–411.

Rhyu MR et al. Aqueous extract of *Schizandra chinensis* fruit causes endothelium-dependent and -independent relaxation of isolated rat thoracic aorta. Phytomedicine 13.9–10 (2006): 651–657.

Schutgens F et al. The influence of adaptogens on ultraweak biophoton emission: a pilot-experiment. Phytotherapy Research 23.8 (2009): 1103–8.

Seok YM et al. Effects of gomisin A on vascular contraction in rat aortic rings. Naunyn-Schmiedeberg's Archives Of Pharmacology 383.1 (2011): 45–56.

Shi YM et al. Schicagenins A-C: three cagelike nortriterpenoids from leaves and stems of *Schisandra chinensis*. Organic Letters. 13.15 (2011): 3848–51.

Shin SS et al. The Korean traditional medicine Gyeongshingangjeehwan inhibits adipocyte hypertrophy and visceral adipose tissue accumulation by activating PPARα actions in rat white adipose tissues. Journal Of Ethnopharmacology 127.1 (2010): 47–54.

Slaninova I et al. Dibenzocyclooctadiene lignans overcome drug resistance in lung cancer cells — Study of structure-activity relationship. Toxicology in Vitro 23.6 (2009): 1047–54.

Smejkal K et al. Evaluation of the antiradical activity of *Schisandra chinensis* lignans using different experimental models. Molecules 15.3 (2010): 1223–31.

Sohn D et al. Elevation of intracavernous pressure and NO-cGMP activity by a new herbal formula in penile tissues of spontaneous hypertensive male rats. Journal of Ethnopharmacology 120.2 (2008): 176–80.

Song JX et al. Protective effects of dibenzocyclooctadiene lignans from *Schisandra chinensis* against beta-amyloid and homocysteine neurotoxicity in PC12 cells. Phytotherapy Research 25.3 (2011): 435–43.

Song, QY et al. Eleven new highly oxygenated triterpenoids from the leaves and stems of *Schisandra chinensis*. Organic & Biomolecular Chemistry 11.7 (2013): 1251–8.

Stacchiotti A et al. Schisandrin B stimulates a cytoprotective response in rat liver exposed to mercuric chloride. Food and Chemical Toxicology 4711 (2009): 2834–40.

Stacchiotti A et al. Different role of Schisandrin B on mercury-induced renal damage in vivo and in vitro. Toxicology 286.1–3 (2011): 48–57.

Steele M et al. Cytoprotective properties of traditional Chinese medicinal herbal extracts in hydrogen peroxide challenged human U373 astroglia cells. Neurochemistry International 62.5 (2013): 522–9.

Su T et al. Effects of unprocessed versus vinegar-processed *Schisandra chinensis* on the activity and mRNA expression of CYP1A2, CYP2E1 and CYP3A4 enzymes in rats. Journal Of Ethnopharmacology 146.1 (2013).

Szeto YT et al. In vitro antioxidation activity and genoprotective effect of selected Chinese medicinal herbs. American Journal of Chinese Medicine 39.4 (2011): 827–38.

Takeda S et al. Effects of TJN-101, a lignan compound isolated from Schisandra fruits, on liver fibrosis and on liver regeneration after partial hepatectomy in rats with chronic liver injury induced by CCl4. Nippon Yakurigaku Zasshi 90.1 (1987): 51–65.

Takimoto Y et al. Gomisin N in the herbal drug gomishi (*Schisandra chinensis*) suppresses inducible nitric oxide synthase gene via C/EBPβ and NF-kB in rat hepatocytes. Nitric Oxide 28.0 (2013): 47–56.

Tang SH et al. The protective effect of schisandra lignans on stress-evoked hepatic metastases of P815 tumor cells in restraint mice. Journal of Ethnopharmacology 134.1 (2011): 141–6.
Tsi D, Tan A. Evaluation on the combined effect of Sesamin and Schisandra extract on blood fluidity. Bioinformation 2.6 (2008): 249–252.
Waiwut P et al. Gomisin N enhances TNF-α-induced apoptosis via inhibition of the NF-κB and EGFR survival pathways. Molecular and Cellular Biochemistry 350.1–2 (2011): 169–75.
Waiwut P et al. Gomisin A enhances tumor necrosis factor-α-induced G1 cell cycle arrest via signal transducer and activator of transcription 1-mediated phosphorylation of retinoblastoma protein. Biological & Pharmaceutical Bulletin 35.11 (2012): 1997–2003.
Wan CK et al. Gomisin A alters substrate interaction and reverses P-glycoprotein-mediated multidrug resistance in HepG2-DR cells. Biochem Pharmacol 72.7 (2006): 824–837.
Wan C et al. Inhibition of cytochrome P450 3A4 activity by schisandrol A and gomisin A isolated from Fructus Schisandrae chinensis. Phytomedicine 17.8–9 (2010): 702–5.
Wang J. Study on the bacteriostatic and bactericidal activity of extract from *Schisandra chinensis*. Journal of Anhui Agricultural Sciences 16.83 (2008).
Wang HJ & Chiang BH. Anti-diabetic effect of a traditional Chinese medicine formula. Food & Function 3.11 (2012): 1161–9.
Wang M, et al. High throughput screening and antioxidant assay of dibenzo[a,c]cyclooctadiene lignans in modified-ultrasonic and supercritical fluid extracts of *Schisandra chinensis* Baill by liquid chromatography-mass spectrometry and a free radical-scavenging method. Journal of separation science 31.8 (2008): 1322–32.
Wang W et al. Sedative and hypnotic effects of each extract of Fructus Schisandrae in mice. Journal of Jiangsu University 2.9 (2008a).
Wang W et al. Effects of *Schisandra chinensis* Baill extract on anti-hypoxia and anti-fatigue in Mice. Journal of Inner Mongolia University for Nationalities 6.23 (2008b).
Wang B et al. Effects of *Schisandra chinensis* (Wuweizi) constituents on the activity of hepatic microsomal CYP450 isozymes in rats detected by using a cocktail probe substrates method. Acta pharmaceutica Sinica 46.8 (2011): 922.
Wang SD et al. Xiao-Qing-Long-Tang attenuates allergic airway inflammation and remodeling in repetitive *Dermatogoides pteronyssinus* challenged chronic asthmatic mice model. Journal of Ethnopharmacology 142.2 (2012): 531–8.
Wei B et al. Development of a UFLC-MS/MS method for simultaneous determination of six lignans of *Schisandra chinensis* (Turcz.) Baill. in rat plasma and its application to a comparative pharmacokinetic study in normal and insomnic rats. Journal of Pharmaceutical and Biomedical Analysis 77.0 (2013): 120–7.
Wen-qiang W. Study on in vitro antimicrobial effect of four Chinese herb medicines. Journal of Anhui Agricultural Sciences 6.83 (2009).
Xie X et al. Effects of Schisandra on behavioral learning and hippocampal AChE activity in ovariectomized mice. Journal of South China Normal University 3.24 (2010).
Xie Y et al. Integral pharmacokinetics of multiple lignan components in normal, CCl4-induced hepatic injury and hepatoprotective agents pretreated rats and correlations with hepatic injury biomarkers. Journal of Ethnopharmacology 131.2 (2010): 290–9.
Xin H et al. Effects of *Schisandra sphenanthera* extract on the pharmacokinetics of tacrolimus in healthy volunteers. British Journal of Clinical Pharmacology 64.4 (2007): 469–75.
Xin H et al. Effects of *Schisandra sphenanthera* extract on the pharmacokinetics of midazolam in healthy volunteers. British Journal of Clinical Pharmacology 67.5 (2009): 541–546.
Xu C et al. Inhibitory effect of *Schisandra chinensis* leaf polysaccharide against L5178Y lymphoma. Carbohydrate Polymers 88.1 (2012): 21–5.
Xu X, et al. Schizandrin prevents dexamethasone-induced cognitive deficits. Neurosci Bull. 2012 Oct;28(5):532–40
Xv G et al. Hypoglycemic effects of a water-soluble polysaccharide isolated from *Schisandra chinensis* (Turcz.) Baill in alloxan-induced diabetic mice. Journal of Biotechnology 136.0 (2008): S725.
Yamada S, et al. Preventive effect of gomisin A, a lignan component of shizandra fruits, on acetaminophen-induced hepatotoxicity in rats. Biochem Pharmacol 46.6 (1993): 1081–1085.
Yan F et al. Synergistic hepatoprotective effect of *Schisandrae* lignans with *Astragalus* polysaccharides on chronic liver injury in rats. Phytomedicine 16.9 (2009): 805–13.
Yang L et al. Study on immunological activity of coarse polysaccharides from ethanol-insoluble residue of Schisandra. Food Science 6.89 (2008).
Yang, J et al. Inhibitory effect of schisandrin on spontaneous contraction of isolated rat colon. Phytomedicine 18.11 (2011a): 998–1005.
Yang, J et al. Relaxant effects of *Schisandra chinensis* and its major lignans on agonists-induced contraction in guinea pig ileum. Phytomedicine 18.13 (2011b): 1153–60.
Yang SH et al. Schisandrin enhances dendrite outgrowth and synaptogenesis in primary cultured hippocampal neurons. Journal of the Science of Food and Agriculture 91.4 (2011): 694–702.
Yang X et al. Screening vasoconstriction inhibitors from traditional Chinese medicines using a vascular smooth muscle/cell membrane chromatography-offline-liquid chromatography-mass spectrometry. Journal of Separation Science 34.19 (2011): 2586–93.
Yang J et al. *Schisandra chinensis* reverses visceral hypersensitivity in a neonatal-maternal separated rat model. Phytomedicine: International Journal Of Phytotherapy And Phytopharmacology 19.5 (2012): 402–8.
Yao HT et al. Shengmai San reduces hepatic lipids and lipid peroxidation in rats fed on a high-cholesterol diet. Journal of Ethnopharmacology 116.1 (2008): 49–57.
Yao Q et al. Induction effects of the different processed Fructus schisandrae Chinensis on the hepatic microsomal cytochrome P450 in rats. West China Journal of Pharmaceutical Sciences 3.19 (2011).
Yasukawa K et al. Gomisin A inhibits tumor promotion by 12-*O*-tetradecanoylphorbol-13-acetate in two-stage carcinogenesis in mouse skin. Oncology 49.1 (1992): 68–71.
Yasukawa K et al. Gomisin A inhibits tumor promotion by 12-o-tetra-decanoylphorbol-13-acetate in two-stage carcinogenesis in mouse skin. Oncology 49.1 (2009): 68–71.
Ye C et al. Extraction optimization of polysaccharides of Schisandrae Fructus and evaluation of their analgesic activity. International Journal of Biological Macromolecules 57.1 (2013): 291–96.
Yim TK, Ko KM. Schisandrin B protects against myocardial ischemia-reperfusion injury by enhancing myocardial glutathione antioxidant status. Mol Cell Biochem 196.1–2 (1999): 151–156.
Yim SY et al. Gomisin N isolated from *Schisandra chinensis* significantly induces anti-proliferative and pro-apoptotic effects in hepatic carcinoma. Molecular Medicine Reports 2.5 (2009): 725–32.
Yoo HH et al. Effects of schisandra lignans on P-glycoprotein-mediated drug efflux in human intestinal Caco-2. Planta Med 73.5 (2007): 444–450.
Yu C et al. Identification of novel pregnane X receptor activators from traditional Chinese medicines. Journal of Ethnopharmacology 136.1 (2011): 137–43.
Yuezhen L. Effects of the different concentration Schisandrin B including multiplication and apoptosis in human gastric cancer cell line MGC-803. Journal of Mudanjiang Medical University 4.2 (2010).
Zeng KW et al. Schisandrin B exerts anti-neuroinflammatory activity by inhibiting the Toll-like receptor 4-dependent MyD88/IKK/NF-kB signaling pathway in lipopolysaccharide-induced microglia. European Journal of Pharmacology 692.1–3 (2012): 29–37.
Zhang Y & Li PP. Evaluation of estrogenic potential of Shu-Gan-Liang-Xue decoction by dual-luciferase reporter based bioluminescent measurements in vitro. Journal Of Ethnopharmacology 126.2 (2009): 345–9.
Zhang J, et al. Dibenzocyclooctadiene lignans from Fructus Schisandrae Chinensis improve glucose uptake in vitro. Natural Product Communications 5.2 (2010): 231–4.
Zhang N et al. Studies on chemical constituents of leaf of *Schisandra chinensis* and inhibitory effect of schizandrin on activation of microglia induced by LPS. Chinese Journal of Medicinal Chemistry 20.2 (2010): 110–5.
Zhang M et al. *Schisandra chinensis* fruit extract attenuates albuminuria and protects podocyte integrity in a mouse model of streptozotocin-induced diabetic nephropathy. Journal of Ethnopharmacology 141.1 (2012): 111–8.
Zhao T et al. Anti-diabetic effects of polysaccharides from ethanol-insoluble residue of *Schisandra chinensis* (Turcz.) Baill on alloxan-induced diabetic mice. Chemical Research in Chinese Universities 29.1 (2013a): 99–102.
Zhao T et al. Antitumor and immunomodulatory activity of a water-soluble low molecular weight polysaccharide from *Schisandra chinensis* (Turcz.) Baill. Food and Chemical Toxicology 55.0 (2013b): 609–16.
Zhu M et al. Evaluation of the protective effects of *Schisandra chinensis* on phase I drug metabolism using a CCl4 intoxication model. J Ethnopharmacol 67.1 (1999): 61–68.
Zhu M et al. Improvement of phase I drug metabolism with *Schisandra chinensis* against CCl4 hepatotoxicity in a rat model. Planta Med 66.6 (2000): 521–525.
Zhu S et al. Protective effect of schisandrin B against cyclosporine A-induced nephrotoxicity in vitro and in vivo. The American Journal of Chinese Medicine 40.3 (2012): 551–66.

Selenium

HISTORICAL NOTE During his travels in the 13th century, Marco Polo first reported what is thought to be selenium toxicity in grazing animals. He observed that certain grazing areas in China were associated with horses developing diseased hooves (Hendler & Rorvik 2001). It is now known that parts of China have the highest selenium soil concentrations in the world and diseased hooves were likely to be due to selenium toxicity. It was not until nearly 500 years later, in 1817, that selenium was actually discovered (Tinggi 2003), and the fact that it is essential in mammals was not discovered until 1957 (Navarro-Alarcon & Lopez-Martinez 2000). In 1979, the importance of selenium in human nutrition was further reinforced when Chinese researchers reported that selenium supplementation prevented the development of Keshan disease, a cardiomyopathy seen in children living in selenium-replete areas, and New Zealand workers reported a clinical response to selenium supplementation in a selenium-depleted patient (Shils et al 2006).

BACKGROUND AND RELEVANT PHARMACOKINETICS

Selenium is an essential trace element that enters the food chain through incorporation into plants from the soil. Selenium is mainly present in the form of selenite in acid soils, which is poorly assimilated by crops, whereas for alkaline soils it is in the form of selenate, which is more soluble and assimilated by crops. When taken in supplement form, animal and human trials demonstrate that bioavailability of organic forms of selenium (Se-methionine and Se-cysteine) is higher than that obtained for inorganic forms (selenite and selenate) (Navarro-Alarcon & Lopez-Martinez 2000).

The variation in selenium content of adult humans living in different parts of the world is testimony to the influence of the natural environment on the selenium content of soils, crops and human tissues. According to a WHO report, adults in New Zealand have approximately 3 mg selenium in their bodies and a daily intake of about 30 gm (100 gm/day is common) compared with 14 mg body content in some Americans and a daily intake around 100 g/day in North America. Intakes in Europe are in the range of 30 to 60 g/day.

Selenium is readily absorbed, especially in the duodenum and also in the caecum and colon. Vitamins A, E and C can modulate selenium absorption, and there is a complex relationship between selenium and vitamin E that has not been entirely elucidated for humans (Bates 2005). Selenium enters the body in two major forms: Se-methionine, which is derived from plants, and Se-cysteine, which is mainly derived from animal selenoproteins (Shils et al 2006). Metabolism is complex and occurs via several routes for the different selenoproteins. Se-methionine enters the methionine pool where it undergoes the same fate as methionine until catabolised. Once the selenium from Se-methionine is liberated by the trans-sulfuration pathway in the liver or kidney, it is able to be used by peripheral cells. Ingested selenite, selenate and selenocysteine are metabolised to selenide. Urinary excretion accounts for 50–60% of total excretion of selenium and homeostasis is achieved through regulation in the kidney. Volatile forms of selenium are exhaled when intake is very high and presents a significant route of excretion at this level.

CHEMICAL COMPONENTS

In human tissues, it is found as either L-selenomethionine or L-selenocysteine.

FOOD SOURCES

Most dietary selenium is in the form of selenomethionine which is virtually completely bioavailable. The amount of selenium in a food greatly depends on the amount of selenium in the soil where it was grown. As such, a single food plant can vary greatly in its selenium content. By contrast, animal and marine sources tend to have more consistent selenium content. In general, the most concentrated food sources are brewer's yeast, wheatgerm, meats, fish and seafood, Brazil nuts, garlic and organ meats.

DEFICIENCY SIGNS AND SYMPTOMS

Selenium deprivation reduces the activity of selenium-dependent enzymes and has widespread effects. Characteristic signs of selenium deficiency have not been described in humans, but very low selenium status is a factor in the aetiologies of a juvenile cardiomyopathy (Keshan disease) and a chondrodystrophy (Kashin-Beck disease) that occur in selenium-deficient regions of China.

Low selenium status has been associated with:

- loss of immunocompetence (Ongele et al 2002)
- increased risk of developing certain cancers (Clark et al 1998)
- reduced male fertility (Scott et al 1998, Xu et al 2003)
- poorer prognosis in HIV infection and AIDS (Baum et al 1997, Campa et al 1999)
- greater incidence of depression, anxiety, confusion and hostility (Rayman 2000)
- compromised thyroid hormone metabolism (particularly when iodine deficiency is also present) (Gartner et al 2002)
- asthma and atopy (Kadrabova et al 1996, Misso et al 1996, Omland et al 2002)

- rheumatoid arthritis (Zamamiri-Davis et al 2002)
- possibly, increased inflammatory processes (Zamamiri-Davis et al 2002)
- changes to drug-metabolising enzymes, including the cytochrome P450 system, with some activities increasing and others decreasing (Shils et al 2006).

Low selenium status may contribute to the aetiology of several diseases, while in others this state exacerbates disease progression, such as in HIV infection.

People at risk of marginal selenium deficiency include those living in areas of low environmental selenium, such as some regions of New Zealand, people receiving long-term total parenteral nutrition (TPN), low-protein diet associated with phenylketonuria and hyperphenylalaninaemia, alcoholics, and those with liver cirrhosis, hepatitis C virus infection, malabsorption syndromes, cystic fibrosis, coeliac disease and AIDS (Procházková et al 2013).

MAIN ACTIONS

Antioxidant

Selenium is an integral part of thioredoxin reductase and the glutathione peroxidases and therefore is intimately involved in the body's antioxidant systems. These enzymes are involved in controlling tissue levels of free radical molecules and maintain cell-mediated immunity.

Chemopreventative

Chemoprotective effects of selenium have been identified through RCTs and by experimental studies of selenium and known carcinogens in the development of specific cell lines. Several mechanisms have been postulated to explain the chemopreventive effect of selenium, including protection against oxidative damage, alterations to immune and metabolic systems, alterations to carcinogen metabolism, production of cytotoxic selenium metabolites, inhibition of protein synthesis, stabilisation of genetic material facilitating DNA repair by activation of p53, inhibition of nuclear factor-kappa B (NF-kappa B) and stimulation of apoptosis (Christensen et al 2007, Chun et al 2006, Clark et al 1996, El Bayoumy 2001, Schrauzer 2000, Seo et al 2002). One study demonstrated that combining vitamin E succinate and methylselenic acid produces a synergistic effect on cell growth suppression, primarily mediated by augmenting apoptosis (Zu & Ip 2003).

In humans, the chemopreventive effect is strongest for individuals with the lowest selenium status; however, it is still unclear whether low selenium status is implicated in the aetiology of cancer or whether it produces a state of increased susceptibility to the effects of carcinogens.

Immunomodulation

Confirmed in both animal studies and human trials, immunomodulation is in part due to improved activation and proliferation of B-lymphocytes and enhanced T-cell function (Gazdik et al 2002a, 2002b, Hawkes et al 2001, Kiremidjian-Schumacher & Roy 1998, Ongele et al 2002). A role for selenoprotein S in immune response has been proposed, with a study observing dose-dependent increased expression following influenza vaccine in selenium-supplemented adults (Goldson et al 2011). Interestingly, selenium concentrations significantly decrease during stages of acute infection, suggesting increased use and/or excretion or decreased absorption during this period (Sammalkorpi et al 1988).

Thyroid hormone modulation

Selenium is required for normal thyroid hormone synthesis, activation and metabolism (Sher 2001). Three different selenium-dependent iodothyronine deiodinases (types I, II, and III) can both activate and inactivate thyroid hormone, making selenium an essential element for normal development, growth and metabolism through the regulation of thyroid hormones. However, it should be noted that selenium supplementation across a number of studies has been found to have no effect on thyroid hormone concentrations (Combs et al 2009, Hawkes et al 2008, Thomson et al 2011). In a randomised controlled trial of elderly UK residents (n = 501), supplementation with selenium (100–300 mcg/day) did not have any significant effects on thyroid function despite significant increases in plasma selenium concentration (Rayman et al 2008). A small, statistically significant increase in T3 was observed in males; however, this did not correlate with a corresponding decrease in thyroid stimulating hormone, thus the clinical relevance on this increase in questionable (Combs et al 2009).

OTHER ACTIONS

Male fertility

Reduced selenium levels have been observed in infertile males, regardless of inflammatory status, which in turn has been associated with reduced percentage of normal sperm (Türk et al 2013). Selenium is required for testosterone synthesis, normal sperm maturation and sperm motility (Rayman & Rayman 2002). Two clinical studies have confirmed this association (Scott et al 1998, Vezina et al 1996) and identified selenium supplements as able to increase sperm motility. The effect of selenium in spermatogenesis may be due to several mechanisms, including the activity of the selenium-dependent enzyme phospholipid hydroperoxide glutathione peroxidase (GPX4) (Flohe 2007), altering oxidative stress-mediated apoptosis in germ cells (Kaushal & Bansal 2007a, 2007b), and the modulation of transcription factor NF-kappaB (Shalini & Bansal 2006, 2007a). Interestingly, animal studies suggest that detrimental effects on fertility are associated with either too little or excessive selenium intake (Shalini & Bansal 2007b, 2008).

Anti-inflammatory

Selenium deficiency produces a significantly increased COX-2 protein expression, as well as higher PGE_2 levels, according to one in vitro study

(Zamamiri-Davis et al 2002). It has also been theorised that selenium may decrease leukotriene production (McCarty 1984). In vivo tests have identified anti-inflammatory activity in the lung with selenium, which is thought to relate to an increase in glutathione levels and immune parameters (Jeong et al 2002).

Reduces heavy metal toxicity

Selenium protects against toxicity of some heavy metals, such as cadmium, arsenic, lead, silver and mercury (Berry & Galle 1994, Bolkent et al 2008, Chuang et al 2007, El-Sharaky et al 2007, El-Shenawy & Hassan 2008, Li et al 2012, Lindh et al 1996, Navarro-Alarcon & Lopez-Martinez 2000, Yiin et al 1999a, 1999b, 2000, 2001). A physiological role for selenium in counteracting heavy metal poisoning has been proposed (Shils et al 2006). It appears that the form of selenium is important, as inorganic selenium has been shown to enhance the toxic effects of inorganic arsenic by increasing its retention in tissues and suppressing its metabolism in vitro (Styblo & Thomas 2001).

Antiatherogenic activity

Selenium supplementation reduces high-fat diet-induced atherosclerosis, according to an in vivo study (Kang et al 2001). In healthy subjects fed a test meal high in lipid hydroperoxides, selenium supplementation counteracted the postprandial synthesis of the atherogenic form of LDL (Natella et al 2007). By contrast, no association between toenail selenium and markers of subclinical atherosclerosis were found in a longitudinal study over an 18-year period (n = 3112) (Xun et al 2010).

According to studies with experimental models, beneficial effects on lipid metabolism are due to significant up-regulation of LDL receptor activity and mRNA expression (Dhingra & Bansal 2006a), and down-regulation of hypercholesterolaemia-induced changes in apolipoprotein B (apoB) and 3-hydroxy 3-methylglutaryl coenzyme A (HMG-CoA) reductase expression during experimental hypercholesterolaemia (Dhingra & Bansal 2006b).

Bone health

In healthy, euthyroid postmenopausal women, increased plasma selenium levels and selenoprotein P was associated with increased bone mineral density and reduced bone turnover (Hoeg et al 2012).

CLINICAL USE

Deficiency states: prevention and treatment

Traditionally, selenium supplementation has been used to treat deficiency or prevent deficiency in conditions such as malabsorption syndromes. In addition, the elderly are at increased risk of selenium deficiency. Poor levels are negatively associated with subjective indicators of quality of life (QOL) in older people, such as self-perceived health, chewing ability, physical activity (Gonzalez et al 2007), muscle strength (Beck et al 2007, Lauretani et al 2007) and cognitive function (Akbaraly et al 2007, Gao et al 2007). Supplementation in this population where deficiency has been demonstrated is warranted.

Cancer: prevention and possible adjunct to treatment

The first suggestion of a correlation between low selenium intake and increased cancer incidence arose in the 1970s, an observation which has been supported over time. However, it appears that selenium alone is not the only factor responsible for the protective effect. As such, it is not surprising that a recent Cochrane review determined that no reliable conclusions can be drawn regarding low selenium exposure and increased risk of cancer (Dennert et al 2011). The authors recommend that in many cases, results from available trials should be interpreted cautiously due to potential for confounding, bias and limited heterogeneity.

Chemoprevention

Collectively, evidence available from a range of human, animal and cell-based studies supports a protective role for selenium against the development of cancer; however, results are not always consistent. Further research is required to better determine characteristics of responders, optimal dosage and dose forms. Populations who live in low-selenium environments and have low selenium intakes tend to have higher cancer mortality rates. However, the results from epidemiological studies have been less consistent and show that the effect may be strongest in males.

Total cancer incidence and mortality

In a follow-up to the Linxian General Population Nutrition Intervention Trial, patients who received selenium in combination with vitamin E and beta-carotene had a lower overall mortality (HR 0.95, 95% CI 0.91–0.99) than placebo 10 years after the end of active intervention (Qiao et al 2009).

Several large-scale studies, including the Nutritional Prevention of Cancer (NPC) Trial and the Third National Health and Nutrition Examination Survey (NHANES III), have found that 200 mcg/day selenium is associated with reduced total cancer incidence and cancer mortality (Bleys et al 2008, Clark et al 1998, Reid et al 2008). Specifically, the NPC trial was a large multi-centre, double-blind randomised controlled trial (RCT) (n = 1312) of patients with a history of basal cell or squamous cell carcinoma which investigated the effects of 200 mcg/day selenium (as 500 mg brewer's yeast). Findings from this study suggest that while supplementation in this population did not alter future incidence of skin cancer, it significantly reduced total cancer mortality, total cancer incidence by 37% and the incidences of lung, colorectal and prostate cancers by 46%, 58% and 63%, respectively (Clark et al 1998). Further studies on this population suggest the protective effect of selenium may be restricted to people with low baseline plasma levels, and most pronounced for colorectal cancer and current smokers, whereas protective effects in prostate cancer were further restricted to lower baseline levels of prostate-specific antigen (PSA: ≤4 ng/mL) (Duffield-Lillico et al 2002, 2003, Reid et al 2002, 2006). Although 200 mcg/day selenium was associated with a lowered cancer incidence of 25%, this protective effect was not seen when a double dose was used (Reid et al 2008). At the 12-year follow-up of the NHANES III trial, both all-cause and cancer mortality were found to be reduced with increasing serum selenium levels up to <130 ng/mL, but a gradual increase in mortality was seen at higher levels exceeding 150 ng/mL (Bleys et al 2008).

Liver cancer

A trial involving 130,471 individuals living in a high-risk area for viral hepatitis and liver cancer (Quidong, China) found that table salt enriched with sodium selenite reduced the incidence of liver cancer by 35% during the 8-year follow-up period, whereas no changes were observed for the control groups (Yu et al 1997). Additionally, incidences of liver cancer began to rise after withdrawal of selenium supplementation. Patients with hepatocellular carcinoma had significantly lower serum selenium levels (along with iron, copper, and zinc) compared to those in the control group. The researchers speculated that lower levels of these minerals may act as biomarkers of the increased severity of viral hepatic damage (Lin et al 2006).

Prostate cancer

While much epidemiological and clinical data suggest that selenium may prevent prostate cancer, not all studies have shown a protective effect.

The Selenium and Vitamin E Cancer Prevention Trial (SELECT) (n = 35,533) determined that selenium (200 mcg/day) with or without concomitant vitamin E supplementation did not prevent prostate cancer among healthy men over age 50 (Se without vitamin E HR 1.09; Se with vitamin E HR 1.05) (Klein et al 2011). Secondary analyses corroborated these primary findings (Se without vitamin E HR 1.04; Se with vitamin E HR 1.05) (Lippman et al 2009). Similarly, among participants in the Prostate Cancer Prevention trial, secondary analysis found no association between selenium, either through dietary intake or supplementation, and risk of prostate cancer (Kristal et al 2010). A recent phase III randomised, double-blinded, placebo-controlled trial found that compared to placebo, selenium supplementation had no effect on incidence of prostate cancer in men (n = 699) who were at high risk of the disease (200 mcg/day HR 0.94; 400 mcg/day HR 0.90) (Algotar et al 2013).

Peters et al (2007) observed that there was no inverse association between prediagnostic serum selenium concentration and the risk of prostate cancer in a large cohort study with 724 cases and 879 matched controls. However, higher serum selenium levels may reduce prostate cancer risk in men who reported a high intake of vitamin E, in multivitamin users and in smokers (Peters et al 2007). Another prospective cohort study, the Vitamins And Lifestyle (VITAL) study, investigated the association of vitamin E and selenium supplementation with prostate cancer. No association was found between long-term selenium supplementation (average of 10 years) and prostate cancer risk, with an average intake of >50 microgram/day compared to non-users. Supplementation for longer than an average of 10 years, however, was associated with a statistically non-significant reduction in prostate cancer among older men (≥ 70 years) (Peters et al 2008).

Selenium supplementation has been found to have no significant effect on prostate cancer in a number of populations, men with localised non-metastatic prostate cancer not receiving active treatment (Stratton et al 2010), men with high-grade prostatic intraepithelial neoplasia (HGPIN) (Fleshner et al 2011, Marshall et al 2011). Subset analysis of the study by Marshall and colleagues (2011) found a non-significant reduced risk in men receiving selenium verses placebo in the lowest quartile of baseline plasma selenium, suggesting that future studies on this population alone may be of benefit.

By contrast, a large case-control study involved 33,737 males and identified an association between higher selenium status and a reduced risk of prostate cancer (Yoshizawa et al 1998). The study showed that men consuming the most dietary selenium (assessed indirectly by measuring toenail selenium levels) developed 65% fewer cases of advanced prostate cancer than those with the lowest intake.

Strong evidence for a protective effect of selenium against prostate cancer comes from the Nutritional Prevention of Cancer (NPC) trial, as described above, in which the incidence of prostate cancer was reduced in the selenium group by two-thirds as compared to placebo. Further follow-up has revealed that selenium supplementation continues to show a marked reduction on the incidence of prostate cancer with strongest effects seen in men with a PSA <4 ng/mL and those with the lowest serum selenium levels at study entry (Duffield-Lillico et al 2003). It is interesting to note that the NPC trial was conducted in an area with low soil selenium content, and this may in part explain the conflicting results in studies conducted in various countries around the world.

A meta-analysis of 20 epidemiological studies found an inverse association between selenium levels (assessed in studies by serum, plasma and toenail) and risk of prostate cancer (Brinkman et al 2006). This supports the findings of an earlier meta-analysis of 16 studies (Etminan et al 2005). Similarly, in a prospective, case-control study (n = 130), men with newly diagnosed prostate cancer had significantly lower serum selenium compared to healthy controls (66.3 microgram/L versus 77.5 microgram/L, respectively). An increase of 10 microgram/L in serum selenium concentration was associated with a significant decrease in risk of prostate cancer (Pourmand et al 2008).

Stomach and oesophageal cancers

A Cochrane review of five trials found that selenium appears to show significant beneficial effects against gastrointestinal cancer incidence (RR 0.59); however, four of these had a high risk of bias, therefore further RCTs are warranted (Bjelakovic et al 2008).

A large study of nearly 30,000 people demonstrated a protective effect for a combination of selenium, beta-carotene and vitamin E against the development of cancer of the gastric cardia and oesophagus (Mark et al 2000). Supplementation also reduced the cancer mortality rate compared with those not receiving supplementation. Protective effects on total cancer deaths developed slowly, appearing after 1 year of treatment, and the effect on stomach cancer appeared after 2 years. Gene–selenium interactions may influence an individual's susceptibility to oesophageal cancer. Individuals with polymorphisms in aldehyde dehydrogenase-2 Lys/Lys, X-ray repair cross-complementing 1399 Gln/Gln or Gln/Arg alleles, glutathione S-transferase isoenzyme Ile/Ile genotype or p53 (tumour suppressor gene) Pro/Pro genotype who consumed a low-selenium diet were at the greater risk of oesophageal squamous cell carcinoma, especially when combined with tobacco and alcohol intake (Cai et al 2006a, 2006b).

The protective role of selenium on gastric cancer risk may occur only in those with low baseline selenium. In a study where the levels of selenium were relatively high in both cases and controls, the lowest risk of gastric cancer was found in those with the lowest quartile of selenium level (assessed by toenail levels), whereas those with the highest risk were in the second highest quartile (Koriyama et al 2008).

Colorectal cancer

The incidence of colorectal adenomas, the precursor to most colorectal cancers, may be reduced by selenium. An inverse association between selenium and adenomas has been found in numerous studies, particularly among smokers and those with low baseline serum or plasma selenium (Clark et al 1993, Connelly-Frost et al 2006, Fernandez-Banares et al 2002, Jacobs et al 2004, Peters et al 2006, Reid et al 2006, Russo et al 1997). However, others have reported no association in risk (Early et al 2002, Wallace et al 2003). Compared to age-matched healthy controls, patients with colorectal cancer were found to have statistically lower serum selenium levels. Furthermore, a higher level of selenium was present in the cancerous tissue than in healthy tissue, though it is unclear whether this is the reason for the decreased selenium in the serum or whether the decreased serum levels occur prior to the development of colorectal cancer (Charalabopoulos et al 2006).

Premalignant skin lesions

Increased selenium status may reduce the incidence of arsenic-related premalignant skin lesions (Chen et al 2007, Huang et al 2008). This is consistent with several observational studies that found a protective association between plasma selenium level and the risk of non-melanoma skin cancer (Breslow et al 1995, Clark et al 1984, Karagas et al 1997). Long-term selenium supplementation may exert a protective effect against arsenic-induced premalignant skin lesions by reversing some of the changes in gene expression (Kibriya et al 2007).

Female reproductive

Selenium status measured by plasma levels and erythrocyte glutathione peroxidase activity was significantly lower in patients with cancer or benign neoplasia of the reproductive tract (uterus or ovary). Furthermore, examination of tissue margins of the tumours following surgery revealed significantly higher selenium concentrations compared to healthy tissue margins of healthy tissue. This suggests a protective role of selenium in the development of these reproductive tumours and a compensatory up-regulation of antioxidant defence systems in tumours due to persistent oxidative stress (Piekutowski et al 2007).

Oral cancer

Selenium levels are significantly associated with risk of oral squamous cell carcinoma, with lower levels found in patients compared to both healthy controls and those with precancerous lesions (oral submucous fibrosis and oral leucoplakia) (Khanna & Karjodkar 2006).

Lymphoma

In combination with chemotherapy, supplementation of selenium (as sodium selenite, 0.2 mg/kg/day) was found to have a synergistic effect, as observed through increased percentage of apoptotic lymphoma cells, reduced cervical and axillary lymphadenopathy, decreased splenic size and decreased bone marrow infiltration (Asfour et al 2009). This suggests that selenium may be a useful adjunct treatment in patients with non-Hodgkin's lymphoma; however, further studies are required with increased sample size and power to fully determine the effect of selenium supplementation.

Lung cancer

A randomised, double-blind, placebo-controlled, phase III trial, which looked at selenium supplementation in patients with resected stage I non-small-cell lung cancer found that while selenium (200 mcg/day for 48 months) was safe and well tolerated, it did not provide any significant benefit over placebo in the prevention of secondary primary tumours (Karp et al 2013).

Reducing radiotherapy-related adverse effects

In a multicentre, phase III clinical trial, selenium supplementation during radiotherapy for cerival and uterine cancers was found to be effective to reduce frequency and severity of radiotherapy-induced diarrhea in cervical and uterine cancers (Muecke et al 2010, 2013).

Reducing mortality from HIV infection

Selenium appears to be important in HIV infection, with plasma selenium a strong predictor of disease outcome in both adults and children (Baum & Shor-Posner 1998, Baum et al 1997, Campa et al 1999).

Low selenium status is common in HIV-positive patients and associated with a decline in Th (CD4) cell counts (Bates 2005). Low selenium is also associated with an increased incidence of mycobacterial diseases in HIV-1-seropositive drug users (Dworkin 1994, Dworkin et al 1986, 1989, Shor-Posner et al 2002).

In a double-blind, randomised, placebo-controlled trial, selenium supplementation (200 microgram/day) for 9 months suppressed the progression of HIV-1 viral burden and indirectly improved CD4 counts in adult HIV-infected men and women (Hurwitz et al 2007). One small intervention trial using low-dose selenium supplements (80 microgram/day with 25 mg vitamin E) over 2 months showed an improvement in general symptoms, but no alterations to immunological or haemotological parameters (Cirelli et al 1991).

In antiretroviral therapy-naïve adults, the combination of selenium with multivitamins over 24 months significantly reduced the risk of immune decline and morbidity association with HIV infection; however, neither selenium nor multivitamins alone resulted in any statistically significant changes (Baum et al 2013).

The protective role of selenium in HIV-infected pregnant women is less clear. A 2012 Cochrane review determined that while selenium may improve child survival and reduce maternal diarrhoeal morbidity, it did not delay maternal HIV progression or improve pregnancy outcomes (Siegfried et al 2012).

One study found that low plasma selenium status was associated with increased risk of intrapartum transmission of HIV, risk of fetal and child mortality and the risk of small-for-gestational age (Kupka et al 2005). Selenium supplementation (200 mcg/day) during pregnancy in an RCT was also associated with reduced diarrhoeal morbidity risk by 40% (RR 0.60, 95% CI 0.42–0.84) in HIV-infected women (Kupka et al 2009). By contrast, in a randomised, double-blind, placebo-controlled trial, 200 microgram/day of selenium during and after pregnancy did not improve HIV disease progression, fetal mortality, prematurity or small-for-gestational age birth. Supplementation may, however, improve child survival after 6 weeks (Kupka et al 2008).

Selenium and selenium-dependent glutathione peroxidase (GSH-Px) are important for antioxidant protection and reducing oxidative damage in HIV. Antioxidant defences are increased in selenium-replete HIV patients due to the increase in oxidative stress induced by the infection (Stephensen et al 2007). However, in those with poor selenium levels and subsequently reduced GSH-Px defences, the increased oxidative stress may increase HIV progression (Ogunro et al 2006).

Cardiovascular disease prevention

While a number of epidemiological studies have implicated a role for selenium in reducing cardiovascular disease mortality a recent Cochrane review of 12 RCTs (n = 19,715) found that of the data available, current evidence does not support the use of selenium for the primary prevention of cardiovascular disease (Rees et al 2013). A 2006 meta-analysis found that while analysis of RCTs had suggested there were no significant changes in coronary events following selenium supplementation, when analysing observational studies, 11 out of 14 cohort studies and 9 out of 11 case-control studies found an overall positive effect associated with selenium (Flores-Mateo et al 2006). These discrepancies may be due to observational studies, including selenium in combination with other vitamins/minerals, which may have confounded results.

No significant primary preventive effect was seen for selenium supplementation (200 microgram/day) and incidence of cardiovascular disease, myocardial infarction, stroke or all cardiovascular disease mortality in the NPC study (Stranges et al 2006). Lack of association was confirmed when analyses were further stratified by tertiles of baseline plasma selenium concentrations. Selenium has also been found to have no significant effect on endothelial function or pheripheral artery responsiveness in a randomised placebo-controlled trial of healthy men (Hawkes & Laslett 2009).

Many of the studies investigating selenium and cardiovascular disease have been conducted in European countries that have a lower selenium intake compared to countries such as the United States. It is possible that selenium is most effective at preventing cardiovascular disease in areas with intake levels less than those in the United States (Bleys et al 2008). The dose used in studies may also affect findings, with Bleys et al (2008) identifying that serum selenium levels below 120 ng/mL were associated with reduced cardiovascular and coronary heart disease mortality, while levels above this showed no statistically significant effect (Bleys et al 2008). It has been suggested that low selenium status may contribute to the development of hypertension. In a cross-sectional longitudinal study involving 710 Flemish subjects with an average baseline blood pressure of 130/77 mmHg, an inverse relationship was found between blood selenium and blood pressure in men at follow-up (median of 5.2 years). A 20-microgram/L higher baseline blood selenium concentration was associated with a 37% lower risk of developing high-normal BP or hypertension. No association was found in women (Nawrot et al 2007).

In non-Hodgkin's lymphoma patients receiving selenium supplementation as an adjunct to chemotherapy, supplementation prevented reductions in cardiac ejection fractions seen in patients who received chemotherapy alone, suggesting a possible cardioprotective effect (Asfour et al 2009).

Dyslipidaemia

Randomised, placebo-controlled, parallel-group study (n = 501) identified that selenium supplementation (100–300 mcg/day) had a beneficial effect on lipid profile in persons aged 60–74 years. Reductions at all doses were seen for total cholesterol and non-HDL cholesterol; however, improvement was seen at 300 mcg/day selenium only in HDL cholesterol (Rayman et al 2011).

Compared to premenopausal women, postmenopausal women had lower erythrocyte selenium levels, which were associated with significantly higher levels of total cholesterol, triglycerides and LDL cholesterol. This association remained after controlling for age, smoking status and body mass index (Karita et al 2008). Further studies with increased sample size and across a wider age range is recommended.

Diabetes

The relationship between selenium and diabetes is complex. It has been proposed that the association between selenium and cardiometabolic outcomes is U-shaped, with potential harm possible outside of the physiological range (Rayman & Stranges 2013, Zhou et al 2013). Inconsistent evidence available for selenium and its role in diabetes may be a result of differences in biomarker specificity, variability between trial subjects in baseline selenium status as well as inherent variations between population, age or racial groups (Rayman & Stranges 2013).

Selenium and selenoproteins appears to be involved in several key aspects of pancreatic beta-cell and islet function, increasing insulin content and secretion (Campbell et al 2008). Compared to healthy controls, diabetic patients have been found to have lower selenium levels (assessed by toenail levels) (Rajpathak et al 2005). Supplementation with selenium in diabetic patients has been found to reduce activation of NF-kappa B and levels of oxidative stress, and thus may help to prevent vascular complications (Faure et al 2004). Selenium has also been found to inhibit high glucose- and high insulin-induced expression of adhesion molecule via modulation of p38 pathway, and may therefore help to prevent the development of atherosclerosis in diabetics (Zheng et al 2008).

A randomised, double-blind, placebo-controlled trial (n = 84) determined that selenium supplementation (200 mcg/day) significantly lowered fasting serum insulin levels after 6 weeks, and, in combination with L-arginine (5 g/day), reduced the fasting nitric oxide concentration (Alizadeh et al 2012).

However, some evidence suggests that chronically high selenium levels in selenium-replete populations may increase the risk of developing diabetes. Results from the NHANES III found that those in the highest quintile of serum selenium had a statistically significant increased prevalence of diabetes compared with those in the first quintile (Bleys et al 2007). Similarly, secondary analysis of the NPC trial found that 200 microgram/day of selenium for an average of 7.7 years did not prevent diabetes and statistically significantly increased the risk of type 2 diabetes compared to the placebo group (Stranges et al 2007).

Selenium may play a protective role in gestational diabetes. A cross-sectional study involving 178 pregnant women (24–28 weeks of gestation) found a significant inverse correlation between selenium and blood glucose levels in patients with gestational diabetes mellitus or glucose intolerance having lower serum selenium levels compared to healthy controls (Kilinc et al 2008). This supports similar findings (Al-Saleh et al 2004, 2007, Bo et al 2005, Hawkes et al 2004, Molnar et al 2008, Tan et al 2001).

Adiposity

Associations between selenium and adiposity have been identified through a number of studies. A cross-sectional analysis of the National Diet and Nutrition Survey from the United Kingdom identified an inverse association between plasma selenium and waist circumference, and a positive association between red blood cell waist-to-hip ratio, although causality and underlying mechanisms were not investigated (Spina et al 2013).

Respiratory diseases

Asthma

Despite a number of observational studies suggesting that asthma, respiratory symptoms and ventilatory function may be associated with lowered circulatory selenium status and glutathione peroxidase activity (Devereux & Seaton 2005, Hasselmark et al 1990, Kadrabova et al 1996, Misso et al 1996, Omland et al 2002), a small number of intervention studies have been conducted, producing mixed results (Gazdik et al 2002a, 2002b, Hasselmark et al 1993).

Meta-analysis of data from a case-control study involving 569 asthmatic patients and 576 healthy controls in 14 European centres found no overall effect between plasma selenium levels and the risk of asthma (Burney et al 2008). These results are similar to those from a randomised, double-blind, placebo-controlled trial involving 197 asthmatic subjects given either a selenium supplement (high-selenium yeast preparation of 100 microgram) daily or placebo for 6 months. While the baseline plasma selenium levels increased by 48% in the treatment group, there was no significant difference between the groups with regard to either the primary outcome (asthma-related QOL score) or the secondary outcomes, including lung function, asthma symptom scores, peak flow and bronchodilator usage (Shaheen et al 2007).

A small randomised, double-blind study (n = 24) of patients with intrinsic asthma found that while

100 mcg sodium selenite daily for 14 weeks significantly increased serum selenium and platelet glutathione peroxidase activity, no significant improvements over baseline in any clinical parameters were observed (Hasselmark et al 1993). By contrast, a small pilot study of 17 asthmatics dependent on corticosteroid medication found that a dose of 200 microgram selenium daily taken over a 96-week period reduced both inhaled and systemic corticosteroid requirements. The same study observed selenium supplementation enhancing immunity (Gazdik et al 2002a, 2002b).

Selenium appears to have a protective role in reducing childhood wheezing. Low plasma selenium levels during early pregnancy and in the neonate have been found to increase the risk of early childhood wheezing, although this positive association was no longer found at the age of 5 (Devereux et al 2007). Similarly, in a study of 61 children aged 0.3–5 years with no atopic history, lower serum selenium levels were found in those with frequent wheezing compared with those in healthy controls, and selenium levels were significantly correlated with the number of wheezing episodes experienced in the previous year. This protective effect may be due to preventing the progression of respiratory infections, which subsequently contribute to the development of wheezing (Kocabas et al 2006).

UPPER RESPIRATORY TRACT INFECTION — IN COMBINATION

Echinacea purpurea in combination with selenium, zinc and ascorbic acid, but not *E. purpurea* alone, in chronic obstructive pulmonary disease patients with upper-respiratory tract infection significantly reduced severity and duration of infection compared to placebo. Further studies are warranted to determine the role of selenium within this multiple micronutrient supplementation (Isbaniah et al 2011).

Autoimmune thyroiditis

Selenium appears to play an important role in the health of thyroid gland function and the prevention of disease. In a study of differences in selenium levels between those with thyroid disease and those without, selenium levels were significantly decreased in those with both benign thyroid disease (subacute and silent thyroiditis) and malignant thyroid disease (follicular and papillary thyroid carcinoma) compared to healthy controls (Moncayo et al 2008). Similarly in a study of patients with Graves' disease, those with the highest serum selenium levels (>120 microgram/L) were more likely to be in disease remission (Wertenbruch et al 2007). Following 6 months selenium treatment (100 microgram twice daily), patients with mild Graves' orbitopathy were found to have a slowed disease progression and an increased quality of life compared to placebo in a randomised, controlled, clinical trial (Marcocci et al 2011). These data suggest selenium may be of benefit in those patients with Graves' disease.

Selenium supplementation may improve inflammatory activity in chronic autoimmune thyroiditis patients, as evidenced by a significant reduction in the concentration of thyroid peroxidase antibodies (TPO-Ab) to 63.8% in selenium-supplemented subjects versus 88% (P = 0.95) in placebo subjects (Gartner et al 2002). The randomised study of 70 females (mean age 47.5 years) compared 200 microgram sodium selenium daily orally for 90 days to placebo. A follow-up crossover study of 47 patients from the initial 70 was conducted for a further 6 months (Gartner & Gasnier 2003). The group that continued to take sodium selenite (200 microgram/day) experienced further significant decreases, whereas the group that ceased selenium use experienced a significant increase. The patients who received 200 microgram sodium selenite after placebo also experienced a significant decrease in levels of TPO-Ab.

A recent Cochrane review of four RCTs found that selenium supplementation in Hashimoto's thyroiditis determined that currently there was insufficient evidence to support use of selenium in this disorder (van Zuuren et al 2013). A total of 463 participants across four RCTs (279 selenium treated, 184 controls) were included in the meta-analysis, with duration of treatment ranging from 3 to 18 months. The Cochrane review concluded that there is a need for high-quality RCTs to properly evaluate the effects of selenium in this population, with three currently ongoing studies that may aid in clarifying current evidence.

In a prospective study of 80 patients with Hashimoto's thyroiditis receiving 200 microgram selenium (as selenomethionine) there was a significant 9.9% decrease in TPO-Ab levels after 6 months. In those patients who continued to take the selenium for another 6 months TPO-Ab levels decreased by another 8%, while those who ceased treatment experienced a 4.8% increase (Mazokopakis et al 2007).

Rheumatoid arthritis (RA)

Selenium supplements have been used in RA because of its antioxidant activity and the observation that some patients with RA have been reported with low selenium status (O'Dell et al 1991, Rosenstein & Caldwell 1999). One double-blind, placebo-controlled intervention study of 55 patients with moderate RA found that both placebo and selenium appeared to have significant effects on a number of symptoms; however, only selenium significantly improved arm movements and sense of wellbeing (Peretz et al 2001).

Lowered male fertility

Xu et al (2003) identified a significantly positive correlation between selenium levels and sperm density, sperm number, sperm motility and sperm viability in human volunteers. Similarly, Akinloye et al (2005) reported a significant inverse correlation between serum selenium level and sperm count and serum testosterone, and seminal plasma selenium with spermatozoa motility, viability and morphology (Akinloye et al 2005). Supplementation with selenium in selenium-replete subfertile men has been shown to improve sperm motility and the chance of successful conception in over half the treated patients (Scott et al 1998). When taken with vitamin E over 6 months, selenium produces a statistically significant increase in sperm motility, per cent live and per cent normal spermatozoa, with effects reversing after supplement cessation (Vezina et al 1996). Although results are encouraging, particularly for subfertile men with low selenium status, some studies have found no effect of selenium supplementation (Hawkes et al 2009, Iwanier & Zachara 1995).

General immune enhancement

Several intervention trials of either double-blind or open design have shown that selenium supplementation can enhance immune function and decrease the risk of developing certain infections in selenium-replete subjects, healthy adults and the elderly (Girodon et al 1999, Kiremidjian-Schumacher et al 1994, Roy et al 1994, Yu et al 1989).

The largest was a 3-year study of 20,847 people that showed substituting conventional table salt with table salt fortified with sodium selenite significantly reduced the incidence of viral hepatitis compared with controls provided with normal table salt (Yu et al 1989).

Critically ill patients

Selenoproteins play an important role in the immunomodulation of critically ill patients, and low levels of plasma selenium have been associated with increased markers of oxidative stress, risk of organ failure and higher mortality rates. Clinical trials of selenium supplementation in critically ill patients however have produced mixed results. A recent systematic review and meta-analysis found that selenium supplementation (≤500 microgram/day) may be associated with a beneficial effect on 28-day mortality in critically ill patients. However, it should be acknowledged that due to several factors relating to study quality, the authors state that further evaluation is required before routine adjuvant use of selenium is recommended in a clinical setting (Landucci et al 2014).

The long-term effect of selenium on mortality remains unclear. A 2011 RCT (n = 502) found selenium supplementation did not affect the risk of developing a new infection, 6-month mortality, length of stay, days of antibiotic use or modified sepsis-related organ failure assessment (Andrews et al 2011). One possible explanation suggested for negative findings is sodium selenite having a direct pro-oxidant action in these patients (Forceville 2007).

Daily infusion of 1600 microgram Se (as selenite) over 10 days was also found to significantly decrease incidence of hospital-acquired pneumonia, including early ventilator-associated pneumonia, in critically ill patients with SIRS (Manzanares et al 2011).

Mood elevation and reduced anxiety

Considering that low dietary intake of selenium has been linked with greater incidence of anxiety, depression and tiredness, several research groups have investigated whether higher dietary intake or selenium supplementation will elevate mood and/or reduce anxiety. Currently, results are equivocal; however, it appears that selenium-replete individuals are most likely to respond to supplementation, if a response is observed.

A randomised double-blind placebo-controlled trial of primigravida women (n = 166) found that 100 microgram/day selenium supplementation was associated with reduced symptoms of depression compared to those receiving placebo in the 8 weeks following delivery (Mokhber et al 2011).

Simiarly, an early double-blind, crossover study showed that short-term selenium supplementation (100 microgram/day for 5 weeks) significantly elevated mood and decreased anxiety, depression and tiredness, with effects most marked in people with low dietary intake (Benton & Cook 1991). A study of 30 selenium-replete men who were fed either a low (32.6 microgram/day) or a high (226.5 microgram/day) selenium diet for 15 weeks found that the mood of those with the higher selenium intake improved, whereas mood worsened with low intake (Finley & Penland 1998 as reported in Rayman 2005). Alternatively, another study involving 11 men of adequate selenium intake failed to show effects on mood when high (356 microgram/day) and low (13 microgram/day) selenium diets were followed for 99 days (Hawkes & Hornbostel 1996). Similarly, a large (n = 448) 2-year randomised study also failed to find evidence that additional selenium enhanced mood or any of its subscales, despite significant increases in plasma selenium levels (Rayman et al 2006). This study compared the effects of 100, 200 or 300 microgram/day of selenium to placebo for effects on mood and QOL. Selenium supplementation was given as high-selenium yeast, SelenoPrecise (Pharma Nord, Vejle, Denmark).

Reducing morbidity in preterm babies

Preterm infants are born with slightly lower selenium and glutathione peroxidase concentrations than full-term infants and have low hepatic stores of selenium. In very preterm infants, low selenium concentrations have been associated with an increased risk of chronic neonatal lung disease and retinopathy of prematurity (Darlow & Austin 2003). Although the full consequences of low selenium concentrations in this population are not fully known, observation from animal studies has found an association between selenium deficiency and increased susceptibility to oxidative lung injury. This has special significance for sick, very preterm infants as they are exposed to many possible sources of oxygen radical products, including high concentrations of inspired oxygen. A Cochrane review of three randomised studies that reported outcomes on 297 infants receiving selenium supplements and 290 control infants concluded that selenium supplementation in very preterm infants is associated with benefit in terms of a reduction in one or more episodes of late-onset sepsis, but is not associated with improved survival, a reduction in neonatal chronic lung disease or retinopathy of prematurity (Darlow & Austin 2003). It should be noted that most of the evidence derives from research conducted in New Zealand, a country with low soil and population selenium concentrations, and may not be readily translated to other populations. In one study, despite preterm infants having lower selenium levels compared to term infants, selenium levels did not correlate with chronic lung disease or septicaemia (Loui et al 2008).

OTHER USES

Used in combination with other antioxidants or administered intravenously, selenium has been used in pancreatitis and as adjunctive therapy in cancer patients.

Supplementation of selenium with coenzyme Q10 and vitamin E has been found to improve clinical conditions associated with severe psoriasis, including reduced oxidative stress markers in both plasma and lesional epidermis (Kharaeva et al 2009).

Oral sodium selenite (350 microgram/m^2 body surface area) was given daily for 4–6 weeks to 52 patients with extensive, persistent or progressive lymphoedema from radiation and resulted in the majority experiencing some reduction in oedema (Micke et al 2002). A further study (Micke et al 2003) of 48 patients found that sodium selenite supplementation had a positive effect on secondary lymphoedema caused by radiation therapy alone or by irradiation after surgery. The group consisted of 12 patients with oedema of the arm and 36 with oedema of the head and neck region. Increased dietary intake of selenium over 1 year was found to be positively correlated with capillary recruitment in skin of healthy men ($P = 0.038$), suggesting it may have a role in microvascular function and health (Buss et al 2013). In patients with leukaemia, undergoing allogenic haematopoietic stem cell transplantation, selenium treatment was found to reduce the incidence of oral mucositis, as well as the duration of objective oral mucositis compared to placebo (Jahangard-Rafsanjani et al 2013).

Cancer treatment often induces toxicity associated with the oxidative damage to normal cells. A Cochrane review of selenium in the prevention of side effects associated with cancer treatment (Dennert & Horneber 2006) found only three trials that met inclusion criteria. One study found a lower incidence of recurrent erysipela infections of lymphoedematous upper limbs after breast cancer treatment in the selenium group, with a second study finding reduced facial swelling in selenium-treated patients in a 2-week period following surgical tumour resection. Preliminary results from another study suggest a lower incidence of diarrhoea in those receiving pelvic radiotherapy. On the whole, the authors concluded that there was still insufficient evidence to support selenium supplementation to reduce adverse effects of tumour-specific chemotherapy.

In an animal model, moderate selenium supplementation increased the total antioxidant activity leading to a lower generation of reactive oxygen metabolites, which helped to counteract the cardiotoxicity associated with the chemotherapeutic drug Adriamycin (Danesi et al 2006).

DOSAGE RANGE

The Therapeutic Goods Act altered the allowed amount of selenium in listed products to be raised to 150 microgram. Supplements containing selenium carry the following caution on their label: 'This product contains selenium which is toxic in high doses. A daily dose of 150 microgram for adults of selenium from dietary supplements should not be exceeded.'

Australian RDI

Children

- 1–3 years: 25 microgram
- 4–8 years: 30 microgram
- 9–13 years: 50 microgram

14–18 years

- Boys: 70 microgram
- Girls: 60 microgram

Adults

- Males >18 years: 70 microgram
- Females >18 years: 60 microgram
- Pregnancy: 65 microgram
- Lactation: 75 microgram

According to clinical studies

- Asthma: 100–200 microgram/day of sodium selenite.
- Cancer prophylaxis: 200 microgram/day selenium (supplied as 500 mg brewer's yeast).
- Infertility: 100 microgram/day.
- Mood disturbances: 100 microgram/day.
- Post myocardial infarction: selenium-rich yeast 100 microgram/day.
- Rheumatoid arthritis: 200 microgram/day.
- Autoimmune thyroiditis: 200 microgram/day sodium selenite.
- HIV-positive status: 80 microgram/day has been used but it is most likely that higher doses are required.

TOXICITY

Long-term ingestion of excessive levels of selenium (>1000 microgram/day) may produce fatigue, depression, arthritis, hair or fingernail loss, garlicky breath or body odour and gastrointestinal disorders or irritability (Fan & Kizer 1990). Chronic low-level overexposure has been associated with lethargy, dizziness, motor weakness and paraesthesia (Vinceti et al 2013).

ADVERSE REACTIONS

Nausea, vomiting, nail changes, irritability and fatigue have been reported.

The organic form of selenium found in high-selenium yeast is often preferred because it is less toxic.

The National Health and Medical Research Council of Australia states that selenium intake should not exceed 600 microgram/day.

SIGNIFICANT INTERACTIONS

Cisplatin

Selenium may reduce associated nephrotoxicity, myeloid suppression and weight loss, according to in vitro and in vivo tests (Camargo et al 2001, Ohkawa et al 1988) — potentially beneficial interaction.

Heavy metals (e.g. mercury, lead, arsenic, silver and cadmium)

Selenium reduces toxicity of heavy metals such as mercury, lead, arsenic, silver and cadmium by forming inert complexes — beneficial interaction.

Practice points/Patient counselling

- Selenium is a trace element that is essential for health.
- Low selenium states have been associated with a variety of conditions, such as cardiovascular disease, cancer, asthma, atopy, male subfertility, rheumatoid arthritis, depression and anxiety and compromised immune function.
- High-intensity sports training has been associated with a reduction in plasma selenium levels (Wang et al 2012).
- Studies have identified selenium deficiency in a significant number of people with the HIV infection and suggested a link between selenium levels and mortality rate.
- It is also involved in the detoxification of some heavy metals and xenobiotics.
- Selenium-enriched yeast is the safest way to supplement the diet, but other forms are also used.

CONTRAINDICATIONS AND PRECAUTIONS

Sensitivity to selenium.

PREGNANCY USE

Considered safe in usual dietary doses; safety at higher levels is unknown.

PATIENTS' FAQs

What will this supplement do for me?

Adequate selenium intake, and in some cases supplementation may reduce the risk of developing certain cancers and heart disease and help to improve a range of conditions such as rheumatoid arthritis, asthma, autoimmune thyroiditis, male subfertility, depression and anxiety.

When will it start to work?

If a protective effect is to occur with selenium against cancer or cardiovascular disease, the effect appears to develop slowly over several years' consistent intake.

Are there any safety issues?

High intakes of selenium above 1000 microgram/day have been associated with a number of adverse effects and should be avoided.

REFERENCES

Akbaraly TN et al. Plasma selenium over time and cognitive decline in the elderly. Epidemiology 18.1 (2007): 52–58.

Akinloye O et al. Selenium status of idiopathic infertile Nigerian males. Biol Trace Elem Res 104.1 (2005): 9–18.

Al-Saleh E et al. Maternal-fetal status of copper, iron, molybdenum, selenium and zinc in patients with gestational diabetes. J Matern Fetal Neonatal Med 16.1 (2004): 15–21.

Al-Saleh E et al. Maternal-foetal status of copper, iron, molybdenum, selenium and zinc in obese gestational diabetic pregnancies. Acta Diabetol 44.3 (2007): 106–113.

Algotar AM et al. Phase 3 clinical trial investigating the effect of selenium supplementation in men at high-risk for prostate cancer. Prostate 73.3 (2013): 328–335.

Alizadeh M et al. Effect of L-arginine and selenium added to a hypocaloric diet enriched with legumes on cardiovascular disease risk factors in women with central obesity: a randomized, double-blind, placebo-controlled trial. Ann Nutr Metab 60.2 (2012): 157–168.

Andrews PJ et al. Randomised trial of glutamine, selenium, or both, to supplement parenteral nutrition for critically ill patients. BMJ 342 (2011): d1542.

Asfour IA et al. High-dose sodium selenite can induce apoptosis of lymphoma cells in adult patients with non-Hodgkin's lymphoma. Biol Trace Elem Res 127.3 (2009): 200–210.

Bates CJ. Selenium. In: Benjamin C (ed), Encyclopedia of human nutrition., Oxford: Elsevier, 2005, pp. 118–125.

Baum MK, Shor-Posner G. Micronutrient status in relationship to mortality in HIV-1 disease. Nutr Rev 56.1 (1998): S135–S139.

Baum MK et al. Effect of micronutrient supplementation on disease progression in asymptomatic, antiretroviral-naive, HIV-infected adults in Botswana: a randomized clinical trial. JAMA 310.20 (2013): 2154–2163.

Baum MK et al. High risk of HIV-related mortality is associated with selenium deficiency. J Acquir Immune Defic Syndr Hum Retrovirol 15.5 (1997): 370–374.

Beck J et al. Low serum selenium concentrations are associated with poor grip strength among older women living in the community. Biofactors 29.1 (2007): 37–44.

Benton D, Cook R. The impact of selenium supplementation on mood. Biol Psychiatry 29.11 (1991): 1092–1098.

Berry JP, Galle P. Selenium-arsenic interaction in renal cells: role of lysosomes. Electron microprobe study. J Submicrosc Cytol Pathol 26.2 (1994): 203–210.

Bjelakovic G et al. Antioxidant supplements for preventing gastrointestinal cancers. Coch DB Syst Rev 2008 (2008): CD004183.

Bleys J, Navas-Acien A, Guallar E. Serum selenium and diabetes in U.S. adults. Diabetes Care 30.4 (2007): 829–834.

Bleys J et al. Serum selenium levels and all-cause, cancer, and cardiovascular mortality among US adults. Arch Intern Med 168.4 (2008): 404–410.

Bo S et al. Gestational hyperglycemia, zinc, selenium, and antioxidant vitamins. Nutrition 21.2 (2005): 186–191.

Bolkent S et al. Effects of vitamin E, vitamin C, and selenium on gastric fundus in cadmium toxicity in male rats. Int J Toxicol 27.2 (2008): 217–222.

Breslow RA et al. Serological precursors of cancer: malignant melanoma, basal and squamous cell skin cancer, and prediagnostic levels of retinol, beta-carotene, lycopene, alpha-tocopherol, and selenium. Cancer Epidemiol Biomarkers Prev 4.8 (1995): 837–842.

Brinkman M et al. Are men with low selenium levels at increased risk of prostate cancer? Eur J Cancer 42.15 (2006): 2463–2471.
Burney P et al. A case-control study of the relation between plasma selenium and asthma in European populations: a GAL2EN project. Allergy 63.7 (2008): 865–871.
Buss C et al. Long-term dietary intake of selenium, calcium, and dairy products is associated with improved capillary recruitment in healthy young men. Eur J Nutr 52.3 (2013): 1099–1105.
Cai L et al. Dietary selenium intake, aldehyde dehydrogenase-2 and X-ray repair cross-complementing 1 genetic polymorphisms, and the risk of esophageal squamous cell carcinoma. Cancer 106.11 (2006a): 2345–2354.
Cai L et al. Dietary selenium intake and genetic polymorphisms of the GSTP1 and p53 genes on the risk of esophageal squamous cell carcinoma. Cancer Epidemiol Biomarkers Prev 15.2 (2006b): 294–300.
Camargo SM et al. Oral administration of sodium selenite minimizes cisplatin toxicity on proximal tubules of rats. Biol Trace Elem Res 83.3 (2001): 251–262.
Campa A et al. Mortality risk in selenium-deficient HIV-positive children. J Acquir Immune Defic Syndr Hum Retrovirol 20.5 (1999): 508–513.
Campbell SC et al. Selenium stimulates pancreatic beta-cell gene expression and enhances islet function. FEBS Lett 582.15 (2008): 2333–2337.
Charalabopoulos K et al. Low selenium levels in serum and increased concentration in neoplastic tissues in patients with colorectal cancer: correlation with serum carcinoembryonic antigen. Scand J Gastroenterol 41.3 (2006): 359–360.
Chen Y et al. A prospective study of blood selenium levels and the risk of arsenic-related premalignant skin lesions. Cancer Epidemiol Biomarkers Prev 16.2 (2007): 207–213.
Christensen MJ et al. High selenium reduces NF-kappaB-regulated gene expression in uninduced human prostate cancer cells. Nutr Cancer 58.2 (2007): 197–204.
Chuang HY et al. A case-control study on the relationship of hearing function and blood concentrations of lead, manganese, arsenic, and selenium. Sci Total Environ 387.1–3 (2007): 79–85.
Chun JY et al. Mechanisms of selenium down-regulation of androgen receptor signaling in prostate cancer. Mol Cancer Ther 5.4 (2006): 913–918.
Cirelli A et al. Serum selenium concentration and disease progress in patients with HIV infection. Clin Biochem 24.2 (1991): 211–214.
Clark LC et al. Decreased incidence of prostate cancer with selenium supplementation: results of a double-blind cancer prevention trial. Br J Urol 81.5 (1998): 730–734.
Clark LC et al. Effects of selenium supplementation for cancer prevention in patients with carcinoma of the skin: a randomized controlled trial (Nutritional Prevention of Cancer Study Group). JAMA 276.24 (1996): 1957–1963.
Clark LC et al. Plasma selenium concentration predicts the prevalence of colorectal adenomatous polyps. Cancer Epidemiol Biomarkers Prev 2.1 (1993): 41–46.
Clark LC et al. Plasma selenium and skin neoplasms: a case-control study. Nutr Cancer 6.1 (1984): 13–21.
Combs GF Jr et al. Effects of selenomethionine supplementation on selenium status and thyroid hormone concentrations in healthy adults. Am J Clin Nutr 89.6 (2009): 1808–1814.
Connelly-Frost A et al. Selenium, apoptosis, and colorectal adenomas. Cancer Epidemiol Biomarkers Prev 15.3 (2006): 486–493.
Danesi F et al. Counteraction of adriamycin-induced oxidative damage in rat heart by selenium dietary supplementation. J Agric Food Chem 54.4 (2006): 1203–1208.
Darlow BA, Austin NC. Selenium supplementation to prevent short-term morbidity in preterm neonates. Cochrane Database Syst Rev 4 (2003): CD003312.
Dennert G et al. Selenium for preventing cancer. Coch DB Syst Rev 5 (2011): CD005195.
Dennert G, Horneber M. Selenium for alleviating the side effects of chemotherapy, radiotherapy and surgery in cancer patients. Cochrane Database Syst Rev 3 (2006): CD005037.
Devereux G et al. Early childhood wheezing symptoms in relation to plasma selenium in pregnant mothers and neonates. Clin Exp Allergy 37.7 (2007): 1000–1008.
Devereux G, Seaton A. Diet as a risk factor for atopy and asthma. J Allergy Clin Immunol 115.6 (2005): 1109–1117.
Dhingra S, Bansal MP. Hypercholesterolemia and LDL receptor mRNA expression: modulation by selenium supplementation. Biometals 19.5 (2006a): 493–501.
Dhingra S, Bansal MP. Modulation of hypercholesterolemia-induced alterations in apolipoprotein B and HMG-CoA reductase expression by selenium supplementation. Chem Biol Interact 161.1 (2006b): 49–56.
Duffield-Lillico AJ et al. Selenium supplementation, baseline plasma selenium status and incidence of prostate cancer: an analysis of the complete treatment period of the Nutritional Prevention of Cancer Trial. BJU Int 91.7 (2003): 608–612.
Duffield-Lillico AJ et al. Baseline characteristics and the effect of selenium supplementation on cancer incidence in a randomized clinical trial: a summary report of the Nutritional Prevention of Cancer Trial. Cancer Epidemiol Biomarkers Prev 11.7 (2002): 630–639.
Dworkin BM. Selenium deficiency in HIV infection and the acquired immunodeficiency syndrome (AIDS). Chem Biol Interact 91.2–3 (1994): 181–186.
Dworkin BM et al. Reduced cardiac selenium content in the acquired immunodeficiency syndrome. J Parenter Enteral Nutr 13.6 (1989): 644–647.
Dworkin BM et al. Selenium deficiency in the acquired immunodeficiency syndrome. J Parenter Enteral Nutr 10.4 (1986): 405–407.
Early DS et al. Selenoprotein levels in patients with colorectal adenomas and cancer. Am J Gastroenterol 97.3 (2002): 745–748.
El Bayoumy K. The protective role of selenium on genetic damage and on cancer. Mutat Res 475.1–2 (2001): 123–139.
El-Sharaky AS et al. Protective role of selenium against renal toxicity induced by cadmium in rats. Toxicology 235.3 (2007): 185–193.
El-Shenawy SM, Hassan NS. Comparative evaluation of the protective effect of selenium and garlic against liver and kidney damage induced by mercury chloride in the rats. Pharmacol Rep 60.2 (2008): 199–208.
Etminan M et al. Intake of selenium in the prevention of prostate cancer: a systematic review and meta-analysis. Cancer Causes Control 16.9 (2005): 1125–1131.
Fan AM, Kizer KW. Selenium: Nutritional, toxicologic, and clinical aspects. West J Med 153.2 (1990): 160–167.
Faure P et al. Selenium supplementation decreases nuclear factor-kappa B activity in peripheral blood mononuclear cells from type 2 diabetic patients. Eur J Clin Invest 34.7 (2004): 475–481.
Fernandez-Banares F et al. Serum selenium and risk of large size colorectal adenomas in a geographical area with a low selenium status. Am J Gastroenterol 97.8 (2002): 2103–2108.
Finley W, Penland JG. Adequacy or deprivation of dietary selenium in healthy men: clinical and psychological findings. J Trace Elem Exp Med 11 (1998): 1–27.
Fleshner NE et al. Progression from high-grade prostatic intraepithelial neoplasia to cancer: a randomized trial of combination vitamin-E, soy, and selenium. J Clin Oncol 29.17 (2011): 2386–2390.
Flohe L. Selenium in mammalian spermiogenesis. Biol Chem 388.10 (2007): 987–995.
Flores-Mateo G et al. Selenium and coronary heart disease: a meta-analysis. Am J Clin Nutr 84.4 (2006): 762–773.
Forceville X. Effects of high doses of selenium, as sodium selenite, in septic shock patients: a placebo-controlled, randomized, double-blind, multi-center phase II study–selenium and sepsis. J Trace Elem Med Biol 21 (Suppl 1) (2007): 62–65.
Gao S et al. Selenium level and cognitive function in rural elderly Chinese. Am J Epidemiol 165.8 (2007): 955–965.
Gartner R et al. Selenium supplementation in patients with autoimmune thyroiditis decreases thyroid peroxidase antibodies concentrations. J Clin Endocrinol Metab 87.4 (2002): 1687–1691.
Gartner R, Gasnier BC. Selenium in the treatment of autoimmune thyroiditis. Biofactors 19.3–4 (2003): 165–170.
Gazdik F et al. The influence of selenium supplementation on the immunity of corticoid-dependent asthmatics. Bratisl Lek Listy 103.1 (2002b): 17–21.
Gazdik F et al. Decreased consumption of corticosteroids after selenium supplementation in corticoid-dependent asthmatics. Bratisl Lek Listy 103.1 (2002a): 22–25.
Girodon F et al. Impact of trace elements and vitamin supplementation on immunity and infections in institutionalized elderly patients: a randomized controlled trial. MIN. VIT. AOX. geriatric network. Arch Intern Med 159.7 (1999): 748–754.
Goldson AJ et al. Effects of selenium supplementation on selenoprotein gene expression and response to influenza vaccine challenge: a randomised controlled trial. PLoS One 6.3 (2011): e14771.
Gonzalez S et al. Life-quality indicators in elderly people are influenced by selenium status. Aging Clin Exp Res 19.1 (2007): 10–15.
Hasselmark L et al. Lowered platelet glutathione peroxidase activity in patients with intrinsic asthma. Allergy 45.7 (1990): 523–527.
Hasselmark L et al. Selenium supplementation in intrinsic asthma. Allergy 48.1 (1993): 30–36.
Hawkes WC, Hornbostel L. Effects of dietary selenium on mood in healthy men living in a metabolic research unit. Biol Psychiatry 39.2 (1996): 121–128.
Hawkes WC, Laslett LJ. Selenium supplementation does not improve vascular responsiveness in healthy North American men. Am J Physiol Heart Circ Physiol 296.2 (2009): H256–262.
Hawkes WC et al. Selenium supplementation does not affect testicular selenium status or semen quality in North American men. J Androl 30.5 (2009): 525–533.

Hawkes WC et al. High-selenium yeast supplementation in free-living North American men: no effect on thyroid hormone metabolism or body composition. J Trace Elem Med Biol 22.2 (2008): 131–142.

Hawkes WC et al. Plasma selenium decrease during pregnancy is associated with glucose intolerance. Biol Trace Elem Res 100.1 (2004): 19–29.

Hawkes WC et al. The effects of dietary selenium on the immune system in healthy men. Biol Trace Elem Res 81.3 (2001): 189–213.

Hendler S, Rorvik D. PDR for nutritional supplements. Montvale NJ: Thomson Healthcare Publishers (2001).

Hoeg A et al. Bone turnover and bone mineral density are independently related to selenium status in healthy euthyroid postmenopausal women. J Clin Endocrinol Metab 97.11 (2012): 4061–4070.

Huang Z et al. Low selenium status affects arsenic metabolites in an arsenic exposed population with skin lesions. Clin Chim Acta 387.1–2 (2008): 139–144.

Hurwitz BE et al. Suppression of human immunodeficiency virus type 1 viral load with selenium supplementation: a randomized controlled trial. Arch Intern Med 167.2 (2007): 148–154.

Isbaniah F et al. Echinacea purpurea along with zinc, selenium and vitamin C to alleviate exacerbations of chronic obstructive pulmonary disease: results from a randomized controlled trial. J Clin Pharm Ther 36.5 (2011): 568–576.

Iwanier K, Zachara BA. Selenium supplementation enhances the element concentration in blood and seminal fluid but does not change the spermatozoal quality characteristics in subfertile men. J Androl 16.5 (1995): 441–447.

Jacobs ET et al. Selenium and colorectal adenoma: results of a pooled analysis. J Natl Cancer Inst 96.22 (2004): 1669–1675.

Jahangard-Rafsanjani Z et al. The efficacy of selenium in prevention of oral mucositis in patients undergoing hematopoietic SCT: a randomized clinical trial. Bone Marrow Transplant 48.6 (2013): 832–836.

Jeong DW et al. Protection of mice from allergen-induced asthma by selenite: prevention of eosinophil infiltration by inhibition of NF-kappa B activation. J Biol Chem 277.20 (2002): 17871–17876.

Kadrabova J et al. Selenium status is decreased in patients with intrinsic asthma. Biol Trace Elem Res 52.3 (1996): 241–248.

Kang BP, Mehta U, Bansal MP. Selenium supplementation protects from high fat diet-induced atherogenesis in rats: role of mitogen stimulated lymphocytes and macrophage NO production. Indian J Exp Biol 39.8 (2001): 793–797.

Karagas MR et al. Risk of squamous cell carcinoma of the skin in relation to plasma selenium, alpha-tocopherol, beta-carotene, and retinol: a nested case-control study. Cancer Epidemiol Biomarkers Prev 6.1 (1997): 25–29.

Karita K et al. Associations of blood selenium and serum lipid levels in Japanese premenopausal and postmenopausal women. Menopause 15.1 (2008): 119–124.

Karp DD et al. Randomized, double-blind, placebo-controlled, phase III chemoprevention trial of selenium supplementation in patients with resected stage I non-small-cell lung cancer: ECOG 5597. J Clin Oncol 31.33 (2013): 4179–4187.

Kaushal N, Bansal MP. Dietary selenium variation-induced oxidative stress modulates CDC2/cyclin B1 expression and apoptosis of germ cells in mice testis. J Nutr Biochem 18.8 (2007a): 553–564.

Kaushal N, Bansal MP. Inhibition of CDC2/Cyclin B1 in response to selenium-induced oxidative stress during spermatogenesis: potential role of Cdc25c and p21. Mol Cell Biochem 298.1–2 (2007b): 139–150.

Khanna SS, Karjodkar FR. Circulating immune complexes and trace elements (Copper, Iron and Selenium) as markers in oral precancer and cancer: a randomised, controlled clinical trial. Head Face Med 2 (2006): 33.

Kharaeva Z et al. Clinical and biochemical effects of coenzyme Q10, vitamin E, and selenium supplementation to psoriasis patients. Nutrition 25.3 (2009): 295–302.

Kibriya MG et al. Changes in gene expression profiles in response to selenium supplementation among individuals with arsenic-induced pre-malignant skin lesions. Toxicol Lett 169.2 (2007): 162–176.

Kilinc M et al. Evaluation of serum selenium levels in Turkish women with gestational diabetes mellitus, glucose intolerants, and normal controls. Biol Trace Elem Res 123.1–3 (2008): 35–40.

Kiremidjian-Schumacher L, Roy M. Selenium and immune function. Z Ernahrungswiss 37 (Suppl 1) (1998): 50–56.

Kiremidjian-Schumacher L et al. Supplementation with selenium and human immune cell functions. II: Effect on cytotoxic lymphocytes and natural killer cells. Biol Trace Elem Res 41.1–2 (1994): 115–127.

Klein EA et al. Vitamin E and the risk of prostate cancer: the Selenium and Vitamin E Cancer Prevention Trial (SELECT). JAMA 306.14 (2011): 1549–1556.

Kocabas CN et al. The relationship between serum selenium levels and frequent wheeze in children. Turk J Pediatr 48.4 (2006): 308–312.

Koriyama C et al. Toenail selenium levels and gastric cancer risk in Cali. Colombia. J Toxicol Sci 33.2 (2008): 227–235.

Kristal AR et al. Diet, supplement use, and prostate cancer risk: results from the prostate cancer prevention trial. Am J Epidemiol 172.5 (2010): 566–577.

Kupka R et al. Effect of Selenium Supplements on Hemoglobin Concentration and Morbidity among HIV-1–Infected Tanzanian Women. Clin Infect Dis 48.10 (2009): 1475–1478.

Kupka R et al. Randomized, double-blind, placebo-controlled trial of selenium supplements among HIV-infected pregnant women in Tanzania: effects on maternal and child outcomes. Am J Clin Nutr 87.6 (2008): 1802–1808.

Kupka R et al. Selenium status, pregnancy outcomes, and mother-to-child transmission of HIV-1. J Acquir Immune Defic Syndr 39.2 (2005): 203–210.

Landucci F et al. Selenium supplementation in critically ill patients: A systematic review and meta-analysis. J Crit Care 29.1 (2014): 150–156.

Lauretani F et al. Association of low plasma selenium concentrations with poor muscle strength in older community-dwelling adults: the InCHIANTI Study. Am J Clin Nutr 86.2 (2007): 347–352.

Li YF et al. Organic selenium supplementation increases mercury excretion and decreases oxidative damage in long-term mercury-exposed residents from Wanshan, China. Environ Sci Technol 46.20 (2012): 11313–11318.

Lin CC et al. Selenium, iron, copper, and zinc levels and copper-to-zinc ratios in serum of patients at different stages of viral hepatic diseases. Biol Trace Elem Res 109.1 (2006): 15–24.

Lindh U, Danersund A, Lindvall A. Selenium protection against toxicity from cadmium and mercury studied at the cellular level. Noisy-le-grand: Cell Mol Biol 42.1 (1996): 39–48.

Lippman SM et al. Effect of selenium and vitamin E on risk of prostate cancer and other cancers: the Selenium and Vitamin E Cancer Prevention Trial (SELECT). JAMA 301.1 (2009): 39–51.

Loui A et al. Selenium status in term and preterm infants during the first months of life. Eur J Clin Nutr 62.3 (2008): 349–355.

Manzanares W et al. High-dose selenium reduces ventilator-associated pneumonia and illness severity in critically ill patients with systemic inflammation. Intensive Care Med 37.7 (2011): 1120–1127.

Marcocci C et al. Selenium and the course of mild Graves' orbitopathy. N Engl J Med 364.20 (2011):1920–1931.

Mark SD et al. Prospective study of serum selenium levels and incident esophageal and gastric cancers. J Natl Cancer Inst 92.21 (2000): 1753–1763.

Marshall JR et al. Phase III trial of selenium to prevent prostate cancer in men with high-grade prostatic intraepithelial neoplasia: SWOG S9917. Cancer Prev Res (Phila) 4.11 (2011): 1761–1769.

Mazokopakis EE et al. Effects of 12 months treatment with L-selenomethionine on serum anti-TPO levels in patients with Hashimoto's thyroiditis. Thyroid 17.7 (2007): 609–612.

McCarty M. Can dietary selenium reduce leukotriene production? Med Hypotheses 13.1 (1984): 45–50.

Micke O et al. Selenium in the treatment of radiation-associated lymphedema. In: Prog Radio-Oncol VII Proc, 2002: 533–546.

Micke O et al. Selenium in the treatment of radiation-associated secondary lymphedema. Int J Radiat Oncol Biol Phys 56.1 (2003): 40–49.

Misso NL et al. Reduced platelet glutathione peroxidase activity and serum selenium concentration in atopic asthmatic patients. Clin Exp Allergy 26.7 (1996): 838–847.

Mokhber N et al. Effect of supplementation with selenium on postpartum depression: a randomized double-blind placebo-controlled trial. J Matern Fetal Neonatal Med 24.1 (2011): 104–108.

Molnar J et al. Serum selenium concentrations correlate significantly with inflammatory biomarker high-sensitive CRP levels in Hungarian gestational diabetic and healthy pregnant women at mid-pregnancy. Biol Trace Elem Res 121.1 (2008): 16–22.

Moncayo R et al. The role of selenium, vitamin C, and zinc in benign thyroid diseases and of selenium in malignant thyroid diseases: Low selenium levels are found in subacute and silent thyroiditis and in papillary and follicular carcinoma. BMC Endocr Disord 8 (2008): 2.

Muecke R et al. Impact of treatment planning target volumen (PTV) size on radiation induced diarrhoea following selenium supplementation in gynecologic radiation oncology — a subgroup analysis of a multicenter, phase III trial. Radiat Oncol 8 (2013): 72.

Muecke R et al. Multicenter, phase 3 trial comparing selenium supplementation with observation in gynecologic radiation oncology. Int J Radiat Oncol Biol Phys 78.3 (2010): 828–835.

Natella F et al. Selenium supplementation prevents the increase in atherogenic electronegative LDL (LDL minus) in the postprandial phase. Nutr Metab Cardiovasc Dis 17.9 (2007): 649–656.

Navarro-Alarcon M, Lopez-Martinez MC. Essentiality of selenium in the human body: relationship with different diseases. Sci Total Environ 249.1–3 (2000): 347–371.

Nawrot TS et al. Blood pressure and blood selenium: a cross-sectional and longitudinal population study. Eur Heart J 28.5 (2007): 628–633.

O'Dell JR et al. Serum selenium concentrations in rheumatoid arthritis. Ann Rheum Dis 50.6 (1991): 376–378.

Ogunro PS et al. Plasma selenium concentration and glutathione peroxidase activity in HIV-1/AIDS infected patients: a correlation with the disease progression. Niger Postgrad Med J 13.1 (2006): 1–5.

Ohkawa K et al. The effects of co-administration of selenium and cis-platin (CDDP) on CDDP-induced toxicity and antitumour activity. Br J Cancer 58.1 (1988): 38–41.

Omland O et al. Selenium serum and urine is associated to mild asthma and atopy: The SUS study. J Trace Elem Med Biol 16.2 (2002): 123–127.

Ongele EA et al. Effects of selenium deficiency in the development of trypanosomes and humoral immune responses in mice infected with Trypanosoma musculi. Parasitol Res 88.6 (2002): 540–545.

Peretz A, Siderova V, Neve J. Selenium supplementation in rheumatoid arthritis investigated in a double blind, placebo-controlled trial. Scand J Rheumatol 30.4 (2001): 208–212.

Peters U et al. Vitamin E and selenium supplementation and risk of prostate cancer in the Vitamins and lifestyle (VITAL) study cohort. Cancer Causes Control 19.1 (2008): 75–87.

Peters U et al. Serum selenium and risk of prostate cancer — a nested case-control study. Am J Clin Nutr 85.1 (2007): 209–217.

Peters U et al. High serum selenium and reduced risk of advanced colorectal adenoma in a colorectal cancer early detection program. Cancer Epidemiol Biomarkers Prev 15.2 (2006): 315–320.

Piekutowski K et al. The antioxidative role of selenium in pathogenesis of cancer of the female reproductive system. Neoplasma 54.5 (2007): 374–378.

Pourmand G et al. Serum selenium level and prostate cancer: a case-control study. Nutr Cancer 60.2 (2008): 171–176.

Procházková D et al. Controlled diet in phenylketonuria and hyperphenylalaninemia may cause serum selenium deficiency in adult patients: the Czech experience. Biol Trace Elem Res 154.2 (2013): 178–184.

Qiao Y-L et al. Total and Cancer Mortality After Supplementation With Vitamins and Minerals: Follow-up of the Linxian General Population Nutrition Intervention Trial. J Natl Cancer Inst 101.7 (2009): 507–518.

Rajpathak S et al. Toenail selenium and cardiovascular disease in men with diabetes. J Am Coll Nutr 24.4 (2005): 250–256.

Rayman MP. Selenium in cancer prevention: a review of the evidence and mechanism of action. Proc Nutr Soc 64.4 (2005): 527–542.

Rayman MP. The importance of selenium to human health. Lancet 356.9225 (2000): 233–241.

Rayman MP, Stranges S. Epidemiology of selenium and type 2 diabetes: Can we make sense of it? Free Radical Bio Med 65 (2013): 1557–1564.

Rayman MP et al. Effect of supplementation with high-selenium yeast on plasma lipids: a randomized trial. Ann Intern Med 154.10 (2011): 656–665.

Rayman MP et al. Randomized controlled trial of the effect of selenium supplementation on thyroid function in the elderly in the United Kingdom. Am J Clin Nutr 87.2 (2008): 370–378.

Rayman M et al. Impact of selenium on mood and quality of life: a randomized, controlled trial. Biol Psychiatry 59.2 (2006): 147–154.

Rayman MP, Rayman MP. The argument for increasing selenium intake. Proc Nutr Soc 61.2 (2002): 203–215.

Rees K et al. Selenium supplementation for the primary prevention of cardiovascular disease. Coch DB Syst Rev 1 (2013): CD009671.

Reid ME et al. Selenium supplementation and colorectal adenomas: an analysis of the nutritional prevention of cancer trial. Int J Cancer 118.7 (2006): 1777–1781.

Reid ME et al. Selenium supplementation and lung cancer incidence: an update of the nutritional prevention of cancer trial. Cancer Epidemiol Biomarkers Prev 11.11 (2002): 1285–1291.

Reid ME et al. The nutritional prevention of cancer: 400 mcg per day selenium treatment. Nutr Cancer 60.2 (2008): 155–163.

Rosenstein ED, Caldwell JR. Trace elements in the treatment of rheumatic conditions. Rheum Dis Clin North Am 25.4 (1999): 929–935: viii.

Roy M et al. Supplementation with selenium and human immune cell functions. I. Effect on lymphocyte proliferation and interleukin 2 receptor expression. Biol Trace Elem Res 41.1–2 (1994): 103–114.

Russo MW et al. Plasma selenium levels and the risk of colorectal adenomas. Nutr Cancer 28.2 (1997): 125–129.

Sammalkorpi K et al. Serum selenium in acute infections. Infection 16.4 (1988): 222–224.

Schrauzer GN. Anticarcinogenic effects of selenium. Cell Mol Life Sci 57.13–14 (2000): 1864–1873.

Scott R et al. The effect of oral selenium supplementation on human sperm motility. Br J Urol 82.1 (1998): 76–80.

Seo YR, Kelley MR, Smith ML. Selenomethionine regulation of p53 by a ref1-dependent redox mechanism. Proc Natl Acad Sci U S A 99.22 (2002): 14548–14553.

Shaheen SO et al. Randomised, double blind, placebo-controlled trial of selenium supplementation in adult asthma. Thorax 62.6 (2007): 483–490.

Shalini S, Bansal MP. Dietary selenium deficiency as well as excess supplementation induces multiple defects in mouse epididymal spermatozoa: understanding the role of selenium in male fertility. Int J Androl 31.4 (2008): 438–449.

Shalini S, Bansal MP. Alterations in selenium status influences reproductive potential of male mice by modulation of transcription factor NFkappaB. Biometals 20.1 (2007a): 49–59.

Shalini S, Bansal MP. Co-operative effect of glutathione depletion and selenium induced oxidative stress on API and NFkB expression in testicular cells in vitro: insights to regulation of spermatogenesis. Biol Res 40.3 (2007b): 307–17.

Shalini S, Bansal MP. Role of selenium in spermatogenesis: differential expression of cjun and cfos in tubular cells of mice testis. Mol Cell Biochem 292.1–2 (2006): 27–38.

Sher L. Role of thyroid hormones in the effects of selenium on mood, behavior, and cognitive function. Med Hypotheses 57.4 (2001): 480–483.

Shils M et al (eds). Modern nutrition in health and disease. Baltimore: Lippincott Williams and Wilkins, 2006. Available at: Clinicians health channel gateway.ut.ovid.com/gw1/ovidweb.cgi (accessed 13-06-06).

Shor-Posner G et al. Impact of selenium status on the pathogenesis of mycobacterial disease in HIV-1-infected drug users during the era of highly active antiretroviral therapy. J Acquir Immune Defic Syndr 29.2 (2002): 169–173.

Siegfried N et al. Micronutrient supplementation in pregnant women with HIV infection. Coch DB Syst Rev 2012 (2012): CD009755.

Spina A et al. Anthropometric indices and selenium status in British adults: The U.K. National Diet and Nutrition Survey. Free Radical Bio Med 65 (2013): 1315–1321.

Stephensen CB et al. Glutathione, glutathione peroxidase, and selenium status in HIV-positive and HIV-negative adolescents and young adults. Am J Clin Nutr 85.1 (2007): 173–181.

Stranges S et al. Effects of long-term selenium supplementation on the incidence of type 2 diabetes: a randomized trial. Ann Intern Med 147.4 (2007): 217–223.

Stranges S et al. Effects of selenium supplementation on cardiovascular disease incidence and mortality: secondary analyses in a randomized clinical trial. Am J Epidemiol 163.8 (2006): 694–699.

Stratton MS et al. Oral selenium supplementation has no effect on prostate-specific antigen velocity in men undergoing active surveillance for localized prostate cancer. Cancer Prev Res (Phila) 3.8 (2010): 1035–1043.

Styblo M, Thomas DJ. Selenium modifies the metabolism and toxicity of arsenic in primary rat hepatocytes. Toxicol Appl Pharmacol 172.1 (2001): 52–61.

Tan M et al. Changes of serum selenium in pregnant women with gestational diabetes mellitus. Biol Trace Elem Res 83.3 (2001): 231–237.

Thomson CD et al. Minimal impact of excess iodate intake on thyroid hormones and selenium status in older New Zealanders. Eur J Endocrinol 165.5 (2011): 745–752.

Tinggi U. Essentiality and toxicity of selenium and its status in Australia: a review. Toxicol Lett 137.1–2 (2003): 103–110.

Türk S et al. Male infertility: Decreased levels of selenium, zinc and antioxidants. J Trace Elem Med Biol (2013) Corrected proof.

van Zuuren EJ et al. Selenium supplementation for Hashimoto's thyroiditis. Coch DB Syst Rev 6 (2013): CD010223.

Vezina D et al. Selenium-vitamin E supplementation in infertile men: Effects on semen parameters and micronutrient levels and distribution. Biol Trace Elem Res 53.1–3 (1996): 65–83.

Vinceti M et al. Selenium neurotoxicity in humans: Bridging laboratory and epidemiologic studies. Toxicol Letters (2013) Corrected proof.

Wallace K et al. Prediagnostic serum selenium concentration and the risk of recurrent colorectal adenoma: a nested case-control study. Cancer Epidemiol Biomarkers Prev 12.5 (2003): 464–467.

Wang L et al. Effects of high-intensity training and resumed training on macroelement and microelement of elite basketball athletes. Bio Trace Elem Res 149.2 (2012): 148–154.

Wertenbruch T et al. Serum selenium levels in patients with remission and relapse of Graves' disease. Med Chem 3.3 (2007): 281–284.

Xu DX et al. The associations among semen quality, oxidative DNA damage in human spermatozoa and concentrations of cadmium, lead and selenium in seminal plasma. Mutat Res 534.1–2 (2003): 155–163.

Xun P et al. Longitudinal association between toenail selenium levels and measures of subclinical atherosclerosis: the CARDIA trace element study. Atherosclerosis 210.2 (2010): 662–667.

Yiin SJ et al. Cadmium-induced liver, heart, and spleen lipid peroxidation in rats and protection by selenium. Biol Trace Elem Res 78.1–3 (2000): 219–230.

Yiin SJ et al. Cadmium induced lipid peroxidation in rat testes and protection by selenium. Biometals 12.4 (1999a): 353–359.

Yiin SJ et al. Cadmium-induced renal lipid peroxidation in rats and protection by selenium. J Toxicol Environ Health A 57.6 (1999b): 403–413.
Yiin SJ et al. Lipid peroxidation in rat adrenal glands after administration cadmium and role of essential metals. J Toxicol Environ Health A 62.1 (2001): 47–56.
Yoshizawa K et al. Study of prediagnostic selenium level in toenails and the risk of advanced prostate cancer. J Natl Cancer Inst 90.16 (1998): 1219–1224.
Yu SY et al. Chemoprevention trial of human hepatitis with selenium supplementation in China. Biol Trace Elem Res 20.1–2 (1989): 15–22.
Yu SY, Zhu YJ, Li WG. Protective role of selenium against hepatitis B virus and primary liver cancer in Qidong. Biol Trace Elem Res 56.1 (1997): 117–124.
Zamamiri-Davis F et al. Nuclear factor-kappaB mediates over-expression of cyclooxygenase-2 during activation of RAW 264.7 macrophages in selenium deficiency. Free Radic Biol Med 32.9 (2002): 890–897.
Zheng HT et al. Selenium inhibits high glucose- and high insulin-induced adhesion molecule expression in vascular endothelial cells. Arch Med Res 39.4 (2008): 373–379.
Zhou J et al. Selenium and diabetes—Evidence from animal studies. Free Radical Biol Med 65 (2013): 1548–1556.
Zu K, Ip C. Synergy between selenium and vitamin E in apoptosis induction is associated with activation of distinctive initiator caspases in human prostate cancer cells. Cancer Res 63.20 (2003): 6988–6995.

Shark cartilage

HISTORICAL NOTE Shark cartilage became a popular supplement in the 1980s, largely based around the claim that sharks rarely get cancer and therefore must have some protection against the disease. By 1995, the annual world market for shark-cartilage products exceeded US$30 million and dozens of shark cartilage products were available in retail stores and usually sold as food supplements (Ernst 1998). Over the past few decades, progress has been made in identifying various naturally occurring molecules in avascular tissue, such as cartilage, which exhibit antiangiogenic properties and could be investigated as treatments in cancer. Shark cartilage is one such tissue and numerous shark cartilage derivatives and extracts have been investigated for effects on tumours, including squalamine lactate, AE-941 and U-995. Previously, much work had been conducted with bovine cartilage, which also exhibits anti-angiogenic properties, although to a lesser extent.

CHEMICAL COMPONENTS

Shark cartilage is mainly composed of proteins, calcium, phosphorus, water, collagen and proteoglycans, chiefly chondroitin sulfates. Collagen imparts tensile strength and proteoglycans impart resilience to cartilage.

MAIN ACTIONS

Analgesic and anti-inflammatory

Both analgesic and anti-inflammatory activities have been reported for shark cartilage preparations in animal studies (Fontenele et al 1996, 1997). The mechanism of action is unknown; however, tests with the opioid antagonist naloxone have found it does not involve the opioid system (Fontenele et al 1997). One mechanism of action suggested is that shark cartilage significantly inhibits IL-1-induced PGE_2 synthesis (Pearson et al 2007).

Suppression of airway inflammation, by downregulating vascular endothelial growth factor, was demonstrated in an animal model, suggesting a possible novel therapeutic application to treat bronchial asthma. This research was carried out with a marine cartilage pharmaceutical formula called Neovastat (AE-941) (Lee et al 2005, Lee & Chung 2007).

There is also research indicating that shark cartilage might be useful for some but not all inflammatory conditions. A number of different commercial shark cartilage extracts were tested and found to induce TH1 type inflammatory cytokines. In addition, the acid extracts of shark cartilage tested produced higher amounts of TNF (alpha) than the other aqueous extracts. As well as stimulating a TH1 response, the cartilage extracts appeared to inhibit TH2 cells, which may be useful for hypersensitive individuals who would benefit from downregulation of the IgE response (Merly et al 2007).

Anti-angiogenic

Neovastat and shark cartilage extract (SCE) are preparations with demonstrated antiangiogenesis activity occurring via multiple mechanisms (Patra & Sandell 2012).

Shark cartilage extract appears to block the two main pathways that contribute to the process of angiogenesis, matrix metalloproteases and the vascular endothelial growth factor signalling pathway (Anon 2004). The effect is due to several different constituents that have been isolated from shark cartilage and identified as exerting anti-angiogenic activity (Bargahi & Rabbani-Chadegani 2008, Dupont et al 1998, Gonzalez et al 2001, Rabbani-Chadegani et al 2008, Shen et al 2001, Sheu et al 1998, Zheng et al 2007) in various experimental models.

Neovastat, a shark cartilage preparation containing a mix of water soluble components, also demonstrates antiangiogenic activity in various models. A concentration-dependent inhibition of cell proliferation in human umbilical vein endothelial and bovine endothelial cells has been observed. It also inhibited angiogenesis induced by basic fibroblast growth factor (FGF) in the chicken chorioallantoic membrane model and also significantly retarded vascularisation of bFGF-containing Matrigel implanted in mice after oral administration (Dupont et al 2002).

Antineoplastic effects

Due to its anti-angiogenic activity, shark cartilage has been investigated for antineoplastic effects. In one study, oral administration of powdered shark cartilage significantly delayed the development of papillary and solid tumours in a murine renal tumour model in experimental animals (Barber et al 2001). Shark cartilage proteoglycan was found to inhibit pancreatic carcinogenesis when administered to hamsters for 50 days (Kitahashi et al 2006). Neovastat has demonstrated activity against lung metastases in the murine Lewis lung carcinoma model and when Neovastat (0.5 mL/day) was used with a suboptimal dose of cisplatin (2 mg/kg, IP) a greater anti-metastatic effect was observed by exerting a protective activity against cisplatin-induced body weight loss and myelosuppression (Dupont et al 2002).

Immunostimulant

Shark cartilage stimulates cellular and humoral immune responses as demonstrated in vitro (Bargahi et al 2011). A complex mixture of constituents is responsible for the immunostimulating properties of shark cartilage, according to in vitro research (Kralovec et al 2003). Of these, a protein fraction composed of two proteins with molecular weights of approximately 14 and 15 kDa have exhibited the most immunostimulatory effects (Hassan et al 2005).

OTHER ACTIONS

Antibiotic

Squalamine, isolated from dogfish shark cartilage, is a broad-spectrum antibiotic with activity against protozoa, fungi and both Gram-positive and Gram-negative bacteria (Moore et al 1993).

Antioxidant

Antioxidant activity has been demonstrated in vitro (Gomes et al 1996).

Fibrinolytic

Fibrinolytic activity of a shark cartilage extract was demonstrated in an in vitro study (Ratel et al 2005).

CLINICAL USE

One of the most studied shark cartilage preparations is known as Neovastat (or AE-941), which is a mix of water-soluble components derived from shark cartilage prepared by a proprietary manufacturing process developed by Aeterna Laboratories (Quebec, Canada). The few studies conducted with shark cartilage preparations have been disappointing from a clinical perspective.

Osteoarthritis

Based on its analgesic and anti-inflammatory activities, shark cartilage has been used to relieve symptoms in osteoarthritis (OA). To date, no clinical studies are available to determine its effectiveness; however, positive results have been obtained in several clinical studies for one of its constituents, chondroitin sulfate (see *Chondroitin* monograph for details).

Cancer

Shark cartilage used to be a popular supplement with cancer patients, although results from the few clinical trials conducted using shark cartilage in people with advanced cancers have generally been disappointing. Several theories have been proposed to explain the lack of correlation between the highly promising in vitro and in vivo studies and the clinical trials conducted to date, mainly calling into question the bioavailability of shark cartilage and the key active constituents responsible for the anti-angiogenic effect (de Mejia & Dia 2010).

One study of 60 people with advanced, previously treated cancer (breast, colorectal, lung, prostate, non-Hodgkin's lymphoma, brain) failed to demonstrate an effect for orally administered shark cartilage (1 g/kg) on tumour growth or QOL (Miller et al 1998). A larger study of 83 patients with advanced breast and colorectal cancers, which was published in 2005, also found that shark cartilage failed to improve survival or QOL (Loprinzi et al 2005). This study was a two-arm, randomised, placebo-controlled, double-blind, clinical trial. Of note, there was a high drop-out rate as only half the patients receiving shark cartilage powder continued with treatment beyond 1 month and only 10% were still using the treatment by 6 months. It was thought that gastrointestinal symptoms may have contributed to the poor patient compliance.

Several smaller preliminary studies have produced positive results, with some patients experiencing less tumour progression and weight loss, improved appetite or decreased pain. Unfortunately, details of these studies are difficult to locate and much remains unanswered, such as doses used, time frames for use and criteria for improvement.

S

Investigation with Neovastat (AE-941), a standardised shark cartilage extract, has produced more promising results and demonstrated inhibitory effects on the growth and metastasis of tumours; however, research has mainly been conducted in animal models (Hassan et al 2005). One clinical study conducted with Neovastat did report a significant survival advantage for the patients with unresectable stage IIIA, IIIB or IV non-small-cell lung cancers receiving treatment (Hassan et al 2005). Similarly, an open-label, multicentre study testing four different strengths of Neovastatin (30, 60, 120, or 240 mL/day) in 80 patients with histologically confirmed lung cancer reported a significant survival advantage for patients receiving doses >2.6 mL/kg/

day (which correspond to approximately 180 mL/day in a 70-kg patient) compared to patients receiving lower doses (median, 6.1 months vs 4.6 months; $P = 0.026$). Interestingly, no tumour response was observed in this study (Latreille et al 2003). The treatment was considered well tolerated and the most common side effects were nausea (9%), pruritus (5%), anorexia (4%), and vomiting (4%).

A Phase II trial tested two different doses of Neovastat (60 or 240 mL/day) given twice daily in patients with solid tumours (renal cell carcinoma) who were refractory to standard treatment (Batist et al 2002). A survival analysis conducted on 22 patients with a primary diagnosis of refractory RCC found a significant relationship between dose and survival; the median survival time was significantly longer (16.3 versus 7.1 months; $P = 0.01$) in patients treated with Neovastat 240 mL/day ($n = 14$) compared with patients receiving 60 mL/day ($n = 8$). The treatment was well tolerated and the most common side effect was taste alteration (14%).

In contrast, a double-blind RCT of patients with breast or colorectal carcinoma considered uncurable but receiving standard care compared a shark cartilage product to placebo given three to four times each day. Data on a total of 83 evaluable patients revealed there were no differences in overall survival between patients groups or in QOL beyond placebo (Loprinzi et al 2005).

More recently in 2010, Lu et al conducted a double blind RCT involving people with unresectable stage III non-small cell lung cancer who were treated with chemoradiotherapy (Lu et al 2010). Unfortunately, the study was unable to recruit a sufficient number of people to meet the sample size target making results difficult to interpret. All volunteers received both chemotherapy (either carboplatin and paclitaxel, or cisplatin and vinorelbine) and chest radiotherapy. Treatment with Neovastatin + standard treatment ($n = 188$) failed to significantly alter overall survival beyond placebo ($n = 191$). Additionally, there were no differences between the groups for time to progression, progression-free survival, and tumour response rates and no protection against toxic effects attributable to chemoradiotherapy.

OTHER USES

There is one case report of a man with Kaposi's sarcoma whose lesion disappeared after taking shark cartilage (3.75–4.5 g/day for 9 months) (Hillman et al 2001).

DOSAGE RANGE

Depending on the purity of the supplement, 500–4500 mg/day in divided doses.

Various doses of cartilage have been used in different studies, ranging from 2.5 mg to 100 g/day (Simone et al 1998).

Practice points/Patient counselling

- Shark cartilage is mainly composed of calcium, phosphorus, water, collagen and proteoglycans, chiefly chondroitin sulfates.
- Anti-angiogenic, antineoplastic, immunostimulant and broad-spectrum antibiotic activities have been reported in preliminary studies.
- Both analgesic and anti-inflammatory activities have been reported for shark cartilage preparations in animal studies, most likely due to its chondroitin content. As a result, it is used to relieve symptoms in arthritic conditions.
- It is a popular supplement among cancer patients; however, the few clinical trials conducted so far with people with advanced cancers have generally produced negative results, suggesting no benefit.
- Its use is contraindicated in people with seafood allergy, and in pregnancy. Do not use 3 weeks before and 6 weeks after surgery, or in children or teenagers still experiencing growth.

Clinical note — Angiogenesis and tumour growth

Angiogenesis is defined as the formation of new capillary blood vessels from existing microvessels and is a process regulated by inducers and inhibitors. It is critical for development, reproduction and repair and dominates many pathological conditions (Folkman 2003). In 1971, the hypothesis that tumour growth is angiogenesis-dependent was first proposed and since then, the study of angiogenesis inhibitors in cancer research has developed. It has now been demonstrated that solid tumours that exceed 1–2 mm in diameter require new blood vessels or angiogenesis to feed their growth (Patra & Sandell 2012). They secrete angiogenic substances to set up an internal network of blood vessels to support further growth and there is a correlation between tumour microvessel density and the risk of metastases. In the absence of angiogenesis, tumour growth is restricted to a microscopic size and tumour cells do not shed into the circulation. Cartilage is an avascular tissue and therefore must contain substances which prevent blood vessel growth, making it a prime target for anti-angiogenesis research.

ADVERSE REACTIONS

The most common side effects reported in clinical trials are: taste alteration (14%), nausea (9%), pruritus (5%), anorexia (4%) and vomiting (4%).

SIGNIFICANT INTERACTIONS

Controlled studies and sufficient reliable information are not available to predict or determine interactions.

CONTRAINDICATIONS AND PRECAUTIONS

Contraindicated in people with seafood allergy.

Do not use 3 weeks before until 6 weeks after surgery, or in children or teenagers still experiencing growth.

Hypercalcaemia: Due to the high calcium content of this supplement, it should be used with caution in people with hypercalcaemia.

PREGNANCY USE

Although not scientifically investigated in this population, it is not recommended in pregnancy or lactation based on theoretical considerations.

PATIENTS' FAQs

What will this supplement do for me?

Shark cartilage has a number of different actions, such as anti-inflammatory, antibiotic, anti-tumour and pain-relieving effects. However, these have not been confirmed in controlled human studies. As a result, it is difficult to determine what effects will be experienced.

When will it start to work?

Due to the lack of human research, this is unknown.

Are there any safety issues?

Shark cartilage products are not to be used in people with seafood allergy or in pregnancy. They should not be used by children or teenagers still experiencing growth or 3 weeks before and for 6 weeks after surgery.

REFERENCES

Anon. AE 941. Drugs R D 5.2 (2004): 83–89.

Barber R et al. Oral shark cartilage does not abolish carcinogenesis but delays tumor progression in a murine model. Anticancer Res 21.2A (2001): 1065–1069.

Bargahi A et al. Effect of shark cartilage derived protein on the NK cells activity. Immunopharmacol Immunotoxicol 33.3 (2011): 403–409.

Bargahi A, Rabbani-Chadegani A. Angiogenic inhibitor protein fractions derived from shark cartilage. Biosci Rep 28.1 (2008): 15–21.

Batist G et al. 2002. Neovastat (AE-941) in refractory renal cell carcinoma patients: report of a phase II trial with two dose levels. Ann. Oncol., 13, (8) 1259–1263.

Couzin J. Beefed-up NIH center probes unconventional therapies. Science 282.5397 (1998): 2175–2176.

de Mejia EG, Dia VP. The role of nutraceutical proteins and peptides in apoptosis, angiogenesis, and metastasis of cancer cells. Cancer Metastasis Rev 29.3 (2010): 511–528.

Dupont E et al. Antiangiogenic and antimetastatic properties of Neovastat (AE-941), an orally active extract derived from cartilage tissue. Clin Exp.Metastasis 19.2 (2002): 145–153.

Dupont E et al. Antiangiogenic properties of a novel shark cartilage extract: potential role in the treatment of psoriasis. J Cutan Med Surg 2.3 (1998): 146–152.

Ernst E. Shark cartilage for cancer? Lancet 351.9098 (1998): 298.

Folkman J. Angiogenesis and apoptosis. Semin Cancer Biol 13.2 (2003): 159–167.

Fontenele JB et al. Anti-inflammatory and analgesic activity of a water-soluble fraction from shark cartilage. Braz J Med Biol Res 29.5 (1996): 643–646.

Fontenele JB et al. The analgesic and anti-inflammatory effects of shark cartilage are due to a peptide molecule and are nitric oxide (NO) system dependent. Biol Pharm Bull 20.11 (1997): 1151–1154.

Gomes EM et al. Shark-cartilage containing preparation protects cells against hydrogen peroxide induced damage and mutagenesis. Mutat Res 367.4 (1996): 204–208.

Gonzalez RP et al. Demonstration of inhibitory effect of oral shark cartilage on basic fibroblast growth factor-induced angiogenesis in the rabbit cornea. Biol Pharm Bull 24.2 (2001): 151–154.

Hassan ZM et al. Low molecular weight fraction of shark cartilage can modulate immune responses and abolish angiogenesis. Int Immunopharmacol 5.6 (2005): 961–970.

Hillman JD et al. Treatment of Kaposi sarcoma with oral administration of shark cartilage in a human herpesvirus 8-seropositive, human immunodeficiency virus-seronegative homosexual man. Arch Dermatol 137.9 (2001): 1149–1152.

Kitahashi T et al. Inhibition of Pancreatic Carcinogenesis by Shark Cartilage Proteoglycan in Hamsters. Exp Toxicol Pathol 19.4 (2006): 179–184.

Kralovec JA et al. Immunomodulating principles from shark cartilage. Part 1. Isolation and biological assessment in vitro. Int Immunopharmacol 3.5 (2003): 657–669.

Latreille J et al. Phase I/II trial of the safety and efficacy of AE-941 (Neovastat) in the treatment of non-small-cell lung cancer. Clin Lung Cancer 4.4 (2003): 231–236.

Lee SY et al. Neovastat (AE-941) inhibits the airway inflammation and hyperresponsiveness in a murine model of asthma. J Microbiol 43.1 (2005): 11–16.

Lee SY, Chung SM. Neovastat (AE-941) inhibits the airway inflammation via VEGF and HIF-2 alpha suppression. Vascul Pharmacol 47.5–6 (2007): 313–18.

Loprinzi CL et al. Evaluation of shark cartilage in patients with advanced cancer: a North Central Cancer Treatment Group trial. Cancer, 104.1 (2005): 176–182.

Lu C et al. Chemoradiotherapy with or without AE-941 in stage III non-small cell lung cancer: a randomized phase III trial. J Natl Cancer Inst 102.12 (2010): 859–865.

Merly L et al. Induction of inflammatory cytokines by cartilage extracts. Int Immunopharmacol 7.3 (2007): 383–391.

Miller DR et al. Phase I/II trial of the safety and efficacy of shark cartilage in the treatment of advanced cancer. J Clin Oncol 16.11 (1998): 3649–3655.

Moore KS et al. Squalamine: an aminosterol antibiotic from the shark. Proc Natl Acad Sci USA 90.4 (1993): 1354–1358.

Patra D, Sandell LJ Antiangiogenic and anticancer molecules in cartilage. Expert Rev Mol Med 14 (2012): e10.

Pearson W et al. Anti-inflammatory and chondroprotective effects of nutraceuticals from Sasha's Blend in a cartilage explant model of inflammation. Mol Nutr Food Res 51.8 (2007): 1020–1030.

Rabbani-Chadegani A et al. Identification of low-molecular-weight protein (SCP1) from shark cartilage with anti-angiogenesis activity and sequence similarity to parvalbumin. J Pharm Biomed Anal 46.3 (2008): 563–567.

Ratel D et al. Direct-acting fibrinolytic enzymes in shark cartilage extract: Potential therapeutic role in vascular disorders. Thrombosis Research 115.1–2 (2005): 143–152.

Shen XR et al. SCAIF80, a novel inhibitor of angiogenesis, and its effect on tumor growth. Sheng Wu Hua Xue Yu Sheng Wu Wu Li Xue Bao (Shanghai) 33.1 (2001): 99–104.

Sheu JR et al. Effect of U-995, a potent shark cartilage-derived angiogenesis inhibitor, on anti-angiogenesis and anti-tumor activities. Anticancer Res 18.6A (1998): 4435–4441.

Simone CB et al. Shark cartilage for cancer. Lancet 351.9113 (1998): 1440.

Zheng L et al. A novel polypeptide from shark cartilage with potent anti-angiogenic activity. Cancer Biol Ther 6.5 (2007): 775–780.

Shatavari

HISTORICAL NOTE There are approximately 300 species of 'asparagus' (derived from the Greek word for 'stalk' or 'shoot'), including the popular European vegetable *Asparagus officinalis*. The medicinal use of *Asparagus racemosus* (shatavari) has been recorded in traditional systems of medicine such as Ayurveda, Unani and Siddha (Bopana & Saxena 2007). It is a different form of asparagus from *Asparagus officinalis*. Shatavari, meaning 'she who possesses a hundred husbands', is often considered an aphrodisiac (Sharma et al 2000) and a 'female tonic'. It is recommended in Ayurvedic texts for the prevention and treatment of gastric ulcers and dyspepsia; for threatened miscarriage and as a galactogogue; and is known as a 'rasayana' (a substance that promotes general physical and mental wellbeing by improving defence mechanisms and vitality) (Goyal et al 2003). Demand for shatavari in combination with destructive harvesting techniques and deforestation has resulted in the plant becoming 'endangered' in its natural habitat (Bopana & Saxena 2007).

OTHER NAMES

Asparagus bush, Inli-chedi, Kairuwa, Majjigegadde, Narbodh, Norkanto, Philli-gaddalu, Satavari, Satawar, Shatmuli, Shimaishadavari, Toala-gaddalu, wild asparagus

BOTANICAL NAME/FAMILY

Asparagus racemosus Willd. (family Asparagaceae [previously Liliaceae, subfamily Asparagae]) (Goyal et al 2003)

It should be differentiated from numerous other species reported in the scientific literature, including *A. acutifolius*, *A. adscendens*, *A. africanus*, *A. curillus*, *A. dumosus*, *A. filicinus*, *A. gonoclados*; and from *A. officinalis* (the stalks of which are consumed as a vegetable).

PLANT PART USED

Root

CHEMICAL COMPONENTS

Steroidal saponins (shatavarins VI–X); saponins (shatavarin I [or asparoside B], shatavarin IV [or asparinin B, a glycoside of sarsasapogenin], shatavarin V, immunoside and schidigera saponin D5 [or asparanin A] (Hayes et al 2008); isoflavones (Saxena & Chourasia 2001), racemofuran, asparagamine A and racemosol (Wiboonpun et al 2004), ascorbic acid (vitamin C) (Visavadiya & Narasimhacharya 2005). Sarsasapogenin and kaempferol have also been isolated from the woody portion of the roots (Bopana & Saxena 2007). However, a recent study (Kumeta et al 2013) revealed that *A. racemosus* does not contain pyrrolo[1,2-a]azepine alkaloid, asparagamine A as reported in previous studies. Kumeta et al (2013) report that studies that identified aspargamine A may have wrongly identified stemonia plants as *A. racemosus*.

Steroidal saponins (racemosides A, B and C) have also been isolated from the fruit (Mandal et al 2006). Shatavaroside A (1) and shatavaroside B (2) have been isolated from the root (Sharma et al 2009). Quercetin, rutin and hyperoside have been identified in the flowers and fruits, and diosgenin and quercetin-3 glucuronide in the leaves (Bopana & Saxena 2007). More recently, an isoflavone, 8-methoxy-5,6,4'-trihydroxyisoflavone-7-O-β-D-glucopyranoside, has been found in *A. racemosus* roots (Negi et al 2010).

MAIN ACTIONS

Adaptogenic (modulates stress response)

In Ayurvedic medicine herbs are usually used in combination and shatavari is used in approximately 64 Ayurvedic formulations. Research is usually conducted with herbal combinations containing shatavari, thereby making it difficult to ascertain the pharmacological and clinical effects of the individual herb (Bopana & Saxena 2007).

A polyherbal formula, known as EuMil, which contains standardised extracts of *A. racemosus* in combination with *Withania somnifera*, *Ocimum sanctum* and *Emblica officinalis*, ameliorates chronic stress-induced neurochemical perturbations and normalises noradrenaline, dopamine and 5-hydroxytryptamine (5HT) levels in animal experiments (Bhattacharya et al 2002). Other animal studies using EuMil have demonstrated attenuation of stress-induced glucose intolerance and immunosuppression, increased male sexual behaviour, and improvements in depression and cognitive dysfunction (Muruganandam et al 2002). These results were also found in a similar polyherbal known as Siotone, containing *A. racemosus*, *Withania somnifera*, *Ocimum sanctum*, *Tribulus terrestris* and shilajit (a composted plant exudate high in minerals) (Bhattacharya et al 2000). Methanolic extract of shatavari has demonstrated physiological modulation of stress pathways by reducing plasma corticosterone and noradrenaline (norepinephrine) in animal models, thus indicating shatavari's possible adaptogenic effect (Krishnamurthy et al 2013). Whether these results are consistent in humans, and which herbs they are attributed to, has not yet been established.

Digestive effects

Early studies suggested that shatavari could improve digestion by increasing levels of amylase and lipase (Dange et al 1969). A small study of eight healthy males using a crossover design found that oral administration of dried shatavari root had similar effects on gastric emptying time to the antiemetic drug metoclopramide, a synthetic dopamine antagonist which is used in dyspepsia to promote gastric emptying (Dalvi et al 1990). Animal experiments using oral doses of shatavari have also reversed the effects of cisplatin on gastric emptying, while normalising cisplatin-induced intestinal hypermotility (Rege et al 1999).

Antiulcerogenic

Antiulcerogenic activity comparable to a standard antiulcer drug ranitidine (30 mg/kg/day orally) has been demonstrated in rats. Treatment with a crude extract of shatavari (100 mg/kg/day orally) for fifteen days significantly reduced indomethacin (NSAID)-induced ulceration when compared with the control group. The effect appeared to be related to an inhibition of hydrochloric acid and protection of the gastric mucosa (Bhatnagar & Sisodia 2006). Early studies demonstrated that shatavari could relieve pain and burning due to duodenal ulceration and proposed that these effects may be due to: an increase in the secretion and viscosity of gastric mucus; formation of a shatavari–mucus complex at the base of the ulcer, providing protection from corrosive agents; prolongation of the life span of mucosal cells and/or a cytoprotective effect similar to that of prostaglandins (Goyal et al 2003). Some of these hypotheses have been supported by further research. The antiulcerogenic effect of oral administration of a methanolic extract of fresh shatavari root (25–100 mg/kg) twice daily for 5 days was studied on different gastroduodenal ulcer models in rats (Sairam et al 2003). Doses of 50 mg/kg twice daily demonstrated significant protection against acute gastric ulceration induced by 'cold restraint stress, pyloric ligation, aspirin plus pyloric ligation, and duodenal ulcers induced by cysteamine' and promoted healing of acetic acid-induced chronic gastric ulceration after 10 days of treatment. An effect was not demonstrated for aspirin- or ethanol-induced gastric ulcers. The effect was believed to be due to an increase in mucus secretion, cellular mucus, the life span of cells, as well as a significant antioxidant effect (Sairam et al 2003).

Immunomodulation

In in vitro studies *A. racemosus* increased the phagocytic and killing capacity of macrophages in a dose-dependent manner (up to 200 mg/kg) (Rege & Dahanukar 1993), and an aqueous extract of *A. racemosus* activated T-cells in vivo. Experimental models in mice have demonstrated the immunostimulating properties of *A. racemosus*, inhibiting the leucopenia associated with cyclophosphamide by inducing leucocytosis with neutrophilia (Thatte & Dahanukar 1988). Animal studies have demonstrated that oral administration of *A. racemosus* inhibited some of the deleterious effects of ochratoxin A suppression of chemotactic activity and production of IL-1 and TNF-alpha by macropahges, and also induced excess production of TNF-alpha in animals that did not receive ochratoxin A (Dhuley 1997). It also appears to reduce intraperitoneal adhesions induced by caecal rubbing by increasing the activity of macrophages (Rege et al 1989), and may act as an immunoadjuvant in animals immunised with diphtheria, tetanus, pertussis (DTP) vaccine, increasing antibody titres to *Bordetella pertussis* and providing improved immunoprotection on challenge (Gautam et al 2004).

Two steroidal saponins, shatavaroside A and shatavaroside B, extracted from the root of *A. racemosus* exhibited a dose-dependent and potent immunostimulant activity at low concentrations (5 ng/mL) in vitro (Sharma et al 2013).

Antibacterial and anti-leishmanial

In vitro studies using different concentrations (50, 100, 150 microgram/mL) of the methanolic extract of shatavari root demonstrated considerable antibacterial efficacy against: *Escherichia coli*, *Shigella dysenteriae*, *Shigella sonnei*, *Shigella flexneri*, *Vibrio cholerae*, *Salmonella typhi*, *Salmonella typhimurium*, *Pseudomonas putida*, *Bacillus subtilis* and *Staphylococcus aureus* (Mandal et al 2000b). Another in vitro study using aqueous and ethylacetate extracts of shatavari roots demonstrated antibacterial activity against Gram-negative *Alcaligenes* with the ethyl acetate extract having stronger effects (Phatak et al 2011).

A constituent of *A. racemosus* fruit, racemoside A, exhibits potent anti-leishmanial activity against the dangerous visceral form of leishmaniasis (Dutta et al 2007).

Hormonal activity

The steroidal saponins (shatavarins) contained in *A. racemosus* may help explain some of the hormonal effects demonstrated in animal models. An alcoholic extract of shatavari root (300 mg/kg bodyweight) was administered orally to pregnant female albino rats during days 1–15 of gestation. The results suggested an oestrogenic effect on the mammary glands and genital organs (Pandey et al 2005). Tests with animal models indicate shatavari competitively blocks the effect of oxytocin, thereby inhibiting oxytocin-induced uterine contraction in rabbits, rats and guinea pigs (Gaitonde & Jetmalani 1969). This action appears to be due to the asparagamine, a polycyclic alkaloid (Sekine et al 1994).

Galactagogue

Galactagogue activity has been demonstrated in animal models (Patel & Kanitkar 1969, Sabnis et al 1968). One study of weaning rats found shatavari treatment increased the weight of mammary glands, inhibited involution of lobulo-alveolar tissue and maintained milk secretion (Sabnis et al 1968). It has been proposed that this effect may be due to the action of released corticoids and prolactin (Goyal et al 2003). Oral treatment with a shatavari root capsule (60 mg/kg body weight/day for 30 days) has also been shown to significantly elevate prolactin levels in a double-blind randomised controlled trial (RCT) of lactating mothers indicating the effect is clinically significant at this dose (Gupta et al 2011).

Antidiarrhoeal

Ethanol and aqueous extracts (200 mg/kg) of shatavari root have been shown to inhibit castor oil-induced diarrhoea, and PGE_2 induced enteropooling (excessive secretion of water and electrolytes); and reduced gastrointestinal motility in rats (Venkatesan et al 2005). A recent study, in which ethanol extract of *A. racemosus* was administered to mice to inhibit castor oil-induced diarrhoea confirmed the previous results showing a delay in the onset of diarrhoea as well as a reduced frequency of defecation at the dose of 250 to 500 mg/kg body weight compared to the standard drug loperamide (Karmakar et al 2012).

Antioxidant and hepatoprotective

A. racemosus contains known antioxidant compounds, including ascorbic acid, polyphenols and flavonoids (Visavadiya & Narasimhacharya 2005). Antioxidant properties have also been identified for racemofuran, asparagamine A and racemosol (Wiboonpun et al 2004). In vitro experiments have demonstrated antioxidant effects comparable to that of glutathione and ascorbic acid in inhibiting lipid peroxidation and protein oxidation (Kamat et al 2000). Animal models confirmed the inhibition of lipid peroxidation and also showed an increase in antioxidant enzymes (superoxide dismutase, catalase) and ascorbic acid (Bhatnagar et al 2005, Visavadiya & Narasimhacharya 2005). An alcoholic extract of shatavari root significantly reduces elevated levels of alanine transaminase (ALT), aspartate transaminase (AST) and alkaline phosphatase (ALP) in vivo (Muruganandan et al 2000). *A. racemosus* extract administered in isoniazid induced hepatotoxicity in mice at 50 mg/kg body weight for 21 days showed hepatoprotective effects indicated by an improved liver function profile ($P < 0.05$) and inhibition of cytochrome P4502EI (CYP2EI). The study suggests that *A. racemosus* inhibits production of free radicals and *A. racemosus* acts as a scavenger by inhibiting CYP2EI activity.

Cardiovascular effects

Studies using different animal models indicate various effects on heart function. Goyal et al (2003) found lower doses of shatavari root produce a positive inotropic and chronotropic effect on frog's heart, with higher doses causing cardiac arrest. The extract was also found to produce hypotension in cats (attenuated by atropine) indicating a cholinergic mechanism; and a slight increase in bleeding time in rabbits (Goyal et al 2003).

Studies with animal models have indicated lipid-lowering activity for *A. racemosus* (Visavadiya et al 2009, Zhu et al 2010). In one study, a 5% and 10% dose of *A. racemosus* root powder administered to hypercholesterolaemic rats on a normal diet or hypercholesterolaemic diet respectively for 4 weeks, showed reduction in hepatic lipid profile, increased excretion of faecal cholesterol and increased hepatic HMG-CoA reductase activity. These effects have been attributed to the presence of phytosterols, saponins, flavonoids, ascorbic acid and polyphenols in *A. racemosus* (Visavadiya et al 2009).

Neuroprotective

Oxidative stress and excitotoxicity are considered to be major mechanisms of neuronal cell death in neurodegenerative disorders such as Alzheimer's and Parkinson's diseases. Experimental studies have demonstrated that shatavari extract may attenuate oxidative damage, elevating glutathione peroxidase (GPx) activity and glutathione (GSH) content; and could result in a protective effect on kainic acid (KA)-induced excitotoxicity (Parihar & Hemnani 2004).

A methanolic extract of *A. racemosus* root administered to test animals at 100 mg/kg body weight daily for 30 days and subjected to 3 hours of swim stress showed higher total normal cell counts in the hippocampus compared to rats subjected to the swim stress test without active treatment, suggesting a potential neuroprotective activity (Saxena et al 2010).

Antidepressant

Antidepressant activity has been demonstrated in vivo. A methanolic extract of *A. racemosus* root (MAR) (standardised to saponins 62.2% w/w) was given to rats in doses of 100, 200 and 400 mg/kg daily for 7 days. The results show that MAR decreased immobility in forced swim tests (FST) and increased avoidance response in learned helplessness tests (LH), indicating antidepressant activity. Effects were thought to be mediated through the serotonergic and noradrenergic systems, and augmentation of antioxidant defences (Singh et al 2009). A methanolic extract of *A. racemosus* demonstrated inhibition of cholinesterase and monoamine oxidase (MAO) activities in vivo (Meena et al 2011). The saponin content in the extract was thought to be responsible for the observed activity.

Antineoplastic

An extract of shatavari root has been reported to reduce the incidence of DMBA (7,12-dimethyl benz(a)anthracene)-induced mammary cancer in female rats (Rao 1981). The effect is thought to be due to properties that render the mammary epithelium refractory to the carcinogen. Clinical implications remain to be tested.

Rats pretreated with aqueous extract of *A. racemosus* showed no p53+ foci while rats not receiving *A. racemosus* showed p53+ foci on immunohistochemical staining indicating that *A. racemosus* has the potential to prevent hepatocarcinogenesis induced by diethylnitrosamine (Agarwal et al 2008). Isolated shatavarin IV with shatavarin rich fraction has shown anticancer activity in vitro against human breast cancer, human colon adenocarcinoma and human kidney carcinoma cell lines (Mitra et al 2012). In this study, oral administration of isolated shatavarin IV at doses of 250 and 500 mg/kg body weight to cancer-induced mice showed reduction in tumour volume, per cent increase in body weight and packed cell volume, suggesting anticancer activity (Mitra et al 2012).

Antilithic

An ethanolic extract of shatavari inhibited experimentally-induced urinary lithiasis (stone formation) in vivo (Christina et al 2005). Administration of shatavari reduced elevated urinary concentrations of calcium, oxalate and phosphate, which contribute to stone formation, and increased urinary concentration of magnesium, which is thought to be protective. Elevated serum creatinine was also reduced. Similar results were obtained in another animal study (Jagannath et al 2012). However, there is little evidence on antilithic activity of *A. racemosus* in clinical trials.

Antitussive

Strong antitussive activity has been demonstrated in animal models. A methanolic extract of shatavari root (200 and 400 mg/kg orally) showed significant antitussive activity on sulfur dioxide-induced cough in mice. The dose-dependent cough inhibition (40.0 and 58.5%, respectively) was comparable to that of 10–20 mg/kg codeine phosphate (36.0 and 55.4%, respectively) (Mandal et al 2000a).

Analgesic

Ethanolic extract of *A. racemosus* in acetic acid-induced writhing model in mice showed 52.39% ($P < 0.05$) and 67.47% ($P < 0.05$) writhing inhibition at doses of 250 and 500 mg/kg body weight suggesting analgesic activity of shatavari (Karmakar et al 2012).

Antihyperglycaemic

Administering ethanol extracts of *A. racemosus* roots orally in diabetic and healthy rats showed improved glucose tolerance by suppressing post-prandial sucrose load. Daily oral administration of *A. racemosus* extracts in type 2 diabetic rats over a period of 28 days resulted in decreased serum glucose and increased pancreatic insulin indicating that *A. racemosus* inhibits carbohydrate absorption therefore *A. racemosus* can be a potentially useful antidiabetic nutritional adjuvant. However, the hyperglycaemic potential of *A. racemosus* needs to be tested in human clinical studies (Hanna et al 2012).

CLINICAL USE

Shatavari has not been subjected to extensive clinical testing so most information is derived from traditional use and in vivo experiments, thereby providing biological plausibility for some of its uses.

Stress

Currently, evidence to support the use of shatavari as a sole agent for reducing the deleterious effects of stress on the body is limited. Animal studies using polyherbal formulations (Mukherjee et al 2011), such as EuMil (Bhattacharya et al 2002, Muruganandam et al 2002) and Siotone (Bhattacharya et al 2000), have shown some promise, but further research is required.

Dyspepsia

Shatavari root is used in Ayurvedic medicine for the treatment of dyspepsia. This may in part be due to improved digestion via increased levels of amylase and lipase (Dange et al 1969), and its ability to promote gastric emptying in a manner comparable to metoclopramide (Goyal et al 2003), and to normalise intestinal hypermotility (Rege et al 1999).

Gastrointestinal ulcers

In animal models, shatavari has been shown to reduce the incidence and increase the rate of healing of ulcers (Samarakoon et al 2011); while also relieving the pain and burning associated with duodenal ulceration (Goyal et al 2003). Antiulcerogenic activity of a crude extract of shatavari (100 mg/kg/day orally) has been found to be comparable to a standard antiulcer drug ranitidine (30 mg/kg/day orally) in rats. The effect may be related to an inhibition of hydrochloric acid and protection of the gastric mucosa (Bhatnagar & Sisodia 2006). Studies investigating ulcer healing activity of shatavari seem to use poly-herbal formulations (Samarakoon et al 2011), which poses a limitation on interpreting the role of shatavari as a single herb in ulcer healing.

Prevention of infection

In vitro and animal experiments have demonstrated positive effects on immunity (particularly on the activity of macrophages) (Rege et al 1989, Rege & Dahanukar 1993) as well as antibacterial effects against *Escherichia coli*, *Shigella dysenteriae*, *Shigella sonnei*, *Shigella flexneri*, *Vibrio cholerae*, *Salmonella typhi*, *Salmonella typhimurium*, *Pseudomonas putida*, *Bacillus subtilis* and *Staphylococcus aureus* (Mandal et al 2000b). Shatavari has also shown antibacterial activity against *Alcaligenes* (Phatak et al 2011). Further research is required in clinical trials to ascertain whether these effects can be demonstrated in humans.

OTHER USES

Hormonal disturbances in women

Traditionally shatavari is used as a 'rejuvenative tonic' for females and for lowered libido and infertility in both sexes (Sharma et al 2011). Due to its oestrogenic effects it is often used by herbalists for the treatment of conditions related to low oestrogen, including some presentations of PMS and menopause; and to re-establish normal ovulation and menstruation patterns (Trickey 2003). Human trials have demonstrated positive results for dysfunctional uterine bleeding, dysmenorrhoea, PMS and menopausal symptoms, however these studies used the polyherbal formulations EveCare and Menosan which contain *A. racemosus* (Bopana & Saxena 2007) so it is difficult to ascertain the role played by shatavari alone.

Promoting lactation

Shatavari root is used traditionally in Ayurvedic medicine to increase milk production and secretion during lactation (Sharma et al 2011). Early animal studies support this use (Sabnis et al 1968, Patel & Kanitkar 1969). Whether shatavari increases prolactin levels and consequently improves lactation remains difficult to determine from the evidence as most studies used it as part of a herbal combination. Previously, polyherbal combinations including *A. racemosus* Ricalex (Alphali Pharmaceutical Ltd, Ahmednagar) (Joglekar et al 1967) and Lactare (TIK Pharma, Chennai) have been shown to increase milk production in women complaining of poor milk supply (Goyal et al 2003). In contrast, a placebo-controlled RCT of 64 lactating women in India found a herbal combination galactagogue formula (including shatavari 15%) had no effect on prolactin levels or lactation compared to placebo (Sharma et al 1996). Since shatavari was only one component of the formulas tested, it is not possible to identify the contribution of shatavari to these results.

Positive results were obtained in a more recent double-blind, randomised, parallel group clinical trial ($n = 60$) which found that use of a shatavari root capsule (60 mg/kg body weight/day) for a duration of 30 days resulted in a 33% increase in prolactin levels compared to an increase of 9.5% in the control group among women aged 20–40 years having trouble lactating and with infants up to 6 months of age (Gupta & Shaw 2011). The galactogogue activity was attributed to the possible steroidal saponins in *A. racemosus*. Although, this study did not find any acute toxicity on oral administration of shatavari, the long-term toxicity of shatavari is not clearly understood and needs further investigation (Mortel & Mehta 2013).

Diarrhoea

Shatavari root is used traditionally in Ayurvedic medicine for the treatment of diarrhoea and dysentery. Ethanol and aqueous extracts of shatavari root have demonstrated antidirrhoeal effect by reducing gastrointestinal motility in animal studies (Venkatesan et al 2005, Karmakar et al 2012). Human studies are warranted to confirm these effects.

DOSAGE RANGE

Fluid extract (1:2): 30–60 mL/week (Australian manufacturer's recommendations).

ADVERSE REACTIONS

No significant adverse events or biochemical liver dysfunction was noted in a randomised controlled trial of shatavari (Sharma et al 1996). Due to the saponin content, gastric irritation may occur in some individuals.

Practice points/Patient counselling

- In Ayurvedic medicine shatavari is used in approximately 64 Ayurvedic polyherbal formulations. As much of the current research focuses on these preparations, it is difficult to ascertain the pharmacological and clinical effects of the individual herb.
- Shatavari may exert beneficial effects on digestion by increasing levels of lipase and amylase, promoting gastric emptying, normalising intestinal motility and protecting against ulceration.
- Shatavari is used, often in combination with other herbs, to improve milk production in lactating women, although human data supporting this effect are currently lacking. More promising was a recent study using shatavari as a stand-alone treatment.
- Animal models suggest that the steroidal saponins contained in *A. racemosus* may exert some hormonal effects, which may account for its reputation as a female tonic and aphrodisiac.
- As teratogenicity has recently been demonstrated in rats, caution should be exercised in pregnancy until more is known about effects in humans.
- Demand for shatavari in combination with destructive harvesting techniques and deforestation has resulted in the plant becoming 'endangered' in its natural habitat.

SIGNIFICANT INTERACTIONS

As controlled studies are not available, interactions are currently speculative and based on evidence of pharmacological activity. No evidence could be located that suggested any negative drug interactions.

Metoclopramide

As shatavari root was found in animal studies to have similar effects on gastric emptying time to the antiemetic drug metoclopramide (a synthetic dopamine antagonist), an additive effect is possible (Dalvi et al 1990, Sharma et al 2011).

Diphtheria, tetanus, pertussis (DTP) vaccine

Experimental studies have suggested a possible immunoadjuvant effect in animals immunised with diphtheria, tetanus, pertussis (DTP) vaccine, increasing antibody titres to *Bordetella pertussis* and providing improved immunoprotection on challenge (Gautam et al 2004). Beneficial effects possible.

CONTRAINDICATIONS AND PRECAUTIONS

No toxic effects or mortality have been observed with doses ranging from 50 mg/kg to 1 g/kg for 4 weeks, and acute and subacute (15–30 day) toxicity studies have not detected any changes in results of vital organ function tests. The LD_{50} is >1 g/kg (Rege et al 1999).

As inhibition of hydrochloric acid has been proposed as a possible factor contributing to the antiulcer effects of shatavari (Bhatnagar & Sisodia 2006), those with hypochlorhydria may need to be observed.

Herbs with theoretical oestrogenic effects may not be suitable for those with or at risk of oestrogen-dependent tumours. However, the clinical significance is unclear.

The Commission E has approved the use of *A. officinalis* root in irrigation therapy for inflammatory diseases of the urinary tract and for prevention of kidney stones; however, this should be avoided if oedema exists due to functional heart or kidney disorders (Blumenthal et al 2000). Similar cautions might be expected for *A. racemosus*.

PREGNANCY USE

Although shatavari has been used traditionally to promote conception and for threatened miscarriage, teratogenicity has been demonstrated in rats at doses of 100 mg/kg/day for 60 days (Goel et al 2006). Caution should be exercised in pregnancy until more is known about effects in humans. Little evidence is available about the safe use of shatavari in breast-feeding; however, what is available suggests no significant side effects (Sharma et al 1996).

PATIENTS' FAQs

What will this herb do for me?

It is difficult to determine what effects shatavari will display when used as a sole treatment, as it is most often tested as part of a polyherbal combination formula. The herbal combinations containing shatavari have a myriad of uses, such as improving digestion, promoting lactation and increasing libido. Shatavari root is used traditionally in Ayurvedic medicine for the treatment of diarrhoea and dysentery, gastric ulcers and dyspepsia, threatened miscarriage and as a galactogogue.

When will it start to work?

This is difficult to estimate as the majority of human trials have been conducted with polyherbal preparations containing shatavari and not with shatavari as a sole treatment.

Are there any safety issues?

Caution should be exercised in pregnancy until more is known about the potential teratogenic effects.

REFERENCES

Agrawal A et al. The effect of the aqueous extract of the roots of Asparagus racemosus on hepatocarcinogenesis initiated by diethylnitrosamine. Phytother Res 22.9 (2008): 1175–1182.

Bhatnagar M et al. Antiulcer and antioxidant activity of Asparagus racemosus Willd and Withania somnifera Dunal in rats. Ann N Y Acad Sci 1056 (2005): 261–278.

Bhatnagar M, Sisodia SS. Antisecretory and antiulcer activity of Asparagus racemosus Willd. against indomethacin plus phyloric ligation-induced gastric ulcer in rats. J Herb Pharmacother 6.1 (2006): 13–20.

Bhattacharya A et al. Effect of poly herbal formulation, EuMil, on neurochemical perturbations induced by chronic stress. Indian J Exp Biol 40.10 (2002): 1161–1163.

Bhattacharya SK et al. Adaptogenic activity of Siotone, a polyherbal formulation of Ayurvedic rasayanas. Indian J Exp Biol 38.2 (2000): 119–128.

Blumenthal M et al (eds). Herbal medicine expanded Commission E monographs. Austin, TX: Integrative Medicine Communications, 2000.

Bopana N, Saxena S. Asparagus racemosus—ethnopharmacological evaluation and conservation needs. J Ethnopharmacol 110.1 (2007): 1–15.

Christina AJ et al. Antilithiatic effect of Asparagus racemosus Willd on ethylene glycol-induced lithiasis in male albino Wistar rats. Methods Find Exp Clin Pharmacol 27.9 (2005): 633–638.

Dalvi SS et al. Effect of Asparagus racemosus (Shatavari) on gastric emptying time in normal healthy volunteers. J Postgrad Med 36.2 (1990): 91–94.

Dange PS et al. Amylase and lipase activities in the root of Asparagus racemosus. Planta Med 17.4 (1969): 393–395.

Dhuley JN. Effect of some Indian herbs on macrophage functions in ochratoxin A treated mice. J Ethnopharmacol 58.1 (1997): 15–20.

Dutta A et al. Racemoside A, an anti-leishmanial, water-soluble, natural steroidal saponin, induces programmed cell death in Leishmania donovani. J Med Microbiol 56 Pt 9 (2007): 1196–1204.

Gaitonde BB, Jetmalani MH. Antioxytocic action of saponin isolated from Asparagus racemosus Willd (Shatavari) on uterine muscle. Arch Int Pharmacodyn Ther 179.1 (1969): 121–129.

Gautam M et al. Immunoadjuvant potential of Asparagus racemosus aqueous extract in experimental system. J Ethnopharmacol 91.2–3 (2004): 251–255.

Goel RK et al. Teratogenicity of Asparagus racemosus Willd. root, a herbal medicine. Indian J Exp Biol 44.7 (2006): 570–573.

Goyal RK et al. Asparagus racemosus—an update. Indian J Med Sci 57.9 (2003): 408–414.

Gupta M, Shaw B. A double-blind randomized clinical trial for evaluation of galactogogue activity of Asparagus racemosus Willd. Iranian J Pharmacolog Res 10.1, (2011): 167–172.

Hanna JMA et al. Antihyperglycaemic activity of Asparagus racemosus roots is partly mediated by inhibition of carbohydrate digestion and absorption, and enhancement of cellular insulin action. Brit J Nutr 107.09 (2012): 1316–1323.

Hayes PY et al. Steroidal saponins from the roots of Asparagus racemosus. Phytochemistry 69.3 (2008): 796–804.

Jagannath N et al. Study of antiurolithiatic activity of Asparagus racemosus on albino rats. Indian J Pharmacol 44.5(2012): 576–579.

Joglekar GV et al. Galactogogue effect of Asparagus racemosus. Preliminary communication. Indian Med J 61.7 (1967): 165.

Kamat JP et al. Antioxidant properties of Asparagus racemosus against damage induced by gamma-radiation in rat liver mitochondria. J Ethnopharmacol 71.3 (2000): 425–435.

Karmakar UK et al. Cytotoxicity, Analgesic and Antidiarrhoeal Activities of Asparagus racemosus. J Appl 12.6 (2012): 581–586.

Krishnamurthy B et al. Asparagus racemosus modulates the hypothalamic–pituitary–adrenal axis and brain monoaminergic systems in rats. Nutr Neurosci 16.6 (2013): 255–261.

Kumeta Y et al. Chemical analysis reveals the botanical origin of shatavari products and confirms the absence of alkaloid asparagamine A in Asparagus racemosus. J Nat Med 67(2013): 168 173.

Mandal D et al. Steroidal saponins from the fruits of Asparagus racemosus. Phytochemistry 67.13 (2006): 1316–1321.

Mandal SC, Kumar CKA et al. Antitussive effect of Asparagus racemosus root against sulfur dioxide-induced cough in mice. Fitoterapia 71.6 (2000a): 686–689.

Mandal SC, Nandy A et al. Evaluation of antibacterial activity of Asparagus racemosus willd. root. Phytother Res 14.2 (2000b): 118–119.
Meena J et al. Asparagus racemosus competitively inhibits in vitro the acetylcholine and monoamine metabolizing enzymes. Neurosci Lett 503.1(2011): 6–9.
Mitra SK et al. Shatavarins (containing Shatavarin IV) with anticancer activity from the roots of Asparagus racemosus. Ind J Pharmcol 44.6 (2012): 732.
Mortel M, Mehta SD. Systematic review of the efficacy of herbal galactogogues. J Hum Lact 29.2 (2013): 154–62.
Muruganandam AV et al. Effect of poly herbal formulation, EuMil, on chronic stress-induced homeostatic perturbations in rats. Indian J Exp Biol 40.10 (2002): 1151–1160.
Muruganandan S et al. Studies on the immunomodulant and antihepatotoxic activities of Asparagus racemosus root extract. J Med Aromat Plant Sci 22 (2000): 49–52.
Negi JS et al. Chemical constituents of Asparagus. Pharmacogn Rev 4.8 (2010): 215.
Pandey SK et al. Effect of Asparagus racemosus rhizome (Shatavari) on mammary gland and genital organs of pregnant rat. Phytother Res 19.8 (2005): 721–724.
Parihar MS, Hemnani T. Experimental excitotoxicity provokes oxidative damage in mice brain and attenuation by extract of Asparagus racemosus. J Neural Transm 111.1 (2004): 1–12.
Patel AB, Kanitkar UK. Asparagus racemosus willd–form bordi, as a galactogogue, in buffaloes. Indian Vet J 46.8 (1969): 718–721.
Phatak K et al. In Vitro Antibacterial activity of some Medicinal plants against the bacterial strain–Alcaligenes. Int J Basic App Res 1 (2011): 88–92.
Rao AR. Inhibitory action of Asparagus racemosus on DMBA-induced mammary carcinogenesis in rats. Int J Cancer 28.5 (1981): 607–610.
Rege NN et al. Adaptogenic properties of six rasayana herbs used in Ayurvedic medicine. Phytother Res 13.4 (1999): 275–291.
Rege NN et al. Immunotherapeutic modulation of intraperitoneal adhesions by Asparagus racemosus. J Postgrad Med 35.4 (1989): 199–203.
Rege NN, Dahanukar SA. Quantitation of microbicidal activity of mononuclear phagocytes: an in vitro technique. J Postgrad Med 39.1 (1993): 22–25.
Sabnis PB et al. Effects of alcoholic extracts of Asparagus racemosus on mammary glands of rats. Indian J Exp Biol 6.1 (1968): 55–57.
Sairam K et al. Gastroduodenal ulcer protective activity of Asparagus racemosus: an experimental, biochemical and histological study. J Ethnopharmacol 86.1 (2003): 1–110.
Samarakoon SMS et al. Experimental evaluation of gastroprotective and adaptogenic activity of Amalakayas Rasayana and its vehicle (ghee and honey). Sri Lanka J Indig Med 1.2 (2011): 51–54.
Saxena G et al. Neuroprotective Effects of Asparagus Racemosus Linn Root Extract: An Experimental and Clinical Evidence. Ann Nuerol Sci 14.3 (2010): 57–63.
Saxena VK, Chourasia S. A new isoflavone from the roots of Asparagus racemosus. Fitoterapia 72.3 (2001): 307–309.
Sekine T et al. Structure of asparagamine A, a novel polycyclic alkaloid from Asparagus racemosus. Chem Pharm Bull 42 (1994): 1360.
Sharma K et al. Asparagus racemosus (Shatavari): a versatile female tonic. Int J Pharm Biol Arch 2.3 (2011): 855–863.
Sharma P et al. Database on medicinal plants used in Ayurveda, Volume I. New Delhi: Central Council for Research in Ayurveda and Siddha (2000): 418–30.
Sharma S et al. Randomized controlled trial of Asparagus racemosus (Shatavari) as a lactogogue in lactational inadequacy. Indian Pediatr 33.8 (1996): 675–677.
Sharma U et al. Immunomodulatory active steroidal saponins from *Asparagus racemosus*. Med Chem Res (2013) 22: 573–579.
Sharma U et al. Steroidal saponins from Asparagus racemosus. Chem Pharm Bull 57.8 (2009): 890–893.
Singh GK et al. Antidepressant activity of Asparagus racemosus in rodent models. Pharmacol Biochem Behav 91.3 (2009): 283–690.
Thatte UM, Dahanukar SA. Comparative study of immunomodulating activity of Indian medicinal plants, lithium carbonate and glucan. Methods Find Exp Clin Pharmacol 10.10 (1988): 639–644.
Trickey R. Women, Hormones and the menstrual cycle, 2nd edn. Sydney: Allen & Unwin, 2003.
Venkatesan N et al. Anti-diarrhoeal potential of Asparagus racemosus wild root extracts in laboratory animals. J Pharm Pharm Sci 8.1 (2005): 39–46.
Visavadiya N, Narasimhacharya A. Hypolipidemic and antioxidant activities of Asparagus racemosus in hypercholesteremic rats. Indian J Pharmacol 37.6 (2005): 376–380.
Visavadiya NP et al. Asparagus root regulates cholesterol metabolism and improves antioxidant status in hypercholesteremic rats. Evidence Based Complement Alt Med, 6.2 (2009): 19–26.
Wiboonpun N et al. Identification of antioxidant compound from Asparagus racemosus. Phytother Res 18.9 (2004): 771–773.
Zhu X et al. Hypolipidaemic and hepatoprotective effects of ethanolic and aqueous extracts from Asparagus officinalis L. by-products in mice fed a high-fat diet. J Sci Food Agric 90.7 (2010): 1129–1135.

Slippery elm

HISTORICAL NOTE The dried inner bark of the slippery elm tree was a popular remedy used by many Native American tribes, and subsequently taken up by European settlers. It was mixed with water and applied topically to treat wounds, bruises and skin irritations, and used internally for sore throat, coughs and gastrointestinal conditions. When mixed with milk, it was used as a nutritious gruel for children and convalescents. It also gained a reputation as an effective wound healer among soldiers during the American Civil War. From 1820 until 1960, it was listed in the US Pharmacopeia as a demulcent, emollient and antitussive (Ulbricht & Basch 2005). The name 'slippery elm' refers to the slippery consistency of the inner bark when it comes into contact with water.

COMMON NAME

Slippery elm

OTHER NAMES

American elm, Indian elm, moose elm, red elm, sweet elm, winged elm

BOTANICAL NAME/FAMILY

Ulmus fulvus or *Ulmus rubra* (family Ulmaceae)

According to current botanical nomenclature, it should now be referred to as *Ulmus rubra*.

PLANT PART USED

Dried inner bark

CHEMICAL COMPONENTS

The inner bark chiefly contains mucilage (various hexoses, pentoses, methylpentoses), glucose, polyuronides, tannins, galacturonic acid, L-rhamnose, D-galactose, starches, fat, phytosterols, sesquiterpenes, oxalate acid, flavonoids, salicyclic acid, capric acid, caprylic acid, decanoic acid and cholesterol (Beveridge et al 1969, Duke 2003, IM Gateway Database

2003, Newell et al 1996, Rousseau & Watts 2012). The bark provides 2740 kcal/kg. It contains a variety of nutritional factors, such as glucose, calcium, iron, vitamin C, thiamine, zinc, magnesium and potassium, providing support for its traditional use as a nutritious gruel.

> ***Clinical note — Mucilages***
> Mucilages are hydrophilic structures, capable of trapping water, which causes them to swell in size and develop a gel-like consistency. The gels tend to have soothing properties and can be broken down by bowel flora when taken internally (Mills & Bone 2000). Mucilages are known to have beneficial effects on burns, wounds and ulcers when applied externally and on gastric inflammation, irritations and diarrhoea when taken internally.

MAIN ACTIONS

The pharmacological actions of slippery elm have not been significantly investigated in clinical studies. Therefore, information is generally based on what is known about key constituents found within the herb.

Soothes irritated and inflamed tissue

The large amount of mucilage found in slippery elm bark will coat the surface of mucous membranes or wounds and sores when it comes in contact with water, and form a gel-like layer. Mucilaginous medicinal plants, such as slippery elm, have beneficial effects on burns, wounds, ulcers, external and internal inflammations and irritations (Morton 1990). They provide a moist, protective barrier which can soothe and promote healing.

Nutritive demulcent

A number of constituents, such as starch, glucose, calcium, iron, vitamin C, thiamine, zinc, magnesium and potassium are present in slippery elm, making it a source of many nutritional factors (Duke 2003).

Antioxidant

In vitro studies show a free radical-scavenging activity that may relate to its anti-inflammatory action (Langmead et al 2002). Compounds with antioxidant activity are sometimes investigated for their tumoricidal activity; however an in vitro study found slippery elm to exhibit only weak tumoricidal properties (Mazzio & Soliman 2009).

CLINICAL USE

The therapeutic effectiveness of slippery elm has not been significantly investigated under clinical trial conditions, so evidence is derived from traditional, in vitro and animal studies.

Gastrointestinal conditions

Based on traditional evidence, slippery elm is taken internally to relieve the symptoms of gastritis, acid dyspepsia, gastric reflux, peptic ulcers, irritable bowel syndrome (IBS) and Crohn's disease.

It is widely accepted that, when orally ingested, the mucilage forms a physical barrier protecting the oesophageal and stomach walls from the damaging effects of stomach acid and possibly also exerting mild anti-inflammatory activity locally. Currently, clinical research is not available to determine the effectiveness of slippery elm in these conditions; however, anecdotally the treatment appears to be very successful and patients report rapid improvement in upper gastrointestinal symptoms.

Solid-dose tablets and capsules are used in the treatment of lower gastrointestinal conditions such as diarrhoea, where it is believed the fibre will slow down gastric transit time and act as a bulking agent. Although clinical studies are not available to determine its effectiveness, the high mucilaginous content and presence of tannins in the herb provide a theoretical basis for its use.

IN COMBINATION

A small, open pilot study investigated the use of a herbal formula containing slippery elm in the treatment of 31 patients with IBS, with promising results. Twenty-one patients with diarrhoea-predominant or alternating bowel habit IBS were given the herbal formula containing slippery elm (4.5 g), powdered bilberry fruit (10.0 g), agrimony (3.0 g) and cinnamon (1.5 g) twice daily for 3 weeks. Ten patients with constipation-predominant IBS were given a herbal formula containing slippery elm (7.0 g), lactulose (3.0 g), oat bran (2.0 g) and licorice root (1.5 g) twice daily for 3 weeks. The diarrhoea-predominant or alternating bowel habit IBS group reported no improvements in bowel habit, although they did report a significant improvement in a number of IBS symptoms, including straining, abdominal pain, bloating, flatulence and global IBS symptoms. There was a significant improvement in bowel habits in the constipation-predominant IBS group, with a 20% increase in bowel movement frequency and improvements in stool consistency, and IBS symptoms, including reductions in straining, abdominal pain, bloating and global IBS symptom severity (Hawrelak & Myers 2010). While some of these results are promising, the role of slippery elm in achieving the reported benefits is unclear. Further research is required to expand upon the findings of this pilot study.

Dermatitis and wounds

Slippery elm has also been used as a topical agent to soothe irritated and/or inflamed skin conditions, wounds and burns and to draw out boils and abscesses (Fisher & Painter 1996). When applied, it forms a protective gel-like layer, which is considered to have soothing properties.

Laryngeal 'soothing' effect

A single oral dose of 3 g of slippery elm taken in warm water as a tea had no 'soothing' effect according to a randomised, controlled, single-blind study of 24 volunteers without pharyngeal or laryngeal complaints (Rousseau & Watts 2012). A 'soothing' effect was defined as 'when the [tissue] surface feels as if it were coated with something, such as a layer of protective covering'. Further research should be conducted testing the preparation in people with current inflammation and discomfort.

OTHER USES

Traditionally, slippery elm is used to treat bronchitis, cystitis and intestinal parasites. Externally, it has been used to treat gout, inflamed joints and toothache (Fisher & Painter 1996).

> ***Clinical note — Essiac tea***
> Slippery elm is one of the key ingredients in Essiac tea, which was reportedly developed by the Ojibwa tribe of Canada and named after an Ontario nurse (Rene Caisse) to whom the formula for the herbal tea was given by an Ojibwa healer in 1922 (Smith & Boon 1999). It is used to treat a variety of diverse conditions, such as allergies, hypertension and osteoporosis. The tea is made up of a mixture of four herbs, *Arctium lappa* (burdock root), *Rumex acetosella* (sheep sorrel), *Ulmus rubra* (slippery elm) and *Rheum officinale* (rhubarb) and is considered to possess antioxidant and, possibly, anticancer activities (Leonard et al 2006). As a result, it is used widely by North American cancer patients during chemo- and radiotherapies (Cheung et al 2005) for reduction in symptoms associated with cancer treatment and as a possible adjunctive treatment. In vitro tests with Essiac have identified anticancer activity, although its effects in vivo are controversial and evidence of efficacy is anecdotal (Leonard et al 2006). A recent study demonstrated that Essiac tea effectively scavenges several types of radicals and possesses DNA-protective effects (Leonard et al 2006). A retrospective cohort study of 510 women with breast cancer found that Essiac did not improve quality-of-life scores or mood (Zick et al 2006). Daily doses of Essiac range from 12 to 114 mL, with the average dose being 43.6 mL, corresponding to doses recommended on popular products. Duration of treatment ranged from 1 to 28 months, with the average being 11.1 months. The formula was well tolerated, with only two women reporting minor adverse events, while many women reported beneficial effects. In contrast, an in vitro study found Essiac tea stimulated the growth of human breast cancer cells via both oestrogen receptor-dependent and oestrogen receptor-independent mechanisms (Kulp et al 2006). Patients and health practitioners should consider these findings when making clinical decisions regarding treatment protocols.

DOSAGE RANGE

Owing to insufficient data available from clinical studies, doses have been derived from Australian manufacturers' recommendations.

> ***Practice points/Patient counselling***
> - Slippery elm inner bark is a highly mucilaginous substance, which has been traditionally used as a topical application to soothe irritated and inflamed skin conditions and promote wound healing.
> - It is used internally to soothe an irritated throat and is often combined with antiseptic herbs.
> - Slippery elm is used to provide symptomatic relief in acid dyspepsia, gastrointestinal reflux and inflammatory bowel diseases, but has not been scientifically studied to any significant extent.
> - Overall, slippery elm has not been significantly investigated in clinical studies, so most information is derived from traditional sources and the known activity or key constituents.

Gastrointestinal symptoms

- One to two capsules containing 150 mg of slippery elm before meals.
- Fluid extract (60%): 5 mL three times daily.
- Half a teaspoon of slippery elm bark powder is mixed with one cup of hot water and taken up to three times daily. For added flavouring, cinnamon or nutmeg can be added.

External use

- Mix the coarse powdered bark with enough boiling water to make a paste and use as a poultice (Hoffman 1983).

TOXICITY

Insufficient reliable information is available.

ADVERSE REACTIONS

Insufficient reliable information is available.

SIGNIFICANT INTERACTIONS

Controlled studies are unavailable, but interactions are theoretically possible with some medicines.

Since slippery elm forms an inert barrier over the gastrointestinal lining, it may theoretically alter the rate and/or extent of absorption of medicines with a narrow therapeutic range (e.g. barbiturates, digoxin, lithium, phenytoin, warfarin). The clinical significance of this is unclear. Separate doses by 2 hours.

CONTRAINDICATIONS AND PRECAUTIONS

Insufficient reliable information is available.

PREGNANCY USE

It is likely to be safe, but safety is still to be established.

PATIENTS' FAQs

What will this herb do for me?

The inner bark of slippery elm is highly mucilaginous, meaning that it forms a thick gel-like substance when combined with water. Traditionally, it has been used internally to relieve symptoms of dyspepsia and inflamed bowel conditions and topically to soothe irritated skin and promote wound healing.

When will it start to work?

Whether used internally for upper gastrointestinal symptoms (such as reflux and dyspepsia) or applied topically to irritated skin, it should theoretically provide quick symptomatic relief; however, research to confirm this is not available.

Are there any safety issues?

Although slippery elm has not been scientifically investigated, the US Food and Drug Administration has approved it as a safe demulcent substance.

REFERENCES

Beveridge RJ et al. Some structural features of the mucilage from the bark of *Ulmus fulvus*. Carbohydr Res 9 (1969): 429–439.

Cheung S, et al. Antioxidant and anti-inflammatory properties of ESSIAC and Flor-essence. Oncol Rep 14 (2005): 1345–1350.

Duke JA. Dr Duke's phytochemical and ethnobotanical databases. Beltsville, MD: US Department of Agriculture–Agricultural Research Service–National Germplasm Resources Laboratory, Beltsville Agricultural Research Center, 2003. Available online: www.ars-grin.gov/duke (accessed March, 2008).

Fisher C, Painter G. Materia Medica for the southern hemisphere. Auckland: Fisher-Painter Publishers, 1996.

Hawrelak JA, Myers, SP. Effects of two natural medicine formulations on irritable bowel syndrome symptoms: a pilot study. The Journal of Alternative and Complementary Medicine 16.10 (2010):1065–71.

Hoffman D. The new holistic herbal. Dorset: Element Books, 1983.

IM Gateway Database. Slippery elm review. Available online: www.imgateway.com (accessed May 2003).

Kulp KS et al. Essiac and Flor-Essence herbal tonics stimulate the in vitro growth of human breast cancer cells. Breast cancer research and treatment 98.3 (2006): 249–59.

Langmead L et al. Antioxidant effects of herbal therapies used by patients with inflammatory bowel disease: an in vitro study. Aliment Pharmacol Ther 16.2 (2002): 197–205.

Leonard SS et al. Essiac tea: scavenging of reactive oxygen species and effects on DNA damage. J Ethnopharmacol 103.2 (2006): 288–296.

Mazzio EA, & Soliman KFA. In vitro screening for the tumoricidal properties of international medicinal herbs. Phytotherapy Research, 23.3 (2009): 385–98.

Mills S, Bone K. Principles and practice of phytotherapy. London: Churchill Livingstone, 2000.

Morton, JF. Mucilaginous plants and their uses in medicine. Journal of Ethnopharmacology 29.3 (1990): 245–66.

Newell CA, et al. Herbal medicines: a guide for health care professionals. London, UK: Pharmaceutical Press, 1996.

Rousseau B, Watts CR. Slippery elm, its biochemistry, and use as a complementary and alternative treatment for laryngeal irritation. Journal of Investigational Biochemistry, 1.1 (2012): 17–23.

Smith M, Boon HS. Counseling cancer patients about herbal medicine. Patient Educ Couns 38 (1999): 109–120.

Ulbricht CE, Basch EM. Natural standard herb and supplement reference. St Louis: Mosby, 2005.

Zick SM et al. Trial of Essiac to ascertain its effect in women with breast cancer (TEA-BC). J Altern Complement Med 12.10 (2006): 971–980.

Soy

HISTORICAL NOTE Soybeans were one of the first crops grown by humans and have been consumed for approximately 5000 years in China, where they are regarded as both a food and a medicine. During the Chou dynasty (1134–246 BC), fermentation techniques were developed to produce tempeh, miso and tamari soy sauce, with tofu being invented around the second century BC. Soy first reached the West as imported soy sauce, and soybean cultivation began in the 1770s, primarily for animal feed. It was not until World War I that soy became a significant crop for human consumption (Natural Standard Patient Monograph 2005). Soy protein was first produced in the 1930s for its functional properties and used as a pigment binder for paper, as a foam for fire extinguishers and as a fibre for making artificial silk before being used as a food supplement in the 1960s.

S

COMMON NAME

Glycine max

OTHER NAMES

Glycine max, Glycine soja, Dolichos soja, Glycine gracilis, Glycine hispida, Phaseolus max, Soja hispida, Soja max

BOTANICAL NAME/FAMILY

Glycine max (family Fabaceae [Leguminosae])

PLANT PART USED

Bean

CHEMICAL COMPONENTS

Soybeans are a high-nutrient food containing up to 40% protein. Soy protein contains all of the essential amino acids in sufficient quantities to act as a sole protein source (Yimit et al 2012).

Soy is a major food source of phyto-oestrogens (isoflavones and lignans), with each gram of soy protein containing approximately 3.5 mg of isoflavones (Hamilton-Reeves et al 2010), including glycosides of genistein, daidzein and glycitein (Cederroth et al 2012, Napora et al 2011). Soy also contains the lignans secoisolariciresinol, matairesinol, syringaresinol, lariciresinol, isolariciresinol and pinoresinol (Peterson et al 2010), as well as soy lecithin (a phospholipid containing linoleic and linolenic acid), vitamin E (in its four isomeric forms as alpha, beta, gamma and delta-tocopherol), oligosaccharides, the phytosterols beta-sitosterol, campesterol and stigmasterol, phytates and protease inhibitors, inositol hexaphosphate, saponins and oligosaccharides (Cederroth & Nef 2009).

Soybeans are usually consumed as fermented and non-fermented soy foods such as miso, tempeh and tofu as well as whole soybeans, soy nuts, soy milk or soy cheese. In addition soy flour is a common ingredient in foods, beverages and condiments (Larkin et al 2008). Wide variability has been reported in the total amount of isoflavones in commercial soy products (Nurmi et al 2002).

Theories of whether cooking soy is more beneficial are still unclear as cooking increases some compounds in soy, such as daidzin, genistin, daidzein and antioxidants, but decreases genistein (Dong et al 2012).

MAIN ACTIONS

Trials have reported improvements in vasomotor symptoms, osteoporosis (as measured by increasing bone mineral density), prostate cancer and the cardiovascular risk biomarkers.

Daidzein, an isoflavone found in soy, is metabolised to the more metabolically active equol and O-desmethylangolensin (O-DMA) by intestinal bacteria (Cederroth et al 2012). In vitro studies have shown strains of *Eubacterium ramulus* and *Clostridrium* spp. produce O-DMA. Recently a strain from clostridrium was isolated in human faeces and shown to produce O-DMA (Frankfield 2011). Following soy or daidzein consumption, approximately 30–50% of the human population produce equol, and approximately 80–90% produce O-DMA. The significance of this is uncertain, despite some studies suggesting that the ability to produce equol and O-DMA may be associated with reduced risk of certain diseases, including breast and prostate cancers (Atkinson et al 2005, Frankfield 2011).

The mechanisms for the clinical effects of soy are yet to be fully evaluated (Balk et al 2005, Setchell & Cassidy 1999). Predicting the effects of isoflavones in vivo is difficult because the route of administration, chemical form of the phyto-oestrogen, its metabolism, bioavailability, half-life, timing and level of exposure, intrinsic oestrogenic state and the non-hormonal secondary mediated actions of isoflavones may all influence their biological and clinical effects (Setchell & Cassidy 1999).

Oestrogen receptor/hormonal modulation

Soy isoflavones and lignans share structural similarities with oestrogen and are referred to as phyto-oestrogens and/or selective oestrogen receptor modulators (SERMs) (Cederroth et al 2012, Wei et al 2012). The oestrogenic effects of soy are postulated to contribute to protective effects against cardiovascular disease (CVD), cancer and menopausal symptoms (Napora et al 2011). Although a review of 861 studies on the effects of phyto-oestrogens suggests that they are indeed biologically active in humans (Knight & Eden 1996), major gaps in knowledge still exist regarding the effects of phyto-oestrogen supplements on bone diseases, various cancers, menopausal symptoms and cognitive function (Gratten 2013, Lu et al 2001, Stark & Madar 2002).

The order of oestrogenic activity from soy isoflavones in in vivo assays is glycitein > genistein > daidzein (Carmignani et al 2012, PDRHealth 2004). Soy isoflavone glycosides bind weakly to both oestrogen receptors, with the binding affinity of genistein, dihydrogenistein and equol being comparable to the binding affinity of 17-beta-oestradiol (Cederroth et al 2012, Morito et al 2001).

Isoflavones have complex actions that may be tissue-specific and may act as partial oestrogen agonists and antagonists, as well as having non-classical effects on plasma membranes and cell signalling pathways (Barrett 2006, Setchell & Cassidy 1999).

Interestingly, soy has a greater affinity for the oestrogen beta-receptor than the alpha-receptor (Carmignani et al 2012). The beta-receptor is found in brain (Weiser et al 2008), bone and vascular epithelia, tissues in which isoflavones purportedly have activity. To a lesser extent, the beta-receptor is also found in the dome of the bladder (Ablove et al 2009, Setchell & Cassidy 1999).

Genistein has been found to have an oestrogen-like effect on the serum lipid profile, having a particular effect on CYP19 in the liver (Ye et al 2009). However, in a double-blind, placebo-controlled trial in 40 healthy postmenopausal women aged 50–75 years, 40 g of soy protein containing 118 mg isoflavones did not produce biologically significant oestrogenic effects on coagulation, fibrinolysis or endothelial function (Teede et al 2005).

Hormonal effects in men

To date the evidence on soy and male reproductive health is unclear and requires further longer-term studies (Cederroth et al 2012). A meta-analysis found no significant effects of soy protein or isoflavone intake on measures of bioavailable testosterone concentrations in men. This included testosterone, sex hormone-binding globulin, free testosterone and free androgen index (Hamilton-Reeves et al 2010).

Cardiovascular disease

There are many potential mechanisms by which soy isoflavones may improve cardiovascular outcomes, including reduction in total cholesterol, low-density lipoprotein (LDL), high-density lipoprotein (HDL), triglycerides, lipoprotein A, blood pressure (Rebholz et al 2013) and endothelial function (Cano et al 2010). While soy has anti-inflammatory properties, there appears to be little effect on reducing C-reactive protein (CRP), other inflammatory markers (Bakhtiary et al 2012) or homocysteine (Marini et al 2010). However study results are limited and inconclusive (Rebholz et al 2013) and reducing vascular inflammation and homocysteine concentrations are unlikely to be the mechanisms by which soy reduces the risk of CVD (Greany et al 2008).

It has been postulated that soy isoflavones influence nitric oxide-dependent vasorelaxation. However, in a small randomised controlled trial (n = 24), postmenopausal women with high-normal blood pressure and a body mass index <30 were supplemented with 80 mg of soy per day (or placebo) for 6 weeks. The study found no change in nitric oxide, arginine or rulline flux from baseline measures (Wong et al 2012). Conversely, in an earlier study, postmenopausal women (n = 22) received a low-fat test meal, with or without 80 mg isoflavones (containing both genistein and daidzein), in random order 1 week apart. Flow-mediated dilatation and plasma nitric oxide concentrations were greater in the treatment group compared with control, demonstrating that isoflavones have an acute effect on endothelial function in postmenopausal women. This suggests possible effects on endothelial function. Furthermore, the anti-inflammatory and vasodilatory actions of nitric oxide may potentially retard atherosclerosis development in postmenopausal women, but large, robustly designed, randomised, controlled dietary intervention trials are required to confirm this. It should also be noted that 80 mg is a relatively large dose of isoflavones compared with dietary intakes of between 30 and 50 mg/day in Asian countries such as China and Japan, although not so large as to be a physiological impossibility (Hall et al 2008).

Additional mechanisms include an inhibition of proinflammatory cytokines, cell adhesion proteins and inducible nitric oxide production, potential reduction in the susceptibility of the LDL particle to oxidation, inhibition of platelet aggregation and an improvement in vascular reactivity (Rimbach et al 2008).

Consumption of soy protein may also produce cardiovascular benefits through various mechanisms, including the low methionine content reducing serum homocysteine concentration (Nagata et al 2003), reduction of the insulin/glucagon ratio (Imani et al 2009, Napora et al 2011, Sanchez & Hubbard 1991) and downregulation of the hepatic transcription factor sterol regulatory element binding protein-1, which in turn reduces lipotoxicity in the liver (Torres et al 2006). Other possible mechanisms include: regulation of hepatic lipid metabolism through upregulation of LDL receptors and increase in bile acid secretion (Potter 1995), although the mechanisms are unclear (Maki et al 2010), reducing hepatic fatty acid and triglyceride biosynthesis and increasing fatty acid oxidation (Tovar et al 2005), preventing the transfer of fatty acids to extra adipose tissues by increasing the adipocyte hormone adiponectin (Nagasawa et al 2003) and increasing bile acid secretion and bacterial conversion of cholesterol to the non-absorbable coprostanol (Huff & Carroll 1980).

Soybean protein has been shown to reduce E-selectin and leptin levels (Rebholz et al 2013). Soy protein peptides may also act to decrease intestinal cholesterol absorption and bile acid uptake, reduce aortic accumulation of cholesterol esters and suppress food intake and gastric emptying by increasing cholecystokinin and inhibiting angiotensin-converting enzyme (Torres et al 2006).

It is unclear how soy exerts its beneficial effects on lipid metabolism or exactly which components are most active. It is suspected that these include soy protein, bioactive peptides, interaction of isoflavones within the intact soy matrix or other compounds (Cassidy & Hooper 2006, Torres et al 2006). It is reported that isolated soy protein that maintains the native protein structure is more effective in reducing serum lipids than denatured protein (Hoie et al 2007). Soy protein is also reported to have beneficial effects on renal function, with suggestions that the isoflavones genistein and daidzein reduce glomerular damage by protecting LDL from oxidation and the high arginine content acts as a precursor for nitric oxide, thus improving renal flow (Torres et al 2006).

There may be variations in the response to soy and its components in different population groups. Greater isoflavone intake is associated with better vascular endothelial function and lower carotid atherosclerotic burden in people at high risk of cardiovascular events (Chan et al 2007). Soy supplementation improves endothelial function in renal transplant patients (Cupisti et al 2007) and soy isoflavones improve systemic arterial compliance in perimenopausal and menopausal women (Nestel et al 1997). Soy protein, regardless of isoflavone content, modulates serum lipid ratios in a direction beneficial for CVD risk in healthy young men (McVeigh et al 2006) and soy consumption is associated with decreased carotid intima media thickness and plasma lipids, with the association being stronger for men than women (Zhang et al 2008). Interestingly, studies have revealed improvements in biomarkers such as LDL-cholesterol and CRP in those with plasma S-equol levels of >5–10 ng/mL (Jackson et al 2011), so individuals may vary in their response to soy and its components.

Antiosteoporotic

There has been speculation that the oestrogenic effects of soy isoflavone may help prevent osteoporosis (Cvejić et al 2012). Recent systematic reviews of over 30 studies suggest that soy protein prevents bone loss and inhibits excretion of urinary deoxypyridinoline. In human trials, 35 g/day soy protein for 12 weeks was found to significantly reduce urinary deoxypyridinoline and increase total alkaline phosphatase in a small study of 15 women aged 45–64 years (Roudsari et al 2005). However further studies are required to address the clinical effect of soy isoflavones on bone turnover markers and bone alkaline phosphatase (Taku et al 2011, Wei et al 2012).

Anticancer

Soy phyto-oestrogens are converted by gut bacteria to derivatives with weak oestrogenic and antioxidant properties, and epidemiological studies suggest that the highest plasma levels of their metabolites are found in individuals living in countries or regions with a low incidence of both cancer and CVD (Cederroth et al 2012, Jackson et al 2011). Although soy phyto-oestrogens have been implicated in soy's anticarcinogenic activity, a causal relationship to disease prevention is hypothetical, as the exact mechanisms have not been fully elucidated (Adlercreutz 2002a, 2002b).

There are multiple mechanisms by which soy protein may protect against cancer, as there is evidence for soy isoflavones having oestrogenic, anti-oestrogenic, antioxidant and antiproliferative activities (Leclerq & Jacquot 2014, Zhang et al 2012). Soy also contains other putative anticarcinogenic compounds, such as lignans, saponins, phytates, protease inhibitors and phytosterols (Cederroth & Nef 2009), and it is possible that soy consumption may be a marker for other dietary factors that provide anticancer properties.

Soy isoflavones inhibit transcription factors and genes that are essential for tumour cell growth (Hillman & Singh-Gupta 2011). Both in vitro and in vivo studies have shown genistein (the main active compound found in soy) inhibits cell growth of malignant tumours (Hillman & Singh-Gupta 2011). In vitro experiments also have shown that isoflavones inhibit the activity of aromatase and 17β-hydroxysteroid dehydrogenases involved in the synthesis of oestradiol from circulating androgens and oestrones (Brooks & Thompson 2005, Chi et al 2013, Lacey et al 2005).

The effects of soy on oestrogen metabolism and synthesis may contribute to the anticancer activity, as studies have shown that oestrogen inhibits cancer cell proliferation by promoting a more beneficial 2-OH E1:16-alpha-OH E1 ratio (Morimoto et al 2012).

Furthermore, soy phyto-oestrogens may influence cancer growth through effects on oestrogen receptors, through inhibition of tyrosine and other protein kinases, and aromatase enzymes, alteration of growth factor activity and inhibition of angiogenesis (Cederroth et al 2012, Nynca et al 2013). In terms of initiation or progression of breast cancer, soy isoflavones may have a protective effect due to their ability to inhibit the local production of oestrogens from circulating precursors in breast tissue (Kang et al 2010).

After menopause, oestrogens are synthesised in peripheral tissue and exert their effects locally. In vitro studies have shown that isoflavones inhibit aromatase activity, which is thought to have a protective action against breast cancer formation (Kang et al 2010).

Genistein is the most studied of the phyto-oestrogens and has weak oestrogenic activity but is not fully understood (Nynca et al 2013, Yuan-Jing et al 2009). It has also been found to cause apoptosis in cancer cells (Hillman & Singh-Gupta 2011), stimulate several antioxidative enzymes, such as catalase, superoxide dismutase, glutathione peroxidase and reductase, induce tumour cell differentiation, downregulate the epidermal growth factor receptor and erbB2/Neu receptors in cancer cells, and also possibly inhibit tumour cell invasion by inhibiting matrix metallopeptidase-9 (92 kDa type IV collagenase) (Adlercreutz 2002a, 2002b). Genistein and daidzein were shown to suppress breast cancer genes *BRCA1* and *BRCA2* after a 3-day incubation period (Satih et al 2009, Yuan et al 2012).

Genistein is also reported to inhibit angiogenesis, DNA topoisomerase II, protein tyrosine kinases, aromatase, nuclear factor-kappaB and to downregulate transforming growth factor-beta and stimulate the sex hormone-binding globulin (Cederroth & Nef 2009, PDRHealth 2004). Isoflavones have also been shown to inhibit the activity of aromatase (CYP19), thus decreasing oestrogen biosynthesis and producing antioestrogenic effects, which may be important in breast and prostate cancers (Li et al 2011).

Soy isoflavones also demonstrate a variety of oestrogen-independent activities, and some of them are directly associated with the suppression of the invasive behaviour of breast cancer cells (Korde et al 2009). Furthermore, it is suggested that variability in xenobiotic metabolising enzymes and the effect of flavonoid ingestion on enzyme activity may contribute to individual variations in susceptibility to diseases such as cancer (Moon et al 2006).

Although in vitro and animal models point to several pathways by which isoflavones may reduce the incidence of cancer (Rosenberg Zand et al 2002), and experimental evidence also exists for an inhibitory effect of soy bran on prostate cancer growth and of isolated lignans on colon cancer (Adlercreutz 2002a, 2002b), clinical trial data supporting this are still lacking.

Evidence on whether isoflavones are preventive or therapeutic in cancer treatment is inconclusive and unclear, as some in vitro and in vivo studies suggest that isoflavones may induce oestrogen-dependent cancers. Longer-term trials (>4 years) are required to investigate this possibility (Bhoo-Pathy et al 2013, Hooper et al 2010).

OTHER ACTIONS

Antioxidant

Oxygen stress is believed to contribute to menopause and degenerative changes associated with ageing and it is suggested that antioxidants, such as soy isoflavones, may help to protect mitochondria against premature oxidative damage (Larkin et al 2008). Although several clinical trials have suggested that soy intake decreases oxidative stress and that soy isoflavones, such as genistein, have antioxidant properties in vitro, results of supplementation in clinical trials are inconclusive. Furthermore, diets relatively high in soy protein or soy-derived isoflavones are reported to have little effect on plasma antioxidant capacity or biomarkers of oxidative stress (Vega-Lopez et al 2005). In equol producers, S-equol may prevent the oxidation of LDL (Jackson et al 2011). Hwang et al (2000) have reported that equol may act synergistically with ascorbic acid to inhibit the metal-induced oxidation of LDL.

Cognitive function

Soy isoflavones may mimic the actions and functions of oestrogen on the brain, and they have been shown to have positive effects on cognitive function in females, whereas results in males are inconsistent. Soy isoflavones, and particularly genistein, have been suggested to influence cognitive function via an oestrogen receptor-mediated pathway and via the inhibition of tyrosine kinase; however, definitive data are still lacking (Sumien et al 2013).

CLINICAL USE

Soy protein and soy isoflavones have been the subject of much scientific investigation in recent decades. Several epidemiological studies have shown beneficial effects with high-dose isoflavones in menopausal symptoms, CVD (specifically atherosclerosis and stroke), reducing risk of breast and prostate cancer, possible improvements in bone health and neurodegeneration (Dhananjaya et al 2012, Patisaul & Jefferson 2010). Similarly, soy protein has demonstrated health benefits, chiefly in CVD prevention (via improving lipid profiles) (Anderson & Bush 2011).

Menopausal symptoms

The natural oestrogen receptor activity of soy isoflavones is popularly considered an alternative to controversial hormone replacement therapy for postmenopausal women (Sliva 2005).

In regard to hot flushes, the effects of phyto-oestrogens are still far from being fully understood. However, in general, studies show isoflavones can reduce the frequency and severity of vasomotor symptoms. Women with a higher consumption of isoflavones tend to have less frequent and less severe hot flushes and night sweats (Bedell et al 2014, Moreira et al 2014). The North American Menopause Society in 2011 also concluded that soy-based isoflavones are modestly effective in relieving menopausal symptoms and supplements providing higher proportions of genistein or increases in S( ) equol may provide more benefits.

While many people focus on the potential effects of isoflavones on hot flushes, there is also clinical trial evidence that isoflavones significantly improve sleep efficiency and reduce sleep disturbances in postmenopausal women. One double-blind study showed that 80 mg isoflavones over 4 months was significantly superior to placebo and another showed that doses of either 52 mg or 104 mg daily of isoflavones over 12 months were effective (Drews et al 2007b, Hachul et al 2011).

Determining an optimal dose is difficult; however, it is generally believed that at least 40–104 mg/day of total soy isoflavones is sufficient. This dose is consistent with intakes in countries that consume soy as a staple, and is also the level at which clinical endocrine effects can be seen in premenopausal women (Bedell et al 2014). Whether an individual responds to isoflavones is thought to partly depend on their ability to effectively biotransform daidzein to equol in the intestines, as equol has an oestrogenic activity several magnitudes greater than diadzein, a major metabolite of soy isoflavones (Jackson et al 2011). The conversion is mediated by intestinal bacteria and factors such as diet, antibiotic use and illness will affect the equol-producing ability of an individual (Bedell et al 2014).

Unfortunately, making a definitive conclusion as to whether soy isoflavones reduce the frequency and severity of hot flushes is more complex, as meta-analyses tend to group various soy interventions together, making interpretation difficult. For instance, a 2010 meta-analysis of 19 studies concluded that, even though the overall combined results showed a significant tendency in favour of soy, it was still difficult to establish conclusive results given the high heterogeneity of the studies (Bolanos et al 2010). The studies in the analysis were randomised controlled trials, including a placebo arm, and of a 12-week treatment duration. The intervention was loosely described as 'soy dietary supplement', 'soy extract' or 'isoflavone concentrate' (genistein or daidzein), with greatest results seen for the soy concentrate intervention.

A 2011 systematic review and meta-analysis investigating soy extracts, hormone replacement therapy and hot flushes concluded that both interventions are efficacious in reducing hot flushes in postmenopausal women when compared to placebo (Bolanos-Diaz et al 2011). To tease out the results further, a comparison study was analysed which found that daily hot flushes reduced by 22% with genistein concentrate treatment compared to a 53% reduction with daily oestrogen-progestogen therapy compared to placebo over 12 weeks. As such, while both treatments are effective, isoflavones are a weaker treatment.

A recent Cochrane systematic review of 30 studies looking at phyto-oestrogen treatment of vasomotor symptoms for peri- and postmenopausal women showed that soy extract preparations globally demonstrated mixed results; however, three placebo-controlled studies conducted from 2002 to 2008 showed a significant reduction in flush frequency: 61%, 74% and 50% compared with placebo (21%, 43% and 38% reduction respectively) (Villaseca 2012). Additionally, significant improvements in vasomotor symptoms have been described in the more recent placebo-controlled trials with soy products.

An older systematic review and meta-analysis that included 17 trials found that isoflavone supplementation significantly reduced hot flushes, with the percentage reduction being related to the number of baseline flushes per day and the dose of isoflavone studied (Howes et al 2006). More recent studies have also reported that isoflavone supplementation reduces hot flushes (Eden 2012). In an Australian randomised controlled trial, 60 postmenopausal women were supplemented with 90 mg of soy isoflavone, 1 mg oestradiol or placebo. After 16 weeks of therapy there was a significant improvement in hot flushes and urogenital symptoms in the soy and oestradiol groups, although there was no statistically significant difference with respect to the overall Menopause Rating Scale or psychological symptoms (Carmignani et al 2012).

One of the largest studies conducted to determine whether soy isoflavones have a favourable effect on hot flushes was the Soy Phytoestrogens as Replacement Estrogens (SPARE) study in 2004, funded by the US National Institutes of Health. This was a double-blinded, single-centre randomised controlled trial involving 248 healthy women with the onset of menopause within 5 years of enrolment who received either daily soy isoflavones (200 mg) or placebo for 2 years (Chalupka 2011). There was no significant difference between the soy group and placebo group regarding hot flush symptoms after 2 years; however this study did not attempt to differentiate between reduced frequency and reduced intensity. As Bedell et al (2014) point out, studies that make the distinction between frequency and severity of hot flushes tend to produce positive results. The example they give is a study by Drews et al (2007a), which involved 169 postmenopausal women and showed treatment with 104 mg of isoflavones daily reduced both the frequency and the intensity of hot flushes. This study also noted that treatment significantly decreased sleep disturbances ($P < 0.05$) and decreased headache, dizziness, arthrosis pain, tiredness, palpitation and breathlessness ($P < 0.05$). In addition, treatment with Soyfem (a standardised isoflavone extract) improved the variability and moderation of depressive mood ($P < 0.05$) (Drews et al 2007a).

Theories explaining inconsistent results

Although some trial data seem to support the efficacy of isoflavones in reducing the incidence and severity of hot flushes, other studies have not found any difference between the isoflavone recipients and the controls (Lethaby et al 2010). These inconsistent results may be due to insufficient sample size, variations in the isoflavone type, content or delivery form of the preparations used or varying responses in different population groups. To add to the confusion, the source of isoflavones is not always reported and the composition and dose of soy supplements and isoflavone content vary considerably between studies, which makes comparisons and interpretations difficult (Low Dog 2005).

Another key factor which is thought to affect response rates is whether an individual can effectively produce equol from daidzein, a metabolite of soy isoflavones (Jackson et al 2011). This is clinically relevant since the oestrogen agonist potency of equol is much greater than its precursor, daidzein. Equol thus serves as the reference compound associated with the health benefits of isoflavone consumption (Bedell et al 2014).

Clinical note — What are phyto-oestrogens?

Phyto-oestrogens are constituents found in plants which have a similar chemical structure to oestradiol (E2).

They have a phenolic ring which means they can bind to oestrogen receptors. They also have a molecular weight similar to E2 and can work as either agonists or antagonists at oestrogen receptor sites. The cellular effects of phyto-oestrogens are influenced by many factors, including concentration, receptor status, presence or absence of endogenous oestrogens and the target tissue (Moreira et al 2014).

There are four main classes of phyto-oestrogens: isoflavones, lignans, coumestans and stilbenes. Isoflavones from soy and soy derivatives are the most common phyto-oestrogens and genistein and daidzein are the most studied. Lignans are the most prevalent phyto-oestrogens in nature and many are commonly found in the human diet, such as in oilseeds, flaxseed and grains such as wheat, rye and oat and in various types of berries. Coumestans and stilbenes are less abundant in the diet and are less well studied. Coumestrol is a coumestan found in clover and alfalfa sprouts and in lower concentrations in lima bean and sunflower seeds, among other sources, whereas resveratrol is the most studied stilbene, being present in grapes, peanuts and cranberries (Moreira et al 2014). All phyto-oestrogens are SERMs and each has a profile of action of its own (Bedell et al 2014).

Cardiovascular disease

Both soy-derived isoflavones and soy protein have been investigated for potential benefits in CVD. A meta-analysis of 43 randomised controlled trials concluded that soy protein was protective against CVD due to beneficial effects on lipid profiles (Anderson & Bush 2011). In addition, substantial data from epidemiological surveys and nutritional interventions in humans and animals indicate that soy protein reduces serum total and LDL cholesterol and triglycerides, as well as hepatic cholesterol and triglycerides (Torres et al 2006). Based on this data, the US Food and Drug Administration has approved a food label health claim stating that a diet with a daily intake of 25 g of soy protein and low in saturated fat and cholesterol may reduce the risk of heart disease (Balk et al 2005). This claim, however, is based largely on studies demonstrating beneficial effects on lipids and other biomarkers rather than hard end points (Anderson & Bush 2011, Cassidy & Hooper 2006).

A recent Cochrane review (five randomised controlled trials) concluded that there is no evidence to suggest that isoflavones have any impact on improving lipid profiles (Qin et al 2013). Despite this, other effects of benefit in CVD have been reported. For example, a reduction in the risk of both cerebral and myocardial infarctions was reported in a cohort study of Japanese women with a high consumption of isoflavones (Kokubo et al 2007). In addition, the World Health Organization CARDIAC study determined the relationship between the mortality rate of coronary heart disease and the consumption of soy products and isoflavones. It was shown that individuals in China and Japan who excreted >10 mmol isoflavones daily experienced a lower rate of coronary heart disease (<100 events per 100,000 people) than those with <1 mmol/day (>500 events per 100,000 people) (Jackson et al 2011, Yamori 2007).

Some population groups may have a better response to soy than others. For instance, thoughts surround an increased risk of CVD amongst postmenopausal women, which may in part be due to a reduction in ovarian function (Cano et al 2010).

Limitations surround many clinical trials, making it difficult to ascertain the true effects of isoflavones on cardiovascular health. Small populations and inconsistent soy forms and doses are the main reasons for such a diverse difference in results.

Hypercholesterolaemia

A meta-analysis of 43 randomised controlled trials concluded that, on average, a daily intake of 30 g of soy protein per day was protective against CVD, showing a significant reduction in lipoproteins. LDL-cholesterol was reduced by 5.5% and triglycerides by 10%, with a slight (3%) increase in HDL (Anderson & Bush 2011). Soy isoflavones do not appear to be as effective as soy protein, as demonstrated by a Cochrane review which reported on five randomised controlled trials (n = 208, 104 each in intervention and control groups) which ranged in length from 3 to 6 months and investigated the effect of isoflavone versus placebo on lipid profiles (Qin et al 2013). Overall the authors concluded a lack of substantive evidence for isoflavone use in lowering cholesterol in hypercholesterolaemic patients. When compared with placebo, two trials (Aubertin-Leheudre et al 2007, Dewell 2002) showed a small but significant effect on triglycerides in the isoflavone group (mean difference −0.46 mmol/L: 95% confidence interval −0.84 to −0.09; P = 0.02; n = 52), but no significant difference was found on total cholesterol, LDL-cholesterol and HDL-cholesterol between the treatment and control group. The review reported a potential risk of high (or unclear) level of bias and relatively low participant numbers.

A number of other systematic reviews have been conducted over the years, with varying conclusions (Balk et al 2005, Cassidy & Hooper 2006, Dewell et al 2006, Reynolds et al 2006, Taku et al 2008, Yang et al 2011, Zhan & Ho 2005).

Dyslipidaemia is more prevalent amongst females, particularly postmenopausal, due to endocrine changes and physiological mechanisms (Bakhtiary et al 2012). In a 12-week randomised controlled trial 75 women aged 60–70 and diagnosed with metabolic syndrome were given 35 g of soy nuts per day, 35 g per day soy protein (textured soy protein) or placebo. Both soy groups had improved lipid profiles and apolipoprotein. Significant decreases in serum total cholesterol were also observed in both treatment groups compared with the control group (P < 0.005). Comparison of results between treatment groups showed soy nuts were more beneficial. Soy nuts significantly improved LDL-cholesterol, very-low-density-lipoprotein cholesterol and ApoB100 levels (P < 0.05). Changes in total cholesterol, HDL-cholesterol, fibrinogen, CRP and blood pressure were not significant between treatment and control groups (Bakhtiary et al 2012). A study investigated the effects of traditional fermented soybean products on body mass index, reproductive hormones, lipids and glucose among 60 postmenopausal Thai women. Along with their usual diet, the experimental group (n = 31) were supplemented for 6 months with approximately 60 mg of isoflavone per day from traditional fermented soybean products. Favourable effects on progesterone and cholesterol were found, while oestradiol, glucose and triglycerides were not affected. Interestingly, a decrease of oestradiol and an increase of glucose were found in the control group (Sapbamrer et al 2013). Another randomised controlled trial (n = 389) found an improvement in lipid profiles and a reduction in CVD in postmenopausal women. However, both arms of the study were on restricted diets and were supplemented with therapeutic doses of calcium and vitamin D and either 54 mg genistein or placebo (Marini et al 2010).

Blood pressure

In addition to possible effects on lipids, epidemiological data suggest that soy may affect blood pressure. A systematic review of 11 randomised controlled trials concluded that doses of 65–153 mg soy isoflavones improved blood pressure in hypertensive patients but had no effect on normotensive subjects (Liu et al 2012). Another review supports these findings, concluding that there was a positive effect on systolic (SBP) but not diastolic blood pressure (DBP) (Kyoko et al 2010), although several earlier reviews found no evidence of a reduction in blood pressure (Balk et al 2005, Rosero Arenas et al 2008). Further studies are required to confirm these findings.

The Shanghai Women's Health Study was one of the more influential epidemiological studies supporting the role of soy in blood pressure reduction. In this observational study of 45,694 participants, aged 40–70 years, with no history of hypertension, diabetes or CVD, the intake of soy foods over 2–3 years was inversely associated with both SBP and DBP, particularly among elderly women. Results of this study found that, compared to women consuming less than 2.5 g/day of soy, consumption of more than 25 g/day was associated with a significant reduction in SBP of 1.9 mmHg and a significant reduction in DBP of 0.9 mmHg, and that the inverse association between soy consumption and blood pressure became stronger with increasing age, with significant reductions of 4.9 mmHg for SBP and 2.2 mmHg for DBP in women aged over 60 years (Yang et al 2005). Once again, equol producers may experience more favourable responses than non-producers (Kreijkamp-Kaspers et al 2005).

Diabetes and diabetic nephropathy

Replacing animal protein with soy protein has been found to improve various disease markers in patients with type 1 or type 2 diabetes (Yang et al 2011).

Although there are positive results with the use of soy to improve blood glucose levels, a meta-analysis that included 24 trials (n = 1518) using soy isoflavones concluded that soy consumption did not significantly affect measures of glycaemic control and there was no improvement in overall fasting glucose or insulin levels (Liu et al 2011). However, in subgroup analysis, a favourable change in fasting glucose concentrations was observed in the studies that utilised whole-soy foods or a soy diet (Liu et al 2011).

Interventions which increase dietary soy intake have revealed a number of potential benefits, including improvements in HbA_{1C}, a reduction in weight and in sulfonylureas and metformin use in type 2 diabetes patients (Li et al 2005); and improvements in glycaemic control and lipid profiles in obese individuals (Deibert et al 2004). It may also be of benefit in diabetic nephropathy, with several small studies showing possible improvements in glomerular filtration rate in young adults with type 1 diabetes mellitus (Stephenson et al 2005); reduced urinary albumin and improved lipid profiles in males with type 2 diabetes and nephropathy (Teixeira et al 2004); and improved renal function and lipid profile in patients with type 2 diabetes and nephropathy (Azadbakht et al 2003).

Cancer prevention

High levels of phyto-oestrogens (lignans and isoflavonoids) are frequently associated with low risk of breast, prostate and colon cancers, and breast cancer and multiple epidemiological studies have identified an inverse relationship between soy consumption and cancer risk (Badger et al 2005, Trock et al 2006, Wu et al 2008b). For example, in a cohort study of over 73,000 Chinese women who consumed either dietary isoflavones or soy protein, only 546 case reports of breast cancer were recorded, suggesting that soy protein and/or isoflavone consumption may be protective (Lee et al 2009). The protective effect of soy food consumption was reiterated in 2011 by the North American Menopause Society, which concluded that soy foods generally appear to be breast cancer-protective and recommended moderate lifelong dietary soy consumption as part of a healthy lifestyle. They confirmed that, based on the latest evidence, soy food consumption is associated with lower risk of breast and endometrial cancer in observational studies, and soy food consumption or intervention in women does not promote breast cancer growth or cancer recurrence. However, specific recommendations regarding breast cancer survivors and soy or isoflavone consumption could not be reached, as studies in humans imply a null or protective effect, whereas animal studies indicate potential for risk.

It has been suggested that the protective effect is most pronounced for women of Asian background, as a 2011 meta-analysis of 14 studies of breast cancer incidence found that consumption of soy isoflavones was associated with reduced risk of breast cancer incidence (relative risk 0.89); however, the effect was limited to Asian populations, and did not apply to Western populations (Dong & Qin 2011). Encouragingly, a 2011 meta-analysis revealed that, overall, soy may reduce the mortality and morbidity of cancer incidence and increase survival rates (Hillman & Singh-Gupta 2011). Furthermore, soy intake after cancer diagnosis has been associated with reduced mortality and recurrence (Hillman & Singh-Gupta 2011).

In any investigation on the role of soy and its anticancer properties, there are several variables that need to be acknowledged and considered both within the design of any studies, and within systematic reviews and meta-analyses. Some of these variables include different types and amounts of soy consumed amongst different populations. For example, Asian diets generally contain greater amounts of soy compared with Western populations. Thus when a mix of both Asian and Western population-based studies is analysed in the one meta-analysis or systematic review, this requires attention and consideration (Morimoto et al 2012, Wu et al 2008a). Another confounding factor is that Western lifestyle may influence cancer risk due to dietary choices that are independent of soy consumption (Morimoto et al 2012, Wu et al 2008a). Effects are likely to be dose-dependent (Wu et al 2008a). The timing may also be important with reviews suggesting soy may be beneficial if consumed in early life before puberty or during adolescence (Adlercreutz 2002a, 2002b). A further study suggests that the protective effect of soy differs by receptor status, with reduced risk being evident in women who are oestrogen and progesterone receptor-positive and HER2 receptor-negative (Suzuki et al 2008).

Most recently, in a randomised controlled trial of 82 premenopausal women, a low- and high-soy-based diet was compared over 6 months. Following a wash-out period, the participants crossed over to the alternative diet for a further 6 months. The participants were Asian, American and Caucasian. In the high-soy group, participants consumed two daily servings of soy foods per week. In the low-soy group participants consumed less than three servings of soy-based foods per week. Assessment of intake was done using 24-hour diet recall and through urinary analysis to assess the level of isoflavones. The study observed a possible influence of two daily soy food servings on urinary oestrogen excretion; however there was little or no change in oestrone, oestradiol and oestriol. There was a small statistically significant benefit for soy as a protective measure against breast cancer, due to the ability of soy to modify oestrogen metabolism, resulting in a lower exposure to carcinogenic metabolites (Morimoto et al 2012).

Prostate cancer

Soy proteins, common in the Asian diet, have been shown to inhibit prostate cancer cell growth (Kurahashi et al 2008, Sonn et al 2005). Prostatic tissue appears to readily accumulate potentially anticancerous isoflavones (Gardner et al 2009) and in vitro studies support findings of soy being protective against prostate cancer (Dong et al 2012). For instance, genistein appears to suppress cyclooxygenase-2 pathways, which is often seen to be a leading cause of prostate cancer (Swami et al 2009).

In an epidemiological study of over 82,000 men, legume intake was associated with a moderate reduction in prostate cancer risk but this was unrelated to isoflavone content (Park et al 2008), while a case-controlled study suggests that isoflavones might be an effective dietary protective factor against prostate cancer in Japanese men (Nagata et al 2007). In randomised controlled trials in men aged 50–80 years, 12 months' supplementation with 83 mg/day isoflavones did not alter serum levels of prostate-specific antigen in healthy men (Adams et al 2004), while 60 mg/day of soy isoflavone did alter serum prostate-specific antigen and free testosterone in some men with early-stage prostate cancer (Kumar et al 2004). In another randomised controlled trial involving 29 men with prostate cancer and scheduled to undergo a radical prostatectomy, supplementation with bread containing 50 g of soy grits was found to significantly reduce prostate-specific antigen levels (Dalais et al 2004). A recent randomised controlled trial was unable to demonstrate effects of 20 g of soy protein isolate on the recurrence of prostate cancer following radical prostatectomy (Bosland et al 2013).

Lung cancer

In non-smoking women, an inverse relationship has been observed between lung cancer survival and soy food consumption prior to diagnosis (Yang et al 2013). Compared with the median intake of soy food, fully adjusted hazard ratios for total mortality were lower in those with the highest soy intake versus the lowest (90th percentile hazard ratio 0.89 vs 10th percentile hazard ratio 1.81).

> ***Clinical note — Soy and breast cancer patients***
>
> As isoflavones exert oestrogen-like activity, there is some concern about their use in women with a history of breast cancer. When phyto-oestrogens bind to either alpha or beta oestrogen receptors they initiate cell differentiation (Leclercq & Jacquot 2014). They are also reported to increase cortisol, and activate or interfere with some neurotransmitters (Leclercq & Jacquot 2014). Genistein has been shown to stimulate oestrogen-mediated tumour cell growth and induce aromatase activity (van Duursen et al 2011). There are also concerns that soy constituents may interfere with tamoxifen therapy and encourage cancer cell proliferation (Chi et al 2013).
>
> The NSW Cancer Council supports the consumption of soy foods in the diet as part of the national dietary guidelines to eat a diet high in plant-based foods. The current position statement from the Australian Cancer Council does not recommend or support the use of supplements such as soy protein isolates or isoflavone capsules for healthy men and women to prevent cancer. There is evidence to suggest that women with existing breast cancer or past breast cancer should be cautious in consuming large quantities of soy foods or phyto-oestrogen supplements (Cancer Council 2009). However, according to current research, soy consumption may be protective against postmenopausal (but not necessarily premenopausal) breast cancer (Wada et al 2013) and may lower the recurrence of breast cancer, especially in postmenopausal women (Chi et al 2013, Guha 2009, Shu et al 2009). Soy isoflavones consumed at levels comparable to those in Asian populations may reduce the risk of cancer recurrence in women receiving tamoxifen therapy and do not appear to interfere with tamoxifen efficacy (Guha 2009).
>
> A study on children supports the use of dietary soy in reducing breast cancer risk in later life. Although the results are not strong, they are promising and are encouraging for further research in childhood exposure to soy (Korde et al 2009).

Osteoporosis prevention and bone mass

Despite a small number of conflicting studies, the body of evidence available indicates a positive relationship between soy isoflavones and bone health (Bedell et al 2014). Inconsistencies were mainly seen in early studies, whereas the majority of those conducted in the last decade that followed participants for longer time intervals tended to demonstrate a positive effect on bone mineral density.

A 2013 systematic review of studies investigating isoflavones confirmed that in vitro and animal studies show a positive effect on increasing bone mineral density and decreasing bone turnover resorption markers (Castelo-Branco & Soveral 2013, Wei et al 2012). The effect of soy isoflavones on bone mineral density is mediated by equol production, reproductive status, supplement type, isoflavone dose and intervention duration. As such, a key factor is how efficiently an individual produces equol, and equol producers seem to have a more positive response to isoflavone intervention and diets, which could help maintain peak bone mass in premenopausal women. Whether isoflavones in perimenopausal women attenuate bone loss in the menopausal transition is insufficiently studied but current results are promising. In the postmenopausal period, isoflavones may present a modest benefit but their clinical relevance in preventing osteoporotic fractures remain to be determined (Castelo-Branco & Soveral 2013).

It seems that in both animal and human studies the route of administration, the dose and, in animal studies, the type of animal all seem to affect the results (Patisaul & Jefferson 2010). In humans, effects appear to become more significant when more than 90 mg/day of isoflavones is consumed for at least 6 months (Castelo-Branco & Cancelo Hidalgo 2011, Ma et al 2008, Wei et al 2012). More specifically, the effect of isoflavones appears greatest for lumbar spine bone mineral density but not hip, femoral neck and trochanter bone mineral density in menopausal women (Taku et al 2010, 2011). The meta-analysis of clinical studies by Taku et al (2011) investigating bone turnover concluded that, while soy had no specific therapeutic effect on bone, it did significantly decrease urine deoxypyridinoline and increase bone mineral density, reducing the risk of fracture in menopausal women (Taku et al 2011). Previously, Zhang et al (2005) had suggested that the association between soy or isoflavone consumption and fracture risk was more pronounced among women in early menopause (Zhang et al 2005).

The effect may also be life stage-specific and dependent on the number of oestrogen receptors and the endogenous hormone milieu. Perimenopausal and early menopausal women may therefore be more receptive to the therapeutic effects of isoflavones on bone loss prior to the diminution of oestrogen receptors that occurs in the postmenopausal years (Wei et al 2012).

The most recent negative study was a double-blind randomised controlled trial which found that daily administration of tablets containing 200 mg of soy isoflavones for 2 years did not prevent bone loss amongst women who were aged 45–60 years and within 5 years of menopause (Levis et al 2011). Unfortunately, the study did not investigate the role of equol producers or non-producers in achieving this negative result.

Cognitive function

To date, the body of evidence does not suggest that soy isoflavones have a beneficial effect on cognitive function.

A recent randomised controlled trial in 350 menopausal women who were given 25 g of isoflavones for 30 months showed no significant change in cognition, although there was a possible improvement in visual memory (Henderson et al 2012). A systematic review of soy therapy in postmenopausal woman which included 12 randomised controlled trials found that there was no improvement in cognition; however, the review has several major limitations and should be interpreted accordingly (Clement et al 2011). Only one trial (Ho et al 2007) adequately satisfied all the methodological criteria outlined by the Cochrane collaboration tool for risk of bias assessment. In this study isoflavone supplementation, at 80 mg/day given for 6 months, did not improve cognitive function in generally healthy Chinese postmenopausal women (Clement et al 2011).

In contrast, in a small randomised controlled trial, 34 healthy males and females who were supplemented with 100 mg soy isoflavone for 6 months found that treatment resulted in improvements in all areas of cognition, including visual and spatial memory, construction, fluency, speeded dexterity and motor planning (Gleason et al 2009).

Most studies on soy and cognition have been conducted on menopausal women and previous reviews have identified factors such as variation in the composition of phyto-oestrogen interventions and the heterogeneous characteristics of study populations as contributing to discrepant results (Zhao & Brinton 2007).

OTHER USES

Soy infant formula

Soy has been used as an alternative for cow's milk in infant feeding for more than 30 years and may account for as much as 25% of infant formula (Badger et al 2009, Mendez et al 2002). Soy formula is commonly used for infants with cow's milk allergy and there is evidence to suggest that soy milk may be effective in reducing infant colic (Garrison & Christakis 2000). There are few studies, however, examining the effects of phyto-oestrogens in infants. Infants consuming soy formula may be exposed to 6–11 mg/kg/day of phyto-oestrogens and have plasma levels of isoflavones an order of magnitude higher than adults consuming soy foods (Andres et al 2012).

There are inconsistent results from epidemiological studies comparing soy and cow's milk formula during infancy and age of menarche. One study reported no clinically significant difference in age at menarche (Strom et al 2001) between the two formulas, while another reported that those who received soy formula early in life (≤4 months to ≥6 months of age) had earlier menarche (Adgent et al 2011).

Unfortunately, studies assessing the long-term effects of soy-based formulas are limited. There are methodological flaws in the studies available for review, limited by small sample size and variation in the amount and form of soy used (Cederoth et al 2012). There are suggestions that soy-based formulas may exceed the recommended daily intake (RDI) of nutrients, which in itself is not a concern, given that the RDIs are generally the minimum required to prevent deficiency diseases. However, of greater concern is the processing of soy, and whether it leads to heavy-metal contamination (Ljung et al 2011). Furthermore, due to the high phyto-oestrogen levels in soy, the effect on long-term reproductive health requires further research (Badger et al 2009).

Seasonal allergic rhinitis

Polysaccharides from soy sauce have been shown to have antiallergic activities in vitro and in vivo, and an 8-week double-blind study involving 51 subjects with seasonal allergic rhinitis found that oral supplementation with 600 mg of soy polysaccharides was effective in significantly improving symptom scores such as sneezing, nasal stuffiness and hindrance of daily life, as well as significantly improving the appearance and state of the nasal mucosa (Kobayashi 2005, Kobayashi et al 2005).

Premenstrual syndrome

Isolated soy protein containing 68 mg/day (aglycone equivalents) soy isoflavones was found to significantly improve specific premenstrual syndrome symptoms, including headache, breast tenderness, cramps and swelling in a seven-menstrual cycle, double-blind, placebo-controlled, crossover intervention study in 23 women (Bryant et al 2005).

DOSAGE RANGE

Soy foods contain variable amounts of isoflavones. Soy flour contains 1.3 mg/g of isoflavones; tofu contains 0.4 mg/g, soy milk 0.25 mg/g, tempeh 0.4 mg/g, miso 0.92 mg/g, soy sauce 0.023 mg/g, soybean paste 0.57 mg/g and soy cheese 0.05 mg/g (Coward et al 1993). Soy isoflavones are also available in some functional food products. Although soy oils and lecithin are used in many food ingredients, the typical Western diet provides negligible isoflavones, whereas Asian diets typically contain 20–50 mg of isoflavones (Nagata et al 1998, Hall et al 2008). The optimal dose required to have clinical effects is yet to be established; however, it is suggested that optimal soy protein and isoflavone intakes are 15–20 g/day and 50–90 mg/day, respectively, with 25–30 g/day recommended for cholesterol reduction (Anderson & Bush 2011, Messina 2008).

TOXICITY

Soy and soy isoflavones are considered non-toxic in the doses that are generally consumed as foods. Soy may interfere with the absorption of synthetic thyroid hormone, and there is a theoretical concern based on in vitro and animal data that soy foods may increase the risk of developing clinical hypothyroidism in individuals with compromised thyroid function and/or whose iodine intake is marginal (Messina & Redmond 2006). Soy food consumers should ensure their intake of iodine is adequate, although studies suggest that soy isoflavones in a protein matrix do not significantly influence circulating thyroid hormones in healthy young men (Dillingham et al 2007).

Although the phyto-oestrogens may have hormonal activity, they have relatively short half-lives of approximately 6–8 hours, which is contrasted with the environmental xeno-oestrogens that may persist for years in fat tissue and hence bioaccumulate (Setchell & Cassidy 1999).

ADVERSE REACTIONS

There is little suggestion of adverse effects of soy or isoflavones at physiological doses, although soy isoflavone supplements have induced gastrointestinal discomfort and menstrual complaints (Cassidy & Hooper 2006). Unconjugated soy isoflavones appear to be safe and well tolerated in healthy postmenopausal women at doses of 900 mg/day (Pop et al 2008).

There is a case report of a 60-year-old man having gynaecomastia and breast tenderness along

Practice points/Patient counselling

- Soy is a component of many foods and a nutritious source of complete, high-quality protein.
- There are many different types and formulations of soy and people may react differently to soy products depending on their diet and the activity of their gut bacteria.
- In countries where people regularly consume soy products there appears to be a lower incidence of CVD, menopausal symptoms and some cancers such as breast and prostate cancer.
- The most active agents in soy are the isoflavones, which are used to treat menopausal symptoms and improve bone health.
- Soy isoflavones are generally shown to have a modest effect, reducing the frequency and severity of hot flushes and improving sleep when taken by menopausal women with sleep disturbances. There is some encouraging evidence that they may improve bone health, but this is not yet conclusive.
- Although there has not been much research on the use of soy in infants, there do not appear to be any adverse effects from feeding infants soy formula.
- The long-term benefits of soy may relate to the lifetime exposure to soy products.

with high oestradiol levels due to soy milk consumption (Martinez & Lewi 2008).

There are structural similarities between birch pollen and soy allergens, leading to allergic cross-reactions (Kleine-Tebbe et al 2008) and the potential for anaphylaxis (Jacquenet et al 2008).

SIGNIFICANT INTERACTIONS

It has been suggested that isoflavones can inhibit the oxidative and conjugative metabolism of drugs in vitro and interact with transporters such as P-glycoprotein; however, their ability to interact with drugs remains uncertain until clinical studies can confirm these findings (Evans 2000).

Antibiotics

Antibiotic administration blocks metabolism of isoflavones to equol through inhibition of the intestinal microflora, whereas a high carbohydrate milieu increases intestinal fermentation and results in more extensive biotransformation of phyto-oestrogens (Setchell & Cassidy 1999). The biotransformation of diadzein (an isoflavone metabolite) to equol in the gut by microflora is considered important for clinical responsiveness.

Calcium, magnesium, zinc, copper and iron

Soy contains phytic acid, which may bind with certain minerals, such as calcium, magnesium, manganese, zinc, copper and iron, reducing their availability (PDRHealth 2004). Separate by 2–3 hours.

Tamoxifen

Animal studies have shown that soy enhances the therapeutic effects of tamoxifen, as both have SERM actions (Mishra et al 2011). Additionally, in vivo studies suggest that the isoflavone daidzein may enhance the effect of tamoxifen against breast cancer patients, burden and incidence (Charalambous et al 2013).

Usual dietary intake levels appear safe; however, the safety of concentrated extracts is yet to be established (see Clinical note — Soy and breast cancer patients, above).

While the soy isoflavone genistein may theoretically compete with tamoxifen for oestrogen receptors, thereby reducing drug efficacy, a meta-analysis of five cohort studies found no safety concerns with using soy isoflavones to reduce the recurrence of breast cancer, especially oestrogen-positive tumours (Chi et al 2013). A study found that soy isoflavones consumed at levels comparable to those in Asian populations may reduce the risk of cancer recurrence in women receiving tamoxifen therapy and, importantly, does not appear to interfere with tamoxifen efficacy. Furthermore, it suggests there is no evidence to indicate that soy foods are unsafe in breast cancer patients (Guha 2009) — possible beneficial effect under professional supervision.

PREGNANCY USE

Soy is likely to be safe when used as a food; however, pregnant women and nursing mothers should avoid the use of high dose soy isoflavone supplements pending long-term safety studies.

PATIENTS' FAQs

What will this supplement do for me?

Soy is a nutritious food and a good source of high-quality, complete protein that appears to have beneficial effects on cholesterol, and possible activity protecting against various cancers and CVD. Soy isoflavones modestly reduce the frequency and severity of hot flushes in menopause. They have been shown to improve sleep quality amongst menopausal women with sleep disturbances.

When will it start to work?

Clinical studies suggest the lipid-lowering effects of soy protein take between 6 and 12 weeks to appear. Reduction in hot flush frequency and severity may take up to 12 weeks and any positive effects on bone health take 6–12 months to be seen.

Are there any safety issues?

Soy is generally considered safe when taken as a food source or protein substitute; however, soy isoflavone supplements should be taken with caution in pregnancy, and safety remains unclear in those with breast cancer or prostate cancer.

REFERENCES

Ablove TS et al. Effects of endogenous ovarian estrogen versus exogenous estrogen replacement on blood flow and ERα and ERβ levels in the bladder. Reproductive Sciences 16.7 (2009) 657–664.

Adams K et al. Soy isoflavones do not modulate prostate-specific antigen concentrations in older men in a randomized controlled trial. Cancer Epidemiol Biomarkers Prev 13.4 (2004): 644–648.

Adgent MA, et al. Early-life soy exposure and age at menarche. Paediatric and Perinatal Epidemiology. 26.2 (2011): 163–175.

Adlercreutz H. Phytoestrogens and breast cancer. J Steroid Biochem Mol Biol 83 (2002a): 113–18.

Adlercreutz H. Phyto-oestrogens and cancer. Lancet Oncol 3.6 (2002b): 364–73.

Anderson JW & Bush HM. Soy protein effects on serum lipoproteins: a quality assessment and meta-analysis of randomized controlled studies. Journal of the American College of Nutrition 30.2 (2011) 79–91.

Atkinson C, et al. Gut bacterial metabolism of the soy isoflavone daidzein: exploring the relevance to human health. Exp Biol Med. 2005;230:155–170.

Aubertin-Leheudre M, et al. Effect of 6 months of exercise and isoflavone supplementation on clinical cardiovascular risk factors in obese postmenopausal women: a randomized, double-blind study. Menopause 2007;14(4):624–9.

Azadbakht L et al. Beneficiary effect of dietary soy protein on lowering plasma levels of lipid and improving kidney function in type II diabetes with nephropathy. Eur J Clin Nutr 57.10 (2003): 1292–1294.

Badger TM et al. Soy protein isolate and protection against cancer. J Am Coll Nutr 24.2 (2005): 146S–9S.

Badger TM, et al. The health implication of soy infant formula. The American Journal of Clinical Nutrition 89.5 (2009) 1668S-1672S.

Bakhtiary A, et al. Effects of soy on metabolic biomarkers of cardiovascular disease in elderly women with metabolic syndrome. Archives of Iranian Medicine 15.8 (2012) 462–468.

Balk E et al. Effects of soy on health outcomes. Evidence Report/Technology Assessment (Summary). Report no. 126. Agency for Healthcare Research and Quality (2005): 1–8.

Barret JR. The science of soy, what do we really know? Environmental Health Perspectives 114.6 (2006) 353–358.

Bedell, S., et al. 2014. The pros and cons of plant estrogens for menopause. J Steroid Biochem. Mol. Biol., 139, 225–236.

Bhoo-Pathy N, et al. Breast cancer research in Asia: adopt or adapt Western knowledge? European Journal of Cancer 49.3 (2013) 703–709.
Bolanos, R., et al. 2010. Soy isoflavones versus placebo in the treatment of climacteric vasomotor symptoms: systematic review and meta-analysis. Menopause., 17, (3) 660–666.
Bolanos-Diaz, R., et al. 2011. Soy extracts versus hormone therapy for reduction of menopausal hot flushes: indirect comparison. Menopause., 18, (7) 825–829.
Bosland MC, et al. Effect of soy protein isolate supplementation on biochemical recurrence of prostate cancer after radical prostatectomy: a randomized trial. JAMA. 2013 Jul 10;310(2):170–8.
Brooks JD, Thompson LU (2005). Mammalian lignans and genistein decrease the activities of aromatase and 17beta-hydroxysteroid dehydrogenase in MCF-7 cells. J Steroid Biochem Mol Biol, 94, 461–7.
Bryant M et al. Effect of consumption of soy isoflavones on behavioural, somatic and affective symptoms in women with premenstrual syndrome. Br J Nutr 93.5 (2005): 731–739.
Cancer Council. Available online: www.cancercouncil.com.au/editorial.asp?pageid=2350&fromsearch=yes (accessed 17-03-09).
Cano A, et al. Isoflavones and cardiovascular disease. Maturitas 67 (2010) 219–226.
Carmignani LO, et al. The effect of dietary soy supplementation compared to estrogen and placebo on menopausal symptoms: a randomized control trial. Maturitas 67 (2012) 262–269.
Cassidy A, Hooper L. Phytoestrogens and cardiovascular disease. J Br Menopause Soc 12.2 (2006): 49–56.
Castelo-Branco, C. & Cancelo Hidalgo, M.J. 2011. Isoflavones: effects on bone health. Climacteric., 14, (2) 204–211.
Castelo-Branco, C. & Soveral, I. 2013. Phytoestrogens and bone health at different reproductive stages. Gynecol. Endocrinol., 29, (8) 735–743.
Cederroth CR, Nef S. Soy, phytoestrogens and metabolism: a review. Mollecular & Cellular Endocrinology 304 (2009) 30–42.
Cederroth CR et al. Soy, phytoestrogens and their impact on reproductive health. Molecular and Cellular Endocrinology 355 (2012): 192–200.
Chalupka, S. 2011. Soy isoflavones for the prevention of menopausal symptoms and bone loss — a safe and effective alternative to estrogen? AAOHN.J, 59, (11) 504.
Chan YH et al. Isoflavone intake in persons at high risk of cardiovascular events: implications for vascular endothelial function and the carotid atherosclerotic burden. Am J Clin Nutr 86.4 (2007): 938–945.
Charalambous C, et al. Equol enhances tamoxifen's anti-tumor activity by induction of caspase-mediated apoptosis in MCF-7 breast cancer cells. BMC Cancer 13 (2013) 238.
Chi F, et al. Post-diagnosis soy food intake and breast cancer survival. A meta-analysis of cohort studies. Asian Pacific Journal of Cancer Prevention 14.4 (2013) 2407–2412.
Clement YN, et al. Effects of herbal and dietary supplements on cognition in menopause: a systematic review. Maturitas 68 (2011) 256–263.
Coward L et al. Genistein, daidzein, and their beta-glycoside conjugates — Antitumor isoflavones in soybean foods from American and Asian diets. J Agric Food Chem 41.11 (1993): 1961–1967.
Cupisti A et al. Soy protein diet improves endothelial dysfunction in renal transplant patients. Nephrol Dial Transplant 22.1 (2007): 229–234.
Cvejić J, et al. Phytoestrogens: estrogene-like phytochemicals. Studies in Natural Products Chemistry 38 (2012) 1–35.
Dalais F et al. Effects of a diet rich in phytoestrogens on prostate-specific antigen and sex hormones in men diagnosed with prostate cancer. Urology 64.3 (2004): 510–5115.
Deibert P et al. Weight loss without losing muscle mass in pre-obese and obese subjects induced by a high-soy-protein diet. Int J Obes Relat Metab Disord 28.10 (2004): 1349–1352.
Dewell A, et al. The effects of soy- derived phytoestrogens on serum lipids and lipoproteins in moderately hypercholesterolemic postmenopausal women. Journal of Clinical Endocrinology and Metabolism 2002;87 (1):118–21.
Dewell A et al. Clinical review a critical evaluation of the role of soy protein and isoflavone supplementation in the control of plasma cholesterol concentrations. J Clin Endocrinol Metab 91.3 (2006): 772–780.
Dhananjaya K, et al. Insilico studies of daidzein and genistein with human estrogen receptor-α. Asian Pacific Journal of Tropical Biomedicine (2012) S1747-S1753.
Dillingham BL et al. Soy protein isolates of varied isoflavone content do not influence serum thyroid hormones in healthy young men. Thyroid 17.2 (2007): 131–137.
Dong, J.Y. & Qin, L.Q. 2011. Soy isoflavones consumption and risk of breast cancer incidence or recurrence: a meta-analysis of prospective studies. Breast Cancer Res. Treat., 125, (2) 315–323.
Dong X, et al. Apoptopic effects of cooked and in vitro digested soy on human prostate cancer. Food Chemistry 135 (2012) 1643–1652.
Drews, K., et al. 2007a. [Efficacy of standardized isoflavones extract (Soyfem) (52–104 mg/24h) in moderate and medium-severe climacteric syndrome]. Ginekol. Pol., 78, (4) 307–311.
Drews, K., et al. 2007b. [The safety and tolerance of isoflavones (Soyfem) administration in postmenopausal women.] Ginekol. Pol., 78, (5) 361–365.
Eden JA. Phytoestrogens for menopausal symptoms: a review. Maturitas 72.2 (2012) 157–159.
Evans A. Influence of dietary components on the gastrointestinal metabolism and transport of drugs. Ther Drug Monit 22.1 (2000): 131–136.
Frankfield CL. O-Desmethylangolensin: the importance of equol's lesser known cousin to human health. Advances in Nutrition 2 (2011) 317–324.
Gardner, CD, et al. Prostatic soy isoflavone concentrations exceed serum levels after dietary supplementation. Prostate. 2009 May 15; 69(7): 719–726.
Garrison MM, Christakis DA. A systematic review of treatments for infant colic. Pediatrics 106 (1 Pt 2) (2000): 184–190.
Gleason CE, et al. A preliminary study of the safety, feasibility and cognitive efficacy of soy isoflavone supplements in older men and women. Age and Ageing 38.1 (2009) 86–93.
Grattan BJ. Plant sterols as anticancer nutrients: evidence for their role in breast cancer. Nutrients 5 (2013) 359–387.
Greany KA, et al. Consumption of isoflavone-rich soy protein does not alter homocystein or markers of inflammation in postmenopausal women. European Journal of Clinic Nutrition 62.12 (2008) 1419–1425.
Guha N. Soy isoflavones and risk of cancer recurrence in a cohort of breast cancer survivors: the Life After Cancer Epidemiology study. Breast Cancer Res Treat 118.2 (2009) 395–405.
Hachul, H., et al. 2011. Isoflavones decrease insomnia in postmenopause. Menopause., 18, (2) 178–184.
Hall, W L, et al. A meal enriched with soy isoflavones increases nitric oxide-mediated vasodilation in healthy postmenopausal women. The Journal of Nutrition, 138.7 (2008): 1288–1292.
Hamilton-Reeves JM et al. Clinical studies show no effects of soy protein or isoflavones on reproductive hormones in med: results of a meta-analysis. Fertility & Sterility 94.3 (2010): 997–1007.
Henderson VW et al. Long-term soy isoflavone supplementation and cognition in women, A randomized controlled trial. Neurology 78 (2012): 1841–1848.
Hillman GG & Singh-Gupta V. Soy isoflavones sensitize cancer cells to radiotherapy. Free Radical Biology & Medicine 51 (2011) 289–298.
Ho SC et al Effects of soy isoflavone supplementation on cognitive function in Chinese postmenopausal women: a double-blind, randomized controlled trial. Menopause, 14 (3) (2007), pp. 489–499.
Hoie LH et al. Cholesterol-lowering effects of a new isolated soy protein with high levels of nondenaturated protein in hypercholesterolemic patients. Adv Ther 24.2 (2007): 439–447.
Hooper L, et al. Effects of isoflavones on breast density in pre and post menopausal women: a systematic review and meta-analysis of randomized controlled trials. Human Reproductive Update 16.6 (2010) 745–769.
Howes LG et al. Isoflavone therapy for menopausal flushes: a systematic review and meta-analysis. Maturitas 55.3 (2006): 203–211.
Huff MW, Carroll KK. Effects of dietary protein on turnover, oxidation, and absorption of cholesterol, and on steroid excretion in rabbits. J Lipid Res 21.5 (1980): 546–548.
Hwang J, et al. Synergistic inhibition of LDL oxidation by phyto-estrogens and ascorbic acid. Free Radic Biol Med. 2000;29:79–89.
Imani H, et al. Effects of soy consumption on oxidative stress, blood homocystein, coagulation factors and phosphorus in peritoneal dialysis patients. J Renal Nutr 19.5 (2009); 389–395.
Jackson RL et al. Emerging evidence of the health benefits of S-equol, an estrogen receptor β agonist. Nutrition Reviews 69.8 (2011) 432–448.
Jacquenet S et al. Severe anaphylaxis to soymilk: an increase of prevalence? Report of the Allergy Vigilance network. Revue Francaise d'Allergologie et d'Immunologies Clinique 48.6 (2008): 456–458.
Kang X, et al. Effect of soy isoflavones on breast cancer recurrence and death for patients receiving adjuvant endocrine therapy. Canadian Medication Association Journal 182.17 (2010) 1857–1862.
Kleine-Tebbe J et al. Soy allergy due to cross reactions to major birch pollen allergen Bet v 1. Allergologie 31.8 (2008): 303–313.
Knight DC, Eden JA. A review of the clinical effects of phytoestrogens. Obstet Gynecol 87(5 Pt 2) (1996): 897–904.
Kobayashi M. Immunological functions of soy sauce: hypoallergenicity and antiallergic activity of soy sauce. J Biosci Bioeng 100.2 (2005): 144–151.
Kobayashi M et al. Shoyu polysaccharides from soy sauce improve quality of life for patients with seasonal allergic rhinitis a double-blind placebo-controlled clinical study. Int J Mol Med 15.3 (2005): 463–467.
Kokubo Y, et al. Association of dietary intake of soy, beans and isoflavone with risk of cerebral and myocardial infarctions in Japanese

S

populations: the Japan public health centre-based (JPHC) study cohort I. Circulation 116.22 (2007) 2553–2562.

Korde LA, et al. Childhood soy intake and breast cancer risk in Asian American women. Cancer Epidemiology, Biomarkers & Prevention 18 (2009) 1050–1059.

Kreijkamp-Kaspers S et al. Randomized controlled trial of the effects of soy protein containing isoflavones on vascular function in postmenopausal women. Am J Clin Nutr 81.1 (2005): 189–195.

Kumar N et al. The specific role of isoflavones in reducing prostate cancer risk. Prostate 59.2 (2004): 141–147.

Kurahashi N et al. Plasma isoflavones and subsequent risk of prostate cancer in a nested case-control study: The Japan Public Health Center. J Clin Oncol 26.36 (2008): 5923–59229.

Kyoko T et al. Effects of soy isoflavone extract supplements on blood pressure in adult humans: Systematic review and meta-analysis of randomized placebo-controlled trials. J Hypertension 28.10 (2010): 1971–1982.

Lacey M, et al (2005). Dose-response effects of phytoestrogens on the activity and expression of 3beta-hydroxysteroid dehydrogenase and aromatase in human granulosa-luteal cells. J Steroid Biochem Mol Biol, 96, 279–86.

Larkin TA, et al. The key importance of soy isoflavone bioavailability to understanding health benefits. Clinical Reviews in Food, Science & Nutrition 48.6 (2008) 538–552.

Leclercq G & Jacquot Y. Interactions of isoflavones and other plant derived estrogens with estrogen receptors for prevention and treatment of breast cancer — considerations concerning related efficacy and safety. Journal of Steroid Biochemistry & Molecular Biology 139 (2014): 237–244.

Lee SA et al. Adolescent and adult soy food intake and breast cancer risk: results from the Shanghai Women's Health Study. American Journal of Clinical Nutrition 89.6 (2009): 1920–1926.

Lethaby A, et al. Phytoestrogens for vasomotor menopausal symptoms (review). The Cochrane Collaboration 11 (2010).

Levis S, et al. Soy isoflavones in the prevention of menopausal bone loss and menopausal symptoms: a randomized, double-blind trial. Arch Intern Med. 2011;171(15):1363–1369.

Li Z et al. Long-term efficacy of soy-based meal replacements vs an individualized diet plan in obese type II DM patients: relative effects on weight loss, metabolic parameters, and C-reactive protein. Eur J Clin Nutr 59.3 (2005): 411–418.

Li F, et al. Dietary flavones and flavonones display differential effects on aromatase (CYP19) transcription in the breast cancer cells MCF-7. Molecular and Cellular Endocrinology 344 (2011) 51–58.

Liu ZM, et al. Effects of soy intake on glycemic control: a meta-analysis of randomized controlled trials. The American Journal of Clinical Nutrition 93.5 (2011) 1092–1101.

Liu XX et al. Effect of soy isoflavones on blood pressure: A meta-analysis of randomized control. Nutrition, Metabolism & Cardiovascular Diseases (2012) 22, 463–470.

Ljung K et al. High concentrations of essential and toxic elements in infant formula and infant foods – A matter of concern. Food Chemistry, Elsevier, 2011 online

Low Dog T. Menopause: a review of botanical dietary supplements. Am J Med 118 (Suppl) 12B (2005): 98S–108S.

Lu LJ et al. Phytoestrogens and healthy aging: gaps in knowledge. A workshop report [comment]. Menopause 8.3 (2001): 157–170.

Ma DF et al. Soy isoflavone intake increases bone mineral density in the spine of menopausal women: meta-analysis of randomized controlled trials. Clin Nutr 27.1 (2008): 57–64.

Maki KC, et al. Effects of soy protein on lipoprotein lipids and fecal bile acid excretion in men and women with moderate hypercholesterolemia. Journal of Clinic Lipidology 4.6 (2010) 531–542.

Marini H, et al. Efficacy of genistein aglycone on some cardiovascular risk factors and homocysteine levels: a follow up study. Nutrition, Metabolism & Cardiovascular Diseases 20 (2010) 332–340.

Martinez J, Lewi JE. An unusual case of gynecomastia associated with soy product consumption. Endocr Pract 14.4 (2008): 415–4118.

McVeigh BL et al. Effect of soy protein varying in isoflavone content on serum lipids in healthy young men. Am J Clin Nutr 83.2 (2006): 244–251.

Mendez MA et al. Soy-based formulae and infant growth and development: a review. J Nutr 132.8 (2002): 2127–2130.

Messina M. Investigating the optimal soy protein and isoflavone intakes for women: a perspective. Womens Health 4.4 (2008): 337–356.

Messina M, Redmond G. Effects of soy protein and soybean isoflavones on thyroid function in healthy adults and hypothyroid patients: a review of the relevant literature. Thyroid 16.3 (2006): 249–258.

Mishra R et al. Glycine soya diet synergistically enhances the suppressive of tamoxifen and inhibits tamoxifen-promoted hepatocarinogenesis in 7,12-dimethylbenz[α]anthracene-induced rat mammary tumor model. Food & Chemical Toxicology 49 (2011): 434–440.

Moon YJ et al. Dietary flavonoids: effects on xenobiotic and carcinogen metabolism. Toxicol In Vitro 20.2 (2006): 187–210.

Moreira, A.C., et al. 2014. Phytoestrogens as alternative hormone replacement therapy in menopause: What is real, what is unknown. The Journal of Steroid Biochemistry and Molecular Biology, 143, 61–71.

Morimoto Y, et al. Urinary estrogen metabolites during a randomized soy trial. Nutrition & Cancer — an International Journal 64.2 (2012) 307–314.

Morito K et al. Interaction of phytoestrogens with estrogen receptors alpha and beta. Biol Pharm Bull 24.4 (2001): 351–356.

Nagasawa A et al. Divergent effects of soy protein diet on the expression of adipocytokines. Biochem Biophys Res Commun 311.4 (2003): 909–914.

Nagata C et al. Decreased serum total cholesterol concentration is associated with high intake of soy products in Japanese men and women. J Nutr 128.2 (1998): 209–213.

Nagata C et al. Soy product intake is inversely associated with serum homocysteine level in premenopausal Japanese women. J Nutr 133.3 (2003): 797–800.

Nagata Y et al. Dietary isoflavones may protect against prostate cancer in Japanese men. J Nutr 137.8 (2007): 1974–1979.

Napora JK et al. High dose insoflavones do not improve metabolic and inflammatory parameters in androgen deprived men with prostate cancer. J Androl 32.1 (2011) 40–48.

Natural Standard Patient Monograph. Herbal/plant therapies: Soy (*Glycine max* [L.] Merr.) 2005. Available online: www.naturalstandard.com/naturalstandard/monographs/herbssupplements/patient-soy.asp (accessed 18-08-06).

Nestel P et al. Soy isoflavones improve systemic arterial compliance but not plasma lipids in menopausal and perimenopausal women. Arterioscler Thromb Vasc Biol 17.12 (1997): 3392–3398.

North American Menopause Society 2011. The role of soy isoflavones in menopausal health Menopause., 18, (7) 732–753.

Nurmi T et al. Isoflavone content of the soy based supplements. J Pharm Biomed Anal 28.1 (2002): 1–111.

Nynca A, et al. Effects of the phytoestrogens, genistein and protein tyrosine kinase inhibitor-dependent mechanisms on steroidogensesis and estrogen receptor expression in porcine granulosa cells of medium follicles. Domestic Animal Endocrinology 44 (2013) 10–18.

Park SY et al. Legume and isoflavone intake and prostate cancer risk: the Multiethnic Cohort Study. Int J Cancer 123.4 (2008): 927–932.

Patisaul HB & Jefferson W. The pros and cons of phytoestrogens. Frontiers in Neuroendocrinology 31 (2010) 400–419.

PDRHealth [online]. Soy Isoflavones. Thomson Healthcare, 2004. Available online: http://www.pdrhealth.

Peterson J, et al. Dietary lignans: physiology and potential for cardiovascular disease risk reduction. Nutrition Reviews 68.10 (2010) 571–603.

Pop EA et al. Effects of a high daily dose of soy isoflavones on DNA damage, apoptosis, and estrogenic outcomes in healthy postmenopausal women: a phase I clinical trial. Menopause 15 (4 Pt 1) (2008): 684–692.

Potter SM. Overview of proposed mechanisms for the hypocholesterolemic effect of soy. J Nutr 125.3 (1995): 606S–11S.

Qin Y, et al. Isoflavones for hypercholesterolaemia in adults (review). The Cochrane Collaboration 6 (2013).

Rebholz CM, et al. Effect of soybean protein on novel cardiovascular disease risk factors: a randomized controlled trial
. European Journal of Clinical Nutrition 67 (2013) 58–63.

Reynolds K et al. A meta-analysis of the effect of soy protein supplementation on serum lipids. Am J Cardiol 98.5 (2006): 633–640.

Rimbach G et al. Dietary isoflavones in the prevention of cardiovascular disease — a molecular perspective. Food Chem Toxicol 46.4 (2008): 1308–1319.

Rosenberg Zand RS, et al. Flavonoids and steroid hormone-dependent cancers. J Chromatogr B 777.1–2 (2002): 219–232.

Rosero Arenas M et al. Usefulness of phytooestrogens in reduction of blood pressure. Systematic review and meta-analysis. Aten Primaria 40.4 (2008): 177–186.

Roudsari AH et al. Assessment of soy phytoestrogens' effects on bone turnover indicators in menopausal women with osteopenia in Iran: a before and after clinical trial. Nutr J 4 (2005): 30.

Sanchez A, Hubbard RW. Plasma amino acids and the insulin/glucagon ratio as an explanation for the dietary protein modulation of atherosclerosis. Med Hypotheses 36.1 (1991): 27–32.

Sapbamrer R, et al. Effects of dietary traditional fermented soybean on reproductive hormones, lipids, and glucose among postmenopausal women in northern Thailand. Asia Pac J Clin Nutr. 2013;22(2): 222–8.

Satih S, et al. Expression analyses of nuclear receptor genes in breast cancel cell lines exposed to spy phytoestrogens after BRCA2 knockdown by TaqMan low-density array (TLDA). Journal of Molecular Signaling 4.3 (2009).

Setchell KDR, Cassidy A. Dietary isoflavones: biological effects and relevance to human health. J Nutr 129.3 (1999): 758S–67S.

Shu XO, et al. Soy food and breast cancer survival. Journal of the American Medical Association 302.22 (2009) 2437–2443.
Sliva D. Soy isoflavones and the invasiveness of breast cancer. Agric Food Industry Hi-Tech 16.1 (2005): 40–41.
Sonn GA et al. Impact of diet on prostate cancer: a review. Prostate Cancer Prostatic Dis 8.4 (2005): 304–310.
Stark A, Madar Z. Phytoestrogens: a review of recent findings. J Pediatr Endocrinol Metab 15.5 (2002): 561–572.
Stephenson TJ et al. Effect of soy protein-rich diet on renal function in young adults with insulin-dependent diabetes mellitus. Clin Nephrol 64.1 (2005): 1–111.
Strom BL, et al. Exposure to soy-based formula in infancy and endocrinological and reproductive outcomes in young adulthood. JAMA. 2001;286(7):807–14.
Sumien N, et al. Does phytoestrogen supplementation affect cognition differentially in males and females? Brain Research 1514 (2013) 123–127.
Suzuki T et al. Effect of soybean on breast cancer according to receptor status: a case-control study in Japan. Int J Cancer 123.7 (2008): 1674–1680.
Swami, S, et al. Inhibition of prostaglandin synthesis and actions by genistein in human prostate cancer cells and by soy isoflavones in prostate cancer patients. International Journal of Cancer 124.9 (2009) 2050–2059.
Taku K et al. Effects of extracted soy isoflavones alone on blood total and LDL cholesterol: meta-analysis of randomized controlled trials. Ther Clin Risk Manag 4.5 (2008): 1097–1103.
Taku K, et al. Effects of soy isoflavone supplements in bone turnover markers in menopausal women: systematic review and meta-analysis of randomized controlled trials. Bone 47 (2010) 413–423.
Taku K, et al. Soy isoflavones for osteoporosis: an evidence based approach. Maturitas 70 (2011) 333–338.
Teede HJ et al. Dietary soy containing phytoestrogens does not activate the hemostatic system in postmenopausal women. J Clin Endocrinol Metab 90.4 (2005): 1936–1941.
Teixeira SR et al. Isolated soy protein consumption reduces urinary albumin excretion and improves the serum lipid profile in men with type 2 diabetes mellitus and nephropathy. J Nutr 134.8 (2004): 1874–1880.
Torres N et al. Regulation of lipid metabolism by soy protein and its implication in diseases mediated by lipid disorders. J Nutr Biochem 17.6 (2006): 365–373.
Tovar AR et al. Soy protein reduces hepatic lipotoxicity in hyperinsulinemic obese Zucker fa/fa rats. J Lipid Res 46.9 (2005): 1823–1832.
Trock BJ et al. Meta-analysis of soy intake and breast cancer risk. J Natl Cancer Inst 98.7 (2006): 459–471.
van Duursen MB, et al. Genistein induces breast cancer-associated aromatase and stimulates estrogen dependent tumor cell growth in vitro breast cancer model. Toxicology 289 (2011) 67–73.
Vega-Lopez S et al. Plasma antioxidant capacity in response to diets high in soy or animal protein with or without isoflavones. Am J Clin Nutr 81.1 (2005): 43–49.
Villaseca, P. 2012. Non-estrogen conventional and phytochemical treatments for vasomotor symptoms: what needs to be known for practice. Climacteric., 15, (2) 115–124.
Wada K, et al. Soy isoflavone intake and breast cancer risk in Japan: from the Takayama study. Int J Cancer. 2013 Aug 15;133(4):952–60.
Wei P, et al. Systematic review of soy isoflavone supplements on osteoporosis in women. Asian Pacific Journal of Tropical Medicine (2012) 243–248.
Weiser, MJ, et al. Estrogen receptor beta in the brain: from form to function. Brain Res Rev 57.2 (2008) 309–320.
Wong WW, et al. Effect of soy isoflavone supplementation on nitric oxide metabolism and blood pressure in menopausal women. American Journal of Clinical Nutrition 95.6 (2012) 1487–1494.
Wu AH, et al. Epidemiology of soy exposure and breast cancer risk. British Journal of Cancer 98 (2008a) 9–14.
Wu AH et al. Soy intake and breast cancer risk in Singapore Chinese Health Study. Br J Cancer 99.1 (2008b): 196–200.
Yamori Y. Cardiac study and dietary intervention study. In: Sugnao M, ed. Soy in Health and Disease Prevention. Boca Raton, FL: CRC Press; 2007:107–119.
Yang G et al. Longitudinal study of soy food intake and blood pressure among middle-aged and elderly Chinese women. Am J Clin Nutr 81.5 (2005): 1012–10117.
Yang B, et al. Systematic review and meta-analysis of soy products consumption in patients with type 2 diabetes mellitus. Asian Pacific Journal of Clinical Nutrition 20.4 (2011) 593–602.
Yang G, et al. Prediagnosis soy food consumption and lung cancer survival in women. J Clin Oncol. 2013 Apr 20;31(12):1548–53.
Ye L, et al. The soy isoflavone genistein induces estrogen synthesis in an extragonadal pathway. Molecular & Cellular Endocrinology 302 (2009) 73–80.
Yimit D et al. Effects of soybean peptide on immune function, brain function, and neurochemistry in healthy volunteers. Nutrition 28 (2012): 154–159.
Yuan-Jing F, et al. Genistein synergizes with RNA interference inhibiting surviving for inducing DU-145 of prostate cancer cells to apoptosis. Cancer Letters 284.2 (2009) 189–197.
Zhan S, Ho SC. Meta-analysis of the effects of soy protein containing isoflavones on the lipid profile. Am J Clin Nutr 81.2 (2005): 397–408.
Zhang X et al. Prospective cohort study of soy food consumption and risk of bone fracture among postmenopausal women. Arch Intern Med 165.16 (2005): 1890–1895.
Zhang B et al. Greater habitual soyfood consumption is associated with decreased carotid intima-media thickness and better plasma lipids in Chinese middle-aged adults. Atherosclerosis 198.2 (2008): 403–411.
Zhang TF, et al. Positive effects of soy isoflavone food on survival of breast cancer patients in China. Asian Pacific Journal of Cancer Prevention 13 (2012) 479–482.
Zhao L, Brinton RD. WHI and WHIMS follow-up and human studies of soy isoflavones on cognition. Expert Rev Neurother 7.11 (2007): 1549–1564.

St John's wort

HISTORICAL NOTE St John's wort (SJW) has been used medicinally since ancient Greek times when, it is believed, Dioscorides and Hippocrates used it to rid the body of evil spirits. Since the time of the Swiss physician Paracelsus (*c.* 1493–1541), it has been used to treat neuralgia, anxiety, neurosis and depression. Externally, it has also been used to treat wounds, bruises and shingles. The name 'St John's wort' is related to its yellow flowers, traditionally gathered for the feast of St John the Baptist, and the term 'wort' is the old English word for plant. SJW has enjoyed its greatest popularity in Europe and comprises 25% of all antidepressant prescriptions in Germany (Schrader 2000). In the past few decades, its popularity has grown in countries such as Australia and the United States.

OTHER NAMES

Amber, balsana, devil's scourge, goatweed, hardhay, hartheu, herb de millepertuis, hierba de San Juan, hypericum, iperico, johanniskraut, klamath weed, konradskraut, millepertuis, rosin rose, sonnenwend-kraut, St Jan's kraut, tipton weed, witch's herb

BOTANICAL NAME/FAMILY

Hypericum perforatum (family Clusiaceae or Guttiferae)

PLANT PARTS USED

Aerial parts, flowering tops

CHEMICAL COMPONENTS

Naphthodianthrones (including hypericin and pseudohypericin). Flavonoids, mostly hyperoside, rutin, quercitrin, isoquercitrin, quercetin and kaempferol, phenolics, including hyperforin, procyanidins, essential oil, sterols (beta-sitosterol), vitamins C and A, xanthones and choline.

> ***Clinical note — Pharmacologically important constituents***
>
> It has generally been considered that most of the pharmacological activities of SJW are attributable to hypericin and the flavonoid constituent, hyperforin. Besides contributing to the antidepressant activity, hypericin is the primary constituent responsible for the photosensitivity reactions reported with high intakes. Hyperforin is also a major contributor to the herb's antidepressant activity (Butterweck et al 2003a, Mennini & Gobbi 2004) and considered the main constituent responsible for inducing the cytochrome P-glycoprotein (P-gp) and thereby producing drug interactions. Besides this, it demonstrates many other pharmacological effects, such as antibacterial, anti-inflammatory and antineoplastic activities. Components previously considered void of activity have also been identified as important for pharmacological activity. For example, both procyanidin B2 and hyperoside increase the oral bioavailability of hypericin by 58% and 34%, respectively, and therefore, its clinical effects (Butterweck et al 2003b). A report published in June 2003 demonstrated that an extract devoid of both hyperforin and hypericin still exhibited antidepressant activity (Butterweck et al 2003a). Other constituents with antidepressant activity were identified and include hyperoside, isoquercitrin and miquelianin, and the 3-*O*-galactoside, 3-*O*-glucoside and 3-*O*-glucuronide of quercetin.
>
> Manufactured products will vary in the concentrations and proportions of the different plant constituents present because these are influenced by the plant's place of origin, its harvest time and drying, extraction processes and storage conditions. Hyperforin, in particular, can be present in variable concentrations because it is unstable in light, air and most organic solvents (Mennini & Gobbi 2004). This is extremely important to remember when comparing studies, as variations in chemical composition could be responsible for differences in results. It also provides a rationale for lack of interchangeability between brands.

MAIN ACTIONS

SJW has demonstrated multiple mechanisms of action, due to the presence of multiple active constituents. Research has been undertaken to identify the key constituents responsible for each mechanism of action. Often, the resulting activity is due to a combination of phytochemicals and cannot be ascribed to a single chemical entity.

Antidepressant

Although SJW has been investigated extensively in scientific studies, there are still many questions about its pharmacology and mechanisms of action.

Collectively, the data show that SJW extract exerts significant pharmacological activity within several neurochemical systems believed to be implicated in the pathophysiology of depression. Recent investigations reveal that hyperforin and other constituents (e.g. adhyperforin, hypericins, flavanol glycosides) act synergistically through both pharmacodynamic and pharmacokinetic mechanisms to alleviate depression (Nahrstedt & Butterweck 2010). The synergistic antidepressive effects have been observed in vitro and in vivo (Fiebich et al 2011).

Inhibits synaptic reuptake of several neurotransmitters

Preclinical animal studies have found that SJW inhibits the synaptic reuptake system for serotonin, noradrenaline and dopamine (Nathan 1999, Wonnemann et al 2001). Studies using specific isolated constituents have demonstrated potent uptake inhibition of gamma-aminobutyric acid (GABA) and L-glutamate in vivo (Bilia et al 2002, Chatterjee et al 1998). These effects appear to be non-competitive, dose-dependent and mediated via sodium channels (Roz & Rehavi 2004).

Studies with hyperforin have shown that it does not interact directly with uptake transporters but instead acts by reducing the pH gradient across the synaptic vesicle membrane, resulting in diffusion of uncharged monoamines out of the vesicular compartment into the cytoplasm. The increase in cytoplasmic concentration decreases the transmembrane gradient of the neurotransmitters, causing an 'apparent' inhibition of synaptosomal uptake by hyperforin. Additionally, hyperforin elevates intracellular sodium concentration, thereby inhibiting gradient-driven neurotransmitter reuptake (Beerhues 2006). This is a novel mechanism of action, which differs from conventional antidepressant drugs.

Although hyperforin is the main constituent responsible for these effects, tests now show that a number of others are also involved (Gobbi et al 2001), such as adhyperforin, which has demonstrated a strong inhibitory effect on neurotransmitter uptake, and the oligomeric procyanidin fraction, which has demonstrated weak to moderate effects (Wonnemann et al 2001).

GABA receptor binding

SJW extracts have been shown to bind at GABA-A and -B receptors, to inhibit GABA reuptake, to evoke GABA release from synaptosomes and to exert an anxiolytic effect that is blocked by the benzodiazepine antagonist flumazenil (Perfumi et al 2002).

Upregulation of serotonin receptors

SJW significantly upregulates both 5-HT_{1A} and 5-HT_{2A} receptors and has a significant affinity for opiate sigma receptors, which may contribute to the antidepressant effect (Teufel-Mayer & Gleitz 1997).

Dopamine beta-hydroxylase inhibition

Studies on isolated constituents showed that hypericin and pseudohypericin can inhibit the enzyme dopamine beta-hydroxylase in vitro (Bilia et al 2002).

Inhibition of catechol-*O*-methyltransferase

This has been demonstrated in test tube studies (Thiede & Walper 1994).

Suppresses interleukin-6 (IL-6) synthesis

Various extracts from SJW produce a potent and dose-dependent inhibition of substance P-induced IL-6 synthesis (Fiebich et al 2001), which may also contribute to the herb's overall antidepressant effect.

Monoamine oxidase (MAO) inhibition

Inhibition of MAO by hypericin demonstrated in vitro was believed to be the primary mode of action; however, this has not been confirmed in several subsequent studies that have shown only weak inhibitory activity at doses in excess of usual therapeutic levels (Di Carlo et al 2001).

Anxiolytic

Several in vivo studies confirm the anxiolytic effects of SJW extract (Beijamini & Andreatini 2003, Jakovljevic et al 2000, Vandenbogaerde et al 2000). Activity at the GABA receptors and an increase in circulating GABA levels are likely to be involved. Whether the effect is clinically significant is unclear, as a recent systematic review concluded that there is insufficient evidence to conclude that SJW monotherapy is an effective anxiolytic treatment (Lakhan & Vieira 2010).

Cognitive effects

SJW extracts and hyperforin improve cognitive function in experimental models (Kiewert et al 2004); however, clinical studies have been less convincing (Siepmann et al 2002, Timoshanko et al 2001). In vivo studies with hyperforin have found that it induces the release of acetycholine from cholinergic terminals in the hippocampus and striatum, providing an explanation for the observed effects. Preventive administration of *Hypericum perforatum* (350 mg/kg orally) counteracted the working-memory impairments caused by repeated stress in male Wistar rats. The herb significantly improved hippocampus-dependent spatial working memory in comparison with control ($P < 0.01$) and alleviated some other negative effects of stress on cognitive functions (Trofimiuk & Braszko 2008). Interestingly, a small trial ($n = 20$) reported that smokers' cognitive function may benefit from taking SJW (Remotiv, ZE117) while on nicotine replacement therapy (Nicabate CQ) (Camfield et al 2013).

Neuroprotective

A 2010 review of neurobiological effects of hyperforin and its potential role in Alzheimer's disease indicates that it has several mechanisms which are of relevance, including the ability to disassemble amyloid-beta aggregates in vitro, decrease of astrogliosis and microglia activation, as well as improving spatial memory in vivo (Griffith et al 2010). A recent in vivo study confirmed that mainly hyperforin and quercetin appear to be involved in the neuroprotective action of SJW standardised extracts (Gómez Del Rio et al 2013).

Anticonvulsant effects

A study in mice showed that SJW methanolic extract increased latency of seizure in the pretreated group (50 mg/kg) against seizure induced by picrotoxin. The higher dose of extract (200 mg/kg) significantly decreased the duration of seizure and death latency (Etemad et al 2011).

Effects on alcohol and food intake

Several reports indicate comorbidity between depression and ethanol abuse and that depressive disorders and ethanol abuse may be associated with similar changes in the activity of central neurotransmitters (Markou et al 1998). In vivo studies using SJW in animal models of alcoholism have found that it does not alter food and water intake, or the pharmacokinetics of alcohol, but a reduction in ethanol intake occurs (Panocka et al 2000).

In a model of binge eating (brought upon by stress and food restrictions), treatment with 250 and 500 mg/kg of SJW dry extract decreased the binge-eating episode (Micioni Di Bonaventura et al 2012).

Effects on morphine withdrawal syndrome

A study in morphine-dependent rats suggests that SJW extract is capable of reducing the symptoms of opiate withdrawal. Its effectiveness may be equivalent to clonidine in reducing the opiate withdrawal syndrome (Feily & Abbasi 2009).

Anti-inflammatory and analgesic

SJW extract and several of its various isolated constituents have demonstrated effects on inflammation and pain pathways in different in vitro and animal models (Jakovljevic et al 2000, Raso et al 2002).

It potently inhibits binding to mu-, delta- and kappa-opioid receptors (Simmen et al 1998). In vivo tests also identify modulation of cyclooxygenase-2 (COX-2) expression for hypericum extract (Raso et al 2002). Studies with the isolated constituent hyperforin have shown that it potently inhibits COX-1 and 5-lipo-oxygenase in vitro (Albert et al 2002), and also demonstrates high effectiveness in vivo (Feisst et al 2009).

A more recent study found that hyperforin inhibits microsomal prostaglandin E_2 synthase-1 and suppresses prostaglandin E_2 formation in vivo (Koeberle et al 2011). Quercetin and other flavonoids contribute to the anti-inflammatory effect. Hyperoside (quercetin-3-O-galactoside) seems to exert its anti-inflammatory activity through the suppression of nuclear factor-κB activation, as detected in mouse peritoneal macrophages (Kim et al 2011).

A dried extract of SJW, as well as purified hyperforin and hypericin, induced a prolonged antinociception effect that persisted for 120 minutes after administration. The persistent thermal and chemical antinociception of SJW was mainly mediated by protein kinase C-inhibiting mechanisms (Galeotti et al 2010). Similarly, a single oral dose of a SJW dried extract (5 mg/kg orally) produced prolonged relief from pain hypersensitivity in vivo. Moreover, preventive SJW administration increased the latency to induction of hyperalgesia and reduced the duration of the painful symptomatology in a migraine model (Galeotti et al 2013a). Subsequently, hypericin was identified as a key component responsible for reversing nitric oxide-induced nociceptive hypersensitivity, whereas hyperforin and flavonoids were ineffective (Galeotti et al 2013b).

Anticancer effects

Hypericin, the photoactive compound of *Hypericum perforatum*, is probably the most powerful photosensitiser found in nature (Kacerovska et al 2008). It has minimal toxicity but exhibits potent photo-damaging effects in the presence of light (Olivo et al 2006). It is known to generate a high yield of singlet oxygen and other reactive oxygen species that are associated with photo-oxidative cellular damage (Karioti & Bilia 2010). The application of photodynamic therapy (PDT) with hypericin for the treatment of cancers such as recurrent mesothelioma and skin cancer has been validated in clinical trials. It may also have potential as a photodynamic agent in the treatment of nasopharyngeal cancer according to in vitro and in vivo models (Kacerovska et al 2008).

Hyperforin also exhibits antineoplastic potential based on the sum of its anticarcinogenic, antiproliferant, proapoptotic, anti-invasive and antimetastatic effects (Medina et al 2006). Hyperforin has been shown to effectively decrease the proliferation rates of a number of mammalian cancer cell lines, induce apoptosis of tumour cells and inhibit angiogenesis both in vitro and in vivo. For example, under hyperforin treatment in vivo, the growth of Kaposi's sarcoma — a highly angiogenic tumour — is strongly inhibited, with the resultant tumours reduced in size and vascularisation as compared with controls. Hyperforin inhibits neutrophil and monocyte chemotaxis in vitro and angiogenesis in vivo induced by angiogenic chemokines (CXCL8 or CCL2) (Lorusso et al 2009).

Besides hypericin and hyperforin, polyphenolic procyanidin B2 has also demonstrated an inhibitory effect on the growth of leukaemia cells, brain glioblastoma cells and normal human astrocytes in vitro (Hostanska et al 2003). Further, the inhibitory effects on leukaemic cell growth were synergistically strengthened when hypericin and hyperforin were tested together.

Antiretroviral, antifungal and antibacterial

Alcoholic SJW extracts (methanolic/ethanolic) have more pronounced antibacterial activity than aqueous extracts (Saddiqe et al 2010). The key antibacterial compound isolated to date from SJW is hyperforin, which has a higher antibacterial activity against Gram-positive than Gram-negative bacteria. More recently, a study found that an SJW extract was effective at inhibiting five non-pathogenic *Mycobacterium* isolates and *Bacillus subtilis*, but not *Escherichia coli*. Hyperforin isolated from this extract was more effective than hypericin or pseudohypericin (Mortensen et al 2012). This supports an earlier paper which identified hyperforin as a key constituent demonstrating antibacterial activities (Medina et al 2006).

Hyperforin exhibits effective antibacterial activity against methicillin-resistant *Staphylococcus aureus* and other Gram-positive bacteria, but no growth-inhibitory effect on Gram-negative bacteria or *Candida albicans* (Schempp et al 1999).

In a recent animal study SJW reduced the lung index and viral titre of mice infected with influenza A virus, decreasing mortality and prolonging the mean survival time (Xiuying et al 2012).

Although in vitro and studies in animal models have identified antiretroviral activity for hypericin and pseudohypericin (Meruelo et al 1988), two clinical trials could not confirm these effects, even when larger doses of hypericin were administered (Gulick et al 1999, Jacobson et al 2001).

The mechanism involved is not known; however, it is suspected to involve direct inactivation of the virus or prevention of virus shedding, budding or assembly at the cell membrane (Meruelo et al 1988). The presence of light is an important requirement for antiretroviral activity to be demonstrated, as the effect appears to be photoactivated (Hudson et al 1993, Miskovsky 2002).

Cardiovascular effects

New in vivo research revealed that SJW significantly lowered total cholesterol and low-density lipoprotein (LDL) cholesterol when tested in healthy rats. It significantly inhibited weight gain in high-fat-fed rats, and in fructose-fed rats, SJW normalised the dyslipidaemia induced by fructose feeding and improved the insulin sensitivity (Husain et al 2011a). The same authors showed that SJW significantly reduced elevated blood glucose levels in diabetic rats and exerted a significant anxiolytic effect in this test group (Husain et al 2011b). A significant decrease in blood glucose levels was also observed after 1 week's administrations of SJW extract (125 and 250 mg/kg) to streptozotocin-diabetic rats. It also improved their dysregulated metabolic parameters (Can et al 2011).

Hypolipidaemic activity and antiatherosclerotic effects were also seen in another study utilising hypercholesterolaemic rabbits being treated with hydroalcoholic SJW extract (150 mg/kg). The effect appeared to be stronger than that of lovastatin (10 mg/kg) (Asgary et al 2012).

Previously, SJW extracts were identified as inhibitors of adipogenesis of 3T3-L1 cells and shown to inhibit insulin-sensitive glucose uptake in mature fat cells. The same authors subsequently found that SJW extract limits the differentiation of pre-adipocytes and significantly induces insulin resistance in mature fat cells. These effects were not mediated by hyperforin and hypericin (Richard et al 2012)

Gastrointestinal effects

SJW exhibits antispasmodic activity, according to research conducted with an experimental animal model (Jakovljevic et al 2000), most likely mediated via GABA activity. Among the chemical constituents of SJW extract tested, hyperforin and, to a lesser extent, the flavonoids kaempferol and quercetrin inhibited acetylcholine-induced contractions in an animal model (Capasso et al 2008). SJW has a direct inhibitory effect on smooth muscle and could also possibly modulate gastric neurotransmission. A more recent in vivo irritable bowel syndrome study showed that SJW extract diminished the recruitment of inflammatory cells and tumour necrosis factor-α following restraint stress not in a dose-dependent manner and inhibited small-bowel and colonic transit acceleration like loperamide, but had minimal effect on gastric emptying (Mozaffari et al 2011).

OTHER ACTIONS

No clinically significant effect on platelet aggregation has been identified (Beckert et al 2007).

Induction of CYP3A4 activity in the intestinal wall

Human studies have identified CYP3A4 and 2C19 induction effects for standard SJW extracts (e.g. LI 160), but no effects on CYP1A2, CYP2C9 or CYP2D6 (Durr et al 2000, Gurley et al 2008a, Jiang et al 2004, Wang et al 2001, 2004a). Human studies have failed to identify significant CYP3A4, 2D6, 2C9, 1A2 or 2C19 induction for low-hyperforin SJW extracts, such as ZE 117, using the appropriate probe drugs (Arold et al 2005, Madabushi et al 2006, Mueller et al 2004).

Hyperforin is a potent ligand for the pregnane X receptor, an orphan nuclear receptor that regulates expression of the CYP3A4 mono-oxygenase (Moore et al 2000). Although it is considered the chief constituent responsible for the pharmacokinetic interactions reported, there are other, less potent constituents in SJW, which also modulate cytochrome enzymes (Obach 2000).

Results from an open-label clinical study suggest that the effects of standard SJW (LI 160) on CYP3A4 enzymes may be biphasic, where the initial dose leads to a minor inhibition, followed by significant induction during long-term use (Rengelshausen et al 2005). Clinical studies indicate that CYP3A activity returns progressively to the basal level approximately 1 week after cessation of SJW administration (Imai et al 2008).

Increases levels of intestinal P-glycoprotein

SJW extract produced a 3.8-fold increase of intestinal P-gp expression in vivo (Durr et al 2000). Hyperforin has been identified as the key constituent responsible for P-gp induction effects (Tian et al 2005), although in vitro tests suggest other less potent constituents also exist, such as quercetin, hypericin, biapigenin and kaempferol (Patel et al 2004, Weber et al 2004).

Once again, low-hyperforin SJW extracts do not appear to significantly induce P-gp (Arold et al 2005, Madabushi et al 2006, Mueller et al 2004).

In vitro and in vivo tests further indicate that P-gp effects caused by standard SJW (LI 160) are biphasic, with an initial inhibitory effect followed by induction after longer exposure (Rengelshausen et al 2005, Wang et al 2004a).

Decreases levels of P-glycoprotein at blood–brain barrier

Newer research shows that SJW extract and the constituents hyperforin, hypericin and quercetin decreased P-gp transport activity at the blood–brain barrier in a dose- and time-dependent manner. SJW extract and hyperforin directly inhibited P-gp activity, whereas hypericin and quercetin modulated transporter function through a mechanism involving protein kinase C (Ott et al 2010).

CLINICAL USE

SJW is one of the most clinically tested herbal medicines available. As a result, we have an understanding of the key mechanisms of action, clinical effects, safety issues and also how it compares to standard pharmaceutical treatments. Its strong evidence base provides a good rationale for every clinician to consider its use where appropriate. Various SJW extracts have been tested in clinical trials. Some trials conducted with SJW used a 0.3% hypericin water and alcohol extract, known as LI 160. Most newer studies use different preparations, such as WS 5573 (standardised to hyperforin) or ZE 117 (a low-hyperforin concentration preparation).

S

Depression

Overall, SJW preparations are mainly used for mood disorders in modern-day practice, although it demonstrates benefits for other indications. There is now strong evidence from several meta-analyses to conclude that SJW extract is an effective treatment in mild, moderate and major depressive disorder with efficacy comparable to tricyclic and selective serotonin reuptake inhibitor (SSRI) antidepressant drugs (Cipriani et al 2012, Linde et al 2005a, 2009, Nahas & Sheikh 2011, Sarris & Kavanagh 2009). Additionally, SJW is well tolerated and associated with fewer side effects than pharmaceutical antidepressants. There is also evidence indicating that it reduces relapse.

Clinical note — The Hamilton Depression Scale (HDS)

The HDS is an observer-rated scale that focuses mainly on somatic symptoms of depression. Although the original version included 21 items, a similar version using 17 items is more commonly used in clinical trials. Most studies using the HDS report the number of 'treatment responders' (patients achieving a score less than 10 and/or less than 50% of the baseline score) (Linde et al 2005a).

Mild to moderate depression

SJW has shown efficacy as a successful treatment for mild to moderate depression in numerous double-blind, placebo-controlled trials, confirmed by several meta-analyses and systematic reviews. Moreover, the clinical guidelines for the management of major depressive disorder in adults published by the Canadian Network for Mood and Anxiety Treatments (CANMAT) conclude that level 1 evidence supports SJW in mild to moderate depressive disorder (Ravindran et al 2009).

A 2005 Cochrane review analysed data from 37 double-blind, randomised studies (n = 4925) that used monopreparations of SJW over a treatment period of at least 4 weeks (Linde et al 2005a). It concluded that SJW extracts were superior to placebo for improving symptoms and SJW produced effects similar to synthetic antidepressants (tricyclic antidepressants [TCAs] and SSRIs) in adults with mild to moderate depression. The same conclusion was found in a later systematic review (Sarris & Kavanagh 2009).

Kasper et al (2008a) reanalysed data from a subset of patients (n = 217) suffering from an acute episode of mild depression from controlled trials testing SJW extract WS 5570 from the 2005 Cochrane review. The analysis shows that SJW extract WS 5570 has a meaningful beneficial effect during acute treatment of patients suffering from mild depression and leads to a substantial increase in the probability of remission. The studies tested three different doses — 600, 900 or 1200 mg/day — or placebo for 6 weeks. Patients receiving active treatment with WS 5570 experienced decreases in the HDS total score by an average of 10.8 (600 mg/day), 9.6 (900 mg/day), and 10.7 (1200 mg/day) points between the pre-treatment baseline value and the end of acute treatment, compared to 6.8 points in the placebo group. All differences were significant. The rates of responders were 73%, 64%, 71% and 37% for WS 5570 600 mg/day, 900 mg/day and 1200 mg/day and placebo, respectively.

Since then, a long-term, open, multicentre study testing 500 mg/day of SJW ZE117 extract over 52 weeks found that the herbal treatment produced a significant reduction in depression scores (HDS) and was associated with a lower side effect rate than for standard antidepressants, thereby confirming earlier results (Brattström 2009).

Melzer et al (2010) conducted a different type of trial in an attempt to see whether using SJW in a real practice setting, where patients were taking multiple medications and required individualised dosing, would still be effective in the treatment of depression. This open-label, German study (n = 1778, from 304 centres) utilised Helarium-425 capsules from Bionorica, Neumarkt, Germany, at different doses, individualised for the patient. The mean daily dose was 822.5 ± 205.4 mg dry ethanolic *Hypericum* extract at admission (range 425–1700 mg) and 754.4 ± 231.1 mg at the last visit. The most commonly prescribed dosage schedules were an intake twice or three times daily. Used in this way by outpatients, SJW treatment was effective as an antidepressant in the management of depression in daily practice and lower age and shorter duration of the disorder were associated with significantly better outcomes (Melzer et al 2010). The herbal drug was well tolerated, and no new or serious adverse drug reactions were identified. More specifically, the SJW treatment was an extract with 255–285 mg dry ethanolic extract per coated tablet, standardised to hypericin 0.3% and a hyperforin content of 2–3%, or Helarium-425 with 425 mg dry ethanolic extract per capsule (DER 3.5–6 : 1) or Helarium-425, which is standardised to hypericin 0.1–0.3% and has a hyperforin content of maximum 6%, flavonoid/rutoside minimum 6% in the extract.

Major depression

Although a 2005 Cochrane review stated that SJW shows only minimal benefits over placebo in major depression (Linde et al 2005a), an updated 2009 Cochrane systematic review has concluded that SJW extracts: (1) are superior to placebo in patients with major depression; (2) are similarly effective as standard antidepressants (SSRIs and TCAs); and (3) have fewer side effects than standard antidepressants (Linde et al 2009). A total of 29 randomised controlled trials (RCTs) were evaluated (n = 5489), including 18 comparisons with placebo and 17 comparisons with synthetic standard antidepressants. The standard antidepressants used as active comparators were fluoxetine (six trials, dosage 20–40 mg), sertraline (four trials, 50–100 mg), imipramine (three trials, dosage 100–150 mg), citalopram (one trial, 20 mg), paroxetine (one trial, 20–40 mg), maprotiline (one trial, 75 mg) and amitriptyline (one trial, 75 mg). Most trials used a dose range 500–1200 mg/day of SJW.

More recently, another double-blind, placebo-controlled, randomised study was conducted which involved 100 patients with moderate severity of major depression and vegetative features of atypical depression (Mannel et al 2010). The SJW extract LI 160 (600 mg/day) given over 8 weeks was significantly superior to placebo for producing an antidepressant effect (HDS) and also improved hypersomnolence. In addition, the secondary outcome variables were significantly improved by SJW treatment. These were the depression subscore of the Patient Health Questionnaire, the Clinical Global Impression (CGI), a patient's satisfaction scale and the Hamilton Anxiety Scale.

This result is clinically important as the effects of standard antidepressants over placebo are modest and, although SSRIs are better tolerated than older antidepressant drugs (such as monoamine oxidase inhibitors), side effects are still common.

Comparative studies

SJW vs SSRIs

SJW is as effective as the newer generation of antidepressants but with fewer adverse events and better tolerability. The most recent Cochrane review found no significant differences between SJW and SSRIs in the proportion of people responding (12 RCTs) and active treatment with SJW resulted in significantly fewer drop-outs due to side effects compared with SSRIs (11 RCTs, 1769 people). There were no significant differences between groups in the reporting of adverse effects, although the result was of borderline significance (nine RCTs, 1641 people; $P = 0.048$) (Cipriani et al 2011, Linde et al 2009). Similarly, a meta-analysis of SJW trials (13 controlled trials) in major depressive disorder found that SJW does not differ from SSRIs according to efficacy and adverse events. Once again, there were fewer drop-outs due to adverse events in the SJW group (Rahimi et al 2009).

A comparative analysis by Kasper et al (2010b) between paroxetine and SJW extract WS 5570 revealed a 10–38-fold higher adverse events rate for the synthetic comparator.

Citalopram

A double-blind study (n = 388) found SJW extract (900 mg daily of extract STW3-VI) to be as effective as citalopram (20 mg daily) in moderate depression (Gastpar et al 2006). Both antidepressants were significantly more effective than placebo. Significantly more adverse events were documented in the citalopram group (53.2%) than for SJW (17.2%) or placebo (30%). In contrast, a subsequent three-arm RCT (n = 81) found that neither SJW (810 mg/day, extract not further described) nor citalopram (20 mg/day) showed a statistically significant effect over placebo in the treatment of minor depression over a 12-week period. The authors state that both treatments were associated with a significant number of adverse effects during the treatment. However, the prevalence of adverse effects reported in the placebo arm was higher (91.3%) than in the SJW (84.6%) arm, confirming Gastpar's study (Rapaport et al 2011).

Sertraline

To study the long-term efficacy of SJW, a cohort of 124 participant 'responders' continued treatment after week 8, until week 26. They were randomly assigned SJW (900–1500 mg), sertraline (50–100 mg) or matching placebo during this extension phase. At week 26, the outcome was equivocal; although both SJW and sertraline were still therapeutically effective, a pronounced 'placebo effect' impeded calling a significant result at week 26 (Sarris et al 2012a).

SJW vs TCAs

The most recent Cochrane review found no significant differences between SJW and TCAs in the proportion of people responding (five RCTs in total, of which three RCTs used imipramine, one RCT used amitriptyline and one RCT used maprotiline). Additionally, significantly fewer participants withdrew for any reason or due to side effects with SJW treatment compared to older antidepressants (three RCTs, imipramine; one RCT, amitriptyline; one RCT, maprotiline) and significantly fewer reported any adverse effects (Cipriani et al 2011, Linde et al 2009). Importantly, SJW is not associated with orthostatic hypotension, a common adverse effect associated with TCAs and related drugs, the older MAO inhibitors and serotonin-noradrenaline reuptake inhibitors (SNRIs) (Darowski et al 2009).

SJW vs SSRI and SNRI and others (mirtazapine)

A Cochrane review analysing citalopram vs other antidepressants for depression found that SJW was equally effective as citalopram, mirtazapine or venlafaxine. They also found that citalopram was associated with a higher rate of patients experiencing side effects than SJW (odds ratio 1.69, 95% confidence interval 1.01–2.83; one trial, 258 participants). It was shown that citalopram was associated with a higher rate of patients experiencing gastrointestinal problems or vertigo (Cipriani et al 2012).

Clinical note — Which extracts are effective?

Since the constituents of SJW extract differ between the individual manufacturers, the efficacy cannot be extrapolated from one extract to another. Three RCTs have favourably compared low-hyperforin extracts (ZE 117) to fluoxetine or imipramine, suggesting that the absence of hyperforin does not hinder the antidepressant effect (Friede et al 2001, Schrader 2000, Woelk 2000). In a subsequent review of trials included in the clinical studies above, WS 5572, LI 160, WS 5570 and ZE 117 SJW extracts have all shown significantly greater efficacy than placebo and similar efficacy and better tolerability than standard antidepressant drugs (Kasper et al 2010a).

Paediatric use

Results from a postmarketing surveillance study of 101 children under 12 years with mild to moderate depression have suggested that SJW may be an effective and well-tolerated treatment in this population (Hubner & Kirste 2001). The number of doctors rating effectiveness of treatment with SJW as 'good' or 'excellent' was 72% after 2 weeks, 97% after 4 weeks and 100% after 6 weeks and ratings

> ***Clinical note — Is SJW cost-effective?***
> A recent study reports on using the Markov model to estimate the health and economic impacts of SJW versus antidepressants. Outcomes were treatment costs, quality-adjusted life years and net monetary benefits. SJW was shown to be a cost-effective alternative to generic antidepressants (Solomon et al 2011, 2013).
> Similarly, a report commissioned by the National Institute of Complementary Medicine in Australia and undertaken by Access Economics concluded that, based on analyses of RCTs for SJW, it was found to be cost-effective and produced a cost saving compared to standard antidepressants for patients with mild to moderate depression (Access Economics 2010). More specifically, with treated mild and moderate depression estimated to affect 339,752 Australians in 2009, there could be around $50 million per annum in potential savings from switching to SJW from standard antidepressants.
> In the sensitivity analysis, SJW dominated standard antidepressants for mild to moderate depression because it is cheaper than standard antidepressants and fewer patients withdraw from SJW than from standard antidepressants. Even if the unit cost of SJW was the same as that of standard antidepressants, SJW would remain dominant due to the lower changeover rates compared to standard antidepressants.

by parents were similar. Although encouraging, it is difficult to interpret the clinical significance of the results, as there was no placebo group and the final evaluation included only 76% of the initial sample. A subsequent study by Findling and colleagues (2003) evaluated the use of SJW in 33 children aged 6–16 years in an open-label design for 8 weeks, also finding good results. The initial dose was 150 mg three times daily and could be titrated up to 300 mg three times daily. Using the Children's Depression Rating Scale, 76% of the patients clinically improved and 93% continued therapy at the end of the study.

An 8-week open pilot study was conducted with SJW (300 mg three times daily) in 26 adolescents with major depressive disorder (Simeon et al 2005). The subjects were aged 12–17 years (mean 14.8 years). Only 11 patients completed the study; 9 (82%) of them showed significant clinical improvement based on CGI change scores. Of the 15 patients (58%) who did not complete the study, 8 patients were non-compliant and 7 patients were discontinued because of persisting or worsening depression. The interpretation of these results is difficult due to a large drop-out rate.

Preventing relapse of depression

A double-blind, placebo-controlled, multicentre trial conducted by Kasper et al (2008b) evaluated the efficacy and safety of hypericum extract WS 5570 in preventing relapse during 6 months' continuation treatment and 12 months' long-term maintenance treatment after recovery from an episode of recurrent depression. After 6 weeks of single-blind treatment with 3 × 300 mg/day WS 5570, patients with score ≤2 on item 'Improvement' of the CGI scale and an HDS total score decrease ≥50% versus baseline were randomised to 3 × 300 mg/day WS 5570 or placebo for 26 weeks. This provided a total of 426 patients in the next study phase. Treatment with WS 5570 showed more favourable HDS and Beck Depression Inventory time courses and greater overall improvement (CGI) than controls. In long-term maintenance treatment, a pronounced prophylactic effect of WS 5570 was observed in patients with an early onset of depression as well as in those with a high degree of chronicity. Adverse event rates under WS 5570 were comparable to placebo.

A reanalysis of data obtained from a total of 154 patients responders, in a multicentre RCT after 6 weeks of treatment for an episode of moderate depression with either 20 mg citalopram or 900 mg SJW extract STW 3-VI, showed that SJW extract STW 3-VI is more efficient in lowering the relapse and recurrence rates of responders, when compared to citalopram and placebo. In addition, duration of response was increased in the group treated with SJW extract STW 3-VI (Singer et al 2011).

Postnatal depression

A 2009 systematic review found no clinically important results about the effects of SJW in postnatal depression (Craig & Howard 2009).

Obsessive-compulsive disorder (OCD)

Treatment with a fixed dose of 450 mg of SJW containing 0.3% hypericin twice daily over 12 weeks improved the condition in 5 of 12 patients, according to an open study (Taylor & Kobak 2000). Two recent systematic reviews, however, concluded that controlled studies suggest that SJW is ineffective in treating OCD (Camfield et al 2011, Sarris et al 2012b).

Autism

SJW was only modestly effective in the short-term treatment of irritability in some patients with autistic disorder in an open pilot study of three male participants (Niederhofer 2009).

Seasonal affective disorder (SAD)

Wheatley (1999) found that people with mild to moderate SAD experienced significant improvements with anxiety, loss of libido and insomnia after 8 weeks' treatment with SJW. The test group receiving SJW extract (Kira 300 mg) three times daily plus light therapy experienced superior sleep compared with the group receiving SJW as standalone treatment.

Clinical note — Relative safety of SJW compared with pharmaceutical antidepressants

Much has been made of the known or suspected risks associated with the use of SJW, with far too little discussion focusing on the decisive question of its relative safety compared with pharmaceutical antidepressants. It has been estimated that approximately 1 in 30,000 people using SJW will experience an adverse reaction, including those attributed to drug interactions (Schulz 2006). An overview of 16 postmarketing surveillance studies involving different SJW preparations and 34,804 patients found that side effect incidence varied from 0 to 2.8% in short-term studies (4–6 weeks) and 3.4–5.7% in long-term studies (52 weeks) (Linde & Knuppel 2005). Gastrointestinal symptoms, sensitivity to light and other skin conditions and agitation were the most commonly reported side effects and were generally described as mild. The review found that serious side effects or interactions were not reported by any study. Taking this into account, the incidence of side effects to SJW is approximately 10-fold lower than for conventional antidepressants (SSRIs) (Schulz 2006). The most common adverse event among spontaneous reports is photosensitivity, which is estimated to occur in 1 in 300,000 treated cases. This can occur with a dose of 5–10 mg/day hypericin, which is 2–4-fold higher than the recommended dose. SJW has no significant effect on blood pressure or heart rate (Siepmann et al 2002), making it a safer choice than TCAs in patients with cardiovascular disease. It also lacks anticholinergic activity, so side effects such as dry mouth, urinary retention and blurred vision do not occur. In addition, the common side effects reported for SSRIs, such as anorexia, insomnia, sexual dysfunction, excessive sweating and visual disturbance, have not been reported for SJW. Similarly to all standard antidepressants, SJW can interact with other medicines and needs to be judiciously prescribed.

Polyneuropathy

Although SJW is sometimes used for nerve pain, a randomised, double-blind, crossover study of 54 patients identified a trend towards lower total pain score with SJW treatment, although none of the individual pain ratings was significantly changed (Sindrup et al 2001). The dose of SJW used provided 2.7 mg/day total hypericin and was taken over 5 weeks.

Menopause: psychological and psychosomatic symptoms

A 2013 meta-analysis has concluded that *Hypericum perforatum* L. extracts and its combination with other herbs were significantly superior to placebo in the treatment of menopause (Liua et al 2013). Importantly, SJW treatment had fewer side effects than the placebo arms of the studies analysed.

It appears that its effects are seen after at least 8 weeks of treatment, according to a placebo-controlled study showing SJW was an effective treatment for the vasomotor symptoms of perimenopausal or postmenopausal women (n = 100) (Abdali et al 2010). Other symptoms may also respond, as was seen in another study using SJW (160 mg effervescent tablet, Goldaru, three times a day), which significantly decreased psychomental changes, sleep disorders and vasomotor symptoms in 30 menopausal women throughout the third and the sixth week of the study (Fahami et al 2010). An early study not only confirmed that menopausal symptoms reduced or disappeared completely in the majority of women (76.4% by patient evaluation and 79.2% by doctor evaluation) but sexual wellbeing also improved in 80% of cases (Grube et al 1999). The study used 900 mg hypericum (Kira 300 mg three times daily) in the 12-week study.

A review of the evaluations given by women assessed in the VITamins And Lifestyle (VITAL) cohort (n = 35,016), of whom n = 880 had invasive breast cancer, found no risks associated with taking SJW for menopausal symptoms (Brasky et al 2010).

IN COMBINATION

SJW and black cohosh

A fixed combination of isopropanolic black cohosh (Remifemin; standardised to 1 mg triterpene glycosides) and ethanolic SJW (standardised to 0.25 mg total hypericin) was tested in 301 women with menopausal symptoms with pronounced psychological symptoms (Uebelhack et al 2006). The double-blind, randomised study found that 16 weeks of herbal treatment produced a significant 50% reduction in the Menopause Rating Scale score compared to 20% with placebo and a significant 42% reduction in the HDS score compared to only 13% in the placebo group.

A second study testing the effectiveness of combined SJW and black cohosh found that combination therapy was superior to stand-alone black cohosh therapy for the treatment of climacteric mood symptoms in general practice (Briese et al 2007). This was a prospective, controlled, open-label observational study which involved 6141 women attending 1287 outpatient gynaecologists in Germany.

A 2012 review similarly concluded that the combination of black cohosh and SJW showed an improvement of climacteric complaints in comparison to placebo, whereas most of the studies that compared black cohosh monotherapy with placebo did not show significant effects (Laakmann et al 2012).

SJW and chaste tree

The herbal combination of SJW and *Vitex agnus-castus* (chaste tree) was not found to be superior to placebo for the treatment of menopausal symptoms in an RCT with 93 women (van Die et al 2009a).

Perimenopause

Symptomatic perimenopausal women aged 40–65 years who experience hot flushes (three or more per day) may experience significant improvements to menopause-specific quality of life using SJW extract (900 mg t.i.d.) according to a double-blind, placebo-controlled study (Al-Akoum et al 2009). After 3 months of treatment, herbal treatment was significantly better than placebo for menopause-specific quality of life and also provided significant improvements for self-reported sleep problems. No significant effects were seen at 6 weeks, indicating that the effects have slow onset.

IN COMBINATION

SJW and chaste tree

It has been suggested that some of the symptoms typically attributed to menopause may be more related to premenstrual syndrome (PMS) than menopause, as perimenopausal women appear to be more prone to PMS-like symptoms, or at least to tolerate them less well. An RCT (n = 14, late perimenopausal women) conducted over 16 weeks found that the herbal combination was superior to placebo for total PMS-like scores ($P = 0.02$), PMS-depression ($P = 0.006$), and PMS-craving clusters ($P = 0.027$) and produced a significant reduction in anxiety ($P = 0.003$) and flushes ($P = 0.002$) (van Die et al 2009b).

Premenstrual syndrome

An early open study in patients with PMS found that a low dose of 300 mg SJW daily produced significant reductions in all outcome measures. The degree of improvement in overall PMS scores between baseline and the end of the trial was 51%, with over two-thirds experiencing at least a 50% decrease in symptom severity (Stevinson & Ernst 2000). Similarly, a 2009 systematic review concluded that SJW shows some benefit in PMS (Whelan et al 2009).

In a subsequent study Canning et al (2010) reported that SJW was more effective than placebo in the treatment of PMS. By measuring levels of serum sex hormones and inflammatory cytokines, they also excluded inflammatory or hormone regulation as a possible mechanism of action. Another subsequent RCT (n = 170 women with PMS for at least 6 months) showed that those receiving SJW (tablets, standardised to 680 mg of hypericin per day) had significantly lower PMS scores compared with baseline and placebo. The biggest improvements in score occurred for crying (71%) and depression (52%) (Ghazanfarpour et al 2011).

Attention-deficit hyperactive disorder (ADHD)

A double-blind RCT found that SJW (300 mg three times daily of *H. perforatum* standardised to 0.3% hypericin) was ineffective for the symptomatic treatment of ADHD in children (Weber et al 2008). The study involved 54 children aged 6–17 years who met *Diagnostic and Statistical Manual of Mental Disorders* (Fourth Edition) criteria for ADHD by structured interview and was conducted over 8 weeks. Two subsequent reviews have also concluded that SJW is ineffective in ADHD (Rucklidge et al 2009, Sarris et al 2011).

Nervous agitation in children

IN COMBINATION

A multicentre, prospective observational study with 115 children aged between 6 and 12 years tested a herbal combination of SJW, valerian root and passionflower root dry extract for 4 weeks. According to the parents, a distinct improvement was observed in children who had attention problems, showed social withdrawal and/or were anxious/depressive. Based on the doctors' assessment, 82–94% of the affected children responded as they showed no or just mild symptoms at the end of the treatment period, an observation based on evaluated symptoms such as depression, school/examination anxieties, further anxieties, sleeping problems and different physical problems. Therapeutic success was not influenced by additional medication or therapies and treatment was well tolerated (Trompetter et al 2013).

Smoking cessation

Preliminary evidence from experimental models suggested that SJW may be of use in reducing nicotine withdrawal signs, although more recent research indicates no effect on abstinence rates. In the study, SJW significantly and dose-dependently reduced the total nicotine abstinence score (Catania et al 2003). In contrast, a placebo-controlled blinded RCT (n = 143) which tested 900 mg SJW or placebo tablets taken 2 weeks prior and 2 weeks after the quit day did not find that SJW increased absolute quit rates or affected withdrawal symptoms (Parsons et al 2009). Similarly, a placebo-controlled blinded RCT (n = 118) which tested 300 mg SJW, 600 mg SJW or placebo tablets three times daily also did not find that SJW increased smoking abstinence rates (Sood et al 2010).

Herpes infection

Based on its antiviral activity, SJW is also used clinically in the treatment of herpesvirus infections. One study of unknown design found that oral extract LI 160 (over a period of 3 months) reduced the frequency and severity of episodes of recurrent herpes labialis and herpes genitalis (Mannel et al 2000).

Topical use

SJW extract is used in a variety of skin conditions based on effects such as increased skin hydration, reduced the transepidermal water loss and promoted keratinocyte differentiation. For further information on the underlying mechanisms of these effects, please refer to Casetti et al (2011).

Atopic dermatitis

A cream containing SJW extract (standardised to 1.5% hyperforin) was shown to reduce the intensity of eczematous lesions when used twice daily in a prospective, double-blind study (Schempp et al 2003). Beneficial effects were already observed at the first visit, which was on day 7. A review evaluating plants for their effects in skin diseases also concluded that SJW appears promising for atopic dermatitis (Reuter et al 2010).

Treatment of acute and contused injuries

No controlled studies are available, but anti-inflammatory, analgesic and bactericidal activities provide a theoretical basis for its use.

Commission E approves the topical use of oily SJW preparations for this indication (Blumenthal et al 2000).

Herpes simplex 1 and 2

IN COMBINATION

A single-use, topical formulation containing copper sulfate pentahydrate and SJW (Dynamiclear) was compared to topical 5% aciclovir cream in an RCT (n = 149) for the treatment of herpes simplex virus type 1 and 2 lesions in adult patients. The SJW formulation was well tolerated and more effective in reducing burning, stinging, pain, erythema and vesiculation (Clewell et al 2012).

Myalgia

Although no controlled studies are available, anti-inflammatory and analgesic activities provide a theoretical basis for its use in this condition.

Commission E approves the topical use of oily SJW preparations for this indication (Blumenthal et al 2000).

First-degree burns

Although no controlled studies are available, anti-inflammatory, analgesic and bactericidal activities provide a theoretical basis for its use in this condition.

Commission E approves the topical use of oily SJW preparations for this indication (Blumenthal et al 2000).

Plaque-type psoriasis

SJW ointment applied twice daily for 4 weeks may be effective in reducing psoriasis area severity index scores in mild plaque-type psoriasis (Najafizadeh et al 2012).

Ultraviolet (UV)-protective effects

SJW cream significantly reduced UVB-induced erythema as opposed to the vehicle when tested on 20 volunteers in a randomised, double-blind, vehicle-controlled study (Meinke et al 2012).

Caesarean section

A placebo-controlled study of 144 volunteers supports the use of SJW ointment (applied three times daily for 16 days) following caesarean section to promote wound healing, improve scar formation and reduce pain and pruritus (Samadi et al 2010).

Diabetic foot

IN COMBINATION

A case report exists describing the successful use of an extract of SJW and neem oil (*Azadirachta indica*) for foot wounds with exposed bone in a patient with bilateral advanced diabetic ulcers (Labichella 2013).

Venous ulcers

IN COMBINATION

The therapeutic effects of the ointment Herbadermal (extracts of garlic, SJW and calendula) was tested over a 7-week period in 25 patients with ulceration of the lower leg (no longer than 2 months or recurrent ulceration during the last 6 months). The percentage of epithelialisation was 99.1% without significant effects on the microbial flora (Kundaković et al 2012).

Scalp wounds

IN COMBINATION

A retrospective, non-controlled analysis suggests that a mixture of SJW oil and neem oil (*Azadirachta indica*) is a therapy that is very simple to use, safe and potentially effective for the treatment of scalp wounds with exposed bone (Läuchli et al 2012).

Photodynamic therapy

A prospective study aimed at investigating the efficacy of PDT with topical application of an extract of *H. perforatum* in actinic keratosis, basal cell carcinoma (BCC) and morbus Bowen (carcinoma in situ) was conducted with 34 patients (8 with actinic keratoses, 21 with BCC and 5 with Bowen's disease) (Kacerovska et al 2008). Hypericum extract was applied on the skin lesions under occlusion and followed by irradiation with 75 J/cm^2 of red light 2 hours later. The treatment was performed weekly for 6 weeks on average. The percentage of complete clinical response was 50% for actinic keratoses, 28% in patients with superficial BCC and 40% in patients with Bowen's disease. There was only a partial remission seen in patients with nodular BCCs. A complete disappearance of tumour cells was found in the histological preparation of 11% of patients with superficial BCCs and 80% in the patients with Bowen's disease. Unfortunately, the combined treatment was poorly tolerated, as all patients complained of burning and painful sensations during irradiation.

S

OTHER USES

In practice, SJW is also used to treat fibrositis, nervous exhaustion, sciatica and gastrointestinal conditions, such as oesophagitis and peptic ulcers. Traditionally, SJW has been used for wound healing, as a diuretic, for melancholy, as pain relief, treatment for snake bites, for bedwetting in children, and in malaria and psychosis.

DOSAGE RANGE

- Dried herb: 2–5 g/day.
- Liquid extract (1:2): 3–6 mL/day.

Clinical note — PDT for tumour cells

PDT involves the administration of a photosensitiser, which is taken up and stored within tumour cells, followed by light irradiation with a specific wavelength, giving rise to irreversible tissue destruction (Kacerovska et al 2008). It is aimed at destroying tumour cells without damaging the surrounding normal tissues (Agostinis et al 2002). This combination approach results in the production of cytotoxic oxygen singlets within the tumour that cause irreversible cellular damage and tumour destruction.

- Tincture (1:5): 7.5–15 mL/day.
- Standardised extract containing 1.0–2.7 mg total hypericin daily.
- It is advised that patients using SJW long-term should have their doses reduced slowly when discontinuing its use.

External use

- Oily macerate: Macerate flowering tops in olive oil for several weeks and stir often, then drain through a gauze. Store in a dark bottle out of direct light. Apply oil directly to the affected area. To promote extraction of flavonoids, store in a sunny area for 6 weeks (oil will turn red).

According to clinical studies

Doses are for dried herb or equivalent.

- Mild to moderate depression: adult — doses ranging from 350 to 1800 mg/day have been used; children (aged 6–12 years) — 200–400 mg/day in divided doses.
- Major depression: 500 mg–1800 mg/day in divided doses.
- OCD: 450 mg twice daily of an extract containing 0.3% hypericin.
- Menopausal symptoms: 900 mg/day in divided doses.
- PMS: 300 mg/day (standardised to 900 mcg hypericin).
- SAD: 900 mg/day in divided doses.

Several pharmaceutical-grade preparations of SJW are commercially available, typically extracted from dried aerial parts. LI 160, produced by Lichtwer Pharma, Berlin, Germany, is standardised to contain 0.3% hypericin derivatives and 1–4% hyperforin. It is normally sold as 300 mg capsules. Similarly, the STEI 300 extract, produced by Steiner Arzneimittel of Berlin, Germany, contains 0.2–0.3% hypericin and pseudohypericin and 2–3% hyperforin. Capsules contain 350 mg of extract.

The extracts WS 5570, WS 5572 and WS 5573 are produced by Dr Willmar Schwabe Pharmaceuticals, Karlsruhe, Germany. In contrast to the previously mentioned extracts WS 5570 and WS 5572 contain a higher hyperforin amount (5–6%), whereas WS 5573 contains only low hyperforin levels (0.5%). WS 5570 is an 80% ethanolic extract of SJW with a plant-to-extract ratio of between 3:1 and 3:1–7:1. Tablets contain 300 or 600 mg of extract. The product WS 5572 has similar hyperforin and hypericin profiles to WS 5570, but has a plant-to-extract ratio of between 2.5:1 and 5:1.

In contrast, the hyperforin content of Ze 117 is only 0.2%, much lower than that of other products. Ze 117 is produced by Zeller, Switzerland. It is a 50% ethanolic extract with a herb-to-extract ratio of 4:1–7:1. The dosage of Ze 117 is 500 mg/day.

Helarium-425, produced by Bionorica, Neumarkt, Germany, contains 425 mg SJW 60% ethanolic extract with a plant-to-extract ratio of 3.5–6:1 (Kienow et al 2011).

Clinical note — Mechanisms responsible for reported interactions

Based on the herb's pharmacology, there are several mechanisms by which it may interact with drugs. Considering that SJW has significant serotonin reuptake inhibitor activity and significantly upregulates both 5-HT_{1A} and 5-HT_{2A} receptors, concomitant use of drugs that elevate serotonin levels, such as TCAs or SSRIs, may result in additive or synergistic effects and increase the risk of serotonergic syndrome. As the constituent hyperforin has a significant and selective induction effect on CYP3A4 and 2C19 activity (Durr et al 2000, Wang et al 2001) and induces the drug transporter P-gp, a number of pharmacokinetic interactions are possible with those drugs that are substrates for CYP3A4 or 2C19 and/or rely on P-gp transport. Refer to Chapter 8 for further information on interactions with herbs and natural supplements.

ADVERSE REACTIONS

It has been estimated that approximately 1 in 30,000 people using SJW will experience an adverse reaction, including those attributed to drug interactions (Schulz 2006). The incidence of side effects to SJW is approximately 10-fold lower than for conventional antidepressants (SSRIs). According to an overview of 16 postmarketing surveillance studies, gastrointestinal symptoms, sensitivity to light and other skin conditions and agitation were the most commonly reported side effects and were generally described as mild (Linde & Knuppel 2005). Recent reviews confirm earlier studies stating that adverse effects from SJW are infrequent and minor (Posadzki et al 2013).

Photosensitivity (unlikely at therapeutic doses)

The most common adverse event among spontaneous reports is photosensitivity, which is estimated to occur in 1 in 300,000 treated cases. This can occur with a dose of 5–10 mg/day hypericin, which is 2–4-fold higher than the recommended dose. Commission E has noted the possibility of photosensitivity reactions, particularly in fair-skinned people.

SIGNIFICANT INTERACTIONS

SJW is one of the few herbal medicines that has been subjected to controlled studies in order to determine the significance of its interaction with numerous drugs, which are mainly due to CYP450 enzyme induction and the induction of P-gp (Colalto 2010), and therefore mainly pharmacokinetic in nature (Tsai et al 2012). Although this can be reassuring, the clinical significance of many interactions is still unpredictable because of the variable chemical composition of products (Steinhoff 2012).

Hyperforin is a key mediator of SJW's antidepressive action and mainly responsible for the herb's drug interaction potential. It is a high-affinity ligand for human pregnane X receptor, an orphan nuclear receptor selectively expressed in the liver and intestine that mediates the induction of XME and efflux transporter gene transcription, resulting in decreased oral bioavailability, enhanced systemic clearance and reduced drug efficacy for many drugs.

Most SJW extracts are currently standardised to contain 3% hyperforin, yet several clinical studies have demonstrated that SJW extracts containing less than 1% hyperforin (e.g. ZE 117 extract) are both effective and less likely to produce clinically relevant pharmacokinetic herb-drug interactions (Arold et al 2005, Mai et al 2004, Mueller et al 2009).

Please also note that the enzyme induction may be unmasked after the withdrawal of a combination of SJW (a potent CYP3A inducer with a potent CYP3A inhibitor, e.g. ritonavir) leading to substantial drops in drug exposure of CYP3A substrates (e.g. midazolam). This may require substantial dose adjustments, particularly of orally administered drugs (Hafner et al 2010).

Alprazolam

Decreases serum levels of alprazolam via CYP induction. Monitor for signs of reduced drug effectiveness and adjust the dose if necessary or avoid.

Amitriptyline

Although SJW decreases serum levels of amitriptyline via CYP induction in vivo (Johne et al 2002), theoretically it could also induce increases in serotonin availability, which has an opposite effect; the clinical outcome of these two interacting mechanisms is unknown — monitor for signs of changed drug effectiveness and adjust the dose if necessary or avoid concurrent use.

Antidepressants (SSRIs and SNRIs)

Increased risk of serotonin syndrome possible; however, increased antidepressant activity is also possible with appropriate doses — avoid concurrent use unless under medical supervision, so that doses may be altered appropriately.

Anticonvulsants

Phenobarbitone, phenytoin: SJW may increase drug metabolism, resulting in reduced drug efficacy — avoid concurrent use unless under medical supervision, so that doses may be altered appropriately.

Antineoplastic drugs

Irinotecan imatinib mesylate: plasma levels decreased (He et al 2010, Mathijssen et al 2002) (see Chapter 10 for more information on the safety of complementary medicines and cancer). Reduction of toxicity — the combination might be of benefit (Rahimi & Abdollahi 2012).

Atorvastatin

SJW reduces the efficacy of atorvastatin, so lipid-lowering effects are compromised, according to a clinical study which tested a product called Movina (containing 300 mg of *Hypericum perforatum*), taken as one tablet twice daily (Andren et al 2007).

Bupropion

SJW decreased, to a statistically significant extent, the plasma concentrations of bupropion, probably by increasing the clearance of bupropion — avoid (Lei et al 2010).

Cisplatin

Cisplatin-induced histological abnormality of the kidney was blocked by pretreatment with SJW in vivo (Shibayama et al 2007). Total and free cisplatin concentration in serum was not influenced by SJW treatment, suggesting that this may be a beneficial interaction under professional supervision.

Clopidogrel

SJW might represent a valid option to increase the antiplatelet effect of clopidogrel in non-responders and/or hyporesponders. For example, SJW increased platelet inhibition by enhancement of CYP3A4 metabolic activity for clopidogrel in hyporesponsive volunteers (Lau et al 2011), and a recent study showed that residual platelet reactivity improved with SJW during the first month post percutaneous coronary intervention (Trana et al 2013).

Cyclosporin

Decreases plasma levels of cyclosporin significantly within 3 days of concomitant use via CYP induction (Bauer et al 2003) — avoid concurrent use.

A pharmacokinetic study with kidney graft recipients suggests that the effect is not significant when low-hyperforin products are used (Madabushi et al 2006).

Digoxin

Decreases serum digoxin levels significantly within 10 days of concomitant use (Johne et al 1999), chiefly due to induction of the P-gp. The interaction between digoxin and SJW in humans has been confirmed more recently by Gurley et al (2008) and is clinically significant — monitor patient for signs of reduced drug effectiveness and adjust the dose if necessary or avoid concurrent use.

Fexofenadine

In rats, SJW (1 g/kg) enhanced the elimination of fexofenadine, an antihistamine and P-gp substrate, into the bile when given once daily for 14 days (Turkanovic et al 2009).

Finasteride

SJW treatment for 2 weeks induced the metabolism of finasteride and caused a reduced plasma exposure of the drug (Lundahl et al 2009). A case report reported on an increased prostate-specific antigen value for a man who had started SJW 900 mg/day 10 weeks prior to the test and who was previously well controlled on finasteride (Lochner & Kirch 2011).

Gliclazide

Treatment with SJW significantly increases the apparent clearance of gliclazide, which is independent of CYP2C9 genotype, according to a crossover clinical study (Xu et al 2008). People with diabetes receiving this combination should be closely monitored to evaluate possible signs of reduced efficacy.

HIV non-nucleoside transcriptase inhibitors

Decreases serum levels — avoid concurrent use.

Etravirine — potential effect (Kakuda et al 2011)

Rilpivirine (Sharma & Saravolatz 2013).

HIV protease inhibitors

Decreases serum levels — avoid concurrent use.

Indinavir

Oral administration of either 150 or 300 mg/day SJW for 15 days significantly reduced indinavir plasma levels in rats. This interaction was attributable to the induction of indinavir metabolism by SJW (Ho et al 2009).

Ketamine

SJW greatly decreased the exposure to oral S-ketamine in healthy volunteers. Although this decrease was not associated with significant changes in the analgesic or behavioural effects of ketamine in the present study, usual doses of S-ketamine may need adjustment if used concomitantly with SJW (Peltoniemi et al 2012) — use with caution.

Methadone

Decreases serum levels via CYP induction — avoid concurrent use (Eich-Hochli et al 2003).

Methotrexate

Coadministration of 300 and 150 mg/kg of SJW significantly increased the systemic exposure and toxicity of methotrexate (Yang et al 2012).

Midazolam

Decreases serum levels of midazolam via CYP induction — monitor for signs of reduced drug effectiveness and adjust the dose if necessary or avoid.

Nifedipine

SJW was shown to induce nifedipine metabolism in vivo (Wang et al 2007) — monitor for signs of reduced drug effectiveness and adjust the dose if necessary or avoid.

Non-steroidal anti-inflammatory drugs (etoricoxib)

Decreases serum levels of the drug via CYP induction in vivo — avoid coadministration (Radwan et al 2012).

Omeprazole

Decreases serum levels via CYP induction (Wang et al 2004b) — monitor for signs of reduced drug effectiveness and adjust the dose if necessary or avoid.

Oral contraceptives

Breakthrough bleeding has been reported, which can indicate decreased effectiveness of oral contraceptives. In 2003, a controlled study confirmed that standard doses of SJW cause an induction of ethinyl oestradiol–norethindrone metabolism, consistent with increased CYP3A activity (Hall et al 2003) — use this combination with caution.

In 2002, a pharmacokinetic study found no significant interaction between low-hyperforin SJW and low-dose oral contraceptives (Madabushi et al 2006). This has been confirmed in a further clinical study using an SJW extract (Ze 117) with low hyperforin content on the pharmacokinetics of ethinyl oestradiol and 3-ketodesogestrel (Will-Shahab et al 2009) — low-hyperforin extracts appear to be safe.

Oxycodone

SJW greatly reduced the plasma concentrations of oral oxycodone — avoid (Nieminen et al 2010).

Pegylated interferon-alpha (peginterferon-α)

The combination of peginterferon-α and SJW (taken for 6 weeks during 8 weeks' drug treatment) resulted in severe acute hepatitis in a 61-year-old woman. After 6 months of prednisone treatment, the liver function tests returned to baseline levels — avoid combination (Piccolo et al 2009).

Psoralen plus UVA therapy

High-dose hypericin may increase sensitivity to UV radiation — caution is advised.

Simvastatin

Decreases serum levels of simvastatin via CYP induction (Sugimoto et al 2001) — monitor for signs of reduced drug effectiveness and adjust the dose if necessary (no interaction is expected with pravastatin).

Tacrolimus

Decreases serum levels of tacrolimus via CYP induction (Mai et al 2003) — avoid this combination.

Verapamil

Decreases serum levels of verapamil via CYP induction — monitor for signs of reduced drug effectiveness and adjust the dose if necessary.

Warfarin

Metabolism of warfarin is chiefly by CYP2C9, and a minor metabolic pathway is CYP3A4, so theoretically it may interact with SJW. A clinical study found no change to international normalised ratio (INR) or platelet aggregation (Jiang et al 2004), but there are case reports suggesting that SJW may lower the INR. Caution is advised — monitor INR.

Zolpidem

Repeated administration of SJW decreases the plasma concentration of zolpidem, probably by enhancing CYP3A4 activity (Hojo et al 2011) — avoid.

CONTRAINDICATIONS AND PRECAUTIONS

People with fair skin undergoing UV treatment or with conditions which would be adversely affected by high UV exposure should use high doses of SJW with caution.

A case study reported on the occurrence of radiation-induced optic neuropathy, which may have been the result of radiosensitisation by temozolomide, which could have been strengthened by the hypericin the patient was also taking (Schreiber et al 2010).

People with cancer and undergoing treatment

Hypericum extract, by inducing both CYP3A4 and P-gp, can reduce the plasma concentrations of different antineoplastic agents such as imatinib, irinotecan and docetaxel, thus reducing the clinical efficacy of these drugs. Although these interactions are often predictable, the concomitant use of hypericum extract should be avoided in cancer patients taking interacting medications (Caraci et al 2011).

PREGNANCY AND LACTATION USE

A systematic review of the literature for evidence on the use, safety and pharmacology of SJW focusing on issues pertaining to pregnancy found there is in vitro evidence from animal studies that SJW during pregnancy does not affect cognitive development nor cause long-term behavioural defects, but may lower offspring birth weight (Dugoua et al 2006). A prospective study investigated 54 SJW-exposed pregnancies and 108 pregnancies in the two comparator groups (the second group was taking other pharmacological therapy for depression and a third group of healthy women was not exposed to any known teratogens). The rates of major malformations were similar across the three groups, and were not different from the 3–5% risk expected in the general population. The live birth and prematurity rates were also not different among the three groups (Moretti et al 2009).

A recent study comparing the effects of 7.5 mg/kg fluoxetine and 100 mg/kg SJW showed that maternal exposure to fluoxetine but not SJW could interfere with reproductive parameters in adult male rats (Vieira et al 2013). However, encouragingly, safe doses in pregnant women have not yet been determined. In practice, SJW is not recommended in pregnancy.

SJW appears to be relatively safe in lactation (Dugoua et al 2006, Howland 2010). A systematic review, which reported the results of observational studies, found weak evidence that SJW use during lactation did not affect maternal milk production or infant weight. However, in a few cases, it may cause infant colic, drowsiness or lethargy (Linde et al 2005b). A more recent review identified three studies in which SJW was used by breastfeeding mothers (one case report, one open-label and one cohort study). No adverse effects were reported for mothers and infants for any of these studies (Budzynska et al 2012).

S

PATIENTS' FAQS

What will this herb do for me?

SJW is an effective treatment for mild, moderate and severe depression and it reduces the risk of relapse. Its antidepressant effects are similar to pharmaceutical antidepressant drugs; however, it is better tolerated with fewer side effects. It may also be useful for PMS symptoms, in SAD and OCD and for menopausal and premenopausal women with psychological and psychosomatic symptoms. The oily preparations are also used topically to treat burns, injuries, allergic dermatitis and muscle pain.

When will it start to work?

It often starts to exert beneficial effects in depression within 2–4 weeks of continuous use; however, maximal effects in other conditions may take longer.

Are there any safety issues?

SJW is well tolerated and has far fewer side effects than pharmaceutical antidepressant drugs, but it can interact with a number of different medications. Patients with clinically diagnosed depression should be under the care of a healthcare professional.

Practice points/Patient counselling

- SJW contains numerous constituents with pharmacological activity, including antidepressant, analgesic, anti-inflammatory, antispasmodic, anxiolytic, antineoplastic, antiviral and bactericidal activities.
- The efficacy of SJW in the treatment of mild-to-moderate major depressive disorders is well established through numerous clinical studies. The most commonly studied extract is LI 160, although others have also been tested (e.g. WS 5573 [standardised to hyperforin], ZE 117 [a low-concentration hyperforin preparation], WS 550 and STW3-V1). Clinical effects are comparable to TCAs and SSRIs; it also reduces the incidence of depression relapse.
- With regard to safety, SJW is better tolerated than standard antidepressants (SSRIs and TCAs); however, it still needs to be prescribed judiciously to avoid interactions. Patients with clinically-diagnosed depression should be under the care of a healthcare professional.
- Low-hyperforin-containing SJW extracts do not have the same interaction potential as standard SJW extracts and may present a safer option for some individuals.
- Preliminary human studies have suggested a possible role in PMS, SAD, OCD and in menopausal and premenopausal women with psychological and psychosomatic symptoms.
- Oily preparations have been used topically to treat burns, acute and contused injuries, atopic dermatitis and myalgia.

REFERENCES

Abdali K, et al. Effect of St John's wort on severity, frequency, and duration of hot flashes in premenopausal, perimenopausal and postmenopausal women: a randomized, double-blind, placebo-controlled study. Menopause. 2010 Mar;17(2):326–31.

Agostinis P et al. Hypericin in cancer treatment: more light on the way. Int J Biochem Cell Biol 34.3 (2002): 221–241.

Al-Akoum M et al. Effects of *Hypericum perforatum* (St. John's wort) on hot flashes and quality of life in perimenopausal women: a randomized pilot trial. Menopause 16.2 (2009): 307–14.

Albert D et al. Hyperforin is a dual inhibitor of cyclooxygenase-1 and 5-lipoxygenase. Biochem Pharmacol 64.12 (2002): 1767–1775.

Andren L, et al. Interaction between a commercially available St. John's wort product (Movina) and atorvastatin in patients with hypercholesterolemia. Eur J Clin Pharmacol 63.10 (2007): 913–9116.

Arold G et al. No relevant interaction with alprazolam, caffeine, tolbutamide, and digoxin by treatment with a low-hyperforin St John's wort extract. Planta Med 71.4 (2005): 331–337.

Asgary S, et al. Effect of hydroalcoholic extract of *Hypericum perforatum* on selected traditional and novel biochemical factors of cardiovascular diseases and atherosclerotic lesions in hypercholesterolemic rabbits: A comparison between the extract and lovastatin. J Pharm Bioallied Sci. 2012 Jul;4(3):212–8.

Bauer S et al. Alterations in cyclosporin A pharmacokinetics and metabolism during treatment with St John's wort in renal transplant patients. Br J Clin Pharmacol 55.2 (2003): 203–211.

Beckert BW et al. The effect of herbal medicines on platelet function: an in vivo experiment and review of the literature. Plast Reconstr Surg 120.7 (2007): 2044–2050.

Beerhues L. Hyperforin. Phytochemistry 2006; 67: 2201–2207.

Beijamini V, Andreatini R. Effects of *Hypericum perforatum* and paroxetine on rat performance in the elevated T-maze. Pharmacol Res 48.2 (2003): 199–207.

Bilia AR, et al. St John's wort and depression: efficacy, safety and tolerability: an update. Life Sci 70.26 (2002): 3077–3096.

Blumenthal M, et al (eds), Herbal medicine: expanded Commission E monographs. Austin, TX: Integrative Medicine Communications, 2000.

Brasky TM, et al. Specialty supplements and breast cancer risk in the VITamins And Lifestyle (VITAL) Cohort. Cancer Epidemiol Biomarkers Prev. 2010 Jul;19(7):1696–708.

Brattström A Long-term effects of St. John's wort (*Hypericum perforatum*) treatment: a 1-year safety study in mild to moderate depression. Phytomedicine 2009;16(4):277–83.

Briese V et al. Black cohosh with or without St. John's wort for symptom-specific climacteric treatment — results of a large-scale, controlled, observational study. Maturitas 57.4 (2007): 405–414.

Budzynska K, et al. Systematic review of breastfeeding and herbs. Breastfeed Med. 2012;7(6):489–503.

Butterweck V et al. Step by step removal of hyperforin and hypericin: activity profile of different *Hypericum* preparations in behavioral models. Life Sci 73.5 (2003a): 627–39.

Butterweck V et al. Plasma levels of hypericin in presence of procyanidin B2 and hyperoside: a pharmacokinetic study in rats. Planta Med 69.3 (2003b): 189–92.

Camfield DA, et al. Nutraceuticals in the treatment of obsessive compulsive disorder (OCD): a review of mechanistic and clinical evidence. Prog Neuropsychopharmacol Biol Psychiatry. 2011 Jun 1;35(4):887–95.

Camfield DA, et al. The Neurocognitive Effects of *Hypericum perforatum* Special Extract (Ze 117) during Smoking Cessation. Phytother Res. (2013): 27: 1605–1613..

Can ÖD, et al. Effects of treatment with St. John's Wort on blood glucose levels and pain perceptions of streptozotocin-diabetic rats. Fitoterapia. 2011 Jun;82(4):576–84.

Canning S, et al. The efficacy of *Hypericum perforatum* (St John's wort) for the treatment of premenstrual syndrome: a randomized, double-blind, placebo-controlled trial. CNS Drugs. 2010 Mar;24(3):207–25.

Capasso R et al. Inhibitory effect of the herbal antidepressant St. John's wort (*Hypericum perforatum*) on rat gastric motility. Naunyn Schmiedebergs Arch Pharmacol 376.6 (2008): 407–

Caraci, F., et al. 2011. Metabolic drug interactions between antidepressants and anticancer drugs: focus on selective serotonin reuptake inhibitors and hypericum extract. Curr.Drug Metab, 12, (6) 570–577.

Casetti F, et al. Dermocosmetics for dry skin: a new role for botanical extracts. Skin Pharmacol Physiol. 2011;24(6):289–93.

Catania MA et al. *Hypericum perforatum* attenuates nicotine withdrawal signs in mice. Psychopharmacology (Berl) 169.2 (2003): 186–189.

Chatterjee SS et al. Hyperforin as a possible antidepressant component of hypericum extracts. Life Sci 63.6 (1998): 499–510.

Cipriani A, et al., Depression in adults: drug and physical treatments. Clin Evid (Online). (2011) 2011: 1003.

Cipriani A, et al. Citalopram versus other anti-depressive agents for depression. Cochrane Database Syst Rev. (2012) 7: CD006534.

Clewell A, et al. Efficacy and tolerability assessment of a topical formulation containing copper sulfate and *Hypericum perforatum* on patients with herpes skin lesions: a comparative, randomized controlled trial. J Drugs Dermatol. 2012 Feb;11(2):209–15.

Colalto C Herbal interactions on absorption of drugs: Mechanisms of action and clinical risk assessment. Pharmacol Res. 2010 Sep;62(3):207–27.

Craig M, Howard L. Postnatal depression. Clin Evid (Online). 2009 Jan 26;2009. pii: 1407.

Darowski A, et al. Antidepressants and falls in the elderly. Drugs Aging. 2009;26(5):381–94.

Di Carlo G et al. St John's wort: Prozac from the plant kingdom. Trends Pharmacol Sci 22.6 (2001): 292–297.

Dugoua JJ et al. Safety and efficacy of St. John's wort (hypericum) during pregnancy and lactation. Can J Clin Pharmacol 13.3 (2006): e268–e276.

Durr D et al. St John's Wort induces intestinal P-glycoprotein/MDR1 and intestinal and hepatic CYP3A4. Clin Pharmacol Ther 68.6 (2000): 598–604.

Eich-Hochli D et al. Methadone maintenance treatment and St John's Wort: a case report. Pharmacopsychiatry 36.1 (2003): 35–37.

Etemad L, et al. Investigation of *Hypericum perforatum* extract on convulsion induced by picrotoxin in mice. Pak J Pharm Sci. 2011 Apr;24(2):233–6.

Fahami F, et al. A comparative study on the effects of *Hypericum perforatum* and passion flower on the menopausal symptoms of women

referring to Isfahan city health care centers. Iran J Nurs Midwifery Res. 2010 Fall;15(4):202–7.
Feily A, Abbasi N. The inhibitory effect of *Hypericum perforatum* extract on morphine withdrawal syndrome in rat and comparison with clonidine. Phytother Res. 2009 Nov;23(11):1549–52.
Feisst C, et al. Hyperforin is a novel type of 5-lipoxygenase inhibitor with high efficacy in vivo. Cell Mol Life Sci. 2009 Aug;66(16):2759–71.
Fiebich B, et al. Inhibition of substance P-induced cytokine synthesis by St John's wort extracts. Pharmacopsychiatry 34 (Suppl 1) (2001): S26–S28.
Fiebich BL, et al. Pharmacological studies in an herbal drug combination of St. John's Wort (*Hypericum perforatum*) and passion flower (*Passiflora incarnata*): in vitro and in vivo evidence of synergy between *Hypericum* and *Passiflora* in antidepressant pharmacological models. Fitoterapia. 2011 Apr;82(3):474–80.
Findling R, et al. An open-label study of St. John's wort in juvenile depression. J Am Acad Child Adolesc Psychiatry 2003;42:908–14.
Friede M, et al. Differential therapy of mild to moderate depressive episodes (ICD-10 F 32.0; F 32.1) with St John's wort. Pharmacopsychiatry 34 (Suppl 1) (2001): S38–S41.
Galeotti N, Ghelardini C. St. John's wort relieves pain in an animal model of migraine. Eur J Pain. 2013a Mar;17(3):369–81.
Galeotti N, Ghelardini C. Reversal of NO-induced nociceptive hypersensitivity by St. John's wort and hypericin: NF-κB, CREB and STAT1 as molecular targets. Psychopharmacology (Berl). 2013b May;227(1):149–63.
Galeotti N, et al A prolonged protein kinase C-mediated, opioid-related antinociceptive effect of St John's Wort in mice. J Pain. 2010 Feb;11(2):149–59.
Gastpar M, et al. Comparative efficacy and safety of a once-daily dosage of hypericum extract STW3-VI and citalopram in patients with moderate depression: a double-blind, randomised, multicentre, placebo-controlled study. Pharmacopsychiatry 39.2 (2006): 66–75.
Ghazanfarpour M, et al. *Hypericum perforatum* for the treatment of premenstrual syndrome. Int J Gynaecol Obstet. 2011 Apr;113(1):84–5.
Griffith TN, et al. Neurobiological effects of Hyperforin and its potential in Alzheimer's disease therapy. Curr Med Chem. 2010;17(5):391–406.
Gobbi M et al. In vitro binding studies with two *Hypericum perforatum* extracts (hyperforin, hypericin and biapigenin) on 5-HT6, 5-HT7, GABA(A)/benzodiazepine, sigma, NPY-Y1/Y2 receptors and dopamine transporters. Pharmacopsychiatry 34 (Suppl 1) (2001): S45–S48.
Gómez Del Rio MA, et al. Neuroprotective properties of standardized extracts of *Hypericum perforatum* on rotenone model of Parkinson's disease. CNS Neurol Disord Drug Targets. (2013) 12: 665–679.
Grube B, et al. St John's Wort extract: efficacy for menopausal symptoms of psychological origin. Adv Ther 16.4 (1999): 177–186.
Gulick RM et al. Phase I studies of hypericin, the active compound in St John's Wort, as an antiretroviral agent in HIV-infected adults AIDS Clinical Trials Group Protocols 150 and 258. Ann Intern Med 130.6 (1999): 510–5114.
Gurley BJ et al. Clinical assessment of CYP2D6-mediated herb-drug interactions in humans: effects of milk thistle, black cohosh, goldenseal, kava kava, St. John's wort, and Echinacea. Mol Nutr Food Res 52.7 (2008a): 755–63.
Gurley BJ et al. Gauging the clinical significance of P-glycoprotein-mediated herb-drug interactions: comparative effects of St. John's wort, Echinacea, clarithromycin, and rifampin on digoxin pharmacokinetics. Mol Nutr Food Res 52.7 (2008b): 772–9.
Hafner V, et al. Effect of simultaneous induction and inhibition of CYP3A by St John's Wort and ritonavir on CYP3A activity. Clin Pharmacol Ther. 2010 Feb;87(2):191–6.
Hall SD et al. The interaction between St John's wort and an oral contraceptive. Clin Pharmacol Ther 74.6 (2003): 525–535.
Ho YF, et al. Effects of St. John's wort extract on indinavir pharmacokinetics in rats: differentiation of intestinal and hepatic impacts. Life Sci. 2009 Aug 12;85(7–8):296–302.
Hojo Y, et al. Drug interaction between St John's wort and zolpidem in healthy subjects. J Clin Pharm Ther. 2011 Dec;36(6):711–5.
Hostanska K et al. Hyperforin a constituent of St John's wort (*Hypericum perforatum* L) extract induces apoptosis by triggering activation of caspases and with hypericin synergistically exerts cytotoxicity towards human malignant cell lines. Eur J Pharm Biopharm 56.1 (2003): 121–132.
Howland RH. Update on St. John's Wort J Psychosoc Nurs Ment Health Serv. 2010 Nov;48(11):20–4.
Hubner WD, Kirste T. Experience with St John's Wort (*Hypericum perforatum*) in children under 12 years with symptoms of depression and psychovegetative disturbances. Phytother Res 15.4 (2001): 367–370.
Hudson JB, et al. The importance of light in the anti-HIV effect of hypericin. Antiviral Res 20.2 (1993): 173–178.
Husain GM, et al. Hypolipidemic and antiobesity-like activity of standardised extract of *Hypericum perforatum* L. in rats. ISRN Pharmacol. 2011a;2011:505247.
Husain GM, et al. Beneficial effect of *Hypericum perforatum* on depression and anxiety in a type 2 diabetic rat model. Acta Pol Pharm. 2011b;68(6):913–8.
Imai H et al. The recovery time-course of CYP3A after induction by St John's wort administration. Br J Clin Pharmacol 65.5 (2008): 701–707.
Jacobson JM et al. Pharmacokinetics, safety, and antiviral effects of hypericin, a derivative of St John's wort plant, in patients with chronic hepatitis C virus infection. Antimicrob Agents Chemother 45.2 (2001): 517–524.
Jakovljevic V et al. Pharmacodynamic study of *Hypericum perforatum* L. Phytomedicine 7.6 (2000): 449–453.
Jiang X et al. Effect of St John's wort and ginseng on the pharmacokinetics and pharmacodynamics of warfarin in healthy subjects. Br J Clin Pharmacol 57.5 (2004): 592–599.
Johne A et al. Pharmacokinetic interaction of digoxin with an herbal extract from St John's wort (*Hypericum perforatum*). Clin Pharmacol Ther 66.4 (1999): 338–345.
Johne A et al. Decreased plasma levels of amitriptyline and its metabolites on comedication with an extract from St John's wort (*Hypericum perforatum*). J Clin Psychopharmacol 22.1 (2002): 46–54.
Kacerovska D et al. Photodynamic therapy of nonmelanoma skin cancer with topical *Hypericum perforatum* extract — a pilot study. Photochem Photobiol 84.3 (2008): 779–785.
Kakuda TN, et al. Pharmacokinetic interactions between etravirine and non-antiretroviral drugs. Clin Pharmacokinet. 2011 Jan;50(1):25–39.
Karioti A, Bilia AR. Hypericins as potential leads for new therapeutics. Int J Mol Sci. 2010 Feb 4;11(2):562–94.
Kasper S et al. Efficacy of St. John's wort extract WS 5570 in acute treatment of mild depression: a reanalysis of data from controlled clinical trials. Eur Arch Psychiatry Clin Neurosci 258.1 (2008a): 59–63.
Kasper S et al. Continuation and long-term maintenance treatment with *Hypericum* extract WS 5570 after recovery from an acute episode of moderate depression — a double-blind, randomized, placebo controlled long-term trial. Eur Neuropsychopharmacol 18.11 (2008b): 803–13.
Kasper, S., et al 2010a. Efficacy and tolerability of *Hypericum* extract for the treatment of mild to moderate depression. Eur. Neuropsychopharmacol. 20, 747–765.
Kasper, S., et al 2010b. Better tolerability of St. John's wort extract WS 5570 compared to treatment with SSRIs: a reanalysis of data from controlled clinical trials in acute major depression. Int. Clin. Psychopharmacol. 25, 204–213.
Kiewert C et al. Stimulation of hippocampal acetylcholine release by hyperforin, a constituent of St John's Wort. Neurosci Lett 364.3 (2004): 195–198.
Kim SJ, et al Anti-inflammatory activity of hyperoside through the suppression of nuclear factor-κB activation in mouse peritoneal macrophages. Am J Chin Med. 2011;39(1):171–81.
Koeberle A, et al. Hyperforin, an Anti-Inflammatory Constituent from St. John's Wort, Inhibits Microsomal Prostaglandin E(2) Synthase-1 and Suppresses Prostaglandin E(2) Formation in vivo. Front Pharmacol. 2011 Feb 18;2:7.
Kundaković T, et al. Treatment of venous ulcers with the herbal-based ointment Herbadermal®: a prospective non-randomized pilot study. Forsch Komplementmed. 2012;19(1):26–30.
Laakmann E, et al. Efficacy of *Cimicifuga racemosa*, *Hypericum perforatum* and *Agnus castus* in the treatment of climacteric complaints: a systematic review. Gynecol Endocrinol. 2012 Sep;28(9):703–9.
Labichella ML The use of an extract of *Hypericum perforatum* and *Azadirachta indica* in advanced diabetic foot: an unexpected outcome. BMJ Case Rep. (2013) 2013: pii:bcr2012007299..
Lakhan SE, Vieira KF. Nutritional and herbal supplements for anxiety and anxiety-related disorders: systematic review. Nutr J. 2010 Oct 7;9:42.
Lau WC, et al. The effect of St John's Wort on the pharmacodynamic response of clopidogrel in hyporesponsive volunteers and patients: increased platelet inhibition by enhancement of CYP3A4 metabolic activity. J Cardiovasc Pharmacol. 2011 Jan;57(1):86–93.
Läuchli S, et al. Post-surgical scalp wounds with exposed bone treated with a plant-derived wound therapeutic. J Wound Care. 2012 May;21(5):228, 230, 232–3.
Lei HP, et al. Effect of St. John's wort supplementation on the pharmacokinetics of bupropion in healthy male Chinese volunteers. Xenobiotica. 2010 Apr;40(4):275–81.
Linde K, Knuppel L. Large-scale observational studies of hypericum extracts in patients with depressive disorders: a systematic review. Phytomedicine 12.1–2 (2005): 148–157.
Linde K et al. St John's wort for depression. Cochrane Database Syst Rev 2 (2005a): CD000448.
Linde K, et al. St John's wort for depression: meta-analysis of randomised controlled trials. Br J Psychiatry 2005b;186:99–107.
Linde K, et al St John's wort for major depression. Cochrane Database Syst Rev 2009;(4):CD000448.
Liua, Y.R., et al 2013. *Hypericum perforatum* L. preparations for menopause: a meta-analysis of efficacy and safety. Climacteric Dec 27 (epub ahead of print).

Lochner S, Kirch W Does St. John's wort interact with finasteride? Dtsch Med Wochenschr. 2011 Aug;136(34–35):1746.

Lorusso G, et al Mechanisms of Hyperforin as an anti-angiogenic angioprevention agent. Eur J Cancer. 2009 May;45(8):1474–84.

Lundahl A, et al. The effect of St. John's wort on the pharmacokinetics, metabolism and biliary excretion of finasteride and its metabolites in healthy men. Eur J Pharm Sci. 2009 Mar 2;36(4–5):433–43.

Madabushi R et al. Hyperforin in St John's wort drug interactions. Eur J Clin Pharmacol 62.3 (2006): 225–233.

Mai I et al. Impact of St John's wort treatment on the pharmacokinetics of tacrolimus and mycophenolic acid in renal transplant patients. Nephrol Dial Transplant 18.4 (2003): 819–822.

Mai I, et al. Hyperforin content determines the magnitude of the St John's wort cyclosporine drug interaction. Clin Pharmacol Ther 2004; 76: 330–340 383.

Mannel M, et al. Oral hypericum extract LI 160 is an effective treatment of recurrent herpes genitalis and herpes labialis: 3rd International Congress on Phytomedicine. Phytomedicine 7 (II) (2000).

Mannel M, et al. St. John's wort extract LI160 for the treatment of depression with atypical features — a double-blind, randomized, and placebo-controlled trial. J Psychiatr Res. 2010 Sep;44(12):760–7.

Markou A, et al. Neurobiological similarities in depression and drug dependence: a self-medication hypothesis. Neuropsychopharmacology 18.3 (1998): 135–174.

Mathijssen RH et al. Effects of St John's wort on irinotecan metabolism. J Natl Cancer Inst 94.16 (2002): 1247–1249.

Medina MA et al. Hyperforin: more than an antidepressant bioactive compound?. Life Sci 79.2 (2006): 105–111.

Meinke MC, et al. In vivo photoprotective and anti-inflammatory effect of hyperforin is associated with high antioxidant activity in vitro and ex vivo. Eur J Pharm Biopharm. 2012 Jun;81(2):346–50.

Melzer J, et al. A hypericum extract in the treatment of depressive symptoms in outpatients: an open study. Forsch Komplementmed. 2010 Mar;17(1):7–14.

Mennini T, Gobbi M. The antidepressant mechanism of *Hypericum perforatum*. Life Sci 75.9 (2004): 1021–1027.

Meruelo D, et al. Therapeutic agents with dramatic antiretroviral activity and little toxicity at effective doses: aromatic polycyclic diones hypericin and pseudohypericin. Proc Natl Acad Sci U S A 85.14 (1988): 5230–5234.

Micioni Di Bonaventura MV, et al. Effect of *Hypericum perforatum* Extract in an Experimental Model of Binge Eating in Female Rats. J Obes. 2012;2012:956137.

Miskovsky P. Hypericin: a new antiviral and antitumor photosensitizer: mechanism of action and interaction with biological macromolecules. Curr Drug Targets 3.1 (2002): 55–84.

Moore LB et al. St John's wort induces hepatic drug metabolism through activation of the pregnane X receptor. Proc Natl Acad Sci U S A 97.13 (2000): 7500–7502.

Moretti ME, et al Evaluating the safety of St. John's Wort in human pregnancy. Reprod Toxicol. 2009 Jul;28(1):96–9.

Mortensen T, et al. Investigating the effectiveness of St John's wort herb as an antimicrobial agent against mycobacteria. Phytother Res. 2012 Sep;26(9):1327–33.

Mozaffari S, et al. Effects of *Hypericum perforatum* extract on rat irritable bowel syndrome. Pharmacogn Mag. 2011 Jul;7(27):213–23.

Mueller SC et al. Effect of St John's wort dose and preparations on the pharmacokinetics of digoxin. Clin Pharmacol Ther 75.6 (2004): 546–557.

Mueller SC et al. No clinically relevant CYP3A induction after St. John's wort with low hyperforin content in healthy volunteers. Eur J Clin Pharmacol 65.1 (2009): 81–87.

Nahas R, Sheikh O. Complementary and alternative medicine for the treatment of major depressive disorder. Can Fam Physician. 2011 Jun;57(6):659–63.

Nahrstedt A, Butterweck V. Lessons learned from herbal medicinal products: the example of St John's wort. J Nat Prod 2010; 73: 1015–1021.

Najafizadeh P, et al. The evaluation of the clinical effect of topical St Johns wort (*Hypericum perforatum* L.) in plaque type psoriasis vulgaris: a pilot study. Australas J Dermatol. 2012 May;53(2):131–5.

Nathan P. The experimental and clinical pharmacology of St John's Wort (*Hypericum perforatum* L). Mol Psychiatry 4.4 (1999): 333–338.

Niederhofer H. St John's Wort treating patients with autistic disorder. Phytother Res. 2009 Nov;23(11):1521–3.

Nieminen TH, et al. St John's wort greatly reduces the concentrations of oral oxycodone. Eur J Pain. 2010 Sep;14(8):854–9.

Obach RS. Inhibition of human cytochrome P450 enzymes by constituents of St John's Wort, an herbal preparation used in the treatment of depression. J Pharmacol Exp Ther 294.1 (2000): 88–95.

Olivo M, et al. Hypericin lights up the way for the potential treatment of nasopharyngeal cancer by photodynamic therapy. Curr Clin Pharmacol 1.3 (2006): 217–222.

Ott M, et al. St. John's Wort constituents modulate P-glycoprotein transport activity at the blood-brain barrier. Pharm Res. 2010 May;27(5):811–22.

Panocka I et al. Effects of *Hypericum perforatum* extract on ethanol intake, and on behavioral despair: a search for the neurochemical systems involved. Pharmacol Biochem Behav 66.1 (2000): 105–111.

Parsons A, et al. A proof of concept randomised placebo controlled factorial trial to examine the efficacy of St John's wort for smoking cessation and chromium to prevent weight gain on smoking cessation. Drug Alcohol Depend. 2009 Jun 1;102(1–3):116–120.

Patel J et al. In vitro interaction of the HIV protease inhibitor ritonavir with herbal constituents: changes in P-gp and CYP3A4 activity. Am J Ther 11.4 (2004): 262–277.

Peltoniemi MA, et al St John's wort greatly decreases the plasma concentrations of oral S-ketamine. Fundam Clin Pharmacol. 2012 Dec;26(6):743–50.

Perfumi M et al. Blockade of gamma-aminobutyric acid receptors does not modify the inhibition of ethanol intake induced by *Hypericum perforatum* in rats. Alcohol Alcohol 37.6 (2002): 540–546.

Piccolo P, et al. Severe drug induced acute hepatitis associated with use of St John's wort (*Hypericum perforatum*) during treatment with pegylated interferon α. BMJ Case Rep. 2009;2009.

Posadzki P, et al. Adverse effects of herbal medicines: an overview of systematic reviews. Clin Med. 2013 Feb;13(1):7–12.

Radwan MA, et al Pharmacokinetics and cardiovascular effect of etoricoxib in the absence or presence of St. John's Wort in rats. Arzneimittelforschung. 2012 Jul;62(7):313–8.

Rahimi R, Abdollahi M. An update on the ability of St. John's wort to affect the metabolism of other drugs. Expert Opin Drug Metab Toxicol. 2012 Jun;8(6):691–708.

Rahimi R, et al. Efficacy and tolerability of *Hypericum perforatum* in major depressive disorder in comparison with selective serotonin reuptake inhibitors: a meta-analysis. Prog Neuropsychopharmacol Biol Psychiatry 33.1 (2009): 118–127.

Rapaport MH, et al. The treatment of minor depression with St. John's Wort or citalopram: Failure to show benefit over placebo. Journal of Psychiatric Research 2011;45(7):931–41.

Raso GM et al. In-vivo and in-vitro anti-inflammatory effect of Echinacea purpurea and *Hypericum perforatum*. J Pharm Pharmacol 54.10 (2002): 1379–1383.

Ravindran AV, et al Canadian Network for Mood and Anxiety Treatments (CANMAT) Clinical guidelines for the management of major depressive disorder in adults. V. Complementary and alternative medicine treatments. J Affect Disord. 2009 Oct;117 Suppl 1:S54–64.

Rengelshausen J et al. Opposite effects of short-term and long-term St John's wort intake on voriconazole pharmacokinetics. Clin Pharmacol Ther 78.1 (2005): 25–33.

Reuter J, et al. Botanicals in dermatology: an evidence-based review. Am J Clin Dermatol. 2010;11(4):247–67.

Richard AJ, et al. St. John's Wort inhibits insulin signaling in murine and human adipocytes Biochim Biophys Acta. 2012 Apr;1822(4):557–63.

Roz N, Rehavi M. Hyperforin depletes synaptic vesicles content and induces compartmental redistribution of nerve ending monoamines. Life Sci 75.23 (2004): 2841–2850.

Rucklidge JJ, et al. Nutrient supplementation approaches in the treatment of ADHD. Expert Rev Neurother. 2009 Apr;9(4):461–76.

Saddiqe Z, et al. A review of the antibacterial activity of *Hypericum perforatum* L. J Ethnopharmacol. 2010 Oct 5;131(3):511–21.

Samadi S, et al The effect of *Hypericum perforatum* on the wound healing and scar of cesarean. J Altern Complement Med. 2010 Jan;16(1):113–7.

Sarris J, Kavanagh DJ. Kava and St John's wort: current evidence for use in mood and anxiety disorders. J Altern Complement Med. 2009;15(8):827–836.

Sarris J, et al Complementary medicines (herbal and nutritional products) in the treatment of Attention Deficit Hyperactivity Disorder (ADHD): a systematic review of the evidence. Complement Ther Med. 2011a Aug;19(4):216–27.

Sarris J, et al. St John's wort (*Hypericum perforatum*) versus sertraline and placebo in major depressive disorder: continuation data from a 26-week RCT. Pharmacopsychiatry. 2012a Nov;45(7):275–8.

Sarris J, et al. Complementary medicine, self-help, and lifestyle interventions for obsessive compulsive disorder (OCD) and the OCD spectrum: a systematic review. J Affect Disord. 2012b May;138(3):213–21.

Schempp CM et al. Antibacterial activity of hyperforin from St John's wort against multiresistant *Staphylococcus aureus* and Gram-positive bacteria. Lancet 353.9170 (1999): 2129.

Schempp CM et al. Topical treatment of atopic dermatitis with St John's wort cream: a randomized, placebo controlled, double-blind half-side comparison. Phytomedicine 10 Suppl 4 (2003): 31–7.

Schrader E. Equivalence of St John's wort extract (Ze 117) and fluoxetine: a randomized, controlled study in mild-moderate depression. Int Clin Psychopharmacol 15.2 (2000): 61–68.

Schreiber S, et al Bilateral posterior RION after concomitant radiochemotherapy with temozolomide in a patient with glioblastoma multiforme: a case report. BMC Cancer. 2010 Oct 1;10:520.

Schulz V. Safety of St. John's Wort extract compared to synthetic antidepressants. Phytomedicine 13.3 (2006): 199–204.

Sharma M, Saravolatz LD. Rilpivirine: a new non-nucleoside reverse transcriptase inhibitor. J Antimicrob Chemother. 2013 Feb;68(2):250–6.

Shibayama Y et al. Effect of pre-treatment with St John's Wort on nephrotoxicity of cisplatin in rats. Life Sci 81.2 (2007): 103–108.

Siepmann M et al. The effects of St John's wort extract on heart rate variability, cognitive function and quantitative EEG: a comparison with amitriptyline and placebo in healthy men. Br J Clin Pharmacol 54.3 (2002): 277–282.

Simeon J et al. Open-label pilot study of St John's wort in adolescent depression. J Child Adolesc Psychopharmacol 15.2 (2005): 293–301.

Simmen U et al. *Hypericum perforatum* inhibits the binding of mu- and kappa-opioid receptor expressed with the Semliki Forest virus system. Pharm Acta Helv 73.1 (1998): 53–56.

Sindrup SH et al. St John's wort has no effect on pain in polyneuropathy. Pain 9.3 (2001): 361–365.

Singer A, et al. Duration of response after treatment of mild to moderate depression with Hypericum extract STW 3-VI, citalopram and placebo: a reanalysis of data from a controlled clinical trial. Phytomedicine. 2011 Jun 15;18(8–9):739–42.

Solomon D, et al. Potential of St John's Wort for the treatment of depression: the economic perspective. Aust N Z J Psychiatry. 2011 Feb;45(2):123–30.

Solomon D, et al Economic evaluation of St. John's wort (*Hypericum perforatum*) for the treatment of mild to moderate depression. J Affect Disord. 2013 Jun;148(2–3):228–34.

Sood A, et al. A randomized clinical trial of St. John's wort for smoking cessation. J Altern Complement Med. 2010 Jul;16(7):761–7.

Steinhoff B., Current perspectives on herb-drug interactions in the European regulatory landscape. Planta Med. 2012 Sep;78(13):1416–20.

Stevinson C, Ernst E. A pilot study of *Hypericum perforatum* for the treatment of premenstrual syndrome. Br J Obstet Gynaecol 107.7 (2000): 870–876.

Sugimoto K et al. Different effects of St John's wort on the pharmacokinetics of simvastatin and pravastatin. Clin Pharmacol Ther 70.6 (2001): 518–524.

Taylor LH, Kobak KA. An open-label trial of St John's Wort (*Hypericum perforatum*) in obsessive-compulsive disorder. J Clin Psychiatry 61.8 (2000): 575–578.

Teufel-Mayer R, Gleitz J. Effects of long-term administration of hypericum extracts on the affinity and density of the central serotonergic 5-HT1A and 5-HT2A receptors. Pharmacopsychiatry 30 (Suppl 2) (1997): 113–1116.

Thiede HM, Walper A. Inhibition of MAO and COMT by hypericum extracts and hypericin. J Geriatr Psychiatry Neurol 7 (Suppl 1) (1994): S54–S56.

Tian R et al. Functional induction and de-induction of P-glycoprotein by St John's wort and its ingredients in a human colon adenocarcinoma cell line. Drug Metab Dispos 33.4 (2005): 547–554.

Timoshanko A et al. A preliminary investigation on the acute pharmacodynamic effects of hypericum on cognitive and psychomotor performance. Behav Pharmacol 12.8 (2001): 635–640.

Trana C, et al. St. John's Wort in patients non-responders to clopidogrel undergoing percutaneous coronary intervention: a single-center randomized open-label trial (St. John's Trial). J Cardiovasc Transl Res. 2013 Jun;6(3):411–4.

Trofimiuk E, Braszko JJ. Alleviation by *Hypericum perforatum* of the stress-induced impairment of spatial working memory in rats. Naunyn Schmiedebergs Arch Pharmacol 376.6 (2008): 463–471.

Trompetter I, et al. Herbal triplet in treatment of nervous agitation in children. Wien Med Wochenschr. 2013 Feb;163(3–4):52–7.

Tsai HH, et al. Evaluation of documented drug interactions and contraindications associated with herbs and dietary supplements: a systematic literature review. Int J Clin Pract. 2012 Nov;66(11):1056–78.

Turkanovic J, et al. Effect of St John's wort on the disposition of fexofenadine in the isolated perfused rat liver. J Pharm Pharmacol. 2009 Aug;61(8):1037–42.

Uebelhack R et al. Black cohosh and St. John's wort for climacteric complaints: a randomized trial. Obstet Gynecol 107.2 (2006): 247–255.

Vandenbogaerde A et al. Evidence that total extract of *Hypericum perforatum* affects exploratory behavior and exerts anxiolytic effects in rats. Pharmacol Biochem Behav 65.4 (2000): 627–633.

van Die MD, et al *Hypericum perforatum* with Vitex agnus-castus in menopausal symptoms: a randomized, controlled trial. Menopause. 2009a Jan-Feb;16(1):156–63.

van Die MD, et al. Effects of a combination of *Hypericum perforatum* and Vitex agnus-castus on PMS-like symptoms in late-perimenopausal women: findings from a subpopulation analysis. J Altern Complement Med. 2009b Sep;15(9):1045–8.

Vieira ML, et al Could maternal exposure to the antidepressants fluoxetine and St. John's Wort induce long-term reproductive effects on male rats? Reprod Toxicol. 2013 Jan;35:102–7.

Wang EJ, et al. Quantitative characterization of direct P-glycoprotein inhibition by St John's wort constituents hypericin and hyperforin. J Pharm Pharmacol 56.1 (2004a): 123–8.

Wang LS et al. St John's wort induces both cytochrome P450 3A4-catalyzed sulfoxidation and 2C19-dependent hydroxylation of omeprazole. Clin Pharmacol Ther 75.3 (2004b): 191–7.

Wang XD et al. Rapid and simultaneous determination of nifedipine and dehydronifedipine in human plasma by liquid chromatography-tandem mass spectrometry: application to a clinical herb-drug interaction study. J Chromatogr B Analyt Technol Biomed Life Sci 852.1–2 (2007): 534–544.

Wang Z et al. The effects of St John's wort (*Hypericum perforatum*) on human cytochrome P450 activity. Clin Pharmacol Ther 70.4 (2001): 317–326.

Weber CC et al. Modulation of P-glycoprotein function by St John's wort extract and its major constituents. Pharmacopsychiatry 37.6 (2004): 292–298.

Weber W et al. *Hypericum perforatum* (St John's wort) for attention-deficit/hyperactivity disorder in children and adolescents: a randomized controlled trial. JAMA 299.22 (2008): 2633–2641.

Wheatley D. Hypericum in seasonal affective disorder (SAD). Curr Med Res Opin 15.1 (1999): 33–37.

Whelan AM, et al Herbs, vitamins and minerals in the treatment of premenstrual syndrome: a systematic review. Can J Clin Pharmacol. 2009 Fall;16(3):e407–29.

Will-Shahab L et al. St John's wort extract (Ze 117) does not alter the pharmacokinetics of a low-dose oral contraceptive. Eur J Clin Pharmacol 65.3 (2009): 287–294.

Woelk H. Comparison of St John's wort and imipramine for treating depression: randomised controlled trial. BMJ 321.7260 (2000): 536–539.

Wonnemann M et al. Evaluation of synaptosomal uptake inhibition of most relevant constituents of St John's wort. Pharmacopsychiatry 34 (Suppl 1) (2001): S148–S151.

Xiuying P, et al. Therapeutic efficacy of *Hypericum perforatum* L. extract for mice infected with an influenza A virus. Can J Physiol Pharmacol. 2012 Feb;90(2):123–30.

Xu H et al. Effects of St John's wort and CYP2C9 genotype on the pharmacokinetics and pharmacodynamics of gliclazide. Br J Pharmacol 153.7 (2008): 1579–1586.

Yang SY, et al St. John's wort significantly increased the systemic exposure and toxicity of methotrexate in rats. Toxicol Appl Pharmacol. 2012 Aug 15;263(1):39–43.

St Mary's thistle

HISTORICAL NOTE St Mary's thistle has a long history of traditional use since ancient times. Over the centuries, it has been touted as a remedy for snakebite, melancholy, liver conditions and promoting lactation. The name 'milk thistle' derives from its characteristic spiked leaves with white veins which, according to legend, were believed to carry the milk of the Virgin Mary.

OTHER NAMES

Carduus marianus, cardo blanco, cardo de burro, chandon marie, holy thistle, lady's milk, lady's thistle, Mariendistel, Marian thistle, Mary thistle, milk thistle, silybum, true thistle.

BOTANICAL NAME/FAMILY

Silybum marianum (family [Compositae] Asteraceae)

PLANT PART USED

Ripe seed

CHEMICAL COMPONENTS

Often silymarin is referred to as the active constituent of seeds from St Mary's thistle, but in fact it is a complex of at least seven flavonolignans, one flavonoid taxifolin and a bioflavonoid quercetin. The principal component of silymarin is silybin (more commonly referred to as silibinin), which makes up more than 50% of silymarin and is regarded as one of the most biologically active constituents (Jacobs et al 2002). Silibinin is not a single compound either, but rather a mixture of two diastereoisomers, silybin A and silybin B (Kroll et al 2007). Other flavonolignans include isosilybin, silychristin and silydianin, all of which exist as diastereoisomers. A new flavonolignan, silyamandin, was discovered in St Mary's thistle preparations (MacKinnon et al 2007). St Mary's thistle seeds also contain a fixed oil comprising linoleic, oleic and palmitic acids, tocopherol and sterols, including cholesterol, campesterol, stigmasterol and sitosterol.

MAIN ACTIONS

Silymarin has confirmed antioxidant (Aghazadeh et al 2011, Gazák et al 2010, Morazzoni & Bombardelli 1995, Shaker et al 2010), antifibrotic (Hernandez-Gea & Friedman 2011, Trappoliere et al 2009, Tzeng et al 2013), anti-inflammatory (Aghazadeh et al 2011, El-Zayadi et al 2005, Morishima et al 2010, Polyak et al 2007), hepatoprotective (Ferenci et al 1989, Fraschini et al 2002, Lieber et al 2003), antihypercholesterolaemic (Krecman et al 1998), antihyperglycaemic (Velussi et al 1997), immunomodulatory (Polyak et al 2007) and antiviral (Ahmed-Belkacem et al 2010, Ferenci et al 2008, Neumann et al 2010, Polyak et al 2007) pharmacological actions in vitro, in vivo and in human studies.

Hepatoprotective

Hepatoprotection is defined as several non-mutually exclusive biological activities including antiviral, antioxidant, anti-inflammatory and immunomodulatory functions (Polyak et al 2013).

Silymarin and silibin exert some of these mechanisms and have hepatoprotective effects (Abenavoli et al 2010). In particular, *Silybum marianum* achieves many of its pharmacological actions via its antioxidant mechanisms.

Specifically, in regards to *Amanita phalloides* (death cap mushroom) poisoning cases, silibinin as Legalon SIL appears to exert its hepatoprotective effects by competitive inhibition of amatoxin binding and uptake by hepatocytes (Jacobs et al 2002) and by the reduction of enterohepatic recirculation through the modulation of bile flow. Adjunct to these mechanisms, silibinin reduces the oxidative stress, consequent to necrotic cell death caused by amatoxin poisoning with anti-inflammatory and antifibrotic downstream effects. Silibinin also reduces damage through inhibition of TNF-α and helps recovery through the stimulation of protein synthesis for repair in damaged liver cells (Mengs et al 2012).

It has therefore been postulated that *Silybum marianum* protects the liver by preventing the uptake of toxins and viruses through the stabilisation of cell membranes, reducing the oxidative stress caused by the metabolism of toxins and reducing hepatic inflammation, fibrosis and aiding hepatic repair and regeneration (Polyak et al 2010).

The mechanisms of membrane stability have been researched in detail. Silymarin and silibinin alter the structure of hepatocyte cell membranes by being incorporated into the hydrophobic–hydrophilic interface of the microsomal bilayer (Parasassi et al 1984). Silibinin interacts with the surface rather than deeper regions of the bilayer, and therefore does not change significantly the biophysical properties of the deeper membrane regions (Wesolowska et al 2007). Additionally, inhibition of cyclic adenosine monophosphate (AMP)-dependent phosphodiesterase by silibinin has been shown in vitro, which results in increased cAMP and stabilisation of lysosomal membranes (Koch et al 1985).

Toxin blockade

Protection of liver cells has been demonstrated against the following substances in vitro or in vivo:

- Carbon tetrachloride-induced liver cirrhosis (Chrungoo et al 1997, Mourelle et al 1989, Muriel & Mourelle 1990, Tsai et al 2008).
- Ethanol (Das & Vasudevan 2006).
- Paracetamol-induced liver peroxidation (Chrungoo et al 1997, Muriel et al 1992).
- Cyclosporin (von Schonfeld et al 1997).
- Phenothiazine (Palasciano et al 1994).
- Butyrophenone (Palasciano et al 1994).
- Erythromycin (Davila et al 1989).
- Amitriptyline and nortriptyline (Davila et al 1989).
- Oestradiol (Morazzoni & Bombardelli 1995).
- *Amanita phalloides* (Floersheim 1976, Vogel et al 1984).
- Tacrine (Galisteo et al 2000).
- Iron overload (Choi 2012, Masini et al 2000, Pietrangelo et al 1995).
- Benzo(a)pyrene-induced lung cancer (Kiruthiga et al 2007).

CHELATES IRON AND DECREASES IRON EXCESS

Silybum marianum interacts with iron in a number of ways. Excess iron increases oxidative stress and

Silybum marianum exerts antioxidant activity thereby decreasing the pathological consequences of excessive oxidative stress. *Silybum marianum* acts indirectly to reduce iron-induced damage by protecting the mechanisms, such as the expression of hepcidin, that regulates iron uptake (Choi 2012) and directly chelating iron to reduce its absorption (Hutchinson et al 2010) and reactivity (Borsari et al 2001).

Antioxidant

In vivo research suggests the key mechanisms of action responsible for the antioxidant activity of silymarin are:

- direct activity via redox reactions;
- indirect activity by inhibiting the activity of free radical producing enzymes; and
- indirect activity achieved by upregulating endogenous, antioxidant enzyme systems such as Nrf2 (Son et al 2008) and glutathione (Kim et al 2012, Lu et al 2010a).

In vivo research involving rats with induced-steatohepatitis found that treatment with *Silybum marianum* decreased the oxidative stress marker malondialdehyde (MDA) by 45%, while glutathione (GSH) was increased by 65% and TNF-α lowered by 47% all relative to the control group (Aghazadeh et al 2011).

Anti-inflammatory

The anti-inflammatory activity of silymarin is due to several different mechanisms, such as antioxidant and membrane-stabilising effects, and inhibition of the production or release of inflammatory mediators, such as arachidonic acid metabolites. Inhibitory activity on lipo-oxygenase, cyclo-oxygenase (COX) and prostaglandin (PG) synthetase has been demonstrated in several in vitro assays and animal studies (Alarcon de la Lastra et al 1992, Dehmlow et al 1996, Fiebrich & Koch 1979, Rui et al 1990, Zhao et al 1999). Furthermore, silymarin inhibits NF-kappaB signalling and suppresses tumour necrosis factor (TNF)-alpha, nitric oxide synthase (iNOS) and interleukin (IL)-1 (Agarwal et al 2006, Kim et al 2012, Polyak et al 2007).

Antifibrotic

Silymarin and silibinin demonstrate antifibrotic activity in a variety of preclinical models via multiple mechanisms of action.

Silymarin reduces markers for collagen accumulation in the liver and exerts antifibrotic activity, according to an animal model of liver fibrosis (Boigk et al 1997). Oral silibinin (25–50 microM) dose-dependently inhibited the transforming growth factor beta (TGF-β)-induced de novo synthesis of pro-collagen I directly, by reducing platelet derived growth factor (PDGF)-induced cell proliferation, and indirectly, by de novo reduction of TGF-β-induced synthesis of collagen type 1 in human hepatic stellate cells (Trappoliere et al 2009). This finding was confirmed in thioacetamide-induced hepatic fibrosis, where silibinin downregulated hepatic MMP-2, MMP-13, TIMP-1, TIMP-2, AP-1, KLF6, TGFβ1, αSMA and COL-α1 (Chen et al 2012).

A silibinin-phosphatidylcholine complex (silibinin 200 mg per kg) taken for five weeks caused an improvement in liver steatosis and inflammation and reduced the levels of plasma insulin and TNF-α. These effects were associated with a reduction in membrane lipid peroxidation, decreased free radical release and restoration of GSH levels (Haddad et al 2011).

Oral silymarin reduced steatohepatitis, raised nuclear translocation of nuclear factor erythroid 2-r elated factor 2 (Nrf2), and reduced tumour necrosis factor (TNF)-α mRNA expression in the liver in insulin-resistant rats, suggesting its antifibrotic effect is achieved through anti-inflammatory, antioxidant and hepatoprotective effects (Kim et al 2012).

Antitumour effects

A variety of mechanisms attributed to silymarin show it has promise in the prevention and/or treatment of several different cancers.

Oxidative stress (OS) in chronic disease accelerates inflammation, fibrosis and necrosis, through damage to proteins, DNA, lipids, sensitising redox-regulated necrotic and inflammatory cell signalling pathways, affecting gene expression (Finkel & Holbrook 2000) and causing mitochondrial dysfunction and pathology (Kung et al 2011, Pias & Aw 2002, Pias et al 2003, Polyak et al 2007). Therefore it has been suggested that by ameliorating OS and inflammation, silymarin could theoretically have a role in reducing disease progression and cancer incidence (Ting et al 2013).

In vivo and in vitro research with silibinin has identified an ability to reduce proliferation and angiogenesis, and to promote cell cycle arrest and apoptosis (Agarwal et al 2013, Deep & Agarwal 2010, Kauntz et al 2012b, Li et al 2010, Zeng et al 2011). Recent in vitro studies have shown that silibinin also possesses strong anti-invasive and anti-metastatic efficacy (Agarwal et al 2013, Deep & Agarwal 2010).

At this stage, most studies investigating mechanisms of action and effects in cancer have been conducted in vivo and in vitro, whereas human trials are limited (Li et al 2010). There have also been preclinical trials in humans to investigate suitable doses, treatment safety and improvements in bioavailability with phytosome-based preparations (Flaig et al 2010).

Silibinin has been shown to regulate multiple cellular proliferative pathways in cancer cells, including receptor tyrosine kinases, androgen receptor, STATs, NF-κB, cell cycle regulatory and apoptotic signalling pathways in vivo and in vitro (Li et al 2010). In prostate cancer, in mice, silymarin treatment down-regulates androgen receptor, epidermal growth factor receptor, and nuclear factor-κB mediated signalling and induces cell cycle arrest (Deep & Agarwal 2007). Kim et al (2009) showed in in vitro studies that silibinin can prevent the degradation of certain proteins in breast cancer. By studying the effects of silibinin on matrix metalloproteinases (MMPs), whose abnormal expression is associated with carcinoma and vascular endothelial growth factor (VEGF) which is expressed by malignant and non-malignant cells, they propose that this constituent is a possible candidate for the therapy of tumour metastasis and angiogenesis. The action responsible appears to be inhibition of 12-*O*-tetradecanoyl phorbol-13-acetate (TPA)-induced MMP and VEGF expression in breast cancer cells (Kim et al 2009).

In colon carcinogenesis, in rats, silibinin shifted the disturbed balance between cell renewal and cell death through potent proapoptotic, anti-inflammatory and multi-targeted effects at the molecular level. The study concluded that the effective reduction of pre-neoplastic lesions by silibinin supports its use as a natural agent for colon cancer chemoprevention (Kauntz et al 2012a).

Brain, neuroprotective activity

Silymarin has been shown to reduce sepsis-induced lung and brain injury, partially through its antioxidant effects, inhibition of neutrophil infiltration and regulation of inflammatory mediator release (Nencini et al 2007, Toklu et al 2008). Additionally, pre-treatment with silymarin, but not silibinin, dose-dependently reduced cerebral ischaemic/reperfusion induced brain infarction by 16–40% and improved neurological deficits in rats through antioxidant and anti-inflammatory mechanisms (Hou et al 2010). Another study in rats pre-treated with silymarin found it slowed neuronal injury in focal cerebral ischaemia and enabled functional recovery close to the baseline. Similar to previous studies, the authors suggest that the neuroprotective potential of silymarin is mediated through its antioxidative and anti-apoptotic properties (Raza et al 2011).

According to an in vitro study, silibinin may have potential as both a preventive and an active treatment for Alzheimer's disease as it reduced the formation of amyloid plaque and also protected cells from amyloid plaque-induced oxidative stress in a dose-dependent manner (Yin et al 2011).

Nephroprotective effect

In vitro experiments with kidney cells damaged by paracetamol, cisplatin or vincristin demonstrate that administration of silibinin before or after the chemical-induced injury can lessen or avoid the nephrotoxic effects (Sonnenbichler et al 1999). Animal studies have confirmed the nephroprotective effect for cisplatin-induced injury (Karimi et al 2005). In one study, the effects of cisplatin on glomerular and proximal tubular function as well as proximal tubular morphology were totally or partly ameliorated by silibinin (Gaedeke et al 1996). In an in vivo study, silymarin significantly decreased gentamicin-induced nephrotoxicity when used as a single agent and when used in combination with vitamin E in comparison to the placebo group. Serum creatinine concentrations, but not urea concentrations, were significantly lower (Varzi et al 2007).

Gastroprotective effect

St Mary's thistle extract produces a dose-dependent antiulcerogenic activity against indomethacin-induced ulcers, which can be histologically confirmed, according to research with test animals (Khayyal et al 2001). This is associated with reduced acid output, increased mucin secretion, increased PGE_2 release and decreased leukotriene release. Experiments with silymarin have found it to be effective in the prevention of gastric ulceration induced by cold-restraint stress in rats (Alarcon de la Lastra et al 1992) and postischaemic gastric mucosal injury (Alarcon de la Lastra et al 1995).

IN COMBINATION

A herbal formulation known as STW 5, containing extracts of milk thistle fruit and eight other herbs (bitter candy tuft, lemon balm leaf, chamomile flower, caraway fruit, peppermint leaf, licorice root, angelica root and greater celandine) produced antiulcerogenic activity against indomethacin-induced gastric ulcers in rats as well as antisecretory and cytoprotective activities (Khayyal et al 2001). In addition, it was shown that STW 5 lowered the gastric acidity as effectively as commercial antacid preparations (i.e. Rennie, Talcid, Maaloxan), prevented secondary hyperacidity more effectively and, additionally, inhibited serum gastrin levels in rats (Khayyal et al 2006).

Antidiabetic effect

In type 2 diabetes (T2DM) amyloid deposits contribute to the dysfunction of β-cells and the loss of β-cell mass in T2DM patients. In vitro silibinin reduces the formation of amyloid deposits and enhances the viability of pancreatic β cells (Cheng et al 2012).

In vivo research showed that silibinin exerts pronounced effects on liver carbohydrate metabolism. The metabolic pathways that contribute to glycaemia maintenance, i.e. gluconeogenesis in the fasted condition and glycogenolysis and glycolysis in the fed condition, were both reduced by silibinin corroborating the role of the liver in the antihyperglycaemic effect of silibinin (Colturato et al 2012).

Antiviral effect

Silybum marianum, particularly silymarin and intravenous silibinin, block hepatitis C virus (HCV) infection and proliferation in vitro by blocking viral fusion, viral entry, viral RNA and protein synthesis, and virus transmission (Ahmed-Belkacem et al 2010, Blaising & Pecheur 2013, McClure et al 2012, Morishima et al 2010, Polyak et al 2007, 2010, 2013, Wagoner et al 2010, 2011). This mechanism would also apply to other viruses such as vesicular stomatitis virus, reovirus, and the influenza virus (McClure et al 2012). Guedj et al (2012) confirmed in vivo that intravenous silibinin may block both viral infection and viral production/release dose-dependently.

Intravenous silibinin reduced HCV RNA in previous non-responders to pegylated interferon and ribavirin in a clinical study (Ferenci et al 2008) and prevented HCV RNA re-infection after liver transplantation (Beinhardt et al 2011, Marino et al 2013, Neumann et al 2010). Intravenous silibinin has also been found to inhibit HIV in human cell lines (McClure et al 2012), previously confirmed in a HCV/HIV co-infected patient (Payer et al 2010).

Mast-cell stabilisation

Silibinin has shown mast-cell stabilisation activity in vivo (Lecomte 1975), which was confirmed some years later and found to be dose-dependent (Fantozzi et al 1986).

Asthma

Allergic asthma is a chronic inflammatory disease regulated by coordination of T-helper2 (Th2) type cytokines and inflammatory signal molecules. Previously, silymarin has been shown to exert protective effects in the early phase of asthma, most likely due to its influence on histamine release (Breschi et al 2002). More recently, research with an animal model of asthma showed that pretreatment with silibinin prevented the development of airway hyperresponsiveness, significantly inhibited airway inflammatory cell recruitment and peribronchiolar inflammation and reduced the production of various cytokines in bronchoalveolar fluid (Choi et al 2012).

Cytochromes

Effects on Phase I CYP450

There has been extensive investigation into the effects of various St Mary's thistle preparations on various cytochromes. Human studies with standard St Mary's thistle preparations have identified no clinically significant effect on cytochromes CYP 1A2, 2D6, 3A4 whereas 2C9 appears most vulnerable to inhibition (Gurley et al 2012, Hackett et al 2013, Hermann & von Richter 2012). The lack of effect may be due to poor bioavailability (Goey et al 2013). If this is the case, then preparations with greater bioavailability still require testing to confirm that clinically significant drug interactions are absent. Additionally, the use of isolated silymarin and silibinin preparations could produce different results (Loguercio & Festi 2011).

Tests with an animal model suggest inhibition of CYP 1A1 however human studies have not confirmed the findings (Kiruthiga et al 2013).

Effects on phase II conjugation pathways

Phytochemicals such as silymarin can increase levels of Nrf2 either by stimulating its release or inhibiting its proteolytic breakdown. Activated Nrf2 translocates into the nucleus where it interacts with small MAF family proteins bound to the antioxidant response element (ARE), allowing transcription of target genes including those that regulate antioxidant and phase II enzymes (Kim et al 2012, Son et al 2008).

An in vitro study on cardiomyocytes with a product called Protandim (*Bacopa monniera, Silybum marianum, Withania somnifera, Camellia sinensis* and *Curcuma longa*) resulted in nuclear accumulation of Nrf2, upregulation of key endogenous phase II antioxidant enzymes, and Nrf2-dependent protection of cardiomyocytes from apoptosis after an oxidative stress (Reuland et al 2012).

P-glycoprotein

No clinically significant effects are seen for St Mary's thistle preparations and P-gp (Gurley et al 2006a, 2006b, Hermann & von Richter 2012), despite an earlier in vitro study which identified that silymarin inhibited P-glycoprotein (P-gp) ATPase activity in such a way as to suggest direct interaction with P-gp substrate binding (Zhang & Morris 2003).

OTHER ACTIONS

Cholesterol lowering

Cholesterol reduction has been demonstrated for silymarin in three studies of rats fed a highcholesterol diet (Krecman et al 1998, Shaker et al 2010, Sobolova et al 2006).

Although the mechanism of action is unknown, it has been suggested that inhibition of HMG-CoA reductase (Skottova & Krecman 1998a) and inhibition of cholesterol absorption from dietary sources (Sobolova et al 2006) are involved. Considering that the herb also contains phytosterols, these too may play a role in cholesterol reduction.

CLINICAL USE

In practice, St Marys thistle is commonly used for treating digestive disorders and any indication whereby improved liver function or liver protection may be a benefit. Milk thistle fruits have a positive European Scientific Cooperative on Phytotherapy (ESCOP) monograph for the following therapeutic indications: toxic liver damage; supportive treatment in patients with chronic inflammatory liver conditions and hepatic cirrhosis (ESCOP 2009).

Dyspepsia

St Mary's thistle is commonly used to treat dyspeptic complaints, such as loss of appetite, poor digestion and upper gastrointestinal discomfort. Animal studies have identified a dose-dependent increase in bile flow and bile salt secretion for silymarin, achieved by stimulating the synthesis of bile salts (Crocenzi et al 2000). Silymarin has been found to impact on bile salt synthesis, bile secretion, biotransformation of cholestatic compounds and changes in transported expression and activity (Crocenzi & Roma 2006).

Commission E approves the use of crude milk thistle preparations for dyspeptic complaints (Blumenthal et al 2000).

Toxic liver damage

Mushroom poisoning (*Amanita phalloides*)

One of the best-documented uses of milk thistle is in the treatment of poisoning by the mushroom *Amanita phalloides.* Nausea, vomiting, abdominal cramps and severe diarrhoea usually occur 8–12 hours after ingestion, with extensive hepatic necrosis occurring 1–2 days later. A mortality rate of 20–30% has been observed but can be as high as 50% in children under 10 years of age (Floersheim et al 1982).

Since intervention studies would be unethical, a review of case reports and studied mechanisms of action are used as evidence to support its use.

A review of 154 cases of *Amanita phalloides* poisoning in Germany (1983–1992) showed a mortality rate of 15.2% in non-silibinin treated cases ($n = 38$) compared to 8.3% in patients treated with silibinin ($n = 116$) (Saller et al 2008). A more recent review of nearly 1500 documented cases concluded that the overall mortality in patients treated with Legalon SIL is less than 10% in comparison to more than 20% when using penicillin or a combination of silibinin and penicillin. Mengs et al (2012) recommend a daily dose of 20 mg silibinin/kg via continuous infusion over 24 hours, following a single loading dose of 5 mg silibinin/kg and to start treatment as soon as possible.

At the Poison Information Centre, Vienna, Austria; if silibinin is administered within 48 hours of poisoning, only mild to moderate liver injury is observed ($n = 18$) (Hruby et al 1983). After 48 hours, if left untreated, severe liver damage, coagulation disorders and coma are likely to occur. Hruby administered four divided doses of silibinin intravenously, each dose consisting of 20–50 mg/kg body weight/day; the dose varied depending on the severity of intoxication (Hruby et al 1983).

Silymarin protects against the *Amanita phalloides* toxins, α-amanita and phalloidin, by inhibiting the toxins binding to cell receptors by competitive inhibition of hepatocyte-specific OATP2 transporters; their uptake and interaction with cell components; binding with nuclear receptors and inhibiting protein synthesis and cell repair (Ferenci et al 1989, Hackett et al 2013). As silymarin reduces the uptake of toxins into cells, the earlier it is administered after exposure, the better the protective effects (Hruby et al 1983, Mengs et al 2012).

> ***Clinical note — Hepatic fibrosis***
>
> Hepatic fibrosis is a pathological wound-healing process that occurs when the liver is injured chronically, such as in chronic alcohol abuse. The oxidative metabolite of ethanol, acetaldehyde, often in conjunction with viral or metabolic liver disease, is implicated as the major cause for liver fibrogenesis, which ultimately leads to cirrhosis (Schuppan et al 1995). Antifibrotic and antiviral interventions, which interrupt the continuous process of wound healing in the liver, are being investigated as strategies to prevent or reverse liver cirrhosis (Poynard et al 2009).

Environmental toxins and drugs

In animals, milk thistle reduces acute liver injury caused by paracetamol (Ali et al 2001, Muriel et al 1992), carbon tetrachloride (Favari & Perez-Alvarez 1997, Letteron et al 1990), radiation (Hakova & Misurova 1996, Kropacova et al 1998), iron overload (Masini et al 2000, Pietrangelo et al 1995), phenylhydrazine (Valenzuela & Guerra 1985) and D-galactosamine (Tyutyulkova et al 1981, 1983).

One randomised, double-blind study involving 222 patients showed that silymarin improves the tolerability of tacrine without altering the drug's cognitive effects (Allain et al 1999). Two other clinical trials have documented the effectiveness of silymarin in improving or preventing hepatotoxicity from chronic administration of phenothiazines or butyrophenone.

Supportive treatment in chronic liver diseases

Milk thistle fruits have a positive European Scientific Cooperative on Phytotherapy (ESCOP) monograph for supportive treatment in patients with chronic inflammatory liver conditions and hepatic cirrhosis (ESCOP 2009).

Numerous clinical trials have been conducted with St Mary's thistle preparations in various chronic liver diseases. The most studied treatments are Legalon (Madaus Corporation, Cologne, Germany) and silipide (Inverni Della Beffa Research and Development Laboratories, Milan, Italy), designed to improve oral absorption of silymarin.

A 1998 clinical review of St Mary's thistle concluded that it may be effective in improving the clinical courses of both acute and chronic viral, drug-induced, toxin-induced and alcoholic hepatitis (Flora et al 1998). A systematic review of efficacy for St Mary's thistle in chronic liver diseases stated that data are still too limited to detect a substantial benefit on mortality or recommend the herb in liver disease (Jacobs et al 2002).

Twelve clinical studies were located in which researchers have attempted to clarify the role of St Mary's thistle in the treatment of various liver diseases (Angulo et al 2000, Benda et al 1980, Buzzelli et al 1993, Ferenci et al 1989, Loguercio et al 2007, Lucena et al 2002, Magliulo et al 1978, Par et al 2000, Pares et al 1998, Salmi & Sarna 1982, Trinchet et al 1989, Velussi et al 1997). Much of the research focuses on the different forms of hepatitis and alcoholic liver cirrhosis with doses ranging from 100 to 300 mg three times daily, usually given in a standardised extract of 70–80% silymarin. Overall, results have been mixed, with nine trials showing generally positive results and three negative, suggesting that milk thistle is effective in only some forms of liver disease.

Alcoholic liver disease

A 2005 Cochrane review of 13 randomised clinical trials and a 2007 Cochrane review of 18 randomised clinical trials assessed milk thistle in 915 and 1088 patients, respectively, looking at its effect in alcoholic and/or hepatitis B or C virus liver diseases (Rambaldi et al 2005, 2007). The authors stated in both reviews that the methodological quality of the trials was low and that milk thistle versus placebo or no intervention had no significant effect on complications of liver disease or liver histology, and that milk thistle was not associated with a significantly increased risk of adverse events.

In comparison to the 2005 review, which concluded that liver-related mortality was significantly reduced by milk thistle in patients with alcoholic liver disease, the 2007 review found that liver-related mortality was significantly reduced by milk thistle in all trials, but not in high-quality trials (Rambaldi et al 2005, 2007).

A review of 36 papers concluded that silymarin may have a role in the treatment of liver cirrhosis, especially alcoholic cirrhosis. In five trials of patients with liver cirrhosis (n = 602), a significant but small (7%) reduction of liver-related mortality (not corrected for study duration) was attained with silymarin (Saller et al 2001). These findings were confirmed in a recent meta-analysis by the same author (Saller et al 2008).

Acute viral hepatitis

Several studies have investigated the use of milk thistle in this disease, reporting beneficial effects on serological outcomes (Bode et al 1977, Magliulo et al 1978, Tkacz & Dworniak 1983). However, these early studies were not clearly blinded.

More recently, a randomised, double-blind, placebo-controlled clinical trial involving 105 subjects with acute hepatitis (hepatitis A, B, C and E) patients tested a commercial St Mary's thistle product (Legalon 140 mg three times daily) taken for four weeks. The silymarin group had faster resolution of symptoms related to biliary retention, dark urine (P = 0.013), jaundice (P = 0.02) and scleral icterus (P = 0.043). However, the primary outcome measure of normalisation of bilirubin and hepatic enzymes did not differ between the herbal and placebo groups (El-Kamary et al 2009).

Hepatitis C infection

A 2003 systematic review of medicinal herbs for HCV infection concluded that compared with placebo, none of the herbs showed effects on HCV RNA or liver enzymes, except for the constituent silybin, which showed a significant reduction of serum aspartate aminotransferase (AST) and gamma-glutamyltranspeptidase levels in one trial (Liu et al 2003).

In a 4-week randomised, controlled clinical trial (n = 34) using 160 mg of milk thistle three times a day, AST, alanine aminotransferase (ALT) and viral load values decreased from baseline levels after 4 weeks although the effect was not significant. In comparison, values for ALT and viral load showed a significant increase in the control group over the same period. When treatment and control groups were then compared, a significant difference was observed for ALT and AST, but not for viral load (Torres et al 2004). Similarly, a 2005 review concluded that silymarin decreases serum AST and ALT levels, but does not seem to affect viral load or liver histology (Mayer et al 2005).

A randomised, double-blind, placebo-controlled, crossover study (n = 24) where subjects received 12 weeks treatment with 600 or 1200 mg milk thistle daily, viral load, ALT levels and quality of life scores (short-form (SF)-36) were not significantly different to placebo (Gordon et al 2006).

As part of the hepatitis C Antiviral Long-Term Treatment Against Cirrhosis (HALT-C) trial (n = 1145 participants), involving people with advanced chronic hepatitis C, non-responders to prior antiviral therapy continued taking pegylated interferon treatment with the addition of oral silymarin therapy; however, no changes to ALT and viral load were observed with adjunctive herbal treatment. Silymarin therapy did significantly lower liver-related symptoms and improved QOL parameters such as fatigue, nausea, liver pain, anorexia, muscle and joint pain, as well as general health (Seeff et al 2008).

Non-responders to pegylated interferon and ribavirin were treated with increasing doses of intravenous (IV) silibinin (Legalon, SIL; Madaus) (Ferenci et al 2008). A dose-dependent reduction of HCV RNA was achieved. Patients were given 15 or 20 mg/kg/day IV silibinin for 14 days, and 280 mg oral silymarin three times per day combined with pegylated interferon and ribavirin therapy from day 8. At week 12, 50% (7/14) previous non-responders had undetectable HCV RNA (Ferenci et al 2008). Despite the small numbers and lack of a control group, this was the first time that silibinin (intravenously) had shown a direct anti-HCV activity in chronic hepatitis C patients (Ferenci et al 2008). It identifies a new pharmacological action for silibinin in humans and provides useful information about effective doses of intravenous silibinin and oral silymarin. It is of clinical significance, because adding pegylated interferon and ribavirin to intravenous silibinin showed greater efficacy than silibinin or pegylated interferon and ribavirin alone, suggesting a synergistic effect.

A review found no evidence for a beneficial effect of oral silymarin on the progression of viral hepatitis, especially hepatitis C (Saller et al 2008). Negative results were also obtained in a 2012 double-blind placebo-controlled trial testing oral Legalon (420 mg or 700 mg three times a day) in people with chronic hepatitis C (CHC). The study of 154 CHC patients found treatment with silymarin for 24 weeks produced no significant change in serum ALT levels during or after the trial, compared to placebo. Additionally, other markers of advanced liver disease such as serum bilirubin, albumin and platelet counts were the same (Fried et al 2012).

The recent use of intravenous silibinin prevented HCV RNA re-infection after orthotopic liver transplantation (Neumann et al 2010). Neumann and colleagues (2010) started silibinin infusions (1400 mg daily for 14 days) administered eight hours after orthotopic liver transplantation, when HCV RNA levels measured 182 IU/mL. Three days later HCV RNA became undetectable (<15 IU/mL) and remained so 168 days later (Neumann et al 2010).

IN COMBINATION

More recently, a randomised, double-blind, placebo-controlled trial of 118 chronic hepatitis C participants showed that treatment with silymarin (720 mg silybin per day) and 12 vitamin and phytochemical based antioxidants achieved a higher rate of ALT normalisation compared to placebo ($P = 0.02$) or silymarin ($P = 0.003$) at Week 24. There was also a significant improvement in overall mental wellbeing (mental component summary scale) in the active treatment group (Salmond et al 2010).

A review concluded that silymarin 'is reasonable' to be employed as an adjunct therapy for alcoholic and grade Child A liver cirrhosis (Saller et al 2008).

Non-alcoholic fatty liver disease (NAFLD)

A phase III, double-blind clinical trial assessing the effects of silybin plus phosphatidylcholine on patients with nonalcoholic fatty liver disease showed positive outcomes over the 12-month treatment program. Patients were given Realsil, which is comprised of 94 mg silymarin, 194 mg phosphatidylcholine and 89.28 mg vitamin E acetate 50%. The study showed that there was substantial normalisation in ALT, AST and glutamyl-transpeptidase levels over the trial period. Blood glucose was 31% lower in the treatment group compared to placebo suggesting positive improvements in insulin resistance. Liver histology improvement was also noted via ultrasound (lobular inflammation, ballooning and fibrosis). In all measurements the active treatment group outperformed controls. It is suspected that the herb's antioxidant activity is chiefly responsible for the beneficial effects observed (Loguercio et al 2012).

IN COMBINATION

In 2013, another study was published testing silymarin (twice daily) in NAFLD producing positive results. The open study involved 72 patients who were on a restricted diet for 3 months and a food supplement containing vitamin E, L-glutathione, L-cysteine, L-methionine and *Silybum marianum* (Epaclin 3.5 g) taken twice a day. This treatment regimen reduced the biochemical, inflammatory and ultrasonic indices of hepatic steatosis and some parameters indicative of early stage of atherosclerosis (Cacciapuoti et al 2013). In particular, Steato test significantly ($P < 0.001$) reduced from baseline (0.71 ± 0.07) to the end of treatment (0.40 ± 0.05), ALT serum levels ($P < 0.01$) fell from a mean level of 109.48 ± 4.4 to 75.12 ± 3.3 U/L and AST recorded at baseline (72.39 ± 8.4 U/L) also significantly reduced ($P < 0.05$) after silymarin and diet (48.65 ± 3.2 U/L) (Cacciapuoti et al 2013).

Clinical note — What is NAFLD?

Non-alcoholic fatty liver disease is the most common silent liver disease worldwide. It is characterised by fat accumulation in the liver (steatosis) and alterations in liver biochemical tests in people who do not consume high amounts of alcohol. Importantly, there are no obvious symptoms of disease. It has been estimated that the prevalence of NAFLD in Western countries is 20–30%. Obesity, type 2 diabetes and hyperlipidaemia are often associated with NAFLD (Cacciapuoti et al 2013).

Diabetes

Silymarin has also been investigated in people with type 2 diabetes both with and without cirrhosis. Velussi et al (1997) investigated whether long-term treatment with silymarin is effective in reducing lipoperoxidation and insulin resistance in diabetic patients with cirrhosis. The 6-month open trial found that silymarin treatment had several benefits. After the first month's treatment, fasting glucose levels showed a progressive and significant decline that, interestingly, did not lead to an increase in the frequency of hypoglycaemic episodes. Other observations revealed decreased glucosuria and levels of glycosylated haemoglobin also decreased significantly, indicating an overall improvement in glucose control. The dose used was 600 mg/day silymarin.

A 4-month randomised, double-blind, placebo-controlled trial in 51 type 2 diabetes patients receiving silymarin (200 mg three times daily) as an adjunct treatment to their conventional therapy showed a significant decrease in HbA_{1C}, fasting blood glucose, total cholesterol, LDL and triglyceride levels compared with placebo as well as with values at the beginning of the study in each group (Huseini et al 2006). Another randomised, double-blind, placebo-controlled trial of 4 months' duration involving 59 subjects with type 2 diabetes compared treatment with 200 mg silymarin/day plus 10 mg glibenclamide to placebo plus glibenclamide vs glinenclamide alone. The silymarin group had significant reductions in both fasting and postprandial glucose levels, HbA_{1C} and BMI compared to the placebo (Hussain 2007). A meta-analysis found the pooled mean difference (in the above two studies) in HbA_{1C} and fasting glucose were −1.92% ($P = 0.008$) and −38.05 mg/dL ($P < 0.009$) in silymarin plus conventional treatment vs placebo plus conventional treatment (Suksomboon et al 2011). This meta-analysis concluded that treatment with *Silybum marianum* may improve glycaemic control in T2DM and called for further high quality studies to better elucidate the effects of these herbs on glycaemic control (Suksomboon et al 2011).

OTHER USES

Traditionally, the seeds have been used to treat jaundice, hepatitis, haemorrhoids and psoriasis, as a tonic for nursing mothers, and as a general 'liver-cleansing' agent.

Haemochromatosis

St Mary's thistle may have benefits in this condition, based on its mechanisms of action. Hutchinson et al suggested that silybin could chelate iron in the neutral pH of the duodenum and reduce the absorption of iron postprandially which they demonstrated in a crossover study with 10 people with haemochromatosis. Consumption of 140 mg of silybin with a meal resulted in a reduction in the postprandial increase in serum iron (AUC ± SE) compared with water (silybin 1726.6 ± 346.8 vs water 2988.8 ± 167; $P < 0.05$) and tea (silybin 1726.6 ± 346.8 vs tea 2099.3 ± 223.3; $P < 0.05$) (Hutchinson et al 2010).

Hypercholesterolaemia

In clinical practice, it is not unusual to find treatment with St Mary's thistle at the higher end of the dose range results in cholesterol-lowering effects. Several in vivo studies confirm that St Mary's thistle increases LDL cholesterol clearance and raises HDL cholesterol levels; however, only one clinical trial is available to determine whether the effect is clinically significant (Krecman et al 1998, Skottova & Krecman 1998b, Somogyi et al 1989). An open trial involving 14 subjects with type 2 hyperlipidaemia found that treatment with silymarin (420 mg/day) slightly reduced total cholesterol and HDL cholesterol levels (Somogyi et al 1989).

Cancer prevention and treatment

In the past two decades, silybin has demonstrated remarkable anti-cancer as well as cancer chemopreventive efficacy in preclinical cell culture and animal models of several cancer models including skin, breast, lung, bladder (Zeng et al 2011), colon, prostate, lung and kidney carcinomas (Deep & Agarwal 2010, Niture et al 2014). Silybin has also been tested in human phase I–II pilot clinical trials, where it was reported to be well tolerated and showed plasma and target-tissue bioavailability, though limited (Agarwal et al 2013, Flaig et al 2007, 2010).

Topical application of silymarin provided significant protection against different stages of UVB-induced skin carcinogenesis in mouse skin tumourigenesis models (Ahmad et al 1998, Lahiri-Chatterjee et al 1999).

A randomised, double-blind, placebo-controlled study of 37 men, 2–3 months after radical prostatectomy were randomised to receive 570 mg of silymarin and 240 mcg selenium ($n = 19$) or placebo ($n = 18$) daily for 6 months. The combination of silymarin and selenium significantly reduced two markers of lipid metabolism associated with prostate cancer (PCa) progression, LDL and total cholesterol which suggests that silymarin and selenium may be effective in reducing PCa progression (Vidlar et al 2010).

Chemotherapy support

Whether silymarin is a useful treatment to prevent organ toxicity due to chemotherapy remains to be tested. Based on its anti-inflammatory, antioxidant and hepatoprotective mechanisms, it could prove useful (Comelli et al 2007, Greenlee et al 2007). In a case of hepatotoxicity during chemotherapy which did not resolve with supportive care, there was an immediate response to milk thistle at 280 mg twice daily (McBride et al 2012).

Besides lowering toxicity, silybin strongly sensitises human prostate carcinoma cells to doxorubicin, cisplatin, carboplatin, and mitoxantrone-induced growth inhibition and apoptotic death. Similar synergistic effects of silybin with doxorubicin and cisplatin have also been reported in various other cancer cell lines (Agarwal et al 2013, Greenlee et al 2007). Further research is warranted to determine its role in practice and identify any safety issues.

Obsessive compulsive disorder

In a pilot randomised, double-blind trial of 35 adults with obsessive compulsive disorder (OCD) designed to compare the efficacy of silymarin to fluoxetine, both interventions provided equal and highly significant reductions on Yale-Brown Scale for OCD (Y-BOCS) ($P = 0.0001$). Patients were randomly assigned to receive either capsules of the *Silybum marianum* (600 mg/day taken in 200 mg capsules 3 times a day) or fluoxetine (30 mg/day taken in 10 mg capsules three times a day). There was also no significant difference between the two groups in terms of observed side effects (Sayyah et al 2010). Camfield suggests this effect is achieved through silibinin's inhibition of monoamine oxidase activity (Mazzio et al 1998) which increases serotonin levels in the cortex (Osuchowski et al 2004) and was shown to ameliorate decreases in dopamine and serotonin in the prefrontal cortex and hippocampus associated with methamphetamine abuse (Camfield et al 2011, Lu et al 2010b).

S

> ***Clinical note — Cisplatin***
> Cisplatin is one of the most active cytotoxic agents in the treatment of testicular cancer, head and neck, gastrointestinal, cervical, lung and bladder cancer. However, its clinical use is associated with side effects, such as severe nausea, ototoxicity, neurotoxicity and nephrotoxicity (Giacomelli et al 2002).

Pharmacokinetics of silymarin

Silymarin has low solubility in water and has poor oral bioavailability, similar to other flavonolignans, and undergoes rapid excretion (Loguercio & Festi 2011). Following oral administration, silymarin undergoes phase I and phase II metabolism, especially phase II conjugation reactions, forming chiefly monoglucuronides detectable in human plasma and in urine two hours after ingestion (Calani et al 2012). It undergoes multiple conjugation reactions and is primarily excreted into bile and urine (Pradhan & Girish 2006, Venkataramanan et al 2006, Wen et al 2008, Wu et al 2009).

A pharmacokinetic dosing study identified that oral doses of between 140 mg and 560 mg of silymarin resulted in increases in plasma silibinin A and silibinin B only whereas a higher dose of 700 mg silymarin resulted in six silymarin flavonolignans being detected in the plasma (Hawke et al 2010).

Due to its poor water solubility, research has been undertaken to find methods of improving silymarin bioavailability. This includes creating different preparations of more soluble derivatives of silybin creating silymarin nanoparticles, using a semisolid dispersion system and phytosomes of phosphatidylcholine as emulsifying agents (Filburn et al 2007, Hsu et al 2012, Hussein et al 2012, Loguercio & Festi 2011).

Efforts to improve silymarin bioavailability are important to obtain better clinical outcomes. For example, poor bioavailability with oral silymarin is correlated with liver inflammation (Hawke et al 2010, Loguercio & Festi 2011, Schrieber et al 2008). This supports the results and comments from the HALT-C trial (Freedman et al 2011). Ferenci's study (Ferenci et al 1989) and *A. phalloides* poisoning (Hruby et al 1983) showed that early administration of more bioavailable silymarin has better hepatoprotective activity.

To overcome oral bioavailability issues, intravenous silibinin has also been investigated. This method of use has recently been applied to patients with chronic hepatitis C, successfully clearing hepatitis C virus (HCV) infection in some patients even in monotherapy (Esser-Nobis et al 2013) and has also been successfully used to treat amatoxin poisoning (Mengs et al 2012).

DOSAGE RANGE

Studies show that the dose; route of administration; treatment duration; patient's diagnosed condition and any comorbidities; the inflammatory stage in the disease process (Loguercio & Festi 2011) and the genotype of the virus in HCV (Huber et al 2005) all impact the efficacy of silymarin treatment in liver disease. In summary:

- To show benefits in hepatic necroinflammation: 450 mg/day silymarin for 12 months achieved ALT normalisation in 15% of the CHC patients in a randomised study (El-Zayadi et al 2005);
- To improve liver histology: 420 mg/day silymarin for 41 months (mean) is required in alcoholic cirrhosis (Child-Pugh A, 5–7) (Fehér et al 1989, Ferenci et al 1989);
- To elicit antioxidant effects: 600 mg/day silymarin for 12 months reduced malondialdehyde in diabetic cirrhotics (Velussi et al 1997); and
- To elicit direct anti-HCV activity: 1400 mg/day intravenous silibinin administered for 14 days is needed (Biermer et al 2010, Ferenci et al 2008, Neumann et al 2010).

In most clinical trials the effective daily doses of silymarin range from 420 to 600 mg (Saller et al 2008). To obtain a midpoint of 500 mg of silymarin from a 1:1 herbal extract, assuming 1 mL of herbal extract contains 25 mg of silymarin, then 20 mL/day of the *Silybum marianum* extract is required. This is a higher level than is normally recommended in clinical practice.

- Liquid extract (1:1): 4–9 mL/day (Mills & Bone 2000).
- Silybin-phytosome: 13 g daily (Flaig et al 2007).

TOXICITY

Extremely low

Hawke et al (2010) showed that oral doses up to 2100 mg oral silymarin were non-toxic. Toxicity studies in rats and mice have shown that silymarin, even at daily doses as high as 2500–5000 mg/kg, produced no adverse toxic effects (Madaus 1989). In a 12-month study in rats and dogs given up to 2500 mg/day, no signs of toxicity were seen. Milk thistle products with a standardised content of silymarin (70–80%) were found to be safe for up to 41 months of usage (Francine 2005). Safety was further confirmed after comprehensive in vitro studies concluded that interference or heptatotoxicity of the dry extract from *S. marianum* at the recommended maximum daily dose of four Hepar-Pasc tablets, equivalent to 210 mg silibinin, is unlikely, and is to be considered safe (Doehmer et al 2011).

ADVERSE REACTIONS

Milk thistle is considered safe and well-tolerated when taken within the recommended dose range (Post-White et al 2007). A review of studies involving more than 7000 participants identified three cases of serious adverse reactions (two anaphylaxis and one gastroenteritis symptoms) (Jacobs et al 2002). In one clinical trial, patients with colorectal adenocarcinoma who received silipide (silybin with phosphatidylcholine) at dosages of 360, 720 or 1440 mg daily for 7 days found the administration of silipide to be safe (Hoh et al 2006). Another clinical trial (n = 13) reported hyperbilirubinaemia in 9/13 patients and increased ALT in 1/13 patients using silybin-phytosome (Flaig et al 2007), whereas all other trials reported only rare adverse events (Gordon et al 2006, Rainone 2005, Torres et al 2004), mostly gastrointestinal symptoms, even for intravenously administered silymarin (Ferenci et al 2008). Reviews concluded that silymarin has an excellent safety profile (Dryden et al 2006, Rainone 2005, Sagar 2007).

Overall, adverse effect frequency was the same as for placebo and had a low frequency, ranging from 2% to 12% in controlled trials. In practice, loose bowels and gastrointestinal symptoms have been reported.

SIGNIFICANT INTERACTIONS

In vitro studies using a standardised dry extract from *Silybum marianum* (Hepar-Pasc) state that according to FDA regulations, drug–drug interactions are possible for CYP2C8 and CYP2C9 but not likely, and are remote for CYP2C19, CYP2D6, and CYP3A4 (Doehmer et al 2011, Kiruthiga et al 2013). Although in vitro and some animal studies (Kiruthiga et al 2013) show possible drug interactions with silymarin these are not replicated in clinical interactions (Hackett et al 2013). A prospective human study of standard milk thistle extracts (non-phytosome) concluded that on the basis of current clinical data, the drug interaction risk for milk thistle products is minimal (Gurley et al 2012).

Cisplatin

Preliminary research has shown this combination may reduce toxic effects, yet enhance antitumour activity — theoretically adjunctive use may be beneficial when used under professional supervision however further research is required to confirm benefits (Agarwal et al 2013, Greenlee et al 2007).

Doxorubicin

Silymarin reduces cardiotoxicity and possibly chemosensitises resistant cells to anthracyclines — theoretically adjunctive use may be beneficial when used under professional supervision (Agarwal et al 2013, Greenlee et al 2007).

Hepatotoxic substances

General hepatoprotective effects reported for silymarin — adjunctive use may be beneficial when used under professional supervision.

CONTRAINDICATIONS AND PRECAUTIONS

Contraindicated in people with known allergy to the Asteraceae (Compositae) family of plants. One case of exacerbation of haemochromatosis due to ingestion of milk thistle has been reported (Whittington 2007); however, the association between herbal intake and outcome reported is unlikely (Kidd 2008).

PREGNANCY USE

An in vivo study concluded that silibinin was safe when used by pre-eclamptic pregnant women (Giorgi et al 2012). A review of four studies found no evidence of adverse effects in mothers and their offspring for silymarin when used by pregnant women with intrahepatic cholestasis, alcoholic and non-alcoholic liver cirrhosis, chronic and acute viral hepatitis, drug-induced liver toxicity, fatty degeneration of the liver (Hess 2013).

PATIENTS' FAQs

What will this herb do for me?

St Mary's thistle may improve digestion, particularly of fatty foods, and afford protection against the toxic effects of a number of drugs and environmental poisons. It is also used as supportive treatment in chronic liver diseases and high-cholesterol states.

When will it start to work?

This varies, depending on the indication.

Are there any safety issues?

St Mary's thistle is considered a very safe and well-tolerated herb. The most common side effects relate to gastrointestinal symptoms such as loose bowels.

Practice points/Patient counselling

- St Mary's thistle has hepatoprotective activity and has been shown to reduce the hepatotoxic effects of a variety of environmental toxins and medicines, such as paracetamol, erythromycin, carbon tetrachloride and death cap mushrooms (*Amanita phalloides* poisoning).
- It has direct and indirect antioxidant activities, accelerates the regeneration of hepatocytes after liver damage, has significant gastroprotective and nephroprotective activities, anti-inflammatory and antihistamine activities, and anti-tumour effects according to in vitro and animal studies.
- Numerous clinical studies have investigated its effects in a variety of liver diseases, many producing promising results however it's still too early to suggest the herb is used as routine treatment in chronic liver diseases. An individualised approach is best.
- In clinical practice, it is used to treat dyspepsia, toxic liver damage, as supportive therapy in chronic liver diseases and hypercholesterolaemia.
- Preliminary evidence suggests a possible role as adjunctive therapy with cisplatin and as a skin cancer preventive agent when applied topically.
- Dose and route of administration of silymarin preparations are important considerations in management of liver disease.

S

REFERENCES

Abenavoli, L., et al. (2010) Milk thistle in liver diseases: past, present, future. Phytother Res, 24, 1423–32.

Agarwal, C., et al. (2013) Anti-cancer efficacy of silybin derivatives — a structure-activity relationship. PLoS One, 8, e60074.

Agarwal R et al. Anticancer potential of silymarin: from bench to bed side. Anticancer Res 26.6B (2006): 4457–4498.

Aghazadeh, S., et al. (2011) Anti-apoptotic and anti-inflammatory effects of *Silybum marianum* in treatment of experimental steatohepatitis. Exp Toxicol Pathol, 63, 569–74.

Ahmad N et al. Skin cancer chemopreventive effects of a flavonoid antioxidant silymarin are mediated via impairment of receptor tyrosine kinase signaling and perturbation in cell cycle progression. Biochem Biophys Res Commun 247.2 (1998): 294–301.

Ahmed-Belkacem, A., et al. (2010) Silibinin and related compounds are direct inhibitors of hepatitis C virus RNA-dependent RNA polymerase. Gastroenterology, 138, 1112–22.

Alarcon de la Lastra AC et al. Gastric anti-ulcer activity of silymarin, a lipoxygenase inhibitor, in rats. J Pharm Pharmacol 44.11 (1992): 929–931.

Alarcon de la Lastra AC et al. Gastroprotection induced by silymarin, the hepatoprotective principle of *Silybum marianum* in ischemia-reperfusion mucosal injury: role of neutrophils. Planta Med 61.2 (1995): 116–1119.

Ali BH, et al. Effect of the traditional medicinal plants *Rhazya stricta, Balanitis aegyptiaca* and *Haplophylum tuberculatum* on paracetamol-induced hepatotoxicity in mice. Phytother Res 15.7 (2001): 598–603.

Allain H et al. Aminotransferase levels and silymarin in de novo tacrine-treated patients with Alzheimer's disease. Dement Geriatr Cogn Disord 10.3 (1999): 181–185.

Angulo P et al. Silymarin in the treatment of patients with primary biliary cirrhosis with a suboptimal response to ursodeoxycholic acid. Hepatology 32.5 (2000): 897–900.

Beinhardt, S., et al. (2011) Silibinin monotherapy prevents graft infection after orthotopic liver transplantation in a patient with chronic hepatitis C. J Hepatol, 54, 591–2; author reply 592-3.

Benda L et al. The influence of therapy with silymarin on the survival rate of patients with liver cirrhosis (author's transl). Wien Klin Wochenschr 92.19 (1980): 678–683.

Biermer, M., et al. (2010) Silibinin as a rescue treatment for HCV-infected patients showing suboptimal virologic response to standard combination therapy. J Hepatol, 52, S16.

Blaising, J. & Pecheur, E. I. (2013) Lipids: a key for hepatitis C virus entry and a potential target for antiviral strategies. Biochimie, 95, 96–102.

Blumenthal M, et al. (eds). Herbal medicine: expanded commission E monographs. Austin, TX: Integrative Medicine Communications, 2000.

Bode JC, et al. [Silymarin for the treatment of acute viral hepatitis? Report of a controlled trial. (author's transl)] Med Klin 72.12 (1977): 513–5118.

Boigk G et al. Silymarin retards collagen accumulation in early and advanced biliary fibrosis secondary to complete bile duct obliteration in rats. Hepatology 26.3 (1997): 643–649.

Borsari M et al. Silybin, a new iron-chelating agent. J Inorg Biochem 85.2–3 (2001): 123–129.

Breschi MC et al. Protective effect of silymarin in antigen challenge- and histamine-induced bronchoconstriction in in vivo guinea-pigs. Eur J Pharmacol 437.1–2 (2002): 91–95.

Buzzelli G et al. A pilot study on the liver protective effect of silybin-phosphatidylcholine complex (IdB1016) in chronic active hepatitis. Int J Clin Pharmacol Ther Toxicol 31.9 (1993): 456–460.

Cacciapuoti, F., et al. 2013. Silymarin in non alcoholic fatty liver disease. World J Hepatol., 5, (3) 109–113.

Calani, L., et al. 2012. Absorption and metabolism of milk thistle flavanolignans in humans. Phytomedicine, 20, (1) 40–46.

Camfield, D. A., et al. (2011) Nutraceuticals in the treatment of obsessive compulsive disorder (OCD): a review of mechanistic and clinical evidence. Prog Neuropsychopharmacol Biol Psychiatry, 35, 887–95.

Chen, I. S., et al. (2012) Hepatoprotection of silymarin against thioacetamide-induced chronic liver fibrosis. J Sci Food Agric, 92, 1441–7.

Cheng, B., et al. (2012) Silibinin inhibits the toxic aggregation of human islet amyloid polypeptide. Biochem Biophys Res Commun, 419, 495–9.

Choi, J. (2012) Oxidative stress, endogenous antioxidants, alcohol, and hepatitis C: pathogenic interactions and therapeutic considerations. Free Radic Biol Med, 52, 1135–50.

Choi, Y.H., et al. 2012. Silibinin attenuates allergic airway inflammation in mice. Biochem.Biophys.Res.Commun., 427, (3) 450–455.

Chrungoo VJ, et al. Silymarin mediated differential modulation of toxicity induced by carbon tetrachloride, paracetamol and D-galactosamine in freshly isolated rat hepatocytes. Indian J Exp Biol 35.6 (1997): 611–6117.

Colturato, C. P., et al. (2012) Metabolic effects of silibinin in the rat liver. Chem Biol Interact, 195, 119–32.

Comelli MC et al. Toward the definition of the mechanism of action of silymarin: activities related to cellular protection from toxic damage induced by chemotherapy. Integr Cancer Ther 6.2 (2007): 120–129.

Crocenzi FA, Roma MG. Silymarin as a new hepatoprotective agent in experimental cholestasis: new possibilities for an ancient medication. Curr Med Chem 13.9 (2006): 1055–1074.

Crocenzi FA et al. Effect of silymarin on biliary bile salt secretion in the rat. Biochem Pharmacol 59.8 (2000): 1015–1022.

Das SK, Vasudevan DM. Protective effects of silymarin, a milk thistle (*Silybum marianum*) derivative on ethanol-induced oxidative stress in liver. Indian J Biochem Biophys 43.5 (2006): 306–311.

Davila JC, et al. Protective effect of flavonoids on drug-induced hepatotoxicity in vitro. Toxicology 57.3 (1989): 267–286.

Deep, G. & Agarwal, R. (2007) Chemopreventive efficacy of silymarin in skin and prostate cancer. Integr Cancer Ther, 6, 130–45.

Deep, G. & Agarwal, R. (2010) Antimetastatic efficacy of silibinin: molecular mechanisms and therapeutic potential against cancer. Cancer Metastasis Rev, 29, 447–63.

Dehmlow C, et al. Scavenging of reactive oxygen species and inhibition of arachidonic acid metabolism by silibinin in human cells. Life Sci 58.18 (1996): 1591–1600.

Doehmer, J., et al. (2011) Assessment of a dry extract from milk thistle (*Silybum marianum*) for interference with human liver cytochrome-P450 activities. Toxicol In Vitro, 25, 21–7.

Dryden GW, et al. Polyphenols and gastrointestinal diseases. Curr Opin Gastroenterol 22.2 (2006): 165–170.

El-Kamary, S. S., et al. (2009) A randomized controlled trial to assess the safety and efficacy of silymarin on symptoms, signs and biomarkers of acute hepatitis. Phytomedicine, 16, 391–400.

El-Zayadi, A. R., et al. (2005) Non-interferon-based therapy: an option for amelioration of necro-inflammation in hepatitis C patients who cannot afford interferon therapy. Liver Int, 25, 746–51.

ESCOP (2009) ESCOP Monographs :The Scientific Foundation for Herbal Medicinal Products Supplement 2009, Stuttgart, Thieme.

Esser-Nobis, K., et al. 2013. Analysis of hepatitis C virus resistance to silibinin in vitro and in vivo points to a novel mechanism involving nonstructural protein 4B. Hepatology, 57, (3) 953–963.

Fantozzi R et al. FMLP-activated neutrophils evoke histamine release from mast cells. Agents Actions 18.1–2 (1986): 155–158.

Favari L, Perez-Alvarez V. Comparative effects of colchicine and silymarin on CCl4-chronic liver damage in rats. Arch Med Res 28.1 (1997): 11–117.

Fehér J et al. Liver-protective action of silymarin therapy in chronic alcoholic liver diseases. Orv Hetil 130.51 (1989): 2723–2727.

Ferenci P et al. Randomized controlled trial of silymarin treatment in patients with cirrhosis of the liver. J Hepatol 9.1 (1989): 105–113.

Ferenci P et al. Silibinin is a potent antiviral agent in patients with chronic hepatitis C not responding to pegylated interferon/ribavirin therapy. Gastroenterology 135.5 (2008): 1561–1567.

Fiebrich F, Koch H. Silymarin, an inhibitor of lipoxygenase. Experientia 35.12 (1979): 1548–1560.

Filburn CR, et al. Bioavailability of a silybin-phosphatidylcholine complex in dogs. J Vet Pharmacol Ther 30.2 (2007): 132–138.

Finkel, T. & Holbrook, N. J. (2000) Oxidants, oxidative stress and the biology of ageing. Nature, 408, 239–47.

Flaig TW et al. A phase I and pharmacokinetic study of silybin-phytosome in prostate cancer patients. Invest New Drugs 25.2 (2007): 139–146.

Flaig, T. W., et al. (2010) A study of high-dose oral silybin-phytosome followed by prostatectomy in patients with localized prostate cancer. Prostate, 70, 848–55.

Floersheim GL. Antagonistic effects against single lethal doses of *Amanita phalloides*. Naunyn Schmiedebergs Arch Pharmacol 293.2 (1976): 171–174.

Floersheim GL et al. Clinical death-cap (*Amanita phalloides*) poisoning: prognostic factors and therapeutic measures. Analysis of 205 cases. Schweiz Med Wochenschr 112.34 (1982): 1164–1177.

Flora K et al. Milk thistle (*Silybum marianum*) for the therapy of liver disease. Am J Gastroenterol 93.2 (1998): 139–143.

Francine R. Milk thistle. Am Fam Physician 72 (2005): 1285.

Fraschini, F., et al. (2002) Pharmacology of Silymarin. Clin Drug Investig, 22, 51–65.

Freedman, N. D., et al. (2011) Silymarin use and liver disease progression in the Hepatitis C Antiviral Long-Term Treatment against Cirrhosis trial. Aliment Pharmacol Ther, 33, 127–137.

Fried, M. W., et al. (2012) Effect of silymarin (milk thistle) on liver disease in patients with chronic hepatitis C unsuccessfully treated with interferon therapy: a randomized controlled trial. JAMA, 308, 274–82.

Gaedeke J et al. Cisplatin nephrotoxicity and protection by silibinin. Nephrol Dial Transplant 11.1 (1996): 55–62.

Galisteo M et al. Hepatotoxicity of tacrine: occurrence of membrane fluidity alterations without involvement of lipid peroxidation. J Pharmacol Exp Ther 294.1 (2000): 160–167.

Gazák, R., et al. (2010) Antioxidant and antiviral activities of silybin fatty acid conjugates. Eur J Med Chem, 45, 1059–67.

Giacomelli S et al. Silybin and its bioavailable phospholipid complex (IdB 1016) potentiate in vitro and in vivo the activity of cisplatin. Life Sci 70.12 (2002): 1447–1459.

Giorgi, V. S., et al. (2012) Silibinin modulates the NF-kappab pathway and pro-inflammatory cytokine production by mononuclear cells from preeclamptic women. J Reprod Immunol, 95, 67–72.

Goey, A. K., et al. (2013) Relevance of in vitro and clinical data for predicting CYP3A4-mediated herb-drug interactions in cancer patients. Cancer Treat Rev.

Gordon A et al. Effects of *Silybum marianum* on serum hepatitis C virus RNA, alanine aminotransferase levels and well-being in patients with chronic hepatitis C. J Gastroenterol Hepatol 21.2 (2006): 275–280.

Greenlee H et al. Clinical applications of *Silybum marianum* in oncology. Integr Cancer Ther 6.2 (2007): 158–65.

Guedj, J., et al. (2012) Understanding silibinin's modes of action against HCV using viral kinetic modeling. J Hepatol, 56, 1019–24.

Gurley BJ et al. Effect of milk thistle (*Silybum marianum*) and black cohosh (*Cimicifuga racemosa*) supplementation on digoxin pharmacokinetics in humans. Drug Metab Dispos 34.1 (2006a): 69–74.

Gurley B et al. Assessing the clinical significance of botanical supplementation on human cytochrome P450 3A activity: comparison of a milk thistle and black cohosh product to rifampin and clarithromycin. J Clin Pharmacol 46.2 (2006b): 201–13.

Gurley, B. J., et al. (2012) Pharmacokinetic herb-drug interactions (part 2): drug interactions involving popular botanical dietary supplements and their clinical relevance. Planta Med, 78, 1490–514.

Hackett, E. S., et al. (2013) Milk thistle and its derivative compounds: a review of opportunities for treatment of liver disease. J Vet Intern Med, 27, 10–6.

Haddad, Y., et al. (2011) Antioxidant and hepatoprotective effects of silibinin in a rat model of nonalcoholic steatohepatitis. Evid Based Complement Alternat Med, 2011, nep164.

Hakova H, Misurova E. Therapeutical effect of silymarin on nucleic acids in the various organs of rats after radiation injury. Radiats Biol Radioecol 36.3 (1996): 365–370.

Hawke, R. L., et al. (2010) Silymarin ascending multiple oral dosing phase I study in noncirrhotic patients with chronic hepatitis C. J Clin Pharmacol, 50, 434–49.

Hermann, R. & von Richter, O. (2012) Clinical evidence of herbal drugs as perpetrators of pharmacokinetic drug interactions. Planta Med, 78, 1458–77.

Hernandez-Gea, V. & Friedman, S. L. (2011) Pathogenesis of liver fibrosis. Annu Rev Pathol, 6, 425–56.

Hess, H. M. (2013) 23 — Herbs and Alternative Remedies. Clinical Pharmacology During Pregnancy. Waltham MA, Academic Press.

Hoh C et al. Pilot study of oral silibinin, a putative chemopreventive agent, in colorectal cancer patients: silibinin levels in plasma, colorectum, and liver and their pharmacodynamic consequences. Clin Cancer Res 12.9 (2006): 2944–2950.

Hou, Y. C., et al. (2010) Preventive effect of silymarin in cerebral ischemia-reperfusion-induced brain injury in rats possibly through impairing NF-kappaB and STAT-1 activation. Phytomedicine, 17, 963–73.

Hruby, K., et al. (1983) Chemotherapy of *Amanita phalloides* poisoning with intravenous silibinin. Hum Toxicol, 2, 183–95.

Hsu, W.C., et al. 2012. Characteristics and antioxidant activities of silymarin nanoparticles. J Nanosci.Nanotechnol., 12, (3) 2022–2027.

Huber, R., et al. (2005) Oral silymarin for chronic hepatitis C — a retrospective analysis comparing three dose regimens. Eur J Med Res, 10, 68–70.

Huseini HF et al. The efficacy of *Silybum marianum* (L.) Gaertn. (silymarin) in the treatment of type II diabetes: a randomized, double-blind, placebo-controlled, clinical trial. Phytother Res 20.12 (2006): 1036–1039.

Hussain, S. A. (2007) Silymarin as an adjunct to glibenclamide therapy improves long-term and postprandial glycemic control and body mass index in type 2 diabetes. J Med Food, 10, 543–7.

Hussein A, El-Menshawe S, Afouna M (2012) Enhancement of the in vitro dissolution and in vivo oral bioavailability of silymarin from liquid-filled hard gelatin capsules of semisolid dispersion using Gelucire 44/14 as a carrier. Pharmazie 67, 209–214.

Hutchinson, C., et al. (2010) The iron-chelating potential of silybin in patients with hereditary haemochromatosis. Eur J Clin Nutr, 64, 1239–41.

Jacobs BP et al. Milk thistle for the treatment of liver disease: a systematic review and meta-analysis. Am J Med 113.6 (2002): 506–515.

Karimi G, et al. Cisplatin nephrotoxicity and protection by milk thistle extract in rats. Evid Based Complement Altern Med 2.3 (2005): 383–386.

Kauntz, H., et al. (2012a) Silibinin, a natural flavonoid, modulates the early expression of chemoprevention biomarkers in a preclinical model of colon carcinogenesis. Int J Oncol, 41, 849–54.

Kauntz, H., et al. (2012b) The flavonolignan silibinin potentiates TRAIL-induced apoptosis in human colon adenocarcinoma and in derived TRAIL-resistant metastatic cells. Apoptosis, 17, 797–809.

Khayyal MT et al. Antiulcerogenic effect of some gastrointestinally acting plant extracts and their combination. Arzneimittelforschung 51.7 (2001): 545–553.

Khayyal MT et al. Mechanisms involved in the gastro-protective effect of STW 5 (Iberogast) and its components against ulcers and rebound acidity. Phytomedicine 13 (Suppl 5) (2006): 56–66.

Kidd R. Exacerbation of hemochromatosis by ingestion of milk thistle. Can Fam Physician 54.2 (2008): 182; author reply 182–3.

Kim, M., et al. (2012) Silymarin suppresses hepatic stellate cell activation in a dietary rat model of non-alcoholic steatohepatitis: analysis of isolated hepatic stellate cells. Int J Mol Med, 30, 473–9.

Kim, S., et al. (2009) Silibinin prevents TPA-induced MMP-9 expression and VEGF secretion by inactivation of the Raf/MEK/ERK pathway in MCF-7 human breast cancer cells. Phytomedicine, 16, 573–80.

Kiruthiga PV et al. Protective effect of silymarin on erythrocyte haemolysate against benzo(a)pyrene and exogenous reactive oxygen species (H2O2) induced oxidative stress. Chemosphere 68.8 (2007): 1511–15118.

Kiruthiga, P. V., et al. (2013) Silymarin prevents benzo(a)pyrene-induced toxicity in Wistar rats by modulating xenobiotic-metabolizing enzymes. Toxicol Ind Health 0748233713475524.

Koch HP, et al. Silymarin: potent inhibitor of cyclic AMP phosphodiesterase. Methods Find Exp Clin Pharmacol 7.8 (1985): 409–413.

Krecman V et al. Silymarin inhibits the development of diet-induced hypercholesterolemia in rats. Planta Med 64.2 (1998): 138–142.

Kroll DJ, et al. Milk thistle nomenclature: why it matters in cancer research and pharmacokinetic studies. Integr Cancer Ther 6.2 (2007): 110–1119.

Kropacova K, et al. Protective and therapeutic effect of silymarin on the development of latent liver damage. Radiats Biol Radioecol 38.3 (1998): 411–4115.

Kung, G., et al. (2011) Programmed necrosis, not apoptosis, in the heart. Circ Res, 108, 1017–36.

Lahiri-Chatterjee M et al. A flavonoid antioxidant, silymarin, affords exceptionally high protection against tumor promotion in the SENCAR mouse skin tumorigenesis model. Cancer Res 59.3 (1999): 622–632.

Lecomte J. General pharmacologic properties of silybin and silymarin in the rat. Arch Int Pharmacodyn Ther 214.1 (1975): 165–176.

Letteron P et al. Mechanism for the protective effects of silymarin against carbon tetrachloride-induced lipid peroxidation and hepatotoxicity in mice: evidence that silymarin acts both as an inhibitor of metabolic activation and as a chain-breaking antioxidant. Biochem Pharmacol 39.12 (1990): 2027–2034.

Li, L., et al. (2010) Targeting silibinin in the antiproliferative pathway. Expert Opin Investig Drugs, 19, 243–55.

Lieber, C. S., et al. (2003) Silymarin retards the progression of alcohol-induced hepatic fibrosis in baboons. J Clin Gastroenterol, 37, 336–9.

Liu J et al. Medicinal herbs for hepatitis C virus infection: a Cochrane hepatobiliary systematic review of randomized trials. Am J Gastroenterol 98.3 (2003): 538–544.

Loguercio, C. & Festi, D. (2011) Silybin and the liver: from basic research to clinical practice. World J Gastroenterol, 17, 2288–301.

Loguercio C et al. The effect of a silybin-vitamin e-phospholipid complex on nonalcoholic fatty liver disease: a pilot study. Dig Dis Sci 52.9 (2007): 2387–2395.

Loguercio, C., et al (2012) Silybin combined with phosphatidylcholine and vitamin E in patients with nonalcoholic fatty liver disease: a randomized controlled trial. Free Radic Biol Med, 52, 1658–65.

Lu, J. M., et al. (2010a) Chemical and molecular mechanisms of antioxidants: experimental approaches and model systems. J Cell Mol Med, 14, 840–60.

Lu, P., et al. (2010b) Silibinin attenuates cognitive deficits and decreases of dopamine and serotonin induced by repeated methamphetamine treatment. Behav Brain Res, 207, 387–93.

Lucena MI et al. Effects of silymarin MZ-80 on oxidative stress in patients with alcoholic cirrhosis: results of a randomized, double-blind, placebo-controlled clinical study. Int J Clin Pharmacol Ther 40.1 (2002): 2–8.

MacKinnon SL et al. Silyamandin, a new flavonolignan isolated from milk thistle tinctures. Planta Med 73.11 (2007): 1214–12116.

Madaus. Legalon booklet. Cologne: Madaus, 1989, pp 3–42. (As cited in Combest WL. Milk thistle. US Pharmacist 23.9 (1998).)

Magliulo E, et al. Results of a double blind study on the effect of silymarin in the treatment of acute viral hepatitis, carried out at two medical centres (author's transl). Med Klin 73.28–29 (1978): 1060–1065.

Marino, Z., et al. (2013) Intravenous silibinin monotherapy shows significant antiviral activity in HCV-infected patients in the peri-transplantation period. J Hepatol, 58, 415–20.

Masini A et al. Iron-induced oxidant stress leads to irreversible mitochondrial dysfunctions and fibrosis in the liver of chronic iron-dosed gerbils: the effect of silybin. J Bioenerg Biomembr 32.2 (2000): 175–182.

Mayer KE, et al. Silymarin treatment of viral hepatitis: a systematic review. J Viral Hepat 12.6 (2005): 559–567.

Mazzio, E. A., et al. (1998) Food constituents attenuate monoamine oxidase activity and peroxide levels in C6 astrocyte cells. Planta Med, 64, 603–6.

McBride, A., et al. (2012) *Silybum marianum* (milk thistle) in the management and prevention of hepatotoxicity in a patient undergoing reinduction therapy for acute myelogenous leukemia. J Oncol Pharm Pract, 18, 360–5.

McClure, J., et al. (2012) Silibinin inhibits HIV-1 infection by reducing cellular activation and proliferation. PLoS One, 7, e41832.

Mengs, U., et al. (2012) Legalon(R) SIL: the antidote of choice in patients with acute hepatotoxicity from amatoxin poisoning. Curr Pharm Biotechnol, 13, 1964–70.

Mills S, Bone K. Principles and practice of phytotherapy. London: Churchill Livingstone, 2000.

Morazzoni P, Bombardelli E. *Silybum marianum* (*Carduus marianus*). Fitoterapia 66 (1995): 3–42.

Morishima, C., et al. (2010) Silymarin inhibits in vitro T-cell proliferation and cytokine production in hepatitis C virus infection. Gastroenterology, 138, 671–81, 681.e1–2.

Mourelle M et al. Prevention of CCL4-induced liver cirrhosis by silymarin. Fundam Clin Pharmacol 3.3 (1989): 183–191.

Muriel P, Mourelle M. Prevention by silymarin of membrane alterations in acute CCl4 liver damage. J Appl Toxicol 10.4 (1990): 275–279.

Muriel P et al. Silymarin protects against paracetamol-induced lipid peroxidation and liver damage. J Appl Toxicol 12.6 (1992): 439–442.

Nencini C, et al. Protective effect of silymarin on oxidative stress in rat brain. Phytomedicine 14.2–3 (2007): 129–135.

Neumann, U. P., et al. (2010) Successful prevention of hepatitis C virus (HCV) liver graft reinfection by silibinin mono-therapy. J Hepatol, 52, 951–2.

Niture, S. K., et al. (2014) Regulation of Nrf2-an update. Free Radic Biol Med 66: 36–44.

Osuchowski, M. F., et al. (2004) Alterations in regional brain neurotransmitters by silymarin, a natural antioxidant flavonoid mixture, in BALB/c mice. Pharm Biol 42, 384–9.

Palasciano G et al. The effect of silymarin on plasma levels of malondialdehyde in patients receiving long-term treatment with psychotropic drugs. Curr Ther Res 55 (1994): 537–545.

Par A et al. Oxidative stress and antioxidant defense in alcoholic liver disease and chronic hepatitis C. Orv Hetil 141.30 (2000): 1655–1659.

Parasassi T et al. Drug-membrane interactions: silymarin, silybin and microsomal membranes. Cell Biochem Funct 2.2 (1984): 85–88.

Pares A et al. Effects of silymarin in alcoholic patients with cirrhosis of the liver: results of a controlled, double-blind, randomized and multicenter trial. J Hepatol 28.4 (1998): 615–621.

Payer, B. A., et al. (2010) Successful HCV eradication and inhibition of HIV replication by intravenous silibinin in an HIV-HCV coinfected patient. J Clin Virol, 49, 131–3.

Pias, E. K. & Aw, T. Y. (2002) Early redox imbalance mediates hydroperoxide-induced apoptosis in mitotic competent undifferentiated PC-12 cells. Cell Death Differ, 9, 1007–16.

Pias, E. K., et al. (2003) Differential effects of superoxide dismutase isoform expression on hydroperoxide-induced apoptosis in PC-12 cells. J Biol Chem, 278, 13294–301.

Pietrangelo A et al. Antioxidant activity of silybin in vivo during long-term iron overload in rats. Gastroenterology 109.6 (1995): 1941–1949.

Polyak SJ et al. Inhibition of T-cell inflammatory cytokines, hepatocyte NF-kappaB signaling, and HCV infection by standardized Silymarin. Gastroenterology 132.5 (2007): 1925–1936.

Polyak, S. J., et al H. (2010) Identification of hepatoprotective flavonolignans from silymarin. Proc Natl Acad Sci U S A, 107, 5995–9.

Polyak, S. J., et al. (2013) Silymarin for HCV infection. Antivir Ther. 18: 141–147.

Post-White J, et al. Advances in the use of milk thistle (*Silybum marianum*). Integr Cancer Ther 6.2 (2007): 104–109.

Poynard, T., et al. (2009) Peginterferon alfa-2b and ribavirin: effective in patients with hepatitis C who failed interferon alfa/ribavirin therapy. Gastroenterology, 136, 1618–28.e2.

Pradhan SC, Girish C. Hepatoprotective herbal drug, silymarin from experimental pharmacology to clinical medicine. Indian J Med Res 124.5 (2006): 491.

Rainone F. Milk thistle. Am Fam Physician 72.7 (2005): 1285–1288.

Rambaldi A et al. Milk thistle for alcoholic and/or hepatitis B or C liver diseases–a systematic cochrane hepato-biliary group review with meta-analyses of randomized clinical trials. Am J Gastroenterol 100.11 (2005): 2583–2591.

Rambaldi A, et al. Milk thistle for alcoholic and/or hepatitis B or C virus liver diseases. Cochrane Database Syst Rev 4 (2007): CD003620.

Raza, S. S., et al. (2011) Silymarin protects neurons from oxidative stress associated damages in focal cerebral ischemia: a behavioral, biochemical and immunohistological study in Wistar rats. J Neurol Sci, 309, 45–54.

Reuland, D. J., et al. (2012) Upregulation of phase II enzymes through phytochemical activation of Nrf2 protects cardiomyocytes against oxidant stress. Free Radic Biol Med, 56C, 102–111.

Rui YC et al. Effects of silybin on production of oxygen free radical, lipoperoxide and leukotrienes in brain following ischemia and reperfusion. Zhongguo Yao Li Xue Bao 11.5 (1990): 418–421.

Sagar SM. Future directions for research on *Silybum marianum* for cancer patients. Integr Cancer Ther 6.2 (2007): 166–173.

Saller R, et al. The use of silymarin in the treatment of liver diseases. Drugs 61.14 (2001): 2035–2063.

Saller R et al. An updated systematic review with meta-analysis for the clinical evidence of silymarin. Forsch Komplementmed 15.1 (2008): 9–20.

Salmi HA, Sarna S. Effect of silymarin on chemical, functional, and morphological alterations of the liver. A double-blind controlled study. Scand J Gastroenterol 17.4 (1982): 517–521.

Salmond, S. J., et al. (2010) Hep573 study–a randomised double-blind placebo-controlled trial of silymarin alone or combined with antioxidants in chronic hepatitis C. Proceedings of Digestive Diseases Week, AASLD. New Orleans, LA, Gastroenterology.

Sayyah, M., et al. (2010) Comparison of *Silybum marianum* (L.) Gaertn. with fluoxetine in the treatment of Obsessive-Compulsive Disorder. Prog Neuropsychopharmacol Biol Psychiatry, 34, 362–5.

Schrieber SJ et al. The pharmacokinetics of silymarin is altered in patients with hepatitis C virus and nonalcoholic fatty liver disease and correlates with plasma caspase-3/7 activity. Drug Metab Dispos 36.9 (2008): 1909–1916.

Schuppan D et al. Alcohol and liver fibrosis: pathobiochemistry and treatment. Z Gastroenterol 33.9 (1995): 546–550.

Seeff LB et al. Herbal product use by persons enrolled in the hepatitis C Antiviral Long-Term Treatment Against Cirrhosis (HALT-C) Trial. Hepatology 47.2 (2008): 605–612.

Shaker, E., et al. (2010) Silymarin, the antioxidant component and *Silybum marianum* extracts prevent liver damage. Food Chem Toxicol, 48, 803–6.

Skottova N, Krecman V. Dietary silymarin improves removal of low density lipoproteins by the perfused rat liver. Acta Univ Palacki Olomuc Fac Med 141 (1998a): 39–40.

Skottova N, Krecman V. Silymarin as a potential hypocholesterolaemic drug. Physiol Res 47.1 (1998b): 1–7.

Sobolova L et al. Effect of silymarin and its polyphenolic fraction on cholesterol absorption in rats. Pharmacol Res 53.2 (2006): 104–112.

Somogyi A et al. Short term treatment of type II hyperlipoproteinaemia with silymarin. Acta Med Hung 46.4 (1989): 289–295.

Son, T. G., et al. (2008) Hormetic dietary phytochemicals. Neuromolecular Med, 10, 236–46.

Sonnenbichler J et al. Stimulatory effects of silibinin and silicristin from the milk thistle *Silybum marianum* on kidney cells. J Pharmacol Exp Ther 290.3 (1999): 1375–1383.

Suksomboon, N., et al. (2011) Meta-analysis of the effect of herbal supplement on glycemic control in type 2 diabetes. J Ethnopharmacol, 137, 1328–33.

Ting, H., et al. (2013) Molecular mechanisms of silibinin-mediated cancer chemoprevention with major emphasis on prostate cancer. AAPS J, 15, 707–16.

Tkacz B, Dworniak D. [Sylimarol in the treatment of acute viral hepatitis]. Wiad Lek 36.8 (1983): 613–6116.

Toklu HZ et al. Silymarin, the antioxidant component of *Silybum marianum*, prevents sepsis-induced acute lung and brain injury. J Surg Res 145.2 (2008): 214–222.

Torres M et al. Does *Silybum marianum* play a role in the treatment of chronic hepatitis C? P R Health Sci J 23 (2 Suppl) (2004): 69–74.

Trappoliere, M., et al. (2009) Silybin, a component of silymarin, exerts anti-inflammatory and anti-fibrogenic effects on human hepatic stellate cells. J Hepatol, 50, 1102–11.

Trinchet JC et al. Treatment of alcoholic hepatitis with silymarin: a double-blind comparative study in 116 patients. Gastroenterol Clin Biol 13.2 (1989): 120–124.

Tsai JH et al. Effects of silymarin on the resolution of liver fibrosis induced by carbon tetrachloride in rats. J Viral Hepat 15.7 (2008): 508–514.

Tyutyulkova N et al. Hepatoprotective effect of silymarin (Carsil) on liver of D-galactosamine treated rats: biochemical and morphological investigations. Methods Find Exp Clin Pharmacol 3.2 (1981): 71–77.

Tyutyulkova N et al. Effect of silymarin (Carsil) on the microsomal glycoprotein and protein biosynthesis in liver of rats with experimental galactosamine hepatitis. Methods Find Exp Clin Pharmacol 5.3 (1983): 181–184.

Tzeng, J. I., et al. (2013) Silymarin decreases connective tissue growth factor to improve liver fibrosis in rats treated with carbon tetrachloride. Phytother Res. 27: 1023–1028.

Valenzuela A, Guerra R. Protective effect of the flavonoid silybin dihemisuccinate on the toxicity of phenylhydrazine on rat liver. FEBS Lett 181.2 (1985): 291–294.

Varzi HN et al. Effect of silymarin and vitamin E on gentamicin-induced nephrotoxicity in dogs. J Vet Pharmacol Ther 30.5 (2007): 477–481.

Velussi M et al. Long-term (12 months) treatment with an anti-oxidant drug (silymarin) is effective on hyperinsulinemia, exogenous insulin need and malondialdehyde levels in cirrhotic diabetic patients. J Hepatol 26.4 (1997): 871–879.

Venkataramanan R, et al. In vitro and in vivo assessment of herb drug interactions. Life Sci 78.18 (2006): 2105–2115.

Vidlar, A., et al. (2010) The safety and efficacy of a silymarin and selenium combination in men after radical prostatectomy — a six

month placebo-controlled double-blind clinical trial. Biomed Pap Med Fac Univ Palacky Olomouc Czech Repub, 154, 239–44.
Vogel G et al. Protection by silibinin against *Amanita phalloides* intoxication in beagles. Toxicol Appl Pharmacol 73.3 (1984): 355–362.
von Schonfeld J, et al. Silibinin, a plant extract with antioxidant and membrane stabilizing properties, protects exocrine pancreas from cyclosporin A toxicity. Cell Mol Life 53.11–12 (1997): 917–920.
Wagoner, J., et al. (2010) Multiple effects of silymarin on the hepatitis C virus lifecycle. Hepatology, 51, 1912–21.
Wagoner, J., et al. (2011) Differential in vitro effects of intravenous versus oral formulations of silibinin on the HCV life cycle and inflammation. PLoS One, 6, e16464.
Wen Z et al. Pharmacokinetics and metabolic profile of free, conjugated, and total silymarin flavonolignans in human plasma after oral administration of milk thistle extract. Drug Metab Dispos 36.1 (2008): 65–72.
Wesolowska O et al. Influence of silybin on biophysical properties of phospholipid bilayers. Acta Pharmacol Sin 28.2 (2007): 296–306.
Whittington C. Exacerbation of hemochromatosis by ingestion of milk thistle. Can Fam Physician 53.10 (2007): 1671–1673.
Wu JW, et al. Drug–drug interactions of silymarin on the perspective of pharmacokinetics. J Ethnopharmacol 121.2 (2009): 185–193.
Yin, F., et al. (2011) Silibinin: a novel inhibitor of Abeta aggregation. Neurochem Int, 58, 399–403.
Zeng, J., et al. (2011) Chemopreventive and chemotherapeutic effects of intravesical silibinin against bladder cancer by acting on mitochondria. Mol Cancer Ther, 10, 104–16.
Zhang S, Morris ME. Effect of the flavonoids biochanin A and silymarin on the P-glycoprotein-mediated transport of digoxin and vinblastine in human intestinal Caco-2 cells. Pharm Res 20.8 (2003): 1184–1191.
Zhao J et al. Significant inhibition by the flavonoid antioxidant silymarin against 12-O-tetradecanoylphorbol 13-acetate-caused modulation of antioxidant and inflammatory enzymes, and cyclooxygenase 2 and interleukin-1alpha expression in SENCAR mouse epidermis: implications in the prevention of stage I tumor promotion. Mol Carcinog 26.4 (1999): 321–333.

Stinging nettle

HISTORICAL NOTE Stinging nettle has been used since ancient times, with Dioscorides and Galen in ancient Greece reporting diuretic and laxative effects for nettle leaf. Roman troops were thought to flail themselves with the stinging nettle to keep warm. It is also widely used for gynaecological complaints by North American Indians and in Ayurvedic medicine in India (Blumenthal et al 2000). The Latin root of *urtica* is *uro*, meaning 'I burn', indicative of the small stings caused by the hairs on the leaves of nettle when contact is made with the skin.

OTHER NAMES

Common nettle, brenessel, brennesselkraut, brennesselwurzel, urtica ortie, great stinging nettle, haarnesselkraut, haarnesselwurzel, ortica, ortie, otriga.

BOTANICAL NAME/FAMILY

Urtica dioica (family Urticaceae)

PLANT PARTS USED

Aerial parts and root

CHEMICAL COMPONENTS

Constituents found within the leaf include vitamins A and C, B group, K, beta-carotene, calcium and potassium, phosphorus, chlorophyll, magnesium and tannins, flavonoids, sterols and amines (US Department of Agriculture 2003). Various constituents' levels will vary with the age of the plants at harvest time, the season of harvest and the cut used. For example, beta-carotene is more concentrated in older plants. Iron and manganese content are higher in the leaves of young plants whereas nickel and lead are the lowest in older plants. There is a seasonal variation in the concentration of tannin and chlorophyll in the plant. The leaves contain a higher concentration of calcium and magnesium than the roots but are not affected by the age of the plant (Upton 2013).

Constituents found chiefly in the root include polysaccharides, lectins, lignans, fatty acids, terpenes and coumarin (Ernst et al 2001).

MAIN ACTIONS

Anti-inflammatory and analgesic

In vitro studies have identified anti-inflammatory activity for *Urtica* extract (Obertreis et al 1996a, 1996b, Riehemann et al 1999). The mechanism of action has not been fully elucidated, but test tube studies have demonstrated inhibitory effects on NF-kappaB activation and partial inhibitory effects on cyclo oxygenase and 5-lipoxygenase-derived reactions. Additionally, isolated phenolic acid from nettle has been shown to inhibit leukotriene B_4 synthesis in a concentration-dependent manner in vitro.

Although extensive investigation has not been conducted in humans to confirm anti-inflammatory mechanisms, one study of 20 volunteers showed that oral ingestion of 1.34 g nettle extract for 3 weeks significantly decreased lipopolysaccharide-stimulated tumour necrosis factor-alpha (TNF-alpha) and interleukin-1 beta (IL-1-beta) when tested ex vivo but had no effects on cytokine levels (Teucher et al 1996).

In vitro data have shown that nettle leaf extract (IDS 30) reduces the induction of primary T-cell responses and TNF-alpha in T-cell-mediated diseases such as rheumatoid arthritis (Broer & Behnke 2002). Faecal IL-1-beta and TNF-alpha concentrations were significantly reduced in mice with induced Crohn's disease treated with IDS 30 (Konrad et al 2005). Mice treated with nettle extract

S

displayed fewer histological changes and general disease symptoms. The authors conclude that the effect may be due to a decrease in TH1 response and may constitute a new treatment option for prolonging remission in inflammatory bowel disease.

A recent study investigating different stinging nettle preparations for anti-inflammatory activity found lipophilic extracts had stronger activity than the traditional tinctures (water, methanol, ethanol), thereby suggesting clinical effects may be more likely with these forms (Johnson et al 2013).

Hypotensive and diuretic

When administered intravenously to test animals, *Urtica* extract exerts an acute hypotensive action accompanied by diuretic and natriuretic effects (Tahri et al 2000). It is uncertain whether the same effects are seen with oral administration.

A review of in vitro and in vivo studies concluded that the hypotensive action of *U. dioica* is due in part to negative inotropic activity and a vasodilatory effect (Testai et al 2002).

Antihyperglycaemic

A 33% reduction in blood glucose was noted in rats administered 250 mg/kg of nettle leaf extract orally, 30 minutes before glucose loading (Bnouham et al 2003). Nettle was shown to decrease glucose absorption in the small intestine of rats under anaesthesia; however, administration of 500 mg/kg failed to modify blood glucose levels in alloxan-induced diabetic rats.

A six-fold increase in blood insulin levels occurred after intravenous administration of a nettle leaf fraction in streptozotocin-diabetic rats, with a corresponding drop in blood sugar levels as compared to control (Farzami et al 2003). Details of the isolated fraction were not given.

Antiproliferative effects on prostate cells

Nettle extract has shown antiproliferative effects on prostate cells; however, the exact mechanism of action has not been fully elucidated (Lichius & Muth 1997, Lichius et al 1999). Results from several in vitro studies suggest that a combination of mechanisms is responsible. It seems likely that sex hormone binding globulin (SHBG), aromatase, epidermal growth factor and prostate steroid membrane receptors are involved in the antiprostatic effect, but less likely that 5-alpha reductase or androgen receptors are involved (Chrubasik et al 2007).

Prostate cancer

One study found that a methanolic extract of stinging nettle roots slows the progression of prostate cancer in both an in vivo model and an in vitro system (Konrad et al 2000). One study involving 20 males with prostatic adenoma found that treatment for 7 days with nettle produced a significant drop in zinc level, thought to be a result of altering zinc-testosterone metabolism and diminishing zinc secretion in adenomatous tissue (Romics & Bach 1991).

Antiviral

A lectin extracted from nettle had inhibitory effects against HIV-1, HIV-2, human cytomegalovirus, respiratory syncytial virus and influenza A virus in vitro (Balzarini et al 1992).

Antioxidant

Nettle has shown potent antioxidant activity in a range of in vitro tests (Gulcin et al 2004): 50, 100 and 250 microgram inhibited peroxidation of linoleic acid by 39%, 66% and 98%, respectively, as compared to 30% inhibition demonstrated by 60 microgram/mL of alpha-tocopherol.

In the same study, nettle was shown to scavenge free radicals, hydrogen peroxide and superoxide anion radicals and to chelate heavy metals. Ozen and Korkmaz (2003) reported that constituents from nettle can regulate glutathione reductase, glutathione peroxidase, superoxide dismutase and catalase in vivo.

The fixed oil of nettle has demonstrated strong antioxidant activity in mice treated with carbon tetrachloride, by decreasing lipid peroxidation and increasing antioxidant status (Kanter et al 2003). Nettle extract is significantly effective in preventing fibrosis in liver tissue from carbon tetrachloride damage in vivo (Turkdogan et al 2003). Dried nettle added to the diet of rats decreased cerebral free radicals after forced-swim tests (Toldy et al 2005).

Antioxidant activity has also been demonstrated in humans. An alcoholic extract of stinging nettle was tested fror effects on oxidative stress in 50 volunteers with type 2 diabetes. The test dose of 100 mg kg(-1) of nettle extract of body weight taken for 8 weeks resulted in a significant increase in Total Antioxidant Capacity (TAC) and superoxide dismutase (SOD) compared to the control group ($P < 0.05$) (Namazi et al 2012).

Hepatoprotective

Treatment with stinging nettle effectively protected against aflatoxin-induced hepatotoxicity, as evidenced by decreased aspartate aminotransferase (AST), alanine aminotransferase (ALT) and gamma glutamyl transpeptidase (GGT) levels, and hepatic lipid peroxidation and elevated the antioxidants' levels in an animal model (Yener et al 2009). These findings were confirmed by histological observation. One mechanism proposed to account for this observation is nettle-maintained antioxidant enzyme activity (superoxide dismutase, catalase and glutathione reductase) which protected against hepatotoxic effects induced by aflatoxin. Comparisons between groups revealed the untreated animals experienced a significant decrease in antioxidant enzyme activity, whereas no significant changes were seen with co-administration of nettle treatment.

CLINICAL USE

Different parts of the nettle herb have been used for different indications, notably the whole herb and the root. More recently, fresh, freeze-dried leaves have also been used. Some evidence comes from traditional usage; however, most recent research efforts have investigated various nettle preparations in urological and rheumatological conditions.

Arthritic conditions

Traditionally, nettle herb and leaf have been used to treat painful joint diseases, but scientific investigation has only just begun to determine whether there is a demonstrable benefit with its use.

One randomised, double-blind crossover study involving 27 patients with osteoarthritic pain at the base of the thumb or index finger compared topical applications of stinging nettle leaf with placebo, used daily for 1 week. After a 5-week washout period, treatments were then reversed. Nettle application used for 1 week showed reduction in pain and disability and produced significantly superior results to placebo (Randall et al 2000). An open study of 17 patients reporting beneficial effects with the nettle sting of *U. dioica* showed that a transient urticarial rash can be associated with topical use (Randall et al 1999). It is suspected that a counterirritant effect is chiefly responsible.

Most recently, a randomised, controlled, single-blind pilot study of 42 adults with knee pain and taking NSAIDs or analgesics (presumed osteoarthritis) investigated the feasibility of conducting research to determine the effect of the sting of *Urtica dioica*, for chronic knee pain (Randall et al 2008). Patients were instructed to apply a specific number of nettle (*Urtica dioica*) leaves to the affected area, or placebo intervention with *Urtica galeopsifolia* daily for 1 week. The effect of *U. dioica* did not appear to be superior to the control treatment; however, the authors suggested several possible interpretations of this negative result. Importantly, during the study it was found that the choice of placebo was poor as *Urtica galeopsifolia* had a stinging irritant effect similar to stinging nettle. Next, there was the possibility of inadequate treatment as researchers found it difficult to supply well-grown nettles in late season, and not all patients used as many leaves as recommended. Finally, the study may have been underpowered to detect a statistical difference between groups.

A large, multi-centre, post-marketing surveillance review including 8955 patients (5953 females, 2920 males) suffering from osteoarthritis ($n = 7935$) or rheumatoid arthritis ($n = 1550$) also investigated the effects of 1340 mg of stinging nettle extract (IDS23) over 3 weeks as mono- or co-treatment (Ramm & Hansen 1997 as reported in Upton 2013). Fifty per cent of the patients were pretreated with NSAIDs (82% diclofenac), while 8% received other treatments.

Treatment with IDS23 resulted in 5% improvement in pain at rest, 45% improvement in pain during movement and 38% improvement in physical impairment. In 38% of the patients NSAID consumption was reduced by 50% whereas for 28% of patients there was no change to NSAID requirements and in 8% additional NSAIDs were necessary. There was no difference in the score improvement (rest, movement, physical impairment) between patients pretreated with NSAIDs and those not pretreated.

There was a low incidence (1.2%) of adverse effects reported during treatment, which mainly consisted of gastrointestinal discomfort.

Nettle, fish oils and vitamin E

In combination, treatment of fish oils, vitamin E and *Urtica dioica* (concentrations not stated) was compared to placebo in a double-blind, randomised study of 81 volunteers with OA of the knee or hip (Jacquet et al 2009). The treatment product known as Phytalgic was taken for 3 months. The active treatment group had a significantly-reduced requirement for analgesics and NSAIDs compared to controls and significantly-different WOMAC scores indicating symptomatic benefits. While these results are promising, the role of the stinging nettle ingredient is unknown and concerns have been raised about detection bias.

Clearly, further clinical research is required to clarify the effectiveness of *Urtica dioica* in musculoskeletal conditions.

Commission E approved stinging nettle as supportive therapy for rheumatic ailments when used internally or applied externally (Blumenthal et al 2000).

Benign prostatic hyperplasia (BPH)

Clinical trials have used many different nettle extracts in liquid or oral dose forms utilising root preparations. The Bazoton products (Kanoldt) have been most commonly investigated; however, there has also been some investigation with extracts including Urtica plus (Osterholz/Schwarzpharma), Urtica APS (Zyma/Novartis), Prostatin (Abbott), Prostaherb (Cesra), and Prosta Truw (Truw).

According to a 2007 systematic review, at least 40,000 men with BPH have been treated with various nettle root preparations in 34 clinical studies (Chrubasik et al 2007). Twenty-four studies were open and uncontrolled, two studies were open and controlled and six were randomised controlled studies. All studies evaluated methanolic nettle root extracts. Overall, available evidence indicates that methanolic nettle extracts are effective in BPH. Most studies report decreased residual urine volume, increased maximal urinary flow and improvements in symptom scores compared to placebo. Significant improvements in prostate size have also been reported in some open trials (ESCOP 1996–97). Further randomised studies are required to determine the significance and magnitude of these effects. Commission E approved the use of *Urtica* root for difficulty in urination in BPH stages 1 and 2 (Blumenthal et al 2000).

IN COMBINATION

In practice, nettle root preparations are often prescribed in combination with other herbal medicines, such as saw palmetto or pygeum. Several clinical trials have investigated combination products which are more reflective of practice, overall producing positive results.

Nettle and pygeum

In one study, 134 patients with BPH were randomly assigned an *Urtica* and *Pygeum* preparation (300 mg *Urtica dioica* root extract combined with 25 mg *Pygeum africanum* bark extract) or a preparation containing half that dose under double-blind test conditions for 8 weeks. Both treatments significantly increased urine flow, and reduced residual urine and nocturia after 28 days, whereas after 56 days further significant decreases were found in residual urine (half-dose group) and in nocturia (both groups) (Krzeski et al 1993).

Nettle and saw palmetto extract

In 1995, an open, prospective, multicentre observational study involving 419 specialist urological practices investigated the efficacy and tolerability of a saw palmetto and nettle combination in 2080 patients with BPH (Schneider et al 1995). Herbal treatment was seen to improve pathological findings and obstructive and irritative symptoms. Both efficacy and tolerability were assessed by doctors as very good or good and most patients reported an improvement in general quality of life (QOL) and reduction in symptoms of BPH.

A randomised, multicentre double-blind study involving 543 patients with early stage BPH found that a combination of nettle and saw palmetto extract was as effective as finasteride at increasing maximum urinary flow and improving International Prostate Symptom Scores (IPSS) after 24 weeks' treatment, which continued to improve by week 48 (Sokeland 2000). Improvement in QOL scores was similarly observed with both treatments, regardless of prostate size. Overall, the two treatments only differed in regard to adverse reaction incidence, with the herbal combination much better tolerated (Sokeland & Albrecht 1997). A 2003 review concluded that a combination of nettle and saw palmetto is safe and effective for the treatment of lower urinary tract symptoms associated with BPH, comparable to the alpha-blocker tamsulosin (Bondarenko et al 2003).

A randomised, placebo-controlled, double-blind, multicentre trial in 2005 further demonstrated the effectiveness of saw palmetto fruit (160 mg) and nettle root (120 mg) for lower urinary tract symptoms due to prostate enlargement (Lopatkin et al 2005): 257 men aged 50 years or more were randomised to take either two capsules of the study medication (320 mg saw palmetto and 240 mg nettle root) daily or placebo for 24 weeks. Men on the treatment experienced a 35% reduction in symptoms — most notably intermittency, hesitancy, urgency and nocturia — compared to 24% for placebo. At the end of the 24-week period, an open trial was conducted for an additional 24 weeks and all men were given the herbal medicine. Those previously taking placebo reported significant improvements when switched to the study medication.

Allergic rhinitis

A double-blind randomised study showed that a freeze-dried preparation of nettles improved global assessments of allergic rhinitis after 1 week's therapy (Mittman 1990).

Nutritional tonic

Due to the presence of a range of vitamins and minerals, including iron, the stinging nettle herb is used as a nutritional tonic and to increase energy. It is used as a steamed green vegetable, pureed ingredient in soup or as a tea.

An open study involving 10 healthy women drinking 1 L of strained stinging nettle tea for 12 days found significant increase in vitamin B_{12} blood levels, an increase in red cell folate and iron binding capacity. There was no noted change in ferritin levels. The tea was made from 15 g of herb in 1 L of boiling water, cooled for 4 to 8 hours before consumption (Burgess & Baillie 1999).

OTHER USES

Stinging nettle has also been used in various preparations for diarrhoea, dysentery and diseases of the colon, internal bleeding, chronic skin eruptions such as eczema and discharges.

Practice points/Patient counselling

- Preliminary research has demonstrated anti-inflammatory, analgesic and antiviral activities for nettle.
- Several test tube studies have shown that it reduces prostate cell proliferation and slows the progression of prostate cancer in both an in vivo model and an in vitro system.
- The aerial parts are most commonly used to relieve symptoms of arthritis, whereas the root is used for BPH symptom relief.
- There is evidence that stinging nettle extracts provide significant symptom relief in BPH and some studies indicate a possible reduction in prostate size. In practice, nettle root preparations are often prescribed in combination with other herbal medicines, such as saw palmetto or pygeum.
- Application of nettle leaf for 1 week reduced pain and disability in osteoarthritis according to one double-blind study; however, larger studies have not been performed to confirm the effects.
- One double-blind study found that nettle reduced symptoms of allergic rhinitis.
- Studies using nettle root in combination with saw palmetto or pygeum have shown positive results in BPH.

DOSAGE RANGE

Leaf

- Dry extract: 0.6–2.1 g/day in divided doses; or
- Liquid extract (1:2): 15–40 mL/week.
- Tincture (1:5, 25% ethanol): 6 mL up to 3 times daily.
- Freeze-dried powder : 300–600 mg up to 3 times daily.

Root

4–9 mL daily of 1:2 liquid extract, although Commission E recommend 4–6 g/day cut root for symptoms of BPH, doses up to 18 g/day have been used (www.phytotherapies.org June 2003).

TOXICITY

Insufficient reliable evidence is available.

ADVERSE REACTIONS

One report states that gastrointestinal discomfort, allergic reactions, urticaria, pruritus, oedema and decreased urine volume are possible with oral use (Ernst et al 2001).

Clinical studies in BPH with herbal combinations containing nettle have found that only 0.72–3.7% experience mild adverse effects.

Clinical note — What causes the sting?

A frequent cause of contact urticaria is skin exposure to the stinging nettle. The urticaria is accompanied by a stinging sensation lasting longer than 30 minutes. The hairs of the leaves of the stinging nettle plant *Urtica dioica* contain acetylcholine histamine, 5-hydroxytryptamine (serotonin) and small amounts of leukotrienes B_4 and C_4 (Czarnetzki et al 1990). It is recommended to wear rubber or plastic gloves when handling and processing dried or fresh material to avoid irritation due to direct contact. Much of the irritating contents of the stinging hairs are dissipated upon extraction, drying and cooking, but not all. This means skin irritation can still occur when handling properly dried material (Upton 2013).

SIGNIFICANT INTERACTIONS

Controlled studies are not available; therefore, interactions are based on evidence of activity and are largely theoretical and speculative.

Diuretic medicines

Potentiated effects are theoretically possible — observe patients taking this combination.

Antihypertensive medicines

Additive effects are theoretically possible — observe patients taking antihypertensives concurrently.

Finasteride

Additive effects are theoretically possible, although the interaction may be beneficial.

CONTRAINDICATIONS AND PRECAUTIONS

People with known sensitivities or allergies to stinging nettle should use this herb cautiously.

The leaves have a powerful topical counter-irritant effect and can cause blistering and wheal and flare. People handling or processing dried or fresh material should wear rubber or plastic gloves to avoid irritation due to direct contact with skin. Irritation can still occur with properly dried materials (Upton 2013).

PREGNANCY USE

Use of nettle during pregnancy is contraindicated because of its effects on hormones (WHO 2003). It is suggested to be used with caution in the first trimester (Upton 2013).

PATIENTS' FAQs

What will this herb do for me?

Nettle leaf may reduce pain in osteoarthritis when applied topically for 1 week, whereas oral preparations of nettle root in combination with saw palmetto or pygeum reduce symptoms of BPH. Internal preparations may also reduce symptoms of allergic rhinitis, according to one human study.

When will it start to work?

Topical applications of the leaf in osteoarthritis have been shown to work after 1 week, whereas benefits in BPH require at least 28 days' treatment.

Are there any safety issues to be concerned about?

Local application of nettle can be irritating and cause contact urticaria, but preparations taken internally seem generally well tolerated.

S

REFERENCES

Balzarini J et al. The mannose-specific plant lectins from Cymbidium hybrid and Epipactis helleborine and the (N-acetylglucosamine) n-specific plant lectin from Urtica dioica are potent and selective inhibitors of human immunodeficiency virus and cytomegalovirus replication in vitro. Antiviral Res 18.2 (1992): 191–207.

Blumenthal M et al (eds), Herbal medicine: expanded commission E monographs. Austin, TX: Integrative Medicine Communications, 2000.

Bnouham M et al. Antihyperglycemic activity of the aqueous extract of Urtica dioica. Fitoterapia 74.7–8 (2003): 677–681.

Bondarenko B et al. Long-term efficacy and safety of PRO 160/120 (a combination of sabal and urtica extract) in patients with lower urinary tract symptoms (LUTS). Phytomedicine 10 (Suppl 4) (2003): 53–55.

Broer J, Behnke B. Immunosuppressant effect of IDS 30, a stinging nettle leaf extract, on myeloid dendritic cells in vitro. J Rheumatol 29.4 (2002): 659–666.

Burgess I, Baillie N. Iron tonics — what really works? In: International Conference 99; Herbal Medicine Practice & Science; 1999. p. 25 as reported in Upton, R. Stinging nettle leaf, extraordinary vegetable medicine. J Herb Med, 39 (2013).

Chrubasik JE et al. A comprehensive review on the stinging nettle effect and efficacy profiles. Part II: Urticae radix. Phytomedicine 14.7–8 (2007): 568–579.

Czarnetzki BM et al. Immunoreactive leukotrienes in nettle plants (Urtica urens). Int Arch Allergy Appl Immunol 91.1 (1990): 43–46.

Ernst E et al. The desktop guide to complementary and alternative medicine: an evidence-based approach. St Louis: Mosby, 2001.
European Scientific Cooperative on Phytotherapy (ESCOP). Urticae radix. Monographs on the uses of plant drugs. Fascicule 2. Exeter, UK: ESCOP, 1996–1997: 4–5.
Farzami B et al. Induction of insulin secretion by a component of Urtica dioica leaf extract in perifused Islets of Langerhans and its in vivo effects in normal and streptozotocin diabetic rats. J Ethnopharmacol 89.1 (2003): 47–53.
Gulcin I et al. Antioxidant, antimicrobial, antiulcer and analgesic activities of nettle (Urtica dioica L.). J Ethnopharmacol 90.2–3 (2004): 205–215.
Jacquet A et al. Phytalgic, a food supplement, vs placebo in patients with osteoarthritis of the knee or hip: a randomised double-blind placebo-controlled clinical trial. Arthritis Res Ther 11.6 (2009): R192.
Johnson TA et al. Lipophilic stinging nettle extracts possess potent anti-inflammatory activity, are not cytotoxic and may be superior to traditional tinctures for treating inflammatory disorders. Phytomedicine, 20.2 (2013): 143–147.
Kanter M et al. Effects of Nigella sativa L. and Urtica dioica L. on lipid peroxidation, antioxidant enzyme systems and some liver enzymes in CCl4-treated rats. J Vet Med A Physiol Pathol Clin Med 50.5 (2003): 264–268.
Konrad A et al. Ameliorative effect of IDS 30, a stinging nettle leaf extract, on chronic colitis. Int J Colorectal Dis 20.1 (2005): 9–17.
Konrad L et al. Antiproliferative effect on human prostate cancer cells by a stinging nettle root (Urtica dioica) extract. Planta Med 66.1 (2000): 44–47.
Krzeski T et al. Combined extracts of Urtica dioica and Pygeum africanum in the treatment of benign prostatic hyperplasia: double-blind comparison of two doses. Clin Ther 15.6 (1993): 1011–1020.
Lichius JJ et al. Antiproliferative effect of a polysaccharide fraction of a 20% methanolic extract of stinging nettle roots upon epithelial cells of the human prostate (LNCaP). Pharmazie 54.10 (1999): 768–771.
Lichius JJ, Muth C. The inhibiting effects of Urtica dioica root extracts on experimentally induced prostatic hyperplasia in the mouse. Planta Med 63.4 (1997): 307–310.
Lopatkin N et al. Long term efficacy and safety of a combination of sabal and urtica extract for lower urinary tract symptoms — a placebo controlled, double-blind, multicentre trial. World J Urol 23 (2005): 139–146.
Mittman P. Randomized, double-blind study of freeze-dried Urtica dioica in the treatment of allergic rhinitis. Planta Med 56.1 (1990): 44–47.
Namazi N et al. The effect of hydro alcoholic nettle (Urtica dioica) extract on oxidative stress in patients with type 2 diabetes: a randomized double-blind clinical trial. Pak J Biol Sci 15.2 (2012): 98–102.
Obertreis B et al. Anti-inflammatory effect of Urtica dioica folia extract in comparison to caffeic malic acid. Arzneimittelforschung 46.1 (1996a): 52–6.
Obertreis B et al. Ex-vivo in-vitro inhibition of lipopolysaccharide stimulated tumor necrosis factor-alpha and interleukin-1 beta secretion in human whole blood by extractum urticae dioicae foliorum. Arzneimittelforschung 46.4 (1996b): 389–94.
Ozen T, Korkmaz H. Modulatory effect of Urtica dioica L. (Urticaceae) leaf extract on biotransformation enzyme systems, antioxidant enzymes, lactate dehydrogenase and lipid peroxidation in mice. Phytomedicine 10.5 (2003): 405–415.
Ramm S, Hansen C. Arthrse: Brennesselblätter-Extrakt IDS23 spart NSAR ein. Jatros Ortho 1997;12:29–33 as reported in Upton, R. Stinging nettle leaf, extraordinary vegetable medicine. J Herb Med, 39. (2013).
Randall C et al. Nettle sting of Urtica dioica for joint pain–an exploratory study of this complementary therapy. Complement Ther Med 7.3 (1999): 126–131.
Randall C et al. Randomized controlled trial of nettle sting for treatment of base-of-thumb pain. J R Soc Med 93.6 (2000): 305–309.
Randall C et al. Nettle sting for chronic knee pain: a randomised controlled pilot study. Complement Ther Med, 16.2 (2008): 66–72.
Riehemann K, Behnke B, Schulze-Osthoff K. Plant extracts from stinging nettle (Urtica dioica), an antirheumatic remedy, inhibit the proinflammatory transcription factor NF-kappaB. FEBS Lett 442.1 (1999): 89–94.
Romics I, Bach D. Zn, Ca and Na levels in the prostatic secretion of patients with prostatic adenoma. Int Urol Nephrol 23.1 (1991): 45–49.
Schneider HJ et al. Treatment of benign prostatic hyperplasia. Results of a treatment study with the phytogenic combination of Sabal extract WS 1473 and Urtica extract WS 1031 in urologic specialty practices. Fortschr Med 113.3 (1995): 37–40.
Sokeland J. Combined sabal and urtica extract compared with finasteride in men with benign prostatic hyperplasia: analysis of prostate volume and therapeutic outcome. BJU Int 86.4 (2000): 439–442.
Sokeland J, Albrecht J. Combination of Sabal and Urtica extract vs. finasteride in benign prostatic hyperplasia (Aiken stages I to II). Comparison of therapeutic effectiveness in a one year double-blind study. Urologe A 36.4 (1997): 327–333.
Tahri A et al. Acute diuretic, natriuretic and hypotensive effects of a continuous perfusion of aqueous extract of Urtica dioica in the rat. J Ethnopharmacol 73.1–2 (2000): 95–100.
Testai L et al. Cardiovascular effects of Urtica dioica L. (Urticaceae) roots extracts: in vitro and in vivo pharmacological studies. J Ethnopharmacol 81.1 (2002): 105–109.
Teucher T et al. Cytokine secretion in whole blood of healthy subjects following oral administration of Urtica dioica L. plant extract. Arzneimittelforschung 46.9 (1996): 906–910.
Toldy A et al. The effect of exercise and nettle supplementation on oxidative stress markers in the rat brain. Brain Res Bull 65.6 (2005): 487–493.
Turkdogan MK et al. The role of Urtica dioica and Nigella sativa in the prevention of carbon tetrachloride-induced hepatotoxicity in rats. Phytother Res 17.8 (2003): 942–946.
Upton, R. Stinging nettle leaf, extraordinary vegetable medicine. J Herb Med, 39. 2013.
US Department of Agriculture. Phytochemical database. Agricultural Research Service–National Germplasm Resources Laboratory. Beltsville, Maryland: Beltsville Agricultural Research Center, 2003.
World Health Organization. Department of Essential Drugs and Medicines (EDM). Essential Drugs and Medicines Policy. Geneva: WHO, 2003.
Yener Z et al. Effects of Urtica dioica L. seed on lipid peroxidation, antioxidants and liver pathology in aflatoxin-induced tissue injury in rats. Food and Chemical Toxicology 47.2 (2009): 418–424.

Taurine

BACKGROUND AND RELEVANT PHARMACOKINETICS

Taurine occurs as one of the most abundant free amino acids in a wide variety of animal tissues; it is mostly absent from plants (Bouckenooghe et al 2006). In humans and other mammals, the highest taurine concentrations are found in heart, retina, spleen and bone marrow (Timbrell et al 1995). Blood cells such as platelets and leucocytes are also very rich in taurine.

Traditionally taurine has been regarded as an end product of methionine metabolism. Other pathways for taurine biosynthesis exist but they have not been fully characterised and in mammals the cysteine sulfinate pathway seems to be the major pathway (Brosnan & Brosnan 2006).

There is marked variation in taurine biosynthesis in different organs and it is species- and age-dependent. The activity of cysteine sulfinic acid decarboxylase, a key enzyme in the biosynthesis of taurine from cysteine (Lambert 2004), is low in the liver and brain of human fetuses, infants and adults. The extent to which taurine can be synthesised by humans is unknown at present.

Taurine does not undergo any major metabolic biotransformation, although a small amount is deaminated to isethionic acid. As taurine is metabolically inert, free taurine is readily excreted in the urine. The kidney is the major organ involved in regulating taurine levels (Chesney et al 1985, Rozen & Scriver 1982) and excess dietary taurine is excreted in the urine (Sturman 1988).

A small amount of taurine is also degraded by intestinal bacteria to sulfate, which is absorbed from the intestine and excreted in urine. The high tissue taurine levels in both mature and newborn animals have led to much speculation about possible roles of taurine in brain, retina, heart and skeletal muscle (Grimble 2006).

CHEMICAL COMPONENTS

2-Aminoethanesulfonic acid

FOOD SOURCES

Taurine does not need to be supplied in the human diet as it can be derived indirectly from dietary precursors. Dietary taurine is found preformed in considerable quantities in meat, fish and seafood (Roe & Weston 1965). Daily intake of preformed taurine can be 40–400 mg/day (Hayes & Trautwein 1994, Rana & Sanders 1986). Taurine can become a conditionally essential nutrient when there are limited dietary and precursor amino acid supplies, biosynthetic enzymes or their cofactors are deficient, or there is excessive loss, such as in conditions characetrised by digestive malabsorption (e.g. cystic fibrosis).

DEFICIENCY SIGNS AND SYMPTOMS

Deficiency

Taurine deficiency is associated with cardiomyopathy, renal dysfunction, developmental abnormalities, pancreatic β-cell malfunction and severe damage to retinal neurons (Ripps & Shen 2012). Children receiving parenteral nutrition without supplemental taurine develop low taurine plasma levels and neuronal (especially retinal) dysfunction, which can be counteracted by taurine supplementation (Geggel et al 1985).

This was previously detected as degeneration of the retina in taurine-deficient cats (Knopf et al 1978). The animals showed growth retardation and developed retina degeneration that eventually led to blindness. The retina degeneration could be prevented or reversed by the addition of preformed taurine to the diet, but not by feeding methionine or cysteine.

Taurine deficiency has been reported in parenteral nutrition as taurine is not routinely added to parenteral formulations (Lloyd & Gabe 2007).

Taurine deficiency can present in infants with cholestatic disease and this can be prevented by parenteral supplementary taurine; extensive gastrointestinal surgery can also result in taurine deficiency due to increased loss of bile acids (Lloyd & Gabe 2007, Schneider et al 2006). It has also been found that people with cystic fibrosis frequently have taurine deficiency due to bile acid malabsorption. Low levels have also been found in people with heart failure.

MAIN ACTIONS

Taurine is one of the most abundant amino acids in the brain, retina, muscle tissue and organs throughout the body, although it is not incorporated into proteins (Ripps & Shen 2012). Many studies report that taurine is involved in a wide variety of biological processes, although the exact mechanisms of action are usually not well defined. The evidence that taurine is essential to human nutrition remains unclear: dietary taurine has been shown to play an important part in maintaining body taurine pools.

Taurine has been proposed to have numerous roles, such as a membrane stabiliser, a substrate for the formation of bile salts, a neurotransmitter/neuromodulator, an intracellular osmolyte involved in cell volume regulation and an antioxidant, and may have a number of other roles, including immunomodulation and growth modulator (Bouckenooghe et al 2006, Huxtable 1992, 1996, Ripps & Shen 2012).

Eye function and health

All ocular tissues contain taurine, which is critical for photoreceptor development in the retina and acts as a cytoprotectant against stress-related neuronal damage and other pathological conditions. Supplementation can inhibit light-induced lipid peroxidation, and thereby protect isolated rod outer segments from photic damage (Ripps & Shen 2012).

Bile acid conjugation

Despite extensive studies on the proposed functions of taurine, the only well-defined role for taurine is conjugation with bile acids. Taurine is preferentially conjugated with bile acids in the liver, forming predominantly taurocholic acid, prior to excretion in the bile (Bouckenooghe et al 2006). Bile acids have an important role in the emulsification of dietary fat. The regulation of cholesterol and bile acid homeostasis is mediated by CYP7A1, which has become a biomarker for cholesterol metabolism (Chen et al 2012).

OTHER ACTIONS

Taurine has many of the same characteristics as neurotransmitters, but evidence of a taurine-specific receptor has yet to be identified (Ripps & Shen 2012). Animal studies indicate that taurine supplementation may result in lower plasma lipid levels (Murakami et al 2002) and improve insulin sensitivity (Anuradha & Balakrishnan 1999, Nakaya et al 2000).

The compound taurine chloramine (Tau-Cl) is reported to act as an antioxidant; it is produced when hypochlorous acid, produced in the 'oxidant burst' of stimulated neutrophils and monocytes, interacts with taurine (Grimble 2006). Studies report that Tau-Cl downregulates the production of pro-inflammatory mediators and also has antibacterial properties (Schuller-Levis & Park 2004).

Cell membrane stabilisation

Taurine reportedly acts as a modulator of membrane excitability in the central nervous system by inhibiting the release of other neurotransmitters and decreasing mitochondrial release of calcium (Grimble 2006, Muramatsu et al 1978).

Osmoregulation

It has been suggested that taurine plays an important role in osmoregulation due to its biophysical and biochemical properties (Huxtable 1992); however, this characteristic may be significant in some species and not in others.

Calcium modulation

Taurine is a modulator of intra- and extracellular calcium levels and is able both to increase Ca^{2+} availability and to resist Ca^{2+} overload, depending on the circumstances (Bradford & Allen 1996).

Xenobiotic conjugation

Taurine can conjugate with xenobiotics, and animal studies indicate that this is to a varying degree, being dependent on the animal species (Nakashima et al 1982).

Neuroprotective

Taurine has been shown to prevent mitochondrial dysfunction in neurons and to protect against endoplasmic reticulum stress associated with neurological disorders (Kumari et al 2013).

CLINICAL USE

Deficiency: treatment and prevention

Taurine deficiency has not been significantly investigated in humans, so the information is generally derived from in vitro and animal studies. Taurine deficiency may be reflected by low plasma levels and these can be normalised by supplementary taurine.

Growth and development

Findings from animal studies have shown that maternal diet supplemented with taurine during late gestation resulted in higher fetal plasma taurine levels and the offspring had increased postnatal growth, although the mechanism for this has not been elucidated (Hultman et al 2007).

Adult humans have a low activity of hepatic cysteine sulfinic acid decarboxylase and infants, especially premature infants, possess even lower enzyme activity. It has therefore been suggested that infants and particularly premature infants may have a greater requirement for preformed taurine than adults (Sturman 1975).

A systemic review by Verner et al (2009) assessed the effect of supplemental taurine versus no supplementation on the growth and development of preterm or low-birth-weight infants who were fed via enteral and parenteral nutrition. The authors identified nine small studies in which supplemental taurine was given with formula milk via enteral feeding in eight studies and supplemental taurine via parenteral nutrition in one study. Meta-analyses of these randomised or quasi-randomised controlled trials showed that supplemental taurine did not result in improved outcomes. However, the infants in these studies were clinically stable and the majority were greater than 30 weeks' gestational age at birth, and it may be that taurine requirements are different among infants who are ill or in other subgroups.

Cardiovascular disease (CVD)

Various studies have indicated reduced CVD risk from supplementary taurine intake alone or in combination with omega-3 polyunsaturated fatty acids (PUFA) (Militante & Lombardini 2004, Mizushima et al 1997). Studies by Yamori et al (2001, 2006) found that urinary taurine excretion was the most significant single factor to correlate inversely with ischaemic heart disease (IHD) mortality and they also highlighted the benefits of combined taurine and omega-3 fatty acids with respect to IHD mortality.

Elvevoll et al (2008) studied hypolipidaemic and antiatherogenic effects of taurine and omega-3 fatty acids in 75 healthy adults in a 7-week double-blind and parallel intervention trial where one group received omega-3 PUFA, eicosapentaenoic acid (EPA) and docosahexaenoic acid (DHA) (1.1 g EPA + DHA/day) and the second group received both omega-3 and taurine (425 mg/day). The results of this study demonstrated the beneficial effect of omega-3 combined with taurine, producing significant reductions in total cholesterol, low-density lipoprotein cholesterol and apolipoprotein (apo) B in the omega-3 + taurine group compared to the omega-3 group alone.

Taurine supplementation has also been reported to have a beneficial effect on plasma homocysteine levels in a study of 22 healthy middle-aged women aged 40.3 ± 4.7 years (range 33–54 years) who were provided with 3 g taurine per day for 4 weeks; the levels of plasma homocysteine and serum thiobarbituric acid reaction products were significantly decreased (Ahn 2009). In contrast, a recent prospective case–control study nested in the New York University Women's Health Study of 223 cases of coronary heart disease (1986–2006) and age and menopausal status-matched controls (median age 58 years at baseline) found no association between serum taurine levels and coronary heart disease risk (Wójcik et al 2013).

Hypertension

In a randomised controlled study of 31 borderline hypertensive adults and normal adults, 6 g taurine was given daily for 7 days; although the normal subjects did not experience any effects, the intervention group experienced a significant decrease in blood pressure and serum catecholamines (Fujita et al 1987).

In another randomised controlled trial of 11 healthy adult males taking 6 g taurine/day in the presence of a high-fat, high-cholesterol diet for 3 weeks, there was no change in blood pressure but there was a significant increase in very-low-density lipoproteins and triglycerides (Mizushima et al 1996).

Heart failure

Patients suffering from CHF have suboptimal taurine levels together with impaired myocardial energy production, myocyte calcium overload, and increased oxidative stress. Taurine plays an important role in the prevention of these conditions, so it is reasonable to suspect that supplemental taurine could have a beneficial role in HF management. Several small studies confirm it is a promising treatment, but further research is required. Oral taurine supplementation (2 g twice daily) improves left ventricular function in people with heart failure (New York Heart Association [NYHA] class II-IV). The study of 24 patients found that treatment was effective in 19 of the 24 patients after 4–8 weeks of active treatment. In addition, 13 of the 15 patients designated as NYHA functional class III or IV before receiving taurine could be designated as class II after they completed the study (Azuma et al 1983).

Following this, a double-blind, randomised, crossover study was performed with 14 patients with congestive heart failure receiving standard care also receiving taurine or placebo for 4 weeks (Azuma et al 1985). Compared with placebo, taurine significantly improved the NYHA functional class ($P < 0.02$), pulmonary crackles ($P < 0.02$) and chest film abnormalities ($P < 0.01$). Pre-ejection period (corrected for heart rate) decreased from 148 ± 14 ms before taurine treatment to 137 ± 12 ms after taurine ($P < 0.001$), and the quotient pre-ejection period/left ventricular ejection time decreased from 47 ± 9 to 42 ± 8% ($P < 0.001$).

In a 1992 study, oral taurine (3 g/day) was found to be more effective than low-dose coenzyme Q10 (30 mg/day) for improving systolic left ventricular function after 6 weeks in a double-blind study of 17 patients with congestive heart failure secondary to ischaemic or idiopathic dilated cardiomyopathy, whose ejection fraction assessed by echocardiography was less than 50% (Azuma et al 1992).

In a randomised, single-blind, placebo-controlled clinical study involving 29 patients with heart failure, oral taurine supplementation of 500 mg three times a day taken for 2 weeks significantly improved exercise performance compared to placebo (Beyranvand et al 2011). Taurine supplementation resulted in increased exercise time, metabolic equivalents and exercise distance.

Obesity

In a small randomised controlled trial, 15 healthy overweight adults were treated with 3 g taurine/day for 7 weeks, resulting in a significant decrease in serum triglycerides, although there was no change in high-density lipoprotein cholesterol or fasting glucose (Zhang et al 2004a). In a somewhat larger study of 30 overweight or obese non-diabetic young subjects, taurine supplementation (3 g/day; 1 g × 3 times/day) over a 7-week period resulted in a beneficial effect on lipid metabolism and a decrease in body weight (Zhang et al 2004b).

Diabetes

In animal studies taurine appears to exert a positive effect on insulin resistance and the complications of diabetes mellitus, including retinopathy, nephropathy, neuropathy, atherosclerosis and cardiomyopathy, independently of hypoglycaemic effect in several animal models (Ito et al 2012). However, human studies do not altogether support a role for taurine in the management of diabetes. Numerous studies have reported mixed findings regarding the effectiveness of taurine supplementation. Most studies have been small-scale with insufficient numbers of patients, and the mechanisms of reported beneficial effects remain to be elucidated. A study of 22 patients with type 2 diabetes mellitus (T2DM) who were treated with 3 g taurine/day for 4 months found no effect on glycated haemoglobin A_{1C} or fasting glucose (Chauncey et al 2003). Likewise, a double-blinded, randomised, crossover study of 20 non-diabetic subjects who were overweight first-degree relatives of T2DM patients received a daily supplementation of 1.5 g taurine or placebo; the results of this study showed that taurine supplement did not exert any effect on blood lipid levels or insulin secretion or sensitivity in subjects with both genetic and some non-genetic factors predisposing them to T2DM (Brøns et al 2004). Similarly, Spohr et al (2005) showed that taurine supplementation had no effect on platelet aggregation in 20 healthy men with a predisposition to T2DM. A study by Franconi et al (1995) looking at 1.5 g/day of taurine supplementation for 90 days in 39 patients with insulin-dependent diabetes mellitus, with healthy age- and sex-matched subjects, found that taurine reduced platelet aggregation in patients with diabetes whereas aggregation was not affected in the controls. In a recent randomised, double-blind, crossover study, Moloney et al (2010) reported that taurine supplementation was beneficial regarding early detectable endothelial dysfunction in young men with type 1 diabetes: male patients (under 30 years of age) with type 1 diabetes and no evidence of macrovascular or microvascular disease were provided with 1.5 g/day taurine (500 mg three times daily) for 14 days. Taurine supplementation was reported to reverse the augmentation index, a marker of arterial stiffness, and restored conduit vessel dysfunction.

T

Epilepsy

Several studies have investigated the role of taurine supplementation in the management of seizure disorders, overall producing inconsistent results. In some studies, patients with severe intractable epilepsy were administered taurine either orally or intravenously, varying in both duration and dose (from 200 mg/day and up to 21 g/day), making comparisons difficult. Additionally, most studies were uncontrolled and flawed with regard to methodology, thereby hindering accurate interpretation

(Fariello et al 1985). Some studies reported a reduction in seizure frequency (Takahashi & Nakane 1978), whereas others did not observe any benefit (Mantovani & DeVivo 1979).

The optimal dose of taurine supplementation in the management of epilepsy may be in the range of 100–500 mg/day, with a study by Gaby (2007) noting loss of antiseizure activity in some patients when the dose was increased to above 1.5 g/day. According to this study, beneficial effects are relatively short-lasting and are not maintained beyond a few weeks of treatment. Additional studies are required to clarify the role of taurine supplementation in practice.

Liver disease

Taurine supplementation has been reported to ameliorate liver injury and improve liver function. In a small study of 24 patients with chronic hepatitis, 12 patients (average age 58 years: range 46–75 years) were given 2 g taurine three times a day for 3 months, and then treatment was stopped for 1 month and 12 patients (control group; an average of 58 years: 41–78 years) were given a placebo without taurine for 4 months. Taurine supplementation resulted in a significant decrease ($P < 0.05$) in the activities of alanine aminotransferase and aspartate aminotransferase and likewise thiobarbituric acid reaction product values were also significantly affected (Hu et al 2008).

Exercise and sport

A number of small studies have reported that taurine supplementation may be useful for exercise performance and/or reducing muscle soreness and damage; however further research is required before a definitive conclusion can be made. It is most likely for this reason that it is included in many 'energy' and 'sports' drinks.

In a randomised, double-blind, crossover study, taurine supplementation was reported to significantly improve exercise performance of eight well-trained competitive male middle-distance runners (age 19.9 ± 1.2 years). Active treatment consisted of 1000 mg taurine taken 2 hours prior to a simulated 3-km time trial on a treadmill and resulted in significant differences in the overall 3-km time trial performance ($P = 0.013$) (Balshaw et al 2013). A recent randomised study of 21 male participants (mean age 21 ± 6 years; $n = 11$ taurine group and $n = 10$ placebo group) reported that 14 days of taurine supplementation resulted in less muscle damage and better performance after eccentric exercise (three sets until exhaustion, with eccentric exercise of the elbow flexors on the Scott bench, 80% one repetition maximum) (da Silva et al 2014).

In contrast, in a double blind study, Rutherford et al (2010) found no effect of a smaller acute dose of taurine (1.66 g) on endurance time trial performance and whole-body metabolism in well-trained cyclists. Supplementation of taurine 1 hour before 90 minutes of submaximal cycling followed by an ~25-minute time trial was not effective in improving performance. The differences in the effects of taurine on exercise performance across studies may be due to methodological differences, including factors such as size of the taurine dose, ingestion timing and varying exercise protocols.

Taurine has been shown to attenuate delayed-onset muscle soreness and muscle damage induced by high-intensity exercise in 36 untrained male volunteers. The combination of 2.0 g taurine and 3.2 g branched-chain amino acids three times a day for 2 weeks prior to and 4 days after elbow flexion eccentric exercise was superior to single or placebo supplementation (Ra et al 2013).

Practice points/Patient counselling

- Taurine can be readily obtained by eating meat, fish and seafood.
- Most people are able to produce taurine naturally; however, young infants are limited in their ability to produce taurine and obtain their dietary taurine from either breast milk or supplemented milk formulas.
- Plasma taurine levels can be low in some illnesses and conditions (such as sepsis) and can be restored with supplementary taurine.
- At present there is no evidence to prove the benefit of taking taurine during breastfeeding.
- Traditionally taurine has been used in CVD, hypertension and hyperlipidaemia. Several small studies indicate that there may be significant benefits for people with congestive heart failure.
- 'Energy' soft drinks may contain taurine as well as caffeine, although the potential interactions between these two ingredients have not been determined.

DOSAGE RANGE

Taurine is administered orally, usually in divided doses; adult dosage is generally 500 mg to 3 g daily and paediatric dosage 250 mg to 1 g daily, and these are dependent on the size and age of the child.

There appear to be very few health concerns regarding taurine supplementation, although safety has been of interest recently because of the high intakes that can be easily consumed from some sports drinks (Munro & Renwick 2006).

TOXICITY

In a risk assessment by Shao and Hathcock (2008), the following recommendations have been made: no observed adverse effect level and lowest observed adverse effect level >10 g taurine/day; observed safe level 3 g/day; upper level for supplements: 3 g/day.

ADVERSE REACTIONS

Taurine administration appears to be safe, even at higher doses. Children should be monitored for any adverse side effects and supplementation ceased if any adverse effects develop.

At dosages of 2 g/day, patients with psoriasis experienced intense temporary itching (Kendler

1989); dosages of 1.5 g taurine/day caused nausea, headache, dizziness and gait disturbances in some epileptic patients (Van Gelder et al 1975). Recently a case was reported of a 33-year-old female who experienced anaphylaxis due to taurine-containing drinks. The response was due to ingestion of synthetic taurine, as confirmed by an oral challenge test. In contrast the patient had no signs or symptoms of an adverse reaction after ingesting 1500 mg natural taurine (Lee et al 2013).

SIGNIFICANT INTERACTIONS

Controlled studies are not available and at present there are no known drug interactions with taurine.

CONTRAINDICATIONS AND PRECAUTIONS

High doses of taurine (10 g/day for 6 months) have been taken without any major side effects (Durelli et al 1983); the longest duration recorded has been 1 year (Colombo et al 1988). Many commercially-available energy drinks contain substantial amounts of supplementary taurine (1000 mg/L) and, as there is very little information about the effects of these doses, the young, people who are immunocompromised, pregnant and nursing mothers should consult a relevant health professional before excessive intake. People with psoriasis and epilepsy should avoid high intakes of taurine.

PREGNANCY USE

At present there is no evidence to prove the benefit of taking supplementary taurine during pregnancy.

PATIENTS' FAQs

What will this supplement do for me?

Decreased plasma levels can be normalised by taurine supplementation. There is some evidence that taurine may be a useful treatment in CVD and heart failure and possibly enhance physical exercise performance.

When will it start to work?

Plasma taurine levels can increase within a week of taking supplementary taurine.

Are there any safety issues?

Generally taurine supplementation has a good safety profile.

REFERENCES

Ahn CS. Effect of taurine supplementation on plasma homocysteine levels of the middle-aged Korean women. Adv Exp Med Biol. 643 (2009):415–22.

Anuradha CV, Balakrishnan SD. Taurine attenuates hypertension and improves insulin sensitivity in the fructose-fed rat, an animal model of insulin resistance. Can J Physiol Pharmacol 77.10 (1999): 749–754.

Azuma, J., et al. 1983. Therapy of congestive heart failure with orally administered taurine. Clin Ther., 5, (4) 398–408.

Azuma, J., et al 1985. Therapeutic effect of taurine in congestive heart failure: a double-blind crossover trial. Clin Cardiol., 8, (5) 276–282.

Azuma, J., et al 1992. Usefulness of taurine in chronic congestive heart failure and its prospective application. Jpn.Circ. J, 56, (1) 95–99.

Balshaw TG, et al. The effect of acute taurine ingestion on 3-km running performance in trained middle-distance runners. Amino Acids. 44(2) (2013):555–61.

Beyranvand MR, et al. Effect of taurine supplementation on exercise capacity of patients with heart failure. J Cardiol. 57(3) (2011):333–7.

Bouckenooghe T, et al. Is taurine a functional nutrient? Curr Opin Clin Nutr Metab Care 9 (2006): 728–733.

Bradford RW, Allen HW. Taurine in health and disease. J Adv Med 9 (1996): 179–199.

Brøns C et al. Effect of taurine treatment on insulin secretion and action, and on serum lipid levels in overweight men with a genetic predisposition for type II diabetes mellitus. Eur J Clin Nutr 58 (2004): 1239–1247.

Brosnan JT, Brosnan ME. The sulphur-containing amino acids: an overview. J Nutr 136 (2006): 1636S–40S.

Chauncey KB et al. The effect of taurine supplementation on patients with type 2 diabetes mellitus. Adv Exp Med Biol 526 (2003): 91–96.

Chen, W., et al. (2012). The effect of taurine on cholesterol metabolism. Mol Nutr Food Res, 56(5), 681–690.

Chesney RW, et al. Renal cortex taurine content regulates renal adaptive response to altered dietary intake of sulfur amino acids. J Clin Invest 76 (1985): 2213–2221.

Colombo C et al. Effect of taurine supplementation on fat and bile acid absorption in patients with cystic fibrosis. Scand J Gastroenterol 143 (Suppl) (1988): 151–156.

da Silva LA, et al. Effects of taurine supplementation following eccentric exercise in young adults. Appl Physiol Nutr Metab. 2014 Jan;39(1):101–4.

Durelli L et al. The treatment of myotonia: evaluation of chronic oral taurine therapy. Neurology 33 (1983): 599–603.

Elvevoll EO et al. Seafood diets: hypolipidemic and antiatherogenic effects of taurine and n–3 fatty acids. Atherosclerosis 200 (2008): 396–402.

Fariello RG, et al. Taurine and related amino acids in seizure disorders — current controversies. Prog Clin Biol Res 179 (1985): 413–424.

Franconi et al. Plasma and platelet taurine are reduced in subjects with insulin-dependent diabetes mellitus: effects of taurine supplementation. Am J Clin Nutr 61 (1995): 1115–1119.

Fujita T et al. Effects of increased adrenomedullary activity and taurine in young patients with borderline hypertension. Circulation 75 (1987): 525–532.

Gaby AR. Natural approaches to epilepsy. Altern Med Rev 12.1 (2007): 9–24.

Geggel HS et al. Nutritional requirements for taurine in patients receiving long-term parenteral nutrition. N Engl J Med 312 (1985): 142–146.

Grimble RF. The effects of sulfur amino acid intake on immune function in humans. J Nutr 136 (2006): 1660S–5S.

Hayes KC, Trautwein EA. Taurine. Modern nutrition in health and disease. Lea and Febiger, 1994 pp. 477–85.

Hu YH, et al. Dietary amino acid taurine ameliorates liver injury in chronic hepatitis patients. Amino Acids. 35(2) (2008):469–73.

Hultman K et al. Maternal taurine supplementation in the late pregnant rat stimulates postnatal growth and induces obesity and insulin resistance in adult offspring. J Physiol 579.3 (2007): 823–833.

Huxtable RJ. Physiological actions of taurine. Physiol Rev 72 (1992): 101–163.

Huxtable RJ. Taurine. Past, present, and future. Adv Exp Med Biol 403 (1996): 641–650.

Ito, T., et al. (2012). The potential usefulness of taurine on diabetes mellitus and its complications. Amino Acids, 42(5), 1529–1539.

Kendler BS. Taurine: an overview of its role in preventive medicine. Prev Med 18 (1989): 79–100.

Knopf K et al. Taurine: an essential nutrient for the cat. J Nutr 108.5 (1978): 773–778.

Kumari, N., et al. (2013). Taurine and its neuroprotective role. Adv Exp Med Biol, 775, 19–27.

Lambert IH. Regulation of the cellular content of the organic osmolyte taurine in mammalian cells. Neurochem Res 29 (2004): 27–63.

Lee SE, et al. A case of taurine-containing drink induced anaphylaxis. Asia Pac Allergy.3(1) (2013):70–3.

Lloyd DA, Gabe SM. Managing liver dysfunction in parenteral nutrition. Proc Nutr Soc 66.4 (2007): 530–538.

Mantovani J, DeVivo DC. Effects of taurine on seizures and growth hormone release in epileptic patients. Arch Neurol 36 (1979): 672–674.

Militante JD, Lombardini JB. Dietary taurine supplementation: hypolipidemic and antiatherogenic effects. Nutr Res 24 (2004): 787–801.

Mizushima S et al. Effects of oral taurine supplementation on lipids and sympathetic nerve tone. Adv Exp Med Biol 403 (1996): 615–622.

Mizushima S et al. Fish intake and cardiovascular risk among middle-aged Japanese in Japan and Brazil. J Cardiovasc Risk 4 (1997): 191–199.

Moloney MA, et al. Two weeks taurine supplementation reverses endothelial dysfunction in young male type 1 diabetics. Diab Vasc Dis Res. 7(4) (2010):300–10.

Munro IC, Renwick AG. The 5th workshop on the adequate intake of dietary amino acids: general discussion 2. J Nutr 136 (2006): 1755S–7S.

Murakami S et al. Effect of taurine on cholesterol metabolism in hamsters: up-regulation of low density lipoprotein (LDL) receptor by taurine. Life Sci 70.20 (2002): 2355–66.

Muramatsu M et al. A modulating role of taurine on release of acetylcholine and norepinephrine from neuronal tissues. Jpn J pharmacol 28.2 (1978): 259–68.
Nakashima T, et al. Therapeutic effect of taurine administration on carbon tetrachloride-induced hepatic injury. Jpn J Pharmacol 32 (1982): 583–589.
Nakaya Y et al. Taurine improves insulin sensitivity in the Otsuka Long-Evans Tokushima Fatty rat, a model of spontaneous type 2 diabetes. Am J Clin Nutr 71.1 (2000): 54–8.
Ra, S. G., et al. Additional effects of taurine on the benefits of BCAA intake for the delayed-onset muscle soreness and muscle damage induced by high-intensity eccentric exercise. Adv Exp Med Biol 776 (2013): 179–87.
Rana SK, Sanders TA. Taurine concentrations in the diet, plasma, urine and breast milk of vegans compared with omnivores. Br J Nutr 56 (1986): 17–27.
Ripps, H., & Shen, W. (2012). Review: Taurine: A "very essential" amino acid. Mol Vis, 18, 2673–2686.
Roe DA, Weston MO. Potential significance of free taurine in the diet. Nature 205 (1965): 287–288.
Rozen R, Scriver CR. Renal transport of taurine adapts to perturbed taurine homeostasis. Proc Natl Acad Sci U S A 79 (1982): 2101–2105.
Rutherford JA, et al. The effect of acute taurine ingestion on endurance performance and metabolism in well-trained cyclists. Int J Sport Nutr Exerc Metab. 20(4) (2010):322–9.
Schneider SM et al. Taurine status and response to intravenous taurine supplementation in adults with short-bowel syndrome undergoing long-term parenteral nutrition: a pilot study. Br J Nutr 96 (2006): 365–370.
Schuller-Levis GB, Park E. Taurine and its chloramine: modulators of immunity. Neurochem Res 29.1 (2004): 117–126.
Shao A, Hathcock JN. Risk assessment for the amino acids taurine, L-glutamine and L-arginine. Reg Tox Pharmol 50 (2008): 376–399.
Spohr C et al. No effect of taurine on platelet aggregation in men with a predisposition to type 2 diabetes mellitus. Platelets 16.5 (2005): 301–305.
Sturman JA. Taurine in the brain and liver of the developing human and monkey. J Neurochem 25.6 (1975): 831–85.
Sturman JA. Taurine in development. J Nutr 118 (1988): 1169–1176.
Takahashi R, Nakane Y. Clinical trial of taurine in epilepsy. In: Barbeau A, Huxatable RJ (eds). Taurine and neurological disorders. New York, NY: Raven Press, 1978, pp 375–385.
Timbrell JA, et al. The in vivo and in vitro protective properties of taurine. Gen Pharmacol 26 (1995): 453–462.
Van Gelder NM et al. Biochemical observations following administration of taurine to patients with epilepsy. Brain Res 94 (1975): 297 306.
Verner AM, et al. Effect of taurine supplementation on growth and development in preterm or low birth weight infants. Cochrane Database of Systematic Reviews. 4 (2009): Art. No.: CD006072.
Wójcik OP, et al. Serum taurine and risk of coronary heart disease: a prospective, nested case-control study. Eur J Nutr. 52(1) (2013):169–78.
Yamori Y et al. Distribution of twenty-four hour urinary taurine excretion and association with ischemic heart disease mortality in 24 populations of 16 countries: results from the WHO-CARDIAC Study. Hypertens Res 24 (2001): 453–457.
Yamori Y et al. Male cardiovascular mortality and dietary markers in 25 population samples of 16 countries. J Hypertens 24 (2006): 1499–1505.
Zhang M et al. Effects of taurine supplementation on VDT work induced visual stress. Amino Acids 26 (2004a): 59–63.
Zhang M et al. Beneficial effects of taurine on serum lipids in overweight or obese non-diabetic subjects. Amino Acids 26 (2004b): 267–71.

Tea tree oil

HISTORICAL NOTE The Bundjalong Australian Aboriginal people of northern New South Wales knew of the medicinal qualities of this plant's leaves for many centuries and used it to treat burns, cuts and insect bites. It was not until the 1700s that it became known in the Western world as 'tea tree' because Captain Cook found its aromatic leaves an enjoyable substitute for real tea. The first official report of its medicinal use appeared in the *Medical Journal of Australia* in 1930, when a Sydney surgeon wrote of its impressive wound-healing and antiseptic qualities (Murray 1995). In modern times, tea tree oil has become widely accepted as a standard treatment for wounds and minor skin infections.

COMMON NAME

Tea tree

OTHER NAMES

Australian tea tree oil, melaleuca, melasol, narrow-leaved paperbark, paperbark tree oil, punk tree, ti tree oil

BOTANICAL NAME/FAMILY

Melaleuca alternifolia (family Myrtaceae)

PLANT PARTS USED

Essential oil from leaves and branches

CHEMICAL COMPONENTS

Tea tree oil contains almost 100 components, of which the majority are monoterpenes and their alcohol-related derivatives (Pazyar et al 2012). Active constituents include cineole, alpha-cadinine, terpinenes, pinenes, alpha-terpineol, aromadendrene, terpinenols and terpinolene (Duke 2003). The constituent 1,8-cineole appears to be responsible for the undesirable allergenic effects sometimes observed with tea tree oil products (Pazyar et al 2012).

Antibacterial and antiparasitic

In vitro studies have demonstrated that tea tree oil has activity against a wide range of bacterial species such as *Corynebacterium* spp., *Escherichia coli*, including extended-spectrum beta-lactamase strains, *Enterococcus* spp., including vancomycin-resistant strains, *Klebsiella pneumoniae*, *Micrococcus* spp. (*M. luteus*, *M. varians*), *Propionibacterium acnes*, *Streptococcus pyogenes*, *Pseudomonas aeruginosa*, *Acinetobacter baumannii*, *Staphylococcus* spp. (*S. aureus*, including methicillin-resistant strains (MRSA), *S. capitis*, *S. epidermidis*, *S. haemolyticus*, *S. hominis*, *S. marcescens*, *S. saprophyticus*, *S. warneri* and *S. xylosus*) (Bagg et al 2006, Carson et al 2006, Concha et al 1998, De Mondello et al 2003, Hada et al 2001, Messager et al 2005, Murray 1995, Papadopoulos et al 2006, Tortorano et al

2008, Warnke et al 2012) and against the protozoa, *Trichomonas vaginalis* (Azimi et al 2011).

It is suggested that the antibacterial activity of tea tree is due to its ability to effectively bind to the bacterial cell wall (Chung et al 2007). Tea tree oil disrupts the permeability barrier of cell membrane structures of microorganisms and denatures the proteins (Carson et al 2002, Cox et al 2000, Gustafson et al 1998, Tao & Zhang 2006). This activity is similar to pharmaceutical disinfectants such as chlorhexidine and quaternary ammonium compounds.

Purified components have been found to have greater antibacterial and fungicidal activities than the whole oil, with terpinen-4-ol being the most active constituent, displaying strong antimicrobial and anti-inflammatory properties (Loughlin et al 2008, Pazyar et al 2012, Terzi et al 2007).

Antifungal

Tea tree oil demonstrates antifungal activity against *Candida* species according to in vitro and in vivo studies (Agarwal et al 2010, Mondello et al 2003, Ramage et al 2012). Antifungal activity has also been demonstrated against other yeasts and fungi, including *Fusarium graminearum, F. culmorum, Pyrenophora graminea* (Williamson et al 2007) and *Pityrosporum ovale* (Satchell et al 2002a), and other dermatophytes (Pazyar & Yaghoobi 2012).

Antiviral

An in vitro study has identified activity against herpes simplex virus types 1 and 2 (Schnitzler et al 2001). Tea tree oil has also been shown to be effective in treating hand warts caused by human papillomavirus (Millar & Moore 2008) as well as inhibiting viral replication of Influenza A/PR/8 in vitro (Garozza et al 2011).

Oestrogenic and antiandrogenic activities

Studies in human cell lines have indicated that tea tree oil has oestrogenic and antiandrogenic activities. These actions may have contributed to the effective treatment of cases of prepubertal gynaecomastia, with topical use (Henley et al 2007).

Anticancer activity

In vitro data suggest that tea tree oil may confer antitumour activity by inhibiting growth of melanoma cells, including drug-resistant cells (Bozzuto et al 2011). A murine study reported that topical application of tea tree oil (10%) had a cytotoxic effect on tumour cells, while simultaneously activating local immune response mechanisms (Ireland et al 2012).

Other actions

Tea tree oil is reported to have anti-inflammatory activity (Carson et al 2006) and animal studies have demonstrated that inhalation of tea tree oil has both anti-inflammatory and immunomodulatory actions that are likely to be mediated by the hypothalamic-pituitary axis (Golab & Skwarlo-Sonta 2007). The anti-inflammatory action of the constituent terpinen-4-ol, including inhibition of tumour necrosis factor-α, interleukin-1 (IL-1), IL-8 and prostaglandin E_2, may prove useful in the treatment of psoriasis (Pazyar & Yaghoobi 2012); however, clinical studies have yet to be conducted.

CLINICAL USE

Topical tea tree oil preparations have been investigated in a number of clinical studies, either as the oil itself or as an ingredient of gels, creams or ointments. In vitro studies suggest that the penetration of topical tea tree oil components through the skin is limited, therefore local effects should be expected with little systemic response (Cross et al 2008).

Acne vulgaris

A randomised, double-blind, placebo-controlled study of 60 patients found that a topical 5% tea tree oil gel was an effective treatment for mild to moderate acne vulgaris (Enshaieh et al 2007). This result is supported by a single-blind, randomised clinical trial involving 124 patients with mild to moderate acne which showed that a similar gel significantly improved the condition and reduced the number of acne lesions. These benefits were similar to those produced by 5% benzoyl peroxide lotion, but the tea tree oil gel was better tolerated and produced fewer side effects (Bassett et al 1990).

Athlete's foot, tinea pedis

Two randomised, double-blind studies have tested three different strengths of tea tree oil cream (10%, 25% and 50% w/w) for both symptom relief and curative effects in tinea pedis (Satchell et al 2002a, Tong et al 1992). Based on these studies, it appears that there is a dose-response as the higher concentrations of tea tree oil cream performed better than the lowest-tested concentration. Symptom relief was achieved for most patients; however, none of the tested preparations achieved negative mycology in all cases.

The first study involved 104 subjects with tinea pedis (athlete's foot) and compared 10% w/w tea tree oil cream to 1% tolnaftate or placebo creams (Tong et al 1992). In this study, significantly more tolnaftate-treated patients (85%) than tea tree oil- (30%) and placebo-treated (21%) patients showed conversion to negative culture at the end of therapy. However, tea tree oil cream reduced symptoms as effectively as tolnaftate 1%. A more recent randomised, double-blind, controlled study by the same group used two preparations of more concentrated tea tree oil (25% and 50% w/w) for the treatment of interdigital tinea pedis in 158 patients over 4 weeks (Satchell et al 2002a). In the 50% tea tree oil group, 68% of patients had a significant response and 64% achieved negative mycology. In the 25% tea tree group, 72% of patients responded and 50% were cured. The placebo responder rates were 39% and 31%, respectively, with 3% of patients using tea tree developing dermatitis.

It has been suggested that the fungicidal activity of tea tree and other essential oils can be enhanced using footbaths heated to 42°C (Inouye et al 2007).

Toenail infection (onychomycosis)

A randomised, double-blind multicentre study involving 177 volunteers found that 6 months' treatment with 1% clotrimazole solution (applied twice daily) or 100% tea tree oil (applied twice daily) produced similar results, improving nail appearance and associated symptoms (Buck et al 1994). Additionally, 3 months after either treatment ceased, continued improvement or complete resolution was observed in approximately half of participants. Another randomised, double-blind, placebo-controlled study investigated the effects of a combined tea tree oil (5%) and butenafine hydrochloride (2%) cream in chronic toenail onychomycosis and found that, after 6 weeks, 80% of patients achieved a cure with active treatment compared with none using placebo cream (Syed et al 1999).

MRSA infection

Tea tree oil has been shown to have activity against MRSA and coagulase-negative *Staphylococci* (Brady et al 2006, Loughlin et al 2008), providing a basis for research in this area. Clinical trials with 5% tea tree oil body wash, 10% cream and 4% nasal ointment have been conducted, producing encouraging results. As yet, no definitive conclusions can be made about the best forms, concentrations and treatment regimens necessary to prevent and/or treat MRSA infection.

Washing with a 5% tea tree oil for 5 days has been shown to be effective in removing MRSA on the skin (Dryden et al 2004) and tea tree oil has been effectively used against biofilm formation on tympanostomy tubes in vitro (Park et al 2007). A combination of 4% tea tree oil nasal ointment and 5% tea tree oil body wash was found to be superior to the standard 2% mupirocin nasal ointment and triclosan body wash used for the eradication of MRSA (Caelli et al 2000).

While the study by Caelli et al (2000) suggests tea tree is more effective than mupirocin, other studies have shown it to be effective, but not superior to this standard treatment for MRSA (Bradley 2011). A review reported on two randomised controlled trials (n = 30, n = 224), both of which demonstrated that tea tree oil was effective, although not to the same extent as mupirocin. In the larger trial, 224 patients were given either mupirocin 2% nasal ointment, chlorhexidine gluconate 4% soap and silver sulfadiazine 1% cream or tea tree 10% cream and tea tree 5% body wash for 5 days (Dryden et al 2004). Rates of MRSA clearance were similar: 41% in the tea tree group and 49% using standard treatment. Mupirocin was significantly more effective at clearing nasal carriage (78%) than tea tree cream (47%), although tea tree treatment was more effective than both chlorhexidine and silver sulfadiazine at clearing superficial skin sites and skin lesions.

An uncontrolled case study series (n = 12) reported that an aqueous solution of tea tree oil (3.3%) was unsuccessful in eradicating MRSA from wounds, with none of the 12 participants being MRSA-negative after treatment. The study also reported that use of tea tree oil did not inhibit healing (Edmondson et al 2011).

Overall, tea tree oil may be an effective antimicrobial agent when appropriately used at bactericidal concentrations; however it remains to be seen whether its application at sublethal concentrations may contribute to the development of antibiotic resistance in human pathogens (McMahon et al 2007).

Vaginitis and cervicitis

Limited clinical data and results from in vitro studies support the use of tea tree oil for vaginitis and cervicitis caused by *Trichomonas vaginalis* (Azimi et al 2011, Jandourek et al 1998, Vila & Canigueral 2006).

An open study found that intravaginal application of tampons saturated in a diluted emulsified solution successfully healed vaginitis and cervicitis (n = 130) caused by *T. vaginalis*. A combination of vaginal pessaries containing 0.2 g tea tree oil inserted nightly and daily douching with 0.4% tea tree oil in water resulted in clinical cure from trichomonal vaginitis (Peña 1962). Positive results from in vitro studies provide further support for this indication. There is now a need to confirm these results under double-blind conditions.

A case report shows that a 5-day course of 200 mg tea tree oil in a vegetable oil base inserted into the vagina may also be successful at treating vaginal candidiasis, with eradication of anaerobic bacterial vaginosis being confirmed after 1 month (Blackwell 1991). While further clinical evidence is lacking, in vitro studies demonstrate that tea tree oil is moderately effective against *Candida albicans* (Agarwal et al 2010).

Cystitis

A randomised, double-blind study investigated the effects of tea tree oil, administered as 8 mg essential oil (taken three times daily) in an enteric-coated capsule, in 26 women with chronic idiopathic colibacillary cystitis (Belaiche 1988). After the 6-month test period, 54% of women receiving active treatment were symptom-free compared with only 15% receiving placebo. Although symptom-free, 50% of women in the tea tree group still showed evidence of infection.

Gingivitis

Tea tree oil was as effective as chlorhexidine against *Streptococcus mutans*, the bacteria that causes gingivitis, in a controlled study of 30 individuals (Groppo et al 2002). A more recent double-blind, randomised, longitudinal study evaluated and compared the effects of tea tree oil gel (2.5%) and chlorhexidine gel (0.2%) in 49 patients with severe chronic gingivitis (Soukoulis & Hirsch 2004). Subjects brushed with the tea tree, chlorhexidine or placebo gel twice daily for a period of 8 weeks. Tea tree oil significantly reduced the papillary bleeding index and gingival index, but did not reduce plaque.

Dandruff

Tea tree oil may be effective for improving, but not eradicating, dandruff according to a randomised, single-blind, parallel-group study (Satchell et al 2002b). In the study, tea tree oil shampoo (5%) was compared to placebo in 126 patients with mild to moderate dandruff over 4 weeks (Satchell et al 2002b). The tea tree oil group achieved a 41% improvement as compared to 11% in the placebo group, with no adverse effects.

Head lice eradication

In test tube studies, topical application of tea tree oil was extremely effective against head lice, with 93% of lice and 83% of eggs destroyed (Veal 1996). In a more recent in vitro study, a 1% concentration of tea tree oil was found to be effective against head lice, with 100% mortality within 30 minutes (Di Campli et al 2012). Phenols, phenolic ethers, ketones and oxides appear to be the major toxic components responsible for this activity. Using a mite chamber assay, tea tree oil was also found to be effective against both head lice and dust mites (Williamson et al 2007).

While these in vitro studies and anecdotal evidence provide some basis for its clinical use, large double-blind, clinical trials have yet to be conducted (Centre 2008).

Dermatitis

Tea tree oil has been shown to reduce the severity of induced experimental contact dermatitis due to nickel sulfate and perform better than either zinc oxide or clobetasone butyrate (Wallengren 2011). Tea tree oil was tested at a 20% and 50% concentration. Similar efficacy was reported at both strengths; however there was a higher incidence of erythema at the higher dose, suggesting that the 20% dose is preferable.

Tea tree oil-containing cream may also be an effective treatment for dermatitis in dogs according to two studies. Tea tree oil cream (10%) was applied, twice daily, for 4 weeks to 53 dogs suffering from chronic dermatitis, allergic dermatitis, interdigital pyoderma, acral lick dermatitis and skinfold pyoderma (Fitzi et al 2002). At the end of the trial, 82% of the animals had a good or very good response to treatment with most symptoms disappearing, although two dogs experienced local irritation. Another trial by the same research team again evaluated the tea tree cream and blinded the study with a commercial skin care cream (Reichling et al 2004). Fifty-seven dogs were involved in this study and similar results were obtained, with drastically reduced dermatitis in 71% of animals as compared to 41% using the control cream. A local reaction was reported in one dog.

OTHER USES

Herpes

Since tea tree oil exhibits antiviral activity in vitro, tea tree oil preparations have been used in the treatment of genital herpes simplex virus. Clinical trials investigating tea tree oil for this indication are not available, so it is unknown whether effects are clinically significant.

Hair follicle mite eradication (ocular demodicosis)

Clinical research indicates a possible role for tea tree oil in the treatment of blepharitis and ocular discomfort caused by the ectoparasite *Demodex*. A randomised study involving 281 patients with symptoms of eye discomfort, who had tested positive for ocular *Demodex* infestation, were treated with weekly lid scrubs at the clinic with tea tree oil 50%, combined with twice-daily home use of an eyelid scrub that included tea tree oil 10% or weekly clinic and twice-daily home use of an eyelid scrub without tea tree oil, for a period of 4 weeks. The study was limited by poor compliance; however a 37.5% eradication rate of *Demodex* was reported in a subgroup of the treatment group who showed good compliance (use of scrub >10 times/week) (Koo et al 2012).

This finding supports those from an earlier retrospective review of 11 cases, in which eyelid scrub with 50% tea tree oil combined with daily lid hygiene and tea tree shampoo for 4 weeks was observed to effectively eradicate the hair follicle mite *Demodex folliculorum* and result in subjective and objective improvements (Gao et al 2007).

Wart eradication

There is a case report that daily topical application of 100% tea tree oil for 12 days successfully eradicated warts on the hand of a paediatric patient (Millar & Moore 2008).

Oral candidiasis

Results from an animal study suggest that tea tree oil and its constituent terpinen-4-ol may decrease the symptom score in oral candidiasis in azole-resistant strains of *Candida albicans* (Ninomiya et al 2012). This encouraging result requires testing in humans to further determine efficacy.

Idiopathic hirsutism

Preliminary evidence suggests that a combination of tea tree and lavender oil as a spray may offer some benefit in women with mild idiopathic hirsutism. One small study involving 24 women showed that application of tea tree and lavender oil for 3 months reduced hair diameter in areas affected by hirsutism, compared to no change in the placebo group. It was proposed that this was due to antiandrogenic properties found in tea tree and lavender essential oils (Tirabassi et al 2013).

Practice points/patient counselling

- Tea tree has multiple actions, including antibacterial, antiviral, antiparasitic, antifungal and anti-inflammatory.
- Tea tree preparations may be effective as treatments for gingivitis, *Candida albicans* or *Trichomonas vaginalis* vaginitis and cervicitis, cystitis, head lice, blepharitis and contact dermatitis according to available research; however further clinical research is required to clarify its role.
- 100% tea tree oil is a safe and effective alternative to clotrimazole for the treatment of toenail onychomycosis.
- 5% tea tree oil gel has been shown to significantly improve acne vulgaris, with effects similar to 5% benzoyl peroxide lotion.
- 10% tea tree oil preparation is effective at treating dermatitis in dogs.
- Clinical evidence supports the use of tea tree oil preparations in MRSA infection.
- Tea tree oil should not be ingested and a test patch is advised before widespread topical application.

DOSAGE RANGE

Tea tree oil is used in a variety of forms, such as gels, creams, ointments, oral rinses, soaps, shampoos and paints. Minimum bactericidal concentrations are generally 0.25%.

- Onychomycosis: 100% essential oil applied twice daily for months.
- Tinea pedis: 10% essential oil in cream base applied twice daily.
- Acne: 5% essential oil in cream or gel base applied daily.
- Contact dermatitis: 20–50% tea tree oil preparation.
- Dermatitis in dogs: 10% preparation applied twice daily for 4 weeks.
- Dandruff: 5% tea tree oil shampoo daily for at least 4 weeks.
- Gingivitis: 2.5% oral gel — brush teeth with preparation twice daily for 8 weeks.
- MRSA: 2–4% nasal ointment and 5% tea tree oil body wash used for 5 days.
- Vaginitis (*Candida albicans* or *Trichomonas vaginalis*): intravaginally applied tampons saturated in a 1% emulsified solution, vaginal pessaries containing 0.2 g essential oil.
- Cervicitis (*Candida albicans* or *Trichomonas vaginalis*): intravaginally applied tampons saturated in a 20% emulsified solution.

TOXICITY

Tea tree oil should not be orally ingested, based on a risk of toxicity. Although no deaths have been reported in the literature (Hammer et al 2006), accidental ingestion has resulted in confusion, disorientation, general malaise and coma, according to case reports.

One case has been reported of an infant ingesting less than 10 mL of 100% oil; this resulted in confusion and an inability to walk within 30 minutes, followed by a full recovery within 5 hours (Jacobs & Hornfeldt 1994).

ADVERSE REACTIONS

Anecdotal evidence from almost 80 years of use suggests that the topical use of the oil is relatively safe, and that adverse events are minor, self-limiting and occasional (Hammer et al 2006). Skin irritation, contact dermatitis, linear immunoglobulin A disease and erythema multiforme-like reactions are possible in sensitive individuals (Hammer et al 2006, Pazyar et al 2012, Posadzki et al 2012, Williams et al 2007). It has been suggested that this is underreported and that tea tree oil should be included in patch testing. Oxidised monoterpenes, such as ascaridole, are likely to be the sensitising agents (Bakker 2011, Reichling et al 2006) as tea tree oil from freshly opened products elicits no or weak reactions. It is therefore suggested that patch testing needs to be done with oxidised tea tree oil (Rutherford et al 2007).

Three cases of prepubertal gynaecomastia have been reported in boys who had used topical products containing lavender and tea tree oils, with the gynaecomastia resolving after the products were discontinued (Henley et al 2007).

SIGNIFICANT INTERACTIONS

None known.

CONTRAINDICATIONS AND PRECAUTIONS

Caution should be exercised if applying the oil to eczematous or inflamed skin as it may cause irritation. It is suggested that a small amount be first applied to a test patch, to determine whether irritation will occur, as contact dermatitis has been reported.

PREGNANCY USE

Insufficient reliable information is available to determine safety.

PATIENTS' FAQs

What will tea tree oil do for me?

Tea tree oil is an antiseptic substance that is effective against a wide range of common bacterial and fungal organisms. It also has antiviral, antiparasitic and anti-inflammatory actions. Scientific evidence shows that it is an effective treatment for acne and fungal infections of the toenails and feet. There is preliminary evidence that it might be useful in *Trichomonas vaginalis* vaginitis and cervicitis, cystitis, gingivitis, head lice, blepharitis and MRSA infection.

When will it start to work?

This will depend on the indication it is being used to treat. In some cases, clinical tests are not available, so it is uncertain when, if any, effects are seen.

Are there any safety issues?

Tea tree oil should not be ingested orally and used with caution on inflamed and sensitive skin.

REFERENCES

Agarwal V, et al. Effect of plant oils on *Candida albicans*. J Microbiol Immunol Infect 43.5 (2010):447–451.

Azimi H et al. A comprehensive review of vaginitis phytotherapy. Pakistan Journal of Biological Sciences 14.21 (2011):960–966.

Bagg J et al. Susceptibility to *Melaleuca alternifolia* (tea tree) oil of yeasts isolated from the mouths of patients with advanced cancer. Oral Oncol 42.5 (2006): 487–492.

Bakker CV. Ascaridole, a sensitizing component of tea tree oil, patch tested at 1% and 5% in two series of patients. Contact Dermatitis 65 (2011):239–248

Bassett IB, et al. A comparative study of tea-tree oil versus benzoylperoxide in the treatment of acne. Med J Aust 153.8 (1990): 455–458.

Belaiche P. Letter to the editor. Phytother Res 2 (1988): 157.

Blackwell AL. Tea tree oil and anaerobic (bacterial) vaginosis. Lancet 337.8736 (1991): 300.

Bozzuto G et al. Tea tree oil might combat melanoma. Planta Medica 77.1 (2011):54–6

Bradley SF. MRSA colonisation (eradicating colonisation in people with active/invasive infection. Clinical Evidence 1. (2011):923

Brady A et al. In vitro activity of tea-tree oil against clinical skin isolates of methicillin-resistant and -sensitive *Staphylococcus aureus* and coagulase-negative staphylococci growing planktonically and as biofilms. J Med Microbiol 55.10 (2006): 1375–1380.

Buck DS, et al. Comparison of two topical preparations for the treatment of onychomycosis: *Melaleuca alternifolia* (tea tree) oil and clotrimazole. J Fam Pract 38.6 (1994): 601–605.

Caelli M et al. Tea tree oil as an alternative topical decolonization agent for methicillin-resistant *Staphylococcus aureus*. J Hosp Infect 46.3 (2000): 236–237.

Carson CF, et al. Mechanism of action of *Melaleuca alternifolia* (tea tree) oil on *Staphylococcus aureus* determined by time-kill, lysis, leakage, and salt tolerance assays and electron microscopy. Antimicrob Agents Chemother 46.6 (2002): 1914–1920.

Carson CF, et al. *Melaleuca alternifolia* (tea tree) oil: a review of antimicrobial and other medicinal properties. Clin Microbiol Rev 19.1 (2006): 50–62.

Centre NP. Management of head lice in primary care. MeReC Bulletin 18.4 (2008): 1–7.

Chung KH et al. Antibacterial activity of essential oils on the growth of *Staphylococcus aureus* and measurement of their binding interaction using optical biosensor. J Microbiol Biotechnol 17.11 (2007): 1848–1855.

Concha JM, et al. 1998 William J. Stickel Bronze Award: Antifungal activity of *Melaleuca alternifolia* (tea-tree) oil against various pathogenic organisms. J Am Podiatr Med Assoc 88.10 (1998): 489–492.

Cox SD et al. The mode of antimicrobial action of the essential oil of *Melaleuca alternifolia* (tea tree oil).J Appl Microbiol 88.1 (2000): 170–175.

Cross SE et al. Human skin penetration of the major components of Australian tea tree oil applied in its pure form and as a 20% solution in vitro. Eur J Pharm Biopharm 69.1 (2008): 214–222.t

De Mondello F et al. In vitro and in vivo activity of tea tree oil against azole-susceptible and –resistant human pathogenic yeasts. J Antimicrob Chemother 51.5 (2003): 1223–1229.

Di Campli E et al. Activity of tea tree oil and nerolidol alone or in combination against *Pediculus capitus* (head lice) and its eggs. Parasitology Research 111.5 (2012):1985–92

Dryden MS, et al. A randomized, controlled trial of tea tree topical preparations versus a standard topical regimen for the clearance of MRSA colonization. J Hosp Infect 56.4 (2004): 283–286.

Duke JA. Dr Duke's Phytochemical and Ethnobotanical Databases. US Department of Agriculture–Agricultural Research Service–National Germplasm Resources Laboratory. Beltsville Agricultural Research Center, Beltsville, MD, 2003. Available online: www.ars-grin.gov/duke.

Edmondson M et al. Uncontrolled, open-label, pilot study of tea tree (*Melaleuca alternifolia*) oil solution in the decolonisation of methicillin-resistant *Staphylococcus aureus* positive wounds and its influence on wound healing. Int Wound J. 8.4. (2011):375–84

Enshaieh S et al. The efficacy of 5% topical tea tree oil gel in mild to moderate acne vulgaris: a randomized, double-blind placebo-controlled study. Indian J Dermatol Venereol Leprol 73.1 (2007): 22–25.

Fitzi J et al. Phytotherapy of chronic dermatitis and pruritus of dogs with a topical preparation containing tea tree oil (Bogaskin). Schweiz Arch Tierheilkd 144.5 (2002): 223–231.

Gao YY et al. Clinical treatment of ocular demodecosis by lid scrub with tea tree oil. Cornea 26.2 (2007): 136–143.

Garozza A et al. Activity of *Melaleuca alternifolia* (tea tree) oil on Influenza virus A/PR/8: Study on the mechanism of action. Antiviral Res 89 (2011):83–88.

Golab M, Skwarlo-Sonta K. Mechanisms involved in the anti-inflammatory action of inhaled tea tree oil in mice. Exp Biol Med (Maywood) 232.3 (2007): 420–426.

Groppo FC et al. Antimicrobial activity of garlic, tea tree oil, and chlorhexidine against oral microorganisms. Int Dent J 52.6 (2002): 433–437.

Gustafson JE et al. Effects of tea tree oil on *Escherichia coli*. Lett Appl Microbiol 26.3 (1998): 194–198.

Hada T et al. Comparison of the effects in vitro of tea tree oil and plaunotol on methicillin-susceptible and methicillin-resistant strains of *Staphylococcus aureus*. Microbios 106 (Suppl 2) (2001): 133–141.

Hammer KA et al. A review of the toxicity of *Melaleuca alternifolia* (tea tree) oil. Food Chem Toxicol 44.5 (2006): 616–625.

Henley DV et al. Prepubertal gynecomastia linked to lavender and tea tree oils. N Engl J Med 356.5 (2007): 479–485.

Inouye S et al. Combined effect of heat, essential oils and salt on the fungicidal activity against *Trichophytonmenta grophytes* in foot bath. Nippon Ishinkin Gakkai Zasshi 48.1 (2007): 27–36.

Ireland DJ et al. Topically applied *Melaleuca alternifolia* (tea tree) oil causes direct anti-cancer cytotoxicity in subcutaneous tumour bearing mice. Journal of Dermatological Science 67 (2012):120–129.

Jacobs MR, Hornfeldt CS. Melaleuca oil poisoning. J Toxicol Clin Toxicol 32.4 (1994): 461–464.

Jandourek A et al. Efficacy of melaleuca oral solution for the treatment of fluconazole refractory oral candidiasis in AIDS patients. AIDS 12.9 (1988): 1033–1037.

Koo H et al Ocular surface discomfort and *Demodex*: effect of tea tree oil eyelid scrub in *Demodex* blepharitis. J Korean Med Sci 27 (2012):1574–1579.

Loughlin R et al. Comparison of the cidal activity of tea tree oil and terpinen-4-ol against clinical bacterial skin isolates and human fibroblast cells. Lett Appl Microbiol 46.4 (2008): 428–433.

McMahon MA et al. Habituation to sub-lethal concentrations of tea tree oil (*Melaleuca alternifolia*) is associated with reduced susceptibility to antibiotics in human pathogens. J Antimicrob Chemother 59.1 (2007): 125–127.

Messager S et al. Assessment of the antibacterial activity of tea tree oil using the European EN 1276 and EN 12054 standard suspension tests. J Hosp Infect 59.2 (2005): 113–125.

Millar BC, Moore JE. Successful topical treatment of hand warts in a paediatric patient with tea tree oil (*Melaleuca alternifolia*). Complement Ther Clin Pract 14.4 (2008): 225–227.

Mondello F et al. In vitro and in vivo activity of tea tree oil against azole-susceptible and -resistant human pathogenic yeasts. J Antimicrob Chemother. 51.5 (2003):1223–9

Murray M. The healing power of herbs. Rocklin, CA: Prima Health, 1995.

Ninomiya K et al. The essential oil of *Melaleuca alternifolia* (tea tree oil) and its main component, terpinen-4-ol protect mice from experimental oral candidiasis. Biological and Pharmaceutical Bulletin 35.6 (2012):861–865

Papadopoulos CJ et al. Susceptibility of *Pseudomonas* to *Melaleuca alternifolia* (tea tree) oil and components. J Antimicrob Chemother 58.2 (2006): 449–451.

Park H et al. Antibacterial effect of tea-tree oil on methicillin-resistant *Staphylococcus aureus* biofilm formation of the tympanostomy tube: an in vitro study. In Vivo 21.6 (2007): 1027–1030.

Pazyar N. Yaghoobi R. Tea tree oil as a novel antipsoriasis weapon. Skin Pharmacol Physiol 25 (2012):162–163.

Pazyar N et al. A review of applications of tea tree oil in dermatology.International Journal of Dermatology(2012) 52: 784–790.

Peña EF. Melaleuca alternifolia oil. Its use for trichomonal vaginitis and other vaginal infections. Obstet Gynecol 19.6 (1962): 793–795.

Posadzki P, et al. Adverse effects of aromatherapy: a systematic review of case reports and case series. Int J Risk Saf Med 24 (2012):147–161.

Ramage G. et al. Antifungal, cytotoxic, and immunomodulatory properties of tea tree oil and its derivative components: potential role in management of oral candidosis in cancer patients. Frontiers in Microbiology. 3.220(2012):1–8

Reichling J et al. Topical tea tree oil effective in canine localised pruritic dermatitis: a multi-centre randomised double-blind controlled clinical trial in the veterinary practice. Deutsch Tierarztl Wochenschr 111.10 (2004): 408–414.

Reichling J, et al. [Australian tea tree oil (*Melaleuca eaetheroleum*). Pharmaceutical quality, efficacy and toxicity.] AustralischesTeebaumöl (*Melaleuca eaetheroleum*).Pharmazeutische Qualität, Wirksamkeit und Toxizität 18.4 (2006): 193–200.

T

Rutherford T et al. Allergy to tea tree oil: retrospective review of 41 cases with positive patch tests over 4.5 years. Australas J Dermatol 48.2 (2007): 83–87.
Satchell AC et al. Treatment of interdigital tinea pedis with 25% and 50% tea tree oil solution: a randomized, placebo-controlled, blinded study. Aust J Dermatol 43.3 (2002a): 175–8.
Satchell AC et al. Treatment of dandruff with 5% tea tree oil shampoo. J Am Acad Dermatol 47.6 (2002b): 852–5.
Schnitzler P, et al. Antiviral activity of Australian tea tree oil and eucalyptus oil against herpes simplex virus in cell culture. Pharmazie 56.4 (2001): 343–347.
Soukoulis S, Hirsch R. The effects of a tea tree oil-containing gel on plaque and chronic gingivitis. Aust Dent J 49.2 (2004): 78–83.
Syed TA et al. Treatment of toenail onychomycosis with 2% butenafine and 5% *Melaleuca alternifolia* (tea tree) oil in cream. Trop Med Int Health 4.4 (1999): 284–287.
Tao FY, Zhang XM. Progress on mechanism of antimicrobial activity of tea tree oil. Chinese Journal of Antibiotics 31.5 (2006): 261–266.
Terzi V et al. In vitro antifungal activity of the tea tree (*Melaleuca alternifolia*) essential oil and its major components against plant pathogens. Lett Appl Microbiol 44.6 (2007): 613–6118.
Tirabassi G et al. Possible efficacy of lavender and tea tree oils in the treatment of young women affected by mild idiopathic hirsutism. Journal of Endocrinological Investigation 36.1 (2013):50–54
Tong MM, et al. Tea tree oil in the treatment of tinea pedis. Australas J Dermatol 33.3 (1992): 145–149.
Tortorano AM et al. In vitro activity of conventional antifungal drugs and natural essences against the yeast-like alga Prototheca. J AntimicrobChemother 61.6 (2008): 1312–13114.
Veal L. The potential effectiveness of essential oils as a treatment for headlice, Pediculus humanus capitis. Complement Ther Nurs Midwifery 2.4 (1996): 97–101.
Vila R, Canigueral S. [The essential oil of *Melaleuca alternifolia* in the treatment of vulvovaginitis.] Ginecología y obstetricia clínica 7.2 (2006): 87–95.
Wallengen J. Tea tree oil attenuates experimental contact dermatitis. Arch Dermatol Res 303 (2011):333–338.
Warnke PH et al. The ongoing battle against multi-resistant strains: In-vitro inhibition of hospital-acquired MRSA, VRE, *Pseudomonas*, ESBL *E. coli* and *Klebsiella* species in the presence of plant-derived antiseptic oils. Journal of Cranio-Maxillo-Facial Surgery (2012):1–6.
Williams JD, et al. Recurrent allergic contact dermatitis due to allergen transfer by sunglasses. Contact Dermatitis 57.2 (2007): 120–121.
Williamson EM, et al. An investigation and comparison of the bioactivity of selected essential oils on human lice and house dust mites. Fitoterapia 78.7–8 (2007): 521–525.

Thyme

HISTORICAL NOTE Although thyme has been used as a cooking spice for centuries in Europe, it is also used medicinally to treat common infections, coughs, bronchitis and asthma. Red thyme oil has been used as an antimicrobial agent since the 16th century (Bahadoran et al 2010). The 17th-century herbalist Nicholas Culpeper recommended thyme for whooping cough, gout, stomach pains and shortness of breath. It was also used in perfumes and embalming oils. In medieval times the plant was seen as imparting courage and vigour (Blumenthal et al 2000).

COMMON NAME

Thyme

OTHER NAMES

Common thyme, garden thyme, farigola, folia thymi, gartenthymian, herba thymi, almindelig timian, thym, thymian, thymianblätter, timo

BOTANICAL NAME/FAMILY

Thymus vulgaris (family Lamiaceae)

PLANT PARTS USED

Leaves and flowering tops

CHEMICAL COMPONENTS

The primary constituents are the volatile oils (1–2.5%), which include phenols (0.5%), namely thymol (30–70%), eugenol and carvacrol (3–15%), also flavonoids, apigenin, luteolin and saponins and tannins. Rosmarinic acid, caffeic acid and calcium are also found in significant quantities (Chohan et al 2012, Duke 2003). The herb also contains bitter principles and salicylates.

MAIN ACTIONS

Although thyme has not been significantly investigated in human studies, there has been some investigation into the activity of several of its constituents, in particular, thymol and carvacrol and the volatile oil component of the herb. It is not known whether results obtained for these constituents are representative for the crude herb, but they provide some further understanding. Both the essential oil and thymol are ingredients in many proprietary products.

Antitussive and antispasmodic effects

These actions have been attributed to the phenolic compounds in thyme (WHO 2003). Antispasmodic effects on guinea pig trachea and ileum have been demonstrated for these constituents and for the whole extract of thyme (Engelbertz et al 2008).

Expectorant

The saponin content is believed to have expectorant activity, as demonstrated in animal studies. An in vivo trial has demonstrated improved expectoration and mucociliary clearance (Wienkotter et al 2007).

Analgesic

In vivo research suggests that *Thymus vulgaris* extract has an inhibitory effect on pain sensation; however, the mechanism of action remains unknown (Taherian et al 2009).

Antibacterial

Both the extract and essential oil exhibit antibacterial activity against a wide range of bacteria. This is chiefly due to the eugenol, thymol and carvacrol constituents.

Extract

Thyme extract has demonstrated activity of thyme extract against *Escherichia coli, Listeria monocytogenes, Streptococcus mutans* and *Salmonella enterica* in vitro (Burt et al 2005, 2007, Fabian et al 2006, Friedman et al 2002, Hammad et al 2007, Schelz et al 2006, Solomakos et al 2008). Aqueous thyme extract also has a significant inhibitory effect on *Helicobacter pylori*, reducing both its growth and its potent urease activity in vitro (Tabak et al 1996).

Essential oil

The essential oil of thyme also has potent antibacterial properties as demonstrated in vitro against a wide range of pathogens, including clinical bacterial strains of *Staphylococcus, Enterococcus, Escherichia* and *Pseudomonas* genera, *Clostridium botulinum, Haemophilus influenzae, Klebsiella pneumoniae, Salmonella typhi, Brochothrix thermosphacta* and *P. acnes* (Kalemba & Kunicka 2003, Schmidt et al 2012, Sienkiewicz et al 2011, Zu et al 2010). *T. vulgaris* essential oil also exhibits better inhibitory effects against *H. pylori* than essential oil from *Eucalyptus globulus* (Esmaeili et al 2012).

In vitro tests have also identified antibacterial activity against four Gram-negative food-borne bacteria (*Escherichia coli, Salmonella abony, Pseudomonas aeruginosa* and *P. fragi*) (Schmidt et al 2012).

Multi-drug resistant bacteria

Emerging in vitro evidence suggests that thyme essential oil has activity against multidrug resistant strains of *Staphylococcus, Enterococcus, Escherichia*, and *Pseudomonas* genus (Sienkiewicz et al 2012). Thyme essential oil may enter the extracellular matrix, cell membrane or cell wall of bacterial biofilms, eradicating bacteria within biofilms with greater efficiency than certain antibiotics (Kavanaugh & Ribbeck 2012).

Thyme extract and essential oil potentiates the antibacterial effects of tetracycline against methicillin-resistant *Staphylococcus aureus* in vitro (Fujita et al 2005, Warnke et al 2009, Sienkiewicz et al 2011). The antibacterial activity of thyme essential oil against antibiotic resistance strains (such as MRSA) is probably due to the significant content of thymol (48.1%) (Tohidpour et al 2010).

Antifungal

The essential oil of thyme has exhibited antifungal activity against *Candida albicans* (Kalemba & Kunicka 2003). The constituents thymol and eugenol have demonstrated antifungal activity by establishing the ability to alter the cell wall and membrane of the yeasts *Saccharomyces cervisiae* and *Candida albicans* (Bennis et al 2004, Braga et al 2007a, 2007b). *Thymus vulgaris* is also likely to have significant potential for the biological control of fungi in food (Centeno et al 2010).

Azole resistance

Thymol and carvacrol found in thyme appear to exert a synergistic antifungal effect with the azole antimycotic fluconazole against *Candida* spp. according to in vitro research. Both constituents exhibited a high potency to block drug transporter pumps in resistant strains thereby restoring the sensitivity of resistant *Candida* isolates to fluconazole as well as having direct fungicidal activity (Ahmad et al 2013).

Antiviral

Thyme oil demonstrates antiviral activity against HSV-1, HSV-2 and an aciclovir-resistant strain of the virus (Koch et al 2007, Nolkemper et al 2006, Schnitzler et al 2007). One study found that the oil decreased plaque formation by more than 90% when preincubated with HSV-2; however, no effect was observed when the oil was added prior to infection or after the absorption stage (Koch et al 2007). It was suggested that thyme essential oil interferes with the viral envelope.

Antioxidant

Thyme and thymol exhibit significant antioxidant activity according to both in vitro and in vivo research. Several in vitro studies have investigated the antioxidant effects of thyme (Braga et al 2006a, Chizzola et al 2008, Lee et al 2005, Tsai et al 2011). One study found that eugenol, carvacrol, thymol and 4-allylphenol (5 mcg/mL) all inhibited the oxidation of hexanal for a period of 30 days, demonstrating potent antioxidant activity comparable to alpha-tocopherol (Lee et al 2005). Other research reveals that thyme had significant antioxidant effects in a N-nitrosodiethylamine-induced oxidative stress model in rats (Rana & Soni 2008), and that thyme essential oil exhibited a dose-dependent protective effect against aflatoxin-induced toxicity in rats (El-Nekeety et al 2011). Thyme aqueous extract has been shown to increase the activity of glutathione peroxidase in serum, liver and brain tissue of rats exposed to alcohol toxicity indicating an ability to increase antioxidant capacity in vivo (Shati & Elsaid 2009).

The polyphenol content of thyme is most likely to be responsible for its antioxidant activity.

Anticancer

In vitro research reveals that thyme essential oil inhibits human head and neck squamous cell carcinoma growth in vitro (Sertel et al 2011). It also exhibits cytotoxicity against human prostate carcinoma (PC-3), human lung carcinoma (A549) and human breast cancer (MCF-7) cell lines with strongest effects against PC-3 (Zu et al 2010).

Astringent

The tannin content of the herb is chiefly responsible for its astringent activity.

Anthelmintic/antiparasitic

Thymol possesses anthelmintic activity, demonstrated in vitro (Newell et al 1996). In vitro research also shows that Iranian thyme essential oil is effective against trophozoites of *E. histolytica*, when compared to metronidazole (Behnia et al 2008).

Anti-inflammatory

Dietary ingestion of the culinary herb thyme together with research using thyme oil and the constituent thymol have all identified anti-inflammatory effects. Thymol has demonstrated anti-inflammatory effects in vitro by reducing elastase (Braga et al 2006b). Moreover, thyme essential oil has shown to have anti-inflammatory effects in vivo. Carvacrol, which is present in thyme oil, exhibits an inhibitory effect on leucocyte migration (Fachini-Queiroz et al 2012) and has been shown to reduce TNF-α, IL-1β, and IL-8 secretion levels of THP-1 cells in vitro (Tsai et al 2011).

One study investigated the impact of both cooking and digestion on its biological and health promoting properties. The researchers found that thyme significantly decreased IL-8 release via inhibition of, and protection against, the action of H_2O_2 or TNFα (Chohan et al 2012).

IN COMBINATION

A combination of oregano and thyme essential oils has been shown to reduce inflammation in trinitrobenzene sulfonic acid (TNBS)-induced colitis in vivo (Bukovska et al 2007). A dose of 0.2% thyme and 0.1% oregano led to a reduction in IL-1 beta, IL-6, GM-CSF and TNFalpha. The oils also decreased mortality rate, increased body weight and reduced histological damage (Bukovska et al 2007).

OTHER ACTIONS

Thyme may possess antithrombotic properties (Naemura et al 2008).

CLINICAL USE

Thyme has not been significantly investigated in controlled studies, therefore information is generally derived from evidence of activity and traditional use.

Respiratory tract infections

Thyme extract has been used to treat the common cold, bronchitis, laryngitis and tonsillitis. It is orally ingested or used in a gargle for local activity. The herb's significant antibacterial activity provides a biological basis for its use.

Bronchitis — in combination

Encouraging data have been reported for chronic bronchitis treated by thyme in combination with other herbs in large ($n > 3000$) comparative clinical trials, although no data are available for thyme as a stand-alone treatment (Ernst et al 1997). A combination of thyme and primrose root (1 mL five times/day) has been found to be beneficial in both double-blind and single-blind trials (Gruenwald et al 2005, 2006). The double-blind, placebo-controlled, randomised, multicentre trial in 150 outpatients with acute bronchitis found that 58.7% of participants in the treatment group were symptom-free at the end of the 7 to 9 days compared to 5.3% in the placebo group (Gruenwald et al 2005). A double-blind, placebo-controlled, multicentre study investigated the efficacy of the same combination in 361 outpatients with acute bronchitis or severe cough (Kemmerich 2007). The combination successfully reduced coughing fits by 67.1% compared to 51.3% on days 7 to 9 ($P < 0.0001$). The active group reported a 50% reduction in coughing on average 2 days earlier than the placebo group. The singular effect of thyme in this formula, however, is uncertain.

A postmarketing surveillance study investigated the effects of a different mixture containing thyme and ivy as a syrup (Bronchipret Saft) in 1234 children and adolescents with acute bronchitis (Marzian 2007). Coughing fits reduced by 81.3% by day 10 and the responder rates for the various age groups were 92.0 to 96.5%. The singular effect of thyme in this formula however is uncertain.

Thyme is approved by Commission E in the treatment of bronchitis, whooping cough and upper respiratory tract catarrh (Blumenthal et al 2000).

Candida vaginitis — *in combination*

A prospective, single-blind, two-stage clinical trial involving 64 women found that a topical cream containing garlic and thyme was as effective as clotrimazole treatment for candidal vaginitis (Bahadoran et al 2010). Treatment was used for 7 nights by both groups. Clinical symptoms were decreased by at least 50% in more than 83% of women using the herbal cream compared to 92% in the clotrimazole group, but the difference was not significantly different.

Diarrhoea

The astringent properties of thyme provides a theoretical basis for its application in this condition.

Gastritis and dyspepsia

The bitter principles present in the herb and its antispasmodic activity provide a theoretical basis for its use in these conditions.

Skin disinfection (topical use)

Thyme extract has been used topically for infection control in minor wounds. The herb's antimicrobial and astringent activity provides a theoretical basis for this use.

OTHER USES

Traditionally, it has been used to aid in labour and delivery, promote menstruation and topically for warts and inflamed swellings (Fisher & Painter

1996). It has also been used to treat enuresis in children.

DOSAGE RANGE

Internal use

- Fluid extract (1 : 1): 1–2 mL up to three times a day.
- Fluid extract (1 : 2): 15–40 mL/week.
- Tincture (1 : 5): 2–6 mL three times daily.
- Infusion of dried herb: 1–4 g three times daily.

External use

- 5% infusion used as a compress.

It has been used together with garlic in a vaginal cream to treat vaginitis caused by *Candida* infection; however, the research report does not specify the concentration of these ingredients (Bahadoran et al 2010).

ADVERSE REACTIONS

The volatile oil is considered an irritant topically and can cause nausea and vomiting, headache, dizziness, convulsions, cardiac or respiratory arrest if taken internally (Newell et al 1996). As such, the crude herb is considered far safer.

Contact dermatitis reactions have been reported with topical use (Lorenzi et al 1995).

SIGNIFICANT INTERACTIONS

Thyme may induce enzymes in phase one and two detoxification in the liver (Sasaki et al 2005). The clinical significance of this is unknown.

CONTRAINDICATIONS AND PRECAUTIONS

Contraindicated in people who are allergic to the Lamiaceae (Labiatae) family of plants. Other cautions are gastritis, enterocolitis and congestive heart failure (Ernst et al 2001).

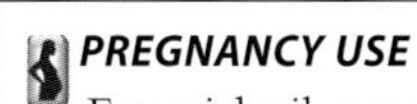

PREGNANCY USE

Essential oil not recommended in pregnancy.

PATIENTS' FAQs

What will this herb do for me?

When taken internally, thyme is used to treat bronchitis, symptoms of the common cold, diarrhoea and dyspepsia. It is also used as an antiseptic gargle for sore throats and can be diluted and applied externally to minor wounds.

Thyme has strong antibacterial activity and antifungal actions and is used as a treatment for common infections such as bronchitis and upper respiratory tract infections. It is also used as a food preservative, for relieving symptoms of dyspepsia and diarrhoea.

When will it start to work?

The lack of human studies for this herb make it difficult to determine when effects will start to occur.

Are there any safety issues?

Thyme should not be used by people allergic to the Lamiaceae (Labiatae) family of plants or in pregnancy, and it should be used with caution in gastritis, enterocolitis and congestive heart failure.

Practice points/Patient counselling

- Thyme is an aromatic and medicinal plant that has been used in traditional medicine, in phytopharmaceutical preparations, as a food preservative, and as an aromatic ingredient.
- Although thyme is used as a cooking spice, it is also used medicinally to treat common upper respiratory tract infections, coughs, bronchitis and asthma, dyspepsia and diarrhoea.
- Thyme extract is used as a gargle for pharyngitis or applied topically (5% dilution) as a compress to wounds due to its antimicrobial and astringent activities.
- Thyme has significant antibacterial and antifungal activity against a wide range of microorganisms. Preliminary evidence suggests activity against azole-resistant candida and multidrug resistant strains of *Staphylococcus, Enterococcus, Escherichia* and *Pseudomonas* genus.
- Thyme has not been significantly investigated in controlled trials, so much information is based on traditional use or evidence of activity.
- Thyme has antispasmodic, antimicrobial, antitussive, astringent and anthelmintic activities as demonstrated in vitro or in animal studies.

REFERENCES

Ahmad A et al. Reversal of efflux mediated antifungal resistance underlies synergistic activity of two monoterpenes with fluconazole. Eur J Pharm Sci 48.1–2 (2013): 80–86.

Bahadoran P et al. Investigating the therapeutic effect of vaginal cream containing garlic and thyme compared to clotrimazole cream for the treatment of mycotic vaginitis. Iran J Nurs Midwifery Res. Dec; 15 (Suppl 1) (2010): 343–349.

Behnia M et al. Inhibitory effects of Iranian Thymus vulgaris extracts on in vitro growth of Entamoeba histolytica. Korean J Parasitol. 46.3 (2008): 153–156.

Bennis S et al. Surface alteration of Saccharomyces cerevisiae induced by thymol and eugenol. Lett Appl Microbiol 38.6 (2004): 454–458.

Blumenthal M et al. (eds). Herbal medicine: expanded Commission E monographs. Austin, TX: Integrative Medicine Communications, 2000.

Braga PC et al. Antioxidant potential of thymol determined by chemiluminescence inhibition in human neutrophils and cell-free systems. Pharmacology 76.2 (2006a): 61–68.

Braga PC et al. Anti-inflammatory activity of thymol: inhibitory effect on the release of human neutrophil elastase. Pharmacology 77.3 (2006b): 130–136.

Braga PC et al. Eugenol and thymol, alone or in combination, induce morphological alterations in the envelope of Candida albicans. Fitoterapia 78.6 (2007a): 396–400.

Braga PC et al. Inhibitory activity of thymol against the formation and viability of Candida albicans hyphae. Mycoses 50.6 (2007b): 502–506.

Bukovska A et al. Effects of a combination of thyme and oregano essential oils on TNBS-induced colitis in mice. Mediators Inflamm (2007): 23296.

Burt SA et al. Increase in activity of essential oil components carvacrol and thymol against Escherichia coli O157:H7 by addition of food stabilizers. J Food Prot 68.5 (2005): 919–926.

Burt SA et al. Carvacrol induces heat shock protein 60 and inhibits synthesis of flagellin in Escherichia coli O157:H7. Appl Environ Microbiol 73.14 (2007): 4484–4490.

Centeno S et al. Antifungal activity of extracts of Rosmarinus officinalis and Thymus vulgaris against Aspergillus flavus and A. ochraceus. Pak J Biol Sci. 13.9 (2010): 452–5.
Chizzola R, Michitsch H, Franz C. Antioxidative properties of Thymus vulgaris leaves: comparison of different extracts and essential oil chemotypes. J Agric Food Chem 56.16 (2008): 6897–6904.
Chohan M et al. An investigation of the relationship between the anti-inflammatory activity, polyphenolic content, and antioxidant activities of cooked and in vitro digested culinary herbs. Oxid Med Cell Longev. (2012): 627843.
Duke JA. Dr Duke's phytochemical and ethnobotanical databases. US Department of Agriculture–Agricultural Research Service–National Germplasm Resources Laboratory. Beltsville Agricultural Research Center, Beltsville, MD. Online. Available: www.ars-grin.gov/duke 9 June 2003.
El-Nekeety AA et al. Antioxidant properties of Thymus vulgaris oil against aflatoxin-induce oxidative stress in male rats. Toxicon. 57.(7–8) (2011): 984–991.
Engelbertz J et al. Thyme extract, but not thymol, inhibits endothelin-induced contractions of isolated rat trachea. Planta Med 74.12 (2008): 1436–1440.
Ernst E et al. Acute bronchitis: effectiveness of Sinupret. Comparative study with common expectorants in 3,187 patients. Fortschr Med 115.11 (1997): 52–53.
Ernst E et al. The desktop guide to complementary and alternative medicine: An evidence-based approach. St Louis: Mosby, 2001.
Esmaeili D, Mobarez AM, Tohidpour A. Anti-helicobacter pylori activities of shoya powder and essential oils of thymus vulgaris and eucalyptus globulus. Open Microbiol J. 6 (2012):65–69.
Fabian D et al. Essential oils — their antimicrobial activity against Escherichia coli and effect on intestinal cell viability. Toxicol In Vitro 20.8 (2006): 1435–1445.
Fachini-Queiroz FC et al. Effects of Thymol and Carvacrol, Constituents of Thymus vulgaris L. Essential oil, on the Inflammatory Response. Evid Based Complement Alternat Med. (2012): 657026.
Fisher C, Painter G. Materia Medica for the Southern Hemisphere. Auckland: Fisher-Painter Publishers, 1996.
Friedman M, Henika PR, Mandrell RE. Bactericidal activities of plant essential oils and some of their isolated constituents against Campylobacter jejuni, Escherichia coli, Listeria monocytogenes, and Salmonella enterica. J Food Prot 65.10 (2002): 1545–1560.
Fujita M et al. Remarkable synergies between baicalein and tetracycline, and baicalein and beta-lactams against methicillin-resistant Staphylococcus aureus. Microbiol Immunol 49.4 (2005): 391–396.
Gruenwald J et al. Efficacy and tolerability of a fixed combination of thyme and primrose root in patients with acute bronchitis. A double-blind, randomized, placebo-controlled clinical trial. Arzneimittelforschung 55.11 (2005): 669–676.
Gruenwald J et al. Evaluation of the non-inferiority of a fixed combination of thyme fluid and primrose root extract in comparison to a fixed combination of thyme fluid extract and primrose root tincture in patients with acute bronchitis. A single-blind, randomized, bi-centric clinical trial. Arzneimittelforschung 56.8 (2006): 574–581.
Hammad M et al. Inhibition of Streptococcus mutans adhesion to buccal epithelial cells by an aqueous extract of Thymus vulgaris. Int J Dent Hyg 5.4 (2007): 232–235.
Kalemba D, Kunicka A. Antibacterial and antifungal properties of essential oils. Curr Med Chem 10.10 (2003): 813–829.
Kavanaugh NL, Ribbeck K. Selected antimicrobial essential oils eradicate Pseudomonas spp. and Staphylococcus aureus biofilms. Appl Environ Microbiol. 78.11 (2012): 4057–4061.
Kemmerich B. Evaluation of efficacy and tolerability of a fixed combination of dry extracts of thyme herb and primrose root in adults suffering from acute bronchitis with productive cough. A prospective, double-blind, placebo-controlled multicentre clinical trial. Arzneimittelforschung 57.9 (2007): 607–615.
Koch C et al. Inhibitory effect of essential oils against herpes simplex virus type 2. Phytomedicine 15.1–2 (2007): 71–78.
Lee S et al. Identification of volatile components in basil (Ocimum basilicum L.) and thyme leaves (Thymus vulgaris L.) and their antioxidant properties. Food Chem 91 (2005): 131–137.
Lorenzi S et al. Allergic contact dermatitis due to thymol. Contact Dermatitis 33.6 (1995): 439–440.
Marzian O. Treatment of acute bronchitis in children and adolescents. Non-interventional postmarketing surveillance study confirms the benefit and safety of a syrup made of extracts from thyme and ivy leaves. MMW Fortschr Med 149.11 (2007): 69–74.
Naemura A et al. Long-term intake of rosemary and common thyme herbs inhibits experimental thrombosis without prolongation of bleeding time. Thromb Res 122.4 (2008): 517–522.
Newell CA et al. Herbal medicines: a guide for health care professionals. London: The Pharmaceutical Press, 1996.
Nolkemper S et al. Antiviral effect of aqueous extracts from species of the Lamiaceae family against Herpes simplex virus type 1 and type 2 in vitro. Planta Med 72.15 (2006): 1378–1382.
Rana P, Soni G. Antioxidant potential of thyme extract: alleviation of N-nitrosodiethylamine-induced oxidative stress. Hum Exp Toxicol 27.3 (2008): 215–221.
Sasaki K et al. Thyme (Thymus vulgaris L.) leaves and its constituents increase the activities of xenobiotic-metabolizing enzymes in mouse liver. J Med Food 8.2 (2005): 184–189.
Schelz Z et al. Antimicrobial and antiplasmid activities of essential oils. Fitoterapia 77.4 (2006): 279–285.
Schmidt E et al Chemical composition, olfactory analysis and antibacterial activity of Thymus vulgaris chemotypes geraniol, 4-thujanol/ terpinen-4-ol, thymol and linalool cultivated in southern France. Nat Prod Commun 7.8 (2012): 1095–1098.
Schnitzler P et al. Susceptibility of drug-resistant clinical herpes simplex virus type 1 strains to essential oils of ginger, thyme, hyssop, and sandalwood. Antimicrob Agents Chemother 51.5 (2007): 1859–1862.
Sertel S et al. Cytotoxicity of Thymus vulgaris essential oil towards human oral cavity squamous cell carcinoma. Anticancer Res. 31.1 (2011): 81–87.
Shati AA, Elsaid FG. Effects of water extracts of thyme (Thymus vulgaris) and ginger (Zingiber officinale Roscoe) on alcohol abuse. Food Chem Toxicol. 47.8 (2009): 1945–1949.
Sienkiewicz M et al Antibacterial activity of thyme and lavender essential oils. Med Chem 7.6 (2011): 674–689.
Sienkiewicz M et al. The antimicrobial activity of thyme essential oil against multidrug resistant clinical bacterial strains. Microb Drug Resist. 18.2 (2012): 137–148.
Solomakos N et al. The antimicrobial effect of thyme essential oil, nisin, and their combination against Listeria monocytogenes in minced beef during refrigerated storage. Food Microbiol 25.1 (2008): 120–127.
Tabak M et al. In vitro inhibition of Helicobacter pylori by extracts of thyme. J Appl Bacteriol 80.6 (1996): 667–672.
Taherian AA et al. Antinociceptive effects of hydroalcoholic extract of Thymus vulgaris. Pak J Pharm Sci. 22.1 (2009): 83–89.
Tohidpour A et al. Antibacterial effect of essential oils from two medicinal plants against Methicillin-resistant Staphylococcus aureus(MRSA). Phytomed. 17.2 (2010):142–145.
Tsai ML et al. Antimicrobial, antioxidant, and anti-inflammatory activities of essential oils from five selected herbs. Biosci Biotechnol Biochem. 75.10 (2011): 1977–1983.
Warnke PH et al. The battle against multi-resistant strains: Renaissance of antimicrobial essential oils as a promising force to fight hospital-acquired infections. J Craniomaxillofac Surg. .7 (2009): 392–397.
Wienkotter N et al. The effect of thyme extract on beta2-receptors and mucociliary clearance. Planta Med 73.7 (2007): 629–635.
World Health Organization Department of Essential Drugs and Medicines Policy (EDM). Essential drugs and medicines policy: Herba Thymi. Geneva: WHO, 2003, pp 259–66.
Zu Y et al. Activities of ten essential oils towards Propionibacterium acnes and PC-3, A-549 and MCF-7 cancer cells. Molecules 15.5 (2010): 3200–3210.

Tribulus

HISTORICAL NOTE Widely distributed in the Mediterranean region, Middle East and southern Africa, tribulus is an important plant used in traditional Ayurvedic, Arabic and Chinese medicine. Different parts of the tribulus plant are used to treat a variety of conditions, such as cough, colicky spasms, diarrhoea, haemorrhage, cardiovascular disease, rheumatic pain, gout, various kidney disorders, including kidney stones, and as an insect repellent.

COMMON NAME

Tribulus

OTHER NAMES

Al-gutub, cat's-head, devil's-thorn, devil's-weed, goathead, puncture vine, qutiba

BOTANICAL NAME/FAMILY

Tribulus terrestris (family Zygophyllaceae)

PLANT PARTS USED

Leaf or fruit

CHEMICAL COMPONENTS

Different parts of the plant contain different constituents in varying ratios. Chemical constituents extracted from tribulus include phenolic compounds, saponins, sterols and alkaloids (Hammoda et al 2013). Overall, the steroidal saponin content is considered the most important and includes constituents such as protodioscin, diosgenin, yamogenin, epismilagenin, tigogenin, neotigogenin, gitogenin and neogitogenin (Miles et al 1994). New steroidal saponins continue to be isolated from extracts of tribulus fruit (Chen et al 2012, Hammoda et al 2013, Huang et al 2003, Su et al 2008, 2009, Xu et al 2008, Zhangh et al 2011). The significance of this is yet to be determined. Beta-sitosterol, vitamin C, potassium and calcium are also found in the herb (Li et al 1998). Two major alkaloids have been identified: harmane and norharmane (Bourke et al 1992).

Of the steroidal saponins, protodioscin is considered the chief constituent responsible for the plant's effects on libido and sexual functioning. Preliminary observations suggest that *Tribulus terrestris* grown in different soils does not consistently produce this constituent and considerable variations have been identified in commercial products (Ganzera et al 2001). Steroidal saponins consist of a furostanol- or spirostanol-based aglycone and an oligosaccharide attached to a steroid nucleus. Steroidal saponins are very common in the plant kingdom and are natural components in many foods, such as asparagus, garlic and oats.

MAIN ACTIONS

Tribulus has not undergone significant clinical investigation; therefore, evidence of activity primarily derives from animal and in vitro studies. Additionally, some studies have investigated the pharmacological effects of the isolated saponin content.

Increases libido and enhances sexual function

Administration of tribulus extracts to animals improves libido and increases sexual behaviour and spermatogenesis.

Results from a 2002 animal study have produced positive results suggestive of aphrodisiac activity (Gauthaman et al 2002). The study compared the effects of subcutaneous testosterone, an orally administered tribulus extract containing protodioscin (45% dry weight) or placebo over 8 weeks in castrated rodents. Both testosterone and tribulus treatments significantly improved sexual behaviour compared with controls, although testosterone was the more effective treatment.

A follow-up study by the same research team added further data (Gauthaman et al 2003). In this study, rats were treated with 2.5, 5 and 10 mg/kg once daily for 8 weeks. The results showed a considerable increase in sexual behaviour and slight weight gain compared to controls. Interestingly, the results were more pronounced at the lower dose range.

Tribulus standardised to 20% saponins was administered to sexually sluggish male rats (50 mg/kg body weight and 100 mg/kg body weight). A dose-dependent improvement in sexual behaviour was observed with the treatment as characterised by an increase in mount frequency, intromission frequency and penile erection index, as well as a decrease in mount latency, intromission latency and ejaculatory latency. The enhancement of sexual behaviour was more prominent on chronic administration of tribulus (Singh et al 2012).

The exact mechanism by which tribulus influences sexual behaviour is not known, but increasing androgenic status and nitric oxide (NO) release have been proposed to be chiefly responsible (Gauthaman et al 2002). More specifically, some reports have suggested that increases in dehydroepiandrosterone (DHEA) and testosterone are possible (Adimoelja 2000, Gauthaman et al 2002). The constituent protodioscin is considered the most important for this action and has been reported to directly convert to DHEA (McKay 2004). Additionally, ex vivo tests have observed proerectile effects with protodioscin due to increased release of NO from the endothelium and nitronergic nerve endings (Adaikan et al 2000). Hormonal effects of tribulus were tested in primates, rabbits and rats. Administration of tribulus demonstrated a statistically significant increase in testosterone and DHEA levels in the primates, an increase of these hormones in rabbits, but very little increase in rats (Gauthaman & Ganesan 2008). Animal studies show that chronic administration more favourably enhances sexual function compared with acute dosing (Singh et al 2012).

Whether these hormonal effects are seen in humans remains unclear. One study investigated the influence of tribulus extract on androgen metabolism in 21 healthy 20–36-year-old men. Testosterone, androstenedione and luteinising hormone (LH) levels in the serum were measured 24 hours before supplementation, and at 24, 72, 240, 408 and 576 hours after supplementation. No significant differences were observed between the supplemented groups at two different concentrations (10 mg or 20 mg/kg body weight daily) and placebo (Neychev & Mitev 2005). Longer clinical trials measuring androgen-enhancing activity of tribulus are required to validate these actions.

Hormone modulation

Saponins from tribulus appear to increase follicle-stimulating hormone (FSH) in women, which in turn increases levels of oestradiol (Mills & Bone 2000). The presence of steroidal saponins could be responsible for intrinsic hormonal activity by directly stimulating female endocrine-sensitive tissues; however, studies in ovariectomised rats showed that this plant was not able to stimulate endocrine-sensitive tissues, including the uterus and vagina, indicating a lack of oestrogenic activity in vivo (Mazaro-Costa et al 2010). Comparatively, a luteinising effect of tribulus has been demonstrated in polycystic ovaries in vivo. After supplementation with tribulus, ovarian cysts significantly decreased and the number of corpora lutea and primary and secondary follicles significantly increased compared with placebo in a rat model. The results suggest that tribulus may also increase LH (Dehghan et al 2012).

Antimicrobial

Antimicrobial activity of organic and aqueous extracts from fruits, leaves and roots of *Tribulus terrestris* were tested. The most active extract against both Gram-negative and Gram-positive bacteria was ethanol extract of the fruits against *Bacillus subtilis, Bacillus cereus, Corynebacterium diphtheriae* and *Proteus vulgaris*. The strongest antifungal activity was against *Candida albicans* (Al-Bayati & Al-Mola 2008). Another study extracted and identified two saponins from tribulus, and demonstrated potent antifungal activity against *C. albicans*. Saponins appear to exert their antifungal action by damaging the cell membrane, causing leakage of cellular material. They may also inhibit fungal hyphae (Zhang et al 2006). More recently, tribulus fruiting body extract has been used in the process of synthesising silver nanoparticles — a novel nanotechnology approach. The antibacterial property of synthesised nanoparticles was observed in multidrug-resistant bacteria, including *Streptococcus pyogenes, Pseudomonas aeruginosa, Escherichia coli, Bacillus subtilis* and *Staphylococcus aureus* (Gopinath et al 2012).

Diuretic

A large oral dose of 5 g/kg tribulus was shown to have greater diuretic activity than frusemide 120 mg/kg in vivo (Al Ali et al 2003). The dose required for this effect does not appear to be clinically practical.

Urolithic

With regard to kidney stones, tribulus has been found to decrease the amount of urinary oxalate in rats (Sangeeta et al 1994) and produce significant dose-dependent protection against experimentally induced uroliths in animal studies (Anand et al 1994, Sangeeta et al 1994). Experimental studies further found that tribulus was effective in preventing the deposition of crystals on glass beads in the urinary bladder of rats, dissolving phosphate-type calculi in an in vitro model, and dissolving uric acid and cystine stones to some extent (Prasad et al 2007). In vitro studies using human urine suggest that the diuretic properties of tribulus may be the most crucial mechanism for preventing urinary stone formation (Joshi et al 2005). More recent research demonstrated that extract of dried tribulus exhibited a concentration-dependent inhibition on the growth of calcium oxalate crystals. In addition, when epithelial renal cells were injured by exposure to oxalate for 72 hours, tribulus extract prevented cell injury in a dose-dependent manner. These results suggest that tribulus may not only prevent growth of calcium oxalate crystals, but also has a cytoprotective role (Aggarwal et al 2010).

Antispasmodic

A dose-dependent antispasmodic activity causing a significant decrease in peristaltic movements has been demonstrated with the isolated saponin content of tribulus (Arcasoy et al 1998).

Cardioprotective activity

Tribulus is shown to have some cardioprotective actions (Ojha et al 2008). A Chinese report of successful treatment of angina pectoris with the saponin content of tribulus suggests that the preparation dilates coronary arteries and improves coronary circulation (Wang et al 1990). A triterpene saponin of tribulus may play a role in cardiocyte survival during chemical hypoxia–ischaemia, as demonstrated in vitro (Sun et al 2008).

In another study 10 mg/kg/day of the aqueous extract of the fruit has shown antihypertensive effects in an animal trial when compared to control. The authors concluded that effects are possibly due to inhibition of angiotensin-converting enzyme activity (Sharifi et al 2003). More recent research demonstrates that the antihypertensive effect appears to result from a direct arterial smooth-muscle relaxation, possibly involving NO release and membrane hyperpolarisation (Phillips et al 2006). Tribulus saponins not only lowered serum lipidaemia, but also relieved left ventricular remodelling, and improved cardiac function in the early stage after myocardial infarct in a hyperlipidaemia mouse model (Guo et al 2007). The mechanism of action is suggested to be a reduction in cardiac muscle cell apoptosis by regulating protein expressions (Guo et al 2006).

A study undertaken in rabbits found tribulus significantly lowered serum lipid profiles and decreased endothelial cellular surface damage and rupture. Results also suggested tribulus may partially repair the endothelial dysfunction resulting from hyperlipidaemia (Tuncer et al 2009).

OTHER ACTIONS

Experiments with healthy mice have found that *Tribulus terrestris* significantly inhibits gluconeogenesis, influences glycometabolism and reduces triglyceride and total cholesterol levels (Li et al 2001).

Tribulus demonstrates some protection against oxidative stress in rats with induced diabetes (Amin et al 2006) and the saponins are found to have a hypoglycaemic action.

An in vitro test has also identified cyclooxygenase-2 inhibition activity (Hong et al 2002), suggesting possible anti-inflammatory actions. An animal study using a percolated extract of the fruits of tribulus at a dose of 100 mg/kg showed a significant analgesic effect compared to the control group with a lower gastric ulcerogenicity than indomethacin (Heidari et al 2007). Diabetic rats exhibited significant hyperalgesia after treatment with standardised aqueous extract of tribulus, through modulation of oxidative stress and inflammatory cytokine release (Ranjithkumar et al 2013). Two isolated constituents, tribulosin and beta-sitosterol-D-glucoside, have shown anthelminthic activity in vitro against *Caenorhabditis elegans* (Deepak et al 2002).

Protection against mercury-induced nephrotoxicity was demonstrated with 7 days' administration of tribulus fruit extract (6 mg/kg body weight) in an animal study (Kavitha & Jagadeesan 2006).

CLINICAL USE

Evaluation of the efficacy of tribulus is hampered by the lack of quality clinical trials. The trials that are available tend to use small sample sizes, lack placebo groups and often test a combination of herbs. Nonetheless, the evidence so far is promising and warrants larger controlled trials using tribulus independently of other herbal and nutritional supplements.

Increases libido and enhances sexual function

The observed pharmacological effects on androgen status and results from animal models indicating an aphrodisiac activity (Gauthaman et al 2002) and increase in sexual behaviour (Gauthaman et al 2003; Singh et al 2012) provide a theoretical basis for the use of tribulus. Unfortunately, clinical trials using stand-alone tribulus treatment have not been published to determine its effects in humans.

IN COMBINATION

A formula Tradamixina (containing 150 mg of alga *Ecklonia bicyclis*, 396 mg of *Tribulus terrestris* and 144 mg of D-glucosamine and *N*-acetyl-D-glucosamine per capsule) was tested in a double-blind randomised controlled trial involving 70 male patients experiencing low libido. The formula was taken as two capsules daily and compared to tadalafil 5 mg/daily. After 2 months the combination product produced a significant increase in serum total testosterone levels (230 ± 18 ng/dL vs 671 ± 14 ng/dL) and free testosterone levels (56 ± 2.4 pg/mL vs 120 ± 3.9 pg/mL) ($P < 0.005$), while those taking tadalafil had a small non-significant increase in both markers. Both groups showed improved scores in the International Index of Erectile Function (IIEF) and Sexual Quality of Life Questionnaire-Male. The combination formula improved libido in aged males without the side effects of tadalafil (Iacono et al 2012a).

Erectile dysfunction

IN COMBINATION

A mixture of nine oriental herbs, including tribulus, was evaluated using both in vitro and in vivo experiments on laboratory animals and demonstrated an improvement in sexual activity and erectile function (Park 2006). The same formula was tested in 150 men with erectile dysfunction in an observational study. The formulation was administered as two capsules daily for 2 months. IIEF scores increased in the treated group by 78% in the mild erectile dysfunction group, 80% in the moderate erectile dysfunction group, and 108% in the severe erectile dysfunction group compared with the baseline. The mean IIEF scores amongst all patients indicated a significant improved in erectile dysfunction after 2 months (Iacono et al 2011).

Ergogenic aid

Tribulus has been touted as a natural anabolic supplement or ergogenic aid, capable of producing large gains in strength and lean muscle mass in 5–28 days. The observed pharmacological effects on androgen status provide a theoretical basis for this activity; however, clinical trials have produced disappointing results.

A small, randomised, placebo-controlled study found that treatment with tribulus (3.21 mg/kg body weight daily) had no effects on body composition and exercise performance in resistance-trained men after 8 weeks (Antonio et al 2000). The study has been criticised by some athletes, as the dose of tribulus tested was very low and not indicative of the doses used in real life. A more recent randomised controlled trial by Rogerson et al (2007) compared the effects of tribulus extract (450 mg/day) to placebo in 22 Australian elite male rugby league players during their preseason training period. The double study was conducted over 5 weeks and found that muscular strength and fat-free mass increased significantly in both groups, with no advantage seen for tribulus treatment. Additionally, no significant differences were seen for urinary testosterone/epitestosterone ratio compared with placebo. Once again, the trial has been criticised as using subtherapeutic doses which do not reflect manufacturer recommendations or current use.

A study undertaken in two females found tribulus 500 mg three times daily for 2 days had no impact on endogenous testosterone metabolism and was well below the cut-off values defined by the World Anti-Doping Agency (Saudan et al 2008).

Menopausal symptoms

Saponins from tribulus appear to increase FSH in women, which in turn increases levels of oestradiol (Mills & Bone 2000). The primary site of action of steroidal saponins is probably the hypothalamus (Trickey 1998). In postmenopausal women, steroidal saponin-containing herbs like tribulus have been used to alleviate oestrogen withdrawal symptoms. Clinical studies are unavailable to determine whether the effect is significant.

Kidney stones

A human trial was conducted with a herbal combination containing *Tribulus terrestris* and another Ayurvedic herb, *Bergenia ligulata*, in the treatment of 14 patients with renal calculi and 16 patients with ureteric calculi. A total of 28.57% of patients with renal calculi and 75% patients with ureteric calculi passed their calculi completely and in other patients, there was a marked or partial expulsion of calculi along with changes in the shapes and sizes of calculi (Prasad et al 2007). The role of tribulus in achieving these results is unknown.

Benign prostatic hyperplasia (BPH)

Tribulus has been included in combination formulas for the relief of symptoms of BPH. Standardised extracts of *Murraya koenigii* and *Tribulus terrestris* leaves were compared against tamsulosin in a double-blind randomised controlled trial involving 46 men >50 years. Patients received either the plant drug in a dose of two capsules twice daily or tamsulosin 400 mcg once daily for 12 weeks with two interim follow-up visits at the end of 4 and 8 weeks. The exact dose of the herbs was not disclosed. Median International Prostate Symptom Score (IPSS) declined from 17.0 (12.0–19.0) to 9.0 (5.0–13.0) with the plant drug and from 14.0 (11.0–18.0) to 8.0 (6.0–13.0) with tamsulosin after 12 weeks of treatment. The decline was individually significant in both groups (both $P < 0.001$). The herbal combination proved effective for the symptomatic treatment of BPH; however, larger trials beyond 12 weeks are required to confirm these results (Sengupta et al 2011).

The compound Tradamixina plus *Serenoa repens* (80 mg of alga *Ecklonia bicyclis*, 100 mg of *Tribulus terrestris* and 100 mg of D-glucosamine and *N*-acetyl-D-glucosamine plus 320 mg of *Serenoa repens*) was administered daily for 2 months in 100 patients with lower urinary tract symptoms or BPH. Results showed a statistically significant difference in IPSS scores, quality of life index and BPH impact index. A decrease in overall prostate-specific antigen scores was also observed (Iacono et al 2012b).

It remains to be determined how much of a contribution tribulus makes in these clinical trials.

OTHER USES

Traditionally, the acidic fruits are thought to be cooling and are used for painful micturition, urinary disorders, kidney stone prevention and impotence, whereas the leaves are thought to possess tonic, diuretic and anti-inflammatory properties and are used to increase menstrual flow. Interestingly, preliminary research into the pharmacological actions of tribulus or its constituents provides some support for several of these uses.

DOSAGE RANGE

In Australia, preparations containing both the fruit and the root are available that are standardised to saponin content. As no clinical studies are available, the manufacturers' recommended dose is included here, which is 2–30 g/day.

- Leaf: 750–1500 mg/day of extract standardised to contain 45% protodioscin.

TOXICITY

Although toxicity levels in humans are not known, extensive grazing on tribulus by sheep produces a syndrome known as 'staggers', which is characterised by nervous and muscular locomotor disturbances (Bourke 1984). Outbreaks are repeatedly associated with drought periods during which sheep graze on large areas of *Tribulus terrestris* for many months at a time (Bourke 1995, Glastonbury et al 1984). Investigation with isolated harmane and norharmane found naturally in tribulus has found these constituents to be responsible for the 'staggers' syndrome (Bourke et al 1992).

Hepatogenous photosensitivity has also been reported among sheep grazing on *Tribulus terrestris* for long periods (Bourke 1984, Glastonbury et al 1984, McDonough et al 1994, Miles et al 1994, Tapia et al 1994, Wilkins et al 1996). A small animal study examined the clinical, laboratory and pathological findings of this disease in sheep and concluded that tribulus was responsible for hepatogenous photosensitivity (Aslani et al 2003). Laboratory and pathology tests found significantly increased white blood cells, bilirubin, total serum protein and plasma fibrinogen, and histological findings showed crystalloid materials in the bile ducts with hepatocyte degeneration. A year later, the same research team found very similar results in goats (Aslani et al 2004).

A case report describes a male patient who developed hepatotoxicity, nephrotoxicity and neurotoxicity after consuming tribulus water in an attempt to pass kidney stones; he consumed 2 L over 2 days. The patient presented having had two episodes of seizure preceded by severe weakness in the lower limbs, malaise and poor appetite. His vital signs were normal except for rising blood pressure to 180/110 mmHg, very high serum aminotransferases and creatinine levels. The patient's symptoms resolved after he was treated with anticonvulsant, antihypertensive and prednisolone medication, and haemodialysis treatment (Talasaz et al 2010). This reaction has been described in animals grazing long term on tribulus; however no other reports have been described relating to toxicity in animal or human trials. This report did not detail the exact quantity of tribulus taken, or how it was extracted. There was no testing performed to confirm the product had not been adulterated.

ADVERSE REACTIONS

Gastrointestinal disturbance may occur in sensitive individuals due to the saponin content.

SIGNIFICANT INTERACTIONS

Controlled studies are not available and currently no interactions are known.

Practice points/Patient counselling

- Tribulus has been used traditionally in various parts of the world to treat colicky spasms, diarrhoea, cardiovascular disease and various kidney disorders, including kidney stones, and as an insect repellent.
- Tribulus has not undergone significant clinical testing, so much information is speculative and based on animal and test tube studies.
- Popular as an aphrodisiac, some research suggests that it increases levels of DHEA, testosterone and NO release, providing a theoretical basis for this activity. Until controlled studies are available, it is uncertain whether these effects are clinically significant.
- Tribulus is also popular among athletes as an ergogenic aid and to increase muscle strength; however, clinical studies using low-dose tribulus have not supported this use. Larger controlled studies testing higher doses for longer periods that are reflective of real-world use are required to determine its efficacy.
- Emerging studies propose it may have an impact in combination with other herbs for the treatment of BPH.

CONTRAINDICATIONS AND PRECAUTIONS

People with androgen-sensitive tumours should avoid use.

Warfarin

A herbal combination of *Tribulus terrestris, Panax ginseng* and *Avena sativa* was reported to significantly increase international normalised ratio values in two patients prescribed warfarin. It is unknown if the tribulus contributed to this effect (Turfan et al 2012).

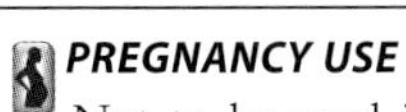

PREGNANCY USE

Not to be used in pregnancy.

PATIENTS' FAQs

What will this herb do for me?

Preliminary research suggests that this herb increases androgen levels and improves sexual function, but human studies are not available to confirm these effects.

When will it start to work?

This is unknown. Animal models indicate chronic use is more effective than short-term use.

Are there any safety issues?

Pregnant and lactating women and people with androgen-sensitive tumours should avoid use.

REFERENCES

Adaikan PG et al. Proerectile pharmacological effects of *Tribulus terrestris* extract on the rabbit corpus cavernosum. Ann Acad Med Singapore 29.1 (2000): 22–26.

Adimoelja A. Phytochemicals and the breakthrough of traditional herbs in the management of sexual dysfunctions. Int J Androl 23 (Suppl 2) (2000): 82–84.

Aggarwal A, et al (2010). Diminution of oxalate induced renal tubular epithelial cell injury and inhibition of calcium oxalate crystallization in vitro by aqueous extract of *Tribulus terrestris*. International Braz J Urol 36(4): 480–488; discussion 488, 489.

Al Ali M et al. *Tribulus terrestris*: preliminary study of its diuretic and contractile effects and comparison with *Zea mays*. J Ethnopharmacol 85.2–3 (2003): 257–260.

Al-Bayati FA, Al-Mola HF. Antibacterial and antifungal activities of different parts of *Tribulus terrestris* L. growing in Iraq. J Zhejiang Univ Sci B 9.2 (2008): 154–159.

Amin A et al. The protective effect of *Tribulus terrestris* in diabetes. Ann N Y Acad Sci 1084 (2006): 391–401.

Anand R et al. Activity of certain fractions of *Tribulus terrestris* fruits against experimentally induced urolithiasis in rats. Indian J Exp Biol 32.8 (1994): 548–552.

Antonio J et al. The effects of *Tribulus terrestris* on body composition and exercise performance in resistance-trained males. Int J Sport Nutr Exerc Metab 10.2 (2000): 208–215.

Arcasoy HB et al. Effect of *Tribulus terrestris* L. saponin mixture on some smooth muscle preparations: a preliminary study. Boll Chim Farm 137.11 (1998): 473–475.

Aslani MR et al. Experimental *Tribulus terrestris* poisoning in sheep: clinical, laboratory and pathological findings. Vet Res Commun 27.1 (2003): 53–62.

Aslani MR et al. Experimental *Tribulus terrestris* poisoning in goats. Small Ruminant Res 51 (2004): 261–267.

Bourke CA. Staggers in sheep associated with the ingestion of *Tribulus terrestris*. Aust Vet J 61.11 (1984): 360–363.

Bourke CA. The clinical differentiation of nervous and muscular locomotor disorders of sheep in Australia. Aust Vet J 72.6 (1995): 228–234.

Bourke CA, et al. Locomotor effects in sheep of alkaloids identified in Australian *Tribulus terrestris*. Aust Vet J 69.7 (1992): 163–165.

Deepak M et al. Tribulosin and beta-sitosterol-D-glucoside, the anthelmintic principles of *Tribulus terrestris*. Phytomedicine 9.8 (2002): 753–756.

Dehghan A, et al (2012). Alternative treatment of ovarian cysts with *Tribulus terrestris* extract: a rat model. Reproduction in domestic animals = Zuchthygiene 47(1): e12–15.

Ganzera M, et al. Determination of steroidal saponins in *Tribulus terrestris* by reversed-phase high-performance liquid chromatography and evaporative light scattering detection. J Pharm Sci 90.11 (2001): 1752–1758.

Gauthaman K, Ganesan AP. The hormonal effects of *Tribulus terrestris* and its role in the management of male erectile dysfunction — an evaluation using primates, rabbit and rat. Phytomedicine 15.1–2 (2008): 44–54.

Gauthaman K, et al. Aphrodisiac properties of *Tribulus terrestris* extract (Protodioscin) in normal and castrated rats. Life Sci 71.12 (2002): 1385–1396.

Gauthaman K et al. Sexual effects of puncturevine (*Tribulus terrestris*) extract (protodioscin): an evaluation using a rat model. J Altern Complement Med 9.2 (2003): 257–265.

Glastonbury JR et al. A syndrome of hepatogenous photosensitisation, resembling geeldikkop, in sheep grazing *Tribulus terrestris*. Aust Vet J 61.10 (1984): 314–3116.

Gopinath V, et al (2012). Biosynthesis of silver nanoparticles from *Tribulus terrestris* and its antimicrobial activity: a novel biological approach. Colloids and surfaces. B, Biointerfaces 96: 69–74.

Guo Y, et al. Effect of xinnao shutong capsule on cardiac muscle cell apoptosis and protein expressions of Bcl-2 and Bax in hyperlipidemia rats after myocardial infarction (article in Chinese, abstract in English). Zhongguo Zhong Xi Yi Jie He Za Zhi 26.6 (2006): 541–544.

Guo Y et al. Effects of *Tribuli* saponins on ventricular remodeling after myocardial infarction in hyperlipidemic rats. Am J Chin Med 35.2 (2007): 309–316.

Hammoda HM, et al (2013). Chemical constituents from *Tribulus terrestris* and screening of their antioxidant activity. Phytochemistry 92: 153–159.

Heidari MR et al. The analgesic effect of *Tribulus terrestris* extract and comparison of gastric ulcerogenicity of the extract with indomethacine in animal experiments. Ann N Y Acad Sci 1095 (2007): 418–427.

Hong CH et al. Evaluation of natural products on inhibition of inducible cyclooxygenase (COX-2) and nitric oxide synthase (iNOS) in cultured mouse macrophage cells. J Ethnopharmacol 83.1–2 (2002): 153–159.

Huang JW et al. Terrestrinins A and B, two new steroid saponins from *Tribulus terrestris*. J Asian Nat Prod Res 5.4 (2003): 285–290.

Iacono F, et al (2012a). Sexual asthenia: Tradamixina versus Tadalafil 5 mg daily. BMC surgery 12 Suppl 1: S23.
Iacono F, et al (2012b). Observational study: daily treatment with a new compound "Tradamixina" plus serenoa repens for two months improved the lower urinary tract symptoms. BMC surgery 12 Suppl 1: S22.
Joshi VS et al. Inhibition of the growth of urinary calcium hydrogen phosphate dihydrate crystals with aqueous extracts of *Tribulus terrestris* and *Bergenia ligulata*. Urol Res 33.2 (2005): 80–86.
Kavitha AV, Jagadeesan G. Role of *Tribulus terrestris* (Linn.) (Zygophyllacea) against mercuric chloride induced nephrotoxicity in mice, *Mus musculus* (Linn.). J Environ Biol 27.2 Suppl (2006): 397–400.
Li JX et al. Tribulusamide A and B, new hepatoprotective lignanamides from the fruits of *Tribulus terrestris*: indications of cytoprotective activity in murine hepatocyte culture. Planta Med 64.7 (1998): 628–631.
Li M et al. Effect of the decoction of *Tribulus terrestris* on mice gluconegenesis. Zhong Yao Cai 24.8 (2001): 586–588.
Mazaro-Costa R, et al (2010). Medicinal plants as alternative treatments for female sexual dysfunction: utopian vision or possible treatment in climacteric women? journal of sexual medicine 7(11): 3695–3714.
McDonough SP et al. Hepatogenous photosensitization of sheep in California associated with ingestion of *Tribulus terrestris* (puncture vine). J Vet Diagn Invest 6.3 (1994): 392–395.
McKay D (2004). Nutrients and botanicals for erectile dysfunction: examining the evidence. Alternative medicine review 9(1): 4–16.
Miles CO et al. Photosensitivity in South Africa. VII. Chemical composition of biliary crystals from a sheep with experimentally induced geeldikkop. Onderstepoort J Vet Res 61.3 (1994): 215–222.
Mills SB, Bone K. Principles and Practice of Phytotherapy: modern herbal medicine. Edinburgh: Churchill Livingstone, 2000.
Neychev VK, Mitev VI (2005). The aphrodisiac herb *Tribulus terrestris* does not influence the androgen production in young men. Journal of ethnopharmacology 101(1–3): 319–323.
Ojha SKNM et al. Chronic administration of *Tribulus terrestris* Linn. extract improves cardiac function and attenuates myocardial infarction in rats. International Journal of Pharmacology 4.1 (2008): 1–10.
Park SW. Effect of SA1, a herbal formulation, on sexual behavior and penile erection. Biol Pharm Bull 29.7 (2006): 1383–1386.
Phillips OA, et al. Antihypertensive and vasodilator effects of methanolic and aqueous extracts of *Tribulus terrestris* in rats. J Ethnopharmacol 104.3 (2006): 351–355.
Prasad KVSRGSD, Bharathi K. Herbal drugs in urolithiasis — a review. Pharmacognosy Reviews 1.1 (2007): 175–179.
Ranjithkumar R, et al (2013). Standardized aqueous *Tribulus terristris* (nerunjil) extract attenuates hyperalgesia in experimentally induced diabetic neuropathic pain model: role of oxidative stress and inflammatory mediators. Phytotherapy research 27:1646–1657.
Rogerson S et al. The effect of five weeks of *Tribulus terrestris* supplementation on muscle strength and body composition during preseason training in elite rugby league players. J Strength Cond Res 21.2 (2007): 348–353.
Sangeeta D et al. Effect of *Tribulus terrestris* on oxalate metabolism in rats. J Ethnopharmacol 44.2 (1994): 61–66.
Saudan C, et al (2008). Short term impact of *Tribulus terrestris* intake on doping control analysis of endogenous steroids. Forensic science international 178(1): e7–10.
Sengupta G, et al (2011). Comparison of *Murraya koenigii*- and *Tribulus terrestris*-based oral formulation versus tamsulosin in the treatment of benign prostatic hyperplasia in men aged >50 years: a double-blind, double-dummy, randomized controlled trial. Clinical therapeutics 33(12): 1943–1952.
Sharifi AM, et al. Study of antihypertensive mechanism of *Tribulus terrestris* in 2K1C hypertensive rats: role of tissue ACE activity. Life Sci 73.23 (2003): 2963–2971.
Singh S, et al (2012). Evaluation of the aphrodisiac activity of *Tribulus terrestris* Linn. in sexually sluggish male albino rats. Journal of pharmacology & pharmacotherapeutics 3(1): 43–47.
Su L et al. Steroidal saponins from *Tribulus terrestris*. Steroids 74.4–5 (2008): 399–403.
Su L et al. Two new steroidal saponins from *Tribulus terrestris*. J Asian Nat Prod Res 11.1 (2009): 38–43.
Sun W, et al. A triterpene saponin from *Tribulus terrestris* attenuates apoptosis in cardiocyte via activating PKC signalling transduction pathway. J Asian Nat Prod Res 10.1–2 (2008): 39–48.
Talasaz AH, et al (2010). *Tribulus terrestris*-induced severe nephrotoxicity in a young healthy male. Nephrology, dialysis, transplantation 25(11): 3792–3793.
Tapia MO, et al. An outbreak of hepatogenous photosensitization in sheep grazing *Tribulus terrestris* in Argentina. Vet Hum Toxicol 36.4 (1994): 311–3113.
Trickey R. Women, hormones & the menstrual cycle. St Leonards, NSW, Australia: Allen & Unwin, 1998.
Tuncer MA, et al. (2009). Influence of *Tribulus terrestris* extract on lipid profile and endothelial structure in developing atherosclerotic lesions in the aorta of rabbits on a high-cholesterol diet. Acta histochemica 111(6): 488–500.
Turfan M, et al (2012). [A sudden rise in INR due to combination of *Tribulus terrestris*, *Avena sativa*, and *Panax ginseng* (*Clavis panax*)]. Turk Kardiyoloji Dernegi arsivi : Turk Kardiyoloji Derneginin yayin organidir 40(3): 259–261.
Wang B, et al. 406 cases of angina pectoris in coronary heart disease treated with saponin of *Tribulus terrestris*. Zhong Xi Yi Jie He Za Zhi 10.2 (1990): 68, 85–87.
Wilkins AL et al. Photosensitivity in South Africa. IX. Structure elucidation of a beta-glucosidase-treated saponin from *Tribulus terrestris*, and the identification of saponin chemotypes of South African *T. terrestris*. Onderstepoort J Vet Res 63.4 (1996): 327–334.
Xu TH et al. Two new furostanol saponins from *Tribulus terrestris* L. J Asian Nat Prod Res 10.5–6 (2008): 419–423.
Zhang JD, et al. (2006). Antifungal activities and action mechanisms of compounds from *Tribulus terrestris* L. Journal of ethnopharmacology 103(1): 76–84.

Tulsi

HISTORICAL NOTE The tulsi plant is regarded by Hindus as the holiest of all plants and within Ayurveda, tulsi is known as 'The Incomparable One', 'Mother Medicine of Nature', and 'The Queen of Herbs' (Singh et al 2010). Tulsi is revered as being without equal for both its medicinal and spiritual properties. Every part of the plant including the surrounding soil is revered and considered sacred and many Hindi households have tulsi plants growing in special places in their home, typically in an ornate earthen pot in a courtyard where evening and morning prayers are held.

Within Ayurveda, tulsi is regarded as one of the most esteemed plants that regulates the three doshas, and serves as an 'elixir of life' that promotes longevity. As a potent adaptogen, tulsi is recommended to be taken over long periods to prevent and treat diseases such as anxiety, cough, asthma, malaria, fever, diarrhoea, dysentery, arthritis, eye diseases, otalgia, indigestion, hiccups, vomiting, gastropathy, cardiopathy, genitourinary disorders, lumbago, skin diseases, leucoderma, ringworm, insect, snake and scorpion bites and verminosis (Gupta et al 2002, Maheshwari et al 2012, Mohan et al 2011, Mondal et al 2009, Pattanayak et al 2010, Singh et al 2010).

COMMON NAME

Tulsi (Hindi), *Ocimum sanctum* (Latin for 'sacred fragrant lipped basil') or *Ocimum tenuiflorum* (Latin for 'basil with small flowers') also known as Tulasi in Tamil and Holy or Sacred Basil in English. There are different cultivars of tulsi including purple leaf

(Krishna), green leaf (Rama) and wild forest (Vana) tulsi

BOTANICAL NAME/FAMILY

Genus species: *Ocimum sanctum* Family: Lamiaceae

PLANT PARTS USED

The whole plant including leaves, stem, flower, root, seeds and oil are all used medicinally.

GROWING/STORAGE

Tulsi grows as a herbaceous shrub growing up to 1–2 m high.

Like any medicinal plant optimal cultivation, harvesting, preservation and storage methods are required to preserve tulsi's medicinal value and it is suggested that tulsi should be grown in rural areas free from environmental pollution and employing organic methods (Singh et al 2010). This is supported by the finding of toxic elements at almost twice the concentration in tulsi leaves grown in polluted compared to unpolluted areas (Singh & Mittal 2003).

The tradition of revering the soil in which tulsi grows is supported by recent research that found that endophytic fungi from tulsi roots have in vivo hepatoprotective activity (Shukla et al 2012). Tulsi growth is also reported to double when plants are inoculated with *Glomus intraradices* (arbuscular mycorrhizal fungus) and *Azospirillum lipoferum,* a Plant Growth-Promoting Rhizobacteria (Padmavathi & Ranjini 2011) and yields of tulsi oil have been found to increase with cutting (Zheljazkov et al 2008).

Concerns about product quality in European 'Tulsi' products have been raised by reports of a high frequency of substitution with surrogate herbs such as *Ocimum basilicum* (Jürges et al 2009). This may be addressed using HPLC fingerprints to ensure batch-to-batch quality assurance along with adulteration and safety evaluation of standardised extracts (Chanda et al 2013). Microscopical assays have also been used to reliably identify dried or fragmented specimens and discriminate surrogate species from true tulsi (Jürges et al 2009). The quality of tulsi products is also influenced by storage and packaging with a significant effect on fresh weight loss, phenolic compounds, shelf life and anti-oxidant activity (Boonyakiat & Boonprasom 2010). Polyethylene bags packed with ethylene absorbents has been recommended to maintain the quality of stored tulsi (Wongs-Aree & Jirapong 2007).

CHEMICAL COMPONENTS

Tulsi is highly aromatic with a clove-like odour arising from its high eugenol content (Dutt 1939, Kumar et al 2013, Maimes 2004). Tulsi contains various phytochemicals and has a high antioxidant content with constituents that include alkaloids, glycosides, flavonoids, tannins, terpenoids and saponins along with nutrients such as vitamins A and C, zinc, calcium, iron and chlorophyll (Boonyakiat & Boonprasom 2010, Maimes 2004, Padalia & Verma 2011, Shafqatullah et al 2013, Singh et al 2010).

Tulsi leaves contain high levels of ursolic acid and oleanolic acid which account for many medicinal activities (Sarkar et al 2012, Verma & Joshi 2005) with the ursolic acid content of dried leaf powder being up to 11% (Vetal et al 2012) as well as being found in tulsi roots (Zaffer Ahmad et al 2012). Tulsi oil contains many volatile monoterpenes (51.1%) and sesquiterpene hydrocarbons (27.5%) with major constituents including phenolic compounds such as eugenol (up to 71%) and carvacrol (3%) and rosmarinic acid which have antioxidant and anti-inflammatory properties (Dutt 1939, Chanda et al 2013, Kumar et al 2013, Raju et al 1999). Non-phenolic constituents including methyl eugenol (8–45%) (Gbolade & Lockwood 2008, Raseetha Vani et al 2009, Zheljazkov et al 2008), which exhibits antioxidant and free radical scavenging activities (Sathaye & Redkar 2012). Other constituents include methyl chavicol, eucalyptol, α-humulene, humulene-epoxide II, (−)-*trans*-caryophyllene, α-*trans*-bergamotene, and γ-cadinene (Zheljazkov et al 2008), along with anti-stress agents ocimumoside A and ocimumoside B (Ahmad et al 2012b, Gupta et al 2007b).

As with many herbs, chemical components and subsequent biological activity vary with cultivar type (Wangcharoen & Morasuk 2007), plant part used (Shafqatullah et al 2013), preparation method (Mondal et al 2007), growing location (Johnson 2012) and season (Raseetha Vani et al 2009) and storage conditions (Boonyakiat & Boonprasom 2010, Wongs-Aree & Jirapong 2007). For example, the antioxidant capacity of red holy basil was found to be higher than white or green holy basil (Merai et al 2003, Wangcharoen & Morasuk 2007) and the saponin content of stems is higher than leaves (Shafqatullah et al 2013, Shetty et al 2006).

The components, biological activity and amounts of oil obtained from fresh and dried leaves have been found to differ greatly according to cultivar and preparation technique. Up to nine times more eugenol (antibacterial component) has been found in fresh leaves and more β-caryophyllene and caryophyllene oxide (antifungal components) in dried leaves (Mondal et al 2007). The oil content of fresh leaves is reported to be 0.31 mL/100 g (Sathaye & Redkar 2012) with the oil in dried leaves ranging from 0.17 to 0.50% (Zheljazkov et al 2008).

Tulsi is reported to contain copper, nickel, zinc, potassium and sodium in trace amounts (Narendhirakannan et al 2005) and to contain more zinc, magnesium and calcium than tea and to not hyper-accumulate toxic metals such as chromium and lead (Dash et al 2008). It is suggested that trace elements in tulsi may serve as an indicator of environmental pollution as concentrations of potentially toxic elements such as cadmium, caesium, chromium, mercury, scandium and selenium were found to be almost twice as high in tulsi leaves grown in polluted compared to unpolluted areas (Singh & Mittal 2003).

MAIN ACTIONS

Tulsi is one of the most important herbs in Ayurveda and is used extensively in several other ancient systems of medicine including Greek, Roman, Siddha and Unani, where it is valued for its broad spectrum of pharmacological activity and therapeutic actions and wide margin of safety.

Tulsi's actions have been documented in extensive in vitro and in vivo research and a few human studies and recent reviews suggest that these actions are extensive and include: antimicrobial (including antibacterial, antiviral, antifungal, antiprotozoal, antimalarial, anthelmintic), mosquito repellent, antidiarrhoeal, antioxidant, anticataract, anti-inflammatory, chemopreventive, radioprotective, hepato-protective, neuro-protective, cardio-protective, anti-diabetic, anti-hypercholesterolaemic, anti-hypertensive, anticarcinogenic, analgesic, anti-pyretic, anti-allergic, immunomodulatory, central nervous system depressant, memory enhancer, anti-asthmatic, anti-tussive, diaphoretic, anti-thyroidic, anti-fertility, anti-ulcer, anti-emetic, anti-spasmodic, anti-arthritic, adaptogenic/anti-stress, anti-cataract, anti-leucodermal and anticoagulant activities (Gupta et al 2002, Mahajan et al 2012, Mohan et al 2011, Mondal et al 2009, Pandey & Madhuri 2010, Pattanayak et al 2010, Prakash & Gupta 2005).

Adaptogenic antifatigue / anti-stress

In rodent stress models, treatment with tulsi normalises many of the physiological and biochemical changes associated with physical fatigue and stress. In forced-swim tests an aqueous suspension of 70% alcoholic extract of tulsi is reported to enhance aerobic glucose metabolism and improve swimming time, body weight, lipid peroxidation, and normalise biochemical parameters with lowering of malondialdehyde and lactic acid levels in rat liver and muscle (Venu Prasad & Khanum 2012). Similar results are observed in mice supplemented with an ethanolic extract of tulsi leaves, with improved swim duration and normalisation of cold-restraint stress-induced biochemical changes (Anju 2011). A methanolic tulsi leaf extract, in combination with extracts from *Withania somnifera* root and *Zingiber officinalis* rhizome, was further found to have significant corrective effect on swimming-induced oxidative damage on rat cardiac, skeletal and brain tissues (Misra et al 2006).

Pretreatment with ocimumoside A and B prevented both restraint-induced and chronic unpredictable stress-induced changes in the monoaminergic and anti-oxidant systems in the frontal cortex, striatum and hippocampus of rats with an efficacy similar to that of standard antistress (*Panax quinquefolium*) and antioxidant (melatonin) drugs (Ahmad et al 2012b, Singh et al 2010). Posttreatment with aqueous tulsi extract further protected different regions of the rat brain against the detrimental effect of restraint-induced stress with reduced lipid peroxidation, and normalisation of nucleic acids and proteins (Tabassuma et al 2009) while hydroalcoholic tulsi extracts protected rat heart from chronic-restraint stress-induced changes (Sood et al 2006).

Reduction of noise stress

Broadband white noise exposure is often used as an experimental model for stress that results in changes in immune response, neurotransmitter levels and ECG responses, along with increased corticosterone levels and oxidative stress in discrete brain regions. Tulsi extracts have been shown to significantly attenuate the effects of acute and chronic, noise-induced oxidative stress on rat brains (Samson et al 2006, 2007), normalise noise-induced changes in plasma corticosterone levels (Archana & Namasivayam 2002, Dwivedi 1997, Sembulingam et al 1997) and prevent noise stress-induced ECG changes (Sembulingam & Sembulingam 2005).

Ethanolic extracts of tulsi have also been found to normalise the action of noradrenaline, adrenaline, dopamine, and serotonin in discrete regions of the brains of rats exposed to chronic noise stress (Ravindran et al 2005) and reverse acute noise-induced reductions in total acetylcholine content and increases in acetylcholinesterase activity in rat cerebral cortex, corpus striatum, hypothalamus and hippocampus (Sembulingam et al 2005). Tulsi has further been shown to reverse or prevent noise-stress-induced changes in immune parameters of rats (Sembulingam et al 1999) with normalisation of leucocyte levels, thymus weight, antibody titre, spleen weight, neutrophil function and cell count (Archana & Namasivayam 2000).

Antidepressant / anxiolytic

Tulsi has been shown to have antianxiety and antidepressant properties in experimental rodent models (Chatterjee et al 2011, Raghavendra et al 2009, Tabassum et al 2010). Ursolic acid from tulsi leaves has been shown to have anxiolytic activity comparable to diazepam (Pemminati et al 2011) and tulsi has demonstrated antidepressant activity comparable to imipramine in animal models of depression (Moinuddin et al 2011, Sakina et al 1990).

Ethanol and chloroform extracts of tulsi stem and leaf are effective in preventing tonic convulsions induced by transcorneal electroshock (Jaggi et al 2003) and an ethanol extract of tulsi leaves has been shown to prolong the pentobarbitone-induced lost reflex time, decrease the severity and recovery time of electroshock and pentylenetetrazole-induced convulsions, and decreased apomorphine-induced fighting time and ambulation in 'open field' studies in mice. The extract also lowered immobility in a manner comparable to imipramine in rodent forced swimming behavioural despair models. This action was blocked by haloperidol and sulpiride and enhanced with the potent D_2-receptor agonist bromocryptine, suggesting an action on dopaminergic neurones (Sakina et al 1990).

A methanol extract of tulsi roots has demonstrated minor tranquilliser activity in rodents

(Mukherjee et al 2009) with central nervous stimulant properties and/or anti-stress activity comparable to the antidepressant desipramine (Maity et al 2000). In a human study of 35 psychiatric patients with generalised anxiety disorders 500 mg of tulsi twice daily for 30 or 60 days significantly attenuated the disorders and their associated stress and depression (Bhattacharyya et al 2008).

Anti-inflammatory

Tulsi extracts including fresh leaves (Ankur & Sheetal 2012), essential oil (Singh & Majumdar 1995a, 1995b, 1997), ethanol extracts of callus and leaf tissue (Singh & Jaggi 2003), lyophilised aqueous extract (Fernández et al 2004), and extracted eugenol (Thakur & Pitre 2009) have been shown to have anti-inflammatory activity in both acute and chronic inflammatory animal models including carrageenan-induced paw oedema (Ankur & Sheetal 2012, Fernández et al 2004, Singh 1998, Singh & Majumdar 1995a, 1997, Thakur & Pitre 2009), turpentine oil-induced joint oedema (Singh & Majumdar 1996), PGE_2, leukotriene and arachidonic acid-induced paw oedema (Singh 1998), cotton pellet granuloma (Fernández et al 2004), turpentine oil-induced granuloma pouch and formalin-induced oedema models (Ankur & Sheetal 2012).

Tulsi oil has further been demonstrated to significantly inhibit the rise in protein concentration and dye leakage in peritoneal fluid in experimentally induced peritoneal inflammation in mice and carrageenan-induced pleurisy in rats, with significant inhibition of leucocyte migration, vascular permeability and leucocyte migration following an inflammatory stimulus (Singh & Majumdar 1999a). Tulsi has also been shown to significantly reduce hydroxyl free radical-induced lipid peroxidation associated with copper sulfate toxicity (Shyamala & Devaki 1996).

The anti-inflammatory activity of tulsi is attributed to its eugenol (Thakur & Pitre 2009) and linoleic acid content and the inhibition of both the cyclooxygenase and lipoxygenase pathways of arachidonate metabolism (Singh 1998, Singh & Majumdar 1997). This is indicated by its activity in inflammation models that are insensitive to selective cyclooxygenase inhibitors (Singh et al 1996) and the anti-inflammatory effects of tulsi have been assessed as similar to non-steroidal anti-inflammatory drugs such as phenylbutazone (Singh & Majumdar 1995a), ibuprofen, naproxen, aspirin (Kelm et al 2000) and indomethacin (Kalabharathi et al 2011).

Antioxidant

The antioxidant properties of tulsi are attributed to peroxidase (Anbuselvi et al 2013) and a high content of phenolic compounds (Sundaram et al 2012) including eugenol, luteolin and apigenin (Dutta et al 2007) with red tulsi being reported to have significantly higher total phenolic content and antioxidant capacity than white tulsi (Merai et al 2003, Wangcharoen & Morasuk 2007).

Tulsi's antioxidant properties are demonstrated in vitro by free radical (Juntachote & Berghofer 2005, Sundaram et al 2012) superoxide anion, 1,1diphenyl-2-picrylhydrazyl and nitric oxide scavenging activity as well as by anti-lipid peroxidation, Fe^{2+} chelation and reducing power assays (Juntachote & Berghofer 2005 Rege et al 2012, Saiful Islam et al 2011). Tulsi is also documented to enhance endogenous anti-oxidant defences in vitro through increasing levels of glutathione and other anti-oxidant molecules and induction of endogenous anti-oxidant enzymes (Shivananjappa & Joshi 2012).

In animal studies hydro-alcoholic tulsi extracts have been found to reduce lipid peroxidation, increase reduced glutathione content and superoxide dismutase and catalase in normal and immune-compromised rats (Gupta et al 2007a) and protect against lipid peroxidation in experimentally-induced anaemic-hypoxia oxidative stress in rabbits (Jyoti et al 2007, Sethi et al 2003). Experimental evidence further suggests that the antioxidant properties of tulsi may serve to protect against the damaging effects of cerebral (Ahmad et al 2012a, Yanpallewar et al 2004) and cardiac ischaemia (Arya et al 2006, Panda & Naik 2009, Sharma et al 2001, Sood et al 2005) and protect against cataracts (Gupta et al 2005, Halder et al 2009, Sharma et al 1998) and swimming stress- (Anju 2011, Misra et al 2006, Venu Prasad & Khanum 2012) and restraint stress-induced oxidative damage (Tabassum et al 2010), as well as ameliorating sciatic nerve transection-induced peripheral neuropathy in rats (Muthuraman et al 2008) and reducing acute and chronic cocaine-mediated oxidative stress in mice.

Reducing agent for nanoparticle processing

The antioxidant properties of tulsi

Tulsi extracts have been shown to have high anti-oxidative stability at neutral and acidic pH, and exhibit strong dose-dependent superoxide anion scavenging activity, Fe^{2+} chelating activity, and reducing power (Juntachote & Berghofer 2005). The reducing power of aqueous tulsi leaf extracts has been used as a novel reductant and stabiliser for rapid and ecofriendly biosynthesis of stable nanoparticles of silver (Mallikarjuna et al 2011, Patil et al 2012, Singhal et al 2011, Subba Rao et al 2013), gold (Philip & Unni 2011) and platinum (Soundarrajan et al 2012).

Silver nanoparticles (AgNPs) stabilised by Tulsi leaf extract were found to have enhanced antimicrobial activity against well-known pathogenic strains, namely *Staphylococcus aureus* and *E. coli* with the nanoparticles being found to be stabilised by eugenols, terpenes, and other aromatic compounds present in the aqueous extract (Ramteke et al 2013) although the room-dried stem and root of OS has also been used (Ahmad et al 2009, 2010). Tulsi has also been shown to inhibit corrosion of mild steel in hydrochloric acid (Kumpawat et al 2010,

Shyamala & Kasthuri 2011) and zinc in sulfuric acid (Sharma et al 2009).

Hepatoprotection

Tulsi extracts have been shown to have protective effects against a wide range of toxic insults in numerous in vitro and in vivo models. The hepatoprotective effects of tulsi is attributed to its anti-oxidative potency with aqueous extracts producing significant dose-dependent reductions in lipid peroxidation and butylparaben-induced changes in non-enzymatic and enzymatic antioxidants (Shah & Verma 2012).

Tulsi is reported to mitigate against the toxic effects of common pesticides including restoration of endocrine and histopathological abnormalities induced by rogor AQ (Verma et al 2007), protection against chlorpyrifos-induced genotoxicity (Khanna et al 2011) and experimental endosulfan-induced immunotoxicity (Bharath et al 2011) and attenuation of immunotoxicity and oxidative stress produced by lindane (Mediratta et al 2008).

Further in vivo evidence suggests that tulsi can protect against the toxic effects of pharmaceuticals and other chemicals, including reduction of hepatorenal toxicity caused by paracetamol in mice (Makwana & Rathore 2011), hepatotoxicity induced by anti-tubercular drugs (Ubaid et al 2003) and meloxicam in rats (Mahaprabhu et al 2011) and protection against paracetamol-induced liver damage in rats that is enhanced by co-administration with silymarin (Lahon & Das 2011). In other mouse studies, tulsi is reported to prevent haloperidol-induced extrapyramidal side effects (Pemminati et al 2007), protect against ethanol-induced oxidative stress (Bawankule et al 2008) and provide hepatoprotection from exposure to carbon tetrachloride (Enayatallah et al 2004).

Cancer protection

Tulsi extract is seen to provide protection against chemical carcinogenesis in various animal models. This activity is suggested to act at least in part via tulsi's anti-oxidant properties (Prakash & Gupta 2000) with elevation of glutathione levels and decrease in lipid peroxidation and heat shock protein expression as well as by modulating phase I and II detoxification enzymes and inhibiting anti-proliferative activity (Rastogi et al 2007). This is supported by evidence that alcoholic tulsi leaf extract significantly elevates liver enzymes important in the detoxification of carcinogens and mutagens including cytochrome p-450, cytochrome b5, aryl hydrocarbon hydroxylase, and glutathione S-transferase. Tulsi also significantly elevates extra-hepatic glutathione-S-transferase and reduced glutathione levels in mice liver, lung, and stomach tissues (Banerjee et al 1996) as well as reducing the extent of lipid and protein oxidation, upregulating antioxidant defences and inhibiting 9,10-dimethylbenz-a-anthracene (DMBA)-induced genotoxicity and oxidative stress in rats (Manikandan et al 2007). Tulsi leaf extracts have also been found to reduce DMBA-DNA adduct formation in rat hepatocytes (Prashar et al 1998) and produce a dose-dependent decrease in the genotoxic damage of cyproterone acetate on human lymphocytes (Siddique et al 2007).

Further evidence of tulsi's chemo-preventive activity comes from various animal cancer models. Topical treatment with an ethanolic extract of tulsi leaves is reported to reduce tumour incidence, and the cumulative number of papillomas in DMBA-induced skin papillomagenesis in mice (Prashar et al 1994, Prashar & Kumar 1995). Oral administration of fresh tulsi leaf paste, aqueous and ethanolic extracts have also demonstrated in vivo activity against DMBA-induced hamster buccal pouch carcinogenesis with reduced incidence of papillomas and squamous cell carcinomas and increased survival rate (Karthikeyan et al 1999b).

Animal studies also suggest that tulsi is effective in enhancing oxidant-antioxidant status, cell proliferation, apoptosis and angiogenesis in rat forestomach carcinogenesis models (Manikandan et al 2008). Tulsi has also been found to reduce tumour volume and increase survival in mice bearing Sarcoma-180 solid tumours (Karthikeyan et al 1999a), increase survival times and restore haematological parameters in Ehrlich Ascites Carcinoma treated mice (Saiful Islam et al 2011), induce apoptosis in squamous cervical cancer cell lines (Jha et al 2012) and reduce the number of azoxymethane-induced colon tumours in rats (Gajula et al 2009, 2010).

Antitumour and antimetastatic properties of tulsi are further suggested by induction of apoptosis in human non-small cell lung carcinoma cells in vitro and inhibition of growth of Lewis lung carcinoma in vivo (Magesh et al 2009). Antimetastatic properties are also suggested by inhibition of cell adhesion and invasion and cytotoxicity against Lewis lung carcinoma associated with dose-dependent enhancement of anti-oxidative enzymes such as superoxide dismutase, catalase and glutathione peroxidase (Kim et al 2010).

Radiation protection

Tulsi extracts have been demonstrated to have radio-protective effects and reduce the oxidative and chromosomal damage induced by gamma radiation, and radioactive iodine in various in vitro and in vivo models. Polysaccharides isolated from tulsi have been found to have scavenged reactive oxygen species and prevent gamma radiation-mediated cell deaths in mouse splenocytes and prevent radiation-induced oxidative damage to liposomal lipids and plasmid DNA (Subramanian et al 2005).

Aqueous tulsi extracts are reported to be more radio-protective than alcoholic extracts with greater survival enhancement in mice exposed to whole-body gamma radiation (Devi & Ganasoundari 1995). A 50% alcoholic aqueous tulsi extract has demonstrated anti-melanoma and radio-protective activity with significant reduction in tumour volume and survival rate of mice with B16F10 metastatic melanoma cell line-induced metastasis. The extract also reduced radiation-induced chromosomal damage and increased glutathione activity after lethal doses of gamma radiation (Monga et al 2011). Ursolic acid from tulsi is also reported to enhance radiation-induced apoptosis in cancer cell lines and inhibit tumourigenesis in B16F10 melanoma cells implanted into mice, suggesting that it may be used as a radio-sensitiser and enhance therapeutic efficacy of radio therapy in a variety of human cancers (Koh et al 2012).

The free radical-inhibiting activity of tulsi flavonoids is reported to be significantly greater than dimethylsulfoxide (Ganasoundari et al 1997, Uma Devi et al 2000) and low doses of the water-soluble flavonoids orientin and vicenin from tulsi have been shown to scavenge free radicals and protect against radiation-induced cellular damage and significantly reduce lipid peroxidation and enhance glutathione and anti-oxidant enzymes activity in mice bone marrow (Uma Devi et al 1998, 2000, Uma Devi & Ganasoundari 1999) and human lymphocytes (Vrinda 2001). Pretreatment with tulsi flavonoids also leads to a significant reduction in the percentage of aberrant metaphases and other aberrations in bone marrow cells of irradiated mice (Ganasoundari et al 1997, Uma Devi et al 1998). Tulsi further provides mice protection against death from radiation-induced gastrointestinal and bone marrow syndrome (Uma Devi et al 1999) as well as preventing radiation-induced bone marrow damage at clinically-relevant radiation doses (Nayak & Uma Devi 2005).

Pretreatment with tulsi also provides a radio-protective effect after exposure to high-dose radioactive iodine (^{131}I) in rats (Joseph et al 2011). Similarly, in mice exposed to radioactive iodine tulsi produced significant reductions in lipid peroxidation in kidneys and salivary glands and less depletion of reduced glutathione in liver (Bhartiya et al 2006) as well as normalisation of salivary gland weight when given in conjunction with turmeric and vitamin E (Bhartiya et al 2010). Tulsi flavonoids are further reported to significantly increase glucose-6-phosphate dehydrogenase in neutrophils from oral cancer patients given radiation (Reshma et al 2008) and enhance glutathione in erythrocytes of irradiated oral cancer patients (Reshma et al 2005).

Heavy-metal toxicity

Animal evidence suggests that tulsi offers significant protection against lead, arsenic, cadmium, chromium and mercury toxicity. Tulsi has been found to protect against lead toxicity with normalisation of biochemical and haematological parameters in cockerels (Prakash et al 2009a, 2009b) and rats (Akilavalli et al 2011, Karamala et al 2011, Sujatha et al 2012) and significant dose-dependent protective effects on lead-induced brain damage (Sujatha et al 2011) and liver injury (Akilavalli et al 2011). Further evidence suggests that Tulsi leaf extract reduces arsenic-induced oxidative stress and assists in the depletion of arsenic from blood, liver and kidneys, suggesting a use for tulsi during chelating therapy with a thiol chelator (Sharmila Banu et al 2009). Tulsi has also been shown to protect against cadmium-induced toxicity with significant decreases in anti-oxidant enzyme activity and ascorbate levels (Ramesh & Satakopan 2010).

Tulsi leaf extract also has protective effects against chromium- and mercury-induced genetic damage as revealed in cytogenetic assays using *Allium cepa* root tip cells, with lower doses of the leaf extract being found to be more effective than higher doses (Babu & Maheswari 2006). Tulsi also provides protection against mercuric chloride-induced toxicity in mice (Kumar Sharma et al 2002) with pre- and posttreatment of tulsi leaf extract protecting against renal damage against mercuric chloride-induced toxicity (Sharma et al 2005).

Antidiabetic

Tulsi has been found to have effective anti-diabetic activity in human trials (Agrawal et al 1996, Devra et al 2012, Kochhar et al 2009, Rai et al 1997b) as well as in numerous in vitro (Hannan et al 2006) and animal models, including studies on rats (Chattopadhyay 1993, Eshrat & Mukhopadhyay 2006, Hussain et al 2001, Muralikrishnan et al 2012, Reddy et al 2008, Singh et al 2012, Suanarunsawat & Songsak 2005, Vats et al 2004), mice (Dusane & Joshi 2012, Gholap & Kar 2004, Vats et al 2004), rabbits (Gupta et al 2006) and the first report on fish as a diabetes model where an aqueous extract of tulsi produced a dose-dependent drop in serum glucose levels in hyperglycaemic tilapia (Arenal et al 2012).

Studies on streptozotocin-induced diabetic rats have reported that aqueous tulsi extracts reduce fasting blood glucose, serum lipid profile and lipid peroxidation products, improve glucose tolerance and increase anti-oxidant enzymes activity (Hussain et al 2001, Muralikrishnan et al 2012), reduce plasma glucose and HbA_{1C}, and improve retinal changes on angiography (Eshrat & Mukhopadhyay 2006). Further studies on streptozotocin-induced diabetic mice provide evidence of glucosidase inhibition and islet-cell protection (Dusane & Joshi 2012). Tulsi's antidiabetic actions include stimulatory effects on insulin secretion (Hannan et al 2006), potentiation of the action of exogenous insulin (Chattopadhyay 1993) and hypoglycaemic, antiperoxidative and cortisol-lowering activity, leading to the suggestion that it may potentially regulate corticosteroid-induced diabetes mellitus (Gholap & Kar 2004).

Further studies on streptozotocin-induced diabetic rats using alcoholic tulsi extracts provide evidence of dose-dependent hypoglycaemic effects and antihyperglycaemic effects (Chattopadhyay 1993, Vats et al 2004, Zaffer Ahmad et al 2012) along with reversal of diabetic induction, protection of renal glomerular filtration and liver function (Suanarunsawat & Songsak 2005), correction of dyslipidaemia (Zaffer Ahmad et al 2012) and normalisation of carbohydrate metabolism enzymes such as glucokinase, hexokinase and phosphofructokinase (Vats et al 2004).

Tulsi extracts have been further shown to prevent weight gain, hyperglycaemia, hyperinsulinaemia, hypertriglyceridaemia and insulin resistance in rats fed a diabetogenic diet (Chattopadhyay 1993, Reddy et al 2008) and to significantly reduce fasting blood sugar, uronic acid, total amino acids, total cholesterol, triglyceride, phospholipids and total lipids in diabetic rats (Rai et al 1997a). Tulsi extracts have also been observed to have antidiabetic activity and reduce lipid levels in alloxan-induced diabetic rats (Patil et al 2011) and in combination with *Pterocarpus marsupium* (Indian kino tree), tulsi has been shown to restore endogenous anti-oxidant levels in alloxan-induced diabetic rats to the pre-diabetic status and rectify dyslipidaemia (Singh et al 2012). Fresh tulsi leaves have also been found to significantly lower blood glucose and improve the antioxidant status of alloxan-induced diabetic rabbits (Sethi et al 2004), although rabbits displayed not hypoglycaemic effect with tulsi essential oil (Gupta et al 2006).

In randomised, controlled human trials involving patients with noninsulin-dependent diabetes mellitus, supplementation with tulsi leaves is reported to decrease fasting and postprandial blood glucose, improve lipid profiles (Agrawal et al 1996, Rai et al 1997b) and reduce diabetic symptoms such as polydypsia, polyurea, polyphagia and tiredness, sweating, burning feet, itching and headache (Kochhar et al 2009). The results of a randomised controlled trial of tulsi in people with metabolic syndrome further suggest that tulsi supplementation not only helps to control blood glucose, but also improves blood pressure and lipid profile (Devra et al 2012).

Lipid lowering

Tulsi extracts including aqueous and alcoholic leaf extracts as well as tulsi essential oil have been observed to have lipid-lowering effects in a number of animal models including rats fed high-cholesterol diet (Suanarunsawat et al 2009, 2010a, 2010b, 2011), alloxan-induced diabetic rats (Patil et al 2011), healthy rabbits (Dahiya et al 2011, Sarkar et al 1994) and hypercholesterolaemic rabbit models (Khanna et al 2010, Samak et al 2007) as well as in a small human trial (Verma et al 2012). The lipid-lowering and cardio-protective effects of tulsi are attributed to a rise of bile acid synthesis using cholesterol as precursor, and antioxidative activity protecting the liver from hypercholesterolaemia (Suanarunsawat et al 2011) along with the suppression of liver lipid synthesis (Suanarunsawat et al 2009).

Administration of tulsi leaves or aqueous or ethanolic leaf extracts to healthy and/or hypercholesterolaemic rabbits is reported to bring about significant lowering of serum total cholesterol, triglyceride and LDL-cholesterol levels and significant increases in the HDL-cholesterol (Ashok et al 2007, Dahiya et al 2011, Khanna et al 2010, Sarkar et al 1994) with associated anti-atherogenic effects (Samak et al 2007) and dose-dependent liver and aortic tissue protection from hypercholesterolaemia-induced peroxidative damage (Geetha et al 2004). Similar lipid-lowering effects with tulsi have been observed in rats fed high-cholesterol diets (Suanarunsawat et al 2011) and in alloxan-induced diabetic rats (Patil et al 2011). Administration of tulsi essential oil is also reported to produce significant lipid-lowering effects in rats (Suanarunsawat et al 2009, 2010a, 2010b) and rabbits (Gupta et al 2006) fed high-cholesterol diets.

Antimicrobial

Tulsi has been traditionally used for its bactericidal, fungicidal, pesticidal and medicinal values and recent evidence suggests that constituents such as eugenol, methyl chavicol, linalool, isoeugenol, and methyl isoeugenol all contribute to activity against many pathogenic fungi and bacteria as well as stored grain insects, pests and mosquitoes (Vasudevan et al 1999).

Antibacterial

While no human trials have been published, there is evidence to suggest that tulsi may have potential to help in the treatment of various human infections including urinary tract infections (Ali & Dixit 2012), skin and wound infections (Geeta et al 2001, Singh et al 2005), typhoid fever (Goel et al 2010a, Mandal et al 2012, Parag et al 2010), cholera (Geeta et al 2001, Parag et al 2010), tuberculosis (Farivar et al 2006), gonorrhoea (Shokeen et al 2005), acne (Sawarkar et al 2010, Viyoch 2006) and *Klebsiella* and cryptococcal pneumonia (Geeta et al 2001, Saini et al 2009).

Tulsi essential oil also exhibits broad-spectrum antibacterial activity (Rajeswara Rao et al 2011) including activity against *Staphylococcus aureus, Bacillus pumilus* and *Pseudomonas aeruginosa* (Singh et al 2005). The methanol, ethanol and chloroform extracts of tulsi have shown antimicrobial activity comparable with standard antibiotics against common human pathogens such as *Bacillus subtilis, Staphylococcus aureus, Staphylococcus saprophyticus, Escherichia coli, Proteus vulgaris* and *Klebsiella pneumoniae, Pseudomonas aeruginosa, B. subtilis* (Deo et al 2011, Kamble & Deshmukh 2008, Kumar et al 2012, Sagar & Thakur 2012, Sharma et al 2012) as well as activity against commensal bacteria such as *Lactobacillus, Staphylococcus epidermidis* and *Citrobacter* (Kumar et al 2012). The flavanoids, orientin and vicenin, obtained from tulsi leaves have also been shown to have synergistic antibacterial activity against organisms causing human urinary tract infections such as *Escherichia coli, Proteus, Staphylococcus aureus, Staphylococcus cohnii* and *Klebsiella pneumoniae* (Ali & Dixit 2012).

Antifungal

Tulsi essential oil has broad-spectrum antifungal activity (Kumar et al 2013, Rajeswara Rao et al

2011). This has led to suggestions that it may be used to prevent biodeterioration of herbal raw materials (Kumar et al 2013) and spoilage of food stuffs during storage (Kumar et al 2010). Tulsi oil's broad anti-fungal action has been assessed as superior to some prevalent synthetic antifungals against at least 12 commonly-occurring fungi and has been shown to inhibit aflatoxin B_1 production (Kumar et al 2010). Tulsi has also been found to have comparable anti-fungal activity to the standard fungicide carbendazim against *Pyricularia grisea* Sacc. which causes rice blast disease in greenhouse and field conditions and to retain this activity over a 24-month storage period (Tewari 1995, Upadhyaya et al 2012).

Tulsi oil has in vitro activity against fungal pathogens including *Candida* species (Amber et al 2010, Deo et al 2011, Khan et al 2010a, 2010b) with selective fungicidal activity against fluconazole-sensitive and fluconazole-resistant *Candida* isolates (Amber et al 2010). Linalool is assessed as the most active constituent (Khan et al 2010a, 2010b) and ethanolic extracts of tulsi leaves has also been found to have anti-cryptococcus activity when combined with *Cassia alata* extract (Ranganathan & Balajee 2000). Tulsi also has fungicidal activity against clinically isolated dermatophytes (Balakumar et al 2011) with petroleum ether extract, but not aqueous extract, exhibiting broad-spectrum activity against human pathogenic dermatophytes such as *Trichophyton mentagrophytes*, *T. tonsurans* and opportunistic fungi such as *Candida albicans, Trichosporon beigelii* (Das et al 2010) and *Malassezia furfur* (Chandra et al 2011).

Antimalarial

Tulsi ethanolic leaf extract has been found to have excellent in vitro anti-plasmodial activity against *Plasmodium falciparum* without producing chemical injury to erythrocytes. It is suggested that this anti-plasmodial activity might be due to the presence of alkaloids, glycosides, flavonoids, phenols, saponins, triterpenoids, proteins, resins, steroids and tannins and that the ethanolic leaf extracts of tulsi contains lead compounds for the development of antiplasmodial drugs (Inbaneson et al 2012).

Tulsi oil as well as leaf extracts have also been found to have larvicidal activity against dengue, malaria, and filariasis-transmitting mosquito larvae including activity against larvae of *A. aegypti* as well as *C. quinquefasciatus* (Anees 2008, Gbolade & Lockwood 2008, Krishan et al 2007, Rajamma et al 2011, Verma Prashant et al 2006).

Anti-parasitic

Tulsi essential oil and its constituent eugenol have shown potent in vitro anthelmintic activity against the roundworm *Caenorhabditis elegans* (Asha et al 2001) but not against the flatworm *Fasciola gigantica* (Jeyathilakan et al 2010). Compounds isolated from tulsi also showed potent leishmanicidal activity (Suzuki et al 2009). Tulsi oil and its petroleum ether extract also demonstrate selective insecticide activity, being highly toxic against the silkworm parasite *E. sorbillans* and comparatively less toxic to the silk worm *Antheraea assama* larvae (Bora & Khanikor 2011).

Anti viral

Dichloromethane and methanol extracts of tulsi has anti-herpes simplex virus activity at various steps of the viral multiplication cycle (Yucharoen et al 2011). Dry tulsi leaves are also reported to enhance immune activity in poultry infected with infectious bursal disease virus (Sadekar et al 1998).

Immune enhancement

Tulsi seed oil has been shown to modulate both humoral and cell-mediated immune responsiveness in non-stressed and stressed animals as evidenced by increases in anti-sheep red blood cell antibody titre and a decrease in percentage histamine release from peritoneal mast cells of sensitised rats (humoral immune responses), and decrease in footpad thickness and percentage leucocyte migration inhibition (cell-mediated immune responses). The inhibition of these responses by the central benzodiazepine receptor antagonist flumazenil has led to the suggestion that this immunomodulatory action is mediated by GABAergic pathways (Mediratta et al 2002).

In a myelosuppressed mice model, treatment with methanolic tulsi extracts resulted in significant increases in bone marrow cellularity, total WBC count and haemoglobin concentration along with raised antibody titre and production of TNF-α, IL-2, IFN-γ and IL-4 and reduced production of IL-1β and NF-κB (Hemalatha et al 2011). Similarly, in a cyclophosphamide-induced immunosuppression rat model, tulsi significantly increased lymphocyte proliferation (Tripathi et al 2008). In vitro and in vivo studies in rats further suggest that aqueous tulsi leaf extract has stimulatory effects on T and B lymphocytes with enhanced ability of spleen cells to secrete IL-2 (Goel et al 2010c).

The immunomodulatory effects of tulsi have been further demonstrated in a double-blinded, randomised, controlled, crossover trial on healthy human volunteers (n = 24) which reported that ethanolic extracts of leaves of tulsi for 4 weeks resulted in statistically significant increases in the levels of interferon-γ, interleukin-4, T-helper cells and NK cells (Mondal et al 2011).

Further evidence for the immunomodulatory effects of tulsi comes from aquaculture studies. Treatment with tulsi has been shown to increase survival, growth and weight and enhance antibody response and phagocytic activity in fingerlings of common carp (*Cyprinus carpio*) (Pavaraj et al 2011) and Indian carp (*Catla catla*) (Chitra & Krishnaveni 2011) exposed to *Aeromonas hydrophila* bacteria. Similar immunostimulatory effects were observed with increased disease resistance and stimulation of both antibody response and neutrophil activity in tilapia exposed to *Aeromonas hydrophila* (Logambal et al 2000). These studies suggest that tulsi may be an effective immunostimulant and maintain finfish health in intensive freshwater aquaculture where loss of fish production from infectious disease is a major constraint (Chitra & Krishnaveni 2011, Harikrishnan 2008, Logambal et al 2000, Pavaraj et al 2011).

Cognitive enhancement

Tulsi exhibits cognition enhancement, antidepressant and anxiolytic activity in Alzheimer's disease models in rats, with improved reference memory, working memory, spatial learning and anti-oxidant activity (Raghavendra et al 2009). Tulsi extracts are also reported to have memory-enhancing effects in restraint stress-induced memory impaired rats (Kumar et al 2007) and to significantly decrease acetylcholinesterase activity and improve passive avoidance tasks in experimentally-induced cognitive dysfunction (Giridharan et al 2011). Tulsi is also reported to have memory-enhancing and anti-amnesic effects in mice (Dokania et al 2011) and ameliorate the amnesic effect of scopolamine and ageing-induced memory deficits (Joshi & Parle 2006a, 2006b).

OTHER ACTIONS

Diuretic

Tulsi extracts have been shown to have diuretic activity similar to that of the loop diuretic frusemide in healthy rats (Pai et al 2013).

Aphrodisiac

An ethanolic extract of tulsi demonstrated aphrodisiac activity with significant and sustained increase in the sexual activity of normal male mice (Pande & Pathak 2009).

Anti-hypotensive

Tulsi oil has been observed to have a hypotensive effect in anaesthetised dogs attributed to its peripheral vasodilatory action (Singh et al 2001).

Anticoagulant

Tulsi oil was observed to increase blood-clotting time with the effect attributed to inhibition of platelet aggregation comparable to aspirin (Singh et al 2001).

Antipyretic

Tulsi oil has been observed to reduce typhoid-paratyphoid A/B vaccine-induced pyrexia in rodents with antipyretic activity deemed to be similar to that of aspirin (Singh & Majumdar 1995). The antipyretic activity of tulsi oil is attributed to prostaglandin inhibition and peripherally acting analgesic activity (Singh et al 2007).

CLINICAL USES

Tulsi and related basil species are commonly used as culinary herbs to enhance the taste and nutrition of many food preparations around the world (Singh et al 2010). Despite a wide variety of reported uses, the clinical uses of tulsi are mainly based on traditional use and supported by preclinical research. Currently there are very few published human trials that document the clinical benefits of tulsi other than a handful of trials in patients with diabetes or metabolic syndrome and a few studies investigating its use as a mouthwash and for dealing with stress.

Adaptogen / stress

Tulsi has been traditionally used to assist in dealing with the stresses of daily life and promote general health, wellbeing and longevity. Tulsi is a potent adaptogen with a unique combination of anti-oxidant, anti-inflammatory, antimicrobial and other actions that combine to help the body and mind adapt and cope with a wide range of physical, emotional, chemical and infectious stresses and restore physiological and psychological functions to a normal healthy state (Anbuselvi et al 2013, Maheshwari et al 2012, Singh et al 2010).

Recent evidence attests to tulsi's ability to protect against stress and reduce physical fatigue in multiple experimental animal models (Maheshwari et al 2012) and these studies are supported by a recent 6-week, randomised, double-blind, placebo-controlled study involving 150 people that found that tulsi extract significantly improved general stress scores as well as symptoms such as forgetfulness, frequent feeling of exhaustion, and sexual and sleep problems of recent origin (Saxena et al 2012).

Air travel

The unique combination of wide-ranging pharmacological activities makes tulsi one of the most suited herbs to help in the prevention and improvement of air travel health problems (Singh & Gilca 2008). There are various levels of evidence that tulsi has adaptogenic, anti-microbial, antiradiation, anti-oxidant, anticoagulant, anti-inflammatory, anti-restrain- and noise-stress, immune and cognitive enhancement activity. These actions may help address many issues faced by modern air travellers such as infection, fatigue, thrombosis, and dealing with anxiety, restraint, noise, hypoxia, radiation, industrial chemicals and poor sleep.

Metabolic syndrome / diabetes

Tulsi has shown efficacy in improving the glucose and lipid profiles of diabetic patients in a number of human clinical trials. In a 1-month trial with 27 NIDDM patients on hypoglycaemic drugs, supplementation with tulsi powder was seen to significantly lower blood glucose and glycated proteins as well as reducing triglycerides and total and LDL and VLDL cholesterol levels (Rai et al 1997b). In a further randomised, placebo-controlled, single-blind, crossover trial, treatment with tulsi leaves was seen to produce significant decreases in fasting and postprandial blood glucose levels and improve mean total cholesterol levels (Agrawal et al 1996).

More recently, a randomized controlled trial of 100 patients with metabolic syndrome found that

5 mL of tulsi extract twice daily for three months improved clinical and biochemical parameters of metabolic syndrome with significantly reduced blood glucose, blood pressure and improved lipid profile (Devra et al 2012). A further 3-month study of 99 males with NIDDM reported that 2 g of tulsi leaf powder, neem leaf powder or both showed significant reduction in diabetic symptoms such as polydypsia, polyurea, polyphagia and tiredness, sweating, burning feet, itching and headache and non-significant improvements in anthropometric parameters with the greatest effect seen with combination treatment (Kochhar et al 2009).

Ischaemic heart disease and stroke

The antioxidant properties of tulsi, including augmentation of endogenous antioxidants and suppression of oxidative stress are suggested to contribute to potential prophylactic and therapeutic uses in ischaemic heart disease. Tulsi has been shown to have cardioprotective effects against isoproterenol-induced myocardial necrosis in rats (Arya et al 2006, Sharma et al 2001, Sood et al 2005).

The anti-inflammatory, antioxidant and cognition-enhancing properties of tulsi also suggest a role in treating cerebral reperfusion injury and cerebrovascular insufficiency based on rat models of cerebrovascular insufficiency and dementia. Tulsi has been shown to reduce brain injury after middle cerebral artery occlusion (Ahmad et al 2012a) and protect against cerebral reperfusion injury and cerebral hypoperfusion functional disturbances such as exploratory behaviour and memory as well as and structural changes such as cellular oedema, gliosis and perivascular inflammatory infiltrate in rats (Yanpallewar et al 2004).

Pain

Alcoholic tulsi leaf extracts have demonstrated analgesic activity in mice models that suggest both centrally and peripherally mediated anti-nociceptive actions involving an interplay between various neurotransmitter systems (Khanna & Bhatia 2003). Further studies using tulsi seed oil in experimental pain models in rodents suggest that tulsi seed oil has peripheral rather than centrally-mediated analgesic activity as analgesia with tulsi was not associated with an increase in pain threshold (Singh & Majumdar 1995a). Tulsi has also been shown to reduce oxidative stress and calcium levels in rats and ameliorate sciatic nerve transection-induced peripheral neuropathy (Muthuraman et al 2008) and vincristine-induced neuropathic pain, suggesting a role in chemotherapy induced-painful neuropathy (Kaur et al 2010).

Arthritis

The anti-inflammatory, antioxidant and analgesic properties of tulsi all suggest a role in arthritis and tulsi oil has been found to have significant antiarthritic activity in animal models including formaldehyde- or adjuvant-induced arthritis and turpentine-induced joint edema (Singh & Majumdar 1996, Singh et al 2007).

Cataract

Tulsi delays the onset and subsequent maturation of cataract in naphthalene-induced cataract in rabbits and galactose-induced cataracts in rats (Sharma et al 1998). Aqueous tulsi extracts have further been shown to protect against selenite-induced cataract development in rat pups and morphological and biochemical changes in isolated rat lenses, with a significant increase in anti-oxidant enzyme levels, preservation of normal lens protein profile and inhibition of protein insolubilisation (Gupta et al 2005). Tulsi is also reported to protect against hydrogen peroxide-induced cytotoxic changes in human lens epithelial cells (Halder et al 2009).

Allergy / asthmatic

Tulsi has been shown to have anti-asthmatic activity in animals with inhibition of preconvulsive dyspnoea in guinea pigs (Singh & Agrawal 1991, Sridevi et al 2009). A 50% ethanol extract of fresh leaves, volatile oil extracted from fresh leaves and fixed oil from the seeds, but not a 50% ethanol extract of dried leaves, is reported to significantly protect guinea pigs against histamine- and acetylcholine-induced pre-convulsive dyspnoea as well as inhibiting carrageenan-, serotonin-, histamine- or PGE_2-induced hind paw oedema (Singh & Agrawal 1991).

Tulsi leaf extracts have also been shown to have anti-anaphylactic and anti-allergic activity with mast cell stabilisation, suppression of IgE, and inhibition of release of inflammatory mediators in rat and guinea pig models (Sridevi et al 2009). Mast cell stabilisation has also been demonstrated with ursolic acid from tulsi leaves (Rajasekaran et al 1989) and with tulsi ethanolic extract and isolated flavonoidal fraction (Choudhary 2010).

Ulcer

Extracts of tulsi have been shown to have anti-ulcer and ulcer healing activity in many different animal models including aspirin-, indomethacin-, alcohol-, histamine-, reserpine-, serotonin-, acetic acid-, meloxicam-, cold restraint-, pyloric ligation-, and stress-induced ulceration in experimental animal models (Dharmani et al 2004, Kath & Gupta 2006, Mahaprabhu et al 2011, Singh & Majumdar 1999a). Tulsi's anti-ulcer effects are attributed to the reduction of offensive factors such as acid-pepsin secretion and lipid peroxidation and the enhancement of gastric defensive factors such as mucin secretion, cellular mucus, longevity of mucosal cells (Dharmani et al 2004, Goel et al 2005, Sairam et al 2000, Singh & Majumdar 1999a).

Wound healing

Tulsi has many pharmacological actions that suggest a role in wound healing including antioxidant, anti-inflammatory, analgesic and antimicrobial activity. It is suggested that the combination of anti-inflammatory, analgesic and antibacterial activities in a single herb is unique to tulsi (Singh et al 2007) and that tulsi may be particularly suited to the management of staphylococcal wound infections (Singh et al 2005), abnormal healing and hypertrophic scars (Shetty et al 2008).

Alcoholic and aqueous tulsi extract have been shown to reduce oxidative stress and significantly increase wound-breaking strength, percent wound contraction, granulation tissue weight, hydroxyproline, hexuronic acid, hexosamines, superoxide dismutase, catalase, reduce glutathione and significantly decrease lipid peroxidation in experimental incision, excision and dead space wounds in rats (Shetty et al 2006, 2008). Application of tulsi extract in petroleum jelly is also reported to enhance early wound healing and elevate TNF-α production in rats (Goel et al 2010b).

Antifertility / antiandrogenic

Tulsi is reported to have anti-fertility effects (Sethi et al 2010) although very few workers have explored the detailed effects of tulsi on the reproductive system (Ahmed et al 2002b). A benzene extract of tulsi leaves is reported to have a reversible antiandrogenic effect in rats (Ahmed et al 2002a) and extremely high doses of an oil extract of tulsi leaves (300 mg/kg) is reported to reduce reproductive function and fertility in male rats and rabbits (Narayana 2011, Parandin & Haeri Rohani 2010, Sethi et al 2010) and there is an early report of tulsi leaves having antizygotic, anti-implantation and early abortifacient effect in women and in experimental animals (Vora 1969).

Mouth wash

The broad antibacterial and antifungal activity of tulsi has led to suggestions that it may serve as a herbal mouth wash (Kothari et al 2006, Kukreja & Dodwad 2012). Tulsi is said to be good for treating halitosis and mouth ulcers (Malik et al 2012) and ethanolic extracts of tulsi have demonstrated in vitro antimicrobial activity against *Streptococcus mutans* with maximal effect at 4% concentration (Agarwal et al 2010). In a controlled crossover study involving 45 school children, twice-daily rinsing with tulsi extract was as effective as 0.2% chlorhexidine and Listerine in reducing the salivary *S. mutans* levels (Agarwal & Nagesh 2011). Another trial involving 50 subjects randomised to either chlorhexidine or a Ayurvedic multiherbal mouthwash containing tulsi along with other herbs such as cloves, neem, triphala and licorice, found the herbal mouthwash was preferred for its taste and convenience of use, and acted as a potent plaque inhibitor, although not quite as effective as chlorhexidine (Malhotra et al 2011). In a further randomised controlled trial involving 60 participants the Ayurvedic multiherbal mouthwash twice daily for 15 days was found to be as effective as chlorhexidine and more effective than Listerine in preventing plaque and gingivitis (Maimes 2004).

Hand sanitiser

In addition to serving as a mouthwash, tulsi has been used as a herbal hand sanitiser in combination with *Eucalyptus globulus* leaf and has been found to be more effective than a standard reference against *E. coli, Pseudomonas aeuroginosa, Staphylococcus aureus, Bacillus subtilis* and *Sacchromyces cerevisiae* and *Candida albicans* (Wani et al 2013).

OTHER USES

Bioremediation of contaminated air and soil

Tulsi plants may be used to reduce air pollution and hundreds of thousands of tulsi plants have been planted around the Taj Mahal in Agra to help protect the iconic marble building from environmental pollution damage (Sethi et al 2010, Vora 1969). It has also been suggested that Tulsi may be used to bioremediate contaminated soil while still serving as a source of essential oil as tulsi plants may accumulate arsenic without detectable amounts appearing in the oil (Siddiqui et al 2012).

Water treatment

Tulsi has demonstrated anti-microbial activity against many water-borne pathogens including *Escherichia coli, Salmonella typhi, Pseudomonas pyocyaneus, Vibrio cholerae, Shigella dysenteriae* and *Proteus vulgaris* within specified contact time (Parag et al 2010). The broad spectrum antimicrobial properties of tulsi against pathogenic Gram-positive and Gram-negative bacteria have led to suggestions that tulsi may be used for water purification (Parag et al 2010) as well as in the food industry to prevent spoilage (Mishra & Mishra 2011).

Tulsi may be also used to remove fluoride in water and therefore prevent fluorosis, which causes dental and skeletal decay and is endemic in at least 25 countries. It is reported that 75 mg of fresh leaves added to 100 mL of water with a fluoride concentration of 5 ppm removed nearly 95% of the fluoride in 20 minutes and that boiling or shaking a handful of stems and dried tulsi leaves will decontaminate 20 litres of water with a removal efficiency of 74–78% (Maheshwari et al 2012).

Food and herb preservation

The anti-oxidant properties of tulsi may also have uses in food storage and preservation with dried tulsi powder reducing lipid oxidation in cooked ground pork (Juntachote et al 2006, 2007), extending the oxidative stability of ghee (Merai et al 2003) and doubling the non-refrigerated shelf-life of tofu (Anbarasu & Vijayalakshmi 2007). Tulsi essential oil has broad-spectrum anti-fungal activity (Kumar et al 2013, Rajeswara Rao et al 2011) and this has led to suggestions that it may be used to prevent biodeterioration of herbal raw materials (Kumar et al 2013) and spoilage of foodstuffs during storage (Kumar et al 2010). Tulsi oil's broad antifungal action has been assessed as superior to some prevalent synthetic antifungals against at least 12 commonly occurring fungi and has been shown to inhibit aflatoxin B_1 production (Kumar et al 2010). Tulsi has also been found to have comparable antifungal activity to the standard fungicide carbendazim against *Pyricularia grisea* Sacc. which causes rice blast disease in greenhouse and field conditions and to retain this activity over a 24-month storage period (Tewari 1995, Upadhyaya et al 2012).

Animal rearing

Tulsi has also been shown to be effective against many animal pathogens. Intramammary infusion of aqueous extract of tulsi leaf has been found to reduce subclinical bovine mastitis and enhance lysosomal enzymes-content of milk polymorphonuclear cells (Mukherjee 2006, Mukherjee et al 2005). Tulsi and garlic have also been found to have in vitro activity against mixed bacterial cultures causing infectious endometritis in repeat breeding crossbred cows (Kumar et al 2011). Tulsi supplementation was also seen to enhance feed intake, nutrient utilisation, body weight gain and feed conversion efficiency in a 3-month trial in goats (Deka 2009) and to increase survival, growth and weight of fish in freshwater aquaculture systems (Chitra & Krishnaveni 2011, Logambal et al 2000, Pavaraj et al 2011).

DOSAGE

It is suggested the best way to use tulsi is raw as a fresh whole herb rather than as extracts. If fresh whole herbs are not available, tulsi can be given as 300–600 mg of dried leaves daily for prevention, or 600–1800 mg in divided doses as therapy. Tulsi is often recommended for prolonged periods with increased stamina and immunological resistance taking up to one month to take effect. It is often recommended to consume a few fresh tulsi leaves each day and tulsi can also be consumed regularly for prolonged periods of time as a caffeine-free herbal tea that is considered an instant energy provider, staminator and life-long tonic for all ages (Singh et al 2010).

Physicochemical and sensory testing of a functional drink suggests that a preparation of 10% tulsi extract and 5% hill lemon (galgal) juice was adjudged best and had a storage stability of 6 months (Barwal et al 2009). It has been suggested that tulsi seeds can act as a natural super-disintegrant that can be used in the formulation of fast-melt tablets that disintegrate instantaneously within the mouth and can be consumed without water (Malik et al 2012).

TOXICITY

Tulsi has been used for generations for its ability to detoxify and it is not reported to have any toxic effects. Tulsi is reported to have an extremely wide safety margin with the ratio between the lethal (LD_{50}) and effective (ED_{50}) doses being more than 300 (Singh et al 2010).

Acute and subacute toxicity experiments in rats of three standardised tulsi extracts found the extracts were well tolerated, with no adverse changes in mortality, morbidity, gross pathology, body weight, and biochemical parameters (Chanda et al 2013). Tulsi oil is not cytotoxic to mammalian cells (Zheljazkov et al 2008) and the LD_{50} is reported to be 42.5 mL/kg, with long-term use of oil at 3 mL/kg not producing any untoward effects in rats (Singh & Majumdar 1995a, Singh et al 2007).

ADVERSE REACTIONS

Tulsi has a long history of traditional use with no reports of adverse effects.

SIGNIFICANT INTERACTIONS

There are no reports of any significant interactions with tulsi. As tulsi has anti-diabetic and anti-platelet actions there is a theoretical possibility of interactions with anti-coagulant or anti-diabetic medications but such interactions have not been reported.

PREGNANCY USE

Very few workers have explored the detailed effects of tulsi on the reproductive system and there is very little reliable information on the use of tulsi in pregnancy. High doses of tulsi are best avoided in pregnancy and although tulsi is traditionally used throughout pregnancy in Africa (Malan & Neuba 2011), there is some animal evidence to suggest that high doses of tulsi may have antifertility and abortifacient effects (Ahmed et al 2002b).

Practice points/Patient counselling

- Tulsi is considered unique amongst medicinal herbs for its wide variety of actions and ability to treat and prevent a range of diverse conditions.
- Tulsi can be taken as a dried herb, herbal tea or fresh leaves and is recommended for regular ongoing use to assist in adaptation to stress of daily life and promote health and longevity.
- Tulsi may help address many issues faced by modern air travellers such as infection, fatigue, thrombosis, and dealing with anxiety, restraint, noise, hypoxia, radiation, industrial chemicals and poor sleep.

PATIENTS' FAQs

What will this herb do for me?

Tulsi may enhance the ability to cope with a variety of different stresses, help prevent and treat a wide range of diseases and promote longevity when taken over long periods of time.

When will it start to work?

The stamina enhancing effects may take a week to one month to develop. Regular use is said to bestow a range of benefits and give appreciable improvement is health lasting for a month or more after discontinuation (Singh et al 2010).

Are there any safety issues?

Tulsi appears to be extremely safe and has been used for countless generations in different cultures and systems of medicine without any specific safety concerns. There is a theoretical possibility that tulsi's anti-platelet actions may interact with anti-coagulant medications or cause bleeding with surgery and that tulsi's anti-diabetic action may interact with hypoglycaemic medications but such interactions have not been reported. High doses of tulsi are best avoided in pregnancy.

REFERENCES

Agarwal, P. and L. Nagesh (2011). 'Comparative evaluation of efficacy of 0.2% chlorhexidine, Listerine and Tulsi extract mouth rinses on salivary *Streptococcus mutans* count of high school children-RCT.' *Contemporary Clinical Trials* **32**(6): 802–808.

Agarwal, P., et al (2010). 'Evaluation of the antimicrobial activity of various concentrations of Tulsi (*Ocimum sanctum*) extract against *Streptococcus mutans*: An in vitro study.' *Indian Journal of Dental Research* **21**(3): 357–359.

Agrawal, P., et al (1996). 'Randomized placebo-controlled, single blind trial of holy basil leaves in patients with noninsulin-dependent diabetes mellitus.' *International Journal of Clinical Pharmacology and Therapeutics* **34**(9): 406–409.

Ahmad, N., et al (2009). *Ocimum mediated biosynthesis of silver nanoparticles*. Proceedings of the ICMENS 09 Fifth International Conference on MEMS NANO and Smart Systems. Washington, DC: IEEE Computer Society, pp. 80–84.

Ahmad, N., et al (2010). 'Rapid synthesis of silver nanoparticles using dried medicinal plant of basil.' *Colloids and Surfaces B: Biointerfaces* **81**(1): 81–86.

Ahmad, A., et al (2012a). '*Ocimum sanctum* attenuates oxidative damage and neurological deficits following focal cerebral ischemia/reperfusion injury in rats.' *Neurological Sciences*: 1–9.

Ahmad, A., et al (2012b). 'Restraint stress-induced central monoaminergic & oxidative changes in rats & their prevention by novel *Ocimum sanctum* compounds.' *Indian Journal of Medical Research* **135**(4): 548–554.

Ahmed, M., et al (2002a). 'Reversible anti-fertility effect of benzene extract of *Ocimum sanctum* leaves on sperm parameters and fructose content in rats.' *Journal of Basic and Clinical Physiology and Pharmacology* **13**(1): 51–59.

Ahmed, M., et al (2002b). 'Effects of *Ocimum sanctum* (Tulsi) on the reproductive system: An updated review.' *Biomedical Research* **13**(2–3): 63–67.

Akilavalli, N., et al (2011). 'Hepatoprotective activity of *Ocimum sanctum* Linn. against lead induced toxicity in Albino rats.' *Asian Journal of Pharmaceutical and Clinical Research* **4**(SUPPL. 2): 84–87.

Ali, H. and S. Dixit (2012). 'In vitro antimicrobial activity of flavanoids of *Ocimum sanctum* with synergistic effect of their combined form.' *Asian Pacific Journal of Tropical Disease* **2**(SUPPL.1): S396–S398.

Amber, K., et al (2010). 'Anticandidal effect of *Ocimum sanctum* essential oil and its synergy with fluconazole and ketoconazole.' *Phytomedicine* **17**(12): 921–925.

Anbarasu, K. and G. Vijayalakshmi (2007). 'Improved shelf life of protein-rich tofu using *Ocimum sanctum* (tulsi) extracts to benefit Indian rural population.' *Journal of Food Science* **72**(8): M300–M305.

Anbuselvi, S., et al (2013). 'Purification and characterstics of peroxidase from two varities of tulsi and neem.' *Research Journal of Pharmaceutical, Biological and Chemical Sciences* **4**(1): 648–654.

Anees, A. M. (2008). 'Larvicidal activity of *Ocimum sanctum* Linn. (Labiatae) against *Aedes aegypti* (L.) and *Culex quinquefasciatus* (Say).' *Parasitology Research* **103**(6): 1451–1453.

Anju (2011). 'Adaptogenic and anti-stress activity of *Ocimum sanctum* in mice.' *Research Journal of Pharmaceutical, Biological and Chemical Sciences* **2**(3): 670–678.

Ankur, K. and S. Sheetal (2012). 'Evaluation of anti-inflammatory effect of fresh tulsi leaves (*Ocimum sanctum*) against different mediators of inflammation in albino rats.' *International Journal of Pharmaceutical Sciences Review and Research* **14**(2): 119–123.

Archana, R. and A. Namasivayam (2000). 'Effect of *Ocimum sanctum* on noise-induced changes in immune parameters.' *Pharmacy and Pharmacology Communications* **6**(3): 145–147.

Archana, R. and A. Namasivayam (2002). 'A comparative study of different crude extracts of *Ocimum sanctum* on noise stress.' *Phytotherapy Research* **16**(6): 579–580.

Arenal, A., et al (2012). 'Aqueous extract of *Ocimum tenuiflorum* decreases levels of blood glucose in induced hyperglycemic tilapia (*Oreochromis niloticus*).' *Asian Pacific Journal of Tropical Medicine* **5**(8): 634–637.

Arya, D. S., et al (2006). 'Myocardial salvaging effects of *Ocimum sanctum* in experimental model of myocardial necrosis: A haemodynamic, biochemical and histoarchitectural assessment.' *Current Science* **91**(5): 667–672.

Asha, M. K., et al (2001). 'Anthelmintic activity of essential oil of *Ocimum sanctum* and eugenol.' *Fitoterapia* **72**(6): 669–670.

Ashok, P., et al (2007). 'Effect of aqueous alcoholic extract of *Hibiscus sabdariffa* L. and *Ocimum sanctum* L. on plasma triglycerides in wistar rats.' *Journal of Natural Remedies* **7**(1): 155–159.

Babu, K. and K. C. U. Maheswari (2006). 'In vivo studies on the effect of *Ocimum sanctum* L. leaf extract in modifying the genotoxicity induced by chromium and mercury in Allium root meristems.' *Journal of Environmental Biology* **27**(1): 93–95.

Balakumar, S., et al (2011). 'Antifungal activity of *Ocimum sanctum* Linn. (Lamiaceae) on clinically isolated dermatophytic fungi.' *Asian Pacific Journal of Tropical Medicine* **4**(8): 654–657.

Banerjee, S., et al (1996). 'Modulatory influence of alcoholic extract of *Ocimum* leaves on carcinogen-metabolizing enzyme activities and reduced glutathione levels in mouse.' *Nutrition and Cancer* **25**(2): 205–217.

Barwal, V. S., et al (2009). 'Quality evaluation of functional drinks prepared from hill lemon (*Citrus pseudolimon*) and basil (*Ocimum sanctum*).' *Journal of Food Science and Technology* **46**(6): 601–603.

Bawankule, D. U., et al (2008). 'Protective effect of *Ocimum sanctum* on ethanol-induced oxidative stress in swiss albino mice brain.' *Toxicology International* **15**(2): 121–125.

Bharath, B. K., et al (2011). 'Imuuno-modulatory effect of *Ocimum sanctum* against endosulfan induced immunotoxicity.' *Veterinary World* **4**(1): 25–27.

Bhartiya, U. S., et al (2006). 'Protective effect of *Ocimum sanctum* L after high-dose ^{131}iodine exposure in mice: An in vivo study.' *Indian Journal of Experimental Biology* **44**(8): 647–652.

Bhartiya, U. S., et al (2010). 'Effect of *Ocimum sanctum*, turmeric extract and vitamin E supplementation on the salivary gland and bone marrow of radioiodine exposed mice.' *Indian Journal of Experimental Biology* **48**(6): 566–571.

Bhattacharyya, D., et al (2008). 'Controlled programmed trial of *Ocimum sanctum* leaf on generalized anxiety disorders.' *Nepal Medical College journal : NMCJ* **10**(3): 176–179.

Boonyakiat, D. and P. Boonprasom (2010). Effect of vacuum cooling and packaging on physico-chemical properties of 'Red' holy basil. *Chiang Mai University Journal* **877**: 419–426.

Bora, D. and B. Khanikor (2011). 'Selective toxicity of Ageratum conyzoides and *Ocimum sanctum* against *Exorista sorbillans* (Diptera:Tachinidae) and *Antheraea ussama* (Lepidoptera: Saturniidae).' *National Academy Science Letters* **34**(1–2): 9–14.

Chanda, D., et al (2013). 'Application of HPLC fingerprints for defining in vivo safety profile of Tulsi (*Ocimum sanctum*).' *Medicinal Chemistry Research* **22**(1): 219–224.

Chandra, R., et al (2011). 'Detection of antimicrobial activity of *Oscimum sanctum* (Tulsi) & trigonella foenum graecum (Methi) against some selected bacterial & fungal strains.' *Research Journal of Pharmaceutical, Biological and Chemical Sciences* **2**(4): 809–813.

Chatterjee, M., et al (2011). 'Evaluation of ethanol leaf extract of *Ocimum sanctum* in experimental models of anxiety and depression.' *Pharmaceutical Biology* **49**(5): 477–483.

Chattopadhyay, R. R. (1993). 'Hypoglycemic effect of *Ocimum sanctum* leaf extract in normal and streptozotocin diabetic rats.' *Indian Journal of Experimental Biology* **31**(11): 891–893.

Chitra, G. and N. Krishnaveni (2011). 'Immunostimulatory effect of *Ocimum sanctum* leaf extract on the indian major carp, Catla Catla.' *Plant Archives* **11**(1): 213–214.

Choudhary, G. P. (2010). 'Mast cell stabilizing activity of *Ocimum sanctum* leaves.' *International Journal of Pharma and Bio Sciences* **1**(2).

Dahiya, K., et al (2011). 'Effect of *Ocimum sanctum* on homocysteine levels and lipid profile in healthy rabbits.' *Archives of Physiology and Biochemistry* **117**(1): 8–11.

Das, J., et al (2010). 'In vitro evaluation of *Ocimum sanctum* leaf extract against dermatophytes and opportunistic fungi.' *Asian Journal of Microbiology, Biotechnology and Environmental Sciences* **12**(4): 781–784.

Dash, K., et al (2008). 'UV photolysis-assisted digestion of tea (*Camellia sinensis*) and tulsi (*Ocimum sanctum*) and their infusions: Comparison of available trace elements.' *Atomic Spectroscopy* **29**(2): 56–62.

Deka, R. S. (2009). 'Influence of tulsi (*Ocimum sanctum*) and ashwagandha (*Withania somnifera*) supplementation on production of organic meat in goats.' *Veterinary Practitioner* **10**(1): 57–59.

Deo, S. S., et al (2011). 'Antimicrobial activity and HPLC fingerprinting of crude ocimum extracts.' *E-Journal of Chemistry* **8**(3): 1430–1437.

Devi, P. U. and A. Ganasoundari (1995). 'Radioprotective effect of leaf extract of Indian medicinal plant *Ocimum sanctum*.' *Indian Journal of Experimental Biology* **33**(3): 205–208.

Devra, D. K., et al (2012). 'Effect of tulsi (*Ocimum sanctum* Linn) on clinical and biochemical parameters of metabolic syndrome.' *Journal of Natural Remedies* **12**(1): 63–67.

Dharmani, P., V. et al (2004). 'Evaluation of anti-ulcerogenic and ulcer-healing properties of *Ocimum sanctum* Linn.' *Journal of Ethnopharmacology* **93**(2–3): 197–206.

Dokania, M., et al (2011). 'Effect of *Ocimum sanctum* extract on sodium nitrite-induced experimental amnesia in mice.' *Thai Journal of Pharmaceutical Sciences* **35**(3): 123–130.

Dusane, M. B. and B. N. Joshi (2012). 'Islet protective and insulin secretion property of *Murraya koenigii* and *Ocimum tenuflorum* in streptozotocin-induced diabetic mice.' *Canadian Journal of Physiology and Pharmacology* **90**(3): 371–378.

Dutt, S. (1939). 'Chemical examination of the essential oil of *Ocimum sanctum* Linn.' *Proceedings of the Indian Academy of Sciences — Section A* **9**(1): 72–77.

Dutta, D., et al (2007). 'Modulatory effect of distillate of *Ocimum sanctum* leaf extract (Tulsi) on human lymphocytes against genotoxicants.' *Biomedical and Environmental Sciences* **20**(3): 226–234.

Dwivedi, S. (1997). 'Effect of *Ocimum sanctum* linn on noise induced changes in plasma corticosterone level [1].' *Indian Journal of Physiology and Pharmacology* **41**(4): 429–430.

Enayatallah, S. A. M., et al (2004). 'A study of hepatoprotective activity of *Ocimum sanctum* (Krishna tulas) extracts in chemically induced liver damage in albino mice.' *Journal of Ecophysiology and Occupational Health* **4**(1–2): 89–96.

Eshrat M, H. and A. K. Mukhopadhyay (2006). 'Effect of *Ocimum sanctum* (Tulsi) and vitamin E on biochemical parameters and retinopathy in streptozotocin induced diabetic rats.' *Indian Journal of Clinical Biochemistry* **21**(2): 181–188.

Farivar, T. N., et al (2006). 'Anti tuberculosis effect of *Ocimum sanctum* extracts in in vitro and macrophage culture.' *Journal of Medical Sciences* **6**(3): 348–351.

Fernández, P. B., et al (2004). 'Anti-inflammatory effect of lyophilized aqueous extract of *Ocinum tenuiflorum* on rats.' *Efecto antiinflamatorio del extracto acuoso liofilizado de Ocimum tenuiflorum L. en ratas* **23**(4): 492–497.

Gajula, D., et al (2009). 'Determination of total phenolics, flavonoids and antioxidant and chemopreventive potential of basil (*Ocimum basilicum* L. and *Ocimum tenuiflorum* L.).' *International Journal of Cancer Research* **5**(4): 130–143.

Gajula, D., et al (2010). 'Basil (*Ocimum basilicum* and *Ocimum tenuiflorum*) reduces Azoxymethane induced colon tumors in fisher 344 male rats.' *Research Journal of Phytochemistry* **4**(3): 136–145.

Ganasoundari, A., et al (1997). 'Protection against radiation-induced chromosome damage in mouse marrow by *Ocimum sanctum*.' *Mutation Research — Fundamental and Molecular Mechanisms of Mutagenesis* **373**(2): 271–276.

Gbolade, A. A. and G. B. Lockwood (2008). 'Toxicity of *Ocimum sanctum* L. essential oil to *Aedes aegypti* Larvae and its chemical composition.' *Journal of Essential Oil-Bearing Plants* **11**(2): 148–153.

Geeta, D. M. et al (2001). 'Activity of *Ocimum sanctum* (the traditional Indian medicinal plant) against the enteric pathogens.' *Indian Journal of Medical Sciences* **55**(8): 434–438, 472.

Geetha, R. et al (2004). 'Inhibition of lipid peroxidation by botanical extracts of *Ocimum sanctum*: In vivo and in vitro studies.' *Life Sciences* **76**(1): 21–28.

Gholap, S. and A. Kar (2004). 'Hypoglycaemic effects of some plant extracts are possibly mediated through inhibition in corticosteroid concentration.' *Pharmazie* **59**(11): 876–878.

Giridharan, V. V., et al (2011). '*Ocimum sanctum* Linn. Leaf extracts inhibit acetylcholinesterase and improve cognition in rats with experimentally induced dementia.' *Journal of Medicinal Food* **14**(9): 912–919.

Goel, R. K., et al (2005). 'Effect of standardized extract of *Ocimum sanctum* Linn. on gastric mucosal offensive and defensive factors.' *Indian Journal of Experimental Biology* **43**(8): 715–721.

Goel, A., et al (2010a). 'Effect of *Ocimum sanctum* on the development of protective immunity against *Salmonella typhimurium* infection through cytokines.' *Asian Pacific Journal of Tropical Medicine* **3**(9): 682–686.

Goel, A., et al (2010b). 'Wound healing potential of *Ocimum sanctum* linn. with induction of tumor necrosis-α.' *Indian Journal of Experimental Biology* **48**(4): 402–406.

Goel, A., et al (2010c). 'Immunomodulating property of *Ocimum sanctum* by regulating the IL-2 production and its mRNA expression using rat's splenocytes.' *Asian Pacific Journal of Tropical Medicine* **3**(1): 8–12.

Gupta, S. K., et al (2002). 'Validation of traditional claim of Tulsi, *Ocimum sanctum* Linn. as a medicinal plant.' *Indian Journal of Experimental Biology* **40**(7): 765–773.

Gupta, S. K., et al (2005). '*Ocimum sanctum* modulates selenite-induced cataractogenic changes and prevents rat lens opacification.' *Current Eye Research* **30**(7): 583–591.

Gupta, S., et al (2006). 'Antidiabetic, antihypercholesterolaemic and antioxidant effect of *Ocimum sanctum* (Linn) seed oil.' *Indian Journal of Experimental Biology* **44**(4): 300–304.

Gupta, D. K., et al (2007a). 'Evaluation of antioxidant activity of *Ocimum sanctum* and *Emblica officinaux* in rats.' *Indian Journal of Animal Sciences* **77**(7): 563–565.

Gupta, P., et al (2007b). 'Constituents of *Ocimum sanctum* with antistress activity.' *Journal of Natural Products* **70**(9): 1410–1416.

Halder, N., et al (2009). '*Ocimum sanctum* extracts attenuate hydrogen peroxide induced cytotoxic ultrastructural changes in human lens epithelial cells.' *Phytotherapy Research* **23**(12): 1734–1737.

Hannan, J. M. A., et al (2006). '*Ocimum sanctum* leaf extracts stimulate insulin secretion from perfused pancreas, isolated islets and clonal pancreatic β-cells.' *Journal of Endocrinology* **189**(1): 127–136.

Harikrishnan R B. C. (2008). 'In vitro and in vivo studies of the use of some medicinal herbals against the pathogen *Aeromonas hydrophila* in goldfish.' *J Aquat Anim Health* **20**(3): 165–176.

Hemalatha, R., et al (2011). 'Immunomodulatory activity and Th1/Th2 cytokine response of *Ocimum sanctum* in myelosuppressed swiss albino mice.' *Trends in Medical Research* **6**(1): 23–31.

Hussain, E. H. M. A., et al (2001). 'Hypoglycaemic, hypolipidemic and antioxidant properties of tulsi (*Ocimum sanctum* linn) on streptozotocin induced diabetes in rats.' *Indian Journal of Clinical Biochemistry* **16**(2): 190–194.

Inbaneson, S. J., et al (2012). 'In vitro antiplasmodial effect of ethanolic extracts of traditional medicinal plant *Ocimum* species against *Plasmodium falciparum*.' *Asian Pacific Journal of Tropical Medicine* **5**(2): 103–106.

Jaggi, R. K., et al (2003). 'Anticonvulsant potential of holy basil, *Ocimum sanctum* Linn., and its cultures.' *Indian Journal of Experimental Biology* **41**(11): 1329–1333.

Jeyathilakan, N., et al (2010). 'Anthelmintic activity of essential oils of *Cymbopogon citratus* and *Ocimum sanctum* on fasciola gigantica, in vitro.' *Journal of Veterinary Parasitology* **24**(2): 151–154.

Jha, A. K., et al (2012). 'Ethanolic extracts of *Ocimum sanctum*, *Azadirachta indica* and *Withania somnifera* cause apoptosis in SiHa cells.' *Research Journal of Pharmaceutical, Biological and Chemical Sciences* **3**(2): 557–562.

Johnson, M. (2012). 'Studies on intra-specific variation in a multipotent medicinal plant *Ocimum sanctum* Linn. using isozymes.' *Asian Pacific Journal of Tropical Biomedicine* **2**(1 SUPPL.): S21–S26.

Joseph, L. J., et al (2011). 'Radioprotective effect of *Ocimum sanctum* and amifostine on the salivary gland of rats after therapeutic radioiodine exposure.' *Cancer Biotherapy and Radiopharmaceuticals* **26**(6): 737–743.

Joshi, H. and M. Parle (2006a). 'Cholinergic basis of memory improving effect of *Ocimum tenuiflorum* Linn.' *Indian Journal of Pharmaceutical Sciences* **68**(3): 364–365.

Joshi, H. and M. Parle (2006b). 'Evaluation of nootropic potential of *Ocimum sanctum* Linn. in mice.' *Indian Journal of Experimental Biology* **44**(2): 133–136.

Juntachote, T. and E. Berghofer (2005). 'Antioxidative properties and stability of ethanolic extracts of Holy basil and Galangal.' *Food Chemistry* **92**(2): 193–202.

Juntachote, T., et al (2006). 'The antioxidative properties of Holy basil and Galangal in cooked ground pork.' *Meat Science* **72**(3): 446–456.

Juntachote, T., et al (2007). 'Antioxidative effect of added dried Holy basil and its ethanolic extracts on susceptibility of cooked ground pork to lipid oxidation.' *Food Chemistry* **100**(1): 129–135.

Jürges, G., et al (2009). 'Development and validation of microscopical diagnostics for 'Tulsi' (*Ocimum tenuiflorum* L.) in ayurvedic preparations.' *European Food Research and Technology* **229**(1): 99–106.

Jyoti, S., et al (2007). 'Antistressor activity of *Ocimum sanctum* (Tulsi) against experimentally induced oxidative stress in rabbits.' *Methods and Findings in Experimental and Clinical Pharmacology* **29**(6): 411–416.

Kalabharathi, H. L., et al (2011). 'Anti inflammatory activity of fresh tulsi leaves (*Ocimum sanctum*) in albino rats.' *International Journal of Pharma and Bio Sciences* **2**(4): 45–50.

Kamble, R. D. and A. M. Deshmukh (2008). 'Antimicrobial activity of *Ocimum sanctum* extracts on common human pathogens.' *Asian Journal of Microbiology, Biotechnology and Environmental Sciences* **10**(4): 873–877.

Karamala, S. K., et al (2011). 'Hematobiochemical changes of lead poisoning and amelioration with *Ocimum sanctum* in wistar albino rats.' *Veterinary World* **4**(6): 260–263.

Karthikeyan, K., et al (1999a). 'Anticancer activity of *Ocimum sanctum*.' *Pharmaceutical Biology* **37**(4): 285–290.

Karthikeyan, K., et al (1999b). 'Chemopreventive effect of *Ocimum sanctum* on DMBA-induced hamster buccal pouch carcinogenesis.' *Oral Oncology* **35**(1): 112–119.

Kath, R. K. and R. K. Gupta (2006). 'Antioxidant activity of hydroalcoholic leaf extract of *Ocimum sanctum* in animal models of peptic ulcer.' *Indian Journal of Physiology and Pharmacology* **50**(4): 391–396.

Kaur, G., et al (2010). 'Exploring the potential effect of *Ocimum sanctum* in vincristine-induced neuropathic pain in rats.' *Journal of Brachial Plexus and Peripheral Nerve Injury* **5**(1).

Kelm, M. A., et al (2000). 'Antioxidant and cyclooxygenase inhibitory phenolic compounds from *Ocimum sanctum* Linn.' *Phytomedicine* **7**(1): 7–13.

Khan, A., et al (2010a). '*Ocimum sanctum* essential oil and its active principles exert their antifungal activity by disrupting ergosterol biosynthesis and membrane integrity.' *Research in Microbiology* **161**(10): 816–823.

Khan, A., et al (2010b). 'Antifungal activities of *Ocimum sanctum* essential oil and its lead molecules.' *Natural Product Communications* **5**(2): 345–349.

Khanna, N. and J. Bhatia (2003). 'Antinociceptive action of *Ocimum sanctum* (Tulsi) in mice: Possible mechanisms involved.' *Journal of Ethnopharmacology* **88**(2–3): 293–296.

Khanna, N., et al (2010). 'Comparative effect of *Ocimum sanctum*, *Commiphora mukul*, folic acid and ramipril on lipid peroxidation in experimentally-induced hyperlipidemia.' *Indian Journal of Experimental Biology* **48**(3): 299–305.

Khanna, A., et al (2011). 'Role of *Ocimum sanctum* as a genoprotective agent on chlorpyrifos-induced genotoxicity.' *Toxicology International* **18**(1): 9–13.

Kim, S. C., et al (2010). 'Ethanol extract of *Ocimum sanctum* exerts anti-metastatic activity through inactivation of matrix metalloproteinase-9 and enhancement of anti-oxidant enzymes.' *Food and Chemical Toxicology* **48**(6): 1478–1482.

Kochhar, A., et al (2009). 'Effect of supplementation of Tulsi (*Ocimum sanctum*) and Neem (*Azadirachta indica*) leaf powder on diabetic symptoms, anthropometric parameters and blood pressure of non insulin dependent male diabetics.' *Studies on Ethno-Medicine* **3**(1): 5–9.

Koh, S. J., et al (2012). 'Sensitization of ionizing radiation-induced apoptosis by ursolic acid.' *Free Radical Research* **46**(3): 339–345.

Kothari, S. K., et al (2006). 'Antimicrobial activity of essential oil of methyl eugenol rich *Ocimum tenuiflorum* L.F. (Syn. *O. sanctum* L.).' *Indian Drugs* **43**(5): 410–415.

Krishan, V., et al (2007). 'Mosquito larvicidal activity of *Ocimum sanctum* on *Culex quinquefasciatus*.' *Biosciences Biotechnology Research Asia* **4**(2): 717–720.

Kukreja, B. J. and V. Dodwad (2012). 'Herbal mouthwashes — A gift of nature.' *International Journal of Pharma and Bio Sciences* **3**(2): P46–P52.

Kumar, R. S., et al (2007). 'Effect of *Ocimum sanctum* (Linn) extract on restraint stress induced behavioral deficits in male wistar rats.' *Pharmacologyonline* **3**: 394–404.

Kumar, A., et al (2010). 'Chemical composition, antifungal and antiaflatoxigenic activities of *Ocimum sanctum* L. essential oil and its safety assessment as plant based antimicrobial.' *Food and Chemical Toxicology* **48**(2): 539–543.

Kumar, S., et al (2011). 'Antibacterial properties of garlic and tulsi in repeat breeding crossbred cows.' *Indian Veterinary Journal* **88**(1): 28–30.

Kumar, P., et al (2012). 'Antimicrobial potential of leaf and callus tissue extracts of *Ocimum sanctum*.' *Annals of Biology* **28**(2): 83–86.

Kumar, A., et al (2013). 'Antifungal evaluation of *Ocimum sanctum* essential oil against fungal deterioration of raw materials of *Rauvolfia serpentina* during storage.' *Industrial Crops and Products* **45**: 30–35.

Kumar Sharma, M., et al (2002). '*Ocimum sanctum* aqueous leaf extract provides protection against mercury induced toxicity in Swiss albino mice.' *Indian Journal of Experimental Biology* **40**(9): 1079–1082.

Kumpawat, N., et al (2010). 'A comparative study of corrosion inhibition efficiency of stem and leaves extract of *Ocimum sanctum* (Holy Basil) for mild steel in HCl solution.' *Protection of Metals and Physical Chemistry of Surfaces* **46**(2): 267–270.

Lahon, K. and S. Das (2011). 'Hepatoprotective activity of *Ocimum sanctum* alcoholic leaf extract against paracetamol-induced liver damage in Albino rats.' *Pharmacognosy Research* **3**(1): 13–18.

Logambal, S. M., et al (2000). 'Immunostimulatory effect of leaf extract of *Ocimum sanctum* Linn. in *Oreochromis mossambicus* (Peters).' *Hydrobiologia* **430**(1–3): 113–120.

Magesh, V., et al (2009). '*Ocimum sanctum* induces apoptosis in A549 lung cancer cells and suppresses the in vivo growth of lewis lung carcinoma cells.' *Phytotherapy Research* **23**(10): 1385–1391.

Mahajan, N., et al (2012). 'A phytopharmacological overview on *Ocimum* species with special emphasis on *Ocimum sanctum*.' *Biomedicine and Preventive Nutrition*.

Mahaprabhu, R., et al (2011). 'Ameliorative effect of *Ocimum sanctum* on meloxicam induced toxicity in wistar rats.' *Toxicology International* **18**(2): 130–136.

Maheshwari, R., et al. (2012). 'Usage of Holy Basil for Various Aspects.' *Bulletin of Environment, Pharmacology and Life Sciences* **1**(10): 67–69.

Maimes, S. (2004). Maimes Report on Holy Basil. Rochester New Hampshire, SALAM Research Centre.

Maity, T. K., et al (2000). 'Effect of *Ocimum sanctum* roots extract on swimming performance in mice.' *Phytotherapy Research* **14**(2): 120–121.

Makwana, M. and H. S. Rathore (2011). 'Prevention of hepatorenal toxicity of acetaminophen with *Ocimum sanctum* in mice.' *International Journal of Pharmacy and Technology* **3**(1): 1385–1396.

Malan, D., Neuba, DFR. (2011). 'Traditional Practices and Medicinal Plants Use during Pregnancy by Anyi-Ndenye Women (Eastern Co^te d'Ivoire).' *African Journal of Reproductive Health* **15**(1): 85–94.

Malhotra, R., et al (2011). 'Comparison of the effectiveness of a commercially available herbal mouthrinse with chlorhexidine gluconate at the clinical and patient level.' *Journal of Indian Society of Periodontology* **15**(4): 349–352.

Malik, K., et al (2012). '*Ocimum sanctum* seeds, a natural superdisintegrant: formulation and evaluation of fast melt tablets of nimesulide.' *Polimery w medycynie* **42**(1): 49–59.

Mallikarjuna, K., et al (2011). 'Green synthesis of silver nanoparticles using *Ocimum* leaf extract and their characterization.' *Digest Journal of Nanomaterials and Biostructures* **6**(1): 181–186.

Mandal, S., et al (2012). 'Enhancing chloramphenicol and trimethoprim in vitro activity by *Ocimum sanctum* Linn. (Lamiaceae) leaf extract against *Salmonella enterica* serovar Typhi.' *Asian Pacific Journal of Tropical Medicine* **5**(3): 220–224.

Manikandan, P., et al (2007). '*Ocimum sanctum* Linn. (Holy Basil) ethanolic leaf extract protects against 7,12-dimethylbenz[a]anthracene-induced genotoxicity, oxidative stress, and imbalance in xenobiotic-metabolizing enzymes.' *Journal of Medicinal Food* **10**(3): 495–502.

Manikandan, P., et al (2008). 'Combinatorial chemopreventive effect of *Azadirachta indica* and *Ocimum sanctum* on oxidant-antioxidant status, cell proliferation, apoptosis and angiogenesis in a rat forestomach carcinogenesis model.' *Singapore Medical Journal* **49**(10): 814–822.

Mediratta, P. K., et al (2002). 'Evaluation of immunomodulatory potential of *Ocimum sanctum* seed oil and its possible mechanism of action.' *Journal of Ethnopharmacology* **80**(1): 15–20.

Mediratta, P. K., et al (2008). 'Attenuation of the effect of lindane on immune responses and oxidative stress by *Ocimum sanctum* seed oil (OSSO) in rats.' *Indian Journal of Physiology and Pharmacology* **52**(2): 171–177.

Merai, M., et al (2003). 'Extraction of Antioxygenic Principles from Tulsi Leaves and their Effects on Oxidative Stability of Ghee.' *Journal of Food Science and Technology* **40**(1): 52–57.

Mishra, P. and S. Mishra (2011). 'Study of antibacterial activity of *Ocimum sanctum* extract against gram positive and gram negative bacteria.' *American Journal of Food Technology* **6**(4): 336–341.

Misra, D. S., et al (2006). 'Protective response of methanolic extract of *Ocimum sanctum*, *Withania somnifera* and *Zingiber officinalis* on swimming-induced oxidative damage on cardiac, skeletal and brain tissues in male rat: A duration dependent study.' *International Journal of Pharmacology* **2**(6): 647–655.

Mohan, L., et al (2011). '*Ocimum sanctum* linn (TULSI) — an overview.' *International Journal of Pharmaceutical Sciences Review and Research* **7**(1): 51–53.

Moinuddin, G., et al (2011). 'Comparative pharmacological evaluation of *Ocimum sanctum* and imipramine for antidepressant activity.' *Latin American Journal of Pharmacy* **30**(3): 435–439.

Mondal, S., et al (2007). Antimicrobial activities of essential oils obtained from fresh and dried leaves of *Ocimum sanctum* (L.) against enteric bacteria and yeast. *Acta Hort* **756**: 267–269.

Mondal, S., et al (2009). 'The science behind sacredness of Tulsi (*Ocimum sanctum* linn.).' *Indian Journal of Physiology and Pharmacology* **53**(4): 291–306.

Mondal, S., et al (2011). 'Double-blinded randomized controlled trial for immunomodulatory effects of Tulsi (*Ocimum sanctum* Linn.) leaf extract on healthy volunteers.' *Journal of Ethnopharmacology* **136**(3): 452–456.

Monga, J., et al (2011). 'Antimelanoma and radioprotective activity of alcoholic aqueous extract of different species of *Ocimum* in C 57BL mice.' *Pharmaceutical Biology* **49**(4): 428–436.

Mukherjee, R. (2006). 'Antibacterial and therapeutic potential of *Ocimum sanctum* in bovine sub clinical mastitis.' *Indian Veterinary Journal* **83**(5): 522–524.

Mukherjee, R., et al (2005). 'Immunotherapeutic potential of *Ocimum sanctum* (L) in bovine subclinical mastitis.' *Research in Veterinary Science* **79**(1): 37–43.

Mukherjee, J., et al (2009). 'CNS activity of the methanol extract obtained from the roots of *Ocimum sanctum* linn.' *Pharmacologyonline* **2**: 673–685.

Muralikrishnan, G., et al (2012). 'Protective effects of *Ocimum sanctum* on lipid peroxidation and antioxidant status in streptozocin-induced diabetic rats.' *Natural Product Research* **26**(5): 474–478.

Muthuraman, A., et al (2008). 'Ameliorative effects of *Ocimum sanctum* in sciatic nerve transection-induced neuropathy in rats.' *Journal of Ethnopharmacology* **120**(1): 56–62.

Narayana, D. B. A. (2011). 'Effect of Tulsi (*Ocimum sanctum* Linn) on sperm count and reproductive hormones in male albino rabbits.' *International Journal of Ayurveda Research* **2**(1): 64.

Narendhirakannan, R., et al. (2005). 'Mineral content of some medicinal plants used in the treatment of diabetes mellitus.' *Biol Trace Elem Res.* **103**(2): 109–115.

Nayak V and P. Uma Devi (2005). 'Protection of mouse bone marrow against radiation-induced chromosome damage and stem cell death by the *Ocimum* flavonoids orientin and vicenin.' *Radiation Research* **163**(2): 165–171.

Padalia, R. C. and R. S. Verma (2011). 'Comparative volatile oil composition of four *Ocimum* species from northern India.' *Natural Product Research* **25**(6): 569–575.

Padmavathi, T. and R. Ranjini (2011). 'Effect of arbuscular mycorrhizal fungi on the growth of *Ocimum sanctum* and glomalin a soil related protein.' *Research Journal of Biotechnology* **6**(4): 44–50.

Pai, P. G., et al (2013). 'Evaluation of diuretic activity of ethanolic extract of *Ocimum sanctum* (L.) in Wistar albino rat.' *Research Journal of Pharmaceutical, Biological and Chemical Sciences* **4**(1): 533–538.

Panda, V. S. and S. R. Naik (2009). 'Evaluation of cardioprotective activity of Ginkgo biloba and *Ocimum sanctum* in rodents.' *Alternative Medicine Review* **14**(2): 161–171.

Pande, M. and A. Pathak (2009). 'Effect of ethanolic extract of *Ocimum gratissimum* (ram tulsi) on sexual behaviour in male mice.' *International Journal of PharmTech Research* **1**(3): 468–473.

Pandey, G. and S. Madhuri (2010). 'Pharmacological activities of *Ocimum sanctum* (Tulsi): A review.' *International Journal of Pharmaceutical Sciences Review and Research* **5**(1): 61–66.

Parag, S., et al (2010). 'Antibacterial activity of *Ocimum sanctum* Linn. and its application in water purification.' *Research Journal of Chemistry and Environment* **14**(3): 46–50.

Parandin, R. and S. A. Haeri Rohani (2010). 'Effect of the oil extract of *Ocimum gratissimum* leaves on the reproductive function and fertility of adult male rats.' *Journal of Applied Biological Sciences* **4**(2): 1–4.

Patil, R., et al (2011). 'Isolation and characterization of anti-diabetic component (bioactivity-guided fractionation) from *Ocimum sanctum* L. (Lamiaceae) aerial part.' *Asian Pacific Journal of Tropical Medicine* **4**(4): 278–282.

Patil, R. S., et al (2012). 'Bioinspired synthesis of highly stabilized silver nanoparticles using *Ocimum tenuiflorum* leaf extract and their antibacterial activity.' *Spectrochimica Acta — Part A: Molecular and Biomolecular Spectroscopy* **91**: 234–238.

Pattanayak, P., et al (2010). '*Ocimum sanctum* Linn. A reservoir plant for therapeutic applications: An overview.' *Pharmacognosy Reviews* **4**(7): 95–105.

Pavaraj, M., et al (2011). 'Development of immunity by extract of medicinal plant *Ocimum sanctum* on common carp *Cyprinus carpio* (L.).' *Research Journal of Immunology* **4**(1): 12–18.

Pemminati, S., et al (2007). 'Effect of ethanolic leaf extract of *Ocimum sanctum* on haloperidol-induced catalepsy in albino mice.' *Indian Journal of Pharmacology* **39**(2): 87–89.

Pemminati, S., et al (2011). 'Anxiolytic effect of acute administration of ursolic acid in rats.' *Research Journal of Pharmaceutical, Biological and Chemical Sciences* **2**(3): 431–437.

Philip, D. and C. Unni (2011). 'Extracellular biosynthesis of gold and silver nanoparticles using Krishna tulsi (*Ocimum sanctum*) leaf.' *Physica E: Low-Dimensional Systems and Nanostructures* **43**(7): 1318–1322.

Prakash, J. and S. K. Gupta (2000). 'Chemopreventive activity of *Ocimum sanctum* seed oil.' *Journal of Ethnopharmacology* **72**(1–2): 29–34.

Prakash, P. and N. Gupta (2005). 'Therapeutic uses of *Ocimum sanctum* Linn (Tulsi) with a note on eugenol and its pharmacological actions: A short review.' *Indian Journal of Physiology and Pharmacology* **49**(2): 125–131.

Prakash, A., et al (2009a). 'Impact of lead on clinicohematological parameters after dietary oral administration and protective efficacy of tulsi (*Ocimum sanctum*) in cockerels.' *Indian Journal of Animal Research* **43**(3): 173–177.

Prakash, A., et al (2009b). 'Ameliorative efficacy of tulsi in lead toxicity in cockerels.' *Indian Veterinary Journal* **86**(4): 344–346.

Prashar, R. and A. Kumar (1995). 'Chemopreventive action of *Ocimum sanctum* on 2,12-dimethylbenz(a)anthracene DMBA-induced papillomagenesis in the skin of mice.' *International Journal of Pharmacognosy* **33**(3): 181–187.

Prashar, R., et al (1994). 'Chemopreventive action by an extract from *Ocimum sanctum* on mouse skin papillomagenesis and its enhancement of skin glutathione S-transferase activity and acid soluble sulfhydryl level.' *Anti-Cancer Drugs* **5**(5): 567–572.

Prashar, R., et al (1998). 'Inhibition by an extract of *Ocimum sanctum* of DNA-binding activity of 7,12-dimethylbenz[a]anthracene in rat hepatocytes in vitro.' *Cancer Letters* **128**(2): 155–160.

Raghavendra, M., et al (2009). 'Role of *Ocimum sanctum* in the experimental model of Alzheimer's disease in rats.' *International Journal of Green Pharmacy* **3**(1): 6–15.

Rai, V., et al (1997a). 'Effect of Tulasi (*Ocimum sanctum*) leaf powder supplementation on blood sugar levels, serum lipids and tissue lipids in diabetic rats.' *Plant Foods for Human Nutrition* **50**(1): 9–16.

Rai, V., et al (1997b). 'Effect of *Ocimum sanctum* leaf powder on blood lipoproteins, glycated proteins and total amino acids in patients with non-insulin-dependent diabetes mellitus.' *Journal of Nutritional and Environmental Medicine* **7**(2): 113–118.

Rajamma, A. J., et al (2011). 'Comparative larvicidal activity of different species of *Ocimum* against *Culex quinquefasciatus*.' *Natural Product Research* **25**(20): 1916–1922.

Rajasekaran, M., et al (1989). 'Mast cell protective activity of ursolic acid — A triterpene from the leaves of *Ocimum sanctum* L.' *Journal of Drug Development* **2**(3): 179–182.

Rajeswara Rao, B. R., et al (2011). 'Chemical and biological diversity in fourteen selections of four *Ocimum* species.' *Natural Product Communications* **6**(11): 1705–1710.

Raju, P. M., et al (1999). 'Volatile constituents of the leaves of *Ocimum sanctum* L.' *Journal of Essential Oil Research* **11**(2): 159–161.

Ramesh, B. and V. N. Satakopan (2010). 'Antioxidant activities of hydroalcoholic extract of *Ocimum sanctum* against cadmium induced toxicity in rats.' *Indian Journal of Clinical Biochemistry* **25**(3): 307–310.

Ramteke, C., et al (2013). 'Synthesis of silver nanoparticles from the aqueous extract of leaves of *Ocimum sanctum* for enhanced antibacterial activity.' *Journal of Chemistry*.

Ranganathan, S. and S. A. M. Balajee (2000). 'Anti-Cryptococcus activity of combination of extracts of *Cassia alata* and *Ocimum sanctum*.' *Mycoses* **43**(7–8): 299–301.

Raseetha Vani, S., et al (2009). 'Comparative study of volatile compounds from genus *Ocimum*.' *American Journal of Applied Sciences* **6**(3): 523–528.

Rastogi, S., et al (2007). 'Protective effect of *Ocimum sanctum* on 3-methylcholanthrene, 7,12-dimethylbenz(a)anthracene and aflatoxin B1 induced skin tumorigenesis in mice.' *Toxicology and Applied Pharmacology* **224**(3): 228–240.

Ravindran, R., et al (2005). 'Noise-stress-induced brain neurotransmitter changes and the effect of *Ocimum sanctum* (Linn) treatment in albino rats.' *Journal of Pharmacological Sciences* **98**(4): 354–360.

Reddy, S. S., et al (2008). 'Prevention of insulin resistance by ingesting aqueous extract of *Ocimum sanctum* to fructose-fed rats.' *Hormone and Metabolic Research* **40**(1): 44–49.

Rege, A. A., et al (2012). 'In vitro lipid peroxidation inhibitory and anti-arthritic activities of some Indian medicinal plants.' *Indian Drugs* **49**(6): 31–35.

Reshma, K., et al (2005). 'Effect of ocimum flavonoids as a radioprotector on the erythrocyte antioxidants in oral cancer.' *Indian Journal of Clinical Biochemistry* **20**(1): 160–164.

Reshma, K., et al (2008). 'Radioprotective effects of ocimum flavonoids on leukocyte oxidants and antioxidants in oral cancer.' *Indian Journal of Clinical Biochemistry* **23**(2): 171–175.

Sadekar, R. D., et al (1998). 'Immunomodulating effect of *Ocimum sanctum* linn. Dry leaf powder on humoral immune response in poultry naturally infected with IBD virus.' *Indian Veterinary Journal* **75**(1): 73–74.

Sagar, A. and I. Thakur (2012). 'Antibacterial activity of *Ocimum sanctum* (Linn.), *Murraya koenigii* (Linn.) spreng and *Artemisia vulgaris* (Linn.).' *Plant Archives* **12**(1): 377–381.

Saiful Islam M., et al (2011). 'In vitro antioxidant and anti-neoplastic activities of *Ocimum sanctum* leaves in Ehrlich Ascites Carcinoma bearing mice.' *International Journal of Cancer Research* **7**(3): 209–221.

Saini, A., et al (2009). 'Induction of resistance to respiratory tract infection with Klebsiella pneumoniae in mice fed on a diet supplemented with tulsi (*Ocimum sanctum*) and clove (*Syzgium aromaticum*) oils.' *Journal of Microbiology, Immunology and Infection* **42**(2): 107–113.

Sairam, K., et al (2000). 'Effect of *Ocimum sanctum* Linn on peptic ulcers and gastric mucosal offensive and defensive factors.' *Biomedicine* **20**(4): 260–267.

Sakina, M. R., et al (1990). 'Preliminary psychopharmacological evaluation of *Ocimum sanctum* leaf extract.' *Journal of Ethnopharmacology* **28**(2): 143–150.

Samak, G., et al (2007). 'Hypolipidemic efficacy of *Ocimum sanctum* in the prevention of atherogenesis in male albino rabbits.' *Pharmacologyonline* **2**: 115–127.

Samson, J., et al (2006). 'Biogenic amine changes in brain regions and attenuating action of *Ocimum sanctum*in noise exposure.' *Pharmacology Biochemistry and Behavior* **83**(1): 67–75.

Samson, J., et al (2007). 'Oxidative stress in brain and antioxidant activity of *Ocimum sanctum* in noise exposure.' *NeuroToxicology* **28**(3): 679–685.

Sarkar, A., et al (1994). 'Changes in the blood lipid profile after administration of *Ocimum sanctum* (Tulsi) leaves in the normal albino rabbits.' *Indian Journal of Physiology and Pharmacology* **38**(4): 311–312.

Sarkar, D., et al (2012). 'Rapid identification of molecular changes in tulsi (*Ocimum sanctum* Linn) upon ageing using leaf spray ionization mass spectrometry.' *Analyst* **137**(19): 4559–4563.
Sathaye, S. and R. G. Redkar (2012). 'Determination of polyphenolic content and antioxidant activities of essential oil of *Ocimum sanctum*, L.' *Research Journal of Pharmaceutical, Biological and Chemical Sciences* **3**(2): 964–976.
Sawarkar, H. A., et al (2010). 'Development and biological evaluation of herbal anti-acne gel.' *International Journal of PharmTech Research* **2**(3): 2028–2031.
Saxena, R. C., et al (2012). 'Efficacy of an extract of *Ocimum tenuiflorum* (OciBest) in the management of general stress: A double-blind, placebo-controlled study.' *Evidence-based Complementary and Alternative Medicine* **2012**; 2012: 894509.
Sembulingam, K. and P. Sembulingam (2005). 'Effect of *Ocimum sanctum* Linn on noise induced changes in electrocardiogram.' *Biomedicine* **25**(2): 58–63.
Sembulingam, K., et al (1997). 'Effect of *Ocimum sanctum* Linn on noise induced changes in plasma corticosterone level.' *Indian Journal of Physiology and Pharmacology* **41**(2): 139–143.
Sembulingam, K., et al (1999). 'Effect of *Ocimum sanctum* linn on changes in leucocytes of albino rats induced by acute noise stress [1].' *Indian Journal of Physiology and Pharmacology* **43**(1): 137–140.
Sembulingam, K., et al (2005). 'Effect of *Ocimum sanctum* Linn on the changes in central cholinergic system induced by acute noise stress.' *Journal of Ethnopharmacology* **96**(3): 477–482.
Sethi, J., et al (2003). 'Protective effect of tulsi (*Ocimum sanctum*) on lipid peroxidation in stress induced by anemic hypoxia in rabbits.' *Indian Journal of Physiology and Pharmacology* **47**(1): 115–119.
Sethi, J., et al (2004). 'Evaluation of hypoglycemic and antioxidant effect of *Ocimum sanctum*.' *Indian Journal of Clinical Biochemistry* **19**(2): 152–155.
Sethi, J., et al. (2010). 'Effect of tulsi (*Ocimum sanctum* Linn.) on sperm count and reproductive hormones in male albino rabbits.' *International Journal of Ayurved Research* **1**(4): 208–210.
Shafqatullah, et al (2013). 'Comparative analyses of *Ocimum sanctum* stem and leaves for phytochemicals and inorganic constituents.' *Middle East Journal of Scientific Research* **13**(2): 236–240.
Shah, K. and R. J. Verma (2012). 'Protection against butyl p-hydroxybenzoic acid induced oxidative stress by *Ocimum sanctum* extract in mice liver.' *Acta Poloniae Pharmaceutica — Drug Research* **69**(5): 865–870.
Sharma, P., et al (1998). 'Anti-cataract activity of *Ocimum sanctum* on experimental cataract.' *Indian Journal of Pharmacology* **30**(1): 16–20.
Sharma, M., et al (2001). 'Cardioprotective potential of *Ocimum sanctum* in isoproterenol induced myocardial infarction in rats.' *Molecular and Cellular Biochemistry* **225**(1–2): 75–83.
Sharma, M. K., et al (2005). 'Protection against mercury-induced renal damage in Swiss albino mice by *Ocimum sanctum*.' *Environmental Toxicology and Pharmacology* **19**(1): 161–167.
Sharma, S. K., et al (2009). 'Inhibitory effects of *Ocimum tenuiflorum* (Tulsi) on the corrosion of zinc in sulphuric acid: A green approach.' *Rasayan Journal of Chemistry* **2**(2): 332–339.
Sharma, A., et al (2012). 'Antimicrobial activity of plant extracts of *Ocimum tenuiflorum*.' *International Journal of PharmTech Research* **4**(1): 176–180.
Sharmila Banu, G., et al (2009). 'Effects of leaves extract of *Ocimum sanctum* L. on arsenic-induced toxicity in Wistar albino rats.' *Food and Chemical Toxicology* **47**(2): 490–495.
Shetty, S., et al (2006). 'Wound healing activity of *Ocimum sanctum* linn with supportive role of antioxidant enzymes.' *Indian Journal of Physiology and Pharmacology* **50**(2): 163–168.
Shetty, S., et al (2008). 'Evaluation of antioxidant and wound healing effects of alcoholic and aqueous extract of *Ocimum sanctum* Linn in rats.' *Evidence-based Complementary and Alternative Medicine* **5**(1): 95–101.
Shivananjappa, M. and M. Joshi (2012). 'Aqueous extract of tulsi (*Ocimum sanctum*) enhances endogenous antioxidant defenses of human hepatoma cell line (HepG2).' *Journal of Herbs, Spices and Medicinal Plants* **18**(4): 331–348.
Shokeen, P., et al (2005). 'Preliminary studies on activity of *Ocimum sanctum*, *Drynaria quercifolia*, and *Annona squamosa* against *Neisseria gonorrhoeae*.' *Sexually Transmitted Diseases* **32**(2): 106–111.
Shukla, S. T., et al (2012). 'Hepatoprotective and antioxidant activities of crude fractions of endophytic fungi of *Ocimum sanctum* Linn. in rats.' *Oriental Pharmacy and Experimental Medicine* **12**(2): 81–91.
Shyamala, A. C. and T. Devaki (1996). 'Studies on peroxidation in rats ingesting copper sulphate and effect of subsequent treatment with *Ocimum sanctum*.' *Journal of Clinical Biochemistry and Nutrition* **20**(2): 113–119.
Shyamala, M. and P. K. Kasthuri (2011). 'A comparative study of the inhibitory effect of the extracts of *Ocimum sanctum*, *Aegle marmelos*, and *Solanum trilobatum* on the corrosion of mild steel in hydrochloric acid medium.' *International Journal of Corrosion* **2011**; 2011: 129647.
Siddique, Y. H., et al (2007). 'Anti-genotoxic effect of *Ocimum sanctum* L. extract against cyproterone acetate induced genotoxic damage in cultured mammalian cells.' *Acta Biologica Hungarica* **58**(4): 397–409.
Siddiqui, F., et al (2012). 'Arsenic accumulation in *Ocimum* spp. and its effect on growth and oil constituents.' *Acta Physiologiae Plantarum*: 1–9.
Singh, S. (1998). 'Comparative evaluation of antiinflammatory potential of fixed oil of different species of *Ocimum* and its possible mechanism of action.' *Indian Journal of Experimental Biology* **36**(10): 1028–1031.
Singh, S. and S. S. Agrawal (1991). 'Anti-asthmatic and anti-inflammatory activity of *Ocimum sanctum*.' *International Journal of Pharmacognosy* **29**(4): 306–310.
Singh, N. and M. Gilca (2008). 'Tulsi — A potential protector againts air travel health problems.' *Natural Product Radiance* **7**(1): 54–57.
Singh, B. and R. K. Jaggi (2003). 'Antiinflammatory effect of *Ocimum sanctum* Linn. and its cultures.' *Indian Journal of Pharmaceutical Sciences* **65**(4): 425–428.
Singh, S. and D. K. Majumdar (1995a). 'Analgesic activity of *Ocimum sanctum* and its possible mechanism of action.' *International Journal of Pharmacognosy* **33**(3): 188–192.
Singh, S. and D. K. Majumdar (1995b). 'Anti-inflammatory and antipyretic activities of *Ocimum sanctum* fixed oil.' *International Journal of Pharmacognosy* **33**(4): 288–292.
Singh, S. and D. K. Majumdar (1996). 'Effect of fixed oil of *Ocimum sanctum* against experimentally induced arthritis and joint edema in laboratory animals.' *Pharmaceutical Biology* **34**(3): 218–222.
Singh, S. and D. K. Majumdar (1997). 'Evaluation of antiinflammatory activity of fatty acids of *Ocimum sanctum* fixed oil.' *Indian Journal of Experimental Biology* **35**(4): 380–383.
Singh, S. and D. K. Majumdar (1999a). 'Effect of *Ocimum sanctum* fixed oil on vascular permeability and leucocytes migration.' *Indian Journal of Experimental Biology* **37**(11): 1136–1138.
Singh, P. and V. K. Mittal (2003). 'Trace elements in typical herbs as an indicator of environmental pollution.' *Indian Journal of Environmental Protection* **23**(10): 1114–1119.
Singh, S., et al (1996). 'Evaluation of anti-inflammatory potential of fixed oil of *Ocimum sanctum* (Holybasil) and its possible mechanism of action.' *Journal of Ethnopharmacology* **54**(1): 19–26.
Singh, S., et al (2001). 'Effect of *Ocimum sanctum* fixed oil on blood pressure, blood clotting time and pentobarbitone-induced sleeping time.' *Journal of Ethnopharmacology* **78**(2–3): 139–143.
Singh, S., et al (2005). 'Antibacterial activity of *Ocimum sanctum* L. fixed oil.' *Indian Journal of Experimental Biology* **43**(9): 835–837.
Singh, S., et al (2007). 'Biological activities of *Ocimum sanctum* L. fixed oil-an overview.' *Indian Journal of Experimental Biology* **45**(5): 403–412.
Singh, N., et al. (2010). Tulsi: The mother medicine of nature. Lucknow, International Institutue of Herbal Medicine.
Singh, P. K., et al (2012). 'Therapy with methanolic extract of *Pterocarpus marsupium* Roxb and *Ocimum sanctum* Linn reverses dyslipidemia and oxidative stress in alloxan induced type I diabetic rat model.' *Experimental and Toxicologic Pathology* **64**(5): 441–448.
Singhal, G., et al (2011). 'Biosynthesis of silver nanoparticles using *Ocimum sanctum* (Tulsi) leaf extract and screening its antimicrobial activity.' *Journal of Nanoparticle Research* **13**(7): 2981–2988.
Sood, S., et al (2005). 'Chronic oral administration of *Ocimum sanctum* Linn. augments cardiac endogenous antioxidants and prevents isoproterenol-induced myocardial necrosis in rats.' *Journal of Pharmacy and Pharmacology* **57**(1): 127–133.
Sood, S., et al (2006). 'Effect of *Ocimum sanctum* Linn. on cardiac changes in rats subjected to chronic restraint stress.' *Journal of Ethnopharmacology* **108**(3): 423–427.
Soundarrajan, C., et al (2012). 'Rapid biological synthesis of platinum nanoparticles using *Ocimum sanctum* for water electrolysis applications.' *Bioprocess and Biosystems Engineering* **35**(5): 827–833.
Sridevi, G., et al (2009). 'Pharmacological basis for antianaphylactic, antihistaminic and mast cell stabilization activity of *Ocimum sanctum*.' *Internet Journal of Pharmacology* **7**(1).
Suanarunsawat, T. and T. Songsak (2005). 'Anti-hyperglycaemic and anti-dyslipidaemic effect of dietary supplement of white *Ocimum sanctum* Linnean before and after STZ-induced diabetes mellitus.' *International Journal of Diabetes and Metabolism* **13**(1): 18–23.
Suanarunsawat, T., et al (2009). 'Anti-lipidemic actions of essential oil extracted from *Ocimum sanctum* L. leaves in rats fed with high cholesterol diet.' *Journal of Applied Biomedicine* **7**(1): 45–53.
Suanarunsawat, T., et al (2010a). 'Antioxidant activity and lipid-lowering effect of essential oils extracted from *Ocimum sanctum* L. leaves in rats fed with a high cholesterol diet.' *Journal of Clinical Biochemistry and Nutrition* **46**(1): 52–59.
Suanarunsawat, T., et al (2010b). 'Anti-hyperlipidemic and cardioprotective effects of *Ocimum sanctum* L. fixed oil in rats fed a high fat diet.' *Journal of Basic and Clinical Physiology and Pharmacology* **21**(4): 387–400.

Suanarunsawat, T., et al (2011). 'Lipid-lowering and antioxidative activities of aqueous extracts of *Ocimum sanctum* L. leaves in rats fed with a high-cholesterol diet.' *Oxidative Medicine and Cellular Longevity*. **2011**: 962025.
Subba Rao, Y., et al (2013). 'Green synthesis and spectral characterization of silver nanoparticles from *Lakshmi tulasi* (*Ocimum sanctum*) leaf extract.' *Spectrochimica Acta — Part A: Molecular and Biomolecular Spectroscopy* **103**: 156–159.
Subramanian, M., et al (2005). 'Antioxidant and radioprotective properties of an *Ocimum sanctum* polysaccharide.' *Redox Report* **10**(5): 257–264.
Sujatha, K., et al (2011). 'Ultrastructural and histopathological studies in lead acetate induced neurotoxicity in wistar albino rats and its amelioration with *Ocimum sanctum* (OS) a leaf extract.' *International Journal of Pharma and Bio Sciences* **2**(4): 295–304.
Sujatha, K., et al (2012). 'Chronic lead toxicity in wistar albino rats and its amelioration with *Ocimum sanctum*.' *Indian Veterinary Journal* **89**(8): 113–115.
Sundaram, R. S., et al (2012). 'Investigation of standardized ethanolic extract of *Ocimum sanctum* linn. (holy basil) leaves for its in vitro antioxidant potential and phenolic composition.' *Asian Journal of Chemistry* **24**(4): 1819–1824.
Suzuki, A., et al (2009). 'Leishmanicidal active constituents from nepalese medicinal plant tulsi (*Ocimum sanctum* L.).' *Chemical and Pharmaceutical Bulletin* **57**(3): 245–251.
Tabassum, I., et al (2010a). 'Effects of *Ocimum sanctum* and *Camellia sinensis* on stress-induced anxiety and depression in male albino *Rattus norvegicus*.' *Indian Journal of Pharmacology* **42**(5): 283–288.
Tabassum, I., et al (2010b). 'Protective effect of *Ocimum sanctum* and *Camellia sinensis* on stress-induced oxidative damage in the central nervous system of *Rattus norvegicus*.' *Research Journal of Pharmaceutical, Biological and Chemical Sciences* **1**(4): 120–134.
Tabassuma, I., et al (2009). 'Protective effect of *Ocimum sanctum* on lipid peroxidation, nucleic acids and protein against restraint stress in male albino rats.' *Biology and Medicine* **1**(2): 42–53.
Tewari, S. N. (1995). '*Ocimum sanctum* L., a botanical fungicide for rice blast control.' *Tropical Science* **35**(3): 263–273.
Thakur, K. and K. S. Pitre (2009). 'Anti-inflammatory activity of extracted eugenol from *Ocimum sanctum* L. leaves.' *Rasayan Journal of Chemistry* **2**(2): 472–474.
Tripathi, A. K., et al (2008). 'Immunomodulatory activity of *Ocimum sanctum* and its influence on cyclophosphamide induced immunosupression.' *Indian Journal of Animal Sciences* **78**(1): 33–36.
Ubaid, R. S., et al (2003). 'Effect of *Ocimum sanctum* (OS) leaf extract on hepatotoxicity induced by antitubercular drugs in rats [1].' *Indian Journal of Physiology and Pharmacology* **47**(4): 465–470.
Uma Devi, P. and A. Ganasoundari (1999). 'Modulation of glutathione and antioxidant enzymes by *Ocimum sanctum* and its role in protection against radiation injury.' *Indian Journal of Experimental Biology* **37**(3): 262–268.
Uma Devi, P., et al (1998). 'A comparative study of radioprotection by *Ocimum* favonoids and synthetic aminothiol protectors in the mouse.' *British Journal of Radiology* **71**(JULY): 782–784.
Uma Devi, P., et al (1999). 'In vivo radioprotection by ocimum flavonoids: Survival.' *Radiation Research* **151**(1): 74–78.
Uma Devi, P., et al (2000). 'Radiation protection by the *Ocimum* flavonoids orientin and vicenin: Mechanisms of action.' *Radiation Research* **154**(4): 455–460.
Upadhyaya, S., et al (2012). 'Integrated management of foliar blast through ecofriendly formulated product, Oscext-e developed from *Ocimum sanctum* ethanolic extract.' *Archives of Phytopathology and Plant Protection* **45**(19): 2290–2300.
Vasudevan, P., et al (1999). 'Bioactive botanicals from basil (*Ocimum* sp.).' *Journal of Scientific and Industrial Research* **58**(5): 332–338.
Vats, V., et al (2004). 'Ethanolic extract of *Ocimum sanctum* leaves partially attenuates streptozotocin-induced alterations in glycogen content and carbohydrate metabolism in rats.' *Journal of Ethnopharmacology* **90**(1): 155–160.
Venu Prasad, M. P. and F. Khanum (2012). 'Antifatigue activity of Ethanolic extract of *Ocimum sanctum* in rats.' *Research Journal of Medicinal Plant* **6**(1): 37–46.
Verma, J. K. and A. V. Joshi (2005). 'HPTLC method for the determination of ursolic acid from *Ocimum sanctum* Linn. (Tulsi) leaves and its formulations.' *Indian Drugs* **42**(10): 650–653.
Verma, P., et al (2007). 'Protective effect of *Ocimum sanctum* leaf extracts against rogor induced ovarian toxicity in *Clarias batrachus* (Linn).' *Journal of Ecophysiology and Occupational Health* **7**(3–4): 177–184.
Verma, A. K., et al (2012). 'Biochemical studies on serum Hb, Sugar, Urea and lipid profile under influence of *Ocimum sanctum* L in aged patients.' *Research Journal of Pharmacy and Technology* **5**(6): 791–794.
Verma Prashant, R., et al (2006). 'Larvicidal activity of *Artemisia nilagirica* (Clarke) Pamp. and *Ocimum sanctum* Linn. A preliminary study.' *Journal of Natural Remedies* **6**(2): 157–161.
Vetal, M. D., et al (2012). 'Extraction of ursolic acid from *Ocimum sanctum* leaves: Kinetics and modeling.' *Food and Bioproducts Processing* **90**(4): 793–798.
Viyoch, J., et al. (2006). 'Evaluation of in vitro antimicrobial activity of Thai basil oils and their micro-emulsion formulas against *Propionibacterium acnes*.' *Int J Cosmet Sci* **28**(2): 1467–2494.
Vora SB, et al. (1969). 'Antifertility screening of plants Part III. Effect of six indigenous plants on early pregnancy in albino rats.' *Indian J Med Res* **57**: 893–899.
Vrinda B, U. D. P. (2001). 'Radiation protection of human lymphocyte chromosomes in vitro by orientin and vicenin.' *Mutat Res* **498**(1–2): 39–46.
Wangcharoen, W. and W. Morasuk (2007). 'Antioxidant capacity and phenolic content of holy basil.' *Songklanakarin Journal of Science and Technology* **29**(5): 1407–1415.
Wani, N. S., et al (2013). 'Formulation and evaluation of herbal sanitizer.' *International Journal of PharmTech Research* **5**(1): 40–43.
Wongs-Aree, C. and C. Jirapong (2007). Active modified atmospheres affecting quality of holy Basil. *Acta Hort* **746**: 461–466.
Yanpallewar, S. U., et al (2004). 'Evaluation of antioxidant and neuroprotective effect of *Ocimum sanctum* on transient cerebral ischemia and long-term cerebral hypoperfusion.' *Pharmacology Biochemistry and Behavior* **79**(1): 155–164.
Yucharoen, R., et al (2011). 'Anti-herpes simplex virus activity of extracts from the culinary herbs *Ocimum sanctum* L., *Ocimum basilicum* L. and *Ocimum americanum* L.' *African Journal of Biotechnology* **10**(5): 860–866.
Zaffer Ahmad, M., et al (2012). 'Anti-diabetic activity of *Ocimum sanctum* L. roots and isolation of new phytoconstituents using two-dimensional nuclear magnetic resonance spectroscopy.' *Journal of Pharmacognosy and Phytotherapy* **4**(6): 75–85.
Zheljazkov, V. D., et al (2008a). 'Yield and composition of *Ocimum basilicum* L. and *Ocimum sanctum* L. grown at four locations.' *HortScience* **43**(3): 737–741.
Zheljazkov, V. D., et al (2008b). 'Content, composition, and bioactivity of the essential oils of three basil genotypes as a function of harvesting.' *Journal of Agricultural and Food Chemistry* **56**(2): 380–385.

Turmeric

HISTORICAL NOTE Turmeric is a perennial herb, yielding a rhizome that produces a yellow powder that gives curry its characteristic yellow colour and is used to colour French mustard and the robes of Hindu priests. It has been used in Hindu religious ceremonies, and Hindus also apply a mixture of turmeric and sandalwood powder on their foreheads (Jagetia & Aggarwal 2007). Turmeric was probably first cultivated as a dye, and then as a condiment and cosmetic. It is often used as an inexpensive substitute for saffron in cooking and in the 13th century Marco Polo marvelled at its similarities to saffron. In Chinese medicine, turmeric was used in the treatment of inflammatory and digestive disorders and was also used in tooth powder or paste (Anonymous 2001). In Ayurvedic medicine, it was used to treat a wide variety of disorders, including rheumatism, skin conditions, inflammation, intestinal worms, hepatic disorders, biliousness, dyspepsia, diarrhoea, constipation and colic (Jagetia & Aggarwal 2007). In addition to its use in cardiovascular disease and gastrointestinal disorders, research has focused on turmeric's antioxidant, hepatoprotective, anti-inflammatory, anticarcinogenic and antimicrobial properties

(Anonymous 2001). Curcumin was first discovered from the rhizomes of turmeric by Harvard College laboratory scientists Vogel and Pelletier and published in 1815 (Gupta et al 2013). Turmeric is believed to promote the flow of *qi* (Jagetia & Aggarwal 2007).

COMMON NAME

Turmeric

OTHER NAMES

Chiang-huang, curcuma, curcumae longae rhizoma, curcuma rhizome, e zhu, haldi, haridra, Indian saffron, jiang huang, jiang huang curcumae rhizoma, turmeric rhizome, turmeric root, yellow root, yu jin, zedoary

BOTANICAL NAME/FAMILY

Curcuma longa (family Zingiberaceae [ginger])

PLANT PART USED

Dried secondary rhizome (containing not less than 3% curcuminoids calculated as curcumin and not less than 3% volatile oil, calculated on dry-weight basis).

CHEMICAL COMPONENTS

Turmeric rhizome contains 5% phenolic curcuminoids (diarylheptanoids), which give turmeric the yellow colour. The most significant curcuminoid is curcumin (diferuloylmethane). It also contains up to 5% essential oil, including sesquiterpene (e.g. Zingiberene), sesquiterpene alcohols, sesquiterpene ketones, and monoterpenes.

Turmeric also contains immune-stimulating polysaccharides, including acid glucans known as ukonan A, B and C (Evans & Trease 2002).

MAIN ACTIONS

Most research has focused on a series of curcumin constituents found in turmeric. Many of the animal studies involve parenteral administration as oral turmeric or curcumin was considered less active because curcumin is poorly absorbed by the gastrointestinal tract and only trace amounts appear in the blood after oral intake (Ammon & Wahl 1991). Curcumin possesses anti-inflammatory, antioxidant, immuno-modulatory, wound-healing, anti-proliferative and antimicrobial activities (Dulbecco & Savarino 2013). Curcumin may, however, have significant activity in the gastrointestinal tract, and systemic effects may take place as a consequence of local gastrointestinal effects or be associated with metabolites of the curcuminoids.

ANTIOXIDANT

Studies have shown that turmeric, as well as curcumin, has significant antioxidant activity (Ak & Gulcin 2008, Bengmark 2006, Menon & Sudheer 2007, Shalini & Srinivas 1987, Soudamini et al 1992). Turmeric not only exerts direct free radical scavenging activity, it also appears to enhance the antioxidant activity of endogenous antioxidants, such as glutathione peroxidase, catalase and quinine reductase. Curcumin has been shown to induce phase II detoxification enzymes (glutathione peroxidase, glutathione reductase, glucose-6-phosphate dehydrogenase and catalase) (Iqbal et al 2003). Additionally, its antioxidant effects are 10-fold more potent than ascorbic acid or resveratrol (Song et al 2001). In addition to curcumin, turmeric contains the antioxidants protocatechuic acid and ferulic acid, and exhibits significant protection to DNA against oxidative damage in vitro (Kumar et al 2006).

Turmeric's antioxidant activity may protect against damage produced by myocardial and cerebral ischaemia (Al-Omar et al 2006, Fiorillo et al 2008, Shukla et al 2008) and diabetes (Farhangkhoee et al 2006, Jain et al 2006, Kowluru & Kanwar 2007). Turmeric has been shown to restore myocardial antioxidant status, inhibit lipid peroxidation and protect against ischaemia–reperfusion-induced myocardial injuries in two animal studies (Fiorillo et al 2008, Mohanty et al 2004). The mechanism is likely to be due to curcumin's antioxidant and anti-inflammatory effects. Curcumin has also been found to prevent protein glycosylation and lipid peroxidation caused by high glucose levels in vitro (Jain et al 2006) and to improve diabetic nephropathy (Srinivasan 2005) and retinopathy (Kowluru & Kanwar 2007). Turmeric has also been shown to suppress cataract development and collagen cross-linking, promote wound healing, and lower blood lipids and glucose levels (Jain et al 2006, Panchatcharam et al 2006).

Anti-inflammatory

There have been a large number of studies examining the anti-inflammatory effects of curcumin. There is strong molecular evidence published for curcumin's potency to target multiple inflammatory diseases (Henrotin et al 2013). Turmeric is a dual inhibitor of the arachidonic acid cascade. Curcumin has been shown to exert anti-inflammatory effects via phospholipase, lipo-oxygenase, COX-2, leukotrienes, thromboxane, prostaglandins, nitric oxide (NO), collagenase, elastase, hyaluronidase, monocyte chemoattractant protein-1, IFN-inducible protein, TNF-α and IL-12 (Chainani-Wu 2003, Lantz et al 2005, Rao 2007). Due to its anti-inflammatory effects, curcumin has shown promise in many chronic disorders such as arthritis, allergies, arteriosclerosis, colitis, diabetes, respiratory disorders, hepatic injury, pancreatic disease, intestinal disorders, eye diseases, neurodegenerative diseases and various cancers (Aggarwal et al 2007, Bengmark 2006).

The anti-inflammatory effect of curcumin was tested in adjuvant-induced chronic inflammation rats, where it was found that curcumin significantly reduced C-reactive protein, TNF-α, IL-1 and NO, with no significant changes observed in PGE_2 and leukotriene B_4 levels or lymphocyte proliferation (Banerjee et al 2003). Curcumin has also been shown to inhibit inflammation in experimental pancreatitis via inhibition of NF-κB and activator protein-1 in two rat models (Gukovsky et al 2003).

NF-kappa-B inhibition

The many and varied effects of curcumin may be partly associated with the inhibition of the transcription factor, nuclear factor-kappa beta (NF-κB), and induction of heat shock proteins (HSP). NF-κB is a transcription factor pivotal in the regulation of inflammatory genes and is also closely associated with the heat shock response, which is a cellular defence mechanism that confers broad protection against various cytotoxic stimuli. Inhibition of NF-κB may reduce inflammation and protect cells against damage (Chang 2001) and curcumin has been found to attenuate experimental colitis in animal models through a mechanism correlated with the inhibition of NF-κB (Salh et al 2003). The clinical significance of this is unclear.

Gastrointestinal effects

Hepatoprotective

Extracts of both turmeric and curcumin have been found to prevent and improve carbon tetrachloride-induced liver injury, both in vivo and in vitro (Abu-Rizq et al 2008, Deshpande et al 1998, Fu et al 2008, Kang et al 2002, Wu et al 2008). Curcumin also protects against dimethylnitrosamine-induced liver injury (Farombi et al 2008), reverses aflatoxin-induced liver damage in experimental animals (Soni et al 1992) and effectively suppresses the hepatic microvascular inflammatory response to lipopolysaccharides in vivo (Lukita-Atmadja et al 2002). An ethanol-soluble fraction of turmeric was shown to contain three antioxidant compounds — curcumin, demethoxycurcumin and bisdemethoxycurcumin — which exert similar hepatoprotective activity to silybin and silychristin in vitro (Song et al 2001).

Several different mechanisms may contribute to turmeric's hepatoprotective activity. Curcumin has been shown to prevent lipoperoxidation of subcellular membranes in a dosage-dependent manner, due to an antioxidant mechanism (Quiles et al 1998) and turmeric may also protect the liver via inhibition of NF-κB (see above), which has been implicated in the pathogenesis of alcoholic liver disease. Curcumin also appears to chelate hepatic and serum iron in vivo (Jiao et al 2006, 2009). Iron is pro-oxidant to the liver, which may be problematic during hepatic disease. Recent research also suggests that curcumin may be useful in preventing hepatic fibrosis caused by chronic liver disease (Fu et al 2008, O'Connell & Rushworth 2008). Curcumin also blocks endotoxin-mediated activation of NF-κB and suppresses the expression of cytokines, chemokines, COX 2 and iNOS in Kupffer cells (Nanji et al 2003).

Cholagogue and hypolipidaemic

The extracts of turmeric and curcumin have shown dose-dependent hypolipidaemic activity in vivo (Asai & Miyazawa 2001, Babu & Srinivasan 1997, Keshavarz 1976, Manjunatha & Srinivasan 2007a, 2007b, Ramirez-Tortosa et al 1999, Soudamini et al 1992). One in vivo study suggests that curcumin may stimulate the conversion of cholesterol into bile acids, and therefore increase the excretion of cholesterol (Srinivasan & Sambaiah 1991). A further study demonstrated that supplementation with turmeric reduces fatty streak development and oxidative stress (Quiles et al 2002). Curcumin also increases LDL receptor mRNA (Peschel et al 2007). Oral curcumin has also been shown to stimulate contraction of the gall bladder and promote the flow of bile in healthy subjects (Rasyid & Lelo 1999).

Antispasmodic

Curcuminoids exhibit smooth muscle relaxant activity possibly mediated through calcium channel blockade, although additional mechanisms cannot be ruled out (Gilani et al 2005). Curcuminoids produced antispasmodic effects on isolated guinea pig ileum and rat uterus by receptor-dependent and independent mechanisms (Itthipanichpong et al 2003).

Cancer

Curcumin has been studied for its wide-ranging effects on tumourigenesis, angiogenesis, apoptosis and signal transduction pathways (Gururaj et al 2002, Mohan et al 2000, Thaloor et al 1998). It is known to inhibit oncogenesis during both the promotion and the progression periods in a variety of cancers (Anto et al 1996, Kuttan et al 1985, Menon et al 1999, Ruby et al 1995). Curcumin was found to possess chemopreventive effects against cancers of the skin, stomach, colon, prostate, and breast, as well as oral cancer in mice.

Chemoprevention

Chemoprevention refers to reversing, suppressing or preventing the process of carcinogenesis. Carcinogenesis results from the accumulation of multiple sequential mutations and alterations in nuclear and cytoplasmic molecules, culminating in invasive neoplasms. These events have traditionally been separated into three phases: initiation, promotion and progression. Typically, initiation is rapid, whereas promotion and progression can take many years. Ultimately, chemoprevention aims at preventing the growth and survival of cells already committed to becoming malignant (Gescher et al 1998, 2001).

T

Curcumin has been found to inhibit the invasion, proliferation and metastasis of various cancers in vivo (Kunnumakkara et al 2008). Curcumin has been found to effectively block carcinogen-induced skin (Azuine & Bhide 1992), colon (Rao et al 1995a, 1995b, 1995c, 1999) and liver (Chuang et al 2000) carcinogenesis in animals. It has been suggested that the chemoprotective activity of curcumin occurs via changes in enzymes involved in both carcinogen bioactivation and oestrogen metabolism. This is supported by the findings that curcumin treatment produced changes in CYP1A, CYP3A and GST in mice (Valentine et al 2006) and alleviated the CCl_4-induced inactivation of CYPs 1A, 2B, 2C and 3A isozymes in rats, possibly through its antioxidant properties, without inducing hepatic CYP (Sugiyama et al 2006).

Oral curcumin inhibited chemically-induced skin carcinogenesis in mice (Huang et al 1992) and curcumin prevented radiation-induced mammary and pituitary tumours in rats (Inano & Onoda 2002). Curcumin and genistein (from soybeans) inhibited the growth of oestrogen-positive human breast MCF-7 cells induced individually or by a mixture of the pesticides endosulfane, dichlorodiphenyltrichloroethane (DDT) and chlordane, or 17-beta oestradiol (Verma et al 1997). Another study found that curcumin inhibited breast cancer metastases in immunodeficient animals (Bachmeier et al 2007). This may be due to the ability of curcumin to reduce NF-κB and therefore downregulate the two inflammatory cytokines CXCL1 and CXCL2 (Bachmeier et al 2008).

Apoptosis

Apoptosis (programmed cell death) plays a crucial role in regulating cell numbers by eliminating damaged or cancerous cells. Curcumin has been shown to induce apoptosis in many different cancer cell lines, including breast, leukaemia, lymphoma, melanoma, ovarian, colorectal, lung and pancreatic in vitro (Kim et al 2001, Kuo et al 1996, Li et al 2007, Lin et al 2007, Lev-Ari et al 2006, Marin et al 2007, Skommer et al 2006, 2007, Tian et al 2008). Curcumin has also increased apoptosis in breast and ovarian cancers in vivo (Bachmeier et al 2007, Lin et al 2007). Curcumin has been demonstrated to induce apoptosis in human basal cell carcinoma cells associated with the p53 signalling pathway, which controls intracellular redox status, levels of oxidation-damaged DNA and oxidative stress-induced apoptosis (Jee et al 1998). Curcumin has also been found to induce apoptosis in human mutant p53 melanoma cell lines and block the NF-κB cell survival pathway and suppress the apoptotic inhibitor known as XIAP. Because melanoma cells with mutant p53 are strongly resistant to conventional chemotherapy, curcumin may overcome the chemoresistance of these cells and provide potential new avenues for treatment (Bush et al 2001).

Curcumin has also been found to inhibit prostate cancer cell growth in mice (Dorai et al 2001) and decrease proliferation and induce apoptosis in androgen-dependent and androgen-independent prostate cancer cells in vitro. This was found to be mediated through modulation of apoptosis suppressor proteins and interference with growth factor receptor signalling pathways (Dorai et al 2000). However, in a further study with rats curcumin did not prevent prostate carcinogenesis (Imaida et al 2001).

Antiproliferative

Reduction in proliferation and/or increased apoptosis will lead to tumour regression; however, a more potent effect will be achieved if the two mechanisms occur simultaneously. Curcumin has been shown to do this. The inhibition of cell proliferation is partly related to inhibition of various kinases, such as protein kinase and phosphorylase kinase (Reddy & Aggarwal 1994), and inhibition of several oncogenes and transcription factors. For example, turmeric inhibited epidermal growth factor receptor (EGF-R) signalling via multiple mechanisms, including downregulation of the EGF-R protein, inhibition of intrinsic EGF-R tyrosine kinase activity and inhibition of ligand-induced activation of the EGF-R (Dorai et al 2000). These mechanisms may be particularly important in preventing prostate cancer cells from progressing to a hormone refractory state (Dorai et al 2000). Curcumin has also been found to suppress the growth of multiple breast cancer cell lines and deplete p185neu, the protein product of the HER2/neu proto-oncogene, which is thought to be important in human carcinogenesis (Hong et al 1999).

Antimetastatic

Curcumin demonstrated the ability to reduce lung metastases from melanoma cells in mice. The activity of curcumin is varied. In cell adhesion assays, curcumin-treated cells showed a dose-dependent reduction in their binding to four extracellular matrix proteins (binding to proteins is associated with the spreading of the cancer). Another study found that curcumin effectively suppressed COX-2, vascular endothelial growth factor and intercellular adhesion molecules, while enhancing the expression of antimetastatic proteins, tissue inhibitor metalloproteases-2, non-metastatic gene 23 and E-cadherin, a transmembrane protein that plays an important role in cell adhesion (Kuttan et al 2007). Curcumin-treated cells showed a marked reduction in the expression of integrin receptors (integrins functionally connect the cell interior with the extracellular matrix, another process necessary for metastases).

Chemotherapy

Curcumin enhanced the cytotoxicity of chemotherapeutic agents in prostate cancer cells in vitro by inducing the expression of certain androgen receptor and transcription factors and suppressing NF-κB activation (Hour et al 2002). Curcumin enhanced the antitumour effect of cisplatin against fibrosarcoma (Navis et al 1999), fluorouracil and oxaliplatin in colorectal cancer (Du et al 2006, Li et al 2007) and gemcitabine and paclitaxel in bladder cancer (Kamat et al 2007). Curcumin also attenuated multidrug resistance in a non-small cell lung cancer cell line (Andjelkovic et al 2008) and acted as a radiosensitiser for cervical cancer in vitro (Javvadi et al 2008).

Curcumin, however, was found to significantly inhibit cyclophosphamide-induced tumour regression in an in vivo model of human breast cancer. It is suspected that this occurred as a result of inhibition of free radical generation and blockade of JNK function. As such, curcumin intake should be limited in people undergoing treatment for breast cancer with cyclophosphamide until further investigation can clarify the significance of these findings (Somasundaram et al 2002).

Immunomodulation

Curcumin administration was found to significantly increase the total white blood cell count and circulating antibodies in mice. A significant increase in macrophage phagocytic activity was also observed in curcumin-treated animals (Antony et al 1999). However, curcumin has also been demonstrated to have some immunosuppressive activity. Curcumin inhibits PAR2- and PAR4-mediated human mast cell activation by blocking the ERK pathway (Baek et al 2003).

An in vivo study using a cardiac transplant model found that curcumin also significantly reduced expression of IL-2, IFN-gamma and granzyme B (a serine protease associated with the activity of killer T-lymphocytes and NK cells) and increased mean survival time. Curcumin was further shown to work synergistically with the antirejection drug cyclosporin (Chueh et al 2003).

Curcumin also modulates other interleukins and has been shown in vitro to be a potent inhibitor of the production of the pro-inflammatory cytokine IL-8, thereby reducing tumour growth and carcinoma cell viability. Curcumin not only inhibited IL-8 production but also inhibited signal transduction through IL-8 receptors (Hidaka et al 2002) and inhibited cell proliferation, cell-mediated cytotoxicity and cytokine production most likely by inhibiting NF-κB target genes (Gao et al 2004).

Cardiovascular effects

Antiplatelet

Curcumin has been shown to inhibit platelet aggregation in vivo (Chen et al 2007, R Srivastava et al 1985, 1986) and in vitro (Jantan et al 2008, KC Srivastava 1989, KC Srivastava et al 1995). The anticoagulant effect of curcumin is weaker than that of aspirin, which is four-fold more potent than curcumin in treatment of collagen- and noradrenaline-induced thrombosis. Curcumin 100 mg/kg and aspirin 25 mg/kg resulted in 60% protection from thrombosis (Srivastava et al 1985).

Anti-atherogenic

A hydro-ethanolic extract of turmeric was found to decrease LDL oxidation, lower the oxidation of erythrocyte and liver membranes, as well as have a vitamin E-sparing effect in rabbits fed a diet high in saturated fat and cholesterol (Mesa et al 2003, Ramirez-Tortosa et al 1999). The atheroscleroprotective potential of turmeric was further demonstrated by an animal study that found turmeric lowered blood pressure and reduced the atherogenic properties of cholesterol (Zahid Ashraf et al 2005). Curcumin also inhibits the proliferation and migration of vascular smooth muscle cells in vitro (Yang et al 2006).

Many in vivo studies have investigated the effects of dietary curcumin on blood cholesterol in diabetic animals (Babu & Srinivasan 1997, Manjunatha & Srinivasan 2007a, 2007b, Pari & Murugan 2007). The two Manjunatha and Srinivasan studies found that curcumin significantly lowered plasma cholesterol, but only lowered hepatic cholesterol in animals with normal baseline cholesterol. Additionally, hepatic alpha-tocopherol and glutathione levels and serum glutathione peroxidase and glutathione transferase were increased. Babu and Srinivasan (1997) also found a significant decrease in blood triglyceride and phospholipid levels. In a parallel study in which diabetic animals were maintained on a high cholesterol diet, curcumin lowered cholesterol and phospholipid and countered the elevated liver and renal cholesterol and triglyceride levels seen in the diabetic animals (Babu & Srinivasan 1997).

Wound healing

Wound healing is a highly ordered process, requiring complex and coordinated interactions involving peptide growth factors, of which transforming growth factor-beta (TGF-beta) is one of the most important. Nitric oxide is also an important factor in healing, and its production is regulated by iNOS. Topical application of curcumin accelerated wound healing in normal and diabetic rats. The wound healing is partly associated with the regulation of the growth factor TGF-beta-1 and iNOS (Mani et al 2002). Curcumin's wound-healing ability has been confirmed in several other animal studies (Sidhu et al 1998, Sidhu et al 1999). Wounds of animals treated with curcumin showed earlier re-epithelialisation, improved neovascularisation, increased migration of various cells, including dermal myofibroblasts, fibroblasts and macrophages into the wound bed, and a higher collagen content (Sidhu et al 1999). It appears to be effective when used orally or as a local application.

Curcumin has also demonstrated powerful inhibition against hydrogen peroxide damage in human keratinocytes and fibroblasts (Phan et al 2001) and pretreatment with curcumin significantly enhanced the rate of wound contraction, decreased mean wound-healing time, increased synthesis of collagen, hexosamine, DNA and NO and improved fibroblast and vascular densities in full thickness wounds in mice exposed to whole-body gamma-radiation (Jagetia & Rajanikant 2004).

Antibacterial/Antimicrobial

Curcumin is a highly pleiotropic molecule that was first shown to exhibit antibacterial activity in 1949 (Gupta et al 2013). Turmeric is used as an antimicrobial for preserving food (Jayaprakasha et al 2005) and has been found to have antifungal activity, as well as inhibiting aspergillus growth and aflatoxin production in feeds (Gowda et al 2004).

Curcumin has also been found to have dose-dependent, antiprotozoan activity against *Giardia lamblia* with inhibition of parasite growth and adherent capacity, induction of morphological alterations and apoptosis-like changes in vitro (Perez-Arriaga et al 2006). Curcumin has also shown in vitro and in vivo activity against malaria, with inhibition of growth of chloroquine-resistant *Plasmodium falciparum* in vitro and enhancement of survival in mice infected with *P. berghei* (Reddy et al 2005).

OTHER ACTIONS

Curcumin's anti-inflammatory and antioxidant actions may be useful in preventing neurodegenerative diseases, such as Alzheimer's disease and Parkinson's disease, and curcumin has been found to target multiple pathogenic cascades in preclinical models (transgenic and amyloid infusion models) of Alzheimer's disease (Cole et al 2005, Calabrese et al 2006). Curcumin has also been found to dose-dependently inhibit neuroglial proliferation, with low doses being as effective as higher doses, given a longer period of treatment (Ambegaokar et al 2003). It may also enhance immune clearance of amyloidosis in the brain (Zhang et al 2006).

Theracurmin, a highly absorptive curcumin dispersed with colloidal nanoparticles, recently exhibited an inhibitory action against alcohol intoxication after drinking in humans. This was shown by the reduced acetaldehyde concentration of the blood (Sasaki et al 2011).

Curcumin (20 mg/kg body weight) treatment significantly inhibited chemical (ovalbumin)-induced airway constriction and airway hyperreactivity in an animal model of asthma (Ram et al 2003), thereby inidcating potential anti-asthma effects.

Curcumin inhibits P-glycoprotein in numerous in vitro studies (Anuchapreeda et al 2002, Limtrakul et al 2004, Nabekura et al 2005). The clinical significance of this observation has yet to be determined.

CLINICAL USE

In practice, turmeric and the various curcuminoids are used in many forms and administered via various routes. This review will focus mostly on those methods of use that are commonly used and preparations, such as oral dose forms and topical applications. Turmeric may be used as a single therapeutic agent or in combination with other herbal medicines or nutrients, such as the omega-3 polyunsaturated fatty acids. There is strong molecular evidence published for curcumin's potency to target multiple inflammatory diseases (Henrotin et al 2013).

Arthritis

Curcumin is one of the most promising natural ingredients in the treatment of arthritis. It exhibits several mechanisms of action which make it an excellent candidate. In vitro studies have shown that curcumin inhibits NF-κB activation and translocation induced by IL-1β and the consequent expression of NF-κB induced pro-inflammatory genes, COX-2 and VEGF (Henrotin et al 2013). In a randomised, controlled, double-blind study, curcumin 1200 mg/day was compared with phenylbutazone in subjects with rheumatoid arthritis (RA).

Rheumatoid arthritis

Curcumin was found to be effective in improving morning stiffness, walking time and joint swelling; however, the effects of phenylbutazone were stronger (Deodhar et al 1980). A more recent randomised study involving 45 patients with active RA found that treatment with curcumin (500 mg/day) was more effective than diclofenac sodium (50 mg/day) for reducing the Disease Activity Score (DAS) 28, together with tenderness and swelling, as measured by the American College of Rheumatology (ACR) criteria (Chandran & Goel 2012). In particular, the treatment was safe and well tolerated.

Osteoarthritis

A proprietary complex of curcumin with soy phosphatidylcholine (Meriva, Indena SpA), which corresponded to 200 mg curcumin daily, was shown to decrease the global WOMAC score by 58% ($P < 0.05$) at 3 months, increase walking distance and significantly reduce C-reactive protein levels in volunteers with osteoarthritis, thereby indicating a significant anti-inflammatory effect. In comparison, the control group only experienced very modest effects (Belcaro et al 2010b). To test the long-term effects of curcumin treatment, a follow-up study of 100 people with OA was conducted, which showed significant improvements to both the clinical and biochemical end points for Meriva (1 gm/day) compared to controls at 8 months (Belcaro et al 2010a). The WOMAC score was decreased by more than 50%, whereas treadmill-walking performance was increased almost threefold. From a biochemical perspective, serum inflammatory biomarkers such as IL-1β,IL-6, soluble CD40 ligand, soluble vascular cell adhesion molecule-1, and erythrocyte sedimentation rate were also significantly decreased in the treatment group. Of particular importance, there was a significant decrease in the requirement for NSAIDs and reduced gastrointestinal complications.

IN COMBINATION

Curcumin combined with boswellia, withania and zinc produced a significant drop in pain and disability in osteoarthritis (OA) of the knee in a randomised, double-blind, placebo-controlled crossover study of 42 patients (Kulkarni et al 1991); however, the contribution of curcumin to these results is unknown.

Cancer

Epidemiological data suggest that curcumin consumption reduces the rate of colorectal cancer (Hergenhahn et al 2002) and curcumin has wide-ranging chemopreventive activity in preclinical carcinogenic models (Plummer et al 2001), most notably for gastrointestinal cancers (Ireson et al 2001). In 1987 Kuttan et al treated 62 patients with external cancerous lesions with topical curcumin and found remarkable symptomatic relieving activity (Kuttan et al 1987). There was a reduction in smell, itching, lesion size and pain. Interestingly, the effect lasted for several months in most patients. Since then, curcumin, either alone or in combination with other agents, has demonstrated potential against colorectal cancer, pancreatic cancer, breast cancer, prostate cancer, multiple myeloma, lung cancer, oral cancer, and head and neck squamous cell carcinoma (HNSCC) (Gupta et al 2013).

Curcumin appears to be a well-tolerated adjunctive treatment option for patients with pancreatic cancer. Twenty-five participants took 8 g of curcumin daily. Despite significant inter-patient variations in blood curcumin levels, NF-κB, COX-2 and phosphorylated signal transducer and activator of transcription 3 were all downregulated in peripheral blood mononuclear cells (Dhillon et al 2008).

In a phase 1 study, curcumin taken orally for 3 months at a starting dose of 500 mg/day was found to produce histological improvement in cases of bladder cancer, oral leucoplakia, intestinal metaplasia of the stomach, cervical intraepithelial neoplasm and Bowen's disease (Cheng et al 2001).

An ethanol extract of turmeric, as well as an ointment of curcumin, was found to produce remarkable symptomatic relief in patients with external cancerous lesions (Kuttan et al 1987) and there are clinical reports to suggest that curcumin could be safe and effective in the treatment of idiopathic inflammatory orbital pseudotumours (Lal et al 2000).

Curcumin has a potential use in breast cancer as it has been found to inhibit the migratory activity of breast cancer cells, proliferative rate, adhesion, and invasion through down-regulating the expression of NF-κB p65 (Liu & Chen 2013). Cell proliferation assays have shown that curcumin exhibited anti-proliferative effects on MDA-MB-231 and BT-483 breast cancer cells in a time- and dose-dependent manner. Curcumin decreased matrix metalloproteinases-1 expression in MDA-MB231 and BT-483 breast cancer cells. Down-regulation of NF-κB inducing genes (NF-κB p65) was also observed (Liu et al 2009). Curcumin may provide a clinically useful tool for the suppression of vascular endothelial growth factor (VEGF) in tumour cells. It has been found that curcumin suppressed breast tumour angiogenesis by negating osteopontin or medroxyprogesterone acetate-induced VEGF expression. Curcumin was found to inhibit α6β4 signalling and functions by altering intracellular localisation of α6β4, and prevented its association with signalling receptors such as the epidermal growth factor receptor (EGFR) and Protein Kinase B (Akt). In addition, the combination of epigallocatechin gallate (EGCG) and curcumin is efficacious in both in vitro and in vivo models of ERα-breast cancer. In these processes, the regulation of VEGFR-1 may play a key role in the antitumour activities (Liu & Chen 2013). Poly (ADP-ribose) polymerase 1 (PARP-1) plays a significant role in cellular protection against radiation. Targeting PARP-1 may provide an effective way of maximising the therapeutic value of curcumin and antioxidants for cancer prevention (Liu & Chen 2013). More research needs to be conducted for the potential use of curcumin in breast cancer patients.

Cardiovascular disease

Effects of curcumin on risk factors for atherosclerosis were investigated in a 6-month randomised, double-blind, placebo-controlled clinical trial (Chuengsamarn et al 2014).

Hyperlipidaemia

Turmeric may be associated with a decrease in the risk of cardiovascular disease and an intake of 200 mg of a hydro-ethanolic extract of turmeric may decrease total blood lipid peroxides as well as HDL- and LDL-lipid peroxidation, in addition to normalising plasma fibrinogen levels and apolipoprotein B/apolipoprotein A ratio (Miquel et al 2002).

A placebo-controlled, randomised, double-blind study investigated the effects of curcumin on the serum lipids in 36 elderly men and women (Baum et al 2007). The participants were randomised to receive 4 g/day of curcumin, 1 g/day of curcumin or placebo for 6 months. Neither active product significantly altered triglyceride or cholesterol levels at 1 or at 6 months. It was noted that the curcumin concentration was greater after capsule administration of curcumin compared to that of powder administration.

In an open trial, 10 healthy volunteers received 500 mg/day of curcumin for 7 days. A significant decrease in the level of serum lipid peroxides (33%), increase in HDL cholesterol (29%) and a decrease in total serum cholesterol (11.63%) were noted. It also reduced serum lipid peroxides (Soni & Kuttan 1992). In a subsequent study, a 45-day intake (by healthy individuals 27–67 years of age) of a turmeric hydro-alcoholic extract at a daily dose equivalent to 20 mg of curcumin resulted in a significant decrease in serum lipid peroxides (Ramirez-Bosca et al 1995). A daily intake of turmeric equivalent to 20 mg of curcumin for 60 days also decreased peroxidation of both HDL and LDL in 30 healthy volunteers ranging in age from 40 to 90 years. The effect was quite striking in the persons with high baseline values of peroxidised compounds in these lipoproteins, although no apparent change took place in the persons having low baseline values (Ramirez et al 1997). Larger trials are needed to test the efficacy of turmeric in dyslipidaemia.

Diabetes

Turmeric has been used for the treatment of diabetes in Ayurvedic and traditional Chinese medicine (Zhang et al 2013). A systematic review suggests that curcumin could favourably affect most of the leading aspects of diabetes, such as insulin resistance, hyperglycaemia, hyperlipidaemia, and islet apoptosis and necrosis, as well as diabetes-related liver disorders, adipocyte dysfunction, neuropathy, nephropathy, and vascular diseases. Increased inflammation and levels of circulating ROS have been identified in the progression of diabetes. Potential mechanisms in the treatment of diabetes include antioxidant, anti-inflammatory (reduced IL-6, NF-κB, TNFα) and delayed islet ROS production. The authors conclude that studies need to be carried out in humans to confirm the potential of curcumin in limitation of diabetes and other associated disorders.

A 9-month randomised, double-blind, placebo-controlled trial in a prediabetic population showed that curcumin significantly lowered the number of prediabetic individuals who eventually developed type 2 diabetes (16.4% vs 0%) (Chuengsamarn et al 2012). HbA_{1C}, fasting plasma glucose (FPG), and oral glucose tolerance test (OGGT) measured at 2 hours were significantly lower in the curcumin-treated group when compared with the placebo group ($P < 0.01$) in all visits at 3, 6 and 9 months. The curcumin-treated group showed a lower level of homeostasis model assessment-insulin resistance (HOMA-IR) (3.22 vs. 4.04; $P < 0.001$). In addition, the curcumin treatment appeared to improve overall function of β-cells, with very minor adverse effects.

Dyspepsia/peptic ulcers

A randomised, controlled, double-blind, prospective, multicentre pilot study compared the effects of dried extracts of greater celandine and turmeric with placebo in 76 patients with colicky abdominal pain in the right upper quadrant due to biliary dyskinesia. Abdominal pain was reduced more quickly with active treatment; however, other symptoms such as fullness, nausea and vomiting did not respond (Niederau & Gopfert 1999). Another randomised, placebo-controlled, double-blind study that investigated the efficacy of turmeric for treatment of dyspepsia and flatulence in 116 adult patients with acidic dyspepsia, flatulent dyspepsia or atonic dyspepsia found that 87% of patients receiving turmeric responded compared to 53% receiving placebo (Thamlikitkul et al 1989).

In a study of 24 patients with duodenal or gastric ulcers varying between 0.5 and 1.5 cm in diameter, 300 mg of turmeric given five times daily, 30–60 minutes before meals, at 4 pm and at bedtime, successfully healed 48% of ulcers after 4 weeks and 76% after 12 weeks. Of 20 patients who had erosion gastritis and dyspepsia, the same treatment produced a satisfactory reduction in abdominal pain and discomfort after the first and second week (Prucksunand et al 2001). Turmeric has also been positively compared to a liquid antacid for the treatment of gastric ulcer in a controlled clinical trial (Kositchaiwat et al 1993).

Irritable bowel syndrome (IBS)

Turmeric extract shows promise in the symptomatic treatment of IBS, according to a partially blinded, randomised study by Bundy et al (2004). The study of 207 volunteers with diagnosed IBS complying with the Rome II criteria were randomly assigned to receive either 72 mg or 144 mg of turmeric a day or placebo for 8 weeks (Bundy et al 2004). The group receiving the lower dose (72 mg/day) experienced a significant 53% decrease in irritable bowel symptoms, whereas higher treatment (144 mg/day) resulted in a 60% decrease when compared to placebo ($P < 0.001$). Abdominal discomfort was also reduced by 22% and 25% of patients in the 72 mg and 144 mg groups, respectively ($P < 0.001$). Approximately two-thirds of the participants in the active groups reported overall symptom improvement and had better quality-of-life scores.

Inflammatory bowel disease

An open-label pilot study has produced preliminary data to suggest that curcumin may be effective in inflammatory bowel disease (Holt et al 2005). Five patients with Crohn's disease received 360 mg of curcumin three times a day for 1 month, followed by four times a day for another 2 months. The Crohn's disease activity index (CDAI), C-reactive protein (CRP) and erythrocyte sedimentation rate (ESR) fell significantly in four out of five patients. Five patients with ulcerative proctitis were also enrolled and received 550 mg of curcumin twice a day for 1 month, then three times a day for another month. Overall, stool quality was greatly improved and frequency was significantly reduced. Two patients were able to eliminate their concomitant medications altogether, while another two patients were able to reduce them. The CRP and ESR also returned to within normal limits by the cessation of the study.

A randomised, double-blind, multicentre trial of 89 patients examined the efficacy of curcumin as a maintenance therapy in ulcerative colitis (Hanai et al 2006). Patients in the active group received 1 g of curcumin, twice a day (e.g. 1 g after breakfast and 1 g after the evening meal) with sulfasalazine or mesalazine as compared to placebo plus sulfasalazine or mesalazine. At the end of the study period, 4.7% of patients in the curcumin group relapsed during treatment compared to 20.5% in the placebo group ($P = 0.040$). The clinical activity index ($P = 0.038$) and endoscopic index ($P = 0.0001$) were also significantly improved. This is a promising result that may have great clinical significance.

Ophthalmology

Studies demonstrate the potential therapeutic role and efficacy of curcumin in eye relapsing diseases, such as dry eye syndrome, allergic conjunctivitis, anterior uveitis, glaucoma, maculopathy, and ischaemic and diabetic retinopathy (Pescosolido et al 2013). Curcumin treatment has resulted in a partial, but significant, inhibition of neuronal and vascular damage during ischaemic or oxidative stress, angiogenesis, and inflammatory diseases. The mechanism by which curcumin induces its effects is yet to be fully elucidated. A number of studies have shown its relevance as a potent anti-inflammatory and immunomodulating agent. In addition, curcumin with its pleiotropic activities can modulate the expression and activation of many cellular regulatory proteins such as chemokines, interleukins, haematopoietic growth factors, and transcription factors, which in turn inhibit cellular inflammatory responses and protect cells (Pescosolido et al 2013).

Psoriasis

A phase 2, non-blind, open-label trial investigated the effect of curcuminoid C3 complex (500 mg, 3 capsules three times a day) in 12 patients with plaque psoriasis for 12 weeks followed by a 4-week observation period (Kurd et al 2008). Results were poor with the intention-to-treat analysis response rate only reaching 16.7%. Of the eight patients who completed the trial, two participants responded with good results (83% and 88% improvement in symptoms); however, this could be due to a placebo effect. Overall, the medication was well tolerated with only mild side effects being reported, due to either gastrointestinal upset or hot flushing.

Topical curcumin reduced the severity of active, untreated psoriasis as assessed by clinical, histological and immunohistochemical criteria in an observational study of 10 patients. Curcumin was also found to decrease phosphorylase kinase, which is involved in signalling pathways, including those involved with cell migration and proliferation (Heng et al 2000). Topical administration of curcumin also induced normal skin formation in the modified mouse tail test (Bosman 1994). The effects are thought to be due to immune-modulating, anti-inflammatory and cyclo-oxygenase inhibitory actions. The downregulation of pro-inflammatory cytokines supports the view that turmeric antioxidants may exert a favourable effect on psoriasis-linked inflammation. Moreover, because IL-6 and IL-8 are growth factors for keratinocytes, their inhibition by those antioxidants may reduce psoriasis-related keratinocyte hyperproliferation (Miquel et al 2002).

OTHER USES

Chronic anterior uveitis

An open study of 32 patients found that orally administered curcumin improved symptoms and reduced recurrences of chronic anterior uveitis (a condition often associated with other autoimmune disorders) with an efficacy comparable to corticosteroid therapy, yet without significant side effects (Lal et al 1999).

Oral submucous fibrosis

Turmeric extract 3 g, oil 600 mg and oleoresin 600 mg effectively relieved symptoms and reduced the number of micronuclei (a sign of damage to the DNA and chromosomal integrity) in circulating lymphocytes and oral mucosal cells in patients with oral submucous fibrosis, a debilitating disease of the oral cavity mainly caused by chewing betel nut or tobacco (Hastak et al 1997).

Reducing alcohol intoxication

Theracurmin exhibited an inhibitory action against alcohol intoxication after drinking in humans, as evidenced by the reduced acetaldehyde concentration of the blood (Sasaki et al 2011).

DOSAGE RANGE

Internal use

- Tablet formulas are available, singular or in combination with other anti-inflammatory/antioxidant herbs, where the curcuminoids are formulated with phosphatidylcholine (phospholipid) to increase the relative absorption.
- Powdered turmeric: 1.5–3 g/day in water or cooking.
- Liquid extract (1:1) in 45% ethanol: 5–15 mL/day.
- Powdered extract standardised to 95% curcumin: 100–300 mg/day. Higher doses used for arthritis.

Due to its low solubility, oral bioavailability (Henrotin et al 2013; Pescosolido et al 2013) and systemic bioavailability (Henrotin et al 2013), the biomedical potential of curcumin is not easily realised unless it is taken in a bioavailable form such as theracurmin or Meriva (Indena TM). Multiple approaches are needed to overcome this limited solubility and poor bioavailability of curcumin. Some of these approaches include the synthesis of curcuminoids and development of novel formulations of curcumin, such as emulsions, sustained released tablets (Pescosolido et al 2013), nanoparticles and liposomal encapsulation (Pescosolido et al 2013, Zhang et al 2013).

Theracurmin is a highly absorptive curcumin dispersed with colloidal nanoparticles. Healthy human volunteers were administered orally 30 mg of Theracurmin or curcumin powder. The area under the blood concentration-time curve of Theracurmin was 27-fold higher than that of curcumin powder (Sasaki et al 2011). Something to note is the difference in particle size of Theracurmin vs curcumin (mean particle size (D50% diameter) was 0.19 mcm and 22.75 mcm, respectively). Water dispersion studies observed homogenised very small particles in the Theracurmin sample, while the curcumin powder showed crystal aggregates with various sizes around several dozen micrometres (Sasaki et al 2011).

Dose-escalating studies have indicated the safety of curcumin at doses as high as 12 g/day over 3 months (Gupta et al 2013). Pharmacologically, curcumin does not show any dose-limiting toxicity when it is administered at doses of up to 8 g/day for three months (Pescosolido et al 2013).

External use

- Turmeric powder of standardised powdered extract applied as a paste or poultice — half a cup of turmeric combined with 1 teaspoon of carbonate of soda and then mixed with hot water to make a paste; spread on gauze and apply to affected area.

ADVERSE REACTIONS

The safety of dietary curcumin is demonstrated by the fact that it has been consumed for centuries at levels of up to 10 mg/day by people in certain countries (Ammon & Wahl 1991). Curcumin was non-toxic to humans in doses up to 8000 mg/day when taken by mouth for 3 months (Cheng et al 2001). Multiple other human trials have also found it to be safe with no alteration of liver or renal function tests (Chainani-Wu 2003, Prucksunand et al 2001, Ramirez-Bosca et al 1995, Ramirez et al 1997, Sharma et al 2001). Nausea and diarrhoea are possible effects of curcumins ranging from 0.45 to 3.6 g/day when taken for 1 to 4 months. This also caused an increase in serum alkaline phosphatase and lactate dehydrogenase contents in human participants (Sharma et al 2004).

Large doses of turmeric powder may cause gastrointestinal irritation in some persons (Shankar et al 1980), and very high dosages have been shown to reduce fertility in male rats (human equivalent doses would be 35 g turmeric/70 kg adult) (Bhagat & Purohit 2001). Normal therapeutic dosages of turmeric are not expected to affect fertility. Contact dermatitis has been reported (Hata et al 1997), as has a single case of anaphylaxis (Robinson 2003).

SIGNIFICANT INTERACTIONS

Controlled studies are not available, so interactions are based on evidence of activity and are largely theoretical and speculative.

Antiplatelet drugs

Turmeric has a theoretical interaction with antiplatelet drugs; antiplatelet properties have been demonstrated for curcumin, therefore it may produce an additive effect. The clinical significance of this interaction is unclear and likely to be dose-dependent.

Anticoagulants

Theoretically, high-dose turmeric preparations may increase the risk of bleeding when used together with anticoagulant drugs — caution is advised.

Cyclophosphamide

Animal studies suggest that curcumin may reduce drug efficacy — avoid.

CONTRAINDICATIONS AND PRECAUTIONS

Turmeric is contraindicated in bile duct obstruction (Blumenthal et al 2000) and high doses are probably best avoided in males and females wanting to conceive.

Curcumin is also contraindicated in breast cancer patients treated with cyclophosphamide until the significance of an in vivo model of breast cancer, which found that curcumin reduced the tumour regression effects of chemotherapy, is clarified (Somasundaram et al 2002).

Due to antiplatelet activity and possible increased risk of bleeding, use of concentrated extracts should be suspended 1 week prior to major surgery; however, usual dietary intakes are likely to be safe.

PREGNANCY AND LACTATION USE

When used as a spice, this herb is most likely to be safe; however, the safety of therapeutic doses has not been established. Turmeric has been demonstrated not to be mutagenic in vitro (Nagabhushan & Bhide 1986) or to be teratogenic in mice (Garg 1974, Vijayalaxmi 1980). Constituents and/or metabolites of turmeric and curcumin were transferred to suckling pups, but no ill effect on the offspring was reported.

Practice points/Patient counselling

- In Ayurvedic medicine, turmeric is used to strengthen the overall energy of the body, relieve gas, dispel worms, improve digestion, regulate menstruation, dissolve gallstones, relieve arthritis and purify the blood (Blumenthal et al 2000).
- In Traditional Chinese medicine (TCM), turmeric is used for bruises, sores, ringworm, chest pain, toothache and jaundice. Turmeric was also recommended for abdominal pain, mass formation in the abdomen and amenorrhoea (Blumenthal et al 2000).
- Turmeric is commonly used in foods and is likely to be a safe and healthy addition to the diet.
- Turmeric has been shown to have antioxidant, anti-inflammatory and anti-atherosclerotic activities; however, further clinical evidence is needed before it can be recommended to treat specific conditions.
- Clinical evidence suggests that turmeric may provide benefit for people with dyspepsia, peptic ulcer, hyperlipidaemia and arthritis and there is emerging evidence to suggest that turmeric may help prevent a number of cancers as well as being useful as an adjuvant in cancer treatment.

PATIENTS' FAQs

What will this herb do for me?

In countries where people use turmeric extensively in cooking (generally in curries), the intake seems to be associated with a lower level of certain chronic conditions, possibly including cancer, gastrointestinal diseases and arthritis. There have been some encouraging studies supporting this. Curcumin has shown promising effects for symptomatic relief in numerous inflammatory conditions such as rheumatoid arthritis, osteoarthritis, inflammatory bowel disease, IBS, peptic ulcer, psoriasis and in various cancers, diabetes and eye conditions. Ideally, oral use of preparations where bioavailability has been improved is likely to give the best results.

When will it start to work?

In some studies, the effect began to be noticed after 2 weeks. However, as most of the conditions where turmeric may be beneficial are chronic in nature, treatment with turmeric should be considered long term.

Are there any safety issues?

Turmeric is considered very safe at normal dietary or therapeutic dosages with turmeric extracts. High doses are generally not recommended during pregnancy or for those wanting to conceive.

REFERENCES

Abu-Rizq HA et al. Cyto-protective and immunomodulating effect of Curcuma longa in Wistar rats subjected to carbon tetrachloride-induced oxidative stress. Inflammopharmacology 16.2 (2008): 87–95.

Aggarwal BB et al. Curcumin: the Indian solid gold. Adv Exp Med Biol 595 (2007): 1–75.

Ak T, Gulcin I. Antioxidant and radical scavenging properties of curcumin. Chem Biol Interact 174.1 (2008): 27–37.

Al-Omar FA et al. Immediate and delayed treatments with curcumin prevents forebrain ischemia-induced neuronal damage and oxidative insult in the rat hippocampus. Neurochem Res 31.5 (2006): 611–618.

Ambegaokar SS et al. Curcumin inhibits dose-dependently and time-dependently neuroglial cell proliferation and growth. Neuroendocrinol Lett 24.6 (2003): 469–473.

Ammon HP, Wahl MA. Pharmacology of Curcuma longa. Planta Med 57.1 (1991): 1–7.

Andjelkovic T et al. Synergistic effects of the purine analog sulfinosine and curcumin on the multidrug resistant human non-small cell lung carcinoma cell line (NCI-H460/R). Cancer Biol Ther 7.7 (2008): 1024–32.

Anonymous. Curcuma longa (turmeric) Monograph. Altern Med Rev 6 Suppl (2001): S62–6.

Anto RJ et al. Antimutagenic and anticarcinogenic activity of natural and synthetic curcuminoids. Mutat Res 370.2 (1996): 127–131.

Antony S et al. Immunomodulatory activity of curcumin. Immunol Invest 28.5–6 (1999): 291–303.

Anuchapreeda S et al. Modulation of P-glycoprotein expression and function by curcumin in multidrug-resistant human KB cells. Biochem Pharmacol 64.4 (2002): 573–582.

Asai A, Miyazawa T. Dietary curcuminoids prevent high-fat diet-induced lipid accumulation in rat liver and epididymal adipose tissue. J Nut 131.11 (2001): 2932–2935.

Azuine MA, Bhide SV. Chemopreventive effect of turmeric against stomach and skin tumors induced by chemical carcinogens in Swiss mice. Nutr Cancer 17.1 (1992): 77–83.

Babu PS, Srinivasan K. Hypolipidemic action of curcumin, the active principle of turmeric (Curcuma longa) in streptozotocin induced diabetic rats. Mol Cell Biochem 166.1–2 (1997): 169–175.

Bachmeier B et al. The chemopreventive polyphenol Curcumin prevents hematogenous breast cancer metastases in immunodeficient mice. Cell Physiol Biochem 19.1–4 (2007): 137–152.

Bachmeier BE et al. Curcumin downregulates the inflammatory cytokines CXCL1 and 2 in breast cancer cells via NFkappaB. Carcinogenesis 29.4 (2008): 779–789.

Baek OS et al. Curcumin inhibits protease-activated receptor-2 and -4-mediated mast cell activation. Clin Chim Acta 338.1–2 (2003): 135–141.

Banerjee M et al. Modulation of inflammatory mediators by ibuprofen and curcumin treatment during chronic inflammation in rat. Immunopharm Immunotoxicol 25.2 (2003): 213–224.

Baum L et al. Curcumin effects on blood lipid profile in a 6-month human study. Pharmacol Res 56.6 (2007): 509–514.

Belcaro G et al. Efficacy and safety of Meriva®, a curcumin-phosphatidylcholine complex, during extended administration in osteoarthritis patients. Altern Med Rev 15.4 (2010a): 337–344.

Belcaro G et al. Product-evaluation registry of Meriva®, a curcumin-phosphatidylcholine complex, for the complementary management of osteoarthritis. Panminerva Med 52.2 Suppl 1 (2010b): 55–62.

Bengmark S. Curcumin, an atoxic antioxidant and natural NFkappaB, cyclooxygenase-2, lipooxygenase, and inducible nitric oxide synthase inhibitor: a shield against acute and chronic diseases. JPEN J Parenter Enteral Nutr 30.1 (2006): 45–51.

Bhagat M, Purohit A. Antifertility effects of various extracts of Curcuma longa in male albino rats. Indian Drugs 38.2 (2001): 79–81.

Blumenthal M et al. (eds). Herbal medicine: expanded commission E monographs. Austin, TX: Integrative Medicine Communications, 2000.

Bosman B. Testing of lipoxygenase inhibitors, cyclooxygenase inhibitors, drugs with immunomodulating properties and some reference antipsoriatic drugs in the modified mouse tail test, an animal model of psoriasis. Skin Pharmacol 7.6 (1994): 324–334.

Bundy R et al. Turmeric extract may improve irritable bowel syndrome symptomology in otherwise healthy adults: a pilot study. J Altern Complement Med 10.6 (2004): 1015–1018.

Bush JA et al. Curcumin induces apoptosis in human melanoma cells through a Fas receptor/caspase-8 pathway independent of p53. Exp Cell Res 271.2 (2001): 305–314.

Calabrese V et al. Redox regulation of cellular stress response in neurodegenerative disorders. Ital J Biochem 55.3–4 (2006): 263–282.

Chainani-Wu N. Safety and anti-inflammatory activity of curcumin: a component of turmeric (Curcuma longa). J Altern Complement Med 9.1 (2003): 161–168.

Chandran B & Goel A. A randomized, pilot study to assess the efficacy and safety of curcumin in patients with active rheumatoid arthritis. Phytother Res 26.11 (2012): 1719–1725.

Chang DM. Curcumin: a heat shock response inducer and potential cytoprotector. Crit Care Med 29.11 (2001): 2231–2232.

Chen HW et al. Pretreatment of curcumin attenuates coagulopathy and renal injury in LPS-induced endotoxemia. J Endotoxin Res 13.1 (2007): 15–23.

Cheng AL et al. Phase I clinical trial of curcumin, a chemopreventive agent, in patients with high-risk or pre-malignant lesions. Anticancer Res 21.4B (2001): 2895–2900.

Chuang SE et al. Curcumin-containing diet inhibits diethylnitrosamine-induced murine hepatocarcinogenesis. Carcinogenesis 21.2 (2000): 331–335.

Chueh S-CJ et al. Curcumin enhances the immunosuppressive activity of cyclosporine in rat cardiac allografts and in mixed lymphocyte reactions. Transplant Proc 35.4 (2003): 1603–1605.

Chuengsamarn S et al. Curcumin extract for prevention of type 2 diabetes. Diabetes Care. 35.11 (2012): 2121–2127.

Chuengsamarn S et al. Reduction of atherogenic risk in patients with type 2 diabetes by curcuminoid extract: a randomized controlled trial. J Nutr Biochem. 25.2 (2014): 144–150.

Cole GM et al. Prevention of Alzheimer's disease: Omega-3 fatty acid and phenolic anti-oxidant interventions. Neurobiol Aging 26 Suppl 1 (2005): 133–136.

Deodhar SD et al. Preliminary study on antirheumatic activity of curcumin (diferuloyl methane). Indian J Med Res 71 (1980): 632–634.

Deshpande UR et al. Protective effect of turmeric (Curcuma longa L.) extract on carbon tetrachloride-induced liver damage in rats. Indian J Exp Biol 36.6 (1998): 573–577.

Dhillon N et al. Phase II trial of curcumin in patients with advanced pancreatic cancer. Clin Cancer Res 14.14 (2008): 4491–4499.

Dorai T et al. Therapeutic potential of curcumin in human prostate cancer. III. Curcumin inhibits tyrosine kinase activity of epidermal growth factor receptor and depletes the protein. Mol Urol 4.1 (2000): 1–6.

Dorai T et al. Therapeutic potential of curcumin in human prostate cancer. III. Curcumin inhibits proliferation, induces apoptosis, and inhibits angiogenesis of LNCaP prostate cancer cells in vivo. Prostate 47.4 (2001): 293–303.

Du B et al. Synergistic inhibitory effects of curcumin and 5-fluorouracil on the growth of the human colon cancer cell line HT-29. Chemotherapy 52.1 (2006): 23–28.

Dulbecco P, Savarino V. Therapeutic potential of curcumin in digestive diseases. World J Gastroenterol. 19.48 (2013): 9256–9270.

Evans W, Trease D. Pharmacognosy, 15th edn, Edinburgh: WS Saunders, 2002.

Farhangkhoee H et al. Differential effects of curcumin on vasoactive factors in the diabetic rat heart. Nutr Metab (Lond) 3 (2006): 27.

Farombi EO et al. Curcumin attenuates dimethylnitrosamine-induced liver injury in rats through Nrf2-mediated induction of heme oxygenase-1. Food Chem Toxicol 46.4 (2008): 1279–1287.

Fiorillo C et al. Curcumin protects cardiac cells against ischemia-reperfusion injury: effects on oxidative stress, NF-kappaB, and JNK pathways. Free Radic Biol Med 45.6 (2008): 839–846.

Fu Y et al. Curcumin protects the rat liver from CCl4-caused injury and fibrogenesis by attenuating oxidative stress and suppressing inflammation. Mol Pharmacol 73.2 (2008): 399–409.

Gao X et al. Immunomodulatory activity of curcumin: suppression of lymphocyte proliferation, development of cell-mediated cytotoxicity, and cytokine production in vitro. Biochem Pharmacol 68.1 (2004): 51–61.

Garg SK. Effect of Curcuma longa (rhizomes) on fertility in experimental animals. Planta Med 26.3 (1974): 225–227.

Gescher A et al. Cancer chemoprevention by dietary constituents: a tale of failure and promise. Lancet Oncol 2 (2001): 371–379.

Gescher A et al. Suppression of tumour development by substances derived from the diet: mechanisms and clinical implications. Br J Clin Pharmacol 45.1 (1998): 1–2.

Gilani AH et al. Pharmacological basis for the use of turmeric in gastrointestinal and respiratory disorders. Life Sci 76.26 (2005): 3089–3105.

Gowda NKS et al. Effect of some chemical and herbal compounds on growth of Aspergillus parasiticus and aflatoxin production. Animal Feed Sci Technol 116.3–4 (2004): 281–291.

Gukovsky I et al. Curcumin ameliorates ethanol and nonethanol experimental pancreatitis. Am J Physiol Gastrointest Liver Physiol 284.147-1 (2003): G85–95.

Gupta SC et al. Therapeutic roles of curcumin: lessons learned from clinical trials. AAPS J. 15.1 (2013): 195–218.

Gururaj A et al. Molecular mechanisms of anti-angiogenic effect of curcumin. Biochem Biophys Res Commun 297.4 (2002): 934–942.
Hanai H et al. Curcumin maintenance therapy for ulcerative colitis: randomized, multicenter, double-blind, placebo-controlled trial. Clin Gastroenterol Hepatol 4.12 (2006): 1502–1506.
Hastak K et al. Effect of turmeric oil and turmeric oleoresin on cytogenetic damage in patients suffering from oral submucous fibrosis. Cancer Lett 116.2 (1997): 265–269.
Hata M et al. Allergic contact dermatitis from curcumin (turmeric). Contact Dermatitis 36.2 (1997): 107–108.
Heng MCY et al. Drug-induced suppression of phosphorylase kinase activity correlates with resolution of psoriasis as assessed by clinical, histological and immunohistochemical parameters. Br J Dermatol 143.5 (2000): 937–949.
Henrotin Y et al. Curcumin: a new paradigm and therapeutic opportunity for the treatment of osteoarthritis: curcumin for osteoarthritis management. Springerplus. 2.1 (2013): 56.
Hergenhahn M et al. The chemopreventive compound curcumin is an efficient inhibitor of Epstein-Barr virus BZLF1 transcription in Raji DR-LUC cells. Mol Carcinogen 33.3 (2002): 137–145.
Hidaka H et al. Curcumin inhibits interleukin 8 production and enhances interleukin 8 receptor expression on the cell surface: impact on human pancreatic carcinoma cell growth by autocrine regulation. Cancer 95.6 (2002): 1206–1214.
Holt PR, Katz S, Kirshoff R. Curcumin therapy in inflammatory bowel disease: a pilot study. Dig Dis Sci 50.11 (2005): 2191–2193.
Hong RL, Spohn WH, Hung MC. Curcumin inhibits tyrosine kinase activity of p185neu and also depletes p185neu. Clin Cancer Res 5.7 (1999): 1884–1891.
Hour T-C et al. Curcumin enhances cytotoxicity of chemotherapeutic agents in prostate cancer cells by inducing p21WAF1/CIP1 and C/EBPbeta expressions and suppressing NF-kappaB activation. Prostate 51.3 (2002): 211–218.
Huang M-T et al. Inhibitory effects of curcumin on tumor initiation by benzo[a]pyrene and 7,12-dimethylbenz[a]anthracene. Carcinogenesis 13.11 (1992): 2183–2186.
Imaida K et al. Lack of chemopreventive effects of lycopene and curcumin on experimental rat prostate carcinogenesis. Carcinogenesis 22 (2001): 467–472.
Inano H, Onoda M. Radioprotective action of curcumin extracted from Curcuma longa LINN: inhibitory effect on formation of urinary 8-hydroxy-2'-deoxyguanosine, tumorigenesis, but not mortality, induced by gamma-ray irradiation. Int J Radiat Oncol Biol Phys 53 (2002): 735–743.
Iqbal M et al. Dietary supplementation of curcumin enhances antioxidant and phase II metabolizing enzymes in ddY male mice: possible role in protection against chemical carcinogenesis and toxicity. Pharmacol Toxicol 92.1 (2003): 33–38.
Ireson C et al. Characterization of metabolites of the chemopreventive agent curcumin in human and rat hepatocytes and in the rat in vivo, and evaluation of their ability to inhibit phorbol ester-induced prostaglandin E2 production. Cancer Res 61.3 (2001): 1058–1064.
Itthipanichpong C et al. Antispasmodic effects of curcuminoids on isolated guinea-pig ileum and rat uterus. J Med Assoc Thai 86 Suppl 2 (2003): S299–309.
Jagetia GC, Aggarwal BB. 'Spicing up' of the immune system by curcumin. J Clin Immunol 27.1 (2007): 19–35.
Jagetia GC, Rajanikant GK. Role of curcumin, a naturally occurring phenolic compound of turmeric, in accelerating the repair of excision wound, in mice whole-body exposed to various doses of [gamma]-radiation. J Surg Res 120.1 (2004): 127–138.
Jain SK, Rains J, Jones K. Effect of curcumin on protein glycosylation, lipid peroxidation, and oxygen radical generation in human red blood cells exposed to high glucose levels. Free Radic Biol Med 41.1 (2006): 92–96.
Jantan I et al. Inhibitory effect of compounds from Zingiberaceae species on human platelet aggregation. Phytomedicine 15.4 (2008): 306–309.
Javvadi P et al. The chemopreventive agent curcumin is a potent radiosensitizer of human cervical tumor cells via increased reactive oxygen species production and overactivation of the mitogen-activated protein kinase pathway. Mol Pharmacol 73.5 (2008): 1491–1501.
Jayaprakasha GK et al. Chemistry and biological activities of C. longa. Trends Food Sci Technol 16.12 (2005): 533–548.
Jee S-H et al. Curcumin induces a p53-dependent apoptosis in human basal cell carcinoma cells. J Invest Dermatol 111.4 (1998): 656–661.
Jiao Y et al. Iron chelation in the biological activity of curcumin. Free Radic Biol Med 40.7 (2006): 1152–1160.
Jiao Y et al. Curcumin, a cancer chemopreventive and chemotherapeutic agent, is a biologically active iron chelator. Blood 113.2 (2009): 462–469.
Kamat AM, Sethi G, Aggarwal BB. Curcumin potentiates the apoptotic effects of chemotherapeutic agents and cytokines through down-regulation of nuclear factor-kappaB and nuclear factor-kappaB-regulated gene products in IFN-alpha-sensitive and IFN-alpha-resistant human bladder cancer cells. Mol Cancer Ther 6.3 (2007): 1022–1030.
Kang H-C et al. Curcumin inhibits collagen synthesis and hepatic stellate cell activation in-vivo and in-vitro. J Pharm Pharmacol 54.1 (2002): 119–126.
Keshavarz K. The influence of turmeric and curcumin on cholesterol concentration of eggs and tissues. Poultry Sci 55.3 (1976): 1077–1083.
Kim MS, Kang HJ, Moon A. Inhibition of invasion and induction of apoptosis by curcumin in H-ras-transformed MCF10A human breast epithelial cells. Arch Pharm Res 24.4 (2001): 349–354.
Kositchaiwat C, Kositchaiwat S, Havanondha J. Curcuma longa Linn. in the treatment of gastric ulcer comparison to liquid antacid: a controlled clinical trial. J Med Assoc Thai 76.11 (1993): 601–605.
Kowluru RA, Kanwar M. Effects of curcumin on retinal oxidative stress and inflammation in diabetes. Nutr Metab (Lond) 4 (2007): 8.
Kulkarni RR et al. Treatment of osteoarthritis with a herbomineral formulation: a double-blind, placebo-controlled, cross-over study. J Ethnopharmacol 33.1–2 (1991): 91–95.
Kumar GS et al. Free and bound phenolic antioxidants in amla (Emblica officinalis) and turmeric (Curcuma longa). J Food Comp Anal 19.5 (2006): 446–452.
Kunnumakkara AB, Anand P, Aggarwal BB. Curcumin inhibits proliferation, invasion, angiogenesis and metastasis of different cancers through interaction with multiple cell signaling proteins. Cancer Lett 269.2 (2008): 199–225.
Kuo M-L, Huang T-S, Lin J- K. Curcumin, an antioxidant and anti-tumor promoter, induces apoptosis in human leukemia cells. Biochem Biophys Acta Mol Basis Dis 1317.2 (1996): 95–100.
Kurd SK et al. Oral curcumin in the treatment of moderate to severe psoriasis vulgaris: A prospective clinical trial. J Am Acad Dermatol 58.4 (2008): 625–631.
Kuttan G et al. Antitumor, anti-invasion, and antimetastatic effects of curcumin. Adv Exp Med Biol 595 (2007): 173–184.
Kuttan R et al. Potential anticancer activity of turmeric (Curcuma longa). Cancer Lett 29.2 (1985): 197–202.
Kuttan R et al. Turmeric and curcumin as topical agents in cancer therapy. Tumori 73.1 (1987): 29–31.
Lal B et al. Efficacy of curcumin in the management of chronic anterior uveitis. Phytother Res 13.4 (1999): 318–322.
Lal B et al. Role of curcumin in idiopathic inflammatory orbital pseudotumours. Phytother Res 14.6 (2000): 443–447.
Lantz RC et al. The effect of turmeric extracts on inflammatory mediator production. Phytomedicine 12.6–7 (2005): 445–452.
Lev-Ari S et al. Inhibition of pancreatic and lung adenocarcinoma cell survival by curcumin is associated with increased apoptosis, down-regulation of COX-2 and EGFR and inhibition of Erk1/2 activity. Anticancer Res 26.6B (2006): 4423–4430.
Li L et al. Liposomal curcumin with and without oxaliplatin: effects on cell growth, apoptosis, and angiogenesis in colorectal cancer. Mol Cancer Ther 6.4 (2007): 1276–1282.
Limtrakul P, Anuchapreeda S, Buddhasukh D. Modulation of human multidrug-resistance MDR-1 gene by natural curcuminoids. BMC Cancer 4 (2004): 13.
Lin YG et al. Curcumin inhibits tumor growth and angiogenesis in ovarian carcinoma by targeting the nuclear factor-kappaB pathway. Clin Cancer Res 13.11 (2007): 3423–3430.
Liu D, Chen Z. The effect of curcumin on breast cancer cells. J Breast Cancer. 16.2 (2013): 133–137.
Liu Q et al. Curcumin inhibits cell proliferation of MDA-MB-231 and BT-483 breast cancer cells mediated by down-regulation of NFkappaB, cyclinD and MMP-1 transcription. Phytomedicine. 16.10 (2009): 916–922.
Lukita-Atmadja W et al. Effect of curcuminoids as anti-inflammatory agents on the hepatic microvascular response to endotoxin. Shock 17.5 (2002): 399–403.
Mani H et al. Curcumin differentially regulates TGF-beta1, its receptors and nitric oxide synthase during impaired wound healing. Biofactors 16.1–2 (2002): 29–43.
Manjunatha H, Srinivasan K. Hypolipidemic and antioxidant effects of curcumin and capsaicin in high-fat-fed rats. Can J Physiol Pharmacol 85.6 (2007b): 588–596.
Manjunatha H, Srinivasan K. Hypolipidemic and antioxidant effects of dietary curcumin and capsaicin in induced hypercholesterolemic rats. Lipids 42.12 (2007a): 1133–1142.
Marin YE et al. Curcumin downregulates the constitutive activity of NF-kappaB and induces apoptosis in novel mouse melanoma cells. Melanoma Res 17.5 (2007): 274–283.
Menon LG, Kuttan R, Kuttan G. Anti-metastatic activity of curcumin and catechin. Cancer Lett 141.1–2 (1999): 159–165.
Menon VP, Sudheer AR. Antioxidant and anti-inflammatory properties of curcumin. Adv Exp Med Biol 595 (2007): 105–125.
Mesa MD et al. Oral administration of a turmeric extract inhibits erythrocyte and liver microsome membrane oxidation in rabbits fed with an atherogenic diet. Nutrition 19.9 (2003): 800–804.
Miquel J et al. The curcuma antioxidants: Pharmacological effects and prospects for future clinical use: a review. Arch Gerontol Geriatr 34.1 (2002): 37–46.
Mohan R et al. Curcuminoids inhibit the angiogenic response stimulated by fibroblast growth factor-2, including expression of matrix metalloproteinase gelatinase B. J Biol Chem 275.14 (2000): 10405–10412.
Mohanty I et al. Protective effects of Curcuma longa on ischemia-reperfusion induced myocardial injuries and their mechanisms. Life Sci 75.14 (2004): 1701–1711.

Nabekura T et al. Effects of dietary chemopreventive phytochemicals on P-glycoprotein function. Biochem Biophys Res Commun 327.3 (2005): 866–870.

Nagabhushan M, Bhide SV. Nonmutagenicity of curcumin and its antimutagenic action versus chili and capsaicin. Nutr Cancer 8.3 (1986): 201–210.

Nanji AA et al. Curcumin prevents alcohol-induced liver disease in rats by inhibiting the expression of NF-kappaB-dependent genes. Am J Physiol Gastrointest Liver Physiol 284.2 47–2 (2003): G321–327.

Navis I, Sriganth P, Premalatha B. Dietary curcumin with cisplatin administration modulates tumour marker indices in experimental fibrosarcoma. Pharmacol Res 39.3 (1999): 175–179.

Niederau C, Gopfert E. [The effect of chelidonium- and turmeric root extract on upper abdominal pain due to functional disorders of the biliary system: Results from a placebo-controlled double-blind study]. Med Klin 94.8 (1999): 425–430.

O'Connell MA, Rushworth SA. Curcumin: potential for hepatic fibrosis therapy? Br J Pharmacol 153.3 (2008): 403–405.

Panchatcharam M et al. Curcumin improves wound healing by modulating collagen and decreasing reactive oxygen species. Mol Cell Biochem 290.1–2 (2006): 87–96.

Pari L, Murugan P. Antihyperlipidemic effect of curcumin and tetrahydrocurcumin in experimental type 2 diabetic rats. Ren Fail 29.7 (2007): 881–889.

Perez-Arriaga L et al. Cytotoxic effect of curcumin on Giardia lamblia trophozoites. Acta Tropica 98.2 (2006): 152–161.

Peschel D, Koerting R, Nass N. Curcumin induces changes in expression of genes involved in cholesterol homeostasis. J Nutr Biochem 18.2 (2007): 113–119.

Pescosolido N. Curcumin: Therapeutical Potential in Ophthalmology. Planta Med. 2013 Dec 9. [Epub ahead of print].

Phan T-T et al. Protective effects of curcumin against oxidative damage on skin cells in vitro: Its implication for wound healing. J Trauma-Injury Infect Crit Care 51.5 (2001): 927–931.

Plummer SM et al. Clinical development of leukocyte cyclooxygenase 2 activity as a systemic biomarker for cancer chemopreventive agents. Cancer Epidemiol Biomarkers Prev 10.12 (2001): 1295–1299

Prucksunand C et al. Phase II clinical trial on effect of the long turmeric (Curcuma longa Linn) on healing of peptic ulcer. Southeast Asian J Trop Med Public Health 32.1 (2001): 208–215.

Quiles JL et al. An ethanolic-aqueous extract of Curcuma longa decreases the susceptibility of liver microsomes and mitochondria to lipid peroxidation in atherosclerotic rabbits. Biofactors 8.1–2 (1998): 51–57.

Quiles JL et al. Curcuma longa extract supplementation reduces oxidative stress and attenuates aortic fatty streak development in rabbits. Arterioscler Thromb Vasc Biol 22.7 (2002): 1225–1231.

Ram A, Das M, Ghosh B. Curcumin attenuates allergen-induced airway hyperresponsiveness in sensitized guinea pigs. Biol Pharm Bull 26.7 (2003): 1021–1024.

Ramirez BA et al. Effects of the antioxidant turmeric on lipoprotein peroxides: Implications for the prevention of atherosclerosis. Age 20.3 (1997): 165–168.

Ramirez-Bosca A et al. Antioxidant Curcuma extracts decrease the blood lipid peroxide levels of human subjects. Age 18.4 (1995): 167–169.

Ramirez-Tortosa MC et al. Oral administration of a turmeric extract inhibits LDL oxidation and has hypocholesterolemic effects in rabbits with experimental atherosclerosis. Atherosclerosis 147.2 (1999): 371–378.

Rao CV et al. Chemoprevention of colon cancer by dietary curcumin. Ann NY Acad Sci 768 (1995b): 201–204.

Rao CV et al. Chemoprevention of colon carcinogenesis by dietary curcumin, a naturally occurring plant phenolic compound. Cancer Res 55.2 (1995c): 259–266.

Rao CV et al. Chemoprevention of colon carcinogenesis by phenylethyl-3-methylcaffeate. Cancer Res 55.11 (1995a): 2310–2315.

Rao CV et al. Chemoprevention of colonic aberrant crypt foci by an inducible nitric oxide synthase-selective inhibitor. Carcinogenesis 20.4 (1999): 641–644.

Rao CV. Regulation of COX and LOX by curcumin. Adv Exp Med Biol 595 (2007): 213–226.

Rasyid A, Lelo A. The effect of curcumin and placebo on human gall-bladder function: an ultrasound study. Aliment Pharmacol Ther 13.2 (1999): 245–249.

Reddy RC et al. Curcumin for malaria therapy. Biochem Biophys Res Commun 326.2 (2005): 472–474.

Reddy S, Aggarwal BB. Curcumin is a non-competitive and selective inhibitor of phosphorylase kinase. FEBS Lett 341.1 (1994): 19–22.

Robinson DM. Anaphylaxis to turmeric. J Allergy Clin 111.1 Suppl 2 (2003): S100.

Ruby AJ et al. Anti-tumour and antioxidant activity of natural curcuminoids. Cancer Lett 94.1 (1995): 79–83.

Salh B et al. Curcumin attenuates DNB-induced murine colitis. Am J Physiol Gastrointest Liver Physiol 285.1 (2003): G235–243.

Sasaki H et al. Innovative preparation of curcumin for improved oral bioavailability. Biol Pharm Bull. 34.5 (2011): 660–665.

Shalini VK, Srinivas L. Lipid peroxide induced DNA damage: protection by turmeric (Curcuma longa). Mol Cell Biochem 77.1 (1987): 3–10.

Sharma RA et al. Phase I clinical trial of oral curcumin: biomarkers of systemic activity and compliance. Clin Cancer Res 10.20 (2004): 6847–6854.

Shankar TN et al. Toxicity studies on turmeric (Curcuma longa): Acute toxicity studies in rats, guinea pigs and monkeys. Indian J Exp Biol 18.1 (1980): 73–75.

Sharma RA et al. Pharmacodynamic and pharmacokinetic study of oral Curcuma extract in patients with colorectal cancer. Clin Cancer Res 7.7 (2001): 1894–1900.

Shukla PK et al. Anti-ischemic effect of curcumin in rat brain. Neurochem Res 33.6 (2008): 1036–1043.

Sidhu GS et al. Curcumin enhances wound healing in streptozotocin induced diabetic rats and genetically diabetic mice. Wound Repair Regen 7.5 (1999): 362–374.

Sidhu GS et al. Enhancement of wound healing by curcumin in animals. Wound Repair Regen 6.2 (1998): 167–177.

Skommer J, Wlodkowic D, Pelkonen J. Cellular foundation of curcumin-induced apoptosis in follicular lymphoma cell lines. Exp Hematol 34.4 (2006): 463–474.

Skommer J, Wlodkowic D, Pelkonen J. Gene-expression profiling during curcumin-induced apoptosis reveals downregulation of CXCR4. Exp Hematol 35.1 (2007): 84–95.

Somasundaram S et al. Dietary curcumin inhibits chemotherapy-induced apoptosis in models of human breast cancer. Cancer Res 62.13 (2002): 3868–3875.

Song E-K et al. Diarylheptanoids with free radical scavenging and hepatoprotective activity in vitro from Curcuma longa. Planta Med 67.9 (2001): 876–877.

Soni KB, Kuttan R. Effect of oral curcumin administration on serum peroxides and cholesterol levels in human volunteers. Indian J Physiol Pharmacol 36.4 (1992): 273–275.

Soni KB, Rajan A, Kuttan R. Reversal of aflatoxin induced liver damage by turmeric and curcumin. Cancer Lett 66.2 (1992): 115–121.

Soudamini KK et al. Inhibition of lipid peroxidation and cholesterol levels in mice by curcumin. Indian J Physiol Pharmacol 36.4 (1992): 239–243.

Srinivasan K, Sambaiah K. The effect of spices on cholesterol 7 alpha-hydroxylase activity and on serum and hepatic cholesterol levels in the rat. Int J Vitamin Nutr Res 61.4 (1991): 364–369.

Srinivasan K. Spices as influencers of body metabolism: an overview of three decades of research. Food Res Int 38.1 (2005): 77–86.

Srivastava KC et al. Curcumin, a major component of food spice turmeric (Curcuma longa), inhibits aggregation and alters eicosanoid metabolism in human blood platelets. Prostaglandins Leukot Essent Fatty Acids 52.4 (1995): 223–227.

Srivastava KC. Extracts from two frequently consumed spices — cumin (Cuminum cyminum) and turmeric (Curcuma longa) — inhibit platelet aggregation and alter eicosanoid biosynthesis in human blood platelets. Prostaglandins Leukot Essent Fatty Acids 37.1 (1989): 57–64.

Srivastava R et al. Anti-thrombotic effect of curcumin. Thromb Res 40.3 (1985): 413–417.

Srivastava R et al. Effect of curcumin on platelet aggregation and vascular prostacyclin synthesis. Arzneimittel-Forschung 36.4 (1986): 715–717.

Sugiyama T et al. Selective protection of curcumin against carbon tetrachloride-induced inactivation of hepatic cytochrome P450 isozymes in rats. Life Sci 78.19 (2006): 2188–2193.

Thaloor D et al. Inhibition of angiogenic differentiation of human umbilical vein endothelial cells by curcumin. Cell Growth Differ 9.4 (1998): 305–312.

Thamlikitkul V et al. Randomized double blind study of Curcuma domestica Val for dyspepsia. J Med Assoc Thai 72.11 (1989): 613–620.

Tian B et al. Effects of curcumin on bladder cancer cells and development of urothelial tumors in a rat bladder carcinogenesis model. Cancer Lett 264.2 (2008): 299–308.

Valentine SP et al. Curcumin modulates drug metabolizing enzymes in the female Swiss Webster mouse. Life Sci 78.20 (2006): 2391–2398.

Verma SP, Salamone E, Goldin B. Curcumin and genistein, plant natural products, show synergistic inhibitory effects on the growth of human breast cancer MCF-7 cells induced by estrogenic pesticides. Biochem Biophys Res Commun 233.3 (1997): 692–696.

Vijayalaxmi. Genetic effects of turmeric and curcumin in mice and rats. Mutat Res 79.2 (1980): 125–132.

Wu SJ et al. Curcumin or saikosaponin a improves hepatic antioxidant capacity and protects against CCl4-induced liver injury in rats. J Med Food 11.2 (2008): 224–229.

Yang X et al. Curcumin inhibits platelet-derived growth factor-stimulated vascular smooth muscle cell function and injury-induced neointima formation. Arterioscler Thromb Vasc Biol 26.1 (2006): 85–90.

Zahid Ashraf M et al. Antiatherosclerotic effects of dietary supplementations of garlic and turmeric: Restoration of endothelial function in rats. Life Sci 77.8 (2005): 837–857.

Zhang DW et al. Curcumin and Diabetes: A Systematic Review. Evid Based Complement Alternat Med. (2013): 636053.

Zhang L et al. Curcuminoids enhance amyloid-beta uptake by macrophages of Alzheimer's disease patients. J Alzheimers Dis 10.1 (2006): 1–7.

Tyrosine

HISTORICAL NOTE Tyrosine has been used by the military in the United States and the Netherlands to counter the stressful effects of cold, prolonged and excessive physical activity. It also appears to improve cognition and performance in soldiers under psychologically stressful conditions and has been scientifically shown to improve physical and mental endurance (Deijen et al 1999).

BACKGROUND AND RELEVANT PHARMACOKINETICS

Tyrosine is a conditionally essential aromatic amino acid. It can be consumed through the diet or synthesised in the body from phenylalanine, except in phenylketonurics. Human studies also indicate that people with chronic renal failure have impaired conversion of phenylalanine to tyrosine, leading to low tyrosine and higher phenylalanine levels in plasma and other tissues (Kopple 2007). This is because the kidney plays a major role in the uptake of phenylalanine and its hydroxylation and release as tyrosine. L-Tyrosine is absorbed in the small intestine by active transport and transported to the liver, where it is involved in a number of biochemical reactions, such as protein synthesis and oxidative catabolic reactions. L-Tyrosine that is not metabolised in the liver is distributed via the systemic circulation to various tissues in the body where it is involved in the synthesis of a number of catecholamines and hormones (Hendler & Rorvik 2001), incorporated into protein structures or deaminated for gluconeogenesis. Peak plasma tyrosine levels occur 2 hours after administration and remain elevated for 6–8 hours (Glaeser et al 1979).

There is some question as to tyrosine's ability to cross the blood–brain barrier and this may explain some of the negative results demonstrated in clinical trials. In vivo studies demonstrate that concentrations in the brain are influenced by protein ingested, not only in a single meal, but also when the protein content of the diet is modified over longer periods (Peters & Harper 1985). Proper flow is dependent upon the ratio of tyrosine to other large neutral amino acids (phenylalanine, tryptophan, methionine, leucine, isoleucine and valine) that compete for uptake by transporter proteins (Glaeser et al 1979).

A rat study has demonstrated that combining the essential fatty acid alpha-linolenic acid with L-tyrosine, via a special bond, produces an active biological molecule with potent dopaminergic activity, suggesting that alpha-linolenic acid may play a dual role as a carrier for tyrosine and as a membrane- and receptor-improving agent (Yehuda 2002). In addition, in vivo research has determined that tyrosine nitration in brain proteins is exacerbated by low levels of vitamin D in the blood stream, leading to alterations in glucose metabolism and mitochondrial changes. Cognition was improved in subjects with normal vitamin D status, indicating that vitamin D is an important antioxidant cofactor in the normal functioning of tyrosine (Keeney et al 2013).

CHEMICAL COMPONENTS

L-Tyrosine is the form generally used. Tyrosine is also known as beta-(*para*-hydroxyphenyl) alanine, alpha-amino-*para*-hydroxyhydrocinnamic acid and (*S*)-alpha-amino-4-hydroxybenzenepropanoic acid.

FOOD SOURCES

Good dietary sources include soy products, chicken, fish, almonds, avocados, bananas, dairy products, meat, eggs, nuts, beans, oats, wheat, lima beans, pumpkin seeds, sesame seeds and fermented foods such as yoghurt and miso.

DEFICIENCY SIGNS AND SYMPTOMS

The following have been associated with low levels of tyrosine:

- Depression
- Low blood pressure
- Low body temperature
- Restless legs syndrome
- Hypothyroidism.

MAIN ACTIONS

Neurotransmitter and hormone production

Many of the pharmacological actions of tyrosine relate to its role as a precursor for a number of neurotransmitters and hormones. Tyrosine forms dihydroxyphenylalanine (DOPA), which is then converted to dopamine, and this, in turn, forms noradrenaline and adrenaline. Folate, vitamins B_3, B_6, B_{12} and C, iron, copper and other nutrients are required for the metabolism of tyrosine to catecholamines.

The rate of synthesis and release of monoamine neurotransmitters (serotonin) and catecholamines (dopamine, noradrenaline and adrenaline) in the brain are directly modified by the availability of their amino acid precursors tryptophan, phenylalanine and tyrosine. The availability of these amino acid precursors is largely dependent on physiological and pathophysiological factors and others that compete with them for a common transporter across the blood–brain barrier (the large neutral amino acids or LNAAs). As a result, factors which affect the amino acid precursors from crossing the blood–brain barrier in sufficient levels can affect brain function (Fernstrom & Fernstrom 2007). It has been suggested that, under some circumstances (such as when catecholamine neurons are firing rapidly), insufficient amino acid transport is most likely to affect brain function (Parker & Brotchie 2011).

Interestingly, tyrosine supplementation (or loading) does not always have a clinical effect: some in vivo research has demonstrated that excess tyrosine in the brain or cerebrospinal fluid samples does not always reflect enhanced catecholamine synthesis or turnover, possibly due to feedback mechanisms or substrate inhibition (Badawy et al 2010). Tyrosine and sometimes its precursor phenylalanine are converted into dopamine and noradrenaline. L-tyrosine undergoes hydroxylation into L-3, 4-dihyroxyphenylalanine (L-DOPA) in the presence of a rate-limiting catalytic enzyme, tyrosine hydroxylase and its cofactors, including Fe^{2+}, O_2 and tetrahydropteridine. Further, L-DOPA undergoes decarboxylation to form dopamine, and then to noradrenaline in some neurons (Lakhan & Vieira 2008, Ruhé et al 2007). Elevating tyrosine concentrations in brain catecholamine neurons (particularly dopamine and noradrenaline neurons) can stimulate neurotransmitter production in actively firing neurons but not in those that are quiescent or firing slowly (Fernstrom 2000). Therefore tyrosine plays an essential role in the body as a precursor to the catecholamine neurotransmitters, as illustrated above, and although the biochemical pathways are well understood, the effects on brain function are not.

Thyroid hormones

As tyrosine is a precursor for the synthesis of thyroid hormones, it is involved in the regulation of basal metabolic rate, oxygen use, cellular metabolism, growth and development (Tortora & Grabowski 1996).

Tyrosine undergoes iodination to form monoiodotyrosine (T_1), a second iodination produces diiodotyrosine (T_2), and these combine to produce the active thyroid hormones known as triiodothyronine (T_3) and tetraiodothyronine or thyroxine (T_4) (Tortora & Grabowski 1996).

Tyrosine is also involved in the production of other compounds, such as melanin, enkephalins and some types of oestrogen (Haas 1992, Tortora & Grabowski 1996).

Antioxidant

L-Tyrosine, a monophenolic amino acid, demonstrates antioxidant activity in various assays, including 1,1-diphenyl-2-picryl-hydrazyl (DPPH) free radical scavenging, 2,2'-azino-bis(3-ethylbenzothiazoline-6-sulfonic acid) (ABTS) radical scavenging, superoxide anion radical scavenging, hydrogen peroxide scavenging, total ferric ion reducing power and metal chelating on ferrous ion activities, as well as inhibition of lipid peroxidation of linoleic acid emulsion (Gulcin 2007).

CLINICAL USE

Clinical trials tend to investigate tyrosine in combination with other amino acids, typically LNAAs, which are tryptophan, phenylalanine, valine, leucine and isoleucine or in combination with the branched-chain amino acids (BCAAs: valine, leucine and isoleucine). Conditions which have an underlying dopaminergic-based pathology, such as Parkinson's disease, phenylketonuria, reward deficiency syndrome and depression, have received particular attention.

Phenylketonuria

In phenylketonuria (PKU), a severe deficiency of phenylalanine hydroxylase prevents the conversion of phenylalanine to tyrosine, resulting in a build-up of phenylalanine, which may cause severe mental retardation and a deficiency of tyrosine. PKU is treated by restricting the dietary intake of natural protein and substituting a protein source that lacks phenylalanine but is fortified with tyrosine. Unfortunately, free tyrosine supplementation has not always been shown to consistently improve neuropsychological function in PKU; this is possibly because tyrosine levels naturally fluctuate through the day and increases in plasma tyrosine levels are not sustained, so brain influx remains suboptimal despite tyrosine supplementation (Kalsner et al 2001). In practice, plasma tyrosine levels need to be monitored for diurnal variation (normal: 45 micromol/L) and biochemical evidence of tyrosine deficiency should be established before tyrosine supplementation is considered (Poustie & Rutherford 2000, van Spronsen et al 2001).

Due to the fact that tyrosine deficiency is typical in PKU patients, current guidelines recommend high-tyrosine protein supplementation from the time when a PKU infant starts weaning (MacDonald et al 2012). Infant formulas can include up to three times the concentration of phenylalanine compared to breast milk, therefore caution should be taken when using formulas in infants with PKU (Feillet & Agostoni 2010). The PKU diet is difficult to maintain in adolescence and adult life, and new strategies have been suggested, such as the supplementation of LNAAs as an alternative to phenylalanine restriction (Giovannini et al 2012). The use of the LNAA therapy has been shown to improve amino acid profiles as well as increase tyrosine and tryptophan concentrations in the blood, which are precursors for dopamine and serotonin (Koch et al 2003). A short-term double-blind placebo controlled study, using LNAA supplementation in patients with PKU, showed a lowering of blood phenylalanine concentration by an average of 39% from baseline (Matalon et al 2007). An LNAA blend with tyrosine as the primary ingredient was also found to increase the synthesis of melatonin in patients with PKU (Yano et al 2013). Significant associations have been demonstrated in correlation analyses between depressive symptoms and long-term high-phenylalanine, low-tyrosine (indicating poor dietary control) or low-tyrosine diets in adolescents (Sharman et al 2012). Further studies are required to determine the value of additional tyrosine supplementation in depressed patients with PKU.

Cognitive function in PKU

Tyrosine supplementation (100 mg/kg/day) taken over 4 weeks is not sufficient to counteract the decline in cognitive function seen when people with PKU relax or stop their dietary regimen, according to a double-blind, placebo-controlled crossover study (Pietz et al 1995). However, a later double-blind study found that, when people with PKU maintain their restricted diet and medications, the addition of LNAA had a beneficial effect on executive functioning (Schindeler et al 2007). Subjects adding LNAA supplementation to their usual management experienced significant improvements in executive functions, particularly in verbal generativity and flexibility when compared to the placebo group.

Enhanced cognition

Therapeutically, tyrosine supplements are used to enhance levels of its derivatives and, therefore, improve cognitive function.

One double-blind randomised controlled trial found that treatment with L-tyrosine (150 mg/kg) following one night's sleep loss significantly reduced the usual performance decline on a psychomotor task compared to placebo (Neri et al 1995). There was also a significant reduction in lapse probability on a high-event-rate vigilance task and the cognitive improvement effects lasted approximately 3 hours after dosing.

IN COMBINATION

Other randomised controlled trials have compared the effects of a balanced amino acid drink with one lacking in tyrosine and phenylalanine and shown that tyrosine-depleted individuals experienced impaired spatial recognition memory and spatial working memory and an increase in plasma prolactin levels (Harmer et al 2001, McTavish et al 2005). Subjective feedback indicated that the participants felt better on the amino acid drink containing tyrosine compared to the other, although ratings of depression and other aspects of cognitive function were unchanged (Harmer et al 2001).

Depression

Tyrosine is a popular supplement in mild depression, due to its role as a precursor to both dopamine and noradrenaline and the fact that tyrosine depletion may play a role in the pathogenesis of depression.

Whether or not tyrosine deficiency is a causative factor or consequence in depression remains poorly understood. Two studies have been conducted which suggest an association between low tyrosine levels and depression. One recent study compared serum levels of various neurotransmitter precursors between 60 hospitalised patients with major depressive disorder and 110 healthy volunteers and found that people with major depressive disorder had lower serum levels of tyrosine than controls (Sa et al 2012). Previously, an early study compared plasma tyrosine levels of 38 endogenous depressed patients with those of neurotic depressive and schizophrenic patients as well as healthy controls at four different time points during the day (Benkert et al 1971). A significant decrease in the 11 a.m. tyrosine level in the endogenous depressives was observed when compared with the other three groups; however, the 8 a.m. tyrosine concentration was similar for all.

Whether tyrosine supplementation has a major effect on mood and depression is still unclear as interventional clinical studies have produced inconsistent results (Parker & Brotchie 2011). The studies have tended to be small and relatively short, usually 4 weeks at most, making any definitive conclusions difficult from the available evidence. It also appears possible that some patients are more likely to be affected by fluctuations in tyrosine levels than others. This was suggested in a meta-analysis which reviewed eight acute phenylalanine / tyrosine depletion studies and suggested that such depletion (of noradrenaline and dopamine) did not decrease mood in healthy controls but did have such a mood effect in vulnerable patients who are in remission and are still in receipt of antidepressant medication (Ruhé et al 2007).

One study found that tyrosine- and phenylalanine-depleted individuals became less content and more apathetic than those given a balanced amino acid mixture (McLean et al 2004). However, a separate study in individuals with a past history of recurrent depression found that tyrosine depletion did not alter objective or subjective measures of mood (McTavish et al 2005), although plasma prolactin levels did increase and performance on a spatial recognition memory task was impaired (McTavish et al 2005). One prospective, randomised, double-blind, placebo-controlled trial of 65 subjects with major depression comparing L-tyrosine (100 mg/kg/day), imipramine (2.5 mg/kg/day) and placebo for 4 weeks failed to confirm an antidepressant effect for tyrosine (Gelenberg et al 1990). A small, double-blind placebo-controlled study involving 14 outpatients with major depression found that tyrosine (100 mg/kg/day) taken for 4 weeks led to remission in four (of six) people whereas three people (of eight) receiving placebo experienced remission (Gelenberg et al 1980).

In contrast, another early study involving patients with signs of dopamine-dependent depression found that treatment with oral tyrosine (3200 mg/day) caused an immediate improvement in mood, as judged by clinical impression and objective test scores (Montgomery–Asperg Depression Rating Scale) and sleep parameters from day 1 of treatment (Mouret et al 1988a).

Attention-deficit hyperactivity disorder (ADHD)

There is insufficient research to determine whether supplementation with tyrosine in ADHD produces any benefits. Many of the amino acids needed by the body to manufacture neurotransmitters, such as phenylalanine, tyrosine and tryptophan, are found to be low in the blood of adults and children with ADHD, and tyrosine has been shown to be beneficial for attention in two reviews of treatments for adults with ADHD (Arnold et al 2013, Pellow et al 2011).

An 8-week open trial of L-tyrosine in 12 adults with attention-deficit disorder (residual type) demonstrated benefits at 2 weeks; however tolerance developed after 6 weeks, rendering the treatment ineffectual (Reimherr et al 1987). Previous studies had reported similar effects (Wood et al 1985).

IN COMBINATION

A retrospective single-blinded pilot study of 85 paediatric patients demonstrated significant improvements when supplemented over 8–10 weeks with a mix of tyrosine, tryptophan and other cofactors, including vitamin C, B vitamins and selenium (Hinz et al 2011a).

Reward deficiency syndrome

Tyrosine depletion appears to affect reward-based processing (McLean et al 2004) and tests involving reward/punishment processing are affected by dopamine depletion (Roiser et al 2005). A lack of dopamine receptors and/or dopamine depletion states have been implicated in a number of conditions or destructive behaviours thought to be caused by poorly functioning biochemical reward systems. Individuals tend to be at risk of multiple addictive, impulsive and compulsive behavioural problems, such as severe alcoholism, cocaine, heroin, marijuana and nicotine addiction, pathological gambling, sex addiction, chronic violence, posttraumatic stress disorder, risk-taking behaviours and antisocial behaviour. As such, the use of tyrosine as a precursor to dopamine has a theoretical basis for use in this condition (Blum et al 2000).

Molecular genetic studies are implicating the gene for the D_2 dopamine receptor (DRD_2) as well as other genes in reward deficiency syndrome and in obesity, leading to excessive craving behaviour (Blum et al 2008, Chen et al 2008). One review concluded that utilising natural dopaminergic repletion therapy to promote long-term dopaminergic activation would ultimately lead to a common, safe and effective modality to treat reward deficiency syndrome behaviours, including substance use disorders, ADHD, obesity and other reward-deficient aberrant behaviors (Chen et al 2008). However, achieving amino acid balance can be difficult; therefore many trials have used a combination of amino acids in the treatment protocol.

Tyrosine is part of a treatment program known as neuroadaptogen amino acid therapy, which has been researched in 27 human clinical trials, including double- and triple-blind placebo-controlled evaluations. Along with D- and L-phenylalanine, L-tryptophan, L-glutamine, chromium, pyridoxine and the herbs passionflower and rhodiola, this formula has been shown to promote the release of dopamine at the reward sites of the brain (Chen et al 2011).

Reward deficiency syndrome has also been proposed as a possible mechanism explaining the tendency to drug and alcohol addiction in schizophrenia (Green et al 1999). To date, no large controlled studies are available to determine the clinical effects of tyrosine supplementation in this condition.

Drug withdrawal

Tyrosine has been used to aid in the withdrawal of cocaine, caffeine and nicotine. Anecdotal reports and animal studies suggest it is successful; however, large controlled studies are not available to determine clinical significance.

L-tyrosine supplementation has been considered because chronic cocaine use is believed to cause catecholamine depletion and cocaine withdrawal has been associated with major depression. To date, results from trials using tyrosine as a stand-alone treatment during cocaine withdrawal have produced disappointing results (Chadwick et al 1990, Galloway et al 1996). Although untested as yet, the effects of tyrosine may be of most assistance where a deficiency of dopamine D_2 receptors is suspected, such as in reward deficiency syndrome.

Stress adaptation

Physical and emotional stress can impair performance and memory. In order to reduce the adverse effects of stress on these functions, improvements in stress adaptation are sought, including through the use of supplements such as tyrosine. Tyrosine appears to enhance the release of catecholamines when neurons are firing at an increased rate due to stress, but not at their basal rates (Young 2007). Several clinical studies have explored the effects of tyrosine in volunteers exposed to stressful situations, generally producing positive results on some parameters (see 'Clinical note: allostatic responses to stress' in the Siberian ginseng monograph for more information about stress adaptation).

A number of studies have been conducted by the US and Dutch military, so extrapolation to other population groups should be made with caution.

Tyrosine supplementation was found to reduce the effects of stress and fatigue on cognitive performance in a study conducted with a group of 21 cadets during a demanding military combat training course. Subjects received a protein-rich drink containing (2 g) tyrosine five times daily or a carbohydrate-rich drink with the same amount of calories (255 kcal). Assessments on day 6 of the course showed that the tyrosine group performed better on a memory and a tracking task than the control group and further experienced a decrease in systolic blood pressure; however, no effects on mood were observed (Deijen et al 1999).

Other studies indicate that high-dose tyrosine (150 mg/kg) may also improve some aspects of performance and help sustain working memory when multitasking in stressful situations. One placebo-controlled trial involving 20 people found that administration of tyrosine significantly enhanced accuracy and working memory during the

T

multiple-task battery 1 hour after ingestion. However, tyrosine did not significantly alter performance on the arithmetic, visual or auditory tasks during the multiple task, or modify any performance measures during the simple task battery (Thomas et al 1999).

Cold stress and heat stress

Similar results were obtained in another controlled trial that investigated the effects of tyrosine (150 mg/kg) on memory tasks in cold (4°C) conditions. Two hours after ingesting L-tyrosine, matching accuracy significantly improved in the cold and was at the same level as administration of either tyrosine or placebo at a comfortable 22°C (Shurtleff et al 1994). Two small trials have shown that tyrosine supplementation (total 300 mg/kg) alleviates working memory decrements induced by cold exposure (~10°C) (Mahoney et al 2007) and may also improve the psychomotor task of marksmanship (O'Brien et al 2007).

Other beneficial effects have been obtained with tyrosine supplementation in volunteers exposed to cold stress. A double-blind, placebo-controlled, crossover study found that tyrosine (100 mg/kg) could protect humans from some of the adverse consequences of a 4.5 hour exposure to cold and hypoxia. Tyrosine significantly decreased symptoms, adverse moods and performance impairment in subjects who exhibited average or greater responses to these environmental conditions (Banderet & Lieberman 1989).

A pilot study of 10 healthy males from the Indian army in a double-blind crossover trial showed that administration of 6.5 g tyrosine 90 minutes prior to a 90-minute exposure at 45°C + 30% humidity increased the catecholamine levels and reduced the impairment of cognitive performance during heat exposure. Serum levels of catecholamines and reaction time testing were improved in the tyrosine group (Kishore et al 2013).

OTHER USES

Hepatocellular carcinoma

In patients with hepatocellular carcinoma (HCC), tyrosine and BCAA supplementation reduces the frequency of early recurrence of HCC after hepatic resection or radiofrequency thermal ablation (Ichikawa et al 2013, Nishikawa et al 2013). A recent multicentre open clinical trial (n = 247) tested the supplementation of 5.5–12 g/day tyrosine/BCAAs to cirrhosis patients without HCC with an average observation/supplementation period of 728 days (Kawaguchi et al 2014). Key findings included that tyrosine/BCCA supplementation significantly reduced all-cause mortality, and significantly reduced the risk of hepatocarcinogenesis. A significant predictor of HCC development in this study was a low BCAA:tyrosine ratio, possibly due to insulin resistance (a significant risk factor for HCC) caused by a low BCAA:tyrosine ratio (Kawaguchi et al 2011). In addition, bacterial infection (the cause of 25% of the deaths in the non-BCAA group) was not a cause of death in the BCAA-supplemented group at all (Kawaguchi et al 2014). This reinforces previous research that reported a preventive effect of BCAAs on bacterial infections in liver transplant recipients via upregulation of immune cell functioning (Shirabe et al 2011).

Premenstrual syndrome

Although tyrosine is used to reduce symptoms of irritability, depression and fatigue associated with premenstrual syndrome, this is largely based on theoretical considerations and the observation that a significant reduction in tyrosine levels occurs during the premenstrual period, according to one study (Menkes et al 1994).

This study further found that tryptophan depletion caused a significant aggravation of premenstrual symptoms, particularly irritability, and symptom magnitude was correlated with reduction in tryptophan relative to other amino acids.

Reproductive effects

Although no controlled studies are available, tyrosine is sometimes used for lowered libido as it indirectly increases testosterone and dopamine levels, both factors important in this condition. Five female lambs with delayed puberty who received a single oral dose of L-tyrosine (100 mg/kg body weight) exhibited significantly higher progesterone concentrations than a control group. Three came into heat and two became pregnant compared to none in the control group (El-Battawy 2006).

Parkinson's disease

The process of Parkinson's disease (degeneration of the postsynaptic neurons of the substantia nigra) is associated with depletion of dopamine, tyrosine and tyrosine hydroxylase, noradrenaline and serotonin. Parkinson's disease depletion of these neurotransmitters is compounded by further depletion with L-dopa (Charlton 1997). As noted in the literature, administration of only L-dopa or improperly balanced L-dopa further depletes tyrosine and other amino acids (Hinz et al 2011b). In addition, the depletion of tyrosine by L-dopa would have an impact on other systems where tyrosine acts as a precursor, such as with thyroid hormones. Administration of tyrosine has been shown to increase dopamine production in the central nervous system of patients with Parkinson's disease (Growdon et al 1982), and in addition, multiple case studies have demonstrated that patients taking L-dopa require a minimum administration of 5000–6000 mg/day of tyrosine to prevent significant urinary dopamine fluctuations (Hinz et al 2011b).

Weight loss

Tyrosine supplements have been used in weight loss, based on biochemical considerations and in vivo research, suggesting tyrosine could potentially suppress appetite and stimulate brown adipose tissue due to its enhancement of noradrenaline synthesis.

Additionally, as a precursor for thyroid hormones it may also increase the basal metabolic rate.

Schizophrenia

Whether tyrosine is helpful with or hinders cognitive functioning in schizophrenia is yet to be determined. Theoretically, some have cautioned against the use of tyrosine due to the possibility of a significant increase in neurotransmitter synthesis and cognitive functioning (Cass & Holford 2001); however studies also show that aberrant tyrosine kinetics in patients with schizophrenia might be associated with cognitive dysfunction — a core feature of schizophrenia. It has been noted that, in patients with schizophrenia, cognitive dysfunction was found to be related to a high affinity of tyrosine to transport-binding sites in fibroblasts but not to the transport capacity, so therefore despite the fact that tyrosine binds strongly to receptors, the actual transport and conversion to dopamine are low in these patients (Wiesel et al 2005).

Cognitive enhancement in Alzheimer's dementia and traumatic brain injury

Clinical studies have shown that cognitively impaired subjects have significant levels of mitochondrial dysfunction and oxidative protein damage. In particular, tyrosine nitration is a common early indicator/biomarker of cognitive impairment, including those with an ageing brain, and of age-related neurodegenerative disorders such as Alzheimer's dementia (Butterfield et al 2007). The oxidative stress-induced modification of tyrosine residues can elicit significant changes in protein structure and function which, in some cases, may contribute to biological ageing and age-related pathologies such as neurodegeneration (Feeney & Schoenich 2012).

Clinical research is not available to determine the effects of modified tyrosine intake.

Fatigue

Fatigue is a common feature associated with a range of chronic and/or progressive conditions, interfering with normal activities and general quality of life. Patients with chronic liver diseases such as primary biliary cirrhosis often suffer from profound fatigue, and research has confirmed that aberrant tyrosine metabolism and plasma amino acid concentrations are a feature of fatigued patients when compared to healthy controls, whereby a significant and independent association has been documented between lower tyrosine levels and all measures of fatigue (ter Borg et al 2005). Further studies are required to confirm these findings.

Low tyrosine levels have been identified in subjects with chronic fatigue syndrome, suggesting a possible role for supplementation in this condition (Georgiades et al 2003)

Narcolepsy

Abnormalities of the dopaminergic system are thought to be part of the underlying aetiology of this disorder, therefore tyrosine is used on the theoretical basis that an increase in dopamine levels will produce an improvement (Roufs 1990).

A randomised, double-blind, placebo-controlled study of L-tyrosine (9 g/day for 4 weeks) that tests this theory has been conducted in 10 subjects with narcolepsy and cataplexy. While receiving tyrosine, subjects reported feeling less tired, less drowsy and more alert; however, ratings of daytime drowsiness, cataplexy, sleep paralysis, nighttime sleep, overall clinical response and measurements of multiple sleep latency and tests of speed and attention did not detect a significant difference with placebo (Elwes et al 1989). An earlier trial of longer duration, however, reported that within 6 months all eight participants were free from daytime sleep attacks and cataplexy (Mouret et al 1988b).

Nemaline myopathy

Five patients (four infants and one adolescent) with nemaline myopathy (the most common congenital myopathy, characterised by facial and bulbar weakness, resulting in eating difficulties, recurrent aspiration and poor control of oral secretions) received L-tyrosine (250–3000 mg/day). All infants experienced an initial decrease in sialorrhoea and an increase in energy levels. The adolescent experienced improved strength and exercise tolerance (Ryan et al 2008).

DOSAGE RANGE

- As tyrosine is considered to be a non-essential amino acid, there is no specific recommended daily intake. The typical dose in clinical trials appears to be 100–150 mg/kg. Divided dosing may be beneficial as levels remain above baseline for 6–8 hours following administration.
- Depression, premenstrual syndrome and chronic fatigue: 500–1000 mg before meals three times daily.
- Stress: 1500 mg/day in divided doses.
- Decreased libido, Parkinson's disease, drug detoxification and weight loss: 1–2 g/day in divided doses.
- Natural stimulant: 500–1000 mg on an empty stomach first thing in the morning.
- Alertness following sleep deprivation: 150 mg/kg/day.
- As individual sensitivity to tyrosine can vary, it is recommended to start at 100 mg/day and gradually increase dose (Cass & Holford 2001).

T

ADVERSE REACTIONS

Adverse reactions include migraine headache, mild gastric upset, nausea, headache, fatigue, heartburn, arthralgia, insomnia and nervousness (Hendler & Rorvik 2001).

High blood pressure may occur in susceptive individuals — hypertensive patients taking tyrosine should be monitored closely.

Practice points/Patient counselling

- Tyrosine is a conditionally essential amino acid that is ingested from the diet or produced from phenylalanine in the body.
- Many of the pharmacological actions of tyrosine relate to its role as a precursor to a number of neurotransmitters and thyroid hormones.
- Protein sources enriched with tyrosine but lacking in phenylalanine are used in PKU.
- Tyrosine supplements are used to improve cognitive function, in the management of depression or reward deficiency syndrome associated with noradrenaline or dopamine depletion, and to enhance stress adaptation systems.
- Due to its effects on neurotransmitters, it may elevate blood pressure in susceptible people when taken in high doses, and increase the effects of amphetamines, ephedrine, phenylpropanolamine, thyroxine and pharmaceutical antidepressants.

SIGNIFICANT INTERACTIONS

Amphetamine, ephedrine, phenylpropanolamine

L-Tyrosine (200 and 400 mg/kg) has been shown to increase the side effect of anorexia caused by phenylpropanolamine, ephedrine and amphetamine in a dose-dependent manner in rats (Hull & Maher 1990) — observe patients using this combination.

Antidepressant drugs

Monoamine oxidase inhibitors (MAOIs), tricyclic antidepressants or selective serotonin reuptake inhibitors: theoretically, concurrent use may result in elevated blood pressure and/or enhanced antidepressant effects. In the case of MAOIs, some tyrosine may be metabolised to tyramine and concurrent use with MAOIs may lead to a hypertensive crisis.

Tyrosine should be avoided unless under medical supervision.

Central nervous system stimulants

Tyrosine is a precursor to a number of neurotransmitters, so additive effects may occur — caution.

Oestrogens and antiandrogen therapy

Oestrogens and antiandrogen therapies have been shown to decrease plasma levels of tyrosine by up to 18.3% after 4 and 12 months in transsexual patients, therefore supplementation may be suggested (Giltay et al 2008).

Levodopa

L-Dopa competes with tyrosine for uptake, therefore concurrent use may decrease the uptake of both substances, reducing efficacy (Awad 1984, DiPiro et al 1999, Riederer 1980) — avoid unless under medical supervision.

Morphine sulfate

L-Tyrosine potentiates morphine-induced analgesia by 154% (Hull et al 1994) and 200 mg/kg significantly potentiated the antinocicieptive action of morphine in mice, although L-tyrosine alone did not produce a significant antinociceptive effect (Ali 1995). Observe patients taking tyrosine and morphine sulfate concurrently — there is a potential beneficial interaction.

Thyroid hormone medication

Additive effects are possible because tyrosine is a precursor to thyroid hormones — observe patients taking tyrosine concurrently with thyroid hormone medication.

CONTRAINDICATIONS AND PRECAUTIONS

- Malignant melanoma: a theoretical concern exists that tyrosine supplementation may promote the division of cancer cells (McArdle et al 2001). Tyrosine is contraindicated until safety is established.
- Manic conditions: caution exists due to the theoretical possibility that tyrosine may significantly increase neurotransmitter synthesis (Cass & Holford 2001), and until further studies are undertaken, monitoring is recommended.
- Hyperthyroidism and Graves' disease: theoretically tyrosine may aggravate these conditions as it is a precursor to thyroxine (van Spronsen et al 2001).
- Alkaptonuria and tyrosinaemia (inborn errors of tyrosine metabolism).
- Hypertension: use tyrosine with caution at high dose.
- Ecstasy users should be aware that MDMA increases the concentration of tyrosine in the brain, causing long-term depletion of serotonin (Breier et al 2006).

PREGNANCY USE

High-dose supplements should be used with caution in pregnancy.

PATIENTS' FAQs

What will this supplement do for me?
Tyrosine supplementation appears to increase the levels of important brain chemicals and thyroid hormones. As such, it may elevate mood and alertness, and enhance the body's ability to deal with stress.

When will it start to work?
Although some research suggests that effects begin within 1–2 hours, it may take up to 1 week for maximal effects to be seen.

Are there any safety issues?
Theoretically, tyrosine may increase blood pressure in susceptible individuals and also interact with a number of medicines, such as pharmaceutical antidepressants and thyroid treatment. It is also not recommended in pregnancy.

REFERENCES

Ali BH. The effect of L-tyrosine on some anti-nociceptive and non-nociceptive actions of morphine in mice. Gen. Pharmac. 26.2 (1995):407–09.

Arnold LE et al Attention-Deficit/Hyperactivity Disorder: dietary and nutritional treatments. Child Adolesc Psychiatric Clin N Am 22 (2013): 381–402.

Awad AG. Diet and drug interactions in the treatment of mental illness: a review. Can J Psychiatry 29 (1984): 609–613.

Badawy AAB et al. Specificity of the acute tryptophan and tyrosine plus phenylalanine depletion and loading tests I. Review of biochemical aspects and poor specificity of current amino acid formulations. Int J Tryptophan Res 3 (2010): 23–34.

Banderet LE, Lieberman HR. Treatment with tyrosine, a neurotransmitter precursor, reduces environmental stress in humans. Brain Res Bull 22.4 (1989): 759–762.

Benkert, O., et al. 1971. Altered tyrosine daytime plasma levels in endogenous depressive patients. Arch.Gen.Psychiatry, 25, (4) 359–363 available from: PM:5116991.

Blum K et al. Reward deficiency syndrome: a biogenetic model for the diagnosis and treatment of impulsive, addictive, and compulsive behaviors. J Psychoactive Drugs 32 (Suppl i–iv) (2000): 1–1112.

Blum K et al. Dopamine D2 Receptor Taq A1 allele predicts treatment compliance of LG839 in a subset analysis of pilot study in the Netherlands. Gene Ther Mol Biol Vol 12 (2008):129–140.

Breier JM, et al. L-tyrosine contributes to (+)-3,4-methylenedioxymethamphetamine-induced serotonin depletions. J Neurosci 26.1 (2006): 290–299.

Butterfield DA et al. Elevated levels of 3-nitrotyrosine in brain from subjects with amnestic mild cognitive impairment: Implications for the role of nitration in the progression of Alzheimer's disease. Brain Research 1148 (2007): 243–248.

Cass H, Holford P. Natural highs. London: Piatkus, 2001, p 100.

Chadwick MJ, et al. A double-blind amino acids, L-tryptophan and L-tyrosine, and placebo study with cocaine-dependent subjects in an inpatient chemical dependency treatment center. Am J Drug Alcohol Abuse 16.3–4 (1990): 275–286.

Charlton C. Depletion of nigrostriatal and forebrain tyrosine hydroxylase by S-adenosyl methionine: A model that may explain the occurrence of depression in Parkinson's disease. Life Sci. 61.5 (1997): 495–502.

Chen TJ et al. Neurogenetics and clinical evidence for the putative activation of the brain reward circuitry by a neuroadaptagen: proposing an addiction candidate gene panel map. J Psychoactive Drugs. 43 (2011): 108–127.

Deijen JB et al. Tyrosine improves cognitive performance and reduces blood pressure in cadets after one week of a combat training course. Brain Res Bull 48.2 (1999): 203–209.

DiPiro JT et al (eds), Pharmacotherapy: A pathophysiologic approach, 4th edn, Stamford: Appleton & Lang, 1999.

El-Battawy KA. Reproductive and endocrine characteristics of delayed pubertal ewe-lambs after melatonin and L-tyrosine administration. Reprod Domest Anim 41.1 (2006): 1–4.

Elwes RD et al. Treatment of narcolepsy with L-tyrosine: double-blind placebo-controlled trial. Lancet 2.8671 (1989): 1067–1069.

Feeney MB, Schoenich C. Tyrosine modifications in aging. Antioxid. Redox Signaling 17 (2012): 1571–1579.

Feillet F Agostoni C. Nutritional issues in treating phenylketonuria. J Inherit Metab Dis 33 (2010): 659–664.

Fernstrom JD. Can nutrient supplements modify brain function? Am J Clin Nutr 71.6 (2000): 1669–725.

Fernstrom JD & Fernstrom MH. Tyrosine, phenylalanine, and catecholamine synthesis and function in the brain. J. Nutr. 137 (2007): 1539S–15.

Galloway GP et al. A historically controlled trial of tyrosine for cocaine dependence. J Psychoactive Drugs 28.3 (1996): 305–309.

Gelenberg, A.J., et al. 1980. Tyrosine for the treatment of depression. Am J Psychiatry, 137, (5) 622–623.

Gelenberg AJ et al. Tyrosine for depression: a double-blind trial. J Affect Disord 19.2 (1990): 125–132.

Georgiades E et al. Chronic fatigue syndrome: new evidence for a central fatigue disorder. Clin Sci (Lond) 105.2 (2003): 213–2118.

Giltay EJ et al. Effects of sex steroids on the neurotransmitter- specific aromatic amino acids phenylalanine, tyrosine, and tryptophan in transsexual subjects. Neuroendocrinology 88 (2008): 103–110.

Giovannini M et al. Phenylketonuria: nutritional advances and challenges. Nutr & Metab 9 (2012): 7.

Glaeser BS, et al. Elevation of plasma tyrosine after a single oral dose of L-tyrosine. Life Sci 25.3 (1979): 265–271.

Green AI et al. Clozapine for comorbid substance use disorder and schizophrenia: do patients with schizophrenia have a reward-deficiency syndrome that can be ameliorated by clozapine? Harv Rev Psychiatry 6.6 (1999): 287–296.

Growdon JH et al. Effects of oral L-tyrosine administration on CSF tyrosine and homovanillic acid levels in patients with Parkinson's disease. Life Sci 30 (1982): 827–832.

Gulcin I. Comparison of in vitro antioxidant and antiradical activities of L-tyrosine and L-Dopa. Amino Acids 32.3 (2007): 431–438.

Haas EM. Staying healthy with nutrition. Berkeley, CA: Celestial Arts, 1992, p 51.

Harmer CJ et al. Tyrosine depletion attenuates dopamine function in healthy volunteers. Psychopharmacology (Berl) 154.1 (2001): 105–111.

Hendler SS, Rorvik D (eds). PDR for nutritional supplements. Montvale, NJ: Medical Economics Co., 2001.

Hinz M et al. Treatment of attention deficit hyperactivity disorder with monoamine amino acid precursors and organic cation transporter assay interpretation. Neuropsych Dis Treat (2011a): 31–38.

Hinz M et al. Amino acid management of Parkinson's disease: a case study Int J of Gen Med 4 (2011b): 165–174.

Hull KM, Maher TJ. L-Tyrosine potentiates the anorexia induced by mixed-acting sympathomimetic drugs in hyperphagic rats. J Pharmacol Exp Ther 255.2 (1990): 403–409.

Hull KM, et al. L-tyrosine potentiation of opioid-induced analgesia utilizing the hot-plate test. J Pharmacol Exp Ther 269.3 (1994): 1190–1195.

Ichikawa K et al. Oral supplementation of branched-chain amino acids reduces early recurrence after hepatic resection in patients with hepatocellular carcinoma: a prospective study. Surg Today 43 (2013): 720–726.

Kalsner LR et al. Tyrosine supplementation in phenylketonuria: diurnal blood tyrosine levels and presumptive brain influx of tyrosine and other large neutral amino acids. J Pediatr 139.3 (2001): 421–427.

Kawaguchi T et al. Branched-chain amino acids as pharmacological nutrients in chronic liver disease. Hepatology 54 (2011):1063–1070.

Kawaguchi T et al Branched-chain amino acids prevent hepatocarcinogenesis and prolong survival of patients with cirrhosis. Clin Gastro Hepatol (2014); 12: 1012–1018.

Keeney JTR et al. Dietary vitamin D deficiency in rats from middle to old age leads to elevated tyrosine nitration and proteomics changes in levels of key proteins in brain: Implications for low vitamin D-dependent age-related cognitive decline. Free Radical Biology and Medicine 65 (2013): 324–334.

Kishore K et al Tyrosine ameliorates heat induced delay in event related potential P300 and contingent negative variation. Brain and Cognition 83 (2013): 324–329.

Koch R, et al. Large neutral amino acid therapy and phenylketonuria: a promising approach to treatment. Mol Genet Metab 2003, 79:110–113.

Kopple JD. Phenylalanine and tyrosine metabolism in chronic kidney failure. J. Nutr. 137 (2007): 1586S–1590S

Lakhan SE, Vieira KF Nutritional therapies for mental disorders Nutrition J 7 (2008):2–10.

MacDonald A et al Weaning infants with phenylketonuria: a review. J Hum Nutr Diet. 25 (2012): 103–110.

Mahoney CR et al. Tyrosine supplementation mitigates working memory decrements during cold exposure. Physiol Behav 92.4 (2007): 575–582.

Matalon R et al. Double blind placebo control trial of large neutral amino acids in treatment of PKU: effect on blood phenylalanine. J Inherit Metab Dis 30 (2007):153–158.

McArdle L et al. Protein tyrosine phosphatase genes downregulated in melanoma. J Invest Dermatol 117.5 (2001): 1255–1260.

McLean A et al. The effects of tyrosine depletion in normal healthy volunteers: implications for unipolar depression. Psychopharmacology (Berl) 171.3 (2004): 286–297.

McTavish SF et al. Lack of effect of tyrosine depletion on mood in recovered depressed women. Neuropsychopharmacology 30.4 (2005): 786–791.

Menkes DB, et al. Acute tryptophan depletion aggravates premenstrual syndrome. J Affect Disord 32.1 (1994): 37–44.

Mouret J et al. L-tyrosine cures, immediate and long term, dopamine-dependent depressions. Clinical and Polygraphic Studies 306.3 (1988a): 93–98: C R Acad Sci III [in French].

Mouret J et al. Treatment of narcolepsy with L-tyrosine. Lancet 2.8626–7 (1988b): 1458–1459.

Neri DF et al. The effects of tyrosine on cognitive performance during extended wakefulness. Aviat Space Environ Med 66.4 (1995): 313–3119.

Nishikawa H et al. The effect of long-term supplementation with branched-chain amino acid granules in patients with hepatitis C virus-related hepatocellular carcinoma after radiofrequency thermal ablation. J Clin Gastroenterol 47(2013):359–366.

O'Brien C et al. Dietary tyrosine benefits cognitive and psychomotor performance during body cooling. Physiol Behav 90.2–3 (2007): 301–307.

Parker G, Brotchie H. Mood effects of the amino acids tryptophan and tyrosine. Acta Psychiatr Scand 124 (2011): 417–426

Pellow J et al. Complementary and alternative medical therapies for children with attention-deficit/ hyperactivity disorder (ADHD) Alt Med Rev 16.4 (2011):323–337.

Peters JC, Harper AE. Adaptation of rats to diets containing different levels of protein: effects on food intake, plasma and brain amino acid concentrations and brain neurotransmitter metabolism. J Nutr. 115 (1985):382–98.

Pietz, J., et al. 1995. Effect of high-dose tyrosine supplementation on brain function in adults with phenylketonuria. J Pediatr., 127, (6) 936–943.

Poustie VJ, Rutherford P. Tyrosine supplementation for phenylketonuria. Cochrane Database Syst Rev 2 (2000): CD001507.
Reimherr FW et al. An open trial of L-tyrosine in the treatment of attention deficit disorder, residual type. Am J Psychiatry 144.8 (1987): 1071–1073.
Riederer P. L-Dopa competes with tyrosine and tryptophan for human brain uptake. Nutr Metab 24.6 (1980): 417–423.
Roiser JP et al. The subjective and cognitive effects of acute phenylalanine and tyrosine depletion in patients recovered from depression. Neuropsychopharmacology 30.4 (2005): 775–785.
Roufs JB. L-Tyrosine in the treatment of narcolepsy. Med Hypotheses 33.4 (1990): 269–273.
Ruhé HG et al Mood is indirectly related to serotonin, norepinephrine and dopamine levels in humans: a meta-analysis of monoamine depletion studies. Mol Psychiatry 12.4 (2007):331–359.
Ryan MM et al. Dietary L-tyrosine supplementation in nemaline myopathy. J Child Neurol 23.6 (2008): 609–613.
Sa M et al. Simultaneous determination of tyrosine, tryptophan and 5-hydroxytryptamine in serum of MDD patients by high performance liquid chromatography with fluorescence detection. Clinica Chimica Acta 413 (2012): 973–977.
Schindeler S et al. The effects of large neutral amino acid supplements in PKU: an MRS and neuropsychological study. Mol Genet Metab 91 (2007):48–54.
Sharman R et al. Depressive symptoms in adolescents with early and continuously treated phenylketonuria: Associations with phenylalanine and tyrosine levels. Gene 504.2 (2012): 288–291.
Shirabe K et al. Beneficial effects of supplementation with branched-chain amino acids on postoperative bacteremia in living donor liver transplant recipients. Liver Transpl 17 (2011): 1073–1080.
Shurtleff D et al. Tyrosine reverses a cold-induced working memory deficit in humans. Pharmacol Biochem Behav 47.4 (1994): 935–941.
ter Borg PCJ et al. The relation between plasma tyrosine concentration and fatigue in primary biliary cirrhosis and primary sclerosing cholangitis BMC Gastroenterology 5 (2005):11–18.
Thomas JR et al. Tyrosine improves working memory in a multitasking environment. Pharmacol Biochem Behav 64.3 (1999): 495–500.
Tortora GJ, Grabowski SR. Principles of anatomy and physiology. New York: Harper Collins, 1996 pp 128, 522.
van Spronsen FJ, et al. Phenylketonuria: tyrosine supplementation in phenylalanine restricted diets. Am J Clin Nutr 73 (2001): 153–157.
Wiesel FA et al. Kinetics of tyrosine transport and cognitive functioning in schizophrenia. Schizophrenia Res 74.1 (2005): 81–89.
Wood DR, et al. Amino acid precursors for the treatment of attention deficit disorder, residual type. Psychopharmacol Bull 21.1 (1985): 146–149.
Yano S et al. Large neutral amino acid supplementation increases melatonin synthesis in phenylketonuria: a new biomarker. J.Pediatrics 162.5 (2013):999–1003.
Yehuda S. Possible anti-Parkinson properties of *N*-([alpha]-linolenoyl) tyrosine: A new molecule. Pharmacol Biochem Behav 72.1–2 (2002): 7–11.
Young SN. L-tyrosine to alleviate the effects of stress? J Psychiatry Neurosci 32.3 (2007): 224.

Valerian

HISTORICAL NOTE The sedative effects of valerian have been recognised for over 2000 years, having been used by Hippocrates and Dioscorides in ancient Greece. Over the past 500 years, valerian has been widely used in Europe for nervousness or hysteria and also to treat dyspepsia and flatulence. Legend has it that the Pied Piper put valerian in his pockets to attract the rats out of Hannover. Valerian was widely used by the Eclectic physicians and listed in the United States Formulary until 1946.

COMMON NAME

Valerian and Mexican Valerian

OTHER NAMES

All-heal, amantilla, balderbrackenwurzel, baldrian, baldrianwurzel, fragrant valerian, heliotrope, herbe aux chats, katzenwurzel, phu germanicum, phu parvum, valeriana, wild valerian

BOTANICAL NAME/FAMILY

Valeriana officinalis, *Valeriana edulis* (family Valerianaceae)

PLANT PART USED

Rhizome

CHEMICAL COMPONENTS

Valtrates, didrovaltrates, isovaltrates, monoterpenes, sesquiterpenes, caffeic, gamma-amino butyric and chlorogenic acids, beta-sitosterol, methyl 2-pyrrolketone, choline, tannins, gum, alkaloids, a resin. Essential oils (0.5–2%) in the plant contain the compounds bornyl acetate and the sesquiterpene derivatives valerenic acid, valeranone and valerenal.

The chemical composition of valerian varies greatly depending on such factors as plant age and growing conditions. Processing and storage of the herb also affects its constituents, such as the iridoid esters, which are chemically unstable.

MAIN ACTIONS

Anxiolytic and hypnotic

Both in vivo and numerous clinical studies confirm sedative or hypnotic activity for valerian (Ammer & Melnizky 1999, Balderer & Borbely 1985, Della Loggia et al 1981, Donath et al 2000, Dorn 2000, Gerhard et al 1996, Gessner & Klasser 1984, Leathwood & Chauffard 1985, Leuschner et al 1993, Lindahl & Lindwall 1989, Schulz et al 1994, Wheatley 2001). Anxiolytic activity has been demonstrated, most recently seen with a valerian extract with high valerenic acid concentration (Felgentreff et al 2012). Antidepressant activity has been seen most recently with an ethanolic extract of valerian (Phytofin Valerian 368) in an experimental model (Hattesohl et al 2008).

Extensive pharmacological research has been conducted to identify the main active constituents responsible for these effects. It is apparent that multiple components are at work and several neurobiological mechanisms underlie these actions. Recent in vivo testing has identified that the chief component responsible for the anxiolytic activity of valerian is the valerenic acid content (Felgentreff et al 2012). In the study, two extracts of valerian were tested with different valerenic acid ratios. A stronger anxiolytic effect was seen in test animals for the higher concentration extract (12:1) compared to a lower ratio extract (1 : 1.5). Binding studies confirmed an affinity to GABAergic binding sites. In an in vitro cell culture model, valerenic acid and its derivatives, acetoxyvalerenic acid and hydroxyvalerenic acid, were shown to cross the blood–brain barrier (BBB) to a slower extent than the GABAA modulator diazepam. Valerenic acid was the slowest to permeate in the study, followed by hydroxyvalerenic acid and acetoxyvalerenic acid. The research suggested that these compounds do not cross into the CNS by passive diffusion and instead are transported over the BBB by an as yet unknown transport system (Neuhaus et al 2008).

In vitro tests so far have demonstrated that valerian stimulates the release of GABA, inhibits GABA reuptake and may modulate GABA activity at GABAA receptors (Ortiz et al 1999, Santos et al 1994). The sesquiterpenic acids (valerenic acid and acetoxyvalerenic acid) seem to be at least partly responsible for this effect. This was discovered when a valerian ethyl acetate extract containing high levels of valerenic acid exhibited strong enhancement of GABA receptor activation, whereas the removal of sesquiterpenic acids from the extract led to a loss of GABA enhancement (Trauner et al 2008).

An alternative explanation for the anxiolytic properties of valerian may be CNS depression via inhibition of glutamate receptors as suggested by in vitro and animal models (Del Valle-Mojica et al 2011a, 2011b, 2012). There is also evidence of agonist effects at the human A_1 adenosine receptor for the methanolic extract (Schumacher et al 2002).

Antispasmodic, vasorelaxant and anti-convulsant

Both in vitro and in vivo studies provide evidence of antispasmodic activity on smooth muscle using various models (Hazelhoff et al 1982, Occhiuto et al 2009, Estrada-Soto et al 2010, Rezvani et al 2010). Valerian extracts and valepotriates in aqueous and ethanolic extracts exhibited antispasmodic activity as demonstrated by decreasing uterine contractility in isolated human uterine muscle. The effect occurred in a concentration-dependent manner and is thought to be due to calcium-channel blocker activity (Occhiuto et al 2009). *Valeriana edulis* demonstrated a significant concentration-dependent vasorelaxant activity on isolated rat aorta which also appeared to be due to a calcium-channel blocker mechanism (Estrada-Soto et al 2010). Antiepileptic activity was observed for an aqueous extract of valerian (500 mg/kg) which reduced seizure activity in rats. The mechanism of action was thought to be activation of the adenosine system (Rezvani et al 2010).

OTHER ACTIONS

A pharmacokinetic study with healthy adults found that typical doses of valerian are unlikely to produce clinically significant effects on the CYP2D6 or CYP3A4 pathways of metabolism (Donovan et al 2004). These results were confirmed in another human pharmacokinetic study that found no evidence of valerian affecting CYP3A4/5, CYP1A2, CYP2E1 and CYP2D6 activity (Gurley et al 2005). There is some in vitro evidence that suggests valerian may increase glucuronidation via the UDP-glucuronosyltransferase (UGT) enzymes. However, this has not been confirmed in humans (Mohamed et al 2010, 2011).

CLINICAL USE

In practice, valerian is rarely used as a stand-alone treatment and is often combined with other sedatives or relaxant herbs, such as chamomile, passionflower, skullcap, lemon balm and hops.

Insomnia

Numerous randomised controlled trials (RCTs) have investigated the effects of different valerian preparations as a treatment for insomnia. Some studies have involved people with confirmed sleep disturbances and others involved healthy subjects with no sleep problems. Treatment time-frames varied from acute (1 dose) to longer term (over 1 month) and doses have varied considerably. Some studies use only subjective data such as self-reported sleep quality whereas others use objective measures such as polysomnographs. Additionally, some studies use herbal combinations which include valerian, whereas other use valerian alone as monotherapy. As a result, interpreting the evidence is difficult.

Overall, the research suggests that valerian improves the subjective quality of sleep and may reduce sleep latency, enabling people to fall asleep a little more quickly. It generally shows no significant effect among people without sleep disturbances. Some research also suggests that best results are obtained with continuous use after several days to weeks and in some studies, a herbal combination of valerian with lemon balm or hops is more effective than placebo.

Findings from a pharmacokinetic study indicate that valerian has a short period of activity as it demonstrated that valerenic acid (a pharmacologically active marker compound for valerian) was increased in serum within an hour of ingestion, reached maximal levels between 1 and 2 hours, then fell with a marked decrease within 4 hours and no detectable levels observed after 8 hours (Anderson et al 2005). This pharmacokinetic pattern is also consistent with the finding that valerian does not produce residual morning sedation.

A number of different valerian products have been studied in clinical trials (e.g. Baldosedron, Baldrien-Dispert, Euvegal, Harmonicum Much, Seda-Kneipp, Sedonium, Valdispert, Valverde and Valerina Nutt). The LI 156 valerian extract is one of the most studied.

One of the first major systematic reviews was conducted by Stevinson and Ernst (2000), who identified 19 studies involving valerian treatment that were published prior to May 1999. Of these, nine were chosen for inclusion because they were randomised, measured sleep parameters and tested single ingredient valerian products. Three studies considered the cumulative effects of long-term use of valerian, whereas six investigated the effects of single-dose treatment. Two of the three studies investigating repeated administration of valerian found that effects were established by 2 weeks. The most rigorous placebo-controlled study showed that valerian LI 156 (600 mg) produced improvement on nearly all measures between weeks 2 and 4 (Vorbach et al 1996 as reported by Stevinson & Ernst 2000). The 4-week study involved 121 volunteers and assessed clinical effectiveness using four validated rating scales. At the end of the study, valerian was rated better than placebo on the Clinical Global Impression Scale, and at study conclusion (day 28) 66% of patients rated valerian effective, compared to 26% with placebo. Of the six studies investigating acute effects, valerian produced positive results in three whereas in the other three it was no better than placebo.

Interpretation of study results is difficult because of varying research methodologies. For example, some studies used surveys whereas others used EEG readings; some were conducted at home and others in hospitals or sleep laboratories, and pre-bedtime variables (e.g. caffeine consumption) were not fully controlled. Additionally, some studies used healthy volunteers with no sleep disturbances with little scope to observe further improvements. Since then, several other studies have been published.

In 2007, a comprehensive systematic review conducted by Taibi et al identified 37 separate studies of which 29 were controlled trials which evaluated valerian for both efficacy and safety, and eight were open-label trials which evaluated for safety only (Taibi et al 2007). The search was not limited to English language publications, thereby identifying many additional studies published by European research groups, including 17 studies published in German. The review evaluated data from RCTs and trials of other designs that investigated ethanolic extracts of valerian, aqueous extracts of valerian and valerian herbal combination treatments in people with sleep disturbances and in those who were considered healthy.

Six randomised, double-blind studies of an ethanolic extract of valerian (mainly LI 156 Sedonium) at a dosage between 300 and 600 mg before bedtime were assessed (Taibi et al 2007). Two studies measured polysomnographic outcomes and four collected only subjective measures of sleep quality. Overall, the ethanolic extract was not found to significantly affect objective or subjective sleep outcomes compared to placebo, however it did improve subjective sleep quality ratings in a manner similar to benzodiazepines. If we assume benzodiazepines perform better than placebo, then this is a positive outcome.

Seven studies evaluated the effects of aqueous preparations of valerian (Valdispert, Dixa SA Switzerland) at doses ranging from 400 mg/night to 450 mg three times daily (Taibi et al 2007). Four studies involved healthy subjects, two were of elderly people with sleep disturbances and one study was of people with difficulties in sleep onset. Once again, methodologies were highly varied. Only one study excluded volunteers with medical conditions that could contribute to poor sleep. As may be expected with such variations, results were mixed. The two studies involving elderly volunteers produced contradictory results, whereas reduced subjective latency was demonstrated in people with sleep onset disturbances. Healthy volunteers appeared to gain no benefit from the treatment.

Five further studies used valerian extracts which were standardised to valepotriate content (Taibi et al 2007). Three of these studies used *V. edulis* (one used Harmonicum Much) as a source of valepotriates and one used *V. wallichii* (Valmane). The dose of valepotriates varied from 60 to 120 mg and one preparation of *V. officinalis* used a preparation standardised to 450 mg of valerenic acid (Mediherb, Queensland, Australia). While methodologies varied considerably, overall standardised extracts appeared to reduce sleep disturbances when compared to placebo. A dose of 100 mg valepotriates taken three times a day was found to significantly improve sleep quality ratings in people withdrawing from benzodiazepines when compared to placebo. Additionally, 60 to 120 mg valepotriates was similarly effective in people who had reported disturbed sleep.

Valerian herbal combinations

In the 2007 systematic review by Taibi et al, 10 studies evaluating valerian herbal combinations were reviewed. Four studies tested valerian–lemon balm and six studies tested valerian–hops in combination (Taibi et al 2007). The studies using valerian–lemon balm combinations were shown to reduce sleep latency and increase sleep quality in people suffering sleep disturbances, whereas no change was observed in healthy subjects. In contrast, studies with valerian–hops combinations found no significant improvements using polysomnographic equipment or subjective sleep outcomes (Taibi et al 2007). The hops–valerian treatments used were ZE 91019 (Alluna) or another product sHova (extraction unknown).

In 2007, a later randomised placebo controlled study was published that compared a valerian–hops combination (Ze 91019) to valerian monotherapy (Ze 911) (Koetter et al 2007). The herbal combination treatment contained the same amount of valerian (500 mg) as monotherapy, thereby allowing researchers to evaluate what contribution hops (120 mg) would make to the outcomes measured. Volunteers suffering from non-organic insomnia were given either treatment or placebo for 4 weeks. In contrast to previous studies cited by Taibi et al, the valerian–hops combination was significantly superior to placebo in reducing sleep latency, improving clinical global impression scores and increasing slow-wave sleep, while the single valerian extract failed to show benefits beyond placebo.

A 2008 randomised placebo-controlled double-blinded trial ($n = 42$) investigating a combined preparation of valerian and hops (Dormeasan) found that the time spent in deeper sleep was significantly higher for the active treatment group compared to the placebo group ($P < 0.01$) (Dimpfel et al 2008). The treatment was administered 15 minutes before an 8-hour EEG recording to a group of poor sleepers, as identified by a validated sleep questionnaire (Schlaffragebogen SF-B). An un-medicated first night was used as a reference and compared to a second night where volunteers received either treatment. The findings between the reference and medication night in regards to time spent in deeper sleep were also statistically significant ($P < 0.01$). This suggests that a single dose preparation may be effective in achieving deeper sleep. The dose used was 2 mL of a liquid extract (a 1 : 10 fresh-plant tincture of *Valeriana officinalis* radix equivalent to 460 mg plus a 1 : 12 fresh-plant tincture of *Humulus lupulus* strobilus equivalent to 460 mg in 61% ethanol).

Valerian monotherapy

A 2010 meta-analysis analysed results from 18 RCTs where valerian was used as monotherapy compared to placebo (Fernández-San-Martín et al 2010). Studies varied greatly in design with variations in sample size, population groups, diagnostic criteria, dosage and follow-up times. The outcome measures were improved sleep quality with a dichotomic variable, improved sleep quality identified through visual analogue scales and improved sleep latency (measured via polysomnography or self-reporting questionnaires). Analysis found that valerian did not demonstrate statistical significance in improving sleep latency, but did improve sleep quality when the outcome was measured as a dichotomous variable, but not using a visual analogue scale. This indicates that participants taking valerian subjectively perceived greater sleep quality however this was not confirmed with quantitative measurements. Adverse effects between valerian and placebo were comparable with the exception of diarrhoea. Diarrhoea was more frequent in patients taking Valerian (18%) compared with those taking a placebo (8%, $P = 0.02$).

Restless legs syndrome and insomnia

Whether valerian improves sleep quality and symptoms in people with restless legs syndrome (RLS) is unclear according to this triple-blind, placebo-controlled RCT (Cuellar et al 2009). Thirty-seven volunteers were treated for 8 weeks with either valerian capsules twice daily (800 mg dried *Valeriana officinalis radix* equivalent to 1.16 mg valerenic acid/day) or placebo. The primary aim was to assess sleep quality using the Pittsburgh Sleep Quality Index and sleepiness using the Epworth Sleepiness Scale. The secondary aim was to assess changes in RLS symptom severity using the International RLS Symptom Severity Scale. Although the treatment group displayed a greater improvement in the majority of RLS symptoms and sleep quality, the findings were not statistically significant.

POST-MENOPAUSAL WOMEN WITH INSOMNIA

A 2010 triple-blind, controlled trial involving 100 postmenopausal women aged 50 to 60 years experiencing insomnia found that more women treated with valerian capsules (Sedamin 530 mg concentrated valerian root extract per capsule) twice daily for 4 weeks experienced improved sleep quality (30%) compared to those taking placebo (4%; $P < 0.001$) (Taavoni et al 2011). The improvement in sleep quality was based on changes to the Pittsburgh Sleep Quality index, a self-rated questionnaire assessing subjective sleep quality, latency, duration, sleep disturbances, use of sleep medication and daytime dysfunction.

In contrast, a small ($n = 16$) randomised, double-blind, crossover, controlled trial of healthy women aged 55–80 years with insomnia, valerian capsules (300 mg of a concentrated *Valeriana officinalis* L. root extract Nature's Resource standardised to contain 0.8% valerenic acid /day) taken 30 minutes before bedtime for 2 weeks has no significant effect on sleep latency, sleep efficiency, wake after sleep onset or self-rated sleep quality (Taibi et al 2009). Interestingly, there was a significant increase (+17.7 ± 25.6 minutes, $P = 0.02$) in nocturnal wakefulness in the valerian group compared to placebo (+6.8 ± 26.4 minutes, NS) which the authors attributed to a paradoxical stimulating effect as cited in the traditional literature (Bone 2003). Side effects were minor and did not differ significantly between valerian and placebo. The study used results gathered over 9 nights in the laboratory using a self-reported morning sleep questionnaire and polysomnographic recordings and at home by daily self-reported sleep logs and actigraphy.

Comparisons with benzodiazepines

Three randomised studies have compared valerian monotherapy with benzodiazepine drugs. One double-blind trial found that subjects treated with either 600 mg valerian (ethanolic extract) or 10 mg oxazepam experienced significantly improved sleep, with no statistically significant differences detected between the treatments (Dorn 2000). Another study comparing the immediate sedative effects and residual effects of a valerian and hops preparation, a sole valerian preparation, flunitrazepam and placebo found that subjective perceptions of sleep quality were improved in all treatment groups; however, only flunitrazepam treatment impaired performance the morning after, as assessed both objectively and subjectively (Gerhard et al 1996). Furthermore, 50% of subjects receiving flunitrazepam reported mild side-effects compared with only 10% from the other groups.

A 2002 double-blind randomised trial compared the effects of valerian extract LI 156 (Sedonium)

600 mg/day to 10 mg oxazepam over 6 weeks in 202 patients with non-organic insomnia (Ziegler et al 2002). The multicentre trial took place at 24 study centres in Germany and found that valerian treatment was at least as efficacious as oxazepam, with both treatments improving sleep quality. Subjectively, 83% of patients receiving valerian rated it as 'very good' compared with 73% receiving oxazepam.

Children

The efficacy and tolerability of a valerian and lemon balm combination (Euvegal forte) was tested in a large, open, multicentre study of 918 children (aged under 12 years) with restlessness and nervous sleep disturbance (dyssomnia) (Muller & Klement 2006). Both investigators' and parents' ratings revealed a reduction in the severity of symptoms for most patients. The study reported that 81% of children with dyssomnia experienced an improvement and 70% of children with restlessness improved. Treatment was generally rated as good or very good and considered well tolerated. Each Euvegal forte tablet consisted of 160 mg valerian root dry extract (*Valeriana officinalis* L.) with a drug-extract ratio of 4–5 : 1 (extraction solvent ethanol 62% v/v) and 80 mg lemon balm leaf dry extract (*Melissa officinalis*) with a drug-extract ratio of 4–6 : 1 (extraction solvent ethanol 30% v/v). The standard dosage of Euvegal forte (4 tablets daily) was used by 75% of patients and chosen by the investigator.

Anxiety and psychological stress states

Less investigation has taken place to determine the role of valerian as a treatment for anxiety states.

A randomised study found that low-dose valerian (100 mg) reduced situational anxiety without causing sedation (Kohnen & Oswald 1988). Positive results were also obtained in a smaller open study of 24 patients suffering from stress-induced insomnia who found treatment (valerian 600 mg/day for 6 weeks) significantly reduced symptoms of stress and insomnia (Wheatley 2001). Another randomised trial compared the effects of a preparation of valepotriates (mean daily dose 81.3 mg) with diazepam (mean daily dose 6.5 mg) and placebo in 36 outpatients with GAD under double-blind conditions (Andreatini et al 2002). After 4 weeks' treatment, all groups had significant reductions in Hamilton anxiety (HAM-A) scale scores; however, only those receiving valepotriates or diazepam showed a significant reduction in the psychic factor of HAM-A.

Kava kava is a herbal medicine also used in the treatment of anxiety and found to be effective in clinical studies (Pittler & Ernst 2002). A study that compared the effects of kava kava to valerian and placebo in a standardised mental stress test found that both herbal treatments reduced systolic blood pressure, prevented a stress-induced rise in heart rate and decreased self-reported feelings of stress (Cropley et al 2002).

A 2006 Cochrane review concluded there is insufficient evidence to draw any conclusions about the efficacy or safety of valerian compared with placebo or diazepam for anxiety disorders (Miyasaka et al 2006). RCTs involving larger samples and comparing valerian with placebo or other interventions used to treat of anxiety disorders, such as antidepressants, are needed.

Obsessive-Compulsive Disorder (OCD)

High dose valerian treatment may have a role to play in OCD, according to a placebo-controlled RCT. Thirty-one adult outpatients who met the DSM-IV-TR criteria for OCD received valerian capsules (765 mg/day of concentrated dried valerian extract/day) or placebo for 8 weeks. Patients were assessed using the Yale-Brown Obsessive-Compulsive Scale (Y-BOCS) at weeks 2, 4, 6 and 8. Assessment at weeks 4, 6 and 8 found the treatment group displayed significantly lower scores compared to the placebo group ($P = 0.043$, $P = 0.07$, $P = 0.00$). In regards to frequency of side effects, no significant difference was found between the groups. However, there was a greater incidence of somnolence with valerian treatment compared to placebo ($P = 0.02$) (Pakseresht et al 2011).

Muscle spasm, cramping and dysmenorrhoea

Valerian preparations have long been used to treat a wide variety of gastrointestinal disorders associated with spasms such as diarrhoea, colic and irritable bowel syndrome. It has also been used to relieve cramping in dysmenorrhoea. Valerian is likely to exert some degree of antispasmodic activity based on its pharmacological actions.

Recently, a double-blind, randomised clinical trial involving 100 female students experiencing moderate to severe dysmenorrhoea found valerian treatment provided some significant benefits compared to placebo (Mirabi et al 2011). The study compared a valerian preparation (containing 255 mg of powdered valerian root per capsule) or placebo capsules which were taken 3 times daily for the first 3 days of each cycle and continued for two menstrual cycles. Pain severity was measured three times daily using a visual analogue scale (VAS) and a multidimensional verbal scoring system was used to assess the severity of associated symptoms (fatigue, lack of energy, nausea and vomiting, diarrhoea, headache, mood swings and syncope). Active treatment reduced pain severity from 7.45 out of 10 at baseline to 1.99 in the second cycle compared to the placebo group, where the change was from 7.06 to 4.41. The duration of pain in the intervention cycles was also shorter in the valerian group ($P = 0.01$). No statistically significant differences were seen in the severity of associated systemic symptoms, with the exception of syncope ($P = 0.006$).

OTHER USES

Fibromyalgia

One randomised study, which was investigator blinded, tested the effects of whirl baths with plain water or with water containing pine oil or valerian on pain, disturbed sleep and tender point count in 30 outpatients with generalised fibromyalgia. Valerian significantly improved wellbeing and sleep, together with decreasing tender point count, whereas baths with pine oil worsened pain and plain water baths reduced pain but had no effect on wellbeing and sleeplessness (Ammer & Melnizky 1999).

Benzodiazepine withdrawal

Although no clinical studies are available, the herb is also used in practice to reduce dependency on benzodiazepine drugs. Valerian is prescribed together with other herbal medicines and psychological counselling while the benzodiazepine dose is slowly reduced.

DOSAGE RANGE

- Infusion of dried root: 3–9 g/day.
- Liquid extract (1:2): 2–6 mL/day.
- Tincture (1:5): 5–15 mL/day.
- When used for insomnia, valerian should be taken approximately 1 hour prior to bedtime.

According to clinical studies

- Anxiety: 100 mg–600 mg/day of the dried root or valepotriates (mean daily dose 81.3 mg).
- Insomnia: doses above 600 mg/day of dried root taken 1 hour before bedtime. Ethanolic extract of valerian: 300–600 mg before bedtime. Aqueous preparations of valerian: 400 mg/night to 450 mg three times daily. Standardised extracts: 60–120 mg valepotriates or 450 mg of valerenic acid before bedtime.
- For benzodiazepine withdrawal: 100 mg valepotriates taken three times daily.
- Fibromyalgia: Bath — 20 mL liquid extract (ratio not specified) per 200 L of 36–37°C water, three times per week.

TOXICITY

A combined extract of *Valeriana officinalis, Passiflora incarnata* and *Crataegus oxyacantha* demonstrated no toxicity, genotoxicity or mutagenicity in rats, mice and dogs at high doses over 180 days (Tabach et al 2009). According to one case report, a dose of valerian taken at approximately 20-fold the recommended therapeutic dose appears to be benign (Willey et al 1995).

Hepatotoxicity

Two rare idiosyncratic reactions of valerian-associated hepatotoxicty have been reported. A 27-year-old woman displayed epigastric pain and fatigue for 2 weeks along with raised liver enzymes while taking a 300 mg capsule twice a day for the prior 3 months (Valerian Root, Mason Vitamins) (Cohen et al 2008). Another case report of hepatotoxicity in a 50-year-old woman was reported who had taken valerian tea for 3 weeks (5 cc extract of valerian root thrice weekly), along with consuming 10 tablets of vaimane (containing 125 mg dry valerian extract / tablet). The woman was asymptomatic, but routine blood tests revealed elevated liver enzymes and bilirubin along with inflammation on liver biopsy and a diagnosis of drug-induced hepatitis was made. Over 10 months her transaminase levels returned to normal. The patient did not undergo a rechallenge with valerian and the case report did not mention any preexisting health conditions, concomitant medications or state whether the valerian was tested to rule out adulteration, contamination or substitution (Vassiliadis et al 2009). It is not clear in either case whether the herbal treatment was tested for authenticity or contamination, making interpretation difficult.

ADVERSE REACTIONS

As with numerous pharmaceutical sedatives, next morning somnolence is a possible side-effect of therapy; however, evidence from two human studies suggests this is not associated with valerian use (Gerhard et al 1996, Kuhlmann et al 1999). Additionally, evidence from a pharmacokinetic study indicates this is highly unlikely.

Vivid dreams were reported in one study; however, this is considered rare by clinicians (Wheatley 2001).

Paradoxical stimulating effects have been observed in clinical practice and in one study of postmenopausal women; however, this also appears to be rare (Mills & Bone 2000).

Occasionally, headache and gastrointestinal symptoms have been reported (Ernst et al 2001).

Practice points/Patient counselling

- It appears scientific evidence supports the use of valerian as a treatment for insomnia; however, it appears that ongoing use may be more effective than single-dose use and effects on sleep progress over several weeks. It is often used together with other herbs for better effect, such as lemon balm and hops.
- It appears to be best suited to reducing sleep latency (i.e. time taken until falling asleep) and improves subjective assessments of sleep. Therefore valerian may be more effective for sleep onset insomnia than sleep maintenance insomnia.
- There is no evidence of next-day somnolence or significant adverse effects.
- Valerian may also relieve symptoms of stress and anxiety, with several studies observing effects similar to benzodiazepines; however, further research is required.
- Due to its pungent odour, solid-dose forms may be preferable.

SIGNIFICANT INTERACTIONS

Pharmaceutical sedatives / benzodiazepines

Theoretically, potentiation effects may occur at high doses; however, this has not been tested under clinical conditions — observe patients taking valerian concurrently with pharmaceutical sedatives. This interaction may be beneficial under professional supervision.

There is a case report of a 40-year-old male taking lorazepam (2 mg/24 hours) for 2 months without side effects and then self-medicating with valerian (*Valeriana officinalis*) and passionflower (*Passiflora incarnata*) infusion (dose unknown) for 2 nights. On the third night he took 3 tablets at 1-hour intervals before going to sleep (containing 300 mg of valerian and 380 mg of passionflower extract/tablet). This was repeated on the fourth night and strong handshaking, dizziness and palpitations were experienced, followed by a heavy drowsiness that made him fall asleep. These symptoms disappeared when the herbal treatment was discontinued. While this effect may be due to the herbal medicine increasing the inhibitory activity of benzodiazepines binding to the GABA receptors, until the preparation can be tested, causality remains unclear (Carrasco et al 2009).

Alcohol

RCTs have shown no potentiation effects with alcohol use (Ernst et al 2001).

Haloperidol

In a rat study, oxidative stress parameters in the liver were increased when haloperidol was taken in combination with valerian via a significant increase in lipid peroxidisation levels (enhanced oxidation of thiobarbituric acid reactive species and dichlorofluorescein reactive species, as well as an inhibition of hepatic d-ALA-D activity). The significance in humans is unknown — observe patients taking valerian concurrently with haloperidol (Dalla Corte et al 2008).

CONTRAINDICATIONS AND PRECAUTIONS

No known contraindications. Care should be taken when driving a car or operating heavy machinery when high doses are used.

PREGNANCY USE

No restrictions are known; however, safety has not been well established in pregnancy. No significant negative effects have been reported in toxicological tests with animals and none reported in clinical studies (Upton 1999). A combined extract of *Valeriana officinalis, Passiflora incarnata* and *Crataegus oxyacantha* in rats did not alter the oestrus cycle, did not affect fertility and did not induce teratogenesis in the offspring born from females treated during the entire pregnancy (Tabach et al 2009).

PATIENTS' FAQs

What will this herb do for me?

Valerian is classified as a mild, sedative herbal medicine. It can reduce the time it takes to fall asleep at night, improve the way people feel about their quality of sleep and may also relieve stress and anxiety during the day. When added to a bath, it may increase relaxation, wellbeing and reduce some forms of pain.

When will it start to work?

For some, valerian works within an hour of the first dose; however, research suggests it works best after several weeks of regular use for insomnia.

Are there any safety issues?

From the available evidence, next-day drowsiness is uncommon and physical addiction highly unlikely. Taking high doses during the day may increase drowsiness, so care is needed when driving a car or operating heavy machinery.

REFERENCES

Ammer K, Melnizky P. Medicinal baths for treatment of generalized fibromyalgia. Forsch Komplementarmed 6.2 (1999): 80–85.

Anderson G et al. Pharmacokinetics of valerenic acid after administration of valerian in healthy subjects. [abstract]. In: Pharmacokinetics of valerenic acid after administration of valerian in healthy subjects 19.9 (2005): 801–803.

Andreatini R et al. Effect of valepotriates (valerian extract) in generalized anxiety disorder: a randomized placebo-controlled pilot study. Phytother Res 16.7 (2002): 650–654.

Balderer G, Borbely AA. Effect of valerian on human sleep. Psychopharmacology (Berl) 87.4 (1985): 406–409.

Bone K. A clinical guide to blending liquid herbs: herbal formulations for the individual patient. St. Louis: Churchill Livingstone, 2003.

Carrasco MC et al. Interactions of Valeriana officinalis L. and Passiflora incarnata L. in a patient treated with lorazepam. Phytother Res 23.12 (2009):1795–1796.

Cohen DL, Del Toro Y. A case of valerian-associated hepatotoxicity. J Clin Gastroenterol 42.8 (2008): 961–962.

Cuellar NG, Ratcliffe SJ. Does valerian improve sleepiness and symptom severity in people with restless legs syndrome? Altern Ther Health Med. 15.2 (2009): 22–28.

Cropley M et al. Effect of kava and valerian on human physiological and psychological responses to mental stress assessed under laboratory conditions. Phytother Res 16.1 (2002): 23–27.

Del Valle-Mojica LM, Ortíz JG. Anxiolytic properties of Valeriana officinalis in the zebrafish: a possible role for metabotropic glutamate receptors. Planta Med 78.16(2012): 1719–1724.

Del Valle-Mojica LM et al. Selective Interactions of Valeriana officinalis Extracts and Valerenic Acid with [H] Glutamate Binding to Rat Synaptic Membranes. Evid Based Complement Alternat Med. (2011a): 403591.

Del Valle-Mojica LM et al. Aqueous and Ethanolic Valeriana officinalis Extracts Change the Binding of Ligands to Glutamate Receptors. Evid Based Complement Alternat Med. (2011b): 891819.

Dalla Corte CL et al. Potentially adverse interactions between haloperidol and valerian. Food Chem Toxicol 46.7 (2008): 2369–2375.

Della Loggia R et al. Evaluation of the activity on the mouse CNS of several plant extracts and a combination of them. Riv Neurol 51.5 (1981): 297–310.

Dimpfel W, Suter A. Sleep improving effects of a single dose administration of a valerian/hops fluid extract - a double blind, randomized, placebo-controlled sleep-EEG study in a parallel design using electrohypnograms. Eur J Med Res 13.5 (2008): 200–204.

Donath F et al. Critical evaluation of the effect of valerian extract on sleep structure and sleep quality. Pharmacopsychiatry 33.2 (2000): 47–53.

Donovan JL et al. Multiple night-time doses of valerian (Valeriana officinalis) had minimal effects on CYP3A4 activity and no effect on CYP2D6 activity in healthy volunteers. Drug Metab Dispos 32.12 (2004): 1333–1336.

Dorn M. Efficacy and tolerability of Baldrian versus oxazepam in non-organic and non-psychiatric insomniacs: a randomized, double-blind, clinical, comparative study. Forsch Komplementarmed Klass Naturheilkd 7.2 (2000): 79–84.

Ernst E et al. The desktop guide to complementary and alternative medicine: An evidence-based approach. St Louis: Mosby, 2001.

Estrada-Soto S et al. Vasorelaxant effect of Valeriana edulis ssp. procera (Valerianaceae) and its mode of action as calcium channel blocker. J Pharm Pharmacol 62.9 (2010):1167–1174.

Felgentreff F et al. Valerian extract characterized by high valerenic acid and low acetoxy valerenic acid contents demonstratesanxiolytic activity. Phytomedicine 19.13 (2012):1216–1222.

Fernández-San-Martín et al. Effectiveness of Valerian on insomnia: a meta-analysis of randomized placebo-controlled trials. Sleep Med 11.6 (2010): 505–511.
Gerhard U et al. Vigilance-decreasing effects of 2 plant-derived sedatives. Schweiz Rundsch Med Prax 85.15 (1996): 473–481.
Gessner B, Klasser M. Studies on the effect of Harmonicum Much on sleep using polygraphic EEG recordings. Z Elektroenzephalog Elektromyogr Verwandte Geb 15.1 (1984): 45–51.
Gurley BJ et al. In vivo effects of goldenseal, kava kava, black cohosh, and valerian on human cytochrome P450 1A2, 2D6, 2E1, 3A4/5 phenotypes. Clin Pharmacol Ther 77.5 (2005): 415–426.
Hattesohl M et al. Extracts of Valeriana officinalis L. s.l. show anxiolytic and antidepressant effects but neither sedative nor myorelaxant properties. Phytomedicine 15.1–2 (2008): 2–15.
Hazelhoff B, Malingre TM, Meijer DK. Antispasmodic effects of valeriana compounds: an in-vivo and in-vitro study on the guinea-pig ileum. Arch Int Pharmacodyn Ther 257.2 (1982): 274–287.
Koetter U et al. A randomized, double blind, placebo-controlled, prospective clinical study to demonstrate clinical efficacy of a fixed valerian hops extract combination (Ze 91019) in patients suffering from non-organic sleep disorder. Phytother Res 21.9 (2007): 847–851.
Kohnen R, Oswald WD. The effects of valerian, propranolol, and their combination on activation, performance, and mood of healthy volunteers under social stress conditions. Pharmacopsychiatry 21.6 (1988): 447–448.
Kuhlmann J et al. The influence of valerian treatment on reaction time, alertness and concentration in volunteers. Pharmacopsychiatry 32.6 (1999): 235–241.
Leathwood PD, Chauffard F. Aqueous extract of valerian reduces latency to fall asleep in man. Planta Med 2 (1985): 144–148.
Leuschner J et al. Characterisation of the central nervous depressant activity of a commercially available valerian root extract. Arzneimittelforschung 43.6 (1993): 638–641.
Lindahl O, Lindwall L. Double blind study of a valerian preparation. Pharmacol Biochem Behav 32.4 (1989): 1065–1066.
Mills S, Bone K. Principles and practice of phytotherapy. London: Churchill Livingstone, 2000.
Mirabi P et al. Effects of valerian on the severity and systemic manifestations of dysmenorrhea. Int J Gynaecol Obstet 115.3 (2011): 285–288.
Miyasaka LS et al. Valerian for anxiety disorders. Cochrane Database Syst Rev 4 (2006): CD004515.
Mohamed MF et al. Inhibitory effects of commonly used herbal extracts on UGT1A1 enzyme activity. Xenobiotica 40.10 (2010): 663–669.
Mohamed ME, Frye RF. Effects of herbal supplements on drug glucuronidation. Review of clinical, animal, and in vitro studies. Planta Med 77.4 (2011): 311–321.
Muller SF, Klement S. A combination of valerian and lemon balm is effective in the treatment of restlessness and dyssomnia in children. Phytomedicine 13.6 (2006): 383–387.
Neuhaus W et al. Transport of a GABAA receptor modulator and its derivatives from Valeriana officinalis L. s. l. across an in vitro cellculture model of the blood-brain barrier. Planta Med 74.11 (2008): 1338–1344.
Occhiuto F et al. Relaxing effects of Valeriana officinalis extracts on isolated human non-pregnant uterine muscle. J Pharm Pharmacol 61.2 (2009): 251–256.
Ortiz JG et al. Effects of Valeriana officinalis extracts on [3H]flunitrazepam binding, synaptosomal [3H]GABA uptake, and hippocampal [3H]GABA release. Neurochem Res 24.11 (1999): 1373–1378.
Pakseresht S et al. Extract of valerian root (Valeriana officinalis L.) vs. placebo in treatment of obsessive-compulsive disorder: a randomized double-blind study. J Complement Integr Med 8.1 (2011): Article 32.
Pittler MH, Ernst E. Kava extract for treating anxiety. Cochrane Database Syst Rev 2 (2002): CD003383.
Rezvani ME et al. Anticonvulsant effect of aqueous extract of Valeriana officinalis in amygdala-kindled rats: possible involvement of adenosine. J Ethnopharmacol 127.2 (2010): 313–318.
Santos MS et al. Synaptosomal GABA release as influenced by valerian root extract: involvement of the GABA carrier. Arch Int Pharmacodyn Ther 327.2 (1994): 220–231.
Schulz H et al. The effect of valerian extract on sleep polygraphy in poor sleepers: a pilot study. Pharmacopsychiatry 27.4 (1994): 147–151.
Schumacher B et al. Lignans isolated from valerian: identification and characterization of a new olivil derivative with partial agonistic activity at (A)1 adenosine receptors. J Nat Prod 65.10 (2002): 1479–1485.
Stevinson C, Ernst E. Valerian for insomnia: a systematic review of randomized clinical trials. Sleep Med 1.2 (2000): 91–99.
Taavoni S et al. Effect of valerian on sleep quality in postmenopausal women: a randomized placebo-controlled clinical trial. Menopause 18.9 (2011): 951–955.
Tabach R et al. Preclinical toxicological assessment of a phytotherapeutic product –CPV (based on dry extracts of *Crataegus oxyacantha L., Passiflora incarnata L.,* and *Valeriana officinalis L.*). Phytother Res 23.1 (2009): 33–40.
Taibi DM et al. A systematic review of valerian as a sleep aid: safe but not effective. Sleep Med Rev 11.3 (2007): 209–230.
Taibi DM et al. A randomized clinical trial of valerian fails to improve self-reported, polysomnographic, and actigraphic sleep in older women with insomnia. Sleep Med 10.3 (2009): 319–328.
Trauner G et al. Modulation of GABAA receptors by valerian extracts is related to the content of valerenic acid. Planta Med 74.1 (2008):19–24.
Upton R (eds). Valerian root, Santa Cruz: American Herbal Pharmacopoeia, 1999.
Vassiliadis T et al. Valeriana hepatotoxicity. Sleep Med 10.8 (2009): 935.
Wheatley D. Kava and valerian in the treatment of stress-induced insomnia. Phytother Res 15.6 (2001): 549–551.
Willey LB et al. Valerian overdose: a case report. Vet Hum Toxicol 37.4 (1995): 364–365.
Ziegler G et al. Efficacy and tolerability of valerian extract LI 156 compared with oxazepam in the treatment of non-organic insomnia: a randomized, double-blind, comparative clinical study. Eur J Med Res 7.11 (2002): 480–486.

Vitamin A

HISTORICAL NOTE In ancient Egypt and Greece, physicians recommended the liver of an ox to cure night blindness. Although this could be interpreted as applying the liver locally, it could also refer to ingesting some, which would have provided a good source of vitamin A and proven to be a cure for night blindness caused by deficiency (Shils et al 2006). Modern-day scientific research into vitamin A began in 1913, with its discovery at both Yale and Wisconsin Universities. Researchers at both sites independently noticed that the substance could promote survival and growth of young animals. Since then, each decade has brought important new discoveries about vitamin A. The period from the 1960s to the 1980s was particularly fruitful, as several proteins essential for transport and metabolism of vitamin A were isolated and purified. During the 1980s, another major discovery was made when a link between childhood mortality and subclinical deficiency was identified. Vitamin A research continues to interest a wide spectrum of researchers and influence public health initiatives.

BACKGROUND AND RELEVANT PHARMACOKINETICS

The term 'vitamin A' refers to a family of fat-soluble dietary compounds that are structurally related to retinol, and share its biological function. Vitamin A is found in foods as itself or as a precursor, which is converted into vitamin A in the body. The precursors, known as carotenes, are found in deep yellow, green and red-coloured plants.

Retinyl esters, retinol or carotenoids from the diet, or supplements, are hydrolysed in the small intestine where they are absorbed as retinol into the mucosal cells (Miller et al 1998). Entering the body within the lipid core of chylomicrons, they are transported through lymph to blood, where it then recycles between plasma and tissues numerous times, before arriving at the liver. The liver performs three key tasks in relation to vitamin A. It is responsible for regulating the secretion of retinol to specific transport proteins known as 'retinol-binding proteins', it serves as a major storage organ and is the major site of vitamin A catabolism. Vitamin A metabolites are excreted mainly through the faeces and urine.

The body has a good capacity for vitamin A storage; however, its ability to rapidly dispose of excess vitamin A is quite limited (Shils et al 2006), with the efficacy of beta-carotene conversion to retinol in humans found to decrease with increasing dietary dose (Novotny et al 2010). This may explain why vitamin A can accumulate to toxic levels when intake greatly exceeds requirements.

This monograph will focus on preformed vitamin A and retinoic acid only. Further information about the carotenoids can be found in other monographs.

FOOD SOURCES

Preformed vitamin A (retinyl esters) is chiefly found in foods of animal origin, such as liver, red meat and eggs, as well as in fish, milk, butter and cream. A number of studies have proposed use of beta-carotene-rich orange sweet potato to improve vitamin A status in deficient African countries (Hotz et al 2012a, 2012b).

Cooking can destroy up to 40% of the vitamin A content of food (Wahlqvist et al 1997).

DEFICIENCY SIGNS AND SYMPTOMS

- Night blindness, which can progress to complete blindness if left untreated
- Keratinisation of epithelial surfaces, causing them to dry and harden
- Poor dental health
- Compromised immune function
- Reduced reproductive capabilities.

Primary deficiency

Primary deficiency is caused by prolonged dietary deprivation. In large areas of the world, vitamin A deficiency is endemic, causing widespread blindness and mortality (Sklan 1987).

Secondary deficiency

Secondary deficiency can develop when absorption, storage or transport is reduced or carotene is not adequately converted to vitamin A. Conditions associated with risk of secondary deficiency include malabsorption syndromes, such as coeliac disease and cystic fibrosis (CF), pancreatic disease, duodenal bypass, congenital partial obstruction of the jejunum, obstruction of the bile ducts, giardiasis, diabetes and kwashiorkor.

MAIN ACTIONS

Vitamin A is an essential nutrient required for life and serves two very different biological functions. First, in the form of retinaldehyde, it constitutes the light-sensitive component of the retina, rhodopsin, and second, in the form of retinoic acid, it activates a large number of transcription factors (McCaffery & Drager 1993).

Antioxidant vs pro-oxidant activity

Vitamin A exhibits free radical scavenging properties and is generally considered an antioxidant molecule. Vitamin A bound to protein kinase C is an essential cofactor in redox activation of the mitochondrial signalling pathway (Acin-Perez et al 2010, Hoyos et al 2012).

Despite this, in vivo evidence has demonstrated that, at high doses, vitamin A elicits pro-oxidant effects, including increased superoxide production, mitochondrial redox dysfunction and increased oxidative and nitrosative stress in rat brains (Behr et al 2012, de Oliveria et al 2008, 2009, 2012). Pro-oxidant activity associated with vitamin A supplementation has been noted in several other rat models, including the neonatal lung (Pasquali et al 2010), kidney, liver and plasma (Schnorr et al 2011).

Growth and development

Vitamin A is essential for embryonic growth, with crucial roles in the induction of neurogenesis and control of neuronal patterning (Shearer et al 2012). Deficiency, as well as excess, has been shown to be teratogenic in animal studies, suggesting the same may be true in humans. It is currently unclear whether vitamin A itself or one of its metabolites or both are responsible for the teratogenic effects seen with high exposure (Miller et al 1998).

Vitamin A is also necessary for healthy bone formation and osteoblastogenesis. In vivo, vitamin A deficiency was associated with delayed bone healing in mice and the suppression of osteoblast differentiation-related genes (Tanaka et al 2010).

Immune function and maintenance of epithelial surfaces

Vitamin A maintains the health of epithelial cells in the body, which form an important barrier to infection, and the function of the immune system. Despite limited human studies, there is an increasing body of evidence from animal studies to suggest that adequate vitamin A status is an important factor for the maintenance of T-cell function and the prevention of prolonged inflammatory reactions (Ross 2012). Vitamin A stores in healthy men have been positively associated with several measures of innate immune activity, including natural killer (NK) and NK T cells and monocyte oxidative burst (Ahmed et al 2009).

A pilot study also found that vitamin A supplementation increased yellow fever virus (YFV)- and tetanus toxin-specific immune responses, including lymphocyte proliferation and production of YFV-specific interleukin-5 (IL-5), IL-10 and tumour necrosis factor-alpha (Ahmed et al 2008).

Comparably, studies in animal models and cell lines show that vitamin A and related retinoids play a major role in immunity, including expression of mucins and keratins, lymphopoiesis, production of antibodies, and the function of neutrophils, NK cells, macrophages, T lymphocytes and B lymphocytes (Liu et al 2014, Semba 1999).

In vivo, a vitamin A-deficient diet was shown to alter rat intestinal microflora, as well as alter mucin dynamics, downregulate defensin 6 expression and upregulate Toll-like receptor expression, ultimately interfering with the integrity of the gastrointestinal mucosal barrier (Amit-Romach et al 2009). It has also been shown to potentiate antibody responses and lymphocyte proliferation in response to antigens, reduce intestinal inflammation and restore the integrity and function of mucosal surfaces (Dong et al 2010, Semba 1994).

Vision

Vitamin A is involved in ocular health and function in two distinct ways. First, in the form of retinaldehyde, it is an essential component of rhodopsin and is necessary for maintaining vision (Wahlqvist et al 1997). Deficiency states initially cause a reversible night blindness that can progress to complete blindness due to photoreceptor degeneration (McCaffery & Drager 1993). Second, as retinoic acid, it maintains normal differentiation of cells in the conjunctiva, cornea and other ocular structures, with deficiency resulting in xerophthalmia (dry eye) and corneal ulceration. In xerophthalmia, the cells lining the cornea lose their ability to produce mucus, and therefore lubrication of the eye becomes compromised. Dirt particles that eventually enter the eye are more easily able to scratch the surface, increasing the risk of infection and, ultimately, blindness.

In vivo, retinyl palmitate eye drops (1500 IU/mL) in conjunction with antibiotics were shown to promote corneal healing through inhibition of vascular endothelial growth factor-A, matrix metalloproteinase-9 and transforming growth factor-β, as well as activation of thrombospondin 2, compared to antibiotics alone in rats subjected to corneal alkali burn injury (Kim et al 2012). A rat model of obesity-associated retinal degradation, dietary supplementation with oral vitamin A was found to modulate expression of retinal genes in obese rats, which corroborated with immunohistochemical and histological data showing improved retinal health compared to non-supplemented rats (Tiruvalluru et al 2013).

Chemoprevention

Studies in cell culture and animal models have documented the capacity for natural and synthetic retinoids to reduce carcinogenesis significantly in skin, breast, liver, colon, cervical, prostate and other sites (Ross 1999). The mechanism of action responsible has not been fully elucidated, but several theories exist. It has been known since early in the 20th century that vitamin A deficiency can induce metaplastic changes to epithelial cells (De Luca et al 1997). Retinoic acid is thought to act as an inhibitor of carcinogenesis by interfering with promotion rather than with initiation, which may be blocked by inhibition of proliferation, stimulation of differentiation or induction of apoptosis (Niles 2000). Other research suggests it may also inhibit the final stage when malignant conversion of a benign tumour to a carcinoma occurs (De Luca et al 1997).

Cognitive development and function

Pregnancy-related vitamin A deficiency in rats was found to affect postnatal expression of retinoic acid receptor-α and *N*-methyl-D-aspartate receptor unit 1 in the hippocampus (Zhang et al 2011). When subjected to water maze tests, pups from vitamin A-deficient dams had significantly reduced capacity for spatial learning, short-term memory, long-term memory and the ability to learn new things. A derivative of vitamin A has also been found to suppress hippocampal cellular proliferation, resulting in disturbed hippocampal-dependent learning in mice (Crandall et al 2004).

In vivo, vitamin A deficiency has been associated with circadian rhythm and circadian-dependent genes in a number of studies. In rats, vitamin A deficiency was shown to affect circadian expression in the hippocampus through the modification of rhythmic profiles of retinoic acid receptors (Navigatore-Fonzo et al 2013). Similarly, within the rat hippocampus, vitamin A deficiency was associated with modulation of the cognition-related genes, brain-derived neurotrophic factor and RC3, as well as affecting the circadian oscillation of a number of clock proteins (Golini et al 2012).

Conversely, a model of vitamin A supplementation at 9000 IU/kg over 28 days found increased α-synuclein content, impaired mitochondrial electron transport chain activity and increased superoxide production in both rat substantia nigra and striatum (de Oliveria et al 2009).

These studies implicate a role for vitamin A in modulation of central nervous system activity, including memory and learning, and warrant further investigation.

V

Promotion of aortic valve calcification

A recent study found that long-term dietary intake of vitamin A resulted in aortic valve stenosis and leaflet calcification in vivo (Huk et al 2013). This study suggests those patients on chronic vitamin A or vitamin A-derivative therapy, or who have dietary hypervitaminosis A, may be at increased risk of developing calcific aortic valve disease.

Alterations to spermatogenesis

A comprehensive in vivo study identified the effects of a chronic vitamin A-deficient diet on sperm health in mice (Boucheron-Houston et al 2013). This study identified that the earliest measurable effects were seen after 12 weeks, whereby expression of retinoic acid receptors and retinol-binding protein were reduced. Subsequent direct and indirect effects of vitamin A deficiency included the arrest of germ cell differentiation, increased germ cell apoptosis, altered spermatogonia transcriptome profile and disruption of somatic cell organisation.

CLINICAL USE

Deficiency: prevention and treatment

Traditionally, vitamin A supplementation has been used to treat deficiency or prevent deficiency in conditions associated with risk of vitamin A deficiency, such as diabetes, hyperthyroidism, protein deficiency, intestinal infections and infestations and CF.

Paediatrics

Reducing infection severity

Vitamin A deficiency impairs systemic immunity and increases the incidence and severity of infections during childhood, particularly measles and infectious diarrhoea (Chen et al 2013). There is also evidence to suggest that infectious diseases, such as measles, depress serum retinol concentrations, by >30% according to one study (Enwonwu & Phillips 2004). This phenomenon does not just occur in undernourished populations. A study of well-nourished children in the United States with measles identified that 50% had concurrent vitamin A deficiency (Arrieta et al 1992). A 2010 Cochrane review determined that vitamin A supplementation in infants reduced the incidence of diarrhoea (relative risk [RR] 0.85) and measles morbidity (RR 0.50); however there was no significant effect of vitamin A supplementation on cause-specific mortality of measles, respiratory disease or meningitis (Imdad et al 2010).

It is suspected that infectious diseases influence retinol metabolism through mechanisms that are more complex than simple loss of retinol stores (Enwonwu & Phillips 2004). Impaired synthesis of retinol-binding protein and transthyretin and decreased expression of the receptors for retinoic acid could also be responsible. As such, the use of vitamin A in the treatment of infectious disease is not limited to developing countries, but may also have application in well-nourished populations.

In areas where vitamin A deficiency may be present, the World Health Organization (WHO) recommends administration of an oral dose of 200,000 IU (or 100,000 IU in infants) of vitamin A per day for 2 days to children with measles (D'Souza & D'Souza 2002a, 2002b). It has also been recommended that prophylactic vitamin A supplements be given to all infants and young children (0–59 months), pregnant women and postpartum women, 6 weeks after delivery, in these same areas (Ross 2002). A randomised, triple-blinded controlled trial found that postpartum supplementation of breastfeeding mothers (n = 276) with 400,000 IU of vitamin A did not confer any additional benefits over use of 200,000 IU vitamin A on risk of child developing fever, diarrhoea, otitis, acute respiratory infections or the need for antibiotic treatment over a 6-month period (Fernandes et al 2012).

According to a 2005 Cochrane review, the WHO recommendation of two large doses of vitamin A does successfully lower the risk of death from measles in hospitalised children under the age of 2 years, but not in all children with measles (Huiming et al 2005).

Reducing secondary infections associated with measles

A meta-analysis of six clinical trials found a 47% reduction in the incidence of croup in children with measles who were treated with 200,000 IU of vitamin A on two consecutive days. One study in the analysis reported a 74% reduction in the incidence of otitis media, but this was not confirmed in others. A statistically significant decrease in the duration of diarrhoea, pneumonia, hospital stay and fever was also observed (D'Souza & D'Souza 2002a).

Reducing childhood mortality in neonates

It has been estimated that a 23–30% reduction in young child mortality is possible with improvements in vitamin A status. This is most marked for deaths due to acute gastroenteritis and measles, but not acute respiratory infections or malaria (Ramakrishnan & Martorell 1998), and is particularly the case for older preschool children, whereas the effect on infants is less clear.

In neonates, data from meta-analyses are conflicting in terms of the benefit or harm associated with vitamin A supplementation and risk of mortality. A 2011 Cochrane review determined that data from seven trials (51,446 neonates) suggested a potential benefit of supplementing neonates with vitamin A at birth in reducing mortality in the first half of infancy in developing countries (Haider et al 2011). However, due to wide confidence intervals, small number of studies and the existence of highly conflicting trial data, the authors have recommended cautious interpretation of the findings (Haider et al 2011). In contrast, a 2011 Cochrane review of 18 trials determined that there was no convincing evidence to suggest vitamin A supplementation within the first 6 months of infancy reduced infant morbidity or mortality in low and middle incomes (Gogia & Sachdev 2011). Discrepancies between these two analyses may be due to Haider and colleagues focusing on data only from developing countries.

When stratified by sex-specific effects, a 2010 meta-analysis found no overall benefit but had confidence intervals (Kirkwood et al 2010b). This is consistent with studies which have found trends for harm associated with vitamin A use both in girls only (Benn et al 2008, 2010) and in boys only (Malaba et al 2005). It has been suggested that inconsistencies observed may be a result of non-specific interactions with routine vaccinations, the administration of which generally coincides with vitamin A administration (Benn et al 2009a, 2009b).

Reducing childhood mortality in infants

In contrast to neonatal data, evidence for vitamin A supplementation in infants aged 6 months to 5 years is much stronger. A 2010 Cochrane review of 43 trials (n = 215,633) found a reduced risk of all-cause mortality for vitamin A compared with control (RR 0.76, 95% confidence interval [CI] 0.69–0.83). While the study concluded that further placebo-controlled trials were likely to be unnecessary, studies which compared different doses and delivery mechanisms for vitamin A were warranted (Imdad et al 2010).

In areas of endemic vitamin A deficiency, vitamin A supplementation was not found to lower the incidence of illness such as diarrhoea, dysentery or fever; however, it did reduce mortality, with fewer case fatalities in young children with these diseases compared to placebo (Tielsch et al 2007). In newborn infants supplemented with 50,000 IU of vitamin A, all-cause mortality at 6 months was reduced by 15% (Klemm et al 2008).

Reducing febrile neutropenia

In a cohort of 49 children with cancer, those with plasma retinol levels below 20 mcg/dL at diagnosis had a greater risk of developing episodes of febrile neutropenia compared to children with higher vitamin A status (Wessels et al 2008).

Very-low-birth-weight (VLBW) infants

Supplementing VLBW infants with intramuscularly administered vitamin A is associated with a reduction in death or oxygen requirement at 1 month of age (Darlow & Graham 2007).

Reducing renal scarring secondary to pyelonephritis

An open-label randomised controlled trial (n = 61) found that, in children aged 1 month to 10 years, the treatment of acute pyelonephritis with routine antibiotics and vitamin A supplements significantly reduced the worsening of lesions and development of renal scarring at 6-month follow-up (Sobouti et al 2013). Similarly, a single intramuscular injection of vitamin A (25,000 IU in infants <12 months; 50,000 IU in >12 months) in conjunction with routine antibiotics reduced renal scarring at 3-month follow-up compared to antibiotics alone in first-time cases of pyelonephritis (Ayazi et al 2011).

Reducing risk of bronchopulmonary dysplasia in premature newborns

Compared to receipt of inhaled nitric oxide alone, the combination of inhaled nitric oxide with vitamin A supplementation in premature newborns with respiratory failure reduced the incidence of bronchopulmonary dysplasia and death following bronchopulmonary dysplasia (Gadhia et al 2014). At 1-year follow-up, mental development in infants who had received nitric oxide and vitamin A was significantly improved compared to those who had received nitric oxide alone. No effect of vitamin A supplementation was seen in premature newborns who did not receive inhaled nitric oxide.

Reducing infection-associated hearing loss

While a cluster randomised, double-blinded, placebo-controlled trial found no difference in the prevalence of middle-ear infection in preschool children receiving vitamin A supplements vs placebo, a follow-up study found that children who had ear discharge in early childhood had a 42% reduced risk of hearing loss (odds ratio [OR] 0.58, 95% CI 0.37–0.92) (Schmitz et al 2012).

Reducing the risk of HIV transmission from mother to infant

The dominant mode of acquisition of HIV infection for children is mother-to-child transmission. Currently, this results in more than 2000 new paediatric HIV infections each day worldwide. A 2009 systematic review of randomised controlled trials (n = 7528 women) found that there was no evidence of an effect of either prenatal or postnatal vitamin A supplementation on the risk of mother-to-child transmission of HIV (RR 1.06, 95% CI 0.89–1.26) (Kongnyuy et al 2009). This is in agreement with a 2011 Cochrane review, which analysed results from five trials, which enrolled 7528 HIV-infected pregnant women, and found no evidence to support the use of vitamin A supplementation for this indication (Wiysonge et al 2011). One benefit that was identified for vitamin A supplementation was an improvement in infant birth weight. Neither maternal nor neonatal vitamin A supplementation significantly affected the overall mortality of children exposed to HIV by 2 years of age. Interestingly, in infants who were HIV-negative at baseline but positive by 6 weeks of age, supplementation reduced mortality by 28%, whereas in infants who did not become HIV-positive by 6 weeks, supplementation doubled the risk of mortality by age 2 years. It has been suggested that vitamin A supplementation may have increased viral load among babies who subsequently became infected during breastfeeding, but this remains untested (Humphrey et al 2006b).

Fetal growth

Low levels of vitamin A impair fetal growth. In a cross-sectional study on 100 neonate–mother pairs, lower placental and neonatal levels of vitamin A were associated with prematurity and intrauterine growth retardation (Agarwal et al 2008). However, supplementation with either vitamin A or β-carotene did not affect birth weight, infant length or head, arm and chest circumference compared to placebo in a trial of 13,709 Bangladeshi newborns (Christian et al 2013). Gestational age and preterm birth rate were also found to be unaffected by supplementation.

Congenital malformations

A case-control study determined that, in normal-weight mothers, intake of dietary vitamin A below the recommended levels during pregnancy was associated with a significantly increased risk of offspring having congenital diaphragmatic hernia (Beurskens et al 2013).

Despite this finding, due to limited sample size, study design and acknowledged teratogenicity of vitamin A, it is still recommended that women avoid supplementation unless on the advice of a medical professional.

Risk of schizophrenia in fetus

Data from the Prenatal Determinants of Schizophrenia study suggested that low maternal vitamin A levels during the second trimester of pregnancy were associated with threefold increased risk of schizophrenia spectrum disorders following adjustments for age and maternal education (OR 3.04, 95% CI 1.06–8.79). No association between schizophrenia spectrum disorders and maternal vitamin A status was observed in the third trimester (Bao et al 2012). The clinical relevance or causality of this association is unclear.

Cancer prevention

Most forms of cancer arise from cells that are influenced by vitamin A (Wardlaw et al 1997). Combined with its antioxidant and immunomodulatory activities, vitamin A has been considered as a potential chemopreventive agent. Research thus far using cell cultures and animal models has identified the ability for natural and synthetic retinoids to reduce carcinogenesis significantly in skin, breast, liver, colon, prostate and other sites (Krinsky 2002). A look at the literature shows that impressive treatment results have mainly been obtained for synthetic retinoids and the relationship between natural vitamin A ingestion and cancer is less clear in humans.

In a cohort study of 3254 Japanese subjects aged from 39 to 85 years, high serum levels of carotenoids were associated with reduced mortality rates of cancer of all sites or of cardiovascular disease, while high serum levels of beta-carotene, total carotene, provitamin A and total carotenoids reduced risk of colorectal cancer or stroke at follow-up after 11.7 years. Serum retinol and tocopherols, however, were not associated with a reduction in risk of mortality from cancer or cardiovascular disease (Ito et al 2006).

Prostate cancer

Despite numerous large-scale studies, there is conflicting evidence surrounding the role of vitamin A and its derivatives on prostate cancer risk, with support for positive, negative and null effects. Due to these inconsistencies, studies designed at clarifying the underlying biological mechanisms of the vitamin A-prostate cancer association are required. A Finnish randomised, double-blind, placebo-controlled trial investigating cancer incidence in adult male smokers (n = 29,133) found that, at baseline, subjects in the highest quintile of serum alpha-tocopherol had improved prostate cancer survival after 3 years (hazard ratio [HR] 0.26, 95% CI 0.09–0.71) (Watters et al 2009). No effects on survival were seen with baseline serum beta-carotene, baseline serum retinol or supplemental beta-carotene. Similarly, a nested case-control study within the Prostate, Lung, Colorectal, and Ovarian Cancer Screening Trial (692 prostate cancer cases, 844 controls) found that, although serum retinol concentrations were not associated with overall prostate cancer risk, the highest versus lowest concentrations of serum retinol were associated with a 42% reduction in risk of aggressive prostate cancer (P = 0.02) (Schenk et al 2009).

Conversely, a large prospective 3-year study in the Alpha-Tocopherol, Beta-Carotene Cancer Prevention Study cohort (n = 22,843) found that men with higher retinol concentrations at baseline were more likely to develop prostate cancer (HR 1.19, 95% CI 1.03–1.36) (Mondul et al 2011). In the Carotene and Retinol Efficacy Trial, which tested a daily dose of 30 mg beta-carotene and 25,000 IU retinyl palmitate in smokers, secondary outcomes analysis found that men in the intervention arm who used additional supplements also had an increased risk of aggressive prostate cancer (RR 1.52, 95% CI 1.03–2.24) (Neuhouser et al 2009).

It should be noted that several large studies nested within multicentre trials have also found no associations between the plasma concentrations of carotenoids, retinol or tocopherols and overall prostate cancer risk or more risk of more aggressive prostate cancer phenotypes (Beilby et al 2010, Gilbert et al 2012, Key et al 2007). A cohort study of 1985 men previously exposed to asbestos found that, while increasing the intake of vitamin C-rich vegetables such as peppers and broccoli was associated with reduced risk of prostate cancer, vitamin A intake (supplement of 7.5 mg retinol daily) did not lower risk (Ambrosini et al 2008).

Gastric cancer

In a large nested case–control study of patients with gastric cancer, a higher plasma concentration of beta-cryptoxanthin, zeaxanthin, retinol and alpha-tocopherol was associated with a significantly lower risk of developing gastric cancer (Jenab et al 2006). A high intake of vitamin A, alpha-carotene and beta-carotene was associated with a reduced risk of gastric cancer in a prospective cohort study of 82,002 Swedish adults. However, no protective effect was found from beta-cryptoxanthin, lutein and zeaxanthin or lycopene intake (Larsson et al 2007).

In contrast, studies in Japanese cohorts have yielded conflicting results. A prospective study of Japanese community-dwelling subjects (n = 2467) found that, over 14 years, increased dietary intake of vitamin A was associated with increased incidence of gastric cancer, irrespective of location or histological type of cancer (Miyazaki et al 2012). A larger study among 36,745 Japanese subjects (aged 40–69) with *Helicobacter pylori* infection did not find a statistically significant association between plasma levels of retinol or lutein/zeaxanthin, lycopene, alpha- or gamma-tocopherol and the risk of gastric cancer (Persson et al 2008). Due to the limited generalisability of these studies (small isolated population and disease-specific subjects respectively), the effects of vitamin A on gastric cancer in Japanese populations remain unclear.

Lung cancer

A number of epidemiological studies have identified an inverse association between risk of lung cancer and serum carotenoid levels, but intervention studies have produced conflicting results. In general, vitamin A is supplied together with carotenoids, making it difficult to determine the role of vitamin A as a stand-alone agent. (See Beta-carotene monograph for further discussion.) The pooled analysis of the primary data from eight prospective studies involving 430,281 subjects found those with the highest quintile of intake of vitamins A, C and E and folate from food only had a statistically significant 28% reduction in the risk of lung cancer compared to those in the lowest quintile. This protective effect was lost, however, after adjusting for multiple risk factors for lung cancer, including smoking habits (Cho et al 2006). In a case-controlled study involving 333 patients diagnosed with primary lung cancer, however, a significantly lower risk of lung cancer was associated with a higher intake of vitamin A, alpha-carotene and beta-carotene-rich food. Interestingly, no protective effect was observed for vitamin A consumed as supplements (Jin et al 2007). In patients exposed to blue asbestos, low plasma retinol levels were associated with increased risk of developing mesothelioma and lung cancer (Alfonso et al 2006). Patients with lung cancer have been found to have similar levels of retinol but lower levels of serum metabolites retinyl palmitate and retinoic acid levels compared to healthy controls, suggesting retinol metabolism may be impaired in these patients (Moulas et al 2006).

Cervical cancer

Meta-analysis of 15 trials (n = 12,136) determined that vitamin A intake was associated with a reduced cervical cancer risk (OR 0.59, 95% CI 0.49–0.72); however this analysis did not contain any randomised controlled trials or cohort studies; thus confirmation of this trend is still required using large high-quality trials (Zhang et al 2012).

A 2013 Cochrane review determined that retinoids are not effective in causing regression of severe cervical intraepithelial neoplasm (CIN3); however limited evidence suggests they may have some effect in moderate cervical intraepithelial neoplasm (CIN2) (Helm et al 2013). The review also stated that data for mild cervical intraepithelial neoplasm (CIN1) were currently inadequate to determine the effect of retinoids.

Other cancers

Vitamin A intake, including supplements and dietary sources, was inversely associated with risk of non-Hodgkin's lymphoma among 154,363 postmenopausal women in the Women's Health Initiative study (HR 0.83, 95% CI 0.69–0.99) (Kabat et al 2012).

A nested case-control study within the Multiethnic Cohort Study found that there was no significant association between plasma carotenoids, tocopherols or retinol in women with breast cancer compared to healthy controls (Epplein et al 2009). In a prospective cohort study involving 89,835 women aged between 40 and 59 years, dietary intake of carotenoids or vitamins A, C or E was not found to be associated with a reduced risk of ovarian cancer (Silvera et al 2006). While a prospective study of 88,759 women and 47,828 men found the intake of vitamins A and C from food was inversely associated with the risk of renal cell cancer in men, the total retinol intake from sources such as supplements, liver, vitamin A-fortified milk and cereals was not associated with a reduction in risk. The beneficial effects may possibly be due to other protective nutrients or chemicals in carotenoid-containing foods (Lee et al 2006).

Adjunct in chemotherapy

Vitamin A (350,000–500,000 IU/day) was randomly allocated to patients in a group of 100 with metastatic breast carcinoma treated by chemotherapy (Israel et al 1985). Patients supplemented with vitamin A showed a greater than twofold increase in the complete response compared to controls (38% vs 15%; $P < 0.02$). Among chemotherapy responders in both groups, the projected 43-month survival rate was 93% in vitamin A-supplemented responders vs 30% in non-supplemented responders ($P < 0.02$).

Infections

Urinary tract

A placebo-controlled, double-blinded study involving 24 patients found a single dose of 200,000 IU vitamin A in addition to antimicrobial therapy significantly reduced recurrent urinary tract infections. In the treatment group, the rate of infection reduced to 0.12 attacks/month in the first 6-month period, and 0.29 attacks/month in the second 6-month period, compared to 0.47 attacks/month and 0.44 attacks/month respectively in the control group (Yilmaz et al 2007).

Lower respiratory tract

A 2008 Cochrane systematic review of nine randomised controlled trials involving 33,179 children examined the effectiveness and safety of vitamin A in preventing acute lower respiratory tract infections (LRTIs) in children up to 7 years old. Six studies used megadose vitamin A (100,000–206,000 IU) (every 4 months for a year or as once off), while four studies used low-dose vitamin A (5000 IU daily, 10,000 IU weekly, 8333 IU weekly, and 20,000 IU or 45,000 IU every 2 months). Most studies did not find a beneficial effect on LRTI. While two studies found vitamin A supplementation prevented acute LRTIs in children with low serum retinol or those with a poor nutritional status, unexpectedly, three studies found vitamin A was associated with negative outcomes, including an increased incidence of acute LRTI, and increased symptoms of cough, fever and rapid breathing. The authors concluded that the effect of vitamin A was influenced by the child's nutritional status or weight, with supplementation increasing the acute LRTI episodes in 'normal' children (Chen et al 2008).

HIV

The Zimbabwe Vitamin A for Mothers and Babies (ZVITAMBO) project examined the effects of a vitamin A supplementation on serum retinol concentration, and mortality and morbidity among HIV-positive and HIV-negative postpartum women. A single 400,000 IU dose of vitamin A given during the immediate postpartum period had no effect on maternal mortality of both HIV-negative and -positive women after 2 years compared to placebo. Among HIV-positive women, the supplementation reduced clinic visits for treatment for malaria, cracked and bleeding nipples, pelvic inflammatory disease and vaginal infection, but did not lower overall rates of hospitalisation. While vitamin A deficiency was more common among HIV-positive women, serum levels of retinol were unresponsive to supplementation, except in those with a CD4 count of less than 200 cells × 10^6/L (Zvandasara et al 2006). In a subsample of HIV-negative women enrolled in ZVITAMBO trial, a single dose of 400,000 IU vitamin A within 96 hours postpartum did not reduce the incidence of HIV infection; however, HIV-negative women with low vitamin A levels (serum retinol < 0.7 micromol/L) were 10.4 times more likely to acquire HIV. In women with low vitamin A who received supplementation, there was a slightly (non-significantly) lower incidence of HIV (Humphrey et al 2006a).

Bacterial vaginosis

In a cluster-randomised, placebo-controlled trial, the weekly supplementation of vitamin A or β-carotene in women (n = 1812) from early-stage pregnancy reduced the prevalence and incidence of bacterial vaginosis during the third trimester and at 3 months postpartum compared to placebo (Christian et al 2013).

Hepatitis C virus

A recent study found a strong association between chronic hepatitis C virus infection and serum vitamin A deficiency ($P < 0.0001$). The presence of this deficiency in patients was found to be a strong predictor for non-response to interferon-based antiviral therapy, thus further study to determine whether increasing serum vitamin A levels can modulate responsiveness to therapy is warranted (Bitteto et al 2013).

Other infections

Children with acute upper respiratory tract infection and acute upper respiratory tract infection with wheezing were found to have lower serum retinol levels compared to healthy controls (Amaral et al 2013). Whether this association was a result of poorer health status overall or a result of vitamin A's effects on airway function is unclear.

A randomised placebo-controlled trial (n = 154) found that supplementation with a single 200,000 IU vitamin A dose plus 15 mg zinc/day for 8 weeks did not affect treatment outcomes, including smear time, culture conversion, weight gain or radiological resolutions, in patients with pulmonary tuberculosis (Visser et al 2011).

Vitamin A supplementation has also been associated with reduced incidence of *Giardia* spp. infections (Lima et al 2010).

> ***Clinical note — Retinitis pigmentosa***
> Retinitis pigmentosa describes a group of hereditary retinal dystrophies, characterised by the early onset of night blindness, followed by a progressive loss of the visual field. The underlying pathology is a defect that alters the function of the rod photoreceptor cell and subsequent degeneration of these cells (van Soest et al 1999).

Dermatology

Numerous clinical studies have shown beneficial effects of vitamin A or its derivatives on skin diseases such as acne, psoriasis, ichthyoses, keratodermas, skin cancers, lichen planus and ultraviolet-induced skin damage and photoageing (Futoryan & Gilchrest 1994). Currently, most research has been conducted with synthetic retinoid derivatives and is not representative of the effects of natural vitamin A. In a study of 100 newly diagnosed, untreated acne patients (mean age 21 years), plasma levels of both vitamin A and vitamin E were found to be significantly lower compared to age-matched healthy controls. An inverse relationship was also found between plasma vitamin A concentrations and the severity of the acne (El-Akawi et al 2006).

Topical vitamin A improves the appearance of older skin, and may also increase its resistance to injury and ability to heal. A 9-month, double-blind randomised placebo-controlled trial (n = 48) found that 0.1% retinol topical application once daily significantly improved wrinkles under the eyes, fine lines and skin tone evenness compared to an equivalent application containing no retinol in Caucasian women aged 41–60 (Bellemère et al 2009). This study determined that the 0.1% retinol product promoted keratinocyte proliferation ex vivo and in vivo, and induced epidermal thickening ex vivo. Similarly, a lotion containing 0.4% retinol was tested in a 6-month randomised controlled trial involving 36 elderly subjects aged between 80 and 96 years. The lotion was applied three times a week to left or right upper arm, with a lotion without retinol used on the other arm. The retinol-treated skin had fewer fine wrinkles and reduced roughness compared to the skin treated with the non-retinol lotion. The effects are due to an increase in glycosaminoglycan, which helps the skin retain water, and increased collagen production (Kafi et al 2007).

Ophthalmological diseases

Retinitis pigmentosa

A 2013 Cochrane review of three trials (n = 866) determined that currently there is no clear evidence for the benefit of using vitamin A with or without fish oils for treatment of retinitis pigmentosa (Rayapudi et al 2013). Due to limited trials included and inadequate power to detect clinically relevant changes, it was recommended in this review that future studies look to address these shortcomings.

It is thought that vitamin A transport or the retention capacity of the retina is abnormal in retinitis pigmentosa, or defects in the pigment epithelium involving vitamin-associated proteins occurs (Sharma & Ehinger 1999).

Xerophthalmia

Xerophthalmia is responsible for at least half of all cases of measles-associated blindness and is the cause of at least half a million cases of paediatric blindness worldwide (Sommer 1998). This condition is associated with vitamin A deficiency and protein malnutrition.

Dry-eye syndrome

An open-label randomised controlled trial (n = 300 eyes) found that retinyl palmitate (0.05%, four times per day) significantly improved blurred vision, tear film break-up time and impression cytological findings after 3 months compared to an 'artificial tears' control (0.5% carboxymethylcellulose, four times per day) in the treatment of refractory dry-eye syndrome (Kim et al 2009).

Retinopathy of prematurity

A double-blind, randomised controlled trial (n = 89) found that vitamin A supplementation (10,000 IU for three times a week for 6–12 doses) in infants born at less than 32 weeks' gestation did not affect plasma retinol between groups, but did increase retinal sensitivity by 36 weeks' postmenstrual age (Mactier et al 2012).

Reducing morbidity and mortality of pregnant women

It has been suggested that vitamin A supplements in pregnancy may improve outcomes, including maternal mortality and morbidity. Studies to date are conflicting. While some large-scale analyses have determined no benefit in the reduction of morbidity and mortality (Hurt et al 2013, West et al 2011), others suggest that vitamin A has benefit in specific populations which have high prevalence of gestational night blindness and very high risk of maternal mortality (Kirkwood et al 2010a, West et al 1999, 2010).

A 2010 Cochrane review of 16 trials found that vitamin A supplementation does not affect the risk of maternal mortality (RR 0.78, 95% CI 0.55–1.10) or perinatal mortality (van den Broek et al 2010). It was also determined that vitamin A had no effect on a number of neonatal outcomes, including neonatal mortality, stillbirth, neonatal anaemia, preterm birth or the risk of having a low-birth-weight baby. One trial from Nepal found that vitamin A supplementation reduced the risk of maternal night blindness (RR 0.70, 95% CI 0.60–0.82). Benefits to anaemia were also found in vitamin A-deficient populations and in women with HIV.

On the whole, current evidence does not support use of vitamin A supplementation during 'normal' pregnancy. Further clarification of the specific subset populations who would benefit from supplementation is recommended.

Vitamin A during or after pregnancy has not been found to reduce postpartum mortality in HIV-positive women. (See discussion under Infections: HIV, above.)

Leucoplakia

A Cochrane review of treatments for the prevention of malignant transformation of leucoplakia identified five randomised controlled trial involving 245 patients which tested vitamin A and retinoids (used topically or as oral treatment), and one study each for beta-carotene and lycopene. While these studies failed to demonstrate prevention of malignant transformation of leucoplakia, they were associated with a small but significant rate of clinical resolution when compared with placebo or absence of treatment. Retinoic acid and lycopene may also result in histological improvement, though results were based on only a small number of patients. Adverse effects were reported in studies using 13-*cis*-retinoic acid (1–2 mg/kg/day), and high-dose vitamin A (300,000 IU per week) (Lodi et al 2006).

Asthma

A study evaluated serum vitamin A concentrations in 26 well-nourished Japanese children with asthma (mean age of 5.5 years) with C-reactive protein concentration <0.6 mg/dL, to exclude the acute-phase response. Mean serum vitamin A concentrations were significantly lower in asthmatic children compared to controls, and there was also a significant correlation between C-reactive protein and serum vitamin A concentrations in children with asthma (Mizuno et al 2006). This observation was also reported in a case–control study involving 96 subjects which found low serum levels of vitamin A (and lycopene) were associated with an increased risk of bronchial asthma (Riccioni et al 2007).

Based on in vivo work, it has been suggested that vitamin A deficiency during pregnancy at a critical point in fetal development can result in chronic airway hyperresponsiveness (Chen et al 2014). This study identified that retinoic acid plays a crucial role in restricting airway smooth-muscle differentiation during murine lung development, with disruption of this process via vitamin A deficiencies resulting in altered airways expression of smooth-muscle markers that persisted postnatally. Vitamin A has also been shown to modify collagen IV and laminin chain composition in weanling rat pup airways following deficiency, which is only partly reversible with retinoic acid supplementation (Esteban-Pretel et al 2013).

Lung function in cystic fibrosis

Patients with CF may have impaired absorption of fat-soluble vitamins such as vitamin A. Some studies indicate vitamin A status is associated with respiratory health in patients with CF. Whether supplemental vitamin A has any benefits in CF is still speculative. A Cochrane systematic review did not find any eligible randomised or quasi-randomised controlled trials, and could not provide any firm conclusions on the effects (beneficial or harmful) of supplementation with vitamin A (O'Neil et al 2008). Previously, a small study involving 38 patients with stable CF (mean age of 15.3 years) found a significant correlation between serum vitamin A concentrations and lung function measurements, including forced expiratory volume in 1 second, forced vital capacity and peak expiratory flow (Aird et al 2006). Similarly, a retrospective study found CF patients with reduced vitamin A and E levels (even within the normal range) had increased incidence of pulmonary exacerbations (evaluated by a scale of clinical status, including symptoms and chest examination findings) (Hakim et al 2007). It is possible the antioxidant activity of vitamin A reduces oxidative damage to lung tissues and in this way provides some protection in CF. While patients with CF and pancreatic insufficiency are at increased risk of deficiency of fat-soluble vitamins, including vitamin A, two studies examining vitamin A status in CF patients found CF patients had higher intake and serum retinol levels compared to those without CF (Graham-Maar et al 2006, Maqbool et al 2008). Monitoring may be required to prevent excessive vitamin A supplementation.

Osteoporosis

Whether high-dose vitamin A supplementation increases the risk of osteoporosis remains unclear.

Evidence supporting the association comes from cell studies, animal studies and some, but not all, human observational studies. Four large, prospective observational studies reported a positive association between vitamin A intake and osteoporosis and fracture rates (Feskanich et al 2002, Melhus et al 1998, Michaelsson et al 2003, Promislow et al 2002). These studies suggested that the amount needed to reduce bone density may be as low as 1500 retinol equivalents (RE), although vitamin A is normally regarded as safe in amounts up to 3000 RE (Penniston & Tanumihardjo 2006). In contrast, numerous studies have failed to find a significant association (Ambrosini et al 2013, Barker et al 2005, Houtkooper et al 1995, Kaptoge et al 2003, Kawahara et al 2002, Rejnmark et al 2004, Sowers & Wallace 1990, Wolf et al 2005). In a study comparing vitamin A intake, serum vitamin A and bone turnover markers in postmenopausal women, no statistical differences were found between those with osteoporosis compared with those without (Penniston et al 2006). The inconsistency in results may be partly due to the difficulty in accurately assessing vitamin A intake and status, as well as the multiple variables influencing bone health (Ribaya-Mercado & Blumberg 2007).

Anaemia

Vitamin A and iron are interdependent nutrients, with iron required for the metabolism of vitamin A and maintenance of circulating levels of retinol, and vitamin A required for the mobilisation of iron from its stores for use in haemoglobin synthesis. Some studies have found improving vitamin A status in deficient individuals improves anaemia (Al-Mekhlafi et al 2013, Berger et al 2007, Hyder et al 2007, Zimmermann et al 2006). This is thought to be due to the involvement of vitamin A in regulation of iron regulator proteins, and the subsequent expression of iron metabolism genes (Jiang et al 2012). In a double-blind, randomised trial, 81 children (77% with low vitamin A status) received either vitamin A (200,000 IU) or placebo at baseline and again after 5 months. After 10 months, compared to the placebo group, the vitamin A-treated group had increased levels of retinol, increased haemoglobin and mean corpuscular volume and decreased the serum transferrin receptors, indicating improved iron-deficient erythropoiesis. Prevalence of anaemia in the treated group decreased from 54% to 38%. Ferritin levels in the vitamin A group were also decreased, suggesting vitamin A increased mobilisation of hepatic iron stores (Zimmermann et al 2006). In a study comparing the impact of vitamin A on the health of children aged 12–59 months in rural Indonesia, it was found that those who had not received their vitamin A treatment in the previous 6 months were significantly more likely to be anaemic, underweight, wasted and have higher rates of diarrhoea and fever than children who received vitamin A (Berger et al 2007).

Alternatively, some studies found no association between iron deficiency and vitamin A. In a randomised controlled trial in central Africa, 700 pregnant women (2–24 weeks' gestation) with haemoglobin <11.0 g/dL were treated with either vitamin A (5000 IU or 10,000 IU) or placebo, plus iron (60 mg elemental iron as ferrous sulfate), folate (0.25 mg) and sulfadoxine/pyrimethamine for antimalarial prophylaxis until delivery. While women in the vitamin A-treated groups were less likely to have depleted vitamin stores at the end of the pregnancy, there were no significant differences in anaemia, severe anaemia and iron status compared with the placebo group. This population was thought to be less vitamin A-deficient compared with Asian countries such as Indonesia and Nepal, where positive results have previously been found (van den Broek et al 2006). Similarly, a randomised, placebo-controlled trial conducted with mothers and their infants in Zimbabwe observed no effect on haemoglobin or anaemia levels evaluated 8–14 months after supplementation (400,000 IU for mothers and 50,000 IU for infants) (Miller et al 2006). In a double-blind trial involving HIV-1-infected pregnant women from Tanzania, subjects were randomised to receive daily supplements of 30 mg beta-carotene + 5000 IU preformed vitamin A only, multivitamins (vitamins B, C and E), preformed vitamin A and beta-carotene plus multivitamins, or placebo. All women also received iron and folate supplements during pregnancy. While haemoglobin concentrations significantly improved in women in the multivitamin group and their children, those in the beta-carotene and vitamin A-only group did not significantly differ from placebo (Fawzi et al 2007).

In children with sickle cell anaemia, 12-month supplementation of vitamin A with the recommended doses for healthy children, based on age and sex, did not improve serum retinol concentration (Dougherty et al 2012). This suggests that higher doses may be required in this population, although more research is required.

Mortality risk

In a Cochrane systematic review, the effect of antioxidant supplements on mortality in primary or secondary prevention randomised clinical trials was evaluated; vitamin A used as sole treatment or in combination with other antioxidants (15 trials, mean dose of 20,219 IU) had no significant effect on mortality. In fact, after excluding the high-bias risk, trials analysis found vitamin A significantly increased mortality in five trials (Bjelakovic et al 2008). This finding requires further investigation to confidently rule out the possible effect of confounders.

Deficiency as a predictor for coronary events

The PRIME study prospectively evaluated European men aged 50–59 (n = 9758) who were free from coronary heart disease at baseline over 5 years

> ***Clinical note — Vitamin A toxicity in two young children***
>
> In 2001, a report of two children admitted to hospital with symptoms of vitamin A toxicity was published in the *Medical Journal of Australia*. One case involved a 2-year-old girl with anorexia, lethargy and leg pain, an erythematous rash over her back and elbows and irritability. All symptoms resolved over 2 weeks following withdrawal of the supplement. The second case involved a child who had previously been prescribed oral etretinate by a dermatologist (for an unspecified period of time), which was ceased 3 months prior to vitamin A supplementation. In both cases, the dose of vitamin A taken was in excess of that provided by standard over-the-counter products (Coghlan & Cranswick 2001).

(Gey et al 2010). The study found that plasma retinol levels below 601 mcg/L in a fifth of men placed them at a threefold relative risk of developing coronary heart disease. Due to the limited number of control subjects, confirmation of these findings in a larger population is warranted.

OTHER USES

Vitamin A has also been used in the treatment of menorrhagia and premenstrual syndrome, to prevent glaucoma and cataract, and in Crohn's disease, sinusitis and rhinitis.

DOSAGE RANGE

- Vitamin A activity is expressed as a unit called microgram RE (Miller et al 1998): 1 microgram RE = 1 mcg all-*trans* retinol or 6 mcg all-*trans* beta-carotene or 3.33 international units (IU) of vitamin A or 1 mcg RE is equivalent in activity to 1.78 mcg of retinyl palmitate and 10 IU activity from beta-carotene.

Recent changes to the Therapeutic Goods Act regarding vitamin A require the following statement be included on the labels of vitamin A preparations for internal use:

> The recommended adult daily intake of vitamin A from all sources is 700 microgram RE (2330 IU) for women, and 900 microgram RE (3000 IU) for men.
>
> WARNING — when taken in excess of 3000 microgram RE daily, vitamin A may cause birth defects.
>
> If you are pregnant, or considering becoming pregnant, do not take vitamin A supplements without consulting your doctor or pharmacist.

Australian recommended daily intake (in mcg RE)

Children

- 1–3 years: 300 mcg/day
- 4–8 years: 400 mcg/day

V

- 9–13 years: 600 mcg/day
- Girls, 14–18 years: 700 mcg/day
- Boys, 14–18 years: 900 mcg/day.

Adults

- Females: 700 mcg/day
- Males: 900 mcg/day
- Upper level of intake: 3000 mcg/day.

Pregnancy

- <18 years: 700 mcg/day
- >18 years: 800 mcg/day
- Lactation: 1100 mcg/day
- Deficiency without corneal changes: 10,000–15,000 IU/day for 1–2 weeks, until clinical improvement is apparent
- General treatment doses: 10,000–50,000 IU/day have been used short term.

According to clinical studies

- Reducing secondary infection in children with measles: 200,000 IU of vitamin A on two consecutive days when vitamin A deficiency may be present (not to be consumed at this dose long-term)
- Retinitis pigmentosa: 15,000 IU/day.

TOXICITY

Cumulative toxicity is possible when doses greater than 100,000 IU are ingested long-term. Acute toxicity is very difficult to induce in adults, as doses above 2,000,000 IU are required (Hendler & Rorvik 2001).

Early signs of toxicity include dry rough skin, cracked lips, coarse hair, sparse hair, alopecia of eyebrows, diplopia, dryness of the mucous membranes, desquamation, bone and joint pain, fatigue and malaise, nausea and vomiting and psychological changes mimicking depression and schizophrenia.

Later signs include irritability, increased intracranial pressure and headache, dizziness, liver cirrhosis, fibrosis, vomiting, haemorrhage and coma (Miller et al 1998).

People with chronic renal disease typically have elevated plasma retinol levels and therefore may be at greater risk of toxicity if supplementation is used. It is important to note that beta-carotene is not associated with teratogenic effects or vitamin A toxicity and is considered a far safer nutrient.

ADVERSE REACTIONS

In general, doses of vitamin A that do not exceed physiological requirements have no adverse effects. A Cochrane review determined that there was an increased risk of vomiting within the first 48 hours following vitamin A supplementation (Imdad et al 2010).

SIGNIFICANT INTERACTIONS

Chemotherapeutic agents

Adjunctive treatment may improve drug response — consider individual patient characteristics, form and presentation of cancer, drugs used before administration — use only under professional supervision.

Cholestyramine

Reduces vitamin A absorption — increase dietary intake of vitamin A-rich foods or consider supplementation with long-term use.

Colchicine

Colchicine may interfere with vitamin A absorption and homeostasis — co-administer for beneficial interaction.

HMG-CoA reductase inhibitor drugs (statins)

These drugs increase the serum levels of vitamin A, the clinical significance of which is unclear — observe patients taking this combination (Muggeo et al 1995).

Isotretinoin

Toxicity may be increased — avoid this combination.

Minocycline

Long-term vitamin A use with this drug increases the risk of pseudotumour cerebri — use with caution.

Oral contraceptives

Increased vitamin A levels occur in oral contraceptive pill users due to longer storage in the liver

Practice points/Patient counselling

- Vitamin A is a fat-soluble antioxidant that is chiefly stored in the liver.
- It is involved in maintaining vision and healthy immune function; it is necessary for growth and development, reproductive capability and healthy epithelial cell function.
- It is used to treat and prevent deficiency states, and there is clinical evidence that supplementation reduces the incidence and severity of infections during childhood, particularly measles and infectious diarrhoea, reduces the incidence of croup and otitis media in children with measles, and may be useful in retinitis pigmentosa.
- Vitamin A deficiency is widespread in some countries, increasing the risk of childhood infectious disease, mortality and deficiency-associated blindness.
- While primary vitamin A deficiency is less common in Western countries, there are a number of drugs and surgical procedures, including bariatric surgery, which can result in secondary deficiency occurring.
- Excessive vitamin A supplementation can induce a toxicity state that can have serious, sometimes irreversible, consequences.

(Tyrer 1984) — use caution with large doses of retinol.

Orlistat

Reduces vitamin A levels — increase dietary intake of vitamin A-rich foods or consider supplementation with long-term use.

Tetracyclines

Adjunctive use may increase side effects such as headaches, pseudotumour cerebri — avoid.

CONTRAINDICATIONS AND PRECAUTIONS

Doses greater than 10,000 IU/day long-term should be used with caution.

People with liver or renal disease, alcoholism or severe osteoporosis should use vitamin A supplements with caution.

PREGNANCY USE

In the United States, sources state that doses up to 10,000 IU/day are safe in pregnancy, but Australian authorities recommend that supplements containing ≥2500 IU of vitamin A per dose must have pregnancy warning statements on their labels. Excessive use of vitamin A during pregnancy has been associated with heart defects in vivo (Feng et al 2013).

It is important to note that beta-carotene, found naturally in plants, is not associated with teratogenic effects or vitamin A toxicity.

The teratogenicity of 13-*cis*-retinoic acid, a synthetic derivative of vitamin A available in Australia as Roaccutane, is well established and that substance is contraindicated in pregnancy.

PATIENTS' FAQs

What will this vitamin do for me?

Vitamin A is essential for health and is involved in many different biochemical processes in the body. Some research has suggested that it reduces the incidence and severity of some infectious diseases in children. Vitamin A or its synthetic derivatives have also been used in many skin conditions, such as acne, psoriasis, ultraviolet-induced skin damage and photoageing and the treatment of some cancers.

When will it start to work?

This will depend on the form of vitamin A being used and the indication it is being used to treat.

Are there any safety issues?

Taking high doses of vitamin A long-term can cause side effects and is contraindicated in pregnancy.

REFERENCES

Acin-Perez R et al. Control of oxidative phosphorylation by vitamin A illuminates a fundamental role in mitochondrial energy homoeostasis. FASEB J 24.2 (2010): 627–636.

Agarwal K et al. Factors affecting serum vitamin A levels in matched maternal-cord pairs. Indian J Pediatr 75.5 (2008): 443–446.

Ahmed SM et al. Men with low vitamin A stores respond adequately to primary yellow fever and secondary tetanus toxoid vaccination. J Nutr 138.11 (2008): 2276–2283.

Ahmed SM et al. Markers of innate immune function are associated with vitamin A stores in men. J Nutr 139.2 (2009): 377–385.

Aird FK et al. Vitamin A and lung function in CF. J Cyst Fibros 5.2 (2006): 129–131.

Alfonso HS et al. Plasma vitamin concentrations and incidence of mesothelioma and lung cancer in individuals exposed to crocidolite at Wittenoom, Western Australia. Eur J Cancer Prev 15.4 (2006): 290–294.

Al-Mekhlafi HM et al. Effects of vitamin a supplementation on iron status indices and iron deficiency anaemia: a randomized controlled trial. Nutrients 6.1 (2013): 190–206.

Amaral CT et al. Vitamin A deficiency alters airway resistance in children with acute upper respiratory infection. Pediatr Pulmonol 48.5 (2013): 481–489.

Ambrosini GL et al. Fruit, vegetable, vitamin A intakes, and prostate cancer risk. Prostate Cancer Prostatic Dis 11.1 (2008): 61–66.

Ambrosini GL et al. No dose-dependent increase in fracture risk after long-term exposure to high doses of retinol or beta-carotene. Osteoporos Int 24.4 (2013): 1285–1293.

Amit-Romach E et al. Bacterial population and innate immunity-related genes in rat gastrointestinal tract are altered by vitamin A-deficient diet. J Nutr Biochem 20.1 (2009): 70–77.

Arrieta AC et al. Vitamin A levels in children with measles in Long Beach, California. J Pediatr 121.1 (1992): 75–78.

Ayazi P et al. The effect of vitamin A on renal damage following acute pyelonephritis in children. Eur J Pediatr 170.3 (2011): 347–350.

Bao YY et al. Low maternal retinol as a risk factor for schizophrenia in adult offspring. Schizophr Res 137.1–3 (2012): 159–165.

Barker ME et al. Serum retinoids and beta-carotene as predictors of hip and other fractures in elderly women. J Bone Miner Res 20.6 (2005): 913–920.

Behr GA et al. Increased cerebral oxidative damage and decreased antioxidant defenses in ovariectomized and sham-operated rats supplemented with vitamin A. Cell Biol Toxicol 28.5 (2012):317–330.

Beilby J et al. Serum levels of folate, lycopene, β-carotene, retinol and vitamin E and prostate cancer risk. Eur J Clin Nutr 64.10 (2010): 1235–1238.

Bellemère G et al. Antiaging action of retinol: from molecular to clinical. Skin Pharmacol Physiol 22.4 (2009): 200–209.

Benn CS et al. Effect of 50,000 IU vitamin A given with BCG vaccine on mortality in infants in Guinea-Bissau: randomised placebo controlled trial. BMJ 336.7658 (2008):1416–1420.

Benn CS et al. Does vitamin A supplementation interact with routine vaccinations? An analysis of the Ghana Vitamin A Supplementation Trial. Am J Clin Nutr 90.3 (2009a): 629–639.

Benn CS et al. The effect of high-dose vitamin A supplementation administered with BCG vaccine at birth may be modified by subsequent DTP vaccination. Vaccine 27.11 (2009b): 2891–2898.

Benn CS et al. Vitamin A supplementation and BCG vaccination at birth in low birthweight neonates: two by two factorial randomised controlled trial. BMJ 340 (2010): c1101.

Berger S et al. Malnutrition and morbidity are higher in children who are missed by periodic vitamin A capsule distribution for child survival in rural Indonesia. J Nutr 137.5 (2007): 1328–1333.

Beurskens LWJE et al. Dietary vitamin A intake below the recommended daily intake during pregnancy and the risk of congenital diaphragmatic hernia in the offspring. Birth Defects Res A Clin Mol Teratol 97.1 (2013): 60–66.

Bitteto D et al. Vitamin A deficiency is associated with hepatitis C virus chronic infection and with unresponsiveness to interferon-based antiviral therapy. Hepatology 57.3 (2013): 925–933.

Bjelakovic G et al. Antioxidant supplements for prevention of mortality in healthy participants and patients with various diseases. Cochrane Database Syst Rev 2 (2008): CD007176.

Boucheron-Houston C et al Long-term vitamin A deficiency induces alteration of adult mouse spermatogenesis and spermatogonial differentiation: direct effect on spermatogonial gene expression and indirect effects via somatic cells. J Nutr Biochem 24.6 (2013): 1123–1135.

Chen H et al. Vitamin A for preventing acute lower respiratory tract infections in children up to seven years of age. Cochrane Database Syst Rev 1 (2008): CD006090.

Chen K et al. Effect of simultaneous supplementation of vitamin A and iron on diarrheal and respiratory tract infection in preschool children in Chengdu City, China. Nutrition 29.10 (2013):1197–1203.

Chen F et al. Prenatal retinoid deficiency leads to airway hyperresponsiveness in adult mice. J Clin Invest 124.2 (2014): 801–811.

Cho E et al. Intakes of vitamins A, C and E and folate and multivitamins and lung cancer: a pooled analysis of 8 prospective studies. Int J Cancer 118.4 (2006): 970–978.

Christian P et al. Effects of vitamin A and β-carotene supplementation on birth size and length of gestation in rural Bangladesh: a cluster-randomized trial. Am J Clin Nutr 97.1 (2013): 188–194.

Coghlan D, Cranswick NE. Complementary medicine and vitamin A toxicity in children. Med J Aust 175.4 (2001): 223–224.

Crandall J et al. 13-*cis*-retinoic acid suppresses hippocampal cell division and hippocampal dependent learning in mice. Proc Natl Acad Sci U S A 101.14 (2004): 5111–5116.

Darlow BA, Graham PJ. Vitamin A supplementation to prevent mortality and short and long-term morbidity in very low birthweight infants. Cochrane Database Syst Rev 4 (2007): CD000501.

De Luca L et al. The role of vitamin in differentiation and skin carcinogenesis. J Nutr Biochem 8 (1997): 426–437.

De Oliveria MR et al. Impaired redox state and respiratory chain enzyme activities in the cerebellum of vitamin A-treated rats. Toxicol 253.1–3 (2008): 125–130.

De Oliveria MR et al. Evaluation of the effects of vitamin A supplementation on adult rat substantia nigra and striatum redox and bioenergetic states: Mitochondrial impairment, increased 3-nitrotyrosine and α-synuclein, but decreased D2 receptor contents. Prog Neuro-Psychoph 33.2 (2009): 353–362.

De Oliveria MR et al. The effects of vitamin A supplementation for 3 months on adult rat nigrostriatal axis: increased monoamine oxidase enzyme activity, mitochondrial redox dysfunction, increased β-amyloid(1–40) peptide and TNF-α contents, and susceptibility of mitochondria to an in vitro H2O2 challenge. Brain Res Bull 87.4–5 (2012): 432–444.

Dong P et al. Expression of retinoic acid receptors and retinoid X receptors in normal and vitamin A deficient adult rat brain. Nutrition 26.7–8 (2010):740–745.

Dougherty KA et al. No improvement in suboptimal vitamin A status with a randomized, double-blind, placebo-controlled trial of vitamin A supplementation in children with sickle cell disease. Am J Clin Nutr 96.4 (2012): 932–940.

D'Souza RM, D'Souza R. Vitamin A for preventing secondary infections in children with measles: a systematic review. J Trop Pediatr 48.2 (2002a): 72–7.

D'Souza RM, D'Souza R. Vitamin A for treating measles in children. Cochrane Database Syst Rev 1 (2002b): CD001479.

El-Akawi Z, et al. Does the plasma level of vitamins A and E affect acne condition? Clin Exp Dermatol 31.3 (2006): 430–434.

Enwonwu CO, Phillips RS. Increased retinol requirement in acute measles infection in children: an hypothesis on role of hypercortisolemia. Nutr Res 24.3 (2004): 223–227.

Epplein M et al. Plasma carotenoids, retinol, and tocopherols and postmenopausal breast cancer risk in the Multiethnic Cohort Study: a nested case-control study. Breast Cancer Res 11.4 (2009): R49.

Esteban-Pretel G et al. Vitamin A deficiency disturbs collagen IV and laminin composition and decreases matrix metalloproteinase concentrations in rat lung. Partial reversibility by retinoic acid. J Nutr Biochem 24.1 (2013): 137–145.

Fawzi WW et al. Multivitamin supplementation improves hematologic status in HIV-infected women and their children in Tanzania. Am J Clin Nutr 85.5 (2007): 1335–1343.

Feng Y et al. Alteration in methylation pattern of GATA-4 promoter region in vitamin A-deficient offspring's heart. J Nutr Biochem 24.7 (2013): 1373–1380.

Fernandes TF et al. Effect on infant illness of maternal supplementation with 400 000 IU vs 200 000 IU of vitamin A. Pediatrics 129.4 (2012): e960–966.

Feskanich D et al. Vitamin A intake and hip fractures among postmenopausal women. JAMA 287.1 (2002): 47–54.

Futoryan T, Gilchrest BA. Retinoids and the skin. Nutr Rev 52.9 (1994): 299–310.

Gadhia MM et al. Effects of early inhaled nitric oxide therapy and vitamin A supplementation on the risk for bronchopulmonary dysplasia in premature newborns with respiratory failure. J Pediatr (2014); 164: 744–748.

Gey KF et al. Low plasma retinol predicts coronary events in healthy middle-aged men: The PRIME Study. Atherosclerosis 208.1 (2010): 270–274.

Gilbert R et al. Associations of circulating retinol, vitamin E, and 1,25-dihydroxyvitamin D with prostate cancer diagnosis, stage, and grade. Cancer Causes Control 23.11 (2012):1865–1873.

Gogia S & Sachdev HS. Vitamin A supplementation for the prevention of morbidity and mortality in infants six months of age or less. Cochrane DB Syst Rev 2011 (2011): CD007480.

Golini RS et al. Daily patterns of clock and cognition-related factors are modified in the hippocampus of vitamin A-deficient rats. Hippocampus 22.8 (2012): 1720–1732.

Graham-Maar RC et al. Elevated vitamin A intake and serum retinol in preadolescent children with cystic fibrosis. Am J Clin Nutr 84.1 (2006): 174–182.

Haider BA et al. Neonatal vitamin A supplementation for the prevention of mortality and morbidity in term neonates in developing countries. Cochrane DB Syst Rev 2011 (2011): CD006980.

Hakim F et al. Vitamins A and E and pulmonary exacerbations in patients with cystic fibrosis. J Pediatr Gastroenterol Nutr 45.3 (2007): 347–353.

Helm CW et al. Retinoids for preventing the progression of cervical intra-epithelial neoplasia. Cochrane DB Syst Rev 2013 (2013). CD003296.

Hendler SS, Rorvik D (eds). PDR for nutritional supplements. Montvale, NJ: Medical Economics, 2001.

Hotz C et al. A large-scale intervention to introduce orange sweet potato in rural Mozambique increases vitamin A intakes among children and women. Br J Nutr 108.1 (2012a): 163–176.

Hotz C et al. Introduction of β carotene-rich orange sweet potato in rural Uganda resulted in increased vitamin A intakes among children and women and improved vitamin A status among children. J Nutr 142.10 (2012b): 1871–1880.

Houtkooper LB et al. Nutrients, body composition and exercise are related to change in bone mineral density in premenopausal women. J Nutr 125.5 (1995): 1229–1237.

Hoyos R et al. Hiding in plain sight: Uncovering a new function of vitamin A in redox signaling. BBA Mol Cell Biol L 1821.1 (2012): 241–247.

Huiming Y, et al. Vitamin A for treating measles in children. Cochrane Database Syst Rev 4 (2005): CD001479.

Huk DJ et al. Increased dietary intake of vitamin A promotes aortic valve calcification in vivo. Arterioscler Thromb Vasc Biol 33.2 (2013): 285–293.

Humphrey JH et al. HIV incidence among post-partum women in Zimbabwe: risk factors and the effect of vitamin A supplementation. AIDS 20.10 (2006a): 1437–46.

Humphrey JH et al. Effects of a single large dose of vitamin A, given during the postpartum period to HIV-positive women and their infants, on child HIV infection. HIV-free survival, and mortality. J Infect Dis 193.6 (2006b): 860–871.

Hurt L et al. Effect of vitamin A supplementation on cause-specific mortality in women of reproductive age in Ghana: a secondary analysis from the ObaapaVitA trial. Bull World Health Organ 91.1 (2013): 19–27.

Hyder SM et al. A multiple-micronutrient-fortified beverage affects hemoglobin, iron, and vitamin A status and growth in adolescent girls in rural Bangladesh. J Nutr 137.9 (2007): 2147–2153.

Imdad A et al. Vitamin A supplementation for preventing morbidity and mortality in children from 6 months to 5 years of age. Cochrane DB Syst Rev 2010 (2010): CD008524.

Israel L et al. [Vitamin A augmentation of the effects of chemotherapy in metastatic breast cancers after menopause. Randomized trial in 100 patients.] Ann Med Interne (Paris) 136.7 (1985): 551–4.

Ito Y et al. A population-based follow-up study on mortality from cancer or cardiovascular disease and serum carotenoids, retinol and tocopherols in Japanese inhabitants. Asian Pac J Cancer Prev 7.4 (2006): 533–546.

Jenab M et al. Plasma and dietary carotenoid, retinol and tocopherol levels and the risk of gastric adenocarcinomas in the European prospective investigation into cancer and nutrition. Br J Cancer 95.3 (2006): 406–415.

Jiang S et al. Vitamin A deficiency aggravates iron deficiency by upregulating the expression of iron regulatory protein-2. Nutrition 28.3 (2012): 281–287.

Jin YR et al. Intake of vitamin A-rich foods and lung cancer risk in Taiwan: with special reference to garland chrysanthemum and sweet potato leaf consumption. Asia Pac J Clin Nutr 16.3 (2007): 477–488.

Kabat GC et al. Intake of antioxidant nutrients and risk of non-Hodgkin's lymphoma in the Women's Health Initiative. Nutr Cancer 64.2 (2012): 245–254.

Kafi R et al. Improvement of naturally aged skin with vitamin A (retinol). Arch Dermatol 143.5 (2007): 606–612.

Kaptoge S et al. Effects of dietary nutrients and food groups on bone loss from the proximal femur in men and women in the 7th and 8th decades of age. Osteoporos Int 14.5 (2003): 418–428.

Kawahara TN et al. Short-term vitamin A supplementation does not affect bone turnover in men. J Nutr 132.6 (2002): 1169–1172.

Key TJ et al. Plasma carotenoids, retinol, and tocopherols and the risk of prostate cancer in the European Prospective Investigation into Cancer and Nutrition study. Am J Clin Nutr 86.3 (2007): 672–681.

Kim EC et al. A comparison of vitamin A and cyclosporine A 0.05% eye drops for treatment of dry eye syndrome. Am J Opthamol 147.2 (2009): 206–213.

Kim EC et al. The wound healing effects of vitamin A eye drops after a corneal alkali burn in rats. Acta Opthamol 90.7 (2012):e540–e546.

Kirkwood B et al. Effect of vitamin A supplementation on maternal survival. Lancet 375.9726 (2010a): 1640–1649.

Kirkwood B et al. Neonatal vitamin A supplementation and infant survival. Lancet 376.9753 (2010b): 1643–1644.

Klemm RD et al. Newborn vitamin A supplementation reduced infant mortality in rural Bangladesh. Pediatrics 122.1 (2008): e242–e250.
Kongnyuy EJ et al. A systematic review of randomized controlled trials of prenatal and postnatal vitamin A supplementation of HIV-infected women. Int J Gynecol Obstet 104.1 (2009): 5–8.
Krinsky NI. Vitamin A. Oregon: Linus Pauling Institute, 2002.
Larsson SC et al. Vitamin A, retinol, and carotenoids and the risk of gastric cancer: a prospective cohort study. Am J Clin Nutr 85.2 (2007): 497–503.
Lee JE et al. Intakes of fruits, vegetables, vitamins A, C, and E, and carotenoids and risk of renal cell cancer. Cancer Epidemiol Biomarkers Prev 15.12 (2006): 2445–2452.
Lima AA et al. Effects of vitamin A supplementation on intestinal barrier function, growth, total parasitic, and specific *Giardia* spp infections in Brazilian children: a prospective randomized, double-blind, placebo-controlled trial. J Pediatr Gastroenterol Nutr 50.3 (2010): 309–315.
Liu X et al. Gestational vitamin A deficiency reduces the intestinal immune response by decreasing the number of immune cells in rat offspring. Nutrition 30.3 (2014): 350–357.
Lodi G et al. Interventions for treating oral leukoplakia. Cochrane Database Syst Rev 4 (2006): CD001829.
Mactier H et al. Vitamin A supplementation improves retinal function in infants at risk of retinopathy of prematurity. J Pediatr 160.6 (2012): 954–959.e1.
Malaba LC et al. Effect of postpartum maternal or neonatal vitamin A supplementation on infant mortality among infants born to HIV-negative mothers in Zimbabwe. Am J Clin Nutr 81.2 (2005): 454–460.
Maqbool A et al. Vitamin A intake and elevated serum retinol levels in children and young adults with cystic fibrosis. J Cyst Fibros 7.2 (2008): 137–141.
McCaffery P, Drager UC. Retinoic acid synthesis in the developing retina. Adv Exp Med Biol 328 (1993): 181–190.
Melhus H et al. Excessive dietary intake of vitamin A is associated with reduced bone mineral density and increased risk for hip fracture. Ann Intern Med 129.10 (1998): 770–778.
Michaelsson K et al. Serum retinol levels and the risk of fracture. N Engl J Med 348.4 (2003): 287–294.
Miller RK et al. Periconceptional vitamin A use: how much is teratogenic? Reprod Toxicol 12.1 (1998): 75–88.
Miller MF et al. Effect of maternal and neonatal vitamin A supplementation and other postnatal factors on anemia in Zimbabwean infants: a prospective, randomized study. Am J Clin Nutr 84.1 (2006): 212–222.
Miyazaki M et al. Dietary vitamin A intake and incidence of gastric cancer in a general Japanese population: the Hisayama Study. Gastric Cancer 15.2 (2012): 162–169.
Mizuno Y et al. Serum vitamin A concentrations in asthmatic children in Japan. Pediatr Int 48.3 (2006): 261–264.
Mondul AM et al. Serum retinol and risk of prostate cancer. Am J Epidemiol 173.7 (2011): 813–821.
Moulas AN et al. Serum retinoic acid, retinol and retinyl palmitate levels in patients with lung cancer. Respirology 11.2 (2006): 169–174.
Muggeo M et al. Serum retinol levels throughout 2 years of cholesterol-lowering therapy. Metabolism 44.3 (1995): 398–403.
Navigatore-Fonzo LS et al. Retinoic acid receptors move in time with the clock in the hippocampus. Effect of a vitamin-A-deficient diet. J Nutr Biochem 24.5 (2013): 859–867.
Neuhouser ML et al. Dietary supplement use and prostate cancer risk in the Carotene and Retinol Efficacy Trial. Cancer Epidemiol Biomarkers Prev 18.8 (2009): 2202–2206.
Niles RM. Recent advances in the use of vitamin A (retinoids) in the prevention and treatment of cancer. Nutrition 16.11–12 (2000): 1084–1089.
Novotny JA et al. β-carotene conversion to vitamin A decreases as the dietary dose increases in humans. J Nutr 140.5 (2010): 915–918.
O'Neil C, et al. Vitamin A supplementation for cystic fibrosis. Cochrane Database Syst Rev 1 (2008): CD006751.
Pasquali MA et al. Vitamin A supplementation to pregnant and breastfeeding female rats induces oxidative stress in the neonatal lung. Reprod Toxicol 30.3 (2010): 452–456.
Penniston KL, Tanumihardjo SA. The acute and chronic toxic effects of vitamin A. Am J Clin Nutr 83.2 (2006): 191–201.
Penniston KL et al. Serum retinyl esters are not elevated in postmenopausal women with and without osteoporosis whose preformed vitamin A intakes are high. Am J Clin Nutr 84.6 (2006): 1350–1356.
Persson C et al. Plasma levels of carotenoids, retinol and tocopherol and the risk of gastric cancer in Japan: a nested case-control study. Carcinogenesis 29.5 (2008): 1042–1048.
Promislow JH et al. Retinol intake and bone mineral density in the elderly: the Rancho Bernardo Study. J Bone Miner Res 17.8 (2002): 1349–1358.
Ramakrishnan U, Martorell R. The role of vitamin A in reducing child mortality and morbidity and improving growth. Salud Publica Mex 40.2 (1998): 189–198.
Rayapudi S et al. Vitamin A and fish oils for retinitis pigmentosa (Review). The Cochrane Collaboration. The Cochrane Library 12 (2013).
Rejnmark L et al. No effect of vitamin A intake on bone mineral density and fracture risk in perimenopausal women. Osteoporos Int 15.11 (2004): 872–880.
Ribaya-Mercado JD, Blumberg JB. Vitamin A: is it a risk factor for osteoporosis and bone fracture? Nutr Rev 65.10 (2007): 425–438.
Riccioni G et al. Plasma lycopene and antioxidant vitamins in asthma: the PLAVA study. J Asthma 44.6 (2007): 429–432.
Ross AC. Vitamin A and retinoids. In: Shils M (Ed.), Modern Nutrition in Health and Disease, 9th edn. Baltimore: Williams & Wilkins, 1999, pp. 305–327.
Ross DA. Recommendations for vitamin A supplementation. J Nutr 132.9 Suppl (2002): 2902–6s.
Ross AC. Vitamin A and retinoic acid in T cell-related immunity. Am J Clin Nutr 96.5 (2012): 1166S–1172S.
Schenk JM et al. Serum retinol and prostate cancer risk: a nested case-control study in the prostate, lung, colorectal, and ovarian cancer screening trial. Cancer Epidemiol Biomarkers Prev 18.4 (2009): 1227–1231.
Schmitz J et al. Vitamin A supplementation in preschool children and risk of hearing loss as adolescents and young adults in rural Nepal: randomised trial cohort follow-up study. BMJ 344 (2012): d7962.
Schnorr CE et al. The effects of vitamin A supplementation to rats during gestation and lactation upon redox parameters: Increased oxidative stress and redox modulation in mothers and their offspring. Food Chem Toxicol 49.10 (2011): 2645–2654.
Semba RD. Vitamin A, immunity, and infection. Clin Infect Dis 19.3 (1994): 489–499.
Semba RD. Vitamin A and immunity to viral, bacterial and protozoan infections. Proc Nutr Soc 58.3 (1999): 719–727.
Sharma RK, Ehinger B. Management of hereditary retinal degenerations: present status and future directions. Surv Ophthalmol 43.5 (1999): 427–444.
Shearer KD et al. A vitamin for the brain. Trends Neurosci 35.12 (2012): 733–741.
Shils M et al (eds). Modern nutrition in health and disease. Baltimore: Lippincott Williams & Wilkins, 2006. Available at: Clinicians Health Channel gateway.ut.ovid.com (accessed 21-06-06).
Silvera SA et al. Carotenoid, vitamin A, vitamin C, and vitamin E intake and risk of ovarian cancer: a prospective cohort study. Cancer Epidemiol Biomarkers Prev 15.2 (2006): 395–397.
Sklan D. Vitamin A in human nutrition. Prog Food Nutr Sci 11.1 (1987): 39–55.
Sobouti B et al. The effect of vitamin E or vitamin A on the prevention of renal scarring in children with acute pyelonephritis. Pediatr Nephrol 28.2 (2013): 277–283.
Sommer A. Xerophthalmia and vitamin A status. Prog Retin Eye Res 17.1 (1998): 9–31.
Sowers MF, Wallace RB. Retinol, supplemental vitamin A and bone status. J Clin Epidemiol 43.7 (1990): 693–699.
Tanaka K et al. Deficiency of vitamin A delays bone healing process in association with reduced BMP2 expression after drill-hole injury in mice. Bone 47.6 (2010): 1006–1012.
Tielsch JM et al. Newborn vitamin A dosing reduces the case fatality but not incidence of common childhood morbidities in South India. J Nutr 137.11 (2007): 2470–2474.
Tiruvalluru M et al. Vitamin A supplementation ameliorates obesity-associated retinal degeneration in WNIN/Ob rats. Nutrition 29.1 (2013): 298–304.
Tyrer LB. Nutrition and the pill. J Reprod Med 29.7 Suppl (1984): 547–550.
van den Broek NR et al. Randomised trial of vitamin A supplementation in pregnant women in rural Malawi found to be anaemic on screening by HemoCue. BJOG 113.5 (2006): 569–576.
van den Broek NR et al. Vitamin A supplementation during pregnancy for maternal and newborn outcomes. Cochrane DB Syst Rev 2010 (2010): CD008666.
van Soest S et al. Retinitis pigmentosa: defined from a molecular point of view. Surv Ophthalmol 43.4 (1999): 321–334.
Visser ME et al. The effect of vitamin A and zinc supplementation on treatment outcomes in pulmonary tuberculosis: a randomized controlled trial. Am J Clin Nutr 93.1 (2011): 93–100.
Wahlqvist M et al. Food and nutrition. Sydney: Allen & Unwin, 1997.
Watters JL et al. Associations between alpha-tocopherol, beta-carotene, and retinol and prostate cancer survival. Cancer Res 69.9 (2009): 3833–3841.
Wardlaw G et al. Contemporary nutrition, 3rd edn. Dubuque: Brown and Benchmark, 1997.
Wessels G et al. The effect of vitamin A status in children treated for cancer. Pediatr Hematol Oncol 25.4 (2008): 283–290.

West KP Jr et al. Double blind, cluster randomized trial of low dose supplementation with vitamin A or beta carotene on mortality related to pregnancy in Nepal. BMJ 318.7183 (1999): 570–575.
West KP Jr et al. Effect of vitamin A supplementation on maternal survival. Lancet 376.9744 (2010): 873–874.
West KP Jr et al. Effects of vitamin A or beta carotene supplementation on pregnancy-related mortality and infant mortality in rural Bangladesh: a cluster randomized trial. JAMA 305.19 (2011): 1986–1995.
Wiysonge CS et al. Vitamin A supplementation for reducing the risk of mother-to-child transmission of HIV infection. Cochrane Database Syst Rev 2011 (2011): CD003648.
Wolf RL et al. Lack of a relation between vitamin and mineral antioxidants and bone mineral density: results from the Women's Health Initiative. Am J Clin Nutr 82.3 (2005): 581–588.
Yilmaz A et al. Adjuvant effect of vitamin A on recurrent lower urinary tract infections. Pediatr Int 49.3 (2007): 310–3113.
Zhang X et al. Effect of marginal vitamin A deficiency during pregnancy on retinoic acid receptors and *N*-methyl-D-aspartate receptor expression in the offspring of rats. J Nutr Biochem 22.12 (2011): 111–1120.
Zhang X et al. Vitamin A and risk of cervical cancer: A meta-analysis. Gynecol Oncol 124.2 (2012): 366–373.
Zimmermann MB et al. Vitamin A supplementation in children with poor vitamin A and iron status increases erythropoietin and hemoglobin concentrations without changing total body iron. Am J Clin Nutr 84.3 (2006): 580–586.
Zvandasara P et al. Mortality and morbidity among postpartum HIV-positive and HIV-negative women in Zimbabwe: risk factors, causes, and impact of single dose postpartum vitamin A supplementation. J Acquir Immune Defic Syndr 43.1 (2006): 107–116.

Vitamin B_1

HISTORICAL NOTE The Chinese medical book *Neiching* describes beriberi in 2697 BC, but it was not known for a long time that vitamin B_1 deficiency was responsible. The neurological symptoms such as leg weakness characteristic of thiamin deficiency were also recorded in the 1890s in chicks fed a diet of polished rice. In 1912, thiamin was isolated from rice bran and in the mid-1930s the structure of vitamin B_1 was determined (Gropper & Smith 2013). Since it was found not to contain an amine group, the 'e' was dropped from its name (thiamine → thiamin).

BACKGROUND AND RELEVANT PHARMACOKINETICS

Vitamin B_1 is a water-soluble compound required by all tissues. It is also known as thiamin (previously thiamine), anti-beriberi factor, antineuritic factor and its active coenzyme form, thiamin diphosphate (TDP), also called thiamin pyrophosphate (TPP). Thiamin's phosphate ester functions as a coenzyme and its ability to shift between different degrees of phosphorylation makes it a key nutrient in energy pathways.

There are two sources of thiamin: dietary and bacterial, which is synthesised by normal intestinal microflora. Thiamin is absorbed, predominantly in the jejunum and ileum as free (unphosphorylated) thiamin, by a saturable rate-limiting transport mechanism and may be passive or active. Passive absorption occurs at high concentrations, while at physiological levels, two active thiamin transporters, ThTr1 and ThTr2, are utilised. The activity of these transporters is inhibited by alcohol. The absorption of thiamin in the gastrointestinal tract can also be impaired by the presence of naturally occurring antithiamin factors such as thiaminases, found in raw fish, and polyhydroxyphenols, found in coffee, tea, blueberries, red cabbage and Brussels sprouts (Groff & Gropper 2009). Interestingly, calcium and magnesium exacerbate the effect of the polyhydroxyphenols. Conversely, thiamin preservation in the gastrointestinal tract is enhanced by vitamin C and citric acid (Gropper & Smith 2013).

Thiamin is transported via the portal circulation, travelling in plasma either free, bound to albumin, or as thiamin monophosphate, to the liver, where it is phosphorylated to its TDP coenzyme form (80% total body thiamin), which is also its most active state. Magnesium is required as a cofactor for this conversion/activation while alcohol has an inhibitory effect. Thiamin is taken up into brain by a blood–brain barrier transporter and via cerebrospinal fluid (CSF) (Fernstrom & Fenstrom 2013). Thiamin is excreted mainly by the kidneys. Thiamin is found in high concentrations in skeletal muscle, heart, liver, kidneys and brain and its half-life is approximately 15 days (Singleton & Martin 2001).

CHEMICAL COMPONENTS

Thiamin (vitamin B_1) is a water-soluble substance, composed of two heterocyclic moieties, substituted thiazole and pyrimidine rings joined by a methylene bridge (Rapala-Kozik 2011). It does not contain an amine group, as originally postulated.

FOOD SOURCES

Thiamin found in plant foods exists in its free form, while 95% of thiamin found in animal foods occurs primarily as TDP (Gropper & Smith 2013).

Brewer's yeast, lean meat and legumes are considered the richest sources of thiamin. Other sources include cereals, grains, pasta, wheat germ, soy milk, seeds and peanuts.

It is possible to lose up to 85% of the thiamin content in meat through cooking and canning, and up to 60% from cooking vegetables (Tanphaichitr 1999); cooking foods in water will further exacerbate the loss (Gropper & Smith 2013). There is also loss through refining of grains and polishing of rice (where the germ and bran have been removed, leaving only the endosperm). However, in Australia the fortification of wheat flour used for making bread with thiamin is mandatory to compensate for this loss (FSANZ 2012). Thiamin is not stable in alkaline environments; a pH of 8 or above destroys its activity (Gropper & Smith 2013).

DEFICIENCY SIGNS AND SYMPTOMS

The body only stores a small amount of thiamin and signs of deficiency tend to develop within 15–18 days of restricted intake.

Despite an expansive understanding of the role of thiamin at the cellular level, many aspects of the pathophysiological manifestations of thiamin deficiency remain unexplained (Gropper & Smith 2013). Beriberi (*beri* means weakness) is the classic deficiency state. General early or subclinical deficiency signs and symptoms include fatigue, weakness, rigidity (due to corresponding increase in lactic acid production), poor memory, sleep disturbances, chest wall pain, anorexia, abdominal discomfort and constipation. Other characteristic signs and symptoms include retarded growth, oedema, cardiomyopathy, bradycardia, heart failure and peripheral neuropathy (Combs 2012).

There are four forms of beriberi: dry, wet, acute and cerebral, otherwise known as Wernicke-Korsakoff syndrome. Dry beriberi is associated with muscle weakness and wasting, especially of the lower limbs, peripheral neurological changes and nerve conduction problems that may lead to symmetrical foot drop with calf tenderness (Gropper & Smith 2013). In addition to neurological changes, wet beriberi is associated with cardiovascular changes such as cardiomegaly and tachycardia. It is characterised by peripheral vasodilation, oedema due to sodium and water retention, increased cardiac output and myocardial failure, which can become fatal in severe cases. Acute beriberi occurs most commonly in infants and is associated with nausea and vomiting, convulsions, lactic acidosis, tachycardia and cardiomegaly; acute attacks may result in death if thiamin deficiency is not rapidly corrected.

Cerebral beriberi involves alterations to ocular and cognitive function secondary to bilateral symmetrical brain lesions in the paraventricular grey matter, producing ataxia, which can also be fatal. Ophthalmoplegia (paralyisis of the ocular muscles), nystagamus (involuntary, constant eyeball movement) and ataxia are the recognised triad of symptoms of Wernicke's encephalopathy. People with alcohol dependency are particularly at risk due to reduced consumption of food (thus thiamin intake), decreased absorption (Gropper & Smith 2013) and increased requirements due to decreased liver function (which impairs TDP formation).

Additionally, Wernicke–Korsakoff syndrome has been reported in several other conditions, such as hyperemesis gravidarum, hyperemesis due to gastroplasty (Kuhn et al 2012), acute psychosis after gastric bypass (Walker & Kepner 2012), gastric lap band (Becker et al 2012) and bariatric surgery (Lu'o'ng & Nguyen 2011, Sriram et al 2012), hyperthyroidism and inadequate parenteral nutrition (Bonucchi et al 2008, Gardian et al 1999, Ogershok et al 2002, Seehra et al 1996, Spruill & Kuller 2002, Tan & Ho 2001, Togay-Isikay et al 2001, Toth & Voll 2001). A 2007 case report of thrombocytopenia in a patient with Wernicke–Korsakoff syndrome, responsive to thiamin repletion, has introduced the possibility that this may constitute an unusual feature of the deficiency picture (Francini-Pesenti et al 2007).

While it is well recognised that the brain, heart and neuronal tissue are classically affected by thiamin deficiency, a recent in vivo study has found evidence of an endogenous self-preservation mechanism for brain and heart tissue that becomes established within 4 weeks of a thiamin-deficient diet (Klooster et al 2013). After this period, brain tissue transketolase activity remained constant and TDP (TPP) levels were significantly conserved in brain and heart tissue. The authors have suggested that other tissues could be suffering thiamin deficiency despite the absence of classical beriberi or Wernicke-Korsakoff syndrome (Lu'o'ng & Nguyen 2011, Sriram et al 2012). The length of time by which this self-preservation response can be effective during periods of low thiamin intake remains to be tested.

Clinical note — Thiamin deficiency is not uncommon in the elderly

Several observational studies have reported that thiamin deficiency is not uncommon in the elderly. A study of 118 elderly hospital patients identified a moderate deficiency incidence of 40% (Pepersack et al 1999). Similar results were obtained in another survey, where marginal thiamin deficiency had an incidence of 31% and frank deficiency of 17% in 36 non-demented elderly patients admitted to an acute geriatric unit. Delirium occurred in 32% of patients with normal thiamin status and 76% of thiamin-deficient patients ($P < 0.025$), although one or more other possible causes for delirium were present in all cases (O'Keeffe et al 1994). The importance of including thiamin deficiency in diagnostic work-ups of at-risk individuals is underscored by the high mortality rate in Wernicke–Korsakoff syndrome (10–20%), reported to be the direct result of underdiagnosis (Bonucchi et al 2008). Similarly, it is important to keep in mind that there is significant interindividual variability in both susceptibility to thiamin deficiency and its consequences (Al-Nasser et al 2006).

Preliminary research suggests that inadequate intake could also increase susceptibility to neurodegeneration, particularly in aged organisms (Nixon et al 2006, Pitkin & Savage 2004).

Primary deficiency

Primary deficiency is caused by inadequate dietary intake of thiamin, particularly in people subsisting mainly on highly polished rice (de Montmollin et al

> ***Clinical note — Thiamin food fortification in Australia and New Zealand***
> Australia New Zealand Food Standards Code, Standard 2.1.1 Amendment No. 111 2009 Cereals and Cereal Products, defines 'a number of products composed of cereals, qualifies the use of the term "bread", and requires the mandatory fortification of flour for bread making with thiamin in Australia' (Australian Government Comlaw 2009).

2002) or unfortified refined grain products. Insufficient intake may also occur in anorexia. Historically, those receiving total parenteral nutrition (TPN) without adequate additional thiamin were at risk of a primary deficiency. Current TPN formulae include 3 mg thiamin (Merck Manual Professional 2009).

Secondary deficiency

Secondary deficiency is caused by an increased requirement, as in hyperthyroidism, pregnancy, lactation, fever, acute infection, increased carbohydrate intake, folate deficiency, malabsorption states, hyperemesis, prolonged diarrhoea, strenuous physical exertion, breastfeeding, adolescent growth and states of impaired utilisation such as severe liver disease, alcoholism, chronic haemodialysis, diabetes (types 1 and 2) and people taking loop diuretics long-term. Additionally, pyruvate dehydrogenase deficiency can result in deficiency (Beers & Berkow 2003, Thornalley et al 2007, Wardlaw et al 1997, Wahlqvist et al 2002). Alternatively, latent primary thiamin deficiencies produce overt clinical features when the patient is exposed to thiamin metabolism stressors, such as those listed above, e.g. pregnancy, surgery (Al-Nasser et al 2006).

MAIN ACTIONS

Coenzyme

Carbohydrate and branched-chain amino acid metabolism.

Thiamin serves as a cofactor for several enzymes involved in carbohydrate catabolism, including pyruvate dehydrogenase complex, where TDP/TPP converts pyruvate to acetyl CoA (Fattal-Valevski 2011), transketolase and alpha-ketoglutarate, and for the branched-chain alpha-keto acid dehydrogenase complex that is involved in amino acid catabolism (Singleton & Martin 2001). Some of these enzymes are also important in brain oxidative metabolism (Molina et al 2002).

Neurotransmitter biosynthesis

Thiamin is involved in the biosynthesis of a number of neurotransmitters, including acetylcholine and gamma-aminobutyric acid. As TTP, it may also be involved in nerve impulse transmission (Gropper & Smith 2013).

DNA

Thiamin is involved in the synthesis of DNA precursors, therefore its use is increased in people with tumours.

Neuropsychological actions and neurodegenerative diseases

Thiamin is taken up into brain by a blood–brain barrier transporter and via CSF (Fernstrom & Fenstrom 2013). It is involved in neurotransmitter biosynthesis and is required for neurotransmission, nerve conduction, blood CSF barrier functionality and muscle action.

In the form of TTP, it plays an essential role in the physiology of the nervous system as it concentrates in nerve and muscle cells and activates membrane ion channels. TTP represents the smallest percentage of thiamin forms in humans; however, its phosphorylation of key regulatory proteins and the activation of high-conductance anion channels in nerve cells demonstrate its vital role in nervous system physiology (Gangolf et al 2010, Rapala-Kozik 2011). Thiamin deficiency leads to impaired oxidative metabolism due to impaired thiamin-dependent enzyme activity, and subsequently results in a multitude of negative events in the brain, including oxidative stress, lactic acidosis, blood–brain barrier disruption, decreased glucose utilisation and inflammation (Jhala & Hazell 2011). The consequence of such impaired metabolism alters brain function and can result in structural damage, neurodegeneration and, ultimately, neuronal cell loss (Jhala & Hazell 2011, Rapala-Kozik 2011).

Severe thiamin deficiency in the nervous tissue of animals reduces TPP levels and causes loss of coordinated muscle control. Upon correcting thiamin levels these anomalies are reversed, suggesting no permanent neural damage or destruction (Fernstrom & Fenstrom 2013). However, evidence from animal studies suggests that impaired blood CSF barrier function, secondary to thiamin deficiency, allows passage of neuroactive substances into the brain, damaging the choroid plexus (Nixon et al 2006). In Wernicke-Korsakoff syndrome, selective damage of mammillary bodies, the thalamus and pons has been observed, and analysis at the cellular level shows microglial activation and astrocyte proliferation (Hazell 2009, Hazell et al 1998, Rapala-Kozik 2011, Wang & Hazell 2010). Furthermore, in Wernicke-Korsakoff syndrome, the activity of all TDP-dependent enzymes is reduced, which in turn leads to decreased glutamate, aspartate and gamma-aminobutyric acid production, mitochondrial disintegration, lactate accumulation, acidosis and ultimately neuronal cell loss (Rapala-Kozik 2011).

Energy production

The B vitamins collectively function as coenzymes particularly involved in mitochondrial energy production. TDP, specifically, is utilised as a cofactor in pyruvate dehydrogenase, alpha-ketoglutarate dehydrogenase and branched-chain alpha-keto acid dehydrogenase. Evidence suggests that impaired mitochondrial energy production and decreased antioxidant activity, secondary to thiamin deficiency, may be responsible for the neuronal damage associated with this deficiency.

Antioxidant

While thiamin does not have any direct free radical scavenging activity, it has been postulated that, in thiamin deficiency, the neuronal damage and cellular energy depletion may be due to oxidative stress; high nitric oxide synthase production and formation of peroxynitrites have been observed and may be responsible for the deactivation of ketoglutarate dehydrogenase (Gibson & Blass 2007, Huang et al 2010, Rapala-Kozik 2011).

Mood

In addition to thiamin's important roles in neurotransmitter production, neurotransmission and nerve conduction, a deficiency of thiamin impedes the brain's ability to utilise glucose for energy. Subsequent manifestations include a plethora of neuropsychological effects, including mental depression, anxiety, irritability, apathy, poor concentration, forgetfulness and dementia. An early study found that as little as 50 mg/day thiamin per day for 2 months improved thiamin status in deficient individuals and was associated with greater mental clarity (Benton et al 1997).

CLINICAL USE

Many of the clinical uses of thiamin supplements are conditions thought to arise from a marginal deficiency, but some indications are based on the concept of high-dose supplements acting as therapeutic agents. In practice, vitamin B_1 is usually recommended in combination with other B group vitamins.

Deficiency: treatment and prevention

Thiamin supplements are traditionally used to treat or prevent thiamin deficiency states in people at risk (see Secondary deficiency, above).

Hyperemesis

Although thiamin supplementation will not reduce the symptoms of hyperemesis, it may be necessary in cases of hyperemesis gravidarum and hyperemesis due to gastroplasty and gastric lap band surgery in order to avoid deficiency, which has been infrequently reported in these situations. Permanent multifocal neurological dysfunction has been reported in women, including adolescent women, within 3 months of undergoing gastroplasty and gastric lap band surgery and reporting hyperemesis (Becker et al 2012, Kuhn et al 2012, Towbin et al 2004, Walker & Kepner 2012). It may be precipitated in part by intravenous (IV) fluids containing dextrose, and is more commonly seen when the patient's liver transaminases are elevated, which may contribute to the encephalopathy (Becker et al 2012, Francini-Pesenti et al 2007, Gardian et al 1999, Kuhn et al 2012; Seehra et al 1996, Spruill & Kuller 2002, Tan & Ho 2001, Togay-Isikay et al 2001, Toth & Voll 2001, Welsh 2005).

Alcoholism

In alcoholism, a state of decreased intake, absorption, utilisation and increased requirement for thiamin occurs, necessitating increased intakes to avoid deficiency states (D'Amour et al 1991). In cases of Wernicke's encephalopathy, monitoring of thiamin status and prophylactic IV treatment will inhibit the progression to Korsakoff's psychosis (Thomson & Marshall 2005). Ongoing research has revealed that the cerebellar neurotoxicity associated with excess alcohol is more likely to be mediated predominantly by thiamin deficiency than by direct ethanol cytotoxicity, as previously believed (Mulholland et al 2005); however, there is growing evidence of a strong negative synergy between the two that extends well beyond the increased need for thiamin as a result of alcohol consumption (Nixon et al 2006). In the treatment of Wernicke's encephalopathy, two studies have found IV or intramuscular (IM) administration of 100–500 mg of thiamin over 30 minutes for 3 days necessary to sufficiently raise plasma thiamin levels, and improve thiamin uptake and transport across the blood–brain barrier (Francini-Pesenti et al 2009, Sechi & Serra 2007).

Total parenteral nutrition

Several case reports show that patients who have received TPN without proper replacement of thiamin are at risk of developing deficiency signs and Wernicke's encephalopathy (Francini-Pesenti et al 2007, Hahn et al 1998, van Noort et al 1987, Vortmeyer et al 1992, Zak et al 1991). Preliminary evidence suggests that current TPN formulations are not sufficient to ensure thiamin repletion in all patients (Francini-Pesenti et al 2009).

Hyperthyroidism

Although a somewhat rare sequela, a handful of case reports describe Wernicke–Korsakoff's syndrome in patients suffering thyrotoxicosis (Bonucchi et al 2008).

Surgical patients

Several case reports detailing Wernicke's encephalopathy in surgical patients highlight why this patient group should be considered 'high-risk' for thiamin deficiency: malnutrition, high stress levels, vomiting and ileus all increase thiamin requirements substantially (Al-Nasser et al 2006, Francini-Pesenti et al 2007). Several authors suggest that thiamin deficiency may be latent in the preoperative patient, with surgery or postoperative TPN precipitating clinical manifestation, and consequently recommend preoperative screening for thiamin status (Al-Nasser et al 2006).

Acute alcohol withdrawal

Several guidelines for the support of alcohol withdrawal recommend a dose of 100 mg thiamin administered IV or IM before routine administration of dextrose-containing solutions (Adinoff et al 1988, Erstad & Cotugno 1995).

Alzheimer's disease (AD)

Thiamin status has been investigated and found, amongst other nutrients, to have an inverse relationship with cognitive function in the elderly (Nourhashemi et al 2000). More specifically, AD has been associated with reduced plasma levels of thiamin, according to several clinical studies (Gold et al 1995, 1998, Molina et al 2002). One study analysing cerebral cortex samples from autopsied patients with AD found slight reductions in TDP levels compared with matched controls (Mastrogiacoma et al 1996). Others have demonstrated reduced activities of thiamin-dependent enzymes, together with a strong correlation between these reductions and the extent of the dementia pathology in autopsied brains (Gibson & Blass 2007). Proposed mechanisms for the relationship between thiamin and AD are varied, ranging from its role as an antioxidant and its critical contribution to the Krebs cycle to its involvement in the production of acetylcholine, disturbances of which have all been implicated in AD pathology (Bubber et al 2004, Butterfield et al 2002, Gibson & Blass 2007, Kruse et al 2004). Animal research points towards the shared features of thiamin deficiency and AD pathology in the brain, in particular, with increased oxidative stress and inflammation precipitating neuronal loss in specific brain areas and concomitant promotion of plaque formation (Karuppagounder et al 2009).

Investigation with high-dose thiamin supplementation in this population has produced mixed results (Blass et al 1988, Meador et al 1993, Mimori et al 1996). One double-blind, placebo-controlled, crossover study showed that a dose of 3000 mg thiamin/day produced higher global cognitive ratings, as assessed by the Mini-Mental State Examination, compared with a niacinamide placebo. However, there were no changes to clinical state and behavioural ratings (Blass et al 1988). Another clinical study of unknown design found positive results with a dose ranging between 3 and 8 g/day of thiamin (Meador et al 1993), whereas a long-term study using high-dose supplementation produced negative results (Mimori et al 1996).

Although promising overall, a 2001 Cochrane review stated that it is still not possible to draw any conclusions about the effectiveness of thiamin supplementation in AD (Rodriguez-Martin et al 2001). In practice, it is often used as part of a broad-spectrum approach with other B group vitamins in age-related cognitive decline; however, further research is required to determine whether this method produces more consistent results, particularly as an adjunct to standard pharmaceutical treatments (Gibson & Blass 2007).

Diabetes

Given thiamin's essential role in the key carbohydrate metabolic enzymes transketolase, pyruvate dehydrogenase and alpha-ketoglutarate dehydrogenase and the glucose toxicity that occurs secondary to thiamin deficiency (Nixon et al 2006), there is growing interest in the therapeutic potential of this nutrient in diabetes. Preliminary research of thiamin status in diabetic patients reveals significantly high rates of deficiency (≈75% of type 1 and 2 diabetics), secondary to greatly increased renal losses (Thornalley et al 2007). It has been suggested that reduced thiamin availability may exacerbate diabetic metabolic dysfunction, particularly with respect to microvascular complications. This finding adds to the evidence produced earlier in test tube studies demonstrating that thiamin improves endothelial function, while protecting against insulin-mediated vascular smooth-muscle cell proliferation (Arora et al 2006).

In diabetes, benfotiamine, a synthetic derivative of thiamin (see section on Supplemental forms, below), induces key thiamin-dependent enzymes of the pentose shunt to reduce accumulation of toxic metabolites, including advanced glycation end products (Gibson et al 2013).

An investigation into high-dose thiamin (100 mg taken three times daily) over 3 months in a small sample of type 2 diabetes mellitus patients with microalbuminuria demonstrated reversal of early-stage nephropathy in the treatment group, without altering glycaemic control, dyslipidaemia or blood pressure (Rabbani et al 2009). Another study employing thiamin, this time in IV form, improved endothelium-dependent vasodilation in hyperglycaemic patients (both diabetic and non-diabetic); however, the mechanism of action remains unclear (Arora et al 2006).

Thiamin status in non-diabetic patients is typically assessed by the well-validated red blood cell transketolase activity test. However, an established limitation in this test is its inaccuracy in diabetic patients, complicating accurate assessment in this population (Thornalley et al 2007).

Congestive heart failure (CHF)

A large trial published in 2006 confirmed that the incidence of thiamin deficiency is notable amongst CHF patients (Hanninen et al 2006). These results were echoed by a more recent review in which the majority of studies reflect a general trend of increased risk of thiamin deficiency amongst this patient group compared with individuals free from the condition (McKeag et al 2012). It is suspected that patients with existing heart failure are at increased risk of thiamin deficiency because of diuretic-induced depletion, advanced age, malnutrition and/or periods of hospitalisation. A cross-sectional study reported that approximately one-third of hospitalised patients with heart failure had tissue levels suggestive of thiamin deficiency (Keith et al 2009).

Clinical note — The link between glucose metabolism, Alzheimer's dementia and thiamin

A continuous supply of glucose is essential for normal brain function and a key feature and biomarker of progression of AD is reduced glucose metabolism (Gibson et al 2013). Changes in brain glucose metabolism occur decades before the development of symptoms (Reiman et al 2004). In a multicentre, longitudinal neuroimaging study (Alzheimer Disease Neuroimaging Initiative: ADNI) launched in 2004, in which 819 adult subjects, 55–90 years old, were investigated, it was found that brain glucose utilisation was the best predictor of developing and progressing from mild cognitive impairment to AD (Jack et al 2010).

Thiamin-dependent processes responsible for glucose metabolism are diminished in brains of AD patients at autopsy and have been correlated with worse outcomes on dementia rating scales (Gibson et al 2013). Furthermore, thiamin deficiency exacerbates plaque formation and impairs memory in animal studies, while benfotiamine diminishes plaques and reverses memory deficits. Despite the linkages between diminished glucose metabolism in the brain and AD, why glucose metabolism is diminished remains elusive.

While a 2001 review concluded that there was insufficient evidence from large trials to confirm thiamin as a corrective treatment in CHF, a number of small interventional studies have assessed the effect of thiamin supplementation in patients with CHF, with promising results. In one pilot study of 6 patients treated with IV thiamin, such that their thiamin status returned to normal, there was increased left ventricular ejection fraction (LVEF) in 4 of 5 patients studied by electrocardiograph (Seligmann et al 1991). A randomised, placebo-controlled, double-blind study of 30 patients compared the effects of IV thiamin (200 mg/day) to placebo over 1 week followed by oral thiamin (200 mg/day) taken for 6 weeks. In the 27 patients completing the full 7-week intervention, LVEF rose by 22%. Other positive results have been reported from similar studies (Hanninen et al 2006). The current position of key researchers in this area is that, together with other micronutrients critical for myocardial energy production and control of oxidative stress (e.g. taurine), thiamin inadequacy is likely to exacerbate myocyte dysfunction and loss in this condition, making repletion an important therapeutic objective (Allard et al 2006).

IN COMBINATION

A Cochrane review of vitamin B complex for treating peripheral neuropathy, which included 13 studies (11 parallel RCTs and two quasi-randomised trials) involving 741 participants (488 treated with vitamin B alone) with alcoholic or diabetic neuropathy, concluded there are limited data and the evidence is insufficient to determine whether vitamin B complex is beneficial or harmful in these populations (Ang et al 2008).

One study using benfotiamine (see section on Supplemental forms, below), however, showed possible short-term benefit from 8-week treatment compared to placebo (Woelk et al 1998). Only 30 participants were treated with the oral benfotiamine in this study at a dosage of 320 mg/day during weeks 1–4 and 120 mg benfotiamine/day during weeks 5–8 (one capsule t.i.d.). Within the 8-week study period, benfotiamine led to a significant improvement of the threshold of vibration perception at the great toe, motor function and the overall symptom score. Marked improvement occurred in both pain and coordination (Woelk et al 1998). However, the strength of this evidence is weakened by the lack of other larger positive trials since this time.

Dysmenorrhoea

A Cochrane review of herbal and dietary therapies for primary and secondary dysmenorrhoea concluded that thiamin is an effective treatment when taken at 100 mg/day, although this conclusion is tempered slightly by its basis in only one large randomised controlled trial (Proctor & Murphy 2009). That trial was a randomised, double-blind, placebo-controlled, crossover design conducted over 5 months in 556 women and procured a positive improvement in >90% of the treatment cycle versus <1% in the placebo phase. The improvements observed during treatment appeared to have lasting effects, even after cessation of supplementation, for up to 3 months (Gokhale 1996). Due to the dramatic 'success' of this study, it has attracted scepticism regarding its methodology; certainly a question is why, with such positive results, an attempt to replicate the findings has not been undertaken since the mid-1990s (Fugh-Berman & Kronenberg 2003).

Epilepsy

A randomised, placebo-controlled trial involving 72 epileptic patients who had received long-term phenytoin treatment alone or in combination with phenobarbitone found that administration of thiamin (50 mg/day) over 6 months improved neuropsychological functions in both verbal and non-verbal IQ testing (Botez et al 1993). This study, interestingly, also found both folate supplementation (also typically depleted by the medication) and placebo ineffective. A 2009 Cochrane review investigating the role of B vitamins in controlling certain types of seizures found that thiamin supplementation improved neuropsychological functions related to psychomotor speed, visuospatial abilities, selective attention and verbal abstracting ability; however the sample was small and the authors concluded there is insufficient evidence that B vitamins improve seizure control or prevent harmful side effects of antiepileptic drugs in epileptic patients (Ranganathan & Ramaratnam 2009).

OTHER USES

Cataracts

A case-controlled study of 72 patients found that thiamin supplementation reduced the incidence of cortical, nuclear and mixed cataracts (Leske et al 1991).

Coma

A general approach to patients presenting to hospital with coma is to ensure adequate oxygenation, blood flow and treatment with hypertonic glucose and thiamin (Alguire 1990, Buylaert 2000).

Mortality in the elderly

In a recent study, higher intakes of vitamins B_1 and B_6 observed amongst Taiwanese elders were associated with increased survival rates by up to 10 years (Huang et al 2012). The Taiwanese Elderly Nutrition and Health Survey (1999–2000) interviewed 747 participants aged 65 years and over. Dietary and biochemical data were collected at baseline. Survivorship was determined until 31 December 2008. Controlled for confounders, and relative to the lowest tertile of vitamin B_1 or B_6 intakes, the hazard ratios (95% confidence interval) for tertile 3 were 0.74 (0.58–0.95) and 0.74 (0.57–0.97) (both $P < 0.05$). The authors concluded that deficiencies of vitamin B_1 and B_6 were found to be clearly predictive of mortality in elderly Taiwanese.

Polycystic ovarian syndrome

Insulin resistance is a key clinical feature in polycystic ovarian syndrome. Given the importance of thiamin in carbohydrate metabolism, it may suggest an important clinical role for thiamin in polycystic ovarian syndrome and improved insulin sensitivity (Hechtman 2011).

Tumour proliferation

In advanced cancer, thiamin deficiency, along with many other micronutrients, frequently occurs. However TPP is involved in ribose synthesis, required for cellular replication, and hence the concern about a proliferative role ensues. In a metabolic control analysis in vivo, a high stimulatory effect on tumour growth of 164% was found for thiamin doses at 25 times the recommended dietary allowance (RDA) compared to controls. However, in the same study when thiamin supplementation was 2500 times the RDA for mice, the opposite effect was observed and a 10% inhibition of tumour growth was recognised. This effect was heightened, resulting in a 36% decrease, when thiamin supplementation was administered from the 7th day prior to tumour inoculation (Comin-Anduix et al 2001). Human research is urgently needed in order to elucidate any potential benefits or risks for thiamin in cancer.

Clinical note — No protection against insect bites

One claim that has been around for many years is that high oral doses of certain B vitamins could act as a deterrent to insects such as mosquitoes. Principally, the myth has centred on thiamin. A review of prophylaxis against insect bites found that neither topical application nor oral dosing of thiamin is an effective preventive strategy (Rudin 2005).

IN COMBINATION

The B group vitamins function as coenzymes in energy production and are a popular supplement taken by the public to lessen the impact of 'stress' and provide an energy boost. In one study, thiamin 10 mg/day significantly increased appetite, energy intake, body weight and general wellbeing and decreased fatigue, compared with placebo in a group of 80 randomly chosen women from a population with known marginal deficiency (Smidt et al 1991). Thiamin supplementation also tended to reduce daytime sleep time, improve sleep patterns and increase activity.

Fibromyalgia

Studies have detailed thiamin metabolism disorders in fibromyalgia patients (Eisinger et al 1994, Juhl 1998). Due to its importance in energy production, it is suggested that any subsequent deficiencies due to the metabolic alteration may negatively impact energy production, potentially exacerbating the fatigue already prevalent in fibromyalgia sufferers.

HIV

Several neuropathological reports have described brain lesions characteristic of Wernicke's encephalopathy in patients with AIDS. One study found a 23% prevalence of thiamin deficiency in AIDS patients with no history of alcohol abuse (Butterworth et al 1991), which may correlate with symptoms of fatigue and lethargy related to HIV. Another study found a decreased progression to AIDS from HIV in patients replete in vitamins B and C (Tang et al 1993).

Neurogenic impotence

A dose of 25 mg thiamin taken orally resulted in normalisation of erection in a man with a history of chronic alcoholism and erectile dysfunction of 1 year's duration (Tjandra & Janknegt 1997). However, more recent evidence discussing the causes of neurogenic impotence suggests that thiamin deficiency is relatively rare (Finsterer 2005).

Maple syrup urine disease

Of four paediatric patients with maple syrup urine disease, three responded to thiamin therapy with a reduction in concentration of plasma and urinary branched-chain amino and keto acids (Fernhoff et al 1985).

IN COMBINATION

B vitamins were investigated for reducing sensitivity to painful stimuli in mice (Franca et al 2001), whereby thiamin and pyridoxine (50–200 mg/kg intraperitoneally [IP]) or riboflavin (3–100 mg/kg IP) induced an antinociceptive effect, not changed by naloxone (10 mg/kg IP), indicating that activity is not mediated by opiate pathways. The authors state that the B vitamins' antinociceptive effect may involve inhibition of the synthesis and/or action of inflammatory mediators. Furthermore, in an animal study the therapeutic effects of glucosamine hydrochloride and chondroitin sulfate as chondroprotection were enhanced by the addition of fursultiamine, a thiamin derivative, in the treatment of osteoarthritis (Kobayashi et al 2005).

Optic neuropathy

Several case reports suggest this condition can be caused by thiamin deficiency and successfully treated with supplementation. One case report of a man developing optic neuropathy as a result of receiving TPN without thiamin for 4 weeks found that supplementation with thiamin reversed the condition (Suzuki et al 1997). Two cases of symmetrical, bilateral optic neuropathy associated with thiamin deficiency were successfully treated with thiamin supplementation.

Fertility, preconception and health of the offspring

An animal study investigated the effects of thiamin deficiency in newly developing neuronal cells, reporting cellular membrane damage, apoptosis and irregular and ectopic cells (Ba 2008). The same paper postulates that thiamin repletion may stabilise neurons and prevent cellular death.

Another animal study by the same author investigated the impact of alcohol consumption and thiamin deficiency in the developing central nervous system (Ba 2011). Neurotoxicity caused by maternal thiamin deficiency during pre-, peri- and postnatal stages was compared with neurotoxicity caused by chronic maternal alcohol intake alone and finally compared with the combined effects. Neurodevelopmental abilities in the offspring were then measured. Both thiamin deficiency and ethanol exposure interfered with periods of intense cellular proliferation prenatally, and with cellular differentiation, synaptogenesis, axonogenesis and myelinogenesis during peri- and postnatal stages, producing neurofunctional alterations. Furthermore, perinatal effects of thiamin deficiency on primary cellular differentiation in the developing central nervous system were similar to those caused by alcohol exposure (Ba 2011).

Due to the imperative role of thiamin in female reproductive function, cellular differentiation and proliferation, and normal hormonal processes during gestation, a deficiency of thiamin during pregnancy may be implicated in an increased risk of miscarriage (Ba 2009). A limitation of this evidence is that the majority of investigations have been animal-based.

DOSAGE RANGE

- Prevention of deficiency (adult Australian recommended dietary intake [RDI]): 1.1–1.2 mg/day
- Treatment of marginal deficiency states: 5–30 mg/day
- Critical deficiency: 50–100 mg IV or IM for 7–14 days, after which oral doses are used (Tanphaichitr 1999)
- Therapeutic dose: generally 5–150 mg/day, atypical therapeutic doses >3 g daily
- CHF: when indicated, 100 mg twice daily IV for 1–2 weeks, then 200 mg/day orally
- Dysmenorrhoea: 100 mg/day orally
- Support of alcohol withdrawal: 100 mg given IV or IM
- Fatigue (when marginal deficiency likely): 10 mg/day
- Type 2 diabetes mellitus: 100 mg three times daily
- Wernicke's encephalopathy: 100–500 mg (IV or IM) over 30 minutes for 3 days
- Mental depression: 50 mg/day for 2 months
- Mood disorders: 10 mg/day with marginal deficiency.

Australian RDI

- Females >13 years: 1.1 mg/day.
- Males >13 years: 1.2 mg/day.

TOXICITY

Toxicity does not occur with oral thiamin as it is rapidly excreted by the kidneys (Tanphaichitr 1999), although there is some evidence that toxicity can occur with very large doses given parenterally (Jacobs & Wood 2003).

ADVERSE REACTIONS

Thiamin is well tolerated.

SUPPLEMENTAL FORMS

Thiamin hydrochloride is the most common form used in supplements, which consist of 89% thiamin and 11% HCl.

Benfotiamine is an *Allium*-derived, lipid-soluble derivative of thiamin that has better bioavailability than water-soluble salts. It is the preferred form in the treatment of alcoholic and diabetic neuropathies (Ang et al 2008, Stracke et al 1996) where supplementation with thiamin or benfotiamine in rat models revealed that equivalent doses of thiamin have a fivefold lower bioavailability than benfotiamine. Its higher cellular bioavailability is due to the thiazole ring that allows easier passage across cell membranes (Balakumar et al 2010).

Oral supplements are non-toxic, but should be used with caution in patients with cancer (Comin-Anduix et al 2001). (See Tumour proliferation section, above, and Cancer section, below.)

SIGNIFICANT INTERACTIONS

Antibiotics

Antibiotics can reduce the endogenous production of B group vitamins by gastrointestinal flora, theoretically resulting in lowered B vitamin levels. The clinical significance of this is unclear — increase intake of vitamin B_1-rich foods or consider supplementation.

Coffee, tea, blueberries, red cabbage and Brussels sprouts

Reduce the absorption of oral thiamin — separate doses by 2 hours (Groff & Gropper 2009).

Vitamin C and citric acid

May enhance oral bioavailability of thiamin (Gropper & Smith 2013).

Iron

Iron precipitates thiamin, thereby reducing its absorption — separate doses by 2 hours.

Loop diuretics

Chronic use may result in lowered levels of vitamin B_1 — increase intake of vitamin B_1-rich foods or consider long-term supplementation.

Other B vitamins

Thiamin deficiency commonly occurs in conjunction with poor B_2 and B_6 status (Jacobs & Wood 2003).

Sulfites

Concomitant intake may inactivate thiamin, which has been reported in TPN solutions (Bowman & Nguyen 1983).

Tannins

Tannins precipitate thiamin, thereby reducing its absorption — separate doses by 2 hours.

Horsetail (*Equisetum arvense*)

Theoretically, horsetail may destroy thiamin in the stomach due to the presence of a thiaminase-like compound found in the herb. Those who have a pre-existing thiamin deficiency or are at risk of thiamin deficiency may be advised to avoid concurrent use of horsetail (Shils et al 2005).

CONTRAINDICATIONS AND PRECAUTIONS

Cancer

There is some evidence of thiamin being associated with nucleic acid ribose synthesis of tumour cells in its biologically activated form (Boros 2000). In a metabolic control analysis in vivo in mice, a high stimulatory effect was observed with thiamin doses of 25 times the RDA on tumour growth of 164%, when compared to controls. However, in the same study, when thiamin supplementation was 2500 times the RDA for mice, the opposite effect was observed and a 10% inhibition of tumour growth was recognised (Comin-Anduix et al 2001).

As such, whether thiamin has any effect on tumour formation in humans remains unclear.

PREGNANCY USE

Safe during pregnancy and lactation.

Practice points/Patient counselling

- Thiamin is necessary for healthy functioning and is involved in carbohydrate and protein metabolism, the production of DNA and several neurotransmitters and nerve and muscle functions.
- Supplements are used to treat deficiency or prevent secondary deficiency in people at risk (e.g. alcoholism, malabsorption syndromes, hyperemesis, chronic diarrhoea, hyperthyroidism, pregnancy, lactation, fever, acute infection, folate deficiency, strenuous physical exertion, breastfeeding, adolescent growth, severe liver disease and chronic use of loop diuretics). There is a higher incidence of deficiency in people with CHF; however, it is not known whether correction of the deficiency will improve disease symptoms.
- High-dose thiamin supplements relieve symptoms of dysmenorrhoea, according to one large randomised controlled trial.
- Additionally, some early research has found an association between AD and low plasma thiamin levels, with supplementation producing some benefits; however, further investigation is still required.
- Some research has also suggested a potential use for thiamin in the improvement of vibration perception, motor function, pain and coordination associated with peripheral neuropathy. Further research is necessary.
- Oral supplements are non-toxic, but high doses should be used with caution in patients with cancer.

PATIENTS' FAQs

What will this vitamin do for me?

Thiamin is necessary for healthy functioning and is involved in carbohydrate and protein metabolism, the production of DNA and several brain chemicals and nerve and muscle functions. Supplements are taken to avoid deficiency states that can occur, for instance, in alcoholism, extreme vomiting, chronic diarrhoea or malabsorption syndromes. In high doses, it may relieve symptoms of painful menstruation and may be a useful adjunct in CHF.

When will it start to work?

Thiamin supplements can have dramatic effects on deficiency states within 24 hours. The response time for other conditions, such as dysmenorrhoea and CHF, also appears to be reasonably fast. Within two menstrual cycles, supplementation produced marked reductions in dysmenorrhoea, and CHF patients treated for only 7 weeks showed positive responses.

Are there any safety issues?

Taken orally, thiamin is considered non-toxic. People with cancer should consult with their doctor before taking high-dose thiamin supplements.

REFERENCES

Adinoff B et al. Acute ethanol poisoning and the ethanol withdrawal syndrome. Med Toxicol Adverse Drug Exp 3.3 (1988): 172–196.

Alguire PC. Rapid evaluation of comatose patients. Postgrad Med 87.6 (1990): 223–233: 8.

Allard ML, et al. The management of conditioned nutritional requirements in heart failure. Heart Fail Rev 11.1 (2006): 75–82.

Al-Nasser B, et al. Lower limb neuropathy after spinal anesthesia in a patient with latent thiamin deficiency. J Clin Anesth 18.8 (2006): 624–627.

Ang CD, et al. Vitamin B for treating peripheral neuropathy. Cochrane Database Syst Rev, 2008. CD004573.

Arora S et al. Thiamin (vitamin B_1) improves endothelium-dependent vasodilatation in the presence of hyperglycemia. Ann Vasc Surg 20.5 (2006): 75–82.

Australian Government ComLaw (2009) http://www.comlaw.gov.au /Details/F2009C00811. Viewed 20th April, 2013.

Ba A. Metabolic and structural role of thiamin in nervous tissue. Cell Mol Neurobiol 2008:28(7):943–53.

Ba A Alcohol and B_1 vitamin deficient-related stilbirths. J Maternal Foetal Neonatal Med, 2009;22(5):452–7.

Ba A Comparative effects of alcohol and thiamin deficiency on the developing central nervous system. Behavioural Brain Research 225 (2011) 235–242.

Balakumar, P., et al. The multifaceted therapeutic potential of benfotiamine. Pharmacological Research 61(2010)., 482–488.

Becker DA., et al. Dry beriberi and Wernicke's encephalopathy following gastric lap band surgery. Journal of Clinical Neuroscience 19 (2012) 1050–1052.

Beers MH, Berkow R (eds). The Merck manual of diagnosis and therapy, 17th edn. Whitehouse, NJ: Merck, 2003.

Benton D., et al. Thiamin supplementation mood and cognitive functioning. Psychopharmacology (1997) 129: 66–71.

Blass JP et al. Thiamin and Alzheimer's disease: a pilot study. Arch Neurol 45.8 (1988): 833–835.

Bonucchi J et al. Thyrtoxicosis associated Wernicke's encephalopathy. J Gen Intern Med 23.1 (2008): 106–109.

Boros LG. Population thiamin status and varying cancer rates between western. Asian and African countries. Anticancer Res 20.3B (2000): 2245–2248.

Botez MI et al. Thiamin and folate treatment of chronic epileptic patients: a controlled study with the Wechsler IQ scale. Epilepsy Res 16.2 (1993): 157–163.

Bowman BB, Nguyen P. Stability of thiamin in parenteral nutrition solutions. J Parenter Enteral Nutr 7.6 (1983): 567–568.

Bubber P, et al. Tricarboxylic acid cycle enzymes following thiamin deficiency. Neurochem Int 45.7 (2004): 1021–1028.

Butterfield DA et al. Nutritional approaches to combat oxidative stress in Alzheimer's disease. J Nutr Biochem 13.8 (2002): 444–461.

Butterworth RF et al. Thiamin deficiency and Wernicke's encephalopathy in AIDS. Metab Brain Dis 6.4 (1991): 207–212.

Buylaert WA. Coma induced by intoxication. Acta Neurol Belg 100.4 (2000): 221–224.

Combs GF Jr. The Vitamins (Fourth Edition). Chapter 10 — Thiamin. 2012, Pages 261–276. London: Elsevier

ComõÂn-Anduix BA, et al. The effect of thiamin supplementation on tumour proliferation A metabolic control analysis study. Eur. J. Biochem. 268, 4177–4182 (2001).

D'Amour ML, et al. Abnormalities of peripheral nerve conduction in relation to thiamin status in alcoholic patients. Can J Neurol Sci 18.2 (1991): 126–128.

de Montmollin D et al. Outbreak of beri-beri in a prison in West Africa. Trop Doct 32.4 (2002): 234–236.

Eisinger J., et al. Glycolysis abnormalities in fibromyalgia. J Am Coll Nutr 1994;24(2):144–8.

Erstad BL, Cotugno CL. Management of alcohol withdrawal. Am J Health Syst Pharm 52.7 (1995): 697–709.

Fattal-Valeski, A. Thiamin (vitamin B_1). Journal of Evidence-Based Complementary & Alternative Medicine 16 (1):12–20, 2011.

Fernhoff PM et al. Thiamin response in maple syrup urine disease. Pediatr Res 19.10 (1985): 1011–1016.

Fernstrom JD and Fenstrom MH Biology, metabolism, and nutritional requirements. In: Brain and Nervous System, 2013. Amsterdam: Elsevier.

Finsterer J. Mitochondrial neuropathy. Clin Neurol Neurosurg 107.3 (2005): 181–186.

Franca DS., et al. B vitamins induce an antinociceptive effect in the acetic acid and formaldehyde models of nociception in mice. European Journal of Pharmacology Volume 421, Issue 3, 15 June 2001, Pages 157–164.

Francini-Pesenti F et al. Wernicke's encephalopathy during parenteral nutrition. J Parenter Enteral Nutr 31.1 (2007): 69–71.

Francini-Pesenti F et al. Wernicke's syndrome during parenteral feeding: Not an unusual complication. Nutrition 2009a;25(2):142–146.

Francini-Pesenti F, et al. Wernicke's syndrome during parenteral feeding: not an unusual complication, Nutrition, 2009b; 25:142–46.

FSANZ Food Standards New Zealand and Australia (2012). http:// www.foodstandards.gov.au/consumerinformation/fortification.cfm

Fugh-Berman A, Kronenberg F. Complementary and alternative medicine (CAM) in reproductive-age women: a review of randomized controlled trials. Reprod Toxicol 17.2 (2003): 137–152.

Gangolf, M., et al Thiamin triphosphate synthesis in rat brain occurs in mitochondira and is coupled to the respiratory chain. The Journal of Biological Chemistry, (2010), 285, 583–594.

Gardian G et al. Wernicke's encephalopathy induced by hyperemesis gravidarum. Acta Neurol Scand 99.3 (1999): 196–198.

Gibson GE, Blass JP. Thiamin-dependent processes and treatment strategies in neurodegeneration. Antioxid Redox Signal 9.10 (2007): 1605–1619.

Gibson GE, et al. Abnormal thiamin-dependent processes in Alzheimer's disease. Lessons from diabetes. Molecular and Cellular Neuroscience 55 (2013) 17–25.

Gokhale LB. Curative treatment of primary (spasmodic) dysmenorrhoea. Indian J Med Res 103 (1996): 227–231.

Gold M, et al. Plasma and red blood cell thiamin deficiency in patients with dementia of the Alzheimer's type. Arch Neurol 52.11 (1995): 1081–1086.

Gold M et al. Plasma thiamin deficiency associated with Alzheimer's disease but not Parkinson's disease. Metab Brain Dis 13.1 (1998): 43–53.

Groff, J., Gropper, S. Advanced nutrition and human metabolism, 5th edition. Belmont, CA: Wadsworth, Cengage Learning, 2009.

Gropper, S., Smith, J Advanced nutrition and human metabolism, 6th edition. Belmont CA: Wadsworth, Cengage Learning, 2013.

Hahn JS et al. Wernicke encephalopathy and beriberi during total parenteral nutrition attributable to multivitamin infusion shortage. Pediatrics 101.1 (1998): E10.

Hanninen SA et al. The prevalence of thiamin deficiency in hospitalized patients with congestive heart failure. J Am Coll Cardiol 47.2 (2006): 354–361.

Hazell, A. S. Astrocytes are a major target in thiamin deficiency and Wernicke's encephalopathy. Neurochemistry International (2009) 55, 129–135.

Hazell, A. S., et al. Mechanisms of neuronal cell death in Wernicke's encephalopathy. Metabolic Brain Disease (1998). 13, 97–122.

Hechtman, L. Clinical naturopathic medicine. Chatswood, NSW: Churchill Livingstone, Elsevier, 2011.

Huang, H. M., et al. (2010). Thiamin and oxidants interact to modify cellular calcium stores. Neurochemical Research 35, 2107–2116.

Huang, Y, et al. Prediction of all-cause mortality by B group vitamin status in the elderly. Clinical Nutrition 31 (2012) 191–198.

Jack Jr., C.R., et al 2010. Hypothetical model of dynamic biomarkers of the Alzheimer's pathological cascade. Lancet Neurol. 9, 119–128.

Jacobs P, Wood L. Hematology of malnutrition. II: Vitamin B_1. Disease-a-Month 49.11 (2003): 646–652.

Jhala SS & Hazell A S. Modeling neurodegenerative disease pathophysiology in thiamine deficiency: consequences of impaired oxidative metabolism. Neurochemistry International 58; 2011: 248–260.

Juhl JH. Fibromyalgia and the serotonin pathway. Altern Med Rev 1998;3(5):367–75.

Karuppagounder SS et al. Thiamin deficiency induces oxidative stress and exacerbates the plaque pathology in Alzheimer's mouse model. Neurol Aging 2009; 30: 1587–1600.

Keith ME., et al. B-Vitamin deficiency in hositalised patients with heart failure. Journal of American Dietetic Association, 2009; 109: 1406–1410.

Klooster, A., et al. Are brain and heart tissue prone to the development of thiamin deficiency? Alcohol (2013) 1–7.

Kobayashi T., et al. Fursultiamine, a vitamin B_1 derivative, enhances chondroprotective effects of glucosamine hydrochloride and chondroitin sulfate in rabbit experimental osteoarthritis. Inflamm Res 2005;54(6):249–55.

Kuhn AL., et al. Vitamin B_1 in the treatment of Wernicke's encephalopathy due to hyperemesis after gastroplasty. Journal of Clinical Neuroscience 19 (2012) 1303–1305.

Kruse M et al. Increased brain endothelial nitric oxide synthase expression in thiamin deficiency: relationship to selective vulnerability. Neurochem Int 45.1 (2004): 49–56.

Leske MC et al. The lens opacities case-control study: risk factors for cataract. Arch Ophthalmol 109.2 (1991): 244–251.
Lu'o'ng, K. V., & Nguyen, L. T. (2011). Role of thiamin in Alheimer's disease. American Journal of Alzheimer's Disease and Other Dementias, 26, 588e598.
Mastrogiacoma F et al. Brain thiamin, its phosphate esters, and its metabolizing enzymes in Alzheimer's disease. Ann Neurol 39.5 (1996): 585–591.
McKeag NA., et al. The role of micronutrients in heart failure. Journal of the Academy of Nutrition and Dietetics, 2012; 112: 870–886.
Meador K et al. Preliminary findings of high-dose thiamin in dementia of Alzheimer's type. J Geriatr Psychiatry Neurol 6.4 (1993): 222–229.
Mimori Y, et al. Thiamin therapy in Alzheimer's disease. Metab Brain Dis 11 (1996): 89–94.
Molina JA et al. Cerebrospinal fluid levels of thiamin in patients with Alzheimer's disease. J Neural Transm 109.7–8 (2002): 1035–1044.
Mulholland PJ et al. Thiamin deficiency in the pathogenesis of chronic ethanol-associated cerebellar damage in vitro. Neuroscience 135.4 (2005): 1129–1139.
Nixon PF et al. Choroid plexus dysfunction: the initial event in hyperglycemia. Ann Vasc Surg 20.5 (2006): 653–658.
Nourhashemi S et al. Alzheimer disease: protective factors. Am J Clin Nutr 71.2 (2000): 643–649s.
Ogershok PR et al. Wernicke encephalopathy in nonalcoholic patients. Am J Med Sci 323.2 (2002): 107–111.
O'Keeffe ST et al. Thiamin deficiency in hospitalized elderly patients. Gerontology 40.1 (1994): 18–24.
Pepersack T et al. Clin relevance of thiamin status amongst hospitalized elderly patients. Gerontology 45.2 (1999): 96–101.
Pitkin SR, Savage LM. Age-related vulnerability to diencephalic amnesia produced by thiamin deficiency: the role of time of insult. Behav Brain Res 148.1–2 (2004): 93–105.
Proctor M & Murphy PA. Herbal and dietary therapies for primary and secondary dysmenorrhoea. Cochrane Database Syst Rev 2001 (2009): CD002124.
Rabbani N et al. High dose thiamin therapy for patients with type 2 diabetes and microalbuminuria: a randomized, double-blind-placebo controlled pilot study. Diabetologia (2009): 52: 208–212.
Ranganathan LN., Ramaratnam S. Vitamins for epilepsy. Cochrane Database of Syst Rev (2009), Issue 2: CD004304.
Rapala-Kozik M. Vitamin B_1 (thiamin): a cofactor for enzymes involved in the main metabolic pathways and an environmental stress protectant. Advances in Botanical Research, Vol 58, 2011; 37–91.
Reiman, E.M., et al 2004. Functional brain abnormalities in young adults at genetic risk for late-onset Alzheimer's dementia. Proc. Natl. Acad. Sci. U. S. A. 101, 284–289.
Rodriguez-Martin JL, et al. Thiamin for Alzheimer's disease. Cochrane Database Syst Rev 2 (2001): CD001498.
Rudin W. Protection against insect bites. Ther Umsch 62.11 (2005): 713–7118.
Sechi G, Serra A. Wernicke's encephalopathy: new clinical setting and recent advances in diagnosis and management. Lancet Neurol, 2007; 6:442–55.
Seehra H et al. Wernicke's encephalopathy after vertical banded gastroplasty for morbid obesity. BMJ 312.7028 (1996): 434.
Seligmann H et al. Thiamin deficiency in patients with congestive heart failure receiving long-term furosemide therapy: a pilot study. Am J Med 91 (1991): 151–155.
Shils ME, et al. Modern nutrition in health and disease. 10th edn. Baltimore, MD: Lippincott Williams & Wilkins; 2005, 2146.
Singleton CK, Martin PR. Molecular mechanisms of thiamin utilization. Curr Mol Med 1.2 (2001): 197–207.
Smidt LJ et al. Influence of thiamin supplementation on the health and general well-being of an elderly Irish population with marginal thiamin deficiency. J Gerontol 46.1 (1991): M16–M22.
Spruill SC, Kuller JA. Hyperemesis gravidarum complicated by Wernicke's encephalopathy. Obstet Gynecol 99.5 (2002): 875–877.
Sriram, K., et al. (2012). Thiamin in nutrition therapy. Nutrition in Clinical Practice, 27, 41e50.
Stracke H, et al. A benfotiamine-vitamin B combination in treatments of diabetic polyneuropathy. Experimental and Clinical Endocrinology and Diabetes 1996;104(4):311–6.
Suzuki S et al. Optic neuropathy from thiamin deficiency. Intern Med 36.7 (1997): 532.
Tan JH, Ho KH. Wernicke's encephalopathy in patients with hyperemesis gravidarum. Singapore Med J 42.3 (2001): 124–125.
Tang AM., et al. Dietary micronutrient intake and risk of progression to acquired immunodeficiency syndrome (AIDS) in human immunodeficiency virus type-1 (HIV-1) infected homosexual men. Am J Epidemiol 1993;138:937–51.
Tanphaichitr V. Thiamin. In: Shils M (ed.), Modern nutrition in health and disease. Baltimore: Lippincott Williams & Wilkins, 1999.
The Merck Manual Professional, reviewed 2009. http://www.merckmanuals.com/professional/nutritional_disorders/nutritional_support/total_parenteral_nutrition_tpn.html#v883534. Viewed online 20th April, 2013.
Thomson AD, Marshall EJ. The natural history and pathophysiology of Wernicke's encephalopathy and Korsakoff's psychosis. Alcohol 41.2 (2005): 151–158.
Thornalley PJ et al. High prevalence of low plasma thiamin concentration in diabetes linked to a marker of vascular disease. Diabetologia 50.10 (2007): 2164–2170.
Tjandra BS, Janknegt RA. Neurogenic impotence and lower urinary tract symptoms due to vitamin B_1 deficiency in chronic alcoholism. J Urol 157.3 (1997): 954–955.
Togay-Isikay C, et al. Wernicke's encephalopathy due to hyperemesis gravidarum: an under-recognised condition. Aust NZ J Obstet Gynaecol 41.4 (2001): 453–456.
Toth C, Voll C. Wernicke's encephalopathy following gastroplasty for morbid obesity. Can J Neurol Sci 28.1 (2001): 89–92.
Towbin, A., et al. Beri beri after gastric bypass surgery in adolescence. J Pediatr 2004; 145:263–7.
van Noort BA et al. Optic neuropathy from thiamin deficiency in a patient with ulcerative colitis. Doc Ophthalmol 67.1–2 (1987): 45–51.
Vortmeyer AO, et al. Haemorrhagic thiamin deficient encephalopathy following prolonged parenteral nutrition. J Neurol Neurosurg Psychiatry 55.9 (1992): 826–829.
Wahlqvist M et al. Food and nutrition. Sydney: Allen & Unwin, 2002.
Walker J & Kepner A. Wernicke's encephalopathy presenting as acute psychosis after gastric bypass. The Journal of Emergency Medicine, Vol 43, No 5, pp. 811–814, 2012.
Wang, D. and Hazell, A. S. Microglial activation is a major contributor to neurologic dysfunction in thiamin deficiency. Biochemical and Biophysical Research Communications (2010). 402, 123–128.
Wardlaw G et al. Contemporary nutrition. 3rd edn. Brown and Benchmark, Dubuque, 1997.
Welsh A. Hyperemesis, gastrointestinal and liver disorders in pregnancy. Curr Obstet Gynaecol 15.2 (2005): 123–131.
Woelk H, et al. Benfotiamine in treatment of alcoholic polyneuropathy: an 8-week randomized controlled study (BAP I study). Alcohol and Alcoholism 1998;33(6):631–8.
Zak J III et al. Dry beriberi: unusual complication of prolonged parenteral nutrition. J Parenter Enteral Nutr 15.2 (1991): 200–201.

Vitamin B_2 — riboflavin

BACKGROUND AND RELEVANT PHARMACOKINETICS

Riboflavin was first discovered in 1917 and was originally referred to as vitamin G in the United States. Its name reflects both its structure and colour: *ribo* refers to the presence of a ribose-like side chain, and *flavus* is Latin for yellow (Gropper & Smith 2013). Structurally, it consists of a flavin isoalloxazine ring and a sugar alcohol side chain, ribitol.

Riboflavin is a water-soluble B group vitamin that is sensitive to light (including sunlight) and alkali conditions. It is resistant to heat, oxidation and acid; therefore most means of sterilisation, canning and cooking do not affect the riboflavin content of foods (Combs 2012).

Dietary B_2 occurs in three forms: flavin adenine dinucleotide (FAD), flavin mononucleotide (FMN) and riboflavin phosphate (see Food sources section, below). Prior to absorption these forms must all be freed to riboflavin, which requires specific gastrointestinal phosphatase enzymes for these conversions.

Riboflavin uptake occurs mainly in the proximal part of the small intestine and involves a specialised, saturable, energy-dependent, Na^+-independent carrier-mediated system, riboflavin transporter 2 (RFT2). Adaptive changes alter the number and/or activity of carriers, e.g. when large pharmacological doses of riboflavin are ingested, absorption occurs via simple diffusion. Approximately 95% of riboflavin from food is absorbed (Food and Nutrition Board 1998). There is evidence that bioavailability is optimal at 25 mg peak plasma levels, and doses in excess of this are poorly absorbed.

Absorption is enhanced by the presence of bile and the consumption of fresh foods and impeded by the presence of divalent metals (zinc, iron, copper and manganese), whereas alcohol has an inhibitory effect.

Once absorbed, much of the riboflavin is converted back into one of its active forms, as a component of two primary coenzymes, FAD (40%) and FMN (10%). Both of these belong to the class known as the flavin coenzymes (flavoenzymes, flavoproteins), which are active in redox reactions involving hydrogen transfer and consequently important for the body's energy production. The various forms are transported in blood by plasma proteins, including albumin, fibrinogen and immunoglobulins (Gropper & Smith 2013). Free riboflavin is the form that crosses most cell membranes and, in the case of the liver, calcium or calmodulin regulates riboflavin uptake. The liver, kidneys and heart contain the greatest concentrations of riboflavin.

FOOD SOURCES

There are two sources of riboflavin: dietary and bacterial; the latter, produced by normal gastrointestinal microflora, is dependent upon the type of diet consumed, with higher synthesis resulting from intake of vegetable-based diets than from meat-based diets (Said 2004).

Riboflavin is found in a wide variety of foods, especially those of animal origin. Milk and milk products such as cheese are thought to contribute the most dietary riboflavin, providing about one-half of total intake (Combs 2012, Gropper & Smith 2013). Other main food sources are organ meats, especially liver, eggs, legumes, yeast products (including Vegemite), almonds, wheatgerm, wild rice and mushrooms. It is also found to a lesser extent in fruits, vegetables and cereal grains. Refined grains are enriched with riboflavin due to its loss from the milling process that removes the bran and germ, resulting in a loss of about two-thirds of the riboflavin content (Gropper & Smith 2013). Maximum loss during cooking is 75% (Wahlqvist 2002).

Milk, eggs and enriched cereal grains contain either free or protein-bound riboflavin, while in most other foods it predominantly exists as its coenzyme derivatives or phosphorus-bound riboflavin.

DEFICIENCY SIGNS AND SYMPTOMS

Acute deficiency of riboflavin, known as ariboflavinosis, seldom occurs in isolation and is usually associated with a deficiency of other B group vitamins (Gropper & Smith 2013).

Primary deficiency

Primary deficiency is associated with inadequate dietary intake, such as vegetarianism and poor consumption of milk and other animal products (Combs 2012). Primary deficiency is reported to be more common in the elderly and adolescent girls.

Secondary deficiency

Secondary deficiencies can develop in chronic diarrhoea, liver disease, chronic alcoholism, alcohol and drug use, including use of the oral contraceptive pill, adrenal or thyroid hormone insufficiency, hyperthyroid, anorexia nervosa and postoperative situations in which total parenteral nutrition solutions lack riboflavin. In most cases, riboflavin deficiency is accompanied by other vitamin deficiencies, such as deficiencies of vitamin B_6, niacin and folic acid. Drugs that impair riboflavin absorption or utilisation by inhibiting the conversion of the vitamin to the active coenzymes include tricyclic antidepressants, chemotherapy drugs and psychotropic agents. There is also evidence suggesting an apparent increase in riboflavin requirements with increased physical exercise.

Signs and symptoms of deficiency

The body's 'storage capacity' is sufficient to provide riboflavin for 2–6 weeks when riboflavin is inadequate.

Initial symptoms of riboflavin deficiency are often non-specific and include weakness, fatigue, mouth pain, angular stomatitis, cheilosis and personality changes. In animals, general signs of anorexia, impaired growth and reduced efficiency of feed utilisation have occurred.

Clinical symptoms of deficiency appear after 3–4 months of inadequate intake. Because of the fundamental role of riboflavin in metabolism, deficiency manifestations initially occur in tissues with high and rapid cellular turnover, such as epithelial tissue and skin (Combs 2012). This will account for many of the early deficiency signs, including:

- Angular stomatitis, cold sores and cheilosis
- Glossitis (inflammation of the tongue), magenta tongue (Lo 1984)
- Red or bloody (hyperaemic) and swollen (oedematous) mouth or oral cavity
- Failure to grow in children
- Ocular and visual disturbances, with symptoms such as burning, itching, sensitivity to light and conjunctivitis

- Scaly and greasy dermatitis affecting the nasolabial folds, ears, eyelids, scrotum and labia majora (Lo 1984)
- Inflammatory skin conditions — desquamative dermatitis, seborrhoeic dermatitis
- Hair loss
- Poor wound healing
- Anaemia
- Peripheral nerve dysfunction (neuropathy).

MAIN ACTIONS

Riboflavin is involved in many different biological processes and is essential for maintaining health. The flavoproteins are central to carbohydrate, protein and lipid metabolism, are involved in adenosine triphosphate production, and are essential for immune function, tissue repair processes and general growth (required for the healthy growth of skin, nails and hair). Riboflavin extends the life of red blood cells and plays a key role in fatty acid oxidation and the metabolism of several other B vitamins. In particular, riboflavin activates vitamin B_6 and folate, which are essential cofactors in neurotransmitter formation and metabolism (Gropper & Smith 2013).

Coenzyme functions

Riboflavin exerts its functions as two flavin enzymes (flavoenzymes), FAD and FMN. These coenzymes are essential in carbohydrate, amino acid and lipid metabolism.

Flavoenzymes exhibit a range of redox potentials, acting as oxidising agents because of their ability to accept a pair of hydrogen atoms (Gropper & Smith 2013). Consequently, FMN and FAD function as coenzymes in cellular antioxidant protection and for a variety of oxidative enzyme systems (Combs 2012). Riboflavin increases intracellular levels of reduced glutathione (an essential antioxidant in itself) and maintains the glutathione redox cycle as part of the FAD-dependent enzyme glutathione reductase (Combs 2012). Other flavoproteins provide reducing equivalents to neutralise reactive oxygen species (free radicals).

CLINICAL USE

A number of clinical trials have been conducted in which patients presenting with different conditions have subsequently been found to have riboflavin deficiency. Treating the deficiency in some of these cases has been shown to improve the initial presenting condition.

Wound healing

Riboflavin deficiency lengthens the time to epithelialisation of wounds, slows the rate of wound contraction and reduces the tensile strength of incision wounds in vivo. Total collagen content is also significantly decreased, suggesting riboflavin deficiency will slow down wound-healing rate (Lakshmi et al 1989).

Migraine headaches: prophylaxis

Three clinical studies of varying design have found that treatment with high-dose riboflavin (400 mg) can reduce the frequency of migraines; however, one double-blind study that used it in combination with magnesium and feverfew failed to show any superior effects over low-dose riboflavin (25 mg) alone.

The first was an open pilot study testing the effects of 400 mg riboflavin over 3 months in 49 patients. The mean global improvement after therapy was 68.2% (Schoenen et al 1994). Based on these results, a second study with 55 subjects was conducted using a 3-month, randomised, placebo-controlled design, with similar positive findings (Schoenen et al 1998). Riboflavin treatment produced positive results, with 59% of the treatment group experiencing a reduction in migraine frequency of at least 50%. Using an intention-to-treat analysis, riboflavin was superior to placebo in reducing attack frequency ($P = 0.005$) and headache days ($P = 0.012$) and the number needed to treat for effectiveness was 2.3. More recently, a 2004 open-label study retested the same high dose of vitamin B_2 over 6 months, once again producing a significant reduction in headache frequency, from 4 days/month at baseline to 2 days/month after 3 and 6 months of treatment ($P < 0.05$). Use of abortive drugs reduced from 7 units/month to 4.5 units/month; however, the duration and intensity of each episode did not change significantly (Boehnke et al 2004).

Finally, a randomised, double-blind, controlled study using a combination of vitamin B_2 (400 mg), magnesium (300 mg) and feverfew (100 mg) failed to show benefits over riboflavin 25 mg alone, with both groups experiencing comparable significant reductions in number of migraines, migraine day and migraine index; however, in neither group was frequency successfully reduced by more than 50%, which was the primary outcome (Maizels et al 2004). Interestingly, the response obtained was greater than the placebo response reported in other migraine prophylaxis trials.

A Cochrane review intervention protocol (Exposito et al 2009) states there is no single theory or hypothesis that can explain all the phenomena that occur with migraines; therefore the manner in which riboflavin might prevent migraine headaches is also not clear (Bajwa & Sabahat 2008, as cited in Exposito et al 2009). Despite this, it is frequently suggested that where mitochondrial dysfunction and impaired metabolism are causal in migraine pathogenesis, riboflavin appears to be useful in its management (Maizels et al 2004, Markley 2012, Sandor 2005, Schoenen et al 1998). High-dose riboflavin assists in promoting cellular mitochondrial metabolism, thereby improving some headache symptomatology (Woolhouse 2005). These studies are important, as riboflavin displays high tolerance with a high index of safety and relatively few side effects.

Migraine prophylaxis in children

The first study to evaluate the efficacy of riboflavin for migraine prophylaxis in children was a randomised, double-blind study of 200 mg/day versus placebo in 48 children. No differences were found in primary efficacy measure (number of patients achieving a 50% or greater reduction in the number of migraine attacks per 4 weeks) nor secondary outcome measures (mean severity of migraine per day, mean duration of migraine, days with nausea or vomiting, analgesic use and adverse effects). The authors concluded that riboflavin is not an effective therapy for preventing migraine in children. A high placebo responder rate was also seen, with implications for other studies of paediatric migraine (MacLennan et al 2008). Similar negative findings were produced in another small study by Bruijn et al (2010); however, the authors did find a significant difference ($P = 0.04$) in the reduction of mean frequency of tension-type headaches in favour of riboflavin treatment.

A retrospective study of migraine prophylaxis in 41 paediatric and adolescent patients, who received higher riboflavin doses (200 or 400 mg/day for 3, 4 or 6 months), however, reported significantly decreased attack frequency and intensity ($P < 0.01$) during treatment. Additionally, during follow-up, 68.4% of cases had a 50% or greater reduction in frequency of attacks and 21% in intensity. The authors concluded riboflavin to be a well-tolerated, effective and low-cost prophylactic treatment in children and adolescents suffering from migraine (Condo et al 2009).

From these studies, it is perhaps evident that riboflavin has a positive prophylaxis effect in the reduction of attack frequency and intensity with higher doses (200–400 mg) combined with longer treatment times (more than 4 weeks). The effect of taking a daily riboflavin supplement from the adult studies was maximal after 3 months (Breen 2003). It would suggest further studies of longer duration are required.

> ***Clinical note — Causes of migraine***
>
> Numerous theories exist to explain the underlying pathology of migraine headache. One theory proposes a deficit of mitochondrial energy metabolism, as patients with migraine show decreased brain mitochondrial energy reserve between attacks. Interestingly, patients with mitochondrial encephalomyopathy, lactic acidosis and stroke-like episodes (MELAS) exhibit impaired mitochondrial energy metabolism, producing migraine-like headaches, which are in part ameliorated by prophylactic B_2 (Magis et al 2007).
>
> Accordingly, riboflavin coenzyme Q10 and lipoic acid, as enhancers of mitochondrial energy efficiency, have been tested for prophylactic activity in migraine and appear to be promising agents (Magis et al 2007, Markley 2012, Schoenen et al 1994). Recent studies in experimental models add to our knowledge of the actions of riboflavin in migraine, with confirmation that it produces antinociception and anti-inflammatory effects. The analgesic activity observed is independent of opioid mechanisms (Granados-Soto et al 2004).

> ***Clinical note — Age-related cataract and antioxidants***
>
> Age-related cataract is an important public health problem, because approximately 50% of the 30–50 million cases of blindness worldwide result from leaving the condition untreated (Jacques 1999). The mechanisms that bring about a loss in transparency include oxidation, osmotic stress and chemical adduct formation (Bunce et al 1990). Besides traditional risk factors such as diabetes, nutrient deficiency is also being considered, particularly nutrients with antioxidant properties.

Comparative trial

A 4-month clinical trial comparing riboflavin supplementation (400 mg/day) with beta-adrenergic antagonists (metoprolol 200 mg/day and bisoprolol 10 mg/day) found that both treatments significantly decreased the frequency of migraine headache and improved the clinical symptoms of migraine headache (Sandor et al 2000). Analysis of their effects on cortical potentials showed that the two treatments achieve these results by working through different mechanisms.

Age-related cataract prevention

Cataract was shown to be associated with riboflavin deficiency in animals in the 1930s and subsequently with deficiencies of amino acids, vitamins and some minerals (Wynn & Wynn 1996). This has been confirmed in human studies, in which lens opacities have been associated with lower levels of riboflavin, vitamins A, C and E, iron and protein status (Leske et al 1995, Mares-Perlman et al 1995).

Glutathione reductase is a key enzyme involved in lens protection. Riboflavin levels indirectly influence glutathione reductase activity, increasing the ability of the lens to deal with free radical formation (Head 2001). One study documented severe glutathione reductase deficiency in 23% of human lens epithelium specimens, possibly reflecting a dietary deficiency of riboflavin (Straatsma et al 1991). Another study found that a significant number of people with cataracts have inactive epithelial glutathione reductase (Horwitz et al 1987).

A large cross-sectional survey of 2873 volunteers aged 49–97 years detected a link between dietary vitamin supplement and a lower incidence of both nuclear and cortical cataract. Vitamin A, niacin, riboflavin, thiamine, folate and vitamin B_{12} all appeared to be protective, either in isolation or as constituents of multivitamin preparations (Kuzniarz et al 2001).

A sample of 408 women from the Nurses' Health Study aged 52–74 years at baseline participated in a 5-year study that assessed nutrient intake and the degree of nuclear density (opacification). Findings revealed that the geometric mean 5-year change in nuclear density was inversely associated with the intake of riboflavin (P = 0.03) and thiamin (P = 0.04), and most significantly with the duration of vitamin E supplement use (P = 0.006) (Jacques et al 2005).

The evidence currently suggests that higher intakes of riboflavin protect against the progression of age-related lens opacification.

Congestive heart failure

A recent review of micronutrients in heart failure summarised several observational studies investigating riboflavin status (McKeag et al 2012). While the authors state the results are inconclusive, one recent study they included produced significant findings. This study measured riboflavin and pyridoxine levels in 100 patients with heart failure (as defined by Framingham criteria). The percentage of individuals with evidence of riboflavin deficiency was 27% (erythrocyte gluthathione reductase activity coefficient >1.2) and this was significantly higher in patients with heart failure compared with controls (27.0% vs 2.2%; P = 0.001) (Keith et al 2009). More research needs to be conducted in this area to determine if this could be a cause or consequence of the disease.

> ***Clinical note — Vitamin B_2 deficiency and protracted malaria recovery?***
>
> In a study of 35 of 64 children suffering malarial infection, riboflavin was assessed by measuring erythrocyte glutathione reductase activity (Das et al 1988). Interestingly, in the riboflavin-deficient group, the median parasite count was in fact lower than the non-deficient group; however, the correlation between activity coefficient and parasite count was significant (R = −0.49). Therefore the recovery process was slower in the deficient group, even though they had a relatively lower parasite count. The authors have thus inferred that riboflavin deficiency leads to inhibition of growth and multiplication of plasmodia. Its beneficial effects in malaria infection need further evaluation.

Anticarcinogenesis

Riboflavin deficiency may cause protein and DNA damage and prevent cellular differentiation in the G1 phase of cellular division, according to cell culture studies (Manthey et al 2006, as cited by Gropper & Smith 2013).

Riboflavin deficiency has been reported to enhance carcinogenesis (Combs 2012). In a rat study the formation of single-strand breaks in nuclear DNA was more pronounced on a riboflavin-deficient diet compared to that on a normal diet (Webster et al 1973). The introduction of riboflavin reversed this trend. The authors suggest that, as DNA damage and its altered repair may relate to carcinogenesis, modulation of these parameters by riboflavin suggests a potential chemopreventive role for this vitamin.

The proposed mechanism of action is that a decrease in riboflavin produces a reduction in antioxidant protection, increasing the activation of carcinogens and oxidative DNA damage. While clinical data relative to this possibility are few, recently an inverse relationship has been found between riboflavin status and cancer risk in three observational studies (de Vogel et al 2008 as cited by Combs 2012). The cancers were specifically oesophageal squamous cell cancer and colorectal cancer. More research is required in these areas.

Breast cancer

The majority of studies investigating the protective role of B vitamins in breast cancer have focused on folate, B_6 and B_{12}. Several case-controlled studies have reported protective associations (Chen et al 2005, Lajous et al 2006, Larsson et al 2007, Yang et al 2013), while cohort studies have shown inconsistent results (Cho et al 2007, Ericson et al 2007, Shrubsole et al 2011, Stevens et al 2010). Two of these studies also included an investigation of the role of riboflavin and found no risk reduction with B_2 (Shrubsole et al 2011, Yang et al 2013).

Breast cancer — adjunctive treatment to tamoxifen

Riboflavin's importance is recognised in a range of terminal disease states, most notably in breast cancer, where its cellular absorption is significantly enhanced (Bareford et al 2008). Based on its established antioxidant properties, its role in maintaining epithelial integrity, and its influence on prostaglandin synthesis and glutathione metabolism (Premkumar et al 2008a), vitamin B_2 (10 mg) has been tested in combination with coenzyme Q10 (100 mg) and niacin (50 mg) (known as CORN) together with tamoxifen in breast cancer patients. The results have consistently demonstrated augmenting actions — enhanced manganese superoxide dismutase expression, resulting in prevention of cancer cell proliferation (Premkumar et al 2008b), reduction of lipid peroxides (which are elevated in breast cancer and associated with tumour promotion) (Yuvaraj et al 2008), reduced tumour markers carcinoembryonic antigen (CEA) and CA15-3 and reduced serum cytokines (interleukin-1 [IL-1]-beta, IL-6, IL-8, tumour necrosis factor-alpha and vascular endothelial growth factor) (Premkumar et al 2008a). In addition to this, CORN supplementation reduced proangiogenic markers, with a corresponding increase in antiangiogenic markers. Given that the growth and metastasising capacity of any tumour (but particularly of breast tumours) are dependent upon angiogenesis, this could represent a means to improved prognoses (Premkumar et al 2008a). Finally, CORN supplementation was shown to moderate some of the negative side effects of tamoxifen treatment, with normalisation of lipid and lipoproteins following 90 days of treatment in postmenopausal breast cancer patients (Yuvaraj et al 2007).

Clinical note — Riboflavin carrier protein: a new marker to predict breast cancer

Interestingly, studies have shown that riboflavin carrier protein (RCP), an oestrogen-inducible protein that occupies a key position in riboflavin metabolism, is elevated in women with breast cancer. Oestrogen-inducible proteins such as RCP are upregulated and secreted into circulation in animal models and in women with neoplastic breast disease (Karande et al 2001). In a prospective blinded study, serum RCP levels were significantly elevated in women with breast cancer (n = 52) as compared with control subjects (n = 50; 6.06 ± 7.27 ng/mL vs 0.70 ± 0.19 ng/mL [mean ± SD], respectively; P < 0.0001). Furthermore, a serum RCP level of ≥1.0 ng/mL was highly predictive of the presence of breast cancer, detecting 88% of tumours in stages I–II and 100% of tumours in stages III–IV (Rao et al 1999). In another double-blind study, pre- and postmenopausal women with clinically diagnosed early and advanced breast cancer were compared with controls. This study also revealed that serum RCP levels in cycling breast cancer patients were three- to fourfold higher (P < 0.01) than in normal counterparts (Karande et al 2001). This difference in circulatory RCP levels is further magnified to nine- to 11-fold (P < 0.005) at the postmenopausal stage. Additionally, rising RCP levels are positively correlated with disease progression, as significantly higher RCP concentrations (P < 0.005) are encountered in patients with advanced (compared with early) metastasising breast cancer. A more recent study also noted elevated levels of RCP in breast cancer pathways, and the authors suggest it as a new marker to predict early-stage breast cancer (Shigemizu et al 2012). The current research is not suggesting any clear role, either preventive or causative, of riboflavin and breast cancer.

Role in folate and pyridoxine metabolism and the methylation pathologies

Effective one-carbon metabolism relies on nutrients beyond folate, B_6 and B_{12} — most notably B_2, which, although attracting significantly less research attention, is critical. Riboflavin, as FAD, is the cofactor for methylenetetrahydrofolate reductase (MTHFR), a key enzyme of the folate activation pathway, catalysing the interconversion of 5,10-methylene tetrahydrofolate and 5-methyltetrahydrofolate-converting folate into its active form (Bates 2013, Powers 2003, 2005, Sharp et al 2008). Consistent with this, there is emerging evidence of substantial interplay between folate and riboflavin in conditions previously associated principally with folate deficiency or ameliorated by folate treatment. For example, plasma levels of vitamin B_2 and homocysteine have been shown to correlate; that is, high homocysteine levels have in fact been found to be low in subjects with low riboflavin status (Combs 2012, de Vogel et al 2008, Ganji & Kafai 2004), especially in individuals with the MTHFR C677TT genotype (McNulty et al 2006).

Of several single-nucleotide polymorphisms affecting MTHFR, the best known are the C699T and A1298C variants. The first displays thermolability and lowered reductase activity exaggerated by the loss of FAD cofactor (Allen & Prentice 2013). Preliminary studies employing combinations of folate (400 mcg) and riboflavin (5 mg) have demonstrated improved efficacy over folate alone, for example in colorectal cancer (Powers 2005).

Additionally, high doses of folate alone have been reported to modestly but significantly reduce vitamin B_2 levels (Powers 2005). Taken together with the knowledge that riboflavin is central to pyridoxine metabolism (McCormick 2000), there is growing interest in the therapeutic potential of riboflavin in pathologies associated with poor methylation.

Fertility and pregnancy

Fetal and embyronic development require adequate riboflavin status (Karande et al 2001). In a 2010 study of mice, low dietary riboflavin status negatively affected embryonic growth and cardiac development (Chan et al 2010), with a greater incidence of delayed embryos and lower embryonic weights (P < 0.05, two-factor analysis of variance). The number of embryos with ventricular septal defects was significantly greater in the riboflavin-deficient mice (P < 0.005, Fisher's exact test).

Similarly, in humans, a case-controlled family study of 276 mothers of children with congenital heart defects has shown that mothers consuming a diet high in saturated fat and low riboflavin and niacin during the preconception period markedly increased the risk of congenital heart defects in the offspring (Smedts et al 2008). Thus, it has been extrapolated that ensuring adequate riboflavin status during preconception and pregnancy may prevent such complications.

A prospective cohort study of 1461 pregnancies found that low-birth-weight offspring are more common in women consuming diets low in vitamin C, riboflavin, pantothenic acid and sugars, even after adjustment for deprivation index, smoking, marital status and parity (Haggarty et al 2009).

Postpartum depression (PPD)

A prospective study of 865 Japanese women investigated the role of riboflavin consumption during pregnancy with risk of PPD (Miyake et al 2006). In this study, PPD was identified when subjects had an Edinburgh Postnatal Depression Scale score of ≥9 between 2 and 9 months postpartum. A total of 121 developed PPD and the results indicated that riboflavin adequacy reduced the risk of PPD (multivariate odds ratio 0.53, 95% confidence interval 0.29–0.95, P_{trend} = 0.55). The authors concluded that moderate consumption of riboflavin may be protective, e.g. 10–50 mg/day.

Pre-eclampsia

In a prospective study, 154 women at increased risk of pre-eclampsia were observed until delivery (Wacker et al 2000). Riboflavin deficiency was consistently found in 33.8%. The incidence of deficiency rose towards the end of the pregnancy, from 27.3% at 29–36 weeks' gestation compared with 53.3% at over 36 weeks. In the riboflavin-deficient group, mothers were 28.8% more likely to develop pre-eclampsia than in the riboflavin-adequate group (7.8%; $P < 0.001$, odds ratio 4.7). The authors concluded that riboflavin deficiency should be considered a possible risk factor for pre-eclampsia.

However, these results were not duplicated in a randomised, placebo-controlled, double-blind trial where a protective effect was not demonstrated in high-risk pregnant women supplemented with 15 mg of riboflavin (Neugebauer et al 2006). Such variability in results may be due to differences in study design and, in this study, the supplemental dose may be inadequate given that therapeutic levels of riboflavin ranges are 10–200 mg.

Sickle cell anaemia

Riboflavin supplementation (5 mg twice daily for 8 weeks) in patients with sickle cell anaemia resulted in improved haematological measurements compared with controls, suggesting that riboflavin enhances erythropoiesis (Ajayi et al 1993).

Rheumatoid arthritis

One study has suggested that patients with higher pain scores and active disease are at significantly greater risk of riboflavin deficiency than those with inactive disease (Mulherin et al 1996). In this study of 91 patients, pain score, articular index, C-reactive protein and erythrocyte sedimentation rate were all increased in those patients exhibiting riboflavin deficiency (all $P < 0.02$). It is unclear whether riboflavin deficiency influences pain threshold or is a result of the disease.

Osteoarthritis

B vitamins were investigated for reducing sensitivity to painful stimuli in mice (Franca et al 2001), whereby thiamin and pyridoxine (50–200 mg/kg, intraperitoneally [IP]) or riboflavin (3–100 mg/kg IP) induced an antinociceptive effect, not changed by naloxone (10 mg/kg IP). The authors state the B vitamins' antinociceptive effect may involve inhibition of the synthesis and/or action of inflammatory mediators. Furthermore, in an animal study the therapeutic effects of glucosamine hydrochloride and chondroitin sulfate as chondroprotective were enhanced by the addition of fursultiamine, a thiamine derivative, in the treatment of osteoarthritis (Kobayashi et al 2005).

OTHER USES

Riboflavin is also used to treat carpal tunnel syndrome and acne, although only case reports are available (Folkers et al 1984).

HIV/AIDS

A decreased progression of HIV to AIDS has been found in patients replete with vitamins B and C (Tang et al 1993).

DOSAGE RANGE

- Migraine prevention: 400 mg/day, taken for at least 3 months.
- Treating deficiency states: 10–20 mg/day until symptoms resolve or B_2 assays improve.
- Therapeutic levels: 10–200 mg/day.
- As an adjunct to tamoxifen in breast cancer treatment: 10 mg/day together with coenzyme Q10 100 mg/day and niacin 50 mg/day — based on preliminary evidence.
- Postpartum depression: 10–50 mg/day may be protective in at risk women.

Australian recommended dietary intake

<70 years

- Women: 1.1 mg/day.
- Men: 1.3 mg/day.

>70 years

- Women: 1.3 mg/day.
- Men: 1.6 mg/day.

Intake of vitamin B_2 causes a characteristic bright yellow-orange discolouration to urine.

TOXICITY

Riboflavin is considered an extremely safe supplement. Even at the high doses (e.g. 400 mg) used in some trials, no adverse effects are noted and riboflavin remains non-toxic.

ADVERSE REACTIONS

General side effects noted in trials using high doses were reasonably uncommon, but included diarrhoea and polyuria (Bianchi et al 2004). One case of anaphylaxis has been reported (Ou et al 2001).

SIGNIFICANT INTERACTIONS

Certain medicines can increase the body's requirements for riboflavin.

Antibiotics

Antibiotic drugs can reduce endogenous production of B group vitamins — increase intake of vitamin B_2.

Oral contraceptive pill

The oral contraceptive pill may increase demand for vitamin B_2 (Pelton et al 2000) — consider increasing intake with long-term use.

Tricyclic antidepressants

Reduce the absorption of riboflavin — may increase riboflavin requirements (Pelton et al 2000).

Amitryptyline

Increases the renal excretion of riboflavin (Bianchi et al 2004) — consider increased dietary intake with long-term use.

CONTRAINDICATIONS AND PRECAUTIONS

None known.

PREGNANCY USE

Considered safe.

Practice points/Patient counselling

- Vitamin B_2 deficiency signs include poor wound healing, hair loss, greasy dermatitis, ocular disturbances, failure to grow in children, angular stomatitis, cold sores, cracked lips and magenta tongue.
- Besides inadequate intake, deficiency can also result from chronic diarrhoea, liver disease and chronic alcoholism.
- There is some evidence suggesting that high-dose supplements (400 mg daily) significantly reduce the frequency of migraine headaches.
- Preliminary evidence suggests that regular supplementation with a multivitamin may also reduce the risk of developing cataracts.
- Supplementation results in a characteristic yellow-orange discolouration of urine.

PATIENTS' FAQs

What will this vitamin do for me?

Vitamin B_2 is essential for health and is involved in many different biochemical processes in the body. Research has suggested that, when taken in high doses, it can significantly reduce the incidence of migraine headaches.

When will it start to work?

Deficiency is reversed rapidly with supplementation. If using riboflavin to prevent migraine headaches, 3–4 months' treatment is required to see significant effects.

Are there any safety issues?

The vitamin is considered a safe nutrient.

REFERENCES

Ajayi OA et al. Clinical trial of riboflavin in sickle cell disease. East Afr Med J 70.7 (1993): 418–421.

Allen L H & Prentice A. Encyclopedia of Human Nutrition (Third Edition) 2013. Amsterdam: Academic Press, Elsevier p. 162.

Bajwa ZH, Sabahat A. Pathophysiology, clinical manifestations, and diagnosis of migraine in adults. UpToDate 2008. Available at www.uptodate.com.

Bareford LM et al. Intracellular processing of riboflavin in human breast cancer cells. Mol Pharm 5.5 (2008): 839–848.

Bates CJ Encyclopedia of Human Nutrition. 3rd edn, Cambridge UK, 2013, pp. 158–165.

Bianchi A et al. Role of magnesium, coenzyme q10, riboflavin, and vitamin B_{12} in migraine prophylaxis. Vitamins Hormones 69 (2004): 297–312.

Boehnke C et al. High-dose riboflavin treatment is efficacious in migraine prophylaxis: an open study in a tertiary care centre. Eur J Neurol 11.7 (2004): 475–477.

Breen C. High dose riboflavin for prophylaxis of migraine. Can Fam Physician 2003;49:1291–3.

Bruijn J, et al. Medium-dose riboflavin as a prophylactic agent in children with migraine: A preliminary placebo-controlled, randomized, double-blind, cross-over trial. Cephalalgia December 2010 vol. 30 no. 12 1426–1434.

Bunce GE et al. Nutritional factors in cataract. Annu Rev Nutr 10 (1990): 233–254.

Chen J, et al. (2005) One-carbon metabolism, MTHFR polymorphisms, and risk of breast cancer. Cancer Res 65: 1606–1614.

Cho E, et al (2007) Nutrients involved in one-carbon metabolism and risk of breast cancer among premenopausal women. Cancer Epidemiology, Biomarkers & Prevention 16: 2787–2790.

Combs G. The Vitamins: Considering the Individual Vitamins. London: Elsevier 2012 pp 277–289.

Condo M, et al. Riboflavin prophylaxis in pediatric and adolescent migraine. J Headache Pain 2009 Oct;10(5):361–5.

Das BS, et al. Riboflavin deficiency and severity of malaria. Eur J Clin Nutr. 1988 Apr;42(4):277–83.

De Vogel S et al. Dietary folate, methionine, riboflavin, and vitamin B-6 and risk of sporadic colorectal cancer. J Nutr 138.12 (2008): 2372–2378.

Ericson U, et al (2007) High folate intake is associated with lower breast cancer incidence in postmenopausal women in the Malmo Diet and Cancer cohort [see comment]. Am J Clin Nutr 86: 434–443.

Exposito JA, et al. Riboflavin (vitamin B_2) for the prevention of migraine (Protocol). Cochrane Database of Systematic Reviews 2009, Issue 3. Art. No.: CD007889.

Folkers K et al. Enzymology of the response of the carpal tunnel syndrome to riboflavin and to combined riboflavin and pyridoxine. Proc Natl Acad Sci USA 81.22 (1984): 7076–7078.

Food and Nutrition Board. Dietary reference intakes for thiamin, riboflavin, niacin, vitamin B_6, folate, vitamin B_{12}, pantothenic acid, biotin and choline. Washington DC: National Academy Press, 1998 pp 87–122.

Franca DS., et al. B vitamins induce an antinociceptive effect in the acetic acid and formaldehyde models of nociception in mice. European Journal of Pharmacology Volume 421, Issue 3, 15 June 2001, Pages 157–164.

Granados-Soto V et al. Riboflavin reduces hyperalgesia and inflammation but not tactile allodynia in the rat. Eur J Pharmacol 492.1 (2004): 35–40.

Gropper, S., Smith, J Advanced Nutrition and Human Metabolism, 6th Edition. Belmont CA: Wadsworth, Cengage Learning, 2013.

Haggarty P, et al. Diet and deprivation in pregnancy. British Journal of Nutrition (2009), 102, 1487–1497.

Head KA. Natural therapies for ocular disorders, part two: cataracts and glaucoma. Altern Med Rev 6.2 (2001): 141–166.

Horwitz J et al. Glutathione reductase in human lens epithelium: FAD induced in vitro activation. Curr Eye Res 6.10 (1987): 1249–1256.

Jacques PF. The potential preventive effects of vitamins for cataract and age-related macular degeneration. Int J Vitam Nutr Res 69.3 (1999): 198–205.

Jacques PF et al. Long-term nutrient intake and 5-year change in nuclear lens opacities. Arch Ophthalmol 123.4 (2005): 517–526.

Karande A A, et al. Riboflavin carrier protein: A serum and tissue marker for breast carcinoma. International Journal of Cancer 2001; 95:277–281.

Keith ME, et al. B-vitamin deficiency in hospitalized patients with heart failure. J Am Diet Assoc. 2009;109(8): 1406–1410.

Kuzniarz M et al. Use of vitamin supplements and cataract: the Blue Mountains Eye Study. Am J Ophthalmol 132.1 (2001): 19–26.

Lajous M, et al (2006) Folate, vitamin B_6, and vitamin B_{12} intake and the risk of breast cancer among Mexican women. Cancer Epidemiol Biomarkers Prev 15: 443–448.

V

Lakshmi R et al. Skin wound healing in riboflavin deficiency. Biochem Med Metab Biol 42.3 (1989): 185–191.
Larsson SC, et al (2007) Folate and risk of breast cancer: a meta-analysis. J Natl Cancer Inst 99: 64–76.
Leske MC et al. Biochemical factors in the lens opacities: Case-control study (The Lens Opacities Case-Control Study Group). Arch Ophthalmol 113.9 (1995): 1113–11119.
Lo CS. Riboflavin status of adolescents in southern China: Average intake of riboflavin and clinical findings. Med J Aust 141.10 (1984): 635 637.
MacLennan SC, et al. High-dose riboflavin for migraine prophylaxis in children: a double-blind, randomized, placebo-controlled trial. Child Neurol November 2008 vol. 23 no. 11 1300–1304.
Magis D et al. A randomized double-blind placebo-controlled trial of thioctic acid in migraine prophylaxis. Headache 47.1 (2007): 52–57.
Maizels M et al. A combination of riboflavin, magnesium, and feverfew for migraine prophylaxis: a randomized trial. Headache 44.9 (2004): 885–890.
Manthey K, et al. Riboflavin deficiency causes protein and DNA damage in HepG2 cells, triggering arrest in G1 phase of the cell cycle. J Nutr Biochem, 2006 17:250–256.
Mares-Perlman JA et al. Diet and nuclear lens opacities. Am J Epidemiol 141.4 (1995): 322–334.
Markley HG. CoEnzyme Q10 and riboflavin: the mitochondrial connection. Headache: The Journal of Head and Face Pain 2012 52(2):81–87.
McCormick DB. A trail of research on cofactors: an odyssey with friends. J Nutr 130 (2S Suppl) (2000): 323S–330S.
McKeag NA., et al. The role of micronutrients in heart failure. Journal of the Academy of Nutrition and Dietetics, 2012; 112: 870–886.
McNulty H et al. Riboflavin lowers homocysteine in individuals homozygous for the MTHFR 677C →T polymorphism. Circulation 113.1 (2006): 74–80.
Miyake Y, et al. Dietary folate and vitamins B_{12}, B_6, and B_2 intake and the risk of postpartum depression in Japan: The Osaka Maternal and Child Health Study. Journal of affective disorders 2006:96(1–2): 133–138.
Mulherin DM et al. Glutathione reductase activity, riboflavin status, and disease activity in rheumatoid arthritis. Ann Rheum Dis 55.11 (1996): 837–840.
Neugebauer J, et al. Riboflavin supplementation and pre-eclampsia. International Journal of Gynecology & Obstetrics 2006;92(2):136–7.
Ou LS et al. Anaphylaxis to riboflavin (vitamin B_2). Ann Allergy Asthma Immunol 87.5 (2001): 430–433.
Pelton R et al. Drug-induced nutrient depletion handbook 1999–2000. Hudson, OH: Lexi-Comp, 2000.
Powers HJ. Riboflavin (vitamin B_2) and health. Am J Clin Nutr 77.6 (2003): 1352–1360.
Powers HJ. Interaction among folate, riboflavin, genotype, and cancer, with reference to colorectal and cervical cancer. J Nutr 135 (12 Suppl) (2005): 2960S–6S.
Premkumar VG et al. Anti-angiogenic potential of coenzyme Q10, riboflavin and niacin in breast cancer patients undergoing tamoxifen therapy. Vascul Pharmacol 48.4–6 (2008a): 191–201.
Premkumar VG et al. Co-enzyme Q10, riboflavin and niacin supplementation on alteration of DNA repair enzyme and DNA methylation in breast cancer patients undergoing tamoxifen therapy. Br J Nutr 100.6 (2008b): 1179–82.
Rao PN, et al. Elevation of serum riboflavin carrier protein in breast cancer. Cancer Epidemiol Biomarkers Prev. 1999 Nov;8(11):985–90.
Said HM. Recent advances in carrier-mediated intestinal absorption of water-soluble vitamins. Annu Rev Physiol 66 (2004): 419–446.
Sandor PS et al. Prophylactic treatment of migraine with beta-blockers and riboflavin: differential effects on the intensity dependence of auditory evoked cortical potentials. Headache 40.1 (2000): 30–35.
Schoenen J et al. High-dose riboflavin as a prophylactic treatment of migraine: results of an open pilot study. Cephalalgia 14.5 (1994): 328–329.
Schoenen J et al. Effectiveness of high-dose riboflavin in migraine prophylaxis. A randomized controlled trial. Neurology 50.2 (1998): 466–470.
Sharp L et al. Polymorphisms in the methylenetetrahydrofolate reductase (MTHFR) gene, intakes of folate and related B vitamins and colorectal cancer: a case-control study in a population with relatively low folate intake. Br J Nutr 99.2 (2008): 379–389.
Shigemizu D, et al. (2012) Using functional signatures to identify repositioned drugs for breast, myelogenous leukemia and prostate cancer. PLoS Comput Biol 8(2): e1002347.
Shrubsole MJ, et al. Dietary B vitamin and methionine intakes and breast cancer risk among Chinese women.Am J Epidemiol. 2011 May 15;173(10):1171–82.
Smedts HP, et al. Maternal intake of fat, riboflavin and nicotinamide and the risk of having offspring with congenital heart defects. Eur J Nutr 2008;47(7):357–365.
Stevens VL, et al (2010) Folate and other one-carbon metabolism-related nutrients and risk of postmenopausal breast cancer in the Cancer Prevention Study II Nutrition Cohort. Am J Clin Nutr 91: 1708–1715.
Straatsma BR et al. Lens capsule and epithelium in age-related cataract. Am J Ophthalmol 112.3 (1991): 283–296.
Tang AM., et al. Dietary micronutrient intake and risk of progression to acquired immunodeficiency syndrome (AIDS) in human immunodeficiency virus type-1 (HIV-1) infected homosexual men. Am J Epidemiol 1993;138:937–51.
Wacker J et al. Riboflavin deficiency and preeclampsia. Obstet Gynecol 96.1 (2000): 38–44.
Wahlqvist M (ed) Food and nutrition. Sydney: Allen & Unwin, 2002.
Webster, R. P., et al. (1973). Modulation of carcinogen-induced DNA damage and repair enzyme activity by dietary riboflavin. Cancer Res. 33, 1997.
Woolhouse M. Migraine and tension headaches: a complementary and alternative medicine approach. Australian Family Physician 2005;34:647–51.
Wynn M, Wynn A. Can improved diet contribute to the prevention of cataract? Nutr Health 11.2 (1996): 87–104.
Yang D, et al. Dietary intake of folate, B-vitamins and methionine and breast cancer risk among Hispanic and non-Hispanic white women. 2013 PLoS ONE 8(2): e54495.
Yuvaraj S et al. Ameliorating effect of coenzyme Q10, riboflavin and niacin in tamoxifen-treated postmenopausal breast cancer patients with special reference to lipids and lipoproteins. Clin Biochem 40.9–10 (2007): 623–628.
Yuvaraj S et al. Augmented antioxidant status in tamoxifen treated postmenopausal women with breast cancer on co-administration with coenzyme Q10, niacin and riboflavin. Cancer Chemother Pharmacol May 61.6 (2008): 933–941.

Vitamin B_5 — pantothenic acid

BACKGROUND AND RELEVANT PHARMACOKINETICS

The Greek word *pantos* means 'everywhere'. As the name pantothenic acid implies, B_5 is widely distributed, present in nearly all plant and animal foods. Relatively unstable, it is sensitive to heat, freezing, canning and cooking and both acid and alkali, and considerable amounts are lost through the milling of cereal grains. The intestine is exposed to two sources of pantothenic acid: dietary and bacterial. Current research suggests that bacterial synthesis may be more dominant and important in ruminant species (Bates 1998).

Pantothenic acid is absorbed in the jejunum by passive diffusion at high concentrations, but at low concentrations it requires a sodium-dependent multivitamin transporter. Both biotin and lipoic acid share the multivitamin transporter. A study of placental tissue demonstrated that biotin uses the same transport mechanisms as pantothenic acid, which may indicate competition between these two nutrients in other tissues (Bates 1998).

Between 40% and 63% of pantothenic acid is bioavailable from the gastrointestinal tract, an amount that decreases to 10% when doses 10-fold greater than the recommended daily intake are taken (Gropper & Smith 2013). Rapid absorption seems to occur after oral doses, and increased tissue levels of coenzyme A (CoA) and other metabolites can occur within 6 hours. In leucocytes both CoA and pantothenic acid levels increase between 6 and 24 hours following oral ingestion (Kelly 2011).

In circulation, pantothenic acid is primarily found intracellularly in the red blood cells with a small amount in plasma. Organ uptake is via the same sodium-dependent multivitamin transporter and it is found as pantothenic acid, 4-phosphopantothenic acid and pantetheine in cells (Gropper & Smith 2013). The organ with the highest concentration of pantothenic acid is the liver, followed by the adrenal cortex, which reflects the large requirements of these tissues and is indicative of the biochemical role of the vitamin's coenzyme derivatives. There are contrasting opinions about whether a genuine storage capacity exists for this vitamin; however, if there is any at all, the consensus is that pantothenic acid is 'stored' in very limited amounts and in those tissues with the greatest requirements (Groff & Gropper 2009). Most pantothenic acid is used to synthesise or resynthesise CoA, which is found in high concentrations in the liver, adrenal gland, kidneys, brain and heart (Gropper & Smith 2013).

Following its absorption into cells, it can be converted to CoA or acyl carrier proteins (ACP), both of which are essential cofactors in fatty acid synthesis (Kelly 2011).

CHEMICAL COMPONENTS

Pantothenic acid is an amide and consists of β-alanine and pantoic acid joined by a peptide bond. In supplements, it is often found as calcium pantothenate.

FOOD SOURCES

The most concentrated sources are meats (especially liver), egg yolk, broad beans, legumes and potatoes, but it is also found in many other foods, such as whole grains, milk, peanuts, broccoli, avocado, mushroom and apricots. Royal jelly from bees also provides substantial amounts (Gropper & Smith 2013). Up to 50% can be lost through cooking (Wahlqvist 2002).

Approximately 85% occurs in food as a component of CoA, which is hydrolysed to pantothenic acid or pantethine during digestion.

DEFICIENCY SIGNS AND SYMPTOMS

Due to its widespread occurrence of pantothenate in foods, deficiencies are considered unlikely, and more often in conjunction with multiple nutrient deficiencies, as would occur in generalised malnutrition (Gropper & Smith 2013). Because pantothenic acid deficiency is so rare, most information regarding its signs and symptoms comes from experimental research in animals or cases of severe malnutrition. The deficiency picture appears to be generalised and species-specific (Bates 1998). Preliminary studies in humans using competitive analogues of pantothenic acid have produced the following symptoms:

- 'Burning feet syndrome': this affects the lower legs and is characterised by a sensation of heat (Gropper & Smith 2013, Kohlmeier 2003, Whitney 2011)
- Vomiting, fatigue, weakness, restlessness, dizziness, sleeplessness and irritability (Gropper & Smith 2013; Kohlmeier 2003)
- Neurological disturbances (Whitney et al 2011)
- Gastrointestinal disturbances, ulcers, abdominal distress (Hechtman 2012, Whitney et al 2011)
- Muscular weakness, burning cramps, paraesthesia (tingling sensation of toes and feet) (Hechtman 2012, Kohlmeier 2003)
- Loss of immune (antibody) function and increased susceptibility to infections (Kohlmeier 2003)
- Dermatitis, achromotrichia, alopecia (The Vitamins 2012)
- Adrenal hypofunction, with an inability to respond appropriately to stress. In late-stage deficiency, the adrenals atrophy and morphological damage occurs (Kelly 2011)
- Insensitivity to adrenocorticotrophic hormone
- Increased sensitivity to insulin.

Some conditions that have been associated with increased requirements are:

- Alcoholism (due to typically low intakes of vitamin B complex) (Gropper & Smith 2013)
- Diabetes mellitus (as a result of increased excretion) (Gropper & Smith 2013)
- Inflammatory bowel diseases (due to decreased vitamin absorption) (Gropper & Smith 2013).

MAIN ACTIONS

Pantothenic acid is involved in a myriad of important chemical reactions in the body as a result of its involvement in CoA and ACP.

Coenzyme function

CoA and the Krebs cycle

Numerous metabolic activities depend on adequate availability of pantothenate. Pantothenic acid is required for CoA synthesis and most pantothenate-dependent reactions use CoA as the universal donor and acceptor of acetyl and acyl groups (Kohlmeier 2003).

As part of CoA, pantothenate participates extensively in the metabolism of carbohydrate, lipids and protein (Gropper & Smith 2013). It plays a pivotal role in cellular respiration, the oxidation of fatty acids and acetylation of other molecules, so as to enable transportation. Together with thiamine, riboflavin and niacin, it is involved in the oxidative decarboxylation of pyruvate and alpha-ketoglutarate in the Krebs cycle and ultimately is important for energy storage and release (Gropper & Smith 2013).

Acyl carrier protein

Pantothenic acid functions in the body as a component of the acylation factors, CoA and 4'-phosphopantetheine (the prosthetic group for ACP) (Gropper & Smith 2013, Kohlmeier 2003). A few reactions use 4'-phosphopantetheine; most of these are related to lipid synthesis (Kohlmeier 2003).

Indirect antioxidant effects

New in vitro research supports an indirect antioxidant role for pantothenic acid through its ability to increase cellular adenosine triphosphate, which in turn creates increased levels of free glutathione and enhanced protection of cells against peroxidative damage (Slyshenkov et al 2004).

ADRENAL CORTEX FUNCTION AND NEUROTRANSMITTER SYNTHESIS

Pantothenic acid is essential in controlling stress and the ability to cope with stressful events, due to its involvement in the synthesis of the neurotransmitter acetylcholine. It plays an important role in adrenal function and, as CoA, is needed for proper adrenal cortex function and the synthesis of steroid hormones, namely cortisone. A consistent finding in animal studies conducted in the 1950s is that a deficiency of pantothenic acid initially causes adrenal hypertrophy, followed by progressive morphological and functional changes to the adrenal gland, resulting in adrenal hypofunction and an impaired stress response (Hurley & Morgan 1952, Kelly 2011).

Other functions

Pantothenate is required in the production of many secondary metabolites such as polyisoprenoid-containing compounds (e.g. ubiquinone, squalene and cholesterol), steroid hormones, vitamin D and bile acids, acetylated compounds such as *N*-acetylglucosamine, *N*-acetylserotonin, acetylcholine, and prostaglandins and prostaglandin-like compounds (Kelly 2011).

Pantothenic acid, thiamine, riboflavin and niacin participate in the oxidative decarboxylation of alpha-ketoglutarate to succinyl-CoA, an intermediate used with glycine to synthesise haem (Gropper & Smith 2013).

Lipid lowering

Pantethine, a metabolite of pantothenic acid, has been investigated in several clinical studies and found to exert significant lipid-lowering activity (Coronel et al 1991, Donati et al 1986, Gaddi et al 1984), with a 2005 study producing a 50% inhibition of fatty acid synthesis and an 80% inhibition of cholesterol synthesis (McRae 2005).

The mechanism of action relates to reduced insulin resistance and activation of lipolysis in serum and adipose tissue, according to in vivo research (Naruta & Buko 2001). Additionally, inhibition of HMG-CoA reductase, as well as more distal enzymes in the cholesterol synthetic pathway, is likely to be responsible (McCarty 2001).

As part of CoA, pantothenic acid is essential for the formation of acetyl CoA, an important substrate in the catabolism of fatty acids. Fat accumulation has been shown to increase with pantothenic acid deficiency, and refeeding pantothenic acid to rats originally fed a pantothenic acid-deficient diet decreased tissue fat (Shibata et al 2013).

Wound healing

Both oral and topical administration has been shown to accelerate closure of wounds and increase strength of scar tissue in vivo (Plesofsky 2002, Vaxman et al 1990). Both in vitro and in vivo studies reveal that topical dexpanthenol, the stable alcoholic analogue of pantothenic acid, induces activation of fibroblast proliferation, which contributes to accelerated re-epithelialisation in wound healing (Ebner et al 2002).

CLINICAL USE

Although pantothenic acid has been investigated in some studies, most investigation has occurred with several of its derivatives, chiefly an alcoholic analogue of pantothenic acid called dexpanthenol (Bepanthen; see below) and pantethine.

Deficiency states: prevention and treatment

Due to the widespread occurrence of pantothenate in foods, deficiencies are considered unlikely, and more often in conjunction with multiple nutrient deficiencies, as would occur in generalised malnutrition (Gropper & Smith 2013). Traditionally, pantothenic acid is recommended, together with other vitamin B complex nutrients, to treat generalised malnutrition or prevent deficiency in conditions such as alcoholism, diabetes mellitus and malabsorption syndromes (Gropper & Smith 2013). The interference from some prescription drugs (antimetabolites) may also interfere with pantothenate absorption and lead to deficiencies (Kohlmeier 2003).

Enhances wound healing

Pantothenic acid has been both used as an oral supplement and applied topically in a cream base to enhance wound healing; it has been shown to accelerate closure of wounds and increase strength of scar tissue in experimental animals (Plesofsky 2002, Vaxman et al 1990). Furthermore, fibroblast content of scar tissue has been shown to significantly increase following injections of pantothenate (20 mg/kg of body weight/24 hours) for 3 weeks (Aprahamian et al 1985). Skin dehydration and irritation have been found to be reduced with the use of dexapanthenol, a pantothente derivative (Biro et al 2003).

Although these results are encouraging, there has been little investigation in humans. One double-blind randomised controlled trial testing the effects of vitamin C (1000 mg) and pantothenic acid (200 mg) supplements over a 21-day period showed increased fibroblast proliferation but no significant alteration to wound healing during recovery from surgical tattoo removal (Vaxman et al 1995).

Topical use

In a randomised, double-blind trial in Mumbai, 207 women 30–60 years of age with epidermal hyperpigmentation were recruited and randomly assigned to apply a test or control facial lotion containing 4% niacinamide, 0.5% panthenol and 0.5% tocopheryl acetate to the face daily for 10 weeks (Jerajani et al 2010). Women who used the test lotion reportedly experienced significantly reduced hyperpigmentation, improved skin tone evenness, appearance of lightening of skin and positive effects on skin texture from as early as 6 weeks. Some evidence of a beneficial effect on barrier function was also observed. The authors state that these results concur with previous positive findings for topical niacinamide (Bissett 2002, Bissett et al 2005, Draelos et al 2005, Hakozaki et al 2002, Matts et al 2002) and panthenol (Biro et al 2003, Ebner et al 2002).

Bepanthen is a well-known dermatological preparation containing dexpanthenol, an alcoholic analogue of pantothenic acid. It has been investigated in numerous studies and found to act like a moisturiser, activate fibroblast proliferation, accelerate re-epithelialisation in wound healing, have anti-inflammatory activity against ultraviolet-induced erythema and reduce itch (Ebner et al 2002). Under double-blind study conditions, epidermal wounds treated with dexpanthenol emulsion showed a reduction in erythema, and more elastic and solid tissue regeneration. Another randomised, prospective, double-blind, placebo-controlled study published in 2003 investigated the efficacy of topical dexpanthenol as a protectant against skin irritation. The study involved 25 healthy volunteers who were treated with a topical preparation containing 5% dexpanthenol or a placebo and then exposed to sodium lauryl sulfate 2% twice daily over 26 days. Treatment with topical dexpanthenol provided protection against skin irritation, whereas a statistically significant deterioration was observed in the placebo group (Biro et al 2003).

Although Bepanthen is commonly used in radiotherapy departments to ameliorate acute radiotherapy skin reactions, a prospective study of 86 patients undergoing radiotherapy showed that topical use of Bepanthen did not improve skin reactions under these conditions (Lokkevik et al 1996). In an animal study by Dorr et al (2005), negative results were similarly obtained and it is not currently recommended for individuals undergoing radiotherapy.

Acne vulgaris

One hundred Chinese patients diagnosed with acne vulgaris (45 males and 55 females) were given oral pantothenic acid, 10 g a day in four divided doses, and a cream consisting of 20% by weight of pantothenic acid to apply to the affected areas four to six times a day. Within 1–2 days sebum production was noticeably reduced, frequency of new acne eruptions began to decline and existing lesions started to regress within 1–2 weeks. Patients who were categorised as suffering moderate-severity acne reported complete control of acne after 8 weeks with only occasional new eruptions, while in more severe cases complete control occurred after 6 months (Leung 1995b). The author notes that daily doses of 15–20 g/day of pantothenic acid did produce faster results in severe cases and a maintenance dose was 1–5 g/day of pantothenic acid.

Interestingly, it has been shown that dexpanthenol cream can help treat some mucocutaneous adverse reactions caused by isotretinoin, a chemotherapeutic drug used to treat acne (Romiti & Romiti 2002, as cited by Kelly 2011).

Nasal spray

A randomised controlled trial of 48 outpatients diagnosed with rhinitis sicca anterior found that dexpanthenol nasal spray is an effective symptomatic treatment for this condition (Kehrl & Sonnemann 1998). Two years later, another randomised controlled trial compared the effects of xylometazoline-dexpanthenol nasal spray versus xylometazoline nasal spray over a 2-week period in 61 patients with rhinitis after nasal surgery (Kehrl & Sonnemann 2000); it showed that the combination of xylometazoline-dexpanthenol nasal spray was significantly superior to the other treatment and well tolerated.

More recent studies support this emerging trend and point towards a reduction in ciliary and cytotoxic effects from nasal decongestants when 5% dexpanthenol is concurrently administered (Klocker et al 2003).

Elevated cholesterol and triglyceride levels

Several clinical studies confirm that pantethine, a metabolite of pantothenic acid, exerts significant lipid-lowering activity (Coronel et al 1991, Donati et al 1986, Gaddi et al 1984).

One double-blind study of 29 patients found that 300 mg of pantethine taken three times daily resulted in significant reductions to plasma total cholesterol, low-density lipoprotein (LDL) cholesterol and triglycerides, and an increase in high-density lipoprotein (HDL) cholesterol levels (Gaddi et al 1984).

A 2005 review analysed results from 28 clinical trials encompassing a pooled population of 646 hyperlipidaemic patients who were supplemented with a mean dose of 900 mg pantethine over an average trial length of 12.7 weeks (McRae 2005). The results of these studies suggest a response to pantethine that is time-dependent, with progressively greater reductions in LDL cholesterol and triacylglycerols between month 1 and 9. The most impressive results were observed at 9 months, with a reduction of total cholesterol by 20.5%, LDL cholesterol by 27.6% and triacylglycerols by 36.5% from baseline. Although minor increases were observed in HDL levels in the early stages of most trials, longer-term studies suggested that this is not sustained.

Of the trials studied, 22 were conducted in Italy and all were conducted between 1981 and 1991. The authors point out that no further clinical trials were published, and concluded that evidence to date has yielded positive and promising results, and further research is warranted.

Obesity and weight loss

An investigation of vitamin B_5 for weight loss was conducted with 100 Chinese volunteers (40 male) aged 15–55 years, following a strict calorie-controlled diet and supplemented with 2.5 g of pantothenic acid four times a day. The average weight loss was found to be 1.2 kg per week. Ketone bodies in urine were monitored regularly and were found to be absent in most circumstances and therefore did not explain the weight loss. While feelings of neither hunger nor weakness were reported, a sense of wellbeing was observed. To maintain the weight loss, the subjects required 1–3 g/day along with continual strict dietary advice. The author attributes the success to the role of CoA in carbohydrate, fat and protein metabolism, and its key role in the biosynthesis of many lipids and steroids (Leung 1995a). However, in the absence of a control group, the weight loss that occurred could be attributed to the calorie-controlled diet rather than the inclusion of pantothenic acid.

IN COMBINATION

Similarly, a double-blind, randomised, parallel-group, placebo-controlled study carried out on a product containing *Garcinia cambogia* extract with calcium pantothenate (standardised for the content of hydroxycitric acid and pantothenic acid) and extracts of *Matricaria chamomilla, Rosa damascena, Lavandula officinalis* and *Cananga odorata,* on body weight in overweight and obese volunteers during a 60-day treatment period found that the average reduction in body weight for the treatment group (n = 30) was 4.67% compared with 0.63% for placebo (n = 28; $P < 0.0001$). Weight losses of ≥3 kg were recorded for 23 subjects in the treatment group and only one in the placebo group (Toromanyan et al 2007).

OTHER USES

Pantothenic acid has been used for many other indications, but controlled studies to determine whether treatment is effective are lacking.

Stress

As vitamin B_5 is essential for adrenal cortex function and the synthesis of steroid hormones, it is often used together with other B vitamins during times of stress in order to improve the body's response and restore nutrient levels. In continual deficiency, a progressive morphological and functional degradation of the adrenal glands may occur, resulting in adrenal hypofunction, and an inability to respond to stress appropriately (Hurley & Morgan 1952, Kelly 2011, Melampy et al 1951). If pantothenic acid is supplied early enough after deficiency has been induced (i.e. before adrenal exhaustion occurs), the response to stress can be improved (Kelly 2011).

Clinical note — Could pantothenic acid be an antiageing nutrient?

A contemporary theory of ageing implicates mitochondrial functional decline, or 'oxidative decay' of the mitochondria, as a major contributor. In light of this hypothesis, nutrients that possess a critical role in the mitochondria are being re-examined to determine their ability to prevent ageing in humans. The focus has been on pantothenic acid, biotin, lipoic acid, iron and zinc, because deficiencies of these micronutrients have been implicated in increased mitochondrial oxidation (Ames et al 2005, Atamna 2004). In addition, those with antioxidant capabilities are of particular interest, such as pantothenic acid, lipoic acid and zinc.

Because of the numerous nutrients implicated in mitochondrial health and disease, a broad-based multivitamin should be considered instead of a single-nutrient supplement for populations at increased risk of poor nutrition, such as the elderly, young, poor and obese (Ames et al 2005).

Life extension in animals supplemented with B_5 has been shown in several older studies (Gardner 1948a, 1948b, Pelton & Williams 1958). The first of these studies investigated the chemical components of royal jelly, a well-recognised antiageing supplement. Using *Drosophila melanogaster* (common fruit fly) as the testing medium, it was found that pantothenic acid was the primary antiageing factor (Gardner 1948a). In a follow-up study, the combination of biotin, pyridoxine and sodium yeast nucleate was shown to lengthen lifespan in *D. melanogaster,* and was further extended with pantothenic acid (Gardner 1948b). Furthermore, the mean lifespan for mice given 300 mcg/day supplementary calcium pantothenate was 653.1 days and that for the control mice was 549.8 days. The statistical difference between the two groups is $P = 0.05$ (t-test), 0.01 (U-test).

Clinical note — Could vitamin B_5 prevent neural tube defects?

Ongoing evidence from animal studies suggests that pantothenic acid may have a preventive role against neural tube defects independently of folic acid (Dawson et al 2006). Pharmaceuticals such as valproic acid that increase the risk of neural tube defect offspring have been shown also to reduce hepatic concentrations of CoA, an effect attenuated by coadministration of pantothenic acid. While the role of B_5 in neural tube closure remains unknown, it appears that it exerts actions both overlapping with and independent of folate.

Interestingly, a large number of experiments from the 1950s (Dumm & Ralli 1953, Dumm et al 1955, Ershoff 1953, Hurley & Morgan 1952, Melampy et al 1951, Ralli & Dumm 1953) attempted to elicit the impact of pantothenic acid deficiency on adrenal function and stress response in animals; however, little research has been done since. One study in 2008 demonstrated that pantothenic acid enhanced the basal levels of corticosterone (and progesterone) in adrenal cells of male rats that had pantothenic acid (0.03%) added to their drinking water for 9 weeks. Increased sensitivity to stimulation with adrenocorticotrophic hormone and a slight non-significant increase in adrenal gland weight in the pantothenic acid group were also observed (Jaroenporn et al 2008).

Ulcerative colitis (UC)

In a pilot study of 3 patients, it was hypothesised that topically administered dexpanthenol may be beneficial in increasing tissue levels of CoA, improving fatty acid oxidation and ameliorating UC (Loftus et al 1997). It was proposed that a possible cause of UC is a block in the conversion of pantothenic acid to CoA, which reduces colonic CoA activity levels, inhibits short-chain fatty acid oxidation and contributes to distal UC. The patients received 4 weeks of dexpanthenol (1000 mg) enemas and the authors concluded that, despite increases in urinary pantothenic acid output, the treatment was ineffective (Loftus et al 1997). With such a minute sample size in this pilot study, further research is required to more appropriately ascertain its effectiveness. Interestingly, conditions of ulcers and colitis negatively impact the status and excretion rates of pantothenate (Bates 2013).

Coeliac disease

In 1972, a letter to the editor of the *British Medical Journal* suggested the use of pantothenic acid in patients with coeliac disease who respond only partially to a gluten-free diet as they may benefit from the administration of pantothenic acid (Monro 1972). Coeliac disease is a permanent enteropathy of the small bowel and may be characterised by ulceration and stricture formation, leading to narrowing and scarring. The author explains that pantothenic acid deficiency can produce atrophy of the small intestinal mucosa in animal species; in many species ulceration of the gastric and intestinal mucosa can occur, and this destruction may occur despite the sufferer consuming a gluten-free diet. Furthermore, Monro explains that 'pseudohypoadrenalism' and carbohydrate metabolism derangement with glucose intolerance are common features of both coeliac disease and pantothenic acid deficiency, suggesting a potential role in the management of these symptoms with pantothenic acid administration (Monro 1972).

Lupus erythematosus

The evidence for the use of pantothenic acid in persons with lupus erythematosus dates back to the 1950s. Kelly (2011) cites a study (Welsh 1954) that showed efficacy in lupus treatment using pantothenic acid (10–15 g/day) with 1500–3000 IU/day of vitamin E for 19 months.

One study administered doses of 10 g/day pantothenic acid, 2 g of vitamin C, 500 mg of B_1, 200 mg of B_6, 2 mg of B_{12} and two tablets of Super B and two tablets of multivitamins with minerals per day to females with systemic lupus erythematosus. After 4 weeks of treatment, there were varying degrees of improvement, particularly in fatigue. Later follow-up showed that the incidence of fever was decreased and no major flares were noted. In many cases, the original systemic lupus erythematosus medications could gradually be reduced (Leung 2004). More research needs to be conducted.

Ergogenic aid and athletic performance

Based on its role in carbohydrate metabolism as CoA, vitamin B_5 has been used to increase stamina and athletic performance.

Whether pantothenic acid supplementation improves overall exercise performance remains unclear. One study showed that blood lactate levels and oxygen consumption were decreased in endurance runners during prolonged exercise at 75% maximal oxygen uptake ($\dot{V}O_{2max}$) (Litoff et al 1985). However, the time for highly trained distance runners to reach the point of exhaustion when taking 1 g/day of pantothenic acid for 2 weeks did not increase (Nice et al 1984).

In a randomised, double-blind, counterbalanced design study, cyclists ingesting either a placebo or a combination of 1 g of allithiamin (vitamin B_1 derivative) and 1.8 g of a 55%/45% pantethine/pantothenic acid compound for 7 days did not demonstrate any improvements in exercise metabolism or performance when completing a 2000-metre time trial (Webster 1998). Similarly, 1.5 g/day pantothenic acid and cysteine supplementation did not increase resting muscle CoA content, fuel selection or exercise performance in 8 males who cycled at 75% $\dot{V}O_{2max}$ until exhaustion (Wall et al 2012).

Reducing drug toxicity

Preliminary research in animal models shows that pantothenic acid reduces the toxicity effects of kanamycin and carbon tetrachloride and, when combined with carnitine, protects against valproate toxicity (Moiseenok et al 1984, Nagiel-Ostaszewski & Lau-Cam 1990, Thurston & Hauhart 1992).

Female alopecia — ineffective

According to a study of 46 women with symptoms of diffuse alopecia, calcium pantothenate (200 mg/day) over 4–5 months does not cause a significant improvement in this condition (Brzezinska-Wcislo 2001).

Testicular endocrinology, sperm motility and male fertility

In one study, the physiological roles of pantothenic acid on testicular endocrinology and sperm motility were investigated in 3-week-old male rats that were fed a B_5-free diet or a 0.0016% pantothenic acid diet (control) for 7 weeks. In the B_5-deficient group, sperm motility was significantly reduced, plasma concentrations of testosterone and corticosterone were significantly lower and testicular weight was significantly higher (Yamamoto et al 2009).

Female fertility

A prospective cohort study of 1461 pregnancies found that low-birth-weight offspring were more common in women consuming diets low in vitamin C, riboflavin, pantothenic acid and sugars, even after adjustment for deprivation index, smoking, marital status and parity (Haggarty et al 2009).

DOSAGE RANGE

Australian adequate intake

- Women: 4 mg/day (NHMRC nutrient reference values 2007).
- Men: 6 mg/day (NHMRC nutrient reference values 2007).
- Adults: 5 mg/day (Gropper & Smith 2013).
- Pregnancy: 5 mg/day (NHMRC nutrient reference values 2007) or 6 mg/day (Gropper & Smith 2013).
- Lactation: 6 mg/day (NHMRC nutrient reference values 2007) or 7 mg/day (Gropper & Smith 2013).
- Therapeutic dose: 20–500 mg/day.

According to clinical studies

- Wound healing: dexpanthenol cream 5% applied to affected areas up to two times daily (Biro et al 2003).
- Acne vulgaris: 15–20 g/day of pantothenic acid for 6 months for severe acne (Leung 1995b).
- Acne vulgaris: 1–5 g/day of pantothenic (Leung 1995b) acid maintenance dose.
- Lipid lowering: pantethine 300 mg three times daily (McRae 2005).

TOXICITY

No toxicity level known.

ADVERSE REACTIONS

Pantothenic acid is well tolerated, but contact dermatitis has been reported with topical dexpanthenol.

SIGNIFICANT INTERACTIONS

Antibiotics

Under in vitro conditions, experimental work from the 1950s suggests that pantothenic acid may interfere with the ability of some antibiotics (aureomycin, erythromycin and streptomycin) to inhibit the growth of certain microorganisms.

It has been speculated that these antibiotics might reduce endogenous production of vitamin B_5 by gastrointestinal flora or its downstream coenzymes (CoA or ACP); supplying pantothenic acid overcomes this enzyme inhibition (Watanabe et al 2010, as cited by Kelly 2011).

Oral contraceptive pill

Taking the oral contraceptive pill may increase the requirement for pantothenic acid. Increase vitamin B_5-rich foods or consider supplementation (Plesofsky 2002).

Isotretinoin

A single study reports that a 5% dexpanthenol cream can help treat mucocutaneous adverse reactions caused by using isotretinoin for acne (Romiti & Romiti 2002).

Acetylcholinesterase inhibitor drugs

A theoretical concern exists that pantothenic acid, since it is involved in the biosynthesis of acetylcholine, might increase the effects of acetylcholinesterase inhibitor drugs (Kelly 2011).

CONTRAINDICATIONS AND PRECAUTIONS

None known.

PREGNANCY USE

Considered safe when ingested at usual dietary doses.

PATIENTS' FAQs

What will this vitamin do for me?

Vitamin B_5 is essential for health and is used for many different conditions; for example, it is often used as part of a vitamin B complex supplement to aid the body during times of stress. In many of its uses research is not available to determine whether it is effective. Research generally supports its use in wound healing and in the form of pantethine to reduce cholesterol levels.

When will it start to work?

Pantethine reduces cholesterol levels within 2 months; however, optimal results are achieved with 9 months of supplementation. Xylometazoline-dexpanthenol nasal spray reduces symptoms of rhinitis within 2 weeks. It is not known how quickly the vitamin starts to work in most other conditions.

Are there any safety issues?

Pantothenic acid and pantethine are considered safe substances and are generally well tolerated.

Practice points/Patient counselling

- Deficiency is extremely rare, as pantothenic acid is widely distributed and present in nearly all plant and animal foods. Those at risk of reduced vitamin status are alcoholics, diabetics and people with malabsorption syndromes.
- Pantethine reduces total cholesterol levels significantly, according to controlled studies in both healthy and diabetic people.
- Dexpanthenol cream acts like a moisturiser, activates fibroblast proliferation, accelerates re-epithelialisation in wound healing, has anti-inflammatory activity against ultraviolet-induced erythema and reduces itch. When used in a nasal spray, it reduces symptoms of rhinitis.
- Vitamin B_5 supplements are commonly used together with other B vitamins during times of stress in order to improve the body's response and restore nutrient levels.
- Vitamin B_5 has also been used as adjunctive treatment for inflammatory conditions, such as dermatitis and asthma, as an ergogenic aid, to treat alopecia and to restore colour to greying hair, although no controlled studies are available to determine effectiveness in these conditions.

REFERENCES

Ames BN et al. Mineral and vitamin deficiencies can accelerate the mitochondrial decay of aging. Mol Aspects Med 26.4–5 (2005): 363–378.

Aprahamian M, et al. Effects of supplemental pantothenic acid on wound healing: experimental study in rabbit. Am J Clin Nutr 1985;41(3):578–89.

Atamna H. Heme, iron, and the mitochondrial decay of ageing. Age Res Rev 3.3 (2004): 303–318.

Bates CJ. Pantothenic acid. In: Physiology, dietary sources and requirements, Encyclopedia of human nutrition. St Louis: Elsevier, 1998, pp 1511–1515.

Bates CJ. Pantothenic acid. Encyclopedia of human nutrition. Elsevier, 2013 pp1–5.

Biro K et al. Efficacy of dexpanthenol in skin protection against irritation: a double-blind, placebo-controlled study. Contact Dermatitis 49.2 (2003): 80–84.

Bissett D. Topical niacinamide and barrier enhancement. Cutis 2002;70:8–12.

Bissett DL, et al. Niacinamide: A B vitamin that improves aging facial skin appearance. Dermatol Surg 2005;31:860–5.

Brzezinska-Wcislo L. Evaluation of vitamin B6 and calcium pantothenate effectiveness on hair growth from clinical and trichographic aspects for treatment of diffuse alopecia in women. Wiad Lek 54.1–2 (2001): 11–118.

Coronel F et al. Treatment of hyperlipemia in diabetic patients on dialysis with a physiological substance. Am J Nephrol 11.1 (1991): 32–36.

Dawson JE, et al. Folic acid and pantothenic acid protection against valproic acid-induced neural tube defects in CD-1 mice. Toxicol & App Pharmacol 211 (2006): 124–132.

Donati C et al. Pantethine improves the lipid abnormalities of chronic hemodialysis patients: results of a multicenter clinical trial. Clin Nephrol 25.2 (1986): 70–74.

Dorr W et al. Effects of dexpanthenol with or without Aloe vera extract on radiation-induced oral mucositis: preclinical studies. Int J Radiat Biol 81.3 (2005): 43–50.

Dumm ME, Ralli EP. Factors influencing the response of adrenalectomized rats to stress. Metabolism 1953;2:153–164.

Dumm ME, et al. Factors influencing adrenal weight and adrenal cholesterol in rats following stress. J Nutr 1955;56:517–531.

Draelos ZD, et al. Niacinamide-containing facial moisturizer improves skin barrier and benefits subjects with rosacea. Cutis 2005;76: 135–41.

Ebner F et al. Topical use of dexpanthenol in skin disorders. Am J Clin Dermatol 3.6 (2002): 427–433.

Ershoff BF. Comparative effects of pantothenic acid deficiency and inanition on resistance to cold stress in the rat. J Nutr 1953;49:373–385.

Gaddi A et al. Controlled evaluation of pantethine, a natural hypolipidemic compound, in patients with different forms of hyperlipoproteinemia. Atherosclerosis 50.1 (1984): 73–83.

Gardner TS. The use of *Drosophila melanogaster* as a screening agent for longevity factors; pantothenic acid as a longevity factor in royal jelly. J Gerontol 1948a;3:1–8.

Gardner TS. The use of *Drosophila melanogaster* as a screening agent for longevity factors; the effects of biotin, pyridoxine, sodium yeast nucleate, and pantothenic acid on the life span of the fruit fly. J Gerontol 1948b;3:9–13.

Groff JL, Gropper SS. Advanced nutrition and human metabolism, 3rd edn. Belmont, CA: Wadsworth, 2009.

Gropper, S., Smith, J Advanced nutrition and human metabolism, 6th edition. Belmont CA: Wadsworth, Cengage Learning, 2013.

Haggarty P, et al. Diet and deprivation in pregnancy. British Journal of Nutrition (2009), 102, 1487–1497.

Hakozaki T, et al. The effect of niacinamide on reducing cutaneous pigmentation and suppression of melanosome transfer. Br J Dermatol 2002;147:20–31.

Hechtman, L. Clinical Naturopathic Medicine. Revised Edition. Churchill Livingstone, Elsevier, 2012.

Hurley LS, Morgan AF. Carbohydrate metabolism and adrenal cortical function in the pantothenic acid-defi- cient rat. J Biol Chem 1952;195:583–590.

Jaroenporn S, et al. Effects of pantothenic acid supplementation on adrenal steroid secretion from male rats. Biol Pharm Bull 2008;31:1205–1208.

Jerajani HR,et al. The effects of a daily facial lotion containing vitamins B3 and E and provitamin B5 on the facial skin of Indian women: A randomized, double-blind trial. Indian Journal of Dermatology, Venereolgy and Leprology 2010;76(1):20–26.

Kehrl W, Sonnemann U. Dexpanthenol nasal spray as an effective therapeutic principle for treatment of rhinitis sicca anterior. Laryngorhinootologie 77.9 (1998): 506–512.

Kehrl W, Sonnemann U. Improving wound healing after nose surgery by combined administration of xylometazoline and dexpanthenol. Laryngorhinootologie 79.3 (2000): 151–154.

Kelly, G S. Pantothenic acid. Alternative Medicine Review 2011;16(3):263–274.

Klocker N et al. The protective effect of dexpanthenol in nasal sprays. First results of cytotoxic and ciliary-toxic studies in vitro. Laryngorhinootologie 82.3 (2003): 177–182.

Kohlmeier, M. Nutrient Metabolism. Food science and technology. International series. London: Elsevier 2003.

Leung LH. Pantothenic acid as a weight-reducing agent: fasting without hunger, weakness and ketosis. Med Hypotheses 1995a;44:403–405.

Leung LH. Pantothenic acid deficiency as the pathogenesis of acne vulgaris, Med Hypotheses 1995b;44:490–492.

Leung LH. Systemic lupus erythematosus: a combined deficiency disease. Medical Hypotheses 62 (6) 2004, 922–924.

Litoff D, et al. Effects of pantothenic acid supplementation on human exercise. Med Sci Sports Exerc 1985;17:287.

Loftus EV Jr, et al. Dexpanthenol enemas in ulcerative colitis: a pilot study. Mayo Clin Proc 1997;72:616–620.

Lokkevik E et al. Skin treatment with bepanthen cream versus no cream during radiotherapy: a randomized controlled trial. Acta Oncol 35.8 (1996): 1021–1026.

Matts PJ, et al. A review of the range of effects of niacinamide in human skin. Int Fed Soc Cosmet Chem Mag 2002;5:285–90.

McCarty MF. Inhibition of acetyl-CoA carboxylase by cystamine may mediate the hypotriglyceridemic activity of pantethine. Med Hypotheses 56.3 (2001): 314–317.

McRae MP. Treatment of hyperlipoproteinemia with pantethine: A review and analysis of efficacy and tolerability. Nutr Res 25.4 (2005): 319–333.

Melampy RM, et al. Effect of pantothenic acid deficiency upon adrenal cortex, thymus, spleen, and circulating lymphocytes in mice. Proc Soc Exp Biol Med 1951;76:24–27.

Moiseenok AG et al. Antitoxic properties of pantothenic acid derivatives, precursors of coenzyme A biosynthesis, with regard to kanamycin. Antibiotiki 29.11 (1984): 851–855.

Monro J. Pantothenic acid and coeliac disease. Br Med J 1972; 4: 112–113.

Nagiel-Ostaszewski I, Lau-Cam CA. Protection by pantethine, pantothenic acid and cystamine against carbon tetrachloride-induced hepatotoxicity in the rat. Res Commun Chem Pathol Pharmacol 67.2 (1990): 289–292.

Naruta E, Buko V. Hypolipidemic effect of pantothenic acid derivatives in mice with hypothalamic obesity induced by aurothioglucose. Exp Toxicol Pathol 53.5 (2001): 393–398.

V

Nice C, et al. The effects of pantothenic acid on human exercise capacity. J Sports Med 1984;24:26–29.
Pelton RB, Williams RJ. Effect of pantothenic acid on the longevity of mice. Proc Soc Exp Biol Med 1958;99:632–633.
Plesofsky N. Pantothenic acid. Oregon: Linus Pauling Institute, 2002.
Ralli EP, Dumm ME. Relation of pantothenic acid to adrenal cortical function. Vitam Horm 1953;11:133–158.
Romiti R, Romiti N. Dexpanthenol cream significantly improves mucocutaneous side effects associated with isotretinoin therapy. Pediatr Dermatol 2002;19:368.
Shibata K, et al. Pantothenic acid refeeding diminishes the liver, perinephrical fats, and plasma fats accumulated by pantothenic acid deficiency and/or ethanol consumption. Nutrition 2013:1–6.
Slyshenkov VS et al. Pantothenic acid and pantothenol increase biosynthesis of glutathione by boosting cell energetics. FEBS Lett 569.1–3 (2004): 169–172.
Thurston JH, Hauhart RE. Amelioration of adverse effects of valproic acid on ketogenesis and liver coenzyme A metabolism by cotreatment with pantothenate and carnitine in developing mice: possible clinical significance. Pediatr Res 31.4 (1992): 419–423.
Toromanyan E, et al. Efficacy of Slim339 in reducing body weight of overweight and obese human subjects. Phytother Res 2007;21:1177–1181.
Vaxman F et al. Improvement in the healing of colonic anastomoses by vitamin B_5 and C supplements: Experimental study in the rabbit. Ann Chir 44.7 (1990): 512–520.
Vaxman F et al. Effect of pantothenic acid and ascorbic acid supplementation on human skin wound healing process. A double blind, prospective and randomized trial. Eur Surg Res 27.3 (1995): 158–166.
Wahlqvist M (ed). Food and nutrition. Sydney: Allen & Unwin, 2002.
Wall B T, et al. Acute pantothenic acid and cysteine supplementation does not affect muscle coenzyme A content, fuel selection, or exercise performance in healthy humans. J Appl Physiol 2012; 112:272–278.
Watanabe T, et al. Dietary intake of seven B vitamins based on a total diet study in Japan. J Nutr Sci Vitaminol (Tokyo) 2010;56:279–286.
Webster MJ. Physiological and performance responses to supplementation with thiamin and pantothenic acid derivatives. Eur J Appl Physiol Occup Physiol 1998;77:486–491.
Welsh AL. Lupus erythematosus: treatment by combined use of massive amounts of pantothenic acid and vitamin E. AMA Arch Derm Syphilol 1954;70:181–198.
Yamamoto, T. et al. The effect of pantothenic acid on testicular function in male rats. Journal of Veterinary Medical Science 2009 71 No. 11 1427–1432.

Vitamin B_6

BACKGROUND AND RELEVANT PHARMACOKINETICS

Vitamin B_6 as pyridoxine was first isolated in 1938. Pyridoxal and pyridoxamine were later identified in the mid-1940s (Gropper & Smith 2013). In total, there are six different vitamin B_6 forms — pyridoxine, pyridoxal, pyridoxamine and their phosphorylated derivatives, pyridoxine phosphate (PNP), pyridoxal phosphate (PLP) and pyridoxamine phosphate (PMP), all of which are found in food. PLP is the active coenzyme important for amino acid metabolism.

For absorption, phosphorylated forms are hydroysed (dephosphorylated) to the free forms (pyridoxine, pyridoxal, pyridoxamine) by zinc-dependent alkaline phosphatase. (However, at high-ingested concentrations, the phosphorylated forms may be absorbed without dephosphorylation.)

Absorption of vitamin B_6 takes place in the jejunum by a passive, non-saturable process. The more acidic the environment, the greater is the absorption. Pyridoxine, pyridoxal and pyridoxamine are transported in the plasma and red blood cells to the liver, where they are metabolised predominantly to PLP. In all, 60–90% of vitamin B_6 found in systemic blood is in the form of PLP. Prior to cellular uptake, it must be enzymatically hydrolysed to free pyridoxal again, as extrahepatic tissues uptake only unphosphorylated forms (Gropper & Smith 2013). It is mainly stored in muscle tissue, and ultimately metabolised and excreted via the kidneys.

CHEMICAL COMPONENTS

Vitamin B_6 is a water-soluble vitamin and has six vitamer forms, of which pyridoxine hydrochloride is the main form, found in supplements and used to fortify foods, as it is particularly stable (Combs 2012). Pyridoxine is the alcohol form, pyridoxal the aldehyde form and pyridoxamine the amine form, each with a 5′-phosphate derivative (Gropper & Smith 2013).

> ***Clinical note — Marginal B_6 deficiency***
> Although frank deficiency is rare, marginal deficiency appears to be common. One study found that 100% of 174 university students tested had some degree of vitamin B_6 deficiency (Shizukuishi et al 1981). A larger survey of 11,658 adults found that 71% of males and 90% of females did not meet the recommended daily intake (RDI) requirements for B_6 (Kant & Block 1990).

FOOD SOURCES

All six forms of vitamin B_6 are found in food. Vitamin B_6 is widely distributed in animal and plant foods. Plant foods contain mainly pyridoxine, PNP and a conjugated pyridoxine glycoside, while animal products, such as sirloin steak, salmon and chicken, are the richest sources of pyridoxal, pyridoxamine, PLP and PMP (Gropper & Smith 2013). It occurs in the highest concentrations in meats (organ meats, beef, chicken, pork), salmon, wholegrain products, legumes, eggs, vegetables, some fruits (bananas) and nuts (Combs 2012, Gropper & Smith 2013). Per milligram, Vegemite is one of the richest sources.

On average, the bioavailability of vitamin B_6 from the most commonly consumed foods is between 61% and 92%. Prolonged heating, milling and refining grains and food storage contribute to substantial loss (Gropper & Smith 2013). Up to 40% can be lost through cooking (Wahlqvist 1997); however, more recent sources suggest a variation of up to 70% (Combs 2012). Plant-derived foods lose very little vitamin B_6 from cooking, as they contain the most stable pyridoxine, whereas animal foods that contain mostly pyridoxal and pyridoxamine lose substantial amounts (Combs 2012).

DEFICIENCY SIGNS AND SYMPTOMS

Clinical signs and symptoms are non-specific because this vitamin is necessary for the proper functioning of over 60 enzymes (Pelton et al 2000, Wahlqvist 1997). Signs of deficiency can occur within 2–3 weeks of reduced intake, but may take up to 2½ months to develop (Gropper & Smith 2013). In adults with B_6 deficiency, chiefly dermatological, circulatory and neurological changes develop. In adults with chronic deficiency, a subacute or chronic neuropathy develops. In most cases, chronic deficiency is a result of the long-term use of vitamin B_6 antagonists such as isoniazid, hydralazine and penicillamine. Sensory symptoms appear first in the distal portion of the feet and then spread proximally to the knees and hands if medicine use continues (So & Simon 2012). In children, the central nervous system (CNS) is also affected. Signs and symptoms include:

- Seborrhoeic rash/dermatitis (similar to that seen in pellagra) on face, neck, shoulders and buttocks (Gropper & Smith 2013)
- Weakness, sleeplessness and fatigue
- Angular stomatitis and glossitis, and cheilosis (Combs 2012, Gropper & Smith 2013)
- Sideroblastic anaemia
- Hypochromic, microcytic anaemia due to impaired haem production (Gropper & Smith 2013)
- Impaired cell-mediated immunity and increased susceptibility to infection (Combs 2012)
- Renal calculi
- Elevated homocysteine levels (Lakshmi & Ramalakshmi 1998)
- Impaired niacin production from tryptophan (Combs 2012, Gropper & Smith 2013)
- Impaired glucose tolerance (Combs 2012)
- CNS effects such as irritability, confusion, lethargy, clinical depression, peripheral neuropathy, elevated seizure activity and convulsions (particularly in children) (Combs 2012, Gropper & Smith 2013), abnormal brain wave patterns and nerve conduction
- Birth defects such as cleft palate (associated with elevated homocysteine) (Weingaertner et al 2005).

Pyridoxine deficiency has also been associated with premature coronary artery disease and with impaired oxidative defence mechanisms (Miner et al 2001).

Primary deficiency

Primary deficiency is rare because this vitamin is widely available in many foods. Groups at risk of deficiency include breastfed babies born with low plasma B_6 levels, the elderly, those who consume large quantities of alcohol and individuals who are on dialysis due to abnormal vitamin loss (Groff & Gropper 2009).

Secondary deficiency

This may result from malabsorption syndromes, cancer, liver cirrhosis and alcoholism, hyperthyroidism, congestive heart failure or use of medicines that affect B_6 status or activity such as isoniazid, hydralazine, penicillamine, theophylline, monoamine oxidase inhibitors (Beers & Berkow 2003, Bratman & Kroll 2000, Wardlaw 1997), corticosteroids (promote vitamin B_6 loss), anticonvulsants (inhibit vitamin B_6 activity) and the oral contraceptive pill (Gropper & Smith 2013).

MAIN ACTIONS

Coenzyme

In the form of PLP, vitamin B_6 is associated with >100 enzymes and predominantly involved in amino acid metabolism (Gropper & Smith 2013) All except one amino acid, proline, rely on vitamin B_6 for their biosynthesis and catabolism (Combs 2012).

It is an important coenzyme in the biosynthesis of the neurotransmitters gamma-aminobutyric acid (GABA), dopamine and serotonin (Gerster 1996). It is also involved in protein metabolism, haemoglobin synthesis, gluconeogenesis, lipid metabolism, niacin formation, immune system processes, nucleic acid synthesis and hormone modulation (Bratman & Kroll 2000, Combs 2012, Wardlaw 1997).

Homocysteine

Homocysteine is formed from the essential amino acid methionine and about 50% is then remethylated to methionine via steps that require folic acid and vitamin B_{12}. Vitamin B_6 is required for another metabolic pathway and is a cofactor for cystathionine beta-synthase, which mediates the transformation of homocysteine to cystathionine (Wilcken & Wilcken 1998).

Serotonin, adrenaline and noradrenaline

Pyridoxine is required for the synthesis of many neurotransmitters, including serotonin, adrenaline and noradrenaline. It is a cofactor for the enzyme 5-hydroxytryptophan decarboxylase, which is involved in one of the steps that converts tryptophan to serotonin (Pelton et al 2000) and tyrosine carboxylase that converts tyrosine to dopamine, adrenaline and noradrenaline (Combs 2012). Deficiency states are therefore associated with alterations to mood and other psychological disturbances.

Niacin synthesis

Vitamin B_6 is a required cofactor for kynureninase and transaminases required for tryptophan conversion to niacin (Combs 2012).

Antioxidant

B_6 has been shown both in vitro and in vivo to display antioxidant activity (Anand 2005, Ji et al 2006, Kannan & Jain 2004, Matxain et al 2007).

Antitumour

In vitro and in vivo experiments have found evidence of some antitumour action on a number of cell lines, including breast and pituitary cells (Ren & Melmed 2006, Shimada et al 2005, 2006).

Reducing diabetic complications

According to Jain (2007), animal studies show that B_6 may reduce the incidence of several diabetic complications, such as retinopathy, nephropathy and dyslipidaemia. It is thought that advanced glycation end products (AGEs) contribute to the development of diabetic nephropathy and other diabetes complications, and, according to in vivo research, pyridoxamine (from the B_6 group of compounds) exerts antioxidant and anti-AGE action in the kidneys (Tanimoto et al 2007). The anti-AGE action of PLP was confirmed in a diabetic rat model, where it prevented the progression of nephropathy (Nakamura et al 2007).

OTHER ACTIONS

Pyridoxine displayed a protective effect against neurotoxicity induced by glutamate in vivo, which may prove useful in hypoxic-ischaemic brain injury (Buyukokuroglu et al 2007). Another animal study indicated that neuroprotective activity preventing ischaemic damage may be due to a GABA-inhibitory effect (Hwang et al 2007).

Immune-stimulant actions, with an increase in T-helper and T-lymphocyte cells, were found in critically ill patients to whom B_6 was administered (Cheng et al 2006).

Myelin formation

PLP is required for the synthesis of sphingolipids for myelin sheath formation (Ang et al 2008).

Gene expression

In its non-coenzyme role, vitamin B_6 has been shown to affect gene expression by binding to DNA and modulating steroid hormones (including progesterone, androgens and oestrogens), binding to regulatory DNA regions (Oka 2001).

CLINICAL USE

Vitamin B_6 supplementation is used to treat a large variety of conditions and is mostly prescribed in combination with other B group vitamins.

Deficiency

It is traditionally used to treat vitamin B_6 deficiency.

Premenstrual syndrome (PMS)

Vitamin B_6 supplementation is used in doses beyond RDI levels for the treatment of PMS. A 1999 systematic review of nine clinical trials involving 940 patients with PMS supports this use, finding that doses up to 100 mg/day are likely to be of benefit in treating symptoms and PMS-related depression (Wyatt et al 1999). Another double-blind randomised controlled trial of 94 patients taking a dose of 40 mg B_6 twice a day found that active treatment significantly decreased PMS symptoms during the luteal phase. Benefits were most pronounced for mood and psychiatric symptoms (Kashanian et al 2008).

Comparative study

One randomised double-blind study compared the effects of pyridoxine (300 mg/day), alprazolam (0.75 mg/day), fluoxetine (10 mg/day) or propranolol (20 mg/day) in four groups of 30 women with severe PMS (Diegoli et al 1998). In this study, fluoxetine produced the best results (a mean reduction of 65.4% in symptoms), followed by propranolol (58.7%), alprazolam (55.6%), pyridoxine (45.3%) and placebo (39.4–46.1%). Symptoms responding well to pyridoxine were tachycardia, insomnia, acne and nausea (Diegoli et al 1998). Another comparative study of 60 women tested 100 mg of B_6 against bromocriptine and a placebo over 3 months. Both active treatments produced a significant reduction in symptoms compared to the control group; however, vitamin B_6 treatment was slightly more effective than bromocriptine and produced fewer side effects (Sharma et al 2007).

More recently, a systematic review investigated the role of herbs, vitamins and minerals advocated in the treatment of PMS and/or premenstrual dysphoric disorder (PMDD) to determine their efficacy in reducing the severity of PMS/PMDD symptoms (Whelan et al 2009). Data support the use of calcium for PMS, and suggest that chasteberry and vitamin B_6 may be effective (Whelan et al 2009).

Dysmenorrhoea

A Cochrane review of herbal and dietary therapies for primary and secondary dysmenorrhoea found one small trial with B_6 that showed it was more effective at reducing pain than both placebo (in this case ibuprofen) and a combination of magnesium and vitamin B_6 (Davis 1988) but, due to poor reporting of data, this was not included in the meta-analysis (Proctor & Murphy 2009).

Pregnancy

Vitamin B_6 has been associated with some benefits during pregnancy; however, more research is required to understand the role of B_6 supplementation in this population.

A 2006 Cochrane Review investigated the clinical effects of vitamin B_6 oral capsules or lozenges during pregnancy and/or labour to see whether there were any changes to Apgar score, birth weight, incidence of pre-eclampsia or preterm birth (Thaver et al 2006). Five trials (1646 women) were included. Vitamin B_6 as oral capsules or lozenges resulted in decreased risk of dental decay in pregnant women. A small trial showed reduced mean birth weights with vitamin B_6 supplementation, and no significant differences in the risk of eclampsia, pre-eclampsia or low Apgar scores at 1 minute between supplemented and non-supplemented groups. No differences were found in Apgar scores at 1 or 5 minutes, or breast milk production between controls and women receiving oral or intramuscular loading doses of pyridoxine at labour (Thaver et al 2006). The authors concluded there were not enough data to be able to make any useful assessments, and further research is required. Furthermore, three of the five studies were from the 1960s (Hillman et al 1962, 1963, Swartwout et al 1960); the other two were from the 1980s (Schuster et al 1984, Temesvari et al 1983). More updated information is required.

A more recent systematic review evaluated the risks and benefits of interventions with vitamins B_6, B_{12} and C during pregnancy on maternal, neonatal and child health and nutrition outcomes (Dror & Allen 2012). In this meta-analysis based on three small studies, vitamin B_6 supplementation had a significant positive effect on birth weight; however, there were no significant effects on other neonatal outcomes, including preterm birth, low birth weight and perinatal morbidity and mortality.

Homocysteine and recurrent miscarriages

A 2012 study assessed homocysteine levels and pregnancy outcomes in 50 cases of recurrent miscarriage. Active treatment consisted of B_{12} 1500 mcg, vitamin B_6 10 mg and folic acid 5 mg daily taken throughout the pregnancy (n = 25) or during the first trimester only (n = 25). Following treatment with the B group vitamins, homocysteine levels decreased by 37%. Miscarriage rate in patients with hyperhomocysteinaemia was 26.6% compared with 11.4% in patients with normal homocysteine. The authors concluded that hyperhomocysteinaemia was associated with a 2.5-fold increased risk of miscarriage (Agarwal et al 2012).

Morning sickness

A systematic review investigated the effectiveness and safety of a range of treatments for nausea and vomiting in early pregnancy and suggested there was low-quality evidence to support B_6 versus placebo for nausea but not vomiting (Festin 2009). A Cochrane review in 2010 of 27 trials with 4042 women investigated the outcomes of vitamin B_6 supplementation, ginger and conventional drug therapy in reducing nausea and vomiting in early pregnancy (Matthews et al 2010). Two studies of 416 women compared vitamin B_6 with placebo (Sahakian et al 1991, Vutyavanich et al 1995) and showed that vitamin B_6 supplementation reduced nausea after 3 days. A well-designed, double blind, randomised, controlled trial had similar results but over a 3-week period (Smith & Crowther 2005). It is unclear whether vomiting frequency also reduced, due to the heterogeneity of studies.

In the same review, the comparative effectiveness of ginger and vitamin B_6 for nausea and vomiting in early pregnancy found both interventions significantly reduced nausea and vomiting scores (P < 0.05, P < 0.001 respectively) (Chittumma et al 2007, Sripramote & Lekhyananda 2003). Two other studies (Ensiyeh & Sakineh 2009, Smith et al 2004) report improvements in vomiting frequency, nausea and retching (Matthews et al 2010). In an experimental study of 60 pregnant women experiencing nausea and/or vomiting (prior to the 12th week of gestation), 30 women were given 10 mg of vitamin B_6 and 30 were given 1.28 mg for 2 weeks to investigate the outcome on Pregnancy-Unique Quantification of Emesis and nausea (PUQE) score. Plasma B_6 concentration was significantly increased in both groups (P < 0.05), and the higher supplementation group had a greater decrease in PUQE score (Wibowo et al 2012), suggesting that the 10 mg dose of vitamin B_6 is effective in reducing both nausea and vomiting in early-stage pregnancy.

Another study (Bsat et al 2001) looked at the effectiveness of three different antiemetics (metoclopramide with vitamin B_6, prochlorperazine and promethazine). The authors report that approximately 65%, 38% and 40% of women in each group, respectively, responded that they felt better on the third day of treatment. The authors conclude that their results favour pyridoxine-metoclopromide over the other two regimens.

Based on current research, vitamin B_6 appears to be effective in reducing both nausea and vomiting in early stages of pregnancy in a number of individual clinical trials. Its effectiveness is equivalent to that of ginger and may occur within 3 days of starting supplementation. Furthermore, the combination of metoclopramide with vitamin B_6 appears to be more effective than other conventional treatment (prochlorperazine and promethazine), and this effect may also begin within 3 days of treatment. Although a number of the trials showed benefit of B_6 overall, the authors concluded there was limited evidence from trials to support the use of pharmacological agents, including vitamin B_6 (Matthews et al 2010).

Heart disease

A growing body of evidence in contemporary studies has suggested a subtle relationship between heart failure and micronutrient status (McKeag et al 2012). While the authors state the results are inconclusive, one recent study reviewed by them showed potentially significant results. This observational study measured riboflavin and pyridoxine levels in 100 patients (mean age 67.1 years, 58% males) with heart failure (as defined by Framingham criteria). It was found that the percentage of patients with evidence of pyridoxine deficiency was significantly higher in patients with heart failure (38.0% vs 19.0%; P = 0.02) (Keith et al 2009). Whether low B_6 is a causative factor or consequence of disease remains to be clarified.

Elevated homocysteine levels

In practice, the relative safety and affordability of combined vitamin B supplementation (B_{12}, folic acid and B_6) make it an attractive recommendation in people with familial hyperhomocysteinaemia. Whether lowering total homocysteine improves cardiovascular mortality and morbidity is questionable, as recent large-scale clinical trials and meta-analyses have failed to demonstrate any benefits for B group vitamins (including B_6) in reducing overall cardiovascular risk, despite showing a reduction in homocysteine levels (Albert et al 2008, Clarke et al 2007, CTSUESU 2006, den Heijer et al 2007, Mann et al 2008, Marcus et al 2007, Ray et al 2007). Negative results were obtained yet again in a 2013 Cochrane intervention review which evaluated the clinical effectiveness of homocysteine-lowering interventions (in the form of supplements of vitamin B_6, B_9 and B_{12}) at reducing the incidence of myocardial infarction, stroke or all-cause mortality as compared to placebo.

Twelve randomised controlled trials involving 47,429 participants both with and without preexisting cardiovascular disease were included in the review, which concluded that the interventions did not significantly affect non-fatal or fatal myocardial infarction (pooled relative risk [RR] 1.02), stroke (pooled RR 0.91) or death by any cause (pooled RR 1.01) as compared with placebo (Martí-Carvajal et al 2013).

Failure of combined B vitamin therapy to reverse inflammatory processes associated with atherogenesis may partly explain the negative results (Bleie et al 2007). The consistent findings of an association between elevated plasma total homocysteine levels and vascular risk are yet to be fully explained; however, it is possible that the association is a consequence rather than a cause of disease (Toole et al 2004).

Venous thrombosis (VT)

A systematic review and meta-analysis investigated the association between B group vitamins and VT (Zhou et al 2012), given that a homocysteine-independent role for B group vitamins on VT development has been reported. In this review, significant standardised mean differences were obtained for plasma folic acid and vitamin B_{12}, suggesting that reduced levels of folic acid and vitamin B_{12} may be independent risk factors of VT. Moreover, a qualitative systematic review indicated that low level of vitamin B_6 was an independent risk factor of VT (Zhou et al 2012). Further prospective clinical studies are needed to provide additional evidence on the clinical benefits of B group vitamin supplementation for VT.

IN COMBINATION

In a 12-week, open-label, randomised, placebo-controlled trial, 85 hypertriglyceridaemic (triglycerides >150 mg/dL) males were randomised to one of five groups and given lysine (1 g/day), vitamin B_6 (50 mg/day), lysine (1 g/day) plus vitamin B_6 (50 mg/day), carnitine (1 g/day) or placebo for 12 weeks. Results showed that nutritional supplementation was associated with a significant reduction in total cholesterol by 10%. Additionally, plasma triglycerides were reduced by 36.6 mg/dL at 6 weeks compared with an increase of 18 mg/dL in the placebo group, although not statistically significant (Hlais et al 2012). The role of B_6 itself is unclear in achieving this result.

Reducing thromboembolism

A prospective cohort study of 757 patients experiencing first venous thromboembolism found that patients with lower plasma B_6 had a 1.8-fold higher risk of recurrence than those with higher levels of B_6 (Hron et al 2007). In contrast, no risk reduction was found in a secondary analysis of the HOPE-2 trial, which included over 5000 individuals with known cardiovascular disease or diabetes who were given a daily supplement of folic acid (2.5 mg), B_6 (50 mg) and B_{12} (1 mg) or a placebo for 5 years. In this analysis, vitamin therapy reduced homocysteine levels; however, it did not reduce the risk of venous thromboembolism, deep-vein thrombosis or pulmonary embolism (Ray et al 2007).

Improving outcomes after heart transplantation

Cardiac transplantation represents a potentially life-saving procedure for patients with end-stage cardiac disease. Short-term survival is improving because of improved immunosuppression, but long-term survival remains limited by an aggressive form of atherosclerosis known as transplant coronary artery disease (Miner et al 2001).

A randomised, double-blind placebo-controlled study showed that pyridoxine supplementation (100 mg/day) taken for 10 weeks improved endothelial function as assessed by flow-mediated dilatation in cardiac transplant recipients (Miner et al 2001). Interestingly, homocysteine levels remained unchanged with treatment, suggesting that other mechanisms are responsible.

IN COMBINATION

A randomised, double-blind, placebo-controlled study of 50 patients who were perceived to be at risk of cerebral ischaemia received B_6 (25 mg), folate (2.5 mg) and B_{12} (0.5 mg) or a placebo daily for a year. The study found that supplementation significantly reduced carotid intima-media thickness, which is a marker of atherosclerotic changes (Till et al 2005). In contrast, another small, double-blind, randomised and placebo-controlled trial of 30 individuals with a history of ischaemic stroke found that long-term treatment over 3.9 years with similar dosages of B_6 and B_{12} to the previous trial and slightly less folate (2 mg) produced no differences in carotid intima-media thickness and endothelial function (Potter et al 2007).

Cancer

A number of studies have investigated whether low B_6 may be associated with a higher prevalence of certain cancers and if higher levels have a chemopreventive effect. Some studies have focused on B_6 alone but often it is included as part of an investigation into the effects of folic acid, B_{12}, methionine and B_6 as a combination.

Theoretically, adequate B_6, B_{12}, folate and methionine might have a chemopreventive effect due to their roles in the one-carbon metabolism pathway, which is critical for DNA synthesis, methylation and repair (Harris et al 2012), and by reducing inflammation, cell proliferation and oxidative stress (Zhang et al 2013).

Ovarian cancer

The association between folate, methionine, vitamin B_6, vitamin B_{12} and alcohol among 1910 women with ovarian cancer and 1989 controls from a case-control study was conducted. An inverse association between dietary vitamin B_6 (covariate-adjusted odds ratio [OR] 0.76, 95% confidence interval [CI] 0.64–0.92; P_{trend} = 0.002) and methionine intake (covariate-adjusted OR 0.72, 95% CI 0.60–0.87; P_{trend} < 0.001) and ovarian cancer risk was found. The association with dietary vitamin B_6 was strongest for serous borderline (covariate-adjusted OR 0.49, 95% CI 0.32–0.77; P_{trend} = 0.001) and serous invasive (covariate-adjusted OR 0.74, 95% CI 0.58–0.94; P_{trend} = 0.012) subtypes. The authors concluded that methionine and especially vitamin B_6 may lower ovarian cancer risk (Harris et al 2012).

Breast cancer

The association of prediagnostic plasma concentrations of PLP with postmenopausal breast cancer risk was investigated in a case–control study of 706 cases and 706 controls. Women with higher plasma PLP concentrations had a 30% reduced risk of invasive breast cancer (CI 0.50–0.98) as compared with women with low PLP (P_{trend} = 0.02). The results suggest that higher circulating levels of vitamin B_6 are associated with a reduced risk of invasive postmenopausal breast cancer. The authors suggest a role for vitamin B_6 in the prevention of postmenopausal breast cancer, although further research is required (Lurie et al 2012).

The majority of studies investigating the protective role of B vitamins in breast cancer have focused on folate, B_6 and B_{12}. Several case-controlled studies have reported protective associations (Chen et al 2005, Larsson et al 2007, Lajous et al 2006, Yang et al 2013) while cohort studies have shown inconsistencies in results (Cho et al 2007, Ericson et al 2007, Shrubsole et al 2011, Stevens et al 2010). One investigated the association between dietary intakes of folate, B_2, B_6, B_{12} and methionine for breast cancer risk in Hispanic and non-Hispanic white women in the United States. Higher intakes of folate, B_{12} and methionine were associated with a lower risk of breast cancer; however there was no risk reduction with vitamin B_6 or B_2 (Yang et al 2013).

Other researchers, using the prospective cohort Shanghai Women's Health Study (1997–2008), including 718 Chinese breast cancer cases, investigated folate, B_6, B_{12}, niacin, riboflavin and methionine intakes and their association with breast carcinogenesis and again found no specific benefit from vitamin B_6 (Shrubsole et al 2011).

Bladder cancer

In an attempt to find a link between dietary components and incidence of bladder cancer, diet was assessed for 912 patients with bladder cancer and 873 controls by Garcia-Closas et al (2007). Individuals in the highest quintile for B_6 intake had a 40% reduced risk of bladder cancer compared with those in the lowest quintile.

Colorectal cancer

Current evidence suggests high dietary vitamin B_6 intake is associated with a reduced risk of colorectal cancer. One large longitudinal population study (n = 61; 433 women aged 40–76 years) used a food frequency questionnaire with a follow-up over 14.8 years and found that high dietary vitamin B_6 was associated with lower colorectal cancer risk, with protective effects most notably seen in women who drank alcohol (Larsson et al 2005). Similarly, a case-control study of 2028 people with colorectal cancer and 2722 controls confirmed a dose-dependent protective effect of B_6, with strongest protective effects observed for the highest intake and in people aged over 55 years (Theodoratou et al 2008). Another large population study of both men and women further confirmed that low dietary B_6 was associated with an increased risk in colorectal cancer, but the effect was specific for men and not for women. Protective effects were strongest in men with higher alcohol intake. These findings were from the large Japan Public Health Center-based Prospective Study, from which there were 526 cases of colorectal cancer (Ishihara et al 2007). A randomised controlled trial also found that high levels of plasma B_6 may be protective against colorectal adenomas (Figueiredo et al 2008).

A systematic review with meta-analysis of prospective studies assessed the association of vitamin B_6 intake or blood levels of PLP (the active form of vitamin B_6) with risk of colorectal cancer (Larsson et al 2010). Nine studies focused on vitamin B_6 intake and four studies on blood PLP levels. The pooled RRs of colorectal cancer for the highest vs lowest category of vitamin B_6 intake and blood PLP levels were 0.90 (95% CI 0.75–1.07) and 0.52 (95% CI 0.38–0.71), respectively. There was heterogeneity among studies of vitamin B_6 intake but not among studies of blood PLP levels. The risk of colorectal cancer decreased by 49% for every 100 pmol/mL increase in blood PLP levels (RR 0.51). Vitamin B_6 intake and blood PLP levels were inversely associated with the risk of colorectal cancer in this meta-analysis (Larsson et al 2010).

Another later study evaluated whether higher vitamin B_6 intake in the remote past is strongly associated with a lower risk of colorectal cancer than intake in the recent past. Vitamin B_6 intake was assessed every 4 years for up to 28 years using validated food frequency questionnaires from 86,440 women in the Nurses' Health Study and 44,410 men in the Health Professionals Follow-up Study. Total vitamin B_6 intake was significantly associated with an approximately 20–30% lower risk of colorectal cancer in age-adjusted results but these significant associations became attenuated and non-significant after adjustment for other colorectal cancer risk factors. Additionally, results did not differ by cancer subsite, source of vitamin B_6 (food or supplement) or intake of alcohol and folate (Zhang et al 2012).

Conversely, a randomised, double-blind, placebo-controlled trial of 5442 female health professionals at high risk for cardiovascular disease examined the effect of a combination pill of folic acid (2.5 mg), vitamin B_6 (50 mg) and vitamin B_{12} (1 mg) or placebo on the occurrence of colorectal adenoma. This study included 1470 participants who were followed up for as long as 9.2 years and underwent an endoscopy at any point during follow-up. The results indicated no statistically significant effect of the combination treatment on incidence of colorectal adenoma among this population. The risk of colorectal adenoma was similar among participants receiving treatment (24.3%, 180 of 741 participants) vs placebo (24.0%, 175 of 729 participants) (multivariable adjusted RR 1.00) (Song et al 2012).

Observational studies of dietary or dietary plus supplementary intake of vitamin B_6 and colorectal cancer risk have been inconsistent, with most studies reporting non-significant positive or inverse associations (Zhang et al 2013). However, a 30–50% reduction in colorectal cancer risk has been consistently reported in published studies where high circulating plasma levels of active vitamin B_6 (plasma POP) have been found. Zhang et al (2013) suggest that the discrepancy in the results may be due to dietary-based versus plasma-based studies, but why this is the case remains elusive. The age of vitamin B_6 repletion and the effect of repletion at different life stages, suboptimal levels, differing subtypes of colorectal cancer and genetic variants may also influence the results and explain such variations (Zhang et al 2013).

Lung cancer prognosis and vitamin B_6

The bioactive form of B_6, produced by pyridoxal kinase, has been found to exacerbate cisplatin-(cytotoxic agent used to treat non-small-cell lung cancer) mediated DNA damage and sensitise cancer cell lines to apoptosis, both in vitro and in vivo. Furthermore, low pyridoxal kinase activity, and thus low bioactive vitamin B_6, has been associated with poor disease outcome. The authors suggest pyridoxal kinase expression may be a marker for risk stratification in non-small-cell lung cancer patients (Galluzzi et al 2012).

Carpal tunnel syndrome (CTS)

It has been suspected that vitamin B_6 deficiency may play a role in the development of CTS, as several studies have found that patients with CTS and pyridoxine deficiency respond to supplementation (Ellis et al 1991). More recent evidence now casts doubt on the usefulness of B_6 supplementation in CTS. A 2002 review found no benefit with pyridoxine treatment in CTS (Gerritsen et al 2002). Similarly, a 2007 systematic review of treatments for CTS concluded that there was moderately strong evidence to suggest that B_6 was ineffective in the treatment of the condition (Piazzini et al 2007).

Autism

Overall, there is some research which suggests that supplementation with pyridoxine in combination with other nutrients, mainly magnesium, may improve some features of autism (Kuriyama et al 2002, Mousain-Bosc et al 2006, Pfeiffer et al 1995); however, larger trials with rigorous methodology are required before a more definitive conclusion can be made.

In 1997, a small, 10-week, double-blind, placebo-controlled trial found that an average dose of 638.9 mg pyridoxine and 216.3 mg magnesium oxide was ineffective in ameliorating autistic behaviours (Findling et al 1997). More recently, combination treatment with magnesium and B_6 was shown to improve symptoms such as social interaction, communication and general behaviour in autism (Mousain-Bosc et al 2006).

In a 2006 Cochrane systematic review, one study (Kuriyama et al 2002) concluded that pyridoxine was associated with improvement in verbal IQ scores; however it only included eight subjects and was a short-term study for 4 weeks. Overall, the review found that the quality and small sizes of the studies posed problems in evaluating the evidence that led to their conclusion that B_6-Mg therapy could not be recommended (Nye & Brice 2005). This review has been edited with no change to conclusions and republished in 2009. However, more current research needs to be conducted, including investigations on the clinical significance of the reduction in urinary dicarboxylic acid in autism.

Several studies have sought to explain how vitamin B_6 supplementation may provide benefits in this population.

Several studies have observed dietary deficiencies of vitamin B_2, vitamin B_6 and magnesium in autism (Kałuzna-Czaplinska et al 2009, Lakshmi Priya & Geetha 2011, Marlowe et al 1984, Xia et al 2010).

Increased homocysteine levels have been associated with autism (Kaluzna-Czaplinska et al 2013) as well as high levels of urinary dicarboxylic acids (an important marker of metabolism, energy production, intestinal dysbiosis and nutritional status in autistic children) (Kałuzna-Czaplinska et al 2011). Homocysteine levels can be lowered with a combination of vitamins B_6, B_{12} and folate; however it remains unclear whether this effect translates into a clinical benefit. Supplementation with magnesium (200 mg/day), pyridoxine (500 mg/day) and riboflavin (20 mg/day) for 3 months is able to reduce excretion of urinary dicarboxylic acid according to a study of 30 autistic children (Kałuzna-Czaplinska et al 2011). In this study, parents of the children being treated observed improvements in eye contact and the ability to concentrate, suggesting a possible clinical improvement.

Adams et al (2006) found that children with autism spectrum disorder had very high plasma levels of B_6 (without supplementation) compared to other children and suggested this may have occurred because of low activity of pyridoxal kinase to convert pyridoxine into PLP, which is the active cofactor for dozens of enzymatic reactions, including the formation of neurotransmitters. This may explain why high doses of B_6 seem necessary to produce benefits.

IN COMBINATION

A Cochrane review of vitamin B complex for treating peripheral neuropathy, which included 13 studies (11 parallel randomised controlled trials and two quasi-randomised trials) involving 741 participants (488 treated with vitamin B complex and 253 treated with placebo or another substance) with alcoholic or diabetic neuropathy, concluded there are only limited data, and the evidence is insufficient to determine whether vitamin B complex is beneficial or harmful (Ang et al 2008). Within this review, however, one trial suggested that 4-week treatment with high doses of oral vitamin B complex (thiamin 25 mg/daily and pyridoxine 50 mg/daily) was more efficacious than lower doses (1 mg each of thiamin and pyridoxine) in short-term reduction of pain, composite impairments, paraesthesiae and neuropathic symptoms (Abbas & Swai 1997). It is not clear if the results were due to the thiamin or pyridoxine or the combination. Given the age of this study, further investigations need to be conducted to attempt to elucidate similar findings.

Seizures

A study found that vitamin B_6-responsive seizures decrease or disappear following high-dose oral B_6 treatment (Ohtahara et al 2011). Vitamin B_6-responsive seizures or epilepsy are associated predominantly with West syndrome, but may also include Lennox-Gastaut syndrome, grand mal or partial motor seizures. In the study, 216 consecutive cases of West syndrome in children aged from 3 months to 5 years with both idiopathic and symptomatic seizures with organic brain lesions were administered high-dose B_6 and had an overall response rate of 13.9%. In responsive patients, long-term seizure and mental outcomes were noted. An increasing dose of 30 to 50–100 mg daily showed a slight clinical response, while doses of 100–400 mg/daily showed dramatic clinical improvements, with effects being noted within 1 week of treatment (Ohtahara et al 2011). In some cases the need for conventional antiepileptic medication was reduced.

This latter finding increases in significance and relevance in the clinical management of seizure control. A study found that 16/33 patients (48%) taking inducing antiepileptic drugs (AED) (phenytoin and carbamazepine) developed a vitamin B_6 deficiency compared with 9% in the control group. Of those that switched to non-inducing AED (levetiracetam, lamotrigine or topiramate), 21% were B_6-deficient (Mintzer et al 2012). The authors concluded that treatment with inducing AEDs commonly causes vitamin B_6 deficiency that is often severe.

Convulsions during a febrile episode

Two randomised trials have been conducted in children, producing conflicting results. One study of 65 children who had been admitted to hospital with febrile convulsions showed that a dose of 2–10 mg/kg PLP daily (orally or intravenously) produced a 100% success rate, whereas 43% in the control group experienced repeated convulsions (Kamiishi et al 1996). A second randomised trial found that a lower dose of 20 mg twice daily did not alter the incidence of febrile convulsions compared with placebo (McKiernan et al 1981).

Symptomatic treatment for stress

The term 'stress', as used by the public, is a subjective one and often described in different ways. One theoretical model that has been developed to predict psychological stress includes measures of life stressors, social support and coping style. Using this model, pyridoxine deficiency has been identified as a significant predictor of increased overall psychological stress during bereavement. More specifically, pyridoxine deficiency is significantly associated with increases in depression, fatigue and confused mood levels, but not with those of anxiety, anger or vigour (Baldewicz et al 1998).

One explanation is that pyridoxine is involved in neurotransmitter biosynthesis, such as GABA and serotonin, and therefore deficiency states that are associated with mood disturbances are improved with consequent supplementation (McCarty 2000).

Cognitive performance/Alzheimer's disease

Whether vitamin B_6 supplementation provides benefits in cognitive function and Alzheimer's disease (AD) remains to be clarified. It has gained some attention as a cheap and safe method of reducing homocysteine, which is implicated in the aetiology of AD and cognitive dysfunction; however, findings are equivocal.

One systematic review evaluated data from 16 studies that investigated the association between cognitive function in the elderly and B_6, folate and B_{12}. An association was found between folate and cognition in AD, but no association was found for vitamins B_6 or B_{12}. However, the authors suggested that heterogeneity in the methodology of the studies made interpretation problematic (Raman et al 2007).

A similar research group doing a systematic review of 14 trials found that most studies were small and of low quality. They found that three studies of B_6 and six trials of combined B vitamins revealed no effect, despite different dosages, on cognitive function. Only one of the trials found a significant improvement using B_6 to improve long-term memory. The review concluded that there was insufficient evidence to support a positive effect of B_6 on cognition. The reviewers suggested that larger, well-designed trials are needed to assess different groups of the population for any association between B_6 and cognitive function (Balk et al 2007).

A Cochrane systematic review on vitamin B_6 and cognition found no evidence for short-term benefit of vitamin B_6 in improving mood (depression, fatigue and tension symptoms) or cognitive functions (Malouf & Grimley Evans 2003). The review included two trials only (Bryan et al 2002, Deijen et al 1992) that used a double-blind, randomised, placebo-controlled design and involved 109 healthy older people. No trials of vitamin B_6 involving people with cognitive impairment or dementia were found, which may explain the negative results.

The development of cognitive impairment has been linked to elevated plasma homocysteine (Ford & Almeida 2012). A systematic review and meta-analysis of 19 randomised controlled trials was conducted to determine the effects of vitamins B_6, B_{12} and folic acid (commonly recognised homocysteine-lowering B vitamins) in individuals with and without cognitive impairment. It was found that these B vitamins, either alone or in combination, did not show an improvement in cognitive function for individuals with or without cognitive impairment. It remains to be established if prolonged treatment with B vitamins can reduce the risk of dementia in later life (Ford & Almeida 2012).

Homocysteine and Alzheimer's disease

According to one systematic review published in 2008, evidence is strong to suggest high homocysteine is a risk factor for AD and further randomised controlled trials are warranted to evaluate the association between B_6, folate, B_{12}, homocysteine levels and AD (Van Dam & Van Gool 2008).

Brain matter

Investigation of a healthy elderly population found a relationship between greater B_6 supplement intake and greater grey-matter volume (Erickson et al 2008). Another study with Alzheimer's patients found that low B_6 levels in patients were associated with white-matter lesions in the brain (Mulder et al 2005). The clinical significance of these findings remains to be clarified.

It has also been theorised that inflammation may be implicated in AD and dementia and that C-reactive protein, as a marker for systemic inflammation, may be a risk factor. A study of 85 individuals discovered that, where C-reactive protein was elevated, this was related to low B_6 levels and cerebral atrophy (Diaz-Arrastia et al 2006). This anti-inflammatory effect of B_6 may explain its possible role in neurodegenerative diseases; another interesting observation came from a study with older men, where levels of beta-amyloid levels were reduced with B_6, folate and B_{12} (Flicker et al 2008).

Schizophrenia

It has been suggested that high levels of homocysteine contribute to the pathogenesis of schizophrenia and the complex metabolic regulation of homocysteine that could be disrupted in schizophrenia (Petronijevic et al 2008).

To test whether supplementation could benefit this population, Levine et al (2006) conducted a randomised controlled trial of 42 schizophrenic patients with plasma homocysteine levels > 15 micromol/L. Treatment with oral folic acid, vitamin B_{12} and pyridoxine for 3 months reduced homocysteine and, more importantly, significantly improved clinical symptoms as measured by the Positive and Negative Syndrome Scale and neuropsychological tests overall, in particular the Wisconsin Card Sort (Levine et al 2006).

Tardive dyskinesia (TD)

TD is a significant clinical problem. Vitamin B_6 is a potent antioxidant and has a role in almost all of the possible mechanisms that are thought to be associated with the appearance of TD (Lerner et al 2007). To test whether supplementation would have any benefits, a 26-week, double-blind, placebo-controlled trial was conducted with 50 inpatients who had DSM-IV diagnoses of schizophrenia or schizoaffective disorder and TD. The randomised study found treatment with vitamin B_6 (1200 mg/day) significantly reduced symptoms of TD compared to a placebo.

Parkinson's disease (PD)

A higher dietary intake of vitamin B_6 was associated with a significantly decreased risk of PD, probably through mechanisms unrelated to homocysteine metabolism, according to findings from the Rotterdam Study — a prospective, population-based cohort study of people aged 55 years and older (de Lau et al 2006). The association between dietary intake of folate, vitamin B_{12} and vitamin B_6 and the risk of incident PD among 5289 participants was evaluated. After a mean follow-up of 9.7 years, the authors identified 72 participants with incident PD. Stratified analyses showed that this association was restricted to smokers. No association was observed for dietary folate and vitamin B_{12}.

Hyperhomocysteinaemia has been reported repeatedly in PD patients; the increase, however, seems mostly related to the methylated catabolism of L-dopa, the main pharmacological treatment of PD (Martignoni et al 2007).

OTHER USES

Vitamin B_6 supplements are effective for treating hereditary sideroblastic anaemia and refractory seizures in newborns, caused by pyridoxine withdrawal after delivery. Vitamin B_6 supplements have been used to prevent diabetic retinopathy and kidney stones, and to treat symptoms of vertigo, allergy to monosodium glutamate, asthma, photosensitivity and pervasive developmental disorders with hypersensitivity to sound. Women taking the oral contraceptive pill sometimes use supplemental B_6 to relieve mood disturbances and restore vitamin status. Whether supplementation has benefits in these circumstances remains unknown.

A small trial has shown some future potential clinical use in renal transplant patients with high homocysteine levels and endothelial dysfunction. A dose of folate (5 mg/day), B_6 (50 mg/day) and B_{12} (1000 mcg/day) was given to stable renal transplant patients for 6 months and homocysteine levels decreased and endothelial function was improved compared to the control patients (Xu et al 2008). Further trials are needed to confirm this finding.

Dream states

Many have suspected that pyridoxine supplements taken at night are able to influence dream states and sleep, causing disruption in some people. The results of a 2002 double-blind, placebo-controlled crossover study support this observation (Ebben et al 2002). Pyridoxine supplementation (250 mg) taken before bedtime was shown to significantly influence dream salience scores (a composite score containing measures for vividness, bizarreness, emotionality and colour), starting on the first night of treatment.

Leg cramps during pregnancy

A study of 84 pregnant women with leg cramps found that a combination of vitamin B_1 (100 mg/day) and B_6 (40 mg/day) improved symptoms 7.5-fold, and this was a better result than given by treatment with calcium carbonate (Sohrabvand et al 2006).

Irritable bowel syndrome (IBS)

In a cross-sectional study, IBS symptom score and dietary intake were assessed in 17 subjects with diagnosed IBS according to the Rome II criteria. The mean dietary intake was found to be 0.9 mg/day, below the recommended intake of 1.6 mg daily for men and 1.2 mg daily for women. The results indicated a high symptom score was associated with low vitamin B_6 intake (P = 0.0002) (Ligaarden & Farup 2011). This was a preliminary study, and the authors recognise the possibility of a type II error due to the small study group. However, this study may have clinical implications in the treatment and improvement of IBS symptoms with B_6 therapy, especially if given at therapeutic doses (minimum 5–25 mg to improve deficiency states). Further investigations need to be conducted to ascertain such possibilities.

Mortality in the elderly

A recent study identified that higher intakes of vitamins B_1 and B_6 observed among Taiwanese elders were associated with increased survival rates in this population by up to 10 years (Huang et al 2012). The Taiwanese Elderly Nutrition and Health Survey (1999–2000) provided data from 1747 participants 65 years and older. Dietary and biochemical data were collected at baseline and survivorship was determined until 31 December 2008. After controlling for confounders, a significant difference in mortality was found when comparing people in the lowest tertile to the highest tertile for both B_1 and B_6 dietary intakes (hazard ratios 0.74 and 0.74 respectively). The authors concluded that deficiencies of vitamin B_1 and B_6 were found to be clearly predictive of mortality in elderly Taiwanese.

DOSAGE RANGE

- Prevention of deficiency: Australian RDI for adults and children > 8 years: 1–1.7 mg/day.
- Treatment of deficiency: 5–25 mg/day.
- Morning sickness: 30–75 mg/day, sometimes taken as 25 mg three times daily. In clinical practice, monitored doses of 150 mg daily are often used.
- Symptoms of PMS: 100–500 mg/day.
- Elevated homocysteine levels: 100 mg/day (usually taken with B_{12} and folic acid).
- Leg cramps in pregnancy: vitamin B_1 100 mg/day and B_6 40 mg/day.
- Schizophrenic people with TD: vitamin B_6 (1200 mg/day).

TOXICITY

Symptoms of toxicity include paraesthesia, hyperaesthesia, bone pain, muscle weakness, numbness and fasciculation, most marked at the extremities (Dalton & Dalton 1987, Diegoli et al 1998). Some symptoms include unsteady gait, numbness of the hands and feet and impaired tendon reflexes. Excessive doses of vitamin B_6 cause degeneration of the dorsal root ganglia in the spinal cord, loss of myelination and degeneration of sensory fibres in the peripheral nerves.

The dose and time frame at which toxicity occurs vary significantly between individuals. Studies involving large population groups using 100–150 mg/day have shown minimal or no toxicity in 5–10-year studies, whereas studies of women self-medicating for PMS, taking 117 ± 92 mg for 2.9 ± 1.9 years, have reported increased incidence of peripheral neuropathy (Bernstein 1990, Dalton & Dalton 1987).

ADVERSE REACTIONS

Pyridoxine is considered non-toxic, although nausea and vomiting, headache, paraesthesia, sleepiness and low-serum folic acid levels have been reported.

Supplements taken at night may result in more vivid dreams and, for some individuals, disrupted sleep (Ebben et al 2002).

SIGNIFICANT INTERACTIONS

Amiodarone

Pyridoxine may increase the risk of drug-induced photosensitivity. Exercise caution with patients taking pyridoxine and amiodarone concurrently.

Antibiotics

Destruction of gastrointestinal flora can decrease endogenous production of vitamin B_6. Increase intake of vitamin B_6-rich foods or consider supplementation with long-term drug treatment.

Hydralazine

Hydralazine may induce B_6 deficiency according to a clinical study. Increased intake may be required with long-term drug therapy.

Isoniazid

Isoniazid increases vitamin B_6 requirements. Increase intake of vitamin B_6-rich foods or consider supplementation with long-term drug treatment.

L-dopa (without carbidopa)

In people with PD, L-dopa can cause hyperhomocysteinaemia, the extent of which is influenced by B vitamin status. To maintain normal plasma homocysteine concentrations, the B vitamin requirements are higher in L-dopa-treated patients than in those not on L-dopa therapy. B vitamin supplements may be warranted for PD patients on L-dopa therapy (Miller et al 2003).

Oral contraceptives

Oral contraceptives increase vitamin B_6 requirements. Increase intake of vitamin B_6-rich foods or consider supplementation with long-term drug treatment.

Penicillamine

This drug increases vitamin B_6 requirements. Increase intake of vitamin B_6-rich foods or consider supplementation.

Phenobarbitone, phenytoin

Vitamin B_6 supplements may lower plasma levels and efficacy of these drugs. Monitor for drug effectiveness, and exercise caution when these drugs are being taken concurrently.

Theophylline

May induce pyridoxine deficiency. Increased intake may be required with long-term drug therapy.

CONTRAINDICATIONS AND PRECAUTIONS

Monitor long-term use of high-dose pyridoxine supplements (>100 mg, although this level varies between individuals).

PREGNANCY USE

Pyridoxine supplements are commonly used during pregnancy to reduce symptoms of morning sickness, suggesting safety when used in appropriate doses.

Practice points/Patient counselling

- Vitamin B_6 is available in many foods; however, several surveys suggest that inadequate intakes are common.
- Deficiency can manifest with psychological symptoms of depression, irritability and confusion, and physical symptoms of lethargy, dermatitis, angular stomatitis, glossitis and impaired immunity.
- Overall, clinical research supports the use of vitamin B_6 supplements in relieving mild to moderate symptoms of PMS (particularly breast tenderness and mood disturbance), nausea in pregnancy and as a treatment for hyperhomocysteinaemia (usually with folate and B_{12}).
- Preliminary evidence suggests regular high dietary B_6 intake may have a protective effect in colorectal, breast, bladder and ovarian cancer risk, incidence of improvement of IBS symptomatology and possibly all-cause mortality.
- There is conflicting evidence as to whether vitamin B_6 supplements improve symptoms of CTS and autism (combined with magnesium), and whether they prevent febrile convulsions in children.
- Pyridoxine should not be used in high doses for the long term, as this can induce toxicity.

PATIENTS' FAQs

What will this vitamin do for me?

Vitamin B_6 is essential for the body's normal functioning. It has been used to treat many different conditions; however, scientific evidence generally supports its use in only a few conditions (e.g. morning sickness, mild to moderate PMS and elevated homocysteine levels).

When will it start to work?

This will depend on what is being treated. With regard to PMS symptoms, effects may take two to three menstrual cycles, whereas for morning sickness effects can be seen within 2–3 days.

Are there any safety issues?

High doses should not be taken for the long term, as this can cause toxicity.

REFERENCES

Abbas ZG, Swai ABM. Evaluation of the efficacy of thiamine and pyridoxine in the treatment of symptomatic diabetic peripheral neuropathy. East African Medical Journal 1997;74(12):803–8.

Adams JB et al. Abnormally high plasma levels of vitamin B_6 in children with autism not taking supplements compared to controls not taking supplements. J Altern Complement Med 12.1 (2006): 59–63.

Agarwal N, et al. Response of therapy with vitamin B_6, B_{12} and folic acid on homocystein level and pregnancy outcome in hyperhomocysteinaemia with unexplained recurrent abortions. International journal of Gynaecology and Obstetrics, 2012; 119(3): S759.

Albert CM et al. Effect of folic acid and B vitamins on risk of cardiovascular events and total mortality among women at high risk for cardiovascular disease: a randomized trial. JAMA 299.17 (2008): 2027–2036.

Anand SS. Protective effect of vitamin B_6 in chromium-induced oxidative stress in liver. J Appl Toxicol 25.5 (2005): 440–443.

Ang CD, et al. Vitamin B for treating peripheral neuropathy. Cochrane Database Syst Rev, 2008. CD004573.

Baldewicz T et al. Plasma pyridoxine deficiency is related to increased psychological distress in recently bereaved homosexual men. Psychosom Med 60.3 (1998): 297–308.

Balk EM et al. Vitamin B_6, B_{12}, and folic acid supplementation and cognitive function: a systematic review of randomized trials. Arch Intern Med 167.1 (2007): 21–30.

Beers MH, Berkow R (eds). The Merck manual of diagnosis and therapy, 17th edn. Whitehouse, NJ: Merck, 2003.

Bernstein AL. Vitamin B_6 in clinical neurology. Ann NY Acad Sci 585 (1990): 250–260.

Bleie O et al. Homocysteine-lowering therapy does not affect inflammatory markers of atherosclerosis in patients with stable coronary artery disease. J Intern Med 262.2 (2007): 141–272.

Bratman S, Kroll D. Natural health bible. Rocklin, CA: Prima Health, 2000.

Bryan J, et al. Short term folate vitamin B_{12} or vitamin B_6 supplementation slightly affects memory performance but not mood in women of various ages. Journal of Nutrition 2002;132(6):1345–56.

Bsat F, et al. Randomized study of three common outpatient treatments for nausea and vomiting of pregnancy [abstract]. American Journal of Obstetrics and Gynecology 2001;185(6 Suppl): S181.

Buyukokuroglu ME et al. Pyridoxine may protect the cerebellar granular cells against glutamate-induced toxicity. Int J Vitam Nutr Res 77.5 (2007): 336–340.

Chen J, et al. (2005) One-carbon metabolism, MTHFR polymorphisms, and risk of breast cancer. Cancer Res 65: 1606–1614.

Cheng CH et al. Vitamin B_6 supplementation increases immune responses in critically ill patients. Eur J Clin Nutr 60.10 (2006): 1207–1213.

Chittumma P, et al. Comparison of the effectiveness of ginger and vitamin B_6 for treatment of nausea and vomiting in early pregnancy: a randomized double-blind controlled trial. J Med Assoc Thai 90.1 (2007): 15–20.

Cho E, et al (2007) Nutrients involved in one-carbon metabolism and risk of breast cancer among premenopausal women. Cancer Epidemiology, Biomarkers & Prevention 16: 2787–2790.

Clarke R et al. Effects of B-vitamins on plasma homocysteine concentrations and on risk of cardiovascular disease and dementia. Curr Opin Clin Nutr Metab Care 10.1 (2007): 32–9.

Combs GF Jr. The Vitamins (Fourth Edition) Chapter 13 — Vitamin B_6. 2012, Pages 309–323. London: Elsevier

CTSUESU (Clinical Trial Service Unit and Epidemiological Studies Unit, Oxford, United Kingdom). Homocysteine-lowering trials for prevention of cardiovascular events: A review of the design and power of the large randomized trials. Am Heart J 151.2 (2006): 282–287.

Dalton K, Dalton MJ. Characteristics of pyridoxine overdose neuropathy syndrome. Acta Neurol Scand 76.1 (1987): 8–11.

Davis LS. Stress, vitamin B_6 and magnesium in women with and without dysmenorrhea: a comparison and intervention study [dissertation]. Austin (TX): University of Texas at Austin, December 1988.

Deijen JB, et al. Vitamin B_6 supplementation in elderly men effects on mood memory performance and mental effort. Psychopharmacology 1992;109(4):489–96.

De Lau LM et al. Dietary folate, vitamin B_{12}, and vitamin B_6 and the risk of Parkinson disease. Neurology 67.2 (2006): 315–3118.

Den Heijer MH et al. Homocysteine lowering by B vitamins and the secondary prevention of deep vein thrombosis and pulmonary embolism: A randomized, placebo-controlled, double-blind trial. Blood 109.1 (2007): 139–144.

Diaz-Arrastia R et al. P1-163: C-reactive protein in aging and Alzheimer's disease: Correlation with cerebral atrophy and low plasma vitamin B6. Alzheimers Dement 2.3, Supplement 1 (2006): S143.

Diegoli MS et al. A double-blind trial of four medications to treat severe premenstrual syndrome. Int J Gynaecol Obstet 62.1 (1998): 63–67.

Dror DK, Allen LH. Paediatric and Perinatal Epidemiology, 2012, 26 (Suppl. 1), 55–74.

Ebben M et al. Effects of pyridoxine on dreaming: a preliminary study. Percept Mot Skills 94.1 (2002): 135–140.

Ellis JM et al. A deficiency of vitamin B_6 is a plausible molecular basis of the retinopathy of patients with diabetes mellitus. Biochem Biophys Res Commun 179.1 (1991): 615–6119.

Ensiyeh J, Sakineh MAC. Comparing ginger and vitamin B_6 for the treatment of nausea and vomiting in pregnancy: a randomised controlled trial. Midwifery 2009;25(6):649–53.

Erickson KI et al. Greater intake of vitamins B_6 and B_{12} spares gray matter in healthy elderly: A voxel based morphometry study. Brain Res 1199 (2008): 20–26.

Ericson U, et al (2007) High folate intake is associated with lower breast cancer incidence in postmenopausal women in the Malmo Diet and Cancer cohort [see comment]. Am J Clin Nutr 86: 434–443.

Festin, M Nausea and vomiting in early pregnancy. Clinical Evidence 2009;06:1405.

Figueiredo CJ et al. Vitamins B_2, B_6, and B_{12} and risk of new colorectal adenomas in a randomized trial of aspirin use and folic acid supplementation. Cancer Epidemiol Biomarkers Prev 17.8 (2008): 2136–2145.

Findling RL et al. High-dose pyridoxine and magnesium administration in children with autistic disorder: an absence of salutary effects in a double-blind, placebo-controlled study. J Autism Dev Disord 27.4 (1997): 467–478.

Flicker L et al. B-vitamins reduce plasma levels of beta amyloid. Neurobiol Aging 29.2 (2008): 303–305.

Ford AH, Almeida OP. Effect of homocysteine lowering treatment on cognitive function: a systematic review and meta-analysis of randomized controlled trials. J Alzheimers Dis. 2012;29(1):133–49.

Galluzzi L, et al. Prognostic impact of vitamin B_6 metabolism in lung cancer. Cell Reports 2012; 2:257–269.

Garcia-Closas R et al. Food, nutrient and heterocyclic amine intake and the risk of bladder cancer. Eur J Cancer 43.11 (2007): 1731–1740.

Gerritsen AA et al. Conservative treatment options for carpal tunnel syndrome: a systematic review of randomised controlled trials. J Neurol 249.3 (2002): 272–280.

Gerster H. The importance of vitamin B_6 for development of the infant: Human medical and animal experiment studies. Ernahrungswiss 35.4 (1996): 309–317.

Groff JL, Gropper SS. Advanced nutrition and human metabolism. Belmont, CA: Wadsworth, 2009.

Gropper, S., Smith, J Advanced nutrition and human metabolism, 6th edition. Belmont, CA: Wadsworth, Cengage Learning, 2013.

Harris, H. R., et al. (2012), Folate, vitamin B_6, vitamin B_{12}, methionine and alcohol intake in relation to ovarian cancer risk. Int. J. Cancer, 131: E518–E529.

Hillman RW, et al. The effects of pyridoxine supplements on the dental caries experience of pregnant women. American Journal of Clinical Nutrition 1962;10:512–5.

Hillman R, et al. Pyridoxine supplementation during pregnancy. Clinical and laboratory observations. American Journal of Clinical Nutrition 1963;12:427–30.

Hlais S, et al. Effect of lysine, vitamin B_6, and carnitine supplementation on the lipid profile of male patients with hypertriglyceridemia: a 12-week, open-label, randomized, placebo-controlled trial. Clinical Therapeutics, 2012; 34:8.

Hron G et al. Low vitamin B_6 levels and the risk of recurrent venous thromboembolism. Haematologica 92.9 (2007): 1250–1253.

Huang, Y, et al. Prediction of all-cause mortality by B group vitamin status in the elderly. Clinical Nutrition 31 (2012) 191–198.

Hwang IK et al. Time course of changes in pyridoxal 5'-phosphate (vitamin B_6 active form) and its neuroprotection in experimental ischemic damage. Exp Neurol 206.1 (2007): 114–125.

Ishihara J et al. Low intake of vitamin B-6 is associated with increased risk of colorectal cancer in Japanese men. J Nutr 137.7 (2007): 1808–1814.

Jain S. Vitamin B_6 supplementation and complications of diabetes. Metab 56.2 (2007): 168–1071.

Ji Y et al. Pyridoxine prevents dysfunction of endothelial cell nitric oxide production in response to low-density lipoprotein. Atherosclerosis 188.1 (2006): 84–94.

Kałużna-Czaplińska J, et al. Nutritional deficiencies in children an example of autistic children. Nowa Pediatria 2009;4:94–100.

Kałużna-Czaplińska J, et al. Vitamin supplementation reduces the level of homocysteine in the urine of autistic children. Nutr Research 31, 2011; 318–321.

Kaluzna-Czaplinska, J., et al. 2013. A focus on homocysteine in autism. Acta Biochim.Pol., 60, (2) 137–142.

Kamiishi A et al. A clinical study of the effectiveness of vitamin B_6 for the prevention of repeated convulsions during one febrile episode. Brain Dev 18 (1996): 471–478.

Kannan K, Jain SK. Effect of vitamin B_6 on oxygen radicals, mitochondrial membrane potential, and lipid peroxidation in H_2O_2-treated U937 monocytes. Free Radic Biol Med 36.4 (2004): 423–428.

Kant AK, Block G. Dietary vitamin B-6 intake and food sources in the US population: NHANES II, 1976–1980. Am J Clin Nutr 52.4 (1990): 707–716.

Kashanian M et al. The evaluation of the effectiveness of pyridoxine (vitamin B_6) for the treatment of premenstrual syndrome: A double blind randomized clinical trial. Eur Psychiatry 23 Supplement 2 (2008): S381.

Keith ME, et al. B-vitamin deficiency in hospitalized patients with heart failure. J Am Diet Assoc. 2009;109(8): 1406–1410.

Kuriyama S, et al. Pyridoxine treatment in a subgroup of children with pervasive developmental disorders. Developmental Medicine & Child Neurology, 2002, 44:283–286.

Lajous M, et al (2006) Folate, vitamin B(6), and vitamin B(12) intake and the risk of breast cancer among Mexican women. Cancer Epidemiol Biomarkers Prev 15: 443–448.

Lakshmi AV, Ramalakshmi BA. Effect of pyridoxine or riboflavin supplementation on plasma homocysteine levels in women with oral lesions. Natl Med J India 11.4 (1998); as cited by Court S. A controlled trial of pyridoxine supplementation in children with febrile convulsions. Clin Pediatr 20.3 (1981): 208–11.

Lakshmi Priya MD, Geetha A. Level of trace elements (copper, zinc, magnesium and selenium) and toxic elements (lead and mercury) in the hair and nail of children with autism. Biol Trace Elem Res 2011; 142: 142–158.

Larsson SC et al. Vitamin B_6 intake, alcohol consumption, and colorectal cancer: A longitudinal population-based cohort of women. Gastroenterology 128.7 (2005): 1830–1837.

Larsson SC, et al (2007) Folate and risk of breast cancer: a meta-analysis. J Natl Cancer Inst 99: 64–76.

Larsson SC, et al. Vitamin B_6 and risk of colorectal cancer: a meta-analysis of prospective studies. JAMA. 2010;303(11):1077–1083.

Lerner V et al. Vitamin B_6 treatment for tardive dyskinesia: a randomized, double-blind, placebo-controlled, crossover study. J Clin Psychiatry 68.11 (2007): 1648–1654.

Levine J et al. Homocysteine-reducing strategies improve symptoms in chronic schizophrenic patients with hyperhomocysteinemia. Biol Psychiatry 60.3 (2006): 265–269.

Ligaarden S C & Farup R G. Low intake of vitamin B_6 is associated with irritable bowel syndrome symptoms. Nutrition Research 31 (2011) 356–361.

Lurie, G, et al. Prediagnositic plasma pyridoxal 5-phosphate (Vitamin B_6) levels and invasive breast carcinoma risk: the multiethnic cohort. Cancer Epidemiol Biomarkers Prev 2012; 21(11); 1942–8.

Malouf R, Grimley Evans J. Vitamin B_6 for cognition. Cochrane Database of Systematic Reviews 2003, Issue 4. Art. No.: CD004393.

Mann JF et al. Homocysteine lowering with folic acid and B vitamins in people with chronic kidney disease — results of the renal Hope-2 study. Nephrol Dial Transplant 23.2 (2008): 645–53.

Marcus J et al. Homocysteine lowering and cardiovascular disease risk: lost in translation. Can J Cardiol 23.9 (2007): 707–10.

Marlowe M, et al. Decreased magnesium in the hair of autistic children. J Orthomol psychiatry 1984;13:117–22.

Martí-Carvajal AJ, et al. Homocysteine-lowering interventions for preventing cardiovascular events. Cochrane Database of Systematic Reviews 2013, Issue 1. Art. No.: CD006612.

Martignoni E et al. Homocysteine and Parkinson's disease: a dangerous liaison? J Neurol Sci 257.1–2 (2007): 31–37.

Matthews A, et al. Interventions for nausea and vomiting in early pregnancy. Cochrane Database of Systematic Reviews 2010, Issue 9. Art. No.: CD007575.

Matxain JM et al. Theoretical study of the reaction of vitamin B_6 with 1O2. Chemistry 13.16 (2007): 4636–4642.

McCarty MF. High-dose pyridoxine as an 'anti-stress' strategy. Med Hypotheses 54.5 (2000): 803–807.

McKeag NA., et al. The role of micronutrients in heart failure. Journal of the Academy of Nutrition and Dietetics, 2012; 1.12: 870–886.

McKiernan J et al. A controlled trial of pyridoxine supplementation in children with febrile convulsions. Clin Pediatr (Phila) 20.3 (1981): 208–211.

Miller JW et al. Effect of L-dopa on plasma homocysteine in PD patients: relationship to B-vitamin status. Neurology 60.7 (2003): 1125–1129.

Miner SE et al. Pyridoxine improves endothelial function in cardiac transplant recipients. J Heart Lung Transplant 20.9 (2001): 964–969.

Mintzer S, et al. B-Vitamin deficiency in patients treated with antiepileptic drugs. Epilepsy & Behavior 24 (2012) 341–344.

Mousain-Bosc M et al. Improvement of neurobehavioral disorders in children supplemented with magnesium-vitamin B_6. II. Pervasive developmental disorder-autism. Magnes Res 19.1 (2006): 53–62.

Mulder C et al. Low vitamin B_6 levels are associated with white matter lesions in Alzheimer's disease. J Am Geriatr Soc 53.6 (2005): 1073–1074.

Nakamura S et al. Pyridoxal phosphate prevents progression of diabetic nephropathy. Nephrol Dial Transplant 22.8 (2007): 2165–2174.

Nye C, Brice A. Combined vitamin B_6-magnesium treatment in autism spectrum disorder. Cochrane Database Syst Rev 4 (2005): CD003497.

Ohtahara S, et al. Vitamin B_6 treatment of intractable seizures. Brain & Development 33 (2011) 783–789.

Oka T. Modulation of gene expression by vitamin B_6. Nutr Res Rev. 2001; 14:257–65.

Pelton R et al. Drug-induced nutrient depletion handbook 1999–2000. Hudson, OH: Lexi-Comp, 2000.

Petronijevic ND et al. Plasma homocysteine levels in young male patients in the exacerbation and remission phase of schizophrenia. Prog Neuropsychopharmacol Biol Psychiatry 32.8 (2008): 1921–1926.

Pfeiffer SI et al. Efficacy of vitamin B_6 and magnesium in the treatment of autism: a methodology review and summary of outcomes. J Autism Dev Disord 25.5 (1995): 481–493.

Piazzini DB et al. A systematic review of conservative treatment of carpal tunnel syndrome. Clin Rehabil 21.4 (2007): 299–314.

Potter K et al. Long-term treatment with folic acid, vitamin B_6 and vitamin B_{12} does not improve vascular structure or function: A randomised double-blind placebo-controlled trial. Heart Lung Circ 16 Supplement 2 (2007): S168.

Proctor M & Murphy PA. Herbal and dietary therapies for primary and secondary dysmenorrhoea. Cochrane Database Syst Rev 2001 (2009): CD002124.

Raman G et al. Heterogeneity and lack of good quality studies limit association between folate, vitamins B-6 and B-12, and cognitive function. J Nutr 137.7 (2007): 1789–1794.

Ray JG et al. Homocysteine-lowering therapy and risk for venous thromboembolism: a randomized trial. Ann Intern Med 146.11 (2007): 761–767.

Ren SG, Melmed S. Pyridoxal phosphate inhibits pituitary cell proliferation and hormone secretion. Endocrinology 147.8 (2006): 3936–3942.

Sahakian V, et al. Vitamin B_6 is effective therapy for nausea and vomiting of pregnancy: a randomized, double-blind placebo-controlled study. Obstetrics & Gynecology 1991;78:33–6.

Schuster K, et al. Effect of maternal pyridoxine-HCl supplementation on the vitamin B-6 status of mother and infant and on pregnancy outcome. Journal of Nutrition 1984;114:977–88.

Sharma P et al. Role of bromocriptine and pyridoxine in premenstrual tension syndrome. Indian J Physiol Pharmacol 51.4 (2007): 368–374.

Shimada D et al. Effect of high dose of pyridoxine on mammary tumorigenesis. Nutr Cancer 53.2 (2005): 202–207.

Shimada D et al. Vitamin B_6 suppresses growth of the feline mammary tumor cell line FRM. Biosci Biotechnol Biochem 70.4 (2006): 1038–1040.

Shizukuishi S et al. Distribution of vitamin B_6 deficiency in university students. Tokyo: J Nutr Sci Vitaminol 27.3 (1981) 193–7.

Shrubsole MJ, et al. Dietary B vitamin and methionine intakes and breast cancer risk among Chinese women. Am J Epidemiol. 2011 May 15;173(10):1171–82.

Smith C, Crowther C. Ginger was as effective as vitamin B_6 in improving symptoms of nausea and vomiting in early pregnancy. Evidence-based Obstetrics & Gynecology 7.2 (2005): 60–61.

Smith C, et al. A randomized controlled trial of ginger to treat nausea and vomiting in pregnancy. Obstetrics & Gynecology 2004; 103(4):639–45.

So Y, Simon R. Chapter 57 Deficiency diseases of the nervous system. in Bradley's Neurology in Clinical Practice, 6th edn. Philadelphia, PA: Saunders, 2012.

Sohrabvand F et al. Vitamin B supplementation for leg cramps during pregnancy. Int J Gynaecol Obstet 95.1 (2006): 48–49.

Song, Y, et al. Effect of combined folic acid, vitamin B_6, and vitamin B_{12} on colorectal adenoma. JNCI J Natl Cancer Inst (2012) 104 (20): 1562–1575.

Sripramote M, Lekhyananda N. A randomized comparison of ginger and vitamin b6 in the treatment of nausea and vomiting in pregnancy. Journal of the Medical Association of Thailand 2003;86:846–53.

Stevens VL, et al (2010) Folate and other one-carbon metabolism-related nutrients and risk of postmenopausal breast cancer in the Cancer Prevention Study II Nutrition Cohort. Am J Clin Nutr 91: 1708–1715.

Swartwout JR, et al. Vitamin B_6, serum lipids and placental arteriolar lesions in human pregnancy. A preliminary report. American Journal of Clinical Nutrition 1960;8:434–44.

Tanimoto M et al. Effect of pyridoxamine (K-163), an inhibitor of advanced glycation end products, on type 2 diabetic nephropathy in KK-Ay/Ta mice. Metabolism 56.2 (2007): 160–167.

Temesvari P, et al. Effects of an antenatal load of pyridoxine (vitamin B_6) on the blood oxygen affinity and prolactin levels in newborn infants and their mothers. Acta Paediatrica Scandinavica 1983;72: 525–9.

Thaver D, et al. Pyridoxine (vitamin B_6) supplementation in pregnancy. Cochrane Database of Systematic Reviews 2006, Issue 2. Art. No.: CD000179.

Theodoratou E et al. Dietary vitamin B_6 intake and the risk of colorectal cancer. Cancer Epidemiol Biomarkers Prev 17.1 (2008): 171–182.

Till U et al. Decrease of carotid intima-media thickness in patients at risk to cerebral ischemia after supplementation with folic acid, vitamins B_6 and B_{12}. Atherosclerosis 181.1 (2005): 131–135.
Toole JF et al. Lowering homocysteine in patients with ischaemic stroke to prevent recurrent stroke, myocardial infarction and death. JAMA 291 (2004): 565–75.
Van Dam F, Van Gool WA. Hyperhomocysteinemia and Alzheimer's disease: A systematic review. Arch Gerontol Geriatr 48.3 (2008): 425–430.
Vutyavanich T, et al. Pyridoxine for nausea and vomiting of pregnancy: a randomized, double-blind, placebo-controlled trial. American Journal of Obstetrics and Gynecology 1995;173:881–4.
Wahlqvist M (ed). Food and nutrition. Sydney: Allen & Unwin, 1997.
Wardlaw G. Contemporary nutrition, 3rd edn. Madison, WI: Brown and Benchmark, 1997.
Weingaertner J et al. Initial findings on teratological and developmental relationships and differences between neural tube defects and facial clefting: First experimental results. J Cranio-Maxillofacial Surg 33.5 (2005): 297–300.
Whelan AM, et al. Herbs, vitamins and minerals in the treatment of premenstrual syndrome: a systematic review. Can J Clin Pharmacol. 2009 Fall;16(3):e407–29.
Wibowo N, et al. Vitamin B_6 supplementation in pregnant women with nausea and vomiting. International Journal of Gynecology and Obstetrics 116, 2012: 206–210.
Wilcken DE, Wilcken B. B vitamins and homocysteine in cardiovascular disease and aging. Ann NY Acad Sci 854 (1998): 361–370.
Wyatt KM et al. Efficacy of vitamin B-6 in the treatment of premenstrual syndrome: systematic review. BMJ 318.7195 (1999): 1375–1381.
Xia W, et al. A preliminary study on nutritional status and intake in Chinese children with autism. Eur J Pediatr 2010;169: 1201–6.
Xu T et al. Treatment of hyperhomocysteinemia and endothelial dysfunction in renal transplant recipients with B vitamins in the Chinese population. J Urol 179.3 (2008): 1190–1194.
Yang D, et al. Dietary intake of folate, B-vitamins and methionine and breast cancer risk among Hispanic and Non-Hispanic white women. 2013 PLoS ONE 8(2): e54495.
Zhang X, et al. Prospective cohort studies of vitamin B_6 intake and colorectal cancer incidence: modification by time? Cancer Epidemiol Biomarkers Prev March 2012; 21; 560.
Zhang X-H, et al Vitamin B_6 and colorectal cancer: Current evidence and future directions. World J Gastroenterol 2013; 19(7): 1005–1010.
Zhou K, et al Association between B-group vitamins and venous thrombosis: systematic review and meta-analysis of epidemiological studies. Journal of Thrombosis and Thrombolysis 2012, Volume 34, Issue 4, pp 459–467.

Vitamin B_{12}

BACKGROUND AND RELEVANT PHARMACOKINETICS

Vitamin B_{12} (cobalamin) is a water-soluble vitamin obtained mostly from animal protein products in the diet. In the stomach gastric acid is required to liberate protein-bound cobalamin, which is then immediately bound to R-binders (glycoproteins) that protect it from being denatured. When the contents of the stomach reach the duodenum, the R-binders are partially digested by pancreatic proteases, releasing them to bind to intrinsic factor (a glycoprotein), which is secreted by the parietal cells of the gastric mucosa. This complex is then absorbed in the terminal ileum and transported to cells, where it carries out its metabolic function, or to the liver, where it is stored until required (FAO/WHO 2002, Oh & Brown 2003). An alternative method of absorption, which is independent of intrinsic factor, also appears to exist and accounts for the absorption of approximately 1% of large oral doses (> 300 mcg) of B_{12} (Elia 1998). Absorption via intrinsic factor is limited to about 1.5–2.0 mcg/meal owing to limited receptor capacity (FAO/WHO 2002).

> ***Clinical note — Nori: a source for vegetarians***
>
> While the majority of non-meat sources of vitamin B_{12} do not contain the biologically active form, it is possible to get B_{12} from some non-meat foods. In fact, improvements in B_{12} status have been observed following the ingestion of nori (seaweed). Nori is said to contain as much B_{12} as liver (Croft et al 2005), approximately 55–59 mcg/100 g dry weight. Five different biologically active vitamin B_{12} compounds have been identified in nori: cyanocobalamin, hydroxycobalamin, sulfitocobalamin, adenosylcobalamin and methylcobalamin (Takenaka et al 2001); the source of B_{12} appears to be bacteria (Croft et al 2005).

CHEMICAL COMPONENTS

Vitamin B_{12} is the largest of the B vitamins and is a complex structure containing a central cobalt atom. There are five forms of B_{12}: cyanocobalamin (a synthetic form that has a cyanide attached to the cobalt), hydroxycobalamin (hydroxyl group attached to the cobalt; it is produced for parenteral administration), aquacobalamin (water group bound to the cobalt) and the coenzymatically active forms (methylcobalamin and 5-deoxyadenosylcobalamin), in which a methyl group or a 5-deoxyadenosyl group is bound to the cobalt atom (FAO/WHO 2002, Freeman et al 1999).

FOOD SOURCES

Vitamin B_{12} is found in lamb's liver, sardines, oysters, egg yolk, fish, beef, kidney, cheese and milk. Up to 10% is lost in cooking (Wahlqvist 2002). Fortified breakfast cereals are also available.

Vitamin B_{12} bioavailability significantly decreases with increasing intake as the intrinsic factor-mediated intestinal absorption system is estimated to be saturated at about 1.5–2.0 mcg/meal for healthy adults with normal gastrointestinal function. The bioavailability of vitamin B_{12} from different sources is variable: fish (42%), lamb (56–89%), chicken (61–66%) and eggs (<9%) (Watanabe 2007).

Plants do not contain B_{12} because they have no cobalamin-dependent enzymes (Croft et al 2005). Most microorganisms, including bacteria and algae, synthesise B_{12}, which then makes its way into the food chain (FAO/WHO 2002). Human intestinal bacteria also synthesise B_{12}, but this is not absorbed to any considerable extent (Wahlqvist 2002). Vegans living in situations with more stringent hygiene are therefore more likely to develop deficiencies.

DEFICIENCY SIGNS AND SYMPTOMS

Vitamin B_{12} deficiencies manifest primarily as haematological and neurological disturbances. The elderly are particularly at risk, with vitamin B_{12} deficiency estimated to affect 10–15% of individuals over the age of 60 years (Baik & Russell 1999).

- Haemotological: macrocytic (megaloblastic) anaemia, pancytopenia (leucopenia, thrombocytopenia); symptoms may include lethargy, dyspnoea, anorexia, weight loss and pallor (Wahlqvist 2002).
- Neurological disturbances: paraesthesias, ataxia, optic neuropathy (reversible), peripheral neuropathy and demyelination of the corticospinal tract and dorsal columns (subacute combined systems disease).
- Psychological disturbances: impaired memory, irritability, depression, personality change, dementia, delirium and psychosis (Lee 1999, Lindenbaum et al 1988). A case report of vitamin B_{12} deficiency presenting as obsessive compulsive disorder has been described (Sharma & Biswas 2012).
- Various gastrointestinal symptoms can also develop, such as loss of appetite, intermittent constipation and diarrhoea, glossitis and abdominal pain.
- Folic acid supplementation may mask an underlying B_{12} deficiency, leading to the progression of neurological symptoms.

Primary deficiency

People at risk are those living in India, Central and South America, and selected areas in Africa (Stabler & Allen 2004), strict vegetarians and vegans, breastfed infants of vegetarian mothers with low B_{12} stores, elderly patients with 'tea and toast diets' and chronic alcoholics. Vitamin B_{12} deficiency exists more commonly among vegans than vegetarians, with depletion or deficiency of vitamin B_{12} found to occur irrespective of demographic, place of residency, age or type of vegetarian diet (Pawlak et al 2013). Approximately 62% of pregnant vegetarians are B_{12}-deficient as are 25–86% of vegetarian children, 21–41% of vegetarian adolescents and 11–90% of elderly vegetarians.

As vitamin B_{12} is stored to a considerable extent, even after complete depletion of food-ingested cobalamin, clinically relevant deficiencies will usually only develop after 5–10 years (Schenk et al 1999). This time frame increases to an average of approximately 18 years in strict vegetarians when intrinsic factor secretion is intact (Babior 1996). In this case, some enterohepatic recycling of cobalamin should occur in the distal ileum (Howden 2000).

Secondary deficiency

Vitamin B_{12} deficiency is more likely to result from inadequate absorption, defects in vitamin B_{12} metabolism or gastrointestinal disorders than a lack of dietary intake.

- Pernicious anaemia: an autoimmune condition affecting gastric parietal cells that produce intrinsic factor; common cause of megaloblastic anaemia, especially in persons of European or African descent (Stabler & Allen 2004).
- Methylmalonic acidaemia: inherited defect in B_{12} metabolism.
- Congenital absence of transcobalamin II.
- Medications that reduce gastric acidity (e.g. H_2 blockers and proton pump inhibitors [PPIs]).
- Atrophic gastritis/gastric atrophy: probably due to a decrease in acid output and intrinsic factor production (Schenk et al 1999). Gastric atrophy is more common in the elderly.
- Intestinal resection of the part of the ileum where absorption takes place or gastric resection, which affects the parietal cells and in turn production of intrinsic factor.
- Achlorhydria (Termanini et al 1998).
- Pancreatic insufficiency: the cobalamin-R-protein complex is split by pancreatic enzymes in the duodenum (Festen 1991).
- Ileal dysfunction (Howden 2000): may affect absorption at this site.
- Crohn's disease, irritable bowel disease, coeliac disease: reduced absorption.
- Bacteria and parasites in the intestine may also compete for B_{12}.
- Radiotherapy for rectal cancer: causes a rapid and persistent decrease in B_{12} status, as reflected by reduced serum B_{12} combined with increased serum methylmalonic acid (MMA) (Gronlie Guren et al 2004).
- Nitrous oxide may induce or potentiate B_{12} deficiency myelopathy (Hathout & El-Saden 2011).

The elderly deserve a separate mention as a population at risk of deficiency because of both primary and secondary causes, such as poor dietary intake, failure to separate vitamin B_{12} from food protein, inadequate absorption, utilisation and storage, as well as drug–food interactions leading to malabsorption and metabolic inactivation (Bradford & Taylor 1999, Dharmarajan et al 2003). Subtle signs of deficiency may include lethargy, weight loss and dementia (Dharmarajan et al 2003).

Elevated B_{12} levels

Elevated levels of serum cobalamin may be a sign of a serious, even life-threatening, disease such as chronic myelogenous leukaemia, promyelocytic leukaemia, polycythaemia vera, hypereosinophilic syndrome, acute hepatitis, cirrhosis, hepatocellular carcinoma and metastatic liver disease. Elevated B_{12} levels, therefore, warrant a full diagnostic workup to assess the presence of disease (Ermens et al 2003).

Liver failure mortality

A prospective study of patients with acute-on-chronic liver failure (n = 105) found that elevated vitamin B_{12} levels on hospital admission were associated with increased severity of liver disease and 3-month mortality rate (Dou et al 2012).

> ***Clinical note — Testing for vitamin B_{12} deficiency***
> Numerous studies have indicated that serum B_{12} levels are an inadequate guide to B_{12} status (Briddon 2003, Carmel 1988, Kapadia 2000, Karnaze & Carmel 1990, Termanini et al 1998). The use of this test has led to poorly defined reference intervals for serum B_{12} (Briddon 2003), potentially delaying the diagnosis and allowing the progression of B_{12} deficiency. Approximately 50% of patients with subclinical disease have normal serum B_{12} levels and older patients present with neurological and psychiatric symptoms without haematological findings. In addition, use of the oral contraceptive pill may affect test results (Bor 2004). As a result, this method of testing has lost favour as an adequate measure of B_{12} status. A combination of two tests appears to be more conclusive. Elevated levels of total homocysteine in serum and plasma reflect deficiencies of either folate or B_{12}. MMA is a more specific marker of cobalamin function, but renal insufficiency may affect the results of this test. Therefore, a combination of the two is probably the clearest indicator (Bjorke Monsen & Ueland 2003, FAO/WHO 2002, Kapadia 2000). Preliminary evidence also suggests that overnight fasting urinary MMA concentrations correlate strongly with serum MMA; however, further investigations are required to confirm the application of this test in various populations (Kwok et al 2004). While the use of such markers may improve the assessment of B_{12} deficiency, establishing the cause of deficiency should also be part of the diagnostic approach (Schneede & Ueland 2005).

MAIN ACTIONS

Important cofactor

Vitamin B_{12} is essential for the normal function of all cells. It affects cell growth and replication, the metabolism of carbohydrates, lipids and protein and is involved in fatty acid and nucleic acid synthesis. It is also involved in the production of red blood cells in bone marrow, and activates folacin coenzymes for red blood cell production.

Homocysteine reduction

Methylcobalamin aids in the conversion of homocysteine to methionine by the action of methionine synthase, transferring a methyl group from methylfolate (folic acid).

After conversion from homocysteine, methionine is then converted to *S*-adenosyl-L-methionine (SAMe), important for methylation reactions and protein synthesis. An increase in homocysteine levels and decrease in SAMe levels have been implicated in depression and may also contribute to the neurological symptoms seen in pernicious anaemia (IMG 2003).

Nervous system

Vitamin B_{12} is involved in the synthesis of protein structures in the myelin sheath and nerve cells. As methylation is required for the production of myelin basic protein, a reduction in B_{12} and SAMe will result in demyelination of peripheral nerves and the spinal column (subacute combined degeneration; FAO/WHO 2002).

Immune system

Vitamin B_{12} acts as an immunomodulator for cellular immunity (Tamura et al 1999).

Liver

Vitamin B_{12} deficiency results in decreased serine dehydratase (SDH) and tyrosine aminotransferase activities in rat livers (Ebara et al 2008). In dimethylnitrosamine-induced liver injury in mice, vitamin B_{12} decreased the blood levels of aspartate aminotransferase and alanine aminotransferase, suggesting a possible hepatoprotective effect (Isoda et al 2008).

Antioxidant capacity

Recent studies have identified that vitamin B_{12} and its cobalamin-based derivatives are powerful antioxidants at pharmacological concentrations (Birch et al 2009, Moreira et al 2011, Weinburg et al 2009).

CLINICAL USE

Vitamin B_{12} supplementation is administered using various routes, such as intravenous and oral doses. This review will focus on oral supplementation as this is the form generally used by the public and is available over the counter. It is sometimes used in combination with other B group vitamins, in particular B_6 and folate.

Deficiency: treatment and prevention

Traditionally, vitamin B_{12} supplementation has been used to treat deficiency or prevent it in conditions such as pernicious anaemia and atrophic gastritis, but special consideration should be given to the elderly, who are at high risk.

Pernicious anaemia

Pernicious anaemia is caused by a deficiency of intrinsic factor, leading to malabsorption of vitamin B_{12}. Signs and symptoms include pallor, glossitis, weakness and neurological symptoms, including paraesthesias of the hands and feet, decreased deep-tendon reflexes and loss of sensory perception and motor controls (neurological symptoms may be irreversible). In more progressed conditions confusion, memory loss, moodiness, psychosis and delusional behaviour may be present. Achlorhydria and gastric mucosal atrophy may also occur, further complicating the condition.

Uncomplicated pernicious anaemia is characterised by mild or moderate megaloblastic anaemia without leucopenia, thrombocytopenia or neurological symptoms. In more advanced cases urgent parenteral administration of vitamin B_{12} and folic acid (typically 100 mcg of cyanocobalamin and 1–5 mg of folic acid) is given intramuscularly, as well as blood transfusions.

Atrophic gastritis

Elderly patients with atrophic gastritis appear to have higher rates of vitamin B_{12} deficiency ($P < 0.01$) which responds to B_{12} supplementation (Lewerin et al 2008).

Infants

In infants, severe vitamin B_{12} deficiency can cause neurological symptoms, including irritability, failure to thrive, apathy, anorexia and developmental regression which responds well to supplementation (Dror & Allen 2008). A large cohort study (n = 2001) found that vitamin B_{12} levels at birth did not affect asthma or eczema-related outcomes between birth and age 6 (van der Valk et al 2013).

Elderly

Vitamin B_{12} deficiency is common in the elderly, with estimates as high as 43% (Wolters et al 2004). Poor vitamin B_{12} status has been associated with vascular disease, depression, impaired cognitive performance and dementia. Elderly patients (>60 years) should be monitored for evidence of B_{12} deficiency (a minimum threshold of 220–258 pmol/L [300–350 pg/mL] is desirable in the elderly) and general supplementation with vitamin B_{12} (> 50 mcg/day) should be considered (Wolters et al 2004). Significantly higher doses may be required to correct deficiency. A randomised, parallel-group, double-blind, dose-finding trial found that the lowest dose of oral cyanocobalamin required to normalise mild vitamin B_{12} deficiency in the elderly is 647–1032 mcg/day, more than 200-fold the recommended dietary allowance (Eussen et al 2005). Conversely another randomised controlled trial (RCT) reported that even low doses of B_{12} could improve the vitamin status in elderly people with food-bound vitamin B_{12} malabsorption. The dose required to increase mean serum vitamin B_{12} by 37 pmol/L was 5.9 mcg/day (95% confidence interval [CI] 0.9–12.1) (Blacher et al 2007). In another study of elderly people with malabsorption taking 1000 mcg/day of crystalline cyanocobalamin for 1 month, 85% of subjects normalised their serum cobalamin concentrations, and all subjects corrected their initial macrocytosis and had medullar regeneration with a mean increase in reticulocyte count (Andres et al 2006). While hearing loss has been associated with poor B_{12} status in the elderly, short-term supplementation has so far failed to show benefits (Park et al 2006).

Pemetrexed treatment

To reduce the incidence of adverse effects, pretreatment with folate and vitamin B_{12} is recommended prior to treatment with pemetrexed, an antifolate chemotherapeutic used in non-small-cell lung cancer (Molina & Adjei 2003). No significant difference in adverse effects was noted in a trial which compared duration of folate and vitamin B_{12} (5–14 days versus less than 4 days: Kim et al 2013).

Hyperhomocysteinaemia

Vitamin B_{12} alone may not be sufficient to normalise elevated homocysteine levels (Yajnik et al 2007). As a result, vitamin B_{12} is often recommended in combination with folic acid and vitamin B_6 in conditions for which homocysteine is implicated as a possible causative factor.

> ***Clinical note — Oral forms are effective***
>
> Vitamin B_{12} is often given parenterally as an intramuscular injection, based on the understanding that oral doses will not be efficacious in cases of malabsorption.
>
> There is now considerable evidence that oral vitamin B_{12} therapy is comparable in efficacy to parenteral therapy, even when intrinsic factor is not present or in other diseases affecting absorption (Andres et al 2005a, 2005b, Castelli et al 2011, Delpre et al 1999, Oh & Brown 2003, Roth & Orija 2004, Vidal-Alaball et al 2005, Wellmer et al 2006). A 2005 Cochrane review suggested that 2000 mcg/day of oral vitamin B_{12} or 1000 mcg initially daily then weekly and monthly may be as effective as intramuscular injections in obtaining short-term haematological and neurological responses in vitamin B_{12}-deficient patients (Vidal-Alaball et al 2005). As rare cases of anaphylaxis may occur with parenteral administration, oral therapy is also considered a safer option with improved cost and compliance (Bilwani et al 2005, Bolaman et al 2003). At doses of 500 mcg/day, correction of serum B_{12} levels is likely to occur within 1 week to 1 month, with correction of haematological abnormalities after at least 3 months (Andres et al 2005b).

Cardiovascular protection

In practice, the relative safety and affordability of combined vitamin B supplementation (B_{12}, folic acid and B_6) make it an attractive recommendation in people with familial hyperhomocysteinaemia. Whether lowering total homocysteine improves cardiovascular mortality and morbidity is questionable, as large-scale clinical trials and meta-analyses have failed to demonstrate any benefits for either B_{12} alone or in combination for reducing overall cardiovascular risk, despite showing a reduction in homocysteine levels (Albert et al 2008, Clarke et al 2007, Mann et al 2008, Marcus et al 2007, Ray et al 2007). Furthermore, a 2013 Cochrane systematic review concluded that there was insufficient evidence to support the use of homocysteine-lowering interventions, including vitamin B_{12}, to prevent cardiovascular events (Martí-Carvajal et al 2013).

Failure of combined B vitamin therapy to reverse inflammatory processes associated with atherogenesis may partly explain the negative results (Bleie et al 2007). The consistent findings of an association between elevated plasma total homocysteine levels and vascular risk is yet to be fully explained; however it is possible that the association is a consequence rather than a cause of disease (Toole et al 2004).

Cardiovascular disease

There is very limited evidence from cohort studies that vitamin B_{12} deficiency predisposes for cardiovascular disease or diabetes according to a systematic review (Rafnsson et al 2011). As such, current data do not support the use of vitamin B_{12} supplementation to reduce the risk of either of these diseases. An intervention study, VITATOPS, was a randomised, double-blind, placebo-controlled trial (n = 8164), which also found that daily administration of B_{12} in combination with folic acid and vitamin B_6 did not reduce the incidence of major vascular events such as stroke or transient ischaemic attacks (TIAs) in elderly patients with a recent history of stroke or TIA (VITATOPS Trial Study Group 2010).

Renal transplant recipients

Although studies investigating the effects of vitamin B_{12} as a stand-alone treatment in this condition are not available, several clinical studies have produced conflicting evidence for the use of combination vitamin B treatment (vitamin B_{12}, folic acid and B_6).

An RCT involving 56 renal transplant patients found that vitamin supplementation with folic acid (5 mg/day), vitamin B_6 (50 mg/day) and vitamin B_{12} (400 mcg/day) for 6 months reduced the progression of atherosclerosis. Patients taking the vitamin combination experienced a significant decrease in homocysteine levels and carotid intima media thickness, which is reflective of early atherosclerosis (Marcucci et al 2003). In another trial, 36 stable renal transplant recipients with hyperhomocysteinaemia received a similar combination of 5 mg folic acid and 50 mg B_6, in addition to either 1000 mcg B_{12} or placebo per day for 6 months. Supplementation decreased blood homocysteine and improved endothelium-dependent and independent vasodilation responses (Xu et al 2008). Despite these preliminary findings, combined therapy using even higher doses (40 mg folic acid, 100 mg B_6 and 2 mg B_{12}) did not improve survival (448 vitamin group deaths vs 436 placebo group deaths) (hazard ratio 1.04; 95% CI 0.91–1.18) or reduce the incidence of vascular disease (myocardial infarct, stroke and amputations) in patients with advanced chronic kidney disease or end-stage renal disease (Jamison et al 2007).

Restenosis after percutaneous coronary intervention

An RCT found that vitamin B_{12} (cyanocobalamin, 400 mcg/day), folic acid (1 mg/day) and vitamin B_6 (pyridoxine hydrochloride, 10 mg/day) taken for 6 months significantly decreased the incidence of major adverse events, including restenosis after percutaneous coronary intervention (Schnyder et al 2002).

Neural tube defects

Vitamin B_{12} is required to cleave folate, without which folate is not effective, and postpartum analysis of serum B_{12} levels has shown an increased risk of neural tube defects in women with low B_{12} status (Groenen et al 2004, Ray & Blom 2003, Suarez et al 2003). Some authors have called for combined fortification of food with folic acid and vitamin B_{12} because there are concerns about masking B_{12} deficiency (Czernichow et al 2005).

Noise-induced hearing loss

Homocysteine levels are significantly higher in subjects with noise-induced hearing loss as compared to healthy controls (Gok et al 2004) and elevated plasma B_{12} levels appear to play a protective role (Quaranta et al 2004).

Recurrent abortion

There appears to be a correlation between low serum B_{12} levels, increased homocysteine levels and early or very early recurrent abortion in some women (Reznikoff-Etievant et al 2002, Zetterberg et al 2002). One small study of five women with a history of very early recurrent abortion found that vitamin B_{12} supplementation resulted in four normal pregnancies (Reznikoff-Etievant et al 2002). Further research is required to investigate possible benefits.

Osteoporosis — inconclusive

Elevated homocysteine levels have been suggested as a risk factor for osteoporosis (Herrmann et al 2005); however, this remains uncertain. A meta-analysis of six studies identified that vitamin B_{12} and homocysteine levels were significantly increased in postmenopausal osteoporotic women compared to controls (Zhang et al 2014), whereas a more recent meta-analysis found no association between homocysteine, folate or vitamin B_{12} with bone mineral density in women (van Wijngaarden et al 2013). A small intervention study of women over 65 years of age (n = 31) with elevated homocysteine levels found that treatment with the combination of vitamin B_{12} and folate had no significant effect on bone turnover or bone health (Keser et al 2013).

Depression

Elevation of homocysteine and low levels of vitamin B_{12} and folate are commonly seen in depression (Coppen & Bolander-Gouaille 2005). Observational studies have found as many as 30% of patients hospitalised for depression to be deficient in vitamin B_{12} (Hutto 1997). A cross-sectional study of 700 community-living, physically disabled women over the age of 65 years found that vitamin B_{12}-deficient women were twice as likely to be severely depressed as non-deficient women (Penninx et al 2000). Similarly, a recent Finnish study found that, in subjects aged 45–74 years, vitamin B_{12} level was associated with melancholic depressive symptoms, but not with non-melancholic depressive symptoms (Seppälä et al 2013).

A study of 225 hospitalised acutely ill older patients receiving 400 mL of an oral nutritional supplement (106 subjects) or placebo (119 subjects) daily for 6 weeks reported significant increases in plasma vitamin B_{12} concentrations and red cell folate, and a decrease in depression scores (Gariballa & Forster 2007). Whether the study cohort were B_{12}-deficient at baseline was not clear.

AIDS and HIV

Low vitamin B_{12} levels are often observed in patients infected with HIV type 1 (Remacha & Cadafalch 1999, Remacha et al 1993). One study identified deficiency in 10–35% of all patients seropositive for HIV, presumably as a result of decreased intake, intestinal malabsorption and/or abnormalities in plasma-binding proteins or antagonism by the drug azidothymidine. Importantly, as serum cobalamin levels declined, progression to AIDS increased and neurological symptoms worsened.

Adjuvant treatment in hepatitis C infection

The combination of vitamin B_{12} with standard treatment significantly improved viral response compared to standard treatment only in antiviral-naïve patients with chronic hepatitis C virus infection (Rocco et al 2013).

Cognitive impairment and dementia

More than 77 cross-sectional studies including more than 34,000 subjects have reported a significant association between low blood levels of folate and B_{12} (or high levels of homocysteine) and prevalent dementia. The association has been described for different types of cognitive impairment, including vascular dementia, Alzheimer's disease and mild cognitive impairment; however, it is not clear whether low B_{12} was a cause or consequence of dementia (Vogel et al 2009). A positive association between serum homocysteine levels and incidence of dementia has also been described in a recent meta-analysis of eight cohort studies ($n = 8669$; odds ratio 1.50; 95% CI 1.13–2.00) (Wald et al 2011).

Despite this possible association, few interventional studies using B_{12} supplementation have been conducted. A systematic review reports on six RCTs utilising B_{12} supplementation for effects on cognitive function; however, the range of doses and administration forms together with cognitive status of volunteers and measures used make interpretation difficult (Vogel et al 2009). Overall, the review concludes that there is insufficient evidence to suggest vitamin B_{12} supplementation to improve cognitive decline or incidence of dementia but also states there are several confounding factors to consider. Unfortunately, few studies considered taking fasting B_{12} blood samples at baseline: the possibility of misclassification of study subjects as cognitive-impaired (or demented) or healthy and classing subjects with normal scores on cognitive tests as healthy even though they have Alzheimer's disease at the preclinical state are other confounding factors.

This is important to bear in mind when considering that, while some interventional studies are negative, there are also positive studies showing that supplementation with vitamin B_{12} significantly reversed impaired mental function in individuals with pre-existing low levels (Healton et al 1991, Miller 2003, Refsum & Smith 2003, Tripathi et al 2001, Weir & Scott 1999).

Interestingly, women in the highest quartile of plasma vitamin B_{12} levels during midlife scored significantly higher on cognitive function tests in later years and were cognitively equivalent to those 4 years younger (Kang & Grodstein 2005). Another study of 370 non-demented 75-year-olds found a twofold increased risk of developing Alzheimer's dementia in subjects with low serum levels of vitamin B_{12} and folate over a 3-year period (Wang et al 2001).

Diabetic neuropathy

According to a 2005 review of seven RCTs, vitamin B_{12} supplementation may improve pain and paraesthaesia in patients with diabetic neuropathy (Sun et al 2005). The studies cited, however, were generally of low quality and more research is required to confirm these results and determine whether positive effects are due to the correction of deficiency or to alteration of abnormal metabolism.

Sleep disorders

A preliminary study investigated the effects of randomly assigned methyl- and cyanocobalamin on circadian rhythms, wellbeing, alertness and concentration after 14 days in 20 healthy subjects (Mayer et al 1996). Methylcobalamin supplementation led to a significant decrease in daytime melatonin levels, improved sleep quality, shorter sleep cycles, increased feelings of alertness, better concentration and a feeling of waking up refreshed in the morning. It appeared that methylcobalamin was significantly more effective than cobalamin.

Tinnitus

A group of 113 army personnel (mean age 39 years) exposed to military noise was studied, of which 57 had chronic tinnitus and noise-induced hearing loss

(Shemesh et al 1993). Of this subset, 47% also had vitamin B_{12} deficiency. Treatment with vitamin B_{12} supplementation produced some improvement in tinnitus and associated symptoms.

OTHER USES

Human trials have shown vitamin B_{12} levels to be low in people with recurrent aphthous stomatitis, suggesting a possible aetiological factor (Piskin et al 2002). An inhalation of vitamin B_{12} mixed solution has been shown to be effective for the treatment of acute radiation-induced mucosal injury (Chen & Shi 2006).

Prostate cancer risk — no association

A large-scale population-based study (n = 317,000) found no association with vitamin B_{12} levels and prostate cancer risk (de Vogel et al 2013).

Erythema nodosum

A case report exists of a 38-year-old female diagnosed with erythema nodosum and B_{12} deficiency whose symptoms resolved completely without recurrence following vitamin B_{12} therapy (Volkov et al 2005). Testing for deficiency may be advised in such cases.

Atopic dermatitis

A novel use for B_{12} in a topical cream for atopic dermatitis was tested in a prospective, randomised, placebo-controlled phase III multicentre trial involving 49 patients. Subjects applied the B_{12} cream twice daily to one side of the body and a placebo cream to the contralateral side, according to the randomisation scheme, for 8 weeks. The B_{12} cream was reported to significantly improve the extent and severity of atopic dermatitis and was considered safe and very well tolerated (Stucker et al 2004).

Multiple sclerosis

Multiple sclerosis (MS) and vitamin B_{12} deficiency share common inflammatory and neurodegenerative characteristics and low or decreased levels of vitamin B_{12} have been demonstrated in MS patients and may correlate with early onset (<18 years) (Miller et al 2005). Considering vitamin B_{12} is a cofactor, and myelin formation has important immunomodulatory and neurotrophic effects (Loder et al 2002, Miller et al 2005, Sandyk & Awerbuch 1993), a theoretical basis exists for its use in MS.

Amyotrophic lateral sclerosis (ALS)

Early evidence suggests a possible benefit for long-term ultra-high-dose methylcobalamin (administered intravascularly or intramuscularly) for sporadic or familial cases of ALS (motor neuron disease) (Izumi & Kaji 2007); however, large-scale clinical trials are required to assess the efficacy and safety of this treatment.

Schizophrenia

An improvement in the negative symptoms of schizophrenia was seen following daily vitamin B_{12} (400 mcg) and folic acid (2 mg) supplementation during a 16-week multicentre RCT (Roffman et al 2013). Treatment response was affected by genetic variation in folic acid absorption. The effect of vitamin B_{12} in the absence of folic acid was not investigated.

DOSAGE RANGE

Australian recommended daily intake

- Adult >13 years: 2.4 mcg/day.
- Pregnancy: 2.6 mcg/day.
- Lactation: 2.8 mcg/day.
- Requirements may be higher for elderly people with impaired digestion or absorption.
- Sublingual cyanocobalamin: 1000–2000 mcg/day taken 30 min before breakfast.
- Pernicious anaemia: generally, vitamin B_{12} 1000 mcg intramuscularly 2–4 times weekly is given until haematological abnormalities are corrected, and then it is given once monthly. Alternatively, oral B_{12} can be given in very large doses (0.5–2 mg/day). Correction of haematological abnormalities usually occurs within 6 weeks of treatment, but neural improvement may take up to 18 months.
- Homocysteine lowering: 0.5 mg/day (Dusitanond et al 2005).

Note: Sublingual cobalamin is the preferred oral form for many practitioners, with methylcobalamin also becoming available in some regions.

ADVERSE REACTIONS

Although adverse effects to parenteral cobalamin have been reported, oral supplements appear to be well tolerated (Branco-Ferreira et al 1997, Hillman 1996).

SIGNIFICANT INTERACTIONS

Carbamazepine

In studies with children, long-term carbamazepine use led to a decrease in vitamin B_{12} levels (Karabiber et al 2003) — observe for signs and symptoms of B_{12} deficiency. Increased intake may be required with long-term therapy.

Colchicine

The use of colchicine may reduce the absorption of orally administered vitamin B_{12} — monitoring of serum B_{12} concentration is recommended, particularly if there is a history of deficiency.

Gastric acid inhibitors: PPI and H_2 receptor antagonists

Gastric acid is required to liberate protein-bound cobalamin. Therefore, vitamin B_{12} concentration may be decreased when gastric acid is markedly suppressed for prolonged periods (Laine et al 2000, Schenk et al 1999, Termanini et al 1998). Studies have shown that omeprazole therapy acutely decreases cyanocobalamin absorption in a dose-dependent manner

(Marcuard et al 1994, Saltzman et al 1994) and deficiency may occur with long-term use (Valuck & Ruscin 2004). Additionally, a large-scale 2013 case-control study found that use of PPIs or H_2 receptor antagonists for 2 years or more was associated with an increased risk of vitamin B_{12} deficiency (Lam et al 2013). It should be noted that vitamin B_{12} supplements do not suffer the same fate, as they are not bound to protein — observe for signs and symptoms of B_{12} deficiency; vitamin B_{12} supplements may be required with long-term therapy.

Hydrochlorothiazide

There are a number of medications that have the ability to increase homocysteine levels, such as hydrochlorothiazide (Westphal et al 2003), therefore concurrent use of vitamin B_{12} (with folic acid) may be a useful adjunct — potential beneficial interaction.

Lithium

Lithium administration may result in a decrease in serum B_{12} concentration; however, the clinical significance of these findings is not yet clear (Cervantes et al 1999). Beneficial interaction is possible.

Metformin

In patients with type 2 diabetes, metformin has been shown to reduce levels of vitamin B_{12} (and folate) and increase homocysteine (Sahin et al 2007). This effect was not demonstrated in women with polycystic ovary syndrome who were taking metformin and receiving vitamin B_{12} and folate substitution, a daily oral multivitamin tablet, and dietary and lifestyle advice (Carlsen et al 2007). Supplementation may be beneficial.

Oral contraceptive pill

Users of the oral contraceptive pill showed significantly lower concentrations of cobalamin than controls in a 2003 clinical study (Sutterlin et al 2003). However, it would appear that this may be due to an effect on B_{12}-binding proteins in serum affecting test results, because total homocysteine and MMA markers were unchanged and no symptoms of deficiency were present (Bor 2004) — observe for signs and symptoms of B_{12} deficiency and conduct testing if deficiency is suspected.

Phenobarbitone and phenytoin

One clinical study reports that combined long-term use of phenobarbitone and phenytoin resulted in significantly increased serum levels of vitamin B_{12} (Dastur & Dave 1987) — observe patients taking this combination.

Prednisolone

Decreased vitamin B_{12} levels have been reported in the cerebrospinal fluid and serum of MS patients following high-dose (1000 mg daily for 10 days) intravenous methylprednisolone (Frequin et al 1993). Given the suggested importance of B_{12} in MS sufferers, a beneficial interaction is possible.

Sodium valproate

Administration of sodium valproate has been shown to increase plasma vitamin B_{12} concentrations, with one study citing increases of over 50% of baseline (Gidal et al 2005).

Tetracycline antibiotics

B complexes containing B_{12} may significantly reduce the bioavailability of tetracycline hydrochloride (Omray 1981) — separate doses by at least 2 hours.

Practice points/Patient counselling

- Vitamin B_{12} (cobalamin) is a water-soluble vitamin obtained mostly from animal protein products in the diet.
- There is considerable evidence that oral vitamin B_{12} therapy is comparable in efficacy to parenteral therapy, even when intrinsic factor is not present or in other diseases affecting absorption.
- As numerous studies have indicated that serum B_{12} levels are an inadequate guide to B_{12} status, a combination of total homocysteine and MMA is probably the clearest indicator, although discrepancies can still occur.
- Vitamin B_{12} deficiencies manifest primarily as haematological and neurological disturbances and are estimated to affect 10–15% of individuals over the age of 60 years.
- Traditionally, supplementation is recommended to treat deficiency states or prevent them in people at risk, such as in pernicious anaemia or atrophic gastritis.
- When administered together with folic acid and vitamin B_6 (pyridoxine), vitamin B_{12} is used to reduce homocysteine levels. In this way, vitamin B_{12} is sometimes recommended in conditions where homocysteine is implicated as a possible causative factor.
- Some evidence has shown supplementation can be useful in HIV and AIDS, depression, tinnitus and cognitive impairment when low vitamin B_{12} levels are also present. Preliminary evidence also suggests a possible role for supplementation in diabetic retinopathy and sleep disturbances.
- There are several commonly prescribed pharmaceutical medicines that can reduce vitamin B_{12} absorption when used long-term.

CONTRAINDICATIONS AND PRECAUTIONS

- Parenteral cyanocobalamin given for vitamin B_{12} deficiency caused by malabsorption should be given intramuscularly or by the deep subcutaneous route — never intravenously.
- Folic acid supplementation may mask a B_{12} deficiency.
- Treatment with cyanocobalamin should be avoided in cases of altered cobalamin metabolism or deficiency associated with chronic cyanide intoxication (Freeman et al 1999).

PREGNANCY USE

Vitamin B_{12} is considered safe in pregnancy.

Low-dose vitamin B_{12} (1–18 mcg/day) does not appear to impact on the circulating level of serum cobalamins or its binding proteins in lactating women (Morkbak et al 2007). If required, higher doses may need to be utilised.

PATIENTS' FAQs

What will this vitamin do for me?

Vitamin B_{12} is essential for healthy growth, development and health maintenance. It will reverse signs and symptoms of deficiency and can alleviate symptoms of tinnitus, poor memory, depression and HIV and AIDS when low vitamin B_{12} levels are also present. There is also some research suggesting some positive effects in diabetic retinopathy and sleep disturbances.

When will it start to work?

In cases of pernicious anaemia, the classical deficiency state, correction of blood abnormalities occurs within 6 weeks; however, correction of nervous system changes is slower and may take up to 18 months.

Are there any safety issues?

Vitamin B_{12} is considered a very safe nutrient.

REFERENCES

Albert CM et al. Effect of folic acid and B vitamins on risk of cardiovascular events and total mortality among women at high risk for cardiovascular disease: a randomized trial. JAMA 299.17 (2008): 2027–2036.

Andres E et al. Food-cobalamin malabsorption in elderly patients: Clinical manifestations and treatment. Am J Med 118.10 (2005a): 1154–1159.

Andres E et al. Usefulness of oral vitamin B_{12} therapy in vitamin B_{12} deficiency related to food-cobalamin malabsorption: Short and long-term outcome. Eur J Intern Med 16.3 (2005b): 218.

Andres E et al. Hematological response to short-term oral cyanocobalamin therapy for the treatment of cobalamin deficiencies in elderly patients. J Nutr Health Aging 10.1 (2006): 3–6.

Babior BM. Metabolic aspects of folic acid and cobalamin. In: Beutler E et al (eds). Williams haematology, 5th edn. New York: McGraw-Hill, 1996: 380–393.

Baik HW, Russell RM. Vitamin B_{12} deficiency in the elderly. Annu Rev Nutr 19 (1999): 357–377.

Bilwani F et al. Anaphylactic reaction after intramuscular injection of cyanocobalamin (vitamin B_{12}): a case report. J Pak Med Assoc 55.5 (2005): 217–2119.

Birch CS et al. A novel role for vitamin B12: Cobalamins are intracellular antioxidants in vitro. Free Radic Biol Med 47.2 (2009): 184–188.

Bjorke Monsen AL, Ueland PM. Homocysteine and methylmalonic acid in diagnosis and risk assessment from infancy to adolescence. Am J Clin Nutr 78.1 (2003): 7–21.

Blacher J et al. Very low oral doses of vitamin B_{12} increase serum concentrations in elderly subjects with food-bound vitamin B_{12} malabsorption. J Nutr 137.2 (2007): 373–378.

Bleie O et al. Homocysteine-lowering therapy does not affect inflammatory markers of atherosclerosis in patients with stable coronary artery disease. J Intern Med 262.2 (2007): 244–253.

Bolaman Z et al. Oral versus intramuscular cobalamin treatment in megaloblastic anemia: A single-center, prospective, randomized, open-label study. Clin Ther 25.12 (2003): 3124–3134.

Bor MV. Do we have any good reason to suggest restricting the use of oral contraceptives in women with pre-existing vitamin B_{12} deficiency? Eur J Obstet Gynecol Reprod Biol 115.2 (2004): 240–241.

Bradford GS, Taylor CT. Omeprazole and vitamin B_{12} deficiency. Ann Pharmacother 33.5 (1999): 641–643.

Branco-Ferreira M et al. Anaphylactic reaction to hydroxycobalamin. Allergy 52 (1997): 118–1119.

Briddon A. Homocysteine in the context of cobalamin metabolism and deficiency states. Amino Acids 24.1–2 (2003): 1–12.

Carlsen SM et al. Homocysteine levels are unaffected by metformin treatment in both nonpregnant and pregnant women with polycystic ovary syndrome. Acta Obstet Gynecol Scand 86.2 (2007): 145–150.

Carmel R. Pernicious anemia. The expected findings of very low serum cobalamin levels, anemia, and macrocytosis are often lacking. Arch Intern Med 148.8 (1988): 1712–1714.

Castelli MC et al. Comparing the efficacy and tolerability of a new daily oral vitamin B12 formulation and intermittent intramuscular vitamin B12 in normalizing low cobalamin levels: a randomized, open-label, parallel-group study. Clin Ther 33.3 (2011): 358–371.

Cervantes P et al. Vitamin B_{12} and folate levels and lithium administration in patients with affective disorders. Biol Psychiatry 45.2 (1999): 214–221.

Chen XL, Shi YS. [Effect of vitamin B_{12} mixed solution inhalation for acute radiation-induced mucosal injury.] Nan Fang Yi Ke Da Xue Xue Bao 26.4 (2006): 512–5114.

Clarke R et al. Effects of B-vitamins on plasma homocysteine concentrations and on risk of cardiovascular disease and dementia. Curr Opin Clin Nutr Metab Care 10.1 (v) (2007): 32–9.

Coppen A, Bolander-Gouaille C. Treatment of depression: time to consider folic acid and vitamin B_{12}. J Psychopharmacol 19.1 (2005): 59–65.

Croft MT et al. Algae acquire vitamin B_{12} through a symbiotic relationship with bacteria. Nature 438.7064 (2005): 90–93.

Czernichow S et al. Case for folic acid and vitamin B_{12} fortification in Europe. Semin Vasc Med 5.2 (2005): 156–162.

Dastur DK, Dave UP. Effect of prolonged anticonvulsant medication in epileptic patients: serum lipids, vitamins B_6, B_{12}, and folic acid, proteins, and fine structure of liver. Epilepsia 28.2 (1987): 147–159.

Delpre G et al. Sublingual therapy for cobalamin deficiency as an alternative to oral and parenteral cobalamin supplementation. Lancet 354.9180 (1999): 740.

de Vogel S et al. Serum folate and vitamin B12 concentrations in relation to prostate cancer risk — a Norwegian population-based nested case-control study of 3000 cases and 3000 controls within the JANUS cohort. Int J Epidemiol 42.1 (2013): 201–210.

Dharmarajan TS, et al. Vitamin B_{12} deficiency. Recognizing subtle symptoms in older adults. Geriatrics 58.3 (2003): 30–34, 37–8.

Dou JF et al. Serum vitamin B12 levels as indicators of disease severity and mortality of patients with acute-on-chronic liver failure. Clin Chim Acta 413.23–24 (2012): 1809–1812.

Dror DK, Allen LH. Effect of vitamin B_{12} deficiency on neurodevelopment in infants: current knowledge and possible mechanisms. Nutr Rev 66.5 (2008): 250–255.

Dusitanond P et al. Homocysteine-lowering treatment with folic acid, cobalamin, and pyridoxine does not reduce blood markers of inflammation, endothelial dysfunction, or hypercoagulability in patients with previous transient ischemic attack or stroke: a randomized substudy of the VITATOPS trial. Stroke 36.1 (2005): 144–146.

Ebara S et al. Vitamin B_{12} deficiency results in the abnormal regulation of serine dehydratase and tyrosine aminotransferase activities correlated with impairment of the adenylyl cyclase system in rat liver. Br J Nutr 99.3 (2008): 503–510.

Elia M. Oral or parenteral therapy for B_{12} deficiency. Lancet 352 (1998): 1721–1722.

Ermens AAM, et al. Significance of elevated cobalamin (vitamin B_{12}) levels in blood. Clin Biochem 36.8 (2003): 585–590.

Eussen SJ et al. Oral cyanocobalamin supplementation in older people with vitamin B_{12} deficiency: a dose-finding trial. Arch Intern Med 165.10 (2005): 1167–1172.

FAO/WHO (Food and Agriculture Organization/World Health Organization). Vitamin B_{12}: Report of a joint FAO/WHO expert consultation. Rome: WHO, 2002.

Festen HP. Intrinsic factor secretion and cobalamin absorption: Physiology and pathophysiology in the gastrointestinal tract. Scand J Gastroenterol Suppl 188 (1991): 1–7.

Freeman AG et al. Sublingual cobalamin for pernicious anaemia. Lancet 354.9195 (1999): 2080.

Frequin ST et al. Decreased vitamin B_{12} and folate levels in cerebrospinal fluid and serum of multiple sclerosis patients after high-dose intravenous methylprednisolone. J Neurol 240.5 (1993): 305–308.

Gariballa S, Forster S. Effects of dietary supplements on depressive symptoms in older patients: a randomised double-blind placebo-controlled trial. Clin Nutr 26.5 (2007): 545–551.

Gidal BE et al. Blood homocysteine, folate and vitamin B-12 concentrations in patients with epilepsy receiving lamotrigine or sodium valproate for initial monotherapy. Epilepsy Res 64.3 (2005): 161–166.

Gok U et al. Comparative analysis of serum homocysteine, folic acid and vitamin B_{12} levels in patients with noise-induced hearing loss. Auris Nasus Larynx 31.1 (2004): 19–22.

Groenen PMW et al. Marginal maternal vitamin B_{12} status increases the risk of offspring with spina bifida. Am J Obstet Gynecol 191.1 (2004): 11–17.

Gronlie Guren M et al. Biochemical signs of impaired cobalamin status during and after radiotherapy for rectal cancer. Int J Radiat Oncol Biol Phys 60.3 (2004): 807–813.

Hathout L and El-Saden S. Nitrous oxide-induced B_{12} deficiency myelopathy: Perspectives on the clinical biochemistry of vitamin B_{12}. J Neurol Sci 301.1–2 (2011): 1–8.

Healton EB et al. Neurologic aspects of cobalamin deficiency. Medicine (Baltimore) 70.4 (1991): 229–45.

Herrmann et al. Homocysteine: a newly recognized risk factor for osteoporosis. Clin Chem Lab Med 43.10 (2005): 1111–1117.

Hillman RS. Hematopoietic agents: growth factors, minerals, and vitamins. In: Hardman JG (eds). The pharmacological basis of therapeutics. New York: McGraw-Hill, 1996, pp 1311–40.

Howden C. Vitamin B_{12} levels during prolonged treatment with proton pump inhibitors. J Clin Gastroenterol 30.1 (2000): 29–33.

Hutto BR. Folate and cobalamin in psychiatric illness. Compr Psychiatry 38.6 (1997): 305–314.

IMG (Integrative Medicine Gateway). Unity Health 2001–06. Available at: www.imgateway.net (accessed 2003).

Isoda K et al. Hepatoprotective effect of vitamin B_{12} on dimethylnitrosamine-induced liver injury. Biol Pharm Bull 31.2 (2008): 309–311.

Izumi Y, Kaji R. [Clinical trials of ultra-high-dose methylcobalamin in ALS.] Brain Nerve 59.10 (2007): 1141–1147.

Jamison RL et al. Effect of homocysteine lowering on mortality and vascular disease in advanced chronic kidney disease and end-stage renal disease: a randomized controlled trial. JAMA 298.10 (2007): 1163–1170.

Kang JH, Grodstein F. Mid-life plasma folate and vitamin B_{12} levels and cognitive function in older women. Alzheimer Dementia 1.1 (Suppl 1) (2005): 28.

Kapadia C. Cobalamin [vitamin B_{12}] deficiency; Is it a problem for our aging population and is the problem compounded by drugs that inhibit gastric acid secretion? J Clin Gastroenterol 30.1 (2000): 4–6.

Karabiber H et al. Effects of valproate and carbamazepine on serum levels of homocysteine, vitamin B_{12}, and folic acid. Brain Dev 25.2 (2003): 113–1115.

Karnaze DS, Carmel R. Neurologic and evoked potential abnormalities in subtle cobalamin deficiency states, including deficiency without anemia and with normal absorption of free cobalamin. Arch Neurol 47.9 (1990): 1008–1012.

Keser I et al. Folic acid and vitamin B12 supplementation lowers plasma homocysteine but has no effect on serum bone turnover markers in elderly women: a randomized, double-blind, placebo-controlled trial. Nutr Res 33.3 (2013): 211–219.

Kim YS et al. The optimal duration of vitamin supplementation prior to the first dose of pemetrexed in patients with non-small-cell lung cancer. Lung Cancer 81.2 (2013): 231–235.

Kwok T et al. Use of fasting urinary methylmalonic acid to screen for metabolic vitamin B_{12} deficiency in older persons. Nutrition 20.9 (2004): 764–768.

Laine L et al. Review article: potential gastrointestinal effects of long-term acid suppression with proton pump inhibitors. Aliment Pharmacol Ther 14.6 (2000): 651–658.

Lam JR et al. Proton pump inhibitor and histamine 2 receptor antagonist use and vitamin B12 deficiency. JAMA 310.22 (2013): 2435–2442.

Lee GR. Pernicious anemia and other causes of vitamin B_{12} (cobalamin) deficiency. In: Lee GR et al (eds). Wintrobe's clinical hematology, 10th edn. Baltimore: Williams & Wilkins, 1999, pp 941–964.

Lewerin C et al. Serum biomarkers for atrophic gastritis and antibodies against *Helicobacter pylori* in the elderly: Implications for vitamin B_{12}, folic acid and iron status and response to oral vitamin therapy. Scand J Gastroenterol 43.9 (2008): 1050–1056.

Lindenbaum J et al. Neuropsychiatric disorders caused by cobalamin deficiency in the absence of anemia or macrocytosis. N Engl J Med 318 (1988): 1720–1728.

Loder C et al. Treatment of multiple sclerosis with lofepramine, L-phenylalanine and vitamin B(12): mechanism of action and clinical importance: roles of the locus coeruleus and central noradrenergic systems. Med Hypotheses 59.5 (2002): 594–602.

Mann JF et al. Homocysteine lowering with folic acid and B vitamins in people with chronic kidney disease–results of the renal Hope-2 study. Nephrol Dial Transplant 23.2 (2008): 645–653.

Marcuard SP et al. Omeprazole therapy causes malabsorption of cyanocobalamin (vitamin B_{12}). Ann Intern Med 120.3 (1994): 211–215.

Marcucci R et al. Vitamin supplementation reduces the progression of atherosclerosis in hyperhomocysteinemic renal-transplant recipients. Transplantation 75.9 (2003): 1551–1555.

Marcus J et al. Homocysteine lowering and cardiovascular disease risk: lost in translation. Can J Cardiol 23.9 (2007): 707–710.

Martí-Carvajal AJ et al. Homocysteine lowering interventions for preventing cardiovascular events. Cochrane Database Syst Rev (2013) CD006612.

Mayer G et al. Effects of vitamin B_{12} on performance and circadian rhythm in normal subjects. Neuropsychopharmacology 15.5 (1996): 456–464.

Miller AL. The methionine-homocysteine cycle and its effects on cognitive diseases. Altern Med Rev 8.1 (2003): 7–19.

Miller A et al. Vitamin B_{12}, demyelination, remyelination and repair in multiple sclerosis. J Neurol Sci 233.1–2 (2005): 93–97.

Molina JR and Adjei AA. The role of pemetrexed (Alimta, LY231514) in lung cancer therapy. Clin Lung Cancer 5.1 (2003): 21–27.

Moreira ES et al. Vitamin B_{12} protects against superoxide-induced cell injury in human aortic endothelial cells. Free Radic Biol Med 51.4 (2011): 876–883.

Morkbak AL et al. A longitudinal study of serum cobalamin and its binding proteins in lactating women. Eur J Clin Nutr 61.2 (2007): 184–189.

Oh RC, Brown DL. Vitamin B_{12} deficiency. Am Fam Physician 67.5 (2003): 979.

Omray A. Evaluation of pharmacokinetic parameters of tetracycline hydrochloride upon oral administration with vitamin C and B complex. Hindustan Antibiot Bull 23.VI (1981): 33–37.

Park S et al. Age-related hearing loss, methylmalonic acid, and vitamin B_{12} status in older adults. J Nutr Elder 25.3–4 (2006): 105–120.

Pawlak R et al. How prevalent is vitamin B(12) deficiency among vegetarians? Nutr Rev 71.2 (2013): 110–117.

Penninx BW et al. Vitamin B (12) deficiency and depression in physically disabled older women: epidemiologic evidence from the Women's Health and Aging Study. Am J Psychiatry 157.5 (2000): 715–721.

Piskin S et al. Serum iron, ferritin, folic acid, and vitamin B_{12} levels in recurrent aphthous stomatitis. J Eur Acad Dermatol Venereol 16.1 (2002): 66–67.

Quaranta A et al. The effects of 'supra-physiological' vitamin B_{12} administration on temporary threshold shift. Int J Audiol 43.3 (2004): 162–165.

Rafnsson SB et al. Is a low blood level of vitamin B12 a cardiovascular and diabetes risk factor? A systematic review of cohort studies. Eur J Nutr 50.2 (2011): 97–106.

Ray JG, Blom HJ. Vitamin B_{12} insufficiency and the risk of fetal neural tube defects. Q J Med 96.4 (2003): 289–295.

Ray JG et al. Homocysteine-lowering therapy and risk for venous thromboembolism: a randomized trial. Ann Intern Med 146.11 (2007): 761–767.

Refsum H, Smith AD. Low vitamin B-12 status in confirmed Alzheimer's disease as revealed by serum holotranscobalamin. J Neurol Neurosurg Psychiatry 74.7 (2003): 959–961.

Remacha AF, Cadafalch J. Cobalamin deficiency in patients infected with the human immunodeficiency virus. Semin Hematol 36.1 (1999): 75–87.

Remacha AF et al. Vitamin B_{12} transport proteins in patients with HIV-1 infection and AIDS. Haematologica 78.2 (1993): 84–88.

Reznikoff-Etievant MF et al. Low vitamin B(12) level as a risk factor for very early recurrent abortion. Eur J Obstet Gynecol Reprod Biol 104.2 (2002): 156–159.

Rocco A et al. Vitamin B12 supplementation improves rates of sustained viral response in patients chronically infected with hepatitis C virus. Gut 62.5 (2013): 766–773.

Roffman JL et al. Randomized multicenter investigation of folate plus vitamin B12 supplementation in schizophrenia. JAMA Psychiatry 70.5 (2013): 481–489.

Roth M, Orija I. Oral vitamin B_{12} therapy in vitamin B_{12} deficiency. Am J Med 116.5 (2004): 358.

Sahin M et al. Effects of metformin or rosiglitazone on serum concentrations of homocysteine, folate, and vitamin B_{12} in patients with type 2 diabetes mellitus. J Diabetes Complications 21.2 (2007): 118–123.

Saltzman JR et al. Effect of hypochlorhydria due to omeprazole treatment or atrophic gastritis on protein-bound vitamin B_{12} absorption. J Am Coll Nutr 13.6 (1994). 584–591.

Sandyk R, Awerbuch GI. Vitamin B_{12} and its relationship to age of onset of multiple sclerosis. Int J Neurosci 71.1–4 (1993): 93–99.

Schenk BE et al. Atrophic gastritis during long-term omeprazole therapy affects serum vitamin B_{12} levels. Aliment Pharmacol Ther 13.10 (1999): 1343–1346.

Schneede J, Ueland PM. Novel and established markers of cobalamin deficiency: complementary or exclusive diagnostic strategies. Semin Vasc Med 5.2 (2005): 140–155.

Schnyder G et al. Effect of homocysteine-lowering therapy with folic acid, vitamin B_{12}, and vitamin B_6 on clinical outcome after

percutaneous coronary intervention: the Swiss Heart study: a randomized controlled trial. JAMA 288.8 (2002): 973–979.
Seppälä J et al. Association between vitamin b12 levels and melancholic depressive symptoms: a Finnish population-based study. BMC Psychiatry 13.1 (2013): 145.
Sharma V and Biswas D. Cobalamin deficiency presenting as obsessive compulsive disorder: case report. Gen Hosp Psychiatry 34.6 (2012): 578e7–578e8.
Shemesh Z et al. Vitamin B_{12} deficiency in patients with chronic tinnitus and noise-induced hearing loss. Am J Otolaryngol 14.2 (1993): 94–99.
Stabler SP, Allen RH. Vitamin B_{12} deficiency as a worldwide problem. Annu Rev Nutr 24 (2004): 299–326.
Stucker M et al. Topical vitamin B_{12}: a new therapeutic approach in atopic dermatitis-evaluation of efficacy and tolerability in a randomized placebo-controlled multicentre clinical trial. Br J Dermatol 150.5 (2004): 977–983.
Suarez L et al. Maternal serum B_{12} levels and risk for neural tube defects in a Texas-Mexico border population. Ann Epidemiol 13.2 (2003): 81–88.
Sun Y, et al. Effectiveness of vitamin B_{12} on diabetic neuropathy: systematic review of clinical controlled trials. Acta Neurol Taiwan 14.2 (2005): 48–54.
Sutterlin MW et al. Serum folate and Vitamin B_{12} levels in women using modern oral contraceptives (OC) containing 20 μg ethinyl estradiol. Eur J Obstet Gynecol Reprod Biol 107.1 (2003): 57–61
Takenaka S et al. Feeding dried purple laver (nori) to vitamin B_{12}-deficient rats significantly improves vitamin B_{12} status. Br J Nutr 852 (2001): 699–70.
Tamura J et al. Immunomodulation by vitamin B_{12}: augmentation of CD8+ T lymphocytes and natural killer (NK) cell activity in vitamin B_{12}-deficient patients by methyl-B_{12} treatment. Clin Exp Immunol 116.1 (1999): 28–32.
Termanini B et al. Effect of long-term gastric acid suppressive therapy on serum vitamin B_{12} levels in patients with Zollinger-Ellison syndrome. Am J Med 104.5 (1998): 422–430.
Toole JF et al. Lowering homocysteine in patients with ischemic stroke to prevent recurrent stroke, myocardial infarction, and death: the Vitamin Intervention for Stroke Prevention (VISP) randomized controlled trial. JAMA 291.5 (2004): 565–575.
Tripathi M et al. Serum cobalamin levels in dementias. Neurol India 49.3 (2001): 284–286.
Valuck RJ, Ruscin JM. A case-control study on adverse effects: H2 blocker or proton pump inhibitor use and risk of vitamin B_{12} deficiency in older adults. J Clin Epidemiol 57.4 (2004): 422–428.
van der Valk et al. Neonatal folate, homocysteine, vitamin B12 levels and methylenetetrahydrofolate reductase variants in childhood asthma and eczema. Allergy 68.6 (2013): 788–795.
van Wijngaarden JP et al. Vitamin B12, folate, homocysteine, and bone health in adults and elderly people: a systematic review with meta-analyses. J Nutr Metab (2013) 2013: 486186.
Vidal-Alaball J et al. Oral vitamin B_{12} versus intramuscular vitamin B_{12} for vitamin B_{12} deficiency. Cochrane Database Syst Rev 3 (2005): CD004655.
VITATOPS Trial Study Group. B vitamins in patients with recent transient ischaemic attack or stroke in the VITAmins TO Prevent Stroke (VITATOPS) trial: a randomised, double-blind, parallel, placebo-controlled trial. Lancet Neurol 9.9 (2010): 855–865.
Vogel T et al. Homocysteine, vitamin B12, folate and cognitive functions: a systematic and critical review of the literature. Int J Clin Pract 63.7 (2009): 1061–1067.
Volkov I, et al. Successful treatment of chronic erythema nodosum with vitamin B_{12}. J Am Board Fam Pract 18.6 (2005): 567–569.
Wahlqvist ML (ed.). Food and nutrition, 2nd edn. Sydney: Allen & Unwin, 2002, p 260.
Wald DS et al. Serum homocysteine and dementia: Meta-analysis of eight cohort studies including 8669 participants. Alzheimers Dement 7.4 (2011): 412–417.
Wang HX et al. Vitamin B(12) and folate in relation to the development of Alzheimer's disease. Neurology 56.9 (2001): 1188–1194.
Watanabe F. Vitamin B_{12} sources and bioavailability. Exp Biol Med (Maywood) 232.10 (2007): 1266–1274.
Weinburg JB et al. Inhibition of nitric oxide synthase by cobalamins and cobinamides. Free Radic Biol Med 46.12 (2009): 1626–1632.
Weir GD, Scott MJ. Brain function in the elderly: role of vitamin B_{12} and folate. Br Med Bull 55.3 (1999): 669.14.
Wellmer J et al. [Oral treatment of vitamin B_{12} deficiency in subacute combined degeneration]. Nervenarzt 77.10 (2006): 1228–1231.
Westphal S et al. Antihypertensive treatment and homocysteine concentrations. Metabolism 52.3 (2003): 261–263.
Wolters M, et al. Cobalamin: a critical vitamin in the elderly. Prev Med 39.6 (2004): 1256–1266.
Xu T et al. Treatment of hyperhomocysteinemia and endothelial dysfunction in renal transplant recipients with B vitamins in the Chinese population. J Urol 179.3 (2008): 1190–1194.
Yajnik CS et al. Oral vitamin B_{12} supplementation reduces plasma total homocysteine concentration in women in India. Asia Pac J Clin Nutr 16.1 (2007): 103–109.
Zetterberg H et al. The transcobalamin codon 259 polymorphism influences the risk of human spontaneous abortion. Hum Reprod 17.12 (2002): 3033–3036.
Zhang H et al. Association of homocysteine, vitamin B12, and folate with bone mineral density in postmenopausal women: a meta-analysis. Arch Gynecol Obstet (2014) 289: 10039.

Vitamin C

HISTORICAL NOTE Vitamin C deficiency has been known for many centuries as scurvy, a potentially fatal condition, dreaded by seamen in the 15th century, who were often forced to subsist for months on diets of dried beef and biscuits. It was also described by the European crusaders during their numerous sieges. In the mid-1700s Lind was the first doctor to conduct systematic clinical trials of potential cures for scurvy, identifying oranges and lemons as successful treatments (Bartholomew 2002). However, it was not until 1928 that vitamin C (then known as antiscorbutic factor) was isolated, leading to mass production in the mid-1930s.

BACKGROUND AND RELEVANT PHARMACOKINETICS

Vitamin C is an essential water-soluble nutrient for humans and required in the diet on a regular basis, as we are one of few species of animals that cannot synthesise it. This is because humans lack the enzyme L-gulonolactone oxidase, which is required for the conversion of glucose into vitamin C (Braunwald et al 2003).

The bioavailability of ascorbic acid is dependent on both intestinal absorption and renal excretion. Vitamin C, consumed either in the diet or as dietary supplements, is absorbed by the epithelial cells of the small intestine by the sodium vitamin C co-transporter 1 (SVCT1) and subsequently diffuses into the surrounding capillaries and then passes into the circulatory system (Li & Schellhorn 2007). Ultimately, the degree of absorption depends on the dose ingested and decreases as the dose increases.

Clinical note — Differences between major forms of vitamin C supplements

Here is a brief summary of the most common forms found in over-the-counter supplements.

- Ascorbic acid. The major dietary form of vitamin C.
- Mineral ascorbates (also known as non-acid vitamin C). These are buffered forms of vitamin C and believed to be less irritating to the stomach than ascorbic acid. Sodium ascorbate and calcium ascorbate are the most common forms. When mineral salts are taken, both the ascorbic acid and the mineral are absorbed. For example, sodium ascorbate generally provides 131 mg of sodium per 1000 mg of ascorbic acid, and calcium ascorbate provides 114 mg of calcium per 1000 mg of ascorbic acid.
- Vitamin C with bioflavonoids. Many bioflavonoids are antioxidant substances and are added to some vitamin C preparations in the belief that this increases the bioavailability or efficacy of vitamin C. Typically, the bioflavonoids are sourced from citrus fruits.
- Ascorbyl palmitate. A fat-soluble form of vitamin C formed by esterification with palmitic acid and most often used in topical creams.

This is because, at low concentrations, most vitamin C is absorbed in the small intestine and reabsorbed from the renal tubule, but at high concentrations SVCT1 becomes saturated, which, combined with ascorbate-mediated SVCT1 downregulation, limits the amount of ascorbic acid absorbed from the intestine and reabsorbed from the kidney (Li & Schellhorn 2007). For this reason, oral vitamin C is best absorbed when it is ingested in small doses at regular intervals. Complete plasmatic saturation occurs at 1000 mg daily with a concentration of around 100 microM (Verrax & Buc Calderon 2008). Pectin and zinc are also able to impair oral absorption. These limitations are bypassed with the use of intravenously administered vitamin C, which can achieve much higher plasma levels than oral administration.

Following its absorption, ascorbic acid is ubiquitously distributed in the cells of the body. Within the body, the highest levels of ascorbic acid are found in the adrenal glands, the white blood cells, skeletal muscles and the brain, especially in the pituitary gland (Verrax & Buc Calderon 2008). Interestingly, the brain is the most difficult organ to deplete of ascorbate. As a polar compound with a relatively large molecular weight, vitamin C cannot readily cross the cell membrane by simple diffusion. The flux of vitamin C in and out of the cell is controlled by specific mechanisms, including facilitated diffusion and active transport, which are mediated by distinct classes of membrane proteins such as facilitative glucose transporters (GLUT) and SVCT respectively (Li & Schellhorn 2007). Once in cells, dehydroascorbic acid (the oxidised form of ascorbate) is rapidly reduced to ascorbate (Harrison & May 2009). Eventually it is metabolised in the liver, filtered by the kidneys and excreted in the urine. The biological half-life of vitamin C is 8–40 days (NHMRC 2006).

Clinical note — Deficiencies in smokers

It is well established that smokers have lowered vitamin C status than non-smokers and therefore have higher requirements for vitamin C. Vitamin C status is inversely related to cigarette use (Cross & Halliwell 1993). The depletion of plasma ascorbic acid associated with cigarette smoking was first described in the late 1930s. Reports have shown that low ascorbic acid concentrations in the plasma, leucocytes and urine of both male and female cigarette smokers are associated with increased numbers and activity of neutrophils, which suggests increased utilisation and lower intake, or reduced bioavailability, of vitamin C in smokers than in non-smokers (Northrop-Clewes & Thurnham 2007).

CHEMICAL COMPONENTS

Vitamin C exists as both its reduced form (L-ascorbic acid) and its oxidised form (L-dehydroascorbic acid). The two forms interchange in the body in a reversible equilibrium.

FOOD SOURCES

Vitamin C is found in many different fruits and vegetables. The most concentrated food sources are blackcurrants, sweet green and red peppers, hot red peppers, green chilli peppers, oranges and fresh orange juice, and strawberries. Other good sources are watermelon, papaya, citrus fruits, cantaloupe, mango, cabbage, cauliflower, broccoli and tomato juice. In practice, vegetables may be a more important source of vitamin C than fruits because they are often available for longer periods during the year.

The vitamin C content of food is strongly influenced by many factors, such as season, transportation, shelf-life, storage conditions and storage time, cooking techniques and chlorination of water (FAO/WHO 2002). Cutting or bruising food will reduce its vitamin C content; however, blanching or storing at low pH will preserve it.

Up to 100% of the vitamin C content of food can be destroyed during cooking and storing because the vitamin is sensitive to light, heat, oxygen and alkali (Wahlqvist 2002). Additionally, using too much water during cooking can leach the vitamin from food and further reduce its vitamin C content.

DEFICIENCY SIGNS AND SYMPTOMS

In adults, scurvy remains latent for 3–6 months after reducing dietary intake to less than 10 mg/day

(Beers & Berkow 2003). It manifests when the body pools fall below 300–400 mg (NHMRC 2006). Many of the features of frank vitamin C deficiency (scurvy) result from a defect in collagen synthesis.

Early symptoms are:

- weakness
- fatigue and listlessness
- muscular weakness
- petechial haemorrhages and ecchymoses (bruising)
- swollen gums
- poor wound healing and the breakdown of recently healed wounds
- poor appetite and weight loss
- emotional changes such as irritability and depression
- vague myalgias and arthralgias
- congested hair follicles.

Symptoms of more severe deficiency are:

- fever
- drying of the skin and mucous membranes
- susceptibility to infection
- bleeding gums and loosening of teeth
- oedema of the lower extremities
- anaemia
- joint swelling and tenderness, due to bleeding around or into the joint
- oliguria
- pain in the extremities
- haemorrhage
- convulsions
- shock
- eventually death if left untreated.

Although frank deficiency is uncommon in Western countries, marginal deficiency states are not uncommon.

Primary deficiency

This occurs if there is an inadequate dietary intake, which is often caused by a combination of poor cooking and eating habits. It occurs in areas of urban poverty, during famine and war, in young children fed exclusively on cow's milk for a prolonged period, in the institutionalised or isolated elderly, and in chronic alcoholics (Pimentel 2003, Richardson et al 2002). One Australian hospital identified that 73% of all new admissions had hypovitaminosis C and 30% had levels suggestive of scurvy (Richardson et al 2002).

Secondary deficiency

Factors that increase nutritional requirements include cigarette smoking, pregnancy, lactation, thyrotoxicosis, acute and chronic inflammatory diseases, major surgery and burns, infection and diabetes (Beers & Berkow 2003, FAO/WHO 2002, Hendler & Rorvik 2001, Wahlqvist 2002). Decreased vitamin C absorption in achlorhydria and increased excretion in chronic diarrhoea also increase the risk of deficiency, particularly when combined with poor dietary intake.

MAIN ACTIONS

Vitamin C is an electron donor (reducing agent or antioxidant), and this accounts for most of its biochemical and molecular functions. It is involved in many biochemical processes in the body, such as:

- energy release from fatty acids
- metabolism of cholesterol
- reduction of nitrosamine formation in the stomach
- formation of thyroid hormone
- carnitine biosynthesis
- modulation of iron and copper absorption
- corticosteroid biosynthesis
- protection of folic acid reductase, which converts folic acid to folinic acid
- collagen biosynthesis
- tyrosine biosynthesis and catabolism
- neurotransmitter biosynthesis.

The main actions of vitamin C are summarised below.

Antioxidant and pro-oxidant

At physiological concentrations, vitamin C is the most effective aqueous antioxidant in plasma, interstitial fluids and soluble phases of cells. As such, it is one of the most important water-soluble antioxidant substances in the body, acting as a potent free radical scavenger in the plasma, protecting cells against oxidative damage caused by reactive oxygen species (ROS). It scavenges free radical oxygen and nitrogen species such as superoxide, hydroxyl, peroxyl and nitroxide radicals and non-radical reactive species such as singlet oxygen, peroxynitrite and hypochlorite (FAO/WHO 2002, Hendler & Rorvik 2001). Besides having a direct antioxidant function, it also indirectly increases free radical scavenging by regenerating vitamin E (Vatassery 1987) and maintaining glutathione in reduced form. Much of the vitamin's physiological role stems from its very strong reducing power (high redox potential) and its ability to be regenerated using intracellular reductants such as glutathione, nicotinamide adenine dinucleotide and nicotinamide adenine dinucleotide phosphate (Chaudière & Ferrari-Iliou 1999).

In the presence of oxidised metal ions (e.g. Fe^{3+}, Cu^{2+}), high concentrations of ascorbic acid can have pro-oxidant functions at least in vitro, thereby promoting oxidative damage to DNA. The effect does not appear to be significant under normal physiological conditions in vivo; however, when used at higher pharmacological concentrations (0.3–20 mmol/L), ascorbic acid displays transition metal-independent pro-oxidant activity, which is more profound in cancer cells than healthy cells and causes cell death (Li & Schellhorn 2007).

Whether vitamin C functions as an antioxidant or pro-oxidant is determined by at least three factors: (1) the redox potential of the cellular environment; (2) the presence/absence of oxidised metal ions; and (3) the local concentrations of ascorbate (Li & Schellhorn 2007).

Maintenance of connective tissue

Vitamin C maintains the body's connective tissue and is essential for the formation of collagen, the major fibrous element of blood vessels, skin, tendon, cartilage and teeth (Morton et al 2001). If collagen is produced in the absence of vitamin C, it is unstable and cannot form the triple helix required for normal tissue structure. Vitamin C is involved in the biosynthesis of other substances important for connective tissue, such as elastin, proteoglycans, bone matrix, fibronectin and elastin-associated fibrillin (Hall & Greendale 1998).

These effects have been harnessed by the dermatological and cosmetic industries and are the rationale for producing topically applied products containing vitamin C.

Collagen stability

Vitamin C is necessary for the synthesis of collagen proteins, whereby it is involved in the hydroxylation of specific prolyl and lysyl residues of the unfolded procollagen chain. These reactions are catalysed by the enzymes prolyl 4-hydroxylase and prolyl 3-hydroxylase, which stabilise collagen molecules, and lysyl hydroxylase enzyme, responsible for collagen molecule cross-linking (Ochiai et al 2006, Traikovich 1999). In vivo and in vitro studies have explored topical vitamin C effects on melanogenesis and ageing.

Brain and nerve function

Ascorbate is involved in neurotransmitter synthesis. It is a cofactor required for the biosynthesis of noradrenaline from dopamine and hydroxylation of tryptophan to produce serotonin. It also acts as a modulator of glutaminergic, cholinergic and GABAergic transmission (Bornstein et al 2003, FAO/WHO 2002, Harrison & May 2009). Furthermore, it is involved in neural maturation and acts as a neuroprotective agent (Harrison & May 2009),

Immunostimulant

Ascorbic acid affects the immune system in several different ways and there is abundant evidence that the immune system is sensitive to circulating levels of vitamin C. Ascorbic acid modulates T-cell gene expression, specifically affecting genes involved with signalling, carbohydrate metabolism, apoptosis, transcription and immune function. It can also stimulate the production of interferons, the proteins that protect cells against viral attack and stimulate the synthesis of humoral thymus factor and antibodies of the immunoglobulin G (IgG) and IgM classes (Combs 2012).

Both in vivo and in vitro studies provide evidence of immunostimulant effects, generally at doses beyond recommended dietary intake (RDI) levels (Hendler & Rorvik 2001). In high doses, it is a potent immunomodulator and is preferentially cytotoxic to neoplastic cells. Vitamin C enhances the activity of natural killer cells in vivo and also both B- and T-cell activity (Drisko et al 2003).

Leucocytes maintain high levels of ascorbate which are correlated with their function. In fact, leucocyte ascorbate levels are 20–100 times higher than plasma levels. The uptake occurs via active transport which is temperature- and energy-dependent. Many infections and inflammatory diseases lower plasma and neutrophil ascorbate levels. Clinically, an association exists between recurrent infections and impaired neutrophil function. Adequate ascorbate nutrition improves several aspects of neutrophil activity, especially chemotaxis, proliferation and motility. Vitamin C can enhance neutrophil chemotaxis and motility, even in healthy individuals (Combs 2012, Muggli 1998).

In addition to these direct effects on the immune system, the antioxidant properties of vitamin C play a role. When neutrophils are activated during infection, they release free radicals. However, neutrophils are susceptible to free radical damage themselves. Protection against auto-oxidation is afforded by ascorbic acid together with other antioxidants and is essential during the mobilisation of host defences. Apart from its own effects, vitamin C helps immune function indirectly by protecting the antioxidant capacity of vitamin E, which is an immune-enhancing nutrient in its own right (Muggli 1998).

Antihistamine

Ascorbic acid is involved in histamine metabolism, acting with Cu^{2+} to inhibit its release and enhance its degradation (Combs 2012).

An inverse association has been identified between blood histamine levels and vitamin C status in humans (Johnston et al 1996). In that study, increasing vitamin C status with supplements (up to 250 mg/day) over 3 weeks was shown to decrease histamine levels. It is unclear whether single, high-dose supplementation also affects histamine levels, as two studies using 2 g doses have produced conflicting results (Bucca et al 1990, Johnston et al 1992).

Anticancer

In millimolar concentrations, vitamin C is selectively cytotoxic to many cancer cell lines and has in vivo anticancer activity when administered alone or together with other agents (Hoffer et al 2008). Importantly, pharmacological concentrations of ascorbic acid (0.3–20 mmol/L) are required to find evidence of cytotoxicity in vitro and in vivo, whereas physiological concentrations of ascorbic acid (0.1 mmol/L) do not have any effect on either tumour or normal cells (Li & Schellhorn 2007). The most reliable method of achieving these high doses is with intravenous (IV) administration of vitamin C and not via the oral route, which has limited absorption (Padayatty et al 2006). The effect is clearly dose-dependent and mediated via several mechanisms, such as immunomodulation, inhibition of cell division and growth, gene regulation and induction of apoptosis. One mechanism of cytotoxicity demonstrated in several models is the ability of ascorbate at pharmacological concentrations to exert pro-oxidant activity, generating hydrogen peroxide-dependent cytotoxicity towards a variety of cancer cells in vitro and in vivo without adversely affecting normal cells (Chen et al 2008, Tamayo & Richardson 2003).

Much investigation has been undertaken to understand how preferential cytotoxicity is achieved; however, the mechanisms are still largely unknown. For example, studies with radioactive-labelled vitamin C have found that tumour cells accumulate more vitamin C than healthy cells, whereas other studies have reported no differences in intracellular concentrations (Prasad et al 2002). There is also some preliminary evidence of synergistic cytotoxic effects and decreased drug toxicity with some pharmaceutical anticancer agents (Giri et al 1998).

One theory proposed to explain the preferential targeting of tumour cells relates to their overexpression of facilitative GLUTs (Gatenby & Gillies 2004) and dehydroascorbic acid, transported by GLUTs, accumulating within the tumour cells, which enables intracellular hydrogen peroxide levels to increase (Chen et al 2005, Verrax & Buc Calderon 2008, Zhang et al 2001). Other intrinsic properties of cancer cells may also be involved, such as reduced concentrations of antioxidant enzymes (e.g. catalase and superoxide dismutase) and increased intracellular transitional metal availability, both of which further augment free radical production (Li & Schellhorn 2007). Alternatively, it has been suggested that extracellular ascorbate is the source of this anticancer effect and is more important than intracellular vitamin C.

There are a number of factors that may be contributing to the inconsistent results obtained to date, such as the variable characteristics of the subjects studied, type of infecting virus, lack of control for dietary vitamin C intake and differences in measures of outcomes. Clearly, further investigation is required to clarify many issues surrounding the use of vitamin C supplements for upper respiratory tract infections (URTIs). In practice, naturopaths often recommend megadoses of vitamin C (taken frequently, in small amounts), which are well beyond the doses investigated so far, and often report good results. Although anecdotal, it is interesting to note that little research has investigated this method.

Modulation of gene expression

Many transcription factors, such as NF-κB, AP-1 or peroxisome proliferator-activated receptors, are redox-regulated, and moderate amounts of oxidative stress are known both to modulate gene expression and to signal transduction cascades by affecting kinases, phosphatases as well as Ca^{2+} signalling. L-ascorbic acid may modulate relatively unspecific gene expression by affecting the redox state of transcription factors and of enzymes involved in signal transduction (Table 1).

OTHER ACTIONS

High oral doses (4–12 g/day in divided doses) can acidify urine.

Ascorbic acid greatly enhances iron bioavailability from food. Within the body, ascorbic acid promotes the utilisation of haem iron, which appears to involve enhanced incorporation of iron into its intracellular storage form, ferritin. This effect involves facilitation of ferritin synthesis and enhanced ferritin stability (Combs 2012).

Vitamin C can also interact with other nutritional metals, reducing their toxicity, such as selenium, nickel, lead, vanadium and cadmium. This is achieved by interacting with them to create a reduced form which is poorly absorbed or more rapidly excreted (Combs 2012).

CLINICAL USE

Vitamin C is an important biological antioxidant and has been a popular nutritional supplement for decades. It is administered as intramuscular or IV injections and used topically and orally. This review will chiefly focus on oral and topical use, as these are the forms of vitamin C most commonly used by the public.

Deficiency: prevention and treatment

Traditionally, vitamin C supplements are used both to treat and to prevent deficiency. Treatment may include 250 mg vitamin C daily and encouragement to eat fresh fruits and vegetables on a regular basis (Kumar et al 2002), or 100 mg taken 3–5 times daily until 4000 mg has been reached (Braunwald et al 2003). Some deficiency symptoms start to respond within 24 hours, although most take from several weeks to months to resolve completely.

Iron-deficiency anaemia

Ascorbic acid is a potent enhancer of iron absorption. Vitamin C facilitates iron absorption by forming soluble complexes and may be used with an iron supplement and nutritious diet in the treatment of iron-deficiency anaemia. It is specifically helpful in increasing absorption of iron from plant-based foods. It is also recommended for women with menorrhagia in order to reduce the risk of iron deficiency.

Dermatological uses

Vitamin C is used as an oral supplement or topical application in a number of dermatological conditions.

Wound healing

Vitamin C is important for effective wound healing, as deficiency contributes to fragile granulation tissue and therefore impairs the wound-healing process (Russell 2001).

In vitro studies with skin graft samples have demonstrated that vitamin C extends cellular viability, promotes formation of an epidermal barrier and promotes engraftment (Boyce et al 2002). In this way, vitamin C is used to enhance wound healing before surgery has commenced.

TABLE 1 KNOWN OR PUTATIVE GENES AND ENZYMATIC ACTIVITIES RESPONSIVE TO L-ASCORBIC ACID

Gene	Cellular process involved	Mechanism	Expression/activity with L-ascorbic acid
h1-Calponin	VSMC phenotypic modulation	?	↑
h-Caldesmon	VSMC phenotypic modulation	?	↑
SM22α	VSMC phenotypic modulation	?	↑
α-SM actin	VSMC phenotypic modulation	?	↑
Collagen I	Matrix production	Transcription, mRNA stability	↑
Collagen III	Matrix production	Transcription, mRNA stability	↑
Elastin	Elasticity of arterial wall, VSMC phenotypic modulation	mRNA stability	↓
MMP2	Matrix degradation	?	↓
TIMP1	Inhibits matrix degradation	?	↑
Calponin 1	VSMC phenotypic modulation	?	↑
Myosin heavy chain-1	VSMC phenotypic modulation	?	↑
GATA4	Cardiac development	?	↑
Nkx2.5	Cardiac development	?	↑
ANF	Regulation of cardiac and vascular tone	?	↑
eNOS	Vascular homeostasis	Increased intracellular Ca^{2+}	↑
Prolyl hydroxylase	Stability and secretion of collagen	Cofactor	↑
ICAM-1	Cell adhesion	?	↓
Enzymes involved in carnitine synthesis	Fatty acid metabolism	Cofactor (epsilon-*N*-trimethyllysine hydroxylase and gamma-butyrobetaine hydroxylase)	↑

VSMC, vascular smooth-muscle cell.
Adapted from Villacorta et al (2007).

Numerous case reports of surgical and dental patients generally suggest a use for vitamin C supplementation in doses beyond RDI as a means of enhancing the rate of wound healing (Ringsdorf & Cheraskin 1982). One early double-blind study found that vitamin C (500 mg twice daily) resulted in a significant mean reduction in pressure sore area of 84% after 1 month compared with 43% in the placebo group (Taylor et al 1974). The mean rates of healing were 2.47 cm^2 for vitamin C and 1.45 cm^2 for the placebo.

Photo-damaged skin

Two double-blind studies investigating the effects of topical preparations of vitamin C on photo-damaged skin have demonstrated good results after 3 months' use (Fitzpatrick & Rostan 2002, Humbert et al 2003). One study tested a topical application of 5% vitamin C in a cream base, whereas the other used a newly formulated vitamin C complex having 10% ascorbic acid (water-soluble) and 7% tetrahexyldecyl ascorbate (lipid-soluble) in an anhydrous polysilicone gel base.

Prevention of sunburn

One controlled study found oral vitamin C (2000 mg/day) in combination with vitamin E (1000 IU/day) had a protective effect against sunburn after 8 days' treatment in human subjects (Eberlein-Konig et al 1998). Similar results have been obtained for topical vitamin C preparations in several animal models (Darr et al 1992, 1996, JY Lin et al 2003) and a small human study (Keller & Fenske 1998). The latter found that application of an aqueous 10% L-ascorbic acid solution after ultraviolet B (UVB) radiation produced a significant reduction in the minimal erythema dose and a less intense erythematous response than controls.

As with many nutrients, studies associating dietary vitamin intake and disease risk are difficult to interpret. This is because it is difficult to separate the effects of the individual vitamin from the effects of other components in the diet. Where possible, an effort has been made to include information that will help in the interpretation of this type of data.

Hyperpigmentation

The beneficial effects of vitamin C on skin hyperpigmentation and ageing are mostly attributed to its antioxidant properties and key role in collagen production. The efficacy of vitamin C in hyperpigmentation disorders has been investigated in small studies, mostly as an adjunctive therapy. Hwang et al (2009) studied the efficacy of a formulation containing 25% L-ascorbic and a chemical penetration enhancer for the treatment of melasma. A 16-week open-label trial was conducted and 40 subjects were involved. The skin was assessed every month, and results showed significant decrease in pigmentation with the treatment. Espinal-Perez et al (2004) conducted a double-blind randomised trial comparing 5% L-ascorbic acid and 4% hydroquinone for melasma treatment. They concluded L-ascorbic acid to have beneficial effects on hyperpigmentation with minimal side effects, and therefore, to be a viable single or adjunctive long-term therapy for melasma (Espinal-Perez et al 2004). Results show that vitamin C has the ability to significantly improve abnormal skin pigmentation caused by chronic UV radiation exposure, including melasma.

Antiageing

Vitamin C antioxidant properties contribute to its antiageing effect as well, since ROS are known to interfere with fibroblasts and to destroy collagen and connective tissue structures. Vitamin C is a well-known potential antiageing agent due to its antioxidant effect and major role in collagen production (Humbert et al 2003, Park et al 2009, Taniguchi et al 2012, Traikovich 1999). A 3-month randomised double-blind vehicle-controlled study was conducted to determine the efficacy of topical vitamin C in photo-damaged skin. Clinical assessment showed significant improvement in many features, including fine wrinkles, tactile roughness, laxity and tone. Self-assessment questionnaire demonstrated that 84.2% of the subjects preferred the side treated with vitamin C. Photographic assessment showed vitamin C-treated skin to have 57.9% greater improvement compared to controls and optical profilometry analysis demonstrated improvement with active treatment up to 73.7% greater than control (Traikovich 1999).

Upper respiratory tract infections

Vitamin C is widely used both to prevent and to treat common URTIs, such as the common cold and influenza, largely based on its effects on the immune system, its ability to reduce histamine levels and the observations that the gastrointestinal absorption of vitamin C increases in the common cold (suggesting an increased demand for this nutrient) and that vitamin C concentrations in the plasma and leucocytes rapidly decline during infection (Wilson et al 1976, Wintergerst et al 2006). Although extremely popular, its usefulness in these conditions is widely debated.

A meta-analysis of 29 trials involving 11,306 participants was undertaken to assess the risk ratio (RR) of developing a cold while taking vitamin C regularly over the study period (Hemilä & Chalker 2013). To be eligible for inclusion, at least 200 mg daily of vitamin C was required and each study needed to have a placebo arm. The most promising results were obtained for children and athletes. Five trials involving a total of 598 marathon runners, skiers and soldiers on subarctic exercises yielded a pooled RR of 0.48, indicating that regular vitamin C supplementation significantly reduced the incidence of the common cold in this population. For the studies involving children, using a dose of 1–2 g/daily, vitamin C shortened the duration of colds by 18% and also reduced the severity of the cold infection. In regard to the general adult community (n = 10708), the pooled RR was 0.97, indicating similar effects to placebo and the duration was only slightly reduced, by 8% (3–12%), and in children by 14% (7–21%). Overall, the review concluded that routine vitamin C supplementation did not reduce the incidence of colds in the general population, yet vitamin C may be useful for people exposed to brief periods of severe physical exercise.

It has been suggested that the dose used may affect the magnitude of the benefit, there being on average greater benefit from ≥2 g/day compared to 1 g/day of vitamin C. In five studies with adults administered 1 g/day of vitamin C, the median decrease in cold duration was only 6%, whereas in two studies with children administered 2 g/day the median decrease was four times higher, 26% (Hemilä 1999).

Vitamin C taken in combination with zinc may be more successful, according to clinical trials. Both nutrients play a role in immune function and dietary intakes can be low. When the results of two double-blind, randomised, placebo-controlled trials utilising a combination of 1000 mg vitamin C plus 10 mg zinc in patients with the common cold are pooled together, the combination was significantly more efficient than placebo at reducing rhinorrhoea over 5 days of treatment. Furthermore, symptom relief was quicker and the product was well tolerated (Maggini et al 2012).

Reduction in all-cause mortality

Several studies have identified an inverse association between plasma ascorbate levels, vitamin C intake and all-cause mortality. This means that low serum ascorbic acid levels are associated with higher all-cause mortality and in some studies, higher cardiovascular disease (CVD) mortality and cancer mortality.

In the Western Electric Company study, data on diet and other factors were obtained in 1958 and 1959 for a cohort of 1556 employed middle-aged men and an inverse association between vitamin C and mortality was identified (Pandey et al 1995). The next year, a prospective cohort study conducted with 725 older adults also identified an inverse relationship between vitamin C blood concentrations and total mortality during a 12 year follow-up (Sahyoun et al 1996). Similar results were obtained in the large European Prospective Investigation into Cancer and Nutrition (EPIC)-Norfolk study of 19,496 men and women aged 45–79 years (Khaw et al 2001). Plasma ascorbate concentration was inversely related to mortality from all causes, and from CVD and ischaemic heart disease in both men and women. Risk of mortality in the group with the highest intake was about half that of the low intake group and was independent of age, systolic blood pressure (SBP), serum cholesterol, cigarette smoking, diabetes or supplement use.

The Second National Health and Nutrition Examination Survey (NHANES II) mortality study further confirmed the inverse association between plasma ascorbate and risk of dying from all causes; however, this study identified a gender difference (Loria et al 2000). After adjustments for race, educational level, number of cigarettes smoked at baseline, serum total cholesterol, SBP, body mass index, diabetes status and alcohol consumption, men in the lowest serum ascorbate quartile (serum ascorbate concentrations <28.4 micromol/L) had a 57% higher risk of dying from any cause than did men in the highest quartile (>73.8 micromol/L). Additionally, men in the lowest serum ascorbate quartile had double the risk of dying from cancer than those in the highest quartile after adjustment for age. The dose corresponds to approximately 60 mg/day vitamin C. In contrast, among women no association was observed between quartiles of serum ascorbate concentration and total mortality or mortality from CVD or cancer.

As an extension to this, Simon et al (2001) identified that, amongst the 8453 Americans aged ≥ 30 years at baseline in the NHANES II, low serum ascorbic acid levels were marginally associated with an increased risk of fatal CVD and significantly associated with an increased risk for all-cause mortality (Simon et al 2001). Conversely, people with normal to high serum ascorbic acid levels had a marginally significant 21–25% decreased risk of fatal CVD (P for trend = 0.09) and a 25–29% decreased risk of all-cause mortality (P for trend < 0.001) compared to people with low level. Low serum ascorbic acid levels were also a risk factor for cancer death in men, but unexpectedly were associated with a decreased risk of cancer death in women. In other words, among men, normal to high serum ascorbic acid levels were associated with an approximately 30% decreased risk of cancer deaths, whereas such serum ascorbic acid levels were associated with an approximately twofold increased risk of cancer deaths among women.

A gender difference was also reported in the NHANES I Epidemiologic Follow-up Study (NHEFS) (Enstrom et al 1992). Vitamin C intakes >50 mg/day plus regular supplement use were associated with reduced mortality, compared with intakes <50 mg/day in men, but apparently not in women.

Prevention of cardiovascular disease

The association between vitamin C and CVD prevention is still unclear, although several themes are emerging as evidence accumulates.

In general, epidemiological studies show that low vitamin C intake is associated with higher CVD mortality and risk of heart failure and conversely higher levels are associated with lower risk, whereas interventional studies are less consistent (Carr & Frei 1999, Houston 2005, Khaw et al 2001, Knekt et al 2004, Kushi et al 1996, Lopes et al 1998, MRC/BHF 2002, Ness et al 1996, Nyyssonen et al 1997, Osganian et al 2003).

For example, subjects in NHANES I with the highest vitamin C intakes showed less cardiovascular death (standardised mortality ratio, 0.66; 95% confidence limits, 0.53–0.83) than subjects with lower estimated vitamin C intakes (Enstrom et al 1992). In the NHANES III survey of 8453 Americans, low serum ascorbic acid levels were marginally associated with an increased risk of fatal CVD (Simon et al 2001). A study by Toohey et al (1996) provides some rationale for the coronary heart disease (CHD)-preventive effects seen. In their trial, a significant inverse correlation was found between plasma ascorbic acid levels and both systolic (P < 0.0001) and diastolic blood pressure (DBP) (P < 0.03), and between plasma ascorbic acid and serum total cholesterol (P < 0.03), low-density lipoprotein (LDL)-cholesterol (LDL-C) (P < 0.004), and the ratio of LDL-cholesterol to high-density lipoprotein (HDL)-cholesterol (LDL-C:HDL-C) (P < 0.004). Serum HDL-cholesterol was positively related to plasma ascorbic acid (P < 0.05). When multiple regression analysis was applied, ascorbic acid was shown to be a significant independent contributor to the prediction of blood pressure and LDL-C concentration (Toohey et al 1996).

More recently, the European Prospective Investigation into Cancer and Nutrition study in Norfolk, United Kingdom, identified that the risk of heart failure decreased with increasing plasma vitamin C; the hazard ratios comparing each quartile with the lowest were 0.76 (95% confidence interval [CI] 0.65–0.88), 0.70 (95% CI 0.60–0.81) and 0.62 (95% CI 0.53–0.74) in age- and sex-adjusted analyses (P for trend < 0.0001) (Pfister et al 2011). This means that, for every 20 micromol/L increase in plasma vitamin C concentration, there was an accompanying 9% relative reduction in risk of heart failure after adjustment for age, sex, smoking, alcohol consumption, physical activity, occupational social class, educational level, SBP, diabetes, cholesterol concentration and body mass index, with similar result if adjusting for interim CHD. The study analysed results from 9187 healthy men and 11,112 women aged 39–79 years.

Possible mechanisms

Ascorbic acid is inversely related to several risk factors and indicators of atherosclerotic CVD, including hypertension and elevated concentrations of LDL, acute-phase proteins and haemostatic factors (Price et al 2001). More specifically, vitamin C inhibits oxidative modification of LDL cholesterol directly through free radical scavenging activity according to in vitro data, and indirectly by increasing glutathione and vitamin E concentrations within cell membranes. This has been demonstrated against the pro-oxidant combination of homocysteine and iron (Alul et al 2003) and may have implications for other diseases such as Alzheimer's dementia.

Other evidence suggests that other mechanisms are also likely to be involved. Vitamin C is linked to endothelial function and glucose metabolism. It improves endothelial dysfunction in smokers, renal transplant recipients, patients with CVD after a fatty meal, people with intermittent claudication diabetes and those with hypertension (Kaufmann et al 2000, Ling et al 2002, Silvestro et al 2002, Solzbach et al 1997, Williams et al 2001), but not in healthy elderly people (Singh et al 2002). It is also required for collagen synthesis and metabolism, and has been shown to reduce arterial stiffness and platelet aggregation in healthy male volunteers, smokers and non-smokers, and diabetics (Schindler et al 2002, Wilkinson et al 1999). These effects are often observed with doses several times higher than current RDI levels. In vivo studies further indicate that vitamin C decreases carotid wall thickness, downregulates inducible nitric oxide (NO) synthase expression, normalises gene expression of antioxidant enzymes and inhibits plaque maturation (Kaliora et al 2006).

A 1997 review of epidemiological studies showed some inverse associations between SBP, DBP or both and vitamin C plasma concentration or intake (Ness et al 1997). Three more recent studies have supported this finding (Bates et al 1998, Block 2002, Block et al 2001). Four intervention studies investigated the effects of vitamin C supplementation, with three producing positive results (Duffy et al 1999, Fotherby et al 2000, Galley et al 1997, Ghosh et al 1994). The doses used were typically 250 mg twice daily for a period of 6–8 weeks, although effects have been reported after 4 weeks' treatment. The negative study by Ghosh et al showed a significant reduction in both SBP and DBP with ascorbic acid. This became non-significant when compared with the placebo responses, although the placebo and ascorbic acid groups were not evenly matched for baseline plasma ascorbate concentration.

Additionally, plasma ascorbate concentrations have been shown to be inversely correlated to pulse rate in one cross-sectional study involving 500 subjects (Bates et al 1998).

Nitrate tolerance

Preliminary studies seem to support the role of vitamin C in attenuating the development of nitrate tolerance. Three human studies have found that vitamin C administration prevents the development of nitrate tolerance (Bassenge et al 1998, Watanabe et al 1998a, 1998b). Although the mechanism responsible is not yet known, results from a double-blind study using an acute dose of 2 g have suggested that vitamin C is likely to protect NO from inactivation by oxygen free radicals (Wilkinson et al 1999), which could in part explain its observed effects.

Myocardial infarction (MI)

Two prospective studies in men have suggested that ascorbic acid deficiency and marginal deficiency predict subsequent MI, independently of classical risk factors. The first, a 5-year prospective population study of 1605 middle-aged Finnish men, free of coronary disease at baseline, found that a significantly higher percentage (13.2%) of the 91 men with baseline plasma vitamin C concentrations less than 11.4 micromol/L (2.0 mg/L) experienced MI, compared with men with higher plasma vitamin C levels (Nyyssonen et al 1997). These results are particularly impressive because low plasma ascorbate was the strongest risk factor of all the measured factors. The second, a 12-year follow-up study, revealed a significantly increased relative risk of ischaemic heart disease and stroke at initially low plasma levels of vitamin C (<22.7 micromol/L), independently of vitamin E and of the classical cardiovascular risk factors (Gey et al 1993).

In contrast, one smaller study involving 180 male patients with a first acute MI, but no recent angina, failed to detect an association between low plasma concentration of vitamin C and the risk of acute MI (Riemersma et al 2000). Similarly, analysis from the NHANES III survey, which involved 7658 men and women, found that among participants who reported no alcohol consumption, serum ascorbic acid concentrations were not independently associated with CVD prevalence (Simon & Hudes 1999). Among participants who consumed alcohol, serum ascorbic acid concentrations consistent with tissue saturation (1.0–3.0 mg/dL) were associated with a decreased prevalence of angina (multivariate odds ratio (OR) 0.48; 95% CI 0.23–1.03%; P for trend = 0.06), but were not significantly associated with MI or stroke prevalence.

Clinical studies involving vitamin C supplementation

Interventional studies with supplements have been performed; however, many use vitamin C in combination with other nutrients such as vitamin E,

V

making it difficult to assess the contribution of vitamin C alone.

One review which analysed studies that only used supplemental vitamin C produced encouraging results. Knekt et al (2004) analysed results from nine prospective studies and a 10-year follow-up whereby 4647 major incident CHD events occurred in 293,172 subjects who were free of CHD at baseline (Knekt et al 2004). They found that people with higher supplemental vitamin C intake had a lower CHD incidence. Compared with subjects who did not take supplemental vitamin C, those who took >700 mg supplemental vitamin C daily had a relative risk of CHD incidence of 0.75 (0.60, 0.93; P for trend < 0.001). Interestingly, dietary intake of antioxidant vitamins was only weakly related to a reduced CHD risk after adjustment for potential non-dietary and dietary confounding factors and, compared with subjects in the lowest dietary intake quintiles for vitamins E and C, those in the highest intake quintiles had relative risks of CHD incidence of 0.84 (95% CI 0.71–1.00; $P = 0.17$) and 1.23 (95% CI 1.04–1.45; $P = 0.07$), respectively.

IN COMBINATION

The Women's Antioxidant Cardiovascular Study tested the effects of vitamin C (500 mg daily), vitamin E (600 IU every other day) and beta-carotene (50 mg every other day) on the combined outcome of MI, stroke, coronary revascularisation or CVD death among 8171 female health professionals at increased risk. Participants were 40 years of age or older, with a prior history of CVD or three or more CVD risk factors, and were followed for an average 9.4 years. The study's factorial design enabled a comparison to be made between individual test agents as well as combination therapy. Overall, there was no significant effect for the individual nutrients vitamin C, vitamin E or beta-carotene on the primary combined end point, or on the individual secondary outcomes of MI, stroke, coronary revascularisation or CVD death. A marginally significant reduction in the primary outcome with active vitamin E was observed among the prespecified subgroup of women with prior CVD (RR = 0.89, $P = 0.04$). With regard to combination therapy, people receiving both vitamins C and E experienced fewer strokes ($P = 0.03$), but there were no other significant findings (Cook et al 2007).

Effects on blood pressure

Although epidemiological evidence and prospective clinical trials point strongly to a role of vitamin C in reducing blood pressure in hypertensive and normotensive subjects, controlled studies have been inconsistent (Houston 2005). Interpretation of these results is difficult, as some studies lack a control group, have no baseline readings, use variable vitamin C doses and population characteristics, and do not report serum vitamin C or oxidative stress status. Overall, it appears that doses between 100 mg and 1000 mg of vitamin C daily are required for a reduction in blood pressure, with greater reduction in SBP than DBP and greater response in people with higher initial value.

There is a large body of evidence that ROS produced during myocardial ischaemia and reperfusion play a crucial role in myocardial damage and endothelial dysfunction. As a result, there has been some investigation to determine whether antioxidant supplementation (chiefly vitamins C and E) may improve the clinical outcome of patients with acute MI and limit the size of the infarct.

According to a large, randomised, double-blind, multicentre trial of 800 patients (mean age 62 years) with acute MI and receiving standard care, co-treatment with vitamin C (1000 mg/12 hours infusion) followed by 1200 mg/day orally and vitamin E (600 mg/day) for 30 days resulted in significantly less frequent incidence of reinfarction and other post-MI complications compared to a placebo (14% versus 19% respectively) (Jaxa-Chamiec et al 2005). Another randomised, double-blind, placebo-controlled study of 37 patients with acute MI investigated the effects of starting supplementation with vitamins C and E (600 mg/day each) on the first day of symptoms and continuing for a further 14 days (Bednarz et al 2003). Active treatment resulted in significantly lower exercise-induced QT-interval dispersion compared to a placebo, although baseline QT dispersion was similar in both groups. A prospective, randomised study of 61 patients further suggests that oral vitamin C administration (1 g/day) could be beneficial for patients at higher thrombotic risk post-MI, such as those with diabetes (Morel et al 2003).

Postmenopausal cardiovascular health

Across multiple large clinical trials, vitamin C supplementation, alone or in combination with vitamin E and betacarotene, appears to be ineffective at secondary prevention of CHD in pre- and postmenopausal women (Bjelakovic et al 2007, Cook et al 2007, Heart Protection Study Collaborative Group 2002, Waters et al 2002). However, observational studies evaluating vitamin C for primary prevention of CHD have found conflicting results in women (Gale et al 1995, Osganian et al 2003).

Cancer: prevention and treatment

One of the most important modifiable determinants of cancer risk is diet. Several research panels and committees have independently concluded that high fruit and vegetable intake decreases the risk of many types of cancer and, because vitamin C is present in large quantities in these foods, it is plausible that the reduction in cancer risk associated with the consumption of fruits and vegetables may be, at least in part, attributable to dietary vitamin C (Li & Schellhorn 2007).

Prevention

Epidemiological evidence of a protective effect of dietary vitamin C for non-hormone-dependent cancers is strong (Block 1991a, 1991b). The majority

Clinical note — Vitamin C for cancer: a historical perspective

More than three decades ago, the well-known team of Ewan Cameron and Linus Pauling started investigating the effects of high doses of continuous IV vitamin C and oral supplements in treating advanced, incurable cancer. The idea of using vitamin C was born out of the recognition that the outcome of every cancer is determined to a significant extent by the individual's inherent resistance, which in turn is influenced by the availability of certain nutritional factors such as ascorbic acid (Cameron 1982). They have published the results of several trials that have shown enhanced quality of life for some terminal patients and also improvements in objective markers. As a result, a protocol for the use of vitamin C in the treatment of cancer has been developed at the Vale of Leven Hospital, Scotland, the chief site of Cameron and Pauling's investigations (Cameron 1991). The protocol emphasises the importance of using an initial course of IV ascorbate, followed by a maintenance oral dose. Although their results are encouraging, they have been criticised because randomised double-blind principles were not adopted.

of studies in which a dietary vitamin C intake was calculated have identified a statistically significant protective effect, with high intake conferring approximately a twofold protective effect compared with low intake. In general, most have shown that higher intakes of vitamin C are associated with decreased incidence of cancers of the mouth, throat and vocal cords, oesophagus and stomach, pancreas, colon, rectum, renal cell and lung (Cohen & Bhagavan 1995, FAO/WHO 2002, Jenab et al 2006, Negri et al 2000, You et al 2000). More recently, a case-control study of men in New York found that a higher intake of vitamin C was associated with reduced risk of prostate cancer (McCann et al 2005).

Two other large studies have identified inverse associations between dietary vitamin C and breast cancer risk (Michels et al 2001, Zhang et al 1999). More specifically, the Nurses' Health Study, which involved 83,234 women, detected a strong inverse association between total vitamin C from foods and breast cancer risk among premenopausal women with a positive family history of breast cancer (Zhang et al 1999). Those who consumed an average of 205 mg/day of vitamin C from foods had a 63% lower risk of breast cancer than those who consumed an average of 70 mg/day. A large Swedish population-based prospective study that comprised 59,036 women found that high dietary intakes of ascorbic acid (mean intake 110 mg/day) reduced the risk of breast cancer among women who were overweight and/or had a high intake of linoleic acid (Michels et al 2001).

More recently, a case–control study nested within the EPIC study identified an inverse risk of gastric cancer in the highest versus lowest quartile of plasma vitamin C (Jenab et al 2006). The inverse association was more pronounced in subjects consuming higher levels of red and processed meats, a factor that may increase endogenous *N*-nitroso compound production. It has been proposed that vitamin C protects against gastric cancer because it inhibits carcinogenic *N*-nitroso compound production in the stomach and acts as a free radical scavenger.

Overall, it appears that the protective effect is dose-dependent, with studies finding significant cancer risk reductions in people consuming at least 80–110 mg of vitamin C daily in the long term (Carr & Frei 1999).

Clinical studies

One of the first published studies by Cameron and Pauling (1974) was a phase I–II study in 50 patients with advanced, untreatable malignancies, in which both subjective and objective markers were evaluated. They observed that 27 patients failed to respond to treatment; however, three patients experienced stabilisation of disease, tumour regression occurred in five patients and tumour haemorrhage and necrosis occurred in four patients. Two years later, the same research team published a report that compared the survival rates of 100 terminal cancer patients given supplemental ascorbate as part of their routine management with 1000 patients who were not given the supplement, and observed the mean survival time to be more than 4.2 times longer for the ascorbate subjects (>210 days) than for the controls (50 days) (Cameron & Pauling 1976).

In subsequent years, two randomised, placebo-controlled studies investigating the effects of oral vitamin C supplementation (10 g/day) in terminal cancer patients failed to detect a significant difference in outcome (Creagan et al 1979, Moertel et al 1985). These two studies are often cited as evidence disproving the benefits of vitamin C in cancer treatment; however, the different routes of administration investigated in these studies is an important factor central to the discrepant results (Padayatty & Levine 2000). Maximal plasma vitamin C concentrations achievable by oral administration are limited by the kidney, which eliminates excess ascorbic acid through renal excretion, whereas IV injection bypasses the renal absorptive system, resulting in elevated plasma concentrations to high levels. As such, it has been argued that only IV administration of high-dose ascorbate can produce millimolar plasma concentrations that are toxic to many cancer cell lines.

Scientific interest in the interaction between ascorbic acid and cancer has been reawakened in recent years, with new evidence that in millimolar concentrations (only achievable after parenteral administration) vitamin C is selectively cytotoxic to many neoplastic cell lines, potentiates cytoxic agents and demonstrates anticancer activity alone and in combination with other agents in tumour-bearing rodents (Hoffer et al 2008). Simultaneously, theoretical interest has arisen in the potential of redox-active molecules like menadione, trolox and ascorbic acid to modify cancer biology, especially when administered with cytotoxic drugs.

Intravenous vitamin C

IV administration of vitamin C achieves much higher plasma and urine concentrations than oral dosing and has been proposed as the only viable means of achieving the high concentrations required to induce the antitumour effects exhibited by the vitamin (Padayatty et al 2004). Case studies suggest that this approach can improve patient wellbeing and, in some cases, reduce tumour size and improve survival (Padayatty et al 2006, Riordan et al 2005).

A safety study conducted in 2005 involved 24 late-stage terminal cancer patients who were administered continuous vitamin C infusions of 150–710 mg/kg/day for up to 8 weeks (Riordan et al 2005). This treatment regimen increased plasma ascorbate concentrations to a mean of 1.1 mmol/L and was considered relatively safe. The most common side effects reported were nausea, oedema and dry mouth or skin, and two 'possible' adverse events occurred. One was a patient with a history of renal calculi who developed a kidney stone after 13 days of treatment, and another was a patient who experienced hypokalaemia after 6 weeks. Interestingly, the majority of patients were vitamin C-deficient before treatment.

Clinical trials for phases I and II are currently being conducted using intravenously administered vitamin C in patients with solid tumours. The phase I study was primarily conducted to determine a recommended phase II dose, with secondary objectives to define any toxic effects, detect any preliminary antitumour effects and monitor for preservation of or improvement in quality of life. In the first phase I trial published in 2008, patients with advanced cancer or haematological malignancy were assigned to sequential cohorts infused with 0.4, 0.6, 0.9 and 1.5 g ascorbic acid/kg body weight three times weekly, delivered intravenously (Hoffer et al 2008). This protocol achieved plasma ascorbic acid concentrations of >10 microM for more than 4 hours, which is considered sufficient to induce cancer cell death according to in vitro research. In addition, all patients were provided with a daily multivitamin tablet (Centrum Select, Wyeth) and 400 IU D-alpha-tocopherol twice daily with meals, and, on non-infusion days, 500 mg ascorbic acid twice daily to obviate large shifts in plasma ascorbic acid concentrations. No unusual biochemical or haematological abnormalities were observed, and there were no changes in the social, emotional or functional parameters of quality of life in any cohort. Unlike in the previous case series by Cameron and Pauling (1974), in which acute tumour haemorrhage and necrosis were reported, these effects were not seen in this study (Hoffer et al 2008). Researchers concluded that the promise of ascorbic acid in the treatment of advanced cancer may lie in its combination with cytotoxic agents, where high concentrations might modify either toxicity or response. A phase I–II clinical trial is being planned that will combine IV ascorbic acid with chemotherapy as a first-line treatment in advanced-stage non-small-cell lung cancer, using the dose determined from this study.

Based on the available evidence of antitumour mechanisms and these case reports, further research into this approach is clearly warranted.

Adjunct to oncology treatments

Whether vitamin C improves or hinders responses to standard oncology treatment has been the focus of intense debate for many decades. There are in vitro studies showing that vitamin C can enhance the antitumour activity of cisplatin and doxorubicin (Abdel-Latif et al 2005, Kurbacher et al 1996, Reddy et al 2001, Sarna & Bhola 1993). In vivo evidence shows vitamin C enhances the effectiveness of 5-fluorouracil, doxorubicin, cyclophosphamide and vincristine (Lamson & Brignall 2000, Nagy et al 2003), whereas other studies find no change in drug effect. Although these results are promising, no large randomised studies are available to confirm their significance in humans.

Most recently, vitamin C inactivated the effects of bortezomib, a new proteasome inhibitor approved by the US Food and Drug Administration for the treatment of patients with relapsed multiple myeloma (Zou et al 2006). Interestingly, drug inactivation was not achieved through antioxidative mechanisms.

Evidence from experimental models suggests that vitamin C may also reduce drug toxicity in a dose-dependent manner (Giri et al 1998, Greggi Antunes et al 2000).

Breast cancer

There is limited evidence to support the use of vitamin C in the primary prevention of total cancer incidence, including breast cancer (Lin et al 2009, Moorman et al 2001, Poulter et al 1984). One of the largest studies in women found that vitamin C (500 mg daily) had no effect on the incidence of cancer after 9.4 years of follow-up (Lin et al 2009).

While vitamin C may not significantly reduce the risk of breast cancer, reduced risk of mortality was reported for vitamin C supplements taken after diagnosis, according to a recent meta-analysis of 10 prospective studies (Harris et al 2014). Harris et al (2014) found that postdiagnosis vitamin C supplement use was associated with a reduced risk of mortality. Dietary vitamin C intake was also statistically significantly associated with a reduced risk of total mortality and breast cancer-specific mortality. The studies involved 17,696 breast cancer cases and found the summary RR for postdiagnosis vitamin C supplement use was 0.81 for total mortality (95% CI 0.72–0.91) and 0.85 for breast cancer-specific mortality (95% CI 0.74–0.99). The summary RR for a 100 mg/day increase in dietary vitamin C intake was 0.73 for total mortality (95% CI 0.59–0.89) and 0.78 for breast cancer-specific mortality (95% CI 0.64–0.94) (Harris et al 2014).

Oral cancer

A recent systematic review showed that the pro-oxidant activity of pharmacological ascorbic acid is a part of its dose-dependent bimodal activity and is a result of the proposed Fenton mechanism. In vitro, animal and ex vivo studies of pharmacological ascorbic acid have yielded meritorious results proving vitamin C as an effective cytotoxic agent against oral neoplastic cells with potentially no harming effects on normal cells (Putchala et al 2013).

> ***Clinical note — The debate continues ... to vitamin C or not?***
> One research group based at the University of Colorado has produced evidence that suggests that vitamin C and other antioxidant nutrients may not only protect healthy cells from damage, but also improve the antitumour effects of standard treatment (Gottlieb 1999). They are currently conducting further research to identify how cell selectivity occurs, but propose that cancer cells may have lost the normal homeostatic regulatory mechanism that stops excessive concentrations of antioxidants from entering the cell. As intracellular levels rise, a series of reactions occurs, resulting in growth inhibition and cell death. Another group at Memorial Sloan Kettering Cancer Center (Gottlieb 1999) argues that tumours already contain higher levels of ascorbic acid than normal cells and have identified a mechanism to explain this observation. As such, they advocate against the use of vitamin C when cytotoxic agents that rely on free radical production are being used (see Chapter 10 for further discussion).

Prevention of cataracts

Ascorbate has long been known to accumulate in tears and other biofluids, such as cerebrospinal fluid relative to plasma (Patterson & O'Rourke 1987), and lowered levels of vitamin C in the eye have been associated with increased oxidative stress in the human cornea (Shoham et al 2008). Ascorbic acid is thought to be a primary substrate in ocular protection because of its high concentration in the eye. Within the cell, vitamin C helps to protect membrane lipids from peroxidation by recycling vitamin E (May 1999). It is present at high concentrations in vitreous humour (Hanashima & Namiki 1999), cornea (Brubaker et al 2000) and tear film (Dreyer & Rose 1993).

Numerous observational and prospective clinical studies have been performed to examine the effect on cataracts of vitamin C alone or in combination with other antioxidants. Several epidemiological studies have identified an association between vitamin C and cataract incidence (Ferrigno et al 2005, Jacques & Chylack Jr 1991, Jacques et al 1988, Valero et al 2002); however, studies investigating whether supplementation is protective have produced mixed results (Chasan-Taber et al 1999, Chylack et al 2002, Hammond & Johnson 2002, Jacques et al 1997, 2001, Kuzniarz et al 2001, Seddon et al 1994, Taylor et al 2002).

Results from the Harvard Nurses' Health Study, Physicians' Health Study, the Beaver Dam Eye Study and the Australian Blue Mountains study suggest that if protective effects are to be seen, they are most likely when vitamin C is taken for a long period (5–10 years or more) and/or used as part of a multivitamin combination (Kuzniarz et al 2001, Mares-Perlman et al 2000, Seddon et al 1994, Taylor et al 2002).

It is suspected that vitamin C protects the lens of the eye from oxygen-related damage over time by both direct free radical scavenging activity and indirect activity. This is achieved primarily by protecting endogenous alpha-tocopherol (the major lipid-soluble antioxidant of retinal membranes) against oxidation induced by UV radiation and by regenerating it (Stoyanovsky et al 1995).

Diabetes

Vitamin C has several actions that provide a basis for its use in diabetes. It has been reported to lower erythrocyte sorbitol concentrations (important for preventing complications in type 1 diabetes), improve endothelial function (important for slowing atherosclerosis) and reduce blood pressure (Beckman et al 2001, Cunningham 1998). Plasma vitamin C levels seem to play a role in the modulation of insulin activity in aged healthy or diabetic subjects (Paolisso et al 1994) and are inversely related to glycosylated haemoglobin. Additionally, increased free radical production has been reported in patients with diabetes mellitus as a result of hyperglycaemia, which directly induces oxidative stress (Ceriello et al 1998).

Blood glucose

At this stage there are few studies that test the effects of supplemental vitamin C on plasma glucose levels directly. Although one early study demonstrated that an oral dose of 1500 mg vitamin C reduces plasma glucose levels in patients with type 2 diabetes (Sandhya & Das 1981), no further published studies confirm this result.

Endothelial function

The results of studies investigating the role of vitamin C on endothelial function in diabetes have attracted interest.

A double-blind, placebo-controlled study demonstrated that chronic oral vitamin C supplementation (500 mg/day) in type 2 diabetes significantly lowered arterial blood pressure and improved arterial stiffness compared with a placebo (Mullan et al 2002). After 1 month's treatment, SBP fell from 142.1 to 132.3 mmHg, mean pressure from 104.7 to 97.8 mmHg, DBP from 83.9 to 79.5 mmHg and peripheral pulse pressure from 58.2 to 52.7 mmHg, whereas placebo had no effect.

A randomised study of women with a history of gestational diabetes showed that ascorbic acid supplementation resulted in a significant improvement of endothelium-dependent flow-mediated dilatation, with no effect seen for a placebo (Lekakis et al 2000).

However, a randomised, double-blind, placebo-controlled study of vitamin C (800 mg/day for 4 weeks) concluded that high-dose oral vitamin C therapy resulted in incomplete replenishment of vitamin C levels and does not improve endothelial dysfunction and insulin resistance in type 2 diabetes (Chen et al 2006).

The mechanism of action appears to involve several steps, such as reduction in LDL oxidation, enhanced endothelial NO synthase activity and NO bioavailability and reduced insulin resistance, which can cause endothelium-dependent, NO-mediated vasodilation.

Eye health

Diabetes mellitus is associated with a number of ocular complications that can eventually lead to blindness. Vitamin C is found in high concentration in the eye and is thought to be important for protection against free radicals. This may have special significance for people with diabetes mellitus, as most studies have found that their circulating vitamin C levels are at least 30% lower than in people without the disease (Peponis et al 2002). Furthermore, a systematic review (Lee et al 2010) assessing five hospital-based, cross-sectional studies consistently reported that diabetic patients with retinopathy had lower vitamin C levels than those without retinopathy (Ali & Chakraborty 1989, Gupta & Chari 2005, Gurler et al 2000, Rema et al 1995, Sinclair et al 1992).

According to a 2008 Cochrane systematic review (Lopes de Jesus et al 2008) investigating the effectiveness of vitamin C in diabetic retinopathy, no research to date has adequately examined the treatment of diabetic retinopathy with vitamin C or superoxidase dismutase, so it remains unknown whether the intervention has a significant impact on the progress of this complication.

Because of its safety, cost-effectiveness and generally encouraging results, a strategy of adding 200–600 mg of vitamin C to a healthy diet is worth considering for individuals with diabetes type 1 or 2.

Pneumonia

Three prophylactic trials found a statistically significant (80% or greater) reduction in pneumonia incidence in the vitamin C group. These trials were assessed in a recent Cochrane review, which concluded that the prophylactic use of vitamin C to prevent pneumonia should be further investigated in populations who have a high incidence of pneumonia, especially if dietary vitamin C intake is low (Hemilä & Louhiala 2013).

> ***Clinical note — Do asthmatic lungs need more antioxidant protection?***
> In 1999, Kelly et al found that people with mild asthma have low levels of antioxidant nutrient vitamins E and C in their lung lining fluid, even though blood levels of these vitamins may be normal or increased. This observation, together with other factors, indicated that the asthmatic lung is exposed to greater oxidative stress in people with asthma than in non-asthmatics. The researchers suggested that the inflammatory cells in the lungs of asthmatic patients generate more free radical species than those in healthy people, adding to bronchoconstriction, increased mucus secretion and increased airways responsiveness. Given that oral supplementation in asthma has produced inconsistent results, chief researcher Frank Kelly suggests that future studies should focus on other administration forms, such as vitamin C inhalers (personal communication, Melbourne, 1998).

Asthma

Vitamin C is the major antioxidant present in the extracellular fluid lining of the lung, where it protects against both endogenous free radicals (produced as a byproduct of inflammation) and environmental free radicals (such as ozone in air pollution). Theoretically, it may be of benefit in reducing symptoms of inflammatory airway conditions such as asthma, and may also be beneficial in reducing exercise-induced bronchoconstriction.

According to many epidemiological studies, dietary intake of vitamin C-rich foods or serum ascorbate is associated with improved lung function in both asthmatic and normal subjects (Devereux & Seaton 2005, Kelly 2005, McDermoth 2000). Oxygen metabolites can play a direct or indirect role in the modulation of airway inflammation. Many studies suggest that superoxide dismutase and free radical scavengers in the blood are significantly lower in asthma, and document a correlation between asthmatic severity and ROS products in asthmatic subjects (Shanmugasundaram 2001, Vural 2000). Not surprisingly, low blood concentrations of vitamin C have been found in mildly asthmatic subjects (Rahman 2006).

Despite a theoretical basis for its use in lung diseases such as asthma, its value in this disease is controversial. A 2001 Cochrane review of three studies concluded that current evidence is insufficient to recommend a specific role for vitamin C in the treatment of asthma and that a large-scale randomised controlled trial (RCT) is required to clarify its role (Kaur et al 2001). This was repeated in a Cochrane review published in 2004 that included new data from a study of 201 adults taking inhaled corticosteroids and came to a similar conclusion, stating that evidence is currently conflicting (Ram et al 2004).

A recent Cochrane review (Milan et al 2013) concluded that there is insufficient evidence to provide a robust assessment on the use of vitamin C in the management of asthma or exercise-induced bronchoconstriction. There was some indication that vitamin C was helpful in exercise-induced breathlessness in terms of lung function and symptoms; however, as these findings were provided only by small studies, more research is required before a conclusive recommendation can be made. Three human studies have produced positive results when vitamin C was used as pretreatment in doses ranging from 500 mg to 2000 mg (Cohen et al 1997, Miric & Haxhiu 1991, Schachter & Schlesinger 1982).

Asthma and atopy in children

A systematic review and meta-analysis (Nurmatov et al 2011) assessed 14 papers reviewing the association between vitamin C and asthma or atopic outcomes in children. While some of the studies showed some improvement in wheeze or allergy symptomatology overall, the body of evidence was judged to be methodologically weak and the possible effectiveness of vitamin C to prevent atopic outcomes remains unclear.

Bone mineral density (BMD)

Although the relationship between calcium, vitamin D and BMD is well known, other nutrients, such as vitamin C, are also critical for bone development, repair and maintenance (Ilich et al 2003). Epidemiological studies have demonstrated a positive association between BMD and intake of vitamin C (Hall & Greendale 1998, Leveille et al 1997). Low vitamin C intakes have been associated with a decline in BMD specifically at the femoral neck and total hip (Hall & Greendale 1998).

Data collected from 13,080 adults enrolled in NHANES III from 1988 to 1994 have identified an association between dietary and serum ascorbic acid, BMD and bone fracture (Simon & Hudes 2001). Dietary ascorbic acid intake was independently associated with BMD among premenopausal women and postmenopausal women without a history of smoking or oestrogen use. Additionally, fracture risk fell by 49% in postmenopausal women (with a history of smoking and oestrogen use) who had high serum vitamin C levels.

Vitamin C supplementation

Two controlled studies have investigated the effects of long-term vitamin C supplementation in postmenopausal women and found that it increases BMD (Hall & Greendale 1998, Morton et al 2001). Both studies identified a positive association with BMD in postmenopausal women with dietary calcium intakes of at least 500 mg or those taking calcium supplements. The effect was especially marked in those women taking calcium supplements and concurrent hormone replacement therapy.

The daily dose taken was generally in excess of the RDI and ranged from 100 mg to 5000 mg. More specifically, one study found that, for each 100 mg increment in dietary vitamin C intake, there was an associated increase of 0.017 g/cm^2 in BMD (femoral neck and total hip), and for those women with calcium intakes above 500 mg/day the increment increased to 0.019 g/cm^2 in BMD per 100 mg vitamin C.

An Australian study of 533 randomly selected women determined that vitamin C supplements may suppress bone resorption in non-smoking postmenopausal women (Pasco et al 2006).

In contrast to these results, no effect on BMD was observed for dietary or supplemental vitamin C in the Women's Health Initiative Observational Study and Clinical Trial, which involved 11,068 women aged 50–79 years (Wolf et al 2005). However, a significant beneficial interaction was observed between total vitamin C and hormone replacement therapy on total body, femoral neck, spine and total hip BMD.

Animal studies have detected an improved healing response in bone fractures with supplemental vitamin C, suggesting a further role in fracture healing (Yilmaz et al 2001).

Sports

Vitamin C supplementation is often used by athletes in order to improve recovery, restore immune responses, enhance wound healing and counteract oxidative stress and changes to adrenal hormones and inflammatory responses. It is often taken together with other antioxidant vitamins and minerals, such as vitamin E and zinc. One placebo-controlled study has shown that 20 mg of ascorbic acid twice daily over 14 days has some modest beneficial effects on recovery from unaccustomed exercise (Thompson et al 2001); however, no studies have reported improved performance for vitamin C supplementation.

Prevention of postendurance exercise infections

Athletes often use vitamin C supplements to prevent infections, as strenuous training and physiological stress appear to increase the body's need for vitamin C to a level above the usual RDI (Schwenk & Costley 2002). Additionally, the risk of infection after an intense aerobic training session or competition (such as a marathon) is increased (Jeurissen et al 2003).

A 2004 Cochrane review that analysed results from six trials involving a total of 642 marathon runners, skiers and soldiers on subarctic exercises found regular vitamin C supplementation significantly reduced the incidence of the common cold, supporting its use in this population (Douglas et al 2004).

Alterations to neurotransmitters and adrenal hormones

Several studies have been conducted with ultramarathon runners to investigate whether vitamin C supplementation, usually in doses of 1500 mg/day, is able to restore exercise-induced changes to neurotransmitters, adrenal hormones or inflammatory responses (Nieman et al 2000, Peters et al 2001a, 2001b). Overall, it appears that high-dose vitamin C supplements taken at least 7 days before racing do have some effect.

One study involving 45 ultramarathon runners found that doses of 1500 mg vitamin C taken for 7 days before the race, on the day of the race and for 2 days following the race significantly attenuated exercise-induced elevations in cortisol, adrenaline and interleukin-10 (IL-10) and IL-1 receptor antagonist levels compared with a placebo (Peters et al 2001a); however, the effect was transient.

Male infertility

A relationship between infertility and the generation of ROS has been established and extensively studied. Alterations in the testicular microenvironment and haemodynamics can increase production of ROS and/or decrease local antioxidant capacity, resulting in generation of excessive oxygen species. A large number of studies have elucidated the effects of increased oxygen species in the serum, semen and testicular tissues of patients.

Vitamin C (ascorbic acid), a major antioxidant found in extracellular fluid, is present in seminal fluid at a high concentration compared with that in blood plasma (364 versus 40 microM) and is present in detectable amounts in sperm (Patel & Sigman 2008). In infertile men, vitamin C has been found in reduced quantity in the seminal plasma (Lewis et al 1997). An association between oxidative stress and sperm DNA fragmentation has been identified and has led to studies looking for changes in semen DNA fragmentation as an outcome rather than just changes in semen parameters.

A review of the literature reveals that interventional studies have produced promising but inconsistent results and incomplete reporting of study outcomes. Sometimes changes to semen parameters are noted, but there is little or no information about successful pregnancies or characteristics of the study population, thereby hindering accurate interpretation of results. Clearly further research is required to better evaluate the effects of vitamin C in male fertility.

An RCT of 75 fertile, heavy smokers compared placebo to two different doses of vitamin C (200 mg and 1000 mg) and found that both supplemented groups experienced a significant improvement in sperm concentration, morphology and viability (Dawson et al 1992).

A randomised, placebo-controlled trial found that treatment with oral vitamin C and E of men with unexplained infertility associated with elevated sperm DNA fragmentation led to decreased DNA fragmentation without a change in semen parameters (Greco et al 2005b).

In an uncontrolled study of 38 men with an elevated percentage of fragmented spermatozoa (15%) and one prior failed intracytoplasmic sperm injection (ICSI) attempt, oral supplementation with vitamins E and C demonstrated a significant improvement in pregnancy rate (48.2% vs 6.9%) and implantation rate (19.6% vs 2.2%) when compared with their prior ICSI attempt (Greco et al 2005a).

A systematic review on the effect of oral antioxidants on male infertility evaluated results from 17 RCTs including a total of 1665 men, which differed in the populations studied and type, dosage and duration of antioxidants used. None of the studies assessed vitamin C as a single oral agent; however, when reviewing the effectiveness of vitamin C in conjunction with other antioxidants, the results were as follows. Sperm motility improved in two out of five studies (Omu et al 2008, Scott et al 1998), sperm concentration improved in one out of five studies (Galatioto et al 2008) and sperm DNA fragmentation index was reduced in two out of two studies (Greco et al 2005a, Omu et al 2008). However, sperm morphology did not improve in any of the five studies. Pregnancy rate after ICSI was significantly improved in the treatment group in one study ($P = 0.046$) (Tremellen et al 2007).

Pregnancy

A Cochrane systematic review evaluated results from five RCTs involving 766 women in which vitamin C supplementation was used (Rumbold & Crowther 2005). No difference was seen between women supplemented with vitamin C alone or in combination with other supplements compared with placebo for the risk of stillbirth, perinatal death, birth weight or intrauterine growth restriction. In regard to preterm birth, women supplemented with vitamin C were at increased risk compared to placebo. No difference was seen between women supplemented with vitamin C compared with placebo for the risk of neonatal death whereas a reduced incidence of pre-eclampsia was found with supplementation when using a fixed-effect model.

More recently, another three systematic reviews and meta-analyses concluded that combined vitamin C and E supplementation did not decrease the risk of pre-eclampsia and should not be offered to gravidas for the prevention of pre-eclampsia or other pregnancy-induced hypertensive disorders (Ahmet et al 2010, Conde-Agudelo et al 2011, Rossi & Mullin 2011).

Alzheimer's disease (AD)

A systematic review and meta-analysis reviewed eight RCTs, including a cohort of 223 people diagnosed with AD (da Silva et al 2013). Four studies showed statistically significantly lower plasma levels of vitamin C than in controls (unrelated to the classic malnourishment that is common in patients with AD). However, whether this means AD patients have increased oxidative stress and therefore increased antioxidant requirements which would benefit from vitamin C supplementation remains to be tested.

Periodontal disease

Nishida et al (2000) used data from the NHANES III study, which identified a statistically significant, albeit weak, association between decreased dietary vitamin C intake and increased risk of periodontal disease (OR 1.19). More recently, it was reported from the same NHANES III study that higher serum antioxidant levels were associated with lower ORs of severe periodontitis, with an OR of 0.53 for vitamin C (Chapple et al 2007). In a population of 413 non-institutionalised active older adults in Japan, a significant but weak association was found between serum vitamin C levels and clinical attachment loss (grade of severity of periodontal disease) (Amarasena et al 2005). Clinical attachment loss was 4% greater in subjects with lower serum vitamin C levels compared with subjects with higher serum vitamin C levels. The association was independent of other covariates, including smoking and random blood sugar levels. This result is in accordance with the findings from another study investigating the association of serum vitamin C levels with serology of periodontitis in a random subsample of Finnish and Russian men (Pussinen et al 2003).

Complex regional pain syndrome (CRPS)

A 2013 systematic review and meta-analysis assessed the use of high-dose vitamin C for CRPS (Shibuya et al 2013). Use of high-dose vitamin C has been recommended by the Evidence Based Guidelines for Type 1 CRPS for wrist fractures (oral administration of 500 mg of vitamin C per day for 50 days from the date of the injury) (Perez et al 2010). Quantitative synthesis showed a relative risk of 0.22 when daily vitamin C of at least 500 mg was initiated immediately after the extremity surgery or injury and continued for 45–50 days. A routine, daily administration of vitamin C may therefore be beneficial in foot and ankle surgery or injury to avoid CRPS.

Adjunct therapy for haemodialysis patients

Recent research highlights that vitamin C can potentiate the mobilisation of iron from inert tissue stores, and facilitates the incorporation of iron into protoporphyrin in haemodialysis patients being treated with epoetin. Eighteen published studies in the past decade have addressed this issue (Attallah et al 2006, Chan et al 2005, Deira et al 2003, Gastaldello et al 1995, Giancaspro et al 2000, Hörl 1999, Keven et al 2003, CL Lin et al 2003, Macdougall 1999, Mydlik et al 2003, Nguyen 2004, Sezer et al 2002, Taji et al 2004, Tarng & Huang 1998, Tarng et al 1999a, 1999b, 2004, Tovbin et al 2000).

Administration of IV vitamin C to haemodialysis patients with functional iron deficiency may promote better anaemia control and iron utilisation and has also been used successfully in patients with iron overload (Tarng & Huang 1998, Tarng et al 1999a, 1999b). Current recommendations for maintenance of haemodialysis patients advise supplementation with ascorbic acid 75–90 mg daily (Fouque et al 2007) during dialysis. In addition to the potential benefits of vitamin C for anaemia management, the importance of adequate vitamin C with regard to improving cardiovascular outcomes in haemodialysis patients is also the subject of research. A study by Deicher and colleagues of 138 haemodialysis patients examined baseline levels of plasma vitamin C and followed the cohort for occurrence of cardiovascular events (Deicher et al 2005). Results showed that low total vitamin C plasma concentrations (less than 32 micromol/L) were associated with an almost fourfold increased risk for fatal and major non-fatal cardiovascular events compared with haemodialysis patients who had higher plasma vitamin C levels (greater than 60 micromol/L).

OTHER USES

Vitamin C is used for numerous indications, although many have not been significantly studied, such as irritable bowel syndrome, osteoarthritis, menopausal hot flushes, cervical dysplasia, prevention of Alzheimer's dementia, allergies, treatment of lead toxicity and reducing delayed-onset muscle soreness.

Vitamin C supplements have also been used as part of antioxidant combination therapy in HIV. Preliminary research has shown that some antioxidant combinations reduce oxidative stress (Jaruga et al 2002), induce immunological and virological effects that might be of therapeutic value (Muller et al 2000) and produce a trend towards a reduction in viral load in HIV (Allard et al 1998).

For heroin withdrawal, high doses of oral ascorbic acid and vitamin E may ameliorate the withdrawal syndrome of heroin addicts after 4 weeks' treatment, according to one study (Evangelou et al 2000).

DOSAGE RANGE

Australian and New Zealand RDI

Infants

- 0–6 months: 25 mg.
- 7–12 months: 30 mg.

Children

- 1–8 years: 35 mg.
- 9–18 years: 40 mg.

Adults

- >19 years: 45 mg.

Pregnancy

- <19 years: 55 mg.
- >19 years: 60 mg.

V

Lactation

- <19 years: 80 mg.
- >19 years: 85 mg.

Deficiency

- 100 mg taken 3–5 times daily until 4000 mg has been administered, followed by a maintenance dose of 100 mg/day and encouragement to eat a diet with fresh fruit and vegetables.
- In cases of acute infection, complementary and alternative medicine practitioners frequently recommend vitamin C in doses of 1000 g (or more), to be taken in divided doses every few hours until loose bowels are experienced, otherwise known as 'bowel tolerance'. The rationale behind this dosage regimen is that body requirements during infection are dramatically increased, and not only does high-dose vitamin C meet these needs, but also maximum vitamin C absorption is attained when it is taken in divided doses rather than one large amount.

According to clinical studies

- Asthma: 500–2000 mg before exercise.
- Cancer: 10–100 g/day IV.
- CVD prevention: up to 1000 mg/day long-term.
- BMD: 750 mg/day long-term.
- Cataract protection: 500 mg/day long-term.
- Diabetes: 0.5–3 g/day long-term.
- Histamine-lowering effects: 250 mg to 2 g/day for several weeks.
- Respiratory infection: at least 2 g/day.
- Sunburn protection: oral vitamin C (2000 mg/day) in combination with vitamin E (1000 IU/day).
- Urinary acidification: 4–12 g taken in divided doses every 4 hours.

ADVERSE REACTIONS

Adverse effects of oral vitamin C include loose bowels and diarrhoea with high-dose supplements; however, the dose at which this occurs varies between individuals and also varies for each individual at different times.

SIGNIFICANT INTERACTIONS

Aluminium-based antacids

Vitamin C increases the amount of aluminium absorbed. Separate doses by at least 2 hours.

Aspirin

Aspirin may interfere with both absorption and cellular uptake mechanisms for vitamin C, thereby increasing vitamin C requirements (observed in animal and human studies). Increased vitamin C intake may be required with long-term therapy (Basu 1982).

Chitosan

According to a preliminary study in rats, taking vitamin C in combination with chitosan might provide additional benefit in lowering cholesterol. Potentially beneficial interaction.

Cisplatin

Vitamin C enhanced the antitumour activity of cisplatin in several in vitro tests (Abdel-Latif et al

Clinical note — Is the kidney stone risk overstated?

Most kidney stones consist of calcium oxalate, and higher urinary oxalate increases the risk of calcium oxalate nephrolithiasis (Taylor & Curhan 2007). Four mechanisms have been identified that account for increased oxalate excretion: increased dietary intake of oxalate, abnormally increased intestinal absorption of oxalic acid, a deficiency of oxalate-degrading bacteria (in particular *Oxalobacter formigenes*) and increased endogenous production of oxalate. Vitamins C and B_6 are both involved in the metabolic pathway of oxalate. While 40% of dietary vitamin C undergoes a non-enzymatic conversion to oxalate, vitamin B_6 has the opposite effect and metabolises oxalate (Gill & Rose 1985). Since vitamin C has been shown in some (but not all) studies to increase urinary oxalate, researchers speculated that it might have a detrimental role in increasing the risk of kidney stone formation.

Reports of a possible link between ascorbic acid and kidney stones started to appear in the literature in the 1980s (Griffith et al 1986, Power et al 1984). These findings have been challenged by several studies carried out in humans and in experimental animals since that time. In 1994, researchers discovered that vitamin C (in doses as high as 10 g/day) does not increase the amount of oxalate produced in the body in non-stone-forming people (Wandzilak et al 1994). Instead, urine tests used to detect oxalate levels were actually detecting oxalate formed by the conversion of ascorbate during the test procedure. As such, urine oxalate levels tested by this method do not genuinely represent in vivo oxalate when ascorbate is involved. Three studies that followed found no association between vitamin C intake and kidney stone risk. Two prospective studies of more than 85,000 women and 45,000 men found that doses ranging from less than 250 mg/day to more than 1500 mg/day taken over 6–14 years did not correlate with occurrence of kidney stones (Curhan et al 1996, 1999). The third was a controlled study measuring oxalate excretion and several other biochemical and physicochemical risk factors associated with calcium oxalate urolithiasis (Auer et al 1998, Curhan et al 1996, 1999).

Based on the available evidence, it appears unlikely that vitamin C supplements increase the risk of nephrolithiasis in the general population, particularly if they are used in the short to medium term.

2005, Reddy et al 2001, Sarna & Bhola 1993) and reduced drug toxicity in experimental models (Giri et al 1998, Greggi Antunes et al 2000). Potentially beneficial but difficult to assess.

Corticosteroids

Corticosteroids may increase the requirement for vitamin C based on in vitro and in vivo data (Chowdhury & Kapil 1984, Levine & Pollard 1983). Increased intake may be required with long-term drug therapy.

> ***Clinical note — Does vitamin C interact with the oral contraceptive pill?***
> In 1981 a case was reported of a woman who had experienced heavy breakthrough bleeding as a result of stopping vitamin C supplementation while taking the oral contraceptive pill (Morris et al 1981). At the time, it was suspected that vitamin C in high doses increases the bioavailability of oestrogen and raises blood concentrations due to competition for sulfation (resulting in reduced drug metabolism) (Back & Orme 1990). Therefore, ceasing supplement use would have the opposite effect and potentially cause breakthrough bleeding, as reported in this case. Since then, further investigation has been conducted to evaluate whether this interaction is clinically significant. In 1993 a placebo-controlled study was conducted with 37 women and found that 1000 mg of vitamin C does not lead to an increased systemic bioavailability of ethinyl oestradiol, and therefore the purported interaction is unlikely to be of any clinical importance (Zamah et al 1993).

Cyanocobalamin

Vitamin C can reduce absorption of cyanocobalamin. Separate doses by at least 2 hours.

Cyclophosphamide

Vitamin C enhanced the therapeutic drug effect in vivo (Lamson & Brignall 2000). Potentially beneficial but difficult to assess.

Doxorubicin

Vitamin C enhanced the therapeutic drug effect and reduced drug toxicity in vivo (Lamson & Brignall 2000). Potentially beneficial but difficult to assess.

Etoposide

Vitamin C enhanced the antitumour activity of etoposide in vitro (Reddy et al 2001). Potentially beneficial but difficult to assess.

Fluorouracil

Vitamin C enhanced the antitumour activity of 5-fluorouracil in vitro and in vivo (Abdel-Latif et al 2005, Nagy et al 2003). Potentially beneficial but difficult to assess.

Iron

Vitamin C increases the absorption of iron. Potentially beneficial interaction.

L-Dopa

A case report of co-administration with vitamin C suggests this may reduce drug side effects (Sacks & Simpson 1975). Beneficial interaction.

Tamoxifen

Vitamin C enhanced the antitumour activity in vitro (Lamson & Brignall 2000). Potentially beneficial but difficult to assess.

Vincristine

Vitamin C enhanced the drug's effect in vivo (Lamson & Brignall 2000). Potentially beneficial but difficult to assess.

PS-341 (bortezomib, Velcade)

This is a proteasome inhibitor approved by the US Food and Drug Administration for the treatment of patients with relapsed multiple myeloma. Vitamin C inactivated drug activity in vitro (Zou et al 2006). Avoid until safety can be established.

> ***CONTRAINDICATIONS AND PRECAUTIONS***
> In patients who are sensitive to iron overload, vitamin C supplementation may exacerbate iron toxicity by mobilising iron reserves. As such, vitamin C supplementation should be used with caution by people with erythrocyte glucose-6-phosphate dehydrogenase deficiency, haemochromatosis, thalassaemia major or sideroblastic anaemia.

Intravenous vitamin C

A dose-response study involving patients with solid tumours receiving high-dose IV vitamin C found virtually all the side effects that occurred were consistent with the side effects attending the rapid infusion of any high-osmolarity solution. The symptoms were preventable by encouraging patients to drink fluids before and during the infusion. Indeed, rather than provoking fluid overload, ascorbic acid acted like an osmotic diuretic which could induce volume depletion if patients did not compensate by increasing their voluntary fluid intake. Therefore, contraindications to the infusion of very-high-osmolarity ascorbic acid infusions are the same as for other osmotic diuretics: anuria, dehydration, severe pulmonary congestion or pulmonary oedema and a fixed low cardiac output (Hoffer et al 2008).

Laboratory tests

Supplemental vitamin C can affect the results of numerous laboratory tests and should be stopped prior to:

- carbamazepine
- lactate dehydrogenase

- serum aspartate transaminase
- serum bicarbonate
- serum cholesterol
- serum creatinine
- serum creatine kinase
- serum HbA_{1C}
- serum phosphate
- serum triglycerides
- serum urea nitrogen
- stool guiac
- theophylline
- urine 17-hydroxy corticosteroids
- urine 17-ketosteroids
- urine amphetamine
- urine and serum bilirubin
- urine and serum glucose
- urine and serum uric acid
- urine barbiturate
- urine beta-hydroxybutyrate
- urine iodide
- urine oxalate
- urine paracetamol
- urine protein.

Practice points/Patient counselling

- Vitamin C is an essential nutrient for humans, as we are one of the few animal species that cannot synthesise it endogenously.
- Although vitamin C is found widely in fruit and vegetables, up to 100% can be destroyed during cooking and storing, as it is sensitive to light, heat, oxygen and alkali.
- Although frank deficiency is uncommon in Western countries, marginal deficiency states are not uncommon, particularly in young children fed exclusively on cow's milk for a prolonged period, the institutionalised or isolated elderly, chronic alcoholics, the urban poor and cigarette smokers.
- Vitamin C generally acts as an antioxidant and is involved in a myriad of biochemical processes in the body, such as neurotransmitter and hormone synthesis, maintenance of connective tissue, immune function and adrenal function.
- Many, but not all, studies have found a protective effect for dietary vitamin C intake on CVD and cancer incidence, emphasising the importance of adequate dietary intake of fresh fruit and vegetables.
- Oral vitamin C supplements have been investigated in many different conditions. Positive results have been obtained in some of these studies, such as for reducing incidence of the common cold in children, CHD prevention, prevention of several CVDs and BMD. Positive effects on mortality have been reported when vitamin C intake is increased after a diagnosis of breast cancer; however, use as a cancer treatment remains controversial. There are also possible benefits for bone density and cataract incidence and increasing intake after a diagnosis of breast cancer.
- Research shows that long-term supplements do not increase the risk of kidney stones and do not interact with oral contraceptives.

PREGNANCY USE

Vitamin C is safe in pregnancy; however, it is recommended to not exceed the therapeutic dose nor abruptly cease supplementation.

PATIENTS' FAQs

What will this vitamin do for me?

Vitamin C is necessary for health and wellbeing. Supplements have also been used for a variety of indications and in some cases shown to have benefits.

When will it start to work?

Studies have found that dietary or supplemental vitamin C may be required for at least 10 years before protection against heart disease or cancer incidence is detected. However, other benefits may be experienced more quickly, depending on the dose used and indication. Research also indicates that increasing vitamin C intake after a diagnosis of breast cancer may reduce mortality.

Are there any safety issues?

Vitamin C is considered very safe, although high doses may induce reversible loose bowels or diarrhoea. Supplements should be taken only under medical supervision by people with erythrocyte glucose-6-phosphate dehydrogenase deficiency, haemochromatosis, thalassaemia or sideroblastic anaemia.

REFERENCES

Abdel-Latif MM et al. Vitamin C enhances chemosensitization of esophageal cancer cells in vitro. J Chemother 17 (2005): 539–549.

Ahmet, B, et al Combined Vitamin C and E Supplementation for the Prevention of Preeclampsia: A Systematic Review and Meta-Analysis, Obstet Gynecol Surv, 2010 Oct 65(10):653–67.

Ali SM, Chakraborty SK. Role of plasma ascorbate in diabetic microangiopathy. Bangladesh Med Res Counc Bull 1989;15:47–59.

Allard JP et al. Effects of vitamin E and C supplementation on oxidative stress and viral load in HIV-infected subjects. AIDS 12.13 (1998): 1653–1659.

Alul RH et al. Vitamin C protects low-density lipoprotein from homocysteine-mediated oxidation. Free Radic Biol Med 34.7 (2003): 881–891.

Amarasena N, et al. Serum vitamin C–periodontal relationship in community-dwelling elderly Japanese. J Clin Periodontol 2005;32:93–7.

Attallah N et al. Effect of intravenous ascorbic acid in hemodialysis patients with EPOhyporesponsive anemia and hyperferritinemia. Am J Kidney Dis 47 (2006): 644–654.

Auer BL, et al. The effect of ascorbic acid ingestion on the biochemical and physicochemical risk factors associated with calcium oxalate kidney stone formation. Clin Chem Lab Med 36.3 (1998): 143–147.

Back DJ, Orme ML. Pharmacokinetic drug interactions with oral contraceptives. Clin Pharmacokinet 18.6 (1990): 472–484.

Bartholomew M. James Lind's treatise of the scurvy (1753). Postgrad Med J 78.925 (2002): 695–696.

Bassenge E et al. Dietary supplement with vitamin C prevents nitrate tolerance. J Clin Invest 102.1 (1998): 67–71.

Basu TK. Vitamin C–aspirin interactions. Int J Vitam Nutr Res Suppl 23 (1982): 83–90.

Bates CJ et al. Does vitamin C reduce blood pressure? Results of a large study of people aged 65 or older. J Hypertens 16.7 (1998): 925–932.

Beckman JA et al. Ascorbate restores endothelium-dependent vasodilation impaired by acute hyperglycemia in humans. Circulation 103.12 (2001): 1618–1623.

Bednarz B et al. Antioxidant vitamins decrease exercise-induced QT dispersion after myocardial infarction. Kardiol Pol 58 (2003): 375–379.

Beers MH, Berkow R (eds). The Merck manual of diagnosis and therapy, 17th edn. Whitehouse, NJ: Merck, 2003.

Bjelakovic G, et al. Mortality in randomized trials of antioxidant supplements for primary and secondary prevention. Systematic Review and Meta-Analysis. J Am Med Assoc 2007;297:842–57.

Block G. Epidemiologic evidence regarding vitamin C and cancer. Am J Clin Nutr 54.6 (Suppl) (1991a): 1310–14S.

Block G. Vitamin C and cancer prevention: the epidemiologic evidence. Am J Clin Nutr 53.1 (Suppl) (1991b): 270–82S.

Block G. Ascorbic acid, blood pressure, and the American diet. Ann NY Acad Sci 959 (2002): 180–187.

Block G et al. Ascorbic acid status and subsequent diastolic and systolic blood pressure. Hypertension 37.2 (2001): 261–267.

Bornstein SR et al. Impaired adrenal catecholamine system function in transgenic mice with deficiency of the ascorbic acid transporter (SVCT2). FASEB J 17 (2003): 1928–1930.

Boyce ST et al. Vitamin C regulates keratinocyte viability, epidermal barrier, and basement membrane in vitro, and reduces wound contraction after grafting of cultured skin substitutes. J Invest Dermatol 118.4 (2002): 565–572.

Braunwald E et al (ed). Harrison's principles of internal medicine. New York: McGraw Hill, 2003.

Brubaker RF et al. Ascorbic acid content of human corneal epithelium. Investig Ophthalmol Vis Sci 41 (2000): 1681–1683.

Bucca C et al. Effect of vitamin C on histamine bronchial responsiveness of patients with allergic rhinitis. Ann Allergy 65.4 (1990): 311–314.

Cameron E. Vitamin C and cancer: an overview. Int J Vitam Nutr Res Suppl 23 (1982): 115–127.

Cameron E. Protocol for the use of vitamin C in the treatment of cancer. Med Hypotheses 36.3 (1991): 190–194.

Cameron E, Pauling L. The orthomolecular treatment of cancer. I. The role of ascorbic acid in host resistance. Chem Biol Interact 9.4 (1974): 273–283.

Cameron E, Pauling L. Supplemental ascorbate in the supportive treatment of cancer: Prolongation of survival times in terminal human cancer. Proc Natl Acad Sci USA 73.10 (1976): 3685–3689.

Carr AC, Frei B. Toward a new recommended dietary allowance for vitamin C based on antioxidant and health effects in humans. Am J Clin Nutr 69.6 (1999): 1086–1107.

Ceriello A et al. Antioxidant defences are reduced during the oral glucose tolerance test in normal and non-insulin-dependent diabetic subjects. Eur J Clin Invest 28.4 (1998): 329–333.

Chan D, et al. Efficacy and safety of oral versus intravenous ascorbic acid for anemia in hemodialysis patients. Nephrology (Carlton) 10 (2005): 336–40.

Chapple IL, et al. The prevalence of inflammatory periodontitis is negatively associated with serum antioxidant concentrations. J Nutr 2007;137:657–64.

Chasan-Taber L et al. A prospective study of vitamin supplement intake and cataract extraction among U.S. women. Epidemiology 10.6 (1999): 679–684.

Chaudière J, Ferrari-Iliou R. Intracellular antioxidants: from chemical to biochemical mechanisms. Food Chem Toxicol 37 (1999): 949–962.

Chen Q et al. Pharmacologic ascorbic acid concentrations selectively kill cancer cells: action as a pro-drug to deliver hydrogen peroxide to tissues. Proc Natl Acad Sci USA 102 (2005): 13604–13609.

Chen H et al. High-dose oral vitamin C partially replenishes vitamin C levels in patients with type 2 diabetes and low vitamin C levels but does not improve endothelial dysfunction or insulin resistance. Am J Physiol Heart Circ Physiol 290.1 (2006): H137–H145.

Chen Q, et al. Pharmacologic doses of ascorbate act as a prooxidant and decrease growth of aggressive tumor xenografts in mice. Proc Natl Acad Sci USA 105 (2008): 11105–11109.

Chowdhury AR, Kapil N. Interaction of dexamethasone and DHEA on testicular ascorbic acid and cholesterol in prepubertal rat. Arch Andriol 12.1 (1984): 65–7; as cited in Pelton R et al. Drug-induced nutrient depletion handbook 1999–2000. Hudson, OH: Lexi-Comp, 2000.

Chylack LT Jr. et al. The Roche European American Cataract Trial (REACT): a randomized clinical trial to investigate the efficacy of an oral antioxidant micronutrient mixture to slow progression of age-related cataract. Ophthal Epidemiol 9.1 (2002): 49–80.

Cohen M, Bhagavan HN. Ascorbic acid and gastrointestinal cancer. J Am Coll Nutr 14.6 (1995): 565–578.

Cohen HA et al. Blocking effect of vitamin C in exercise-induced asthma. Arch Pediatr Adolesc Med 151.4 (1997): 367–370.

Combs Jr, G. F. 2012, "Chapter 9 — Vitamin C," In Combs GF (ed.) The Vitamins, Fourth Edition. San Diego: Academic Press, pp. 233–259.

Conde-Agudelo A, et al. Supplementation with vitamins C and E during pregnancy for the prevention of preeclampsia and other adverse maternal and perinatal outcomes: a systematic review and metaanalysis. Am J Obstet Gynecol 2011;204:503.e1–12.

Cook NR, et al. A randomized factorial trial of vitamins C and E and beta carotene in the secondary prevention of cardiovascular events in women: results from the Women's Antioxidant Cardiovascular Study. Arch Intern Med 2007;167:1610–8.

Creagan ET et al. Failure of high-dose vitamin C (ascorbic acid) therapy to benefit patients with advanced cancer: A controlled trial. N Engl J Med 301.13 (1979): 687–690.

Cross CE, Halliwell B. Nutrition and human disease: how much extra vitamin C might smokers need? Lancet 341 (1993): 1091.

Cunningham JJ. The glucose/insulin system and vitamin C: implications in insulin-dependent diabetes mellitus. J Am Coll Nutr 17.2 (1998): 105–108.

Curhan GC et al. A prospective study of the intake of vitamins C and B6, and the risk of kidney stones in men. J Urol 155.6 (1996): 1847–1851.

Curhan GC et al. Intake of vitamins B6 and C and the risk of kidney stones in women. J Am Soc Nephrol 10.4 (1999): 840–845.

Darr D et al. Topical vitamin C protects porcine skin from ultraviolet radiation-induced damage. Br J Dermatol 127.3 (1992): 247–253.

Darr D et al. Effectiveness of antioxidants (vitamin C and E) with and without sunscreens as topical photoprotectants. Acta Derm Venereol 76.4 (1996): 264–268.

da Silva, SL, et al Plasma nutrient status of patients with Alzheimer's disease: Systematic review and meta-analysis, Alzheimer's & Dementia, (2013)1–18.

Dawson EB et al. Effect of ascorbic acid supplementation on the sperm quality of smokers. Fertil Steril 58 (1992): 1034–1039.

Deicher, R.; et al. (2005) Low Total Vitamin C Plasma Level Is a Risk Factor for Cardiovascular Morbidity and Mortality in Hemodialysis Patients. J Am Soc Nephrol, Vol.16,No.6,pp. 1811–1818

Deira J et al. Comparative study of intravenous ascorbic acid versus low-dose desferrioxamine in patients on hemodialysis with hyperferritinemia. J Nephrol 16 (2003): 703–709.

Devereux G, Seaton A. Diet as a risk factor for atopy and asthma. J Allergy Clin Immunol 115 (2005): 1109–1117.

Douglas RM et al. Vitamin C for preventing and treating the common cold. Cochrane Database Syst Rev 2 (2004): CD000980.

Dreyer R, Rose RC. Lacrimal gland uptake and metabolism of ascorbic acid. Proc Soc Exp Biol Med 202 (1993): 212–2116.

Drisko JA et al. The use of antioxidant therapies during chemotherapy. Gynecol Oncol 88.3 (2003): 434–439.

Duffy SJ et al. Treatment of hypertension with ascorbic acid. Lancet 354.9195 (1999): 2048–2049.

Eberlein-Konig B et al. Protective effect against sunburn of combined systemic ascorbic acid (vitamin C) and d-alpha-tocopherol (vitamin E). J Am Acad Dermatol 38.1 (1998): 45–48.

Enstrom JE et al. Vitamin C intake and mortality among a sample of the United States population. Epidemiology 3 (1992): 194–202.

Espinal-Perez LE, et al. A double-blind randomized trial of 5% ascorbic acid vs. 4% hydroquinone in melasma. Int J Dermatol 2004;43:604e7.

Evangelou A et al. Ascorbic acid (vitamin C) effects on withdrawal syndrome of heroin abusers. In Vivo 14.2 (2000): 363–366.

FAO/WHO (Food and Agriculture Organization/World Health Organization). Report of a Joint FAO/WHO Expert Consultation, Bangkok, Thailand. FAO/WHO: Rome, 2002.

Ferrigno L et al. Associations between plasma levels of vitamins and cataract in the Italian–American Clinical Trial of Nutritional Supplements and Age-Related Cataract (CTNS): CTNS Report #2. Ophthal Epidemiol 12 (2005): 71–80.

Fitzpatrick RE, Rostan EF. Double-blind, half-face study comparing topical vitamin C and vehicle for rejuvenation of photodamage. Dermatol Surg 28.3 (2002): 231–236.

Fotherby MD et al. Effect of vitamin C on ambulatory blood pressure and plasma lipids in older persons. J Hypertens 18.4 (2000): 411–411.

Fouque, D.; et al. (2007) EBPG Guideline on Nutrition. Nephrol Dial Transplant, Vol.22, Suppl. 2,pp. ii45–ii87.

Galatioto, G.P., et al., 2008. May antioxidant therapy improve sperm parameters of men with persistent oligospermia after retrograde embolization for varicocele? World J. Urol. 26, 97–102.

Gale CR, et al. Vitamin C and risk of death from stroke and coronary heart disease in cohort of elderly people. Br Med J 1995;310:1563–6.

Galley HF et al. Combination oral antioxidant supplementation reduces blood pressure. Clin Sci (Lond) 92.4 (1997): 361–365.

Gastaldello K et al. Resistance to erythropoietin in iron-overloaded haemodialysis patients can be overcome by ascorbic acid administration. Nephrol Dial Transplant 10 (Suppl) (1995): 44–47

Gatenby R, Gillies R. Why do cancers have high aerobic glycolysis? Nat Rev Cancer 4 (2004): 891–899.

Gey KF et al. Poor plasma status of carotene and vitamin C is associated with higher mortality from ischemic heart disease and stroke: Basel Prospective Study. Clin Invest 71.1 (1993): 3–6.

Ghosh SK et al. A double-blind, placebo-controlled parallel trial of vitamin C treatment in elderly patients with hypertension. Gerontology 40.5 (1994): 268–272.

Giancaspro V et al. Intravenous ascorbic acid in hemodialysis patients with functional iron deficiency (a clinical trial). J Nephrol 13 (2000): 444–449.

Gill HS, Rose GA. Idiopathic hypercalciuria. Urate and other ions in urine before and on various long term treatments. Urol Res 13.6 (1985): 271–275.

Giri A et al. Vitamin C mediated protection on cisplatin induced mutagenicity in mice. Mutat Res 421 (1998): 139–148.

Gottlieb N. Cancer treatment and vitamin C: the debate lingers. J Natl Cancer Inst 91 (1999): 2073–2075.

Greco E et al. Efficient treatment of infertility due to sperm DNA damage by ICSI with testicular spermatozoa. Hum Reprod 20 (2005a): 226–30.

Greco E et al. Reduction of the incidence of sperm DNA fragmentation by oral antioxidant treatment. J Androl 26 (2005b): 349–53.

Greggi Antunes LM et al. Protective effects of vitamin C against cisplatin-induced nephrotoxicity and lipid peroxidation in adult rats: a dose-dependent study. Pharmacol Res 41 (2000): 405–411.

Griffith HM et al. A case-control study of dietary intake of renal stone patients. I. Preliminary analysis. Urol Res 14.2 (1986): 67–74.

Gupta MM, Chari S. Lipid peroxidation and antioxidant status in patients with diabetic retinopathy. Indian J Physiol Pharmacol 2005;49:187–92.

Gurler B, et al. The role of oxidative stress in diabetic retinopathy. Eye 2000;14:730–5.

Hall SL, Greendale GA. The relation of dietary vitamin C intake to bone mineral density: results from the PEPI study. Calcif Tissue Int 63.3 (1998): 183–189.

Hammond BR Jr., Johnson MA. The Age-Related Eye Disease Study (AREDS). Nutr Rev 60 (2002): 283–288.

Hanashima C, Namiki H. Reduced viability of vascular endothelial cells by high concentration of ascorbic acid in vitreous humor. Cell Biol Int 23 (1999): 287–298.

Harris HR, et al . Vitamin C and survival among women with breast cancer: a meta-analysis. Eur J Cancer. 2014 May;50(7):1223–31

Harrison FE, May JM. Vitamin C function in the brain: vital role of the ascorbate transporter SVCT2. Free Rad Bio Med 46.6 (2009): 719–730.

Heart Protection Study Collaborative Group, MRC/BHF Heart Protection Study of antioxidant vitamin supplementation in 20536 high-risk individuals: a randomized placebo-controlled trials. Lancet 2002;360:23

Hemilä, H. Vitamin C supplementation and common cold symptoms: factors affecting the magnitude of the benefit. Medical hypotheses 52[2], 171–178. 1-2-1999.

Hemilä H, Chalker E. Vitamin C for preventing and treating the common cold. Cochrane Database of Systematic Reviews 2013, Issue 1. Art. No.: CD000980.

Hemilä H, Louhiala P. Vitamin C for preventing and treating pneumonia. Cochrane Database of Systematic Reviews 2013, Issue 8. Art. No.: CD005532.

Hendler SS, Rorvik D (eds). PDR for nutritional supplements. Montvale, NJ: Medical Economics, 2001.

Hoffer L et al. Phase I clinical trial of i.v. ascorbic acid in advanced malignancy. Ann Oncol 19.12 (2008): 2095.

Hörl WH. Is there a role for adjuvant therapy in patients being treated with epoetin? Nephrol Dial Transplant 14 (Suppl) (1999): 50–60.

Houston MC. Nutraceuticals, vitamins, antioxidants, and minerals in the prevention and treatment of hypertension. Prog Cardiovasc Dis 47 (2005): 396–449.

Humbert PG et al. Topical ascorbic acid on photoaged skin: Clinical, topographical and ultrastructural evaluation: double-blind study vs placebo. Exp Dermatol 12.3 (2003): 237–244.

Hwang SW, et al. Clinical efficacy of 25% L-ascorbic acid (C'ensil) in the treatment of melasma. J Cutan Med Surg 2009;13(2):74e 81.

Ilich JZ et al. Bone and nutrition in elderly women: protein, energy, and calcium as main determinants of bone mineral density. Eur J Clin Nutr 57.4 (2003): 554–565.

Jacques PF, Chylack LT Jr. Epidemiologic evidence of a role for the antioxidant vitamins and carotenoids in cataract prevention. Am J Clin Nutr 53 (1991): 352–355S.

Jacques PF et al. Nutritional status in persons with and without senile cataract: blood vitamin and mineral levels. Am J Clin Nutr 48 (1988): 152–158.

Jacques PF et al. Long-term vitamin C supplement use and prevalence of early age-related lens opacities. Am J Clin Nutr 66 (1997): 911–9116.

Jacques PF et al. Long-term nutrient intake and early age-related nuclear lens opacities. Arch Ophthalmol 119.7 (2001): 1009–1019.

Jaruga P et al. Supplementation with antioxidant vitamins prevents oxidative modification of DNA in lymphocytes of HIV-infected patients. Free Radic Biol Med 32.5 (2002): 414–420.

Jaxa-Chamiec T et al. Antioxidant effects of combined vitamins C and E in acute myocardial infarction: The randomized, double-blind, placebo controlled, multicenter pilot Myocardial Infarction and VITamins (MIVIT) trial. Kardiol Pol 62 (2005): 344–350.

Jenab M et al. Plasma and dietary vitamin C levels and risk of gastric cancer in the European Prospective Investation into Cancer and Nutrition (EPIC-EURGAST). Carcinogenesis 27.11 (2006): 2250–2257.

Jeurissen A et al. [The effects of physical exercise on the immune system]. Ned Tijdschr Geneeskd 147.28 (2003): 1347–1351.

Johnston CS et al. Antihistamine effect of supplemental ascorbic acid and neutrophil chemotaxis. J Am Coll Nutr 11.2 (1992): 172–176.

Johnston CS et al. Vitamin C depletion is associated with alterations in blood histamine and plasma free carnitine in adults. J Am Coll Nutr 15.6 (1996): 586–591.

Kaliora AC et al. Dietary antioxidants in preventing atherogenesis. Atherosclerosis 187 (2006): 1–17.

Kaufmann PA et al. Coronary heart disease in smokers: vitamin C restores coronary microcirculatory function. Circulation 102.11 (2000): 1233–1238.

Kaur B et al. Vitamin C supplementation for asthma. Cochrane Database Syst Rev 4 (2001): CD000993.

Keller KL, Fenske NA. Uses of vitamins A, C, and E and related compounds in dermatology: A review. J Am Acad Dermatol 39 (1998): 611–625.

Kelly FJ. Vitamins and respiratory disease: antioxidant micronutrients in pulmonary health and disease. Proc Nutr Soc 64 (2005): 510–526.

Kelly FJ et al. Altered lung antioxidant status in patients with mild asthma. Lancet 354.9177 (1999): 482–483.

Keven K et al. Randomized, crossover study of the effect of vitamin C on EPO response in hemodialysis patients. Am J Kidney Dis 41 (2003): 1233–1239.

Khaw KT et al. Relation between plasma ascorbic acid and mortality in men and women in EPIC-Norfolk prospective study: a prospective population study. European Prospective Investigation into Cancer and Nutrition. Lancet 357.9257 (2001): 657–663.

Knekt P et al. Antioxidant vitamins and coronary heart disease risk: A pooled analysis of 9 cohorts. Am J Clin Nutr 80 (2004): 1508–1520.

Kumar P et al. Clinical medicine, 5th edn. London: WB Saunders, 2002.

Kurbacher CM et al. Ascorbic acid (vitamin C) improves the antineoplastic activity of doxorubicin, cisplatin, and paclitaxel in human breast carcinoma cells in vitro. Cancer Lett 103 (1996): 183–189.

Kushi LH et al. Dietary antioxidant vitamins and death from coronary heart disease in postmenopausal women. N Engl J Med 334 (1996): 1156–1162.

Kuzniarz M et al. Use of vitamin supplements and cataract: the Blue Mountains eye study. Am J Ophthalmol 132 (2001): 19–26.

Lamson DW, Brignall MS. Antioxidants and cancer therapy II: quick reference guide. Altern Med Rev 5 (2000): 152–163.

Lee, CTC, et al Micronutrients and Diabetic Retinopathy – A Systematic Review, Ophthalmology 2010;117:71–78

Lekakis JP et al. Short-term oral ascorbic acid improves endothelium-dependent vasodilatation in women with a history of gestational diabetes mellitus. Diabetes Care 23.9 (2000): 1432–1434.

Leveille SG, et al. Dietary vitamin C and bone mineral density in postemenopausal women in Washington State, USA. J Epidemiol Commun Health 1997;51:479–85.

Levine MA, Pollard HB. Hydrocortisone inhibition of ascorbic acid transport by Chromaffin cells. FEBS Lett 158.1 (1983): 13408; as cited in Pelton R et al. Drug-induced nutrient depletion handbook 1999–2000. Hudson, OH: Lexi-Comp, 2000.

Lewis SE et al. Comparison of individual antioxidants of sperm and seminal plasma in fertile and infertile men. Fertil Steril 67 (1997): 142–147.

Li Y, Schellhorn HE. New Developments and Novel Therapeutic Perspectives for Vitamin C. J Nutr 137.10 (2007): 2171–2184.

Lin CL et al. Low dose intravenous ascorbic acid for erythropoietin-hyporesponsive anemia in diabetic hemodialysis patients with iron overload. Ren Fail 25 (2003): 445–453.

Lin JY et al. UV photoprotection by combination topical antioxidants vitamin C and vitamin E. J Am Acad Dermatol 48.6 (2003): 866–874.

Lin J, et al. Vitamins C and E and beta carotene supplementation and cancer risk: a randomized controlled trial. J Natl Cancer Inst 2009;101:14–23.

Ling L et al. Vitamin C preserves endothelial function in patients with coronary heart disease after a high-fat meal. Clin Cardiol 25.5 (2002): 219–224.

Lopes C et al. [Diet and risk of myocardial infarction: A case-control community-based study]. Acta Med Port 11.4 (1998): 311–3117.

Lopes de Jesus CC, et al. Vitamin C and superoxide dismutase (SOD) for diabetic retinopathy. Cochrane Database of Systematic Reviews 2008, Issue 1. Art. No.: CD006695.

Loria CM et al. Vitamin C status and mortality in US adults. Am J Clin Nutr 72 (2000): 139–145.

Macdougall IC. Metabolic adjuvants to erythropoietin therapy. Miner Electrolyte Metab 25 (1999): 357–364.

Maggini, S., et al. 2012. A combination of high-dose vitamin C plus zinc for the common cold. J Int.Med Res., 40, (1) 28–42.

Mares-Perlman JA et al. Vitamin supplement use and incident cataracts in a population-based study. Arch Ophthalmol 118.11 (2000): 1556–1563.

May JM. Is ascorbic acid an antioxidant for the plasma membrane? FASEB J 13 (1999): 995–1006.

McCann SE et al. Intakes of selected nutrients, foods, and phytochemicals and prostate cancer risk in western New York. Nutr Cancer 53 (2005): 33–41.

McDermoth JH. Antioxidant nutrients: current dietary recommendations and research update. J Am Pharm Assoc 40 (2000): 785–799.

Michels KB et al. Dietary antioxidant vitamins, retinol, and breast cancer incidence in a cohort of Swedish women. Int J Cancer 91.4 (2001): 563–567.

Milan SJ, et al. Vitamin C for asthma and exercise-induced bronchoconstriction. Cochrane Database of Systematic Reviews 2013, Issue 10. Art. No.: CD010391.

Miric M, Haxhiu MA. Effect of vitamin C on exercise-induced bronchoconstriction. Plucne Bolesti 43.1–2 (1991): 94–97.

Moertel CG et al. High-dose vitamin C versus placebo in the treatment of patients with advanced cancer who have had no prior chemotherapy: A randomized double-blind comparison. N Engl J Med 312.3 (1985): 137–141.

Moorman PG, et al. Vitamin supplement use and breast cancer in a North Carolina population. Publ Health Nutr 2001;4(3):821–7.

Morel O et al. Protective effects of vitamin C on endothelium damage and platelet activation during myocardial infarction in patients with sustained generation of circulating microparticles. J Thromb Haemost 1 (2003): 171–177.

Morris JC et al. Interaction of ethinyl estradiol with ascorbic acid in man. BMJ 283 (1981): 503. Cited online: www.micromedex.com.

Morton DJ et al. Vitamin C supplement use and bone mineral density in postmenopausal women. J Bone Miner Res 16.1 (2001): 135–140.

MRC/BHF. Heart protection study of antioxidant vitamin supplementation in 20,536 high-risk individuals: a randomised placebo-controlled trial. Lancet 360.9326 (2002): 23–33.

Mullan BA et al. Ascorbic acid reduces blood pressure and arterial stiffness in type 2 diabetes. Hypertension 40.6 (2002): 804–809.

Muggli, R. 1998, “Vitamin C and the Immune System,” In: Delves PJ (ed.) Encyclopedia of Immunology, Second Edition. Oxford: Elsevier, pp. 2491–2494.

Muller F et al. Virological and immunological effects of antioxidant treatment in patients with HIV infection. Eur J Clin Invest 30.10 (2000): 905–914.

Mydlik M et al. Oral use of iron with vitamin C in hemodialyzed patients. J Ren Nutr 13 (2003): 47–51.

Nagy B et al. Chemosensitizing effect of vitamin C in combination with 5-fluorouracil in vitro. In Vivo 17 (2003): 289–292.

Negri E et al. Selected micronutrients and oral and pharyngeal cancer. Int J Cancer 86.1 (2000): 122–127.

Ness AR et al. Vitamin C and cardiovascular disease: a systematic review. J Cardiovasc Risk 3.6 (1996): 513–521.

Ness AR et al. Vitamin C and blood pressure: an overview. J Hum Hypertens 11.6 (1997): 343–350.

Nguyen TV. Oral ascorbic acid as adjuvant to epoetin alfa in hemodialysis patients with hyperferritinemia. Am J Health-Syst Ph 61 (2004): 2007–2008.

NHMRC (National Health & Medical Research Council). Nutrient reference values for Australia and New Zealand. Canberra: NHMRC, 2006.

Nieman DC et al. Influence of vitamin C supplementation on cytokine changes following an ultramarathon. J Interferon Cytokine Res 20.11 (2000): 1029–1035.

Nishida M, et al. Dietary vitamin C and the risk for periodontal disease. J Periodontol 2000;71:1215–23.

Northrop-Clewes CA, Thurnham DI. Monitoring micronutrients in cigarette smokers. Clin Chim Acta 377 (2007): 14–38.

Nurmatov, U, et al. Nutrients and foods for the primary prevention of asthma and allergy: Systematic review and meta-analysis, J Allergy Clin Immunol 2011;127:724–33.

Nyyssonen K et al. Vitamin C deficiency and risk of myocardial infarction: prospective population study of men from eastern Finland. BMJ 314.7081 (1997): 634–638.

Ochiai Y, et al. A new lipophilic pro-vitamin C, tetra-isopalmitoyl ascorbic acid (VC-IP), prevents UV-induced skin pigmentation through its anti-oxidative properties. J Dermatol Sci 2006;44:37e44.

Omu, A.E., et al., 2008. Indication of the mechanisms involved in improved sperm parameters by zinc therapy. Med. Princ. Pract. 17, 108–116.

Osganian SK et al. Vitamin C and risk of coronary heart disease in women. J Am Coll Cardiol 42.2 (2003): 246–252.

Padayatty SJ, Levine M. Reevaluation of ascorbate in cancer treatment: emerging evidence, open minds and serendipity. J Am Coll Nutr 19.4 (2000): 423–425.

Padayatty SJ et al. Vitamin C pharmacokinetics: implications for oral and intravenous use. Ann Intern Med 140 (2004): 533–537.

Padayatty SJ et al. Intravenously administered vitamin C as cancer therapy: three cases. CMAJ 174 (2006): 937–942.

Pandey DK et al. Dietary vitamin C and beta-carotene and risk of death in middle-aged men: The Western Electric Study. Am J Epidemiol 142 (1995): 1269–1278.

Paolisso G et al. Plasma vitamin C affects glucose homeostasis in healthy subjects and in non-insulin-dependent diabetics. Am J Physiol 266.2 Pt 1 (1994): E261–E268.

Park HJ, et al. Vitamin C attenuates ERK signaling to inhibit the regulation of collagen production by LL-37 in human dermal fibroblasts. Exp Dermatol 2009;19:e258e64

Pasco JA et al. Antioxidant vitamin supplements and markers of bone turnover in a community sample of nonsmoking women. J Womens Health 15 (2006): 295–300.

Patel SR, Sigman M. Antioxidant therapy in male infertility. Urol Clin N Am 35 (2008): 319–330.

Patterson CA, O’Rourke MC. Vitamin C levels in human tears. Arch Opthalmol 105 (1987): 376–377.

Peponis V et al. Protective role of oral antioxidant supplementation in ocular surface of diabetic patients. Br J Ophthalmol 86.12 (2002): 1369–1373.

Perez RS, et al. Evidence based guidelines for complex regional pain syndrome type 1. BMC Neurol 10:20, 2010.

Peters EM et al. Vitamin C supplementation attenuates the increases in circulating cortisol, adrenaline and anti-inflammatory polypeptides following ultramarathon running. Int J Sports Med 22.7 (2001a): 537–43.

Peters EM et al. Attenuation of increase in circulating cortisol and enhancement of the acute phase protein response in vitamin C-supplemented ultramarathoners. Int J Sports Med 22.2 (2001b): 120–126.

Pfister, R., et al. 2011. Plasma vitamin C predicts incident heart failure in men and women in European Prospective Investigation into Cancer and Nutrition-Norfolk prospective study. Am Heart J, 162, (2) 246–253.

Pimentel L. Scurvy: Historical review and current diagnostic approach. Am J Emerg Med 21.4 (2003): 328–332.

Poulter JM, et al. Ascorbic acid supplementation and five year survival rates in women with early breast cancer. Acta Vitaminol Enzymol 1984;6:175–82.

Power C et al. Diet and renal stones: a case-control study. Br J Urol 56.5 (1984): 456–459.

Prasad KN et al. Pros and cons of antioxidant use during radiation therapy. Cancer Treat Rev 28 (2002): 79–91.

Price KD et al. Hyperglycemia-induced ascorbic acid deficiency promotes endothelial dysfunction and the development of atherosclerosis. Atherosclerosis 158.1 (2001): 1–12.

Pussinen PJ, et al. Periodontitis is associated with a low concentration of vitamin C in plasma. Clin Diagn Lab Immunol 2003;10:897–902.

Putchala, MC, et al. Ascorbic acid and its pro-oxidant activity as a therapy for tumours of oral cavity – A systematic review, Arch Oral Bio 58(2013)563–574

Rahman I. Oxidant and antioxidant balance in the airways and airway diseases. Eur J Pharmacol 533 (2006): 222–239.

Ram FS et al. Vitamin C supplementation for asthma. Cochrane Database Syst Rev 3 (2004): CD000993.

Reddy VG et al. Vitamin C augments chemotherapeutic response of cervical carcinoma HeLa cells by stabilizing P53. Biochem Biophys Res Commun 282 (2001): 409–415.

Rema M, et al. Does oxidant stress play a role in diabetic retinopathy? Indian J Ophthalmol 1995;43:17–21.

Richardson TI et al. Will an orange a day keep the doctor away? Postgrad Med J 78.919 (2002): 292–294.

Riemersma RA et al. Vitamin C and the risk of acute myocardial infarction. Am J Clin Nutr 71.5 (2000): 1181–1186.

Ringsdorf J, Cheraskin E. Vitamin C and human wound healing. Oral Surg Oral Med Oral Pathol 53 (1982): 231–236.

Riordan HD et al. A pilot clinical study of continuous intravenous ascorbate in terminal cancer patients. Puerto Rica Health Sci J 24 (2005). 269–276.

Rossi, AC, Mullin, PM, Prevention of pre-eclampsia with low-dose aspirin or vitamins C and E in women at high or low risk: a systematic review with meta-analysis, European Journal of Obstetrics & Gynecology and Reproductive Biology 158 (2011) 9–16.

Rumbold A, Crowther CA. Vitamin C supplementation in pregnancy. Cochrane Database of Systematic Reviews 2005, Issue 1. Art. No.: CD004072.

Russell L. The importance of patients’ nutritional status in wound healing. Br J Nurs 10.6 (Suppl) (2001): S42–4, S49.

Sacks W, Simpson GM. Ascorbic acid in levodopa therapy (Letter). Lancet 1.7905 (1975): 527. Cited online at: www.micromedex.com.

Sahyoun NR et al. Carotenoids, vitamins C and E, and mortality in an elderly population. Am J Epidemiol 144 (1996): 501–511.

Sandhya P, Das UN. Vitamin C therapy for maturity onset diabetes mellitus: relevance to prostaglandin involvement. IRCS I Med Sci 9 (1981): 618.

Sarna S, Bhola RK. Chemo-immunotherapeutical studies on Dalton's lymphoma in mice using cisplatin and ascorbic acid: synergistic antitumor effect in vivo and in vitro. Arch Immunol Ther Exp (Warsz) 41 (1993): 327–333.

Schachter EN, Schlesinger A. The attenuation of exercise-induced bronchospasm by ascorbic acid. Ann Allergy 49.3 (1982): 146–151.

Schindler TH et al. [Effect of vitamin C on platelet aggregation in smokers and nonsmokers]. Med Klin 97.5 (2002): 263–269.

Schwenk TL, Costley CD. When food becomes a drug: nonanabolic nutritional supplement use in athletes. Am J Sports Med 30.6 (2002): 907–916.

Scott, R., et al., 1998. The effect of oral selenium supplementation on human sperm motility. Br. J. Urol. 82, 76–80.

Seddon JM et al. The use of vitamin supplements and the risk of cataract among US male physicians. Am J Public Health 84 (1994): 788–792.

Sezer S et al. Intravenous ascorbic acid administration for erythropoietin hyporesponsive anemia in iron loaded hemodialysis patients. Artif Organs 26 (2002): 366–370.

Shanmugasundaram KR. Excessive free radical generation in the blood of children suffering from asthma. Clin Chim Acta 305 (2001): 107–114.

Shibuya, N, et al. Efficacy and Safety of High-dose Vitamin C on Complex Regional Pain Syndrome in Extremity Trauma and Surgery-Systematic Review and Meta-Analysis, J Foot Ankl Surg, 52(2013)62–66.

Shoham A et al. Oxidative stress in diseases of the human cornea. Free Radical Biology and Medicine 45.8 (2008): 1047–1055.

Silvestro A et al. Vitamin C prevents endothelial dysfunction induced by acute exercise in patients with intermittent claudication. Atherosclerosis 165.2 (2002): 277–283.

Simon, J.A. & Hudes, E.S. 1999. Serum ascorbic acid and cardiovascular disease prevalence in U.S. adults: the Third National Health and Nutrition Examination Survey (NHANES III). Ann.Epidemiol., 9, (6) 358–365

Simon JA, Hudes ES. Relation of ascorbic acid to bone mineral density and self-reported fractures among US adults. Am J Epidemiol 154.5 (2001): 427–433.

Simon, J.A., et al. 2001. Relation of serum ascorbic acid to mortality among US adults. J Am Coll. Nutr., 20, (3) 255–263.

Sinclair AJ, et al. An investigation of the relationship between free radical activity and vitamin C metabolism in elderly diabetic subjects with retinopathy. Gerontology 1992;38:268 –74.

Singh N et al. Effects of a 'healthy' diet and of acute and long-term vitamin C on vascular function in healthy older subjects. Cardiovasc Res 56.1 (2002): 118–125.

Solzbach U et al. Vitamin C improves endothelial dysfunction of epicardial coronary arteries in hypertensive patients. Circulation 96.5 (1997): 1513–15119.

Stoyanovsky DA et al. Endogenous ascorbate regenerates vitamin E in the retina directly and in combination with exogenous dihydrolipoic acid. Curr Eye Res 14.3 (1995): 181–189.

Taji Y et al. Effects of intravenous ascorbic acid on erythropoiesis and quality of life in unselected hemodialysis patients. J Nephrol 17 (2004): 537–543.

Tamayo C, Richardson MA. Vitamin C as a cancer treatment: state of the science and recommendations for research. Altern Ther Health Med 9 (2003): 94–101.

Taniguchi M, et al. Anti-oxidative and antiaging activities of 2-O-a-glucopyranosil-L-ascorbic acid on human dermal fibroblasts. Eur J Pharmacol 2012;674:126e31.

Tarng DC, Huang TP. A parallel, comparative study of intravenous iron *versus* intravenous ascorbic acid for erythropoietin hyporesponsive anaemia in haemodialysis patients with iron overload. Nephrol Dial Transplant 13 (1998): 2867–2872.

Tarng DC, et al. Erythropoietin hyporesponsiveness: from iron deficiency to iron overload. Kidney Int 55 (Suppl) (1999a): S107–18.

Tarng DC et al. Intravenous ascorbic acid as an adjuvant therapy for recombinant erythropoietin in hemodialysis patients with hyperferritinemia. Kidney Int 55 (1999b): 2477–86.

Tarng DC, et al. Effect of intravenous ascorbic acid medication on serum levels of soluble transferrin receptor in hemodialysis patients. J Am Soc Nephrol 15 (2004): 2486–2493.

Taylor EN, Curhan GC. Oxalate intake and the risk for nephrolithiasis. J Am Soc Nephrol 18.7 (2007): 2198–2204.

Taylor TV et al. Ascorbic acid supplementation in the treatment of pressure-sores. Lancet 304 (1974): 544–546.

Taylor A et al. Long-term intake of vitamins and carotenoids and odds of early age-related cortical and posterior subcapsular lens opacities. Am J Clin Nutr 75.3 (2002): 540–549.

Thompson D et al. Prolonged vitamin C supplementation and recovery from demanding exercise. Int J Sport Nutr Exerc Metab 11.4 (2001): 466–481.

Toohey, L., et al. 1996. Plasma ascorbic acid concentrations are related to cardiovascular risk factors in African-Americans. J Nutr., 126, (1) 121–128.

Tovbin D et al. Effectiveness of erythropoiesis on supervised intradialytic oral iron and vitamin C therapy is correlated with Kt/V and patient weight. Clin Nephrol 53 (2000): 276–282.

Traikovich SS. Use of topical ascorbic acid and its effects on photodamaged skin topography. Arch Otolaryngol Head Neck Surg 1999;125:1091e8.

Tremellen, K., et al., 2007. A randomized control trial of an antioxidant (Menevit) on pregnancy outcome during IVF-ICSI treatment. Aust. NZ J. Obstet. Gynaecol. 47, 216–221.

Valero MP et al. Vitamin C is associated with reduced risk of cataract in a Mediterranean population. J Nutr 132.6 (2002): 1299–1306.

Vatassery GT. In vitro oxidation of alpha-tocopherol (vitamin E) in human platelets upon incubation with unsaturated fatty acids, diamide and superoxide. Biochim Biophys Acta 926.2 (1987): 160–169.

Verrax J, Buc Calderon B. The controversial place of vitamin C in cancer treatment, Biocehem Pharmacol 76 (2008): 1644–1652.

Villacorta L, et al. Regulatory role of vitamins E and C on the extracellular matrix components of the vascular system. Mol Asp Med 28 (2007): 507–537.

Vural H. Serum and red blood cell antioxidant status in patients with bronchial asthma. Can Respir J 7 (2000): 476–480.

Wahlqvist M (ed). Food and nutrition, 2nd edn. Sydney: Allen & Unwin, 2002.

Wandzilak TR et al. Effect of high dose vitamin C on urinary oxalate levels. J Urol 151.4 (1994): 834–837.

Watanabe H et al. Randomized, double-blind, placebo-controlled study of the preventive effect of supplemental oral vitamin C on attenuation of development of nitrate tolerance. J Am Coll Cardiol 31.6 (1998a): 1323–1329.

Watanabe H et al. Randomized, double-blind, placebo-controlled study of ascorbate on the preventive effect of nitrate tolerance in patients with congestive heart failure. Circulation 97.9 (1998b): 886–891.

Waters DD, et al. Effects of hormone replacement therapy and antioxidant vitamin supplements on coronary atherosclerosis in postmenopausal women: a randomized controlled trial. J Am Med Assoc 2002;288:2432–40.

Wilkinson IB et al. Oral vitamin C reduces arterial stiffness and platelet aggregation in humans. J Cardiovasc Pharmacol 34.5 (1999): 690–693.

Williams MJ et al. Vitamin C improves endothelial dysfunction in renal allograft recipients. Nephrol Dial Transplant 16.6 (2001): 1251–1255.

Wilson CW et al. The metabolism of supplementary vitamin C during the common cold. J Clin Pharmacol 16.1 (1976): 19–29.

Wintergerst ES et al. Immune-enhancing role of vitamin C and zinc and effect on clinical conditions. Ann Nutr Metab 50 (2006): 85–94.

Wolf RL et al. Lack of a relation between vitamin and mineral antioxidants and bone mineral density: results from the Women's Health Initiative. Am J Clin Nutr 82 (2005): 581–588.

Yilmaz C et al. The contribution of vitamin C to healing of experimental fractures. Arch Orthop Trauma Surg 121.7 (2001): 426–428.

You WC et al. Gastric dysplasia and gastric cancer: *Helicobacter pylori*, serum vitamin C, and other risk factors. J Natl Cancer Inst 92.19 (2000): 1607–1612.

Zamah NM et al. Absence of an effect of high vitamin C dosage on the systemic availability of ethinyl estradiol in women using a combination oral contraceptive. Contraception 48.4 (1993): 377–391.

Zhang S et al. Dietary carotenoids and vitamins A, C, and E and risk of breast cancer. J Natl Cancer Inst 91.6 (1999): 547–556.

Zhang W et al. Synergistic cytotoxic action of vitamin C and vitamin K3. Anticancer Res 21 (2001): 3439–3444.

Zou W et al. Vitamin C inactivates the proteasome inhibitor PS-341 in human cancer cells. Clin Cancer Res 12 (2006): 273–280.

Vitamin D

HISTORICAL NOTE Vitamin D was identified as a nutrient in the early 1900s, when it was first realised that cod liver oil had an antirachitic effect in infants.

Is vitamin D really a vitamin?

Many characteristics of the vitamin D molecules vary substantially from the orthodox definition of a vitamin (Dusso et al 2005, NHMRC 2006, Vieth 2006) in that they:

- are not essential in the diet of all individuals, given adequate sun exposure (Dusso et al 2005, Holick 2008, Nowson & Margerison 2001, Nowson et al 2012)
- are structurally steroid derivatives (Gropper et al 2009, Valdivielso et al 2009)
- are inherently biologically inactive and require hydroxylation to produce the active form (Holick 2005, Kemmis et al 2006, Prietl et al 2013)
- produce $1,25(OH)_2D$, which is a steroidal hormone (Dusso et al 2005)
- require vitamin D receptors (VDR) on cell surfaces, a member of the steroid receptor superfamily, to convey most, if not all, of their actions (Dusso et al 2005, Holick 2004, Hossein-nezhad & Holick 2013).

These discoveries and others have precipitated a revolution in vitamin D research over the last two decades (Dusso et al 2005, Holick 2004, 2005, Nowson et al 2012).

BACKGROUND AND RELEVANT PHARMACOKINETICS

The name 'vitamin D' actually refers to several related fat-soluble vitamin variants, all of which are sterol (cholesterol-like) substances. It is a pleiotropic steroid hormone, with its role being in the regulation of calcium and phosphorus levels (Zittermann et al 2014), involvement in vascular biology (Valdivielso et al 2009), bone mineralisation (Nowson et al 2012) and immunomodulation (Clancy et al 2013, Prietl et al 2013). Research over the last two decades has suggested that vitamin D has a role in autoimmune disease, cardiovascular disease, certain cancers, cognitive decline, depression, pregnancy complications, allergy, frailty and potential fetal epigenetics and brain development (Abrams et al 2013, Eyles et al 2013, Hossein-nezhad & Holick 2013, Liu et al 2013).

Cholecalciferol (D_3) is the form found in animal products and fish oils, whereas ergocalciferol (D_2) is the major synthetic form of provitamin D typically found in supplements and fortified foods; however, other forms also exist. These ingested forms have 50–80% bioavailability and enter the lymphatic circulation from the small intestine following emulsification by bile salts, and promote the absorption of calcium and phosphate from the gut (Nowson et al 2012).

Vitamin D (D_3) is also produced in the body through the conversion of a cholesterol-based precursor, 7-dehydrocholesterol, which is produced in the sebaceous glands of the skin. Exposure to sunlight (ultraviolet B [UVB]) converts this precursor into cholecalciferol over a 2–3-day period. Prolonged exposure to UVB can inactivate some of the newly formed vitamin D and its precursors, so that eventually a state of equilibrium is reached between vitamin D synthesis and catabolism. Therefore, short periods of sun exposure are considered more efficacious than long periods (Working Group 2005, 2012). Some vitamin D is stored in adipose tissue and can be mobilised during periods when exposure to sunlight is reduced or shortages develop (Nowson & Margerison 2002, Nowson et al 2012). This has implications for obesity research. Vitamin D and its metabolites are primarily excreted through bile, and the degraded active form is removed via the kidney. Losses are believed to be minor, owing to both reabsorption of vitamin D derivatives via the enterohepatic recirculation and limited filtration at the kidneys (Kohlmeier 2003). Parathyroid hormone (PTH), calcium, phosphorus and magnesium are involved in the regulation of vitamin D metabolism.

Traditionally associated with bone health, the identification of VDRs on a large and diverse number of cells has precipitated significant reconsideration of this nutrient (Dusso et al 2005, Holick 2004, 2006). VDRs are present in most tissues and cells in the body, including the brain, vascular smooth muscle, prostate, breast and macrophages (Hossein-nezhad & Holick 2013, Nowson et al 2012), and we now understand that vitamin D possesses two distinct action pathways dependent upon the site of bioactivation (Dusso et al 2005, Holick 2006). Renal hydroxylation of 25(OH)D produces $1,25(OH)_2D$, primarily responsible for its traditional endocrine actions. In this two-step process, high-capacity cytochromes in the liver convert initially to D's major circulating form, 25-hydroxycholecalciferol (inactive) — 25(OH)D, and then further hydroxylation in the proximal tubular epithelial cells of the kidneys, to the biological active form: 1,25-dihydroxycholecalciferol — $1,25(OH)_2D$, also known as calcitriol. This conversion is performed by CYP27B1 (25OH-1α-hydroxylase) (Clancy et al 2013, Nowson et al 2012). By contribution to regulation of extracellular calcium and phosphate homeostasis and through interaction with PTH,

V

mineralisation of the skeleton is promoted, and regulation of muscle function (Angeline et al 2013). Importantly, as stated (Hossein-nezhad & Holick 2013, Nowson et al 2012), almost every nucleated cell expresses the VDR, and additionally, many extrarenal tissues have the capacity to make 1,25$(OH)_2$D. This is suggestive that vitamin D not only operates by the classical endocrine pathways, but through autocrine and paracrine pathways as well, implying that there are local synthesis and actions. This extrarenal bioactivation, by immune, prostate, breast, colon, beta and skin cells, however, results in non-genomic responses, characterised as autocrine rather than endocrine effects (Dusso et al 2005, Holick 2006, Kemmis et al 2006, Valdivielso et al 2009). Production of 1,25$(OH)_2$D at these sites does not fall under the same tight regulatory control as renal 1-alpha-hydroxylase (Dusso et al 2005, Kemmis et al 2006). This means that increasing concentrations of 25(OH)D provide a substrate for extrarenal bioactivation, with the rate of conversion mainly reliant upon local factors such as cytokines, which act to protect the internal cells from microbial invaders (Clancy et al 2013, Holick 2005, Lips 2006). Monocyte-macrophages contain CYP27B1, which enables intracellular production of active vitamin D, promoting an intracrine effect, which, by contrast to renal conversion, is not regulated by Ca^{2+} levels (Clancy et al 2013). It is instead driven by immune components such as chemokines like interferon-gamma (IFN-gamma) and Toll-like receptors (TLRs), which gives vitamin D the ability to act independently on the immune system. Its destruction by catabolic enzyme 24-hydroxylase (CYP24A1) is also initiated by its activation to the active form, but not in macrophages, which results in a prolonged signalling of vitamin D, which may provide insight into the potential mechanism of action in fighting intracellular organisms such as tuberculosis (Clancy et al 2013).

CHEMICAL COMPONENTS

Cholecalciferol (D_3) is considered to be the most important dietary form and is identical to the form produced in the body. Ergocalciferol (D_2) is produced by fungi and yeasts and is rare in the diet, but a common supplemental/fortificant form (Nowson & Margerison 2002, Nowson et al 2012). Some authors suggest that D_2 should not be classified as a nutrient, given that it has no natural place in human biology (Trang et al 1998, Vieth 2006) and, while both D_2 and D_3 were previously considered to be equipotent as supplements (FAO/WHO 2002, Nowson & Margerison 2002, Prietl et al 2013, Wahlqvist 2002), recent exploration of this issue points to marked discrepancies in favour of D_3. D_2 also comes under the names 1-alpha-OHD_2, calcifediol, calciferol, dihydrotachysterol, ergocalciferolum and ergosterol; D_3 may be referred to as 1-alpha-OHD_3, alfacalcidiol, calcitriol or rocaltrol (Micromedex 2003).

Quantification of any of the vitamin D forms is expressed in either international units (IU) or micrograms. The conversion is: 1 mcg = 40 IU.

Are all vitamin D forms alike?

Coincident with the recognition of 25(OH)D as the key marker of individual vitamin D status, the ability of cholecalciferol (D_3) and ergocalciferol (D_2) to increase serum levels of this marker has been compared (Trang et al 1998). Results from these studies reveal a 70% greater increase in serum 25(OH)D in response to cholecalciferol (D_3). Hypothesised reasons for this difference are based upon the distinct metabolic handling of the two different forms. D_3 demonstrates higher affinity for D-binding protein, making it less likely to be excreted in bile (Armas et al 2004, Dusso et al 2005, Hossein-nezhad & Holick 2013); D_3 produces more potent metabolites and is converted into 25(OH)D up to five times faster than D_2 (FSANZ 2007, Houghton & Vieth 2006, Trang et al 1998). The results of another study showed that serum 25(OH)D increases in response to D_2 supplementation were not sustained, and in fact fell below baseline values over 14 days, while the serum levels of those supplemented with D_3 continued to rise throughout the same period (Armas et al 2004). In addition to these concerns, the stability and purity of D_2 preparations are questionable (Houghton & Vieth 2006). This is confirmed by a recent systematic review reporting on 144 cohorts from 94 independent studies from 1990 to 2012. The review found that, in all four cohorts where D_2 was the supplement used, a decline in circulating 25(OH)D was observed. Further, in three of the four cohorts where D_2 and D_3 were reported separately, while an overall decline in 25(OH)D was noted, it is of interest that circulating $25(OH)D_2$ increased significantly, but seemingly at the expense of $25(OH)D_3$, which showed a marked decline (Zittermann et al 2014).

These findings have major ramifications for the interpretation of vitamin D research and the clinical implementation of such protocols. Every piece of vitamin D research must now be considered in the light of the supplemental form used. Clinically D_3's improved potency translates to significantly lower dose requirements, in the vicinity of 2.5–10 times less (FSANZ 2007, Houghton & Vieth 2006), compared with a D_2-based product (Glendenning 2002). Zittermann et al's (2014) review calculated that D_3 supplementation, compared with D_2, corresponded to an average increase of 20.19 nmol/L in circulating 25(OH)D. The review also found that concomitant calcium supplementation incurred a significant decrease in circulating 25(OH)D levels by an average of 6.34 nmol/L. Body weight, age and baseline circulating levels of 25(OH)D also impacted on circulating levels of 25(OH)D, with 54% of variability in levels being explained by these factors. Body weight was the main factor contributing more than one-third of the variance; however all these variables should be considered when reviewing or implementing the evidence, or planning new trials. The Working Group (2012) also discusses the concern of the effect of obesity on dosage regimens. Vitamin D enters adipose tissue and may not be readily available unless there is fat breakdown, which may result in lower circulating vitamin D following oral supplementation.

FOOD SOURCES

Small amounts are found in fatty fish, such as herring, salmon, tuna and sardines, beef and liver, butter, eggs and fortified foods such as margarine and milk (Gropper et al 2009). Cod liver oil is also a good source. Notably, meat products also contain some 25(OH)D, which is five times more active than D_3 (Nowson & Margerison 2001); however, the vitamin D content of all animal products is dependent upon the individual animal's vitamin D status and the use of fortified feed (Mattila et al 2004). There is therefore concern that, as a consequence of modern agricultural and aquacultural practices, vitamin D content is in decline, as demonstrated by a study which revealed a 75% decrease in the vitamin D content of farmed compared to wild salmon (Lu et al 2007). Naturally occurring D_2 is found only in mushrooms.

Current vitamin D fortification practices in Australia provide very little supplementation of D_3 in mandatory fortification (including edible oil spreads and table margarine) and voluntary fortification (modified and skim milks, powdered milk, yoghurt, cheese, butter, legume- and cereal-based analogue beverages) (FSANZ 2011, Nowson & Margerison 2001). There is one specially supplemented milk product in Australia that provides 200 IU per 250 mL serving. However dietary fortifications are not mandated as they are in other countries such as the United States and Canada, and remain an inadequate source of supplementation (Working Group 2012). Australian diet studies reveal that fortified margarine and edible oil spreads make the largest single contribution to vitamin D consumption (28–53%) (NHMRC 2006, Nowson & Margerison 2001). An Australian study found that average dietary consumption of vitamin D was 1.2 mcg/day and that only 7.9% of this sample took vitamin D supplements (van der Mei et al 2007).

DEFICIENCY SIGNS AND SYMPTOMS

Although the traditional understanding of hypovitaminosis D revolves around its critical role in calcium metabolism, the extensive presence of VDR throughout the body is providing the impetus for further research into actions, deficiency states and therapeutic applications (Gropper et al 2009). Its role in vascular biology and cardiovascular health in particular has been a focus of clinical studies in recent years. Some clinical studies have linked low levels of vitamin D metabolites with higher incidence of congestive heart failure and increases in mortality (Valdivielso et al 2009). Several studies have looked into the relationship between chronic kidney disease and vitamin D status (Palmer et al 2007). However, in the expert opinion piece by Valdivielso et al (2009), the importance of vitamin D research in relation to vascular effects has been highlighted. The authors state that a causal relationship has been established in several basic science experiments between vitamin D and cardiovascular diseases (atherosclerosis, hypertension, arterial dysfunction, left ventricular hypertrophy). Equally, nephrology research has shown a great deal of interest due to the low levels of calcidiol and calcitriol seen in patients with chronic kidney disease, and with a higher mortality rate. With targeted trials to evaluate therapeutic levels of vitamin D to control secondary hyperparathyroidism, and cardiovascular disease, which is the major cause of death, vitamin D status is an important marker for these two patient populations (Valdivielso et al 2009). These authors, however, caution against the routine use of vitamin D supplementation in healthy humans where no deficit exists, with the idea of a U-shaped curve of benefit in metabolite levels for individuals.

Primary deficiency

Unlike many other vitamins, vitamin D is not only ingested through the diet but also produced and stored in the body. As such, endogenous production, which is reliant on adequate exposure to sunlight, will greatly influence whether deficiency states develop. It has been estimated that exposing the skin to UVB radiation produces approximately 90% of the vitamin D_3 (cholecalciferol) that is bioavailable in the body. Currently, the National Health and Medical Research Council (NHMRC) reports that it is almost impossible to get sufficient vitamin D from dietary sources alone, stressing the importance of UVB exposure (NHMRC 2006, Working Group 2012).

Deficiency more prevalent than once thought

Inadequate vitamin D among Australians is now recognised as a substantial concern, given the significant percentage demonstrating a combination of poor dietary intake and inadequate sun exposure, according to the 2012 position statement released by the Working Group of the Australian and New Zealand Bone and Mineral Society, Endocrine Society of Australia and Osteoporosis Australia. This working group cites epidemiological data that estimate 31% of adults in Australia have inadequate vitamin D status, which they define as <50 nmol/L, and up to 50% of women during winter and spring (Nowson et al 2012).

V

Ongoing epidemiological research in Australia supports this view and has identified the wider community at risk of mild deficiency, with the results of numerous studies supporting this proposition. Using a cut-off of ≤50 nmol/L for serum 25(OH)D, vitamin D insufficiency has been found to affect >40% of healthy adults in Queensland (Kimlin et al 2007, van der Mei et al 2007), >65% Tasmanians (van der Mei et al 2007) and up to 74% of general medical inpatients (Chatfield et al 2007) — including 54% of the last group, who were taking vitamin D supplements. A study of maternal and neonatal levels in Sydney revealed that 15% of mothers (at 23–32 weeks' gestation) and 11% of neonates met the criteria for overt vitamin D deficiency (≤25 nmol/L) (Bowyer et al 2009). These rates increase dramatically if the reference range for optimal serum 25(OH)D is raised, as has been proposed in the scientific literature (Dawson-Hughes et al 2005, Vieth et al 2001, 2004). One group of researchers reanalysed population data based on the proposed cut-off of ≤80 nmol/L (Dawson-Hughes et al 2005, Heaney 2006, Holick 2005) and found that 70% of their sample of healthy Australians would, using this definition, be below optimal (van der Mei et al 2007).

More recently, in 2014, a cohort of community-dwelling elective cardiothoracic surgical patients attending the Alfred Hospital in Melbourne, Australia, was found to have a high prevalence of suboptimal vitamin D (Braun et al 2014). When fasting serum samples were taken on the day of surgery, 92.5% of patients had vitamin D levels <75 nmol/L, 67.5% had levels <60 nmol/L, 52.5% had levels between 30 and 59 nmol/L and 15% had levels <30 nmol/L (Braun et al 2014). The implications for surgical outcomes, healing and future cardiovascular events remain to be investigated.

Factors associated with lower 25(OH)D levels in Australia include:

- seasonal effects, with winter–early spring demonstrating peak incidence (Bowyer et al 2009, Chatfield et al 2007, Kimlin et al 2007, McGillivray et al 2007, van der Mei et al 2007)
- increasing latitude (Angeline et al 2013, Nowson et al 2012, van der Mei et al 2007)
- increasing skin pigmentation (Kimlin et al 2007, Nowson et al 2012), with one study calculating an odds ratio (OR) of 2.7 for dark skin (Bowyer et al 2009)
- non-Australian birthplace: OR 2.2 (Erbas et al 2008)
- hospitalisation, and institutionalisation and age (Bruyere et al 2009).

The institutionalised elderly are of particular concern, as their exposure to sunlight is often restricted and they have an estimated twofold reduction in capacity of the skin to produce D_3 (Wilson et al 1991), compromised final conversion in the kidneys, reduced tissue response and further reductions to calcium absorption independently of these pathways (Bouillon et al 1997, FAO/WHO 2002). The increasing risk with age is clearly demonstrated by the results of a Tasmanian study, which revealed that, although only 8% of 8-year-olds were considered vitamin D-deficient, deficiency escalated with increasing age to peak at 85% for people aged 60 years (RACGP 2003).

At the other end of the age spectrum, a 2-year surveillance of infants presenting with vitamin D deficiency-related problems at the Monash Medical Centre in Clayton, Victoria, found that the 13 infants admitted to hospital all had migrant parents and were predominantly or exclusively breastfed (Pillow et al 1995). This is a dangerous combination, with dark-skinned migrants at a significantly greater risk of deficiency (Bowyer et al 2009, Erbas et al 2008), particularly women who are veiled (OR 21.7) (Bowyer et al 2009, Grover & Morley 2001, Nowson & Margerison 2002, Wigg et al 2006), and breast milk is recognised as a poor source of vitamin D (Andiran et al 2002). Australian research demonstrates that recently immigrated infants or first-generation offspring of immigrant parents, especially Indian, Middle Eastern, African and Polynesian, are a key at-risk group: 40% of infants aged 4–12 months were found to be deficient (Nozza & Rodda 2001, Robinson et al 2006) and 87% of sampled East African children (0–17 years) living in Melbourne recorded serum 25(OH)D levels ≤50 nmol/L (McGillivray et al 2007).

Other populations at risk include obese individuals (Arunabh et al 2003, Blum et al 2008, Harris & Dawson-Hughes 2007, Hossein-nezhad & Holick 2013), psychiatric patients (Berk et al 2007), individuals with an intellectual disability (estimated deficiency prevalence 50–60%) (Vanlint et al 2008) and those observing requirements of modest clothing (Zittermann et al 2014).

Secondary deficiency

Malabsorption states such as coeliac disease, Crohn's disease, gastrectomy, intestinal resection, chronic cholestasis, cystic fibrosis and pancreatic disorders increase the risk of deficiency (Hendler & Rorvik 2001, Kumar & Clark 2002, Nowson et al 2012).

The use of certain anticonvulsants and chronic administration of glucocorticoids increase the risk of vitamin D deficiency. Several rare hereditary forms of rickets develop because the body cannot process (metabolise) vitamin D normally (Beers & Berkow 2003). Chronic liver disease will obstruct the first hydroxylation reaction, and end-stage kidney disease results in negligible conversion of 25(OH)D into 1,25(OH)D (Kumar & Clark 2002, Micromedex 2003). One large study also demonstrated that levels of serum 25(OH)D are inversely correlated with percentage of body fat and, as such, morbidly obese individuals have increased requirements (Arunabh et al 2003).

Signs and symptoms of deficiency

The previously determined serum concentrations of 25(OH)D believed to be indicative of deficiency (<20–25 nmol/L) are considered outdated (Gomez et al 2003). It is now apparent that much higher concentrations, deemed 'suboptimal' status, have deleterious effects (Dawson-Hughes et al 2005, Heaney 2006, Holick 2005, Nowson & Margerison 2002). Indications of deficiency include:

- alopecia with dilated hair follicles and dermal cysts (Dusso et al 2005)
- anaemia, decreased bone cellularity and extramedullary erythropoiesis (Brown et al 1999)
- cardiomegaly (Dusso et al 2005, Holick 2005, Valdivielso et al 2009)

Clinical note — The vitamin D dilemma

Between 80% and 100% of our vitamin D needs can be met through adequate sun exposure, with dietary intake only required to meet the shortfall (Nowson & Margerison 2001, 2002, Nowson et al 2012, Samanek et al 2006). Quantifying this shortfall, however, is complex and individualistic, as multiple variables influence the rate of endogenous production, such as age, weight, season, latitude, time of day, part of body exposed to sunlight and use of sunscreen. Researchers estimate that full-body sun exposure in Australia, sufficient to induce mild erythema (minimal erythemal dose), is equivalent to consuming 15,000 IU orally, and that exposure of around 15% of the body surface (arms and hands or equivalent) for a third of a minimal erythemal dose, near the middle of the day, will produce about 1000 IU (25 mcg) (Working Group 2005, 2012). Hence, we have the dilemma: while the majority of public health messages continue to promote sun protection, there is growing media coverage of the negatives associated with this and advocacy for exposure to UVB in order to prevent vitamin D deficiency (Scully et al 2008). The successful Slip Slop Slap campaign in Australia, which encourages covering up and reduced sun exposure, appears at odds with the vitamin D message and may have put many Australians at risk of poor vitamin D status. Australian research concurs with this, indicating that the public health message battle is currently being won by 'sun protection', with only 15% of surveyed Australians agreeing with the statement that 'sun protection may result in not having enough vitamin D' (Janda et al 2007).

Clearly, revision of the current public health messages regarding both vitamin D and safe sunlight exposure has been required for some time. In response, work has been undertaken to develop a message of compromise (Nowson & Margerison 2002, Working Group 2005, 2012), and the development of a vitamin D index, similar to a UV index, has been proposed (van der Mei et al 2007). Evidence from a study by Samanek et al (2006) supports the concept that safe sun exposure can yield vitamin D adequacy. Their research concluded that from October to March only 10–15 minutes of unprotected exposure to 15% of the body outside of the hours of 10 a.m. to 3 p.m. was sufficient; however, during other seasons, up to 1 hour of exposure was required. In addition to this, the authors themselves acknowledge that calculations were based on existing serum values, which have been widely contested by other researchers (Gomez et al 2003). In view of some of these concerns, the new NHMRC vitamin guidelines released in 2006 are now recommending an increased adequate intake of vitamin D, particularly for adults aged over 50 years. The guidelines also suggest varying lengths of time for sun exposure for different skin types in order to achieve adequate levels. Whether these initiatives are sufficient to prevent deficiency in the community remains to be seen. The Working Group (2012) recommendations range from 5 minutes exposure in Townsville, 7 minutes in Sydney, to 9 minutes in Hobart over the summer, and 16 min to 29 min for the rest of the year. They state that those with darker skin are likely to require exposure three to six times longer than suggested values, and those at risk of deficiency include very fair-skinned people who avoid exposure, those who may have clothing that blocks exposure, as well as those with chronic illness, or who are confined indoors.

- cardiovascular disease (atherosclerosis, hypertension, arterial dysfunction, left ventricular hypertrophy) (Valdivielso et al 2009)
- chronic kidney disease increased mortality from cardiovascular causes (Valdivielso et al 2009)
- chronic fatigue syndrome (deficiency may be misdiagnosed as this) (Holick 2004, Schinchuk & Holick 2007)
- chronic lower-back pain (Al Faraj & Al Mutairi 2003)
- excess PTH secretion and parathyroid hyperplasia
- fibromyalgia (it is estimated that 40–60% of patients diagnosed with this condition are actually suffering from vitamin D deficiency) (Holick 2004, 2005, Schinchuk & Holick 2007)
- hypertension (Dusso et al 2005, Forman et al 2007, Holick 2005)
- impaired glucose-mediated insulin secretion (Brown et al 1999)
- increased risk of fracture in the elderly (not limited to vitamin D's influence on bone mass)
- increased susceptibility to mycobacterial and viral infections (Dusso et al 2005)
- peripheral vascular disease with claudication (may be misdiagnosed or confounding factor) (Holick 2005)
- rickets and osteomalacia
- osteopenia and osteoporosis
- sarcopenia — skeletal muscle weakness and atrophy (Dusso et al 2005, Visser et al 2003)
- stunting.

Deficiency also significantly increases the risk of:

- autoimmunity, including multiple sclerosis (MS) (including increased severity of pre-existing cases) (Dusso et al 2005, Hall & Juckett 2013, Holick 2004), diabetes type 1 (Clancy et al 2013, Cooper et al 2011, Holick 2006) and inflammatory bowel disease (Hewison 2011, Holick 2004)
- cancer — breast, prostate, colon and skin cancers are among the 20 different cancer types demonstrating an inverse relationship with vitamin D levels (Holick 2004)
- heart failure in patients with cardiovascular disease (Holick 2005, Valdivielso et al 2009)

- non-insulin-dependent diabetes mellitus in high-risk populations — some studies (Pittas et al 2007), but not all (Reis et al 2007), show positive association
- pre-eclampsia — particularly if hypovitaminosis D is present at <22 weeks (Bodnar et al 2007, Hossein-nezhad & Holick 2013).

MAIN ACTIONS

Whereas vitamin D is considered a fat-soluble vitamin, its active metabolite 1,25$(OH)_2D_3$ is considered to be more like a steroid hormone, because it can be produced by the body and moves through the systemic circulation to reach target tissues via receptors both at the cell membrane and at the nuclear receptor proteins. Vitamin D possesses two distinct action pathways dependent upon the site of bioactivation (Clancy et al 2013, Dusso et al 2005, Holick 2006). Renal hydroxylation of 25(OH)D produces 1,25$(OH)_2D$, primarily responsible for its traditional endocrine actions mentioned, as well as playing a role in intestinal detoxification and calcium absorption (Kutuzova & DeLuca 2007, Nowson et al 2012), healthy insulin secretion (Brown et al 1999, Dusso et al 2005, Mathieu & Badenhoop 2005) and blood pressure control, via inhibition of renin production and blunting cardiomyocyte hypertrophy (Dusso et al 2005, Holick 2005, Simpson et al 2007, Valdivielso et al 2009).

Extrarenal bioactivation, by immune, prostate, breast, colon, beta and skin cells, however, results in non-genomic responses characterised as autocrine rather than endocrine effects (Dusso et al 2005, Hewison 2011, Holick 2006, Kemmis et al 2006). These autocrine effects include controlling immune function (especially anti-inflammatory), cellular growth, maturation, differentiation and apoptosis (Dusso et al 2005, Hewison 2011, Holick 2005, Kemmis et al 2006, Lips 2006) as well as photoprotection (Dixon et al 2007), explaining vitamin D's role in immune function and cancer prevention.

Regulation of calcium and phosphorus levels

In conjunction with PTH, which is released under conditions of low calcium levels, vitamin D can stimulate calcium and phosphorus absorption in the intestines, reabsorption in the kidneys and release of calcium from the bones back into the blood. 1,25$(OH)_2D_3$ in turn is regulated by PTH, calcium, phosphorus and 1,25$(OH)_2D_3$ itself (Wahlqvist 2002). To achieve the maximal efficiency of vitamin D-induced intestinal calcium transport, the serum 25(OH)D concentrations must be at least 78 nmol/L (30 ng/mL). In deficiency, intestinal absorption of calcium can be halved in adults (Hossein-nezhad & Holick 2013, Holick 2004).

Modelling and remodelling of bone

Besides influencing bone by maintaining calcium and phosphorus homeostasis, vitamin D may also contribute to bone health in other ways.

One pathway involves binding of 1,25$(OH)_2D_3$ to DNA to promote transcription of specific mRNA, which codes for osteocalcin. Osteocalcin is then secreted by the osteoblasts, which bind calcium in new bone (Gropper et al 2009). Vitamin D also appears to play a role in oestrogen biosynthesis by increasing expression of the aromatase enzyme gene. It has demonstrated a synergistic effect in select tissues with the phyto-oestrogen genistein, with co-administration leading to a prolonged half-life of active vitamin D (Harkness & Bonny 2005, Swami et al 2005).

Cell differentiation, proliferation and growth

Some of the actions already described are the result of the vitamin's capacity to affect cell differentiation, proliferation and growth in many tissues (e.g. differentiation of stem cells into osteoclasts to facilitate bone resorption). Alternatively, 1,25$(OH)_2D_3$ can inhibit proliferation in many cells, including lymphocytes, keratinocytes, mammary, cardiac and both skeletal and smooth-muscle cells. This ability has led to its investigation as a treatment for proliferative disorders such as cancer (Brown et al 1999, Gropper et al 2009, Hossein-nezhad & Holick 2013, Kohlmeier 2003).

Reduction of PTH and regulation of growth of the parathyroid gland

Although PTH regulates the levels of 1,25$(OH)_2D$, its secretion is regulated by vitamin D, calcium and phosphorus. In deficiency, hypersecretion of this hormone can cause excessive growth of the parathyroid gland and secondary hyperparathyroidism (Brown et al 1999, Hewison 2011).

Immunomodulation

Increasing evidence for vitamin D's importance outside its classical role in bone metabolism is emerging. However the use of vitamin D to treat diseases has been used since Hippocrates first prescribed sunlight for tuberculosis (Clancy et al 2013). Vitamin D enhances the immune system's response to both bacterial and viral agents (Grant 2008c), primarily through promoting differentiation and activity of the macrophages, which means that immune responses can be tailored through the appropriate cell response (Brown et al 1999), but also through the induction of cathelicidin (Maalouf 2008). Vitamin D influences the cytokine production of immune cells, suppressing the release of interleukin-2 (IL-2), IFN-gamma and TNF-alpha, products of the Th1 line of cells, thereby reducing the propensity for a range of autoimmune conditions (Thien et al 2005). This reflects its propensity for inhibiting adaptive immunity while potentiating the innate response (Bikle 2008). There is speculation that, through this mechanism, vitamin D will promote a Th2 dominance and may predispose to the atopic diathesis. Supporting evidence comes from two studies that reveal supplementation with vitamin D in early life to be a potential precipitator of allergic disease (Hyppönen et al 2001); however, in other scenarios (e.g. autoimmunity) this effect would be considered to be therapeutic (Smolders et al 2008). In recent years, data have increasingly linked vitamin D deficiency with Th1 autoimmune disorders (Clancy et al 2013), such as MS, type 1 diabetes and Crohn's disease, suggesting a significant impact of vitamin D on immune function. Even increased susceptibility to infectious diseases, such as tuberculosis, is thought to have a link to low vitamin D levels (Hewison 2012). In a symposium paper from the Proceedings of the Nutrition Society, Hewison (2012) discusses that cells from the immune system are capable of converting the precursor 25-hydroxyvitamin D to the active 1,25-dihydroxyvitamin D, which stimulates a macrophage response to this active form in an antimicrobial fashion. Additionally, regulation of the maturation of antigen-presenting dendritic cells (DCs) occurs, from which vitamin D may control T-lymphocyte (T-cell) function. T cells, however, also have a direct response capacity to the active form of vitamin D in the activation of suppressor regulatory T cells. This suggests an immune adaptive response as well as innate immunity. Its influence on cytokine inflammatory markers, as mentioned above, may indicate a protective effect by reducing prolonged exposure to inflammation (Hewison 2012). Prietl et al (2013) also suggest that vitamin D-metabolising enzymes and VDRs, present in many cell types, are expressed extensively in immune cells, including antigen-presenting cells, T cells, B cells and monocytes, and purport that this not only modulates innate immune cells, but promotes a more tolerogenic immunological state.

OTHER ACTIONS

Our current understanding of the role of vitamin D appears to be only part of the picture. Ongoing discovery of previously unidentified receptors on tissues continues to broaden our understanding of its diverse effects. Recently, Nowson et al (2012), in the Working Group paper, state that almost every nucleated cell expresses the VDR, and that many extrarenal tissues have the capacity to make $1,25(OH)_2D$. This suggests evidence for not only classical endocrine operation, but also autocrine and paracrine pathways, which suggests vitamin D's role and importance in local synthesis and actions. This has major implications for vitamin D research and therapeutic value.

Haematopoietic tissues

VDRs have been identified on haematopoietic and lymphoid cells, suggesting the role of vitamin D in blood cell development and immune system function. The biologically active form of vitamin D, calcitriol, exerts an effect on erythropoiesis and bone cellularity. Calcitriol activates the VDRs, which appear to be the mediator of vitamin D's action, and may have a role in homing lymphoid cells to specific tissues. It has been found that VDRs are ubiquitous in human tissue, and that the gene for VDR, with its various polymorphisms (encoded on chromosome 12) and differences in transcription effects, is responsible for at least some of the variability among individuals, not only in vitamin D absorption and status, but in biologically diverse ways, such as adult height, bone mineral density and susceptibility to diseases such as tuberculosis (Hall & Juckett 2013).

Vitamin D has also been shown to inhibit clonal cell proliferation in some leukaemia lines and to promote leucocyte differentiation (Brown et al 1999). VDRs are expressed in various cells such as monocytes, thymocytes, activated B and T lymphocytes, as well as haematopoietic precursors in the haematopoietic system. The presence on activated lymphocytes suggests that there is an immune modulation role on differentiated cells. Changes in inflammatory cytokine profiles in VDR knockout mice suggest vitamin D's role in mediating inflammation (Hall & Juckett 2013). The expression of VDR on isolated DCs from lymphoid tissue further confirms the role of vitamin D in immunoregulation (Hewison 2012). DCs are critical in the adaptive immune response, in the establishment of immunological memory, and have the ability to induce a primary immune response in T lymphocytes (Wieder 2003). Treatment with 1,25(OH)2D has been shown to suppress DC maturation, specifically in the myeloid DC, which is responsible for T-cell activation, and promote the more tolerogenic plasmacytoid DC (Hewison 2012).

Muscle function

Vitamin D maintains muscle strength and has an effect on skeletal muscle and smooth muscle, with proximal muscle weakness being a common feature of deficiency (Hossein-nezhad & Holick 2013). Early work performed in 1975 demonstrated a relationship between vitamin D and muscle function. Birge and Haddad found that phosphate regulation within the muscle cell promoted maintenance of muscle metabolism and function. In 2004, Holick suggested a link between fibromyalgia and vitamin D deficiency, with 40–60% of cases presenting with generalised muscle weakness and pain being estimated as undiagnosed hypovitaminosis. More recently, with VDR being identified on smooth-muscle cells, and with vitamin D's classic role in calcium and phosphate homeostasis, there are major implications for skeletal muscle function as well as smooth muscle in the respiratory, cardiovascular and reproductive systems. Cannell and colleagues (2009) describe the binding of $1,25(OH)_2D_3$ to the VDR, leading to gene transcription and increased cell protein synthesis and growth. Further, Bischoff-Ferrari et al (2004) show an age-related decline of VDR expression in muscle tissue, and abnormal development of muscle fibres and maturation have been demonstrated in VDR knockout mice (Minasyan et al 2009).

V

The cellular effect of vitamin D can be seen in a variety of cellular signalling cascades. Principal among them is the mitogen-activated protein kinase signalling pathway, which initiates muscle tissue cell genesis, proliferation and differentiation (Angeline et al 2013). Disruption of this pathway in deficient murine models and subsequent supplementation showed an increase in muscle mass through increased protein synthesis. Interestingly, however, exercise-induced muscle cell apoptosis was reduced in these animals (Cannell et al 2009, Ceglia 2009). Further clinical trials should be implemented to elucidate the implications of this effect.

The US Preventive Services Task Force report concluded that vitamin D supplementation is effective in preventing falls in community-dwelling adults over 65 years, but the evidence is less convincing about primary fracture prevention (Moyer 2013). With a demonstrated age-related decline in VDR expression (Bischoff-Ferrari et al 2004), and Minasyan et al's (2009) finding that their VDR knockout mice with abnormal muscle fibre development and maturation also showed poorer motor and balance function, the role of vitamin D in muscle health and strength may play at least a part in falls prevention and therefore fracture risk reduction in the elderly.

Vascular function

Local production of calcitriol acts as a regulator of certain cell functions. In both endothelial and vascular smooth muscle, the VDR activity suggests that vitamin D acts via an endocrine pathway as a regulator of vascular function. VDR is expressed in cells throughout the vascular system, including vascular smooth-muscle cells, endothelial cells and cardiomyocytes, which all produce CYP27B1 to convert into the active form calcitriol. Calcitriol has been shown to exhibit anti-inflammatory properties, through local control of cytokines, and also exhibit an inhibitory effect on vascular smooth-muscle cell proliferation, and help to regulate the renin-angiotensin system (Shapses & Manson 2011). Vitamin D has been found to exert a direct effect on the myocardium: $1,25(OH)_2D_3$ controls hypertrophy in cardiac monocytes and, together with 25(OH)D, improves the left ventricular function in patients with cardiomyopathies (Brown et al 1999). Cardiovascular pathology is the leading cause of death in patients with chronic kidney disease, and there is a relationship between cardiovascular health and vitamin D status. Metabolite levels are associated with a higher incidence of congestive heart failure and increases in mortality (Valdivielso et al 2009). Vitamin D deficiency has also been linked to an increased risk of developing incident hypertension (Forman et al 2007, Wang et al 2008). Observational studies have suggested considerable benefits from vitamin D dietary intake and supplementation; however, clinical trial evidence for hypertension and diabetes is inconsistent, and in subanalysis potentially suggests a benefit for those with the lowest levels of circulating vitamin D, and a potential detriment for normotensive individuals, or those with adequate circulating 25(OH)D levels, suggesting a U-shaped curve of benefit. While biological plausibility exists, the data have been less compelling in human subjects compared with animal models (Shapses & Manson 2011, Valdivielso et al 2009). Confounding factors such as obesity, age and exercise levels need to be considered in conducting robust large-scale randomised controlled trials (RCTs) with cardiovascular outcomes as the primary measure.

Pancreatic function

Vitamin D is essential for normal insulin secretion, as demonstrated in both animals and humans, and VDRs have been found in pancreatic beta cells, whose function improves following vitamin D repletion (Alemzadeh et al 2008, Mathieu & Badenhoop 2005, Palomer et al 2008). Enhanced insulin synthesis may be due to vitamin D's role in controlling intracellular calcium flux in islet cells which facilitates conversion of proinsulin to insulin, exocytosis of insulin and beta-cell glycolysis (Brown et al 1999, Palomer et al 2008). Vitamin D also modulates insulin receptor gene expression (Palomer et al 2008).

Brain function

Evidence over the past 10–15 years confirms that the steroid hormone vitamin D is essential for normal homeostasis and development of the brain (Eyles et al 2013). The data implicate $1,25(OH)_2D$ in the biosynthesis of neurotrophic factors, contribution to brain detoxification pathways with increased glutathione and reduced nitric oxide, neuroprotective effects, induction of glioma cell death and involvement in neurotransmitter synthesis, including acetylcholine and the catecholamines (Garcion et al 2002). The VDR and 1-alpha-hydroxylase activity has been demonstrated in specific brain regions (e.g. the hypothalamus), implying a potential role for vitamin D as a neuroactive hormone (Berk et al 2007, Eyles et al 2014, Obradovic et al 2006, Vieth et al 2004). There is also increasing evidence of vitamin D's modulation of several neurotransmitters, such as acetylcholine, catecholamines and serotonin (Jorde et al 2006, Obradovic et al 2006). Preliminary studies in rats have demonstrated an antiepileptic action (Kalueff & Tuohimaa 2005). Tentative links are being made between the aetiology/pathophysiology of Parkinson's disease and poor vitamin D status (Johnson 2001, Kim et al 2005). The extensive and interesting work of the Australian group of Eyles and colleagues has been presented in a series of papers, and has outlined the varied and far-reaching implications of vitamin D deficiency and absence in the developing fetal brain (Byrne et al 2005, Cui et al 2010, Eyles et al 2003, 2011, 2013, 2014, Harms et al 2011). Vitamin D affects an array of cellular functions, and the group has described in experimental mouse and rat models the effects of induced extreme deficiency, and developmental absence of vitamin D. These models show: a less differentiated brain;

changes to neurotrophic factor expression; cytokine regulation; neurotransmitter synthesis; intracellular calcium signalling; antioxidant activity; greater number of proliferating cells (which elongates the shape of the developing brain); less apoptosis (further influencing distribution and shape of brain); expression of genes/proteins; structure and metabolism; and a reduction in factors associated with neuronal maturation (Eyles et al 2003, 2011, 2014). Additionally the group has demonstrated a persistent effect into adulthood of altered brain anatomy in structure and function (Eyles et al 2013), and neurochemistry (Eyles et al 2012) for fetuses exposed to deficiency or absence of vitamin D.

VDRs are shown to be nucleic in fetal life and readily apparent in the brain, although in lower amount than the more usual target organs of the gut and kidneys. However, in adulthood VDRs are demonstrated to be in the plasma membrane and more prominent in the gut and kidney, suggesting a change in function with maturation of the organs (Eyles et al 2014). Vitamin D deficiency has been linked to developmental psychiatric disorders, such as autism spectrum disorder, schizophrenia and Parkinson's disease, in observational and epidemiological studies (Eyles et al 2014). Correlations with greater risk associated with increasing latitude, seasonal variation as well as darker skin pigmentation in migrant groups have been well established for risk of schizophrenia (Cantor-Graae & Selten 2005, Davies et al 2003), depression (Byrne et al 2005), and are emerging for autism spectrum disorder (Cannell 2008, Grant & Soles 2009).

CLINICAL USE

Vitamin D is administered using various routes and can be prescribed as either a supplement or a drug, largely depending on dose and administration route. This review will focus on oral supplementation of D_2 or D_3 only and will not cover the variety of analogues that continue to be extensively studied. For many conditions that appear to require high doses, the race is on to develop and trial pharmaceutical analogues that retain, in particular, the antiproliferative nature of the vitamin, but are low-calcaemic in order to minimise the associated toxicity seen at such doses.

Deficiency states

Frank vitamin D deficiency in infancy or childhood produces rickets, which results from reduced sun exposure, deficient diet or metabolic or malabsorptive diseases. Vitamin D deficiency results in inadequate calcium and phosphorus levels for bone mineralisation (Beers & Berkow 2003). Diagnosis is confirmed with X-ray and serum assay of 25(OH)D. When occurring in adults, it is called osteomalacia, and its first presentation is often as chronic lower-back pain (Al Faraj & Al Mutairi 2003).

Defective vitamin D metabolism may be another cause, and consequently deficiency will not respond to standard oral treatment. In this situation, extremely high doses may be required, which should be monitored carefully for toxicity (Beers & Berkow 2003).

Pregnancy and lactation supplementation

Vitamin D's role in pregnancy is extremely complex, and points to its importance not only in establishing a pregnancy, but also in fetal and neonatal growth and development (Hossein-nezhad & Holick 2013). Vitamin D appears to be critical both to musculoskeletal and neurological growth and to the development of the infant. A recent Cochrane review, including six trials and reporting on a total of 1023 women, concluded that supplementation with vitamin D significantly improved women's vitamin D levels. The clinical significance of this finding and the potential use of vitamin D supplementation as a part of routine antenatal care are yet to be determined. (De-Regil et al 2012). The authors reported that data from three trials indicated that women who received vitamin D supplementation were slightly less likely to have a low-birth-weight (<2500 g) baby. However, no difference was apparent with regard to: pre-eclampsia; gestational diabetes; impaired glucose tolerance; caesarean section; gestational hypertension; or death in the mothers. For the newborns there was no difference in: preterm birth; stillbirth; neonatal death; neonatal admission to intensive care unit; low Apgar score; or neonatal infection (De-Regil et al 2012). In a study by Merewood and colleagues (2009), a strong association was found between vitamin D deficiency and increased risk of caesarean section. When all other factors were controlled for, having serum 25(OH)D <37.5 nmol/L increased the odds of having a caesarean delivery by 3.84. Women who had the highest serum 25(OH)D levels had the lowest risk of requiring a caesarean delivery. The authors hypothesise that, given that muscles contain VDRs, and that suboptimal muscle performance and weakness are associated with low serum 25(OH)D, this may be responsible for a potential failure to spontaneously begin labour or failure to progress in labour. Also, given the role of 25(OH)D in calcium regulation, this may also affect the action of smooth muscle required for efficient labour initiation and effective contractions (Merewood et al 2009).

An Australian study investigated the well-documented seasonal variation in birth weight to determine the parameters of anthropometric changes associated with this seasonal variation (McGrath et al 2005). Comparison of over 350,000 mean monthly birth weights of neonates at more than 37 weeks' gestation revealed that overall size, length, head size and skinfold thickness all display seasonal variation, but in particular greater limb length occurred with winter/spring births. Earlier animal studies imply that this may be a consequence of hypertrophy of the cartilage growth plates due to prenatal hypovitaminosis D (McGrath et al 2005).

Whether pregnant women require additional supplementation has been investigated in some studies. Trials involving more than 500 women conducted by Marya et al (1981, 1987), not included in the Cochrane Register review, have demonstrated statistically significant increased fetal birth weight, reduced prevalence of hypocalcaemia and hypophosphataemia, detected in both maternal and cord blood, and reduced blood pressure in non-toxaemic women. Additional evidence suggests a preventive role for a range of autoimmune conditions in the offspring when prenatal vitamin D levels are adequate (Holick 2004).

There is greater consensus regarding the need for vitamin D supplementation during lactation; breast milk is recognised as a poor source of this vitamin and infants are largely dependent on stored vitamin D acquired in utero (Andiran et al 2002, De-Regil et al 2012).

Children

The optimal regimen in relation to both route and dose of vitamin D for at-risk children remains controversial and is based on studies of limited size (Huh & Gordon 2008). The most common recommendation for infants is to supplement with D_2 or D_3 at 1000–2000 IU/day and up to 4000 IU/day in children older than 1 year. The US Institute of Medicine released a report in 2010 recommending dietary intakes of 400 IU/day for healthy infants and 600 IU for healthy children. The target circulating level of 25(OH)D was set at 50 nmol/L. This does not take into account the requirements for acutely or chronically unwell infants and children (Abrams et al 2013).

Treatment of deficiencies secondary to malabsorptive syndromes

Numerous studies have confirmed a high prevalence (25–75%) of hypovitaminosis D in patients with coeliac disease, Crohn's disease, small-bowel resection or cystic fibrosis. A positive correlation between low vitamin D status and clinical consequences, such as reduced bone mineral density and osteopenia, has been demonstrated in most studies. Interestingly, trials investigating the benefits of oral vitamin D supplements (400–800 IU/day) found limited success in patients. Owing to the theoretical advantage of supplementation in conditions associated with poor nutrient absorption, larger trials involving higher doses or different forms are expected to determine the most effective treatment (Abrams et al 2013, Buchman 1999, Congden et al 1981, Hanly et al 1985, Hoffmann & Zeitz 2000, Jahnsen et al 2002). A study of children with cystic fibrosis demonstrated 25(OH)D levels that were consistently >50 nmol/L with an average dose of 1405 IU/day.

Reducing all-cause mortality

Several large studies have identified an association between serum 25(OH)D concentrations and all-cause and cause-specific mortality, finding that, in particular, vitamin D deficiency (25(OH)D concentration <30 nmol/L) mortality was strongly associated with mortality from all causes, cardiovascular diseases, cancer and respiratory diseases (Schottker et al 2013, 2014). One German study investigated concentrations of 25(OH)D in 9578 people who were followed up over 9.5 years. For those people with vitamin D deficiency (<30 nmol/L) or insufficiency (30–50 nmol/L) was significantly increased (1.71 [1.43, 2.03] and 1.17 [1.02, 1.35], respectively) compared with that of subjects with sufficient 25(OH)D concentrations (>50 nmol/L). Vitamin D deficiency was also associated with increased cardiovascular mortality (1.39: 95% CI 1.02–1.89), cancer mortality (1.42: 95% CI 1.08–1.88) and respiratory disease mortality (2.50: 95% CI 1.12–5.56). The association of 25(OH)D concentrations with all-cause mortality proved to be a non-linear inverse association with risk that started to increase at 25(OH)D concentrations <75 nmol/L (Schottker et al 2013). Chowdery et al (2014) also concluded that evidence from observational studies indicates inverse associations of circulating 25-hydroxyvitamin D with risks of death due to cardiovascular disease, cancer and other causes. In particular, supplementation with vitamin D_3 significantly reduces overall mortality among older adults (Chowdhury et al 2014). The conclusion was based on study-specific relative risks from 73 cohort studies (849,412 participants) and 22 randomised controlled trials (vitamin D given alone versus placebo or no treatment; 30,716 participants). These were meta-analysed using random effects models and grouped by study and population characteristics.

The same group continued to explore the relationship in a larger study that involved a meta-analysis of individual participant data of eight prospective cohort studies from Europe and the United States. This involved data from 26,018 men and women aged 50–79 years. Comparing bottom versus top quintiles for vitamin D, a pooled risk ratio of 1.57 (95% CI 1.36–1.81) for all-cause mortality was observed. Risk ratios for cardiovascular mortality were similar in magnitude to that for all-cause mortality in subjects both with and without a history of cardiovascular disease at baseline. With respect to cancer mortality, an association was only observed among subjects with a history of cancer (risk ratio, 1.70: 1.00–2.88). Interestingly, no strong age, sex, season or country-specific differences were detected. The authors concluded that, despite levels of 25(OH)D strongly varying with country, sex and season, the association between 25(OH)D level and all-cause and cause-specific mortality was remarkably consistent (Schottker et al 2014).

Cancer prevention

In the 1930s it was reported that US navy personnel exposed to high-level UVB showed higher rates of skin cancer but lower rates of cancer malignancies (Giovannucci 2008, Grant 2008a). World Health Organization data from as early as 1955 have demonstrated latitudinal gradients in cancer mortality rates for breast, colon, lung, prostate, rectal and renal cancer (Grant 2008a); however, the hypothesis linking UVB, vitamin D and cancer was not formally proposed until 1980. Since this time, ongoing epidemiological evidence has demonstrated in both single and multiple-country studies that there is increasing cancer incidence or mortality with increasing distance from the equator (Garland et al 1999, Grant 2008a). Both advancing age and ethnicity have also been positively correlated with these cancers and this has been similarly explained in relation to reduced UVB exposure. Further epidemiological support comes from the inverse relationship between prospective serum 25(OH)D levels and cancer risk, season of cancer diagnosis and survival time and lower rates of cancer in high fish-consuming countries such as Iceland and Japan (Giovannucci 2008, Grant 2008a). In 2002 Grant identified 14 cancers for which there was strong evidence to support vitamin D sensitivity, including breast, colon, ovarian, prostate and rectal forms. Recently, Hossein-nazhad & Holick (2013) have outlined evidence to support the hypothesis of vitamin D's ability to regulate microRNA and its effect in several cancer cell lines, tissues and sera. They also suggest that local conversion of 25(OH)D in healthy cells in the colon, breast and prostate can help prevent malignancy. This prevention may occur due to 25(OH)D's capacity to induce cellular maturation, induce apoptosis and inhibit angiogenesis (Hewison 2011). Additionally, 25(OH)D may act to enhance the genes which control cellular proliferation and active detoxifying enzymes (Eyles et al 2013, Hossein-nazhad & Holick 2013).

Evidence from an interventional study of calcium (1400–1500 mg/day), alone or with vitamin D_3 (1100 IU/day), versus a placebo over 4 years supports a chemoprotective role for vitamin D (Lappe et al 2007). The study, involving 1179 women >55 years old, was primarily designed to assess reductions in fracture incidence, but upon further analysis also demonstrated significant risk reduction (relative risk [RR] 0.40) for all cancer incidence in the combined calcium and vitamin D group. When the analysis was restricted to those cancers diagnosed only after the first year of treatment, the RR became 0.23. While the group receiving calcium alone also demonstrated a reduced risk, the researchers speculate that this may not be robust and conclude that vitamin D is the key variable in reduced incidence of all cancer. Given the ability of vitamin D to inhibit abnormal proliferation, facilitate apoptosis, attenuate growth signals and reduce angiogenesis around tumours, its chemoprotective potential continues to be enthusiastically investigated through both in vitro studies and RCTss (Giovannucci 2008, Grant 2008a, Hossein-nazhad & Holick 2013). Risk reduction via protection against viral infections has also recently been hypothesised (Grant 2008b, Hewison 2012).

Improving cancer prognosis

According to a systematic review of 26 clinical studies, evidence now suggests that circulating 25-OHD levels may be associated with better prognosis in patients with breast and colorectal cancer (Toriola et al 2014).

Colorectal cancer and prevention of adenomatous polyps

Evidence of vitamin D's chemoprotective effect is strongest in relation to colorectal cancer (Giovannucci 2008) and comes from several different lines of investigation (Garland et al 1991, Giovannucci 2008, Grant & Garland 2004, Holt 2008, Holt et al 2002, Theodoratou et al 2008). A 2004 review of more than 20 epidemiological studies of vitamin D and colorectal cancer concluded that the overwhelming majority of studies have demonstrated an inverse relationship between dietary intake, serum 25(OH)D and incidence (Garland et al 2004). An estimate of daily requirements needed for prevention has been formulated using the data from the studies, suggesting that an oral intake of >1000 IU/day of vitamin D or serum 25(OH)D levels of >33 ng/mL (82 nmol/L) could reduce the risk of colorectal cancer by as much as 50%. Most intervention studies to date, however, have focused on calcium supplementation. Interestingly, some of these show that calcium's protective effect against recurrent adenomas is largely restricted to individuals with baseline serum 25(OH)D above the median (≈ 29 ng/mL). These data, together with later findings (Mizoue et al 2008), strongly point to a synergism between calcium and vitamin D for colorectal cancer and recurring adenoma risk reduction (Grau et al 2003, Holt 2008, Oh et al 2007, Theodoratou et al 2008).

An often-cited negative finding comes from the Women's Health Initiative (WHI), in which women supplemented with 1000 mg calcium and 400 IU vitamin D per day failed to demonstrate reduced cancer rates; however, several authors have published major criticisms of the study that include the inadequate dose of vitamin D administered and the time frame (Giovannucci 2008, Grant 2008a, Holt 2008). Reanalysis of the WHI findings has also elucidated oestrogen's critical modifying effect upon both nutrients, whereby higher oestrogen levels of both menstruating and postmenopausal women taking hormone replacement therapy negate calcium's otherwise protective effect (Ding et al 2008). Explanations for this phenomenon include competitive binding between vitamin D and oestrogen (Ding et al 2008, Oh et al 2007). Two recent meta-analyses reporting on more than 2000 participants each have shown a significant decrease in the risk of colorectal and rectal cancer in an inverse relationship with circulating levels of 25(OH)D (Chung et al 2011, Lee et al 2011). Stubbins et al (2012) show that the active form of vitamin D targets a β-catenin pathway by upregulating key tumour suppressor genes, which promote an epithelial phenotype. This is only possible when there is adequate VDR expression. This could provide useful targets for therapeutic administration.

Current evidence for a combined protective role of calcium, either dietary or supplemental, and vitamin D, particularly in men and postmenopausal women not taking hormone replacement therapy, is strong and further elucidation of the independent and combined effects of these nutrients will assist in the development of preventive protocols. Stubbins et al (2012) suggest that the recommended dietary intake should be increased to 2000 IU to target and increase serum 25(OH)D levels to above 30 ng/mL.

Prostate

Vitamin D's relationship to cancer is least clear with respect to prostate cancer, with inconsistent findings from numerous studies (Giovannucci 2008, Li et al 2007, Mucci & Spiegelman 2008). The belief that increased calcium, dairy consumption and vitamin D levels could increase risk has dominated, with epidemiological evidence from a number of substantial studies, including the Helsinki Heart Study, involving 19,000 men. This study showed that increased levels of circulating $1,25(OH)_2D_3$ and low levels of 25(OH)D are inversely associated with prostate cancer, in both incidence and aggressiveness, and are associated with an earlier age of onset (Chen & Holick 2003, Mucci & Spiegelman 2008). However, evidence of the potentially protective effects of increased serum 25(OH)D and $1,25(OH)_2D$ continue to emerge (Li et al 2007), while more comprehensive investigations of the relationship between dietary vitamin D intake and risk fail to show any effect (Huncharek et al 2008), largely due to globally poor intakes. Several explanations for these contrasting findings have been proposed, including that vitamin D status many years prior to diagnosis may be more predictive and relevant than levels just before or following diagnosis (Giovannucci 2008, Mucci & Speigelman 2008). In a recent review of ecological studies, there was strong evidence for a correlation with solar UVB irradiance and 15 types of neoplasms, and weaker, but significant, evidence of nine other types of cancer, including prostate (Grant 2012).

Experimental research with vitamin D has produced interesting results. Prostate cancer cells in vitro respond to vitamin D_3 with reduced proliferation, increased differentiation and apoptosis. More recently, reduced activity of the 1-alpha-hydroxylase enzyme in cancerous prostate cells when compared to healthy prostate tissue was discovered, resulting in a reduced ability to convert vitamin D to its active form. Therefore, prostates with cancer display partial resistance to the tumour-suppressing activity of $1,25(OH)_2D_3$ (Ma et al 2004). Clinical trials using supplemental vitamin D at various stages of prostate cancer have yielded inconsistent results (Miller 1999).

Breast

Normal breast cells produce $1,25(OH)_2D$, which in turn may contribute to healthy mammary function, inducing differentiation, inhibiting proliferation and modulating immune responses (Perez-Lopez 2008). VDRs in mammary tissue have also been shown to oppose oestrogen-driven proliferation of cells (Welsh et al 2003). In addition, there is growing epidemiological evidence to suggest an inverse association between vitamin D and breast cancer (Grant 2006, 2008c, 2012, Mohr et al 2008, Perez-Lopez 2008), with increasing UVB exposure reported to produce a RR of between 0.67 and 0.85 (Perez-Lopez 2008). One study that involved 179 breast cancer patients and 179 controls assessed vitamin D status of patients and polymorphisms of vitamin D, and identified an inverse relationship, possibly as high as sevenfold, between 25(OH)D levels and breast cancer risk (Lowe et al 2005). Interestingly, from a population-based case-control study in Ontario, there is evidence to suggest that sun exposure between the ages of 10 and 19 years is particularly protective against subsequent breast cancer diagnoses (Perez-Lopez 2008). This implies that vitamin D status may be especially important during breast development.

A more recent investigation of the effect of UVB exposure on breast cancer incidence in 107 countries also confirmed that increased UVB exposure is independently protective, with age-standardised incidence rates substantially higher at latitudes distant from the equator (Mohr et al 2008). The same study demonstrated that the protective effect was evident at serum levels above 22 ng/mL. Another study revealed that women with serum 25(OH)D $\geq$ 50 ng/mL halve their risk of breast cancer compared to those below this cut-off level (Perez-Lopez 2008).

A large meta-analysis of dietary studies initially failed to find a relationship between vitamin D intake and breast cancer risk. Restricting studies to only those with intakes > 400 IU/day, however, revealed a trend towards risk reduction with increasing vitamin D intake (RR 0.92) (Gissel et al 2008).

Autoimmune diseases

Autoimmune status is affected by multifactorial inputs: environmental contribution, as well as a genetic predisposition, and exposure to epidemiological risk factors are all key influencers of a person's immune state. Increasing prevalence of autoimmune disorders as well as geographical and seasonal variations have led to investigations of vitamin D insufficiency as a potential key factor. Autoimmune diseases such as type 1 diabetes mellitus (T1DM), MS, systemic lupus erythematosus (SLE), rheumatoid arthritis, Crohn's disease and other inflammatory bowel disease have been linked to significant epidemiological data which suggest associations with vitamin D (Hewison 2011, Prietl et al 2013). Treatment with calcitriol in animal models has shown to have preventive effects, or amelioration of disease (Bock et al 2012; Hewison 2011). Further, Bock et al (2012) present animal data from vitamin D-deficient or VDR knockout mice, showing increased inflammation and increased susceptibility to autoimmune disorders such as

T1DM and Crohn's disease. Interestingly, they also demonstrate disturbed T-cell function, such as homing, and a lack of host protection from bacterial invasion and infection. Hall and Juckett (2013) elucidate the mechanism of action. Inflammatory cytokines, such as IL-2 and IFN-γ, stimulate a cellular immune response termed Th1, whereas IL-4, IL-6 and IL-10 drive a humoral immune response, termed Th2. Stimulation of VDR tends to favour the inflammatory mediating Th2 response by suppressing IFN-γ, which is implicated in innate and adaptive immunity, as well as autoimmune disease, when uncontrolled. Hewison (2011) also discusses regulation of cytokine synthesis and apoptosis of inflammatory cells with therapeutic administration of calcitriol in MS model mice.

Type 1 diabetes mellitus

Vitamin D deficiency has been linked to both types of diabetes mellitus, but the largest volume of evidence relates to an inverse association between prenatal and infant vitamin D levels and a child's overall risk of developing T1DM (Bailey et al 2007, Hyppönen et al 2001, 2010, Littorin et al 2006, Prietl et al 2013, Zipitis & Akobeng 2008). Incidence rates vary widely according to geographical location related to latitude. It is hypothesised that vitamin influences T1DM pathogenesis by reducing lymphocyte proliferation and cytokine production through immunomodulatory actions (Melamed & Kumar 2010). International epidemiological data confirm this marked geographical pattern of increasing incidence with increasing latitudes, together with significantly greater rates of diagnosis in autumn and winter (Svensson et al 2009, Zipitis & Akobeng 2008). In addition, assessment of T1DM patients reveals significantly lower 25(OH)D than age-matched controls. Given that the beta-cell destruction of T1DM frequently begins in infancy, with diagnosis typically occurring when 80% of cells have already been destroyed, much focus has been placed on the environmental and nutritional influences in early life as potential aetiological factors. Greer et al (2007) found in Australia that adolescents with newly diagnosed T1DM had a three times higher risk of having levels below 20 ng/mL than controls.

One birth cohort study published in the *Lancet* in 2001 involved the offspring of 12,055 pregnant Finnish women who gave birth in 1966. The families were assessed for vitamin D supplementation in the infant's first year of life and then the child was followed until 31 years of age to account for subsequent diagnoses of T1DM. It was shown that treatment of children with 2000 IU/day vitamin D from 1 year of age decreased the risk of developing the disease by 80% through the next 20 years; furthermore, children from the same cohort who were vitamin D-deficient at 1 year old had a fourfold increased risk of developing T1DM (Hyppönen et al 2001). Similar findings have been demonstrated in animal models, with pretreatment with $1,25(OH)_2D$ being effective in mitigating or preventing the onset of T1DM (Palomer et al 2008).

A case-control study conducted in Norway that involved 545 Norwegian children up to 15 years old with T1DM retrospectively assessed their cod liver oil and vitamin D use from birth to 12 months old. Children who had been given cod liver oil five times a week had a 26% lower incidence of the disease, whereas other forms of vitamin D appeared to bear no relationship (Stene & Joner 2003). Although this does not adequately assess vitamin D as a sole treatment agent and is not conclusive, it adds to the growing body of evidence implicating vitamin D in a preventive role against diabetes.

A meta-analysis of five studies of vitamin D supplementation in infancy, including the above two, concluded that supplementation during an infant's first year appears to be associated with a significant risk reduction for the development of T1DM later in life (OR 0.71) (Zipitis & Akobeng 2008). Current evidence points to the superiority of cod liver oil as a delivery form, but a lack of specific detail in many of the studies means that optimal dose, duration of supplementation and timing cannot currently be elucidated.

Research into the role of vitamin D metabolism genes demonstrates a consistent genetic predisposition to lower vitamin D metabolism and the risk of T1DM. Cooper and colleagues (2011) have shown consistent results indicating that circulating levels of calcitriol vary seasonally and are under the same genetic control as the normal population, but three key metabolism genes (CYP27B1, DHCR7 and CYP2R1) are much lower in those with T1DM. This indicates that there is a genetic role leading to vitamin D deficiency in T1DM, which has implications for the efficacy of supplementation and the dosages required in this population.

Seasonal variation suggests that the pathophysiology is multifactorial. Hewison (2011) indicates that low vitamin D status is linked to risk of developing T1DM, and that supplementation provides a protective effect. In knockout model mice, those under dietary restriction of vitamin D showed increased severity of disease. Further, genetic investigation reveals that polymorphic variations in genes for various aspects of vitamin D metabolisms and signalling affect diabetes susceptibility. In particular, the presence of specific VDR gene alleles is protective (Ramos-Lopez et al 2006), and variations in CYP27BI (conversion enzyme) impacts on susceptibility (Bailey et al 2007).

Type 2 diabetes mellitus (T2DM)

Epidemiological studies suggest that vitamin D deficiency places some populations (e.g. non-Hispanic blacks) at a higher risk of insulin resistance, impaired glucose homeostasis and metabolic syndrome (Palomer et al 2008). The mechanisms for this effect remain speculative, including suppression of PTH, reducing calcium influx and therefore limiting lipogenesis. Other theories relate to vitamin D's immunomodulatory actions. A range of elevated inflammatory markers has been identified to predate the onset of T2DM and many of these appear to be downregulated by vitamin D, but direct evidence of this pathogenetic path is currently lacking (Palomer et al 2008, Shapses & Manson 2011). The relationship between diabetes and vitamin D, however, is likely to be a bidirectional one, with low levels of functioning insulin impairing bioactivation of vitamin D, and poor vitamin D status impeding correct insulin release and function.

Consistent evidence of an inverse relationship between serum 25(OH)D and adiposity highlights another domain of potential overlap and potential confounding between hypovitaminosis D and T2DM (Alemzadeh et al 2008, Palomer et al 2008). Consequently, vitamin D deficiency is common in T2DM patients (Sugden et al 2008). One study revealed that three-quarters of obese adolescents had levels <50 nmol/L, with a positive correlation between poor vitamin D status and glucose dysregulation (Alemzadeh et al 2008), while 49% of adult T2DM patients in another study demonstrated vitamin D deficiency (Sugden et al 2008). A meta-analysis concurs with these findings, while also adding calcium to the equation; it calculates an OR of 0.82 for incident T2DM among individuals with low vitamin D status, calcium or dairy intake (Pittas et al 2007).

Vitamin D supplementation in patients with mild T2DM and in non-diabetic patients with vitamin D deficiency can improve insulin secretion in response to oral glucose loads, but it is ineffective in patients with established or severe T2DM (Palomer et al 2008). In one clinical trial, 1332 IU/day oral vitamin D was administered for 1 month to 10 adult women with T2DM. Corresponding changes were observed in first-phase insulin secretion (34.3% increase) and serum 25(OH)D levels. Improvements observed in second-phase insulin secretion and insulin resistance were deemed non-significant (Borissova et al 2003). A more recent pilot study employed a single high dose of D_2 (100,000 IU) to vitamin D-deficient T2DM patients; this resulted in improved endothelial function, as evidenced by a highly significant reduction in systolic blood pressure. The proposed mechanisms for this effect are many and varied but remain hypothetical at this time (Sugden et al 2008). Intravenous administration of vitamin D to patients with gestational diabetes produces a transient reduction in both fasting glucose and insulin, suggesting improved insulin sensitivity rather than secretion (Palomer et al 2008).

It is important to note that single high-dose vitamin D actually increases blood glucose levels in patients with diabetes (Palomer et al 2008). While there is some biological plausibility for the role of vitamin D in the treatment of T2DM, and positive findings from observational studies, the results from clinical studies have been inconsistent, and insufficient to make recommendations (Maxwell & Wood 2011, Shapses & Manson 2011, Valdivielso et al 2009). There is some evidence to support a beneficial effect in people with very low levels of circulating 25(OH)D, but some evidence also points to a potential increase in risk at the highest levels, representing a U-shaped curve of effect (Shapses & Manson 2011). Pooled analysis shows inconsistent results; however results for insulin sensitivity seem to be more positive (Maxwell & Wood 2011, Shapses & Manson 2011). Well-designed large RCTs, with prespecified outcomes for T2DM, insulin resistance and cardiovascular outcomes, are required to establish whether vitamin D is effective for the treatment of these metabolic disorders.

Hypoparathyroidism

Vitamin D in combination with calcium has established benefits in the treatment of hypoparathyroidism, by promoting homeostasis of calcium, phosphorus, 25(OH)D and PTH levels (Hewison 2011, Mimouni et al 1986, Nowson et al 2012).

Secondary hyperparathyroidism

In a controlled study of 100 postmenopausal women with confirmed vitamin D deficiency (<18 nmol), supplementation with combination calcium and low-dose vitamin D showed more significant reductions in PTH levels over the 90-day trial period than supplementation with calcium alone (Deroisy et al 2002).

Hypophosphataemia

A combination of high-dose vitamin D and phosphorus results in improved phosphorus and calcium balance in these patients (Lyles et al 1982).

Osteoporosis and fracture prevention

One of the main functions of vitamin D is to maintain serum calcium and phosphorus levels in order to maintain healthy metabolic functions, transcription regulation and bone metabolism (Hossein-nezhad & Holick 2013). Both serum 25(OH)D and $1,25(OH)_2D$ levels are low in osteoporotic patients (Cranney et al 2008, Hunter et al 2000, Wilson et al 1991); however, conclusions regarding improvement of bone health with vitamin D supplementation alone have been mixed and largely hampered by methodological issues (e.g. accurate vitamin D assessment, accounting for and discriminating between different vitamin D sources, extricating effects of vitamin D from those of calcium) (Cranney et al 2008). A 2008 systematic review that included 17 RCTs of either D_2 or D_3 supplementation (300–2000 IU/day) in postmenopausal women or older men has found consistent evidence of a protective effect of D_3 at doses of ≥700 IU/day in combination with calcium (500–1200 mg/day) (Cranney et al 2008). Notably, however, vitamin D at these doses provided no additional benefits in black populations. A meta-analysis of 29 RCTs conducted in 63,897 individuals ≥50 years over an average of 3.5 years also concluded that calcium alone (≥1200 mg/day) or in combination with vitamin D (≥800 IU/day) reduced the risk of fracture by 12–24%, and reduced bone loss by 0.54% at the hip and 1.19% at the spine (Tang et al 2007). The greatest improvements were noted specifically in the elderly, institutionalised, underweight and calcium-deficient. In addition, an Australian trial that investigated the administration to 120 women aged 70–80 years of 1200 mg/day of calcium alone or in combination with 1000 IU vitamin D over 5 years yielded beneficial effects on bone mineral density and bone turnover markers for both treatment groups, with evidence of more sustained improvements in those also taking vitamin D (Zhu et al 2008). In a recent pooled analysis of the evidence, Bischoff-Ferrari et al (2012) state that doses of 20–50 mcg/day (800–2000 IU/day) have been demonstrated to prevent osteoporotic fractures in the elderly, and recommendations from the European Society for Clinical and Economic Aspects of Osteoporosis and Osteoarthritis state that up to 250 mcg (10,000 IU) daily is considered to be safe in this patient population (Rizzoli et al 2013).

Another study comparing the combined effects of calcium (500 mg/day) with either oral vitamin D_2 (700 IU/day) or calcitriol over 3 years demonstrated a protective effect of vitamin D_2 on the spine but not on the hip (Zofkova & Hill 2007).

Serum 25(OH)D levels in postmenopausal women are inversely associated with fracture risk, independent of number of falls, physical functionality, frailty and other associated risks (Cauley et al 2008). These data reveal that individuals with baseline serum levels <47.5 nmol/L have an increased risk of hip fracture rate over the next 7 years of 1.71 compared to those with values >70.7 nmol/L. Other studies of similar design concur with these results, while producing different cut-off values. Studies investigating vitamin D supplementation for fracture prevention in osteoporosis have produced some positive results. In the context of adequate or supplemented calcium, a 60% reduction in the incidence of peripheral fractures was observed by Cosman (700–800 IU/day), with a 40% reduction in hip fracture incidence specifically (Cosman 2005). A systematic review of 15 RCTs involving mostly D_3 supplementation (300–800 IU/day) found a non-significant reduction in fractures; however, methodological limitations, including the relatively low dose, could be a confounding issue (Cranney et al 2008).

One study has investigated the bone mineral density effects of co-supplementing silicon with calcium and vitamin D. In an RCT of 136 predominantly postmenopausal osteopenic women, 1000 mg calcium, 20 mcg vitamin D and 3 mg, 6 mg or 12 mg silicon in the form of orthosilicic acid was administered daily for 12 months to the treatment group. These subjects demonstrated significantly greater type I collagen, indicative of increased bone synthesis, compared to those receiving the placebo (Spector et al 2008). There was also a trend of decreasing resorption with increasing silicon dose.

The mechanisms behind vitamin D's bone actions are not limited to the suppression of PTH and improved calcium balance alone; evidence also exists of direct inhibition of bone resorption and reduced inflammatory markers. The active calcitriol interacts with its VDR in the small intestine to increase the efficiency of intestinal calcium and phosphorus absorption. It also interacts with VDR in osteoblasts to stimulate a receptor activator of the ligand of NF-κB, which works to produce immature preosteoclasts, stimulating them to become mature bone-resorbing osteoclasts, which then remove calcium and phosphorus from the bone to maintain blood calcium and phosphorus levels. In the kidneys, calcitriol stimulates calcium reabsorption from the glomerular filtrate (Hossein-nezhad & Holick 2013). There is also speculation regarding vitamin D's potentially positive effects on lean body mass, which would then convey an anabolic effect via increased mechanical load (Cauley et al 2008, Zofkova & Hill 2007).

Reducing falls in the elderly

The most recent recommendations from the Australian Working Group recognise vitamin D deficiency as an independent predictor of falls in older people, and have summarised the evidence for insufficient vitamin D and its association with impaired balance, increased muscle mass loss, lower-extremity muscle weakness, and impaired strength and physical function (Nowson et al 2012). Poor vitamin D status (e.g. low serum 25(OH)D, compromised VDR numbers or binding affinity, colder seasons) is independently associated with an increased risk of falling in the elderly, particularly in those aged 65–75 years (Prince et al 2008, Richy et al 2008, Snijder et al 2006) and in some studies with poorer physical performance generally (Brunner et al 2008). A 2004 review of double-blind RCTs of vitamin D in elderly populations concluded that vitamin D supplementation reduced the risk of falling by more than 20%. The results were significant only in women and appeared to be independent of calcium administration, type of vitamin D and duration of therapy (Bischoff-Ferrari et al 2006). More recent research has suggested an even greater effect, but the degree of risk reduction varies between studies. According to a double-blind randomised trial involving 64 institutionalised elderly women (age range 65–97 years; mean 25(OH)D levels 16.4 ng/mL), treatment with 1200 mg/day calcium plus 800 IU/day D_3 over 3 months reduced the rate of falls by 60% compared with calcium supplementation alone (Bischoff-Ferrari et al 2006). An Australian study of community-based women aged 70–90 years with baseline serum 25(OH)D < 24 ng/mL found that D_2 (1000 IU/day) in combination with 1000 mg calcium citrate over 1 year reduced falls by 19% (Prince et al 2008). An interesting finding was the marked seasonal variation in efficacy, with vitamin D's protective effect evident in winter/spring (months exhibiting increased risk of falls generally) but not in summer/autumn. This has been attributed to the decline in serum 25(OH)D during these months and has also been postulated as an explanation for the lack of effect seen in some larger long-term studies. The researchers also concluded that a serum level of <24 ng/mL is predictive of individuals who may benefit from vitamin D supplementation in this context.

In 2007 a pilot study of an osteopenic/osteoporotic elderly female population (≥65 years) investigated the possible additional clinical benefits of 3 months' exercise training and increased protein intake on top of year-long calcium and vitamin D supplementation (500–1000 mg/day and 400–800 IU/day, respectively) (Swanenburg et al 2007). Although the number of falls reduced dramatically in both groups, the group undertaking exercise training demonstrated greater and more sustained risk reduction (e.g. 100% at 6 months versus 40%). This multipronged approach appears promising and warrants further investigation. A systematic review funded by the US Office of Dietary Supplements of the National Institute of Health and the Agency for Healthcare Research and Quality included 14 RCTs of vitamin D for fall prevention and concluded that there was consistent evidence of benefit (OR 0.89) (Cranney et al 2008).

As a result of the accumulating evidence, routine vitamin D administration has been recommended for those institutionalised or housebound elderly who are already at risk of deficiency (Nowson et al 2012, Sambrook & Eisman 2002). The findings of an Australian study, however, suggest there are a significant number of community-dwelling elderly with sufficiently low vitamin D status who might also benefit from routine vitamin D (Prince et al 2008). One additional consideration is the best delivery form, with a comparative meta-analysis demonstrating superior results from vitamin D analogues, e.g. alfacalcidol and calcitriol, when compared to oral vitamin D (Richy et al 2008). These analogues, which override renal regulation of vitamin D bioactivation, may be particularly indicated in individuals who take high-dose glucocorticoids, exhibit impaired renal function or chronic inflammation, or who have T1DM.

In a recent systematic review on vitamin D supplementation on muscle strength, gait and balance in older adults, Muir and Montero-Odasso (2011) found that there was a significant improvement in postural sway, time to complete the timed up-and-go test for lower-extremity strength and balance with 800–1000 IU supplementation per day. They conclude that there were consistently demonstrated beneficial effects of vitamin D supplementation on strength and balance; however, gait was not affected.

In 2013, the American Geriatrics Society Workgroup on Vitamin D supplementation for Older Adults (American Workgroup) has recommended supplementation at 4000 IU/day to reduce the risk of falls and fractures for those with no underlying risk of hypercalcaemia. This larger dose recommendation is based on: the population's potential decreased adherence compared with trial participants, and increased requirement due to age and sun exposure likelihood.

Anticonvulsant-induced osteomalacia

Preliminary evidence has shown vitamin D to be an effective treatment for this condition; however, much emphasis has been placed on establishing the most superior form of D, D_2 or D_3, as they exhibit important metabolic differences in these patients (Hartwell et al 1989, Tjellesen et al 1985, 1986). More recent evidence suggests that the resultant bone disease in patients treated with anticonvulsant drugs mostly demonstrates bone remodelling rather than decreased mineralisation, some with significant turnover of bone, with manifest features of osteomalacia. Prophylactic vitamin D_3 supplementation of up to 2000 IU/day is recommended, and up to 2000–4000 IU/day in patients exhibiting osteopenic/osteoporotic disorders (Drezner 2004).

Hepatic and renal osteodystrophy

Both chronic liver disease and those conditions exhibiting end-stage renal disease result in compromised hydroxylation of vitamin D to produce its active metabolite. It has been reported that 50% of patients with chronic liver disease, especially those with primary or secondary biliary cirrhosis, present with associated osteodystrophy. This frequently leads to a vitamin D deficiency and manifests most commonly as metabolic bone disorders, hypocalcaemia and secondary hyperparathyroidism (Wills & Savory 1984). The resultant hypovitaminosis D can result in bone loss, cardiovascular disease, immune suppression and increased mortality in patients with end-stage kidney failure (Andress 2006). Consequently, correction of this deficiency has been one of many first-line treatments in these situations.

Although vitamin D_2 supplementation in combination with calcium, phosphorus and magnesium (where indicated) has shown some success in those patients with hepatic osteodystrophy (Compston et al 1979, Long & Wills 1978), recent trials and emerging research implicate other factors in the aetiology of these sequelae (Klein et al 2002, Suzuki et al 1998). As such, therapy with D_2 may need to be reviewed.

The treatment of renal osteodystrophy is reliant upon only the active forms or analogues of vitamin D, and natural supplementation is ineffective because of the inability to convert these precursors into 1,25-alpha-$(OH)_2D$ (Kim & Sprague 2002). In a recent Cochrane review of vitamin D for chronic kidney disease, it was found that, although the evidence was insufficiently powered to make clear recommendations, it did seem that vitamin D suppresses PTH in people with chronic kidney disease, but treatment was associated with clinically relevant serum elevations in both phosphorus and calcium. Observational data suggest improved survival rates in this population, but large RCTs are required to confirm these results.

Localised and systemic scleroderma

Although patients suffering from scleroderma do not show compromised D synthesis (Matsuoka et al 1991), vitamin D_3 has been investigated as a therapeutic agent to moderate the excessive proliferation and collagen production typically seen in this condition. An in vitro study assessing the action of vitamin D_3 on the behaviour of affected fibroblasts has confirmed a non-selective antiproliferative action (Boelsma et al 1995).

To date, clinical studies have produced mixed results. Clinical trials focusing on generalised scleroderma have involved small numbers and produced promising results, such as increased joint mobility, reduced induration and increased extensibility of the skin, with benefits lasting at least 1 year after discontinuation of treatment (Caca-Biljanovska et al 1999, Hulshof et al 1994). However, the largest RCT involving 27 patients (the majority of whom suffered a localised condition) found that treatment over 9 months with a similar dose of D_3 failed to produce any significant changes in any of the assessment criteria (Hulshof et al 2000). These results suggest that different therapies may be required for the two conditions; however, larger controlled studies are needed to confirm those positive results from the preliminary open trials. Pelago et al (2010) have criticised previous trials for dosage regimens being too low (40 IU/day) to demonstrate the potential benefits. Larger well-controlled randomised studies are required.

Prevention and treatment of infections and tuberculosis

The potential immune-enhancing effect of vitamin D was first described indirectly in 1849, when cod liver oil was attributed with being one of the most efficacious agents in the treatment of pulmonary tuberculosis (Maalouf 2008). However, the treatment of tuberculosis with sunlight was prescribed by Hippocrates. It is now understood that $1,25(OH)_2D$ is a potent suppressor for *Mycobacterium tuberculosis* proliferation in human monocytes (Hewison 2011). It was demonstrated under gene array analysis that macrophage expression of the converting enzyme CYP27B1 and the VDR was induced by the activation of TLR 2/1, which is a pathogen recognition receptor for Gram-positive bacteria and *M. tuberculosis* (Liu et al 2006). This antibacterial activity is, however, not restricted to macrophages and monocytes. Vitamin D-medicated induction by intracrine synthesis also induces the expression of the gene for cathelicidin (LL-37), which is an antimicrobial peptide that produces 1,25(OH)D only in primates (Hewison 2011, Reinholz et al 2012). The production or transcription of LL-37 is stimulated by the $1,25(OH)D_2$-VDR complex, and its bacterial killing response can be enhanced by simply increasing the precursor 25(OH)D. Studies conducted by Liu et al (2006) demonstrate this capacity, where the serum from vitamin D-deficient individuals produced lower levels of LL-37 following activation by TLR 2/1 compared with individuals who were vitamin D-sufficient.

Hewison (2011) describes the role of vitamin D, which has also been shown to promote increased levels of autophagy, and the formation of associated autophagosomes. These are known to be important for intracellular isolation of pathogens and their subsequent eradication by antibacterial proteins (Hewison 2011).

Remarkably, in spite of mounting evidence regarding the vast and potent immunomodulatory effects of vitamin D, the evidence supporting its use in the prevention and treatment of infections has not progressed substantially and the small number of in vivo studies conducted in this area possess marked methodological weaknesses. The most robust evidence to date comes from a small study of 67 patients with pulmonary tuberculosis, who received 10,000 IU/day in addition to standard antimycobacterial treatment and showed higher rates of sputum conversion and radiological improvement as a result. Several post hoc analyses of vitamin D supplementation studies using other primary outcomes (e.g. fracture) have revealed trends of decreasing infections, colds and flu for those individuals taking a minimum of 800 IU/day (Grant 2008b, Maalouf 2008). In a recent Australian study (D-Health), in a secondary analysis it was found that there was a 28% non-significant reduction in antibiotic use in the vitamin D group compared to the placebo group during the study period. When the data were stratified for age, there was a significant reduction in antibiotic use in the high-dose >70-year-old group, with an RR of 0.53. Dosages were high, at 60,000 IU/month (Tran et al 2014).

This is an area of potential growth and promise. Large clinical trials with primary antibacterial outcomes are required.

Depression

Patients with primary hyperparathyroidism, which secondarily impedes the bioactivation of vitamin D and raises serum calcium, frequently present with depressive disorders that normalise following successful PTH lowering (Hoogendijk et al 2008). Rodents deficient in VDR demonstrate mood abnormalities that include increased anxiety (Hoogendijk et al 2008, Jorde et al 2006, Obradovic et al 2006), and the presence of both VDR and 1-alpha-hydroxylase activity in specific brain regions (e.g. hypothalamus) implies a potential role for vitamin D as a neuroactive hormone (Berk et al 2007, Obradovic et al 2006, Vieth et al 2004). There is also increasing evidence of vitamin D's modulation of several neurotransmitters, such as acetylcholine, catecholamines and serotonin (Jorde et al 2006, Obradovic et al 2006). Yet in spite of such strong theoretical underpinning, concerted research into the links between vitamin D and mood has only recently begun in earnest.

Recent epidemiological data reveal a strong independent inverse relationship between serum 25(OH)D and both depression scores and cognitive impairment in elderly subjects (Hoogendijk et al 2008, Johnson et al 2008, Wilkins et al 2006), premenstrual syndrome, seasonal affective disorder, non-specific mood disorder and major depressive disorder in women (Murphy & Wagner 2008), depression and anxiety in fibromyalgia patients (Armstrong et al 2007), depression rating scores on the Beck Depression Inventory in overweight and obese patients (Jorde et al 2008) and significantly lower vitamin D levels in patients with uni- and bipolar depression compared with matched controls (Berk et al 2007).

Initial interventional studies of vitamin D supplementation produced mixed findings in depression, seasonal affective disorder and general wellbeing; however, notably low doses were used (400 IU/day over short durations and in small samples), which may partly explain this lack of effect in some studies (Berk et al 2007, Hoogendijk et al 2008, Lansdowne & Provost 1998). More recent study designs have attempted to account for such shortcomings and have produced more consistent results (Jorde et al 2008, Vieth et al 2004). In two studies, thyroid outpatients with low vitamin D status during summer received either 600 or 4000 IU/day over the following 6 months (a placebo treatment was deemed unethical, given confirmation of hypovitaminosis D of all subjects at baseline). When vitamin D status and wellbeing questionnaires were repeated the following winter, improvements in mood and self-reported health were noted, particularly in those patients taking 4000 IU/day and those with the lowest serum concentrations at baseline. Another study of 441 overweight and obese individuals, only some of whom had vitamin D deficiency, found that supplementation with either 40,000 IU/week or 20,000 IU per week in combination with 500 mg/day calcium over 1 year produced significant reductions in depression rating scores (Jorde et al 2008). The greatest effects were evident in those with higher depression scores at baseline and were independent of both body mass index and initial serum 25(OH)D values. Another study of elderly women supplemented with 800 IU/day and 1000 mg/day calcium, however, failed to produce improvements on mental health scores (Dumville et al 2006).

Vieth et al (2004) comment that previous studies have suggested gender-specific mood effects of vitamin D, with women being more susceptible to seasonally-dependent mood lability and more responsive to supplementation. They also identify many potential modulating influences upon vitamin D's mood effects, which future researchers must take into consideration in addition to baseline 25(OH)D: season, dose, duration, age and sex. More well-designed research is needed in this area to clarify the real therapeutic potential of vitamin D in depressed mood.

In a systematic review of the evidence to date, while high-quality trial data are still largely unavailable, the authors conclude that this is an association evident between vitamin D deficiency and depression. They examined a total of 31,424 participants in case-control, cross-sectional and cohort studies, and found lower vitamin D levels in depressed individuals compared with controls (standard mean difference = 0.60), and an increased OR of depression in the group with the lowest vitamin D levels versus the highest group in the cross-sectional studies of 1.31, or an increase of 31%, and an increase in the hazard ratio of lowest versus highest in the cohort studies (hazard ratio = 2.21). However, for establishing more robust causal relationship data, RCTs are needed (Anglin 2013).

Clinical note — A link between vitamin D and schizophrenia?

The epidemiological correlation between babies born in winter and spring and an increased prevalence of schizophrenia has been a long-established phenomenon and presented many riddles for researchers (Eyles et al 2013, Kendell & Adams 2002). The association has also been observed in cities where air pollution reduces UV irradiation, and, more recently, a 7–10-fold increased risk has been identified in second-generation dark-skinned migrants. These observations have led to the emergence of a neurodevelopmental theory of schizophrenia, which suggests that low prenatal vitamin D interferes with brain development by interacting with D-responsive/susceptible genes to create the currently recognised polygenic effects of schizophrenia (Mackay-Sim et al 2004).

A significant progression of this theory was made at the Queensland Centre for Schizophrenic Research, led by Professor John McGrath. The centre's work has taken the level of evidence beyond the early epidemiological findings, with research being conducted to assess the impact of vitamin D deficiency on animal brains and in vitro cultures. Research has also been conducted to measure third-trimester serum 25(OH)D levels in schizophrenic and schizo-affective mothers, while investigating the impact of vitamin D supplementation prior to 1 year of age in the infants and the subsequent risk reduction for the disease in later life (McGrath et al 2003, 2004a, 2004b). Subsequent investigations from the same group (Eyles et al 2013) have furthered the basic science evidence for the developmental basis of vitamin D deficiency and its association with schizophrenia. The evidence to date shows support for this hypothesis, with a consistent positive relationship appearing for males, and evidence pointing towards a stronger relationship in dark-skinned populations compared to fairer-skinned populations.

OTHER USES

Multiple sclerosis

There is strong evidence that vitamin D status is associated with risk of MS (Grant 2006, Kampman

& Brustad 2008, Kragt et al 2009, Hewison 2011, Munger et al 2006, Niino et al 2008, Smolders et al 2008). A variety of observational studies illustrate a relationship between MS incidence and geographical location, with very low prevalence in the equatorial regions and increasing risk with increasing latitude in both hemispheres. Other demonstrated associations with MS incidence include the level of outdoor activity in adolescents and risk of onset later in life, while there is evidence of lower 25(OH)D levels in newly diagnosed patients when compared to controls and in relapsing patients compared to those in remission (Kampman & Brustad 2008, Niino et al 2008, Smolders et al 2008). Evidence is more mixed regarding VDR polymorphisms, month of birth and season of diagnosis.

In spite of these findings, strong evidence linking vitamin D to modulation of MS is currently lacking. A limited number of interventional studies using vitamin D also leave us without a firm conclusion. Some studies, including the Nurses' Health Study, point towards a protective effect in the years following regular supplement use, but the effects of vitamin D are difficult to extricate from other supplemented nutrients. In an open and uncontrolled study of 39 MS patients treated with 1000 IU/day for 6 months, changes in inflammatory markers were observed but clinical benefits were not investigated. The most promising study to date was conducted in 12 patients administered 1000 IU/day over 28 weeks, which reduced the number of gadolinium-enhancing lesions on the magnetic resonance imaging of one subject (Smolders et al 2008).

In the latest Cochrane review of vitamin D for the management of MS (Jagannath et al 2010), only one study was of sufficient quality to be included in the review. The results of this review suggest that there is some evidence of a beneficial effect of vitamin D supplementation, and a relative absence of any adverse events or risk of high serum calcium levels. A single trial assessed outcomes for 49 participants over a 52-week period. The study group (n = 25) were administered with escalating doses of vitamin D, and demonstrated a relative benefit in outcomes such as annualised relapse rate, suppression of T-cell proliferation and higher satisfaction scores. Hewison (2011) reviews evidence for the experimental autoimmune encephalomyelitis mouse model of MS, that shows an increased severity of disease under dietary restrictions of vitamin D, and a protective effect against symptoms when used therapeutically.

Crohn's disease and other inflammatory bowel disease

Crohn's disease is an autoimmune disease marked by an aberrant colonic immune response to enteric bacteria (Hewison 2012). Epidemiological evidence suggests that incidence of Crohn's disease and other inflammatory bowel diseases, in adult and paediatric patients, is related to levels of circulating vitamin D (Vagianos et al 2007). Research by Liu et al (2013) has identified that VDR expression on the intestinal epithelium is substantially reduced in patients with Crohn's disease or ulcerative colitis, and that in the knockout mouse model, gut epithelial VDR signalling has potent anticolitic activity that can be differentiated and is independent of non-epithelial immune VDR actions. Elevation of VDR expression by an approximate factor of 2 was protective against many experimental colitis models.

In another VDR gene knockout mouse study, aberrant gut migration of a specific cytotoxic T cell appears to be linked to an increased risk of inflammatory bowel disease (Yu et al 2008). In a study of vitamin D status in a paediatric population with inflammatory bowel disease, the prevalence of deficiency was reported to be 34.6%. Deficiency was more pronounced in children with darker skin, in winter months and in those not taking vitamin D supplementation (Pappa 2006). Hewison (2012) elucidates the aberrant or inadequate innate immune response of enteric microbiota as initiating an inflammatory adaptive immune response and its consequent damage. The effectiveness of vitamin D therapeutics may well function to both stimulate the innate immune response and suppress the inflammatory adaptive immune response.

Lupus (SLE)

There is growing evidence suggesting an aetiological role for vitamin D in SLE, as in MS and other autoimmune diseases. In addition to epidemiological studies showing low 25(OH)D in SLE patients compared to healthy controls, and inverse correlations between vitamin D status and disease severity, individuals with this condition are identified as being at high risk of vitamin D deficiency because of a range of factors (Cutolo & Otsa 2008, Kamen & Aranow 2008). These factors include increased photosensitivity, renal involvement impeding bioactivation and evidence of anti-D antibodies in select patient subsets. Data from animal and in vitro studies also point to vitamin D as an effective treatment, in particular reversing the characteristic immune abnormalities, while experimentally-induced deficiencies exacerbate clinical features. Additionally, given that SLE is a B-cell-related disorder, studies demonstrating the effect of 1,25(OH)D on VDR-expressing B cells indicate a suppression of proliferation and immunoglobulin production, and with the identification that B cells have a capacity to express CYP27B1 to activate conversion of vitamin D, this highlights the potential role of vitamin D in disorders such as SLE (Hewison 2012). Interventional studies in SLE patients are now required to confirm this indication.

Psoriasis

As a regulator of cellular growth and differentiation in various tissues, vitamin D has been investigated in psoriasis. The active form of vitamin D and its analogues have been found to suppress growth and stimulate the terminal differentiation of keratinocytes. Schauber et al (2011) have found that vitamin D may ameliorate the symptoms of psoriasis when treated with the antimicrobial peptide cathelicidin, whose production in the skin is stimulated by vitamin D.

Vaginal atrophy

Animal studies have revealed the presence of VDR in the cells lining the vagina (Yildirim et al 2004a). Given the established role of vitamin D in regulating growth and differentiation of tissues, especially those lining stratified squamous epithelium, a possible role for vitamin D in the prevention and treatment of vaginal atrophy associated with menopause is being considered (Yildirim et al 2004b). A number of studies involving co-administration with calcium have produced some positive results; however, a trial of calcium and D_3 (500 mg/day and 400 IU/day, respectively) used as a replacement for transdermal oestrogen replacement therapy in menopausal women over 1 year revealed an objective worsening of vaginal atrophy (Checa et al 2005). Dose, however, may be an issue.

DOSAGE RANGE

Acceptable daily intake (ADI)

The NHMRC vitamin guidelines released in 2006 make the following recommendations for ADI:

- Children and adults < 50 years: 200 IU/day.
- Adults 51–70 years: 400 IU/day.
- Adults over 70 years: 600 IU/day.

The ADI is based on the amount of vitamin D required to maintain serum 25(OH)D at a level of at least 27.5 nmol/L with minimal sun exposure. The level has been raised in the 51–70-year age group to account for the reduced capacity of the skin to produce vitamin D with ageing. The higher level recommended in the over-70-years group was made because this group tends to have less exposure to sunlight.

In a recent systematic review, recommendations were made on a 'per kg of body weight' dosage. The review found that up to 34.5% of variation in circulating 25(OH)D could be explained by body weight. The authors also found that type of supplement (D_3 or D_2), age, concomitant calcium intake and baseline 25(OH)D could explain further variations in circulating levels (Zittermann et al 2014).

According to clinical studies

(D_3 supplemental form unless otherwise indicated.)

- Uncomplicated rickets: 1600 IU/day for the first month, gradually reducing the dose to 400 IU.
- Osteomalacia: 36,000 IU/day with calcium supplementation.
- Rickets and osteomalacia due to defective metabolism: 50,000–300,000 IU/day.
- Pregnancy supplementation: two large doses of 600,000 IU in the seventh and eighth months (Marya et al 1981).
- Reduction in fractures associated with osteoporosis: prevention of fractures has resulted from as little as 200 IU/day in combination with calcium, but the most effective dose is ≥800 IU/day in combination with ≥1200 mg/day calcium.
- Reduction in falls: 1000 IU/day in combination with 1000 mg/day calcium.
- Hyperparathyroidism: 2.5–6.25 mg/day.
- Hepatic osteodystrophy: 4000 IU/day.
- Anticonvulsant osteomalacia: 4000 IU D_2/day for 105 days, followed by 1000 IU/day.
- Systemic scleroderma: 0.75–1.25 mcg D_3/day for 6 months.

TOXICITY

Toxic ingestion of prescribed forms of vitamin D or excessive dietary consumption of either D_2 or D_3 has been reported in the vicinity of 50,000–100,000 IU/day or 10,000 IU/day taken routinely for several months. Obtaining such enormous amounts from unfortified foods is improbable. Traditionally the toxicity picture of vitamin D has been attributed to a secondary hypercalcaemia, which manifests as anorexia, nausea, vomiting, polyuria, muscle pain, unusual tiredness, dry mouth, persistent headache and secondary polydipsia. Over extended periods of time, this state of hypervitaminosis can result in metastatic calcification of soft tissues, including kidney, blood vessels, heart and lungs. Symptoms and signs at this later stage include cloudy urine, pruritus, drowsiness, weight loss, sensitivity to light, hypertension, arrhythmia, fever and abdominal pain. Toxic levels cannot be obtained from excessive sun exposure (FAO/WHO 2002, Gropper et al 2009). More recent research into vitamin D pharmacokinetics, however, points towards 25(OH)D's ability at high doses to displace $1,25(OH)_2D$ from VDR, therefore increasing free concentrations of the active form and subsequent gene transcription (Jones 2008).

ADVERSE REACTIONS

High doses of supplements may induce the following:

- arterial calcification
- arrhythmia
- gastrointestinal distress, including nausea, vomiting and constipation
- hypercalcaemia
- nephrotoxicity, manifesting as polyuria, polydipsia and nocturia.

SIGNIFICANT INTERACTIONS

Only those interactions relevant to the oral supplemental forms of vitamin D will be reviewed.

A number of pharmacokinetic and pharmacodynamic interactions are possible with vitamin D and a range of medicines and minerals.

Antituberculosis drugs

Drugs such as rifampicin and isoniazid have been reported to induce catabolism of vitamin D and in some cases manifest as reduced levels of metabolites. This may represent a concern in those patients already at risk of poor vitamin D status (Harkness & Bratman 2003).

Calcium channel blockers

Vitamin D supplementation may reduce the effectiveness of these drugs. Use with caution unless under medical supervision (Harkness & Bratman 2003).

Glucocorticoids

In high doses, these drugs directly inhibit vitamin D-mediated calcium uptake in the gastrointestinal tract and through unknown mechanisms may deplete levels of active vitamin D (Wilson et al 1991). During long-term therapy with either oral or inhaled corticosteroids, calcium and vitamin D supplementation should be considered.

Ketoconazole

This drug reduces the conversion of vitamin D to its active forms. Increased vitamin D intake may be required with long-term drug use.

Lipid-lowering drugs

Drugs such as cholestyramine and colestipol may compromise the absorption of all fat-soluble vitamins. To avoid the interaction, administer the supplement at least 1 hour prior to or 4–6 hours after ingestion of the drug (Harkness & Bratman 2003). Conversely, long-term use of statins is associated with increased 25(OH)D levels via an unknown mechanism (Aloia et al 2007).

Magnesium

Either an excess or inadequate level of magnesium can impact on vitamin D status. The final hydroxylation step to $1,25(OH)_2D_3$ is dependent upon magnesium and a deficiency would compromise this. However, high levels of magnesium, mimicking calcium, can suppress PTH secretion, also suppressing the activation phase (Groff & Gropper 2005). Therefore magnesium levels within the normal range will enhance activation of vitamin D to its active form.

Mineral oil

Mineral oil impairs absorption of all fat-soluble nutrients and may therefore deplete oral intake of vitamin D sources. Separate doses by at least 2 hours.

Oestrogens

Vitamin D works synergistically with oestrogens to prevent bone loss. Interaction is beneficial.

Orlistat

Although orlistat has been shown to reduce the absorption of some fat-soluble nutrients, its effect on vitamin D specifically remains unclear. Concurrent supplementation of a multivitamin with D is advised. Separate doses by a minimum of 4 hours either side of ingestion of orlistat (Harkness & Bratman 2003).

Phenytoin and valproate

The anticonvulsants induce catabolism of vitamin D through liver induction and prolonged use is associated with increased risk of developing rickets and osteomalacia.

Practice points/Patient counselling

- Vitamin D has a critical role in bone growth and development, but also has diverse roles throughout the body, including inhibiting abnormal proliferation of cells.
- Most vitamin D is endogenously produced through sun exposure and an activation process that involves both the liver and the kidneys; food sources represent a secondary and often unreliable source. Those groups in the community who have restricted sun exposure are at the greatest risk of a deficiency, including the elderly, newborns, institutionalised, adolescents and young children with marginal calcium intake during rapid growth periods, and those with dark skins.
- In the prevention of falls and prevention or treatment of osteoporosis, vitamin D supplements are most commonly given in combination with other nutrients, such as calcium.
- Other uses for vitamin D include: supplementation during pregnancy to increase fetal levels; correction of deficiencies that may result from medications or malabsorptive diseases such as coeliac disease, Crohn's disease and cystic fibrosis; as a protective agent against breast, prostate and colorectal cancer; and for a variety of metabolic bone disorders. Evidence suggests that higher circulating vitamin D levels may also be associated with better prognosis in patients with breast and colorectal cancer and vitamin D supplementation, reducing mortiality in the elderly.

CONTRAINDICATIONS AND PRECAUTIONS

- Hypersensitivity to vitamin D.
- Hypercalcaemia.
- Not to be taken in sarcoidosis or hyperparathyroidism without medical supervision.
- Possible interference with the action of calcium channel blockers.
- High doses require medical supervision in patients with arteriosclerosis and heart disease.
- High doses capable of inducing hypercalcaemia may precipitate arrhythmias in patients taking digitalis.

PREGNANCY USE

Vitamin D supplements as either D_2 or D_3 are exempt from pregnancy classification by the Therapeutic Goods Administration, which reflects their safety in pregnancy and lactation (Australian Drug Evaluation Committee 1999).

PATIENTS' FAQs

What will this vitamin do for me?

Vitamin D is essential for health and wellbeing. It plays a critical role in regulating calcium and phosphorus levels in the body, and is important for healthy bones and preventing abnormal cell changes, which may increase the risk of some cancers. Optimal levels of vitamin D appear to be associated with reduced mortality and supplementation for reducing mortality in the elderly.

When will it start to work?

This will depend on the condition being treated. In uncomplicated rickets, serum levels should begin to rise in 1–2 days, and after 3 weeks signs of calcium and phosphorus mineralisation appear on X-ray. For disease prevention, long-term adequate vitamin D status is recommended.

Are there any safety issues?

Vitamin D is considered a safe supplement when used in the recommended doses; however, it may interact with some medicines.

REFERENCES

Alemzadeh R et al. Hypovitaminosis D in obese children and adolescents: relationship with adiposity, insulin sensitivity, ethnicity, and season. Metabolism 57.2 (2008): 183–91.

Al Faraj S, Al Mutairi K. Vitamin D deficiency and chronic low back pain in Saudi Arabia. Spine 28.2 (2003): 177–9.

Aloia JF, et al. Statins and vitamin D. Am J Cardiol 100.8 (2007): 1329.

Andiran N, et al. Risk factors for vitamin D deficiency in breast-fed newborns and their mothers. Nutrition 18 (2002): 47–50.

Andress DL. Vitamin D in chronic kidney disease: A systemic role for selective vitamin D receptor activation. Kidney Int 69.1 (2006): 33–43.

Angeline M et al. The effects of vitamin D deficiency in athletes. Am J Sp Med 41 (2013): 461–464.

Anglin R. Vitamin D deficiency and depression in adults: systematic review and meta-analysis. Brit J Psych 202.2 (2013): 100–107.

Armas LA, et al. Vitamin D2 is much less effective than vitamin D3 in humans. J Clin Endocrinol Metab 89.11 (2004): 5387–91.

Armstrong DJ et al. Vitamin D deficiency is associated with anxiety and depression in fibromyalgia. Clin Rheumatol 26.4 (2007): 551–4.

Arunabh S et al. Body fat content and 25-hydroxyvitamin D levels in healthy women. J Clin Endocrinol Metab 88.1 (2003): 157–61.

Australian Drug Evaluation Committee. Prescribing medicines in pregnancy, 4th edn. Canberra: Therapeutic Goods Administration, 1999.

Bailey R et al. Association of the vitamin D metabolism gene CYP27B1 with type 1 diabetes. Diabetes 56 (2007): 2616–2621.

Beers MH, Berkow R (eds). The Merck manual of diagnosis and therapy, 17th edn. Whitehouse, NJ: Merck, 2003.

Berk M et al. Vitamin D deficiency may play a role in depression. Med Hypotheses 69.6 (2007): 1316–19.

Bikle DD. Vitamin D and the immune system: role in protection against bacterial infection. Curr Opin Nephrol Hypertens 17.4 (2008): 348–52.

Bischoff-Ferrari HA et al. Vitamin D receptor expression in human muscle tissue decreases with age. J Bone Miner Res 19.2 (2004): 265–69.

Bischoff-Ferrari HA et al. Is fall prevention by vitamin D mediated by a change in postural or dynamic balance? Osteoporos Int 17.5 (2006): 656–63.

Blum M, et al. Vitamin D(3) in fat tissue. Endocrine 33.1 (2008): 90–4.

Bodnar L et al. Maternal vitamin D deficiency increases the risk of pre-eclampsia. J Clin Endo Metab 92.9 (2007): 3517–22.

Boelsma E et al. Effects of calcitriol on fibroblasts derived from skin of scleroderma patients. Dermatology 191.3 (1995): 226–33.

Borissova AM et al. The effects of vitamin D3 on insulin secretion and peripheral insulin sensitivity in type 2 diabetic patients. Int J Clin Pract 57.4 (2003): 258–61.

Bouillon R et al. Ageing and calcium metabolism. Baillieres Clin Endocrinol Metab 11.2 (1997): 341–65.

Bowyer L, et al Vitamin D, PTH and calcium levels in pregnant women and their neonates. Clin Endocrinol (Oxf) 70.3 (2009): 372–7.

Braun, L.A., et al (2014) Prevalence of Vitamin D Deficiency Prior to Cardiothoracic Surgery. Heart, Lung and Circulation (0) available from: http://www.sciencedirect.com/science/article/pii/S1443950614001504

Brown A et al. Vitamin D. Am J Phys 277 (1999): F157–75.

Brunner RL et al. Calcium, vitamin D supplementation, and physical function in the Women's Health Initiative. J Am Diet Assoc 108.9 (2008): 1472–9.

Bruyere O et al. Highest prevalence of vitamin D inadequacy in institutionalized women compared with noninstitutionalized women: a case-control study. Women's Health (Lond Engl) 5.1 (2009): 49–54.

Buchman AL. Bones and Crohn's: problems and solutions. Inflamm Bowel Dis 5.3 (1999): 212–227.

Byrne J H et al. The impact of adult vitamin D deficiency on behavior and brain function in male Sprague-Dawley rats. Brain Rd Bull 65.2 (2005): 141–8.

Caca-Biljanovska NG et al. Treatment of generalized morphea with oral 1,25-dihydroxyvitamin D3. Adv Exp Med Biol 455 (1999): 299–304.

Cannell JJ. Autism and vitamin D. Med Hypotheses 70.4 (2008):750–9.

Cannell J et al. Athletic performance and vitamin D. Med Sci Sports Exerc. 41.5 (2009): 1102–1110.

Cantor-Graae E, Selten JP. Schizophrenia and migration: a meta-analysis and review. Am J Psychiatry 162.1 (2005):12–24.

Cauley JA et al. Serum 25-hydroxyvitamin D concentrations and risk for hip fractures. Ann Intern Med 149.4 (2008): 242–50.

Ceglia L. Vitamin D and its role in skeletal muscle. Curr Opin Clin Nutr Metab Care 12.6 (2009): 628–633.

Chatfield S et al. Vitamin D deficiency in general medical inpatients in summer and winter. Intern Med 37 (2007): 377–82.

Checa MA et al. A comparison of raloxifene and calcium plus vitamin D on vaginal atrophy after discontinuation of long-standing postmenopausal hormone therapy in osteoporotic women. A randomized, masked-evaluator, one-year, prospective study. Maturitas 52.1 (2005): 70–7.

Chen TC, Holick MF. Vitamin D prostate cancer prevention and treatment. Trends Endocrinol Metabol 14.9 (2003): 423–431.

Chowdhury R et al. Vitamin D and risk of cause specific death: systematic review and meta-analysis of observational cohort and randomised intervention studies. BMJ 348 (2014): g1903.

Chung M et al. Vitamin D with or without calcium supplementation for the prevention of cancer and fractures: an updated meta-analysis for the U.S. Preventive Services Task Forch. Arm Intern Med. 155.12 (2011): 827–838.

Clancy N et al. Vitamin D and neonatal immune function. J Matern Fetal Neoant Med 26.7 (2013): 639–646.

Compston JE et al. Treatment of osteomalacia associated with primary biliary cirrhosis with parenteral vitamin D2 or 25-hydroxyvitamin D3. Gut 20 (1979): 133–6.

Congden PJ et al. Vitamin status in treated patients with cystic fibrosis. Arch Dis Child 56.9 (1981): 708–14.

Cooper, J et al. Inherited Variation in Vitamin D Genes Is Associated With Predisposition to Autoimmune Disease Type 1 Diabetes. Diabet 60.5 (2011):1624–31.

Cosman F. The prevention and treatment of osteoporosis: a review. Med Gen Med 7.2 (2005): 73.

Cranney A et al. Summary of evidence-based review on vitamin D efficacy and safety in relation to bone health. Am J Clin Nutr 88.2 (2008): 513S–19S.

Cui X, et al. Maternal vitamin D deficiency alters the expression of genes involved in dopamine specification in the developing rat mesencephalon. Neurosci Lett 486.3 (2010): 220–3.

Cutolo M, Otsa K. Review: vitamin D, immunity and lupus. Lupus 17.1 (2008): 6–10.

Davies G, et al. A systematic review and meta-analysis of Northern Hemisphere season of birth studies in schizophrenia. Schizophr Bull 29.3 (2003):587–93.

Dawson-Hughes B et al. Estimates of optimal vitamin D status. Osteoporos Int 16.7 (2005): 713–16.

De-Regil LM et al. Vitamin D supplementation for women during pregnancy. Cochrane Datab Syst Rev. 2 (2012): DOI: 10.1002/14651858.

Deroisy R et al. Administration of a supplement containing both calcium and vitamin D is more effective than calcium alone to reduce secondary hyperparathyroidism in postmenopausal women with low 25(OH) vitamin D circulating levels. Aging Clin Exp Res 14.1 (2002): 13–17.

Ding EL et al. Interaction of estrogen therapy with calcium and vitamin D supplementation on colorectal cancer risk: reanalysis of Women's Health Initiative randomized trial. Int J Cancer 122.8 (2008): 1690–4.

Dixon K et al. In vivo relevance for photoprotection by the vitamin D rapid response pathway. J Steroid 103.3–5 (2007): 451–6.

Drezner MK. Treatment of anticonvulsant drug-induced bone disease. Epilep & Beh 5 (2004) S41–S4.

Dumville JC et al. Can vitamin D supplementation prevent winter-time blues? A randomised trial among older women. J Nutr Health Aging 10.2 (2006): 151–3.

Dusso A, et al. Vitamin D. Am J Physiol Renal Physiol 289 (2005): F8–28.

Erbas B, et al. Suburban clustering of vitamin D deficiency in Melbourne, Australia. Asia Pac J Clin Nutr 17.1 (2008): 63–7.

Eyles D et al. Vitamin D3 and brain development. Neuroscience 118 (2003): 641–653.

Eyles DW et al. Vitamin D in fetal brain development. Seminars in cell & devt boil 22 (2011): 629–636.

Eyles DW et al. Vitamin D, effects on brain development, adult brain function and the links between low levels of vitamin D and neurophychiatric disease. Front Neuroendocrin 34 (2013): 47–64.

Eyles DW et al. Intracellular distribution of the vitamin D receptor in the brain: comparison with classic target tissues and redistribution with development. Neurosci 268 (2014): 1–9.

FAO/WHO (Food and Agriculture Organization/World Health Organization). Report of a joint FAO/WHO expert consultation, Bangkok, Thailand. Rome: FAO/WHO, 2002.

Forman J et al. Plasma 25-hydroxyvitamin D levels and risk of incident hypertension. Hypertension 49.5 (2007): 1063–9.

FSANZ (Food Standards Australia New Zealand). Australia New Zealand Food Standards Code. Report no. 91. Canberra: FSANZ, 2007.

Garcion E et al. New clues about vitamin D functions in the nervous system. Trends Endocrinol Metab 13.3 (2002): 100–5.

Garland CF et al. Can colon cancer incidence and death rates be reduced with calcium and vitamin D? Am J Clin Nutr 54.1 (Suppl) (1991): 193–201S.

Garland CF et al. Calcium and vitamin D: Their potential roles in colon and breast cancer prevention. Ann NY Acad Sci 889 (1999): 107–19.

Garland CF et al. An epidemiologic basis for estimating optimal vitamin D3 intake for colon cancer prevention and a public health recommendation for greater vitamin D intake. AEP 15.8 (2004): 630.

Giovannucci E. Vitamin D status and cancer incidence and mortality. Adv Exp Med Biol 624 (2008): 31–42.

Gissel T et al. Intake of vitamin D and risk of breast cancer — a meta-analysis. J Steroid Biochem Mol Biol 111.3–5 (2008): 195–9.

Glendenning P. Vitamin D deficiency and multicultural Australia. Med J Aust 176.5 (2002): 242–3.

Gomez AC et al. Review of the concept of vitamin D 'sufficiency and insufficiency'. Nefrologia 23.2 (2003): 73–7.

Grant WB. Epidemiology of disease risks in relation to vitamin D insufficiency. Prog Biophys Mol Biol 92.1 (2006): 65–79.

Grant WB. Solar ultraviolet irradiance and cancer incidence and mortality. Adv Exp Med Biol 624 (2008a): 16–30.

Grant WB. Hypothesis — ultraviolet-B irradiance and vitamin D reduce the risk of viral infections and thus their sequelae, including autoimmune diseases and some cancers. Photochem Photobiol 84.2 (2008b): 356–65.

Grant WB. Differences in vitamin-D status may explain black–white differences in breast cancer survival rates. J Natl Med Assoc 100.9 (2008c): 1040.

Grant WB. Ecological studies of the UV-B-vitamin D-cancer hypothesis. Anitcancer Res 32.1 (2012): 223–236.

Grant WB, Garland CF. A critical review of studies on vitamin D in relation to colorectal cancer. Nutr Cancer 48.2 (2004): 115–23.

Grant WB, Soles CM. Epidemiologic evidence supporting the role of maternal vitamin D deficiency as a risk factor for the development of infantile autism. Dermatoendocrin 1.4 (2009):223–8.

Grau MV et al. Vitamin D, calcium supplementation, and colorectal adenomas: results of a randomized trial. J Natl Cancer Inst 95.23 (2003): 1765–71.

Greer RM, et al. Australian children and adolescents with Type 1 diabetes have low vitamin D levels. Med. J. Aust. 187.1 (2007): 59–60.

Groff JL, Gropper SS. Advanced nutrition and human metabolism. Belmont, CA: Wadsworth, 2005.

Gropper SS, et al. Advanced nutrition and human metabolism, 5th edition. Belmont, CA: Wadsworth, 2009.

Grover SR, Morley R. Vitamin D deficiency in veiled or dark-skinned pregnant women. Med J Aust 175 (2001): 251–2.

Hall A and Juckett M. The role of vitamin D in hematologic disease and stem cell transplantation. Nutr 5 (2013): 2206–2221.

Hanly JG et al. Hypovitaminosis D and response to supplementation in older patients with cystic fibrosis. Q J Med 56.219 (1985): 377–85.

Harkness LS, Bonny AE. Calcium and vitamin D status in adolescents: Key roles for bone, body weight, glucose tolerance and estrogen biosynthesis. J Pediatr Adolesc Gynecol 18 (2005): 305–11.

Harkness R, Bratman S. Mosby's handbook of drug–herb and drug–supplements interactions. St Louis: Mosby, 2003.

Harms L et al. Vitamin D and the brain. Best Prac & Res Clin Endocrin & Metab 25 (2011) 657–669

Harris SS, Dawson Hughes B. Reduced sun exposure does not explain the inverse association of 25-hydroxyvitamin D with percent body fat in older adults. J Clin Endocrinol Metab 92.8 (2007): 3155–7.

Hartwell D et al. Metabolism of vitamin D2 and vitamin D3 in patients on anti-convulsant therapy. Acta Neurol Scand 79.6 (1989): 487–92.

Heaney R. Barriers to optimizing vitamin D3 intake for the elderly. J Nutr 136.4 (2006): 1123–5.

Hendler SS, Rorvik D (eds). PDR for nutritional supplements. Montvale, NJ: Medical Economics, 2001.

Hoffmann JC, Zeitz M. Treatment of Crohn's disease. Hepatogastroenterology 47.31 (2000): 90–100.

Holick MF. Vitamin D and health in the 21st century: bone and beyond: sunlight and vitamin D for bone health and prevention of autoimmune diseases, cancers, and cardiovascular disease. Am J Clin Nutr 80.6 (2004):1678–188S.

Holick M. The vitamin D epidemic and its health consequences. J Nutr 135 (2005): 2739S–48S.

Holick M. Vitamin D. In: Shils M (ed.), Modern nutrition in health and disease, 10th edn. Baltimore: Lippincott Williams & Wilkins, 2006, pp 376–95.

Holt PR. New insights into calcium, dairy and colon cancer. World J Gastroenterol 14.28 (2008): 4429–33.

Holt PR et al. Colonic epithelial cell proliferation decreases with increasing levels of serum 25-hydroxy vitamin D. Cancer Epidemiol Biomarkers Prev 11.1 (2002): 113–19.

Hoogendijk WJ et al. Depression is associated with decreased 25-hydroxyvitamin D and increased parathyroid hormone levels in older adults. Arch Gen Psychiatry 65.5 (2008): 508–12.

Hossein-Nezhad A, Holick MF. Vitamin D for health: A global perspective. Mayo Clinic Proc 88 (2013): 720–55.

Houghton LA, Vieth R. The case against ergocalciferol (vitamin D2) as a vitamin supplement. Am J Clin Nutr. 84.4 (2006): 694–7.

Huh SY, Gordon CM. Vitamin D deficiency in children and adolescents: epidemiology, impact and treatment. Rev Endocr Metab Disord 9.2 (2008): 161–70.

Hulshof MM et al. Oral calcitriol as a new therapeutic modality for generalized morphea. Arch Dermatol 130.10 (1994): 12990–3.

Hulshof MM et al. Double-blind, placebo-controlled study of oral calcitriol for the treatment of localized and systemic scleroderma. J Am Acad Dermatol 43.6 (2000): 1017–23.

Huncharek M, et al. Dairy products, dietary calcium and vitamin D intake as risk factors for prostate cancer: a meta-analysis of 26,769 cases from 45 observational studies. Nutr Cancer 60.4 (2008): 421–41.

Hunter D et al. A randomized controlled trial of vitamin D supplementation on preventing postmenopausal bone loss and modifying bone metabolism using identical twin pairs. J Bone Miner Res 15.11 (2000): 2276–83.

Hyppönen E et al. Vitamin D and increasing incidence of type 1 diabetes-evidence for an association? Diabet Obes Metab 12 (2010): 737–743.

Hyppönen E et al. Intake of vitamin D and risk of type 1 diabetes: a birth-cohort study. Lancet 358 (2001): 1500–3.

Jagannath V et al. Vitamin D for the management of multiple sclerosis. Cochrane Datab Syst Rev. 12 (2010): DOI:10.1002/14651858.

Jahnsen J et al. Vitamin D status, parathyroid hormone and bone mineral density in patients with inflammatory bowel disease. Scand J Gastroenterol 37.2 (2002): 192–9.

Janda M et al. Sun protection messages, vitamin D and skin cancer: out of the frying pan and into the fire? MJA 186.2 (2007): 52–3.

Johnson S. Micronutrient accumulation and depletion in schizophrenia, epilepsy, autism and Parkinson's disease? Med Hypotheses 56.5 (2001): 641–5.

Johnson MA et al. Age, race and season predict vitamin D status in African American and white octogenarians and centenarians. J Nutr Health Aging 12.10 (2008): 690–5.

Jones G. Pharmacokinetics of vitamin D toxicity. Am J Clin Nutr 88.2 (2008): 582S–6S.

Jorde R et al. Neuropsychological function in relation to serum parathyroid hormone and serum 25-hydroxyvitamin D levels. The Tromsø study. J Neurol 253.4 (2006): 464–70.

Jorde R et al. Effects of vitamin D supplementation on symptoms of depression in overweight and obese subjects: randomized double blind trial. J Intern Med 264.6 (2008): 599–609.

Kalueff AV, Tuohimaa P. Vitamin D: an antiepileptic neurosteroid hormone? Eur Neuropsychopharmacol 15 (Suppl 3) (2005): S618.

Kamen D, Aranow C. Vitamin D in systemic lupus erythematosus. Curr Opin Rheumatol 20.5 (2008): 532–7.

Kampman MT, Brustad M, Vitamin D: a candidate for the environmental effect in multiple sclerosis — observations from Norway. Neuroepidemiology 30.3 (2008): 140–6.

Kemmis C et al. Human mammary epithelial cells express CYP27B1 and are growth inhibited by 25-hydroxyvitamin D-3, the major circulating form of vitamin D-3. J Nutr 136 (2006): 887–92.

Kendell RE, Adams W. Exposure to sunlight, vitamin D and schizophrenia. Schizophrenia Res 54 (2002): 193–8.

Kim G, Sprague SM. Use of vitamin D analogs in chronic renal failure. Adv Renal Replace Ther 9.3 (2002): 175–83.

Kim JS et al. Association of vitamin D receptor gene polymorphism and Parkinson's disease in Koreans. J Korean Med Sci J 20.3 (2005): 495–8.

Kimlin M et al. Does a high UV environment ensure adequate vitamin D status? J Photochem Photobiol B 89.2–3 (2007): 139–47.

Klein GL et al. Hepatic dystrophy in chronic cholestasis: evidence for a multifactorial etiology. Pediatr Transplant 6.2 (2002): 136–40.

Kohlmeier M. Nutrient metabolism. London: Academic Press, 2003.
Kumar P, Clark M. Clinical medicine, 5th edn. London: WB Saunders, 2002.
Kutuzova G, DeLuca H. 1,25-dihydroxyvitamin D(3) regulates genes responsible for detoxification in intestine. Toxicol Appl Pharmacol 218 (2007): 37–44 (abstract).
Lansdowne AT, Provost SC. Vitamin D3 enhances mood in healthy subjects during winter. Psychopharmacology (Berl) 135.4 (1998): 319–23.
Lappe J et al. Vitamin D and calcium supplementation reduces cancer risk: results of a randomized trial. AJCN 85.6 (2007): 1586–91.
Lee JE et al. Circulating levels of vitamin D and colon and rectal cancer the Physicians' Health Study and a meta-analysis of prospective studies. Cancer Prev Res. 4.5 (2011): 735–743.
Li H et al. A prospective study of plasma vitamin D metabolites, vitamin D receptor polymorphisms, and prostate cancer. PLoS Med 4.3 (2007): e103.
Lips P. Vitamin D physiology. Prog Biophys Mol Biol 92.1 (2006): 4–8.
Littorin, B et al. Lower levels of plasma 25-hydroxyvitamin D among young adults at diagnosis of autoimmune type 1 diabetes compared with control subjects: Results from the nationwide Diabetes Incidence Study in Sweden (DISS). Diabetologia 49 (2006): 2847–2852.
Liu PT et al. Toll-like receptor triggering of a vitamin D-mediated human antimicrobial response. Science 311 (2006): 1770–1773.
Long RG, Wills MR. Hepatic osteodystrophy. Br J Hosp Med 20.3 (1978): 312–21.
Lowe C et al. Plasma 25-hydroxy vitamin D concentrations, vitamin D receptor genotype and breast cancer risk in a UK Caucasian population. Eur J Cancer 41 (2005): 1164–9.
Lu Z et al. An evaluation of the vitamin D3 content in fish: Is the vitamin D content adequate to satisfy the dietary requirement for vitamin D? J Steroid Biochem Mol Biol 103.3–5 (2007): 642–4.
Lyles KW et al. The efficacy of vitamin D2 and oral phosphorus therapy in X-linked hypophosphatemic rickets and osteomalacia. J Clin Endocrinol Metab 54 (1982): 307–15.
Ma JF et al. Mechanisms of decreased vitamin D 1 alpha hydrolase activity in prostate cancer cells. Mol Cell Endocrinol 221 (2004): 67–74.
Maalouf NM. The noncalciotropic actions of vitamin D: recent clinical developments. Curr Opin Nephrol Hypertens 17.4 (2008): 408–15.
Mackay-Sim A et al. Schizophrenia, vitamin D, and brain development. Int Rev Neurobiol 59 (2004): 351–80.
Marya RK et al. Effects of vitamin D supplementation in pregnancy. Gynecol Obstet Invest 12.3 (1981): 155–61.
Marya RK et al. Effect of calcium and vitamin D supplementation on toxaemia of pregnancy. Gynecol Obstet Invest 24.1 (1987): 38–42.
Mathieu C, Badenhoop K. Vitamin D and type 1 diabetes mellitus: state of the art. Trends Endocrinol Metab 16.6 (2005): 262–6.
Mattila P et al. Effect of vitamin D2- and D3-enriched diets on egg vitamin D content, production, and bird condition during an entire production period. Poult Sci 83.3 (2004): 433–40.
Matsuoka LY et al. Cutaneous vitamin D3 formation in progressive systemic sclerosis. J Rheumatol 18.8 (1991): 1196–8.
McGillivray G, et al. High prevalence of asymptomatic vitamin D and iron deficiency in East African immigrant children and adolescents living in a temperate climate. Arch Dis Child 92.12 (2007): 1088–93.
McGrath J et al. Low maternal vitamin D as a risk factor for schizophrenia: a pilot study using banked sera. Schizophrenia Res 63 (2003): 73–8.
McGrath JJ et al. Vitamin D3-implications for brain development. Steroid Biochem Mol Biol 89–90.1–5 (2004a): 557–60.
McGrath JJ et al. Vitamin D supplementation during the first year of life and risk of schizophrenia: a Finnish birth cohort study. Schizophrenia Res 67 (2004b): 237–45.
McGrath JJ et al. Seasonal fluctuations in birth weight and neonatal limb length: does prenatal vitamin D influence neonatal size and shape? Early Hum Dev 81 (2005): 609–18.
Melamed M & Kumar J. Low levels of 25-hydroxyvitamin D in the pediatric populations: prevalence and clinical outcomes. Pediatric Health 4.1 (2010): 89–97.
Merewood A, et al. Association between Vitamin D Deficiency and Primary Cesarean Section. J Clin Endorin Metab 94.3 (2009): 940–945.
Micromedex. Vitamin D. Thomson 2003. Available online at: www.micromedex.com.
Miller GJ. Vitamin D and prostate cancer: Biologic interactions and clinical potentials. Cancer Metastasis Rev 17 (1999): 353–60.
Mimouni F et al. Vitamin D2 therapy of pseudohypoparathyroidism. Clin Pediatr 25 (1986): 49–52.
Minasyan A et al Vestibular dysfunction in vitamin D receptor mutant mice. J Steroid Biochem Mol Biol 114.3–5 (2009): 161–166.
Mizoue T et al. Calcium, dairy foods, vitamin D, and colorectal cancer risk: the Fukuoka Colorectal Cancer Study. Cancer Epidemiol Biomarkers Prev 17.10 (2008): 2800–7.
Mohr SB et al. Relationship between low ultraviolet B irradiance and higher breast cancer risk in 107 countries. Breast J 14.3 (2008): 255–60.
Mucci LA, Spiegelman D. Vitamin D and prostate cancer risk — a less sunny outlook? J Natl Cancer Inst 100.11 (2008): 759–61.
Munger KL et al. Serum 25-hydroxyvitamin D levels and risk of multiple sclerosis. JAMA 296 (2006): 2832–2838.
Murphy PK, Wagner CL. Vitamin D and mood disorders among women: an integrative review. J Midwifery Women's Health 53.5 (2008): 440–6.
NHMRC (National Health & Medical Research Council). Nutrient reference values for Australia and New Zealand. Canberra, Australia Government of Health & Ageing, 2006.
Niino M et al. Therapeutic potential of vitamin D for multiple sclerosis. Curr Med Chem 15.5 (2008): 499–505.
Nowson C, Margerison C. Vitamin D status of Australians: impact of changes to mandatory fortification of margarine with vitamin D. Melbourne: Deakin University, 2001.
Nowson CA, Margerison C. Vitamin D intake and vitamin D status of Australians. Med J Aust 177.3 (2002): 149–52.
Nozza J, Rodda C. Vitamin D deficiency in mothers of infants with rickets. MJA 175 (2001): 253–5.
Obradovic D et al. Cross-talk of vitamin D and glucocorticoids in hippocampal cells. J Neurochem 96.2 (2006): 500–9.
Oh K et al. Calcium and vitamin D intakes in relation to risk of distal colorectal adenoma in women. Am J Epidemiol 165.10 (2007): 1178–86.
Palmer SC et al. Meta-analysis: vitamin D compounds in chronic kidney disease. Ann Intern Med 147 (2007): 840–53.
Palomer X et al. Role of vitamin D in the pathogenesis of type 2 diabetes mellitus. Diabetes Obes Metab 10.3 (2008): 185–97.
Pappa H. Vitamin D Status in Children and Young Adults With Inflammatory Bowel Disease. Pediatr 118.5 (2006): 1950–62.
Perez-Lopez FR. Sunlight, the vitamin D endocrine system, and their relationships with gynaecologic cancer. Maturitas 59.2 (2008): 101–13.
Pillow JJ et al. Vitamin D deficiency in infants and young children born to migrant parents. J Paediatr Child Health 31.3 (1995): 180–4.
Pittas A et al. The role of vitamin D and calcium in type 2 diabetes. A systematic review and meta-analysis. J Clin Endo Metab 92.6 (2007): 2017–29.
Prietl B et al. Vitamin D and immune function. Nutr 5 (2013): 2502–2521.
Prince RL et al. Effects of ergocalciferol added to calcium on the risk of falls in elderly high-risk women. Arch Intern Med 168.1 (2008): 103–8.
RACGP (Royal Australian College of General Practitioners). Proceedings of the RACGP Conference, Hobart, October 2003.
Ramos-Lopez E et al. Protection from type 1 diabetes by vitamin D receptory haploytpes. Ann N Y Acad Sci 1079 (2006): 327–334.
Reinholz, M, et al. Cathelicidin LL-37: An Antimicrobial Peptide with a Role in Inflammatory Skin Disease. Ann Dermatol. 24.2 (2012): 126–135.
Reis J et al. Vitamin D, parathyroid hormone levels, and the prevalence of metabolic syndrome in community-dwelling older adults. Diabetes Care 30.6 (2007): 1549–55.
Richy F, et al. Differential effects of D-hormone analogs and native vitamin D on the risk of falls: a comparative meta-analysis. Calcif Tissue Int 82.2 (2008): 102–7.
Robinson P et al. The re-emerging burden of rickets: a decade of experience in Sydney. Arch Dis Child 91 (2006): 564–8.
Samanek AJ et al. Estimates of beneficial and harmful sun exposure times during the year for major Australian population centres. Med J Aust 184.7 (2006): 338–41.
Sambrook PN, Eisman JA. Osteoporosis prevention and treatment. Med J Aust 172 (2002): 226–9.
Schauber J et al. Taming psoriasis with vitamin D. Sci Trans Med 3 (2011): 82ra38.
Schinchuk L, Holick M. Vitamin D and rehabilitation: improving functional outcomes. Nutr Clin Prac 22 (2007): 297–304.
Schottker, B., et al. 2013. Strong associations of 25-hydroxyvitamin D concentrations with all-cause, cardiovascular, cancer, and respiratory disease mortality in a large cohort study. Am J Clin Nutr., 97, (4) 782–793.
Schottker, B., et al. 2014. Vitamin D and mortality: meta-analysis of individual participant data from a large consortium of cohort studies from Europe and the United States. BMJ, 348, g3656.
Scully M, et al. Trends in news coverage about skin cancer prevention, 1993–2006: Increasingly mixed messages for the public. Aust N Z J Public Health 32.5 (2008): 461–6.
Simpson RU, et al. Characterization of heart size and blood pressure in the vitamin D receptor knockout mouse. J Steroid Biochem Mol Biol 103.3–5 (2007): 521–4.
Smolders J et al. Vitamin D as an immune modulator in multiple sclerosis, a review. J Neuroimmunol 194.1–2 (2008): 7–17.
Snijder MB et al. Vitamin D status in relation to one-year risk of recurrent falling in older men and women. J Clin Endocrinol Metab 91 (2006): 2980–5.
Spector TD et al. Choline-stabilized orthosilicic acid supplementation as an adjunct to calcium/vitamin D3 stimulates markers of bone formation in osteopenic females: a randomized, placebo-controlled trial. BMC Musculoskelet Disord 9 (2008): 85.
Stene LC, Joner G. Use of cod liver oil during first year of life is associated with a lower risk of childhood-onset type 1 diabetes: a large

population-based, case-control study. Am J Clin Nutr 78.6 (2003): 1128–34.
Sugden JA et al. Vitamin D improves endothelial function in patients with Type 2 diabetes mellitus and low vitamin D levels. Diabet Med 25.3 (2008): 320–5.
Suzuki K et al. Hepatic osteodystrophy. Nippon Rinsho 56.6 (1998): 1604–8.
Svensson J et al. Danish Childhood Diabetes Registry. Long-term trends in the incidence of type 1 diabetes in Denmark: the seasonal variation changes over time. Pediatr Diabetes 2008 Nov 24 (Epub ahead of print). Available online at: http://www.ncbi.nlm.nih.gov/pubmed/19175901?ordinalpos=1&itool=EntrezSystem2.PEntrez.Pubmed.Pubmed_ResultsPanel.Pubmed_DefaultReportPanel.Pubmed_RVDocSum.
Swami S et al. Genistein potentiates the growth inhibitory effects of 1,25-dihydroxyvitamin D3 in DU145 prostate cancer cells: role for the direct inhibition of CYP24 enzyme activity. Mol Cell Endocrinol 241 (2005): 49–61.
Swanenburg J et al. Effects of exercise and nutrition on postural balance and risk of falling in elderly people with decreased bone mineral density: randomized controlled trial pilot study. Clin Rehabil 21.6 (2007): 523–34.
Tang BM et al. Use of calcium or calcium in combination with vitamin D supplementation to prevent fractures and bone loss in people aged 50 years and older: a meta-analysis. Lancet 370.9588 (2007): 657–66.
Theodoratou E et al. Modification of the inverse association between dietary vitamin D intake and colorectal cancer risk by a FokI variant supports a chemoprotective action of Vitamin D intake mediated through VDR binding. Int J Cancer 123.9 (2008): 2170–9.
Thien R et al. Interactions of 1 alpha,25-dihydroxyvitamin D3 with IL-12 and IL-4 on cytokine expression of human T lymphocytes. J Allergy Clin Immunol 116 (2005): 683–90.
Tjellesen L et al. Different actions of vitamin D2 and D3 on bone metabolism in patients treated with phenobarbitone/phenytoin. Calcif Tissues Int 37.3 (1985): 218–22.
Tjellesen L et al. Different metabolism of vitamin D2/D3 in epileptic patients treated with phenobarbitone/phenytoin. Bone 7.5 (1986): 337–42.
Toriola AT et al. Circulating 25-hydroxyvitamin D levels and prognosis among cancer patients: a systematic review. Cancer Epidemiol Biomarkers Prev 23.6 (2014): 917–933.
Tran B et al. Effect of vitamin D supplementation on antibiotic use: a randomized controlled trial. Amer J Clin Nutr 99.1 (2014): 156–61.
Trang HM et al. Evidence that vitamin D3 increases serum 25-hydroxyvitamin D more efficiently than does vitamin D2. Am J Clin Nutr 68.4 (1998): 854–8.
Vagianos, K et al. Nutrition assessment of patients with inflammatory bowel disease. J parenteral & ent nutr, 31.4 (2007): 311–319.
Valdivielso JM, et al. Vitamin D and the vasculature: can we teach an old drug new tricks? Expert Opin. Ther Targets 13.1 (2009): 29–38.
van der Mei IA et al. The high prevalence of vitamin D insufficiency across Australian populations is only partly explained by season and latitude. Environ Health Perspect 115.8 (2007): 1132–9.
Vanlint S, et al. Vitamin D and people with intellectual disability. Aust Fam Physician 37.5 (2008): 348–51.
Vieth R. Critique of the considerations for establishing the tolerable upper intake level for vitamin D: critical need for revision upwards. J Nutr 136 (2006): 1117–22.
Vieth R, et al. Efficacy and safety of vitamin D intake exceeding the lowest observed adverse effect level. AJCN 73 (2001): 288–94.
Vieth R et al. Randomized comparison of the effects of the vitamin D3 adequate intake versus 100 mcg (4000 IU) per day on biochemical responses and the wellbeing of patients. Nutr J 19.3 (2004): 8.
Visser M, et al. Low vitamin D and high parathyroid hormone levels as determinants of loss of muscle strength and muscle mass (sarcopenia): The Longitudinal Aging Study Amsterdam. J Clin Endo Metab 88.12 (2003): 5766–72.
Wahlqvist ML (ed). Food and nutrition, 2nd edn. Sydney: Allen & Unwin, 2002.
Wang TJ et al. Vitamin D deficiency and risk of cardiovascular disease. Circulation 117 (2008): 503–11.
Welsh JE et al. Vitamin D3 receptor as a target for breast cancer prevention. J Nutr 133 (2003): 2425–33S.
Wieder E. Dendritic Cells: A basic overview. Int Soc Cell Ther (2003).
Wigg A et al. A system for improving vitamin D nutrition in residential care. MJA 185.4 (2006): 195–8.
Wilkins CH et al. Vitamin D deficiency is associated with low mood and worse cognitive performance in older adults. Am J Geriatr Psychiatry 14.12 (2006): 1032–40.
Wills MR, Savory J. Vitamin D metabolism and chronic liver disease. Ann Clin Lab Sci 14.3 (1984): 189–97.
Wilson JD et al. Harrison's principles of internal medicine, 12th edn. New York: McGraw-Hill, 1991.
Working Group (of the Australian and New Zealand Bone and Mineral Society, Endocrine Society of Australia and Osteoporosis Australia). Vitamin D and adult bone health in Australia and New Zealand: a position statement. Med J Aust 182.6 (2005): 281–5.
Yildirim B et al. The effect of postmenopausal vitamin D treatment on vaginal atrophy. Maturitas 49 (2004a): 334–7.
Yildirim B et al. Immunohistochemical detection of 1,25-dihydroxyvitamin D receptor in rat epithelium. Fertil Steril 82.6 (2004b): 1602–8.
Yu S et al. Failure of T cell homing, reduced CD4/CD8αα intraepithelial lymphocytes and inflammation in the gut of vitamin D receptor KO mice. Proc Natl Acad Sci USA 105 (2008): 20834–20839.
Zhu K et al. Effects of calcium and vitamin D supplementation on hip bone mineral density and calcium-related analytes in elderly ambulatory Australian women: a five-year randomized controlled trial. J Clin Endocrinol Metab 93.3 (2008): 743–9.
Zipitis CS, Akobeng AK. Vitamin D supplementation in early childhood and risk of type 1 diabetes: a systematic review and meta-analysis. Arch Dis Child 93.6 (2008): 512–17.
Zittermann A et al. Vitamin D supplementation, body weight and human serum 25-hydroxyvitamin D response: a systematic review. Eur J Nutr 53 (2014): 367–374.
Zofkova I, Hill M. Long-term 1,25(OH)2 vitamin D therapy increases bone mineral density in osteopenic women. Comparison with the effect of plain vitamin D. Aging Clin Exp Res 19.6 (2007): 472–7.

Vitamin E

HISTORICAL NOTE Vitamin E was first discovered in 1922 at the University of California in Berkeley, when it was observed that rats required the nutrient in order to maintain their fertility (Evans 1925). In this way, vitamin E became known as the antisterility vitamin, which is reflected in its name, as *tokos* and *pherein* are the Greek words for 'offspring' and 'to bear or bring forth' (Saldeen & Saldeen 2005). Although considered an essential nutrient, it was not until the mid-1960s that deficiency states in humans were first identified (McDowell 2000). More specifically, deficiency was detected in children with fat malabsorption syndromes, and defects in genetic hepatic alpha-tocopherol transfer protein (Shils 1999, Traber et al 2006, Wahlqvist 2002). Most fat-soluble vitamins (A, D and K) have defined roles in human metabolism. However, vitamin E does not present an actual role; rather it is utilised in deficiency states, and is seen in malabsorptive and in genetic disorders. It is an antioxidant functioning via peroxyl radical-scavenging actions protecting membranous lipoproteins and polyunsaturated fats. Vitamin E depends on a complex network of other antioxidants and antioxidant enzymes to maintain efficacy and therefore rarely acts alone, as demonstrated by many journal papers (Blaner 2013, McDowell 2000, Saldeen & Saldeen 2005). Most of the research regarding vitamin E has been on alpha-tocopherols, with approximately 1% investigating tocotrienols (Wong 2012). This makes vitamin E as a single prescriptive supplement difficult to evaluate in human studies, rendering many studies equivocal (Blaner 2013, Traber et al 2006).

V

BACKGROUND AND RELEVANT PHARMACOKINETICS

Vitamin E is a collective term relating to all antioxidant activities of tocol and tocotrienol derivatives (Blaner 2013). Alpha-tocopherol is absorbed from the intestinal lumen and is dependent upon adequate fat digestion. After micellisation, it enters the lymphatic circulation and then the systemic circulation, where it is transported in chylomicrons. Breakdown of chylomicrons in the blood releases some vitamin E, which is then taken up by circulating lipoproteins such as low-density lipoprotein (LDL) and high-density lipoprotein (HDL). The remaining vitamin E is transported via chylomicron remnants to the liver. Here, the RRR alpha-tocopherol form is preferentially secreted back into the circulation in very-low-density lipoprotein (VLDL). It is suspected that hepatic alpha-tocopherol transfer protein is responsible for discriminating between the different types of tocopherol at this point (with the natural form preferentially taken up). Vitamin E is ultimately delivered to tissues when chylomicrons and VLDL are broken down by lipoprotein lipase. Vitamin E transported by LDL is also taken up by tissues via the LDL receptor. The bulk of vitamin E is stored in adipose tissue, although some storage also occurs in cell membranes, such as the plasma mitochondrial and microsomal membranes of the heart, muscles, testes, uterus, adrenal and pituitary glands, and blood (Borel 2013). Vitamin E molecules cannot be recycled. The inactive oxidated end product conjugates entering bile, and is mainly excreted in the faeces and urine, although the skin has also been implicated in its evacuation via sebaceous secretions (Shils 1999, Traber et al 2006). The efficiency of vitamin E absorption varies from 17% to roughly 79%, has an unknown saturation point, is enhanced by the presence of dietary lipids and is dependent upon adequate fat digestion, involving effective secretion of free fatty acids, monoglycerides and bile acids (Traber et al 2006).

CHEMICAL COMPONENTS

To date, there are eight identified naturally occurring compounds — 'tocochromanols' — collectively known as vitamin E 'vitamers', that display the biological activity of RRR-alpha-tocopherol, alpha-, beta-, gamma- and delta-tocopherol; and alpha-, beta-, gamma- and delta-tocotrienol. They all share the same chromanol structure and are divided into two classes: tocopherols (saturated side chain with 16 carbons) and tocotrienols (unsaturated side chain with 16 carbons). The various vitaminers cannot be interconverted by the body, and RRR-alpha-tocopherol is the most biologically active form meeting human requirements (Blaner 2013, Colombo 2010, Traber et al 2006). The human diet generally provides a mixture of compounds with vitamin E activity (Bender 2003). Natural vitamin E consists of four forms — alpha-, beta-, gamma- and delta-tocotrienol — and is labelled as 'D' forms. The synthetic forms are labelled 'dl' or 'all-*rac*' for clarification (Colombo 2010).

Relative strengths of the various forms of vitamin E

The relative strength of the different forms of vitamin E can be expressed as either alpha-tocopherol equivalents (alpha-TE) or international units (IU). One alpha-TE (IU) represents the activity of 1 mg RRR-alpha-tocopherol (D-alpha-tocopherol representing the highest biopotency), and the alpha-TE of natural forms of vitamin E can be calculated using mathematical calculations as follows. The number of milligrams of beta-tocopherol should be multiplied by 0.5, gamma-tocopherol by 0.1 and alpha-tocotrienol by 0.3, whereas any of the synthetic all-*rac*-alpha-tocopherols (DL-alpha-tocopherol) should be multiplied by 0.74 (FAO/WHO 2002).

More commonly, activity is described in terms of IU, where 1 mg of synthetic all-*rac*-alpha-tocopherol (DL-alpha-tocopherol) acetate is equivalent to 1 IU vitamin E. Relative to this, 1 mg of DL-alpha-tocopherol is equal to 1.1 IU, 1 mg of D-alpha-tocopherol acid succinate is equal to 1.21 IU and 1 mg of D-alpha-tocopherol acetate is equal to 1.36 IU (Table 1). The natural form of D-alpha-tocopherol has the highest biopotency, which is equal to at least 1.49 IU (Meydani & Hayes 2003).

FOOD SOURCES

Vitamin E is found in various forms in both animal and plant foods. The richest food sources of vitamin E are cold-pressed vegetable oils, with safflower oil being the highest source. Good alternative sources are wheatgerm oil, sunflower oil, and nuts and seeds, particularly almonds and sunflower seeds. Non-lipid sources include spinach, kale, sweet potatoes, yams, egg yolk, liver, soya beans, asparagus and dairy products such as butter and milk. Higher tocopherol sources are found in olive oil, soya bean, corn and sunflower oils. Higher tocotrienol lipid sources include palm oil, coconut oil and cocoa butter, with non-lipid forms such as rice bran, legumes, and the bran and germ portions of cereal grains such as rice, barley and oats (Colombo 2010, NUTTAB 2010).

TABLE 1	EQUIVALENCE TABLE	
1 mg	DL-alpha tocopherol — synthetic	1 IU
1 mg	DL-alpha-tocopherol	1.1 IU
1 mg	D-alpha-tocopherol acid succinate	1.21 IU
1 mg	D-alpha-tocopherol acetate	1.36 IU
1 mg	D-alpha-tocopherol	1.49 IU

Similar to all fat-soluble vitamins, vitamin E is susceptible to oxidation and destruction during food preparation and storage, frying, processing, bleaching, milling and freezing. Therefore processed foods may not confer adequate intakes (Whitney et al 2011).

Fortified foods

Fortified foods contain esterified vitamin E (alpha-tocopherol acetate and succinate) prolonging the shelf-life and protecting its antioxidant property. It is suggested that the body efficiently hydrolyses and absorbs esters; however there is little supportive evidence (Leonard et al 2004).

Clinical note — Free radicals, antioxidant recycling and the antioxidant network

Oxygen-containing free radicals (such as the hydroxyl radical, superoxide anion radical, hydrogen peroxide, oxygen singlet and nitric oxide radical) are highly reactive species, capable of damaging biologically important molecules such as DNA, proteins, carbohydrates and lipids. Antioxidants can break the destructive cascade of reactions initiated by free radicals by converting them into harmless derivatives.

The term 'oxidative stress' refers to an imbalance of pro-oxidants over antioxidants. The term 'antioxidant capacity' is a measure of the sum of available endogenous and exogenous defence mechanisms that work synergistically to restore and maintain the oxidative balance. During the process of maintaining oxidative balance, antioxidants such as vitamin E become oxidised themselves. Other antioxidants, such as ubiquinone, ascorbate and glutathione, are then involved in recycling vitamin E back to its unoxidised state, allowing it to continue neutralising free radical molecules (Sen & Packer 2000). When these other antioxidants become oxidised in turn, they are also regenerated to their antioxidant forms by yet others, such as alpha-lipoic acid and cysteine. In this way, the recycling of various antioxidants occurs in an orchestrated manner. The interactions between antioxidant substances have been described as the 'antioxidant network', which comprises four parts that work together to provide a continuous defence against free radical damage (De Vita et al 2005). These are:

1. enzymes that destroy or detoxify common oxidants (e.g. catalase, glutathione peroxidase, which needs selenium)
2. antioxidant vitamins, notably vitamins E and C, and coenzyme Q10, which are continuously recycled, as discussed earlier
3. dietary antioxidants or phytochemicals (e.g. carotenoids, polyphenols and allyl sulfides).
4. proteins that sequester iron and copper so that free forms do not exist in the body.

The antioxidant network provides a basis for recommending combinations of foods and antioxidant nutrients to provide maximal benefits, rather than single entities in high doses.

DEFICIENCY SIGNS AND SYMPTOMS

Owing to the widespread availability of vitamin E in the food chain, it is generally accepted that primary vitamin E deficiency is rare; however, due to alpha-tocopherol transfer protein deficiency it does occur in genetic abnormalities, lipoprotein synthesis defects, fat malabsorpative syndromes and possibly with total parenteral nutrition. It may also manifest in low-birth-weight infants given infant formula or cow's milk with low vitamin E levels, diseases such as cystic fibrosis, Crohn's disease, cholestatic liver disease, pancreatitis and biliary obstruction. Due to the malabsorption of fats, people with conditions such as those listed may sometimes require water-soluble forms of vitamin E, e.g. tocopherol polyethylene glycol-1000 succinate (NIH 2013). Individuals limiting their dietary fat intake thereby reduce both vitamin E availability and absorption (Shils 1999, Traber et al 2006).

Ultimately, it is tissue uptake, local oxidative stress levels and polyunsaturated fat content that influence whether symptoms of deficiency develop.

Symptoms of deficiency tend to be vague and difficult to diagnose because of the nutrient's widespread actions, but the following signs and symptoms have been reported in humans (FAO/WHO 2002, Meydani & Hayes 2003, Traber et al 2006):

- haemolytic anaemia
- immunological abnormalities
- neurological disturbances (e.g. peripheral neuropathies and ataxia)
- platelet dysfunction
- leakage of muscle enzymes such as creatine kinase and pyruvate kinase into plasma
- increased levels of lipid peroxidation products in plasma.

Retinal degeneration

It is possible that there is an increased usage of vitamin E in intense physical training, in smokers and in polluted environments; however further research is needed (Dunford & Doyle 2012, Packer 2002).

MAIN ACTIONS

Vitamin E is an electron donor (reducing agent or antioxidant), and many of its biochemical and molecular functions can be accounted for by this function. It is involved in many biochemical processes in the body, but its most important biological function is that of an antioxidant and working within the antioxidant network. The actions of the electron donor activity relate to maintenance of membrane integrity in body tissue, providing protection from destructive reactive oxidation species, particularly during inflammation and tissue injury (Mittal et al 2014, Traber et al 2006).

Antioxidant

Vitamin E is considered to be one of the most important and potent lipid-soluble antioxidants, due to its oxidative inhibitory action, protecting cell membranes against lipid peroxidation. It prevents free radical damage to the polyunsaturated fatty acids (PUFAs) within the phospholipid layer of each cell membrane and oxidation of LDL. It has been estimated that, for every 1000–2000 molecules of phospholipid, one molecule of vitamin E is present for antioxidant defence (Rizvi et al 2014).

This is achieved by reacting with free radical molecules and forming a tocopheroxyl radical, which then leaves the cell membrane. Upon entering the aqueous environment outside the membrane, it reacts with vitamin C (or other hydrogen donors, such as glutathione) to become reduced and, therefore, regenerated (Vatassery 1987). In this way, vitamin E activity is influenced by what has been called the 'antioxidant network', which restores vitamin E to its unoxidised state, ready to act as an antioxidant many times over (see Clinical note for more information).

Taking a larger perspective, the collective antioxidant action at each cell membrane protects the body's tissues and organs from undue oxidative stress. Prolonged and/or excessive exposure to free radicals has been implicated in many conditions, such as cardiovascular disease (CVD), cancer initiation and promotion, degenerative diseases and ageing in general (FAO/WHO 2002, Rizvi et al 2014).

Regulates immunocompetence

Vitamin E increases humoral antibody production, resistance to bacterial infections, cell-mediated immunity, the T-lymphocyte response, tumour necrosis factor production and natural killer cell activity, thereby playing a role in immunocompetence. It also decreases prostaglandin E_2 production and therefore reduces its immunosuppressive effects and decreases levels of lipid peroxides that can adversely affect immune function. It is now considered an antiangiogenic vitamer due to the mediating effect on growth factor-alpha. Alpha, gamma and delta tocopherols have various actions in the inhibition of cancer, each having its own biochemical pathway in halting cancer growth (Meydani 1995, Rizvi et al 2014, Takahaski et al 2009).

OTHER ACTIONS

- Regulates vascular smooth-muscle cell proliferation
- Inhibits smooth-muscle cell proliferation by inhibiting protein kinase C activity
- Inhibits phospholipase A_2 activity, suppressing arachidonic acid metabolism
- Antiplatelet activity has been demonstrated in vitro, but in vivo tests have been inconsistent for D-alpha-tocopherol
- Modulates vascular function by regulating the enzymatic activities of endothelial nitric oxide synthase and NAD(P)H oxidase (Ulker et al 2003)
- Analgesic activity: most likely mediated via inhibitory effects on cyclooxygenase-2 and 5-lipoxygenase
- Promotes wound healing
- Exerts neuroprotective effects
- Gene regulation. Vitamin E modulates genes involved in cholesterol homeostasis, atherosclerosis, inflammatory pathways and cellular trafficking, including of synaptic vesicular transport and the synthesis pathways of neurotransmitters (Brigelius-Flohe 2009, Munteanu et al 2004).

More specifically, vitamin E regulates genes encoding proteins involved in apoptosis (CD95L, Bcl2-L1), cell cycle regulation (p27, cyclin D1, cyclin E), cell adhesion (E-selectin, L-selectin, intercellular adhesion molecule-1, vascular cell adhesion molecule-1, integrins), cell growth (connective tissue growth factor), extracellular matrix formation/degradation (collagen alpha-1(1), glycoprotein IIb, matrix metalloproteinase-1 [MMP-1, MMP-19), inflammation (interleukin-1β [IL-1β], IL-2, IL-4, transforming growth factor-beta), lipoprotein receptors (CD36, SR-BI, SR-AI/II, LDL receptor), transcriptional control (peroxisome proliferator-activated receptor-gamma), metabolism (CYP3A4, HMG-CoA reductase, gamma-glutamylcysteine synthetase), and other processes (leptin, a beta-secretase in neurons, tropomyosin), activation of the cellular retinoic acid-binding protein II (Brigelius-Flohe 2009).

Cell signalling

Under in vitro conditions efficiency of vitamin E is involved in the upregulation of Christmas factor, increasing blood coagulation and catalysing an increased conversion of testosterone to 5-alpha dihydrotestosterone, simultaneously upregulating enzymatic activity involved in the rate limitation of glutathione synthesis (Rimbach et al 2010).

Telomere length

In co-administration with vitamin C, vitamin E was associated with longer telomere production (in women), demonstrated by both foods containing the antioxidants and supplemental forms (Xu et al 2009).

CLINICAL USE

Although vitamin E supplementation is used to correct or prevent deficiency states, most uses are based on the concept of high-dose supplements acting as therapeutic agents to either prevent or treat various health conditions. The Scientific Committee of Food set a tolerable upper intake level for D-alpha tocopherol of 300 mg/day in adults. However, there are numerous clinical trials which have used higher doses and not shown any serious adverse effects. The Joint Expert Committee on Food additives suggests an acceptable daily intake at 0.15–2.0 mg/kg/day. These intakes are likely to have individual response differences dependent on uptake

(Colombo 2010). In recent years, accumulating evidence has suggested that gamma tocopherol, mixed tocopherols and tocotrienols may have properties superior to alpha tocopherol and are being scientifically investigated.

Deficiency: prevention and treatment

Traditionally, vitamin E supplementation has been used to treat or prevent deficiency in conditions such as genetic abnormalities with alpha-tocopherol transfer protein, apolipoprotein B, or microsomal triglyceride transfer protein; and to treat fat malabsorption syndromes (e.g. chronic cholestasis, cystic fibrosis, short-bowel syndromes such as Crohn's disease, chronic steatorrhoea, coeliac disease, chronic pancreatitis and total parenteral nutrition) (Traber et al 2006).

Cardiovascular disease

Oxidative stress has been shown to play an integral role in the formation, progression and rupture of the atherosclerotic plaque via modification of proteins and DNA, alteration of gene expression, promotion of inflammation and endothelial dysfunction, enhancement of surface adhesion molecule expression, LDL oxidation, MMP production and consequently plaque rupture (Katsiki & Manes 2009). Vitamin E in the form of mixed tocopherols has an inhibitory effect on platelet aggregation and adhesion, and smooth-muscle cell proliferation has an anti-inflammatory effect on monocytes, improves endothelial function and decreases lipid peroxidation (Kaul et al 2001, Rizvi et al 2014). Based on these observations and evidence, largely from epidemiological studies, investigation of various antioxidant substances, in particular vitamin E, has been conducted to determine their role in primary and/or secondary prevention of CVD.

Vitamin E also modulates the expression of genes that are involved in atherosclerosis (e.g. scavenger receptors, integrins, selectins, cytokines, cyclins) (Munteanu et al 2004). Its ability to reduce oxidative stress, both directly and indirectly as part of the antioxidant network, is of particular importance as oxidation of LDL is a key process in atherogenesis, enhancing foam cell and early lesion formation (Terentis et al 2002).

In animal cell lines tocotrienols inhibit cholesterol synthesis, suppressing the key enzyme in sterologenic pathways 3-hydroxy-3-methylglutaryl CoA reductase enzyme. This has an effect of downregulating cholesterol biosynthesis in the liver. In humans, a study of tocotrienols combined with lovastatin (cholesterol-lowering medication) lowered cholesterol through different mechanisms. The outcome suggested that the combined therapy was effective, avoiding some of the detrimental effects of statin medication (Colombo 2010, McAnally et al 2007).

Based on these observations and evidence, largely from epidemiological studies, investigation of various antioxidant substances, in particular vitamin E, has been conducted to determine their role in primary and/or secondary prevention of CVD.

Epidemiological and clinical studies

Many epidemiological studies have observed an inverse association between cardiovascular disease (CVD) and dietary intake of vitamin E that contains mainly gamma tocopherol and alpha tocopherol; however, the results from intervention studies are more controversial. In humans, some clinical trials have reported a clear association between the reduction in the relative risk of CVD with high intake or supplementation of Vitamin E, whereas others have shown no association. The genetic background, type of vitamin E and dose used, baseline levels and dietary habits of test volunteers may have contributed to the different results and deserve further study. It was back in 1946 when a Canadian doctors first reported that vitamin E could protect against coronary heart disease; however, it was not until the results of two very large human studies were published nearly 50 years later that the greater scientific community and the public started to take note of vitamin E. In 1993, the prospective Nurses' Health Study and the Health Professionals' Follow-up study both reported that, compared to non-users, vitamin E supplementation at a dose of at least 100 IU for at least 2 years significantly reduced the risk of coronary disease by an estimated 40% (Rimm et al 1993, Stampfer et al 1993).

The prospective Nurses' Health Study followed 87,245 women aged 34–59 years without known coronary disease over 8 years and found that those women with the highest intake of vitamin E had the lowest relative risk of non-fatal myocardial infarction (MI) or death from coronary disease, compared to those with the lowest intake (Stampfer et al 1993). Interestingly, short-term use or dietary intake alone did not produce the same significant reduction. The Health Professionals' Follow-up study observed 39,910 men aged 40–75 years over 4 years and produced similar results, finding that long-term vitamin E (at least 100 IU/day) significantly reduced the relative risk of coronary disease compared to non-users (Rimm et al 1993).

Subsequently, a double-blind study conducted at Cambridge University, UK, and published in 1996 supported these results, but further suggested that higher doses could produce benefits more quickly and more dramatically (Stephens et al 1996). The placebo-controlled randomised study known as the Cambridge Heart Antioxidant Study (CHAOS) involved 2002 patients with angiographically proven coronary atherosclerosis, and compared the effects of two different strengths of alpha-tocopherol supplementation (400 IU and 800 IU) and a placebo over a median of 510 days. Treatment with either dose of vitamin E was seen to reduce the risk of cardiovascular death and non-fatal MI by over 75%, with effects established after 12 months.

In 1999, results from the large Gruppo Italiano per lo Studio della Sopravvivenza nell'Infarto miocardico (GISSI) trial were published, which were less convincing. However, the trial used synthetic vitamin E at a lower dose than the previously positive CHAOS study (Albert et al 1999, GISSI 1999). The trial, which involved 11,324 patients who had recently survived MI (<3 months), investigated the effects of three different treatment protocols compared to a placebo: 1 g omega-3 fatty acid/day, 300 IU synthetic vitamin E/day, fish oils plus vitamin E/day or a placebo. The four groups were observed for nearly 4 years for CVD morbidity and mortality. Results showed that the fish oil treatment groups had significantly decreased combined end points of death, non-fatal MI and stroke over this time, whereas the vitamin E treatment produced little effect. The trial has since been criticised because the form of vitamin E used was synthetic and the dose was relatively low compared to doses in other studies involving patients with pre-existing disease.

To date, 27 different randomised controlled trials (RCTs) in the peer-reviewed literature have evaluated the effects of vitamin E in people at risk of CVD or with clinically diagnosed CVD (Katsiki & Manes 2009). The larger studies — GISSI (1999), Women's Antioxidant Cardiovascular Study (WACS) and Alpha-Tocopherol Beta-Carotene (ATBC) cancer prevention study — have resulted in several published papers as researchers analyse effects in subgroups or results are re-evaluated using different models, with respect to the GISSI 2006 study, which tested the same daily intervention with slightly different patient characteristics (post-MI vs post-MI without congestive heart failure at baseline). Overall, eight RCTs have tested vitamin E as a sole treatment, five studies have studied vitamin E in combination with vitamin C supplementation, and 11 have used multiple vitamin combinations, which included vitamin E. Nine studies combined beta-carotene with vitamin E or in a multivitamin combination. The dose of vitamin E administered in the studies varies considerably, from 55 IU to 1,200 IU daily, and in at least nine studies, synthetic vitamin E was used. In general, studies using natural vitamin E tend to produce positive results, showing a benefit on cardiovascular outcomes, however, inconsistent results still remain. Additionally, RCTs conducted in people with established CVD were more likely to report a cardioprotective effect than primary prevention studies (Table 2). Most recently, new data has emerged that allows identification of a specific target population for vitamin E supplementation, namely patients with diabetes mellitus and the haptoglobin genotype 2-2 as being more likely to respond (Vardi et al 2013).

Restenosis

Restenosis is a major limitation to the long-term success of angioplasty. Therefore, measures that prevent or delay this occurrence are being investigated to extend the beneficial effects of the procedure.

While studies in experimental models have shown that vitamin E helps to stabilise atherosclerotic plaque after angioplasty and favours vascular remodelling (Orbe et al 2003), clinical trials to date have produced disappointing results.

An early double-blind study using oral synthetic vitamin E (1200 IU) for 4 months found that treatment did not significantly reduce the rate of restenosis after percutaneous transluminal coronary angioplasty, with restenosis defined as >50%. However, minor reductions were noted (treatment group 35.5% vs control group 47.5%) which did not reach statistical significance (DeMaio et al 1992, Vardi et al 2013).

In the Multivitamin Prevention (MVP) trial, Tardif et al (1997) aimed to decrease the incidence and severity of restenosis after coronary angioplasty (317 patients). The patients were randomly assigned one of four different treatments: (1) a combination of vitamins, including vitamin E (30,000 IU beta-carotene, 500 mg vitamin C and 700 IU vitamin E 2000 IU); (2) placebo; (3) probucol and MVP combination; or (4) probucol 500 mg. Treatment was given 1 month prior to surgery and 6 months post-surgery at a dose of twice daily, unless procedure-related complications were noted. Additionally all patients received an extra 1000 mg of probucol, and 2000 IU of vitamin E or placebo 12 hours prior to angioplasty. It was found that probucol treatment was the most effective in reducing restenosis (mean ± SD); there was a reduction in luminal diameter 6 months > angioplasty 0.12 ± 0.41 mm in the probucol group, 0.22 ± 0.46 mm in the combined treatment group, 0.33 ± 0.51 mm in the multivitamin alone group, and 0.38 ± 0.50 mm in the placebo group.

Angina pectoris

Low-dose vitamin E supplements (50 mg/day) produce a minor decrease in the incidence of angina pectoris in smokers without previous coronary heart disease, according to an RCT (Rapola et al 1996). A smaller study of 29 subjects with variant angina identified six patients who did not respond to calcium channel blockers and had lower plasma levels than normal, but who responded positively to supplementation with 300 mg/day vitamin E. Treatment resulted in a significantly reduced incidence of angina episodes (Miwa et al 1996). Several years later, the same research group identified a transcardiac reduction in plasma vitamin E concentrations concomitant with lipid peroxide formation, suggesting that oxidative stress and vitamin E depletion may be involved in the pathogenesis of coronary artery spasm (Kusama et al 2011, Miwa et al 1999).

Nitrate tolerance

Nitroglycerin (NTG) is utilised to prevent vasoconstriction in the acute treatment of angina, acute MI, pulmonary oedema and severe arterial hypertension. One limitation of treatment is that nitrate tolerance

TABLE 2 SUMMARY OF POSITIVE FINDINGS FROM RANDOMISED STUDIES OF VITAMIN E IN PRIMARY OR SECONDARY CARDIOVASCULAR DISEASE (CVD) PREVENTION

Name of study	Prevention goal	Number of subjects	Characteristics	Daily intervention	Findings
CHAOS (Stephens et al 1996)	Secondary	2002	Coronary disease	Natural vitamin E (400 IU or 800 IU)	Vitamin E reduced risk of cardiovascular death and non-fatal MI by over 75%
SPACE (Boaz et al 2000)	Secondary	2198	End-stage renal disease — people on haemodialysis with pre-existing cardiovascular event	Natural vitamin E (800 IU)	Vitamin E caused a 50% reduction in cardiac events
CLAS (Azen et al 1996)	Secondary	146	Non-smoking 40–59-year-old men with previous coronary artery bypass graft surgery	Vitamin E (< or >100 IU) and vitamin C (< or >250 mg)	Higher vitamin E intake was associated with less carotid intima media thickness progression compared with low vitamin E users in people not treated with colestipol
DeMaio et al (1992)	Secondary	100	Restenosis	Dl tocopherol 1200 IU/day	35.5% reduction in restenosis versus 47.5% not statistically significant
ASAP (Salonen et al 2003)	Primary	520	Smoking/ non-smoking men and postmenopausal women aged 45–69 years with elevated serum cholesterol	Twice daily either (136 IU) of D-alpha-tocopherol, 250 mg of slow-release vitamin C, a combination of these, or a placebo, for 3 years	The proportion of men with progression of carotid atherosclerosis was reduced by 74% with combination of vitamins E and C compared to the placebo; no significant effect was seen in women
ASAP follow-up (Salonen et al 2003)	Primary	520	Smoking/ non-smoking men and postmenopausal women aged 45–69 years with elevated serum cholesterol	Twice daily (136 IU) D-alpha-tocopherol, 250 mg of slow-release vitamin C, or a placebo, for 6 years	Effect was still significant after a further 3 years: combined vitamins E and C continued to slow down atherosclerotic progression in hypercholesterolaemic men
ATBC (Rapola et al 1996)	Primary: incidence of angina pectoris	29,134	Finnish male smokers aged 50–69 years with no history of MI	Synthetic vitamin E (55 IU), beta-carotene (20 mg), or both, or a placebo	Vitamin E was associated with a minor decrease in incidence of angina pectoris
ATBC (Virtamo et al 1998)	Primary and secondary	29,134	Finnish male smokers aged 50–69 years with no history of MI	Synthetic vitamin E (55 IU), beta-carotene (20 mg), or both, or a placebo	Vitamin E decreased incidence of primary major coronary events by 4%; no effect on incidence of non-fatal MI; vitamin E decreased incidence of fatal coronary heart disease by 8%

V

TABLE 2 SUMMARY OF POSITIVE FINDINGS FROM RANDOMISED STUDIES OF VITAMIN E IN PRIMARY OR SECONDARY CARDIOVASCULAR DISEASE (CVD) PREVENTION *(continued)*

Name of study	Prevention goal	Number of subjects	Characteristics	Daily intervention	Findings
ATBC (subset) (Leppala et al 2000)	Primary: prevention of incident and fatal subarachnoid, intracerebral haemorrhage, cerebral infarction and stroke	29,134	Finnish male smokers aged 50–69 years with no history of MI	Synthetic vitamin E (55 IU), beta-carotene (20 mg), or both, or a placebo	Vitamin E prevented ischaemic stroke in high-risk hypertensive patients
St Francis (Arad et al 2005)	Primary	1005	Asymptomatic calcium scores >80th percentile	Atorvastatin 20 mg/day, vitamin C 1 g/day, vitamin E 1000 IU/day, aspirin 81 mg/day	Arteriosclerotic CVD event rate decreased 6.9% vs 9.9%
VEAPS (Hodis et al 2002)	Primary	353	LDL >3.37 mmol/L	DL-alpha-tocopherol 400 IU/day	Coronary carotid intimal thickness did not change, circulating LDL reduced
ATIC (Nanyakkara et al 2007)	Primary	93	Mild to moderate chronic kidney failure	Alpha-tocopherol, pravastatin and homocysteine-lowering therapy, consecutively introduced	Significant decrease in intima media thickness, endothelial dysfunction, albuminuria; no effect on renal output
IEISS (Singh et al 1996)	Secondary	125	Patients with suspected acute MI	Vitamin E (400 mg), vitamin A (50,000 IU), vitamin C (1000 mg), beta-carotene (25 mg)	Treatment reduced mean infarct size, angina pectoris and total arrhythmias; poor left ventricular function occurred less often with antioxidants; cardiac end points were significantly less in the antioxidant group (20.6% vs 30.6%, respectively)
Fang et al (2002)	Secondary	40	After cardiac transplantation	Twice-daily vitamin C (500 mg) plus vitamin E (400 IU)	Supplementation with vitamins C and E retarded early progression of transplant-associated coronary arteriosclerosis compared to the placebo
WACS (Cook et al 2007)	Secondary	8171	Women with CVD or at least three risk factors	Vitamin C (500 mg/day), natural vitamin E (600 IU every other day) and beta-carotene (50 mg every other day)	Vitamin E significantly reduced incidence of stroke and produced a marginally significant reduction in the primary outcome (a combination of MI, stroke, coronary revascularisation or CVD death) in a prespecified subgroup of women with prior CVD

TABLE 2 SUMMARY OF POSITIVE FINDINGS FROM RANDOMISED STUDIES OF VITAMIN E IN PRIMARY OR SECONDARY CARDIOVASCULAR DISEASE (CVD) PREVENTION *(continued)*

Name of study	Prevention goal	Number of subjects	Characteristics	Daily intervention	Findings
SPACE (Boaz et al 2000)	Secondary	196	-	DL-alpha-tocopherol 800 IU/day	Relative risk 0.46 in composite MI, ischaemic stroke, peripheral vascular disease and unstable angina

CHAOS, Secondary Prevention with Antioxidants of Cardiovascular disease in Endstage renal disease; MI, myocardial infarction; SPACE, Secondary Prevention with Antioxidants of Cardiovascular disease in Endstage renal disease; CLAS, Cholesterol Lowering Atherosclerosis Study; ASAP, Antioxidant Supplementation in Atherosclerosis Prevention; ATBC, Alpha-Tocopherol Beta-Carotene; VEAPS, Vitamin E Atherosclerosis Prevention Study; LDL, low-density lipoprotein; ATIC, Anti-oxidant Therapy in Chronic renal insufficiency; IEISS, Indian Experiment of Infarct Survival Study; WACS, Women's Antioxidant Cardiovascular Study; SPACE, Secondary Prevention with Antioxidants of Cardiovascular disease in Endstage renal disease.

develops with continuous use of NTG over time (Klemenska & Beresewicz 2009). Vitamin E supplements (200 mg three times daily) prevented nitrate tolerance when given concurrently with transdermal nitroglycerin (NTG 10 mg/24 hours) according to one randomised, placebo-controlled study in which 24 patients with ischaemic heart disease were compared with 24 healthy volunteers over a 6-day period (Watanabe et al 1997).

In animal studies of rats with angina pectoris, research indicates that continuous NTG infusion causes a time-dependent vitamin E depletion in plasma and tissue. Vitamin E dietary supplementation (0.5 g/kg) administered to the animals delayed the onset of, and extent of, tolerance, demonstrating vitamin E is beneficial in the prevention of nitrate tolerance (Minamiyama et al 2006). Yasue et al (2008) concur with animal study findings in that human trials demonstrate plasma vitamin E levels are low in coronary spasm disorders, with vasoconstriction causing oxygen free radical degradation. This suggests that vitamin E's antioxidant properties may be of use; however further trials are needed.

Hypertension

Vitamin E supplementation may reduce blood pressure and LDL oxidation and improve endothelial dysfunction in hypertension, according to clinical research.

An early double-blind, placebo-controlled study found that DL-alpha-tocopherol nicotinate (3000 mg) significantly reduced systolic blood pressure (SBP) from 151.0 to 139.2 mmHg within 4–6 weeks in hypertensive subjects; however, diastolic blood pressure (DBP) remained unchanged (Iino et al 1977). More recently, long-term vitamin E (200 IU/day) was shown to decrease SBP by 24% in mildly hypertensive patients compared with a 1.6% reduction with a placebo, according to a triple-blind placebo-controlled study conducted over 27 weeks (Boshtam et al 2002). The study involved 70 hypertensive patients (SBP 140–160 mmHg; DBP 90–100 mmHg) aged 20–60 years without other cardiovascular risk factors. Besides reducing SBP, DBP was reduced by 12.5% compared to 6.2% with a placebo.

Some studies have revealed that hypertensive patients have a higher susceptibility to LDL oxidation than normotensive subjects and, therefore, increased atherogenic potential. One study measured the effect of vitamin E (400 IU/day) on the resistance of LDL to oxidation in 47 volunteers (Brockes et al 2003). Comparisons made before and after 2 months' supplementation showed that vitamin E caused a significant increase in the lag time in normotensive and hypertensive patients, ultimately bringing hypertensive patients up to the same point as the healthy controls.

All-cause mortality (ACM)

There is substantial research indicating benefits for vitamin E supplementation in the treatment and prevention of various diseases, but regardless of these benefits, three meta-analyses have drawn the conclusion that vitamin E supplementation increases ACM (Bjelakovic et al 2007, 2013, Miller et al 2005). These findings have been unexpected and widely criticised, as they are based on the results of smaller studies of variable quality, often involving people with chronic disease and sometimes testing vitamin E as part of a multinutritional intervention and not as a stand-alone treatment. Based on recent reanalysis of the data by Berry et al (2009) and Gerss and Kopcke (2009), which are discussed below, the evidence is not convincing that vitamin E supplementation increases mortality.

In 2005, Miller et al published a meta-analysis of the dose–response relationship between vitamin E supplementation and total mortality using data from 19 RCTs consisting of a large study population (n = 135,967). A dose–response analysis showed a statistically significant relationship between vitamin E dosage and ACM. The authors suggested caution with doses of 400 IU/day or higher, while acknowledging that the high-dose studies (≥400 IU/day) analysed in the report were often small and performed in patients with chronic diseases.

TABLE 3 SUMMARY OF NEGATIVE FINDINGS FROM RANDOMISED STUDIES OF VITAMIN E IN PRIMARY OR SECONDARY CARDIOVASCULAR DISEASE (CVD) PREVENTION

Name of study	Prevention goal	Number of subjects	Characteristics	Daily intervention	Results
GISSI (Albert et al 1999)	Secondary	11,324	Post-MI	Synthetic vitamin E (300 mg/day), fish oils (1 g/day), combination of fish oil and vitamin E, or a placebo	There was no significant reduction in the combined end points of death, non-fatal MI and stroke
GISSI (Marchioli et al 2006)	Secondary	8415	Post-MI patients without CHF at baseline	Synthetic vitamin E (300 mg/day), fish oils (1 g/day), combination of fish oil and vitamin E, or a placebo	Vitamin E treatment was associated with a significant 50% increase of CHF in patients with left ventricular dysfunction (ejection fraction <50%)
HOPE (Yusuf et al 2000)	Primary and secondary	9541	2545 women and 6996 men 55 years of age or older who were at high risk of cardiovascular events because they had CVD or diabetes in addition to one other risk factor	Natural vitamin E (400 IU), and a placebo or angiotensin-converting-enzyme inhibitor (ramipril), or both	There was no significant effect on the primary outcome, which was a composite of MI, stroke and death from cardiovascular causes
MICRO-HOPE (Lonn et al 2005)	Secondary	3654	Middle-aged and elderly people with diabetes and CVD and/or additional coronary risk factor(s)	Vitamin E (400 IU) for an average of 4.5 years	Vitamin E had no effect on CV outcomes or nephropathy
PPP (de Gaetano 2001)	Primary	4495	Those at risk of CVD: people with hypertension, hypercholesterolaemia, diabetes, obesity, family history of premature MI or the elderly	Vitamin E (300 mg)	There was no significant reduction in CV events
ATBC (subset) (Rapola et al 1997)	Secondary	1862	Finnish male smokers with previous MI	Synthetic vitamin E (55 IU), beta-carotene (20 mg), or both, or a placebo	Risk of fatal coronary heart disease increased in groups receiving either beta-carotene or vitamin E and beta-carotene. There was a non-significant trend of increased deaths in the vitamin E group

This meta-analysis has several serious flaws and has been criticised on a number of accounts, inspiring over 40 letters to the journal's editor and hundreds of emails and telephone calls to the authors (Jialal & Devaraj 2005b). In summary, these responses centre on six major flaws. First, results from 12 clinical studies that reported fewer than 10 deaths each were excluded from the meta-analysis, which created the appearance of bias and would have given an artificial weight to studies in which more people died. Second, the meta-analysis included trials of different designs, treatment times, doses, combinations and end points. Pooling information together from such heterogeneous studies was considered inappropriate. Third, subjects in many studies had significant chronic diseases, such as Parkinson's

TABLE 3 SUMMARY OF NEGATIVE FINDINGS FROM RANDOMISED STUDIES OF VITAMIN E IN PRIMARY OR SECONDARY CARDIOVASCULAR DISEASE (CVD) PREVENTION *(continued)*

Name of study	Prevention goal	Number of subjects	Characteristics	Daily intervention	Results
HPS (Parkinson Study Group 2002)	Secondary	20,536	High CVD risk: coronary disease, other occlusive arterial disease, or diabetes	Vitamin E (600 mg), vitamin C (250 mg), beta-carotene (20 mg)	There were no significant differences in all-cause mortality, or in deaths due to vascular or non-vascular causes; no significant reduction in incidence of non-fatal MI, coronary death, non-fatal or fatal stroke or coronary or non-coronary revascularisation
MVP (Tardif et al 1997)	Secondary: aimed to decrease incidence and severity of restenosis after angioplasty	317	Before and after coronary angioplasty	One month before angioplasty and for 6 months afterwards: multivitamins (30,000 IU beta-carotene, 500 mg vitamin C, and 700 IU vitamin E) twice daily and/or probucol, or a placebo 12 hours before angioplasty given an extra 1000 mg probucol, 2000 IU vitamin E, or both, or a placebo	Multivitamin ineffective at reducing the rate of restenosis
WAVE (Waters et al 2002)	Secondary	423	Postmenopausal women	Vitamin E 400 IU/day plus vitamin C 500 mg BID, HRT or placebo	Increased risk of death, MI and stroke
SUVIMAX (Zureik et al 2004)	Primary	1162	Healthy population	Vitamin C (120 mg), vitamin E (30 mg), beta-carotene (6 mg), selenium (100 mcg), and zinc (20 mg)	There was no beneficial effect on carotid atherosclerosis and arterial stiffness
PHS 11 (Sesso et al 2008)	Primary	14,641	Male >50 years old /94.9% were CVD-free at enrolment	Alpha-tocopherol 400 IU every other day, vitamin C or placebo	No effect on CV outcomes: associated with increased risk of haemorrhagic stroke

GISSI, Gruppo Italiano per lo Studio della Sopravvivenza nell'Infarto miocardico; MI, myocardial infarction; CHF, congestive heart failure; HOPE, Heart Outcomes Prevention Evaluation; PPP, Primary Prevention Project; ATBC, Alpha-Tocopherol Beta-Carotene; HPS, Heart Protection Study; MVP, Multivitamin Prevention; WAVE, Women's Angiographic Vitamin and Estrogen; HRT, hormone replacement therapy; PHS 11, Physician's Health Study 11.

V

disease (PD), end-stage renal disease, coronary artery disease, diabetes mellitus and Alzheimer's dementia (AD), which would have influenced their mortality risk. This also means that the results do not necessarily apply to healthy adults taking these supplements. Fourth, studies used different forms of vitamin E (natural and synthetic) and sometimes used vitamin E in combination with other nutrients; however, results of all these studies were pooled and not separated. Furthermore, subject adherence to the treatment protocol was considered in only one study (CHAOS). Lastly, the use of some statistical models has been questioned.

In 2007, Bjelakovic et al conducted a meta-analysis using data from 68 randomised trials involving 232,606 adults that compared beta-carotene,

Clinical note — Confusing results for vitamin E

To date, many in vitro, animal and epidemiological studies support the use of vitamin E in the prevention of CVD (Clarke & Armitage 2002). However, intervention studies are equivocal. Many factors could account for the lack of benefit on the primary end point in the majority of trials (Linus Pauling Institute 2008).

Dose selection

A closer look at the evidence shows that dose selection varies enormously, from levels just above the recommended dietary intake (RDI: 50 mg/day) to large doses of 2000 IU/day. Clinical research reveals that a daily dose of at least 400 IU is required for LDL to become less susceptible to oxidation (Brockes et al 2003, Miller et al 2005) and an effective threshold dose may be as high as 800 IU/day (Jialal & Devaraj 2005a, Traber et al 2006). However an RCT review suggests that a dose relationship with mortality exists with supplementation over 150 IU/day (Miller et al 2005). More recently, Colombo (2010) suggests a beneficial dose should reach 0.15–2.0 mg/kg body weight per day.

Biomarkers of oxidative stress

Just as the statin trials investigate subjects with high cholesterol levels rather than the general population, it can reasonably be assumed that antioxidant treatment is best suited to those people with increased oxidative stress rather than the general population, yet researchers consistently fail to consider this as a biochemical basis for patient inclusion (Meagher 2003). The levels of oxidised amino acids in urine and plasma can reflect those in tissues and identify people with high levels of oxidative stress; this may be one method of subject selection (Heinecke 2002). Brack et al (2013) suggest in both chronic and acute disease, such as CVD, amongst others, multiple abnormalities can be found, where a broad-spectrum approach to measuring numerous antioxidant profiles, including vitamin E status, is warranted (Niki 2014).

Type of supplement

In the specific case of vitamin E, the form of tocopherol used is crucial, as synthetic forms have less biological activity than RRR D-alpha-tocopherol. According to a 2002 FAO/WHO report, cross-country correlations between coronary heart disease mortality in men and the supply of vitamin E homologues across 24 European countries show a highly significant ($P < 0.001$) correlation for D-alpha-tocopherol, whereas all other forms of vitamin E do not achieve statistical significance.

In the last few years, it has further been proposed that the lack of efficacy of commercial tocopherol preparations in some clinical trials may be due to the absence of other natural tocopherols, primarily gamma- and delta-tocopherol. Preliminary studies provide some support for this view (Jialal & Devaraj 2005a, Saldeen & Saldeen 2005). Studies using different mixtures of alpha-, beta-, gamma- and delta-tocopherol have found that a mixture of gamma-, delta- and alpha-tocopherol with the ratio of 5:2:1 have a much better antioxidant effect than alpha-tocopherol alone. This mixture is similar to that found in nature. In human and animal studies, the mixed tocopherol preparation also had much more favourable effects on constitutive NO synthase and superoxide dismutase activity than alpha-tocopherol, and in a rat model was more effective in decreasing platelet aggregation and inhibiting thrombus formation. A mixed tocopherol preparation is also superior to alpha-tocopherol in terms of myocyte protection (Chen et al 2002). Similarly, Yoshida et al (2003) sustain a similar view. This view is not supported by Niki et al (2014) who remain steadfast in the view that alpha-tocopherol alone exerts antioxidant effects in vivo and in vitro. It is important to note that, in diets rich in mixed tocopherols such as Mediterranean diets, there is a lower incidence of heart disease; however this may be due to many other nutrient and lifestyle factors (Roehm 2009).

Plasma vitamin E levels

The measurement of plasma vitamin E levels in the supplemented groups has been inconsistent in studies, so it is uncertain whether levels significantly rose in response to treatment and subjects were compliant. For example, in the CHAOS, Antioxidant Supplementation in Atherosclerosis Prevention (ASAP), ASAP follow-up and Secondary Prevention with Antioxidants of Cardiovascular disease in Endstage renal disease (SPACE) studies, a significant increase in plasma antioxidant levels was reported and all studies found a benefit on the primary end point, whereas measurement of plasma levels has been inconsistent in the negative studies (Jialal & Devaraj 2005a).

Clearly, the optimal form/s, dosage regimen, duration of use and subpopulation best suited to primary and secondary preventive treatment still need to be clarified with future trials.

Identifying responders

New data is emerging to suggest that the specific target population for vitamin E supplementation appears to be patients with excessive oxidative stress, such as those undergoing haemodialysis and those with diabetes mellitus and the haptoglobin genotype 2-2 as likely responders (Vardi et al. 2013).

vitamin A, vitamin C (ascorbic acid), vitamin E and selenium, either singly or combined, to a placebo or to no intervention. When all trials of antioxidant supplements were pooled, there was no significant effect on mortality for vitamin E given singly in high (≥1000 IU) or low dose (<1000 IU). After exclusion of high-bias risk (studies with heterogeneity) and selenium trials, vitamin E given singly or combined with other antioxidants significantly increased mortality, with an estimate of increased mortality of about 5%. A closer look at the details of the study reveals that, of the 815 trials originally identified, 405 trials were excluded from the meta-analysis because mortality was zero (n = 40,000). Vitamin E was administered in doses ranging from 10 to 5000 IU daily, and populations studied were either healthy (primary prevention trials) or had a variety of established diseases such as cancer, CVD, renal disease, hepatitis, systemic lupus erythematosus, heart failure, cirrhosis, gastritis, MI or macular degeneration.

Gerss and Kopcke (2009) concur that the use of different methodological approaches yields contradictory results, with some statistical models finding an association and others not. They used the same data as that described in the Miller et al study (2005). The meta-analysis was augmented with 2495 additional participants receiving vitamin E doses from 136 to 5000 IU/day. Moreover in two of the originally included trials, the updated results of mortality at longer periods of follow-up were made available.

More specifically, hierarchical logistic regression analyses confirmed the former results, showing an increased mortality of patients receiving high-dose vitamin E, whereas application of a traditional methodological approach to meta-regression found that in certain trials increased mortality was not due to high-dose vitamin E, but could be explained by a higher proportion of male subjects in comparison to other trials (Gerss & Kopcke 2009). Overall, the causal relationship of vitamin E supplementation and increased ACM is questionable and, in particular, high-dose vitamin E supplementation cannot be regarded as 'proven' to increase mortality.

Similar findings were obtained by Berry et al (2009), who applied a Bayesian meta-analytical method to synthesise results from previous clinical trials of vitamin E. They used data from studies in the Miller et al (2005) meta-analysis, appended by 10 more recent studies, and concluded that vitamin E intake is unlikely to affect ACM, regardless of dose.

Re-evaluation of data from the original Framingham Heart Study has also failed to find an association between vitamin E supplementation and increased risk of ACM (Dietrich et al 2009). The Framingham Heart Study (n = 4270) began enrolling in 1948 to investigate the association between supplemental vitamin E and the 10-year incidence of CVD and ACM. Eleven per cent of people participating in the study used vitamin E supplements at baseline and the most commonly consumed dose was 300–500 IU/day. In all statistical models, age, diabetes and treatment for blood pressure were significant positive predictors of CVD and ACM, whereas no statistically significant associations were found between vitamin E supplement intake and CVD and ACM. In secondary analyses, the associations of vitamin E dose and duration of use with CVD and ACM were assessed. Once again, no statistically significant associations were observed in any of the analyses for CVD or ACM. The effects of potential confounders, such as use of aspirin, anticholesterol treatment and multivitamins, were minimised using multivariate models which did not change the results.

In a further attempt to suggest the effects of supplementation of beta-carotene, vitamin A, and vitamin E singly or in combination on increased ACM, Bjelakovic et al (2013) included 53 RCTs involving 241,883 participants. Meta-regression analysis revealed that doses of >15 mg of vitamin E increased mortality significantly. In rebuttal, Hemilä (2013: not peer-reviewed) states that the increase in ACM by 3% based on a pooling of studies does not correspond to an individual level analysis. The latest ATBC studies confirm the statement made by Hemilä casting doubt on the significance of the review by Bjelakovic et al (2013) (Kataja-Tuomola et al 2010, Lynch et al 2012).

Clinical note — LDL oxidation and vitamin E

Oxidative stress affects lipid metabolism by producing an oxidised LDL that has greater atherogenic potential than its original form. In the past, attention focused on investigating various antioxidants, such as vitamin E, for their ability to prevent LDL oxidation. In recent years, researchers have started to focus on identifying the biological oxidants responsible for initiating oxidation of LDL within the human arterial wall and on a better understanding of what makes oxidised LDL proatherogenic. In 2003, in vitro testing with LDL discovered that myeloperoxidase is a pathway that promotes LDL oxidation in the human artery wall, although others are also likely to exist. It is noteworthy that vitamin E failed to inhibit LDL oxidation by myeloperoxidase in vitro (Heinecke 2003), although it does reduce LDL oxidation in animals and humans when given in doses well above RDI (Brockes et al 2003). Oil palm vitamin E (tocopherols 70% and tocotrienols 30%) reduced atherogenesis in a recent animal model trial (Che Anishas et al 2014). In earlier studies the effect of palm oil vitamin E in humans suggests its use in lowering LDL and protecting HDL levels (Mukherjee & Mitra 2009). Supplemental forms of tocopherols are available from a palm oil source.

Clinical note — Neurodegenerative disease and oxidative stress

Neurodegenerative diseases are defined by the progressive loss of specific neuronal cell populations and are associated with protein aggregates. A growing body of evidence suggests that oxidative stress plays a key role in the pathophysiology of neurodegenerative disorders such as AD and PD. Reactive oxygen species are known to cause cell damage by way of three main mechanisms: lipid peroxidation, protein oxidation and DNA oxidation. Cells have developed several defence and repair mechanisms to deal with oxidative stress, and antioxidants such as vitamin E represent the first line of defence. In addition to its antioxidant properties, vitamin E can act as an anti-inflammatory agent, which may also be neuroprotective, and it regulates specific enzymes, thus changing the properties of membranes. The central nervous system is especially vulnerable to free radical damage because, compared to other tissues, it has a high oxygen consumption rate, abundant lipid content and a relative deficit in antioxidant systems. While it remains unclear whether oxidative stress is the primary initiating event associated with neurodegeneration or a secondary effect related to other pathological pathways, a growing body of evidence implicates it as being involved in the propagation of cellular injury (Ricciarelli et al 2007).

Parkinson's disease

Based on experimental and clinical data, it is well established that oxidative stress and lipid peroxidation are increased in the substantia nigra of people with PD and this may play an important role in the disease's aetiology. Vitamin E has therefore been the focus of research as a potential treatment. Using both in vitro and in vivo experimental model systems for PD, studies have demonstrated both vitamin E-mediated protection and lack of protection (Fariss & Zhang 2003). Similarly, inconsistent results have been obtained for vitamin E supplementation in the prevention and treatment of clinical PD. An open study using high doses of both tocopherol (3200 IU/day) and ascorbic acid (3000 mg/day) delayed the use of levodopa or dopamine agonists for 2 years in subjects with early PD (Fahn 1992). In contrast, the Deprenyl and Tocopherol Antioxidative Therapy of Parkinsonism (DATATOP) study found no effect on the progression of disability with a dose of alpha-tocopherol 2000 IU/day (Parkinson Study Group 1996). The same study found that vitamin E had no effect on mortality (Parkinson Study Group 1998). A meta-analysis six case-control, one cohort study and a cross-sectional study of several vitamins and the risk of PD found that vitamin E demonstrated a protective role seen in both high (less significant and warranting further trials) and moderate intakes, suggesting that vitamin E has a neuroprotective role attenuating risk (Mahyar et al 2005).

Alzheimer's dementia and cognitive decline

Alzheimer's disease occurs due to protein oxidation and lipid peroxidation. Beta amyloid proteins undergo oxidative stress via hydrogen peroxide, leading to neuronal death and decline into the disease. Vitamin E may block hydrogen peroxide production, slowing progression of cytotoxicity, resulting in reduced beta amyloid cell death (animal studies) (Rizvi et al 2014). The current standard of care for pharmacological management of the cognitive and functional disabilities of AD consists of a cholinesterase inhibitor and sometimes the addition of high-dose vitamin E (Bonner & Peskind 2002). The inclusion of vitamin E is largely based on a 1997 double-blind study that compared a large dose of synthetic vitamin E (1000 IU twice daily) with selegiline (5 mg twice daily) and placebo in a group of patients with moderately severe AD. The 2-year study found that vitamin E significantly slowed down the progression of the disease, delayed institutionalisation and increased survival rate (Sano et al 1997). In contrast to the positive 1997 study, a study involving 769 subjects with possible or probable AD using the same dose found no significant effects in patients with mild cognitive impairment and no change in the rate of progression to AD over a 3-year period (Petersen et al 2005).

Despite this, positive results were again achieved in a double-blind RCT which found that supplementation with alpha-tocopherol in mild to moderate AD was effective in slowing functional decline and decreasing caregiver burden (Dysken et al 2014). The study involved 613 patients with mild to moderate AD who received 2000 IU/day of alpha-tocopherol (n = 152), 20 mg/day memantine (n = 155), the combination (n = 154) or placebo (n = 152). Over a mean follow-up of 2.27 years, Alzheimer's Disease Co-operative Study — Activities of Daily Living (ADCS-ADL) inventory scores declined by 3.15 units (95% confidence interval [CI], 0.92–5.39; adjusted $P = 0.03$) less in the alpha-tocopherol group compared with the placebo group. In the memantine group, these scores declined 1.98 units less (95% CI, –0.24 to 4.20; adjusted $P = 0.40$) than the placebo group's decline. This change in the alpha-tocopherol group translates into a delay in clinical progression of 19% per year compared with placebo or a delay of approximately 6.2 months over the follow-up period.

Recent research suggests that in fact gamma-tocopherol may be more important than previously suspected in AD. A study by Morris et al (2014) found gamma-tocopherol concentrations were associated with lower amyloid load ($P = 0.002$) and lower neurofibrillary tangle severity ($P = 0.02$), whereas concentrations of alpha-tocopherol were not associated with AD neuropathology, except as modified by gamma-tocopherol. High alpha-tocopherol was associated with higher amyloid load when gamma-tocopherol levels were low and with lower amyloid levels when gamma-tocopherol levels were high (*P* for interaction = 0.03). Brain concentrations of gamma- and alpha-tocopherols may be associated with AD neuropathology in interrelated, complex ways (Morris et al 2014).

Prevention

Higher plasma vitamin E levels are associated with a significantly reduced risk of cognitive impairment and dementia in older adults. Protection is most consistently seen with vitamin E from food sources, but not always from vitamin E supplements (Cherubini et al 2005, Engelhart et al 2002, Morris et al 2005). Intervention studies using supplements have produced mixed results and focus on alpha-tocopherol only. The Cache County Study was a large study of 4740 people aged 65 years or older that found a combination of vitamins E (400 IU/day) and C (500 mg/day) taken for at least 3 years was associated with a reduced incidence of AD (Zandi et al 2004). No protective effects were seen when vitamin E or C was taken alone. In the Honolulu/Asia Aging Study, long-term use of vitamin E and C supplements was associated with an 88% reduction in the frequency of subsequent vascular dementia and appeared to improve cognitive function in later life; however, a protective effect against AD was not observed (Masaki et al 2000). A lack of association between dietary or supplemental vitamin E and risk of AD in elderly subjects was also found in the Washington Heights/Inwood Columbia Aging Project (WHICAP), which involved 980 older subjects (Luchsinger et al 2003). It must be noted that dietary intakes were assessed in this study with a limited food frequency questionnaire, which is likely to be less accurate than the more detailed surveys used in some other studies.

Immunity in the elderly

Immune cell function is influenced by the oxidant and antioxidant balance, so antioxidant supplements have been investigated clinically for their ability to enhance immune responses (Meydani et al 1998). Increased markers of T-cell-mediated immunity were enhanced with all doses of synthetic vitamin E tested, according to a randomised, double-blind study of 78 healthy elderly subjects. Doses used were 60, 200 and 800 mg/day for 4 months, with best overall responses obtained with the 200 mg dosage (Meydani et al 1997). Rizvi et al (2014) state that supplementation enhances immunity in the elderly, correlating higher plasma vitamin E levels with reduced number of infections over a 3-year period. Enhanced vaccine antibody response with no adverse side effects was also observed, with other authors stating that vitamin E improves resistance to respiratory infections in the aged (Rizvi et al 2014, Wu & Meydani 2008).

Common cold and respiratory disease

Low-dose vitamin E supplementation (50 mg/day) was found to reduce the incidence of the common cold by 28% in a subgroup of men enrolled in the ATBC cancer prevention study (Hemila et al 2006). Participants were older city-dwelling men (≥ 65 years) who smoked only 5–14 cigarettes/day. More recently, researchers re-evaluated the data and found that the effect of vitamin E diverged, depending on location of dwelling and smoking status. Among city-dwelling men considered to be low–moderate-level smokers (5–14 cigarettes/day), vitamin E significantly reduced common-cold risk, whereas among those smoking more and living away from cities, vitamin E increased common-cold risk. It appears that different modifying factors have an influence on whether vitamin E supplementation has beneficial or harmful effects. The ATBC study correlated vitamin E with a 14% higher incidence of pneumonia in smokers of five cigarettes a day aged 50–69 years over a 6-year period (Hemila & Kaprio 2008).

Haemodialysis (HD)

HD increases oxidative stress and triggers atherosclerosis and dialysis-related amyloidosis (Masatomi Sasaki 2006). Vitamin E supplementation may offer several benefits to patients on HD, who typically experience high levels of oxidative stress, as there is some evidence that supplementation reduces oxidative stress and LDL oxidability in this population (Badiou et al 2003, Diepeveen et al 2005, Galli et al 2001, Giray et al 2003). The SPACE study by Boaz et al (2000) found that high-dose vitamin E supplementation (natural vitamin E 800 IU/day) caused a 50% reduction in cardiac events. This is a highly significant outcome and worthy of further investigation.

HD patients also experience cramps, which appeared to respond to vitamin E supplementation according to a placebo-controlled, double-blind study of 60 subjects (Khajehdehi et al 2001). Treatment with a vitamin E dose of 400 mg/day for 8 weeks resulted in a 54% reduction in cramps, which increased to a 97% reduction when combined with vitamin C (250 mg/day). The benefits were not significantly associated with age, sex, aetiology of end-stage renal disease, serum electrolytes or HD duration, but showed a positive correlation (*P* = 0.01) with the type of therapy used.

According to one small study, vitamin E supplementation (500 mg/day) allowed for a reduction in erythropoietin dose (from 93 to 74 IU/kg/week) while maintaining stable haemoglobin concentrations (Cristol et al 1997).

Intradialytic hypotension is a condition plaguing diabetic HD patients where SBP may drop by up to 20% during treatment. In a small unrandomised trial of 62 diabetic HD patients, vitamin E-bonded polysulfone membrane dialysers were utilised to observe SBP. Two groups entered the trial. The groups were divided into those with very low SBP (28) requiring medication and those with low SBP (34) who were not medicated. Both groups demonstrated significantly improved SBP at 3 months (Koremoto 2012).

Premenstrual syndrome (PMS)

Treatment with D-alpha-tocopherol (400 IU/day) over three menstrual cycles significantly alleviated some affective and physical symptoms of PMS according to one randomised double-blind study (London et al 1987). Symptoms of anxiety, food craving and depression responded to active treatment, whereas effects on other measured parameters such as weight gain were not significant.

An earlier study of 75 women with benign breast disease found that D-alpha-tocopherol (150–600 IU/day) significantly decreased some symptoms of PMS compared with placebo; however, the study involved subjective patient evaluation, which may have influenced the findings (London et al 1983). Women who suffer from PMS do not statistically differ from other women in regard to biochemical deficiency. In a study of 62 women who presented with moderate to severe forms of PMS, cohorts were given either vitamin E 400 IU/day or placebo and both groups demonstrated significant benefits in physical and mental symptoms. Further observation and cross-over studies are obviously needed (Mandana et al 2013).

Dysmenorrhoea

According to two randomised placebo-controlled studies, taking 200 IU vitamin E twice daily or 500 IU daily, starting 2 days before menstruation and continuing for the first 3 days of bleeding, seems to reduce menstrual pain severity and duration and to decrease blood loss in teenage girls with primary dysmenorrhoea (Ziaei et al 2001, 2005). Beneficial effects can be seen after 2 months and reach maximal effect after 4 months.

Intermittent claudication

A Cochrane review of five placebo-controlled studies including a total of 265 volunteers (average age 57 years) concluded that, although further research is required to determine its effectiveness, vitamin E may have beneficial effects in intermittent claudication with no serious side effects (Kleijnen & Mackerras 2000). Treatment duration varied from 12 weeks to 18 months, and dosage regimens varied between the studies, which were considered generally small and of poor quality. A closer look at the evidence suggests that doses of at least 600 IU/day for a minimum of 12 weeks are required.

Since then a double-blind RCT testing vitamin E (400 IU/day) found no beneficial effects on perceived pain or treadmill-walking duration in people with claudication (Collins et al 2003).

A small study of 16 patients with stable claudication revealed that administration of vitamin E (200 mg/day) and vitamin C (500 mg/day) for 4 weeks reduces oxidative stress in this population, and therefore may also have an effect on the remote ischaemia-reperfusion damage (Wijnen et al 2001). Although mentioned as a possible supplement in the treatment of intermittent claudication, no further trials have been conducted (Brass 2013).

Cancer

Most of the epidemiological evidence suggests that vitamin E and other antioxidants decrease the incidence of certain cancers. Based on these observations, numerous prospective and intervention studies have been conducted in various populations. Very often, vitamin E is used in combination with other antioxidant nutrients, and sometimes the form of tocopherol administered is not stated, making it difficult to interpret study findings.

A review that systematically evaluated the scientific literature using guidelines developed by the US Preventative Services Task Force concluded that there is evidence to suggest that those individuals with higher serum vitamin E levels or who are receiving vitamin E supplementation have a decreased risk of some cancers, including lung, prostate, stomach and gastrointestinal carcinoma (Sung et al 2003). As can be expected, study design, differing treatment dose (nutritional levels or higher), form of vitamin used and population studied (general or high-risk) had an influence on outcomes. Since then, several new studies have been published that cast doubt on the cancer-protective effects of vitamin E for the general population. However, it seems likely that certain subpopulations (e.g. the poorly nourished) may benefit, and that lifestyle factors modify responses to supplementation (e.g. smoking). Research further suggests that differences in telomere length may be another factor affecting individuals' responses to vitamin E supplements (Shen et al 2009).

The role of vitamin E in cancer prevention remains controversial. The Cancer Institute of New Jersey states that gamma- and delta-tocopherols are preventive in prostate, lung, breast and colon cancer. Alpha-tocopherols had no effect. The Heart Outcomes Prevention Evaluation — The Ongoing Outcomes (HOPE-TOO) trial and the Women's Health Study found no significant reduction in risk with daily doses of 400–600 IU (Rizvi et al 2014).

All cancers

A large study of nearly 30,000 subjects was carried out in Linxian, China. It tested four combinations of vitamins and minerals (retinol and zinc; riboflavin and niacin; vitamin C and molybdenum; and beta-carotene, vitamin E and selenium) over a 5-year period in a population with a persistently low intake of several micronutrients (Blot et al 1995). Although no statistically significant effect on cancer incidence was achieved by any intervention, secondary analysis showed that the combination of selenium, beta-carotene and alpha-tocopherol was associated with a statistically significant lower total mortality rate, a 13% reduction (borderline significant) in total cancer mortality rate and a statistically significant lower mortality rate from stomach cancer (a major cancer in Linxian).

Results from the SUVIMAX study suggest that the protective effects of vitamin E may be gender-specific (Zureik et al 2004). In this trial, antioxidant supplementation (vitamin C 120 mg, vitamin E 30 mg, beta-carotene 6 mg, selenium 100 mcg and zinc 20 mg) was associated with a lower cancer incidence in men, but not in women. It is possible that men in the SUVIMAX trial benefited from supplementation due to their lower baseline levels of antioxidants.

More recently four large studies have found that vitamin E supplementation has no protective effect against cancer incidence. The Medical Research Council/British Heart Foundation study of 20,536 UK adults aged 40–80 years with coronary disease, other occlusive arterial disease or diabetes found that a daily antioxidant supplement containing 600 mg vitamin E, 250 mg vitamin C and 20 mg beta-carotene produced no significant reduction in the incidence of cancer or ACM (Parkinson Study Group 2002). The HOPE-TOO study, which used long-term natural vitamin E (400 IU/day) as a stand-alone supplement, failed to find a protective effect against cancer incidence or cancer deaths in people with pre-existing vascular disease or diabetes mellitus (Lonn et al 2005). Long-term use of natural vitamin E (600 IU) taken on alternate days provided no overall benefit for cancer incidence or total mortality in a large randomised study involving 39,876 healthy women of at least 45 years of age (Lee et al 2005).

Results from 7627 women free of cancer at baseline in the WACS found that long-term use (average 9.4 years) of vitamin C (500 mg/day), natural vitamin E (600 IU every other day) and beta-carotene (50 mg every other day) was not significantly associated with lowered incidence of total cancer or cancer mortality for any of the tested antioxidants (O'Donnell et al 2009).

When data were evaluated for effects on site-specific cancers, women receiving vitamin E supplements had a reduced risk (but not statistically significant) for colorectal cancer compared with the placebo group. This was largely due to a reduced risk of colon cancer. However, there was no statistically significant association of vitamin E supplementation with rectal or other cancers. Further subgroup analysis revealed that women in the vitamin E supplement group who currently smoked or had smoked in the past had lower rates of cancer death than those who never smoked. The *Cancer Prevention Research Journal* suggests that, at a nutritional level, all forms of vitamin E are protective against cancer. However supplementation has not been proven to reduce cancer incidence and supplementation did not alter cancer progression or prevention (Chung 2012). However in the Selenium and vitamin E Cancer Prevention Trial (SELECT 2008 and 2011 update) for prevention of prostate cancer, statistical significance was reached with a 17% relative increase in prostate cancer compared to placebo, whereas the selenium alone or E and selenium supplementation were not statistically significant (National Cancer Institute (NIH) 2014).

Urinary tract cancer

Analysis of data from the ATBC cancer prevention study, which tested synthetic vitamin E (50 mg/day) and beta-carotene (20 mg/day) in male Finnish smokers aged 50–69 years (n = 29,133), found neither supplement affected the incidence of urothelial cancer or of renal cell cancer (Virtamo et al 2000). Jacobs et al (2002) assessed the US Cancer Prevention Study II, where vitamin C and E supplements were trialled, to determine reduced risk in bladder cancer. In the E group regular supplementation use ≥10 years demonstrated a reduced risk of bladder cancer mortality whereas shorter-duration supplementation did not prove beneficial. In a large epidemiological study plasma alpha-tocopherol and gamma-tocopherol with vitamin A were assessed. Researchers from Texas University suggest that gamma-tocopherol is not protective in isolation (Hernandez et al 2004). In the groups where plasma levels of all three nutrients were higher there was a reduction in the risk associated with bladder cancer, leading to the conclusion that there is a potentially protective effect in combination treatment (Liang et al 2008).

Respiratory tract cancers

Smoking and alcohol consumption are the major risk factors for upper aerodigestive tract cancers, and observational studies indicate a protective role for fruits, vegetables and antioxidant nutrients (Wright et al 2007). Analysis of data from the ATBC cancer prevention study testing long-term supplementation with synthetic vitamin E (50 mg/day) and beta-carotene (20 mg/day) in male Finnish smokers aged 50–69 years (n = 29,133) found no effect of either agent on the overall incidence of any upper aerodigestive tract cancer nor any effect on mortality from these neoplasms. In animal models oesophageal squamous cell carcinoma was visibly reduced by supplementation of selenium and vitamin E (80 IU/kg) in diet; this has yet to be proven in human trials (Yang et al 2012).

Breast cancer

Mixed results have been obtained for vitamin E in the primary prevention of breast cancer, although a 2003 study has detected a modest protective effect against recurrence of breast cancer and disease-related mortality in postmenopausal women previously diagnosed with the disease (Fleischauer et al 2003). Protective effects were established after 3 years' use, according to the study.

In a single study Chamras et al (2005) found a dose-responsive inhibition of cell proliferation in oestrogen receptor-positive cells. This trial is hopeful as the cell proliferation was reduced by 69–84%; vitamin E altered the expression of oestrogen receptor cells. This suggests that vitamin E may inhibit oestrogen receptor-positive cell growth and alter cellular response to oestrogen.

Ovarian cancer

Vitamin E supplements were protective against the incidence of ovarian cancer whereas consumption of antioxidants from diet was unrelated to risk according to another study (Fleischauer et al 2001). In analyses combining antioxidant intake from diet and supplements, vitamins C (>363 mg/day) and E (>75 mg/day) were associated with significant protective effects. In a human case-controlled study in Korean ovarian cancer patients, women with the highest tertile group for both alpha-tocopherol and gamma-tocopheral plasma levels presented >72% overall reduced risk compared to the lowest tertile group (Jeong et al 2009).

Colorectal cancer

Colorectal cancers are highly prevalent, with Australian levels reaching >12,000 diagnosed per year (ABS 2005). Studies investigating the association between vitamin E and incidence of colorectal cancer have produced inconsistent results. Prospective studies have shown that high serum levels of vitamin E are protective; however, only one of three intervention studies has produced positive results (Stone & Papas 1997). These results are difficult to interpret, as the studies have been criticised for not adequately distinguishing between cancer incidence and adenoma recurrence.

In the WACS (n = 7627), women receiving natural vitamin E (600 IU every other day) had a reduced risk (but not statistically significant) of colorectal cancer compared with the placebo group. This was largely because of a reduced risk of colon cancer; however, there was no statistically significant association of vitamin E supplementation with rectal or other cancers (O'Donnell et al 2009). The ATBC study also detected a somewhat lower incidence of colorectal cancer in the alpha-tocopherol arm compared with the no alpha-tocopherol arm, but this was not statistically significant (Virtamo et al 2000).

The World Cancer Research Fund (2011) suggests that vitamin E does not present with significant evidence of reduced incidence or prevalence of colorectal cancer. In a recent systematic review, although there was a concession that observational studies suggest vitamin E may be protective, experimental studies have had inconsistent results. From four studies Arain and Qadeer (2010) state that vitamin E as a primary prevention of colorectal cancer does not reduce incidence. In another review of dietary supplements where two trials regarding vitamin E were assessed, the conclusion remains steadfast (Posadzki et al 2013).

Prostate cancer

The ATBC cancer prevention study provided information about the incidence of prostate cancer with long-term use of synthetic alpha-tocopherol (50 mg), beta-carotene (20 mg), both agents or a placebo daily for 5–8 years (Albanes et al 2000). One of the most striking outcomes was a 32% decrease in the incidence of prostate cancer for volunteers receiving vitamin E (n = 14,564) compared to those not receiving it (n = 14,569) and a 41% reduction in mortality among men using vitamin E. Neither agent had any effect on the time interval between diagnosis and death (Heinonen et al 1998). The preventive effect of vitamin E on prostate cancer incidence was observed to be long-term according to later analysis of postintervention effects (Virtamo et al 2003).

One study has identified a decrease in serum androgen concentrations associated with long-term alpha-tocopherol supplementation, suggesting this may be one of the factors contributing to the observed reduction in incidence and mortality of prostate cancer (Hartman et al 2001). In contrast, SELECT (National Cancer Institute (NIH) 2014) determined that, in combination with selenium, there was an increased risk of prostate cancer with vitamin E. More specifically, there were 17% more prostate cancer cases diagnosed in the group of men assigned to take 400 IU of vitamin E (and no selenium) daily compared to the men taking two placebos (no vitamin E and no selenium), after an average of 7 years — 5.5 of the years on supplements followed by 1.5 years not taking supplements. Importantly, the vast majority of all of the cancers that were screened were very early-stage disease, and the rate of advanced or aggressive cancers in the vitamin E group was no higher than in the placebo group. Several theories have been proposed to explain the differences in results, such as a U-shaped response curve, where very low or very high blood levels of a nutrient are harmful but more moderate levels are beneficial. In other words, while the ATBC dose may have been preventive, the SELECT dose may have been too large to have a prevention benefit (http://www.cancer.gov/newscenter/qa/2008/selectqa).

Pancreatic cancer

Higher alpha-tocopherol concentrations may play a protective role in pancreatic carcinogenesis in male smokers, according to the ATBC cancer prevention study, which found that men with the highest serum tocopherol levels had a lower pancreatic cancer risk (highest compared with lowest quintile) (Stolzenberg-Solomon et al 2009). Polyunsaturated fat, a putative pro-oxidant nutrient, modified the association such that the inverse alpha-tocopherol association was most pronounced in subjects with a high polyunsaturated fat intake. Gong et al (2010) suggest that a positive association was noted in high intakes of monounsaturated palmitoleic and oleic fatty acids and polyunsaturated linolenic acid with vitamin C. In the study of a large population-based case-control study in San Francisco, it was found that vitamin C and vitamin E together or alone may reduce the risk of pancreatic cancer.

Adjunct with cisplatin

Bove et al (2001) made the observation that the neurotoxic presentation associated with cisplatin use was similar to that of vitamin E deficiency. They hypothesised that cumulative cisplatin use could induce vitamin E deficiency if patients' levels were not sufficiently high throughout treatment. To test the theory they started by measuring vitamin E in the plasma of five patients who developed severe neurotoxicity after cisplatin treatment and in another group of five patients before and after two or four cycles of cisplatin treatment. This produced preliminary data that supported the theory that inadequate vitamin E due to cisplatin treatment could be responsible for the peripheral nerve damage induced by free radicals (Bove et al 2001). Following this, four clinical trials were conducted where it was concluded that the incidence of chemotherapy-induced peripheral neuropathy was significantly reduced with vitamin E supplementation (Wolf et al 2008). Oral vitamin E (300 mg/day), taken before cisplatin treatment and continued for 3 months after cessation of treatment, significantly reduced the incidence and severity of neurotoxicity according to a randomised study (n = 47), in which the incidence of neurotoxicity was significantly lower in the group receiving vitamin E (30.7%) compared to those receiving the placebo (85.7%; $P < 0.01$) (Pace et al 2003). Shortly afterwards, Argyriou et al (2005) conducted a randomised study of 31 patients with cancer treated with six courses of cumulative cisplatin, paclitaxel or their combination regimens. Only 25% of patients randomly assigned to receive oral vitamin E (600 mg/day) during chemotherapy and for 3 months after its cessation developed neurotoxicity, compared to 73% in the control group. A year later, in another randomised study, 30 patients scheduled to receive six courses of cumulative cisplatin-based regimens were randomly allocated to receive either vitamin E (600 mg/day) during chemotherapy and for 3 months after its cessation or no adjunctive therapy (controls). This study again found a significantly reduced incidence of neurotoxicity with vitamin E (21.4%) compared to controls (68.5%) ($P = 0.026$) (Argyriou et al 2006).

While no data were included on the long-term survival of the patients involved, studies undertaken have failed to show a detrimental effect from combining vitamin E with chemotherapy (Ladas et al 2004, Pace et al 2003).

Arthritis

High-dose vitamin E supplements may be effective in relieving pain in osteoarthritis (OA) and rheumatoid arthritis (RA), according to several double-blind studies, with some studies finding that the effects are as strong as with diclofenac. Vitamin E supplements have been studied in people with OA, RA, spondylitis ankylosis, spondylosis and psoriatic arthritis. Comparisons have been made to placebos and non-steroidal anti-inflammatory drugs (NSAIDs).

Osteoarthritis

According to an early crossover study (Machtey & Ouaknine 1978), 52% of OA patients experienced less pain when treated with vitamin E (600 mg/day) compared to a placebo. Several years later, a double-blind randomised study of 50 volunteers with OA confirmed these findings and showed that vitamin E (400 IU/day) was significantly superior to a placebo in relieving pain, increasing mobility and reducing analgesic requirements (Blankenhorn 1986). Symptoms of pain at rest, during movement or with applied pressure all responded to treatment with vitamin E.

Vitamin E supplementation (500 IU/day) did not alter the loss of cartilage volume in knee OA according to a 2-year, double-blind, randomised, placebo-controlled study of 138 patients (American College of Rheumatology clinical and radiographic criteria) (Wluka et al 2002). Additionally, symptoms did not improve. Vitamin E also failed to alleviate symptoms in a shorter, 6-month double-blind study using the same dose (Brand et al 2001) and symptoms of pain, stiffness and function did not change at the 1-, 3- or 6-month assessments.

Research has continued in recent years, so that by 2007 a systematic review by Canter et al (2007) identified a total of seven RCTs that tested vitamin E in OA: four trials compared the treatment with a placebo, two tested against diclofenac and one against vitamin A. Of these, two placebo-controlled trials demonstrated the effectiveness of vitamin E for pain. One trial was considered methodologically weak, but the second was more robust and indicated greater effectiveness both for the whole patient sample and for a subgroup with OA of the knee and hip. Haflah et al's (2009) findings suggest that a dose of 400 mg/day has a potential role in reducing the symptoms of OA of the knee and may be as effective as glucosamine. This is in contrast to two earlier studies that involved patients with OA of the knee and produced largely negative results. Two equivalence trials comparing vitamin E to diclofenac produced more positive outcomes and suggested similar effectiveness for the two treatments, with one study reporting a statistically significant superiority of vitamin E over diclofenac (Canter et al 2007). The authors of the review have claimed that variable methodological rigour does not yet allow a definitive conclusion to be made about the effectiveness of vitamin E in OA. Further trials are needed; however it appears that the supplement of palm vitamin E is safe to use.

Rheumatoid arthritis

According to several double-blind studies, a dose of 1200 mg/day vitamin E significantly reduces pain symptoms in people with RA, but not always morning stiffness.

A double-blind study of 42 RA patients who received vitamin E (600 mg twice a day) over 12 weeks showed that pain parameters were significantly decreased with active treatment compared to a placebo (Edmonds et al 1997). The same study also found no change in the Ritchie Articular Index, duration of morning stiffness, swollen joint count or laboratory parameters with vitamin E supplementation compared to a placebo. A further study using the same dose detected a significant inverse correlation between vitamin E levels and pain score, whereas morning stiffness and sedimentation rate were not affected (Scherak & Kolarz 1991).

Edmonds et al (1997) enrolled 42 patients with RA in a double-blind randomised study in which alpha-tocopherol (600 mg twice a day) was compared to a placebo for 12 weeks. While laboratory measures of inflammatory activity and oxidative modification were unchanged with active treatment, pain parameters were significantly decreased after vitamin E treatment when compared with the placebo, suggesting that vitamin E may exert a small but significant analgesic activity independently of a peripheral anti-inflammatory effect. More recently, a combination of standard treatment (intramuscular methotrexate, oral sulfasalazine and indomethacin suppository at night) and vitamin E (400 mg three times daily) was compared to standard treatment and a combination of antioxidants or to standard treatment alone (Helmy et al 2001). Standard treatment started to produce tangible improvements after 2 months, whereas additional treatment with either vitamin E or antioxidants improved symptoms more quickly (after 1 month). Karlson et al (2008) suggest in a primary prevention Women's Health Study of females >45 years (randomised, double-blind, controlled) that, while inflammatory laboratory measures were unchanged in the active treatment group, pain parameters demonstrated significantly decreased levels after vitamin E treatment at 600 IU on alternate days. Although no significant associations were found in the primary end point in the prevention of RA, there was a suggestion of an inverse association with vitamin E treatment and seropositive RA; however it did not reach statistical significance. As seropositive RA is the more severe phenotype, this deserves further study. The limitations of the study were numerous, as discussed by the authors; larger numbers are needed to detect the risk reductions in seropositive and negative RA and inflammatory polyarthritis, due to previous findings of other authors reporting 28–56% reduction in risk with vitamin E supplement use (Cerhan et al 2003). In a systematic review of natural alternatives to RA treatment, McFarlane et al (2010) also suggest that vitamin E alleviates pain with no reported changes in laboratory measures of inflammation.

Comparisons with pharmaceutical medication

After 3 weeks' treatment with either high-dose vitamin E (400 mg RRR-alpha-tocopherol acetate three times daily) or diclofenac sodium, a significant improvement in all assessed clinical parameters was observed in hospitalised patients with established chronic RA (n = 85), according to a randomised, double-blind parallel-group trial (Wittenborg et al 1998). Duration of morning stiffness, grip strength and the degree of pain, assessed by a 10-cm visual analogue scale, reduced significantly with vitamin E as well as with diclofenac. Both treatments were considered to be equally effective by patients and doctors.

Menopausal symptoms

According to a review published by the Mayo Clinic in the United States, behavioural changes in conjunction with vitamin E (800 IU/day) are a reasonable initial approach for menopausal women with mild symptoms that do not interfere with sleep or daily function (Shanafelt et al 2002). The recommendation is based on a double-blind, randomised, placebo-controlled, crossover clinical trial that found that vitamin E (800 IU/day) was more effective than a placebo in controlling hot flushes in breast cancer survivors. Benefits have been confirmed in another double-blind, placebo-controlled trial, which found that treatment with 400 IU vitamin E daily significantly reduced hot flush severity and daily frequency as reported by participants (Ziaei et al 2007).

Male infertility

Lipid-soluble antioxidants such as vitamin E have been studied for their effects in male reproductive physiology because the membranes of germ cells and spermatozoa are very sensitive to oxidation (Bhardwaj et al 2000, Bolle et al 2002).

According to three of four studies, oral vitamin E supplementation can effectively treat some forms of male infertility (Geva et al 1996, Kessopoulou et al 1995, Rolf et al 1999, Suleiman et al 1996). Doses varied from 200 to 800 mg/day.

Kessopoulou et al (1995) compared vitamin E (600 mg/day) to a placebo over 3 months in 30 healthy men with high levels of reactive oxygen species generation in semen and a normal female partner. The randomised, crossover study found that active treatment improved zona binding, thereby showing that vitamin E significantly improved the in vitro function of human spermatozoa. Geva et al (1996) studied men enrolled in an in vitro fertilisation program who previously had had low fertilisation rates, and treated them with oral vitamin E (200 mg/day) for 3 months. After the first month, fertilisation rates increased significantly, from 19% to 29%. The same year, Suleiman et al (1996) treated asthenospermic patients with oral vitamin E, which significantly decreased the malondialdehyde concentration in spermatozoa and improved sperm motility. Of the 52 treated males, 11 (21%) impregnated their spouses; nine of the spouses successfully continued to have normal-term deliveries, whereas two aborted in the first trimester. No pregnancies were reported in the spouses of the placebo-treated patients.

The negative study used high-dose oral vitamin C (1000 mg/day), and vitamin E (800 mg/day) was tested over 56 days in 31 men with asthenozoospermia (<50% motile spermatozoa) and normal or only moderately reduced sperm concentration (>7 × 10^6 spermatozoa/mL) (Rolf et al 1999). Most recent studies combine vitamin E (400 IU/day) with selenium (and/or vitamin C) and are positively correlated with increased fertility and oligoasthenozoopermia syndrome; however it is not known whether vitamin E alone would have been just as effective (Kobori et al 2014, Moslemi & Tavanbakhsh 2011).

Dermatological conditions

Vitamin E is used both as an oral supplement and as a topical preparation in a variety of dermatological conditions. It is a popular ingredient in many moisturising preparations used to: alleviate dry and cracked skin; assist in the repair of abrasions, burns, grazes and skin lesions; prevent stretch marks; and diminish scar tissue. Vitamin E oil is used as a stand-alone preparation or incorporated into a cream or ointment base for these purposes.

Sunburn protection

Topical application of 1% alpha-tocopherol provided significant protection against erythema and sunburn in an experimental model. When combined with 15% ascorbic acid, the protective effect was enhanced (Lin et al 2003). Further improvements were seen when ferulic acid was added to the alpha-tocopherol (1%) and ascorbic acid (15%) solution, as this substance improves chemical stability of the antioxidants and doubles the photoprotective effect (Lin et al 2005).

Once again, it appears that not all forms of vitamin E exert a significant protective effect (McVean & Liebler 1999). According to an in vivo study, a 5% dispersion of alpha-tocopherol, gamma-tocopherol or delta-tocopherol in a neutral cream vehicle produced a statistically significant inhibition of thymine dimer formation, whereas alpha-tocopherol acetate and alpha-tocopherol methyl ether had no effect. Further research revealed that gamma-tocopherol and delta-tocopherol were five- to 10-fold less potent than alpha-tocopherol (McVean & Liebler 1997).

A comparison between topical vitamins E and C has demonstrated that vitamin E affords better protection against ultraviolet B radiation, whereas vitamin C is superior against ultraviolet A radiation (Baumann & Spencer 1999).

Although most research has focused on topical use, oral administration of a combination of high-dose vitamins E and C increases the threshold to erythema. The first study to show that the systemic administration of vitamins E and C reduces the sunburn reaction in humans was a small, double-blind, placebo-controlled trial that used ascorbic acid (2 g/day) combined with D-alpha-tocopherol (1000 IU/day) (Eberlein-Konig et al 1998). The effect was seen after 8 days. The next to show reduction of the sunburn reaction was a 50-day study of 40 volunteers (20–47 years old), which showed that supplemental vitamin E (2 g/day) and C (3 g/day) protected against sunburn and resulted in increased vitamin E levels in keratinocytes (Fuchs & Kern 1998). This was once again confirmed in a controlled study of 45 healthy volunteers (Mireles-Rocha et al 2002). The doses used were lower in this study: 1200 IU/day of D-alpha-tocopherol in combination with vitamin C (2 g/day).

Scar tissue

Although vitamin E is widely used to diminish the appearance of scars, a small double-blind study of 15 patients who had undergone skin cancer removal found that applying an emollient preparation known as Aquaphor with added vitamin E after surgery either had no effect or worsened the appearance of scars compared to Aquaphor alone (Baumann & Spencer 1999). A larger study of 80 people with hypertrophic scars and keloids found that treatment with vitamin E and silicone gel sheets was successful in scar treatment (Palmieri et al 1995). After 2 months, 95% of patients receiving vitamin E and gel sheet treatment had improved by 50%, whereas 75% had improved by 50% without vitamin E.

Type 1 diabetes

Although the Heart Outcomes Prevention Evaluation (HOPE) study involving 3654 people with diabetes failed to detect a preventive effect for long-term vitamin E (400 IU/day) on CVD outcomes or nephropathy (Jain et al 1996, Lonn et al 2002), it is known that both types of diabetes demonstrate increased free radicals. It could be rationalised that the antioxidant effect on lipid peroxidation would be of some use; however metabolic parameters do not appear to improve in type 1 patients after vitamin E supplementation. There are limited trials and cohorts are relatively small (Gupta et al 2011).

Type 2 diabetes

In type 2 diabetes there is a similar increased production of free radicals as displayed in type 1 diabetes. Plasma measures of vitamin E are found to be lower in a small group of 52, with 36.2% diabetics with low alpha-tocopherol <12 micromol/L, 32.7% with a low alpha-tocopherol. Larger epidemiological and longitudinal studies are needed to confirm the use of vitamin E supplementation in this group (Illison et al 2011).

Chronic hepatitis C

According to a 2004 systematic review, significant improvements in biochemical responses were seen for vitamin E compared to a placebo (Coon & Ernst 2004). The authors report on one placebo-controlled trial in which a statistically significant reduction in liver enzyme (alanine aminotransferase [ALT]) was observed during vitamin E treatment but reductions were not consistent for all patients and complete normalisation of ALT levels did not occur. In the Middle East, where hepatitis C genotype is prevalent, ribavirin when used with pegylated interferon induces anaemia. Supplemental vitamin E 1000 IU/day demonstrated a protective impact on neutrophils and platelet counts, ameliorating the effect of haemolysis associated with ribavirin administration (Assem 2011).

Asthma and atopy

Studies have consistently demonstrated beneficial associations between dietary vitamin E and ventilatory function, and a few have demonstrated beneficial associations with asthma and atopy (Devereux & Seaton 2005). However, benefits do not extend to vitamin E supplements, as a randomised study (*n* = 72) using natural vitamin E (500 mg/day) over 6 weeks found no clinical benefit in subjects with mild to moderate asthma (Pearson et al 2004).

Age-related macular degeneration (AMD)

According to a review of RCTs comparing antioxidant vitamin and/or mineral supplement to controls, there is no evidence that antioxidant (vitamin E or beta-carotene) supplementation prevents AMD. However, there is evidence that supplementation with antioxidants (beta-carotene 15 mg, vitamin C 500 mg and vitamin E 400 IU) and zinc (elemental 80 mg) daily slows down the progression to advanced AMD and visual acuity loss in people with signs of the disease (Evans 2008). People with AMD, or early signs of the disease, may experience some benefit from taking supplements as used in the Age-Related Eye Disease Study (AREDS) (Sackett & Schenning 2002). Christen et al (2012) conducted an 8-year trial in well-nourished doctors of 400 IU every other day and vitamin C 500 mg/day. There appeared to be no beneficial or harmful effect on the risk of incidence of AMD. The dose for vitamin E was much lower than in the AREDS, at 400 IU/daily. Although this represents the largest study of its kind, it is not unreasonable to conclude that the dose was not high enough to exert effect and that the men were already nutritionally replete and perhaps at less risk.

Neurogenerative disease

Vitamin E supplementation may slow the rate of motor decline early in the course of Huntington's disease, according to a randomised, double-blind, placebo-controlled study of high-dose D-alpha-tocopherol treatment (Peyser et al 1995). The study of 73 patients with Huntington's disease found that treatment with D-alpha-tocopherol had no effect on neurological and neuropsychiatric symptoms in the treatment group overall; however, post hoc analysis revealed a significant selective therapeutic effect on neurological symptoms for patients early in the course of the disorder.

It now seems that the role of vitamin E has been established as essential for neurological function. In a recent review vitamin E was validated in the treatment of disorders of the central nervous system, specifically the use of vitamin E in the prevention or cure of Huntington's disease, tardive dyskinesia, amyotrophic lateral sclerosis (motor neuron disease [MND]), PD and AD (the last discussed earlier). Many trials for the use of vitamin E in the nervous system have been too small or the dose of vitamin E has been too low. Imounan et al (2012) suggest that in many neuropathic disorders vitamin E is revealing an important role.

OTHER USES

Oral supplements have been used to prevent or treat many other conditions, such as exercise-induced tissue damage, some types of senile cataracts, epilepsy and fibromyalgia.

Vitamin E prophylaxis in premature babies significantly reduces the risk of stage 3+ retinopathy by 52%, according to a 1997 meta-analysis of six randomised studies (Raju et al 1997).

Infusions of vitamin E are being investigated as a means of preventing ischaemic reperfusion injury in liver and heart surgery (Bartels et al 2004, Jaxa-Chamiec et al 2005).

DOSAGE RANGE

The body's requirement for vitamin E changes according to the amount and type of fat eaten in the diet. For example, vitamin E requirements increase when there is a high intake of PUFAs (Wahlqvist 2002).

Many scientists believe it is difficult for an individual to consume more than 15 mg/day of alpha-tocopherol from food alone, without also increasing fat intake above recommended levels.

Recommendations for adults (Australian adequate intake)

Adequate intake is used when there is insufficient scientific evidence derived from approximations of intakes in groups or a group of possibly healthy people (NHMRC 2014). It is at best a guide, not a therapeutic dose, and will not suffice where frank deficiency is observed.

- Men > 18 years: 10 mg/day alpha-tocopherol.
- Women > 18 years: 7 mg/day alpha-tocopherol.
- Upper level of intake: 300 mg/day alpha-tocopherol.
- Deficiency treatment: 800–1200 mg/day.

According to clinical studies

Both natural and synthetic forms of vitamin E have been evaluated in clinical trials at different doses and durations, and sometimes in combination with other nutrients that also exhibit antioxidant properties.

Unless stated, dosages are for natural vitamin E (alpha-tocopherol).

- Alzheimer's disease: 2000 IU/day synthetic alpha-tocopherol.
- Anaemia in HD: 500 mg/day.
- Angina pectoris: 50–300 mg/day.
- Antioxidant effects: 400 IU/day.
- Cancer, to reduce cisplatin-induced neurotoxicity: oral vitamin E (600 mg/day) during chemotherapy and for 3 months after its cessation.
- Cerebral infarction prevention: 50 mg/day synthetic vitamin E.
- Colorectal cancer prevention: 50 mg/day long-term.
- CVD: primary prevention: 100–260 IU/day long-term (benefits uncertain with supplementation).
- CVD: secondary prevention: 100–800 IU/day long-term (benefits most likely in people with low baseline vitamin E and higher oxidative stress, e.g. people on haemodialysis and diabetics).
- Carotid atherosclerosis, slowing progression: 136 IU twice daily and vitamin C 250 mg (slow-release) twice daily.
- Dementia prevention: 400 IU/day alpha-tocopherol plus vitamin C 500 mg/day.
- HD, associated cramps: 400 mg/day alpha-tocopherol plus vitamin C 250 mg/day.
- Hypertension: 200 IU/day long-term.
- Immune system support in the elderly: 200 mg/day.
- Intermittent claudication: 600–1600 IU/day.
- Ischaemic stroke prevention in high-risk hypertension: 50 mg/day.
- Male infertility: 200–800 mg/day.
- Menopausal symptoms: 800 IU/day.
- Nitrate tolerance prevention: 200 mg three times daily.
- OA: 1200 IU/day.
- Ovarian cancer: >75 mg/day.
- Premenstrual symptoms: 400–600 IU/day.
- Prostate cancer prevention: 50 mg/day (200 mg detrimental).
- Retinopathy of prematurity: 100 mg/kg/day.
- RA: 1200 IU/day.
- Sunburn protection: 1000 IU/day up to 2000 mg/day plus vitamin C 2000–3000 mg/day.

TOXICITY

Vitamin E is relatively non-toxic. It is not stored as readily in the body as other fat-soluble vitamins and up to 60–70% of a daily dose is excreted in the faeces. Doses as high as 3200 mg/day have been used for 12 years with few adverse effects (Fariss & Zhang 2003).

In April 2000, the Food and Nutrition Board of the Institute of Medicine in the United States set an upper tolerable limit of 1500 IU of RRR-alpha tocopherol as the highest dose unlikely to result in haemorrhage in most adults.

ADVERSE REACTIONS

Adverse effects are dose-related and tend to occur only at very high supplemental doses (>1200 IU/day); they include diarrhoea, flatulence, nausea and heart palpitations. Doses above this level should be used only under professional supervision.

SIGNIFICANT INTERACTIONS

Considering vitamin E is a fat-soluble vitamin, any medication that reduces the absorption of fats in the diet will also reduce the absorption of vitamin E. These include cholestyramine, colestipol, isoniazid, mineral oil, orlistat and sucralfate.

Oral contraceptive pill

A very small cross-sectional study suggests the oral contraceptive pill significantly lowered coenzyme Q10, and alpha-tocopherol levels. Further studies are needed (Palan et al 2006).

HMG-CoA reductase inhibitors (statins)

The effect of statins on lowering blood lipid levels of vitamin E has been suggested as a risk factor in the development of statin-associated myopathy. Further studies are warranted (Galli et al 2010).

Chloroquine

According to in vitro research, vitamin E inhibits drug uptake in human cultured fibroblasts. The clinical significance of this observation is unknown. Observe patients taking this combination (Scuntaro et al 1996).

Chlorpromazine

According to in vitro research, vitamin E inhibits drug uptake in human cultured fibroblasts. The clinical significance of this observation is unknown — observe patients taking this combination (Scuntaro et al 1996).

Cisplatin

A review of four clinical trials testing the effects of the combination of vitamin E with cisplatin has shown that in all trials the incidence of chemotherapy-induced peripheral neuropathy was significantly reduced (Wolf et al 2008). Beneficial interaction, but should be used under professional supervision.

Warfarin

Contradictory results have been obtained in clinical studies that have investigated whether vitamin E affects platelet aggregation or coagulation. A dose of 1200 IU/day (800 mg of D-alpha-tocopherol) taken for 28 days had no effect on platelet aggregation or coagulation according to one clinical study (Morinobu et al 2002). Similarly, a second clinical study found that a lower dose of 600 mg (900 IU) of RRR-alpha-tocopherol taken daily for 12 weeks did not alter coagulation activity (Kitagawa & Mino 1989). In contrast, increased risk of gingival bleeding at doses of 50 mg/day was found by another study (Liede et al 1998).

Overall, it appears that people with reduced levels of vitamin K may be more susceptible to the effects of vitamin E, potentiating warfarin activity.

Practice points/Patient counselling

- Vitamin E is actually a generic term used to describe any chemical entity that displays the biological activity of RRR-alpha-tocopherol, the most abundant form found in nature. The 'natural' form is the most potent of all eight forms of vitamin E, although there is evidence that other tocopherols also exhibit significant beneficial effects.
- It is involved in myriad biochemical processes such as immunocompetence and neurological function, but its most important biological function is that of an antioxidant.
- Vitamin E is used for many different indications. There is evidence to suggest that supplementation may be useful in:
  - secondary CVD prevention, although effects are inconsistent
  - slowing down progression of AD, although effects are inconsistent
  - enhancing immune function in the elderly• preventing anaemia and treating cramps in patients on HD
  - reducing PMS, dysmenorrhoea and menopause symptoms
  - reducing pain in OA and RA
  - improving some forms of male infertility
  - reducing risk of stage 3+ retinopathy in premature babies
  - preventing ischaemic stroke in high-risk hypertensive patients
  - reducing incidence of some cancers, although effects are inconsistent
  - preventing sunburn (when used with vitamin C)
  - slowing down carotid atherosclerosis (when used with vitamin C)
  - reducing blood pressure
  - reducing nitrate tolerance
  - reducing cisplatin-induced neurotoxicity.
- Oral supplements have been used to prevent or treat many other conditions, such as exercise-induced tissue damage, some types of senile cataracts, epilepsy and fibromyalgia.
- It is a popular ingredient in many moisturising preparations used to: alleviate dry and cracked skin; assist in the repair of abrasions, burns, grazes and skin lesions; prevent stretch marks; and diminish scar tissue. Vitamin E oil is used as a stand-alone preparation or incorporated into a cream or ointment base for these purposes.
- People with impaired coagulation, inherited bleeding disorders, a history of haemorrhagic stroke or vitamin K deficiency, or who are at risk of pulmonary embolism or thrombophlebitis should use high-dose supplements under medical supervision.

Until further research can clarify whether the interaction is clinically significant for most people, it is recommended that prothrombin time ratio, or international normalised ratio, should be closely monitored upon the addition and withdrawal of treatment with high-dose vitamin E supplements.

Doxorubicin

One study found that oral DL-alpha-tocopherol acetate (1600 IU/day) prevented doxorubicin-induced alopecia (Wood 1985). The same dose of oral DL-alpha-tocopherol acetate failed to prevent alopecia after doxorubicin treatment following mastectomy for breast cancer (Martin-Jimenez et al 1986). It also failed to prevent alopecia in a second study of 20 patients with different types of solid tumours (Perez et al 1986). Possible beneficial interaction but difficult to assess.

Nitrates

Oral vitamin E prevented nitrate tolerance when given concurrently with transdermal nitroglycerin (10 mg/24 hours), according to one randomised placebo-controlled study (Watanabe et al 1997). Beneficial interaction possible.

NSAIDs and simple analgesics

Vitamin E may enhance the pain-modifying activity of drugs. Beneficial interaction possible; drug dosage may require modification.

Propranolol

According to in vitro research, vitamin E inhibits drug uptake in human cultured fibroblasts. The clinical significance of this observation is unknown. Observe patients taking this combination (Scuntaro et al 1996).

CONTRAINDICATIONS AND PRECAUTIONS

Vitamin E is considered to be a safe substance.

People with impaired coagulation, inherited bleeding disorders, a history of haemorrhagic stroke, vitamin K deficiency or at risk of pulmonary embolism or thrombophlebitis should use high-dose supplements under medical supervision.

Although it was thought that people with hypertension wanting to take supplements should start with low doses, evidence does not support the concern that high-dose supplements will significantly elevate blood pressure. Suspend use of high doses (>1000 IU/day) 1 week before major surgery.

PREGNANCY USE

Vitamin E is considered to be safe in pregnancy.

PATIENTS' FAQs

What will this vitamin do for me?

Vitamin E is essential for health and wellbeing. It is involved in many important biological processes in the body and may prevent serious diseases such as heart disease and some cancers; however, people with these conditions should seek professional advice. It is also used to reduce symptoms in common conditions such as arthritis, PMS and menopause. Vitamin E supplements enhance immune function in the elderly and may slow the progression of AD. Oral supplements have been used to prevent or treat many other conditions, such as exercise-induced tissue damage, some types of senile cataracts, epilepsy and fibromyalgia.

When will it start to work?

This depends largely on the reason for taking the supplement. In the case of disease prevention, studies suggest that long-term use is necessary (i.e. 2–3 years or longer). When using vitamin E to reduce symptoms, effects have generally been seen within 3 months.

Are there any safety issues?

People with impaired coagulation, inherited bleeding disorders, a history of haemorrhagic stroke or vitamin K deficiency, or who are at risk of pulmonary embolism or thrombophlebitis should use high-dose supplements under medical supervision. Additionally, vitamin E can interact with some medicines, so professional advice is recommended when using high-dose supplements.

REFERENCES

ABS 2005 Mortality and Morbidity: Colorectal Cancer. [Online] http://www.abs.gov.au/AUSSTATS/abs@.nsf/94713ad445ff1425ca25682000192af2/89be997ee1e35bd6ca25703b0080ccbd!OpenDocument [Accessed 10th may 2014].

Albanes D et al. Effects of supplemental alpha-tocopherol and beta-carotene on colorectal cancer: results from a controlled trial (Finland). Cancer Causes Control 11.3 (2000): 197–205.

Albert CM et al. Moderate alcohol consumption and the risk of sudden cardiac death among US male physicians. Circulation 100.9 (1999): 944–950.

Arad YLA, et al 2005. Treatment of asymptomatic adults with elevated coronary calcium scores with atorvastin, vitamin C, and vitamin E: the St Francis Heart Study randomized clinical trial. J Am Coll Cardiol 46: 166–172.

Arain MA, Qadeer A, 2010. Systematic review on 'vitamin E and prevention of colorectal cancer'. Pak J Pharm Sci 23;2:125–30.

Argyriou AA, et al. 2005. Vitamin E for prophylaxis against chemotherapy induced neuropathy: a randomized controlled trial. Neurology 64:26–31.

Assem, YM, (2011) Impact of pentoxifylline and vitamin E on Ribavirin-induced haemolytic anaemia in chronic hepatitis C patients: an Egyptian survey. Int J Hepatol: 530949.

Azen SP et al. Effect of supplementary antioxidant vitamin intake on carotid arterial wall intima-media thickness in a controlled clinical trial of cholesterol lowering. Circulation 94.10 (1996): 2369–2372.

Badiou S et al. Vitamin E supplementation increases LDL resistance to ex vivo oxidation in hemodialysis patients. Int J Vitam Nutr Res 73.4 (2003): 290–296.

Bartels M et al. Pilot study on the effect of parenteral vitamin E on ischemia and reperfusion induced liver injury: A double blind, randomized, placebo-controlled trial. Clin Nutr 23.6 (2004): 1360–1370.

Baumann LS, Spencer J. The effects of topical vitamin E on the cosmetic appearance of scars. Dermatol Surg 25.4 (1999): 311–3115.

Bender DA, 2003. Nutritional biochemistry of vitamins. 2nd edn. University College of London. Cambridge University Press.

Berry D, et al. Bayesian model averaging in meta-analysis: Vitamin E supplementation and mortality. Clin Trials 6.1 (2009): 28–41.

Bhardwaj A et al. Status of vitamin E and reduced glutathione in semen of oligozoospermic and azoospermic patients. Asian J Androl 2.3 (2000): 225 228.

Bjelakovic G et al. Mortality in randomized trials of antioxidant supplements for primary and secondary prevention: Systematic review and meta-analysis. JAMA 297.8 (2007): 842–857.

Bjelakovic G, et al 2013. Meta-regression analyses, meta-analyses, and trial sequential analyses of the effects of supplementation with beta-carotene, vitamin A and vitamin E singly or in different combinations on all-cause mortality: do we have evidence for lack of harm? PLOS ONE 8:9 e74558

Blaner WS, 2013. Vitamin E: the enigmatic one! Journal of Lipid Research, 54:2293–2294.

Blankenhorn G. Clinical effectiveness of Spondyvit (vitamin E) in activated arthroses. A multicenter placebo-controlled double-blind study. Z Orthop Ihre Grenzgeb 124.3 (1986): 340–343.

Blot WJ et al. The Linxian trials: Mortality rates by vitamin-mineral intervention group. Am J Clin Nutr 62.6 (Suppl) (1995): 1424S–6S.

Boaz M et al. Secondary Prevention with Antioxidants of Cardiovascular disease in Endstage renal disease (SPACE): randomised placebo-controlled trial. Lancet 356.9237 (2000): 1213–1218.

Bolle P et al. The controversial efficacy of vitamin E for human male infertility. Contraception 65.4 (2002): 313–315.

Bonner LT, Peskind ER. Pharmacologic treatments of dementia. Med Clin North Am 86.3 (2002): 657–674.

Boshtam M et al. Vitamin E can reduce blood pressure in mild hypertensives. Int J Vitam Nutr Res 72.5 (2002): 309–314.

Bove L et al. A pilot study on the relation between cisplatin neuropathy and vitamin E. J Exp Clin Cancer Res 20.2 (2001): 277–280.

Brack m, et al 2013. Distinct profiles of systemic biomarkers of oxidative stress in chronic human pathologies: Cardiovascular, psychiatric, neurodegenerative, rheumatic, infectious, neoplasmic and endogrinological diseases. Advances in Bioscience and Biotechnology, 2013, 4, 331–339.

Brand C et al. Vitamin E is ineffective for symptomatic relief of knee osteoarthritis: A six month double blind, randomised, placebo controlled study. Ann Rheum Dis 60.10 (2001): 946–949.

Brass EP, 2013. Intermittent Claudication: New targets for drug development. Drugs 73:999–1014.

Brigelius-Flohe R. Vitamin E: the shrew waiting to be tamed. Free Radic Biol Med 46.5 (2009): 543–554.

Brockes C et al. Vitamin E prevents extensive lipid peroxidation in patients with hypertension. Br J Biomed Sci 60.1 (2003): 5–8.

Canter PH, et al The antioxidant vitamins A, C, E and selenium in the treatment of arthritis: a systematic review of randomized clinical trials. Rheumatology (Oxford) 46.8 (2007): 1223–33.

Cerhan JR, et al 2003. Antioxidant micronutrients and risk of rheumatoid arthritis in a cohort of older women. Am J Epidemiol. 157(4):345–54.

Chamras H, et al 2005. Novel interactions of vitamin E and estrogen in breast cancer. Nutr Cancer 52:1;43–48.

Che Anishas C, et al 2014. Oil palm phenolics and vitamin E reduce atherosclerosis in rabbits, Journal of Functional Foods, 7; 550: 1756–4646.

Chen H et al. Mixed tocopherol preparation is superior to alpha-tocopherol alone against hypoxia-reoxygenation injury. Biochem Biophys Res Commun 291.2 (2002): 349–353.

Cherubini A et al. Vitamin E levels, cognitive impairment and dementia in older persons: the InCHIANTI study. Neurobiol Aging 26.7 (2005): 987–994.

Christen WG, et al 2012. Vitamins E and C and medical record confirmed age related macular degeneration in a randomized trial of male physicians. Ophthalmology 119:8;1642–1649.

Clarke R, Armitage J. Antioxidant vitamins and risk of cardiovascular disease. Review of large-scale randomised trials. Cardiovasc Drugs Ther 16.5 (2002): 411–415.

Collins EG et al. Pole striding exercise and vitamin E for management of peripheral vascular disease. Med Sci Sports Exerc 35.3 (2003): 384–393.

Colombo ML, 2010. An update on vitamin E, tocopherol and tocotrienol perspectives. Molecules, 15: 2103–2113.

Cook NR et al. A randomized factorial trial of vitamins C and E and beta carotene in the secondary prevention of cardiovascular events in women: Results from the Women's Antioxidant Cardiovascular Study. Arch Intern Med 167.15 (2007): 1610–1618.

Coon JT, Ernst E. Complementary and alternative therapies in the treatment of chronic hepatitis C: A systematic review. J Hepatol 40.3 (2004): 491 500.

Cristol JP et al. Erythropoietin and oxidative stress in haemodialysis: Beneficial effects of vitamin E supplementation. Nephrol Dial Transplant 12.11 (1997): 2312–23117.

De Gaetano G. Low-dose aspirin and vitamin E in people at cardiovascular risk: A randomised trial in general practice: Collaborative Group of the Primary Prevention Project. Lancet 357.9250 (2001): 89–95.

DeMaio SJ et al. Vitamin E supplementation, plasma lipids and incidence of restenosis after percutaneous transluminal coronary angioplasty (PTCA). J Am Coll Nutr 11.1 (1992): 68–73.
Devereux G, Seaton A. Diet as a risk factor for atopy and asthma. J Allergy Clin Immunol 115.6 (2005): 1109–1117.
De Vita VT, et al (eds). Cancer: principles and practice in oncology, 7th edn. Philadelpia: Lippincott, Williams and Wilkins, 2005
Diepeveen SH et al. Effects of atorvastatin and vitamin E on lipoproteins and oxidative stress in dialysis patients: a randomised-controlled trial. J Intern Med 257.5 (2005): 438–445.
Dietrich M et al. Vitamin E supplement use and the incidence of cardiovascular disease and all-cause mortality in the Framingham Heart Study: Does the underlying health status play a role? Atherosclerosis 205.2 (2009): 549–553.
Dunford M, Doyle J, 2012. Nutrition for sport and exercise, 3rd edn. Cengage learning.
Dysken, M.W., et al 2014. Effect of vitamin E and memantine on functional decline in Alzheimer disease: the TEAM-AD VA cooperative randomized trial. JAMA, 311, (1) 33–44.
Eberlein-Konig B et al. Protective effect against sunburn of combined systemic ascorbic acid (vitamin C) and d-[alpha]-tocopherol (vitamin E). J Am Acad Dermatol 38.1 (1998): 45–48.
Edmonds SE et al. Putative analgesic activity of repeated oral doses of vitamin E in the treatment of rheumatoid arthritis: Results of a prospective placebo controlled double blind trial. Ann Rheum Dis 56.11 (1997): 649–655.
Engelhart MJ et al. Dietary intake of antioxidants and risk of Alzheimer disease. JAMA 287.24 (2002): 3223–3229.
Evans, H.M. Invariable occurrence of male sterility with dietaries lacking fat soluble vitamin E. Proc. Natl. Acad. Sci. U.S.A. 1925: 11,373.
Evans J. Antioxidant supplements to prevent or slow down the progression of AMD: a systematic review and meta-analysis. Eye 22.6 (2008): 751–760.
Fahn S. A pilot trial of high-dose alpha-tocopherol and ascorbate in early Parkinson's disease. Ann Neurol 32 (Suppl.) (1992): S128–S132.
Fang JC et al. Effect of vitamins C and E on progression of transplant-associated arteriosclerosis: A randomised trial. Lancet 359.9312 (2002): 1108–1113.
FAO/WHO (Food and Agriculture Organization/World Health Organization). Vitamin E. In: Report of a Joint FAO/WHO Expert Consultation, Bangkok, Thailand. Rome: FAO/WHO, 2002.
Fariss MW, Zhang JG. Vitamin E therapy in Parkinson's disease. Toxicology 189.1–2 (2003): 129–146.
Fleischauer AT et al. Dietary antioxidants, supplements, and risk of epithelial ovarian cancer. Nutr Cancer 40.2 (2001): 92–98.
Fleischauer AT et al. Antioxidant supplements and risk of breast cancer recurrence and breast cancer-related mortality among postmenopausal women. Nutr Cancer 46.1 (2003): 15–22.
Fuchs J, Kern H. Modulation of UV-light-induced skin inflammation by d-alpha-tocopherol and l-ascorbic acid: A clinical study using solar simulated radiation. Free Radic Biol Med 25.9 (1998): 1006–1012.
Galli F et al. Vitamin E, lipid profile, and peroxidation in hemodialysis patients. Kidney Int Suppl 78 (2001): S148–S154.
Galli, F., et al. 2010. Do statins cause myopathy by lowering vitamin E levels? Med Hypotheses. 74(4):707–709.
Gerss J, Kopcke W. The questionable association of vitamin E supplementation and mortality — inconsistent results of different meta-analytic approaches. Cell Mol Biol 55 Suppl (2009): OL1111–20.
Geva E et al. The effect of antioxidant treatment on human spermatozoa and fertilization rate in an in vitro fertilization program. Fertil Steril 66.3 (1996): 430–434.
Giray B et al. The effect of vitamin E supplementation on antioxidant enzyme activities and lipid peroxidation levels in hemodialysis patients. Clin Chim Acta 338.1–2 (2003): 91–98.
GISSI. Dietary supplementation with n-3 polyunsaturated fatty acids and vitamin E after myocardial infarction: results of the GISSI-Prevenzione trial (Gruppo Italiano per lo Studio della Sopravvivenza nell'Infarto miocardico). Lancet 354.9177 (1999): 447–455.
Gong, Z, et al 2010. Intake of fatty acids and antioxidants and pancreatic cancer in a large population-based case-control study in the San Francisco Bay area. Int J Cancer. 127(8):1893–1904
Gupta S, et al 2011. Vitamin E supplementation may ameliorate oxidative stress in type 1 diabetes mellitus patients. Clin. Lab,Vol.57, No.5–6, pp.379–386
Haflah HM, et al 2009. Effects of palm vitamin E on osteoarthritis. Saudi Med 30:11; 1432–1437
Hartman TJ et al. Effects of long-term alpha-tocopherol supplementation on serum hormones in older men. Prostate 46.1 (2001): 33–38.
Heinecke JW. Oxidized amino acids: culprits in human atherosclerosis and indicators of oxidative stress. Free Radic Biol Med 32.11 (2002): 1090–1101.
Heinecke JW. Oxidative stress: new approaches to diagnosis and prognosis in atherosclerosis. Am J Cardiol 91.3A (2003): 12–16A.
Heinonen OP et al. Prostate cancer and supplementation with alpha-tocopherol and beta-carotene: incidence and mortality in a controlled trial. J Natl Cancer Inst 90.6 (1998): 440–446.
Hemilä H, 2013. Vitamin E may significantly increase and decrease mortality in some population groups [Comment]. PloS One, vol 8, e74558.
Hemila H, Kaprio J, 2008. Vitamin E supplementation and pneumonia risk in males who initiated smoking at an early age: effect modification by body weight and dietary vitamin C. Nutr J 7:33.
Hemila H et al. The effect of vitamin E on common cold incidence is modified by age, smoking and residential neighborhood. J Am Coll Nutr 25.4 (2006): 332–339.
Hernandez, L. M., et al. 2004. 95th Annual Meeting of the American Association for Cancer Research. Orlando, Florida, USA. March 27–31.
Hodis HN et al. Alpha-tocopherol supplementation in healthy individuals reduces low-density lipoprotein oxidation but not atherosclerosis: The Vitamin E Atherosclerosis Prevention Study (VEAPS). Circulation 106.12 (2002): 1453–1459.
Iino K et al. A controlled, double-blind study of dl-alpha-tocopheryl nicotinate (Juvela-Nicotinate) for treatment of symptoms in hypertension and cerebral arteriosclerosis. Jpn Heart J 18.3 (1977): 277–286.
Illison, V. K, et al 2011. The Relationship between plasma alpha-tocopherol concentration and vitamin E intake in patients with type 2 diabetes mellitus. Int J Vitam Nutr Res. 81(1):12–20.
Imounan F, et al 2012. Vitamin E in ataxia and neurodegenerative diseases: A review. World Journal of Neuroscience, 2;217–222.
Institute of Medicine, 2000. Food and Nutrition Board. Dietary Reference Intakes: Vitamin C, Vitamin E, Selenium, and Carotenoids. Washington, DC: National Academy Press.
Jacobs, E J, et al. 2002. Vitamin C and vitamin E supplement use and bladder cancer mortality in a large cohort of US men and women. American Journal of Epidemiology. 156(11):1002–1010.
Jain SK et al. Effect of modest vitamin E supplementation on blood glycated hemoglobin and triglyceride levels and red cell indices in type I diabetic patients. J Am Coll Nutr 15.5 (1996): 458–461.
Jaxa-Chamiec T et al. Antioxidant effects of combined vitamins C and E in acute myocardial infarction: The randomized, double-blind, placebo-controlled, multicenter pilot Myocardial Infarction and VITamins (MIVIT) trial. Kardiol Pol 62.4 (2005): 344–350.
Jeong, N. H, et al., 2009. Plasma carotenoids, retinol and tocopherol levels and the risk of ovarian cancer. Acta Obstet Gynecol Scand. 88(4):457–462.
Jialal I, Devaraj S. Scientific evidence to support a vitamin E and heart disease health claim: research needs. J Nutr 135.2 (2005a): 348–53.
Jialal I, Devaraj S. High-dosage vitamin E supplementation and all-cause mortality. Ann Intern Med 143.2 (2005b): 155.
Karlson EW, et al 2008. Vitamin E in the Primary prevention of Rheumatoid Arthritis: The Women's Health Study. Arthritis Rhuem.59:11;1189–1595
Kataja-Tuomola MJ, et al 2010. Effects of alpha-tocopherol and beta carotene supplementation on macrovascular complications and total mortality from diabetes: Results of the ATBC Study. 42 ;3: 178–186.
Katsiki N, Manes C. Is there a role for supplemented antioxidants in the prevention of atherosclerosis? Clinical Nutrition 28.1 (2009): 3–9.
Kaul N et al. Alpha-tocopherol and atherosclerosis. Exp Biol Med 226.1 (2001): 5–12.
Kessopoulou E et al. A double-blind randomized placebo cross-over controlled trial using the antioxidant vitamin E to treat reactive oxygen species associated male infertility. Fertil Steril 64.4 (1995): 825–831.
Khajehdehi P et al. A randomized, double-blind, placebo-controlled trial of supplementary vitamins E, C and their combination for treatment of haemodialysis cramps. Nephrol Dial Transplant 16.7 (2001): 1448–1451.
Kitagawa M, Mino M. Effects of elevated d-alpha(RRR)-tocopherol dosage in man. J Nutr Sci Vitaminol (Tokyo) 35.2 (1989): 133–42.
Kleijnen J, Mackerras D. Vitamin E for intermittent claudication. Cochrane Database Syst Rev 2 (2000): CD000987.
Klemenska E, Beresewicz A, 2009. Bioactivation of organic nitrates and the mechanism of nitrate tolerance. Cardiology Journal 16;1: 11–19
Kobori Y, et al 2014. Antioxidant cosupplementation therapy with vitamin C, vitamin E, and coenzyme Q10 in patients with oligoasthenozoospermia. Arch Ital Urol Andol 86;1
Kusama Y, et al 2011. Review: Variant angina and coronary artery spasm: The clinical spectrum, pathophysiology and management. J Nippon Med Sch;78:1.
Lee IM et al. Vitamin E in the primary prevention of cardiovascular disease and cancer: The Women's Health Study: a randomized controlled trial. ACC Curr J Rev 14.10 (2005): 10–111.
Leonard, SW, et al 2004. Vitamin E bioavailability from fortified breakfast cereal is greater than that from encapsulated supplements. The American Journal of Clinical Nutrition, 79:1, 86–92.
Leppala JM et al. Vitamin E and beta carotene supplementation in high risk for stroke: a subgroup analysis of the Alpha-Tocopherol, Beta-Carotene Cancer Prevention Study. Arch Neurol 57.10 (2000): 1503–1509.

Liang, D, et al 2008. Plasma vitamins E and A and risk of bladder cancer: a case-control analysis. Cancer Causes Control. 19:98
Liede KE et al. Increased tendency towards gingival bleeding caused by joint effect of alpha-tocopherol supplementation and acetylsalicylic acid. Ann Med 30.6 (1998): 542–546.
Lin JY et al. UV photoprotection by combination topical antioxidants vitamin C and vitamin E. J Am Acad Dermatol 48.6 (2003): 866–874.
Lin FH et al. Ferulic acid stabilizes a solution of vitamins C and E and doubles its photoprotection of skin. J Invest Dermatol 125.4 (2005): 826–832.
Linus Pauling Institute. Research newsletter – Spring/Summer 2008: 'Fatally Flawed' clinical trials of vitamin E. Oregan State University. [Online] http://lpi.oregonstate.edu/ss08/itamin.html [Accessed 2nd May 2014].
London RS et al. Evaluation and treatment of breast symptoms in patients with the premenstrual syndrome. J Reprod Med 28.8 (1983): 503–508.
London RS et al. Efficacy of alpha-tocopherol in the treatment of the premenstrual syndrome. J Reprod Med 32.6 (1987): 400–404.
Lonn E et al. Effects of vitamin E on cardiovascular and microvascular outcomes in high-risk patients with diabetes: results of the HOPE study and MICRO-HOPE substudy. Diabetes Care 25.11 (2002): 1919–1927.
Lonn E et al. Effects of long-term vitamin E supplementation on cardiovascular events and cancer: a randomized controlled trial. JAMA 293.11 (2005): 1338–1347.
Luchsinger JA et al. Antioxidant vitamin intake and risk of Alzheimer disease. Arch Neurol 60.2 (2003): 203–208.
Lynch SM, et al 2012. Abstract 13: Teleomere length and pancreatic cancer in the alpha-topherol beta carotene cancer prevention (ATBC) study. Cancer Epidemiol Biomarkers Prev. 21; 13.
Machtey I, Ouaknine L. Tocopherol in osteoarthritis: a controlled pilot study. J Am Geriatr Soc 26.7 (1978): 328–330.
Mahyar E, et al 2005. Intake of vitamin E, vitamin C and carotenoids and the risk of Parkinson's disease: A meta-analysis. The Lancet Neurology 4.6:362–5
Mandana Z, et al 2013. Evaluation the effect of vitamin E on treatment of premenstrual syndrome: A clinical randomized trial. Research and Reviews: Journal of Medical and Health Sciences 2:4.
Marchioli R et al. Vitamin E increases the risk of developing heart failure after myocardial infarction: Results from the GISSI-Prevenzione trial. J Cardiovasc Med (Hagerstown) 7.5 (2006): 347–350.
Martin-Jimenez M et al. Failure of high-dose tocopherol to prevent alopecia induced by doxorubicin. N Engl J Med 315.14 (1986): 894–895.
Masaki KH et al. Association of vitamin E and C supplement use with cognitive function and dementia in elderly men. Neurology 54.6 (2000): 1265–1272.
Masatomi Sasaki MS 2006. Development of vitamin E modified polysulfone membrane dialyzers. J Artif Organs 9:50–60.
McAnally, J.A, et al 2007. Tocotrienols potentiate lovastatin- mediated growth suppression in vitro and in vivo. Exp. Biol. Med. 232: 523–531
McDowell LR. (2000) Vitamins in animal and human nutrition. 2nd edn. Ames: Iowa State University Press, p156.
McFarlane GJ et al., 2010. Evidence for the efficacy of complementary and alternative medicines in the management of rheumatoid arthritis: systematic review. Rheumatology 50:9;1672–1683.
McVean M, Liebler DC. Inhibition of UVB induced DNA photodamage in mouse epidermis by topically applied alpha-tocopherol. Carcinogenesis 18.8 (1997): 1617–1622.
McVean M, Liebler DC. Prevention of DNA photodamage by vitamin E compounds and sunscreens: roles of ultraviolet absorbance and cellular uptake. Mol Carcinog 24.3 (1999): 169–176.
Meagher EA. Treatment of atherosclerosis in the new millennium: is there a role for vitamin E? Prev Cardiol 6.2 (2003): 85–90.
Meydani M. Vitamin E. Lancet 345.8943 (1995): 170–175.
Meydani M, Hayes KC. (2003) Vitamin E. Available online at: http. jn.nutrition.org (accessed 02-06-03).
Meydani SN et al. Vitamin E supplementation and in vivo immune response in healthy elderly subjects. A randomized controlled trial. JAMA 277.17 (1997): 1380–1386.
Meydani SN et al. Antioxidant modulation of cytokines and their biologic function in the aged. Z Ernahrungswiss 37 (Suppl 1) (1998): 35–42.
Miller ER III et al. Meta-analysis: high-dosage vitamin E supplementation may increase all-cause mortality. Ann Intern Med 142.1 (2005): 37–46.
Minamiyama Y et al. Vitamin E deficiency accelerates nitrate tolerance via a decrease in cardiac P450 expression and increased oxidative stress. Free Radic Biol Med 40.5 (2006): 808–816.
Mireles-Rocha H et al. UVB photoprotection with antioxidants: Effects of oral therapy with d-alpha-tocopherol and ascorbic acid on the minimal erythema dose. Acta Derm Venereol 82.1 (2002): 21–24.
Mittal M, et al 2014. Reactive oxygen species in inflammation and tissue injury. Antioxid Redox. Signal. 20(7): 1126–1167.
Miwa K et al. Vitamin E deficiency in variant angina. Circulation 94.1 (1996): 14–118.
Miwa K et al. Consumption of vitamin E in coronary circulation in patients with variant angina. Cardiovasc Res 41.1 (1999): 291–298.
Morinobu T et al. The safety of high-dose vitamin E supplementation in healthy Japanese male adults. J Nutr Sci Vitaminol (Tokyo) 48.1 (2002): 6–9.
Morris MC et al. Relation of the tocopherol forms to incident Alzheimer disease and to cognitive change. Am J Clin Nutr 81.2 (2005): 508–514.
Morris, M.C., et al 2014. Brain tocopherols related to Alzheimer's disease neuropathology in humans. Alzheimers Dement. doi: 10.1016/j. jalz.2013.12.015.
Moslemi, M. K, Tavanbakhsh S, 2011. Selenium-vitamin E supplementation in infertile men: effects on semen parameters and pregnancy rate. Int J Gen Med. 4:99–104.
Mukherjee S, and Mitra A, 2009. Health effects of palm oil. J Human Ecol 26:3: 197–203
Munteanu A et al. Anti-atherosclerotic effects of vitamin E: myth or reality? J Cell Mol Med 8.1 (2004): 59–76.
Nanyakkara PW et al. Effect of a treatment strategy consisting of pravastatin, vitamin E, and homocysteine lowering on carotid intima-media thickness, endothelial function and renal function in patients with mild to moderate chronic kidney disease: results from the Anti-odixant Therapy in Chronic Renal Insufficiency (ATIC) study. Arch Intern Med 167: 1262–1270.
National Cancer Institute (NIH) 2014 Selenium and Vitamin E Cancer Prevention Trial (SELECT). http://www.cancer.gov/newscenter/qa/2008/selectqa
NHMRC Nutrient Reference Values for Australia and New Zealand. Vitamin E Background. http://www.nrv.gov.au/nutrients/vitamin-e [Accessed 1st May 2014].
NIH (2013): Office of Dietary Supplements [Online], Vitamin E: Fact Sheet for Health Professionals. http://ods.od.nih.gov/factsheets/VitaminE-HealthProfessional/.[Accessed 06 May 14].
NUTTAB. 2010. Database Online. [Online] Available at: http://www.foodstandards.gov.au/science/monitoringnutrients/nutrientables/nuttab/Pages/default.aspx. [Accessed 06 May 14].
O'Donnell ME et al. The effects of cilostazol on exercise-induced ischaemia-reperfusion injury in patients with peripheral arterial disease. Eur J Vasc Endovasc Surg 37.3 (2009): 326–335.
Orbe J et al. Antioxidant vitamins increase the collagen content and reduce MMP-1 in a porcine model of atherosclerosis: Implications for plaque stabilization. Atherosclerosis 167.1 (2003): 45–53.
Packer L (2002), Handbook of antioxidants. Marcel Dekker Inc [Online]. NY 1016 Available at: http://lpi.oregonstate.edu/infocenter/vitamins/vitaminE/. [Accessed 07 May 14].
Palan, P. R., et al. 2006. Effects of menstrual cycle and oral contraceptive use on serum levels of lipid-soluble antioxidants. Am J Obstet Gynecol. 194(5):35–38.
Palmieri B et al. Vitamin E added silicone gel sheets for treatment of hypertrophic scars and keloids. Int J Dermatol 34.7 (1995): 506–509.
Parkinson Study Group. Impact of deprenyl and tocopherol treatment on Parkinson's disease in DATATOP patients requiring levodopa: Parkinson Study Group. Ann Neurol 39.1 (1996): 37–45.
Parkinson Study Group. Mortality in DATATOP: A multicenter trial in early Parkinson's disease. Parkinson Study Group. Ann Neurol 43.3 (1998): 318–325.
Parkinson Study Group. MRC/BHF Heart Protection Study of antioxidant vitamin supplementation in 20,536 high-risk individuals: A randomised placebo-controlled trial. Lancet 360.9326 (2002): 23–33.
Pearson PJK et al. Vitamin E supplements in asthma: A parallel group randomised placebo controlled trial. Thorax 59.8 (2004): 652–656.
Perez JE et al. High-dose alpha-tocopherol as a preventive of doxorubicin-induced alopecia. Cancer Treat Rep 70.10 (1986): 1213–12114.
Petersen RC et al. Vitamin E and donepezil for the treatment of mild cognitive impairment. N Engl J Med 352.23 (2005): 2379–2388.
Posadzki P, et al 2013. Dietary supplements and prostate cancer: a systematic review of double-blind, placebo-controlled randomised clinical trials, Maturitas, 75;2: 125–130.
Raju TN et al. Vitamin E prophylaxis to reduce retinopathy of prematurity: a reappraisal of published trials. J Pediatr 131.6 (1997): 844–850.
Rapola JM et al. Effect of vitamin E and beta carotene on the incidence of angina pectoris: A randomized, double-blind, controlled trial. JAMA 275.9 (1996): 693–698.
Rapola JM et al. Randomised trial of alpha tocopherol and beta-carotene supplements on incidence of major coronary events in men with previous myocardial infarction. Lancet 349.9067 (1997): 1715–1720.
Ricciarelli R et al. Vitamin E and neurodegenerative diseases. Mol Aspects Med 28.5–6 (2007): 591–606.
Rimbach G, et al 2010. Gene regulatory activity of a- tocopherol. Molecules 2010, 15, 1746–1761.
Rimm EB et al. Vitamin E consumption and the risk of coronary heart disease in men. N Engl J Med 328.20 (1993): 1450–1456.

V

Rizvi S, et al 2014. The Role of Vitamin E in Human Health and Some Diseases. Sultan Qaboos Univ Med J. 14(2): e157–e165.

Roehm E, 2009. The evidence based Mediterranean diet reduces coronary heart disease risk, and plant derived monounsaturated fats may reduce coronary heart disease risk. Am J Clin Nutr 90.3:697–698.

Rolf C et al. Antioxidant treatment of patients with asthenozoospermia or moderate oligoasthenozoospermia with high-dose vitamin C and vitamin E: A randomized, placebo-controlled, double-blind study. Hum Reprod 14.4 (1999): 1028–1033.

Sackett CS, Schenning S. The age-related eye disease study: the results of the clinical trial. Insight 27.1 (2002): 5–7.

Saldeen K, Saldeen T 2005. Importance of tocopherols beyond alpha tocopherol: evidence from animal and human studies. Nutrition Research. 2005: 25; 877–889.

Salonen RM et al. Six-year effect of combined vitamin C and E supplementation on atherosclerotic progression: the Antioxidant Supplementation in Atherosclerosis Prevention (ASAP) Study. Circulation 107.7 (2003): 947–953.

Sano M et al. A controlled trial of selegiline, alpha-tocopherol, or both as treatment for Alzheimer's disease: The Alzheimer's Disease Cooperative Study. N Engl J Med 336.17 (1997): 1216–1222.

Scherak O, Kolarz G. Vitamin E and rheumatoid arthritis. Arthritis Rheum 34.9 (1991): 1205–1206.

Scuntaro I et al. Inhibition by vitamin E of drug accumulation and of phospholipidosis induced by desipramine and other cationic amphiphilic drugs in human cultured cells. Br J Pharmacol 119.5 (1996): 829–834.

Sen C, Packer L. Thiol homeostasis and supplements in physical exercise. Am J Clin Nutr 72 (s) (2000): 653–69s.

Sesso HD, et al 2008. Vitamins E and C in the prevention of cardiovascular disease in men: the Physician's Health Study 11 randomized controlled trial. JAMA 300: 2123–2133.

Shanafelt TD et al. Pathophysiology and treatment of hot flashes. Mayo Clin Proc 77.11 (2002): 1207–1218.

Shen J et al. Telomere length, oxidative damage, antioxidants and breast cancer risk. Int J Cancer 124.7 (2009): 1637–1643.

Shils M (ed). Modern nutrition in health and disease, 9th edn. Baltimore: Lippincott Williams & Wilkins, 1999.

Singh RB et al. Usefulness of antioxidant vitamins in suspected acute myocardial infarction (the Indian experiment of infarct survival-3). Am J Cardiol 77.4 (1996): 232–236.

Stampfer MJ et al. Vitamin E consumption and the risk of coronary disease in women. N Engl J Med 328.20 (1993): 1444–1449.

Stephens NG et al. Randomised controlled trial of vitamin E in patients with coronary disease: Cambridge Heart Antioxidant Study (CHAOS). Lancet 347.9004 (1996): 781–786.

Stolzenberg-Solomon RZ et al. Vitamin E intake, alpha-tocopherol status, and pancreatic cancer in a cohort of male smokers. Am J Clin Nutr 89.2 (2009): 584–591.

Stone WL, Papas AM. Tocopherols and the etiology of colon cancer. J Natl Cancer Inst 89.14 (1997): 1006–1014.

Suleiman SA et al. Lipid peroxidation and human sperm motility: protective role of vitamin E. J Androl 17.5 (1996): 530–537.

Sung L et al. Vitamin E: the evidence for multiple roles in cancer. Nutr Cancer 46.1 (2003): 1–14.

Takahashi S, et al 2009. Suppression of prostate cancer in a transgenic rat model via gamma-tocopherol activation of caspase signaling. Prostate. 69(6):644–51.

Tardif JC et al. Probucol and multivitamins in the prevention of restenosis after coronary angioplasty. Multivitamins and Probucol Study Group. N Engl J Med 337.6 (1997): 365–372.

Terentis AC et al. Vitamin E oxidation in human atherosclerotic lesions. Circ Res 90.3 (2002): 333–339.

Traber, MG, et al 2006. Vitamin E: Nutrition in Health and Disease. 10th edn. Baltimore, MD: Lippincott Williams & Wilkins.

Ulker S et al. Vitamins reverse endothelial dysfunction through regulation of eNOS and NAD(P)H oxidase activities. Hypertension 41.3 (2003): 534–539.

Vardi M, et al 2013. Vitamin E in the prevention of cardiovascular disease: the importance of proper patient selection. Journal of lipid research 54: 2013.

Vatassery GT. In vitro oxidation of alpha-tocopherol (vitamin E) in human platelets upon incubation with unsaturated fatty acids, diamide and superoxide. Biochim Biophys Acta 926.2 (1987): 160–169.

Virtamo J et al. Effect of vitamin E and beta carotene on the incidence of primary nonfatal myocardial infarction and fatal coronary heart disease. Arch Intern Med 158.6 (1998): 668–675.

Virtamo J et al. Effects of supplemental alpha-tocopherol and beta-carotene on urinary tract cancer: Incidence and mortality in a controlled trial (Finland). Cancer Causes Control 11.10 (2000): 933–939.

Virtamo J et al. Incidence of cancer and mortality following alpha-tocopherol and beta-carotene supplementation: A postintervention follow-up. JAMA 290.4 (2003): 476–485.

Wahlqvist ML (ed). Food and nutrition, 2nd edn. Sydney: Allen & Unwin, 2002.

Watanabe H et al. Randomized, double-blind, placebo-controlled study of supplemental vitamin E on attenuation of the development of nitrate tolerance. Circulation 96.8 (1997): 2545–2550.

Waters DD, et al. 2002. Effects of hormone replacement therapy and antioxidant vitamin supplements on coronary atherosclerosis in postmenopausal women: a randomized controlled trial. JAMA. 288: 2432–2440.

Whitney E, et al 2011. A Understanding of Nutrition Australia and New Zealand. 2nd ed. Australia: Cengage Learning.

Wijnen MH et al. Antioxidants reduce oxidative stress in claudicants. J Surg Res 96.2 (2001): 183–187.

Wittenborg A et al. Effectiveness of vitamin E in comparison with diclofenac sodium in treatment of patients with chronic polyarthritis. Z Rheumatol 57.4 (1998): 215–221.

Wluka AE et al. Supplementary vitamin E does not affect the loss of cartilage volume in knee osteoarthritis: a 2 year double blind randomized placebo controlled study. J Rheumatol 29.12 (2002): 2585–2591.

Wolf S et al. Chemotherapy-induced peripheral neuropathy: Prevention and treatment strategies. Eur J Cancer 44.11 (2008): 1507–1515.

Wood LA. Possible prevention of adriamycin-induced alopecia by tocopherol. N Engl J Med 312.16 (1985): 1060.

World Cancer Research Fund International 2011. Colorectal Cancer. [Online] http://www.wcrf.org/cancer_research/cup/colorectal_cancer.php [Accessed 8th May 2014]

Wright ME et al. Effects of alpha-tocopherol and beta-carotene supplementation on upper aerodigestive tract cancers in a large, randomized controlled trial. Cancer 109.5 (2007): 891–898.

Wu D, Meydani SN, 2008. Age-associated changes in immune and inflammatory responses: impact of vitamin E intervention. J Leukoc Biol. 84:4: 900–914.

Xu Q1, et al 2009. Multivitamin use and telomere length in women. Am J Clin Nutr. 89(6):1857–63.

Yang CS, et al 2012. Does vitamin E prevent or promote cancer. Cancer Prev Res 5:701.

Yang, H, et al 2012. Time selective chemoprevention of vitamin E and selenium on esophageal carcinogenesis in rats: the possible role of nuclear factor kappaB signaling pathway. Int J Cancer. 131;7:1517–1527.

Yasue H, et al. Coronary artery spasm-Clinical features, diagnosis, pathogenesis, and treatment. Journal of Cardiology 2008:51:1;2–7.

Yusuf S et al. Vitamin E supplementation and cardiovascular events in high-risk patients: The Heart Outcomes Prevention Evaluation Study Investigators. N Engl J Med 342.3 (2000): 154–160.

Zandi PP et al. Reduced risk of Alzheimer disease in users of antioxidant vitamin supplements: The Cache County Study. Arch Neurol 61.1 (2004): 82–88.

Ziaei S et al. A randomised placebo-controlled trial to determine the effect of vitamin E in treatment of primary dysmenorrhoea. BJOG 108.11 (2001): 1181–1183.

Ziaei S, et al. A randomised controlled trial of vitamin E in the treatment of primary dysmenorrhoea. BJOG 112.4 (2005): 466–469.

Ziaei S, et al. The effect of vitamin E on hot flashes in menopausal women. Gynecol Obstet Invest 64.4 (2007): 204–207.

Zureik M et al. Effects of long-term daily low-dose supplementation with antioxidant vitamins and minerals on structure and function of large arteries. Arterioscler Thromb Vasc Biol 24.8 (2004): 1485–1491.

Wild yam

HISTORICAL NOTE Wild yams have made a significant contribution as a root crop to tribal people in some parts of the world, such as Nepal. They are usually consumed boiled, steamed, baked or fried. Many different forms and cultivars of the wild edible yam species are available in different areas, and it is likely that these differ in composition and nutritional values. Traditionally, wild yams have also been used as medicine and are believed to exert antispasmodic, anti-inflammatory and autonomic nervous system-relaxant effects. Wild yam is a source of diosgenin, the raw material originally used to produce progesterone in the laboratory.

COMMON NAME

Wild yam

OTHER NAMES

Atlantic yam, barbasco, China root, colic root, devil's bones, Mexican yam, natural DHEA, rheumatism root, wild Mexican yam, yuma

BOTANICAL NAME/FAMILY

Discorea composita, D. floribunda, D. mexicana, D. macrostachya, D. villosa (family Dioscoreaceae [yams])

PLANT PART USED

Root and rhizome

CHEMICAL COMPONENTS

The root of the wild yam contains diosgenin, dioscin, dioscorin and a range of vitamins and minerals such as vitamin C, beta-carotene, vitamins B_1, B_2 and B_3, iron, magnesium, potassium, selenium and zinc (USDA 2003), along with polyphenols (Bhandari & Kawabata 2004). Although diosgenin can be converted to dihydroepiandosterone (DHEA) and other steroid compounds in the laboratory, and has been used for commercial production of these compounds, this conversion does not occur in the human body. Additionally, wild yam does not contain progesterone or any other active steroid hormones.

MAIN ACTIONS

Hormonal actions

The evidence of a hormonal action with wild yam varies. Wild yam extract may enhance oestradiol binding to oestrogen receptors and induce transcription activity in oestrogen-responsive cells (Park et al 2009), and diosgenin has been observed to have an oestrogenic action on mouse mammary epithelium (Aradhana Rao & Kale 1992). In contrast, in an oestrogen competition assay using human breast cancer cell, diosgenin was found to cause an acute, endothelium-independent coronary artery relaxation, but did not interact with oestrogen or progesterone receptors (Au et al 2004), and extracts with an upper limit of 3.5% diosgenin have been found to have no oestrogenic activity (Hooker 2004).

One study looking at steroid hormone-regulated gene expression using an in vitro tissue culture indicator system suggests that wild yam extract does not have significant oestrogenic or progesteronal activity, but rather weak antioestrogenic and/or antiandrogenic activities (Rosenberg Zand et al 2001). A further study suggests that wild yam extract suppresses progesterone synthesis without direct effects on oestrogen or progesterone receptors (Zava et al 1998). In an in vivo study, supplementation with diosgenin protected the kidney from morphological changes associated with ovariectomy (Tucci & Benghuzzi 2003) and produced a significant decrease in the cortical and medullary adrenal areas of ovariectomised rats (Benghuzzi et al 2003).

There is in vitro evidence that diosgenin upregulates vascular endothelial growth factor A and promotes angiogenesis in pre-osteoblast-like cells via pathways involving oestrogen receptors (Men et al 2005).

Cholagogue

There appears to be more consistent evidence for wild yam's effect on bile flow. Diosgenin has been shown to increase biliary secretion of cholesterol (Accatino et al 1998, Yamada et al 1997) and prevent oestrogen-induced bile flow suppression in rats (Accatino et al 1998), as well as increase elimination of indomethacin and reduce indomethacin-induced intestinal inflammation (Yamada et al 1997).

OTHER ACTIONS

Traditionally, wild yam is also believed to exert antispasmodic, anti-inflammatory and autonomic nervous system-relaxant effects (Fisher & Painter 1996). Wild yam exhibits significant antioxidant activity (Bhandari & Kawabata 2004). Wild yam has also demonstrated potential cytotoxic action against certain cancer cell lines in animal and in vitro models (Saekoo et al 2010, Tong et al 2012).

CLINICAL USE

The therapeutic effectiveness of wild yam has not been significantly investigated under clinical trial conditions, so evidence is derived from traditional, in vitro and animal studies.

Clinical note — The major influence of wild yam on modern medicine

The Mexican wild yam has had a major influence on drug development and modern medical practice, although few people are familiar with the story and misunderstandings abound.

In the late 1930s scientists entering the field of sex endocrinology were confronted with the sober reality that they were dealing with research materials (animal glands) that needed to be sourced from slaughterhouses and were not readily available in sufficient quantities (Soto Laveaga 2005). Eventually, female urine was identified as a better source of hormones and provided an alternative. As pharmaceutical companies embarked upon large-scale hormone production, it became apparent that a cheaper and more abundant source of raw materials would need to be found; hence, a search through the plant kingdom ensued.

The American chemist Russell Marker identified that saponins in plants could be chemically modified to produce steroids and that sex hormones could be synthesised using yams (Soto Laveaga 2005). For several years he tried unsuccessfully to direct pharmaceutical companies to use Mexico as a source of wild yams, but the general perception was that Mexico was too politically unstable and unsophisticated. Over time, changes in the infrastructure of the Mexican countryside coincided with further chemical discoveries, and wild yam root picking became a financial panacea to previously unemployed peasants in yam-rich areas. By the 1950s, scientists at the pharmaceutical company Upjohn had found a way to convert diosgenin to progesterone, then to hydrocortisone and finally cortisone, thereby reinforcing the importance of wild yam as a source of raw materials for steroid drugs. Considering the importance of these events, it could be said that wild yams revolutionised the world of modern medicine.

At one stage Mexican wild yams provided up to 90% of the world's raw material for steroid drug synthesis, but this has steadily fallen owing to the rapid increase in demand for larger quantities and Mexico's reduced ability to produce wild yam tubers (Soto Laveaga 2005).

Menopausal symptoms and other female reproductive conditions

Although wild yam has been a popular treatment for menopausal symptoms, there is scarce clinical research supporting its use for these indications.

Wild yam has been used as a 'natural alternative' to oestrogen replacement therapy, to treat postmenopausal vaginal dryness, premenstrual syndrome and osteoporosis, and to increase energy and libido in men and women, as well as for breast enlargement. The use of wild yam as a natural progesterone appears misguided, because diosgenin is not converted to progesterone, DHEA or other steroid hormones in vivo. One small, double-blind, placebo-controlled crossover trial of topical wild yam extract showed no effect on menopausal symptoms (Komesaroff et al 2001). The study involved 23 healthy women suffering menopausal symptoms. Each woman was randomly assigned the active cream or matching placebo for 3 months, after which no significant changes to symptoms or physical health measurements were recorded.

It is possible that other yams have beneficial effects in treating menopausal symptoms. For example, a double-blind, placebo-controlled trial found that regular oral ingestion of purple yam (*Diascorea alata*) significantly improved menopausal symptoms (Hsu et al 2011). The study involved 50 otherwise healthy symptomatic menopausal women, randomised to receive either 12 mg dried yam extract or placebo for a period of 12 months. The women were followed up at 1, 6 and 12 months; with improvement noted from 6 months and best results at 12 months. Significant improvements were noticed for symptoms of anxiety, insomnia, 'excitability' and musculoskeletal pain.

OTHER USES

Wild yam has been used traditionally as an antispasmodic for treating diverticulosis, gallbladder colic, painful menstruation, cramp, nausea in pregnancy and rheumatoid arthritis, and for increasing energy (Fisher & Painter 1996). It may also be useful when combined with other herbs for irritable bowel syndrome (Abascal & Yarnell 2005).

DOSAGE RANGE

- Decoction of dried root: 2–4 g three times daily.
- Tincture (1:5): 2–10 mL three times daily.
- Liquid extract (1:2): 3–6 mL/day.

TOXICITY

Considering that wild yams are widely consumed as food by several tribal groups, it appears that dietary ingestion is non-toxic. After assessment with short-term toxicity tests, dermal irritation tests, a sensitisation test, an ocular irritation test, a rat uterotropic assay and genotoxicity tests, wild yam was deemed safe for use in cosmetic products (Hooker 2004). An in vivo study demonstrated that high doses of wild yam (0.79 g/kg/day) induced significant increases in kidney, and to a lesser extent liver, fibrotic markers (Wojcikowski et al 2008). While serological markers did not indicate decreased organ function, the researchers concluded that long-term use of wild yam would not be advisable in patients with compromised kidney function, or when taking nephrotic agents.

ADVERSE REACTIONS

In large doses, wild yam may cause nausea, vomiting and diarrhoea.

SIGNIFICANT INTERACTIONS

Insufficient reliable data are available to determine whether interactions may occur.

CONTRAINDICATIONS AND PRECAUTIONS

None known.

PREGNANCY USE

Likely to be safe when consumed in dietary amounts; however, safety is not known when used in larger quantities.

PATIENTS' FAQs

What will this herb do for me?
Although wild yam has been used medicinally to treat menopausal symptoms, there is scientific evidence showing it is ineffective.

When will it start to work?
This cannot be answered based on scientific evidence.

Are there any safety issues?
Given that it is consumed as food, usual dietary intakes may be considered safe.

Practice points/Patient counselling

- Wild yam is a popular root vegetable in some parts of the world.
- It was a popular ingredient in commercial herbal formulas for menopausal women; however, scientific research has since found it does not improve menopausal symptoms.
- Wild yam has been touted as having progesteronal and/or oestrogenic activity, but current evidence suggests this is unlikely.
- There is no clinical or scientific evidence to support the use of wild yam in the treatment of conditions of the female reproductive system.
- Wild yam root may be useful as an antispasmodic. Its use as a source of naturally occurring sex hormones appears misguided.

REFERENCES

Abascal K, Yarnell E. Combining herbs in a formula for irritable bowel syndrome. Altern Complement Ther 11.1 (2005): 17–23.

Accatino L et al. Effects of diosgenin, a plant-derived steroid, on bile secretion and hepatocellular cholestasis induced by estrogens in the rat. Hepatology 28.1 (1998): 129–140.

Aradhana Rao AR, Kale RK. Diosgenin: a growth stimulator of mammary gland of ovariectomized mouse. Indian J Exp Biol 30.5 (1992): 367–370.

Au ALS et al. Activation of iberiotoxin-sensitive, Ca^{2+}-activated K^+ channels of porcine isolated left anterior descending coronary artery by diosgenin. Eur J Pharmacol 502.1–2 (2004): 123–133.

Benghuzzi H et al. The effects of sustained delivery of diosgenin on the adrenal gland of female rats. Biomed Sci Instrument 39 (2003): 335–340.

Bhandari MR, Kawabata J. Organic acid, phenolic content and antioxidant activity of wild yam (*Dioscorea* spp.) tubers of Nepal. Food Chem 88.2 (2004): 163–168.

Fisher C, Painter G. Materia Medica for the Southern Hemisphere. Auckland: Fisher-Painter Publishers, 1996.

Hooker E. Final report of the amended safety assessment of *Dioscorea villosa* (Wild yam) root extract. Int J Toxicol 23 (Suppl 2) (2004): 49–54.

Hsu C et al. The assessment of efficacy of *Diascorea alata* for menopausal symptom treatment in Taiwanese women. Climacteric 14 (2011): 132–139.

Komesaroff PA et al. Effects of wild yam extract on menopausal symptoms, lipids and sex hormones in healthy menopausal women. Climacteric 4.2 (2001): 144–150.

Men LY et al. Diosgenin induces hypoxia-inducible factor-1 activation and angiogenesis through estrogen receptor-related phosphatidylinositol 3-kinase/Akt and p38 mitogen-activated protein kinase pathways in osteoblasts. Mol Pharmacol 68.4 (2005): 1061–1073.

Park M et al. Estrogen Activities and the Cellular Effects of Natural Progesterone from Wild Yam Extract in MCF-7 Human Breast Cancer Cells. Am J Chin Med 37.1 (2009): 159–167.

Rosenberg Zand RS, et al. Effects of natural products and nutraceuticals on steroid hormone-regulated gene expression. Clin Chim Acta 312.1–2 (2001): 213–2119.

Saekoo J et al. Cytotoxic effect and its mechanism of dioscorealide B from *Dioscorea membranacea* against breast cancer cells. J Med Assoc Thai 93 (2010): S277-S282.

Soto Laveaga G. Uncommon trajectories: steroid hormones, Mexican peasants, and the search for a wild yam. Studies in History and Philosophy of Science Part C: Studies in History and Philosophy of Biological and Biomedical Sciences 36.4 (2005): 743–760.

Tong Q et al. Cytotoxicity and apoptosis-inducing effect of steroidal saponins from *Dioscorea zingiberensis* Wright against cancer cells. Steroids 77 (2012): 1219–1227.

Tucci M, Benghuzzi H. Structural changes in the kidney associated with ovariectomy and diosgenin replacement therapy in adult female rats. Biomed Sci Instrument 39 (2003): 341–346.

USDA (US Department of Agriculture. Phytochemical Database). Agricultural Research Service—National Germplasm Resources Laboratory. Beltsville, MD: Beltsville Agricultural Research Center, 2003.

Wojcikowski K et al. *Dioscorea villosa* (wild yam) induces chronic kidney injury via pro-fibrotic pathways. Food Chem Toxicol 46 (2008): 3122–3131.

Yamada T et al. Dietary diosgenin attenuates subacute intestinal inflammation associated with indomethacin in rats. Am J Physiol 273.2 (Part 1) (1997): G355–G364.

Zava DT, et al. Estrogen and progestin bioactivity of foods, herbs, and spices. Proc Soc Exp Biol Med 217.3 (1998): 369–378.

Willow bark

HISTORICAL NOTE This herb has been used as a therapeutic agent since ancient times, with some reports of its use around 500 BC in ancient China as a treatment for pain and fever, and around 400 BC by Hippocrates, who recommended the bark be chewed for relief of fever and pain (Hedner & Everts 1998). Willow bark was also used traditionally as an anti-inflammatory agent (Drummond et al 2013). As centuries passed, herbalists continued to prescribe the bark for many conditions, and by the 18th century it was widely used as an antipyretic and analgesic (Hedner & Everts 1998). In a report published in 1763 (Stone 1763), willow bark (dried, pulverised and dispersed in tea or water) was given to 50 patients. At a dose of 1 dram (1.8 g), it cured their fever. During the late 1820s, French and German scientists extracted the glycosidic constituents, including salicin (Hedner & Everts 1998). The oxidation of salicin yields salicylic acid, which was produced in the mid-1800s but had limited clinical use due to the gastric irritation it caused. In 1853 a French chemist neutralised salicylic acid to create acetylsalicylic acid, but had no interest in marketing it and abandoned his discovery. A Bayer chemist called Hoffmann rediscovered acetylsalicylic acid in 1897 as a better-tolerated treatment for his father's rheumatoid arthritis and within 2 years it was marketed by Bayer under the trade name of Aspirin (Setty & Sigal 2005). Since then it has become one of the most successful medicines in history. The health benefits may be due to the polyphenol constituents in willow bark. Polyphenols are known for their antioxidative and anti-inflammatory characteristics (Drummond et al 2013). Although many believe aspirin was synthesised from the salicin found in willow bark, it was actually from the salicin found in another herb, meadowsweet, that aspirin was developed.

OTHER NAMES

White willow bark, brittle willow, bay willow, crack willow, purple willow, silberweide, violet willow

While white willow (*Salix alba*) is the willow species most commonly used for medicinal purposes, crack willow (*S. fragilis*), purple willow (*S. purpurea*) and violet willow (*S. daphnoides*) are all salicin-rich and are sometimes sold under the label of willow bark (Setty & Sigal 2005).

BOTANICAL NAME/FAMILY

Salix alba (family Salicaceae)

PLANT PART USED

Bark

CHEMICAL COMPONENTS

The ethyl acetate fraction contains a high amount of polyphenols, whereas the ethanol fraction contains a high amount of salicin and salicin derivatives while having a comparatively low polyphenol content (Ulrich-Merzenich et al 2012), phenolic glycosides (mainly salicylates including salicin and its derivatives), tannins (mainly catechin, tannins, some gallontannins and condensed tannins [procyanidins]), lignans and flavonoids.

With polyphenols (e.g. proanthocyanidins) and flavonoids identified as fractions contributing to the efficacy of willow bark, future research should be directed towards the identification of the constituents or combination of constituents mainly responsible for the observed effects of willow bark (Nahrstedt et al 2007).

Two pharmacokinetic studies have been conducted and confirm that maximal serum levels of salicylic acid are reached within 2 hours of oral administration (Schmid et al 2001b). In one study, testing an oral willow bark extract containing 240 mg salicin, salicylic acid was the major metabolite of salicin detected in the serum (86% of total salicylates), as well as salicyluric acid (10%) and gentisic acid (4%). In a second study testing a dose of willow bark extract (equivalent to 240 mg of total salicin), serum levels of catechol and salicylic acid were measured via high-performance liquid chromatography analysis with a peak concentration of 13.3 microM (1.5 mg/L) for catechol at 1.2 hours and no catechol after 24 hours. Maximum salicylic acid concentrations of 24.5 microM (3.4 mg/L) were reached at 2.7 hours (Knuth et al 2013).

MAIN ACTIONS

Anti-inflammatory and analgesic effects

Clinical studies using willow bark preparations standardised to salicin content have shown anti-inflammatory and analgesic activity (Chrubasik et al 2000, 2001a, 2001b, Mills et al 1996, Schmid et al 2000). In vitro studies have demonstrated that *Salix* extract inhibits cyclooxygenase-2 (COX-2)-mediated prostaglandin E_2 release and that it is a weak inhibitor of proinflammatory cytokines (Fiebich & Chrubasik 2004). While salicin is considered the main analgesic constituent, it is now thought that other constituents, such as tannins, flavonoids and salicin esters, may contribute to its overall effect (Schmid et al 2001a). In addition, the flavonoids and polyphenols contribute to the potent willow bark analgesic and anti-inflammatory effect (Vlachojannis et al 2011).

The effect of a standardised willow bark extract (STW 33-I), containing 23–26% salicin and a high polyphenol content, and its fractions A–E was investigated in a rat model. Two dosage levels of STW 33-I were compared with anti-inflammatory doses of acetylsalicylic acid, as a non-selective COX inhibitor, and celecoxib, as a selective COX-2 inhibitor. On an mg/kg basis, the extract was at least as effective as acetylsalicylic acid in reducing inflammatory exudates and in inhibiting leucocytic infiltration as well as in preventing the rise in cytokines. In addition, STW 33-I was more effective than acetylsalicylic acid in suppressing leukotrienes, but equally effective in suppressing prostaglandins. STW 33-I was more effective than acetylsalicylic acid in reducing COX-2 (Khayyal et al 2005). STW 33-I was found to have in vitro anti-inflammatory effects on lipopolysaccharide-stimulated human monocytes and differentiated macrophages. In addition, there was a significant lowering of intracellular tumour necrosis factor-α (TNF-α) content along with a proapoptotic effect in non-activated monocytes. Apoptosis in monocytes is inhibited by microbial products such as lipopolysaccharide, or by certain inflammatory cytokines such as interferon-γ. Real-time polymerase chain reaction revealed that 10 mcg/mL STW 33-I exhibited a significant inhibitory effect on the COX-2 (30–55%) and TNF-α expression (75–85%) ($P < 0.01$) (Bonaterra et al 2010). An aqueous extract of willow bark showed significant reduction in TNF-α-induced adhesion molecule intercellular adhesion molecule-1 (ICAM-1) expression in human microvascular endothelial cells without showing cytotoxic effects. The ethyl acetate extract of willow bark, containing a variety of phenols from different structural classes (particularly catechol), exhibited the most pronounced reduction in ICAM-1 expression (Freischmidt et al 2012). It is suggested that willow bark extract does not damage the gastrointestinal mucosa, probably due to a gastroprotective constituent in the extract. An ethanol extract of willow bark containing 12% salicin in a dose of up to 120 mg/kg did not produce any mucosal lesions in rats, whereas 9 of 10 aspirin-treated rats (100 mg/kg aspirin) showed stomach lesions (Vlachojannis et al 2011).

Antioxidant effects

A standardised willow bark extract (STW 33-I) was examined in a rat model. The extract raised GSH (reduced glutathione) levels, an effect which helps to limit lipid peroxidation. Higher doses of the extract also reduced malondialdehyde levels and raised superoxide dismutase activity (Khayyal et al 2005). Willow bark extract has been found to reduce oxidative stress in human umbilical vein endothelial cells as well as increase antioxidant enzyme expression by activating nuclear factor erythroid 2-related factor 2 (Ishikado et al 2013).

Antidepressant effects

Ulrich-Merzenich and colleagues (2012) investigated whether a standardised willow bark preparation would have an effect in a standard model of depression, the forced swimming test in male Sprague-Dawley rats, compared to the tricyclic antidepressant imipramine. Studies were accompanied by gene expression analyses. The 4-week treatment of willow bark (15 and 60 mg/kg body weight) increased the serotonin concentration in the hippocampus significantly, whereas the concentration of 5-hydroxyindole acetic acid decreased (willow bark: 15 and 30 mg/kg body weight), showing a slower serotonin turnover (5-hydroxyindole acetic acid/serotonin [$P < 0.05$]). Imipramine (15 mg/kg) also showed a slower serotonin turnover ($P < 0.05$). In the willow bark group, the transcript for the 5-HT receptor 1A was downregulated, whereas in the imipramine group, the transcripts for the 5-HT receptors 1A, 1F, 3A and 5B were downregulated.

OTHER ACTIONS

Heat shock protein (HSP) 47, derived from the serpin family of proteins, interacts transiently with procollagen during its folding, assembly and transport (Nizard et al 2004). An in vitro study tested the effect of willow bark on HSP 47 expression on old and young donor normal human fibroblasts. The dermal cells were prepared by means of facial liftings from 20- and 70-year-old healthy female donors. Treatment with an aqueous solution of willow bark on young donor cells induced no clear increase of HSP 47 level. However, a significant increase was observed when treatment was performed on 70-year-old donor cells. This level was approximately similar to the level of control young donor cells.

CLINICAL USE

In clinical practice, willow bark is generally used as a symptomatic treatment in osteoarthritic conditions and lower-back pain.

Arthritis

Osteoarthritis

Four randomised double-blind trials have investigated the efficacy of willow bark in people with osteoarthritis, with the two earlier studies finding that herbal treatment produced symptom-relieving effects superior to a placebo (Biegert et al 2004, Mills et al 1996, Schmid et al 2000). Seventy-eight subjects were randomly assigned willow bark extract (240 mg salicin/day) or a placebo over a 2-week period, after which active treatment was found to produce a statistically significant improvement (Schmid et al 2000). Mills et al (1996), testing willow bark in 82 patients with chronic arthritic pain, also found active treatment produced a statistically significant alleviation of pain symptoms. The effectiveness and tolerance of willow bark extract compared to conventional therapies were tested in patients with knee or hip pain in a cohort study with a control group. This open, observational study included 90 patients treated with a standardised willow bark extract preparation (equivalent to 240 mg salicin daily) and a reference group of 41 patients with a standard therapy prescribed by a doctor, and 8 patients with a combination of the two. Both the doctors and the patients judged the effectiveness in both groups to be comparable. After 6 weeks, the effectiveness and tolerance of the willow bark extract were better than conventional therapy. No adverse events were recorded in the willow bark group (Beer & Wegener 2008).

These findings contrast with earlier studies in which willow bark failed to reduce Western Ontario and McMaster Universities Arthritis Index (WOMAC) pain scores better than a placebo in a trial on 127 outpatients with painful hip or knee osteoarthritis (Biegert et al 2004). Patients were randomised to receive willow bark extract, corresponding to 240 mg of salicin/day, diclofenac 100 mg/day or a placebo. Treatment with diclofenac produced the strongest pain-reducing effects (WOMAC scores decreased by 47%) compared with willow bark (17% reduction) and the placebo (10% reduction), with the difference between willow bark extract and placebo not statistically significant.

Rheumatoid arthritis

Willow bark extract (corresponding to 240 mg salicin/day) failed to significantly reduce pain in people with active rheumatoid arthritis, according to a small, double-blind, randomised study of 26 volunteers (Biegert et al 2004). The main outcome measure used was each patient's assessment of pain rated on a 100-mm visual analogue scale.

IN COMBINATION

A placebo-controlled, randomised, double-blind trial investigated the effects of a supplement on joint pain for 8 weeks (Nieman et al 2013). The daily supplement contained glucosamine sulfate (1500 mg), methylsufonylmethane (500 mg), white willow bark extract (standardised to 15% salicin) (250 mg), *Boswellia serrata* extract (standardised to 65% boswellic acid) (125 mg), ginger root concentrate (50 mg), turmeric root extract (50 mg), cayenne 40 m HU (50 mg) and hyaluronic acid (4.0 mg). The subjects in the study reported knee pain (74.2%), upper-limb joint pain (55.7%), hip pain (41.2%), lower-limb joint pain (24.7%) and back pain (18.6%). Joint pain severity was assessed biweekly using the 12-point Likert visual scale from the symptom logs. Joint pain reduction became apparent by the fourth week in the supplement group. Furthermore, joint pain severity was significantly reduced in the supplement group compared to placebo at 8 weeks (WOMAC, interaction effect $P = 0.025$). The most significant results were in subjects reporting knee pain. This was shown by reductions in joint pain symptom severity for the supplement compared to placebo (interaction effect, $P = 0.0125$). Decreases in WOMAC total ($P = 0.018$) and pain ($P = 0.014$), function index ($P = 0.027$), and stiffness ($P = 0.081$) scores were greater for the supplement compared to placebo. Systemic inflammation biomarkers and the 6-minute walk test did not differ significantly between groups. The supplement had no adverse symptoms or negative effects on general metabolism and liver and kidney function.

Lower-back pain

Two randomised studies have investigated the use of oral white willow bark in people with acute episodes of chronic non-specific low-back pain (Chrubasik et al 2000, 2001a). According to a 2006 Cochrane systematic review, there is moderate evidence that a daily dose of 240 mg salicin from an extract of *S. alba* reduces pain more than either a placebo or a daily dose of 120 mg of salicin in the short term for individuals with acute episodes of chronic non-specific low-back pain (Gagnier et al 2006).

One randomised, placebo-controlled study involving 210 patients with chronic lower-back pain found that 39% of those treated with 240 mg salicin became pain-free after 4 weeks compared with 6% in the placebo group. This response was achieved after 1 week (Chrubasik et al 2000). Similar results were achieved in an open trial conducted over 18 months that compared willow bark extract containing 120 mg or 240 mg salicin with what the authors term 'conventional treatment' in 451 people with acute exacerbations of lower-back pain. Those receiving 240 mg salicin experienced the best results, with 40% becoming pain-free after 4 weeks, compared to 19% in the 120 mg salicin group and 18% in the control group (Chrubasik et al 2001b).

Comparative trial with rofecoxib

No significant differences in pain-relieving effects were found between white willow bark, standardised to provide a daily dose of 240 mg salicin, and 12.5 mg of the synthetic COX-2 inhibitor rofecoxib according to a randomised trial of individuals with acute episodes of chronic non-specific low-back pain (Chrubasik et al 2001a). With regard to rescue treatments, the percentage of patients requiring non-steroidal anti-inflammatory drugs (NSAIDs), tramadol or both was 10% for the willow bark group and 13% for the rofecoxib group. Approximately 90% of doctors and patients rated either treatment as effective and close to 100% rated either treatment as acceptable.

Given that some pharmaceutical treatments used in the management of pain and inflammatory conditions are costly, such as the newer COX-2 inhibitors, Chrubasik et al (2001b) also compared the cost savings associated with the use of willow bark. A dose of 120 mg salicin/day from willow bark reduced overall patient spending on additional drugs by about 35–50%. In comparison, 240 mg salicin/day produced superior pain relief that resulted in even less reliance on supplementary treatments, but savings were outweighed by the extra cost of the higher dose.

In a systematic review of the same studies, Gagnier et al (2007) concluded there is moderate-level evidence to support the acute and short-term use of willow bark for pain at daily doses standardised to 120 mg or 240 mg salicin, where it has relative equivalence to 12.5 mg per day of rofecoxib. Most recently, a 2009 systematic review (Vlachojannis et al 2009) of studies ranging from 2 to 6 weeks in length concluded that ethanolic willow bark extract was a promising analgesic in the treatment of low-back pain with a low incidence of adverse events. There was a dose-dependent effect where an extract with 240 mg of salicin in the daily dosage was more effective than that of 120 mg.

Musculoskeletal pain

In a multicentre study, a total of 436 patients with musculoskeletal disorders were treated with STW 33-I (daily administration of the equivalent of 240 mg salicylic alcohol derivates) alone (61.5%) or in combination with other analgesics (28.9% of the patients received additional NSAIDs [mainly diclofenac and ibuprofen], 3.9% additionally NSAIDs and opioids and 5.7% additionally other medication). Of the 436 participants, 56% had osteoarthritis, 60% had back pain, 34% had osteoarthritis and back pain,

15% had fibromyalgia, 9% had osteoarthritis with back pain and fibromyalgia, 6% had soft-tissue rheumatism, 8% had rheumatoid arthritis and 18% reported other conditions. During the visits the global pain intensity was rated by patients on a visual analogue scale and the global efficacy of treatment was rated by doctors on a five-point Likert scale. The mean reductions in the pain intensity scale were significant ($P < 0.01$) after 3 weeks and clinically relevant at the end of the study. Of the patients available for the last rating after 24 weeks, 60% had a nearly complete or partial remission (rating 0–1) of their symptoms compared to 27.1% after 3 weeks. The relative reductions of the weekly means of the daily patient self-rated scores of the pain were between 33% and 44% of the baseline values during the course of the study (Uehleke et al 2013).

Fever and headaches

The known activity of salicylate constituents in willow bark provides support for its use as symptomatic treatment in fever and headaches. Commission E has approved willow bark for these indications (Blumenthal et al 2000). Despite this, only one clinical study has been conducted exploring the effectiveness of willow bark for headaches, but it was used in combination with the herb feverfew, so the efficacy of stand-alone treatment remains unknown (Shrivastava et al 2006).

IN COMBINATION

A prospective, open-label study was performed in 12 patients diagnosed with migraine without aura. Twelve weeks' treatment with feverfew (*Tanacetum parthenium*, 300 mg) plus willow bark (300 mg) twice daily was shown to reduce attack frequency and intensity, with 70% of patients having a reduction of at least 50%. Attack duration also decreased significantly in all patients. Self-assessed general health, physical performance, memory and anxiety also improved by the end of the study. The treatment was well tolerated and no adverse events occurred (Shrivastava et al 2006).

OTHER USES

An in vitro study that examined the effects of the main groups of compounds (salicylalcohol derivates, flavonoids, proanthocyanidins) and salicin isolated from willow bark extract BNO 1455 found that all compounds exerted antiproliferative activity, inhibited cell growth and promoted apoptosis in human colon and lung cancer cell lines, irrespective of their COX-selectivity (Hostanska et al 2007).

DOSAGE RANGE

- Tincture (1:1): 1–2 mL three times daily.
- Decoction: 1–3 g finely chopped herb in 1 cup of cold water, brought to the boil then reduced to simmer for 5 minutes, drunk 3–4 times daily.
- The European Scientific Co-operative on Phytomedicine (ESCOP) monograph recommends a daily dose of willow bark equivalent to 120–240 mg total salicin (Nahrstedt et al 2007).

> ***Clinical note — Lack of significant haematological effects***
>
> It has largely been assumed that willow bark alters platelet aggregation and increases bleeding time, in much the same way as aspirin. Whether this is in fact correct and clinically significant has been investigated by Krivoy et al (2001). The clinical study found that consumption of *Salicis cortex* extract (containing 240 mg salicin per daily dose) only minimally affected platelet aggregation compared to a cardioprotective dose of acetylsalicylate (up to 100 mg/day). The particular preparation studied produced a total serum salicylate concentration bioequivalent to only 50 mg acetylsalicylate.

According to clinical studies

- Osteoarthritic joint pain and inflammation — willow bark preparations standardised to total salicin content and providing 240 mg daily in divided doses.
- Acute episodes of chronic non-specific low-back pain — willow bark preparations standardised to total salicin content and providing 240 mg daily in divided doses.

ADVERSE REACTIONS

None reported. Theoretically, the tannin and salicylate content may cause gastrointestinal disturbances, but willow bark extract contains a gastroprotective principle (Vlachojannis et al 2011). In rare cases allergic skin reaction may occur (Cameron et al 2009).

SIGNIFICANT INTERACTIONS

Controlled studies are not available, therefore interactions are based on evidence of pharmacological activity and clinical significance is uncertain.

Anticoagulants

Although a clinical study found that consumption of salicin 240 mg/day produced minimal effects on platelet aggregation, higher doses may have a significant effect. Exercise caution with high doses >240 mg salicin/day. In a prospective, longitudinal study, patients completed a 16-week diary by recording bleeding events and exposure to factors previously reported to increase the risk of bleeding and supratherapeutic international normalised ratios, including CM consumption. This study identified that the use of willow bark was associated with an increased risk of self-reported bleeding in patients using warfarin (Shalansky et al 2007). Controlled studies are now warranted to confirm whether oral willow bark preparations induce clinically significant changes to bleeding.

Salicylate drugs

Theoretically, concurrent use may result in additive effects, although this has yet to be tested. Observe patients taking this combination.

Aspirin

Theoretically, willow bark may enhance the anti-inflammatory and antiplatelet effects at doses above salicin 240 mg/day. Since salicylic acid concentrations after 100 mg aspirin impair platelet aggregation but those after willow bark with 240 mg salicin almost not, it remains to be established if salicylic acid derivatives have a different effect on blood clotting (Vlachojannis et al 2011). Observe patients taking this combination; beneficial interaction may be possible.

An increased risk of bleeding is theoretically possible with high doses >240 mg salicin. Observe.

NSAIDs

A reduction in drug requirements may be possible with the use of white willow bark for lower-back pain. Beneficial interaction is possible.

CONTRAINDICATIONS AND PRECAUTIONS

Commission E states that there is no evidence that willow bark preparations should be contraindicated in small children because of the risk of Reye's syndrome, as the salicylates in the herb are metabolised differently from those in aspirin.

Owing to the relatively high concentration of salicylates in this herb, it should not be used by people with salicylate sensitivity.

PREGNANCY USE

It is generally not advised to recommend salicylate-containing medicines during pregnancy or lactation, although no restrictions are known for willow bark directly.

Practice points/Patient counselling

- Evidence from several randomised controlled trials suggests that willow bark is an effective treatment for relieving pain in chronic backache and osteoarthritis.
- The results of one clinical study suggest it is as effective as 12.5 mg of the synthetic COX-2 inhibitor rofecoxib when used at a daily dose of 240 mg salicin.
- People using willow bark may find they have lowered requirements for traditional anti-inflammatory medicines such as NSAIDs.
- Currently, there is no evidence to suggest gastrointestinal side effects or significant platelet inhibition.
- Due to its salicylate content, people with salicylate sensitivity should avoid use of willow bark.

PATIENTS' FAQs

What will this herb do for me?
Scientific studies have found that willow bark is a useful treatment for relieving pain in osteoarthritis and chronic backache. It may also relieve symptoms of headache and fever.

When will it start to work?
Studies using willow bark preparations in diseases characterised by joint pain have found that effects start within 1 week of use.

Are there any safety issues?
Willow bark appears to be free of major side effects or drug interactions, but it should not be taken by people with salicylate sensitivity.

REFERENCES

Beer AM, Wegener T. Willow bark extract (*Salicis cortex*) for gonarthrosis and coxarthrosis — Results of a cohort study with a control group. Phytomedicine 15.11 (2008): 907–13.

Biegert C et al Efficacy and safety of willow bark extract in the treatment of osteoarthritis and rheumatoid arthritis: results of 2 randomized double-blind controlled trials. J Rheumatol 31.11 (2004): 2121–30.

Blumenthal M, et al. (eds). Herbal medicine: expanded Commission E monographs. Austin, TX: Integrative Medicine Communications, 2000.

Bonaterra GA et al Anti-inflammatory effects of the willow bark extract STW 33-I (Proaktiv(®)) in LPS-activated human monocytes and differentiated macrophages. Phytomedicine. 17.14 (2010): 1106–13.

Cameron M, et al. Evidence of effectiveness of herbal medicinal products in the treatment of arthritis. Part I: Osteoarthritis.Phytother Res. 2009 Nov;23(11):1497–515.

Chrubasik S et al Treatment of low back pain exacerbations with willow bark extract: a randomized double-blind study. Am J Med 109.1 (2000): 9–14.

Chrubasik S et al Treatment of low back pain with a herbal or synthetic anti-rheumatic: a randomised controlled study: willow bark extract for low back pain. Rheumatology (Oxford) 40.12 (2001a): 1388–93.

Chrubasik S et al Potential economic impact of using a proprietary willow bark extract in outpatient treatment of low back pain: an open non-randomized study. Phytomedicine 8.4 (2001b): 241–51.

Drummond EM et al Inhibition of proinflammatory biomarkers in THP1 macrophages by polyphenols derived from chamomile, meadowsweet and willow bark. Phytother Res 27.4 (2013):588–94.

Fiebich BL, Chrubasik S. Effects of an ethanolic salix extract on the release of selected inflammatory mediators in vitro. Phytomedicine 11.2–3 (2004): 135–8.

Gagnier JJ et al Herbal medicine for low back pain. Cochrane Database Syst Rev no. 2 (2006): CD004504.

Gagnier JJ et al Herbal medicine for low back pain: a Cochrane review. Spine 32.1 (2007): 82–92.

Hedner T, Everts B. The early clinical history of salicylates in rheumatology and pain. Clin Rheumatol 17.1 (1998): 17–25.

Hostanska K et al Willow bark extract (BNO1455) and its fractions suppress growth and induce apoptosis in human colon and lung cancer cells. Cancer Detect Prev 31.2 (2007): 129–39.

Ishikado A et al Willow bark extract increases antioxidant enzymes and reduces oxidative stress through activation of Nrf2 in vascular endothelial cells and *Caenorhabditis elegans*. Free Radic Biol Med. 65 (2013): 1506–15.

Khayyal MT et al Mechanisms involved in the anti-inflammatory effect of a standardized willow bark extract. Arzneimittelforschung. 55.11 (2005): 677–87.

Knuth S et al Catechol conjugates are in vivo metabolites of *Salicis cortex*. Planta Med. 79.16 (2013): 1489–94.

Krivoy N et al Effect of *Salicis cortex* extract on human platelet aggregation. Planta Med 67.3 (2001): 209–12.

Mills SY et al Effect of a proprietary herbal medicine on the relief of chronic arthritic pain: a double-blind study. Br J Rheumatol 35.9 (1996): 874–7.

Nahrstedt A et al Willow bark extract: the contribution of polyphenols to the overall effect. Wien Med Wochenschr. 157.13–14 (2007): 348–51.

Nieman DC et al A commercialized dietary supplement alleviates joint pain in community adults: a double-blind, placebo-controlled community trial. Nutr J. 12.1 (2013): 154.

Nizard C et al Heat shock protein 47 expression in aged normal human fibroblasts: modulation by *Salix alba* extract. Ann N Y Acad Sci 1019 (2004):223–7.

Schmid B et al Effectiveness and tolerance of standardized willow bark extract in arthrosis patients. Randomized, placebo controlled double-blind study. Z Rheumatol 59.5 (2000): 314–20.
Schmid B et al Efficacy and tolerability of a standardized willow bark extract in patients with osteoarthritis: randomized placebo-controlled, double blind clinical trial. Phytother Res 15.4 (2001a): 344–50.
Schmid B et al Pharmacokinetics of salicin after oral administration of a standardised willow bark extract. Eur J Clin Pharmacol 57.5 (2001b): 387–91.
Setty AR, Sigal LH. Herbal medications commonly used in the practice of rheumatology: mechanisms of action, efficacy, and side effects. Semin Arthritis Rheum 34.6 (2005): 773–84.
Shalansky S et al Risk of warfarin-related bleeding events and supratherapeutic international normalized ratios associated with complementary and alternative medicine: a longitudinal analysis. Pharmacotherapy. 27.9 (2007): 1237–47.
Shrivastava R, et al. Tanacetum parthenium and *Salix alba* (Mig-RL) combination in migraine prophylaxis: a prospective, open-label study. Clin Drug Investig 26.5 (2006): 287–96.
Stone E. (1763) An account of the success of the bark of the willow in the cure of agues. Philosophical Transactions (1683–1775) 53: 195–200.
Uehleke B et al Willow bark extract STW 33-I in the long term treatment of outpatients with rheumatic pain mainly osteoarthritis or back pain. Phytomedicine. 20.11 (2013): 980–4.
Ulrich-Merzenich G et al Novel neurological and immunological targets for salicylate-based phytopharmaceuticals and for the anti-depressant imipramine. Phytomedicine. 19.10 (2012):930–9.
Vlachojannis JE et al A systematic review on the effectiveness of willow bark for musculoskeletal pain. Phytother Res 23.7 (2009): 897–900.
Vlachojannis J et al Willow species and aspirin: different mechanism of actions. Phytother Res 25.7 (2011):1102–4.

Withania

HISTORICAL NOTE The name ashwagandha (one of the common names for this herb) comes from the Sanskrit, meaning 'horse-like smell'. Apparently, this name not only refers to the smell of the herb but also to its strengthening and aphrodisiac qualities. It is often referred to as 'Indian ginseng' because it is used in much the same way as *Panax ginseng* in traditional Chinese medicine, although it is considered less stimulating. In Ayurvedic medicine it is classified as a 'rasayana', used to promote physical and mental health and improve vitality and longevity (Kulkarni & Dhir 2008).

OTHER NAMES

Ashwagandha (and a variety of spellings, including ashvagandha, ashwaganda, asvagandha), Ayurvedic ginseng, Indian ginseng, winter cherry.

BOTANICAL NAME/FAMILY

Withania somnifera (family Solanaceae)

Sometimes confused with *Physalis alkekengi*, also known as winter cherry, and another related species with known medicinal properties, *Withania coagulans* (Mirjalili et al 2009).

PLANT PARTS USED

Primarily root and leaves, although berry and bark are sometimes used.

CHEMICAL COMPONENTS

Steroidal lactones (comprising 40 withanolides, e.g. withaferin A), 12 alkaloids (including withanine, somniferine, isopelletierine, anaferine, tropine, pseudotropine), flavonoids, saponins, sitoindosides, iron, choline, acylsteryl glucosides, coumarins (scopoletin and aesculetin), triterpene (beta-amyrin), phytosterols (stigmasterol, stigmasterol glucoside, beta-sitosterol and beta-sitosterol glucoside), polysaccharides, Viscosa lactone B, alpha + beta glucose, essential oils (ipuranol, withaniol) (Abou Douh 2002, Kulkarni & Verma 1993, Mills & Bone 2000, Mirjalili et al 2009, Misra et al 2008).

Plants sourced from Sardinia, Italy have significantly higher levels of withaferin A content than those sourced from India or Sicily (Scartezzini et al 2007).

MAIN ACTIONS

Withania and several of its key constituents have been subjected to scientific investigation in vitro and in vivo. While it is important to understand the pharmacological actions of individual components, clinical effects are difficult to predict from these studies as the ultimate effect of the herbal treatment will be a result of many intraherbal interactions.

Adaptogen (modulates stress responses)

Withania has been shown to attenuate the negative effects of chronic stress in rats, including hyperglycaemia, glucose intolerance, increase in plasma corticosteroid levels, gastric ulcerations, male sexual dysfunction, cognitive deficits, immunosuppression and mental depression (Bhattacharya & Muruganandam 2003, Kour et al 2009).

Animal trials have shown that a withanolide-free hydrosoluble fraction of withania reduces the stress response induced both chemically and physically (Singh et al 2003). It suppresses stress-induced increases in dopamine receptors in the corpus striatum and acts as a gamma-aminobutyric acid (GABA)-mimetic agent by binding to GABA receptors (Mehta et al 1991, Upton 2000). Animal studies also suggest an ability to reduce adrenal weight and plasma cortisol levels (Kurandikar et al 1986), thus potentially protecting against the negative effects of elevated cortisol levels in chronic stress and allostasis.

Cognitive enhancement

The potent acetylcholinesterase inhibitory activity of withania in vitro may help to explain its traditional use for improving cognition (Vinutha et al 2007). Memory enhancement has been confirmed by animal studies and appears to be mediated by a cholinergic effect (Dhuley 2001). Increased cortical muscarinic acetylcholine receptor capacity has been observed in animals and humans with extracts of withania (Schliebs et al 1997). Several withanolides exert calcium antagonistic ability, together with anticholinesterase activity, by inhibiting butyrylcholinesterase and acetylcholinesterase enzymes (Choudhary et al 2004, 2005). The presence of choline in the herb may also contribute to the production of acetylcholine and further increase cholinergic effects. Withania extract is also protective of hypobaric hypoxia-induced memory loss and neurodegeneration in rats by modulation of corticosterone levels, via the nitric oxide pathway in the hippocampus (Baitheru et al 2013).

Neuroprotective

Several animal studies indicate the potential for protection of neurons (Ahmed et al 2013, Jain et al 2001), including protection from neuronal injury in Parkinson's disease (Ahmad et al 2005, RajaSankar et al 2009) and promotion of dendrite formation (Tohda et al 2000). One possible explanation is due to the antioxidant properties of withania (Parihar & Hemnani 2003). More recently a mouse model of Parkinson's disease demonstrated the antioxidant actions of *Withania somnifera* root extract on nigrostriatal dopaminergic neurodegeneration and significant improvement in behavioural, physiological and biochemical irregularities (Prakash et al 2013).

In animal experiments withania has been shown to be useful for the treatment of drug-induced dyskinesia (chewing movements, tongue protrusion and buccal tremors) due to reserpine (an antihypertensive and antipsychotic agent no longer available in Australia) and haloperidol (an antipsychotic). In one study, *W. somnifera* root extract (50 and 100 mg/kg) was administered for 4 weeks and dose-dependently reduced reserpine-induced vacuous chewing movements and tongue protrusions, and memory retention deficits in rats. The effect was most likely due to reversal of the drug-induced depletion of glutathione, superoxide dismutase and catalase (Naidu et al 2006). Other researchers support the theory that benefits of withania appear to be due to its antioxidant rather than GABA-mimetic action (Bhattacharya et al 2002, Naidu et al 2003).

In vitro results suggest that withanolide A, withanoside IV and withanoside VI are involved in reconstructing neuronal networks, including axons, dendrites, pre- and postsynapses in the neurons (Kuboyama et al 2002, 2005, Tohda 2008). In vivo, oral withanolide A, withanoside IV and withanoside VI (10 micromol/kg/day for 12 days) have been shown to improve experimentally-induced memory impairment, neurite atrophy and synaptic loss in the cerebral cortex and hippocampus in mice; and withanoside IV (10 micromol/kg/day for 21 days) improves locomotor functions in mice with spinal cord injury (Tohda 2008).

A rat model studying the effect of withanolides A and C in rat neurons with beta-amyloid proteins found they bind with the active motif of the protein, preventing the fibril formation common in Alzheimer's disease (AD) (Jayaprakasam et al 2010). This was confirmed for an aqueous *W. somnifera* extract in a second study in 2012 (Kumar et al 2012).

A 30-day course of a withania extract, semipurified to contain mostly withanolides and withanosides, was administered to middle-aged and old APP/PSI AD transgenic mice, resulting in the eradication of behavioural deficits and amyloid plaque in the hippocampus and cortex of middle-aged mice and significant reductions of both in the old mice (Seghal et al 2011). In 2012 Patil et al demonstrated in rat cortical neurons that withanolide A and Asiatic acid modulated several targets associated with amyloid-beta protein and amyloid-beta precursor protein production, indicating they may be useful in the treatment of AD.

Antioxidant

Withania exerts an indirect antioxidant action in vivo (Bhattacharya et al 1997, 2001). This mechanism is responsible for much of the herb's protective action against organ toxicity, degeneration or injury.

Daily administration of *W. somnifera* root extract increases hepatic glucose-6-phosphatase activity and decreases hepatic lipid peroxidation, most likely by increasing the activity of endogenous antioxidant enzymes (Panda & Kar 1997, 1998, 1999).

In vitro *W. somnifera* inhibits both the lipid peroxidation and the protein oxidative modification induced by copper (Gupta et al 2003). In animal studies the antioxidant actions have been proposed as a possible mechanism for withania, preventing the negative effects of stroke induced by middle cerebral artery occlusion in rats (Choudhary et al 2003). The antioxidant properties may also contribute to the anticataleptic effect noted in studies of haloperidol-induced catalepsy in albino mice (Nair et al 2008) and may protect against the genotoxic potency of commercial-grade malathion, a commonly used insecticide (Bernhardt et al 2011). Pretreatment with withania was also protective in radiation-induced hepatotoxicity in rats via antioxidant mechanisms (Mansour & Hafez 2012).

Increases haematopoiesis

Animal trials indicate that the herb increases haemoglobin and red blood cell levels (Ziauddin et al 1996) and increases haematopoiesis (Aphale et al 1998). The iron content of the herb may further contribute to its role in red blood cell formation.

Immunomodulation

Immunomodulating activity has been demonstrated in vivo for withania, including an increase in white blood cell, platelet and neutrophil counts (Agarwal et al 1999, Davis & Kuttan 2000, Gupta et al 2001,

Ziauddin et al 1996), proliferation of lymphocytes, increased interferon-gamma (Teixeira et al 2006, Yamada et al 2011) and interleukin-2 (IL-2) levels and a reduction in tumour necrosis factor (TNF) (Davis & Kuttan 1999, Yamada et al 2011). The effects on immune function have also been demonstrated clinically in a small study of 5 people who were given 6 mL of withania root extract twice daily for 96 hours, resulting in increases in lymphocytes and natural killer cells from baseline (Mikolai et al 2009).

In animal studies, oral administration of a standardised fluid extract (1 : 1) of withania (30 mg/kg) for 15 days resulted in enhanced T-helper cell (Th1) immunity (increased expression of Th1 cytokines, interferon-gamma and IL-2) with a moderate decline in Th2 (decreased expression of Th2 cytokine IL-4). This effect appeared to be due to withanolide A. The extract also strongly activated macrophage function and no toxicity was noted (Malik et al 2007). Other studies have confirmed an increased expression of Th1 cytokines in chronically stressed (Khan et al 2006) and immunosuppressed mice (Bani et al 2006, Kour et al 2009, Malik et al 2009). Although human trials are required to confirm these effects, withania shows promise for selective Th1/Th2 modulation.

Antibacterial and antifungal activity

Animal and in vitro studies have shown antibacterial effects against *Staphylococcus aureus* (Datta et al 2011), *Listeria monocytogenes, Bacillus anthracis, Bacillus subtilis, Salmonella enteridis* (Akin et al 1986) and *Salmonella typhimurium* (Owais et al 2005). The methanol and hexane extracts of both the leaves and the roots have potent antibacterial activity against *S. typhimurium* and *Escherichia coli* (Arora et al 2004); and the steroidal withanolides from the related species *W. coagulens* have been found to have antifungal activity against *Allescheria boydii, Aspergillus niger, Curvularia lunata, Drechslera rostrata, Epidermophyton floccosum, Microsporum canis, Nigrospora oryzae, Pleurotus ostreatus* and *Stachybotrys atra* (Choudhary et al 1995). *W. somnifera* glycoprotein exerts an antibacterial activity against *Clavibacter michiganensis* and a fungistastic effect against *Aspergillus flavus, Fusarium oxysporum* and *F. verticillioides* (by inhibiting spore germination and hyphal growth) (Girish et al 2006).

Anti-inflammatory activity

Withania extract suppresses the production of pro-inflammatory molecules in many in vitro models. This is partly due to inhibition of transcription factors nuclear factor-kappa B (NF-κB) and activator protein-1 by withanolides (steroidal lactones) (Ichikawa et al 2006, Kaileh et al 2007, Maitra et al 2009, Mulabagal et al 2009, Oh et al 2008, Singh et al 2007). Several withanolides exert selective cyclooxygenase-2 (COX-2) enzyme inhibition (Jayaprakasam & Nair 2003) and withania has been found to decrease alpha-2-macroglobulin, a liver-synthesised plasma protein that increases during inflammation (Anbalagan & Sadique 1985).

Withania rectal gel 1000 mg/kg was applied in an experimental inflammatory bowel disease rat model, resulting in highly significant protection compared to controls ($P < 0.001$) upon histological examination (Pawar et al 2011). Additionally, withaferin A reduces the microglial inflammatory response via downregulation of lipolysaccharide-induced COX-2 expression and prostaglandin E_2 production, believed to occur at least partially through STAT 1/3 inhibition (Min et al 2011). In pulmonary epithelial cells withaferin A inhibits TNF-α, downregulating NF-κB (Oh et al 2009). Withaferin A has also been compared to indomethacin in an experimental mouse model of induced inflammation, pyrexia and gastric ulceration. Withaferin A significantly reduced inflammation and pyrexia at 20/30 mg/kg and without causing gastric damage at 30/40 mg/kg, as compared to indomethacin 20 mg/kg, which caused significant gastric ulceration (Sabina et al 2009).

A reduction in the erythrocyte sedimentation rate has also been noted in a double-blind clinical trial of 50–59-year-old males (Kupparajan et al 1980).

Chondroprotective

Withania root powder has demonstrated chondroprotective effects in vitro (human osteoarthritic cartilage matrix), inhibiting the gelatinase activity of collagenase type 2 enzyme and exerting a significant short-term chondroprotective effect in a subset (50%) of patient samples (Sumantran et al 2007). A more recent study had similar results (Ganesan et al 2011). In vivo the root powder rectified biochemical changes resulting from experimentally induced arthritis in rats (Rasool & Varalakshmi 2007). Associated with arthritis were increased levels of lipid peroxides, glycoproteins and urinary constituents; and depletion of antioxidant status and bone collagen. These biochemical alterations were ameliorated significantly by oral administration of *W. somnifera* root powder (1000 mg/kg body weight) in test animals. It should be noted, however, that the high dose used (1000 mg/kg body weight) is not likely to be reproducible in human trials.

Anticancer (antineoplastic and chemoprevention)

Some research has been conducted with withania; however most has focused on the component withaferin A, which has multiple mechanisms of action.

In vitro studies have determined that withania extracts possess cell cycle disruption and antiangiogenic activity (Mathur et al 2006). Withania stimulates the production of cytotoxic T lymphocytes in vivo and in vitro, and may prevent or reduce tumour growth (Choudhary et al 2010, Davis & Kuttan 2002, Jayaprakasam et al 2003, Malik et al 2008). In animal models, withania was found to prevent skin carcinoma induced by ultraviolet B radiation (Mathur et al 2004) and forestomach tumours (Padmavathi et al 2005); reduce the incidence, number and size of tumours; and counteract the associated decrease in body weight (Singh et al 1986).

The withaferin A fraction appears to exert antiangiogenic activity (Mohan et al 2004) and antigenotoxic effects on bone marrow (Panjamurthy et al 2008), and may be partly responsible for the antineoplastic effects observed in both in vitro and in vivo studies (Uma Devi et al 1995, 1996). The antioxidant effects aid in the prevention of DNA damage by mutagens (Khanam & Devi 2005) and this, in combination with detoxifying properties, anti-inflammatory and immunomodulatory effects, determined in animal studies, is likely to contribute to its chemopreventive action (Prakash et al 2001, 2002).

Because several genes that regulate cellular proliferation, carcinogenesis, metastasis and inflammation are regulated by NF-κB, the ability of withanolides to inhibit activation of NF-κB and NF-κB-regulated gene expression may partly explain the role of withania in enhancing apoptosis and inhibiting invasion and osteoclastogenesis (Grover et al 2011b, Ichikawa et al 2006).

Further investigation of withaferin A in apoptosis demonstrates that it induces endoplasmic reticulum stress via mediation of reactive oxygen species (ROS) (Choi et al 2011) and the modulation of heat shock protein 90 client complexes involved in protein folding (Grover et al 2011a, Yu et al 2010), leading to protein disruption and apoptosis. Um et al (2012) have also demonstrated that the downregulation of the STAT 3 signalling pathway may play a role in apoptosis, as might microtubule disruption (Grin et al 2012, Thaiparambil et al 2011). Withaferin A may also induce apoptosis in cervical cancer cells by downregulating human papillomavirus oncogenes E6/7 and restoring the p53 pathway (Munagala et al 2011). Breast cancer cell lines have also been studied with withaferin A, inducing apoptosis via ROS inhibition of mitochondrial respiration, survivin protein suppression, microtubule disassembly, inhibition of STAT 3 signalling pathways and antioestrogen effects (Hahm et al 2011, Lee et al 2010, Thaiparambil et al 2011). Additionally, studies have found that NOTCH2 and NOTCH4 involved in breast cancer cell migration were inhibited (Lee et al 2012).

Anxiolytic and antidepressant

Animal studies have found that glycowithanolides exert anxiolytic effects comparable to those of lorazepam, and antidepressant effects comparable to those of the antidepressant drug imipramine (SK Bhattacharya et al 2000). Anxiolytic and antidepressant activities have also been demonstrated for the withania root extract (WS 100, 200 or 500 mg/kg) and potentiation of diazepam at subtherapeutic doses (WS 50 mg/kg) has been demonstrated (Gupta & Rana 2007). Recently, a double-blind, randomised study confirmed significant anxiolytic and antidepressant activity after 60 days of treatment with an oral root extract standardised to at least 5% withanolide content (Chandrasekhar et al 2012).

Blood glucose control

Withania extract (200 and 400 mg/kg) was administered orally once daily for 5 weeks in a type 2 diabetes experimental model. The treatment reduced elevated levels of blood glucose, HbA_{1C} and insulin, and improved glucose tolerance and insulin sensitivity (Anwer et al 2008). Similar results have been seen in animal models that further suggest an antioxidant-related effect (Anwer et al 2012, Udayakumar et al 2009, 2010). In experimental in vitro models, withania (especially the ethanolic extract) has shown effects comparable to metformin in preventing the formation of advanced glycation end products, which are implicated in the pathogenesis of diabetes mellitus (Babu et al 2007).

Cardioprotective

Cardioprotective effects have been noted in animal studies (Dhuley 2000, Mohanty et al 2004), significantly reducing myocardial injury after ischaemia and reperfusion (Gupta et al 2004). These effects are most likely to be due to restoration of the myocardial oxidant–antioxidant balance and the marked antiapoptotic properties of withania (Mohanty et al 2008). Cardioprotective effects were also observed against doxorubicin-induced cardiotoxicity in vivo when pretreatment with a standardised withania extract (300 mg/kg; 1.5% withanolides) was administered before drug exposure (doxorubicin 10 mg/kg) (Hamza et al 2008). The alkaloids are considered to be sedative and reduce blood pressure and heart rate (Chevallier 1996, Malhotra et al 1965a). The withanolides have a chemical structure similar to cardiac glycosides and have demonstrated mild ionotropic and chronotropic effects on the heart (Roja et al 1991, Tripathi et al 1996).

Antihypercholesterolaemic

High doses of withania root powder (0.75 and 1.5 g/day) produced significant decreases in total lipids (–40.54%; –50.69%), cholesterol (–41.58%; –53.01%) and triglycerides (–31.25%; –44.85%); and significant increases in high-density lipoprotein cholesterol levels (+15.10%; +17.71%) in an experimental model of hypercholesterolaemia. Additionally, treatment resulted in significant decreases in HMG-CoA reductase activity and bile acid content in the liver of these animals, and there was a trend towards increased excretion of bile acid (+22.43%; +28.52%), cholesterol (+14.21%; +17.68%) and neutral sterol (+12.40%; +18.85%). Lipid peroxidation also decreased significantly (–35.29%; –36.52%) (Visavadiya & Narasimhacharya 2007). The doses used in this study may not be feasible in humans.

Thyroid modulating

An in vivo study reported that daily administration of *W. somnifera* root extract enhanced serum thyroxine concentration (Panda & Kar 1998, 1999). Withania 1.4 g/kg returned triiodothyronine/thyroxine levels to normal in metformin-induced hypothyroidism in type 2 diabetic mice (Jatwa & Kar 2009). Note that this dose is unlikely to be safely achieved in practice. There is one case report of thyrotoxicosis in a 32-year-old woman attributed to a withania-containing herbal capsule (van der Hooft et al 2005), so caution is advised.

Sexual enhancer

Traditionally used for this purpose, one double-blind clinical trial found that a dose of 3 g taken daily for 1 year improved the sexual performance of 71.4% of healthy ageing males (Kupparajan et al 1980). Alternatively, animal studies have indicated that very high doses (3000 mg/kg) result in reduced sexual performance (Ilayperuma et al 2002); however, in a randomised study of 95 men with psychogenic erectile dysfunction withania 500 mg given for 60 days was found to be no better than placebo in improving function (Mamidi & Thakar 2011).

OTHER ACTIONS

Hepatoprotective

Animal studies have demonstrated hepatoprotective effects (A Bhattacharya et al 2000, Sudhir et al 1986) and that withania inhibits phase I, and activates phase II and antioxidant enzymes in the liver (Padmavathi et al 2005).

Anticonvulsant

Withania root extract (100 or 200 mg/kg orally) increases seizure threshold in mice. The effect is likely to be due to GABA-A modulation (Kulkarni et al 2008).

Antitussive

A water extract polysaccharide fraction from withania showed reduced coughing efforts in guinea pigs in a manner similar to codeine (Sinha et al 2011).

Blood pressure — no effects

A small, poor-quality study consisted of 51 hypertensive patients (presumed to be stress-related) sampled purposively into two groups: 2 g of withania powder was given in either milk (group I) or water (group II) for 3 months. While there were systolic decreases in group I and diastolic reductions in both groups, neither was statistically significant (Kushwaha et al 2012).

CLINICAL USE

W. somnifera has not undergone significant scientific investigation in humans, therefore much of its use is based on pharmacological effects demonstrated in experimental models or traditional usage. In practice, it is often used in herbal combination treatments as part of the Ayurvedic system of medicine.

Stress adaptation

The pharmacological effects of the herb, which have been well established in animal studies, provide a theoretical basis for its use in situations characterised by stress (Archana & Namasivayam 1999, Bhattacharya & Muruganandam 2003, Dhuley 2000, Grandhi et al 1994).

More specifically, oral administration of an aqueous, standardised extract of *W. somnifera* (in a dose extrapolated from the human dose) has been found to offer protection against experimentally induced biological, physical and chemical stressors (Rege et al 1999).

In one in vivo study, plasma cortisol levels and adrenal weight were significantly lower, while liver weight increased (Kurandikar et al 1986).

(For more information see Clinical note — Allostasis and adaptation to stress in the Siberian ginseng monograph.)

Anxiety and depression

A daily dose of 300 mg of standardised root extract of *W. somnifera* root (KSM-66 ashwagandha extract, Ixoreal Biomed, Hyderabad, India, standardised to withanolide content of at least 5%) was investigated in a double-blind randomised controlled trial (RCT) involving 64 subjects over a period of 60 days. Active treatment resulted in a highly significant reduction in all measures compared to placebo; perceived stress scale 44% vs 5.5% ($P < 0.0001$) and total score for depression anxiety stress scale and the subsets; depression 77% vs 5.2%, anxiety 75.6% vs –4.3%, and stress 64.2 vs 10.4% ($P < 0.0001$). Similarly, significant improvements were seen in all subsets of the general health questionnaire: somatic stress, stress and anxiety, social dysfunction and severe depression ($P < 0.0001$). Additionally, greater serum cortisol reductions were seen with active treatment compared to placebo: 27.9% vs 7.9% ($P < 0.0006$) (Chandrasekhar et al 2012).

The herb's pharmacological effects, such as its GABA-mimetic activity (Mehta et al 1991) and ability to lower cortisol levels (Kurandikar et al 1986), provide a theoretical basis for its use in anxiety states. In vivo studies with withania root extract (WS 100, 200 or 500 mg/kg) confirm its anxiolytic effects and its ability to potentiate diazepam at subtherapeutic doses (WS 50 mg/kg) (Gupta & Rana 2007).

IN COMBINATION

One study used a herbal combination treatment known as Geriforte, which contains primarily *W. somnifera*. The product was taken by 34 subjects with anxiety neurosis, and after 12 weeks significant reductions in the frequency, duration and intensity of symptoms were observed (Ghosal et al 1990).

An RCT of 81 people with moderate to severe anxiety received naturopathic care (dietary counselling, deep-breathing relaxation techniques, multivitamin and withania 300 mg BD) or psychotherapy, the same deep-breathing techniques and placebo. The Beck Anxiety

Inventory (BAI) was the primary outcome measure. In all, 93% of participants were followed for 8 or more weeks, with final BAI scores reducing 56.5% ($P <$ 0.0001) in naturopathic care group and 30.5% in the psychotherapy group ($P < 0.0001$), with a significant difference favouring naturopathic care ($P < 0.003$), where *W. somnifera* was a major treatment (Cooley et al 2009).

Anabolic and weight gain promotion

Both animal and human studies have shown significant improvements in weight gain during the growth phase with the use of withania (Sharma et al 1986, Ziauddin et al 1996). It is suspected that an anabolic effect is responsible. This theory is supported by more recent research which shows that withania can increase testosterone levels (Ahmad et al 2010). Withania-fortified milk (2 g/day for 60 days) has been investigated in children and found to induce weight gain and increase total plasma proteins and haemoglobin levels (Venkatraghaven et al 1980).

Anaemia

The herb is used in the treatment of iron-deficiency anaemia due to its effects on haematopoiesis and natural iron content (Aphale et al 1998, Ziauddin et al 1996). This use has been supported by studies showing increased haemoglobin levels in children, induced by withania.

Attention-deficit hyperactivity disorder (ADHD)

IN COMBINATION

An RCT of 120 children aged 6–12 years tested the effect of a herbal combination including *Withania somnifera, Paeonia alba, Centella asiatica, Spirulina plantensis, Bacopa monniera* and *Melissa officinalis*. The participants met the *Diagnostic and Statistical Manual of Mental Disorders* (fourth edition) (DSM-IV) criteria for ADHD and took the test of variables of attention (TOVA) at baseline and after 4 months of treatment. The active treatment group had a significant improvement in all four subsets of TOVA, compared to placebo ($P < 0.004$) (Katz et al 2011). The 2:1 randomisation of participants to the treatment and placebo groups, with a high drop-out rate in the placebo arm, has affected study quality. Additionally the dose of each herb used within the combination was not reported.

Cancer therapy

The substantial preclinical research conducted to date with withania indicates a potential role in the treatment of cancer as a means of improving survival time and reducing treatment toxicity. Currently, only one clinical study has been conducted with oral withania extract which was used together with chemotherapy in women with breast cancer. The prospective non-randomised open study of 100 women (mean age 50 years) with breast cancer (77% having stage II or III disease) compared treatment with chemotherapy to treatment with chemotherapy and oral withania (2 g three times daily). Fatigue score and quality-of-life scores were monitored before, during and on the final cycle of chemotherapy treatment. Fatigue scores were significantly less, as were seven out of 18 quality-of-life symptoms ($P <$ 0.001), and 24-month survival favoured the treatment group (72% versus 56%), but was no longer statistically significant at median follow-up (26 months: $P < 0.176$) (Biswall et al 2012). Larger RCTs are needed to further explore the potential benefits and limitations of concomitant treatment.

Preclinical research has shown that *W. somnifera* reduces tumour cell proliferation while increasing overall survival time in animal trials. It enhances the effectiveness of radiation therapy while potentially attenuating the undesirable side effects of radio- and chemotherapeutic agents (including cyclophosphamide and paclitaxel) without interfering with the tumour-reducing actions of the drugs (Winters 2006).

Withania has been attributed with antitumour activity (Davis & Kuttan 2002, Jayaprakasam et al 2003), antiangiogenic effects (Mathur et al 2006, Mohan et al 2004) as well as antigenotoxic effects on bone marrow (Panjamurthy et al 2008). The antioxidant effects aid in the prevention of DNA damage by mutagens (Khanam & Devi 2005) and this, in combination with detoxifying properties, anti-inflammatory and immunomodulatory effects, determined in animal studies, is likely to contribute to its chemopreventive action (Prakash et al 2001, 2002).

Animal studies suggest a potential role for withania as an adjunctive treatment during chemotherapy for the prevention of drug-induced bone marrow depression (Davis & Kuttan 1999, Gupta et al 2001).

The ability to stimulate stem-cell proliferation has led to concerns that *W. somnifera* could reduce cyclophosphamide-induced toxicity and therefore reduce its usefulness in cancer therapy (Davis & Kuttan 1998). However, preliminary animal studies indicate that withania could prove to be a potent and relatively safe radiosensitiser and chemotherapeutic agent (Uma Devi 1996, Yang et al 2011). In one animal experiment, pretreatment with a standardised withania extract (300 mg/kg; 1.5% withanolides) attenuated the cardiotoxic side effects of doxorubicin (10 mg/kg) (Hamza et al 2008). In mice, the addition of *W. somnifera* (400 mg/kg orally once weekly for 4 weeks) to paclitaxel treatment (33 mg/kg intraperitoneally once weekly for 4 weeks) may extend its chemotherapeutic effect through modulating protein-bound carbohydrate levels and marker enzymes. The combination may effectively treat benzo(a)pyrene-induced lung cancer by offering protection against damage from ROS and also by suppressing cell proliferation (Senthilnathan et al 2006a).

Diabetes

Preclinical research suggests a hypoglycaemic effect which has been tested for clinical significance in a small study of six people with mild non-insulin-dependent diabetes mellitus. Treatment with withania root extract was used for 30 days and a decrease in blood glucose levels was detected and described as comparable to oral hypoglycaemic medicines (Andallu & Radhika 2000). No further published clinical studies have been located.

Drug and alcohol withdrawal

Withania is used in herbal combination therapy during opiate and alcohol withdrawal. This is based on preclinical research which suggests a potential role; however no clinical studies have been conducted thus far. In animal studies, repeated administration of withania (100 mg/kg) inhibited morphine tolerance and dependence (Kulkarni & Ninan 1997) and reduced neuronal damage during co-administration with chronic morphine use, but not during the withdrawal phase in rats (Kasture et al 2009). An ethanol withdrawal mouse model concluded that withania reduced the number of seizures and anxiety associated with alcohol withdrawal (Ruby et al 2012). It may also be useful in the management of withdrawal-induced anxiety due to chronic ethanol consumption (Gupta & Rana 2008). Another in vivo study found that withania root extract significantly impaired motivation for drinking alcohol, a result probably mediated by GABAB receptors (Peana et al 2014).

Hypercholesterolaemia

Treatment for 30 days with a withania root extract significantly decreased serum cholesterol, triglycerides, low-density lipoproteins and very-low-density lipoproteins in a small open study of six volunteers starting with mildly elevated lipids (Andallu & Radhika 2000). Further clinical research is warranted.

Osteoarthritis

The documented anti-inflammatory, chondroprotective (Rasool & Varalakshmi 2007, Sumantran et al 2007) and antioxidant activities of withania provide some support for its traditional use in arthritis. Arthritis results from dysregulation of proinflammatory cytokines (e.g. TNF and IL-1beta) and enzymes that mediate the production of prostaglandins (e.g. COX-2) and leukotrienes (e.g. lipoxygenase), together with the expression of adhesion molecules and matrix metalloproteinases, and hyperproliferation of synovial fibroblasts. These factors are regulated by the activation of the transcription factor NK-κB, which is inhibited by withanolides (Khanna et al 2007).

Withania root powder (500 and 1000 mg/kg) exerts a potent analgesic effect in rats and appears to retard amplification and propagation of the inflammatory response without causing any gastric damage (Rasool & Varalakshmi 2006). The root powder (1000 mg/kg) has also been shown to rectify biochemical changes resulting from experimentally induced arthritis (Rasool & Varalakshmi 2007). It should be noted, however, that this dose is not likely to be reproducible in human trials.

IN COMBINATION

While no RCT has been conducted with stand-alone withania treatment, several randomised clinical studies have been conducted using herbal combinations which contain withania as one of the ingredients, producing positive results. While promising, the contribution of withania to these results is difficult to determine.

One randomised, double-blind, placebo-controlled, crossover study of 42 patients with osteoarthritis found that a herbal combination treatment consisting of roots of *Withania somnifera*, the stem of *Boswellia serrata*, rhizomes of *Curcuma longa* and a zinc complex (Articulin-F) produced a significant decrease in the severity of pain ($P < 0.001$) and disability score ($P < 0.05$), although radiological assessment did not show any significant changes in either group (Kulkarni et al 1991). Similarly, a double-blind RCT of 90 patients with knee osteoarthritis found treatment with RA-11 (ARTREX, MENDAR), a standardised multiherb Ayurvedic treatment (*Withania somnifera, Boswellia serrata, Zingiber officinale* and *Curcuma longa*), produced a significant reduction in pain compared to placebo ($P < 0.05$) and significant improvement in the WOMAC scores at week 16 and week 32 ($P < 0.01$) and was well tolerated (Chopra et al 2004).

Osteoporosis

An ethanolic extract of withania root markedly prevented bone loss and associated biochemical changes in ovariectomised rats, indicating possible prevention of osteoporosis (Nagareddy & Lakshmana 2006). Controlled trials in humans are currently lacking.

Sleep

As its alkaloids are considered to be sedative and able to reduce blood pressure and heart rate (Chevallier 1996, Malhotra et al 1965a), withania is also used as a treatment for insomnia, although controlled trials are lacking in this area. Compared to diazepam (0.5 mg/kg) alone, the addition of withania root extract (100 mg/kg) to sleep-disturbed mice significantly attenuates the negative consequences of sleep deprivation. These include reduction in body weight, reduced locomotor activity, anxiety and altered antioxidant status (Kumar & Kalonia 2007).

Male infertility

Several recent clinical trials suggest a possible role in male infertility, which needs to be explored further.

A prospective study of 75 infertile (25 normozoospermic, 25 oligozoospermic and 25 asthenozoospermic) but otherwise healthy men (with fertile partners) that had not conceived after 1 year were matched against 75 fertile men (who had at least one pregnancy and normal sperm count) and were given 5 g of withania root powder in milk a day. Sperm concentration and motility were increased in all groups but remained suboptimal in the asthenozoospermic subset. Sperm volume was increased in all ($P < 0.01$) but the asthenozoospermic group, but sperm count per ejaculate was increased in all ($P < 0.01$). Additionally, oxidative biomarkers were all significantly improved ($P < 0.01$), and vitamins A, C, E ($P < 0.01$) and corrected seminal fructose ($P < 0.05$) were all improved from baseline. There were also significant increases in testosterone and luteinising hormone and decreases in follicle-stimulating hormone and prolactin in all treatment groups (Ahmad et al 2010).

In a similar group of men, sperm apoptosis, intracellular ROS, sperm concentration and levels of essential metal ions in seminal plasma (copper, zinc, gold and iron) were measured before and after 3-month treatment with withania powder 5 g/day. Degree of apoptosis and intracellular ROS were significantly reduced from abnormal baselines ($P < 0.05$), while deficient metal ions all increased after treatment ($P < 0.01$) (Shukla et al 2011). A prospective parallel trial by the same authors matched 60 normozoospermic fertile men with 60 normozoospermic infertile men, further divided into 20 men with psychological stress (measured by State Anxiety Index), 20 men who were heavy smokers and 20 men with infertility of unknown origin. Each was administered 5 g/day of powdered withania root for 3 months. After treatment, semen concentration, liquefaction time and motility improved in all groups and pregnancy outcome was 14% overall, but only 10% in the smoking group. Additionally, biomarkers of oxidative stress, the hormones testosterone, luteinising hormone, follicle-stimulating hormone, prolactin and blood cortisol were all significantly improved in all groups (Mahdi et al 2011).

OTHER USES

Traditionally used in convalescence for people who are stressed and both physically and emotionally exhausted, it is considered a non-stimulating tonic allowing for the restoration of vitality.

In rural parts of India, withania is applied topically as an antidote to snakebite. *W. somnifera* glycoprotein inhibits the hyaluronidase activity of cobra (*Naja naja*) and Russell's viper (*Daboia russelii*) venoms, providing some support for this use (Machiah et al 2006). Hyaluronidase activity is involved in rapid spreading of the toxins by destroying the integrity of the extracellular matrix.

Kalani et al (2012) report the case of a 57-year-old woman with non-classical adrenal hyperplasia with androgen excess who self-medicated with withania for 6 months, who showed significant reduction of biochemical markers and reduced hair loss.

DOSAGE RANGE

- Fluid extract (1:1): 20–50 mL/week (Australian manufacturer recommendations).
- Dried root: 3–6 g/day in capsule, milk or tea form.

According to clinical trials

- Anxiety and depression: 300–600 mg/day of withania extract standardised to 5% withanolides.
- Male infertility: 5 g/day in milk of powdered withania root.
- Breast cancer: 2 g oral withania 3 times a day.

ADVERSE REACTIONS

Withania appears well tolerated according to clinical research. Large doses can cause gastrointestinal upset, diarrhoea and vomiting (Tierra 2005).

A case report exists of thyrotoxicosis in a 32-year-old woman after taking a herbal capsule containing withania (van der Hooft et al 2005). Central nervous system and respiratory depression (Malhotra et al 1965b), decreased body temperature (Malhotra et al 1965b), gastrointestinal upset (Lindner 1996), kidney and liver abnormalities (Arseculeratne et al 1985) and fixed drug eruptions (Sehgal et al 2012) have also been noted.

Acute toxicity studies in animals show a good margin of safety with a high therapeutic index (Aphale et al 1998, Prabu et al 2013, Rege et al 1999, Sharada et al 1993, Singh et al 2001, 2003).

In a safety and tolerability study, 18 adults aged 18–30, body mass index 19–30 were administered an aqueous 8:1 extract via capsule in variable increasing doses every 10 days for 30 days in two divided doses (750 mg, 1000 mg and 1250 mg). Only one subject experienced any adverse effects, leaving the study at the lowest dose with increased appetite and libido, hallucination and vertigo. All physical and biochemical parameters remained normal in the rest (Raut et al 2012).

SIGNIFICANT INTERACTIONS

Controlled studies are not available; therefore, interactions are based on evidence of activity and are largely theoretical and speculative.

Antipsychotic/neuroleptic agents

In animal experiments, withania has been shown to be useful in the treatment of drug-induced dyskinaesia (chewing movements, tongue protrusion and buccal tremors) due to reserpine and haloperidol (Bhattacharya et al 2002, Naidu et al 2003, 2006). Beneficial interaction theoretically possible.

Barbiturates

Additive effects are theoretically possible, leading to increased sedation (NMCD 2005, Tierra 2005). Observe patients taking withania and barbiturates concurrently — beneficial interaction possible under medical supervision.

Benzodiazepines

Based on evidence from in vivo models (Kumar & Kalonia 2007), an increased sedative effect is theoretically possible (Upton 2000). Observe patients taking withania and benzodiazepines concurrently. Beneficial interaction theoretically possible under professional supervision.

Chemotherapy

Animal studies suggest a potential role for withania as an adjunctive treatment during chemotherapy. Observe — beneficial interaction theoretically possible — only to be used under professional supervision.

Cyclophosphamide

While the ability to stimulate stem-cell proliferation has led to concerns that *W. somnifera* could reduce cyclophosphamide-induced toxicity and therefore reduce its usefulness in cancer therapy (Davis & Kuttan 1998), preliminary animal studies indicate that withania could prove to be a potent and relatively safe radiosensitiser and chemotherapeutic agent (Uma Devi 1996).

Doxorubicin

In rats pretreatment with a standardised withania extract (300 mg/kg; 1.5% withanolides) attenuates the cardiotoxic side effects of doxorubicin (10 mg/kg) (Hamza et al 2008).

Paclitaxel

In mice the addition of *W. somnifera* (400 mg/kg, orally once weekly for 4 weeks) to paclitaxel (33 mg/kg, intraperitoneally once weekly for 4 weeks) may extend its chemotherapeutic effect through modulating protein-bound carbohydrate levels and marker enzymes. The combination may effectively treat the benzo(a)pyrene-induced lung cancer by offering protection from oxidative damage and also by suppressing cell proliferation (Senthilnathan et al 2006a, 2006b).

Digoxin assays

Withania may modestly interfere with serum digoxin measurements by the fluorescent polarisation immunoassay and other assays (Dasgupta et al 2007, 2008).

Immunosuppressants

The ability to stimulate stem-cell proliferation has led to concerns that *W. somnifera* could reduce the effectiveness of immunosuppressant drugs (Davis & Kuttan 1998). Caution should be exercised with patients taking immunosuppressants concurrently; however, a beneficial interaction may be possible under professional supervision.

Morphine

In animal studies, repeated administration of withania (100 mg/kg) inhibited morphine tolerance and dependence (Kulkarni & Ninan 1997). For this reason it is sometimes used in opiate withdrawal. Theoretically beneficial interaction possible under professional supervision.

Thyroid medication (e.g. levothyroxine)

Additive effects are theoretically possible. An in vivo study reported that daily administration of withania enhanced serum thyroxine concentrations (Upton 2000) and a case report exists of withania-induced thyrotoxicosis (van der Hooft et al 2005) — observe patients taking withania and thyroid medications concurrently.

Practice points/patient counselling

- Withania is an Ayurvedic herbal medicine, also referred to as Indian ginseng or ashwaganda. Scientific human research has only recently begun; however, extensive laboratory investigation and evidence from traditional use provide a guide.
- It is traditionally used for improving stress adaptation responses in people who are both physically and emotionally stressed and exhausted, and during periods of convalescence.
- New clinical research suggests a possible role in treating stress, anxiety and depression.
- Preliminary evidence suggests it increases haematopoiesis, promotes weight gain, reduces anxiety symptoms, increases cognitive function, improves male fertility and exerts a neuroprotective effect. It has shown promise in early investigations in Parkinson's and Alzheimer's disease.
- It has also demonstrated antioxidant, immunomodulating, antineoplastic, antifungal and antibacterial, anti-inflammatory and glucose-lowering activity in animal or test tube studies.
- The herb should not be taken in pregnancy, and should be used with caution in people sensitive to the Solanaceae family of plants.

CONTRAINDICATIONS AND PRECAUTIONS

Use with caution in peptic ulcer disease: withania may cause gastrointestinal irritation (Upton 2000). People who are sensitive to the Solanaceae family should use this herb with caution.

PREGNANCY USE

Western texts urge caution in pregnancy (Lindner 1996) due to a reputed abortifacient activity and antifertility effects noted in early animal studies, despite there being no evidence of fetal damage (Mills & Bone 2005). More recently a 500 mg polyherbal supplement (*Withania somnifera, Tribulus terrestris, Mucuna pruriens* and *Argyreia speciosa*) containing withania 300 mg out of 500 mg total was tested in mice, resulting in an oral toxicity LD_{50} of 5000 mg/kg with a significant improved birth rate, birth number and survival over two generations (Riaz et al 2010). Note that withania is used to support pregnancy and lactation in the Ayurvedic tradition (McGuffin et al 1997, Tirtha & Shiva 2002).

Metformin

Withania may protect type 2 diabetics on metformin from drug-induced hypothyroidism (Jatwa & Kar 2009). A potentially beneficial interaction that should only be used under supervision due to theoretical risk of induced thyrotoxicosis (see above).

PATIENTS' FAQs

What will this herb do for me?

Preliminary scientific research shows beneficial effects in stress, anxiety and depression and possibly some types of male infertility. Most information comes from other research and traditional use which suggests possible roles in improving memory, increasing red blood cell production, increasing immune responses and in convalescence.

When will it start to work?

Symptoms of anxiety and stress improve within 2 months' continual use and male fertility may improve after 4 months. It is not known when other effects start to develop.

Are there any safety issues?

The herb should not be taken in pregnancy, and should be used with caution in people sensitive to the Solanaceae family of plants.

REFERENCES

Abou-Douh AM. New withanolides and other constituents from the fruit of *Withania somnifera*. Arch Pharm (Weinheim) 335.6 (2002): 267–276.

Agarwal R et al Studies on immunomodulatory activity of *Withania somnifera* (Ashwagandha) extracts in experimental immune inflammation. J Ethnopharmacol 67.1 (1999): 27–35.

Ahmad M et al Neuroprotective effects of *Withania somnifera* on 6-hydroxydopamine induced Parkinsonism in rats. Hum Exp Toxicol 24.3 (2005): 137–147.

Ahmad, M. K., et al *Withania somnifera* improves semen quality by regulating reproductive hormone levels and oxidative stress in seminal plasma of infertile males. Fertil Steril 94.3 (2010) 989–96.

Ahmed, M.E., et al Attenuation of oxidative damage-associated cognitive decline by *Withania somnifera* in rat model of streptozotocin-induced cognitive impairment. Protoplasma (2013) 250: 1067–1078.

Akin S et al Antibacterial effects of some higher plants. Gazi Ecz Fak Der 3.1 (1986): 65–80.

Anbalagan K, Sadique J. Int J Crude Drug Res 23 (1985): 177. Cited in: Bone K. Clinical applications of Ayurvedic and Chinese herbs. Warwick, Qld: Phytotherapy Press, 1996.

Andallu, B. & Radhika, B. 2000. Hypoglycemic, diuretic and hypocholesterolemic effect of winter cherry (*Withania somnifera*, Dunal) root. Indian J Exp.Biol., 38, (6) 607–609.

Anwer T et al Effect of *Withania somnifera* on insulin sensitivity in non-insulin-dependent diabetes mellitus rats. Basic Clin Pharmacol Toxicol 102.6 (2008): 498–503.

Anwer T et al. Protective effect of *Withania somnifera* against oxidative stress and pancreatic beta-cell damage in type 2 diabetic rats. Acta Pol Pharm 69.6 (2012): 1095–101.

Aphale AA et al Subacute toxicity study of the combination of ginseng (*Panax ginseng*) and ashwagandha (*Withania somnifera*) in rats: a safety assessment. Indian J Physiol Pharmacol 42.2 (1998): 299–302.

Archana R, Namasivayam A. Antistressor effect of *Withania somnifera*. J Ethnopharmacol 64.1 (1999): 91–93.

Arora S et al The in vitro antibacterial/synergistic activities of *Withania somnifera* extracts. Fitoterapia 75.3–4 (2004): 385–388.

Arseculeratne SN, et al. Studies on medicinal plants of Sri Lanka. Part 14: toxicity of some traditional medicinal herbs. J Ethnopharmacol 13.3 (1985): 323–335.

Babu PV et al Protective effect of *Withania somnifera* (Solanaceae) on collagen glycation and cross-linking. Comp Biochem Physiol B Biochem Mol Biol 147.2 (2007): 308–313.

Baitheru, I., et al *Withania somnifera* root extract ameliorates hypoxia induxed memory impairment in rats. J. Ethnopharm. 145 (2013): 431–441

Bani S et al. Selective Th1 up-regulating activity of *Withania somnifera* aqueous extract in an experimental system using flow cytometry. J Ethnopharmacol 107.1 (2006): 107–115.

Bernhardt, V., et al In vivo genetic damage induced by commercial malathion and the antigenotoxic role of Withanis somnifera. International Journal of Integrative Biology 11.2 (2011): 78:8.

Bhattacharya SK, Muruganandam AV. Adaptogenic activity of *Withania somnifera*: an experimental study using a rat model of chronic stress. Pharmacol Biochem Behav 75.3 (2003): 547–555.

Bhattacharya SK et al Antioxidant activity of glycowithanolides from *Withania somnifera*. Indian J Exp Biol 35.3 (1997): 236–239.

Bhattacharya A et al Effect of *Withania somnifera* glycowithanolides on iron-induced hepatotoxicity in rats. Phytother Res. 14.7 (2000): 568–570.

Bhattacharya SK et al Anxiolytic-antidepressant activity of *Withania somnifera* glycowithanolides: an experimental study. Phytomedicine 7.6 (2000): 463–469.

Bhattacharya A et al Anti-oxidant effect of *Withania somnifera* glycowithanolides in chronic foot shock stress-induced perturbations of oxidative free radical scavenging enzymes and lipid peroxidation in rat frontal cortex and striatum. J Ethnopharmacol 74.1 (2001): 1–6.

Bhattacharya SK et al Effect of *Withania somnifera* glycowithanolides on a rat model of tardive dyskinesia. Phytomedicine 9.2 (2002): 167–170.

Biswal, B. M., et al Effect of *Withania somnifera* (Ashwagandha) on the development of chemotherapy-induced fatigue and quality of life in breast cancer patients. Integr Cancer Ther (2012): 1534735412464551.

Chandrasekhar, K., et al. 2012. A prospective, randomized double-blind, placebo-controlled study of safety and efficacy of a high-concentration full-spectrum extract of ashwagandha root in reducing stress and anxiety in adults. Indian J Psychol.Med, 34, (3) 255–262.

Chevallier A. The encyclopedia of medicinal plants. London, UK: Dorling Kindersley, 1996.

Choi, M.J., et al Endoplasmic reticulum stress mediates withaferin A-induced apoptosis in human renal carcinoma cells. Toxicol In Vitro 25.3(2011) 692–8.

Chopra, A., et al. 2004. A 32-week randomized, placebo-controlled clinical evaluation of RA-11, an Ayurvedic drug, on osteoarthritis of the knees. J Clin.Rheumatol., 10, (5) 236–245.

Choudhary MI et al Antifungal steroidal lactones from Withania coagulance. Phytochemistry 40.4 (1995): 1243–1246.

Choudhary G et al Evaluation of *Withania somnifera* in a middle cerebral artery occlusion model of stroke in rats. Clin Exp Pharmacol Physiol 30.5–6 (2003): 399–404.

Choudhary MI et al Cholinesterase inhibiting withanolides from *Withania somnifera*. Chem Pharm Bull, (Tokyo) 52.11 (2004): 1358–61.

Choudhary MI et al Withanolides, a new class of natural cholinesterase inhibitors with calcium antagonistic properties. Biochem Biophys Res Commun 334.1 (2005): 276–287.

Choudhary, M.I., et al Chlorinated and diepoxy withanolidesfrom *Withania somnifera* and their cytotoxic effects against human lung cancer cell line. Phytochem 71 (2010): 2205–09

Cooley K., et al Naturopathic care for anxiety: A randomized controlled trial. Plos one 4.8 (2009): e6628.

Dasgupta A et al Effect of Indian Ayurvedic medicine Ashwagandha on measurement of serum digoxin and 11 commonly monitored drugs using immunoassays: study of protein binding and interaction with Digibind. Arch Pathol Lab Med 131.8 (2007): 1298–1303.

Dasgupta A et al Effect of Asian ginseng, Siberian ginseng, and Indian ayurvedic medicine Ashwagandha on serum digoxin measurement by Digoxin III, a new digoxin immunoassay. J Clin Lab Anal 22.4 (2008): 295–301.

Datta, S., et al Inhibition of the emergence of multi drug resistant *Staphylococcus aureus* by *Withania somnifera* root extracts. Asian Pac J Trop Med 4.11(2011): 917–20.

Davis L, Kuttan G. Suppressive effect of cyclophosphamide-induced toxicity by *Withania somnifera* extract in mice. J Ethnopharmacol 62.3 (1998): 209–214.

Davis L, Kuttan G. Effect of *Withania somnifera* on cytokine production in normal and cyclophosphamide treated mice. Immunopharmacol Immunotoxicol 21.4 (1999): 695–703.

Davis L, Kuttan G. Immunomodulatory activity of *Withania somnifera*. J Ethnopharmacol 71.1–2 (2000): 193–200.

Davis L, Kuttan G. Effect of *Withania somnifera* on CTL activity. J Exp Clin Cancer Res 21.1 (2002): 115–1118.

Dhuley JN. Adaptogenic and cardioprotective action of ashwagandha in rats and frogs. J Ethnopharmacol 70.1 (2000): 57–63.

Dhuley JN. Nootropic-like effect of ashwagandha (*Withania somnifera* L.) in mice. Phytother Res 15.6 (2001): 524–528.

Ganesan, K., et al Protective effect of *Withania somnifera* and *Cardiospermum halicacabum* extracts against collagenolytic degradation of collagen. Applied Biochemistry and Biotechnology 165. 3–4 (2011) 1075–91.

Ghosal S et al Role of an indigenous drug Geriforte on blood levels of biogenic amines and its significance in the treatment of anxiety neurosis. Acta Nerv Super 32.1 (1990): 1–5.

Girish KS et al Antimicrobial properties of a non-toxic glycoprotein (WSG) from *Withania somnifera* (Ashwagandha). J Basic Microbiol 46.5 (2006): 365–374.

Grandhi A, et al. A comparative pharmacological investigation of Ashwagandha and Ginseng. J Ethnopharmacol 44.3 (1994): 131–135.

Grin B, et al. Witaferin A alters intermediate filament organization, cell shape and bevahiour. PLoS One 7.8 (2012): e39065.

Grover, A., et al. Hsp90/Cdc37 Chaperon/co-chaperone complex, a novel junction anticancer target elucidated by the mode of action of herbal drug withaferin A. BMC Bioinformatics 12. (2011a):SUPPL. 1.

Grover, A., et al. Inhibition of the Nemo/ IKKi association complex formation, a novel mechanism associated with NF-κB activation suppression by *Withania somnifera*'s key metaboliye withaferin A. BMC Genomics 11 (2011b): SUPPL. 4.

Gupta GL, Rana AC. Protective effect of *Withania somnifera* dunal root extract against protracted social isolation induced behavior in rats. Indian J Physiol Pharmacol 51.4 (2007): 345–353.

Gupta GL, Rana AC. Effect of *Withania somnifera* Dunal in ethanol-induced anxiolysis and withdrawal anxiety in rats. Indian J Exp Biol 46.6 (2008): 470–475.

Gupta YK et al Reversal of paclitaxel induced neutropenia by *Withania somnifera* in mice. Indian J Physiol Pharmacol 45.2 (2001): 253–257.

Gupta S, et al. *Withania somnifera* (Ashwagandha) attenuates antioxidant defense in aged spinal cord and inhibits copper induced lipid peroxidation and protein oxidative modifications. Drug Metab Drug Interact 19.3 (2003): 211–222.

Gupta SK et al Cardioprotection from ischemia and reperfusion injury by *Withania somnifera*: a hemodynamic, biochemical and histopathological assessment. Mol Cell Biochem 260.1–2 (2004): 39–47.

Hahm, E.R., et al Withaferin A Suppresses estrogen receptor-alpha expression in human breast cancer cells. Mol Carcinog 50.8 (2011): 614–24.

Hamza A et al The protective effect of a purified extract of *Withania somnifera* against doxorubicin-induced cardiac toxicity in rats. Cell Biol Toxicol 24.1 (2008): 63–73.

Ichikawa H et al Withanolides potentiate apoptosis, inhibit invasion, and abolish osteoclastogenesis through suppression of nuclear factor-kappaB (NF-kappaB) activation and NF-kappaB-regulated gene expression. Mol Cancer Ther 5.6 (2006): 1434–1445.

Ilayperuma I, et al. Effect of *Withania somnifera* root extract on the sexual behaviour of male rats. Asian J Androl 4.4 (2002): 295–298.

Jain S et al Neuroprotective effects of *Withania somnifera* Dunn. in hippocampal sub-regions of female albino rat. Phytother Res 15.6 (2001): 544–548.

Jatwa, R., and Kar, A. Amelioration of Metformin-induced hypothyroidism by *Withania somnifera* and *Bauhinia purpura* extracts in type 2 diabetic mice. Phytother Res 23.8 (2009): 1140–5.

Jayaprakasam B, Nair MG. Cyclooxygenase-2 enzyme inhibitory withanolides from *Withania somnifera* leaves. Tetrahedron 59.6 (2003): 841–849.

Jayaprakasam B et al Growth inhibition of human tumor cell lines by withanolides from *Withania somnifera* leaves. Life Sci 74.1 (2003): 125–132.

Jayaprakasam, B., et al Withanamides in *Withania somnifera* fruit protect Pc-12 cells from beta-amyloid responsible for Alzheimer's disease. Phytother Res 24.6 (2010): 859–63.

Kaileh M et al Withaferin a strongly elicits IkappaB kinase beta hyperphosphorylation concomitant with potent inhibition of its kinase activity. J Biol Chem 282.7 (2007): 4253–4264.

Kalani, A., et al Ashwagandha root in the treatment of non-classical adrenal hyperplasia. BMJ Case Rep 2012: doi: 10.1136/bcr-2012-006989.

Kasture, S., et al *Withania somnifera* prevents morphine withdrawal-induced decrease in spine density in nucleus accumbens shell of rats: A confocal laser scanning microscopy study. Neurotox Res 16.4 (2009): 343–55.

Katz, M., et al A compound herbal preparation (CHP) in the treatment of children with ADHD: A randomized controlled trial. J Atten Disord 14.3 (2011): 281–91.

Khan B et al Augmentation and proliferation of T lymphocytes and Th-1 cytokines by *Withania somnifera* in stressed mice. Int Immunopharmacol 6.9 (2006): 1394–1403.

Khanam S, Devi K. Antimutagenic activity of Ashwagandha. J Nat Remed 5.2 (2005): 126–131.

Khanna D et al Natural products as a gold mine for arthritis treatment. Curr Opin Pharmacol 7.3 (2007): 344–351.

Kour, K., et al Restoration of stress-induced altered T cell function and corresponding cytokines patterns by withanolide A. Int Immunpharmacol 9.10 (2009): 1137–44.

Kuboyama T et al Axon- or dendrite-predominant outgrowth induced by constituents from Ashwagandha. Neuroreport 13.14 (2002): 1715–1720.

Kuboyama T, et al. Neuritic regeneration and synaptic reconstruction induced by withanolide A. Br J Pharmacol 144.7 (2005): 961–971.

Kulkarni SK, Dhir A. *Withania somnifera*: an Indian ginseng. Prog Neuropsychopharmacol Biol Psychiatry 32.5 (2008): 1093–1105.

Kulkarni SK, Ninan I. Inhibition of morphine tolerance and dependence by *Withania somnifera* in mice. J Ethnopharmacol 57.3 (1997): 213–217.

Kulkarni SK, Verma A. Aswagandha and brahmi: nootropic and de-addiction profile of psychotropic indigenous plants. Drugs Today 29.4 (1993): 257–263.

Kulkarni, R.R., et al. 1991. Treatment of osteoarthritis with a herbomineral formulation: a double-blind, placebo-controlled, cross-over study. J Ethnopharmacol., 33, (1–2) 91–95.

Kulkarni SK et al Effect of *Withania somnifera* Dunal root extract against pentylenetetrazol seizure threshold in mice: possible involvement of GABAergic system. Indian J Exp Biol 46.6 (2008): 465–469.

Kumar A, Kalonia H. Protective effect of *Withania somnifera* Dunal on the behavioral and biochemical alterations in sleep-disturbed mice (Grid over water suspended method). Indian J Exp Biol 45.6 (2007): 524–528.

Kumar, S. et al. An aqueous extract of *Withania somnifera* roots inhibits amyloid beta fibril formation in vitro. Phytother Res 26.1 (2012) 113–7.

Kupparajan K et al J Res Ayu Sid 1 (1980): 247. Cited in: Bone K. Clinical Applications of Ayurvedic and Chinese Herbs. Warwick, Qld: Phytotherapy Press, 1996.

Kurandikar et al Indian Drugs 23 (1986): 123. Cited in: Bone K. Clinical Applications of Ayurvedic and Chinese Herbs. Warwick, Qld: Phytotherapy Press, 1996.

Kushwaha, S., et al Effect of Ashwagandha (*Withania somnifera*) root powder supplementation in treatment of hypertension. Ethno Med 2.6 (2012): 111–115.

Lee, J., et al Withaferin A inhibits actvation of signal transducer and activator of transcription 3 in human breast cancer cells. Carcinogenesis 31.11(2010): 1991–8.

Lee, J., et al Withaferin A causes activation of notch2 and notch4 in human breast cancer cells. Beast Cancer Res Treat 136.1 (2012): 45–56.

Lindner S. *Withania somnifera*. Aust J Med Herbalism 8.3 (1996): 78–82.

Machiah DK et al A glycoprotein from a folk medicinal plant, *Withania somnifera*, inhibits hyaluronidase activity of snake venoms. Comp Biochem Physiol C Toxicol Pharmacol 143.2 (2006): 158–161.

Mahdi, A. A., et al *Withania somnifera* improves semen quality in stress-related male infertility. Evid Based Complement Alternat Med 2011 http://dx.doi.org/10.1093%2Fecam%2Fnep138

Maitra, R., et al Inhibition of NF kappa B by natural product withaferin A in cellular models of cystic fibrosis inflammation. J Inflamm (Lond) 6 (2009):15.

Malhotra CL et al Studies on Withania — ashwagandha, Kaul. Part IV: The effect of total alkaloids on the smooth muscles. Indian J Physiol Pharmacol 9.1 (1965a): 9–15.

Malhotra CL et al Studies on *Withania* — ashwagandha, Kaul. Part V: The effect of total alkaloids (ashwagandholine) on the central nervous system. Indian J Physiol Pharmacol 9.3 (1965b): 127–136.

Malik F et al A standardized root extract of *Withania somnifera* and its major constituent withanolide-A elicit humoral and cell-mediated immune responses by up regulation of Th1-dominant polarization in BALB/c mice. Life Sci 80.16 (2007): 1525–1538.

Malik, F., et al Immune modulation and apoptosis induction:Two sides of antitumoural activity of a standardized herbal formulation of *Withania somnifera*. Euro J of Cancer 45 (2009): 1494–1509.

Mamidi, P., and Thakar, A. B. Efficacy of ashwagandha (*Withania somnifera* Dunal. Linn.) in the management of psychogenic erectile dysfunction. Ayu 32.3 (2011):322–8.

Mathur S et al The treatment of skin carcinoma, induced by UV B radiation, using 1-oxo-5[beta], 6[beta]-epoxy-witha-2-enolide, isolated from the roots of *Withania somnifera*, in a rat model. Phytomedicine 11.5 (2004): 452–460.

Mathur R et al Evaluation of the effect of *Withania somnifera* root extracts on cell cycle and angiogenesis. J Ethnopharmacol 105.3 (2006): 336–341.

Mehta AK et al Pharmacological effects of *Withania somnifera* root extract on GABA receptor complex. Indian J Med Res 94(B) (1991): 312–3115.

Mikolai, J., et al In vivo effects of ashwaghanda (*Withania somnifera*) extract on the activation of lymphocytes. J Altern Complement Med 15.4 (2009): 423–30.

Mills S, Bone K. Principles and practice of phytotherapy. London: Churchill Livingstone, 2000.

Mills S, Bone K. Withania. In: The essential guide to herbal safety. St Louis: Elsevier, 2005, p 631.

Min, K., et al Withaferin A down-regulates lipopolysaccharide-induced cyclooxygenase-2 expression and PGE2 production through inhibition of STAT1/3 activation in microglial cells. International Immunopharmacology 11(2011) 1137–1142.

Mirjalili, M.H., et al Steroidal lactones from *Withania somnifera*, an ancient plant for novel medicine. Molecules 14.7 (2009): 2373–93.

Misra L et al Withanolides from *Withania somnifera* roots. Phytochemistry 69.4 (2008): 1000–1004.

Mohan R et al Withaferin A is a potent inhibitor of angiogenesis. Angiogenesis 7.2 (2004): 115–122.

Mohanty I et al Mechanisms of cardioprotective effect of *Withania somnifera* in experimentally induced myocardial infarction. Basic Clin Pharmacol Toxicol 94.4 (2004): 184–190.

Mohanty IR et al *Withania somnifera* provides cardioprotection and attenuates ischemia-reperfusion induced apoptosis. Clin Nutr 27.4 (2008): 635–642.

Mulabagal, V. et al Withanolide sulfoxide from aswagandha roots inhibits nuclear transcription factor-kappa B, cyclooxygenase and tumour cell proliferation. Phytother Res 23.7 (2009): 987–92.

Munagala, R., et al Withaferin A induces p53-dependent apoptosis by repression of HPV oncogenes and up-regulation of tumour suppressor proteins in human cervical cancer cells. Carcinogenesis 32.11 (2011): 1697–705.

Nagareddy PR, Lakshmana M. *Withania somnifera* improves bone calcification in calcium-deficient ovariectomized rats. J Pharm Pharmacol 58.4 (2006): 513–5119.

Naidu PS, et al. Effect of *Withania somnifera* root extract on haloperidol-induced orofacial dyskinesia: possible mechanisms of action. J Med Food 6.2 (2003): 107–114.

Naidu PS et al Effect of *Withania somnifera* root extract on reserpine-induced orofacial dyskinesia and cognitive dysfunction. Phytother Res 20.2 (2006): 140–146.

Nair V et al Effect of *Withania somnifera* root extract on haloperidol-induced catalepsy in albino mice. Phytother Res 22.2 (2008): 243–246.

NMCD (Natural Medicines Comprehensive Database). Withania. Available online from: http://www.naturaldatabase.com 10 November 2005.

Oh, J.H., et al Withaferin A inhibits iNOS expression and nitrix oxide production by Akt inactivation and down-regulating LPS-induced activity of NF –κB in RAW 364.7 cells. Euro J Pharmacol. 599 (2008):11–17.

Oh, J.H., et al Withaferin A inhibits tumor necrosis factor –α- induced expression of cell adhesion molecules by inactivation of Akt and NF-κB in human pulmonary cells. International Immunopharmacoloy 9 (2009) 614–619.

Owais M et al Antibacterial efficacy of *Withania somnifera* (ashwagandha) an indigenous medicinal plant against experimental murine salmonellosis. Phytomedicine 12.3 (2005): 229–235.

Padmavathi B et al Roots of *Withania somnifera* inhibit forestomach and skin carcinogenesis in mice. Evidence Based Complement Altern Med 2.1 (2005): 99–105.

Panda S, Kar A. Evidence for free radical scavenging activity of Ashwagandha root powder in mice. Indian J Physiol Pharmacol 41.4 (1997): 424–426.

Panda S, Kar A. Changes in thyroid hormone concentrations after administration of ashwagandha root extract to adult male mice. J Pharm Pharmacol 50.9 (1998): 1065–1068.

Panda S, Kar A. *Withania somnifera* and Bauhinia purpurea in the regulation of circulating thyroid hormone concentrations in female mice. J Ethnopharmacol 67.2 (1999): 233–239.

Panjamurthy K et al Protective role of withaferin-A on 7,12-dimethylbenz(a)anthracene-induced genotoxicity in bone marrow of Syrian golden hamsters. J Biochem Mol Toxicol 22.4 (2008): 251–258.

Parihar MS, Hemnani T. Phenolic antioxidants attenuate hippocampal neuronal cell damage against kainic acid induced excitotoxicity. J Biosci 28.1 (2003): 121–128.

Patil, S., et al Withanolide A and asiatic acid modulate multiple targets associated with amyloid precursor protein and amyloid protein clearance. Journal of Natural Products 73.7 (2012): 1196–202.

Pawar, P., et al Rectal gel application of *Withania somnifera* root extract expounds anti-inflammaotry and muco-restorative activity in TNBS- induced inflammatory bowel disease. BMC Complement ALtern Med 11.34 (2011): doi: 10.1186/1472-6882-11-34

Peana AT et al. Effects of *Withania somnifera* on oral ethanol self-administration in rats. Behav Pharmacol 25.7 (2014): 618–628.

Prabu, P.C., et al Acute and sub-acute oral toxicity assessment of the hydroalcoholic eztract of *Withania somnifera* roots in wistar rats. Phytother Res (2013): 27: 1169–1178.

Prakash J et al Chemopreventive activity of *Withania somnifera* in experimentally induced fibrosarcoma tumours in Swiss albino mice. Phytother Res 15.3 (2001): 240–244.

Prakash J, et al. *Withania somnifera* root extract prevents DMBA-induced squamous cell carcinoma of skin in Swiss albino mice. Nutr Cancer 42.1 (2002): 91–97.

Prakash, J., et al neuroprotective role of *Withania somnifera* root extract in Maneb-Paraquat induced mouse model of Parkinsonism. Neurochem Res 38.5 (2013): 972–80.

RajaSankar, S., et al *Withania somnifera* root extract improves catecholamines and physiological abnormalities seen in a Parkinson's disease mouse model. J Ethnopharmacol 125.3 (2009): 369–73.

Rasool M, Varalakshmi P. Suppressive effect of *Withania somnifera* root powder on experimental gouty arthritis: An in vivo and in vitro study. Chem Biol Interact 164.3 (2006): 174–180.

Rasool M, Varalakshmi P. Protective effect of *Withania somnifera* root powder in relation to lipid peroxidation, antioxidant status, glycoproteins and bone collagen on adjuvant-induced arthritis in rats. Fundam Clin Pharmacol 21.2 (2007): 157–164.

Raut, A. A., et al Exploratory study to evaluate tolerability, safety, and activity of ashwagandha (*Withania somnifera*) in healthy volunteers. J Ayurveda Integr Med 3.3 (2012): 111–4.

Rege NN, et al. Adaptogenic properties of six rasayana herbs used in Ayurvedic medicine. Phytother Res 13.4 (1999): 275–291.

Riaz, A., et al Assessment of acute toxicity and reproductive capability of a herbal combination. Pak J of Pharm. Sci. 23.3 (2010): 291–294.

Roja G, et al. Tissue cultures of *Withania somnifera*: morphogenesis and withanolide synthesis. Phytother Res 5.4 (1991): 185–1887.

Scartezzini P et al Genetic and phytochemical difference between some Indian and Italian plants of *Withania somnifera* (L.) Dunal. Nat Prod Res 21.10 (2007): 923–932.

Schliebs R et al Systemic administration of defined extracts from *Withania somnifera* (Indian Ginseng) and Shilajit differentially affects cholinergic but not glutamatergic and GABAergic markers in rat brain. Neurochem Int 30.2 (1997): 181–190.

Sehgal VN et al. Fixed drug eruption caused by ashwagandha (*Withania somnifera*): A widely used ayurvedic drug. Skin Med 10.1 (2012): 48–49.

Senthilnathan P et al Chemotherapeutic efficacy of paclitaxel in combination with *Withania somnifera* on benzo(a)pyrene-induced experimental lung cancer. Cancer Sci 97.7 (2006a): 658–64.

Senthilnathan P et al Stabilization of membrane bound enzyme profiles and lipid peroxidation by *Withania somnifera* along with paclitaxel on benzo(a)pyrene induced experimental lung cancer. Mol Cell Biochem 292.1–2 (2006b): 13–17.

Sharada AC, et al. Toxicity of *Withania somnifera* root extract in rats and mice. Int J Pharmacogn 31.3 (1993): 205–212.

Sharma S, et al. Indian Drugs 23.3 (1986): 133–9. Cited in Mills S, Bone K. Principles and practice of phytotherapy. London: Churchill Livingstone, 2000.

Shukla, K.K, et al, *Withania somnifera* improves semen quality by combating oxidative stress and cell death and improving essential metal concentrations. Reprod Biomed Online 22.5 (2011): 421–27.

Singh N et al Int J Crude Drug Res 24 (1986): 90. Cited in: Bone K. Clinical applications of Ayurvedic and Chinese herbs. Warwick, Qld: Phytotherapy Press, 1996.

Singh B et al Adaptogenic activity of a novel, withanolide-free aqueous fraction from the roots of *Withania somnifera* Dun. Phytother Res 15.4 (2001): 311–3118.

Singh B, et al. Adaptogenic activity of a novel withanolide-free aqueous fraction from the roots of *Withania somnifera* Dun. Part II. Phytother Res 17.5 (2003): 531–536.

Singh D et al *Withania somnifera* inhibits NF-kappaB and AP-1 transcription factors in human peripheral blood and synovial fluid mononuclear cells. Phytother Res 21.10 (2007): 905–913.

Sinha, S., et al In vivo anti-tussive activity and structural features of a polysaccharide fraction from water extracted *Withania somnifera*. J Ethnopharmacol 134.2 (2011): 510–13

Sudhir S et al Pharmacological studies on leaves of *Withania somnifera*. Planta Med 52.1 (1986): 61–63.

Sumantran VN et al Chondroprotective potential of root extracts of *Withania somnifera* in osteoarthritis. J Biosci 32.2 (2007): 299–307.

Teixeira ST et al Prophylactic administration of *Withania somnifera* extract increases host resistance in *Listeria monocytogenes* infected mice. Int Immunopharmacol 6.10 (2006): 1535–1542.

Thaiparambil, J. T., et al Withaferin A inhibits breast cancer invasion and metastasis at sub-cytotoxic doses by inducing vimentin disassembly and serine 56 phosphorylation. Int J Cancer 129.11 (2011): 2744–55.

Tierra M. Ashwagandha: Wonder Herb of India. Available online from: http://www.planetherbs.com/articles/ashwagandha.htm 8 December 2005.

Tirtha, S. S. & Shiva, T.S.S. The Ayurveda Encyclopedia. B. JainPublishers, 2002.

Tohda C. Overcoming several neurodegenerative diseases by traditional medicines: the development of therapeutic medicines and unraveling pathophysiological mechanisms. Yakugaku Zasshi 128.8 (2008): 1159–1167.

Tohda C, et al. Dendrite extension by methanol extract of Ashwagandha (roots of *Withania somnifera*) in SK-N-SH cells. Neuroreport 11.9 (2000): 1981–1985.

Tripathi AK, et al. Ashwagandha (*Withania somnifera* Dunal (Solanaceae)): A status report. J Med Aromatic Plant Sci 1 (1996): 46–62.

Udayakumar, R. et al Hypoglycaemic and hypolipidaemic effects of *Withania somnifera* root and leaf extracts on alloxan-induced diabetic rats. International Journal of Molecular Sciences 10.5 (2009): 2367–82.

Udayakumar, R., et al Antioxidant effect of dietary supplement *Withania somnifera* L. Reduce blood glucose levels in alloxan-induced diabetic rats. Plant Foods Hum Nutr 65.2(2010): 91–8.

Um, H. J., et al Withaferin A inhibits JAk/Stat3 signaling and induces apoptosis of human renal carcinoma cali cells. Biochem Biophys Res Commun 427.1 (2012) 24–9

Uma Devi P, et al. In vivo growth inhibitory and radiosensitizing effects of withaferin A on mouse Ehrlich ascites carcinoma. Cancer Lett 95.1–2 (1995): 189–193.

Uma Devi P. *Withania somnifera* Dunal (ashwagandha): potential plant source of a promising drug for cancer chemotherapy and radiosensitization. Indian J Exper Biol 34.10 (1996): 927–932.

Upton R (ed.). Ashwagandha root (*Withania somnifera*): Analytical quality control and therapeutic monograph. Am Herbal Pharm (2000): 1–25.

Van der Hooft CS et al [Thyrotoxicosis following the use of ashwagandha]. Ned Tijdschr Geneeskd 149.47 (2005): 2637–2638.

Venkatraghaven S et al J Res Ayu Sid 1 (1980): 370. Cited in: Bone K. Clinical applications of Ayurvedic and Chinese herbs. Warwick, Qld: Phytotherapy Press, 1996.

Vinutha B et al Screening of selected Indian medicinal plants for acetylcholinesterase inhibitory activity. J Ethnopharmacol 109.2 (2007): 359–363.

Visavadiya NP, Narasimhacharya AV. Hypocholesteremic and antioxidant effects of *Withania somnifera* (Dunal) in hypercholesteremic rats. Phytomedicine 14.2–3 (2007): 136–142.

Winters M. Ancient medicine, modern use: *Withania somnifera* and its potential role in integrative oncology. Altern Med Rev 11.4 (2006): 269–277.

Yamada, K., et al A comparison of the immunostimulatory effects of the medicinal herbs Echinacea, Ashwaghanda, and Brahmi. J ethnopharm 137 (2011): 231–235.

Yang, E. S., et al Withaferin A enhances radiation-induced apoptosis in caki cells through induction of reactive oxygen species, Bcl-2 downregulation and Akt inhibition. Chem Biol Interact 190.1 (2011): 9–15.

Yu, Y., et al Withaferin A targets heat shock protein 90 in pancreatic cancer cells. Biochem Pharmacol 79.4 (2010)542–51.

Ziauddin M et al Studies on the immunomodulatory effects of Ashwagandha. J Ethnopharmacol 50.2 (1996): 69–76.

Zinc

BACKGROUND AND RELEVANT PHARMACOKINETICS

Zinc was recognised as being essential for the growth of numerous plant and animal species by the 1960s. However, it was not until a fortuitous meeting in 1961, between the clinical scientist Prasad and a group of young Iranian men with severe growth retardation and hypogonadism, that zinc essentiality in humans was considered (Prasad 2013). A decade of controversy followed, ending with the discovery that zinc deficiency was central to the pathology of acrodermatitis enteropathica, a rare autosomal recessive trait that produces severe multisystem disease shortly after infants start weaning. In 1974 the National Research Council of the National Academy of Sciences finally declared zinc to be essential in human nutrition and established a recommended dietary allowance (RDA) (Prasad 2013). In human nutrition this is a relatively recent discovery and, as such, explains why zinc research is still in its infancy.

Zinc is an essential trace element known to play an important role in all human living cells. The human body contains approximately 2 g zinc in total, distributed across all body tissues and fluids, with 60% found in skeletal muscle and 30% in bone mass (Wahlqvist et al 2002). In spite of being a dietary trace element, it is one of the most abundant elements within cells and a complex homeostatic system maintains cellular zinc concentrations within a narrow range (King 2011). Its wide distribution and diverse roles have attracted the label of the 'ubiquitous nutrient' given by some authors (Hambidge 2000, King & Cousins 2006). Zinc belongs to the class of type II nutrients which are considered the cellular building blocks (Golden 1996, King & Cousins 2006) and therefore zinc, together with the other type II nutrients (essential amino acids, magnesium, potassium, phosphorus, protein and sulfur), is required for the synthesis of any new tissue. They are not stored by the body and are under tight physiological control.

Dietary intake of zinc by healthy adults is 6–15 mg/day; however, less than half of this is absorbed (Beers & Berkow 2003). Zinc absorption is influenced by many factors and adequate dietary intake does not guarantee adequate zinc status. The International Zinc Nutrition Consultative Group (IZiNCG) concludes that the two key dietary influences on zinc bioavailability are phytates and calcium. Foods with high phytate content significantly reduce zinc absorption due to the formation of strong and insoluble complexes (Lonnerdal 2000) and a phytate : zinc molar ratio ≥ 15, e.g. whole grains, seeds and nuts, is reported to render the zinc virtually unobtainable (IZiNCG 2004). In addition to this, calcium in large amounts constitutes the main antagonistic mineral interaction and therefore calcium-rich diets may also precipitate zinc deficiency. Soy protein has been shown to negatively impact zinc bioavailability, above and beyond its phytate content (Lim et al 2013). In contrast, the amount of animal protein in a meal positively correlates to zinc absorption and the amino acids histidine and methionine, and various organic acids present in foods, such as citric, malic and lactic acids, can also increase absorption. As such, zinc, similarly to iron, is best absorbed from animal food sources (King 2003). These combined factors may partly explain why vegetarians are at risk of low zinc status, a finding reported in a 2013 meta-analysis of 26 studies (Foster et al 2013).

Zinc absorption is a saturable process occurring in the small intestine principally via ZIP4, ZnT1 and, to a lesser extent, DMT1 (the shared divalent metal transporter) and CTR1 (primarily a copper transporter) (Espinoza et al 2012, King 2010, 2011); however, there is evidence of unregulated paracellular uptake with very high doses. Regulated zinc uptake is influenced by current dietary intake of the mineral, i.e. as the total amount of zinc ingested increases, the fractional uptake decreases. This adjustment to high intakes is particularly apparent when single doses >20 mg are administered (Tran et al 2004). Several papers report that zinc bioavailability from supplements is significantly better than from food; however, longer-term studies have revealed that this diminishes over a few days of consecutive dosing, due to compensatory downregulation of zinc transporters, and quickly becomes comparable with the fractional absorption seen with food (Hambidge et al 2010, King 2010, Tran et al 2004). Studies assessing bioavailability using disparate methods and sources have produced contrasting figures, from 46% to 74% (Tran et al 2004). A recent study evaluating average uptake from a standard Brazilian diet which controlled for phytate levels found that, while bioavailability varied from 11% to 47%, mean uptake was 30% (Ribeiro et al 2013).

Zinc homeostasis principally occurs in the gastrointestinal tract, whereby zinc uptake is balanced with endogenous zinc losses (Hambidge et al 2010, King 2010) which are estimated to total 0.5–3 mg/day. Other losses occur via urine and skin (0.5–0.7 mg) and semen (1 mg/ejaculate) (Lim et al 2013). When dietary zinc intake is insufficient, the body's homeostatic response is to minimise zinc losses and increase gastrointestinal absorption. As there is only a small zinc pool within the body, deficiency features develop quickly if dietary intake remains low. In growing children, deficiency signs and/or symptoms can develop within days, whereas for adults, this happens in a few weeks. Once zinc intake is increased, repletion can occur quickly, with rapid improvement of the clinical picture within days of supplementation (King 2011). Metallothionein (MT) is a cysteine-rich molecule found all over the body which can bind ≤7 zinc molecules, as well as other metals such as copper and cadmium. Gut and pancreatic MT concentrations respond readily to changes in dietary zinc; for example, high intakes induce MT synthesis and limit zinc absorption by binding zinc within the enterocyte and inhibiting basolateral transfer. Low dietary zinc produces a decline in pancreatic and renal MT, facilitating the decline in faecal and urinary zinc losses (King 2011).

Zinc is mainly an intracellular nutrient; little is found in the cytoplasm or found 'free' (loosely bound). This is likely due to its role in second-messenger systems, which means zinc levels need to be tightly regulated (primarily via MT) and largely sequestered inside organelles (Lazarczyk & Favre 2008).

Typically, only 5% of body zinc is found extracellularly (King 2011). Inflammatory processes and increased glucocorticoids can cause redistribution of zinc, leading to sequestration by the liver and adipocytes (Ferro et al 2011). Two recent studies investigating altered zinc homeostasis in obesity (Feitosa et al 2013, Ferro et al 2011) found evidence of lower erythrocyte zinc, while Feitosa et al demonstrated an inverse relationship specifically with tumour necrosis factor-alpha (TNF-alpha), consistent with the hypothesis that chronic inflammation in obesity will negatively impact zinc homeostasis.

Lastly, zinc homeostasis is altered in the elderly due to both higher intracellular levels of MT and defective zinc influx transporters, ultimately producing less available free intracellular zinc (Mocchegiani et al 2011).

CHEMICAL COMPONENTS

Zinc sulfate and gluconate are the most common forms of zinc found in commercially produced supplements. There is growing research on other forms, such as zinc picolinate and methionine and carnosine complexes, the latter specifically for gastrointestinal complaints. There is currently a lack of human research comparing the bioavailability of these forms; however, animal studies suggest that zinc sulfate is approximately twice as bioavailable as zinc oxide (in dogs, horses and rabbits), while zinc methionine and zinc propionate also produced significant increases in plasma zinc (Andermann & Dietz 1982, Wedekind & Lowry 1998, Wedekind et al 1992, 1994, Wichert et al 2002).

FOOD SOURCES

Meat, liver, eggs and seafood (especially oysters and shellfish) are the best sources both quantitatively and qualitatively. While zinc is also found in nuts, legumes, whole grains and seeds, the high phytate content (stored phosphate) of these foods makes them an inferior source. Phytates can be reduced through fermentation or sprouting, which in turn would improve zinc bioavailability in these foods. Other dietary sources include miso, tofu, brewers' yeast, mushrooms and green beans. It has been reported that, while zinc is found as organic complexes in meats, it is presented as inorganic salts in plant foods (Lim et al 2013) and this may in part explain the superior bioavailability of zinc from animal products and seafood.

DEFICIENCY SIGNS AND SYMPTOMS

Severe deficiency is rarely seen in industrialised countries, but marginal deficiency and inadequate intakes are not uncommon. According to a large national survey conducted in the United States of over 29,000 people, only 55.6% had adequate zinc intakes (based on total intakes of >77% of the 1989 US recommended daily intake (RDI) levels). Young children aged 1–3 years, female adolescents and older people aged ≥71 years had the lowest percentage of 'adequate' zinc intake, and were identified at greatest risk of deficiency (Briefel et al 2000).

Due to its important role in growth and development, zinc deficiency is characterised by impaired growth (linear growth velocity, weight or body composition) (Hambidge 2000). This will produce overt presentations in those life stages and tissues, necessitating rapid replication and turnover for health (Hambidge 2000), e.g. embryos, early childhood, adolescence, immune cells, epidermal and gastrointestinal tissue (Hambidge 2000, IZiNCG 2004, King 2000, King & Cousins 2006, Mahomed et al 1993), but often indiscernible pictures outside of these.

The clinical picture of mild zinc deficiency is subtle, ambiguous, idiosyncratic (Golden 1996, Hambidge 2000) and notoriously difficult to diagnose (Golden 1996, Wood 2000). King (2011) reminds us that, being a type II nutrient, zinc deficiency evokes sophisticated conservation mechanisms to limit endogenous losses and a metabolic adaptation to reduce the high-demand pathways for zinc such as growth and immunity. Altogether this can rapidly produce non-specific signs of metabolic or clinical dysfunction, such as malaise and apathy. Another prominent zinc researcher says, 'the ubiquity and versatility of zinc in subcellular metabolism suggest that zinc deficiency may well result in a generalised impairment of many metabolic functions' (Hambidge 2000, p 1345S).

Signs and symptoms of deficiency

Most consistently reported

- Anorexia, impaired sense of taste and smell
- Slowed growth and development
- Delayed sexual maturation, hypogonadism, hypospermia and menstrual problems
- Dermatitis, particularly around the body's orifices, as seen in acrodermatitis enteropathica
- Alopecia
- Chronic and severe diarrhoea
- Immune system deficiencies and increased susceptibility to infection, including bacterial, viral and fungal
- Impaired wound healing due to decreased collagen synthesis
- Night blindness; swelling and clouding of the corneas
- Behavioural disturbances such as mental fatigue and depression (King 2003).

Less consistently reported

- Erectile dysfunction
- Anergy
- Glossitis
- Nail dystrophy
- Hypopigmented hair
- Photophobia
- Photic injury
- Swelling and clouding of the corneas
- Reduced serum testosterone in males
- Reduced alcohol clearance
- Hyperammonaemia
- Impaired protein synthesis.

Zinc deficiency in pregnancy is associated with the following (Bedwal & Bahuguna 1994, Prasad 1996):

- Increased maternal morbidity, pre-eclampsia and toxaemia
- Prolonged gestation
- Inefficient labour
- Atonic bleeding
- Increased risk of abortion and stillbirths
- Teratogenicity
- Low-birth-weight infants
- Diminished attention in the newborn and poorer motor function at 6 months (Higdon 2003).

PRIMARY DEFICIENCY (Table 1)

Primary deficiency occurs as a result of inadequate intake, with greatest risks seen in vegetarians and individuals consuming high-phytate diets. This is particularly the case in many developing countries, with the World Health Organization estimating that suboptimal zinc nutrition affected nearly half the world's population in 2002 (Mistry & Williams 2011).

In developed countries, phytate levels are greatest in 'healthy high-fibre diets' with greater intake of wholegrains and legumes and can provide in excess of 1000 mg phytic acid/day. Hambidge et al (2010) used a mathematical model to determine that the RDA would need to be doubled for such individuals. A study of 20 women with type 2 diabetes consuming a high-fibre diet (1194 ± 824 mg/day) found that this was a risk factor for zinc deficiency (Foster et al 2013). Recently a systematic review and meta-analysis of 26 studies examining the zinc status of vegetarians concluded that both dietary zinc intake and serum zinc were significantly lower in this group, with particular at-risk sub-groups being females, vegans and those living in developing countries (Foster et al 2013). As zinc is a type II nutrient (see Clinical note — Measuring zinc status is difficult), which is essential for cellular growth, the life stages that are most at risk of deficiency include childhood, adolescence and pregnancy.

SECONDARY DEFICIENCY

Factors which interfere with zinc absorption (i.e. malabsorption), distribution (i.e. inflammation), retention (i.e. weight loss), excretion (e.g. antihypertensive drugs) or significantly increase requirements (i.e. specific infections or periods of growth) can all play a part in producing a secondary zinc deficiency, as per the following (Gehrig & Dinulos 2010):

- Acrodermatitis enteropathica, a rare autosomal recessive defect in zinc transporters that manifests rapidly as severe zinc deficiency in infants after weaning
- Anorexia nervosa
- Antihypertensive medication (in particular angiotensin-converting enzyme inhibitors, angiotensin II receptor blockers and thiazide diuretics) (Braun & Rosenfeldt 2013)

TABLE 1 COMMON FEATURES OF MILD, MODERATE AND SEVERE ZINC DEFICIENCIES (PRASAD 2013)

Mild deficiency	Moderate deficiency	Severe deficiency
↓ Serum testosterone	Growth retardation	Growth retardation
Oligospermia	Male adolescent hypogonadism	Male adolescent hypogonadism
↓ Natural killer cell activity	Rough skin	Bullous pustular dermatitis, especially around orifices and extremities
↓ Interleukin-2 activity	↓ Appetite	Blepharitis, conjunctivitis
↓ T-helper cells	Mental lethargy	Photophobia
↓ Serum thymulin activity	Delayed wound healing	Alopecia
Hyperammonaemia	Cell-mediated immune dysfunction	Diarrhoea and changes to small intestinal villi
Hypogeusia (impaired taste)	Abnormal neurosensory changes	Weight loss
↓ Dark adaptation		Emotional disorders, e.g. irritability, emotional instability
↓ Lean body mass		↓ Healing of ulcers
		Death

- Breastfeeding
- Chronic alcoholism
- Malabsorption syndromes, e.g. Crohn's and coeliac disease (CD), ulcerative colitis, cystic fibrosis
- Renal impairments and dialysis
- Extensive cutaneous burns
- Hepatic or pancreatic insufficiency
- HIV infection
- Intestinal bypass procedures — percentage zinc absorption decreases significantly from 32.3% to 13.6% at 6 months after gastric bypass, with partial correction at 18 months (Ruz et al 2011)
- Prematurity with low zinc storage
- Penicillamine or chlorothiazide therapy
- *Yersinia enterocolitica* infection (Gehrig & Dinulos 2010)
- Obesity and cardiometabolic syndrome — redistribution due to chronic inflammation (Feitosa et al 2013, Ferro et al 2011, Foster & Samman 2012).

MAIN ACTIONS

Cofactor in many biochemical reactions

In humans, zinc metalloenzymes outnumber all the other trace mineral-dependent enzymes combined, with between 70 and 200 present in humans (Gropper et al 2009), found across all six different enzyme classes (Hambidge 2000). Consequently, zinc is involved in myriad chemical reactions that are important for normal body functioning, such as carbohydrate metabolism, protein and DNA synthesis, protein digestion, bone metabolism and endogenous antioxidant systems (Merck 2009, Wahlqvist et al 2002, Wardlaw et al 1997).

At the cellular level, zinc's functions can be divided into three categories: catalytic, structural and regulatory (King 2003, 2011). In its catalytic capacity, zinc metalloenzymes are defined as those apometalloenzymes which are dependent upon the binding of zinc for their activity, such as alkaline phosphatase. Structural roles are evident in a range of proteins, enzymes, e.g. CuZn, superoxide dismutase (SOD) and biomembranes. Of particular note is the zinc finger motif, which allows zinc to be bound in a tetrahedral complex with two cysteines within the protein.

Zinc's contribution as an intra- and intercellular regulatory ion continues to emerge and includes its profound role in gene expression, whereby zinc binds to a metal-binding transcription factor and a metal response element in the promoter of the regulated gene to stimulate transcription (King 2011). Other regulatory roles include receptor-mediated signal transduction, neurotransmitter release from synaptic vesicles, packaging of insulin into pancreatic granules and subsequent release, antigen-dependent T-cell activation and insulin-like growth factor receptor binding (Hambidge 2000, King 2011, King & Cousins 2006).

Growth and development

Zinc is essential for the formation of biomembranes and zinc finger motifs found in DNA transcription factors (Semrad 1999) and, belonging to the type II nutrient class, is required for the building of all new tissues (King 2011). Additionally, several studies of children with growth retardation and zinc deficiency have confirmed that repletion leads to increased levels and activity of growth hormone and insulin-like growth factor and insulin-like growth factor-binding proteins (Prasad 2013).

Normal immune responses

Zinc is involved in many aspects of immunological function. It is essential for the normal development

Clinical note — Measuring zinc status is difficult

According to the scientific evidence, there is currently no means of assessing zinc status in humans (particularly with respect to the detection of marginal deficiency states) that has demonstrated absolute accuracy, and the identification of such a test has been flagged as an area requiring urgent research (Bales et al 1990, Hambidge 2000, IZiNCG 2004, Wood 2000). The assessment of zinc in orthodox medicine currently utilises serum or plasma assays (Gropper et al 2009, IZiNCG 2004, Wood 2000). Principally validated as a tool to assess zinc adequacy of populations (IZiNCG 2004, Wood 2000), serum/plasma zinc lacks the sensitivity to accurately ascertain the zinc status of the individual, with decreased values reflective of end-stage depletion only (Gordon et al 1982, Gropper et al 2009, Hambidge 2000, 2003, IZiNCG 2004, Wood 2000). Multiple established confounding variables include diurnal variation, concomitant infections and inflammation, acute stress and trauma, haemodilution of pregnancy, low serum albumin, high white blood cell counts and the concomitant use of hormones and steroids (King & Cousins 2006, Wood 2000). Each of these scenarios is susceptible to producing false negatives, underpinning concerns regarding the specificity of serum/plasma zinc assessment (Hambidge 2003, Hotz et al 2003). In addition to this, data from the National Health and Nutrition Examination Survey (NHANES II) revealed significant differences in the mean values of 'healthy individuals' dependent on age and sex alone (IZiNCG 2004). In spite of these documented limitations, this test remains the first-line assay in orthodox medicine.

A range of other biochemical indices have been used to assess zinc, including red (Kenney et al 1984, Prasad 1985) and white blood cells (Bunker et al 1987, Prasad 1985), platelets (Baer & King 1984), hair (Bunker et al 1987, Erten et al 1978, Hambidge 2003, McBean et al 1971, McKenzie 1979), nails (McKenzie 1979), saliva (Bales et al 1990, Freeland-Graves et al 1981, Greger & Sickles 1979), sweat (Baer & King 1984, Eaton et al 2004) and urinary concentrations (Hambidge 2003, McKenzie 1979, Prasad 1985). All represent static measures and, as such, lack the sensitivity required to account for zinc's dynamic and complex homeostasis (Gropper et al 2009). Many researchers believe that an accurate indicator of zinc nutriture will therefore also need to be dynamic, similar to using ferritin as a marker for iron status (Hambidge 2000, 2003, Wood 2000) and measurement of both serum and erythrocyte metallothienein seems a likely candidate (King 2011).

One area of functional zinc assessment extensively researched since the 1970s is taste acuity testing (Gibson 1990, Gibson et al 1989, Henkin et al 1975b). Hypogeusia is recognised as an early indicator of zinc deficiency (Buzina et al 1980, Gibson 1990, Henkin et al 1975a, Kosman & Henkin 1981, Tanaka 2002, Wright et al 1981) and is believed to be the result of compromised gustin activity, a carbonic anhydrase zinc metalloenzyme which facilitates differentiation, growth and turnover of taste buds (Gibson et al 1989, Henkin et al 1975b, 1977, Law et al 1987, Thatcher et al 1998). The zinc taste response test (also known as the Bryce-Smith taste test) is a popular measure among naturopathic practitioners. It relies on patients detecting a taste after oral administration of 5–10 mL of a zinc sulfate heptahydrate solution. Delayed taste perception or lack of taste recognition is interpreted as a zinc deficiency state. This method is not particularly accurate and is hampered by variations in patients' subjective sense of taste and the fact that agents other than zinc influence taste perception. Clinical studies with zinc taste tests have confirmed the inconsistency of the results (Birmingham et al 2005, Eaton et al 2004, Garg et al 1993, Mahomed et al 1993) and a literature review of the zinc taste test, that remains popular in Australia and some other countries, reached the same conclusions (Gruner & Arthur 2012).

and function of cells, for mediating non-specific immunity such as neutrophils, monocytes and natural killer cells and for affecting the development of acquired immunity and T-lymphocyte function. Deficiency primarily impacts on T-lymphocyte function, reducing both peripheral numbers and thymic cells, compromising function of the T-helper and cytotoxic cells and reducing serum levels of thymulin and T-helper subset 1 cell cytokines, e.g. interleukin-2 and interferon-gamma. In addition, zinc depletion rapidly diminishes antibody and cell mediated responses in both humans and animals, altogether leading to increased opportunistic infections and mortality rates (Fraker et al 2000, Prasad 2009, 2013).

Animal models have shown that suboptimal zinc intake over 30 days can lead to 30–80% loss in defence capacity and that this occurs significantly earlier than changes in serum or plasma values (Prasad 2013). Investigation using a human model has demonstrated that even mild deficiency in humans adversely affects T-cell functions (Prasad 1998). Conversely, high-dose zinc supplementation (20-fold RDI) can also produce immune dysfunction due to an induced copper deficiency.

A key area of research interest currently relates to zinc's influence on cytokine production. Zinc is regarded as a key anti-inflammatory nutrient due to its ability to both reduce the source of oxidative stress, reactive oxygen species (ROS), and control the body's inflammatory response by reducing nuclear factor-kappaB (NF-κB), TNF-alpha and interleukin-beta (Feitosa et al 2013, Overbeck et al 2008, Prasad 2009, 2013). It is important to note, however, the new evidence of negative zinc redistribution that occurs in chronic inflammation that would hamper this anti-inflammatory role (Feitosa et al 2013).

Gastrointestinal structure and function

Numerous animal studies demonstrate the deleterious effects of zinc deficiency on villi (atrophy, reduced height), crypt cells (reduced number and depth), mucosal cells (increased apoptosis), tissue integrity (increased ulceration, disruption of junctional complexes and cytoskeleton disorganisation in $CaCo_2$ cells) and immune response (increased inflammation) (Scrimgeour & Condlin 2009, Tran et al 2011). Secondary to this is clear evidence of impaired function, including reduced expression of the brush border disaccharidases. New animal research suggests that, in part, these actions require not just adequate zinc but healthy levels of MT. Importantly, zinc supplementation (in individuals with normal MT production) corrects these observed gastrointestinal tract anomalies (Tran et al 2011).

Neurological function

Central nervous system zinc is found predominantly in the brain, specifically the hippocampus, amygdala and cortex, where it possesses both catalytic (cofactors) and regulatory roles (Szewczyk et al 2008). While 95% of brain zinc is bound to metalloproteins, the remainder is found in presynaptic vesicles. Neurons that contain these are known as zinc-enriched neurons (ZEN) (Frederickson & Danscher 1990, Frederickson & Moncrieff 1994, Frederickson et al 2000, Szewczyk et al 2008). Cerebellar ZEN are primarily associated with gamma-aminobutyric acid (GABA) neurotransmission, whereas in the other regions they are found in glutamate-producing neurons. Zinc therefore has the ability to inhibit both GABA and glutaminergic receptors, making it a candidate for neuronal excitability modulation. It also potentially plays an important role in synaptic plasticity (Szewczyk et al 2008). Other general actions include the stabilisation of certain stored macromolecules in presynaptic vesicles, the inhibition of GSK3 phosphorylation, which leads to increased brain-derived neurotrophic factor (BDNF) levels, and its anti-inflammatory functions, which are all important for the health and function of the brain.

Specific neurotransmitter actions include potent dopamine transporter inhibition, which allows dopamine to stay and engage with receptors longer within the synapse. Zinc is now considered an important regulator of dopamine transporter function (Stockner et al 2013). There is also evidence of zinc modulating serotonin uptake in vitro (Szewczyk et al 2008).

Prostate health

The prostate contains the highest zinc concentration of any soft tissue in humans. The concentration of zinc found in the prostate differs between the four lobes and is tightly regulated according to their different functions. The peripheral lobes hold the highest concentration and this relates to their central role in secretion of prostatic fluid, which contains ≈500 mcg/mL of zinc compared with plasma, 1–2 mcg/mL. With ageing, the zinc content of both the prostate and its fluid declines, a factor which has been linked with declining fertility. Beyond acting as a reservoir for the high zinc needs of prostatic fluid, zinc also plays an important role in making citrate available, which is also found in large amounts in prostatic fluid and zinc is at unusually high levels within prostatic mitochondria (unknown reason). Lastly, zinc has an antimicrobial role within the fluid and the greater gland itself (Kelleher et al 2011).

Low prostatic zinc has been linked to prostate disease and, while there is evidence of some dysregulation of zinc within the gland in these individuals, dietary zinc deficiency alone has been associated with increased DNA damage in the prostate during oxidative stress. This becomes a vicious circle, in that the greater the oxidative stress, the greater the prostate's need for zinc (Kelleher et al 2011).

Fertility

Zinc is important for both male and female fertility. In adult males, the testis and prostate have the highest concentration of zinc of any organ in the body (Bedwal & Bahuguna 1994). In moderate to severe zinc deficiency male hypogonadism has been well-documented (Prasad 2013). Zinc in humans is necessary for the formation and maturation of spermatozoa, for ovulation and for fertilisation (Favier 1992). Studies generally have shown a positive correlation between seminal zinc levels and sperm counts and motility. As an antioxidant, zinc protects vulnerable sperm from excess ROS, heavy metals, fluoride, cigarette smoke and heat (Sankako et al 2012, Talevi et al 2013, Yamaguchi et al 2009). An in vivo model of acute dietary zinc deficiency revealed that a zinc-deficient diet for 3–5 days pre-ovulation (preconception) dramatically disrupted oocyte chromatin methylation and preimplantation development (Tian & Diaz 2013). Zinc also has multiple actions on the metabolism of androgen hormones, oestrogen and progesterone, and these, together with the prostaglandins and nuclear receptors for steroids, are all zinc finger proteins.

Pregnancy and lactation

Zinc is recognised as being a key nutrient during embryogenesis, fetal growth and development (Donangelo & King 2012, Mistry & Williams 2011). Severe deficiency results in a range of devastating outcomes, including multiple fetal malformations, growth retardation or death, embryonic death and potentially life-threatening complications in both pregnancy and delivery (Chaffee & King 2012, Donangelo & King 2012). The consequences of mild to moderate deficiency are less clear, although most studies demonstrate reduced birth weights and some found increased prematurity, possibly secondary to maternal infection. There is also specific interest in zinc's antioxidant and anti-inflammatory roles in pregnancy and prevention of pre-eclampsia and fetal growth restriction, both of which have oxidative stress as an essential component (Chen et al 2012, Mistry & Williams 2011).

While it has been reported that zinc requirements in pregnancy would theoretically necessitate an 18–36% increase in dietary intake, most pregnant women do not increase zinc consumption (Donangelo & King 2012). This has led researchers to conclude that the primary means of meeting these higher zinc needs is via homeostatic adjustment; however, the exact mechanisms remain unclear and fail to completely compensate when zinc intake is significantly inadequate.

Similarly, zinc is essential for healthy mammary gland function, specifically the expansion and reduction of mammary tissue dependent upon stage of pregnancy and lactation, differentiation into secretory tissue, proliferation of the mammary epithelial cells which line the acini and transfer nutrients into milk, and milk secretion (Kelleher et al 2011). When milk zinc levels are compromised, this results in failure to thrive, diarrhoea, irritability and dermatitis in the infant (Kelleher et al 2011). Zinc losses in breast milk are significant, e.g. mean 1.35 mg/day, and if this was to be met by diet alone, a 50% increase in zinc intake would be required; however, limited evidence points to some adaptive mechanisms such as increased intestinal absorptive capacity, reduced faecal losses and increased renal conservation. The greatest contribution to maternal zinc during the postpartum period is speculated to be through resorption of trabecular bone. During 6 months of exclusive breastfeeding, 4–6% of maternal bone mass is lost, and this would contribute about 20% of the breast milk zinc during this period (Donangelo & King 2012).

Antioxidant

Zinc limits oxidant-induced damage in a number of indirect ways. It protects against vitamin E depletion, controls vitamin A release, contributes to the structure of the antioxidant enzyme extracellular SOD, restricts endogenous free radical production, maintains tissue concentrations of MT, is a possible scavenger of free radicals, antagonising both iron and copper levels, and stabilises membrane structure (DiSilvestro 2000, Rai et al 2013). It was observed to decrease lipid peroxidation and protect mononuclear cells from TNF-alpha-induced NF-kappa-B activation associated with oxidative stress (Prasad et al 2004).

Supporting glycaemic control

Zinc pancreatic concentrations are very high, negatively impacted by deficiency and, not surprisingly, zinc possesses multiple related roles, including the processing, storage, secretion and action of insulin in β cells. In fact, as insulin and zinc are co-stored within the dense core vesicles (DCVs), when insulin is exocytosed (released), a substantial amount of ionic zinc is also released into local circulation, with important autocrine and paracrine effects on nearby cells (Li 2013, O'Halloran et al 2013), including 'switching off' glucagon release from the pancreatic α cells (Kelleher et al 2011). The co-storage of zinc and insulin within β cells appears critical, such that polymorphisms that reduce expression of the zinc transporters expressed on these DCVs are associated with significantly reduced insulin secretion, increased HbA_{1C} and an increased risk of type 2 diabetes (Chimienti 2013). Zinc is also an essential cofactor for insulin degradation, peripheral insulin signalling and several key zinc finger transcription factors are required for β-cell development and insulin gene expression (Kelleher et al 2011, O'Halloran et al 2013). Furthermore, zinc is necessary for activity of several gluconeogenic enzymes, including phosphoenolpyruvate carboxykinase, making zinc central in glucose metabolism regulation (Kelleher et al 2011).

Interestingly, another zinc-dependent enzyme, called insulin-responsive aminopeptidase (IRAP), is colocalised with GLUT4 transporters on cell membranes, with both upregulating in response to insulin (Kelleher et al 2011). Although the exact action of IRAP is yet to be elucidated, its membrane expression in muscle cells and adipocytes is reduced in type 2 diabetes, just like the GLUT4s, suggesting a strong link between zinc signalling and insulin activity.

Suboptimal zinc status decreases insulin secretion from the pancreas while during severe deficiency hyperglycaemia and hyperinsulinaemia can manifest (Kelleher et al 2011) and zinc supplementation has been shown to ameliorate some physiological aspects of diabetes.

CLINICAL USE

Most of the clinical uses of zinc supplements are for conditions thought to arise from a marginal zinc deficiency, but some indications are based on the concept that high-dose zinc supplements act as a therapeutic agent above and beyond the point of repletion.

Deficiency

Traditionally, zinc supplementation has been used to treat or prevent deficiency in conditions such as acrodermatitis enteropathica, anorexia nervosa, malabsorption syndromes, conditions associated with chronic, severe diarrhoea, alcoholism and liver cirrhosis, diabetes, HIV and AIDS, recurrent infections, severe burns, after major surgery, Wilson's disease and sickle cell anaemia. Zinc supplements are also popular among athletes in order to counteract zinc losses that occur through perspiration. There are numerous supplementation and fortification schemes which include zinc in developing countries, where deficiency is most prevalent.

Common cold

Oral zinc supplements, lozenges, nasal sprays and gels have been investigated in the prevention and treatment of the common cold. It has been demonstrated that a transient increase in zinc concentrations in and around the nasal cavity prevents rhinovirus binding to cells and disrupts infection (Novick et al 1996) and/or modulates inflammatory cytokines and histamine release, as well as astringes the trigeminal nerve, to reduce cold symptoms (Kurugöl et al 2007, Science et al 2012). There is also evidence to suggest that zinc inhibits viral replication and speculation regarding zinc's ability to change the activities of different transcription factors and thus the expression patterns of cellular and viral genes (Lazarczyk & Favre 2008).

Zinc's administration via a lozenge form appears particularly important regarding its efficacy in upper respiratory tract infections (URTIs). A prolific researcher in this area explains this via the 'mouth-nose biologically closed electric circuit' (BCEC) (Eby & Halcomb 2006). The BCEC moves electrons from the nose into the mouth and, in response to the electron flow, moves positively charged metal ions, such as ionic zinc, from the mouth into the nose, where it then exerts its key virucidal actions via competing with rhinoviruses for attachment to the intracellular adhesion molecule-1 receptor in nasal epithelium (Singh & Das 2013). If correct, this underscores the importance of using 'free' or ionic forms of zinc in the lozenge, rather than tightly bound ones (see Oral supplements, below).

Acute treatment

Nasal preparations

At least three placebo-controlled studies indicate that intranasal preparations containing zinc have benefits in the treatment of the common cold; however safety issues regarding transient anosmia limit its use in practice.

Administration of a zinc sulfate (0.12%) nasal spray reduced the total symptom score significantly better than placebo, according to a double-blind randomised controlled trial involving 160 people. The same treatment had no effect on the duration of cold symptoms or mean time to resolution (Belongia et al 2001). Two other placebo-controlled trials showed that zinc in a nasal gel formulation significantly reduced cold duration compared with placebo when used within 24–48 hours of symptom onset (Hirt et al 2000, Mossad 2003). The active nasal gel spray contained 33 mmol/L zinc gluconate and was administered as one dose per nostril four times daily until symptoms resolved or for a maximum of 10 days. Symptoms that responded included nasal drainage, hoarseness and sore throat (Mossad 2003).

Despite these promising results, concerns have been raised regarding temporary anosmia secondary to use of the zinc gluconate nasal preparations (Duncan-Lewis et al 2011). Based on consumer reports, in 2009 the US Food and Drug Administration issued a warning against the use of zinc nasal preparations, which were subsequently removed from the US market. The safety of these preparations has been the subject of debate between industry and government

Anosmia has been reported in animal models following the application of nasal zinc chloride or sulfate preparations and a more recent study which nasally irrigated rats with zinc gluconate further confirmed temporary anosmia compared with placebo. While the sensory loss is only transient and the mechanism remains unclear, any sensory loss is worrying (Duncan-Lewis et al 2011, Hemila 2011).

Oral supplements

According to two meta-analyses, zinc lozenges (≥75 mg/day) significantly reduce symptom duration compared to placebo in the acute treatment of URTIs but not symptom severity (Science et al 2012, Singh & Das 2013). Ideally, lozenges should be taken every 2 hours and started as soon as symptoms arise, thereby reducing symptom duration by about 1.65 days in adults (95% confidence interval −2.50 to −0.81) (Science et al 2012). They should not be taken with any food or beverage which may limit zinc absorption or ionisation (see Background and relevant pharmacokinetics, above).

While the body of evidence is positive, some adult studies do not demonstrate benefits, which may be due to differences in study methodology and whether zinc in the test preparation is accompanied by other ingredients which affect its release and/or absorption, such as citrate, tartrate, sorbitol or glycine, which decrease the level of free zinc ion (Hemila 2011). Since zinc ionisation is considered an important step in the clinical effectiveness of zinc, this is of particular concern. Ideally, future researchers should pay careful attention to exact lozenge composition in order to minimise this confounding factor (Hemila 2011, Silk & LeFante 2005). It has also been suggested that zinc lozenges be allowed to completely dissolve in the mouth without chewing and that citrus fruits or juices be avoided 30 minutes before or after dissolving each lozenge to avoid negating the therapeutic effects of zinc (Silk & LeFante 2005).

An updated Cochrane review of 16 double-blind randomised controlled trials (n = 1357) investigating zinc administration ≥75 mg/day for acute treatment of URTIs concluded there was a significant mean reduction in symptom duration compared to placebo ($P = 0.003$) and a smaller proportion of symptomatic individuals after 7 days in treatment groups; however, there was no significant difference in the severity of cold symptoms (Singh & Das 2013). Due to the heterogeneity of the studies, the authors urge caution regarding their calculated average estimates. Another 2013 systematic review and meta-analysis tried to improve upon the Cochrane methodology, including 17 trials (n = 2121) of oral zinc administration within 3 days of URTI symptom onset. They too concluded that, although no significant difference in symptom severity was evident, there was a mean reduction in duration (mean difference [MD] −1.65 days, 95% confidence interval [CI] −2.50 to −0.81). A subgroup analysis revealed that the effect was only significant in adults (MD −2.63, 95% CI −3.69 to −1.58) and was restricted to studies using a zinc acetate form and when administered at higher doses, e.g. ≥75 mg/day. The authors speculate that the lack of significance in paediatric cohorts is due to lower doses, reduced frequency of administration and alternative forms used, e.g. syrups rather than lozenges. Their findings would suggest that the impact of zinc administration on reducing URTI duration has previously been underestimated in studies that fail to attend to these important details (Science et al 2012).

An earlier systematic review focused specifically on zinc lozenges in acute URTI treatment, with all but one study conducted in adults (Hemila 2011). This review demonstrates, and argues convincingly for the merit of, several differences in statistical analysis. Firstly, the authors make the point that URTI symptom duration is highly variable independent of any treatment, and, as such, is more logical to calculate via relative effect on duration, rather than an absolute, e.g. percentage rather than days. When calculated like this, the authors found the evidence strengthened for zinc lozenge efficacy. The review also presents an extended discussion of lozenge dose and form, most notably pointing out that there is a sevenfold difference in total daily zinc dose across the included studies. Subgroup analysis found no effect was evident in the five trials using <75 mg/day. In contrast, the majority of studies using >75 mg/day demonstrated positive effects. The review also found greater reductions in symptom duration with zinc acetate (mean −42%, 95% CI 35–48) compared with other forms (mean effect −20%, 95% CI 12–28). These findings were recently echoed by Science et al (2012).

Prevention of colds

There is relatively little research dedicated to determining whether long-term zinc supplementation reduces URTI incidence. A 2013 Cochrane review included only two studies investigating zinc as a prophylactic treatment (n = 394) and concluded there was very low-level evidence of efficacy; however, the studies differed in many key variables, e.g, dose, form, duration of administration and still collectively produced an incident rate ratio of 0.64 (P = 0.006) (Singh & Das 2013). Critics of this review suggest that bias has insufficiently been accounted for and therefore the effect of zinc has possibly been overstated (Peters et al 2012).

In children

A recent double-blind randomised controlled trial not included in the Cochrane review of 100 8–13-year-old children showed that administration of zinc *bis*-glycinate 15 mg once a day for 3 months was not sufficient to reduce the incidence of URTIs but did reduce symptom severity and duration associated with colds if an URTI developed, as compared to placebo (Rerksuppaphol & Rerksuppaphol 2013).

In the elderly

Both zinc deficiency, due to poor dietary intake and altered homeostasis, and impaired cell-mediated immunity are commonly reported in the elderly (>55 years) and have been used to explain the increased infection rates observed in this population. A double-blind randomised controlled trial involving 50 healthy elderly subjects found that the majority had a marginal zinc deficiency and 35% were below the cut-off for frank deficiency, as measured via plasma zinc at baseline (Prasad et al 2007). Participants taking zinc gluconate supplements (45 mg/day) for 12 months experienced a significant reduction in infection incidence compared to placebo (88% vs 29%), with protective effects evident against URTIs (12% vs 24%), the common cold (10% vs 40%) and influenza (0% vs 12%). Also of note, while no individual in the treatment group experienced more than one infection in the 12-month period, six individuals taking placebo had two infections, and three subjects had three or more infections during the same period. Inflammatory cytokines and markers of oxidative stress were also investigated in this study, confirming zinc's role as both an anti-inflammatory and antioxidant in the elderly. Prior studies using much smaller zinc doses (15–20 mg/day) in multivitamin and mineral combinations failed to demonstrate efficacy in this cohort (Avenell et al 2005, Girodon et al 1999, Hemila 2011).

There is ongoing research interest in the relationship between zinc status and senescence, with preliminary in vivo studies pointing to zinc dysregulation being a key factor in the increasing inflammation and reduced immunocompetence seen with ageing (Mocchegiani et al 2011, Wong et al 2013).

Pneumonia

Worldwide, pneumonia is the leading cause of paediatric morbidity and mortality and approximately 95% of the pneumonia-related deaths occur in developing countries where zinc deficiency is most prevalent (Shah et al 2012). Several studies have investigated both prevention and treatment of paediatric pneumonia using zinc supplementation, usually as an adjunct to standard treatment.

Prevention

Supplemental zinc (70 mg/day) significantly reduced the incidence of pneumonia (relative risk [RR] 0.83) compared to placebo and significantly reduced

Z

mortality (P = 0.013) in a randomised controlled trial of 1665 poor, urban children aged < 12 months. In addition, active treatment resulted in a 49% decrease in the incidence of severe pneumonia and reduced URTI by 8% and reactive airways disease (bronchiolitis) by 12% (Brooks et al 2005).

Serum zinc concentrations have been shown to negatively correlate with pneumonia incidence in a study of nursing-home residents, prompting researchers to consider zinc as a potential prophylactic in this population also; however, there are currently no randomised controlled trials (Overbeck et al 2008).

Active treatment

In terms of acute treatment, positive findings include the study by Brooks et al (2004) — a randomised controlled trial involving 270 children aged between 6 and 12 months, hospitalised with pneumonia, which found that those given 20 mg/day of zinc (as acetate) experienced significant reductions in recovery time from severe pneumonia. Overall hospital stay duration was also reduced when used with standard antimicrobial therapy (Brooks et al 2004). Results from a similarly designed study, however, failed to corroborate zinc as an effective treatment (Bose et al 2006).

It is possible that the lack of differentiation between bacterial and non-bacterial pneumonia in these studies is an important feature. Another study which investigated the efficacy of adjunctive zinc treatment (10 mg zinc sulfate administered twice daily) in paediatric patients (<2 years) hospitalised for severe pneumonia identified that zinc supplementation in bacterial pneumonia had detrimental effects which were not seen in non-bacterial cases (Coles et al 2007). Further research is not available to confirm these results.

A Cochrane review includes four trials of zinc given as an adjunct to standard antimicrobial therapy in children (n = 3267) aged 2–35 months suffering with severe and non-severe pneumonia (Haider et al 2011). The studies by Brooks et al (2004) and Bose et al (2006) were included along with two other moderately-sized trials. All four studies tested 20 mg elemental zinc per day, except that by Valentiner-Branth et al (2010), who administered only 10 mg/day for <12 months. Duration of treatment varied from as little as 5 days to >14 days (discharge). The reviewers concluded that there was no significant reduction in clinical recovery in the groups receiving adjunctive zinc; however, none of the studies identified whether the aetiology was bacterial or viral, which, according to the findings of Coles et al (2007), limits the meaningfulness of these conclusions.

A 2012 meta-analysis of seven studies (n = 1066), including many of the ones already discussed, concludes that zinc supplementation fails to produce significant reductions in recovery time from paediatric pneumonia. The authors acknowledge several limitations of the review, including lack of distinction between bacterial and viral aetiologies (Das et al 2012). They also suggest that future studies should consider higher doses given the absence of adverse reactions and standardise definitions, recovery parameters, timing and doses of zinc before drawing definitive conclusions.

Since these two reviews were published, two other key studies have been conducted which provide additional insight. A Ugandan study of 352 children aged 6–59 months (Srinivasan et al 2012) provides us with a well-thought-out methodology, clearly taking into account the findings of recent research in this area, such as that by Coles et al (2007). Zinc gluconate was administered (<12 months received 10 mg/day, >12 months 20 mg/day) to the treatment group for 7 days. Both placebo and treatment groups also received vitamin A, in line with World Health Organization recommendations. Baseline plasma zinc levels were lower than seen in other studies (e.g. 4.4 micromol/L [1.3–8.0]) and the researchers confirmed that 17.7% of the sample were HIV-positive (highly active antiretroviral treatment-naïve). Interestingly, while zinc failed to reduce recovery time, it significantly reduced mortality (18.8% in placebo versus 6.7%; RR 0.3). This protective effect seen across the treatment group on further analysis was found to be greatest amongst the HIV-positive children (11% in placebo vs 0%; RR 0.2). Additionally, children with either bacterial or viral pneumonia when treated with zinc demonstrated reduced mortality; the majority of cases (75.5%) had a viral cause. The number needed to treat in order to save one life was 13 and, poignantly, the authors comment that this comes at a meagre cost of US$4.

Another study of adjunctive zinc (20 mg/day sulfate; administered for a maximum of 14 days) in paediatric (2–24 months) pneumonia (n = 550) where baseline plasma zinc averaged ≈9 micromol/L found that, in spite of significant increases in plasma zinc levels in the treatment group (4.3 ± 5.6 micromol), there was no significant reduction in time to recovery overall (Wadhwa et al 2013). Further analysis revealed that children diagnosed with very severe pneumonia at baseline did exhibit increased recovery time with zinc supplementation and there was a non-significant trend of reduced treatment failure in this subgroup.

Age-related macular degeneration (ARMD)

Both dietary and supplemental zinc have been investigated in the prevention and/or delayed progression of ARMD. This is not surprising as evidence that lifetime oxidative stress plays an important role in the development of ARMD is now compelling (Hogg & Chakravarthy 2004). ARMD is thought to be the result of free radical damage to photoreceptors within the macula, and therefore it is suspected that inefficient macular antioxidant systems play a role in disease development. After ageing, smoking is the next significant risk factor and a direct association between risk and the number of cigarettes smoked has been reported (Coleman et al 2008, Wills et al 2008a). Smokers have four times greater retinal cadmium concentrations than non-smokers and the associated morphological changes are reasonably consistent with ARMD pathology (Wills et al 2008a).

A 2005 study found that high dietary intake of zinc, beta-carotene and vitamins C and E was associated with a 35% reduced risk in elderly persons (van Leeuwen et al 2005). Similarly, the Blue Mountains Eye Study, an Australian prospective population-based cohort study conducted over 10 years, demonstrated protective effects of lutein and zeaxanthin, but also found that those individuals consuming the highest zinc had an RR of 0.56 for any ARMD and 0.54 for early ARMD compared with all other participants (Tan et al 2008). An interesting study has revealed that increased lifetime exposure to blue light appears to amplify the risk of low dietary antioxidants and zinc (Fletcher et al 2008). Originally it was believed that zinc simply acts as an antioxidant in this condition, yet ongoing discussions of zinc's possible actions in the prevention of this aetiology has produced new hypotheses.

A comparison of zinc and copper concentrations within the retinal pigment epithelium and choroid complex of eye donor subjects previously suffering from ARMD and those without the condition has revealed a 23–24% reduction in these metals in afflicted subjects (Erie et al 2009). Furthermore, in vitro studies confirm that zinc and copper, as well as manganese (the latter being most potent), effectively prevent the intracellular concentration of cadmium in retinal tissues and hence modulate its toxicity (Satarug et al 2008, Wills et al 2008b). Taken together, the knowledge that zinc and copper supplementation, in combination with antioxidants, has delayed progression of ARMD points towards a critical role for metal homeostasis in retinal health.

A 2006 Cochrane review assessed the effects of antioxidant vitamin and/or mineral supplementation on the progression of ARMD and found that evidence of effectiveness is currently dominated by one large trial that showed modest benefit in people with moderate to severe signs of the disease (Evans 2002). The study the authors refer to is the Age-Related Eye Disease Study (AREDS 2001), which showed that high-dose vitamins C and E, beta-carotene and zinc supplementation delayed the progression from intermediate to advanced disease by 25% over 5 years. The 11-centre, double-blind, prospective study involved 3640 volunteers aged between 55 and 80 years who were randomly divided into four treatment groups, receiving either antioxidant supplements (500 mg vitamin C, 400 IU vitamin E, and 15 mg beta-carotene daily), zinc oxide and cupric oxide (80 mg elemental zinc, 2 mg elemental copper daily), antioxidants plus zinc, or placebo. This treatment effect appeared to persist following 5 additional years of follow-up after the clinical trial was stopped. The AREDS formulation became the standard of care for persons who are at high risk for ARMD (Chew 2013); however, the actual contribution of zinc to this result is unknown (see Lutein monograph for more information about ARMD).

A more recent randomised controlled trial tested supplementation with zinc monocysteine (25 mg elemental zinc twice daily) as a stand-alone treatment to 80 ARMD patients over 6 months (Newsome 2008). Those in the treatment group experienced improved visual acuity, contrast sensitivity and reduced macular light flash recovery time when compared with the placebo group, with some benefits evident 3 months into the treatment.

Overall, current evidence suggests that zinc supplementation, either alone or in combination with other antioxidants, may help to prevent ARMD in those at least at moderate risk and delay progression of this condition in those suffering the early stages. Additional evidence suggests that genetic factors may be important when determining who will best respond to this treatment. Retrospective analyses of the AREDS study demonstrated a strong interaction between those individuals whose progression of the condition was delayed by zinc supplementation and the presence of the complement factor H genotype (Klein et al 2008, Lee & Brantley 2008). Substantiation of these findings could assist in the improved targeting of ARMD nutritional therapies.

Herpes simplex virus (HSV) infection

Various topical zinc applications have been studied, producing encouraging results in reducing the incidence, severity and duration of symptoms in HSV infection.

In a study of 90 volunteers with diagnosed genital herpes, three different concentrations of liquid zinc sulfate (1%, 2% and 4%) were compared. The strongest concentration (4%) gave the lowest risk of recurrence over a 6-month test period compared to the others or a control group using only distilled water (Mahajan et al 2013). The treatments were applied with a cotton bud to genital herpetic lesions every 5 days for a month, then every 10 days for 2 months and finally every 15 days for 3 months. This protective effect has also been demonstrated in vivo for topical zinc acetate (0.5–1%) in a carrageenan-based gel applied locally for 7 days prior to vaginal or rectal exposure to the virus (Kenney et al 2013).

A double-blind randomised controlled trial of 46 people with facial and circumoral herpes infection showed that prompt application of a zinc oxide and glycine cream every 2 hours reduced recovery time from 6.5 to 5 days. The people using active treatment also experienced a reduction in the overall severity of signs and symptoms, particularly blistering, soreness, itching and tingling, compared to controls. The only side effects reported were a burning and itching sensation (Godfrey et al 2001). Previously, another double-blind randomised controlled trial showed that a zinc sulfate (1%) gel applied every few hours resulted in 50% of patients with HSV-1 becoming symptom-free by day 5 compared to only 35% in the placebo group (Kneist et al 1995). Another study of 200 volunteers with herpes simplex found that a lower dose of only 0.25% zinc sulfate solution, started within 24 hours of lesion appearance and applied 8–10 times daily, cleared lesions within 3–6 days (Finnerty 1986). Not surprisingly, a randomised controlled trial using a far lower dose of 0.05% or 0.025% zinc sulfate found no effects on frequency, duration or severity of herpes attacks, suggesting that stronger concentrations are required for effectiveness (Graham et al 1985).

According to an experimental study using zinc oxide, the attachment of HSV-2 to target cells is inhibited by the presence of zinc (Antoine et al 2012). In vitro studies also confirm that zinc can inhibit the replication of HSV; however, the concentration required is much higher than possible in a physiological context (Overbeck et al 2008).

Interestingly, new research suggests that people with recurrent HSV-1 have significantly lower salivary zinc levels compared to healthy controls and that levels are lowest in the acute phase compared to the convalescent phase (Khozeimeh et al 2012).

Diabetes mellitus (type 1 and 2)

Zinc is abundant in the pancreas due to extensive roles in both its endocrine and exocrine functions. During deficiency, this is one of the few tissues that demonstrates reduced concentrations (Islam & Loots 2007). Limited data derived from both epidemiological studies and animal models suggest that increased dietary zinc intake may be protective against the development of both types of diabetes (Bolkent et al 2009, Islam & Loots 2007, Sun et al 2009). It is suspected that zinc may have a protective role due to its antioxidant activity, both directly and indirectly, via MT induction (Islam & Loots 2007). Decreasing oxidative stress may protect beta cells from damage and therefore assist in maintaining normal insulin secretion.

Zinc supplementation is sometimes used to avoid deficiency, a state synonymous with both type 1 and type 2 diabetes due to a combination of increased losses and reduced uptake (Chimienti 2013, Cunningham et al 1994). While animal studies have demonstrated improved glucose management with zinc, the results from human studies are less consistent (Chimienti 2013). It remains unclear whether simply addressing zinc deficiency or using high-dose zinc to induce other effects will be beneficial in the clinical management of diabetes, its complications or its prevention, as evidence from both animal and human studies has produced varying results (Baydas et al 2002, Cunningham et al 1994, Farvid et al 2004, Gupta et al 1998, Niewoehner et al 1986, Roussel et al 2003, Tobia et al 1998).

Several intervention studies utilising oral zinc have produced positive results in populations with type 1 diabetes, with evidence of reduced HbA_{1C} amongst individuals in the treatment group (30 mg/day elemental zinc for 3 months) when compared to controls (Al-Maroof & Al-Sharbatti 2006), improved blood lipid profiles following 12 weeks of zinc treatment (100 mg/day zinc sulfate) in another study (Partida-Hernández et al 2006) and improved glycaemic control and diabetic neuropathy in 20 patients administered 660 mg/day zinc sulfate over 6 weeks (Hayee et al 2005). Interestingly, new research has identified a fourth autoantibody common to type 1 diabetes which is made against the zinc transporter unique to islet cells (ZnT8) and therefore impairs zinc accumulation within the DCVs, making altered zinc regulation a potential cause (Chimienti 2013, O'Halloran et al 2013). Incredibly, since the 1930s it was known that the pancreas of diabetics contained only half of the zinc found in healthy individuals (Chimienti 2013).

Zinc supplementation to address the secondary multisystem effects of type 1 diabetes has been investigated with regard to vascular changes in mice. In control genetic type 1 diabetes mice, significant increases in aortic oxidative damage, inflammation, fibrosis and thickness were observed; however, in mice receiving $ZnSO_4$ 5 mg/kg over 3 months these changes were completely prevented, reportedly due to upregulation of both MT and Nrf2 (Miao et al 2013). In vitro studies of human endothelial cells have produced similar findings.

With respect to type 2 diabetes, a prospective, double-blind, clinical interventional study of 56 obese women with normal glucose tolerance randomised subjects to treatment with zinc, 30 mg/day, or placebo for 4 weeks (Marreiro et al 2002). Zinc treatment decreased insulin resistance from 5.8 to 4.3 and insulin decreased from 28.8 to 21.2 mU/mL, but was unchanged in the placebo group. These results are particularly noteworthy because the women were not zinc-deficient, suggesting a therapeutic role for zinc. Another small study of metformin-resistant patients with type 2 diabetes administered zinc (zinc acetate 50 mg/day) in combination with melatonin (10 mg/day) ± metformin to two treatment groups and placebo to a third (Hussain et al 2006). This combined treatment proved effective in improving fasting and postprandial glucose levels and augmented the action of the hypoglycaemic drug.

Zinc deficiency has been established as an independent risk factor for fatal coronary heart disease events in a large cohort of patients with type 2 diabetes, with serum zinc values < 14.1 micromol/L associated with 20.8% patients with fatal events versus 12.8% ($P < 0.001$) (Sarmento et al 2013, Soinio et al 2007). Studies investigating zinc's potential for reducing these secondary deleterious effects are still emerging. One randomised double-blind crossover study of 50 patients with type 2 diabetes with microalbuminuria, administered 30 mg/day elemental zinc over 3 months, revealed a significant reduction in homocysteine levels (from 13.71 ± 3.84 micromol/L to 11.79 ± 3.06 micromol/L;

$P < 0.05$), a cardiovascular inflammatory mediator, while improving folate and B_{12} status. Other proposed protective effects are via both general anti-inflammatory and antioxidant actions as well as via MT induction (Miao et al 2013).

Regarding diabetic retinopathy, hypothesised protective mechanisms include zinc's inhibition of vascular endothelial growth factor, involved in the initiation and progression of neovascularisation and vascular leakage in diabetic retinopathy; however, clinical studies are lacking to date (Miao et al 2013).

Further studies with larger sample sizes are required to validate zinc as an effective treatment in type 1 and 2 diabetes and elucidate the optimal dosing and administration regimen. There is currently a study under way in Sri Lanka investigating zinc supplementation in prediabetics which may also further our knowledge in this area (Ranasinghe et al 2013).

Clinical note — Zinc deficiency and diabetes

Diabetes affects zinc homeostasis in many ways and is associated with increased urinary loss, decreased absorption and decreased total body zinc (Chausmer 1998, Cunningham et al 1994). The role of zinc and zinc deficiency in diabetes and its complications or prevention is currently unclear. It has been suggested that deficiency may exacerbate destruction of islet cells in type 1 diabetes and may adversely affect the synthesis, storage and secretion of insulin, a process that requires zinc. Furthermore, evidence indicates that patients with type 1 diabetes have a higher concentration of free radicals than healthy controls; this is due to increased oxidant production and/or decreased efficiency of endogenous antioxidant systems (Davison et al 2002). It is suspected that deficiency of key micronutrients (i.e. zinc, copper, manganese and selenium), which are integral components of important antioxidant systems, may be partly responsible.

Wound healing

Zinc is an essential cofactor in both wound healing and immune function. Therefore, zinc deficiency retards both fibroplasia and epithelialisation, and results in delayed wound healing in spite of maintained skin stores of zinc, except in instances of severe concomitant protein restriction (Lansdown et al 2007). Zinc supplements are used to restore zinc status in cases of wound healing associated with malnutrition and deficiency. Additionally, zinc administered orally or topically to wounds can promote healing and reduce infection, according to one major review (Lansdown 1996).

Oral application

In 2001, a randomised study demonstrated that oral zinc sulfate significantly improved healing of cutaneous leishmaniasis (Sharquie et al 2001). Results showed that the cure rate for a dose of 2.5 mg/kg was 83.9%, for 5 mg/kg it was 93.1% and for 10 mg/kg it was 96.9%, whereas no lesions showed any sign of healing in the control group. The results of several studies suggest a specific role for oral zinc in surgical wound repair (Lansdown et al 2007). Zinc redistribution and sequestration in the liver occur following both surgical trauma and infection. The corresponding reduction in serum zinc may then impair the individual's healing capacity, as demonstrated in a study of 80 total hip replacement patients (mean age 66 years), in whom serum zinc levels were significantly related to rates of infection and dehiscence (Lansdown et al 2007). Similarly, an interventional study of pre- and postoperative zinc infusion (30 mg/day) in patients undergoing major vascular reconstructive surgery attenuated the anticipated decline in serum zinc and produced significantly fewer wound-healing complications than placebo.

Topical application

Theoretically, topical zinc treatment is most suited to human wound healing that necessitates epithelialisation, e.g. suction blister wound, superficial small incision and split-thickness skin graft donor sites. While clinical trials have demonstrated its efficacy in relation to treatment of leg ulcers, pressure ulcers, diabetic foot ulcers and burn wounds (Lansdown et al 2007), one study also demonstrated that *Staphylococcus aureus* was cultured significantly less frequently in zinc oxide-treated wounds, which points to the additional antiseptic action. Topical zinc oxide promotes cleansing and re-epithelialisation of ulcers and reduces the risk of infection and deterioration of ulcers compared with placebo, according to one double-blind trial of leg ulcer patients with low serum zinc levels (Agren 1990). Evidence from animal and in vitro research suggests that topically applied zinc solution is more effective when combined with iron than when used alone, and can effectively enhance healing in acute partial-thickness and second-degree burn wounds (Feiner et al 2003). The form of zinc used topically may be of marked importance, with some studies investigating high concentrations of zinc sulfate delaying healing and increasing dermal inflammatory cell infiltration (Lansdown et al 2007). Preparations such as zinc oxide may be more suitable than readily water-soluble forms, providing a sustained release of bioavailable zinc at non-cytotoxic levels. Interestingly, pharmacopoeias attribute various zinc forms with different qualities/actions, e.g. zinc sulfate is regarded as a local astringent and antiseptic, insoluble zinc oxide as a mild antiseptic, astringent and protective agent, particularly indicated in inflamed skin and wounds.

Arterial and venous leg ulcers

Chronic leg ulcer patients often exhibit abnormal zinc metabolism and depressed serum concentrations (Lansdown et al 2007). A 2000 Cochrane review assessed six placebo-controlled trials of zinc sulfate supplementation (≈220 mg administered three times daily) in arterial and venous leg ulcers and concluded that, overall, there is no evidence of a beneficial effect on the number of ulcers healed. However, there is some evidence that oral zinc might improve healing of venous ulcers in people with low serum zinc levels (Wilkinson & Hawke 2000).

Double-blind studies producing encouraging results have used oral zinc (600 mg/day) combined with topical treatment and compression bandages (Haeger & Lanner 1974, Hallbook & Lanner 1972).

Acne and other skin conditions

Over the past two to three decades, tetracyclines and macrolide antibiotics have been widely prescribed for the treatment of acne; however, resistance has been reported, especially to erythromycin and clindamycin, with cross-resistance being widespread among strains of *Propionibacterium acnes* and increasing (Iinuma et al 2011). As a result, non-antibiotic treatments such as topical/oral zinc preparations have been investigated as both alternatives and adjunctive therapy.

Overall, there is increasingly consistent clinical evidence of the efficacy of zinc (both oral and topical) for the treatment of acne, showing it can improve skin condition. However, definitive conclusions are hampered by some poor-quality studies. Some studies utilise zinc supplementation in combination with other nutrients, making it difficult to ascertain the role of zinc but providing clinical guidance nonetheless.

Surprisingly, it is only recently that epidemiological research has demonstrated lower plasma zinc in acne patients ($P < 0.001$) and that blood zinc (and vitamin E) correlates with acne severity (Ozuguz et al 2014). Dietary analysis was not performed in this study, which still leaves the question of whether the low zinc is the cause or consequence of acne.

Oral supplementation

Numerous studies have been conducted investigating the effects of zinc supplementation in acne vulgaris (Dreno et al 1989, 1992, 2001, Goransson et al 1978, Hillstrom et al 1977, Orris et al 1978, Verma et al 1980, Weimar et al 1978, Weismann et al 1977). Doses between 90 mg and 200 mg (30 mg elemental zinc) daily taken over 6–12 weeks have been associated with generally positive results, whereas larger doses tend to be poorly tolerated.

Two double-blind studies have compared the effects of oral zinc supplementation with two antibiotic medicines, minocycline or oxytetracycline, over 3 months (Cunliffe et al 1979, Dreno et al 1989). Zinc sulfate (135 mg) was as effective as oxytetracycline after 12 weeks' use, decreasing acne scores by 65% in one study, whereas the same dose was not as effective as minocycline (500 mg) in the second study. An open study involving 30 subjects with inflammatory acne found that a lower dose of oral zinc gluconate (30 mg) taken daily reduced the number of inflammatory lesions after 2 months, regardless of whether *P. acnes* was present (Dreno et al 2005).

Both oral and topical zinc have also been investigated as an adjunct to antibiotic therapy under laboratory conditions. When administered in combination with erythromycin, it inhibits erythromycin-resistant propionibacteria according to two in vitro studies (Dreno et al 2005, Oprica et al 2002).

IN COMBINATION

A more recent open-label observational study involving 48 subjects with moderate acne vulgaris, treated with a zinc antioxidant combination (equivalent to 15 mg elemental zinc, 60 mg vitamin C, 15 IU vitamin E and 0.13 mg chromium) administered over 12 weeks produced a 79% response rate. Although a large clinical improvement (80–100%) was reported, particularly with respect to reduced inflammatory features, the absence of a control group and blinding of the intervention detract from the positive findings (Sardana & Garg 2010). Similarly, another open-label trial with positive findings in acne patients adds little to our evidence base for zinc, given the intervention was a multivitamin mineral containing forms of zinc and other minerals with poor bioavailability, i.e. oxides (Shalita et al 2012).

Topical application

A number of studies have investigated the effects of a topical erythromycin–zinc acetate (≈1.2%) formulation (Bojar et al 1994, Feucht et al 1980, Habbema et al 1989, Morgan et al 1993, Pierard & Pierard-Franchimont 1993, Pierard-Franchimont et al 1995, Schachner et al 1990).

Statistically significant effects have been observed within the first 12 weeks of treatment for acne severity grades, and for papule, pustule and comedo counts, with the effect of the combination superior to preparations containing erythromycin alone (Habbema et al 1989, Schachner et al 1990). A systematic review of acne treatments also concluded that topical erythromycin–zinc appears to be more effective than the antibiotic alone for the treatment of both inflammatory and non-inflammatory lesions (Purdy & de Berker 2011).

A 2013 review of 29 studies investigating zinc and acne concluded that there is inconsistent or limited quality patient-centred evidence for either oral or topical treatment with zinc; however, the review was funded and partly written by Galderma, a manufacturer of non-zinc-based acne treatments, thereby requiring confirmation by other researchers (Brandt 2013).

Human studies have identified antibacterial activity against *Propionibacterium* spp. in short-term treatment, which is mostly attributed to zinc (Fluhr et al 1999) and sebosuppressive effects (Pierard & Pierard-Franchimont 1993). New in vitro research, building on prior successful studies using topical ascorbic acid derivatives, has found superior antimicrobial activity in zinc ascorbate compared with other ascorbates, e.g. 0.064% concentration compared with 5%

(Iinuma et al 2011). The study also confirms an additive effect when combined with some topical antibiotics (i.e. erythromycin and clindamycin) and, perhaps more impressively, demonstrated that zinc ascorbate was effective as a stand-alone treatment in inhibiting the proliferation of antibiotic-resistant strains of *P. acnes* (minimum inhibitory concentration 640 mcg/mL). The same researchers have shown topical zinc ascorbate similarly possesses potent antimicrobial activity against *Staphylococcus aureus* and, to a lesser extent, *Escherichia coli*, Gram-negative bacteria that typically act in concert with *P. acnes* in acne vulgaris. Again this is seen at significantly lower concentrations than with other ascorbate derivatives and ascorbic acid alone (Iinuma & Tsuboi 2012). Both zinc and ascorbic acid's capacity to inhibit ROS production (SOD-like activity) is speculated as an important attribute in acne treatment, with previous research demonstrating that elevated ROS and impaired SOD are characteristic features in acne patients, leading to an excess inflammatory response.

Reduced male fertility

Zinc deficiency leads to several clinical signs, such as decreased spermatogenesis, altered sperm morphology and impaired male fertility and, given zinc's pivotal role in DNA transcription, this is not surprising. Furthermore, zinc finger proteins are critical to the genetic expression of steroid hormone receptors. Together with zinc's additional antiapoptotic and antioxidant actions, these effects make zinc a promising contributor to healthy sperm (Ebisch et al 2007). The relationship between zinc concentrations in seminal fluid and semen fertility, however, remains somewhat unclear.

When zinc deficiency is not present, a 2002 survey found no statistically significant relationship between zinc in seminal plasma or serum and semen quality or local antisperm antibody of the immunoglobulin G (IgG) or IgA class (Eggert-Kruse et al 2002). Furthermore, zinc levels did not influence sperm capacity to penetrate cervical mucus in vitro or in vivo, nor affect subsequent fertility. However, a study of Chinese men (aged 20–59 years) revealed that, when serum zinc concentration was low, the risk of asthenozoospermia increased and the Cu/Zn ratio was higher in those with progressive motility abnormalities (Yuyan et al 2008).

In contrast to this, a small number of both animal (Kumar et al 2006) and human supplementation studies (Ebisch et al 2006) have produced positive results. The latter study, involving 40 subfertile and 47 fertile men treated for 26 weeks with 66 mg/day zinc sulfate and 5 mg/day folic acid or placebo, produced a 74% increase in normal sperm count in the subfertile subjects; however, more studies with larger sample sizes and measurement of pregnancy outcomes are required to substantiate these preliminary findings. In spite of this relative paucity of randomised controlled trial evidence, a trend of treatment has begun. A recent review of antioxidant supplementation in the treatment of idiopathic oligoasthenoteratospermia observes that, while elevated ROS is undoubtedly damaging to spermatids and mature spermatozoa and is implicated in male infertility, antioxidant treatment including zinc, which has become widely accepted, is yet to be established as efficacious (Agarwal & Sekhon 2010).

Impotence

In men, zinc deficiency may lead to impaired testosterone synthesis, resulting in hypogonadism and impotency. One placebo-controlled study has investigated whether oral zinc supplementation improves erectile dysfunction. The study involved 20 uraemic haemodialysis patients and showed that 6 months' treatment with oral zinc acetate (25 mg elemental zinc) taken twice daily 1–2 hours before meals resulted in greater libido, improved potency and more frequent intercourse compared to placebo (Mahajan et al 1982). Active treatment also resulted in significant increases in plasma zinc, serum testosterone and sperm count and decreases in serum levels of luteinising hormone and follicle-stimulating hormone.

Attention-deficit hyperactivity disorder (ADHD)

Zinc deficiency has been implicated in the pathogenesis of ADHD from numerous perspectives. With a critical role in neurological development and evidence of impaired learning and depressed psychomotor retardation in deficiency states, zinc may constitute a direct aetiological cause (Black 2003, Fanjiang & Kleinman 2007). An interesting longitudinal paediatric study found that children with malnutrition (protein, zinc and iron deficiencies) at 3 years of age demonstrated higher externalisation behaviour problems at 8, 11 and 17 years, when compared to replete children (Liu & Raine 2006), with this trifecta of deficiencies, a particularly common combination in young children.

Hypotheses of indirect actions of zinc deficiency include negative behavioural effects mediated via impaired fatty acid metabolism, blockage of the dopamine transporter to increase synaptic concentrations and through the exacerbation of heavy-metal effects.

In 1990, Arnold et al observed that boys aged 6–12 years with ADHD and a higher baseline hair zinc level had better responses to amphetamine therapy than children with hair concentrations indicative of mild zinc deficiency. At the time, it was suggested that poor/non-responders to drug therapy and those presenting with suboptimal zinc status would require zinc supplementation instead of amphetamine treatment to address the condition. Since then, numerous controlled studies have identified that children with ADHD have lower zinc tissue levels (serum, red cells, hair, urine, nails) than normal children (Arnold & DiSilvestro 2005). It is not certain why this occurs, but it may result from not sitting for long enough to consume a balanced diet, picky eating, stimulant-related appetite suppression, malabsorption or biochemical changes.

Recently it has been suggested that zinc may be a proxy of poor diet quality in this group (Ghanizadeh & Berk 2013). Zinc status has also been also shown to correlate with the amplitude and latency of select brain waves, suggesting that zinc may particularly influence information processing in ADHD children (Yorbik et al 2008).

Three early double-blind studies, all conducted in Middle Eastern populations, investigated whether oral zinc supplementation has a beneficial effect in ADHD, producing promising results. One randomised study involving 400 Turkish children with a mean age of 9.6 years found that treatment with 150 mg zinc sulfate (equivalent to 40 mg of elemental zinc) daily for 12 weeks resulted in significant reductions in hyperactive, impulsive and impaired socialisation features, but not in reducing attention deficiency symptoms, as assessed by the ADHD scale (Bilici et al 2004). A significant difference between zinc and placebo was evident by week 4 ($P = 0.01$). Older children with low zinc and free fatty acid levels and high body mass index responded best to treatment.

A second placebo-controlled trial used a combination of 55 mg zinc sulfate (equivalent to 15 mg elemental zinc) and methylphenidate (1 mg/kg) daily for 6 weeks in Iranian children aged 5–11 years and reported significant benefits with the combination (Akhondzadeh et al 2004). Zinc (15 mg/day elemental) or placebo was administered to 218 grade three students in a low-income district of Turkey over 10 weeks, resulting in a reduced prevalence of clinically significant ratings of attention deficit and hyperactivity in the treatment group (Uçkardeş et al 2009). As all of these early studies were conducted in Middle Eastern countries where zinc deficiency is particularly prevalent, researchers were keen to see results of studies conducted in other regions and the chance arose with an American three-phased pilot study published in 2011 (Arnold et al 2011).

Being a pilot study, the numbers are small ($n = 52$, with only 28 assigned to zinc); however, the methodology is regarded as substantially superior to prior studies, including more comprehensive zinc assessment both pre- and posttreatment. The first phase was essentially a single-blind 8-week trial of zinc (15 mg/day as glycinate) compared with placebo, while the second phase added in open-label amphetamine (dosage according to body weight), maintained over 2 weeks. The third phase, which lasted 3 weeks, allowed clinicians to closely monitor and accordingly titrate the dose of amphetamine with no change to the zinc or placebo from the first phase. The findings were that zinc supplementation was not effective either alone or as an adjunct to amphetamines in the management of ADHD; however, it did reduce the effective dose necessary of the stimulant medication. What is particularly interesting about this study, the negative findings of which are given a lot of weight in a recent review by Ghanizadeh & Berk (2013), is the low zinc dose used and the subsequent failure to raise serum zinc in the supplemented group. In fact, in the third phase the researchers doubled this dose in 8 subjects, which produced greater improvements both on serum levels and behaviour ratings, begging the question of whether the dose administered to the majority was inadequate.

Somewhat similarly, two longer-term studies (6 months) conducted in Mexico and Guatemala failed to find a positive effect from zinc supplementation. However, in both instances, zinc oxide (a poorly absorbed form) was used to provide only 10 mg elemental zinc per day and there were numerous other confounding variables, e.g. lead intoxication (Kordas et al 2005) and lack of diagnostic criteria and selection for ADHD children only (DiGirolamo et al 2010).

The aforementioned systematic review includes the American study by Arnold and two of the mid-Eastern trials, ultimately concluding that there is insufficient evidence of efficacy for zinc in the management of ADHD and recommending that future studies correct for methodological flaws of the past (Ghanizadeh & Berk 2013). Until there is research of a higher standard with consistent outcomes, the case for zinc in ADHD is promising but requires further investigation to determine optimal dosage, treatment regimens and what symptoms are most likely to respond.

Depression

Zinc deficiency has been investigated as a contributing factor to the development of depression. Zinc supplementation has also been investigated as a treatment in depression, most commonly as an adjunctive therapy taken with standard pharmaceutical agents, for which there is positive evidence.

Epidemiological evidence has revealed an inverse relationship between serum zinc and depression-rating scores in depressed patients (Nowak et al 2005, Siwek et al 2010), the elderly (Marcellini et al 2006) and postpartum women (Wojcik et al 2006). Inadequate dietary intake has also been correlated with increased depression rates, particularly amongst women, in an American food frequency study (Maserejian et al 2012). A meta-analysis of 17 epidemiological studies ($n = 1643$ depressed individuals and 804 controls) investigating zinc levels and depression adds further weight to this association (Swardfager et al 2013), with 16 studies demonstrating a relationship. While meta-analysis found the actual difference in plasma/serum zinc to be small — approximately −1.85 micromol/L lower in depressed compared with control individuals ($P < 0.00001$) — the effect size increased in individuals with more severe depression, inpatients and studies with more robust methodology. It is important to note that these lower levels were typically still within the established reference range. While associations do not prove causality, there is also an increasing body of evidence piecing together how zinc might convey such antidepressant effects.

Zinc supplementation produces antidepressant-like effects in animal tests and models such as the forced-swim test and can augment the action of orthodox antidepressants in these scenarios (Nowak et al 2005). Theories regarding zinc's aetiological role in depression traditionally centred on its inhibition of *N*-methyl-D-aspartate receptor function and regulation of both hippocampal and cortical glutaminergic circuits and, interestingly, suicide victims demonstrate a statistically significant 26% decrease in zinc's antagonistic potency in hippocampal tissue, suggestive of an aberrant interaction between this mineral and the receptor underlying the psychopathology (Nowak et al 2003). There is current interest in the increased inflammatory markers evident in depressed individuals, which would, through redistribution of zinc, potentially create a pseudodeficiency (Marcellini et al 2006, Nowak et al 2005) and, via zinc's roles in both immunity generally and antioxidant defence specifically, improve with supplementation (Swardfager et al 2013, Szewczyk et al 2011). Other theories regarding mechanisms include zinc's capacity to increase synaptic dopamine levels (Stockner et al 2013), its critical role in fatty acid metabolism (Swardfager et al 2013), increased neural plasticity, increased hippocampal BDNF RNA and inhibition of the GSK-3 enzyme (Szewczyk et al 2008).

In spite of growing interest in zinc's antidepressant potential, there have been limited published interventional studies to date. Twenty patients with unipolar depression had an improved response to antidepressant medication when it was taken with zinc aspartate supplements (equivalent to 25 mg elemental daily), according to a small, double-blind pilot study (Nowak et al 2003). Significantly greater reductions in Hamilton Depression Rating Scale scores were achieved with zinc treatment compared to placebo by the 6th week and maintained until the end of the 12-week study. The same research group published the results of a study very similar in design, using ≈140 mg imipramine and 25 mg supplemental zinc ($n = 30$), compared with imipramine and placebo in the control group ($n = 30$) over 12 weeks, also with positive findings (Siwek et al 2009), and in a follow-up publication were able to show that treatment-resistant subjects had lower serum zinc (−14%) when compared with those subjects responsive to treatment, as did those who had had depression for a longer duration. They also found that serum zinc increased in all responders whether supplemented or not, concurrent with remission and a negative correlation between serum zinc and ratings on the Montgomery-Asberg Depression Rating Scale at the study's conclusion in all subjects (Siwek et al 2010). Based on their findings, Siwek et al go as far as to say that changes in serum zinc can be viewed as a state marker of depression and remission. A 2012 review paper which includes the Nowak et al and Siwek et al studies, as well as two others, concludes that there is consistent evidence of zinc's efficacy as an adjunct to antidepressants but less certainty as a stand-alone treatment (Lai et al 2012).

Diarrhoea

An updated 2013 Cochrane review of oral zinc treatment for paediatric diarrhoea which analysed results from 18 randomised controlled trials (n = 6165) concluded that zinc supplementation consistently reduced the duration and volume of both acute and persistent diarrhoea within a few days (for example, by day 3 of the intervention: RR 0.69, 95% CI 0.59–0.81; 1073 children, two trials) (Lazzerini & Ronfani 2013). While zinc-treated children were significantly more likely to experience vomiting as an adverse reaction to the supplement, it was concluded that the benefits of the treatment outweighed this side effect.

Typically, the intervention consisted of 10 mg/day of zinc, as a sulfate, acetate or gluconate salt, administered in a single or divided dose over 2 weeks to children aged 1 month to 5 years presenting with acute or persistent diarrhoea or dysentery. It is important to note that all except three of these trials were conducted in countries considered to be at high risk of widespread zinc deficiency and in such instances, due to the high rates of malnourishment, the RDA for zinc for <5-year-olds jumps to 2–4 mg/kg compared with only 3–5 mg/day in developed countries. Interestingly, however, there was no effect from geographical location, background zinc deficiency, supplemental form or general nutritional status. This review found no benefit in children less than 6 months old and it remains unclear at this time whether morbidity rates were impacted in children of any age.

Coeliac disease

Untreated coeliac patients demonstrate increased turnover and losses of intestinal zinc, although the mechanisms behind this appear to be greater than malabsorption alone (Tran et al 2011). In fact, researchers claim that zinc deficiency is the earliest and most pronounced nutritional issue in untreated CD adults (Scrimgeour & Condlin 2009), and researchers investigating zinc status in children undergoing investigation for CD concluded that a low serum zinc should be a prompt in this cohort for small-bowel biopsy (Hogberg et al 2009). A study of zinc homeostasis in children with CD found a correlation between impaired disaccharide digestion, reduced fractional zinc absorption and reduced zinc status and suggested that treated CD patients with ongoing gastrointestinal derangement are key candidates for zinc deficiency (Tran et al 2011). Interestingly, zinc is a potent inhibitor of the tissue transglutaminase (tTG) type 2 enzyme, therefore in zinc deficiency this will lead to greater activation of tTG, ultimately increasing the inflammation and villi atrophy at the core of CD pathology (Scrimgeour & Condlin 2009, Stenberg et al 2008). Recent research adds to concerns of zinc deficiency in the CD population, in finding that a gluten-free diet provides inadequate zinc levels for most individuals, therefore making supplementation a necessity (Shepherd & Gibson 2013). To date there are no published studies investigating the benefits of zinc supplementation in CD.

Crohn's disease

Zinc is important in the maintenance of gastrointestinal barrier function. Research has revealed that patients with inflammatory bowel disease with low mucosal zinc levels typically accumulate neutrophils in epithelial crypts and the intestinal lumen, resulting in the formation of crypt abscesses, which constitute a serious complication of the disease (Scrimgeour & Condlin 2009). Although reduced zinc status has long been associated with chronic diarrhoea and Crohn's disease (Sturniolo et al 1980), the results from a small open study demonstrated that oral zinc sulfate (110 mg three times daily) resolved intestinal permeability problems in people with increased permeability and decreased relapse rates (Sturniolo et al 2001). Given animal and human evidence suggesting that the supplemental form, zinc carnosine, has particular injury/ulcer-preventing actions (Mahmood et al 2007, Watari et al 2013), some researchers speculate whether this may be especially indicated in patients with inflammatory bowel disease (Scrimgeour & Condlin 2009).

Anorexia nervosa

Evidence suggests zinc deficiency may be intimately involved with anorexia nervosa, if not as an initiating cause, then as an accelerating or 'sustaining' factor for abnormal eating behaviours that may deepen the pathology of the anorexia in relation to neurological, immunological and metabolic aberrations (McClain et al 1992, Saito et al 2007, Shay & Mangian 2000). Zinc status is compromised due to an inadequate zinc intake, with supplementation (50 mg elemental zinc/day) shown to decrease depression and anxiety, stop body weight loss and improve weight gain (Katz et al 1987, Safai-Kutti 1990). According to one randomised, double-blind, placebo-controlled trial, 100 mg of zinc gluconate (14 mg/day elemental) doubled the rate of subjects with anorexia nervosa increasing their body mass index compared to placebo (Birmingham et al 1994); however, two other studies in a similiar cohort administered 50 mg zinc/day failed to show any improvement over placebo in weight gain (Flament et al 2012). Results from a series of animal studies suggest that zinc may stimulate food intake in short-term zinc-deficient rats through the afferent vagus nerve, with subsequent effects on hypothalamic peptides, such as increased expression of neuropeptide Y and orexin (Suzuki et al 2011). Accordingly, some key researchers advocate for routine prescribing of zinc for a minimum of 2 months in all anorexia nervosa patients (Birmingham & Gritzner 2006), in spite of reviewers concluding there is inadequate evidence to support this practice (Flament et al 2012).

Recent research has highlighted significantly greater serum zinc in recovered individuals when compared with those who remain ill; however, this is speculated to be largely due to altered dietary intake (Zepf et al 2012a) and, although leptin levels also increase during remission, a small epidemiological study failed to find a correlation between these two phenomena (Zepf et al 2012b).

Improves taste perception

Dysfunctional taste perception, or dysgeusia, is a condition that can at the least affect quality of life and occasionally can become life-threatening. Research into the aetiology of taste impairment has revealed a long list of possible causes and contributing factors, including various pathologies and drugs (Brown & Toma 1986, Deems et al 1991, Ikeda et al 2005, Kettaneh et al 2005, Osaki et al 1996, Rareshide & Amedee 1989, Zverev 2004). The pioneer of research in zinc-related taste acuity, Henkin, concluded in 1976 that zinc could not explain all cases of taste impairment (Henkin et al 1976). A subsequent review concurred: 'depletion of zinc can lead to decreased taste acuity but decreased taste acuity is not necessarily associated with depletion of zinc' (Catalanotto 1978).

Impaired gustatory function in the elderly is also well established (Bales et al 1986, Bartoshuk 1989, Deems et al 1991, Greger 1977, Greger & Geissler 1978, Ikeda et al 2005, Kettaneh et al 2005, Sandstead et al 1982, Schiffman 1983), particularly in relation to salt perception (Bales et al 1986, Greger & Sickles 1979, Sandstead et al 1982). Although zinc status also characteristically declines with age (Bales et al 1986, Greger 1977, Greger & Geissler 1978, Sandstead et al 1982), many studies have failed to demonstrate a consistent correlation between the two phenomena. While this has been challenged by the findings of a study (Stewart-Knox et al 2005), previous large-scale studies of elderly patients presenting with hypogeusia or ageusia have indicated that zinc deficiency represents the sole cause in <40% of elderly patients (Deems et al 1991, Ikeda et al 2005). Other major causes of taste impairment in this age group include the effect of medications and systemic diseases (Deems et al 1991, Ikeda et al 2005, Schiffman 1983). Consequently, confirmation of zinc deficiency in patients with taste impairment is necessary in order to determine the suitability of zinc as a treatment.

Several interventional studies investigating zinc as a treatment for taste impairment have produced generally positive findings. Zinc supplementation of 140 mg of zinc gluconate (20 mg/day elemental) in 50 patients with idiopathic dysgeusia improved gustatory function when compared with placebo (Heckmann et al 2005). In another study of 109 patients with idiopathic taste impairment, including some with low serum zinc, subjects were randomly assigned to either placebo or one of three zinc treatment groups: 17 mg/day, 34 mg/day or 68 mg/day zinc carnosine for 12 weeks (Sakagami et al 2008).

Only those patients receiving 68 mg/day demonstrated significantly improved gustatory sensitivity over placebo. Two studies focusing specifically on improving taste perception in the elderly (Ikeda et al 2008, Stewart-Knox et al 2008) have been successful, particularly in relation to increased salt sensitivity and in the former study achieved a 74% response rate for improved gustatory function generally. However, benefit was only evident at doses ≥30 mg/day elemental zinc presented either as a gluconate or as a carnosine complex (Aliani et al 2013).

In contrast, treatment with zinc sulfate (45 mg three times daily) concomitant with and 1 month following radiotherapy treatment in patients suffering from head and neck cancers did not prevent taste alterations typically associated with this treatment and previously speculatively linked with poor zinc status (Halyard et al 2007). A more recent double-blind randomised controlled trial investigating zinc supplementation (50 mg elemental per day as a sulfate) over 3 months in taste disorders of patients receiving chemotherapy ($n = 58$) also failed to demonstrate any beneficial effect over placebo (Lyckholm et al 2012). Limitations of this study include the informal assessment of taste and lack of baseline zinc assessment, with the researchers concluding that more studies are necessary. New areas of research are investigating relationships between zinc status and specific genetic polymorphisms that impact taste (Noh et al 2013).

Tinnitus

In addition to its many diverse neurological roles, zinc has specifically been shown to modulate synaptic function in the cochlear nucleus through its involvement with glutamate receptors (Coehlo et al 2007). Also required for production of Cu/Zn SOD, the most abundant antioxidant enzyme in this tissue, zinc has a critical role in its healthy function through control of oxidation and the large amounts of generated ROS. There is also evidence that a deficiency of Cu/Zn SOD potentiates ear hair cell degeneration secondary to excessive oxidative damage. Other recent theories regarding zinc's role include its role in the structure of carbonic anhydrase, which removes free radicals in the vascular stria of the cochlea, and its ability to alter the endocochlear potential, altering cochlear electrophysiology (Ferreira et al 2009). In 1987, a report was published suggesting a link between reduced zinc status and intermittent head noises in people suffering with tinnitus (Gersdorff et al 1987). This has been further investigated in several studies; however, the poorly defined patient groups and use of serum zinc as the means of measuring zinc status make interpretation of results difficult to assess (Coehlo et al 2007). Results from these studies, however, suggest a non-significant trend of lower serum zinc values for patients suffering this condition compared to healthy controls.

In 1991 Paaske et al reported the results of a double-blind randomised controlled trial of 48 patients with tinnitus that failed to find a significant effect on symptoms with sustained-release zinc sulfate tablets. Of note, only one subject had low serum zinc levels. A study of 111 subjects aged 20 59 years found that individuals with tinnitus who had normal hearing had significantly lower serum zinc levels than controls, whereas zinc levels were normal for those with accompanying hearing loss (Ochi et al 2003). In addition, a significant correlation between average hearing sensitivity and serum zinc level was observed. Yetiser et al (2002) investigated serum zinc levels and response to supplementation in 40 patients with severe tinnitus of various origins. Some relief in tinnitus symptoms was reported by 57.5% of all subjects who received 220 mg of zinc daily for 2 months; however, the effect was considered minor. When results were divided by age, a different finding emerged, as 82% of people over 50 years of age experienced an improvement on the tinnitus scale compared to only 48% of younger subjects. There was no correlation between severity of tinnitus and serum zinc levels. Zinc supplementation (50 mg/day) was further studied in a randomised, placebo-controlled trial involving 41 Turkish patients with tinnitus of no known cause. Active treatment for 2 months produced clinically favourable progress in 46.4% of subjects; however, this result was not statistically significant (Arda et al 2003).

A review of these studies concluded that, although hampered by methodological weaknesses, zinc treatment may be beneficial in some tinnitus sufferers and, while an optimal dose for zinc has yet to be elucidated, most successful designs have employed 50–66 mg/day of elemental zinc in divided doses (Coehlo et al 2007). A randomised double-blind placebo-controlled cross-over trial designed by Coehlo et al tried to address the limitations of previous studies (Coehlo et al 2013). In a total sample size of 94, individuals were administered zinc 50 mg/day or placebo for a duration of 4 months followed by a 1-month wash-out and then treatment with the other for the same period. Final analysis revealed that 5% of individuals found their tinnitus improved with zinc and 2% with placebo, the difference being not statistically significant. Subsequently these authors concluded that zinc is not an effective treatment in tinnitus.

Warts

Oral zinc sulfate (10 mg/kg) supplements administered in three divided doses per day (up to 600 mg/day) for 2 months completely cleared recalcitrant viral warts in 87% of patients, according to a single-blind, placebo-controlled trial of 80 volunteers with at least 15 viral warts that were resistant to other treatments (Al Gurairi et al 2002). Warts were completely cleared in 61% of patients after 1 month of treatment, whereas none of the patients receiving placebo reported a successful response and some developed new warts. In both placebo and treatment groups, the drop-out rates were high: 50% and

45%, respectively. Interestingly, patients in the treatment group with low serum zinc baseline levels (mean 62.4 mcg/100 mL) reportedly exhibited no signs or symptoms of deficiency and zinc serum levels failed to rise in the patients who remained resistant to zinc therapy. Treatment with high-dose zinc supplements was accompanied by nausea and in some cases vomiting and mild epigastric pain, although these symptoms were described as mild and transient. A similar intervention was employed in a 2011 open-label study of 31 individuals with non-genital recurring warts with the same dose of zinc sulfate administered over 2 months. While 58% of subjects had deficient serum zinc at baseline, 50% were classed as responders, with full resolution of the warts and no recurrences within a 6-month follow-up (Mun et al 2011).

Wilson's disease

Due to the fact that zinc blocks copper absorption and increases its elimination in people with Wilson's disease, zinc supplementation is a common treatment in this condition. Patients with diagnosed Wilson's disease have increased hepatic glutathione and reduced oxidation when supplemented with zinc sulfate (220 mg three times daily) for 3 months, compared with those using penicillamine (Farinati et al 2003).

OTHER USES

Reducing the risk of cancer

Epidemiological studies suggest that zinc deficiency may be associated with increased risk of cancer (Prasad & Kucuk 2002). Research into mechanisms behind zinc and cancer prevention are being actively pursued via both in vitro (Hong et al 2012) and in vivo research and a key topic of discussion centres around evidence of zinc dysregulation in both prostate and breast cancer (Alam & Kelleher 2012, Ho et al 2011). As yet, however, there are no clinical trials or clear clinical directives from this research.

HIV and AIDS

Given zinc deficiency most profoundly compromises T-cell function, interest in zinc treatment for HIV and AIDS has been ongoing. Low plasma zinc concentration occurs in HIV infection, especially with advancing illness (Wellinghausen et al 2000). The balance of evidence favours the view that a low plasma zinc level is a marker for disease progression (Siberry et al 2002). A series of small interventional studies have produced mixed results, some demonstrating improved immune markers and reduced opportunistic infections (Mocchegiani et al 1995, Zazzo et al 1989), while others suggesting either no therapeutic effect or increased risk of progression from HIV to AIDS (Tang et al 1996). These contrasting findings have been speculatively attributed to differences in baseline zinc status amongst subjects. One author points out that antiretroviral treatment has been shown to counteract zinc deficiency and therefore administering zinc to individuals taking this medication may enhance the risk of zinc toxicity and its associated immune impairment (Overbeck et al 2008). A small pilot study (n = 31) looked specifically at zinc supplementation in the treatment of immune discordance (defined as complete viral suppression without a rise in $CD4^+$ counts, which is associated with increased morbidity and mortality) amongst HIV-positive patients (Asdamongkol et al 2013). While the results found that 39% of these individuals had deficient plasma zinc, this is not strikingly dissimilar from the incidence in the general HIV population. They also reported that zinc supplementation (15 mg/day as a chelate for 6 months) resulted in increases in $CD4^+$ counts; however, due to the small numbers and lack of control group, their findings are weakened.

In a well-designed larger randomised placebo-controlled study of 231 HIV-positive adults, the treatment group received 12 mg (females) or 15 mg (males) zinc daily for 18 months. In comparison to placebo, zinc treatment was found to reduce the rate of immunological failure, defined as any $CD4^+$ count <200 cells/mm^3 fourfold (RR = 0.24; P < 0.002) and also significantly reduced the occurrence of diarrhoea (OR = 0.4; P = 0.019) (Baum et al 2010).

A 2010 Cochrane review, which does not include the studies cited here, included just two trials in adults (n = 559) and two in children (n = 128) and concluded that zinc supplementation is yet to be established as a beneficial adjunct in HIV management, except in the instance of prevention of diarrhoea in children, where there is a significant decrease in those treated with zinc (P = 0.001) (Irlam et al 2013). One of the limitations, however, of this review is the disparate nature of the HIV populations (from pregnant women to those suffering protracted diarrhoea), as well as heterogeneous design.

Malaria

Duggan et al (2005) identified low plasma zinc levels in children with acute malaria, including a significant correlation between evidence of illness severity, C-reactive protein levels and zinc status; however, this may be an artifact of the acute-phase effects on zinc homeostasis, rather than indicative of genuine depletion (Overbeck et al 2008). Similarly, a recent cross-sectional survey of children in Laos revealed a surprising inverse relationship between serum zinc and anti-*Plasmodium falciparum* IgG antibodies (e.g. an increase of 1 mcg/dL in serum zinc equated with −0.453 in antibody titre, P = 0.003) in individuals with active malaria; however, low zinc secondary to inflammation is flagged as a possible confounding variable by the researchers (Akiyama et al 2013).

Zinc supplementation (10 mg elemental) randomly allocated to preschool children residing in a malaria-endemic region of Papua New Guinea for

6 days a week over 46 weeks reduced morbidity due to *P. falciparum* (Shankar et al 2000). Further studies have produced contradictory findings in relation to zinc's capacity to prevent malaria, while studies of treatment regimens that include zinc as an adjuvant to standard chemotherapy have found no benefit (Overbeck et al 2008). A 2011 review into zinc treatment and the prevention of both morbidity and mortality in <5 years old in developing countries included four studies wherein zinc supplementation was assessed for effect on malaria incidence and found the pooled data failed to reach statistical significance (RR = 0.92; P = 1.04) (Yakoob et al 2011). Similarly, with regard to malaria-related mortality, there was a 10% non-significant reduction in association with zinc supplementation (RR = 0.90; P = 1.06).

IN COMBINATION

Subsequent to this review a study designed to investigate whether zinc adds to the preventive effects of vitamin A supplementation in malaria morbidity in Ghana infants administered either a one-off dose of 100,000 IU (<12 months old)/200,000 IU (>12 months old) vitamin A alone (n = 88) or additional elemental zinc of 10 mg/day for 6 months (n = 87) (Owusu-Agyei et al 2013). Follow-up was also performed 6 months after the conclusion of the supplementation phase. Results show a further 27% reduction in uncomplicated malaria incidence in those infants administered zinc (P = 0.03), which equates to reducing incidence from 62.5% in the vitamin A group to 46% in the combined treatment group. The combined intervention, however, failed to have any statistically significant impact on the incidence of other key morbidities such as diarrhoea, pneumonia and severe malaria over vitamin A alone: the reason for this is unknown. It is perhaps noteworthy that the change in plasma zinc from baseline to end point did not reach statistical significance in the supplemented group.

Alzheimer's dementia

There is significant ongoing discussion about the role of zinc deficiency in Alzheimer's disease in the scientific literature. Epidemiological studies have produced some mixed results (da Silva et al 2013, Kyumcu et al 2013, Szewczyk 2013), which may well be the result of disparate methodologies for assessment.

Cognitive performance was temporarily improved after 3 months of zinc supplementation (zinc chelate 15 mg) taken twice daily by six subjects with Alzheimer's disease (Potocnik et al 1997). Although the initial improvement was not maintained in this small open study, a modest cognitive improvement on psychometric testing was observed at 12 months for the four patients evaluated. A double-blind study tested 150 mg of a new zinc formulation per day (unknown elemental zinc content) or placebo for 6 months given to 58 subjects, 29 with Alzheimer's disease and 29 age- and sex-matched controls (Brewer & Kaur 2013). Zinc supplementation was found to raise serum zinc and reduce free copper as anticipated, but cognitive effects were limited to a non-significant trend towards improvement. Post hoc analysis, however, of those subjects >70 years in the treatment group (n = 14) revealed a significant cognitive benefit on all three tests (P = 0.067). While the researchers report these to be 'exciting' results, they also concede that the small sample size and need for post hoc analysis mean that much larger and better-designed studies are necessary to confirm their findings.

DOSAGE RANGE

Australian RDI

Children

- 1–3 years: 3 mg/day
- 4–8 years: 4 mg/day
- 9–13 years: 6 mg/day
- Males 14–18 years: 13 mg/day
- Females 14–18 years: 7 mg/day.

Adults

- Males >18 years: 14 mg/day
- Females >18 years: 8 mg/day.

Pregnancy

- <19 years: 10 mg/day
- ≥19 years: 11 mg/day.

Deficiency

- 25–50 mg elemental zinc daily.

According to clinical studies

- Common cold — zinc acetate lozenges are the most effective (free of sorbitol, mannitol or citric acid).
- Adults: 9–24 mg elemental zinc dissolved in the mouth, without chewing, every 2 hours for acute treatment. Total daily dose should provide ≥75 mg of elemental zinc.
- School-aged children: zinc acetate lozenges four times daily for acute treatment.
- It is recommended that citrus fruits or juices be avoided 30 minutes before or after dissolving each lozenge to avoid negating the effects of zinc.
- Improved immune function in elderly — 45 mg/day elemental zinc as zinc gluconate.
- Common cold — nasal gel sprays are no longer recommended due to the high incidence of temporary anosmia associated with their use.
- Pneumonia — 70 mg/day prophylactically or 20 mg/day in children suffering acute infection — especially in non-bacterial cases.
- Malaria — 10 mg/day elemental zinc.
- ARMD — zinc oxide (equivalent to 80 mg elemental zinc), together with 500 mg vitamin C, 400 IU vitamin E, taken daily, or 50 mg/day of zinc as zinc monocysteine as stand-alone treatment.
- ADHD — 30–40 mg elemental zinc daily.

- Depression – 25 mg elemental zinc per day.
- Type 1 diabetes — 30 mg/day (type of zinc unknown).
- Type 2 diabetes — 50 mg/day zinc acetate.
- Wound healing — 2.5 mg/kg zinc sulfate daily: zinc oxide form preferable topically.
- Leg ulcers — 600 mg zinc sulfate daily.
- Male fertility — 60 mg/day of zinc sulfate and 5 mg/day as folic acid.
- Acne vulgaris — 90–200 mg (50 mg elemental) daily.
- Crohn's disease — 110 mg zinc sulfate taken three times daily. However, a zinc carnosine preparation may be more appropriate.
- Diarrhoea — 10–20 mg/day elemental zinc in children between 6 months and 5 years for 2 weeks. Note: this dose was used in populations with a high prevalence of zinc deficiency.
- Herpes infection — 4% zinc sulfate solution applied via a cotton bud every 5 days for a month, then every 10 days for 2 months and finally every 15 days for 3 months.
- Anorexia nervosa — 14–50 mg elemental zinc daily.
- Dysgeusia — 20 mg/day elemental zinc as zinc gluconate and 68 mg/day as zinc carnosine.
- Tinnitus — 50–200 mg daily of zinc (salt unknown). Unclear benefit.
- Warts — 10 mg/kg zinc sulfate taken orally in three divided doses (up to 600 mg/day) for 1–2 months.

TOXICITY

Signs of toxicity are nausea, vomiting, diarrhoea, fever and lethargy and have been observed after ingestion of 4–8 g zinc according to a 2002 World Health Organization report. Single doses of 225–450 mg of zinc usually induce vomiting (King 2003).

Doses of zinc ranging from 100 to 150 mg/day interfere with copper metabolism and cause hypocuprinaemia, red blood cell microcytosis and neutropenia if used long-term.

ADVERSE REACTIONS

Mild gastrointestinal distress has been reported at doses of 50–150 mg/day of supplemental zinc (King 2003). According to a randomised, double-blind study, zinc gluconate glycine lozenge (104 mg, equivalent to 13.3 mg ionic zinc) taken every 3–4 hours is well tolerated (Silk & Lefante 2005). Of the side effects that were reported, dry mouth and a burning sensation on the tongue were probably related to use, whereas symptoms of nausea, dizziness, lightheadedness and upset stomach were considered as possibly related.

SIGNIFICANT INTERACTIONS

Calcium

High levels of dietary calcium impair zinc absorption in animals, but it is uncertain whether this occurs in humans — separate doses by 2 hours.

Angiotensin-converting enzyme inhibitors, angiotensin II receptor blockers and thiazide diuretics

These drugs reduce zinc status, most likely due to increased urinary excretion of zinc (Braun and Rosenfeldt 2013). Increased zinc intake may be required with long-term drug treatment.

Coffee

Coffee reduces zinc absorption — separate intakes by 2 hours (Pecoud et al 1975).

Copper

High zinc intakes (100–150 mg/day) interfere with copper metabolism and can cause hypocuprinaemia with long-term use. Avoid using high-dose zinc supplements long-term, or increase intake of copper.

Folate

Folate intake may reduce zinc levels — observe patient for signs and symptoms of zinc deficiency with long-term folate supplementation.

Iron

Supplemental (38–65 mg/day elemental) iron decreases zinc absorption (King 2003) — separate doses by 2 hours.

Non-steroidal anti-inflammatory drugs

Zinc interacts with non-steroidal anti-inflammatory drugs by forming complexes with these drugs (Dendrinou-Samara et al 1998) — separate dose by 2 hours.

Tetracyclines and quinolones

Complex formation between zinc and tetracycline results in reduced absorption of both substances with potential reduction in efficacy — separate dose by 2 hours.

Thiazide and loop diuretics

These diuretics increase urinary zinc loss — monitor for signs and symptoms of zinc deficiency with long-term drug use. Increased zinc intake may be required with long-term therapy.

Methylphenidate

The efficacy of this drug is improved by supplementation with zinc sulfate (15 mg elemental zinc) for 6 weeks in children with ADHD. There is no change to side effects reported (Akhondzadeh et al 2004).

Vaccinations

Zinc acetate improved seroconversion of vibriocidal antibodies in children given a cholera vaccination (Albert et al 2003) in both faecal and serum titres (Karlsen et al 2003).

Radiotherapy

Radiotherapy reduces plasma zinc levels (Ertekin et al 2004). Supplementation may be required with intensive radiotherapy treatment.

Interferon-alpha/ribavirin

Interferon-alpha and ribavirin treatment for hepatitis C patients is not affected by zinc supplementation (Ko et al 2005).

Orlistat

Orlistat has no significant effect on zinc levels (Zhi et al 2003).

Tricyclic antidepressants and selective serotonin reuptake inhibitors (SSRIs)

Zinc supplementation (25 mg elemental zinc daily) improves the efficacy of antidepressants such as tricyclic antidepressants and SSRIs after 2 weeks of intervention (Nowak et al 2003) — beneficial interaction possible.

CONTRAINDICATIONS AND PRECAUTIONS

Amiloride reduces zinc excretion and can lead to zinc accumulation (Reyes et al 1983). Therefore, supplementation should be used with caution.

PREGNANCY USE

Zinc is safe in pregnancy and may improve fetal heart rate in zinc-deficient mothers (in conjunction with iron and folic acid) (Merialdi et al 2004).

Practice points/Patient counselling

- Zinc is involved in many chemical reactions that are important for normal body functioning and it is essential for health and wellbeing.
- Although zinc supplements are traditionally used to treat deficiency, they are also used to prevent deficiency in conditions associated with low zinc status or deficiency, such as acrodermatitis enteropathica, anorexia nervosa, malabsorption syndromes, conditions associated with chronic diarrhoea, alcoholism, liver cirrhosis, diabetes, HIV and AIDS, recurrent infections, severe burns, postsurgery and sickle cell anaemia.
- Zinc supplements are also popular among athletes in order to counteract zinc loss that occurs through perspiration.
- Zinc lozenges have been used to prevent and treat the symptoms of the common cold and oral supplements have been used to treat acne vulgaris, improve wound healing and chronic leg ulcers, resolve intestinal permeability problems and reduce recurrences in Crohn's disease, treat recalcitrant warts, reduce symptoms of tinnitus and improve ADHD.
- Topical applications of zinc have been used to treat acne vulgaris (in combination with erythromycin) and herpes simplex and to promote wound healing.
- Numerous interactions exist between other minerals, foods and medicines and zinc.

PATIENTS' FAQs

What will this supplement do for me?
Zinc is found in every cell of the body and is essential for health and wellbeing. Some studies have found that supplements are not only useful to treat and prevent deficiency, but may also be useful in conditions such as the common cold, poor wound healing and leg ulcers, diabetes, Crohn's disease, acne vulgaris, warts, ADHD and tinnitus. Topical preparations may be useful in acne vulgaris (with erythromycin), herpes infection and chronic wounds.

When will it start to work?
This depends on the indication (refer to monograph for more details).

Are there any safety issues?
Used in high doses, zinc can cause nausea, vomiting, gastrointestinal discomfort and, if used long-term, reduce copper levels. Zinc also interacts with a number of other minerals, foods and medicines.

REFERENCES

Agarwal, A., & Sekhon, L. H. (2010). The role of antioxidant therapy in the treatment of male infertility. Hum Fertil (Camb), 13(4), 217–225.

Age-Related Eye Disease Study. A randomized, placebo-controlled, clinical trial of high-dose supplementation with vitamins C and E, beta-carotene, and zinc for age-related macular degeneration and vision loss: AREDS report no. 8. Arch Ophthalmol 119.10 (2001): 1417–36.

Agren MS. Studies on zinc in wound healing. Acta Derm Venereol Suppl (Stockh) 154 (1990): 1–36.

Akhondzadeh S, et al. Zinc sulfate as an adjunct to methylphenidate for the treatment of attention deficit hyperactivity disorder in children: a double blind and randomized trial. BMC Psychiatry 4.1 (2004): 9.

Akiyama, T., et al. (2013). Association between serum zinc concentration and the *Plasmodium falciparum* antibody titer among rural villagers of Attapeu Province, Lao People's Democratic Republic. Acta Trop, 126(3), 193–197.

Alam, S., & Kelleher, S. L. (2012). Cellular mechanisms of zinc dysregulation: a perspective on zinc homeostasis as an etiological factor in the development and progression of breast cancer. Nutrients, 4(8), 875–903.

Albert MJ et al. Supplementation with zinc, but not vitamin A, improves seroconversion to vibriocidal antibody in children given an oral cholera vaccine. J Infect Dis 187.6 (2003): 909–13.

Al Gurairi FT, et al. Oral zinc sulphate in the treatment of recalcitrant viral warts: randomized placebo-controlled clinical trial. Br J Dermatol 146 (2002): 423–31.

Aliani, M., et al. (2013). Zinc deficiency and taste perception in the elderly. Crit Rev Food Sci Nutr, 53(3), 245–250.

Al-Maroof RA, Al-Sharbatti SS. Serum zinc levels in diabetic patients and effect of zinc supplementation on glycemic control of type 2 diabetics. Saudi Med J 27.3 (2006): 344–50.

Antoine, T.E., et al. 2012. Prophylactic, therapeutic and neutralizing effects of zinc oxide tetrapod structures against herpes simplex virus type-2 infection. Antiviral Res., 96, (3) 363–375.

Arda HN et al. The role of zinc in the treatment of tinnitus. Otol Neurotol 24 (2003): 86–9.

Arnold LE, DiSilvestro RA. Zinc in attention-deficit/hyperactivity disorder. J Child Adolesc Psychopharmacol 15 (2005): 619–27.

Arnold LE et al. Does hair zinc predict amphetamine improvement of ADD/hyperactivity? Int J Neurosci 50 (1990): 103–7.

Arnold, L. E., et al. (2011). Zinc for attention-deficit/hyperactivity disorder: placebo-controlled double-blind pilot trial alone and combined with amphetamine. J Child Adolesc Psychopharmacol, 21(1), 1–19.

Asdamongkol, N., et al. (2013). Low plasma zinc levels and immunological responses to zinc supplementation in HIV-infected patients with immunological discordance after antiretroviral therapy. Jpn J Infect Dis, 66(6), 469–474.

Baer MT, King JC. Tissue zinc levels and zinc excretion during experimental zinc depletion in young men. Am J Clin Nutr 39 (1984): 556–70.

Bales CW et al. The effect of age on plasma zinc uptake and taste acuity. Am J Clin Nutr 44 (1986): 664–9.

Bales CW et al. Zinc, magnesium, copper, and protein concentrations in human saliva: age- and sex-related differences. Am J Clin Nutr 51.3 (1990): 462–9.

Bartoshuk LM. Taste. Robust across the age span? Ann N Y Acad Sci 561 (1989): 65–75.

Baum, M.K., et al. 2010. Randomized, controlled clinical trial of zinc supplementation to prevent immunological failure in HIV-infected adults. Clin Infect.Dis., 50, (12) 1653–1660

Baydas B, et al. Effects of oral zinc and magnesium supplementation on serum thyroid hormone and lipid levels in experimentally induced diabetic rats. Biol Trace Elem Res 88.3 (2002): 247–53.

Bedwal RS, Bahuguna A. Zinc, copper and selenium in reproduction. Experientia 50.7 (1994): 626–40.

Beers MH, Berkow R (eds). The Merck manual of diagnosis and therapy, 17th edn. Whitehouse, NJ: Merck, 2003.

Belongia EA, et al. A randomized trial of zinc nasal spray for the treatment of upper respiratory illness in adults. Am J Med 111.2 (2001): 103–8.

Bilici M et al. Double-blind, placebo-controlled study of zinc sulfate in the treatment of attention deficit hyperactivity disorder. Prog Neuropsychopharmacol Biol Psychiatry 28 (2004): 181–90.

Birmingham CL, Gritzner S. How does zinc supplementation benefit anorexia nervosa? Eat Weight Disord 11.4 (2006): e109–11.

Birmingham CL, et al. Controlled trial of zinc supplementation in anorexia nervosa. Int J Eat Disord 15.3 (1994): 251–5.

Birmingham CL et al. Reliability of the AccuSens Taste Kit(c) in patients with eating disorders. Eat Weight Disord 10.2 (2005): e45–8.

Black MM. The evidence linking zinc deficiency with children's cognitive and motor functioning. J Nutr 133 (5 Suppl 1) (2003): 1473S–6S.

Bojar RA et al. Inhibition of erythromycin-resistant propionibacteria on the skin of acne patients by topical erythromycin with and without zinc. Br J Dermatol 130.3 (1994): 329–36.

Bolkent S et al. The influence of zinc supplementation on the pancreas of streptozotocin-diabetic rats. Dig Dis Sci. 2009; 54: 2583–2587.

Bose A et al. Efficacy of zinc in the treatment of severe pneumonia in hospitalized children <2 y old. Am J Clin Nutr 83.5 (2006): 1089–96.

Brandt, S. (2013). The clinical effects of zinc as a topical or oral agent on the clinical response and pathophysiologic mechanisms of acne: a systematic review of the literature. J Drugs Dermatol, 12(5), 542–545.

Braun, L.A. & Rosenfeldt, F. 2013. Pharmaco-nutrient interactions — a systematic review of zinc and antihypertensive therapy. Int.J Clin Pract., 67, (8) 717–725.

Briefel RR et al. Zinc intake of the U.S. population: findings from the third National Health and Nutrition Examination Survey, 1988–1994. J Nutr 130 (2000): 1367–73S.

Brooks WA et al. Zinc for severe pneumonia in very young children: double-blind placebo-controlled trial. Lancet 363.9422 (2004): 1683–8.

Brooks WA et al. Effect of weekly zinc supplements on incidence of pneumonia and diarrhoea in children younger than 2 years in an urban, low-income population in Bangladesh: randomized controlled trial. Lancet 366.9490 (2005): 999–1004.

Brown JE, Toma RB. Taste changes during pregnancy. Am J Clin Nutr 43.3 (1986): 414–8.

Bunker VW et al. Metabolic balance studies for zinc and copper in housebound elderly people and the relationship between zinc balance and leukocyte zinc concentrations. Am J Clin Nutr 46 (1987): 353–9.

Buzina R et al. Zinc nutrition and taste acuity in school children with impaired growth. Am J Clin Nutr 33.11 (1980): 2262–7

Catalanotto F. The trace metal zinc and taste. Am J Clin Nutr 31 (1978): 1098–103.

Chausmer AB. Zinc, insulin and diabetes. J Am Coll Nutr 17.2 (1998): 109–15.

Coehlo CB, et al. Hyperacusis, sound annoyance, and loudness hypersensitivity in children. Progress in Brain Research. Elsevier; 2007: 279–85.

Coehlo, C., et al. (2013). Zinc to treat tinnitus in the elderly: a randomized placebo controlled crossover trial. Otol Neurotol, 34(6), 1146–1154.

Coleman HR et al. Age-related macular degeneration. Lancet 372.9652 (2008): 1835–45.

Coles CL et al. Infectious etiology modifies the treatment effect of zinc in severe pneumonia. Am J Clin Nutr 86.2 (2007): 397–403.

Cunliffe WJ et al. A double-blind trial of a zinc sulphate/citrate complex and tetracycline in the treatment of acne vulgaris. Br J Dermatol 101.3 (1979): 321–5.

Cunningham JJ et al. Hyperzincuria in individuals with insulin-dependent diabetes mellitus: concurrent zinc status and the effect of high-dose zinc supplementation. Metabolism 43.12 (1994): 1558–62.

Davison GW et al. Exercise, free radicals, and lipid peroxidation in type 1 diabetes mellitus. Free Radic Biol Med 33.11 (2002): 1543–51.

Deems DA et al. Smell and taste disorders, a study of 750 patients from the University of Pennsylvania Smell and Taste Center. Arch Otolaryngol Head Neck Surg 117.5 (1991): 519–28.

Dendrinou-Samara C et al. Anti-inflammatory drugs interacting with Zn(II), Cd(II) and Pt(II) metal ions. J Inorg Biochem 71.3–4 (1998): 171–9.

DiGirolamo, A. M., et al. (2010). Randomized trial of the effect of zinc supplementation on the mental health of school-age children in Guatemala. Am J Clin Nutr, 92(5), 1241–1250.

DiSilvestro RA. Zinc in relation to diabetes and oxidative disease. J Nutr 130 (5S Suppl) (2000): 1509–11S.

Dreno B et al. Low doses of zinc gluconate for inflammatory acne. Acta Derm Venereol 69.6 (1989): 541–3.

Dreno B et al. Zinc salts effects on granulocyte zinc concentration and chemotaxis in acne patients. Acta Derm Venereol 72.4 (1992): 250–2.

Dreno B et al. Multicenter randomized comparative double-blind controlled clinical trial of the safety and efficacy of zinc gluconate versus minocycline hydrochloride in the treatment of inflammatory acne vulgaris. Dermatology 203.2 (2001): 135–40.

Dreno B et al. Effect of zinc gluconate on *Propionibacterium acnes* resistance to erythromycin in patients with inflammatory acne: in vitro and in vivo study. Eur J Dermatol 15 (2005): 152–5.

Duggan C et al. Plasma zinc concentrations are depressed during the acute phase response in children with falciparium malaria. J Nutr 135.4 (2005): 802.

Eaton K, et al. Diagnosing human zinc deficiency. A comparison between the Bryce-Smith test and sweat mineral analysis. J Nutr Environ Med 14.2 (2004): 83–7.

Ebisch IM et al. Does folic acid and zinc sulphate intervention affect endocrine parameters and sperm characteristics in men? Int J Androl 29.2 (2006): 339–45.

Ebisch IM et al. The importance of folate, zinc and antioxidants in the pathogenesis and prevention of subfertility. Hum Reprod Update 13.2 (2007): 163–74.

Eby GA, Halcomb WW. Ineffectiveness of zinc gluconate nasal spray and zinc orotate lozenges in common-cold treatment: a double-blind, placebo-controlled clinical trial. Alt Ther Health Med 12.1 (2006): 34–8.

Eggert-Kruse W et al. Are zinc levels in seminal plasma associated with seminal leukocytes and other determinants of semen quality? Fertil Steril 77.2 (2002): 260–9.

Erie JC et al. Reduced zinc and copper in the retinal pigment epithelium and choroid in age-related macular degeneration. Am J Ophthalmol 147.2 (2009): 276–282.e1.

Ertekin MV et al. The effects of oral zinc sulphate during radiotherapy on anti-oxidant enzyme activities in patients with head and neck cancer: a prospective, randomized, placebo-controlled study. Int J Clin Pract 58.7 (2004): 662–8.

Erten J et al. Hair zinc levels in healthy and malnourished children. Am J Clin Nutr 31 (1978): 1172–4.

Evans JR. Antioxidant vitamin and mineral supplements for age-related macular degeneration. Cochrane Database Syst Rev 2 (2002): CD000254.

Fanjiang G, Kleinman RE. Nutrition and performance in children. Curr Opin Clin Nutr Metab Care 10.3 (2007): 342–7.

Farinati F et al. Zinc treatment prevents lipid peroxidation and increases glutathione availability in Wilson's disease. J Lab Clin Med 141.6 (2003): 372–7.

Farvid MS et al. The impact of vitamin and/or mineral supplementation on lipid profiles in type 2 diabetes. Diabetes Res Clin Pract 65.1 (2004): 21–8.

Favier AE. The role of zinc in reproduction: Hormonal mechanisms. Biol Trace Elem Res 32 (1992): 363–82.

Feiner AM et al. Evaluation of the effects of a zinc/iron solution on the migration of fibroblasts in an in-vitro incisional wound healing model. Wounds 15.4 (2003): A23–34.

Ferreira, G. D., et al. (2009). Vestibular evaluation using videonystagmography of chronic zinc deficient patients due to short bowel syndrome. Braz J Otorhinolaryngol, 75(2), 290–294.

Feucht CL et al. Topical erythromycin with zinc in acne: a double-blind controlled study. J Am Acad Dermatol 3.5 (1980): 483–91.

Finnerty EF. Topical zinc in the treatment of herpes simplex. Cutis 37.2 (1986): 130–1.

Flament, M. F., et al. (2012). Evidence-based pharmacotherapy of eating disorders. Int J Neuropsychopharmacol, 15(2), 189–207.

Fletcher AE et al. Sunlight exposure, antioxidants, and age-related macular degeneration. Arch Ophthalmol 126.10 (2008): 1396–403.

Fluhr JW et al. In-vitro and in-vivo efficacy of zinc acetate against propionibacteria alone and in combination with erythromycin. Zentralbl Bakteriol 289.4 (1999): 445–56.

Foster, M., et al. 2013. Effect of vegetarian diets on zinc status: a systematic review and meta-analysis of studies in humans. J Sci. Food Agric., 93, (10) 2362–2371

Fraker PJ et al. The dynamic link between the integrity of the immune system and zinc status. J Nutr 130 (2000): 1399–406S.

Frederickson CJ, Danscher G. Zinc-containing neurons in hippocampus and related CNS structures. Prog Brain Res 83 (1990): 71–84.

Frederickson CJ, Moncrieff DW. Zinc-containing neurons. Biol Signals 3.3 (1994): 127–39.

Frederickson CJ et al. Importance of zinc in the central nervous system: the zinc-containing neuron. J Nutr 130 (5S Suppl) (2000): 1471S–83S.
Freeland-Graves J et al. Salivary zinc as an indicator of zinc status in women fed a low-zinc diet. Am J Clin Nutr 34 (1981): 312–21.
Garg HK, et al. Zinc taste test in pregnant women and its correlation with serum zinc level. Indian J Physiol Pharmacol 37.4 (1993): 318–22.
Gersdorff M et al. A clinical correlation between hypozincemia and tinnitus. Arch Otorhinolaryngol 244 (1987): 190–3.
Ghanizadeh, A., & Berk, M. (2013). Zinc for treating of children and adolescents with attention-deficit hyperactivity disorder: a systematic review of randomized controlled clinical trials. Eur J Clin Nutr, 67(1), 122–124.
Gibson R. Principles of nutritional assessment. New York: Oxford University; 1990.
Gibson RS et al. A growth-limiting, mild zinc deficiency syndrome in some southern Ontario boys with low height percentiles. Am J Clin Nutr 49 (1989): 1266–73.
Godfrey, H.R., et al. 2001. A randomized clinical trial on the treatment of oral herpes with topical zinc oxide/glycine. Altern. Ther. Health Med, 7, (3) 49–56
Golden M. Severe malnutrition. In: Weatherall D, Ledingham J, Warrell D, editors. Oxford textbook of medicine. 3rd edn. Oxford, UK: Ford Medical Publications; 1996. Vol. 1 pp. 1278–85.
Goransson K, et al. Oral zinc in acne vulgaris: a clinical and methodological study. Acta Derm Venereol 58.5 (1978): 443–8.
Gordon P et al. Effect of acute zinc deprivation on plasma zinc and platelet aggregation in adult males. Am J Clin Nutr 35 (1982): 113–9.
Graham RM, et al. Low concentration zinc sulphate solution in the management of recurrent herpes simplex infection. Br J Dermatol 112.1 (1985): 123–4.
Greger J. Dietary intake and nutritional status in regard to zinc of institutionalized aged. J Gerontol 32.5 (1977): 549–53.
Greger JL, Geissler AH. Effect of zinc supplementation on taste acuity of the aged. Am J Clin Nutr 31.4 (1978): 633–7.
Greger JL, Sickles VS. Saliva zinc levels: potential indicators of zinc status. Am J Clin Nutr 32 (1979): 1859–66.
Gropper S, et al. Advanced nutrition and human metabolism. 5th edn. Belmont: Wadsworth Thomson Learning; 2009.
Gupta R et al. Oral zinc therapy in diabetic neuropathy. J Assoc Physicians India 46.11 (1998): 939–42.
Habbema L et al. A 4% erythromycin and zinc combination (Zineryt) versus 2% erythromycin (Eryderm) in acne vulgaris: a randomized, double-blind comparative study. Br J Dermatol 121.4 (1989): 497–502.
Haeger K, Lanner E. Oral zinc sulphate and ischaemic leg ulcers. Vasa 3.1 (1974): 77–81.
Hallbook T, Lanner E. Serum-zinc and healing of venous leg ulcers. Lancet 2.7781 (1972): 780–2.
Halyard MY et al. Does zinc sulfate prevent therapy-induced taste alterations in head and neck cancer patients? Results of phase III double-blind, placebo-controlled trial from the North Central Cancer Treatment Group (N01C4). Int J Radiat Oncol Biol Phys 67.5 (2007): 1318–22.
Hambidge M. Human zinc deficiency. J Nutr 130 (2000): 1344S–9S.
Hambidge C. Biomarkers of trace mineral intake and status. J Nutr 133. Suppl 3 (2003): 948S–55S.
Hayee MA, et al. Diabetic neuropathy and zinc therapy. Bangladesh Med Res Counc Bull 31.2 (2005): 62–7.
Heckmann SM et al. Zinc gluconate in the treatment of dysgeusia: a randomized clinical trial. J Dent Res 84.1 (2005): 35–8.
Henkin RI et al. A syndrome of acute zinc loss. Cerebellar dysfunction, mental changes, anorexia, and taste and smell dysfunction. Arch Neurol 32.11 (1975a): 745–51.
Henkin RI, et al. Estimation of zinc concentration of parotid saliva by flameless atomic absorption spectrophotometry in normal subjects and in patients with idiopathic hypogeusia. J Lab Clin Med 86.1 (1975b): 175–80.
Henkin RI et al. A double blind study of the effects of zinc sulfate on taste and smell dysfunction. Am J Med Sci 272.3 (1976): 285–99.
Henkin RI et al. Fractionation of human parotid saliva proteins. J Biol Chem 253.20 (1977): 7556–65
Higdon J. An evidence-based approach to vitamins and minerals. New York: Thieme, 2003: 197–205.
Hillstrom L et al. Comparison of oral treatment with zinc sulphate and placebo in acne vulgaris. Br J Dermatol 97.6 (1977): 681–4.
Hirt M, et al. Zinc nasal gel for the treatment of common cold symptoms: a double-blind, placebo-controlled trial. Ear Nose Throat J 79.10 (2000): 778–80, 782.
Ho, E., et al. (2011). Dietary factors and epigenetic regulation for prostate cancer prevention. Adv Nutr, 2(6), 497–510.
Hogberg, L., et al. (2009). Serum zinc in small children with coeliac disease. Acta Paediatr, 98(2), 343–345.
Hogg, R. & Chakravarthy, U. 2004. AMD and micronutrient antioxidants. Curr.Eye Res., 29, (6) 387–401
Hong, S. H., et al. (2012). Induction of apoptosis of bladder cancer cells by zinc-citrate compound. Korean J Urol, 53(11), 800–806.
Hotz C et al. Assessment of the trace element status of individuals and populations: the example of zinc and copper. J Nutr 133 (2003): 1563S–8S
Hussain SA et al. Effects of melatonin and zinc on glycemic control in type 2 diabetic patients poorly controlled with metformin. Saudi Med J 27.10 (2006): 1483–8.
Iinuma, K., & Tsuboi, I. (2012). Zinc ascorbate has superoxide dismutase-like activity and in vitro antimicrobial activity against *Staphylococcus aureus* and *Escherichia coli*. Clin Cosmet Investig Dermatol, 5, 135–140.
Iinuma, K., et al. (2011). Susceptibility of *Propionibacterium acnes* isolated from patients with acne vulgaris to zinc ascorbate and antibiotics. Clin Cosmet Investig Dermatol, 4, 161–165.
Ikeda M et al. Taste disorders: a survey of the examination methods and treatment used in Japan. Acta Otolaryngol 125 (2005): 1203–10.
Ikeda M et al. Causative factors of taste disorders in the elderly, and therapeutic effects of zinc. J Laryngol Otol 122.2 (2008): 155–60.
Irlam, J. H., et al. (2013). Micronutrient supplementation for children with HIV infection. Cochrane Database Syst Rev, 10, CD010666.
Islam MS, Loots du T. Diabetes, metallothionein, and zinc interactions: a review. Biofactors 29.4 (2007): 203–12.
IZiNCG. Assessment of the risk of zinc deficiency in populations and options for its control. Food Nutr Bull 25 (2004): S91–S204.
Karlsen TH et al. Intestinal and systemic immune responses to oral cholerz toxoid B subunit whole-cell vaccine administered during zinc supplementation. Infect Immun 71.7 (2003): 3909–13.
Katz RL et al. Zinc deficiency in anorexia nervosa. J Adolesc Health Care 8.5 (1987): 400–6.
Kenney MA et al. Erythrocyte and dietary zinc in adolescent females. Am J Clin Nutr 39 (1984): 446–51.
Kenney, J., et al. (2013). A modified zinc acetate gel, a potential nonantiretroviral microbicide, is safe and effective against simian-human immunodeficiency virus and herpes simplex virus 2 infection in vivo. Antimicrob Agents Chemother, 57(8), 4001–4009.
Kettaneh A et al. Clinical and biological features associated with taste loss in internal medicine patients. A cross-sectional study of 100 cases. Appetite 44.2 (2005): 163–9.
Khozeimeh, F., et al. (2012). Comparative analysis of salivary zinc level in recurrent herpes labialis. Dent Res J (Isfahan), 9(1), 19–23.
King JC. Determinants of maternal zinc status during pregnancy. Am J Clin Nutr 71 (5 Suppl) (2000): 1334S–43S.
King J. Zinc. Oregon: The Linus Pauling Institute, 2003.
King J, Cousins R. Zinc. In: Shils M, et al. editors. Modern nutrition in health and disease. 10th edn. Baltimore: Lippincott Williams & Wilkins; 2006. pp. 271–85.
Klein ML et al. CFH and LOC387715/ARMS2 genotypes and treatment with antioxidants and zinc for age-related macular degeneration. Ophthalmology 115.6 (2008): 1019–25
Kneist W, et al. Clinical double-blind trial of topical zinc sulfate for herpes labialis recidivans. Arzneimittelforschung 45.5 (1995): 624–6.
Ko W-S et al. The effect of zinc supplementation on the treatment of chronic hepatitis C patients with interferon and ribavirin. Clin Biochem 38 (2005): 614–20.
Kordas, K., et al. (2005). Iron and zinc supplementation does not improve parent or teacher ratings of behavior in first grade Mexican children exposed to lead. J Pediatr, 147(5), 632–639.
Kosman DJ, Henkin RI. Erythrocyte zinc in patients with taste and smell dysfunction. Am J Clin Nutr 34.1 (1981): 118–9.
Kumar N et al. Effect of different levels and sources of zinc supplementation on quantitative and qualitative semen attributes and serum testosterone level in crossbred cattle (*Bos indicus* x *Bos taurus*) bulls. Reprod Nutr Dev 46.6 (2006): 663–75.
Kurugöl Z, et al. Effect of zinc sulfate on common cold in children: randomized, double blind study. Pediatr Int 49.6 (2007): 842–7.
Lai, J., et al. (2012). The efficacy of zinc supplementation in depression: systematic review of randomised controlled trials. J Affect Disord, 136(1–2), e31–39.
Lansdown AB. Zinc in the healing wound. Lancet 347.9003 (1996): 706–7.
Lansdown AB et al. Zinc in wound healing: theoretical, experimental, and clinical aspects. Wound Repair Regen 15.1 (2007): 2–16.
Law JS et al. Human salivary gustin is a potent activator of calmodulin-dependent brain phosphodiesterase. Proc Natl Acad Sci U S A 84 (1987): 1674–8.
Lazzerini, M., & Ronfani, L. (2013). Oral zinc for treating diarrhoea in children. Cochrane Database Syst Rev, 1, CD005436.
Lee AY, Brantley MA. C and LOC387715/ARMS2 genotypes and antioxidants and zinc therapy for age-related macular degeneration. Pharmacogenomics 9.10 (2008): 1547–50.
Liu J, Raine A. The effect of childhood malnutrition on externalizing behavior. Curr Opin Pediatr 18.5 (2006): 565–70.

Lonnerdal B. Dietary factors influencing zinc absorption. J Nutr 130 (2000): 1378–83S.

Lyckholm, L., et al. (2012). A randomized, placebo controlled trial of oral zinc for chemotherapy-related taste and smell disorders. J Pain Palliat Care Pharmacother, 26(2), 111–114.

Mahajan SK et al. Effect of oral zinc therapy on gonadal function in hemodialysis patients: a double-blind study. Ann Intern Med 97 (1982): 357–61.

Mahajan, B. B., et al. (2013). Herpes genitalis — Topical zinc sulfate: An alternative therapeutic and modality. Indian J Sex Transm Dis, 34(1), 32–34.

Mahmood, A., et al. (2007). Zinc carnosine, a health food supplement that stabilises small bowel integrity and stimulates gut repair processes. Gut, 56(2), 168–175.

Mahomed K et al. Failure to taste zinc sulphate solution does not predict zinc deficiency in pregnancy. Eur J Obstet Gynecol Reprod Biol 48.3 (1993): 169–75.

Marcellini F et al. Zinc status, psychological and nutritional assessment in old people recruited in five European countries: Zincage study. Biogerontology 7.5–6 (2006): 339–45.

Marreiro DN et al. Abstracts 1644-P, 569-P. In: Proceedings of the American diabetes association annual meeting, June 16–17, 2002.

Maserejian, N. N., et al. (2012). Low dietary or supplemental zinc is associated with depression symptoms among women, but not men, in a population-based epidemiological survey. J Affect Disord, 136(3), 781–788.

McBean L et al. Correlation of zinc concentrations in human plasma and hair. Am J Clin Nutr 24 (1971): 506–9.

McClain CJ et al. Zinc status before and after zinc supplementation of eating disorder patients. J Am Coll Nutr 11.6 (1992): 694–700.

McKenzie JM. Content of zinc in serum, urine, hair, and toenails of New Zealand adults. Am J Clin Nutr 32 (1979): 570–9.

Merialdi M et al. Randomized controlled trial of prenatal zinc supplementation and the development of fetal heart rate. Am J Obstet Gynecol 190.4 (2004): 1106–12.

Mocchegiani E et al. Benefit of oral zinc supplementation as an adjunct to zidovudine (AZT) therapy against opportunistic infections in AIDS. Int J Immunopharmacol 17.9 (1995): 719–27

Morgan AJ et al. The effect of zinc in the form of erythromycin-zinc complex (Zineryt lotion) and zinc acetate on metallothionein expression and distribution in hamster skin. Br J Dermatol 129.5 (1993): 563–70.

Mossad SB. Effect of zincum gluconium nasal gel on the duration and symptom severity of the common cold in otherwise healthy adults. QJM 96.1 (2003): 35–43.

Mun, J. H., et al. (2011). Oral zinc sulfate treatment for viral warts: an open-label study. J Dermatol, 38(6), 541–545.

Newsome DA. A randomized, prospective, placebo-controlled clinical trial of a novel zinc-monocysteine compound in age-related macular degeneration. Curr Eye Res 33.7 (2008): 591–8.

Niewoehner CB et al. Role of zinc supplementation in type II diabetes mellitus. Am J Med 81.1 (1986): 63–8.

Noh, H., et al. (2013). Salty taste acuity is affected by the joint action of alphaENaC A663T gene polymorphism and available zinc intake in young women. Nutrients, 5(12), 4950–4963.

Novick SG et al. How does zinc modify the common cold? Clinical observations and implications regarding mechanisms of action. Med Hypotheses 46 (1996): 295–302.

Nowak G et al. Effect of zinc supplementation on antidepressant therapy in unipolar depression: a preliminary placebo-controlled study. Pol J Pharmacol 55.6 (2003): 1143–7.

Nowak G, et al. Zinc and depression. An update. Pharmacol Rep 57 (2005): 713–8.

Ochi K et al. Zinc deficiency and tinnitus. Auris Nasus Larynx 30 (Suppl) (2003): S25–8.

Oprica C, et al. Overview of treatments for acne. Dermatol Nurs 14 (2002): 242–6.

Orris L et al. Oral zinc therapy of acne. Absorption and clinical effect. Arch Dermatol 114.7 (1978): 1018–20.

Osaki T et al. Clinical and physiological investigations in patients with taste abnormality. J Oral Pathol Med 25.1 (1996): 38–43.

Overbeck S, et al. Modulating the immune response by oral zinc supplementation: a single approach for multiple diseases. Arch Immunol Ther Exp (Warsz) 56.1 (2008): 15–30.

Owusu-Agyei, S., et al. (2013). Impact of vitamin A with zinc supplementation on malaria morbidity in Ghana. Nutr J, 12, 131.

Ozuguz, P., et al. (2013). Evaluation of serum vitamins A and E and zinc levels according to the severity of acne vulgaris. Cutan Ocul Toxicol.

Paaske PB et al. Zinc in the management of tinnitus: Placebo-controlled trial. Ann Otol Rhinol Laryngol 100 (1991): 647–9.

Partida-Hernández G et al. Effect of zinc replacement on lipids and lipoproteins in type 2-diabetic patients. Biomed Pharmacother 60.4 (2006): 161–8.

Pecoud A, et al. Effect of foodstuffs on the absorption of zinc sulfate. Clin Pharmacol Ther 17.4 (1975): 469–74.

Pierard GE, Pierard-Franchimont C. Effect of a topical erythromycin-zinc formulation on sebum delivery. Evaluation by combined photometric-multi-step samplings with Sebutape. Clin Exp Dermatol 18.5 (1993): 410–3.

Pierard-Franchimont C et al. A double-blind controlled evaluation of the sebosuppressive activity of topical erythromycin-zinc complex. Eur J Clin Pharmacol 49.1–2 (1995): 57–60.

Potocnik FC et al. Zinc and platelet membrane microviscosity in Alzheimer's disease: the in vivo effect of zinc on platelet membranes and cognition. S Afr Med J 87.9 (1997): 1116–9.

Prasad A. Laboratory diagnosis of zinc deficiency. J Am Coll Nutr 4.6 (1985): 591–8.

Prasad AS. Zinc deficiency in women, infants and children. J Am Coll Nutr 15.2 (1996): 113–20.

Prasad AS. Zinc and immunity. Mol Cell Biochem 188.1–2 (1998): 63–9.

Prasad, A.S. 2013. Discovery of human zinc deficiency: its impact on human health and disease. Adv.Nutr., 4, (2) 176–190

Prasad AS, Kucuk O. Zinc in cancer prevention. Cancer Metastasis Rev 21.3–4 (2002): 291–5.

Prasad AS et al. Antioxidant effect of zinc in humans. Free Radic Biol Med 37.8 (2004): 1182–90.

Prasad AS et al. Zinc supplementation decreases incidence of infections in the elderly: effect of zinc on generation of cytokines and oxidative stress. Am J Clin Nutr 85.3 (2007): 837–44.

Purdy, S., & de Berker, D. (2011). Acne vulgaris. Clin Evid (Online), 2011.

Rareshide E, Amedee R. Disorders of taste. J La State Med Soc 141.9 (1989): 9–11.

Reyes AJ et al. Urinary zinc excretion, diuretics, zinc deficiency and some side-effects of diuretics. S Afr Med J 64.24 (1983): 936–41.

Roussel A-M et al. Antioxidant effects of zinc supplementation in Tunisians with type 2 diabetes mellitus. J Am Coll Nutr 22.4 (2003): 316–21.

Safai-Kutti S. Oral zinc supplementation in anorexia nervosa. Acta Psychiatr Scand Suppl 361 (1990): 14–17.

Saito H et al. Malnutrition induces dissociated changes in lymphocyte count and subset proportion in patients with anorexia nervosa. Int J Eat Disord 40.6 (2007): 575–9.

Sakagami M et al. A zinc-containing compound, Polaprezinc, is effective for patients with taste disorders: randomized, double-blind, placebo-controlled, multi-center study. Acta Otolaryngol 26 (2008): 1–6.

Sandstead HH et al. Zinc nutriture in the elderly in relation to taste acuity, immune response, and wound healing. Am J Clin Nutr 36 (5 Suppl) (1982): 1046–59.

Sardana, K., & Garg, V. K. (2010). An observational study of methionine-bound zinc with antioxidants for mild to moderate acne vulgaris. Dermatol Ther, 23(4), 411–418.

Satarug S et al. Prevention of cadmium accumulation in retinal pigment epithelium with manganese and zinc. Exp Eye Res 87.6 (2008): 587–93.

Schachner L et al. Topical erythromycin and zinc therapy for acne. J Am Acad Dermatol 22.2 (1990): 253–60.

Schiffman S. Mechanisms of disease (first of two parts). N Engl J Med 308.21 (1983): 1275–9.

Scrimgeour, A. G., & Condlin, M. L. (2009). Zinc and micronutrient combinations to combat gastrointestinal inflammation. Curr Opin Clin Nutr Metab Care, 12(6), 653–660.

Semrad CE. Zinc and intestinal function. Curr Gastroenterol Rep 1.5 (1999): 398–403.

Shalita, A. R., et al. (2012). Inflammatory acne management with a novel prescription dietary supplement. J Drugs Dermatol, 11(12), 1428–1433.

Shankar AH et al. The influence of zinc supplementation on morbidity due to *Plasmodium falciparum*: a randomized trial in preschool children in Papua New Guinea. Am J Trop Med Hyg 62.6 (2000): 663–9.

Sharquie KE et al. Oral zinc sulphate in the treatment of acute cutaneous leishmaniasis. Clin Exp Dermatol 26.1 (2001): 21–6.

Shay NF, Mangian HF. Neurobiology of zinc-influenced eating behavior. J Nutr 130 (5S Suppl) (2000): 1493–9S.

Shepherd, S. J., & Gibson, P. R. (2013). Nutritional inadequacies of the gluten-free diet in both recently-diagnosed and long-term patients with coeliac disease. J Hum Nutr Diet, 26(4), 349–358.

Siberry GK, et al. Zinc and human immunodeficiency virus infection. Nutr Res 22.4 (2002): 527–38.

Silk R, LeFante C. Safety of zinc gluconate glycine (Cold-Eeze) in a geriatric population: a randomized, placebo-controlled, double-blind trial. Am J Ther 12 (2005): 612–7.

Siwek, M., et al. (2009). Zinc supplementation augments efficacy of imipramine in treatment resistant patients: a double blind, placebo-controlled study. J Affect Disord, 118(1–3), 187–195.

Siwek, M., et al. (2010). Serum zinc level in depressed patients during zinc supplementation of imipramine treatment. J Affect Disord, 126(3), 447–452.

Stenberg, P., et al. (2008). Transglutaminase and the pathogenesis of coeliac disease. Eur J Intern Med, 19(2), 83–91.

Stewart-Knox B et al. Zinc status and taste acuity in older Europeans: the Zenith study. Eur J Clin Nutr 59 (Suppl 2) (2005): S31–6.
Stewart-Knox BJ et al. Taste acuity in response to zinc supplementation in older Europeans. Br J Nutr 99.1 (2008): 129–36.
Stockner, T., et al. (2013). Mutational analysis of the high-affinity zinc binding site validates a refined human dopamine transporter homology model. PLoS Comput Biol, 9(2), e1002909.
Sturniolo GC et al. Zinc absorption in Crohn's disease. Gut 21.5 (1980): 387–91.
Sturniolo GC et al. Zinc supplementation tightens leaky gut in Crohn's disease. Inflamm Bowel Dis 7.2 (2001): 94–8.
Sun Q et al. A prospective study of zinc intake and risk of type 2 diabetes in women. Diabetes Care. 2009; 32: 629–634.
Suzuki, H., et al. (2011). Zinc as an appetite stimulator — the possible role of zinc in the progression of diseases such as cachexia and sarcopenia. Recent Pat Food Nutr Agric, 3(3), 226–231.
Swardfager, W, et al. (2013). Potential roles of zinc in the pathophysiology and treatment of major depressive disorder. Neuroscience & Biobehavioral Reviews, 37(5), 911–929.
Szewczyk, B. (2013). Zinc homeostasis and neurodegenerative disorders. Front Aging Neurosci, 5, 33.
Szewczyk, B., et al. (2008). Antidepressant activity of zinc and magnesium in view of the current hypotheses of antidepressant action. Pharmacol Rep, 60(5), 588–589.
Szewczyk, B., et al. (2011). The role of zinc in neurodegenerative inflammatory pathways in depression. Prog Neuropsychopharmacol Biol Psychiatry, 35(3), 693–701.
Tan JS et al. Dietary antioxidants and the long-term incidence of age-related macular degeneration: the Blue Mountains Eye Study. Ophthalmology 115.2 (2008): 334–41.
Tanaka M. Secretory function of the salivary gland in patients with taste disorders or xerostomia: correlation with zinc deficiency. Acta Otolaryngol Suppl 546 (2002): 134–41.
Tang AM, et al. Effects of micronutrient intake on survival in human immunodeficiency virus type 1 infection. Am J Epidemiol 143.12 (1996): 1244–56.
Thatcher B et al. Gustin from human partod saliva is carbonic anhydrase VI. Biochem Biophys Res Commun 250 (1998): 635–41.
Tobia MH et al. The role of dietary zinc in modifying the onset and severity of spontaneous diabetes in the BB Wistar rat. Mol Genet Metab 63.3 (1998): 205–13.
Tran, C. D., et al. (2011). Zinc homeostasis and gut function in children with celiac disease. Am J Clin Nutr, 94(4), 1026–1032.
Uçkardeş Y et al. Effects of zinc supplementation on parent and teacher behaviour rating scores in low socioeconomic level Turkish primary school children. Acta Paediatr 2009; 98: 731–736.
van Leeuwen R et al. Dietary intake of antioxidants and risk of age-related macular degeneration. JAMA 294 (2005): 3101–7.
Verma KC, et al. Oral zinc sulphate therapy in acne vulgaris: a double-blind trial. Acta Derm Venereol 60.4 (1980): 337–40.
Wahlqvist M et al. Food and nutrition. 2nd edn. Sydney: Allen & Unwin, 2002.
Wardlaw GM et al. Contemporary nutrition: issues and insights. 3rd edn. Boston: McGraw-Hill, 1997.
Watari, I., et al. (2013). Effectiveness of polaprezinc for low-dose aspirin-induced small-bowel mucosal injuries as evaluated by capsule endoscopy: a pilot randomized controlled study. *BMC Gastroenterol*, 13, 108.
Weimar VM et al. Zinc sulfate in acne vulgaris. Arch Dermatol 114.12 (1978): 1776–8.
Weismann K, et al. Oral zinc sulphate therapy for acne vulgaris. Acta Derm Venereol 57.4 (1977): 357–60.
Wellinghausen N et al. Zinc serum level in human immunodeficiency virus-infected patients in relation to immunological status. Biol Trace Elem Res 73.2 (2000): 139–49.
Wilkinson EA, Hawke CI. Oral zinc for arterial and venous leg ulcers. Cochrane Database Syst Rev 2 (2000): CD001273.
Wills NK et al. Cadmium accumulation in the human retina: effects of age, gender, and cellular toxicity. Exp Eye Res 86.1 (2008a): 41–51.
Wills NK et al. Copper and zinc distribution in the human retina: relationship to cadmium accumulation, age, and gender. Exp Eye Res 87.2 (2008b): 80–8.
Wojcik J et al. Antepartum/postpartum depressive symptoms and serum zinc and magnesium levels. Pharmacol Rep 58 (2006): 571–6.
Wood RJ. Assessment of marginal zinc status in humans. J Nutr 130 (2000): 1350–4S.
World Health Organization. Zinc: report of a joint FAO/WHO expert consultation, Bangkok, Thailand: WHO, 2002.
Wright A et al. Experimental zinc depletion and altered taste perception for NaCl in young adult males. Am J Clin Nutr 34.5 (1981): 848–52.
Yakoob, M. Y., et al. (2011). Preventive zinc supplementation in developing countries: impact on mortality and morbidity due to diarrhea, pneumonia and malaria. BMC Public Health, 11 Suppl 3, S23.
Yetiser S, et al. The role of zinc in management of tinnitus. Auris Nasus Larynx 2002; 29(4):329–333.
Yorbik O et al. Potential effects of zinc on information processing in boys with attention deficit hyperactivity disorder. Prog Neuropsychopharmacol Biol Psychiatry 32.3 (2008): 662–7.
Yuyan L et al. Are serum zinc and copper levels related to semen quality? Fertil Steril 89.4 (2008): 1008–11.
Zazzo JF et al Effect of zinc on the immune status of zinc-depleted AIDS related complex patients. Clin Nutr 8.5 (1989): 259–61.
Zepf, F. D., et al. (2012a). Differences in zinc status and the leptin axis in anorexic and recovered adolescents and young adults: a pilot study. Food Nutr Res, 56. doi: 10.3402/fnr.v56i0.10941
Zepf, F. D., et al. (2012b). Differences in serum zn levels in acutely ill and recovered adolescents and young adults with anorexia nervosa — a pilot study. Eur Eat Disord Rev, 20(3), 203–210.
Zhi J, et al. The effect of short-term (21-day) orlistat treatment on the physiologic balance of six selected macrominerals and microminerals in obese adolescents. J Am Coll Nutr 22.5 (2003): 357–62.
Zverev YP. Effects of caloric deprivation and satiety on sensitivity of the gustatory system. BMC Neurosci 5 (2004): 5

APPENDIX 1

GLOSSARY AND ABBREVIATIONS

Abortifacient–Substance used to terminate a pregnancy.
ACE–angiotensin-converting enzyme.
ACM–all-cause mortality.
ACTH–adrenocorticotrophic hormone.
Active constituents–Chemical components that exhibit pharmacological activity and contribute to the agent's overall therapeutic effects.
Acute–Beginning abruptly; sharp and intense; subsiding after a short period.
Adaptogen–Innocuous agent, non-specifically increasing resistance to physical, chemical, environmental, emotional or biological factors ('stressors') and having a normalising effect independent of the nature of the pathological state.
ADHD–attention deficit hyperactivity disorder.
ADI–acceptable daily intake.
Adjuvant–Substance added to a mixture to enhance the effect of the main ingredient.
ADR–adverse drug reaction.
ADRAC–Adverse Drug Reactions Advisory Committee (Australia).
Adverse reaction–Unintended harmful, undesirable or seriously unpleasant response to a medicine at doses intended for prophylaxis, diagnosis or therapeutic effect.
Aerial parts–All parts of a plant that are above the ground. Very often, plants that have useful aerial parts are harvested when flowering (e.g. St John's wort — *Hypericum perforatum* of the Hypericaceae family).
Agonist–Substance that binds to and activates a receptor, thereby causing a response.
Alkaloid–Naturally occurring cyclic organic compound containing nitrogen in a negative oxidation state, which has limited distribution in living organisms. Based on their structures, alkaloids are divided into several subgroups: non-heterocyclic alkaloids and heterocyclic alkaloids, which are again divided into 12 major groups according to their basic ring structure. They tend to have marked physiological effects in vivo (e.g. morphine, codeine, nicotine).
Allostatic responses–Changes that occur in the body in order to adapt and respond to physical or psychological change (e.g. standing, sitting, stress). They are critical to survival, have broad boundaries and involve the sympathetic nervous system and the hypothalamus–pituitary–adrenal axis.
ALT–alanine aminotransferase.
Amino acid–Organic compound composed of one or more basic amino groups and one or more acidic carboxyl groups; form the basic structural units of protein.
AMP–adenosine monophosphate.
Analgesic–Substance that relieves the symptoms of pain.
ANF–atrial natriuretic factor.
Antagonist–Substance that binds to a receptor (blocking others from doing so), but does not activate it, causing a diminished response.
Anthelmintic–Substance that destroys or assists in the expulsion of intestinal worms.
Anthocyanins–Compounds responsible for the bright colours of most flowers and fruits; water-soluble pigments that occur as glycosides and their aglycones (anthocyanidins) and have significant antioxidant activity.
Anti-allergic–Substance that reduces the allergic response (e.g. antihistamine activity or mast-cell stabilisation).
Anti-asthmatic–Substance that prevents asthma attacks and/or reduces their severity.
Anti-emetic–Substance or procedure that prevents or alleviates nausea and vomiting.
Anticholinergic–Agent that blocks cholinergic receptors (e.g. atropine), which results in inhibition of transmission of parasympathetic nerve impulses.
Anticoagulant–Substance that prevents or delays blood coagulation (e.g. warfarin).
Antidiabetic–Substance that aids in blood glucose management or improves management of diabetes via other mechanisms.
Antigen–Substance that the body recognises as foreign and to which it can evoke an immune response; often it is a protein.

Antimicrobial–Substance that kills microorganisms or inhibits their growth or replication.
Antioxidant–Substance that inhibits or delays the oxidation of a second substance; also described as scavenging free-radical molecules.
Antiplatelet–Substance that inhibits platelet aggregation and thereby prolongs bleeding time (e.g. aspirin).
Antipruritic–Substance or procedure that relieves or prevents itching.
Antipyretic–Substance or procedure that reduces fever.
Antispasmodic–Substance that reduces smooth muscle spasms.
Antitussive–Substance that suppresses the cough reflex.
Anxiolytic–Substance used to treat and relieve anxiety states.
Apolipoprotein–Protein on the surface of lipoproteins that may bind to receptors, activate enzymes involved in lipoprotein metabolism and provide structure.
Apoptosis–Programmed cell death.
ARMD–age-related macular degeneration.
AST–aspartate aminotransferase.
Astringent–Substance that precipitates proteins, causes vasoconstriction and constriction of mucous membranes, and reduces cell permeability when applied topically.
ATP–adenosine triphosphate.
Bark–Outermost protective layer of a tree trunk, formed by layers of living cells just above the wood itself. There are usually high concentrations of the active ingredients in the bark (e.g. cinnamon from *Cinnamomum camphora* of the Lauraceae family).
Bioavailability–Proportion of an administered dose that reaches the systemic circulation intact.
Bitter tonic–Herbs with a bitter taste, which are used to stimulate the upper gastrointestinal tract (i.e. stomach, liver, pancreas). They stimulate appetite and digestive function.
BMD–bone mineral density.
BMI–body mass index.
BPH–benign prostatic hypertrophy.
Bulb–Fleshy structure made up of numerous layers of bulb scales, which are leaf bases. Bulbs that are popular for medicinal use include onion and garlic (*Allium cepa* and *A. sativum*, respectively, both of the Liliaceae family).
BZM–bortezomib.
CAM–complementary and alternative medicine.
Cardioprotective–Substance that protects the heart from damage by toxins or ischaemia (oxygen deficiency).
Carminative–Substance that relieves flatulence, abdominal distension, spasm and discomfort by relaxing the intestinal muscles and sphincters.
Carotenoid–Group of red, yellow or orange highly unsaturated pigments found naturally in foods. Some are converted to vitamin A in the body and most exhibit antioxidant properties.
CFS–chronic fatigue syndrome.
Chelation–Chemical interaction of a metal ion with another substance, which results in the formation of a molecular complex with the metal firmly bound and isolated.
Chemoprevention–Substance or intervention that reduces the incidence of cancer.
Cholagogue–Substance that stimulates the release of stored bile from the gall bladder.
Choleretic–Substance that stimulates both the production and the flow of bile.
Chronic–Persisting for a long period of time.
Chylomicrons–Large particles that transport dietary cholesterol and fatty acids from the gastrointestinal tract to the liver.
CMEC–Complementary Medicines Evaluation Committee.
CMs–complementary medicines.
CNS–central nervous system.
Cognitive activator–Substance or procedure that stimulates the mental processes such as memory, judgment, reasoning and comprehension.
Cohort study–Study concerning a specific population that shares a common characteristic (e.g. same age, same gender).
Cold extraction–Process in which plant material is extracted in a solvent of differing polarity at room temperature, enabling maximum extraction of most components.
Contraindication–Any factor that makes it undesirable or dangerous to administer a medicine or perform a procedure on a specific patient.
Corticosteroids–Steroidal hormones that are synthesised and released from the adrenal cortex; includes both glucocorticoids and mineralocorticoids.
COX–cyclo-oxygenase.
CPI–consumer product information.
CRP–C-reactive protein.
Crude herb–Raw plant before it is processed or dried.
CVD–cardiovascular disease.
Cytochrome P450 (CYP)–Proteins involved in extra-mitochondrial electron transfer, chiefly in the liver and during detoxification. There are many CYPs; they are named by the root symbol CYP, followed by a number for family, a letter for subfamily, and another number for the specific gene.
DBP–diastolic blood pressure.
Debridement–Removal of foreign objects, damaged tissue, cellular debris and dirt from a wound or burn to prevent infection and promote healing.
Decoction–Aqueous medicine made from an extract of water-soluble substances, usually with the aid of boiling water.
Decongestant–Substance or procedure that reduces or eliminates congestion and swelling, usually of mucous membranes.

Demulcent–Substance that soothes and reduces irritation of tissues such as skin or mucous membranes.
DHA–docosahexaenoic acid.
DHEA–dehydroepiandrosterone.
Diuretic–Substance that modifies kidney function to increase the rate of urine flow.
DMBA–7,12-dimethylbenz[a]anthracene.
Double-blind study–Study in which neither the test subject nor the clinician knows whether a placebo or active medicine is being administered. The substances are often identifiable by a code that is revealed after results are obtained. This method is widely used in clinical studies to confer greater objectivity.
DSM-IV–*Diagnostic and Statistical Manual [of Mental Health Disorders]*, 4th edn.
EAR–estimated average requirement.
EBM–evidence-based medicine.
ECG–electrocardiogram.
EEG–electroencephalogram.
EGCG–epigallocatechin-3-gallate.
Emmenagogue–Substance that increases the strength and frequency of uterine contractions, and initiates and promotes menstrual flow (some are also abortifacients).
Emollient–Substance that softens tissue and reduces irritation, usually of the skin and mucous membranes.
Endogenous–Originating from within the body; synthesised by the body.
Epidemiological study–Study of occurrence and distribution of disease in large human populations.
Ergogenic aid–Substance that improves energy utilisation with the expectation that it will enhance physical performance.
Erythropoiesis–Process of erythrocyte production in the bone marrow.
ESADDI–estimated safe and adequate daily dietary intake.
ESCOP–European Scientific Cooperative on Phytotherapy.
ESR–erythrocyte sedimentation rate.
Essential amino acids–Eight amino acids that are required for health and must be obtained from the diet: isoleucine, leucine, lysine, methionine, phenylalanine, threonine, tryptophan and valine.
Essential fatty acids (EFA)–Polyunsaturated acids that are required for growth and general health and must be obtained from the diet (e.g. omega-3 EFAs found in fish oils).
Essential oil–Volatile oils usually extracted from plants through a process of either steam distillation or microwave extraction. They consist of terpenes (mono and sesquiterpenoids and coumarins) and are of considerable importance as active ingredients (e.g. peppermint oil from *Mentha* × *piperita* from the Lamiaceae family).
Expectorant–Substance that promotes the expulsion of mucus, fluids or sputum from the respiratory tract.
Extract–Substance prepared by the use of solvents or evaporation to separate it from the original material.
Fatty oils–Non-volatile, insoluble oils pressed from either the seeds or the fruits of a plant (e.g. olive oil).
FDA–Food and Drug Administration (USA).
FEV_1–forced expiratory volume in 1 second.
Flavonoids–Compounds responsible for the colour of flowers, fruits and sometimes leaves. The name derives from the Latin *flavus*, meaning yellow. Some may contribute to the colour as co-pigment. Flavonoids protect the plant from UV damage and play a role in reproduction by attracting pollinators.
Flowers–Commonly used in medicine (e.g. cloves (*Syzygium aromaticum*, Myrtaceae family), chamomile (*Chamomilla recutita*, Asteraceae family) and marigold (*Calendula officinalis*, Asteraceae family)).
Fluid extract–Hydro-ethanolic extract of crude herbal material with a drug solvent ratio of 1:1 or 1:2 (e.g. 1 part herb to 1 or 2 parts solvent).
Free radical–Unstable organic compound with at least one unpaired electron.
Fresh plant tincture–Herbal extract made from fresh plant instead of dried material.
Fruit–Most commonly used seeds are anis (*Pimpinella anisum*) and fennel (*Foeniculum vulgare*), both of the Apiaceae family. In some instances, the fruit peel is used specifically (e.g. citrus spp, from the Rutaceae family).
FSH–follicle stimulating hormone.
FVC–forced vital capacity.
GABA–gamma-aminobutyric acid.
GAD–generalised anxiety disorder.
Galactogogue–Substance that promotes the production and flow of breast milk.
GI–glycaemic index.
GLUT–glucose transporters.
Glycoside–Sugar-containing compound with a glycone (sugar) and aglycone (non-sugar) components that can be cleaved on hydrolysis.
GSH–glutathione.
Gum–Solids consisting of mixtures of polysaccharides that are water-soluble and are partially digested by humans. Gums sometimes flow from a damaged plant stem as a defence mechanism or sometimes as a protective system against the invasion of bacteria and fungi. Well-known examples are gum arabic (*Acacia senegal*, Leguminosae), and aloe gel (*Aloe vera*, Liliaceae family: gum mixed with water).
Gy–gray (unit of radiation).
Haemostasis–Physiological process that stops bleeding (i.e. vessel constriction, platelet plug formation and blood coagulation).
HbA_{1C}–haemoglobin A_{1C}.
HBeAg–hepatitis B early antigen.
HDL–high-density lipoprotein.
Hepatoprotective–Substance that reduces or prevents liver damage; protects against the destructive effect of hepatotoxins.

High-performance liquid chromatography–Very popular and widely used method for the analysis and isolation of bioactive natural products.
HIV–human immunodeficiency virus.
HMG-CoA–3-hydroxy-3-methylglutaryl coenzyme A.
HPA–hypothalamus–pituitary–adrenal [axis].
HRT–hormone replacement therapy.
HSV–herpes simplex virus.
Hypnotic–Substance that induces sleep or the feeling of dreamy sleepiness.
Hypoglycaemic–Substance that reduces blood glucose levels.
Hypolipidaemic–Substance that reduces blood levels of lipids (e.g. cholesterol, triglycerides).
Iatrogenic–Condition caused by medical or surgical treatment or diagnostic procedures.
IBS–irritable bowel syndrome.
IFN–interferon.
Ig–immunoglobulin.
IL–interleukin.
IM–integrative medicine.
Immunomodulation–Substance that alters the immune response; also described as having a balancing effect on immune responses.
Immunostimulant–Substance that augments the immune response.
Immunosuppressant–Substance that inhibits the immune response.
Infused oil–Herbal extract using a fixed oil as the solvent.
Infusion (herbal)–Herbal tea prepared by pouring boiling water over plant parts and steeping for a short time.
iNOS–inducible nitric oxide synthase.
Inotrope–Substance that has an effect on the force of myocardial contractility. A positive inotrope increases the force of contraction whereas a negative inotrope decreases the force of contraction.
INR–international normalised ratio.
Interaction–Pharmacological interaction is said to occur when the response to one medicine varies from what is usually predicted because another substance has altered the response. An interaction may lead to drug toxicity or a loss of drug effect; however, it can also be manipulated to benefit the patient by improving outcomes, reducing side effects or reducing drug dose and costs.
IO–integrative oncology.
IP–intraperitoneal.
IQ–intelligence quotient.
Ischaemia–Oxygen deficiency.
IV–intravenous.
IVF–in vitro fertilisation.
Laxative–Substance that causes bowel evacuation.
LD_{50}–median lethal dose.
LDL–low-density lipoprotein.
LH–luteinising hormone.
LOHAS–lifestyles of health and sustainability.
Maceration–Method of herbal extraction in which cut herb is soaked in solvent (such as cold water) for a period of time before draining, straining and pressing.
Meta-analysis–Quantitative statistical procedure for combining the results of independent studies to better analyse the efficacy of a specific treatment.
Mineral–Compound containing a non-metal, metal, radical or phosphate required for proper body functioning and health maintenance.
Mineral oil–Faecal softener and laxative.
MND–motor neuron disease.
MOA–monoamine oxidase.
MRL–maximum residue level.
MRSA–methicillin-resistant *Staphylococcus aureus*.
MSSA–methicillin-sensitive *Staphylococcus aureus*.
MTHFR–methylenetetrahydrofolate reductase.
Mucilage–Sticky mixture of carbohydrates produced by plant cell activity. Herbs with a high mucilaginous content are often used as demulcents (e.g. *Ulmus fulvus* (slippery elm), *Althea officinalis* (marshmallow)).
Mucolytic–Substance that dissolves or destroys mucus.
Myocardial infarction (MI)–Necrosis (death) of a portion of the heart muscle; also called a heart attack.
NAD–nicotinamide adenine dinucleotide.
NADPH–nicotinamide adenine dinucleotide phosphate.
Narrow therapeutic index (NTI)–The dose required to produce a toxic effect in 50% of test animals (TD_{50}) is close to the dose required to produce an effective therapeutic response in 50% of test animals (ED_{50}); NTI drugs are particularly susceptible to adverse interactions (e.g. digoxin).
Nervine–Substance that exerts a relaxant effect; described as nourishing and strengthening the nervous system.
Neurotransmitter–Chemical that acts as a messenger, enabling transmission of nerve impulses across synapses and neuromuscular junctions. The most important are acetylcholine, catecholamines (noradrenaline, adrenaline and dopamine), serotonin, some amino acids and neuro-active peptides.
NK–natural killer [cell].
NO–nitric oxide.
NSAID–non-steroidal anti-inflammatory drug.
Nutritive–Substance that contains numerous nutrients such as vitamins, minerals, carbohydrates and fats.
NYHA–New York Heart Association [classification].
OA–osteoarthritis.
OCP–oral contraceptive pill.
OS–oxygen species.
OTC–over-the-counter.
Oxytocic–Substance that exerts similar effects to oxytocin (i.e. stimulates smooth muscle, usually of the uterus, to contract).

P-glycoprotein (P-gp)–P-gp is a transport protein found on the surface of hepatocytes, renal tubular epithelial cells, epithelial cells in the intestine, and placenta and capillary epithelial cells in the brain. It has a counter-transport activity (i.e. can transport medicines from the blood back into the gastrointestinal tract, thereby reducing bioavailability).
PCOS–polycystic ovaries syndrome.
PEF–peak expiratory flow.
Peri-operative–Pertaining to the time of surgery.
PG–prostaglandin.
Pharmacodynamics–Study of the effects of drugs on living organisms.
Pharmacokinetics–Study of the actions of drugs within the body (i.e. absorption, distribution, metabolism and excretion, onset of action and duration of effect).
Phytochemical–Naturally occurring chemical found in a plant.
Phytotherapy–Study and application of plant medicine; a modern term used to describe scientifically investigated and validated herbal medicine.
Placebo–Harmless inactive substance that does not contain an active medicine; used in clinical studies for comparison with medicines suspected of exerting a clinical effect to determine whether in fact a significant response does occur.
PMS–premenstrual syndrome.
PO–per os (oral).
Polypharmacy–Use of many medicines by a patient with one or more health conditions.
Polysaccharide–Carbohydrate polymer formed from three or more sugar molecules.
Postprandial–After a meal.
Poultice–Paste made from crushed fresh plant, either mixed with oil or alcohol or simply made in water and applied to the parts of the body.
PPI–proton-pump inhibitors.
ppm–parts per million.
Prospective study–Study designed to determine the relationship between a condition and a characteristic shared by some members of a group. Usually the population selected is healthy at the beginning of the study and is observed over a period of time for the development of certain conditions in the different subgroups (e.g. smokers and non-smokers).
PTH–parathyroid hormone.
PUFA–polyunsaturated fatty acid.
PUVA–psoralen ultraviolet A.
QOL–quality of life.
RA–rheumatoid arthritis.
RAST–radioallergosorbent test.
RCT–randomised controlled trial.
RDA–recommended daily allowance.
RDI–recommended daily intake.
Resin–Excreted from specialised cells or ducts in plants, this consists of a mixture of essential oils and polymerised terpenes; usually insoluble in water. Well-known examples include frankincense (*Boswellia sacra*) and myrrh (*Commiphora molmol*), both of the Burseraceae family.
Restorative–Restores or renews a person's state of health or consciousness to normal.
Rhizome–Root; underground fleshy stem that grows horizontally and acts as food storage for the plant.
Risk factor–Factor that increases a person's susceptibility to an unwanted, unpleasant or unhealthy event or disease.
Root–Fleshy or woody, usually underground, part of a plant; may be fibrous (e.g. *Urtica dioica* or *U. radix* of the Urticaceae family, stinging nettle), solid (e.g. *Glycyrrhiza glabra* of the Leguminosae family, licorice) or fleshy (e.g. *Harpagophytum procumbens* of the Pedaliaceae family, devil's claw).
ROS–reactive oxygen species.
Salicylate–Substance that contains or is derived from salicylic acid.
Saponin–Vast group of glycosides that occur in many plants; dissolve in water and form a soapy solution when shaken; used in demulcents.
SBP–systolic blood pressure.
SC–subcutaneous.
Seeds–Contained in the fruit and used medicinally (e.g. fennel seed, *Foeniculum vulgare*: Apiaceae).
SLE–systemic lupus erythematosus.
SSRI–selective serotonin reuptake inhibitor.
SVCT–sodium vitamin C co-transporters.
Synergistic–Several components acting or working together in a coordinated manner to produce an effect greater than that of the sum of the individual effects.
Tannin–Substance that forms a precipitate with proteins, nitrogenous bases, polysaccharides and some alkaloids and glycosides (e.g. *Camellia sinensis*, the herb commonly used to make 'tea', is a rich source of tannins).
TCM–traditional Chinese medicine.
TGA–Therapeutic Goods Administration (Australia).
Th–T helper cell.
Therapeutic index–Measure of the safety of a medicine based upon the dose required to produce a toxic effect in 50% of test animals (TD_{50}) divided by the dose required to produce an effective therapeutic response in 50% of test animals (ED_{50}); i.e. $TI = TD_{50}/ED_{50}$.
Thin layer chromatography–Analytical method using glass or aluminium plates precoated with the sorbent (e.g. silica gel) to separate a compound mixture according to the polarity of its components.
Tincture–Hydro-ethanolic extraction of crude herbal material; usually extracted in the ratio of 1:5 (1 part herb to 5 parts solvent). Glyceride tinctures may be prepared by using glycerol rather than alcohol.
TNF–tumour necrosis factor.

TPN–total parenteral nutrition.
TSH–thyroid stimulating hormone.
URTI–upper respiratory tract infection.
UTI–urinary tract infection.
UV–ultraviolet.
VAS–visual analogue scale.
VDR–vitamin D receptors.
Vitamin–Organic compound essential to life. With few exceptions, vitamins cannot be synthesised in the body and must be obtained from the diet.
VLDL–very low-density lipoprotein.
WOMAC–Western Ontario and McMasters University Osteoarthritis Index.
WSR–whole systems research.

APPENDIX 2

HERB/NUTRIENT–DRUG INTERACTIONS

ASSUMPTIONS MADE WHEN COLLATING AND ASSESSING INFORMATION FOR THIS TABLE

- Information is compiled from the 132 monographs included in this book.
- The clinical significance of many interactions is still unknown because controlled trials are lacking in most cases. In these instances, interactions are based on evidence of pharmacological activity and case reports, and have a sound theoretical basis, although remain to be tested.
- All information refers to oral dose forms unless otherwise specified.
- Information is correct at the time of writing; however, because of the ever-expanding knowledge base developing in this area, new research is constantly being published.
- The interaction table is provided as a guide only and should not replace the use of professional judgement. It has been developed to assist clinicians when advising patients.

USING THIS GUIDE IN PRACTICE

- Refer to Chapter 8: Interactions with Herbal and Natural Medicines for background information.
- Commonly used prescription and over-the-counter medications are organised by therapeutic class and subclass and are listed alphabetically.
- Common names have been used when referring to herbs.
- Refer to the original monograph for more information about a particular substance.

RECOMMENDATIONS

Avoid — there may be insufficient information available to be able to advise using the two substances safely together, so avoid until more is known. The drug may have a narrow therapeutic index and there is sufficient evidence to suggest that the interaction may be clinically significant. Consider an alternative treatment that is unlikely to produce an undesirable interaction.

Avoid use unless under medical supervision — harmful effects of the potential interaction can be avoided if doses are altered appropriately under professional supervision or the patient is closely monitored. Some of these interactions can be manipulated to the advantage of the patient. Changes to the dosage regimen may be required for safe combined use.

Caution — the possibility exists of an interaction that may change effects clinically; be aware and monitor. It is prudent to tell patients to be aware and seek advice if they are concerned.

Observe — interaction may not be clinically significant at the usual recommended doses and theoretical; however, the clinician should be alert to the possibility of an interaction.

Beneficial interaction possible — prescribing the interacting substance may improve clinical outcomes; for example, reducing drug requirements, complementing drug effects, reducing drug side-effects, counteracting nutritional deficiencies caused by drugs, alleviating drug withdrawal symptoms and enhancing patient wellbeing.

KEY TO THE TABLE BY HERB/SUPPLEMENT

Herb/Supplement	Pathway	Potential outcome	Recommendation	Evidence/Comments
DRUGS METABOLISED/UTILISED BY				
Cytochrome P450 (e.g. CYP2E1, CYP2D6, CYP2C8, CYP2C9, CYP2C19, CYP3A, CYP3A4)				
Aloe vera	CYP3A4 and CYP2D6	Inhibition	Caution	Aloe vera juice was found to inhibit both CYP3A4 and CYP2D6 by both CYP and non-CYP mechanisms. The estimated IC_{50} inhibition values was suggestive of no major interference in humans, however some degree of caution and acknowledgement should be exercised.
Citrus aurantium	CYP3A	Reduced drug effects	Caution	Theoretically, an interaction exists for CYP 3A and P-glycoprotein substrates, as human studies indicate that the juice made from *Citrus aurantium* (Seville orange) inhibits CYP3A and possibly P-glycoprotein. * More research is required to investigate the effect of *Citrus aurantium* on individual medications.
Cranberry	CYP3A	Reduced drug effects	Caution. Monitor patients taking high-strength cranberry preparations and medicines chiefly metabolised by CYP3A. Special care should be taken if the medicines have a narrow therapeutic index.	Cranberry juice has the potential to inhibit the metabolism of drugs chiefly metabolised by CYP3A isoenzymes. It appears to be dependent on the concentration of three triterpenes (maslinic acid, corosolic acid and ursolic acid) in the juice. These have been identified as the important constituents responsible for inhibiting intestinal CYP3A and most likely explain the inter-brand differences seen in various clinical and preclinical trials.
Golden seal	CYP3A4 and CYP2D6	Inhibition	Caution	Studies in healthy volunteers demonstrated that CYP3A4 and CYP2D6 were significantly down-regulated following goldenseal treatment.
Green tea	CYP3A4	Potential inhibition	Observe. Separate doses by at least 2 hours	In vitro and animal research has shown green tea to inhibit CYP3A4 metabolism and a probable inhibition of intestinal CYP3A4, but clinical relevance is unknown.
Honey	CYP3A4	Altered drug metabolism.	Observe. Separate doses by at least 2 hours.	Oral intake of honey may induce CYP3A4 enzyme activity.
Hops	CYP2C8, CYP2C9, CYP2C19	Altered drug metabolism.	Observe the patient for signs of altered drug effectiveness.	Altered drug effect — cytochrome (CYP) inhibition has been demonstrated in vitro. However, it is unknown whether these effects are clinically significant.
Kava	CYP2E1	Reduced drug absorption	Caution	Inhibition of CYP2E1 has been demonstrated in vivo — serum levels of CYP2E1 substrates may become elevated.
Korean Ginseng	CYP1A, CYP2D6 and CYP3A4	Reduced drug absorption	Caution. Observe for increased drug bioavailability and clinical effects.	Mixed reports exist as to whether ginseng may act as an inhibitor of cytochrome CYP1A. Whether these effects are likely to be clinically significant has not been established.

Licorice	CYP3A4	Reduced drug absorption	Caution. Observe for increased drug bioavailability and clinical effects.	Licorice has been shown to cause a moderate, clinically relevant, induction of CYP3A4. Other constituents have been found to affect various CYP P450 isoforms in vitro. Until studies in humans come to light, the clinical significance of this remains unclear.
Nigella	CYP2B, CYP3A2, CYP2C11, and CYP1A2	Reduced drug absorption	Separate doses by at least 2 hours	Preliminary animal study data suggests that Nigella may be protective against carbon tetrachloride-induced downregulation of Cytochrome P450 enzymes CYP2B, CYP3A2, CYP2C11, and CYP1A2. A potential interaction with drugs with Cytochrome P450 metabolising activity is theoretical and speculative. Further research is required to determine clinical significance.
Peppermint	CYP3A4	Increased oral bioavailability	Observe	Peppermint may increase the oral bioavailability of certain drugs by inhibition of CYP3A4-mediated drug metabolism, which has been demonstrated in vitro but not in test animals. Although these studies seem to suggest that peppermint may modulate drug-metabolising enzymes, the clinical significance of this is unknown and requires further investigation.
Quercetin	CYP1A1, CYP1A2, CYP3A4	Altered metabolism	Carefully monitor the concurrent use of all drugs chiefly metabolised by CYP1A1, CYP1A2, CYP3A4	Possible inhibition of CYP1A1, CYP1A2 activity should be considered when prescribing. According to a recent crossover RCT, 500 mg of oral quercetin significantly induces CYP3A4.
Rhodiola	CYP3A4	Raised drug serum levels	Caution. Monitor the concurrent use of all drugs chiefly metabolised by CYP3A4	In vitro tests reveal that Rhodiola extract inhibits CYP 3A4; this has also been suggested in vivo — clinical significance is unknown. Until further tests have been conducted, caution is advised when concurrently using medicines chiefly metabolised by CYP3A4 as the interaction could result in raised drug serum levels.
Schisandra	CYP3A4 substrates	Increased serum levels of drugs chiefly metabolised by CYP 3A4	Avoid, unless already under medical care	Increased serum levels of drugs chiefly metabolised by CYP 3A4 are possible, based on current evidence. Practitioners are advised to carefully monitor patients that are already taking drugs that are CYP3A4 substrates to avoid inducing drug side effects caused by increased serum levels. Schisandra should not be prescribed together with CYP3A4 substrates that have a narrow therapeutic index in order to avoid inducing drug toxicity.

Continued

2

Herb/Supplement	Pathway	Potential outcome	Recommendation	Evidence/Comments
P-glycoprotein				
Citrus aurantium	P-glycoprotein	Reduced drug effects	Caution	Theoretically, an interaction exists for CYP 3A and P-glycoprotein substrates, as human studies indicate that the juice made from *Citrus aurantium* (Seville orange) inhibits CYP3A and possibly P-glycoprotein. *More research is required to investigate the effect of *Citrus aurantium* on individual medications.
Quercetin	P-glycoprotein	Altered metabolism	Carefully monitor the concurrent use of all drugs chiefly metabolised by P-glycoprotein	Possible modulation of P-glycoprotein activity should be considered when prescribing. According to a recent crossover RCT, 500 mg of oral quercetin significantly induces CYP3A4.
Rhodiola	Drugs metabolised by P-glycoprotein substrates	Potential altered metabolism	Observe	In vitro tests reveal that Rhodiola extract inhibits P-glycoprotein — clinical significance is unknown.
Rosemary	Drugs dependent on P-glycoprotein transport	Potential altered metabolism	Observe	Theoretically, increased drug uptake can occur with those drugs dependent on P-glycoprotein transport. The clinical significance of this finding remains to be tested, although it has been suggested that this activity may be used to enhance the effects of chemotherapeutic agents.
Schisandra	P-glycoprotein substrates	Serum levels of P-gp substrates could be increased	Avoid, unless already under medical care	Based on current evidence, it appears that P-gp inhibition is possible. As a result, serum levels of P-gp substrates could be increased. Practitioners are advised to carefully monitor patients who are already taking drugs that are P-gp substrates to avoid inducing drug side effects caused by increased serum levels. Schisandra should not be prescribed together with P-gp substrates that have a narrow therapeutic index in order to avoid inducing drug toxicity.
Soy	P-glycoprotein substrates	Altered metabolism	Caution	It has been suggested that isoflavones can inhibit the oxidative and conjugative metabolism of drugs in vitro and interact with transporters such as P-glycoprotein; however, their ability to interact with drugs remains uncertain until clinical studies can confirm these findings.
Other (e.g. OATP1A2, UGT1A3)				
Bergamot	Organic anion-transporting polypeptide 1A2 (OATP1A2)	Possible reduced drug effects	Observe	Theoretical concern about possible interactions due to the presence of naringin in bergamot. This constituent is also found in grapefruit juice and while it does not have any appreciable effect on cytochromes, it may inhibit OATP1A2.

Schisandra	Drugs metabolised by UGT1A3	Altered metabolism	Avoid, unless already under medical care	Deoxyschizandrin and schisantherin A have demonstrated an inhibitory effect on UDP-glucuronosyltransferase 1A3 (UGT1A3) in vitro. This suggests a potential for herb–drug interactions between Schisandra and drugs that mainly undergo UGT1A3-mediated 12 metabolism, however, the effect has not been confirmed clinically.
ALLERGIC DISORDERS				
Antihistamines				
Antihistamines and mast-cell-stabilising drugs	Albizia	Additive effects	Beneficial interaction possible	Both in vitro and in vivo tests have reported significant mast-cell-stabilisation effects similar to those of cromoglycate.
	Baical skullcap	Additive effects	Beneficial interaction possible	Luteolin and baicalein have been shown to inhibit IgE antibody-mediated immediate- and late-phase allergic reactions in mice.
	Perilla	Additive effects	Observe	Perilla seed extract has been shown to inhibit histamine release from mast cells in a dose-dependent manner — drug dosage may need modification.
	St John's wort	Increased elimination of drug	Observe. Monitor drug requirements	In rats, SJW enhanced the elimination of fexofenadine, an antihistamine and P-glycoprotein substrate, into the bile when given once daily for 14 days.
ANALGESIA				
Narcotic analgesics				
Codeine	Adhatoda	Additive effects	Beneficial interaction possible	Theoretically will increase antitussive effects of drug.
	Kava	Additive effects	Caution	Increased CNS depression theoretically possible.
Morphine	Kava	Additive effects	Caution	Increased CNS depression theoretically possible.
	Tyrosine	Additive effects	Observe patients taking tyrosine and morphine sulfate concurrently — potential beneficial interaction.	Tyrosine potentiates morphine-induced analgesia by 154% in mice. Suggestive of a clinically relevant effect but not confirmed
	Withania	Reduced morphine tolerance/ dependence	Beneficial interaction possible with professional supervision	In animal studies, repeated administration of withania (100 mg/kg) inhibited morphine tolerance and dependence, so it is sometimes used in opiate withdrawal.

Continued

Herb/Supplement	Pathway	Potential outcome	Recommendation	Evidence/Comments
Oxycodone	St John's wort	Reduced plasma concentrations of oxycodone	Avoid	St John's wort greatly reduced the plasma concentrations of oral oxycodone.
Simple analgesics and antipyretics				
Simple analgesics and antipyretics	Meadowsweet	Additive effects	Observe Beneficial interaction possible	Additive anti-inflammatory and analgesic effects theoretically possible.
	Nigella	Additive effects	Beneficial interaction possible	Potentiation effects are possible when using black seed at high doses based on animal models. Clinical significance unknown.
	Vitamin E	Additive effects	Beneficial interaction possible Drug dosage may require modification	Vitamin E may enhance the pain-modifying effects of drug in RA.
	Willowbark	Additive effects	Observe Beneficial interaction possible	Additive anti-inflammatory and analgesic effects theoretically possible.
Aspirin	Grapeseed extract	Increased bruising and bleeding	Observe Beneficial interaction possible	Theoretically may enhance antiplatelet and anti-inflammatory activity of aspirin.
	Licorice	Reduce gastro-irritant effects of drug therapy	Observe Beneficial interaction possible	Co-administration with licorice may reduce gastro-irritant effects induced by drug therapy — potentially beneficial interaction. Whether the effect is clinically significant for licorice remains to be determined — use high doses with caution.
	Meadowsweet	Increased bruising and bleeding	Observe Beneficial interaction possible	Theoretically may enhance anti-inflammatory and antiplatelet effects.
	Policosanol	Increased bruising and bleeding	Observe	Doses >10 mg/day may inhibit platelet aggregation.
	Vitamin C	Decreased vitamin C effects	Beneficial interaction	Aspirin may interfere with both absorption and cellular uptake mechanisms for vitamin C, thereby increasing vitamin C requirements, as observed in animal and human studies. Increased vitamin C intake may be required with long-term therapy.
	Willowbark	Increased bruising and bleeding	Observe Beneficial interaction possible Caution with high-dose (> 240 mg salicin daily)	Theoretically may enhance anti-inflammatory and antiplatelet effects. Although a clinical study found that consumption of salicin 240 mg/day produced minimal effects on platelet aggregation, higher doses may have a significant effect.
Paracetamol	Andrographis	Reduced side-effects	Beneficial interaction possible	May exert hepatoprotective activity against liver damage induced by paracetamol.

	Garlic	Reduced side-effects	Beneficial interaction possible	May exert hepatoprotective activity against liver damage induced by paracetamol.
	Quercetin	Reduced side-effects	Beneficial interaction possible	May exert hepatoprotective activity against liver damage induced by paracetamol.
	St Mary's thistle	Reduced side-effects	Beneficial interaction possible	May exert hepatoprotective activity against liver damage induced by paracetamol.
	SAMe	Reduced side-effects	Beneficial interaction possible	May exert hepatoprotective activity against liver damage induced by paracetamol.
	Schisandra	Reduced side-effects	Beneficial interaction possible	May exert hepatoprotective activity against liver damage induced by paracetamol.
Salicylate drugs	Willowbark	Additive effects	Observe Beneficial interaction possible	Additive anti-inflammatory and analgesic effects theoretically possible.
CARDIOVASCULAR SYSTEM				
Anti-angina agents				
Nitroglycerin/ glyceryl trinitrate (e.g. anginine)	Vitamin E	Prevention of drug tolerance	Beneficial interaction possible	Oral vitamin E prevented nitrate tolerance when given concurrently with transdermal nitroglycerin (10 mg/24 h) according to one randomised placebo-controlled study.
Anti-arrhythmic agents				
	Astragalus	Additive effects	Observe	Additive effects are theoretically possible with IV administration of astragalus, based on positive inotropic activity identified in clinical studies; the clinical significance of these findings for oral dose forms is unknown.
	Devil's claw	Additive effects	Observe	Devil's claw has demonstrated anti-arrhythmic activity, but interaction is theoretical and clinical significance is unclear.
	Hawthorn	Additive effects	Observe	Hawthorn has demonstrated anti-arrhythmic activity in vitro and in vivo, but interaction is theoretical and clinical significance is unclear.
	Magnesium	Additive effects	Observe	High-dose oral magnesium has demonstrated anti-arrhythmic activity according to one clinical trial.
Amiodarone	Vitamin B_6	Increased side effects	Caution	Pyridoxine may increase the risk of drug-induced photosensitivity. Exercise caution with patients taking pyridoxine and amiodarone concurrently.

Continued

Herb/Supplement	Pathway	Potential outcome	Recommendation	Evidence/Comments
Anticoagulants, antiplatelets				
Monitor bleeding time and signs and symptoms of excessive bleeding				
Anticoagulants (e.g. warfarin)	Alpha Lipoic Acid	Potential bruising and bleeding	Observe — monitor bleeding time	ALA reduces platelet reactivity in vitro. It is uncertain whether the effect is clinically significant — observe patients taking these agents together.
	Andrographis	Increased bruising and bleeding	Caution — monitor bleeding time	Andrographolide clinically confirmed to inhibit platelet-activating-factor-induced platelet aggregation. However, andrographis used together with warfarin did not produce any significant effects on the pharmacokinetics of warfarin, and had even less effect on its pharmacodynamics in vivo.
	Baical Skullcap	Increased risk of bleeding	Caution	Increased risk of bleeding is theoretically possible.
	Bilberry	Increased bruising and bleeding	Caution with high-dose (>170 mg) anthocyanadins unless under medical supervision	Dose is particularly high and not relevant to clinical practice.
	Carnitine	Increased bruising and bleeding	Caution — monitor bleeding time and signs and symptoms of excessive bleeding	According to one case report, L-carnitine 1 g/day may potentiate the anticoagulant effects of acenocoumarol.
	Celery	Increased bruising and bleeding	Observe with concentrated extracts	Although it contains naturally occurring coumarins, interaction is unlikely.
	Chitosan	Increased bruising and bleeding	Avoid	Chitosan may potentiate warfarin by inhibiting absorption of fat-soluble vitamin K.
	Chondroitin	Increased bruising and bleeding	Observe with high-dose supplements	Theoretical risk; not observed in clinical trials.
	Coenzyme Q10	Reduced drug effects theoretically possible with high doses	Caution	A double-blind crossover study found that oral CoQ10 100 mg/day had no significant effect on INR or warfarin levels; however, in vivo tests using 10 mg/kg/day CoQ10 decreased serum concentrations of warfarin by increasing drug metabolism.
	Cranberry	Increased bruising and bleeding	Caution	Based on case reports. Until the interaction can be better understood, patients taking warfarin with cranberry juice should continue to monitor their INR changes and signs and symptoms of bleeding.
	Devil's claw	Increased bruising and bleeding	Caution	Case reports suggest possible anticoagulant activity.

	Evening primrose oil	Increased bruising and bleeding	Caution with high-dose supplements	Gamma-linoleic acid in evening primrose oil affects prostaglandin synthesis, leading to inhibition of platelet aggregation — clinical significance is unknown.
	Fenugreek	Increased bruising and bleeding	Observe	Contains naturally occurring coumarins, but a placebo-controlled study found no effect on platelet aggregation, fibrinogen or fibrinolytic activity.
	Feverfew	Increased bruising and bleeding	Observe	Although feverfew inhibits platelet aggregation in vitro and in vivo, no effects were seen in a clinical study.
	Fish oils	Increased bruising and bleeding	Caution with doses <12 g Avoid with very high doses (>12 g) unless under medical supervision	Bleeding time is increased at doses of 12 g/day, according to a clinical study.
	Garlic	Increased bruising and bleeding	Avoid at high dose (>4 g) unless under medical supervision	Large doses may increase INR.
	Ginger	Increased bruising and bleeding	Avoid at high dose (>10 g) unless under medical supervision	Inhibits platelet aggregation at high doses.
	Ginkgo biloba	Increased bruising and bleeding	Caution	Although case reports suggest possible anticoagulant effect, two recent clinical studies indicate no effect on pharmacokinetics, pharmacodynamics or clinical effects of warfarin.
	Glucosamine	Possible increased risk of bruising and bleeding	Caution	Case reports exist of glucosamine and glucosamine/chondroitin combinations increasing bruising, bleeding and INR among people taking warfarin.
	Ginseng — Korean	Increased bruising and bleeding	Avoid unless under medical supervision	Inhibits platelet aggregation both in vitro and in vivo; clinical significance unknown.
	Ginseng — Siberian	Increased bruising and bleeding	Observe	In vivo study demonstrated that an isolated constituent in Siberian ginseng has anticoagulant activity and a clinical trial found a reduction in blood coagulation induced by intensive training in athletes — whether these effects also occur in non-athletes is unknown.

Continued

2

Herb/Supplement	Pathway	Potential outcome	Recommendation	Evidence/Comments
	Goji	Increased bruising and bleeding	Caution	Case reports exist in the literature, suggesting an interaction between warfarin and goji is possible; however, causality remains unclear as it is unknown whether the suspected products were tested for authenticity and presence of contaminants.
	Grapeseed extract	Increased bruising and bleeding	Caution	Inhibits platelet aggregation in vitro — clinical significance unknown.
	Green tea	Reduced drug effects	Caution with high doses	A case report of excessive intake (2.25–4.5 L green tea daily) was reported to inhibit warfarin activity and decrease INR.
	Guarana	Increased bruising and bleeding	Caution	In vitro and in vivo research has identified antiplatelet activity.
	Horse chestnut	Possible increased risk of bruising and bleeding	Observe	Properly prepared HCSE should not contain aesculin and should not carry the risk of antithrombin activity. The clinical significance is unclear.
	Horseradish	Increased bruising and bleeding risk	Observe with high-dose supplements	Although it contains coumarins, interaction unlikely, but this has not been established clinically.
	Licorice	Increased bruising and bleeding	Caution with high doses	Isoliquiritigenin inhibits platelet aggregation, and glycyrrhizin inhibits prothrombin, according to in vitro and in vivo tests — clinical significance unknown.
	Maca	Theoretical interactions	Observe. Separate doses by 2 hours	Theoretical interactions have been suggested to be plausible in people taking anticoagulants. However, there are no reported drug interactions.
	Meadowsweet	Increased bruising and bleeding	Observe	In vitro tests have indicated anticoagulant activity — clinical significance unknown.
	Myrrh	Increased bruising and bleeding	Observe with myrrh preparations Caution with guggul preparations	Guggul inhibited platelet aggregation in vitro and in a clinical study, so concurrent use may theoretically increase the risk of bleeding — implications for *Commiphora molmol* use unclear.
	Nigella	Theoretical interactions	Caution	Theoretical interaction predicted based on antiplatelet, anticoagulant and conversely coagulant effects observed in vitro and in vivo. Clinical significance unknown.
	Noni	Decreased drug effects	Caution	There is one case report of noni juice consumption causing resistance to warfarin. Further investigation is required to determine the certainty of this causal association.
	Policosanol	Increased bruising and bleeding	Caution with doses >10 mg daily	Current evidence is contradictory, as one study failed to detect an interaction between policosanol and warfarin, but others have found that doses >10 mg/day may inhibit platelet aggregation.

	Psyllium	Decreased drug absorption	Separate doses by at least 1 hour	Soluble fibre may decrease the bioavailability of coumarin derivatives.
	Red clover	Increased bruising and bleeding	Observe	Red clover contains coumarin, which could theoretically exert anticoagulant activity and therefore increase the clinical effects of warfarin. Observe patients taking red clover and anticoagulants concurrently.
	Rosemary	Increased bruising and bleeding	Caution	Rosemary demonstrates antithrombotic activity in vitro and in vivo.
	Slippery elm	Altered rate and/or extent of absorption	Caution. Separate doses by 2 hours	Controlled studies are unavailable, but interactions are theoretically possible with some medicines. Slippery elm forms an inert barrier over the gastrointestinal lining and may theoretically alter the rate and/or extent of absorption of medicines with a narrow therapeutic range (e.g. warfarin). The clinical significance of this is unclear.
	St John's wort	Decreased drug effects	Avoid unless under medical supervision to monitor for signs of reduced drug effectiveness and adjust dose if necessary Prothrombin time or INR should be closely monitored with addition or withdrawal of St John's wort	Metabolism of warfarin is chiefly by CYP2C9, and a minor metabolic pathway is CYP3A4. St John's wort increases metabolism of drug.
	St Mary's thistle	Increased drug effects	Caution — monitor for signs of increased drug effectiveness	Possible CYP (liver cytochrome) inhibition effects, but conflicting evidence makes evaluation difficult.
	Tribulus	Increased INR values	Observe for changes in INR.	A herbal combination of *Tribulus terrestris*, *Panax ginseng* and *Avena sativa* was reported to significantly increase INR values in two patients prescribed warfarin. It is unknown if the tribulus contributed to this effect.
	Tulsi	Potential interactions based on actions	Observe for interactions	There are no reports of significant interactions with tulsi. As tulsi has anti-platelet actions there is a theoretically possibility of interactions with anti-coagulant medications but such interactions have not been reported.
	Turmeric	Increased bruising and bleeding	Caution with concentrated extracts	Curcumin inhibits platelet aggregation in vitro and in vivo. Theoretically, high-dose turmeric preparations may increase the risk of bleeding when used together with anticoagulant drugs. Clinical significance unknown.

Continued

Herb/Supplement	Pathway	Potential outcome	Recommendation	Evidence/Comments
	Vitamin E	Increased bruising and bleeding	Caution with high-dose supplements (>1000 IU daily) Until clinical significance can be established prothrombin time or INR should be closely monitored with addition or withdrawal of high-dose vitamin E supplements	Clinical studies have produced conflicting results: several found no effects of platelet aggregation or coagulation, although others found an increased bleeding risk People with reduced levels of vitamin K may be more susceptible to the effects of vitamin E potentiating warfarin activity.
	Willowbark	Potential bruising and bleeding	Exercise caution with high doses > 240 mg salicin/day.	Although a clinical study found that consumption of salicin 240 mg/day produced minimal effects on platelet aggregation, higher doses may have a significant effect. The use of willow bark was associated with an increased risk of self-reported bleeding in patients using warfarin. Controlled studies are now warranted to confirm whether oral willowbark preparations induce clinically significant changes to bleeding.
Antiplatelet drugs (e.g. aspirin)	Alpha Lipoic Acid	Potential bruising and bleeding	Observe — monitor bleeding time	ALA reduces platelet reactivity in vitro. It is uncertain whether the effect is clinically significant — observe patients taking these agents together.
	Andrographis	Increased bruising and bleeding	Observe	Andrographis inhibits platelet aggregation, observed in animal and clinical studies.
	Bilberry	Increased bruising and bleeding	Caution with high-dose (>170 mg) anthocyanadins unless under medical supervision	Dose is particularly high and not relevant to clinical practice.
	Evening primrose oil	Increased bruising and bleeding	Observe, although beneficial interaction possible	Theoretically may enhance anti-inflammatory and antiplatelet effects.
	Feverfew	Increased bruising and bleeding	Observe	Although feverfew inhibits platelet aggregation in vitro and in vivo, no effects were seen in a clinical study.
	Fish oils	Additive effects	Observe — beneficial interaction possible under professional supervision	No haemorrhagic effects were seen in a clinical study — theoretical concern.
	Garlic	Increased bruising and bleeding	Caution at doses >4 g/day	
	Ginger	Increased bruising and bleeding	Caution at high dose (>10 g) unless under professional supervision	Inhibits platelet aggregation at very high doses.

	Ginkgo biloba	Increased bruising and bleeding	Observe	Theoretically possible because of platelet-activating-factor inhibitor activity, but three trials cast doubt on the clinical significance of this effect.
	Grapeseed extract	Increased bruising and bleeding	Observe	Theoretically may enhance antiplatelet activity.
	Guarana	Increased bruising and bleeding	Observe	Decreases platelet aggregation.
	Hawthorn	Potential additive effects	Observe	Although *Crataegus laevigata* does not display antiplatelet effects as a stand-alone treatment, this has not been tested in patients with atherothrombotic vascular disease in conjunction with antiplatelet drugs.
	Horse chestnut	Possible increased risk of bruising and bleeding	Observe	Properly prepared HCSE should not contain aesculin and should not carry the risk of antithrombin activity. The clinical significance is unclear.
	Myrrh	Increased bruising and bleeding	Observe	Guggul inhibited platelet aggregation in vitro and in a clinical study, so concurrent use may theoretically increase the risk of bleeding. It is uncertain what implications this observation has for use of *Commiphora molmol*.
	Nigella	Theoretical interactions	Caution	Theoretical interaction predicted based on antiplatelet, anticoagulant and conversely coagulant effects observed in vitro and in vivo. Clinical significance unknown.
	Policosanol	Increased bruising and bleeding	Observe	Increased antiplatelet effects may develop in patients taking aspirin and policosanol concurrently.
	St John's wort	Additive effects	Observe. Monitor drug requirements (interaction may be beneficial)	SJW might represent a valid option to increase the antiplatelet effect of clopidogrel in non- and/or hypo-responders. For example, SJW increased platelet inhibition by enhancement of CYP3A4 metabolic activity for clopidogrel in hypo-responsive volunteers, and a recent study showed that residual platelet reactivity improved with SJW during the first month post percutaneous coronary intervention.
	Tulsi	Potential interactions based on actions	Observe for interactions	There are no reports of significant interactions with tulsi. As tulsi has anti-platelet actions there is a theoretical possibility of interactions with anti-coagulant medications but such interactions have not been reported.

Continued

Herb/Supplement	Pathway	Potential outcome	Recommendation	Evidence/Comments
	Turmeric	Increased bruising and bleeding	Observe with concentrated extracts	Curcumin inhibits platelet aggregation in vitro and in vivo. Turmeric has a theoretical interaction with antiplatelet drugs, therefore it may produce an additive effect — clinical significance unknown.
Aspirin	Grapeseed extract	Additive effects	Beneficial interaction possible	Theoretically may enhance antiplatelet and anti-inflammatory activity of aspirin.
	Meadowsweet	Increased bruising and bleeding	Observe — beneficial interaction possible	Theoretically may enhance anti-inflammatory and antiplatelet effects.
	Policosanol	Increased bruising and bleeding	Observe	Doses >10 mg/day may inhibit platelet aggregation.
	Vitamin C	Decreased vitamin C effects	Observe	Aspirin may interfere with both absorption and cellular uptake mechanisms for vitamin C, thereby increasing vitamin C requirements, as observed in animal and human studies. Increased vitamin C intake may be required with long-term therapy.
	Willowbark	Increased bruising and bleeding	Caution with high dose (>240 mg/day)	Theoretically may enhance anti-inflammatory and antiplatelet effects. Although a clinical study found that consumption of salicin 240 mg/day produced minimal effects on platelet aggregation, higher doses may have a significant effect.
Cilostazol	Ginkgo biloba	Additive effects	Observe. Beneficial interaction possible	Used for intermittent claudication with peripheral arterial disease, adjunctive use with Ginkgo biloba may produce additional benefits based on in vivo.
Clopidogrel	St John's Wort	Additive effects	Observe. Monitor drug requirements (interaction may be beneficial)	SJW might represent a valid option to increase the antiplatelet effect of clopidogrel in non- and/or hypo-responders. For example, SJW increased platelet inhibition by enhancement of CYP3A4 metabolic activity for clopidogrel in hypo-responsive volunteers, and a recent study showed that residual platelet reactivity improved with SJW during the first month post percutaneous coronary intervention.
Antihypertensive agents				
Antihypertensive drugs	Arginine	Additive effects	Caution	Theoretically, additive hypotensive effects may occur — use with caution. Potential benefits under professional supervision.
	Essential fatty acids — omega-3 and omega-6	Increased drug effects	Observe — beneficial interaction possible	Both omega-3 and omega-6 fatty acids exhibit antihypertensive activity.

	Evening primrose oil	Additive effects	Observe — monitor drug requirements (interaction may be beneficial)	Evening primrose oil has been shown to enhance the effects of several antihypertensive drugs, including dihydralazine, clonidine and captopril in rats under experimental conditions.
	Guarana	Antagonistic effects	Caution	Theoretical concern
	Garlic	Additive effects	Caution — monitor drug requirements (interaction may be beneficial)	Clinical trials have shown garlic to reduce blood pressure.
	Hawthorn	Additive effects	Caution — monitor drug requirements (interaction may be beneficial)	Mild antihypertensive activity has been reported with long-term use of hawthorn.
	Licorice	Reduced drug effect	Caution — monitor blood pressure when high-dose licorice preparations are taken for more than 2 weeks	High-dose glycyrrhizin taken long-term can lead to increased blood pressure.
	Maca	Theoretical interactions	Observe. Separate doses by 2 hours	Theoretical interactions have been suggested to be plausible in people taking antihypertensives. However, there are no reported drug interactions.
	Nigella	Additive effects	Observe. Beneficial interaction possible.	A clinical study reported that Nigella reduced blood pressure in patients with mild hypertension.
	Oats (oat-based cereals)	Additive effects	Observe — monitor drug requirements (interaction may be beneficial)	A clinical trial has shown that ingestion of oat-based cereals decreased blood pressure in 73% of hypertensive patients and reduced drug requirements.
	Olive leaf and olive oil	Additive effects	Beneficial interaction possible	
	St John's wort	Altered drug effects	Caution. Monitor for signs of reduced drug effectiveness and adjust the dose if necessary or avoid.	SJW was shown to induce nifedipine metabolism in vivo.
	Stinging nettle	Additive effects	Observe patients taking antihypertensives concurrently	Additive effects are theoretically possible.

Continued

Herb/Supplement	Pathway	Potential outcome	Recommendation	Evidence/Comments
Hydralazine (e.g. Apresoline, Alphapress)	Coenzyme Q10	Reduced CoQ10 serum levels	Beneficial interaction possible	Increased CoQ10 intake may be required with long-term therapy.
	Vitamin B_6 (pyridoxine)	Reduced vitamin B_6 absorption	Separate doses by at least 2 hours	A clinical trial has shown that the drug may induce B_6 deficiency, so increased intake may be required with long-term therapy.
Methyldopa (e.g. Aldomet)	Coenzyme Q10	Reduced CoQ10 serum levels	Beneficial interaction possible	Increased CoQ10 intake may be required with long-term therapy.
ACE inhibitors (e.g. captopril, enalapril)	Iron	Reduced drug effect	Separate doses by at least 2 hours	A small clinical trial found that concomitant iron administration reduced area-under-the-curve plasma levels of unconjugated captopril by 37%.
	Zinc	Reduced zinc levels	Monitor for zinc efficacy and zinc status	These drugs reduce zinc status, most likely due to increased urinary excretion of zinc. Increased zinc intake may be required with long-term therapy.
ACE inhibitors (e.g. Losartan)	Rhodiola	Potential for increased drug serum levels	Avoid	Rhodiola significantly alters the pharmacokinetic properties of losartan after concurrent oral administration to rabbits. The results indicate that rhodiola is likely to inhibit CYP3A4 resulting in increased drug serum levels. Avoid — until further research is available to determine the level of the interaction.
Angiotensin 2 receptor blockers	Zinc	Reduced zinc levels and increased excretion	Monitor for zinc efficacy and zinc status	These drugs reduce zinc status, most likely due to increased urinary excretion of zinc.
Verapamil	St John's wort	Reduces drug levels via increased metabolism	Monitor and adjust dose as necessary under medical supervision	Decreases serum levels of verapamil via CYP induction.
Beta-adrenergic-blocking agents	Coenzyme Q10	Reduced CoQ10 serum levels	Beneficial interaction possible	Increased CoQ10 intake may be required with long-term therapy.
Propranolol	Myrrh	Reduced drug effect	Observe	A clinical trial has shown that guggulipid reduces bioavailability of propranolol. It is uncertain what implications this has for use of *Commiphora molmol.*
	Vitamin E	Reduced drug effect	Observe	According to in vitro research, vitamin E inhibits drug uptake in human cultured fibroblasts — clinical significance unknown.

Calcium-channel blockers (e.g. verapamil)	Calcium	Reduced drug effect/Antagonist	Avoid high-dose supplements unless under medical supervision	Calcium may reduce antihypertensive effect of drug. Can have an antagonistic effect on the desired action of calcium channel blockers.
	Magnesium	Additive effects	Observe — monitor drug requirements (interaction may be beneficial)	A meta-analysis of 20 randomised trials showed that magnesium has a modest antihypertensive activity.
	Vitamin D	Reduced drug effect	Caution unless under medical supervision	
Felodipine	Peppermint oil	Increased drug effects	Caution	Peppermint oil has been shown to increase the oral bioavailability of felodipine in animal studies.
Nifedipine	Ginseng — Korean	Increased drug effects	Caution	Ginseng was found to increase the mean plasma concentration of the calcium channel blocker nifedipine by 53% at 30 minutes in an open trial. Exercise caution.
	St John's wort	Altered drug effects	Caution. Monitor for signs of reduced drug effectiveness and adjust the dose if necessary or avoid.	SJW was shown to induce nifedipine metabolism in vivo.
Diltiazem	Myrrh	Reduced drug effect	Prudent to avoid guggulipid preparations	A clinical trial has shown that guggulipid reduces bioavailability of diltiazem. It is uncertain what implications this has for use of *Commiphora molmol.*
	Quercetin	Increased drug effects	Caution. Use under professional supervision	Increased drug bioavailability observed in vivo.
Antimigraine preparations				
Antimigraine preparations	Coenzyme Q10	Additive effects	Beneficial interaction possible	CoQ10 demonstrated migraine prevention activity in a clinical study.
	Feverfew	Additive effects	Beneficial interaction possible	Feverfew demonstrated migraine prevention activity in several clinical studies, so migraine medication requirements may reduce.
	Vitamin B_2 (riboflavin)	Additive effects	Beneficial interaction possible	Vitamin B_2 has demonstrated migraine prevention activity in several clinical studies.
Clonidine (e.g. Catapres)	Coenzyme Q10	Reduced CoQ10 serum levels	Beneficial interaction possible	In vivo study indicates that clonidine reduces serum CoQ10 levels. Increased CoQ10 intake may be required with long-term therapy.

Continued

2

Herb/Supplement	Pathway	Potential outcome	Recommendation	Evidence/Comments
Cardiac inotropic agents				
Cardiac glycosides	Calcium	May potentiate digoxin toxicity	Caution, unless under medical supervision	Administered concurrently, high-dose calcium may potentiate digoxin toxicity — use this combination with caution unless under medical supervision.
	Hawthorn	Additive effects	Caution — monitor drug requirements (interaction may be beneficial)	Theoretical interaction, as in vitro and in vivo studies indicate that hawthorn has positive inotropic activity. Small clinical study found interaction not clinically significant when digoxin 0.25 mg taken with Hawthorn (WS1442) 450 mg twice daily.
	Psyllium	Decreased drug absorption	Caution. Separate doses by 2 hours	Soluble fibre may decrease the bioavailability of cardiac glycosides.
Digoxin (e.g. Lanoxin) Adverse effects of high-dose digoxin include: nausea, vomiting, diarrhoea, confusion, fainting, palpitations, irregular heart beat, visual disturbances	Aloe vera	Increased drug toxicity	Avoid long-term use of high-dose preparations	Long-term oral use of aloe can deplete potassium levels and reduced potassium status lowers the threshold for drug toxicity.
	Astragalus	Additive effects	Observe patients using high-dose astragalus preparations	Additive effects are theoretically possible with intravenous administration of Astragalus, based on positive inotropic activity identified in clinical studies. The clinical significance of these findings for oral dose forms is unknown.
	Calcium	May potentiate digoxin toxicity	Caution, unless under medical supervision	Administered concurrently, high-dose calcium may potentiate digoxin toxicity — use this combination with caution unless under medical supervision.
	Ginseng — Korean	Interferes with therapeutic drug monitoring for digoxin	Caution — drug assay may produce false-positive results	Ginseng contains glycosides with structural similarities to digoxin, which may interfere with digoxin results.
	Ginseng — Siberian	Interferes with therapeutic drug monitoring for digoxin	Caution — drug assay may produce false-positive results	Refer to Chapter 8 on interactions for further information.
	Guarana	Increased drug toxicity	Avoid long-term use of high-dose preparations	Long-term guarana use can deplete potassium levels and reduced potassium status lowers the threshold for drug toxicity.

	Licorice	Increased drug toxicity	Avoid long-term use of high-dose preparations (>100 mg glycyrrhizin daily >2 weeks) unless under medical supervision	Reduced potassium status lowers the threshold for drug toxicity.
	Quercetin	Increased drug toxicity	Avoid concurrent use	Increased drug bioavailability possible.
	Slippery elm	Altered rate and/or extent of absorption	Caution. Separate doses by 2 hours	Controlled studies are unavailable, but interactions are theoretically possible with some medicines. Slippery elm forms an inert barrier over the gastrointestinal lining and may theoretically alter the rate and/or extent of absorption of medicines with a narrow therapeutic range (e.g. digoxin). The clinical significance of this is unclear.
	St John's wort	Reduced drug effects	Avoid unless under medical supervision Monitor for signs of reduced drug effectiveness and adjust dose if necessary When St John's wort is started or ceased, monitor serum levels and alter drug dosage as required	St John's wort induces CYP enzymes and P-glycoprotein. A clinical trial shows that St John's wort significantly decreases serum levels of drug within 10 days of concomitant use.
Digoxin assays	Withania	Altered test results	Caution. Use under medical care. Monitor test results.	Withania may modestly interfere with serum digoxin measurements by the fluorescent polarisation immunoassay (FPIA) and other assays.
Diuretics				
Caffeine	Calcium	Increases urinary excretion of calcium	Separate doses by 2–3 hours	Caffeine increases urinary excretion of calcium and may affect calcium absorption — ensure adequate calcium intake and monitor for signs and symptoms of deficiency in those with high caffeine intake.
Diuretics	Dandelion leaf	Additive effects	Observe	Theoretically increased diuresis is possible — clinical significance is unknown.
	Elder	Additive effects	Observe	Elderflower has diuretic activity. Increased diuresis is possible with concomitant use.
	Green tea	Additive effects	Observe	Based on the caffeine content of green tea, high intakes of green tea can theoretically increase the diuretic effects of drugs such as frusemide; however, the clinical significance of this is unknown.

Continued

Herb/Supplement	Pathway	Potential outcome	Recommendation	Evidence/Comments
	Guarana	Additive diuretic effects but decreased hypotensive effects of drug	Caution Monitor potassium status	Theoretically increased diuresis and decreased hypotensive effects are possible — clinical significance is unknown.
	Licorice	Increased potassium excretion	Avoid long-term use unless under medical supervision Monitor potassium status	Potassium loss may become significant when licorice is used in high dose (>100 mg glycyrrhizin daily) for longer than 2 weeks.
	Stinging nettle	Additive effects	Observe patients taking this combination	Theoretically increased diuresis is possible — clinical significance is unknown.
Loop diuretics	Magnesium	Increased magnesium excretion	Monitor magnesium efficacy and status — beneficial interaction possible	Increased magnesium intake may be required with long-term therapy.
	Stinging nettle	Additive effects	Observe	Theoretically increased diuresis is possible — clinical significance is unknown.
	Vitamin B_1 (thiamin)	Reduced B_1 levels	Monitor B_1 efficacy and status — beneficial interaction possible	Increased B_1 dietary intake may be required with long-term therapy. Consider long-term supplementation.
	Zinc	Increased urinary zinc excretion	Monitor zinc efficacy and status — beneficial interaction possible	Increased zinc intake may be required with long-term therapy.
Potassium-sparing diuretics	Magnesium	Increased magnesium effects	Observe	
Thiazide diuretics	Calcium	Decreased urinary calcium excretion	Observe Monitor serum calcium and look for signs of hypercalcaemia	Thiazide diuretics decrease urinary excretion of calcium. Monitor serum calcium and look for signs of hypercalcaemia, such as anorexia, polydipsia, polyuria, constipation and muscle hypertonia when using high-dose calcium supplements.
	Magnesium	Increased magnesium excretion	Monitor magnesium efficacy and status — beneficial interaction possible	Increased magnesium intake may be required with long-term therapy.
	Zinc	Increased urinary zinc excretion	Monitor zinc efficacy and status — beneficial interaction possible	Increased zinc intake may be required with long-term therapy.
Hydrochlorothiazide (e.g. Diclotride)	Coenzyme Q10	Reduced CoQ10 serum levels	Beneficial interaction possible	Increased CoQ10 intake may be required with long-term therapy.
	Garlic	Raises drug serum levels	Cautious use under medical supervision	Co-administration may require a reduction in the dose of hydrochlorothiazide due to a pharmacokinetic interaction raising drug serum levels.

	Vitamin B_{12}	Reduces hyper-homocysteinaemia	Beneficial interaction possible in conjunction with folate	Hydrochlorothiazide may increase homocysteine levels.
Hypolipidaemic agents				
Hypolipidaemic agents	Chromium	Additive effects	Observe — monitor drug requirements (interaction may be beneficial)	Clinical trials indicate that chromium reduces total cholesterol levels.
	Garlic	Additive effects	Observe — monitor drug requirements (interaction may be beneficial)	A meta-analysis of 13 clinical trials concluded that garlic significantly reduces total cholesterol levels — effects are described as modest.
	Myrrh	Additive effects	Observe — monitor drug requirements (interaction may be beneficial for guggul preparations)	Guggul has demonstrated cholesterol-lowering activity in several clinical studies.
	Nigella	Additive effects	Observe. Beneficial interaction possible — monitor drug requirements	Black seed has been shown to modulate lipid levels according to clinical trials.
	Oats (oat-based cereals)	Additive effects	Beneficial interaction possible — monitor drug requirements	Clinical trials indicate that oat-based cereals reduce total cholesterol levels.
	Policosanol	Additive effects	Caution, although beneficial interaction possible under medical supervision	Policosanol may theoretically increase cholesterol-lowering effects of statins, but a theoretical concern exists as to whether concurrent use will also increase incidence of adverse effects.
	Vitamin B_3 (niacin)	Additive effects	Beneficial interaction possible — caution with sustained-release form	Several clinical trials confirm the cholesterol-lowering activity of niacin and the safety of niacin with statins, but the sustained-release form may be unsafe.
	Vitamin D	Reduced absorption of vitamin D	Observe. Administer the vitamin D at least 1 hour prior to or 4–6 hours after ingestion of the drug.	Hypolipidaemic agents may compromise the absorption of all fat-soluble vitamins. To avoid the interaction, administer the supplement at least 1 hour prior to or 4–6 hours after ingestion of the drug. Conversely, long-term use of statins is associated with increased 25(OH)D levels via an unknown mechanism.
Cholestyramine (e.g. Questran lite, colestipol [e.g. Colestid])	Beta-carotene	Reduced absorption of beta-carotene	Separate doses by 2 hours	Drugs that reduce fat absorption, such as cholestyramine, colestipol and orlistat, may also reduce absorption of beta-carotene.
	Fat-soluble vitamins (A, D, E, K, beta-carotene)	Reduced vitamin absorption	Separate doses by at least 4 hours and monitor vitamin status	Increased vitamin intake may be required with long-term therapy.

Continued

2

Herb/Supplement	Pathway	Potential outcome	Recommendation	Evidence/Comments
	Folate	Reduced folate absorption	Separate doses by at least 4 hours and monitor iron status	Increased vitamin intake may be required with long-term therapy.
	Iron	Reduced iron absorption	Separate doses by at least 4 hours and monitor iron status	Increased iron intake may be required with long-term therapy.
	Vitamin A	Reduced vitamin A absorption	Separate doses by at least 4 hours and monitor vitamin A status	Reduces vitamin A absorption — increase dietary intake of vitamin A-rich foods or consider supplementation with long-term use.
	Vitamin D	Reduced absorption of vitamin D	Observe. Administer the vitamin D at least 1 hour prior to or 4–6 hours after ingestion of the drug.	Hypolipidaemic agents may compromise the absorption of all fat-soluble vitamins. To avoid the interaction, administer the supplement at least 1 hour prior to or 4–6 hours after ingestion of the drug. Conversely, long-term use of statins is associated with increased 25(OH)D levels via an unknown mechanism.
	Vitamin E	Reduced vitamin absorption	Separate doses by at least 4 hours and monitor vitamin status	Increased vitamin intake may be required with long-term therapy.
Chitosan	Vitamin C	May increase cholesterol-lowering effect	Beneficial interaction possible	
Fibric-acid derivatives (e.g. gemfibrozil)	Beta-carotene		Beneficial interaction possible	There may be a positive interaction between fibrate and natural beta-carotene, which has been found to significantly increase HDL cholesterol levels.
	Coenzyme Q10	Reduced CoQ10 serum levels	Beneficial interaction possible — separate doses by 4 hours	Increased CoQ10 intake may be required with long-term therapy.
HMG-CoA reductase inhibitors (statins)	Carnitine	Additive effects	Beneficial interaction possible	the addition of L-carnitine (2 g/day) to simvastatin therapy (20 mg/day) appears to lower lipoprotein-a serum levels in patients with type 2 diabetes.
	Coenzyme Q10	Reduced CoQ10 serum levels	Beneficial interaction possible	Clinical study indicates several statin drugs reduce CoQ10 levels — increased CoQ10 intake may be required with long-term therapy.
	Red rice yeast	Additive effects	Observe	Red rice yeast products contain low doses of natural statins and, as such, a pharmacodynamic interaction is possible with other statin medications with increased lipid lowering effects.
	St John's wort	Reduced drug effects	Monitor for signs of reduced drug effectiveness and adjust the dose if necessary When St John's wort is started or ceased, monitor serum levels and alter drug dosage as required	SJW reduces the efficacy of atorvastatin, so lipid-lowering effects are compromised.

	Vitamin A	Increased vitamin A activity	Observe	A clinical trial has reported increased serum levels of vitamin A — clinical significance unclear.
	Vitamin B_3 (niacin)	Additive effects	Beneficial interaction possible — caution with sustained-release form	Several clinical trials confirm the cholesterol-lowering activity of niacin and the safety of niacin with statins, but the sustained release form may be less safe.
	Vitamin E	Reduced vitamin E levels	Observe. Monitor for vitamin E deficiency	The effect of statins on lowering blood lipid levels of vitamin E have been suggested as a risk factor in the development of statin-associated myopathy. Further studies are warranted.
Pravastatin (e.g. Pravachol)	Fish oils	Additive effects	Beneficial interaction possible	A clinical trial suggests improved lipid-lowering effects when used concurrently.
Simvastatin (e.g. Lipex, Zocor)	Peppermint oil	Additive effects	Observe — monitor drug requirements (interaction may be beneficial)	Peppermint oil has been shown to increase the oral bioavailability of simvastatin in animal studies.
	St John's wort	Reduced drug effects and serum levels	Monitor for signs of reduced drug effectiveness and adjust the dose if necessary When St John's wort is started or ceased, monitor serum levels and alter drug dosage as required	St John's wort increases metabolism of simvastatin. Decreases serum levels of simvastatin via CYP induction.
	St Mary's thistle	Increased drug effect	Observe — monitor drug requirements	May reduce metabolism of drug resulting in increased serum levels and adverse effects (difficult to evaluate evidence).
CENTRAL NERVOUS SYSTEM				
Anticonvulsants				
Anticonvulsants	Beta-carotene	Reduced plasma beta-carotene	Observe	Epileptic patients who gain weight with valproate therapy have been found to have reduced plasma concentrations of beta-carotene and other fat-soluble antioxidant vitamins.
	Carnitine	Reduced side-effects	Beneficial interaction possible	L-Carnitine deficiency may cause or potentiate valproic acid toxicity, and supplementation is known to reduce the toxicity of valproate as well as symptoms of fatigue — concurrent use is recommended, as a beneficial interaction is possible.
	Folate	Reduced side-effects	Monitor for drug effectiveness Beneficial interaction possible	Requires close supervision to ensure that drug efficacy is not substantially reduced.

Continued

Herb/Supplement	Pathway	Potential outcome	Recommendation	Evidence/Comments
	Ginkgo biloba	Reduced drug effects	Caution — monitor for reduced drug effectiveness	Based on case reports. One report was of a patient taking Dilantin and Depakote and ginkgo, together with other herbal medicines, who suffered a fatal breakthrough seizure, with no evidence of non-compliance with anticonvulsant medications. The autopsy report revealed subtherapeutic serum levels for both anticonvulsants.
	Nigella	Interaction may be beneficial	Observe — monitor drug requirements	Small clinical study shows anticonvulsant effects in epileptic children refractory to their antiepileptic medication. The constituent thymoquinone was reported to reduce sodium valproate-induced hepatotoxicity in one animal study.
	St John's wort	Reduced drug effects	Avoid unless under medical supervision to alter doses appropriately When St John's wort is started or ceased, monitor serum levels and alter drug dosage as required	St John's wort may increase drug metabolism, resulting in reduced drug efficacy.
	Vitamin B_{12}	Additive effect	Observe. Possible beneficial effect	Administration of sodium valproate has been shown to increase plasma vitamin B_{12} concentrations, with one study citing increases of over 50% of baseline.
Carbamazepine (e.g. Tegretol) NTI: signs of overdose include CNS and respiratory depression, hypotension, vomiting, fluid retention	St Mary's thistle	Increased drug effects	Caution — monitor drug requirements	May reduce metabolism of drug resulting in increased serum levels and adverse effects (difficult to evaluate evidence).
	Vitamin B_{12}	Decreased B_{12} levels	Observe for signs and symptoms of B_{12} deficiency Beneficial interaction possible	In studies with children, long-term carbamazepine use led to a decrease in vitamin B_{12} levels. Increased intake may be required with long-term therapy.
Phenobarbitone	Celery	Prolonged action	Caution	Celery juice has been found to prolong the action of phenobarbitone in rats — clinical significance unknown.
	Kava	Increased sedation	Caution	

	Vitamin B_6 (pyridoxine)	Reduced drug effects	Caution — monitor for reduced drug effectiveness	B_6 in high doses may lower plasma levels and efficacy of drug and decrease seizure control. Monitor for drug effectiveness, and exercise caution when these drugs are being taken concurrently.
	Withania	Increased sedation	Observe although beneficial interaction possible	
Phenobarbitone and phenytoin	Kava	Increased sedation	Caution	
	Slippery elm	Altered rate and/or extent of absorption	Caution. Separate doses by 2 hours	Controlled studies are unavailable, but interactions are theoretically possible with some medicines. Slippery elm forms an inert barrier over the gastrointestinal lining and may theoretically alter the rate and/or extent of absorption of medicines with a narrow therapeutic range (e.g. phenytoin). The clinical significance of this is unclear.
	St John's wort	Decreased drug effects (increased drug metabolism)	Avoid — monitor drug requirements. When St John's wort is started or ceased, monitor serum levels and alter drug dosage as required	
	Vitamin B_6 (pyridoxine)	Reduced drug effects	Caution — monitor for reduced drug effectiveness	B_6 in high doses may lower plasma levels and efficacy of drug and decrease seizure control. Monitor for drug effectiveness, and exercise caution when these drugs are being taken concurrently.
	Vitamin B_{12}	Increased serum B_{12} levels	Observe	One clinical study reported that combined long-term use of phenobarbitone and phenytoin resulted in significantly increased serum B_{12} levels — clinical significance unknown.
Phenytoin	Vitamin B_6 (pyridoxine)	Reduced drug effects	Caution — monitor for reduced drug effectiveness	B_6 in high doses may lower plasma levels and efficacy of drug and decrease seizure control. Monitor for drug effectiveness, and exercise caution when these drugs are being taken concurrently.
Phenytoin and valproate	Vitamin D	Reduced side-effects	Beneficial interaction possible	Anticonvulsants induce catabolism of vitamin D through liver induction — prolonged use is associated with increased risk of developing rickets and osteomalacia, therefore increased intake may be useful with long-term therapy.
Sodium valproate	Celery	Reduced side-effects	Observe — beneficial interaction possible	In animal studies, celery was found to have a protective effect against sodium valproate's well established toxicity to the testes and sperm production.

Continued

Herb/Supplement	Pathway	Potential outcome	Recommendation	Evidence/Comments
Antidepressants				
Antidepressants including SSRIs, SNRIs, tricyclics and MAOIs	Albizia	Additive effects	Observe	Increased risk of serotonergic syndrome is theoretically possible, as the herb increases serotonin levels, according to in vivo studies — clinical significance unknown
	Brahmi	Additive effects	Caution until further investigation can confirm.	Serotonergic activity has been identified for Bacopa extracts therefore there is a theoretical increased risk of serotonin syndrome when bacopa is used together with SSRI and SNRI medicines — the clinical significance of the interaction is unclear.
	Ginkgo biloba	Reduced side-effects	Beneficial interaction possible	Reduced sexual dysfunction side-effects reported in a clinical study and may also improve sleep continuity.
	Green tea	Reduced drug effects	Caution	Caution is advised when using highly concentrated supplements with monoamine oxidase inhibitors or dopamimmetic drugs because catechins are metabolised by catechol-O-methyltransferase.
	Maca	Theoretical interactions	Observe. Separate doses by 2 hours	Theoretical interactions have been suggested to be plausible in people taking antidepressants. However, there are no reported drug interactions.
	Rhodiola	Reduced drug effects	Observe	In vitro tests suggest an inhibition of MAO A by Rhodiola extracts, a theoretical interaction exists with MAOI antidepressants. The clinical significance of this and whether other antidepressants may be affected is as yet unclear.
	Saffron	Additive effects	Caution. Use under medical supervision.	Saffron exhibits significant antidepressant activity; concomitant use should be carefully supervised. It is theoretically possible that pharmaceutical antidepressant dosage requirements will decrease with the addition of saffron in therapeutic doses.
	St John's wort	Additive effects	Avoid unless under medical supervision	SJW decreases serum levels of some antidepressants via CYP induction in vivo. Risk of serotonergic syndrome if combined use is not carefully monitored. Avoid concurrent use unless under medical supervision, so that doses may be altered appropriately.
	SAMe	Additive effects	Caution	Theoretically may increase risk of serotonergic syndrome, and a case report exists; however, an experimental study found that brain SAMe levels were significantly reduced after chronic treatment with imipramine.
	Tyrosine	Additive effects	Avoid unless under medical supervision	Tyrosine is a precursor for several neurotransmitters, which theoretically increases risk of serotonin syndrome.

	Vitamin B_2 (riboflavin)	Decreased B_2 levels	Monitor for signs and symptoms of B_2 deficiency Beneficial interaction possible	Tricyclic antidepressants may reduce the absorption of riboflavin. Increased B_2 intake may be required with long-term therapy.
SSRI (Bupropion/ Zyban)	St John's Wort	Decreased plasma concentration. Reduced drug effects	Avoid	SJW statistically significantly decreased plasma concentrations of bupropion, probably by increasing the clearance of bupropion.
MAOIs	Green tea	Reduced drug effects	Caution	Caution is advised when using highly concentrated supplements with monoamine oxidase inhibitors or dopamimetic drugs because catechins are metabolised by catechol-O-methyltransferase.
	Rhodiola	Reduced drug effects	Observe	In vitro tests suggest an inhibition of MAO A by Rhodiola extracts, a theoretical interaction exists with MAOI antidepressants. The clinical significance of this and whether other antidepressants may be affected is as yet unclear.
	Tyrosine	Increased side-effects	Avoid	Some tyrosine may be metabolised to tyramine Concurrent use with MAOIs may lead to hypertensive crisis.
Tricyclic antidepressants	Albizia	Additive effects	Observe	Increased risk of serotonin syndrome is theoretically possible as Albizia increases serotonin levels, according to in vivo studies — clinical significance unknown.
	Andrographis	Reduced side-effects	Beneficial interaction possible	Andrographis may exert hepatoprotective activity against liver damage induced by tricyclic antidepressants.
	Coenzyme Q10	Reduced CoQ10 serum levels	Beneficial interaction possible	Increased CoQ10 intake may be required with long-term therapy.
	SAMe	Additive effects	Caution. Use under medical supervision	Co-administration of SAMe with SSRIs has shown benefits in partial responders and may be a useful combination under professional supervision.
	St John's wort	Additive effects	Avoid unless under medical supervision	Although St John's wort decreases drug plasma levels of tricyclic antidepressants, it may increase available serotonin.
	St Mary's thistle	Reduced side-effects	Beneficial interaction possible	St Mary's thistle may exert hepatoprotective activity against liver damage induced by tricyclic antidepressants.
	Tyrosine	Additive effects	Avoid unless under medical supervision	Tyrosine is a precursor for several neurotransmitters, which theoretically increases risk of serotonin syndrome.
	Vitamin B_2 (riboflavin)	Decreased B_2 levels	Monitor for signs and symptoms of B_2 deficiency Beneficial interaction possible	Tricyclic antidepressants may reduce the absorption of riboflavin. Increased B_2 intake may be required with long-term therapy.

Continued

Herb/Supplement	Pathway	Potential outcome	Recommendation	Evidence/Comments
Imipramine	Vitamin B_3 (niacin)	Additive effects	Beneficial interaction possible	A combination of imipramine with L-tryptophan 6 g/day and niacinamide 1500 mg/day has been shown to be more effective for people with bipolar disorder than imipramine alone.
Antipsychotic agents				
	Withania	Reduced side-effects	Observe — beneficial interaction possible under professional supervision	In animal experiments, withania has been shown to be useful in the treatment of drug-induced dyskinesia (chewing movements, tongue protrusion and buccal tremors) due to reserpine and haloperidol.
Clozapine	Ginkgo biloba	Increased drug effects	Observe — beneficial interaction possible under professional supervision	Ginkgo may enhance the effects of clozapine on negative affect in refractory schizophrenic patients.
Haloperidol (e.g. Serenace)	Ginkgo biloba	Increased drug effects and reduced side-effects	Observe — beneficial interaction possible under professional supervision	Three clinical trials demonstrate that ginkgo increases drug effectiveness.
	Iron	Reduced iron effect	Monitor iron status	May cause decreased blood levels of iron — clinical significance unclear. Increased iron intake may be required with long-term therapy.
	Quercetin	Reduced drug side-effects	Beneficial interaction possible	According to in vivo studies, reduced chewing movements and tongue protrusions (tardive dyskinesia) possible with concurrent use.
	Valerian	Increased side effects and oxidative stress	Observe patient for side effects. Use under medical supervision	In a rat study, oxidative stress parameters in the liver were increased when haloperidol was taken in combination with valerian via a significant increase in lipid peroxidisation levels (enhanced oxidation of thiobarbituric acid reactive species and dichlorofluorescein reactive species as well as an inhibition of hepatic d-ALA-D activity). The significance in humans is unknown.
Phenothiazines (e.g. chlorpromazine, trifluoperazine)	Coenzyme Q10	Reduced drug effects	Beneficial interaction possible	CoQ10 reduces adverse effect this drug class has on CoQ10-related enzymes, NADH oxidase and succinoxidase — beneficial interaction with co-administration.
	Evening primrose oil	Reduced drug effects	Avoid concomitant use until safety can be established	Several case reports suggest that evening primrose oil may reduce seizure threshold and reduce drug effectiveness in patients with schizophrenia treated with phenothiazines.
Chlorpromazine (e.g. Largactil)	Vitamin E	Reduced drug effects	Observe	According to in vitro research, vitamin E inhibits drug uptake in human cultured fibroblasts — clinical significance unknown.

CNS agents				
Acetylcholinesterase inhibitor drugs	Vitamin B_5	Additive effects	Observe. Use under medical supervision.	A theoretical concern exists that pantothenic acid, since it is involved in the biosynthesis of acetylcholine, might increase the effects of acetylcholinesterase inhibitor drugs.
Cholinergic drug Tacrine (e.g. Cognex)	Brahmi	Additive effects	Observe Beneficial interaction possible	Cholinergic activity has been identified for brahmi, so increased drug activity is theoretically possible.
	Ginkgo biloba	Additive effects	Observe Beneficial interaction possible	Cholinergic activity has been identified for ginkgo, so increased drug activity is theoretically possible.
	Lemon balm	Additive effects	Observe Beneficial interaction possible	Cholinergic activity has been identified for lemon balm, so increased drug activity is theoretically possible.
	St Mary's thistle	Reduced side-effects	Beneficial interaction possible	St Mary's thistle may exert hepatoprotective activity against liver damage induced by tacrine.
CNS stimulants	Green tea	Additive effects	Observe	Based on the caffeine content of Green tea, high intakes of green tea can theoretically increase the CNS stimulation effects of drugs such as nicotine and beta-adrenergic agonists (e.g. salbutamol); however, the clinical significance of this is unknown.
	Guarana	Additive effects	Caution	Herb has demonstrated CNS stimulant activity.
	Tyrosine	Additive effects	Caution	Tyrosine is a precursor for several neurotransmitters (theoretical concern).
Methylphenidate (e.g. Ritalin)	Zinc	Additive effects	Observe under medical care	The efficacy of this drug may be improved by supplementation with zinc sulfate (15 mg elemental zinc) for 6 weeks in children with ADHD. There is no change to side effects reported.
Movement disorders				
L-Dopa (levodopa)	Calcium	Reduced drug absorption	Separate doses by 2 hours	L-dopa can form an insoluble complex with calcium.
	Iron	Reduced drug absorption	Separate doses by 2 hours	L-dopa can form an insoluble complex with iron.
	Kava	Reduced drug effects	Avoid unless under medical supervision	Theoretical interaction, as dopamine antagonist effects have been reported for kava.
	Magnesium	Reduced drug absorption	Separate doses by 2 hours	L-dopa can form an insoluble complex with magnesium.

Continued

Herb/Supplement	Pathway	Potential outcome	Recommendation	Evidence/Comments
	Psyllium	Potential increased drug absorption	Observe. Monitor drug effectiveness.	Animal research suggests that concomitant administration of psyllium husks with levodopa results in an improvement in the levodopa kinetic profile with higher final concentrations and a longer plasma half-life.
	SAMe	Reduced drug effects	Observe	SAMe methylates levodopa, which could theoretically reduce the effectiveness of levodopa given for Parkinson's disease; however, the effect has not been observed clinically.
	Tyrosine	Decreased drug and tyrosine effect	Avoid unless under medical supervision	L-dopa competes with tyrosine for uptake, so concurrent use may decrease uptake of both substances, thereby reducing efficacy.
	Vitamin B_6 (pyridoxine)	Reduced drug effects	Observe Monitor for reduced drug effectiveness	Interaction does not occur with combination L-dopa products. In people with Parkinson's disease, L-dopa can cause hyperhomocysteinaemia, the extent of which is influenced by B-vitamin status. To maintain normal plasma homocysteine concentrations, the B-vitamin requirements are higher in L-dopa-treated patients than in those not on L-dopa therapy. B-vitamin supplements may be warranted for PD patients on L-dopa therapy.
	Vitamin C	Reduced side-effects	Beneficial interaction possible	A case report of co-administration with vitamin C suggests this may reduce drug side-effects.
	Zinc	Reduced drug absorption	Separate doses by 2 hours	L-Dopa can form an insoluble complex with zinc.
L-Dopa with carbidopa	Iron	Reduced drug effects	Separate doses by at least 2 hours	May reduce bioavailability of carbidopa and L-dopa.
Sedatives, hypnotics				
CNS sedatives	Eucalyptus	Addictive effects	Caution	Oral ingestion of eucalyptus has been associated with CNS depression, therefore additive effects are theoretically possible.
	Green tea	Reduced drug effects	Observe	Based on the caffeine content of green tea, high intakes of green tea can theoretically decrease the CNS depressant effects of drugs such as benzodiazepines; however, the clinical significance of this is unknown.
	Guarana	Reduced drug effects	Observe	Theoretically guarana may reduce the sedative effects of drug via its CNS stimulation effects; however, an in vivo study found no interaction with pentobarbitone.
	Hops	Additive effects	Caution	

	Kava	Additive effects	Caution Beneficial interaction possible under medical supervision	May be useful in benzodiazepine withdrawal.
	Lavender oil	Additive effects	Observe	
	Passionflower	Additive effects	Caution Beneficial interaction possible under medical supervision	May be useful in benzodiazepine withdrawal.
	St John's wort	Decreased the plasma concentration of zolpidem	Avoid	Repeated administration of SJW decreases the plasma concentration of zolpidem, probably by enhancing CYP3A4 activity.
	Valerian	Additive effects	Caution Beneficial interaction possible under medical supervision	Theoretically, potentiation effects may occur at high doses. May be useful in benzodiazepine withdrawal.
Midazolam (e.g. Hypnovel)	St John's wort	Reduced drug effects	Caution Monitor for signs of reduced drug effectiveness and adjust the dose if necessary	St John's wort may increase drug metabolism and so reduce serum levels of drug.
Barbiturates	Albizia	Additive effects	Caution Beneficial interaction possible under medical supervision	Potentiation of phenobarbitone-induced sleeping was observed in vivo — clinical significance unknown.
	Andrographis	Additive effects	Observe Beneficial interaction possible under medical supervision	Potentiation effects observed in vivo — clinical significance unknown.
	Celery	Additive effects	Caution. Use under medical supervision	Celery juice has been found to prolong the action of pentobarbitone in rats. Use with caution.
	Folate	Reduced drug effects	Caution Monitor for signs of reduced drug effectiveness	Concomitant folic acid use can reduce seizure control.
	Kava	Additive effects	Caution Beneficial interaction possible under medical supervision — monitor drug dosage	Increased sedation.
	Lemon balm	Additive effects	Observe Beneficial interaction possible under medical supervision	Increased sedation.

Continued

Herb/Supplement	Pathway	Potential outcome	Recommendation	Evidence/Comments
	Passionflower	Additive effects	Caution Beneficial interaction possible under medical supervision — monitor drug dosage	Increased sedation.
	Slippery elm	Altered rate and/or extent of absorption	Caution. Separate doses by 2 hours	Controlled studies are unavailable, but interactions are theoretically possible with some medicines. Slippery elm forms an inert barrier over the gastrointestinal lining and may theoretically alter the rate and/or extent of absorption of medicines with a narrow therapeutic range (e.g. barbiturates). The clinical significance of this is unclear.
	St John's wort	Reduced drug effects	Avoid — monitor drug requirements. When St John's wort is started or ceased, monitor serum levels and alter drug dosage as required	St John's wort induces CYP enzymes and P-glycoprotein, so can reduce drug serum levels.
	Valerian	Additive effects	Caution Beneficial interaction possible under medical supervision	Increased sedation.
	Vitamin B_6 (pyridoxine)	Reduced plasma levels and drug effects	Caution Monitor for drug effectiveness	Concomitant B_6 use can reduce seizure control.
	Withania	Additive effects	Observe Beneficial interaction possible under medical supervision	Theoretically may increase sedation.
Benzodiazepines	Chamomile	Additive effects	Observe Beneficial interaction possible under medical supervision	Theoretically an additive effect can occur with concurrent use.
	Kava	Additive effects	Caution Beneficial interaction possible under medical supervision — monitor drug dosage	Combination has been used to ease symptoms of benzodiazepine withdrawal under medical supervision.
	Passionflower	Additive effects	Caution Beneficial interaction possible under medical supervision — monitor drug dosage	Increased sedation. Passiflora may be a useful support during benzodiazepine withdrawal; use under medical supervision.

	St John's wort	Reduced serum levels and drug effects	Observe and caution. Use under medical supervision and monitor for signs of reduced drug effectiveness.	Decreases serum levels of alprazolam via CYP induction. Monitor for signs of reduced drug effectiveness and adjust the dose if necessary or avoid.
		Reduced serum levels and drug effects	Observe and caution. Monitor for signs of reduced drug effectiveness and adjust the dose if necessary or avoid.	Decreases serum levels of midazolam via CYP induction.
	Valerian	Additive effects	Observe Beneficial interaction possible under medical supervision	Combination has been used to ease symptoms of benzodiazepine withdrawal under medical supervision.
	Withania	Additive effects	Observe Beneficial interaction possible under medical supervision	
CONTRACEPTIVE AGENTS				
Combined oral contraceptive agents				
Oral contraceptive pill	Chaste tree	Reduced herb effects	Observe	There has been speculation as to whether chaste tree is effective when OCPs are being taken. Several clinical studies conducted in women taking the OCP have confirmed that chaste tree still reduces symptoms of premenstrual syndrome.
	Folate	Reduced folate levels	Beneficial interaction possible	Folate levels are reduced with long-term use. Increased intake may be required with long-term therapy.
	Licorice	Increased side-effects	Observe Caution with high-dose licorice (>100 mg/day glycyrrhizin) or long-term use (> 2 weeks)	Increased risk of side-effects such as hypokalaemia, fluid retention and elevated blood pressure have been noted in case reports.
	St John's wort	Reduced drug effects	Caution — avoid use with low-dose OCP	Breakthrough bleeding has been reported in 12 cases, which may indicate decreased effectiveness. Caution related to hyperforin.
	Vitamin A	Increased vitamin A levels	Observe. Monitor Vitamin A status	OCP increases serum vitamin A levels.
	Vitamin B_2 (riboflavin)	Reduced vitamin B_2 levels	Observe for signs and symptoms of B_2 deficiency	OCP may increase demand for vitamin B_2. Increased intake may be required with long-term therapy. Supplementation may be required.
	Vitamin B_3 (niacin)	Reduced vitamin B_3 levels	Observe for signs and symptoms of B_3 deficiency	Increased intake may be required with long-term therapy.

Continued

Herb/Supplement	Pathway	Potential outcome	Recommendation	Evidence/Comments
	Vitamin B_5 (pantothenic acid)	Reduced vitamin B_5 levels	Observe for signs and symptoms of B_5 deficiency	Increased intake may be required with long-term therapy. Supplementation may be required.
	Vitamin B_6 (pyridoxine)	Reduced vitamin B_6 levels	Observe for signs and symptoms of B_6 deficiency	OCP may induce pyridoxine deficiency. Increased intake may be required with long-term therapy.
	Vitamin B_{12}	Reduced vitamin B_{12} levels	Observe for signs and symptoms of B_{12} deficiency	OCP users showed significantly lower concentrations of cobalamin than controls in a clinical study. Increased intake may be required with long-term therapy. Observe for signs and symptoms of B_{12} deficiency and conduct testing if deficiency is suspected.
	Vitamin E	Reduced vitamin E levels	Observe for signs and symptoms of vitamin E deficiency	Very small cross sectional study suggests the OCP significantly lowered coenzyme Q10 and alpha tocopherol levels. Further studies are needed.
ENDOCRINE AND METABOLIC DISORDERS				
Adrenal steroid hormones				
Corticosteroids	Calcium	Reduced side-effects. Reduced calcium absorption	Beneficial interaction possible. Ensure adequate calcium intake.	Through inhibiting vitamin D-mediated calcium absorption and increased excretion, overall levels of calcium may be decreased. Increased calcium intake may be required with long-term therapy.
	Chromium	Reduced side-effects	Beneficial interaction possible	Corticosteroids increase urinary losses of chromium, and chromium supplementation has been shown to aid in recovery from steroid-induced diabetes mellitus.
	Licorice	Additive effects	Beneficial interaction possible but patients should be monitored closely for corticosteroid excess	Concurrent use of licorice preparations potentiates the effects of topical and oral corticosteroids (e.g. prednisolone) as glycyrrhizin inhibits the metabolism of prednisolone. Some practitioners use licorice to minimise requirements for, or to aid in withdrawal of, corticosteroid medications.
	Vitamin B_{12}	Decreased vitamin B_{12} levels	Observe for signs and symptoms of B_{12} deficiency. Separate doses by at least 2 hours	Decreased vitamin B_{12} levels have been reported in the cerebrospinal fluid and serum of multiple sclerosis patients following high-dose (1000 mg) intravenous methylprednisolone daily for 10 days.
	Vitamin C	Reduced vitamin C effects	Beneficial interaction possible	May increase requirement for vitamin C. Increased intake may be required with long-term therapy.
	Vitamin D	Reduced vitamin D absorption	Beneficial interaction possible	Increased vitamin D intake may be required with long-term therapy.

Betamethasone	Carnitine	Additive effects	Beneficial interaction possible	RCT has shown that a combination of low-dose betamethasone (2 mg/day) and L-carnitine (4 g/5 days) was more effective in preventing respiratory distress syndrome (7.3% vs 14.5%) and death (1.8% vs 7.3%) in preterm infants than high-dose betamethasone given alone (8 mg/2 days).
Agents affecting calcium and bone metabolism				
Alendronate (e.g. Fosamax) and Etidronate (e.g. Didronel)	Calcium	Reduced drug absorption	Separate doses by at least 2 hours	Calcium may reduce drug absorption; however, adequate calcium is required for optimal drug effects.
	Iron	Reduced drug absorption	Separate doses by at least 2 hours	
	Magnesium	Reduced drug absorption	Separate doses by at least 2 hours	Magnesium may reduce drug absorption; however, adequate magnesium is required for optimal drug effects.
	Zinc	Reduced drug absorption	Separate doses by at least 2 hours	
Glucocorticoids				
	Vitamin D	Reduced vitamin D absorption	Separate doses by at least 2 hours	In high doses, these drugs directly inhibit vitamin-D-mediated calcium uptake in the gastrointestinal tract and through unknown mechanisms may deplete levels of active vitamin D. During long-term therapy with either oral or inhaled corticosteroids, calcium and vitamin D supplementation should be considered.
Gonadal hormones				
Oestrogen	Hops	Additive effects	Observe	Theoretical interaction, based on mild oestrogenic effect of hops.
	Red clover	Reduced drug effects	Observe	Theoretically, if taken in large quantities phyto-oestrogens may compete with synthetic oestrogens for receptor binding — clinical significance unknown.
	Vitamin D	Additive effects	Observe	Vitamin D works synergistically with oestrogens to prevent bone loss.
Oestrogen receptor blockers (Tamoxifen)	Soy	Additive effects	Possible beneficial effect under professional supervision	Animal studies have shown that soy enhances the therapeutic effects of tamoxifen as both have SERM actions. Additionally, in vivo studies suggest that the isoflavone daidzein may enhance the effect of tamoxifen against breast cancer burden and incidence.
	Vitamin C	Additive effects	Observe under medical care. Beneficial interaction possible	Vitamin C enhanced the antitumour activity in vitro.

Continued

Herb/Supplement	Pathway	Potential outcome	Recommendation	Evidence/Comments
Oestrogen and progesterone	Calcium	Additive effects	Beneficial interaction possible	Possible beneficial interaction on bone mineralisation.
	Licorice	Increased side-effects	Observe Caution with high-dose licorice or long-term use (> 2 weeks)	OCP can increase sensitivity to glycyrrhizin side-effects such as hypertension, fluid retention and hypokalaemia.
Oestrogens and anti-androgen therapy	Tyrosine	Decreased plasma levels of tyrosine	Observe. Supplementation under medical supervision.	Oestrogens and anti-androgen therapies have been shown to decrease plasma levels of tyrosine by up to 18.3% after 4 and 12 months in transsexual patients, therefore supplementation may be suggested.
Testosterone	Licorice	Altered testosterone effect	Observe Monitor testosterone levels	Contradictory evidence suggests possible effects on testosterone levels.
Haemopoietic agents				
Erythropoietin	Ginseng — Korean	Enhanced drug effects	Beneficial interaction possible	The total saponin fraction has been shown to promote haematopoiesis — clinical significance for total herb unknown.
	Iron	Enhanced drug effects	Beneficial interaction possible	
	Withania	Enhanced drug effects	Beneficial interaction possible	Animal studies indicate herb increases haematopoiesis — clinical significance unknown.
Human growth hormone				
Human growth hormone	Glutamine	Enhanced nutrient absorption	Beneficial interaction possible	In patients with severe short bowel syndrome, concomitant use of glutamine and human growth hormone may enhance nutrient absorption.
Hypoglycaemic agents				
Hypoglycaemic (e.g. metformin) agents Adverse effects associated with increased hypoglycaemic effects include sweating, hunger, depression, tremor and headaches	Aloe vera	Additive effects	Observe	Oral aloe vera may have hypoglycaemic activity, so additive effects are theoretically possible.
	Alpha Lipoic Acid	Additive effects	Observe	Theoretically, concomitant use may affect glucose control and require medication dosage changes — observe.

	Andrographis	Additive effects	Caution — blood glucose levels should be checked regularly Beneficial interaction possible under professional supervision	Andrographis has hypoglycaemic activity comparable to that of metformin in vivo, so additive effects are theoretically possible.
	Bilberry	Additive effects	Observe	Animal study identified the constituent myrtillin as exerting hypoglycaemic actions — relevance for bilberry unclear.
	Bitter melon	Additive effects	Caution Monitor drug requirements Possible beneficial effect under professional supervision	Theoretically an additive effect is possible, resulting in increased hypoglycaemic effects — caution.
	Chromium	Additive effects	Caution Monitor drug requirements Beneficial interaction possible under professional supervision	Clinical studies have shown that chromium has hypoglycaemic activity in some individuals. Chromium may reduce requirements for hypoglycaemic agents. While a beneficial interaction is possible, this combination should be used with caution and drug requirements monitored and adjusted if necessary by a healthcare professional.
	Cinnamon	Additive effects	Observe — potentially beneficial interaction	Oral ingestion of cinnamon capsules may reduce blood glucose levels, therefore theoretically, an additive effect is possible with concurrent use.
	Damiana	Additive effects	Observe	Additive effects are theoretically possible, with unknown clinical significance.
	Elderflower	Additive effects	Observe	Elderflower has demonstrated hypoglycaemic effects in vitro; the clinical significance of this observation remains unknown, and further research is required.
	Eucalyptus	Additive effects	Caution	If used in combination with oral glucose-lowering conventional or complementary medicines oral by people with diabetes, doses of eucalyptus might contribute to hypoglycaemia. Blood glucose levels should be monitored to detect hypoglycaemia.
	Fenugreek	Additive effects	Caution — blood glucose levels should be checked regularly Beneficial interaction possible under professional supervision	Additive effects are theoretically possible in diabetes and drug dose reductions may be required in some patients.
	Ginseng — Siberian	Additive effects	Observe	Speculation is based on IV use in animal studies and has not been observed in humans with oral dose forms.
	Green tea	Additive effects	Observe	Clinical significance unknown.

Continued

Herb/Supplement	Pathway	Potential outcome	Recommendation	Evidence/Comments
	Gymnema	Additive effects	Caution — blood glucose levels should be checked regularly Beneficial interaction possible	Gymnema may enhance the blood glucose-lowering effects of insulin and hypoglycaemic agents.
	Horse chestnut	Possible additive effects	Observe	Due to possible hypoglycaemic activity, blood glucose levels should be monitored when horse chestnut or HCSE and hypoglycaemic agents are used concurrently. The clinical significance is unclear.
	Myrrh	Additive effects	Caution — blood glucose levels should be checked regularly Beneficial interaction possible	Myrrh has been shown to increase glucose tolerance in both normal and diabetic rats — clinical significance unknown.
	Nigella	Additive effects	Caution — however interaction may be beneficial	Preliminary clinical studies suggest Nigella reduces blood glucose levels and improves glucose tolerance in patients with type 2 diabetes, including those with the co-morbidity in dyslipidaemic patients.
	Oats	Additive effects	Observe. Beneficial interaction possible under supervision.	An uncontrolled pilot study found that oatmeal reduced insulin requirements in hospitalised patients with metabolic syndrome; the effect persisted after a 4-week outpatient period. Insulin requirements should be monitored in patients taking oat beta-glucans as a change to medication dose could be required.
	Olive leaf extract	Additive effects	Beneficial interaction possible — drug dose may need modification	
	Psyllium	Additive effects	Separate doses by 2 hours. Drug dose may need modification	Additive hypoglycaemic effects are theoretically possible.
	Tulsi	Potential interactions based on actions	Observe for interactions	There are no reports of significant interactions with tulsi. As tulsi has anti-diabetic actions there is a theoretically possibility of interactions with anti-diabetic medications but such interactions have not been reported.
	Vitamin B_3 (niacin)	Increased drug requirement	Caution Monitor drug effectiveness	Niacin may affect glycaemic control and increase fasting blood glucose levels, so medication doses may need to be reviewed.
	Vitamin B_{12}	Decreased vitamin B_{12} levels	Observe	In patients with type 2 diabetes, metformin has been shown to reduce levels of vitamin B_{12} (and folate) and increase homocysteine. Increased B_{12} intake may be required with long-term drug use.

	Withania	Reduced side effects	A potentially beneficial interaction that should only be used under supervision due to theoretical risk of induced thyrotoxicosis	Withania may protect type 2 diabetics on metformin from drug-induced hypothyroidism. A potentially beneficial interaction that should only be used under supervision due to theoretical risk of induced thyrotoxicosis.
Gliclazide	St John's wort	Increased clearance of drug	Observe and caution. Closely monitor to evaluate possible signs of reduced efficacy	Treatment with SJW significantly increases the apparent clearance of gliclazide, which is independent of CYP2C9 genotype, according to a crossover clinical study. People with diabetes receiving this combination should be closely monitored to evaluate possible signs of reduced efficacy.
Pioglitazone	Quercetin	Increases the bioavailability of drug	Caution	Quercetin may increase the bioavailability of pioglitazone (Actos). Due to the potential for toxicity, careful monitoring of hepatic and cardiac function is required.
Sulfonylureas	Coenzyme Q10	Reduced adverse effects of sulfonylureas	Observe. Beneficial interaction with co-administration	CoQ10 reduces adverse effects this drug class has on CoQ10-related enzymes. NADH oxidase and low CoQ10 levels have been observed in people with diabetes — beneficial interaction with co-administration.
Thyroid hormones and antithyroid agents				
Levothyroxine (e.g. Oroxine)	Alpha Lipoic Acid	Suppress T4 to T3 conversion	Observe. Separate doses by 2–4 hours	Uncertain interaction exists. When co-administered, ALA may suppress T4 to T3 conversion, decrease total cholesterol, triglycerides, albumin and total protein.
	Calcium	Reduced drug absorption	Separate doses by 2–4 hours	Calcium and thyroxine form an insoluble complex. Calcium administered concurrently may reduce drug absorption, while levothyroxine may block absorption of calcium, e.g. calcium carbonate.
	Celery	Decreased drug effect	Observe	One case report suggests that celery extract may reduce drug effects. Clinical significance unknown.
	Horseradish	Increased drug requirement	Observe Monitor thyroid function. Dose may need to be adjusted	Isothiocyanates may inhibit thyroxine formation and be goitrogenic, although this has not been demonstrated clinically.
	Iron	Decreased drug absorption	Separate doses by 2–4 hours	Iron supplements may decrease absorption of thyroid medication; however, iron deficiency may impair the body's ability to make thyroid hormones.
	Magnesium	Reduced drug absorption	Separate doses by 2–4 hours	Magnesium and thyroxine form an insoluble complex together.
	SAMe	Unknown	Caution	Caution and monitoring may be warranted.

Continued

Herb/Supplement	Pathway	Potential outcome	Recommendation	Evidence/Comments
	Tyrosine	Additive effects	Observe	Additive effects theoretically possible, as tyrosine is a precursor to thyroid hormones.
	Withania	Additive effects	Observe	An in vivo study reported that daily administration of *Withania somnifera* root extract enhanced serum T4 concentration.
	Zinc	Reduced drug absorption	Separate doses by 2–4 hours	Zinc and thyroxine form an insoluble complex together.
EYE				
Glaucoma preparations				
Timolol eye drops	Coenzyme Q10	Reduced side-effects	Beneficial interaction possible	A clinical trial of people with glaucoma found that oral CoQ10 reduced cardiovascular side-effects of timolol eye drops without affecting intraocular pressure.
GASTROINTESTINAL SYSTEM				
Digestive supplements				
Pancreatin	Folate	Reduced folate absorption	Monitor for folate efficacy and folate status	Reduced folate absorption.
Hyperacidity, reflux and ulcers				
Aluminium-based antacids	Calcium	Increased urinary excretion of calcium	Separate doses by 2–3 hours	Aluminium-containing antacids may increase urinary excretion of calcium.
	Vitamin C	Increased aluminium absorption	Separate doses by at least 2 hours	Vitamin C increases the amount of aluminium absorbed.
Antacids	Calcium	Reduced calcium absorption	Separate doses by 2–3 hours	Antacids that raise gastric pH may reduce calcium absorption, especially that of calcium carbonate or calcium phosphate as these salts require an acidic environment for solubilisation before calcium can be absorbed. Aluminium- and magnesium-containing antacids may increase urinary excretion of calcium.
	Cranberry	Increased B_{12} absorption	Beneficial interaction possible	Cranberry juice increases the absorption of vitamin B_{12} when used concurrently with PPI medicines.
	Folate	Reduced folate absorption	Separate doses by 2–3 hours	
	Iron	Reduced iron absorption	Separate doses by at least 2 hours	

	Licorice	May enhance ulcer-healing drug effects	Observe. Beneficial interaction possible	Adjunctive licorice treatment may enhance ulcer-healing drug effects — potentially beneficial interaction.
Antiulcer drugs				
Sucralfate (e.g. Carafate, Ulcyte)	Vitamin E	Reduced vitamin absorption	Separate doses by at least 4 hours Monitor vitamin status	Increased vitamin intake may be required with long-term therapy.
	Calcium	Reduced calcium absorption	Monitor calcium status	Calcium supplementation may be required.
Gastric-acid inhibitors (proton-pump inhibitors [e.g. omeprazole], H_2-receptor antagonists [e.g. ranitidine])	Folate	Reduced folate absorption	Separate doses by 2–3 hours	
	Iron	Reduced drug and iron effect	Monitor for iron efficacy and iron status	Drug reduces gastric acidity and therefore iron absorption.
	Licorice	May enhance ulcer-healing drug effects	Observe. Beneficial interaction possible	Adjunctive licorice treatment may enhance ulcer-healing drug effects — potentially beneficial interaction.
	St John's wort	Decreases serum levels of the drug	Avoid	Decreases serum levels of omeprazole via CYP induction in vivo.
	Vitamin B_{12}	Reduced B_{12} absorption	Beneficial interaction possible Monitor B_{12} status	B_{12} supplementation may be required with long-term therapy.
Helicobacter pylori triple-therapy	Garlic	Additive effects	Interaction may be beneficial	Garlic inhibits growth of *H. pylori* in vitro and in vivo and two studies have shown a synergistic effect with omeprazole.
Laxatives				
	Aloe vera	Additive effects	Caution	Anthraquinones have significant laxative activity and may increase adverse effects of griping.

Continued

2

Herb/Supplement	Pathway	Potential outcome	Recommendation	Evidence/Comments
GENITOURINARY SYSTEM				
Bladder function disorders				
5-alpha-reductase inhibitors (e.g. finasteride [e.g. Proscar])	Pygeum	Additive effects	Beneficial interaction possible	
	Saw palmetto	Additive effects	Beneficial interaction possible	Meta-analyses show that herb is beneficial for BPH and in vitro tests show it may also inhibit 5-alpha-reductase activity.
	St John's wort	Reduced plasma concentration of drug	Caution. Monitor drug requirements under professional care.	SJW treatment for 2 weeks induced the metabolism of finasteride and caused a reduced plasma exposure of the drug. A case report reports on an increased PSA value for a man who had started SJW 900 mg/day,10 weeks prior to the test and who was previously well controlled on finasteride.
	Stinging nettle root	Additive effects	Beneficial interaction possible	Clinical studies show nettle root to improve symptoms of BPH.
IMMUNOLOGY				
Immune modifiers				
Cyclosporin	Baical skullcap	Decreased drug effects	Avoid	A decoction of baical skullcap has been reported to significantly decrease plasma levels of cyclosporin in rats. The co-administration of these two substances should be avoided until further research is available.
	Coriolus versicolor	Decreased drug effects	Avoid	The use of Coriolus versicolor polysaccharopeptides are contraindicated when immune suppression is desired. Polysaccharopeptides reduce the potency of immunosuppressants such as cyclosporin.
	Echinacea	Decreased drug effects	Caution	Theoretically, the immunostimulant activity of the herb may reduce drug effects — clinical significance unknown.
	Goldenseal	Increased drug effects	Caution	RCT conducted with berberine constituent — clinical relevance for goldenseal difficult to assess.
	Licorice	Reduced oral bioavailability	Observe. Monitor cyclosporin levels closely	An in vivo study found that GA induced P-glycoprotein and CYP3A4, resulting in reduced oral bioavailability of cyclosporin — monitor cyclosporin levels closely.

	Nigella	Possible additive and antagonistic effects	Caution. Use under medical supervision.	Based on laboratory and animal studies, black seed displays immunomodulatory activity and may theoretically interact with either immunostimulant or immunosuppressant drugs. Human studies are not available, therefore interactions are currently speculative and based on evidence of pharmacological activity. Clinical significance unknown.
	Peppermint	Additive effects	Avoid unless under medical supervision	Peppermint oil has been shown to increase the oral bioavailability of cyclosporin in animal studies — clinical significance unknown.
	Quercetin	Reduced oral bioavailability	Avoid.	Animal studies demonstrate that co-administration of quercetin significantly decreases the oral bioavailability of cyclosporin.
	Red rice yeast	Potential increased side-effects	Observe	Monacolins are metabolised by the cytochrome P450 system and therefore cyclosporin and other P450 inhibitors have the potential to increase the risk of rhabdomyolysis. This is a theoretical concern only — clinical significance unclear.
	St John's wort	Reduced drug effects	Avoid	Decreases plasma levels significantly within 3 days of concomitant use.
	St Mary's thistle	Reduced drug side-effects but may increase drug effects	Caution	Decreases hepatotoxicity; however, herb may reduce drug metabolism leading to increased effects — clinical significance unknown.
Interferon	Baical skullcap	Increased side-effects	Caution	There have been reports of acute pneumonitis due to a possible interaction between Sho-saiko-to preparation (containing baical skullcap) and interferon, which appears to be due to an allergic–immunological mechanism rather than direct toxicity.
Interferon-alpha	Carnitine	Reduced side-effects	Beneficial interaction possible	Clinical trials with patients being treated with interferon-alpha for hepatitis C found a reduction in fatigue associated with treatment when carnitine 2 g/day was co-administered.
Pegylated Interferon alpha (peginterferon α)	St John's wort	Increased side-effects	Avoid	The combination of peginterferon α and SJW (taken for 6 weeks during 8-week drug treatment) resulted in a severe acute hepatitis in a 61-year-old woman.
Tacrolimus (e.g. Prograf)	St John's wort	Reduced drug effects	Avoid unless under medical supervision	Decreased drug serum levels via CYP induction.
Vaccines				
Influenza virus vaccine	Ginseng — Siberian	Reduced side-effects	Beneficial interaction possible	May reduce the risk of post-vaccine reactions.

Continued

Herb/Supplement	Pathway	Potential outcome	Recommendation	Evidence/Comments
Shatavari	Diphtheria, tetanus, pertussis (DTP) vaccine	Additive effect	Observe. Beneficial effects possible	Experimental studies have suggested a possible immunoadjuvant effect in animals immunised with diphtheria, tetanus, pertussis (DTP) vaccine, increasing antibody titres to *Bordetella pertussis* and providing improved immunoprotection on challenge.
INFECTIONS AND INFESTATIONS				
Antibiotics	Ginger	Possible enhanced absorption of antibiotics	Observe	Ginger may enhance the absorption of antibiotics such as azithromycin, erythromycin, cephalexin when used in doses of between 10 and 30 mg/kg due to the herb's modulating effect on the gastric mucosa; however, the clinical significance of this effect is untested.
	Ginkgo biloba	Increased drug tolerance	Observe	Animal model studies indicate that ginkgo extract EGb 761 reduces oxidative stress induced by bleomycin. This may improve drug tolerance; however, clinical studies have not yet been conducted to test this further.
	Ginseng — Korean	Possible additive effects	Beneficial interaction possible.	In animal studies, the combination of ginseng polysaccharides with vancomycin resulted in a 100% survival rate for animals treated for *Staphylococcus aureus* compared to only 67 or 50% survival in animals treated with ginseng polysaccharides or vancomycin alone. Clinical use in humans has not yet been established.
	Probiotics	Reduced side-effects	Beneficial interaction possible	Reduces gastrointestinal and genitourinary side-effects. A meta-analysis of nine studies found that *Lactobacilli* and *Saccharomyces boulardii* successfully prevent antibiotic-induced diarrhoea. Increase intake with antibiotic therapy.
	Soy	Reduced phyto-oestrogen effect	Observe. Separate doses by 2–3 hours.	Inhibits metabolism of isoflavones to equol through inhibition of intestinal microflora.
	Vitamin B_1 (thiamin)	Reduces endogenous vitamin production	Observe. Separate doses by 2–3 hours.	Antibiotics can reduce the endogenous production of B-group vitamins by gastrointestinal flora. Increase dietary intake or consider supplementation with long-term therapy.
	Vitamin B_2 (Riboflavin)	Reduces endogenous vitamin production	Observe. Separate doses by 2–3 hours.	Antibiotic can reduce endogenous production of B-group vitamins — increase intake of vitamin B_2.
	Vitamin B_5 (pantothenic acid)	Reduces endogenous vitamin production	Observe. Separate doses by 2–3 hours.	Increase dietary intake or consider supplementation with long-term therapy.

Aminoglycosides (e.g. gentamicin)	Magnesium	Decreased magnesium absorption	Caution Monitor for signs and symptoms of magnesium deficiency	Aminoglycosides may deplete magnesium levels and result in neuromuscular weakness. Increased magnesium may be required with long-term therapy.
	Nigella	Reduced side effects	Observe. Beneficial interaction possible	Theoretically protective against gentamicin-induced nephrotoxicity, based on findings in animal studies but the clinical significance is unknown.
Quinolone antibiotics (e.g. norfloxacin [e.g. Noroxin])	Calcium	Reduced drug absorption	Separate antibiotic dose by at least 2 hours before or 4 hours after oral calcium	Drug bioavailability may be reduced by concurrent administration with calcium supplements, reducing drug efficacy and increasing risk of developing bacterial resistance.
	Dandelion	Reduced drug absorption	Separate doses by at least 2 hours	Reduced drug absorption and bioavailability observed in an experimental study.
	Iron	Reduced drug absorption	Separate antibiotic dose by at least 2 hours before or 4–6 hours after oral iron	
	Magnesium	Reduced drug absorption	Separate antibiotic dose by at least 2 hours before or 4 hours after oral magnesium	Magnesium may decrease absorption of fluoroquinolone antibiotics.
	Quercetin	Reduced drug effect	Caution	Theoretical concern based on test tube studies.
	Zinc	Reduced drug and zinc absorption	Separate doses by at least 2 hours	Complex formation between zinc and quinolones results in reduced absorption of both substances, with potential reduction in efficacy.
Tetracycline antibiotics (e.g. minocycline [e.g. Minomycin] doxycycline)	Calcium	Reduced drug and calcium absorption	Separate doses by at least 2 hours	Tetracyclines form insoluble complexes with calcium, thereby reducing its absorption.
	Iron	Reduced drug and iron absorption	Separate doses by at least 4 hours	Tetracyclines form insoluble complexes with iron, thereby reducing its absorption.
	Magnesium	Reduced drug and magnesium absorption	Separate doses by at least 2 hours	Tetracyclines form insoluble complexes with iron, thereby reducing its absorption.
	Vitamin A	Increased side effects	Avoid	Adjunctive use may increase side effects such as headaches, pseudotumour cerebri.

Continued

Herb/Supplement	Pathway	Potential outcome	Recommendation	Evidence/Comments
	Vitamin B_{12}	Reduced drug absorption	Separate doses by at least 2 hours	B complexes containing B_{12} may significantly reduce the bioavailability of tetracycline hydrochloride.
	Zinc	Reduced drug and zinc absorption	Separate doses by at least 2 hours	Complex formation between zinc and tetracycline results in reduced absorption of both substances, with potential reduction in efficacy.
Other antibiotics and anti-infectives (Trimethoprim [e.g. Triprim])	Folate	Reduced folate levels	Caution Monitor folate status with long-term or high-dose therapy Beneficial interaction possible	Trimethoprim is a folate antagonist drug. Increased folate intake may be required with long-term or high-dose therapy.
Anthelmintics (e.g. Albendazole)	Ginseng — Korean	Accelerated drug clearance	Caution. Avoid, unless under medical supervision	Panax ginseng significantly accelerated the intestinal clearance of the anthelmintic albendazole sulfoxide, when co-administered to rats.
Other: Stibanate	Quercetin	Improved efficacy and reduced drug side effects	Observe. Beneficial interaction possible.	Concurrent use of quercetin with the antileishmanial drug stibanate appears to improve the efficacy of the drug and reduce anaemia and parasitaemia associated with the condition.
Antimalarials				
Pyrimethamine (e.g. Daraprim)	Folate	Reduced folate effects	Beneficial interaction possible with folinic acid	Impaired folate utilisation occurs with drug use — supplementation may be required.
Chloroquine (e.g. Chlorquin)	Vitamin E	Reduced drug effects	Observe	According to in vitro research, vitamin E inhibits drug uptake in human cultured fibroblasts — clinical significance unknown.
Antituberculotics and Antileprotics				
Cycloserine and isoniazid	Vitamin B_6 (pyridoxine)	Reduced B_6 levels	Beneficial interaction possible	Drug may induce pyridoxine deficiency. Increased intake may be required with long-term therapy.
Isoniazid	Vitamin B_3 (niacin)	Reduced B_3 levels	Beneficial interaction possible	Prolonged isoniazid therapy (the drug replaces niacinamide in NAD) may induce pellagra. Increased intake may be required with long-term therapy.
	Vitamin B_6	Increase B_6 requirements	Observe. Use under medical care	Isoniazid increases vitamin B_6 requirements. Increase intake of vitamin B_6-rich foods or consider supplementation with long-term drug treatment.
	Vitamin D	Induced catabolism of vitamin D	Observe. Use under medical care	Drugs such as rifampicin and isoniazid have been reported to induce catabolism of vitamin D and in some cases manifest as reduced levels of metabolites. This may represent a concern in those patients already at risk of poor vitamin D status.

	Vitamin E	Reduced vitamin absorption	Separate doses by at least 4 hours and monitor vitamin status	Increased vitamin intake may be required with long-term therapy.
Rifampicin	Vitamin D	Reduced vitamin D levels	Beneficial interaction possible	Increase vitamin D intake with long-term therapy.
Antiviral agents				
Aciclovir	Astragalus	Possible additive effects	Beneficial interaction possible	Possibly enhances antiviral activity against herpes simplex type 1. Adjunctive use may be beneficial.
HIV drugs (e.g. zidovudine [AZT, e.g. Retrovir])	Carnitine	Reduced carnitine levels	Beneficial interaction possible	In vitro studies indicate prevention of muscle damage due to carnitine depletion. Increased intake may be required with long-term therapy.
	Ginseng — Korean	Delay in the development of resistance	Observe. Monitor use under medical supervision.	Long-term intake (60 ± 15 months) of Korean red ginseng in HIV-1-infected patients has been shown to delay the development of resistance mutation to zidovudine.
HIV non-nucleoside transcriptase inhibitors	St John's wort	Reduced drug effects	Avoid	St John's wort increases drug metabolism, thereby reducing drug serum levels.
HIV protease inhibitors (e.g. Indinavir)	St John's wort	Reduced drug effects	Avoid	St John's wort increases drug metabolism, thereby reducing drug serum levels.
Saquinavir	Garlic	Reduced drug effects	Avoid	A clinical study found that garlic reduces serum levels of saquinavir and therefore drug efficacy.
	Quercetin	Potential reduced absorption of drug	Caution under the care of medical supervision	Despite the inhibition of P-glycoprotein by quercetin, co-administration does not appear to alter plasma saquinavir concentrations. There appears to be a substantial inter- and intrasubject variability in saquinavir intracellular concentrations, caution should be exerted until more is known.
MUSCULOSKELETAL SYSTEM				
Non-steroidal anti-inflammatory drugs				
	Celery seed extract	Reduced side-effects	Beneficial	Gastroprotective activity seen in animal model.
	Chamomile	Reduced side-effects	Beneficial interaction	Gastroprotective activity seen in animal model.

Continued

2

Herb/Supplement	Pathway	Potential outcome	Recommendation	Evidence/Comments
	Chondroitin	Additive effects	Beneficial interaction possible Drug dosage may require modification	May enhance the anti-inflammatory effects of the NSAID.
	Colostrum	Reduced side-effects	Beneficial interaction	Gastroprotective activity.
	Devil's claw	Additive effects	Beneficial interaction possible Drug dosage may require modification	May enhance the anti-inflammatory effects of the NSAID.
	Fish oils	Additive effects	Beneficial interaction possible Drug dosage may require modification	May enhance the anti-inflammatory effects of the NSAID and improve symptom relief.
	Ginger	Additive effects	Beneficial interaction possible Drug dosage may require modification	May enhance the anti-inflammatory effects of NSAIDs at high doses.
	Glucosamine	Additive effects	Beneficial interaction possible Drug dosage may require modification	May enhance the anti-inflammatory effects of the NSAID.
	Glutamine	Reduced side-effects	Beneficial interaction	May ameliorate the increased intestinal permeability caused by indomethacin.
	New Zealand (NZ) green-lipped mussel	Additive effects	Beneficial interaction possible. Drug dosage may require modification	Anti-inflammatory activity reported in a c inical study — may enhance the anti-inflammatory effects of the NSAID.
	Nigella	Additive effects	Beneficial interaction possible. Drug dosage may require modification	Based on laboratory and animal studies, black seed displays anti-inflammatory activity and may therefore theoretically interact with nonsteroidal anti-inflammatory agents and COX 2 inhibitors. Human studies are not available, therefore interactions are currently speculative and based on evidence of pharmacological activity, but may theoretically be beneficial.
	SAMe	Additive effects	Beneficial interaction possible Drug dosage may require modification	Anti-inflammatory activity reported in a clinical study — may enhance the anti-inflammatory effects of the NSAID.
	St John's wort	Decreased serum levels of drug	Avoid	Decreases serum levels via CYP induction in vivo.
	Stinging nettle	Additive effects	Beneficial interaction possible Drug dosage may require modification	Anti-inflammatory activity reported in a clinical study — may enhance the anti-inflammatory effects of the NSAID.

	Vitamin E	Additive effects	Beneficial interaction possible Drug dosage may require modification	May enhance the pain-modifying effects of the NSAID when used in high doses for RA.
	Willowbark	Additive effects	Beneficial interaction possible Drug dosage may require modification	May enhance the anti-inflammatory effects of the NSAID.
	Zinc	Reduced absorption	Separate doses by at least 2 hours	Zinc interacts with NSAIDs by forming complexes with these drugs.
NSAIDs (etoricoxib)	St John's wort	Decreased serum levels of drug	Avoid	Decreases serum levels of etoricoxib via CYP induction in vivo.
Aspirin	Grapeseed extract	Additive effects	Observe Beneficial interaction possible	Theoretically may enhance antiplatelet and anti-inflammatory activity of aspirin and may increase risk of bleeding.
	Licorice	Reduce gastro-irritant effects of drug therapy	Observe Beneficial interaction possible	Co-administration with licorice may reduce gastro-irritant effects induced by drug therapy — potentially beneficial interaction. Whether the effect is clinically significant for licorice remains to be determined — use high doses with caution.
	Meadowsweet	Increased bruising and bleeding	Observe Beneficial interaction possible	Theoretically may enhance anti-inflammatory and antiplatelet effects.
	Policosanol	Increased bruising and bleeding	Observe	Doses >10 mg/day may inhibit platelet aggregation.
	Vitamin C	Decreased vitamin C effects	Beneficial interaction	Aspirin may interfere with both absorption and cellular uptake mechanisms for vitamin C, thereby increasing vitamin C requirements, as observed in animal and human studies. Increased vitamin C intake may be required with long-term therapy.
	Willowbark	Increased bruising and bleeding	Observe Beneficial interaction possible Caution with high dose (>240 mg salicin daily)	Theoretically may enhance anti-inflammatory and antiplatelet effects. Although a clinical study found that consumption of salicin 240 mg/day produced minimal effects on platelet aggregation, higher doses may have a significant effect.
Diclofenac sodium (topical)	Licorice	Additive effects	Beneficial interaction possible	In vitro studies have shown that the addition of glycyrrhizin enhanced the topical absorption of diclofenac sodium — significance for licorice unknown.

Continued

Herb/Supplement	Pathway	Potential outcome	Recommendation	Evidence/Comments
Other				
Colchicine	Vitamin A	Altered Vitamin A absorption	Observe	Colchicine may interfere with vitamin A absorption and homeostasis.
	Vitamin B_{12}	Reduced absorption of B_{12}	Observe and monitor B_{12} levels	The use of colchicine may reduce the absorption of orally administered vitamin B_{12} — monitoring of serum B_{12} concentration is recommended, particularly if history of deficiency.
Neuromuscular blockers	Magnesium	Additive effects	Observe	May potentiate effects of neuroblockers.
Sulfasalazine (e.g. Salazopyrin)	Folate	Reduced drug absorption	Separate doses by 2–3 hours	Folic acid can reduce drug absorption.
	Iron	Reduced drug and iron effects	Separate doses by at least 2 hours	May bind together, decreasing the absorption of both.
NEOPLASTIC DISORDERS				
	St John's wort	Reduction of plasma concentrations of various antineoplastic agents	Avoid	By inducing both the CYP3A4 and the P-glycoprotein (P-gp), Hypericum can reduce the plasma concentrations of different antineoplastic agents such as imatinib, irinotecan and docetaxel, thus reducing the clinical efficacy of these drugs. Although these interactions are often predictable, the concomitant use of Hypericum extract should be avoided in cancer patients taking interacting medications.
Chemotherapy	Bilberry	Possible reduction of chemotherapy effectiveness	Observe	An in vitro study using human colon cancer cells showed anthocyanin-rich berry extracts may be protective of DNA damage caused by topoisomorase drugs and therefore may reduce chemotherapy effectiveness. As the concentration required (>50 mcg/mL) to cause this effect is likely greater than could be achieved through oral ingestion, it remains theoretical.
	Ginseng — Korean	Improved treatment tolerance	Caution — possible beneficial interaction under medical supervision	Panax ginseng saponins may reduce nausea and vomiting associated with chemotherapy, radiotherapy and general anaesthetics by antagonising serotonin (5-hydroxytryptamine) type 3A receptors. Ginseng may also help to sensitise cancer cells to chemotherapeutic agents.
	Ginseng — Siberian	Improved treatment tolerance	Caution — possible beneficial interaction under medical supervision	Co-administration may increase drug tolerance and improve immune function. An increased tolerance for chemotherapy and improved immune function has been demonstrated in women with breast and ovarian cancer undergoing chemotherapy treatment. Caution, as co-administration may theoretically reduce drug effects. However, beneficial interaction may be possible under medical supervision.

	Nigella	Possibly enhance anti-tumour activity	Caution — possible beneficial interaction under medical supervision	A theoretical and speculative interaction exists between nigella when used in combination with antineoplastic agents. Cytotoxic, apoptotic and necrotic effects have been observed in laboratory studies with the constituents thymoquinone and alpha-hederin. Theoretically beneficial interactions exist, but further research required to determine significance in humans.
	Pelargonium	Reduced drug effects	Avoid	Theoretically, use of this herb may reduce the effectiveness of immunosuppressant medication — avoid until safety can be established.
	Rosemary	Increased drug effects of P-gp substrates	Caution	Inhibits P-glycoprotein so may affect the bio-availability of P-gp substrates.
	Vitamin A	Reduced vitamin A absorption	Observe and monitor vitamin A status	Reduces vitamin A absorption — increase dietary intake of vitamin A-rich foods or consider supplementation with long-term use.
	Vitamin C	May enhance anti-tumour activity	Beneficial interaction possible	Controversial
	Withania	Reduced side-effects	Observe Beneficial interaction possible under medical supervision	Animal studies suggest a potential role for withania as an adjunctive treatment during chemotherapy for the prevention of drug-induced bone marrow suppression — clinical significance unknown.
Radiotherapy	Zinc	Reduced plasma zinc levels	Monitor zinc levels and use under medical care	Radiotherapy reduces plasma zinc levels. Supplementation may be required with intensive radiotherapy treatment.
Alkylating agents				
Carboplatin	Carnitine	Increased urinary loss	Use combination under professional supervision	Treatment with carboplatin appears to result in marked urinary losses of L-carnitine and acetyl-L-carnitine, most likely due to inhibition of carnitine reabsorption in the kidney.
Cyclophosphamide	Astragalus	Possible reduction of adverse effects	Only use combination under professional supervision	Adjunctive treatment with astragalus may have beneficial effects in regards to improving patient wellbeing and reducing adverse effects associated with treatment such as nausea and vomiting.
	Echinacea	Reduced drug effects	Avoid	Echinacea appears to increase the immunostimulatory effect of low-dose cyclophosphamide, which may be detrimental in autoimmune disease where low doses are used.

Continued

Herb/Supplement	Pathway	Potential outcome	Recommendation	Evidence/Comments
	Rhodiola	Additive effect. Possible reduction of adverse effects	Observe. Use under medical care	Rhodiola rosea root extract synergises the antitumour activity of cyclophosphamide and decreases its hepatotoxicity in an experimental rodent model. Whether the effects are clinically relevant remains to be tested.
	Turmeric	Reduced drug effects	Avoid	Animal studies suggest that curcumin may reduce drug efficacy.
	Vitamin C	Additive effect.	Observe. Use under medical care	Vitamin C enhanced the therapeutic drug effect in vivo.
Immuno-suppressants (e.g. cyclophosphamide)	Withania	Reduced drug effects Reduced side-effects/ toxicity	Caution — possible beneficial interaction	The ability to stimulate stem cell proliferation has led to concerns that withania could reduce cyclophosphamide-induced toxicity, although preliminary animal studies indicate a potential role as a potent and relatively safe radiosensitiser and chemotherapeutic agent. Theoretically it may also decrease the effectiveness of other immunosuppressant drugs.
	Herbs with immunostimulant properties (e.g. echinacea, andrographis, astragalus, baical skullcap, garlic, Ginseng — Korean Ginseng — Siberian)	Reduced drug effects	Observe	Theoretically, immunostimulating agents may reduce drug effectiveness; however, clinical significance is unknown.
Antibiotic cytotoxics				
Docetaxel	Black cohosh	Increased the cytotoxicity of Docetaxel	Avoid	Black cohosh extracts increased the cytotoxicity of Docetaxel. It is advisable that patients undergoing cancer therapy should be made aware that use of black cohosh could alter their response to the agents commonly used to treat breast cancer.
Doxorubicin (e.g. Adriamycin)	Aloe vera	Reduced drug effects	Caution	In vitro evidence suggests that aloe emodin antagonises the cytotoxic effects on both paclitaxel and doxorubicin. While the clinical relevance of this remains unknown, caution should be observed in patients concurrently taking aloe with either of these chemotherapeutic agents.
	Black cohosh	Increased the cytotoxicity of doxorubicin	Avoid	Increased cytotoxicity of doxorubicin in an experimental breast cancer model — while the clinical significance of this finding is unknown, it is recommended patients taking doxorubicin avoid black cohosh until safety can be confirmed.

	Carnitine	Reduced side-effects	Beneficial interaction possible	Animal and human studies suggest that long-term carnitine administration may reduce the cardiotoxic side-effects of Adriamycin. Potentially beneficial interaction; use only under professional supervision.
	Coenzyme Q10	Reduced side-effects	Beneficial interaction possible	Animal and human studies suggest that the cardiotoxic side-effects of Adriamycin are reduced with CoQ10 supplementation.
	Ginkgo biloba	Reduced side-effects	Beneficial interaction possible	In vivo research suggests that ginkgo can prevent doxorubicin-induced cardiotoxicity, although no human studies are available to confirm this.
	Nigella	Reduced side-effects	Observe — beneficial interaction possible	The constituent thymoquinone is theoretically protective against doxorubicin-induced cardiotoxicity and renal toxicity based on findings in animal studies. Clinical significance unknown.
	Quercetin	Reduced side-effects and potentiated antitumour effects	Observe — beneficial interaction possible	When combined with doxorubicin, quercetin potentiated antitumour effects, specifically in the highly invasive breast cancer. Moreover, in non-tumour cells, quercetin reduced doxorubicin cytotoxic side effects. Therefore, it theoretically may have benefits in reducing doxorubicin-mediated toxicity. Further investigation is required to confirm.
	Rhodiola	Reduced side-effects	Observe. Beneficial interaction is possible under clinical supervision	Rhodiola extract has been shown to reduce the liver dysfunction (suggested by a sharp increase in blood transaminase levels) associated with Adriamycin in vivo without affecting the drug's antitumour effects. Theoretically, a beneficial interaction is possible under clinical supervision.
	St Mary's thistle	Reduced side-effects	Observe. Use may be beneficial when used under professional supervision	Silymarin reduces cardiotoxicity and possibly chemosensitises resistant cells to anthracyclines.
	Vitamin C	Reduces side-effects and enhances therapeutic action	Beneficial interaction possible	Vitamin C enhanced the therapeutic drug effect and reduced drug toxicity in vivo. Encouraging — further evidence required.
	Vitamin E	Reduced side-effects	Beneficial interaction possible	One study found that oral DL-alpha tocopheryl acetate (1600 IU/day) prevented doxorubicin-induced alopecia; however, the same dosage failed to prevent alopecia after doxorubicin treatment after mastectomy for breast cancer.

Continued

Herb/Supplement	Pathway	Potential outcome	Recommendation	Evidence/Comments
	Withania	Reduced side-effects	Observe. Beneficial interaction possible	In rats pretreatment with a standardised withania extract (300 mg/kg; 1.5% withanolides) attenuates the cardiotoxic side-effects of doxorubicin (10 mg/kg).
Etoposide	Echinacea	Increased drug effects	Avoid	A recent case study reported a probable interaction of cisplatin and etoposide with echinacea resulting in profound thrombocytopenia requiring platelet transfusion. The authors postulated an interaction via the CYP3A4 enzyme with Echinacea being an inhibitor of CYP3A4 in vitro and etoposide being a substrate of CYP3A4.
	Vitamin C	Increased drug effects	Observe. Use may be beneficial when used under professional supervision	Vitamin C enhanced the antitumour activity of etoposide in vitro.
Antimetabolites				
Methotrexate	Folate	Reduced side-effects but may reduce drug response	Caution in cancer treatment Observe in other conditions	Methotrexate is a folate antagonist drug; supplementation may reduce toxicity. This action may be problematic in cancer treatment and reduce drug response, but beneficial in other uses.
	Nigella	Reduced side-effects	Observe. Beneficial interaction possible	Theoretically, the antioxidant properties of black seed may ameliorate the gastrointestinal adverse effects associated with methotrexate, according to preliminary animal studies. Clinical studies are not yet available.
	Licorice	Additive effects	Caution. Monitor for signs of methotrexate toxicity.	Concurrent administration of methotrexate and either GL or licorice decoction can significantly increase MRT and AUC. Until clarification of this interaction occurs, use combination with caution and monitor for signs of methotrexate toxicity.
	St John's wort	Additive effects and increased toxicity	Caution. Monitor for signs of methotrexate toxicity.	Co-administration of 300 and 150 mg/kg of SJW significantly increased the systemic exposure and toxicity of methotrexate.
Paclitaxel	Licorice	Additive effects	Observe	A constituent of licorice has been demonstrated to significantly potentiate the effects of paclitaxel in vitro — clinical significance for licorice unknown.
	Quercetin	Increased drug effects	Caution	Increased drug bio-availability seen in animal study.

	Withania	Increased/ extended drug effects	Caution	In mice, the addition of Withania (400 mg/kg, orally once weekly for 4 weeks) to paclitaxel (33 mg/kg, intraperitoneally once weekly for 4 weeks) may extend its chemotherapeutic effect through modulating protein-bound carbohydrate levels and marker enzymes. The combination may effectively treat the benzo(a)pyrene-induced lung cancer by offering protection from oxidative damage and also by suppressing cell proliferation.
Immunosuppressant drugs				
	Andrographis	Reduced drug effects	Caution	Immunostimulant activity has been demonstrated in vivo.
	Astragalus	Reduced drug effects	Caution	Due to known immunostimulant effects observed clinically.
	Baical skullcap	Reduced drug effects	Caution	Due to known immunostimulant effects observed clinically.
	Echinacea	Reduced drug effects	Caution	Due to known immunostimulant effects observed clinically.
	Garlic	Reduced drug effects	Caution	Due to known immunostimulant effects observed clinically.
	Ginseng — Korean and Ginseng — Siberian	Reduced drug effects	Caution	Due to known immunostimulant effects observed clinically.
Cisplatin	Black cohosh	Decreased cytotoxicity of cisplatin	Avoid	Decreased cytotoxicity of cisplatin in an experimental breast cancer model — while the clinical significance of this finding is unknown, it is recommended that patients taking cisplatin should avoid black cohosh until safety can be confirmed.
	Carnitine	Reduced side-effects	Beneficial interaction possible under professional supervision	Research into the use of L-carnitine 4 g/day for 7 days showed reduced fatigue from treatment with cisplatin.
	Ginger		Observe. Beneficial interaction possible under professional supervision	Pretreatment has restored testicular antioxidant parameters and sperm motility in cisplatin-induced damage in an animal model. Clinical implications are uncertain; however, potential benefits may be found upon further testing.
	Ginkgo biloba	Reduced side-effects	Beneficial interaction possible under professional supervision	As an antioxidant, Ginkgo may reduce the nephrotoxic effects of cisplatin. Animal model studies have indicated that ginkgo may protect against cisplatin-induced ototoxicity.

Continued

Herb/Supplement	Pathway	Potential outcome	Recommendation	Evidence/Comments
	Nigella	Reduced side-effects	Observe — interaction theoretically beneficial.	Thymoquinone is theoretically protective against cisplatin–induced nephrotoxicity and deleterious drug effects on haemoglobin levels and leucocyte count, based on animal study findings. Synergistic effects were observed when thymoquinone was used in combination with cisplatin in lung cancer cells and in animal models. Clinical significance unknown.
	Quercetin	Increased drug effects	Beneficial interaction theoretically possible under professional supervision	Pre-treatment may sensitise human cervix carcinoma cells to drug according to preliminary research.
	St John's wort	Reduced side-effects	Caution. Pretreatment with SJW under professional supervision may have a beneficial interaction	Cisplatin-induced histological abnormality of the kidney was blocked by pretreatment with SJW in vivo. Total and free cisplatin concentration in serum was not influenced by SJW treatment suggesting that this may be a beneficial interaction under professional supervision.
	St Mary's thistle	Increased drug effects Reduced side-effects	Beneficial interaction possible under professional supervision	Preliminary research has shown that this combination may reduce toxicity effects yet enhance antitumour activity.
	Selenium	Reduced side-effects	Beneficial interaction possible under professional supervision	In vitro and in vivo studies indicate that selenium may reduce drug-associated nephrotoxicity, myeloid suppression and weight loss.
	Vitamin C	Increased drug effects Reduced side-effects	Beneficial interaction possible under professional supervision	Vitamin C enhanced the antitumour activity of cisplatin in several in vitro tests and reduced drug toxicity in experimental models.
	Vitamin E	Reduced side-effects	Beneficial interaction possible under professional supervision	Oral vitamin E (300 mg/day) taken before cisplatin treatment and continued for 3 months significantly reduced the incidence and severity of neurotoxicity, according to a randomised study.
Dasatinib	Magnesium	Potentially beneficial interaction	Observe. Beneficial interaction possible under professional supervision	May increase magnesium blood levels.
Interleukin-2-immunotherapy	Carnitine	Reduced side-effects	Beneficial interaction possible under professional supervision	Clinical trials using L-carnitine (1000 mg/day orally) found that it may successfully prevent cardiac complications during IL-2-immunotherapy in cancer patients with clinically relevant cardiac disorders.
Myelosuppressive chemotherapeutic agents	Echinacea	Potentially beneficial interaction	Potentially beneficial interaction under professional supervision	Use of echinacea between treatment cycles may theoretically improve white cell counts, reduce dose-limiting toxicities on myelopoeisis and improve patient's quality of life.

Proteasome inhibitors				
PS-341 (Bortezomib, Velcade)	Vitamin C	Reduced drug effects	Avoid until safety can be established.	Vitamin C inactivated drug activity in vitro.
Pyrimidine analogues				
Fluorouracil	Vitamin C	Additive effects	Observe under professional supervision	Vitamin C enhanced the antitumour activity of 5-fluorouracil in vitro and in vivo.
Vinca alkaloids				
Vinblastine	Licorice	Additive effects	Observe Beneficial interaction possible under medical supervision	A constituent of licorice has been demonstrated to significantly potentiate the effects of vinblastine in vitro — clinical significance unknown.
Vincristine	Vitamin C	Additive effects	Observe under professional supervision	Vitamin C enhanced the drug's effect in vivo.
NUTRITION				
Anorectics and weight-reducing agents				
Olestra	Lutein and zeaxanthin	Reduced lutein and zeaxanthin absorption	Separate doses by at least 4 hours Monitor lutein and zeaxanthin status	Lutein and zeaxanthin levels have been found to decrease with long-term use of olestra. Increased dietary intake of lutein should be considered.
Orlistat (e.g. Xenical)	Lutein	Reduced lutein absorption	Separate doses by at least 4 hours Monitor lutein status	Long-term use of orlistat leads to reduced plasma levels of lutein due to reduced gastric absorption. Increased dietary intake of lutein should be considered.
	Vitamin A	Reduced vitamin absorption	Separate doses by at least 4 hours Monitor vitamin status	Reduces vitamin A levels. Increased dietary vitamin intake may be required with long-term therapy. Supplementation may be considered with long-term use.
	Vitamin D	Reduced vitamin absorption	Separate doses by at least 4 hours Monitor vitamin status	Increased vitamin intake may be required with long-term therapy.
	Vitamin E	Reduced vitamin absorption	Separate doses by at least 4 hours Monitor vitamin status	Increased vitamin intake may be required with long-term therapy.

Continued

Herb/Supplement	Pathway	Potential outcome	Recommendation	Evidence/Comments
Nutrient–Nutrient interactions				
Alpha Lipoic Acid	Coenzyme Q10	Positive additive effects	Monitor vitamin status	ALA reconstitutes coenzyme Q10 from the oxidised form to an un-oxidised form as part of the antioxidant cycle in humans — beneficial interaction.
	Copper	Reduced absorption/ Chelation	If not using for chelation, separate dose by 3 hours	ALA is a metal chelator and binds to copper in vivo — separate dose by 3 hours, unless this is the desired effect.
	Glutathione	Positive additive effects	Monitor glutathione status	ALA reconstitutes glutathione from the oxidised form to an un-oxidised form as part of the antioxidant cycle in humans — beneficial interaction.
	Manganese	Reduced absorption/ Chelation	Separate dose by 3 hours	ALA is a metal chelator and binds to manganese in vivo.
	Vitamin C	Positive additive effects	Monitor vitamin status	ALA reconstitutes vitamin C from the oxidised form to an un-oxidised form as part of the antioxidant cycle in humans — beneficial interaction.
	Vitamin E	Positive additive effects	Monitor vitamin status	ALA reconstitutes vitamin E from the oxidised form to an un-oxidised form as part of the antioxidant cycle in humans — beneficial interaction.
	Zinc	Reduced absorption/ Chelation	Separate dose by 3 hours	ALA is a metal chelator and binds to zinc in vivo.
Arginine	Lysine	Reduced/ competitive absorption	Caution. Separate dose by 3 hours	Arginine may compete with lysine uptake by tissues. Caution is needed if considering the administration of both amino acids.
Calcium	Iron	Reduced absorption	Separate dose by 2 hours	Concurrent administration of calcium with iron may reduce absorption of both minerals.
	Lysine	Additive effect	Observe. Beneficial interaction	Additive effects may occur as lysine enhances intestinal absorption and reduces renal excretion of calcium.
	Magnesium	Reduced absorption	Separate dose by 2 hours	Magnesium decreases calcium absorption as they compete for the same absorption pathway, however it is unclear if this mineral interaction is clinically significant.
	Zinc	Reduced absorption	Separate dose by 2 hours	Concurrent administration of calcium and zinc may reduce absorption of both minerals, however it is unclear if this is clinically significant, Calcium supplementation has been shown in some studies to increase faecal losses of zinc. Ensure adequate zinc intake and monitor for signs and symptoms of deficiency.

Citric acid	Vitamin B_1	Additive	Beneficial interaction	Citric acid may enhance oral bioavailability of thiamin.
Coenzyme Q10	Vitamin E	Additive	Beneficial interaction	Reconstitutes oxidised vitamin E to its unoxidised form — beneficial interaction with co-administration.
Copper	Zinc	Reduced copper levels	Avoid using high-dose zinc supplements long term, or increase intake of copper.	High zinc intakes (100–150 mg/day) interfere with copper metabolism and can cause hypocuprinaemia with long-term use.
Folate	Zinc	Reduced zinc levels	Observe patients for signs and symptoms of zinc deficiency	At high doses of folate (>15 mg/day), minor zinc depletion may develop.
Iron	Vitamin C	Additive	Beneficial interaction	Vitamin C increases the absorption of iron.
	Zinc	Decreases zinc absorption	Separate dose by 2 hours	Supplemental (38–65 mg/day elemental) iron decreases zinc absorption.
Lysine	Calcium	Additive effect	Observe. Beneficial interaction	Lysine enhances intestinal absorption and decreases renal excretion of calcium.
Magnesium	Calcium	Increased renal excretion	Monitor for signs and symptoms of calcium deficiency	If magnesium intake is excessive, calcium levels decline due to inhibition of PTH release and increased renal excretion. There is additional redistribution with impaired calcium influx and release from intracellular stores. Magnesium can also bind calcium-binding sites and mimic its actions.
	Potassium	Magnesium deficiency leads to increased renal excretion	Monitor for signs and symptoms of potassium deficiency	Hypomagnesaemia results in hypokalaemia due to increased potassium efflux from cells and renal excretion. Magnesium supplementation may be required.
	Vitamin D	Altered metabolism of vitamin D	Monitor for signs and symptoms of both magnesium and vitamin D deficiency	Either an excess or inadequate level of magnesium can impact on vitamin D status. The final hydroxylation step to $1,25(OH)2D_3$ is dependent upon magnesium and a deficiency would compromise this. However, high levels of magnesium, mimicking calcium, can suppress PTH secretion, also suppressing the activation phase. Therefore magnesium levels within the normal range will enhance activation of vitamin D to its active form.
Phosphorus	Calcium	Increased excretion	Monitor for signs and symptoms of deficiency	Excess intake (soft drinks, meat consumption) can increase urinary excretion of calcium — ensure adequate calcium intake and monitor for signs and symptoms of deficiency.
Quercetin	Iron	Reduced absorption and increased chelation	Separate dose by 2 hours	Quercetin is a powerful iron chelator so should not be ingested at the same time as iron supplements or iron rich foods to avoid reducing absorption.

Continued

Herb/Supplement	Pathway	Potential outcome	Recommendation	Evidence/Comments
Selenium	Iodine	Additive effects	Beneficial interaction	Selenium facilitates the conversion of T4 to T3 and is also responsible for the only iodine recycling pathway of the body through the action of the deiodinases on excess or unnecessary thyroid hormones to release the iodine.
Vitamin B_1	Vitamins B_2 and B_6	Concurrent deficiencies	Observe and correct deficiencies	Thiamin deficiency commonly occurs in conjunction with poor B_2 and B_6 status.
	Iron	Reduces B_1 absorption	Separate dose by 2 hours	Iron precipitates thiamin, thereby reducing its absorption.
Vitamin C	Vitamin B_1	Additive	Beneficial interaction	Vitamin C may enhance oral bioavailability of thiamin.
	Iron	Additive	Beneficial interaction	Vitamin C increases the absorption of iron.
Vitamin D	Magnesium	Altered metabolism of vitamin D	Monitor for signs and symptoms of both magnesium and vitamin D deficiency	Either an excess or inadequate level of magnesium can impact on vitamin D status. The final hydroxylation step to 1,25(OH)2D_3 is dependent upon magnesium and a deficiency would compromise this. However, high levels of magnesium, mimicking calcium, can suppress PTH secretion, also suppressing the activation phase. Therefore magnesium levels within the normal range will enhance activation of vitamin D to its active form.
Zinc	Calcium	Impaired zinc absorption	Separate dose by 2 hours	High levels of dietary calcium impair zinc absorption in animals, but it is uncertain whether this occurs in humans.
	Copper	Reduced copper levels	Avoid using high-dose zinc supplements long term, or increase intake of copper.	High zinc intakes (100–150 mg/day) interfere with copper metabolism and can cause hypocuprinaemia with long-term use.
	Folate	Reduced zinc levels	Observe patient for signs and symptoms of zinc deficiency with long-term folate supplementation.	Folate intake may reduce zinc levels.
	Iron	Decreases zinc absorption	Separate dose by 2 hours	Supplemental (38–65 mg/day elemental) iron decreases zinc absorption.
POISONING, TOXICITY AND DRUG DEPENDENCE				
Agents used in drug dependence				
Methadone	Kava	Additive effects	Caution	Increased sedation theoretically possible.
	St John's wort	Reduced drug effects	Avoid	Decreases serum levels via CYP induction.

Detoxifying agents, antidotes				
Penicillamine (e.g. D-penamine)	Calcium	Reduced drug effects	Separate doses by 2 hours	Combination forms insoluble complex.
	Iron	Reduced drug and iron effects	Separate doses by at least 2 hours. Do not suddenly withdraw iron	Sudden withdrawal of iron during penicillamine use has been associated with penicillamine toxicity and kidney damage.
	Magnesium	Reduced drug effects	Separate doses by 2 hours	Combination forms insoluble complex.
	Vitamin B_6 (pyridoxine)	Reduced B_6 effect	Beneficial interaction possible	Drug may induce pyridoxine deficiency — increase intake with long-term therapy. Consider supplementation in long-term use under medical supervision.
	Zinc	Reduced drug effects	Separate doses by 2 hours	Combination forms insoluble complex.
RESPIRATORY SYSTEM				
Broncospasm relaxants				
Ephedrine	Tyrosine	Increased side-effects	Observe	Tyrosine (200 and 400 mg/kg) has been shown to increase side effects of anorexia caused by ephedrine and amphetamine in a dose-dependent manner in rats — clinical significance unknown.
	Nigella	Additive effects	Observe. Beneficial interaction possible	Black seed has been shown to have anti-asthmatic effects according to preliminary human study. Adjunctive use may be beneficial.
Theophylline	Coenzyme Q10	Potential interactions	Observe. Monitor for signs of reduced drug effectiveness	An animal study suggests significant changes to the pharmacokinetics of theophylline such as time to peak concentration, half-life and distribution following treatment with CoQ10. While there is very limited research, there may be possible interactions.
	St John's wort	Reduced drug effects	Monitor for signs of reduced drug effectiveness and adjust the dose if necessary	Decreased drug serum levels.
	Vitamin B_6 (pyridoxine)	Reduced B_6 levels	Beneficial interaction possible	Drug may induce pyridoxine deficiency. Increased intake may be required with long-term therapy.

Continued

2

Herb/Supplement	Pathway	Potential outcome	Recommendation	Evidence/Comments
Expectorants, antitussives, mucolytics and decongestants				
	Adhatoda	Increased drug effects	Observe	Results from animal studies show that *Adhatoda vasica* extract exerts considerable antitussive activity when administered orally and is comparable to codeine when cough is due to irritant stimuli.
Phenyl-propanolamine (found in Neo-Diophen)	Tyrosine	Increased side-effects	Observe	Tyrosine (200 and 400 mg/kg) has been shown to increase side-effects of anorexia caused by phenylpropanolamine in a dose-dependent manner in rats — clinical significance unknown.
SKIN				
Acne, keratolytics and cleansers				
Isotretinoin (e.g. Roaccutane)	Vitamin A	Additive effects	Avoid	Isotretinoin is a vitamin A derivative, so adverse effects and toxicity may be increased.
	Vitamin B_5	Reduced adverse reaction	Observe	A single study reports that a 5% dexpanthenol cream can help treat mucocutaneous adverse reactions caused by using isotretinoin for acne.
Psoriasis, seborrhoea and ichthyosis				
Ketoconazole (e.g. Nizoral)	Vitamin D	Reduced vitamin D effects	Beneficial interaction possible	Ketoconazole reduces the conversion of vitamin D to its active forms. Increased intake may be required with long-term therapy.
Topical corticosteroids				
Topical corticosteroids (e.g. hydrocortisone)	Aloe vera (topical)	Additive effects	Beneficial interaction possible	In addition to its own anti-inflammatory effects, animal studies have shown that aloe vera increases the absorption of hydrocortisone by hydrating the stratum corneum, inhibits hydrocortisone's antiwound-healing activity and increases wound tensile strength.
OTHER				
Alcohol	Andrographis	Reduced side-effects	Beneficial interaction possible	May reduce hepatic injury.
	Ginseng — Korean	Reduced side-effects	Beneficial interaction possible	May reduce hepatic injury.
	Kava	Additive effects	Observe	Potentiation of CNS sedative effects have been reported in an animal study; however, one double-blind, placebo-controlled study found no additive effects on CNS depression or safety-related performance.

	Magnesium	Increased urinary excretion of magnesium	Separate by at least 2 hours	Alcohol consumption results in increased urinary losses of magnesium. Additional magnesium may be necessary with higher chronic ingestion of alcohol.
	St Mary's thistle	Reduced side-effects	Beneficial interaction possible	May reduce hepatic injury.
	SAMe	Reduced side-effects	Beneficial interaction possible	May reduce hepatic injury caused by such agents as paracetamol, alcohol and oestrogens.
	Schisandra	Reduced side-effects	Beneficial interaction possible	May reduce hepatic injury.
Aloe vera	Vitamins C and E	Additive effects	Beneficial interaction possible	Concurrent prescription of oral Aloe vera (both gel and latex) with vitamins C and E shows improved absorption and increased plasma life of vitamin concentration for both vitamins when taken together.
Amphetamines	Tyrosine	Increased side effects	Observe patients using this combination.	L-Tyrosine (200 and 400 mg/kg) has been shown to increase the side-effect of anorexia caused by phenylpropanolamine, ephedrine and amphetamine in a dose-dependent manner in rats.
Anaesthetics	Ginseng — Korean	Improved treatment tolerance	Caution — possible beneficial interaction under medical supervision	Panax ginseng saponins may reduce nausea and vomiting associated with chemotherapy, radiotherapy and general anaesthetics by antagonising serotonin (5-hydroxytryptamine) type 3A receptors. Ginseng may also help to sensitise cancer cells to chemotherapeutic agents.
Anaesthetics (e.g. Ketamine)	St John's wort	Reduced drug effects	Caution. Use under medical supervision	SJW greatly decreased the exposure to oral S-ketamine in healthy volunteers. Although this decrease was not associated with significant changes in the analgesic or behavioural effects of ketamine in the present study, usual doses of S-ketamine may become ineffective if used concomitantly with SJW.
Blueberries	Vitamin B_1	Reduced absorption	Separate doses by at least 2 hours	Reduce the absorption of oral thiamin.
Brussel sprouts	Vitamin B_1	Reduced absorption	Separate doses by at least 2 hours	Reduce the absorption of oral thiamin.

Continued

Herb/Supplement	Pathway	Potential outcome	Recommendation	Evidence/Comments
Chitosan	B-group vitamins	Reduced absorption	Observe. Separate doses by at least 2 hours	In vitro studies using fluorescence and ultraviolet–visible absorption measurements have shown vitamin B_2 and B_{12} interact with chitosan in an acid-aqueous environment replicate of the stomach. These studies suggest chitosan may inhibit the absorption of these nutrients; however, the degree of clinical significance is unknown.
	Fat-soluble nutrients	Reduced absorption	Observe. Separate doses by at least 2 hours	Given chitosan's capacity to bind dietary fats and reduce their absorption, chitosan can also affect the absorption of fat-soluble vitamins.
	Vitamin C	Additive	Beneficial interaction possible	According to a preliminary study in rats, taking vitamin C together with chitosan might provide additional benefit in lowering cholesterol.
Cocoa	Iron	Reduced absorption	Separate doses by at least 2 hours	Polyphenols may reduce iron absorption, with a cocoa beverage containing 100–400 mg total polyphenols per serving having been shown to reduce iron absorption by approximately 70%.
Coffee	Vitamin B_1	Reduced absorption	Separate doses by at least 2 hours	Reduce the absorption of oral thiamin.
Dopamine antagonists	Chaste tree	Reduced drug effects	Observe	Reduced drug effects theoretically possible.
Ecstasy	Tyrosine	Increased concentration of tyrosine in the brain causing long-term depletion of 5-HT.	Avoid	Ecstasy users should be aware that MDMA increases the concentration of tyrosine in the brain causing long-term depletion of 5-HT.
Ephedrine	Tyrosine	Increased side effects	Observe patients using this combination.	L-Tyrosine (200 and 400 mg/kg) has been shown to increase the side-effect of anorexia caused by phenylpropanolamine, ephedrine and amphetamine in a dose-dependent manner in rats.
Fenugreek	Iron	Reduced absorption	Separate doses by at least 2 hours	Frequent use of fenugreek can inhibit iron absorption.
Fibre, including guar gum	*All medications	Reduced absorption	Separate doses by at least 2 hours	May delay or decrease absorption of medications. *More research is required to investigate the effect of fibre on individual medications.
	Calcium	Reduced absorption	Separate doses by at least 2 hours	May delay or decrease absorption of calcium.

Goitrogens	Iodine	Inhibition	Separate intake of iodine and goitrogens where possible	Interferes with iodine utilisation, uptake into the thyroid or thyroid hormone production.
Grapeseed extract	Iron and iron-containing preparations	Decreased iron absorption.	Separate doses by at least 2 hours	Decreased iron absorption. Tannins can bind to iron, forming insoluble complexes.
Green tea	Iron and iron-containing preparations	Decreased iron absorption.	Observe. Separate doses by at least 2 hours.	Tannins found in *Camellia sinensis* can bind to iron and reduce its absorption. Protein and iron have also been found to interact with tea polyphenols and decrease their antioxidant effects in vitro.
Hepatotoxic drugs	Andrographis	Reduced side-effects	Beneficial interaction possible	May exert hepatoprotective activity against liver damage induced by drugs such as paracetamol and tricyclic antidepressants.
	Garlic	Reduced side-effects	Beneficial interaction possible	May exert hepatoprotective activity against liver damage induced by drugs such as paracetamol.
	Nigella	Reduced side-effects	Beneficial interaction possible	Based on animal studies, black seed appears to confer hepatoprotective effects against a number of agents. A theoretically beneficial interaction exists, but further research required to determine significance in humans and with other hepatotoxic drugs.
	Quercetin	Reduced side-effects	Beneficial interaction	Hepatoprotective activity.
	St Mary's thistle	Reduced side-effects	Beneficial interaction possible	May exert hepatoprotective activity against liver damage induced by drugs such as paracetamol.
	SAMe	Reduced side-effects	Beneficial interaction possible	May exert hepatoprotective activity against liver damage induced by drugs such as paracetamol, alcohol.
	Schisandra	Reduced side-effects	Beneficial interaction possible	May exert hepatoprotective activity against liver damage induced by drugs such as paracetamol.
Horsetail (*Equisetum arvense*)	Vitamin B_1	Reduced absorption	Observe. Avoid if pre-existing thiamin deficiency.	Theoretically, horsetail may destroy thiamin in the stomach due to the presence of a thiaminase-like compound found in the herb. Those that have a pre-existing thiamin deficiency or are at risk of thiamin deficiency may be advised to avoid concurrent use of horsetail.
Lutein	Vitamin C	Additive effects	Beneficial interaction	Lutein showed increased antioxidant efficacy with vitamin C in an animal study. A small in vivo study showed 2000 mg of vitamin C enhanced the absorption of lutein.
	Vitamin E	Additive effects	Beneficial interaction	Vitamin E showed increased antioxidant efficacy with lutein according to an animal study.

Continued

Herb/Supplement	Pathway	Potential outcome	Recommendation	Evidence/Comments
Licorice	Potassium	Reduced effect of potassium supplementation	Separate doses by at least 2 hours Observe the patient for signs of potassium deficiency.	Licorice may reduce the effect of potassium supplementation. In many cases potassium supplementation may be beneficial in reducing the hypokalaemic side effects of licorice.
Lipophilic drugs	Chitosan	Reduced drug absorption	Separate doses by at least 2 hours	Binds to dietary fats and reduces their absorption and so can also affect the absorption of lipophilic drugs.
Lithium	Fibre	Decreased bioavailability and absorption	Separate doses by at least 1–2 hours	Soluble fibre may decrease the bioavailability of lithium.
	Psyllium	Decreased bioavailability and absorption	Separate doses by at least 1–2 hours	Soluble fibre may decrease the bioavailability of lithium.
	Slippery elm	Potential decreased bioavailability and absorption	Separate doses by at least 2 hours	Since slippery elm forms an inert barrier over the gastrointestinal lining, it may theoretically alter the rate and/or extent of absorption of medicines with a narrow therapeutic range (e.g. barbiturates, digoxin, lithium, phenytoin, warfarin). The clinical significance of this is unclear.
	Vitamin B_{12}	Decreased B_{12} concentration	Observe. Separate doses by at least 2 hours	Lithium administration may result in a decrease in serum B_{12} concentration; however, the clinical significance of these findings is not yet clear.
Meadowsweet	Iron	Reduced iron absorption	Separate doses by at least 2 hours	The tannin content of meadowsweet potentially forms an insoluble complex with iron reducing its absorption.
Mineral oil	Vitamin D	Reduced vitamin D absorption	Separate doses by at least 2 hours	Mineral oil impairs absorption of all fat-soluble nutrients and may therefore deplete oral intake of vitamin D sources.
Nigella	Iron	Increased iron status	Beneficial interaction	Increased iron status possible with consumption of black seed, based on limited animal study. Clinical significance is unknown, but theoretically beneficial in iron deficiency.
Phenylpropanolamine (norephedrine and norpseudoephedrine)	Tyrosine	Increased side effects	Observe patients using this combination.	L-Tyrosine (200 and 400 mg/kg) has been shown to increase the side-effect of anorexia caused by phenylpropanolamine, ephedrine and amphetamine in a dose-dependent manner in rats.
Phytosterols	Lutein	Reduced lutein absorption	Separate doses by at least 2 hours	High dietary intake of phytosterol esters (6.6 g/day) reduced plasma levels of lutein by 14% in a small clinical trial; however, this was reversed by increasing fruit and vegetable intake.

Psyllium	Calcium	Decreased bioavailability and absorption	Separate doses by at least 1–2 hours	Animal studies suggest that soluble fibre from sources of purified psyllium negatively impact calcium balance by decreasing the bioavailability of calcium from the diet. Psyllium and other soluble fibre supplements should be taken at least 1 hour before or after calcium.
	Lithium	Decreased bioavailability and absorption	Separate doses by at least 1–2 hours	Soluble fibre may decrease the bioavailability of lithium.
	Minerals	Decreased bioavailability and absorption	Separate doses by at least 1–2 hours	Given the known capacity of psyllium husks to decrease the absorption of calcium, it would be prudent to avoid co-administration of psyllium husks with any vitamin or mineral supplement.
	Vitamin B_{12}	Decreased bioavailability and absorption	Separate doses by at least 1–2 hours	Soluble fibre may decrease the bioavailability of vitamin B_{12}.
	Vitamins	Decreased bioavailability and absorption	Separate doses by at least 1–2 hours	Given the known capacity of psyllium husks to decrease the absorption of calcium, it would be prudent to avoid co-administration of psyllium husks with any vitamin or mineral supplement.
PUVA therapy	Celery	Additive effects	Caution	While celery has been found to contain psoralens, celery extract does not seem to be photosensitising, even after ingestion in large amounts; however, it may increase the risk of phototoxicity with concurrent PUVA therapy.
	St John's wort	Additive effects	Caution	Hypericin may increase sensitivity to UV radiation.
Raspberry leaf	Calcium	Decreased absorption	Separate doses by at least 2 hours	Due to its high tannin content, raspberry leaf may decrease absorption of calcium, as well as some drugs.
	Iron	Decreased absorption	Separate doses by at least 2 hours	Due to its high tannin content, raspberry leaf may decrease absorption of iron, as well as some drugs.
	Magnesium	Decreased absorption	Separate doses by at least 2 hours	Due to its high tannin content, raspberry leaf may decrease absorption of magnesium, as well as some drugs.
Red cabbage	Vitamin B_1	Reduced absorption	Separate doses by at least 2 hours	Reduce the absorption of oral thiamin.
Red rice yeast	Coenzyme Q10	May reduce endogenous production of Coenzyme Q10	Observe. When supplementing coenzyme Q10, separate doses by at least 2 hours	Similar to statin medications, Red rice yeast may reduce endogenous production of CoQ10 — a 3-month trial of CoQ10 supplementation may be worth considering with long-term use of red rice yeast in people complaining of fatigue.

Continued

2

Herb/Supplement	Pathway	Potential outcome	Recommendation	Evidence/Comments
Rosemary	Iron	Inhibition of absorption	Observe. Separate doses by 2 hours.	Rosemary extracts are widely used as an antioxidant to preserve foods; however, the phenolic-rich extracts may reduce the uptake of dietary iron.
Sage	Calcium	Reduced absorption	Observe. Separate doses by 2 hours.	Due to the tannin content, sage may reduce the absorption of calcium.
	Iron	Reduced absorption	Observe. Separate doses by 2 hours.	Due to the tannin content, sage may reduce the absorption of iron.
	Magnesium	Reduced absorption	Observe. Separate doses by 2 hours.	Due to the tannin content, sage may reduce the absorption of magnesium.
SAMe	Betaine	Additive effects	Observe.	In studies supplementing mice with betaine, significant increases in SAMe were observed with a three-fold elevation of the activity of methionine adenosyltransferase.
Selenium	Heavy metals (e.g. mercury, lead, arsenic, silver and cadmium)	Reduces toxicity of heavy metals	Observe. Beneficial interaction	Selenium reduces toxicity of heavy metals such as mercury, lead, arsenic, silver and cadmium by forming inert complexes.
Shatavari	Metoclopramide	Additive effect	Observe. Beneficial interaction	Shatavari root was found in animal studies to have similar effects on gastric emptying time to the antiemetic drug metoclopramide (a synthetic dopamine antagonist); an additive effect is possible.
Slippery elm	Lithium	Altered rate and/or extent of absorption	Caution. Separate doses by 2 hours	Controlled studies are unavailable, but interactions are theoretically possible with some medicines. Slippery elm forms an inert barrier over the gastrointestinal lining and may theoretically alter the rate and/or extent of absorption of medicines with a narrow therapeutic range (e.g. lithium). The clinical significance of this is unclear.
Soy	Calcium	Reduced absorption	Caution. Separate doses by 2–3 hours	Soy contains phytic acid, which may bind with calcium reducing availability.
	Copper	Reduced absorption	Caution. Separate doses by 2–3 hours	Soy contains phytic acid, which may bind with copper reducing availability.
	Iodine	Inhibition of absorption	Separate intake of iodine and goitrogens where possible	Ingestion of soy appears to inhibit iodine absorption to some extent (particularly when presented in its thyroxine form in the gut) and also high levels of the isoflavones, genistein and daidzein, can inhibit T3 and T4 production.
	Iron	Reduced absorption	Caution. Separate doses by 2–3 hours	Soy contains phytic acid, which may bind with iron reducing availability.

	Magnesium	Reduced absorption	Caution. Separate doses by 2–3 hours	Soy contains phytic acid, which may bind with magnesium reducing availability.
	Manganese	Reduced absorption	Caution. Separate doses by 2–3 hours	Soy contains phytic acid, which may bind with manganese reducing availability.
	Tamoxifen	Additive effects	Possible beneficial effect under professional supervision	Animal studies have shown that soy enhances the therapeutic effects of tamoxifen as both have SERM actions. Additionally, in vivo studies suggest that the isoflavone daidzein may enhance the effect of tamoxifen against breast cancer burden and incidence.
	Zinc	Reduced absorption	Caution. Separate doses by 2–3 hours	Soy contains phytic acid, which may bind with zinc reducing availability.
	Thyme	Clinical significance unknown	Observe	Thyme may induce enzymes in phase one and two detoxification in the liver. The clinical significance of this is unknown.
Tannins	Vitamin B_1	Reduced absorption and increased precipitation	Observe. Separate doses by 2–3 hours	Tannins precipitate thiamin, thereby reducing its absorption.
Vaccinations	Zinc	Improved seroconversion of vibriocidal antibodies	Possible beneficial effect under professional supervision	Zinc acetate improved seroconversion of vibriocidal antibodies in children given a cholera vaccination in both faecal and serum titres.

APPENDIX 3

GUIDE TO THE SAFE USE OF COMPLEMENTARY MEDICINES DURING THE PREOPERATIVE PERIOD

This table is intended to provide clinicians with some guidance when advising patients due for surgery about the safe use of complementary medicines (CMs). It is limited to the CMs reviewed in this book, especially those that are known or suspected to increase bleeding or interact with drugs commonly used in the perioperative period. The recommendations are conservative and not likely to be relevant to many low-risk or minor surgical procedures, but it is imperative that each patient be individually assessed before surgery.

CMs are listed alphabetically by common name. The comments section includes a brief description of the type of evidence available to support the recommendation; more detailed information is given in the individual monographs. Several different recommendations are possible. Sometimes there is a recommendation to suspend use 1–2 weeks before surgery, which should provide ample time for bleeding rates to return to normal or potential interactions to be avoided. This is most likely an overestimation of the actual time required. Please note that coumarin-containing and salicylate-containing herbs have not been included in the table unless they have demonstrated antiplatelet or anticoagulant effects in animal or human studies. Sometimes the recommendations are dose dependent; in other cases CM use appears safe but there is a theoretical concern.

It is acknowledged that, in practice, not all surgical patients will be able to follow these recommendations. In situations where bleeding would be a serious complication and a 1-week minimum deferment is not possible, tests of haemostasis prior to surgery should be considered.

It must be reiterated that the clinical relevance of some interactions and adverse effects is unknown and controlled studies in surgical patients are not available. However, it would seem prudent for healthcare providers to become familiar with these medicines, in order to advise patients appropriately and to anticipate, manage or avoid adverse events during the perioperative period.

Common name	Botanical name (where applicable)	Comments	Recommendation
Andrographis	*Andrographis paniculata*	Andrographolide inhibits platelet-activating-factor-induced platelet aggregation in a dose-dependent manner (confirmed clinically) (Amroyan et al 1999, Zhang et al 1994).	Suspend use 1 week before surgery.
Baical skullcap	*Scutellaria baicalensis*	There is a theoretical risk of anticoagulant activity; not observed in clinical trials.	Use under observation, but likely to be safe.
Evening primrose oil (EPO)	Omega-6 essential fatty acids or omega-6 fatty acids	Gamma linolenic acid in EPO affects PG synthesis, leading to inhibition of platelet aggregation — clinical significance unknown.	Suspend use of high-dose concentrated products 1 week before surgery; however, safety is difficult to assess.

Common name	Botanical name (where applicable)	Comments	Recommendation
Feverfew	*Tanacetum parthenium*	Evidence is contradictory as to whether feverfew inhibits platelet aggregation. Inhibition of platelet aggregation has been observed in several in vitro studies (Groenewegen & Heptinstall 1990, Marles et al 1992, Voyno-Yasenetskaya et al 1988); however, a small human study found no effects on platelet aggregation (Biggs et al 1982).	Use under observation but likely to be safe
Fish oils	Omega-3 essential fatty acids or omega-3 fatty acids	Multiple clinical studies conducted in surgical patients with no significant increase in bleeding observed (Harris 2007). Some benefits reported (see monograph). Bleeding times increased at very high doses of 12 g/day of omega-3 fatty acids (Harris et al 1990).	Usual therapeutic doses are safe according to systematic review of use in surgical patients. Suspend use of high-dose products (12 g/day and higher) 1 week before surgery.
Garlic	*Allium sativum*	Inhibition of platelet aggregation is clinically significant — two cases of postoperative bleeding after excessive dietary intake have been reported (Burnham 1995, German et al 1995). One clinical study found reduced haematocrit values and plasma viscosity (Jung et al 1991).	Usual dietary intakes are likely to be safe. Suspend use of concentrated extracts (> 7 g) 1 week before surgery.
Ginger	*Zingiber officinale*	Standard intake likely to be safe. Oral doses of 4 g/day did not alter platelet aggregation or fibrinogen levels in one clinical study, whereas a high dose of 10 g/day significantly reduced platelet aggregation in another clinical study (Bordia et al 1997).	Usual dietary and therapeutic intakes are likely to be safe. Suspend use of high-dose (10 g/day) concentrated extracts 1 week before surgery.
Ginkgo	*Ginkgo biloba*	At least 10 clinical studies have found no significant effect on bleeding or platelets; however, rare cases of bleeding have been reported. One escalating dose study found that doses of 120 mg, 240 mg or 480 mg given daily for 14 days did not alter platelet function or coagulation (Bal Dit et al 2003).	Use under observation but likely to be safe.
Ginseng — Korean	*Panax ginseng*	Herb inhibits platelet aggregation according to both in vitro and animal studies, but clinical significance unknown. In contrast, the total saponin fraction has been shown to promote haemopoiesis by stimulating proliferation of human granulocyte-macrophage progenitors (Niu et al 2001).	Suspend use 1 week before surgery; however, safety is difficult to assess.
Ginseng — Siberian	*Eleutherococcus senticosus*	Siberian ginseng constituent 3,4-dihydroxybenzoic acid has demonstrated antiplatelet activity in vivo.	Suspend use 1 week before surgery; however, safety is difficult to assess.
Goji	*Lycium barbarum*	Inhibition of platelet aggregation in vitro — clinical significance unknown. Not demonstrated in human studies	Use under observation but likely to be safe.
Green tea	*Camellia sinensis*	Shown to exert antiplatelet aggregation and antithrombogenic activities. A case report of excessive daily intake 2.5–4.5 L/day decreased INR.	Usual dietary intake likely to be safe.

3

Continued

Common name	Botanical name (where applicable)	Comments	Recommendation
Guarana	*Paullinia cupana*	In vitro and in vivo research have identified antiplatelet activity (Bydlowski et al 1991).	Suspend use of concentrated extracts 1 week before surgery.
Kava Kava	*Piper methysticum*	Increased sedation due to significant CNS-depressant effects possible. Inhibition of CYP2E1 has been demonstrated in vivo therefore serum levels of CYP2E1 substrates may become elevated (e.g. the anaesthetic drugs). halothane isoflurane methoxyflurane	Suspend use of concentrated extract 1 week before surgery in cases when drug interactions possible.
Licorice root	*Glycyrrhiza glabra*	Isoliquiritigenin inhibits platelet aggregation (Tawata et al 1992) and glycyrrhizin inhibits prothrombin (Francischetti et al 1997) according to in vitro tests — clinical significance unknown.	Usual dietary intakes likely to be safe. Concentrated extracts should be used with caution.
Meadowsweet	*Filipendula ulmaria*	In vitro and in vivo tests have identified anticoagulant activity (Liapina & Koval'chuk 1993) — clinical significance of these findings is unknown.	Suspend use of concentrated extracts 1 week before surgery.
Myrrh	*Commiphora molmol*	Guggul inhibits platelet aggregation in vitro and in a clinical study (Bordia & Chuttani 1979).	Suspend use of guggul preparations 1 week before surgery.
Policosanol		Doses of 10 mg/day and greater reduce platelet aggregation, according to clinical studies (Arruzazabala et al 2002, Castano et al 1999). Effect of 20 mg/day is similar to aspirin 100 mg stat.	Suspend use of doses 10 mg/day or greater 1 week before surgery.
Rosemary	*Rosmarinus officinalis*	Rosemary demonstrates antithrombotic activity in vitro and in vivo, possibly through inhibition of platelets. Clinical significance unknown.	Suspend use of concentrated extracts 1 week before surgery; however, clinical significance difficult to assess.
Shark cartilage		Substance displays anti-angiogenic properties, which could theoretically hinder healing.	Suspend use of supplement 1 week before surgery and until postoperative healing is complete (approx 6 weeks).
St John's wort	*Hypericum perforatum*	Use of herb for more than 2 weeks can induce pharmacokinetic interactions with CYP3A4 and P-gp substrates. This will result in reduced therapeutic responses to these drugs e.g. alprazolam cyclosporin digoxin midazolam morphine nortriptyline warfarin	Do not cease use unless under supervision to avoid inducing drug interaction — consider patient benefits vs potential risks. **Caution:** Withdrawal effects possible as SSRI-like activity is reduced and CYP and P-gp induction is removed — therapeutic failure of herb and possible drug toxicity.

Common name	Botanical name (where applicable)	Comments	Recommendation
Turmeric root	*Curcuma longa*	Curcumin inhibits platelet aggregation in vivo (Srivastava et al 1985, 1986, Chen et al 2007) and in vitro (Srivastava 1989, Srivastava et al 1995, Jantan et al 2008). The anticoagulant effect of curcumin is weaker than that of aspirin — clinical significance unknown.	Usual dietary intakes likely to be safe.
Vitamin E	Alpha-tocopherol	Contradictory results have been obtained in clinical studies that have investigated whether vitamin E affects platelet aggregation or coagulation. A dose of 1200 IU/day (800 mg of D-alpha-tocopherol) taken for 28 days had no effects on platelet aggregation or coagulation, according to one clinical study (Morinobu et al 2002). Similarly, a second clinical study found the lower dose of 600 mg (900 IU) of RRR-alpha-tocopherol taken daily for 12 weeks did not alter coagulation activity (Kitagawa et al 1989). Alternatively, increased risk of gingival bleeding at doses of 50 mg/day was found by another study (Liede et al 1998).	Usual therapeutic doses are likely to be safe. Suspend use of high-dose supplements (> 1000 IU/day) 1 week before surgery; however, safety is difficult to assess.
Willow bark	*Salix* spp	Although it has been assumed that willow bark affects platelet aggregation owing to its salicylate content, one clinical study found that consumption of *Salicis cortex* (240 mg salicin daily) produced minimal effects on platelet aggregation (Krivoy et al 2001).	Use under observation but likely to be safe.

REFERENCES

Amroyan E et al. Inhibitory effect of andrographolide from Andrographis paniculata on PAF-induced platelet aggregation. Phytomedicine 6.1 (1999): 27–31.

Arruzazabala ML et al. Antiplatelet effects of policosanol (20 and 40 mg/day) in healthy volunteers and dyslipidaemic patients. Clin Exp Pharmacol Physiol 29.10 (2002): 891–7.

Bal Dit C et al. No alteration in platelet function or coagulation induced by EGb761 in a controlled study. Clin Lab Haematol 25.4 (2003): 251–3.

Biggs MJ et al. Platelet aggregation in patients using feverfew for migraine. Lancet 2.8301 (1982): 776.

Bordia A et al. Effect of ginger (Zingiber officinale Rosc.) and fenugreek (Trigonella foenumgraecum L.) on blood lipids, blood sugar and platelet aggregation in patients with coronary artery disease. Prostaglandins Leukot Essent Fatty Acids 56.5 (1997): 379–84.

Bordia A, Chuttani SK. Effect of gum guggulu on fibrinolysis and platelet adhesiveness in coronary heart disease. Indian J Med Res 70 (1979): 992–6.

Burnham BE. Garlic as a possible risk for postoperative bleeding. Plast Reconstr Surg 95.1 (1995): 213.

Bydlowski SP et al. An aqueous extract of guarana (Paullinia cupana) decreases platelet thromboxane synthesis. Braz J Med Biol Res 24.4 (1991): 421–4.

Castano G et al. Effects of policosanol and pravastatin on lipid profile, platelet aggregation and endothelemia in older hypercholesterolemic patients. Int J Clin Pharmacol Res 19.4 (1999): 105–16.

Chen HW et al. Pretreatment of curcumin attenuates coagulopathy and renal injury in LPS-induced endotoxemia. J Endotoxin Res 13.1 (2007): 15–23.

Francischetti IM et al. Identification of glycyrrhizin as a thrombin inhibitor. Biochem Biophys Res Commun 235.1 (1997): 259–63.

German K et al. Garlic and the risk of TURP bleeding. Br J Urol 76.4 (1995): 518.

Groenewegen WA, Heptinstall S. A comparison of the effects of an extract of feverfew and parthenolide, a component of feverfew, on human platelet activity in-vitro. J Pharm Pharmacol 42.8 (1990): 553–7.

Harris WS et al. Fish oils in hypertriglyceridemia: a dose-response study. Am J Clin Nutr 51.3 (1990): 399–406.

Harris WS. Expert opinion: omega-3 fatty acids and bleeding-cause for concern? Am J Cardiol 99.6A (2007): 44C–6C.

Jantan I et al. Inhibitory effect of compounds from Zingiberaceae species on human platelet aggregation. Phytomedicine 15.4 (2008): 306–9.

Jung EM et al. Influence of garlic powder on cutaneous microcirculation: A randomized placebo-controlled double-blind cross-over study in apparently healthy subjects. Arzneimittelforschung 41.6 (1991): 626–30.

Kitagawa M, Mino M. Effects of elevated d-alpha(RRR)-tocopherol dosage in man. J Nutr Sci Vitaminol (Tokyo) 35.2 (1989): 133–42.

Krivoy N et al. Effect of salicis cortex extract on human platelet aggregation. Planta Med 67.3 (2001): 209–12.

Liapina LA, Koval'chuk GA. A comparative study of the action on the hemostatic system of extracts from the flowers and seeds of the meadowsweet (Filipendula ulmaria (L.) Maxim.). Izv Akad Nauk Ser Biol 4 (1993): 625–8.

Liede KE et al. Increased tendency towards gingival bleeding caused by joint effect of alpha-tocopherol supplementation and acetylsalicylic acid. Ann Med 30.6 (1998): 542–6.

Marles RJ et al. A bioassay for inhibition of serotonin release from bovine platelets. J Nat Prod 55.8 (1992): 1044–56.

Morinobu T et al. The safety of high-dose vitamin E supplementation in healthy Japanese male adults. J Nutr Sci Vitaminol (Tokyo) 48.1 (2002): 6–9.

Niu YP et al. Effects of ginsenosides Rg1 and Rb1 on proliferation of human marrow granulocyte-macrophage progenitor cells. Zhongguo Shi Yan Xue Ye Xue Za Zhi 9.2 (2001): 178–80.

Srivastava KC et al. Curcumin, a major component of food spice turmeric (Curcuma longa) inhibits aggregation and alters eicosanoid metabolism in human blood platelets. Prostaglandins Leukot Essent Fatty Acids 52.4 (1995): 223–7.

Srivastava KC. Extracts from two frequently consumed spices – cumin (Cuminum cyminum) and turmeric (Curcuma longa) – inhibit platelet aggregation and alter eicosanoid biosynthesis in human blood platelets. Prostaglandins Leukot Essent Fatty Acids 37.1 (1989): 57–61.

Srivastava R et al. Anti-thrombotic effect of curcumin. Thromb Res 40.3 (1985): 413–17.

Srivastava R et al. Effect of curcumin on platelet aggregation and vascular prostacyclin synthesis. Arzneimittel-Forschung 36.4 (1986): 715–17,

Tawata M et al. Anti-platelet action of isoliquiritigenin, an aldose reductase inhibitor in licorice. Eur J Pharmacol 212.1 (1992): 87–92.

Voyno-Yasenetskaya TA et al. Effects of an extract of feverfew on endothelial cell integrity and on cAMP in rabbit perfused aorta. J Pharm Pharmacol 40.7 (1988): 501–2.

Zhang YZ et al. [Study of Andrographis paniculata extracts on antiplatelet aggregation and release reaction and its mechanism]. Zhongguo Zhong Xi Yi Jie He Za Zhi 14.1 (1994): 28–30, 34, 35.

3

APPENDIX 4

CLINICAL USE AND SAFETY OF VITAMINS AND MINERALS

Clinical use and safety of vitamins

Vitamin	Australian and New Zealand RDI for adults (>18 years)	Dose range used in practice	Major uses (oral or topical forms)	Cautions	Side effects	Toxicity
A	Women: 700 mcg Men: 900 mcg	10,000–50,000 IU/day orally in divided doses Not recommended for more than 2 weeks without medical supervision	Treating deficiency Prevention of secondary deficiency (e.g. coeliac disease, cystic fibrosis, pancreatic disease) Reducing severity of infectious diseases in children Dermatology — many uses Adjunct to chemotherapy Slowing progression of retinitis pigmentosa Osteoporosis Anaemia	Hypersensitivity Pregnancy Hypervitaminosis A Retinoid analogue use Lactation Chronic renal failure or liver disease	**Early signs** Dry rough skin and mucous membranes, desquamation Coarse sparse hair, alopecia of eyebrows Diplopia Bone and joint pain **Later signs** Irritability Increased intracranial pressure and headache Dizziness Hepatotoxicity	Cumulative toxicity if > 100,000 IU long term. Acute toxicity possible if > 2,000,000 IU. The recommended adult daily amount of vitamin A from all sources is 2500 IU. Taking more than 8000 IU a day during pregnancy may cause birth defects.
B_1 (thiamin)	Women: 1.1 mg Men: 1.2 mg	5–3000 mg	Treating deficiency Prevention of secondary deficiency (e.g. hyperemesis and malabsorption states) Acute alcohol withdrawal Alzheimer's dementia Dysmenorrhoea Congestive heart failure Diabetes	Hypersensitivity	Well tolerated	Non-toxic
B_2 (riboflavin)	Women: 1.1 mg (<70 yrs: 1.3 mg) Men: 1.3 mg (>70 yrs: 1.6 mg)	10–400 mg/day	Treating deficiency Prevention of secondary deficiency (e.g. chronic diarrhoea, liver disease, chronic alcoholism) Prevention of migraine headaches Reducing incidence of both nuclear and cortical cataract Wound healing Pyridoxine metabolism Breast cancer adjunct to tamoxifen	Hypersensitivity	Generally well tolerated, but rare side effects include diarrhoea and polyuria.	Non-toxic

Continued

Clinical use and safety of vitamins *continued*

Vitamin	Australian and New Zealand RDI for adults (>18 years)	Dose range used in practice	Major uses (oral or topical forms)	Cautions	Side effects	Toxicity
B_3 (niacin)	Women: 11 mg Men: 12 mg	1500–2000 mg crystalline niacin or sustained-release forms daily	Treating deficiency Pellagra Prevention of secondary deficiency (e.g. anorexia nervosa) Hypercholesterolaemia and hypertriglyceridaemia Syndrome X Tryptophan deficiency Diabetes	Hypersensitivity Diabetes Peptic ulcer disease Gout Hepatitis Liver function should be monitored and patients observed for symptoms of myopathy.	Flushing is a common side effect (not with nicotinamide). Night-time administration, extended-release (ER) niacin or concurrent administration of aspirin can reduce these effects. Palpitations, chills, pruritus, GIT upset and cutaneous tingling.	Tachycardia, chills, sweating, shortness of breath, nausea, vomiting, myalgias, hepatotoxicity. ER niacin is considered the safest form.
B_5 (pantothenic acid)	Women: 4 mg/day Men: 6 mg/day	200–300 mg/day	Deficiency rare Prevention of secondary deficiency (e.g. malabsorption syndrome, alcoholism, diabetes, OCP and IBD) Enhanced wound healing Hypercholesterolaemia Prevention of NTD Female alopecia		Well tolerated Contact dermatitis from topical application	No toxicity level known

B_6 (pyridoxine)	Women: 1.3 mg (> 50 yrs: 1.5 mg) Men: 1.3 mg (> 50 yrs: 1.7 mg)	5–1200 mg/day	Treating deficiency Prevention of secondary deficiency (e.g. malabsorption syndromes, cancer, liver cirrhosis and alcoholism, hyperthyroidism) Relieving symptoms of PMS and morning sickness Leg cramps of pregnancy Hyperhomocysteinaemia (often with folic acid and vitamin B_{12}) Reducing thromboembolism Improved outcomes after heart transplant Reducing repeated febrile convulsions in children Autism (with magnesium) Stress Cognitive performance/ Alzheimer's disease Schizophrenia Tardive dyskinesia Parkinson's disease	Hypersensitivity Long-term use of high-dose pyridoxine supplements (>100 mg, although this level varies between individuals) should be used with caution.	Nausea, vomiting, headache, paraesthesias, sleepiness and low serum folic acid levels have been reported. If taken at night, may induce vivid dreams.	Paraesthesia, hyperaesthesia, bone pain, muscle weakness, numbness and fasciculation most marked at the extremities Unsteady gait, numbness of hands and feet, impaired tendon reflexes. Excess doses of B_6 can cause degeneration of the dorsal root ganglia in the spinal cord, loss of myelination and degeneration of sensory fibres in the peripheral nerves. Dose and time frame at which toxicity occurs varies significantly between individuals. Studies involving large populations found minimal or no toxicity with 100–150 mg/day over 5–10 years, whereas women self-medicating for PMS taking 117 ± 92 mg for 2.9 ± 1.9 years have reported increased incidence of peripheral neuropathy.

Continued

Clinical use and safety of vitamins *continued*

Vitamin	Australian and New Zealand RDI for adults (>18 years)	Dose range used in practice	Major uses (oral or topical forms)	Cautions	Side effects	Toxicity
B_{12} (cobalamin)	Adult > 13 years: 2.4 mcg/day	0.5–2000 mg/day	Treating deficiency: primary deficiency (vegans and vegetarians, breast-fed infants of vegetarian mothers, elderly patients and alcoholics) Prevention of secondary deficiency (e.g. atrophic gastritis, achlorhydria, pancreatic insufficiency, Crohn's disease, bacterial or parasitic infestations) Pernicious anaemia Hyperhomocysteinaemia (with B_6 and folate) Cardiovascular protection Prevention of NTD Recurrent abortion Depression HIV infection Cognitive impairment Diabetic retinopathy Sleep disorders Tinnitus Multiple sclerosis Motor neuron disease (MND) (amyotrophic lateral sclerosis)	Hypersensitivity Avoid in cases of altered cobalamin metabolism or deficiency associated with chronic cyanide intoxication.	None known	Well-tolerated
Folate	Adults: 400 mcg/day Up to 1 mg/day in deficiency states	1–30 mg/day	Treating deficiency Prevention of secondary deficiency (e.g. malabsorption syndromes such as coeliac and Crohn's disease, HIV infection), MTHFR gene polymorphism Preconception care and pregnancy (prevention of neural tube defects) Hyperhomocysteinaemia Cardiovascular disease protection	Hypersensitivity Use may mask B_{12} deficiency by correcting the apparent microcytic anaemia without altering the potential for or progression of neurological damage.	Doses > 5 mg/day: generalised urticaria, nausea, flatulence and bitter taste in the mouth, and some CNS activation in the form of irritability and excitability, altered sleep pattern.	Non-toxic

			Cognitive impairment Anticonvulsant-induced folate deficiency Depression Schizophrenia Reducing incidence of cancer Periodontal disease Vitiligo Topical: periodontal disease			
C	45 mg	250–12,000 mg/day orally in divided doses More used when administered IV	Treating deficiency Prevention of secondary deficiency (e.g. heavy smokers, achlorhydria, chronic diarrhoea, major surgery) Treating iron deficiency anaemia (with iron) Prevention and treatment of common URTI such as colds and influenza and mild allergic responses Prevention and adjunctive treatment of cardiovascular disease and cancer Management of diabetes and asthma Atopy Prevention of cataracts Male infertility Adjunct for haemodialysis patients Oral and topical forms used for various dermatological conditions (e.g. wound healing, photo-aged skin, prevention of sunburn (with vitamin E)	Hypersensitivity Increases iron, and decreases copper, absorption Glucose-6-phosphate dehydrogenase deficiency Haemochromatosis Thalassaemia major Sideroblastic anaemia Renal impairment Interacts with numerous laboratory tests (e.g. serum cholesterol and triglycerides and urinary oxalate; refer to monograph)	None expected if <3000–4000 mg/day, but this varies between individuals Gastrointestinal upset: nausea, diarrhoea, flatulence, distension Hyperoxaluria and renal stones now considered doubtful	Considered non-toxic

Continued

Clinical use and safety of vitamins *continued*

Vitamin	Australian and New Zealand RDI for adults (>18 years)	Dose range used in practice	Major uses (oral or topical forms)	Cautions	Side effects	Toxicity
D	Children & adults <50 yrs: 200 IU/day Adults 51–70 yrs: 400 IU/day Adults >70 yrs: 600 IU/day	400–300,000 IU/day	Treating deficiency Inadequate sun exposure or poor dietary intake Prevention of secondary deficiency (e.g. malabsorption states) Hypoparathyroidism (with calcium) Hypophosphataemia (with phosphorus) Prevention of bone fracture and osteoporosis (with calcium) Hepatic and renal osteodystrophy Scleroderma Cancer Diabetes Prevention and treatment of infections Depression Multiple sclerosis Lupus	Hypersensitivity Hypercalcaemia Sarcoidosis Hyperparathyroidism SLE Vitamin D toxicity Pregnancy Lactation Renal failure Use of cardiac glycosides, thiazide diuretics, calcium-channel blockers	Not seen with doses <2400 IU/day Doses >3800 IU: hypercalcaemia, soft tissue calcification Fatigue, headache, nausea, vomiting, metallic taste, abdominal cramps, myalgia, tinnitus, arthralgia, constipation, polyuria, polydipsia	Caution when using high doses regularly. Between 50,000 and 100,000 IU/day: signs of hypercalcaemia 50,000–200,000 IU/day: nausea, vomiting, anorexia, polyuria, muscle pain Calcification of soft tissue and organs, cardiac arrhythmias Toxic levels cannot be obtained from sun exposure.

E	Women: 7 mg alpha-tocopherol Men: 10 mg alpha-tocopherol	50–3200 IU/day	Treating deficiency Prevention of secondary deficiency (e.g. malabsorption syndromes, cystic fibrosis) Prevention of cardiovascular disease, certain cancers, ischaemic stroke in high-risk hypertensive patients, nitrate tolerance Enhancing immune function in the elderly Reducing incidence of common cold Slowing progression of Alzheimer's dementia Improving symptoms in PMS, dysmenorrhoea, menopause, intermittent claudication Reducing pain in OA and RA Cancer Age-related macular degeneration Huntington's disease Treating some forms of male infertility Oral and topical use for many dermatological states Scar tissue Prevention or treatment of many other conditions, such as exercise-induced tissue damage, some types of senile cataracts, epilepsy and fibromyalgia	Hypersensitivity People with impaired coagulation, inherited bleeding disorders, history of haemorrhagic stroke, vitamin K deficiency or at risk of pulmonary embolism or thrombophlebitis Suspend use of supplements 1–2 weeks before major surgery.	Adverse effects are dose-related and tend to occur only at very high doses (> 1200 IU/day) Side effects include diarrhoea, flatulence, nausea and heart palpitations Increased risk of bleeding if vitamin K deficiency present	Vitamin E is relatively non-toxic. Doses as high as 3200 mg/day have been used for 12 years without signs of toxicity.

Clinical use and safety of minerals ***continued***

Mineral	Australian and New Zealand RDI for adults (>18 years)	Dose range used in practice	Major uses (oral or topical forms)	Cautions	Side effects	Toxicity
Calcium	Adults: < 70 yrs: 1000 mg/day > 70 yrs: 1300 mg/day	100–2000 mg/day	Treating deficiency Prevention of secondary deficiency (e.g. achlorhydria and malabsorption syndromes), more common in elderly Prevention of osteoporosis, pre-eclampsia, maintenance of bone density, colorectal cancer Symptoms of PMS Hypertension and hyperlipidaemia Dyspepsia Weight loss Nephrolithiasis Dry eye	Hypersensitivity Hyperparathyroidism Hypercalcaemia Renal impairment or kidney disease Sarcoidosis or other granulomatous diseases only under medical supervision	Gastrointestinal discomfort, nausea, loss of appetite, constipation, flatulence, metallic taste, muscle weakness	Increased serum calcium level may be associated with hypotonia, depression, lethargy and coma. Prolonged hypercalcaemic state, especially if normal or elevated serum phosphate, can precipitate ectopic calcification of blood vessels, joints, gastric mucosa, cornea and renal tissue.
Chromium	Women: 25 mcg Men: 35 mcg	50–1000 mcg	Treating deficiency Diabetes Hypoglycaemia Hyperlipidaemia Obesity Atypical depression Polycystic ovary syndrome Syndrome X Exercise aid Prevention of myocardial infarction	Hypersensitivity	Irritability and insomnia have been reported with chromium yeast supplementation. Chromium picolinate is well tolerated.	Chromium IV is used in industry and is highly toxic, whereas Cr III, which is used in supplements, is well tolerated.

Iodine	Adults: 150 mcg/day	0.5–6 mg	Treating deficiency Secondary deficiency (high consumption of goitrogens combined with low iodine intake) Preventing deficiency in high-risk groups including in utero, pregnancy, infancy Prevention of ADHA Fibrocystic breast disease Breast cancer Mastalgia	Hypersensitivity Thyroid conditions	Symptoms of iodine hypersensitivity are fever, painful joints, lymph node enlargement, eosinophilia, urticaria, angio-oedema, cutaneous and mucosal haemorrhage and fatal peri-arteritis.	Chronic iodine toxicity when intake is > 2 mg/day. Symptoms: brassy taste in mouth, burning sensation in mouth and throat, increased salivation, gastric irritation, abdominal pain, nausea, vomiting and diarrhoea Acneiform skin lesions, pulmonary oedema, depression Chronic ingestion > 500 mcg/day by children → increased thyroid size
Iron	Women: 19 to menopause: 18 mg Post-menopause: 8 mg Men: 8 mg	10–100 mg/day	Treating deficiency Prevention of secondary deficiency (e.g. menorrhagia, cystic fibrosis) Unexplained fatigue without anaemia Improving athletic performance Pregnancy Postpartum anaemia Cognitive function ADHD	Hypersensitivity Haemochromatosis Haemosiderosis Iron-loading anaemias (thalassaemia, sideroblastic anaemia) Liquid iron preparations can discolour teeth (brush teeth after use)	Gastrointestinal disturbances such as nausea, diarrhoea, constipation, heartburn, upper gastric discomfort Preliminary evidence indicates iron may be implicated in the pathogenesis of various disease states. Therefore, supplementation is indicated only with demonstrated biological need.	Haemochromatosis can develop from long-term excessive intake Iron toxicity causes severe organ damage and death The most pronounced effects are haemorrhagic necrosis of the gastrointestinal tract and liver damage.

Continued

Clinical use and safety of minerals *continued*

Mineral	Australian and New Zealand RDI for adults (>18 years)	Dose range used in practice	Major uses (oral or topical forms)	Cautions	Side effects	Toxicity
Magnesium	Women: 310 mg > 30 yrs: 320 mg Men: 400 mg > 30 yrs 420 mg	200–1200 mg/day	Treating deficiency Prevention of secondary deficiency (e.g. inflammatory bowel diseases, diabetes, hyperthyroidism, elevated cortisol) Alleviating symptoms of coronary heart disease, reducing hypertension, reducing plasma lipid levels, reducing incidence of arrhythmias in congestive heart failure Prevention of migraine headache, premenstrual headache, PMS, dysmenorrhoea, osteoporosis ADHD, autism spectrum disorders Kidney stone prevention Asthma Diabetes Dyspepsia Constipation Chronic leg cramps Leg cramps in pregnancy	Hypersensitivity Renal failure and heart block (unless pacemaker present)	**Most common** Diarrhoea and gastric irritation; usually not seen at doses <350 mg/day (elemental) Doses of inorganic magnesium >350 mg/day may be associated with adverse effects. Dividing doses will maximise bioavailability and reduce side effects. Overuse of magnesium hydroxide or magnesium sulfate may cause deficiencies of other minerals or lead to toxicity. **Other side effects** Decreased heart rate, hypotension, muscle weakness	Most commonly seen in patients with renal insufficiency. Symptoms: muscle weakness, sedation, ECG changes, confusion, hypotension
Selenium	Women: 60 mcg Men: 70 mcg	80–200 mcg/day	Treating deficiency Prevention of secondary deficiency (e.g. cirrhosis, malabsorption syndromes, cystic fibrosis, coeliac disease, HIV infection) Reducing total cancer incidence and mortality (especially lung, colorectal and prostate cancers), adjunctive treatment HIV infection Cardiovascular disease Autoimmune thyroiditis Diabetes	Hypersensitivity NHMRC upper level of intake is 400 mcg/day	Nausea, vomiting, nail changes, irritability, fatigue Organic form of selenium found in high-selenium yeast is less toxic and safer than other forms.	Long-term use of excessive doses (> 1000 mcg/day) can produce fatigue, depression, arthritis, hair or fingernail loss, garlicky breath or body odour, gastrointestinal disorders and irritability.

			Symptoms of RA, asthma Male infertility Immune enhancement Anxiety and depression Reducing morbidity in preterm infants			
Zinc	Women: 8 mg/day Men: 14 mg/day	25–200 mg/day	Treating deficiency Prevention of secondary deficiency (e.g. cirrhosis, malabsorption syndromes, severe burns, major surgery) Treating the common cold and reducing symptoms Age related macular degeneration Diabetes Enhancing wound healing (e.g. leg ulcers) Decreasing relapse rates in Crohn's disease Decreasing incidence of pneumonia Arterial and venous leg ulcers Male infertility Impotence ADHD Depression Diarrhoea Anorexia nervosa Tinnitus Warts Acne vulgaris Topical herpes simplex infection	Hypersensitivity	Mild gastrointestinal upset at doses of 50–150 mg/day	Single doses of 225–450 mg usually induce vomiting Nausea, vomiting, diarrhoea, fever and lethargy have been observed after ingestion of 4–8 g. Doses ranging from 100 to 150 mg/day interfere with copper metabolism and cause hypocupraemia, red blood cell microcytosis and neutropenia if used long term.

NOTE

Mutivitamins. Overall, acute toxicity is unlikely with combination vitamin supplements unless huge amounts have been ingested. In the case of toxicity or side-effects, signs and symptoms will relate to the individual nutrient ingested. In general, gastrointestinal symptoms such as discomfort, nausea and diarrhoea are the most frequent adverse effects.

Special care. Of all the nutrients listed, extra special care must be taken when supplementing with vitamins A and D and the mineral iron. The forms of selenium and niacin used in practice also have a major influence on their safety profile and should be taken into consideration.

RDI. For more details regarding RDI for specific age groups: www.nhmrc.gov.au/publications/synopses/n35syn.htm

For further information, refer to individual monographs.

INDEX

Page numbers followed by 't' indicate tables, and 'b' indicate boxes.

C

K

L

N

X

Y

Z